Handbook of
COSMETIC AND
PERSONAL CARE ADDITIVES

Handbook of
COSMETIC AND
PERSONAL CARE ADDITIVES

**An International Guide to More Than 15,000 Products
by Trade Name, Function, Composition and Manufacturer**

Compiled by

Michael and Irene Ash

Gower

Published by
Gower Publishing Limited
Gower House
Croft Road
Aldershot
Hampshire GU11 3HR
England

Gower
Old Post Road
Brookfield
Vermont 05036
U.S.A.

British Library Of Cataloguing in Publication Data
Handbook of Cosmetic and Personal Care Additives: International Guide to More Than 15,000 Products by Trade Name, Function, Composition and Manufacturer
  I. Ash, Michael   II. Ash, Irene
  668

Library of Congress Cataloging-in-Publication Data
Ash, Michael
    Handbook of cosmetic and personal care additives : an international guide to more than 15,000 products by trade name, function, composition and manufacturer / compiled by Michael and Irene Ash.
    984 p. 23.4 cm
    Includes index.
    1. Cosmetics—Additives.   2. Toilet preparations—Additives.
    I. Ash, Irene. II. Title
    TP983.A82 1994   94-2689
    668´.5—dc20   CIP

ISBN 0-566-07470-2

Typeset in Arial Narrow by Synapse Information Resources, Inc.

Printed and Bound in Great Britain by Hartnolls Limited, Bodmin, Cornwall.

Contents

Preface

This reference work describes more than 15,000 trade name additive ingredients that are used for the formulation of cosmetic and personal care products. Entries contain extensive information gathered from more than 750 world-wide manufacturers and their branches, distributors, and trade magazines.

The cosmetic and personal care industries encompass a diversity of products including: body and face lotions, creams, and salves; deodorants and antiperspirants; sunscreens and tanning aids; make-up preparations (face powder, lipstick, mascara, eye shadows and liners, nail products); hair preparations (shampoos, conditioners, coloring rinses and dyes, waving solutions); bath preparations and soaps; shaving preparations; oral care products; and fragrances. Choosing optimal ingredients in the overall process of marketing and developing new and improved products is a monumental task. This reference coalesces the necessary research into a single source and expedites material selection for the user by cross-referencing trade name products by function, chemical composition, CAS number, and EINECS number.

An important feature of this book is the inclusion of historical tracing for both trade name products and their manufacturers. Former names for trade name products are included in the entries. The Appendix contains both a listing of products that are discontinued, redesignated, no longer standard, or not verified; and a listing of companies that have been acquired by other chemical manufacturers.

The book is divided into four sections:

Part I—*Trade Name Reference* contains over 15,000 alphabetical entries of trade name cosmetic and personal care ingredients. Each entry references its manufacturer, chemical composition, associated CAS and EINECS identifying numbers, general properties, applications and functions, toxicology, and compliance and regulatory information as provided by the manufacturer and other sources.

Part II—*Trade Name Functional Cross-Reference* contains an alphabetical listing of major cosmetic and personal care functional categories. Over 40 categories are included, e.g., anticaking agents, emollients, enzymes, film formers, fragrances, moisture barriers, nutritive additives, suncare additives, thickeners, waxes, etc. Each functional category entry is followed by an alphabetical listing of the trade name products that have that functional attribute.

Part III—*Chemical Component Cross-Reference* contains an alphabetical listing of cosmetic and personal care chemical compounds. Each chemical entry lists the trade name products that are equivalent to the chemical compound or contains that chemical compound as the trade name product's major chemical constituent. Wherever possible CAS (Chemical Abstract Service) numbers and EINECS (European Inventory of Existing Commercial Chemical Substances) numbers are included. The CTFA (Cosmetic, Toiletry, and Fragrance Association) adopted names for the chemical entry have been updated in most instances to the newly established INCI (International Nomenclature Ingredients) names. Synonyms for the chemical compounds are grouped with the entry and many synonyms are cross-referenced back to the main entry.

Part IV—*Manufacturers Directory* contains detailed contact information for the manufacturers of the more than 15,000 trade name products referenced in this handbook. Wherever possible telephone, telefax, and telex numbers, toll-free 800 numbers, and complete mailing addresses are included for each manufacturer.

The Appendix includes the following references:

CAS Number-to-Trade Name Cross-Reference orders many trade names found in Part I by identifying CAS numbers; it should be noted that trade names may contain more than one chemical component and the associated CAS numbers in this section refer to each trade name product's primary chemical component.

CAS Number-to-Chemical Cross-Reference orders chemical compounds found in Part III by CAS numbers.

EINECS Number-to-Trade Name Cross-Reference orders many trade names found in Part I by identifying EINECS numbers that refer to each trade name product's primary chemical component as well.

EINECS Number-to-Chemical Cross-Reference orders chemical compounds found in Part III by EINECS numbers.

Trade Name Status Reference lists discontinued, redesignated, nonstandard, or unverified trade name products.

This book is the culmination of many months of research, investigation of product sources, and sorting through a variety of technical data sheets and brochures acquired through personal contacts and correspondences with major chemical manufacturers world-wide as well as trade journals. We are especially grateful to Roberta Dakan for her skills in chemical information database management. Her tireless efforts have been instrumental in the production of this reference.

M. & I. Ash

NOTE:

The information contained in this reference is accurate to the best of our knowledge; however, no liability will be assumed by the publisher for the correctness or comprehensiveness of such information. The determination of the suitability of any of the products for prospective use is the responsibility of the user. It is herewith recommended that those who plan to use any of the products referenced seek the manufacturer's instructions for the handling of that particular chemical.

Abbreviations

abs.	absolute
ABS	acrylonitrile-butadiene-styrene
absorp.	absorption
act.	active
adsorp.	adsorption
agric.	agricultural
agrochem.	agrochemical
AMP	2-amino -2-methyl-1- propanol
AMPD	aminomethyl propanediol
anhyd.	anhydrous
APHA	American Public Health Association
applic(s).	application(s)
aq.	aqueous
ASA	acrylic-styrene-acrylonitrile
ASTM	American Society for Testing and Materials
atm	atmosphere
aux.	auxiliary
avail.	available
avg.	average
BGA	Federal Republic of Germany Health Dept. certification
BHA	butylated hydroxyanisole
BHT	butylated hydroxytoluene
biodeg.	biodegradable
blk.	black
b.p.	boiling point
BP	British Pharmacopeia
br., brn.	brown
brnsh.	brownish
Btu	British thermal unit
C	degrees Centigrade
CAS	Chemical Abstracts Service
CC	closed cup
cc	cubic centimeter(s)
CCl_4	carbon tetrachloride
CFR	U.S. Code of Federal Regulations
char.	characteristic
chel.	chelation
chem.	chemical
CHDM	cyclohexanedimethanol
cm	centimeter(s)
cm^3	cubic centimeter(s)
CMC	carboxymethylcellulose, critical Micelle concentration
COC	Cleveland Open Cup
compat.	compatible
compd.	compound
conc.	concentrated, concentration
cosolv.	cosolvent
cp	centipoise(s)
CP	Canadian Pharmacopeia
cps	centipoise(s)
cryst.	crystalline, crystallization
cs, cst, or cSt	centistoke(s)
CTFA	Cosmetic, Toiletry and Fragrance Association
ctks	centistoke(s)

DEA	diethanolamide, diethanolamine
dec.	decomposes
decomp.	decomposition
dens.	density
deriv.	derivative(s)
DIA	diisopropyl adipate
diam.	diameter
DIBA	dihydroxyisobutylamine
dielec.	dielectric
disp.	dispersible, dispersion
dissip.	dissipation
dist.	distilled
distort.	distortion
dk.	dark
DMDM	dimethylol dimethyl
DMSO	dimethyl sulfoxide
DNA	deoxyribonucleic acid
DOT	Department of Transportation
DTPA	diethylene triamine pentaacetic acid
DVB	divinylbenzene
DW	distilled water, deionized water
EC	European Community
EEC	European Economic Community
EINECS	European Inventory of Existing Commercial Chemical Substances
elec.	electrical
EO	ethylene oxide
EP	extreme pressure
EP	European Pharmacopoeia
EPA	Environmental Protection Agency
equip.	equipment
esp.	especially
EVA	ethylene vinyl acetate
F	degrees Fahrenheit
FCC	Food Chemicals Codex
FDA	Food and Drug Administration
FD&C	Foods, Drugs, and Cosmetics
FG	food grade
flamm.	flammable, flammability
f.p.	freezing point
ft	foot, feet
F-T	Fischer-Tropsch
G	giga
g	gram(s)
gal	gallon(s)
G-H	Gardner-Holdt
GLY	glycine
gr.	gravity
gran.	granules, granular
GRAS	generally recognized as safe
grn.	green
h	hour(s)
HC	hydrocarbon
HCl	hydrochloride, hydrochloric acid
HEDTA	hydroxyethylenediamine triacetic acid
Hg	mercury
HLB	hydrophilic lipophilic balance
hyd.	hydroxyl

hydrog.	hydrogenated
i.b.p.	initial boiling point
INCI	International Nomenclature Cosmetic Ingredient
incl.	including
incompat.	incompatible
inj.	injection
inorg.	inorganic
insol.	insoluble
Int'l.	International
IPA	isopropyl alcohol, isopropanol
IPM	isopropyl myristate
IPP	isopropyl palmitate
ISO	International Standards Organization
IU	international units
JCID	Japanese Cosmetic Ingredients Dictionary
JP	Japanese Pharmacopoeia
JSCI	Japanese Standard of Cosmetic Ingredients
k	kilo
kg	kilogram(s)
KU	Krebs units
l	liter(s)
lb	pound(s)
LD50	lethal dose 50%
LDPE	low-density polyethylene
liq.	liquid
lt.	light
Ltd.	Limited
M	mole, mega
m	milli or meter(s)
m-	meta
MA	maleic anhydride
max.	maximum
mbar	millibar
MEA	monoethanolamine, monoethanolamide
mech.	mechanial
med.	medium
MEK	methyl ethyl ketone
mfg.	manufacture
mg	milligram(s)
MIBK	methyl isobutyl ketone
microcryst.	microcrystalline
min	minute(s)
min.	mineral, minimum
MIPA	monoisopropanolamine, monoisopropanolamide
misc.	miscible
mixt.	mixture(s)
ml	milliliter(s)
mm	millimeter(s)
mN	millinewton(s)
m.p.	melting point
mPa·s	millipascal-seconds
m.w.	molecular weight
N	normal
nat.	natural
NC	nitrocellulose
need.	needles
NF	National Formulary

nm	nanometer
no.	number
nonflamm.	nonflammable
nonyel.	nonyellowing
NR	isoprene rubber (natural)
NTA	nitrilotriacetic acid
NV	nonvolatiles
o-	ortho
OC	open crucible
org.	organic
OTC	over-the-counter
o/w	oil-in-water
p-	para
Pa	Pascal
PABA	p-aminobenzoic acid
PCA	2-pyrrolidone-5-carboxylic acid
PEG	polyethylene glycol
PEI	polyethylenimine
petrol.	petroleum
PG	propylene glycol
pH	hydrogen-ion concentration
pkg.	packaging
P-M	Pensky-Martens
PMCC	Pensky-Martens closed cup
PMOC	Pensky-Martens open cup
PO	propylene oxide
POE	polyoxyethylene, polyoxyethylated
POP	polyoxypropylene, polyoxypropylated
powd.	powder
PP	polypropylene
PPG	polypropylene glycol
ppm	parts per million
pract.	practically
prep.	preparation(s)
prod.	product(s), production
props.	properties
PS	polystyrene
psi	pounds per square inch
pt.	point
PU	polyurethane
PVA	polyvinyl alcohol
PVAc	polyvinyl acetate
PVC	polyvinyl chloride
PVM	polyvinyl methyl ether
PVM/MA	polyvinyl methyl ether/maleic anhydride
PVP	polyvinylpyrrolidone
quat.	quaternary
R&B	Ring & Ball
R.T.	room temperature
rdsh.	reddish
ref.	refractive
resist.	resistance, resistant, resistivity
resp.	respectively
RNA	ribonucleic acid
rpm	revolutions per minute
RT	room temperature
s	second(s)

sapon.	saponification
sat.	saturated
SD	specially denatured
SDA	specially denatured alcohol
SE	self-emulsifying
sec.	secondary
sl.	slightly
sm.	small
soften.	softening
sol.	soluble, solubility
sol'n.	solution
solid.	solidification
solv(s).	solvent(s)
sp.	specific
SPF	sun protection factor
std	standard
Stod.	Stoddard solvent
surf.	surface
SUS	Saybolt Universal Seconds
susp.	suspension
syn.	synthetic
t	tertiary
TBHQ	t-butyl hydroquinone
TCC	Tag closed cup
TDI	toluene diisocyanate
TEA	triethanolamine, triethanolamide
tech.	technical
temp.	temperature
tens.	tensile or tension
tert.	tertiary
thru	through
TIPA	triisopropanolamine
TOC	Tag open cup
typ.	typical
unsat.	unsaturated
USDA	United States Department of Agriculture
USP	Unites States Pharmacopeia
V	volt
VA	vinyl acetate
veg.	vegetable
visc.	viscous, viscosity
VM&P	Varnish Makers and Painters
VOC	volatile organic compounds
vol.	volume
wh.	white
w/o	water-in-oil
wt.	weight
yel.	yellow
ylsh.	yellowish
#	number
%	percent
<	less than
>	greater than
@	at
≈	approximately
α	alpha
β	beta

ε	epsilon
γ	gamma
δ	delta
μ	micron, micrometer

Part I
Trade Name Reference

A

A-611. [ICI Surf. Am.] Hydrog. starch hydrolysate; CAS 68425-17-2; humectant.

A-641. [ICI Am.] Sorbitol; CAS 50-70-4; EINECS 200-061-5; cosmetic/pharmaceutical ingred.

AA USP. [CasChem] Castor oil; CAS 8001-79-4; EINECS 232-293-8; emollient for cosmetic and pharmaceutical purposes; lubricant for food processing (release aid, protective coatings for vitamins, tableting); FDA approval; sol. in alcohols, esters, ethers, ketone, and aromatic solvs.

AB®. [Angus] 2-Amino-1-butanol; CAS 96-20-8; EINECS 202-488-2; pigment dispersant, neutralizing/emulsifying amine, corrosion inhibitor, acid-salt catalyst, pH buffer, chemical and pharmaceutical intermediate, solubilizer; m.w. 89.1; water-sol.; m.p. −2 C; b.p. 178 C; flash pt. 193 F (TCC); pH 11.1 (0.1M aq. sol'n.); 99% conc.

Abesin E. [Fabriquimica] Syn. beeswax, emulsifiable; cosmetic ingred.; acid no. 35-45; iodine no. < 1; sapon. no. 110-130.

Abesin NE. [Fabriquimica] Syn. beeswax; cosmetic ingred.; acid no. < 2; iodine no. < 1; sapon. no. 95-105.

Abex® LIV/30. [Rhone-Poulenc Surf. & Spec.] Ammonium alkylaryl ether sulfate; anionic; emulsifier for emulsion polymerization of acrylic, styrene-acrylic, vinyl acetate; detergent, emulsifier, foam stabilizer, wetting agent in household and industrial detergents, shampoos, bubble baths; liq.; 30% conc.; formerly Geropon® LIV/30.

Abietate de Glycerol. [Prod'Hyg] Glyceryl abietate; CAS 1337-89-9.

Abil® 10-10000. [Goldschmidt AG] Dimethicone; nonionic; conditioner for skin and hair care, sunscreens, tanning creams, or lotions; aftershave, aerosol preparations; colorless liq.; insol. in water; disp. in veg. and min. oils; sp.gr. 0.94-0.98; 100% act.

Abil® AV 20-1000. [Goldschmidt; Goldschmidt AG] Phenyl trimethicone; CAS 2116-84-9; EINECS 218-320-6; nonionic; emollient, conditioner for skin and hair care, sunscreen, tanning creams or lotions; aftershave, aerosol preparations; forms easy spreading film on skin; colorless liq.; sol. in veg. and min. oils; insol. in water; sp.gr. 0.97-1.078; 100% act.

Abil® AV 8853. [Goldschmidt AG] Phenyl trimethicone; CAS 2116-84-9; EINECS 218-320-6; nonionic; emollient providing skin protection, barrier against aq. media; perfume ingred. and fixative; provides improved rub and spreadability, faster penetration; nonsticky; prevents aerosol clogging; colorless liq.; sol. in veg. and min. oils; insol. in water; sp.gr. 0.90-0.94.

Abil® B 8839. [Goldschmidt AG] Cyclomethicone; CAS 69430-24-6; nonionic; conditioner for hair care prods., aerosols, sticks, shaving preparations, deodorants, antiperspirants; colorless liq.; sol. with sl. turbidity in min. and veg. oils; insol. in water; sp.gr. 0.94-0.97; 100% act.

Abil® B 8842. [Goldschmidt] Dimethicone copolyol; non-

ionic; surface active wetting agent, lubricant for soaps, shampoos, shower gels, creams, lotions, and aerosols; refatting agent; improves foam; contributes to compatibility/sheen in shampoos.

Abil® B 8843. [Goldschmidt; Goldschmidt AG] Dimethicone copolyol; CAS 68937-55-3; nonionic; surfactant, conditioner used in personal care prods.; emollient for hair and skin care prods., aerosol shaving lather, deodorants, antiperspirants, creams and lotions, perfumes and colognes; pale liq.; water-sol.; disp. in min. and veg. oils; sp.gr. 1.070; 100% conc.

Abil® B 8847. [Goldschmidt] Dimethicone copolyol.

Abil® B 8851. [Goldschmidt AG] Dimethicone copolyol; CAS 68937-55-3; nonionic; surfactant, conditioner for personal care prods.; emollient for hair and skin care prods., aerosol shaving lather, deodorants, antiperspirants, creams and lotions, perfumes and colognes; pale yel. liq.; water-sol.; disp. in veg. and min. oils; sp.gr. 1.050; 100% conc.

Abil® B 8852. [Goldschmidt AG] Dimethicone copolyol; CAS 68937-55-3; nonionic; surfactant, conditioner for personal care prods.; emollient for hair and skin care prods., aerosol shaving lather, deodorants, antiperspirants, creams and lotions, perfumes and colognes; pale yel. liq.; disp. in water, veg. and min. oils; sp.gr. 1.011; 100% conc.

Abil® B 8863. [Goldschmidt AG] Dimethicone copolyol; nonionic; surface active wetting agent, lubricant for soaps, shampoos, shower gels, creams, lotions, and aerosols; refatting agent; improves foam; contributes to compatibility/sheen in shampoos; amber liq.; sol. in water; disp. in veg. and min. oils; 100% conc.

Abil® B 8873. [Goldschmidt] Dimethicone copolyol; nonionic; surface active wetting agent, lubricant for soaps, shampoos, shower gels, creams, lotions, and aerosols; refatting agent; improves foam; contributes to compatibility/sheen in shampoos.

Abil® B 9806. [Goldschmidt] Cetyl dimethicone copolyol; surfactant, emollient for creams and lotions; emulsifier for cyclomethicone.

Abil® B 9808. [Goldschmidt] Cetyl dimethicone copolyol and hexyl laurate; surfactant, emollient for creams and lotions; emulsifier for cyclomethicone.

Abil® B 9950. [Goldschmidt; Goldschmidt AG] Dimethicone propyl PG-betaine; CAS 102523-96-6; amphoteric; silicone surfactant, conditioner; used in hair and skin care prods.; yel. liq.; sol. with sl. turbidity in water; disp. in veg. and min. oils; sp.gr. 1.078-1.092; 30% conc.

Abil® B 88183. [Goldschmidt; Goldschmidt AG] Dimethicone copolyol; CAS 68937-55-3; nonionic; surfactant used as foam formers and providing lubricating and gloss properties; refatting agent for skin prods.; increases slip in shaving creams; also for shampoos, shower gels, hand cleaners, aerosols, antiperspirants; pale yel. liq.; sol. in water, alcohol, 1,2-propylene glycol; sp.gr. 1.024; visc. 95

3

± 15 mms⁻¹; cloud pt. 71 ± 3 C (4% aq.); ref. index 1.375; surf. tens. 34.5 mN ·m⁻¹ (1% aq.); 50% act.

Abil® B 88184. [Goldschmidt; Goldschmidt AG] Dimethicone copolyol; CAS 68937-55-3; nonionic; surfactant for hair and skin care prods.; anticracking agent for soap bars; pale yel. liq.; sol. in water; sp.gr. 1.04; 100% conc.

Abil® EM-90. [Goldschmidt; Goldschmidt AG] Cetyl dimethicone copolyol; nonionic; surfactant, emollient, conditioner, emulsifier for w/o type creams and lotions, roll-ons, skin treatments, suncare prods., shampoos and conditioners; liq.; HLB 4-6; 100% conc.

Abil® K 4. [Goldschmidt AG] Cyclomethicone; CAS 69430-24-6; nonionic; emollient, conditioner used in hair care prods., aerosols, shaving preparations, deodorants, antiperspirants; colorless liq.; sol. veg. and min. oils; insol. in water; sp.gr. 0.94-0.97; 100% act.

Abil® OSW 12, OSW 13. [Goldschmidt] Cyclomethicone, dimethiconol, dimethicone; glossing and conditioning agent for hair care prods.; moisturizer and protectant for skin care creams and lotions.

Abil® OSW 15. [Goldschmidt] Cyclomethicone, dimethiconol, and dimethicone.

Abil® S201. [Goldschmidt] Sodium poly PG-propyl dimethicone thiosulfate; anionic; hair conditioner and setting lotion; improves gloss and sheen of shampoos, conditioners, mousses, gels, styling aids.

Abil® S255. [Goldschmidt] Sodium PG-propyl thiosulfate dimethicone; conditioner and setting lotion; improves gloss and sheen of shampoos and conditioners.

Abil® WE 09. [Goldschmidt AG] Polyglyceryl-4 isostearate, cetyl dimethicone copolyol, hexyl laurate; nonionic; emulsifier for highly stable w/o emulsions; improves uv protection in sunscreens; for skin care treatment emulsions; pale yel. liq.; sol. in veg. and min. oils; insol. in water; sp.gr. 0.89-0.93; HLB 5.0; 100% conc.

Abil® WS 08. [Goldschmidt AG] Cetyl dimethicone copolyol, cetyl dimethicone, polyglyceryl-3 oleate, hexyl laurate; nonionic; emulsifier for w/o creams and lotions; pale yel. liq.; sol. in min. and veg. oils; insol. in water; sp.gr. 0.87-0.91; HLB 5.0.

Abil®-Quat 3270. [Goldschmidt; Goldschmidt AG] Quaternium-80; CAS 134737-05-6; cationic; conditioner, antistat for shampoos and hair rinses; also refatting agent for skin cleansers; amber clear liq.; sol. in water, alcohol, 1,2-propylene glycol, glycerol; sp.gr. 1.014; visc. 400 ± 100 mm² s⁻¹; flash pt. 90 C; ref. index 1.443; pH 7.2 ± 1 (30% aq.); surf. tens. 31.5 ± 2 g/cm³; 50 ± 1% act.

Abil®-Quat 3272. [Goldschmidt; Goldschmidt AG] Quaternium-80; CAS 134737-05-6; cationic; conditioner, antistat for shampoos and hair rinses; also refatting agent for skin cleansers; amber clear liq.; sol. in water, alcohol, 1,2-propylene glycol, glycerol; sp.gr. 1.008; visc. 1000 ± 200 mm² s⁻¹; flash pt. 90 C; ref. index 1.429; pH 7.2 ± 1 (30% aq.); surf. tens. 44 ± 2 g/cm³; 50 ± 1% act.

Abil®-Wax 2434. [Goldschmidt; Goldschmidt AG] Stearoxy dimethicone; CAS 68554-53-0; nonionic; wax improving applic. and skin care properties of emulsions; spreading and emollient properties for protection against aq. media; water barrier for creams and lotions; pale yel. liq. > 40 C, waxy < 10 C; sol. in cyclomethicone, min. oil, IPM, sunflower seed oil; sp.gr. 0.88 (35 C); m.p. 25 C; pour pt. 20-30 C; flash pt. > 100 C; usage level: 1-5%; 100% act.

Abil®-Wax 2440. [Goldschmidt; Goldschmidt AG] Behenoxy dimethicone; nonionic; wax improving applic. and skin care properties of emulsions; spreading and emollient properties for protection against aq. media; reduces whitening during applic. of creams and lotions; pigment solubilizer; pale yel. waxy solid; disp. in min. oil, IPM, sunflower seed oil; sp.gr. 0.90 (50 FC); m.p. 35 C; pour pt. 30-35 C; flash pt. > 100 C; usage level: 1-5%; 100% act.

Abil®-Wax 9800. [Goldschmidt; Goldschmidt AG] Stearyl dimethicone; nonionic; wax improving color, luster, and spreadability of pigmented prods.; spreading, penetrating, and emollient properties for skin care prods.; wh. waxy liq.; sol. in min. oil, IPM, sunflower seed oil; sp.gr. 0.86 (35 C); pour pt. 20 C; flash pt. > 40 C; usage level: 1-5%; 100% act.

Abil®-Wax 9801. [Goldschmidt; Goldschmidt AG] Cetyl dimethicone; nonionic; wax providing emolliency and applic. benefits for antiperspirants; pigment solubilizer; also for skin care prods.; pale yel. liq. wax; sol. in cyclomethicone, min. oil, IPM, sunflower seed oil; sp.gr. 0.86; pour pt. 10 C; flash pt. 40 C; usage level: 1-5%; 100% act.

Abil®-Wax 9809. [Goldschmidt] Stearyl methicone; CAS 68607-75-0; wax providing water barrier for night creams and protective lotions; sol. in min. oil; m.p. 40 C.

Abil®-Wax 9810. [Goldschmidt] C24-28 alkyl methicone; high m.w. wax used as thickening agent for min. oils and cosmetic esters; water barrier for night creams and protective lotions; provides gloss and smoothness for lipsticks; gels min. oil; m.p. 60 C.

Abil®-Wax 9811. [Goldschmidt] C30-45 alkyl methicone.

Abil®-Wax 9814. [Goldschmidt] Cetyl dimethicone; emollient and spreading agent for cosmetic esters and oils; pigment grinding aid and dispersant esp. for titanium dioxide (prevents reagglomeration); used in sunscreens and pigmented prods. such as pressed powds.

Abiol. [3V-Sigma] Imidazolidinyl urea NF; CAS 39236-46-9; EINECS 254-372-6; preservative for cosmetics; effective against Gram-negative bacteria; active over wide pH range; water-sol.; usage level: 0.2-0.6%.

Ablucols EDP. [Taiwan Surf.] Proprietary blend; high-intensity pearlescent for hair and skin care prods.; easily dispersible at ambient temps.; visc. paste; 32% solids.

Ablumide CDE. [Taiwan Surf.] Cocamide DEA (1:1); CAS 61791-31-9; EINECS 263-163-9; nonionic; foam stabilizer, thickener for shampoos, bubble baths, liq. detergents, toiletries; clear liq.; water-disp.; 100% solids.

Ablumide CDE-G. [Taiwan Surf.] Cocamide DEA; CAS 61791-31-9; EINECS 263-163-9; low-cost equivalent to coco superamide; contains glycerin; foam stabilizer and thickener for personal care prods.; clear liq.; 100% solids.

Ablumide CKD. [Taiwan Surf.] Narrow cut cocamide DEA; CAS 61791-31-9; EINECS 263-163-9; foam stabilizer and thickener for shampoos; conditioning agent; clear liq.; 100% solids.

Ablumide CME. [Taiwan Surf.] Cocamide MEA (1:1); CAS 68140-00-1; EINECS 268-770-2; nonionic; foam builder/ stabilizer for anionic systems, thickener for shampoos, bubble baths, liq. detergents, toiletries; recommended for powd. and stick formulations; conditioning agent; flakes; 100% solids.

Ablumide LDE. [Taiwan Surf.] Lauramide DEA (1:1); CAS 120-40-1; EINECS 204-393-1; nonionic; foam stabilizer, thickener, conditioner for shampoos, bubble baths, liq. detergents, toiletries, hand-laundry detergent; wh. wax; water-disp.; 100% solids.

Ablumide LME. [Taiwan Surf.] Lauramide MEA (1:1); CAS 142-78-9; EINECS 205-560-1; nonionic; foam stabilizer, thickener for shampoos, bubble baths, liq. detergents, toiletries; solid; 95% conc.

Ablumide SME. [Taiwan Surf.] Stearamide MEA (1:1); CAS 111-57-9; EINECS 203-883-2; nonionic; opacifier, thickener for shampoo, cream rinse, bubble bath; solid; 90% conc.

Ablumine 18. [Taiwan Surf.] Alkyl (4% C16, 92% C18) benzyl dimethyl quat.; cationic; conditioner, softener, antistat for human hair, wool, cotton, other cellulosic fibers; paste; 25% act.

Ablumine 1618. [Taiwan Surf.] Stearalkonium chloride; CAS

122-19-0; EINECS 204-527-9; base for hair conditioners; imparts softness, manageability, and antistatic props. to hair; paste; 25% solids.

Ablumine DHT75. [Taiwan Surf.] Distearyldimonium chloride; CAS 107-64-2; EINECS 203-508-2; cationic; base for hair conditioners and creme rinses; imparts softness, manageability, and antistatic props. to hair; emulsifier for creams and lotions; antistat, fabric softener suitable for dryer sheets; soft paste; 75% act.

Ablumine TMC. [Taiwan Surf.] Cetrimonium chloride; CAS 112-02-7; EINECS 203-928-6; base for formulation of hair conditioners and creme rinses; imparts softness and manageability to hair without greasy feel; liq.; 30% solids.

Ablumine TMS. [Taiwan Surf.] Stearyl trimethyl ammonium chloride; CAS 112-03-8; EINECS 203-929-1; base for hair conditioners; liq.; 25% solids in water.

Ablumox CAPO. [Taiwan Surf.] Cocamidopropyl amine oxide; CAS 68155-09-9; EINECS 268-938-5; nonionic; low-irritation emulsifier, foam booster/stabilizer, visc. modifier, detergent, wetting agent, emollient; conditioner and antistat in hair care prods.; liq.; 35% solids.

Ablumox LO. [Taiwan Surf.] Lauramine oxide; CAS 1643-20-5; EINECS 216-700-6; nonionic; low-irritation emulsifier, foam booster/stabilizer, detergent, visc. modifier, wetting agent, detergent, emollient; conditioner and antistat for hair care prods.; liq.; 30% solids.

Ablunol 200ML. [Taiwan Surf.] PEG 200 laurate; CAS 9004-81-3; nonionic; emulsifier, lubricant, dispersing and leveling agent, defoamer used in cosmetic, textile, paint, dyestuffs, and other industrial uses; liq.; HLB 9.5; 100% act.

Ablunol 200MO. [Taiwan Surf.] PEG 200 oleate; CAS 9004-96-0; EINECS 233-293-0; nonionic; emulsifier, lubricant, dispersing and leveling agents used in cosmetic, textile, leather, paint and other industrial uses; liq.; HLB 7.9; 100% act.

Ablunol 200MS. [Taiwan Surf.] PEG 200 stearate; CAS 9004-99-3; EINECS 203-358-8; nonionic; emulsifier, thickener, lubricant, softener, defoamer, dispersing and leveling agent used in cosmetic, textile, paint and other industrial uses; solid; HLB 8.0; 100% act.

Ablunol 400ML. [Taiwan Surf.] PEG 400 laurate; CAS 9004-81-3; nonionic; emulsifier, lubricant, dispersing and leveling agent, defoamer used in cosmetic, textile, paint, dyestuffs, and other industrial uses; liq.; HLB 13.1; 100% act.

Ablunol 400MO. [Taiwan Surf.] PEG 400 oleate; CAS 9004-96-0; nonionic; emulsifiers, lubricants, dispersing and leveling agents used in cosmetic, textile, leather, paint and other industrial uses; liq.; HLB 11.5; 100% act.

Ablunol 400MS. [Taiwan Surf.] PEG 400 stearate; CAS 9004-99-3; nonionic; emulsifier, thickener, lubricant, softener, defoamer, dispersing and leveling agent used in cosmetic, textile, paint and other industrial uses; solid; HLB 11.6; 100% act.

Ablunol 600ML. [Taiwan Surf.] PEG 600 laurate; CAS 9004-81-3; nonionic; emulsifier, lubricant, dispersing and leveling agent, defoamer used in cosmetic, textile, paint, dyestuffs, and other industrial uses; liq.; HLB 15.0; 100% act.

Ablunol 600MO. [Taiwan Surf.] PEG 600 oleate; CAS 9004-96-0; nonionic; emulsifiers, lubricants, dispersing and leveling agents used in cosmetic, textile, leather, paint and other industrial uses; liq.; HLB 13.5; 100% act.

Ablunol 600MS. [Taiwan Surf.] PEG 600 stearate; CAS 9004-99-3; nonionic; emulsifier, thickener, lubricant, softener, defoamer, dispersing and leveling agent used in cosmetic, textile, paint and other industrial uses; solid; HLB 13.6; 100% act.

Ablunol 1000MO. [Taiwan Surf.] PEG 1000 oleate; CAS 9004-96-0; nonionic; emulsifiers, lubricants, dispersing and leveling agents used in cosmetic, textile, paint and other industrial uses; solid; HLB 15.2; 100% conc.

Ablunol 1000MS. [Taiwan Surf.] PEG 1000 stearate; CAS 9004-99-3; nonionic; emulsifiers, lubricants, dispersing and leveling agents used in cosmetic, textile, paint and other industrial uses; solid; HLB 15.2; 100% conc.

Ablunol 6000DS. [Taiwan Surf.] PEG 6000 distearate; CAS 9005-08-7; nonionic; emulsifier, thickener for cosmetic, pigment preparations, textile printing; flake; HLB 19.0; 100% act.

Ablunol CO 5. [Taiwan Surf.] PEG-5 castor oil; CAS 61791-12-6; nonionic; emulsifier, lubricant, antistat; liq.; HLB 4.0.

Ablunol CO 15. [Taiwan Surf.] PEG-15 castor oil; CAS 61791-12-6; nonionic; emulsifier, lubricant, antistat; liq.; HLB 8.5.

Ablunol CO 30. [Taiwan Surf.] PEG-30 castor oil; CAS 61791-12-6; nonionic; emulsifier, lubricant, antistat; liq.; HLB 11.8.

Ablunol DEGMS. [Taiwan Surf.] Diethylene glycol stearate; CAS 9004-99-3; EINECS 203-363-5; nonionic; opacifier, pearlescent for cosmetics, detergents; solid; HLB 3.7.

Ablunol EGDS. [Taiwan Surf.] Glycol distearate; CAS 627-83-8; EINECS 211-014-3; pearlescent, opacifier for emulsions and surfactant preps., shampoos, body cleaners, hand dishwashing detergents, rinses, cosmetics and creams; flake; HLB 1; 100% solids.

Ablunol EGMS. [Taiwan Surf.] Glycol stearate; CAS 111-60-4; EINECS 203-886-9; nonionic; opacifier, pearlescent for cosmetics (emulsions, shampoos, body cleaners, creams), hand dishwashing detergents, rinses; flakes; HLB 2.0; 100% solids.

Ablunol GMS. [Taiwan Surf.] Glyceryl stearate; nonionic; emulsifier for hand creams, lotions, cosmetics; textile lubricant-softener; solid; 100% act.

Ablunol LA-3. [Taiwan Surf.] Laureth-3; CAS 3055-94-5; EINECS 221-280-2; nonionic; emulsifier, dispersant, detergent, wetting agent used in textile processing, cosmetics, metalworking compds., agric., industrial cleaners; liq.; HLB 7.9; 100% act.

Ablunol LA-5. [Taiwan Surf.] Laureth-5; CAS 3055-95-6; EINECS 221-281-8; nonionic; emulsifier, dispersant, detergent, wetting agent used in textile processing, cosmetics, metalworking compds., agric., industrial cleaners; liq.; HLB 10.5; 100% act.

Ablunol LA-7. [Taiwan Surf.] Laureth-7; CAS 3055-97-8; EINECS 221-283-9; nonionic; emulsifier, dispersant, detergent, wetting agent used in textile processing, cosmetics, metalworking compds., agric., industrial cleaners; liq.; HLB 12.1; cloud pt. 28-38 C; 100% act.

Ablunol LA-9. [Taiwan Surf.] Laureth-9; CAS 3055-99-0; EINECS 221-284-4; nonionic; emulsifier, dispersant, detergent, wetting agent used in textile processing, cosmetics, metalworking compds., agric., industrial cleaners; liq.; HLB 13.3; cloud pt. 51-61 C; 100% act.

Ablunol LA-12. [Taiwan Surf.] Laureth-12; CAS 3056-00-6; EINECS 221-286-5; nonionic; emulsifier, dispersant, detergent, wetting agent used in textile processing, cosmetics, metalworking compds., agric., industrial cleaners; liq.; HLB 14.5; cloud pt. 78-88 C; 100% act.

Ablunol LA-16. [Taiwan Surf.] Laureth-16; CAS 9002-92-0; nonionic; emulsifier, dispersant, detergent, wetting agent used in textile processing, cosmetics, metalworking compds., agric., industrial cleaners; semisolid; HLB 15.2; 100% act.

Ablunol LA-40. [Taiwan Surf.] Laureth-40; CAS 9002-92-0; nonionic; emulsifier, dispersant, detergent, wetting agent used in textile processing, cosmetics, metalworking compds., agric., industrial cleaners; solid; HLB 18.0; 100% act.

Ablunol OA-6. [Taiwan Surf.] Oleth-6; CAS 9004-98-2; nonionic; emulsifier for min. oil and cosmetics; liq.; HLB 10.0; 100% act.

Ablunol OA-7. [Taiwan Surf.] Oleth-7; CAS 9004-98-2; nonionic; emulsifier for min. oil and cosmetics; liq.; HLB 10.7; 100% act.

Ablunol S-20. [Taiwan Surf.] Sorbitan laurate; CAS 1338-39-2; nonionic; emulsifier, emulsion stabilizer, thickener for cosmetic, pharmaceutical, food applics.; textile fiber lubricant, softener; antifog agent; oily liq.; oil-sol.; water-disp.; HLB 8.6; 100% act.

Ablunol S-40. [Taiwan Surf.] Sorbitan palmitate; CAS 26266-57-9; EINECS 247-568-8; nonionic; emulsifier, emulsion stabilizer, thickener for cosmetic, pharmaceutical, food applics.; textile fiber lubricant, softener; antifog agent; waxy solid; oil-sol.; HLB 6.7.

Ablunol S-60. [Taiwan Surf.] Sorbitan stearate; CAS 1338-41-6; EINECS 215-664-9; nonionic; emulsifier, emulsion stabilizer, thickener for cosmetic, pharmaceutical, food applics.; textile fiber lubricant, softener; antifog agent; silicone defoamer emulsions; waxy flake; HLB 4.7; 100% act.

Ablunol S-80. [Taiwan Surf.] Sorbitan oleate; CAS 1338-43-8; EINECS 215-665-4; nonionic; emulsifier, emulsion stabilizer, thickener for cosmetic, pharmaceutical, food applics.; textile fiber lubricant, softener; antifog agent; wet processing of syn. PU leather; oily liq.; HLB 4.3; 100% act.

Ablunol S-85. [Taiwan Surf.] Sorbitan trioleate; CAS 26266-58-0; EINECS 247-569-3; nonionic; emulsifier, emulsion stabilizer, thickener for cosmetic, pharmaceutical, food applics.; textile fiber lubricant, softener; antifog agent; oily liq.; HLB 1.8; 100% act.

Ablunol SA-7. [Taiwan Surf.] Steareth-7; CAS 9005-00-9; nonionic; emulsifier for wax and cosmetics; solid; HLB 10.7; 100% act.

Ablunol T-20. [Taiwan Surf.] POE sorbitan laurate; nonionic; o/w emulsifier for cosmetic, pharmaceutical and food applics.; oily liq.; water-sol.; HLB 16.7; 100% solids.

Ablunol T-40. [Taiwan Surf.] POE sorbitan laurate; nonionic; o/w emulsifier for cosmetic, pharmaceutical and food applics.; oily liq.; water-sol.; HLB 15.6; 100% conc.

Ablunol T-60. [Taiwan Surf.] POE sorbitan stearate; nonionic; o/w emulsifier for cosmetic, pharmaceutical and food applics.; oily liq.; water-sol.; HLB 14.9; 100% conc.

Ablunol T-80. [Taiwan Surf.] POE sorbitan oleate; nonionic; o/w emulsifier for cosmetic, pharmaceutical and food applics.; oily liq.; water-sol.; HLB 15.0; 100% conc.

Abluphat MLP-200. [Taiwan Surf.] Monolauryl phosphate; CAS 12751-23-4; EINECS 235-798-1; moderate cleaning and foaming agent, base material for facial foaming cleansers, body shampoos; very mild to human skin; solid; HLB 10.0; 100% solids.

Abluphat MLP-220. [Taiwan Surf.] Monolaureth phosphate; moderate cleaning and foaming agent, base material for facial foaming cleansers, body shampoos; very mild to human skin; paste; HLB 12.5; 100% solids.

Ablusol CDE. [Taiwan Surf.] Cocamide DEA sulfosuccinate monoester; anionic; detergent, foam booster/stabilizer for low irritation shampoos, bubble baths, liq. detergents; liq.; 40% act.

Ablusol DBD. [Taiwan Surf.] DEA dodecylbenzene sulfonate; CAS 26545-53-9; EINECS 247-784-2; anionic; surfactant, emulsifier, wetting agent for bubble bath, shampoos, detergents; liq.; water-sol.; 100% act.

Ablusol DBM. [Taiwan Surf.] Ammonium dodecylbenzene sulfonate; CAS 1331-61-9; EINECS 215-559-8; anionic; surfactant, emulsifier, wetting agent for bubble bath, shampoos, detergents; liq.; water-sol.; 100% act.

Ablusol DBT. [Taiwan Surf.] TEA dodecylbenzene sulfonate; CAS 27323-41-7; EINECS 248-406-9; anionic; surfactant, emulsifier, wetting agent for bubble bath, shampoos, detergents; liq.; water-sol.; 100% act.

Ablusol LA. [Taiwan Surf.] Ethoxylated lauryl alcohol sulfosuccinate monoester; anionic; surfactant for bubble bath, shampoo, skin cleansing preps. where high sudsing and low skin irritation are important; liq.; 40% act.

Ablusol LAE. [Taiwan Surf.] Disodium laureth sulfosuccinate; low-irritation foaming agent for shampoos, bubble bath, and body cleansers; has some conditioning and moisturizing effect; liq.; 40% solids.

Ablusol LDE. [Taiwan Surf.] Lauramide DEA sulfosuccinate monoester; anionic; detergent, foam booster/stabilizer for low irritation shampoos, bubble baths, liq. detergents; liq.; water-sol.; 40% act.

Abluter CPB. [Taiwan Surf.] Cocamidopropyl betaine; amphoteric; foam booster for shampoos; visc. builder; low-irritation skin cleaner; lime dispersant; aids deposition of protein and cationic polymer on the hair; coemulsifier; liq.; 35% solids.

Abluter CPS. [Taiwan Surf.] Cocamidopropyl hydroxysultaine; CAS 68139-30-0; EINECS 268-761-3; amphoteric; high-foaming mild detergent for shampoos and bubble bath; better response to salt than regular betaines; coemulsifier; liq.; 50% solids.

Abluter DCM-2. [Taiwan Surf.] Cocoamphocarboxyglycinate; CAS 68650-39-5; EINECS 272-043-5; amphoteric; high-foaming mild detergent for shampoos and bubble bath; conditioner; liq.; 50% solids.

Abluter LDB. [Taiwan Surf.] Lauryl betaine; CAS 683-10-3; EINECS 211-669-5; amphoteric; high-foaming mild detergent for shampoos and bubble bath; liq.; 35% solids.

Abscents® Deodorizing Powd. [UOP] Organophilic molecular sieve (sodium potassium aluminosilicate); hypoallergenic deodorizing powd. for odor control in unscented personal care prods. (feminine protection, diapers, body/foot powds., deodorants, nonwoven wipes, ostomy prods.); attracts odors and traps them tightly within its porous structure; maintains capability in high humidity or wet conditions; effective against org. acids, ammonia, aldehydes, sulfur compds., ketones, indoles, amines, perspiration, menstrual flow, fecal matter, urine; stable to > 800 C and at pH 3-10; meets Codex requirements; wh. free-flowing dry powd., odorless; particle size 3-5 μ; insol. in water or org. solvs.; sp.gr. 2.0; bulk dens. 33 lb/ft³ (tapped); surf. area > 400 m²/g; oil adsorp. 60 g/100 g; pH 5.0-6.5 (10% slurry); ref. index. 1.45-1.47; toxicology: low acute toxicity by ingestion, skin penetration, dust inhalation; sl. eye irritant; mild vaginal irritant.

Abscents 1000. [UOP] Zeolite.

Abscents 2000. [UOP] Zeolite.

Abscents 5000. [UOP] Zeolite.

A-C® 6. [Allied-Signal/A-C® Perf. Addit.] Polyethylene homopolymer; CAS 9002-88-4; EINECS 200-815-3; additive wax for use in adhesives, ink, floor finishes, paper coatings, personal care, plastics, rubber, textiles, wax blends; gellant for oils in personal care prods.; increases permanency, emolliency, moisture retention, water resist., and thermal stability; film-former, oil or fragrance encapsulator, nonirritating abrasive; prills, powd.; dens. 0.92 g/cc; visc. 375 cps (140 C); drop pt. 106 C; acid no. nil; hardness 4.0 dmm.

A-C® 6A. [Allied-Signal/A-C® Perf. Addit.] Polyethylene homopolymer; CAS 9002-88-4; EINECS 200-815-3; additive wax for use in adhesives, inks, floor finishes, paper coatings, personal care, plastics, rubber, textiles, and wax blends; gellant for oils in personal care prods.; increases permanency, emolliency, moisture retention, water resist., and thermal stability; film-former, oil or fragrance encapsulator, nonirritating abrasive; prills, powd.; dens. 0.92 g/cc; visc. 375 cps (140 C); drop pt. 106

C; acid no. nil; hardness 4.0 dmm.

A-C® 7, 7A. [Allied-Signal/A-C® Perf. Addit.] Polyethylene homopolymer wax; CAS 9002-88-4; EINECS 200-815-3; processing lubricant, melt index modifier, pigment dispersant, mold release aid; external lubricant PVC, color concs., polyolefin flow modifiers; thickener for cosmetic and pharmaceutical gels; powd. (A grades), others prilled or diced; sol. in hot min. oil and fatty esters.

A-C® 8, 8A. [Allied-Signal/A-C® Perf. Addit.] Polyethylene homopolymer; CAS 9002-88-4; EINECS 200-815-3; gellant for oils in personal care prods.; increases permanency, emolliency, moisture retention, water resist., and thermal stability; film-former, oil or fragrance encapsulator, nonirritating abrasive; processing lubricant, melt index modifier, pigment dispersant, mold release aid; external lubricant PVC, color concs., polyolefin flow modifiers; dens. 0.93 g/cc; visc. 400 cps (140 C); drop. pt. 116 C; acid no. nil; hardness 1.0 dmm.

A-C® 9, 9A, 9F. [Allied-Signal/A-C® Perf. Addit.] Polyethylene homopolymer; CAS 9002-88-4; EINECS 200-815-3; gellant for oils in personal care prods.; increases permanency, emolliency, moisture retention, water resist., and thermal stability; film-former, oil or fragrance encapsulator, nonirritating abrasive; processing lubricant, melt index modifier, pigment dispersant, mold release aid; external lubricant PVC, color concs., polyolefin flow modifiers; avg. particle size 220 μ (9A), 110 μ (9F); dens. 0.94 g/cc; visc. 450 cps (140 C); drop. pt. 117 C; acid no. nil; hardness 0.5 dmm.

A-C® 15. [Allied-Signal/A-C® Perf. Addit.] Polyethylene homopolymer; CAS 9002-88-4; EINECS 200-815-3; additive wax for use in inks and personal care prods.; gellant for oils in personal care prods.; increases permanency, emolliency, moisture retention, water resist., and thermal stability; film-former, oil or fragrance encapsulator, nonirritating abrasive; prills; dens. 0.93 g/cc; visc. 125 cps (140 C); drop pt. 109 C; acid no. nil; hardness 2.5 dmm.

A-C® 16. [Allied-Signal/A-C® Perf. Addit.] Polyethylene homopolymer; CAS 9002-88-4; EINECS 200-815-3; gellant for oils in personal care prods.; increases permanency, emolliency, moisture retention, water resist., and thermal stability; film-former, oil or fragrance encapsulator, nonirritating abrasive; dens. 0.91 g/cc; visc. 525 cps (140 C); drop. pt. 102 C; acid no. nil; hardness 5.5 dmm.

A-C® 143. [Allied-Signal/A-C® Perf. Addit.] Ethylene-acrylic acid copolymer; CAS 9010-77-9; gellant for oils in personal care prods.; increases permanency, emolliency, moisture retention, water resist., and thermal stability; film-former, oil or fragrance encapsulator, nonirritating abrasive; dens. 0.94 g/cc; visc. 650 cps (140 C); drop. pt. 92 C; acid no. 120; hardness 11.5 dmm.

A-C® 316, 316A. [Allied-Signal/A-C® Perf. Addit.] Oxidized HDPE homopolymer; CAS 68441-17-8; additive wax for ink, floor finishes, personal care, plastics, textiles, wax blends; gellant for oils in personal care prods.; increases permanency, emolliency, moisture retention, water resist., and thermal stability; film-former, oil or fragrance encapsulator, nonirritating abrasive; gran., powd.; dens. 0.98 g/cc; visc. 8500 cps (150 C); drop pt. 140 C; acid no. 16; hardness < 0.5 dmm.

A-C® 395, 395A. [Allied-Signal/A-C® Perf. Addit.] Oxidized HDPE homopolymer; CAS 68441-17-8; additive wax for use in inks and personal care prods.; gran.; dens. 1.00 g/cc; visc. 2500 cps (150 C); drop pt. 137 C; acid no. 41; hardness < 0.5 dmm.

A-C® 400. [Allied-Signal/A-C® Perf. Addit.] Ethylene/VA copolymer; CAS 24937-78-8; additive wax for use in adhesives, inks, personal care, and wax blends; gellant for oils in personal care prods.; increases permanency, emolliency, moisture retention, water resist., and thermal stability; film-former, oil or fragrance encapsulator, nonirritating abrasive; prills, powd.; dens. 0.92 g/cc; visc. 575 cps (140 C); drop pt. 92 C; hardness 9.5 dmm; 13% VA.

A-C® 400A. [Allied-Signal/A-C® Perf. Addit.] Low m.w. EVA copolymer; CAS 24937-78-8; wax additive for use in adhesives, inks, personal care prods., wax blends; pigment dispersant; PS color concs.; gellant for oils in personal care prods.; increases permanency, emolliency, moisture retention, water resist., and thermal stability; film-former, oil or fragrance encapsulator, nonirritating abrasive; prills, powd.; dens. 0.92 g/cc; visc. 575 cps (140 C); drop pt. 92 C; hardness 9.5 dmm; 13% VA.

A-C® 405M. [Allied-Signal/A-C® Perf. Addit.] EVA copolymer; CAS 24937-78-8; wax additive for adhesives, inks, personal care, wax blends; prills; dens. 0.92 g/cc; visc. 600 cps (140 C); drop pt. 101 C; hardness 5.0 dmm; 8% VA.

A-C® 405S. [Allied-Signal/A-C® Perf. Addit.] EVA copolymer; CAS 24937-78-8; wax additive for adhesives, inks, personal care, wax blends; prills; dens. 0.92 g/cc; visc. 600 cps (140 C); drop pt. 95 C; hardness 7.0 dmm; 11% VA.

A-C® 405T. [Allied-Signal/A-C® Perf. Addit.] EVA copolymer; CAS 24937-78-8; wax additive for adhesives, inks, personal care, wax blends; gellant for oils in personal care prods.; increases permanency, emolliency, moisture retention, water resist., and thermal stability; film-former, oil or fragrance encapsulator, nonirritating abrasive; prills; dens. 0.92 g/cc; visc. 600 cps (140 C); drop pt. 103 C; hardness 4.0 dmm; 6% VA.

A-C® 430. [Allied-Signal/A-C® Perf. Addit.] EVA copolymer; CAS 24937-78-8; gellant for oils in personal care prods.; increases permanency, emolliency, moisture retention, water resist., and thermal stability; film-former, oil or fragrance encapsulator, nonirritating abrasive; wax additive for adhesives, personal care, wax blends; suspending agent for active ingreds. in cosmetic formulations; grease-like; dens. 0.93 g/cc; visc. 600 cps (140 C); drop pt. 80 C.

A-C® 540, 540A. [Allied-Signal/A-C® Perf. Addit.] Ethylene-acrylic acid copolymer; CAS 9010-77-9; plastics lubricant and processing aid, pigment dispersant; internal lubricant PVC, nylon 6, nylon color concs.; for adhesives, floor finishes, personal care, plastics, wax blends; gellant for oils in personal care prods.; increases permanency, emolliency, moisture retention, water resist., and thermal stability; film-former, oil or fragrance encapsulator, nonirritating abrasive; prills, powd.; dens. 0.93 g/cc; visc. 575 cps (140 C); drop pt. 105 C; acid no. 40; hardness 2.0 dmm.

A-C® 580. [Allied-Signal/A-C® Perf. Addit.] Ethylene/acrylic acid copolymer; CAS 9010-77-9; alkali-dispersible additive for recyclable hot-melt and aq. adhesives and coatings; gellant for oils in personal care prods.; increases permanency, emolliency, moisture retention, water resist., and thermal stability; film-former, oil or fragrance encapsulator, nonirritating abrasive; dens. 0.94 g/cc; visc. 650 cps (140 C); drop pt. 102 C; acid no. 75; hardness 4.0 dmm.

A-C® 617, 617A. [Allied-Signal/A-C® Perf. Addit.] Polyethylene homopolymer; CAS 9002-88-4; EINECS 200-815-3; additive wax for use in inks, plastics, rubber, and personal care prods.; thickener for cosmetic and pharmaceutical gels; increases permanency, emolliency, moisture retention, water resist., and thermal stability; film-former, oil or fragrance encapsulator, nonirritating abrasive; prills, powd.; sol. in hot min. oil and fatty esters; dens. 0.91 g/cc; visc. 200 cps (140 C); drop pt. 101 C; acid no. nil; hardness 7.0 dmm.

A-C® 617G. [Allied-Signal/A-C® Perf. Addit.] Polyethylene homopolymer; CAS 9002-88-4; EINECS 200-815-3; gellant for oils in personal care prods.; increases permanency, emolliency, moisture retention, water resist., and thermal stability; film-former, oil or fragrance encapsulator, nonirritating abrasive; dens. 0.91 g/cc; visc. 200 cps (140 C); drop. pt. 102 C; acid no. nil; hardness 7.0 dmm.

A-C® 629, 629A. [Allied-Signal/A-C® Perf. Addit.] Oxidized polyethylene homopolymer; CAS 68441-17-8; additive wax for adhesives, ink, floor finishes, paper coatings, personal care, plastics, textiles, wax blends; processing lubricant, mold release aid; PVC lubricant; gellant for oils in personal care prods.; increases permanency, emolliency, moisture retention, water resist., and thermal stability; film-former, oil or fragrance encapsulator, nonirritating abrasive; prills, powd.; dens. 0.93 g/cc; visc. 200 cps (140 C); drop pt. 101 C; acid no. 15; hardness 5.5 dmm.

A-C® 655. [Allied-Signal/A-C® Perf. Addit.] Oxidized polyethylene homopolymer; CAS 68441-17-8; additive wax for use in adhesives, inks, floor finishes, paper coatings, personal care, plastics, rubber, textiles, and wax blends; prills; dens. 0.93 g/cc; visc. 210 cps (140 C); drop pt. 107 C; acid no. 16; hardness 2.5 dmm.

A-C® 656. [Allied-Signal/A-C® Perf. Addit.] Oxidized polyethylene homopolymer; CAS 68441-17-8; additive wax for use in adhesives, inks, floor finishes, paper coatings, personal care, plastics, and rubber; prills; dens. 0.92 g/cc; visc. 185 cps (140 C); drop pt. 98 C; acid no. 15; hardness 9.0 dmm.

A-C® 1702. [Allied-Signal/A-C® Perf. Addit.] Polyethylene homopolymer; CAS 9002-88-4; EINECS 200-815-3; gellant for oils in personal care prods.; increases permanency, emolliency, moisture retention, water resist., and thermal stability; film-former, oil or fragrance encapsulator, nonirritating abrasive; dens. 0.88 g/cc; visc. 40 cps (140 C); drop. pt. 92 C; acid no. nil; hardness 90.0 dmm (D1321).

A-C® 5120. [Allied-Signal/A-C® Perf. Addit.] Low m.w. ethylene-acrylic acid copolymer; CAS 9010-77-9; alkalidispersible additive for recyclable hot-melt and aq. adhesives and coatings; gellant for personal care and household prods. (cosmetics, protective moisturizers, medications, dental adhesives, deodorizers); dens. 0.94 g/cc; visc. 650 cps (140 C); drop pt. 92 C; acid no. 120; hardness 11.5 dmm.

A-C® 6702. [Allied-Signal/A-C® Perf. Addit.] Oxidized polyethylene; CAS 68441-17-8; gellant for oils in personal care prods.; increases permanency, emolliency, moisture retention, water resist., and thermal stability; film-former, oil or fragrance encapsulator, nonirritating abrasive; dens. 0.85 g/cc; visc. 35 cps (140 C); drop pt. 85 C; acid no. 15; hardness 90.0 dmm (D1321).

Acacia Flower Extract HS 2744 G. [Grau Aromatics] Propylene glycol and acacia extract; botanical extract.

Acacia Glycolysat. [C.E.P.] Propylene glycol, water, black locust extract; botanical extract.

Acacia Oleat M. [C.E.P.] Propylene glycol dicaprylate/dicaprate and black locust extract.

Accomeen C2. [Karlshamns] PEG-2 cocamine; CAS 61791-14-8; nonionic; emulsifier, antistat, surfactant; Gardner 4–6 liq., amine odor; sol. in org. solv.; dens. 7.25 lb/gal; sp.gr. 0.87; 99% act.

Accomeen C5. [Karlshamns] PEG-5 cocamine; CAS 61791-14-8; nonionic; emulsifier, antistat, surfactant; Gardner 4–6 liq., amine odor; sol. in org. solv., water; dens. 8.15 lb/gal; sp.gr. 0.98; 99% act.

Accomeen C10. [Karlshamns] PEG-10 cocamine; CAS 61791-14-8; nonionic; emulsifier, antistat, surfactant; Gardner 4–6 liq., amine odor; sol. in org. solv., water;

dens. 8.3 lb/gal; sp.gr. 1.0; 99% act.

Accomeen C15. [Karlshamns] PEG-15 cocamine; CAS 61791-14-8; nonionic; emulsifier, antistat, surfactant; Gardner 4–6 liq., amine odor; sol. in org. solv.; dens. 8.7 lb/gal; sp.gr. 1.04; 99% act.

Accomeen S2. [Karlshamns] PEG-2 soyamine; CAS 61791-24-0; nonionic; emulsifier, antistat, surfactant; Gardner 5–10 liq.; amine odor; sol. in org. solv.; dens. 7.6 lb/gal; sp.gr. 0.91; surf. tens. 31.3 (0.1%); 99% act.

Accomeen S10. [Karlshamns] PEG-10 soyamine; CAS 61791-24-0; nonionic; emulsifier, antistat, surfactant; Gardner 5–10 liq.; amine odor; sol. in org. solv., water; dens. 8.5 lb/gal; sp.gr. 1.02; 99% act.

Accomeen S15. [Karlshamns] PEG-15 soyamine; CAS 61791-24-0; surfactant.

Accomeen T2. [Karlshamns] PEG-2 tallow amine; CAS 61791-44-4; nonionic; emulsifier, antistat, surfactant, dispersant; Gardner 3–5; amine odor; sol. in org. solv., insol. in water; dens. 7.7 lb/gal; sp.gr. 0.92; 99% act.

Accomeen T5. [Karlshamns] PEG-5 tallow amine; CAS 61791-44-4; nonionic; emulsifier, antistat, surfactant, dispersant; Gardner 3–5; amine odor; sol. in org. solv., insol. in water; 99% act.

Accomeen T15. [Karlshamns] PEG-15 tallow amine; nonionic; emulsifier, antistat, surfactant, dispersant; Gardner 3–5; amine odor; sol. in org. solv., insol. in water; dens. 8.1 lb/gal; sp.gr. 0.97); 99% act.

Accomid 50. [Karlshamns] Palm kernelamide DEA; CAS 73807-15-5; surfactant, thickener.

Accomid C. [Karlshamns] Cocamide DEA (1:1); CAS 61791-31-9; EINECS 263-163-9; nonionic; detergent, emulsifier, visc. builder, foam booster/stabilizer for shampoos, bath prods., liq. soap, liq. detergents, dishwashes; biodeg.; Gardner 4 liq., mild odor; water-sol.; sp.gr. 0.99; dens. 8.3 lb/gal; pH 9-10.5; 98% act.

Accomid PK. [Karlshamns] Palm kernelamide DEA (1:1); CAS 73807-15-5; nonionic; visc. builder, foam booster/stabilizer, emulsifier for shampoos, liq. soaps, dish detergents, bubble bath prods.; Gardner 5 liq.; pH 9–10.6 (10% aq.).

Acconon 200-MS. [Karlshamns] PEG-4 stearate; CAS 9004-99-3; EINECS 203-358-8; nonionic; surfactant used as emulsifier, dispersant, solubilizer, visc. control agent for cosmetics, hair care preps., pharmaceuticals, and industrial applics.; Gardner 4 max. solid; HLB 8; pH 5.5–6.5.

Acconon 400-MO. [Karlshamns] PEG-8 oleate; CAS 9004-96-0; nonionic; emulsifier, dispersant, lubricant, chemical intermediate, solubilizer, visc. control agent; for cosmetics, pharmaceuticals, food, agric., plastics; Gardner 4 max. liq.; sol. in org. solv.; water-disp.; sp.gr. 1.01; dens. 8.4 lb/gal; m.p. < 10 C; HLB 12; pH 5.5–6.5; 99% act.

Acconon 400-MS. [Karlshamns] PEG-8 stearate; CAS 9004-99-3; nonionic; surfactant used as emulsifier, dispersant, solubilizer, visc. control agent for cosmetics, pharmaceuticals, and industrial applics.; Gardner 4 max. solid; HLB 12; pH 5.5–6.5.

Acconon 1300. [Karlshamns] PPG-3-laureth-9; nonionic; surfactant used as emulsifier, dispersant, solubilizer, visc. control agent for cosmetics, pharmaceuticals, and industrial applics.; Gardner 3 max. liq.; sp.gr. 1.016–1.019; dens. 8.35–8.45 lb/gal; HLB 11; cloud pt. 135–145 F; pH 6.0–7.0.

Acconon CA-5. [Karlshamns] PEG-5 castor oil; CAS 61791-12-6; nonionic; surfactant used as emulsifier, dispersant, solubilizer, visc. control agent for cosmetics, pharmaceuticals, and industrial applics.; Gardner 3 max. liq.; HLB 8.0; pH 6.0–7.0.

Acconon CA-9. [Karlshamns] PEG-9 castor oil; CAS 61791-12-6; nonionic; surfactant used as emulsifier, lubricant, dispersant, solubilizer, visc. control agent for cosmetics, pharmaceuticals, and industrial applics.; Gardner 3 max. liq.; water-disp.; HLB 12.0; pH 6-7.

Acconon CA 10. [Karlshamns] PPG-10 cetyl ether; CAS 9035-85-2; emollient.

Acconon CA-15. [Karlshamns] PEG-15 castor oil; CAS 61791-12-6; nonionic; surfactant used as emulsifier, lubricant, dispersant, solubilizer, visc. control agent for cosmetics, pharmaceuticals, and industrial applics.; Gardner 3 max. liq.; water-disp.; HLB 16; pH 6.0–7.0.

Acconon CON. [Karlshamns] PEG-10 propylene glycol glyceryl laurate; nonionic; surfactant used as emulsifier, dispersant, solubilizer, visc. control agent for cosmetics, pharmaceuticals, and industrial applics.; Gardner 2 max. liq.; HLB 10; pH 6.0–7.0.

Acconon E. [Karlshamns] PPG-15 stearyl ether; CAS 25231-21-4; nonionic; surfactant used as emulsifier, dispersant, solubilizer, visc. control agent for cosmetics, pharmaceuticals, and industrial applics.; Gardner 3 max. liq.; HLB 16; pH 6.0–7.0.

Acconon ETG. [Karlshamns] Glycereth-26; CAS 31694-55-0; nonionic; humectant; lubricant for skin care prods., creams, lotions, industrial applics.; Gardner 3 max. liq.; sol. in water, alcohol, ketones, esters; HLB 15; pH 5.5–6.5.

Acconon MA3. [Karlshamns] PPG-3 myristyl ether; CAS 63793-60-2; emollient.

Acconon TGH. [Karlshamns] PEG-20-PPG-10 glyceryl stearate; nonionic; surfactant used as emulsifier, dispersant, solubilizer, visc. control agent, wetting and foaming agent for cosmetics, pharmaceuticals, and industrial applics.; biodeg.; Gardner 3 max. liq., mild odor; HLB 16; pH 6.0–7.0; 100% conc.

Acconon W230. [Karlshamns] Ceteareth-20; CAS 68439-49-6; nonionic; surfactant used as emulsifier, dispersant, solubilizer, visc. control agent for cosmetics, pharmaceuticals, and industrial applics.; Gardner 3 max. solid; HLB 15; pH 6.5–7.5.

Acelan A. [Fabriquimica] Cetyl acetate, acetylated lanolin alcohol; multifunctional cosmetic ingred.; drop pt. 16-20 C; acid no. < 1; iodine no. 6-12; sapon. no. 180-200.

Acelan L. [Fabriquimica] Acetylated lanolin; CAS 61788-48-5; EINECS 262-979-2; multifunctional cosmetic ingred.; drop pt. 30-40 C; acid no. < 3; iodine no. 16-30; sapon. no. 95-125.

Acerola Extract HS 2855 G. [Grau Aromatics] Propylene glycol and bitter cherry extract; botanical extract.

Acetadeps. [Westbrook Lanolin] Acetylated lanolin; CAS 61788-48-5; EINECS 262-979-2; emollient, moisturizer for antiperspirants, baby oils, cleansers, shampoos, hair conditioners, sunscreen; binder for pressed powds.; m.p. 33039; acid no. 3 max.; sapon. no. 100-120; hyd. no. 8 max.

Acetol® 1706. [Henkel/Cospha; Henkel Canada] Cetyl acetate, acetylated lanolin alcohol; water repellent; strongly hydrophobic emollient, penetrant, lubricant, and cosolv. used in hair prods., creams, lotions, bath preps., suntan preps., and baby prods.; lt. yel. liq.; sol. in IPM, min., castor, and olive oil; water-insol.

Acetoquat CTAB. [Aceto] Cetrimonium bromide; CAS 57-09-0; EINECS 200-311-3; cationic; germicide, sanitizing agent; powd.; 95% act.

Acetulan® . [Amerchol] Cetyl acetate, acetylated lanolin alcohol; binder for pressed powds.; emollient, plasticizer, cosolv., NV and sebum solv. for personal care prods.; lubricant for clay, talc, and starch; stabilizer for lanolin; solubilizer in aerosols; penetrant and spreading agent; pale yel. thin oily liq.; odorless; sol. in ethanol, min., castor and veg. oil, IPM, IPP, IPA, silicone, butyl stearate, sulfonated castor oil, ethyl acetate, and org. solv.; insol. in water; sp.gr. 0.850–0.880; visc. 10 cps; acid no. 1.0 max.;

sapon. no. 180–200; hyd. 8.0 max.; pH neutral.

Acidan BC Veg. [Grindsted Prods.] Hydrog. vegetable glycerides citrate; CAS 97593-31-2; EINECS 207-334-9.

Acidan N 12. [Grindsted Prods.] Hydrog. tallow glyceride citrate; CAS 68990-59-0; EINECS 273-613-6; used in emulsions, w/o phase creams and lotions, hair care.

Acidan N 12 Veg. [Grindsted Prods.] Hydrog. vegetable glycerides citrate; CAS 97593-31-2; EINECS 207-334-9.

Acid Mucopolysaccharides. [R.I.T.A.] Hydrolyzed glycosaminoglycans; moisturizer.

Acintol® 2122. [Arizona] Tall oil heads; CAS 61790-12-3; EINECS 263-107-3; surfactant; Gardner 16 solid; sp.gr. 0.92; dens. 7.60 lb/gal; visc. 15 cps (50 C); flash pt. (CC) > 200 F; acid no. 135-155; sapon. no. 105-155; 76.2-68.2% fatty acids.

Acintol® 7002. [Arizona] Tall oil acid; CAS 61790-12-3; EINECS 263-107-3; surfactant; Gardner > 18; sp.gr. 0.97; dens. 7.89 lb/gal; visc. 1600-2000 cps; flash pt. (CC) > 200 F; acid no. 140-142; sapon. no. 179; 76.2-68.2% fatty acids.

AClyn® 201. [Allied-Signal] Ethylene/calcium acrylate copolymer; CAS 26445-96-5.

AClyn® 201A. [Allied-Signal] Ethylene/calcium acrylate copolymer; CAS 26445-96-5; low m.w. ionomers used as processing and performance additives; improves dispersion of additives in plastics; adhesion to variety of substrates; encapsulant for personal care prods.; visc. 5500 cps (190 C); m.p. 102 C; acid no. 42.

AClyn® 246. [Allied-Signal] Ethylene/magnesium acrylate copolymer.

AClyn® 246A. [Allied-Signal] Ethylene/magnesium acrylate copolymer; low m.w. ionomers used as processing and performance additives; improves dispersion of additives in plastics; adhesion to variety of substrates; encapsulant for personal care prods.; visc. 7000 cps (190 C); m.p. 95 C; acid no. nil.

AClyn® 262A. [Allied-Signal/A-C® Perf. Addit.] Ethylene/sodium acrylate copolymer; CAS 25750-82-7; low m.w. ionomer; encapsulant for personal care prods.; visc. 2800 cps (190 C); m.p. 102 C; acid no. 40.

AClyn® 272, 276, 285. [Allied-Signal] Ethylene/sodium acrylate copolymer; CAS 25750-82-7; encapsulant for personal care prods.

AClyn® 272A. [Allied-Signal/A-C® Perf. Addit.] Ethylene/sodium acrylate copolymer; CAS 25750-82-7; low m.w. ionomer; encapsulant for personal care prods.; visc. 1400 cps (190 C); m.p. 105 C; acid no. 20.

AClyn® 276A. [Allied-Signal/A-C® Perf. Addit.] Ethylene/sodium acrylate copolymer; CAS 25750-82-7; low m.w. ionomer; encapsulant for personal care prods.; visc. 70,000 cps (190 C); m.p. 98 C; acid no. nil.

AClyn® 285A. [Allied-Signal/A-C® Perf. Addit.] Ethylene/sodium acrylate copolymer; CAS 25750-82-7; low m.w. ionomer; encapsulant for personal care prods.; visc. 110,000 cps (190 C); m.p. 82 C; acid no. 20.

AClyn® 291, 293, 295. [Allied-Signal] Ethylene/zinc acrylate copolymer.

AClyn® 291A. [Allied-Signal/A-C® Perf. Addit.] Ethylene/zinc acrylate copolymer; low m.w. ionomer; encapsulant for personal care prods.; visc. 5500 cps (190 C); m.p. 102 C; acid no. 40.

AClyn® 293A. [Allied-Signal/A-C® Perf. Addit.] Ethylene/zinc acrylate copolymer; low m.w. ionomer; encapsulant for personal care prods.; visc. 500 cps (190 C); m.p. 101 C; acid no. 30.

AClyn® 295A. [Allied-Signal/A-C® Perf. Addit.] Ethylene/zinc acrylate copolymer; low m.w. ionomer; encapsulant for personal care prods.; visc. 4500 cps (190 C); m.p. 99 C; acid no. nil.

Acrisint 400, 410, 430. [3V-Sigma] Carbomer; emulsifier, thickener, stabilizer, suspending agent used in cosmetics.

Acritamer® 934. [R.I.T.A.] Carbomer 934; emulsifier, dispersing, suspending and visc. agent, gellant for use in systems where sparkling clarity is not essential; stabilizer for w/o and o/w emulsions; suitable for topical pharmaceuticals, cosmetic/personal care, and industrial applics.; wh. fluffy hygroscopic powd.; water-disp.; m.w. 3,000,000; bulk dens. 15 lb/ft³; visc. 2000-5450 cps (0.2%), 26,000-39,500 cps (0.5%); pH 2.7-3.3 (0.5%); toxicology: mildly irritating to eyes; nonirritating to skin, nonsensitizing.

Acritamer® 934P. [R.I.T.A.] Carbomer 934 NF; pharmaceutical grade emulsifier, dispersing, suspending and visc. agent and gellant for use in systems where sparkling clarity is not essential; stabilizer for w/o and o/w emulsions; suitable for topical and oral pharmaceuticals, cosmetic and personal care applics.; wh. fluffy hygroscopic powd.; bulk dens. 15 lb/ft³; visc. 2000-5450 cps (0.2%), 26,000-39,500 cps (0.5%); pH 2.7-3.3 (0.5%); toxicology: mildly irritating to eyes; nonirritating to skin, nonsensitizing.

Acritamer® 940. [R.I.T.A.] Carbomer 940; emulsifier, dispersing, suspending and visc. agent, gellant for use in systems where sparkling clarity or a sharp visc. response is required; stabilizer for w/o and o/w emulsions; suitable for topical pharmaceuticals, cosmetic/personal care, and industrial applics.; wh. fluffy hygroscopic powd.; m.w. 4,000,000; bulk dens. 15 lb/ft³; visc. 15,000-30,000 cps (0.2%), 45,000-70,000 cps (0.5%); pH 2.7-3.3 (0.5%); toxicology: mildly irritating to eyes; nonirritating to skin, nonsensitizing.

Acritamer® 941. [R.I.T.A.] Carbomer 941; emulsifier, dispersing, suspending and visc. agent, gellant for use in systems where ionic strength interferes with proper gellation; stabilizer for w/o and o/w emulsions; suitable for topical pharmaceuticals, cosmetic/personal care, and industrial applics.; wh. fluffy hygroscopic powd.; m.w. 1,250,000; bulk dens. 15 lb/ft³; visc. 2500-6400 cps (0.2%), 5400-11,400 cps (0.5%); pH 2.7-3.3 (0.5%); toxicology: mildly irritating to eyes; nonirritating to skin, nonsensitizing.

Acrymul AM 123R. [Protex] Acrylates copolymer; thickener, stabilizer for cosmetics.

Acrysol® 22 Polymer. [Rohm & Haas Europe] Acrylates/steareth-20 methacrylate copolymer; thickener, stabilizer for sunscreens, lotions, makeup, shampoos, aq. formulations; liq.; usage level: 1-6%; 28% act. in water.

Acrysol® 33 Polymer. [Rohm & Haas Europe] Acrylates copolymer; thickener, stabilizer for sunscreens, lotions, makeup, shampoos, aq. formulations; liq.; usage level: 1-6%; 28% act. in water.

Acrysol® A-1. [Rohm & Haas] Polyacrylic acid; CAS 9003-01-4; emulsifier, thickener.

Acrysol® ICS-1 Thickener. [Rohm & Haas] Acrylates/steareth-20 methacrylate copolymer; thickener for cosmetics.

ACS 60. [Witco/H-I-P] Ammonium cumenesulfonate.; CAS 37475-88-0; EINECS 253-519-1; hydrotrope, solubilizer for personal care applics.

Act II 500 USP. [Luzenac Am.] Talc USP/FCC; CAS 14807-96-6; EINECS 238-877-9; ultrafine high purity talc featuring softness, brightness; wh. extender and antitackifying agent; esp. for aerosol applics.; USP, CTFA, and FCC compliance; powd.; 99.9% thru 400 mesh; median diam. 3.5 μ; tapped dens. 36 lb/ft³; pH 9 (10% slurry).

Actibronze. [Alban Muller; Tri-K Industries] Glucose tyrosinate; amino acid/enzyme complex used as sun-tan facilitator.

Acticel™ 12. [Active Organics] Microcrystalline cellulose; CAS 9004-34-6; porous vehicle permitting high loadings of both aq. and oily prods. while exhibiting exc. compress-

ibility; can be used in conjunction with Actiphytes and Aromaphytes; recommended to enhance texture and applic. of bar soaps, pressed/loose powds.; usage level: 5-50%.

Acticel™ Plus. [Active Organics] Microcrystalline cellulose; CAS 9004-34-6; porous vehicle permitting high loadings of aq. and oily prods.; for incorporating botanical extracts into compressed powds., e.g., eyeshadow and blushers.

Actigen C. [Active Organics] Soluble collagen; CAS 9007-34-5; EINECS 232-697-4; cosmetic protein.

Actigen E. [Active Organics] Hydrolyzed elastin; CAS 100085-10-7; cosmetic protein.

Actiglide™. [Active Organics] Sodium hyaluronate and hydrolyzed glycosaminoglycans; lubricating moisturizer for skin care preps., moisturizing creams, lotions, gels, foundations, eye shadows, eyeliners, and mascaras; colorless to lt. yel. visc. liq., char. odor; sol. in water; sp.gr. 1.02-1.09; pH 4.5-6.5; usage level: 1-35%.

Actiglow™. [Active Organics] Hydrolyzed glycosaminoglycans; skin conditioner for moisturizing lotions, creams, gels, masques, and face packs.

Actiglow™ C. [Active Organics] Hydrolyzed mucopolysaccharides; skin conditioner for moisturizing lotions, creams, gels, masques, and face packs.

Actimoist™. [Active Organics] Sodium hyaluronate sol'n.; CAS 9067-32-7; moisturizer for skin care preps., foundations, moisturizing creams and lotions, eyeshadow, eye liners, mascaras; esp. effective for normal, dry, and sensitive skins.

Actimoist™ Bio-2. [Active Organics] Sodium hyaluronate aq. sol'n. with preservatives (0.5% phenoxyethanol, 0.15% methylparaben); CAS 9067-32-7; natural moisturizer with ideal balance of water absorbing and holding props.; helps maintain the structure, moisture, lubricity, and flexibility of skin tissue; transparent visc. liq., char. odor; sol. in water; m.w. 1,900,000-2,700,000; sp.gr. 0.99-1.01; pH 5.5-6.5; 1% act.

Actimulse 250. [Active Organics] Glyceryl stearate, PEG-69 stearate, and cetearyl alcohol; cosmetics ingred., e.g., for skin lotions.

Actiphyte™. [Active Organics] Extensive range of botanical extracts.

Actiphyte of Acacia. [Active Organics] Propylene glycol, water, acacia extract; botanical extract.

Actiphyte of Alfalfa. [Active Organics] Propylene glycol, water, alfalfa extract; botanical extract.

Actiphyte of Almond. [Active Organics] Propylene glycol, water, sweet almond extract; botanical extract.

Actiphyte of Aloe Vera. [Active Organics] Propylene glycol, water, aloe extract; botanical extract.

Actiphyte of Aloe Vera 10-Fold. [Active Organics] Propylene glycol, water, aloe extract; botanical extract.

Actiphyte of Aloe Vera 20-Fold. [Active Organics] Propylene glycol, water, aloe extract; botanical extract.

Actiphyte of Aloe Vera 40-Fold. [Active Organics] Propylene glycol, water, aloe extract; botanical extract.

Actiphyte of Apple Leaves. [Active Organics] Propylene glycol, water, apple leaf extract; botanical extract.

Actiphyte of Apple Pectin. [Active Organics] Propylene glycol, water, apple pectin extract; botanical extract.

Actiphyte of Apricot Fruit. [Active Organics] Propylene glycol, water, apricot extract; botanical extract.

Actiphyte of Apricot Leaves. [Active Organics] Propylene glycol, water, apricot leaf extract; botanical extract.

Actiphyte of Arbutus. [Active Organics] Propylene glycol, water, arbutus extract; botanical extract.

Actiphyte of Arnica. [Active Organics] Propylene glycol, water, arnica extract; botanical extract.

Actiphyte of Arrowroot. [Active Organics] Propylene glycol, water, arrowroot extract; botanical extract.

Actiphyte of Avocado Fruit. [Active Organics] Propylene glycol, water, avocado extract; botanical extract.

Actiphyte of Avocado Leaves. [Active Organics] Propylene glycol, water, avocado leaf extract; botanical extract.

Actiphyte of Balm Mint. [Active Organics] Propylene glycol, water, balm mint extract; botanical extract.

Actiphyte of Basil. [Active Organics] Propylene glycol, water, basil extract; botanical extract.

Actiphyte of Bee Pollen. [Active Organics] Propylene glycol, water, pollen extract; botanical extract.

Actiphyte of Black Walnut. [Active Organics] Propylene glycol, water, black walnut extract; botanical extract.

Actiphyte of Bran. [Active Organics] Propylene glycol, water, oat bran extract; botanical extract.

Actiphyte of Calendula. [Active Organics] Propylene glycol, water, calendula extract; botanical extract.

Actiphyte of Capsicum. [Active Organics] Propylene glycol, water, capsicum extract; botanical extract.

Actiphyte of Chamomile. [Active Organics] Propylene glycol, water, matricaria extract; botanical extract.

Actiphyte of Chaparral. [Active Organics] Propylene glycol, water, chaparral extract; botanical extract.

Actiphyte of Chrysanthemum. [Active Organics] Propylene glycol, water, chrysanthemum extract; botanical extract.

Actiphyte of Cinnamon. [Active Organics] Propylene glycol, water, cinnamon extract; botanical extract.

Actiphyte of Coconut. [Active Organics] Propylene glycol, water, coconut extract; botanical extract.

Actiphyte of Comfrey. [Active Organics] Propylene glycol, water, comfrey extract; botanical extract.

Actiphyte of Coriander. [Active Organics] Propylene glycol, water, coriander extract; botanical extract.

Actiphyte of Cornsilk. [Active Organics] Propylene glycol, water, corn silk extract; botanical extract.

Actiphyte of Eucalyptus. [Active Organics] Propylene glycol, water, eucalyptus extract; botanical extract.

Actiphyte of Flax Seed. [Active Organics] Propylene glycol, water, linseed extract; botanical extract.

Actiphyte of Garlic. [Active Organics] Propylene glycol, water, garlic extract; botanical extract.

Actiphyte of Ginseng. [Active Organics] Propylene glycol, water, ginseng extract; botanical extract.

Actiphyte of Goldenseal. [Active Organics] Propylene glycol, water, goldenseal root extract; botanical extract.

Actiphyte of Henna. [Active Organics] Propylene glycol, water, henna extract; botanical extract.

Actiphyte of Honeysuckle. [Active Organics] Propylene glycol, water, honeysuckle extract; botanical extract.

Actiphyte of Hops. [Active Organics] Propylene glycol, water, hops extract; botanical extract.

Actiphyte of Irish Moss. [Active Organics] Propylene glycol, water, carrageenan extract; botanical extract.

Actiphyte of Jojoba Meal. [Active Organics] Propylene glycol, water, jojoba extract; botanical extract.

Actiphyte of Lavender. [Active Organics] Propylene glycol, water, lavender extract; botanical extract.

Actiphyte of Lemon Juice. [Active Organics] Propylene glycol, water, lemon juice extract; botanical extract.

Actiphyte of Lemon Peel. [Active Organics] Propylene glycol, water, lemon peel extract; botanical extract.

Actiphyte of Malt. [Active Organics] Propylene glycol, water, barley extract; botanical extract.

Actiphyte of Marigold. [Active Organics] Propylene glycol, water, calendula extract; botanical extract.

Actiphyte of Meadowsweet. [Active Organics] Propylene glycol, water, meadowsweet extract; botanical extract.

Actiphyte of Oat Bran. [Active Organics] Propylene glycol, water, oat bran extract; botanical extract.

Actiphyte of Oat Flour. [Active Organics] Propylene glycol, water, oat extract; botanical extract.

Actiphyte of Olive Leaves. [Active Organics] Propylene glycol, water, olive extract; botanical extract.

Actiphyte of Orange Bioflavonoids. [Active Organics] Propylene glycol, water, orange peel extract; botanical extract.

Actiphyte of Pennyroyal. [Active Organics] Propylene glycol, water, pennyroyal extract; botanical extract.

Actiphyte of Peppermint. [Active Organics] Propylene glycol, water, peppermint extract; botanical extract.

Actiphyte of Rice Bran. [Active Organics] Propylene glycol, water, rice bran extract; botanical extract.

Actiphyte of Rose. [Active Organics] Propylene glycol, water, rose extract; botanical extract.

Actiphyte of Rose Hips. [Active Organics] Propylene glycol, water, rose hips extract; botanical extract.

Actiphyte of Royal Jelly. [Active Organics] Propylene glycol, water, royal jelly extract; botanical extract.

Actiphyte of St. John's Wort. [Active Organics] Propylene glycol, water, hypericum extract; botanical extract.

Actiphyte of Tansy. [Active Organics] Propylene glycol, water, tansy extract; botanical extract.

Actiphyte of Wheat. [Active Organics] Propylene glycol, water, wheat extract; botanical extract.

Actiphyte of Wheat Germ. [Active Organics] Propylene glycol, water, wheat germ extract; botanical extract.

Actiphyte of Wintergreen. [Active Organics] Propylene glycol, water, wintergreen extract; botanical extract.

Actiphyte of Witch Hazel. [Active Organics] Propylene glycol, water, witch hazel extract; botanical extract.

Actiplex™. [Active Organics] Custom-made mixtures of Actiphyte extracts; cosmetic ingreds.

Actiplex™ 745. [Active Organics] Ginseng extract, ginko extract, comfrey extract, arnica extract, and lemon bioflavonoids extract; botanical extract for cosmetics, e.g., skin lotions.

Actiquat™. [Active Organics] Quaternized botanical extract; cationic; ionically bonds with hair and skin for conditioning and shine in hair care prods. and smooth effect and velvety after-feel in skin care prods.; transparent, sl. visc. liq., char. odor; sol. in water; pH 4.5-6.0; usage level: 1-40%.

Actisea™ 100. [Active Organics] Aloe vera gel, algae extract, and hydrolyzed glycosaminoglycans; forms protective hydrophilic barrier to help fortify skin and maintain its natural healing process; bio-chelated minerals and vitamins complement natural sugars.

Active #4. [Blew Chem.] Cocamide DEA and DEA-dodecyl-benzenesulfonate; biodeg. high sudsing surfactant used as base for hand dishwashing detergents, shampoos, bubble baths; wool fulling agent; wetting and dispersing agent; straw visc. liq., bland odor; water-sol.; dens. 8.7 lb/gal; pour pt. 40 F; pH 9 (5%); surf. tens. 30 dynes/cm (0.1%); toxicology: LD50 (rat) 3157 mg/kg; 100% act.

Activegetal™ IPF. [Solabia; Barnet Prods.] (Integral plantes fraiches). Botanical extracts obtained by a process of cryogenics, cyro-grinding, and molecular ultrapressure which preserves active constituents of plants normally lost by heat extraction methods.

Activera™. [Active Organics] Aloe vera gel; full range of prods. for topical and ingestible use; avail. in liq., powd., liq. concs., and oil forms, and in drink forms.

Activera™ 1-1FA (Filtered). [Active Organics] Aloe vera gel; cosmetic and pharmaceutical ingred. where consistent quality and color stability are important; also used as a vegetable drink and juice enhancer; colorless cloudy liq.

Activera™ 1-10. [Active Organics] Aloe vera gel; 10 fold conc. using high vacuum, low heat evaporation process; reconstituted (1:9 conc./deionized water) as clear, opalescent liq. with the same color stability as single strength prod.; honey-like lt. syrup.

Activera™ 1-20. [Active Organics] Aloe vera gel; reconstituted (1:19 conc./deionized water) for use interchangeably with 1-1 and 1-10 prods.; honey-like med. syrup.

Activera™ 1-200 A. [Active Organics] Aloe vera gel; used in veg. drinks, cosmetics, and pharmaceutical mfg.; reconstitute by adding 199 parts of deionized water to 1 part powd. by wt.; eggshell-wh. free-flowing powd.

Activera™ 104. [Active Organics] Aloe vera gel; cosmetic and pharmaceutical ingred. where clarity, color stability, purity, and batch-to-batch consistency are important; colorless clear liq.

Activera™ 106 LIPO M. [Active Organics] Aloe extract; CAS 85507-69-3; used for pure oil or oil and wax formulations, bath oils, suntan oils, and other oil-based prods.; bright yel. oily liq.

Activera™ 107 LIPO C. [Active Organics] Aloe extract; CAS 85507-69-3; used in nail care prods. and lip color prods.; golden-amber oily liq.; sol. in acetone, ethyl acetate, and some oils.

Actrasol EO. [Climax Fluids Additives] Sulfated glyceryl trioleate, sodium neutralized; anionic; surfactant for shampoos, metalworking; liq.; 75% conc.

Aculyn™ 22. [Rohm & Haas] Acrylates/steareth-20 methacrylate copolymer; anionic; thickener and stabilizer for cosmetics and toiletries (hair care prods., hand creams, lotions, waterless hand cleaners); off-wh. milky liq.; alkalisol.; dens. 8.75 lb/gal; visc. 20 cps; pH 3.0; usage level: 1.5-6%; toxicology: LD50 (oral, rat) > 5 g/kg, (dermal, rabbit) 5 g/kg; moderate irritating to eyes; sl. irritating to skin; 30% act. in water.

Acylyn™ 33. [Rohm & Haas] Acrylates copolymer; thickener, stabilizer for sunscreens, lotions, makeup, shampoos, aq. formulations; liq.; usage level: 1-6%; 28% act. in water.

ACumist™ A-12. [Allied-Signal/A-C® Perf. Addit.] Micronized polyethylene; CAS 9002-88-4; EINECS 200-815-3; wax additive for adhesives, inks, personal care, rubber applics.; suspension aid, flatting and texturizing agent, and binder for personal care prods.; micronized powd.; 12 µ avg. particle size; dens. 0.99 g/cc; drop pt. 136 C; acid no. 30; hardness < 0.5 dmm.

ACumist™ A-18. [Allied-Signal/A-C® Perf. Addit.] Micronized polyethylene; CAS 9002-88-4; EINECS 200-815-3; wax additive for adhesives, inks, personal care, and rubber applics.; suspension aid, flatting and texturizing agent, and binder for personal care prods.; micronized powd.; 18 µ avg. particle size; dens. 0.99 g/cc; drop pt. 136 C; acid no. 30; hardness < 0.5 dmm.

ACumist™ B-6. [Allied-Signal/A-C® Perf. Addit.] Micronized polyethylene; CAS 9002-88-4; EINECS 200-815-3; wax additive for adhesives, inks, personal care, rubber applics.; suspension aid, flatting and texturizing agent, and binder for personal care prods.; provides smoother, silkier afterfeel; micronized powd.; 6 µ avg. particle size; dens. 0.96 g/cc; drop pt. 126 C; acid no. nil; hardness < 0.5 dmm.

ACumist™ B-9. [Allied-Signal/A-C® Perf. Addit.] Micronized polyethylene; CAS 9002-88-4; EINECS 200-815-3; wax additive for adhesives, inks, personal care, and rubber applics.; micronized powd.; 9 µ avg. particle size; dens. 0.96 g/cc; drop pt. 126 C; acid no. nil; hardness < 0.5 dmm.

ACumist™ B-12. [Allied-Signal/A-C® Perf. Addit.] Micronized polyethylene; CAS 9002-88-4; EINECS 200-815-3; wax additive for adhesives, inks, personal care, and rubber applics.; suspension aid, flatting and texturizing agent, and binder for personal care prods.; micronized powd.; 12 µ avg. particle size; dens. 0.96 g/cc; drop pt. 126 C; acid no. nil; hardness < 0.5 dmm.

ACumist™ B-18. [Allied-Signal/A-C® Perf. Addit.] Micronized polyethylene; CAS 9002-88-4; EINECS 200-815-3; wax additive for adhesives, inks, personal care, and

rubber applics.; suspension aid, flatting and texturizing agent, and binder for personal care prods.; micronized powd.; 18 µ avg. particle size; dens. 0.96 g/cc; drop pt. 126 C; acid no. nil; hardness < 0.5 dmm.

ACumist™ C-5. [Allied-Signal/A-C® Perf. Addit.] Micronized polyethylene; CAS 9002-88-4; EINECS 200-815-3; wax additive for adhesives, inks, personal care, and rubber applics.; suspension aid, flatting and texturizing agent, and binder for personal care prods.; micronized powd.; 5 µ avg. particle size; dens. 0.95 g/cc; drop pt. 121 C; acid no. nil; hardness 1.0 dmm.

ACumist™ C-9. [Allied-Signal/A-C® Perf. Addit.] Micronized polyethylene; CAS 9002-88-4; EINECS 200-815-3; wax additive for adhesives, inks, personal care, and rubber applics.; suspension aid, flatting and texturizing agent, and binder for personal care prods.; micronized powd.; 9 µ avg. particle size; dens. 0.95 g/cc; drop pt. 121 C; acid no. nil; hardness 1.0 dmm.

ACumist™ C-12. [Allied-Signal/A-C® Perf. Addit.] Micronized polyethylene; CAS 9002-88-4; EINECS 200-815-3; wax additive for adhesives, inks, personal care, and rubber applics.; suspension aid, flatting and texturizing agent, and binder for personal care prods.; micronized powd.; 12 µ avg. particle size; dens. 0.95 g/cc; drop pt. 121 C; acid no. nil; hardness 1.0 dmm.

ACumist™ C-18. [Allied-Signal/A-C® Perf. Addit.] Micronized polyethylene; CAS 9002-88-4; EINECS 200-815-3; wax additive for adhesives, inks, personal care, and rubber applics.; suspension aid, flatting and texturizing agent, and binder for personal care prods.; micronized powd.; 18 µ avg. particle size; dens. 0.95 g/cc; drop pt. 121 C; acid no. nil; hardness 1.0 dmm.

ACumist™ D-9. [Allied-Signal/A-C® Perf. Addit.] Micronized polyethylene; CAS 9002-88-4; EINECS 200-815-3; wax additive for adhesives, inks, personal care, and rubber applics.; micronized powd.; 10 µ avg. particle size; dens. 0.95 g/cc; drop pt. 118 C; acid no. nil; hardness 1.5 dmm.

ACuscrub® 30. [Allied-Signal/A-C® Perf. Addit.] Oxidized polyethylene; CAS 68441-17-8; nonirritating, mild abrasive for personal care prods.; gran.; dens. 0.98 g/cc; drop. pt. 140 C; acid no. 16; hardness < 0.5 dmm.

ACuscrub® 31. [Allied-Signal/A-C® Perf. Addit.] Oxidized polyethylene; CAS 68441-17-8; nonirritating, mild abrasive for personal care prods.; gran.; dens. 0.99 g/cc; drop. pt. 138 C; acid no. 30; hardness < 0.5 dmm.

ACuscrub® 32. [Allied-Signal/A-C® Perf. Addit.] Oxidized polyethylene; CAS 68441-17-8; nonirritating, mild abrasive for personal care prods.; gran.; dens. 1.00 g/cc; drop. pt. 137 C; acid no. 41; hardness < 0.5 dmm.

ACuscrub® 40. [Allied-Signal] Polyethylene; CAS 9002-88-4; EINECS 200-815-3; nonirritating, mild abrasive for personal care prods.; atomized; dens. 0.91 g/cc; drop. pt. 101 C; acid no. nil; hardness 7.0 dmm.

ACuscrub® 41. [Allied-Signal/A-C® Perf. Addit.] Polyethylene; CAS 9002-88-4; EINECS 200-815-3; nonirritating, mild abrasive for personal care prods.; atomized; dens. 0.92 g/cc; drop. pt. 106 C; acid no. nil; hardness 4.0 dmm.

ACuscrub® 42. [Allied-Signal/A-C® Perf. Addit.] Polyethylene; CAS 9002-88-4; EINECS 200-815-3; nonirritating, mild abrasive for personal care prods.; atomized; dens. 0.92 g/cc; drop. pt. 109 C; acid no. nil; hardness 2.5 dmm.

ACuscrub® 43. [Allied-Signal/A-C® Perf. Addit.] Polyethylene; CAS 9002-88-4; EINECS 200-815-3; nonirritating, mild abrasive for personal care prods.; atomized; dens. 0.93 g/cc; drop. pt. 113 C; acid no. nil; hardness 1.0 dmm.

ACuscrub® 44. [Allied-Signal/A-C® Perf. Addit.] Polyethylene; CAS 9002-88-4; EINECS 200-815-3; nonirritating, mild abrasive for personal care prods.; atomized; dens. 0.93 g/cc; drop. pt. 115 C; acid no. nil; hardness 0.5 dmm.

ACuscrub® 50. [Allied-Signal] Oxidized polyethylene; CAS

68441-17-8; mild scrub agent, nonirritating abrasive for personal care prods., waterless hand cleaners; ground; dens. 0.98 g/cc; drop. pt. 140 C; acid no. 16; hardness < 0.5 dmm.

ACuscrub® 51. [Allied-Signal/A-C® Perf. Addit.] Oxidized polyethylene; CAS 68441-17-8; nonirritating, mild abrasive for personal care prods.; ground; dens. 1.00 g/cc; drop. pt. 137 C; acid no. 41; hardness < 0.5 dmm.

ACuscrub® 52. [Allied-Signal/A-C® Perf. Addit.] Polyethylene; CAS 9002-88-4; EINECS 200-815-3; nonirritating, mild abrasive for personal care prods.; ground; dens. 0.93 g/cc; drop. pt. 115 C; acid no. nil; hardness 0.5 dmm.

Acusol® 820. [Rohm & Haas] Acrylic copolymer; detergent polymer, processing aid, thickener, and stabilizer for cosmetics, detergents and cleaners, water treatment, min. processing, other industrial markets; alkali-sol.; m.w. 500,000; pH 3; 30% solids.

Acylan. [Croda Inc.; Croda Chem. Ltd.] Acetylated lanolin; CAS 61788-48-5; EINECS 262-979-2; lipid emollient for personal care and pharmaceutical prods.; forms water-repellent films; Gardner 11 soft solid; bland odor; sol. in min. oil and soft waxy hydrophobic films; m.p. 32–39 C; acid no. 2.0 max.; iodine no. 30 max.; sapon. no. 100–125; hyd. no. 12 max.; usage level: 1-10%; 100% act.

Adeka GH-200. [Asahi Denka Kogyo] PPG-24-glycereth-24; CAS 51258-15-2; emollient.

Adeka PA Series. [Asahi Denka Kogyo] Palmitic acid; CAS 57-10-3; EINECS 200-312-9; used for cosmetics, raw material for surfactants; flakes, liq.; m.p. 58-62 C; iodine no. < 1.

Adeka Carpol DL-30, DL-150. [Asahi Denka Kogyo] Polyoxyalkylene glycol; used for hydraulic fluid oils, heat media, defoamers, cosmetics; water-insol.; visc. 31.2 and 149 cst resp. (40 C).

Adeka Carpol GL-130, GL-320. [Asahi Denka Kogyo] Polyoxyalkylene glycol; used for break fluids, defoamers, cosmetics; water-insol.; visc. 118 and 286 cst resp. (40 C).

Adeka Carpol MH-50, MH-150, MH-1000. [Asahi Denka Kogyo] Polyoxyalkylene glycol; hydraulic fluid oil, lubricant in high/low temp., heat media, lubricant for textile, compressor; mold lubricant for rubber, plastics, cosmetics, cutting oil, break oil, defoamer; water-sol.; visc. 54.6, 135, and 938 cst resp. (40 C).

Adekacol CS, PS, TS. [Asahi Denka Kogyo] Phosphate ester type surfactants; for hair care prods.; stable to acid/alkali at high temp.; anticorrosive; liq.

Adeka Dipropylene Glycol (Cosmetic Grade). [Asahi Denka Kogyo] Dipropylene glycol; for cosmetics use; APHA > 15 color; sp.gr. 1.020-1.030.

Adeka Propylene Glycol (P). [Asahi Denka Kogyo] Propylene glycol; CAS 57-55-6; EINECS 200-338-0; pharmaceutical grade for cosmetics, food additives; APHA > 10 color; sp.gr. 1.037-1.039.

Adekatol DES, DS, HAN, LS, TR, SAN, YES. [Asahi Denka Kogyo] Sulfate type surfactants; anionic surfactants.

ADF Oleile. [Vevy] PPG-25-laureth-25; CAS 37311-00-5.

Adinol CT95. [Croda Chem. Ltd.] Sodium methyl cocoyl taurate; CAS 61791-42-2; anionic; cosmetic and pharmaceutical detergent/emulsifier; wh. paste; 95% min. conc.

Adinol OT16. [Croda Chem. Ltd.] Sodium methyl oleoyl taurate; CAS 137-20-2; EINECS 205-285-7; anionic; biodeg. surfactant, wetting agent, detergent, emulsifier, foamer, dispersant for cosmetic and industrial applics., esp. textile processing; liq.; 16+% conc.

Adma® 8. [Ethyl] Octyldimethylamine; CAS 7378-99-6; cationic; intermediate for quat. ammonium compds., amine oxides, betaines; for household prods., disinfectants, sanitizers, industrial hand cleaners, cosmetics, bubble baths, deodorants; APHA < 10 liq., fatty amine odor; sp.gr. 0.765; f.p. -57 C; amine no. 352; flash pt.

(TCC) 64 C; corrosive; 100% conc.

Adma® 10. [Ethyl] Decyldimethylamine; CAS 1120-24-7; cationic; intermediate for quat. ammonium compds., amine oxides, betaines; for household prods., disinfectants, sanitizers, industrial hand cleaners, cosmetics, bubble baths, deodorants; clear liq., fatty amine odor; sp.gr. 0.778; f.p. -35 C; amine no. 300; flash pt. (TCC) 91 C; corrosive; 100% conc.

Adma® 12. [Ethyl] Dodecyl dimethylamine; CAS 112-18-5; EINECS 203-943-8; cationic; intermediate for quat. ammonium compds., amine oxides, betaines; for household prods., disinfectants, sanitizers, industrial hand cleaners, cosmetics, bubble baths, deodorants; clear liq., fatty amine odor; sp.gr. 0.778; f.p. -22 C; amine no. 259; flash pt. (PM) 114 C; corrosive; 100% conc.

Adma® 14. [Ethyl] Tetradecyl dimethylamine; CAS 112-75-4; EINECS 204-002-4; cationic; intermediate for quat. ammonium compds., amine oxides, betaines; for household prods., disinfectants, sanitizers, industrial hand cleaners, cosmetics, bubble baths, deodorants; clear liq.; sp.gr. 0.794; f.p. -6 C; amine no. 229; flash pt. (PM) 132 C; corrosive; 100% conc.

Adma® 16. [Ethyl] Hexadecyl dimethylamine; CAS 112-69-6; EINECS 203-997-2; cationic; intermediate for quat. ammonium compds., amine oxides, betaines; for household prods., disinfectants, sanitizers, industrial hand cleaners, cosmetics, bubble baths, deodorants; clear liq., fatty amine odor; sp.gr. 0.800; f.p. 8 C; amine no. 206; flash pt. (PM) 142 C; corrosive; 100% conc.

Adma® 18. [Ethyl] Octadecyl dimethylamine; CAS 124-28-7; EINECS 204-694-8; intermediate for mfg. of quaternary ammonium compds. for biocides, textile chems., oilfield chems., amine oxides, betaines, polyurethane foam catalysts, epoxy curing agents; household prods., disinfectants, sanitizers, industrial hand cleaners, cosmetics, bubble baths, deodorants; clear liq., fatty amine odor; sp.gr. 0.807; f.p. 21 C; amine no. 186; flash pt. (PM) 163 C; corrosive; 98% tert. amine.

Adma® 246-451. [Ethyl] Dodecyl dimethylamine (40%), tetradecyl dimethylamine (50%), hexadecyl dimethylamine (10%); cationic; intermediate for quat. ammonium compds., amine oxides, betaines; for household prods., disinfectants, sanitizers, industrial hand cleaners, cosmetics, bubble baths, deodorants; clear liq., fatty amine odor; sp.gr. 0.792; f.p. -13 C; amine no. 238; flash pt. (PM) 114 C; corrosive; 100% conc.

Adma® 246-621. [Ethyl] Dodecyl dimethylamine (65%), tetradecyl dimethylamine (25%), hexadecyl dimethylamine (10%); cationic; intermediate for quat. ammonium compds., amine oxides, betaines; for household prods., disinfectants, sanitizers, industrial hand cleaners, cosmetics, bubble baths, deodorants; clear liq., fatty amine odor; sp.gr. 0.791; f.p. -18 C; amine no. 245; flash pt. (PM) 121 C; corrosive; 100% conc.

Adma® 1214. [Ethyl] Dodecyl dimethylamine (65%), tetradecyl dimethylamine (35%); CAS 112-18-5, 112-75-4; cationic; intermediate for quat. ammonium compds., amine oxides, betaines; for household prods., disinfectants, sanitizers, industrial hand cleaners, cosmetics, bubble baths, deodorants; clear liq., fatty amine odor; sp.gr. 0.791; f.p. -18 C; amine no. 249.2; flash pt. (PM) 121 C; corrosive; 100% conc.

Adma® 1416. [Ethyl] Dodecyl dimethylamine (5%), tetradecyl dimethylamine (60%), hexadecyl dimethylamine (30%), octadecyl dimethylamine (5%); cationic; intermediate for quat. ammonium compds., amine oxides, betaines; for household prods., disinfectants, sanitizers, industrial hand cleaners, cosmetics, bubble baths, deodorants; APHA < 10 liq.; sp.gr. 0.796; amine no. 220; 100% conc.

Adma® WC. [Ethyl] Octyl dimethylamine (7%), decyl dimeth-ylamine (6%), dodecyl dimethylamine (53%), tetradecyl dimethylamine (19%), hexadecyl dimethylamine (9%), octadecyl dimethylamine (6%); cationic; intermediate for quat. ammonium compds., amine oxides, betaines; for household prods., disinfectants, sanitizers, industrial hand cleaners, cosmetics, bubble baths, deodorants; clear liq., fatty amine odor; sp.gr. 0.798; f.p. -22 C; amine no. 249; flash pt. (PM) 102 C; corrosive; 100% conc.

Admox® 14-85. [Ethyl] Myristamine oxide; CAS 3332-27-2; EINECS 222-059-3; for soap bars, shaving creams, fabric softeners, hard surf. cleaners, laundry detergents, oxy-gen bleach powds., toothpaste, agric., automatic dish-wash, cellulose extraction, gasoline additives, bubble baths; solid; m.w. 257; m.p. 40-42 C; flash pt. > 93 C; 87 ± 2% amine oxide.

Admox® 18-85. [Ethyl] Stearamine oxide; CAS 2571-88-2; EINECS 219-919-5; for soap bars, shaving creams, fabric softeners, hard surf. cleaners, laundry detergents, oxy-gen bleach powds., tootphaste, agric., automatic dish-wash, cellulose extraction, gasoline additives, bubble baths; solid; m.w. 313; m.p. 61-62 C; flash pt. > 93 C; 87 ± 2% amine oxide.

Admox® 1214. [Ethyl] Alkyldimethylamine oxide; nonionic; high foaming material to improve foam profile of anionic surfactants; visc. modifier, emollient; liq.; 30% conc.

Adogen® 140D. [Witco/H-I-P] Stearamine.

Adogen® 160D. [Witco/H-I-P] Cocamine; CAS 61788-46-3; EINECS 262-977-1; emulsifier.

Adogen® 163D. [Witco/H-I-P] Lauramine; CAS 124-22-1; EINECS 204-690-6; personal care surfactant.

Adogen® 170D. [Witco/H-I-P] Tallowamine; CAS 61790-33-8; EINECS 263-125-1; emulsifier.

Adogen® 216 SF. [Witco/H-I-P] Dipalmitamine.

Adogen® 240 SF. [Witco/H-I-P] Hydrog. ditallowamine; CAS 61789-79-5; EINECS 263-089-7.

Adogen® 444. [Witco/H-I-P] Palmityl trimethyl ammonium chloride; CAS 112-02-7; EINECS 203-928-6; cationic; specialty quat.; emulsifier, dispersant, cream rinse, fer-mentation aid; Gardner 6 max. liq.; m.w. 319; flash pt. (PM) 58 F; 49–52% quat.

Adogen® MA-102. [Witco/H-I-P] Dimethyl lauramine; CAS 112-18-5; EINECS 203-943-8; surfactant intermediate.

Adogen® MA-104. [Witco/H-I-P] Dimethyl myristamine; CAS 112-75-4; EINECS 204-002-4; surfactant intermedi-ate.

Adogen® MA-106. [Witco/H-I-P] Dimethyl palmitamine; CAS 112-69-6; EINECS 203-997-2; surfactant intermedi-ate.

Adogen® MA-108. [Witco/H-I-P] Dimethyl stearamine; CAS 124-28-7; EINECS 204-694-8; surfactant intermediate.

Adogen® MA-108 SF. [Witco/H-I-P] Dimethyl stearamine; CAS 124-28-7; EINECS 204-694-8; nonionic; neutralizer, conditioner, coemulsifier for personal care prods.; paste; amine no. 188; 99% solids.

Adogen® MA-112 SF. [Witco/H-I-P] Dimethyl behenamine; CAS 215-42-9; nonionic; neutralizer, conditioner, co-emulsifier for personal care prods.; paste; amine no. 156; 99% solids.

Adogen® S-18 V. [Witco/H-I-P] Stearamidopropyl dimethyl-amine; CAS 7651-02-7; EINECS 231-609-1; nonionic; conditioner, antistat, coemulsifier, plasticizer, neutralizer for personal care prods.; off-wh. flakes; amine no. 152; 99% solids.

Adol® 52. [Procter & Gamble] Cetyl alcohol; CAS 36653-82-4; EINECS 253-149-0; cosmetic ingred.

Adol® 52 NF. [Procter & Gamble] Cetyl alcohol; CAS 36653-82-4; EINECS 253-149-0; nonionic; coemulsifier, lubri-cant, foam control agent, cosolvent, plasticizer, stabilizer, emollient, intermediate; for metal lubricants, inks, textiles, emulsions, paper, cosmetics, mineral processing, oil field chemicals, fabric softeners; Lovibond 5Y/0.5R max.; sol. in fatty alcohols, IPA, benzene, trichloroethylene, ac-etone, turpentine, VMP naphtha, kerosene, lt. min. oil; m.w. 247; sp.gr. 0.815 (60/25 C); m.p. 45–50 C; acid no. 1.0 max.; sapon. no. 3.0 max.

Adol® 60. [Procter & Gamble] Behenyl alcohol; CAS 661-19-8; EINECS 211-546-6; lubricant, foam control agent, cosolv., plasticizer, emollient; Lovibond 10Y/1.0R; m.w. 316; sp. gr. 0.79 (100/25 C); acid no. 1.5 max.; iodine no. 6 max.; sapon. no. 3 max.

Adol® 61. [Procter & Gamble] Stearyl alcohol; CAS 112-92-5; EINECS 204-017-6; nonionic; emollient, emulsion sta-bilizer, visc. modifier, conditioner for skin care prods.; opacifier for creams and lotions; also used in emulsifiers, surfactants, wax formulations; wh. cryst. solid; odorless; sol. in IPA, acetone, naphtha, lt. min. oil; m.w. 272; sp.gr. 0.817 (60/25 C); m.p. 56–60 C; acid no. 0.5; sapon. no. 1.0 max.; 100% conc.

Adol® 61 NF. [Procter & Gamble] Stearyl alcohol; CAS 112-92-5; EINECS 204-017-6; emollient, cosmetic/pharma-ceutical raw material.

Adol® 62 NF. [Procter & Gamble] Stearyl alcohol; CAS 112-92-5; EINECS 204-017-6; nonionic; emollient, glass frit binders, waxes, emulsion stabilizers, esters, tertiary amines, surfactants, polymers, chemical intermediate; emollient, emulsion stabilizer, visc. modifier, conditioner cosmetic formulations, skin care prods.; opacifier; Lovibond 5Y/0.54 max. flakes, odorless; sol. in IPA, acetone, naphtha, lt. min. oil; m.w. 272; sp.gr. 0.817 (60/25 C); visc. 42 SSU (210 F); m.p. 56-60 C; b.p. 337–360 C (760 mm, 90%); acid no. 1.0 max.; sapon. no. 3.0 max.; 100% conc.

Adol® 63. [Procter & Gamble] Cetearyl alcohol; nonionic; emulsifiers; prime base for detergents; used in plasticiz-ers, tert. amines, lube oil additives, textile auxiliaries, mold lubricants, polymers, org. synthesis, chemical intermedi-ates; emollient, emulsion stabilizer, visc. modifier, condi-tioner for skin care prods.; opacifier for creams and lotions; Lovibond 5Y/0.5R max. flake; m.w. 268; sp.gr. 0.816 (60/25 C); visc. 44 SSU (210 F); m.p. 48-53 C; b.p. 312-344 C (760 mm, 90%); acid no. 1.0 max.; sapon. no. 3.0 max.; 100% conc.

Adol® 64. [Procter & Gamble] Cetearyl alcohol; emollient, emulsion stabilizer, visc. modifier for skin care prods.; conditioner imparting velvety feel; opacifier for creams and lotions; flakes; m.p. 46-52 C.

Adol® 66. [Procter & Gamble] Isostearyl alcohol; CAS 27458-93-1; EINECS 248-470-8; nonionic; coemulsifier, lubricant, foam control agent, cosolvent, plasticizer, stabi-lizer, emollient, intermediate; for metal lubricants, inks, textiles, emulsions, paper, mineral processing, oil field chemicals, fabric softeners; emollient for skin care prods.; as replacement for oleyl alcohol; Lovibond 5Y/0.5R max. liq.; sol. in fatty alcohols, IPA, benzene, trichlorethylene, acetone, turpentine, VMP naphtha, kerosene, lt. min. oil; m.w. 295; sp.gr. 0.861; cloud pt. 8 C max.; acid no. 1.0 max.; sapon. no. 2.0 max.; 100% conc.

Adol® 80. [Procter & Gamble] Oleyl alcohol; CAS 143-28-2; EINECS 205-597-3; nonionic; coemulsifier, lubricant, foam control agent, cosolvent, plasticizer, stabilizer, emollient, intermediate; for metal rolling oils and lubri-cants, gas scrubbing, printing inks, auto antifreeze, textile dyeing and finishing, emulsion systems, paper pulping, cosmetics, cationic surfactants, min. processing, oil field chemicals, fabric softeners; Lovibond 5Y/0.5R liq.; m.w. 263; sol. in fatty alcohols, IPA, benzene, trichlorethylene, acetone, turpentine, VMP naphtha, kerosene, lt. min. oil; sp.gr. 0.840; cloud pt. 13 C max.; sapon. no. 3.0 max.; 100% conc.

Adol® 85. [Procter & Gamble] Oleyl alcohol; CAS 143-28-2; EINECS 205-597-3; nonionic; emulsifier, lubricant, foam control agent, cosolv., plasticizer, emollient for personal care prods.; Lovibond 3Y/0.3R liq.; m.w. 268; sp.gr. 0.84; acid no. 1.0; iodine no. 85–95; sapon no. 2 max.; cloud pt. 10 C max.; 100% conc.

Adol® 90. [Procter & Gamble] Oleyl alcohol; CAS 143-28-2; EINECS 205-597-3; emollient.

Adol® 90 NF. [Procter & Gamble] Oleyl alcohol; CAS 143-28-2; EINECS 205-597-3; nonionic; cosmetic and pharmaceutical grade emollient imparting smoothness, freshness, and suppleness to the skin; used in lotions, creams, bath oils; coupling agent; plasticizer for hair sprays; lubricant for aerosols; emulsion stabilizer; lt. clear liq., low odor; sol. in ethanol, IPA, benzene, ethyl ether, acetone, turpentine, VM&P naphtha, kerosene, lt. min. oil; m.w. 268; sp.gr. 0.840; b.p. 282–349 C (760 mm, 90%); acid no. 0.5; iodine no. 90; sapon. no. 1.5; hyd. no. 210; cloud pt. 6 C.; 100% conc.

Adol® 320, 330, 340. [Procter & Gamble] Nonionic; emulsifiers, emollients; liq.; 100% conc.

Adol® 520 NF. [Procter & Gamble] Cetyl alcohol; CAS 36653-82-4; EINECS 253-149-0; nonionic; coemulsifier, lubricant, foam control agent, cosolvent, plasticizer, stabilizer, emollient, intermediate; for metal lubricants, inks, textiles, emulsions, paper, cosmetics, mineral processing, oil field chemicals, fabric softeners; emollient, emulsion stabilizer, visc. modifier, conditioner for skin care prods.; opacifier for creams and lotions; APHA 50 max. flake; sol. in fatty alcohols, IPA, benzene, trichlorethylene, acetone, turpentine, VMP naphtha, kerosene, lt. min. oil; m.w. 246; sp.gr. 0.815 (60/25 C); m.p. 45–50 C; solid pt. 48–53 C; acid no. 1.0 max.; sapon. no. 2.0 max.; 100% conc.

Adol® 620 NF. [Procter & Gamble] Stearyl alcohol; CAS 112-92-5; EINECS 204-017-6; nonionic; coemulsifier, lubricant, foam control agent, cosolvent, plasticizer, stabilizer, emollient, intermediate; for metal lubricants, inks, textiles, emulsions, paper, cosmetics, mineral processing, oil field chemicals, fabric softeners; emollient, emulsion stabilizer, visc. modifier, conditioner for skin care prods.; opacifier for creams and lotions; APHA 50 max. flake; sol. in fatty alcohols, IPA, benzene, trichlorethylene, acetone, turpentine, VMP naphtha, kerosene, lt. min. oil; m.w. 267; sp.gr. 0.817 (60/25 C); m.p. 55–60 C; acid no. 2.0 max.; sapon. no. 2.0 max.; 100% conc.

Adol® 630. [Procter & Gamble] Cetearyl alcohol; nonionic; emulsifier, emollient, emulsion stabilizer, visc. modifier, conditioner for skin care prods; opacifier for creams and lotions; flakes; m.p. 48-53 C; 100% conc.

Adol® 640. [Procter & Gamble] Cetearyl alcohol; nonionic; emulsifier, lubricant, foam control agent, cosolv., plasticizer, emollient; APHA 40 max. flake; m.w. 253; sp.gr. 0.82 (50/50 C); m.p. 43–46 C; acid no. 1.0 max.; iodine no. 1.5 max.; sapon. no. 1.0 max.; 100% conc.

Advantage™ CP. [ISP] Vinyl acetate/butyl maleate/isobornyl acrylate copolymer, ethanol SDA-40B; hairspray polymer offering improved hold, stiffness, removability, tactile props., and drying time; pale yel. clear liq.; acid no. 185; 50% ethanol sol'n.

Advantage™ V. [ISP] Vinyl acetate/butyl maleate/isobornyl acrylate copolymer, ethanol SDA-40B; hairspray polymer with faster drying, minimal curl droop; leaves nontacky film on hair; formulated to meet 80% VOC requirements in pumps and aerosols.

AE-1214/3. [Procter & Gamble] Laureth-3; CAS 3055-94-5; EINECS 221-280-2; nonionic; detergent, emulsifier; liq.; 100% act.

AEPD®. [Angus] 2-Amino-2-ethyl-1,3-propanediol; CAS 115-70-8; EINECS 204-101-2; nonionic; pigment dispersant, neutralizing amine, corrosion inhibitor, acid-salt catalyst, pH buffer, chemical and pharmaceutical intermediate, solubilizer; m.w. 119.2; water-sol.; m.p. 37.5 C; b.p. 152 C; flash pt. > 200 F (TCC); pH 10.8 (0.1M aq. sol'n.); 100% conc.

Aerosil® 130. [Degussa; Degussa AG] Silica; filler for plastics and silicone rubbers; thixotrope and thickener in personal care creams.

Aerosil® 200. [Degussa; Degussa AG] Fumed silica; anticaking and free-flow agent with high absorp. capacity; for adhesive, food, cosmetics, paint, paper, film, pesticides, pharmaceuticals, plastics, silicone rubber, inks, sealants industries; thixotrope for greases and min. oils; FDA approved; wh. fluffy powd.; dens. 50 g/l; surf. area 200 m2/g; pH 3.6–4.3 (4% aq. disp.); > 99.8% SiO2.

Aerosil® 255. [Degussa; Degussa AG] Silica.

Aerosil® 300. [Degussa; Degussa AG] Fumed silica; for low thermal syn. powds. used to produce insulation materials; thixotrope, antisettling agent for paints, plastics, sealants, personal care creams; filler for silicone rubber.

Aerosil® 380. [Degussa; Degussa AG] Silica.

Aerosil® R812. [Degussa] Syn. amorphous fumed silica; antisettling, antisag, anticorrosion agent for paints, plastics; suspension and redispersability props. in pharmaceutical/cosmetic aerosols; water repellent props. for lipsticks.

Aerosil® R972. [Degussa; Degussa AG] Syn. amorphous fumed silica; anticaking and free-flow agent for adhesive, elec., cosmetics, paint, pesticides, pharmaceuticals, plastics, inks industries; improves water resist. of greases; water repellent for lipsticks; wh. fluffy powd.; dens. 50 g/l; surf. area 110 m^2/g; pH 3.6–4.3 (4% aq. disp.); > 99.8% SiO$_2$.

Aerosol® 19. [Am. Cyanamid] Disodium N-alkyl sulfosuccinamate; emulsifier, foaming and wetting agent; biodeg.; Gardner 10 clear liq.; water sol.; dens. 8.9 lb/gal; sp.gr. 1.07; surf. tens. 41 dynes/cm; 35% act.

Aerosol® A-102. [Am. Cyanamid; Cyanamid BV] Disodium deceth-6 sulfosuccinate; CAS 39354-45-5; anionic; emulsifier, solubilizer, foamer, dispersant, surfactant, wetting agent; used in emulsion polymerization of PVAc/acrylics, textiles, cosmetics, shampoos, wallboard, adhesives; biodeg.; stable to acid media; colorless to lt. yel. clear liq.; sol. in water, dimethyl sulfoxide; m.w. 614; sp.gr. 1.08; dens. 9.01 lb/gal; visc. 40 cps; f.p. –4 C; flash pt. (Seta CC) > 200 F; acid no. 6 max.; pH 4.5-5.5; surf. tens. 33 dynes/cm; toxicology: LD50 (rat, oral) 30.8 mL/kg, (rabbit, dermal) > 5.0 mL/kg; moderate skin, minimal eye irritation; 30% act. in water.

Aerosol® A-103. [Am. Cyanamid; Cyanamid BV] Disodium nonoxynol-10 sulfosuccinate; CAS 9040-38-4; anionic; emulsifier, solubilizer, wetting agent, surfactant, surf. tens. depressant; used in PVAc acrylic emulsions; textile emulsions, pad-bath additive, textile wetting; cosmetics, shampoos, wallboard, adhesives; colorless to lt. yel. clear liq.; sol. in water, MEK; partly sol. in other polar solvs.; m.w. 854; sp.gr. 1.09; dens. 9.1 lb/gal; visc. 170–190 cps; f.p. –9 C; flash pt. (Seta CC) > 200 F; acid no. 10 max.; pH 4.5-5.5; surf. tens. 34 dynes/cm; toxicology: LD50 (rat, oral) > 10 mL/kg; not appreciably irritating to skin and eyes; 35% act. in water.

Aerosol® MA-80. [Am. Cyanamid; Cyanamid BV] Dihexyl sodium sulfosuccinate; CAS 3006-15-3; EINECS 221-109-1; anionic; dispersant, textile wetting agent, emulsifier, solubilizer, penetrant; used for emulsion polymerization, battery separators, electroplating, ore leaching; germicidal act.; solubilizer for shampoos; not as rapidly biodeg. as Aerosol 18 and 22; APHA 50 max. clear slightly visc. liq.; sol. in water, alcohol, and org. solvs.; sp.gr. 1.13; dens. 9.4 lb/gal; f.p. –28 C; m.p. 199–292 C; flash pt. (Seta

CC) 115 F; surf. tens. 28 dynes/cm; 80% act. in water/alcohol.

Aerosol® NPES 458. [Am. Cyanamid] Ammonium salt of sulfated nonylphenoxy POE ethanol; CAS 9051-57-4; anionic; high foaming surfactant for emulsion polymerization of acrylic, styrene and vinyl acetate systems, dishwashing detergents, germicides, pesticides, general purpose cleaners, cosmetics, and textile wet processing applics.; pale yel. clear liq., alcoholic odor; sol. in water; partly sol. in org. solvs.; m.w. 493; sp.gr. 1.065; dens. 8.9 lb/gal; visc. 100 cps; f.p. < 0 C; flash pt. (PMCC) 83 F; pH 6.5-7.5; surf. tens. 31 dynes/cm; toxicology: LD50 (rat, oral) > 5 g/kg; severe eye, moderate skin irritant; 58% conc. in water/alcohol.

Aerosol® OT-70 PG. [Am. Cyanamid; Cyanamid BV] Sodium dioctyl sulfosuccinate, propylene glycol/water; CAS 577-11-7; EINECS 209-406-4; anionic; wetting agent, surf. tens. depressant, emulsifier, surfactant; for use where high flash required; face and hand creams; biodeg.; clear to slightly yel. liq.; limited water sol.; sol. in org. solv.; sp.gr. 1.09; visc. 200–400 cps; flash pt. (Seta CC) > 200 F; surf. tens. 26 dynes/cm; 70% act.

Aerosol® OT-75%. [Am. Cyanamid; Cyanamid BV] Dioctyl sodium sulfosuccinate; CAS 577-11-7; EINECS 209-406-4; anionic; wetting agent and surf. tens. depressant used in textile, rubber, petrol., paper, metal, paint, plastic, and agric. industries; antistat for cosmetics, dry cleaning detergents, emulsion, plastic, pipelines, and suspension polymerization; emulsifier wax for polish, firefighting, germicide, metal cleaner, mold release agent; dispersant in paints and inks, paper, photography, process aid, rust preventative, soldering flux, wallpaper removal; APHA 100 max. clear visc. liq.; m.w. 444; sol. org. solv.; limited water sol.; sp.gr. 1.09; visc. 200 cps; flash pt. 85 C (OC); acid no. 2.5 max.; surf. tens. 28.7 dynes/cm (0.1% aq.); biodeg.; 75 ± 2% solids in water/alcohol.

Aerosol® OT-B. [Am. Cyanamid; Cyanamid BV] Dioctyl sodium sulfosuccinate, sodium benzoate; anionic; wetting agent, dispersant, solubilizer, adjuvant for agric. chem. wettable powds.; pigment dispersant in plastics; used in face powds. and powd. shampoos; wh. powd.; bulk particle size 15–150 μ; m.w. 444; water-disp.; sp.gr. 1.1; m.p. < 300 C; acid no. 2.5 max.; surf. tens. 28.7 dynes/cm (0.1% aq.); 85% act., 15% sodium benzoate.

Aerothene TT. [Dow] Trichloroethane; CAS 71-55-6; EINECS 200-756-3.

Aethoxal® B. [Henkel/Cospha; Henkel KGaA/Cospha] PPG-5-laureth-5; CAS 68439-51-0; nonionic; superfatting agent, emollient for bath oils, shampoos, skin and personal care prods., pharmaceuticals; biodeg.; pale yel. oily liq.; forms spontaneous emulsion in warm water; oil-sol.; sp.gr. 0.9340-0.9370 (70 C); acid no. 0.5 max.; hyd. no. 84-92; pH 6.5-7.5 (5%); 99–100% conc.

Aethyl-Steriline. [Zimmerli] Ethylparaben; CAS 120-47-8; EINECS 204-399-4; preservative for cosmetics; usage level: 0.08-1.0%.

Afaine™ 35. [McIntyre] Cocamidopropyl betaine (via glyceride); veg.-derived prod. for personal care applics.; liq.; pH 6.0; 35% conc.

Afaine™ 35 HP. [McIntyre] Cocamidopropyl betaine; veg.-derived prod. for personal care applics.; liq.; pH 6.0; 35% conc.

Afaine™ ISA. [McIntyre] Isostearamidopropyl betaine; veg.-derived prod. for personal care applics.; liq.; pH 7.5; 33% conc.

Afaine™ LMB. [McIntyre] Lauramidopropyl betaine; EINECS 224-292-6; veg.-derived prod. for personal care applics.; liq.; pH 6.0; 35% conc.

Afaine™ WGB. [McIntyre] Wheat germamidopropyl betaine; CAS 133934-09-5; veg.-derived prod. for personal care

applics.; liq.; pH 6.5; 34% conc.

Afalene™ 117. [McIntyre] Cocamidopropyl dimethylamine propionate; CAS 68425-43-4; cationic; veg.-derived conditioner for personal care applics.; liq.; pH 7.0; 40% conc.

Afalene™ 216. [McIntyre] Ricinoleamidopropyl dimethylamine lactate; CAS 977012-91-1; cationic; veg.-derived conditioner for personal care applics.; liq.; pH 6.0; 95% conc.

Afalene™ 416. [McIntyre] Isostearamidopropyl dimethylamine lactate; CAS 55852-15-8; cationic; veg.-derived conditioner for personal care applics.; liq.; pH 7.0; 95% conc.

Afalene™ 716. [McIntyre] Wheat germamidopropyl dimethylamine lactate; CAS 124046-40-8; cationic; veg.-derived conditioner for personal care applics.; liq.; pH 7.0; 95% conc.

Afalene™ AFC. [McIntyre] Isostearamidopropyl morpholine lactate; cationic; veg.-derived conditioner for personal care applics.; liq.; pH 5.0; 25% conc.

Afamine™ CAO. [McIntyre] Cocamidopropylamine oxide; CAS 68155-09-9; EINECS 268-938-5; veg.-derived prod. for personal care applics.; liq.; pH 7.0; 30% conc.

Afamine™ CO. [McIntyre] Cocamine oxide; CAS 61788-90-7; EINECS 263-016-9; veg.-derived prod. for personal care applics.; liq.; pH 7.0; 30% conc.

Afamine™ IAO. [McIntyre] Isostearamidopropylamine oxide; veg.-derived prod. for personal care applics.; liq.; pH 7.0; 30% conc.

Afamine™ ISMO. [McIntyre] Isostearamidopropylmorpholine oxide; veg.-derived prod. for personal care applics.; liq.; pH 7.0; 30% conc.

Afamine™ WGO. [McIntyre] Wheat germamidopropylamine oxide; veg.-derived prod. for personal care applics.; gel; pH 7.0; 30% conc.

Afanate™ CP. [McIntyre] Disodium cocamido MIPA sulfosuccinate; CAS 68515-65-1; EINECS 271-102-2; veg.-derived prod. for personal care applics.; liq.; pH 6.0; 40% conc.

Afanate™ EL. [McIntyre] Disodium laureth sulfosuccinate; veg.-derived prod. for personal care applics.; liq.; pH 6.0; 40% conc.

Afanate™ LO. [McIntyre] Disodium lauryl sulfosuccinate; veg.-derived prod. for personal care applics.; paste; pH 6.0; 40% conc.

Afanate™ OD-28. [McIntyre] Disodium oleamido PEG-2 sulfosuccinate; CAS 56388-43-3; EINECS 260-143-1; veg.-derived prod. for personal care applics.; liq.; pH 6.0; 28% conc.

Afanate™ RM. [McIntyre] Disodium ricinoleamido MEA sulfosuccinate; veg.-derived prod. for personal care applics.; liq.; pH 6.0; 40% conc.

Afanate™ UM. [McIntyre] Disodium undecylenamido MEA sulfosuccinate; veg.-derived prod. for personal care applics.; liq.; pH 6.0; 45% conc.

Afanate™ WGD. [McIntyre] Disodium wheatgermamido PEG-2 sulfosuccinate; veg.-derived prod. for personal care applics.; liq.; pH 6.0; 35% conc.

Afdet™ KCS. [McIntyre] Potassium coconate; natural soap for personal care applics.; liq.; pH 10.0; 38% conc.

Afdet™ WGS. [McIntyre] Potassium coconate and TEA wheat germ oil soap; natural soap for personal care applics.; liq.; pH 10.0; 40% conc.

Afmide™ C. [McIntyre] Cocamide DEA; CAS 61791-31-9; EINECS 263-163-9; veg.-derived prod. for personal care applics.; liq.; pH 10.0; 100% conc.

Afmide™ CMA. [McIntyre] Cocamide MEA; CAS 68140-00-1; EINECS 268-770-2; veg.-derived prod. for personal care applics.; flake; pH 10.0; 100% conc.

Afmide™ ISA. [McIntyre] Isostearamide DEA; CAS 52794-79-3; EINECS 258-193-4; veg.-derived prod. for personal care applics.; liq.; pH 10.0; 100% conc.

Afmide™ LLM. [McIntyre] Lauramide DEA; CAS 120-40-1; EINECS 204-393-1; veg.-derived prod. for personal care applics.; liq.; pH 10.0; 100% conc.

Afmide™ LMD. [McIntyre] Lauramide DEA (70% lauric); CAS 120-40-1; EINECS 204-393-1; veg.-derived prod. for personal care applics.; solid; pH 10.0; 100% conc.

Afmide™ LMM. [McIntyre] Lauramide MEA; CAS 142-78-9; EINECS 205-560-1; veg.-derived prod. for personal care applics.; flake; pH 10.0; 100% conc.

Afmide™ PK. [McIntyre] Palmkernelamide DEA; CAS 73807-15-5; veg.-derived prod. for personal care applics.; liq.; pH 10.0; 100% conc.

Afmide™ PKM. [McIntyre] Palmkernelamide MEA; veg.-derived prod. for personal care applics.; flake; pH 10.0; 100% conc.

Afmide™ R. [McIntyre] Ricinoleamide DEA; CAS 40716-42-5; EINECS 255-051-3; veg.-derived prod. for personal care applics.; liq.; pH 10.0; 100% conc.

Afmide™ S. [McIntyre] Soyamide DEA; CAS 68425-47-8; EINECS 270-355-6; veg.-derived prod. for personal care applics.; liq.; pH 10.0; 100% conc.

Afmide™ WGA. [McIntyre] Wheat germamide PEG-2; veg.-derived prod. for personal care applics.; paste; pH 10.0; 100% conc.

Afoteric™ 1C. [McIntyre] Cocoamphoacetate; amphoteric; veg.-derived prod. for personal care applics.; liq.; pH 11.0; 45% conc.

Afoteric™ 1L. [McIntyre] Lauroamphoacetate; amphoteric; veg.-derived prod. for personal care applics.; liq.; pH 10.0; 44% conc.

Afoteric™ 2C. [McIntyre] Cocoamphodiacetate; CAS 68650-39-5; EINECS 272-043-5; amphoteric; veg.-derived prod. for personal care applics.; liq.; pH 11.0; 50% conc.

Afoteric™ 2L. [McIntyre] Lauroamphodiacetate; amphoteric; veg.-derived prod. for personal care applics.; liq.; pH 9.0; 50% conc.

Afoteric™ 2W. [McIntyre] Wheat germamphodiacetate; amphoteric; veg.-derived prod. for personal care applics.; liq.; pH 9.5; 35% conc.

Afoteric™ 151C. [McIntyre] Cocaminopropionic acid; CAS 84812-94-2; EINECS 284-219-9; amphoteric; veg.-derived prod. for personal care applics.; liq.; pH 5.0; 40% conc.

Afoteric™ 151L. [McIntyre] Lauraminopropionic acid; CAS 1462-54-0; EINECS 215-968-1; amphoteric; veg.-derived prod. for personal care applics.; liq.; pH 5.0; 40% conc.

Afoteric™ 160C. [McIntyre] Sodium lauriminodipropionate; CAS 14960-06-6; EINECS 239-032-7; amphoteric; veg.-derived prod. for personal care applics.; liq.; pH 7.0; 38% conc.

Afpro™ WLP. [McIntyre] Wheat germamidopropyl silkhydroxypropyl dimonium chloride; cationic; veg.-derived protein for personal care applics.; liq.; pH 5.0; 38% conc.

Afpro™ WWP. [McIntyre] Wheat germamidopropyl dimethylamine hydrolyzed wheat protein; cationic; veg.-derived protein for personal care applics.; liq.; pH 5.0; 35% conc.

A.F.R. [Laboratoires Sérobiologiques] α Tocopherol, glycoceramides, saccharides, and phospholipids; complex providing anti-free radical activity, anti-lipoperoxide activity; for skin care prods. fighting premature aging; ivory opalescent liq.; disp. in water; usage level: 3-10%.

AFR LS. [Laboratoires Sérobioligiques] Water, mannitol, glycosphingolipids, tocopheryl acetate, lecithin, PEG-36 castor oil, and cholesterol.

Afron 22. [Vevy] MEA-lauryl sulfate, potassium phosphate, magnesium aspartate, PEG-8.

Afrosalt. [Vevy] Sea salt.

Aftershave HS 292. [Alban Muller] Witch hazel, horse chestnut, horsetail, and thyme phytocomplex with propylene glycol; aftershave.

Aftershave LS 692. [Alban Muller] Sunflower seed oil, horse chestnut extract, witch hazel extract, horsetail extract, and thyme extract; aftershave.

Agave Extract HS 2817 G. [Grau Aromatics] Propylene glycol and sisal extract; botanical extract.

Ageflex FM-1. [CPS] Dimethylaminoethyl methacrylate; CAS 2867-47-2; EINECS 220-688-8; detergent and sludge dispersant in lubricants; visc. index improver; flocculant for waste water treatment; retention aid for paper mfg.; acid scavenger in PU foams; corrosion inhibitor; resin and rubber modifier; used in acrylic polishes and paints, hair prep. copolymers, sugar clarification, adhesives, water clarification; APHA 50 clear liq.; very sol. in water; sol. in org. solvs.; m.w. 157.21; visc. 1.38 cst; b.p. 68.5 C (10 mm); f.p. < -60 C; toxicology: poison; harmful if swallowed; severe eye burns and skin irritation; irritating vapor; 99% assay.

Ageflex mDMDAC. [CPS] Dimethyl diallyl ammonium chloride; CAS 7398-69-8; cationic; monomer for synthesis of homo and copolymers used as coagulant and flocculants for water treatment, min. processing, demulsifier for petrol. recovery, elec. conductive paper and coatings, wet and dry str. resins, antistatic additives and coatings, cosmetic additives in hair conditioners, biocides, detergent additives, water-sol. polymers, electrographic paper and film; clear liq.; m.w. 161.68; sp.gr. 1.04; dens. 8.7 lb/gal; visc. 15 cps; pH 6; toxicology: nonhazardous; mildly corrosive; 65% solids.

Agequat 400. [CPS] Polyquaternium-6; CAS 26062-79-3; for personal care formulations incl. hair sprays, shampoos, conditioners, mousses, and rinses; APHA 100 color; sp.gr. 1.08; visc. 10,000 cps; 40% solids.

Agequat 500, -5008. [CPS] Polyquaternium-7; CAS 26590-05-6; for personal care formulations incl. hair sprays, shampoos, conditioners, mousses, and rinses; APHA 50 color; high m.w.; sp.gr. 1.03 and 1.02 resp.; visc. 15,000 and 10,000 cps resp.; 10 and 8.5% solids resp.

Ages 2006K. [Solvay GmbH] Potassium lauryl hydroxypropyl sulfonate.

Ages 2006/Mg. [Solvay GmbH] Magnesium lauryl hydroxypropyl sulfonate.

AGI Talc, BC 1615. [Whittaker, Clark & Daniels] Talc; CAS 14807-96-6; EINECS 238-877-9; cosmetic ingred.

Agnosol 3. [Croda Chem. Ltd.] PEG-3 lanolate; CAS 68459-50-7; emulsifier, solvent.

Agnosol 5. [Croda Chem. Ltd.] PEG-5 lanolate; CAS 68459-50-7; emulsifier, solvent.

Ajicoat SPG. [Ajinomoto] Sodium polyglutamate; CAS 28829-38-1; anionic; surface modifier, coemulsifier, codispersant; solid; 100% conc.

Ajidew A-100. [Ajinomoto] PCA; CAS 98-79-3; EINECS 202-700-3; nat. humectant used in cosmetics, soaps, dentifrices, medicinal supplies, tobacco, cellulose film, paper prods., fiber prods., paints; dyeing agent, softening agent, finishing agent, and antistatic agent; intermediate for synthesis; antistat for hair care prods.; wh. cryst. powd., odorless, sl. acidic taste, nonhygroscopic; m.w. 129.11; m.p. 181 C; pH 1.8-2.2.

Ajidew N-50. [Ajinomoto] Sodium PCA aq. sol'n.; CAS 28874-51-3; EINECS 249-277-1; nat. humectant used in cosmetics, soaps, dentifrices, medicinal supplies, tobacco, cellulose film, paper prods., fiber prods., paints; dyeing agent, softening agent, finishing agent, and antistatic agent; intermediate for synthesis; thickener for shampoos; liq.; pH 6.8-7.4; 50% act.

Ajidew SP-100. [Ajinomoto] Sodium PCA and PCA; nat. humectant used in cosmetics, soaps, dentifrices, medicinal supplies, tobacco, cellulose film, paper prods., fiber prods., paints; additive to dyeing agent, softening agent, finishing agent, and antistatic agent; intermediate for synthesis; wh. cryst.

Akopol R. [Karlshamns] Partially hydrog. soybean and cottonseed oils; fractionated hard butter for use in nontempering confectioner's coatings, vegetable dairy, cosmetics, and pharmaceuticals; Lovibond 3.0 R max.; m.p. 97-101 F.

Akucell CMC. [Robeco] Cellulose gum.

Akypo 23Q38. [Chem-Y GmbH] C12-13 pareth-5 carboxylic acid; CAS 70750-17-3.

Akypo AD 100 SPC. [Chem-Y GmbH] Sodium PEG-3 lauramide carboxylate; anionic; surfactant for mild cosmetic prods.; solid; 100% conc.

Akypo EH 15. [Chem-Y GmbH] Octeth-3 carboxylic acid.

Akypo KA 150 CNV, KA 450 CNV. [Chem-Y GmbH] Special alkyl ether carboxylate; anionic; surfactant for mild cosmetic prods.; liq.; 30% conc.

Akypo NP 70. [Chem-Y GmbH] Nonoxynol-8 carboxylic acid; CAS 3115-49-9; anionic; emulsifier; Gardner 4 liq.; visc. 1500 mPa·s; pH 2-3 (1%); surf. tens. 37 mN/m; 90% conc.

Akypo RCS 60. [Chem-Y GmbH] Ceteareth-7 carboxylic acid; CAS 68954-89-2; surfactant; ylsh. wh. solid; pH 2-3 (1%); surf. tens. 44 mN/m; 90% act.

Akypo RLM 38. [Chem-Y GmbH] Laureth-5 carboxylic acid; surfactant; Gardner 1 liq.; visc. 500 mPa·s; pH 2-3 (1%); surf. tens. 33 mN/m; 90% act.

Akypo RLM 38 NV. [Chem-Y GmbH] Fatty alcohol polyglycol ether carboxylic acid, sodium salt; anionic; detergent for shampoo, liq. soap and foam bath; emulsifier and wetting agent; liq.; toxicology: LD50 (rat, oral) 4 g/kg; 22% conc.

Akypo RLM 45. [Chem-Y GmbH] Laureth-6 carboxylic acid; CAS 68954-89-2; anionic/nonionic; emulsifier, dispersant, superfatting and foam stabilizing agent for emulsion and detergent use, shampoos, bubble baths; Gardner 1 liq.; visc. 500 mPa·s; HLB 11.0; pH 2-3 (1%); surf. tens. 34 mN/m; toxicology: LD50 (rat, oral) 3.5 g/kg; 90% act.

Akypo RLM 45 A. [Chem-Y GmbH] Ammonium laureth-6 carboxylate; for shampoos, hair dye formulations; paste; 85% act.

Akypo RLM 45 N. [Chem-Y GmbH] Sodium laureth-6 carboxylate; CAS 33939-64-9; anionic; detergent for shampoos and bubble baths, hair dye formulations; improves skin in bath, shower and shampoo formulations; paste; 90% act.

Akypo RLM 100. [Chem-Y GmbH] Laureth-11 carboxylic acid; CAS 27306-90-7; anionic/nonionic; emulsifier for cosmetics applics.; foam booster for cleaners, heavy-duty detergent formulations; Gardner 1 liq.; visc. 500 mPa·s; HLB 14.8; pH 2-3 (1%); surf. tens. 38 mN/m; 90% act.

Akypo RLM 100 NV. [Chem-Y GmbH] Sodium laureth-11 carboxylate; CAS 33939-64-9; anionic; surfactant and additive for personal care prods.; liq.; HLB 31.8; 22% conc.

Akypo RLM 130. [Chem-Y GmbH] Laureth-14 carboxylic acid; CAS 68954-89-2; nonionic; emulsifier; Gardner 1 liq.; visc. 2000 mPa·s; HLB 15.9; pH 2-3 (1%); surf. tens. 40 mN/m; 90% conc.

Akypo RLM 160. [Chem-Y GmbH] Laureth-17 carboxylic acid; CAS 27306-90-7; anionic/nonionic; emulsifier; ylsh. wh. solid; pH 2-3 (1%); surf. tens. 47 mN/m; 85% conc.

Akypo RLM 160 N. [Chem-Y GmbH] Sodium laureth-17 carboxylate; CAS 33939-64-9; surfactant.

Akypo RLMQ 38. [Chem-Y GmbH] Laureth-5 carboxylic acid; CAS 68954-89-2; nonionic; emulsifier, dispersant, additive for personal care prods., household and industrial formulas; primary emulsifier for syn. latex; liq.; HLB 10.2; 90% conc.

Akypo RS 60. [Chem-Y GmbH] Steareth-7 carboxylic acid;

CAS 68954-89-2; 59559-30-7; surfactant; ylsh. wh. solid; pH 2-3 (1%); surf. tens. 44 mN/m; 90% act.

Akypo RS 100. [Chem-Y GmbH] Steareth-11 carboxylic acid; CAS 68954-89-2; surfactant; ylsh. wh. solid; pH 2-3 (1%); surf. tens. 45 mN/m; 90% act.

Akypo RT 60. [Chem-Y GmbH] Talloweth-7 carboxylic acid; CAS 68954-89-2; surfactant; ylsh. wh. solid; pH 2-3 (1%); surf. tens. 39 mN/m; 90% act.

Akypogene FP 35 T. [Chem-Y GmbH] TEA cocoate; CAS 61790-64-5; EINECS 263-155-5; anionic; cosmetics surfactant for shower, shampoo and bath formulations, liq. hand cleaner; liq.; 35% conc.

Akypogene HM 8. [Chem-Y GmbH] MEA lauryl sulfate, sodium PEG-6 cocamide carboxylate, disodium laureth sulfosuccinate; anionic; economical surfactant for mfg. of mild shampoos, foam baths, shower baths, liq. soaps not irritating to optic mucosa; liq.; 25% act.

Akypogene HM 12. [Chem-Y GmbH] Sodium C12-13 pareth sulfate, sodium PEG-6 cocamide carboxylate, disodium laureth sulfosuccinate, trideceth-2 carboxamide MEA; anionic; ecnomical surfactant for prep. of mild shampoos, foam baths, shower baths, and liq. soaps not irritating to optic mucosa; liq.; 41% act.

Akypogene ZA 97 SP. [Chem-Y GmbH] Potassium xylene sulfonate, potassium tallate, potassium cocoate; anionic; surfactant blend for liq. soap; liq.; 25% conc.

Akypo®-Muls 400. [Chem-Y GmbH] PEG-9 stearamide carboxylic acid; CAS 90453-59-1; anionic; nontoxic, biodeg. emulsifier for cosmetics, o/w emulsions; sl. brnsh. wax; m.p. 40 C; HLB 12.0; 93% act.

Akypoquat 131. [Chem-Y GmbH] Behenoyl PG-trimonium chloride; CAS 69537-38-8; EINECS 274-033-6; cationic; raw material for cosmetic hair prods., cream rinses; antistat; good wet and dry combing props.; molecule is fully biodeg.; wh. solid; sp.gr. 1.1 kg/l; pH 3.5-4.5; toxicology: nonirritating to eyes; LD50 (rat, oral) 5.2 g/kg; LD50 (rabbit, dermal) > 9 ml/kg; 70% act.

Akypoquat 131 V. [Chem-Y GmbH] Behenoyl PG-trimonium chloride; CAS 69537-38-8; EINECS 274-033-6; cationic; surfactant for mfg. of hair conditioners; paste; 35% act.

Akypoquat 131 VC. [Chem-Y GmbH] Behenoyl PG-trimonium chloride, cetyl alcohol; cationic; biodeg. cosmetics surfactant for prep. of cream rinses, hair conditioners; paste; sp.gr. 1.05 kg/l; pH 3.5-4.5; 48% act., 42% water.

Akypoquat 132. [Chem-Y GmbH] Lauroyl PG-trimonium chloride, hexylene glycol; cationic; raw material for cosmetic hair and skin prods.; molecule is fully biodeg.; opaque paste; sp.gr. 1.1; flash pt. > 100 C; pH 3.5-4.5; 70% act., 17% hexylene glycol.

Akyporox CO 400. [Chem-Y GmbH] PEG-40 hydrog. castor oil; CAS 61788-85-0; nonionic; perfume solubilizer, o/w emulsifier for cosmetic prods.; eliminates oil bath turbidity; paste; m.p. 25 C; cloud pt. > 100 C (1%); surf. tens. 47 mN/m; 100% act.

Akyporox CO 600. [Chem-Y GmbH] PEG-60 hydrog. castor oil; CAS 61788-85-0; nonionic; perfume solubilizer, o/w emulsifier for cosmetic prods.; eliminates oil bath turbidity; solid; m.p. 35 C; cloud pt. > 100 C (1%); surf. tens. 48 mN/m; 100% act.

Akyporox NP 30. [Chem-Y GmbH] Nonoxynol-3; CAS 9016-45-9; nonionic; for hair dye formulations; emulsifier for emulsion polymerization; liq.; 100% act.

Akyporox OP 250V. [Chem-Y GmbH] Octoxynol-25; CAS 9002-93-1; nonionic; emulsifier for emulsion polymerization; perfume solubilizer; Gardner 2 clear liq.; sp.gr. 1.07; visc. 1000 mPa·s; cloud pt. > 100 C (1%); HLB 17.3; pH 8-9 (5%); surf. tens. 40 mN/m; 70% act.

Akyporox RC 200. [Chem-Y GmbH] Ceteth-20; CAS 9004-95-9; nonionic; solubilizer for cosmetic prods.; solid;

sp.gr. 1.1; m.p. 43 C; cloud pt. > 100 C (1%); HLB 15.7; surf. tens. 43 mN/m; 100% act.

Akyporox RLM 22. [Chem-Y GmbH] Laureth-2; CAS 3055-93-4; EINECS 221-279-7; nonionic; emulsifier for mfg. of hair dye formulations; additive for mfg. of snow from spray cans; liq.; oil-sol.; sp.gr. 0.91; HLB 6.3; surf. tens. 29 mN/m; 100% act.

Akyporox RLM 40. [Chem-Y GmbH] Laureth-4; CAS 5274-68-0; EINECS 226-097-1; nonionic; emulsifier for mfg. of hair dye formulations, cosmetic aerosols, oil bath formulations, window cleaners, hand cleaners, heavy-duty detergents; liq.; sp.gr. 0.95; HLB 9.4; surf. tens. 29 mN/m; 100% act.

Akyporox RLM 80V. [Chem-Y GmbH] Laureth-8; CAS 3055-98-9; nonionic; emulsifier for mfg. of cosmetic aerosols, heavy-duty detergents, all-purpose cleaners; liq.; 85% act.

Akyporox RO 90. [Chem-Y GmbH] Oleth-9; CAS 9004-98-2; nonionic; emulsifier, wetting agent for textile prods., metalworking fluids, all-purpose cleaners, hand cleaners, creams and lotions; liq.; sp.gr. 0.99; HLB 12.1; cloud pt. > 60 C (1%); surf. tens. 34 mN/m; 100% act.

Akyporox SAL SAS. [Chem-Y GmbH] Sodium lauryl sulfate; CAS 142-87-0; anionic; detergent, shampoo base, emulsifier for emulsion polymerization; liq.; 28% conc.

Akyposal 23 ST 70. [Chem-Y GmbH] Sodium C12-13 pareth sulfate; anionic; detergent; shampoo base; paste; water-sol.; 70% conc.

Akyposal 40 DAL. [Chem-Y GmbH] Lauryl ether sulfate, amine salt; anionic; surfactant for mild cosmetic prods.; liq.; 40% conc.

Akyposal 100 DAL. [Chem-Y GmbH] TIPA-laureth sulfate; CAS 107600-36-2; anionic; emulsifier for bath oils; suited for anhyd. formulations; biodeg.; yel. clear liq.; sol. in water and oil; sp.gr. 1.0 kg/l; visc. 20,000 mPa·s; pour pt. 10-15 C; pH 4-6 (10%); 96% act.

Akyposal 2010 S. [Chem-Y GmbH] Sodium laureth sulfate, cocamide DEA, glycol distearate; anionic; surfactant, pearling agent, foam stabilizer for cosmetics; biodeg.; wh. opaque thixotropic liq.; visc. 4000 mPa·s; pH 7.5-8.0; 36% conc.

Akyposal 2010 SD. [Chem-Y GmbH] Sodium PEG-6 cocamide carboxylate, glycol distearate; anionic; surfactant, pearling agent for cosmetics; biodeg.; lt. yel. opaque liq.; visc. 7000 mPa·s; pH 6.7-7.0; 41% act.

Akyposal ALS 33. [Chem-Y GmbH] Ammonium lauryl sulfate; CAS 2235-54-3; EINECS 218-793-9; anionic; detergent, emulsifier; shampoo base; used in emulsion polymerization; liq.; 33% conc.

Akyposal DS 28. [Chem-Y GmbH] Sodium laureth sulfate; CAS 68957-18-6; anionic; detergent; shampoo base; liq.; 28% conc.

Akyposal DS 56. [Chem-Y GmbH] Sodium C12-13 pareth sulfate; CAS 68957-18-6; anionic; detergent; shampoo base; liq.; water-sol.; 56% conc.

Akyposal EO 20. [Chem-Y GmbH] Sodium laureth sulfate; anionic; base for shampoos and bubble baths; liq.; 28% conc.

Akyposal EO 20 MW. [Chem-Y GmbH] Sodium laureth sulfate; CAS 9004-82-4; anionic; detergent, base for shampoos and bubble baths, emulsifier for emulsion polymerization; liq.; 28% conc.

Akyposal EO 2067. [Chem-Y GmbH] Sodium laureth sulfate; CAS 9004-82-4; anionic; base for shampoos and bubble baths; liq.; 28% conc.

Akyposal HF 28. [Chem-Y GmbH] Sodium laureth sulfate, magnesium laureth-16 sulfate; anionic; base for mild shampoos and shower prods.; liq.; 28% conc.

Akyposal MGLS. [Chem-Y GmbH] Magnesium lauryl sulfate; CAS 3097-08-3; EINECS 221-450-6; anionic; deter-

gent for shampoos, foam bath; liq.; 28% conc.

Akyposal MLES 35. [Chem-Y GmbH] MEA-laureth sulfate; CAS 68184-04-3; anionic; base, foamer for shampoo and bubble baths; liq.; 35% conc.

Akyposal MLS 30. [Chem-Y GmbH] MEA-lauryl sulfate; CAS 4722-98-9; EINECS 225-214-3; anionic; detergent, shampoo base, shower baths; liq.; 30% conc.

Akyposal NLS. [Chem-Y GmbH] Sodium lauryl sulfate; CAS 151-21-3; EINECS 205-788-1; anionic; detergent; liq.; 31% conc.

Akyposal RLM 56 S. [Chem-Y GmbH] Fatty alcohol ether sulfate; CAS 3088-31-1; anionic; detergent for personal care prods., liq. soaps, dishwashing prods.; liq.; 56% conc.

Akyposal RLM 70. [Chem-Y GmbH] Fatty alcohol ether sulfate; CAS 9004-82-4; anionic; detergent; shampoo base; liq.; water-sol.; 70% conc.

Akyposal TBP 120. [Chem-Y GmbH] Sodium butoxynol-12 sulfate.

Akyposal TIPA 45. [Chemsal] TIPA lauryl sulfate; CAS 66161-60-2; anionic; surfactant for cosmetics, shampoos, shower and foam baths; liq.; 45% conc.

Akyposal TLS 42. [Chem-Y GmbH] TEA-lauryl sulfate; CAS 139-96-8; EINECS 205-388-7; anionic; detergent; base for personal care prods. and car shampoos; foaming agent for agrochemicals and fire extinguishers; liq.; 42% act.

Akyposept B. [Chem-Y GmbH] Benzylhemiformal; CAS 14548-60-8; EINECS 238-588-8.

Akypo®-Soft 45 NV. [Chem-Y GmbH] Sodium laureth-6 carboxylate; CAS 33939-64-9, 53610-02-9; anionic; mild cosmetics surfactant for baby care prods., shampoos, foam baths, medicinal liq. soaps, feminine hygiene prods.; well tolerated by optic mucosa; biodeg.; water-wh. liq., odorless; m.w. 457; sp.gr. 1.0 kg/l; visc. 100 mPa·s; pH 6.5-7.5; toxicology: nonirritant; 22% act. in water.

Akypo®-Soft 100 MgV. [Chem-Y GmbH] Magnesium laureth-11 carboxylate; CAS 99330-44-6; anionic; mild detergent, emulsifier, wetting agent for shampoos, liq. soaps, foam baths, low irritation formulas, feminine hygiene prods.; well tolerated by optic mucosa; biodeg.; water-wh. clear liq.; sp.gr. 1.0 kg/l; visc. 500 mPa·s; pH 5-6; 22% act.

Akypo®-Soft 100 NV. [Chem-Y GmbH] Sodium laureth-11 carboxylate; CAS 68987-89-3; anionic; detergent, emulsifier, wetting agent for shampoos, liq. soaps, foam baths, feminine hygiene prods., low irritation formulas; PU foam for orthopedic use; biodeg.; water-wh. clear liq.; sp.gr. 1.0 kg/l; visc. 100 mPa·s; pH 6.5-7.5; toxicology: nonirritant; 22% act.

Akypo®-Soft 130 NV. [Chem-Y GmbH] Sodium laureth-14 carboxylate; CAS 68987-89-3; anionic; detergent, emulsifier, wetting agent for shampoos, liq. soaps, foam baths, low irritation formulas; liq.; 22% conc.

Akypo®-Soft 160 NV. [Chem-Y GmbH] Sodium laureth-17 carboxylate; CAS 68987-89-3; anionic; detergent, emulsifier, wetting agent for shampoos, liq. soaps, foam baths, low irritation formulas; surfactant for contact lens cleaning fluids; biodeg.; water-wh. clear liq.; sp.gr. 1.0 kg/l; visc. 100 mPa·s; pH 6-7; toxicology: very low eye irritation; 22% act.

Akypo®-Soft KA 250 BV. [Chem-Y GmbH] Sodium PEG-6 cocamide carboxylate; CAS 107628-03-5; anionic; economical surfactant for formulation of mild shampoos, foam baths, shower baths, liq. soaps; mild to skin and eyes; biodeg.; clear sl. ylsh. liq.; sp.gr. 1.1 g/ml; visc. < 500 mPa·s; pH 7.0-8.0; 30% conc.

Akypo®-Soft KA 250 BVC. [Chem-Y GmbH] Sodium PEG-6 cocamide carboxylate; CAS 107628-03-5; anionic; economical surfactant for mild cosmetic prods., mild shampoos, foam baths, shower baths, liq. soaps; biodeg.; clear ylsh., sl. visc. liq.; sp.gr. 1.15 g/ml; visc. 600 mPa·s; f.p. 15 C; pH 7.0-8.0 (10% aq.); 52% act.

Alacen. [New Zealand Milk Prods.] Whey protein; CAS 84082-51-9; cosmetic protein.

Alacid. [New Zealand Milk Prods.] Casein; CAS 9000-71-9; EINECS 232-55-1.

Alanate 110. [New Zealand Milk Prods.] Sodium caseinate; CAS 9005-46-3; emulsifier, stabilizer.

Alanate 351. [New Zealand Milk Prods.] Potassium caseinate; CAS 68131-54-4.

Alaren. [New Zealand Milk Prods.] Casein; CAS 9000-71-9; EINECS 232-55-1.

Alatal. [New Zealand Milk Prods.] Whey protein; CAS 84082-51-9; cosmetic protein.

Albagel 4446. [Whittaker, Clark & Daniels] Bentonite; CAS 1302-78-9; EINECS 215-108-5; thickener.

Albagel Premium USP 4444. [Whittaker, Clark & Daniels] Bentonite; CAS 1302-78-9; EINECS 215-108-5; thickener.

Albagen 4439. [Whittaker, Clark & Daniels] Bentonite; CAS 1302-78-9; EINECS 215-108-5; thickener.

Albalan. [Westbrook Lanolin] Lanolin wax; CAS 68201-49-0; EINECS 269-220-4; nonionic; emollient, emulsifier for face masks, foundations, hair conditioners, lipsticks, sunscreen preps., toilet soaps; binder for pressed powds.; forms stable w/o emulsions; soft wax; m.p. 38-45; HLB 5.0; acid no. 1 max.; iodine no. 18-32; sapon. no. 96-114; 100% conc.

Alberger® . [Akzo Salt] Sodium chloride; crystalline salt refined by Alberger process; used as abrasives, antiseptics, binders, builders, carriers, diluent, freshener, thickener, or ingred. in household prods. (dishwash, dyes, fabric softener, metal polishes, pest control prods., etc); and personal care prods. (bar soap, cosmetics, denture cleaners, first aid prods., mouthwash, shampoo, shave cream, toothpaste, etc.).

Albone® 35 CG. [DuPont] Hydrogen peroxide; CAS 7722-84-1; EINECS 231-765-0; specially stabilized cosmetic grade for prep. of stable dilute sol'ns. for consumer use in cosmetic and pharmaceutical applics. or as laundry bleach; meets USP specs. when properly diluted to 3%; FDA approved; colorless clear liq., sl. pungent odor; sp.gr. 1.133 mg/m³; dens. 9.45 lb/gal; m.p. -33 C; b.p. 108 C (760 mm Hg); pH 2.3-2.8; 35% hydrogen peroxide, 16.5% act. oxygen.

Albone® 50 CG. [DuPont] Hydrogen peroxide; CAS 7722-84-1; EINECS 231-765-0; specially stabilized cosmetic grade for prep. of stable dilute sol'ns. for consumer use in cosmetic and pharmaceutical applics. or as laundry bleach; meets USP specs. when properly diluted to 3%; FDA approved; colorless clear liq., sl. pungent odor; sp.gr. 1.196 mg/m³; dens. 9.98 lb/gal; m.p. -52 C; b.p. 114 C (760 mm Hg); pH 1.5-2.0; 50% hydrogen peroxide, 23.5% act. oxygen.

Albone® 70CG. [DuPont] Hydrogen peroxide; CAS 7722-84-1; EINECS 231-765-0; specially stabilized cosmetic grade for prep. of stable dilute sol'ns. for consumer use in cosmetic and pharmaceutical applics. or as laundry bleach; meets USP specs. when properly diluted to 3%; FDA approved; colorless clear liq., sl. pungent odor; sp.gr. 1.3 mg/m³; dens. 10.75 lb/gal; m.p. -40 C; b.p. 126 C (760 mm Hg); pH 0.4-0.8; 68% hydrogen peroxide, 32.9% act. oxygen.

Alchlordrate. [Universal Preserv-A-Chem] Aluminum chlorohydrate; CAS 1327-41-9; EINECS 215-477-2; antiperspirant active.

AlcoCare® 1000. [Rhone-Poulenc Surf. & Spec.] Surfactant/humectant blend; anionic; provides foam, feel, visc. and mildness to health care formulations; forms stable emul-

sions with many poorly sol. materials without the use of heat; yel./straw; visc. 400 cps; pH 7.0-7.5; usage level: 10-25%; 33.5-40% solids.

AlcoCare® 1010. [Rhone-Poulenc Surf. & Spec.] Anionic surfactant blend; anionic; designed for max. stability when formulated with povidone-iodine in surgical scrubs; yel. liq.; visc. 500 cps; pH 3-4; 22-26% solids.

AlcoCare® 2011. [Rhone-Poulenc Surf. & Spec.] Chloroxylenol PCMX concs.; high foaming antimicrobial conc.; alkali stable; for handwash, surgical scrubs, health care; clear liq.; visc. < 1000 cps; pH 6-7; 39-43% solids, 7% PCMX.

AlcoCare® 2012. [Rhone-Poulenc Surf. & Spec.] Chloroxylenol PCMX conc.; high foaming antimicrobial conc. for handwash, surgical scrubs, health care; clear liq.; visc. < 1000 cps; pH 6-7; 39-43% solids, 7% PCMX.

AlcoCare® 2013. [Rhone-Poulenc Surf. & Spec.] Chloroxylenol PCMX conc.; high foaming antimicrobial conc. for handwash, surgical scrubs, health care; clear liq.; visc. < 1000 cps; pH 6-7; 39-43% solids, 7% PCMX.

AlcoCare® 2115. [Rhone-Poulenc Surf. & Spec.] PCMX/ether complex; antimicrobial; clear/amber liq.; visc. 1225 cps; pH 9.5 (10%); 100% solids, 15% PCMX.

AlcoCare® 2123. [Rhone-Poulenc Surf. & Spec.] PCMX/ether complex; antimicrobial; clear/amber liq.; visc. 1050 cps; pH 9.5 (10%); 100% solids, 23% PCMX.

AlcoCare® 2150. [Rhone-Poulenc Surf. & Spec.] PCMX/ethoxylate complex; antimicrobial; clear/amber liq.; visc. 2350 cps; pH 9.6 (10%); 100% solids, 50% PCMX.

AlcoCare® 3020. [Rhone-Poulenc Surf. & Spec.] Iodine/surfactant conc.; anionic/nonionic; low foaming antimicrobial conc.; acid stable; for surgical scrubs, health care; dk. brn. liq.; visc. 200-1000 cps; pH 2.5-3.8; 2.2-2.7% iodine.

AlcoCare® 3050. [Rhone-Poulenc Surf. & Spec.] Iodine complexed with polyvinyl pyrillodone; starting point for pre-operative patient prep. and surgical scrubs; dk. brn. liq.; visc. 500-1500 cps; pH 2.5-3.5; 3.4-3.7% iodine.

AlcoCare® 6012. [Rhone-Poulenc Surf. & Spec.] Cold mix of two proprietary blends and water, containing 1.75% chloroxylenol; formulated sanitizer conc., antimicrobial; skin cleanser for meat/poultry handling facilities; USDA approval; water-wh. clear liq., char. odor; visc. 700-1500 cps; pH 6.4-7.2.

Alcodet® SK. [Rhone-Poulenc Surf. & Spec.] PEG-8 isolauryl thioether; CAS 9004-83-5; nonionic; emulsifier, wetting agent, detergent, carbon soil and grease cleaners, metal cleaning specialties, textile scouring, insecticide emulsions, paints, hair prods., wood and paper industries; emulsifier for petrol oils, chlorinated solvs., silicones; Gardner 6 max. liq.; sol. in water; sp.gr. 1.03; dens. 8.5 lb/gal; HLB 12.7; cloud pt. 28 C (1% aq.); surf. tens. 31 dynes/cm (0.05%); 100% conc.; formerly Siponic® SK.

Alcolan® . [Amerchol] Petrolatum, sorbitan sesquioleate, and lanolin alcohol; nonionic; w/o emulsifier, emollient base for cosmetic and pharmaceutical emulsions; paste; 100% conc.

Alcolan® 36W. [Amerchol] Lanolin, petrolatum, and sorbitan sesquioleate; nonionic; emulsifier, emollient for cosmetics and pharmaceutical emulsions; paste; 100% conc.

Alcolan® 40. [Amerchol] Petrolatum, lanolin, beeswax, sorbitan sesquioleate, and polysorbate 81; w/o emulsifier, emollient base for cosmetic and pharmaceutical emulsions; paste; 100% conc.

Alcolec® BS. [Am. Lecithin] Single bleached lecithin; CAS 8002-43-5; EINECS 232-307-2; nonionic; w/o emulsifier, wetting and dispersing agent, stabilizer, release and lubricating agent, foam suppressant, solubilizer, and emollient for personal care, food, and industrial applics.; choline source; Gardner 14 liq.; acid no. 32 max.

Alcolec® Extra A. [Am. Lecithin] Lecithin; CAS 8002-43-5; EINECS 232-307-2; nonionic; emulsifier for aq. and oil-based systems, food industry; higher phosphatide content; liq.; 100% conc.

Alcolec® F-100. [Am. Lecithin] De-oiled lecithin; CAS 8002-43-5; EINECS 232-307-2; emulsifier for personal care, industrial, and food applics.; instantizing for milk powd., cake mixes, etc.; choline source; lt. tan/yel. powd.; acid no. 36 max.

Alcolec® Granules. [Am. Lecithin] Lecithin; CAS 8002-43-5; EINECS 232-307-2; nonionic; wetting agent, release agent, emulsifier, stabilizer, diet supplement, in industrial, cosmetics, pharmaceuticals, food applics.; instantizing for milk powd., cake mixes, etc.; choline source; lt. tan/yel. gran.; bland odor and taste; sp.gr. 0.5; acid no. 36 max.; 97% act.

Alcolec® PG. [Am. Lecithin] Lecithin; CAS 8002-43-5; EINECS 232-307-2; o/w emulsifier, moisturizer, and emollient for personal care prods., cosmetics, skin care prods; wetting agent in magnetic tape media; food grade; virtually oil-free; GRAS; kosher approval; sl. yel. waxy gran.

Alcolec® Powder. [Am. Lecithin] Soy phosphatides; nonionic; emulsifier, stabilizer for cosmetics, pharmaceuticals; powd.; 97% conc.

Alcolec® S. [Am. Lecithin] Unbleached lecithin; CAS 8002-43-5; EINECS 232-307-2; nonionic; commercial lecithin emulsifier, wetting and dispersing agent, stabilizer, release and lubricating agent, foam suppressant, solubilizer for food and industrial applics.; choline source; Gardner 17 liq.; acid no. 32 max.

Alcolec® SFG. [Am. Lecithin] An oil-free lecithin containing a high inositol content; CAS 8002-43-5; EINECS 232-307-2; w/o emulsifier for personal care prods.; dough conditioner/volume improver, release aid, lubricant for food applics.; foam suppressant; GRAS; kosher approval; gran.; acid no. 32 max.

Alcolec® Z-3. [Am. Lecithin] Hydroxylated lecithin; CAS 8029-76-3; EINECS 232-440-6; nonionic; wetting agent, emulsifier for personal care products, pharmaceuticals, food use; improves dispersability of fatty powds.; lt. amber liq.; sol. in most fat solv. except acetone; visc. 8000 cps; acid no. < 38.

Alcolec® Z-7. [Am. Lecithin] Hydroxylated lecithin; CAS 8029-76-3; EINECS 232-440-6; emulsifier.

Alcolite. [Guardian Labs] Sodium stearate and stearic acid.

Alcoramnosan. [Vevy] Hydroxyethylcellulose; CAS 9004-62-0; thickener.

Aldehyd 11-11. [Henkel/Cospha] Aroma chemical for cosmetic, personal care, detergent, and cleaning prods.; colorless liq., aldehydic odor; b.p. 90-105 C; flash pt. 86 C.

Aldehyd 13-13. [Henkel/Cospha] Aroma chemical for cosmetic, personal care, detergent, and cleaning prods.; colorless liq., aldehydic odor; b.p. 248-281 C; flash pt. 104 C.

Aldehyde C 14 Soc. Peach (3/010811). [Dragoco] γ-Undecalactone; CAS 104-67-6; EINECS 203-225-4.

Aldehyde C 18 Soc. Coconut (3/010921). [Dragoco] γ-Nonalactone.

Alder Buckthorn HS. [Dragoco] Propylene glycol, buckthorn extract; botanical extract.

Aldo® DC. [Lonza] Propylene glycol dicaprylate/dicaprate; nonionic; coupling agent for mixed solv. systems; emulsifier for food, cosmetic, industrial use; Gardner 2 max. liq.; sol. in ethanol, min. and veg. oil; insol. in water; sp.gr. 0.92; HLB 2 ± 1; iodine no. 0.5 max.; sapon. no. 315-335.; 100% conc.

Aldo® HMS. [Lonza] Glyceryl stearate; CAS 123-94-4; nonionic; emulsifier for w/o systems; stabilizer, consis-

tency builder, emollient in personal care prods.; wh. beads; sol. in ethanol, min. and veg. oil; disp. in water; HLB 2.8; m.p. 61-68 C; sapon. no. 165-175; 52-56% mono content.

Aldo® MLD. [Lonza] Glyceryl laurate SE; nonionic; emulsifier for cosmetic, pharmaceutical and industrial use; cream soft solid; sol. in ethanol, ethyl acetate, toluol, min. and veg. oils, disp. in water; sp.gr. 0.97; m.p. 21-26 C; HLB 6.8; sapon. no. 185-195; pH 7.5-8.5 (5% aq.); 100% conc.

Aldo® MO. [Lonza] Glyceryl oleate; CAS 111-03-5; nonionic; emulsifier, defoamer; yel., soft solid; sol. in ethyl acetate; sp.gr. 0.95; m.p. < 25 C; HLB 3.4; sapon. no. 170-180; pH 4.5-6.5; 100% conc.

Aldo® MOD. [Lonza] Glyceryl oleate SE; nonionic; emulsifier; avail. in animal, veg., food, and Kosher grades; yel. liq.; sol. in toluol, naphtha, min. and veg. oils, disp. in water; sp.gr. 0.95; m.p. < 0 C; HLB 5.0; sapon. no. 141-147; pH 8.5-9.5 (5% aq.); 100% conc.

Aldo® MO FG. [Lonza] Glyceryl mono- and dioleate; nonionic; emulsifier and antifoam for foods; emulsifier, solubilizer for cosmetic, pharmaceutical, and industrial applics.; liq.; HLB 3.0; 100% conc.

Aldo® MR. [Lonza] Glyceryl ricinoleate; CAS 141-08-2; EINECS 205-455-0; nonionic; emulsifier, solubilizer for cosmetic, pharmaceutical and industrial applics.; yel. liq.; sol. in methanol, ethanol, ethyl acetate, toluol, veg. oil, disp. in water; sp.gr. 1.02; m.p. < -8 C; HLB 6.0; sapon. no. 66-69; pH 8.3-9.3; 100% conc.

Aldo® MS. [Lonza] Glyceryl stearate; CAS 123-94-4; nonionic; emulsifier for cosmetic, pharmaceutical and industrial use; wh. beads; sol. hot in methanol, ethanol, toluol, naphtha, min. and veg. oils, disp. in hot water; sp.gr. 0.97; m.p. 57-61 C; HLB 4.0; sapon. no. 158-165; pH 7.6-8.6 (3% aq.); 100% conc.

Aldo® MSA. [Lonza] Glyceryl stearate; CAS 123-94-4; nonionic; emulsifier for o/w personal care prods., cosmetics, pharmaceuticals, industrial use; wh. beads; sol. in ethanol, min. and veg. oil; disp. in water; HLB 11 ± 1; m.p. 56-60 C; sapon. no. 90-100; 100% conc., 17.5% min. mono content.

Aldo® MSC. [Lonza] Glyceryl stearate; CAS 31566-31-1; nonionic; emulsifier, surfactant for cosmetics, toiletries, and pharmaceuticals (creams, lotions, gels, hair conditioners, shampoos, OTC prods., skin/facial treatments); aux. emulsifier for o/w emulsions; lt. tan beads or flakes, mild fatty odor; sol. hot in methanol, ethanol, toluol, naphtha, min. and veg. oils, disp. in hot water; sp.gr. 0.97; m.p. 55-58 C; HLB 3.0; acid no. 6 max.; iodine no. 3 max.; sapon. no. 168-176; flash pt. (COC) 204 C; pH 6 (3%); toxicology: LD50 (rat) > 5000 mg/kg; nonlethal, nontoxic; nonirritating to eyes and skin; 100% conc., 42-48% alpha mono.

Aldo® MSD. [Lonza] Glyceryl stearate SE; CAS 123-94-4; nonionic; emulsifier, solubilizer for cosmetic, pharmaceutical and industrial applics.; wh. beads; sol. hot in methanol, ethanol, toluol, naphtha, min. and veg. oils, disp. in hot water; sp.gr. 0.97; m.p. 56-60 C; HLB 6.0; sapon. no. 140-150; pH 9.2-10.2 (3% aq.); 100% conc.

Aldo® MS LG. [Lonza] Glyceryl stearate; CAS 123-94-4; nonionic; emulsifier for w/o systems; stabilizer, consistency builder, emollient in personal care prods.; wh. beads; sol. in ethanol, min. and veg. oil; disp. in water; HLB 3.3; m.p. 58-62 C; sapon. no. 160-170; 40-45% mono content.

Aldo® MSLG FG. [Lonza] Glyceryl stearate, low glycerin; CAS 31566-31-1; nonionic; food emulsifier and emulsion stabilizer for baked goods, dairy prods., edible oils/shortenings, confectionery, pet foods; slip and antitack agent in hot-melt adhesives, solv. or solventless coatings;

emulsifier for paper defoamers; emulsifier for cosmetic creams, lotions, pastes, and gels; FDA GRAS; wh. beads, bland odor and taste; m.p. 58-62 C; HLB 3; acid no. 2 max.; sapon. no. 162; 40-45 alpha monoglyceride.

Aldo® TC. [Lonza] Caprylic/capric triglyceride; CAS 538-23-8; nonionic; emulsifier for cakes, shortenings, toppings; emollient in cosmetic creams, bath oils, lotions, over-the-counter pharmaceuticals; carrier for oil-soluble antibiotics; lt. yel. clear liq., bland odor; HLB 1.0; acid no. 1 max.; iodine no. 1 max.; sapon. no. 330-360; pH 4.5 (5%); 100% conc.

Aldo® TS. [Lonza] Glyceryl tristearate; CAS 555-43-1; EINECS 209-097-6; nonionic; component of lipsticks, deodorant sticks, gel prods.; binder in household gelled air fresheners and sticks; wh. flakes or beads; m.p. 53 C min.; HLB 2.0; acid no. 4 max.

Aldosperse® L L-20. [Lonza] Sorbitan laurate and polysorbate 20; emulsifier, visc. modifier for cosmetics (shampoos, hair conditioners); emulsifier and binder for textile syn. fiber finishes, acetate tow processing; emulsifier in household waxes, polishes, cleaning formulations; amber liq.; visc. 1500 SUS (100 F); acid no. 3.2-5.7; sapon. no. 108-120; hyd. no. 225-260.

Aldosperse® ML-23. [Lonza] PEG-23 glyceryl laurate; CAS 37324-85-9; nonionic; emulsifier, solubilizer, suspending and dispersing agent used in cosmetics (hair and skin care prods.), textiles (syn. fiber finish oil formulations), household waxes, polish, cleaning formulations; yel. clear liq.; sol. in ethanol, veg. oil; sp.gr. 1.09; visc. 250 cts; HLB 17; acid no. 3 max.; iodine no. < 2; sapon. no. 42-50; hyd. no. 82-97; pH 5 (5%).

Aldosperse® MS-20. [Lonza] PEG-20 glyceryl stearate; CAS 51158-08-8; nonionic; emulsifier, solubilizer, suspending and dispersing agent used in personal care prods., food industry, textiles; wh. soft solid; sol. in ethanol; disp. in water; HLB 13 ± 1; m.p. 32–38 C; acid no. 2; sapon. no. 65–75; hyd. no. 73.

Aldosperse® O-20 FG. [Lonza] 80% Glyceryl stearate, 20% polysorbate 80; nonionic; emulsifier, solubilizer for frozen desserts, cosmetic, pharmaceutical, and industrial applics.; bead; HLB 5.0; 100% conc.

ALE-56. [Union Carbide] Amino bispropyl dimethicone.

Alfalfa Herb Extract HS 2967 G. [Grau Aromatics] Propylene glycol, alfalfa extract; botanical extract.

Alfol® 16. [Vista] Cetyl alcohol; CAS 36653-82-4; EINECS 253-149-0; detergent intermediate; emollient used in cosmetics; plastics additive; wh. waxy solid; typ. fatty alcohol odor; sol. in alcohol, acetone, ether; water-insol.; dens. 6.77; sp.gr. 0.813; visc. 6.77; m.p. 117 C; b.p. 604 C; 98.9% act.

Alfol® 18. [Vista] Stearyl alcohol; CAS 112-92-5; EINECS 204-017-6; surfactant intermediate; emollient used in cosmetics; plastics additive; wh. waxy solid; typ. fatty alcohol odor; sol. in alcohol, acetone, ether; water-insol.; dens. 6.71; sp.gr. 0.8075; visc. 13.5; m.p. 135 C; b.p. 640 C; 98.7% act.

Alfol® 22+. [Vista] C22 and higher linear alcohols; biodeg. detergent intermediate; lubricant, defoamer; emollient; used in fuel oil; waxes and polishers used in paper pulp defoamers; wh. solid; sol. in alcohol, acetone, ether; water-insol.; 100% conc.

Alfol® 610. [Vista] C6-C10 linear primary alcohol; intermediate for plasticizers, biodeg. surfactants for household, industrial cleaning and personal care prods.; colorless liq.; mild, sweet odor; sol. in alcohol, ether, benzene, insol. in water; dens. 6.92; sp.gr. 0.829; visc. 11.0; m.p. –8 C; b.p. 350 C; 99% act.

Alfol® 610 ADE. [Vista] C6, C8, C10 alcohol blend; chemical intermediate; also for lube oil additives, plasticizers, and surfactant feedstocks for household, industrial, and per-

sonal care cleaners; clear colorless liq.; m.w. 140; 100% conc.

Alfol® 610 AFC. [Vista] C6-C10 linear primary alcohol; biodeg. detergent intermediate for household, industrial and personal care prods.; plasticizer intermediate; liq.; 100% conc.

Alfol® 810. [Vista] C8–C10 linear primary alcohol; intermediate for plasticizers and biodeg. surfactants for household, industrial, and personal care products; colorless liquid; mild, sweet odor; sol. in alcohol, ether, benzene; dens. 6.93; sp.gr. 0.831; visc. 8.9; m.p. 7 C; b.p. 400 C; 99% act.

Alfol® 1012 HA. [Vista] C10-C12 linear primary alcohol; as lubricants in polymer processing, metal rolling and forming, emollients/lubricants for cosmetics, defoamers; intermediate for surfactants for cosmetic, household, and industrial use, esters for additives for plastics, rubber, metalworking, lubricants, and quaternaries for germicides and fabric softeners; colorless clear liq.; m.w. 164; sp.gr. 0.834; visc. 10.4 cSt (100 F); m.p. 35-40 F; b.p. 425-525 F; iodine no. 0.04; sapon. no. 0.1; hyd. no. 343; flash pt. (PM) 237 F; 99.8% conc.

Alfol® 1014 CDC. [Vista] C10-C14 linear primary alcohol; as lubricants in polymer processing, metal rolling and forming, emollients/lubricants for cosmetics, defoamers; intermediate for surfactants for cosmetic, household, and industrial use, esters for additives for plastics, rubber, metalworking, lubricants, and quaternaries for germicides and fabric softeners; colorless clear liq.; m.w. 186; sp.gr. 0.836; visc. 12.5 cSt (100 F); m.p. 41-45 F; b.p. 450-545 F; iodine no. 0.07; sapon. no. 0.1; hyd. no. 302; flash pt. (PM) 250 F; 99% conc.

Alfol® 1214. [Vista] C12–C14 linear primary alcohol; biodeg. lubricants in polymer processing, metal rolling and forming, emollients/lubricants for cosmetics, defoamers; intermediate for surfactants for cosmetic, household, and industrial use, esters for additives for plastics, rubber, metalworking, lubricants, and quaternaries for germicides and fabric softeners; colorless clear liq.; sweet, typ. fatty alcohol odor; sol. in alcohol, acetone, ether; water-insol.; m.w. 198; sp.gr. 0.838; dens. 7.0; visc. 14.3 cSt (100 F); m.p. 70-75 F; b.p. 518-575 F; iodine no. 0.05; sapon. no. 0.1; hyd. no. 284; flash pt. (PM) 265 F; 99.5% act.

Alfol® 1214 GC. [Vista] C12-C14 linear primary alcohol; biodeg. lubricants in polymer processing, metal rolling and forming, emollients/lubricants for cosmetics, defoamers; intermediate for surfactants for cosmetic, household, and industrial use, esters for additives for plastics, rubber, metalworking, lubricants, and quaternaries for germicides and fabric softeners; colorless clear liq.; m.w. 195; sp.gr. 0.838; visc. 14.3 cSt (100 F); m.p. 70-75 F; b.p. 518-575 F; iodine no. 0.05; sapon. no. 0.18; hyd. no. 287; flash pt. (PM) 265 F; 99% act.

Alfol® 1216. [Vista] C12–C16 linear alcohols; CAS 68855-56-1; lubricants in polymer processing, metal rolling and forming, emollients and lubricants for cosmetics, defoamers; intermediate for surfactants for cosmetic, household, and industrial applications, esters for additives for plastics, rubber, metalworking, lubricants, and quaternaries for germicides and fabric softeners; colorless clear liq., sweet, typ. fatty alcohol odor; sol. in alcohol, acetone, ether; water-insol.; m.w. 203; sp.gr. 0.84; dens. 7.0; visc. 14.5 cSt (100 F); m.p. 63-70 F; b.p. 514-592 F; iodine no. 0.1; sapon. no. 0.5; hyd. no. 276; flash pt. (PM) 265 F; 99% act.

Alfol® 1216 CO. [Vista] C12-C14 linear primary alcohol; lubricants in polymer processing, metal rolling and forming, emollients/lubricants for cosmetics, defoamers; intermediate for surfactants for cosmetic, household, and industrial use, esters for additives for plastics, rubber, metalworking, lubricants, and quaternaries for germicides and fabric softeners; colorless clear liq.; m.w. 198; sp.gr. 0.84; visc. 14.5 cSt (100 F); m.p. 63-70 F; b.p. 529-590 F; iodine no. 0.08; sapon. no. 0.18; hyd. no. 284; flash pt. (PM) 265 F; 99.7% act.

Alfol® 1218 DCBA. [Vista] C12–C18 linear primary alcohol; lubricants in polymer processing, metal rolling and forming, emollients/lubricants for cosmetics, defoamers; intermediate for surfactants for cosmetic, household, and industrial use, esters for additives for plastics, rubber, metalworking, lubricants, and quaternaries for germicides and fabric softeners; colorless clear liq.; m.w. 214; sp.gr. 0.84; visc. 15.0 cSt (100 F); m.p. 68-73 F; b.p. 525-660 F; iodine no. 0.11; sapon. no. 0.18; hyd. no. 262; flash pt. (PM) 275 F; 99.6% act.

Alfol® 1412. [Vista] C12-C14 linear primary alcohol; lubricants in polymer processing, metal rolling and forming, emollients/lubricants for cosmetics, defoamers; intermediate for surfactants for cosmetic, household, and industrial use, esters for additives for plastics, rubber, metalworking, lubricants, and quaternaries for germicides and fabric softeners; wh. solid; m.w. 205; sp.gr. 0.839; visc. 14.4 cSt (100 F); m.p. 72-75 F; b.p. 525-585 F; iodine no. 0.1; sapon. no. < 1; hyd. no. 274; flash pt. (PM) 270 F; 99.7% act.

Alfol® 1416 GC. [Vista] C14-16 linear primary alcohol; as lubricants in polymer processing, metal rolling and forming, emollients/lubricants for cosmetics, defoamers; intermediate for surfactants for cosmetic, household, and industrial use, esters for additives for plastics, rubber, metalworking, lubricants, and quaternaries for germicides and fabric softeners; wh. solid; m.w. 222; sp.gr. 0.822 (100/100 F); visc. 11.5 cSt (100 F); m.p. 95-99 F; b.p. 582-638 F; iodine no. < 0.04; sapon. no. < 1; hyd. no. 253; flash pt. (PM) 305 F; 99.8% conc.

Alfol® 1418 DDB. [Vista] C14, C16, C18 alcohol blend; as lubricants in polymer processing, metal rolling and forming, emollients/lubricants for cosmetics, defoamers; intermediate for surfactants for cosmetic, household, and industrial use, esters for additives for plastics, rubber, metalworking, lubricants, and quaternaries for germicides and fabric softeners; wh. solid; m.w. 243; sp.gr. 0.819 (110/110 F); visc. 14.6 cSt (110 F); m.p. 97-102 F; b.p. 598-659 F; iodine no. 0.6; sapon. no. 0.5; hyd. no. 231; flash pt. (PM) 290 F; 99.9% act.

Alfol® 1418 GBA. [Vista] C14-C18 linear primary alcohol; as lubricants in polymer processing, metal rolling and forming, emollients/lubricants for cosmetics, defoamers; intermediate for surfactants for cosmetic, household, and industrial use, esters for additives for plastics, rubber, metalworking, lubricants, and quaternaries for germicides and fabric softeners; wh. solid; m.w. 227; sp.gr. 0.835 (100/100 F); m.p. 97-102 F; b.p. 598-660 F; iodine no. < 0.7; sapon. no. < 1; hyd. no. 247; flash pt. (PM) 305 F; 99.8% conc.

Alfol® 1618. [Vista] C16–C18 linear primary alcohol; biodeg. lubricants in polymer processing, metal rolling and forming, emollients/lubricants for cosmetics, defoamers; intermediate for surfactants for cosmetic, household, and industrial use, esters for additives for plastics, rubber, metalworking, lubricants, and quaternaries for germicides and fabric softeners; wh. waxy solid; typ. fatty alcohol odor; sol. in water, alcohol, chloroform, ether, benzene, glacial acetic acid; sp.gr. 0.840 (60/60 F); dens. 6.81; visc. 15 cSt (122 F); m.p. 110-120 F; b.p. 628-662 F; iodine no. 0.15; sapon. no. 0.07; hyd. no. 219; flash pt. (PM) 325 F; 99.6% act.

Alfol® 1618 CG. [Vista] C16-C18 linear primary alcohol; biodeg. lubricants in polymer processing, metal rolling and forming, emollients/lubricants for cosmetics, defoam-

ers; intermediate for surfactants for cosmetic, household, and industrial use, esters for additives for plastics, rubber, metalworking, lubricants, and quaternaries for germicides and fabric softeners; wh. solid; m.w. 266; sp.gr. 0.820 (120/120 F); visc. 13.7 cSt (140 F); m.p. 110-120 F; b.p. 630-670 F; iodine no. 0.15; sapon. no. 0.07; hyd. no. 211; flash pt. (PM) 340 F; 99.6% act.

Alfol® 1618 GC. [Vista] C16-18 linear primary alcohol; as lubricants in polymer processing, metal rolling and forming, emollients/lubricants for cosmetics, defoamers; intermediate for surfactants for cosmetic, household, and industrial use, esters for additives for plastics, rubber, metalworking, lubricants, and quaternaries for germicides and fabric softeners; wh. solid; m.w. 263; sp.gr. 0.820 (140/140 F); m.p. 110-120 F; b.p. 630-670 F; iodine no. 0.8; sapon. no. 0.5; hyd. no. 213; flash pt. (PM) 325 F; 99.8% conc.

Alfonic® 1012-2.5. [Vista] C10-12 pareth-2.5; nonionic; biodeg. surfactant and emulsifier for household laundry detergents, shampoos, industrial/institutional cleaners, hard surf. cleaners, personal care prods. (creams, lotions, lipsticks, ointments, and makeup), transportation cleaners; foaming agent for wallboard, sheetrock; solvent degreaser; APHA 5 clear liquid; sol. in hydrocarbons; sparingly soluble in water; m.w. 274; sp.gr. 0.918; visc. 13 cSt (100 F); m.p. 23-30 F; HLB 8; hyd. no. 203; pour pt. 23 F; flash pt. (PM) 285 F; pH 6.8 (1% aq.); formerly Alfonic 1012-40.

Alfonic® 1214-GC-2. [Vista] C12-14 pareth-1.9; biodeg. surfactant, emulsifier for household laundry detergents, shampoos, industrial/institutional cleaners, hard surf. cleaners, personal care prods. (creams, lotions, lipsticks, ointments, makeup), transportation cleaners; foaming agent for wallboard, sheetrock; solv. degreaser; APHA 10 clear liq.; sol. in hydrocarbons; sparingly sol. in water; m.w. 284; sp.gr. 0.900; visc. 14.6 cSt (104 F); m.p. 45-51 F; HLB 6; hyd. no. 201; pour pt. 45 F; cloud pt. 56 F (1% aq.); flash pt. (PM) 280 F; pH 6.9 (1% aq.); formerly Alfonic 1214-GC-30.

Alfonic® 1216-1.5 [Vista] C12-16 pareth-1.3; CAS 68551-12-2; nonionic; biodeg. surfactant, emulsifier for household laundry detergents, shampoos, industrial/institutional cleaners, hard surf. cleaners, personal care prods. (creams, lotions, lipsticks, ointments, makeup), transportation cleaners; foaming agent for wallboard, sheetrock; solv. degreaser; APHA 10 clear liq.; sol. in hydrocarbons; sparingly sol. in water; m.w. 258; sp.gr. 0.869; visc. 17 cSt (100 F); m.p. 37-40 F; HLB 4.4; hyd. no. 222; pour pt. 39 F; cloud pt. 41 F (1% aq.); flash pt. (PM) 260 F; pH 6.7 (1% aq.); 100% conc.; formerly Alfonic 1216-22.

Alfonic® 1216-CO-2. [Vista] C12-16 pareth-1.9; nonionic; biodeg. surfactant, emulsifier for household laundry detergents, shampoos, industrial/institutional cleaners, hard surf. cleaners, personal care prods. (creams, lotions, lipsticks, ointments, makeup), transportation cleaners; foaming agent for wallboard, sheetrock; solv. degreaser; APHA 10 clear liq.; sol. in hydrocarbons; sparingly sol. in water; m.w. 280; sp.gr. 0.902; visc. 15 cSt (100 F); m.p. 45-51 F; HLB 6.0; hyd. no. 200; pour pt. 45 F; flash pt. (PM) 297 F; pH 7.2 (1% aq.); 100% conc.; formerly Alfonic 1216-30.

Alfonic® 1412-3. [Vista] C14-12 pareth-3.1; CAS 68439-50-9; nonionic; biodeg. surfactant, emulsifier for household laundry detergents, shampoos, industrial/institutional cleaners, hard surf. cleaners, personal care prods. (creams, lotions, lipsticks, ointments, makeup), transportation cleaners; foaming agent for wallboard, sheetrock; solv. degreaser; APHA 10 clear liq.; sol. in hydrocarbons; sparingly sol. in water; m.w. 341; sp.gr. 0.918; visc. 20 cSt (100 F); m.p. 46-56 F; HLB 8.0; hyd. no. 170; pour pt. 46

F; cloud pt. 54 F (1% aq.); flash pt. (PM) 320 F; pH 6.8 (1% aq.); 100% act.; formerly Alfonic 1412-40.

Alginic Acid FCC. [Meer] Alginic acid; CAS 9005-32-7; EINECS 232-680-1; tablet binder for pharmaceutical and health food industries; conforms to FCC; wh. to off-wh. free-flowing powd., ≥ 95% thru 80 mesh; visc. 5-50 cps (1%); pH 1.5-3.5 (1%); usage level: 0.4-1.0%.

Algisium. [Exsymol] Sodium mannuronate methylsilanol.

Algisium-C. [Exsymol; Biosil Tech.] Methylsilanol mannuronate; provides cutaneous hydration, lipolytic action, skin regeneration and maintenance, for cosmetic and health prods., milks, emulsions, creams, lotions, anti-aging formulations; pale yel. sl. opalescent liq., odorless; misc. with water; insol. in alcohols, glycols, hexane; sp.gr. 1.0; b.p. 100 C; pH 5.5; usage level: 4-6%; toxicology: nontoxic.

Algon DS 6000. [Auschem SpA] PEG-150 distearate; CAS 9005-08-7; personal care surfactant.

Algon LA 40. [Auschem SpA] PEG-4 laurate; CAS 9004-81-3; nonionic; emulsifier for cosmetic and pharmaceutical preps.; liq.; HLB 12.2; 100% conc.

Algon LA 80. [Auschem SpA] PEG-8 laurate; CAS 9004-81-3; nonionic; emulsifier for cosmetic and pharmaceutical preps.; liq.; HLB 13.0; 100% conc.

Algon OL 60. [Auschem SpA] PEG-6 oleate; CAS 9004-96-0; nonionic; emulsifier for cosmetic and pharmaceutical preps.; liq.; HLB 13.0; 100% conc.

Algon OL 70. [Auschem SpA] PEG-7 oleate; CAS 9004-96-0; nonionic; emulsifier for cosmetic and pharmaceutical preps.; liq.; HLB 10.4; 100% conc.

Algon OL 90. [Auschem SpA] PEG-9 oleate; CAS 9004-96-0; personal care surfactant.

Algon ST 50. [Auschem SpA] PEG-5 stearate; CAS 9004-99-3; nonionic; emulsifier for cosmetic and pharmaceutical preps.; paste; HLB 9.0; 100% conc.

Algon ST 80. [Auschem SpA] PEG-8 stearate; CAS 9004-99-3; nonionic; emulsifier for cosmetic and pharmaceutical preps.; paste/solid; HLB 11.1; 100% conc.

Algon ST 100. [Auschem SpA] PEG-10 stearate; CAS 9004-99-3; nonionic; emulsifier for cosmetic and pharmaceutical preps.; solid; HLB 11.5; 100% conc.

Algon ST 200. [Auschem SpA] PEG-20 stearate; CAS 9004-99-3; nonionic; emulsifier for cosmetic and pharmaceutical preps.; solid; HLB 14.0; 100% conc.

Algon ST 400. [Auschem SpA] PEG-40 stearate; CAS 9004-99-3; nonionic; emulsifier for cosmetic and pharmaceutical preps.; flakes; HLB 16.9; 100% conc.

Algon ST 500. [Auschem SpA] PEG-50 stearate; CAS 9004-99-3; nonionic; emulsifier for cosmetic and pharmaceutical preps.; flakes; HLB 17.9; 100% conc.

Algon ST 1000. [Auschem SpA] PEG-100 stearate; CAS 9004-99-3; nonionic; emulsifier for cosmetic and pharmaceutical preps.; flakes; HLB 18.8; 100% conc.

Alkamide® 327. [Rhone-Poulenc Surf. & Spec.] Lauramide DEA; CAS 120-40-1; EINECS 204-393-1; nonionic; foam and visc. modifier for personal care prods.; clear yel. liq.

Alkamide® 1195. [Rhone-Poulenc Surf. & Spec.] Lauramide DEA; CAS 120-40-1; EINECS 204-393-1; nonionic; superfatting agent and thickener for toiletries; clear liq.

Alkamide® 2204. [Rhone-Poulenc Surf. & Spec.] 2:1 Cocamide DEA; CAS 61791-31-9; EINECS 263-163-9; nonionic-anionic; detergent, rust inhibitor; base for hand soap, floor cleaners, all-purpose cleaners, wax strippers; amber visc. liq.; low odor; water sol.; 100% act.

Alkamide® 2204A. [Rhone-Poulenc Surf. & Spec.] 2:1 Fatty acid alkanolamide; anionic/nonionic; detergent; more readily disp. in aq. systems than Alkamide 2204; liq.; 100% conc.

Alkamide® C-5. [Rhone-Poulenc Surf. & Spec.] PEG-5 cocamide; CAS 61791-08-0; nonionic; thickener, foam

stabilizer, and emulsifier for formulated detergents and cosmetics; tan paste; sol. in aromatic solv., perchloroethylene; disp. in water; pH 10.0-11.5 (5% DW); formerly Alkamidox C-5.

Alkamide® C-212. [Rhone-Poulenc Surf. & Spec.] Cocamide MEA (1:1); CAS 68140-00-1; EINECS 268-770-2; nonionic; thickener, foam builder and stabilizer for soap or syn. based washing powds., shampoos, liq. soaps, facial cleansers, bath gels, and bubble baths; cream-colored flakes; 100% act.; 95% amide.; formerly Cyclomide C-212.

Alkamide® CDE. [Rhone-Poulenc Surf. & Spec.] Cocamide DEA; CAS 68603-42-9; EINECS 263-163-9; nonionic; detergent, emulsifier, stabilizer, thickener, foam stabilizer for personal care and detergent prods.; lt. amber liq.; low odor; sol. in detergent systems, aromatic and chlorinated aliphatic solvent, petroleum solvent, mineral oils; water-dispersible; sp.gr. 1.04; dens. 1.0 g/ml; pH 8-11 (1% DW); 90% act.

Alkamide® CDM. [Rhone-Poulenc Surf. & Spec.] Cocamide DEA.; CAS 68603-42-9; EINECS 263-163-9; nonionic; emulsifier, thickener, foam stabilizer for liq. shampoos, bubble baths, liq. detergents; liq.; 100% conc.

Alkamide® CDO. [Rhone-Poulenc Surf. & Spec.] Cocamide DEA; CAS 68603-42-9; EINECS 263-163-9; nonionic; detergent, emulsifier, foam stabilizer, thickener for personal care and detergent prods.; lt. amber liq.; low odor; sol. in aromatic and chlorinated aliphatic solv., petrol. solv.; min. oils, water; sp.gr. 1.04; dens. 1.0 g/ml; pH 8-11 (1% DW); 82% act.

Alkamide® CL63. [Rhone-Poulenc Surf. & Spec.] Cocamide DEA; CAS 61791-31-9; EINECS 263-163-9; nonionic; detergent, thickener, emulsifier, foam stabilizer in toiletry and cleaning preparations; amber clear to cloudy liq.; sol. in detergent systems, aromatic and chlorinated aliphatic solv., petrol. solv., min. oils; water-disp.; sp.gr. 1.03-1.05; dens. 1.0 g/ml; pH 8-11 (1% DW); 92% act.

Alkamide® CME. [Rhone-Poulenc Surf. & Spec.] Cocamide MEA; CAS 68140-00-1; EINECS 268-770-2; nonionic; detergent, foam boosters, visc. builder, opacifier for liq. and powd. detergents, shampoos; wh. waxy solid; sol. in detergent systems, various solv., min. oils; m.p. 56 C; 95% act.

Alkamide® DC-212. [Rhone-Poulenc Surf. & Spec.] Cocamide DEA (2:1) and diethanolamine; CAS 68603-42-9; nonionic; visc. booster, foaming agent, emulsifier, dispersant, detergent used in cosmetic and laundry prods.; amber liq.; 100% act.; formerly Cyclomide DC-212.

Alkamide® DC-212/S. [Rhone-Poulenc Surf. & Spec.] Cocamide DEA (1:1); CAS 68603-42-9; EINECS 263-163-9; nonionic; emulsifier, thickener, foam stabilizer and visc. booster with low cloud pt.; for liq. soaps, shampoos, bath gels, bubble baths, facial cleansers, liq. detergents; liq.; 100% act.; 85% amide.; formerly Cyclomide DC-212/S.

Alkamide® DC-212/SE. [Rhone-Poulenc Surf. & Spec.] 1:1 Cocamide DEA; CAS 68603-42-9; EINECS 263-163-9; nonionic; detergent, foam stabilizer, thickener, foam booster in shampoos and detergent formulations; liq.; 100% act.; 95% amide.; formerly Cyclomide DC-212/SE.

Alkamide® DIN-100. [Rhone-Poulenc Surf. & Spec.] Lauric/ linoleic diethanolamide; nonionic; thickener, foam stabilizer for toiletries, cosmetics, and detergents; liq.; 100% conc.

Alkamide® DIN-295/S. [Rhone-Poulenc Surf. & Spec.] Linoleamide DEA (1:1); CAS 68425-47-8; nonionic; foam booster, emulsifier, visc. builder, thickener for shampoos, industrial cleaners; conditioning to hair; liq.; 100% conc.; formerly Cyclomide DIN295/S.

Alkamide® DL-203/S. [Rhone-Poulenc Surf. & Spec.] 1:1 Lauramide DEA; CAS 120-40-1; EINECS 204-393-1; nonionic; foam stabilizer, visc. and detergency booster for cosmetic prods. (shampoos, liq. soaps, facial cleansers, bath gels, bubble baths); superfatting agent; lubricant for metalworking fluids; off-wh. cryst. solid; sol. in oil and water; pour pt. 60 C; 95% act.; formerly Cyclomide DL-203/S.

Alkamide® DL-207/S. [Rhone-Poulenc Surf. & Spec.] 1:1 Lauramide DEA; CAS 120-40-1; EINECS 204-393-1; nonionic; foam booster/stabilizer, visc. builder, wetting agent, superfatting agent for shampoos, liq. soaps, facial cleansers, bath and toiletries; off-wh. liq., wh. paste; 100% act.; 95% amide.; formerly Cyclomide DL-207/S.

Alkamide® DO-280. [Rhone-Poulenc Surf. & Spec.] 2:1 Oleamide DEA and diethanolamine; CAS 93-83-4; nonionic; emulsifier for sol. oils; corrosive inhibitor; liq.; 100% conc.; formerly Cyclomide DO-280.

Alkamide® DO-280/S. [Rhone-Poulenc Surf. & Spec.] 1:1 Oleamide DEA; CAS 93-83-4; EINECS 202-281-7; nonionic; thickening and superfatting agent, emulsifier, for lotion shampoos; liq.; 100% act.; 85% amide.; formerly Cyclomide DO-280/S.

Alkamide® DS-280/S. [Rhone-Poulenc Surf. & Spec.] Stearamide DEA (1:1); CAS 93-82-3; EINECS 202-280-1; nonionic; visc. builder, thickener, foam booster, dispersant for nonionic and cationic systems, shampoos, facial cleansers, bath preps., industrial cleaners; emulsifier, corrosion inhibitor, lubricant for metalworking fluids; conditioner for hair and skin care prods.; liq.; sol. in oil and water; dens. 8.33 lb/gal; pour pt. 36 C; flash pt. > 200 C; 95% conc.; formerly Cyclomide DS-280/S.

Alkamide® HTDE. [Rhone-Poulenc Surf. & Spec.] Stearamide DEA; CAS 93-82-3; EINECS 202-280-1; nonionic; detergent, thickener, visc. builder, emulsifier for kerosene, veg. and min. oil, microcryst. wax; cream-colored waxy solid; low odor; sol. in min. spirits, aromatic solvs., perchloroethylene; water-disp.; m.p. 50–55 C; pH 8–11 (1%); 90% act.

Alkamide® KD. [Rhone-Poulenc Surf. & Spec.] Cocamide DEA (1:1); CAS 68603-42-9; EINECS 263-163-9; nonionic; foam booster/stabilizer and visc. builder for shampoos, liq. soaps, facial cleansers, bath gels, and bubble baths; visc. builder, foam booster/stabilizer for industrial, institutional and household cleaners; pale yel. liq.; 100% act.; 95% amide.; formerly Cyclomide KD.

Alkamide® L7DE. [Rhone-Poulenc Surf. & Spec.] Lauric-myristic DEA (1:1); nonionic; detergent, foam booster/stabilizer, superfatting and thickening agent for toiletry and cleaning formulations; fortifier for perfumes in soaps; wh. paste, liq. > 25 C; low odor; sol. in min. spirits, aromatic solv., perchloroethylene; water-disp.; sp.gr. 1.03–1.05; m.p. 34 C; pH 8–11 (1% DW); 92% act.

Alkamide® L9DE. [Rhone-Poulenc Surf. & Spec.] Lauramide DEA, high purity; CAS 120-40-1; EINECS 204-393-1; nonionic; detergent, emulsifier, foam stabilizer and booster, thickener for toiletry and cleaning applics., industrial and household detergents; wh. waxy solid, liq. > 25 C; low odor; sol. in aromatic and chlorinated solvs., min. oils; sp.gr. 1.04; f.p. 25 C; m.p. 51 C; 92% act.

Alkamide® LE. [Rhone-Poulenc Surf. & Spec.] 1:1 Lauramide DEA; CAS 120-40-1; EINECS 204-393-1; nonionic; visc. booster, foam stabilizer in shampoo; liq.; 100% conc.; formerly Cyclomide LE.

Alkamide® S-280. [Rhone-Poulenc Surf. & Spec.] Stearamide MEA (1:1); CAS 111-57-9; EINECS 203-883-2; nonionic; viscosifier for industrial cleaners; skin protectant in toilet bars, creams, lotions, pastes; off-wh. flakes; 100% act.; 95% amide.; formerly Cyclomide S-280.

Alkamide® SDO. [Rhone-Poulenc Surf. & Spec.] Soyamide DEA; CAS 68425-47-8; EINECS 270-355-6; nonionic; foam stabilizer, visc. builder, and superfatting agent for toiletries, cutting and sol. oils, textiles, household and industrial cleaners, corrosion inhibitor; amber visc. liq.; low odor; sol. in min. oil and spirits, perchloroethylene; water-disp.; sp.gr. 1.04; dens. 1.0 g/ml; pH 8–11 (1%); 100% conc.

Alkamuls® 400-DO. [Rhone-Poulenc Surf. & Spec.] PEG-8 dioleate; CAS 9005-07-6; nonionic; emulsifier, solubilizer, lubricant, wetting agent for cosmetic, textile, metalworking, and agric. uses; clear, amber liq.; sol. in min. spirits and oil, aromatic solv, perchloroethylene; water-disp.; sp.gr. 0.97–0.99; dens. 8.163 lb/gal; HLB 7.2; sapon. no. 105–115; 100% act.

Alkamuls® 400-MO. [Rhone-Poulenc Surf. & Spec.] PEG-9 oleate; CAS 9004-96-0; nonionic; emulsifier for fats, wetting agent, dispersant, lubricant used in dairy industry, cosmetic, metalworking, and industrial applics.; amber clear liquid; sol. in min. oil; disp. in water; sp.gr. 1.01–1.03; dens. 8.497 lb/gal; HLB 11.0; flash pt. > 200 C; 100% act.

Alkamuls® 600-DO. [Rhone-Poulenc Surf. & Spec.] PEG-12 dioleate; CAS 9005-07-6; nonionic; dispersant, emulsifier for o/w emulsions; for cosmetic, metalworking, and industrial use; amber liq.; sol. in min. spirits, aromatic solvs., perchloroethylene; disp. in min. oil; sp.gr. 1.01–1.03; dens. 8.497 lb/gal; HLB 10.0; sapon. no. 99–104; flash pt. > 200 C; 100% act.

Alkamuls® B. [Rhone-Poulenc Surf. & Spec.] PEG-33 castor oil; CAS 61791-12-6; nonionic; emulsifier, dispersant for textiles, metallurgy, metal degreasing, personal care prods.; dye leveler, fabric softener; liq.; HLB 11.5; 96% conc.; formerly Rhodiasurf B.

Alkamuls® BR. [Rhone-Poulenc Surf. & Spec.] PEG-33 castor oil; CAS 61791-12-6; nonionic; emulsifier, dispersant for textiles, metallurgy, metal degreasing, personal care prods.; dye leveler, fabric softener; visc. liq.; 96% conc.; formerly Rhodiasurf BR.

Alkamuls® CO-15. [Rhone-Poulenc Surf. & Spec.] PEG-15 castor oil; CAS 61791-12-6; nonionic; emulsifier, dispersant, detergent, wetting agent, defoamer, antistat; liq.; 100% conc.; formerly Alkasurf® CO-15.

Alkamuls® EGDS. [Rhone-Poulenc Surf. & Spec.] Glycol distearate pure; CAS 627-83-8; EINECS 211-014-3; thickener, opacifier, pearlizing agent used in shampoos and cosmetic lotions; wh. flakes; m.p. 61 C; sapon. no. 195.; formerly Cyclochem® EGDS.

Alkamuls® EGMS. [Rhone-Poulenc Surf. & Spec.] Glycol stearate; CAS 111-60-4; EINECS 203-886-9; nonionic; detergent, emulsifier for liq. soaps, bar soaps, creams and lotions, facial cleansers, bath preps., toiletries; 100% conc.

Alkamuls® EGMS/C. [Rhone-Poulenc Surf. & Spec.] Ethylene glycol monostearate; CAS 111-60-4; EINECS 203-886-9; nonionic; visc. booster, opacifying and pearlescing agent for liq. cosmetic and detergent compds.; wh. flakes; insol. in water; m.p. 56 C; HLB 2.9; sapon. no. 174–184.; formerly Cyclochem EGMS.

Alkamuls® EL-620. [Rhone-Poulenc Surf. & Spec.] PEG-30 castor oil; CAS 61791-12-6; nonionic; detergent, emulsifier, wetting agent, pigment dispersant, antistat, lubricant, solubilizer for industrial/household cleaners, cosmetics, pharmaceuticals, metalworking fluids, leather, pesticides, herbicides, paper industries; FDA, EPA compliance; lt. brn. clear liq.; sol. in water, acetone, CCl_4, alcohols, veg. oil, ethers, toluene, xylene; sp.gr. 1.04–1.05; dens. 8.705 lb/gal; visc. 600–1000 cps; HLB 12.0; cloud pt. 42 C (1% aq.); flash pt. 291–295 C; surf. tens. 41 dynes/; 100% conc.; formerly Emulphor® EL-620.

Alkamuls® EL-620L. [Rhone-Poulenc Surf. & Spec.] PEG-30 castor oil; CAS 61791-12-6; nonionic; emulsifier, dispersant, softener, rewetting agent, lubricant, emulsion stabilizer, dyeing assistant, antistat, and solubilizer for textiles, wet-strength papers, fat liquoring, emulsion paints, oleoresinous binders, glass-reinforced plastics, PU foams, perfumes, cosmetics; low dioxane; EPA compliance; liq.; HLB 12.0; 10% act.; formerly Emulphor® EL-620L.

Alkamuls® EL-630. [Rhone-Poulenc Surf. & Spec.] PEG-36 castor oil; CAS 61791-12-6; personal care surfactant.

Alkamuls® EL-719. [Rhone-Poulenc Surf. & Spec.] PEG-40 castor oil; CAS 61791-12-6; nonionic; emulsifier, wetting agent for industrial/household cleaners; dispersant for pigments; for pesticides, paper, leather, plastics, paint, textile and cosmetics industries; emulsifier for vitamins and drugs; FDA, EPA compliance; liq.; sol. in water, acetone, CCl$_4$, alcohols, veg. oil, ether, toluene, xylene; sp.gr. 1.06-1.07; dens. 8.9-9.0 lb/gal; visc. 500-800 cps; HLB 13.6; cloud pt. 80 C (1% aq.); flash pt. 275-279 C; surf. tens. 38 dynes/cm (0.1%); 96% act.; formerly Emulphor® EL-719.

Alkamuls® GMS/C. [Rhone-Poulenc Surf. & Spec.] Glyceryl stearate; CAS 31566-31-1; nonionic; emulsifier, wetting agent for cosmetic, agric., textile industries; coupler used to bind waxes together; emollient and thickener in cosmetic creams; flake; water-disp.; m.p. 58-63 C; HLB 3.4; 100% conc.; formerly Cyclochem GMS, Dermalcare® GMS.

Alkamuls® L-9. [Rhone-Poulenc Surf. & Spec.] PEG-9 laurate; CAS 9004-81-3; EINECS 203-359-3; nonionic; emulsifier, coemulsifier for cosmetic and toiletry preps.; defoamer, leveling agent for latex paints; dispersant for dyes and pigments; yel. liq. to paste; sol. in aromatic solv., perchloroethylene; disp. in water; dens. 1.03 g/ml; HLB 12.8; sapon. no. 91-101; 100% conc.; formerly Alkasurf® L-9.

Alkamuls® LVL. [Rhone-Poulenc Surf. & Spec.] Lauryl lactate; CAS 6283-92-7; EINECS 228-504-8; personal care emollient.

Alkamuls® MM/M. [Rhone-Poulenc Surf. & Spec.] Myristyl myristate; CAS 3234-85-3; EINECS 221-787-9; emollient, moisturizer, lubricant, and conditioner for hair and skin care prods.; visc. builders and gelling/stiffening agents for makeup and deodorant applics.; off-wh. flake; m.p. 37-39 C; sapon. no. 130; formerly Dermalcare® MM/M, Cyclochem MM/M.

Alkamuls® MST. [Rhone-Poulenc Surf. & Spec.] Myristyl stearate; CAS 17661-50-6; EINECS 241-640-2; emollient.

Alkamuls® PE/400. [Rhone-Poulenc Surf. & Spec.] PEG 400 laurate; CAS 9004-81-3; nonionic; wetting agent for emulsion paints; PVC visc. depressant; grease improver in cosmetics; liq.; 100% conc.; formerly Soprophor PE/400.

Alkamuls® PEG 300 DS. [Rhone-Poulenc Surf. & Spec.] PEG-6 distearate; CAS 9005-08-7; emulsifier.

Alkamuls® PEG 400 DS. [Rhone-Poulenc Surf. & Spec.] PEG-8 distearate; CAS 9005-08-7; personal care surfactant.

Alkamuls® PEG 600 DS. [Rhone-Poulenc Surf. & Spec.] PEG-12 distearate; CAS 9005-08-7; personal care surfactant.

Alkamuls® PETS. [Rhone-Poulenc Surf. & Spec.] Pentaerythrityl tetrastearate; CAS 115-83-3; EINECS 204-110-1; lubricant wax providing high heat stability in lubricants; emulsifier for nat. waxes in cosmetics.

Alkamuls® PSML-20. [Rhone-Poulenc Surf. & Spec.] Polysorbate 20; CAS 9005-64-5; nonionic; emulsifier, solubilizer, antistat, visc. modifier, lubricant for textiles, cosmetics, pharmaceuticals; yel. liq.; sol. water, aromatic solvs.; dens. 1.1 g/ml; HLB 16.7; sapon. no. 40-50; 97% act.

Alkamuls® PSMO-5. [Rhone-Poulenc Surf. & Spec.] Polysorbate 81; CAS 9005-65-6; nonionic; emulsifier, solubilizer, antistat, lubricant for paint, food, cosmetic, insecticides, herbicides, fungicides, textiles, cutting oils; amber liq. to paste; sp.gr. 1.0 g/ml; dens. 8.330 lb/gal; HLB 10; sapon. no. 96-104; flash pt. > 200 C; 100% act.

Alkamuls® PSMO-20. [Rhone-Poulenc Surf. & Spec.] Polysorbate 80; CAS 9005-65-6; nonionic; emulsifier, wetting agent for cosmetic, food, agric. applics.; coemulsifier for aliphatic alcohols, petrol. oils, fats, solvs., waxes; yel. liq.; water-sol.; HLB 15; 97% act.

Alkamuls® PSMS-20. [Rhone-Poulenc Surf. & Spec.] Polysorbate 60; CAS 9005-67-8; nonionic; wetting agent, emulsifier for cosmetic and food applics., textiles, paper coatings; fiber-to-metal lubricant for fibers and yarns; yel. visc. liq., gel on standing; typ. odor; water disp.; dens. 1.1 g/ml; HLB 14.9; sapon. no. 45-55; 97% act.

Alkamuls® PSTO-20. [Rhone-Poulenc Surf. & Spec.] Polysorbate 85; CAS 9005-70-3; nonionic; emulsifier for cosmetic and food applics.; textile and leather lubricant; amber liq.; typ. odor; water disp.; dens. 1.0 g/ml; HLB 11; sapon. no. 80-95; 97% act.

Alkamuls® S-6. [Rhone-Poulenc Surf. & Spec.] PEG-6 stearate; CAS 9004-99-3; nonionic; coemulsifier, softener, lubricant for textile processing; emulsifier for cosmetic, pharmaceutical and food applics.; wax; 99% conc.; formerly Rhodiasurf S-6.

Alkamuls® SDG. [Rhone-Poulenc Surf. & Spec.] PEG-2 stearate; CAS 106-11-6; EINECS 203-363-5; nonionic; emollient, moisturizer, lubricant for skin and hair care systems; solid; m.p. 43-47 C; 100% conc.; formerly Dermalcare SDG.

Alkamuls® SEG. [Rhone-Poulenc Surf. & Spec.] Ethylene glycol monostearate; CAS 111-60-4; EINECS 203-886-9; nonionic; opacifier and pearling agent for shampoos, creams, liq. hand soaps, liq. detergents; emulsion stabilizer, visc. builder; flake; m.p. 55-60 C; 100% conc.; formerly Cyclochem® SEG.

Alkamuls® SML. [Rhone-Poulenc Surf. & Spec.] Sorbitan laurate; CAS 1338-39-2; nonionic; emulsifier for oils and fats in cosmetic, metalworking and industrial oil prods.; corrosion inhibitor; antistat for PVC; amber liq.; typ. odor; disp. in water; moderately sol. most alcohols, veg. and min. oils; sp.gr. 1.05 (60 F); dens. 8.330 lb/gal; HLB 8.6; sapon. no. 160-170; hyd. no. 320-350; flash pt. > 200 C; 100% act.

Alkamuls® SMO. [Rhone-Poulenc Surf. & Spec.] Sorbitan oleate; CAS 1338-43-8; EINECS 215-665-4; nonionic; emulsifier, coupling agent, wetting agent for medicants; petrol. oils, fats, and waxes in the industrial, textile, metalworking, and cosmetic industries; textile and leather lubricant and softener; corrosion inhibitor; amber liq.; sol. in most veg., min. oils, aromatic solv., perchloroethylene; insol. in water; sp.gr. 1.0; dens. 8.330 lb/gal; HLB 4.3; sapon. no. 145-160; hyd. no. 193-210; flash pt. > 200 C; 100% act.

Alkamuls® SMS. [Rhone-Poulenc Surf. & Spec.] Sorbitan stearate; CAS 1338-41-6; EINECS 215-664-9; nonionic; emulsifier and coupling agent; used to prepare silicone defoamer emulsions for industrial applics., paraffin wax emulsions for processing paper coatings; textile process lubricant; internal PVC film lubricant; cosmetics; foods; cream flakes; sol. (10%) in aromatic solv., perchloroethylene; dens. 1.0 g/ml; HLB 4.7; sapon. no 147-157; hyd. no. 235-260; 98.5% act.

Alkamuls® SS. [Rhone-Poulenc Surf. & Spec.] Stearyl stearate; CAS 2778-96-3; EINECS 220-476-5; emollient, moisturizer, lubricant, and conditioner for hair and skin care prods.; visc. builders and gelling/stiffening agents for makeup and deodorant applics.; off-wh. flake; water-insol.; m.p. 53-55 C; sapon. no. 110; formerly Cyclochem® SS, Dermalcare® SS.

Alkamuls® ST-40. [Rhone-Poulenc Surf. & Spec.] PEG-40 stearate; CAS 9004-99-3; emulsifier.

Alkamuls® T-20. [Rhone-Poulenc Surf. & Spec.] Polysorbate 20; CAS 9005-64-5; nonionic; emulsifier, solubilizer, antistat and lubricant for textile industry; solubilizer for essential oils; raw material for no-tears shampoo; liq.; 100% conc.; formerly Soprofor T/20.

Alkamuls® T-60. [Rhone-Poulenc Surf. & Spec.] PEG-20 sorbitan stearate; CAS 9005-67-8; nonionic; emulsifier, solubilizer, antistat and lubricant for textile industry; solubilizer for essential oils; raw material for no-tears shampoo; paste; 100% conc.; formerly Soprofor T/60.

Alkamuls® T-65. [Rhone-Poulenc Surf. & Spec.] Sorbitan tristearate, ethoxylated; nonionic; emulsifier, solubilizer, antistat and lubricant for textile industry; solubilizer for essential oils; raw material for no-tears shampoo; solid; 100% conc.; formerly Soprofor T/65.

Alkamuls® T-85. [Rhone-Poulenc Surf. & Spec.] PEG-20 sorbitan trioleate; CAS 9005-70-3; nonionic; emulsifier, solubilizer, antistat and lubricant for textile industry; solubilizer for essential oils; raw material for no-tears shampoo; liq.; 100% conc.; formerly Soprofor T/85.

Alkamuls® VR/50. [Rhone-Poulenc Surf. & Spec.] PEG-200 glyceryl stearate; nonionic; thickener for no-tears shampoo; visc. control; liq.; 50% conc.; formerly Soprofor VR/50.

Alkanet LS. [Alban Muller] Sunflower seed oil, alkanet extract; botanical extract.

Alkanolamine 144. [Dow] Triethanolamine; CAS 102-71-6; EINECS 203-049-8; used in surfactants, cosmetics/toiletries, metalworking fluids, textile chemicals, gas conditioning chemicals, agric. intermediates, and cement grinding aids; sp.gr. 1.1205; dens. 9.35 lb/gal; visc. 600.7 cps; f.p. 21 C; b.p. 340 C (760 mm Hg); flash pt. (COC) 350 F; fire pt. 420 F; ref. index 1.4839.

Alkanolamine 244. [Dow] Triethanolamine; CAS 102-71-6; EINECS 203-049-8; used in surfactants, cosmetics/toiletries, metalworking fluids, textile chemicals, gas conditioning chemicals, agric. intermediates, and cement grinding aids; sp.gr. 1.1205; dens. 9.35 lb/gal; visc. 600.7 cps; f.p. 21 C; b.p. 340 C (760 mm Hg); flash pt. (COC) 350 F; fire pt. 420 F; ref. index 1.4839.

Alkanolamine 244 Low Freeze Grade. [Dow] Triethanolamine; CAS 102-71-6; EINECS 203-049-8; used in surfactants, cosmetics/toiletries, metalworking fluids, textile chemicals, gas conditioning chemicals, agric. intermediates, and cement grinding aids; sp.gr. 1.1205; dens. 9.35 lb/gal; visc. 600.7 cps; f.p. 21 C; b.p. 340 C (760 mm Hg); flash pt. (COC) 350 F; fire pt. 420 F; ref. index 1.4839.

Alkaquat® DMB-451-50, DMB-451-80. [Rhone-Poulenc Surf. & Spec.] Benzalkonium chloride; CAS 61789-71-7; cationic; wetting agent, emulsifier, biocide, disinfectant for use in beverage industry, dairy industry, food processing, water treatment, paper industry, pest control, preservatives, antidandruff rinses, general disinfection and sanitization for hospitals, laundries; pale-yel. liq.; sol. in water, ethanol, acetone, aliphatic solv.; sp.gr. 0.96; surf. tens. 33 dynes/cm (1%); 50 and 80% act.

Alkasil® NE 58-50. [Rhone-Poulenc Surf. & Spec.] Silicone polyalkoxylate block copolymer; nonionic; nonhydrolyzable surfactant; intermediate for prod. of rigid PU foams; also used in cosmetics, toiletries, textiles, coatings, and as release agent; colorless to lt. amber liq.; 100% act.

Alkasil® NEP 73-70. [Rhone-Poulenc Surf. & Spec.] Silicone polyalkoxylate block copolymer; nonionic; nonhydrolyzable surfactant; intermediate for prod. of rigid PU foams; also used in cosmetics, toiletries, textiles, coat-

ings, and as release agent; lower visc. and f.p. than 58-50 for improved handling and convenience; colorless to lt. amber liq.; 100% act.

Alkasil® NEPCA 250-185. [Rhone-Poulenc Surf. & Spec.] Dimethicone copolyol.

Alkasurf® NP-1. [Rhone-Poulenc Surf. & Spec.] Nonoxynol-1; EINECS 248-762-5; nonionic; emulsifier and dispersing agent for petroleum oils; coemulsifier and retardant in hair care formulations; defoamer; liq.; sol. in min. oil and spirits, aromatic solv, perchloroethylene; insol. in water; dens. 0.99; HLB 4.6; pH 5-8 (5% DW); 99.0% min. act.

Alkasurf® NP-4. [Rhone-Poulenc Surf. & Spec.] Nonoxynol-4; CAS 9016-45-9; nonionic; emulsifier, detergent, dispersant, intermediate, stabilizer; plasticizer, antistat for plastics, surfactants, household, industrial, and cosmetic use, fat liquoring, cutting and sol. oils; lt. liq.; low odor; water insol.; sp.gr. 1.02; HLB 9; 100% act.

Alkasurf® NP-6. [Rhone-Poulenc Surf. & Spec.] Nonoxynol-6; CAS 9016-45-9; nonionic; emulsifier, coemulsifier, oil-sol. dispersant; used for household and industrial cleaners; intermediate; plasticizer and antistat for plastics; emulsifier for min. oils; insecticides, fungicides, herbicides; fat liquoring; making of cutting and sol. oils; dispersing waxes, pigments, resins; printing; preparation of emulsified paint; lt. liq.; low odor; oil-sol., water insol.; sp.gr. 1.04; HLB 11; 100% act.

Alkasurf® NP-8. [Rhone-Poulenc Surf. & Spec.] Nonoxynol-8; CAS 9016-45-9; nonionic; detergent, wetting agent, emulsifier; lt. liq.; low odor; water sol.; sp.gr. 1.05; HLB 12; 100% act.

Alkasurf® NP-12. [Rhone-Poulenc Surf. & Spec.] Nonoxynol-12; CAS 9016-45-9; nonionic; surfactant for household and industrial cleaning formulations; liq.; HLB 13.9; 100% conc.

Alkasurf® NP-15. [Rhone-Poulenc Surf. & Spec.] Nonoxynol-15; CAS 9016-45-9; nonionic; detergent, wetting agent, emulsifier; lt. paste; low odor; water sol.; sp.gr. 1.07; HLB 15; 100% act.

Alkasurf® NP-30, 70%. [Rhone-Poulenc Surf. & Spec.] Nonoxynol-30; CAS 9016-45-9; nonionic; solubilizer, coemulsifier for highly polar substances; liq.; HLB 17.1; 70% conc.

Alkasurf® NP-40, 70%. [Rhone-Poulenc Surf. & Spec.] Nonoxynol-40; CAS 9016-45-9; nonionic; wetting agent, stabilizer, penetrant, emulsifier, dispersant; lt. liq.; low odor; water sol.; f.p. 50-60F; HLB 17.6; 70% act.

Alkaterge®-E. [Angus] Ethyl hydroxymethyl oleyl oxazoline; CAS 68140-98-7; EINECS 268-820-3; amphoteric; detergent, emulsifier, wetting agent, antifoamer, antioxidant; used in salt, soap, paper, textiles, and metal cleaners; emulsion stabilizer; acid acceptor; pigment grinding and disp.; cosmetic and personal care raw material; Gardner 15 max. clear liq.; sol. in most org. liq., slight sol. in water; sp.gr. 0.9; dens. 7.74 lb/gal; visc. 155 cp; f.p. –31 C; flash pt. > 200 F; surf. tens. 40 dynes/cm; HLB 4.0-5.0; 70% conc.

Allantoin. [Sutton Labs] Allantoin; CAS 97-59-6; EINECS 202-592-8; skin protectant.

Allantoin. [3V-Sigma] Allantoin; CAS 97-59-6; EINECS 202-592-8; skin protectant.

Allantoin Powd. No. 1015. [Rona; E. Merck] Allantoin; CAS 97-59-6; EINECS 202-592-8; skin protectant.

All-Natural Nail Polish Remover. [Aventura Industries] Dimethyl glutarate, dimethyl succinate, dimethyl adipate, and butyrolactone.

Almolan AE. [Alma Chimica] Cetearyl alcohol, ceteareth-3, and hydrog. tallow glycerides.

Almolan HL. [Alma Chimica] Hydrog. lanolin; CAS 8031-44-5; EINECS 232-452-1; emollient.

Almolan LIS. [Alma Chimica] Cetearyl alcohol, min. oil,

lanolin alcohol, and cholesterol.

Almondermin® . [Laboratoires Sérobiologiques] Uronic mucilages extracted from marshmallow, linseed, and sweet almond; emollient, moisturizer, softener; increases skin elasticity; for facial care, body care, sun care, anti-aging, makeup, and hair care prods.; ivory colloidal syrupy liq.; disp. in water; usage level: 3-7%.

Almondermin® LS. [Laboratoires Sérobiologiques] Linseed extract, SD alcohol 39-C, althea extract, sweet almond extract, and xanthan gum.

Almond Oil. [Arista Industries; Tri-K Industries] Sweet almond oil; penetrant, softener, and moisturizer for skin and hair care prods., body oils, sun tan oils, massage oils; carrier for other materials; clear oily liq., odorless, bland taste; insol. in water; sp.gr. 0.910-0.915; congeal pt. < 18 C; iodine no. 95-105; sapon. no. 190-197; ref. index 1.463-1.466 (40 C); toxicology: nonhazardous, nonirritating; 0.05% moisture.

Aloe HS. [Alban Muller] Propylene glycol, aloe extract; botanical extract.

Aloe Con UP 10. [Florida Food Prods.] Aloe vera gel, ultra purified grade; used for cosmetic creams and lotions, shampoo rinses, therapeutic prods., clear gels, beverages; Gardner 3 max. liq.; pH 4.0-5.0; 5% solids.

Aloe Con UP 40. [Florida Food Prods.] Aloe vera gel, ultra purified grade; used for cosmetic creams and lotions, shampoo rinses, therapeutic prods., clear gels, beverages; Gardner 3 max. liq.; pH 4.0-5.0; 20% solids.

Aloe-Con UP-200. [Florida Food Prods.] Freeze-dreid aloe vera gel, ultra purified grade; used for cosmetic creams and lotions, shampoo rinses, therapeutic prods., clear gels, beverages; Gardner 3 max. powd.; pH 4.0-5.0; 100% solids.

Aloe Con WG 10. [Florida Food Prods.] Aloe vera whole gel; used for cosmetic creams and lotions, shampoo rinses, therapeutic prods., clear gels, beverages; lt. tan, typ. aloe flavor; pH 4.0-5.0; 5 ± 1% solids.

Aloe Con WG 40. [Florida Food Prods.] Aloe vera whole gel; used for cosmetic creams and lotions, shampoo rinses, therapeutic prods., clear gels, beverages; lt. tan, typ. aloe flavor; pH 4.0-5.0; 20 ± 1% solids.

Aloe Con WG 200. [Florida Food Prods.] Aloe vera whole gel; used for cosmetic creams and lotions, shampoo rinses, therapeutic prods., clear gels, beverages; lt. tan, typ. aloe flavor; pH 4.0-5.0; 100% solids.

Aloe Con WLG 10. [Florida Food Prods.] Aloe vera whole leaf gel; used for cosmetic creams and lotions, shampoo rinses, therapeutic prods., clear gels, beverages; Gardner 3 max. liq.; pH 4.0-5.0; 5% solids.

Aloe Con WLG 200. [Florida Food Prods.] Freeze-dried aloe vera whole leaf gel; used for cosmetics, clear gels, beverages, pharmaceuticals, and health supplements; sl. tan free-flowing powd.; pH 3.5-5.5 (1:199); 7% moisture.

Aloe Extract #101. [Florida Food Prods.] Aloe extract; CAS 85507-69-3; cosmetic ingred.

Aloe Extract #102. [Florida Food Prods.] Petrolatum and aloe extract.

Aloe Extract #103. [Florida Food Prods.] Lanolin oil and aloe extract.

Aloe Extract #104. [Florida Food Prods.] Isopropyl myristate and aloe extract.

Aloe Extract #105. [Florida Food Prods.] Octyl palmitate and aloe extract.

Aloe Extract HS 2386 G. [Grau Aromatics] Propylene glycol and aloe extract; botanical extract.

Aloe Extract Special. [Novarom GmbH] Propylene glycol and aloe extract; botanical extract.

Aloe Extract Vera. [Ichimaru Pharcos] Water, butylene glycol, alcohol, and aloe extract.

Aloe Flower Extract PG. [Tri-K Industries] Propylene glycol,

water, and aloe flower extract; botanical extract.

Aloe Gel Stabilized. [Terry Labs] Aloe vera gel; moisturizer, soothing/healing aid for personal care.

Aloe Phytogel 1:199 Powd. [Lipo] Aloe vera gel; moisturizer, soothing/healing aid for personal care.

Aloe-Phytogel 199 Powd. [Bio-Botanica] Aloe vera gel; moisturizer, soothing/healing aid for personal care.

Aloe Vera Aqueous Extract Conc. [Terry Labs] Aloe extract; CAS 85507-69-3; cosmetic ingred.

Aloe Vera Conc. 40 Fold. [Meer] Aloe vera gel; moisturizer, soothing/healing aid for personal care.

Aloe Vera Freeze Dried Powd. 200:1. [Aloecorp] Aloe vera gel; moisturizer, soothing/healing aid for personal care.

Aloe Vera Gel. [Provital; Centerchem] Aloe vera gel; moisturizer, soothing/healing aid for personal care.

Aloe Vera Gel 1:1. [Aloecorp] Aloe vera gel; moisturizer, soothing/healing aid for personal care.

Aloe Vera Gel 1:1. [Agro-Mar; Tri-K Industries] Aloe vera gel; ingred. for sun care prods.; colorless opaque/translucent liq., typ. vegetable odor, slicky tangy taste; completely water-sol.; sp.gr. 1.002-1.008; b.p. 210 F; pH 3.5-5.5; protect from freezing; 1.25% max. solids.

Aloe Vera Gel 1:1 Decolorized. [Aloecorp] Aloe vera gel; moisturizer, soothing/healing aid for personal care.

Aloe Vera Gel 1:1 With Pulp. [Aloecorp] Aloe vera gel; moisturizer, soothing/healing aid for personal care.

Aloe Vera Gel 1:2. [Bio-Botanica] Aloe vera gel; moisturizer, soothing/healing aid for personal care.

Aloe Vera Gel 1:2. [Lipo] Aloe vera gel; moisturizer, soothing/healing aid for personal care.

Aloe Vera Gel 1:10. [Lipo] Aloe vera gel; moisturizer, soothing/healing aid for personal care.

Aloe Vera Gel 1:10 Conc. [Bio-Botanica] Aloe vera gel; moisturizer, soothing/healing aid for personal care.

Aloe Vera Gel 1:50. [Lipo] Aloe vera gel; moisturizer, soothing/healing aid for personal care.

Aloe Vera Gel 1:50 Conc. [Bio-Botanica] Aloe vera gel; moisturizer, soothing/healing aid for personal care.

Aloe Vera Gel 1:100. [Lipo] Aloe vera gel; moisturizer, soothing/healing aid for personal care.

Aloe Vera Gel 1:100 Conc. [Bio-Botanica] Aloe vera gel; moisturizer, soothing/healing aid for personal care.

Aloe Vera Gel 10:1, 40:1. [Tri-K Industries] Aloe vera gel; ingred. for sun care prods.

Aloe Vera Gel 10:1 Decolorized. [Aloecorp] Aloe vera gel; moisturizer, soothing/healing aid for personal care.

Aloe Vera Gel Conc. 10:1. [Aloecorp] Aloe vera gel; moisturizer, soothing/healing aid for personal care.

Aloe Vera Gel Conc. 40:1. [Aloecorp] Aloe vera gel; moisturizer, soothing/healing aid for personal care.

Aloe Vera Gel Conc. 40:1 Decolorized. [Aloecorp] Aloe vera gel; moisturizer, soothing/healing aid for personal care.

Aloe Vera Gel CS. [Terry Labs] Aloe vera gel; moisturizer, soothing/healing aid for personal care.

Aloe Vera Gel CS 10. [Terry Labs] Aloe vera gel; moisturizer, soothing/healing aid for personal care.

Aloe Vera Gel CS 40. [Terry Labs] Aloe vera gel; moisturizer, soothing/healing aid for personal care.

Aloe Vera Gel DC. [Terry Labs] Aloe vera gel; moisturizer, soothing/healing aid for personal care.

Aloe Vera Gel DC 10. [Terry Labs] Aloe vera gel; moisturizer, soothing/healing aid for personal care.

Aloe Vera Gel DC 40. [Terry Labs] Aloe vera gel; moisturizer, soothing/healing aid for personal care.

Aloe Vera Gel TEX. [Novarom GmbH] Aloe vera gel; moisturizer, soothing/healing aid for personal care.

Aloe Vera Gel Filtered. [Apree] Aloe vera gel; moisturizer, soothing/healing aid for personal care.

Aloe Vera Gel Single Fold. [Meer] Aloe vera gel; moisturizer, soothing/healing aid for personal care.

Aloe Vera Gel Unfiltered. [Apree] Aloe vera gel; moisturizer, soothing/healing aid for personal care.
Aloe Vera Juice. [Warren Labs] Aloe vera gel; moisturizer, soothing/healing aid for personal care.
Aloe Vera Lipo-Quinone Extract. [Terry Labs] Aloe extract; CAS 85507-69-3; cosmetic ingred.
Aloe Vera Oil. [Agro-Mar; Tri-K Industries] Aloe vera oil; emollient leaving shiny, nongreasy film and soft feel on skin; vehicle for pigmented preps., blending agent and solubilizer for waxes and resins; ingred. for cosmetics, toiletries, sun care prods., pharmaceuticals; pale yel. clear to hazy oil, char. vegetable-type odor; sp.gr. 0.86 ± 0.04; b.p. 590 F; acid no. 3 max.; sapon. no. 10 max.; toxicology: nonhazardous.
Aloe Vera Oil 0030X. [Aloecorp] Isopropyl palmitate, isopropyl myristate, and aloe extract.
Aloe Vera Oil 0040X. [Aloecorp] Safflower oil and aloe extract.
Aloe Vera Polysaccharide#0179121B01. [Terry Labs] Aloe extract; CAS 85507-69-3; cosmetic ingred.
Aloe Vera Powd. 200:1. [Tri-K Industries] Aloe vera oil; ingred. for sun care prods.
Aloe Vera Powd. 200XXX Extract-Microfine. [Agro-Mar; Tri-K Industries] Aloe vera gel; rapidly dissolving ingred. for cosmetic, health and pharmaceutical industries; off-wh. to lt. beige powd., mild vegetable odor; 100% water-sol.; pH 3.5-6.5 (0.5% aq.); material extremely slick when wet; toxicology: dust may cause irritation on direct/prolonged contact with eyes or skin; 7.5-8.5% moisture.
Aloe Vera Powd. A 1-200. [Apree] Aloe vera gel; moisturizer, soothing/healing aid for personal care.
Aloe Vera Pulp. [Aloecorp] Aloe vera gel; moisturizer, soothing/healing aid for personal care.
Aloe Vera Spray Dried Powd. [Aloecorp] Aloe vera gel; moisturizer, soothing/healing aid for personal care.
Aloe Vera Whole Leaf Dried Powd. [Aloecorp] Aloe; CAS 8001-97-6; film-former, moisturizer for skin care prods.
Alomucin. [Aruba Aloe Balm] Aloe vera gel; moisturizer, soothing/healing aid for personal care.
Alowcape Liq. B-7. [Ichimaru Pharcos] Water, butylene glycol, and aloe extract.
Alo-X-11. [Warren Labs] Aloe vera gel; moisturizer, soothing/healing aid for personal care.
Aloxe MG-20. [Alzo] Methyl gluceth-20; CAS 68239-43-0; moisturizer.
Aloxicoll® L. [Giulini] Aluminum chlorohydrate; CAS 1327-41-9; EINECS 215-477-2; mild astringent or more powerful antiperspirant for cosmetic formulations; pale yel. liq.; pH 4.0-4.4 (15%); usage level: 25% max.; toxicology: nontoxic; does not cause dermatological irritation; 50% act.
Aloxicoll® PC. [Giulini] Aluminum chlorohydrate; CAS 1327-41-9; EINECS 215-477-2; mild astringent or more powerful antiperspirant for cosmetic aerosol formulations; wh. powd.; 99% < 75 µm controlled particle size; pH 4.0-4.4 (15%); very hygroscopic; usage level: 25% max.; toxicology: nontoxic; does not cause dermatological irritation.
Aloxicoll® PF. [Giulini] Aluminum chlorohydrate; CAS 1327-41-9; EINECS 215-477-2; mild astringent or more powerful antiperspirant for nonaerosol cosmetic formulations, such as sticks and roll-on antiperspirants; wh. fine powd.; 100% < 75 µm particle size; pH 4.0-4.4 (15%); very hygroscopic; usage level: 25% max.; toxicology: nontoxic; does not cause dermatological irritation.
Aloxicoll® PSF. [Giulini] Aluminum chlorohydrate; CAS 1327-41-9; EINECS 215-477-2; mild astringent or more powerful antiperspirant for nonaerosol cosmetic formulations, such as sticks and roll-on antiperspirants; wh. superfine powd.; 100% < 38 µm particle size; pH 4.0-4.4 (15%); very hygroscopic; usage level: 25% max.; toxicol-

ogy: nontoxic; does not cause dermatological irritation.
Alpha W 6 Pharma Grade. [Wacker-Chemie GmbH] α-Cyclodextrin; CAS 7585-39-9; EINECS 231-493-2; complex hosting guest molecules; increases the sol. and bioavailability of other substances; masks flavor, odor, or coloration; stabilizes against light, oxidation, heat, and hydrolysis; turns liqs. or volatiles into stable solid powds.; for use in pharmaceuticals, cosmetics, toiletries, foods; wh. cryst. powd.; sol. 14.5 g/100 ml in water; m.w. 972; > 98% act.
Alpha-Elastin. [Koken] Hydrolyzed elastin; CAS 100085-10-7; cosmetic protein.
Alphafil 200 USP. [Luzenac Am.] Talc USP; CAS 14807-96-6; EINECS 238-877-9; high purity soft talc with very low abrasiveness, exc. color, brightness, and softness; glidant, lubricant, film enhancer, diluent, filler, antitackifying agent for pharmaceuticals; powd.; 99% thru 200 mesh; median diam. 10 µ; tapped dens. 61 lb/ft³; pH 8 (10% slurry).
Alphafil 500 USP. [Luzenac Am.] Talc USP; CAS 14807-96-6; EINECS 238-877-9; high purity, extra-fine soft talc with very low abrasiveness, exc. color, brightness, and softness; glidant, lubricant, film enhancer, diluent, filler, antitackifying agent, opacifier, extender pigment for pharmaceuticals; powd.; 99.98% thru 400 mesh; median diam. 4 µ; tapped dens. 39 lb/ft³; pH 9 (10% slurry).
Alpha-Step® ML-40. [Stepan; Stepan Canada; Stepan Europe] Sodium methyl 2-sulfolaurate and sodium ethyl 2-sulfolaurate; anionic; biodeg. surfactant, detergent, foaming agent, hydrotrope for dishwashing liqs., fine fabric washes, hard surf. cleaners, and bubble baths; scouring, leveling, coupling and foaming agent for textiles; metalworking formulations; yel. clear liq.; pH 7.0 (1%); 38% act.
Alpinamed. [Sederma] Fresh plant extracts prepared with mixts. of water, propylene glycol, and ethanol; cosmetic ingreds.; sol. in water, ethanol.
Alpinamed Balm. [Sederma] Extract of fresh balm (Melissa officinalis) containing tannins, essential oils, flavone glycosides; astringent for cosmetic toners, sensitive skin preps., aftershave and shave preps.; ylsh.-brn. liq., aromatic citrin-like odor; sp.gr. 1.000-1.020; ref. index 1.3858-1.3878; pH 5.0-6.0; usage level: 2-10%.
Alpinamed Burdock. [Sederma] Extract of fresh burdock roots (Arcitum lappa) containing tannins, essential oils, mucilage, inulin, polyacethylene, resin; anti-dandruff agent, antibacterial, astringent for hair and scalp treatment cosmetics; yel.-brn. liq., light earthy odor; sp.gr. 1.000-1.020; ref. index 1.3875-1.3895; pH 5.5-6.5; usage level: 2-10%.
Alpinamed Chamomile. [Sederma] Extract of fresh flowering herbs (Matricaria chamomilla) containing bisabolol, flavonoids, amino acids; regenerating and calming agent for anti-inflammatory cosmetic preps. (e.g., for puffy eyes), sun and after-sun prods.; yel. liq., pleasant odor; sp.gr. 1.000-1.020; ref. index 1.3844-1.3864; pH 5.0-6.0; usage level: 2-6%.
Alpinamed Ivy. [Sederma] Extract of fresh leaves (Hedera helix) containing saponins, glycosides, and tannins; vasoconstrictor and anti-inflammatory for cosmetics, fragile capillary treatment, aftershaves, anti-blotch treatment, sensitive skin treatment, after-sun preps.; sp.gr. 1.000-1.020; ref. index 1.3904-1.3924; pH 5.0-6.0; usage level: 1-3%.
Alpinamed Sage. [Sederma] Extract of fresh leaves (Salvia officinalis) containing essential oils, tannins, saponins, and glycosides; astringent and anti-perspirant agent for toiletries, antiperspirants, and deodorants; yel.-greenish liq., aromatic odor; sp.gr. 1.000-1.015; ref. index 1.3889-1.3909; pH 5.0-6.0; usage level: 2-6%.
Alpinamed Witch Hazel. [Sederma] Extract of fresh leaves

(*Hamamelis virginiana*) containing tannins, essential oils, and gallic acid; astringent, microcirculation regulator, healing and soothing agent for after-sun treatment, aftershaves, scalp treatment, anti-blotch treatment, refresheners, tonics, and toners; yel.-brn. liq., pleasant odor; sp.gr. 1.010-1.025; ref. index 1.3893-1.3913; pH 4.0-5.0; usage level: 2-15%.

Alpine Talc USP BC 127. [Whittaker, Clark & Daniels] Talc; CAS 14807-96-6; EINECS 238-877-9; cosmetic ingred.

Alrosperse 11P Flake. [Ciba-Geigy] Fatty acid amide; nonionic; emulsifier, lubricant used in hair rinses, hand modifiers for textiles, spreading agent in paste waxes and polishes; off-wh., waxy flake.

Alscoap LE-240. [Toho Chem. Industry] TEA alkyl ether sulfate; anionic; foaming agent, base material for hair shampoos; liq.; 40% conc.

Alscoap LN-40, LN-90. [Toho Chem. Industry] Sodium lauryl sulfate; CAS 151-21-3; EINECS 205-788-1; anionic; foaming agent, detergent, base for shampoos, detergents, toothpaste; polymerization emulsifier for syn. resins and latex; liq. and powd. resp.; 40 and 90% conc.

Alscoap M-3S. [Toho Chem. Industry] Higher syn. alcohol ether sodium sulfate; foaming agent, base material for liq. shampoos; liq.

Alscoap SS-90. [Toho Chem. Industry] Alkyl ether sulfate/ coconut diethanolamide blend; anionic/nonionic; detergent for formulated hair shampoo; pale yel. paste; 90% act.

Alscoap TA-40. [Toho Chem. Industry] TEA-laureth sulfate; CAS 27028-82-6; personal care surfactant.

Altalc 200 USP. [Luzenac Am.] Talc; CAS 14807-96-6; EINECS 238-877-9; exc. color and purity; for pharmaceutical and cosmetic applics. incl. baby powds., medicated foot powds.; glidant, lubricant, pigment carrier.

Altalc 400 USP. [Luzenac Am.] Talc; CAS 14807-96-6; EINECS 238-877-9; glidant, lubricant, diluent, filler; high purity; for eye shadows, antiperspirants, as host material for surf. modifiers, carrier for citric acid for gum bases.

Altalc 500 USP. [Luzenac Am.] Talc USP/FCC; CAS 14807-96-6; EINECS 238-877-9; high purity, ultrafine talc with very consistent particle size ideal for tableting applics.; diluent, glidant, antitackifying agent, TiO_2 extender pigment; suitable for aerosols; powd.; 99.9% thru 400 mesh; median diam. 4 μ; tapped dens. 38 lb/ft^3; pH 9 (10% slurry).

Althea Liq. [Ichimaru Pharcos] Water, butylene glycol, and althea extract.

Altriform S. [Zschimmer & Schwarz] Aluminum formate; CAS 7360-53-4; EINECS 230-898-1.

Aludone®. [UCIB; Barnet Prods.] Aluminum PCA; CAS 59792-81-3; EINECS 261-931-8; astringent, antiseptic; peripheral antiperspirant; for spray or stick deodorants, shower gel, hair comb-out balm; wh.-cream powd., odorless; sol. in water; m.w. 411.3; usage level: 0.2-20%; toxicology: nontoxic; nonirritating to skin; sl. irritating to eyes.

Alumina, Activated 4082. [Whittaker, Clark & Daniels] Alumina.

Alumina, Calcined 612. [Whittaker, Clark & Daniels] Alumina.

Alumina, Tabular 635. [Whittaker, Clark & Daniels] Alumina.

Alumina Trihydrate 617. [Whittaker, Clark & Daniels] Alumina.

Aluminum Hydroxychloride 23. [Hoechst Celanese/Colorants & Surf.] Aluminum chlorohydrate; CAS 1327-41-9; EINECS 215-477-2; antiperspirant active.

Aluminum Hydroxychloride 47. [Hoechst Celanese/Colorants & Surf.] Aluminum chlorohydrate; CAS 1327-41-9; EINECS 215-477-2; antiperspirant active.

Aluminum Oxide C. [Degussa] Alumina; free-flow and anticaking agent; aids in reducing electrostatic charges of powder substances for personal care and elec. industry; wh. fluffy powd.; dens. 60 g.; surf. area 100 m^2/g; pH 4–5 (4% aq. disp.); > 99.6 Al_2O_3.

Alumystique™. [U.S. Cosmetics] Metal soap; surface treatment to enhance cosmetic prods.; exc. skin adhesion, smoother, wetter feel; good hydrohobicity; superior binding props.; mixes well with oils.

Alutrat. [Vevy] Aluminum citrate; CAS 813-92-3.

Amanduline. [Silab] Hydrolyzed sweet almond protein.

Amberlite® IRA-68. [Rohm & Haas] Acrylic; weakly basic anion exchange resin for industrial water treatment, pharmaceutical, chem. and food processing industries.

Ambroxan. [Henkel/Cospha; Henkel Canada] 8-α-12-oxido-13,14,15,16 tetra-norlabdane; fragrance raw material for personal care and detergent prods.; wh. cryst., ambergris odor; b.p. 120 C; flash pt. 161 C.

Amercell® Polymer HM-1500. [Amerchol] Nonoxynyl hydroxyethylcellulose; nonionic; nontacky thickener for aq. sol'ns., surfactant, emulsion stabilizer, film-former; substantive to skin and hair; for body lotions, moisturizers, hydroalcoholic prods., sun lotions, hair conditioners, mousses, liq. makeup; free-flowing gran. powd.; water-sol.; toxicology: LD50 (acute oral) > 5 g/kg (10% aq.); minor eye irritant; nonirritating to skin.

Amerchol® 400. [Amerchol; Amerchol Europe] Petrolatum, lanolin alcohol, cetyl alcohol, lanolin, stearone; nonionic; aux. emulsifier, emulsion stabilizer for o/w and w/o systems, incl. pigmented makeup, lipsticks, pharmaceuticals; moisturizing emollient with barrier props., lubricant for pigmented systems; lt. cream soft solid, pract. odorless; HLB 9.0; m.p. 49–50 C; acid no. 1.5; sapon. no. 8; 100% conc.

Amerchol® BL. [Amerchol; Amerchol Europe] Lanolin, min. oil, and lanolin alcohol; nonionic; absorp. base, aux. emulsifier and stabilizer for o/w systems, conditioner, w/o emollient, moisturizer for cosmetics and pharmaceuticals (lotions, night creams, pomades, ointments); yel.-amber semisolid, slight char. sterol odor; oil sol.; HLB 8.0; acid no. 2.0 max.; sapon. no. 60–70; 100% conc.

Amerchol® C. [Amerchol; Amerchol Europe] Petrolatum, lanolin, lanolin alcohol; nonionic; absorp. base, aux. emulsifier and stabilizer for o/w systems, conditioner, emollient, moisturizer for cosmetics and pharmaceuticals (creams, ointments, dermatologicals, lotions), textile finishes; pale yel.-cream soft solid, slight, char. sterol odor; oil sol.; HLB 9.5; m.p. 40–46 C; acid no. 1.0 max.; sapon. no. 10–20; 100% conc.

Amerchol® CAB. [Amerchol; Amerchol Europe] Petrolatum, lanolin alcohol; nonionic; emollient, w/o emulsifier, moisturizer, stabilizer, plasticizer for therapeutic ointments, burn preparations, dermatological prods., hypoallergenic preparations, cosmetics, pharmaceuticals, absorp. bases, bar soaps, textile finishes; pale cream soft solid, faint, char. sterol odor; oil sol.; HLB 9.0; m.p. 40–46 C; acid no. 1 max.; sapon. no. 1.0 max.; 100% conc.

Amerchol® H-9. [Amerchol; Amerchol Europe] Petrolatum, lanolin, lanolin alcohol; nonionic; emollient, w/o emulsifier, penetrant, stabilizer, absorp. base for cosmetics, pharmaceutical ointments, burn ointments, dermatologicals; plasticizer; pale yel. soft solid, slight, char. sterol odor; oil sol.; HLB 9; m.p. 55–62 C; acid no. 1 max.; sapon. no. 15–27; 100% conc.

Amerchol® L-99. [Amerchol; Amerchol Europe] Min. oil, lanolin alcohol; nonionic; absorp. base, w/o emulsifier, stabilizer, conditioner, nontacky emollient, moisturizer for creams and lotions, hair and skin preparations, dermatological specialties; lt. yel. oily liq., faint char. sterol odor; oil misc.; sp.gr. 0.855–0.875; HLB 8; acid no. 2 max.; sapon. no. 2 max.; 100% conc.

Amerchol L-101® . [Amerchol] Min. oil, lanolin alcohol; nonionic; emollient, penetrant, w/o emulsifier, moisturizer, softener, stabilizer for cosmetics, creams, makeup, hair dressing, pharmaceuticals, aerosols, baby prods., textile finishes; wetting and dispersing agent for pigmented prods.; plasticizer for hair sprays; pale yel. oily liq., faint char. sterol odor; oil sol.; sp.gr. 0.840–0.860; visc. 20–30 cps; HLB 8; acid no. 1 max.; sapon. no. 1 max.; 100% conc.

Amerchol® L-500. [Amerchol] Min. oil, lanolin alcohol, octyldodecanol; nonionic; aux. w/o emulsifier, stabilizer, emollient, moisturizer, conditioner for hair and skin prods., creams, lotions, makeup, aerosols, cleansing creams, lipstick, cold creams, pharmaceutical vehicles, baby toiletries; amber thick liq. to semisolid; oil-misc.; HLB 6; acid no. 2 max.; sapon. no. 5 max.; 100% conc.

Amerchol® RC. [Amerchol] Petrolatum, lanolin alcohol, stearyl alcohol, and stearone; lubricating base, moisturizer, aux. emulsifier, stabilizer, emollient, conditioner for creams, lotions, pigmented makeup, ointments; aids pigment disp., color definition; pale ivory soft solid, slight char. sterol odor; misc. with common oil phase ingred.; m.p. 55–64 C; HLB 9.0; acid no. 2 max.; sapon. no. 10 max.

Amerlate® LFA. [Amerchol; Amerchol Europe] Lanolin acid; CAS 68424-43-1; EINECS 270-302-7; anionic; emulsifier, stabilizer, emollient for fatty acid systems, aerosol shave creams, cream shampoos, wax systems, household prods.; pigment dispersant; increases tack and plasticity of wax films; ylsh.-tan firm, waxy solid; mild, waxy odor; m.p. 55–62 C acid no. 130–150; sapon. no. 170–190; 100% conc.

Amerlate® P. [Amerchol; Amerchol Europe] Isopropyl lanolate; CAS 63393-93-1; EINECS 264-119-1; nonionic; conditioner, penetrant, lubricant, moisturizer, emollient, w/o emulsifier, stabilizer, opacifier for cosmetics and pharmaceuticals; pigment dispersant; wetting agent and dispersant for solids; plasticizer for wax and pigment systems; yel. buttery solid, faint char. odor; HLB 9; acid no. 18 max.; sapon. no. 130–155; 100% act.

Amerlate® W. [Amerchol; Amerchol Europe] Isopropyl lanolate; CAS 63393-93-1; EINECS 264-119-1; nonionic; dispersant/wetting agent for pigments in personal care prods., pharmaceuticals; emulsifier, softener, lubricant, emollient; yel. buttery solid; faint char. odor; insol. in water; HLB 9; acid no. 18 max.; sapon. no. 135–165; hyd. no. 35–55; 100% act.

Amerlate® WFA. [Amerchol; Amerchol Europe] Lanolin acid; CAS 68424-43-1; EINECS 270-302-7; anionic; emulsifier, stabilizer for emulsions, aerosols, shampoos; stabilizer for conventional soap emulsions; wets and disperses pigments in makeups; ylsh.-tan waxy solid, mild waxy odor; misc. with warm min. oil, IPP, IPM, castor oil; m.p. 60 C; acid no. 120; sapon. no. 165; 100% conc.

Ameroxol® OE-2. [Amerchol; Amerchol Europe] Oleth-2; CAS 9004-98-2; nonionic; solubilizer, emulsifier, dispersant, stabilizer, lipophilic cosolv. for creams and lotions, shampoos, and detergents, fluid and gelled transparent emulsions, fragrance prods., and aerosols; pale straw-colored clear liq.; bland odor; sol. in min. oil, isopropyl esters, anhyd. ethanol; HLB 5.0; acid no. 0.2 max.; sapon. no. 2 max.; pH 4.5–7.0; 100% conc.

Ameroxol® OE-5. [Amerchol] Oleth-5; CAS 9004-98-2; emulsifier, stabilizer, solubilizer for cosmetics and toiletries; hazy to cloudy liq., bland odor; acid no. 1 max.; iodine no. 37-49; sapon. no. 2 max.; hyd. no. 113-128; pH 4.5-7.5 (3% aq.).

Ameroxol® OE-10. [Amerchol; Amerchol Europe] Oleth-10; CAS 9004-98-2; nonionic; emulsifier, stabilizer, solubilizer for cosmetics and toiletries; broad electrolyte and pH tolerance; wh. semisolid; bland odor; sol. in ethanol, water, hydroalcoholics, glycols; HLB 12; cloud pt. 47–55 C; acid no. 0.5 max.; sapon. no. 2 max.; pH 4.5–7.0 (10% aq.); 100% conc.

Ameroxol® OE-20. [Amerchol; Amerchol Europe] Oleth-20; CAS 9004-98-2; nonionic; emulsifier, stabilizer, solubilizer for cosmetics and toiletries; wh. waxy solid; bland odor; sol. in ethanol, water, hydroalcoholics, glycols; HLB 15; cloud pt. 87–93 C; acid no. 0.5 max.; sapon. no. 2 max.; pH 4.5–7.0 (10% aq.); 100% conc.

Amersil® DMC-20. [Amerchol] Dimethicone copolyol; nonionic; used for hair spray applics.; Gardner 1 max. clear liq.; sp.gr. 1.03-1.05; visc. 1000-1300 cSt; cloud pt. 39-45 C; pH 5.5-8.0.

Amersil® DMC-287. [Amerchol] Dimethicone copolyol; used for hair glosses, hair sprays; pract. colorless, clear liq., mild char. odor; sol. in water and alcohol; visc. 1750 cSt; cloud pt. 38 C; surf. tens. 28 mN/m (0.1%).

Amersil® DMC-357. [Amerchol] Dimethicone copolyol; used for shampoos, hair glosses, hair sprays; pract. colorless, clear liq., mild char. odor; sol. in water and alcohol; visc. 600 cSt; cloud pt. 89 C; surf. tens. 29 mN/m (0.1%).

Amersil® DMC-500. [Amerchol] Dimethicone copolyol; nonionic; used for cosmetic creams and lotions, hair glossing, hair sprays; must be emulsified; Gardner 5 max. clear liq.; visc. 100-200 cSt; pH 5.5-8.0.

Amersil® DMC-604. [Amerchol] Dimethicone copolyol; nonionic; emollient used for facial prods. for night repair; also for hair spray applics.; Gardner 2 max. clear liq.; visc. 300-800 cSt; pH 5.5-8.0.

Amersil® L-45 Grades. [Amerchol] Dimethicone; used for shampoos, skin creams and lotions, as glossing agent for hair.

Amersil® L-45/10. [Amerchol] Dimethicone; used for shampoos, skin creams and lotions, as glossing agent for hair; clear liq.; sp.gr. 0.931-0.939; visc. 9-11 cSt; acid no. 0.05 max.; flash pt. 325 F min.; ref. index 1.397-1.401.

Amersil® L-45/20. [Amerchol] Dimethicone; used for shampoos, skin creams and lotions, as glossing agent for hair; clear liq.; sp.gr. 0.946-0.954; visc. 18-22 cSt; acid no. 0.05 max.; flash pt. 400 F min.; ref. index 1.398-1.402.

Amersil® L-45/50. [Amerchol] Dimethicone; used for shampoos, skin creams and lotions, as glossing agent for hair; clear liq.; sp.gr. 0.956-0.964; visc. 47.5-52.5 cSt; acid no. 0.05 max.; flash pt. 535 F min.; ref. index 1.400-1.404.

Amersil® L-45/100. [Amerchol] Dimethicone; used for shampoos, skin creams and lotions, as glossing agent for hair; clear liq.; sp.gr. 0.962-0.970; visc. 95-105 cSt; acid no. 0.05 max.; flash pt. 575 F min.; ref. index 1.4005-1.4045.

Amersil® L-45/200. [Amerchol] Dimethicone; used for shampoos, skin creams and lotions, as glossing agent for hair; clear liq.; sp.gr. 0.964-0.972; visc. 190-210 cSt; acid no. 0.05 max.; flash pt. 575 F min.; ref. index 1.4013-1.4053.

Amersil® L-45/350. [Amerchol] Dimethicone; used for shampoos, skin creams and lotions, as glossing agent for hair; clear liq.; sp.gr. 0.965-0.973; visc. 332.5-367.5 cSt; acid no. 0.05 max.; flash pt. 575 F min.; ref. index 1.4013-1.4053.

Amersil® L-45/500. [Amerchol] Dimethicone; used for shampoos, skin creams and lotions, as glossing agent for hair; clear liq.; sp.gr. 0.967-0.975; visc. 475-525 cSt; acid no. 0.05 max.; flash pt. 575 F min.; ref. index 1.4013-1.4053.

Amersil® L-45/1000. [Amerchol] Dimethicone; used for shampoos, skin creams and lotions, as glossing agent for hair; clear liq.; sp.gr. 0.967-0.975; visc. 940-1050 cSt; acid no. 0.05 max.; flash pt. 600 F min.; ref. index 1.4013-1.4053.

Amersil® L-45/12500. [Amerchol] Dimethicone; used for shampoos, skin creams and lotions, as glossing agent for hair; clear liq.; sp.gr. 0.970-0.978; visc. 11,875-13,125 cSt; acid no. 0.05 max.; flash pt. 600 F min.; ref. index 1.4015-1.4055.

Amersil® L-45/60000. [Amerchol] Dimethicone; used for shampoos, skin creams and lotions, as glossing agent for hair; clear liq.; visc. 57,000-63,000 cSt; acid no. 0.05 max.; flash pt. 600 F min.

Amersil® ME-358. [Amerchol] Cyclomethicone and dimethicone copolyol; nonionic; emulsifier for prep. of water-in-silicone oil for personal care prods.; liq.; HLB 5.0; 100% conc.

Amersil® Simethicone EM. [Amerchol] Simethicone; antifoam for skin creams.

Amersil® VS-7158. [Amerchol] Cyclomethicone; CAS 69430-24-6; emollient for antiperspirants and deodorants; volatile silicones evaporate quickly; clear liq., low odor.

Amersil® VS-7207. [Amerchol] Cyclomethicone; CAS 69430-24-6; emollient for antiperspirants and deodorants; volatile silicones evaporate quickly; clear liq., low odor.

Amersil® VS-7349. [Amerchol] Cyclomethicone; CAS 69430-24-6; emollient for antiperspirants and deodorants; volatile silicones evaporate quickly; clear liq., low odor.

Ami Bioprotector. [Alban Muller; Tri-K Industries] Oak apple extract; soothing prod. for cosmetics field.

Amical® 48. [Angus] Diiodomethyl p-tolyl sulfone; mildewcide, fungicide for latex paints, emulsions, caulks, adhesives and sealants, and in lumber, construction, home improvement, textile, cosmetics, and automotive industries; FDA clearance for food pkg. adhesives; avail. as fine tan powd. and visc. lt. tan liq. disp.; insol. in water; sp.gr. 2.20 g/cc (powd.); m.p. 147-150 C (powd.); 95% (powd.) and 44-50% act. (liq.).

Amical® 50. [Angus] Diiodomethyl p-tolyl sulfone with color suppressant; see Amical 48; also preservative for latex paints; for color-critical applics.; tan fine powd. and visc. lt. tan liq. disp.; sol. (mg/ml): 1000 mg in dimethyl formamide, 350 mg in acetone, 263 mg in n-propyl acetate, 220 mg in tributyl phosphate, 182 mg in methyl Cellosolve, 114 mg in Carbitol acetate, 80 mg in benzene, 75 mg in Cellosolve acetate, 58 mg in dibutyl phthalate, 43 mg in toluene, 33 mg.in xylene, 0.1 mg.in water; sp.gr. 1.96 g/cc (powd.); 75% (powd.) and 37-43% act. (liq.).

Amical® Flowable. [Angus] Diiodomethyl-p-tolyl sulfone aq. suspension; CAS 20018-09-1; EINECS 243-468-3; preservative, mildewcide, algicide for polymeric systems, esp. latex paints, caulks, adhesives, leather, cosmetics; lt. gray finely divided suspension; sol. 0.1 mg/l in water; sp.gr. 1.32-1.33; dens. 11.05 lb/gal; visc. 600-1000 cps; b.p. 100 C; f.p. 0 C; pH 7.0-8.5; 40% act. in water.

Amide CD 2:1. [Hysan] Cocamide DEA, diethanolamine.

Amide CMA-2. [Berol Nobel AB] PEG-2 coco MEA; thickener producing stable foam for personal care formulations; Hazen 500 max. paste; sol. in water; dens. 970 kg/m³; visc. 250 mPa·s; HLB 4.9; pH 10 (1%); surf. tens. 30 mN/m; Ross Miles foam 115 mm (initial); 100% act.

Amide RMA-2. [Berol Nobel AB] PEG-2 rapeseedamide; thickener, foaming agent for personal care formulations; Hazen 500 max. paste; sol. in water; dens. ≈ 950 kg/m³; visc. ≈ 125 mPa·s; HLB 4.1; pH 10.5 (1%); surf. tens. 32 mN/m; Ross Miles foam 20 mm (initial); 100% act.

Amidex AME. [Chemron] Acetamide MEA; CAS 142-26-7; EINECS 205-530-8; nonionic; antistat, humectant, conditioner for skin and hair prods.; water-wh. liq.; 70% conc.

Amidex CE. [Chemron] Cocamide DEA (1:1); CAS 61791-31-9; EINECS 263-163-9; nonionic; detergent, thickener, visc. builder, foam stabilizer for shampoos, cleaners, bubble baths, industrial cleaners, car shampoos, dishwashes, drycleaning detergents, waterless cleaners, solv. cleaners; yel. liq.; 100% conc.

Amidex CIPA. [Chemron] Cocamide MIPA; CAS 68333-82-4; EINECS 269-793-0; nonionic; antidefatting surfactant; for shampoos, skin cleansers, bubble baths; waxy flake; 100% conc.

Amidex CME. [Chemron] Cocamide MEA; CAS 68140-00-1; EINECS 268-770-2; nonionic; visc. builder, foam enhancer for personal care prods., soap systems, syn. powd. detergents, liq. dishwashing formulations; waxy flake; 100% conc.

Amidex CP. [Chemron] Capramide DEA (1:1); CAS 136-26-5; EINECS 205-234-9; nonionic; flash foaming detergent, wetting agent for use in pigmented personal care systems; pale yel. liq.; 100% conc.

Amidex KD. [Chemron] Cocamide DEA (1:1); CAS 61791-31-9; EINECS 263-163-9; nonionic; surfactant for ethoxy sulfate systems; yields high stable viscosities at low conc.; flash foamer, foam stabilizer; for gelled shampoos, bath gels, liq. soaps, facial cleansers; pale yel. liq.; 100% conc.

Amidex KDO. [Chemron] Cocamide DEA (1:1); CAS 61791-31-9; EINECS 263-163-9; nonionic; visc. builder, flash foamer, foam stabilizer for shampoos, bath and cleansing prods.; amber liq.; 100% conc.

Amidex KME. [Chemron] Cocamide MEA; CAS 68140-00-1; EINECS 268-770-2; nonionic; foam builder, visc. booster, stabilizer for personal care prods., syn. powd. and liq. detergent systems; waxy flake; 100% conc.

Amidex LD. [Chemron] Lauramide DEA (1:1); CAS 120-40-1; EINECS 204-393-1; nonionic; thickener, visc. builder, foam booster/stabilizer, detergent, emulsifier; for household, institutional and industrial cleaners, personal care prods.; waxy solid; 100% conc.

Amidex LD-8. [Chemron] Lauramide DEA (1:1); CAS 120-40-1; EINECS 204-393-1; nonionic; visc. builder, foam booster; remains liq. at relatively low temps.; pale yel. liq.; 80% conc.

Amidex LIPA. [Chemron] Lauramide MIPA; CAS 142-54-1; EINECS 205-541-8; nonionic; mild, low melting, fully active foam booster/stabilizer; for shampoo and detergent systems; waxy flake; 100% conc.

Amidex LMMEA. [Chemron] Lauramide MEA; CAS 142-78-9; EINECS 205-560-1; nonionic; visc. builder, foam booster; for bath prods., shampoos, skin cleansers; waxy flake; 100% conc.

Amidex LN. [Chemron] Linoleamide DEA (1:1); CAS 56863-02-6; EINECS 260-410-2; nonionic; thickener, foam builder, emulsifier, conditioner; substantive to hair; for bath and skin care prods., shampoos, conditioners; amber liq.; 100% conc.

Amidex O. [Chemron] Oleamide DEA (1:1); CAS 93-83-4; EINECS 202-281-7; nonionic; thickener, emulsifier, lubricant, conditioner; for shampoos, min. oil emulsions; compatible with hair dye systems; amber liq.; 100% conc.

Amidex PK. [Chemron] Palmkernelamide DEA (1:1); CAS 73807-15-5; nonionic; visc. builder and foamer for conditioning shampoos, mousses, styling gels; yel. liq.; 100% conc.

Amidex RC. [Chemron] Ricinoleamide DEA (1:1); CAS 40716-42-5; EINECS 255-051-3; nonionic; low foaming surfactant with wetting and softening props.; emulsifier with lubricity; for hair conditioners, shampoos, skin creams and lotions; amber liq.; 100% conc.

Amidex S. [Chemron] Soyamide DEA (1:1); CAS 68425-47-8; EINECS 270-355-6; nonionic; foamer, visc. builder, emulsifier with skin feel props.; for shower and facial cleansers, liq. soaps, bath gels; amber liq.; 100% conc.

Amidex SE. [Chemron] Stearamide DEA (1:1); CAS 93-82-

3; EINECS 202-280-1; nonionic; thickener, emulsifier for personal care prods. incl. cold wave neutralizers, veg. oil emulsions, conditioning shampoos and mousses; solid; 100% conc.

Amidex SME. [Chemron] Stearamide MEA; CAS 111-57-9; EINECS 203-883-2; nonionic; thickener, emulsifier for min. oil and veg. oil systems; for toiletry bars, creams, lotions; waxy flake; 100% conc.

Amido Betaine C. [Zohar Detergent Factory] Coconut amido alkyl betaine; amphoteric; component of nonirritating shampoos, conditioning shampoos, bubble baths; industrial foamer; liq.; 35% conc.

Amido Betaine C-45. [Zohar Detergent Factory] Coconut amido alkyl betaine; amphoteric; component of nonirritating shampoos, conditioning shampoos, bubble baths; industrial foamer; liq.; 45% conc.

Amido Betaine C Conc. [Zohar Detergent Factory] Coconut amido alkyl betaine; amphoteric; component of nonirritating shampoos, conditioning shampoos, bubble baths; industrial foamer.

Amido Betaine-L. [Zohar Detergent Factory] Lauramidopropyl betaine; EINECS 224-292-6; amphoteric; component of nonirritating shampoos and bubble baths; industrial foamer; liq.; 35% conc.

Amidox® C-2. [Stepan; Stepan Canada] PEG-3 cocamide; CAS 61791-08-0; nonionic; emulsifier, detergent, wetting agent for dishwashing detergents, shampoos, emulsions; textile wetting and leveling agent; emulsifier for fragrances and essential oils; visc. and foam enhancer for shampoos, hand soaps, bath prods.; Gardner 5 pasty liq.; sol. in ethanol, xylene; disp. in water; pH 10.0–11.5 (1% aq.); 100% act.

Amidox® C-5. [Stepan; Stepan Canada] PEG-6 cocamide; CAS 61791-08-0; nonionic; emulsifier, detergent, wetting agent for dishwashing detergents, shampoos, emulsions; textile wetting and leveling agent; emulsifier for fragrances and essential oils; visc. and foam enhancer for shampoos, hand soaps, bath prods.; Gardner 5 liq.; sol. in ethanol, xylene, water; pH 10.0–11.5 (1% aq.); 100% act.

Amidox® L-2. [Stepan; Stepan Canada] PEG-3 lauramide; CAS 26635-75-6; nonionic; emulsifier, detergent, wetting agent for dishwashing detergents, shampoos, emulsions; Gardner 3 waxy solid; pH 10.0–11.5 (1% aq.); 100% conc.

Amidox® L-5. [Stepan; Stepan Canada] PEG-5 lauramide; CAS 26635-75-6; nonionic; emulsifier, detergent, wetting agent for dishwashing detergents, shampoos, emulsions; emulsifier for fragrances and essential oils; visc. and foam enhancer for shampoos, hand soaps, bath prods.; Gardner 6 max. clear visc. liq.; sol. in water, ethanol, xylene; pH 10.0–11.5 (1% aq.); 100% conc.

Amidroxy. [Alban Muller; Tri-K Industries] Fruit extracts; provides light peeling and moisturizing chars. for cosmetics.

Amiema MA-OD. [Nihon Emulsion] Octyldodecyl N-myristoyl-N-methyl alanate; oil-phase cosmetics ingred.; pale yel. liq.; misc. with fatty acid esters and hydrocarbons; HLB 0.

Amiema MA-OL. [Nihon Emulsion] Oleyl N-myristoyl-N-methyl alanate; oil-phase cosmetics ingred.; pale yel. liq.; misc. with fatty acid esters and hydrocarbons; HLB 0.

Amifat P-30. [Ajinomoto; Ajinomoto USA] PCA glyceryl oleate; nonionic; biodeg. surfactant used as emulsifier with superfatting and antistatic props. in personal care prods.; very mild to skin and eyes; paste; HLB 7.0; 100% conc.

Amigel. [Alban Muller; Tri-K Industries] Sclerotium gum; natural gellifying agent for cosmetic field; stable at pH 3-10.

Amihope LL-11. [Ajinomoto] Lauroyl lysine; CAS 52315-75-0; EINECS 257-843-4; amphoteric; biodeg. surface modi-

fier, coemulsifier, codispersant; in cosmetics (lipsticks, foundations, creams/lotions, hair care prods.), medical, painting and other fields; filler for ink and paint; chelating agent; wh. fine powd.; insol. in almost all solvs. except strong acidic and alkaline sol'ns.; sol. in water @ pH < 1 and > 12; sp.gr. 1.2; toxicology: LD50 (oral, mice) > 5.0 g/kg; nonirritating to skin and eyes; nonsensitizing; 100% conc.

Amilon. [Ikeda] Silica, lauroyl lysine; provides smooth touch, ease of use in mfg. due to high temp. stability, and compatibility with parabens; for pressed powds., eyeshadow; wh. spherical powd., char. odor.

AMI Nail Bioregenerator. [Alban Muller; Tri-K Industries] Contains D-panthenol; nail care ingred.

Amine 2HBG. [Berol Nobel AB] Di(hydrog. tallow) amine; CAS 61788-45-2; EINECS 262-976-6; cationic; surfactant intermediate; for pour pt. depressant formulations for diesel fuel, paper chem. aux., personal care prods.; off-wh. solid; sol. in alcohols, chloroform, other hydrocarbons; m.w. 509; dens. 810 kg/m³; visc. 11 cP (70 C); set pt. 60-67 C; iodine no. 3 max.; flash pt. 220 C; toxicology: skin and severe eye irritant; 88% conc.

Amine 2M14D. [Berol Nobel AB] Dimethyl tetradecylamine; CAS 68439-70-3; cationic; surfactant intermediate; end prods. incl. quaternaries and amine oxides for detergent, disinfectant and cosmetic formulations; liq.; sol. in alcohols and chloroform; insol. in water; dens. 800 kg/m³; m.p. -7 C; iodine no. 2 max.; 96% conc.

Amine 2M16D. [Berol Nobel AB] Dimethyl hexadecyl amine; CAS 68037-93-4; cationic; surfactant intermediate; quaternized end prods. used in cosmetic formulations; liq.; sol. in alcohols, chloroform; insol. in water; dens. 800 kg/m³; m.p. 8 C; iodine no. 3 max.; 96% conc.

Amine 2M18D. [Berol Nobel AB] Dimethyl octadecyl amine; CAS 124-28-7; EINECS 204-694-8; cationic; surfactant intermediate; quaternized end prods. used in cosmetic formulations; liq.; sol. in alcohols and chloroform; insol. in water; dens. 800 kg/m³; m.p. 30 C; iodine no. 4 max.; 96% conc.

Amine 2M1214D. [Berol Nobel AB] N,N-Dimethyl dodecyl tetradecylamine; chemical intermediate; end prods. incl. quaternaries and amine oxides used in disinfectant and cosmetic applics.; sol. in alcohols, chloroform; insol. in water; dens. 800 kg/m³; m.p. -10 C; iodine no. 2 max.; 96% conc.

Amine 2M1218D. [Berol Nobel AB] N,N-Dimethyl cocamine; CAS 61788-93-0; EINECS 263-020-0; chemical intermediate; end prods. incl. quaternaries and amine oxides used in detergent and cosmetic applics.; sol. in alcohols, chloroform; insol. in water; dens. 800 kg/m³; m.p. -10 C; iodine no. 10 max.; 96% conc.

Amine 2MKKD. [Berol Nobel AB] Dimethyl coco amine; CAS 61788-93-0; EINECS 263-020-0; cationic; surfactant intermediate; quaternized end prods. used as textile auxs.; betaines for cosmetic applics.; liq.; sol. in alcohols, chloroform; insol. in water; dens. 800 kg/m³; m.p. -15 C; iodine no. 10 max.; 96% conc.

Amine 12. [Berol Nobel AB] N-Dodecylamine; CAS 2016-57-1; EINECS 204-690-6; chemical intermediate; ethoxylated end-prods. used in detergent, cosmetic, and agric. applics.; Gardner 3 max. color; sol. in alcohols, chloroform, and other hydrocarbons; pract. insol. in water; m.w. 185; dens. 800 kg/m³; visc. 4 cP (30 C); set pt. 22-23 C; iodine no. 1; amine no. 185-190; flash pt. 115 C; toxicology: skin and eye irritant; 97% primary amine.

Amine 12-98D. [Berol Nobel AB] n-Dodecylamine; CAS 2016-57-1; EINECS 204-690-6; cationic; emulsifier; chemical intermediate; ethoxylated or guanidated end-prods. used in detergent, cosmetic, and agric. formulations; APHA 80 max. solid; sol. in alcohols, chloroform, other hydrocarbons; pract. insol. in water; m.w. 185; dens. 800 kg/m³; visc. 4 cP (30 C); set pt. 22-23 C; flash pt. 115 C; toxicology: skin and eye irritant; 99% primary amine.

Amine 16D. [Berol Nobel AB] n-Hexadecylamine; CAS 143-27-1; EINECS 205-596-8; cationic; emulsifier; chemical intermediate; end prods. such as quaternary ammonium compds. used as bactericides and in shampoo formulations; Gardner 1 max. solid; sol. in alcohols, chloroform; insol. in water; dens. 800 kg/m³; m.p. 39-40 C; iodine no. 2 max.; 98% primary amine.

Amine 18-90. [Berol Nobel AB] N-Octadeylamine; CAS 124-30-1; EINECS 204-695-3; chemical intermediate; ethoxylated end-prods. used in detergent, cosmetic and agric. applics.; APHA 300 max. color; sol. in alcohols, chloroform, other hydrocarbons; pract. insol. in water; m.w. 267; dens. 810 kg/m³; visc. 4 cP (60 C); set pt. 49-56 C; flash pt. > 150 C; toxicology: skin and eye irritant; 96% primary amine.

Amine 18-90 D. [Berol Nobel AB] N-Octadeylamine; CAS 124-30-1; EINECS 204-695-3; chemical intermediate; ethoxylated end-prods. used in detergent, cosmetic and agric. applics.; APHA 80 max. color; sol. in alcohols, chloroform, other hydrocarbons; pract. insol. in water; m.w. 267; dens. 810 kg/m³; visc. 4 cP (60 C); set pt. 50-60 C; iodine no. 2 max.; flash pt. > 150 C; toxicology: skin and serious eye irritant; 98.5% primary amine.

Amine 18-95. [Berol Nobel AB] N-Octadeylamine; CAS 124-30-1; EINECS 204-695-3; chemical intermediate; ethoxylated end-prods. used in detergent, cosmetic and agric. applics.; Gardner 1 max. color; sol. in alcohols, chloroform, other hydrocarbons; pract. insol. in water; m.w. 269; dens. 810 kg/m³; visc. 4 cP (60 C); set pt. 49-56 C; iodine no. 3 max.; flash pt. > 150 C; toxicology: skin and serious eye irritant; 97% primary amine.

Amine KKD. [Berol Nobel AB] Cocamine; CAS 61788-46-3; EINECS 262-977-1; cationic; emulsifier, corrosion inhibitor; chemical intermediate producing ethoxylates and guanidated end prods. used in detergent, cosmetic, and agric. applics.; Gardner 1 max. liq.; sol. in alcohols, chloroform; insol. in water; dens. 800 kg/m³; m.p. 15-20 C; iodine no. 12 max.; 97% primary amine.

Amine M2HBG. [Berol Nobel AB] Methyl di-(hydrogenated tallow) amine; CAS 61788-63-4; EINECS 262-991-8; cationic; surfactant intermediate; paste; 96% conc.

4-Aminobenzoic Acid, Pure, No. 102. [Rona; E. Merck] PABA; pharmaceutical active.

Amino-Collagen-25, -40. [Maybrook] Collagen amino acids; CAS 9105-54-7; substantivity agent, penetrant, moisturizer for skin and hair care prods., esp. conditioners, shampoos, styling and setting prods., nutritive skin prods.; amber clear liq., char. odor; pH 6.5-7.5; 20-28% solids.

Aminodermin CLR. [Dr. Kurt Richter; Henkel/Cospha] Sulfur rich amino acid conc.; conditioner for structurally damaged and oily hair, dandruff shampoos, oily skin care prods.; wh. powd.

Aminoefaderma. [Vevy] PEG-4 proline linolenate, PEG-4 proline linoleate, propylene glycol.

Aminofoam C. [Croda Inc.; Croda Chem. Ltd.] TEA-lauroyl animal collagen amino acids; anionic; mild protein surfactant, detergent, conditioner for skin and hair care cleansing systems, shaving creams; lt. amber liq.; water-sol.; m.w. 550; usage level: 2-10%; 40% act.

Aminofoam C Potassium Salt. [Croda Chem. Ltd.] Potassium lauroyl collagen amino acids.

Aminofoam K. [Croda Inc.] TEA-lauroyl animal keratin amino acids; anionic; mild protein surfactant, foaming agent for shampoos, conditioners, facial cleansers; lt. amber liq.; water-sol.; m.w. 550; usage level: 2-10%; 40% act.

Aminofoam Soya. [Croda Chem. Ltd.] Potassium lauroyl hydrolyzed soy protein.

Amino Gluten MG. [Croda Inc.] Maize gluten amino acids, sodium chloride; conditioner for skin creams and lotions and hair conditioners; humectant for cosmetics and pharmaceuticals; amber liq.; m.w. 150; water-sol.; usage level: 0.2-3%; 15% act. in water.

Aminol A-15. [Chem-Y GmbH] Trideceth-2 carboxamide MEA; nonionic; biodeg. cosmetics surfactant, thickener, foam stabilizer; exc. dermatological props.; yel. liq., turns sl. turbid below 15 C; sp.gr. 0.95 kg/l; visc. 200 mPa·s; pH 5.5-7.5 (10%); toxicology: very sl. eye irritant at 10-15% active matter; 97% conc.

Aminol CA-2. [Finetex] Ricinoleamide DEA; CAS 40716-42-5; EINECS 255-051-3; nonionic; softening agent for textiles, low-foaming emulsifier, dispersant for dyes and oils, cosmetic emulsions; liq.; 100% conc.

Aminol CM, CM Flakes, CM-C Flakes, CM-D Flakes. [Finetex] Cocamide MEA; CAS 68140-00-1; EINECS 268-770-2; nonionic; soap additive, foam booster/stabilizer, thickener for toiletry, household prods., hair shampoos; solid, flakes; 100% conc.

Aminol COR-2C. [Finetex] Cocamide DEA and diethanolamine; nonionic; foam booster/stabilizer, thickener, emulsifier for w/o emulsions, cosmetic applics.; liq.; 100% conc.

Aminol COR-4C. [Finetex] Cocamide DEA; CAS 61791-31-9; EINECS 263-163-9; nonionic; foam booster, stabilizer, emulsifier, thickener, detergent for cosmetic applics.; liq.; 100% conc.

Aminol HCA. [Finetex] Cocamide DEA; CAS 61791-31-9; EINECS 263-163-9; nonionic; foam booster/stabilizer in shampoos and household detergents; liq.; 100% conc.

Aminol KDE. [Chem-Y GmbH] Cocamide DEA; CAS 68603-42-9; EINECS 263-163-9; nonionic; foam booster/stabilizer, superfatting agent for personal care prods.; solubilizer for perfumes, veg. oils; clear yel. liq.; sp.gr. 1.0; visc. 1200 mPa·s; cloud pt. < 7 C; pH 9.5-10.5 (1% aq.); 100% conc.

Aminol LM-30C, LM-30C Special. [Finetex] Lauramide DEA; CAS 120-40-1; EINECS 204-393-1; nonionic; foam booster/stabilizer in personal care and household prods.; liq.; 100% conc.

Aminol N. [Chem-Y GmbH] PEG-4 rapeseedamide; CAS 85536-23-8; nonionic; biodeg. cosmetics surfactant, thickener; for shower bath, foam bath, shampoo, soap gel, and other surfactant formulations; clear liq.; visc. 500 mPa·s; pH 9.0-10.5 (10% in water/ethanol 1:1); 90% conc.

Aminolan. [Fabriquimica] Fatty aminocarboxylate; cosmetic ingred.; pH 7.5-8.5 (5%); 48-55% solids.

Amino-Silk SF. [Maybrook] Silk amino acids; CAS 977077-71-6; substantive protein for elegant skin and hair preps.; penetrant, moisturizer; amber clear liq., faint char. odor; sol. in water; pH 4.5-7.5; 14-20% solids.

Aminoxid A 4080. [Goldschmidt; Goldschmidt AG] Cocamine oxide; CAS 61788-90-7; EINECS 263-016-9; nonionic; surfactant for acid and alkali-stable formulations; liq.; 30% conc.

Aminoxid WS 35. [Goldschmidt; Goldschmidt AG] Cocamidopropylamine oxide; CAS 68155-09-9; EINECS 268-938-5; nonionic; detergent, emulsifier, wetting agent, softener, foam stabilizer for detergent preparations, cosmetic and pharmaceutical emulsions; amber liq.; pH 5-7; 35% act.

Amiox. [Alban Muller] Rosemary extract; natural antioxidizing agent for cosmetics.

Ami-Pearl Conc. [Nihon Emulsion] Mixt. of acylglutamate and pearling agent; pearling agent for liq. cleaners, hair shampoos, and body shampoos; cream-colored visc. liq.

Ami-Pearl TS. [Nihon Emulsion] Mixt. of acylglutamate and pearling agent; pearling agent for liq. cleaners, hair shampoos, and body shampoos; cream-colored visc. liq.

Amisoft CA. [Ajinomoto] Cocoyl glutamic acid; biodeg. mild surfactant for facial and body cleansers, shampoo, bar soap, children's and dermatological prods.; crystal; insol. in water @ 40 C.

Amisoft CK-11. [Ajinomoto; Ajinomoto USA] Potassium cocoyl glutamate; biodeg. mild surfactant for facial and body cleansers, shampoo, bar soap, children's and dermatological prods.; powd./flake; pH 5.3 (1% , 40 C).

Amisoft CS-11. [Ajinomoto; Ajinomoto USA] Sodium cocoyl glutamate; CAS 68187-32-6; EINECS 269-087-2; anionic; biodeg., nonirritating, high foaming detergent, emollient, bacteriostat for facial and body cleansers, shampoo, bar soap, children's and dermatological prods.; powd./flake; pH 5.5 (1% , 40 C); 100% conc.

Amisoft CT-12. [Ajinomoto; Ajinomoto USA] TEA-cocoyl glutamate aq. sol'n.; CAS 68187-29-1; EINECS 269-084-6; anionic; emulsifier for cosmetics, facial and body cleansers, shampoo, bar soap, children's and dermatological prods.; nonirritating high foaming detergent, emollient, bacteriostat; biodeg.; liq.; pH 5.4 (1% , 40 C); 100% act.

Amisoft GS-11. [Ajinomoto; Ajinomoto USA] Sodium hydrog. tallow glutamate, sodium cocoyl glutamate; anionic; biodeg. emulsifier for cosmetics, facial and body cleansers, shampoo, bar soap, children's and dermatological prods.; nonirritating high foaming detergent, emollient, bacteriostat; powd./flake; pH 6.6 (1% , 40 C); 100% act.

Amisoft HA. [Ajinomoto] Hydrog. tallowoyl glutamic acid; biodeg. mild surfactant for facial and body cleansers, shampoo, bar soap, children's and dermatological prods.; crystals; insol. in water @ 40 C.

Amisoft HS-11. [Ajinomoto; Ajinomoto USA] Sodium hydrog. tallow glutamate; CAS 38517-23-6; anionic; emulsifier for cosmetics, facial and body cleansers, shampoo, bar soap, children's and dermatological prods.; nonirritating high foaming detergent, emollient, bacteriostat; biodeg.; powd./flake; pH 6.9 (1% , 40 C); 100% act.

Amisoft HS-21. [Ajinomoto] Disodium hydrog. tallow glutamate; anionic; biodeg. mild surfactant for facial and body cleansers, shampoo, bar soap, children's and dermatological prods.; powd.; pH 9.0 (1% , 40 C).

Amisoft HT-12. [Ajinomoto] TEA-hydrog. tallow glutamate; emulsifier for cosmetics; liq.; 20% act.

Amisoft LS-11. [Ajinomoto; Ajinomoto USA] Sodium lauroyl glutamate; CAS 29923-31-7; anionic; biodeg. emulsifier for cosmetics; nonirritating high foaming detergent, emollient, bacteriostat; for facial and body cleansers, shampoo, bar soap, children's and dermatological prods.; powd./flake; pH 5.3 (1% , 40 C); 100% act.

Amisoft LT-12. [Ajinomoto] TEA-lauroyl glutamate aq. sol'n.; EINECS 258-046-1; biodeg. mild surfactant, emulsifier for cosmetics, facial and body cleansers, shampoo, bar soap, children's and dermatological prods.; liq.; pH 5.2 (1% , 40 C); 30% act.

Amisoft MS-11. [Ajinomoto; Ajinomoto USA] Sodium myristoyl glutamate; EINECS 253-981-4; anionic; biodeg. nonirritating high foaming detergent, emollient, bacteriostat for facial and body cleansers, shampoo, bar soap, children's and dermatological prods.; powd./flake; pH 6.1 (1% , 40 C); 100% conc.

Amisol™ 406-N. [Lucas Meyer] Lecithin, glycerin, propylene glycol, glyceryl oleate.

Amisol™ 634. [Lucas Meyer] Cocamidopropylamine oxide and lecithin.

Amisol™ 638. [Lucas Meyer] Sodium lauryl sulfate and lecithin.

Amisol™ 688. [Lucas Meyer] Lecithin, cocamide DEA, glycerin.

Amisol™ 4135. [Lucas Meyer] Lecithin, polysorbate 20, sorbitan laurate, propylene glycol stearate, propylene glycol laurate; emulsifier, emollient, conditioning agent for cosmetics and toiletries (skin lotions, liq. and cake makeup, foundation creams, soap prods., hair and scalp preps., skin creams); stabilizes emulsions over wide pH range; Gardner 14 max. liq., almost odorless; acid no. 27 max.; 2% max. moisture.

Amisol™ HS-2. [Lucas Meyer] Sulfated castor oil, lecithin, propylene glycol, and PEG-12 oleate.

Amisol™ HS-3 US. [Lucas Meyer] Sulfated castor oil, lecithin, propylene glycol, PEG-12 oleate; wetting and dispersing agent, coemulsifier, fluidizing factor, emollient, moisturizer, conditioner for cosmetics, skin lotions, hair and scalp preps., clear shampoos, body deodorants, liq. detergents and soaps; lt. colored free-flowing translucent liq., pract. odorless; sp.gr. 1.02-1.05; pH 6.0-9.5; 55-68% moisture.

Amisol™ HS-6. [Lucas Meyer] PEG-6 laurate, lecithin, propylene glycol.

Amisol™ MS-10. [Lucas Meyer] Lecithin, polysorbate 21; emollient, fatting and softening agent imparting typical smooth feel to skin; foam stabilizer, detergency enhancer; produces emulsions of greater stability with resist. to variations in pH; for syn. detergents and soaps, shampoos, shaving creams; emulsifier and wetting agent in foods; lt. amber free-flowing liq., almost odorless; sol. in most fatty oils; readily water-disp.; usage level: 1-3%; 100% act.

Amisol™ MS-12 BA. [Lucas Meyer] Lecithin, polysorbate 20, polysorbate 60, and sorbitan laurate; emulsifier for preparing w/o emulsions for aq. food and nonfood systems; Gardner 14 max. color; disp. in water; visc. 8000 cps max.; acid no. 28 max.; 100% act.

Amisol Nail Strengthener. [Lucas Meyer] Sulfated castor oil, lecithin, propylene glycol, and PEG-12 oleate.

Amiter LGOD. [Ajinomoto; Ajinomoto USA; Nihon Emulsion] Dioctyldodecyl lauroyl glutamate; CAS 82204-94-2; EINECS 279-917-5; nonionic; oily surfactant used in personal care prods.; high affinity to skin and hair; JCID compliance; pale yel. oily liq.; HLB 0; 100% conc.

Amiter LGOD-2. [Ajinomoto; Ajinomoto USA; Nihon Emulsion] Dioctyldodeceth-2 lauroyl glutamate; nonionic; SE oil-phase base for shampoos, hair conditioners, and other hair care prods.; JCID compliance; pale yel. oily liq.; HLB 1.7; 100% conc.

Amiter LGOD-5. [Nihon Emulsion] Dioctyldodeceth-5 lauroyl glutamate; SE oil-phase base for shampoos, hair conditioners, and other hair care prods.; JCID compliance; pale yel. oil; HLB 5.

Amiter LGS-2. [Ajinomoto; Ajinomoto USA; Nihon Emulsion] Disteareth-2 lauroyl glutamate; nonionic; SE waxy material, oil-phase emulsifier, superfatting agent for cosmetic cleansing foams; JCID compliance; cream-colored wax; HLB 2; 100% conc.

Amiter LGS-5. [Ajinomoto; Ajinomoto USA; Nihon Emulsion] Disteareth-5 lauroyl glutamate; nonionic; SE waxy material; oil-phase emulsifier, emulsion stabilizer, and superfatting agent in cosmetic cleansing foams; JCID compliance; cream-colored soft wax; HLB 5.4; 100% conc.

Amiter SG-OD. [Nihon Emulsion] Di(2-octyldodecyl) N-stearoyl-L-glutamate; surfactant for cosmetic goods with high affinity to skin or hair; pale yel. oil; HLB 0.

Ammonyx® 4. [Stepan; Stepan Canada] Stearalkonium chloride; CAS 122-19-0; EINECS 204-527-9; cationic; emulsifier, conditioner, softener, emollient for cosmetics; paste; sp.gr. 0.99; flash pt. > 200 F; 18% act.

Ammonyx® 4B. [Stepan; Stepan Canada] Stearalkonium chloride; CAS 122-19-0; EINECS 204-527-9; cationic; emulsifier, conditioner, softener, emollient for cosmetics;

paste; sp.gr. 0.99; flash pt. > 200 F; 18% act.

Ammonyx® 485. [Stepan; Stepan Canada] Stearalkonium chloride; CAS 122-19-0; EINECS 204-527-9; cationic; emulsifier, conditioner, softener, emollient for cosmetics; paste; sp.gr. 0.45; flash pt. 122 F; 85% act.

Ammonyx® 4002. [Stepan; Stepan Canada] Stearalkonium chloride; CAS 122-19-0; EINECS 204-527-9; cationic; emulsifier, conditioner, softener, emollient for cosmetics; powd.; sp.gr. 0.52; flash pt. 170 F; 95% act.

Ammonyx® CA-Special. [Stepan; Stepan Canada] Stearalkonium chloride; CAS 122-19-0; EINECS 204-527-9; conditioner, softener, emollient for hair rinses, skin prods.; cationic emulsifier; paste; 22% act.

Ammonyx® CDO. [Stepan; Stepan Canada] Cocamidopropylamine oxide; CAS 68155-09-9; EINECS 268-938-5; amphoteric; wetting, foaming agent, foam stabilizer, conditioner for bubble baths, bath oils, dishwashing, hair color systems, softeners, cleansers; liq.; sp.gr. 1.02; flash pt. > 200 F; 30% act.

Ammonyx® CETAC. [Stepan; Stepan Canada] Cetrimonium chloride; CAS 112-02-7; EINECS 203-928-6; cationic; emulsifier, conditioner, softener, emollient for cosmetics; liq.; sp.gr. 0.93; flash pt. > 200 F; 26% act.

Ammonyx® CETAC-30. [Stepan; Stepan Canada] Cetrimonium chloride; CAS 112-02-7; EINECS 203-928-6; cationic; emulsifier, conditioner, softener, emollient for cosmetics; liq.; sp.gr. 0.93; 30% act.

Ammonyx® CO. [Stepan; Stepan Canada] Palmitamine oxide; CAS 7128-91-8; EINECS 230-429-0; amphoteric; conditioner, detergent, foam stabilizer, visc. builder used in cosmetic, household, and janitorial prods.; wetting agent in conc. electrolyte sol'ns.; textile lubricant, emulsifier, wetter, dye dispersant; liq.; sp.gr. 0.96; flash pt. > 200 F; 30% act.

Ammonyx® DMCD-40. [Stepan; Stepan Canada] Lauramine oxide; CAS 1643-20-5; EINECS 216-700-6; cationic; wetting, foaming agent, foam stabilizer for cosmetic, home and janitorial prods.; liq.; sp.gr. 0.91; flash pt. 86 F; 40% act.

Ammonyx® KP. [Stepan; Stepan Canada] Olealkonium chloride; CAS 37139-99-4; EINECS 253-363-4; cationic; conditioner, antistat in clear hair rinses; liq.; sp.gr. 0.98; flash pt. > 200 F; 52% min. solids.

Ammonyx® LKP. [Stepan; Stepan Canada] Olealkonium chloride; CAS 37139-99-4; EINECS 253-363-4; cationic; conditioner, antistat for clear hair rinses; extremely light colored version for use in water-wh. conditioners; lt.-colored liq.; 50% act.

Ammonyx® LO. [Stepan; Stepan Canada] Lauramine oxide; CAS 1643-20-5; EINECS 216-700-6; amphoteric; foamer/foam stabilizer, conditioner, wetting agent, visc. builder, grease emulsifier for shampoos, bath prods., fine fabric cleaners, hard surf. cleaners containing acids or bleach, dishwash, shaving creams, lotions; textile lubricant, emulsifier, dye dispersant; liq., sp.gr. 0.96; flash pt. > 200 F; 30% act.

Ammonyx® MCO. [Stepan; Stepan Canada] Myristamine oxide; CAS 3332-27-2; EINECS 222-059-3; amphoteric; foamer/foam stabilizer, conditioner, visc. builder, and wetting agent for shampoos, bubble baths, hand soaps, and conditioners; liq.; 30% conc.

Ammonyx® MO. [Stepan; Stepan Canada] Myristamine oxide; CAS 3332-27-2; EINECS 222-059-3; amphoteric; wetting and foaming agent, foam stabilizer, conditioner, wetting agent for cosmetics, home and janitorial prods.; textile lubricant, emulsifier, wetter, dye dispersant; liq.; sp.gr. 0.96; flash pt. > 200 F; 29–31% amine oxide.

Ammonyx® OAO. [Stepan; Stepan Canada] Oleamine oxide; CAS 14351-50-9; EINECS 238-311-0; amphoteric; wetting agent, foam booster/stabilizer, conditioner, visc.

builder for shampoos, bubble baths, hand soaps, conditioners; liq.; 50% act.

Ammonyx® SO. [Stepan; Stepan Canada] Stearamine oxide; CAS 2571-88-2; EINECS 219-919-5; amphoteric; conditioner, detergent, foam stabilizer, visc. builder, conditioner, emulsifier used in cosmetic, household, and janitorial prods.; wetting agent in conc. electrolyte sol'ns.; textile lubricant, emulsifier, wetter, dye dispersant; paste; sp.gr. 0.99; flash pt. > 200 F; 25% act.

Amniotic Fluid LAS. [Laboratoires Sérobiologiques] Amniotic fluid.

Amojell Petrolatum Amber, Dark, Snow White. [Amoco Lubricants] Petrolatum; EINECS 232-373-2; emollient, ointment base.

Amonyl 265 BA. [Seppic] Coco-betaine; CAS 68424-94-2; EINECS 270-329-4; amphoteric; detergent for shampoo; liq.; 30% conc.

Amonyl 380 BA. [Seppic] Cocamidopropyl betaine; amphoteric; detergent for shampoos; liq.; 30% conc.

Amonyl 440 NI. [Seppic] Cocamidopropyl betaine; ultra mild surfactant for cosmetics use; 37% conc.

Amonyl 675 SB. [Seppic] Cocamidopropylhydroxysultaine; CAS 68139-30-0; EINECS 268-761-3; nonionic; mild surfactant for shampoos; liq.; 50% act.

Amonyl BR 1244. [Seppic] Lauralkonium bromide; CAS 7281-04-1; EINECS 230-698-4; germicide; liq.

Amonyl DM. [Seppic] Quaternium-82; cationic; high active cosmetic ingred. for use in conditioning shampoos and hair rinses; liq.; 95% act.

AMP. [Angus] 2-Amino-2-methyl-1-propanol; CAS 124-68-5; EINECS 204-709-8; nonionic; emulsifier, catalyst; dispersant for pigments and latex paints; corrosion inhibitor; stabilizer; resin solubilizer; cosmetic and personal care applics.; APHA 20 solid; m.w. 89.14; sp.gr. 0.928; dens. 7.78; visc. 102 cp (30 C); m.p. 30 C; b.p. 165 C; flash pt. 172 F; 100% act.

AMPD. [Angus] 2-Amino-2-methyl-1,3-propanediol; CAS 115-69-5; EINECS 204-100-7; pigment dispersant, neutralizing amine, corrosion inhibitor, acid-salt catalyst, pH buffer, chemical and pharmaceutical intermediate; solubilizer or emulsifier system component in personal care prods.; raw material in hypoallergenic prods.; m.w. 105.1; sol. 250 g/100 ml water; m.p. 109 C; b.p. 151 C; pH 10.8 (0.1M aq. sol'n.); toxicology: LD50 (oral, mice) 3.5 g/kg; irritating to eyes, skin on prolonged contact; 99% conc.

Amphisol®. [Givaudan-Roure; Bernel] DEA-cetyl phosphate; CAS 61693-41-2; anionic; skin-friendly emulsifier and emulsion stabilizer for cosmetic/pharmaceutical creams/lotions; FDA, EEC, and Japanese compliances; wh. to off-wh. powd., pract. odorless to weakly fatty odor; sol. in water, oil; m.w. 427.6; acid no. 230-255; pH 6.0-7.5 (1% aq. disp.); usage level: 1-3%.

Amphisol® K. [Givaudan-Roure; Bernel] Potassium cetyl phosphate; CAS 19035-79-1; EINECS 242-769-1; anionic; emulsifier, stabilizer for cosmetic/pharmaceutical creams and lotions; stable over wide pH range; FDA, EEC, and Japanese compliances; colorless solid; sol. in water, oil; usage level: 1-3%.

Ampho B11-34. [Karlshamns] Complex coco betaine; CAS 68424-94-2; EINECS 270-329-4; amphoteric; detergent, wetting and foaming agent, solubilizer for organics and inorganics; biodeg.; liq.; 30% conc.

Ampho T-35. [Karlshamns] Complex tallow ammonium carboxylate; amphoteric; detergent, wetting and foaming agent, solubilizer for organics and inorganics; biodeg.; liq.; 60% conc.

Amphocerin® E. [Henkel KGaA/Cospha] Cetearyl alcohol, lanolin alcohol, and hydrog. peanut oil; w/o emulsifier and consistency factor for cosmetics; sl. yel. waxy substance; solid. pt. 40-44 C; acid no. 1 max.; iodine no. 45-55; sapon.

no. 110-120; hyd. no. 75-85.

Amphocerin® K. [Henkel/Cospha; Henkel KGaA/Cospha] Cetearyl alcohol, lanolin, hydrog. peanut oil, veg. oil, min. oil, petrolatum; cream base for mfg. of lt. and smooth creams and ointments of the w/o type; translucent wax; acid no. < 1; iodine no. 35 max.; sapon. no. 70.

Ampholak 7CX. [Berol Nobel AB] Cocoamphopolycarboxyglycinate; CAS 97659-53-5; EINECS 307-458-3; amphoteric; med. to high foaming surfactant for detergent applics., nonirritating toiletries, liq. soap, washing-up liqs.; clear liq.; misc. with water; dens. 1150 kg/m³; visc. 100 mPa·s max.; pour pt. -20 C; pH 9.0±0.5 (20%); surf. tens. 38 mN/m (0.1%); 39-41% conc.

Ampholak 7CX/C. [Berol Nobel AB] Cocoamphopolycarboxyglycinate; CAS 97659-53-5; EINECS 307-458-3; amphoteric; substantive cosmetic ingred.; improves skin feel, detoxifies anionics, produces rich lather; mild to skin and eyes; biostatic activity; used for shampoos, liq. soaps, body care prods.; clear liq.; sol. in water; poorly sol. in org. solvs.; dens. 1170 kg/m³; visc. 100 mPa·s max.; pour pt. -22 C; pH 8.5-9.5; surf. tens. 38 mN/m (0.1%); Ross-Miles foam 150 mm (initial, 50 C, 0.05%); 39-41% solids.

Ampholak 7TX. [Berol Nobel AB] Tallowamphopolycarboxyglycinate; CAS 97659-53-5; EINECS 307-458-3; amphoteric; med. foaming detergent used in detergent applics., nonirritating toiletries, cosmetics, shampoos, liq. soaps; reduces irritation of anionics; softening agent; clear liq.; misc. with water; dens. 1150 kg/m³; visc. 100 mPa·s max.; pour pt. -15 C; pH 9.0±0.5 (20%); surf. tens. 44 mN/m (0.1%); 39-41% conc.

Ampholak 7TX/C. [Berol Nobel AB] Tallowamphopolycarboxyglycinate; CAS 97659-53-5; EINECS 307-458-3; amphoteric; used in detergents, shampoos, liq. soaps, body care prods.; conditioner in shampoos; softener; biostatic activity; reduces irritation of anionics; readily biodeg.; clear liq.; sol. in water, poorly sol. in org. solvs.; dens. 1150 kg/m³; visc. 100 mPa·s max.; pour pt. -15 C; pH 8.5-9.5; surf. tens. 44 mN/m (0.1%); Ross-Miles foam 160 mm (initial, 0.05% , 50 C); 39-41% solids.

Ampholak 7TX-SD 55. [Berol Nobel AB] Tallowamphopolycarboxyglycinate; CAS 97659-53-5; EINECS 307-458-3; detergent, softener for laundry and hard surf. cleaners; also for cosmetics; wh. free-flowing fine powd.; sol. in water; dens. 340 kg/m³; pH 101.5±1.0 (20%); surf. tens. 39 mN/m (0.1%); 93% solids.

Ampholak 7TX-T. [Berol Nobel AB] Tallowamphopolycarboxyglycinate; CAS 97659-53-5; EINECS 307-458-3; amphoteric; detergent, softener for detergent applics., cosmetics, shampoos, liq. soaps; reduces irritation of anionics; conditioner in shampoos; clear liq.; misc. with water; dens. 1130 kg/m³; visc. 100 mPa·s max.; pour pt. -15 C; pH 9.0±0.5 (20%); surf. tens. 39 mN/m (0.1%); 39-41% conc.

Ampholak 7TY. [Berol Nobel AB] Tallowamphopolycarboxypropionic acid; CAS 97488-62-5; EINECS 306-998-7; amphoteric; low foaming surfactant for alkaline cleaners, toiletries; clear liq.; misc. with water; dens. 1038 kg/m³; visc. 100 mPa·s; pour pt. 4 C; pH 4.5±1.0 (20%); surf. tens. 45 mN/m (0.1%); 30-32% conc.

Ampholak BCA-30. [Berol Nobel AB] Cocamidopropyl betaine; CAS 70851-07-9; amphoteric; foam booster, visc. regulator, mild surfactant, thickener for liq. soaps, washing-up liqs., toiletries; 34-36% conc.

Ampholak MDX-1. [Berol Nobel AB] Blend of amphoteric surfactants; amphoteric; designed for mild washing up liqs.; reduces irritation to skin from anionics; bacteriostatic props.; preservative for formulations; clear liq.; misc. with water; dens. 1100 kg/m³; visc. 100 mPa·s max.; pour pt. -5 C; pH 9.0 ± 1 (20%); surf. tens. 38 mN/m (0.1%); 39 ±

1% solids.

Ampholak MSX-1. [Berol Nobel AB] Blend of amphoteric surfactants; amphoteric; mild foaming agent for personal care prods. (shampoos, foam baths, liq. soaps, body care prods.); reduces irritation to eyes and skin of anionics; bacteriostatic props.; preservative for formulations; readily biodeg.; clear liq.; sol. in water; poorly sol. in org. solvs.; dens. 1110 kg/m³; visc. 100 mPa·s max.; pour pt. -5 C; pH 9.0 ± 1; surf. tens. 38 mN/m (0.1%); Ross-Miles foam 175 mm (initial, 0.05% , 50 C); 39 ± 1% solids.

Ampholak MSX-2. [Berol Nobel AB] Blend; amphoteric; mild foaming agent for personal care prods.; produces rich lather, provides gentle cleaning in shampoos, liq. soaps, body care prods.; clear liq.; sol. in water; poorly sol. in org. solvs.; dens. 1130 kg/m³; visc. 250 mPa·s max.; pour pt. -20 C; pH 8.0-10.0; surf. tens. 35 mN/m (0.1%); Ross-Miles foam 180 mm (initial, 50 C, 0.05%); 38-41% solids.

Ampholak XCO-30. [Berol Nobel AB] Disodium cocoamphodiacetate; CAS 68650-39-5; EINECS 272-043-5; amphoteric; med. foaming surfactant for toiletries, nonirritating shampoos, acid hard surf. cleaners; detoxifies anionics; readily biodeg.; clear liq.; misc. with water, ethanol, poorly sol. in org. solvs.; dens. 1140 kg/m³; visc. 400 mPa·s max.; pour pt. -18 C; pH 8-9; surf. tens. 34 mN/m (0.1%); Ross-Miles foam 170 mm (initial, 0.05% , 50 C); 38-41% solids.

Ampholak XCO-40. [Berol Nobel AB] Sodium cocoamphoacetate; CAS 68608-65-1; EINECS 271-793-0; surfactant for toiletry prods., esp. nonirritant shampoos with exc. cold storage stability; clear liq.; misc. with water, ethanol; dens. 1175 kg/m³; visc. 500 mPa·s max.; pour pt. -30 C; pH 9.0 ± 1.0; 49-51% solids.

Ampholak XO7. [Berol Nobel AB] Oleoamphocarboxyglycinate; CAS 97659-53-5; EINECS 307-458-3; amphoteric; med. foaming, multipurpose cleaner component; for nonirritating toiletries, conditioners, liq. soap, as softener; clear liq.; misc. with water; dens. 1150 kg/m³; visc. 100 mPa·s max.; pour pt. -15 C; pH 9.0±0.5 (20%); surf. tens. 35.8 mN/m (0.1%); 39-41% conc.

Ampholak XO7/C. [Berol Nobel AB] Oleoamphopolycarboxyglycinate; CAS 97659-53-5; EINECS 307-458-3; med. foaming conditioner with biostatic activity for skin and hair care prods. (shampoos, liq. soaps, body care prods.); detoxifies anionics; clear liq.; sol. in water, poorly sol. in org. solvs.; dens. 1150 kg/m³; visc. 100 mPa·s max.; pour pt. -15 C; pH 8.5-9.5; surf. tens. 35.8 mN/m (0.1%); Ross-Miles foam 160 mm (initial, 0.05% , 50 C); 39.0-40.5% solids.

Ampholak XTP. [Berol Nobel AB] N-Tallowamidopolyamino-polygincate; for detergent applics., cosmetics, shampoos, liq. soaps; conditioner in shampoos; softergent in detergent formulations; anti-irritant for anionics; clear liq.; misc. with water; dens. 1154 kg/m³; visc. 30 mPa·s max.; pH 9.0 ± 0.5 (20%); surf. tens. 45 mN/m (0.1%); 41% min. solids.

Ampholak YCE. [Berol Nobel AB] Cocoiminodipropionate; CAS 97659-50-2; EINECS 307-455-7; amphoteric; med. foaming surfactant for industrial alkaline cleaners, cosmetic preps. (shampoos, liq. soaps); hydrotrope; lime soap dispersant; provides corrosion protection; readily biodeg.; clear liq.; sol. in water, limited sol. in org. solvs.; dens. 1050 kg/m³; visc. 150 mPa·s max.; pour pt. -8 C; pH 6.0-7.0; surf. tens. 38 m/m (0.1%); Ross-Miles foam 150 mm (initial, 0.05% , 50 C); 29-31% conc.

Ampholan® D197. [Harcros UK] Cocamidopropyl betaine; amphoteric; high foaming surfactant used in personal care prods. , shampoos, bath prods., personal hygiene prods., hand cleaners; stable to high concs. of electrolyte and hard water; straw clear liq.; sp.gr. 1.044; visc. 45 cst; flash pt. (COC) > 100 C; pH 5.5; 30% act.

Ampholan® E210. [Harcros UK] Cocodimethyl betaine; CAS 68424-94-2; EINECS 270-329-4; amphoteric; foaming agent, thickener; liq.

Ampholan® U 203. [Harcros UK] Cocoiminodipropionate; CAS 97659-50-2; EINECS 307-455-7; amphoteric; detergent, foaming and stabilizing agent, dispersant, hydrotrope; pale amber liq.; char. odor; water sol.; sp.gr. 1.035; visc. 132 cs; flash pt. > 200 F (COC); pour pt. < 0 C; pH 6.0–8.0 (1% aq); 30% act.

Ampholysat Bois De Panama. [C.E.P.] Water, cocobetaine, and quillaja extract.

Ampholysat Moelle. [C.E.P.] Water, coco-betaine, and spinal cord extract.

Ampholyt™ JA 140. [Hüls Am.; Hüls AG] Sodium lauroamophoacetate; amphoteric; mild surfactant for cosmetics, shampoos, baby and child care prods., detergents, strongly alkaline industrial cleaners; good foaming props.; yel. sl. cloudy liq.; visc. 120 mPa·s; clear pt. 5 C; pH 8-9 (1% aq.); 32-34% act.

Ampholyt™ JB 130. [Hüls Am.; Hüls AG] Cocamidopropyl betaine; amphoteric; surfactant for cosmetics, detergents, hair shampoos, foam baths, shower foams, liq. soaps; ylsh. clear liq.; visc. 20 mPa·s; clear pt. -1 C; pH 4-6 (1% aq.); 29-31% act.

Ampholyte KKE-70. [Berol Nobel AB] Coco alkyl aminopropionic acid; CAS 84812-94-2; EINECS 284-219-9; amphoteric; surfactant for detergents, toiletries; emulsifier, dispersant, corrosion inhibitor; 70% conc.

Amphomer® 4910. [Nat'l. Starch] Octylacrylamide/acrylates/butylaminoethyl methacrylate copolymer; CAS 70801-07-9; amphoteric; hair fixative resin for maximum curl; for aerosol and pump hair sprays, setting lotions, conditioners, spritzes, and cosmetics; wh. powd.; sol. in anhyd. ethanol, IPA; when neutralized, sol. in water; 3% volatiles.

Amphomer® LV-71. [Nat'l. Starch] Octyl acrylamide/acrylates/butylaminoethyl methacrylate copolymer; CAS 70801-07-9; amphoteric; hair fixative resin enhancing stiffness, holding and moisture resist.; for hair sprays, spritzes, spray gels, setting lotions, mousses; wh. fine powd.; sol. in ethanol, IPA; insol. in water; 3% volatiles.

Amphoram® CP1. [Ceca SA] N-Coco amino propionic acid in hydroalcoholic sol'n.; CAS 1462-54-0; amphoteric; base for low-irritation shampoos; detergents, foaming agents; wetting and dispersing agent for pigments and fillers in aq. or org. media; inks mfg.; Gardner ≤ 10 clear to turbid liq.; sp.gr. 098 kg/m³; visc. 150 mm²/s; solid. pt. 3 C; acid no. 125-140; cloud pt. 3 C; flash pt. 15 C; 65% conc.

Amphosol® CA. [Stepan; Stepan Canada; Stepan Europe] Cocamidopropyl betaine; amphoteric; mild conditioner, detergent, wetting agent, visc. builder, foam enhancer/stabilizer, base for cosmetics (shampoos, bubble baths, liq. hand soaps) and household and industrial liq. detergents; straw clear liq.; pH 5.0 (10%); 30% act.

Amphosol® CG. [Stepan; Stepan Canada] Cocamidopropyl betaine; amphoteric; foam booster/stabilizer, visc. builder, wetting agent, and lime soap dispersant; used in shampoos, bubble baths, liq. hand soaps, and liq. detergents; amber clear liq.; pH 4.5–6.5; 29–31% act.

Amphosol® DM. [Stepan Europe] Alkyl betaine; amphoteric; mild foaming, conditioning, thickening base for shampoos, foam baths, liq. soaps, household and industrial cleaners; bacteriostatic; stable in acid systems; water-wh. to pale yel. liq.; 30% act.

Amphoteen 24. [Berol Nobel AB] Lauryl betaine; CAS 683-10-3; EINECS 211-669-5; amphoteric; foam boosting/stabilizing surfactant, emulsifier, dispersant for low-irritation shampoos, household cleaners, industrial and institutional cleaners, washing-up liqs., hard surf. cleaners,

vehicle cleaners; chlorine-stable; clear liq.; sol. in water, poorly sol. in org. solvs.; dens. 1060 kg/m³; visc. 50 mPa·s; pour pt. -18 C; pH 6.5-7.5; surf. tens. 33 mN/m (0.1%); Ross-Miles foam 170 mm (initial, 0.05% , 50 C); 29-31% act.

Amphoteen BCA-30. [Berol Nobel AB] Cocoamidopropyl betaine; CAS 70851-07-9; EINECS 274-923-4; foam enhancer, visc. builder, thickener; used in shampoos and washing-up liqs.; clear liq.; misc. with water; dens. 1040 kg/m³; visc. 16 mPa·s; pour pt. -4 C; pH 7.0 ± 1.0 (20%); surf. tens. 35 mN/m (0.1%); 34-36% solids.

Amphoteen BCM-30. [Berol Nobel AB] Cocoalkyl dimethyl betaine; CAS 68424-94-2; EINECS 270-329-4; surfactant for low irritation shampoos and dishwashing liqs.; clear liq.; misc. with water; dens. 1030 kg/m³; visc. 20 mPa·s; pour pt. -10 C; pH 7.0 ± 1 (20%); surf. tens. 35 mN/m (0.1%); 29-31% act.

Amphoteen BTH-35. [Berol Nobel AB] Tallow bis (hydroxyethyl) betaine; CAS 61791-25-1; EINECS 274-845-0; surfactant for low irritation shampoos and dishwashing liqs.; thickener for household acidic cleaners; stable over wide pH range; clear liq.; sol. in water; poorly sol. in org. solvs.; dens. 1040 kg/m³; visc. 5000 mPa·s; pH 5.0-6.0; surf. tens. 30 mN/m (0.1%); Ross-Miles foam 135 mm (initial, 0.05% , 50 C); 40-44% solids.

Amphotensid 9M. [Zschimmer & Schwarz] Disodium cocoamphodiacetate and sodium laureth sulfate; amphoteric; detergent for personal care, hair shampoos, and bath prods.; liq.; 30% conc.

Amphotensid B4. [Zschimmer & Schwarz] Cocamidopropyl betaine; amphoteric; surfactant for cosmetics, shampoos, baby prods., bath prods., detergents; liq.; 30% conc.

Amphotensid GB 2009. [Zschimmer & Schwarz] Disodium cocoamphodiacetate; CAS 68650-39-5; EINECS 272-043-5; amphoteric; detergent used in personal care prods., shampoos, baby cosmetics, hand soaps, bath preps.; fluid; 38% conc.

Amphoterge® J-2. [Lonza] Disodium caproamphodiacetate; CAS 7702-01-4; EINECS 231-721-0; amphoteric; wetting agent and detergent for personal care and industrial applics.; liq.; visc. 236 cps; pour pt. < -10 C; pH 8.5; surf. tens. 26.4 dynes/cm (0.1%); Draves wetting 30 s; 50% conc.

Amphoterge® K. [Lonza] Sodium cocoamphopropionate; CAS 68919-41-5; amphoteric; detergents used in shampoos, skin cleansers, dishwashing; salt-free; liq.; visc. 186 cps; pour pt. 2 C; pH 9.8; surf. tens. 31.9 dynes/cm (0.1%); Draves wetting 48 s; 40% conc.

Amphoterge® K-2. [Lonza] Disodium cocoamphodipropionate; amphoteric; detergents used in shampoos, skin cleansers, dishwashing, heavy duty liq. cleaners; liq.; visc. 76 cps; pour pt. 0 C; pH 9.6; surf. tens. 38.6 dynes/cm (0.1%); Draves wetting 180 s; 40% conc.

Amphoterge® KJ-2. [Lonza] Disodium caproamphodipropionate; amphoteric; salt-free version; wetting agent, detergent for personal care and industrial applics.; liq.; visc. 50 cps; pour pt. -2 C; pH 9.6; surf. tens. 27.5 dynes/cm (0.1%); Draves wetting 83 s; 40% conc.

Amphoterge® L Special. [Lonza] Disodium lauroamphodiacetate; CAS 14350-97-1; EINECS 238-306-3; amphoteric; mild shampoo conc.; liq.; 37% solids.

Amphoterge® S. [Lonza] Sodium stearoamphoacetate; CAS 30473-39-3; EINECS 250-215-0; amphoteric; surfactant, textile softener; used in creme rinses; biodeg.; paste; 25% conc.

Amphoterge® SB. [Lonza] Sodium cocoamphohydroxypropyl sulfonate; CAS 68604-73-9; EINECS 271-705-0; amphoteric; surfactant used in detergent and cosmetic applic.; liq.; visc. 26 cps; pour pt. -5 C; pH 7.5 (1%); surf. tens. 33.2 dynes/cm (0.1%); Draves wetting 17 s; 45%

conc.

Amphoterge® W. [Lonza] Sodium cocoamphoacetate; amphoteric; surfactant for mild shampoos, skin cleansers, heavy duty cleaners, dishwashing preps.; liq.; visc. 564 cps; pour pt. 8 C; pH 9.8; surf. tens. 28.5 dynes/cm (0.1%); Draves wetting 22 s; 46% conc.

Amphoterge® W-2. [Lonza] Disodium cocoamphodiacetate; CAS 68650-39-5; EINECS 272-043-5; amphoteric; surfactant for nonirritating shampoos and skin cleansers, heavy duty liq. cleaners; gel to visc. liq.; visc. 96,000 cps; pour pt. < -10 C; pH 8.2 (20%); surf. tens. 28.5 dynes/cm (0.1%); Draves wetting 22 s; 52% conc.

Amphoteric L. [Exxon/Tomah] Coco deriv.; amphoteric; detergent, foam stabilizer/booster, wetting agent, mild surfactant for liq. detergents, shampoos, hand soaps, mech. foaming systems, dishwash; stable in mildly acid and alkaline media; lt. amber liq.; sp.gr. 1.04; pour pt. 35 F; pH 5–8 (5%); surf. tens. 33 dynes/cm (0.1%); 35% min. act.

Amphoteric N. [Exxon/Tomah] Sodium C12–15 alkoxypropyl iminodipropionate; amphoteric; high foam wetting agent, coupler for shampoos, hand soaps, alkaline and acid cleaners, mech. foaming systems; corrosion inhibitor in metalworking lubricants; visc. builder; fire fighting foams; lt. amber clear liq.; sol. in glycols, water, alcohol; sp.gr. 1.04; pH 6-9 (5%); surf. tens. 33 dynes/cm (0.1%); 35% solids in water.

Amtolide. [Hercules/PFW] Acetyl hexamethyl tetralin and acetyl hexamethyl indan.

Amyx A-25-S 0040. [Clough] Stearyl dimethyl benzyl ammonium chloride; CAS 122-19-0; EINECS 204-527-9; cationic; conditioner, softener, and emollient for hair rinses, skin creams, and lotions; emulsifier; paste; 25% min. act.

Amyx CDO 3599. [Clough] Cocamidopropylamine oxide; CAS 68155-09-9; EINECS 268-938-5; nonionic; mild high foaming surfactant, foam booster/stabilizer, wetting agent, hair conditioner for personal care, household, and janitorial prods.; liq.; 30-32% conc.

Amyx CO 3764. [Clough] Cetamine oxide; CAS 7128-91-8; EINECS 230-429-0; cationic in acid media; mild high foaming surfactant, foam booster/stabilizer, conditioner for personal care, household, and janitorial prods.; paste; 29-31% act.

Amyx LO 3594. [Clough] Lauramine oxide; CAS 1643-20-5; EINECS 216-700-6; cationic in acid media; mild high foaming surfactant, foam booster/stabilizer, wetting agent, grease emulsifier for personal care, household and janitorial prods.; liq.; 29-31% conc.

Amyx SO 3734. [Clough] Stearamine oxide; CAS 2571-88-2; EINECS 219-919-5; cationic in acid media; mild high foaming surfactant, foam booster/stabilizer, conditioner, emulsifier for personal care, household, and janitorial prods.; paste; 24.5-26.5% act.

Amyx ST 3837. [Clough] Cetearyl alcohol, PEG-40 hydrog. castor oil, stearalkonium chloride; conc. for prep. of hair conditioners; paste; 25-27% act.

Anatol. [Lanaetex Prods.] Lanolin alcohol; CAS 8027-33-6; EINECS 232-430-1; cosmetic ingred.

Angelica HS. [Alban Muller] Propylene glycol, angelica extract; botanical extract.

Anhydrous Citric Acid. [Haarmann & Reimer] Citric acid; CAS 77-92-9; EINECS 201-069-1.

Anhydrous Emcompress® . [Mendell] Dibasic calcium phosphate anhydrous USP/BP; CAS 7757-93-9; for production of pharmaceutical tablets; avg. particle size 136 μ; dens. (tapped) 0.7 g/cc.

Anhydrous Lanolin Grade 1. [Westbrook Lanolin] Lanolin B.P./Ph.Eur.; CAS 8006-54-0; EINECS 232-348-6; emulsifier, emollient for cleansers, face masks, shampoos, night creams, shaving preps., sunscreens, toilet soaps;

binder for pressed powds.; m.p. 38-44 C; acid no. 1 max.; sapon. no. 90-105.

Anhydrous Lanolin Grade 2. [Westbrook Lanolin] Lanolin B.P./Ph.Eur.; CAS 8006-54-0; EINECS 232-348-6; emollient, moisturizer, emulsifier for shampoos, sunscreen preps., toilet soaps; binder for pressed powds.; m.p. 38-44 C; acid no. 1 max.; sapon. no. 90-105.

Anhydrous Lanolin P.80. [Westbrook Lanolin] Anhydrous lanolin, pesticide-reduced; CAS 8006-54-0; EINECS 232-348-6; nonionic; emulsifier, emollient, moisturizer for pharmaceuticals and cosmetics (baby creams, cleansers, eye preps., foundation, lipstick, sunscreen preps.); soft solid; m.p. 38-44 C; HLB 4.5; acid no. 1 max.; sapon. no. 90-105; 100% conc.

Anhydrous Lanolin P.95. [Westbrook Lanolin] Anhydrous lanolin, pract. pesticide-free; CAS 8006-54-0; EINECS 232-348-6; nonionic; emulsifier, emollient, moisturizer for pharmaceuticals and cosmetics (baby creams, cleaners, eye preps., foundation, lipstick, sunscreen preps.); soft solid; m.p. 38-44 C; HLB 4.5; acid no. 1 max.; sapon. no. 90-105; 100% conc.

Anhydrous Lanolin P.95RA. [Westbrook Lanolin] Anhydrous lanolin; CAS 8006-54-0; EINECS 232-348-6; nonionic; hypo-allergenic grade emollient, moisturizer, emulsifier for pharmaceuticals and cosmetics (baby creams, cleansers, eye preps., foundation, hypo-allergenic cosmetics, lipstick, sunscreen preps.); soft solid; m.p. 38-44 C; HLB 4.5; acid no. 1 max.; sapon. no. 90-105; 100% conc.

Anhydrous Lanolin Superfine. [Westbrook Lanolin] Lanolin B.P./Ph.Eur.; CAS 8006-54-0; EINECS 232-348-6; emulsifier, emollient for baby creams/lotions, cleansers, eye preps., face masks, foundations, shampoos, conditioners, night creams, sunscreen preps., toilet soaps; binder for pressed powds.; m.p. 38-44 C; acid no. 1 max.; sapon. no. 90-105.

Anhydrous Lanolin USP. [Protameen] Lanolin; CAS 8006-54-0; EINECS 232-348-6; emollient.

Anhydrous Lanolin USP Cosmetic. [Fanning] Lanolin; CAS 8006-54-0; EINECS 232-348-6; emollient maintaining skin hydration; forms protective films on skin; for baby preps., pharmaceutical ointments, lipstick, shave cream, protective creams and lotions, makeup, hair spray plasticizer, shampoos, sunscreens, burn aids, pet prods.; EP and slip agent for metalworking/rust preventative coatings; plasticizer/lubricant in adhesives; in textile lubricants, printing inks; waterproofing agent for leather; pale yel. tenacous, unctuous substance, faint char. odor; m.p. 36-42 C; iodine no. 18-36.

Anhydrous Lanolin USP Cosmetic AA. [Amerchol] Lanolin; CAS 8006-54-0; EINECS 232-348-6; emollient.

Anhydrous Lanolin USP Cosmetic Grade. [R.I.T.A.] Lanolin USP; CAS 8006-54-0; EINECS 232-348-6; provides emolliency, water absorp., emulsification, emulsion stabilization, and pigment dispersion to cosmetics, pharmaceuticals, topical formulations; Gardner 9+ max. color; m.p. 38-44 C; iodine no. 18-36; sapon. no. 93-107; usage level: 0.1-50%.

Anhydrous Lanolin USP Deodorized AAA. [Amerchol] Lanolin; CAS 8006-54-0; EINECS 232-348-6; emollient.

Anhydrous Lanolin USP Pharmaceutical. [Fanning] Lanolin; CAS 8006-54-0; EINECS 232-348-6; emollient maintaining skin hydration; forms protective films on skin; for baby preps., pharmaceutical ointments, lipstick, shave cream, protective creams and lotions, makeup, hair spray plasticizer, shampoos, sunscreens, burn aids, pet prods.; EP and slip agent for metalworking/rust preventative coatings; plasticizer/lubricant in adhesives; in textile lubricants, printing inks; waterproofing agent for leather; pale yel. tenacous, unctuous substance, faint char. odor; m.p.

36-42 C; iodine no. 18-36.

Anhydrous Lanolin USP Pharmaceutical. [Amerchol] Lanolin; CAS 8006-54-0; EINECS 232-348-6; emollient.

Anhydrous Lanolin USP Pharmaceutical Grade. [R.I.T.A.] Lanolin USP; CAS 8006-54-0; EINECS 232-348-6; provides emolliency, water absorp., emulsification, emulsion stabilization, and pigment dispersion to pharmaceuticals, topical formulations; Gardner > 10+ color; m.p. 38-44 C; iodine no. 18-36; sapon. no. 93-107; usage level: 0.1-50%.

Anhydrous Lanolin USP Pharmaceutical Light Grade. [R.I.T.A.] Lanolin USP; CAS 8006-54-0; EINECS 232-348-6; provides emolliency, water absorp., emulsification, emulsion stabilization, and pigment dispersion to pharmaceuticals, topical formulations; Gardner 10+ max. color; m.p. 38-44 C; iodine no. 18-36; sapon. no. 93-107; usage level: 0.1-50%.

Anhydrous Lanolin USP Superfine [Fanning] Lanolin; CAS 8006-54-0; EINECS 232-348-6; emollient maintaining skin hydration; forms protective films on skin; for baby preps., pharmaceutical ointments, lipstick, shave cream, protective creams and lotions, makeup, hair spray plasticizer, shampoos, sunscreens, burn aids, pet prods.; EP and slip agent for metalworking/rust preventative coatings; plasticizer/lubricant in adhesives; in textile lubricants, printing inks; waterproofing agent for leather; pale yel. tenacous, unctuous substance, faint char. odor; m.p. 36-42 C; iodine no. 18-36.

Anhydrous Lanolin USP Ultrafine. [Fanning] Lanolin; CAS 8006-54-0; EINECS 232-348-6; emollient maintaining skin hydration; forms protective films on skin; for baby preps., pharmaceutical ointments, lipstick, shave cream, protective creams and lotions, makeup, hair spray plasticizer, shampoos, sunscreens, burn aids, pet prods.; EP and slip agent for metalworking/rust preventative coatings; plasticizer/lubricant in adhesives; in textile lubricants, printing inks; waterproofing agent for leather; pale yel. tenacous, unctuous substance, faint char. odor; m.p. 36-42 C; iodine no. 18-36.

Anhydrous Lanolin USP X-tra Deodorized. [R.I.T.A.] Lanolin USP; CAS 8006-54-0; EINECS 232-348-6; provides emolliency, water absorp., emulsification, emulsion stabilization, and pigment dispersion to cosmetics, pharmaceuticals, topical formulations; Gardner 8+ max. color; m.p. 38-44 C; iodine no. 18-36; sapon. no. 93-107; usage level: 0.1-50%.

Anionyx® 12S. [Stepan; Stepan Canada] Disodium oleamido PEG-2 sulfosuccinate; CAS 56388-43-3; EINECS 260-143-1; anionic; detergent for personal care prods., bubble baths, low-irritation shampoos, cleansers, dishwashing liqs.; counter-irritant for other surfactants; liq.; sp.gr. 1.05; flash pt. 138 F; 20% act.

Anise LS. [Alban Muller] Sunflower seed oil, anise extract.

Anise Seed Extract HS 2712 G. [Grau Aromatics] Propylene glycol, anise extract; botanical extract.

Annonyx SO. [Stepan; Stepan Canada] Stearamine oxide; CAS 2571-88-2; EINECS 219-919-5; conditioner, emulsifier, visc. modifier, wetting agent, foam booster/stabilizer; paste; 24.5% conc.

Antaron® ET-201. [ISP] PVP/decene copolymer.

Antaron® FC-34. [ISP] Monocarboxyl coco imidazoline compd.; amphoteric; detergent, wetting agent, emulsifier, dispersant, emollient, surfactant; fulling agent for woolen and worsted fabrics; emulsifier for leather processing; ingred. of bubble baths, hair, upholstery, and rug shampoos, liq. dishwashing and hard-surf. detergents; amber clear semivisc. liq.; sol. in water and high electrolyte sol'ns.; surf. tens. 32.0 dynes/cm (0.0155%); > 38% conc.

Antaron® MC-44. [ISP] Dicarboxylic coco imidazoline, sodium salt; amphoteric; emulsifier, solubilizer, coupling

agent for nonirritating shampoos, skin cleaners, other cosmetics, industrial and household cleaners; amber visc. liq.; 38% act.

Antaron® P-904. [ISP] Butylated PVP.

Antaron® PC-37. [ISP] Ethyl PEG-15 cocamine sulfate; amphoteric; shampoo surfactant; solubilizer used in ultra-mild baby and adult conditioning-type shampoos; amber clear slightly visc. liq.; misc. in water, ethanol; sp.gr. 1.15; visc. 1100–1200 cps; surf. tens. 39 dynes/cm (0.1%); biodeg.; 75% act.

Antaron® V-216. [ISP] PVP/hexadecene copolymer; CAS 32440-50-9; cosmetic ingred.

Antaron® V-220. [ISP] PVP/eicosene copolymer; CAS 28211-18-9.

Antaron® WP-660. [ISP] Tricontanyl PVP; waterproofing polymer providing longer wear for personal care prods. (sunscreens, skin creams and lotions, facial makeup, baby care prods., eye and lip pencils, lipsticks, mascara); pigment dispersant; also improves stick integrity in lipsticks; off-wh. flakes; sol. (@ 5%) in min. oil; insol. in ethanol, water; m.p. 58-68 C; HLB 6.0; 98% min. solids.

Antarox® L-64. [Rhone-Poulenc Surf. & Spec.] Poloxamer 184; CAS 9003-11-6; nonionic; defoamer, dispersant, wetting agent, emulsifier, demulsifier, leveling agent, detergent for industrial/household cleaners, hard surf. cleaning, laundry, skin care, emulsion polymerization; liq.; HLB 15.0; pour pt. 16 C; cloud pt. 59 C (1% aq.); 100% conc.; formerly Pegol® L-64.

Antarox® PGP 18-1. [Rhone-Poulenc Surf. & Spec.] Ethoxylated propoxylated glycol; nonionic; surfactant, detergent, emulsifier; liq.; HLB 3.0; 100% conc.; formerly Alkatronic PGP 18-1.

Antarox® PGP 18-2. [Rhone-Poulenc Surf. & Spec.] Ethoxylated propoxylated glycol; nonionic; surfactant, detergent, emulsifier; liq.; HLB 7.0; 100% conc.; formerly Alkatronic PGP 18-2.

Antarox® PGP 18-2LF. [Rhone-Poulenc Surf. & Spec.] Ethoxylated propoxylated glycol; nonionic; surfactant, detergent, emulsifier; liq.; 100% conc.; formerly Alkatronic PGP 18-2LF.

Antarox® PGP 18-8. [Rhone-Poulenc Surf. & Spec.] Ethoxylated propoxylated glycol; nonionic; surfactant, detergent, emulsifier; liq.; HLB 29.0; 100% conc.; formerly Alkatronic PGP 18-8.

Antarox® PGP 23-7. [Rhone-Poulenc Surf. & Spec.] Poloxamer 237; CAS 9003-11-6; nonionic; coemulsifier for cosmetics, toiletries, pulp and paper defoamers; dispersant, visc. control agent; wh. flake; sol. in water, aromatic and chlorinated solvs.; insol. in min. oil and aliphatic solvs.; m.w. 6700-8373; dens. 1.04 g/ml; HLB 24.0; cloud pt. > 100 C (1% aq.); pH 5.0-7.5 (2.5% aq.); foam height 44 mm (0.1%); 99% min. act.; formerly Alkatronic PGP 23-7.

Antex-MP. [Lanaetex Prods.] Glycerin, propylene glycol.

Antex-MPD. [Lanaetex Prods.] Glycerin, propylene glycol, disodium tridecylsulfosuccinate.

Anthoxan. [Henkel] 4-Isopropyl-5, 5-dimethyl-1, 3-dioxane; fragrance raw material for personal care and detergent formulations; colorless liq., herbal odor; b.p. 71 C; flash pt. 53 C.

Anti-MB. [Collaborative Labs] Butylene glycol, glycerin, and chlorphenesin; cosmetic preservative; USA, Japan, and Europe approvals; usage level: 3.5% max.

Antidandruff Agent NOVA. [Novarom GmbH] Ichthammol and piroctone olamine.

Anti-Dandruff Usnate AO. [Cosmetochem] Cocamidopropylamine oxide and lichen extract; a natural antidandruff additive for shampoos.

Anti-Irritant Complex-1. [Cosmetochem] A blend of plant extracts and panthenol; cosmetic specialty offering anti-irritant effect on sensitive skin.

Antil® 141 Liq. [Goldschmidt; Goldschmidt AG] Propylene glycol and PEG-55 propylene glycol oleate; nonionic; cold processable thickener for aq. sol'ns. of surfactants, e.g., shampoos, foam baths, shower preps., liq. soaps; solubilizes essential oils into aq. surfactant systems; pale yel. liq.; disp. in water; sol. in ethanol, 1,2-propylene glycol; insol. in veg. and min. oils; acid no. 5 max.; sapon. no. 10-22; usage level: > 0.5%; 40% act.

Antil® 171. [Goldschmidt] PEG-18 glyceryl glycol dioleococoate; thickener for shampoos, shower and bath preps.; Gardner 5 max. clear to sl. opalescent, low visc. liq.; acid no. 5 max.; sapon. no. 60-80; 85% act.

Antil® 208. [Goldschmidt] Carbomer 208, ethoxylated lauryl alcohol, propylene glycol, water; highly effective thickener for aq. detergent/soap-based prods., shampoos, shower and bath preps., hand cleaners; refatting agent in hair or skin cleansing prods.; solubilizer for oil-sol. actives in aq. preps.; amber oily liq.; visc. 800-1600 mPa·s; solid. pt. 11 C; acid no. < 0.5; sapon. no. 19-27; 80% act.

Antioxidant G-2. [Provital; Centerchem] Min. oil, tocopheryl acetate, ascorbyl palmitate, lecithin; antioxidant.

Antiphlogistic ARO. [Novarom GmbH] Propylene glycol, panthenol, urea, glycyrrhetinic acid, and allantoin.

Antiraghades HS 361, LS 661. [Alban Muller] Horse chestnut, St. John's wort, myrrh phtyocomplex; face care prod. for delicate skin.

Antistatique WL 879. [Gattefosse] Caprylic acid and sorbitol; antistat.

Antistretchmarks HS 338. [Alban Muller] Fenugreek, horsetail, and incense phytocomplex; prod. for stretch marks.

APG® 300 CS. [Henkel/Cospha; Henkel Canada] Decyl polyglucose; nonionic; cosurfactant, aux. foaming agent for mild shampoos and other personal care cleansers; clear visc. liq.; 50% act.

APG® 325 CS. [Henkel/Cospha; Henkel Canada] Decyl polyglucose; nonionic; cosurfactant, aux. foaming agent for mild shampoos and other personal care cleansers; clear visc. liq.; 50% act.

APG® 350 Glycoside. [Henkel/Organic Prods.] Decyl polyglucose.

APG® 500 Glycoside. [Henkel/Organic Prods.] Lauryl polyglucose; CAS 110615-47-9.

APG® 600 CS. [Henkel/Cospha; Henkel Canada] Lauryl polyglucose; nonionic; cosurfactant, visc. modifier and thickener for mild shampoos, other personal care cleansers; clear visc. liq.; pH 5-7; 50% act.

APG® 600 SP. [Henkel/Organic Prods.] Lauryl polyglucose; CAS 110615-47-9.

APG® 625 CS. [Henkel/Cospha; Henkel Canada] Lauryl polyglucose; nonionic; cosurfactant, visc. modifier and thickener for mild shampoos, personal care cleansers; clear visc. liq.; pH 6-8; 50% act.

AP-Grit. [Ichimaru Pharcos] Apricot seed powd.

Apicerol 2/014081. [Dragoco] Petrolatum, min. oil, beeswax, polyglyceryl-2 sesquioleate, lanolin, isopropyl palmitate.

Apifac. [Gattefosse; Gattefosse SA] Polyglyceryl-2 isostearate; nonionic; self-emulsifying base for w/o cosmetic creams (skin care, night care, sun care, hair care); Gardner < 8 waxy solid, faint odor; sol. @ 60 C in veg. and min. oils; partly sol. in ethanol; insol. in water; drop pt. 59-69 C; HLB 6.0; acid no. < 6; iodine no. < 10; sapon. no. 90-110; usage level: 10-15%; toxicology: sl. skin irritant; 100% conc.

Apifil® . [Gattefosse; Gattefosse SA] PEG-8 beeswax; nonionic; structural self-emulsifying base for o/w emulsions in cosmetics and pharmaceuticals; Gardner < 8 waxy solid; weak odor; sol. @ 60 C in chloroform, methylene chloride; sl. sol. in veg. oils; insol. in water, ethanol; m.p. 60-65 C; HLB 5.0; acid no. < 5; iodine no. < 10;

sapon. no. 70-90; usage level: 8-15%; toxicology: LD50 (oral, rat) > 8.5 g/kg; sl. skin irritant, very sl. eye irritant; 100% conc.

Apple HS. [Grau Aromatics] Propylene glycol and apple extract; botanical extract.

Apple Extract HS 1806 AT. [Grau Aromatics] Propylene glycol and apple extract; botanical extract.

Applichem PDP-200. [Application Chems.] Pentadoxynol-200; CAS 40160-92-7.

Apricot Extract HS 2509 G. [Grau Aromatics] Propylene glycol and apricot extract; botanical extract.

Apricot Glycolysat. [C.E.P.] Propylene glycol, water, and apricot extract; botanical extract.

Aquabase. [Westbrook Lanolin] PEG-20 stearate, cetearyl alcohol; nonionic; base for o/w emulsions; emulsifier for baby creams, cleansers, day creams/lotions, foundations, night creams, sunscreen preps.; flake; m.p. 46-53 C; HLB 10.0; acid no. 4 max.; iodine no. 6 max.; sapon. no. 6-17; pH 4-8 (aq. sol'n.).

Aquabase N.F. [Westbrook Lanolin] Cetearyl alcohol and polysorbate 60; emulsifying wax; emulsifier for baby creams/lotions, cleansers, day/night creams, foundations, sunscreen preps.; m.p. 48-52 C; iodine no. 3.5 max.; sapon. no. 14 max.; hyd. no. 178-192; pH 5.5-7.0 (aq. sol'n.).

Aquaderm. [Novarom GmbH] Sodium PCA, sodium lactate, fructose, collagen amino acids, niacinamide, urea, and inositol.

Aquagel. [Ikeda] Carrageenan; CAS 9000-07-1; EINECS 232-524-2; film-former for hair and skin care prods.; provides long retention of hair set, glossiness, dry, smooth touch; sl. ylsh. powd., char. odor; visc. 30-70 cps; pH 6.5-9.5.

Aqualizer EJ. [Kolmar Labs] Polyamino sugar condensate and urea.

Aqualon® Cellulose Gum. [Aqualon] Sodium carboxymethylcellulose, standard, food, and pharmaceutical grades; CAS 9004-32-4; suspending agent for abrasive and polishing agents, and prevents syneresis in toothpaste; rheology control agent in creams and lotions; adhesive and cohesive agent used in denture adhesive and ostomy adhesive prods.; FDA compliance; GRAS; water-sol.

Aqualose L30. [Westbrook Lanolin] PEG-30 lanolin; CAS 61790-81-6; nonionic; emollient, moisturizer, emulsifier, plasticizer, solubilizer; for cleansers, shampoos, nailcare, toilet soaps; wax; water-sol.; drop pt. 40-48 C; HLB 14.0; acid no. 5 max.; sapon. no. 24-40; cloud pt. 68-75 C (aq.); pH 3.5-7.0 (5% aq.); 100% conc.

Aqualose L75. [Westbrook Lanolin] PEG-75 lanolin USP; CAS 61790-81-6; nonionic; emollient, moisturizer, emulsifier for cleansers, foam baths, hair care, shaving preps.; plasticizer in aerosol hairsprays; solubilizer for perfume and germicidal agents, in aftershaves; conditioner for shampoos; superfatting agent for soap; wax; water-sol.; drop pt. 45-52 C; HLB 16.0; acid no. 5 max.; sapon. no. 10-26; cloud pt. 75-83 C (aq.); pH 3.5-7.0 (5% aq.); 100% conc.

Aqualose L75/50. [Westbrook Lanolin] PEG-75 lanolin USP; CAS 61790-81-6; nonionic; emollient, emulsifier; gel; water-sol.; 50% conc.

Aqualose L100. [Westbrook Lanolin] PEG-100 lanolin; CAS 61790-81-6; emollient, moisturizer for cleansers, foam baths/gels; emulsifier and solubilizer for aftershave lotions; also avail. as 50% sol'n.; water-sol.; drop pt. 46-54 C; acid no. 5 max.; sapon. no. 8-22; cloud pt. 76-84 C (aq.); pH 3.5-8.0 (5% aq.).

Aqualose LL100. [Westbrook Lanolin] PPG-40-PEG-60 lanolin oil; nonionic; emollient, emulsifier, solubilizer used in aq. and alcoholic preps. (aftershave lotions, cleanesrs, foam baths/gels); plasticizer for hairsprays; liq.; sol. in water, alcohol; HLB 13.0; acid no. 4 max.; sapon. no. 5-20; cloud pt. 32-40 C (aq.); pH 3.5-8.0 (5% aq.); 100% conc.

Aqualose SLT. [Westbrook Lanolin] Solubilized lanolin oil (lanolin oil, ceteth-14, steareth-14); emollient, moisturizer for aftershave lotions, cleansers, shampoos; solubilizer, carrier for aftershaves, nailcare preps.; paste; water-sol.; drop pt. 35-45 C; acid no. 5 max.; sapon. no. 16-34; pH 3.5-8.0 (5% aq.).

Aqualose SLW. [Westbrook Lanolin] Solubilized lanolin oil (lanolin oil and laneth-20); emollient, moisturizer, solubilizer used in aq. or dilute alcoholic preparations (shampoos, aftershaves, cleansers); solubilizer and carrier for nailcare preps.; paste; water-sol.; drop pt. 42-50 C; acid no. 5 max.; sapon. no. 20-36; pH 3.5-8.0 (5% aq.).

Aqualose W5. [Westbrook Lanolin] Laneth-5; CAS 61791-20-6; emollient, emulsifier.

Aqualose W20. [Westbrook Lanolin] Laneth-20; CAS 61791-20-6; nonionic; plasticizer and solubilizer for hydrophobic substances; emollient, emulsifier, solubilizer for aftershaves, antiperspirants, cleansers, foam baths, shampoos, nailcare; carrier for foam baths, shampoos, nailcare; wax; water-sol.; drop pt. 41-49; acid no. 6 max.; sapon. no. 6-18; cloud pt. 74-82 C (aq.); pH 3.5-7.0 (5% aq.).

Aqualose W20/50. [Westbrook Lanolin] Laneth-20; CAS 61791-20-6; nonionic; emollient, emulsifier; gel; 50% conc.

Aquapalm No. 63841. [Roche] Retinyl palmitate; CAS 79-81-2; EINECS 201-228-5; vitamin supplement.

Aquaphil K. [Westbrook Lanolin] Lanolin and lanolin alcohol; nonionic; emollient, emulsifier with enhanced w/o emulsion stability; for baby creams/lotions, day/night creams, face masks, foundations; soft solid; m.p. 36-42 C; HLB 4.5; acid no. 1 max.; 100% conc.

Aquarez 7. [Eastman] Nail polish formulation utilizing aq. disp. polymers; gives extremely fast drying time, gloss, and durability, exc. moisture vapor transmission, nonyel. of the nail; wh. liq.; visc. < 60 cps; pH 3-5; 44-45% solids.

Aquaron. [Ikeda] Carrageenan; CAS 9000-07-1; EINECS 232-524-2; provides strong reaction to protein; for hair care prods., shampoos; improves tenacity and flexibility of hair, dry combing, and dyeing effect of acidic dyestuffs; ylsh. brn. clear liq., char. odor; visc. 5 cps max.; pH 4.0 ± 0.2; 10% min. solids.

Aquasorb® A250. [Aqualon] Carboxymethylcellulose; CAS 9004-32-4; absorbent for urine, blood, and other body fluids; used in feminine hygiene prods., medical disposables, disposable diapers, wound dressings; wh. to lt. tan powd.; pH 6.5–8.5; 99.5% min. purity.

Aqua-Tein C. [Maybrook] Collagen amino acids, acetamide MEA, propylene glycol; substantive moisturizer, emollient for hair and skin care prods. (shampoos, conditioners, ethnic prods., nutritive eye creams, face creams and lotions); anti-irritant for anionic shampoos; amber clear liq., char. odor; pH 5.5-6.8; 70% min. solids.

Aqua-Tein S. [Maybrook] Acetamide MEA, MEA-hydrolyzed silk, and propylene glycol; substantive, nongreasy emollient, moisture binder, conditioner for hair and skin care prods. (shampoos, conditioners, nutritive shampoos, ethnic prods., nutritive eye creams, face creams/lotions, treatment prods.); amber clear liq., char. odor; pH 5.0-6.0; 46-52% solids.

Aremsol MA. [Ronsheim & Moore] MEA lauryl sulfate; CAS 4722-98-9; EINECS 225-214-3; anionic; base for prep. of liq. shampoos; biodeg.; liq.; 32% conc.

Aremsol MR. [Ronsheim & Moore] MEA lauryl sulfate; CAS 4722-98-9; EINECS 225-214-3; anionic; base for prep. of liq. shampoos; biodeg.; liq.; 32% conc.

Aremsol TA. [Ronsheim & Moore] TEA lauryl sulfate; CAS 139-96-8; EINECS 205-388-7; anionic; base for prep. of liq. shampoos; rapidly biodeg.; liq.; 42% conc.

Argidone®. [UCIB; Barnet Prods.] Arginine PCA; CAS 56265-06-6; EINECS 260-081-5; moisturizing adjuvant for nutritive or generative creams or lotions, skin care and pigmented cosmetics; activates cell metabolism; creamy-wh. powd., odorless; water-sol.; m.w. 303.3; usage level: 0.5-2%; toxicology: nontoxic; nonirritating to skin; very sl. irritating to eyes.

Argobase 125. [Westbrook Lanolin] Lanolin alcohol, min. oil, lauryl alcohol, octyldodecanol; nonionic; emollient, w/o emulsifier used in baby creams/lotions/oils, foam baths/gels, shampoos; lubricant, glossing agent in night creams, sunscreen preps.; liq.; oil-sol.; sp.gr. 0.84-0.87; HLB 3.0; acid no. 1 max.; iodine no. 12 max.; sapon. no. 2 max.; hyd. no. 9-16; 15% conc.

Argobase EU. [Westbrook Lanolin] Lanolin alcohol, min. oil, petrolatum, and paraffin; nonionic; emollient, emulsifier, stabilizer, absorp. base for pharmaceuticals; B.P. wool alcohols ointment; cream-colored paste; m.p. 39-45 C; HLB 4.0; acid no. 0.25 max.; 6% conc.

Argobase EUC 2. [Westbrook Lanolin] Lanolin alcohol, cetearyl alcohol, ozokerite, min. oil, and petrolatum; absorp. base for pharmaceutical ointments; cream/yel. color; acid no. 2 max.; sapon. no. 2 max.

Argobase EU Hydrous. [Westbrook Lanolin] Lanolin alcohol, min. oil, petrolatum, paraffin, and water; absorp. base.

Argobase L1. [Westbrook Lanolin] Lanolin, lanolin alcohol, cetearyl alcohol, min. oil, beeswax, and triethanolamine; nonionic; emollient, emulsifier, stabilizer, absorp. base; used in baby creams/lotions, day/night creams, foundations, toilet soaps; liq.; HLB 4.0; acid no. 2 max.; iodine no. 12 max.; sapon. no. 14-32; 24% conc.

Argobase L2. [Westbrook Lanolin] Lanolin, lanolin wax, lanolin alcohol, min. oil, petrolatum, ozokerite; absorp. base, emollient, moisturizer, emulsifier for baby creams/lotions, day/night creams, foundations, shaving preps.; pale yel.; m.p. 30-38 C; acid no. 1 max.; sapon. no. 32-42.

Argobase MS 5. [Westbrook Lanolin] Sterols and sterol esters lanolin extracts; nonionic; w/o emulsifier, emollient, moisturizer, stabilizer for baby creams, face masks, foundations, night creams; pale yel. paste; HLB 5.0; acid no. 2 max.; sapon. no. 20-30; hyd. no. 12-28; 25% conc.

Argobase S1. [Westbrook Lanolin] Lanolin, lanolin alcohol, cetearyl alcohol, and min. oil; nonionic; emollient, emulsifier, stabilizer, absorp. base; used for baby creams/lotions, day/night creams, face masks, foundations; paste; m.p. 32-40 C; HLB 4.0; acid no. 2 max.; iodine no. 12-28; sapon. no. 55-75; 92% conc.

Argo Brand Corn Starch. [Corn Prods.] Corn starch; CAS 9005-25-8; EINECS 232-679-6; binder, filler, diluent.

Argonol 40. [Westbrook Lanolin] Isobutylated lanolin oil; CAS 85005-47-6; nonionic; w/o emulsifier, emollient, moisturizer for aftershaves, antiperspirants, baby oils, cleansers, foam baths/gels, nailcare, sunscreen preps.; liq.; acid no. 2 max.; sapon. no. 112-132; hyd. no. 16 max.; pour pt. 15 C max.; cloud pt. 17 C max.; 100% conc.

Argonol 50. [Westbrook Lanolin] Lanolin oil; emollient, moisturizer, lubricant for antiperspirants, baby creams/lotions, cleansers, day creams, foam baths/gels, lipsticks, nailcare, sunscreens; binder for pressed powds.; liq.; acid no. 2 max.; sapon. no. 92-118; pour pt. 18 C max.; cloud pt. 21 C max.

Argonol 50 Pharmaceutical. [Westbrook Lanolin] Lanolin oil; emollient, lubricant; liq., odorless; sol. in min. oil.

Argonol 50 Super. [Westbrook Lanolin] Lanolin oil; emollient, moisturizer.

Argonol 60. [Westbrook Lanolin] Lanolin oil; emollient, moisturizer, emulsifier for baby creams, foam baths/gels, lipsticks, sunscreen preps.; emollient and solubilizer for nailcare preps.; liq.; acid no. 2 max.; sapon. no. 85-105;

pour pt. 18 C max.; cloud pt. 32 C max.

Argonol ACE 5. [Westbrook Lanolin] Cetyl acetate, acetylated lanolin alcohol; emollient, moisturizer for baby oils, eye preps., foam baths, sunscreen preps.; lubricant/ glossing aid for hairsprays, lipsticks; binder for lipsticks, pressed powds.; liq.; acid no. 1 max.; iodine no. 8-12; sapon. no. 180-200; hyd. no. 8 max.

Argonol ACE 6. [Westbrook Lanolin] Cetyl acetate and oleyl acetate; emollient, moisturizer for baby oils, sunscreens; lubricant, glossing agent for hairsprays; lubricant and plasticizer for lipsticks; binder for pressed powds.; liq.; acid no. 1 max.; iodine no. 6-12; sapon. no. 185-205; hyd. no. 8 max.

Argonol ISO. [Westbrook Lanolin] Lanolin oil, isopropyl palmitate, oleyl alcohol; emollient, moisturizer for aftershaves, baby oils, foam baths, nailcare, sunscreen preps.; plasticizer for hair sprays; liq.; sp.gr. 0.875-0.900; acid no. 1 max.; iodine no. 11-26; sapon. no. 140-170; cloud pt. 13 C max.

Argonol LFA Dist. [Westbrook Lanolin] Lanolin acid; CAS 68424-43-1; EINECS 270-302-7; emollient.

Argonol RIC2. [Westbrook Lanolin] Lanolin oil, isopropyl palmitate, and castor oil; emollient, moisturizer for cleansers; emollient, binder for lipsticks; lubricant, glossing agent for hair conditioners; liq.; acid no. 1 max.; iodine no. 23-40; sapon. no. 140-170; hyd. no. 8 max.

Argowax Cosmetic Super. [Westbrook Lanolin] Lanolin alcohol; CAS 8027-33-6; EINECS 232-430-1; nonionic; gelling agent, emulsifier, emollient, moisturizer for baby creams/lotions, day/night creams, face masks, foundations, shaving preps., sunscreens; plasticizer for hairsprays; more economical where pharmacopoeia grade material not required; wax, low color and odor; m.p. 50 C min.; HLB 2.6; acid no. 3 max.; sapon. no. 15 max.; 100% conc.

Argowax Dist. [Westbrook Lanolin] Lanolin alcohol, B.P./ Ph.Eur.; CAS 8027-33-6; EINECS 232-430-1; nonionic; gelling agent, w/o emulsifier, emollient, moisturizer for baby creams/lotions, day/night creams, face masks, foundations, sunscreen preps.; plasticizer for hairsprays; lt. wax, sl. odor; m.p. 58 C min.; HLB 2.6; acid no. 2 max.; sapon. no. 12 max.; hyd. no. 120-180; 100% conc.

Argowax LFA Distilled. [Westbrook Lanolin] Lanolin acid; CAS 68424-43-1; EINECS 270-302-7; emollient, moisturizer for shaving creams/soaps, toilet soaps; m.p. 50-60 C; acid no. 138-152; sapon. no. 170-190; hyd. no. 24-46.

Argowax LFA Standard. [Westbrook Lanolin] Lanolin acid; CAS 68424-43-1; EINECS 270-302-7; emollient.

Argowax Standard. [Westbrook Lanolin] Lanolin alcohol BP/ Ph.Eur.; CAS 8027-33-6; EINECS 232-430-1; nonionic; gelling agent, w/o emulsifier, emollient, moisturizer for baby creams, day creams/lotions, face masks, foundations, sunscreen preps.; plasticizer for hairsprays; wax; m.p. 58 C min.; HLB 2.6; acid no. 2 max.; sapon. no. 12 max.; hyd. no. 120-180; 100% conc.

Argus DLTDP. [Witco/Argus] Dilauryl thiodipropionate; CAS 123-28-4; EINECS 204-614-1; antioxidant used for polyoelfins, thermoplastic elastomers, syn. fubber; antioxidant for cosmetics and pharmaceuticals; FDA regulated; wh. free-flowing powd.

Argus DSTDP. [Witco/Argus] Distearyl thiodipropionate; CAS 693-36-7; EINECS 211-750-5; antioxidant for polyolefins and other polymeric systems where long term heat stability is required; also for pharmaceutical and cosmetic prods., oils, greases, and lubricants; FDA regulated.

Aristoflex A. [Hoechst Celanese/Colorants & Surf.] Vinyl acetate/crotonic acid copolymer; CAS 25609-89-6; hair fixative.

Aristoflex A/60% Sol'n. [Hoechst Celanese/Colorants & Surf.] Vinyl acetate/crotonic acid copolymer and isopro-

pyl alcohol; CAS 25609-89-6; hair fixative.

Arlacel® 20. [ICI Spec. Chem.; ICI Surf. Am.; ICI Surf. Belgium] Sorbitan laurate; nonionic; emulsifier for cosmetics, pharmaceuticals; yel. amber liq.; sol. in methanol, ethanol, min., cottonseed and corn oils, ethylene glycol; sp.gr. 1.0; visc. 4250 cps; HLB 8.6; flash pt. > 300 F; 100% act.

Arlacel® 40. [ICI Spec. Chem.; ICI Surf. Am.; ICI Surf. Belgium] Sorbitan palmitate; CAS 26266-57-9; EINECS 247-568-8; nonionic; emulsifier for cosmetics, pharmaceuticals; cream beads; sol. in IPA; sp.gr. 1; HLB 6.7; pour pt. 48 C; flash pt. > 300 F; 100% act.

Arlacel® 60. [ICI Spec. Chem.; ICI Surf. Am.; ICI Surf. Belgium] Sorbitan stearate; CAS 1338-41-6; EINECS 215-664-9; nonionic; emulsifier for cosmetics, pharmaceuticals; cream-colored waxy beads, solid; sol. in IPA; HLB 4.7; flash pt. > 300 F; pour pt. 53 C; 100% act.

Arlacel® 80. [ICI Spec. Chem.; ICI Surf. Am.; ICI Surf. Belgium] Sorbitan oleate; CAS 1338-43-8; EINECS 215-665-4; nonionic; emulsifier for cosmetics, pharmaceuticals; yel. amber oil, liq.; sol. in IPA, min. and cottonseed oils; sp.gr. 1; visc. 1900 cps; HLB 4.3; flash pt. > 300 F; 100% act.

Arlacel® 83. [ICI Spec. Chem.; ICI Surf. Am.; ICI Surf. Belgium] Sorbitan sesquioleate; CAS 8007-43-0; EINECS 232-360-1; nonionic; emulsifier; cosmetic and pharmaceutical grade of Arlacel® C; yel. clear oily liq.; sol. in min. and cottonseed oils, ethanol, IPA; sp.gr. 1; visc 1500 cps; HLB 3.7; flash pt. > 300 F; 100% act.

Arlacel® 85. [ICI Spec. Chem.; ICI Surf. Am.; ICI Surf. Belgium] Sorbitan trioleate; CAS 26266-58-0; EINECS 247-569-3; nonionic; surfactant for cosmetics and pharmaceuticals; yel. amber oily liq.; sol. in IPA, alcohol, min., cottonseed and corn oil; sp.gr. 0.95; visc. 250 cps; HLB 1.8; flash pt. > 300 F; 100% act.

Arlacel® 129. [ICI Surf. Am.; ICI Surf. Belgium] Glyceryl stearate; nonionic; coemulsifier; wh. powd.; HLB 3.2; 100% conc.

Arlacel® 165. [ICI Spec. Chem.; ICI Surf. Am.; ICI Surf. Belgium] Glyceryl stearate, PEG-100 stearate; nonionic; surfactant, emulsifier, thickener, opacifier for household, cosmetics, and allied fields; acid-stable; self-emulsifying; wh. beads; bland odor; disp. in water; HLB 11; flash pt. > 300 F; pour pt. 48 C; 100% act.

Arlacel® 186. [ICI Spec. Chem.; ICI Surf. Am.; ICI Surf. Belgium] Glyceryl oleate, propylene glycol, 0.02% BHA and 0.01% citric acid as preservatives; nonionic; surfactant, emulsifier, thickener for personal care prods.; defoamer for oral pharmaceutical prods.; pale yel. clear liq.; sol. in ethanol, IPA, cottonseed and min. oils; sp.gr. 1; visc. 150 cps; HLB 2.8; flash pt. > 300 F; 100% act.

Arlacel® 481. [ICI Spec. Chem.; ICI Surf. Belgium] Glyceryl sorbitan fatty acid ester, unsat.; nonionic; emulsifier for cosmetic uses; yel. amber wax; HLB 4.5; 100% conc.

Arlacel® 581. [ICI Spec. Chem.; ICI Surf. Belgium] Glycerol sorbitan oleostearate, ethoxylated; nonionic; emulsifier for w/o creams; amber waxy solid; HLB 5; 100% conc.

Arlacel® 582. [ICI Spec. Chem.; ICI Surf. Belgium] Glycerol sorbitan isostearate, ethoxylated; nonionic; emulsifier for w/o creams; amber waxy solid; HLB 5; 100% conc.

Arlacel® 780. [ICI Surf. Belgium] Alkoxylated glyceryl sorbitan hydroxystearate; nonionic; emulsifier for w/o milks; suitable for cold emulsification technique; amber liq.; HLB 4.7; 100% conc.

Arlacel® 986. [ICI Spec. Chem.; ICI Surf. Belgium] Glycerol sorbitan fatty acid ester, sat.; nonionic; emulsifier for w/o creams, and lotions; yel. amber wax; HLB 4.5; 100% conc.

Arlacel® 987. [ICI Spec. Chem.; ICI Surf. Belgium] Sorbitan isostearate; CAS 54392-26-6; nonionic; emulsifier for w/ o cosmetic, creams and lotions; yel. amber liq.; HLB 4.3;

100% conc.

Arlacel® 988. [ICI Spec. Chem.; ICI Surf. Belgium] POE glycerol sorbitan fatty acid ester; nonionic; emulsifier for cosmetic uses; yel. waxy solid; HLB 4.7; 100% conc.

Arlacel® 989. [ICI Spec. Chem.; ICI Surf. Belgium] PEG-7 hydrog. castor oil; CAS 61788-85-0; nonionic; emulsifier and softener for w/o lotions, cosmetic uses; yel. liq., gel; HLB 4.9; 100% conc.

Arlacel® 1689. [ICI Surf. Belgium] Sorbitan oleate and polyglyceryl ricinoleate; nonionic; emulsifier for w/o creams and milks; amber liq.; HLB 3.5; 100% conc.

Arlacel® A. [ICI Spec. Chem.; ICI Surf. Belgium] Mannide oleate; nonionic; surfactant for use in emulsified vaccines of the w/o type; amber liq.; HLB 4.3; 100% conc.

Arlacel® C. [ICI Spec. Chem.; ICI Surf. Am.; ICI Surf. Belgium] Sorbitan sesquioleate; CAS 8007-43-0; EINECS 232-360-1; nonionic; surfactant, w/o emulsifier; amber oily liq.; sol. in min. oil, cottonseed oil, ethanol, IPA; sp.gr. 1.0; visc. 1000 cps; HLB 3.7; flash pt. > 300 F; HLB 3.7; 100% act.

Arlamol® 801. [ICI Surf. UK] Surfactant blend; nonionic; emollient for personal care industry; wh. solid.

Arlamol® D4. [ICI Surf. UK] Octamethylcyclotetrasiloxane; emollient for personal care industry; colorless liq.

Arlamol® DIDA. [ICI Surf. Am.] Diisodecyl adipate; CAS 27178-16-1; EINECS 248-299-9.

Arlamol® DINA. [ICI Surf. Am.] Diisononyl adipate; CAS 33703-08-1; EINECS 251-646-7.

Arlamol® DOA. [ICI Surf. UK] Diester of adipic acid; emollient for personal care industry; colorless liq.

Arlamol® E. [ICI Spec. Chem.; ICI Surf. Am.; ICI Surf. Belgium] PPG-15 stearyl ether with preservatives; CAS 25231-21-4; nonionic; emollient, solv. for personal care prods.; colorless oily liq.; sol. in min. oil, isopropyl esters, cottonseed oil, ethanol, IPA, hexadecyl alcohol; sp.gr. 0.95; visc. 80 cps; pour pt. typ. < 0 C; 100% act.

Arlamol® F. [ICI Australia] PPG-11 stearyl ether; CAS 25231-21-4; nonionic; emollient for personal care industry; colorless liq.; sol. in alcohol, cottonseed and min. oil; insol. in water; visc. 1200 cps.

Arlamol® GM. [ICI Surf. UK] Ethoxylated glyceride; nonionic; emollient/refattening agent for bath and shower prods.; yel. liq.; HLB 15.7; 100% act.

Arlamol® HD. [ICI Surf. UK] Heptamethylnonane; CAS 4390-04-9; EINECS 224-506-8; emollient for personal care industry; colorless liq.

Arlamol® ISML. [ICI Australia] Isosorbide laurate; nonionic; emollient for personal care industry; wh. solid; insol. in water, min. oil; pour pt. 47 C.

Arlamol® M812. [ICI Surf. UK] Short-chain glycerides; emollient for personal care industry; colorless liq.

Arlamol® PAO Series. [ICI Surf. UK] Polydecene; emollient for personal care industry; colorless liq.

Arlamol® PC. [ICI Surf. UK] Branched esters; emollient for personal care industry; colorless liq.

Arlamol® S3, S7. [ICI Spec. Chem.; ICI Surf. UK] PPG-15-stearyl ether and cyclomethicome; emollient used in cosmetic prods.; colorless liq.

Arlasolve® 200. [ICI Spec. Chem.; ICI Surf. Am.] Isoceteth-20; nonionic; surfactant, emulsifier, solubilizer for cosmetics; wh. soft waxy solid; sol. in water, alcohol, propylene glycol; HLB 15.7; pour pt. 36 C.

Arlasolve® 200 Liq. [ICI Spec. Chem.; ICI Surf. Am.; ICI Surf. Belgium] Isoceteth-20; nonionic; surfactant, emulsifier, solubilizer for cosmetics; colorless liq.; sol. in water, propylene glycol, ethanol; sp.gr. 1.0; visc. 1200 cps; HLB 15.7; flash pt. > 230 F.

Arlasolve® DMI. [ICI Spec. Chem.; ICI Surf. Am.] Dimethyl isosorbide; CAS 5306-85-4; EINECS 226-159-8; nonionic; surfactant, emollient, solubilizer for personal care

industry; colorless liq.; sol. in water, alcohol, cottonseed oil, propylene glycol; visc. 6 cps.

Arlatone® 285. [ICI Spec. Chem.; ICI Surf. Belgium] POE castor oil; nonionic; cosmetic grade surfactant, emulsifier, coupling agent, solubilizer for perfumes, fragrances; pale cream semifluid; HLB 14.4; 100% conc.

Arlatone® 289. [ICI Spec. Chem.; ICI Surf. Belgium] POE hydrog. castor oil; nonionic; coupling agent, solubilizer, emulsifier for o/w creams and lotions; pale cream waxy solid; HLB 14.0; 100% conc.

Arlatone® 650. [ICI Spec. Chem.; ICI Surf. UK] Ethoxylated castor oil; vitamin solubilizer; pale yel. liq.; HLB 12.5.

Arlatone® 827. [ICI Spec. Chem.; ICI Surf. UK] Ethoxylated castor oil; nonionic; vitamin solubilizer; yel. liq.; HLB 11.9; 100% act.

Arlatone® 970. [ICI Spec. Chem.; ICI Surf. UK] POE sorbitan fatty acid ester; nonionic; coupling agent, solubilizer for personal care prods.; yel. amber liq.; HLB 14.3; 100% conc.

Arlatone® 975. [ICI Spec. Chem.; ICI Surf. UK] PEG-45 hydrog. castor oil; CAS 61788-85-0; solubilizer for perfumes and essential oils; yel. liq.; HLB 14.0.

Arlatone® 980. [ICI Spec. Chem.; ICI Surf. UK] PEG-35 hydrog. castor oil; CAS 61788-85-0; solubilizer for perfumes and essential oils; yel. liq.; HLB 12.8.

Arlatone® 983. [ICI Spec. Chem.; ICI Surf. UK] POE fatty acid ester; nonionic; emulsifier for personal care prods.; pale cream solid or sprayed; HLB 8.7; 100% conc.

Arlatone® 983S. [ICI Spec. Chem.; ICI Surf. Belgium] POE fatty acid ester; nonionic; emulsifier for o/w creams and lotions; powd.; HLB 8.7; 100% conc.

Arlatone® 985. [ICI Spec. Chem.; ICI Surf. Belgium] Ethoxylated stearyl stearate; nonionic; coemulsifier and visc. stabilizer for o/w milks; pale cream pellets; HLB 7.5; 100% conc.

Arlatone® 2121. [ICI Surf. Belgium] Sorbitan stearate and sucrose cocoate; nonionic; emulsifier for o/w creams and milks; tan flakes; HLB 6.0; 100% conc.

Arlatone® G. [ICI Spec. Chem.; ICI Surf. Am.; ICI Surf. Belgium] PEG-25 hydrog. castor oil; CAS 61788-85-0; nonionic; surfactant, solubilizer, coupling agent, emollient for personal care prods.; formulates clear gels; yel. visc. liq. to soft paste; sol. water, ethanol and IPA; sp.gr. 1.0; visc. 1400 cps; HLB 10.8; flash pt. > 300 F; 100% act.

Arlatone® SCI. [ICI Surf. Am.] Sodium cocoyl isethionate; EINECS 263-052-5; anionic; detergent for personal care prods.; wh. powd.

Arlatone® SCI-70. [ICI Surf. UK] Sodium cocoyl isethionate and palmitostearic acid; surfactant; wh. flakes.

Arlatone® T. [ICI Spec. Chem.; ICI Surf. Am.; ICI Surf. Belgium] PEG-40 sorbitan peroleate; nonionic; emulsifier, solubilizer, antistat, lubricant, spreading agent; for bath oils, household prods., textile industry; yel. liq.; sol. in veg., min. oils, IPM, IPP; water disp.; sp.gr. 1; visc. 175 cps; HLB 9.5; flash pt. > 300F; 100% act.

Arlenfil 4015. [Gattefosse] Triolein PEG-6 esters, ethoxydiglycol, and arnica extract.

Arlex. [ICI Surf. Am.] Sorbitol; CAS 50-70-4; EINECS 200-061-5; cosmetic/pharmaceutical ingred.

Arlypon® F. [Henkel KGaA/Cospha] Laureth-2; CAS 3055-93-4; EINECS 221-279-7; thickener for cosmetics, shampoos, shower baths, bath preps.; water-clear to sl. turbid liq., faint intrinsic odor; hyd. no. 182-188; cloud pt. 4-8 C; pH 6.5-8.0 (1%); usage level: 1-3%; 1% water.

Armeen® 2-10. [Akzo] Didecylamine; CAS 1120-49-6; cationic; surfactant for industrial and personal care use; Gardner 2 max.; sp.gr. 0.84 (20 C); m.p. -10 C; iodine no. 0.5; amine no. 181; flash pt. (PMCC) > 132 C; 93% min. sec. amine.

Armeen® 2-18 [Akzo] Dioctadecylamine; CAS 112-99-2;

cationic; surfactant for industrial and personal care use; Gardner 2 max.; sp.gr. 0.84 (75 C); visc. 11.7 cps (70 C); m.p. 80 C; iodine no. 1; amine no. 107; flash pt. (PMCC) > 149 C; 93% min. sec. amine.

Armeen® 2C. [Akzo] Dicocamine (sec. amine); CAS 61789-76-2; EINECS 263-086-0; cationic; emulsifier, flotation agent, corrosion inhibitor; also for cosmetics; Gardner 2 max. solid; sol. in chloroform, slightly sol. in IPA, toluene, CCl_4, kerosene; sp.gr. 0.793 (60/40 C); visc. 49.1 SSU (60 C); m.p. 104–117 F; pour pt. 80 F; iodine no. 8; amine no. 140; flash pt. (PMCC) > 149 C; 93% sec. amine.

Armeen® 2HT. [Akzo] Di(hydrog. tallow) amine (sec. amine); CAS 61789-79-5; EINECS 263-089-7; cationic; emulsifier, flotation agent, corrosion inhibitor; also for cosmetics; Gardner 2 max. solid; sp.gr. 0.79 (70 C); visc. 10.82 cps (70 C); m.p. 62 C; iodine no. 3; amine no. 110; flash pt. (PMCC) > 149 C; 93% sec. amine.

Armeen® 2S. [Akzo] Disoyamine; surfactant for industrial and personal care use.

Armeen® 2T [Akzo] Ditallowamine; CAS 68783-24-4; cationic; emulsifier, flotation agent, corrosion inhibitor; also for cosmetics; Gardner 2 max.; sp.gr. 0.79 (70 C); visc. 10.32 cps (70 C); m.p. 55 C; iodine no. 30; amine no. 110; flash pt. (PMCC) > 149 C; 93% min. sec. amine.

Armeen® 3-12 [Akzo] Tridodecylamine; CAS 102-87-4; EINECS 203-063-4; cationic; chemical intermediate for mfg. of sol. betaines and quat. ammonium salts; carrier for mfg. of citric acid and oil; also for cosmetics; Gardner 1 max. liq.; sp.gr. 0.82; m.p. -9 C; amine no. 102; flash pt. (PMCC) 190 C; 95% tert. amine.

Armeen® 3-16 [Akzo] Trihexadecylamine; CAS 67701-00-2; cationic; chemical intermediate for mfg. of oil-sol. betaines and quat. ammonium salts; also for cosmetics; Gardner 3 max. solid; m.p. 38 C; amine no. 82; flash pt. (PMCC) > 149 C; 98% tert. amine.

Armeen® 12. [Akzo] Lauramine; CAS 124-22-1; EINECS 204-690-6; surfactant for industrial and personal care use; Gardner 3 max. color; sp.gr. 0.80; visc. 7.37 cps; m.p. 24 C; iodine no. 1; amine no. 294; flash pt. (PMCC) > 149 C; 97% primary amine.

Armeen® 12D. [Akzo; Akzo BV] Lauramine (primary amine); CAS 124-22-1; EINECS 204-690-6; cationic; emulsifier, flotation agent, corrosion inhibitor; lubricant for metal treatment; also for cosmetics; Gardner 1 max. liq.; sol. in methanol, ethanol, acetone, IPA, chloroform, toluene, carbon tetrachloride, kerosene; sp.gr. 0.801; visc. 42.2 SSU; m.p. 24 C; iodine no. 1; amine no. 297; flash pt. (PMCC) > 149 C; pour pt. 80 F; 98% primary amine.

Armeen® 16. [Akzo] Palmitamine; CAS 143-27-1; EINECS 205-596-8; cationic; surfactant for industrial and personal care use; Gardner 3 max. color; sp.gr. 0.79; visc. 6.35 cps; m.p. 48 C; iodine no. 2; amine no. 226; flash pt. (PMCC) > 149 C; 98% primary amine.

Armeen® 16D. [Akzo; Akzo BV] Palmitamine (primary amine); CAS 143-27-1; EINECS 205-596-8; cationic; emulsifier, flotation agent, corrosion inhibitor; also for cosmetics; Gardner 1 max. solid; sol. in methanol, ethanol, IPA, chloroform, toluene, carbon tetrachloride, slightly sol. in acetone, kerosene; sp.gr. 0.789 (60/4 C); visc. 37.5 SSU (55 C); m.p. 100–118 F; iodine no. 2; amine no. 228; pour pt. 100 F; flash pt. (PMCC) > 149 C; 98% primary amine.

Armeen® 18. [Akzo; Akzo BV] Stearamine (primary amine); CAS 124-30-1; EINECS 204-695-3; cationic; emulsifier, flotation agent, corrosion inhibitor, anticaking agent; hard rubber mold release agent; also for cosmetics; Gardner 3 max. solid; sol. in ethanol, IPA, chloroform, toluene, CCl_4, slightly sol. in acetone, kerosene; sp.gr. 0.792 (60/4 C); visc. 45.6 SSU; m.p. 122–133 F; pour pt. 115 F; iodine no. 3; amine no. 202; flash pt. (PMCC) > 149 C; 97% primary

amine.

Armeen® 18D. [Akzo] Stearamine, dist.; CAS 124-30-1; EINECS 204-695-3; cationic; emulsifier, flotation agent, corrosion inhibitor, anticaking agent; rubber processing auxiliary; mold release agent for plastics and rubber; also for cosmetics; Gardner 1 max. solid; sol. in ethanol, IPA, chloroform, toluene, CCl_4, slightly sol. in methanol, kerosene; sp.gr. 0.791–0.792 (60/4 C); visc. 43.7 SSU; m.p. 122–133 F; pour pt. 110 F; iodine no. 3; amine no. 204; flash pt. (PMCC) > 149 C; 98% primary amine.

Armeen® C. [Akzo; Akzo BV] Cocamine (primary amine); CAS 61788-46-3; EINECS 262-977-1; cationic; emulsifier, flotation agent, corrosion inhibitor, stripping agent for paints; also for cosmetics; Gardner 3 max. liq.; sol. in methanol, ethanol, acetone, IPA, chloroform, toluene, CCl_4, kerosene; sp.gr. 0.805; visc. 44.2 SSU (35 C); m.p. 54–59 F; pour pt. 45 F; iodine no. 8; amine no. 272; flash pt. (PMCC) > 149 C; 97% primary amine.

Armeen® CD. [Akzo] Cocamine (primary amine); CAS 61788-46-3; EINECS 262-977-1; cationic; emulsifier, flotation agent, corrosion inhibitor, stripping agent for paints; also for cosmetics; Gardner 1 max. liq.; sol. in methanol, ethanol, acetone, IPA, chloroform, toluene, CCl_4, kerosene; sp.gr. 0.804; visc. 43 SSU (35 C); m.p. 57–63 F; pour pt. 55 F; iodine no. 8 C; amine no. 275; flash pt. (PMCC) > 149 C; 98% primary amine.

Armeen® DM8. [Akzo BV] Tert. amine; cationic; polyurethane catalyst; corrosion inhibitor; chemical intermediate; also for cosmetics; liq.; 98% conc.

Armeen® DM10. [Akzo BV] Tert. amine; cationic; polyurethane catalyst; corrosion inhibitor; chemical intermediate; also for cosmetics; liq.; 98% conc.

Armeen® DM12. [Akzo BV] Tert. amine; cationic; polyurethane catalyst; corrosion inhibitor; chemical intermediate; also for cosmetics; liq.; 98% conc.

Armeen® DM12D. [Akzo] Dimethyl lauramine; CAS 112-18-5; EINECS 203-943-8; cationic; surfactant intermediate; also for cosmetics; yel. liq.; amine odor; water insol.; sp.gr. 0.78; visc. 2.6 cps; f.p. –15 C; b.p. 80–115 C (3 mm Hg); iodine no. 0.5; amine no. 250; flash pt. (PMCC) > 149 C; 98% tert. amine.

Armeen® DM14. [Akzo BV] Tert. amine; cationic; polyurethane catalyst; corrosion inhibitor; chemical intermediate; also for cosmetics; liq.; 98% conc.

Armeen® DM14D. [Akzo] Dimethyl myristamine; CAS 112-75-4; EINECS 204-002-4; cationic; surfactant intermediate; also for cosmetics; yel. liq.; amine odor; water insol.; sp.gr. 0.79; visc. 4.7 cs; f.p. –8 C; b.p. 100–125 C (3 mm Hg); flash pt. 28 C (COC); 98% act.

Armeen® DM16. [Akzo BV] Tert. amine; cationic; polyurethane catalyst; corrosion inhibitor; chemical intermediate; also for cosmetics; liq.; 98% conc.

Armeen® DM16D. [Akzo] Dimethyl palmitamine; CAS 112-69-6; EINECS 203-997-2; cationic; chemical intermediate, raw material for surfactants; also for cosmetics; yel. liq.; amine odor; water insol.; sp.gr. 0.80; visc. 5.4 cps; f.p. 8 C; b.p. 100–136 C (3 mm Hg); iodine no. 0.5; amine no. 198; flash pt. (PMCC) > 149 C; 95% tert. amine.

Armeen® DM18D. [Akzo] Dimethyl stearamine; CAS 124-28-7; EINECS 204-694-8; cationic; chemical intermediate, raw material for surfactants; also for cosmetics; yel. liq., amine odor; water insol.; sp.gr. 0.79; visc. 7.5 cps; f.p. 20 C; b.p. 145–160 C (3 mm Hg); iodine no. 1; amine no. 180; flash pt. (PMCC) > 149 C; 95% tert. amine.

Armeen® DMC. [Akzo BV] Tert. amine; cationic; polyurethane catalyst; corrosion inhibitor; chemical intermediate; also for cosmetics; liq.; 98% conc.

Armeen® DMCD. [Akzo; Akzo BV] Dimethyl cocamine; CAS 61788-93-0; EINECS 263-020-0; cationic; chemical intermediate, raw material for surfactants; also for cosmetics;

yel. liq.; amine odor; water insol.; sp.gr. 0.79; visc. 3.1 cps; b.p. 42–150 C (3 mm); m.p. -22 C; iodine no. 10; amine no. 234; flash pt. (PMCC) > 149 C; 95% tert. amine.

Armeen® DMHT. [Akzo BV] Tert. amine; cationic; polyurethane catalyst; corrosion inhibitor; chemical intermediate; also for cosmetics; liq.; 98% conc.

Armeen® DMHTD. [Akzo; Akzo BV] Dimethyl hydrog. tallow amine; CAS 61788-95-2; EINECS 263-022-1; cationic; chemical intermediate, raw material for surfactants; also for cosmetics; yel. liq.; amine odor; water insol.; sp.gr. 0.80; visc. 7.0 cps; f.p. 18 C; b.p. 100–155 C; iodine no. 1; amine no. 184; flash pt. (PMCC) > 149 C; 95% tert. amine.

Armeen® DMMCD. [Akzo BV] Tert. amine; nonionic; chemical intermediate; solid; 100% conc.

Armeen® DMO. [Akzo BV] Tert. amine; cationic; polyurethane catalyst; corrosion inhibitor; chemical intermediate; also for cosmetics; liq.; 98% conc.

Armeen® DMOD. [Akzo] Oleyl dimethylamine; CAS 28061-69-0; cationic; surfactant intermediate; also for cosmetics; Gardner 1 max. liq.; sp.gr. 0.81; visc. 3.3 cps; m.p. -10 C; iodine no. 60; amine no. 183; flash pt. (PMCC) > 149 C; 95% tert. amine.

Armeen® DMSD. [Akzo] Soyaalkyl dimethylamine; CAS 61788-91-8; EINECS 263-017-4; cationic; surfactant intermediate; also for cosmetics; Gardner 2 max. liq.; sp.gr. 0.81; visc. 3.4 cps; m.p. -10 C; iodine no. 60; amine no. 183; flash pt. (PMCC) > 149 C; 95% tert. amine.

Armeen® DMT. [Akzo BV] Tert. amine; cationic; polyurethane catalyst; corrosion inhibitor; chemical intermediate; also for cosmetics; liq.; 98% conc.

Armeen® DMTD. [Akzo] Tallowalkyl dimethylamine; CAS 68814-69-7; cationic; surfactant intermediate; also for cosmetics; Gardner 1 max. liq.; sp.gr. 0.80 (38 C); visc. 6 cps; m.p. 5 C; iodine no. 42; amine no. 184; flash pt. (PMCC) > 149 C; 95% tert. amine.

Armeen® HT. [Akzo; Akzo BV] (Hydrog. tallow) amine (primary amine); CAS 61788-45-2; EINECS 262-976-6; cationic; emulsifier, flotation agent, corrosion inhibitor, chemical intermediate, anticaking agent; also for cosmetics; Gardner 9 solid; sol. in methanol, ethanol, IPA, chloroform, toluene, CCl$_4$, sp.gr. 0.795 (60/4 C); visc. 47.5 SSU (55 C); m.p. 79–136 F; cloud pt. 115 F; pour pt. 110 F; iodine no. 5; amine no. 207; flash pt. (PMCC) > 149 C; 97% primary amine.

Armeen® HTD. [Akzo; Akzo BV] (Hydrog. tallow) amine (primary amine); CAS 61788-45-2; EINECS 262-976-6; cationic; emulsifier, flotation agent, corrosion inhibitor, chemical intermediate, anticaking agent; also for cosmetics; Gardner 9 solid; sol. in methanol, ethanol, IPA, chloroform, toluene, CCl$_4$, sp.gr. 0.794 (60/4 C); visc. 44.1 SSU (55 C); m.p. 70–120 F; cloud pt. 110 F; pour pt. 100 F; iodine no. 5; amine no. 209; flash pt. (PMCC) > 149 C; 98% primary amine.

Armeen® L8D. [Akzo] 2-Ethylhexylamine, distilled; CAS 104-75-6; cationic; chemical intermediate for vapor phase corrosion inhibitors; also for cosmetics; Gardner 1 max. liq.; sp.gr. 0.79; visc. 4 cps; m.p. < -18 C; iodine no. < 1; amine no. 422; flash pt. (PMCC) 59 C; 98% primary amine.

Armeen® M2-10D. [Akzo] Didecyl methylamine; CAS 7396-58-9; EINECS 230-990-1; cationic; chemical intermediate for water-sol. betaines; catalyst for urethane resins; also for cosmetics; Gardner 1 max. liq.; sp.gr. 0.80; m.p. -4 C; iodine no. 0.5; amine no. 175; flash pt. (PMCC) > 132 C; 97% tert. amine.

Armeen® M2C. [Akzo; Akzo BV] Dicoco methylamine; CAS 61788-62-3; cationic; chemical intermediate; surfactant; for mfg. of oil-sol. betaines and quat. ammonium salts; also for cosmetics; Gardner 2 max. liq.; sp.gr. 0.81 (30 C);

visc. 26 cps (35 C); m.p. -2 C; iodine no. 8; amine no. 137; flash pt. (PMCC) 210 C; 97% tert. amine.

Armeen® M2HT [Akzo; Akzo BV] Dihydrogenated tallow methylamine; CAS 61788-63-4; EINECS 262-991-8; cationic; chemical intermediate; for mfg. of oil-sol. betaines and quat. ammonium salts; also for cosmetics; Gardner 1 max. solid; sp.gr. 0.81 (38 C); visc. 56 cps (30 C); m.p. 38 C; iodine no. 3; amine no. 105; flash pt. (PMCC) > 149 C; 97% tert. amine.

Armeen® N-CMD. [Akzo] N-coco morpholine; catalyst in PU foams; also for cosmetics; Gardner 3 liq.; sol. in acetone, IPA; sp.gr. 0.87; visc. 50 SSU (55 C); m.p. –29/–10 C; pour pt. -10 C; flash pt. 155 C (COC); 97% min. act.

Armeen® O. [Akzo; Akzo BV] Oleamine (primary amine); CAS 112-90-3; EINECS 204-015-5; cationic; emulsifier, wetting agent, corrosion inhibitor, dispersant, chemical intermediate, oil additive; cosmetics; Gardner 8 paste; sol. in acetone, methanol, ethanol, IPA, chloroform; toluene, carbon tetrachloride, kerosene, wh. min. oil; sp.gr. 0.820 (38/4 C); visc. 57.0 SSU; m.p. 50–68 F; flash pt. 320 F; 100% conc.

Armeen® OD. [Akzo] Oleamine (primary amine); CAS 112-90-3; EINECS 204-015-5; cationic; wetting agent, lube oil additive, emulsifier, corrosion inhibitor, cosmetic industry dispersant, chemical intermediate; Gardner 2 paste; water insol.; sp.gr. 0.79 (60 C); visc. 56.6 SSU; m.p. 8–18 C; flash pt. 154 C (COC); 98% act.

Armeen® OL. [Akzo] Oleamine; CAS 112-90-3; EINECS 204-015-5; cationic; emulsifier, flotation agent, corrosion inhibitor; also for cosmetics; Gardner 4 max. paste/liq.; sp.gr. 0.82 (38 C); visc. 8.15 cps (35 C); m.p. 20 C; iodine no. 85; amine no. 202; flash pt. (PMCC) > 149 C; 95% primary amine.

Armeen® OLD. [Akzo] Oleamine, dist.; CAS 112-90-3; EINECS 204-015-5; cationic; emulsifier, flotation reagent, corrosion inhibitor; also for cosmetics; Gardner 1 max. paste/liq.; sp.gr. 0.82 (38 C); visc. 8.15 cps (35 C); m.p. 21 C; iodine no. 85; amine no. 207; flash pt. (PMCC) > 149 C; 98% primary amine.

Armeen® S. [Akzo] Soyamine; CAS 61790-18-9; EINECS 263-112-0; cationic; emulsifier, flotation agent, corrosion inhibitor; also for cosmetics; Gardner 4 max.; sp.gr. 0.81 (38 C); visc. 8.04 cps (35 C); m.p. 29 C; iodine no. 70; amine no. 206; flash pt. (PMCC) > 149 C; 97% primary amine.

Armeen® SD. [Akzo] Soyamine, dist.; CAS 61970-18-9; EINECS 263-112-0; cationic; emulsifier, flotation agent, corrosion inhibitor; also for cosmetics; Gardner 3 paste; sol. in methanol, ethanol, acetone, IPA, chloroform, toluene, CCl$_4$; sp.gr. 0.81 (38/4 C); visc. 46.2 SSU (35 C); m.p. 81–86 F; cloud pt. 85 F; pour pt. 70 F; iodine no. 70; amine no. 208; flash pt. (PMCC) > 149 C; 98% primary amine.

Armeen® SZ. [Akzo BV] Amino acid; amphoteric; wetting agent in alkaline paint strippers, freeze/thaw stable latex emulsions, detergents, cosmetics; liq.; HLB 13.6; 40% conc.

Armeen® T. [Akzo; Akzo BV] Tallowamine (primary amine); CAS 61790-33-8; EINECS 263-125-1; cationic; emulsifier, flotation reagent, corrosion inhibitor, dispersant, anticaking agent, chemical intermediate, cosmetics ingredient; Gardner 11 paste; sol. in IPA, methanol, ethanol, chloroform, toluene, CCl$_4$; sp.gr. 0.813 (38/4 C); visc. 47 SSU (35 C); m.p. 64–117 F; cloud pt. 100 F; pour pt. 70 F; iodine no. 46; amine no. 208; flash pt. (PMCC) > 149 C; 97% primary amine.

Armeen® TD. [Akzo] Tallowamine, dist.; CAS 61790-33-8; EINECS 263-125-1; cationic; emulsifier, flotation agent, corrosion inhibitor; also for cosmetics; Gardner 2 paste; sol. in IPA, methanol, ethanol, chloroform, toluene, CCl$_4$; sp.gr. 0.812 (38/4 C); visc. 45.2 SSU (35 C); m.p. 64–118

F; cloud pt. 102 F; pour pt. 70 F; iodine no. 46; amine no. 210; flash pt. (PMCC) > 149 C; 98% primary amine.

Armeen® Z. [Akzo; Akzo BV] Cocaminobutyric acid; CAS 68649-05-8; EINECS 272-021-5; amphoteric; pigment softening, dispersing agent; antifogging agent, foam booster, stabilizer, wetting agent in alkaline paint strippers, latex emulsions, latex rubber reclamation, inks, plastic films, cosmetics; cooling tower corrosion inhibitor; Gardner 8 pumpable slurry; sol. in water, IPA, ethyl acetate; sp.gr. 0.98; visc. 247 SSU; flash pt. (TCC) 175 F; pour pt. 65 F; pH 6.5–7.5 (10% aq.); 100% conc.

Armid® 18. [Akzo] Stearamide, antiblock agent; CAS 124-26-5; EINECS 204-693-2; internal lubricant and slip agent for processed plastics, coatings, and films; builder, foam visc. stabilizer, and foam booster in syn. detergent formulations, cosmetics; water repellent for textiles; improves dye solubility in printing inks, dyes, carbon paper coatings, and fusible coatings for glassware and ceramics; intermediate for syn. waxes; pigment dispersant; thickener for paint; Gardner 7 flake; water-insol.; sp.gr. 0.52 (100 C); m.p. 99–109 C; flash pt. 225 C; 90% act.

Armid® O. [Akzo] Oleamide; CAS 301-02-0; EINECS 206-103-9; internal lubricant and slip agent for processed plastics, coatings, and films; builder, foam visc. stabilizer, and foam booster in syn. detergent formulations; water repellent for textiles; also release agent in cosmetics, penetrant in paper manufacture; Gardner 7 flake; solid; bland odor; m.w. 279; sol (g/100 ml soln. with heating) 59 g in 95% IPA; 30 g in 95% ethanol; 15 g in acetone and trichloroethylene; 11 g in ethyl acetate and MIBK; insol. in water; sp.gr. 0.830 (100 C); visc. 25 cps; m.p. 68 C; flash pt. 207 C; 90% act.

Armocare® E/C 100. [Akzo] Lauryl dimethylamine oleate; highly substantive emollient imparting slip, conditioning, and lubricity to skin and hair; Gardner 5 max. liq.; sp.gr. 0.863; pour pt. -6.7 C; flash pt. (PMCC) > 190 C; pH 6.8 ± 0.3 (1% aq. IPA).

Armocare® E/C 150. [Akzo] Distearyldimethylamine dimerate; highly substantive emollient imparting slip, conditioning, and lubricity to skin and hair; Gardner 4 max. liq.; sp.gr. 0.891; pour pt. 13 C; flash pt. (PMCC) > 190 C; pH 6.9 ± 0.3 (1% aq. IPA).

Armocare® E/C 151. [Akzo] Dicocodimethylamine dimerate; highly substantive emollient imparting slip, conditioning, and lubricity to skin and hair; Gardner 5 max. liq.; sp.gr. 0.893; pour pt. -1 C; flash pt. (PMCC) > 190 C; pH 6.8 ± 0.3 (1% aq. IPA).

Armocare® E/C 152. [Akzo] Lauryldimethylamine C21 dicarboxylate; highly substantive emollient imparting slip, conditioning, and lubricity to skin and hair; Gardner 6 max. liq.; sp.gr. 0.943; pour pt. 10 C; flash pt. (PMCC) 130 C; pH 6.4 ± 0.3 (1% aq. IPA).

Armocare® PA/11. [Akzo] Ditallowamidoethyl hydroxypropylamine; conditioner for personal care prods.

Armocare® PQ/11. [Akzo] Ditallowamidoethyl hydroxypropylmonium methosulfate; conditioner for personal care prods.

Armotan® ML. [Akzo BV] Sorbitan laurate; CAS 1338-39-2; nonionic; w/o emulsifier; liq.; 100% conc.

Armotan® MO. [Akzo BV] Sorbitan oleate; CAS 1338-43-8; EINECS 215-665-4; nonionic; w/o emulsifier for cosmetic and pharmaceutical preparations, used to make cutting and sol. oils; Gardner 8 liq.; sp.gr. 1.01; visc. 9.5–11 poise; pour pt. –12 C; 100% conc.

Armotan® MP. [Akzo BV] Sorbitan palmitate; CAS 26266-57-9; EINECS 247-568-8; nonionic; w/o emulsifier; waxy substance; 100% conc.

Armotan® MS. [Akzo BV] Sorbitan stearate; CAS 1338-41-6; EINECS 215-664-9; nonionic; w/o emulsifier; cream needle-like; m.p. 51–58 C; > 99% act.

Armotan® NP. [Akzo] Sorbitan palmitate; CAS 26266-57-9; EINECS 247-568-8; emulsifier.

Armotan® PML 20. [Akzo BV] PEG-20 sorbitan laurate; CAS 9005-64-5; nonionic; o/w emulsifier, solubilizer for bath oils; liq.; 100% conc.

Armotan® PMO 20. [Akzo BV] Polysorbate 80; CAS 9005-65-6; 37200-49-0; nonionic; o/w emulsifier; liq.; 100% conc.

Armoteric LB. [Akzo BV] Lauryl betaine; CAS 683-10-3; EINECS 211-669-5; amphoteric; surfactant for shampoo formulations; liq.

Arnica HS. [Novarom GmbH] Propylene glycol and arnica extract; botanical extract.

Arnica LS. [Novarom GmbH] Sunflower seed oil and arnica extract.

Arnica Distillate 2/378370. [Dragoco] Water, SD alcohol 39-C, and arnica extract.

Arnica Extract HS 2397 G. [Grau Aromatics] Propylene glycol and arnica extract; botanical extract.

Arnicaflower Oil PANAROM. [Novarom GmbH] Soybean oil, arnica extract, isopropyl myristate, and tocopherol.

Arnica Oil. [Provital; Centerchem] Sunflower seed oil and arnica extract.

Arnica Oil CLR. [Dr. Kurt Richter; Henkel/Cospha] Arnica extract, soybean oil, tocopherol; emollient, conditioner; protective skin and hair care prods.; herbal creams, oils, and lotions; yel. oil; herbal odor.

Aromaphyte™. [Active Organics] Range of whole plant extracts containing both the oil and water sol. active constituents; permits incorporation of essential oils into aq. surfactant systems, foam baths, shower gels, skin lotions and creams; natural fragrances permit "perfume-free" labeling.

Aromaphyte of Almond. [Active Organics] Propylene glycol, water, sweet almond extract, sweet almond oil; botanical extract.

Aromaphyte of Chamomile. [Active Organics] Propylene glycol, water, matricaria extract, matricaria oil; botanical extract.

Aromaphyte of Orange. [Active Organics] Propylene glycol, water, orange extract, orange oil; botanical extract.

Aromaphyte of Peppermint. [Active Organics] Propylene glycol, water, peppermint extract, peppermint oil; botanical extract.

Aromaplex™. [Active Organics] Blends of individual Aromaphytes; gives a range of aromatherapeutic effects.

Aromox® C/12. [Akzo] Dihydroxyethyl cocamine oxide, IPA; CAS 61791-47-7; EINECS 263-180-1; cationic; wetting agent, emulsifier, stabilizer, antistat, foaming agent for detergents, shampoos, cosmetics, textiles, metal plating, petrol. additives, paper, plastics, rubber; Gardner 2 clear liq.; sp.gr. 0.949; visc. 52 cp; cloud pt. 18 F; flash pt. 82 F; pour pt. 0 F; surf. tens. 33 dynes/cm; biodeg.; 50% act. in aq. IPA.

Aromox® C/12-W. [Akzo; Akzo BV] Dihydroxyethyl cocamine oxide; CAS 61791-47-7; EINECS 263-180-1; cationic; wetting agent, emulsifier, stabilizer, antistat, foaming agent for detergents, shampoos, cosmetics, textiles, metal plating, petrol. additives, paper, plastics, rubber; gel sensitizer for latex foam; biodeg.; Gardner 2 clear liq.; sp.gr. 0.997; visc. 2097 cp; HLB 18.4; flash pt. 212 F; pour pt. 35 F; surf. tens. 30.8 dynes/cm; 40% act. in water.

Aromox® DM14D-W. [Akzo BV] Myristamine oxide; CAS 3332-27-2; EINECS 222-059-3; nonionic; foam stabilizer for detergent and shampoo formulations; thickener; paste; HLB 12.2; 24% conc.

Aromox® DM16. [Akzo] Palmitamine oxide, IPA; CAS 7128-91-8; EINECS 230-429-0; cationic; suds and foam stabilizer for detergent and shampoo formulations; Gardner 1 clear liq.; sp.gr. 0.885; visc. 19 cp; cloud pt. 44 F; flash pt.

47

80 F; pour pt. 0 F; surf. tens. 31.6 dynes/cm; biodeg.; 40% act. in aq. IPA.

Aromox® DMB. [Akzo BV] Amine oxide; nonionic; foam stabilizer for detergent and shampoo formulations; thickener; liq.; 29% conc.

Aromox® DMC. [Akzo] Dimethylcocamine oxide; CAS 61788-90-7; EINECS 263-016-9; cationic; suds and foam stabilizer for detergent and shampoo formulations; liq.; 40% conc.

Aromox® DMCD. [Akzo] Cocamine oxide, IPA; CAS 61788-90-7; EINECS 263-016-9; detergent, thickener for household and cosmetic prods.; Gardner 1 max. liq.; sp.gr. 0.89; HLB 18.6; flash pt. (APCC) 21 C; pH 6–9; 39% min. act.

Aromox® DMC-W. [Akzo] Cocamine oxide; CAS 61788-90-7; EINECS 263-016-9; cationic; suds and foam stabilizer for detergent and shampoo formulations; Gardner 1 clear liq.; sp.gr. 0.971; visc. 17 cp; cloud pt. 34 F; flash pt. > 212 F; pour pt. 35 F; surf. tens. 32.5 dynes/cm; biodeg.; 30% act. in water.

Aromox® DMHT. [Akzo] Dimethyl hydrog. tallow amine oxide; CAS 68390-99-8; detergent, foam stabilizer; Gardner 7 max. liq. to paste; pH 7.0-9.0; flash (Seta) 23 C; 74% quat.

Aromox® DMHTD. [Akzo] Hydrog. tallow dimethylamine oxide; CAS 68390-99-8; cationic; suds and foam stabilizer for detergent and shampoo formulations; Gardner 1 max. liq.; sp.gr. 0.89; flash pt. 29 C (PMCC); 39% min act.

Aromox® DMMC-W. [Akzo] Lauramine oxide; CAS 1643-20-5; EINECS 216-700-6; cationic; wetting agent, emulsifier, foam stabilizer, antistat, foaming agent for detergents, shampoos; Gardner 1 clear liq.; sp.gr. 0.96; visc. 90 cp; cloud pt. 22 F; flash pt. > 212 F; pour pt. 36 F; surf. tens. 31.2 dynes/cm (0.1%); 30% act. in water.

Aromox® DMMCD-W. [Akzo BV] Amine oxide; nonionic; foam stabilizer for detergent and shampoo formulations; thickener; liq.; HLB 18.7; 30% conc.

Aromox® T/12. [Akzo; Akzo BV] Dihydroxyethyl tallow amine oxide, IPA; CAS 61791-46-6; EINECS 263-179-6; nonionic; suds and foam stabilizers for detergent and shampoo formualtions; Gardner 4 clear liq.; sp.gr. 0.94; visc. 77 cp; cloud pt. 60 F; flash pt. 90 F; pour pt. 55 F; surf. tens. 33.0 dynes/cm (0.1%); 50% act. in aq. IPA.

Arosurf® 32-E20. [Witco/H-I-P] PEG-20 oleyl ether; CAS 9004-98-2; nonionic; surfactant, solubilizer, emulsifier, stabilizer for personal care applics.; paste; HLB 11.3; 100% solids.

Arosurf® 42-E6. [Witco/H-I-P] Alkoxylated tallow alcohol; nonionic; emulsifier, detergent base; liq.; 100% conc.

Arosurf® 42-PE10. [Witco/H-I-P] Alkoxylated tallow alcohol; nonionic; low pour pt. detergent for heavy-duty laundry liqs. and personal care prods.; liq.; 100% conc.

Arosurf® 66-E2. [Witco/H-I-P] Isosteareth-2; CAS 52292-17-8; nonionic; emulsifier, emulsion stabilizer, emollient, moisturizer for personal care prods., creams and lotions, cutting oils; o/w and w/o systems; coupling agent, perfume stabilizer; plasticizer; Gardner 1 liq.; m.p. –5 C; HLB 4.6; pH 7 (1% DW); 100% solids.

Arosurf® 66-E10. [Witco/H-I-P] Isosteareth-10; CAS 52292-17-8; nonionic; emulsifier, emulsion stabilizer, emollient, moisturizer for personal care prods., creams and lotions; o/w and w/o systems; coupling agent, detergent; perfume solubilizer for micro emulsions in clear gel formulations; Gardner 1 semisolid; m.p. 22 C; HLB 12.0; pH 7 (1% DW); 100% conc.

Arosurf® 66-E20. [Witco/H-I-P] Isosteareth-20; CAS 52292-17-8; nonionic; emulsion stabilizer, emulsifier, moisturizer, and emollient for creams and lotions; plasticizer; perfume solubilizer for micro emulsions in clear gel formulations; Gardner 1 paste; m.p. 35 C; HLB 15.0; pH 7 (1% DW); 100% solids.

Arosurf® 66-PE12. [Witco/H-I-P] PPG-3-isosteareth-9; nonionic; low cloud pt. emulsifier, emollient, dispersant, bath oil spreading agent, perfume solubilizer; Gardner 1 liq.; m.p. –10 C; HLB 12.2; pH 7 (1% DW); 100% conc.

Arosurf® AA 23. [Witco/H-I-P] Diamine; cationic; asphalt emulsifier for rapid set and mixing grade emulsions; also for personal care applics.; soft solid; sp.gr. 0.84 (35/25 C); dens. 7.0 lb/gal (35 C); m.p. 31 C; pour pt. 31 C; 100% act.

Arosurf® MG-70. [Witco/H-I-P] Primary ether amine; cationic; flotation reagent for the iron mining industry; also for personal care applics.

Arosurf® TA-100. [Witco/H-I-P] Distearyl dimonium chloride; CAS 107-64-2; EINECS 203-508-2; cationic; fabric softener conc., conditioner for home and commerical laundry and textile processing; also for personal care prods.; Gardner 3 max. powd.; m.w. 583; water-disp.; flash pt. (PMCC) > 200 F; 93% quat. min.

Arosurf® TA-101. [Witco/H-I-P] Distearyl dimonium chloride, modified; CAS 107-64-2; EINECS 203-508-2; cationic; fabric softener for commercial and institutional laundries; imparts static control; also for personal care prods.; Gardner 4 max. powd.; disp. in water; bulk dens. 24 lb/ft³; flash pt. (PMCC) > 200 F; 100% solids.

Arova® N. [Hüls AG] 1,4-Dioxacyclohexadecane-5,16-dione; CAS 54982-83-1; fragrance material used in perfumery as a musk component and fixative; good stability in soaps; liq., mild musk odor; m.w. 256.3; dens. 1.059 kg/l; m.p. 19 C; b.p. 340 C; flash pt. 175 C; ≥ 98% purity.

Arquad® 2C-75. [Akzo; Akzo BV] Dicocodimonium chloride, aq. IPA; CAS 61789-77-3; EINECS 263-087-6; cationic; biodeg. emulsifier, foaming, wetting, dispersing agents, corrosion inhibitor, softener, dyeing aid, antistat for textiles, paper, cosmetics; industrial, agriculture, plastics, petrol. industry, acid pickling baths; bactericide, algicide; Gardner 7 semiliq.; sol. in alcohols, benzene, chloroform, CCl₄; disp. in water; m.w. 447; sp.gr. 0.89; HLB 11.4; flash pt. < 80 F; pour pt. 10 F; surf. tens. 30 dynes/cm (0.1%); pH 9; flamm.; 75% act. in aq. IPA.

Arquad® 2HT-75. [Akzo] Quaternium-18, aq. IPA; CAS 61789-80-8; cationic; biodeg. emulsifier, foaming, wetting, dispersing agents, corrosion inhibitor, antistat, bacteriostat for paper softening, household laundry, hair conditioning; soft wh. paste; sol. in alcohols, benzene, chloroform, CCl₄; disp. in water; m.w. 573; sp.gr. 0.87; dens. 7.22 lb/gal; visc. 47.5 cps (120 F); f.p. 95 F; HLB 9.7; flash pt. 112 F; pour pt. 90–100 F; surf. tens. 37 dynes/cm (0.1%); flamm.; 75% act. in aq. IPA.

Arquad® 2S-75. [Akzo] Disoyadimonium chloride.

Arquad® 2T. [Akzo] Ditallowdimonium chloride and IPA.

Arquad® 12-33. [Akzo] Laurtrimonium chloride, IPA; CAS 112-00-5; EINECS 203-927-0; cationic; emulsifier, foaming, wetting, dispersion agents, corrosion inhibitor, antistat for textiles, cosmetics, industrial, agric.; bactericide, algicide; Gardner 7 liq.; m.w. (act.) 263; sp.gr. 0.98; f.p. 5 F; HLB 17.1; flash pt. 140 F; pH 5–8 (10% aq.); biodeg.; 33% act. in aq. IPA.

Arquad® 12-37W. [Akzo] Laurtrimonium chloride; CAS 112-00-5; EINECS 203-927-0; cationic; emulsifier, corrosion inhibitor, textile softener, antistat, hair conditioner and combing aid emulsifier; biodeg.; Gardner 2 max. liq.; sol. in water, alcohols, chloroform, CCl₄; pH 6.5-9; nonflamm.; 35-39% quat. in water.

Arquad® 12-50. [Akzo] Laurtrimonium chloride, IPA; CAS 112-00-5; EINECS 203-927-0; cationic; biodeg. emulsifier, foaming, wetting, dispersing agents, corrosion inhibitor, softener, dyeing aid, antistat for textiles, paper, cosmetics; industrial, agriculture, plastics, petrol. industry, acid pickling baths; bactericide, algicide; gel sensitizer for latex foam; Gardner 1 liq.; sol. in water, alcohols, chloroform, CCl₄; m.w. (act.) 263; sp.gr. 0.89; f.p. 13 F; HLB

48

17.1; flash pt. < 80 F; surf. tens. 33 dynes/cm; pH 5–8 (10% aq.); 50% act. in aq. IPA.

Arquad® 16-25. [Akzo] Cetrimonium chloride, isopropyl alcohol; CAS 112-02-7; EINECS 203-928-6; quat. for personal care prods.

Arquad® 16-25W. [Akzo] Cetrimonium chloride; CAS 112-02-7; EINECS 203-928-6; quat. for personal care prods.

Arquad® 16-29. [Akzo] Cetrimonium chloride; CAS 112-02-7; EINECS 203-928-6; cationic; emulsifier, foaming, wetting, dispersion agents, corrosion inhibitor, antistat for textiles, cosmetics, industrial, agric.; bactericide, algicide; Gardner 6 liq.; m.w. (act.) 319; sp.gr. 0.96; f.p. 61 F; HLB 15.8; flash pt. > 212 F; pH 5–8 (10% aq.); biodeg.; 29% act. in water.

Arquad® 16-29W. [Akzo] Cetrimonium chloride; CAS 112-02-7; EINECS 203-928-6; cationic; emulsifier, corrosion inhibitor, textile softener, antistatic agent, hair conditioner and combing aid emulsifier; biodeg.; Gardner 3 max. liq.; sol. in water, alcohols, chloroform, CCl_4; pH 6-9; nonflamm.; 27-30% quat. in water.

Arquad® 16-50. [Akzo; Akzo BV] Cetrimonium chloride, IPA; CAS 112-02-7; EINECS 203-928-6; cationic; emulsifier, foaming, wetting, dispersing agents, corrosion inhibitor, softener, dyeing aid, antistat for textiles, paper, cosmetics; industrial, agriculture, plastics, petrol. industry, acid pickling baths; bactericide, algicide; rubber to textile bonding agent; biodeg.; Gardner 6 liq.; sol. in water, alcohols, chloroform, CCl_4; m.w. (act.) 319; sp.gr. 0.88; f.p. 61 F; HLB 15.8; flash pt. < 80 F; surf. tens. 34 dynes/cm; pH 5–8 (10% aq.); 49-52% quat. in aq. IPA.

Arquad® 18-50. [Akzo; Akzo BV] Steartrimonium chloride, IPA; CAS 112-03-8; EINECS 203-929-1; cationic; emulsifier, foaming, wetting, dispersing agents, corrosion inhibitor, softener, dyeing aid, antistat for textiles, paper, cosmetics; industrial, agriculture, plastics, petrol. industry, acid pickling baths; bactericide, algicide; dye leveling agent, visc. stabilizer, in lubricant compding.; biodeg.; Gardner 7 liq.; sol. in water, alcohols, chloroform, CCl_4; m.w. (act.) 347; sp.gr. 0.88; HLB 15.7; flash pt. < 80 F; surf. tens. 34 dynes/cm; pH 5–8 (10% aq.); 50% act. in aq. IPA.

Arquad® 316. [Akzo] Tricetylmonium chloride; CAS 52467-63-7.

Arquad® B-50. [Akzo BV] Quat. ammonium compd.; cationic; emulsifier, bactericide, algicide, soil stabilizer, cosmetics ingred., textile antistat, flocculant, fabric softener, decolorizing aid; demulsifier in tetracycline processing; liq.; 50% conc.

Arquad® B-90. [Akzo BV] Quat. ammonium compd.; cationic; emulsifier, bactericide, algicide, soil stabilizer, cosmetics ingred., textile antistat, flocculant, fabric softener, decolorizing aid; demulsifier in tetracycline processing; liq.; 90% conc.

Arquad® B-100. [Akzo] Benzalkonium chloride, aq. IPA; CAS 68391-01-5; cationic; antimicrobial for industrial applics., sec. oil recovery, textiles, cosmetics, pharmaceuticals, sanitizers; Gardner 2 liq.; sol. in acetone, alcohol, most polar solvs., water; m.w. 380; sp.gr. 0.967; pour pt. 0 F; flash pt. (PMCC) 32 C; pH 7–8; 50% act. in aq. IPA.

Arquad® C-33W. [Akzo] Cocotrimonium chloride; CAS 61789-18-2; EINECS 263-038-9; cationic; emulsifier, corrosion inhibitor, textile softener, antistat; hair conditioning and combing aid emulsifier; emulsion-break retardant in cosmetics; biodeg.; Gardner 4 max. liq.; sol. in water, alcohols, chloroform, CCl_4; sp.gr. 0.96; f.p. –3 C; nonflamm.; pH 5–8; 32–35% act. in water.

Arquad® C-50. [Akzo; Akzo BV] Cocotrimonium chloride, IPA; CAS 61789-18-2; EINECS 263-038-9; cationic; biodeg. emulsifier, foaming, wetting, dispersing agents, corrosion inhibitor, softener, dyeing aid, antistat for textiles, paper, cosmetics; industrial, agriculture, plastics,

petrol. industry, acid pickling baths; bactericide, algicide; gel sensitizer for latex foam; Gardner 7 liq.; sol. in water, alcohols, chloroform, CCl_4; m.w. (active) 278; sp.gr. 0.89; f.p. 5 F; HLB 16.5; flash pt. < 80 F; surf. tens. 31 dynes/cm (0.1%); pH 5–8 (10% aq.); 50% act. in aq. IPA.

Arquad® DM14B-90. [Akzo; Akzo BV] Myristyl dimethylbenzyl ammonium chloride dihydrate; CAS 139-08-2; EINECS 205-352-0; cationic; bactericide, fungicide, germicide, disinfectant; cosmetics, textiles, soil stabilization; wh. powd.; 90% act.

Arquad® DMMCB-50. [Akzo; Akzo BV] Alkyl (C12,C14,C16) dimethyl benzyl ammonium chloride; cationic; antistat, flocculant, emulsifier, softener, corrosion inhibitor used in cosmetics, soil stabilization, textiles, fabric softener, fungicide, bactericide; liq.; 50% act.

Arquad® DNHTB-75. [Akzo BV] Lauryl betaine; CAS 683-10-3; EINECS 211-669-5; detergent.

Arquad® DNMCB-50. [Akzo BV] Cocoalkonium chloride; CAS 61789-71-7; EINECS 263-080-8.

Arquad® HC. [Akzo BV] Quaternium-18; CAS 61789-80-8; EINECS 263-090-2; hair conditioner and antistat.

Arquad® HT-50. [Akzo] Hydrog. tallowtrimonium chloride; CAS 61788-78-1; EINECS 263-005-9; emulsifier, conditioner.

Arquad® HTL8-Cl. [Akzo] Stearyl octyldimonium chloride; conditioner for hair care prods.

Arquad® HTL8-MS. [Akzo] Stearyl octyldimonium methosulfate; conditioner for hair care prods.

Arquad® S-50. [Akzo; Akzo BV] Soytrimonium chloride, IPA; CAS 61790-41-8; EINECS 263-134-0; cationic; emulsifier, corrosion inhibitor, textile softener, antistat; hair conditioning and combing aid emulsifier; bitumen emulsions; slime control agent in water systems; biodeg.; Gardner 8 max. liq.; sol. in water, alcohols, chloroform, CCl_4; m.w. 343; sp.gr. 0.89; HLB 15.6; f.p. 20 C; flash pt. (PM) < 80 F; pH 5–8 (10% aq.); 49–52% act. in IPA.

Arquad® T-27W. [Akzo] Tallow trimonium chloride; CAS 8030-78-2; EINECS 232-447-4; biodeg. emulsifier, foaming, wetting, dispersing agents, corrosion inhibitor, softener, dyeing aid, antistat for textiles, paper, cosmetics; industrial, agriculture, plastics, petrol. industry, acid pickling baths; bactericide, algicide; Gardner 3 max. liq.; sol. in water, alcohols, chloroform, CCl_4; m.w. 343; HLB 14.2; pH 5–8 (10% aq.); 26–29% act. in water.

Arquad® T-30. [Akzo BV] Tallowtrimonium chloride; CAS 8030-78-2; EINECS 232-447-4; cosmetic ingred.

Arquad® T-50. [Akzo; Akzo BV] Tallowtrimonium chloride, aq. IPA; CAS 8030-78-2; EINECS 232-447-4; cationic; emulsifier, corrosion inhibitor, textile softener, antistat; hair conditioning and combing aid emulsifier; also used in mfg. of antibiotics; gel sensitizer for latex foam; biodeg.; Gardner 8 max. liq.; sol. in water, alcohols, chloroform, CCl_4; m.w. 340; sp.gr. 0.881; HLB 14.2; flash pt. < 80 F (PM); pour pt. 15–48 F; pH 5–8 (10% aq.); biodeg.; 50% act. in aq. IPA.

Arrectosina. [Vevy] Zinc citrate and propylene glycol citrate.

Artodan CF 40. [Grindsted Prods.] Calcium stearoyl lactylate; CAS 5793-94-2; EINECS 227-335-7; emulsifier.

Artodan SP 55 Kosher. [Grindsted Prods.; Grindsted Prods. Denmark] Sodium stearyl-2-lactylate; CAS 25383-99-7; EINECS 246-929-7; anionic; food emulsifier, dough conditioner, starch complexing agent, bread improver, freeze/thaw emulsions; also for cosmetics/toiletries; sm. beads; HLB 10.0; 100% act.

Aruba Aloe Vera Gel. [Aruba Aloe Balm] Aloe vera gel; moisturizer, soothing/healing aid for personal care.

Ascorbic Acid Ampul Type No. 604065700. [Roche] Ascorbic acid; CAS 50-81-7; EINECS 200-066-2; acidulant for cosmetic applics.

Ascorbic Acid Fine Granular No. 6045655. [Roche] Ascorbic acid USP, FCC; CAS 50-81-7; EINECS 200-066-2; acidulant for cosmetic applics.; fine gran.

Ascorbic Acid Ultra-Fine Powd. No. 604565300. [Roche] Ascorbic acid; CAS 50-81-7; EINECS 200-066-2; acidulant for cosmetic applics.

Ascorbic Acid USP, FCC Type S No. 604566. [Roche] Ascorbic acid USP, FCC; CAS 50-81-7; EINECS 200-066-2; acidulant for cosmetic applics.

Ascorbosilane C. [Exsymol; Biosil Tech.] Ascorbyl methylsilanol pectinate; cosmetic ingred. for anti-aging formulations, after sun bath treatments, superficial burn treatments; colorless to pale yel. sl. opalescent liq.; misc. with water, alcohols, glycols; sp.gr. 1.0; pH 6.0; usage level: 3-4%; toxicology: nontoxic.

Ascorbyl Palmitate No. 60412. [Roche] Ascorbyl palmitate FCC; CAS 137-66-6; EINECS 205-305-4; antioxidant for cosmetics; fat-sol. form of ascorbic acid.

Asebiol® . [Laboratoires Sérobiologiques] Amino acids, sulfur peptides, and vitamin B complex; biotechnological active for oily skin care; regulates sebaceous secretions of acneic skin; amber limpid liq.; water-sol.; usage level: 5-10%.

Asebiol® LS. [Laboratoires Sérobiologiques] Water, hydrolyzed serum protein, hydrolyzed yeast protein, pyridoxine, niacinamide, panthenol, propylene glycol, allantoin, and biotin.

Aseptoform. [R.W. Greeff] Methylparaben; CAS 99-76-3; EINECS 202-785-7; cosmetics preservative.

Asol. [Lucas Meyer] Lecithin fraction; CAS 8002-43-5; EINECS 232-307-2; nonionic; antispatter agent, release agent, emulsifier for food, cosmetics, pharmaceuticals; liq.; 40–100% conc.

Asparlyne. [C.E.P.] Lysine aspartate.

ASU Complex. [Expanchimie] Soybean oil unsaponifiables, avocado oil unsaponifiables.

ATBC. [Morflex] Acetyltri-n-butyl citrate; CAS 77-90-7; EINECS 201-067-0; aq. based pharmaceutical coating.

ATEC. [Morflex] Acetyltriethyl citrate; CAS 77-89-4; EINECS 201-066-5; aq. based pharmaceutical coating.

Ateco. [Herstellung von Naturextrakten GmbH; Lipo] Soluble collagen; CAS 9007-34-5; EINECS 232-697-4; water-binding film-former, moisture regulator used in face creams/masks, collagen ampoules, body lotions, after-sun lotions, hair conditioning treatments; visc. opalescent sol'n., weak intrinsic odor; m.w. 285,000; pH 3.5-4.0; 1% sol'n.

Atelo-Collagen. [Rona; E. Merck] Atelocollagen; CAS 9007-34-5; cosmetic protein.

Atelocollagen M. [Koken] Atelocollagen; CAS 9007-34-5; cosmetic protein.

Atelocollagen MS. [Koken] Atelocollagen; CAS 9007-34-5; cosmetic protein.

Atelocollagen SS. [Koken] Atelocollagen; CAS 9007-34-5; cosmetic protein.

Ateloglycane. [Gattefosse SA] Soluble collagen and glycosaminoglycans complex; biological additive providing moisturization, elasticity, and suppleness to cutaneous tissues and seborrheic flow reduction and improvement to hair; for skin care nutritive prods., capillar prods. (regenerating lotions); liq.

Atlas White Titanium Dioxide. [HK Color Group] Titanium dioxide; CAS 13463-67-7; EINECS 236-675-5; mineral sunscreen.

Atmos 150. [ICI Am.; ICI Surf. UK] Glyceryl stearate; nonionic; surfactant, emulsifier for cosmetic creams and lotions; food emulsifier; antistat for plastics (PP, PS) useful in food pkg.; ivory wh. beads; bland odor and taste; sol. above its m.p. in veg. oils, min. oil, IPA; m.p. 140 F; HLB 3.2; flash pt. > 300 F; 100% conc.

Atmos 300. [ICI Am.; ICI Surf. UK] Glyceryl oleate and

propylene glycol; nonionic; surfactant, emulsifier for cosmetic creams, lotions; food emulsifier; clear yel. liq.; sol. in cottonseed oil, IPA; sp.gr. 0.96; visc. 130 cps; HLB 2.8; flash pt. > 300 F; 100% act.

Atomergic Allantoin. [Atomergic Chemetals] Allantoin; CAS 97-59-6; EINECS 202-592-8; skin protectant.

Atomergic Carboxymethyl Chitin. [Atomergic Chemetals] Sodium carboxymethyl chitin.

Atomergic Carmine. [Atomergic Chemetals] Carmine; CAS 1390-65-4; EINECS 215-724-4; cosmetic colorant.

Atomergic Chitin. [Atomergic Chemetals] Chitin; CAS 1398-61-4; EINECS 215-744-3.

Atomergic Chitosan. [Atomergic Chemetals] Chitosan; CAS 9012-76-4.

Atomergic Cholesterol. [Atomergic Chemetals] Cholesterol; CAS 57-88-5; EINECS 200-353-2; emulsifier, moisturizer.

Atomergic Cocoa Butter. [Atomergic Chemetals] Cocoa butter; CAS 8002-31-1; skin conditioner.

Atomergic Cod Liver Oil. [Atomergic Chemetals] Cod liver oil; CAS 8001-69-2; EINECS 232-289-6.

Atomergic Denatonium Benzoate. [Atomergic Chemetals] Denatonium benzoate; CAS 3734-33-6; EINECS 223-095-2.

Atomergic Denatonium Saccharide. [Atomergic Chemetals] Denatonium saccharide.

Atomergic Hyaluronic Acid. [Atomergic Chemetals] Hyaluronic acid; CAS 9004-61-9; EINECS 232-678-0; cosmetics moisturizer.

Atomergic Imidazolidinyl Urea. [Atomergic Chemetals] Imidazolidinyl urea; CAS 39236-46-9; EINECS 254-372-6; cosmetic preservative.

Atomergic Jojoba Oil. [Atomergic Chemetals] Jojoba oil; CAS 61789-91-1; cosmetic emollient.

Atomergic Lead Acetate. [Atomergic Chemetals] Lead acetate; CAS 301-04-2; EINECS 206-104-4.

Atomergic Propyl Gallate. [Atomergic Chemetals] Propyl gallate; CAS 121-79-9; EINECS 204-498-2; cosmetic antioxidant.

Atomergic Ribonucleic Acid. [Atomergic Chemetals] RNA; CAS 63231-63-0.

Atomergic Royal Jelly. [Atomergic Chemetals] Royal jelly; CAS 8031-67-2.

Atomergic Sodium Chondroitin Sulfate. [Atomergic Chemetals] Sodium chondroitin sulfate; EINECS 232-696-9.

Atomergic Tannic Acid. [Atomergic Chemetals] Tannic acid; CAS 1401-55-4; EINECS 215-753-2.

Atomergic Water Soluble Chitin. [Atomergic Chemetals] Sodium carboxymethyl chitin.

Atomergic Zinc Pyrithione. [Atomergic Chemetals] Zinc pyrithione; CAS 13463-41-7; EINECS 236-671-3; anti-dandruff agent, antimicrobial.

ATP Nucleotides. [Croda Inc.] Propylene glycol, collagen amino acids, adenosine triphosphate; moisturizer; clear liq.; water-sol.; m.w. 150-500; usage level: 1-5%; 5% act.

Atrinon. [Henkel/Cospha] Aroma chemical for cosmetic, personal care, detergent, and cleaning prods.; sl. yel. liq., woody odor; b.p. 82-89 C; flash pt. 123 C.

Atsurf 594. [ICI Surf. Am.; ICI Surf. UK] Glyceryl oleate; emulsifier for personal care and industrial applics.; amber visc. liq.; HLB 3.8.

Attasorb RVM Sorbent. [Engelhard] Attapulgite; CAS 1337-76-4; thickener and suspending agent.

Aubygel X52. [Laserson SA] Carrageenan; CAS 9000-07-1; EINECS 232-524-2; gellant, thickener, suspension stabilizer for cosmetics; forms translucent gels in presence of KCl, NaCl; JSCI and Europe compliance; wh., creamy, or clear beige powd., odorless and tasteless; sol. in water; insol. in oils and org. solvs.; usage level: 1-5%.

Augon 1000. [Vevy] Lecithin; CAS 8002-43-5; EINECS 232-307-2; emulsifier.

Aurantiol®. [BASF AG] Schiff base of hydroxycitronellal and methyl anthranilate; fragrance for cosmetics; sweetly floral.

Autolyzed Silk. [Freeman] Hydrolyzed silk; CAS 96690-41-4; cosmetic protein.

Autolyzed Silk Protein. [Freeman] Hydrolyzed silk; CAS 96690-41-4; cosmetic protein.

Auxina Tricogena. [Vevy] Alcohol, water, coltsfoot extract, yarrow extract, cinchona extract; botanical extract.

Avamid 150. [Mona Industries] Avocadamide DEA, avocado oil; biodeg. SE foam stabilizer, visc. builder, conditioner, lubricant for conditioning shampoos, hair rinses, creams and lotions; imparts smooth, silky feel to skin and hair; clear amber liq.; pH 10.5 (10%); 100% act.

Avanel® S-30. [PPG/Specialty Chem.] Sodium C12-15 pareth-3 sulfonate; anionic; biodeg. mild surfactant, emulsifier for personal care, household, institutional and industrial prods.; stable in presence of hypochlorite and over entire pH range; wh. paste; sol. in water and inorg. sol'ns.; m.w. 420; sp.gr. 1.06; visc. 360 cps (35 C); solid. pt. 25 C; flash pt. 130 F; 35% conc., 5% ethanol.

Avanel® S-35. [PPG/Specialty Chem.] Sodium octoxynol-2 ethane sulfonate; anionic; mild, stable emulsifier for creams, lotions, and liq. soaps; liq.; 28% conc.

Avanel® S-70. [PPG/Specialty Chem.] Sodium C12-15 pareth-7 sulfonate; anionic; biodeg. mild surfactant, wetting agent, and emulsifier for personal care, household, institutional and industrial prods.; stable in presence of hypochlorite and over entire pH range; low irritation, moderate foaming; clear liq., odorless; sol. in water and various inorg. sol'ns.; m.w. 600; sp.gr. 1.07; visc. 270 cps; solid. pt. -1 C; flash pt. 200 F; 35% conc.

Avanel® S-74. [PPG/Specialty Chem.] Sodium alkyl ether sulfonate; anionic; biodeg. mild surfactant, emulsifier for personal care, household, institutional and industrial prods.; stable in presence of hypochlorite and over entire pH range; clear liq., odorless; sol. in water and various inorg. sol'ns.; m.w. 260; sp.gr. 1.10; visc. 30 cps; solid. pt. -8 C; flash pt. 200 F; 35% conc.

Avanel® S-90. [PPG/Specialty Chem.] Sodium C12-15 pareth-9 sulfonate; biodeg. mild surfactant, emulsifier for personal care, household, institutional and industrial prods.; stable in presence of hypochlorite and over entire pH range; clear liq., odorless; sol. in water and various inorg. sol'ns.; m.w. 690; sp.gr. 1.07; visc. 60 cps; solid. pt. -1 C; flash pt. 200 F.

Avanel® S-150. [PPG/Specialty Chem.] Sodium C12-15 pareth-15 sulfonate; anionic; biodeg. mild surfactant, emulsifier with counter-irritant props. for personal care, household, institutional and industrial prods.; stable in presence of hypochlorite and over entire pH range; almost colorless liq., odorless; sol. in water and inorg. sol'ns.; m.w. 950; sp.gr. 1.07; visc. 70 cps; solid. pt. -1 C; flash pt. 200 F; 35% conc.

Avian Sodium Hyaluronate Powd. [Intergen] Sodium hyaluronate; CAS 9067-32-7; moisturizer.

Avian Sodium Hyaluronate Sol'n. [Intergen] Sodium hyaluronate; CAS 9067-32-7; moisturizer.

Avicel PH-101. [FMC] Microcryst. cellulose NF; CAS 9004-34-6; binder, disintegrant, flow aid, and filler for pharmaceuticals and animal health prods.; absorbent; peptizing agent; anticaking agent for oils to make sticky substances free flowing; wh. powd., < 30% +200 mesh; odorless; insol. but disp. in water; pH 5.5-7.0.

Avicel RC-591. [FMC] Microcryst. cellulose, cellulose gum; cosmetic base; lg. surf. area for absorbing ingred. matrix onto RC; opacifier for wh. lotions and creams; adsorbent for dry cream bases and sachets; water-insol.

Avocado Extract HS 2384 G. [Grau Aromatics] Propylene glycol and avocado extract; botanical extract.

Avocado Oil. [Natural Oils Int'l.; Tri-K Industries] Avocado oil; CAS 8024-32-6; EINECS 232-428-0; cosmetic ingred.; pale straw/green clear prod., pleasant odor, bland taste; insol. in water; sp.gr. 0.908-0.920; congeal pt. -5 F; iodine no. 65-95; sapon. no. 177-198; flash pt. 640 F; ref. index 1.460-1.479 (40 C); toxicology: nonhazardous; edible; 0.05% max. moisture.

Avocado Oil. [Provital; Centerchem] Avocado oil; CAS 8024-32-6; EINECS 232-428-0.

Avocado Oil CLR. [Dr. Kurt Richter; Henkel/Cospha] Avocado oil; CAS 8024-32-6; EINECS 232-428-0; emollient; conditioner for protective skin and hair care preparations; ylsh.-grn. to brnsh.-grn. oil; faint char. odor.

Avocado Oil W. [Cosmetochem] PEG-11 avocado glycerides; cosmetic ingred.

Awapuhi Extract. [Bell Flavors & Fragrances] Propylene glycol and white ginger extract; botanical extract.

Azulene 25% WS 2/013000. [Dragoco] PEG-40 castor oil and guaiazulene.

Azulene 50% 2/012990. [Dragoco] Guaiazulene and min. oil; colorant for cosmetics.

Azulene 100% 2/912980. [Dragoco] Guaiazulene; CAS 489-84-9; EINECS 207-701-2; colorant for cosmetics.

B

B-122. [Guardian Labs] Calcium stearate and stearic acid.

B-3279 Cosmetic Brown. [HK Color Group] Iron oxides; cosmetic colorant.

B-3389 Cosmetic Umber. [HK Color Group] Iron oxides and talc; cosmetic colorant.

Babyderme HS 265. [Alban Muller] Propylene glycol, myrrh extract, calendula extract, carrot seed extract, matricaria extract, and sambucus extract; phytocomplex for baby skin care prods.

Babyderme HS 342. [Alban Muller] Propylene glycol, pellitory extract, mallow extract, carrot seed extract, and elm bark extract; phytocomplex for baby skin care.

Babyderme LS 642. [Alban Muller] Sunflower seed oil, pellitory extract, mallow extract, elm bark extract, and carrot seed extract; phytocomplex for baby skin care prods.

Babyderme LS 665. [Alban Muller] Sunflower seed oil, myrrh extract, calendula extract, carrot seed extract, matricaria extract, and sambucus extract; ingred. for baby skin care prods.

Bactericide MB 2/012582. [Dragoco] Butylene glycol, ethylparaben, methylparaben, and propylparaben; antimicrobial.

Bactiphen 2506 G. [Grau Aromatics] Phenoxyethanol, methylparaben, ethylparaben, propylparaben, and butylparaben; antimicrobial.

Balm Mint HS. [Alban Muller] Propylene glycol and balm mint extract; botanical extract.

Balm Mint Oil Infusion. [Novarom GmbH] Peanut oil, balm mint extract, isopropyl myristate, and tocopherol; botanical extract.

Bardac® 2050. [Lonza] Quaternium-24, dioctyldimonium chloride, didecyldimonium chloride; disinfectant, sanitizer, bacteriostat cleared by FDA at only 150 ppm for use in "no rinse" sanitizing sol'ns.; FDA approved; 50% liq.

Bardac® 2250. [Lonza] Didecyldimonium chloride; CAS 7173-51-5; EINECS 230-525-2; disinfectant, sanitizer; 50% liq.

Barlene® 12. [Lonza] Alkyl dimethyl amine; chemical intermediate; personal care additive; liq.; 95% act.

Barlene® 12C. [Lonza] Dimethyl cocamine; CAS 61788-93-0; EINECS 263-020-0; surfactant intermediate.

Barlene® 12S. [Lonza] Dimethyl lauramine; CAS 112-18-5; EINECS 203-943-8; chemical intermediate; personal care additive; liq.; 95% act.

Barlene® 14. [Lonza] Dimethyl myristamine; CAS 112-75-4; EINECS 204-002-4; surfactant intermediate.

Barlene® 14S. [Lonza] Dimethyl myristamine; CAS 112-75-4; EINECS 204-002-4; chemical intermediate; personal care additive; liq.; 95% act.

Barlene® 16S. [Lonza] Cetyl dimethyl amine; CAS 112-69-6; EINECS 203-997-2; chemical intermediate; personal care additive; liq./solid; 95% act.

Barlene® 18S. [Lonza] Stearyl dimethyl amine; CAS 124-28-7; EINECS 204-694-8; chemical intermediate; personal care additive; solid; 95% act.

Barlox® 10S. [Lonza] Decylamine oxide; CAS 2605-79-0; EINECS 220-020-5; nonionic; detergent; visc. builder, emollient; liq.; 30% conc.

Barlox® 12. [Lonza] Cocamine oxide; CAS 61788-90-7; EINECS 263-016-9; nonionic/cationic; detergent; visc. builder, foam stabilizer, emulsifier, conditioner, and emollient for personal care and industrial prods.; liq.; visc. 45 cps; pour pt. 4 C; pH 7.0 (1%); surf. tens. 32.3 dynes/cm (0.1%); Draves wetting 4 s; 30% conc.

Barlox® 14. [Lonza] Myristamine oxide; CAS 3332-27-2; EINECS 222-059-3; nonionic/cationic; detergent; visc. builder, emollient; liq.; visc. 60 cps; pour pt. 2 C; pH 7.0 (1%); surf. tens. 31.0 dynes/cm (0.1%); Draves wetting 5 s; 30% conc.

Barlox® 16S. [Lonza] Cetamine oxide; CAS 7128-91-8; EINECS 230-429-0; biodeg. foam stabilizer, visc. builder, emulsifier, conditioner for personal care and industrial prods.; paste; visc. 27,000 cps; pH 7.0 (1%); surf. tens. 32.4 dynes/cm (0.1%); Draves wetting 9 s; 30% act.

Barlox® 18S. [Lonza] Stearyl dimethyl amine oxide; CAS 2571-88-2; EINECS 219-919-5; biodeg. foam stabilizer, visc. builder, emulsifier, conditioner for personal care and industrial prods.; paste; 25% act.

Barlox® C. [Lonza] Cocamidopropylamine oxide; CAS 68155-09-9; EINECS 268-938-5; nonionic/cationic; foam stabilizer and visc. builder for shampoos, industrial prods.; liq.; visc. 36 cps; pour pt. 4 C; pH 7.0 (1%); surf. tens. 35.4 dynes/cm (0.1%); Draves wetting 27 s; 30% conc.

Barquat® CME-35. [Lonza] Cetethyl morpholinium ethosulfate; CAS 78-21-7; EINECS 201-094-8; antistat, combing aid and detangling agent, textile lubricant, odor counteractant; liq.; 35% act.

Barquat® CT-29. [Lonza] Cetrimonium chloride; CAS 112-02-7; EINECS 203-928-6; coagulating agent in mfg. of antibiotics; liq.; 29% act.

Barquat® MB-50. [Lonza] Benzalkonium chloride; germicide, disinfectant, sanitizer; 50% liq.

Barquat® MB-80. [Lonza] Benzalkonium chloride; germicide, disinfectant, sanitizer; used where a minimum of water is desirable in formulating; 80% liq.

Barquat® MX-50. [Lonza] Myristalkonium chloride; CAS 139-08-2; EINECS 205-352-0; germicide, disinfectant, sanitizer; 50% liq.

Barquat® MX-80. [Lonza] Myristalkonium chloride; CAS 139-08-2; EINECS 205-352-0; germicide, disinfectant, sanitizer; used where a minimum of water is desirable in formulating; 80% liq.

Base 4978. [Gattefosse] Glyceryl stearate and stearic acid.

Base EAC 20. [Sederma] Hydrolyzed glycosaminoglycans; moisturizer.

Base O/W 097. [Les Colorants Wackherr] PEG-2 stearate

SE, ceteareth-25, cetyl alcohol, hydrog. coconut oil, and min. oil.

Base PL 1630. [Gattefosse] PEG-2 stearate, glyceryl stearate, and glyceryl isostearate.

Base WL 2569. [Gattefosse] Paraffin, lanolin wax, and beeswax.

Base W/O 126. [Les Colorants Wackherr] Polysorbate 80, sorbitan oleate, magnesium stearate, and aluminum stearate.

Base Nacrante 1100 AD. [Seppic] Sodium laureth sulfate, cocamide DEA, glycol stearate; personal care surfactant.

Base Nacrante 2078. [Seppic] Cocamidopropyl betaine, cocamide DEA, glycol stearate; foaming base for cosmetic pearlescent preps.; fluid paste; 45% act.

Base Nacrante 6030 CP. [Seppic] Sodium coceth-2 sulfate, triethylene glycol distearate; foaming base for cosmetic pearlescent preps.; fluid paste; 35% act.

Base Nacrante 9578. [Seppic] Sodium laureth sulfate, cocamide DEA, glycol stearate; foaming base for cosmetic pearlescent preps.; fluid paste; 37% act.

BASF Disodium EDTA. [BASF] Disodium EDTA; CAS 139-33-3; EINECS 205-358-3; chelating agent.

Basis LP-20. [Nisshin Oil Mills] Lecithin; CAS 8002-43-5; EINECS 232-307-2; emulsifier.

Basis LP-20H. [Nisshin Oil Mills] Hydrog. lecithin and stearic acid.

Basis LS-60. [Nisshin Oil Mills] Lecithin; CAS 8002-43-5; EINECS 232-307-2; emulsifier.

Basis LS-60H. [Nisshin Oil Mills] Hydrog. lecithin; CAS 92128-87-5; EINECS 295-786-7; moisturizer.

Bayberry Wax Stralpitz. [Strahl & Pitsch] Bayberry wax; CAS 8038-77-5.

Baysilone COM 10,000. [Miles] Cyclomethicone; CAS 69430-24-6; cosmetic ingred.

Baysilone COM 20,000. [Miles] Cyclomethicone; CAS 69430-24-6; cosmetic ingred.

Baysilone Fluid M. [Miles] Dimethicone.

Baysilone Fluid PD 5. [Miles] Phenyl trimethicone; CAS 2116-84-9; EINECS 218-320-6; emollient, conditioner.

Baysilone Fluid PK 20. [Miles] Phenyl trimethicone; CAS 2116-84-9; EINECS 218-320-6; emollient, conditioner.

BB-1. [Research Corp. of Am.] Aluminum hydroxide; CAS 21645-51-2; EINECS 244-492-7; adsorbent and binder.

BBC Mineral Complex. [Bio-Botanica] Alfalfa extract, nettle extract, parsley extract, borage extract, horsetail extract, bladderwrack extract, red raspberry leaf extract, clover blossom extract; botanical extract.

BBC Moisture Trol. [Bio-Botanica] Slippery elm bark, sunflower seed oil, comfrey extract, horsetail extract, oat extract, althea extract, orange flower water, borage extract, chamomile extract, rose extract, peppermint extract.

BBC Relaxing Complex. [Bio-Botanica] Lavender extract, chamomile extract, passionflower extract, peppermint extract, horsetail extract, rose extract.

BBS. [Karlshamns] Partially hydrog. veg. oil; CAS 68334-28-1; EINECS 269-820-6; emollient and emulsifier; m.p. 115-122 F.

BC. [L.A. Salomon] Fuller's earth.

Beaulight A-5000. [Sanyo Chem. Industries] Disodium mono(lauroylethanolamide POE 5) sulfosuccinate; anionic; base materials for shampoos; liq.; 30% conc.

Beaulight ECA. [Sanyo Chem. Industries] Sodium POE 3 tridecylether carboxylate; CAS 68891-17-8; anionic; base materials for shampoos; liq.; 95% conc.

Beaulight ESS. [Sanyo Chem. Industries] Disodium mono(POE 2 alkyl (12-14) sulfosuccinate; CAS 68811-93-3; anionic; base materials for shampoos; liq.; 40% conc.

Beaulight LCA-30D. [Sanyo Chem. Industries] Sodium POE 3 laurylether carboxylate; CAS 33939-64-9; anionic; base

materials for shampoos; liq.; 30% conc.

Beaulight SSS. [Sanyo Chem. Industries] Disodium lauryl sulfosuccinate; CAS 13192-12-6; anionic; base materials for body shampoos; paste; 40% conc.

Bee's Milk. [Koster Keunen] Water (78.5%), beeswax NF (10%), sesame oil NF (10%), lecithin NF, and benzoic acid dispersion; film-former, emollient, conditioner, aq. opacifier, pigment wetter for creams, lotions, shampoos, conditioners, shaving creams, aq. gels; biodeg.; wh. to off-wh. opaque liq., char. odor; particle size < 1000 nm; water-disp.; sp.gr. 0.97-1.030; m.p. 50-55 C; b.p. < 100 C; flash pt. (COC) < 250 C; pH 4.5-6.0; usage level: 1-20%; toxicology: no irritation potential; nontoxic; 17-25% solids.

Beeswax SP 116. [Strahl & Pitsch] Beeswax; wax for personal care prods.

Beeswax SP 125. [Strahl & Pitsch] Beeswax; wax for personal care prods.

Beeswax SP 139. [Strahl & Pitsch] Beeswax; wax for personal care prods.

Beeswax Commercial SP 1142. [Strahl & Pitsch] Beeswax; wax for personal care prods.

Beeswax Semi Bleached SP 752. [Strahl & Pitsch] Beeswax; wax for personal care prods.

Beeswax Synthetic Stralpitz. [Strahl & Pitsch] Synthetic beeswax.

Beeswax White Refined SP 44. [Strahl & Pitsch] Beeswax; wax for personal care prods.

Beeswax White SP 52. [Strahl & Pitsch] Beeswax; wax for personal care prods.

Beeswax White Stralpitz. [Strahl & Pitsch] Beeswax; wax for personal care prods.

Beeswax Yellow Refined SP 6. [Strahl & Pitsch] Beeswax; wax for personal care prods.

Beeswax Yellow SP 57. [Strahl & Pitsch] Beeswax; wax for personal care prods.

Beeswing 1/16. [Mt. Pulaski Prods.] Corn cob meal; filler, absorbent for cosmetics.

Beeswing 3/16. [Mt. Pulaski Prods.] Corn cob meal; filler, absorbent for cosmetics.

Beeswing 3/32. [Mt. Pulaski Prods.] Corn cob meal; filler, absorbent for cosmetics.

Belal. [Belmay] 2,4-Dimethyl-3-cyclohexene carboxaldehyde; CAS 68039-49-6; EINECS 268-264-1.

Beldox. [Belmay] 2-t-Butylcyclohexyl acetate; CAS 88-41-5; EINECS 201-828-7.

Belsil ADM 6041 E. [Wacker-Chemie GmbH] Trimethylsilylamodimethicone, trideceth-6; nonionic/cationic; nonreactive substantive conditioner for hair conditioners and shampoos; clear-opaque liq. emulsion; sol. in water, glycerin, propanediol; sp.gr. 1.00; visc. 3 mm²/s; amine no. 0.12; 17% act.

Belsil ADM 6042 E. [Wacker-Chemie GmbH] Amodimethicone, trideceth-6; nonionic/cationic; reactive substantive conditioner for hair conditioners and shampoos; clear-opaque liq. o/w emulsion; sol. in water, glycerin, propanediol; sp.gr. 1.00; visc. 10 mm²/s; amine no. 0.06; 17% act.

Belsil ADM 6056 E. [Wacker-Chemie GmbH] Amodimethicone, dimethicone, dimethiconol, trideceth-15, and trideceth-5; nonionic; reactive substantive conditioner for hair conditioners and shampoos; milky wh. liq. o/w emulsion; sol. in water, glycerin, propanediol; sp.gr. 0.99; visc. 1000 mm²/s; amine no. 0.08-0.12; 59% act.

Belsil ADM 6057 E. [Wacker-Chemie GmbH] Amodimethicone, cetrimonium chloride, and nonoxynol-10; cationic/nonionic; reactive substantive conditioner for hair conditioners and shampoos; milky wh. o/w liq. emulsion; sol. in water, glycerin, propanediol; sp.gr. 1.0; visc. 200 mm²/s; amine no. 0.05-0.1; 50% act.

Belsil ADM 6059 E. [Wacker-Chemie GmbH] Amodimethicone, trideceth-10, and trideceth-5; nonionic; reactive substantive conditioner for hair conditioners and shampoos; milky wh. liq. o/w emulsion; sol. in water, glycerin, propanediol; sp.gr. 0.99; visc. 50 mm²/s; amine no. 0.05-0.1; 50% act.

Belsil CM 020. [Wacker-Chemie GmbH] Cyclomethicone; CAS 69430-24-6; used in deodorants to replace alcohol and IPM, prevent stickiness of aerosol nozzles and roll-on balls; also for hair and skin care prods. and decorative cosmetics; gives dry, soft, velvety skin feel; colorless clear liq.; sol. in olive oil, lanolin oil, paraffin oil, oleyl oleate, IPA, ethanol, propanediol, IPM; sp.gr. 0.95; visc. 2.0 mm²/s; m.p. 18 C; flash pt. 52 C.

Belsil CM 025. [Wacker-Chemie GmbH] Cyclomethicone; CAS 69430-24-6; used in deodorants to replace alcohol and IPM, prevent stickiness of aerosol nozzles and roll-on balls; also for hair and skin care prods. and decorative cosmetics; gives dry, soft, velvety skin feel; colorless clear liq.; sol. in low-visc. paraffin oil, IPA, ethanol, IPM; sp.gr. 0.95; visc. 2.5 mm²/s; m.p. 12 C; flash pt. 54 C.

Belsil CM 030. [Wacker-Chemie GmbH] Cyclomethicone; CAS 69430-24-6; used in deodorants to replace alcohol and IPM, prevent stickiness of aerosol nozzles and roll-on balls; also for hair and skin care prods. and decorative cosmetics; gives dry, soft, velvety skin feel; colorless clear liq.; sol. in low-visc. paraffin oil, IPA, ethanol, IPM; sp.gr. 0.95; visc. 3.0 mm²/s; m.p. -35 C; flash pt. 61 C.

Belsil CM 040. [Wacker-Chemie GmbH] Cyclomethicone; CAS 69430-24-6; used in deodorants to replace alcohol and IPM, prevent stickiness of aerosol nozzles and roll-on balls; also for hair and skin care prods. and decorative cosmetics; gives dry, soft, velvety skin feel; colorless clear liq.; sol. in oleyl alcohol, decyl oleate, octyldodecanol, low-visc. paraffin oil, IPA, ethanol, IPM; sp.gr. 0.95; visc. 4.0 mm²/s; m.p. -45 C; flash pt. 69 C.

Belsil CM 1000. [Wacker-Chemie GmbH] Cyclomethicone and dimethiconol; film-former used in skin and hair care formulas; gives skin a pleasant, supple feel; results in shiny, sleek hair, and improved dry combing; colorless clear liq.; sp.gr. 0.98-1.0; visc. 4500-5500 mm²/s; flash pt. 76 C; ref. index 1.398-1.401.

Belsil DM 0.65. [Wacker-Chemie GmbH] Dimethicone; used in skin and hair care prods. and decorative cosmetics; enhances suppleness and gives soft, velvety feel to skin; prevents stickiness and increases water resist. of cosmetics; colorless clear liq.; sol. in olive oil, lanolin oil, paraffin oil, oleyl oleate, oleyl alcohol, IPA, ethanol, IPM; sp.gr. 0.76; visc. 0.65 mm²/s; solid. pt. -68 C; flash pt. -1 C; ref. index 1.375.

Belsil DM 35. [Wacker-Chemie GmbH] Dimethicone; used in skin and hair care prods. and decorative cosmetics; enhances suppleness and gives soft, velvety feel to skin; prevents stickiness and increases water resist. of cosmetics; colorless clear prod.; sol. in IPA, IPM; sp.gr. 0.95-0.96; visc. 35 mm²/s; solid. pt. -60 C; flash pt. 250 C; ref. index 1.401-1.402.

Belsil DM 100. [Wacker-Chemie GmbH] Dimethicone; used in skin and hair care prods. and decorative cosmetics; enhances suppleness and gives soft, velvety feel to skin; prevents stickiness and increases water resist. of cosmetics; colorless clear prod.; sol. in IPA, IPM; sp.gr. 0.96-0.97; visc. 100 mm²/s; solid. pt. -55 C; flash pt. 275 C; ref. index 1.402-1.403.

Belsil DM 350. [Wacker-Chemie GmbH] Dimethicone; used in skin and hair care prods. and decorative cosmetics; enhances suppleness and gives soft, velvety feel to skin; prevents stickiness and increases water resist. of cosmetics; colorless clear prod.; sol. in IPA, IPM; sp.gr. 0.96-0.97; visc. 350 mm²/s; solid. pt. -50 C; flash pt. > 300 C; ref. index 1.402-1.403.

Belsil DM 100000. [Wacker-Chemie GmbH] Dimethicone; used in skin and hair care prods. and decorative cosmetics; enhances suppleness and gives soft, velvety feel to skin; prevents stickiness and increases water resist. of cosmetics; colorless clear highly visc. prod.; sol. in IPM; sp.gr. 0.98; visc. 100,000 mm²/s; solid. pt. -40 C; flash pt. > 320 C; ref. index 1.403-1.404.

Belsil DMC 6031. [Wacker-Chemie GmbH] Dimethicone copolyol; wetting aid, emollient, moisturizer, fatting agent improving surface slip in cosmetics; stabilizer for foams and emulsions; plasticizer for hair spray resins; liq.; sol. in castor oil, IPA, ethanol, water, IPM; sp.gr. 1.03; visc. 800-1200 mm²/s; cloud pt. 37-42 C; flash pt. 140 C; ref. index 1.452.

Belsil DMC 6032. [Wacker-Chemie GmbH] Dimethicone copolyol acetate; wetting aid, emollient, moisturizer, fatting agent improving surface slip in cosmetics; stabilizer for foams and emulsions; plasticizer for hair spray resins; solid; sol. in water, IPA, ethanol, IPM; sp.gr. 1.03-1.04; visc. 500-700 mm²/s; cloud pt. 74-84 C; flash pt. 127 C; ref. index 1.430-1.435.

Belsil DMC 6033. [Wacker-Chemie GmbH] Dimethicone copolyol acetate; wetting aid, emollient, moisturizer, fatting agent improving surface slip in cosmetics; stabilizer for foams and emulsions; plasticizer for hair spray resins; liq.; sol. in IPA, ethanol, IPM, PEG-7 glyceryl cocoate; disp. in water; sp.gr. 1.03; visc. 100-300 mm²/s; flash pt. 80 C; ref. index 1.437-1.440.

Belsil DMC 6035. [Wacker-Chemie GmbH] Dimethicone copolyol acetate; wetting aid, emollient, moisturizer, fatting agent improving surface slip in cosmetics; stabilizer for foams and emulsions; plasticizer for hair spray resins; liq.; sol. in water, IPA, ethanol, IPM, PEG-7 glcyeryl cocoate, PEG-75 lanolin oil; sp.gr. 1.11-1.12; visc. 120-260 mm²/s; cloud pt. 35-47 C; flash pt. > 200 C; ref. index 1.454-1.458.

Belsil DMC 6038. [Wacker-Chemie GmbH] Dimethicone copolyol.

Belsil PDM 20. [Wacker-Chemie GmbH] Phenyl-dimethicone; used in skin and hair care prods. and decorative cosmetics; give exc. feel to skin; high penetrating and water repellent props.; imparts suppleness and depth of color to hair; colorless clear liq.; sol. in paraffin oil, oleyl oleate, decyl oleate, IPA, ethanol, IPM; sp.gr. 0.97-1.02; visc. 20 mm²/s; m.p. < -75 C; flash pt. 170 C; ref. index 1.428-1.446.

Belsil PDM 200. [Wacker-Chemie GmbH] Phenyldimethicone; used in skin and hair care prods. and decorative cosmetics; give exc. feel to skin; high penetrating and water repellent props.; imparts suppleness and depth of color to hair; colorless clear liq.; sol. in low-visc. paraffin oil, IPA, ethanol, IPM; sp.gr. 1.03-1.05; visc. 200 mm²/s; m.p. < -60 C; flash pt. 285 C; ref. index 1.445-1.452.

Belsil PDM 1000. [Wacker-Chemie GmbH] Phenyldimethicone; used in skin and hair care prods. and decorative cosmetics; give exc. feel to skin; high penetrating and water repellent props.; imparts suppleness and depth of color to hair; colorless clear liq.; sol. in low-visc. paraffin oil, IPA, ethanol, IPM; sp.gr. 1.04; visc. 1000 mm²/s; flash pt. 300 C; ref. index 1.459-1.463.

Belsil SDM 6021. [Wacker-Chemie GmbH] Dimethicone and stearoxydimethicone; gives nongreasy, soft, velvety feel to skin; enhances gloss and color brightness in decorative cosmetics; good spreading props., protection against aq. media; wh. cryst. wax-like solid; sol. hot in IPA, IPM; sp.gr. 0.84 (50 C); visc. > 15 mm²/s (80 C); m.p. 28-40 C; flash pt. 200 C; ref. index 1.431 (80 C).

Belsil SDM 6022. [Wacker-Chemie GmbH] Dimethicone and stearoxydimethicone; gives nongreasy, soft, velvety feel to skin; enhances gloss and color brightness in decorative cosmetics; good spreading props., protection against aq. media; wh. cryst. wax-like solid; sol. hot in IPM; sp.gr. 0.84 (50 C); visc. > 15 mm²/s (80 C); m.p. 40-50 C; flash pt. 160 C; ref. index 1.426 (80 C).

Benecel® Hydroxypropyl Methylcellulose. [Aqualon] Hydroxypropyl methylcellulose; CAS 9004-65-3.

Benecel® M. [Aqualon] Methyl cellulose; CAS 9004-67-5; nonionic; thickener, stabilizer, rheology control agent, film-former, suspending agent, water-retention aid, binder for food, pharmaceutical, and cosmetic industries; water-sol.; visc. 10-12,000 mPa·s (2% aq.).

Benecel® ME. [Aqualon] Methyl hydroxyethyl cellulose; CAS 9032-42-2; nonionic; thickener, stabilizer, rheology control agent, film-former, suspending agent, water-retention aid, binder for food, pharmaceutical, and cosmetic industries; water-sol.; visc. 100-40,000 mPa·s (2%).

Benecel® MP. [Aqualon] Methylhydroxypropylcellulose; CAS 9004-65-3; nonionic; thickener, stabilizer, rheology control agent, film-former, suspending agent, water-retention aid, binder for food, pharmaceutical, and cosmetic industries; water-sol.; visc. 3–70,000 mPa·s (2%).

Benibana Liq. [Ichimaru Pharcos] Water, alcohol, butylene glycol, and safflower extract; botanical extract.

Benol® . [Witco/Petroleum Spec.] Wh. min. oil NF; lubricant used in food, drug and cosmetic industry; FDA §172.878, 178.3620a; water wh., odorless, tasteless; sp.gr. 0.839-0.855; visc. 18-20 cSt (40 C); pour pt. -7 C; flash pt. 182 C.

Bentex E. [Lanaetex Prods.] Ethyl paraben; CAS 120-47-8; EINECS 204-399-4; cosmetics preservative.

Bentex M. [Lanaetex Prods.] Methyl paraben; CAS 99-76-3; EINECS 202-785-7; cosmetics preservative.

Bentex P. [Lanaetex Prods.] Propylparaben; CAS 94-13-3; EINECS 202-307-7; cosmetics preservative.

Bentolite H. [Southern Clay Prods.] Bentonite; CAS 1302-78-9; EINECS 215-108-5; thickener.

Bentolite H 4430. [Whittaker, Clark & Daniels] Bentonite; CAS 1302-78-9; EINECS 215-108-5; thickener.

Bentolite L. [Southern Clay Prods.] Bentonite; CAS 1302-78-9; EINECS 215-108-5; thickener.

Bentolite WH. [Southern Clay Prods.] Bentonite; CAS 1302-78-9; EINECS 215-108-5; thickener.

Bentone® 27. [Rheox] Stearalkonium hectorite, anhyd.; thixotrope, gellant, thickener for solv.-based coatings, lip and eye care prods, nail lacquers, antiperspirants; suspending agent for pigments and actives; imparts leveling, heat stability, emulsion stability; used for intermediate to high polarity org. systems; creamy wh. powd.; dens. 1.80 g/cc; 100% NV.

Bentone® 34. [Rheox] Quaternium-18 bentonite; CAS 68953-58-2; EINECS 273-219-4; thixotrope, gellant, thickener for solv.-based coatings; lip and eye care prods.; used for intermediate to high polarity org. systems; antiperspirant creams and lotions; very lt. cream powd.; dens. 1.70 g/cc; 100% NV.

Bentone® 38. [Rheox] Quaternium-18 hectorite; CAS 12001-31-9; EINECS 234-406-6; thixotrope, gellant, thickener for solv.-based coatings, lip and eye care prods., creams/lotions, suntan prods., antiperspirants; for low to intermediate polarity org. systems; creamy wh. fine powd.; dens. 1.70 g/cc; 100% NV.

Bentone® EW. [Rheox] Hectorite; CAS 12173-47-6; EINECS 235-340-0; suspending agent, rheological additive, thickener, gellant for water-reducible industrial finishes and inks, cosmetic creams and lotions, antidandruff shampoo, suntan prods., shaving preps., hair conditioners; milky wh. powd.; water-disp.; dens. 2.6 g/cc; 100% NV.

Bentone® Gel CAO. [Rheox] Castor oil, stearalkonium hectorite, and propylene carbonate; rheological additive

providing suspension, flow control, emulsion and thermal stability to lip prods.; lt. buff opaque gel; dens. 8.33 lb/gal; flash pt. (Seta) > 230 F.

Bentone® Gel IPM. [Rheox] IPM, stearalkonium hectorite, and propylene carbonate; rheological additive providing suspension, flow control, emulsion and thermal stability to cosmetic creams/lotions, antiperspirants; lt. buff opaque gel; dens. 7.43 lb/gal; flash pt. (Seta) > 230 F.

Bentone® Gel ISD. [Rheox] Isododecane (87%), quaternium-18 hectorite, and propylene carbonate; rheological additive providing suspension, flow control, emulsion and thermal stability to cosmetic creams/lotions, eye prods., antiperspirants; lt. buff gel; dens. 6.47 lb/gal; flash pt. (Seta) 112 F.; 87% conc.

Bentone® Gel LOI. [Rheox] Lanolin oil, isopropyl palmitate, stearalkonium hectorite, propylene carbonate, propyl paraben; rheological additive providing suspension, flow control, emulsion and thermal stability to lip prods., creams, lotions; dispersant with many cosmetic oils; gold opaque gel; dens. 7.6 lb/gal; flash pt. (Seta) > 230 F.

Bentone® Gel M20. [Rheox] Propylene glycol dicaprate/dicaprylate, quaternium-18 hectorite, and propylene carbonate; rheological additive providing suspension, flow control, emulsion and thermal stability to cosmetic creams and lotions; lt. buff gel; sp.gr. 1.00; flash pt. (PMCC) > 170 F; 1.8% propylene carbonate.

Bentone® Gel MIO. [Rheox] Min. oil, quaternium-18 hectorite, and propylene carbonate; rheological additive providing suspension, flow control, emulsion and thermal stability to lip prods., creams, lotions, hair grooms, suntan prods.; lt. buff opaque gel; dens. 7.29 lb/gal; flash pt. (Seta) > 230 F.

Bentone® Gel MIO A-40. [Rheox] Mineral oil, quaternium-18 hectorite, SDA-40; rheological additive providing suspension, flow control, emulsion and thermal stability to lip prods., creams, lotions, hair grooms, suntan prods.; lt. buff opaque gel; sp.gr. 0.88; dens. 7.31 lb/gal; flash pt. (PMCC) 130 F.

Bentone® Gel SS71. [Rheox] Petrol. distillate, quaternium-18 hectorite, and propylene carbonate; rheological additive providing suspension, flow control, emulsion and thermal stability to eye prods.; lt. buff opaque gel; dens. 7.53 lb/gal; flash pt. (Seta) 135 F.

Bentone® Gel TN. [Rheox] C12-15 alkyl benzoate, stearalkonium hectorite, and propylene carbonate; rheological additive providing suspension, flow control, emulsion and thermal stability to lip prods., creams, lotions, eye prods., antiperspirants; lt. buff gel; sp.gr. 0.96; flash pt. (TCC) > 300 F.

Bentone® Gel TN A-40. [Rheox] C12-15 alkyl benzoate, stearalkonium hectorite, and SDA-40; rheological additive providing suspension, flow control, emulsion and thermal stability to lip prods., creams, lotions, eye prods., antiperspirants.

Bentone® Gel VS-5. [Rheox] Cyclomethicone, quaternium-18 hectorite, SDA-40; rheological additive providing suspension, flow control, emulsion and thermal stability to cosmetic creams and lotions, antiperspirants, eye prods.; lt. beige opaque gel; sp.gr. 1.01; dens. 8.43 lb/gal; flash pt. (Seta) 80 F.

Bentone® Gel VS-5 PC. [Rheox] Cyclomethicone, quaternium-18 hectorite, propylene carbonate; rheological additive providing suspension, flow control, emulsion and thermal stability to cosmetic creams and lotions, antiperspirants, eye prods.; lt. beige gel; sp.gr. 1.00; flash pt. (PMCC) > 170 F.

Bentone® LT. [Rheox] Hectorite and hydroxyethylcellulose; thickener, gellant for water-based coatings; latex paint systems; excellent leveling and flow control; easy dispersing; provides thixotropic visc., pigment suspension, and emulsion stability to cosmetic creams/lotions, eye prods., powd. hair bleach, makeup; milky wh. soft powd.; dens. 1.9 g/cc; 100% NV.

Bentone® MA. [Rheox] Purified hectorite clay; CAS 12173-47-6; EINECS 235-340-0; thickener, rheological additive for antidandruff shampoo, lotions, shave creams, antiperspirants; provides thixotropic visc. and pigment suspension, emulsion stability; wh. color.

Bentone® SD-3. [Rheox] Dihydrog. tallow benzylmonium hectorite; thickener and suspension agent for aromatic systems; lt. cream powd.; sp.gr. 1.60.

Bentonite USP BC 670. [Whittaker, Clark & Daniels] Bentonite; CAS 1302-78-9; EINECS 215-108-5; thickener.

Benzoic Acid Powd. No. 130. [E. Merck] Benzoic acid; CAS 65-85-0; EINECS 200-618-2; cosmetics preservative.

Benzyl Nicotinate No. 6752. [Rona; E. Merck] Benzyl nicotinate; CAS 94-44-0; EINECS 202-332-3.

Bergoxane. [Hercules/PFW] Dimethyl hexahydronaphthyl dihydroxymethyl acetal.

Bermocoll. [Berol Nobel Inc] Hydroxyethyl ethylcellulose.

Bernel® Ester 168. [Bernel] Isocetyl octanoate; emollient with dry, silky feel; FDA, EEC, and Japanese compliances; colorless liq.; oil-sol.; usage level: 2-10%.

Bernel® Ester 2014. [Bernel] Octyldodecyl myristate; rich emollient, pigment disperser, lipstick component; FDA, EEC, and Japanese compliances; colorless liq.; oil-sol.; usage level: 2-15%.

Bernel® Ester CO. [Bernel] Cetyl octanoate; CAS 59130-69-7; EINECS 261-619-1; noncomedogenic emollient; low visc. ester; FDA, EEC, and Japanese compliances; colorless liq.; sol. in oil; usage level: 2-10%.

Bernel® Ester DID. [Bernel] Diisopropyl dimer dilinoleate; emollient, film-former; FDA, EEC, and Japanese compliances; yel. liq.; sol. in oil; usage level: 1-7%.

Bernel® Ester DISM. [Bernel] Diisostearyl malate; CAS 67763-18-2; high visc. emollient for anhyd. systems; FDA, EEC, and Japanese compliances; colorless liq.; sol. in oil; usage level: 2-10%.

Bernel® Ester DOM. [Bernel] Dioctyl maleate; emollient, oxybenzone solubilizer, cleanser and wax solv.; noncomedogenic; imparts shine in hair conditioners; FDA, EEC, and Japanese compliances; colorless liq.; sol. in oil; usage level: 2-10%.

Bernel® Ester EHP. [Bernel] Octyl palmitate; CAS 29806-73-3; EINECS 249-862-1; cost-effective emollient; FDA, EEC, and Japanese compliances; colorless liq.; oil-sol.; usage level: 1-6%.

Bernel® Ester NPDC. [Bernel] Neopentyl dicaprate; light, dry emollient; pigment wetter and binder; FDA, EEC, and Japanese compliances; colorless liq.; oil-sol.; usage level: 2-10%.

Bernel® Ester TOC. [Bernel] Trioctyl citrate; noncomedogenic emollient, pigment wetter; FDA and EEC compliances; yel. liq.; oil-sol.; usage level: 2-10%.

Bernel®OPG. [Bernel] Octyl pelargonate; CAS 59587-44-9; EINECS 261-819-9; dry, nonoily emollient; FDA, EEC, and Japanese compliances; colorless liq.; oil-sol.; usage level: 2-8%.

Berol 452. [Berol Nobel AB] Sodium laureth sulfate; CAS 68891-38-3; anionic; wetting and foaming agent; emulsifier for shampoos, bath preps.; biodeg.; Hazen < 100 clear liq.; sol. in water, ethanol, propylene glycol; disp. in acetone; sp.gr. 1.04; visc. 200 cps; flash pt. > 100 C; surf. tens. 37 dynes/cm (0.1%); pH 6.5–8.0 (1% aq); 27-29% conc.

Berol 480. [Berol Nobel AB] TEA lauryl sulfate; CAS 139-96-8; EINECS 205-388-7; anionic; detergent, foaming agent for hair shampoos, foam baths, hand cleaners; biodeg.; Hazen < 300 soft paste; sol. in propylene glycol and water, disp. in ethanol, trichloroethylene, xylene; sp.gr. 0.97;

flash pt. > 100 C; surf. tens. 37 dynes/cm (0.1%); pH 6.5–8.0 (1% aq.); 39-41% conc.

Be Square® 175. [Petrolite] Microcryst. wax; CAS 63231-60-7; EINECS 264-038-1; plastic wax offering high ductility, flexibility at very low temps.; provides protective barrier properties against moisture vapor and gases; uses incl. hot-melt laminating adhesives and coatings, in antisun-checking agents in rubber goods, elec. insulating agents, leather treating agents, water repellents for textiles, rust-proof coatings, cosmetic ingreds., as plasticizer in crayons, dental compds., chewing gum base, and candles; incl. FDA §172.230, 172.615, 175.105, 175.300, 176.170, 176.180, 176.200, 177.1200, 178.3710, 179.45; amber wax; dens. 0.93 g/cc; visc. 13 cps (99 C); m.p. 83 C; flash pt. 293 C.

Be Square® 185. [Petrolite] Hard microcryst. wax consisting of n-paraffinic, branched paraffinic, and naphthenic hydrocarbons; CAS 63231-60-7; EINECS 264-038-1; wax used in hot-melt coatings and adhesives, cup and paper coatings, printing inks, plastic modification (as lubricant and processing aid), lacquers, paints, and varnishes, as binder in ceramics, for potting in elec./electronic; components, in investment casting, rubber and elastomers (plasticizer, antisunchecking, antiozonant), as emulsion wax size in papermaking, as fabric softener ingred., in cosmetic hand creams and lipsticks; incl. FDA §172.230, 172.615, 175.105, 175.300, 176.170, 176.180, 176.200, 177.1200, 178.3710, 179.45; amber wax; very low sol. in org. solvs.; sp.gr. 0.93; visc. 15 cps (99 C); m.p. 90.5 C.

Be Square® 195. [Petrolite] Hard microcryst. wax consisting of n-paraffinic, branched paraffinic, and naphthenic hydrocarbons; CAS 63231-60-7; EINECS 264-038-1; wax used in adhesives, ceramics, chewing gum, cosmetics, elec., explosives, pkg., paints, polish, printing inks, plastics processing, rustproofing; incl. FDA §172.230, 172.615, 175.105, 175.300, 176.170, 176.180, 176.200, 177.1200, 178.3710, 179.45; wh., amber wax; very low sol. in org. solvs.; sp.gr. 0.93; visc. 15.5 cps (99 C); m.p. 93 C.

Beta W 7. [Wacker-Chemie GmbH] β-Cyclodextrin; CAS 7585-39-9; EINECS 231-493-2; complex hosting guest molecules; increases the sol. and bioavailability of other substances; masks flavor, odor, or coloration; stabilizes against light, oxidation, heat, and hydrolysis; turns liqs. or volatiles into stable solid powds.; for use in pharmaceuticals, cosmetics, toiletries, foods, tobacco, pesticides, textiles, paints, plastics, synthesis, polymers; wh. cryst. powd.; sol. 1.85 g/100 ml in water; m.w. 1135.

Beta Carotene 30% in Veg. Oil No. 65646. [Roche] Beta carotene 500,000 I.U. Vitamin A activity/g; CAS 7235-40-7; EINECS 230-636-6; colorant, antioxidant for cosmetics applics.

BFP 640. [Am. Ingredients/Patco] Mono-diglycerides; emulsifier for pharmaceuticals and cosmetics; ivory wh. plastic; m.p. 102-106 F.

Bicrona®. [Rona] Pearlescent pigments for cosmetics and toiletries.

Bicrona® Carmine. [Rona; E. Merck] Carmine and bismuth oxychloride.

Bicrona® Iron Blue. [Rona; E. Merck] Ferric ammonium ferrocyanide and bismuth oxychloride.

Biju® BNT. [Mearl] Bismuth oxychloride, nitrocellulose, butyl acetate, IPA, stearalkonium hectorite; colorant and pearlescent for frosted cosmetics, nail enamels; high luster; slurry; 60% BiOCl.

Biju® BTD, BXD. [Mearl] Bismuth oxychloride, nitrocellulose, butyl acetate, IPA, toluene, stearalkonium hectorite; colorant and pearlescent for frosted cosmetics, nail enamels; high luster; paste; 25% BiOCl.

Biju® BWD, BWS. [Mearl] Bismuth oxychloride, nitrocellulose, butyl acetate, isopropyl alcohol, toluene; colorant and pearlescent for frosted cosmetics, pearl nail enamel because of brilliance and smoothness; slurry; 25 and 12.5% BiOCl resp.

Biju® BWP. [Mearl] Bismuth oxychloride, nitrocellulose, butyl acetate, IPA, toluene; colorant and pearlescent for frosted cosmetics, nail enamels; high luster; slurry; 60% BiOCl.

Biju® Ultra UNT. [Mearl] Bismuth oxychloride, nitrocellulose, butyl acetate, IPA, stearalkonium hectorite; colorant and pearlescent for frosted cosmetics, nail enamels; very high luster; ioose slurry; 60% BiOCl.

Biju® Ultra UTD, UXD. [Mearl] Bismuth oxychloride, nitrocellulose, butyl acetate, IPA, toluene, stearalkonium hectorite; colorant and pearlescent for frosted cosmetics, nail enamels; very high luster; paste; 25% BiOCl.

Biju® Ultra UWD, UWS. [Mearl] Bismuth oxychloride, nitrocellulose, butyl acetate, IPA, toluene; colorant and pearlescent for frosted cosmetics, nail enamels; very high luster; fluid slurry; 25 and 12.5% BiOCl resp.

Biju® Ultra UWP. [Mearl] Bismuth oxychloride, nitrocellulose, butyl acetate, IPA, toluene; colorant and pearlescent for frosted cosmetics, nail enamels; very high luster; heavy slurry; 60% BiOCl.

Bi-Lite® . [ISP Van Dyk] Bismuth oxychloride-coated mica; pearlescent pigments for cosmetic eye, face, lip, and body make-up and pressed powds.; good luster, transparency; wh.

Bi-Lite® 20, 1070. [ISP Van Dyk] Mica and bismuth oxychloride.

Bi-Lite® R, 1051. [ISP Van Dyk] Mica and bismuth oxychloride.

Bi-Lite® UVR. [ISP Van Dyk] Mica and bismuth oxychloride.

Bi-Lite® Ultralite 3186. [ISP Van Dyk] Mica and bismuth oxychloride.

Bi-Lite® Ultrapress 1082. [ISP Van Dyk] Mica and bismuth oxychloride.

Bi-Lite® Ultrawhite 1084. [ISP Van Dyk] Mica, bismuth oxychloride, and titanium dioxide.

Bio-EPO. [Shiseido] Mortierella oil.

Biobranil 2/948100. [Dragoco] Wheat bran lipids.

Biobranil Watersoluble 2/012600. [Dragoco] Water, wheat bran lipids, propylene glycol, ethoxydiglycol, PEG-40 castor oil, and tocopherol.

BioCare® Polymer HA-24. [Amerchol] Polyquaternium-24, hyaluronic acid; emollient, humectant, conditioner, softener, moisturizer, lubricant for hair and skin; substantive to protein substrates; opalescent visc. liq.

BioCare® SA. [Amerchol] Albumen, hyaluronic acid, dextran sulfate; polymer providing hydration and revitalization to surface skin; lifts wrinkles; substantive to protein substrates; for eye gels, facial treatments, skin toners, makeup, moisturizers, after-sun prods., cleansing lotions.

Biocell S.O.D. [Brooks Industries] Superoxide dismutase; cosmetic ingred.

Biocelose NC-50. [Ikeda] Chitosan lactate; deodorant and antibacterial props. with low irritancy and toxicity; for deodorant lotions, mouthwash, aftershave lotions; sl. ylsh. powd.; pH 4.5-5.3 (1%); 28.5% min. chitosan.

Bio-Chelated Derma-Plex I. [Bio-Botanica] Comfrey extract, plantain extract, sambucus extract, horsetail extract, calendula extract, sage extract, cranesbill extract, ginseng extract, and honey extract.

Biochelated Extract of Lemon Grass. [Lipo] Alcohol and lemongrass extract; botanical extract.

Bio-Chelated Neutral Henna Extract. [Bio-Botanica] Henna extract; botanical extract.

Bio-Chelated Sauna-Derm I. [Bio-Botanica] Comfrey extract, orange peel extract, chamomile extract, althea extract, yarrow extract, fennel extract, licorice extract; botanical extract.

Biochelated Sea Kelp Extract. [Lipo] Alcohol and kelp extract; botanical extract.

Biodermine. [Sederma] Hydrolyzed soy protein and propylene glycol; regulates sebaceous activity and provides revitalizing, firming, toning, and stimulating in skin, face, and body care prods. and for hair care.; pale yel. clear liq., char. odor; sp.gr. 1.010-1.020; ref. index 1.345 ± 0.005; pH 6.5-7.5; usage level: 3-8%.

Biodynes® TRF. [Brooks Industries] Live yeast cell deriv.; promotes wound healing and possesses anti-inflammatory effects for skin care cosmetics.

Biodynes® TRF 5% Sol'n. [Brooks Industries] Live yeast cell deriv.; promotes wound healing and possesses anti-inflammatory effects for skin care cosmetics.; clear liq., low odor.

Biodynes® TRF Ultra-5. [Brooks Industries] Live yeast cell deriv.; moisturizer for skin; minimizes dryness and pain of sunburn and wind chapped skin; clear pale yel. liq., odorless.

Bioecolia® . [Solabia] skin protectant which protects and dynamizes the beneficial resident cutaneous flora and preserves biological equilibrium of cutaneous ecosystems.

Biofloreol Hydrosoluble. [Esperis] Nonoxynol-10 and pollen extract.

Biofloreol Liposoluble. [Esperis] Hydrog. lanolin and pollen extract.

Biofloreol Liq. Liposoluble. [Esperis] Caprylic/capric triglyceride and pollen extract.

BioGir-LAB. [Girindus Chemie] 2-Aminobutanol.

BioGir-MBC. [Girindus Chemie] 4-Methylbenzylidene camphor; CAS 38102-62-4; uv-B filter for cosmetics.

BioGir-PISA. [Girindus Chemie] Phenylbenzimidazole sulfonic acid; CAS 27503-81-7; uv-B filter for cosmetics.

BioLac™. [Barnet Prods.] Lactic acid extract; modifies surface structure of the skin by providing retexturization and stimulation of cell renewal; liq.; pH ≤ 2; usage level: 3-10%; toxicology: caustic to eyes; skin exfoliant.

Bio-Marine Complex SG. [Seporga] A fish skin extract naturally rich in mineral salts, oligo elements, and glycosaminoglycane; cosmetics ingred.

Biomatrix® . [Biomatrix; Amerchol] Hyaluronic acid; CAS 9004-61-9; EINECS 232-678-0; cosmetics moisturizer.

Biomin® Acquacinque Liq. [Brooks Industries] Silicon, zinc, copper, iron, and magneisum glyconucleopeptides; clear filtered version of Biomin Cinque.

Biomin® Ca/P/C. [Brooks Industries] Calcium glycoproteins; biological mineral protein derivs. for cosmetic use; powd.

Biomin® Cinque. [Brooks Industries] Silicon, zinc, copper, iron and magnesium glyconucleopeptides; five essential minerals bound in a complex matrix of a low m.w. peptide/mineral/nucleotide/carbohydrate.

Biomin® Cu/P/C. [Brooks Industries] Copper glycoproteins; biological mineral protein derivs. for cosmetic use; powd.

Biomin® Cu/P/C Liq. [Brooks Industries] Copper glycoproteins; biological mineral protein derivs. for cosmetic use; clear filtered version of Biomin® Cu/P/C; liq.; 5% act.

Biomin® F/P/C. [Brooks Industries] Fluoroglycoproteins; biological mineral protein derivs. for cosmetic use; powd.

Biomin® Fe/P/C. [Brooks Industries] Iron glycoproteins; biological mineral protein derivs. for cosmetic use; powd.

Biomin® Ge/P/C. [Brooks Industries] Germanium glycoproteins; biological mineral protein derivs. for cosmetic use; powd.

Biomin® K/P/C. [Brooks Industries] Potassium glycoproteins; biological mineral protein derivs. for cosmetic use; powd.

Biomin® Marine. [Brooks Industries] Sea minerals yeast deriv.; marine elements in substantive moisturizing form;

for skin care cosmetics; amber liq., low odor; 10% act.

Biomin® Mg/P/C. [Brooks Industries] Magnesium glycoproteins; biological mineral protein derivs. for cosmetic use; powd.

Biomin® Mn/P/C. [Brooks Industries] Manganese glycoproteins; biological mineral protein derivs. for cosmetic use; powd.

Biomin® Se/P/C. [Brooks Industries] Selenopeptides; biological mineral protein derivs. for cosmetic use.; powd.

Biomin® Si/P/C. [Brooks Industries] Silicon glycoproteins; biological mineral protein derivs. for cosmetic use; powd.

Biomin® Z/P/C. [Brooks Industries] Zinc yeast deriv.; biological mineral protein derivs. for cosmetic use.; powd.

Biomin® Z/P/C-20 Liq. [Brooks Industries] Zinc yeast deriv.; biological mineral protein derivs. for cosmetic use; clear filtered version of Biomin Z/P/C; liq.; 20% act.

Bio-Oil GLA-10. [Brooks Industries] Sunflower seed oil, evening primrose oil, borage seed oil, and tocopherol; botanical extract.

Biopeptide CL. [Sederma] An amphiphilic biopeptide in chemically stable form for cosmetic applic.; stimulates collagen synthesis via the liberation of the active tripeptide, glycyl-histidyl-lysine; increased diffusinal affinity for the superficial layers of the skin.

Biopeptide FN. [Sederma] Amphiphilic biopeptide; provides dermal cohesion, firming factor, and epidermal restructuring in skin care prods.

Biopharco CP-12. [Ichimaru Pharcos] Water, butylene glycol, and placental protein.

Biophos 35. [Brooks Industries] Phosphoglycoproteins, adenosine triphosphate, magnesium and potassium glycoprotein; cosmetic ingred. for moisturizing; liq.; 25% act.

Biophytex® . [Laboratoires Sérobiologiques] Propylene glycol, butcherbroom extract, hydrocotyl extract, panthenol, hydrolyzed milk protein, calendula extract, hydrolyzed yeast protein, horse chestnut extract, and licorice extract; soothing phytocomplex providing local anti-inflammatory and anti-irritant action in sun care, after shave, and eye care prods.; amber sl. syrupy liq.; water-sol.; usage level: 3-5%.

Bioplex™ RNA. [Brooks Industries] Propylene glycol, hydrolyzed RNA, hydrolyzed DNA; cosmetic ingred. for skin and hair care prods.; liq., pract. colorless and odorless; water-sol.; 20% act.

Bio-Pol® EA. [Brooks Industries] Sodium C8-16 isoalkylsuccinyl lactoglobulin sulfonate; cosmetic ingred.

Bio-Pol® NCHAP. [Brooks Industries] Sodium coco-hydrolyzed animal protein; CAS 68188-38-5; polyanionic biopolymer acting as mechanical sebum control agent; disperses and reduces tension of oils, improves thixotropy; in cosmetics, reduces oily feel and leaves skin feeling natural; in shampoos and conditioners, controls sticky oily buildup on hair.

Bio-Pol® OE. [Brooks Industries] Sodium C8-16 isoalkyl succinyl lactoglobulin sulfonate; oil-absoring polymer designed to entrap surface oil of the skin; film-former enhancing skin feel; exc. pigment dispersant and color enhancer; liq.; m.w. 100,000; 10% act.

Bio-Pol® OE/SD. [Brooks Industries] Sodium C8-16 isoalkylsuccinyl lactoglobulin sulfonate; cosmetic ingred.

Biopol® TE. [Brooks Industries] Dermal tissular extract; cosmetic ingred. for moisturizing applics.; liq.; 2% act., 1% protein.

Biopolymer HI-13DC. [Grant Industries] Modified heteropolysaccharide; stabilizer for emulsions of solvs. and hydrocarbons in water or brines; for cosmetic and industrial emulsions, pigment and mineral dispersions, cleaning formulations, surface conditioning, corrosion inhibition, visc. reduction of visc. oils, rheology enhancement of polysaccharide sol'ns., deflocculation/floccula-

tion applics.; biodeg.; straw-colored opaque liq., mild odor; m.w. 30,000 max.; sp.gr. 1.01-1.03; pH 7.8-8.6; usage level: 0.1-1.0%; toxicology: nonirritating to human skin @ 0.5%; 9.5-10.5% solids.

Bioprotector AMI. [Alban Muller] Natural ingred. with soothing props. for sun prods.; water-sol.

Biopure 100. [Nipa Labs] Imidazolidinyl urea; CAS 39236-46-9; EINECS 254-372-6; preservative for cosmetics, toiletries, and pharmaceuticals.

Biosil Basics A-30. [Biosil Tech.] Dimethiconol arginate; substantivity agent for hair and skin care prods., e.g., shampoos, rinse-out conditioners, leave-in conditioners, creams and lotions; milky liq.; water-disp.; pH 10-11; usage level: 1-2%; 36-38% solids.

Biosil Basics Amino DL-30. [Biosil Tech.] Panthenol amino dimethicone; substantivity agent for hair care prods., shampoos, rinse-out and leave-in conditioners; milky liq.; water-disp.; pH 6-8; usage level: 1-2%; 37 ± 1% solids.

Biosil Basics DL-30. [Biosil Tech.] Dimethiconol panthenate; conditioner and bodying agent for hair and skin car prods., shampoos, rinse-out and leave-in hair conditioners, creams and lotions; milky liq.; water-disp.; pH 4.3-5.3; usage level: 1-2%; 36-38% solids.

Biosil Basics Fluoro Guerbet 1.0%. [Biosil Tech.] Di(octyldodecyl) fluoro citrate; emollient, pigment dispersant for pigmented prods. and titanium dioxide-based sunscreens; good mold release props. for lipsticks and other stick prods.; improves slip and feel on skin; helps create water barrier; for eye shadow, creams, lotions, gels; oily liq.; sol. @ 5% in safflower oil, castor oil, min. oil, ethanol, oleyl alcohol, octyl palmitate; insol. in water, propylene glycol; sp.gr. 1.01; acid no. 4 max.; sapon. no. 135-165; usage level: 0.5-5%; 0.2% max. moisture.

Biosil Basics Fluoro Guerbet 3.5%. [Biosil Tech.] Di(octyldodecyl) fluoro citrate; emollient, pigment dispersant for pigmented prods. and titanium dioxide-based sunscreens; good mold release props. for lipsticks and other stick prods.; improves slip and feel on skin; helps create water barrier; for eye shadow, creams, lotions, gels; oily liq.; sol. @ 5% in safflower oil, castor oil, min. oil, ethanol, oleyl alcohol, octyl palmitate; insol. in water, propylene glycol; sp.gr. 1.01; acid no. 4 max.; sapon. no. 135-165; usage level: 0.5-5%; 0.2% max. moisture.

Biosil Basics HKP-30. [Biosil Tech.] Dimethiconol keratinate; protein source, conditioner for hair care prods., shampoos, rinse-out and leave-in conditioners, after-permanent wave conditioners, creams, and lotions; milky wh. liq.; water-disp.; pH 5.5-7.5; usage level: 1-2%; 36-38% solids.

Biosil Basics Jasmine Wax S. [Biosil Tech.] Dimethiconol jasminate; wax providing lubrication and softening props. to skin and other substrates; for skin care, sun care, creams, lotions, gels, lipsticks, and eye shadow; buff wax @ 20 C, hazy sel. liq. @ 70 C; insol. in water; usage level: 0.5-5%; 95% min. solids.

Biosil Basics L-30. [Biosil Tech.] Dimethiconol lysinate; substantivity agent for hair and skin care prods., e.g., shampoos, rinse-out conditioners, leave-in conditioners, creams and lotions; milky liq.; water-disp.; pH 10-11; usage level: 1-2%; 36-38% solids.

Biosil Basics L-Cysteine. [Biosil Tech.] Dimethiconol cysteinate; hair care ingred. for shampoos, rinse-out and leave-in condtioners, after permanent wave conditioners, creams and lotions; milky wh. liq.; water-disp.; pH 4-6; usage level: 1-3%; 36-38% solids.

Bio-Soft® D-60. [Stepan] Sodium dodecylbenzenesulfonate; CAS 25155-30-0; EINECS 246-680-4; surfactant.

Bio-Soft® E-200. [Stepan Canada] Laureth-1; CAS 4536-30-5; EINECS 224-886-5; nonionic; emulsifier, detergent, wetting and foam stabilizing; liq.; HLB 4.0; 100% act.

Bio-Soft® E-300. [Stepan Canada] Laureth-2; CAS 3055-93-4; EINECS 221-279-7; nonionic; emulsifier, detergent, wetting and foam stabilizing; liq.; HLB 6.0; 100% act.

Bio-Soft® E-400. [Stepan Canada] C12-15 pareth-3; CAS 68131-39-5; nonionic; emulsifier, detergent, wetting and foam stabilizing; liq.; HLB 8.0; 100% act.

Bio-Soft® EN 600. [Stepan Canada] C12-15 pareth-7; CAS 68131-39-5; nonionic; emulsifier, detergent, wetting and foam stabilizing; liq.; HLB 12.2; 100% act.

Bio-Soft® MT 40. [Stepan Europe] TEA-coco hydrolyzed animal protein; CAS 68952-16-9; anionic; very mild surfactant, conditioner, foaming agent for medicated and conditioning shampoos, creams, baby prods.; amber liq.; 42% act.

Bio-Soft® N-21. [Stepan] TEA-dodecylbenzenesulfonate and cocamide DEA.

Bio-Soft® N-300. [Stepan; Stepan Canada] TEA-dodecylbenzene sulfonate; CAS 27323-41-7; EINECS 248-406-9; anionic; detergent, wetting and foaming agent for dishwash, carwash detergents, oily hair shampoos; effectively removes oil without stripping hair; biodeg.; pale yel. clear liq.; water sol.; dens. 9.0 lb/gal; sp.gr. 1.08; visc. 3200 cps; surf. tens. 38.8 dynes/cm (0.1%); 60% act.

Bio-Soft® TD 400. [Stepan Canada] Trideceth-3; CAS 4403-12-7; EINECS 224-540-3; nonionic; emulsifier; liq.; oil-sol.; HLB 8.0; 100% act.

Bio-Soft® TD 630. [Stepan Canada] Trideceth-8; CAS 24938-91-8; nonionic; emulsifier, detergent; liq.; water-sol.; HLB 12.5; 100% act.

Biosol. [Osaka Kasei] o-Cymen-5-ol; CAS 3228-02-2; EINECS 221-761-7.

Biosulphur Fluid CLR. [Dr. Kurt Richter; Henkel/Cospha] Polysorbate 80 and sulfur; hydro-alcohol solubilized sulfur; conditioner for applic. to skin with excessive sebum secretion; prods. for impure skin, oily hair and dandruff; dk. brn. visc. prod.; 1.6% S.

Biosulphur Powder. [Dr. Kurt Richter; Henkel/Cospha] Micro grained act. sulfur (96.5% S) with protective colloid; CAS 7704-34-9; EINECS 231-722-6; prods. for impure skin, oily hair and dandruff; beige micro-powd.

Bio-Surf PBC-460. [Lonza] Lauryl myristyl dimethyl amine oxides; nonionic/cationic; detergent aid in stabilizing foam; emollient, visc. builder for aq. systems; liq.; 30% conc.

Bio-Terge® 804. [Stepan; Stepan Canada] Sodium C14-16 olefin sulfonate, sodium laureth sulfate, lauramide DEA; anionic; surfactant conc. for hand soaps, bath prods., and shampoos; liq.; 50% act.

Bio-Terge® AS-40. [Stepan; Stepan Canada] Sodium C14-16 olefin sulfonate; CAS 68439-57-6; EINECS 270-407-8; anionic; detergent, foaming agent for personal care (shampoos, hand soaps, bath prods.), commercial and industrial formulations; provides exc. flash foam; biodeg.; contains no phosphates; yel. liquid; water sol.; dens. 8.9 lb/gal; 40% act. in water.

Biowax 754. [Biosil Tech.] Dimethicone copolyol wax; nonionic; wax for cosmetics applics.; wh. wax; water-sol.; flash pt. (PMCC) > 200 F; 100% solids.

Biozan. [Hercules] Xanthan gum; CAS 11138-66-2; EINECS 234-394-2; suspending agent, thickener, emulsifier in slurry explosives, foundry coatings, acid and caustic cleaning compds., cosmetics, pharmaceuticals, oil field chemicals, aq. systems; food grade avail.; water-sol.

Biron® . [Rona] Bismuth oxychloride powds. and dispersions; CAS 7787-59-9; EINECS 232-122-7; pearlescent filler pigments for cosmetics and toiletries, esp. pressed powds., makeup, anhyd. systems.

Biron® B-5. [Rona; E. Merck] Bismuth oxychloride; CAS 7787-59-9; EINECS 232-122-7; pearlescent pigment.

Biron® B-50. [Rona; E. Merck] Bismuth oxychloride; CAS 7787-59-9; EINECS 232-122-7; pearlescent pigment.

Biron® B-50 CO. [Rona; E. Merck] Bismuth oxychloride and castor oil.

Biron® ESQ. [Rona] Bismuth oxychloride powd.; CAS 7787-59-9; EINECS 232-122-7; low opacity, matte pigment with low oil absorp., good compressibility, skin adhesion, and smooth skin feel; for makeup, pressed powds., stick prods., and emulsion, anhyd., and powd. formulations; usage level: 2-30%.

Biron® Fines. [Rona; E. Merck] Bismuth oxychloride; CAS 7787-59-9; EINECS 232-122-7; pearlescent pigment.

Biron® HB. [Rona; E. Merck] Bismuth oxychloride; CAS 7787-59-9; EINECS 232-122-7; pearlescent pigment.

Biron® NLD. [Rona; E. Merck] Bismuth oxychloride and polysorbate 20.

Biron® NLD-SP. [Rona; E. Merck] Bismuth oxychloride; CAS 7787-59-9; EINECS 232-122-7; pearlescent pigment.

Biron® NLY-L-2X AQ. [Rona; E. Merck] Bismuth oxychloride, water, and polysorbate 20.

Biron® NLY-L-2X CO. [Rona; E. Merck] Bismuth oxychloride, castor oil.

Biron® NLY-L-2X MO. [Rona; E. Merck] Bismuth oxychloride, min. oil.

Biron® Silver CO. [Rona; E. Merck] Bismuth oxychloride, castor oil.

α-Bisabolol. [BASF AG] (-)-α-Bisabolol nat. derived from chamomile and (±)-α-bisabolol rac. (synthetic); CAS 515-69-5; EINECS 208-205-9; antiphlogistic (anti-inflammatory) active agent for cosmetics industry for protection and care of sensitive skin, esp. baby/child preps., sunscreen, aftersun, aftershave, and oral hygiene preps.; colorless to sl. ylsh. clear liq., faint floral sweetish odor; sol. in ethanol, 2-propanol, natural, min., and syn. fats and oils; insol. in water and glycerin; toxicology: (-): LD50 (rat) > 15,000 mg/kg; nonirritating to skin, sl. irritating to eyes.

Bismica 46. [Presperse] Mica (60%), bismuth oxychloride (40%); CAS 12001-26-2, 7787-59-9; pearlescent pigment for cosmetics use; JSCI/JCID approved; wh. pearlescent free-flowing powd.; particle size 15-25 μ; 98% min. assay.

Bismica 55. [Presperse] Bismuth oxychloride (50%), mica (50%); CAS 7787-59-9, 12001-26-2; pearlescent pigment for cosmetics; JSCI/JCID approved; wh. pearlescent free-flowing powd.; particle size 15-25 μ; 98% min. assay.

Bismica 596. [Presperse] Bismuth oxychloride (70%), mica (30%); CAS 7787-59-9, 12001-26-2; pearlescent pigment for cosmetics use; JSCI/JCID approved; speckly wh. pearlescent free-flowing powd.; particle size 15-25 μ; 98% min. assay.

Bital® . [Rona] Platy talc coated with bismuth oxychloride; pearlescent pigments for cosmetics and toiletries, esp. loose and pressed powds.; offers good skin feel and adhesion.

Bitrex. [Macfarlan Smith] Denatonium benzoate NF; CAS 3734-33-6; EINECS 223-095-2; aversive (bitter) agent used to minimize danger of prod. ingestion; denaturant for ethanol; wh. gran., odorless; m.w. 446.5; sol. in water, chloroform, IPA; highly sol. in methanol, ethanol; m.p. 163–170 C; pH 6.5–7.5; 99.5–101.0% assay.

Bitter Almond HS. [Alban Muller] Propylene glycol and bitter almond extract; botanical extract.

Bitter Almond LS. [Alban Muller] Sunflower seed oil and bitter almond extract.

Black 103. [Presperse] Iron oxides (90%), bismuth oxychloride (10%); CAS 1309-37-1, 7787-59-9; inorg. colorant for pigmented cosmetics; JSCI/JCID approved.

Black Mica. [Rona; E. Merck] Iron oxides, mica, and titanium dioxide.

Blanc Covachip W 9705. [Les Colorants Wackherr] Titanium dioxide, nitrocellulose, and dibutyl phthalate.

Blanc Covanail W 9737. [Les Colorants Wackherr] Titanium dioxide and acrylates copolymer.

Blanc Covapate W 9765. [Les Colorants Wackherr] Titanium dioxide and castor oil.

Blanc Covasop W 9775. [Les Colorants Wackherr] Titanium dioxide and propylene glycol.

Blandol® . [Witco/Petroleum Spec.] Wh. min. oil N.F.; lubricant used in food, drug, and cosmetic industry; FDA §172.878, 178.3620a; water-wh., odorless, tasteless; sp.gr. 0.839-0.855; visc. 14-17 cSt (40 C); pour pt. -7 C; flash pt. 179 C.

Blanose 7 Types. [Aqualon France] Sodium carboxymethyl cellulose gum, food and pharmaceutical grades; thickener, stabilizer, rheology control agent, film-former, suspending agent, water-retention aid, binder for food, pharmaceutical, toothpaste, and cosmetic industries; FDA, EEC compliance; visc. various grades from 40 to 40,000 mPa·s; pH 6.5-8.5; 99.5% purity.

Blanose 9 Types. [Aqualon France] Sodium carboxymethyl cellulose gum, food and pharmaceutical grades; thickener, stabilizer, rheology control agent, film-former, suspending agent, water-retention aid, binder for food, pharmaceutical, and cosmetic industries; visc. various grades from 2000 to 40,000 mPa·s; pH 6.5-8.5; 99.5% purity.

Blanose 12 Types. [Aqualon France] Sodium carboxymethyl cellulose gum, food and pharmaceutical grades; thickener, stabilizer, rheology control agent, film-former, suspending agent, water-retention aid, binder for food, pharmaceutical, and cosmetic industries; visc. 600-2000 mPa·s; pH 6.5-8.5; 99.5% purity.

Bleached Beeswax. [Will & Baumer] Beeswax; wax for personal care prods.

Blend For Bust Cares HS 201. [Alban Muller] Propylene glycol, fenugreek extract, hops extract, horsetail extract, olibanum extract; botanical extract.

Blend For Chapped Skins HS 361. [Alban Muller] Propylene glycol, hypericum extract, horse chestnut extract, and myrrh extract; botanical extract.

Blend For Delicate Skins HS 215. [Alban Muller] Propylene glycol, olibanum extract, hypericum extract, rose hips extract, and grape extract.

Blend For Deodorant HS 275. [Alban Muller] Propylene glycol, myrrh extract, sage extract, and eucalyptus extract; botanical extract.

Blend For Elderly Skins HS 296. [Alban Muller] Propylene glycol, wheat germ extract, sunflower seed extract, horsetail extract, and myrrh extract; botanical extract.

Blend For Greasy Hair HS 312. [Alban Muller] Propylene glycol, ivy extract, watercress extract, rocket extract; botanical extract.

Blend For Greasy Skin Imperfections HS 315. [Alban Muller] Propylene glycol, rocket extract, ivy extract, myrrh extract, watercress extract; botanical extract.

Blend For Slenderizing Prods. HS 255. [Alban Muller] Propylene glycol, algae extract, ivy extract, and spiraea extract; botanical extract.

Blendmax. [Central Soya] Lysolecithin.

Bleu Covachip W 6700. [Les Colorants Wackherr] Ferric ferrocyanide, nitrocellulose, and dibutyl phthalate.

Bleu Covasop W 6776. [Les Colorants Wackherr] Ultramarines and propylene glycol.

Bleu Covasorb W 6783 A. [Les Colorants Wackherr] Sorbitol and ultramarines.

Bleu De Prusse Micronise W 6805. [Les Colorants Wackherr] Ferric ferrocyanide and talc.

Bleu De Prusse Pur W 745. [Les Colorants Wackherr] Ferric ferrocyanide; CAS 25869-00-5; cosmetic colorant.

Bleu D'Outremer Special. [Les Colorants Wackherr] Ultramarines.

Blonde 90 (Fusion). [Lowenstein] Resorcinol, p-phenylenediamine, 2-nitro-p-phenylenediamine.

Blonde R-50 (Fusion). [Lowenstein] Resorcinol, p-phenylenediamine, 2-nitro-p-phenylenediamine, 4-nitro-o-phenylenediamine.

Blue 135. [Presperse] FD&C blue #1 aluminum lake and bismuth oxychloride; organic colorant for pigmented cosmetics; Japanese approval.

Blue Covapate W 6763. [Les Colorants Wackherr] Castor oil and ultramarines.

Bodaiju Liq. [Ichimaru Pharcos] Water, butylene glycol, and linden extract.

Boisambrene Forte. [Henkel/Cospha] Formaldehyde ethyl cyclododecylacetal; fragrance raw material for personal care and detergent formulations; colorless liq., woody odor; b.p. 94 C; flash pt. 145 C.

Bonarox. [Henkel/Cospha] Aroma chemical for cosmetic, personal care, detergent, and cleaning prods.; colorless liq., fruity odor; b.p. 67-70 C; flash pt. 102 C.

Bovinal-20. [R.I.T.A.] Serum albumin; protein for use in skin and hair care preps.

Bovine Amniotic Liq. [Gattefosse] Amniotic fluid, glycerin, and propylene glycol.

Bovine Fetuin. [Intergen] Glycoproteins.

Bovine Fibronectin Sol'n. [Intergen] Sodium phosphate, urea, and fibronectin.

Bovine Native Insoluble Elastin. [Kelisema Srl; G.F. Secchi] Elastin.

Bovine Serum Albumin Sol'n. [Intergen] Serum albumin.

Bovinol 30. [R.I.T.A.] Serum albumin; whole protein skin, hair, and nail conditioner; amber liq.; 30% sol'n.

BPA-500. [Kobo] Polymethyl methacrylate; CAS 9011-14-7; cosmetic ingred.

Braxicina. [Vevy] Soybean oil and cauliflower unsaponifiables.

Bretol® . [Zeeland] Cetethyldimonium bromide; CAS 124-03-8; EINECS 204-672-8; germicide, detergent.

Brij® 30. [ICI Spec. Chem.; ICI Surf. Am.; ICI Surf. Belgium] Laureth-4; CAS 5274-68-0; EINECS 226-097-1; nonionic; o/w emulsifier, wetting agent for topical cosmetics, household, and industrial applics.; colorless to lt. yel. liq. (may become hazy or form a precipitate); sol. in alcohol, propylene glycol, cottonseed oil; sp.gr. 0.95; visc. 30 cps; HLB 9.7; flash pt. >300 F; 100% conc.

Brij® 30SP. [ICI Spec. Chem.] Laureth-4, preservatives; CAS 5274-68-0; EINECS 226-097-1; nonionic; o/w emulsifier for topical cosmetics; colorless to lt. yel. liq.; sol. in alcohol, propylene glycol, cottonseed oil; sp.gr. 0.95; visc. 30 cps; HLB 9.5; flash pt. >300 F; 100% conc.

Brij® 35. [ICI Spec. Chem.; ICI Surf. Am.; ICI Surf. Belgium] Laureth-23; CAS 9002-92-0; nonionic; emulsifier, wetting agent for personal care, household, and industrial applics.; wh. waxy solid; sol. in water, alcohol, propylene glycol; sp.gr. 1.05; HLB 16.9; flash pt. >300 F; pour pt. 33 C.

Brij® 52. [ICI Spec. Chem.; ICI Surf. Am.; ICI Surf. Belgium] Ceteth-2 (antioxidants added); CAS 9004-95-9; nonionic; emulsifier, wetting agent for topical cosmetics, household and industrial applics.; wh. waxy solid; sol. in alcohol, cottonseed oil, min. oil; HLB 5.3; flash pt. > 300F; pour pt. 33 C; 100% conc.

Brij® 56. [ICI Spec. Chem.; ICI Surf. Am.; ICI Surf. Belgium] Ceteth-10 (antioxidants added); CAS 9004-95-9; nonionic; emulsifier, wetting agent esp. for topical cosmetic applics., household and industrial applics.; solubilizer for fragrances; wh. waxy solid; sol. in alcohol; HLB 12.9; flash pt. > 300F; pour pt. 31 C; 100% conc.

Brij® 58. [ICI Spec. Chem.; ICI Surf. Am.; ICI Surf. Belgium] Ceteth-20 with preservatives; CAS 9004-95-9; nonionic; emulsifier, wetting agent for personal care prods., household and industrial applics.; solubilizer for fragrances; wh. waxy solid; sol. in water, alcohol; HLB 15.7; flash pt. > 300

F; pour pt. 38 C; 100% conc.

Brij® 72. [ICI Spec. Chem.; ICI Surf. Am.; ICI Surf. Belgium] Steareth-2 with preservatives; CAS 9005-00-9; nonionic; emulsifier, wetting agent esp. for topical cosmetics, household and industrial applics.; wh. waxy solid; sol. in alcohol, cottonseed oil; HLB 4.9; flash pt. >300 F; pour pt. 43 C; 100% conc.

Brij® 76. [ICI Spec. Chem.; ICI Surf. Am.; ICI Surf. Belgium] Steareth-10 with preservatives; CAS 9005-00-9; nonionic; o/w emulsifier, wetting agent for topical cosmetics, household and industrial applics.; solubilizer for fragrances; wh. waxy solid; sol. in propylene glycol, ethanol; HLB 12.4; flash pt. > 300 F; pour pt. 38 C; 100% conc.

Brij® 78. [ICI Spec. Chem.; ICI Surf. Am.; ICI Surf. Belgium] Steareth-20 with preservatives; CAS 9005-00-9; nonionic; emulsifier, wetting agent esp. for topical cosmetics, household and industrial applics.; solubilizer for fragrances; wh. waxy solid; sol. in water, alcohol; disp. in cottonseed oil; HLB 15.3; flash pt. > 300 F; pour pt. 38 C; 100% conc.

Brij® 93. [ICI Spec. Chem.; ICI Surf. Am.; ICI Surf. UK] Oleth-2; CAS 9004-98-2; nonionic; surfactant with low color and odor; emulsifier, wetting agent; disperses emollients, perfume oils, and surfactants; esp. for blooming bath oils; also for household and industrial applics.; pale yel. liq.; sol. in alcohol, cottonseed and min. oils, propylene glycol; insol. in water; visc. 30 cps; HLB 4.9.

Brij® 97. [ICI Spec. Chem.; ICI Surf. Am.; ICI Surf. UK] Oleth-10; CAS 9004-98-2; nonionic; o/w emulsifier, wetting agent esp. for cosmetics requiring min. odor and color; also for household and industrial applics.; pale yel. liq.; sol. in water and alcohol; visc. 100 cps; HLB 12.4; flash pt. > 300 F; pour pt. 16 C; 100% conc.

Brij® 98. [ICI Spec. Chem.; ICI Surf. Am.; ICI Surf. Belgium] Oleth-20; CAS 9004-98-2; nonionic; emulsifier, wetting agent for personal care, household, and industrial applics.; solubilizer for fragrances; cream-colored soft waxy solid; sol. in water, alcohol, propylene glycol; HLB 15.3; flash pt. > 300 F; pour pt. 30 C; 100% conc.

Brij® 700. [ICI Spec. Chem.; ICI Surf. Am.; ICI Surf. Belgium] Steareth-100; CAS 9005-00-9; nonionic; emulsifier, wetting agent for cosmetics and pharmaceuticals, stick prods.; oil solubilization; pale yel. solid; sol. in water, alcohol; disp. in cottonseed oil; HLB 18.8; pour pt. 55 C; 100% conc.

Brij® 700S. [ICI Spec. Chem.; ICI Surf. Am.] Steareth-100; CAS 9005-00-9; nonionic; emulsifier, solubilizer, wetting agent for personal care, household, and industrial applics.; wh. solid gran.; sol. in water, alcohol; disp. in cottonseed oil; HLB 18.8; pour pt. 55 C; 100% conc.

Brij® 721. [ICI Spec. Chem.; ICI Surf. Am.; ICI Surf. Belgium] Steareth-21; CAS 9005-00-9; nonionic; emulsifier, wetting agent for personal care, household, and industrial applics.; solubilizer for fragrances; colorless waxy flakes, waxy odor; disp. in water, alcohol, cottonseed oil; HLB 15.5; pour pt. 45 C; flash pt. (PMCC) > 230 F; 100% conc.

Brij® 721S. [ICI Spec. Chem.; ICI Surf. Am.] Steareth-21; CAS 9005-00-9; nonionic; emulsifier, solubilizer, wetting agent for personal care, household, and industrial applics.; wh. solid gran.; disp. in water, alcohol, cottonseed oil; HLB 15.5; pour pt. 45 C; 100% conc.

Brillance 515. [Gattefosse] Apricot kernel oil PEG-6 esters and ethylcellulose.

Brillante. [Luzenac Am.] Pure Italian talc USP; CAS 14807-96-6; EINECS 238-877-9; specially treated for sheer, pearlescent appearance; used in bath and dusting powds., creams, lotions, blushers, and soaps; powd.; 94% thru 200 mesh; median diam. 35 µ; tapped dens. 62 lb/ft³; pH 9 (10% slurry).

Briphos O3D. [Gattefosse] Oleth-3 phosphate; CAS 39464-69-2; personal care surfactant.

Britesil. [PQ Corp.] Sodium silicate; CAS 1344-09-8; EINECS 215-687-4.

Britex C. [Auschem SpA] Ceteth-2; CAS 9004-95-9; nonionic; emulsifier for cosmetics and pharmaceuticals; waxy solid; HLB 5.3; 100% conc.

Britex C 20. [Auschem SpA] Ceteth-2; CAS 9004-95-9; emulsifier.

Britex C 100. [Auschem SpA] Ceteth-10; CAS 9004-95-9; nonionic; emulsifier for cosmetics and pharmaceuticals; solid; HLB 12.9; 100% conc.

Britex C 200. [Auschem SpA] Ceteth-20; CAS 9004-95-9; nonionic; emulsifier for cosmetics and pharmaceuticals; flakes; HLB 15.7; 100% conc.

Britex CO 220. [Auschem SpA] Cetoleth-22; CAS 68920-66-1; nonionic; emulsifier for cosmetics and pharmaceuticals; flakes; HLB 15.9; 100% conc.

Britex CS 110. [Auschem SpA] Ceteareth-11; CAS 68439-49-6; nonionic; emulsifier for cosmetics and pharmaceuticals; flakes; HLB 13.0; 100% conc.

Britex CS 200 B. [Auschem SpA] Ceteareth-20; CAS 68439-49-6; nonionic; emulsifier for cosmetics and pharmaceuticals; BP grade; flakes; HLB 15.5; 100% conc.

Britex CS 250. [Auschem SpA] Ceteareth-25; CAS 68439-49-6; nonionic; emulsifier for cosmetics and pharmaceuticals; flakes; HLB 16.5; 100% conc.

Britex CS 300. [Auschem SpA] Ceteareth-30; CAS 68439-49-6.

Britex CS 1000. [Auschem SpA] Ceteareth-100; CAS 68439-49-6.

Britex EMB. [Auschem SpA] Laureth-9; CAS 3055-99-0; EINECS 221-284-4; personal care surfactant.

Britex EW/BP. [Auschem SpA] Cetearyl alcohol and ceteareth-23.

Britex L 20. [Auschem SpA] Laureth-2; CAS 9002-92-0; EINECS 221-279-7; nonionic; emulsifier for cosmetics and pharmaceuticals; liq.; HLB 6.5; 100% conc.

Britex L 40. [Auschem SpA] Laureth-4; CAS 9002-92-0; EINECS 226-097-1; nonionic; emulsifier for cosmetics and pharmaceuticals; liq.; HLB 9.7; 100% conc.

Britex L 100. [Auschem SpA] Laureth-10; CAS 9002-92-0; nonionic; emulsifier for cosmetics and pharmaceuticals; liq./paste; HLB 14.0; 100% conc.

Britex L 230. [Auschem SpA] Laureth-23; CAS 9002-92-0; nonionic; emulsifier for cosmetics and pharmaceuticals; solid; HLB 16.9; 100% conc.

Britex O 20. [Auschem SpA] Oleth-2; CAS 9004-98-2; nonionic; emulsifier for cosmetics and pharmaceuticals; liq.; HLB 4.9; 100% conc.

Britex O 100. [Auschem SpA] Oleth-10; CAS 9004-98-2; nonionic; emulsifier for cosmetics and pharmaceuticals; liq.; HLB 12.4; 100% conc.

Britex O 200. [Auschem SpA] Oleth-20; CAS 9004-98-2; nonionic; emulsifier for cosmetics and pharmaceuticals; paste/solid; HLB 15.3; 100% conc.

Britex S 20. [Auschem SpA] Steareth-2; CAS 9004-00-9; nonionic; emulsifier for cosmetics and pharmaceuticals; solid; HLB 4.9; 100% conc.

Britex S 100. [Auschem SpA] Steareth-10; CAS 9004-00-9; nonionic; emulsifier for cosmetics and pharmaceuticals; flakes; HLB 12.4; 100% conc.

Britex S 200. [Auschem SpA] Steareth-20; CAS 9004-00-9; nonionic; emulsifier for cosmetics and pharmaceuticals; flakes; HLB 15.3; 100% conc.

Britex TR 120. [Auschem SpA] Trideceth-12; CAS 24938-91-8; nonionic; emulsifier for cosmetics; liq./paste; HLB 14.5; 100% conc.

Britex TR 60. [Auschem SpA] Trideceth-6; CAS 24938-91-8; nonionic; emulsifier for cosmetics; liq.; HLB 11.4; 100% conc.

Britol® . [Witco/Petroleum Spec.] Wh. min. oil USP; emollient, lubricant, binder, carrier, moisture barrier, softener for food processing, pharmaceuticals, cosmetics, and industrial use; FDA §172.878, 178.3620a; water-wh., odorless, tasteless; sp.gr. 0.869-0.885; visc. 56-60 cSt (40 C); pour pt. -15 C; flash pt. 199 C.

Britol® 6NF. [Witco/Petroleum Spec.] White min. oil NF; white oil functioning as binder, carrier, conditioner, defoamer, dispersant, extender, heat transfer agent, lubricant, moisture barrier, plasticizer, protective agent, release agent, and/or softener; used in cosmetics, pharmaceuticals, food, plastics, agric., and paper making applics.; sp.gr. 0.830-0.858; visc. 8.5-10.8 cst (40 C); pour pt. -24 C max.; flash pt. 166 C min.

Britol® 7NF. [Witco/Petroleum Spec.] White min. oil NF; see Britol 6NF; sp.gr. 0.840-0.858; visc. 10.8-13.6 cst (40 C); pour pt. -18 C max.; flash pt. 171 C min.

Britol® 9NF. [Witco/Petroleum Spec.] White min. oil NF; see Britol 6NF; sp.gr. 0.845-0.860; visc. 14.4-16.9 cst (40 C); pour pt. -18 C max.; flash pt. 171 C min.

Britol® 20USP. [Witco/Petroleum Spec.] White min. oil USP; see Britol 6NF; sp.gr. 0.858-0.870; visc. 37.9-40.1 cst (40 C); pour pt. -18 C max.; flash pt. 193 C min.

Britol® 24. [Witco/Petroleum Spec.] Mineral oil; emollient, cosmetic raw material.

Britol® 35USP. [Witco/Petroleum Spec.] White min. oil USP; see Britol 6NF; sp.gr. 0.862-0.880; visc. 65.8-71.0 cst (40 C); pour pt. -15 C max.; flash pt. 216 C min.

Britol® 50USP. [Witco/Petroleum Spec.] White min. oil USP; see Britol 6NF; sp.gr. 0.870-0.890; visc. 91-102.4 cst (40 C); pour pt. -12 C max.; flash pt. 249 C min.

Brocose Q. [Brooks Industries] Hydrog. soyadimoniumhydroxypropyl polyglucose; natural biodeg. quaternary used to condition, soften, and moisturize in hair care prods.

Bromat® . [Zeeland] Cetyl trimethyl ammonium bromide; CAS 57-09-0; EINECS 200-311-3; cationic; surfactant, emulsifier, germicide; effective against Gram-positive bacteria; wh. free-flowing powd., char. odor, astringent bitter taste; sol. in alcohol, chloroform; sl. sol. in ethyl glycol, acetone; m.w. 364.44; soften. pt. 218 C; decomp. pt. 235-240 C; flash pt. (TCC) > 200 F; pH 5-8 (1% aq.); surf. tens. 40 dynes/cm (0.1% aq.); toxicology: LD50 (oral, rabbit) 760 mg/kg; corrosive—causes skin and eye damage in conc. form; 100% conc.

Bromelain 1:10. [Solvay Enzymes] Mixt. of proteases, standardized with lactose; enzyme for hydrolysis of plant and animal proteins to peptides and amino acids; for tenderizer formulations for meat; in baking; pharmaceuticals (wound debriding agent, blood typing studies, digestive aid); fish processing; eliminates protein haze in foods; brewing, fermentation; animal feed supplement; leather bating; paper, photographic, and textile processing; tan to lt. brn. amorphous powd., free of offensive odor and taste; water-sol.

Bromelain Conc. [Solvay Enzymes] Mixt. of proteases; enzyme for hydrolysis of plant and animal proteins to peptides and amino acids; for tenderizer formulations for meat; in baking; pharmaceuticals (wound debriding agent, blood typing studies); fish processing; eliminates protein haze in foods; tan to lt. brn. amorphous powd., free of offensive odor and taste; water-sol.

Bronidox® L. [Henkel/Cospha; Henkel Canada; Henkel KGaA/Cospha] 5-Bromo-5-nitro-1,3-dioxane dissolved in 1,2 propylene glycol; CAS 30007-47-7; EINECS 250-001-7; preservative for shampoos, foam baths, body cleaners, child/baby shampoos, hand cleansers, and all preps. which do not remain on the skin; effective for gram-positive and -negative bacteria and fungi; almost colorless clear liq.; sol. in aq. systems; sp.gr. 1.080-1.090;

cloud pt. 15 C; flash pt. 100 C; ref. index 1.435-1.437; corrosive to metals; usage level: 0.2%; 9.5-10.5% act.

Bronidox® L 5. [Henkel KGaA/Cospha] 5-Bromo-5-nitro-1,3-dioxane dissolved in 1,2 propylene glycol; CAS 30007-47-7; EINECS 250-001-7; preservative for shampoos, foam baths, body cleansers, child/baby shampoos, hand cleaners, and all cosmetics which do not remain on the skin; effective against gram-positive and -negative bacteria and fungi; almost colorless liq.; sol. in aq. systems; sp.gr. 1.055-1.065; cloud pt. < -5 C; flash pt. 100 C; ref. index 1.433-1.435; usage level: 0.4%; 4.5-5.5% act.

Bronodox L. [Universal Preserv-A-Chem] 5-Bromo-5-nitro-1,3-dioxane; CAS 30007-47-7; EINECS 250-001-7; cosmetic preservative.

Bronodox L-5. [Universal Preserv-A-Chem] 5-Bromo-5-nitro-1,3-dioxane and propylene glycol; CAS 30007-47-7; EINECS 250-001-7; cosmetic preservative.

Bronopol. [Angus; Boots Microcheck; Inolex] 2-Bromo-2-nitropropane-1,3-diol; CAS 52-51-7; EINECS 200-143-0; preservative for cosmetics and personal care prods.; wh. or almost wh. cryst. powd.; sol. in water, alcohol, glycols, and polyols.; toxicology: LD50 (acute oral, rat) 324 mg/kg; harmful or fatal if swallowed; eye irritant; not a primary skin irritant; 99-100% purity.

Brookosome® A. [Brooks Industries] Water, phospholipids, and allantoin; liposome for cosmetic applics.; skin protectant and soothing agent; 0.4% act., 10% lipids.

Brookosome® ACEBC. [Brooks Industries] Water, phospholipids, retinyl palmitate, tocopherol, ascorbyl palmitate, and beta-carotene; liposome for cosmetic applics.

Brookosome® ANE. [Brooks Industries] Phospholipids, retinyl palmitate, and tocopheryl acetate; liposome for cosmetics; moisturizer, free radical scavenger; normalizes skin's barrier props.; 10% lipids.

Brookosome® A-Plus. [Brooks Industries] Phospholipids, retinyl palmitate polypeptide; stabilized liposome for cosmetics; 5% act., 10% lipids.

Brookosome® BC. [Brooks Industries] Phospholipids and beta-carotene; liposome for cosmetics; protects skin from damage caused by uv radiation; 0.01% act., 10% lipids.

Brookosome® Biophos. [Brooks Industries] Phospholipids and phosphoglycoproteins; liposome for moisturizing, low-odor cosmetics; rich in the oligoelements lost during exercise; topical applic. produces a revitalized, stimulated, and refreshed feeling; 2% act., 10% lipids.

Brookosome® C. [Brooks Industries] Phospholipids and vitamin C; liposome for cosmetics; free radical scavenger; also capable of reducing melanin to a colorless substance, combatting excessive pigmentation; 0.1% act., 10% lipids.

Brookosome® CS. [Brooks Industries] Phospholipids and chondroitin sulfate; liposome for cosmetic applics.; produces long-lasting moisturing film on the skin; 10% lipids.

Brookosome® CU. [Brooks Industries] Phospholipids and copper glycoproteins; liposome for cosmetics; provides a nontoxic and bioavailable source of copper which as been linked with immune response and cell proliferation; 1% act., 10% lipids.

Brookosome® DHA. [Brooks Industries] Water, phospholipids, and dihydroxyacetone; liposome for cosmetic applics.; 10% act.

Brookosome® DNA/RNA. [Brooks Industries] Phospholipids, DNA, and RNA; liposome for cosmetic applics.; moisturizes and firms the skin; 10% lipids.

Brookosome® E. [Brooks Industries] Water, phospholipids, and tocopheryl acetate; liposome for cosmetic applics.; moisturizer, free radical scavenger combatting lipid peroxidation; 1% act., 10% lipids.

Brookosome® EFA. [Brooks Industries] Phospholipids, omega 6 linoleic acid, omega 3 linolenic acid; moisturizer for skin cosmetics; maintains skin flexibility and barrier function; 1% act., 10% lipids.

Brookosome® Elastin. [Brooks Industries] Phospholipids and hydrolyzed elastin; liposome for cosmetic applics.; moisture binding and film-forming agent; 1% act., 10% lipids.

Brookosome® ELL. [Brooks Industries] Water, phospholipids, brain extract, tocopheryl acetate, retinyl palmitate, and linoleic acid; liposome for cosmetic applics.

Brookosome® EPO. [Brooks Industries] Water, phospholipids, and evening primrose oil; liposome; moisturizer and softener for skin cosmetics; 5% act., 10% lipids.

Brookosome® F. [Brooks Industries] Phospholipids and perfluoropolymethylisopropyl ether; liposome for cosmetics; improves barrier function against a wide range of aggressive agents without impairing aesthetic props. of cosmetic formulations; 1% act., 10% lipids.

Brookosome® FIH. [Brooks Industries] Phospholipids, horsechestnut, ivy and fucus extracts; liposome for cosmetics; increases microcirculation, cell turnover rate, and smoothes the skin; helps fight cellulite; 1% act., 8% lipids.

Brookosome® Fucus. [Brooks Industries] Phospholipids, fucus extract; skin moisturizer for use in slimming creams; derived from succulent giant kelp (*Fucus vesiculosus*).

Brookosome® GSL. [Brooks Industries] Water, phospholipids, and brain extract; liposome for cosmetic applics.; normalizes stratum corneum lipids, preserving the barrier function of the skin and reducing transepidermal water loss; 2% act.

Brookosome® H. [Brooks Industries] Water, phospholipids, and sodium hyaluronate; liposome for cosmetic applics.; moisturizer capable of binding up to 180 times its own weight in water; 0.1% act.

Brookosome® Herbal. [Brooks Industries] Water, phospholipids, horsetail extract, myrrh extract, sunflower seed extract, and wheat germ extract; liposome for cosmetic applics.; stimulates, tones, and conditions the skin; 1% act., 10% lipids.

Brookosome® MPS. [Brooks Industries] Phospholipids and glycosaminoglycans; liposome for skin care prods.; provides long-lasting moisturization; 0.5% act.

Brookosome® MSF. [Brooks Industries] Lecithin and yeast betaglucan; liposome enhancing penetration on skin and retention in the epidermis for a longer lasting effect; macrophage stimulating factor; contributes wound healing props.; for use as topical moisturizer and wrinkle reducer; usage level: 1%; 0.5% act.

Brookosome® MT. [Brooks Industries] Water and phospholipids; liposome for cosmetic applics.; 10% lipids.

Brookosome® P. [Brooks Industries] Water, panthenol, and phospholipids; liposome for cosmetic applics.; moisturizer promoting flexibility in hair, skin, and nails; promotes cellular respiration; 10% act., 10% lipids.

Brookosome® Planell. [Brooks Industries] Phospholipids, squalene, squalane, glycolipids, phytosterol, and tocopherol; plant cell oil liposome; emollient and moisturizer for skin care prods.; normalizes the surface lipids of the skin; 5% act., 10% lipids.

Brookosome® RJ. [Brooks Industries] Phospholipids and royal jelly; liposome for cosmetics; nutritive compd. rich in complex biologicals; 10% act., 10% lipids.

Brookosome® RP. [Brooks Industries] Water, phospholipids, and retinyl palmitate; liposome for cosmetic applics.; normalizes skin's barrier props.; 5% act., 5% lipids.

Brookosome® S. [Brooks Industries] Water, squalane, and phospholipids; liposome for cosmetic applics.; nongreasy emollient, skin conditioner; 10% act., 10% lipids.

Brookosome® SC. [Brooks Industries] Water, phospholipids, and sol. collagen; liposome for moisturizing cosmetics; film-former; 10% act.

Brookosome® SE. [Brooks Industries] Water, phospholipids, and spleen extract; liposome for skin care prods.; increases cellular respiration and oxygen uptake, stimulating and rejuvenating cells of the stratum corneum; 5% act.

Brookosome® Serum. [Brooks Industries] Water, phospholipids, and hydrolyzed serum protein; cationic; liposome for cosmetics; substantive skin conditioning agent, moisturizer; increases flexibility of skin; 10% act.

Brookosome® SOD. [Brooks Industries] Water, lecithin, and superoxide dismutase; stable liposome to help control aging effect in living cells; free radical scavenging enzyme.

Brookosome® TA. [Brooks Industries] Phospholipids, tyrosine, and zinc yeast deriv.; liposome for cosmetic tanning prods., accelerating tanning process; 10% act., 10% lipids.

Brookosome® TE. [Brooks Industries] Water, phospholipids, and thymus extract; liposome for cosmetic applics.; stimulates fibroblast activity.

Brookosome® TRF. [Brooks Industries] Live yeast cell deriv. and phospholipids; tissue respiratory factors promoting wound healing and anti-inflammatory effects on skin; 5% act.

Brookosome® TYE. [Brooks Industries] Water, phospholipids, and thymus extract; liposome for skin care prods.; 5% act.

Brookosome® U. [Brooks Industries] Water, urea, and phospholipids; liposome for cosmetic applics.; promotes wound healing; penetration enhancer; moisturizer; 20% act., 10% lipids.

Brookosome® UV. [Brooks Industries] Phospholipids and octyl methoxycinnamate; liposome for cosmetics; sunscreen providing exc. uv protection; 10% act., 10% lipids.

Brookosome® V. [Brooks Industries] Water, aloe vera gel, and phospholipids; liposome for cosmetic applics.; soothing and moisturizing agent; 90% act., 10% lipids.

Brooksgel 41. [Brooks Industries] PEG-75 lanolin; CAS 61790-81-6; emulsifier, emollient.

Brooksgel 61. [Brooks Industries] PEG-85 lanolin; CAS 61790-81-6; cosmetic ingred.

Brooks Hydrogenated Lanolin. [Brooks Industries] Hydrog. lanolin; CAS 8031-44-5; EINECS 232-452-1; emollient.

Brookswax™ C. [Brooks Industries] Cetearyl alcohol and ceteareth-20; cosmetic ingred.

Brookswax™ D. [Brooks Industries] Cetearyl alcohol, ceteareth-20; emulsifying wax substantive to hair; flaked solid; 100% act.

Brookswax™ G. [Brooks Industries] Stearyl alcohol and ceteareth-20; emollient, cosmetic/pharmaceutical raw material.

Brookswax™ J. [Brooks Industries] Cetearyl alcohol and ceteareth-20; cosmetic ingred.

Brookswax™ Nl. [Brooks Industries] Cetearyl alcohol and ceteareth-20; cosmetic ingred.

Brookswax™ P. [Brooks Industries] Cetearyl alcohol and polysorbate 60; emulsifying wax substantive to hair; flaked solid; 100% act.

Brookswax™ R. [Brooks Industries] Cetearyl alcohol, polysorbate 60, steareth-20, and PEG-150 stearate; cosmetic ingred.

Broom HS. [Alban Muller] Propylene glycol and broom extract; botanical extract.

Broom Glycolysat. [C.E.P.] Propylene glycol, water, and broom extract; botanical extract.

Broom Oleat M. [C.E.P.] Propylene glycol dicaprylate/dicaprate and broom extract; botanical extract.

Broom Tops Extract HS 2645 G. [Grau Aromatics] Propylene glycol and broom extract; botanical extract.

Brophos-3. [Brooks Industries] Oleth-3 phosphate; CAS

39464-69-2; personal care surfactant.

Brophos™ 5C10. [Brooks Industries] PPG-5 ceteth-10 phosphate; CAS 50643-20-4; surfactant, emulsifier substantive to hair; liq.; 100% act.

Brophos™ A. [Brooks Industries] DEA-cetyl phosphate; CAS 61693-41-2; low pH emulsifier for cosmetics use.

Brophos™ OL-2. [Brooks Industries] Oleth-2 phosphate; CAS 39464-69-2; personal care surfactant.

Brophos™ OL-3. [Brooks Industries] Oleth-3 phosphate; CAS 39464-69-2; surfactant, emulsifier substantive to hair; liq.; 100% act.

Brophos™ OL-3N. [Brooks Industries] DEA oleth-3 phosphate; surfactant, emulsifier substantive to hair; thick paste; 100% act.

Brophos™ OL-3NPG. [Brooks Industries] DEA oleth-3 phosphate and propylene glycol; cosmetics emulsifier; free-flowing liq.

Brown 208. [Presperse] Iron oxides (85%), bismuthoxychloride (15%); CAS 1309-37-1, 7787-59-9; inorg. colorant for pigmented cosmetics; JSCI/JCID approved.

Brown GE (Fusion). [Lowenstein] p-Phenylenediamine and m-aminophenol.

Brown R-36 (Fusion). [Lowenstein] Resorcinol, p-phenylenediamine, and o-aminophenol.

Brox AWS. [Brooks Industries] PPG-5-ceteth-20; cosmetic ingred.

Brox HLB-13. [Brooks Industries] Steareth-27; CAS 9005-00-9; personal care surfactant.

Brox OL-2. [Brooks Industries] Oleth-2; CAS 9004-98-2; emulsifier, emollient.

Brox OL-3. [Brooks Industries] Oleth-3; CAS 9004-98-2; emulsifier, emollient.

Brox OL-4. [Brooks Industries] Oleth-4; CAS 9004-98-2; emulsifier, emollient.

Brox OL-5. [Brooks Industries] Oleth-5; CAS 9004-98-2; emulsifier, emollient.

Brox OL-10. [Brooks Industries] Oleth-10; CAS 9004-98-2; emulsifier, emollient.

Brox OL-20. [Brooks Industries] Oleth-20; CAS 9004-98-2; emulsifier.

Brox OL-20 70% Liq. [Brooks Industries] Oleth-20; CAS 9004-98-2; emulsifier.

Brox OL-40. [Brooks Industries] Oleth-40; CAS 9004-98-2; emulsifier.

Brox S-2. [Brooks Industries] Steareth-2; CAS 9005-00-9; personal care surfactant.

Brox S-20. [Brooks Industries] Steareth-20; CAS 9005-00-9; personal care surfactant.

Brox S-30. [Brooks Industries] Steareth-30; CAS 9005-00-9; personal care surfactant.

BTC® 50 USP. [Stepan; Stepan Canada] Benzalkonium chloride; cationic; antimicrobial for hard surf. disinfection, sanitization, deodorization; EPA registered; liq.; sp.gr. 0.96; flash pt. 126 F; 50% act.

BTC® 824. [Stepan; Stepan Canada] Myristalkonium chloride; CAS 139-08-2; EINECS 205-352-0; cationic; antimicrobial for hard surf. disinfection and sanitization; algicide for swimming pools and industrial water treatment; EPA registered; liq.; sp.gr. 0.96; flash pt. 120 F; 50% act.

BTC® 1010. [Stepan; Stepan Canada] Didecyldimonium chloride; CAS 7173-51-5; EINECS 230-525-2; cationic; sanitizer in hard water to 1200 ppm as $CaCO_3$; EPA registered; liq.; water-sol.; sp.gr. 0.89; flash pt. 86 F; 50% act.

BTC® 2125. [Stepan; Stepan Canada] Myristalkonium chloride and quaternium-14; cationic; antimicrobial, hard surf. disinfectant, sanitizer, fungicide for hospitals, public institutions; algicide in swimming pool and industrial water treatment; deodorizer; EPA registered; liq.; sp.gr. 0.97; flash pt. > 200 F; 50% act.

BTC® 2125M. [Stepan; Stepan Canada] Myristalkonium chloride and quaternium-14; cationic; disinfection and sanitization quat. for hospitals, nursing homes, public insitutions; algicide in swimming pool and industrial water treatment; deodorizer; EPA registered; liq.; sp.gr. 0.97; flash pt. > 200 F; 50% act.

BTN. [Vevy] Tridecyl salicylate.

Bubble Breaker® 748. [Witco/H-I-P] Silicone-free blend; defoamer for water-based systems, paints/coatings, personal care formulations; opaque creamy liq.; sol. @ 5% in min. spirits, disp. in water; sp.gr. 0.87; flash pt. (PMCC) > 200 F; pH 9.5; usage level: 0.1-0.5; 100% act.

Bubble Breaker® 900. [Witco/H-I-P] Silicone-free blend; defoamer for water-based systems, paints/coatings, personal care formulations; opaque wh. liq.; sol. @ 5% in min. spirits, disp. in water; sp.gr. 0.89; flash pt. (PMCC) > 200 F; pH 9.4; usage level: 0.1-0.5; 100% act.

Bubble Breaker® 3056A. [Witco/H-I-P] Disp. of reacted silica in hydrocarbon solv.; defoamer used in latex mfg. operations, formulation of water-based paints and adhesives, effluent water, asphalt emulsions, PVC monomer stripping, personal care formulations; opaque oily liq.; sol. @ 5% in min. spirits, disp. in water; sp.gr. 0.89; flash pt. (PMCC) > 200 F; pH 5.0; usage level: 0.01-0.; 100% act.

Bubble Breaker® DMD-1. [Witco/H-I-P] Complex surfactant; nonionic; oilfield surfactant, defoamer; personal care formulations; liq.; sol. in IPA; disp. in water, kerosene, xylene; dens. 8.4 lb/gal; visc. 400 cps; pour pt. < 0 F; pH 10.5.

Bubble Breaker® DMD-2. [Witco/H-I-P] Complex surfactant; nonionic; oilfield surfactant, defoamer; personal care formulations; liq.; sol. in IPA; disp. in water, kerosene, xylene; dens. 8.3 lb/gal; visc. 600 cps; pour pt. < 0 F; pH 10.5.

Bumyr. [Amerchol] Butyl myristate; CAS 110-36-1; EINECS 203-759-8; emollient; cosmetic ingred.; water-wh. liq., pract. odorless; oil-sol.; f.p. 8 C max.; acid no. 1 max.; iodine no. 1 max.; sapon. no. 192-204.

Burco Anionic APS. [Burlington Chem.] Ethoxylated sulfonate; anionic; hypochlorite-stable surfactant, emulsifier for acid and alkaline cleaners, disinfectants, personal care prods., household cleaners, tub and tile cleaners, mildew removers, textile scours, dairy cleaners; stable over entire pH range; clear liq.; m.w. 600; sp.gr. 1.06; visc. 270 cps; pH 6.5-7.5; 35% solids.

Burst RSD-10. [Hydrolabs] Dimethicone silylate.

Burst RSD-30. [Hydrolabs] Dimethicone silylate.

Burtonite V7E. [TIC Gums] Guar gum; CAS 9000-30-0; EINECS 232-536-8; cosmetic thickener.

Busan® 1500. [Buckman Labs] Methenammonium chloride; CAS 76902-90-4; broad-spectrum bactericide for preservation of aq. and aq.-emulsified cosmetic systems; stable over broad pH range; colorless clear liq.; water-sol.; sp.gr. 1.08 g/ml; dens. 8.8 lb/gal; pH 6-8; 18% act.

Busan® 1504. [Buckman Labs] Dimethylhydroxymethylpyrazole; CAS 85264-33-1; broad-spectrum bactericide and fungicide for preservation of aq. and aq.-emulsified cosmetic systems; stable over broad pH range; protein compatible; wh. cryst. powd.; water-sol.; dens. 49.3 g/100 ml; pH 6.1 (4.3%); usage level: 0.01-0.1%; 93% act.

Busan® 1506. [Buckman Labs] Hexahydro-1,3,5-tris(2-hydroxyethyl)-s-triazine; broad-spectrum bactericide for preservation of aq. cosmetic systems; lt. yel. clear liq.; sp.gr. 1.145-1.160 g/ml; dens. 9.6 lb/gal; pH 10.0-10.9; 78.5% act.

Busan® 1507. [Buckman Labs] Poly[oxyethylene (dimethyliminio)ethylene (dimethyliminio)ethylene dichloride] cationic; broad-spectrum bactericide for preservation of aq. and powd. cosmetic systems; effective over broad pH range; colorless to sl. yel. clear liq.; water-sol.; sp.gr. 1.15 g/ml; dens. 9.6 lb/gal; pH 6-7 (100 ppm aq.); 60% act.

Butyl Carbitol®. [Union Carbide] Butoxydiglycol; CAS 112-34-5; EINECS 203-961-6; solvent.

Butyl Cellosolve® . [Union Carbide] Butoxyethanol; CAS 111-76-2; EINECS 203-905-0; solvent.

Butyl Dioxitol. [Shell] Butoxydiglycol; CAS 112-34-5; EINECS 203-961-6; solv. for nitrocellulose, phenolics, Epon resins, alkyds, and acrylics, oils, and dyes; used in lacquers and inks which require slow evaporating solv.; lacquer and enamel formulations requiring improved flow-out and gloss; coupling solv. in preparation of specialized cleaning sol'ns. and cutting oils; coalescing agent in latex paints; component of brake fluids in automotive industry; colorless liq.; mild odor; water-misc.; sp.gr. 0.949–0.952; 0.10% max. water.

Butyl Oxitol. [Shell] Butoxyethanol; CAS 111-76-2; EINECS 203-905-0; solv. for nitrocellulose, alkyds, phenolics, acrylics, Epon resins, nat. resins, dyes, waxes, oils, and org. materials; used in surf. coating formulations such as lacquers and enamels where it imparts gloss and improved leveling chars; coupling agent in cleaners and cutting oils; colorless liq.; mild odor; water-misc.; sp.gr. 0.898–0.901; 0.20% max. water.

Butylparaben NF. [Protameen] Butylparaben; CAS 94-26-8; EINECS 202-318-7; cosmetics preservative.

Butyl Parasept. [Tenneco] Butylparaben; CAS 94-26-8; EINECS 202-318-7; cosmetics preservative.

Butyl Propasol. [Union Carbide] Propylene glycol t-butyl ether; CAS 5131-66-8; EINECS 225-878-4.

Byco A. [Croda Inc.] Gelatin NF; CAS 9000-70-8; EINECS 232-554-6; binder in pharmaceutical tableting; excipient, film former, coating agent; emulsion stabilizer; adjuvant protein in nutritional supplement; wh. powd.; sol. in water; m.w. 4000; bulk dens. 0.25-0.40 g/cc; pH 5.5-6.5 (10% aq.).

Byco C. [Croda Inc.] Gelatin NF; CAS 9000-70-8; EINECS 232-554-6; binder in pharmaceutical tableting; excipient, film-former, coating agent; emulsion stabilizer; adjuvant protein in nutritional supplement; wh. powd.; sol. in water; m.w. 10,000; bulk dens. 0.15-0.30 g/cc; pH 5.5-6.5 (10% aq.); toxicology: LD50 (oral, rat) 5 g/kg.

Byco O. [Croda Inc.] Gelatin NF; CAS 9000-70-8; EINECS 232-554-6; binder in pharmaceutical tableting; excipient, film-former, coating agent; emulsion stabilizer; adjuvant protein in nutritional supplement; wh. powd.; sol. in water; m.w. 1000; bulk dens. 0.25-0.40 g/cc; pH 5.5-6.5 (10% aq.); toxicology: LD50 (oral, rat) 5 g/kg.

C

C-108. [Procter & Gamble] Coconut fatty acid; CAS 67701-05-7; intermediate for mfg. of soaps, amides, esters, alcoholamides, and nonsurfactant applics.; Gardner < 1 liq.; m.w. 207; acid no. 266-274; iodine no. 5 max.; sapon. no. 273; 100% conc.

C-110. [Procter & Gamble] Coconut fatty acid; CAS 67701-05-7; intermediate for mfg. of soaps, amides, esters, alcoholamides, and nonsurfactant applics.; Gardner 3 max. liq.; m.w. 207; acid no. 266-274; iodine no. 12 max.; sapon. no. 272; 100% conc.

Cab-O-Sil® HS-5. [Cabot] Fumed silica.

Cab-O-Sil® L-90. [Cabot] Fumed silica; CAS 112945-52-5; dispersant, anticaking agent for foods, agric. prods., and powds. for cosmetics and coatings industries.

Cab-O-Sil® TS-530. [Cabot] Fumed silica, hexamethyl-disilazane-surface treated; CAS 68909-20-6; reinforcing filler for elastomers; free flow agent for toners and powd. coatings; antisettling agent in coatings; dry powd. carrier for perfumes, pesticides, veterinary prods., etc.

Cachalot® Arachidyl Alcohol AR-20. [M. Michel] Arachidyl alcohol; CAS 629-96-9; EINECS 211-119-4.

Cachalot® Behenyl Alcohol BE-22. [M. Michel] Behenyl alcohol; CAS 661-19-8; EINECS 211-546-6; cosmetic/ pharmaceutical raw material.

Cachalot® C-50. [M. Michel] Cetyl alcohol NF; CAS 36653-82-4; EINECS 253-149-0; emollient used in cosmetics; Hazen 20 color; sol. in acetone, alcohol, aromatic hydrocarbons, carbon disulfide, chloroform, glycol and diglycol ethers; m.w. 241-255; sp.gr. 0.820 (50 C); visc. 7 cps (70 C); m.p. 47-49 C; b.p. 310-330 C; acid no. 0.1 max.; iodine no. 1 max.; sapon. no. 0.5 max.; hyd. no. 225-235; flash pt. 165 C; ref. index 1.4320-1.4322 (70 C).

Cachalot® C-51. [M. Michel] Cetyl alcohol NF; CAS 36653-82-4; EINECS 253-149-0; conditioner, lubricant used in cosmetics; Hazen 25 color; sol. in acetone, alcohol, aromatic hydrocarbons, chloroform, glycol and diglycol ethers; m.w. 241-255; sp.gr. 0.820 (50 C); visc. 7 cps (70 C); m.p. 46-50 C; b.p. 310-340 C; acid no. 0.5 max.; iodine no. 1.5 max.; sapon. no. 1 max.; hyd. no. 225-235; flash pt. 165 C; ref. index 1.4322-1.4324 (70 C).

Cachalot® C-52. [M. Michel] Cetyl alcohol NF; CAS 36653-82-4; EINECS 253-149-0; cosmetic ingred.; Hazen 20 color; m.w. 239-250; sp.gr. 0.820 (50 C); visc. 7 cps (70 C); m.p. 48-49 C; b.p. 310-330 C; acid no. 0.3 max.; iodine no. 0.5 max.; sapon. no. 1 max.; hyd. no. 225-235; flash pt. 165 C; ref. index 1.4319-1.4321 (70 C).

Cachalot® DE-10. [M. Michel] Decyl alcohol; CAS 112-30-1; EINECS 203-956-9; cosmetic and pharmaceutical raw material.

Cachalot® L-90. [M. Michel] Lauryl alcohol; CAS 112-53-8; EINECS 203-982-0; cosmetic and pharmaceutical raw material.

Cachalot® M-43. [M. Michel] Myristyl alcohol; CAS 112-72-1; EINECS 204-000-3; emollient used in cosmetics; Hazen 20 color; sol. in acetone, alcohol, aromatic hydrocarbons, carbon disulfide, chloroform, glycol and diglycol ethers; m.w. 212-220; sp.gr. 0.825 (40 C); visc. 9 cps (50 C); b.p. 280-295 C; solid. pt. 36-38 C; acid no. 0.3 max.; iodine no. 0.3 max.; sapon. no. 0.5 max.; hyd. no. 255-265; flash pt. 150 C; ref. index 1.4334-1.4336 (50 C).

Cachalot® O-3. [M. Michel] Oleyl alcohol; CAS 143-28-2; EINECS 205-597-3; emollient.

Cachalot® O-8. [M. Michel] Oleyl alcohol; CAS 143-28-2; EINECS 205-597-3; emollient.

Cachalot® O-15. [M. Michel] Oleyl alcohol; CAS 143-28-2; EINECS 205-597-3; conditioner, lubricant for cosmetics; corrosion inhibitor additive to lube oils; Hazen 150 color; sol. in acetone, alcohol, aromatic hydrocarbons, chloroform, glycol and diglycol ethers; m.w. 261-274; sp.gr. 0.825 (50 C); visc. 11.2 cps (50 C); b.p. 300-350 C; acid no. 0.2 max.; iodine no. 70-80; sapon. no. 1 max.; hyd. no. 205-220; cloud pt. 18-25 C; flash pt. 170 C; ref. index 1.4567-1.4569.

Cachalot® S-54. [M. Michel] Stearyl alcohol; CAS 112-92-5; EINECS 204-017-6; conditioner, lubricant used in cosmetics; Hazen 25 color; sol. in acetone, alcohol, aromatic hydrocarbons, chloroform, glycol and diglycol ethers; m.w. 267-281; sp.gr. 0.815 (60 C); visc. 9 cps (70 C); m.p. 56-60 C; b.p. 330-350 C; acid no. 0.5 max.; iodine no. 2 max.; sapon. no. 1 max.; hyd. no. 200-220; flash pt. 185 C; ref. index 1.4345-1.4347 (70 C).

Cachalot® S-56. [M. Michel] Stearyl alcohol USP; CAS 112-92-5; EINECS 204-017-6; emollient used in cosmetics; Hazen 20 color; sol. in acetone, alcohol, aromatic hydrocarbons, carbon disulfide, chloroform, glycol and diglycol ethers; m.w. 267-281; sp.gr. 0.815 (60 C); visc. 9 cps (70 C); m.p. 56-58 C; b.p. 330-350 C; acid no. 0.3 max.; iodine no. 1 max.; sapon no. 1 max.; hyd. no. 200-210; flash pt. 190 C; ref. index 1.4347-1.4349 (70 C).

CAE. [Ajinomoto; Ajinomoto USA] PCA ethyl N-cocoyl-L-arginate; cationic; highly biodeg. surfactant, foamer, anti-stat, preservative, antiseptic, germicide, and disinfectant in cosmetics, detergents, dentifrices, medical supplies; strong affinity to hair; hair softener/conditioner, antistat; white crystalline powd.; sol. in water, ethanol, ethyleneglycol; sl. sol. in ethyl acetate, toluene; sol. 5% in water @ 30 C; m.p. 180-185 C; pH 5.0-7.0 (1% aq., 20 C); toxicology: LD50 (oral, mice) 10,750 mg/kg; 100% conc.

Calamide C. [Pilot] Cocamide DEA superamide; CAS 61791-31-9; EINECS 263-163-9; foam stabilizer, emulsifier for liq. dishwash, bubble baths, shampoos, all-purpose cleaners; thickener; imparts mildness.

Calcium Ascorbate FCC No. 60475. [Roche] Calcium ascorbate FCC; sodium-free, acid-free form of vitamin C for cosmetic use.

Calcium Hydroxide USP 802. [Whittaker, Clark & Daniels] Calcium hydroxide; CAS 1305-62-0; EINECS 215-137-3.

Calcium Oxide FCC 801. [Whittaker, Clark & Daniels] Calcium oxide; CAS 1305-78-8; EINECS 215-138-9.

D-Calcium Pantothenate USP, FCC Type SD No. 63924. [Roche] Calcium pantothenate; CAS 137-08-6; EINECS 205-278-9; long-lasting moisturizer for hair and skin care prods.

Calcium Sulfate Anhydrous NF 164. [Whittaker, Clark & Daniels] Calcium sulfate; CAS 7778-18-9; EINECS 231-900-3.

Calendula Oil. [Provital; Centerchem] Sunflower seed oil and calendula extract.

Calendula Oil CLR. [Dr. Kurt Richter; Henkel/Cospha] Soybean oil, calendula extract, tocopherol, emollient, conditioner for herbal creams and lotions for protective care of normal and sensitive skin; emulsified and oily preparations; rdsh.-yel. oil; herbal odor.

Calendula Oil Monarom. [Novarom GmbH] Soybean oil, calendula extract, and tocopherol.

Calenfil 3646. [Gattefosse] Triolein PEG-6 esters, ethoxydiglycol, and calendula extract.

Calester. [Pilot] Alpha sulfo methyl laurate; surfactant for high-quality toilet soaps, laundry detergents, automobile cleaners, spray cleaners, foamers, emulsifiers.

Calfoam ALS-30. [Pilot] Ammonium lauryl sulfate; CAS 2235-54-3; EINECS 218-793-9; surfactant.

Calfoam EA-603. [Pilot] Ammonium laureth sulfate; CAS 32612-48-9; surfactant.

Calfoam ES-30. [Pilot] Sodium laureth sulfate; CAS 9004-82-4; anionic; detergent, foam stabilizer, flash foamer, wetter for detergent systems, personal care prods., wool washing; emulsion polymerization; yel. clear liq.; mild odor; dens. 8.8 lb/gal; pH 8.0; 30% solids.

Calfoam ES-303. [Pilot] Sodium laureth sulfate; personal care surfactant.

Calfoam ES-603. [Pilot] Sodium laureth sulfate; personal care surfactant.

Calfoam NEL-60. [Pilot] Ammonium lauryl ether sulfate; CAS 32612-48-9; anionic; flash foamer, foam stabilizer, detergent, emulsifier, wetter for liq. detergents, bubble baths, shampoos, car washing; lime soap dispersant; clear liq.; faint alcohol odor; sol. in aq. systems; dens. 8.58 lb/gal; pH 7.5; 57.5% act.

Calfoam NLS-30. [Pilot] Ammonium lauryl sulfate; CAS 2235-54-3; EINECS 218-793-9; anionic; mild surfactant base for neutral pH shampoos, bubble baths, rug cleaner formulations, cosmetic emulsifiers, emulsion polymerization; liq.; 30% act.

Calfoam SEL-60. [Pilot] Sodium laureth sulfate; CAS 9004-82-4; anionic; general all-purpose cleaning and wetting for use in bubble baths, shampoos, car washing, liquid detergents; liq.; 60% act.

Calfoam SLS-30. [Pilot] Sodium lauryl sulfate; CAS 151-21-3; EINECS 205-788-1; anionic; mild detergent, foamer for personal care prods.; rug/upholstery shampoos; emulsifier for cosmetics, emulsion polymerization of latex, SBR rubber, polyacrylates, elastomers; foaming agent for foamed rubber; wh. paste; mild odor; pH 8.0; 30% act.

Calfoam TLS-40. [Pilot] TEA-lauryl sulfate; CAS 139-96-8; EINECS 205-388-7; personal care surfactant.

Calgon. [Calgon] Sodium hexametaphosphate; CAS 10124-56-8; EINECS 233-343-1; cosmetic ingred.

Cal-O-Vera 1:1. [Agro-Mar] Aloe vera gel from *Aloe barbadensis miller* with sodium benzoate and citric acid preservatives; used for cosmetic, health, and pharmaceutical applics.; opaque, translucent, colorless liq.; typ. veg. odor; slick, tangy taste; sp.gr. 1.004 ± 0.004; pH 3.5-5.5; 100% act.

Cal-O-Vera 10:1. [Agro-Mar] Aloe vera gel with sodium benzoate and citric acid preservatives; used for cosmetic, health, and pharmaceutical applics.; opaque liq.; typ. veg. odor; slick, tangy taste; sp.gr. 1.004 ± 0.004; pH 3.5-5.5.

Cal-O-Vera 40:1. [Agro-Mar] Aloe vera gel from *Aloe barbadensis miller* with sodium benzoate and citric acid preservatives, and acidifier; used for cosmetic, health, and pharmaceutical applics.; opaque tan liq.; typ. veg. odor; slick, tangy taste; sp.gr. 1.004 ± 0.004; pH 3.5-5.5.

Cal-O-Vera 200XXX Powd. [Agro-Mar] Aloe vera gel from *Aloe barbadensis miller* used for cosmetic, health, and pharmaceutical applics.; also avail. in rapidly dissolving, agglomerated, micro-fine form; off-wh. to lt. beige powd.; pH 3.5-6.5 (reconstituted 200:1).

Calsoft AOS-40. [Pilot] Sodium C14-16 olefin sulfonate; CAS 68439-57-6; EINECS 270-407-8; surfactant for hand soaps, shampoos, hard surf. cleaners, household and industrial cleaners; liq.; 40% act.

Calsoft F-90. [Pilot] Sodium dodecylbenzene sulfonate; CAS 25155-30-0; EINECS 246-680-4; anionic; detergent, emulsifier, wetter for all-purpose and hard surface cleaners, bubble baths, degreasers, laundry powds., textile scouring aids, emulsion polymers, sanitation, emulsion paints, wettable powds., ore flotation, metal pickling; wh. free-flowing flake; water-sol.; dens. 0.45 g/cc; pH 8.0 (1%); 90% act.

Calsoft L-40. [Pilot] Sodium dodecylbenzene sulfonate; CAS 25155-30-0; EINECS 246-680-4; anionic; biodeg. emulsion stabilizer; wetting and foaming agent, detergent, emulsifier for household and industrial detergents, agric. emulsions, dye bath leveling, rug cleaners, bubble baths, ore flotation, and air entrainment in concrete and gypsum board; lt. yel. visc. liq.; water-sol.; sp.gr. 1.07; pH 7.5; 42% solids.

Calsoft L-60. [Pilot] Sodium dodecylbenzene sulfonate; CAS 25155-30-0; EINECS 246-680-4; anionic; biodeg. emulsion stabilizer; wetting and foaming agent, detergent, emulsifier for household and industrial detergents, agric. emulsions, dye bath leveling, rug cleaners, bubble baths, ore flotation, and air entrainment in concrete and gypsum board; washing fruits and vegetables; water-wh. pasty liq.; odorless; dens. 8.7 lb/gal; pH 7.4; 60% solids.

Calsoft LAS-99. [Pilot] Dodecylbenzene sulfonic acid, linear; CAS 27176-87-0; EINECS 248-289-4; anionic; biodeg. detergent, emulsifier, intermediate for liq. and dry detergents, hard surf. cleaners, stripping, wetting, foaming; Klett 50 syrupy liq.; water-sol.; sp.gr. 1.06; dens. 8.83 lb/gal; visc. 1100 cps; 97.5% act.

Calsoft T-60. [Pilot] TEA-dodecylbenzene sulfonate; CAS 27323-41-7; EINECS 248-406-9; anionic; biodeg. detergent, wetting agent, flash foamer; liq. detergents, wool wash compds., cosmetics and shampoos, agric. emulsifiers, industrial cleaners, textile scouring, and car wash compds.; yel. clear visc. liq.; mild odor; dens. 9.1 lb/gal; visc. 2300 cps; pH 5.7; 60% solids.

Calsuds CD-6. [Pilot] Alkylaryl sulfonate/cocamide DEA blend; anionic; conc. base, foam builder/stabilizer, wetting agent, visc. modifier, and emulsifier; used in liq. detergents, shampoos, wool-washing compds., hand, felt, and janitorial cleaners, textile scours, agric. sprays; clear visc. liq.; dens. 8.6 lb/gal; visc. 2100 cps; pH 9.5 (10%); 100% conc.

Camellia Oil. [Ikeda] Camellia oil containing 88.5% oleic acid; nongreasy, nontacky natural oil containing similar sebaceous components of scalp; for hair care treatment; emollient for skin care prods.; pale yel. clear visc. liq.; sp.gr. 0.910-0.915; acid no. 0.1 max.; iodine no. 81-89; sapon. no. 186-196.

Camel-WITE®. [Genstar Stone Prods.] Calcium carbonate; CAS 471-34-1; EINECS 207-439-9; filler for paint, paper, paper coating, PVC, rubber (automotive goods, footwear, medical supplies), thermoplastics, thermosets, and in caulks, glazing compds., ceramics, adhesives, food processing; very wh. dry powd.; 3.0 μ avg. particle dia.;

99.9% finer than 12 μ; 50% finer than 3 μ; 0.08% sol. in water; sp.gr. 2.70–2.71; dens. 22.57 lb/gal solid; bulk dens. 40 lb/ft³ (loose); oil absorp. 15 cc/100 g; ref. index 1.6; pH 9.5 (sat. sol'n.); hardness (Moh) 3.0.

Camofil 4064. [Calgon] Triolein PEG-6 esters, ethoxydiglycol, and chamomile extract.

Camomile Oil Extra. [Novarom GmbH] Caprylic/capric triglyceride and matricaria extract.

Candelilla Wax Cosmetic Grade Stralpitz. [Strahl & Pitsch] Candelilla wax; CAS 8006-44-8; EINECS 232-347-0; wax for cosmetics use.

Candex®. [Mendell] Dextrose with small amounts of higher glucose saccharides; CAS 50-99-7; EINECS 200-075-1; offers sweet, nongritty taste and is easily blended with flavors, lubricants, and other dry additives; exc. flow and compaction props.; for use in chewable tablets, esp. those made by direct compression; wh. porous, spherical granules, sweet noncloying/nongritty taste; avg particle size 218 μ; 30% max. -100 mesh; very sol. in water; dens. (tapped) 0.77 g/ml; pH 3.5 min.

Candex® Plus. [Mendell] Dextrates; CAS 50-99-7; EINECS 200-075-1; vehicle for direct compression and wet granulation of pharmaceutical tablets, incl. chewable tablets; wh. to very sl. off-wh. porous spherical granules, sweet noncloying/nongritty taste; avg. particle size 196 μ; 35% max. -100 mesh; dens. (tapped) 0.82 g/ml max.; pH 4.0-7.5.

Capigen. [Sederma] Hydrolyzed soy protein and 3-aminopropane sulfonic acid; for hair care prods.; regulates seborrhea, reinforces hairs and increases their volume; yel. clear liq., char. odor; sp.gr. 1.010-1.020; ref. index 1.340-1.345; pH 6-7; usage level: 3-15%.

Capigen CG. [Sederma] Water, glycerin, hydrolyzed soy protein, 3-aminopropane sulfonic acid, potassium cyanate, lactoferrin, lactoperoxidase, glucose oxidase; normalizes hyperseborrhea and treats oily hair; brn. clear liq., char. odor; sp.gr. 1.010-1.030; ref. index 1.335-1.355; pH 7-8; usage level: 1-7%; 3-4.5% dry matter.

Capigen CS. [Sederma] Water, glyceryl polymethacrylate, propylene glycol, and hydrolyzed soy protein; dry hair treatment; hydrates scalp and reconstitutes lipidic film of the hair; yel. opalescent liq., char. odor; sp.gr. 1.055-1.070; ref. index 1.355-1.375; pH 5-7; usage level: 1-7%; 65-85% dry matter.

Capilotonique HS 220. [Alban Muller] Propylene glycol, birch leaf extract, fenugreek extract, myrrh extract, lappa extract, and ivy extract; phytocomplex for hair care for oily hair.

Capilotonique HS 226. [Alban Muller] Propylene glycol, sage extract, nettle extract, rosemary extract, and capsicum extract; phytocomplex for hair care for oily hair.

Capilotonique HS 245. [Alban Muller] Propylene glycol, nettle extract, arnica extract, watercress extract, rosemary extract, and sage extract; hair tonic phytocomplex.

Capisome. [Sederma] Water, glycerin, propylene glycol, hydrolyzed soy protein, aminopropane sulfonic acid, and lecithin; regulation vector of excess hair loss; regulates seborrhea; for all hair treatments; pale yel. opalescent liq., char. odor; pH 5.0-6.0; usage level: 5-10%.

Capmul® EMG. [Karlshamns] PEG-20 glyceryl stearate; nonionic; emulsifier, solubilizer forming w/o emulsions; also used to alter HLB; dough conditioner for yeast-raised baked goods; solid; HLB 13.1; 100% conc.

Capmul® GDL. [Karlshamns] Glyceryl dilaurate; CAS 27638-00-2; EINECS 248-586-9; nonionic; emulsifier used in fats and oils; for cosmetics, pharmaceuticals; semisolid; m.p. 28-31 C; HLB 3-4; acid no. 3 max.; iodine no. 20 max.; sapon. no. 215-230.

Capmul® GMO. [Karlshamns] Glyceryl oleate; CAS 111-03-5; nonionic; food emulsifier, wetting control agent; dispersant for pigments, solids; defoamer; emulsifier for cosmetics and pharmaceuticals; semisolid; sol. in org. solvs. and oils; m.p. 25 C max.; HLB 3.4; acid no. 3 max.; iodine no. 75 max.; sapon. no. 160-170; 100% conc.

Capmul® GMS. [Karlshamns] Glyceryl stearate; nonionic; stabilizer; internal lubricant for cosmetics; food emulsifier used in margarine, yeast-raised baked goods; beads, flakes; m.p. 57-62 C; HLB 3.2; acid no. 3 max.; iodine no. 5 max.; sapon. no. 155-165; 100% conc.

Capmul® MCM. [Karlshamns] Glyceryl caprate/caprylate; co-solv. and coupler for org. compds.; w/o emulsifier; for cosmetics, pharmaceuticals; liq.; sol. in oil and alcohol; HLB 5.5-6.0; acid no. 2.5 max.; iodine no. 2 max.; 70% alpha mono.

Capmul® MCM-90. [Karlshamns] Glyceryl caprylate/caprate; w/o emulsifier, solv. for cosmetics, pharmaceuticals; liq.; acid no. 2.5 max.; iodine no. 2 max.; 80+% alpha mono.

Capmul® PGMS. [Karlshamns] Propylene glycol stearate; CAS 1323-39-3; EINECS 215-354-3; personal care surfactant.

Capmul® POE-L. [Karlshamns] Polysorbate 20; CAS 9005-64-5; nonionic; emulsifier, solubilizer forming w/o emulsions; also used to alter HLB; food emulsifier and solubilizer for flavors; Gardner 3 max. liq.; HLB 16.7; acid no. 2 max.; sapon. no. 40-50; hyd. no. 96-108; 100% conc.

Capmul® POE-S. [Karlshamns] Polysorbate 60; CAS 9005-67-8; nonionic; food emulsifier; solubilizer for oils into water systems; Gardner 7 max. liq.; water-sol.; HLB 14.9; acid no. 2 max.; sapon. no. 45-55; hyd. no. 81-96; 100% conc.

Caprol® 2G4S. [Karlshamns] Polyglyceryl-2 tetrastearate; CAS 72347-89-8; nonionic; food emulsifier; opacifier; wax modifier; thickener; solubilizer, clouding agent, crystal growth inhibitor, lip glosser for cosmetics, pharmaceuticals; FDA approved; Gardner 8 max. powd.; sol. in oils, waxes; HLB 2.5; acid no. 6 max.; iodine no. 6 max.; sapon. no. 165-185; 100% conc.

Caprol® 3GO. [Karlshamns] Polyglyceryl-3 oleate; CAS 9007-48-1; nonionic; food emulsifier for frozen desserts, veg. dairy prods., diet spreads; wetting agent for dyes and pigments in cosmetics; defoamer; solubilizer, clouding agent, crystal growth inhibitor, lip glosser for cosmetics, pharmaceuticals; FDA approved; Gardner 7 max. liq.; sol. in org. solvs. and oils; HLB 6.2; acid no. 6 max.; iodine no. 78 max.; sapon. no. 125-150; 100% conc.

Caprol® 3GS. [Karlshamns] Polyglyceryl-3 stearate; EINECS 248-403-2; nonionic; food emulsifier, stabilizer and whipping agent used in frozen desserts and fat reduction; solubilizer, clouding agent, crystal growth inhibitor, lip glosser for cosmetics, pharmaceuticals; FDA approved; Gardner 8 max. powd.; HLB 6.2; acid no. 6 max.; iodine no. 3 max.; sapon. no. 120-135; 100% conc.

Caprol® 6G2O. [Karlshamns] Polyglyceryl-6 dioleate; CAS 76009-37-5; nonionic; food emulsifier for frozen desserts; solubilizer, clouding agent, crystal growth inhibitor, lip glosser for cosmetics, pharmaceuticals; FDA approved; Gardner 10 max. liq.; HLB 8.5; acid no. 6 max.; iodine no. 75 max.; sapon. no. 105-125; 100% conc.

Caprol® 6G2S. [Karlshamns] Polyglyceryl-6 distearate; CAS 34424-97-0; nonionic; food emulsifier for whipped toppings, frozen desserts, coffee whiteners; solubilizer, clouding agent, crystal growth inhibitor, lip glosser for cosmetics, pharmaceuticals; FDA approved; Gardner 10 max. solid; HLB 8.5; acid no. 6 max.; iodine no. 3 max.; sapon. no. 105-125; 100% conc.

Caprol® 10G2O. [Karlshamns] Polyglyceryl-10 dioleate; CAS 33940-99-7; o/w emulsifier, humectant, lubricant; solubilizer, clouding agent, crystal growth inhibitor, lip glosser for cosmetics, pharmaceuticals; also for frozen desserts; FDA approved; Gardner 7 max. liq.; sol. in alcohol; water-disp.; HLB 10.0; acid no. 6 max.; iodine no. 60 max.; sapon. no. 100-120; 100% conc.

Caprol® 10G4O. [Karlshamns] Polyglyceryl-10 tetraoleate; CAS 34424-98-1; EINECS 252-011-7; nonionic; food emulsifier, visc. control, stabilizer, solubilizer, clouding agent, crystal growth inhibitor, lip glosser for cosmetics, pharmaceuticals; FDA approved; Gardner 7 max. liq.; HLB 6.2; acid no. 6 max.; iodine no. 60 max.; sapon. no. 125-150; 100% conc.

Caprol® 10G10O. [Karlshamns] Polyglyceryl-10 decaoleate; CAS 11094-60-3; EINECS 234-316-7; nonionic; food emulsifier, solubilizer, lubricant, and dispersant; solubilizer, clouding agent, crystal growth inhibitor, lip glosser for cosmetics, pharmaceuticals; FDA approved; Gardner 9 max. liq.; sol. in oils and org. solvs.; HLB 3.5; acid no. 8 max.; iodine no. 85 max.; sapon. no. 155-185; 100% conc.

Caprol® 10G10S. [Karlshamns] Polyglyceryl-10 decastearate; CAS 68991-68-5; EINECS 254-495-5; FDA approved; lubricant for thread finishes, wax additive, crystal modifier; thickener; solubilizer, clouding agent, crystal growth inhibitor, lip glosser for cosmetics, pharmaceuticals; Gardner 8 max. liq.; sol. in oils, org. solvs., and waxes; HLB 2.5; acid no. 6 max.; iodine no. 4 max.; sapon. no. 160-180.

Caprol® PGE860. [Karlshamns] Decaglyceryl mono-, dioleate; nonionic; food emulsifier and beverage cloud agent; solubilizer, clouding agent, crystal growth inhibitor, lip glosser for cosmetics, pharmaceuticals; FDA approved; Gardner 10 max. liq.; HLB 11.0; acid no. 6 max.; iodine no. 60 max.; sapon. no. 90-105; 100% conc.

Capsaicin. [Fluka Chemie AG] Capsicum extract; botanical extract.

Captex® 200. [Karlshamns] Propylene glycol dicaprylate/dicaprate; CAS 68583-51-7; carrier, coupler, solv. for flavors, fragrance oil, sol. colorants, vitamins, medicinals, cosmetics; emollient for creams, lotions, makeup; sol. in alcohol, oils, hydrocarbons, ketones; visc. 9-13 mPa·s; acid no. 0.1 max.; iodine no. 0.5; sapon. no. 315-335; cloud pt. -15 C; ref. index 1.4393.

Captex® 300. [Karlshamns] Caprylic/capric triglyceride; CAS 65381-09-1; solv. for colors and perfumes; emollient, moisturizer in cosmetics, toiletries, pharmaceuticals; plasticizer; Gardner 2 max. color; sol. in alcohol, oils, hydrocarbons, ketones; visc. 24-30 mPa·s; acid no. 0.1 max.; iodine no. 0.5; sapon. no. 335-350; cloud pt. < -5 C; ref. index 1.4481.

Captex® 350. [Karlshamns] Caprylic/capric/lauric triglyceride; CAS 68991-68-4; emollient, solv., carrier, fixative, and extender for pharmaceutical, nutritional, and cosmetic applics.; Gardner 2 max. color; visc. 36-42 mPa·s; acid no. 0.1 max.; iodine no. 2; sapon. no. 290-310; cloud pt. 0 C.

Captex® 355. [Karlshamns] Caprylic/capric triglyceride; CAS 65381-09-1; lubricity vehicle for cosmetics and pharmaceuticals; carrier for essential oils, flavors, and fragrances; Lovibond R1.0 max. clear liq.; neutral odor; bland flavor; misc. with most org. solvs. incl. 95% ethanol; sp.gr. 0.92-0.96; visc. 26-32 mPa·s; acid no. 0.1 max.; iodine no. 0.5 max.; sapon. no. 325-345; cloud pt. < -5 C; ref. index 1.4486.

Captex® 800. [Karlshamns] Propylene glycol dioctanoate; CAS 7384-98-7; nonoily lubricant imparting rich feel to skin in cosmetics and pharmaceuticals; carrier for essential oils, flavors; vehicle for vitamins, medicinals, nutritional prods.; APHA 100 max. clear liq.; neutral odor; bland flavor; misc. with most org. solvs. incl. 95% ethanol; visc. 9–13 mPa·s; acid no. 1.0 max.; iodine no. 1.0 max.; sapon. no. 315-335; cloud pt. < -20 C.

Captex® 810A. [Karlshamns] Caprylic/capric/linoleic triglyceride; CAS 67701-28-4; emollient, solv., fixative, and extender in pharmaceutical, nutritional, and cosmetic applics. incl. lipsticks, lip glosses, makeup bases, bath oils, aftershave lotions, aerosols; carrier for flavors and fragrances; Gardner 2 max. color; acid no. 0.1 max.; iodine no. 25; sapon. no. 307-320.

Captex® 810B. [Karlshamns] Caprylic/capric/linoleic triglyceride; CAS 67701-28-4; emollient, solv., fixative, and extender in pharmaceutical, nutritional, and cosmetic applics. incl. lipsticks, lip glosses, makeup bases, bath oils, aftershave lotions, aerosols; carrier for flavors and fragrances; Gardner 2 max. color; visc. 30 cps; acid no. 0.1 max.; iodine no. 55; sapon. no. 280-296; cloud pt. 10 C.

Captex® 810C. [Karlshamns] Caprylic/capric/linoleic triglyceride; CAS 67701-28-4; emollient, solv., fixative, and extender in pharmaceutical, nutritional, and cosmetic applics. incl. lipsticks, lip glosses, makeup bases, bath oils, aftershave lotions, aerosols; carrier for flavors and fragrances; Gardner 2 max. color; acid no. 0.1 max.; iodine no. 75; sapon. no. 257-275.

Captex® 810D. [Karlshamns] Caprylic/capric/linoleic triglyceride; CAS 67701-28-4; emollient, solv., fixative, and extender in pharmaceutical, nutritional, and cosmetic applics. incl. lipsticks, lip glosses, makeup bases, bath oils, aftershave lotions, aerosols; carrier for flavors and fragrances; Gardner 2 max. color; acid no. 0.1 max.; iodine no. 85; sapon. no. 235-253.

Captex® 910A. [Karlshamns] Caprylic/capric/oleic triglyceride; CAS 67701-28-4; emollient, solv., fixative, and extender in pharmaceutical, nutritional, and cosmetic applics. incl. lipsticks, lip glosses, makeup bases, bath oils, aftershave lotions, aerosols; carrier for flavors and fragrances; Gardner 2 max. color; acid no. 0.1 max.; iodine no. 19; sapon. no. 304-318.

Captex® 910B. [Karlshamns] Caprylic/capric/oleic triglyceride; CAS 67701-28-4; emollient, solv., fixative, and extender in pharmaceutical, nutritional, and cosmetic applics. incl. lipsticks, lip glosses, makeup bases, bath oils, aftershave lotions, aerosols; carrier for flavors and fragrances; Gardner 2 max. color; acid no. 0.1 max.; iodine no. 35; sapon. no. 280-296.

Captex® 910C. [Karlshamns] Caprylic/capric/oleic triglyceride; CAS 67701-28-4; emollient, solv., fixative, and extender in pharmaceutical, nutritional, and cosmetic applics. incl. lipsticks, lip glosses, makeup bases, bath oils, aftershave lotions, aerosols; carrier for flavors and fragrances; Gardner 2 max. color; acid no. 0.1 max.; iodine no. 48; sapon. no. 260-275.

Captex® 910D. [Karlshamns] Caprylic/capric/oleic triglyceride; CAS 67701-28-4; emollient, solv., fixative, and extender in pharmaceutical, nutritional, and cosmetic applics. incl. lipsticks, lip glosses, makeup bases, bath oils, aftershave lotions, aerosols; carrier for flavors and fragrances; Gardner 2 max. color; acid no. 0.1 max.; iodine no. 60; sapon. no. 238-250.

Captex® 8000. [Karlshamns] Caprylic triglyceride; CAS 538-23-8; EINECS 208-686-5; nonoily lubricant imparting rich feel to the skin; for cosmetics and pharmaceuticals; carrier for essential oils, flavors; vehicle for vitamins, medicinals, nutritional prods.; APHA 150 max. clear liq.; neutral odor; bland flavor; misc. with most org. solvs. incl. 95% ethanol; visc. 20-28 mPa·s; acid no. 1.0 max.; iodine no. 1.0 max.; sapon. no. 350-365; cloud pt. < -5 C; ref. index 1.4469.

Captex® 8227. [Karlshamns] Triundecanoin; CAS 13552-80-2; EINECS 236-935-8; emollient, solv., fixative, and extender in pharmaceutical, nutritional, and cosmetic applics. incl. lipsticks, lip glosses, makeup bases, bath oils, aftershave lotions, aerosols; carrier for flavors and fragrances; acid no. 3 max.; sapon. no. 270-290; cloud pt. 21 C.

Carbavert. [Henkel/Cospha] Aroma chemical for cosmetic, personal care, detergent, and cleaning prods.; colorless liq., fruity banana-like odor; b.p. 53 C; flash pt. 50 C.

Carbitol® Acetate. [Union Carbide] Ethoxydiglycol acetate; CAS 112-15-2; EINECS 203-940-1; solvent.

Carbopol® 907. [BFGoodrich] Polyacrylic acid; CAS 9003-01-4; anionic; emulsifier, thickener, stabilizer, suspending agent; used for drilling muds, photosensitive emulsions, water treatment, cosmetic and personal care applics., oral prods.; solid; sol. in water, polar solvs., many nonpolar solvs. blends; 100% conc.

Carbopol® 910. [BFGoodrich] Carbomer; anionic; emulsifier, thickener, stabilizer, suspending agent; used for flocking, dip coating, textile back coating; cosmetic and personal care applics., oral prods.; powd.; sol. in water, polar solvs., many nonpolar solvs. blends; 100% conc.

Carbopol® 934P. [BFGoodrich] Carbomer; suspending agent; high purity grade for pharmaceutical industry; for thickening, suspending, and emulsifying; for topical lotions and sustained release tablets; sol. see Carbopol 907.

Carbopol® 940. [BFGoodrich] Carbomer; anionic; emulsifier, thickener, stabilizer, suspending agent used in cosmetic applics., for die-casting and forging lubricants, thixotropic paints; solv. thickening with or without neutralizing; powd.; sol. see Carbopol 907; 100% conc.

Carbopol® 941. [BFGoodrich] Carbomer; anionic; emulsifier, thickener; emulsion stabilization of shampoos, lotions, and thin gels with good clarity; powd.; sol. see Carbopol 907; 100% conc.

Carbopol® 954. [BFGoodrich] Carbomer; emulsifier, thickener, stabilizer, suspending agent used in cosmetics.

Carbopol® 980. [BFGoodrich] Carbomer; emulsifier, thickener, stabilizer, suspending agent used in cosmetics.

Carbopol® 981. [BFGoodrich] Carbomer; emulsifier, thickener, stabilizer, suspending agent used in cosmetics.

Carbopol® 1342. [BFGoodrich] Acrylates/C10-30 alkyl acrylate crosspolymer; emulsifier, stabilizer, moisturizer, thickener, gellant for cosmetic emulsions, skin care prods.; wh. powd.; slightly acetic odor; visc. 10,500–26,900 cP (1%).

Carbopol® 1382. [BFGoodrich] Acrylates/C10-30 alkyl acrylate crosspolymer; emulsifier.

Carbopol® 2984. [BFGoodrich] Carbomer; emulsifier, thickener, stabilizer, suspending agent used in cosmetics.

Carbopol® 5984. [BFGoodrich] Carbomer; emulsifier, thickener, stabilizer, suspending agent used in cosmetics.

Carboset 514. [BFGoodrich] Acrylates copolymer; thickener, stabilizer for cosmetics.

Carboset 525. [BFGoodrich] Acrylic resin; thermoplastic film-forming resin used in protective metal coatings, paints, ceramics, adhesives, textiles, paper, leather, cosmetics, floor polishes, chemical specialties; exc. dispersant, leveling, and binding char.; wh. gran. solid; m.w. 260,000; acid no. 76–85; tens. str. 26.2 MPa; tens. elong. 165%; hardness (Sward) 24; 100% act.

Carboset XL-19X2. [BFGoodrich] Acrylates copolymer; thickener, stabilizer for cosmetics.

Carboset XL-28. [BFGoodrich] Acrylates copolymer; thickener, stabilizer for cosmetics.

Carboset XL-40. [BFGoodrich] Acrylates copolymer; thickener, stabilizer for cosmetics.

Carboset XPD-1616. [BFGoodrich] Acrylates copolymer; thickener, stabilizer for cosmetics.

Carbossalina. [Vevy] Magnesium aspartate and PEG-8.

Carbowax® PEG 300. [Union Carbide] PEG-6; CAS 25322-68-3; EINECS 220-045-1; coupling agent, solv., vehicle, humectant, lubricant, binder, base; used in adhesives, agric., ceramics, chem. intermediates, cosmetics/toiletries, electroplating/electropolishing, food processing, household prods., lubricants, metal fabrication, paints, paper, pharmaceuticals, printing, rubber and elastomers, textiles, wood processing; water-wh. visc. liq.; sol. in water, alcohols, glycerin, glycols; m.w. 285-315; sp.gr. 1.1250; dens. 9.38 lb/gal; visc. 5.8 cSt (99 C); f.p. -15 to -8 C; hyd. no. 356-394; flash pt. (PMCC) > 180 C; ref. index 1.463; pH 4.5-7.5 (5% aq.); surf. tens. 44.5 dynes/cm.

Carbowax® PEG 400. [Union Carbide] PEG-8; CAS 25322-68-3; EINECS 225-856-4; antistat, surfactant intermediate, dye carrier, humectant, lubricant, release agent, plasticizer for adhesives, capsules, ceramic glazes, creams and lotions, deodorant sticks, inks, lipsticks; liq.; sol. in water, methanol, ethanol, acetone, trichloroethylene, Cellosolve®, Carbitol®, dibutyl phthalate, toluene; m.w. 380–420; sp.gr. 1.1254; dens. 9.39 lb/gal; visc. 7.3 cSt (210 F); f.p. 4–8 C; flash pt. (CCC) > 350 F; ref. index 1.465; pH 4.5–7.5 (5% aq.); surf. tens. 44.5 dynes/cm.

Carbowax® PEG 540 Blend. [Union Carbide] PEG-6 and PEG-32 (41:59); base for ointments and suppositories; also for adhesives, agric., ceramics, chem. intermediates, electroplating, household prods., lubricants, metal fabrication, paints, paper, printing, rubber, textiles, wood processing; soft solid; sol. in methylene chloride, 73% in water, 50% in trichloroethylene, 48% in methanol; m.w. 500–600; sp.gr. 1.0930 (60 C); dens. 9.17 lb/gal (55 C); visc. 15.1 cSt (210 F); f.p. 38–41; flash pt. (CCC) > 350 F; pH 4.5–7.5 (5% aq.).

Carbowax® PEG 600. [Union Carbide] PEG-12; CAS 25322-68-3; EINECS 229-859-1; antistat, surfactant intermediate, humectant, lubricant, release agent, plasticizer for adhesives, capsules, ceramic glaze, creams and lotions, dentifrices, deodorant sticks, inks, lipsticks, wood treatment; liq.; sol. in water; m.w. 570–630; sp.gr. 1.1257; dens. 9.40 lb/gal; visc. 10.8 cSt (210 F); f.p. 20–25 C; flash pt. (CCC) > 350 F; ref. index 1.46; pH 4.5–7.5 (5% aq.); surf. tens. 44.5 dynes/cm.

Carbowax® PEG 900. [Union Carbide] PEG-20; CAS 25322-68-3; antistat, surfactant intermediate, lubricant, release agent, ointment and suppository base, plasticizer for adhesives, ceramic glaze, creams and lotions, dentifrices, deodorant sticks, wood treatment; soft solid; sol. 86% in water; m.w. 855-900; sp.gr. 1.0927 (60 C); dens. 9.16 lb/gal (55 C); visc. 15.3 cSt (210 F); f.p. 32–36 ; flash pt. (CCC) > 350 F; pH 4.5–7.5 (5% aq.).

Carbowax® PEG 1000. [Union Carbide] PEG-20; CAS 25322-68-3; antistat, surfactant intermediate, lubricant, release agent, ointment and suppository base, plasticizer for adhesives, ceramic glaze, creams and lotions, dentifrices, deodorant sticks, wood treatment; soft solid; sol. 80% in water; m.w. 950–1050; sp.gr. 1.0926 (60 C); dens. 9.16 lb/gal (55 C); visc. 17.2 cSt (210 F); f.p. 37–40; flash pt. (CCC) > 350 F; pH 4.5–7.5 (5% aq.).

Carbowax® PEG 1450. [Union Carbide] PEG-32; CAS 25322-68-3; antistat, surfactant intermediate, lubricant, release agent for adhesives, ceramic glaze, creams and lotions, dentifrices, deodorant sticks, wood treatment; soft solid or flake; sol. 72% in water; m.w. 1300–1600; sp.gr. 1.0919 (60 C); dens. 9.17 lb/gal (55 C); visc. 26.5 cSt (210 F); f.p. 43–46; flash pt. (CCC) > 350 F; pH 4.5–7.5 (5% aq.).

Carbowax® PEG 3350. [Union Carbide] PEG-75; CAS 25322-68-3; antistat, surfactant intermediate, dye carrier, lubricant, release agent, tablet binder for adhesives, ceramic glaze, creams and lotions, dentifrices, mining, soaps and detergents, tablet coating, toilet bowl cleaners; flake or powd.; sol. 67% in water; m.w. 3000–3700; sp.gr. 1.0926 (60 C); dens. 8.94 lb/gal (80 C); visc. 90.8 cSt (210

F); f.p. 54–58; flash pt. (CCC) > 350 F; pH 4.5–7.5 (5% aq.).

Carbowax® PEG 4600. [Union Carbide] PEG-100; CAS 25322-68-3; antistat, surfactant intermediate, dye carrier, lubricant, release agent, tablet binder for adhesives, ceramic glaze, creams and lotions, mining, soaps and detergents, tablet coating, toilet bowl cleaners; flake or powd.; sol. 65% in water; m.w. 4400–4800; sp.gr. 1.0926 (60 C); dens. 8.95 lb/gal (80 C); visc. 184 cSt (210 F); f.p. 57–61; flash pt. (CCC) > 350 F; pH 4.5–7.5 (5% aq.).

Carbowax® PEG 8000. [Union Carbide] PEG-150; CAS 25322-68-3; antistat, ceramic binder, surfactant intermediate, dye carrier, lubricant, release agent, tablet binder for adhesives, creams and lotions, mining, powd. metallurgy, soaps and detergents, tablet coating, toilet bowl cleaners; flake or powd.; sol. 63% in water; m.w. 7000–9000; sp.gr. 1.0845 (70 C); dens. 8.96 lb/gal (80 C); visc. 822 cSt (210 F); m.p. 60–63; flash pt. (CCC) > 350 F; pH 4.5–7.5 (5% aq.).

Carbowax® Sentry® PEG 300. [Union Carbide] PEG-6, FCC grade; CAS 25322-68-3; EINECS 220-045-1; coupling agent, solv., vehicle, humectant, lubricant, binder, base, bodying agent, dispersant, conditioner for cosmetics/toiletries (antiperspirants, creams/lotions, hand cleaners, toothpaste, makeup, shampoo, shave cream, sunscreens), food processing (citrus coatings, defoamer, pkg. component), pharmaceuticals (coating, binder, plasticizer, and lubricant in tablets), as glycerin replacement; FDA approved; water-wh. visc. liq.; sol. in water, alcohols, glycerin, glycols; m.w. 285-315; sp.gr. 1.1250; dens. 9.38 lb/gal; visc. 5.8 cSt (99 C); f.p. -15 to -8 C; hyd. no. 356-394; flash pt. (PMCC) > 180 C; ref. index 1.463; pH 4.5-7.5 (5% aq.); surf. tens. 44.5 dynes/cm.

Carbowax® Sentry® PEG 400. [Union Carbide] PEG-8, FCC grade; CAS 25322-68-3; EINECS 225-856-4; coupling agent, solv., vehcile, humectant, lubricant, binder, base for cosmetics/toiletries (bath oil, cologne, creams/lotions, toothpaste, hair dressing, lipsticks, makeup, makeup removers, nail polish remover, shampoo, shave cream, soap, sunscreen); food processing (citrus coatings, bodying agent, dispersant, defoamer, pkg. component), pharmaceuticals (coating, binder, plasticizer, and lubricant in tablets); FDA approved; water-wh. visc. liq.; sol. in water, methanol, ethanol, acetone, trichloroethylene, Cellosolve®, Carbitol®, dibutyl phthalate, toluene; m.w. 380-420; sp.gr. 1.1254; dens. 9.39 lb/gal; visc. 7.3 cSt (99 C); f.p. 4-8 C; hyd. no. 267-295; flash pt. (PMCC) > 180 C; ref. index 1.465; pH 4.5-7.5 (5% aq.); surf. tens. 44.5 dynes/cm.

Carbowax® Sentry® PEG 540 Blend. [Union Carbide] PEG-6-32, FCC grade; CAS 25322-68-3; coupling agent, solv., vehicle, humectant, lubricant, binder, base for cosmetics/toiletries (hair dressings, hand cleaners, ointments, antiperspirant, creams/lotions, shaving preps., sunscreens); food processing (citrus coatings, bodying agent, dispersant, defoamer, pkg. component), pharmaceuticals (coating, binder, plasticizer, and lubricant in tablets); FDA approved; wh. soft waxy solid; sol. in methylene chloride, 73% in water, 50% in trichloroethylene, 48% in methanol; m.w. 500-600; sp.gr. 1.0930; dens. 9.17 lb/gal (55 C); visc. 15.1 cSt (99 C); m.p. 38–41 C; hyd. no. 187-224; flash pt. (PMCC) > 180 C; pH 4.5-7.5 (5% aq.).

Carbowax® Sentry® PEG 600. [Union Carbide] PEG-12, FCC grade; CAS 25322-68-3; EINECS 229-859-1; coupling agent, solv., vehicle, humectant, lubricant, binder, base for cosmetics/toiletries (antiperspirnats, colognes, creams/lotions, dentifrices, lipsticks, makeup, shampoo, shave creams, sunscreens); food processing (citrus coatings, bodying agent, dispersant, defoamer, pkg. compo-

nent), pharmaceuticals (coating, binder, plasticizer, and lubricant in tablets); FDA approved; water-wh. visc. liq.; sol. in water, alcohols, glycols; m.w. 570-630; sp.gr. 1.1257; dens. 9.40 lb/gal; visc. 10.8 cSt (99 C); f.p. 20-25 C; hyd. no. 178-197; flash pt. (PMCC) > 180 C; ref. index 1.46; pH 4.5-7.5 (5% aq.); surf. tens. 44.5 dynes/cm.

Carbowax® Sentry® PEG 900. [Union Carbide] PEG-20, FCC grade; CAS 25322-68-3; coupling agent, solv., vehicle, humectant, lubricant, binder, base for cosmetics/toiletries (antiperspirants, creams/lotions, shave creams); food processing (citrus coatings, bodying agent, dispersant, defoamer, pkg. component), pharmaceuticals (coating, binder, plasticizer, and lubricant in tablets); FDA approved; wh. soft waxy solid; sol. 86% in water; m.w. 855-945; sp.gr. 1.0927 (60 C); dens. 9.16 lb/gal (55 C); visc. 15.3 cSt (99 C); m.p. 32-36 C; hyd. no. 119-131; flash pt. (PMCC) > 180 C; pH 4.5-7.5 (5% aq.).

Carbowax® Sentry® PEG 1000. [Union Carbide] PEG-20, FCC grade; CAS 25322-68-3; coupling agent, solv., vehicle, humectant, lubricant, binder, base for cosmetics/toiletries (antiperspirants, creams/lotions, ointments, shave creams); food processing (citrus coatings, bodying agent, dispersant, defoamer, pkg. component), pharmaceuticals (coating, binder, plasticizer, and lubricant in tablets); FDA approved; wh. soft waxy solid; sol. 80% in water; m.w. 950-1050; sp.gr. 1.0926 (60 C); dens. 9.16 lb/gal (55 C); visc. 17.2 cSt (99 C); m.p. 37-40 C; hyd. no. 107-118; flash pt. (PMCC) > 180 C; pH 4.5-7.5 (5% aq.).

Carbowax® Sentry® PEG 1450. [Union Carbide] PEG-32, FCC grade; CAS 25322-68-3; coupling agent, solv., vehicle, humectant, lubricant, binder, base for cosmetics/toiletries (antiperspirants, creams/lotions, ointments, shave creams); food processing (citrus coatings, bodying agent, dispersant, defoamer, pkg. component), pharmaceuticals (coating, binder, plasticizer, and lubricant in tablets); FDA approved; wh. soft waxy solid or flake; sol. 72% in water; m.w. 1300-1600; sp.gr. 1.0919 (60 C); dens. 9.17 lb/gal (55 C); bulk dens. 30 lb/ft^3 (flake); visc. 26.5 cSt (99 C); m.p. 43-46 C; hyd. no. 70-86; flash pt. (PMCC) > 180 C; pH 4.5-7.5 (5% aq.).

Carbowax® Sentry® PEG 3350. [Union Carbide] PEG-75, FCC grade; CAS 25322-68-3; coupling agent, solv., vehicle, humectant, lubricant, binder, base for cosmetics/toiletries (antiperspirants, bath powds., creams/lotions, toothpaste, hair dressing, makeup, nail polish remover, soap); food processing (citrus coatings, bodying agent, dispersant, defoamer, pkg. component), pharmaceuticals (coating, binder, plasticizer, and lubricant in tablets); FDA approved; wh. hard waxy flake or powd.; sol. 67% in water; m.w. 3000-3700; sp.gr. 1.0926 (60 C); dens. 8.94 lb/gal (80 C); bulk dens. 30 lb/ft^3 (flake), 40 lb/ft^3 (powd.); visc. 90.8 cSt (99 C); m.p. 54-58 C; hyd. no. 30-37; flash pt. (PMCC) > 180 C; pH 4.5-7.5 (5% aq.).

Carbowax® Sentry® PEG 4600. [Union Carbide] PEG-100, FCC grade; CAS 25322-68-3; coupling agent, solv., vehicle, humectant, lubricant, binder, base for cosmetics/toiletries (antiperspirants, creams/lotions); food processing (citrus coatings, bodying agent, dispersant, defoamer, pkg. component), pharmaceuticals (coating, binder, plasticizer, and lubricant in tablets); FDA approved; wh. hard waxy flake or powd.; sol. 65% in water; m.w. 4400-4800; sp.gr. 1.0926 (60 C); dens. 8.95 lb/gal (80 C); bulk dens. 30 lb/ft^3 (flake), 40 lb/ft^3 (powd.); visc. 184 cSt (99 C); m.p. 57-61 C; hyd. no. 23-26; flash pt. PMCC) > 180 C; pH 4.5-7.5 (5% aq.).

Carbowax® Sentry® PEG 8000. [Union Carbide] PEG-150, FCC grade; CAS 25322-68-3; coupling agent, solv., vehicle, humectant, lubricant, binder, base for cosmetics/toiletries (antiperspirants, creams/lotions, hair dressing, nail polish remover); food processing (citrus coatings, bodying agent, dispersant, defoamer, pkg. component), pharmaceuticals (coating, binder, plasticizer, and lubricant in tablets); FDA approved; wh. hard waxy flake or powd.; sol. 63% in water; m.w. 7000-9000; sp.gr. 1.0845 (60 C); dens. 8.96 lb/gal (80 C); bulk dens. 30 lb/ft³ (flake), 40 lb/ft³ (powd.); visc. 822 cSt (99 C); m.p. 60-63 C; hyd. no. 13-16; flash pt. (PMCC) > 180 C; pH 4.5-7.5 (5% aq.).

Carbowax® TPEG 990. [Union Carbide] Glycereth-20; CAS 31694-55-0; cosmetic ingred.

Carmine 224. [Presperse] Carmine, bismuth oxychloride; CAS 1390-65-4, 7787-59-9; natural colorant for pigmented cosmetics; JSCI/JCID approved.

Carmine 5297. [Presperse] Carmine; CAS 1390-65-4; EINECS 215-724-4; colorant for pigmented cosmetics; JSCI/JCID approved.

Carmine Ultra-fine. [Presperse] Carmine; CAS 1390-65-4; EINECS 215-724-4; colorant for pigmented cosmetics; JSCI/JCID approved.

Carnation® . [Witco/Petroleum Spec.] Wh. min. oil NF; emollient and lubricant for cosmetic formulations and baby oil; FDA §172.878, 178.3620a; water-wh., odorless, tasteless; sp.gr. 0.837-0.853; visc. 11-14 cSt (40 C); pour pt. -7 C; flash pt. 177 C.

Carnauba Wax NC #2 Stralpitz. [Strahl & Pitsch] Carnauba; CAS 8015-86-9; EINECS 232-399-4; wax for cosmetics use.

Carnauba Wax NC #3 Stralpitz. [Strahl & Pitsch] Carnauba; CAS 8015-86-9; EINECS 232-399-4; wax for cosmetics use.

Carnauba Wax SP 8. [Strahl & Pitsch] Carnauba; CAS 8015-86-9; EINECS 232-399-4; wax for cosmetics use.

Carnitiline. [Sederma] Carnitine, caffeine, hydrolyzed glycoasminoglycans.

Caroat. [Degussa] Potassium caroate.

Carob HS. [Alban Muller] Propylene glycol and carob extract; botanical extract.

Carolane. [Barnet Prods.] Squalane NF; CAS 111-01-3; EINECS 203-825-6; emollient for use in elegant cosmetic formulations; absorption assistant.

Carosulf T-60-L. [Lonza] TEA-dodecylbenzene sulfonate; CAS 27323-41-7; EINECS 248-406-9; personal care surfactant.

Carotene Huileux 10000. [Gattefosse] Apricot kernel oil and beta-carotene.

Carotene Standard RR. [Atomergic Chemetals] Beta-carotene; CAS 7235-40-7; EINECS 230-636-6; cosmetic colorant.

Carraghenate P, Standard, X 2. [Laserson SA] Carrageenan; CAS 9000-07-1; EINECS 232-524-2; gellant, thickener, suspension stabilizer for cosmetics; forms translucent gels in presence of KCl, NaCl; JSCI and Europe compliance; wh., creamy, or clear beige powd., odorless and tasteless; sol. in water; insol. in oils and org. solvs.; usage level: 1-5%.

Carroll 40% Coconut Hand Soap. [Carroll] Potassium coconut oil soap; anionic; for use in hand soaps, shampoos, etc.; liq.; HLB 25.0; 40% conc.

Carrot LS. [Alban Muller] Sunflower seed oil and carrot seed extract.

Carrot Oil. [Provital; Centerchem] Sunflower seed oil, carrot oil, carrot extract, and beta-carotene.

Carrot Oil. [Cosmetochem] Sunflower seed oil, carrot extract, and isopropyl myristate; oily extract containing liposoluble substances from the carrot, i.e., beta-carotene, carotenoids, and tocopherols.

Carrot Oil CLR. [Dr. Kurt Richter; Henkel/Cospha; Henkel Canada] Soybean oil, carrot oil, carrot extract, beta-carotene, tocopherol; nonionic; emollient, conditioner, superfatting agent; emulsified and oily preparations for care of skin and hair, esp. dry skin and scalp; deep red oil;

faint char. odor.

Carrot Oil COS. [Cosmetochem] An oily extract of carrot containing β-carotene, carotinoids, and tocopherols; cosmetic specialty.

Carrot Oil Extra. [Novarom GmbH] Peanut oil, carrot extract, isopropyl myristate, and tocopherol; botanical extract.

Carrots Extract HS 2597 G. [Grau Aromatics] Propylene glycol and carrot extract; botanical extract.

Carsamide® AMEA. [Lonza] Acetamide MEA (1:1); CAS 142-26-7; EINECS 205-530-8; hair conditioner and antistat; liq.; 70% act.

Carsamide® CA. [Lonza] Cocamide DEA (1:1); CAS 61791-31-9; EINECS 263-163-9; nonionic; detergent, dispersant, emulsifier, wetting agent, foam booster, thickener, softener for industrial, cosmetic, and household cleaners; biodeg.; liq.; sol. in water, alcohol, chlorinated and aromatic hydrocarbons, Polysolve, Cellosolves, Carbitols, and natural fats and oils; sp.gr. 1.0; dens. 8.3 lb/gal; 100% act.

Carsamide® CMEA. [Lonza] Cocamide MEA (1:1); CAS 68140-00-1; EINECS 268-770-2; nonionic; foam booster, stabilizer, visc. builder for shampoos and detergents; flake; 100% conc.

Carsamide® O. [Lonza] Oleamide DEA; CAS 93-83-4; EINECS 202-281-7; thickener, foam booster/stabilizer.

Carsamide® SAC. [Lonza] Cocamide DEA (1:1); CAS 61791-31-9; EINECS 263-163-9; nonionic; detergent for industrial, institutional, cosmetic, and household cleaners; dispersant, emulsifier, wetting agent, visc. builder; foam stabilizer for shampoos, bubble baths, detergents; pale amber visc. liq.; mild fatty odor; ol. in water, alcohol, chlorinated and aromatic hydrocarbons, Polysolve, Cellosolves, Carbitols, and natural fats and oils; dens. 8.2 lb/gal; 100% act.

Carsamide® SAL-7. [Lonza] Lauramide DEA (1:1); CAS 120-40-1; EINECS 204-393-1; nonionic; detergent, emulsifier, foaming agent, foam stabilizer, thickener for shampoos, bath prods., household, institutional and industrial detergents; Gardner 2 solid; mild, fatty odor; sol. in alcohol, chlorinated and aromatic hydrocarbons; dens. 8.2 lb/gal; m.p. 104–114 F; biodeg.; 100% conc.

Carsamide® SAL-9. [Lonza] Lauramide DEA (1:1); CAS 120-40-1; EINECS 204-393-1; nonionic; foaming and thickening agent for shampoos, bath prods., detergents; solid; dens. 8.1 lb/gal; biodeg.; 100% conc.

Carsamide® SAL-82. [Lonza] Lauramide DEA; CAS 120-40-1; EINECS 204-393-1; personal care surfactant; clear yel. liq. free from foreign matter; visc. 500 cps.

Carsofoam® 1618. [Lonza] Cetearyl alcohol; bodying agent, visc. modifier for cosmetic, personal care, and household prods.; flakes; m.p. 46 C; acid no. 0.1; flash pt. 163 C.

Carsofoam® BS-I. [Lonza] PEG-80 sorbitan laurate, sodium trideceth sulfate, PEG-150 distearate, disodium lauroamphodiacetate, cocamidopropyl hydroxysultaine, sodium laureth-13 carboxylate; anionic/nonionic/amphoteric; low irritation conc. for baby shampoos which are extremely mild and nonirritating; liq.; 40% conc.

Carsofoam® DEV. [Lonza] Sodium laureth sulfate, cocamide DEA, and cocamidopropyl betaine; surfactant conc. for personal care prods.; imparts rich foam, gentle cleansing, and high visc.; lt. colored clear liq.; sol. 100% in water; pH 8.5-9.0 (10% aq.); 36.5-38.5% act.

Carsofoam® MSP. [Lonza] TEA-lauryl sulfate, cocamide DEA, cocamidopropyl betaine, methyl paraben (0.75%); anionic/amphoteric; shampoo conc. for mild shampoos incl. baby shampoos, acid balanced shampoos, general-purpose shampoos, and gels; lt. yel. hazy liq.; pH 7.3 (10%); 50% act.

Carsofoam® T-60-L. [Lonza] TEA dodecylbenzene sulfonate; CAS 27323-41-7; EINECS 248-406-9; anionic;

high foaming detergent, wetting agent for cosmetic, industrial, and institutional cleaning compds.; biodeg.; Gardner < 5 clear visc. liq.; bland odor; dens. 9.0 lb/gal; pH 7.0–7.6; 60% min. solids.

Carsonol® ALS. [Lonza] Ammonium lauryl sulfate; CAS 2235-54-3; EINECS 218-793-9; anionic; biodeg. high foaming detergent, wetting and emulsifying agent for cosmetics (shampoos, bubble baths, shaving creams, cleansing creams, skin lotions), industrial cleaners, rug/upholstery cleaners, household detergents, veg. scrubbing, auto shampoo, pet shampoo, emulsion polymerization; low color visc. liq., low odor; water-sol.; dens. 8.4 lb/gal; pH 6.5-7.0 (10%); 30% act.

Carsonol® ALS-R. [Lonza] Ammonium lauryl sulfate; CAS 2235-54-3; EINECS 218-793-9; anionic; detergent with high foam, good wetting and emulsifying properties used for cosmetics, chemical specialties; clear visc. liq.; water sol.; dens. 8.4 lb/gal; pH 6.5–7.0 (10%); biodeg.; 29% act.

Carsonol® ALS-S. [Lonza] Ammonium lauryl sulfate; CAS 2235-54-3; EINECS 218-793-9; anionic; biodeg. high foaming surfactant, wetting agent, emulsifier for shampoos, bubble baths, shaving creams, industrial cleaners, foam/dust control, liq. household detergents, automobile shampoos, emulsion polymerization; low salt grade; liq.; 29% act.

Carsonol® ALS Special. [Lonza] Ammonium lauryl sulfate; CAS 2235-54-3; EINECS 218-793-9; anionic; biodeg. high foaming detergent, wetting and emulsifying agent for cosmetics (shampoos, bubble baths, shaving creams, cleansing creams, skin lotions), industrial cleaners, rug/upholstery cleaners, household detergents, veg. scrubbing, auto shampoo, pet shampoo, emulsion polymerization; low color clear liq., low odor; water-sol.; dens. 8.4 lb/gal; pH 6.5-7.0 (10%); 30% act.

Carsonol® AOS. [Lonza] Sodium C14-C16 olefin sulfonate; CAS 68439-57-6; EINECS 270-407-8; surfactant for shampoos, liq. soaps, industrial cleaners; pH 8.0 (5%); 40% act.

Carsonol® BDM. [Lonza] DEA-lauryl sulfate, DEA-lauraminopropionate, and sodium lauraminopropionate; anionic; mild shampoos with conditioning; liq.; 38% conc.

Carsonol® DLS. [Lonza] DEA-lauryl sulfate; CAS 143-00-0; EINECS 205-577-4; anionic; biodeg. detergent, foaming agent, wetting agent, emulsifier for personal care prods. (shampoos, bubble baths, shaving preps., cleansing creams), industrial cleaners, household detergents, pet shampoo, veg. scrubbing, emulsion polymerization; clear liq.; low odor; water sol.; dens. 8.49 lb/gal; pH 7.5–8.5 (10%); 35% act.

Carsonol® MLS. [Lonza] Magnesium lauryl sulfate; CAS 3097-08-3; EINECS 221-450-6; anionic; detergent with high foam, good wetting and emulsifying properties used for cosmetics, chemical specialties, rug and upholstery formulations; visc. liq.; low odor; water-sol.; dens. 8.57 lb/gal; pH 6.5–7.5 (10%); biodeg.; 30% act.

Carsonol® SES-A. [Lonza] Ammonium laureth sulfate; CAS 32612-48-9; anionic; biodeg. surfactant with excellent foaming in hard and soft water, for cosmetic, household, and industrial uses, shampoos, bubble baths, liq. cleaners; liq.; dens. 8.4 lb/gal; pH 6.5–7.5 (10%); 60% act.

Carsonol® SES-S. [Lonza] Sodium laureth sulfate; CAS 9004-82-4; anionic; biodeg. surfactant with excellent foaming in hard and soft water, for cosmetic, household, and industrial uses, liq. carwash, laundry detergents; liq.; dens. 8.8 lb/gal; pH 7.5-9.0 (10%); 60% act.

Carsonol® SLES. [Lonza] Sodium laureth sulfate; CAS 9004-82-4; anionic; surfactant with excellent foaming in hard and soft water, for cosmetic, household, and industrial uses, liq. carwash, laundry detergents; liq.; dens. 8.7 lb/gal; pH 7.5–8.5 (10%); biodeg; 30% act.

Carsonol® SLES-2. [Lonza] Sodium laureth sulfate; anionic; mild biodeg. surfactant with excellent foaming in hard and soft water, for cosmetics (shampoo, bubble bath), liq. detergents, automobile shampoo, household chemical specialties, industrial foaming agents; liq.; dens. 8.63 lb/gal; pH 7.5-8.5 (10%); 30% act.

Carsonol® SLES-3. [Lonza] Sodium laureth sulfate; anionic; mild biodeg. detergent, foaming agent, wetting agent, emulsifier for personal care prods. (shampoos, bubble baths), liq. detergents, automobile shampoo, industrial chemical specialties, industrial foaming agents; liq.; dens. 8.7 lb/gal; pH 7.5-8.5 (10%); 29% act.

Carsonol® SLES-4. [Lonza] Sodium laureth sulfate; personal care surfactant.

Carsonol® SLS. [Lonza] Sodium lauryl sulfate; CAS 151-21-3; EINECS 205-788-1; anionic; biodeg. detergent with high foam, good wetting and emulsifying properties used for cosmetics (shampoos, bubble baths, shaving preps.), industrial cleaners, rug/upholstery shampoos, household detergents, veg. scrubbing, emulsion polymerization; low color liq., low odor; water0sol.; dens. 8.7 lb/gal; pH 7.5-8.5 (10%); 30% act.

Carsonol® SLS Paste B. [Lonza] Sodium lauryl sulfate; CAS 151-21-3; EINECS 205-788-1; anionic; biodeg. detergent with high foam, good wetting and emulsifying properties used for cosmetics, chemical specialties, shampoo bases, textile scouring; paste, low color; low odor; water sol.; dens. 8.8 lb/gal; pH 8.4–8.8 (10%); 30% act.

Carsonol® SLS-R. [Lonza] Sodium lauryl sulfate; CAS 151-21-3; EINECS 205-788-1; anionic; biodeg. detergent, foaming agent, wetting agent, emulsifier for personal care prods., household and industrial cleaners, emulsion polymerization; liq.; 29% act.

Carsonol® SLS-S. [Lonza] Sodium lauryl sulfate; CAS 151-21-3; EINECS 205-788-1; anionic; biodeg. detergent, foaming agent, wetting agent, emulsifier for personal care prods., household and industrial cleaners, emulsion polymerization; liq.; 29% act.

Carsonol® SLS Special. [Lonza] Sodium lauryl sulfate; CAS 151-21-3; EINECS 205-788-1; anionic; biodeg. detergent with high foam, good wetting and emulsifying properties used for cosmetics, industrial cleaners, emulsion polymerization, veg. scrubbing; liq., low color; low odor; water-sol.; dens. 8.7 lb/gal; pH 7.5–8.5 (10%); 30% act.

Carsonol® TLS. [Lonza] TEA-lauryl sulfate; CAS 139-96-8; EINECS 205-388-7; anionic; biodeg. detergent with high foam, good wetting and emulsifying properties used for cosmetics, mild shampoos, bubble baths, chemical specialties, industrial cleaners, emulsion polymerization; clear liq.; low color, odor; water-sol.; dens. 8.7 lb/gal; pH 7.0–7.5 (10%); 40% act.

Carsonon® 144-P. [Lonza] PPG-3 myristyl ether; CAS 63793-60-2; nonionic; lubricant, emollient, solubilizer for cosmetics incl. silicon systems; aids low temp. stability, antistatic and conditioning effects; contributes to mildness and spreading behavior; APHA 35 liq.; hyd. no. 130; 100% act.

Carsonon® 169-P. [Lonza] PPG-10 cetyl ether; CAS 9035-85-2; nonionic; lubricant, emollient, solubilizer for cosmetics incl. silicon systems; aids low temp. stability, antistatic and conditioning effects; contributes to mildness and spreading behavior; APHA 100 liq.; hyd. no. 75; 100% act.

Carsonon® D-5. [Lonza] Isodeceth-5.

Carsonon® L-2. [Lonza] Laureth-2; CAS 3055-93-4; EINECS 221-279-7; emulsifier.

Carsonon® L-3. [Lonza] Laureth-3; CAS 3055-94-5; EINECS 221-280-2; emulsifier.

Carsonon® L-5. [Lonza] Laureth-5; CAS 3055-95-6; EINECS 221-281-8; emulsifier.

Carsonon® L-9. [Lonza] Laureth-9; CAS 3055-99-0;

EINECS 221-284-4; personal care surfactant.

Carsonon® L-12. [Lonza] Laureth-12; CAS 3056-00-6; EINECS 221-286-5; emulsifier.

Carsonon® N-2. [Lonza] Nonoxynol-2; EINECS 248-291-5; personal care surfactant.

Carsonon® N-4. [Lonza] Nonoxynol-4; CAS 9016-45-9; nonionic; emulsifier, detergent, wetting agent, dispersant for household and industrial uses; intermediate; drycleaning detergent; pale liq.; sol. in kerosene, alcohols, aromatic and chlorinated solv., Stod.; sp.gr. 1.02; dens. 8.6 lb/gal; visc. 175-250 cps; flash pt. 500-600 F; pour pt. -5 ± 2 F; solid. pt. -20 ± 2 F; HLB 9.0; 100% act.

Carsonon® N-30. [Lonza] Nonoxynol-30; CAS 9016-45-9; nonionic; emulsifier, stabilizer for emulsion polymerization, oils, fats, waxes, essential oils; pale yel. liq. to semisolid; sp.gr. 1.09; cloud pt. 167–171 F (1%); pH 6.0–7.0 (3%); HLB 17.2; 70% act., 30% water.

Carsonon® N-40. [Lonza] Nonoxynol-40; CAS 9016-45-9; nonionic; emulsifier, stabilizer; wh. to yel. semisolid; cloud pt. 212 F (1%); pH 6.0–7.0 (3%); 70% act., 30% water.

Carsonon® N-100. [Lonza] Nonoxynol-100; CAS 9016-45-9; nonionic; emulsifier, stabilizer; wh. to off-wh. semisolid; water sol.; cloud pt. 212 F (1%); pH 6.0–7.0 (3%); 70% act., 30% water.

Carsoquat® 816-C. [Lonza] Cetearyl alcohol, PEG-40 castor oil, and stearalkonium chloride; cationic; formulated base, cream rinse conc. for personal care prods.; wh. waxy flakes; mild, fatty odor; disp. in water; pH 6.3 (5% disp.); 96% min act.

Carsoquat® 868. [Lonza] Dicetyl dimonium chloride; CAS 1812-53-9; EINECS 217-325-0; cationic; substantive conditioner for hair and skin care prods.; antistat for textiles and other applics.; fabric softener for natural and syn. fibers; pale yel. clear liq.; m.w. 521; sp.gr. 0.86 g/ml; pH 7 (5% solids in 1:1 IPA/water); 68% act. in IPA/water.

Carsoquat® 868-E. [Lonza] Dicetyl dimonium chloride; CAS 1812-53-9; EINECS 217-325-0; cationic; substantive conditioner for hair and skin care prods.; antistat for textiles and other applics.; fabric softener for natural and syn. fibers; pale yel. clear liq.; m.w. 521; sp.gr. 0.86 g/ml; pH 7 (5% solids in 1:1 IPA/water); 68% act. in ethanol.

Carsoquat® 868P. [Lonza] Dicetyl dimonium chloride; CAS 1812-53-9; EINECS 217-325-0; cationic; conditioner for high performance hair conditioners, ethnic hair care sheen spray, and cream rinses; coemulsifier; liq., odorless; pH 7.5 (5% disp.); 68% act. in propylene glycol.

Carsoquat® CB. [Lonza] Cetyl alcohol, glyceryl stearate, dicetyl dimonium chloride, cetrimonium chloride, polysorbate 85, PEG-40 castor oil; cationic; conditioner, emulsifier, softener, emollient for hair rinses, skin creams and lotions; cream rinse conc.; wh. waxy flakes, mild fatty odor; m.p. 55 C; pH 4 (5% disp.); 99% act.

Carsoquat® CT-429. [Lonza] Cetrimonium chloride; CAS 112-02-7; EINECS 203-928-6; cationic; surfactant; conditioner in hair and skin care preparations; antistat; colorless to pale yel. clear liq.; water-sol.; m.w. 319; sp.gr. 0.968; dens. 8.10 lb/gal; pH 3.5-4.5 (2%); 29% act. in water.

Carsoquat® SDQ-25. [Lonza] Stearalkonium chloride (21%), stearyl alcohol (4%), IPA (5%), water (70%); cationic; surfactant, conditioner, softener for cosmetics (cream hair rinse, skin creams and lotions, aerosol hair sprays, hair color rinses), textiles, paper; antistat for natural and syn. fibers; dispersant for pigments and dyestuffs; wh. thick creamy paste; mild, sweet odor; sol. in lower alcohols and glycols; readily disp. in water; dens. 7.9 lb/gal; pour pt. 110-120 F; clear pt. 140 F; pH 3.0–4.0 (1% disp.); 21% act.

Carsoquat® SDQ-85. [Lonza] Stearalkonium chloride; CAS 122-19-0; EINECS 204-527-9; cationic; softener, hair conditioner; wh. waxy flake; mild, sweet odor; water-disp.; m.p. 140 F; pH 5.0–7.0 (0.5%); 85% act.

Carsosulf SXS. [Lonza] Sodium xylene sulfonate; CAS 1300-72-7; EINECS 215-090-9; anionic; coupler, solubilizer for liq. detergent systems and cleaning compd.; biodeg.; nonflamm.; liq.; sp.gr. 1.18–1.22; pH 7.5–10.5; 40% act.

Cartafix U. [Sandoz] PPG-24-PEG-21 tallowaminopropylamine.

Cartaretin F-4. [Sandoz] Adipic acid/dimethylaminohydroxypropyl diethylenetriamine copolymer; cationic; polymer substantive to hair; for shampoo systems; imparts lubricity; sol. in water and certain blends of water and lower alcohols; toxicology: extremely mild.

Cartaretin F-23. [Sandoz] Adipic acid/dimethylaminohydroxypropyl diethylenetriamine copolymer.

Cartilage Mucopolysaccharides E.M.A.C. [Solabia] Hydrolyzed glycosaminoglycans; moisturizer.

Cashmir K-II. [Presperse] Mica and silica; CAS 12001-26-2 and 7631-86-9; provides superior silky smooth skinfeel at economical price; used for pressed and loose powds., pigmented cosmetics.

Castorcet. [Lanaetex Prods.] Castor oil, isocetyl alcohol, and oleyl alcohol; cosmetic ingred.

Castor Oil USP. [United Catalysts] Castor oil; CAS 8001-79-4; EINECS 232-293-8; emollient.

Castorwax® MP-70. [CasChem] Hydrog. castor oil; CAS 8001-78-3; EINECS 232-292-2; wax for anhyd. prods. requiring a soft creamy texture; for cosmetics and pharmaceuticals; FDA approval; m.p. 70 C; acid no. 2; iodine no. 38; sapon. no. 180; hyd. no. 158.

Castorwax® MP-80. [CasChem] Hydrog. castor oil; CAS 8001-78-3; EINECS 232-292-2; release agent; wax used for formulating antiperspirant sticks, suspending aid for aluminum chlorhydrate; FDA approval; wh. flakes; m.p. 80 C; acid no. 2; iodine no. 29; sapon. no. 180; hyd. no. 158; 100% act.

Castorwax® NF. [CasChem] Hydrog. castor oil NF; CAS 8001-78-3; EINECS 232-292-2; wax for pharmaceutical and food applics.; FDA approval; flake.

Catemol 18SA. [Phoenix] Stearamidoethyl ethanolamine; CAS 141-21-9; EINECS 205-469-7; cationic; cosmetic ingred.

Catemol 180-S. [Phoenix] Stearamidopropyl dimethylamine stearate; cationic.

Catemol 220-B. [Phoenix] Behenamidopropyl dimethylamine behenate; CAS 125804-04-8; cationic.

Catemol 360. [Phoenix] Dilinoleamidopropyl dimethylamine; cationic.

Cathelios CL 50. [Ceca SA] Benzalkonium chloride; bactericide, fungicide, antistat for cosmetics use; pale yel. liq.; sp.gr. 1.04-1.06; pH 7-8 (10% aq.); 50 ± 1% act.

Catigene® CT 70. [Phoenix] Cetrimonium methosulfate; CAS 65060-02-8; EINECS 265-352-1.

Catigene® SA 70. [Phoenix] Stearamidopropyl trimonium methosulfate.

Catigene® ST 70. [Phoenix] Steartrimonium methosulfate; CAS 18684-11-2; conditioner.

Catinal HC-100. [Toho Chem. Industry] Cellulosic resin; cationic; conditioning agent for hair shampoo, hair rinse, body soap, body lotion; powd.

Catinal HTB-70. [Toho Chem. Industry] Hexadecyl trimethyl ammonium bromide; CAS 57-09-0; EINECS 200-311-3; base material for hair rinse, antistat, germicide; waxy solid.

Catinal MB-50A. [Toho Chem. Industry] Dodecyl dimethyl benzyl ammonium chloride; CAS 139-07-1; EINECS 205-351-5; cationic; germicide, disinfectant, antistat for medical/pharmaceutical industries; liq.

Catinal OB-80E. [Toho Chem. Industry] Stearyl dimethyl

benzyl ammonium chloride; CAS 122-19-0; EINECS 204-527-9; base material for hair rinses; waxy solid.

Cation LQ. [Sanyo Chem. Industries] N(N'-Lanolin fatty acid amidopropyl) N-ethyl-N,N-dimethyl ammonium ethyl-sulfate; cationic; emulsifier for acid balanced skin moisturizers; conditioning agent for hair; paste; 65% conc.

Cationic Collagen Polypeptides. [Maybrook] Cationic collagen polypeptides; CAS 9007-34-5; substantive film-former for hair and skin care prods. (shampoos, conditioners, mousses, shave preps.); protective colloid effect; clear to sl. hazy visc. liq. or soft gel, mild char. odor; pH 3.5-4.5; 28-32% solids.

Cationic Guar C-261. [Henkel/Cospha; Henkel Canada] Guar hydroxypropyl trimonium chloride; CAS 65497-29-2; cationic; thickener, emulsion stabilizer and additive for shampoos; solid; 100% conc.

Cationico SCL. [Auschem SpA] Benzalkonium chloride.

Cavitron Cyclo-dextrin.™ [Am. Maize Prods.] Cyclodextrin; CAS 7585-39-9; EINECS 231-493-2; host-receptor molecules for binding of guest molecules; molecular encapsulation for use in pharmaceuticals, food, agrichems., chem. processing, cosmetics; protects act. ingreds. against oxidation and decomp., eliminates/reduces undesired taste/odor, and contamination, stabilizes food flavors and fragrances, enhances solubility; avail. as α, β, γ, derivs., and polymers.

Cavitron Cyclodextrin-Sulfated. [Am. Maize Prods.] Sodium cyclodextrin sulfate; CAS 37191-69-8.

C-Base. [Maybrook] Mineral oil, PEG-30 lanolin, and cetyl alcohol; self-emulsifying cosmetic base.

CE-618. [Procter & Gamble] Methyl cocoate; CAS 61788-59-8; EINECS 262-988-1; emollient.

CE-1218. [Procter & Gamble] Methyl laurate; CAS 111-82-0; EINECS 203-911-3; detergent intermediate.

CE-1270. [Procter & Gamble] Methyl laurate; CAS 111-82-0; EINECS 203-911-3; detergent intermediate.

CE-1280. [Procter & Gamble] Methyl laurate; CAS 111-82-0; EINECS 203-911-3; detergent intermediate.

CE-1290. [Procter & Gamble] Methyl laurate; CAS 111-82-0; EINECS 203-911-3; detergent intermediate.

CE-1295. [Procter & Gamble] Methyl laurate; CAS 111-82-0; EINECS 203-911-3; detergent intermediate.

CE-2000. [Siltech] Trioctyldodecyl citrate; CAS 126121-35-5; nonionic; nonsilicone oil phase ingred. for personal care applics.; water-insol.; 100% act.

Cecavon AL 11. [Ceca SA] Aluminum stearate; anticaking and waterproofing agent for inks, greases, stamping, paints, and cosmetics; powd.; dens. 0.40 max.; m.p. 160-165 C; 4.9-5.8% Al.

Cecavon AL 12. [Ceca SA] Aluminum stearate; anticaking and waterproofing agent for inks, greases, stamping, paints, and cosmetics; powd.; dens. 0.30 max.; m.p. 183-187 C; 5.6-6.1% Al.

Cecavon MG 51. [Ceca SA] Magnesium stearate; CAS 557-04-0; EINECS 209-150-3; anticaking agent, for concrete, cosmetics, pharmaceuticals; powd.; dens. 0.20 max.; m.p. 140-145 C; 4.5-5.1% Mg.

Cecavon NA 61. [Ceca SA] Sodium stearate; CAS 822-16-2; EINECS 212-490-5; waterproofing agent, lubricant, gellant, opacifier for paper and cosmetics; powd.; dens. 0.30 max.; m.p. > 200 C; 8.8-9.8% Na.

Cecavon ZN 70. [Ceca SA] Zinc stearate; CAS 557-05-1; EINECS 209-151-9; waterproofing agent, lubricant, gellant, opacifier for rubber, concrete, composites, paints, varnish, cosmetics, pharmaceuticals, molding, and paper applics.; powd.; dens. 0.20 max.; m.p. 125-130 C; 10.2-11% Zn.

Cecavon ZN 71. [Ceca SA] Zinc stearate; CAS 557-05-1; EINECS 209-151-9; waterproofing agent, lubricant, gellant, opacifier for rubber, concrete, composites, paints,

varnish, cosmetics, pharmaceuticals, molding, and paper applics.; powd.; dens. 0.20 max.; m.p. 125-130 C; 10.2-11% Zn.

Cecavon ZN 72. [Ceca SA] Zinc stearate; CAS 557-05-1; EINECS 209-151-9; waterproofing agent, lubricant, gellant, opacifier for rubber, concrete, composites, paints, varnish, cosmetics, pharmaceuticals, molding, and paper applics.; powd.; dens. 0.20 max.; m.p. 125-130 C; 9.8-10.6% Zn.

Cecavon ZN 73. [Ceca SA] Zinc stearate; CAS 557-05-1; EINECS 209-151-9; waterproofing agent, lubricant, gellant, opacifier for rubber, concrete, composites, paints, varnish, cosmetics, pharmaceuticals, molding, and paper applics.; powd.; dens. < 0.20; m.p. 125-130 C; 10.2-10.8% Zn.

Cecavon ZN 735. [Ceca SA] Zinc stearate; CAS 557-05-1; EINECS 209-151-9; waterproofing agent, lubricant, gellant, opacifier for rubber, concrete, composites, paints, varnish, cosmetics, pharmaceuticals, molding, and paper applics.; liq.; sp.gr. 1 ± 0.10; visc. 50-200 mPa·s; 35 ± 2% dry content.

Cedepal TD-403. [Stepan; Stepan Canada] Sodium trideceth sulfate; surfactant, wetting agent, foamer for shampoo, bath prods., mild baby prods.; liq.; 30% act.

Cedepal TD-407. [Stepan; Stepan Canada] Sodium trideceth sulfate; surfactant, wetting agent, foamer for shampoo, bath prods., mild baby prods.; liq.; 73% act.

Cedepal TD-484. [Stepan; Stepan Canada] Sodium trideceth sulfate; surfactant, wetting agent, foamer for shampoo, bath prods., mild baby prods.; liq.; 32% act.

Cegaba. [Siegmar Laboratori Ricerca] Carboxyethyl aminobutyric acid.

Cegesoft® C 17. [Henkel KGaA/Cospha] Myristyl lactate; CAS 1323-03-1; EINECS 215-350-1; emollient; solubilizer for solid and oil-sol. additives; wh. to sl. ylsh. solid, faint intrinsic odor; m.p. 29-34 C; acid no. 5 max.; sapon. no. 180-196.

Cegesoft® C 19. [Henkel KGaA/Cospha] Cetyl lactate; CAS 35274-05-6; EINECS 252-478-7; emollient; solubilizer for solid and oil-sol. additives; solid.

Cegesoft® C 24. [Henkel KGaA/Cospha; Grünau] Octyl palmitate; CAS 29806-73-3; EINECS 249-862-1; used in cosmetic/pharmaceutical skin care preps., sl. fatting emulsions and skin oils; sl. ylsh. clear oil; m.w. 350; sp.gr. 0.855-0.865; visc. 10-15 mPa·s; acid no. 0.5 max.; sapon. no. 148-158; cloud pt. 2 C max.; ref. index 1.446-1.448.

Celanol A.S.L. [Lanaetex Prods.] Isostearyl alcohol and lanolin alcohol.

Celite® 503. [Celite] Diatomaceous earth; CAS 7631-86-9; EINECS 231-545-4; carrier, filler for cosmetics.

Celite® 512. [Celite] Diatomaceous earth; CAS 7631-86-9; EINECS 231-545-4; carrier, filler for cosmetics.

Celite® 521 AW. [Celite] Diatomaceous earth; CAS 7631-86-9; EINECS 231-545-4; carrier, filler for cosmetics.

Celite® 545. [Celite] Diatomaceous earth; CAS 7631-86-9; EINECS 231-545-4; carrier, filler for cosmetics.

Celite® 550. [Celite] Diatomaceous earth; CAS 7631-86-9; EINECS 231-545-4; carrier, filler for cosmetics.

Celite® 560. [Celite] Diatomaceous earth; CAS 7631-86-9; EINECS 231-545-4; carrier, filler for cosmetics.

Celite® 577. [Celite] Diatomaceous earth; CAS 7631-86-9; EINECS 231-545-4; carrier, filler for cosmetics.

Cellactin. [Ichimaru Pharcos] Hydrolyzed hemoglobin.

Cellosize® HEC QP Grades. [Amerchol] Hydroxyethylcellulose; CAS 9004-62-0; water-sol. polymers for use as thickeners in hair conditioners, shampoos, lotions and creams, binder in powds., mascara, eyeliner; suspending aid.

Cellosize® HEC QP-3-L. [Amerchol] Hydroxyethylcellulose; CAS 9004-62-0; water-sol. polymers for use as thickeners in hair conditioners, shampoos, lotions and creams, binder in powds., mascara, eyeliner; suspending aid; wh. powd., mild odor; 98% min. thru 20 mesh; visc. 215-282 cps (5% aq.); pH 6-7 (2% aq.).

Cellosize® HEC QP-40. [Amerchol] Hydroxyethylcellulose; CAS 9004-62-0; water-sol. polymers for use as thickeners in hair conditioners, shampoos, lotions and creams, binder in powds., mascara, eyeliner; suspending aid; wh. powd., mild odor; 98% min. thru 20 mesh; visc. 80-125 cps (2% aq.); pH 6-7 (2% aq.).

Cellosize® HEC QP-100M-H. [Amerchol] Hydroxyethylcellulose; CAS 9004-62-0; water-sol. polymers for use as thickeners in hair conditioners, shampoos, lotions and creams, binder in powds., mascara, eyeliner; suspending aid; wh. powd., mild odor; 98% min. thru 20 mesh; visc. 4400-6600 cps (1% aq.); pH 6-7 (1% aq.).

Cellosize® HEC QP-300. [Amerchol] Hydroxyethylcellulose; CAS 9004-62-0; water-sol. polymers for use as thickeners in hair conditioners, shampoos, lotions and creams, binder in powds., mascara, eyeliner; suspending aid; wh. powd., mild odor; 98% min. thru 20 mesh; visc. 300-400 cps (2% aq.); pH 6-7 (2% aq.).

Cellosize® HEC QP-4400-H. [Amerchol] Hydroxyethylcellulose; CAS 9004-62-0; water-sol. polymers for use as thickeners in hair conditioners, shampoos, lotions and creams, binder in powds., mascara, eyeliner; suspending aid; wh. powd., mild odor; 98% min. thru 20 mesh; visc. 4800-6000 cps (2% aq.); pH 6-7 (2% aq.).

Cellosize® HEC QP-15,000-H. [Amerchol] Hydroxyethylcellulose; CAS 9004-62-0; water-sol. polymers for use as thickeners in hair conditioners, shampoos, lotions and creams, binder in powds., mascara, eyeliner; suspending aid; wh. powd., mild odor; 98% min. thru 20 mesh; visc. 1100-1500 cps (1% aq.); pH 6-7 (1% aq.).

Cellosize® HEC QP-52,000-H. [Amerchol] Hydroxyethylcellulose; CAS 9004-62-0; water-sol. polymers for use as thickeners in hair conditioners, shampoos, lotions and creams, binder in powds., mascara, eyeliner; suspending aid; wh. powd., mild odor; 98% min. thru 20 mesh; visc. 2400-3000 cps (1% aq.); pH 6-7 (1% aq.).

Cellosize® HEC WP Grades. [Amerchol] Hydroxyethylcellulose; CAS 9004-62-0; water-sol. polymers for use as thickeners in hair conditioners, shampoos, lotions and creams, binder in powds., mascara, eyeliner; suspending aid.

Cellosize® Polymer PCG-10. [Amerchol] Hydroxyethylcellulose; CAS 9004-62-0; water-sol. polymers for use as thickeners in hair conditioners, shampoos, lotions and creams, binder in powds., mascara, eyeliner; suspending aid; wh. powd., mild odor; 98% min. thru 20 mesh; visc. 4400-6000 cps (1% aq.); pH 6-7 (1% aq.).

Cellosolve®. [Union Carbide] Ethoxyethanol; CAS 110-80-5; EINECS 203-804-1; solvent.

Cellosolve® Acetate. [Union Carbide] Ethoxyethanol acetate; CAS 111-15-9; EINECS 203-839-2; solvent.

Cellow 940. [Lowenstein] Cellulose-based polymer; visc. builder and film-former for semipermanent hair colors and shampoos.

Celluflow C-25. [Presperse] Cellulose; CAS 9004-34-6; EINECS 232-674-9; cosmetic ingred. with exc. oil absorbancy, moisture retention, high lubricity for powds., emulsions and anhyd. systems; JSCI/JCID approved; wh. to lt. gray fine powd., essentially odorless; particle size 8-10 μ; oil absorp. 91 ml/100 g; bulk dens. 0.6 g/cc; pH 5.0-7.5.

Celluflow TA-25. [Presperse] Cellulose triacetate; CAS 9004-35-7; cosmetic ingred. with exc. oil absorbancy, moisture retention, high lubricity for powds., emulsions and anhyd. systems; JSCI/JCID approved; wh. fine powd., essentially odorless; particle size 6-8 μ; oil absorp. 150 ml/100 g; bulk dens. 0.3 g/cc; pH 6-8.

Cellulase 4000. [Solvay Enzymes] Fungal cellulase derived from *Aspergillus niger*, standardized with lactose; CAS 9012-54-8; EINECS 232-734-4; enzyme for pharmaceuticals (aids digestion of cellulosics), animal feeds, brewing, fruit juices, essential oils and spices, paper and other waste treatment; wh. to lt. tan powd., free of offensive odor and taste; water-sol.; usage level: 0.1-1.0%.

Cellulase Tr Conc. [Solvay Enzymes] Cellulase derived from *Trichoderma reesei*; CAS 9012-54-8; EINECS 232-734-4; enzyme for pharmaceuticals (aids digestion of cellulosics), animal feeds, brewing, fruit juices, essential oils and spices, paper and other waste treatment; lt. tan to wh. powd., free of offensive odor and taste; water-sol.; usage level: 0.1-1.0%.

Cellulinol. [Prod'Hyg] TEA-salicylate, PEG-6, and propylene glycol.

Cellulon. [Weyerhaeuser] Cellulose; CAS 9004-34-6; EINECS 232-674-9; binder, diluent, disintegrant, stabilizer.

Celquat® H-100. [Nat'l. Starch] Polyquaternium-4; cationic; substantive polymer providing gloss and antistat props. to setting lotions, cream rinses, mousses, shampoos, conditioning soaps, skin lotions and creams; tan gran. powd.; sol. in water; visc. 1000 cps (2% aq.); pH 7.2 (2% aq.); 5% volatiles.

Celquat® L-200. [Nat'l. Starch] Polyquaternium-4; cationic; substantive polymer providing gloss and antistat props. to setting lotions, cream rinses, mousses, shampoos, conditioning soaps, skin lotions and creams; tan gran. powd.; sol. in water; visc. 100 cps (2% aq.); pH 7.0 (2% aq.); 5% volatiles.

Celquat® SC-230M. [Nat'l. Starch] Polyquaternium-10; cationic; conditioning polymer imparting lubricity and richness to skin and hair care prods. (shampoos, conditioners, gels, setting lotions, cream rinses, mousses, liq. soaps, skin lotions and creams); tan gran. powd.; readily disp. and sol. in water; insol. in ethanol, IPA; visc. 1500 cps (1% aq.); pH 7 (2% aq.).

Celquat® SC-240. [Nat'l. Starch] Polyquaternium-10; cationic; substantive polymer providing gloss and antistat props. to setting lotions, cream rinses, mousses, shampoos, conditioning soaps, skin lotions and creams; more compat. with anionics; tan gran. powd.; sol. in water; insol. in ethanol, IPA; visc. 400 cps (2% aq.); pH 7.0 (2% aq.); 5% volatiles.

Celquat® SC-240C, 28-6804. [Nat'l. Starch] Polyquaternium-10; conditioner.

Centella Phytosome®. [Indena SpA; Lipo] Complex of centella (hydrocotyl), triterpenes, and soybean phospholipids; skin protectant with moisturizing, smoothing, elasticizing, firming, eutrophic functionality; coadjuvant in external treatment of cellulitis, preps. for aging skin, aftersun prods., dentifrices for sensitive gums, prods. for oral cavity; ylsh.-brn. amorphous powd.; water-disp.; usage level: to 3%.

Centex. [Central Soya] Soy flour; CAS 68513-95-1.

Centrolene® A, S. [Central Soya] Hydroxylated lecithin; CAS 8029-76-3; EINECS 232-440-6; amphoteric; o/w emulsifiers, increased hydrophilic props. for cosmetic applics. incl. hair care; Gardner 11 and 12 resp. heavy-bodied fluid; acid no. 27; 100% conc.

Centrolex® F. [Central Soya] Special grade lecithin; CAS 8002-43-5; EINECS 232-307-2; crystallization control for pharmaceutical suppositories; emulsifier, emollient, pigment dispersant for cosmetics, eyeshadow; antistat adding body and feel to shampoos; yel. powd.; bulk dens. 0.45 g/cc; acid no. 27.

Centrolex® P. [Central Soya] Special grade lecithin; CAS 8002-43-5; EINECS 232-307-2; pigment dispersant for nonaq. cosmetics, coatings, magnetic media; emulsifier and suspending agent for pharmaceuticals; can be easily sterilized and filtered in solvs.; yel. gran.; bulk dens. 0.38 g/cc; acid no. 27.

Centromix® CPS. [Central Soya] Lecithin, polysorbate 80; CAS 8002-43-5; amphoteric; o/w emulsifier; amber fluid; visc. 8500 cP; acid no. 23.

Centromix® E. [Central Soya] Lecithin, ethoxylated mono-diglycerides, propylene glycol; CAS 8002-43-5; EINECS 232-307-2; amphoteric; emulsifier; amber fluid; visc. 6500 cP; acid no. 17.

Centrophase® C. [Central Soya] Special grade lecithin; CAS 8002-43-5; EINECS 232-307-2; amphoteric; wetting agent for lipstick and eyeliner; amber fluid; visc. 1000 cP; acid no. 27.

Centrophase® HR. [Central Soya] Lecithin; CAS 8002-43-5; EINECS 232-307-2; amphoteric; heat resistant multi-functional ingredient; pigment dispersant for aq.-based cosmetics; food substance; lubricant and release agent for heated surfaces; Gardner 13 amber fluid; sol. in liq. veg. and min oil, aliphatic, aromatic and halogenated hydrocarbons, petroleum ether; dens. 1.01 g/cc; visc. 2000 cP; pour pt. 32 F; 52% acetone insol.

Centrophase® HR6B. [Central Soya] Special grade lecithin; CAS 8002-43-5; EINECS 232-307-2; amphoteric; wetting agents; amber fluid; visc. 2500 cP; acid no. 23.

Centrophil® W. [Central Soya] Special grade lecithin; CAS 8002-43-5; EINECS 232-307-2; amphoteric; crystalliza-tion control aid for lipsticks.

Cephalipin. [Pentapharm Ltd; Centerchem] Wheat germ oil and disodium cocoamphodiacetate.

Cephene™. [Rhone-Poulenc Surf. & Spec.] Phenoxy-ethanol; CAS 122-99-6; EINECS 204-589-7; perfume fixative.

Cequartyl™ A. [Rhone-Poulenc Surf. & Spec.] Benzalko-nium chloride; cosmetic ingredient.

Cera-E. [Koster Keunen] Emulsifying wax NF; CAS 97069-99-0; emulsifier and thickener for creams, lotions, sham-poos, conditioners, and makeup; pastilles.

Cera Albalate 101. [Koster Keunen] Behenyl beeswax; CAS 144514-52-3; moisturizer, emollient, gellant producing stable gels with silicone oils for soft feel and lubricity on skin, high spreadability and water repellency; for creams, lotions, makeup, anhyd. gels/lipsticks; usage level: 1-15%.

Cera Albalate 102. [Koster Keunen] Isostearyl behenyl beeswax; CAS 144514-53-4; moisturizer, emollient, gel-lant producing stable gels with silicone oils for soft feel and lubricity on skin, high spreadability and water repellency; for creams, lotions, makeup, anhyd. gels/lipsticks; usage level: 1-15%.

Cera Albalate 103. [Koster Keunen] Hexanediol behenyl beeswax; CAS 144514-54-5; moisturizer, emollient, gel-lant producing stable gels with silicone oils for soft feel and lubricity on skin, high spreadability and water repellency; for creams, lotions, makeup, anhyd. gels/lipsticks; amor-phous solid; m.p. 66-71 C; acid no. < 2; sapon. no. 80-90; usage level: 1-15%.

Cera Albalate 104. [Koster Keunen] Hexanetriol beeswax and behenyl beeswax.

Cera Bellina®. [Koster Keunen] Polyglyceryl-3 beeswax; CAS 136097-93-3; oil gellant, emulsion stabilizer, consis-tency regulator, crystallization inhibitor, pigment disper-sant, thickener, and wetting agent for cosmetic emul-sions, oil gel prods., and decorative cosmetics; gran.; m.p. 63-73 C; acid no. < 1.0; iodine no. 7-11; toxicology: nontoxic; very sl. eye irritant, nonirritating to skin.

Ceraderm S. [Lipoid KG] Brain extract; CAS 90989-78-9.

Cera Euphorbia. [Koster Keunen] Cetearyl candelillate; CAS 138724-54-6; gellant, emollient, stabilizer.

Ceral 10. [Fabriquimica] Cetearyl alcohol, sodium lauryl

sulfate; anionic; self-emulsifying wax BP; emulsifier and thickener for cosmetic emulsions; acid no. < 1; iodine no. < 1; sapon. no. < 1.

Ceral 165. [Fabriquimica] Glyceryl stearate, PEG-100 stear-ate; nonionic; self-emulsifying emulsifier and emollient for cosmetic formulations; acid no. < 6; iodine no. < 2; sapon. no. 90-100.

Ceral CK. [Fabriquimica] Glyceryl stearate SE; anionic; self-emulsifying emulsifier and emollient for cosmetic formula-tions; acid no. 6-10; iodine no. < 3; sapon. no. 150-165.

Ceral EF. [Fabriquimica] Cetearyl alcohol, sodium lauryl sulfate, and ceteareth-20.

Ceral EFN. [Fabriquimica] Cetearyl alcohol, PEG-40 castor oil, and sodium lauryl sulfate; self-emulsifying wax; emul-sifier and thickener for cosmetic emulsions.

Ceral EN 6. [Fabriquimica] Cetearyl alcohol and ceteareth-20; nonionic; Cetomacrogol self-emulsifying wax; emulsi-fier and thickener for cosmetic emulsions; acid no. < 1; iodine no. < 1; sapon. no. < 1.

Ceral G. [Fabriquimica] Stearyl alcohol and ceteareth-20; nonionic; self-emulsifying wax; emulsifier and thickener for cosmetic emulsions; acid no. < 1; iodine no. < 2; sapon. no. < 2.

Ceral LE. [Fabriquimica] Glyceryl stearate and sodium lauryl sulfate; anionic; self-emulsifying emulsifier and emollient for cosmetic formulations; acid no. < 7; iodine no. < 3; sapon. no. 150-160.

Ceral MA. [Fabriquimica] Glyceryl stearate SE; nonionic; self-emulsifying emulsifier and emollient for cosmetic formulations; acid no. < 6; iodine no. < 2; sapon. no. 155-165.

Ceral ME. [Fabriquimica] Glyceryl stearate SE; anionic; self-emulsifying emulsifier and emollient for cosmetic formula-tions; acid no. < 6; iodine no. < 2; sapon. no. 150-160.

Ceral MET. [Fabriquimica] Glyceryl stearate SE; anionic; self-emulsifying emulsifier and emollient for cosmetic formulations; acid no. 16-20; iodine no. < 3; sapon. no. 148-158.

Ceral MEX. [Fabriquimica] Glyceryl stearate SE; anionic; self-emulsifying emulsifier and emollient for cosmetic formulations; acid no. < 10; iodine no. < 3; sapon. no. 150-160.

Ceral ML. [Fabriquimica] Glyceryl stearate and PEG-40 stearate; nonionic; self-emulsifying emulsifier and emol-lient for cosmetic formulations; acid no. < 4; iodine no. < 3; sapon. no. 90-110.

Ceral MN. [Fabriquimica] Glyceryl stearate; emulsifier and emollient for cosmetic formulations; acid no. < 6; iodine no. < 3; sapon. no. 160-175.

Ceral MNT. [Fabriquimica] Glyceryl stearate; emulsifier and emollient for cosmetic formulations; acid no. 16-20; iodine no. < 3; sapon. no. 166-176.

Ceral MNX. [Fabriquimica] Glyceryl stearate; emulsifier and emollient for cosmetic formulations; acid no. < 6; iodine no. < 3; sapon. no. 160-175.

Ceral P. [Fabriquimica] Propylene glycol stearate; CAS 1323-39-3; EINECS 215-354-3; thickener, emulsifier, coemulsifier, and emollient for cosmetics; acid no. < 6; iodine no. < 3; sapon. no. 145-160.

Ceral PA. [Fabriquimica] Propylene glycol stearate SE; thickener, emulsifier, coemulsifier, and emollient for cos-metics; acid no. < 6; iodine no. < 3; sapon. no. 140-155.

Ceral PW. [Fabriquimica] Cetearyl alcohol and ceteareth-20; nonionic; emulsifying wax NF; emulsifier and thickener for cosmetic emulsions; acid no. < 2; iodine no. < 3; sapon. no. 8-20.

Ceral TG. [Fabriquimica] Glyceryl stearate SE; cationic; emulsifier and emollient for cosmetic formulations; acid no. < 6; iodine no. < 3; sapon. no. 150-160.

Ceral TK. [Fabriquimica] Glyceryl stearate and potassium stearate.

Ceral TN. [Fabriquimica] Glyceryl stearate SE; cationic; self-emulsifying emulsifier and emollient for cosmetic formulations; acid no. 32-36; iodine no. < 4; sapon. no. 145-160.

Ceral TP. [Fabriquimica] Propylene glycol stearate SE; thickener, emulsifier, coemulsifier, and emollient for cosmetics; acid no. 16-20; iodine no. < 3; sapon. no. 150-170.

Ceralan® . [Amerchol] Lanolin alcohol; CAS 8027-33-6; EINECS 232-430-1; nonionic; emollient; w/o emulsifier; amber waxy solid, mild char. odor; m.p. 45-60 C; acid no. 3 max.; iodine no. 40-60; sapon. no. 10 max.; hyd. no. 150-175; 100% conc.

Ceramax. [Quest Int'l.] Phospholipids.

Ceram Blanche. [Kawasaki Steel] Boron nitride; CAS 10043-11-5; EINECS 233-136-6.

Ceramide HO3. [Sederma] Trihydroxypalmitamido-hydroxypropyl myristyl ether; epidermal restorer, cell cohesion factor, cutaneous barrier restructurer; reduces dry flaking skin, imparts smoothness, firmness, and moisture retention, and increases formula's affinity to skin; for face, body, sun, and makeup care prods.; off-wh. fine powd., char. odor; m.p. 97-100 C; usage level: 0.5-1%; > 98% purity.

Ceramide II. [Quest Int'l.] Palmitamidohexadecanediol; CAS 129426-19-3.

Ceramides. [Laboratoires Sérobiologiques] Glycero-ceramides; ceramide enriching and reinforcing activity in the superficial epidermal skin layers; for prods. for dry, rough, and sensitive skin, anti-aging, sun care, and hair care; lt. beige powd.; lipo-disp.; usage level: 0.3-1%.

Ceramides LS. [Laboratoires Sérobiologiques] Glyco-sphingolipids, phospholipids, and cholesterol.

Ceranine HCA. [Sandoz] Acetate version of Chemical 39 Base; cationic; emulsifier for skin care prods., softener for laundry/textiles; cream-colored gran.; slight odor; disp. in water; m.p. 71–81 C; 100% act.

Ceranine PN Base. [Sandoz] cationic; emulsifier/conditioner for skin and hair care prods. conferring softening, lubricating and antistatic props.

Ceraphyl® 28. [ISP Van Dyk] Cetyl lactate; CAS 35274-05-6; EINECS 252-478-7; lubricant and emollient for cosmetics and pharmaceuticals; binder for pressed powds.; imparts sheen and silkiness to skin and hair; reduces tack in deodorant sticks; solvent for dyes in lipstick formulas; wh. solid, faint char. odor; sol. @ 5% in min. oil, peanut oil, IPM, oleyl alcohol, and 95% ethanol; partly sol. in water, propylene glycol; sp.gr. 0.893-0.905; HLB 13-15; acid no. 2 max.; sapon. no. 174-189; toxicology: LD50 (oral, rat) > 20 ml/kg; nonirritating to eyes and skin.

Ceraphyl® 31. [ISP Van Dyk] Lauryl lactate; CAS 6283-92-7; EINECS 228-504-8; emollient, skin lubricant, slip agent, binder for pressed powds., lipsticks, hair prods.; also antitack agent in antiperspirants; lt. yel. liq., faint char. odor; sol. in min. oil, peanut oil, 95% ethanol, propylene glycol, and IPM; partly sol. in 70% sorbitol; sp.gr. 0.910-0.922; HLB 10; acid no. 2 max.; sapon. no. 210-225; ref. index 1.4417-1.4456; toxicology: LD50 (oral, rat) > 2 ml/kg; nonirritating to eyes; mild skin irritant.

Ceraphyl® 41. [ISP Van Dyk] C12-15 alkyl lactate; nongreasy emollient for alcoholic and hydroalcoholic skin preps.; reduces tacky, greasy feel in formulations high in petrolatum or min. oil; plasticizer for hair sparys contributing sheen on hair; antitack in antiperspirants; clear to lt. yel. liq.; sol. in aerosol propellants, min. oil, 60% ethanol, propylene glycol, IPM, oleyl alcohol, methylene chloride; partly sol. in water, glycerin; sp.gr. 0.900-0.920; HLB 14; acid no. 2 max.; sapon. no. 195-210; ref. index 1.4430-1.4450; toxicology: LD50 (oral, rat) 21 ± 9.2 ml/kg; moderate eye and skin irritant.

Ceraphyl® 45. [ISP Van Dyk] Dioctyl malate; CAS 56235-92-

8; binder, emollient for cosmetic and hypoallergenic prods.; nongreasy skin feel; fragrance coupler; solubilizer for oxybenzone and other difficult-to-solubilize materials; antitack in carbomer formulations, antiperspirants; hair conditioner; produces clear emollient gels; colorless to pale yel. clear liq., char. mild odor; sol. @ 5% in cyclomethicone, min. oil, IPM, ethanol, dimethicone, hexylene glycol; disp. in propylene glycol; insol. in water; m.w. 358.52; sp.gr. 0.960-0.970; HLB 12; acid no. 5 max.; iodine no. 1 max.; sapon. no. 310 min.; ref. index 1.4480-1.4520; toxicology: LD50 (oral, rat) > 5 g/kg; nonirritating to eyes; not a primary skin irritant; noncomedogenic.

Ceraphyl® 50. [ISP Van Dyk] Myristyl lactate; CAS 1323-03-1; EINECS 215-350-1; lubricant, emollient for skin prods., alcoholic preps., shaving lotions, colognes, makeup, medicated prods., lipsticks; provides soft, silky, water-resist. film on the skin, manageability to hair; water-wh. to pale yel. liq. to soft solid; sol. in peanut oil, min. oil, ethanol, propylene glycol, IPM, oleyl alcohol; partly sol. in 70% sorbitol; insol. in water; sp.gr. 0.892–0.904; HLB 12; acid no. 2 max.; sapon. no. 166–181; toxicology: LD50 (oral, rat) 20 ml/kg; nonirritating to skin.

Ceraphyl® 55. [ISP Van Dyk] Tridecyl neopentanoate; CAS 106436-39-9; emollient for creams and lotions, binder for pressed powds.; imparts nonoily, nonocclusive lubricity and elegant skin feel; improves gloss and spreading in pigmented prods.; lt. yel. clear liq., char. mild odor; sol. @ 5% in corn oil, 95% ethanol, min. oil, IPM, cyclomethicone; insol. in water; m.w. 284; sp.gr. 0.850-0.860; acid no. 2 max.; sapon. no. 190 min.; ref. index 1.4345-1.4365; toxicology: LD50 (oral, rat) > 5 g/kg; minimally irritating to eyes; mildly irritating to skin; noncomedogenic.

Ceraphyl® 60. [ISP Van Dyk] Quaternium-22; CAS 51812-80-7; EINECS 257-440-3; cationic; patented conditioner, emollient, moisturizer, humectant, antistat; highly substantive to skin and hair; imparts rich emollient skin feel in hydroalcoholic sol'ns.; does not impede foaming in shampoo and bubble bath formulas; lt. amber clear liq.; sol. @ 5% in water, 70% ethanol, glycerin, propylene glycol, 70% sorbitol; insol. in min. oil, IPM, 95% ethanol; sp.gr. 1.170-1.210; pH 4.0-5.0; toxicology: LD50 (oral, rat, 6%) > 64 cc/kg; nonirritating to eyes and skin; nonsensitizing; 58-62% solids in water.

Ceraphyl® 65. [ISP Van Dyk] Quaternium-26; CAS 68953-64-0; EINECS 273-222-0; cationic; patented hair conditioner; mild foaming aux. emulsifier with antistatic, antitangle properties for shampoos, rinses and other hair prods.; substantive emollient and emulsifier in skin care prods.; amber clear liq.; sol. @ 5% in water, 70% ethanol, glycerin, propylene glycol; insol. in min. oil, IPM; acid no. 20 max.; alkali no. 25 max.; toxicology: LD50 (oral, rat, 3% aq.) > 20 ml/kg; mild eye irritant; nonirritating to skin; noncomedogenic; 53-63% solids.

Ceraphyl® 70. [ISP Van Dyk] Quaternium-70, propylene glycol; CAS 68921-83-5; patented antitangle, antistatic ingred. used in all types of hair conditioners; aux. emulsifier and substantive emollient for skin creams and lotions; amber soft gel; water-disp.; m.p. 27-32 C; alkali no. 5 max.; sapon. no. 45-60; usage level: 0.5-4%; toxicology: LD50 (oral, rat) > 5 g/kg; mild eye irritant, sl. skin irritant; 48-58% total solids.

Ceraphyl® 85. [ISP Van Dyk] Stearamidopropyl cetearyl dimonium tosylate, propylene glycol; CAS 87616-36-2; cationic; patented hair conditioner; mild foaming aux. emulsifier with antistatic, antitangle properties for shampoos, rinses and other hair prods.; imparts smoothing and emolliency to skin care prods.; also for liq. soap, makeup, emulsions; very low eye irritation; cream-colored waxy solid; sol. @ 5% in oleyl alcohol, ethanol; disp. in water, propylene glycol, glycerin, castor oil; insol. in min. oil; m.p.

44-48 C; acid no. 12 max.; alkali no. 5 max.; sapon. no. 20 max.; toxicology: LD50 (oral, rat) > 5 g/kg; nonirritating to eyes; mild skin irritant; nonsensitizing; 60% act.

Ceraphyl® 140. [ISP Van Dyk] Decyl oleate; CAS 59231-34-4; nonionic; emollient, cosolv., slip agent, lubricant for creams, lotions, moisturizers, skin care prods., bath oils, liq. makeup; binder for pressed powds.; pigment dispersant; wh. to straw-colored liq., char. mild odor; sol. @ 5% in peanut oil, 95% ethanol, IPM, oleyl alcohol; insol. in water; sp.gr. 0.858-0.864; acid no. 5 max.; iodine no. 55-65; sapon. no. 130-145; ref. index 1.4540-1.4560; toxicology: LD50 (oral, rat) > 40 ml/kg; sl. eye irritant; very sl. skin irritant; nonsensitizing; 100% act.

Ceraphyl® 140-A. [ISP Van Dyk] Isodecyl oleate; CAS 59231-34-4; EINECS 261-673-6; nonionic; emollient, cosolv., and solubilizer for cosmetic systems, liq. makeup; binder for pressed powd.; wetting agent for iron oxides; cleansing agent for emulsions; lighter, drier skin feel than Ceraphyl 140; wh. to straw-colored liq., char. mild odor; sol. @ 5% in peanut oil, 95% ethanol, IPM, oleyl alcohol; insol. in water; sp.gr. 0.858-0.864; acid no. 5 max.; iodine no. 50-65; sapon. no. 130-145; ref. index 1.4540-1.4560; toxicology: LD50 (oral, rat) > 40 ml/kg; nonirritating to eyes; mild skin irritant; nonsensitizing; 100% act.

Ceraphyl® 230. [ISP Van Dyk] Diisopropyl adipate; CAS 6938-94-9; EINECS 248-299-9; emollient, coupler for aq. alcoholic systems, shave lotions, hair tonics; imparts spreadability to bath oils, hair pomades; reduces oiliness of min. oil prods.; fragrance solubilizer; plasticizer in hair sprays; colorless clear liq.; sol. @ 5% in min. oil, 50% ethanol, propylene glycol, IPM, oleyl alcohol, 70% sorbitol; water-insol.; sp.gr. 0.950-0.962; acid no. 2 max.; sapon. no. 465-500; ref. index 1.4216-1.4245; toxicology: LD50 (oral, rat) > 20 ± 3 ml/kg; nonirritatng to eyes and skin.

Ceraphyl® 368. [ISP Van Dyk] Octyl palmitate; CAS 29806-73-3; EINECS 249-862-1; nonoily, nonocclusive emollient for sunscreens, emulsions, aerosol antiperspirants, bath oils, liq. makeup; binder for pressed powds., blushers; gloss agent in lipsticks; antitack for antiperspirants; solubilizer for benzophenone-3; water-wh. liq.; sol. @ 5% in min. oil, 95% ethanol, IPM, peanut oil, oleyl alcohol; insol. in water; sp.gr. 0.850-0.856; acid no. 3 max.; sapon. no. 146-156; ref. index 1.4445-1.4465; toxicology: LD50 (oral, rat) > 40 ml/kg; nonirritating to eyes; mild primary skin irritant; nonsensitizing.

Ceraphyl® 375. [ISP Van Dyk] Isostearyl neopentanoate; CAS 58958-60-4; EINECS 261-521-9; mild emollient; binder for pressed powds., blushers; pigment dispersant for eye makeup; improves spreading in highly pigmented prods.; gloss agent in lipsticks; antitack for antiperspirants; pale yel. clear liq.; sol. @ 5% in IPM, oleyl alcohol, 95% ethanol, peanut and min. oils; insol. in water; sp.gr. 0.850-0.870; acid no. 2 max.; sapon. no. 144-165; ref. index 1.4435-1.4475; toxicology: LD50 (oral, rat) > 40 ml/kg; nonirritating to eyes and skin.

Ceraphyl® 424. [ISP Van Dyk] Myristyl myristate; CAS 3234-85-3; EINECS 221-787-9; emollient imparting rich, velvety skin feel to cosmetic emulsions, creams, lotions, makeup; increases visc. of creams and lotions at low concs.; reduces watery feel of low-oil emulsions; melts at body temp.; wh. to sl. yel. waxy solid, bland char. odor; sol. @ 5% in peanut and min. oils, IPM, oleyl alcohol; insol. in water; m.p. 36-39 C; acid no. 3 max.; sapon. no. 120-130; toxicology: LD50 (oral, rat) 8.6 g/kg; minimally irritating to eyes; mild skin irritant; nonsensitizing.

Ceraphyl® 494. [ISP Van Dyk] Isocetyl stearate; CAS 25339-09-7; EINECS 246-868-6; emollient, lubricant for creams and lotions, skin care prods., bath oils, makeup; imparts soft, elegant, nonoily feel; wh. to lt. yel. liq., bland char.

odor; sol. @ 5% in peanut oil, 95% ethanol, IPM, oleyl alcohol; insol. in water; sp.gr. 0.845-0.865; HLB 8; acid no. 5 max.; sapon. no. 95-110; ref. index 1.446-1.456; toxicology: LD50 (oral, rabbit) > 5 g/kg; minimally irritating to eyes; nonirritating to skin.

Ceraphyl® 791. [ISP Van Dyk] Isocetyl stearoyl stearate; CAS 97338-28-8; pigment dispersant, emollient, lubricant, spreading agent for lipsticks, etc.; lt. to straw-colored liq., char. mild odor; sol. @ 5% in min. oil, IPP, IPM, oleyl alcohol, safflower oil; sp.gr. 0.865-0.885; acid no. 10 max.; sapon. no. 132-148; hyd. no. 15 max.; ref. index 1.4560-1.4590; usage level: 2-20%; toxicology: nonirritating, nonsensitizing.

Ceraphyl® 847. [ISP Van Dyk] Octyldodecyl stearoyl stearate; CAS 90052-75-8; EINECS 289-991-0; emollient imparting lubricity and a rich, long-lasting, cushioned feel to the skin; visc. stabilizer for soap-based systems; pigment dispersant and binder in makeup; reduces oily feel of other ingreds.; smooths applic. in lipsticks; lt. to straw-colored liq., char. mild odor; sol. in IPM, safflower oil, min. oil, oleyl alcohol, octyl palmitate; partly sol. in 95% ethanol, propylene glycol, 70% sorbitol; insol. in water; sp.gr. 0.860-0.880; HLB 6; acid no. 10 max.; sapon. no. 115-135; ref. index 1.447-1.467; toxicology: LD50 (oral, rat) > 20 g/kg; nonirritating to eyes and skin.

Ceraphyl® GA. [ISP Van Dyk] Maleated soybean oil; CAS 68648-66-8; emollient for creams and lotions; hair and skin conditioner; clear liq.; sol. in most org. solvs.; water-insol.

Ceraphyl® GA-D. [ISP Van Dyk] Maleated soybean oil, deodorized, 0.1% mixed tocopherols (antioxidant); CAS 68648-66-8; patented moisturizer and skin softener imparting a rich, nongreasy, nontacky, full-bodied, long-lasting feel to the skin; retains emolliency in soap-based systems; refatting agent in detergent systems; suitable for creams, lotions, water-resist. sunscreens, bath oils, nail treatments, hair prods.; amber-yel. visc. oily liq., mild char. odor; sol. @ 5% in dioctyl malate, castor oil, corn oil, IPM; insol. in water; acid no. 43-53; iodine no. 107 max.; sapon. no. 220-250; ref. index 1.4750-1.4850; toxicology: LD50 (oral, rat) > 5 g/kg; nonirritating to eyes; mildly irritating to skin; nonsensitizing, noncomedogenic; 100% act.

Ceraphyl® ICA. [ISP Van Dyk] Isocetyl alcohol; CAS 36311-34-9; EINECS 252-964-9; nongreasy emollient for creams and lotions, pigment dispersant, binder for pressed powds., hair and skin conditioner; reduces tack in deodorant sticks; solv. for lipstick dyes; carrier and extender for flavor and fragrances; ideal for oil-free cosmetics and high-pH applics.; colorless clear liq., low odor; sol. @ 5% in peanut and min. oils, 95% ethanol, IPM, oleyl alcohol, castor oil, cyclomethicone; insol. in water; m.w. 242; sp.gr. 0.830-0.840; HLB 12-14; acid no. 5 max.; iodine no. 10 max.; sapon. no. 10 max.; hyd. no. 195-230; toxicology: LD50 (oral, rat) > 5 g/kg; mild eye and skin irritant; noncomedogenic.

Ceraphyl® IPL. [ISP Van Dyk] Isopropyl linoleate; CAS 22882-95-7; EINECS 245-289-6; superfatting agent for skin, hair, and cleansing prods.; skin conditioner leaving luxurious afterfeel on skin; imparts luster and softness in hair care prods.; reduces dry afterfeel of liq. soap formulas.

Cerasynt® 303. [ISP Van Dyk] Diethylaminoethyl stearate; CAS 3179-81-5; EINECS 221-662-9; cationic; o/w emulsifier for hair care prods. when neutralized with certain acids; visc. builder in hair dyes; pharmaceutical emulsifier; dispersant, wetting agent; straw to amber liq. to semisolid, amine odor; sol. @ 5% in peanut oil, ethanol, IPM, oleyl alcohol; partly sol. in min. oil; gels in glycerin, 70% sorbitol; sp.gr. 0.860-0.880; acid no. 30-40; alkali no. 127-137; sapon. no. 150-160; pH 9.5-10.5 (3%); 100%

conc.

Cerasynt® 840. [ISP Van Dyk] PEG-20 stearate; CAS 9004-99-3; nonionic; hydrophilic emulsifier, visc. builder, stabilizer for o/w creams, lotions, medicated ointments; superfatting agent in shampoos; vehicle for stick prods. melting at body temp.; solid; sol. @ 5% in ethanol; partly sol. in propylene glycol; forms liq. disp. in glycerin, solid disp. in peanut oil, IPM; m.p. 39.5-42.5 C; acid no. 5 max.; iodine no. 0.25 max.; sapon. no. 40-50; 100% conc.

Cerasynt® 945. [ISP Van Dyk] Glyceryl stearate, laureth-23; nonionic; self-emulsifying acid-stable emulsifier, gellant, thickener for cosmetic/pharmaceutical creams and lotions, antiperspirants, depilatories, hair straighteners, cleansing creams; electrolyte tolerant; wh. to cream flakes; partly sol. @ 5% in water, oleyl alcohol; gels in peanut oil; insol. in ethanol, glycerin, propylene glycol, IPM; m.p. 53-55 C; HLB 7-8; acid no. 5 max.; iodine no. 0.5 max.; sapon. no. 142-152; 100% conc.

Cerasynt® D. [ISP Van Dyk] Stearamide MEA-stearate; CAS 14351-40-7; EINECS 238-310-5; nonionic; opacifier, thickener for liq. cream shampoos; aux. emulsifier in hydrocarbon aerosol systems such as shave creams; cream flakes; insol. in water; gels in peanut oil, min. oil, IPM; m.p. 76-82 C; acid no. 10-20; iodine no. 0.5 max.; sapon. no. 97-107; 100% conc.

Cerasynt® GMS. [ISP Van Dyk] Glyceryl stearate; nonionic; sec. o/w emulsifier for creams and lotions; visc. builder for emulsions; wh. to cream flakes; forms visc. disp. in peanut oil, min. oil; insol. in water, 95% ethanol, propylene glycol, IPM; m.p. 56–59 C; HLB 4.0; acid no. 3 max.; iodine no. 2 max.; sapon. no. 162–175; 100% conc.

Cerasynt® IP. [ISP Van Dyk] Glycol stearate and other ingreds.; CAS 111-60-4; EINECS 203-886-9; nonionic; emulsifier, opacifier and pearling agent for lotion shampoos and liq. soaps; minimal foam depression; wh. to cream flake; partly sol. in peanut oil; water-insol.; m.p. 56.5-58.5 C; HLB 3.0; acid no. 5 max.; iodine no. 0.5 max.; sapon. no. 174-184; toxicology: LD50 (oral, rat, 10% in corn oil) > 64 cc/kg; nonirritating to eyes and skin; 100% conc.

Cerasynt® LP. [ISP Van Dyk] Glycol stearate, sodium laureth sulfate, hexylene glycol; opacifier, pearlescent for cold-mix mafg. of shampoos, liq. soaps, and other surfactant prods.; wh. opaque pourable liq.; disp. in water; sp.gr. 1.0 ± 0.4; visc. < 5000 cps; pH 6.5 ± 0.5; usage level: 3-10%; toxicology: minimally irritating to eyes; mildly irritating to skin; 60-70% water.

Cerasynt® M. [ISP Van Dyk] Glycol stearate; CAS 111-60-4; EINECS 203-886-9; nonionic; opacifier, thickener, pearlescent for liq. and cream shampoos, liq. soaps; sec. emulsifier for cosmetics and pharmaceutical creams and lotions; wh. to cream waxy flakes, mild char. odor; partly sol. in peanut oil; insol. in water, min. oil, glycerin, propylene glycol; m.p. 56-60 C; HLB 3.0; acid no. 5 max.; iodine no. 0.5 max.; sapon. no. 185-195; 100% conc.

Cerasynt® MN. [ISP Van Dyk] Glycol stearate SE; CAS 86418-55-5; anionic; opacifier for liq. and cream shampoos; primary emulsifier in cosmetic and pharmaceutical creams and lotions; visc. builder for emulsions containing high percentage of water in aq. phase; wh. to cream flakes; forms liq. disp. in water; insol. in min. oil, ethanol, glycerin, propylene glycol, IPM; m.p. 57-60 C; acid no. 5 max.; iodine no. 0.5 max.; sapon. no. 181-191; 100% conc.

Cerasynt® PA. [ISP Van Dyk] Propylene glycol stearate; CAS 1323-39-3; EINECS 215-354-3; nonionic; opacifier for liq. and cream shampoos; sec. emulsifier for cosmetic lotions and soft creams, liq. and cream makeup; wh. to cream-colored flakes, bland char. odor; sol. @ 5% in peanut and min. oils, IPM, oleyl alcohol; water-insol.; m.p.

35-38 C; HLB 3.0; acid no. 5 max.; iodine no. 0.5 max.; sapon. no. 181-191; toxicology: LD50 (oral, rat) 25.8 g/kg; minimally irritating to eyes; non or mildly irritating to skin; 100% conc.

Cerasynt® Q. [ISP Van Dyk] Glyceryl stearate SE; anionic; emulsifier for soap o/w emulsions, creams and lotions; wh. to cream flakes; sol. @ 5% in oleyl alcohol, partly sol. in water (pH 9), veg. oil, propylene glycol, IPM, 70% ethanol; disp. in min. oil, glycerin, 70% sorbitol; m.p. 57-59 C; acid no. 10 max.; iodine no. 1 max.; sapon. no. 150-160; 100% conc.

Cerasynt® SD. [ISP Van Dyk] Glyceryl stearate; nonionic; aux. emulsifier in cosmetic/pharmaceutical o/w emulsions; opacifier/thickener for liq. and cream shampoos; exc. color, odor, and heat stability; wh. to cream-colored flakes, very mild char. odor; forms solid disp. @ 5% in peant and min. oils; insol. in water, 70% ethanol, glycerin, propylene glycol; m.p. 55-57.5 C; HLB 4.0; acid no. 2 max.; iodine no. 0.5 max.; sapon. no. 165-177; 100% conc.

Cerasynt® WM. [ISP Van Dyk] Glyceryl stearate, stearyl alcohol, and sodium lauryl sulfate; anionic; acid-stable emulsifier for o/w creams, lotions, ointments, antiperspirants; electrolyte tolerance and low pH stability; wh. to cream flakes; forms liq. disp. @ 5% in IPM, solid disp. in water, peanut and min. oils, oelyl alcohol, 70% sorbitol; insol. in ethanol, glycerin, propylene glycol; m.p. 55-57 C; acid no. 5 max.; iodine no. 0.5 max.; sapon. no. 140-150; 100% conc.

Ceresine Wax Cosmetic Stralpitz. [Strahl & Pitsch] Ceresin; CAS 8001-75-0; EINECS 232-290-1; wax for gelling and stabilizing cosmetics.

Ceresine Wax SP 84. [Strahl & Pitsch] Ceresin; CAS 8001-75-0; EINECS 232-290-1; wax for gelling and stabilizing cosmetics.

Cerex EL 150. [Auschem SpA] PEG-15 castor oil; CAS 61791-12-6; personal care surfactant.

Cerex EL 250. [Auschem SpA] PEG-25 castor oil; CAS 61791-12-6; nonionic; solubilizer for essential oils, vitamins, other actives; liq.; HLB 10.8.

Cerex EL 300. [Auschem SpA] PEG-30 castor oil; CAS 61791-12-6; nonionic; solubilizer for essential oils, vitamins, other actives; liq.; HLB 12.5.

Cerex EL 360. [Auschem SpA] PEG-36 castor oil; CAS 61791-12-6; nonionic; solubilizer for essential oils, vitamins, other actives; liq.; HLB 12.9.

Cerex EL 400. [Auschem SpA] PEG-40 castor oil; CAS 61791-12-6; nonionic; solubilizer for essential oils, vitamins, other actives; liq.; HLB 14.4.

Cerex EL 429. [Auschem SpA] PEG-9 ricnoleate; CAS 9004-97-1; nonionic; solubilizer for active ingreds.; liq.; HLB 11.4.

Cerex ELS 50. [Auschem SpA] PEG-5 hydrog. castor oil; CAS 61788-85-0; nonionic; w/o emulsifier for cosmetics and pharmaceuticals; liq.; HLB 4.9.

Cerex ELS 250. [Auschem SpA] PEG-25 hydrog. castor oil; CAS 61788-85-0; nonionic; solubilizer for cosmetic and pharmaceutical applics.; liq.; HLB 10.8.

Cerex ELS 400. [Auschem SpA] PEG-40 hydrog. castor oil; CAS 61788-85-0; nonionic; solubilizer for cosmetic and pharmaceutical applics.; liq.; HLB 14.0.

Cerex ELS 450. [Auschem SpA] PEG-45 hydrog. castor oil; CAS 61788-85-0; nonionic; solubilizer for cosmetic and pharmaceutical applics.; liq.; HLB 14.4.

Cerex U 60. [Auschem SpA] PEG-6 olive oil; CAS 103819-46-1; nonionic; solubilizer, emulsifier for cosmetics; liq.; HLB 10.0.

Cetacene. [Vevy] Acetylated glycol stearate.

Cetaffine. [Laserson SA] Cetyl alcohol; CAS 36653-82-4; EINECS 253-149-0; cosmetic ingred.

Cetal. [Amerchol] Cetyl alcohol NF; CAS 36653-82-4; EINECS 253-149-0; emollient used in emulsions, oils, and makeup; visc. control in emulsions; aux. emulsifier; wh. waxy solid; mild char. odor; m.p. 45–51 C; acid no. 1.0 max.; sapon. no. 2.0.

Cetalox AT. [Witco/H-I-P] Ethoxylated fatty alcohol; nonionic; nonfoaming detergent for personal care prods.; powd.; HLB 17.1.

Cetasal. [Gattefosse] Propylene glycol stearate, stearic acid, TEA-stearate, sulfated castor oil.

Cetats® . [Zeeland] Cetrimonium tosylate; CAS 138-32-9; EINECS 205-324-8.

Cetax 16. [Aquatec Quimica SA] Cetyl alcohol; CAS 36653-82-4; EINECS 253-149-0; emollient, consistency agent for creams and lotions; superfatting agent for hair prods.; base for ointments and creams; flakes; 100% conc.

Cetax 18. [Aquatec Quimica SA] Stearyl alcohol; CAS 112-92-5; EINECS 204-017-6; emollient, consistency agent for creams and lotions; superfatting agent for hair prods.; base for ointments and creams; flakes; 100% conc.

Cetax 50. [Aquatec Quimica SA] Cetyl/stearyl alcohol; CAS 8005-44-5; emollient, consistency agent for creams and lotions; superfatting agent for hair prods.; base for ointments and creams; flakes; 100% conc.

Cetax DR. [Aquatec Quimica SA] Glyceryl stearate and PEG-8 stearate; nonionic; emulsifier for cosmetics; flakes; 100% conc.

Cetax TP. [Aquatec Quimica SA] Stearic acid; CAS 57-11-4; EINECS 200-313-4; intermediate for mfg. of soaps, creams, and lotions; flakes; 100% conc.

Cetina. [Robeco] Cetyl esters and stearamide DEA; CAS 17661-50-6, 93-82-3; nonionic; emulsifying wax, lubricant, emollient providing satiny feel for cosmetic creams, lotions, sticks, and foams; lt. colored flake, bland odor and taste; m.p. 43-50 C; acid no. 0-5; alkali no. 28 max.; sapon. no. 85-100; pH 8.5-10.0 (1%); 100% conc.

Cetinol 1212. [Fabriquimica] Lauryl laurate; CAS 6283-92-7; EINECS 228-504-8; regreasing agent for cosmetic emulsions; acid no. 1; iodine no. 15-20; sapon. no. 115-135.

Cetinol EE. [Fabriquimica] Stearyl stearate; CAS 2778-96-3; EINECS 220-476-5; regreasing agent for cosmetic emulsions; acid no. < 2; iodine no. < 2; sapon. no. 90-105.

Cetinol LA. [Fabriquimica] Cetyl lactate; CAS 35274-05-6; EINECS 252-478-7; regreasing agent for cosmetic emulsions; acid no. < 3; iodine no. < 1; sapon. no. 140-165.

Cetinol LL. [Fabriquimica] Lauryl lactate; CAS 6283-92-7; EINECS 228-504-8; regreasing agent for cosmetic emulsions; acid no. < 3; iodine no. < 1; sapon. no. 170-200.

Cetinol LM. [Fabriquimica] Myristyl lactate; CAS 1323-03-1; EINECS 215-350-1; regreasing agent for cosmetic emulsions; acid no. < 3; iodine no. < 1; sapon. no. 150-170.

Cetinol LU. [Fabriquimica] Cetyl laurate; CAS 20834-06-4; EINECS 244-071-8; regreasing agent for cosmetic emulsions; acid no. < 2; iodine no. < 14; sapon. no. 95-110.

Cetinol MM. [Fabriquimica] Myristyl myristate; CAS 3234-85-3; EINECS 221-787-9; regreasing agent for cosmetic emulsions; acid no. < 1; iodine no. < 15; sapon. no. 100-115.

Cetiol® . [Henkel/Cospha; Henkel Canada; Henkel KGaA/Cospha] Oleyl oleate; CAS 3687-45-4; EINECS 222-980-4; emollient; oily component of strong greasy char., for cosmetic/pharmaceutical skin preps.; carrier for lipid sol. ingreds.; pale yel. clear oil; m.w. 530; sp.gr. 0.861-0.880; visc. 25-30 mPa·s; acid no. 1.0 max.; iodine no. 87-97; sapon. no. 100-110; hyd. no. 12 max.; cloud pt. < 10 C; ref. index 1.4640-1.4660.

Cetiol® 868. [Henkel/Cospha; Henkel Canada; Henkel KGaA/Cospha] Octyl stearate; CAS 91031-48-0; emollient; superfatting oil for o/w and w/o emulsions; for cosmetic/pharmaceutical skin care preps.; pale yel. clear oily liq.; m.w. 390; sp.gr. 0.855-0.865; visc. 14-16 mPa·s; acid no. 0.5 max.; iodine no. 2; sapon. no. 140-150; cloud pt. < 8 C; ref. index 1.447-1.450; 100% act.

Cetiol® 1414E. [Henkel/Cospha; Henkel Canada] Myreth-3-myristate; CAS 59686-68-9; self-emulsifying emollient; cosmetic preparations such as creams, lotions, lipsticks, and blooming bath oils; clear to cloudy liq.; sol. in alcohols, cosmetic oils, glycols, esters, ketones, and aromatics; water-disp.; acid no. 6 max.; sapon. no. 97.

Cetiol® A. [Henkel/Cospha; Henkel Canada; Henkel KGaA/Cospha] Hexyl laurate; CAS 34316-64-8; EINECS 251-932-1; vehicle for lipid-sol. topical act. ingreds. used in skin lubricants, cosmetics, and pharmaceuticals; mild emollient; good spreading props.; solubilizer for lipoid-sol. compds.; superfatting agent for alcoholic hair lotions, shampoos, toilet soap; esp. suitable for aerosols; colorless clear oily liq., odorless; sol. @ 10% in min. and castor oil, IPM, oleyl alcohol, ethyl alcohol-SD 40 (95%), silicone fluid; sp.gr. 0.857-0.861; visc. 6 mPa·s; solid. pt. < 0 C; HLB 12; acid no. 0.2 max.; iodine no. 1; sapon. no. 190-205; hyd. no. 2 max.; cloud pt. < 5 C; flash pt. > 165 C; ref. index 1.438-1.441; 100% act.

Cetiol® B. [Henkel/Cospha; Henkel Canada; Henkel KGaA/Cospha] Dibutyl adipate; CAS 105-99-7; EINECS 203-350-4; emollient; oily component for skin oils, massage oils, sun protection oils, bathing preps., day creams, liq. emulsions; good penetration on skin; solv. for lipoid-sol. substances; superfatting agent and plasticizer for hair sprays; colorless oily liq., faint intrinsic odor; sp.gr. 0.958-0.962; visc. 5-7 mPa·s; solid. pt. < -30 C; acid no. 0.5 max.; iodine no. 1 max.; sapon. no. 420-440; hyd. no. 1 max.; cloud pt. < -25 C; flash pt. 150 C min.; ref. index 1.434-1.437; 100% act.

Cetiol® G16S. [Henkel/Cospha; Henkel Canada] Isocetyl stearate; CAS 25339-09-7; EINECS 246-868-6; emollient, lubricant for cosmetic preparations; lipsticks; clear oily low visc. liq.; sol. in alcohol esters, min. oil; water-insol.; acid no. 1.0 max.; iodine no. 5 max.; sapon. no. 110.

Cetiol® HE. [Henkel/Cospha; Henkel Canada/Cospha] PEG-7 glyceryl cocoate; nonionic; emollient oil, superfatting agent for aq. formulations in personal care prods.; dispersant for biologically act. ingreds.; clear low visc. oil; sol. @ 10%: sol. in water, castor oil, oleyl and ethyl alcohol-SD 40 (95%), ethyl alcohol 3A (70% aq.); dens. 1.050 g/ml; solid. pt. 0 C; cloud pt. < 0 C; acid no. 5 max.; iodine no. 5 max.; sapon. no. 90–100; ref. index 1.460.

Cetiol® J600. [Henkel/Cospha; Henkel Canada; Henkel KGaA/Cospha] Oleyl erucate; CAS 17673-56-2; EINECS 241-654-9; emollient; fatty component for skin creams, liq. emulsions, decorative cosmetics, and hair preps.; jojoba oil substitute; stable to oxidation; pale yel. clear oily liq., very sl. odor; misc. with esters, alcohols, animal, veg., min. fat components; and sp.gr. 0.863-0.868; visc. 40-50 mPa·s; solid. pt. 15 C max.; acid no. 0.5 max.; iodine no. 92 max.; sapon. no. 90-100; hyd. no 10 max.; cloud pt. 20 C max.; ref. index 1.465-1.470; 100% act.

Cetiol® LC. [Henkel/Cospha; Henkel Canada; Henkel KGaA/Cospha] Coco-caprylate/caprate; very dry feeling, penetrating emollient used in personal care prods.; reduces oiliness in creams, lotions, and solid sticks; carrier for oil-sol. actives; superfatting agent for creams, liq. emulsions, bath preps., skin oils, pharmaceutical oils; sl. yel. clear oily liq., pract. odorless; sol. @ 10% in min. and castor oil, IPM, oleyl alcohol, silicone fluid; insol. in water; sp.gr. 0.855-0.860; visc. 9-12 mPa; solid. pt. < 13 C; HLB 9; acid no. 0.2 max.; iodine no. 1 max.; sapon. no. 165-173; hyd. no. 1 max.; cloud pt. 15 C max.; flash pt. > 180 C; ref. index 1.443-1.447.

Cetiol® MM. [Henkel/Cospha; Henkel Canada; Henkel KGaA/Cospha] Myristyl myristate; CAS 3234-85-3;

EINECS 221-787-9; emollient wax ester with superfatting properties; for skin care and decorative stick preps.; improves rub-in of creams; melts near body temp.; wh. waxy solid, faint char. odor; misc. with oils and waxes; m.p. 38-42 C; acid no. 1 max.; iodine no. 1 max.; sapon. no. 120-135; hyd. no. 7 max.

Cetiol® OE. [Henkel/Cospha; Henkel KGaA/Cospha] Dioctyl ether; CAS 629-82-3; dry feel emollient for lt. cosmetic/ pharmaceutical o/w and w/o emulsions; good spreading props.; resist. to hydrolysis; clear liq.; sp.gr. 0.80; visc. 4 mPa·s; acid no. 0.5 max.; sapon. no. 0.1 max.; hyd. no. 0.5 max.; ref. index 1.430.

Cetiol® R. [Henkel/Cospha; Henkel Canada] Trihydroxy methoxystearin; emollient; fatty oil for makeup preparations; castor oil substitute; clear to turbid liq.; acid no. 1 max.; iodine no. 15; sapon. no. 155-165; 100% act.

Cetiol® S. [Henkel/Cospha; Henkel Canada; Henkel KGaA/ Cospha] Dioctylcyclohexane; emollient, superfatting agent; used in cosmetic and pharmaceutical creams and emulsions; colorless clear liq., faint odor; sp.gr. 0.825-0.835; visc. 25 mPa·s; acid no. 0.2 max.; iodine no. 0.5 max.; sapon. no. 0.5 max.; cloud pt. 0 C max.; ref. index 1.455-1.465; 100% act.

Cetiol® SB45. [Henkel/Cospha; Henkel Canada; Henkel KGaA/Cospha] Shea butter; CAS 68424-60-2; emollient, consistency giving agent for o/w and w/o creams and emulsions, makeup; native fatting agent for creams, lotions, anhyd. creams; sun protection props.; sl. ylsh. soft wax; misc. with fatty components; sp.gr. 0.89-0.92; m.p. 42-45 C; acid no. 0.2 max.; iodine no. 70-75; sapon. no. 175-185; usage level: 1-20%; 9-13% unsaponifiables.

Cetiol® SN. [Henkel/Cospha; Henkel Canada; Henkel KGaA/ Cospha] Cetearyl isononanoate; emollient for applic. in skin care, massage and sun protection preparations; oily component with expressed hydrophobic effect; colorless to sl. yel. low visc. oily liq., faint intrinsic odor; sp.gr. 0.853-0.856; visc. 19-22 mPa·s; acid no. 0.2 max.; iodine no. 1 max.; sapon. no. 140-146; hyd. no. 1 max.; cloud pt. 15 C max.; ref. index 1.445-1.450.

Cetiol® T 1500. [Henkel/Cospha] Hydrog. castor oil laurate.

Cetiol® V. [Henkel/Cospha; Henkel Canada; Henkel KGaA/ Cospha] Decyl oleate; CAS 3687-46-5; EINECS 222-981-6; penetrating emollient, carrier for lipid sol. substances used in personal care prods. and pharmaceutical topical applics.; yel. low visc. oily liq.; sol. @ 10%: sol. in min. and castor oil, IPM, oleyl alcohol; insol. in water; dens. 0.86 g/ml; HLB 9; acid no. 1 max.; iodine no. 60; sapon. no. 130-140; solid. pt. < 0 C; flash pt. 240-260 C; cloud pt. < 10 C; ref. index 1.450.

Cetodan. [Grindsted Prods.] Acetylated monoglycerides; nonionic; food emulsifier, aerating agent for shortenings, toppings, cakes; edible coating; plasticizer for chewing gum base; antifoam agent, lubricant, aerator for cosmetic creams and lotions; grades with higher hydrog. levels as moisture barrier; solid, liq.; HLB 1.5; 100% conc.

Cetodan® 95 CO. [Grindsted Prods.] Acetylated palm kernel glycerides.

Cetol® . [Zeeland] Cetalkonium chloride; CAS 122-18-9; EINECS 204-526-3; germicide, surfactant.

Cetomacrogol 1000 BP. [Croda Inc.; Croda Chem. Ltd.] Ceteth-20 BP; CAS 9004-95-9; nonionic; pharmaceutical o/w emulsifier, solubilizer; wetting agent for stick formulations; for depilatories, antiperspirants, conditioning rinses; wh. to off-wh. solid; sol. in water, IPA, propylene glycol; m.w. 1000; HLB 15.7; usage level: 0.5-5%; toxicology: LD50 (oral, rat) 3.6 g/kg; moderate skin irritant, severe eye irritant; 100% conc.

Cetomil. [Fabriquimica] Cetomacrogol BP; nonionic; self-emulsifying wax; emulsifier and thickener for cosmetic emulsions; acid no. < 1; iodine no. < 1; sapon. no. < 1.

Cetostearyl Alcohol BP. [Croda Inc.] Cetearyl alcohol; forms dense cosmetic and pharmaceutical emulsions; thickener and coemulsifier/stabilizer for topical systems; wh. to cream flakes; sol. in min. oil, IPA; sol. warm in propylene glycol; m.p. 45-53 C; acid no. 0.5 max.; iodine no. 3 max.; sapon. no. 1 max.; hyd. no. 208-228; usage level: 2-30%; toxicology: LD50 (oral, rat) > 5 g/kg; mild skin and eye irritant.

Cetostearyl Alcohol NF. [Croda Inc.] Cetearyl alcohol; forms dense cosmetic/pharmaceutical emulsions; thickener and coemulsifier/stabilizer in topical systems; sol. in mi. oil, IPA; sol. warm in propylene glycol; usage level: 2-30%; toxicology: LD50 (oral, rat) > 5 g/kg; mild skin and eye irritant.

Cetrimide. [Zeeland] Cetrimonium bromide; CAS 57-09-0; EINECS 200-311-3; quat. for personal care prods.

Cetrimide BP. [Aceto] Cetyl trimethyl ammonium bromide; CAS 57-09-0; EINECS 200-311-3; antistat in hair conditioners; biocidal applics.; phase transfer catalysis; wh. free-flowing powd., faint char. odor, bitter soapy taste; sol. in alcohol, chloroform; m.w. 365; m.p. 100 C; toxicology: skin dermatitis; dust inhalation is irritating; 94-100% act.

Cetrimide™ BP. [Rhone-Poulenc Surf. & Spec.] Cetrimonium bromide; CAS 57-09-0; EINECS 200-311-3; bactericide and antiseptic for shampoos, liq. soaps, creams and lotions, bath gels, and bubble baths.

C-Flakes. [Karlshamns] Hydrog. cottonseed oil; CAS 68334-00-9; EINECS 269-804-9; lubricant for pharmaceutical tablets; Lovibond R2.5 max.; m.p. 142–146 F; iodine no. 5 max.; sapon. no. 189–198.

CG 10x (Unfiltered and stabilized). [R.I.T.A.] Aloe vera gel; moisturizer, soothing/healing aid for personal care.

Chamomile CL 2/033026. [Dragoco] Water, chamomile extract, PEG-40 hydrog. castor oil, and trideceth-9; botanical extract.

Chamomile Distillate 2/380930. [Dragoco] Water, chamomile extract, SD alcohol 39-C; botanical extract.

Chamomile Extract HS 2382 G. [Grau Aromatics] Propylene glycol and matricaria extract; botanical extract.

Chamomile Extract HS 2779 G. [Grau Aromatics] Propylene glycol and chamomile extract; botanical extract.

Chamomile Oil. [Provital; Centerchem] Sunflower seed oil and matricaria extract.

Chel DM-41. [Ciba-Geigy] Trisodium HEDTA; CAS 139-89-9; EINECS 205-381-9; chelating agent used in bar soaps, photographic developer baths, textiles, and min. separations; yel. clear sol'n.; 41% act.

Chel DTPA. [Ciba-Geigy] Pentetic acid; CAS 67-43-6; EINECS 200-652-8; chelating agent used for stabilizing peroxides, biological preparations, cosmetics, textiles, scale removal, and rare earth separations; wh. cryst. powd.; 98% act.

Chelon 100. [Rhone-Poulenc Basic] Tetrasodium EDTA; CAS 64-02-8; EINECS 200-573-9; chelating agent for heavy metal and alkaline earth ions; pale straw clear aq. sol'n.; sp.gr. 1.31; dens. 10.9 lb/gal; chel. value 102 mg CaCO₃/g (@ pH 11); pH 11.5 (1% aq.); 39% min. act.

Chemal BP 261. [Chemax] Poloxamer 181; CAS 9003-11-6; nonionic; defoamer, emulsifier, demulsifier, dispersant, binder, stabilizer, wetting agent, chemical intermediate; for metalworking, cosmetic, paper, textiles, dishwashing detergents, rinse aids, as lubricant bases; liq.; cloud pt. 24 C (1% aq.); HLB 3.0; 100% act.

Chemal BP-262. [Chemax] Poloxamer 182; CAS 9003-11-6; nonionic; defoamer, emulsifier, demulsifier, dispersant, binder, stabilizer, wetting agent, chemical intermediate; for metalworking, cosmetic, paper, textiles, dishwashing detergents, rinse aids, as lubricant bases; liq.; cloud pt. 30 C (1% aq.); HLB 7.0; 100% act.

Chemal BP-262LF. [Chemax] Difunctional block polymer

ending in primary hydroxyl groups; nonionic; defoamer, emulsifier, demulsifier, dispersant, binder, stabilizer, wetting agent, chemical intermediate; for metalworking, cosmetic, paper, textiles, dishwashing detergents, rinse aids, as lubricant bases; liq.; cloud pt. 28 C (1% aq.); HLB 6.5; 100% act.

Chemal BP-2101. [Chemax] Poloxamer 331; CAS 9003-11-6; nonionic; defoamer, emulsifier, demulsifier, dispersant, binder, stabilizer, wetting agent, chemical intermediate; for metalworking, cosmetic, paper, textiles, dishwashing detergents, rinse aids, as lubricant bases; liq.; cloud pt. 16 C (1% aq.); HLB 1.0; 100% act.

Chemal LA-4. [Chemax] Laureth-4; CAS 5274-68-0; EINECS 226-097-1; nonionic; o/w emulsifier, lubricant, detergent, dispersant, solubilizer, defoamer for cosmetic, household, silicone polish, and mold release prods.; liq.; hyd. no. 150–165; cloud pt. < 25 C (1% aq.); HLB 9.2; 100% conc.

Chemal LA-9. [Chemax] Laureth-9; CAS 3055-99-0; EINECS 221-284-4; nonionic; o/w emulsifier, lubricant, detergent, dispersant, solubilizer, defoamer for cosmetic, household, silicone polish, and mold release prods.; liq.; hyd. no. 90–110; cloud pt. 76 C (1% aq.); HLB 13.3; 100% conc.

Chemal LA-12. [Chemax] Laureth-12; CAS 3056-00-6; EINECS 221-286-5; nonionic; o/w emulsifier, lubricant, detergent, dispersant, solubilizer, defoamer for cosmetic, household, silicone polish, and mold release prods.; liq.; hyd. no. 72–87; 100% conc.

Chemal LA-23. [Chemax] Laureth-23; CAS 9002-92-0; nonionic; o/w emulsifier, lubricant, detergent, dispersant, solubilizer, defoamer for cosmetic, household, silicone polish, and mold release prods.; solid; hyd. no. 40–55; cloud pt. > 100 C (1% aq.); HLB 16.7; 100% conc.

Chemal OA-4. [Chemax] Oleth-4; CAS 9004-98-2; nonionic; dispersant, detergent; emulsifier and solubilizer for topical cosmetic applics.; stabilizer and anticoagulant for natural and syn. latices; emulsifier for waxes used in coating citrus fruit; liq.; cloud pt. < 25 C (1% aq.); HLB 7.9; 100% conc.

Chemal OA-5. [Chemax] Oleth-5; CAS 9004-98-2; nonionic; emulsifier, lubricant, and solubilizer; liq.; 100% conc.

Chemal OA-9. [Chemax] Oleth-9; CAS 9004-98-2; nonionic; dispersant, detergent; emulsifier and solubilizer for topical cosmetic applics.; stabilizer and anticoagulant for natural and syn. latices; emulsifier for waxes used in coating citrus fruit; liq.; cloud pt. 52 C (1% aq.); HLB 11.9; 100% conc.

Chemal OA-10. [Chemax] Oleth-10; CAS 9004-98-2; emulsifier, emollient.

Chemal OA-20. [Chemax] Oleth-20; CAS 9004-98-2; emulsifier.

Chemal OA-20/70CWS. [Chemax] Oleth-20; CAS 9004-98-2; nonionic; emulsifier, lubricant, solubilizer; liq.; cloud pt. > 100 C (1% aq.); HLB 15.3; 70% conc.

Chemal OA-20G. [Chemax] Oleth-20; CAS 9004-98-2; nonionic; dispersant, detergent; emulsifier and solubilizer for topical cosmetic applics.; stabilizer and anticoagulant for natural and syn. latices; emulsifier for waxes used in coating citrus fruit; lubricant; semisolid; cloud pt. > 100 C (1% aq.); HLB 15.3; 100% conc.

Chemal OA-23. [Chemax] Oleth-23; CAS 9004-98-2; emulsifier.

Chemal TDA-3. [Chemax] Trideceth-3; CAS 4403-12-7; EINECS 224-540-3; nonionic; wetting agent, detergent, emulsifier, dispersant, foam stabilizer; solubilizer, penetrant for scouring and dye leveling in textiles, in cleaning and dishwashing compds.; cosmetic and personal care applics.; liq.; cloud pt. < 25 C (1% aq.); HLB 7.9; 100% conc.

Chemal TDA-6. [Chemax] Trideceth-6; CAS 24938-91-8; nonionic; wetting agent, detergent, emulsifier, dispersant, foam stabilizer; solubilizer, penetrant for scouring and dye leveling in textiles, in cleaning and dishwashing compds.; cosmetic and personal care applics.; liq.; cloud pt. < 25 C (1% aq.); HLB 11.4; 100% conc.

Chemal TDA-9. [Chemax] Trideceth-9; CAS 24938-91-8; nonionic; wetting agent, detergent, emulsifier, dispersant, foam stabilizer; solubilizer, penetrant for scouring and dye leveling in textiles, in cleaning and dishwashing compds.; cosmetic and personal care applics.; liq.; cloud pt. 54 C (1% aq.); HLB 13.0; 100% conc.

Chemal TDA-12. [Chemax] Trideceth-12; CAS 24938-91-8; nonionic; wetting agent, detergent, emulsifier, dispersant, foam stabilizer; solubilizer, penetrant for scouring and dye leveling in textiles, in cleaning and dishwashing compds.; cosmetic and personal care applics.; paste; cloud pt. 70 C (1% aq.); HLB 14.5; 100% conc.

Chemal TDA-15. [Chemax] Trideceth-15; CAS 24938-91-8; nonionic; wetting agent, detergent, emulsifier, dispersant, foam stabilizer; solubilizer, penetrant for scouring and dye leveling in textiles, in cleaning and dishwashing compds.; cosmetic and personal care applics.; solid; 100% conc.

Chemal TDA-18. [Chemax] Trideceth-18; CAS 24938-91-8; nonionic; wetting agent, detergent, emulsifier, dispersant, foam stabilizer; solubilizer, penetrant for scouring and dye leveling in textiles, in cleaning and dishwashing compds.; cosmetic and personal care applics.; 100% conc.

Chemax CO-5. [Chemax] PEG-5 castor oil; CAS 61791-12-6; nonionic; emulsifier, lubricant for textiles, cosmetics; pigment dispersant in latex paints, paper; essential oils solubilizer; liq.; oil-sol.; sapon. no. 145; HLB 3.8; 100% conc.

Chemax CO-16. [Chemax] PEG-16 castor oil; CAS 61791-12-6; nonionic; emulsifier for fiber lubricants; cutting oils and hydraulic fluids; clay and pigment dispersant, rewetting agent, softener, dyeing assistant for paint, paper, textile, and leather industries; cosmetics; liq.; water-sol.; sapon. no. 100; HLB 8.6; 100% conc.

Chemax CO-25. [Chemax] PEG-25 castor oil; CAS 61791-12-6; nonionic; emulsifier for industrial lubricants; pigment dispersant in textiles, paint, paper, leather; liq.; sapon. no. 80; HLB 10.8.

Chemax CO-28. [Chemax] PEG-28 castor oil; CAS 61791-12-6; nonionic; emulsifier for industrial lubricants; pigment dispersant in textiles, paint, paper, leather; HLB 11.1.

Chemax CO-30. [Chemax] PEG-30 castor oil; CAS 61791-12-6; nonionic; emulsifier for industrial lubricants; pigment dispersant in textiles, paint, paper, leather; liq.; sapon. no. 73; HLB 11.7; 100% conc.

Chemax CO-36. [Chemax] PEG-36 castor oil; CAS 61791-12-6; nonionic; emulsifier for industrial lubricants; pigment dispersant in textiles, paint, paper, leather; liq.; sapon. no. 68; HLB 12.6.

Chemax CO-40. [Chemax] PEG-40 castor oil; CAS 61791-12-6; nonionic; emulsifier for industrial lubricants; pigment dispersant in textiles, paint, paper, leather; liq.; sapon. no. 61; HLB 12.9; 100% conc.

Chemax CO-80. [Chemax] PEG-80 castor oil; CAS 61791-12-6; nonionic; see Chemax CO-25; solid; sapon. no. 34; HLB 15.8; 100% conc.

Chemax CO-200/50. [Chemax] PEG-200 castor oil; CAS 61791-12-6; nonionic; see Chemax CO-25; liq.; sapon. no. 16; HLB 18.1; 50% conc.

Chemax/DOSS-75E. [Chemax] Dioctyl sodium sulfosuccinate; CAS 577-11-7; EINECS 209-406-4; anionic; wetting and rewetting agent, detergent, emulsifier for emulsion polymerization, cosmetics, textile, agric., detergent formulations; pigment dispersant in paints and inks; solubilizer for drycleaning solvs.; liq.; 75% conc.

Chemax E-200 ML. [Chemax] PEG-4 laurate; CAS 9004-81-3; nonionic; emulsifier for min. and cutting oils; dispersant, detergent, lubricant; coemulsifier and defoamer in water-based coatings; cosmetics ingred.; liq.; sapon. no. 135; HLB 9.3; 100% conc.

Chemax E-200 MO. [Chemax] PEG-5 oleate; CAS 9004-96-0; nonionic; emulsifier for min. and fatty oils, solv.; degreaser, dispersant, detergent, lubricant; metal, textile, cosmetic, plastisol formulations; liq.; oil-sol.; sapon. no. 118; HLB 8.3; 100% conc.

Chemax E-200 MS. [Chemax] PEG-5 stearate; CAS 9004-99-3; nonionic; emulsifier for min. oils and fats used in polishes and metal buffing compds.; dye assistant, lubricant, softener, antistat; for metal lubricants, textiles, cosmetic, plastisol formulations; soft solid; sapon. no. 112; HLB 8.5; 100% conc.

Chemax E-400 ML. [Chemax] PEG-8 laurate; CAS 9004-81-3; nonionic; emulsifier, dispersant, detergent, lubricant; visc. control agent in plastisol formulations; wetting agent and defoamer in latex paint; cosmetics ingred.; liq.; sapon. no. 90; HLB 13.2; 100% conc.

Chemax E-400 MO. [Chemax] PEG-9 oleate; CAS 9004-96-0; nonionic; emulsifier and lubricant for solv. and oils in pesticides and metal cleaners; detergent, dispersant; textile, cosmetics, plastisol formulations; liq.; sapon. no. 85; HLB 11.8; 100% conc.

Chemax E-400 MS. [Chemax] PEG-9 stearate; CAS 9004-99-3; nonionic; lubricant and softener for syn. fibers; dye assistant, antistat, emulsifier; for metal lubricants, textiles, cosmetics, plastisols; soft solid; sapon. no. 87; HLB 12.0; 100% conc.

Chemax E-400 MT. [Chemax] PEG-8 tallate; CAS 61791-00-2; personal care surfactant.

Chemax E-600 ML. [Chemax] PEG-14 laurate; CAS 9004-81-3; nonionic; emulsifier, dispersant, detergent, lubricant; metal, textile, cosmetics, plastisol formulations; liq.; water-sol.; sapon. no. 68; HLB 14.8; 100% conc.

Chemax E-600 MO. [Chemax] PEG-14 oleate; CAS 9004-96-0; nonionic; surfactant used as coemulsifier and lubricant in industrial formulations, cosmetics, metal lubricants, textiles, plastisols; dispersant, detergent; liq.; sapon. no. 65; HLB 13.6; 100% conc.

Chemax E-600 MS. [Chemax] PEG-14 stearate; CAS 9004-99-3; EINECS 233-641-1; nonionic; dye assistant, lubricant, softener, antistat, emulsifier for cosmetic and textile formulations; paste; sapon. no. 62; HLB 13.8; 100% conc.

Chemax E-1000 ML. [Chemax] PEG-20 laurate; CAS 9004-81-3; emulsifier.

Chemax E-1000 MO. [Chemax] PEG-20 oleate; CAS 9004-96-0; nonionic; emulsifier for min. and fatty oils, solv.; degreaser, dispersant, detergent, lubricant; solid; 100% conc.

Chemax E-1000 MS. [Chemax] PEG-20 stearate; CAS 9004-99-3; nonionic; emulsifier for cosmetic and textile formulations; dye assistant, lubricant, softener, antistat; soft solid; water-sol.; sapon. no. 43; HLB 15.7; 100% conc.

Chemax HCO-5. [Chemax] PEG-5 hydrog. castor oil; CAS 61788-85-0; nonionic; emulsifier, lubricant, softener, dispersant; coemulsifier for syn. esters; for cosmetics, plastics, metals, textiles, leather, paint, and paper indutries; liq.; oil-sol.; sapon. no. 142; HLB 3.8; 100% conc.

Chemax HCO-16. [Chemax] PEG-16 hydrog. castor oil; CAS 61788-85-0; nonionic; emulsifier, lubricant, dispersant, softener; for cosmetics, textiles, plastics, metalworking, paint, paper, leather; liq.; sapon. no. 100; HLB 8.6; 100% conc.

Chemax HCO-25. [Chemax] PEG-25 hydrog. castor oil; CAS 61788-85-0; nonionic; emulsifier, lubricant, and softener for cosmetics, plastics, metals, textiles, leather, paint, and paper industries; liq.; sapon. no. 80; HLB 10.8; 100% conc.

Chemax HCO-200/50. [Chemax] PEG-200 hydrog. castor oil; CAS 61788-85-0; nonionic; emulsifier and lubricant for cosmetics, plastics, metals, textiles, paint, paper, leather industries; liq.; water-sol.; sapon. no. 17; HLB 18.1; 50% act.

Chemax NP-1.5. [Chemax] Nonoxynol-1.5; CAS 9016-45-9; EINECS 248-291-5; nonionic; emulsifier, dispersant, detergent, wetting agent, solubilizer, coupler for cosmetics, textile, metalworking, household, industrial, agric., paper, paint, and other industries; liq.; pour pt. –3 F; cloud pt. < 25 C (1% aq.); HLB 4.6.

Chemax NP-4. [Chemax] Nonoxynol-4; CAS 9016-45-9; nonionic; emulsifier, dispersant, detergent, wetting agent, solubilizer, coupler for cosmetics, textile, metalworking, household, industrial, agric., paper, paint, and other industries; liq.; water oil sol.; pour pt. –15 F; cloud pt. < 25 C (1% aq.); HLB 8.9; 100% conc.

Chemax NP-6. [Chemax] Nonoxynol-6; CAS 9016-45-9; nonionic; emulsifier, dispersant, detergent, wetting agent, solubilizer, coupler for cosmetics, textile, metalworking, household, industrial, agric., paper, paint, and other industries; liq.; pour pt. –26 F; cloud pt. < 25 C (1% aq.); HLB 10.9; 100% conc.

Chemax NP-9. [Chemax] Nonoxynol-9; CAS 9016-45-9; nonionic; emulsifier, dispersant, detergent, wetting agent, solubilizer, coupler for cosmetics, textile, metalworking, household, industrial, agric., paper, paint, and other industries; liq.; pour pt. 31 F; cloud pt. 54 C (1% aq.); HLB 13.0; 100% conc.

Chemax NP-10. [Chemax] Nonoxynol-10; CAS 9016-45-9; EINECS 248-294-1; nonionic; emulsifier, dispersant, detergent, wetting agent, solubilizer, coupler for cosmetics, textile, metalworking, household, industrial, agric., paper, paint, and other industries; liq.; pour pt. 49 F; cloud pt. 72 C (1% aq.); HLB 13.5; 100% conc.

Chemax NP-15. [Chemax] Nonoxynol-15; CAS 9016-45-9; nonionic; surfactant, detergent, wetting and rewetting agent, emulsifier in cosmetics, textile, leather, paper, paint, and metal processing; paste; pour pt. 71 F; cloud pt. 96 C (1% aq.); HLB 15.0; 100% conc.

Chemax NP-20. [Chemax] Nonoxynol-20; CAS 9016-45-9; nonionic; see Chemax NP-15; solid; pour pt. 91 F; cloud pt. > 100 C (1% aq.); HLB 16.0.

Chemax NP-30. [Chemax] Nonoxynol-30; CAS 9016-45-9; nonionic; surfactant, detergent, wetting and rewetting agent, emulsifier in cosmetics, textile, leather, paper, paint, and metal processing; solid; pour pt. 109 F; cloud pt. > 100 C (1% aq.); HLB 17.1; 100% conc.

Chemax NP-30/70. [Chemax] Nonoxynol-30; CAS 9016-45-9; nonionic; see Chemax NP-15; liq.; pour pt. 34 F; cloud pt. > 100 C (1% aq.); HLB 17.1.

Chemax NP-40. [Chemax] Nonoxynol-40; CAS 9016-45-9; nonionic; polymerization emulsifier for vinyl acetate and acrylic emulsions; stabilizer for syn. latices; wetting agent in electrolyte sol'ns.; cosmetics surfactant; solid; pour pt. 112 F; cloud pt. > 100 C (1% aq.); HLB 17.8; 100% conc.

Chemax NP-40/70. [Chemax] Nonoxynol-40; CAS 9016-45-9; nonionic; see Chemax NP-40; liq.; pour pt. 46 F; cloud pt. > 100 C (1% aq.); HLB 17.8.

Chemax NP-50. [Chemax] Nonoxynol-50; CAS 9016-45-9; nonionic; see Chemax NP-40; solid; pour pt. 114 F; cloud pt. > 100 C (1% aq.); HLB 18.2.

Chemax NP-50/70. [Chemax] Nonoxynol-50; CAS 9016-45-9; nonionic; see Chemax NP-40; liq.; pour pt. 52 F; cloud pt. > 100 C (1% aq.); HLB 18.2.

Chemax NP-100. [Chemax] Nonoxynol-100; CAS 9016-45-9; nonionic; see Chemax NP-40; solid; pour pt. 122 F; cloud pt. > 100 C (1% aq.); HLB 19.0.

Chemax NP-100/70. [Chemax] Nonoxynol-100; CAS 9016-

45-9; nonionic; see Chemax NP-40; liq.; pour pt. 68 F; cloud pt. > 100 C (1% aq.); HLB 19.0.

Chemax OP-3. [Chemax] Octoxynol-3; CAS 9002-93-1; nonionic; emulsifier, detergent, stabilizer, dispersant, wetting agent; pesticides, floor finishes, cosmetics; liq.; pour pt. –9 F.

Chemax OP-5. [Chemax] Octoxynol-5; CAS 9002-93-1; nonionic; see Chemax OP-3; liq.; oil sol.; pour pt. –15 F; 100% conc.

Chemax OP-7. [Chemax] Octoxynol-7; CAS 9002-93-1; nonionic; detergent comps.; industrial metal cleaning, acid and waterless hand cleaners, floor finishes, cosmetics; liq.; pour pt. 15 F.

Chemax OP-9. [Chemax] Octoxynol-9; CAS 9002-93-1; nonionic; see Chemax OP-7; liq.; pour pt. 45 F; 100% conc.

Chemax OP-30/70. [Chemax] Octoxynol-30; CAS 9002-93-1; nonionic; emulsifier, dispersant, detergent, wetting agent, solubilizer, coupler for cosmetics, textile, metalworking, household, industrial, agric., paper, paint, and other industries; liq.; cloud pt. > 100 C (1% aq.); HLB 17.3; 70% conc.

Chemax OP-40. [Chemax] Octoxynol-40; CAS 9002-93-1; nonionic; emulsifier, detergent, stabilizer, wetting agent, dispersant; cosmetics; solid; 100% conc.

Chemax OP-40/70. [Chemax] Octoxynol-40; CAS 9002-93-1; nonionic; emulsifier for vinyl acetate and acrylate polymerization; cosmetics; liq.; pour pt. 25 F; cloud pt. > 100 C (1% aq.); HLB 17.9; 70% conc.

Chemax PEG 200 DL. [Chemax] PEG-4 dilaurate; CAS 9005-02-1; personal care surfactant.

Chemax PEG 400 DO. [Chemax] PEG-8 dioleate; CAS 9005-07-6; emulsifier and solubilizer for solv., fats, and min. oils; in lubricant, softener, and defoamer formulations for agric., cosmetic, household, leather, metalworking, and textile industries; liq.; oil-sol.; sapon. no. 116; HLB 8.8.

Chemax PEG 400 DT. [Chemax] PEG-8 ditallate; CAS 61791-01-3; surfactant.

Chemax PEG 600 DO. [Chemax] PEG-12 dioleate; CAS 9005-07-6; emulsifier in lubricant, softener, and defoamer formulations for agric., cosmetic, household, leather, metalworking, and textile industries; semiliq.; water-sol.; sapon. no. 102; HLB 10.3.

Chemax PEG 600 DT. [Chemax] PEG-12 ditallate; CAS 61791-01-3; surfactant.

Chembetaine C. [Chemron] Cocamidopropyl betaine; amphoteric; high foaming mild industrial and personal care surfactant; foam and visc. builder; lime soap dispersant; foaming agent for water and acid systems; stable over wide pH range; pale yel. liq.; 35% conc.

Chembetaine CAS. [Chemron] Cocamidopropylhydroxysultaine; CAS 68139-30-0; EINECS 268-761-3; amphoteric; anti-irritant for other surfactants; esp. for baby shampoos and baby bath prods.; detergent for heavy-duty industrial alkaline cleaners (steam cleaners, wax remover, hard surf. cleaner); wetting agent in acid pickling of metals; lime soap dispersant; visc. builder; pale yel. liq.; sol. in soft and hard water, brine and conc. electrolyte sol'ns.; 50% conc.

Chembetaine CB. [Chemron] Coco betaine; CAS 68424-94-2; EINECS 270-329-4; amphoteric; foaming surfactant effective in hard and soft water; mild to hair and skin; for shampoos, soaps, conditioners; pale yel. liq.; 45% conc.

Chembetaine CGF. [Chemron] Cocamidopropyl betaine; amphoteric; high purity, low color surfactant with foam and visc. building props.; for medicated shampoos and conditioners, facial cleansers, bubble baths, bath gels; water-wh. liq.; 35% conc.

Chembetaine L. [Chemron] Lauramidopropyl betaine; EINECS 224-292-6; amphoteric; foam booster; visc. builder; mild surfactant for shower gels, liq. soaps, skin

cleansers, shampoos; water-wh. liq.; 35% conc.

Chembetaine OL. [Chemron] Oleyl betaine; CAS 871-37-4; EINECS 212-806-1; amphoteric; mild, emollient conditioning surfactant; substantive to skin and hair; for shampoos, conditioners, liq. soaps, bath prods.; pale yel. gel; 50% conc.

Chembetaine OL-30. [Chemron] Oleyl betaine; CAS 871-37-4; EINECS 212-806-1; amphoteric; gentle, substantive visc. builder for shampoos, conditioners, mousses; pale yel. gel; 30% conc.

Chembetaine S. [Chemron] Soyamidopropyl betaine; amphoteric; conditioner, foamer, visc. builder for shampoos, conditioners, bath prods.; pale yel. liq.; 35% conc.

Chembetaine TG. [Chemron] Dihydroxyethyl tallow glycinate; amphoteric; conditioner providing nonoily feel and resistance to build-up for cream rinses, shampoos, conditioning mousses, comb-out sprays; pale yel. liq.; 50% conc.

Chemeen 18-2. [Chemax] PEG-2 stearamine; CAS 10213-78-2; EINECS 233-520-3; mild cationic; emulsifier and antistat in cosmetics, textiles, metal buffing, and rubber compds.; lubricant for fiber glass; solid; m.w. 365; HLB 4.8.

Chemeen 18-5. [Chemax] PEG-5 stearamine; CAS 26635-92-7; see Chemeen 18-2; solid; m.w. 540.

Chemeen 18-50. [Chemax] PEG-50 stearamine; CAS 26635-92-7; mild cationic; see Chemeen 18-2; solid; m.w. 2400; HLB 17.8.

Chemeen C-2. [Chemax] PEG-2 cocamine; CAS 61791-14-8; mild cationic; emulsifier, antistat, dye leveler, wetting agent, lubricant, dispersant; substantive to metals, fibers, and clays; suitable for cosmetics; liq.; m.w. 290; HLB 6.1; 100% conc.

Chemeen C-5. [Chemax] PEG-5 cocamine; CAS 61791-14-8; mild cationic; see Chemeen C-2; liq.; m.w. 425; HLB 10.4; 100% conc.

Chemeen C-10. [Chemax] PEG-10 cocamine; CAS 61791-14-8; see Chemeen C-2; liq.; m.w. 645; 100% conc.

Chemeen C-15. [Chemax] PEG-15 cocamine; CAS 61791-14-8; mild cationic; see Chemeen C-2; liq.; m.w. 890; HLB 15.0; 100% conc.

Chemical 39 Base. [Sandoz] Stearamidoethyl ethanolamine; CAS 141-21-9; EINECS 205-469-7; cationic; cosmetic and toiletry base; emulsifying agent for creams and lotions; conditioning/softening additive for hair prods.; lubricant in skin prods.; active ingred. in laundry softener sheets; Gardner 3 color; very slight amine odor; insol. in water; disp. as the amine salt.

Chemical Base 6532. [Sandoz] Stearamidoethyl diethylamine; CAS 16889-14-8; EINECS 240-924-3; cationic; emulsifier, emollient, conditioning agent for skin and hair, shaving creams, hydro-alcoholic lotions, skin creams, cream rinse shampoos; substantive to hair; yel. tan solid; slight odor; m.p. 35–45 C; 100% act.

Chemidex B. [Chemron] Behenamidopropyl dimethylamine; CAS 60270-33-9; EINECS 262-134-8; cationic; substantive surfactant for cream rinses, conditioners, shampoos, creams, and lotions; flakes; 100% act.

Chemidex C. [Chemron] Cocamidopropyl dimethylamine; CAS 68140-01-2; EINECS 268-771-8; cationic; substantive surfactant for cream rinses, conditioners, shampoos, creams, and lotions; soft waxy solid; 100% act.

Chemidex L. [Chemron] Lauramidopropyl dimethylamine; CAS 3179-80-4; EINECS 221-661-3; cationic; substantive surfactant for cream rinses, conditioners, shampoos, creams, and lotions; waxy solid; 100% act.

Chemidex M. [Chemron] Myristamidopropyl dimethylamine; CAS 45267-19-4; EINECS 256-214-1; cationic; substantive surfactant for cream rinses, conditioners, shampoos, creams, and lotions; waxy solid; 100% act.

Chemidex O. [Chemron] Oleamidopropyl dimethylamine; CAS 109-28-4; EINECS 203-661-5; cationic; substantive surfactant for cream rinses, conditioners, shampoos, creams, and lotions; liq.; 100% act.

Chemidex P. [Chemron] Palmitamidopropyl dimethylamine; CAS 39669-97-1; EINECS 254-585-4; cationic; substantive surfactant for cream rinses, conditioners, shampoos, creams, and lotions; waxy solid; 100% act.

Chemidex R. [Chemron] Ricinoleamidopropyl dimethylamine; CAS 20457-75-4; EINECS 243-835-8; cationic; substantive surfactant for cream rinses, conditioners, shampoos, creams, and lotions; liq.; 100% act.

Chemidex S. [Chemron] Stearamidopropyl dimethylamine; CAS 7651-02-7; EINECS 231-609-1; cationic; low irritation emulsifier with substantivity to protein and cellulosic substrates; for cream rinses, conditioners, shampoos, creams, and lotions; flake; 100% conc.

Chemidex SE. [Chemron] Stearamidoethyl dimethylamine; cationic; substantive surfactant for cream rinses, conditioners, shampoos, creams, and lotions; solid; 100% act.

Chemidex SI. [Chemron] Isostearamidopropyl dimethylamine; CAS 67799-04-6; EINECS 267-101-1; cationic; substantive surfactant for cream rinses, conditioners, shampoos, creams, and lotions; liq.; 100% act.

Chemidex SO. [Chemron] Soyamidopropyl dimethylamine; CAS 68188-30-7; cationic; substantive surfactant for cream rinses, conditioners, shampoos, creams, and lotions; liq.; 100% act.

Chemidex T. [Chemron] Tallowamidopropyl dimethylamine; CAS 68425-50-3; EINECS 270-356-1; cationic; substantive surfactant for cream rinses, conditioners, shampoos, creams, and lotions; paste; 100% act.

Chemidex WC. [Chemron] Cocamidopropyl dimethylamine; CAS 68140-01-2; EINECS 268-771-8; cationic; substantive surfactant for cream rinses, conditioners, shampoos, creams, and lotions; liq. to soft paste; 100% act.

Chemie Linz Allantoin. [Chemie Linz N. Am.] Allantoin; CAS 97-59-6; EINECS 202-592-8; skin protectant.

Chemodyne N-Acetyltyrosine. [Chemodyne SA] Acetyl tyrosine; CAS 537-55-3; EINECS 208-671-3.

Chemodyne Tyrosine. [Chemodyne SA] Tyrosine; nutritive additive.

Chemoxide CAW. [Chemron] Cocamidopropylamine oxide; CAS 68155-09-9; EINECS 268-938-5; nonionic; surfactant for mild, low irritation personal care and industrial applics., e.g., shampoos, facial cleansers, bath prods.; foam and visc. builder, emollient over broad pH range; pale yel. liq.; 30% conc.

Chemoxide L. [Chemron] Lauramidopropyl betaine; EINECS 224-292-6; amphoteric; foam booster, visc. builder; mild surfactant; liq.; 35% conc.

Chemoxide LM-30. [Chemron] Lauramine oxide; CAS 1643-20-5; EINECS 216-700-6; nonionic; visc. builder, foam enhancer for household and industrial cleaners, personal care prods.; tolerant to electrolytes for improved hard water performance; water-wh. liq.; 30% conc.

Chemoxide O. [Chemron] Oleamine oxide; CAS 14351-50-9; EINECS 238-311-0; nonionic; thickener, visc. builder; wetting agent for pigments and dyes; used in hair colorants, gels, permanent waves; water-wh. liq.; 30% conc.

Chemoxide SAO. [Chemron] Stearamidopropylamine oxide; CAS 25066-20-0; EINECS 246-598-9; wetting and foaming agent, visc. builder, conditioner, softener for hair; for shampoos, conditioners, mousses; emulsifier in creams and lotions; wh. paste; 25% act.

Chemoxide ST. [Chemron] Stearamine oxide; CAS 2571-88-2; EINECS 219-919-5; conditioner, softener, visc. and foam builder for conditioning shampoos, rinses improving comb-out and manageability; wh. paste; 25% act.

Chemoxide T. [Chemron] Dihydroxyethyl tallowamine oxide; CAS 61791-46-6; EINECS 263-179-6; detergent, wetting agent for low-pH shampoos and conditioners, alkaline media; for use in gels, liqs., or emulsions; clear liq.; 50% act.

Chemoxide TAO. [Chemron] Tallowamidopropylamine oxide; CAS 68647-77-8; EINECS 271-972-3; visc. builder, foam booster; improves manageability and luster in hair; for use in conditioners, sprays, mousses; yel. liq.; 50% act.

Chemoxide WC. [Chemron] Cocamine oxide; CAS 61788-90-7; EINECS 263-016-9; nonionic; visc. builder, foam booster, emollient for shampoos, cleansers, bath prods.; water-wh. liq.; 30% conc.

Chemphos TC-231S. [Chemron] Sodium nonoxynol-9 phosphate; emulsifier, solubilizer, antistat, substantivity agent for hair care prods., perms, straighteners, depilatories; resistant to hydrolysis; clear visc. liq.; 85% act.

Chemphos TC-337. [Chemron] Nonoxynol-20 phosphate; anionic; emulsion polymerization surfactant for vinyl acetate, acrylates, SBR; emulsifier, solubilizer, antistat, substantivity agent for hair care prods., perms, straighteners, depilatories; resistant to hydrolysis; clear visc. liq.; 100% act.

Chemphos TC-341. [Chemron] Nonyl nonoxynol-10 phosphate; CAS 39464-64-7; emulsifier, solubilizer, antistat, substantivity agent for hair care prods., perms, straighteners, depilatories; resistant to hydrolysis; hazy visc. liq.; 100% act.

Chemphos TC-349. [Chemron] Nonyl nonoxynol-15 phosphate; CAS 39464-64-7; emulsifier, solubilizer, antistat, substantivity agent for hair care prods., perms, straighteners, depilatories; resistant to hydrolysis; clear visc. liq.; 90% act.

Chemphos TR-505. [Chemron] Oleth-10 phosphate; CAS 39464-69-2; emulsifier, solubilizer, antistat, substantivity agent for hair care prods., perms, straighteners, depilatories; resistant to hydrolysis; visc. liq.; 100% act.

Chemphos TR-505D. [Chemron] DEA-oleth-10 phosphate; emulsifier, solubilizer, antistat, substantivity agent for hair care prods., perms, straighteners, depilatories; resistant to hydrolysis; visc. liq.; 100% act.

Chemphos TR-510. [Chemron] Laureth-4 phosphate; CAS 39464-66-9; emulsifier, solubilizer, antistat, substantivity agent for hair care prods., perms, straighteners, depilatories; resistant to hydrolysis; clear visc. liq.; 98% act.

Chemphos TR-510S. [Chemron] Sodium laureth-4 phosphate; CAS 42612-52-2; emulsifier, solubilizer, antistat, substantivity agent for hair care prods., perms, straighteners, depilatories; resistant to hydrolysis; clear visc. liq.; 95% act.

Chemphos TR-515. [Chemron] Oleth-3 phosphate; CAS 39464-69-2; emulsifier, solubilizer, antistat, substantivity agent for hair care prods., perms, straighteners, depilatories; resistant to hydrolysis; visc. liq.; 100% act.

Chemphos TR-515D. [Chemron] DEA-oleth-3 phosphate; emulsifier, solubilizer, antistat, substantivity agent for hair care prods., perms, straighteners, depilatories; resistant to hydrolysis; visc. liq.; 100% act.

Chemphos TR-541. [Chemron] Oleth-4 phosphate; CAS 39464-69-2; emulsifier, solubilizer, antistat, substantivity agent for hair care prods., perms, straighteners, depilatories; resistant to hydrolysis; visc. liq.; 100% act.

Chemsalan NLS 30. [Chem-Y GmbH] Sodium lauryl sulfate; CAS 151-21-3; EINECS 205-788-1; anionic; cleaning and foaming agent for hair and body cosmetics, toothpaste, dishwashing, and household cleaners; liq.; 30% conc.

Chemsalan RLM 28. [Chem-Y GmbH] Sodium laureth sulfate; CAS 9004-82-4; anionic; biodeg. surfactant; cleaning and foaming agent for hair and body cosmetics, dishwashing, and household cleaners; clear sl. ylsh. liq.; m.w. 390; visc. 200 mPa·s; pH 6-7; 28% conc.

Chemsalan RLM 56. [Chem-Y GmbH] Sodium laureth sulfate; CAS 9004-82-4; anionic; biodeg. surfactant; cleaning and foaming agent for hair and body cosmetics, dishwashing, and household cleaners; sl. cloudy, lt. ylsh. visc. liq.; m.w. 390; visc. 5000-15,000 mPa·s; pH 6.5-8.0 (10% aq.); 56% conc.

Chemsalan RLM 70. [Chem-Y GmbH] Sodium laureth sulfate; CAS 9004-82-4; anionic; biodeg. surfactant; cleaning and foaming agent for hair and body cosmetics, dishwashing, and household cleaners; sl. ylsh. paste; m.w. 390; pH 6.5-8.5 (10% aq.); 70% conc.

Chemsperse EGDS. [Chemron] Glycol distearate; CAS 627-83-8; EINECS 211-014-3; nonionic; opacifier, conditioner, thickener for shampoos, liq. soaps, creams and lotions; flake; 100% conc.

Chemsperse EGMS. [Chemron] Glycol stearate; CAS 111-60-4; EINECS 203-886-9; nonionic; opacifier, pearlizing agent, thickener for personal care prods. such as shampoos, liq. soaps, creams and lotions; prills; 100% conc.

Chemsperse GMS. [Chemron] Glyceryl stearate; nonionic; emulsifier, thickener, stabilizer, opacifier for personal care prods., vanishing creams, lotions, shampoos, shaving creams; flakes; HLB 2.8; 100% conc.

Chemsperse GMS-PS. [Chemron] Glyceryl stearate, PEG-100 stearate; nonionic; emulsifier for mildly acidic o/w creams and lotions and other o/w prods. containing electrolytes; flake; 100% conc.

Chemsperse GMS-SE. [Chemron] Glyceryl stearate, self-emulsifying; nonionic; emulsifier, stabilizer, emollient, opacifier for netural to sl. alkaline anionic systems; flake; 100% conc.

Cheratina 100%. [Variati] Hydrolyzed keratin.

Ches® 500. [CasChem] Nonfat drymilk, xanthan gum, propylene glycol, alginate, glyceryl stearate, sodium glyceryl oleate phosphate; food grade stabilizer; cold mix emulsifier for cosmetics and pharmaceuticals; cold hot emulsion system; unique ambient temp. emulsifier which yields stable, aesthetic o/w emulsions; powd.; 100% conc.

Chesguar C10, C10R. [Chesham Chem. Ltd.] Guar hydroxypropyltrimonium chloride; CAS 65497-29-2; conditioner and thickener for shampoos, hair conditioners, liq. soaps, bath/shower prods.; stabilizer and conditioner for skin care creams and lotions; visc. 1000-1700 mPa·s (1%); usage level: 0.2-1.0%.

Chesguar C17. [Chesham Chem. Ltd.] Guar hydroxypropyltrimonium chloride; CAS 65497-29-2; conditioner and thickener for shampoos, hair conditioners, liq. soaps, bath/shower prods.; stabilizer and conditioner for skin care creams and lotions; visc. 2000-3000 mPa·s (1%); usage level: 0.2-1.0%.

Chesguar C20, C20R. [Chesham Chem. Ltd.] Guar hydroxypropyltrimonium chloride; CAS 65497-29-2; conditioner and thickener for shampoos, hair conditioners, liq. soaps, bath/shower prods.; stabilizer and conditioner for skin care creams and lotions; visc. 3000-4000 mPa·s (1%); usage level: 0.2-1.0%.

Chesguar HP4. [Chesham Chem. Ltd.] Hydroxypropyl guar; CAS 39421-75-5; nonionic; thickener and stabilizer for water-based cosmetics and toiletries; develops visc. rapidly when the pH is adjusted below 7.0; disp. in cold water; visc. 3600-4200 mPa·s (1%).

Chesguar HP4R. [Chesham Chem. Ltd.] Hydroxypropyl guar; CAS 39421-75-5; nonionic; thickener and stabilizer for water-based cosmetics and toiletries; develops visc. rapidly when the pH is adjusted below 7.0; disp. in cold water; visc. 3600-4200 mPa·s (1%).

Chesguar HP6. [Chesham Chem. Ltd.] Hydroxypropyl guar;

CAS 39421-75-5; nonionic; thickener and stabilizer for water-based cosmetics and toiletries; develops visc. rapidly when the pH is adjusted below 7.0; disp. in cold water; visc. 30,000 mPa·s (2%).

Chimexane AC. [Chimex] DIPA-hydrog. cocoate and DIPA-lanolate.

Chimexane CA. [Chimex] Diethylaminoethyl PEG-5 cocoate.

Chimexane CJ. [Chimex] Methylenebis tallow acetamidodimonium chloride.

Chimexane HA. [Chimex] Hydroxyethyl carboxymethyl cocamidopropylamine.

Chimexane HB. [Chimex] Sodium diethylaminopropyl cocoaspartamide.

Chimexane NF. [Chimex] Polyglyceryl-3 hydroxylauryl ether.

Chimexane NH. [Chimex] Polyglyceryl-2 lanolin alcohol ether.

Chimexane NJ. [Chimex] Polyglyceryl-4-PEG-2 cocamide.

Chimexane NK. [Chimex] Hydroxyceteth-60.

Chimexane NL. [Chimex] Polyglyceryl-3 cetyl ether.

Chimexane NR. [Chimex] Polyglyceryl-3 decyltetradecanol.

Chimexane NS. [Chimex] Lauryl polyglyceryl-6 cetearyl-glycol ether.

Chimin AX. [Auschem SpA] Cocamidopropyl betaine; CAS 61789-40-0; amphoteric; conditioner, emulsifier, detergent for cosmetic use in personal care prods.; liq.; 30% conc.

Chimin BX. [Auschem SpA] Lauryl betaine; CAS 683-10-3; EINECS 211-669-5; amphoteric; dispersant, wetting agent, antistat; soft paste; 40% conc.

Chimin CB. [Auschem SpA] Coco betaine; CAS 85409-25-2; amphoteric; nonirritating surfactant for shampoo, bubble bath; liq.; 30% conc.

Chimin CMO. [Auschem SpA] Cocamidopropylamine oxide; CAS 68155-09-9; EINECS 268-938-5; cosmetic surfactant.

Chimin DOS 70. [Auschem SpA] Sodium di 2-ethylhexyl sulfosuccinate; CAS 577-11-7; EINECS 209-406-4; anionic; wetting agent; liq.; 68% conc.

Chimin IMB. [Auschem SpA] Disodium cocoamphodiacetate; CAS 68650-39-5; EINECS 272-043-5; cosmetic surfactant.

Chimin IMZ. [Auschem SpA] Lauroamphocarboxy glycinate; CAS 14350-97-1; EINECS 238-306-3; amphoteric; mild detergent for shampoos, bubble baths; liq.; 30% conc.

Chimin L. [Auschem SpA] Sodium lauroyl sarcosinate; CAS 137-16-6; EINECS 205-281-5; anionic; mild detergent for shampoos, bubble baths; liq.; 30% conc.

Chimin LE 50. [Auschem SpA] Sodium alkylether sulfate; CAS 911648-56-5; anionic; high foaming raw material for detergency in toiletry preps.; paste; 50% conc.

Chimin LMO. [Auschem SpA] Lauramidopropylamine oxide; CAS 61792-31-2; EINECS 263-218-7; cosmetics surfactant.

Chimin LX. [Auschem SpA] Lauramidopropyl betaine; CAS 4292-10-8; EINECS 224-292-6; amphoteric; mild detergent for shampoos, bubble baths; liq.; 30% conc.

Chimin P10. [Auschem SpA] Alkyl polyphosphate; anionic; wetting and penetrating agent; liq.; 100% conc.

Chimin P45. [Auschem SpA] Sodium alkylpolyglycol ether phosphate; CAS 68071-35-2; anionic; detergent, antistat, wetting agent for textile, paper, cleaners, machine washing, and personal care prods.; liq.; 30% conc.

Chimin P50. [Auschem SpA] Phosphoric acid complex org. ester; nonionic; emulsifier, antistat for use in leather, textile and cosmetic applics.; liq.; sol. in water and solv.; 100% conc.

Chimipal DCL/M. [Auschem SpA] Cocamide DEA; CAS 68603-42-9; EINECS 263-163-9; nonionic; thickener and foam stabilizer, detergent, and shampoo additive; liq.; 100% conc.

Chimipal DE 7. [Auschem SpA] Ethoxylated alkanolamide; nonionic; detergent, foam booster; liq./paste; 100% conc.

Chimipal FV. [Auschem SpA] Ethoxylated monoglyceride; nonionic; superfatting agent in cosmetic preparations; liq.; water-sol.; 100% conc.

Chimipal LDA. [Auschem SpA] Lauramide DEA; CAS 120-40-1; EINECS 204-393-1; nonionic; thickener and foam stabilizer, detergent and shampoo additive; liq.; 100% conc.

Chimipal MC. [Auschem SpA] Cocamide MEA; CAS 68140-00-1; EINECS 268-770-2; nonionic; thickener and foam stabilizer, detergent and shampoo additive; flakes; 100% conc.

Chimipal OLD. [Auschem SpA] Oleamide DEA; CAS 93-83-4; EINECS 202-281-7; nonionic; thickener for shampoos, bubble baths and liq. detergents; liq.; 100% conc.

Chinpi Liq. [Ichimaru Pharcos] Water, alcohol, and bitter orange peel extract; botanical extract.

Chitin Liq. [U.S. Cosmetics] Polysaccharide; cationic; natural material providing moisturizing, smooth feeling, visc., film formation, antistatic effect, heat and pH stability, and skin safety to hair and skin care prods.; liq.; m.w. 6000; usage level: 3-10%.

Chitin Liq. [Ichimaru Pharcos] Carboxymethyl chitin; CAS 52108-64-2.

Chitisol. [Ichimaru Pharcos] Carboxymethyl chitin; CAS 52108-64-2.

Chitoglycan. [Sinerga Srl; Trivent] N-Carboxymethyl chitosan.

Chitomarine. [Sederma] Water, propylene glycol, and chitosan.

Chloracel® 40% Sol'n. [Reheis] Sodium aluminum chlorhydroxy lactate complex; CAS 8038-93-5; deodorant compat. with typical soap-based cologne sticks; clear liq.; 40% act., 8% Al₂O₃, 3% Cl, 5.6% Na.

Chloracel® Solid. [Reheis] Sodium aluminum chlorhydroxy lactate complex; CAS 8038-93-5; deodorant compat. with typical soap-based cologne sticks; wh. free-flowing powd.; 20% Al₂O₃, 7.5% Cl, 14% Na.

Chlorhydrol® 50% Sol'n. [Reheis] Aluminum chlorohydrate; CAS 1327-41-9; EINECS 215-477-2; antiperspirant active; 23.5% Al₂O₃, 8.2% Cl.

Chlorhydrol® Granular. [Reheis] Aluminum chlorohydrate; CAS 1327-41-9; EINECS 215-477-2; antiperspirant active; gran.; 90% min. thru 4 mesh; 47% Al₂O₃, 16.3% Cl.

Chlorhydrol, Impalpable. [Reheis] Aluminum chlorohydrate; CAS 1327-41-9; EINECS 215-477-2; antiperspirant active.

Chlorhydrol® Powd. [Reheis] Aluminum chlorohydrate.; CAS 1327-41-9; EINECS 215-477-2; antiperspirant active; powd., 97% min. thru 100 mesh; 47% Al₂O₃, 16.3% Cl.

Cholecithine. [Rhone-Poulenc] Alcohol and neural extract; botanical extract.

Cholesterol. [Brooks Industries] Cholesterol; CAS 57-88-5; EINECS 200-353-2; emulsifier, moisturizer.

Cholesterol BP. [Solvay Duphar BV] Cholesterol; CAS 57-88-5; EINECS 200-353-2; nonionic; w/o emulsifier, moisturizer for cosmetics; basic raw material for mfg. of liq. crystals; active ingred. in shrimp feed; solid; 91% conc.

Cholesterol NF. [Solvay Duphar BV] Cholesterol; CAS 57-88-5; EINECS 200-353-2; nonionic; w/o emulsifier, moisturizer for cosmetics; basic raw material for steroid hormones; solid; 95% conc.

Cholesterol NF. [Croda Inc.; Croda Chem. Ltd.] Cholesterol; CAS 57-88-5; EINECS 200-353-2; nonionic; moisturizer, emollient, conditioner, primary emulsifier, stabilizer for w/o systems, cosmetics, pharmaceuticals, absorption

bases, ointments; useful in incorporation of drug actives into oils and fats and in mfg. of hydrophilic petrolatum; wh. to pale yel. powd., almost odorless/faint sterol odor; sol. in min. oil, sol. in 1% ethanol, turbid after 2 h; m.p. 147-149 C; HLB 1.0; usage level: 0.1-1%; 100% conc.

Cholesterol NF. [R.I.T.A.] Cholesterol NF; CAS 57-88-5; EINECS 200-353-2; emulsifier, emollient, conditioner, moisturizer, stabilizer, and solubilizer in makeup, lipsticks, skin care prods., bath preps., shampoos, soaps, shave creams, ointments, sun care prods., veterinary prods.; wh. powd.

Chondroitin Sulfate A. [Bioiberica] Sodium chondroitin sulfate; EINECS 232-696-9.

Chotosolbe. [Koyo] Carboxymethyl chitin; CAS 52108-64-2.

Chouji Liq. [Ichimaru Pharcos] Water, alcohol, and clove extract; botanical extract.

Chroma-Lite® . [ISP Van Dyk] Bonded combinations of colored pigments and bismuth oxychloride on mica; low-dusting powds. imparting a subdued satiny luster to pressed powd. prods.

Chroma-Lite® Aqua 4508. [ISP Van Dyk] Mica, bismuth oxychloride, and chromium hydroxide green.

Chroma-Lite® Black 4498. [ISP Van Dyk] Mica, bismuth oxychloride, and iron oxides.

Chroma-Lite® Dark Blue 4501. [ISP Van Dyk] Mica, bismuth oxychloride, and ferric ammonium ferrocyanide.

Chroma-Lite® Magenta 4505. [ISP Van Dyk] Mica, bismuth oxychloride, and carmine.

Chroma-Lite® Violet 4507. [ISP Van Dyk] Mica, bismuth oxychloride, and manganese violet.

Chrome Green 106. [Presperse] Chromium hydroxide (90%), bismuthoxychloride (10%); CAS 1308-38-9, 7787-59-9; inorg. colorant for pigmented cosmetics; JSCI/JCID approved.

Chromoprotulines. [Exsymol; Biosil Tech.] Hydrolyzed vegetable protein, pigmented; CAS 100209-45-8; moisturizer for cosmetics, oily skin care, regeneration and skin treatment, anti-ageing and anti-wrinkle creams; dark blue liq., algal odor; sol. in water; pH 6.0-6.5; usage level: 2-10% of a 4% sol'n.; toxicology: nontoxic.

Chronosphere® G. [Brooks Industries; Polymedia] Polyurethane/acrylate copolymer and glycerin; encapsulated actives for controlled release from anhyd. cosmetic prods.

Chronosphere® Planell® . [Brooks Industries; Polymedia] Polyurethane/acrylate copolymer, squalene, squalane, glycolipids, phytosterols, and tocopherol; encapsulated actives for controlled release from anhyd. cosmetic prods.

Chronosphere® SAL. [Brooks Industries; Polymedia] Polyurethane/acrylate copolymer, salicylic acid; encapsulated actives for controlled release from anhyd. cosmetic prods.

Chronosphere® V-AE. [Brooks Industries; Polymedia] Polyurethane/acrylate copolymer, tocopherol acetate, retinyl palmitate; encapsulated actives for controlled release from anhyd. cosmetic prods.

Chronosponge. [Advanced Polymer Systems] Acrylates copolymer; thickener, stabilizer for cosmetics.

Cirami No. 1. [Alban Muller] Beeswax, candelilla wax, shea butter; natural thickener for cosmetic field.

Circulatory Blend HS 318. [Alban Muller] Propylene glycol, witch hazel extract, cypress extract, butcherbroom extract, and grape leaf extract; phytocomplex for cosmetic prods. for heavy legs.

Cire De Lanol CTO. [Seppic] Ceteareth-33 and cetearyl alcohol; a self-emulsifying wax; cosmetics emulsifier; flakes; 100% act.

Cithrol 2DL. [Croda Chem. Ltd.] PEG-4 dilaurate; CAS 9005-02-1; nonionic; dispersant, w/o emulsifier, wetting agent and co-solv.; used in cosmetic and industrial applics.; paste; HLB 6.0; 97% conc.

Cithrol 2DO. [Croda Chem. Ltd.] PEG-4 dioleate; CAS 9005-

07-6; nonionic; dispersant, w/o emulsifier, wetting agent and co-solv.; used in cosmetic and industrial applics.; liq.; 97% conc.

Cithrol 2ML. [Croda Chem. Ltd.] PEG-4 laurate; CAS 9004-81-3; nonionic; wetting agent, emulsifier, detergent, thickener, solubilizer, dispersant, softener, lubricant, antistat, dye asistant, penetrant for cosmetics, textiles, glass fiber, metal treatment; liq.; m.w. 200; HLB 8.8; sapon. no. 158–168; 100% conc.

Cithrol 2MO. [Croda Chem. Ltd.] PEG-4 oleate; CAS 9004-96-0; EINECS 233-293-0; nonionic; wetting agent, penetrant, detergent, emulsifier, solubilizer, thickening agent, dispersant, textile aux., softener, lubricant for textiles, cosmetics, metalworking; m.w. 200; HLB 6.2; sapon. no. 110–112; 100% conc.

Cithrol 2MS. [Croda Chem. Ltd.] PEG-4 stearate; CAS 9004-99-3; EINECS 203-358-8; nonionic; emulsifier for insecticides and cosmetics, detergent, wetting agent, solubilizer and thickening agent for perfumery, antifrothing agent, foaming agent; m.w. 200; m.p. 39–41 C; HLB 6.3; sapon. no. 110–120; 100% conc.

Cithrol 3MS. [Croda Chem. Ltd.] PEG-6 stearate; CAS 9004-99-3; emulsifier for insecticides, cosmetics and toiletries, detergent, wetting agent, solubilizer and thickening agent for perfumery, antifrothing agent, foaming agent; paste; m.w. 300; m.p. 30–33 C; HLB 10.7; sapon. no. 95–105; 100% conc.

Cithrol 4DL. [Croda Chem. Ltd.] PEG-8 dilaurate; CAS 9005-02-1; nonionic; dispersant, w/o emulsifier, wetting agent and co-solv.; used in cosmetic and industrial applics.; liq.; HLB 10.2; 97% conc.

Cithrol 4DO. [Croda Chem. Ltd.] PEG-8 dioleate; CAS 9005-07-6; nonionic; dispersant, w/o emulsifier, wetting agent and co-solv.; used in cosmetic and industrial applics.; liq.; HLB 8.3; 97% conc.

Cithrol 4DS. [Croda Surf. Ltd.] PEG-8 distearate; CAS 9005-08-7; personal care surfactant.

Cithrol 4ML. [Croda Chem. Ltd.] PEG-8 laurate; CAS 9004-81-3; nonionic; wetting agent, emulsifier, detergent, thickener, solubilizer, dispersant, softener, lubricant, antistat, dye asistant, penetrant for cosmetics, textiles, glass fiber, metal treatment; m.w. 400; HLB 13.1; sapon. no. 92–98; 100% conc.

Cithrol 4MO. [Croda Chem. Ltd.; Croda Surf. Ltd.] PEG-8 oleate; CAS 9004-96-0; nonionic; wetting agent, penetrant, detergent, emulsifier, solubilizer, thickening agent, dispersant, textile aux., softener, lubricant for textiles, cosmetics, metalworking; liq.; m.w. 400; HLB 11.4; sapon. no. 85–93; 100% conc.

Cithrol 4MS. [Croda Chem. Ltd.] PEG-8 stearate; CAS 9004-99-3; nonionic; emulsifier for insecticides and cosmetics, detergent, wetting agent, solubilizer and thickening agent for perfumery, antifrothing agent, foaming agent; paste; m.w. 400; m.p. 31–34 C; HLB 11; sapon. no. 95–105; 100% conc.

Cithrol 6DL. [Croda Chem. Ltd.] PEG-12 dilaurate; CAS 9005-02-1; nonionic; dispersant, w/o emulsifier, wetting agent and co-solv.; used in cosmetic and industrial applics.; liq.; HLB 12.0; 97% conc.

Cithrol 6DO. [Croda Chem. Ltd.] PEG-12 dioleate; CAS 9005-07-6; nonionic; dispersant, w/o emulsifier, wetting agent and co-solv.; used in cosmetic and industrial applics.; liq.; HLB 10.4; 97% conc.

Cithrol 6DS. [Croda Chem. Ltd.] PEG-12 distearate; CAS 9005-08-7; nonionic; antistat in textile finishing; skin care ingred.; solid; HLB 10.8; 97% conc.

Cithrol 6ML. [Croda Chem. Ltd.] PEG-12 laurate; CAS 9004-81-3; nonionic; wetting agent, emulsifier, detergent, thickener, solubilizer, dispersant, softener, lubricant, antistat, dye asistant, penetrant for cosmetics, textiles, glass fiber,

metal treatment, leather treatment; m.w. 600; HLB 16.8; sapon. no. 64–74; 100% conc.

Cithrol 6MO. [Croda Chem. Ltd.] PEG-12 oleate; CAS 9004-96-0; nonionic; wetting agent, penetrant, detergent, emulsifier, solubilizer, thickening agent, dispersant, textile aux., softener, lubricant for textiles, cosmetics, metalworking; liq.; m.w. 600; HLB 13.1; sapon. no. 65–75; 100% conc.

Cithrol 6MS. [Croda Chem. Ltd.] PEG-12 stearate; CAS 9004-99-3; nonionic; emulsifier for insecticides and cosmetics, detergent, wetting agent, solubilizer and thickening agent for perfumery, antifrothing agent, foaming agent; paste; m.w. 600; m.p. 33–35 C; HLB 14; sapon. no. 68–76; 100% conc.

Cithrol 10DL. [Croda Chem. Ltd.] PEG-20 dilaurate; CAS 9005-02-1; nonionic; dispersant, w/o emulsifier, wetting agent and co-solv.; used in cosmetic and industrial applics.; paste; HLB 14.7; 97% conc.

Cithrol 10DO. [Croda Chem. Ltd.] PEG-20 dioleate; CAS 9005-07-6; nonionic; dispersant, w/o emulsifier, wetting agent and co-solv.; used in cosmetic and industrial applics.; liq.; HLB 13.2; 97% conc.

Cithrol 10DS. [Croda Chem. Ltd.] PEG-20 distearate; CAS 9005-08-7; nonionic; antistat in textile finishing; skin care ingred.; solid; HLB 13.7; 97% conc.

Cithrol 10ML. [Croda Chem. Ltd.] PEG-20 laurate; CAS 9004-81-3; nonionic; wetting agent, emulsifier, detergent, thickener, solubilizer, dispersant, softener, lubricant, antistat, dye asistant, and penetrant for cosmetics, textiles, glass fiber, metal treatment; sol. in water, alcohol, polar solv.; m.w. 1000; HLB 18; sapon. no. 51–55; 100% conc.

Cithrol 10MO. [Croda Chem. Ltd.] PEG-20 oleate; CAS 9004-96-0; nonionic; wetting agent, penetrant, detergent, emulsifier, solubilizer, thickening agent, dispersant, textile aux., softener, lubricant for textiles, cosmetics, metalworking; liq.; m.w. 1000; HLB 16.2; sapon. no. 35–40; 100% conc.

Cithrol 10MS. [Croda Chem. Ltd.] PEG-20 stearate; CAS 9004-99-3; nonionic; emulsifier for insecticides and cosmetics, detergent, wetting agent, solubilizer and thickening agent for perfumery, antifrothing agent, foaming agent; solid; m.w. 1000; m.p. 34–40 C; HLB 16; sapon. no. 36–50; 100% conc.

Cithrol 15MS. [Croda Chem. Ltd.] PEG-1500 stearate; nonionic; emulsifier for insecticides and cosmetics, detergent, wetting agent, solubilizer and thickening agent for perfumery, antifrothing agent, foaming agent; solid; m.w. 1500; m.p. 30-41 C; HLB 17; sapon. no. 30–55; 100% conc.

Cithrol 40MS. [Croda Chem. Ltd.] PEG-75 stearate; CAS 9004-99-3; nonionic; emulsifier for insecticides and cosmetics, detergent, wetting agent, solubilizer and thickening agent for perfumery, antifrothing agent, foaming agent; solid; m.w. 4000; m.p. 30–41 C; HLB 18.8; sapon. no. 12–17; 100% conc.

Cithrol 60DS. [Croda Surf. Ltd.] PEG-120 distearate; CAS 9005-08-7; personal care surfactant.

Cithrol DEGMO. [Croda Surf. Ltd.] PEG-2 oleate; CAS 106-12-7; EINECS 203-364-0; personal care surfactant.

Cithrol DGMS N/E. [Croda Chem. Ltd.] Diethylene glycol stearate; CAS 9004-99-3; EINECS 203-363-5; nonionic; w/o emulsifier, dispersant, antistat for skin care prods., textile, paper processing, cutting oils, polishes, emulsion cleaners, rubber latex, wool lubricants; solid; HLB 4.4; 100% conc.

Cithrol DGMS S/E. [Croda Chem. Ltd.] Diethylene glycol stearate SE; CAS 9004-99-3; anionic; w/o emulsifier, dispersant, and antistat for skin care prods., textile, paper processing, cutting oils, polishes, emulsion cleaners, rubber latex, wool lubricants; solid; HLB 5.0; 100% conc.

Cithrol EP. [Croda Surf. Ltd.] Ethyl palmitate.

Cithrol ES. [Croda Surf. Ltd.] Ethyl stearate; CAS 111-61-5; EINECS 203-887-4; emollient, solubilizer for cosmetics.

Cithrol GDL N/E. [Croda Chem. Ltd.] Glyceryl dilaurate; CAS 27638-00-2; EINECS 248-586-9; nonionic; w/o emulsifier, dispersant, antistat for textile, paper processing, cutting oils, polishes, emulsion cleaners, rubber latex, wool lubricants, cosmetics, pharmaceuticals; liq.; HLB 2.0; 100% conc.

Cithrol GDL S/E. [Croda Chem. Ltd.] Glyceryl dilaurate SE; anionic; w/o emulsifier, dispersant, antistat for textile, paper processing, cutting oils, polishes, emulsion cleaners, rubber latex, wool lubricants, cosmetics, pharmaceuticals; liq.; 100% conc.

Cithrol GDO N/E. [Croda Chem. Ltd.] Glyceryl dioleate; CAS 25637-84-7; EINECS 247-144-2; nonionic; emulsifier, coemulsifier, stabilizer, wetting agent, lubricant, and antistat; used in cosmetic, pharmaceutical, industrial, food applics.; liq.; HLB 2.0; 100% conc.

Cithrol GDO S/E. [Croda Chem. Ltd.] Glyceryl dioleate SE; anionic; emulsifier, coemulsifier, stabilizer, wetting agent, lubricant, and antistat; used in cosmetic, pharmaceutical, industrial, food applics.; liq.; HLB 2.9; 100% conc.

Cithrol GDS N/E. [Croda Chem. Ltd.] Glyceryl distearate; CAS 1323-83-7; EINECS 215-359-0; nonionic; emulsifier, coemulsifier, stabilizer, wetting agent, lubricant, and antistat; used in cosmetic, pharmaceutical, industrial, food applics.; solid; HLB 3.4; 100% conc.

Cithrol GDS S/E. [Croda Chem. Ltd.] Glyceryl distearate SE; anionic; emulsifier, coemulsifier, stabilizer, wetting agent, lubricant, and antistat; used in cosmetic, pharmaceutical, industrial, food applics.; solid; HLB 4.2; 100% conc.

Cithrol GML N/E. [Croda Chem. Ltd.] Glyceryl laurate; CAS 142-18-7; EINECS 205-526-6; nonionic; emulsifier, coemulsifier, stabilizer, wetting agent, lubricant, and antistat; used in cosmetic, pharmaceutical, industrial, food applics.; liq.; HLB 4.9; 100% conc.

Cithrol GML S/E. [Croda Chem. Ltd.] Glyceryl laurate SE; anionic; emulsifier, coemulsifier, stabilizer, wetting agent, lubricant, and antistat; used in cosmetic, pharmaceutical, industrial, food applics.; liq.; HLB 5.6; 100% conc.

Cithrol GMM. [Croda Surf. Ltd.] Glyceryl myristate; CAS 589-68-4; cosmetic emulsifier.

Cithrol GMO N/E. [Croda Chem. Ltd.] Glyceryl oleate; CAS 111-03-5; nonionic; emulsifier, coemulsifier, stabilizer, wetting agent, lubricant, and antistat; used in cosmetic, pharmaceutical, industrial, food applics.; liq.; HLB 3.3; 100% conc.

Cithrol GMO S/E. [Croda Chem. Ltd.] Glyceryl oleate SE; anionic; emulsifier, coemulsifier, stabilizer, wetting agent, lubricant, and antistat; used in cosmetic, pharmaceutical, industrial, food applics.; liq.; HLB 4.1; 100% conc.

Cithrol GMR N/E. [Croda Chem. Ltd.] Glyceryl ricinoleate; CAS 141-08-2; EINECS 205-455-0; nonionic; emulsifier, coemulsifier, stabilizer, wetting agent, lubricant, and antistat; used in cosmetic, pharmaceutical, industrial, food applics.; liq.; HLB 2.7; 100% conc.

Cithrol GMR S/E. [Croda Chem. Ltd.] Glyceryl ricinoleate SE; anionic; emulsifier, coemulsifier, stabilizer, wetting agent, lubricant, and antistat; used in cosmetic, pharmaceutical, industrial, food applics.; liq.; HLB 3.6; 100% conc.

Cithrol GMS Acid Stable. [Croda Chem. Ltd.] Glyceryl stearate SE; CAS 31566-31-1; nonionic; emulsifier, coemulsifier, stabilizer, wetting agent, lubricant, and antistat; used in cosmetic, pharmaceutical, industrial, food applics.; solid; HLB 10.9; 100% conc.

Cithrol GMS N/E. [Croda Chem. Ltd.] Glyceryl stearate; CAS 31566-31-1; nonionic; emulsifier, coemulsifier, stabilizer, wetting agent, lubricant, and antistat; used in cosmetic,

pharmaceutical, industrial, food applics.; solid; HLB 3.4; 100% conc.

Cithrol GMS S/E. [Croda Chem. Ltd.] Glyceryl stearate SE; CAS 31566-31-1; anionic; emulsifier, coemulsifier, stabilizer, wetting agent, lubricant, and antistat; used in cosmetic, pharmaceutical, industrial, food applics.; solid; HLB 4.4; 100% conc.

Cithrol GTO. [Croda Surf. Ltd.] Triolein; CAS 122-32-7; EINECS 204-534-7; emollient.

Cithrol L, O Range. [Croda Chem. Ltd.] Polyglycol esters; dispersant for cosmetic and industrial hydrophilic systems; liq., solid; water-sol.

Cithrol PGDO. [Croda Surf. Ltd.] Propylene glycol dioleate; CAS 105-62-4; EINECS 203-315-3; cosmetic ingred.

Cithrol PGML N/E. [Croda Chem. Ltd.] Propylene glycol laurate; CAS 142-55-2; EINECS 205-542-3; nonionic; emulsifier, coemulsifier, stabilizer, wetting agent, lubricant, and antistat; used in cosmetic, pharmaceutical, industrial, food applics.; liq.; HLB 2.7; 100% conc.

Cithrol PGML S/E. [Croda Chem. Ltd.] Propylene glycol laurate SE; anionic; emulsifier, coemulsifier, stabilizer, wetting agent, lubricant, and antistat; used in cosmetic, pharmaceutical, industrial, food applics.; liq.; HLB 3.6; 100% conc.

Cithrol PGMM. [Croda Surf. Ltd.] Propylene glycol myristate; CAS 29059-24-3; EINECS 249-395-3; personal care surfactant.

Cithrol PGMO N/E. [Croda Chem. Ltd.] Propylene glycol oleate; CAS 1330-80-9; EINECS 215-549-3; nonionic; emulsifier, coemulsifier, stabilizer, wetting agent, lubricant, and antistat; used in cosmetic, pharmaceutical, industrial, food applics.; liq.; HLB 3.1; 100% conc.

Cithrol PGMO S/E. [Croda Chem. Ltd.] Propylene glycol oleate SE; anionic; emulsifier, coemulsifier, stabilizer, wetting agent, lubricant, and antistat; used in cosmetic, pharmaceutical, industrial, food applics.; liq.; HLB 3.9; 100% conc.

Cithrol PGMR N/E. [Croda Chem. Ltd.] Propylene glycol ricinoleate; CAS 26402-31-3; EINECS 247-669-7; nonionic; emulsifier, coemulsifier, stabilizer, wetting agent, lubricant, and antistat; used in cosmetic, pharmaceutical, industrial, food applics.; liq.; HLB 2.7; 100% conc.

Cithrol PGMR S/E. [Croda Chem. Ltd.] Propylene glycol ricinoleate SE; anionic; emulsifier, coemulsifier, stabilizer, wetting agent, lubricant, and antistat; used in cosmetic, pharmaceutical, industrial, food applics.; liq.; HLB 3.6; 100% conc.

Cithrol PGMS N/E. [Croda Chem. Ltd.] Propylene glycol stearate; CAS 1323-39-3; EINECS 215-354-3; nonionic; emulsifier, coemulsifier, stabilizer, wetting agent, lubricant, and antistat; used in cosmetic, pharmaceutical, industrial, food applics.; solid; HLB 2.4; 100% conc.

Cithrol PGMS S/E. [Croda Chem. Ltd.] Propylene glycol stearate SE; anionic; emulsifier, coemulsifier, stabilizer, wetting agent, lubricant, and antistat; used in cosmetic, pharmaceutical, industrial, food applics.; solid; HLB 3.2; 100% conc.

Cithrol PR. [Croda Chem. Ltd.] Polyglycerol polyricinoleate; nonionic; w/o emulsifier for veg. oils; liq.; 100% conc.

Cithrol S Range. [Croda Chem. Ltd.] Polyglycol esters; dispersant for cosmetic and industrial hydrophilic systems; liq./solid; water-sol.

Citmol™ 316. [Bernel; Heterene] Triisocetyl citrate; noncomedogenic emollient for cosmetics, cleansing creams; castor oil replacement for lipsticks; pigment dispersant; FDA, EEC compliances; Gardner 1 max. clear visc. liq.; sol. in castor oil, min. oil, safflower oil, octyl palmitate, SD-40 alcohol; acid no. 4 max.; sapon. no. 175-195; hyd. no. 20 max.; usage level: 2-10%.

Citmol 320. [Bernel] Trioctyldodecyl citrate; CAS 126121-35-

5; noncomedogenic, high visc. emollient, film-former, castor oil replacement for lipsticks; FDA, EEC compliances; colorless liq.; oil-sol.; usage level: 2-10%.

Citric Acid USP FCC (Anhyd.) Fine Gran. No. 69941. [Roche] Citric acid USP, FCC; CAS 77-92-9; EINECS 201-069-1; acidulant for cosmetic prods.

Citric Acid USP Fine Granular No. 69941. [Roche] Citric acid; CAS 77-92-9; EINECS 201-069-1.

Citroflex A-4. [Morflex] Acetyl tri-n-butyl citrate; CAS 77-90-7; EINECS 201-067-0; plasticizer for PVC, PVDC, esp. food films, medical articles; APHA 30 max. clear iq., mild odor; m.w. 402.5; sol. in toluene, heptane; sp.gr. 1.045–1.055; visc. 33 cps; flash pt. (COC) 400 F; pour pt. –59 C; ref. index 1.441–1.443; 99% min. ester content.

Citroflex A-6. [Morflex] Acetyl tri-n-hexyl citrate; CAS 24817-92-3; vinyl plasticizer for medical applics. and other toxicologically sensitive areas; APHA 100 max. clear liq., mild odor; m.w. 486; sol. in toluene, heptane; sp.gr. 1.003–1.007; visc. 36 cps; flash pt. (COC) > 500 F; pour pt. –57 C; ref. index 1.445–1.449; 99% min. ester content.

Citroflex B-6. [Morflex] n-Butyryl tri-n-hexyl citrate; CAS 82469-79-2; vinyl plasticizer for medical applics.; APHA 100 max. clear liq., mild odor; m.w. 514; sol. in toluene, heptane; sp.gr. 0.991–0.995; visc. 28 cps; flash pt. (COC) > 500 F; pour pt. –55 C; ref. index 1.444–1.448; 99% min. ester content.

Clar 111. [Clar Sarl] Nonfat dry colostrum.

Clar 120. [Clar Sarl] Colostrum cream.

Clar 142. [Clar Sarl] Colostrum whey.

Clarax. [Belmay] Hexahydrohexamethyl cyclopentabenzopyran and diethyl phthalate.

Clarex® 5XL. [Solvay Enzymes] Pectinase derived from *Aspergillus niger var.*; CAS 9032-75-1; EINECS 232-885-6; enzyme; depectinization of fruit juices, grape processing, jams and jellies, berry processing and wine prod.; extraction of flavors and fragrances; lt. tan to wh. powd., free of offensive odor and taste; water-sol.; usage level: 0.1-1.0%.

Clarex® L. [Solvay Enzymes] Pectinase derived from *Aspergillus niger var.*; CAS 9032-75-1; EINECS 232-885-6; enzyme; depectinization of fruit juices, grape processing, jams and jellies, berry processing and wine prod.; extraction of flavors and fragrances; clear to amber brn. liq.; misc. with water; sp.gr. 1.05-1.15; usage level: 0.1-0.05%.

Claytone 34. [Southern Clay Prods.] Quaternium-18 bentonite; CAS 68953-58-2; EINECS 273-219-4; thixotrope.

Claytone 40. [Southern Clay Prods.] Quaternium-18 bentonite; CAS 68953-58-2; EINECS 273-219-4; thixotrope.

Claytone AF. [Southern Clay Prods.] Stearalkonium bentonite; thixotrope.

Claytone APA. [Southern Clay Prods.] Stearalkonium bentonite; thixotrope.

Claytone GR. [Southern Clay Prods.] Quaternium-18/benzalkonium bentonite.

Claytone HT. [Southern Clay Prods.] Quaternium-18/benzalkonium bentonite.

Claytone PS. [Southern Clay Prods.] Quaternium-18/benzalkonium bentonite.

Claytone XL. [Southern Clay Prods.] Quaternium-18 bentonite; CAS 68953-58-2; EINECS 273-219-4; thixotrope.

Clearcol. [Croda Inc.; Croda Chem. Ltd.] Soluble animal collagen; CAS 9007-34-5; EINECS 232-697-4; protein for moisturizing and conditioning of facial systems where clarity is important; clear to slightly hazy visc. liq.; m.w. 300,000; usage level: 2-20%; 1% act.

Clear Filtered Verajuice-Cold Processed. [Apree] Aloe vera gel; moisturizer, soothing/healing aid for personal care.

Clintonia Borealis Extract Code 9035. [Brooks Industries]

Lily (*Clintonia borealis*) extract; anti-inflammatory props. and pseudohormonal materials; lt. yel.-grn. liq.

Cloisonné®. [Mearl] Mica pigments coated with titanium dioxide and/or iron oxide with carmine, iron blue, etc.; highly lustrous pigments with deep colors produced by combination of light interference and light absorption; for cosmetics and personal care prods.; avail. grades incl. gold, blue, copper, violet, orange, golden bronze, red, rouge flambé, regal gold, cerise flambé, blue flambé.; fine powds.

Cloisonné Blue. [Mearl] Mica, titanium dioxide, and ferric ferrocyanide.

Cloisonné Gold. [Mearl] Mica, titanium dioxide, and iron oxides.

Cloisonné Red. [Mearl] Mica, titanium dioxide, and carmine.

Cloisonné Violet. [Mearl] Mica, titanium dioxide, carmine, and ferric ferrocyanide.

Closyl 30 2089. [Clough] Sodium-N-cocoyl sarcosinate; CAS 61791-59-1; EINECS 263-193-2; anionic; wetting, foaming detergent used in personal care and household prods.; corrosion inhibitor for mild steel; liq.; pH 7.5-9.0; 30–31% conc.

Closyl LA 3584. [Clough] Sodium lauroyl sarcosinate; CAS 137-16-6; EINECS 205-281-5; anionic; soap-like detergent providing wetting and foaming; for personal care and household prods.; corrosion inhibitor for mild steel; liq.; pH 7.5-9.0; 30-31% conc.

CMI 321. [Alban Muller; Tri-K Industries] Purified fraction of green coffee; CAS 84650-00-0; EINECS 283-481-1; uv-B absorber/protective agent, antioxidant, and antibacterial props. and skin stimulation effect; whitish powd., sl. odor, lt. aromatic flavor; sol. in hot water and alcohols; sp.gr. 0.4-0.5; m.p. > 174 C; pH 3-5 (0.1% aq.); usage level: 1-5%; 5% max. moisture.

CMI 324. [Alban Muller] Coffee extract; CAS 84650-00-0; EINECS 283-481-1; anti-uv-B sunscreen.

CMI 400. [Alban Muller] Coffee extract; CAS 84650-00-0; EINECS 283-481-1; anti-uv-B sunscreen.

CMI 550. [Alban Muller; Tri-K Industries] Coffee and wild pansy extract; anti-uv-A and B sunscreen with antioxidant, free radical scavenger, and preservative props.; good substantivity on skin but causes lt. yel. coloration; boosts SPF with syn. sunscreens; yel. powd., char. odor; sl. sol. in cold water; sol. in low bases, alcohols, and glycols; usage level: 1-5%; 90% min. purity.

CMI 551. [Alban Muller; Tri-K Industries] Purified fraction of wild pansy/green coffee; sunscreen props.

CMI 800. [Alban Muller; Tri-K Industries] Wild pansy extract; CAS 84012-42-0; anti-uv-A sunscreen, antioxidant, free radical scavenger, and preservative; good substantivity on skin; boosts SPF of syn. sunscreens; yel. gold powd., char. odor; sl. sol. in cold water; sol. in low bases, alcohols, and glycols; sp.gr. 0.5; usage level: 1-5%; 90% min. purity.

CMI 800. [Alban Muller; Tri-K Industries] Purified fraction of wild pansy; sunscreen props.

CMP-I. [Am. Casein] Milk protein; CAS 9000-71-9; cosmetic protein.

CO-618. [Procter & Gamble] Coconut alcohol; CAS 68425-37-6; EINECS 270-351-4; emollient.

CO-1214. [Procter & Gamble] C12-14 alcohols; CAS 67762-41-8; intermediate for mfg. of alkyl sulfates and ethoxylates, alkyl halides, esters, etc.; water-wh. mobile liq.; sp.gr. 0.823; m.p. 22 C; acid no. 0.1 max.; iodine no. 0.3 max.; sapon. no. 0.5 max.; hyd. no. 280-290; 100% conc.

CO-1670. [Procter & Gamble] Cetearyl alcohol.

CO-1695. [Procter & Gamble] Cetyl alcohol; CAS 36653-82-4; EINECS 253-149-0; emollient, intermediate for mfg. of alkyl sulfates and ethoxylates, alkyl halides, esters, etc.; wh. waxy solid; sp.gr. 0.814 (55 C); m.p. 47-50 C; acid no.

0.5 max.; iodine no. 2 max.; sapon. no. 1 max.; hyd. no. 220-235; 100% conc.

CO-1895. [Procter & Gamble] Stearyl alcohol; CAS 112-92-5; EINECS 204-017-6; emollient, intermediate for mfg. of alkyl sulfates and ethoxylates, alkyl halides, esters, etc.; wh. waxy solid; sp.gr. 0.811 (65 C); m.p. 56-60 C; acid no. 0.5 max.; iodine no. 2 max.; sapon. no. 2 max.; hyd. nno. 200-215; 100% conc.

Coatex 9065 C. [Coatex] Polymethacrylic acid.

CoAxel. [Sederma] Coenzyme A, L-carnitine, and caffeine; cellulite treatment, slimming active ingred. for the cosmetic remodeling of the figure; helps reduce visible or-ange peel appearance associated with cellulite.

Cob Flour #4, 6, 100. [Mt. Pulaski Prods.] Corn cob meal; filler, absorbent for cosmetics.

Cob Grit #1, 2, 3, 8, 150, 3050. [Mt. Pulaski Prods.] Corn cob meal; filler, absorbent for cosmetics.

Coconut Oils® 76, 92, 110. [Stepan/PVO] Coconut oils, refined bleached, deodorized; CAS 8001-31-8; EINECS 232-282-8; base for ice cream coatings, candies, icings; clouding agent for beverages; emollient for creams and lotions; flavor solubilizer; pharmaceutical vehicle.

Cofix. [Cosmetochem] An ingred. for hair setting lotions.

Coflex. [Cosmetochem] A hair spray ingred. which improves the moisture resist. and elasticity of the commonly used resins.

Co-Gell® A2/B270. [Rhone-Poulenc Surf. & Spec.] Min. oil, aluminum isostearates/laurates/palmitates, isopropyl palmitate; stabilizer for continuous phase of w/o emulsion systems and gelling agent for oils and nonaq. fluids; waterproofing, lubricity props.; improved pigment adhe-sion and slip.

Cogilor Amethyst. [Ellis & Everard Personal Care] Ultrama-rine violet; inorganic pigment for cosmetics and toiletries.

Cogilor Aquamarine. [Ellis & Everard Personal Care] Ultra-marine blue; inorganic pigment for cosmetics and toilet-ries.

Cogilor Emerald. [Ellis & Everard Personal Care] Hydrated chromium oxide; inorganic pigment for cosmetics and toiletries.

Cogilor Jade. [Ellis & Everard Personal Care] Anhydrous chrome green; inorganic pigment for cosmetics and toilet-ries.

Cogilor Jet. [Ellis & Everard Personal Care] Black iron oxide; pigment for cosmetics and toiletries.

Cogilor Ochre. [Ellis & Everard Personal Care] Yellow iron oxide; pigment for cosmetics and toiletries.

Cogilor Rose. [Ellis & Everard Personal Care] Ultramine pink; inorganic pigment for cosmetics and toiletries.

Cogilor Rouge. [Ellis & Everard Personal Care] Red iron oxide; pigment for cosmetics and toiletries.

Cogilor Sapphire. [Ellis & Everard Personal Care] Ferric ferrocyanide; CAS 25869-00-5; inorganic pigment for cosmetics and toiletries.

Cogilor Spinel. [Ellis & Everard Personal Care] Manganese violet; CAS 10101-66-3; EINECS 233-257-4; inorganic pigment for cosmetics and toiletries.

Co-Grhetinol. [Maruzen Fine Chems.] Stearyl glycyrrheti-nate; CAS 13832-70-7; anti-inflammatory, anti-allergenic for cosmetics and pharmaceuticals.

Cojoba. [Costec] Jojoba oil; CAS 61789-91-1; cosmetic emollient.

CoKukui. [Costec] Kukui nut oil; cosmetic ingred.

Colan 12. [Lanaetex Prods.] PEG-10 coconut oil complex; cosmetic ingred.

Colan 32. [Lanaetex Prods.] PPG-2 PEG-6 coconut oil complex; cosmetic ingred.

Colladerm Procollagene SC. [Biomex] Soluble collagen; CAS 9007-34-5; EINECS 232-697-4; cosmetic protein.

Colla-Gel AC. [Maybrook] Gelatin; CAS 9000-70-8; EINECS

232-554-6; substantive protein and film-former providing body, sheen, and manageability to hair (styling prods., shampoos, conditioners) and moisturizing and anti-irritancy props. to skin care prods. (creams, lotions, pro-tective creams); clear to sl. hazy visc. liq. or soft gel, char. very mild odor; pH 3.5-4.5; 28-32% solids.

Collagen. [Rona; E. Merck] Soluble collagen; CAS 9007-34-5; EINECS 232-697-4; cosmetic protein.

Collagen. [Grau Aromatics] Collagen; CAS 9007-34-5; EINECS 232-697-4; moisturizing protein.

Collagen 15K. [Brooks Industries] Hydrolyzed mixed gly-cosaminoglycans, hydrolyzed collagen, hydrolyzed der-mal proteins; cosmetic ingred. for moisturizing applics.; lt. tan powd., char. odor; pH 6-8; 93% min. NV.

Collagen BIO-5000. [Bioiberica] Hydrolyzed collagen; CAS 9015-54-7; cosmetic protein.

Collagen-CCK-Complex. [Kelisema Srl; G.F. Secchi] Soluble collagen and potassium cocoate.

Collagen CLR. [Dr. Kurt Richter; Henkel/Cospha; Henkel Canada] Carrier of native sol. collagen in weakly acid hydrophilic medium; CAS 9007-34-5; EINECS 232-697-4; prod. for aging skin, wrinkle and after-sun treatment; lt. nontransparent liq.

Collagen-IMZ Complex. [Kelisema Srl; G.F. Secchi] Soluble collagen and sodium cocoamphoacetate.

Collagen-LSS Complex. [Kelisema Srl; G.F. Secchi] Soluble collagen and sodium lauryl sulfate.

Collagen P. [Provital; Centerchem] Hydrolyzed collagen; CAS 9015-54-7; cosmetic protein.

Collagen S. [Cosmetochem] Hydrolyzed collagen; CAS 9015-54-7; cosmetic protein.

Collagen S.D. [Tri-K Industries] Collagen; CAS 9007-34-5; EINECS 232-697-4; moisturizing protein.

Collagen Amino Acids SF. [ChemMark Development] Col-lagen amino acids; CAS 9105-54-7; moisturizer.

Collagen-Cocoate-Complex V 2037. [Henkel] Potassium cocoyl hydrolyzed collagen; CAS 68920-65-0; cosmetic protein.

Collagen SPO. [Gattefosse] Soluble collagen; CAS 9007-34-5; EINECS 232-697-4; cosmetic protein.

Collagene Lyophilized. [Gattefosse] Collagen; CAS 9007-34-5; EINECS 232-697-4; moisturizing protein.

Collagen Hydrolysate 30%. [Pentapharm Ltd; Centerchem] Hydrolyzed collagen; CAS 9015-54-7; cosmetic protein.

Collagen Hydrolyzate Cosmetic 50. [Maybrook] Hydro-lyzed collagen; CAS 9015-54-7; protein providing protec-tive colloid effect, anti-irritancy, film-forming, substantivity to hair care (styling prods., shampoos, conditioners) and skin care prods. (creams, lotions, shave creams, liq. detergents), dish detergents; amber clear liq., sl. char. odor; pH 6.7-7.3; 48-52% solids.

Collagen Hydrolyzate Cosmetic 55. [Maybrook] Hydro-lyzed collagen; CAS 9015-54-7; protective colloid effect, anti-irritant props.; substantive film-former with dye level-ing effects for skin and hair care prods. (shampoos, conditioners, color treatments, shave creams), liq. soaps, dish detergents; amber clear liq., sl. char. odor; pH 6.0-7.0; 55% min. solids.

Collagen Hydrolyzate Cosmetic N-35. [Maybrook] Hydro-lyzed collagen; CAS 9015-54-7; substantive film-former providing protective colloid effect, anti-irritancy benefits to hair and skin care prods. (styling prods., shampoos, conditioners, skin creams/lotions, shave creams), liq. detergents, dishwash detergents; dye leveling effects for color treatment prods.; lt. amber clear liq., mild char. odor; pH 5.5-6.5; 35% min. solids.

Collagen Hydrolyzate Cosmetic N-55. [Maybrook] Hydro-lyzed collagen; CAS 9015-54-7; protein providing protec-tive colloid effect, anti-irritancy, film-forming, substantivity for hair care (styling prods., shampoos, conditioners), skin care (creams, lotions, shave creams), liq. detergents, dish detergents; lt. amber clear liq., mild char. odor; pH 5.5-6.5; 55% min. solids.

Collagen Hydrolyzate Cosmetic SD. [Maybrook] Hydrolyzed collagen; CAS 9015-54-7; protein providing protective colloid effect, anti-irritancy, film-forming, substantivity for hair care (styling prods., shampoos, conditioners), skin care (creams, lotions, shave creams), liq. detergents, dish detergents; off-wh. powd., bland char. odor; pH 5.5-6.5.

Collagen Masks. [Gattefosse SA] Native fibrous collagen; CAS 9007-34-5; EINECS 232-697-4; skin moisturizing mask for applic. to face, neck, forehead, lips, and eye area; 90% min. act.

Collagen Nativ 1%. [Novarom GmbH] Soluble collagen; CAS 9007-34-5; EINECS 232-697-4; cosmetic protein.

Collagen Native Extra 1%. [Maybrook] Soluble collagen; CAS 9007-34-5; EINECS 232-697-4; moisturizer, film-former for skin care prods.; protective barrier; colorless, clear to sl. hazy visc. liq., sl. char. odor; m.w. 360,000; pH 4 max.; 1.2-2.5% solids.

Collagenol LS/HC-10. [Laboratoires Sérobiologiques] Hydrolyzed collagen; CAS 9015-54-7; cosmetic protein.

Collagenol LS/HC-50. [Laboratoires Sérobiologiques] Hydrolyzed collagen; CAS 9015-54-7; cosmetic protein.

Collagenon. [Vevy] Hydrolyzed collagen; CAS 9015-54-7; cosmetic protein.

Collagen Powd. [Brooks Industries] Collagen; CAS 9007-34-5; EINECS 232-697-4; moisturizing protein.

Collagen Protein WN. [Cosmetochem] Hydrolyzed collagen; CAS 9015-54-7; cosmetic protein.

Collamino™ 25. [Brooks Industries] Collagen amino acids; CAS 9105-54-7; cosmetic ingred.; m.w. 200; 25% act.

Collamino™ 40-SF. [Brooks Industries] Collagen amino acids; CAS 9105-54-7; moisturizer.

Collamino™ Complex. [Brooks Industries] Collagen amino acids, acetamide MEA, propylene glycol; moisturizing cosmetics ingred.; 50% act.

Collamino™ Complex ESC. [Brooks Industries] Collagen amino acids, acetamide MEA, hydrolyzed elastin, propylene glycol, and hydrolyzed silk; cosmetic ingred.

Collamino™ Complex L/O. [Brooks Industries] Lauryloleylmethylamine and collagen amino acids; cationic; conditioning complex for cosmetics; 90% act.

Collamino™ Complex S. [Brooks Industries] Collagen amino acids, acetamide MEA, propylene glycol, and silk amino acids; cosmetic ingred.

Collamino™ Complex SS. [Brooks Industries] Hydrolyzed collagen, hydrolyzed silk, acetamide MEA, and propylene glycol; cosmetic ingred.

Colla-Moist™ CG. [Brooks Industries] Glyceryl collagenate; moisturizing protein complexes for cosmetics; 30% act.

Colla-Moist™ WS. [Brooks Industries] Propylene glycol, hydrolyzed collagen, PPG-12-PEG-65 lanolin oil; moisturizing protein complexes for cosmetics; liq.; 50% act.

Collamoist ZN. [Brooks Industries] Zinc hydrolyzed collagen; cosmetic ingred.

Collapur®. [Grünau; Henkel KGaA/Cospha] Soluble collagen; CAS 9007-34-5; EINECS 232-697-4; protein for cosmetic formulations for skin care; one of the most stable collagens; colorless visc. liq., weak intrinsic odor; pH 3.3-3.7; 1% min. collagen content, 1.5% total solids.

Collapurol® E 1. [Grünau; Henkel KGaA/Cospha] Water, 20% ethanol, and soluble collagen; protein for aq.-alcoholic systems such as aftershaves and face lotions, roll-on deodorant; transparent visc. liq.; sol. in alcohol, aq.-alcoholic systems; pH 4.3-4.7; 1% min. collagen, 1.2% total solids.

Collapuron N. [Henkel] Water and soluble collagen; CAS 9007-34-5; EINECS 232-697-4; cosmetic protein.

Collapuron® DAK. [Grünau; Henkel KGaA/Cospha]

Desamido collagen; CAS 9007-34-5; protein for use in cosmetic formulations, skin and body care prods.; pract. colorless visc. liq., weak intrinsic odor; pH 3.5-3.8; 1.5% collagen content, 2.3% total solids.

Collasol. [Croda Inc.; Croda Chem. Ltd.] Sol. animal collagen; CAS 9007-34-5; EINECS 232-697-4; humectant; hygroscopic film former; conditioner; moisturizer for skin care prods.; off-wh. disp.; m.w. 300,000; pH 4.0; usage level: 2-10%; 3% act.

Collodex. [Dextran Prods.] Lauroyl hydrolyzed collagen.

Colloidal Kaolin NF-Bacteria Controlled. [Whittaker, Clark & Daniels] Kaolin; CAS 1332-58-7; EINECS 296-473-8; cosmetic ingred.

Colorona®. [Rona] Titanium dioxide/mica coated with an additional layer of inorganic or organic pigments; pearlescent pigments for cosmetics and toiletries; more brilliant color effect from mixing of two components.

Colorona® Bordeaux. [Rona; E. Merck] Mica and iron oxides.

Colorona® Bright Gold. [Rona; E. Merck] Mica, titanium dioxide, and iron oxides.

Colorona® Carmine Red. [Rona; E. Merck] Mica, titanium dioxide, and carmine.

Colorona® Copper. [Rona; E. Merck] Mica and iron oxides.

Colorona® Light Blue. [Rona; E. Merck] Mica, titanium dioxide, and ferric ferrocyanide.

Colorona® Magestic Green. [Rona; E. Merck] Titanium dioxide, mica, and chromium oxide greens.

Colorona® Sienna. [Rona; E. Merck] Mica and iron oxides.

Colostrum Clar 101. [Rona; E. Merck] Colostrum.

Combi-Steriline MP. [Zimmerli] Methylparaben, propylparaben; cosmetic preservative; USA, Japan, and Europe approvals; usage level: 0.3-1.0%.

Compactrol®. [Mendell] Calcium sulfate, dihydrate NF; CAS 10101-41-4; tablet and capsule filler for pharmaceutical tablets mfg. by direct compression; wh. to sl. off-wh. powd., odorless; avg. particle size 166 μ; 90% +140 mesh; dens. (tapped) 1.24 g/ml; 100% conc.

Comperlan® 100. [Henkel Canada; Henkel/Cospha; Henkel KGaA/Cospha] Cocamide MEA; CAS 68140-00-1; EINECS 268-770-2; nonionic; foamer, booster for detergents, foam stabilizer, thickener, skin protective in industrial washing-up liqs., protective hand creams, hand cleaners; for bowl cleaners, shampoos; imparts flexibility and strength to cosmetic stick preps.; pale yel. beads, faint fatty odor; sol. in common fatty materials; 100% conc.

Comperlan® CD. [Henkel Canada] Capramide DEA; CAS 136-26-5; EINECS 205-234-9; nonionic; surfactant providing flash foam, no visc. buildup; amber visc. liq.; 98% conc.

Comperlan® COD. [Henkel KGaA/Cospha; Pulcra SA] Cocamide DEA; CAS 61791-31-9; EINECS 263-163-9; foam and visc. increasing agent with emulsifying properties; conditioner for shampoos and other cosmetic and pharmaceutical applics.; solv.; yel. clear liq.; solid. pt. -5 to 5 C; pH 9.5-10.5 (2%); 85% conc.

Comperlan® F. [Henkel KGaA/Cospha] Linoleamide DEA; CAS 56863-02-6; EINECS 260-410-2; nonionic; foam stabilizer and thickener for shampoos; vitamin E substitute; oily visc. liq., specific intrinsic odor; 100% conc.

Comperlan® KD. [Henkel; Henkel Canada; Henkel KGaA/Cospha; Pulcra SA] Cocamide DEA; CAS 61791-31-9; EINECS 263-163-9; nonionic; thickener, foam booster/stabilizer, superfatting agent for personal care prods.; hair conditioner; bright yel. visc. oily liq. or soft paste; pH 8-10; 100% conc.

Comperlan® KDO. [Henkel Canada] 1:1 Cocamide DEA; CAS 61791-31-9; EINECS 263-163-9; nonionic; thickening and foaming agent for personal care prods., cleansers; amber visc. liq.; 100% conc.

Comperlan® LD. [Henkel; Henkel KGaA/Cospha; Pulcra SA] Lauramide DEA superamide; CAS 120-40-1; EINECS 204-393-1; nonionic; foam booster, stabilizer, detergency and visc. builder, emulsifier for personal care prods., household detergents; wh. waxy solid; pH 9.5-10.5 (1%); 100% conc.

Comperlan® LDO, LDS. [Henkel Canada] 1:1 Lauramide DEA; CAS 120-40-1; EINECS 204-393-1; nonionic; foam booster, stabilizer, detergency and visc. builder, emulsifier for personal care prods., bath prods., cleansers; amber visc. liq.; 100% conc.

Comperlan® LMM. [Henkel] Lauramide MEA; CAS 142-78-9; EINECS 205-560-1; personal care surfactant.

Comperlan® LP. [Henkel Canada; Henkel KGaA/Cospha] Lauramide MIPA; CAS 142-54-1; EINECS 205-541-8; nonionic; foam stabilizer, thickener for shampoos and detergents; solid; 100% conc.

Comperlan® LS. [Henkel KGaA/Cospha] Cocamide DEA and laureth-2; emulsifier, thickener, and foam stabilizer for personal care prods.; dissolving intermediates; yel. to golden yel. visc. liq.; pH 9-11 (1%); 65–75% conc.

Comperlan® OD. [Henkel Canada; Henkel KGaA/Cospha] Oleamide DEA; CAS 93-83-4; EINECS 202-281-7; nonionic; foam stabilizer, thickener and superfatting agent for shampoos and bubble bath prods., body cleansers, metal spot removers, engine cleaners; reddish brn. oily liq.; sol. in oils and solvs.; pH 9-10 (1%); 100% conc.

Comperlan® P 100. [Pulcra SA] Cocamide MEA; CAS 68140-00-1; EINECS 268-770-2; nonionic; foamer, thickener, visc. builder for powd. detergents, soaps; dispersant and blending agent for many cosmetic prods.; flakes; 100% conc.

Comperlan® PD. [Henkel/Cospha; Henkel KGaA/Cospha] 2:1 Cocamide DEA; CAS 61791-31-9; EINECS 263-163-9; nonionic; thickener, foam builder/stabilizer for personal care prods., dishwashing agents; coemulsifier for cleaning and metalworking agents; amber visc. liq.; 98% conc.

Comperlan® SD. [Henkel Canada] Cocamide DEA; CAS 61791-31-9; EINECS 263-163-9; nonionic; foamer; liq.; 100% conc.

Comperlan® SDO. [Henkel Canada] Cocamide DEA superamide; CAS 61791-31-9; EINECS 263-163-9; nonionic; foam and visc. builder for personal care prods., cleansers; liq.; 100% conc.

Comperlan® VOD. [Henkel Canada; Henkel KGaA/Cospha] Soyamide DEA; CAS 68425-47-8; EINECS 270-355-6; nonionic; foam and visc. builder with superfatting effect for personal care prods., cleansers; liq.; 100% conc.

Complex GT. [Fabriquimica] Propylene glycol, alcohol, and wheat germ extract; botanical extract.

Complex NR. [C.E.P.] Propylene glycol, water, avocado extract, white lily extract, and soy germ extract; botanical extract.

Complex Relax. [C.E.P.] Propylene glycol, water, artichoke extract, coffee bean extract, celandine extract, passionflower extract, and calendula extract; botanical extract.

Complex T-I, T-II. [Bioiberica] Trachea hydrolysate.

Complex T-I, T-II. [Henley] Hyaluronic acid, sodium chondroitin sulfate, and hydrolyzed collagen.

Complexe AST 1. [C.E.P.] Propylene glycol, blackberry leaf extract, artichoke extract, and lemon extract; botanical extract.

Complexe AV.a. [C.E.P.] Propylene glycol, water, lemon extract, glycine, niacinamide, pyridoxine, and esculin; botanical extract.

Complexe AV.h. [C.E.P.] Corn oil, retinol, tocopherol, arachidonic acid, linoleic acid, and linolenic acid.

Compound 3143F. [Rhone-Poulenc] Sodium C14-16 olefin sulfonate and sodium cocoamphopropionate.

Compound TL. [Rhone-Poulenc] Disodium lauroamphodi-

acetate and sodium trideceth sulfate.

Compritol 888. [Gattefosse] Tribehenin; CAS 18641-57-1; EINECS 242-471-7; emulsifier, emollient.

Compritol 888 ATO. [Gattefosse; Gattefosse SA] Glyceryl behenate; nonionic; food emulsifier and additive for tablet mfg.; solid; drop pt. ≈ 70 C; HLB 2.0; acid no. < 4; iodine no. < 3; sapon. no. 145-165; toxicology: LD50 (oral, rat) > 5 g/kg; 100% conc.

Compritol HD5 ATO. [Gattefosse SA] PEG-8 behenate and tribehenin; tableting agent and lipophilic matrix; drop pt. ≈ 62 C; HLB 5.0; acid no. < 4; iodine no. < 3; sapon. no. 105-125.

Compritol WL 3241. [Gattefosse] Tribehenin; CAS 18641-57-1; EINECS 242-471-7; emulsifier, emollient.

Condipon. [Cosmetochem] Linoleamide DEA, quaternium-52, and polyquaternium-11; cosmetic ingred.

Conditioner P6. [3V-Sigma] Polyquaternium-6; CAS 26062-79-3; conditioner.

Conditioner P7. [3V-Sigma] Polyquaternium-7; CAS 26590-05-6; conditioner.

Controx® KS. [Grünau; Henkel KGaA/Cospha; Henkel Canada] Tocopherol, hydrog. tallow glycerides citrate; antioxidant for syn. oils and fats used in cosmetics; yel.-brownish visc. liq., typ. odor; usage level: 0.02-0.1%; 56% conc.

Controx® VP. [Grünau; Henkel/Cospha; Henkel Canada; Henkel KGaA/Cospha] Lecithin, tocopherol, ascorbyl palmitate, hydrog. tallow glycerides citrate; antioxidant for natural unsat. oils; for cosmetics use; brown paste, typ. odor; usage level: 0.02-0.1%; 17% conc.

Coobato Camomilla. [CGI-Universal Flavors] Propylene glycol, water, and matricaria extract; botanical extract.

Coobato Hamamelis. [CGI-Universal Flavors] Propylene glycol, water, and witch hazel extract; botanical extract.

Coobato Speciale. [CGI-Universal Flavors] Propylene glycol, water, matricaria extract, bitter orange extract, witch hazel extract, and rose extract; botanical extract.

Cooling Agent No. 10. [Takasago Int'l.] Menthoxypropanediol; cooling agent.

Cool-Jel. [Nepera] PEG-crosspolymer.

Copherol® 950LC. [Henkel/Cospha] Tocopherol and cococaprylate/caprate; natural antioxidant and moisturizer for sun protection and skin care prods.; amber clear visc. oil.

Copherol® 1250. [Henkel/Cospha; Henkel Canada; Henkel KGaA/Cospha] Tocopheryl acetate; natural antioxidant, protectant, and moisturizer for sun protection, skin and hair care prods.; clear yel. visc. oil, nearly odorless; usage level: 2-5%; 1250 d-alpha tocophernol USP units.

Copherol® F-1300. [Henkel/Cospha; Henkel Canada; Henkel KGaA/Cospha] D-α-tocopherol; natural antioxidant, protectant, and moisturizer for sun protection and skin and hair care prods.; brownish-red clear visc. oil, mild typ. odor; usage level: 2-5%; 1300 d-alpha-tocopherol USP units.

Copolymer 845. [ISP] PVP/dimethylaminoethylmethacrylate copolymer; CAS 30581-59-0; film-forming resin, substantive conditioner, hair fixative used in personal care prods. (blow-dry conditioners, setting lotions, gels, skin creams, hand lotions, soaps, shaving prods., colognes, deodorants, shampoos); lt. yel. clear visc. liq.; m.w. 1,000,000; pH 7.0; toxicology: LD50 (oral, rat) > 40 g/kg; not primary skin irritants; mild eye irritant; 20% act. in water.

Copolymer 937. [ISP] PVP/dimethylaminoethyl methacrylate copolymer; CAS 30581-59-0; substantive film-forming resin providing conditioning to hair prods., skin creams and lotions; lt. yel. hazy, highly visc. liq.; m.w. 1,000,000; pH 5.6; toxicology: LD50 (oral, rat) > 40 g/kg; not primary skin irritant; mild eye irritant; 20% aq. sol'n.

Copolymer 958. [ISP] PVP/dimethylaminoethyl methacrylate copolymer, ethanol; substantive film-forming resin providing conditioning to hair prods., skin creams and lotions; lt. yel. hazy visc. liq.; m.w. 100,000; pH 6.5; toxicology: LD50 (oral, rat) 14.5 g/kg; not primary skin irritant; moderate eye irritant; 50% ethanol sol'n.

Copolymer VC-713. [Henkel] Vinyl caprolactam/PVP/ dimethylaminoethyl methacrylate copolymer.

CoPrimrose. [Costec] Evening primrose oil; cosmetic ingred.

Coral STar. [Ikeda] Coral sand deriv. containing high calcium and magnesium content; raw material for cosmetics and toiletries; absorbs ingreds. and releases them on skin; for fragranced body powds., makeup, facial cleaners, scrub creams; also as food supplement providing calcium and magnesium; grayish powd., faint char. odor; 90% min. thru 350 mesh; 34% min. Ca, 1.5% min Mg.

Corn Oil, Refined. [Natural Oils Int'l.; Tri-K Industries] Corn oil, refined; CAS 8001-30-7; EINECS 232-281-2; cosmetic ingred.; amber clear oil, bland odor and taste; insol. in water; sp.gr. 0.914-0.921; iodine no. 102-130; sapon. no. 187-193; flash pt. (OC) 580 F; toxicology: nonhazardous; 0.05% max. moisture.

Corn-Pro™ 35. [Brooks Industries] Hydrolyzed corn protein; cosmetic ingredient for skin and hair care prods.; m.w. 1000; 35% act.

Corn Silk Extract HS 2969 G. [Grau Aromatics] Propylene glycol and corn silk extract; botanical extract.

Corona PNL (pure new lanolin). [Croda Inc.] Modified lanolin USP; superfatting emollient, emulsifier for personal care prods.; may be used at 100% conc.; yel. soft solid; m.p. 38-44 C; usage level: 2-10%.

Corona Lanolin. [Croda Chem. Ltd.] Anhyd. lanolin; CAS 8006-54-0; EINECS 232-348-6; nonionic; conditioning emollient, moisturizing agent, cosolv., plasticizer, w/o emulsifier, superfatting agent, wetting/dispersing agent, used in cosmetics, as pharmaceutical base; paste; oil-sol.; 100% conc.

Coronet Lanolin. [Croda Chem. Ltd.] Super refined cosmetic grade lanolin BP; CAS 8006-54-0; EINECS 232-348-6; nonionic; conditioning emollient, moisturizing agent, cosolv., plasticizer, w/o emulsifier, superfatting agent, wetting/dispersing agent, used as pharmaceutical base; minimum odor, color, batch variation in this grade; slightly higher m.p. than USP and BP standards; paste; 100% conc.

Corps Celeri. [Henkel/Cospha] Fragrance raw material for cosmetic, personal care, detergent, and cleaning prods.; colorless liq., aromatic herbal odor; b.p. 108-110 C; flash pt. 118 C.

Cosbiol. [Laserson SA] Squalane; CAS 111-01-3; EINECS 203-825-6; emollient, lubricant.

CoSept 200. [Costec] Quaternium-15; CAS 51229-78-8; EINECS 223-805-0; cosmetic preservative; USA, Europe approvals; usage level: 0.02-0.3%.

CoSept B. [Costec] Butylparaben; CAS 94-26-8; EINECS 202-318-7; preservative for cosmetics; usage level: 0.001-0.2%.

CoSept BNP. [Costec] 2-Bromo-2-nitropropane-1,3-diol; CAS 52-51-7; EINECS 200-143-0; preservative for cosmetics; usage level: 0.01-0.1%.

CoSept E. [Costec] Ethylparaben; CAS 120-47-8; EINECS 204-399-4; preservative for cosmetics; usage level: 0.08-1.0%.

CoSept M. [Costec] Methylparaben; CAS 99-76-3; EINECS 202-785-7; preservative for cosmetics; colorless; usage level: 0.1-1.0%; toxicology: nontoxic.

CoSept P. [Costec] Propylparaben; CAS 94-13-3; EINECS 202-307-7; cosmetic preservative; USA, Japan, Europe approvals; colorless; usage level: 0.02-1.0%; toxicology: nontoxic.

Cosiderm Masks. [Maybrook] Soluble collagen and col-

lagen; CAS 9007-34-5; freeze-dried collagen masks with high water absorp. capacity; upon wetting with water or protein/botanical sol'ns., provides revitalizing treatment improving skin plumping and elasticity.

Cosmedia Guar® C-261. [Henkel/Cospha; Henkel Canada; Henkel KGaA/Cospha] Guar hydroxypropyltrimonium chloride; CAS 65497-29-2; cationic; visc. builder; personal care prod. formulating; substantivity provides hair conditioning; stabilizer and thickener for emulsions and suspensions; antistat for hair and fibers; provides slip to finished formulations; wh. to yel. fine powd., char. intrinsic odor; water-disp.; pH 6.0-7.5 (1% aq.); 93-97% total solids.

Cosmedia® Polymer HSP 1180. [Henkel/Cospha; Henkel Canada] Polyacrylamidomethylpropane sulfonic acid; smooth feel agent for creams, lotions, liq. antiperspirants, shaving creams, soaps, nail polish removers; provides pleasant slip during applic. and lovely talc-like residual feeldisplay; clear visc. liq.

Cosmerlac. [Sandoz Nutrition] Nonfat dry milk; food ingred.

Cosmetic Alumina Hydrate. [HK Color Group] Alumina.

Cosmetic Black Iron Oxide 7075. [Clark Colors] Iron oxides.

Cosmetic Brown Oxide 7144. [Clark Colors] Iron oxides and talc.

Cosmetic Gelatin. [Hormel] Gelatin; CAS 9000-70-8; EINECS 232-554-6; visc. builder and thickening agent forming highly protective films and reducing irritation in personal care prods.; pale yel. powd.; m.w. 150,000; 55% (liq.).

Cosmetic Grade Casein. [Am. Casein] Casein; CAS 9000-71-9; EINECS 232-55-1.

Cosmetic Hydrophobic Black Oxide 9333. [Clark Colors] Iron oxides, min. oil, and methicone.

Cosmetic Hydrophobic Kaolin 9400. [Clark Colors] Kaolin, min. oil, and methicone.

Cosmetic Lanolin. [Fanning] Lanolin; CAS 8006-54-0; EINECS 232-348-6; emollient.

Cosmetic Lanolin. [R.I.T.A.] Lanolin; CAS 8006-54-0; EINECS 232-348-6; emollient.

Cosmetic Lanolin Anhydrous USP. [Croda Inc.] Lanolin; CAS 8006-54-0; EINECS 232-348-6; superfatting emollient, emulsifier for creams, lotions, lipsticks, make-up, sunscreen prods., pharmaceutical ointments, diaper rash preps., hemorrhoidal preps.; lt. amber soft solid; partly sol. in min. oil; m.p. 38-44 C; toxicology: LD50 (oral, rat) > 20 g/kg; mild skin and eye irritant.

Cosmetic Lanolin Anhydrous USP. [Lanaetex Prods.] Lanolin; CAS 8006-54-0; EINECS 232-348-6; cosmetic ingred.

Cosmetic Micro Blend Red Oxide 9268. [Clark Colors] Iron oxides.

Cosmetol® X. [CasChem] Unrefined castor oil USP, with antioxidant; CAS 8001-79-4; EINECS 232-293-8; deodorized specially refined grade of castor oil containing a food grade antioxidant; emollient, pigment wetter, cosolv., lubricant for cosmetics, makeup, antiperspirant sticks; pour pt. -23 C; acid no. 2; iodine no. 86; sapon. no. 180; hyd. no. 164.

Cosmica®. [Mearl] Pigment series where absorption colors are deposited directly on the mica, creating highly intense effects with minimal luster; suitable for most cosmetics.

Cosmocil CQ. [ICI Surf. Am.] Polyaminopropyl biguanide; CAS 27083-27-8; cosmetic preservative.

Cosmol 13. [Nisshin Oil Mills] Octyldodecyl lactate.

Cosmol 41. [Nisshin Oil Mills] Polyglyceryl-2 isostearate.

Cosmol 42. [Nisshin Oil Mills] Polyglyceryl-2 diisostearate.

Cosmol 43. [Nisshin Oil Mills] Polyglyceryl-2 triisostearate; CAS 120486-24-0.

Cosmol 44. [Nisshin Oil Mills] Polyglyceryl-2 tetraisostearate; CAS 121440-30-0.

Cosmol 102. [Nisshin Oil Mills] PPG-7/succinic acid copolymer.

Cosmol 168AR. [Nisshin Oil Mills] Dipentaerythrityl hexahydoxystearate/stearate/rosinate.

Cosmol 168E. [Nisshin Oil Mills] Dipentaerythrityl hexahydoxystearate/isostearate.

Cosmol 168I. [Nisshin Oil Mills] Dipentaerythrityl pentaoctanoate/behenate.

Cosmol 168M. [Nisshin Oil Mills] Dipentaerythrityl hexahydroxystearate.

Cosmol 222. [Nisshin Oil Mills] Diisostearyl malate; CAS 67763-18-2.

Cosmol 525. [Nisshin Oil Mills] Neopentyl glycol dioctanoate; CAS 28510-23-8.

Cosmol 812. [Nisshin Oil Mills] Isostearyl myristate; CAS 72576-81-9.

Cosmol O-42T. [Nisshin Oil Mills] Polyglyceryl-2 dioleate; CAS 9007-48-1; emulsifier.

Cosmopon 35. [Auschem SpA] Sodium lauryl sulfate; CAS 151-21-3; EINECS 205-788-1; anionic; spray-dried wool detergent powd., hand cleaner; paste; 48% conc.

Cosmopon BL. [Auschem SpA] Fatty alkanolamide sulfosuccinate; CAS 68784-08-7; anionic; rug shampoo, bubble bath, conditioner; paste; 50% conc.

Cosmopon BLM. [Auschem SpA] Sodium alkyl sulfosuccinate; anionic; cream shampoos; paste; 30% conc.

Cosmopon BS. [Auschem SpA] Sodium laureth sulfate, sodium lauryl sulfate, and cocamide DEA; anionic/nonionic; formulated bubble bath; liq./paste; 52% conc.

Cosmopon BT. [Auschem SpA] Disodium laureth sulfosuccinate; CAS 39354-45-5; anionic; nonirritating surfactant for baby shampoo and bubble baths; liq.; 40% conc.

Cosmopon HC. [Auschem SpA] MEA-lauryl sulfate, disodium cocamido MEA-sulfosuccinate, and glycol stearate.

Cosmopon LE 50. [Auschem SpA] Sodium laureth sulfate; CAS 9004-82-4; 15826-16-1; anionic; personal care prods. and liq. detergents; paste; sol. in cold water; 50% conc.

Cosmopon ME. [Auschem SpA] MEA-laureth sulfate; cosmetic surfactant and raw material.

Cosmopon MO. [Auschem SpA] MEA lauryl sulfate; CAS 4722-98-9; EINECS 225-214-3; anionic; raw material for liq. detergent; liq.; 32% conc.

Cosmopon MP. [Auschem SpA] Sodium laureth sulfate and glycol stearate; pearling formulated shampoo; liq./paste; 31% conc.

Cosmopon MT. [Auschem SpA] Alkylether sulfate and amides/pearling agent blend; pearling formulated shampoo; liq./paste; 37% conc.

Cosmopon SES. [Auschem SpA] Sodium 2-ethylhexylsulfate; CAS 126-92-1; EINECS 204-812-8; anionic; detergent, wetting agent; liq.; 30% conc.

Cosmopon TR. [Auschem SpA] TEA-lauryl sulfate; CAS 139-96-8; EINECS 205-388-7; anionic; hair shampoo, bubble bath, car wash, liq. hand cleaner; liq.; 40% conc.

Cosmowax J. [Croda Inc.] Cetearyl alcohol and ceteareth-20; nonionic; o/w emulsifier and stabilizer with body, opacity, and conditioning props. for personal care prods., pharmaceutical creams; creamy wh. waxy solid; low odor; HLB 8.5; m.p. 47–55 C; acid no. 0.5 max.; iodine no. 2 max.; sapon. no. 1 max.; usage level: 2-15%; 100% conc.

Cosmowax K. [Croda Inc.] Stearyl alcohol and ceteareth-20; nonionic; emulsifier, stabilizer with body, opacity and conditioning props. for personal care prods. and pharmaceuticals; creamy wh. waxy solid; low odor; HLB 8.0; m.p. 55–63 C; acid no. 0.5 max.; iodine no. 2 max.; sapon. no. 1 max.; usage level: 2-10%; 100% conc.

Cosmowax P. [Croda Inc.] Cetearyl alcohol, ceteareth-20; nonionic; emulsifier, emulsion stabilizer for lotions, creams; wh. to off-wh. flakes; m.p. 46-53 C; usage level:

2-15%.

Costaulon. [Hercules/PFW] Ethyl butyl valerolactone; CAS 67770-79-0; EINECS 267-048-4.

Costausol. [Hercules/PFW] Triethyl citrate and ethyl butyl valerolactone.

Covachip. [Les Colorants Wackherr] Dispersions of minerals and org. pigments in plasticized nitrocellulose chips; cosmetics ingred.

Covacryl IIO, III. [Les Colorants Wackherr] Polyacrylic acid; CAS 9003-01-4; hydrophilic polymers for cosmetics.

Covafluid AMD. [Les Colorants Wackherr] Hydrophobic starch; cosmetics ingred.

Covafluor. [Les Colorants Wackherr] Pigments and wh. minerals coated with perfluoroalkyl phosphate; pigments with water/oil repellency; improve stability, dispersibility, and color development in cosmetic prods.; impart good spreadability; provide resist. to perspiration and sebum in waterproof or long-lasting prods.; provide a nonocclusive coating permeable to oxygen.

Covafresh. [Les Colorants Wackherr] An aq. sol'n. of menthyl lactate; CAS 59259-38-0; EINECS 261-678-3; cooling agent for skin preps.

Covalac. [Les Colorants Wackherr] Lakes of organic and natural dyes; colorants for cosmetics.

Covalim. [Les Colorants Wackherr] Min. oil dispersions; cosmetics ingred.

Covamat. [Les Colorants Wackherr] A blend of pigments and lauroyl lysine; combines the diffraction props. of pyrogenic materials with the reflective props. of a nonpearlizing form of microfine mica; gives a transparent luminance and soft focus effect on the skin.

Covanail. [Les Colorants Wackherr] High pigment conc. nail lacquer concs. in an acrylic base.

Covanor. [Les Colorants Wackherr] Organic pigments for cosmetics use.

Covapate. [Les Colorants Wackherr] Castor oil dispersions; cosmetics ingred.

Covasil. [Les Colorants Wackherr] Pigments and wh. minerals coated with a film of dimethicone; pigments with water repellency; improve dispersion of inorg. pigments and titanium dioxide in powds. and foundations; reduce oil absorp. of pigments; for makeup and other cosmetics.

Covasol. [Les Colorants Wackherr] Water-sol. dyes for cosmetics; includes FDA certified dyes.

Covasop. [Les Colorants Wackherr] Propylene glycol dispersions; cosmetics ingred.

Covasorb. [Les Colorants Wackherr] Sorbitol dispersions; cosmetics ingred.

CoVera. [Costec] Aloe vera gel; moisturizer, soothing/healing aid for personal care.

CoVera Dry. [Costec] Aloe vera gel; cosmetic ingred.

Coverleaf PC-2035. [Ikeda] Sericite plate powd. coated with titanium dioxide; base pigment and uv absorber for pressed powds.; provides best affinity to skin in series; wh. or sl. ylsh. powd.; pH 7.5-9.5 (5% susp.); 27-33% TiO_2.

Coverleaf PC-2055M. [Ikeda] Mica plate powd. coated with titanium dioxide; base pigment and uv absorber providing lighter touch in pressed powds.; wh. or sl. ylsh. powd.; pH 7.5-9.5 (5% susp.); 45-55% TiO_2.

Coverleaf PC-2055T. [Ikeda] Talc plate powd. coated with titanium dioxide; base pigment providing good coverage on skin and lighter touch than conventional titanium dioxide; for pressed powds.; wh. or sl. ylsh. powd.; pH 8.5-10.5 (5% susp.); 45-55% TiO_2.

Covi-Ox® T-30P. [Henkel/Cospha] Tocopherol; antioxidant, vitamin E source.

Covi-Ox® T-50. [Henkel/Cospha; Henkel Canada] Tocopherol; natural antioxidant and blocking agent for cosmetic formulations; brnsh.-red visc. oil; char. odor; b.p. 190–220 C (@ 0.1 mm Hg); 500 mg/g min. total natural tocopherols;

7–9% d-α; 32–38% d-γ and d-β; 10–15% d-δ.

Covi-Ox® T-70. [Henkel/Cospha; Henkel Canada] Tocopherol; natural antioxidant and blocking agent for cosmetics and food industries; brwnsh. red visc. liq.

Covipherol T-75. [Henkel/Cospha; Henkel Canada] Mixed d-tocopherols; antioxidant in food and cosmetic prods.; clear brnsh-red visc. oil.

Covitol 80/20M. [Henkel/Polymers, Fine Chem.] Tocopherol; antioxidant, vitamin E source.

Covitol 1100. [Henkel/Polymers, Fine Chem.] Tocopheryl acetate; antioxidant; pharm. grade natural Vitamin E; 809 mg/g min. assay.

Covitol 1185. [Henkel] Tocopheryl succinate; CAS 4345-03-3; EINECS 224-403-8; antioxidant; pharm. grade natural Vitamin E; wh. gran. powd.; bland odor; 960 mg/g min. assay.

Covitol 1210. [Henkel/Polymers, Fine Chem.] Tocopheryl succinate; CAS 4345-03-3; EINECS 224-403-8; antioxidant; pharm. grade natural Vitamin E; wh. to off-wh. cryst. powd.; 960 mg/g min. assay.

Covitol 1360. [Henkel/Polymers, Fine Chem.] Tocopheryl acetate; antioxidant; pharm. grade natural Vitamin E; yel. clear visc. liq.; m.p. 25 C; 960 mg/g min. assay.

Covitol F-350M. [Henkel/Polymers, Fine Chem.] Tocopherol; antioxidant; pharm. grade natural Vitamin E; cream powd.; 235 mg/g of d-α tocopherol conc. FCC plus 59 mg/g of d-β, d-γ, and d-δ tocopherol FCC.

Covitol F-600. [Henkel/Polymers, Fine Chem.] d-α-Tocopherol conc. FCC; antioxidant; pharm. grade natural Vitamin E; 403 mg/g min. assay.

Covitol F-1000. [Henkel/Polymers, Fine Chem.] Tocopherol; antioxidant; pharm. grade natural Vitamin E; brn.-red clear visc. oil; mild odor; 671 mg/g min. assay.

CPC. [Zeeland] Cetylpyridinium chloride; CAS 123-03-5; EINECS 204-593-9; emulsifier; antibacterial, preservative for cosmetics and pharmaceuticals.

CPC Peptide. [Solabia] Polylysine.

CPC Sumquat 6060. [Zeeland] Cetylpyridinium chloride; CAS 123-03-5; EINECS 204-593-9; emulsifier; antibacterial, and preservative for cosmetics, toiletries, and pharmaceuticals.

CPH-3-SE. [C.P. Hall] Propylene glycol oleate; CAS 1330-80-9; EINECS 215-549-3; personal care surfactant.

CPH-27-N. [C.P. Hall] PEG-4 laurate; CAS 9004-81-3; nonionic; solubilizer and emulsifier; Gardner 3 clear oily liq.; sol. in toluene, kerosene, ethanol, acetone; disp. in water; sp.gr. 0.985; f.p. 5 C; acid no. 4; sapon. no. 139; flash pt. 199 C; ref. index 1.454; 100% conc.

CPH-30-N. [C.P. Hall] PEG-8 laurate; CAS 9004-81-3; emulsifier.

CPH-31-N. [C.P. Hall] Glyceryl oleate; nonionic; antiblocking agent; amber liq.; m.w. 340; sol. in toluene, kerosene, ethanol, acetone, propylene glycol, min. oil; sp.gr. 0.943; f.p. 9 C; HLB 3.7; acid no. 3.0; sapon. no. 168; ref. index 1.467; 100% conc.

CPH-34-N. [C.P. Hall] Glyceryl laurate; CAS 142-18-7; EINECS 205-526-6; cosmetic emulsifier.

CPH-35-N. [C.P. Hall] Glyceryl ricinoleate; CAS 141-08-2; EINECS 205-455-0; emulsifier.

CPH-37-NA. [C.P. Hall] Glycol stearate; CAS 111-60-4; EINECS 203-886-9; emulsifier, opacifier, pearlescent for cosmetics; wh. flake; m.w. 300; sol. in toluene, ethanol, acetone, min. oil; m.p. 57 C; acid no. 3.0; sapon. no. 187.

CPH-40-N. [C.P. Hall] PEG-8 oleate; CAS 9004-96-0; emulsifier.

CPH-41-N. [C.P. Hall] PEG-12 oleate; CAS 9004-96-0; personal care surfactant.

CPH-43-N. [C.P. Hall] PEG-12 laurate; CAS 9004-81-3; nonionic; solubilizer and dispersant; solid; sol. in toluene, kerosene, ethanol, acetone, water; sp.gr. 1.050; HLB

14.6; f.p. 25 C; flash pt. 202 C; acid no. 4.0; sapon. no. 69; ref. index 1.461; 100% conc.

CPH-46-N. [C.P. Hall] PEG-8 oleate; CAS 9004-96-0; emulsifier.

CPH-50-N. [C.P. Hall] PEG-8 stearate; CAS 9004-99-3; emulsifier.

CPH-52-SE. [C.P. Hall] Propylene glycol stearate SE; wh. to cream solid; m.w. 333; sol. in toluene, ethanol, min. oil; disp. hot in water; m.p. 38. C; acid no. 17; sapon. no. 170.

CPH-53-N. [C.P. Hall] Glyceryl stearate.

CPH-79-N. [C.P. Hall] PEG-8 dilaurate; CAS 9005-02-1; personal care surfactant.

CPH-90-N. [C.P. Hall] PEG-20 stearate; CAS 9004-99-3; emulsifier.

CPH-104-DC-SE. [C.P. Hall] PEG-2 stearate SE; CAS 9004-99-3; emulsifier.

CPH-104-DG-SE. [C.P. Hall] PEG-2 stearate SE; CAS 9004-99-3; emulsifier.

CPH-144-N. [C.P. Hall] Glyceryl stearate.

CPH-213-N. [C.P. Hall] PEG-12 dioleate; CAS 9005-07-6; personal care surfactant.

CPH-233-N. [C.P. Hall] PEG-8 oleate; CAS 9004-96-0; emulsifier.

CPH-327-N. [C.P. Hall] PPG-17 dioleate.

CPH-360-N. [C.P. Hall] Glycol distearate; CAS 627-83-8; EINECS 211-014-3; cosmetic ingred.

CPH-361-N. [C.P. Hall] PEG-8 dilaurate; CAS 9005-02-1; personal care surfactant.

CPH-380-N. [C.P. Hall] Stearamide MEA; CAS 111-57-9; EINECS 203-883-2; personal care surfactant, thickener, pearlescent; wh. solid; m.w. 600; sol. in ethanol; partly sol. in hexane, toluene, kerosene, propylene glycol; sp.gr. 0.971; m.p. 80 C; acid no. 17; iodine no. 1.0; sapon. no. 107.

CPH-399-N. [C.P. Hall] Triolein; CAS 122-32-7; EINECS 204-534-7; emollient.

Crafol AP-11. [Pulcra SA] Oleth-3 phosphate; CAS 39464-69-2; anionic; foam stabilizer, antistat, conditioner for cosmetic formulations; detergent and antistat for textile finishing processes; liq.; 100% conc.

Cremao CS-33. [Aarhus Oliefabrik A/S] Palm kernel glycerides.

Cremao CS-34. [Aarhus Oliefabrik A/S] Palm kernel glycerides.

Cremao CS-36. [Aarhus Oliefabrik A/S] Palm kernel glycerides.

Cremeol HF-52, HF-62. [Aarhus Oliefabrik A/S] Hydrog. veg. oil; CAS 68334-28-1; EINECS 269-820-6; emollient, emulsifier.

Cremeol SH. [Aarhus Oliefabrik A/S] Shorea butter.

Cremerol HMG. [Amerchol] Hydroxylated milk glycerides; emollient, aux. emulsifier for personal care prods.; wh. semisolid, char. pleasant odor; sol. in min. oil, castor oil, isopropyl palmitate, caprylic/capric triglyceride; insol. in water, propylene glycol; 100% act.

Cremogen AF. [Haarmann & Reimer] Propylene glycol, ethoxydiglycol, nettle extract, balm mint oil, horse chestnut extract, coltsfoot extract, horsetail extract, birch leaf extract, matricaria extract, sage extract, rosemary extract; botanical extract.

Cremogen M-I 739001. [Haarmann & Reimer] Propylene glycol, ethoxydiglycol, witch hazel extract, matricaria extract, yarrow extract, and arnica extract; botanical extract.

Cremogen Aloe Vera. [Haarmann & Reimer] Propylene glycol, ethoxydiglycol, and aloe extract; botanical extract.

Cremogen Camomile Forte. [Haarmann & Reimer] Propylene glycol, ethoxydiglycol, and matricaria extract; botanical extract.

Cremogen Chamomile 739012. [Haarmann & Reimer] Propylene glycol, ethoxydiglycol, and chamomile extract;

botanical extract.

Cremogen Hamamelis 739008. [Haarmann & Reimer] Propylene glycol, ethoxydiglycol, and witch hazel extract; botanical extract.

Cremogen Hamamelis Dest. 1841 739022. [Haarmann & Reimer] Witch hazel distillate.

Cremogen Pine Needles 739007. [Haarmann & Reimer] Propylene glycol, ethoxydiglycol, pine needle extract; botanical extract.

Cremogen Yarrow 739017. [Haarmann & Reimer] Propylene glycol, ethoxydiglycol, yarrow extract; botanical extract.

Cremophor® A 6. [BASF; BASF AG] Ceteareth-6; CAS 68439-49-6; nonionic; emulsifier for o/w cosmetic preps.; wh. wax; sol. in water, alcohol; drop pt. 41-45 C; HLB 10-12; acid no. < 1; iodine no. < 1; sapon. no. < 3; hyd. no. 115-135; 100% conc.

Cremophor® A 11. [BASF AG] Ceteareth-11; CAS 68439-49-6; nonionic; emulsifier for cosmetic and pharmaceutical preparations; wh. wax; sol. in water, alcohol; sp.gr. 0.964–0.968 (60 C); drop pt. 34-38 C; HLB 12–14; acid no. < 1; iodine no. < 1; sapon. no. < 1; hyd. no. 70-80; pH 6–7; 100% act.

Cremophor® A 25. [BASF; BASF AG] Ceteareth-25; CAS 68439-49-6; nonionic; emulsifier for cosmetic and pharmaceutical preparations; wh. powd.; sol. in water, alcohol; sp.gr. 1.020–1.028 (60 C); drop pt. 44-48 C; HLB 15–17; acid no. < 1; iodine no. < 1; sapon. no. < 3; hyd. no. 35-45; pH 5–7; 100% act.

Cremophor® EL. [BASF; BASF AG] PEG-35 castor oil; CAS 61791-12-6; nonionic; solubilizer, emulsifier used for essential oils, pharmaceuticals, cosmetics, veterinary medicine; pale yel. liq.; sol. in water, ethanol, propanol, ethyl acetate, chloroform, CCl_4, benzene, toluene, and xylene; sp.gr. 1.05–1.06; visc. 700–850 cps; HLB 12–14; acid no. < 2; sapon no. 65–70; ref. index 1.471; pH 6–8 (10% aq.); 100% act.

Cremophor® GO32. [BASF; BASF AG] Polyglyceryl-3 dioleate; CAS 79665-94-4; nonionic; w/o emulsifier for cosmetic emulsions; liq.; 100% conc.

Cremophor® GS32. [BASF; BASF AG] Polyglyceryl-3 distearate; CAS 94423-19-5; w/o emulsifier for nonpolar oils for cosmetics applics.; also forms o/w emulsions; powd.

Cremophor® RH 40. [BASF; BASF AG] PEG-40 hydrog. castor oil; CAS 61788-85-0; nonionic; solubilizer for essential oils and perfumery, emulsifier; for cosmetics and pharmaceuticals; water-wh. visc. liq. or soft paste, very little odor or taste; sol. in water, ethanol, IPA, n-propanol, ethyl acetate, benzene, toluene, and xylene; HLB 14–16; acid no. ≤ 1; iodine no. ≤ 1; sapon. no. 50-60; ynd. no. 60-75; pH 6–7 (10% aq.); toxicology: LD50 (oral, rat) > 16 g/kg; 100% act.

Cremophor® RH 60. [BASF; BASF AG] PEG-60 hydrog. castor oil; CAS 61788-85-0; nonionic; solubilizer, emulsifier for essential oils and perfumes; for cosmetics; wh. visc. liq. or soft paste; sol. in water, ethanol, IPA, n-propanol, ethyl acetate, benzene, toluene, and xylene; HLB 15-17; acid no. ≤ 1; iodine no. ≤ 1; sapon. no. 40-50; hyd. no. 50-70; pH 6-7 (10% aq.); toxicology: LD50 (oral, rat) > 16 g/kg; 100% act.

Cremophor® RH 410. [BASF AG] PEG-40 hydrog. castor oil; CAS 61788-85-0; nonionic; solubilizer and emulsifier for cosmetics and pharmaceuticals; sl. turbid visc. liq.; sol. in water, ethanol, IPA, n-propanol, ethyl acetate, benzene, toluene, and xylene; visc. ≤ 1800 mPa·s; HLB 14–16; acid no. ≤ 1; iodine no. ≤ 1; sapon. no. 45-55; pH 6-7 (10% aq.); 90% act.

Cremophor® RH 455. [BASF AG] PEG-40 hydrog. castor oil and propylene glycol; CAS 61788-85-0; nonionic; solubi-

lizer for essential oils and perfumery, emulsifier; for cosmetics and pharmaceuticals; visc. liq.; sol. in water, ethanol, IPA, n-propanol, ethyl acetate, benzene, toluene, and xylene; visc. 1000–1500 cps; HLB 14–16; acid no. ≤ 1; iodine no. ≤ 1; sapon. no. 45-55; ref. index 1.459-1.464; pH 6-7 (10% aq.); 90% act.

Cremophor® S 9. [BASF; BASF AG] PEG-8 stearate; CAS 9004-99-3; nonionic; emulsifier for o/w type, thickening agent; suspension stabilizer; lubricating and antitack effects; for cosmetics and pharmaceuticals; ylsh. wh. visc. liq.; sol. in water, alcohols, acetone, ethyl acetate, chloroform, benzene, castor oil, and oleic acid; sp.gr. 0.97 (60 C); HLB 12; acid no. 2; sapon. no. 88–98; 100% act.

Cremophor® WO 7. [BASF; BASF AG] PEG-7 hydrogenated castor oil; CAS 61788-85-0; nonionic; emulsifier for cosmetic w/o preps.; visc. liq.; HLB 5.0; 100% conc.

Crestalan A. [Croda Chem. Ltd.] Isopropyl myristate and lanolin oil.

Crestalan B. [Croda Chem. Ltd.] Isopropyl myristate and lanolin oil.

Crestalan CB3910. [Croda Chem. Ltd.] Isopropyl palmitate and lanolin oil.

CR Grit. [Ichimaru Pharcos] Corn cob powd.

Crill 1. [Croda Inc.; Croda Surf. Ltd.] Sorbitan laurate; CAS 1338-39-2; nonionic; emulsifier, pigment dispersant, cosolv., wetting agent, antifoam, visc. reducer, mold release, antiblock agent, corrosion inhibitor, lubricant, antistat; used for cosmetics, food and food pkg., insecticides and herbicides, leather treatment, metalworking fluids, oil slick dispersing, paints and inks, pharmaceuticals, plastics, polishes, textiles; pale yel. clear visc. liq.; sol. in ethanol, oleyl alcohol, min. oil; HLB 8.6; sapon. no. 158-170; 98% conc.

Crill 2. [Croda Inc.; Croda Surf. Ltd.] Sorbitan palmitate; CAS 26266-57-9; EINECS 247-568-8; nonionic; see Crill 1; pale tan hard waxy solid; partially sol. in propylene glycol, ethyl and oleyl alcohols, olive oil, oleic acid; m.p. 46 C; HLB 6.7; sapon. no. 140–150; 98% conc.

Crill 3. [Croda Inc.; Croda Surf. Ltd.] Sorbitan stearate NF; CAS 1338-41-6; EINECS 215-664-9; nonionic; emulsifier, lubricant, antistat; o/w emulsions; cosmetic and pharmaceutical creams and lotions; polishes; insecticides, herbicides; metal cleaners; buffing compds.; textile lubricants; food applics.; pale tan hard waxy solid; low odor; partially sol. in oleyl alcohol, olive oil, oleic acid; insol. in water; m.p. 51–54 C; HLB 4.7; acid no. 5-10; sapon. no. 147–157; hyd. no. 235-260; usage level: 0.5-5%; toxicology: LD50 (oral, rat) > 31 g/kg; nonirritating to eyes; 98% conc.

Crill 4. [Croda Inc.; Croda Surf. Ltd.] Sorbitan oleate NF; CAS 1338-43-8; EINECS 215-665-4; nonionic; w/o emulsifier, wetting agent, pigment dispersant, coupler, antifoam; cosmetic and pharmaceutical applic.; aerosol polishes; insecticidal sprays; inks and surf. coatings; metal working lubricants; cutting oils; textile lubricants; dry cleaning operations; food process antifoam; oil slick dispersant; amber visc. liq.; sol. in ethyl, isopropyl, and oleyl alcohols, min. oil, IPM, olive oil, oleic acid; HLB 4.3; acidno. 5.5-7.5; sapon. no. 147–160; hyd. no. 193-209; usage level: 0.5-5%; toxicology: LD50 (oral, rat) > 40 g/kg; nonirritating to eyes; 98% conc.

Crill 6. [Croda Inc.; Croda Surf. Ltd.] Sorbitan isostearate; CAS 71902-01-7; nonionic; w/o emulsifier, wetting agent, pigment dispersant for creams, lotions, aerosols; pale yel. clear visc. liq.; sol. in min. oil, IPA, olive oil, partly sol. in oleyl alcohol, IPM; HLB 4.7; acid no. 8 max.; sapon. no. 143–153; hyd. no. 220-250; usage level: 0.5-5%; toxicology: LD50 (oral, rat) > 16 g/kg (10% aq.); moderate skin irritant; nonirritating to eyes; 98% conc.

Crill 35. [Croda Inc.; Croda Surf. Ltd.] Sorbitan tristearate;

CAS 26658-19-5; EINECS 247-891-4; nonionic; emulsifier, lubricant, antistat for cosmetic, pharmaceutical, food, and industrial applics.; pale tan hard waxy solid; partly sol. in oleyl alcohol, min. and olive oil, IPM, oleic acid; m.p. 48 C; HLB 2.1; sapon. no. 176–188; 98% conc.

Crill 41. [Croda Chem. Ltd.] Sorbitan tristearate; CAS 26658-19-5; EINECS 247-891-4; emulsifier.

Crill 43. [Croda Inc.; Croda Surf. Ltd.] Sorbitan sesquioleate; CAS 8007-43-0; EINECS 232-360-1; nonionic; w/o emulsifier, wetting agent, pigment dispersant; for cosmetic, pharmaceutical, food, and industrial applics.; amber visc. liq.; sol. in oleyl alcohol, min. and olive oil, oleic acid; HLB 3.7; sapon. no. 149–160; 98% conc.

Crill 45. [Croda Inc.; Croda Surf. Ltd.] Sorbitan trioleate; CAS 26266-58-0; EINECS 247-569-3; nonionic; w/o emulsifier, wetting agent, pigment dispersant; for cosmetic, pharmaceutical, food, and industrial applics.; amber visc. liq.; sol. in oleyl alcohol, min. and olive oil, IPM, oleic acid; HLB 4.3; sapon. no. 172–186; 98% conc.

Crill 50. [Croda Surf. Ltd.] Sorbitan oleate, tech.; CAS 1338-43-8; EINECS 215-665-4; nonionic; emulsifier, dispersant, wetting agent for cosmetic, pharmaceutical, food, and industrial applics.; liq.; 98% conc.

Crillet 1. [Croda Inc.; Croda Chem. Ltd.] Polysorbate 20; CAS 9005-64-5; nonionic; solubilizer, emulsifier, dispersant, wetting agent; often combined with a member of the Crill range in emulsification systems; used in cosmetics, food and food pkg., household prods., insecticides, herbicides, metalworking fluids, paints and inks, pharmaceuticals, textiles; clear, yel. clear liq.; low odor; sol. in water, ethyl and oleyl alcohol, oleic acid; HLB 16.7; sapon. no. 40–51; surf. tens. 38.5 dynes/cm (0.1%); 97% conc.

Crillet 2. [Croda Chem. Ltd.] PEG-20 sorbitan palmitate; CAS 9005-66-7; nonionic; emulsifier, solubilizer, wetting agent for cosmetic, pharmaceutical, food, and industrial applics.; paste; HLB 15.6; 97% conc.

Crillet 3. [Croda Inc.; Croda Chem. Ltd.] Polysorbate 60 NF; CAS 9005-67-8; nonionic; o/w emulsifier for cosmetics and pharmaceuticals, dispersant for insecticides, herbicides, cattle dyes, penetrant, leveling agent, lubricant, antistat; yel. liq. gels to soft solid on cooling; sol. in ethyl, isopropyl, and oleyl alcohol, oleic acid; partly sol. in water; HLB 14.9; acid no. 2 max.; sapon. no. 45–55; hyd. no. 81-96; surf. tens. 42.5 dynes/cm (0.1%); usage level: 0.5-5%; toxicology: LD50 (oral, rat) > 38 g/kg; nonirritating to eyes; 97% conc.

Crillet 4. [Croda Inc.; Croda Chem. Ltd.] Polysorbate 80 NF; CAS 9005-65-6; nonionic; emulsifier, dispersant, solubilizer, lubricant, detergent, antistat, wetting agent for cosmetics, pharmaceuticals, polishes, insecticides, leather degreasing, veterinary prods.; clear yel. amber liq.; faint char. odor; sol. in water, ethyl, isopropyl, and oleyl alcohols, oleic acid; HLB 15.0; acid no. 2 max.; sapon. no. 45-55; hyd. no. 65-80; surf. tens. 42.5 dynes/cm (0.1%); usage level: 0.5-5%; toxicology: LD50 (oral, rat) > 38 g/kg; nonirritating to eyes; 97% conc.

Crillet 6. [Croda Inc.; Croda Chem. Ltd.] PEG-20 sorbitan isostearate; CAS 66794-58-9; nonionic; o/w emulsifier, solubilizer for fragrances and perfumes; for creams, lotions, ointments; improved resistance to oxidation; clear yel. liq.; sol. in water, ethyl, isopropyl, and oleyl alcohols, oleic acid, xylene, trichlorethylene; HLB 14.9; acid no. 2 max.; sapon. no. 40–50; hyd. no. 65-85; surf. tens. 38.6 dynes/cm (0.1%); usage level: 0.5-5%; 97% conc.

Crillet 11. [Croda Chem. Ltd.] PEG-4 sorbitan laurate; CAS 9005-64-5; nonionic; emulsifier, solubilizer, wetting agent for cosmetic, pharmaceutical, food, and industrial applics.; liq.; 97% conc.

Crillet 31. [Croda Chem. Ltd.] Polysorbate 61; CAS 9005-67-8; nonionic; emulsifier, solubilizer, wetting agent for cos-

metic, pharmaceutical, food, and industrial applics.; solid; 97% conc.

Crillet 35. [Croda Chem. Ltd.] Polysorbate 65; CAS 9005-71-4; nonionic; emulsifier, solubilizer, wetting agent for cosmetic, pharmaceutical, food, and industrial applics.; cream/buff waxy solid; sol. in ethyl and oleyl alcohols, oleic acid, trichlorethylene, partly sol. in water; HLB 10.5; sapon. no. 88–98; surf. tens. 42.5 dynes/cm (0.1%); 97% conc.

Crillet 41. [Croda Chem. Ltd.] PEG-5 sorbitan oleate; CAS 9005-65-6; nonionic; emulsifier, solubilizer, wetting agent for cosmetic, pharmaceutical, food, and industrial applics.; liq.; HLB 10.0; 97% conc.

Crillet 45. [Croda Chem. Ltd.] Polysorbate 85; CAS 9005-70-3; nonionic; emulsifier, solubilizer, wetting agent for cosmetic, pharmaceutical, food, and industrial applics.; clear amber visc. liq.; sol. in ethyl and oleyl alcohols, IPM, oleic acid, kerosene, trichlorethylene, butyl stearate; HLB 11.0; sapon. no. 82–95; surf. tens. 41 dynes/cm (0.1%); 97% conc.

Crillon ODE. [Croda Surf. Ltd.] Oleamide DEA; CAS 93-83-4; EINECS 202-281-7; nonionic; emulsifier, stabilizer, skin protectant, lubricant, anti-irritant used in personal care prods.; additive for cutting fluids and sol. cutting oils; liq.

Crodacel QL. [Croda Inc.] Laurdimonium hydroxyethyl cellulose; cationic; conditioner improving foaming for skin and hair care prods.; pale yel. sol'n.; m.w. 10,000; water-sol.; usage level: 1-4%; 20% act.

Crodacel QM. [Croda Inc.] Cocodimonium hydroxyethyl cellulose; cationic; conditioner improving foaming and imparting body to skin and hair care prods.; clear visc. sol'n.; m.w. 10,000; usage level: 1-4%; 20% act.

Crodacel QS. [Croda Inc.] Steardimonium hydroxyethyl cellulose; cationic; conditioner improving foaming and imparting body to skin and hair care prods.; opaque visc. sol'n.; m.w. 10,000; usage level: 1-4%; 20% act.

Crodacid B. [Croda Inc.] Behenic acid; CAS 112-85-6; EINECS 204-010-8; gellant for stick formulations when neutralized; wh. solid; usage level: 0.5-5%.

Crodacid PD3160. [Croda Universal Ltd.] Palmitic acid; CAS 57-10-3; EINECS 200-312-9; surfactant intermediate; soap and cosmetic formulations.

Crodacol A-10. [Croda Inc.] Oleyl alcohol; CAS 143-28-2; EINECS 205-597-3; emollient.

Crodacol C-70. [Croda Inc.] Cetyl alcohol; CAS 36653-82-4; EINECS 253-149-0; sec. emulsifier, thickener, opacifier, and structural agent in anhyd. stick systems; wh. flakes.; usage level: 2-30%.

Crodacol C-90. [Croda Chem. Ltd.] Cetyl alcohol; CAS 36653-82-4; EINECS 253-149-0; cosmetic ingred.

Crodacol C-95NF. [Croda Inc.] Cetyl alcohol NF; CAS 36653-82-4; EINECS 253-149-0; primary structural agent in antiperspirant sticks; emulsion thickener, stabilizer, and coemulsifier for pharmaceutical suppositories, lotions, creams, and ointments; wh. to cream flakes; sol. in IPA; sol. warm in min. oil, propylene glycol; m.p. 45-50 C; acid no. 0.3 max.; iodine no. 3 max.; sapon. no. 1 max.; hyd. no. 218-238; usage level: 2-30%; toxicology: LD50 (oral, rat) > 20 g/kg; mild eye and skin irritant.

Crodacol CS-50. [Croda Inc.; Croda Chem. Ltd.] Cetearyl alcohol; emollient; hair and skin lubricant; wh. to cream flakes; oil-sol.; m.p. 48-54 C; acid no. 0.5 max.; iodine no. 1 max.; sapon. no. 1 max.; hyd. no. 214-222; usage level: 2-30%.

Crodacol GP. [Croda Inc.] Cetearyl alcohol, polysorbate 60, PEG-150 stearate, steareth-20.

Crodacol S-70. [Croda Inc.] Stearyl alcohol; CAS 112-92-5; EINECS 204-017-6; sec. emulsifier, thickener, opacifier, and structural agent in anhyd. stick systems; wh. to cream flakes; m.p. 52-55 C; acid no. 0.5 max.; iodine no. 3 max.; sapon. no. 1 max.; hyd. no. 207-215; usage level: 2-30%.

Crodacol S-95NF. [Croda Inc.; Croda Chem. Ltd.] Stearyl alcohol NF; CAS 112-92-5; EINECS 204-017-6; primary structural agent in antiperspirant sticks; emulsion thickener, stabilizer, and coemulsifier for pharmaceutical suppositories, lotions, creams, and ointments; wh. flakes; sol. in IPA; sol. warm in min. oil, propylene glycol; usage level: 2-30%; toxicology: LD50 (oral, rat) > 5 g/kg; nonirritating to skin; minimal eye irritant.

Crodafos 25 D2 Acid. [Croda Chem. Ltd.] PEG-2 C12-15 ether phosphate; CAS 68071-35-2; anionic; hair conditioner for shampoo formulations; liq.; 99% conc.

Crodafos 25 D5 Acid. [Croda Chem. Ltd.] PEG-5 C12-15 ether phosphate; CAS 68071-35-2; anionic; hair conditioner for shampoo formulations; liq.; 99% conc.

Crodafos 25 D10 Acid. [Croda Chem. Ltd.] PEG-10 C12-15 ether phosphate; CAS 68071-35-2; anionic; hair conditioner for shampoo formulations; paste; 99% conc.

Crodafos 1214A. [Croda Chem. Ltd.] Lauryl phosphate; CAS 12751-23-4; EINECS 235-798-1; detergent, emollient.

Crodafos CAP. [Croda Inc.] PPG-10 cetyl ether phosphate; CAS 111019-03-5; anionic; w/o emulsifier; antistat used in personal care prods.; modifies pH, thickening, emulsifying and suspending props.; enhances hair conditioning; useful for microemulsion systems; yel. clear liq.; sol. in oil, water; usage level: 0.5-3%; 100% conc.

Crodafos CDP. [Croda Chem. Ltd.] Cetyl diethanolamine phosphate; CAS 90388-14-0; anionic; emulsifier and stabilizer for o/w emulsions; powd.; water-disp.; 100% conc.

Crodafos CKP. [Croda Chem. Ltd.] Potassium cetyl phosphate; CAS 19035-79-1; EINECS 242-769-1; emulsifier, stabilizer.

Crodafos CS2 Acid. [Croda Chem. Ltd.] Ceteareth-2 phosphate; anionic; emulsifier and stabilizer for o/w emulsions; solid; 99% conc.

Crodafos CS2N. [Croda Chem. Ltd.] DEA-ceteareth-2 phosphate.

Crodafos CS5 Acid. [Croda Chem. Ltd.] Ceteareth-5 phosphate; anionic; emulsifier and stabilizer for o/w emulsions; solid; 99% conc.

Crodafos CS10 Acid. [Croda Chem. Ltd.] Ceteareth-10 phosphate; anionic; emulsifier and stabilizer for o/w emulsions; solid; 99% conc.

Crodafos G26A. [Croda Chem. Ltd.] Glycereth-26 phosphate.

Crodafos MCA. [Croda Chem. Ltd.] Cetyl phosphate; CAS 3539-43-3; EINECS 222-581-1.

Crodafos N2A. [Croda Chem. Ltd.] Oleth-2 phosphate; CAS 39464-69-2; personal care surfactant.

Crodafos N-3 Acid. [Croda Inc.; Croda Chem. Ltd.] Oleth-3 phosphate; CAS 39464-69-2; anionic; surfactant, conditioner, antistat, o/w emulsifier, gelling agent for surfactants, cosmetics, pharmaceuticals, and toiletries, microemulsion gels; corrosion inhibitor and anti-gelling agent in aerosol antiperspirant systems; amber visc. liq.; sol. in oil, water; acid no. 120-135; iodine no. 45-58; sapon. no. 125-145; pH 1-3 (2% aq.); usage level: 0.5-5%; 100% act.

Crodafos N-3 Neutral. [Croda Inc.; Croda Chem. Ltd.] DEA-oleth-3 phosphate; CAS 58855-63-3; anionic; o/w emulsifier, gelling agent for surfactants and for prep. of clear min. oil gels and microemulsion gels; used in hair relaxers; amber visc. liq.; sol. in oil, water; acid no. 90-100; iodine no. 35-50; pH 6-7 (2% aq.); usage level: 0.5-5%; 100% conc.

Crodafos N-5 Acid. [Croda Chem. Ltd.] Oleth-5 phosphate; CAS 39464-69-2; anionic; emulsifier and stabilizer for o/w emulsions; solid; 99% conc.

Crodafos N5N. [Croda Chem. Ltd.] DEA-oleth-5 phosphate.

Crodafos N-10 Acid. [Croda Inc.; Croda Chem. Ltd.] Oleth-10 phosphate; CAS 39464-69-2; anionic; o/w emulsifier, gelling agent for surfactants, prep. of clear min. oil gels, skin cleansers, clear microemulsion gels; yel. visc. liq.; sol. in oil, water; acid no. 70-100; iodine no. 25-35; sapon. no. 75-115; pH 1-3 (2% aq.); usage level: 0.5-10%; 100% act.

Crodafos N-10 Neutral. [Croda Inc.; Croda Chem. Ltd.] DEA-oleth-10 phosphate; CAS 58855-63-3; anionic; o/w emulsifier, gelling agent for surfactants, prep. of clear min. oil gels, skin cleansers, clear microemulsion gels; yel. visc. liq.; sol. in oil, water; acid no. 65-85; iodine no. 22-32; pH 5.5-7.0 (2% aq.); usage level: 0.5-10%; 100% conc.

Crodafos N20A. [Croda Chem. Ltd.] DEA-oleth-20 phosphate.

Crodafos O2 Acid. [Croda Chem. Ltd.] Oleth-2 phosphate; CAS 39464-69-2; anionic; hair conditioners for shampoo formulations; liq.; 99% conc.

Crodafos O5 Acid. [Croda Chem. Ltd.] Oleth-5 phosphate; CAS 39464-69-2; anionic; hair conditioners for shampoo formulations; liq.; 99% conc.

Crodafos O10 Acid. [Croda Chem. Ltd.] Oleth-10 phosphate; CAS 39464-69-2; anionic; hair conditioners for shampoo formulations; paste; 99% conc.

Crodafos S2A. [Croda Chem. Ltd.] Steareth-2 phosphate.

Crodafos SG. [Croda Inc.; Croda Chem. Ltd.] PPG-5 ceteth-10 phosphate; CAS 50643-20-4; anionic; o/w emulsifier, substantive conditioner, wet comb enhancer for shampoos and cream rinses; thickener, gellant, and pH adjuster for shampoos; corrosion inhibitor; visc. stabilizer for high salt systems; coupling agent for hard-to-solubilize actives; yel. visc. liq., mild char. odor; sol. in water, oil, alcohol, min. oil, oleyl alcohol, isopropyl esters; acid no. 85-105; iodine no. 8 max.; sapon. no. 90-110; pH 1-3 (3%); usage level: 0.5-3%; toxicology: LD50 (rat) 25 g/kg; sl. irritating to eyes and skin; 100% act.

Crodafos T2 Acid. [Croda Chem. Ltd.] Trideceth-2 phosphate; CAS 9046-01-9; anionic; hair conditioners for shampoo formulations; liq.; 99% conc.

Crodafos T5 Acid. [Croda Chem. Ltd.] Trideceth-5 phosphate; CAS 9046-01-9; anionic; hair conditioners for shampoo formulations; liq.; 99% conc.

Crodafos T10 Acid. [Croda Chem. Ltd.] Trideceth-10 phosphate; CAS 9046-01-9; anionic; hair conditioners for shampoo formulations; paste; 99% conc.

Crodalan 0477. [Croda Chem. Ltd.] Lanolin alternative; nonionic; emollient, superfatting agent, w/o emulsifier for cosmetics and pharmaceuticals; paste; 100% conc.

Crodalan AWS. [Croda Inc.; Croda Chem. Ltd.] Polysorbate 80, cetyl acetate, acetylated lanolin alcohol; nonionic; emollient, superfatting agent, conditioner, o/w emulsifier, dispersant, wetting agent, plasticizer, solubilizer used in cosmetics, pharmaceuticals, detergent systems; golden liq.; faint fatty odor; sol. in alcohol, water; sp.gr. 1.02-1.08; acid no. 3 max.; hyd. no. 55-67; pH 5-7 (10% aq.); usage level: 1-5%; 100% act.

Crodalan LA. [Croda Inc.; Croda Chem. Ltd.] Cetyl acetate and cetylated lanolin alcohol; nonionic; emollient, penetrant, wetting agent, conditioner, plasticizer used in cosmetics, pharmaceuticals; pale yel. clear, thin mobile liq.; odorless; sol. in min. oil, esters; cloud pt. 20 C; acid no. 2 max.; iodine no. 10 max.; sapon. no. 180-200; hyd. no. 8 max.; usage level: 2-10%; 100% act.

Croda Lanosterol. [Croda Chem. Ltd.] Lanosterol; CAS 79-63-0; EINECS 201-214-9; cosmetic gellant.

Croda Liq. Base. [Croda Inc.] Min. oil and lanolin alcohol.

Crodamol AB. [Croda Surf. Ltd.] C12-15 alkyl benzoate; CAS 68411-27-8; fine dry emollient, vehicle; solv. and perfume fixative; reduces greasy/oily texture and promotes spreading; for antiperspirants, skin care prods., makeup, sunscreens; colorless to pale straw liq.; sol. in castor oil, corn oil, min. oil, oleyl alcohol, ethanol; sp.gr. 0.92; visc. 13.7 cst.

Crodamol BB. [Croda Chem. Ltd.] Behenyl behenate; CAS 17671-27-1; EINECS 241-646-5; emollient, thickener.

Crodamol BE. [Croda Inc.] Behenyl erucate; CAS 18312-32-8; EINECS 242-201-8; thickening and opacifying agent, emollient, stabilizer, modifier for lipsticks, powd. suspensions; lt. amber waxy solid; oil-sol.; m.p. 43–46 C.; usage level: 1-5%.

Crodamol BM. [Croda Chem. Ltd.] Butyl myristate; CAS 110-36-1; EINECS 203-759-8; emollient.

Crodamol BS. [Croda Surf. Ltd.] Butyl stearate; CAS 123-95-5; EINECS 204-666-5; nonoily emollient; partial replacement for min. and veg. oils in lotions, creams, and salves; plasticizer, gloss aid in hair sprays and nail varnish; improves wetting and sol. of dyestuffs in lipsticks; colorless liq.; sol. in castor oil, corn oil, min. oil, oleyl alcohol, ethanol; sp.gr. 0.853-0.858; visc. 8.9 cst; cloud pt. 20 C.

Crodamol CAP. [Croda Inc.; Croda Surf. Ltd] Cetearyl octanoate; emollient simulating properties of preen gland oil; provides water repellency, promotes spreading, reduces stickiness and occlusivity, imparts smooth afterfeel to skin care and makeup preps.; also for pharmaceuticals (burn creams, acne creams and lotions, antibiotic ointments); clear colorless liq., low odor; sol. in castor oil, corn oil, min. oil, oleyl alcohol, ethanol, IPA; sp.gr. 0.848-0.853; visc. 11.9 cst; cloud pt. 0 C.; usage level: 5-10%; toxicology: LD50 (oral, rat) 13.6 g/kg; moderate skin irritant; nonirritating to eyes.

Crodamol CL. [Croda Surf. Ltd.] Cetyl lactate; CAS 35274-05-6; EINECS 252-478-7; dry emollient for anhyd. makeup and skin care preps.; nongreasy wetting agent; good stability in aq. alcoholic sol'ns.; wh. soft solid to colorless or pale yel. liq.; sol. in castor oil, corn oil, min. oil, oleyl alcohol, ethanol; sp.gr. 1.4433-1.4463 (30 C); m.p. 24 C.

Crodamol CP. [Croda Inc.; Croda Chem. Ltd.] Cetyl palmitate; CAS 540-10-3; EINECS 208-736-6; emollient for replacing spermaceti wax; wh. flakes; oil-sol.; m.p. 50–54 C.; usage level: 3-10%.

Crodamol CSP. [Croda Inc.] Cetearyl palmitate; CAS 85341-79-3; improves feel and body of emulsions; replaces spermaceti wax and beeswax in personal care prods.; Gardner 3 max. wh. flakes; oil-sol.; m.p. 48–52 C; acid no. 1 max.; iodine no. 1 max.; sapon. no. 100–115; usage level: 3-10%.

Crodamol CSS. [Croda Surf. Ltd.] Cetearyl stearate; CAS 93820-97-4; wax-like emollient imparting smooth texture to the skin; produces emulsions with increased visc. and dense, white appearance; modifies consistency and structure in salves and ointments; for cosmetic systems; wh. to off-wh. solid; sol. in min. oil; sol. hot in castor oil, corn oil, oleyl alcohol, ethanol; m.p. 55 C.

Crodamol DA. [Croda Surf. Ltd.] Diisopropyl adipate; CAS 6938-94-9; EINECS 248-299-9; solv. for aromatic oils and perfumes; superfatting agent for aq. alocholic lotions; solv. for lipstick dyestuffs; used for aftershave lotions, colognes, skin fresheners; plasticizer in nail varnish and hair spray; emollient in skin and bath preps.; water-wh. liq., almost odorless; sol. in castor oil, corn oil, min. oil, oleyl alcohol, ethanol; sp.gr. 0.950-0.962; visc. 3.9 cst; f.p. -1 C; acid no. 0.5 max.; sapon. no. 480-500; ref. index 1.422-1.424.

Crodamol DO. [Croda Surf. Ltd.] Decyl oleate; CAS 3687-46-5; EINECS 222-981-6; emollient, lubricant, and penetrant for cosmetics and pharmaceuticals; vehicle for active medicaments; castor oil substitute in lipsticks; straw liq.; bland taste, mild char. odor; sol. in castor oil, corn oil, min.

oil, oleyl alcohol; sp.gr. 0.860-0.870; visc. 15.7 cst.

Crodamol DOA. [Croda Surf. Ltd.] Dioctyl adipate; CAS 103-23-1; EINECS 203-090-1; nonocclusive emollient for skin and makeup preps., antiperspirants, deodorants, bath oils, and sunscreen preps.; colorless liq.; sol. in castor oil, corn oil, min. oil, oleyl alcohol, ethanol; sp.gr. 0.920-0.925; visc. 12.5 cst.

Crodamol GE. [Croda Surf. Ltd.] Glyceryl erucate; CAS 28063-42-5; EINECS 248-812-6.

Crodamol GHS. [Croda Surf. Ltd.] Glyceryl hydroxystearate; CAS 1323-42-8; EINECS 215-355-9; emulsifier, emollient, thickening wax.

Crodamol GTCC. [Croda Surf. Ltd.] Glyceryl tricaprylate/caprate; imparts fine, soft emollience to skin; vehicle and diluent for active ingreds.; substitute for min. hydrocarbon oils in cosmetics and pharamceuticals; exc. dermatological props.; colorless to pale straw liq.; sol. in castor oil, corn oil, min. oil, oleyl alcohol, ethanol; sp.gr. 0.950; visc. 30 cst.

Crodamol ICS. [Croda Surf. Ltd.] Isocetyl stearate; CAS 25339-09-7; EINECS 246-868-6; emollient, lubricant, spreading agent, visc. control aid, and anticrystallization agent for bath oils, creams and lotions; colorless to pale yel. liq.; sol. in castor oil, corn oil, min. oil, oleyl alcohol; sp.gr. 0.850-0.859; visc. 26.5 cst.

Crodamol IPL. [Croda Chem. Ltd.; Croda Surf. Ltd.] Isopropyl laurate; CAS 10233-13-3; EINECS 233-560-1; emollient, plasticizer, and cosolvent for cosmetics; colorless liq.; sol. in castor oil, corn oil, min. oil, oleyl alcohol, ethanol; sp.gr. 0.845-0.852; visc. 3.7 cst.

Crodamol IPM. [Croda Inc.; Croda Chem. Ltd.; Croda Surf. Ltd.] IPM, perfumery grade; CAS 110-27-0; EINECS 203-751-4; spreading agent, emollient, cosolv., and vehicle for cosmetic raw materials; water wh. liq.; odorless.; misc. with veg. and min. oils; sp.gr. 0.847–0.853; visc. 5.3 cst; acid no. 2 max.; ref. index 1.432–1.434; 92% act.

Crodamol IPP. [Croda Chem. Ltd.; Croda Surf. Ltd.] Isopropyl palmitate; CAS 142-91-6; EINECS 205-571-1; emollient, spreading agent, vehicle, and cosolv. for cosmetic applics.; colorless liq.; sol. in castor oil, corn oil, min. oil, oleyl alcohol, ethanol; sp.gr. 0.850-0.855; visc. 7.7 cst.

Crodamol ISNP. [Croda Surf. Ltd.] Isostearyl neopentanoate; CAS 58958-60-4; EINECS 261-521-9; mild emollient imparting a smooth, rich, nongreasy texture to skin; lubricant improving spreading props.; for all skin care prods., neck, face, and eye makeup preps.; stable over wide pH range; pale straw liq., faint char. odor; sol. in castor oil, corn oil, min. oil, oleyl alcohol, ethanol; sp.gr. 0.865; visc. 17.5 cst.

Crodamol JJ. [Croda Surf. Ltd.] Oleyl erucate; CAS 17673-56-2; EINECS 241-654-9; highly lubricating emollient imparting a pleasant smooth texture to the skin; for use alone to simulate properties of jojoba oil or as diluent for natural jojoba; pale yel. liq.; sol. in castor oil, corn oil, min. oil, oleyl alcohol; sp.gr. 0.860-0.865; visc. 34 cst.

Crodamol LL. [Croda Chem. Ltd.; Croda Surf. Ltd.] Lauryl lactate; CAS 6283-92-7; EINECS 228-504-8; emollient for antiperspirants, makeup, hair and skin care prods.; promotes good spreading and wetting chars. and leaves a thin, dry film on the skin and hair; colorless to pale straw liq., faint bland odor; sol. in castor oil, corn oil, min. oil, oleyl alcohol, ethanol; sp.gr. 1.4417-1.4456; visc. 13.9 cst.

Crodamol ML. [Croda Chem. Ltd.; Croda Surf. Ltd.] Myristyl lactate; CAS 1323-03-1; EINECS 215-350-1; emollient improving smoothness and gloss in lipsticks with no tendency to oiliness; tack reducer in antiperspirants; imparts clean, healthy sheen in hair care preps.; colorless to pale yel. liq.; sol. in castor oil, corn oil, min. oil, oleyl alcohol, ethanol; sp.gr. 1.443-1.445; m.p. 13 C.

Crodamol MM. [Croda Inc.; Croda Surf. Ltd.] Myristyl

myristate; CAS 3234-85-3; EINECS 221-787-9; emollient, superfatting agent, visc. builder in emulsions; substitute for spermaceti wax and/or beeswax in cosmetic and pharmaceutical formulations; off-wh. waxy solid.; sol. in min. oil, IPM, IPA, oleyl alcohol; insol. in water; sp.gr. 0.832-0.837 (50 C); m.p. 36–39 C; acid no. 1 max.; sapon. no. 120–130; usage level: 3-10%; toxicology: LD50 (oral, rat) > 5 g/kg; mild skin irritant, minimal eye irritant.

Crodamol MP. [Croda Surf. Ltd.] Myristyl propionate; CAS 6221-95-0; EINECS 226-300-9; emollient.

Crodamol OC. [Croda Chem. Ltd.; Croda Surf. Ltd.] 2-Ethylhexyl cocoate; CAS 92044-87-6; EINECS 295-366-3; modifies occlusivity of other cosmetic materials; fine emollient promoting spreading on skin; reduces tackiness in cosmetics, skin care, makeup, and toiletry preps.; pale yel. liq.; sol. in castor oil, corn oil, min. oil, oleyl alcohol, ethanol; sp.gr. 0.855-0.860; visc. 8.5 cst.

Crodamol OHS. [Croda Surf. Ltd.] 2-Ethylhexyl 12-hydroxystearate; CAS 29383-26-4; rich emollient for creams, lotions, and oils; superfatting agent for detergent compositions such as shampoos, foam baths, liq. and bar soaps; pale yel. liq./off-wh. solid; sol. in castor oil, corn oil, min. oil, oleyl alcohol, ethanol; sp.gr. 0.889-0.895; visc. 77 cst.

Crodamol OO. [Croda Chem. Ltd.; Croda Surf. Ltd.] Oleyl oleate; CAS 3687-45-4; EINECS 222-980-4; emollient, lubricant.

Crodamol OP. [Croda Surf. Ltd.] 2-Ethylhexyl palmitate; CAS 29806-73-3; EINECS 249-862-1; lubricant, spreading agent for makeup, skin and hair care preps.; modifies occlusiveness of creams, ointments, and oils; colorless liq., mild odor; sol. in castor oil, corn oil, min. oil, oleyl alcohol, ethanol; sp.gr. 0.850-0.860; visc. 12.7 cst.

Crodamol OSU. [Croda Surf. Ltd.] Di-2-ethylhexyl succinate; CAS 2915-57-3; EINECS 220-836-1; nonocclusive emollient for skin care prods.; promotes wetting and spreading of other lipophilic substances on skin; gloss aid for hair prods. incl. leave-on conditioners; colorless liq.; sol. in castor oil, corn oil, min. oil, oleyl alcohol, ethanol; sp.gr. 0.930-0.935; visc. 10 cst.

Crodamol PC. [Croda Surf. Ltd.] Propylene glycol dicaprylate; CAS 7384-98-7; EINECS 230-962-9; emollient with exc. spreading props.; imparts pleasant, nonoily lubricity to skin; for bath oils, antiperspirants, lipsticks, skin and hair care prods.; colorless to pale straw liq.; sol. in castor oil, corn oil, min. oil, oleyl alcohol, ethanol; sp.gr. 0.917-0.923; visc. 9.3 cst.

Crodamol PETS. [Croda Surf. Ltd.] Pentaerythrityl tetrastearate; CAS 115-83-3; EINECS 204-110-1; emollient, lubricant.

Crodamol PMP. [Croda Inc.; Croda Surf. Ltd] PPG-2 myristyl ether propionate; emollient, lubricant with dry, lt. greaseless feel; coupling agent; solv. for sunscreen actives; for bath oils, creams, moisturizers, emulsions, pharmaceuticals (burn creams, acne creams and lotions, antibiotic ointments); Gardner 1 max. clear, colorless liq.; very mild char. odor; sol. (1%) in min. oil, IPM, oleyl alcohol, ethanol/water, lanolin, cetyl alcohol; sp.gr. 0.870-0.880; visc. 8.9 cst; cloud pt. -5 C; acid no. 0.5 max.; iodine no. 1.0 max.; sapon. no. 140–155; usage level: 5-20%; toxicology: LD50 (oral, rat) > 5 g/kg; minimal skin irritant, nonirritating to eyes.

Crodamol PTC. [Croda Inc.; Croda Surf. Ltd] Pentaerythritol tetracaprylate/caprate; CAS 68441-68-9; EINECS 270-474-3; lubricant for creams, preshave lotions; reduces tack in clear gel microemulsions; nongreasy emollient for skin care and makeup prods., pharmaceuticals (burn creams, acne creams and lotions, antibiotic ointments); lt. yel. lipophilic visc. liq.; sol. in castor oil, corn oil, min. oil, oleyl alcohol, ethanol.; sp.gr. 0.945-0.955; visc. 50 cst; cloud pt. 10 C; usage level: 1-12%; toxicology: LD50 (oral,

rat) > 5 g/kg; minimal skin irritant, nonirritating to eyes.

Crodamol PTIS. [Croda Inc.; Croda Surf. Ltd] Pentaerythritol tetraisostearate; cosmetic lubricant for creams and lotions; castor oil substitute for makeup; emollient for skin care prods., bath oils; reduces tack in clear gel microemulsions; also for pharmaceuticals (burn creams, acne creams and lotions, antibiotic ointments); lt. amber visc. liq.; sol. in castor oil, corn oil, min. oil, oleyl alcohol; sp.gr. 0.915-0.930; visc. 298 cst; cloud pt. 0 C; usage level: 1-12%; toxicology: LD50 (oral, rat) > 10 g/kg; minimal skin and eye irritant.

Crodamol SS. [Croda Inc.; Croda Surf. Ltd] Cetyl esters; syn. spermaceti NF; emollient and visc. builder for cosmetic and pharmaceutical preparations (burn creams, acne creams and lotions, antibiotic ointments); almost wh. cryst. solid, faint odor; sol. in min. oil; sol. warm in IPA; sp.gr. 0.82–0.84 (50 C); m.p. 43–47 C; acid no. 5 max.; iodine no. 1 max.; sapon. no. 109–120; usage level: 3-10%; toxicology: LD50 (oral, rat) > 5 g/kg; nonirritating to skin, minimal eye irritant.

Crodamol TBC. [Croda Surf. Ltd.] Tributyl citrate; CAS 77-94-1; EINECS 201-071-2.

Crodamol TC. [Croda Surf. Ltd.] Triethyl citrate; CAS 77-93-0; EINECS 201-070-7; cosmetic ingred.

Crodamol TSC. [Croda Surf. Ltd.] Tristearyl citrate; CAS 7775-50-0; EINECS 231-896-3.

Crodamol W. [Croda Inc.; Croda Surf. Ltd] Stearyl heptanoate; CAS 66009-41-4; nongreasy emollient and water repellent for cosmetics and toiletries, esp. stick formulations; melts rapidly on applic. to skin; syn. preen gland wax; also for pharmaceuticals (burn creams, acne creams and lotions, antibiotic ointments); wh. waxy solid; mild odor; sol. in castor oil, corn oil, min. oil, oleyl alcohol, ethanol, IPA; sp.gr. 0.850-0.855; m.p. 23–27 C; usage level: 2-20%; toxicology: LD50 (oral, rat) > 16 g/kg; mild skin and eye irritant.

Crodapearl Liq. [Croda Inc.] Sodium laureth sulfate, glycol MIPA stearate; pearling agent for shampoos, bubble baths, dishwashing liqs.; creamy pearly paste, mild char. odor; pH 7.5-8.5; usage level: 1-5%; 35-40% conc. in water.

Crodapearl NI Liquid. [Croda Inc.] Hydroxyethyl stearamide-MIPA, PPG-5 ceteth-20; nonionic; pearlescent for detergent systems, lotions, gels, clear rinses, bath prods.; wh. soft paste; usage level: 1-5%.

Crodarom Avocadin. [Croda Inc.] Avocado oil unsaponifiables; botanical extract for personal care prods.; pale yel. soft wax, char. odor; acid no. 2 max.; sapon. no. 130-150.

Crodarom Calendula O. [Croda Inc.] Soybean oil, calendula extract, tocopherol; botanical extract of *Flores calendulae* for personal care prods.; helps heal bruises, alleviates skin conditions; clear yel. liq., char. odor; sp.gr. 0.918-0.926; acid no. 0.5-1.0; sapon. no. 180-200; ref. index 1.473-1.476.

Crodarom Carrot O. [Croda Inc.] Peanut oil, carrot extract, isopropyl myristate, tocopherol; botanical extract of *Daucus carota L.* for personal care prods.; conditions reddens and coarse skin; red clear liq., char. odor; sp.gr. 0.880-0.893; acid no. 2 max.; iodine no. 44-68; sapon. no. 185-205; ref. index 1.452-1.460.

Crodarom Chamomile A. [Croda Inc.] Propylene glycol and matricaria extract; botanical extract of *Flores matricariae chamomille L.* for personal care prods.; promotes wound healing, helps relieve effects of eczema; olive-grn. clear liq., char. odor; sp.gr. 1.042-1.052; pH 5.0-6.5; ref. index 1.39-1.40.

Crodarom Chamomile EO. [Croda Inc.] Caprylic/capric triglycerides and matricaria extract; botanical extract of *Flores matricariae chamomille L.* for personal care prods.;

promotes wound healing, helps relieve effects of eczema; lt. blue clear liq., char. odor; sp.gr. 0.94-0.95; acid no. 1 max.; sapon. no. 295-315; ref. index 1.448-1.459.

Crodarom Chamomile O. [Croda Inc.] Caprylic/capric triglycerides and matricaria extract; botanical extract of *Flores matricariae chamomille L.* for personal care prods.; promotes wound healing, helps relieve effects of eczema; bluish-grn. clear liq., char. odor; sp.gr. 0.94-0.95; ref. index 1.448-1.500.

Crodarom Nut O. [Croda Inc.] Peanut oil, min. oil, walnut extract; botanical extract of *Juglans regia L.* for personal care prods.; helps relieve effects of eczema; dk. amber/ brn. clear liq., char. odor; sp.gr. 0.867-0.868; ref. index. 1.466-1.469.

Crodarom St. John's Wort O. [Croda Inc.] Olive oil, hypericum extract; botanical extract of *Hypericum perforatum* for personal care prods.; helps reduce varicose veins, soothes pain of rheumatism; lt. amber clear liq., char. odor; sp.gr. 0.910-0.920; acid no. 5 max.; iodine no. 80-100; sapon. no. 180-220; ref. index 1.468-1.475.

Crodasinic C. [Croda Chem. Ltd.] Cocoyl sarcosine; CAS 68411-97-2; EINECS 270-156-4; cosmetic surfactant.

Crodasinic CS. [Croda Chem. Ltd.] Sodium cocoyl sarcosinate; CAS 61791-59-1; EINECS 263-193-2; personal care surfactant.

Crodasinic L. [Croda Chem. Ltd.] Lauroyl sarcosine; CAS 97-78-9; EINECS 202-608-3; nonionic; salts with detergent props.; lubricants and metal working fluids; also for shampoos and other hair care prods.; solid; oil-sol.; 94% conc.

Crodasinic LS30. [Croda Chem. Ltd.] Sodium N-lauroyl sarcosinate; CAS 137-16-6; EINECS 205-281-5; anionic; foaming, wetting agent and detergent for acidic conditions; corrosion inhibitor; bacteriostat and inhibitor; used in dental care preps., pharmaceuticals, personal care prods., household and industrial applics.; clear liq.; watersol.; 30% act.

Crodasinic LS35. [Croda Chem. Ltd.] Sodium N-lauroyl sarcosinate; CAS 137-16-6; EINECS 205-281-5; anionic; foaming agent, wetting agent, detergent, lubricant, antistat, corrosion inhibitor, bacteriostat, penetrant used in dental, pharmaceutical, shampoos, depilatories, and shaving preparations, food pkg., household and industrial uses; biodeg.; clear liq.; water sol.; 35% act.

Crodasinic LT40. [Croda Chem. Ltd.] TEA lauroyl sarcosinate; CAS 16693-53-1; EINECS 240-736-1; anionic; detergent, foaming agent, wetting agent, dispersant, emulsifier, anticorrosive, foam stabilizing synergist for carpet shampoos, textile and cosmetic detergent systems; liq.; 40% conc.

Crodasinic MS. [Croda Chem. Ltd.] Sodium myristoyl sarcosinate; CAS 30364-51-3; EINECS 250-151-3; personal care surfactant.

Crodasinic O. [Croda Chem. Ltd.] N-Oleoyl sarcosine; CAS 110-25-8; EINECS 203-749-3; nonionic; corrosion inhibitor in oils, fuels, lubricants, greases, surface coatings; for shampoos and hair care prods.; as antifog agent for food pkg. polyolefin films; liq.; 93% conc.

Crodasinic S. [Croda Chem. Ltd.] Stearoyl sarcosine; CAS 142-48-3; EINECS 205-539-7; personal care surfactant.

Croda Solid Base. [Croda Inc.] Petrolatum, lanolin, and lanolin alcohol.

Crodasone W. [Croda Inc.] Hydrolyzed wheat protein polysiloxane copolymer; substantive film-forming copolymer with lubricity, gloss, conditioning props. for hair and skin care prods.; amber visc. liq., char odor; sol. in aq. or aq./ alcoholic systems, glycerin, propylene glycol, surfactant systems; water-sol. above pH 5.5; m.w. 2000; pH 4.0-5.0; 22% act.

Croderm MF. [Croda Inc.] Polyamino sugar condensate,

sodium PCA, and sodium lactate.

Croderol GA 7000. [Croda Universal Ltd.] Glycerin; CAS 56-81-5; EINECS 200-289-5; humectant, conditioner for cosmetics.

Crodesta DKS F10. [Croda Surf. Ltd.] Sucrose mono/di/tri palmitic/stearic acid; CAS 27195-16-0; EINECS 248-317-5; nonionic; emulsifier, wetting agent, dispersant for use in cosmetics, pharmaceuticals; solid; 100% conc.

Crodesta DKS F20. [Croda Surf. Ltd.] Sucrose mono/di/tri palmitic/stearic acid; CAS 27195-16-0; EINECS 248-317-5; nonionic; emulsifier, wetting agent, dispersant for use in cosmetics, pharmaceuticals; solid; 100% conc.

Crodesta DKS F50. [Croda Surf. Ltd.] Sucrose mono/di/tri palmitic/stearic acid; CAS 27195-16-0; EINECS 248-317-5; nonionic; emulsifier, wetting agent, dispersant for use in cosmetics, pharmaceuticals; solid; 100% conc.

Crodesta DKS F70. [Croda Surf. Ltd.] Sucrose mono/di/tri palmitic/stearic acid; CAS 27195-16-0; EINECS 248-317-5; nonionic; emulsifier, wetting agent, dispersant for use in cosmetics, pharmaceuticals; solid; 100% conc.

Crodesta DKS F110. [Croda Surf. Ltd.] Sucrose mono/di/tri palmitic/stearic acid; CAS 25168-73-4; EINECS 246-705-9; nonionic; emulsifier, wetting agent, dispersant for use in cosmetics, pharmaceuticals; solid; 100% conc.

Crodesta DKS F140. [Croda Surf. Ltd.] Sucrose mono/di/tri palmitic/stearic acid; nonionic; emulsifier, wetting agent, dispersant for use in cosmetics, pharmaceuticals; solid; 100% conc.

Crodesta DKS F160. [Croda Surf. Ltd.] Sucrose mono/di/tri palmitic/stearic acid; CAS 25168-73-4; EINECS 246-705-9; nonionic; emulsifier, wetting agent, dispersant for use in cosmetics, pharmaceuticals; solid; 100% conc.

Crodesta F-10. [Croda Inc.; Croda Surf. Ltd.] Sucrose distearate; CAS 27195-16-0; EINECS 248-317-5; nonionic; dispersant, emulsifier, wetting agent, solubilizer, emollient, detergent in cosmetics, toiletries, pharmaceuticals (suntan and baby lotions); creamy wh. powd.; sol. in oil; insol. in water; HLB < 3.0; m.p. 60-68 C; acid no. 5 max.; iodine no. 1 max.; sapon. no. 140-200; hyd. no. 80-130; usage level: 1-3%; 100% act.

Crodesta F-50. [Croda Inc.; Croda Surf. Ltd.] Sucrose distearate; CAS 27195-16-0; EINECS 248-317-5; nonionic; dispersant, emulsifier, wetting agent, solubilizer, emollient, detergent in cosmetics, toiletries, pharmaceuticals, lipsticks; wh. powd.; HLB 6.5; m.p. 74-78 C; acid no. 5 max.; iodine no. 1 max.; sapon. no. 93-153; hyd. no. 419-469; usage level: 3-6%; 100% act.

Crodesta F-110. [Croda Inc.; Croda Surf. Ltd.] Sucrose distearate and sucrose stearate; nonionic; dispersant, emulsifier, wetting agent, solubilizer, detergent in cosmetics, toiletries, pharmaceuticals; thickener and suspending agent; wh. powd.; water-sol.; HLB 12.0; m.p. 72-78 C; acid no. 5 max.; iodine no. 1 max.; sapon. no. 85-145; hyd. no. 475-525; usage level: 3-6%; 100% act.

Crodesta F-140. [Croda Surf. Ltd.] Sucrose stearate and sucrose distearate.

Crodesta F-160. [Croda Inc.; Croda Surf. Ltd.] Sucrose stearate; CAS 25168-73-4; EINECS 246-705-9; nonionic; dispersant, emulsifier, wetting agent, solubilizer, detergent, foaming agent in cosmetics, toiletries, ingestible pharmaceuticals; thickener and suspending agent; wh. powd.; water-sol.; HLB 14.5; m.p. 70-74 C; acid no. 5 max.; iodineno. 1 max.; sapon. no. 75-153; hyd. no. 545-595; usage level: 3-6%; 100% act.

Crodesta SL-40. [Croda Inc.; Croda Surf. Ltd.] Sucrose cocoate; CAS 91031-88-8; nonionic; dispersant, emulsifier, wetting agent, solubilizer, mild detergent, high foaming emollient in cosmetics, toiletries, pharmaceuticals; amber liq.; water-sol.; insol. in oil; HLB 15.0; acid no. 5 max.; iodine no. 1 max.; usage level: 5-20%; 100% conc.

Crodet C10. [Croda Chem. Ltd.] PEG-10 coconut fatty acid; CAS 61791-29-5; nonionic; surfactant for cosmetic and industrial applics.; liq.; 97+% conc.

Crodet L4. [Croda Chem. Ltd.] PEG-4 laurate; CAS 9004-81-3; nonionic; o/w emulsifier for cosmetics and pharmaceutical creams, lotions and ointments, industrial applics., wetting agent, solubilizer for perfumes or aq. alcoholic preparations; dispersant; plasticizer for hair setting sprays; pale straw liq.; sol. in ethyl, oleyl, and cetearyl alcohols, oleic acid; HLB 9.8; sapon. no. 138–150; 97% conc.

Crodet L8. [Croda Chem. Ltd.] PEG-8 laurate; CAS 9004-81-3; nonionic; o/w emulsifier for cosmetics and pharmaceutical creams, lotions and ointments, industrial applics., wetting agent, solubilizer for perfumes or aq. alcoholic preparations; dispersant; plasticizer for hair setting sprays; pale straw liq.; sol. in ethyl, oleyl, and cetearyl alcohols, oleic acid; HLB 12.7; sapon. no. 95–106; 97% conc.

Crodet L12. [Croda Chem. Ltd.] PEG-12 laurate; CAS 9004-81-3; nonionic; o/w emulsifier for cosmetics and pharmaceutical creams, lotions and ointments, industrial applics., wetting agent, solubilizer for perfumes or aq. alcoholic preparations; dispersant; plasticizer for hair setting sprays; pale straw liq.; sol. in water, ethyl, oleyl, and cetearyl alcohols, oleic acid; HLB 14.5; sapon. no. 72–82; 97% conc.

Crodet L24. [Croda Chem. Ltd.] PEG-24 laurate; CAS 9004-81-3; nonionic; o/w emulsifier for cosmetics and pharmaceutical creams, lotions and ointments, industrial applics., wetting agent, solubilizer for perfumes or aq. alcoholic preparations; dispersant; plasticizer for hair setting sprays; off-wh. soft paste; sol. in water, ethyl and cetostearyl alcohol; HLB 16.8; sapon. no. 42–48; 97% conc.

Crodet L40. [Croda Chem. Ltd.] PEG-40 laurate; CAS 9004-81-3; nonionic; o/w emulsifier for cosmetics and pharmaceutical creams, lotions and ointments, industrial applics., wetting agent, solubilizer for perfumes or aq. alcoholic preparations; dispersant; plasticizer for hair setting sprays; off-wh. waxy solid; sol. in water, ethyl and cetostearyl alcohol; HLB 17.9; sapon. no. 26–31; 97% conc.

Crodet L100. [Croda Chem. Ltd.] PEG-100 laurate; CAS 9004-81-3; nonionic; o/w emulsifier for cosmetics and pharmaceutical creams, lotions and ointments, industrial applics., wetting agent, solubilizer for perfumes or aq. alcoholic preparations; dispersant; plasticizer for hair setting sprays; pale yel. waxy solid; sol. in water, ethyl and cetostearyl alcohol; HLB 19.1; sapon. no. 11–15; 97% conc.

Crodet O4. [Croda Chem. Ltd.] PEG-4 oleate; CAS 9004-96-0; EINECS 233-293-0; nonionic; surfactant for cosmetic and industrial applics.; liq.; 97% conc.

Crodet O6. [Croda Chem. Ltd.] PEG-6 oleate; CAS 9004-96-0; emulsifier.

Crodet O8. [Croda Chem. Ltd.] PEG-8 oleate; CAS 9004-96-0; nonionic; surfactant for cosmetic and industrial applics.; liq.; HLB 10.8; 97% conc.

Crodet O12. [Croda Chem. Ltd.] PEG-12 oleate; CAS 9004-96-0; nonionic; surfactant for cosmetic and industrial applics.; liq.; HLB 13.4; 97% conc.

Crodet O23. [Croda Chem. Ltd.] PEG-23 oleate; CAS 9004-96-0; personal care surfactant.

Crodet O24. [Croda Chem. Ltd.] PEG-24 oleate; CAS 9004-96-0; nonionic; surfactant for cosmetic and industrial applics.; paste; HLB 15.8; 97% conc.

Crodet O40. [Croda Chem. Ltd.] PEG-40 oleate; CAS 9004-96-0; nonionic; surfactant for cosmetic and industrial applics.; solid; 97% conc.

Crodet O100. [Croda Chem. Ltd.] PEG-100 oleate; CAS 9004-96-0; nonionic; surfactant for cosmetic and industrial applics.; solid; HLB 18.8; 97% conc.

Crodet S4. [Croda Chem. Ltd.] PEG-4 stearate; CAS 9004-99-3; EINECS 203-358-8; nonionic; o/w emulsifier for cosmetics and pharmaceutical creams, lotions and ointments, industrial applics.; wetting agent, solubilizer for perfumes or aq. alcoholic preparations; dispersant; off-wh. soft paste; sol. in ethyl and oleyl alcohols, oleic acid, ceto stearyl alcohol, arachis oil and isoparaffinic solv.; HLB 7.7; sapon. no. 117–129; 97% conc.

Crodet S8. [Croda Chem. Ltd.] PEG-8 stearate; CAS 9004-99-3; nonionic; o/w emulsifier for cosmetics and pharmaceutical creams, lotions and ointments, industrial applics.; wetting agent, solubilizer for perfumes or aq. alcoholic preparations, dispersant; off-wh. soft paste; sol. in ethyl and oleyl alcohols, oleic acid, ceto stearyl alcohol, arachis oil and isoparaffinic solv.; HLB 10.8; sapon. no. 84–94; 97% conc.

Crodet S12. [Croda Chem. Ltd.] PEG-12 stearate; CAS 9004-99-3; nonionic; o/w emulsifier for cosmetics and pharmaceutical creams, lotions and ointments, industrial applics.; wetting agent, solubilizer for perfumes or aq. alcoholic preparations, dispersant; off-wh. waxy solid; sol. in ethyl, oleyl, and cetostearyl alcohol, water, oleic acide; HLB 13.4; sapon. no. 65–75; 97% conc.

Crodet S24. [Croda Chem. Ltd.] PEG-24 stearate; CAS 9004-99-3; nonionic; o/w emulsifier for cosmetics and pharmaceutical creams, lotions and ointments, industrial applics.; wetting agent, solubilizer for perfumes or aq. alcoholic preparations, dispersant; off-wh. waxy solid; sol. in ethyl and cetostearyl alcohol, water; HLB 15.8; sapon. no. 38–47; 97% conc.

Crodet S40. [Croda Chem. Ltd.] PEG-40 stearate; CAS 9004-99-3; nonionic; o/w emulsifier for cosmetics and pharmaceutical creams, lotions and ointments, industrial applics.; wetting agent, solubilizer for perfumes or aq. alcoholic preparations, dispersant; off-wh. waxy solid; sol. in ethyl and cetostearyl alcohol, water; HLB 16.7; sapon. no. 23–30; 97% conc.

Crodet S50. [Croda Chem. Ltd.] PEG-50 stearate; CAS 9004-99-3; emulsifier.

Crodet S100. [Croda Chem. Ltd.] PEG-100 stearate; CAS 9004-99-3; nonionic; o/w emulsifier for cosmetics and pharmaceutical creams, lotions and ointments, industrial applics.; wetting agent, solubilizer for perfumes or aq. alcoholic preparations, dispersant; off-wh. waxy solid; sol. in ethyl and cetostearyl alcohol, water; HLB 18.8; sapon. no. 10–14; 97% conc.

Crodex A. [Croda Chem. Ltd.] Cetostearyl alcohol and sodium lauryl sulfate; anionic; emulsifying wax BP for pharmaceuticals and cosmetic uses; almost wh. waxy solid; faint char. odor; water-disp.; 100% conc.

Crodex C. [Croda Chem. Ltd.] Cetostearyl alcohol and Cetrimide BP; cationic; emulsifying wax BPC, bactericides, for pharmaceuticals and cosmetics, hair conditioning rinses; almost wh. waxy solid; faint char. odor; water-disp.; 100% conc.

Crodex N. [Croda Chem. Ltd.] Cetostearyl alcohol and ceteth-20; nonionic; emulsifying wax BP, wetting agent, penetrant, emulsifier for most emollient materials in cosmetics and pharmaceuticals; almost wh. waxy solid; faint char. odor; water-disp.; 100% conc.

Crodolene LA1020. [Croda Universal Ltd.] Oleic acid; CAS 112-80-1; EINECS 204-007-1; surfactant intermediate.

Croduret 7. [Croda Chem. Ltd.] PEG-7 hydrog. castor oil; CAS 61788-85-0; emulsifier.

Croduret 10. [Croda Chem. Ltd.] PEG-10 hydrog. castor oil; CAS 61788-85-0; nonionic; emulsifier, solubilizer, emollient, superfatting agent, detergent used for cosmetics, textiles, metalworking fluids, emulsion polymerization, insecticides, herbicides, household detergents; straw-colored liq.; sol. in oleyl alcohol, naphtha, MEK, oleic acid, trichloroethylene; HLB 6.3; cloud pt. < 20 C; sapon. no. 120–130; surf. tens. 37 dynes/cm (0.1%); 100% conc.

Croduret 25. [Croda Chem. Ltd.] PEG-25 hydrog. castor oil; CAS 61788-85-0; personal care surfactant.

Croduret 30. [Croda Chem. Ltd.] PEG-30 hydrog. castor oil; CAS 61788-85-0; emulsifier, solubilizer, emollient, super-fatting agent, detergent for cosmetics, textiles, metal-working fluids, emulsion polymerization, agric., house-hold detergents; straw colored liq.; sol. in water, ethanol, oleyl alcohol, naphtha, MEK, oleic acid, trichloroethylene; HLB 11.6; cloud pt. 48 C; sapon. no. 70–80; surf. tens. 46 dynes/cm (0.1%).

Croduret 40. [Croda Chem. Ltd.] PEG-40 hydrog. castor oil; CAS 61788-85-0; nonionic; emulsifier, solubilizer, emol-lient, superfatting agent, detergent used for cosmetics, textiles, metalworking fluids, emulsion polymerization, insecticides, herbicides, household detergents; off-wh. visc. paste; sol. in water, ethanol, naphtha, MEK, oleic acid, trichloroethylene; HLB 12.9; cloud pt. 62 C; sapon. no. 60–65; surf. tens. 46 dynes/cm (0.1%); 100% conc.

Croduret 50. [Croda Chem. Ltd.] PEG-50 hydrog. castor oil; CAS 61788-85-0; nonionic; solubilizer and emulsifier for cosmetics and pharmaceutical applics.; soft paste; water-sol.; 100% conc.

Croduret 60. [Croda Chem. Ltd.] PEG-60 hydrog. castor oil; CAS 61788-85-0; nonionic; emulsifier, solubilizer, emol-lient, superfatting agent, detergent used for cosmetics, textiles, metalworking fluids, emulsion polymerization, insecticides, herbicides, household detergents; off-wh. stiff paste; sol. in water, ethanol, MEK, oleic acid, trichlo-roethylene; HLB 14.7; cloud pt. 71 C; sapon. no.45–50; surf. tens. 47.5 dynes/cm (0.1%); 100% conc.

Croduret 100. [Croda Chem. Ltd.] PEG-100 hydrog. castor oil; CAS 61788-85-0; nonionic; emulsifier, solubilizer, emollient, superfatting agent, detergent used for cosmet-ics, textiles, metalworking fluids, emulsion polymeriza-tion, insecticides, herbicides, household detergents; off-wh. waxy solid; sol. in water, ethanol, MEK, trichloroeth-ylene; HLB 16.5; cloud pt. 65 C; sapon. no. 25–35; surf. tens. 46.2 dynes/cm (0.1%); 100% conc.

Croduret 200. [Croda Chem. Ltd.] PEG-200 hydrogenated castor oil; CAS 61788-85-0; nonionic; emulsifier, wetting agent, solubilizer, lubricant, antistat; solid; water-sol.; HLB 18.0; 100% conc.

Crodyne BY-19. [Croda Inc.] Pharmaceutical gelatin NF; CAS 9000-70-8; EINECS 232-554-6; protective colloid, moisturizer, conditioner for skin and hair care prods.; humectant, thickener for pharmaceutical and food applics.; buff cryst. powd., bland pleasant odor; water-sol.; m.w. 25,000; visc. 14-18 mps; pH 5.5-6.2 (10%); usage level: 1-5%; toxicology: LD50 (oral, rat) > 5 g/kg; nonirritating to skin and eyes; 85% act.

Crolactil CSL. [Croda Surf. Ltd.] Calcium 2-stearoyl lactylate; CAS 5793-94-2; EINECS 227-335-7; anionic; w/o emulsifier, emollient for skin care and treatment prods.; ingredients in food prods.; off-wh. powd.; HLB 5; sapon. no. 175–250.

Crolactil SISL. [Croda Surf. Ltd.] Sodium isostearoyl lactylate; CAS 66988-04-3; EINECS 266-533-8; anionic; o/w emulsifier, emollient for skin care and treatment prods.; ingredients in food prods.; yel. liq.; HLB 6.5; sapon. no. 210–280.

Crolactil SSL. [Croda Chem. Ltd.] Sodium stearoyl lactylates; CAS 25383-99-7; EINECS 246-929-7; o/w emulsifier, emollient for skin care and treatment prods.; ingredients in food prods.; off-wh. powd.; HLB 6.5; sapon. no. 210–280.

Crolastin. [Croda Inc.] Hydrolyzed animal elastin; CAS 100085-10-7; moisturizer and conditioner for skin care prods. and cleansers; yel. liq.; m.w. 4000; usage level: 1-5%; 30% act.

Crolastin C. [Croda Chem. Ltd.] Hydrolyzed collagen; CAS 9015-54-7; cosmetic protein.

Crolec 4135. [Croda Chem. Ltd.] Modified lecithin; CAS 8002-43-5; EINECS 232-307-2; nonionic; conditioner, superfatting, emulsifier for cosmetics and pharmaceuti-cals; liq.; 100% conc.

Cromeen. [Croda Chem. Ltd.] Substituted alkylamine deriv. lanolin acids; anionic; mild multifunctional surfactant with high foaming, detergency, and emulsifying props.; for shampoos, detergents, and hand cleansing preps., aero-sol skin and shaving foams; soft gel; 45% min. conc.

Cromoist CS. [Croda Inc.] Chondroitin sulfate, hydrolyzed animal protein; moisturizer, conditioner for face and body creams and lotions; clear to slightly hazy visc. sol'n.; m.w. 115,000; usage level: 0.5-5%; 20% act.

Cromoist HYA. [Croda Inc.; Croda Chem. Ltd.] Hydrolyzed animal protein, hyaluronic acid; moisturizer, conditioner for skin care prods., facial creams; amber liq.; m.w. 500,000; usage level: 0.5-2%; 15% act.

Cromoist O-25. [Croda Inc.] Hydrolyzed whole oats; skin care ingred. improving feel props. of creams and lotions, imparting soft, cushiony feel on skin; moisturizer; lt. amber liq., char. odor; sol. in water, glycerin, sodium lauryl sulfate; m.w. 1000; pH 4.0-5.0; usage level: 1-5%; 26% act.

Cromul EM 0685. [Croda Chem. Ltd.] Ceteth-5 and ceteareth-7; nonionic; emulsifier and opacifier for cos-metic and pharmaceutical creams and lotions; soft waxy solid; 100% conc.

Cromul EM 1207. [Croda Chem. Ltd.] Steareth-21; CAS 9005-00-9; nonionic; emulsifier for cosmetic prepara-tions; waxy solid; HLB 15.5; 100% conc.

Cronectin H. [Croda Inc.; Croda Chem. Ltd.] Hydrolyzed fibronectin; CAS 100085-35-6; EINECS 293-509-4; hu-mectant and moisturizing agent for skin creams and lotions; esp. effective in low solids lotions; opalescent low-visc. liq.; m.w. 20,000; usage level: 0.5-6%; 3% act.

Cropepsol 30. [Croda Chem. Ltd.] Hydrolyzed collagen; CAS 9015-54-7; conditioner for skin and hair conditioner; aq. sol'n.

Cropepsol 35. [Croda Chem. Ltd.] Hydrolyzed collagen; CAS 9015-54-7; cosmetic protein.

Cropepsol 50. [Croda Chem. Ltd.] Hydrolyzed collagen; CAS 9015-54-7; cosmetic protein.

Cropepsol SD. [Croda Chem. Ltd.] Hydrolyzed collagen; CAS 9015-54-7; cosmetic protein.

Cropeptide W. [Croda Inc.] Hydrolyzed wheat protein, hydrolyzed wheat starch; film-forming conditioning pro-tein for controlling moisture and strengthening hair; amber clear liq., char. odor; sol. in water, aq./ethanol blends, sodium lauryl sulfate; m.w. 2500; pH 4.0-5.0; 22-26% solids.

Cropeptone 30. [Croda Chem. Ltd.] Hydrolyzed collagen; CAS 9015-54-7; conditioner for skin and hair conditioner; aq. sol'n.

Cropeptone 35. [Croda Chem. Ltd.] Hydrolyzed collagen; CAS 9015-54-7; cosmetic protein.

Cropeptone 50. [Croda Chem. Ltd.] Hydrolyzed collagen; CAS 9015-54-7; cosmetic protein.

Croquat HH. [Croda Inc.] Cocodimonium hydroxypropyl hydrolyzed hair keratin; CAS 68915-25-3; substantive conditioning protein for hair shampoos and conditioners; amber visc. liq., char. odor; water-sol.; m.w. 1000; pH 4.0-6.0; 21% act.

Croquat L. [Croda Inc.; Croda Chem. Ltd.] Laurdimonium hydroxypropyl hydrolyzed collagen; cationic; substantive protein, conditioner for clear rinses, shampoos, conditioners; clear yel. liq.; m.w. 2500; essentially water-sol.; usage level: 0.5-2.5%; 40% act.

Croquat M. [Croda Inc.; Croda Chem. Ltd.] Cocodimonium hydroxypropyl hydrolyzed collagen; cationic; substantive protein, conditioner for shampoos, perms, hair relaxers; clear yel. liq.; m.w. 2500; essentially water-sol.; usage level: 0.5-2.5%; 40% act.

Croquat S. [Croda Inc.; Croda Chem. Ltd.] Steardimonium hydroxypropyl hydrolyzed collagen; cationic; substantive protein, conditioner for cream rinses; yel. paste/gel; partly water-sol.; m.w. 2700; usage level: 0.5-2.5%; 40% act.

Croquat Soya. [Croda Chem. Ltd.] Lauryldimonium hydroxypropyl hydrolyzed soy protein.

Croquat WKP. [Croda Inc.] Cocodimonium hydroxypropyl hydrolyzed keratin; CAS 68915-25-3; cationic; permanent conditioning protein for cream rinses, shampoos, conditioners, perms, nail care prods.; clear amber liq.; water-sol.; m.w. 1000; usage level: 0.25-2%; 30% act. in water.

Crosilk 10,000. [Croda Inc.; Croda Chem. Ltd.] Hydrolyzed silk; CAS 96690-41-4; protein conditioner providing manageability, gloss, texture in hair care prods., moisturizing and protection in skin care prods.; dk. amber liq., sl. char. odor; water-sol.; m.w. 10,000; pH 4.0-6.0; usage level: 0.5-2%; 15% act.

Crosilk Liq. [Croda Inc.; Croda Chem. Ltd.] Silk amino acids; CAS 977077-71-6; conditioner, humectant for skin and hair care prods.; pale amber liq., char. odor; m.w. 90; water-sol.; usage level: 0.2-3%; 15% act., 27-31% total solids.

Crosilk Liq. Complex. [Croda Chem. Ltd.] Hydrolyzed silk; CAS 96690-41-4; cosmetic protein.

Crosilk Powder. [Croda Inc.] Silk powder; CAS 9009-99-8; protein for solid make-up, hair prods. where it absorbs oil, improves leveling, enhances spreading, gives elasticity and lubricity, modifies applic. properties and provides a silky, lustrous appearance; improves pigment binding and stability; lustrous gray/wh. powd., sl. odor; m.w. > 500,000; pH 5.5-7.5 (0.5% disp.); usage level: 1-5%; toxicology: nonirritating; 100% act.

Crosilkquat. [Croda Inc.] Cocodimonium hydroxypropyl silk amino acids; cationic; substantive conditioner and moisturizer with exc. foaming props. for skin and hair conditioners, shampoos, styling mousses, perms and relaxers, night creams and lotions; effective over wide pH range; yel. to pale amber clear liq.; sol. in water, aq./alcoholic mixts., glycerin, propylene glycol; m.w. 320; pH 4.0-5.5; usage level: 0.1-2%; 30% act.

Crosterene SA4310. [Croda Universal Ltd.] Stearic acid; CAS 57-11-4; EINECS 200-313-4; pearlescent in cosmetic creams and lotions; binder; buffing compds., candles, and lubricants; wax-like solids.

Crosterol SFA. [Croda Chem. Ltd.] Petrolatum, min. oil, lanolin alcohol, and glyceryl laurate.

Crosultaine C-50. [Croda Inc.] Cocamidopropyl hydroxysultaine; CAS 68139-30-0; EINECS 268-761-3; amphoteric; foam booster/stabilizer effective over wide range of pH and water hardness; for shampoos, baby shampoos; lime soap dispersant; yel. visc. liq., char. odor; sol. @ 10% in water, ethanol, ethanol/water mixts., propylene glycol, glycerin; pH 6.5-8.5; usage level: 1-10%; 50% act.

Crosultaine E-30. [Croda Inc.] Erucamidopropyl hydroxysultaine; amphoteric; visc. booster and conditioner giving silky feel, comb and static control at levels less than 2% active; improves creaminess and lubricity of lather; lime soap dispersant; yel. to amber gel, char. odor; sol. @ 10% in water, water/ethanol mixts.; disp. in glycerin, propylene glycol; pH 6.5-8.5 (10% in IPA/water 60:40); usage level: 1-10%; 30% act.

Crosultaine T-30. [Croda Inc.] Tallowamidopropyl hydroxysultaine; amphoteric; foam and visc. booster; improves wet combing and hair condition; lime soap dispersant; yel. gel, char. odor; sol. @ 10% in water, ethanol, ethanol/water mixts., propylene glycol, glycerin; pH 6.5-8.5 (10% in IPA/water 60:40); usage level: 1-10%; 30% conc.

Crotein A. [Croda Chem. Ltd.] Hydrolyzed collagen; CAS 9015-54-7; cosmetic protein.

Crotein AD. [Croda Inc.; Croda Chem. Ltd.] AMP-isostearic hydrolyzed collagen; CAS 95032-84-1; protein for use in alcoholic preps., e.g., aerosol hairsprays, skin tonics, pump hairsprays, setting lotions; yel. clear liq.; sp.gr. 0.885-0.900; acid no. 29-39; pH 8.4-92. (10%); 24-26% solids in ethanol/water.

Crotein AD Anhyd. [Croda Inc.] AMP isostearoyl hydrolyzed collagen; CAS 95032-84-1; conditioners for hair preparations, alcohol prods., aerosol hair sprays, skin tonics, setting lotions, aftershaves; yel. clear liq.; m.w. 2000; sp.gr. 0.830-0.850; acid no. 35-50; pH 8.0-9.0 (10%); usage level: 0.1-2.0%; 27-33% solids in ethanol.

Crotein ADW. [Croda Inc.] AMP-isostearoyl hydrolyzed wheat protein; anionic; conditioning protein, film modifier for alcoholic and hydroalcoholic lotions, hair care prods., skin tonics, aftershave, nail preps., quick-breaking foam aerosols; plasticizer for resins in hair prods.; yel. clear liq., alcoholic odor; sol. in water, water/alcohol mixts., glycerin, propylene glycol; m.w. 3000; acid no. 45-60; pH 8.0-9.5; usage level: 0.1-2.0; 36% act.

Crotein ASC. [Croda Inc.] Ethyl ester of hydrolyzed animal protein; CAS 68951-89-3; protein conditioner and film modifier for alcoholic and hydroalcoholic lotions and hair care prods., esp. hard lustrous film prods.; clear lt. amber liq., sl. odor; sol. in water, alcohol; m.w. 2000; sp.gr. 0.890-0.810; acid no. 15-20; pH 6.0-6.5 (10% disp.); usage level: 0.1-0.5%; 20% act.

Crotein ASK. [Croda Inc.] Hydrolyzed animal keratin; CAS 69430-36-0; EINECS 274-001-1; conditioner, film modifier for hair setting/conditioning systems; clear amber liq.; m.w. 2000; sol. in water, alcohol; usage level: 0.1-0.5%; 12% act.

Crotein CAA/SF. [Croda Inc.] Collagen amino acids; CAS 9105-54-7; moisturizer for skin creams and lotions; yel. liq.; m.w. 150; water-sol.; usage level: 0.2-3%; 40% act.

Crotein HKP Powd. [Croda Inc.] Hair keratin amino acids, sodium chloride; amphoteric; substantive conditioner and moisturizer for shampoos, cream rinses; lt. brn. powd.; m.w. 150; water-sol.; usage level: 0.5-2%; 50% act.

Crotein HKP/SF. [Croda Inc.] Keratin amino acids; CAS 68238-35-7; protein conditioner for hair and nail care prods.; pale straw liq.; m.w. 150; compat. with aq. alcohol; usage level: 0.5-2%; 25% act.

Crotein IP. [Croda Inc.; Croda Chem. Ltd.] Isostearoyl hydrolyzed collagen; conditioner for use in solvent-based nail polish and removers; brn. visc. liq.; sol. (@ 10%) in min. oil, ethanol (slight haze); immiscible with water; m.w. 2200; acid no. 180-200; pH 6-8 (10% aq. disp.); usage level: 0.1-0.5%; 100% act.

Crotein IPX. [Croda Inc.] Isostearic hydrolyzed collagen; protein for use in anhyd. preps. such as pomades, brilliantines, and bath oils; brn. visc. liq.; acid no. 130-150; pH 6-8 (10% aq.); 100% act.

Crotein K. [Croda Inc.; Croda Chem. Ltd.] Hydrolyzed keratin; CAS 69430-36-0; EINECS 274-001-1; proteinic conditioner and moisturizer for hair and nail care prods.; lt. tan powd.; m.w. 2000; usage level: 0.5-3%; 60% act.

Crotein Q. [Croda Inc.] Steartrimonium hydroxyethyl hydrolyzed collagen; CAS 111174-62-0; cationic; substantive conditioner, body and gloss agent for hair care preparations; off-wh. powd.; m.w. 12,500; sol. in water; sol. @ 5% in 50% ethanol sol'n.; m.w. 12,000; visc. 15–25 mps

(10%); pH 5.5–6.5 (10%); usage level: 0.5-2.5%; 95% act. min.

Crotein SPA. [Croda Inc.] Hydrolyzed collagen; CAS 9015-54-7; conditioner for hair care preparations; foam stabilizer/booster in shampoo; peptizing aid in shampoos; dye leveling aid in hair dyes and bleaches; also for skin treatment, in depilatories; wh. powd., bland, pleasant odor; m.w. 2000; sol. in 50% ethanol, water; visc. 20–25 mps (10%); pH 5.5–6.5 (10%).; usage level: 0.2-2%; 93% act.

Crotein SPC. [Croda Inc.] Hydrolyzed collagen; CAS 9015-54-7; conditioner for hair care preparations; foam stabilizer/booster in shampoo; peptizing aid in shampoos; dye leveling aid in hair dyes and bleaches; also for skin treatment, in depilatories; wh. powd.; bland, pleasant odor; m.w. 10,000; sol. in 65% ethanol @ 1% solid protein; water-sol.; visc. 40–50 mps (10%); pH 5.5–6.5 (10%).; usage level: 0.2-2%; 93% act.

Crotein SPO. [Croda Inc.] Hydrolyzed collagen; CAS 9015-54-7; used for hair spray formulations; forms a hard clear nontacky film; wh. powd.; bland, pleasant odor; m.w. 1000; sol. in water, 20% ethanol @ 1% solid protein; visc. 15–20 mps (10%); pH 5.5–6.5 (10%).; usage level: 0.2-2%; 93% act.

Crotein WKP. [Croda Inc.] Hydrolyzed keratin; CAS 69430-36-0; EINECS 274-001-1; conditioner for hair prods.; enhanced substantivity to keratinous substrates; pale yel. liq.; m.w. 600; usage level: 0.2-3%; 22% act.

Crothix. [Croda Inc.] Polyol alkoxy ester; nonionic; mild thickener for aq. systems, shampoos, aux. emulsifier and bodying agent for creams and lotions; wh. to off-wh. solid; sol. in aq. surfactant systems; usage level: 0.5-2%.

Crovol A40. [Croda Inc.; Croda Chem. Ltd.] PEG-20 almond glycerides; nonionic; coemulsifier, superfatting agent, emollient, counterirritant, wetting aid, solubilizer, dispersant for skin and hair care prods., soaps, bath oils, astringents, antiperspirants; plasticizer for styling mousses and aq. aerosols; fragrance solubilizer; solubilizer and dispersant for fragrances; emollient and solubilizer for pharmaceutical hydroalcoholic systems and external analgesic prods.; yel. liq.; sol. in ethanol, oleyl alcohol, IPA; partly sol. in min. oil; disp. in water, propylene glycol; HLB 10.0; acid no. 2 max.; sapon. no. 90-100; hyd. no. 155-170; usage level: 1-10%; toxicology: nonirritating to skin and eyes.

Crovol A70. [Croda Inc.; Croda Chem. Ltd.] PEG-60 almond glycerides; nonionic; emulsifier reducing irritation potential of anionic/amphoteric surfactant systems, soap scrubs; emollients for hydroalcoholic systems; wetting agent, solubilizer; yel. soft paste; sol. in water, ethanol, IPA, oleyl alcohol, maize oil; partly sol. in min. oil; HLB 15.0; acid no. 2 max.; sapon. no. 45-55; hyd. no. 70-90; usage level: 1-10%; toxicology: nonirritating to skin and eyes.

Crovol EP-40. [Croda Inc.; Croda Chem. Ltd.] PEG-20 evening primrose glycerides.

Crovol EP-70. [Croda Inc.; Croda Chem. Ltd.] PEG-60 evening primrose glycerides.

Crovol M40. [Croda Inc.; Croda Chem. Ltd.] PEG-20 corn glycerides; nonionic; coemulsifier, superfatting agent, emollient, counterirritant, wetting aid, solubilizer, dispersant for skin and hair care prods., soaps, bath oils, astringents, antiperspirants, pharmaceuticals; plasticizer for styling mousses and aq. aerosols; fragrance solubilizer; yel. liq.; sol. in ethanol, oleyl alcohol, IPA; partly sol. in min. oil; disp. in water, propylene glycol; HLB 10.0; acid no. 2 max.; sapon. no. 90-100; hyd. no. 155-170; usage level: 1-10%; toxicology: nonirritating to skin and eyes.

Crovol M70. [Croda Inc.; Croda Chem. Ltd.] PEG-60 corn glycerides; nonionic; emulsifier reducing the irritation potential of anionic/amphoteric surfactant systems, soap scrubs; emollient for hydroalcoholic systems; wetting agent, fragrance solubilizer; yel. liq. to paste; sol. in water, ethanol, oleyl alcohol, maize oil, IPA; partly sol. in min. oil; disp. in propylene glycol; HLB 15.0; acid no. 2 max.; sapon. no. 45-55; hyd. no. 70-85; usage level: 1-10%; toxicology: nonirritating to eyes; minimal skin irritant.

Crovol PK40. [Croda Inc.; Croda Chem. Ltd.] PEG-12 palm kernel glycerides; nonionic; coemulsifier, superfatting agent, emollient, counterirritant, wetting aid, solubilizer, dispersant for skin and hair care prods., soaps, bath oils, astringents, antiperspirants; plasticizer for styling mousses and aq. aerosols; fragrance solubilizer; off-wh. liq.; sol. in oleyl alcohol, ethanol, maize oil; water-disp.; HLB 9.0; acid no. 2 max.; sapon. no. 130-140; hyd. no. 90-105; usage level: 1-10%.

Crovol PK70. [Croda Inc.; Croda Chem. Ltd.] PEG-45 palm kernel glycerides; nonionic; coemulsifier, superfatting agent, emollient, counterirritant, wetting aid, solubilizer, dispersant for skin and hair care prods., soaps, bath oils, astringents, antiperspirants; plasticizer for styling mousses and aq. aerosols; fragrance solubilizer; wh. soft paste; sol. in water, ethanol, oleyl alcohol; HLB 15.0; acid no. 2 max.; sapon. no. 60-70; hyd. no. 70-85; usage level: 1-10%.

Cryolidone®. [UCIB; Barnet Prods.] Lauryl menthyl PCA; lipophilic cooling and moisturizing agent for cosmetics without menthol odor; for toiletries, skin and hair care prods.; clear sol'n., odorless; insol. in water; usage level: 1%.

Crystal® O. [CasChem] Refined castor oil USP; CAS 8001-79-4; EINECS 232-293-8; emollient, pigment wetter, cosolv., lubricant for cosmetics, makeup, antiperspirant sticks; FDA approval; Gardner 1- color; sp.gr. 0.959; visc. 7.5 stokes; pour pt. -23 C; acid no. 2; iodine no. 86; sapon. no. 180; hyd. no. 164.

Crystal® Crown. [CasChem] Refined castor oil USP, with antioxidant; CAS 8001-79-4; EINECS 232-293-8; emollient, pigment wetter, cosolv., lubricant for cosmetics, makeup, antiperspirant sticks; FDA approval; Gardner 1- color; sp.gr. 0.959; visc. 7.5 stokes; pour pt. -23 C; acid no. 2; iodine no. 86; sapon. no. 180; hyd. no. 164.

Crystal® Crown LP. [CasChem] Castor oil USP; CAS 8001-79-4; EINECS 232-293-8; highly refined cosmetic grade with antioxidant for formulations requiring low peroxide levels; pigment wetting and suspending agent for lipsticks and antiperspirants; m.p. -23 C; acid no. 2; iodine no. 86; sapon. no. 180; hyd. no. 164.

Crystallin Protein. [Sederma] Water, propylene glycol, PEG-8, and crystallins.

Crystalline Beta Carotene No. 65638. [Roche] Beta-carotene; CAS 7235-40-7; EINECS 230-636-6; cosmetic colorant.

Crystosol NF 70. [Witco/H-I-P] Min. oil; emollient, cosmetic raw material.

Crystosol NF 90. [Witco/H-I-P] Min. oil; emollient, cosmetic raw material.

Crystosol USP 200. [Witco/H-I-P] Min. oil; emollient, cosmetic raw material.

Crystosol USP 240. [Witco/H-I-P] Min. oil; emollient, cosmetic raw material.

Crystosol USP 350. [Witco/H-I-P] Min. oil; emollient, cosmetic raw material.

CS-2032. [Crystal] Paraffin; CAS 8002-74-2; EINECS 232-315-6; cosmetic wax.

CS-2037. [Crystal] Paraffin; CAS 8002-74-2; EINECS 232-315-6; cosmetic wax.

CS-2043. [Crystal] Paraffin; CAS 8002-74-2; EINECS 232-315-6; cosmetic wax.

CS-2054. [Crystal] Paraffin; CAS 8002-74-2; EINECS 232-

315-6; cosmetic wax.

CS-2080W. [Crystal] Microcrystalline wax; CAS 63231-60-7; EINECS 264-038-1; cosmetic wax.

CTAC. [Zeeland] Cetrimonium chloride; CAS 112-02-7; EINECS 203-928-6; quat. for personal care prods.

Cuivridone®. [UCIB; Barnet Prods.] Copper PCA; combines moisturizing of PCA with props. of trace metals; antiseborrhoeic and bacteriostatic agent for skin and hair care prods.; powd.; water-sol.; usage level: 0.1-1%.

Cumal. [Mitsubishi Gas] p-Isopropylbenzaldehyde; CAS 122-03-2; EINECS 204-516-9; intermediate for pharmaceuticals, perfumes; colorless liq., aromatic odor; sol. in ethanol, ether, toluene; insol. in water; m.w. 148.2; sp.gr. 0.979; b.p. 235.5 C; acid no. 0.3; flash pt. (COC) 104 C; toxicology: LD50 (oral, rat) 1390 mg/kg; eye and skin irritant; 98.5% purity.

CUPL® PIC. [Heterene; Bernel] PPG-2 isoceteth-20 acetate; CAS 110332-91-7; fragrance solubilizer and o/w emulsifier; FDA, EEC, and Japanese compliances; solid; sol. in water, oil; usage level: 0.5-5.0%.

Cutavit Richter. [Dr. Kurt Richter; Henkel/Cospha] Isopropyl palmitate, tocopherol, linoleic acid, PABA, linolenic acid, retinyl palmitate; complex of vitamins A and E and essential fatty acids in lipopholic medium for dry skin and hair treatments; yel. to reddish-yel. oil.

Cuticulin. [Freeman] Hydrolyzed keratin.

Cutina® AGS. [Henkel Canada] Glycol distearate; CAS 627-83-8; EINECS 211-014-3; pearlescent and opacifier; emulsion shampoos and foam baths; wh. flakes.

Cutina® BW. [Henkel/Cospha; Henkel Canada] Glyceryl hydroxystearate, cetyl palmitate, microcryst. wax, trihydroxystearin; wax for use as beeswax substitute; visc. agent for personal care prods.; pale yel. waxy flakes; m.p. 61-66 C; acid no. 20-26; iodine no. < 5; sapon. no. 110-130.

Cutina® CBS. [Henkel/Cospha; Henkel KGaA/Cospha] Glyceryl stearate, cetearyl alcohol, cetyl palmitate, and cocoglycerides; nonionic; cream base for mfg. of creams and lotions of the o/w type; visc. agent and stabilizer; waxy flakes; m.w. 52-58 C; acid no. 5 max.; sapon. no. 150-165; hyd. no. 170-195; 100% conc.

Cutina® CP. [Henkel/Cospha; Henkel Canada; Henkel KGaA/Cospha] Cetyl palmitate; CAS 95912-87-1; EINECS 208-736-6; syn. spermaceti; consistency factor for creams, ointments, liq. emulsions, fatty makeups, and sticks; wh. waxy coarse flakes; insol. in water; m.p. 50 C; HLB 9; acid no. 1 max.; iodine no. 1 max.; sapon. no. 112-123; ref. index 1.431-1.437.

Cutina® E24. [Henkel Canada; Henkel/Cospha; Henkel KGaA/Cospha] PEG-20 glyceryl stearate; nonionic; o/w emulsifier for mild creams and emulsions for baby and children's preparations, sun preps.; cloudy paste; solid. pt. 18-21 C; sapon. no. 49-54; hyd. no. 76-82; pH 6.0-7.5 (1%); 100% conc.

Cutina® FS 25 Flakes. [Henkel KGaA/Cospha] Palmitic acid and stearic acid; consistency factor after saponification; o/w emulsifier for emulsions and ointments; almost wh. fine flakes, weak char. odor; solid. pt. 49-53 C; acid no. 211-215; iodine no. 1 max.

Cutina® FS 45 Flakes. [Henkel KGaA/Cospha] Palmitic acid, stearic acid; consistency factor after saponification; o/w emulsifier used in cosmetic/pharmaceutical emulsions/ointments; almost wh. fine flakes, weak char. odor; solid. pt. 51-55 C; acid no. 207-210; iodine no. 1 max.

Cutina® GMS. [Henkel/Cospha; Henkel Canada; Henkel KGaA/Cospha] Glyceryl stearate; CAS 67701-33-1; nonionic; nonself-emulsifying cream base for o/w and w/o emulsions; visc. agent for cosmetic/pharmaceutical creams, ointments, sticks; wh. to sl. ylsh. waxy powd.; m.p. 58-60 C; acid no. 2 max.; iodine no. 0.5 max.; sapon.

no. 165-175; 100% conc.

Cutina® HR. [Henkel/Cospha; Henkel Canada; Henkel KGaA/Cospha] Hydrog. castor oil; CAS 8001-78-3; EINECS 232-292-2; lubricant for tablets, high melting consistency giving factor, thickener for oils; caring and decorative cosmetic stick preps., block form makeup; wh. to sl. yel. fine free-flowing powd.; particle size 30% < 10 μ; bulk dens. 350-410 g/l; m.p. 85-88 C; acid no. 3.1 max.; iodine no. < 5; sapon. no. 176-182; hyd. no. 154-162; 99-100% act.

Cutina® KD16. [Henkel Canada; Henkel/Cospha; Henkel KGaA/Cospha] Glyceryl stearate SE; emulsifier, fatting co-agent for o/w ointments and cosmetic creams; base; wh. to sl. waxy compd., faint odor; solid. pt. 55-60 C; acid no. 7 max.; sapon. no. 150-165; hyd. no. 190-220.

Cutina® LM. [Henkel] Castor oil, glyceryl ricinoleate, octyl dodecanol, carnauba, candelilla, and microcryst. waxes, cetyl alcohol, beeswax, and min. oil; wax base for cosmetic stick preparations; yel. wax; slight odor; sp.gr. 0.90; m.p. 70-74 C; sapon. no. 120-130; 100% fatty matter.

Cutina® MD. [Henkel Canada; Henkel KGaA/Cospha] Glyceryl stearate; consistency factor, stabilizer used in ointments, creams, and liq. emulsions; wh. to pale yel. waxy gran.; m.p. 53-57 C; acid no. 6 max.; sapon. no. 165-180; hyd. no. 210-250.

Cutina® TS. [Henkel] PEG-3 distearate; CAS 9005-08-7; nonionic; opacifying and pearly sheen producing wax for shampoos, shower and bath preparations.

Cyanocobalamin USP (Cryst.). [Roche] Vitamin B12; cosmetic ingred.

Cyclamber. [Henkel/Cospha] Fragrance raw material for cosmetic, personal care, detergent, and cleaning prods.; colorless liq., woody odor; b.p. 92-94 C; flash pt. 151 C.

Cyclochem EM 326A. [Witco/H-I-P] Syn. beeswax; cosmetic creams and lotions; wax; m.p. 61-64 C; 100% act.

Cyclochem EM 560. [Witco/H-I-P] Cetearyl alcohol, sodium lauryl sulfate, cetyl esters, and myristyl alcohol; anionic; self-emulsifying wax for cosmetic creams and lotions; wax; m.p. 57-60 C; 100% act.

Cyclogol NI. [Witco/H-I-P] Cetearyl alcohol and ceteareth-20; nonionic; self-emulsifying wax for cosmetic creams and lotions; wax; m.p. 47-49 C; 100% act.

Cyclohexyl Salicylate. [Henkel/Cospha] Fragrance raw material for cosmetic, personal care, detergent, and cleaning prods.; colorless liq., aromatic odor; b.p. 115 C; flash pt. 155 C.

Cyclol SPS. [Witco/H-I-P] Syn. spermaceti; nonionic; spermaceti substitute for cosmetic and pharmaceutical formulations; wax for cosmetic creams and lotions; wax; m.p. 42-50 C; 100% act.

Cycloryl M1. [Rhone-Poulenc] Sodium laureth sulfate, glycol stearate, and cocamide MEA; personal care surfactant.

Cyclosal. [Firmenich] Cyclamen aldehyde; CAS 103-95-7; EINECS 203-161-7.

Cyclovertal. [Henkel/Cospha] 3, 6-Dimethyl-3-cyclohexene-1-carbaldehyde; general fragrance raw material for personal care and detergent applics., gm., fruity notes.; sl. yel. liq., tart odor; b.p. 90 C; flash pt. 65 C.

Cypronat. [Henkel/Cospha] Fragrance raw material for cosmetic, personal care, detergent, and cleaning prods.; colorless liq., honey odor; b.p. 93-97 C; flash pt. 87 C.

Cytochrome C. [Seporga] A protein which acts to transport electrons which play an essential part in the skin's respiratory chain.

Cytochrome Marine. [Seporga] Natural catalysts for the metabolic and respiratory functions of the skin.

Cytoplasmine-1. [Vevy] Water and mushroom extract; botanical extract.

Cytoplasmine-2. [Vevy] Water and yeast extract; CAS 8103-01-2.

D

Dacriosalt. [Vevy] Sea salt.

Daitosol SPA. [Les Colorants Wackherr] An aq. opacifying emulsion for cosmetics.

Damox® 1010. [Ethyl] Didecyl dimethylamine oxide; nonionic; wetting agent, emulsifier, dispersant, visc. modifier, hair conditioner with low foam; liq.; sol. in oil, disp. in water; 80% conc.

Dandelion HS. [Alban Muller] Propylene glycol and dandelion extract; botanical extract.

Dantoin® DMDMH-55. [Lonza] DMDM hydantoin; intermediate; wh. liq.; 55% conc.

Dantoin® DMHF. [Lonza] DMHF; CAS 9065-13-8; intermediate for cosmetics, textiles, and other applics.; wh. solid; m.p. 75 C.

Dantoin® DMHF-75. [Lonza] DMHF; CAS 9065-13-8; intermediate for cosmetics, textiles, and other applics.; hair lacquers and wave sets; film former; clear liq.; sol. in water, alcohol; 75% conc.

Dantoin® MDMH. [Lonza] MDM hydantoin; CAS 116-25-6; EINECS 204-132-1; intermediate for cosmetics and other applics.; preservation and gelation agent; wh. crystals; m.w. 158; m.p. 112 C.

Dantosperse® DHE (5) MO. [Lonza] PEG-5 DEDM hydantoin oleate.

Dar-C. [Darling] Hydrog. tallow acid; CAS 61790-38-3; EINECS 263-130-9; used in bar soaps, cosmetics.

Dariloid® QH. [Kelco] Algin; CAS 9005-38-3; gelling agent, emulsifier and stabilizer in food, pharmaceutical, and industrial applics.

Dascare FSP Liq. [Dasco] Soy protein; CAS 68153-28-6; cosmetic protein.

Dascare HPCH. [Dasco] Hydroxypropyl chitosan; CAS 84069-44-3; film-former for hair care.

Dascare MCCP. [Dasco] Microcryst. cellulose; CAS 9004-34-6; tablet binder, vehicle.

Dascare S.O.D. [Dasco] Superoxide dismutase.

Dascare SWP. [Dasco] Hydrolyzed wheat protein; CAS 70084-87-6; cosmetic protein.

Dascare Bovine Placenta. [Dasco] Placental protein.

Dascare Chitin Liq. [Dasco] Sodium carboxymethyl chitin.

Dascare Micropearl. [Dasco] Rice starch; CAS 9005-25-8; cosmetic ingred.

Dascare Orizanol. [Dasco] Oryzanol; CAS 11042-64-1; uv absorber, antioxidant.

Dascare Oryza-Oil. [Dasco] Rice bran oil; EINECS 271-397-8; cosmetic ingred.

Dascare Royal Jelly Powd. [Dasco] Royal jelly powd.

Dascare Zirconia. [Dasco] Zirconium dioxide; CAS 1314-23-4.

Dascolor Carmine. [Dasco] Carmine; CAS 1390-65-4; EINECS 215-724-4; cosmetic colorant.

Dascolor Chlorophyll. [Dasco] Chlorophyllin-copper complex; CAS 11006-34-1; EINECS 234-242-5.

Daucoil. [Vevy] Carrot oil; CAS 8015-88-1.

Daxad® 30. [Hampshire] Sodium polymethacrylate sol'n.; CAS 25086-62-8; dispersant esp. for pigments in aq. sol'ns.; used in paint formulations, emulsion polymerization, water treatment, agriculture, cosmetic base makeup, industrial cleaners, in large particle suspensions; water-wh. clear liq.; sol. in water systems; sp.gr. 1.15; dens. 9.6 lb/gal; visc. 75 cps max.; pH 10.0; surf. tens. 70 dynes/cm (1%); 25% solids.

Daxad® 31. [Hampshire] Isobutylene maleic anhydride copolymer sol'n.; CAS 26426-80-2; dispersant for aq. systems; used in cosmetic base makeup, latex paints and coatings, enamels, polymerization, leather tanning, and water treatment; pale amber clear liq.; sol. in water systems; sp.gr. 1.11; dens. 9.2 lb/gal; visc. 30 cps; pH 10.0; surf. tens. 50 dynes/cm (1%); 25% total solids.

DEA Commercial Grade. [Dow] Diethanolamine; CAS 111-42-2; EINECS 203-868-0; used in surfactants, cosmetics/toiletries, metalworking fluids, textile chemicals, gas conditioning chemicals, agric. intermediates, adhesives, antistats, coatings, petroleum, polymers, rubber processing, and cement grinding aids; sp.gr. 1.0881 (30/4 C); dens. 9.09 lb/gal (30 C); visc. 351.9 cps (30 C); f.p. 28 C; b.p. 268 C (760 mm Hg); flash pt. (Seta CC) 325 F; fire pt. 300 F; ref. index 1.4750 (30 C).

Dead Sea Bath Salts. [Int'l. Sourcing] Natural hygroscopic materials found in the Dead Sea; for therapeutic baths; wh. cryst. powd., odorless; sol. cloudy 60 g/100 ml in water.

DEA Low Freeze Grade. [Dow] Diethanolamine; CAS 111-42-2; EINECS 203-868-0; used in surfactants, cosmetics/toiletries, metalworking fluids, textile chemicals, gas conditioning chemicals, agric. intermediates, adhesives, antistats, coatings, petroleum, polymers, rubber processing, and cement grinding aids; sp.gr. 1.0881 (30/4 C); dens. 9.09 lb/gal (30 C); visc. 351.9 cps (30 C); f.p. 28 C; b.p. 268 C (760 mm Hg); flash pt. (Seta CC) 325 F; fire pt. 300 F; ref. index 1.4750 (30 C).

Decaprotein. [Vevy] Soy protein and casein.

Decoset-Z. [Decorative Industries] Tosylamide/epoxy resin.

Degras. [Croda Inc.] Woolgrease.

Dehydazol. [Henkel] Cellulose gum.

Dehydol® LS 2 DEO. [Henkel Canada; Henkel KGaA/Cospha; Pulcra SA] Laureth-2; CAS 68439-50-9; EINECS 221-279-7; nonionic; emulsifier, solubilizer for solvs., oils, bases for prod. of sulfates; raw material for cosmetic/pharmaceutical preps., bath oils, waterless hand cleaners, dishwashing, cleansing agent and cold cleaners; water-wh. clear to sl. cloudy liq.; HLB 6.2; hyd. no. 196-204; cloud pt. 5-8 C; pH 6.0-7.5 (1%); 99–100% conc.

Dehydol® LS 3 DEO. [Henkel; Henkel Canada; Henkel KGaA/Cospha] Laureth-3; CAS 68439-50-9; EINECS 221-280-2; nonionic; emulsifier, solubilizer for solvs., oils, bases for prod. of sulfates; raw material for cosmetic/

pharmaceutical preps., oil and cream baths, dishwashing, cleansing agent and cold cleaners; water-wh. clear to sl. cloudy liq.; hyd. no. 173-180; cloud pt. 2-5 C; hyd. no. 173-180; 99–100% conc.

Dehydol® LS 4 DEO. [Henkel KGaA/Cospha] Laureth-4; CAS 68439-50-9; EINECS 226-097-1; nonionic; emulsifier, solubilizer for solvs., oils, bases for prod. of sulfates; raw material for cosmetics/pharmaceutical preps., oil and cream baths, dishwashing, cleansing agent and cold cleaners; water-wh. clear to cloudy liq.; hyd. no. 150-158; cloud pt. 4-10 C; pH 6.0-7.5; 99–100% conc.

Dehydol® PID 6. [Pulcra SA] Laureth-6; CAS 34938-91-8; EINECS 221-282-3; nonionic; emulsifier, wetting agent for industrial, cosmetic, pharmaceutical applics., in high electrolyte concs.; liq.; HLB 11.8; hyd. no. 178-182; pH 6.0-7.5 (1%); 100% conc.

Dehydol® PLT 6. [Pulcra SA] Ethoxylated isotridecanol; CAS 24938-91-8; nonionic; emulsifier, wetting agent for industrial, cosmetic, pharmaceutical applics., in high electrolyte concs.; liq.; HLB 11.7; 100% conc.

Dehydrated Keratine Hydrolysate. [Bretagne Chimie Fine] Hydrolyzed keratin; CAS 69430-36-0; EINECS 274-001-1; cosmetic protein.

Dehymuls® E. [Henkel/Cospha; Henkel Canada; Henkel KGaA/Cospha] Dicocoyl pentaerythrityl distearyl citrate, sorbitan sesquioleate, beeswax, aluminum stearate; anionic; w/o emulsifier with high water absorbency and good resist. to temp. fluctuations; suitable for cosmetics; ylsh. waxy solid; drop pt. 45-60 C; HLB 6.0; iodine no. 20-30; sapon. no. 160-170; 100% conc.

Dehymuls® F. [Henkel Canada; Henkel KGaA/Cospha] Dicocoyl pentaerythrityl distearyl citrate, microcrystalline wax, glyceryl oleate, aluminum stearate, propylene glycol; anionic; w/o emulsifier for creams and emulsions; wh. to sl. yel. wax; m.p. 60-75 C; acid no. 4-10; iodine no. 15-20; sapon. no. 120-140; 100% conc.

Dehymuls® FCE. [Henkel KGaA/Cospha] Dicocoyl pentaerythrityl distearyl citrate; nonionic; emulsifier for w/o emulsions; esp. suited for use with high m.w. emollients and oils; pale yel. flakes; m.p. 42-46 C; acid no. 7 max.; sapon. no. 215-230; hyd. no. 50-60; 100% conc.

Dehymuls® HRE 7. [Henkel/Cospha; Henkel KGaA/Cospha] PEG-7 hydrogenated castor oil; CAS 61788-85-0; nonionic; emulsifier for w/o emulsions for personal care prods.; esp. for low-visc. emulsions; pale yel. cloudy visc. liq., almost odorless; acid no. < 1; sapon. no. 125-140; hyd. no. 110-130; 100% conc.

Dehymuls® K. [Henkel KGaA/Cospha] Petrolatum, decyl oleate, dicocoyl pentaerythrityl distearyl citrate, sorbitan sesquioleate, ceresin, min.oil, beeswax, aluminum stearate; SE ointment base for mfg. of cosmetic and pharmaceutical preparations of the w/o type; wh. to sl. yel. soft waxy solid; solid. pt. 35-50 C; iodine no. 18-23; sapon. no. 75-85; 100% act.

Dehymuls® LS. [Henkel] Dicocoyl pentaerythrityl distearyl citrate, glyceryl oleate, glyceryl stearate, and PEG-5 soya sterol.

Dehymuls® SML. [Henkel KGaA/Cospha] Sorbitan laurate; nonionic; w/o emulsifier and coemulsifier for cosmetic and pharmaceutical applics.; yel. clear liq., pract. odorless; acid no. 4-7; sapon. no. 158-170; hyd. no. 330-358; toxicology: nontoxic.

Dehymuls® SMO. [Henkel KGaA/Cospha] Sorbitan oleate; CAS 1338-43-8; EINECS 215-665-4; nonionic; emulsifier and coemulsifier for w/o cosmetic/pharamceutical ointments and creams; yel.-brn. clear liq.; acid no. 5-8; iodine no. 62-76; sapon. no. 149-160; hyd. no. 193-209; toxicology: nontoxic.

Dehymuls® SMS. [Henkel KGaA/Cospha] Sorbitan stearate; CAS 1338-41-6; EINECS 215-664-9; nonionic; w/o

emulsifier; used in the cosmetic and pharmaceutical industry; wh. to ylsh. flakes; acid no. 5-10; sapon. no. 147-157; hyd. no. 235-260; toxicology: nontoxic.

Dehymuls® SSO. [Henkel KGaA/Cospha] Sorbitan sesquioleate; CAS 8007-43-0; EINECS 232-360-1; nonionic; w/o emulsifier and coemulsifier for waxes and oils for cosmetics and pharmaceuticals; yel.-brn. clear liq., pract. odorless; acid no. 12 max.; iodine no. 65-75; sapon. no. 150-165; hyd. no. 185-215; toxicology: nontoxic.

Dehyquart® A. [Henkel/Cospha; Henkel/Functional Prods.; Henkel KGaA/Cospha] Cetrimonium chloride; CAS 112-02-7; EINECS 203-928-6; cationic; emulsifier for emulsion polymerization, cosmetic creams and lotions; softener, conditioner, bactericide, fungicide, and odor inhibitor in personal care prods.; antistat for hair and fibers; substantive to hair and skin; pale yel. clear liq., typ. odor; pH 5-8; 24% act.

Dehyquart® C. [Henkel/Functional Prods.] Lauryl pyridinium chloride; CAS 104-74-5; EINECS 203-232-2; cationic; surfactant, wetting agent, fungicide, bactericide, and disinfectant used in cleaning formulations and personal care prods.; sequestrant for min. oil industry; wh. paste, powd.; 80–82% act.

Dehyquart® C Crystals. [Henkel/Cospha; Henkel/Functional Prods.] Lauryl pyridinium chloride; CAS 104-74-5; EINECS 203-232-2; cationic; emulsifier in creams and lotions; hair conditioners, skin creams; antistat for hair and fiber; bactericide, fungicide, corrosion inhibitor, sequestrant; conditioner used in personal care prods.; recrystallized powd.; 90–94% act.

Dehyquart® DAM. [Henkel/Functional Prods.] Distearyl dimethyl ammonium chloride; CAS 107-64-2; EINECS 203-508-2; cationic; emulsifier for plastics industry; conditioning component for hair care preparations; antistat; paste; 70–80% act.

Dehyquart® E. [Henkel/Cospha; Henkel Canada; Henkel KGaA/Cospha] Hydroxycetyl hydroxyethyl dimonium chloride; CAS 84643-53-8; cationic; antistat, conditioner for hair treatment, hair conditioners, conditioning shampoos; good adsorption capacity; improves wet and dry combability; compatible with anionic systems; ylsh. clear to sl. turbid liq., mild inherent odor; pH 6.5-7.5; 28% act.

Dehyquart® LDB. [Henkel/Functional Prods.] Lauralkonium chloride; CAS 139-07-1; EINECS 205-351-5; cationic; bactericide and fungicide for disinfectants; emulsifier; external antistat for plastics; liq.; 34–36% conc.

Dehyquart® LT. [Henkel/Functional Prods.] Laurtrimonium chloride; CAS 112-00-5; EINECS 203-927-0; cationic; emulsifier for plastics industry, wetting agent, antistat, bactericide, demulsifier, deodorant, conditioning component for hair care prods.; liq.; 34–36% conc.

Dehyquart® SP. [Henkel/Cospha; Henkel Canada; Henkel KGaA/Cospha] Quaternium-52; CAS 58069-11-7; cationic; emulsifier, conditioning, softening and antistatic agent used in hair conditioners, cream rinses, cationic skin creams and lotions; corrosion inhibitor in metal pkgs. (aerosols); lt. yel. clear low visc. liq.; misc. with water and alcohols; pH 6.9-7.3; 50% act.

Dehyton® AB-30. [Henkel Canada; Henkel KGaA/Cospha; Pulcra SA] Coco-betaine; CAS 68424-94-2; EINECS 270-329-4; amphoteric; detergent, foamer used in personal care prods., liq. shampoos; conditioner, thickener; solubilizer for lauryl sulfates in conc. shampoos; lt. yel. clear liq., mild inherent odor; pH 6.0-7.5; 29-31% act.

Dehyton® G. [Henkel Canada; Henkel KGaA/Cospha; Pulcra SA] Disodium cocoamphodiacetate; CAS 68647-53-0; EINECS 271-957-1; amphoteric; surfactant for mild and conditioning shampoos, bath prods., baby shampoos, skin cleansers, foam baths; yel. clear liq., weak inherent odor; pH 8-9 (10%); 29-31% act.

Dehyton® K. [Henkel KGaA/Cospha] Cocamidopropyl betaine; CAS 61789-40-0; amphoteric; raw material for mfg. of cosmetic/pharmaceutical surfactants, conditioners; lt. yel. clear pumpable liq., mild inherent odor; pH 6.0-7.5; 29-32% act.

Dehyton® PAB-30. [Pulcra SA] Lauryl betaine; CAS 683-10-3; EINECS 211-669-5; amphoteric; high foaming detergent for mild shampoos; solubilizer for lauryl sulfates in conc. shampoos; thickener; liq.; 30% conc.

Dehyton® PG. [Pulcra SA] Disodium cocoamphodiacetate; CAS 68650-39-5; EINECS 272-043-5; amphoteric; foamer, wetting agent for shampoos, foam baths, cosmetics requiring high foaming, mildness; liq.; pH 8-9 (20%); 37-41% act.

Dehyton® PK. [Pulcra SA] Cocamidopropyl betaine; CAS 61789-40-0; amphoteric; high foaming, conditioning detergent for mild shampoos; solubilizer for lauryl sulfates in conc. shampoos; thickener; liq.; pH 4.5-5.5; 29-31.5% act.

Dehyton® PLG. [Pulcra SA] Sodium lauroamphoacetate; CAS 14350-96-0; amphoteric; mild, high foaming surfactant for shampoos, foam baths, cosmetics; liq.; pH 10.0-10.5 (10%); 27.5-31.5% act.

Dehyton® PMG. [Pulcra SA] Sodium lauroamphoacetate; CAS 14350-96-0; amphoteric; raw material for detergents, shampoos, dishwashers, textile softeners, paint emulsifiers, all-purpose washing agents; liq.; pH 9.0-9.5 (20%); 37-41% act.

Dehyton® W. [Henkel] Disodium cocoamphodiacetate; CAS 68650-39-5; EINECS 272-043-5; cosmetic surfactant.

Dekaben. [Zimmerli] Phenoxyethanol, methylparaben, ethylparaben, propylparaben, and butylparaben; cosmetic preservative; USA, Japan, and Europe approvals; usage level: 1%.

Dekacymen. [Jan Dekker BV] 4-Isopropyl-m-cresol; CAS 3228-02-2; EINECS 221-761-7; preservative for cosmetics.

Dekafald. [Jan Dekker BV] DMDM hydantoin; CAS 6440-58-0; EINECS 229-222-8; preservative for cosmetics; usage level: 0.05-0.5%.

Delan 62. [Lanaetex Prods.] Oleth-10, propylene glycol, PEG-10 coconut oil complex; cosmetic ingred.

Delsette. [Hercules] Polyamide resin; hair fixative; imparts improved body and hold to hair; reactive type avail. which is resistant to shampooing; water-sol.

Delsette 101. [Hercules] Adipic acid/epoxypropyl diethylenetriamine copolymer.

Deltyl® Extra. [Givaudan-Roure] Isopropyl myristate; CAS 110-27-0; EINECS 203-751-4; emollient and aux. emulsifier in cosmetics; sol. in alcohol, min., peanut, sesame, olive, and almond oils; water-insol.

Deltyl® Prime. [Givaudan-Roure] Isopropyl palmitate; CAS 142-91-6; EINECS 205-571-1; emollient.

Demaquillant HS 287. [Alban Muller] Propylene glycol, pellitory extract, kidney bean extract, sunflower seed extract, and ivy extract; phytocomplex for facial cleansers.

Demaquillant LS 658. [Alban Muller] Sunflower seed oil, mallow extract, grape extract, and maritime pine extract; phytocomplex for facial cleansers.

Demaquillant LS 687. [Alban Muller] Sunflower seed oil, pellitory extract, faba bean extract, sunflower seed extract, and ivy extract; phytocomplex for facial cleansers.

Demelan HF-12. [Pulcra SA] Blend; anionic/nonionic; conc. for shampoos with superfatting effects; water-sol.; 32% conc.

Demeon D. [Akzo BV] Dimethyl ether; CAS 115-10-6; EINECS 204-065-8; aerosol propellant.

Demol EP. [Kao Corp. SA] Sodium C4-12 olefin/maleic acid copolymer; colorless dispersant for dyestuff and pigment; liq., powd.

Deodorant Richter/K. [Dr. Kurt Richter; Henkel/Cospha] Tetrabromo-o-cresol; combats body odor due to sweat; for deodorant sticks, powds., soaps; ivory powd.

Deo-Usnate. [Cosmetochem] Lichen extract and propylene glycol; CAS 84696-53-7; a natural bactericide and fungicide for cosmetics (deodorants, foot care preps., oral hygiene prods., liq. soaps, skin care creams, lotions); usage level: 0.2-1.0%.

Deproteinated Yeasts. [Sederma] Hydrolyzed yeast.

Deriphat® 151C. [Henkel/Cospha; Henkel Canada] Lauraminopropionic acid; CAS 1462-54-0; EINECS 215-968-1; amphoteric; wetting agent, detergent, emulsifier, corrosion inhibitor; personal care and hard surface cleaners; general-purpose surfactant; high foaming, substantive; Gardner 5 clear liq.; sol. in strong acids, alkalis, ionic systems; sp.gr. 1.03; pH 5.5; 40% solids.

Deriphat® 154. [Henkel/Cospha; Henkel Canada] Disodium N-tallow-β iminodipropionate; CAS 61791-56-8; EINECS 263-190-6; amphoteric; detergent, solubilizer for personal care prods., hard surface cleaning, textiles, emulsion polymerization; good substantivity; wh. powd.; sol. in strong acids, alkalies, and ionic systems; dens. 2 lb/gal; pH 11; 98% solids.

Deriphat® 154L. [Henkel/Cospha; Henkel Canada] Disodium N-tallow β iminodipropionate; CAS 61791-56-8; EINECS 263-190-6; amphoteric; liq. form of Deriphat 154; liq.; 30% conc.

Deriphat® 160. [Henkel/Cospha; Henkel/Functional Prods.; Henkel Canada] Disodium N-lauryl β-iminodipropionate; CAS 3655-00-3; EINECS 222-899-0; amphoteric; detergent, solubilizer, primary emulsifier used in org. and inorg. compds.; emulsion polymerization and stabilization; wetting agent; mild surfactant for hair and skin prods.; wh. powd.; dens. 2.0 lb/gal; 98% solids.

Deriphat® 160C. [Henkel/Cospha; Henkel/Functional Prods.; Henkel Canada] Sodium-N-lauryl β-iminodipropionate; CAS 26256-79-1; amphoteric; detergent, solubilizer, stabilizer; used in petrol. processing, emulsion polymerization, foaming cleaners, personal care prods.; amber clear liq.; sol. in strong acid, alkali, and ionic systems; sp.gr. 1.04; dens. 8.6 lb/gal; pH 7.5; 30% solids.

Dermacol. [Pentapharm Ltd; Centerchem] Soluble collagen; CAS 9007-34-5; EINECS 232-697-4; cosmetic protein.

Dermacryl™ 79. [Nat'l. Starch] Acrylates/octylacrylamide copolymer; highly moisture resist. polymer, occlusive agent, pigment dispersant, and waterproof binder for liq. color cosmetics for skin care applics., waterproofing sunscreens, moisturizing lotions and creams, mascara, eyeliner; wh. powd.; sol. in ethanol, IPA; insol. in water; 3% volatiles.

Dermaffine. [Laserson SA] Oleyl alcohol; CAS 143-28-2; EINECS 205-597-3; emollient.

Dermalcare® 1673. [Rhone-Poulenc Surf. & Spec.] Sodium laureth sulfate, disodium laureth sulfosuccinate, laureth-6 carboxylic acid, cocamidopropyl betaine, and ammonium chloride; high performance base for prep. of ultra-mild face and skin cleanser formulations.

Dermalcare® AC. [Rhone-Poulenc Surf. & Spec.] Alcohol ethoxylate; nonionic; emulsifying wax; waxy solid; HLB 10.4; 100% conc.; formerly Collone AC.

Dermalcare® GMS-165. [Rhone-Poulenc Surf. & Spec.] Glyceryl stearate, PEG 100 stearate; nonionic; emulsifier for o/w creams and lotions; high electrolyte tolerance; flake; m.p. 53–57 C; 100% conc.; formerly Cyclochem GMS-165.

Dermalcare® GMS/SE. [Rhone-Poulenc Surf. & Spec.] Glyceryl stearate SE; anionic; self-emulsifying emulsifier for creams and lotions; flake; m.p. 58–63 C; 100% conc.; formerly Cyclochem GMS/SE.

Dermalcare® HV. [Rhone-Poulenc Surf. & Spec.] Fatty

ester; anionic; emulsifying wax; waxy solid; 100% conc.; formerly Collone HV.

Dermalcare® NI. [Rhone-Poulenc Surf. & Spec.] Cetearyl alcohol, ceteareth-20; nonionic; broad tolerance emulsifier for o/w systems, visc. builder for cosmetic creams, lotions, ointments; flakes; m.p. 48-51 C; 100% conc.; formerly Cyclochem NI; Collone NI.

Dermalcare® POL. [Rhone-Poulenc Surf. & Spec.] Cetearyl alcohol, ceteth-20, and glycol stearate; nonionic; lubricant SE wax, emulsifier for lotions and creams; effective over broad pH range; off-wh. wax; m.p. 48-52 C; 100% conc.; formerly Cyclochem POL.

Dermalcare® SPS. [Rhone-Poulenc Surf. & Spec.] Cetyl esters; nonionic; cosmetic grade emulsifier and emulsion stabilizer for creams, lotions, antiperspirants, creme rinse conditioners, personal care prods.; substitute for natural spermaceti; acid and alkali stable; flake; m.p. 46-48 C; 100% conc.; formerly Cyclochem SPS.

Dermane. [Universal Preserv-A-Chem] Squalane; CAS 111-01-3; EINECS 203-825-6; emollient, lubricant.

Dermane SLO. [Universal Preserv-A-Chem] Shark liver oil; CAS 68990-63-6; EINECS 273-616-2; emollient.

Dermascreen. [Synthelabo-Pharmacie] Water, propylene glycol, and aloe extract; botanical extract.

Dermasome® A. [Microfluidics] Lecithin and allantoin; cosmetic ingred. (allantoin) encapsulated in lipid spheres; for skin care prods.; disp.; particle size 150 nm max.; visc. 50 cps max.; pH 4.5-6.5; 0.4% act.

Dermasome® E. [Microfluidics] Lecithin and tocopheryl acetate; cosmetic ingred. (vitamin E acetate) encapsulated in lipid spheres; for skin care prods.; emulsion; particle size 200 nm max.; visc. 50 cps max.; pH 5.0-7.0; 1% act., 10% lecithin.

Dermasome® EPO. [Microfluidics] Lecithin and evening primrose oil; cosmetic ingred. (evening primrose oil) encapsulated in liq. spheres; for skin care prods.; emulsion; particle size 200 nm max.; visc. 50 cps max.; pH 4.5-6.5; 5% act., 10% lecithin.

Dermasome® H. [Microfluidics] Lecithin and sodium hyaluronate; cosmetic ingred. (sodium hyaluronate) encapsulated in lipid spheres; for skin care prods.; disp.; particle size 100 nm max.; visc. 50 cps max.; pH 4.5-7.5; 0.1% act., 10% lecithin.

Dermasome® MPS. [Microfluidics] Lecithin and mucopolysaccharides; cosmetic ingred. (glycosaminoglycans) encapsulated in liq. spheres; for skin care prods.; dispersion; particle size 100 nm max.; visc. 50 cps max.; pH 4.5-6.5; 0.5% act., 5% lecithin.

Dermasome® MT. [Microfluidics] Lecithin; CAS 8002-43-5; EINECS 232-307-2; water encapsulated in lipid spheres; for skin care prods.; disp.; particle size 100 nm max.; visc. 50 cps max.; 10% lecithin.

Dermasome® P. [Microfluidics] Panthenol and lecithin; cosmetic ingred. (dl-panthenol) encapsulated in lipid spheres; for skin care prods.; disp.; particle size 100 nm max.; visc. 50 cps max.; pH 4.5-6.5; 10% act., 10% lecithin.

Dermasome® RJ. [Microfluidics] Lecithin and royal jelly; cosmetic ingred. (royal jelly) encapsulated in liq. spheres; for skin care prods.; dispersion; particle size 200 nm max.; visc. 50 cps max.; pH 4.5-6.0; 10% act., 10% lecithin.

Dermasome® RP. [Microfluidics] Lecithin and retinyl palmitate; cosmetic ingred. (vitamin A palmitate) encapsulated in liq. spheres; for skin care prods.; emulsion; particle size 200 nm max.; visc. 50 cps max.; pH 5.0-7.0; 5% act., 10% lecithin.

Dermasome® S. [Microfluidics] Squalane and lecithin; cosmetic ingred. (squalane) encapsulated in lipid spheres; for skin care prods.; emulsion; particle size 200 nm max.; visc. 50 cps max.; pH 4.5-6.5; 10% act., 10% lecithin.

Dermasome® SC. [Microfluidics] Lecithin and soluble collagen; cosmetic ingred. (soluble collagen) encapsulated in lipid spheres; for skin care prods.; dispersion; particle size 100 nm max.; visc. 50 cps max.; pH 4.5-6.5; 0.1% act., 10% lecithin.

Dermasome® SE. [Microfluidics] Lecithin and spleen extract; cosmetic ingred. (spleen extract) encapsulated in liq. spheres; for skin care prods.; dispersion; particle size 100 nm max.; visc. 50 cps max.; pH 4.5-6.5; 0.5% act., 5% lecithin.

Dermasome® SOD. [Microfluidics] Lecithin and superoxide dismutase; cosmetic ingred. (superoxide dismutase) encapsulated in lipid spheres; for skin care prods.; dispersion; particle size 150 nm max.; visc. 50 cps max.; pH 4.0-6.0; 0.125% act., 5% lecithin.

Dermasome® TE. [Microfluidics] Lecithin and thymus extract; cosmetic ingred. (thymus extract) encapsulated in liq. spheres; for skin care prods.; dispersion; particle size 100 nm max.; visc. 50 cps max.; pH 4.5-6.5; 0.5% act., 5% lecithin.

Dermasome® TRF. [Microfluidics] Tissue/skin respiratory factors and lecithin; cosmetic ingred. (live yeast cell deriv.) encapsulated in lipid spheres; for skin care prods.; dispersion; particle size 150 nm max.; visc. 50 cps max.; pH 4.5-6.5; 500 units/ml act., 5% lecithin.

Dermasome® U. [Microfluidics] Urea and lecithin; cosmetic ingred. (urea) encapsulated in lipid spheres; for skin care prods.; dispersion; particle size 150 nm max.; visc. 50 cps max.; pH 5.0-7.0; 20% act., 10% lecithin.

Dermasome® V. [Microfluidics] Aloe vera gel and lecithin; cosmetic ingred. (aloe vera) encapsulated in lipid spheres; for skin care prods.; dispersion; particle size 100 nm max.; visc. 50 cps max.; pH 4.5-6.5; 9% act., 10% lecithin.

Dermatan VGF—Viscoelastic Gel Factor. [Seporga] A composition of glycosaminoglycanes in the physiological proportions of the dermis; cosmetics ingred. used to modulate the intercellular salt and water balance.

Dermatan Sulfate. [Bioiberica] Sodium dermatan sulfate.

Dermatein® GSL. [Hormel] Fluid matrix containing glycosphingolipids, phospholipids, and cholesterol; skin lipid for barrier renewal and moisturization; used for night creams, after-shave balms, lip protectants; milky cream-wh. liq., bland lipid odor; pH 4.25–4.75; toxicology: LD50 > 5 g/kg; nontoxic; nonirritating to eyes and skin; 2–3% total solids.

Dermatein® MPS. [Hormel] Hydrolyzed glycosaminoglycans; moisture-binding agent providing elegant silky satiny feel to the skin; ideal for wrinkle preps.; wh. free-flowing powd., bland char. odor; water-sol.; m.w. > 150,000; pH 6.0-6.5 (10%); toxicology: LD50 > 5 g/kg; nontoxic; nonirritating to eyes and skin; 95-98% total solids.

Derma-Vitamincomplex, Oil soluble. [Novarom GmbH] Isopropyl myristate, retinyl palmitate, and tocopherol.

Dermene. [Universal Preserv-A-Chem] Squalene; CAS 111-02-4; EINECS 203-826-1; emollient.

Dermidrol. [Esperis] Sodium PCA; CAS 28874-51-3; EINECS 249-277-1; humectant.

Dermoblock MA. [Alzo] Menthyl anthranilate; CAS 134-09-8; EINECS 205-129-8; uv-A sunscreen; pale to dk. yel. visc. liq., faint sweet aromatic odor; m.w. 275.38; sol. in IPA, min. oil, peanut oil, ethanol; insol. in water; sp.gr. 1.020-1.060; flash pt. (PMCC) > 200 F; sapon. no. 180-210; ref. index 1.532-1.552; toxicology: mild skin or eye irritant on prolonged contact.

Dermoblock OS. [Alzo] Octyl salicylate; CAS 118-60-5; EINECS 204-263-4; uv lt. absorber for sunscreens; colorless to lt. yel. clear liq., typ. bland odor; sol. in min. oil, alcohol; insol. in water; sp.gr. 1.013-1.022; flash pt. (PMCC) > 200 F; ref. index 1.495-1.505; toxicology: mild skin or eye irritant on prolonged contact; 98% purity.

Dermocalmine. [Sederma] Glycerin, water, and hirudinea extract.

Dermoil. [Lanaetex Prods.] Mink oil and lanolin oil; cosmetic ingred.

Dermol 89. [Alzo] Octyl isononanoate; CAS 71566-49-9; EINECS 275-637-2; emollient for skin care and make-up prods.; partial replacement for silicone oils; antitackiness aid in antiperspirants; resin plasticizer for hair sprays; water-wh. clear liq., typ. mild odor; insol. in water; sp.gr. 0.850-0.860; f.p. -34 C; flash pt. (COC) 127 C; acid no. 1 max; sapon. no. 200-215; toxicology: LD50 (acute oral) > 5 kg/g.

Dermol 105. [Bernel] Isodecyl neopentanoate; CAS 60209-82-7; EINECS 262-108-6; dry emollient, low visc. oil; SPF booster; FDA, EEC, and Japanese compliances; colorless liq.; oil-sol.; usage level: 1-10%.

Dermol 108. [Alzo] Isodecyl octanoate; CAS 34962-91-9; emollient for cosmetics; antitackiness aid; Gardner 1 max. liq., mild typ. odor; sol. in min. oil, alcohol; insol. in water; sp.gr. 0.87; b.p. 200 C; flash pt. (COC) 155 C; acid no. 3 max.; sapon. no. 180-220; ref. index 1.43; toxicology: nonhazardous.

Dermol 109. [Alzo] Isodecyl isononanoate; CAS 41395-89-5; emollient.

Dermol 126. [Bernel] Laureth-2 benzoate; emollient, bloomer, wetting agent; compatible with surfactants; FDA, EEC compliance; yel. liq.; sol. in oil, self-emulsifying in water; usage level: 2-10%.

Dermol 138. [Alzo] Tridecyl octanoate.

Dermol 139. [Alzo] Tridecyl isononanoate; CAS 125804-18-4.

Dermol 185. [Bernel] Isostearyl neopentanoate; CAS 58958-60-4; EINECS 261-521-9; emollient, pigment binder, freeze/thaw stabilizer; FDA, EEC, and Japanese compliances; yel. liq.; sol. in oil; usage level: 1-10%.

Dermol 334. [Alzo] Isodecyl octanoate, octyl isononanoate, diethylene glycol diisononanoate, diethylene glycol dioctanoate; Carbopol dispersing aid; dry feel emollient able to replace volatile silicone in elegant cosmetic creams and lotions; reduces tackiness; water-wh. clear liq., mild typ. odor; sol. in min. oil, alcohol; insol. in water; sp.gr. 0.87; f.p. -20 C; b.p. 200 C; acid no. 5 max.; iodine no. 1 max.; sapon. no. 210-250; flash pt. (PM) 145 C; ref. index 1.43 ± 0.01.

Dermol 488. [Alzo] Diethylene glycol dioctanoate.

Dermol 489. [Alzo] Diethylene glycol dioctanoate, diethylene glycol diisononanoate; CAS 72269-52-4, 106-01-4; emollient for cream and lotion formulations; reduces tackiness; dispersant for Carbopol powds.; water-wh. clear liq., typ. odor; sol. in min. oil, alcohol; insol. in water; sp.gr. 0.85; b.p. 170-180 C (4 mm Hg); acid no. 5 max.; sapon. no. 265-285; flash pt. (COC) 260 F; ref. index 1.430-1.440.

Dermol 499. [Alzo] Diethylene glycol diisononanoate; CAS 106-01-4; EINECS 203-353-0.

Dermol 2022. [Alzo] Octyldodecyl behenate; emollient.

Dermol CV. [Fabriquimica] Lauryl oleate; emollient, dermatophilic additive; acid no. < 1; iodine no. 60-75; sapon. no. 100-130.

Dermol DGDIS. [Alzo] Polyglyceryl-2 diisostearate.

Dermol DID. [Alzo] Diisopropyl dimer dilinoleate.

Dermol DISD [Alzo] Diisostearyl dimer dilinoleate; CAS 127358-81-0; emollient for creams, lotions, and makeup; anti-irritant in formulations; yel. clear to sl. hazy liq., mild typ. odor; sol. in higher m.w. alcoholes, esters, ketones, min. oil, aliphatic, aromatic, and chlorinated hydrocarbons, higher glycols; insol. in water; sp.gr. 0.90; f.p. 5 C; b.p. > 390 C; acid no. 3 max.; sapon. no. 85-110; flash pt.

(COC) 170 C; ref. index 1.472.

Dermol EB. [Fabriquimica] Butyl stearate; CAS 123-95-5; EINECS 204-666-5; emollient, dermatophilic additive; plasticizer and solv. for pigments/lipsticks; acid no. < 1; iodine no. < 1; sapon. no. 168-176.

Dermol G-7DI. [Alzo] Glycereth-7 diisononanoate; CAS 125804-15-1.

Dermol G-76. [Alzo] Glycereth-7 benzoate; CAS 125804-12-8; emollient for creams, lotions, bath prods., liq. soaps, hydro-alcoholic sol'ns.; softener and moisturizer for skin; water-wh. to pale yel. clear liq., mild odor; sol. in SDA-40 alcohol, methanol, IPA, ethanol, aldehydes, ketones, propylene glycol; disp. in castor oil, water; sp.gr. 1.17; b.p. 210 c; acid no. 5 max.; flash pt. (COC) 210 C.

Dermol GL-7A. [Alzo] Glycereth-7 triacetate; CAS 57569-76-3; emollient, solubilizer; pale yel. to yel. clear liq., char. odor; sol. in water; m.w. 526; sp.gr. 1.15; b.p. > 200 C; acid no. 2 max.; sapon. no. 315-340; flash pt. (COC) 200 C; ref. index 1.44-1.46.

Dermol ICSA. [Alzo] Isocetyl salicylate; CAS 138208-68-1; emollient; solv. for benzophenone in sunscreen formulations; pale yel. clear liq., sl. typ. odor; sp.gr. 1.02; acid no. 3; sapon. no. 145-160; flash pt. (PMCC) > 200 F; ref. index 1.4865 ± 0.005.

Dermol Jojoba E. [Fabriquimica] Syn. jojoba oil; emollient, dermatophilic additive; acid no. < 1; iodine no. 60-65; sapon. no. 100-110.

Dermol L45. [Alzo] Glycereth-4.5 lactate; CAS 125804-13-9; nonionic; emollient, humectant for hydro/alcoholic formulations, aftershave, body splashes; water-wh. to pale yel. clear visc. liq., mild typ. odor; sol. in water, methanol, IPA; insol. in min. oil; sp.gr. 1.155 ± 0.01; b.p. dec. > 210 C; acid no. 5 max.; sapon. no. 165-185; flash pt. (COC) 210 C.

Dermol M-27. [Alzo] Triundecanoin; CAS 13552-80-2; EINECS 236-935-8; cosmetic ingred.

Dermol MO. [Alzo] Glycereth-7 diisononanoate, diethylene glycol dioctanoate, diethylene glycol diisononanoate; emollient for skin care formulations and lip prods.; replacement for min. oil; water-wh. to pale yel. clear liq., typ. odor; insol. in water; sp.gr. 1.02; b.p. > 200 C; acid no. 3 max.; sapon. no. 138-158; flash pt. (COC) 127 C; ref. index 1.450.

Dermol NS. [Alzo] C12-15 alkyl salicylate.

Dermol OL. [Alzo] Oleyl lactate; CAS 42175-36-0; emollient.

Dermol OO. [Alzo] Octyl oxystearate; CAS 29710-25-6; prevents defatting of skin from harsh surfactants and detergents; for cosmetic and cleansing formulas; binder in pressed powds.; yel. to amber clear to sl. hazy oily liq., mild fatty odor; insol. in water; sp.gr. 0.89; f.p. 12 C; b.p. > 225 C; acid no. 1 max.; iodine no. 3 max.; sapon. no. 140-159; flash pt. (COC) 425 C; ref. index 1.456.

Dermol PSA. [Alzo] Soy sterol acetate.

Dermol QE. [Fabriquimica] Ethyl oleate, ethyl palmitate, ethyl laurate, ethyl myristate, and ethyl linoleate; emollient, dermatophilic additive; acid no. < 1; iodine no. 40-50; sapon. no. 195-195.

Dermol T. [Fabriquimica] Oleic/palmitic/lauric/myristic/linoleic triglyceride; emollient, dermatophilic additive; acid no. < 10; iodine no. 60-70; sapon. no. 200-210.

Dermolan GLH. [Alzo] Glycereth-7.5 hydroxystearate; CAS 138314-11-1; emollient in creams and lotions; self emulsifier; visc. builder for shampoos; conditioner for shampoos; tan semisolid, char. nil odor; misc. with water; sp.gr. 1.15; acid no. 1 max.; sapon. no. 85-110.

Dermoliv. [Alma Chimica] Olive oil unsaponifiables and olive husk oil.

Dermoliv T. [Alma Chimica] Olive oil unsaponifiables and olive husk oil.

Dermonectin. [Vevy] Water, propylene glycol, and hydrolyzed fibronectin; cosmetic ingred.

Dermosaccharides® GY. [Laboratoires Sérobiologiques] Highly purified and conc. glycogen with glycerin; energizer, moisturizer with anti-stress activity; restores defense and repair capability; for anti-aging, antiwrinkle, and sun care prods.; colorless to pale yel. opalescent liq.; water-sol.; usage level: 1-5%.

Dermosaccharides® HC. [Laboratoires Sérobiologiques] Glycerin, water, glycosaminoglycans, and glycogen; epicutaneous hydro-regulator, cell energizer, structuring agent for skin; restores protection, repair, and regeneration capability; used for prods. for anti-aging, antiwrinkle, and skin lacking structuration, firmness, and energy; colorless to pale yel. sl. opalescent liq.; water-sol.; usage level: 1-3%.

Dermosaccharides® SEA. [Laboratoires Sérobiologiques] Glycerin, water, chitin, glycogen, and mannitol; epicutaneous hydro-regulator, cell energizer, structuring agent for skin; restores protection, repair, and regeneration capability; used for prods. for anti-aging, antiwrinkle, and skin lacking structuration, firmness, and energy; colorless to pale yel. sl. opalescent liq.; water-sol.; usage level: 1-3%.

Desamidocollagen K 1.0. [Herstellung von Naturextrakten GmbH; Lipo] Soluble collagen; CAS 9007-34-5; EINECS 232-697-4; water-binding moisture regulator used in skin creams, body lotions, after-sun lotions, hair conditioning treatments; visc. opalescent sol'n., char. intrinsic odor; acid no. 5.5-6.0; pH 3.5-4.0.

Desamidocollagen K 1.5. [Herstellung von Naturextrakten GmbH; Lipo] Soluble collagen; CAS 9007-34-5; EINECS 232-697-4; water-binding moisture regulator used in skin creams, body lotions, after-sun lotions, hair conditioning treatments; visc. opalescent sol'n., char. intrinsic odor; acid no. 0.7-1.2; pH 3.5-4.0.

Desamina. [Vevy] Glucamine; CAS 488-43-7; EINECS 207-677-3.

Desaron. [Herstellung von Naturextrakten GmbH; Lipo] Glycerin, soluble collagen, and sodium hyaluronate; water-binding agent leaving pleasant film on the skin; promotes absorption of oil and fat components of a cream; imparts moisture regulation to hydrogels; visc. opalescent sol'n., char. odor; pH 6.0-7.0.

Desomeen® TA-2. [Witco/H-I-P] PEG-2 tallow amine; CAS 61791-44-4; cationic; emulsifier, dispersant, textile scouring, dyeing assistant, desizing assistant, softener, antistat; personal care formulations; paste; 100% act.

Desomeen® TA-5. [Witco/H-I-P] PEG-5 tallow amine; CAS 61791-44-4; cationic; emulsifier and dispersant; used as textile scouring agents, dyeing assistants, desizing agents, softening agents, antistats, etc.; personal care formulations; liq.; HLB 5.3; cloud pt. 68–74 F; 100% act.

Desomeen® TA-15. [Witco/H-I-P] PEG-15 tallow amine; cationic; emulsifier, dispersant, textile scouring, dyeing assistant, desizing assistant, softener, antistat; personal care formulations; liq.; cloud pt. 172–179 F; 100% act.

Desomeen® TA-20. [Witco/H-I-P] PEG-20 tallow amine; emulsifier, dispersant, textile scouring, dyeing assistant, desizing assistant, softener, antistat; personal care formulations; liq.; cloud pt. 179–181 F (10% NaCl); 100% act.

Desonic® 1.5N. [Witco/H-I-P] Nonoxynol-1 (1.5 EO); EINECS 248-762-5; nonionic; defoamer, detergent, emulsifer for personal care prods.; liq.; oil-sol.; 100% act.

Desonic® 4N. [Witco/H-I-P] Nonoxynol-4; CAS 9016-45-9; nonionic; detergent, emulsifier, defoamer for pesticide, paint, paper, and textile industries, and personal care formulations; liq.; oil-sol.; HLB 8.8; 100% act.

Desonic® 5N. [Witco/H-I-P] Nonoxynol-5; CAS 9016-45-9; nonionic; detergent, surfactant for personal care applics.; liq.; oil-sol.; 100% act.

Desonic® 6D. [Witco/H-I-P] Dodoxynol-6; nonionic; emulsifier for solv. and emulsion cleaners, personal care formulations; liq.; oil-sol.; HLB 10.0; 100% act.

Desonic® 6N. [Witco/H-I-P] Nonoxynol-6; CAS 9016-45-9; nonionic; emulsifier, detergent for personal care applics.; liq.; HLB 10.8; 100% act.

Desonic® 6T. [Witco/H-I-P] Trideceth-6; CAS 24938-91-8; nonionic; low-foam wetting agent, detergent, foamer for mechanical and spray cleaning; pulp, paper, textile industries, personal care formulations; liq.; HLB 11.4; 100% act.

Desonic® 7N. [Witco/H-I-P] Nonoxynol-7; CAS 9016-45-9; EINECS 248-292-0; nonionic; low-foaming surfactant, detergent, emulsifier for personal care applics.; liq.; HLB 11.7; 100% act.

Desonic® 9D. [Witco/H-I-P] Dodoxynol-9; nonionic; emulsifier, detergent for emulsion cleaners, personal care formulations; liq.; cloud pt. 61–64 F; 100% act.

Desonic® 9N. [Witco/H-I-P] Nonoxynol-9; CAS 9016-45-9; nonionic; detergent, wetting agent, emulsifier for textile, paper, metal cleaning, personal care formulations; liq.; HLB 12.8; cloud pt. 127–133 F; 100% act.

Desonic® 9T. [Witco/H-I-P] Trideceth-9; CAS 24938-91-8; nonionic; surfactant for lt. and heavy-duty detergents, textile leveling and scouring, personal care formulations; liq.; cloud pt. 154–170 F; HLB 13.3; 100% act.

Desonic® 10D. [Witco/H-I-P] Dodoxynol-10; nonionic; detergent/wetting agent for industrial and heavy-duty detergents, personal care formulations; liq.; HLB 13.2; cloud pt. 145–153 F; 100% act.

Desonic® 11N. [Witco/H-I-P] Nonoxynol-11; CAS 9016-45-9; nonionic; detergent, wetting agent, emulsifier for textile, paper, metal cleaning, personal care formulations; liq.; HLB 13.6; cloud pt. 158–162 F; 100% act.

Desonic® 12D. [Witco/H-I-P] Dodoxynol-12; nonionic; detergent/wetting agent for industrial and heavy-duty detergents at high temps.; personal care formulations; liq.; cloud pt. 165–174 F; 100% act.

Desonic® 12N. [Witco/H-I-P] Nonoxynol-12; CAS 9016-45-9; nonionic; wetting agent, detergent used with high temp. and electrolytes; personal care formulations; liq.; cloud pt. 176–181 F; 100% act.

Desonic® 12T. [Witco/H-I-P] Trideceth-12; CAS 24938-91-8; nonionic; surfactant for lt.- and heavy-duty detergents; leveling and scouring agent; personal care formulations; liq.; cloud pt. 187–201 F; 100% act.

Desonic® 15N. [Witco/H-I-P] Nonoxynol-15; CAS 9016-45-9; nonionic; detergent, wetting agent at high temps. and electrolyte; metal cleaning; personal care formulations; liq.; cloud pt. 143–149 F (10% NaCl); 100% act.

Desonic® 15T. [Witco/H-I-P] Trideceth-15; CAS 24938-91-8; nonionic; surfactant for lt.- and heavy-duty detergents at high temps.; leveling and scouring agent; personal care formulations; liq.; cloud pt. 156–167 F (10% NaCl); 100% act.

Desonic® 20N. [Witco/H-I-P] Nonoxynol-20; CAS 9016-45-9; nonionic; detergent, wetting agent at high temps. and electrolyte; personal care formulations; solid; cloud pt. 154–162 F (10% NaCl); 100% act.

Desonic® 30C. [Witco/H-I-P] PEG-30 castor oil; CAS 61791-12-6; nonionic; emulsifier, lubricant, dye leveler, antistat, dispersant for textiles; emulsifer for rigid PU foams; softener/rewetter for wet-strength paper; personal care formulations; liq.; HLB 11.7; 100% act.

Desonic® 30N. [Witco/H-I-P] Nonoxynol-30; CAS 9016-45-9; nonionic; emulsifier for fats, oils, waxes; for personal care applics.; solid; HLB 17.1; cloud pt. 159–163 F (10% NaCl); 100% act.

Desonic® 30N70. [Witco/H-I-P] Nonoxynol-30; CAS 9016-45-9; nonionic; emulsifier for fats, oils, waxes; for personal care applics.; liq.; HLB 17.1; cloud pt. 159–163 F (10% NaCl); 70% act.

Desonic®36C. [Witco/H-I-P] PEG-36 castor oil; CAS 61791-12-6; nonionic; emulsifier, lubricant, dye leveler, antistat, dispersant for textiles; emulsifer for rigid PU foams; softener/rewetter for wet-strength paper; personal care formulations; liq.; HLB 12.6; cloud pt. 122–140 F; 100% act.

Desonic® 40N. [Witco/H-I-P] Nonoxynol-40; CAS 9016-45-9; nonionic; surfactant for high temps. and electrolytes; emulsifier; personal care formulations; solid; cloud pt. 165–176 F (10% NaCl); 100% act.

Desonic® 40N70. [Witco/H-I-P] Nonoxynol-40; CAS 9016-45-9; nonionic; emulsifier; surfactant for high temps. and electrolytes; personal care formulations; liq.; cloud pt. 165–176 F (10% NaCl); 70% act.

Desonic® 50N. [Witco/H-I-P] Nonoxynol-50; CAS 9016-45-9; nonionic; emulsifier for waxes, polishes; surfactant for high temps. and electrolytes; personal care formulations; solid; 100% act.

Desonic® 50N70. [Witco/H-I-P] Nonoxynol-50; CAS 9016-45-9; nonionic; emulsifier for waxes, polishes; surfactant for high temps. and electrolytes; personal care formulations; liq.; 70% act.

Desonic®54C. [Witco/H-I-P] PEG-54 castor oil; CAS 61791-12-6; nonionic; emulsifier, lubricant, dye leveler, antistat, dispersant for textiles; emulsifer for rigid PU foams; softener/rewetter for wet-strength paper; personal care formulations; liq.; HLB 14.4; cloud pt. 136–142 F (10% NaCl); 100% act.

Desonic® 100N. [Witco/H-I-P] Nonoxynol-100; CAS 9016-45-9; nonionic; emulsifier for waxes, polishes; surfactant for high temps. and electrolytes; personal care formulations; solid; 100% act.

Desonic® 100N70. [Witco/H-I-P] Nonoxynol-100; CAS 9016-45-9; nonionic; emulsifier for waxes, polishes; surfactant for high temps. and electrolytes; personal care formulations; liq.; 70% act.

Desonic® TDA-9. [Witco/H-I-P] Ethoxylated alcohol; nonionic; wetting agent, degreaser, detergent, and emulsifier for personal care applics.; liq.; 100% conc.

Desophos®5 AP. [Witco/H-I-P] Phosphate ester, free acid; anionic; coupling agent for nonionics in liq. alkaline detergents; moderate foamer; for personal care formulations; liq.; 100% act.

Destressine 2000. [Sederma] Shea butter unsaponifiables, docosahexaenoic acid, eicosapentaenoic acid, tocopheryl acetate, and corn oil unsaponifiables; anti-stress for sensitive skin treatment, protection, and regeneration, face and body care prods.; after-sun preps.; pale beige fatty matter, char. odor; sp.gr. 0.86-0.87; acid no. < 4; iodine no. 40; usage level: 1-4%.

Detergent CR. [Arol Chem. Prods.] Fatty ethanolamine condensate; detergent, wetting agent, emulsifier, thickener, penetrating and leveling agent, for use in textiles, personal care, food, and household prods.; pigment dispersant; pale amber liq.; mild odor; readily sol. in water; sp.gr. 1.01; 100% act.

Detergent Concentrate 840. [Mona Industries] Amido sulfonate complex; nonionic/anionic; high-foaming detergent at low concs.; used in car wash, liq. dishwash, cosmoline cleaners, household and industrial all-purpose cleaners, bubble baths; amber clear liq.; sol. in cold or warm water; sp.gr. 1.05; dens. 8.75 lb/gal; acid no. 90; alkali no. 23; pH 8.7 (10%); 82% conc.

Dew Pearl AH-1. [R.I.T.A.] Guanine; CAS 73-40-5; EINECS 200-799-8; used in biochemical research, cosmetics.

Dew Pearl TS-1. [R.I.T.A.] Guanine and water; CAS 73-40-5; EINECS 200-799-8; used in biochemical research, cosmetics.

Dexpanthenol USP, FCC No. 63909. [Roche] Dex-

panthenol; long-lasting moisturizer for hair and skin care prods.

Dexpearl. [Tomen Am.] Cyclodextrin; CAS 7585-39-9; EINECS 231-493-2; encapsulant.

Dextrol AS-150. [Dexter] Coco-ethyldimonium ethosulfate; CAS 68308-64-5; EINECS 269-662-8.

DF-100. [Chemie Research & Mfg.] Glycerin, grapefruit seed extract, and grapefruit extract.

DHA Melanosponge. [Advanced Polymer Systems] Melanin, dihydroxyacetone, and acrylates copolymer.

DHA Microspheres. [Rona; E. Merck] Dihydroxyacetone, cocoglycerides, stearic acid, and silica.

DHBP Quinsorb 010. [Enterprise] Benzophenone-1; CAS 131-56-6; EINECS 205-029-4; uv absorber.

Diacid 1550. [Westvaco] Cyclocarboxypropyloleic acid; CAS 53980-88-4; EINECS 258-987-1.

Diaformer® Z-301. [Mitsubishi Petrochem.; Sandoz] Methacryloyl ethyl betaine/methacrylates copolymer in ethanol; amphoteric; film-forming polymer for gel hair fixative prods. providing natural hold and feel, antistatic props.; good compat. with gel bases; amber clear visc. liq.; visc. 100-500 cps; pH 6.6-8.6; flamm.; 28-32% solids.

Diaformer® Z-400. [Mitsubishi Petrochem.; Sandoz] Methacryloyl ethyl betaine/methacrylates copolymer in ethanol; amphoteric; film-forming polymer for hair care prods. providing natural hold and feel, antistatic props. (aerosol or pump hairspray, spritz, mousse); deodorized version of Z-AT developed for lightly fragranced or unfragranced prods.; amber clear visc. liq.; visc. 500-2000 cps; pH 7.6-8.6; flamm.; 38-42% solids.

Diaformer® Z-A. [Mitsubishi Petrochem.; Sandoz] Methacryloyl ethyl betaine/methacrylates copolymer in ethanol; amphoteric; film-forming polymer for hair care prods. providing natural hold and feel, antistatic props. (aerosol and pump hairsprays); improved compat. with propellants; for use in formulas with higher propellant levels, exc. curl retention; amber clear visc. liq.; visc. 1000-8000 cps; pH 6.6-8.6; flamm.; 38-42% solids.

Diaformer® Z-AT. [Mitsubishi Petrochem.; Sandoz] Methacryloyl ethyl betaine/methacrylates copolymer in ethanol; amphoteric; film-forming polymer for hair care prods. providing natural hold and feel, antistatic props. (aerosol or pump hairspray, spritz, mousse); good compat. with propellants; amber clear visc. liq.; visc. 500-2000 cps; pH 7.6-8.6; flamm.; toxicology: nonirritating to skin and eyes; 38-42% solids.

Diaformer® Z-SM. [Mitsubishi Petrochem.; Sandoz] Methacryloyl ethyl betaine/methacrylates copolymer in ethanol; amphoteric; film-forming polymer for hair care prods. providing natural hold and feel, antistatic props. (aerosol and pump hairsprays, spritz, setting lotion, mousse); flexible film with softer feel and hold, good propellant compat., good slip for both film and foam; stable in high water content formulations; amber clear visc. liq.; visc. 500-900 cps; pH 7.0-8.5; flamm.; 28-32% solids.

Diaformer® Z-W. [Mitsubishi Petrochem.; Sandoz] Methacryloyl ethyl betaine/methacrylates copolymer in water, 8% ethanol; amphoteric; film-forming polymer for hair care prods. providing natural hold and feel, antistatic props., good conditioning; dispersant for pearling agents; for conditioners, creams rinses, shampoos; amber clear visc. liq.; visc. 300-600 cps; pH 5-7; combustible; 28-32% solids.

Diahold® A-503. [Mitsubishi Petrochem.; Sandoz] AMP-acrylates copolymer in ethanol; anionic; fixative and film-forming polymer for aerosol and pump hairsprays, setting lotions, spritzes; forms hard, glossy films; exc. hair holding performance; compat. with propellants; low visc. in diluted form; amber clear visc. liq.; visc. 500-2000 cps; pH 7.9-

Diamond Quality®

8.9; flamm.; 38-42% solids.

Diamond Quality®. [CasChem] Unrefined castor oil USP; CAS 8001-79-4; EINECS 232-293-8; emollient, pigment wetter, cosolv., lubricant for cosmetics, makeup, antiperspirant sticks; pour pt. -23 C; acid no. 2; iodine no. 86; sapon. no. 180; hyd. no. 164.

Diaquasol. [Solabia] Placental protein, amniotic fluid, hydrolyzed glycosaminoglycans, and arginine PCA.

Diatami. [Alban Muller] Peeling prods. for cosmetics field.

Dichrona®. [Rona] Dual effect pearlescent pigments for cosmetics and toiletries; obtained by coating an interference pigment with an inorganic or organic colorant with a mass tone different from the reflection color of the interference pearl.

Dichrona® BG. [Rona; E. Merck] Titanium dioxide, mica, ferric ferrocyanide.

Dichrona® BR. [Rona; E. Merck] Mica, titanium dioxide, and ferric ferrocyanide.

Dichrona® BY. [Rona; E. Merck] Mica, titanium dioxide, and ferric ferrocyanide.

Dichrona® GY. [Rona; E. Merck] Mica, titanium dioxide, iron oxides, and ferric ferrocyanide.

Dichrona® RB. [Rona; E. Merck] Mica, titanium dioxide, and carmine.

Dichrona® RG. [Rona; E. Merck] Titanium dioxide, mica, and carmine.

Dichrona® RY. [Rona; E. Merck] Mica, titanium dioxide, and carmine.

Dichrona® YB. [Rona; E. Merck] Mica, titanium dioxide, and iron oxides.

Dichrona® YG. [Rona; E. Merck] Titanium dioxide, mica, and iron oxides.

Dichrona® YR. [Rona; E. Merck] Mica, titanium dioxide, and iron oxides.

Dicopamine DP. [Phoenix] Dilinoleamidopropyl dimethylamine dimethicone copolyol phosphate and propylene glycol.

Diglyme. [Ivax] Dimethoxydiglycol; CAS 111-96-6; EINECS 203-924-4.

Dihydral. [Solabia] Placental protein, amniotic fluid, hydrolyzed glycosaminoglycans, and arginine PCA.

Dihydroxyacetone. [Rona] Dihydroxyacetone; CAS 96-26-4; EINECS 202-494-5; skin tanning agent; almost wh. cryst.; sol. in water, ethanol, ether; m.p. 68-71 C; pH 4-6 (5% aq.); usage level: 2-5%; toxicology: LD50 (oral, rat) 16. 0 g/kg.

DIMASPA. [Penn-Squire] Dimethyl aspartic acid; CAS 1115-22-6.

Dimodan LS Kosher. [Grindsted Prods.; Grindsted Prods. Denmark] Glyceryl linoleate; CAS 2277-28-3; EINECS 218-901-4; nonionic; emulsifier for emulsions, face creams and masks; w/o food emulsifier for low-calorie spreads, icing shortenings and cake shortenings; FDA approved; soft plastic; m.p. 40 C; 90% min. monoester.; formerly Grindtek MOL 90.

Dimodan PM. [Grindsted Prods.; Grindsted Prods. Denmark] Glyceryl stearate; nonionic; food emulsifier; starch complexing agent; for margarine, cake shortenings, confectionery coatings; softener for bread; peanut butter stabilizer; also for cosmetics/toiletries; FDA approved; beads; m.p. 70 C; 90% min. monoester.

Dimodan PV. [Grindsted Prods.; Grindsted Prods. Denmark] Hydrog. soybean oil dist. monoglyceride, unsat.; nonionic; food emulsifier, starch complexing agent, antisticking agent; crumb softener for bread; aerating agent in cake mixes and frozen desserts; also for cosmetics/toiletries; beads, powd.; m.p. 72 C; 90% min. monoester.

Dionil® OC. [Hüls Am.; Hüls AG] PEG-3 oleamide; CAS 26027-37-2; 31799-71-0; nonionic; detergent for lt. and

heavy-duty detergents, dishwashing agents, cosmetic preps.; component in textile auxliaries; refatting agent; liq.; cloud pt. 67 (10% in 25% BDG); 100% act.

Dionil® OC/K. [Hüls AG] PEG-4 oleamide; superfatting agent, thickener, and foam stabilizer for hair shampoos, foam baths, shower foams, and liq. soaps; brn. clear liq.; visc. 200 mPa·s; solid. pt. 5 C; clear pt. 15 C; pH 9.5-11.0 (1% aq.).

Dionil® RS. [Hüls Am.; Hüls AG] Fatty acid amide polyglycol ether and ethoxylated alcohols; nonionic; superfatting and preparation agent; liq.; 80% act.

Dionil® S 37. [Hüls Am.; Hüls AG] Fatty acid amide polyglycol ether; nonionic; detergent for lt. and heavy-duty detergents, dishwashing agents, cosmetic preps.; component for textile auxiliaries; wax; 100% conc.

Dionil® SD. [Hüls Am.; Hüls AG] Fatty acid amide polyglycol ether; nonionic; superfatting and preparation agent; wax; 100% conc.

Dionil® SH 100. [Hüls Am.; Hüls AG] PEG-6 oleamide; CAS 26027-37-2; nonionic; detergent for lt. and heavy-duty detergents, dishwashing agents, cosmetic preps., car shampoos; component for textile auxiliaries; good leveling power; liq./paste; 100% act.

Dionil® W 100. [Hüls Am.; Hüls AG] PEG-14 oleamide; CAS 26027-37-2; nonionic; detergent for lt. and heavy-duty detergents, dishwashing agents, cosmetic preps., car shampoos; component for textile auxiliaries; good leveling power; solid; cloud pt. 60 (2% in 10% NaOH); 100% act.

DIPA Commercial Grade. [Dow] Diisopropanolamine; CAS 110-97-4; EINECS 203-820-9; used to produce soaps with good hard surf. detergency, shampoos, pharmaceuticals, emulsifiers, textile specialties, agric. and polymer curing chemicals, adhesives, antistats, coatings, metalworking, petroleum, rubber, gas conditioning chemicals; sp.gr. 0.992 (40/4 C); dens. 8.27 lb/gal (40 C); visc. 870 cps (30 C); f.p. 44 C; b.p. 249 C (760 mm Hg); flash pt. (Seta CC) 276 F; fire pt. 275 C; ref. index 1.4595 (30 C).

DIPA Low Freeze Grade 85. [Dow] Diisopropanolamine; CAS 110-97-4; EINECS 203-820-9; used to produce soaps with good hard surf. detergency, shampoos, pharmaceuticals, emulsifiers, textile specialties, agric. and polymer curing chemicals, adhesives, antistats, coatings, metalworking, petroleum, rubber, gas conditioning chemicals; sp.gr. 0.992 (40/4 C); dens. 8.27 lb/gal (40 C); visc. 870 cps (30 C); f.p. 44 C; b.p. 249 C (760 mm Hg); flash pt. (Seta CC) 276 F; fire pt. 275 C; ref. index 1.4595 (30 C); 15% water.

DIPA Low Freeze Grade 90. [Dow] Diisopropanolamine; CAS 110-97-4; EINECS 203-820-9; used to produce soaps with good hard surf. detergency, shampoos, pharmaceuticals, emulsifiers, textile specialties, agric. and polymer curing chemicals, adhesives, antistats, coatings, metalworking, petroleum, rubber, gas conditioning chemicals; sp.gr. 0.992 (40/4 C); dens. 8.27 lb/gal (40 C); visc. 870 cps (30 C); f.p. 44 C; b.p. 249 C (760 mm Hg); flash pt. (Seta CC) 276 F; fire pt. 275 C; ref. index 1.4595 (30 C); 10% water.

DIPA NF Grade. [Dow] Diisopropanolamine; CAS 110-97-4; EINECS 203-820-9; used to produce soaps with good hard surf. detergency, shampoos, pharmaceuticals, emulsifiers, textile specialties, agric. and polymer curing chemicals, adhesives, antistats, coatings, metalworking, petroleum, rubber, gas conditioning chemicals; sp.gr. 0.992 (40/4 C); dens. 8.27 lb/gal (40 C); visc. 870 cps (30 C); f.p. 44 C; b.p. 249 C (760 mm Hg); flash pt. (Seta CC) 276 F; fire pt. 275 C; ref. index 1.4595 (30 C).

Dipentene No. 122. [Hercules] Dipentene; CAS 138-86-3; EINECS 205-341-0.

Dipsal. [Scher] Dipropylene glycol salicylate; CAS 7491-14-

116

7; uv absorbent for sunscreens; suitable as inhibitor for uv degradation of polymers and dyestuffs; does not deteriorate in contact with perspiration; emollient for toiletries, alcohol lotions, veg. or min.-type prods., and pharmaceutical specialties; suitable for hair applics.; useful to reduce deterioration and discoloration of polymers; yel. clear liq., mild salicylate odor; sol. in most org. solvs.; water-insol.; m.w. 254; sp.gr. 1.165; dens. 9.66 lb/gal; f.p. < -5 C; acid no. 3 max.; iodine no. nil; sapon. no. 225-240; cloud pt. < –5 C; flash pt. (OC) > 160 C; ref. index 1.522.

Disorbene. [Roquette] Dibenzylidene sorbitol; CAS 32647-67-9; EINECS 251-136-4.

Dispal. [Vista] Alumina.

Dispersen-D. [Lanaetex Prods.] Cetearyl alcohol and ceteareth-20; cosmetic ingred.

Dispersen-G. [Lanaetex Prods.] Stearyl alcohol and ceteareth-20; cosmetic ingred.

Dispersen-S. [Lanaetex Prods.] Cetearyl alcohol and polysorbate 60.

Dispex GA40. [Allied Colloids] Ammonium acrylates copolymer.

Disponil FES 92E. [Pulcra SA] Sodium laureth-12 sulfate; CAS 9004-82-4; anionic; surfactant for low-irritation shampoos, emulsion polymerization; liq.; m.w. 830; pH 8.0-9.0 (10%); 29-31% act.

DM Fluid 3000. [Shin-Etsu Silicones] Dimethicone.

DNA LP. [Sederma] DNA; CAS 9007-49-2; cosmetic ingred.

DNA Marine. [Sederma] Propylene glycol, glycerin, water, and DNA; moisturizer and cell repair factor for face care and anti-ageing prods.; yel. sl. visc. liq., char. odor; sp.gr. 1.08-1.10; visc. 200-300 cps; ref. index 1.400±0.005; pH 5.5-6.5; usage level: 2-6%.

Docoil DOS. [Industrial Quimica Lasem] Dioctyl sebacate; CAS 122-62-3; EINECS 204-558-8; emollient.

Docoil Dipa. [Industrial Quimica Lasem] Diisopropyl adipate; CAS 6938-94-9; EINECS 248-299-9; cosmetic ester.

Dodecalene. [Vevy] Tripropylene glycol citrate.

Dodigen 1382, 1383, 5594. [Hoechst AG] Quaternary ammonium salts; cationic; surfactant for penicillin mfg.

Dodigen 1490. [Hoechst AG] Dicoco dimethylammonium chloride; CAS 61789-77-3; EINECS 263-087-6; cationic; surfactant.

Dover 50 A. [Luzenac Am.] Platy talc USP; CAS 14807-96-6; EINECS 238-877-9; extremely platy talc with exc. slip, high brightness and purity, and low oil absorp.; ideal for formulations with sensitive fragrances and pigments; for dusting and pressed powds., antiperspirants, creams, lotions, bath and loose powds.; powd.; 97% thru 200 mesh; median diam. 17 μ; oil absorp. 37; tapped dens. 65 lb/ft³; pH 9 (10% slurry).

Dow 15-200. [Dow] PPG-24 glycereth-24; CAS 9082-00-2; provides solvency, low odor, low irritation, and low toxicity to personal care prods. and cosmetics; liq.; m.w. 2600; sp.gr. 1.063; dens. 8.81 lb/gal; visc. 420 cSt; pour pt. -40 C; flash pt. (PMCC) > 450 F; ref. index 1.460; sp. heat 0.470 cal/g/°C.

Dow 112-2. [Dow] PPG-66 glycereth-12; CAS 9082-00-2; provides solvency, low odor, low irritation, and low toxicity to personal care prods. and cosmetics; liq.; m.w. 4900; sp.gr. 1.028; dens. 8.56 lb/gal; visc. 1000 cSt; pour pt. -18 C; flash pt. (PMCC) 455 F; ref. index 1.455; sp. heat 0.430 cal/g/°C.

Dow B100-1000. [Dow] Polybutylene glycol; provides solvency, low odor, low irritation, and low toxicity to personal care prods. and cosmetics; liq.; sol. in ethanol, IPM, lt. min. oil, cyclomethicone, sunscreens, lactic acid; partly sol. in water, lanolin, stearyl alcohol; m.w. 1000; dens. 8.10 lb/gal; visc. 86.9 cSt (40 C); pour pt. -26 C; flash pt. (PMCC) > 350 F; ref. index 1.4529.

Dow B100-2000. [Dow] Polybutylene glycol; provides sol-

vency, low odor, low irritation, and low toxicity to personal care prods. and cosmetics; liq.; m.w. 2000; dens. 8.09 lb/gal; visc. 209.7 cSt (40 C); pour pt. -26 C; flash pt. (PMCC) > 350 F; ref. index 1.4540.

Dow B100-4800. [Dow] Polybutylene glycol; provides solvency, low odor, low irritation, and low toxicity to personal care prods. and cosmetics; liq.; m.w. 4800; dens. 8.10 lb/gal; visc. 731.4 cSt (40 C); pour pt. -21 C; flash pt. (PMCC) > 350 F; ref. index 1.4551.

Dow E200. [Dow] PEG-4; CAS 25322-68-3; EINECS 203-989-9; used in personal care prods. (makeup, bath preps., toothpaste); liq.; m.w. 200; sp.gr. 1.124; dens. 9.35 lb/gal; visc. 40 cSt; f.p. supercools; flash pt. (PMCC) 340 F; ref. index 1.459; sp. heat 0.524 cal/g/°C.

Dow E300 NF. [Dow] PEG-6 NF; CAS 25322-68-3; EINECS 220-045-1; used in personal care prods. (makeup, bath preps., toothpaste) and pharmaceuticals (ointments for antiseptics and other medicaments, tablet coatings, suppositories, liq. preps., gelatin capsules); liq.; m.w. 300; sp.gr. 1.125; dens. 9.36 lb/gal; f.p. -10 C; visc. 69 cSt; flash pt. (PMCC) > 400 F; ref. index 1.463; sp. heat 0.508 cal/g/°C.

Dow E400 NF. [Dow] PEG-8 NF; CAS 25322-68-3; EINECS 225-856-4; used in pharmaceuticals (ointments for antiseptics and other medicaments, tablet coatings, suppositories, liq. preps., gelatin capsules); clear visc. liq.; m.w. 400; sp.gr. 1.125; dens. 9.36 lb/gal; f.p. 6 C; visc. 90 cSt; flash pt. (PMCC) > 450 F; ref. index 1.465; sp. heat 0.498 cal/g/°C.

Dow E600 NF. [Dow] PEG-12 NF; CAS 25322-68-3; EINECS 229-859-1; used in pharmaceuticals (ointments for antiseptics and other medicaments, tablet coatings, suppositories, liq. preps., gelatin capsules); clear visc. liq.; sol. in water, ethanol, cyclomethicone, sunscreens, lactic acid; m.w. 600; sp.gr. 1.126; dens. 9.37 lb/gal; f.p. 22 C; visc. 131 cSt; flash pt. (PMCC) > 450 F; ref. index 1.466; sp. heat 0.490 cal/g/°C.

Dow E900 NF. [Dow] PEG NF; CAS 25322-68-3; used in pharmaceuticals (ointments for antiseptics and other medicaments, tablet coatings, suppositories, liq. preps., gelatin capsules); wh. waxy solid; m.w. 900; sp.gr. 1.204; f.p. 34 C; visc. 100 cSt (100 F); flash pt. (PMCC) > 450 F.

Dow E1000 NF. [Dow] PEG-20 NF; CAS 25322-68-3; used in pharmaceuticals (ointments for antiseptics and other medicaments, tablet coatings, suppositories, liq. preps., gelatin capsules); wh. waxy solid; m.w. 1000; sp.gr. 1.214; f.p. 37 C; visc. 18 cSt (210 F); flash pt. (PMCC) > 450 F.

Dow E1450 NF. [Dow] PEG-32 NF; CAS 25322-68-3; used in pharmaceuticals (ointments for antiseptics and other medicaments, tablet coatings, suppositories, liq. preps., gelatin capsules); wh. waxy solid; m.w. 1450; sp.gr. 1.214; f.p. 44 C; visc. 29 cSt (210 F); flash pt. (PMCC) > 450 F.

Dow E3350 NF. [Dow] PEG-75 NF; CAS 25322-68-3; used in pharmaceuticals (ointments for antiseptics and other medicaments, tablet coatings, suppositories, liq. preps., gelatin capsules); wh. waxy solid; m.w. 3350; sp.gr. 1.224; f.p. 54 C; visc. 93 cSt (210 F); flash pt. (PMCC) > 450 F.

Dow E4500 NF. [Dow] PEG-100 NF; CAS 25322-68-3; used in pharmaceuticals (ointments for antiseptics and other medicaments, tablet coatings, suppositories, liq. preps., gelatin capsules); wh. waxy solid; m.w. 4500; sp.gr. 1.224; f.p. 58 C; visc. 180 cSt (210 F); flash pt. (PMCC) > 450 F.

Dow E8000 NF. [Dow] PEG-150 NF; CAS 25322-68-3; used in pharmaceuticals (ointments for antiseptics and other medicaments, tablet coatings, suppositories, liq. preps., gelatin capsules); wh. waxy solid; m.w. 8000; sp.gr. 1.224; f.p. 60 C; visc. 800 cSt (210 F); flash pt. (PMCC) > 500 F.

Dow EP530. [Dow] Poloxamer-181; CAS 53637-25-5; provides solvency, low odor, low irritation, and low toxicity to personal care prods. and cosmetics; liq.; m.w. 2000;

sp.gr. 1.017; dens. 8.46 lb/gal; visc. 321 cSt; pour pt. -32 C; flash pt. (PMCC) > 420 F; ref. index 1.452.

Dow L910. [Dow] PPG-14 butyl ether; CAS 9003-13-8; provides solvency, low odor, low irritation, and low toxicity to personal care prods. and cosmetics; liq.; m.w. 910; sp.gr. 0.9833; dens. 8.23 lb/gal; visc. 83 cSt; pour pt. -43 C; flash pt. (PMCC) 345 F; ref. index 1.444.

Dow L1150. [Dow] PPG-18 butyl ether; CAS 9003-13-8; provides solvency, low odor, low irritation, and low toxicity to personal care prods. and cosmetics; liq.; m.w. 1150; sp.gr. 0.9888; dens. 8.28 lb/gal; visc. 115 cSt; pour pt. -40 C; flash pt. (PMCC) > 400 F; ref. index 1.446.

Dow MPEG350. [Dow] PEG-6 methyl ether; CAS 9004-74-4; provides solvency, low odor, low irritation, and low toxicity to personal care prods. and cosmetics; liq.; m.w. 350; sp.gr. 1.097; dens. 9.14 lb/gal; visc. 27 cSt; f.p. 0 C; flash pt. (PMCC) > 350 F; ref. index 1.455.

Dow MPEG550. [Dow] PEG-10 methyl ether; CAS 9004-74-4; provides solvency, low odor, low irritation, and low toxicity to personal care prods. and cosmetics; liq.; m.w. 550; sp.gr. 1.101; dens. 9.17 lb/gal; visc. 56 cSt; f.p. 20 C; flash pt. (PMCC) > 450 F; ref. index 1.461.

Dow MPEG750. [Dow] PEG-16 methyl ether; CAS 9004-74-4; provides solvency, low odor, low irritation, and low toxicity to personal care prods. and cosmetics; solid; m.w. 750; sp.gr. 1.102 (50 C); dens. 9.04 lb/gal (50 C); visc. 53 cSt (100 F); f.p. 30 C; flash pt. (PMCC) > 450 F; ref. index 1.463.

Dow P425. [Dow] PPG-9; CAS 25322-69-4; provides solvency, low odor, low irritation, and low toxicity to personal care prods. and cosmetics; liq.; m.w. 425; sp.gr. 1.007; dens. 8.39 lb/gal; visc. 70 cSt; pour pt. -45 C; flash pt. (PMCC) 330 F; ref. index 1.447; sp. heat 0.477 cal/g/°C.

Dow P1000TB. [Dow] PPG-17; CAS 25322-69-4; provides solvency, low odor, low irritation, and low toxicity to personal care prods. and cosmetics; liq.; m.w. 1000; sp.gr. 1.005; dens. 8.38 lb/gal; visc. 162 cSt; pour pt. -25 C; flash pt. (PMCC) > 360 F; ref. index 1.448; sp. heat 0.461 cal/g/°C.

Dow P1200. [Dow] PPG-20; CAS 25322-69-4; provides solvency, low odor, low irritation, and low toxicity to personal care prods. and cosmetics; liq.; m.w. 1200; sp.gr. 1.007; dens. 8.38 lb/gal; visc. 175 cSt; pour pt. -40 C; flash pt. (PMCC) 345 F; ref. index 1.448; sp. heat 0.459 cal/g/°C.

Dow P2000. [Dow] PPG-26; CAS 25322-69-4; provides solvency, low odor, low irritation, and low toxicity to personal care prods. and cosmetics; liq.; sol. in ethanol, IPM, cyclomethicone, sunscreens, lactic acid; partly sol. in water, lt. min. oil; m.w. 2000; sp.gr. 1.002; dens. 8.34 lb/gal; visc. 300 cSt; pour pt. -30 C; flash pt. (PMCC) 390 F; ref. index 1.449; sp. heat 0.452 cal/g/°C.

Dow P4000. [Dow] PPG-30; CAS 25322-69-4; provides solvency, low odor, low irritation, and low toxicity to personal care prods. and cosmetics; liq.; m.w. 4000; sp.gr. 1.005; dens. 8.36 lb/gal; visc. 800 cSt; pour pt. -26 C; flash pt. (PMCC) 365 F; ref. index 1.450.

Dow PT250. [Dow] PPG glyceryl ether polyglycol; CAS 25791-96-2; provides solvency, low odor, low irritation, and low toxicity to personal care prods. and cosmetics; liq.; m.w. 250; sp.gr. 1.091; dens. 9.07 lb/gal; visc. 850 cSt; pour pt. -18 C; flash pt. (PMCC) 390 F; ref. index 1.459.

Dow PT700. [Dow] PPG-10 glyceryl ether; CAS 25791-96-2; provides solvency, low odor, low irritation, and low toxicity to personal care prods. and cosmetics; liq.; m.w. 700; sp.gr. 1.033; dens. 8.59 lb/gal; visc. 236 cSt; pour pt. -32 C; flash pt. (PMCC) 500 F; ref. index 1.453; sp. heat 0.442 cal/g/°C.

Dow PT3000. [Dow] PPG-55 glyceryl ether; CAS 25791-96-

2; provides solvency, low odor, low irritation, and low toxicity to personal care prods. and cosmetics; liq.; m.w. 3000; sp.gr. 1.010; dens. 8.40 lb/gal; visc. 480 cSt; pour pt. -27 C; flash pt. (PMCC) 430 F; ref. index 1.451; sp. heat 0.445 cal/g/°C.

Dow Corning® 190 Surfactant. [Dow Corning] Dimethicone copolyol; nonionic; silicone surfactant, surf. tens. depressant, wetting agent, emulsifier, foam builder, humectant, softener; used for producing flexible slab stock urethane foam; plasticizer for hair resins; imparts spreadability, lt. nongreasy feel, and detackification to hair sprays, shampoos, skin care lotions, perfumes, shaving soaps; Gardner 2 hazy, low-visc. liq.; sol. in water, ethanol, IPM; disp. in propylene glycol; sp.gr. 1.037; visc. 1500 cst; b.p. > 200 C; HLB 14.4; flash pt. (COC) 121 C; ref. index 1.448; toxicology: nontoxic; 100% conc.

Dow Corning® 193 Surfactant. [Dow Corning] Dimethicone copolyol; nonionic; silicone surfactant, surf. tens. depressant, wetting agent, emulsifier, foam builder, humectant, softener; used for producing flexible slab stock urethane foam; plasticizer for hair resins; imparts spreadability, lt. nongreasy feel, and detackification to hair sprays, shampoos, skin care lotions, perfumes, shaving soaps; Gardner 2 hazy, visc. liq.; sol. in water, alcohol, hydroalcoholic systems, propylene glycol, IPM; sp.gr. 1.07; visc. 465 cs; HLB 13.6; f.p. 50 F; b.p. > 200 C; flash pt. (COC) 149 C; pour pt. 52 F; ref. index 1.454; usage level: 0.1-5.0; toxicology: nontoxic; 100% conc.

Dow Corning® 200 Fluid. [Dow Corning] Dimethicone; foam control agent for nonaq. systems, distillation, resin mfg., asphalt, oil refining, gas-oil separation; water barrier; lubricant, gloss, water repellency, softness agent for hair care prods.; emollient, lubricant in antiperspirants/deodorants; reduces valve clogging in aerosol prods.; emollient for skin lotions and creams; skin protectant; aids spreading and rub-in; clear fluid; sol. in IPM; dilutable in aliphatic, aromatic or chlorinated solvs.; 10 visc. grades: sp.gr. 0.761-0.975; visc. 0.65-12,5000 cst; m.p. < -40 C; b.p. 100- > 200 C; flash pt. (CC) -2 to > 321 C; ref. index 1.375-1.403; toxicology: LD50 (oral, rat) > 35 g/kg; nonirritating to skin on repeated/prolonged contact; transitory eye irritant; 100% act.

Dow Corning® 225. [Dow Corning] Dimethicone; imparts water repellency, hair luster, detackification, and skin protection to cosmetic creams, powds., and aerosols; acts as surface-spreading agent to increase efficacy of other ingreds.; water-wh. liq., odorless, tasteless; sp.gr. 0.94; visc. 9.5 cSt; acid no. 0.01; pour pt. -65 C; flash pt. (OC) 163 C; ref. index 1.395; surf. tens. 20.1 dynes/cm; toxicology: LD50 (oral, rat) > 35 g/kg; transitory eye irritant; nonirritating on prolonged/repeated contact.

Dow Corning® 244 Fluid. [Dow Corning] Cyclomethicone; CAS 69430-24-6; base fluid, vehicle or transient carrier in skin and hair care prods. such as aerosol and roll-on antispirants and deodorants where rapid evaporation is desirable; reduces surf. tens., aids spreading, and promotes leveling of solid pigments; clear liq., odorless; sol. in 190 proof ethanol, lt. min. oil, IPM; insol. in water, propylene glycol; sp.gr. 0.953; visc. 2.5 cst; m.p. 17 C; b.p. 172 C; flash pt. (CC) 55 C; ref. index 1.394; surf. tens. 17.8 dynes/cm.

Dow Corning® 245 Fluid. [Dow Corning] Cyclomethicone; CAS 69430-24-6; base fluid, vehicle or transient carrier for cosmetic and personal care prods.; provides controlled volatility for solid stick cosmetic prods.; reduces surf. tens., aids spreading, promotes leveling of solid pigments; clear liq., odorless; sol. in 190 proof ethanol, lt. min. oil, IPM; insol. in water, propylene glycol; sp.gr. 0.956; visc. 4.2 cst; m.p. < -40 C; b.p. 205 C; flash pt. (CC) 76 C; ref. index 1.397; surf. tens. 18.0 dynes/cm.

Dow Corning® 344 Fluid. [Dow Corning] Cyclomethicone; CAS 69430-24-6; base fluid or vehicle in personal care prods.; lubricant, spreading agent, detackifier for skin cleansers; also for aerosol and roll-on antiperspirants and deodorants where rapid evaporation is desirable; promotes leveling of solid pigments; clear liq., odorless; sol. in 190 proof ethanol, lt. min. oil, IPM; insol. in water, propylene glycol; sp.gr. 0.953; visc. 2.5 cst; m.p. 10 C; b.p. 178 C; flash pt. (CC) 52 C; ref. index 1.394; surf. tens. 19.0 dynes/cm.

Dow Corning® 345 Fluid. [Dow Corning] Cyclomethicone; CAS 69430-24-6; base fluid, vehicle, or transient carrier for cosmetic and personal care prods.; provides controlled volatility for solid stick cosmetic prods.; reduces surf. tens., aids spreading, and promotes leveling of solid pigments; clear liq., odorless; sol. in 190 proof ethanol, lt. min. oil, IPM; insol. in water, propylene glycol; sp.gr. 0.957; visc. 6.0 cst; m.p. < -40 C; b.p. 217 C; flash pt. (CC) 76 C; ref. index 1.398; surf. tens. 20.8 dynes/cm.

Dow Corning® 556 Fluid. [Dow Corning] Phenyltrimethicone; CAS 2116-84-9; EINECS 218-320-6; lubricant, emollient providing water barrier and reducing tackiness in skin and sun care prods., cosmetics, antiperspirants, deodorants, insect repellents, preshaves, hair grooming aids; provides gloss and sheen to hair care prods.; for wax, min. oil, and alcohol-based prods.; APHA 100 max. clear liq.; sol. in 190 proof ethanol, lt. min. oil, IPM, org. solvs.; disp. in propylene glycol; insol. in water; sp.gr. 0.980; visc. 22.5 cst; m.p. < -40 C; b.p. > 200 C; acid no. 0.10; flash pt. (CC) > 121 C; ref. index 1.460; usage level: 1-10%; toxicology: LD50 (oral, rat) > 34.6 g/kg, (dermal, rabbit) > 2 g/kg; nonirritating to skin and eyes.

Dow Corning® 580 Wax. [Dow Corning] Stearoxytrimethylsilane and stearyl alcohol (38%); lubricant for stick cosmetics; imparts feel, occlusiveness, detackification, increased visc., luster, hydrophobicity, and film-forming props. to skin and hair care formulations; ivory soft semicryst. wax; sol. in lt. min. oil; insol. in water, ethanol, propylene glycol; sp.gr. 0.852; m.p. 36-56 C; b.p. > 200 C; acid no. 0.05; cloud pt. 48 C; flash pt. 72 C; toxicology: may cause sl. temporary eye discomfort; non-irritating to skin; nonsensitizing.

Dow Corning® 593 Fluid. [Dow Corning] Dimethicone and trimethylsiloxysilicate; acts as a breathable, protective barrier in skin care and cosmetic applics.; nongreasy lubricant, waterproofing agent for sunscreen creams and lotions; provides detackification, spreadability, and smooth, soft, dry feel; APHA 150 max. clear visc. liq.; sol. in IPM; insol. in water, ethanol, propylene glycol; sp.gr. 1.034; visc. 650 cst; m.p. < -40 C; b.p. 200 C; flash pt. (CC) 200 C; ref. index 1.4089; toxicology: may cause temporary eye discomfort; 100% conc.

Dow Corning® 929. [Dow Corning] Amodimethicone, tallowtrimonium chloride, and nonoxynol-10; cationic; imparts wet and dry combing ease, luster, and resist. to dry fly-away to hair care formulations, esp. for damaged hair; enhances color definition and sheen; also car polish ingred.; milk wh. water-thin liq. emulsion; pH 7.6; toxicology: eye and moderate skin irritant in conc. form; 35% silicone; diluent: water.; formerly Dow Corning EF1-3574B.

Dow Corning® 939. [Dow Corning] Amodimethicone, trideceth-12, and cetrimonium chloride; cationic; conditioner, film-former, and fixative improving wet and dry combing and providing soft feel to hair care prods. incl. mousses, gels, setting lotions, hair fixatives, and perms; milky wh. emulsion; pH 6.5-9.0; 35% silicone.

Dow Corning® 1107 Fluid. [Dow Corning] Methicone; CAS 9004-73-3.

Dow Corning® 1401 Fluid. [Dow Corning] Cyclomethicone and dimethiconol; imparts long-lasting, substantive props. to skin and hair care prods., hair conditioners, facial cosmetics, sunscreens; provides uniform spreading and dry, emollient feel in antiperspirant/deodorant sticks; carrier in skin care prods.; reduces aerosol fogging; clear visc. liq.; sol. in 190 IPM; insol. in water, ethanol, propylene glycol; sp.gr. 0.960; visc. 5000 cst; f.p. -18 C; b.p. 182 C; flash pt. (CC) 52 C; ref. index 1.397; 13% NV.

Dow Corning® 1669. [Dow Corning] Dimethicone, tallowtrimonium chloride, and C11-15 pareth-9; cationic; substantive conditioner for hair conditioners, perms, and styling aids; improves wet and dry combing and feel; wh. water-thin emulsion; pH 6.0; 35% silicone.

Dow Corning® 2501 Cosmetic Wax. [Dow Corning] Dimethicone copolyol; noncomedogenic humectant, foam booster improving spreadability and wetting in cosmetic moisturizing lotions, facial cleansers, protective creams, sun care prods., liq. soaps, shaving creams; reduces tackiness of sticky materials; wh. to sl. yel. wax; sol. in water and ethanol; m.p. 28-34 C; flash pt. > 212 F.

Dow Corning® 2502 Cosmetic Fluid. [Dow Corning] Cetyl dimethicone; cosmetic ingred.

Dow Corning® 2503 Cosmetic Wax. [Dow Corning] Stearyl dimethicone; cosmetic wax.

Dow Corning® 2504 Cosmetic Fluid. [Dow Corning] Stearyl dimethicone; cosmetic ingred.

Dow Corning® 3225C Formulation Aid. [Dow Corning] Cyclomethicone and dimethicone copolyol; nonionic; surfactant for preparing water-in-volatile silicone emulsions used in personal care prods. esp. transparent prods.; reduces tackiness, improves spreadability and wet combing, provides nongreasy feel; emulsifier for aq. aluminum salts, antiperspirants; adds elegant feel to skin care prods.; clear to sl. hazy liq.; sol. in IPM; disp. in water, 190 proof ethanol, lt. min. oil; sp.gr. 0.963; visc. 100-1000 cst; m.p. 10 C; b.p. 178 C; HLB 4.0; flash pt. (CC) 60 C; ref. index 1.398; combustible; toxicology: LD50 (oral, rat) > 10.5 g/kg; nonirritating/nonsensitizing to skin; may cause eye irritation or discomfort; 10.5% conc. in volatile silicone.

Dow Corning® 7224 Conditioning Agent. [Dow Corning] Trimethylsilylamodimethicone, octoxynol-40, isolaureth-6, and propylene glycol; hair conditioning ingred.; emulsion.

Dow Corning® ACH-303. [Dow Corning] Aluminum chlorhydrate; CAS 1327-41-9; EINECS 215-477-2; act. ingred. in antiperspirant and deodorant formulations; sol. in water, methanol, ethanol, propylene glycol, glycerine; 50% conc.

Dow Corning® ACH-323. [Dow Corning] Aluminum chlorhydrate; CAS 1327-41-9; EINECS 215-477-2; for any type of antiperspirant formulation requiring dry, very discrete particle size; impalpable powd.; water-sol.

Dow Corning® ACH-331. [Dow Corning] Aluminum chlorhydrate; CAS 1327-41-9; EINECS 215-477-2; used in suspensoid solid state antiperspirant sticks; super fine powd.; water-sol.

Dow Corning® ACH7-308. [Dow Corning] Aluminum sesquichlorhydrate; act. ingreds. in antiperspirant formulations; beads; sol. in water and 190 proof ethanol.

Dow Corning® ACH7-321. [Dow Corning] Aluminum chlorhydrate; CAS 1327-41-9; EINECS 215-477-2; used in antiperspirant formulations where extremely fine particle size is not required; beads; water-sol.

Dow Corning® AZG-368. [Dow Corning] Aluminum/zirconium tetrachlorohydrex GLY; act. ingred. for all forms of topical antiperspirants; sol. in water and ethanol.

Dow Corning® AZG-369. [Dow Corning] Aluminum/zirconium tetrachlorohydrex GLY; act. ingred. for all forms of topical antiperspirants; sol. see Dow Corning AZG-368.

Dow Corning® AZG-370. [Dow Corning] Aluminum/zirconium tetrachlorohydrex GLY; act. ingred. for all forms of topical antiperspirants; powd.; water-sol.

Dow Corning® MDX-4-4210. [Dow Corning] Vinyldimethicone and silica.

Dow Corning® Q2-1403 Fluid. [Dow Corning] Dimethicone and dimethiconol; forms water-repellent, nonocclusive, silky, lubricious film improving substantivity of active ingreds. in hair conditioners, hand lotions, and cosmetics; clear liq.; sol. in IPM; insol. in water, ethanol, propylene glycol; sp.gr. 0.98; visc. 4000 cst; m.p. < -40 C; b.p. > 200 C; flash pt. (CC) 135 C; ref. index 1.39.

Dow Corning® Q2-5200. [Dow Corning] Laurylmethicone copolyol; water-in-min. oill emulsifier for skin care creams and lotions; less greasy with elegant feel; clear liq.; sol. in 190 proof ethanol, lt. min. oil, IPM; insol. in water, propylene glycol; sp.gr. 0.896; visc. 1000-4500 cst; m.p. -5 C; b.p. > 200 C; flash pt. (CC) 77 C; ref. index 1.452.

Dow Corning® Q2-5220 Resin Modifier. [Dow Corning] Dimethicone copolyol; noncomedogenic spreading agent, wetting agent, emulsifier, lubricant, foam modifier, resin plasticizer, and detackifier for hair care prods.; provides soft feel, reduces soap irritation, and offers exc. foam control in skin care prods.; improves foaming, adds lubrication and glide to shaving prods.; for shampoos, hairsprays, mousses, gels, setting lotions, curl activators, moisturizers, oil sheens, hair dressings; Gardner 2-4 clear liq.; sol. in water, 190 proof ethanol, IPM; disp. in propylene glycol; sp.gr. 1.030; visc. 1000 cst; b.p. > 200 C; flash pt. (CC) 60.6 C; ref. index 1.457; combustible; toxicology: LD50 (oral, rat) > 15.4 g/kg (essentially nontoxic); sl. transient eye irritant; pract. nontoxic skin absorp.

Dow Corning® Q2-5324 Surfactant. [Dow Corning] Dimethicone copolyol; emollient, spreading agent reducing irritancy of surfactants, resin plasticizer, and detackifier for hair care prods.; provides soft feel, reduces soap irritation, and offers exc. foam control in skin care prods.; improves foaming, adds lubrication and glide to shaving prods.; off-wh. to brn. hazy liq.; sol. in 190 proof ethanol, propylene glycol, IPM; disp. in water; sp.gr. 1.040; visc. 600 cst; b.p. > 200 C; flash pt. (CC) 60 C; ref. index 1.454.; combustible; toxicology: LD50 (oral) > 5000 mg/kg; essentially nontoxic; may cause temporary eye discomfort.

Dow Corning® Q2-5434. [Dow Corning] Dimethicone copolyol.

Dow Corning® Q2-7224 Conditioning Additive. [Dow Corning] Trimethylsilylamodimethicone, octoxynol-40, isolaureth-6, and propylene glycol; nonionic; conditioning agent improving wet and dry combing, contributing softness and substantivity, reducing drying time in hair care prods.; esp. effective for damaged hair; milk wh. water-thin emulsion; pH 10.5; toxicology: irritating to skin and eyes in conc. form; 35% silicone, diluent: water.

Dow Corning® Q2-8220 Conditioning Additive. [Dow Corning] Trimethylsilylamodimethicone; conditioning additive; improves wet and dry combing and adds softness, gloss, and substantivity to hair care prods.; reduces damage caused by reactive chemicals; colorless to straw yel. clear to sl. hazy liq.; sol. in IPM; insol. in water, ethanol, propylene glycol; sp.gr. 0.970; visc. 145 cst; m.p. < -40 C; b.p. > 200 C; flash pt. (CC) 76 C; ref. index 1.4065; combustible; toxicology: LD50 (oral, rat) > 5 g/kg (essentially nontoxic); moderate eye irritant; moderate to severe skin irritant.

Dow Corning® Q5-0158A Wax. [Dow Corning] Silicone; water repellent with antistick chars. for cosmetic and skin preps.; soft waxy solid.

Dow Corning® Q5-6038 Polymer Beads. [Dow Corning] Acrylates copolymer and min. oil; abrasive for facial scrubs, sloughing lotions, facial cleansers, skin polishers;

allows release of mineral oil to be absobed by the skin; wh. free-flowing powd.; particle size 200-800 µ; apparent dens. 0.5 g/cc; 35% min. oil.

Dow Corning® Q5-7155 AAZG Powd. [Dow Corning] Aluminum zirconium tetrachlorohydrex GLY.

Dow Corning® Q5-7160 AZAG Powd. [Dow Corning] Aluminum zirconium tetrachlorohydrex GLY; antiperspirant active.

Dow Corning® Q5-7167 AAZG Powd. [Dow Corning] Aluminum zirconium tetrachlorohydrex GLY.

Dow Corning® Q5-7171 AACH Powd. [Dow Corning] Aluminum chlorohydrate; CAS 1327-41-9; EINECS 215-477-2; antiperspirant active.

Dow Corning® Q7-4840. [Dow Corning] Vinyldimethicone and silica.

Dow Corning® QF1-3593A. [Dow Corning] Dimethicone, trimethylsiloxysilicate; emollient with water repellency and low slip for skin care prods.

Dow Corning® X2-1669. [Dow Corning] Dimethicone, tallowtrimonium chloride, pareth-15-9; cationic; enhances conditioning in hair conditoners, perms, colorants, and styling aids; improves wet and dry combing and feel; water-thin emulsion.

Dow Corning® Antifoam 1520-US. [Dow Corning] Silicone emulsion; nonionic; foam control agent for food, beverage mfg., meat/poultry/seafood processing, pharmaceuticals, resin mfg., waste water treatment, adhesives/coatings, metalworking, and textile industries; FDA §173.340, 176.170, 176.180, EPA 40 CFR §180.1001, USDA, kosher approved; milky-wh. thin cream; water-dilutable; sp.gr. 1.0; visc. 6000 cp; pH 4.0; toxicology: may cause temporary eye discomfort; 20% act.

Dow Corning® Antifoam A. [Dow Corning] Simethicone; foam control agent for distillation, resin sizes, textile latex backing, paper, asphalt, lubricants, detergents, pesticides, edible oils, soaps, shampoos; also avail. in food grade; med. off-wh. to gray liq.; 100% act.

Dow Corning® Medical Antifoam A Compound. [Dow Corning] Simethicone; foam control agent.

Dow Corning® Medical Antifoam AF Emulsion. [Dow Corning] Simethicone; foam control agent.

Dow Corning® Medical Antifoam C Emulsion. [Dow Corning] Simethicone; foam control agent.

Dow Corning® Medical Fluid 360. [Dow Corning] Dimethicone.

Dowicide 1. [Dow] o-Phenylphenol; CAS 90-43-7; EINECS 201-993-5; cosmetic preservative; USA, Japan, Europe approvals; usage level: 0.05-0.5%.

Dowicide A. [Dow] Sodium o-phenylphenate; CAS 132-27-4; EINECS 205-055-6; cosmetic preservative; USA, Europe approvals; usage level: 0.05-0.5%.

Dowicil® 200. [Dow] Quaternium-15; CAS 51229-78-8; EINECS 223-805-0; preservative providing broad-spectrum antimicrobial control in aq., anhyd., and emulsion cosmetic systems (hair care, baby prods., shaving prods., liq. hand soaps, sunscreens, surfatants); effective against Gram-positive and Gram-negative bacteria, mold, and yeast; off-wh. hygroscopic powd.; 100% thru 20 mesh; sol. (g/100 g): 127.2 g water, 20.8 g methanol, 18.7 g propylene glycol, 12.6 g glycerin; m.w. 251.2; bulk dens. 25 lb/ft³; usage level: 0.02-0.3%; 94% min. act.

D.P.P.G. [Gattefosse SA] Propylene glycol dipelargonate; CAS 41395-83-9; EINECS 255-350-9; emollient and oily rancidless additive for cosmetic and pharmaceutical preparations; oily liq.; HLB 2.0; acid no. < 0.2; iodine no. < 1; sapon. no. 305-325; toxicology: LD50 (oral, rat) > 16 g/kg; sl. irritating to eyes; nonirritating to skin.

Dracorin 100 SE 2/008479. [Dragoco] Glyceryl stearate and PEG-100 stearate.

Dracorin GMS SE O/W 2/008475. [Dragoco] Glyceryl

stearate SE.

Dragil 2/027011. [Dragoco] Glycol stearate; CAS 111-60-4; EINECS 203-886-9; emulsifier, opacifier, pearlescent for cosmetics.

Dragocid Forte 2/027045. [Dragoco] Ethoxydiglycol, diisopropyl adipate, methylparaben, dehydroacetic acid, propylparaben, and sorbic acid.

Dragoco Farnesol. [Dragoco] Farnesol; CAS 4602-84-0; EINECS 225-004-1.

Dragophos S 2/918501. [Dragoco] Sodium dihydroxycetyl phosphate and isopropyl hydroxycetyl ether.

Dragoplant Arnica 2/034060. [Dragoco] Water, arnica extract, and SD alcohol 39-C.

Dragoplant Balm Mint 2/034050. [Dragoco] Water, balm mint oil, SD alcohol 39-C.

Dragoplant Chamomile 2/034010. [Dragoco] Water, SD alcohol 39-C, and chamomile extract; botanical extract.

Dragoplant Witch Hazel 2/034020. [Dragoco] Water, SD alcohol 39-C, and witch hazel extract.

Dragosantol 2/012681. [Dragoco] Bisabolol; CAS 515-69-5; EINECS 208-205-9.

Dragoxat EH 2/044115. [Dragoco] Octyl octanoate; CAS 7425-14-1; EINECS 231-057-1; emollient.

Drakeol 5. [Penreco] Lt. min. oil NF; CAS 8042-47-5; emollient for hair prods., makeup, makeup removers, pharmaceutical ointments, gelatin capsule lubes, mold release lubricant for foods, egg coatings, fruit/veg. coatings, food pkg. materials, textile lubes, household cleaners and polishes; FDA compliance; sp.gr. 0.831-0.842; dens. 6.89-7.00 lb/gal; visc. 7.6-8.7 cSt (40 C); pour pt. -9 C; flash pt. 154 C; ref. index 1.4600.

Drakeol 6. [Penreco] Lt. min. oil USP; CAS 8042-47-5; base material for hair preps., bath oils, baby oils; FDA compliance; sp.gr. 0.827-0.836; dens. 6.94-7.02 lb/gal; visc. 9.2-10.6 cSt (40 C); pour pt. 15 F; flash pt. 320 F; ref. index 1.4613.

Drakeol 7. [Penreco] Lt. min. oil NF; CAS 8042-47-5; carrier, base ingred. in ointments, lotions, baby oils, sun tan lotions, makeup; solv. and emollient in creams, waterless hand cleaners; protective coating for foods; pigment dispersant, lubricant for plastics; FDA compliance; sp.gr. 0.828-0.843; dens. 6.94-7.08 lb/gal; visc. 10.8-13.6 cSt (40 C); pour pt. -9 C; flash pt. 177 C; ref. index 1.4632.

Drakeol 8. [Penreco] Min. oil; emollient, cosmetic raw material.

Drakeol 9. [Penreco] Lt. min. oil NF; CAS 8042-47-5; base material, carrier for cosmetics; emulsified lubricant for laxatives; pigment dispersant, lubricant for plastics; plasticizer for PS; textile and paper lubricant; FDA compliance; sp.gr. 0.838-0.854; dens. 7.03-7.16 lb/gal; visc. 14.2-17.0 cSt (40 C); pour pt. 09 C; flash pt. 179 C; ref. index 1.4665.

Drakeol 10. [Penreco] Min. oil; emollient, cosmetic raw material.

Drakeol 13. [Penreco] Lt. min. oil NF; CAS 8042-47-5; base ingred. in bath oils, creams and lotions, sunscreens, pharmaceutical topical ointments, food grade lubes and greases, fruit/veg. coatings; FDA compliance; sp.gr. 0.848-0.867; dens. 7.11-7.27 lb/gal; visc. 24.2-26.3 cSt (40 C); pour pt. -9 C; flash pt. 185 C; ref. index 1.4726.

Drakeol 15. [Penreco] Lt. min. oil NF; CAS 8042-47-5; emollient, cosmetic raw material; FDA compliance; sp.gr. 0.850-0.873; dens. 7.13-7.30 lb/gal; visc. 28.1-30.3 cSt (40 C); pour pt. -12 C; flash pt. 188 C; ref. index 1.4740.

Drakeol 19. [Penreco] Min. oil USP; CAS 8042-47-5; primary plasticizer for ethyl cellulose; lubricant for textile/paper; ingred. in cosmetics (creams, lotions, sunscreens, pharmaceuticals (laxatives, topical ointments), foods (lubes/greases, food pkg.), plastics (catalyst carriers); FDA compliance; sp.gr. 0.852-0.876; dens. 7.14-7.31 lb/gal; visc.

34.9-37.3 cSt (40 C); pour pt. -12 C; flash pt. 188 C; ref. index 1.4725.

Drakeol 21. [Penreco] Min. oil USP; CAS 8042-47-5; primary plasticizer for ethyl cellulose; ingred. in cosmetics (creams, lotions, sunscreens), pharmaceuticals (laxatives), foods (lubes/greases, food pkg.), plastics (lubes for PS, PVC, annealing, catalyst carriers), adhesives; FDA compliance; sp.gr. 0.853-0.876; dens. 7.15-7.32 lb/gal; visc. 38.4-41.5 cSt (40 C); pour pt. -12 C; flash pt. 193 C; ref. index 1.4733.

Drakeol 32. [Penreco] Min. oil USP; CAS 8042-47-5; plasticizer; FDA compliance; sp.gr. 0.856-0.876; dens. 7.18-7.35 lb/gal; visc. 60.0-63.3 cSt (40 C); pour pt. -12 C; flash pt. 213 C; ref. index 1.4770.

Drakeol 35. [Penreco] Min. oil USP; CAS 8042-47-5; ingred. in laxatives, cosmetic creams, lotions, sunscreens, foods (bakery pan oils, lubes/greases, food pkg.); plasticizer for PS, ethyl cellulose, PVC, annealing, catalyst carriers, thermoplastic rubber; water repellant for paper; adhesives, household cleaners and polishes; FDA compliance; sp.gr. 0.864-0.881; dens. 7.25-7.35 lb/gal; visc. 65.8-71.0 cSt (40 C); pour pt. -15 C; flash pt. 216 C; ref. index 1.4785.

Drewmulse® 10-10-O. [Stepan/PVO; Stepan Europe] Decaglyceryl decaoleate; CAS 11094-60-3; EINECS 234-316-7; nonionic; emulsifier, solubilizer, dispersant for w/o and o/w emulsions, creams, lotions, for internal, cosmetic, pharmaceutical use; Gardner 8 liq.; sol. in peanut oil, min. oil; HLB 3.0; sapon. no. 165–185.

Drewmulse® 85K. [Stepan/PVO] Glyceryl oleate from tallow and soya; emulsifier for foods (shortenings, icings, breads, dairy, frozen desserts, flavors, essential oils) and pharmaceuticals (vitamins and minerals); lubricant; lt. yel. semiliq.; HLB 3.4; sapon. no. 160–180; 40% alpha mono.

Drewmulse® 200K. [Stepan/PVO; Stepan Europe] Glyceryl stearate; nonionic; emulsifier, emollient, antistat, stabilizer, visc. builder, opacifier for creams, lotions, hair conditioners, foods (breads, chewing gum base, frozen desserts, peanut butter, margarine), pharmaceuticals (suppositories); wh. to beige solid; 100% act.

Drewmulse® 900K. [Stepan/PVO] Glyceryl stearate; nonionic; emulsifier for food industry as dispersing aid, antistaling agent, antistick agent (shortenings, icings, breads, chewing gum base, frozen desserts, peanut butter) and for pharmaceutical suppositories; cream beads; m.p. 138 F; HLB 3.2; sapon. 160–180; 52% alpha mono.

Drewmulse® GMO. [Stepan/PVO] Glyceryl oleate; nonionic; emulsifier, stabilizer and visc. builder in cosmetics and pharmaceuticals, opacifier; Gardner 6 liq.; HLB 3.4; 40–45% conc.

Drewmulse® HM-100. [Stepan/PVO] Glyceryl stearate and PEG-40 stearate; stabilizer and visc. builder in cosmetics and pharmaceuticals, opacifier, esp. effective in antiperspirant formulations; emulsifier for pharmaceutical topical ointments and creams, suppositories; Gardner 2 flake; HLB 8.4; 24% mono.

Drewmulse® POE-SML. [Stepan/PVO] Polysorbate 20; CAS 9005-64-5; nonionic; w/o emulsifier for cosmetics and pharmaceuticals, solubilizer, dispersant, wetting agent, detergent, visc. control agent; liq.; HLB 15.1; sapon. no. 40–51; 100% conc.

Drewmulse® POE-SMO. [Stepan/PVO] Polysorbate 80; CAS 9005-65-6; nonionic; w/o emulsifier for cosmetics and pharmaceuticals, solubilizer, dispersant, wetting agent, detergent, visc. control agent; liq.; HLB 15.0; sapon. no. 45–55.

Drewmulse® POE-SMS. [Stepan/PVO] Polysorbate 60; CAS 9005-67-8; nonionic; w/o emulsifier for cosmetics and pharmaceuticals, solubilizer, dispersant, wetting agent, detergent, visc. control agent; solid; HLB 14.9;

Drewmulse® POE-STS

sapon. no. 45–55.

Drewmulse® POE-STS. [Stepan/PVO] Polysorbate 65; CAS 9005-71-4; nonionic; w/o emulsifier for cosmetics and pharmaceuticals, solubilizer, dispersant, wetting agent, detergent, visc. control agent; solid; HLB 10.5; sapon. no. 88–98.

Drewmulse® SML. [Stepan/PVO] Sorbitan laurate; CAS 1338-39-2; nonionic; w/o emulsifier for cosmetics and pharmaceuticals, solubilizer, dispersant, wetting agent, detergent, visc. control agent; liq.; HLB 8.6; sapon. no. 159–171; 100% conc.

Drewmulse® SMO. [Stepan/PVO] Sorbitan oleate; CAS 1338-43-8; EINECS 215-665-4; nonionic; w/o emulsifier for cosmetics and pharmaceuticals, solubilizer, dispersant, wetting agent, detergent, visc. control agent; liq.; HLB 4.7; sapon. no. 144–156.

Drewmulse® SMS. [Stepan/PVO] Sorbitan stearate; CAS 1338-41-6; EINECS 215-664-9; nonionic; w/o emulsifier for cosmetics and pharmaceuticals, solubilizer, dispersant, wetting agent, detergent, visc. control agent; solid; HLB 2.1; sapon. no. 147–157.

Drewmulse® STS. [Stepan/PVO] Sorbitan tristearate; CAS 26658-19-5; EINECS 247-891-4; nonionic; w/o emulsifier for cosmetics and pharmaceuticals, solubilizer, dispersant, wetting agent, detergent, visc. control agent; solid; HLB 2.1; sapon. no. 170–190.

Drewmulse® TP. [Stepan/PVO] Glyceryl stearate; nonionic; emulsifier, stabilizer, and visc. builder in cosmetics and pharmaceuticals, opacifier; Gardner 4 flake; HLB 2.8; 40% mono.

Drewpol® 3-1-O. [Stepan; Stepan/PVO] Polyglyceryl-3 monooleate; CAS 9007-48-1; nonionic; emulsifier for creams, makeup, lotions, conditioners; food emulsifier; amber clear liq.; HLB 7.0; acid no. 5.0 max.

Drewpol® 6-1-O. [Stepan; Stepan Canada] Polyglyceryl-6 oleate; CAS 9007-48-1; emulsifier for creams, makeups, lotion, conditioners; food emulsifier; amber clear liq.; HLB 8.5; acid no. 6 max.

Drewpol® 10-4-O. [Stepan; Stepan Canada; Stepan Europe] Polyglyceryl-10 tetraoleate; CAS 34424-98-1; EINECS 252-011-7; nonionic; emulsifier, emollient, antistat, stabilizer, visc. builder, opacifier for creams, makeup, lotions, hair conditioners; solubilizer for vitamins, flavors, medicaments; amber clear liq.; HLB 6.0; acid no. 8.0 max.; 100% act.

Drewpol® 10-10-O. [Stepan; Stepan Canada; Stepan Europe] Polyglyceryl-10 decaoleate; CAS 11094-60-3; EINECS 234-316-7; nonionic; emulsifier for creams, makeup, lotions, conditioners; food emulsifier; amber clear liq.; HLB 3.0; acid no. 10.0 max.

Driveron® . [Hüls AG] Methyl-t-butyl ether; cosmetic raw material.

Drivosol® . [Hüls AG] Propane, isobutane, and butane; propellant for cosmetic aerosols with a neutral, weak natural odor; colorless liquefied gas.

Dry Flo® PC. [Nat'l. Starch] Aluminum starch octenyl succinate; CAS 9087-61-0; natural polymer char. by soft, velvety texture, free-flowing props., and extreme resist. to wetting by water; eliminates greasy, oily skinfeel; used for lotions, creams, body powds., makeup, eye liner, mascara, sunscreen, antiperspirants, feminine hygiene sprays, foot powds.; wh. powd.; water-insol.; 12% volatiles.

DSH. [Exsymol] Sodium hyaluronate dimethylsilanol.

D.S.H. C. [Exsymol; Biosil Tech.] Dimethylsilanol hyaluronate; provides skin regeneration, strong hydrating action for cosmetic and health prods. such as milks, emulsions, creams, lotions; pale yel. sl. opalescent liq.; misc. with water, alcohols, glycols; sp.gr. 1.0; pH 5.0; usage level: 4-6%; toxicology: nontoxic.

Duocrome® . [Mearl] Titanium dioxide-coated mica and a thin layer of colored pigment (iron blue, carmine, and/or iron oxide); iridescent colors producing dual-color effects derived from light interference and light absorption; used in cosmetics and personal care prods.; colors incl. blue/red, blue/green, blue/gold, red/blue, red/violet, gold/green, green/blue, etc.; fine lustrous powd.; particle size 6-50 μm; sp.gr. ≈ 3.0.

Duocrome® BG. [Mearl] Mica, titanium dioxide, and ferric ferrocyanide.

Duocrome® GY. [Mearl] Mica, titanium dioxide, iron oxides, and ferric ferrocyanide.

Duocrome® RB. [Mearl] Mica, titanium dioxide, and carmine.

Duocrome® YR. [Mearl] Mica, titanium dioxide, and iron oxides.

Duoquad® O-50. [Akzo] N,N,N′,N′,N′-Pentamethyl-N-octadecenyl-1,3-diammonium dichloride, aq. IPA; CAS 68310-73-6; surfactant for industrial and cosmetic use; Gardner 6 max. liq.; sol. in water, alcohols, chloroform, CCl_4; flash pt. (PMCC) 15 C; pH 6–9; 50% quat. in aq. IPA.

Duoquad® T-50. [Akzo] Tallowdimonium propyltrimonium dichloride, aq. IPA; CAS 68607-29-4; EINECS 271-762-1; cationic; detergent, corrosion inhibitor, metal cleaner; emulsifier for sec. oil recovery; also for cosmetics; Gardner 13 max. liq.; sol. in water, alcohols, chloroform, CCl_4; m.w. 480; sp.gr. 0.90; HLB 14.4; f.p. −20 C; flash pt. (PMCC) 15 C; pH 6–8 (10% aq.); 48–52% act. in aq. IPA.

Durawax #1032. [Frank B. Ross] Methylstyrene/vinyltoluene copolymer, microcryst. wax, and carnauba.

Dur-Em® 114. [Van Den Bergh Foods] Glyceryl oleate; nonionic; emulsifier for personal care prods., foods (icings, cakes, margarine, veg. dairy systems); plastic; HLB 2.8; m.p. 43–49 C; 100% conc.; 40% min. alpha monoglyceride.

Dur-Em® 117. [Van Den Bergh Foods] Glyceryl stearate; nonionic; textile lubricant and finishing agent; emulsifier for cosmetic and pharmaceutical creams and lotions, foods; lubricant for thermoplastics; dispersant for inorg. pigments; bead/flake; HLB 2.8; m.p. 62–65 C; 100% conc.; 40% min. alpha monoglyceride.

Dur-Em® 207E. [Van Den Bergh Foods] Glyceryl stearate SE; nonionic; food emulsifier, emulsifier hydrate for breads, for pharmaceutical, cosmetic uses; wh. powd.; m.p. 140–146 F; HLB 4.2; 100% act.; 50% alpha mono.

Dur-Em® GMO. [Van Den Bergh Foods] Glyceryl oleate; nonionic; solubilizer, dispersant, lubricant, wetting aid, penetrant for foods, personal care prods., dry cleaning bases, paints, and insecticides; HLB 2.8.

Durfax® 20. [Van Den Bergh Foods] Polysorbate 20; CAS 9005-64-5; nonionic; used in personal care and household prods.; food emulsifier; fabric antistat; HLB 16.5; sapon. no. 39–52.

Durfax® 60. [Van Den Bergh Foods] Polysorbate 60; CAS 9005-67-8; nonionic; food emulsifier; personal care prods.; preshave beard lubricant and softener prods.; paste; sol. in water; HLB 14.0; sapon. no. 45–55; 100% conc.

Durfax® 80. [Van Den Bergh Foods] Polysorbate 80; CAS 9005-65-6; nonionic; food emulsifier; personal care prods.; antifog agent in plastics and aerosol furniture polish; liq.; water-sol.; HLB 15.0; sapon. no. 45–55; 100% conc.

Durtan® 20. [Van Den Bergh Foods] Sorbitan laurate; CAS 1338-39-2; nonionic; used in cosmetic, toiletry, and household prods.; fabric antistat and lubricant; HLB 7.4; sapon. no. 158–170.

Dusoran MD. [Solvay Duphar BV] Lanolin alcohols, dist.; CAS 8027-33-6; EINECS 232-430-1; nonionic; w/o emulsifier, stabilizer, softener, emollient for absorption bases, cosmetics, cleansing preps.; lt. yel., waxy solid; sol, in min. oil, abs. and 95% alcohols, chloroform, ether, lt. petrol., toluene; acid no. 2.0; sapon. 8.0; 100% act.

Dymel® 22. [DuPont] Hydrochlorofluorocarbon 22; CAS 75-45-6; EINECS 200-871-9; aerosol propellant; environmentally safe and low in toxicity; only nonflam. liquefied propellant for general aerosol usage; m.w. 86.5; sp.gr. 1.21; b.p. –41.4 F.

Dymel® 142b. [DuPont] Hydrochlorofluorocarbon 142b; CAS 75-68-3; EINECS 200-891-8; aerosol propellant.

Dymel® 152a. [DuPont] Hydrofluorocarbon 152a; CAS 75-37-6; EINECS 200-866-1.

Dymel® A. [DuPont] Dimethyl ether; CAS 115-10-6; EINECS 204-065-8; aerosol propellant; environmentally safe and low in toxicity; low flam.; m.w. 46.1; high sol. in water; misc. with most conventional solvs.; sp.gr. 0.66; b.p. -12.7 F.

Dynacerin® 660. [Hüls Am.; Hüls AG] Oleyl erucate; CAS 17673-56-2; EINECS 241-654-9; jojoba oil substitute; emollient for cosmetic creams and emulsions; yel. liq. wax; sol. in fat solvs.; water-insol.; visc. 15-18 mPa·s (40 C); acid no. 1 max.; iodine no. 85-95; sapon. no. 95-110; sapon. no. 95-110;

Dynasan® 110. [Hüls Am.; Hüls AG] Tricaprin; CAS 621-71-6; EINECS 210-702-0; emollient, tablet lubricant, consistency regulator, nucleating agent, powd. base for cosmetic applics. such as sticks, creams, lotions, powds.; for prep. of margarine, confectionery, milk prods., fruit diets; wh. solid; clear pt. 30 C; acid no. 0.2 max.; iodine no. 1 max.; sapon. no. 295-305.

Dynasan® 112. [Hüls Am.; Hüls AG] Trilaurin; CAS 538-24-

9; EINECS 208-687-0; consistency regulator for cosmetic/pharmaceutical creams, lotions; tablet lubricant, powd. base, nucleating agent in sticks; wh. powd.; clear pt. 45 C; acid no. 0.3 max.; iodine no. 1 max.; sapon. no. 257-266.

Dynasan® 114. [Hüls Am.; Hüls AG] Trimyristin; CAS 555-45-3; EINECS 209-099-7; binder, lubricant for tablets and compressed confectioneries; consistency regulator for creams and lotions; lubricant, powd. base, nucleating agent in sticks; wh. powd./flakes; clear pt. 57 C; acid no. 0.3 max.; iodine no. 1 max.; sapon. no. 230-238.

Dynasan® 116. [Hüls Am.; Hüls AG] Tripalmitin; CAS 555-44-2; EINECS 209-098-1; lubricant, consistency regulator in cosmetic powds., cakes, and production of tablets (pharmaceuticals); powd. and makeup base; nucleating agent in sticks; wh. microcryst. powds.; sol. in ether and benzene; clear pt. 63 C; acid no. 0.5 max.; iodine no. 1 max.; sapon. no. 205-210.

Dynasan® 118. [Hüls Am.; Hüls AG] Tristearin; CAS 555-43-1; EINECS 209-097-6; nonionic; crystallization accelerator in chocolate; lubricant in cosmetic powds., cakes, and prod. of tablets (pharmaceuticals); consistency regulator; nucleating agent in sticks; powd. base; wh. microcryst. powd./flakes; sol. in ether and benzene; clear pt. 71 C; acid no. 0.5 max.; iodine no. 1 max.; sapon. no. 186-192.

Dynasan® P60. [Hüls Am.] Hydrog. palm oil; consistency regulator for creams, lotions, makeup, decorative cosmetics; stabilizer for hindering "oiling out" of an emulsion; wh. to off-wh. powd.; m.p. 58-60 C; acid no. 0.3 max.; iodine no. 3 max.; sapon.no. 190-210.

E

E-2153. [Siltech] Amodimethicone, tallowtrimonium chloride, and nonoxynol-10.

E-2170. [Siltech] Dimethiconol and nonoxynol-10.

EA-209. [Kobo] Ethylene/acrylic acid copolymer; CAS 9010-77-9; cosmetic gellant.

Eastman® AQ 29D. [Eastman] Dispersed thermoplastic polyester; dispersant providing adhesion, bonding, dust suppression, and asbestos mitigation to household adhesives, dyes, hard surf. cleaners, protective coatings, shoe polish, pesticides/herbicides; flocculant for wastewater; detackifier for oily materials; cosmetic film-former (hair spray, mousse, moisturizer, nail polish); ingred. in oil-free cosmetics, hand creams, sun screens; liq.; water-disp.; sp.gr. 1.06; dens. 8.83 lb/gal; visc. 45 cP; pH 5-6; 30% solids in water.

Eastman® AQ 35S. [Eastman] Thermoplastic polyester; dispersant providing adhesion, bonding, dust suppression, and asbestos mitigation to household adhesives, dyes, hard surf. cleaners, protective coatings, shoe polish, pesticides/herbicides; flocculant for wastewater; detackifier for oily materials; cosmetic film-former (hair spray, mousse, moisturizer, nail polish); ingred. in oil-free cosmetics, hand creams, sun screens; clear lt. amber pellet; disp. in water, dimethyl sulfoxide, methylene chloride; m.w. 7000; soften. pt. 35 C; acid no. < 2; hyd. no. < 10.

Eastman® AQ 38D. [Eastman] Dispersed thermoplastic polyester; dispersant providing adhesion, bonding, dust suppression, and asbestos mitigation to household adhesives, dyes, hard surf. cleaners, protective coatings, shoe polish, pesticides/herbicides; flocculant for wastewater; detackifier for oily materials; cosmetic film-former (hair spray, mousse, moisturizer, nail polish); ingred. in oil-free cosmetics, hand creams, sun screens; liq.; water-disp.; sp.gr. 1.06; dens. 8.84 lb/gal; visc. 30 cP; pH 5-6; 25% solids in water.

Eastman® AQ 38S. [Eastman] Diglycol cyclohexanedimethanol isophthalates sulfoisophthalates copolymer; anionic; thermoplastic polyester polymer; dispersant providing adhesion, bonding, dust suppression, and asbestos mitigation to household adhesives, dyes, hard surf. cleaners, protective coatings, shoe polish, pesticides/herbicides; flocculant for wastewater; cosmetic film-former (hair spray, mousse, moisturizer, nail polish); ingred. in oil-free cosmetics, hand creams, sun screens; imparts good holding props. and high sheen in water-based hair sprays; clear lt. amber pellet; disp. in water, cyclohexanone, dimethyl sulfoxide, diethylene glycol; m.w. 10,000; melt visc. 9700 poise (200 C); soften. pt. 38 C; acid no. < 2; hyd. no. < 10; 100% solids.

Eastman® AQ 55S. [Eastman] Diglycol cyclohexanedimethanol isophthalates sulfoisophthalates copolymer; anionic; thermoplastic polyester polymer; dispersant providing adhesion, bonding, dust suppression, and asbes-tos mitigation to household adhesives, dyes, hard surf. cleaners, protective coatings, shoe polish, pesticides/herbicides; flocculant for wastewater; cosmetic film-former (hair spray, mousse, moisturizer, nail polish); ingred. in oil-free cosmetics, hand creams, sun screens; imparts good holding props. and high sheen in water-based hair sprays; high humidity hold; clear, lt. amber pellet; disp. in water, cyclohexanone, methylene chloride, diethylene glycol; m.w. 8000; melt visc. 42,000 poise (200 C); soften. pt. 55 C; acid no. < 2; hyd. no. < 10; 100% act.

Eastman® CAB. [Eastman] Cellulose acetate butyrate; CAS 9004-36-8.

Eastman® CAP. [Eastman] Cellulose acetate propionate.

Eastman® Hydroquinone. [Eastman] Hydroquinone; CAS 123-31-9; EINECS 204-617-8; cosmetics ingred.

Eastman® Vitamin E 4-50. [Eastman] Mixed tocopherols; natural vitamin E source for cosmetics.

Eastman® Vitamin E 4-80. [Eastman] Mixed tocopherols; natural vitamin E source for cosmetics.

Eastman® Vitamin E 5-40. [Eastman] d-α Tocopherol; CAS 59-02-9; natural vitamin E source for cosmetics.

Eastman® Vitamin E 5-67. [Eastman] d-α Tocopherol; CAS 59-02-9; natural vitamin E source for cosmetics.

Eastman® Vitamin E 6-40. [Eastman] d-α Tocopheryl acetate; CAS 7695-91-2; EINECS 231-710-0; natural vitamin E source for cosmetics.

Eastman® Vitamin E 6-81. [Eastman] d-α Tocopheryl acetate; CAS 7695-91-2; EINECS 231-710-0; natural vitamin E source for cosmetics.

Eastman® Vitamin E 6-100. [Eastman] d-α Tocopheryl acetate; CAS 7695-91-2; EINECS 231-710-0; natural vitamin E source for cosmetics.

Eastman® Vitamin E 700. [Eastman] d-α Tocopheryl acetate; CAS 7695-91-2; EINECS 231-710-0; natural vitamin E source for cosmetics; dry form.

Eastman® Vitamin E Succinate. [Eastman] d-α Tocopheryl succinate; CAS 4345-03-3; EINECS 224-403-8; natural vitamin E source for cosmetics; dry form.

Eastman® Vitamin E TPGS. [Eastman] d-α Tocopheryl polyethylene; CAS 9002-96-4; natural vitamin E source for cosmetics; water-sol.

Ebal. [Mitsubishi Gas] p-Ethylbenzaldehyde; CAS 4748-78-1; EINECS 225-268-8; additive for resins; intermediate for pharmaceuticals, fragrances; colorless liq., aromatic odor; sol. in ethanol, ether, toluene; insol. in water; m.w. 134.2; sp.gr. 1.000; b.p. 221 C; m.p. -33 C; acid no. 0.3; flash pt. (COC) 98 C; toxicology: LD50 (oral, rat) 1700 mg/kg; eye and skin irritant; 97.5% purity.

Eccowet® W-50. [Eastern Color & Chem.] Sodium aliphatic ester sulfonate; anionic; wetting agent, penetrant, dispersant, solubilizer, emulsifier, detergent for textiles, metal processing, disinfectants, paints, pigments, wallpaper, rubber cements, adhesives, drycleaning detergents, topical pharmaceuticals, cosmetics; colorless liq.; misc.

with water; sol. in alcohol, glycols, acetones, dilute electrolyte sol'ns. (5%); visc. 55 cps; pH 8.0 ± 0.3 (1%); 50% conc.

Eccowet® W-88. [Eastern Color & Chem.] Sulfonated organic ester; wetting agent, penetrant, dispersant, solubilizer, emulsifier, detergent for textiles, metal processing, disinfectants, paints, pigments, wallpaper, rubber cements, adhesives, drycleaning detergents, topical pharmaceuticals, cosmetics; amber visc. liq.; pH 8.0 ± 0.3 (1%); 21% act.

Edamin S. [Sheffield Prods.] Hydrolyzed casein; CAS 65072-00-6; EINECS 265-363-1; cosmetic protein.

Edenol 302. [Henkel/Cospha; Henkel Canada] Propylene glycol dicaprylate/dicaprate; emollient oil and cosolv. for personal care prods., bath oils, aerosols, antiperspirants; stable vehicle for pigmented cosmetics; yel. low visc. liq.; sol. in alcohols, min. oils, ketones; insol. in water; dens. 0.92 g/ml; HLB 9; solid. pt. < 0 C; acid no. 1 max.; iodine no. 2 max.; sapon. no. 315–335; cloud pt. < 0 C; ref. index 1.435.

Edenor GMS. [Henkel Canada] Glyceryl stearate; nonionic; consistency factor for creams and liq. emulsions; flakes; 100% conc.

Edenor L2SM. [Henkel] Palmitic acid; CAS 57-10-3; EINECS 200-312-9; surfactant intermediate; soap and cosmetic formulations.

Edesal. [Vevy] Isodecyl salicylate.

Edeta®. [BASF AG] Complexing agents for cosmetics industry.

Efaderma. [Vevy] Linoleic acid, linolenic acid, and arachidonic acid.

Efaderma-F. [Vevy] Trilinolein.

Efadermasterolo. [Vevy] Soybean oil, soybean oil unsaponifiables, linoleic acid, linolenic acid, and arachidonic acid.

EFA-Glycerides. [Brooks Industries] Trilinolein, triolein, trilinolenin, and tocopherol; cosmetic ingred.

EFA-Liq. [Brooks Industries] Stabilized omega 6 linoleic acid and omega 3 linolenic acid; natural active lipids for skin care prods.; provides building blocks for cell wall and cellular lipids.

Efamol Evening Primrose Oil. [Efamol] Evening primrose oil.

EFA-Plex. [Brooks Industries] Linoleic acid, myristyl myristate, isopropyl palmitate, linolenic acid, oleic acid, and tocopherol; cosmetic ingred.

EFA-Plexol. [Brooks Industries] Glycerin, linoleic acid, oleic acid, linolenic acid, and tocopherol; cosmetic ingred.

Efevit E. [Fabriquimica] Propylene glycol linoleate and propylene glycol linolenate; emollient, dermatophilic additive; acid no. < 1; iodine no. 80-100; sapon. no. 140-155.

Efevit S. [Fabriquimica] PEG-8 linoleate and PEG-8 linolenate; emollient, dermatophilic additive; acid no. < 1; iodine no. 45-60; sapon. no. 75-85.

Egg White Solids Type P-20. [Henningsen Foods] Albumen; CAS 9006-50-2.

Egg Yolk Solids Type Y-1. [Henningsen Foods] Dried egg yolk.

Eglantineol. [Esperis] Sweet almond oil, corn oil, and rose hips extract.

Eijitsu Extract BG. [Ikeda] Rose fruit extract; anti-inflammatory providing protection against stains and freckles from sun exposure; for skin care creams; yel. amber transparent clear visc. liq., faint char. odor; sp.gr. 1.00-1.10; pH 4.0-5.0; 10% min. solids.

Ektasolve® DB. [Eastman] Butoxydiglycol; CAS 112-34-5; EINECS 203-961-6; solvent for cosmetic and industrial applics.

Ektasolve® DB Acetate. [Eastman] Diethylene glycol butyl ether acetate; CAS 124-17-4; solvent for cosmetic and industrial applics.

Ektasolve® DE. [Eastman] Ethoxydiglycol; CAS 111-90-0; EINECS 203-919-7; solvent for cosmetic and industrial applics.

Ektasolve® DE Acetate. [Eastman] Diethylene glycol ethyl ether acetate; CAS 112-15-2; solvent for cosmetic and industrial applics.

Ektasolve® DM. [Eastman] Diethylene glycol monomethyl ether; CAS 111-77-3; EINECS 203-906-6; evaporating solv. used in brushing lacquers and dye stains; useful in wood stains, printing inks, and dye pastes for textiles; coalescing aid for PVAc latex paints; used in stamp pad and stencil inks; diluent for hydraulic brake fluids; also for cosmetics; water-wh. liq.; agreeable odor; m.w. 120.15; f.p. –85 C; b.p. 191 C min.; water-sol.; sp.gr. 1.023; dens. 1.02 kg/l; ref. index 1.4263; flash pt. 96 C (COC); fire pt. 96 C; > 99% volatiles by vol.

Ektasolve® DP. [Eastman] Diethylene glycol monopropyl ether; CAS 6881-94-3; evaporating, water-misc. solv. used in sol'n. and water-dilutable coatings, cosmetics; act. for many coating materials incl. NC, acrylic copolymers, epoxy resins, chlorinated rubber, and alkyd resins; strong coupling agent with some resin systems in water-dilutable coatings; colorless clear liq.; mild odor; m.w. 148.2; f.p. < –90 C; b.p. 202 C min.; water-sol.; sp.gr. 0.963; dens. 0.96 kg/l; ref. index 1.429; flash pt. 93 C (TCC); fire pt. 103 C; > 99% volatiles by vol.

Ektasolve® EEH. [Eastman] Ethylene glycol 2-ethylhexyl ether; CAS 1559-35-9; solvent for cosmetic and industrial applics.

Ektasolve® EP. [Eastman] Ethylene glycol monopropyl ether; CAS 2807-30-9; slow evaporating solv. used in coatings and cosmetics; useful in waterborne coating systems; coupling solv. for resin/water systems; controls visc. of waterborne resins; effective for NC, acrylic, epoxy, polyamide, and alkyd resins; retarder in coating systems; colorless clear liq.; mild odor; m.w. 104.15; f.p. < –90 C; b.p. 149.5 min.; water-sol.; sp.gr. 0.9125; dens. 0.91 kg/l; ref. index 1.4136; flash pt. 49 C (TCC); fire pt. 56 C; 100% volatiles by vol.

Ektasolve® PM Acetate. [Eastman] Propylene glycol methyl ether acetate; CAS 108-65-6; retarder solvent for cosmetic and industrial applics.; sol. 25.9% in water; dens. 7.91 lb/gal; b.p. 142–147 C; flash pt. 46 C; surf. tens. 26.4 dynes/cm; elec. resist. 6 megohms.

Elacid CLR. [Dr. Kurt Richter; Henkel/Cospha] Elastin partial hydrolysate with elastin specific protein structures in weakly acid hydrophilic medium; cationic; prods. for aging and inelastic skin; clear ylsh. liq.

Elacid Richter. [Dr. Kurt Richter; Henkel/Cospha] cationic; o/w hair conditioner conc. for damaged hair; antistat; ivory paste.

Elastein® 5000. [Hormel] Hydrolyzed elastin; CAS 100085-10-7; exc. film-former enhancing dermal flexibility in skin care systems; clear amber liq.; m.w. 5000.

Elastin. [Koken] Hydrolyzed elastin; CAS 100085-10-7; cosmetic protein.

Elastin. [Provital; Centerchem] Hydrolyzed elastin; CAS 100085-10-7; cosmetic protein.

Elastin 5000. [Hormel] Hydrolyzed elastin; CAS 100085-10-7; cosmetic protein.

Elastin CLR. [Henkel/Cospha; Henkel Canada] Elastin partial hydrolysate; CAS 100085-10-7; for applic. to aging skin whose elastic fibers are becoming brittle; ylsh. clear liq.

Elastin H.P.M. [Solabia] Hydrolyzed elastin; CAS 100085-10-7; cosmetic protein.

Elastin PG 2000. [Herstellung von Naturextrakten GmbH; Lipo] Propylene glycol, hydrolyzed elastin, and soluble collagen; water-binder used in face creams/masks, ampoules, body lotions, after-sun lotions, shampoos, and hair conditioning treatments; yel. visc. opalescent sol'n., weak intrinsic odor; m.w. 5000-30,000; sp.gr. 1.04-1.05; pH 6.5-7.5.

Elastin Hydrolysate COS. [Cosmetochem] Hydrolyzed elastin; CAS 100085-10-7; cosmetic protein.

Elastin (Partialhydrolisate) NOVA. [Novarom GmbH] Hydrolyzed elastin; CAS 100085-10-7; cosmetic protein.

Elastobiol. [Laserson SA] Calf skin extract; elastin peptides providing nutritive and hydrating action on epidermal cells; yel. clear liq.; water-sol.; usage level: 5-10%.

Elastolan LS HE 20. [Laboratoires Sérobiologiques] Hydrolyzed elastin; CAS 100085-10-7; cosmetic protein.

Elastovit. [Variati] Hydrolyzed collagen; CAS 9015-54-7; cosmetic protein.

Elcema® F150, G250, P100. [Degussa] Cellulose NF; CAS 9004-34-6; EINECS 232-674-9; anticaking agent, tabletting aid for pharmaceutical industry; wh. gran. and wh. powd. resp.

Eldew CL-301. [Ajinomoto] Cholesteryl/behenyl/octyldodecyl lauroyl glutamate; emollient for lipstick, skin care creams and lotions, hair treatment, sun care, makeup; provides exc. water permeability, high water-binding capability, and smooth feel to skin; good pigment dispersibility; yields nongreasy, nontacky prods.

Elefac™ I-205. [Bernel] Octyldodecyl neopentanoate; dry emollient, SPF booster, pigment wetter and binder; FDA, EEC, and Japanese compliances; colorless liq.; oil-sol.; usage level: 5-10%.

Eleseryl® SH. [Laboratoires Sérobiologiques] Serum protein; biopolymer providing anti-wrinkle, nutrient, protective, conditioning, softening, and repair props. for sensitive skin; yel. amber liq.; sol. in water; usage level: 3-10%.

Eleseryl® SHT. [Laboratoires Sérobiologiques] Hydrolyzed serum protein; biopeptides providing eutrophic and stimulating effect on dermal and epidermal cells, strengthening of cutaneous elasticity, and emulsification of cutaneous lipids; conditioner, protectant for nutritive, repairing, and anti-age care for skin, hair care prods.; yel. limpid liq.; water-sol.; usage level: 3-10%.

Elespher® . [Laboratoires Sérobiologiques] Marine vegetal (algae) microspheres; entrapment systems with rapid release; carriers of cosmetic actives; hydrating props.; for dry skin with nonstructured microrelief; semifluid gel; hydrophilic; usage level: 3-7%.

Elespher® Almondermin. [Laboratoires Sérobiologiques] Water, linseed extract, sodium hydroxide, SD alcohol 39-C, althea extract, sweet almond extract, algae extract, carbomer, and xanthan gum.

Elespher® Dermosaccharides GY. [Laboratoires Sérobiologiques] Water, glycerin, sodium hydroxide, glycogen, algae extract, and carbomer.

Elespher® Dermosaccharides HC. [Laboratoires Sérobiologiques] Water, glycerin, algae extract, sodium hydroxide, glycosaminoglycans, glycogen, and carbomer.

Elespher® Eleseryl SH. [Laboratoires Sérobiologiques] Water, serum protein, sodium hydroxide, algae extract, and carbomer.

Elesponge® . [Laboratoires Sérobiologiques] Ovoid microparticles of spongious polymeric matrix; microsponge entrapment systems with prolonged release; carriers of cosmetic actives; chronocosmetics; suspension or powd.; disp. in water; usage level: 3-5%.

Elestab® CPN. [Laboratoires Sérobiologiques] Chlorphenesin; CAS 104-29-0; EINECS 203-192-6; preservative for cosmetics; effective against Gram-positive bacteria, fungi, and yeasts; water-sol.

Elestab® HP 100. [Laboratoires Sérobiologiques] Hexamidine diisethionate; CAS 659-40-5; EINECS 211-

533-5; broad-spectrum antimicrobial and preservative for cosmetics; cutaneous asepticizer; used for oily, acneic skin care, oily hair, and antidandruff care; effective against Gram-positive and Gram-negative bacteria; good against yeasts, fungi; wh. microcryst. powd.; water-sol.; usage level: 0.03-0.10%.

Elfacos® BE. [Akzo BV] Behenyl erucate; CAS 18312-32-8; EINECS 242-201-8; emollient.

Elfacos® C26. [Akzo BV] Hydroxyoctacosanyl hydroxystearate; nonionic; consistency regulating agent for w/o emulsions, cosmetic applics.; stabilizer; waxy substance for decorative cosmetics; pellets; 100% conc.

Elfacos® CP. [Akzo BV] Cetyl palmitate; CAS 540-10-3; EINECS 208-736-6; emollient.

Elfacos® DEHS. [Akzo BV] Dioctyl sebacate; CAS 122-62-3; EINECS 204-558-8; emollient.

Elfacos® DO. [Akzo BV] Decyl oleate; CAS 3687-46-5; EINECS 222-981-6; emollient.

Elfacos® E200. [Akzo BV] Methoxy PEG-22/dodecyl glycol copolymer; nonionic; w/o emulsifier with high water-binding capacity; stable to pH and electrolyte; solid; 100% conc.

Elfacos® EGDS. [Akzo BV] Glycol distearate; CAS 627-83-8; EINECS 211-014-3; cosmetic ingred.

Elfacos® EGMS. [Akzo BV] Glycol stearate; CAS 111-60-4; EINECS 203-886-9; emulsifier, opacifier, pearlescent for cosmetics.

Elfacos® EHP. [Akzo BV] Octyl palmitate; CAS 29806-73-3; EINECS 249-862-1; emollient.

Elfacos® EO. [Akzo BV] Ethyl oleate; CAS 111-62-6; EINECS 203-889-5; emollient.

Elfacos® GMO. [Akzo BV] Glyceryl oleate.

Elfacos® GMS. [Akzo BV] Glyceryl stearate.

Elfacos® GMSSE. [Akzo BV] Glyceryl stearate and PEG-100 stearate.

Elfacos® GT 282 L. [Akzo BV] Hydrog. talloweth-60 myristyl glycol.

Elfacos® GT 282 S. [Akzo; Akzo BV] Hydrog. talloweth-60 myristyl glycol.

Elfacos® IPM. [Akzo BV] Isopropyl myristate; CAS 110-27-0; EINECS 203-751-4; emollient.

Elfacos® IPP. [Akzo BV] Isopropyl palmitate; CAS 142-91-6; EINECS 205-571-1; emollient.

Elfacos® OW-100. [Akzo; Akzo BV] Methoxy PEG-17/dodecyl glycol copolymer.

Elfacos® PEG 400 DS. [Akzo BV] PEG-8 distearate; CAS 9005-08-7; personal care surfactant.

Elfacos® PEG 400 ML. [Akzo BV] PEG-8 laurate; CAS 9004-81-3; emulsifier.

Elfacos® PEG 400 MO. [Akzo BV] PEG-8 oleate; CAS 9004-96-0; emulsifier.

Elfacos® PEG 400 MS. [Akzo BV] PEG-8 stearate; CAS 9004-99-3; emulsifier.

Elfacos® PEG 600 DS. [Akzo BV] PEG-12 distearate; CAS 9005-08-7; personal care surfactant.

Elfacos® PEG 600 MS. [Akzo BV] PEG-12 stearate; CAS 9004-99-3; emulsifier.

Elfacos® PEG 1000 MS. [Akzo BV] PEG-20 stearate; CAS 9004-99-3; emulsifier.

Elfacos® PGMS. [Akzo BV] Propylene glycol stearate; CAS 1323-39-3; EINECS 215-354-3; personal care surfactant.

Elfacos® S19. [Akzo BV] PEG-45/dodecyl glycol copolymer.

Elfacos® S137. [Akzo BV] PEG-22/dodecyl glycol copolymer.

Elfacos® ST 9. [Akzo; Akzo BV] PEG-45/dodecyl glycol copolymer; nonionic; stabilizer for w/o emulsions and emollient used in cosmetics; paste; HLB 7.0; 100% conc.

Elfacos® ST 37. [Akzo BV] PEG-22/dodecyl glycol copolymer; nonionic; stabilizer for w/o emulsions and emollient used in cosmetics; liq.; 100% conc.

Elfadent SM 500. [Akzo BV] Hydrated silica; EINECS 215-683-2.

Elfadent SM 514. [Akzo BV] Sodium lauryl sulfate; CAS 151-21-3; EINECS 205-788-1; personal care surfactant.

Elfan® 240. [Akzo BV] Sodium lauryl sulfate; CAS 151-21-3; EINECS 205-788-1; anionic; personal care prods. and lt.-duty detergents; liq.; 30% conc.

Elfan® 240M. [Akzo BV] MEA lauryl sulfate; CAS 4722-98-9; EINECS 225-214-3; anionic; shampoos, bubble baths, lt. duty detergents; liq.; 29% conc.

Elfan® 240T. [Akzo BV] TEA-lauryl sulfate; CAS 139-96-8; EINECS 205-388-7; anionic; shampoos, bubble baths, lt. duty detergents, toothpaste; liq.; 40% conc.

Elfan® 250 TS. [Akzo BV] TEA-C12-15 alkyl sulfate.

Elfan® 280. [Akzo BV] Sodium coco-sulfate; anionic; general purpose heavy duty detergent, industrial, household, personal care uses; yel. paste; water sol. 700 g/l (50 C); sp.gr. 1.05; visc. 8000 cps (50 C); pH 8.5 ± 1; 42% act.

Elfan® 510. [Akzo BV] Disodium tallowamido MEA-sulfosuccinate.

Elfan® 680. [Akzo BV] Oleyl-cetyl alcohol sulfate, sodium salt; anionic; powd. detergent, cleaning agent, textile uses, shampoos, bubble baths, toothpaste; yel.-brn. paste; water sol. < 10 g/l; sp.gr. 1.05; m.p. 40 C; pH 11 ± 1; 50% act.

Elfan® 2240 M. [Akzo BV] MEA-lauryl sulfate; CAS 4722-98-9; EINECS 225-214-3; detergent.

Elfan® 2240 Mg. [Akzo BV] Magnesium lauryl sulfate; CAS 3097-08-3; EINECS 221-450-6; personal care surfactant.

Elfan® A 913. [Akzo BV] Laureth-3 phosphate; CAS 39464-66-9; surfactant.

Elfan® AT 84. [Akzo BV] Sodium cocoyl isethionate; EINECS 263-052-5; surfactant for syndet bars; wh. powd.; bulk dens. ≥ 350 g/l; acid no. 20-33; sapon. no. ≥ 160; pH 4.5-6.0 (10% aq.); 81-86% act.

Elfan® AT 84 G. [Akzo BV] Sodium cocoyl isethionate; EINECS 263-052-5; surfactant for cosmetics and toiletries, esp. mild shampoos, foam baths, baby prods., toothpastes, syndet bars; cream-colored gran.; bulk dens. ≈ 650 g/l; acid no. 20-33; sapon. no. ≥ 160; pH 4.5-6 (10% aq.); 82-86% act.

Elfan® KM 550. [Akzo BV] Alpha olefin sulfonate and lauryl ether sulfate; anionic; personal care prods.; dishwashing detergents, car shampoos and lt.-duty liqs.; liq.; 31% conc.

Elfan® KM 640 Mg. [Akzo BV] Sodium C14-16 olefin sulfonate and magnesium lauryl sulfate.

Elfan® KT 550. [Akzo BV] Sodium coco/hydrog. tallow sulfate; anionic; heavy duty detergent, industrial, household, cosmetic uses; yel. paste; sp.gr. 1.05; visc. 10,000 cps (50 C); pH 8 ± 0.5; 42% act.

Elfan® L 310. [Akzo; Akzo BV] Glycol distearate; CAS 627-83-8; EINECS 211-014-3; anionic; pearlescent for shampoos and bubble baths; lt. yel. solid, flakes; water disp.; sp.gr. 0.96; m.p. 64-66 C; acid no. 6 max.; sapon. no. 200; 100% conc.

Elfan® NS 98 N. [Akzo BV] Sodium nonoxynol-8 sulfate; CAS 9014-90-8; personal care surfactant.

Elfan® NS 213 SL Conc. [Akzo BV] Sodium C12-13 pareth sulfate.

Elfan® NS 232 S Conc. [Akzo BV] Sodium C12-13 pareth sulfate.

Elfan® NS 242. [Akzo BV] Sodium laureth sulfate; CAS 9004-82-4; anionic; surfactant for shampoos, bubble baths, dishwashing, lt. duty detergents, car cleaners, toiletries; liq.; 28% conc.

Elfan® NS 242 A. [Akzo BV] Sodium laureth sulfate; personal care surfactant.

Elfan® NS 242 Conc. [Akzo BV] Sodium laureth sulfate (2.5 EO); CAS 9004-82-4; anionic; detergent, wetting agent used in fire extinguishers and for industrial, household, and cosmetic uses, shampoos, bubble baths, dishwashing, car cleaners, toiletries; yel. paste; water sol. 400 g/l; visc. 30,000 cps; f.p. < 0 C; pH 7-8; 70% act.

Elfan® NS 243 S. [Akzo BV] Sodium laureth sulfate (3 EO); CAS 9004-82-4; anionic; detergent, wetting agent used in fire extinguishers and for industrial, household, and cosmetic uses, shampoos, bubble baths, dishwashing, car cleaners, toiletries; clear liq.; water sol.; sp.gr. 1.04; visc. 50 cps; f.p. < 0 C; pH 6.5-7.5; 28% act.

Elfan® NS 243 S Conc. [Akzo BV] Sodium laureth sulfate (3 EO); CAS 9004-82-4; anionic; detergent, wetting agent used in fire extinguishers and for industrial, household, and cosmetic uses, shampoos, bubble baths, dishwashing, car cleaners, toiletries; yel. paste; water sol.; sp.gr. 1.12; visc. 30,000 cps; f.p. < 0 C; pH 7.5-9.5; 70% act.

Elfan® NS 243 S Mg. [Akzo BV] Magnesium laureth sulfate; CAS 62755-21-9; personal care surfactant.

Elfan® NS 248 S Mg. [Akzo BV] Magnesium laureth-8 sulfate.

Elfan® NS 252 S. [Akzo] Sodium C12-15 pareth sulfate; anionic; detergent, wetting agent for fire extinguishers, industrial, household, and cosmetic uses; wh. liq.; water sol.; sp.gr. 1.05; visc. 150 cps; f.p. < 0 C; pH 6.5-7.5; 28% act.

Elfan® NS 252 S Conc. [Akzo BV] Sodium C12-15 pareth sulfate; anionic; detergent, wetting agent for fire extinguishers, industrial, household, and cosmetic uses; yel. paste; water sol.; sp.gr. 1.11; visc. 30,000 cps; f.p. < 0 C; pH 7.5-9.5; 70% act.

Elfan® NS 252 SL Conc. [Akzo BV] Sodium C12-15 pareth sulfate.

Elfan® NS 423 SH. [Akzo BV] Sodium myreth sulfate; CAS 25446-80-4; EINECS 246-986-8; anionic; detergent for dishwashing, textiles, household, skins; yel. liq.; water sol.; visc. 100 cps; f.p. < 0 C; 28% act.

Elfan® OS 46. [Akzo BV] Sodium C14-16 olefin sulfonate; CAS 68439-57-6; EINECS 270-407-8; anionic; detergent for shampoos, personal care, skin, household and cosmetic cleaners; yel. liq.; water sol.; sp.gr. 1.05; visc. 250 cps; f.p. < 0 C; pH 7-9; 37% act.

Elfan® SG. [Akzo BV] Sodium C14-16 olefin sulfonate, sodium laureth sulfate, lauramide MIPA, glycol distearate, sodium chloride, cocamide MEA, and laureth-8; silver gloss conc., detergent used for pearlescent cosmetics, shampoo base, bubble bath; wh. paste; water disp.; sp.gr. 1.04; visc. 10,000 cps; pH 7.5-9.5; 36% act.

Elfan® SP 400. [Akzo BV] Blend; anionic; for shampoos, bubble baths, dishwashing detergents, car shampoos, lt. duty liqs.; liq.; 40% conc.

Elfan® SP 500. [Akzo BV] Ether sulfate and alkylbenzene sulfonate with a nonionic surfactant; anionic; for shampoos, bubble baths, dishwashing detergents, car shampoos, lt. duty liqs.; yel. liq.; sol. 250 g/l water; sp.gr. 1.05; visc. 5000 cps; f.p. < 0 C; pH 6.5-7.5; 48% conc.

Elfan® WAT. [Akzo BV] TEA dodecylbenzene sulfonate; CAS 27323-41-7; EINECS 248-406-9; anionic; detergent for textile, household, personal care uses; emulsifier for insecticides; yel.-brn. liq.; water sol.; sp.gr. 1.06; visc. 1000 cps; f.p. < 0 C; pH 5.5-6.5; 50% act.

Elfanol® 616. [Akzo BV] Disodium laureth sulfosuccinate; anionic; detergent for cosmetics, shampoos, bubble and baby baths, liq. hand cleaners; clear liq.; water sol.; sp.gr. 1.05; visc. 100 cps; f.p. 0 C; pH 7; 30% act.

Elfanol® 850. [Akzo BV] Disodium cocamido PEG-3 sulfosuccinate; anionic; detergent for shampoos, bubble baths, cosmetics, liq. hand cleaners; yel.-brn. liq.; poor water sol.; sp.gr. 1.06; f.p. 14 C; pH 7; 45% act.

Elfapur® LP 25 SL. [Akzo BV] C12-15 pareth-3; CAS 68131-39-5; cosmetics ingred.

Elfapur® LP 110 SLN. [Akzo BV] C12-15 pareth-11; CAS 68131-39-5; cosmetics ingred.

Elfapur® LT 30 SLN. [Akzo BV] C12-13 pareth-3; CAS 66455-14-9; cosmetics ingred.

Elfapur® LT 65 SLN. [Akzo BV] C12-13 pareth-7; CAS 66455-14-9; cosmetics ingred.

Elfapur® LT 85/9 SLN. [Akzo BV] C12-13 pareth-9; CAS 66455-14-9; cosmetics ingred.

Elfapur® LT 150 SLN. [Akzo BV] C12-13 pareth-15; CAS 66455-14-9; cosmetics ingred.

Elfapur® LT 150 SN. [Akzo BV] C12-13 pareth-15; CAS 66455-14-9; cosmetics ingred.

Elfapur® ML 30 SH. [Akzo] Lauryl polyglycol ether from syn. C12/C14 fatty alcohol; base material for prod. of anionics, cosmetics; yel. liq.; poor water sol.; sp.gr. 1.01; f.p. 5 C; cloud pt. 62–66 C (10% in 25% butyl diglycol); flash pt. (PMCC) 180 C; 97% act.

Elfapur® N 50. [Akzo BV] Nonoxynol-5; CAS 9016-45-9; nonionic; detergent, emulsifier for cosmetics, textiles, household and industrial uses; yel. liq.; poor water sol.; sp.gr. 1.05; f.p. –5 C; cloud pt. 60–62 C (10% in 25% butyl diglycol);flash pt. (PMCC) 90 C; 97% act.

Elfapur® N 70. [Akzo BV] Nonoxynol-7; CAS 9016-45-9; EINECS 248-292-0; nonionic; detergent, emulsifier for cosmetics, textiles, household and industrial uses; yel. liq., gel at 50–70% act.; water sol.; sp.gr. 1.05; f.p. 0 C; cloud pt. 22–24 C (1% aq.);flash pt. (PMCC) 103 C; 97% act.

Elfapur® N 90. [Akzo BV] Nonoxynol-9; CAS 9016-45-9; nonionic; detergent, emulsifier for cosmetics, textiles, household and industrial uses; yel. liq., gel at 50–70% act.; water sol.; sp.gr. 1.06; f.p. 15 C; cloud pt. 60–62 C (1% aq.);flash pt. (PMCC) 114 C; 97% act.

Elfapur® N 120. [Akzo BV] Nonoxynol-12; CAS 9016-45-9; nonionic; detergent, emulsifier for cosmetics, textiles, household and industrial uses; yel. liq., gel at 50–70% act.; water sol.; sp.gr. 1.07; cloud pt. 88–90 C (1% aq.); flash pt. (PMCC) 102 C; 97% act.

Elfapur® N 150. [Akzo BV] Nonoxynol-15; CAS 9016-45-9; nonionic; detergent, emulsifier for cosmetics, textiles, household and industrial uses; yel. liq., gel at 40–70% act.; water sol.; sp.gr. 1.07; cloud pt. 64–66 C (1% in 10% NaCl); flash pt. (PMCC) 94 C; 97% act.

Elfapur® O 80. [Akzo] Oleyl-cetyl alcohol ethoxylate; nonionic; heavy-duty detergent used in textile industry, cosmetics; yel.-brn. liq., gel at 15–90% act.; water sol. 400 g/l; sp.gr. 1.05; m.p. 25–30 C; cloud pt. 44–46 C (1% aq.); 97% act.

Elfapur® O 160. [Akzo] Oleyl-cetyl alcohol polyglycol ether; detergent used in textile industry, cosmetics; water sol. 400 g/l; sp.gr. 1.06; m.p. 29–35 C; cloud pt. 64–66 C (1% in 10% NaCl); 97% act.

Elfapur® R 150. [Akzo BV] PEG-15 castor oil; CAS 61791-12-6; cosmetics ingred.

Elfapur® SP 110 SLN. [Akzo BV] C12-15 pareth-11; CAS 68131-39-5; cosmetics ingred.

Elfapur® T 115. [Akzo BV] Hydrog. talloweth-12; cosmetics ingred.

Elfapur® T 130 S. [Akzo BV] Ceteareth-13; CAS 68439-49-6; cosmetics ingred.

Elfapur® T 250. [Akzo BV] Hydrog. talloweth-25; nonionic; foam controlled heavy-duty detergent powds. for textile use, cosmetics; wh. powd., beads, gel at > 25% act.; water sol. 250 g/l; cloud pt. 77–79 C (1% in 10% NaCl); 98% act.

Elicrisina. [Vevy] Water and everlasting extract; CAS 90045-56-0; botanical extract.

Eltesol® ACS 60. [Albright & Wilson UK] Ammonium cumenesulfonate; CAS 37475-88-0; EINECS 253-519-1; hydrotrope, solubilizer, coupling agent, and visc. modifier in liq. formulations; cloud pt. depressant in detergent formulations; pale pink liq.; dens. 1.10 g/cm³; pH 7.0–8.0 (10% aq.); 60% min. act.

Eltesol® AX 40. [Albright & Wilson UK] Ammonium xylene sulfonate; CAS 26447-10-9; EINECS 247-710-9; anionic; hydrotrope, cloud pt. depressant used in the detergent mfg.; solubilizer, coupler; pale yel. liq.; pH 7–8.5; 41% act.

Eltesol® ST 34. [Albright & Wilson UK] Sodium toluene sulfonate; CAS 657-84-1; anionic; hydrotrope, cloud pt. depressant used in the detergent mfg.; solubilizer, coupler; pale yel. liq.; pH 7–10; 34% act.

Eltesol® ST 40. [Albright & Wilson UK] Sodium toluenesulfonate; CAS 657-84-1; anionic; hydrotrope, solubilizer, coupling agent, and visc. modifier in liq. formulations; cloud pt. depressant in detergent formulations; straw liq.; dens. 1.10 g/cm³; pH 7.0–10.5 (10% aq.); 40.0±1.0% act.

Eltesol® SX 30. [Albright & Wilson UK] Sodium xylene sulfonate; CAS 1300-72-7; EINECS 215-090-9; anionic; hydrotrope, cloud pt. depressant used in the detergent mfg.; solubilizer, coupler; pale yel. liq.; pH 7–10; 30% act.

Eltesol® SX 93. [Albright & Wilson UK] Sodium xylene sulfonate; CAS 1300-72-7; EINECS 215-090-9; anionic; solubilizer and coupling agent in heavy-duty liq. detergents; visc. reducing agent in mfg. of powd. detergents; off wh. powd., pellets; dens. 0.46 g/cc; pH 9–10.5 (3%); 93% act.

Eltesol® TA 65. [Albright & Wilson UK] 65% Toluene sulfonic acid and 1.4% sulfonic acid aq. sol'n.; anionic; curing agent for resins in foundry cores, plastics, coatings; intermediate; catalyst in foundry and chemical industries; hardening agent in plastics; activator for nicotine insecticides; descaling agent in metal cleaning; in electroplating baths; lt. amber clear liq.; dens. 1.2 g/cc; visc. 9–12 cs; 65% conc.

Eltesol® TSX. [Albright & Wilson UK] p-Toluene sulfonic acid monohydrate BP; CAS 70788-37-3; anionic; catalyst for org. synthesis, syn. resins, mfg. of p-cresol, toluene derivs., pharmaceutical prods., dyestuffs; chemical intermediate; wh. to off-wh. cryst.; m.p. 103 C; 97% conc.

Eltesol® TSX/A. [Albright & Wilson UK] p-Toluene sulfonic acid monohydrate; CAS 104-15-4; EINECS 203-180-0; anionic; catalyst for org. synthesis, syn. resins, mfg. of p-cresol, toluene derivs., pharmaceutical prods., dyestuffs; chemical intermediate; curing agent for resins and coatings; wh. crystals; m.p. 103.5 C; 95% act.

Eltesol® TSX/SF. [Albright & Wilson UK] p-Toluene sulfonic acid monohydrate; CAS 104-15-4; EINECS 203-180-0; anionic; catalyst for org. synthesis, syn. resins, mfg. of p-cresol, toluene derivs., pharmaceutical prods., dyestuffs; chemical intermediate; wh. cryst.; m.p. 103.5 C; 98% act.

Elubiol. [Janssen Research Foundation] Dichlorophenyl imidazoldioxolan; CAS 85058-43-1.

Elvanol® 71-30. [DuPont] Fully hydrolyzed PVAL; CAS 9002-89-5; film-forming binder used in adhesives, paper, paperboard sizing and coatings, textiles, films, building prods., hoses, gaskets, emulsification in emulsions and latices, additive for concrete, cement, cosmetics, and food; cosmetic and personal care incl. face masks; wh. gran.; sol. in hot water, ethanol; insol. in cold water; sp.gr. 1.30; dens. 400–432 kg/m3; visc. 28–32 cps (4% aq.); sapon. no. 3–12; ref. index 1.54; pH 5.0–7.0; tens. str. 117 MPa; tens. elong. 10% (break) to 400%; hardness > 100; biodeg.

Elvanol® 75-15. [DuPont] Fully hydrolyzed PVAL; CAS 9002-89-5; visc. stabilizer and imparts gel resistance to aq. sol'ns.; used in, cosmetic and personal care incl. face masks, adhesives, films, paper applic.; binder in cement and ceramic powd.; emulsifier; food pkg. adhesive; cosmetic and personal care incl. face masks; wh. gran.; slurries easily in cold water; visc. 13–15 cps (4% aq.); pH 5.0–7.0; tens. str. 55.2–138 MPa; biodeg.

Elvanol® 85–82. [DuPont] Fully hydrolyzed PVAL; CAS 9002-89-5; used for food pkg. adhesives, films, cosmetic and personal care incl. face masks, and specialty applic.; visc. 25–31 cps (4% aq.); pH 5.0–7.0.

Elvanol® 90-50. [DuPont] Fully hydrolyzed PVAL; CAS 9002-89-5; provides high film strength and binding power in low visc. systems; used in paper and paperboard coating and sizing, adhesives; pigment binder; food additive applic.; cosmetic and personal care incl. face masks; visc. 13–15 cps (4% aq.); pH 5.0–7.0.

Elvanol® HV. [DuPont] Fully hydrolyzed PVAL; CAS 9002-89-5; high-visc. grade, high tensile and adhesive strength, strong resistance to grease and hydrocarbons; used in adhesive, textile, and paper applics.; cosmetic and personal care incl. face masks; wh. gran.; sol. in hot water; Hoeppler falling ball visc. 55–65 cps (4% aq.); pH 5–7 (sol'n.).

Elvax® 40P. [DuPont] Ethylene/VA copolymer; CAS 24937-78-8.

Emalex 102. [Nihon Emulsion] Ceteth-2; CAS 9004-95-9; emulsifier, cleaner, dispersant for cosmetics, esp. creams and lotions; JSCI compliance; wh. soft wax; HLB 3.0.

Emalex 103. [Nihon Emulsion] Ceteth-3; CAS 9004-95-9; emulsifier, cleaner, dispersant for cosmetics, esp. creams and lotions; esp. suited for creamy hair conditioners; JSCI compliance; wh. soft wax; HLB 5.0.

Emalex 105. [Nihon Emulsion] Ceteth-5; CAS 9004-95-9; emulsifier, cleaner, dispersant for cosmetics, esp. creams and lotions; JSCI compliance; wh. soft wax; HLB 7.0.

Emalex 107. [Nihon Emulsion] Ceteth-7; CAS 9004-95-9; emulsifier, cleaner, dispersant for cosmetics, esp. creams and lotions; JSCI compliance; wh. wax; HLB 9.0.

Emalex 110. [Nihon Emulsion] Ceteth-10; CAS 9004-95-9; emulsifier, cleaner, dispersant for cosmetics, esp. creams and lotions; JSCI compliance; wh. wax; HLB 11.0.

Emalex 112. [Nihon Emulsion] Ceteth-12; CAS 9004-95-9; emulsifier, cleaner, dispersant for cosmetics, esp. creams and lotions; JSCI compliance; wh. wax; HLB 12.0.

Emalex 115. [Nihon Emulsion] Ceteth-15; CAS 9004-95-9; emulsifier, cleaner, dispersant for cosmetics, esp. creams and lotions; JSCI compliance; wh. wax; HLB 13.

Emalex 117. [Nihon Emulsion] Ceteth-17; CAS 9004-95-9; emulsifier, cleaner, dispersant for cosmetics, esp. creams and lotions; JSCI compliance; wh. wax; HLB 13.

Emalex 120. [Nihon Emulsion] Ceteth-20; CAS 9004-95-9; emulsifier, cleaner, dispersant for cosmetics, esp. creams and lotions; JSCI compliance; wh. wax; HLB 14.

Emalex 125. [Nihon Emulsion] Ceteth-25; CAS 9004-95-9; emulsifier, cleaner, dispersant for cosmetics, esp. creams and lotions; JSCI compliance; wh. wax; HLB 15.

Emalex 130. [Nihon Emulsion] Ceteth-30; CAS 9004-95-9; emulsifier, cleaner, dispersant for cosmetics, esp. creams and lotions; JSCI compliance; wh. wax; HLB 16.

Emalex 200. [Nihon Emulsion] PEG-2 oleate; CAS 106-12-7; EINECS 203-364-0; personal care surfactant.

Emalex 200 di-AS. [Nihon Emulsion] PEG-4 distearate; CAS 9005-08-7; reforming agent, emulsifier, thickener for cosmetics (creams, lipstick); JCID compliance; wh. wax; HLB 2.

Emalex 200di-IS. [Nihon Emulsion] PEG-4 diisostearate; oil-phase cosmetic ingred.; pale yel. oil; HLB 2.

Emalex 200 di-L. [Nihon Emulsion] PEG-4 dilaurate; CAS 9005-02-1; oil-phase cosmetic ingred., emulsifier for creams, milky lotions, hair conditioners; cleaner, superfatting agent, thickener, reforming agent; pale yel. turbid oil; HLB 4.

Emalex 200 di-O. [Nihon Emulsion] PEG-4 dioleate; CAS 9005-07-6; oil-phase ingred., emulsifier, dispersant with good spreadability for cosmetics, creams, milky lotions, foundations; JCID compliance; pale yel. oil; HLB 2.

Emalex 200 di-S. [Nihon Emulsion] PEG-4 distearate; CAS 9005-08-7; reforming agent, emulsifier, thickener for cosmetics; JCID compliance; wh. wax; HLB 2.

Emalex 218. [Nihon Emulsion] PEG-3 oleate; CAS 9004-96-0; EINECS 233-561-7; surfactant for cosmetics; produces stable emulsions; JSCI compliance; pale yel. oil; HLB 5.

Emalex 300 di-IS. [Nihon Emulsion] PEG-6 diisostearate; emulsifier for cosmetic emulsions, dispersant, reforming agent; pale yel. oil; HLB 4.

Emalex 300 di-L. [Nihon Emulsion] PEG-6 dilaurate; CAS 9005-02-1; oil-phase cosmetic ingred., emulsifier for creams, milky lotions, hair conditioners; cleaner, superfatting agent, thickener, reforming agent; JCID compliance; pale yel. oil; HLB 6.

Emalex 300 di-O. [Nihon Emulsion] PEG-6 dioleate; CAS 9005-07-6; oil-phase ingred., emulsifier, dispersant with good spreadability for cosmetics, creams, milky lotions, foundations; JCID compliance; pale yel. oil; HLB 4.

Emalex 300 di-S. [Nihon Emulsion] PEG-6 distearate; CAS 9005-08-7; reforming agent, emulsifier, thickener for cosmetics (creams, lipstick); JCID compliance; wh. wax; HLB 3.

Emalex 400A. [Nihon Emulsion] PEG-3 stearate; CAS 9004-99-3; EINECS 233-562-2; oil-phase cosmetic ingred., pearlescent, emulsifier, dispersant, emulsion stabilizer, thickener; cream-colored wax; HLB 5.

Emalex 400B. [Nihon Emulsion] PEG-3 stearate; CAS 9004-99-3; EINECS 233-562-2; oil-phase cosmetic ingred., pearlescent, emulsifier, dispersant, emulsion stabilizer, thickener; cream-colored wax; HLB 5.

Emalex 400 di-AS. [Nihon Emulsion] PEG-8 distearate; CAS 9005-08-7; reforming agent, emulsifier, thickener for cosmetics (cream, lipstick); JCID compliance; wh. wax; HLB 5.

Emalex 400 di-IS. [Nihon Emulsion] PEG-8 diisostearate; emulsifier for cosmetic emulsions, dispersant, reforming agent; pale yel. oil; HLB 5.

Emalex 400 di-L. [Nihon Emulsion] PEG-8 dilaurate; CAS 9005-02-1; oil-phase cosmetic ingred., emulsifier for creams, milky lotions, hair conditioners; cleaner, superfatting agent, thickener, reforming agent; JCID compliance; pale yel. oil; HLB 7.

Emalex 400 di-O. [Nihon Emulsion] PEG-8 dioleate; CAS 9005-07-6; oil-phase ingred., emulsifier, dispersant with good spreadability for cosmetics, creams, milky lotions, foundations; JCID compliance; pale yel. oil; HLB 5.

Emalex 400 di-S. [Nihon Emulsion] PEG-8 distearate; CAS 9005-08-7; reforming agent, emulsifier, thickener for cosmetics (creams, lipstick); JCID compliance; cream-colored wax; HLB 5.

Emalex 503. [Nihon Emulsion] Oleth-3; CAS 9004-98-2; emulsifier, dispersant, solubilizer for cosmetics; JSCI compliance; colorless oil; HLB 4.0.

Emalex 506. [Nihon Emulsion] Oleth-6; CAS 9004-98-2; emulsifier, dispersant, solubilizer for cosmetics; JSCI compliance; wh. turbid oil; HLB 8.

Emalex 508. [Nihon Emulsion] Oleth-8; CAS 9004-98-2; emulsifier, dispersant, solubilizer for cosmetics; suitable for hair tonics and hair care prods. as solubilizer for perfumes; JSCI compliance; wh. soft paste; HLB 9.

Emalex 510. [Nihon Emulsion] Oleth-10; CAS 9004-98-2; emulsifier, dispersant, solubilizer for cosmetics; JSCI compliance; wh. soft paste; HLB 10.

Emalex 512. [Nihon Emulsion] Oleth-12; CAS 9004-98-2; emulsifier, dispersant, solubilizer for cosmetics; JSCI compliance; wh. soft wax; HLB 11.

Emalex 515. [Nihon Emulsion] Oleth-15; CAS 9004-98-2; emulsifier, dispersant, solubilizer for cosmetics; JSCI compliance; wh. soft wax; HLB 12.

Emalex 520. [Nihon Emulsion] Oleth-20; CAS 9004-98-2;

emulsifier, dispersant, solubilizer for cosmetics; JSCI compliance; wh. wax; HLB 14.

Emalex 523. [Nihon Emulsion] Oleth-23; CAS 9004-98-2; emulsifier, dispersant, solubilizer for cosmetics; JSCI compliance; wh. wax; HLB 14.

Emalex 550. [Nihon Emulsion] Oleth-50; CAS 9004-98-2; emulsifier, dispersant, solubilizer for cosmetics; JSCI compliance; wh. wax; HLB 18.

Emalex 600 di-AS. [Nihon Emulsion] PEG-12 distearate; CAS 9005-08-7; reforming agent, emulsifier, thickener for cosmetics (creams, lipstick); JCID compliance; wh. wax; HLB 7.

Emalex 600 di-IS. [Nihon Emulsion] PEG-12 diisostearate; emulsifier for cosmetic emulsions, dispersant, reforming agent; pale yel. turbid oil; HLB 7.

Emalex 600 di-L. [Nihon Emulsion] PEG-12 dilaurate; CAS 9005-02-1; oil-phase cosmetic ingred., emulsifier for creams, milky lotions, hair conditioners; cleaner, superfatting agent, thickener, reforming agent; JCID compliance; pale yel. paste; HLB 9.

Emalex 600 di-O. [Nihon Emulsion] PEG-12 dioleate; CAS 9005-07-6; oil-phase ingred., emulsifier, dispersant with good spreadability for cosmetics, creams, milky lotions, foundations; JCID compliance; pale yel. oil; HLB 7.

Emalex 600 di-S. [Nihon Emulsion] PEG-12 distearate; CAS 9005-08-7; reforming agent, emulsifier, thickener for cosmetics (creams, lipstick); JCID compliance; wh. wax; HLB 7.

Emalex 602. [Nihon Emulsion] Steareth-2; CAS 9005-00-9; emulsifier, dispersant, thickener for cosmetics, creams, milky lotions; JSCI compliance; wh. soft wax; HLB 3.

Emalex 603. [Nihon Emulsion] Steareth-3; CAS 9005-00-9; emulsifier, dispersant, thickener for cosmetics, creams, milky lotions; JSCI compliance; wh. soft wax; HLB 4.

Emalex 605. [Nihon Emulsion] Steareth-5; CAS 9005-00-9; emulsifier, dispersant, thickener for cosmetics, creams, milky lotions; JSCI complianceJSCI compliance; wh. soft wax; HLB 6.

Emalex 606. [Nihon Emulsion] Steareth-6; CAS 9005-00-9; emulsifier, dispersant, thickener for cosmetics, creams, milky lotions; JSCI compliance; wh. soft wax; HLB 7.

Emalex 608. [Nihon Emulsion] Steareth-8; CAS 9005-00-9; emulsifier, dispersant, thickener for cosmetics, creams, milky lotions; JSCI compliance; wh. soft wax; HLB 9.

Emalex 611. [Nihon Emulsion] Steareth-11; CAS 9005-00-9; emulsifier, dispersant, thickener for cosmetics, creams, milky lotions; JSCI compliance; wh. wax; HLB 11.

Emalex 615. [Nihon Emulsion] Steareth-15; CAS 9005-00-9; emulsifier, dispersant, thickener for cosmetics, creams, milky lotions; JSCI compliance; wh. wax; HLB 12.

Emalex 620. [Nihon Emulsion] Steareth-20; CAS 9005-00-9; emulsifier, dispersant, thickener for cosmetics, creams, milky lotions; JSCI compliance; wh. wax; HLB 14.

Emalex 625. [Nihon Emulsion] Steareth-25; CAS 9005-00-9; emulsifier, dispersant, thickener for cosmetics, creams, milky lotions; JSCI compliance; wh. wax; HLB 15.

Emalex 630. [Nihon Emulsion] Steareth-30; CAS 9005-00-9; emulsifier, dispersant, thickener for cosmetics, creams, milky lotions; JSCI compliance; wh. wax; HLB 16.

Emalex 640. [Nihon Emulsion] Steareth-40; CAS 9005-00-9; emulsifier, dispersant, thickener for cosmetics, creams, milky lotions; JSCI compliance; wh. wax; HLB 17.

Emalex 703. [Nihon Emulsion] Laureth-3; CAS 3055-94-5; EINECS 221-280-2; emulsifier, penetrant, wetting agent, cleaner, dispersant for cosmetics, creams, milky lotions; JSCI compliance; colorless oil; HLB 6.

Emalex 705. [Nihon Emulsion] Laureth-5; CAS 3055-95-6; EINECS 221-281-8; emulsifier, penetrant, wetting agent, cleaner, dispersant for cosmetics, creams, milky lotions; JSCI compliance; wh. turbid oil; HLB 9.

Emalex 707. [Nihon Emulsion] Laureth-7; CAS 3055-97-8; EINECS 221-283-9; emulsifier, penetrant, wetting agent, cleaner, dispersant for cosmetics, creams, milky lotions; JSCI compliance; wh. turbid oil; HLB 10.

Emalex 709. [Nihon Emulsion] Laureth-9; CAS 3055-99-0; EINECS 221-284-4; emulsifier, penetrant, wetting agent, cleaner, dispersant for cosmetics, creams, milky lotions; paint and itch relieving effect for ointments; JSCI compliance; wh. soft wax; HLB 11.

Emalex 710. [Nihon Emulsion] Laureth-10; CAS 6540-99-4; emulsifier, penetrant, wetting agent, cleaner, dispersant for cosmetics, creams, milky lotions; JSCI compliance; wh. wax; HLB 12.

Emalex 712. [Nihon Emulsion] Laureth-12; CAS 3056-00-6; EINECS 221-286-5; emulsifier, penetrant, wetting agent, cleaner, dispersant for cosmetics, creams, milky lotions; JSCI compliance; wh. wax; HLB 13.

Emalex 715. [Nihon Emulsion] Laureth-15; CAS 9002-92-0; emulsifier, penetrant, wetting agent, cleaner, dispersant for cosmetics, creams, milky lotions; JSCI compliance; wh. wax; HLB 14.

Emalex 720. [Nihon Emulsion] Laureth-20; CAS 9002-92-0; emulsifier, penetrant, wetting agent, cleaner, dispersant for cosmetics, creams, milky lotions; JSCI compliance; wh. wax; HLB 16.

Emalex 725. [Nihon Emulsion] Laureth-25; CAS 9002-92-0; emulsifier, penetrant, wetting agent, cleaner, dispersant for cosmetics, creams, milky lotions; JSCI compliance; wh. wax; HLB 17.

Emalex 730. [Nihon Emulsion] Laureth-30; CAS 9002-92-0; emulsifier, penetrant, wetting agent, cleaner, dispersant for cosmetics, creams, milky lotions; JSCI compliance; wh. wax; HLB 18.

Emalex 750. [Nihon Emulsion] Laureth-50; CAS 9002-92-0; emulsifier, penetrant, wetting agent, cleaner, dispersant for cosmetics, creams, milky lotions; JSCI compliance; wh. wax; HLB 21.

Emalex 800 di-L. [Nihon Emulsion] PEG-16 dilaurate; CAS 9005-02-1; oil-phase cosmetic ingred., emulsifier for creams, milky lotions, hair conditioners; cleaner, superfatting agent, thickener, reforming agent; JCID compliance; cream-colored soft wax; HLB 11.

Emalex 805. [Nihon Emulsion] PEG-5 stearate; CAS 9004-99-3; oil-phase cosmetic ingred., pearlescent, emulsifier, dispersant, emulsion stabilizer; thickener for cleansing foam; JSCI compliance; wh. soft wax; HLB 7.

Emalex 810. [Nihon Emulsion] PEG-10 stearate; CAS 9004-99-3; oil-phase cosmetic ingred., pearlescent, emulsifier, dispersant, emulsion stabilizer; thickener for cleansing foam; JSCI compliance; wh. soft wax; HLB 11.

Emalex 820. [Nihon Emulsion] PEG-20 stearate; CAS 9004-99-3; oil-phase cosmetic ingred., pearlescent, emulsifier, dispersant, emulsion stabilizer; thickener for cleansing foam; JSCI compliance; wh. wax; HLB 14.

Emalex 830. [Nihon Emulsion] PEG-30 stearate; CAS 9004-99-3; oil-phase cosmetic ingred., pearlescent, emulsifier, dispersant, emulsion stabilizer; thickener for cleansing foam; JSCI compliance; wh. wax; HLB 16.

Emalex 840. [Nihon Emulsion] PEG-40 stearate; CAS 9004-99-3; oil-phase cosmetic ingred., pearlescent, emulsifier, dispersant, emulsion stabilizer; thickener for cleansing foam; JSCI compliance; wh. wax; HLB 17.

Emalex 1000 di-L. [Nihon Emulsion] PEG-20 dilaurate; CAS 9005-02-1; oil-phase cosmetic ingred., emulsifier for creams, milky lotions, hair conditioners; cleaner, superfatting agent, thickener, reforming agent; JCID compliance; cream-colored soft wax; HLB 12.

Emalex 1605. [Nihon Emulsion] Ceteth-5; CAS 9004-95-9; emulsifier, dispersant, solubilizer, cleaner, wetting agent for cosmetics, creams, milky lotions, skin lotions; JCID compliance; wh. soft paste; HLB 7.

Emalex 1610. [Nihon Emulsion] Ceteth-10; CAS 9004-95-9; emulsifier, dispersant, solubilizer, cleaner, wetting agent for cosmetics, creams, milky lotions, skin lotions; JCID compliance; wh. soft paste; HLB 11.

Emalex 1615. [Nihon Emulsion] Ceteth-15; CAS 9004-95-9; emulsifier, dispersant, solubilizer, cleaner, wetting agent for cosmetics, creams, milky lotions, skin lotions; JCID compliance; wh. soft wax; HLB 13.

Emalex 1620. [Nihon Emulsion] Ceteth-20; CAS 9004-95-9; emulsifier, dispersant, solubilizer, cleaner, wetting agent for cosmetics, creams, milky lotions, skin lotions; JCID compliance; wh. wax; HLB 14.

Emalex 1625. [Nihon Emulsion] Ceteth-25; CAS 9004-95-9; emulsifier, dispersant, solubilizer, cleaner, wetting agent for cosmetics, creams, milky lotions, skin lotions; JCID compliance; wh. wax; HLB 15.

Emalex 1805. [Nihon Emulsion] Isosteareth-5; CAS 52292-17-8; emulsifier, dispersant, solubilizer, cleaner, wetting agent for cosmetics, creams, milky lotions, skin lotions; JCID compliance; wh. soft paste; HLB 7.

Emalex 1810. [Nihon Emulsion] Isosteareth-10; CAS 52292-17-8; emulsifier, dispersant, solubilizer, cleaner, wetting agent for cosmetics, creams, milky lotions, skin lotions; JCID compliance; wh. soft wax; HLB 10.

Emalex 1815. [Nihon Emulsion] Isosteareth-15; CAS 52292-17-8; emulsifier, dispersant, solubilizer, cleaner, wetting agent for cosmetics, creams, milky lotions, skin lotions; JCID compliance; wh. soft wax; HLB 12.

Emalex 1820. [Nihon Emulsion] Isosteareth-20; CAS 52292-17-8; emulsifier, dispersant, solubilizer, cleaner, wetting agent for cosmetics, creams, milky lotions, skin lotions; JCID compliance; wh. wax; HLB 14.

Emalex 1825. [Nihon Emulsion] Isosteareth-25; CAS 52292-17-8; emulsifier, dispersant, solubilizer, cleaner, wetting agent for cosmetics, creams, milky lotions, skin lotions; JCID compliance; wh. wax; HLB 15.

Emalex 2405. [Nihon Emulsion] PEG-5 decyltetradecyl ether; emulsifier, dispersant, solubilizer, cleaner for cosmetics, creams, milky lotions, skin lotions; wh. soft paste; HLB 5.

Emalex 2410. [Nihon Emulsion] PEG-10 decyltetradecyl ether; emulsifier, dispersant, solubilizer, and cleaner for cosmetics, creams, milky lotions, and skin lotions; wh. paste; HLB 9.

Emalex 2415. [Nihon Emulsion] PEG-15 decyltetradecyl ether; emulsifier, dispersant, solubilizer, and cleaner for cosmetics, creams, milky lotions, and skin lotions; wh. soft wax; HLB 11.

Emalex 2420. [Nihon Emulsion] PEG-20 decyltetradecyl ether; emulsifier, dispersant, solubilizer, and cleaner for cosmetics, creams, milky lotions, and skin lotions; wh. soft wax; HLB 12.

Emalex 2425. [Nihon Emulsion] PEG-25 decyltetradecyl ether; emulsifier, dispersant, and cleaner for cosmetics, creams, milky lotions, and skin lotions; solubilizer for perfumes; wh. soft wax; HLB 14.

Emalex 2505. [Nihon Emulsion] PEG-5 decylpentadecyl ether; emulsifier, solubilizer, cleaner, thickener for cosmetics, creams, milky lotions, skin lotions; wh. soft paste; HLB 5.

Emalex 2510. [Nihon Emulsion] PEG-10 decylpentadecyl ether; emulsifier, solubilizer, cleaner, thickener for cosmetics, creams, milky lotions, skin lotions; wh. paste; HLB 8.

Emalex 2515. [Nihon Emulsion] PEG-15 decylpentadecyl ether; emulsifier, solubilizer, cleaner, thickener for cosmetics, creams, milky lotions, skin lotions; wh. soft wax; HLB 11.

Emalex 2520. [Nihon Emulsion] PEG-20 decylpentadecyl ether; emulsifier, solubilizer, cleaner, thickener for cosmetics, creams, milky lotions, skin lotions; wh. wax; HLB 12.

Emalex 2525. [Nihon Emulsion] PEG-25 decylpentadecyl ether; emulsifier, cleaner, thickener for cosmetics, creams, milky lotions, skin lotions; solubilizer for perfumes; wh. wax; HLB 13.

Emalex 6300 DI-ST. [Nihon Emulsion] PEG-150 distearate; CAS 9005-08-7; thickener, stabilizer for shampoos, hair conditioners, cleansing foams; JCID compliance; wh. flake; HLB 20.

Emalex 6300 M-ST. [Nihon Emulsion] PEG-150 stearate; CAS 9004-99-3; oil-phase cosmetic ingred., thickener for shampoos and hair conditioners; JSCI compliance; wh. flake; HLB 21.

Emalex AF-2. [Nihon Emulsion] Mixt. of nonionic surfactants; nonionic; emulsifier and solubilizer for one-liq. cosmetic aerosols; wh. turbid oil; HLB 7.

Emalex AF-4. [Nihon Emulsion] Mixt. of nonionic surfactants; nonionic; emulsifier and solubilizer for one-liq. cosmetic aerosols; wh. soft wax; HLB 8.

Emalex BHA-5. [Nihon Emulsion] Beheneth-5; emulsifier, dispersant, solubilizer for cosmetics; produces moist, spreading emulsion; JCID compliance; wh. soft wax; HLB 5.

Emalex BHA-10. [Nihon Emulsion] Beheneth-10; emulsifier, dispersant, solubilizer for cosmetics; produces moist, spreading emulsion; JCID compliance; wh. wax; HLB 9.

Emalex BHA-20. [Nihon Emulsion] Beheneth-20; emulsifier, dispersant, solubilizer for cosmetics; produces moist, spreading emulsion; JCID compliance; wh. wax; HLB 13.

Emalex BHA-30. [Nihon Emulsion] Beheneth-30; emulsifier, dispersant, solubilizer for cosmetics; produces moist, spreading emulsion; JCID compliance; wh. wax; HLB 15.

Emalex C-20. [Nihon Emulsion] PEG-20 castor oil; CAS 61791-12-6; emulsifier, solubilizer, dispersant in cosmetics, medical pharmaceuticals; JSCI compliance; pale yel. oil; HLB 9.

Emalex C-30. [Nihon Emulsion] PEG-30 castor oil; CAS 61791-12-6; emulsifier, solubilizer, dispersant in cosmetics, medical pharmaceuticals; JSCI compliance; pale yel. oil; HLB 11.

Emalex C-40. [Nihon Emulsion] PEG-40 castor oil; CAS 61791-12-6; emulsifier, solubilizer, dispersant in cosmetics, medical pharmaceuticals; JSCI compliance; pale yel. oil; HLB 13.

Emalex C-50. [Nihon Emulsion] PEG-50 castor oil; CAS 61791-12-6; emulsifier, solubilizer, dispersant in cosmetics, medical pharmaceuticals; JSCI compliance; pale yel. turbid oil; HLB 14.

Emalex CC-10. [Nihon Emulsion] Cetyl caprate; lipophilic base for cosmetics; pale yel. solid; HLB 0.

Emalex CC-16. [Nihon Emulsion] Cetyl palmitate; CAS 540-10-3; EINECS 208-736-6; lipophilic base for cosmetics; JCID compliance; cream-colored flake; HLB 0.

Emalex CC-18. [Nihon Emulsion] Stearyl stearate; CAS 2778-96-3; EINECS 220-476-5; lipophilic base for cosmetics; JCID compliance; cream-colored wax; HLB 0.

Emalex CC-168. [Nihon Emulsion] Cetyl octanoate; CAS 59130-69-7; EINECS 261-619-1; lipophilic base for cosmetics; squalane substitute; JCID compliance; pale yel. liq.; HLB 0.

Emalex CS-5. [Nihon Emulsion] Choleth-5; emulsifier, solubilizer, dispersant, thickener for cosmetics, creams, milky lotions, skin lotions; emollient for hair care prods.; gloss aid for creams and milky lotions; JCID compliance; pale yel. paste; HLB 6.

Emalex CS-10. [Nihon Emulsion] Choleth-10; CAS 27321-96-6; emulsifier, solubilizer, dispersant, thickener for cosmetics, creams, milky lotions, skin lotions; emollient for hair care prods.; gloss aid for creams and milky lotions; JCID compliance; cream-colored wax; HLB 9.

Emalex CS-15. [Nihon Emulsion] Choleth-15; CAS 27321-96-6; emulsifier, solubilizer, dispersant, thickener for cosmetics, creams, milky lotions, skin lotions; emollient for hair care prods.; gloss aid for creams and milky lotions; JCID compliance; cream-colored wax; HLB 11.

Emalex CS-20. [Nihon Emulsion] Choleth-20; CAS 27321-96-6; emulsifier, solubilizer, dispersant, thickener for cosmetics, creams, milky lotions, skin lotions; emollient for hair care prods.; gloss aid for creams and milky lotions; JCID compliance; cream-colored wax; HLB 13.

Emalex CS-24. [Nihon Emulsion] Choleth-24; CAS 27321-96-6; emulsifier, solubilizer, dispersant, thickener for cosmetics, creams, milky lotions, skin lotions; emollient for hair care prods.; gloss aid for creams and milky lotions; JCID compliance; cream-colored wax; HLB 14.

Emalex CS-30. [Nihon Emulsion] Choleth-30; CAS 27321-96-6; emulsifier, solubilizer, dispersant, thickener for cosmetics, creams, milky lotions, skin lotions; emollient for hair care prods.; gloss aid for creams and milky lotions; JCID compliance; cream-colored wax; HLB 15.

Emalex CWD-2. [Nihon Emulsion] Mixt. of nonionic surfactants; nonionic; emulsifier producing turbid cosmetic goods, e.g., cold perm liqs., enamel removers, and lotions; liq. emulsion; usage level: 5-10%.

Emalex CWD-38. [Nihon Emulsion] Mixt. of nonionic surfactants; nonionic; emulsifier producing turbid cosmetic goods, e.g., cold perm liqs., enamel removers, and lotions; liq. emulsion; usage level: 5-10%.

Emalex CWS-3. [Nihon Emulsion] PEG-3 cetyl ether stearate; SE cosmetic ingred.; hydrophobic component and reforming agent for cosmetics and industrial areas; JCID compliance; cream-colored wax; HLB 0.

Emalex CWS-5. [Nihon Emulsion] PEG-5 cetyl ether stearate; hydrophobic component and reforming agent for cosmetics and industrial areas; JCID compliance; cream-colored wax; HLB 2.

Emalex CWS-7. [Nihon Emulsion] PEG-7 cetyl ether stearate; hydrophobic component and reforming agent for cosmetics and industrial areas; JCID compliance; cream-colored wax; HLB 4.

Emalex CWS-10. [Nihon Emulsion] PEG-10 cetyl ether stearate; hydrophobic component and reforming agent for cosmetics and industrial areas; JCID compliance; cream-colored wax; HLB 6.

Emalex DEG-di-IS. [Nihon Emulsion] PEG-2 diisostearate; oil-phase ingred. for cosmetic emulsions; pale yel. oil; HLB 0.

Emalex DEG-di-L. [Nihon Emulsion] PEG-2 dilaurate; CAS 9005-02-1; EINECS 228-486-1; oil-phase cosmetic ingred., emulsifier for creams, milky lotions, hair conditioners; cleaner, superfatting agent, thickener, reforming agent; JCID compliance; wh. soft wax; HLB 0.

Emalex DEG-di-O. [Nihon Emulsion] PEG-2 dioleate; oil-phase ingred., emulsifier, dispersant with good spreadability for cosmetics, creams, milky lotions, foundations; pale yel. oil; HLB 0.

Emalex DEG-di-S. [Nihon Emulsion] PEG-2 distearate; CAS 109-30-8; EINECS 203-663-6; pearling agent, hydrophobic component, reforming agent, emulsifier, thickener for cosmetics; JCID compliance; wh. wax; HLB 0.

Emalex DEG-m-S. [Nihon Emulsion] PEG-2 stearate; CAS 106-11-6; EINECS 203-363-5; oil-phase cosmetic ingred., pearlescent, emulsifier, dispersant, emulsion stabilizer, thickener; JSCI compliance; wh. wax; HLB 4.

Emalex DISG-2. [Nihon Emulsion] Diglyceryl diisostearate; emulsifier for cosmetics and foods; JCID compliance; pale yel. liq.; HLB 2.

Emalex DISG-3. [Nihon Emulsion] Polyglyceryl-3

diisostearate; CAS 66082-42-6; emulsifier for cosmetics and foods; JCID compliance; pale yel. liq.; HLB 4.

Emalex DISG-5. [Nihon Emulsion] Polyglyceryl-5 diisostearate; emulsifier for cosmetics and foods; pale yel. liq.; HLB 6.

Emalex DISG-10. [Nihon Emulsion] Polyglyceryl-10 diisostearate; CAS 102033-55-6; emulsifier.

Emalex DNP-5. [Nihon Emulsion] Nonyl nonoxynol-5; CAS 9014-93-1; emulsifier, emollient.

Emalex DSG-2. [Nihon Emulsion] Polyglyceryl-2 distearate; emulsifier for cosmetics and foods; cream-colored solid; HLB 2.

Emalex DSG-3. [Nihon Emulsion] Polyglyceryl-3 distearate; CAS 94423-19-5; emulsifier for cosmetics and foods; cream-colored solid; HLB 3.

Emalex DSG-5. [Nihon Emulsion] Polyglyceryl-5 distearate; emulsifier for cosmetics and foods; cream-colored solid; HLB 6.

Emalex DSG-10. [Nihon Emulsion] Polyglyceryl-10 distearate; CAS 12764-60-2.

Emalex EG-2854-IS. [Nihon Emulsion] PEG-4 sorbitol triisostearate; oil-phase base for emulsions; emulsifier for w/o emulsions; pale yel. oil; HLB 1.

Emalex EG-2854-O. [Nihon Emulsion] PEG-4 sorbitol tetraoleate; oil-phase base for emulsions; emulsifier for w/o emulsions; JSCI compliance; pale yel. oil; HLB 0.

Emalex EG-2854-OL. [Nihon Emulsion] PEG-3 sorbitan oleate.

Emalex EG-2854-S. [Nihon Emulsion] PEG-4 sorbitol tristearate; oil-phase base for emulsions; emulsifier for w/o cosmetic emulsions; JCID compliance; cream-colored wax; HLB 1.

Emalex EG-di-L. [Nihon Emulsion] Ethylene glycol dilaurate; CAS 624-04-4; EINECS 210-827-0; oil-phase cosmetic ingred., emulsifier for creams, milky lotions, hair conditioners; cleaner, superfatting agent, thickener, reforming agent; wh. wax; HLB 0.

Emalex EG-di-MPS. [Nihon Emulsion] Ethylene glycol distearate; CAS 627-83-8; EINECS 211-014-3; pearling agent, hydrophobic component, reforming agent, emulsifier, thickener for cosmetics; JCID compliance; wh. wax; HLB 0.

Emalex EG-di-O. [Nihon Emulsion] Ethylene glycol dioleate; CAS 928-24-5; oil-phase ingred., emulsifier, dispersant with good spreadability for cosmetics, creams, milky lotions, foundations; JCID compliance; pale yel. oil; HLB 0.

Emalex EG-di-S. [Nihon Emulsion] Glycol distearate; CAS 627-83-8; EINECS 211-014-3; pearling agent, hydrophobic component, reforming agent, emulsifier, thickener for cosmetics; JCID compliance; wh. flake; HLB 0.

Emalex EG-di-SE. [Nihon Emulsion] Ethylene glycol distearate; CAS 627-83-8; EINECS 211-014-3; pearling agent, hydrophobic component, reforming agent, emulsifier, thickener for cosmetics; JCID compliance; wh. flake; HLB 0.

Emalex EGS-A. [Nihon Emulsion] Ethylene glycol monostearate; CAS 111-60-4; EINECS 203-886-9; oil-phase cosmetic ingred., pearlescent, emulsifier, dispersant, emulsion stabilizer, thickener; clouding agent for shampoos/hair conditioners; JSCI compliance; wh. flake; HLB 2.

Emalex EGS-B. [Nihon Emulsion] Ethylene glycol monostearate; CAS 111-60-4; EINECS 203-886-9; oil-phase cosmetic ingred., pearlescent, emulsifier, dispersant, emulsion stabilizer, thickener; clouding agent for shampoos/hair conditioners; JSCI compliance; wh. flake; HLB 2.

Emalex ET-2020. [Nihon Emulsion] Polysorbate 20; CAS 9005-64-5; nonionic; emulsifier, solubilizer for cosmetics, medical pharmaceuticals; JSCI compliance; pale yel. oil;

HLB 16.

Emalex ET-8020. [Nihon Emulsion] Polysorbate 80; CAS 9005-65-6; emulsifier, solubilizer for cosmetics, medical pharmaceuticals; JSCI compliance; pale yel. oil; HLB 14.

Emalex ET-8040. [Nihon Emulsion] PEG-40 sorbitan oleate; nonionic; emulsifier, solubilizer for cosmetics and medical pharmaceuticals; JCID compliance; pale yel. soft wax; HLB 18.

Emalex FC-1. [Nihon Emulsion] Mixt. of nonionic surfactants; nonionic; emulsifier for cosmetic foundations; wh. wax; HLB 2.

Emalex FC-2. [Nihon Emulsion] Mixt. of nonionic surfactants; nonionic; emulsifier for cosmetic foundations; wh. soft wax; HLB 2.

Emalex FDB-36. [Nihon Emulsion] Sodium lauroyl glutamate and 1,3-butyleneglycol (moisturizing agent); surfactant for cosmetic use; wh. powd.; HLB > 20.

Emalex GM-5. [Nihon Emulsion] PEG-5 glyceryl stearate; emulsifier and thickener for cosmetics, creams, milky lotions, hair conditioners, and facial cleansers; JSCI compliance; cream-colored paste; HLB 8.

Emalex GM-10. [Nihon Emulsion] PEG-10 glyceryl stearate; emulsifier and thickener for cosmetic creams, milky lotions, hair conditioners, and facial cleansers; JSCI compliance; cream-colored paste; HLB 11.

Emalex GM-15. [Nihon Emulsion] PEG-15 glyceryl stearate; emulsifier and thickener for cosmetic creams, milky lotions, hair conditioners, and facial cleansers; JSCI compliance; cream-colored paste; HLB 13.

Emalex GM-20. [Nihon Emulsion] PEG-20 glyceryl stearate; emulsifier, solubilizer for creams and milky lotions; JSCI compliance; cream-colored paste; HLB 14.

Emalex GM-30. [Nihon Emulsion] PEG-30 glyceryl stearate; emulsifier, solubilizer for creams and milky lotions; JSCI compliance; cream-colored wax; HLB 16.

Emalex GM-40. [Nihon Emulsion] PEG-40 glyceryl stearate; emulsifier and solubilizer for cosmetic creams and lotions; JSCI compliance; cream-colored wax; HLB 17.

Emalex GM-6000. [Nihon Emulsion] PEG-60 glyceryl stearate; thickener for shampoos and facial cleansers; JSCI compliance; cream-colored wax; HLB 19.

Emalex GMS-10SE. [Nihon Emulsion] Glyceryl monostearate, SE; surfactant for food, cosmetic and medical pharmaceutical applics.; JSCI compliance; cream-colored wax; HLB 6.

Emalex GMS-15SE. [Nihon Emulsion] Glyceryl monostearate, SE; surfactant for food, cosmetic and medical pharmaceutical applics.; JSCI compliance; cream-colored soft wax; HLB 9.

Emalex GMS-20SE. [Nihon Emulsion] Glyceryl monostearate, SE; surfactant for food, cosmetic and medical pharmaceutical applics.; JSCI compliance; cream-colored wax; HLB 8.

Emalex GMS-25SE. [Nihon Emulsion] Glyceryl monostearate, SE; surfactant for food, cosmetic and medical pharmaceutical applics.; JSCI compliance; cream-colored soft wax; HLB 10.

Emalex GMS-45RT. [Nihon Emulsion] Glyceryl monostearate, SE; surfactant for food, cosmetic and medical pharmaceutical applics.; JSCI compliance; cream-colored wax; HLB 5.

Emalex GMS-50. [Nihon Emulsion] Glyceryl monostearate, SE; surfactant for food, cosmetic and medical pharmaceutical applics.; JSCI compliance; cream-colored wax; HLB 12.

Emalex GMS-55FD. [Nihon Emulsion] Glyceryl monostearate, SE; surfactant for food, cosmetic and medical pharmaceutical applics.; stabilizer, superfatting agent, reforming agent for cleansing foams; JSCI compliance; cream-colored wax; HLB 7.

Emalex GMS-195. [Nihon Emulsion] Glyceryl monostearate, SE; surfactant for food, cosmetic and medical pharmaceutical applics.; JSCI compliance; cream-colored wax; HLB 6.

Emalex GMS-A. [Nihon Emulsion] Glyceryl monostearate; surfactant for food, cosmetic and medical pharmaceutical applics.; JSCI compliance; cream-colored beads; HLB 3.

Emalex GMS-ASE. [Nihon Emulsion] Glyceryl monostearate, SE; surfactant for food, cosmetic and medical pharmaceutical applics.; JSCI compliance; cream-colored beads; HLB 7.

Emalex GMS-B. [Nihon Emulsion] Glyceryl monostearate; surfactant for food, cosmetic and medical pharmaceutical applics.; JSCI compliance; cream-colored beads; HLB 5.

Emalex GMS-P. [Nihon Emulsion] Glyceryl monopalmitate; surfactant for food, cosmetic and medical pharmaceutical applics.; JCID compliance; cream-colored beads; HLB 4.

Emalex GWIS-100. [Nihon Emulsion] Glyceryl mono-isostearate; surfactant for food, cosmetic and medical pharmaceutical applics.; JCID compliance; pale yel. paste; HLB 5.

Emalex GWIS-103. [Nihon Emulsion] PEG-3 glyceryl isostearate; emulsion stabilizer and reforming agent for cosmetic creams, milky lotions, hair conditioners and treatments; pale yel. oil; HLB 5.

Emalex GWIS-105. [Nihon Emulsion] PEG-5 glyceryl isostearate; emulsion stabilizer and reforming agent for cosmetic creams, milky lotions, hair conditioners and treatments; pale yel. oil; HLB 7.

Emalex GWIS-106. [Nihon Emulsion] PEG-6 glyceryl isostearate; emulsion stabilizer and reforming agent for cosmetic creams, milky lotions, hair conditioners and treatments; pale yel. oil; HLB 8.

Emalex GWIS-108. [Nihon Emulsion] PEG-8 glyceryl isostearate; emulsion stabilizer and reforming agent for cosmetic creams, milky lotions, hair conditioners and treatments; pale yel. oil; HLB 9.

Emalex GWIS-110. [Nihon Emulsion] PEG-10 glyceryl isostearate; emulsifier and solubilizer for cosmetic lotions, milky lotions, creams; provides smoothness and good spreading props.; pale yel. oil; HLB 10.

Emalex GWIS-115. [Nihon Emulsion] PEG-15 glyceryl monoisostearate; emulsifier and solubilizer for cosmetic lotions, milky lotions, creams; provides smoothness and good spreading props.; JCID compliance; pale yel. oil; HLB 12.

Emalex GWIS-115(M). [Nihon Emulsion] PEG-15 glyceryl isostearate; emulsifier in alcoholic milky-wh. lotions; JCID compliance; pale yel. oil; HLB 12.

Emalex GWIS-120. [Nihon Emulsion] PEG-20 glyceryl monoisostearate; CAS 69468-44-6; emulsifier and solubilizer for cosmetic lotions, milky lotions, creams; provides smoothness and good spreading props.; JCID compliance; pale yel. oil; HLB 14.

Emalex GWIS-125. [Nihon Emulsion] PEG-25 glyceryl isostearate; emulsifier and solubilizer for cosmetic lotions, milky lotions, creams; provides smoothness and good spreading props.; pale yel. oil; HLB 15.

Emalex GWIS-130. [Nihon Emulsion] PEG-30 glyceryl monoisostearate; CAS 69468-44-6; emulsifier and solubilizer for cosmetic lotions, milky lotions, creams; provides smoothness and good spreading props.; pale yel. oil; HLB 16.

Emalex GWIS-140. [Nihon Emulsion] PEG-40 glyceryl isostearate; emulsifier and solubilizer for cosmetic lotions, milky lotions, creams; provides smoothness and good spreading props.; pale yel. soft paste; HLB 17.

Emalex GWIS-150. [Nihon Emulsion] PEG-50 glyceryl isostearate; emulsifier and solubilizer for cosmetic lotions, milky lotions, creams; provides smoothness and good spreading props.; cream-colored soft wax; HLB 18.

Emalex GWIS-160. [Nihon Emulsion] PEG-60 glyceryl isostearate; emulsifier and solubilizer for cosmetic lotions, milky lotions, creams; provides smoothness and good spreading props.; cream-colored soft wax; HLB 19.

Emalex GWIS-160N. [Nihon Emulsion] PEG-60 glyceryl isostearate; CAS 69468-44-6; personal care emulsifier.

Emalex GWIS-303. [Nihon Emulsion] PEG-3 glyceryl triisostearate; oil-phase cosmetic ingred. for cosmetic creams and milky lotions; stable on prolonged standing; JCID compliance; pale yel. oil; misc. to liq. paraffins, animal or plant fat and waxes; HLB 0.

Emalex GWIS-305. [Nihon Emulsion] PEG-5 glyceryl triisostearate; oil-phase cosmetic ingred. for cosmetic creams and milky lotions; stable on prolonged standing; JCID compliance; pale yel. oil; misc. to liq. paraffins, animal or plant fat and waxes; HLB 0.

Emalex GWIS-310. [Nihon Emulsion] PEG-10 glyceryl triisostearate; emulsifier, dispersant, and reforming agent for cosmetic creams, milky lotions, and hair conditioners; JCID compliance; pale yel. oil; HLB 3.

Emalex GWIS-320. [Nihon Emulsion] PEG-20 glyceryl triisostearate; emulsifier, dispersant, and reforming agent for cosmetic creams, milky lotions, and hair conditioners; JCID compliance; pale yel. oil; HLB 7.

Emalex GWIS-330. [Nihon Emulsion] PEG-30 glyceryl triisostearate; emulsifier, dispersant, and reforming agent for cosmetic creams, milky lotions, and hair conditioners; JCID compliance; pale yel. oil; HLB 10.

Emalex GWIS-340. [Nihon Emulsion] PEG-40 glyceryl triisostearate; solubilizer, thickener, and reforming agent for cosmetic lotions, hair care prods., shampoos, and facial cleansers; JCID compliance; pale yel. soft paste; HLB 11.

Emalex GWIS-350. [Nihon Emulsion] PEG-50 glyceryl triisostearate; solubilizer, thickener, and reforming agent for cosmetic lotions, hair care prods., shampoos, and facial cleansers; JCID compliance; cream-colored soft wax; HLB 13.

Emalex GWIS-360. [Nihon Emulsion] PEG-60 glyceryl triisostearate; solubilizer, thickener, and reforming agent for cosmetic lotions, hair care prods., shampoos, and facial cleansers; JCID compliance; cream-colored soft wax; HLB 14.

Emalex GWO-303. [Nihon Emulsion] PEG-3 glyceryl trioleate; oil-phase cosmetics ingred. for creams and milky lotions; JCID compliance; pale yel. oil; misc. with liq. paraffin, animal or plant fat and waxes; HLB 0.

Emalex GWO-305. [Nihon Emulsion] PEG-5 glyceryl trioleate; oil-phase cosmetics ingred. for creams and milky lotions; JCID compliance; pale yel. oil; misc. with liq. paraffin, animal or plant fat and waxes; HLB 0.

Emalex GWO-310. [Nihon Emulsion] PEG-10 glyceryl trioleate; emulsifier, dispersant, and reforming agent for cosmetic creams, milky lotions, and hair conditioners; JCID compliance; pale yel. oil; HLB 3.

Emalex GWO-320. [Nihon Emulsion] PEG-20 glyceryl trioleate; emulsifier, dispersant, and reforming agent for cosmetic creams, milky lotions, and hair conditioners; JCID compliance; pale yel. oil; HLB 7.

Emalex GWO-330. [Nihon Emulsion] PEG-30 glyceryl trioleate; emulsifier, dispersant, and reforming agent for cosmetic creams, milky lotions, and hair conditioners; JCID compliance; pale yel. oil; HLB 10.

Emalex GWO-340. [Nihon Emulsion] PEG-40 glyceryl trioleate; solubilizer, thickener, and reforming agent for cosmetic lotions, hair care prods., shampoos, and facial cleansers; JCID compliance; pale yel. soft paste; HLB 11.

Emalex GWO-350. [Nihon Emulsion] PEG-50 glyceryl trioleate; solubilizer, thickener, and reforming agent for cosmetic lotions, hair care prods., shampoos, and facial cleansers; JCID compliance; cream-colored soft wax; HLB 12.

Emalex GWO-360. [Nihon Emulsion] PEG-60 glyceryl trioleate; solubilizer, thickener, and reforming agent for cosmetic lotions, hair care prods., shampoos, and facial cleansers; JCID compliance; cream-colored soft wax; HLB 13.

Emalex GWS-204. [Nihon Emulsion] PEG-4 glyceryl distearate; oil-phase cosmetics ingred.; pale yel. soft wax; HLB 1.

Emalex GWS-303. [Nihon Emulsion] PEG-3 glyceryl tristearate; oil-phase cosmetics ingred.; for lipsticks, ointments; JCID compliance; cream-colored wax; HLB 0.

Emalex GWS-304. [Nihon Emulsion] PEG-4 glyceryl tristearate; oil-phase ingred. for lipsticks and ointments; JCID compliance; cream-colored wax; HLB 0.

Emalex GWS-305. [Nihon Emulsion] PEG-5 glyceryl tristearate; oil-phase ingred. for lipsticks and ointments; JCID compliance; cream-colored wax; HLB 0.

Emalex GWS-306. [Nihon Emulsion] PEG-6 glyceryl tristearate; oil-phase ingred. for lipsticks and ointments; JCID compliance; cream-colored wax; HLB 1.

Emalex GWS-310. [Nihon Emulsion] PEG-10 glyceryl tristearate; reforming agent for soap bars, emulsion stabilizer for w/o and o/w cosmetic emulsions; JCID compliance; cream-colored wax; HLB 3.

Emalex GWS-320. [Nihon Emulsion] PEG-20 glyceryl tristearate; reforming agent for soap bars, emulsion stabilizer for w/o and o/w cosmetic emulsions; JCID compliance; cream-colored wax; HLB 7.

Emalex HC-5. [Nihon Emulsion] PEG-5 hydrogenated castor oil; CAS 61788-85-0; nonionic; oil-phase ingred., w/o emulsifier, dispersant for cosmetics and medical prods.; JSCI compliance; pale yel. oil; HLB 3.

Emalex HC-7. [Nihon Emulsion] PEG-7 hydrogenated castor oil; CAS 61788-85-0; nonionic; oil-phase ingred., w/o emulsifier, dispersant for cosmetics and medical prods.; JSCI compliance; pale yel. oil; HLB 5.

Emalex HC-10. [Nihon Emulsion] PEG-10 hydrogenated castor oil; CAS 61788-85-0; nonionic; oil-phase ingred., w/o emulsifier, dispersant for cosmetics and medical prods.; JSCI compliance; pale yel. oil; HLB 6.

Emalex HC-20. [Nihon Emulsion] PEG-20 hydrogenated castor oil; CAS 61788-85-0; nonionic; emulsifier, reforming agent, thickener for creams, milky lotions, hair conditioners, shampoos; solubilizer for oily components and perfumes in alcoholic tonics; JSCI compliance; cream-colored oil; HLB 9.

Emalex HC-30. [Nihon Emulsion] PEG-30 hydrogenated castor oil; CAS 61788-85-0; nonionic; emulsifier, reforming agent, thickener for creams, milky lotions, hair conditioners, shampoos; solubilizer for oily components and perfumes in alcoholic tonics; JSCI compliance; cream-colored soft paste; HLB 11.

Emalex HC-40. [Nihon Emulsion] PEG-40 hydrogenated castor oil; CAS 61788-85-0; nonionic; emulsifier, reforming agent, thickener for creams, milky lotions, hair conditioners, shampoos; solubilizer for oily components and perfumes in alcoholic tonics, oil-sol. vitamins; JSCI compliance; cream-colored soft paste; HLB 12.

Emalex HC-50. [Nihon Emulsion] PEG-50 hydrogenated castor oil; CAS 61788-85-0; nonionic; emulsifier, reforming agent, thickener for creams, milky lotions, hair conditioners, shampoos; solubilizer for oily components and perfumes in alcoholic tonics, oil-sol. vitamins; JSCI compliance; cream-colored soft wax; HLB 13.

Emalex HC-60. [Nihon Emulsion] PEG-60 hydrogenated castor oil; CAS 61788-85-0; nonionic; emulsifier, reforming agent, thickener for creams, milky lotions, hair condi-

cosmetic lotions, hair care prods., shampoos, and facial cleansers; JCID compliance; cream-colored soft wax; HLB 12.

tioners, shampoos; solubilizer for oily components and perfumes in alcoholic tonics, oil-sol. vitamins; JSCI compliance; cream-colored soft wax; HLB 14.

Emalex HC-80. [Nihon Emulsion] PEG-80 hydrogenated castor oil; CAS 61788-85-0; nonionic; emulsifier, reforming agent, thickener for creams, milky lotions, hair conditioners, shampoos; solubilizer for oily components and perfumes in alcoholic tonics; JSCI compliance; cream-colored wax; HLB 16.

Emalex HC-100. [Nihon Emulsion] PEG-100 hydrogenated castor oil; CAS 61788-85-0; nonionic; emulsifier, reforming agent, thickener for creams, milky lotions, hair conditioners, shampoos; solubilizer for oily components and perfumes in alcoholic tonics; JSCI compliance; cream-colored wax; HLB 17.

Emalex HIS-34. [Nihon Emulsion] 2-Hexyldecyl isostearate; lipophilic base for cosmetics; JCID compliance; pale yel. liq.; HLB 0.

Emalex J.J. O-V. [Nihon Emulsion] Jojoba oil; CAS 61789-91-1; stable, natural cosmetics ingred.; JCID compliance; pale yel. liq.; HLB 0.

Emalex K.T.G. [Nihon Emulsion] Caprylic/capric acid triglyceride; CAS 65381-09-1; oil-phase cosmetic ingred.; emollient; JSCI compliance; pale yel. liq.; HLB 1.

Emalex LIP. [Nihon Emulsion] Mixt. of nonionic surfactants; nonionic; base material for lipsticks and other cosmetic sticks; produces good skinfeel; cream-colored wax; HLB 0.

Emalex LWIS-2. [Nihon Emulsion] PEG-2 lauryl ether isostearate; SE cosmetic ingred.; oily base for creams, milky lotions, hair conditioners; good affinity for skin and hair; pale yel. oil; HLB 0.

Emalex LWIS-5. [Nihon Emulsion] PEG-5 lauryl ether isostearate; SE cosmetic ingred.; oily base for creams, milky lotions, hair conditioners; good affinity for skin and hair; pale yel. oil; HLB 3.0.

Emalex LWIS-8. [Nihon Emulsion] PEG-8 lauryl ether isostearate; SE cosmetic ingred.; emulsifier, dispersant, and emulsion stabilizer providing spreading, milky wh. appearance, and gloss; pale yel. turbid oil; HLB 6.

Emalex LWIS-10. [Nihon Emulsion] PEG-10 lauryl ether isostearate; SE cosmetic ingred.; emulsifier, dispersant, and emulsion stabilizer providing spreading, milky wh. appearance, and gloss; pale yel. turbid oil; HLB 7.

Emalex LWS-3. [Nihon Emulsion] PEG-3 lauryl ether stearate; SE cosmetic ingred.; cosmetic and medical ointment base producing good emollient and spreading props.; cream-colored soft wax; HLB 1.

Emalex LWS-5. [Nihon Emulsion] PEG-5 lauryl ether stearate; SE cosmetic ingred.; cosmetic and medical ointment base producing good emollient and spreading props.; cream-colored paste; HLB 3.

Emalex LWS-8. [Nihon Emulsion] PEG-8 lauryl ether stearate; SE cosmetic ingred.; cosmetic and medical ointment base producing good emollient and spreading props.; cream-colored paste; HLB 5.

Emalex LWS-10. [Nihon Emulsion] PEG-10 lauryl ether stearate; SE cosmetic ingred.; cosmetic and medical ointment base producing good emollient and spreading props.; cream-colored soft wax; HLB 7.

Emalex LWS-15. [Nihon Emulsion] PEG-15 lauryl ether stearate; SE cosmetic ingred.; cosmetic and medical ointment base producing good emollient and spreading props.; cream-colored soft wax; HLB 9.

Emalex MSG-2. [Nihon Emulsion] Diglyceryl monostearate; CAS 12694-22-3; EINECS 235-777-7; emulsifier for cosmetics and foods; JCID compliance; cream-colored solid; HLB 7.

Emalex MSG-2MA. [Nihon Emulsion] Diglyceryl monostearate; CAS 12694-22-3; EINECS 235-777-7; emulsifier for cosmetics and foods; JCID compliance; cream-colored solid; HLB 5.

Emalex MSG-2MB. [Nihon Emulsion] Diglyceryl monostearate; CAS 12694-22-3; EINECS 235-777-7; emulsifier for cosmetics and foods; JCID compliance; cream-colored solid; HLB 6.

Emalex MSG-2ME. [Nihon Emulsion] Diglyceryl monostearate; CAS 12694-22-3; EINECS 235-777-7; emulsifier for cosmetics and foods; JCID compliance; cream-colored solid; HLB 7.

Emalex MSG-2ML. [Nihon Emulsion] Diglyceryl monostearate; CAS 12694-22-3; EINECS 235-777-7; emulsifier for cosmetics and foods; JCID compliance; cream-colored solid; HLB 8.

Emalex MTS-30E. [Nihon Emulsion] Phenyl trimethicone; CAS 2116-84-9; EINECS 218-320-6; oil-phase cosmetic ingred. for alcoholic milky-wh. lotions; JSCI compliance; colorless oil; HLB 0; usage level: 2-4%.

Emalex N-83. [Nihon Emulsion] Cocamide DEA; CAS 61791-31-9; EINECS 263-163-9; thickener or bubbling agent in hair shampoos, body shampoos, facial cleansing foams; JSCI compliance; pale yel. oil; HLB 11.

Emalex NN-5. [Nihon Emulsion] Myristamide DEA; CAS 7545-23-5; EINECS 231-426-7; thickener or bubbling agent in hair shampoos, body shampoos, facial cleansing foams; JCID compliance; pale yel. paste; HLB 10.

Emalex NN-15. [Nihon Emulsion] Myristamide DEA; CAS 7545-23-5; EINECS 231-426-7; thickener or bubbling agent in hair shampoos, body shampoos, facial cleansing foams; JCID compliance; pale yel. paste; HLB 12.

Emalex NP-2. [Nihon Emulsion] Nonoxynol-2; EINECS 248-291-5; wetting agent, emulsifier, cleaner, dispersant, foaming agent, solubilizer for cosmetics; JSCI compliance; colorless oil; HLB 5.

Emalex NP-3. [Nihon Emulsion] Nonoxynol-3; CAS 9016-45-9; wetting agent, emulsifier, cleaner, dispersant, foaming agent, solubilizer for cosmetics; JSCI compliance; colorless oil; HLB 6.

Emalex NP-5. [Nihon Emulsion] Nonoxynol-5; CAS 9016-45-9; wetting agent, emulsifier, cleaner, dispersant, foaming agent, solubilizer for cosmetics; JSCI compliance; colorless oil; HLB 8.

Emalex NP-10. [Nihon Emulsion] Nonoxynol-10; CAS 9016-45-9; EINECS 248-294-1; wetting agent, emulsifier, cleaner, dispersant, foaming agent, solubilizer for cosmetics; JSCI compliance; colorless oil; HLB 12.

Emalex NP-11. [Nihon Emulsion] Nonoxynol-11; CAS 9016-45-9; wetting agent, emulsifier, cleaner, dispersant, foaming agent, solubilizer for cosmetics; JSCI compliance; colorless oil; HLB 12.

Emalex NP-12. [Nihon Emulsion] Nonoxynol-12; CAS 9016-45-9; wetting agent, emulsifier, cleaner, dispersant, foaming agent, solubilizer for cosmetics; JSCI compliance; wh. turbid oil; HLB 13.

Emalex NP-13. [Nihon Emulsion] Nonoxynol-13; CAS 9016-45-9; wetting agent, emulsifier, cleaner, dispersant, foaming agent, solubilizer for cosmetics; JSCI compliance; wh. turbid oil; HLB 13.

Emalex NP-15. [Nihon Emulsion] Nonoxynol-15; CAS 9016-45-9; wetting agent, emulsifier, cleaner, dispersant, foaming agent, solubilizer for cosmetics; JSCI compliance; wh. soft paste; HLB 14.

Emalex NP-20. [Nihon Emulsion] Nonoxynol-20; CAS 9016-45-9; wetting agent, emulsifier, cleaner, dispersant, foaming agent, solubilizer for cosmetics; used with Emalex HC-30 as solubilizer for perfumes; JSCI compliance; wh. soft wax; HLB 15.

Emalex NP-25. [Nihon Emulsion] Nonoxynol-25; CAS 9016-45-9; wetting agent, emulsifier, cleaner, dispersant, foaming agent, solubilizer for cosmetics; JSCI compliance; wh.

wax; HLB 16.

Emalex NP-30. [Nihon Emulsion] Nonoxynol-30; CAS 9016-45-9; wetting agent, emulsifier, cleaner, dispersant, foaming agent, solubilizer for cosmetics; JSCI compliance; wh. wax; HLB 17.

Emalex OD-5. [Nihon Emulsion] Octyldodeceth-5; emulsifier, dispersant, solubilizer, cleaner, wetting agent for cosmetics, creams, milky lotions; JCID compliance; wh. soft wax; HLB 6.

Emalex OD-10. [Nihon Emulsion] Octyldodeceth-10; emulsifier, dispersant, solubilizer, cleaner, wetting agent for cosmetics, creams, milky lotions; JCID compliance; wh. soft wax; HLB 10.

Emalex OD-16. [Nihon Emulsion] Octyldodeceth-16; emulsifier, dispersant, solubilizer, cleaner, wetting agent for cosmetics, creams, milky lotions; JCID compliance; wh. soft wax; HLB 12.

Emalex OD-20. [Nihon Emulsion] Octyldodeceth-20; emulsifier, dispersant, solubilizer, cleaner, wetting agent for cosmetics, creams, milky lotions; JCID compliance; wh. wax; HLB 13.

Emalex OD-25. [Nihon Emulsion] Octyldodeceth-25; emulsifier, dispersant, solubilizer, cleaner, wetting agent for cosmetics, creams, milky lotions; JCID compliance; wh. wax; HLB 14.

Emalex OE-6. [Nihon Emulsion] PEG-6 oleate; CAS 9004-96-0; cosmetics surfactant; JSCI compliance; pale yel. oil; HLB 8.

Emalex OE-10. [Nihon Emulsion] PEG-10 oleate; CAS 9004-96-0; cosmetics surfactant; JSCI compliance; pale yel. oil; HLB 11.

Emalex OP-5. [Nihon Emulsion] Octoxynol-5; CAS 9002-93-1; emulsifier, wetting agent, cleaner, dispersant, foaming agent, solubilizer for cosmetics; JSCI compliance; colorless oil; HLB 9.

Emalex OP-8. [Nihon Emulsion] Octoxynol-8; CAS 9002-93-1; emulsifier, wetting agent, cleaner, dispersant, foaming agent, solubilizer for cosmetics; JSCI compliance; colorless oil; HLB 11.

Emalex OP-10. [Nihon Emulsion] Octoxynol-10; CAS 9002-93-1; emulsifier, wetting agent, cleaner, dispersant, foaming agent, solubilizer for cosmetics; solubilizer for aromatic agents; JSCI compliance; colorless oil; HLB 12.

Emalex OP-15. [Nihon Emulsion] Octoxynol-15; CAS 9002-93-1; emulsifier, wetting agent, cleaner, dispersant, foaming agent, solubilizer for cosmetics; JSCI compliance; colorless oil; HLB 14.

Emalex OP-20. [Nihon Emulsion] Octoxynol-20; CAS 9002-93-1; emulsifier, wetting agent, cleaner, dispersant, foaming agent, solubilizer for cosmetics; JSCI compliance; wh. soft wax; HLB 16.

Emalex OP-25. [Nihon Emulsion] Octoxynol-25; CAS 9002-93-1; emulsifier, wetting agent, cleaner, dispersant, foaming agent, solubilizer for cosmetics; JSCI compliance; wh. wax; HLB 17.

Emalex OP-30. [Nihon Emulsion] Octoxynol-30; CAS 9002-93-1; emulsifier, wetting agent, cleaner, dispersant, foaming agent, solubilizer for cosmetics; JSCI compliance; wh. wax; HLB 18.

Emalex OP-40. [Nihon Emulsion] Octoxynol-40; CAS 9002-93-1; emulsifier, wetting agent, cleaner, dispersant, foaming agent, solubilizer for cosmetics; JSCI compliance; wh. wax; HLB 19.

Emalex OP-50. [Nihon Emulsion] Octoxynol-50; CAS 9002-93-1; emulsifier, wetting agent, cleaner, dispersant, foaming agent, solubilizer for cosmetics; JSCI compliance; wh. wax; HLB 21.

Emalex O.T.G. [Nihon Emulsion] Glyceryl trioctanoate; CAS 538-23-8; EINECS 208-686-5; oil-phase cosmetic ingred.; emollient; JCID compliance; colorless liq.; HLB 1.

Emalex PC-6. [Nihon Emulsion] Mixt. of nonionic surfactants; nonionic; stable pearlescent for facial cleansing creams; cream-colored soft wax; HLB 4; usage level: up to 5%.

Emalex PC-7. [Nihon Emulsion] Mixt. of nonionic surfactants; nonionic; stable pearlescent for facial cleansing creams; cream-colored wax; HLB 5; usage level: up to 5%.

Emalex PEIS-3. [Nihon Emulsion] PEG-3 isostearate; CAS 56002-14-3; emulsifier, dispersant, solubilizer for cosmetics; emulsion stabilizer, skin fitness reformer for milky lotions, hair conditioners; pale yel. oil; HLB 5.

Emalex PEIS-6. [Nihon Emulsion] PEG-6 isostearate; CAS 56002-14-3; emulsifier, dispersant, solubilizer for cosmetics; emulsion stabilizer, skin fitness reformer for milky lotions, hair conditioners; JCID compliance; pale yel. oil; HLB 8.

Emalex PEIS-12. [Nihon Emulsion] PEG-12 isostearate; CAS 56002-14-3; emulsifier, dispersant for cosmetics; solubilizer for oily ingreds. and perfumes in lotions; JCID compliance; pale yel. oil; HLB 12.

Emalex PEIS-20. [Nihon Emulsion] PEG-20 isostearate; CAS 56002-14-3; emulsifier, dispersant for cosmetics; solubilizer for oily ingreds. and perfumes in lotions; pale yel. soft wax; HLB 14.

Emalex PG-di-IS. [Nihon Emulsion] Propylene glycol diisostearate; oil-phase cosmetic ingred.; JCID compliance; pale yel. oil; HLB 0.

Emalex PG-di-L. [Nihon Emulsion] Propylene glycol dilaurate; CAS 22788-19-8; EINECS 245-217-3; cosmetic ingred.; pale yel. oil; HLB 0.

Emalex PG-di-O. [Nihon Emulsion] Propylene glycol dioleate; CAS 105-62-4; EINECS 203-315-3; cosmetic ingred.; JSCI compliance; pale yel. oil; HLB 0.

Emalex PG-di-S. [Nihon Emulsion] Propylene glycol distearate; CAS 6182-11-2; EINECS 228-229-3; oil-phase cosmetic ingred.; JCID compliance; wh. wax; HLB 0.

Emalex PGML. [Nihon Emulsion] Propylene glycol monolaurate; CAS 142-55-2; EINECS 205-542-3; nonionic; surfactant for food and cosmetics; emulsion stabilizer for creams, milky lotions, hair conditioners; JCID compliance; pale yel. oil; HLB 4.

Emalex PGMS. [Nihon Emulsion] Propylene glycol monostearate; CAS 1323-39-3; EINECS 215-354-3; nonionic; surfactant for food and cosmetics; emulsion stabilizer for creams, milky lotions, hair conditioners; JSCI compliance; wh. powd.; HLB 2.

Emalex PGO. [Nihon Emulsion] Propylene glycol monooleate; CAS 1330-80-9; EINECS 215-549-3; nonionic; surfactant for food and cosmetics; JCID compliance; pale yel. oil; HLB 2.

Emalex PGS. [Nihon Emulsion] Propylene glycol monostearate; CAS 1323-39-3; EINECS 215-354-3; nonionic; surfactant for food and cosmetics; JSCI compliance; wh. wax; HLB 2.

Emalex PR-3. [Nihon Emulsion] Mixt. of nonionic surfactants; nonionic; emulsifier for hair conditioners; recommended for mixing with cationic surfactants at volume ratios of 1:1 to 1:2 to produce stable, creamy hair conditioners; cream-colored wax; HLB 6.

Emalex PS-1. [Nihon Emulsion] Mixt. of nonionic surfactants; nonionic; base material in hydrophilic transparent hair finishes containing liq. paraffins and squalane; cream-colored soft wax; HLB 12.

Emalex PS-1(S). [Nihon Emulsion] Mixt. of nonionic surfactants; nonionic; base material in hydrophilic transparent hair finishes containing liq. paraffins and squalane; cream-colored soft wax; HLB 13.

Emalex PS-2A. [Nihon Emulsion] Mixt. of nonionic surfactants; nonionic; base material in hydrophilic transparent hair finishes containing animal or plant fats; pale yel. oil; HLB 8.

Emalex PS-2B. [Nihon Emulsion] Mixt. of nonionic surfactants; nonionic; base material in hydrophilic transparent hair finishes containing animal or plant fats; cream-colored soft wax; HLB 14.

Emalex RWIS-105. [Nihon Emulsion] PEG-5 hydrogenated castor oil isostearate; oil-phase component, emulsifier for w/o emulsions, dispersant for hydrophobic components; JCID compliance; cream-colored turbid oil; HLB 2.

Emalex RWIS-110. [Nihon Emulsion] PEG-10 hydrog. castor oil isostearate; oil-phase component, emulsifier for w/o emulsions, dispersant for hydrophobic components; JCID compliance; pale yel. oil; HLB 4.

Emalex RWIS-115. [Nihon Emulsion] PEG-15 hydrog. castor oil isostearate; oil-phase component, emulsifier for w/o emulsions, dispersant for hydrophobic components; JCID compliance; pale yel. oil; HLB 6.

Emalex RWIS-120. [Nihon Emulsion] PEG-20 hydrog. castor oil isostearate; emulsifier and reforming agent for cosmetic creams, milky lotions, and hair conditioners; JCID compliance; pale yel. oil; HLB 7.

Emalex RWIS-130. [Nihon Emulsion] PEG-30 hydrog. castor oil isostearate; emulsifier and reforming agent for cosmetic creams, milky lotions, and hair conditioners; JCID compliance; pale yel. oil; HLB 9.

Emalex RWIS-140. [Nihon Emulsion] PEG-40 hydrog. castor oil isostearate; emulsifier and reforming agent for cosmetic creams, milky lotions, and hair conditioners; JCID compliance; cream-colored paste; HLB 11.

Emalex RWIS-150. [Nihon Emulsion] PEG-50 hydrog. castor oil isostearate; solubilizer for oily components or perfumes; thickener for shampoos and cleansing foams; JCID compliance; cream-colored paste; HLB 12.

Emalex RWIS-160. [Nihon Emulsion] PEG-60 hydrog. castor oil isostearate; solubilizer for oily components or perfumes; thickener for shampoos and cleansing foams; JCID compliance; cream-colored paste; HLB 13.

Emalex RWIS-305. [Nihon Emulsion] PEG-5 hydrogenated castor oil triisostearate; solubilizer for oil-phase ingreds. in cosmetics; emulsifier for w/o emulsions; reforming agent, dispersant for hydrophobic components; pale yel. oil; HLB 0.

Emalex RWIS-310. [Nihon Emulsion] PEG-10 hydrog. castor oil triisostearate; solubilizer for oil-phase ingreds. in cosmetics; emulsifier for w/o emulsions; reforming agent, dispersant for hydrophobic components; pale yel. oil; HLB 1.

Emalex RWIS-315. [Nihon Emulsion] PEG-15 hydrog. castor oil triisostearate; solubilizer for oil-phase ingreds. in cosmetics; emulsifier for w/o emulsions; reforming agent, dispersant for hydrophobic components; pale yel. oil; HLB 3.

Emalex RWIS-320. [Nihon Emulsion] PEG-20 hydrog. castor oil triisostearate; solubilizer for oil-phase ingreds. in cosmetics; emulsifier for w/o emulsions; reforming agent, dispersant for hydrophobic components; pale yel. oil; HLB 4.

Emalex RWIS-330. [Nihon Emulsion] PEG-30 hydrog. castor oil triisostearate; solubilizer for oily components or perfumes; thickener for shampoos, hair conditioners, and other hair care prods.; pale yel. oil; HLB 6.

Emalex RWIS-340. [Nihon Emulsion] PEG-40 hydrog. castor oil triisostearate; solubilizer for oily components or perfumes; thickener for shampoos, hair conditioners, and other hair care prods.; pale yel. soft paste; HLB 8.

Emalex RWIS-350. [Nihon Emulsion] PEG-50 hydrog. castor oil triisostearate; solubilizer for oily components or perfumes; thickener for shampoos, hair conditioners, and other hair care prods.; pale yel. soft paste; HLB 9.

Emalex RWIS-360. [Nihon Emulsion] PEG-60 hydrog. castor oil triisostearate; solubilizer for oily components or per-

fumes; thickener for shampoos, hair conditioners, and other hair care prods.; pale yel. soft paste; HLB 10.

Emalex RWL-120. [Nihon Emulsion] PEG-20 hydrog. castor oil laurate; emulsifier, dispersant, reforming agent for cosmetic creams, milky lotions, hair conditioners; JCID compliance; pale yel. paste; HLB 8.

Emalex RWL-130. [Nihon Emulsion] PEG-30 hydrog. castor oil laurate; emulsifier, dispersant, reforming agent for cosmetic creams, milky lotions, hair conditioners; JCID compliance; pale yel. paste; HLB 10.

Emalex RWL-140. [Nihon Emulsion] PEG-40 hydrog. castor oil laurate; solubilizer, gelling agent, and thickener for cosmetic tonics, hair care prods. of hydrophilic gel type, and shampoos; JCID compliance; cream-colored paste; HLB 11.

Emalex RWL-150. [Nihon Emulsion] PEG-50 hydrog. castor oil laurate; solubilizer, gelling agent, and thickener for cosmetic tonics, hair care prods. of hydrophilic gel type, and shampoos; JCID compliance; cream-colored paste; HLB 12.

Emalex RWL-160. [Nihon Emulsion] PEG-60 hydrog. castor oil laurate; solubilizer, gelling agent, and thickener for cosmetic tonics, hair care prods. of hydrophilic gel type, and shampoos; JCID compliance; cream-colored paste; HLB 13.

Emalex SEF-4. [Nihon Emulsion] Mixt. of nonionic surfactants; nonionic; emulsifier for hair lotions, cleansing lotions, low visc. emulsions; wh. soft wax; HLB 8.

Emalex SEF-8. [Nihon Emulsion] Mixt. of nonionic surfactants; nonionic; emulsifier for hair lotions, cleansing lotions, low visc. emulsions; wh. soft wax; HLB 8.

Emalex SEF-320(A). [Nihon Emulsion] Mixt. of nonionic surfactants; nonionic; emulsifier for cosmetic creams, ointments, highly visc. emulsions; cream-colored wax; HLB 7.

Emalex SG-37. [Nihon Emulsion] Caprylic/capric/stearic triglyceride; oil-phase cosmetic ingred.; exc. waxing material with high emulsifying ability; JCID compliance; wh. soft wax; HLB 0.

Emalex SPE-100S. [Nihon Emulsion] Sorbitan stearate; CAS 1338-41-6; EINECS 215-664-9; oil-phase cosmetic ingred., surfactant; for creams, milky lotions, hair conditioners; JSCI compliance; cream-colored flakes; HLB 8.

Emalex SPE-150S. [Nihon Emulsion] Sorbitan sesquistearate; oil-phase cosmetic ingred., surfactant; for creams, milky lotions, hair conditioners; JSCI compliance; cream-colored wax; HLB 5.

Emalex SPIS-100. [Nihon Emulsion] Sorbitan isostearate; CAS 54392-26-6; oil-phase cosmetic ingred., surfactant; for creams, milky lotions, hair conditioners; JSCI compliance; pale yel. oil; HLB 9.

Emalex SPIS-150. [Nihon Emulsion] Sorbitan sesquiisostearate; oil-phase cosmetic ingred., surfactant; for creams, milky lotions, hair conditioners; JCID compliance; pale yel. oil; HLB 6.

Emalex SPO-100. [Nihon Emulsion] Sorbitan oleate; CAS 1338-43-8; EINECS 215-665-4; oil-phase cosmetic ingred., surfactant; for creams, milky lotions, hair conditioners; JSCI compliance; pale yel. oil; HLB 8.

Emalex SPO-150. [Nihon Emulsion] Sorbitan sesquioleate; CAS 8007-43-0; EINECS 232-360-1; oil-phase cosmetic ingred., surfactant; for creams, milky lotions, hair conditioners; JSCI compliance; pale yel. oil; HLB 5.

Emalex S.T.G. [Nihon Emulsion] Hydrogenated oil; oil-phase cosmetic ingred. with high emulsifying ability; exc. waxing material; JSCI compliance; wh. wax; HLB 0.

Emalex S.T.G.-R. [Nihon Emulsion] Hydrogenated oil; oil-phase cosmetic ingred. with high emulsifying ability; exc. waxing material; JSCI compliance; wh. wax; HLB 0.

Emalex SWS-4. [Nihon Emulsion] PEG-4 stearyl ether

stearate; SE cosmetic ingred.; hydrophobic component and reforming agent for cosmetics and industrial areas; JCID compliance; cream-colored wax; HLB 1.

Emalex SWS-6. [Nihon Emulsion] PEG-6 stearyl ether stearate; SE cosmetic ingred.; hydrophobic component and reforming agent for cosmetics and industrial areas; JCID compliance; cream-colored wax; HLB 3.

Emalex SWS-9. [Nihon Emulsion] PEG-9 stearyl ether stearate; SE cosmetic ingred.; emulsifier, dispersant, and stabilizer for emulsions providing spreading, milky wh. appearance, and water repellency; JCID compliance; cream-colored wax; HLB 5.

Emalex SWS-10. [Nihon Emulsion] PEG-10 stearyl ether stearate; SE cosmetic ingred.; emulsifier, dispersant, and stabilizer for emulsions providing spreading, milky wh. appearance, and water repellency; JCID compliance; cream-colored wax; HLB 6.

Emalex SWS-12. [Nihon Emulsion] PEG-12 stearyl ether stearate; SE cosmetic ingred.; emulsifier, dispersant, and stabilizer for emulsions providing spreading, milky wh. appearance, and water repellency; JCID compliance; cream-colored wax; HLB 7.

Emalex TEG-di-AS. [Nihon Emulsion] PEG-3 distearate; CAS 9005-08-7; pearling agent, superfatting agent, and oil-phse ingred. for cosmetics (shampoos, hair conditioners, cleansing foams, creams); JCID compliance; wh. wax; HLB 1.

Emalex TEG-di-IS. [Nihon Emulsion] PEG-3 diisostearate; cosmetic ingred.; pale yel. oil; HLB 1.

Emalex TEG-di-L. [Nihon Emulsion] PEG-3 dilaurate; CAS 9005-02-1; oil-phase cosmetic ingred., emulsifier for creams, milky lotions, hair conditioners; cleaner, superfatting agent, thickener, reforming agent; wh. soft wax; HLB 3.

Emalex TEG-di-O. [Nihon Emulsion] PEG-3 dioleate; oil-phase ingred., emulsifier, dispersant with good spreadability for cosmetics, creams, milky lotions, foundations; pale yel. oil; HLB 1.

Emalex TEG-di-S. [Nihon Emulsion] PEG-3 distearate; CAS 9005-08-7; pearling agent, hydrophobic component, reforming agent, emulsifier, thickener for cosmetics; JCID compliance; wh. wax; HLB 1.

Emalex TISG-2. [Nihon Emulsion] Diglyceryl triisostearate; CAS 120486-24-0; emulsifier for foods and cosmetics; JCID compliance; pale yel. liq.; HLB 0.

Emalex TPIS-303. [Nihon Emulsion] PEG-3 trimethylolpropane triisostearate; oil-phase cosmetics ingred., emulsifier, solubilizer; offers smooth, clear appearance producing transparent cosmetic prods.; pale yel. oil; HLB 0.

Emalex TPIS-320. [Nihon Emulsion] PEG-20 trimethylolpropane triisostearate; oil-phase cosmetics ingred., emulsifier, solubilizer; offers smooth, clear appearance producing transparent cosmetic prods.; pale yel. oil; HLB 7.

Emalex TPIS-325. [Nihon Emulsion] PEG-25 trimethylolpropane triisostearate; oil-phase cosmetics ingred., emulsifier, solubilizer; offers smooth, clear appearance producing transparent cosmetic prods.; pale yel. oil; HLB 8.

Emalex TPIS-330. [Nihon Emulsion] PEG-30 trimethylolpropane triisostearate; oil-phase cosmetics ingred., emulsifier, solubilizer; offers smooth, clear appearance producing transparent cosmetic prods.; pale yel. turbid oil; HLB 9.

Emalex TPIS-340. [Nihon Emulsion] PEG-40 trimethylolpropane triisostearate; oil-phase cosmetics ingred., emulsifier, solubilizer; offers smooth, clear appearance producing transparent cosmetic prods.; pale yel. soft paste; HLB 11.

Emalex TPIS-350. [Nihon Emulsion] PEG-50 trimethylolpropane triisostearate; oil-phase cosmetics ingred., emulsifier, solubilizer; offers smooth, clear appearance produc-

ing transparent cosmetic prods.; pale yel. soft paste; HLB 12.

Emalex TPM-303. [Nihon Emulsion] PEG-3 trimethylolpropane trimyristate; emulsifier, solubilizer, oil-phase ingred. for cosmetics; reforming agent for creams, milky lotions, hair conditioners; pale yel. oil; HLB 0.

Emalex TPM-305. [Nihon Emulsion] PEG-5 trimethylolpropane trimyristate; emulsifier, solubilizer, oil-phase ingred. for cosmetics; reforming agent for creams, milky lotions, hair conditioners; pale yel. oil; HLB 1.0.

Emalex TPM-308. [Nihon Emulsion] PEG-8 trimethylolpropane trimyristate; emulsifier, solubilizer, oil-phase ingred. for cosmetics; reforming agent for creams, milky lotions, hair conditioners; cream-colored turbid oil; HLB 3.

Emalex TPM-320. [Nihon Emulsion] PEG-20 trimethylolpropane trimyristate; emulsifier, solubilizer, oil-phase ingred. for cosmetics; reforming agent for creams, milky lotions, hair conditioners; pale yel. oil; HLB 8.

Emalex TPM-325. [Nihon Emulsion] PEG-25 trimethylolpropane trimyristate; emulsifier, solubilizer, oil-phase ingred. for cosmetics; reforming agent for creams, milky lotions, hair conditioners; pale yel. oil; HLB 10.

Emalex TPM-330. [Nihon Emulsion] PEG-30 trimethylolpropane trimyristate; emulsifier, solubilizer, oil-phase ingred. for cosmetics; reforming agent for creams, milky lotions, hair conditioners; cream-colored turbid oil; HLB 11.

Emalex TPS-203. [Nihon Emulsion] PEG-3 trimethylolpropane distearate; oil-phase component for hair creams, lipsticks, ointments, cold creams; JCID compliance; cream-colored wax; HLB 0.

Emalex TPS-204. [Nihon Emulsion] PEG-4 trimethylolpropane distearate; oil-phase component for hair creams, lipsticks, ointments, cold creams; cream-colored wax; HLB 1.

Emalex TPS-205. [Nihon Emulsion] PEG-5 trimethylolpropane distearate; oil-phase component for hair creams, lipsticks, ointments, cold creams; cream-colored wax; HLB 2.

Emalex TPS-303. [Nihon Emulsion] PEG-3 trimethylolpropane tristearate; oil-phase cosmetics ingred.; for hair creams, ointments, cold creams; superfatting agent for creamy hair conditoners, cleansing foams; JCID compliance; cream-colored wax; HLB 0.

Emalex TPS-305. [Nihon Emulsion] PEG-5 trimethylolpropane tristearate; oil-phase cosmetics ingred.; for hair creams, ointments, cold creams; superfatting agent for creamy hair conditoners, cleansing foams; cream-colored wax; HLB 0.

Emalex TPS-308. [Nihon Emulsion] PEG-8 trimethylolpropane tristearate; oil-phase cosmetics ingred.; for hair creams, ointments, cold creams; superfatting agent for creamy hair conditoners, cleansing foams; cream-colored wax; HLB 2.

Emalex TPS-310. [Nihon Emulsion] PEG-10 trimethylolpropane tristearate; oil-phase cosmetics ingred.; for hair creams, ointments, cold creams; superfatting agent for creamy hair conditoners, cleansing foams; cream-colored wax; HLB 3.

Emalex TS-8. [Nihon Emulsion] Mixt. of nonionic surfactants; nonionic; solubilizer for perfumes; pale yel. oil; HLB 15.

Emalex VS-31. [Nihon Emulsion] Mixt. of nonionic surfactants; nonionic; solubilizer for oil-sol. vitamins; pale yel. soft paste; HLB 14.

Emalox CG-4. [Nihon Emulsion] Mixt. of nonionic surfactants; nonionic; solubilizer for perfumes; pale yel. oil; HLB 13.

Emcocel® 50M. [Mendell] Microcrystalline cellulose NF/BP; CAS 9004-34-6; tablet binder for pharmaceuticals.

Emcocel® 90M. [Mendell] Microcryst. cellulose NF/BP; CAS 9004-34-6; tablet binder, disintegrant for pharmaceuticals; features low frability, inherent lubricity, enhanced compression of other excipients; avg. particle size 91 µ; 45% min +200 mesh; dens. (tapped) 0.40 g/ml max.; pH 5.5-7.0; 100% conc.

Emcocel® LM. [Mendell] Microcrystalline cellulose NF; CAS 9004-34-6; tablet binder for pharmaceuticals featuring low friability, inherent lubricity, enhanced compression of other excipients, ability to initiate disintegration; conforms to FCC; avg. particle size 51 µ; 30% max. +200 mesh; dens. (tapped) 0.40 g/ml max.; pH 5.5-7.0; 100% conc.

Emcol® 4. [Witco/H-I-P] Stearalkonium chloride; CAS 122-19-0; EINECS 204-527-9; cationic; antistat, substantive conditioner, emollient; wh. paste; water-sol.; sp.gr. 0.99; pH 4.0; 25% solids.

Emcol® 1484. [Witco/H-I-P] Disodium alkylether sulfosuccinate; CAS 39354-45-5; anionic; foaming surfactant for shampoos, other personal care prods.; liq.; 38% conc.

Emcol® 3555. [Witco/H-I-P] Ricinoleamidopropyl dimethylamine lactate; CAS 977012-91-1; conditioner.

Emcol® 4072. [Witco/H-I-P] Disodium hydrog. cottonseed glyceride sulfosuccinate; anionic; cosmetics and toiletries surfactant used as conditioner, emollient, emulsifier; paste; water-sol.

Emcol® 4100M. [Witco/H-I-P] Disodium myristamido MEA-sulfosuccinate; anionic; dispersant, wetting agent, foaming agent, detergent, emulsifier for bubble bath, shampoo, carpet and upholstery cleaners, textiles; wh. creamy semisolid; disp. in water; sp.gr. 1.01; acid no. 4.5; surf. tens. 37.8 dynes/cm (0.05%); pH 6.5 (3% aq.); 38% solids.

Emcol® 4101. [Witco/H-I-P] Disodium ricinoleamido MEA-sulfosuccinate.

Emcol® 4161L. [Witco/H-I-P] Disodium oleamido MIPA sulfosuccinate; CAS 43154-85-4; EINECS 256-120-0; anionic; dispersant, wetting, foam booster/stabilizer, detergent, conditioner, and emulsifying agent for bubble bath, shampoos, cleansers for cosmetics and toiletries; lt. yel. clear liq.; sol. in water; sp.gr. 1.10; flash pt. (PMCC) 93 C; acid no. 6.0; pH 6.5 (3% aq.); surf. tens. 32.6 dynes/cm (0.5%); 38% solids.

Emcol® 4300. [Witco/H-I-P] Disodium C12-15 pareth sulfosuccinate; anionic; dispersant, wetting, foaming, detergent, emulsifying agent for bubble bath, shampoo, cosmetics and toiletries; emulsifier for acrylic, vinyl acetate, vinyl acrylic polymerization; lt. clear liq.; sol. in water; sp.gr. 1.08; visc. 50 cps; acid no. 5.0; pH 6.2 (3% aq.); surf. tens. 29.3 dynes/cm (1%); Ross-Miles foam 162 mm (initial, 1%, 49 C); 33% solids.

Emcol® 4400-1. [Witco/H-I-P] Disodium lauryl sulfosuccinate; anionic; cosmetics and toiletries surfactant used as emulsifier, cleansing, foaming agent, stabilizer; paste; water-sol.

Emcol® 4403. [Witco/H-I-P] Disodium laureth sulfosuccinate; cosmetic surfactant.

Emcol® 4500. [Witco/H-I-P] Sodium dioctyl sulfosuccinate; CAS 577-11-7; EINECS 209-406-4; anionic; dispersant, detergent, wetting, foaming, emulsifying agent; for cosmetics, toiletries, textiles, industrial processing slurries; clear, lt. visc. liq.; sol. in perchloroethylene, CCl₄, kerosene, xylene, Stod.; disp. water and alcohol; sp.gr. 1.10; flash pt. > 93 C; acid no. 3.0; surf. tens. 26.3 dynes/cm (0.05%); pH 6.5 (3% aq.); 70% solids.

Emcol® 5310. [Witco/H-I-P] Disodium lauramido MEA-sulfosuccinate; CAS 25882-44-4; EINECS 247-310-4; cosmetic surfactant.

Emcol® 5315. [Witco/H-I-P] Disodium cocamido MEA-sulfosuccinate; cosmetic surfactant.

Emcol® 5330. [Witco/H-I-P] Disodium undecylenamido MEA-sulfosuccinate.

Emcol® 6613. [Witco/H-I-P] Isostearamidopropyl dimethyl-amine lactate; CAS 55852-15-8; cationic; conditioner for shampoo, cream rinses, clear formulations; liq.; 100% act.

Emcol® 6748. [Witco/H-I-P] Cocamidopropyl betaine; amphoteric; detergent, foam booster/stabilizer, visc. modifier, wetting agent for personal care prods.; Gardner 3 liq.; water-sol.; sp.gr. 1.05; clear pt. 0 C; 35% solids.

Emcol® CBA60. [Witco/H-I-P] Trideceth-7 carboxylic acid.

Emcol® CC-9. [Witco/H-I-P] PPG-9 diethylmonium chloride; CAS 9042-76-6; cationic; dispersant, particle suspension aid, antistat, wetting agent, o/w emulsifier, conditioner, penetrant, lubricant; for cosmetics, toiletries, textiles, industrial slurries; lt. amber clear liq.; sol. in water, IPA; sp.gr. 1.01; flash pt. > 93 C; pH 6.5 (10% aq.); 100% conc.

Emcol® CC-36. [Witco/H-I-P] PPG-25 diethylmonium chloride; cationic; dispersant, particle suspension aid, o/w emulsifier; plasticizer for hair polymers; antistat; skin cleanser for cosmetics; used in dry cleaning systems; industrial processes; lt. amber clear liq.; sol. in water, IPA; sp.gr. 1.01; flash pt. > 93 C; pH 6.7 (10% in 10:6 IPA:water); 100% conc.

Emcol® CC 37-18. [Witco/H-I-P] Coco-betaine; CAS 68424-94-2; EINECS 270-329-4; amphoteric; foaming agent and foam stabilizer for cosmetics and toiletries, specialty cleaning formulations; visc. modifier; liq.; 45% act.

Emcol® CC-42. [Witco/H-I-P] PPG-40 diethylmonium chloride; CAS 9076-43-1; cationic; pigment dispersant, particle suspension aid, emulsifier, solv., conditioner, antistat, lubricant, corrosion inhibitor for toiletries, cosmetics, germicides, syn. fibers and plastics, textiles, industrial processes; ore flotation additive; lt. amber oily liq.; sol. in IPA, acetone, MEK, min. spirits, alcohol; partly sol. in water; sp.gr. 1.01; flash pt. > 200 C (PMCC); pH 6.5; 100% conc.

Emcol® CC-55. [Witco/H-I-P] Polypropoxy quat. ammonium acetate; cationic; antistat; conditioner for hair rinse preparations; emulsifier for cosmetics and textile flame retardants; solv. for phenolic-type germicides for cosmetics and toiletries; antistat for syn. fibers and plastics; fabric conditioner; lubricant for textile and industrial formulations; solv. cleaning and scouring agent; corrosion inhibitor in protective coatings; pigment dispersant in nonaq. media; o/w emulsifier; lt. amber oily liq.; sol. @ 25% in ethanol, IPA, acetone, MEK; water-disp.; sp.gr. 1.02; flash pt. > 93 C (PMCC); pH 6.5; 99% solids.

Emcol® CC-57. [Witco/H-I-P] Polypropoxy quat. ammonium phosphate; cationic; antistat, conditioner, emulsifier, solv., lubricant, solv. cleaning and scouring agent, corrosion inhibitor, and dispersant; used in syn. fibers and plastics, personal care prods., germicides, flame retardants, textile and industrial applic., protective coatings, and pigments; lt. amber oily liq.; sol. in water, ethanol, IPA, acetone, MEK; sp.gr. 1.12; flash pt. > 93 C (PMCC).

Emcol® CDO. [Witco/H-I-P] Cocamidopropylamine oxide; CAS 68155-09-9; EINECS 268-938-5; cosmetic surfactant.

Emcol® CLA-40. [Witco/H-I-P] Laureth-5 carboxylic acid; surfactant.

Emcol® CMCD. [Witco/H-I-P] Sodium cocoamphoacetate; personal care surfactant.

Emcol® Coco Betaine. [Witco/H-I-P] Cocamidopropyl betaine; amphoteric; detergent, foam booster/stabilizer, visc. modifier, wetting agent; Gardner 3 liq.; water-sol.; sp.gr. 1.04; 42% solids.

Emcol® DG. [Witco/H-I-P] Cocamidopropyl betaine; amphoteric; detergent, emulsifier, foaming and wetting agent, visc. builder, foam stabilizer for detergent industry and personal care prods.; lime soap dispersant; Gardner 4 liq.; water-sol.; sp.gr. 1.03; clear pt. 0 C; 36% solids.

Emcol® DMCD-40. [Witco/H-I-P] Lauramine oxide; CAS

1643-20-5; EINECS 216-700-6; personal care surfactant.

Emcol® E-607L. [Witco/H-I-P] Lapyrium chloride; CAS 6272-74-8; EINECS 228-464-1; cationic; emollient, emulsifier, conditioner, foamer, cleanser, substantive agent, deodorant for cosmetics, toiletries, industrial applics.; hair conditioner; wh. to off-wh. cryst. powd.; sol. 37% in water and ethanol, 28% in IPA; surf. tens. 37 dynes/cm (0.1% aq.); pH 3.9 (1% aq.); 97.5% act.

Emcol® E-607S. [Witco/H-I-P] Steapyrium chloride; cationic; emollient, emulsifier, conditioner, foamer, cleanser, substantive agent, deodorant for cosmetics, toiletries, industrial applics.; hair conditioner; wh. to off-wh. powd.; sol. in oil, 2.5% in water; pH 3.4 (1% aq.); 94% act.

Emcol® ISML. [Witco/H-I-P] Isostearamidopropyl morpholine lactate; cationic; cosmetics and toiletries surfactant used as antistat, conditioner, emollient, foaming and substantive agent; nonirritating base for cream rinses and conditioning shampoos; lt. yel. liq.; water-sol.; sp.gr. 1.01; pH 4.5; 25% act.

Emcol® L. [Witco/H-I-P] Lauramine oxide; CAS 1643-20-5; EINECS 216-700-6; cationic; cosmetics and toiletries surfactant used as antistat, cleansing and substantive agent, emollient, lubricant, and visc. builder; detergent and foam booster/stabilizer for industrial detergents; liq.; water-sol.; 25% conc.

Emcol® LO. [Witco/H-I-P] Lauramine oxide; CAS 1643-20-5; EINECS 216-700-6; nonionic; foam booster/stabilizer, visc. modifier; liq.; water-sol.; sp.gr. 0.96.

Emcol® M. [Witco/H-I-P] Myristamine oxide; CAS 3332-27-2; EINECS 222-059-3; cationic; cosmetics and toiletries surfactant used as antistat, cleansing and substantive agent, emollient, lubricant, and visc. builder; detergent and foam booster/stabilizer for industrial detergents; liq.; water-sol.; 25% conc.

Emcol® MO. [Witco/H-I-P] Myristamine oxide; CAS 3332-27-2; EINECS 222-059-3; cosmetic surfactant.

Emcol® NA-30. [Witco/H-I-P] Cocamidopropyl betaine; amphoteric; cosmetics/toiletries surfactant used as antistat, cleansing, foaming, spreading agent, conditioner, foam booster/stabilizer, visc. modifier; lime soap dispersant; Gardner 3 liq.; water-sol.; sp.gr. 1.03; clear pt. 0 C; 36% act.; formerly Emcol 5430.

Emcol® SML. [Witco/H-I-P] Stearamidopropyl morpholine lactate; CAS 55852-14-7; EINECS 259-860-2; conditioner.

Emcol® SO. [Witco/H-I-P] Stearamine oxide; CAS 2571-88-2; EINECS 219-919-5; conditioner, surfactant.

Emcompress®. [Mendell] Dibasic calcium phosphate dihydrate USP/BP; CAS 7789-77-7; excipient, filler for prod. of pharmaceutical tablets by direct compression process; conforms to USP and FCC; wh. free-flowing powd.; avg. particle size 136 µ; 15% max. -200 mesh; readily sol. in dilute hydrochloric and nitric acids; relatively insol. in water and alcohol; dens. (tapped) 0.91 g/ml.

EmCon CO. [Fanning] Castor oil USP; CAS 8001-79-4; EINECS 232-293-8; skin conditioning agent, occlusive solv. for use in lipsticks, eye shadow, blushes, makeup, nail polish; Gardner 1 liq.; sp.gr. 0.957-0.961; acid no. 2 max.; iodine no. 83-88; sapon. no. 176-182; hyd. no. 160-168.

EmCon COCO. [Fanning] Coconut oil; CAS 8001-31-8; EINECS 232-282-8; cosmetic ingred.; Gardner 2 max. liq.; acid no. 0.5 max.; iodine no. 8-12; sapon. no. 260; hyd. no. 3; cloud pt. 22 C.

EmCon COD. [Fanning] Cod liver oil; CAS 8001-69-2; EINECS 232-289-6; cosmetic ingred.; acid no. 1 max.; iodine no. 145-180; sapon. no. 180-192.

EmCon COPA. [Fanning] Balsam copaiba; CAS 8001-61-4; EINECS 232-288-0; moisturizer and lubricant for hair and skin care prods.; colorless liq., char. odor; sp.gr. 0.900;

flash pt. (CC) 100 C; ref. index 1.4966.

EmCon Cotton. [Fanning] Cottonseed oil; CAS 8001-29-4; EINECS 232-280-7; cosmetic ingred.

Emcon E. [Fanning] Mixt. of glycerides, phosphatides, and sterols derived from egg; nonionic; emulsifier, emollient; liq.; 100% conc.

EmCon E-5. [Fanning] Egg oil; CAS 8001-17-0; EINECS 232-271-8; emollient, moisturizer for hair and skin care prods.; w/o emulsifier; superfatting agent, humectant, mold release agent; occlusive agent; yel. liq.; sol. in min. and veg. oils, slightly disp. in most org. solv., insol. water; sp.gr. 0.95; 85.4% triglycerides.

EmCon Eucalyptus. [Fanning] Eucalyptus oil; CAS 8000-48-4; cosmetic ingred.

EmCon Ginger. [Fanning] Ginger oil; CAS 8007-08-7; cosmetic ingred.

EmCon Hazelnut. [Fanning] Hazelnut oil; cosmetic ingred.

EmCon Limnanthes Alba. [Fanning] Meadowfoam seed oil; skin/hair conditioner, occlusive agent for shampoos, makeup, face, body and hand creams and lotions, baby prods., lipsticks, cleansing prods.; Gardner 6 max. color; sol. in castor and min. oils, ethyl acetate, IPM; sl. sol. in glycerin, ethanol; insol. in water; acid no. 0.1 max.; iodine no. 85-100; sapon. no. 165-185; cloud pt. 4.5 C.

EmCon MAC. [Fanning] Macadamia nut oil; cosmetic ingred.

EmCon Olive. [Fanning] Olive oil; CAS 8001-25-0; EINECS 232-277-0; skin and hair conditioning agent, occlusive solv. for shampoos, tonics, cleansing prods., face/body/hand lotions, suntan gels, creams, and lotions; pale straw clear liq., bland odor; sp.gr. 0.910-0.915; acid no. 3.5 max.; iodine no. 79-88; sapon. no. 190-195.

EmCon Orange. [Fanning] Orange oil; CAS 8008-57-9; cosmetic ingred.

EmCon ORO. [Fanning] Orange roughy oil; cosmetic ingred.

EmCon Peanut. [Fanning] Peanut oil; CAS 8002-03-7; EINECS 232-296-4; cosmetic ingred.; Gardner 2 max. liq.; acid no. 0.5 max.; iodine no. 83-105; sapon. no. 185-195; hyd. no. 2; cloud pt. 10 C.

EmCon Rice Bran. [Fanning] Rice bran oil; CAS 68553-81-1; EINECS 271-397-8; skin conditioning agent, occlusive solv. for face powds., cleansing prods., moisturizing creams and lotions; sp.gr. 0.971-0.973; acid no. 0.10 max.; iodine no. 102-110; sapon. no. 185-195.

EmCon Rose. [Fanning] Rose oil; cosmetic ingred.

EmCon Soya. [Fanning] Soybean oil; CAS 8001-22-7; EINECS 232-274-4; cosmetic ingred.; Gardner 1.5 max. liq.; acid no. 0.5 max.; iodine no. 83-87; sapon. no. 185-195; hyd. no. 5; cloud pt. 13 C.

EmCon Spearmint. [Fanning] Spearmint oil; CAS 8008-79-5; cosmetic ingred.

EmCon Tea Tree. [Fanning] Tea tree oil distilled from leaves of *Melaleuca alternifolia*; CAS 68647-73-4; fragrance component, antimicrobial; sp.gr. 0.920-0.930; ref. index 1.472-1.482.

EmCon W. [Fanning] Wheat germ oil; CAS 8006-95-9; skin/hair conditioner, occlusive solv.; for hair conditioners, shampoos, lipsticks, cleansers, moisturizing creams and lotions, skin care prods.; Gardner 10 max. oil; acid no. 0.5 max.; iodine no. 120-135; sapon. no. 180-195.

EmCon Walnut. [Fanning] Walnut oil; CAS 8024-09-7; skin conditioning agent, occlusive solv. for suntan gels, creams, and lotions; clear oil, sl. nutty odor; iodine no. 145-158; sapon. no. 180-200.

Emcosoy®. [Mendell] Soy polysaccharides; CAS 68513-95-1; nonionic; tablet disintegrant for direct compression prep.; wh. to lt. tan gran. powd.; avg. particle size 50 µ; 90% -100 mesh; dens. (tapped) 0.54 g/ml max.; pH 6.5-7.5 (5% slurry).

Emdex®. [Mendell] Dextrates NF [dextrose (95%), isomaltose (2%), gentiobiose (2%), maltose (1%), maltotriose (< 0.1%), panose (< 0.5%)] CAS 50-99-7; EINECS 200-075-1; vehicle for direct compression of pharmaceutical tablets; sweet taste; avg. particle size 211 µ; 25% max. -100 mesh; sol. 100 g/100 ml in water; insol. in alcohol and common org. solvs.; dens. (tapped) 0.77 g/ ml; pH 3.8-5.8.

Emdex® Plus. [Mendell] Dextrates; CAS 50-99-7; EINECS 200-075-1; vehicle for direct compression of pharmaceutical tablets, incl. chewable tablets; free-flowing porous spheres; avg. particle size 211 µ; 30% max. -100 mesh; dens. (tapped) 0.90 g/ml max.; pH 4.5-7.5 (20% aq.).

Emercide® 1199. [Henkel/Cospha; Henkel Canada] Phenoxyethanol and chloroxylenol; liquid preservative system for cosmetics; USA approval; Gardner 1 clear liq., odorless; sol. in triolein, IPA, IPM; disp. in water, min. oil, glycerin; dens. 9.3 lb/gal; pour pt. -10 C; flash pt. 285 F; usage level: 0.3-0.5%; 100% act.

Emeressence® 1150. [Henkel/Organic Prods.] Ethylene brassylate; CAS 105-95-3; EINECS 203-347-8; musk chemical for fragrance or odor masking applics.; Gardner 1 liq.; sol. @ 5% in min. oil, triolein, IPA, IPM; dens. 8.7 lb/ gal; visc. 41 cSt (100 F); pour pt. < 3 C; flash pt. 370 F; 100% act.

Emeressence® 1160 Rose Ether. [Henkel/Organic Prods.] Phenoxyethanol; CAS 122-99-6; EINECS 204-589-7; cosmetic preservative; effective against gram negative microorganisms; liq.; 100% act.

Emerest® 2310. [Henkel/Cospha; Henkel Canada] Isopropyl isostearate; EINECS 250-651-1; low visc. emollient, lubricant for bath oils, creams, lotions, shampoos; binder for pressed powd.; lt. yel. clear liq.; sol. in castor oil, ethanol, IPA, lanolin, min. oil, peanut oil, silicone; acid no. 1 max.; iodine no. 3 max.; sapon. no. 170-180.

Emerest® 2314. [Henkel/Cospha; Henkel Canada] Isopropyl myristate; CAS 110-27-0; EINECS 203-751-4; nonoily emollient for bath oils, makeup, creams, lotions, hair and nail care preps.; sewing thread lubricant; water-wh. clear liq.; sol. 5% in min. oil, toluene, IPA, xylene; water-insol.; dens. 7.1 lb/gal; visc. 4 cSt (100 F); pour pt. –5 C; acid no. 1 max.; iodine no. 1 max.; flash pt. 320 F.

Emerest® 2316. [Henkel/Cospha; Henkel Canada] Isopropyl palmitate; CAS 142-91-6; EINECS 205-571-1; lubricant used for syn. fibers in applics. where low friction is essential; nonoily emollient with exc. spreading props. for cosmetic formulations; high purity; pale yel. clear liq.; sol. 5% in min. oil, toluene, IPA, xylene; insol. in water; dens. 7.1 lb/gal; visc. 6 cSt (100 F); acid no. 1 max.; iodine no. 1 max.; pour pt. 14 C; flash pt. 340 F.

Emerest® 2325. [Henkel/Cospha; Henkel Canada] Butyl stearate; CAS 123-95-5; EINECS 204-666-5; nonionic; emollient in creams and lotions, hair care prods.; dye solubilizer in lipsticks; lubricant; water-wh. clear liq.; sol. 5% in min. oil, toluene, IPA, xylene; water-insol.; dens. 7.1 lb/gal; visc. 7 cSt (100 F); acid no. 1 max.; iodine no. 0.5 max.; pour pt. 18 C; flash pt. 370 F.

Emerest® 2350. [Henkel/Cospha; Henkel Canada] Glycol stearate; CAS 111-60-4; EINECS 203-886-9; nonionic; emulsifier, opacifying and pearlescing agent, thickener, stabilizer used in liq. cosmetic and detergent compds.; wh. waxy solid; sol. @ 5% in IPA, toluol, min. oil, xylene; f.p. 50 C; HLB 2.2; acid no. 4 max.; iodine no. 0.5 max.; sapon. no. 185; flash pt. 390 F; 100% act.

Emerest® 2355. [Henkel/Cospha; Henkel Canada] Glycol distearate; CAS 627-83-8; EINECS 211-014-3; nonionic; emulsifier, opacifier, pearlescent, thickener, stabilizer used in liq. detergent and cosmetic prods.; wh. waxy flakes; sol. 5% in toluene, xylene; disp. in min. oil; insol. in water; f.p. 62 C; HLB 1.3; acid no. 6 max.; iodine no. 1 max.; sapon no. 195; flash pt. 455 F; 100% act.

Emerest® 2380. [Henkel/Cospha; Henkel/Textiles; Henkel

Canada] Propylene glycol stearate; CAS 1323-39-3; EINECS 215-354-3; nonionic; aux. emulsifier, opacifier, pearlescent; for lotions, makeup, textile processing; wh. waxy solid; disp. @ 5% in min. oil, toluene, xylene; insol. in water; dens. 7.3 lb/gal (45 C); HLB 1.8; m.p. 36 C; acid no. 3 max.; iodine no. 0.5 max.; sapon. no. 171-183; flash pt. 470 F; 100% conc.

Emerest® 2384. [Henkel/Cospha; Henkel Canada; Henkel KGaA/Cospha] Propylene glycol isostearate; CAS 68171-38-0; EINECS 269-027-5; solubilizer for fragrances in low alcohol or oil preparations; emollient, stabilizer, and lubricant with dry, nongreasy feel in personal care prods.; lt. yel. clear liq.; sol. in most cosmetic oils, triolein, ethanol, min. oil, toluene, IPA, IPM, xylene; disp. in glycerin; insol. in water; dens. 7.1 lb/gal; visc. 27 cSt (100 F); HLB 1.8; acid no. 4 max.; iodine no. 3 max.; pour pt. < 4 C.

Emerest® 2388. [Henkel/Cospha; Henkel/Textiles; Henkel Canada] Propylene glycol dipelargonate; CAS 41395-83-9; EINECS 255-350-9; lubricant, low visc. emollient with exc. skin penetrating and spreading props. without greasy feel; for preshaves, bath oils, creams and lotions, textile processing; water-wh. liq., odorless; sol. in castor oil, ethanol, IPA, lanolin, min. oil, silicone; dens. 7.6 lb/gal; visc. 11 cSt (100 F); HLB 2.2; acid no. 0.5 max.; iodine no. 1 max.; sapon. no. 305-320; flash pt. 380 F.

Emerest® 2389. [Henkel/Organic Prods.] Propylene glycol isostearate; CAS 68171-38-0; EINECS 269-027-5; solubilizer, cosmetic ingred.

Emerest® 2400. [Henkel/Cospha; Henkel Canada] Glyceryl stearate; nonionic; emulsifier for hand creams, cosmetics, textiles, industrial lubricants, polishes, agric.; lubricant softener for textiles; opacifier and pearling agent; EPA-exempt; wh. flakes; sol. 5% in IPA, hot toluol, hot min. oil; insol. in water; HLB 3.9; m.p. 52-58 C; flash pt. 415 F; acid no. 2.0; iodine no. 2.0; sapon. no. 165-175; flash pt. 415 F; 100% act.

Emerest® 2401. [Henkel/Emery; Henkel/Cospha; Henkel/ Textiles; Henkel Canada] Glyceryl stearate, tech. grade; nonionic; emulsifier and opacifier for hand creams, cosmetics, industrial lubricants, agric., polishes, textiles; EPA-exempt; Gardner 2 beads; sol. @ 5% in IPA, hot toluol, hot min. oil; m.p. 58 C; HLB 3.9; flash pt. 425 F; sapon. no. 153; 100% act.

Emerest® 2407. [Henkel/Emery; Henkel/Cospha; Henkel Canada] Glyceryl stearate SE; nonionic; cosmetic ester; self-emulsifying raw material for emulsions, hair conditioners, creams, lotions, ointments; industrial surfactant for agric. formulation; EPA-exempt; wh. waxy beads; sol. in IPA; sol. hot in min. oil, toluene; disp. in water, xylene; sp.gr. 0.920; m.p. 58 C; HLB 5.1; acid no. 20 max.; iodine no. 1.0 max.; sapon. no. 148–158; cloud pt. < 25 C; flash pt. 385 F.

Emerest® 2410. [Henkel/Cospha; Henkel/Textiles; Henkel Canada] Glyceryl isostearate; nonionic; emollient, lubricant, pearling agent, and w/o emulsifier for creams and lotions, textile applics.; exc. oxidation and color stability; Gardner 2 liq.; sol. @ 5% in min. oil, IPA; insol. in water; dens. 7.8 lb/gal; visc. 260 cSt (100 F); HLB 2.9; acid no. 5 max.; iodine no. 3 max.; sapon. no. 162-172; pour pt. 5 C; flash pt. 400 F; 100% conc.

Emerest® 2421. See Witconol 2421

Emerest® 2423. [Henkel/Cospha; Henkel/Textiles; Henkel Canada] Triolein; CAS 122-32-7; EINECS 204-534-7; nonionic; lubricant, w/o emulsifier for metals, leather, textiles, cosmetics, pharmaceuticals; called syn. olive oil; sulfated form used as softener in leather and textile industries; Gardner 3 liq.; sol. 5% in min. oil, xylene; dens. 7.6 lb/gal; visc. 43 cs; HLB 0.6; pour pt. 9 C; flash pt. 293 C; sapon. no. 197; 100% act.

Emerest® 2452. [Henkel/Cospha; Henkel Canada] Polyglyceryl-3 diisostearate; CAS 66082-42-6; nonionic; emulsifier, solubilizer, dye and pigment wetter; emollient; thickener; solv.; for creams, lotions, lip prods.; amber visc. liq.; sol. @ 5% in min. oil, triolein, IPA, IPM; disp. in glycerin; dens. 8.2 lb/gal; visc. 990 cSt (100 F); HLB 6.7; acid no. 20 max.; iodine no. 0.5 max.; sapon. no. 165-175; pour pt. 4 C; flash pt. 455 F; 100% conc.

Emerest® 2486. [Henkel/Emery; Henkel/Textiles] Pentaerythrityl tetrapelargonate; CAS 14450-05-6; EINECS 238-430-8; nonionic; nongreasy emollient for skin prods.; textile lubricant; lt. yel. clear liq.; sol. @ 5% in min. oil, triolein, IPA, IPM; dens. 8.0 lb/gal; visc. 34 cSt (100 F); HLB 3.3; pour pt. 10 C; flash pt. 550 F; 100% act.

Emerest® 2642. [Henkel/Emery; Henkel/Cospha; Henkel Canada] PEG-8 distearate; CAS 9005-08-7; nonionic; lipophilic waxy surfactant used as emulsifier and thickener in cosmetic, agric. and industrial emulsions; EPA-exempt; Gardner 2 solid; sol. (5%) in min. oil, butyl stearate, glycol trioleate, Stod., xylene; water-disp.; visc. 52 cSt (100 F); HLB 7.5; m.p. 36 C; flash pt. 470 F; cloud pt. < 25 C; 100% conc.

Emerest® 2662. [Henkel/Emery; Henkel/Cospha; Henkel/Textiles; Henkel Canada] PEG-12 stearate; CAS 9004-99-3; nonionic; emulsifier for cosmetic, agric., textile formulations; textile lubricants and softeners; visc. modifier in creams and lotions; EPA-exempt; Gardner 1 solid; sol. 5% in xylene; water-disp.; dens. 8.5 lb/gal; m.p. 40 C; flash pt. 440 F; cloud pt. 55 C; 100% conc.

Emerest® 2701. [Henkel/Organic Prods.] PEG-12 isostearate; CAS 56002-14-3; emulsifier.

Emerest® 2704. [Henkel/Cospha; Henkel Canada] PEG-4 dilaurate; CAS 9005-02-1; nonionic; emulsifier, lubricant, dispersant for bath oils; visc. control agent for creams and lotions; for cosmetic and industrial applics.; yel. clear liq.; sol. @ 5% in min. oil, triolein, IPA; disp. in water, IPM, glycerin; dens. 8.0 lb/gal; visc. 22 cSt (100 F); HLB 7.6; acid no. 10 max.; iodine no. 10 max.; sapon. no. 175-185; pour pt. 0 C; cloud pt. < 25 C; flash pt. 455 F; 100% conc.

Emerest® 2711. [Henkel/Cospha; Henkel Canada] PEG-8 stearate; CAS 9004-99-3; nonionic; emulsifier, thickener for o/w and w/o systems, industrial and cosmetic applics.; Gardner 1 waxy solid; sol. @ 5% in glycerin; disp. in water, min. oil, triolein, IPA, IPM; dens. 8.5 lb/gal (35 C); visc. 57 cSt (100 F); HLB 11.4; m.p. 30 C; acid no. 5 max.; iodine no. 1 max.; sapon. no. 82-92; cloud pt. < 25 C; flash pt. 500 F; 100% conc.

Emerest® 2712. [Henkel/Cospha; Henkel Canada] PEG-8 distearate; CAS 9005-08-7; nonionic; emulsifier, opacifier, thickener for firm creams and high-visc. lotions; for cosmetic and industrial applics.; wh. waxy solid; sol. @ 5% in min. oil, triolein, IPA; disp. in IPM, glycerin; dens. 7.9 lb/gal (53 C); visc. 52 cSt (100 F); HLB 8.1; m.p. 36 C; acid no. 10 max.; iodine no. 1 max.; sapon. no. 115-125; cloud pt. < 25 C; flash pt. 470 F; 100% conc.

Emerest® 2715. [Henkel/Cospha; Henkel/Textiles; Henkel Canada] PEG-40 stearate; CAS 9004-99-3; nonionic; emulsifier, stabilizer, antigellant, lubricant for creams, lotions, shampoos, deodorants, makeup, pharmaceuticals; textile softener; wh. waxy solid or flake; sol. @ 5% in water, IPA; dens. 8.9 lb/gal (50 C); HLB 17.3; m.p. 50 C; acid no. 1 max.; sapon. no. 25-35; cloud pt. 75–81 C (5% saline); flash pt. 515 F; 100% conc.

Emerest® 2717. [Henkel/Organic Prods.] PEG-100 stearate; CAS 9004-99-3; emulsifier, thickener for creams and lotions.

Emericide 1199. [Henkel/Organic Prods.] Phenoxyethanol and chloroxylenol.

Emersol® 110. [Henkel/Emery] Stearic acid; CAS 57-11-4; EINECS 200-313-4; detergent intermediate; opacifier in cosmetics, soaps, emulsifiers, chemical specialties; acid no. 205–210; iodine no. 8–12.

Emersol® 120. [Henkel/Emery] Stearic acid; CAS 57-11-4; EINECS 200-313-4; detergent intermediate; opacifier in cosmetics, soaps, emulsifiers, chemical specialties; acid no. 205-210; iodine no. 5-7.

Emersol® 132 NF Lily®. [Henkel/Emery] Triple pressed stearic acid; CAS 57-11-4; EINECS 200-313-4; detergent intermediate; opacifier in cosmetics, soaps, emulsifiers, chemical specialties; acid no. 205–210; iodine no. 0.5 max.

Emersol® 142. [Henkel/Emery] Palmitic acid; CAS 57-10-3; EINECS 200-312-9; surfactant intermediate; soap and cosmetic formulations.

Emersol® 143. [Henkel/Emery] Palmitic acid; CAS 57-10-3; EINECS 200-312-9; detergent intermediate; opacifier in cosmetics, soaps, emulsifiers, chemical specialties; acid no. 215–223; iodine no. 1 max.

Emersol® 144. [Henkel/Emery] Palmitic acid; CAS 57-10-3; EINECS 200-312-9; surfactant intermediate; soap and cosmetic formulations.

Emersol® 150. [Henkel/Emery] Stearic acid; CAS 57-11-4; EINECS 200-313-4; detergent intermediate; acid no. 197-202; iodine no. 1 max.

Emersol® 210. [Henkel/Emery] Oleic acid; CAS 112-80-1; EINECS 204-007-1; detergent intermediate for personal care, emollient, household and industrial applics.; acid no. 197-204; iodine no. 87-95.

Emersol® 213 NF. [Henkel/Emery] Low-titer oleic acid; CAS 112-80-1; EINECS 204-007-1; detergent intermediate for personal care, emollient, household and industrial applics.; acid no. 199-204; iodine no. 88-95.

Emersol® 221 NF. [Henkel/Emery] Low-titer wh. oleic acid; CAS 112-80-1; EINECS 204-007-1; detergent intermediate for personal care, emollient, household and industrial applics.; acid no. 199-204; iodine no. 88-95.

Emersol® 233 LL. [Henkel/Emery] Oleic acid; CAS 112-80-1; EINECS 204-007-1; detergent intermediate for personal care, emollient, household and industrial applics.; acid no. 200-204; iodine no. 86-90.

Emersol® 315. [Henkel/Emery] Linoleic acid; CAS 60-33-3; EINECS 200-470-9; detergent intermediate for personal care, emollient, household and industrial applics.; acid no. 195-202; iodine no. 145-160.

Emersol® 871. [Henkel/Emery] Isostearic acid; CAS 30399-84-9; detergent intermediate for personal care, emollient, household and industrial applics.; acid no. 175 min.; iodine no. 12 max.

Emersol® 875. [Henkel/Emery] Isostearic acid; CAS 30399-84-9; detergent intermediate for personal care, emollient, household and industrial applics.; acid no. 187-197; iodine no. 3 max.

Emersol® 6313 NF. [Henkel/Emery] Low-titer oleic acid USP/NF; CAS 112-80-1; EINECS 204-007-1; food grade fatty acid; also as binder, defoamer and lubricant for pesticides; detergent intermediate in personal care, emollients, household/industrial detergents; FDA-approved; EPA-exempt; acid no. 201–204; iodine no. 88–93.

Emersol® 6320. [Henkel/Emery] Stearic acid, double pressed; CAS 57-11-4; EINECS 200-313-4; food grade fatty acid; also as binder, defoamer, lubricant in pesticides; detergent intermediate in personal care, emollients, household/industrial detergents; FDA-approved; EPA-exempt; acid no. 205–210; iodine no. 3.5–5.0.

Emersol® 6321 NF. [Henkel/Emery] Low-titer wh. oleic acid UPS/NF; CAS 112-80-1; EINECS 204-007-1; food grade fatty acid; also as binder, defoamer and lubricant for pesticides; detergent intermediate in personal care, emollients, household/industrial detergents; FDA-approved; EPA-exempt; acid no. 201–204; iodine no. 87–92.

Emersol® 6332 NF. [Henkel/Emery] Stearic acid, triple pressed; CAS 57-11-4; EINECS 200-313-4; food grade fatty acid; also as binder, defoamer and lubricant in pesticides; detergent intermediate in personal care, emollients, household/industrial detergents; FDA-approved; EPA-exempt; acid no. 205–211; iodine no. 0.5 max.

Emersol® 6333 NF. [Henkel/Emery] Low-linoleic content oleic acid USP/NF; CAS 112-80-1; EINECS 204-007-1; food grade fatty acid; also as binder, defoamer and lubricant for pesticides; detergent intermediate in personal care, emollients, household/industrial detergents; FDA-approved; EPA-exempt; acid no. 200–204; iodine no. 86–91.

Emersol® 6349. [Henkel/Emery] Stearic acid; CAS 57-11-4; EINECS 200-313-4; food grade fatty acid; also as binder, defoamer and lubricant for pesticides; detergent intermediate in personal care, emollients, household/industrial detergents; FDA-approved; EPA-exempt; acid no. 203–206; iodine no. 0.5 max.

Emersol® 6351. [Henkel/Emery] Stearic acid; CAS 57-11-4; EINECS 200-313-4; food grade fatty acid; also as binder, defoamer and lubricant for pesticides; detergent intermediate in personal care, emollients, household/industrial detergents; FDA-approved; EPA-exempt; acid no. 196-201; iodine no. 1.0 max.

Emersol® 7021. [Henkel/Emery] Oleic acid; CAS 112-80-1; EINECS 204-007-1; food grade kosher fatty acid; detergent intermediate in personal care, emollients, household/industrial detergents; FDA-approved; acid no. 196-204; iodine no. 93-104.

Emerwax® 1251. [Henkel/Cospha; Henkel Canada] Syn. ester wax; for lipsticks, makeup, nail care prods., etc.; Gardner 3 solid; disp. @ 5% in min. oil, triolein, IPM; dens. 8.03 lb/gal (75 C); m.p. 75–80 C; flash pt. 400 F; 100% act.

Emerwax® 1253. [Henkel/Cospha; Henkel Canada] Microcrystalline wax; CAS 63231-60-7; EINECS 264-038-1; beeswax substitute; visc. agent for cosmetic formulations incl. sticks, cold creams, makeup; beeswax substitute; Gardner < 5 solid; disp. @ 5% in min. oil, triolein, IPM; dens. 7.1 lb/gal; m.p. 60–80 C; flash pt. 490 F; 100% act.

Emerwax® 1257. [Henkel/Cospha; Henkel Canada] Emulsifying wax NF; nonionic; emulsifier for cosmetic and pharmaceutical creams and lotions; Gardner < 2 wax; sol. @ 5% in triolein, IPA; disp. in water; dens. 8.1 lb/gal; m.p. 48–52 C; flash pt. 355 F; iodine no. 3.5 max.; sapon. no. 14 max.; 100% act.

Emerwax® 1266. [Henkel/Cospha; Henkel Canada] Cetearyl alcohol and ceteareth-20; nonionic; BP type self-emulsifying base; o/w emulsifier for pharmaceuticals, creams, lotions, antiperspirants, hair care prods., depilatories; wh. waxy solid; sol. in IPA; disp. in min. oil, triolein; dens. 8.0 lb/gal; m.p. 47–55 C; flash pt. 355 F; acid no. 1 max.; iodine no. 2 max.; sapon. no. 5 max.; 100% act.

Emery® 621. [Henkel/Emery] Coconut fatty acid; CAS 61788-47-4; EINECS 262-978-7; detergent intermediate in personal care, emollients, household/industrial detergents; Gardner 5 color; acid no. 258-268; iodine no. 5-16.

Emery® 622. [Henkel/Emery] Coconut acid; CAS 61788-47-4; EINECS 262-978-7; detergent intermediate in personal care, emollients, household/industrial detergents; Gardner 2 color; acid no. 268-276; iodine no. 5-10.

Emery® 625. [Henkel/Emery] Partially hydrog. coconut fatty acid; CAS 68938-15-8; detergent intermediate in personal care, emollients, household/industrial detergents; Gardner 1 color; acid no. 269-273; iodine no. 5 max.

Emery® 626. [Henkel/Emery] Low IV ultra coconut fatty acid; CAS 68938-15-8; detergent intermediate in personal care, emollients, household/industrial detergents; Gardner 1 color; acid no. 270-276; iodine no. 1 max.

Emery® 627. [Henkel/Emery] Low IV, stripped ultra coconut fatty acid; CAS 68937-85-9; detergent intermediate in personal care, emollients, household/industrial detergents; Gardner 1 color; acid no. 252-258; iodine no. 1 max.

Emery® 629. [Henkel/Emery] Stripped coconut fatty acid; detergent intermediate in personal care, emollients, household/industrial detergents; Gardner 1 color; acid no. 253-259; iodine no. 5-10.

Emery® 655. [Henkel/Emery] Myristic acid; CAS 544-63-8; EINECS 208-875-2; detergent surfactant; acid no. 243-246; iodine no. 0.5 max.

Emery® 912. [Henkel/Emery] CP/USP glycerin; CAS 56-81-5; EINECS 200-289-5; skin softener, visc. modifier, flavor enhancer, moisturizer, solv., humectant, thickener, and solubilizer in cosmetics, drug vehicles, food applics., glass, ceramics, agric., and adhesives; EPA-exempt; APHA 20 max. visc. liq.; odorless; sp.gr. 1.2517 min.; pour pt. 18 C; 96.0% min. glycerol.

Emery® 916. [Henkel/Emery] CP/USP glycerin; CAS 56-81-5; EINECS 200-289-5; skin softener, visc. modifier, flavor enhancer, moisturizer, solv., humectant, thickener and solubilizer in cosmetics, drug vehicles, food applics., glass, ceramics, agric., and adhesives; EPA-exempt; APHA 20 max. visc. liq.; odorless; sp.gr. 1.2607 min.; pour pt. 18 C; 99.5% min. glycerol.

Emery® 917. [Henkel/Emery] CP/USP kosher glycerin; CAS 56-81-5; EINECS 200-289-5; skin softener, solubilizer, visc. modifier, flavor enhancer, moisturizer, solv., humectant, thickener and solubilizer in cosmetics, drug vehicles, food applics., glass, ceramics, agric., and adhesives; APHA 10 max. color; sp.gr. 1.2612; 99.7% min. glycerol.

Emery® 918. [Henkel/Emery] CP/USP glycerin; CAS 56-81-5; EINECS 200-289-5; skin softener, visc. modifier, flavor enhancer, moisturizer, solv., humectant, and solubilizer in cosmetics, drug vehicles, and food applics., glass, ceramics, and adhesives; APHA 8 max.; sp.gr. 1.2615; 99.8% min. glycerol.

Emery® 1650. [Henkel/Cospha; Henkel/Textiles; Henkel Canada] Anhyd. lanolin USP; CAS 8006-54-0; EINECS 232-348-6; nonionic; emulsifier, emollient, conditioner, lubricant for cosmetics, hair grooming aids, makeup, nail and sun care prods., textiles; yel. amber paste; sol. @ 5% in IPM; disp. in min. oil, triolein; HLB 10.0; dens. 7.9 lb/gal; m.p. 36–42 C; flash pt. 530 F; 100% conc.

Emery® 1656. [Henkel/Cospha; Henkel/Textiles; Henkel Canada] Anhyd. lanolin USP; CAS 8006-54-0; EINECS 232-348-6; emulsifier, emollient, conditioner, moisturizer, pigment dispersant for pharmaceutical ointments, veterinary prods., industrial hand cleansers, cosmetics, textiles; Gardner < –12 paste; sol. in IPM; disp. in min. oil, triolein; dens. 7.9 lb/gal; m.p. 36–42 C; flash pt. 530 F.

Emery® 1660. [Henkel/Cospha; Henkel Canada] Ultra anhyd. lanolin USP, cosmetic grade; CAS 8006-54-0; EINECS 232-348-6; emulsifier, emollient, conditioner, lubricant, moisturizer, pigment dispersant for lip prods.; yel. amber paste; sol. in IPM; disp. in min. oil, triolein; dens. 7.9 lb/gal; m.p. 38–44 C; flash pt. 460 F.

Emery® 1695. [Henkel/Cospha; Henkel Canada] Propoxylated lanolin wax; nonionic; cosmetic additive for adding shine and stability to anhyd. makeup prods.; solid; 100% conc.

Emery® 1730. [Henkel/Cospha; Henkel Canada] Min. oil and lanolin alcohol; nonionic; liq. absorption base, penetrant, w/o emulsifier, emollient, stabilizer for creams, lotions, makeup, shampoos; provides hypoallergenic skin penetration; yel. to straw colored liq.; sol. in min. oil, triolein, IPA, IPM; dens. 7.4 lb/gal; visc. 39 cSt (100 F); pour pt. 18 C; flash pt. 350 F.

Emery® 1732. [Henkel/Cospha; Henkel Canada] Min. oil and lanolin alcohol; liq. absorption base; emollient, emulsion

stabilizer, moisturizer, emulsifier for creams, lotions, hair dressings, makeup, topical pharmaceutical preps.; yel. to straw colored liq.; sol. in min. oil, triolein, IPA, IPM; disp. in glycerin; dens. 7.2 lb/gal; visc. 15 cSt (100 F); pour pt. < 4 C; flash pt. 360 F.

Emery® 1740. [Henkel/Cospha; Henkel Canada] Petrolatum, lanolin, lanolin oil, and min. oil; nonionic; absorption base; emulsifier for w/o systems, emollient, moisturizer for pharmaceutical ointments and hair prods.; very high water absorp.; yel. to straw colored soft solid; sol. in min. oil, IPM; disp. in triolein; dens. 7.4 lb/gal; m.p. 40–46 C; flash pt. 450 F; 100% conc.

Emery® 1747. [Henkel/Cospha; Henkel Canada] Lanolin/ lanolin alcohol blend in petrolatum base; primary w/o emulsifier, aux. o/w emulsifier; emollient, moisturizer for skin and hair care prods., pharmaceutical ointments; Gardner < 6 solid; sol. in min. oil, IPM; disp. in triolein; dens. 7.4 lb/gal; m.p. 40–46 C; flash pt. 425 F.

Emery® 1780. [Henkel/Cospha; Henkel Canada] Lanolin alcohol; CAS 8027-33-6; EINECS 232-430-1; w/o emulsifier, emollient, visc. builder, stabilizer for emulsions, personal care prods.; straw yel. waxy solid; sol. @ 5% in triolein; dens. 8.2 lb/gal; m.p. 48 C; flash pt. 440 F.

Emery® 1795. [Henkel/Organic Prods.] Lanolin alcohol; CAS 8027-33-6; EINECS 232-430-1; emollient, emulsifier.

Emery® 2423. [Henkel/Emery] Triolein; CAS 122-32-7; EINECS 204-534-7; emollient.

Emery® 5315. [Henkel/Organic Prods.] Disodium cocamido MEA-sulfosuccinate; cosmetic surfactant.

Emery® 5327. [Henkel/Organic Prods.] Disodium laneth-5 sulfosuccinate; CAS 68890-92-6.

Emery® 5412. [Henkel/Organic Prods.] Sodium cocoamphoacetate; personal care surfactant.

Emery® 5418. [Henkel/Organic Prods.] Sodium caprylo- amphoacetate; CAS 13039-35-5; EINECS 235-907-2; wetting agent.

Emery® 6709. [Henkel/Cospha; Henkel Canada] PEG 400; CAS 25322-68-3; EINECS 225-856-4; nonionic; humectant, binder, solv., visc. modifier for personal care prods.; chemical intermediate for coatings, adhesives, lubricants, metalworking, paper mfg., petrol. prod., ceramics, printing, electronics, solvs., cleaners, mold release agent; Gardner < 1 clear, visc. liq.; sol. @ 5% in water, xylene; m.w. 400; dens. 9.4 lb/gal; visc. 45 cSt (100 F); pour pt. 6 C; flash pt. > 350 F; 100% act.

Emery® 6744. [Henkel/Cospha; Henkel/Textiles; Henkel Canada] Cocamidopropyl betaine; amphoteric; surfactant, foamer for personal care prods., shampoos, baby preps., skin cleansers; also for textile applics.; yel. clear liq.; sol. in water; disp. in glycerol trioleate; dens. 8.8 lb/gal; visc. 7 cSt (100 F); pour pt. < -2 C; 35% act.

Emery® 6748. [Henkel/Cospha; Henkel Canada] Cocamidopropyl betaine; amphoteric; surfactant, conditioner, mild foaming agent, visc. control agent; used in hair and bath prods., skin cleaners, specialty cosmetics; Gardner 4 liq.; sol. in water; dens. 8.7 lb/gal; 35% act.

Emery® HP-2050. [Henkel/Cospha; Henkel Canada; Henkel KGaA/Cospha] High purity anhyd. lanolin USP; CAS 8006-54-0; EINECS 232-348-6; coemulsifier, emollient, conditioner, moisturizer, pigment dispersant for personal care prods., pharmaceuticals, creams, lotions, lip and baby care prods.; yel. amber paste, weak intrinsic odor; m.p. 38-44; acid no. 1 max.; iodine no. 18-36; sapon. no. 90-105.

Emery® HP-2060. [Henkel/Cospha; Henkel Canada] High purity ultra anhyd. lanolin; CAS 8006-54-0; EINECS 232-348-6; emulsifier, emollient, conditioner, moisturizer, pigment dispersant for personal care prods., lip prods., and pharmaceuticals; pale yel. amber paste, low odor; m.p. 38-44.

Emery® HP-2095. [Henkel KGaA/Cospha] Lanolin alcohol; CAS 8027-33-6; EINECS 232-430-1; coemulsifier and emollient in creams, lotions, lip and baby care prods.; ylsh. liq., weak intrinsic odor; m.p. 58 C min.; acid no. 2 max.; sapon. no. 12 max.; hyd. no. 120-180.

Emid® 6500. [Henkel/Cospha; Henkel Canada] Cocamide MEA (1:1); CAS 68140-00-1; EINECS 268-770-2; nonionic; thickener, foam stabilizer for shampoos, hair coloring prods., liq. detergents, and rug cleaners; Gardner 8 flaked solid; sol. (5%) in min. oil, butyl stearate, glycerol trioleate, Stod.; water-disp.; dens. 7.5 lb/gal (75 C); m.p. 72 C; acid no. 1; flash pt. 405 F; cloud pt. < 25 C; 100% act.

Emid® 6513. [Henkel/Organic Prods.] Lauramide DEA; CAS 120-40-1; EINECS 204-393-1; personal care surfactant.

Emid® 6515. [Henkel/Cospha; Henkel/Textiles; Henkel Canada] Cocamide DEA (1:1); CAS 61791-31-9; EINECS 263-163-9; nonionic; emulsifier, foam booster and stabilizer; inhibits redeposition of soils; thickener, superfatting agent for shampoos, bubble baths, cleansers, liq. detergents; antiredeposition agent for soils on textiles; Gardner 4 liq.; sol. (5%) in water, butyl stearate, glycerol triolate, Stod., xylene; dens. 8.3 lb/gal; visc. 390 cSt (100 F); acid no. 1; pour pt. 0 C; cloud pt. 370 C; flash pt. 370 F; 100% act.

Emid® 6519. [Henkel/Cospha; Henkel Canada] Lauramide DEA (1:1); CAS 120-40-1; EINECS 204-393-1; foam booster, stabilizer, visc. modifier for personal care prods., soaps, bath additives; Gardner < 5 liq.; sol. @ 5% in water, triolein, IPA, IPM, glycerin; dens. 8.1 lb/gal (50 C); acid no. 1; pour pt. < -10 C; flash pt. 345 F.

Emid® 6521. [Henkel/Emery] Cocamide DEA (2:1); CAS 61791-31-9; EINECS 263-163-9; nonionic/anionic; foam booster, stabilizer, thickener in personal care prods., liq. soaps, bath additives; Gardner < 4 liq.; sol. @ 5% in triolein, IPA, IPM; disp. in water, min. oil; dens. 8.4 lb/gal; visc. 327 cSt (100 F); pour pt. -10 C; cloud pt. < 25 C; flash pt. 345 F.

Emid® 6530. [Henkel/Organic Prods.] Cocamide DEA and diethanolamine.

Emid® 6541. [Henkel/Organic Prods.] Lauramide DEA, diethanolamine; nonionic; emulsifier, foam stabilizer and booster in shampoos and general purpose cleaners; Gardner 3 paste; sol. (5%) in water, Stod., xylene; dens. 8.4 lb/gal; visc. 275 cSt (100 F); pour pt. -15 C; flash pt. 300 F; 100% act.

Emid® 6573. [Henkel/Organic Prods.] Ricinoleamide MEA; CAS 106-16-1; EINECS 203-368-2; personal care surfactant.

Emid® 6590. [Henkel/Cospha; Henkel Canada] Lauramide DEA and propylene glycol; foam booster, visc. modifier for personal care prods., bath additives, liq. soaps; Gardner < 4 liq.; sol. @ 5% in triolein, IPA, glycerin; disp. in water; dens. 8.3 lb/gal; pour pt. < 0 C; flash pt. 375 F.

Emkapol 5000. [ICI Surf. Am.] PEG-100; CAS 25322-68-3; cosmetic ingred.

Emkapol 6000. [ICI Surf. Am.] PEG-135; surfactant, carrier, rheology control agent; wh. solid.

Emkapol 8000. [ICI Surf. Am.] PEG-200; CAS 25322-68-3; surfactant, carrier, rheology control agent; wh. solid.

Emkapol 8500. [ICI Surf. Am.] PEG-200; CAS 25322-68-3; surfactant, carrier, rheology control agent; wh. solid.

Emollient HS 235. [Alban Muller] Propylene glycol, pellitory extract, mallow extract, sambucus extract, and ivy extract; botanical extract.

Emollient HS 238. [Alban Muller] Propylene glycol, wheat germ extract, kidney bean extract, carrot seed extract, watercress extract; botanical extract.

Emollient LS 635. [Alban Muller] Sunflower seed oil, pellitory extract, mallow extract, sambucus extract, and ivy extract; botanical extract.

Emphos™ CS-136. [Witco/H-I-P] Nonoxynol-6 phosphate; anionic; lubricant; antistat; emulsifier for cutting fluids, PVAc, and acrylic film formation; detergent for hard surfaces, metal cleaners, and dry cleaning systems; waterless hand cleaner component; personal care formulations; FDA compliance; clear visc. liq.; sol. in water, ethanol, CCl₄, perchloroethylene, heavy aromatic naphtha, kerosene; sp.gr. 1.09; visc. 4500 cps; pour pt. 18 C; acid no. 28; pH 5.0 (3% aq.); surf. tens. 30.0 dynes/cm (1%); Ross-Miles foam 158 mm (initial, 1%, 49 C); 99% solids.

Emphos™ CS-141. [Witco/H-I-P] Nonoxynol-10 phosphate; CAS 51609-41-7; anionic; electrolyte-compatible lubricant for water-based cutting fluids; detergent for heavy-duty, all-purpose liq. formulations; emulsifier in PVAc and acrylic film formation; textile wetting agent; water-repellent fabric finishing; foaming agent; coupling agent; personal care formulations; FDA compliance; clear visc. liq.; sol. in water, 10% sodium hydroxide, ethanol, CCl₄, perchloroethylene, xylene, heavy aromatic naphtha; sp.gr. 1.12; visc. 4500 cps; pour pt. > 4 C; acid no. 65 (to pH 5.5); 110 (to pH 9.5); pH 2.0 (3% aq.); surf. tens. 35 dynes/cm (1%); Ross-Miles foam 168 mm (initial, 1%, 49 C); 99% solids.

Emphos™ CS-147. [Witco/H-I-P] Alkylaryl ethoxylate phosphate ester; anionic; industrial detergent, o/w emulsifier, lubricant, wetting agent, solubilizer, foaming and coupling agent; personal care formulations; liq.; water-sol.; sp.gr. 1.01; acid no. 87 (to pH 5.5), 150 (to pH 9.5); pH 2.0 (3% aq.).

Emphos™ CS-165. [Witco/H-I-P] Org. phosphate ether; anionic; detergent, emulsifier, dispersant, solubilizer; personal care formulations; liq.

Emphos™ CS-1361. [Witco/H-I-P] Sodium nonoxynol-9 phosphate; anionic; antistat; emulsifier for transparent gels; detergent for hard surfaces, metal cleaners, and drycleaning systems; particle dispersant for aq. systems; coupling agent; wetting agent, dispersant for water-based suspension concs., personal care prods.; clear liq.; sol. @ 25% in water, ethanol, CCl₄, perchloroethylene, aromatic naphtha, kerosene; sp.gr. 1.10; pour pt. 4 C; pH 5.0 (10% aq.); surf. tens. 31 dynes/cm (0.05% aq.); 90% conc.

Emphos™ D70-30C. [Witco/H-I-P] Sodium glyceryl oleate phosphate; anionic; antistat, emollient, emulsifier, substantive agent, and moisture barrier for personal care prods.; aerosol formulation and food processing surfactant; food-grade mold lubricant; liq.; oil-sol.

Emphos™ F27-85. [Witco/H-I-P] Hydrog. veg. glycerides phosphate; CAS 85411-01-4; anionic; emulsifier, mold lubricant, release agent for food use; pigment dispersant in oil-based systems; moisture barrier; personal care formulations; tan soft solid; insol. in water; sp.gr. 1.01; pour pt. 17 C; acid no. 40 (to pH 9.5); pH 6.9 (3% aq.).

Emphos™ PS-21A. [Witco/H-I-P] Alcohol ethoxylate phosphate ester; anionic; detergent base, emulsifier, foaming and wetting agent, lubricant, dispersant; used for detergent industry, industrial surfactants, and personal care formulations; clear liq.; sol. in kerosene, xylene, IPA; water-insol.; sp.gr. 1.05; acid no. 130 (to pH 5.5), 200 (to pH 9.5); flash pt. > 93 C; pH 2.0 (10% aq.).

Emphos™ PS-121. [Witco/H-I-P] Linear alcohol ethoxylate phosphate ester, acid form; anionic; emulsifier/lubricant for cutting fluids; drycleaning detergent with antistat properties; textile wetting and scouring agent; personal care formulations; clear liq.; sol. @ 25% in ethanol, CCl₄, perchloroethylene, xylene, heavy aromatic naphtha, kerosene, min. oil; water-disp.; sp.gr. 1.06; pour pt. < 10 C; acid no. 105 (to pH 5.5); 180 (to pH 9.5); surf. tens. 28.6 dynes/cm (0.05% aq.); pH 2.0 (3% aq.).

Emphos™ PS-220. [Witco/H-I-P] Linear alcohol ethoxylate phosphate ester, acid form; anionic; lubricant; improves lubricity and load bearing of oil-based lubricants; mono-mer/water emulsifier; polymer particle dispersant; emulsifier for caustic sol'ns., aliphatic solvs.; textile antistat; detergent; corrosion inhibitor; personal care formulations; clear liq.; sol. @ 25% in ethanol, CCl₄, perchloroethylene, xylene, heavy aromatic naphtha, kerosene, min. oil; insol. in water; sp.gr. 1.02; pour pt. 10 C; acid no. 105 (to pH 5.5); 185 (to pH 185); surf. tens. 32.3 dynes/cm; pH 2.0 (3% aq.).

Emphos™ PS-222. [Witco/H-I-P] Aliphatic phosphate ester; anionic; emulsifier for pesticide formulations, detergents, hydrotropes and emulsion polymerization; corrosion inhibitor; detergent; dispersant; lubricant; personal care formulations; liq.; sol. in oil, disp. in water; sp.gr. 1.02; acid no. 105 (to pH 5.5), 155 (to pH 9.5); pH 2.4 (3% aq.).

Emphos™ PS-236. [Witco/H-I-P] Alcohol ethoxylate phosphate ester; anionic; detergent base, emulsifier, coupling, foaming and wetting agent, corrosion inhibitor, lubricant, antistat, penetrant, and solubilizer used in the detergent industry, industrial surfactants, textile systems; metal cleaning; emulsion polymerization; personal care formulations; liq.; sol. in naphthenic oils and water; sp.gr. 1.05; acid no. 90 (to pH 5.5), 140 (to pH 9.5); pH 2.0 (3% aq.).

Emphos™ PS-331. [Witco/H-I-P] Aliphatic phosphate ester; anionic; detergent, emulsifier, dispersant, foaming and wetting agent, and solubilizer for use with nonionic surfactants; personal care formulations; liq.; sol. in oil, water; sp.gr. 1.13; acid no. 140 (to pH 5.5), 280 (to pH 9.5); pH 1.8 (3% aq.).

Emphos™ PS-400. [Witco/H-I-P] Linear alcohol ethoxylate phosphate ester, acid form; anionic; polymer particle dispersant; monomer/water emulsifier; textile antistat; also for pesticides, detergents, emulsion polymerization, personal care formulations; lubricant; wetting agent; clear liq.; sol. @ 25% in ethanol, CCl₄, perchloroethylene, xylene, heavy aromatic naphtha, kerosene, min. oil; water-disp.; sp.gr. 1.00; pour pt. > 10 C; acid no. 220 (to pH 5.5), 300 (to pH 9.5); surf. tens. 30.6 dynes/cm (0.05% aq.); pH 2.0 (3% aq.).

Emphos™ TS-230. [Witco/H-I-P] Phenol ethoxylate phosphate ester, acid form; anionic; lubricant; improves lubricity and load-bearing of water-based lubricants; industrial corrosion inhibitor, defoamer, metal processing surfactant for syn. oils; low-foaming hydrotrope for alkaline cleaners; personal care formulations; amber clear liq.; sol. @ 25% in water, 10% sodium hydroxide, ethanol; sp.gr. 1.18; pour pt. < 10 C; acid no. 87 (to pH 5.5); 155 (to pH 9.5); pH 2.0 (3% aq.).

Empicol® 0031/T. [Albright & Wilson UK] DEA-lauryl sulfate; CAS 68585-44-4; anionic; detergent used in personal care prods.; liq.; 34% conc.

Empicol® 0045. [Albright & Wilson UK] Sodium lauryl sulfate; CAS 151-21-3; EINECS 205-788-1; anionic; raw material and foaming agent for toothpaste, shampoos, foam baths; wh. fine powd.; dens. 0.30 g/cm³; pH 9.5–10.5 (1% aq.); 94.0% min. act.

Empicol® 0045V. [Albright & Wilson Am.; Albright & Wilson UK] Sodium lauryl sulfate; CAS 151-21-3; EINECS 205-788-1; anionic; raw material and foaming agent for toothpaste, shampoos, foam baths; wh. needles; 88% conc.

Empicol® 0185. [Albright & Wilson UK] Sodium lauryl sulfate; CAS 151-21-3; EINECS 205-788-1; anionic; detergent, wetting and rewetting agent, emulsifier, dispersant, disintegrator; used in personal care prods., pharmaceuticals, dental care, textile printing inks, agric. and horticultural preps., electroplating baths, medical preps.; wh. powd.; dens. 0.35 g/cm³; pH 9.5–10.5 (1% aq.); 94.0% min. act.

Empicol® 0216. [Albright & Wilson UK] Oleth-3 phosphate;

CAS 39464-69-2; anionic; foam stabilizer, conditioner, and antistatic agent for toiletries; detergent used in textile processing; liq.; 95% conc.

Empicol® 0251/70. [Albright & Wilson UK] Sodium laureth sulfate; personal care surfactant.

Empicol® 0303. [Albright & Wilson UK] Sodium lauryl sulfate BP; CAS 151-21-3; EINECS 205-788-1; anionic; surfactant in toothpaste and pharmaceutical preps.; emulsion polymerization; wh. fine powd.; dens. 0.35 g/cc; pH 8-10 (1% aq.); 95% act.

Empicol® 0303V. [Albright & Wilson UK] Sodium lauryl sulfate BP; CAS 151-21-3; EINECS 205-788-1; anionic; surfactant in toothpaste and pharmaceutical preps.; emulsion polymerization; BP and USP compliance; wh. low-dusting needles; pH 8-10 (1% aq.); 95% conc.

Empicol® 0585/A. [Albright & Wilson Am.] Sodium ethylhexyl sulfate; CAS 126-92-1; EINECS 204-812-8; anionic; surfactant for toiletries; low foam degreasing agent for textiles; liq.; 40% conc.

Empicol® 0758. [Albright & Wilson Am.] Sodium decyl sulfate; anionic; surfactant for toiletries; liq.; 40% conc.

Empicol® 0775. [Albright & Wilson Am.] Sodium lauryl/cetostearyl sulfate; anionic; surfactant for toiletries; liq.; 42% conc.

Empicol® 0775/55. [Albright & Wilson Am.] Sodium lauryl/cetostearyl sulfate; anionic; surfactant for toiletries; liq.; 55% conc.

Empicol® 1220/T. [Albright & Wilson UK] MEA-lauryl sulfate; CAS 4722-98-9; EINECS 225-214-3; detergent.

Empicol® 9060X. [Albright & Wilson Am.] Formulated prod.; pearling/opacifying conc. for toiletries; paste; 40% conc.

Empicol® AL30. [Albright & Wilson Australia] Ammonium lauryl sulfate; CAS 68081-96-9; EINECS 218-793-9; anionic; detergent for shampoos, carpet shampoos, leather processing; amber liq./paste; m.w. 291; visc. 14,000 cs; pH 6-7 (5%); 29% act.

Empicol® AL30/T. [Albright & Wilson UK] Ammonium lauryl sulfate; CAS 2235-54-3; EINECS 218-793-9; anionic; detergent for shampoo, shower prods.; liq.; 30% conc.

Empicol® AL70. [Albright & Wilson UK] Ammonium lauryl sulfate; CAS 68081-96-9; EINECS 218-793-9; anionic; detergent and base used in the cosmetic industry for shampoos, bath prods.; yel. to amber liq. to soft paste; set pt. 25 C; pH 6-7 (2% aq.); 70% conc.

Empicol® ALL. [Albright & Wilson Australia] Ammonium lauryl triethoxy sulfate; anionic; shampoo ingred.; liq.; 25% conc.

Empicol® BSD. [Albright & Wilson UK] Sodium magnesium lauryl ethoxy sulfonate; anionic; base detergent and toiletry raw material; liq.; 26% conc.

Empicol® BSD 52. [Albright & Wilson Am.] Sodium/magnesium laureth sulfate; anionic; surfactant for toiletries; liq.; 52% conc.

Empicol® DA. [Albright & Wilson Australia] DEA-lauryl sulfate; CAS 68585-44-4; anionic; ingred. in personal care prods., automobile cleaners; pale yel. visc. liq.; dilutable in water; sp.gr. 1.05; pH 7.0±0.5 (10% aq.); 34.0 ± 1.0% act.

Empicol® EAA. [Albright & Wilson Am.] Ammonium laureth sulfate; CAS 32612-48-9; anionic; surfactant for toiletries; liq.; 24% conc.

Empicol® EAA70. [Albright & Wilson UK] Ammonium laureth sulfate; CAS 67762-19-0; anionic; detergent and toiletry raw material; base for personal care prods.; liq.; 70% conc.

Empicol® EAB. [Albright & Wilson UK] Ammonium laureth sulfate; CAS 67762-19-0; anionic; detergent and base used in the cosmetic industry; liq.; 23% conc.

Empicol® EAB70. [Albright & Wilson UK] Ammonium laureth sulfate; CAS 67762-19-0; anionic; detergent and raw material for cosmetics, toiletries; liq.; 70% conc.

Empicol® EAB/T. [Albright & Wilson UK] Ammonium laureth sulfate; CAS 32612-48-9; surfactant.

Empicol® EAC. [Albright & Wilson Am.] Ammonium laureth sulfate; CAS 32612-48-9; anionic; surfactant for toiletries; liq.; 25% conc.

Empicol® EAC70. [Albright & Wilson Am.; Albright & Wilson UK] Ammonium laureth sulfate; CAS 32612-48-9; anionic; surfactant in pearly shampoos and shower prods.; amber hazy visc. liq.; set pt. 6 C; pH 6-7 (2% aq.); 70% conc.

Empicol® EAC/T. [Albright & Wilson UK] Ammonium laureth sulfate; CAS 32612-48-9; surfactant.

Empicol® EGB. [Albright & Wilson UK] Magnesium laureth sulfate; CAS 67702-21-4; anionic; detergent and toiletry raw material; liq.; 25% conc.

Empicol® EGC. [Albright & Wilson Am.] Magnesium laureth sulfate; CAS 62755-21-9; anionic; surfactant for toiletries; liq.; 27% conc.

Empicol® EMB. [Albright & Wilson UK] MEA-laureth sulfate; anionic; detergent raw material for shampoos; 30% conc.

Empicol® ESA. [Albright & Wilson UK] Sodium laureth sulfate; CAS 68585-34-2; anionic; detergent and toiletry raw material; liq.; 25% conc.

Empicol® ESA70. [Albright & Wilson UK] Sodium laureth sulfate; CAS 68585-34-2; anionic; detergent and toiletry raw material; liq.; 70% conc.

Empicol® ESB. [Albright & Wilson Australia] Sodium laureth sulfate; CAS 9004-82-4; 68585-34-2; anionic; shampoo ingred.; mild detergent for textile and leather processing; dispersant/emulsifier for emulsion and suspension polymerization; liq.; 28% conc.

Empicol® ESB3. [Albright & Wilson Am.; Albright & Wilson UK] Sodium laureth sulfate; CAS 9004-82-4; 68585-34-2; anionic; base and foam booster/stabilizer for personal care prods.; air entraining agent for construction; colorless-pale yel. liq.; dens. 1.05 g/cm³; visc. 2600 cs (20 C); cloud pt. < 0 C; pH 6.5-7.5 (5% aq.); 27.5 ± 1.0% act.

Empicol® ESB3/D. [Albright & Wilson UK] Sodium laureth sulfate; anionic; base and foam booster/stabilizer for toiletries; colorless liq.; dens. 1.05 g/cm³; visc. 750 cs (20 C); cloud pt. < 0 C; pH 6.5-7.5 (5% aq.); 27% conc.

Empicol® ESB3/M. [Albright & Wilson Am.] Sodium laureth sulfate; anionic; surfactant for toiletries; liq.; 27% conc.

Empicol® ESB70. [Albright & Wilson Am.; Albright & Wilson UK] Sodium laureth sulfate; CAS 68585-34-2; anionic; detergent and toiletry raw material; for shampoos, foam baths; pale straw hazy visc. liq.; dens. 1.1 g/cm³; set pt. 7 C; pH 7.0-9.0 (2% aq.); 68.0 ± 2.0% act.

Empicol® ESB70-AU. [Albright & Wilson Australia] Sodium laureth sulfate; anionic; shampoo ingred.; pale yel. hazy liq.; dens. 1.1 g/cm³; pH 8.0 ± 1.0 (2% aq.); 68.0 ± 2.5% act.

Empicol® ESC/AU. [Albright & Wilson Australia] Sodium laureth sulfate; CAS 68585-34-2; anionic; surfactant used as a base in personal care prods.; pale yel. clear liq.; dilutable in water; sp.gr. 1.05; visc. 140 cP max.; pH 7.2 ± 0.6 (1% aq.); 27.5 ± 1.0% act.

Empicol® ESC3. [Albright & Wilson UK] Sodium laureth sulfate; CAS 68585-34-2; anionic; raw material used in the formulation of personal care prods.; colorless clear liq.; dens. 1.0 g/cm³; visc. 35 cs; cloud pt. 0 C; pH 6.0-8.0 (5% aq.); 28.0 ± 1.0% act.

Empicol® ESC70. [Albright & Wilson Am.] Sodium laureth sulfate; anionic; raw material for toiletries, shampoos, foam baths; pale straw visc. hazy liq.; dens. 1.1 g/cm³; pH 7.0-8.0 (5% aq.); 69.5 ± 2.0% act.

Empicol® ESC70/AU. [Albright & Wilson Australia] Sodium laureth sulfate; anionic; base for personal care prods.; pale yel. visc. liq.; dilutable in water; sp.gr. 1.1; visc. 210

cP max.; cloud pt. 2 C max.; pH 7.2 ± 0.6 (2%); 68.0 ± 2.5% act.

Empicol® ETB. [Albright & Wilson UK] TEA-laureth sulfate; CAS 27028-82-6; anionic; detergent and toiletry raw material; liq.; 30% conc.

Empicol® LM45. [Albright & Wilson UK] Sodium lauryl sulfate; CAS 151-21-3; EINECS 205-788-1; primary act. ingred., detergent, and foaming agent used in personal care and household prods.; wh. paste; dens. 0.95 g/cm³; pH 8.0–10.0 (2% aq.); 45% act.

Empicol® LQ33. [Albright & Wilson Australia] MEA-lauryl sulfate; CAS 68908-44-1; EINECS 225-214-3; anionic; surfactant used in the formulation of personal care prods.; lt. amber clear to opalescent visc. liq.; sp.gr. 1.05; visc. 17 cSt max.; cloud pt. 2 C max.; pH 7.0 ± 0.5 (5% aq.); 33.5% ± 1.0% act.

Empicol® LQ33/T. [Albright & Wilson UK] MEA-lauryl sulfate; CAS 4722-98-9; 68908-44-1; EINECS 225-214-3; anionic; surfactant in the mfg. of personal care prods.; emulsifier in the mfg. of rubber latices and for resins; bactericidal detergents; pale amber visc. liq.; dens. 1.03 g/cm³ visc. 6000 cs; pH 7.0 ± 0.5 (5% aq.); 33.5 ± 1.0% act.

Empicol® LQ70. [Albright & Wilson UK] MEA-lauryl sulfate; CAS 4722-98-9; EINECS 225-214-3; detergent and toiletry raw material; base for personal care prods.; liq.; 70% conc.

Empicol® LS30B. [Albright & Wilson Australia] Sodium lauryl sulfate; CAS 151-21-3; EINECS 205-788-1; base for personal care prods.; pale yel. clear visc. liq.; visc. 800 ± 200 cP; pH 8.5 ± 1.0 (10%); 30.0 ± 1.0% act.

Empicol® LS30P. [Albright & Wilson Australia] Sodium lauryl sulfate; CAS 68585-47-7; anionic; emulsifier, wetting and foaming agent for emulsion polymerization and carpet and upholstery shampoos; base for personal care shampoos; specialty cleaners and industrial processes; pale yel. paste; sp.gr. 1.05; visc. 120 cP max.; pH 7.5 ± 0.7 (10% aq.); 30.0 ± 1.0% act.

Empicol® LX. [Albright & Wilson Am.; Albright & Wilson UK] Sodium lauryl sulfate; CAS 68585-47-4; anionic; emulsifier in the mfg. of plastics, resins, and syn. rubbers; foaming agent for rubber foams, personal care prods., pharmaceuticals, and carpet and upholstery shampoos; lubricant in mfg. of molded rubber goods; wh. powd.; dens. 0.35 g/cm³; pH 9.5–10.5 (1% aq.); 90% act.

Empicol® LX28. [Albright & Wilson Am.; Albright & Wilson UK] Sodium lauryl sulfate; CAS 151-21-3; EINECS 205-788-1; anionic; emulsifier in the mfg. of plastics, resins, and syn. rubbers; foaming agent for rubber foams, personal care prods., toothpaste, and carpet and upholstery shampoos; lubricant in mfg. of molded rubber goods; pale yel. liq., paste; dens. 1.05 g/cm³; pH 8.0–9.5 (5% aq.); 28% act. aq. sol'n.

Empicol® LX100. [Albright & Wilson Am.; Albright & Wilson UK] Sodium lauryl sulfate; CAS 151-21-3; EINECS 205-788-1; anionic; surfactant in toothpaste, pharmaceutical, toiletry preps.; powd.; 97% act.

Empicol® LXS95. [Albright & Wilson UK] Sodium lauryl sulfate; CAS 151-21-3; EINECS 205-788-1; anionic; detergent, foamer, emulsifier used in toothpastes, emulsion polymerization, rubber, pharmaceuticals; wh. powd.; dens 0.35 g/cm³; pH 9.6–10.5 (1% aq.); 94.0% min. act.

Empicol® LXV. [Albright & Wilson Am.; Albright & Wilson UK] Sodium lauryl sulfate; CAS 151-21-3; EINECS 205-788-1; anionic; emulsifier in the mfg. of plastics, resins, and syn. rubbers; foaming agent for rubber foams, personal care prods., toothpaste, and carpet and upholstery shampoos; lubricant in mfg. of molded rubber goods; wh. needles; dens. 0.5 g/cm³; pH 9.5–10.5 (1% aq.); 85% act.

Empicol® LXV100. [Albright & Wilson Am.; Albright & Wilson UK] Sodium lauryl sulfate; CAS 151-21-3; EINECS 205-

788-1; anionic; surfactant in toothpaste, pharmaceutical, and toiletry preps.; needles; 95% act.

Empicol® LXV/D. [Albright & Wilson UK] Sodium lauryl sulfate USP, BP; CAS 151-21-3; EINECS 205-788-1; anionic; emulsifier in the mfg. of plastics and rubbers; foaming agent for rubber foams; lubricant for mfg. of molded rubber goods; also in mfg. of carpet and upholstery shampoos, toiletries, toothpastes; wh. needles; sp.gr. 0.5 g/cc; pH 9.5–10.5 (5% aq.); 90% act.

Empicol® LZ. [Albright & Wilson UK] Sodium lauryl sulfate; CAS 68955-19-1; anionic; detergent, wetting and foaming agent in personal care prods., pharmaceuticals; emulsifier in mfg. of rubbers, plastics, and resins by emulsion polymerization; foaming agent in mfg. of foam rubber goods; lubricant used in plastic goods; wh. powd.; dens. 0.35 g/cm³; pH 9.5–10.5 (1% aq.); 89.0% min. act.

Empicol® LZ/D. [Albright & Wilson UK] Sodium lauryl sulfate BP/USP; CAS 68955-19-1; anionic; surfactant, foaming agent, emulsifier, wetting agent for dental preps., toiletries, rubber, plastics, foam rubber; lubricant in extrusion of plastic goods, e.g., PVC; wh. powd.; sp.gr. 0.35; pH 9.5–10.5 (1% aq.); 90% min. act.

Empicol® LZV. [Albright & Wilson UK] Sodium lauryl sulfate; CAS 68955-19-1; anionic; detergent and foaming agent for shampoos, toothpaste; wh. needles; dens. 0.5 g/cm³; pH 9.5–10.5 (1% aq.); 85.0% min. act.

Empicol® LZV/D. [Albright & Wilson UK] Sodium lauryl sulfate; CAS 151-21-3; EINECS 205-788-1; anionic; surfactant, foaming agent, emulsifier, wetting agent for dental preps., toiletries, rubber, plastics, foam rubber; lubricant in extrusion of plastic goods, e.g., PVC; wh. fine needles; sp.gr. 0.5; pH 9.5–10.5 (1% aq.); 90% min. act.

Empicol® MIPA. [Albright & Wilson Australia] MIPA-lauryl sulfate; CAS 21142-28-9; EINECS 244-238-5; anionic; base for hair shampoos; pale yel. clear visc. liq.; visc. 22 ± 10 s; pH 7.5 ± 0.5 (5%); 30.0 ± 1.0% act.

Empicol® ML 26/F. [Albright & Wilson UK] Magnesium lauryl sulfate; CAS 68081-97-0; anionic; detergent used in the mfg. of shampoos and toothpaste; pale straw liq.; misc. with water; dens. 1.0 g/cc; visc. 150 cs; 26% act.

Empicol® ML30. [Albright & Wilson UK] Magnesium lauryl sulfate; CAS 3097-08-3; EINECS 221-450-6; personal care surfactant.

Empicol® SBB. [Albright & Wilson UK] Disodium cocamide MEA sulfosuccinate; anionic; raw material for toiletries; yel. liq.; dens. 1.10 g/cc; visc. 90 cs (20 C); cloud pt. < 5 C; pH 6-7 (5%); 29% conc.

Empicol® SCC. [Albright & Wilson UK] Disodium lauryl sulfosuccinate; anionic; raw material for toiletries; yel. liq.; may separate; dens. 1.09 g/cc; pH 6-7 (5%); 29% act.

Empicol® SDD. [Albright & Wilson UK] Disodium laureth sulfosuccinate; CAS 37354-45-5; anionic; mild raw material for toiletries and detergents; pale straw liq.; may separate; dens. 1.10 g/cc; visc. 100 cs (20 C); cloud pt. < 2 C; pH 5.5-7 (5%); 40% conc.

Empicol® SEE. [Albright & Wilson UK] Disodium undecylenic monoethanolamide sulfosuccinate; anionic; mild raw material for toiletries and detergents; 25% conc.

Empicol® SFF. [Albright & Wilson UK] Disodium deceth-5 sulfosuccinate; anionic; mild raw material for toiletries and detergents; pale straw free-flowing liq.; dens. 1.09 g/cc; visc. 40 cs (20 C); cloud pt. < 0 C; pH 6-7 (5%); 23% active.

Empicol® SGG. [Albright & Wilson UK] Disodium cocamido PEG-3 sulfosuccinate; anionic; mild raw material for toiletries and detergents; pale straw liq.; may separate; dens. 1.1 g/cc; visc. 150 cs (20 C); pH 6-7 (5%); 30% conc.

Empicol® SHH. [Albright & Wilson UK] Sodium/MEA laureth-2 sulfosuccinate; anionic; mild raw material for toiletries and detergents; colorless to pale straw free-flowing liq.; dens. 1.09 g/cc; visc. 80 cs (20 C); cloud pt. < 5 C; pH 6-

Empicol® SLL

7 (5%); 32% conc.

Empicol® SLL. [Albright & Wilson UK] Disodium lauryl sulfosuccinate; CAS 36409-57-1; anionic; mild raw material for toiletries and detergents; wh. paste; pH 6-7 (5%); 32% conc.

Empicol® SLL/P. [Albright & Wilson UK] Disodium lauryl sulfosuccinate; CAS 36409-57-1; anionic; mild raw material for toiletries and detergents; wh. paste; pH 6-7 (1%); 83% conc.

Empicol® STT. [Albright & Wilson UK] Disodium cetearyl sulfosuccinate; anionic; mild raw material for toiletries and detergents; wh. paste; pH 6-7 (5%); 26% conc.

Empicol® TA40. [Albright & Wilson Australia] TEA-lauryl sulfate; CAS 68908-44-1; anionic; ingred. for personal care prods.; pale yel. clear liq.; pH 7.0 ± 0.5 (5%); 40.0 ± 1.0% act.

Empicol® TA40A. [Albright & Wilson Australia] TEA-lauryl sulfate; CAS 139-96-8; EINECS 205-388-7; base for personal care prods.; water-wh. clear liq.; pH 7.2 ± 0.3 (10%); 40.5–42.0% act.

Empicol® TAS30. [Albright & Wilson UK] Sodium cetearyl sulfate; CAS 68955-20-4; anionic; collector in the beneficiation of minerals by ore flotation; detergent active raw material; cofoaming agent for latex foam compds.; also for shampoos and cosmetic creams; wh./straw paste; dens. 1.10 g/cm³; pH 8.0–10.0 (1%); 30% act. in water.

Empicol® TL40. [Albright & Wilson UK] TEA-lauryl sulfate; CAS 139-96-8; EINECS 205-388-7; detergent used in liq. and lotion shampoos; foam booster for fire fighting; pale yel., clear liq.; misc. with water; dens. 1.025 g/cc; visc. 300 cs; pH 6.8–7.1 (5%); 40% act.

Empicol® TL40/T. [Albright & Wilson UK] TEA-lauryl sulfate; CAS 139-96-8; 68908-44-1; EINECS 205-388-7; anionic; surfactant for personal care prods.; emulsifier in the mfg. of rubber latices; pale yel. clear liq.; dens. 1.08 g/cm³; visc. 45 cs; cloud pt. < 0 C; pH 7.0 ± 0.5 (5% aq.); 41% act. in water.

Empicol® WAK. [Albright & Wilson Australia] Sodium lauryl sulfate; CAS 151-21-3; EINECS 205-788-1; anionic; emulsifier in refining veg. oils; base for personal care prods.; wetting and foaming agent in specialty cleansers and industrial processes; pale yel. clear liq.; sp.gr. 1.050; pH 8.5 ± 0.7 (10% aq.); 35.0 ± 1.0% act.

Empicol® XC35. [Albright & Wilson UK] Sodium laureth sulfate, cocamide DEA, and glycol stearate; anionic/nonionic; pearlescent base for shampoo, bubble bath, liq. soap; formulations should contain preservative; visc. pearly liq.; almost odorless; 35% conc.

Empicol® XPA. [Albright & Wilson UK] Formulated blend; pearlized and opacified conc. for toiletries.

Empigen® 2125-AU. [Albright & Wilson Australia] Soyamide DEA; CAS 68425-47-8; EINECS 270-355-6; nonionic; coactive ingred. in toiletries; liq.; 80% conc.

Empigen® 5089. [Albright & Wilson UK] Laurtrimonium chloride; CAS 112-00-5; EINECS 203-927-0; cationic; bactericide for disinfectant and sanitizer formulations for household, institutional, agric., food processing applics., antiseptic detergents in pharmaceuticals; algicide for swimming pools; wood preservatives; pale yel. liq.; sp.gr. 0.97; pH 5.5–8.5; 34 ± 2% act. in water.

Empigen® 5107. [Albright & Wilson UK] Alkyl dimethylamine betaine; amphoteric; foaming agent/stabilizer, antistat, solubilizer for shampoos, foam baths, latex foam compds., oil prod., alkaline industrial hard surf. cleaners; wetting and coupling agent for cleaners, traffic film removers; pale amber liq.; m.w. 286; sp.gr. 1.04; pH 5–9; 31 ± 2% act. in water.

Empigen® 5509. [Albright & Wilson UK] Cocamino hydroxy sulfobetaine; amphoteric; foam booster, conditioner for shampoos, skin cleansers; liq.; 50% conc.

Empigen® BAC50. [Albright & Wilson UK] Benzalkonium chloride NF; cationic; bactericide for disinfectant and sanitizer formulations for household, institutional, agric., food processing applics., antiseptic detergents in pharmaceuticals; algicide for swimming pools; wood preservatives; masonry biocides; permanent retarders in dyeing of acrylic fibers; phase transfer catalyst; pale straw liq.; misc. with water, alcohol, acetone; sp.gr. 0.99; pH 7–9 (5%); 50% act.

Empigen® BAC50/BP. [Albright & Wilson UK] Benzalkonium chloride BP, NF; cationic; bactericide for disinfectant and sanitizer formulations for household, institutional, agric., food processing applics., antiseptic detergents in pharmaceuticals; algicide for swimming pools; wood preservatives; pale straw liq.; sp.gr. 0.99; pH 7–9 (5%); 50% act.

Empigen® BAC90. [Albright & Wilson UK] Benzalkonium chloride; cationic; bactericide for disinfectant and sanitizer formulations for household, institutional, agric., food processing applics., antiseptic detergents in pharmaceuticals; algicide for swimming pools; wood preservatives; gel; 90% conc.

Empigen® BAC/BP. [Albright & Wilson UK] Benzalkonium chloride.

Empigen® BB. [Albright & Wilson Am.; Albright & Wilson UK] Lauryl betaine; CAS 66455-29-6; amphoteric; foam booster/stabilizer, emulsifier, dispersant, wetting agent, thickening agent, conditioner used for shampoos, detergents, latex foam compds. for carpet backing, industrial applics.; formulation of film removers; stable over wide pH range; pale straw liq.; dens. 1.03 g/cc; cloud pt. < 0 C; pH 7 ± 2 (5% aq.); toxicology: mild to skin; low irritancy to eyes; 30% act.

Empigen® BB-AU. [Albright & Wilson Australia] Cocodimethyl betaine; CAS 66455-29-6; amphoteric; foam booster/stabilizer, thickener, emulsifier, dispersant, wetting and foaming agent; used in personal care prods., industrial and institutional cleaners; pale yel. liq.; sp.gr. 1.04; cloud pt. 1 C max.; pH 8.5 ± 1.0 (5% aq.); 30% act. in water.

Empigen® BCJ-50. [Albright & Wilson UK] Oleyl dimethyl benzyl ammonium chloride; CAS 37139-99-4; EINECS 253-363-4; basic ingred. in personal care prods.; yel. clear liq.; sp.gr. 0.977; visc. 450 cP; cloud pt. < 0 C; pH 4.0 ± 1.0 (1% aq.); 50.0 ± 3.0% quat. act. in water.

Empigen® BS. [Albright & Wilson UK] Cocamidopropyl betaine; foaming agent/stabilizer and antistat for shampoos, foam baths, latex foam compds., oil prod.; wetting and coupling agent for cleaners, traffic film removers; pale straw liq.; m.w. 350; sp.gr. 1.00; pH 4.5–8.0; 30 ± 1% act. in water.

Empigen® BS/AU. [Albright & Wilson Australia] Cocamidopropyl dimethylamine betaine; CAS 61789-40-0; amphoteric; low-irritation foam stabilizer for toiletries; liq.; 30% conc.

Empigen® BS/H. [Albright & Wilson UK] Cocamidopropyl betaine; amphoteric; foaming agent/stabilizer and antistat for shampoos, foam baths, latex foam compds., oil prod.; wetting and coupling agent for cleaners, traffic film removers; colorless/pale sraw liq.; m.w. 350; sp.gr. 1.04; pH 4.5–8.0; 30 ± 1% act. in water.

Empigen® BS/P. [Albright & Wilson UK] Cocamidopropyl betaine; CAS 61789-40-0; amphoteric; foam booster and co-active agent for toiletries and detergents; pale sraw liq.; m.w. 350; sp.gr. 1.00; pH 4.0–8.0; 25.5 ± 1.5% act. in water.

Empigen® CDL30. [Albright & Wilson UK] Lauric imidazoline betaine, modified; amphoteric; detergent used in personal care prods.; liq.

Empigen® CDL60. [Albright & Wilson UK] Disodium lauroamphodiacetate; CAS 68608-66-2; amphoteric; detergent for nonirritating shampoos, skin cleansing, personal care prods.; liq.

Empigen® CDR30. [Albright & Wilson UK] Coconut imidazoline betaine, modified; amphoteric; surfactant used in personal care prods., household and industrial cleaners, textile processing; amber visc. liq.; dens. 1.20 g/cm³; visc. 40,000–180,000 cs; pH 8.2–8.8 (10% aq.).

Empigen® CDR40. [Albright & Wilson UK] Sodium cocoamphoacetate and disodium cocoamphodiacetate; amphoteric; mild detergent for shampoos, skin cleansers, personal care prods., textile processing; liq.

Empigen® CDR60. [Albright & Wilson UK] Sodium cocoamphoacetate; CAS 68334-21-4; amphoteric; mild detergent for shampoos, skin cleansers, personal care prods.; textile processing; liq.; 50% conc.

Empigen® CHB40. [Albright & Wilson UK] Alkyl trimethyl ammonium bromide; cationic; bactericide; liq.; 40% conc.

Empigen® CM. [Albright & Wilson UK] Steartrimonium methosulfate; CAS 18684-11-2; cationic; antistat and conditioning agent for personal care prods.; emulsifier and antistat for industrial use; retarder for dyeing of acrylic fibers; pale straw cloudy liq.; dens. 0.96 g/cm³; flash pt. 40 C; cloud pt. 23 C; pH 6.5–8.5 (5% aq.); 30.0 ± 1.5% act.

Empigen® OB. [Albright & Wilson Am.; Albright & Wilson UK] Lauramine oxide; CAS 1643-20-5; 70592-80-2; EINECS 216-700-6; nonionic; coactive, detergent, antistat, foam booster/stabilizer and visc. modifier for personal care prods., surgical scrubs, fire fighting foam concs., foamed rubbers, bleach additive; solubilizer; pale straw liq.; dens. 0.98 g/cm³; visc. 25 cs (20 C); pH 7.5 ± 0.5 (5% aq.); 30.0 ± 1.5% act.

Empigen® OB/AU. [Albright & Wilson Australia] Coco dimethylamine oxide; CAS 70592-80-2; nonionic; visc. modifier, foam stabilizer for toiletries; liq.; 30% conc.

Empigen® OC. [Albright & Wilson Am.] Alkyl dimethyl amine oxide; nonionic; surfactant; liq.; 30% conc.

Empigen® OH25. [Albright & Wilson Am.; Albright & Wilson UK] n-Myristyl dimethyl amine oxide; CAS 3332-27-2; EINECS 222-059-3; nonionic; foam booster/stabilizer and visc. modifier for shampoos, foam baths, detergents; improves conditioning in shampoos; solubilizer for liq. bleach prods.; pale straw liq.; m.w. 257; sp.gr. 0.99; visc. 800 cs; pH 7.5 ± 0.5 (5% aq.); 25% act.

Empigen® OS/A. [Albright & Wilson Am.; Albright & Wilson UK] Cocamidopropylamine oxide; CAS 68155-09-9; EINECS 268-938-5; nonionic; foam booster/stabilizer and visc. modifier for shampoos, foam baths, detergents; improves conditioning in shampoos; pale straw liq.; m.w. 306; sp.gr. 1.01; visc. 65 cs; pH 6.5–8.00 (5% aq.); 30.5% act.

Empigen® OS/AU. [Albright & Wilson Australia] Cocamidopropyl dimethylamine oxide; CAS 68155-09-9; EINECS 268-938-5; nonionic; visc. modifier, foam stabilizer for toiletries; liq.; 30% conc.

Empigen® OY. [Albright & Wilson Am.; Albright & Wilson UK] PEG-3 lauramine oxide; CAS 59355-61-2; nonionic; detergent, antistat, foam booster/stabilizer for foamed rubbers, fire fighting, bleach additive, shampoos, hair and bath prods.; pale straw liq.; dens. 1.0 g/cm³; visc. 23 cs; pH 6.5 ± 0.5 (5% aq.); 25.0 ± 1.0% act.

Empilan® 2125-AU. [Albright & Wilson UK] Soyamide DEA; CAS 68425-47-8; EINECS 270-355-6; visc. modifier, superfatting agent, and coactive ingred. in personal care prods.; amber clear visc. liq.; sp.gr. 1.01; pH 10.5 ± 1.0 (10% aq.).

Empilan® 2502. [Albright & Wilson UK] Cocamide DEA (1:1); CAS 8051-30-7; EINECS 263-163-9; nonionic; foam booster/stabilizer; liq.; 80% conc.

Empilan® CDE. [Albright & Wilson UK] Cocamide DEA (1:1); CAS 61791-31-9; EINECS 263-163-9; nonionic; foam boosting/stabilizing agent, solubilizer, detergent for use in personal care and detergent prods.; antistat in plastics; softener for leather processing; pale yel. visc. liq.; dens. 1.0 g/cm³; 100% act.

Empilan® CDE/FF. [Albright & Wilson UK] Cocamide DEA; CAS 61791-31-9; EINECS 263-163-9; cosmetic surfactant.

Empilan® CDX. [Albright & Wilson UK] Cocamide DEA; CAS 68603-42-9; EINECS 263-163-9; nonionic; foam booster/stabilizer, solubilizer, and visc. modifier for toiletry and detergent formulations; antistatic agent in plastics; pale yel. visc. liq.; dens. 1.0 g/cm³.

Empilan® CIS. [Albright & Wilson UK] Cocamide MIPA; CAS 68440-05-1; EINECS 269-793-0; nonionic; foam stabilizer, detergent, shampoo additive; cream waxy flake; dens. 0.4 g/cm³; m.p. 46 C; 100% conc.

Empilan® CME. [Albright & Wilson UK] Cocamide MEA; CAS 68140-00-1; EINECS 268-770-2; nonionic; detergent, foam booster/stabilizer in detergent systems; stabilizer for hair and carpet shampoos; base for mfg. of ethoxylated alkylolamides; visc. modifier; cream waxy flake; disp. in hot water; dens. 0.4 g/cm³; m.p. 68 C; 100% act.

Empilan® CM/F. [Albright & Wilson Australia] Cocamide MEA; CAS 68140-00-1; EINECS 268-770-2; nonionic; foam stabilizer, visc. modifier; flake; 85% conc.

Empilan® EGMS. [Albright & Wilson UK] Glycol stearate; CAS 111-60-4; EINECS 203-886-9; nonionic; opacifier/pearling and emulsifying/stabilizing agent in shampoos; emollient; wh. hard, wax-like flake; oil-sol.; m.p. 56 C; 65% diester, 30% monoester.

Empilan® GMS SE32. [Albright & Wilson UK] Glyceryl stearate SE; nonionic; emulsifier; wh. wax-like powd.; m.p. 55–60 C; pH 7–9 (10% aq.); 32.5% min. monoglyceride.

Empilan® KB 2. [Albright & Wilson UK] Laureth-2; CAS 68002-97-1; EINECS 221-279-7; nonionic; emulsifier, foam booster, superfatting agent, used in detergents and emulsifying systems; mortar plasticizer; almost colorless liq.; insol. in cold water; dens. 0.9; visc. 25 cs; 100% act.

Empilan® KB 3. [Albright & Wilson UK] Laureth-3; CAS 68002-97-1; EINECS 221-280-2; nonionic; emulsifier, foam booster, superfatting agent, used in detergents and emulsifying systems; mortar plasticizer; liq.; HLB 8.1; 100% conc.

Empilan® KC 3. [Albright & Wilson UK] Laureth-3; CAS 3055-94-5; EINECS 221-280-2; nonionic; emulsifier, foam booster, superfatting agent, used in detergents and emulsifying systems; liq.; 100% conc.

Empilan® KL 6. [Albright & Wilson UK] Oleth-6; CAS 9004-98-2; nonionic; emulsifier for min. oils in cosmetics, detergent and wetting agents in textile industry; cream soft paste; cold water disp.; dens. 0.9 g/cc; m.p. 35 C; pH 8–10; 100% act.

Empilan® KL 10. [Albright & Wilson UK] Oleth-10; CAS 9004-98-2; nonionic; emulsifier for min. oils in cosmetics, detergent and wetting agents in textile industry; m.p. 40 C; pH 8–10; 100% act.

Empilan® KL 20. [Albright & Wilson UK] Oleth-20; CAS 9004-98-2; nonionic; emulsifier for min. oils in cosmetics, detergent and wetting agents in textile industry; cream soft solid; cold water disp.; dens. 0.9 g/cc; m.p. 42 C; pH 8–10; 100% act.

Empilan® KM 11. [Albright & Wilson UK] Ceteareth-11; CAS 68439-49-6; nonionic; emulsifier, foam control agent in syn. heavy duty detergents, soap additive; dispersant for textile processing; colorless to pale straw paste; 100% act.

Empilan® KM 50. [Albright & Wilson UK] Ceteareth-50; CAS

68439-49-6; nonionic; wetting agent, detergent for industrial/domestic applics.; emulsifier, foam control agent in syn. heavy duty detergents; dispersant for textile processing, polyurethane prod.; colorless to pale straw waxy flake/block; 100% act.

Empilan® LDE. [Albright & Wilson UK] Lauramide DEA (1:1); CAS 120-40-1; EINECS 204-393-1; nonionic; foam booster/stabilizer, solubilizer, thickener, detergent used in shampoos and liq. detergent formulations; antistat for plastics; cream solid; dens. 1.0 g/cm³; 100% act.

Empilan® LDE/FF. [Albright & Wilson UK] Lauramide DEA; CAS 120-40-1; EINECS 204-393-1; personal care surfactant.

Empilan® LDX. [Albright & Wilson UK] Lauramide DEA and diethanolamine; nonionic; foam booster/stabilizer, solubilizer, and visc. modifier for toiletry and detergent formulations; antistatic agent in plastics; cream solid; dens. 1.0 g/cm³; 100% conc.

Empilan® LIS. [Albright & Wilson UK] Lauramide MIPA; CAS 142-54-1; EINECS 205-541-8; nonionic; foam booster/stabilizer for liq. and powd. detergents, shampoos; visc. modifier, base for mfg. of ethoxylated deriv.; cream waxy flake; hot water disp.; dens. 0.4 g/cc; 87.5% act.

Empilan® LME. [Albright & Wilson UK] Lauramide MEA; CAS 142-78-9; EINECS 205-560-1; nonionic; foam booster/stabilizer in detergent systems; stabilizer for hair and carpet shampoos; base for mfg. of ethoxylated alkylolamides; visc. modifier; waxy flake; dens. 0.4 g/cm³; m.p. 85 C; 100% conc.

Empilan® NP9. [Albright & Wilson UK] Nonoxynol-9; CAS 9016-45-9; nonionic; wetting agent, detergent, emulsifier, solubilizer; for agric. emulsifiable and suspension concs., leather processing, emulsion and suspension polymerization; mortar plasticizer; plastics antistat; emulsifier for cosmetic creams and lotions; pale straw soft paste/liq.; dens. 1.0 g/cc; visc. 300 cs; cloud pt. 55 C (1% aq.); 100% act.

Empilan® P7061. [Albright & Wilson UK] EO/PO condensate; nonionic; wetting agent for agric. emulsifiable and suspension concs.; compding. aid for pharmaceuticals; liq.; 100% conc.

Empilan® P7062. [Albright & Wilson UK] EO/PO condensate; nonionic; wetting agent for agric. emulsifiable and suspension concs.; compding. aid for pharmaceuticals; liq.; 100% conc.

Empilan® P7087. [Albright & Wilson UK] EO/PO condensate; nonionic; wetting agent for agric. emulsifiable and suspension concs.; compding. aid for pharmaceuticals; liq.; 100% conc.

Empimin® KSN70. [Albright & Wilson UK] Sodium laureth sulfate (3 EO); CAS 9004-82-4; anionic; detergent raw material for high-quality liq. detergents, textile and leather processing; wetting agent for agric. wettable powds.; emulsifier, dispersant for emulsion polymerization; straw opaque pourable visc. liq.; dens. 1.1 g/cc; set pt. 8 C; pH 7.0–9.0 (2% aq.); 70% aq. sol'n.

Empiphos 4KP. [Albright & Wilson UK] Tetrapotassium pyrophosphate; CAS 7320-34-5; EINECS 230-785-7; detergent builder for liq. detergents; pigment dispersant and stabilizer in emulsion paints; clarifying agent in liq. soaps; mfg. of syn. rubber; boiler water treatment; sol. in water; dens. 75 lb/ ft³; pH 10.3.

Empiwax SK. [Albright & Wilson UK] Cetearyl alcohol and sodium lauryl sulfate; SE wax as o/w emulsifier for pharmaceutical and toilet preparations and ointments; wh. flake; 100% conc.

Empiwax SK/BP. [Albright & Wilson UK] Cetearyl alcohol and sodium lauryl sulfate; SE wax as o/w emulsifier for pharmaceutical and toilet preparations and ointments; complies with B.P. specs. for emulsifying wax; wh. flake;

100% conc.

Empol® 1008. [Henkel/Emery] Dilinoleic acid; CAS 68783-41-5.

Empol® 1024. [Henkel/Emery] Dilinoleic acid; CAS 6144-28-1.

Empol® 1045. [Henkel/Emery] Trilinoleic acid; CAS 68937-90-6.

Emsorb® 2500. [Henkel/Emery; Henkel/Textiles] Sorbitan oleate; CAS 1338-43-8; EINECS 215-665-4; nonionic; coupler, emulsifier, lubricant, and softener for textile fibers, leather, cosmetics, agric., household prods.; for formulating petrol. oils and waxes, natural fats and waxes, and alkyl esters; EPA exempt; Gardner 8 liq.; sol. in min. oil, butyl stearate, Stod., xylene; insol. in water; dens. 8.3 lb/gal; visc. 360 cSt (100 F); HLB 4.6; pour pt. < 0 C; flash pt. 475 F; 100% conc.

Emsorb® 2502. [Henkel/Emery; Henkel/Textiles] Sorbitan sesquioleate; CAS 8007-43-0; EINECS 232-360-1; nonionic; coupler, coemulsifier for o/w systems; emulsifier for w/o systems; household aerosols, cosmetics, agric., industrial and textile oils; EPA exempt; Gardner 6 liq.; sol. in min. oil, butyl stearate, glycerol trioleate, Stod. solv., xylene; insol. in water; dens. 8.2 lb/gal; visc. 475 cSt (100 F); HLB 4.5; pour pt. < 0 C; flash pt. 470 F; 100% conc.

Emsorb® 2503. [Henkel/Emery; Henkel/Textiles] Sorbitan trioleate; CAS 26266-58-0; EINECS 247-569-3; nonionic; coupler, emulsifier, lubricant, and softener for textile fibers and leather, cosmetics, agric., household prods.; for formulating petrol. oils and waxes, natural fats and waxes, and alkyl esters; coemulsifier for min. oil; EPA exempt; Gardner 7 liq.; sol. in min. oil, butyl stearate, glycerol trioleate, Stod. solv., xylene; insol. in water; dens. 7.9 lb/gal; visc. 100 cSt (100 F); HLB 2.1; pour pt. < 0 C; flash pt. 500 F; 100% act.

Emsorb® 2505. [Henkel/Emery] Sorbitan stearate; CAS 1338-41-6; EINECS 215-664-9; nonionic; coupler, hydrophobic emulsifier; coemulsifier for industrial oils, household prods., agric., and cosmetics; textile lubricant; paper and textile processing; EPA exempt; Gardner 4 solid; disp. in butyl stearate, perchloroethylene; insol. in water; HLB 5.2; m.p. 50 C; flash pt. 480 F; 100% conc.

Emsorb® 2507. [Henkel/Emery] Sorbitan tristearate; CAS 26658-19-5; EINECS 247-891-4; nonionic; coupler, emulsifier, lubricant, and softener for textile fibers and leather, cosmetics, agric., household prods.; for formulating petrol. oils and waxes, natural fats and waxes, and alkyl esters; coemulsifier for min. oil; EPA-exempt; Gardner 4 waxy solid; sol. in butyl stearate, perchloroethylene, glycerol trioleate, Stod. solv., xylene; insol. in water; HLB 2.2; m.p. 54 C; flash pt. 480 F; 100% conc.

Emsorb® 2510. [Henkel/Emery] Sorbitan palmitate; CAS 26266-57-9; EINECS 247-568-8; nonionic; coupler, emulsifier for cosmetic, agric. and household prods.; fiber-to-metal lubricant; EPA-exempt; Gardner 8 waxy solid; sol. in oil, Stod. solv., xylene; insol. in water; HLB 6.5; m.p. 47 C; flash pt. 445 F; 100% conc.

Emsorb® 2515. [Henkel/Emery; Henkel/Textiles] Sorbitan laurate; CAS 1338-39-2; nonionic; coupler, emulsifier; used in household specialities, industrial oils, agric., cosmetics, and emulsion polymerization; antifoam properties; EPA-exempt; Gardner 7 liq.; sol. in min. oil, butyl stearate, glycerol trioleate, Stod. solv., xylene; water-disp.; dens. 8.8 lb/gal; visc. 1000 cSt; HLB 8.0; pour pt. 15 C; flash pt. 430 F; cloud pt. < 25 C; 100% conc.

Emsorb® 2720. [Henkel/Cospha; Henkel Canada] Polysorbate 20; CAS 9005-64-5; o/w emulsifier, solubilizer, visc. modifier; used in creams, lotions, shampoos, conditioners, and liq. soaps; Gardner 6 liq.; sol. @ 5% in water, triolein, IPA; dens. 9.2 lb/gal; visc. 160 cSt (100 F); HLB 16.7; acid no. 2 max.; sapon. no. 40-50; pour pt. –10 C;

flash pt. 510 F.

Emsorb® 2721. [Henkel/Cospha; Henkel Canada] PEG-80 sorbitan laurate; CAS 9005-64-5; wetting agent, dispersant, mild cleanser for baby prods.; anti-irritant; Gardner < 6 liq.; sol. @ 5% in water, IPA; dens. 9.2 lb/gal; visc. 500 cSt (100 F); HLB 19.0; pour pt. 15 C; cloud pt. 82.5 C (5% saline); flash pt. 505 F; 72% act. in water.

Emsorb® 2722. [Henkel/Cospha; Henkel Canada] Polysorbate 80; CAS 9005-65-6; nonionic; emulsifier, coemulsifier for cosmetics; dispersant for pigments in makeup; solubilizer for oils, flavors, fragrances; yel. clear liq.; sol. @ 5% in water, triolein, IPA; dens. 9.0 lb/gal; visc. 200 cSt (100 F); HLB 15.0; acid no. 2 max.; sapon. no. 45-55; pour pt. -12 C; flash pt. 505 F.

Emsorb® 2725. [Henkel/Organic Prods.] Polysorbate 80; CAS 9005-65-6; emulsifier.

Emsorb® 2726. [Henkel/Cospha; Henkel Canada] PEG-40 sorbitan diisostearate; emulsifier, solubilizer for oils, flavors, and fragrances in mouthwashes, lipstick, perfumes, germicides, and other polar substances in aq. systems; yel. liq., low odor and taste; sol. in water, alcohol, some cosmetic oils.

Emsorb® 2728. [Henkel/Cospha; Henkel Canada] Polysorbate 60; CAS 9005-67-8; nonionic; o/w emulsifier for cosmetics, hair straighteners, shaving prods., sun care prods.; binder in powds.; with Emsorb 2505 to stabilize wax emulsions; Gardner 3 waxy semisolid; sol. @ 5% in water, IPA; dens. 8.9 lb/gal; visc. 250 cSt (100 F); HLB 15.2; acid no. 2 max.; sapon. no. 45-55; pour pt. 25 C; flash pt. 510 F.

Emsorb® 6900. [Henkel/Emery; Henkel/Textiles] PEG-20 sorbitan oleate; CAS 9005-65-6; nonionic; dispersant for pigments in coatings; solubilizer for oils and fragrances; hydrophilic emulsifier; coemulsifier for petrol. oils, fats, solvs., and waxes in cosmetics, household prods., industrial lubricants, and textile dye carriers; emulsifier for tobacco sucker control concs.; EPA-exempt; Gardner 5 liq.; sol. in water; dens. 9.0 lb/gal; visc. 200 cSt (100 F); HLB 15.0; pour pt. -12 C; flash pt. 535 F; cloud pt. 70 C (5% saline); 100% conc.

Emsorb® 6915. [Henkel/Emery; Henkel/Textiles] PEG-20 sorbitan laurate; CAS 9005-64-5; nonionic; o/w emulsifier and solubilizer of petrol. oils, solvs., and fats; used in cosmetic creams and lotions; visc. modifier in shampoos; emulsifier for dye carriers, antistatic scrooping agent in primary spin finishes, and fiber processing aid in textile industry; agric. formulations; EPA-exempt; Gardner 6 liq.; sol. in water, glycerol trioleate; dens. 9.2 lb/gal; visc. 160 cSt (100 F); HLB 16.5; pour pt. -10 C; flash pt. 510 F; cloud pt. 75–85 C; 100% conc.

Emthox® 2730. [Henkel/Cospha; Henkel Canada] PEG-75 cocoa butter glycerides; nonionic; emollient, humectant, emulsifier for personal care prods.; Gardner 3 paste; sol. @ 5% in water, triolein, IPA; dens. 8.7 lb/gal (50 C); visc. 210 cSt (100 F); m.p. 31–35 C; flash pt. 530 F; 100% conc.

Emthox® 2737. [Henkel/Organic Prods.] PEG-16 hydrog. castor oil; CAS 61788-85-0; emulsifier.

Emthox® 2738. [Henkel/Organic Prods.] PEG-25 hydrog. castor oil; CAS 61788-85-0; personal care surfactant.

Emthox® 5877. [Henkel/Organic Prods.] Laureth-23; CAS 9002-92-0; emulsifier.

Emthox® 5882. [Henkel/Cospha; Henkel Canada] Laureth-4; CAS 5274-68-0; EINECS 226-097-1; nonionic; dispersant for bath oil; emulsifier for creams and lotions; wetting agent; for eye make-up, deodorants, hair coloring prods.; Gardner 1 liq.; sol. @ 5% in min. oil, triolein, IPA, IPM; disp. in water, glycerin; dens. 7.9 lb/gal; visc. 20 cSt (100 F); HLB 9.4; acid no. 10 max.; iodine no. 2 max.; sapon. no. 140-160; cloud pt. < 25 C; flash pt. 355 F; 100% conc.

Emthox® 5885. [Henkel/Cospha; Henkel Canada] Cetear-

eth-20; CAS 68439-49-6; emulsifier, solubilizer for cosmetics, conditioners, depilatories, hair straighteners, sun care prods.; Gardner 1 solid; sol. @ 5% in water, IPA; disp. in min. oil; dens. 7.7 lb/gal; HLB 15.3; m.p. 40 C; cloud pt. 91 C (5% saline).

Emthox® 5967. [Henkel/Cospha; Henkel Canada] Laureth-12; CAS 3056-00-6; EINECS 221-286-5; nonionic; emollient, thickener in shampoos; emulsifier in creams and lotions; solid; HLB 14.0; 100% conc.

Emthox® 6705. [Henkel/Organic Prods.] Phenoxyethanol; CAS 122-99-6; EINECS 204-589-7; preservative.

Emulan®. [Emulan] Mink oil; emollient with high spreading coefficient for skin and hair care formulations requiring good oxidative stability; ingred. in hair holding spray; replacement for sperm oil; avail. in four grades: Super Fine, Light Fraction, Heavy Fraction, and Sable White; liq. (Super Fine, Lt. Fraction), solid (Heavy Fraction, Sable White); sol. in IPM and similar esters, min., animal, and veg. oils, IPA; partly sol. in ethanol; HLB 9.0; cloud pt. 20, 27, 68, and 68 F resp.; ref. index 1.4681 (Super Fine, Lt. Fraction); toxicology: nonirritating to skin and eyes.

Emulan® Mink Wax. [Emulan] Mink wax.

Emulcire 61 WL 2659. [Gattefosse] Cetyl alcohol, ceteth-20, and steareth-20; cosmetic ingred.

Emuldan FP 40. [Grindsted Prods. Denmark] Glyceryl stearate.

Emuldan HA 32/S3. [Grindsted Prods. Denmark] Glyceryl stearate SE.

Emuldan HA 60. [Grindsted Prods. Denmark] Glyceryl stearate.

Emuldan HLT 40. [Grindsted Prods. Denmark] Glyceryl stearate.

Emuldan PK 60. [Grindsted Prods. Denmark] Palm kernel glycerides.

Emulgade® 1000 NI. [Henkel/Cospha; Henkel Canada; Henkel KGaA/Cospha] Cetearyl alcohol and ceteareth-20; nonionic; emulsifying agent, SE o/w base for creams, lotions; esp. suitable for processing cationics; wh. flakes; solid. pt. 48-53 C; acid no. 1 max.; sapon. no. 1 max.; hyd. no. 175-190; ref. index 1.435-1.439; pH 6-8.

Emulgade® C. [Henkel/Cospha; Henkel Canada] Emulsifying wax NF; self-emulsifying raw material for emulsions, hair conditioners, creams, lotions; waxy flakes; acid no. 2 max.; iodine no. 3.5 max.; sapon. no. 14 max.

Emulgade® CL. [Henkel; Henkel Canada; Henkel KGaA/Cospha] Octyl stearate, stearic acid, cetyl palmitate, coconut acid, cetearyl alcohol, glyceryl stearate, potassium stearate, potassium cocoate, sodium stearate, and sodium cocoate; SE cream base, emulsifying agent for creams, lotions; formulated base; waxy flakes.

Emulgade® CL Special. [Henkel] Isopropyl myristate, stearic acid, cetyl palmitate, coconut acid, cetearyl alcohol, glyceryl stearate, potassium stearate, potassium cocoate, sodium stearate, sodium cocoate.

Emulgade® CLB. [Henkel/Cospha] Blend of ester stearates, fatty alcohols, and nonionic emulsifiers; complete base for easy mfg. of o/w creams and lotions; wh. paste.

Emulgade® EO-10. [Pulcra SA] Oleth-25 and cetyl alcohol; self-emulsifying base for prep. of creams and emulsions; flakes.

Emulgade® F. [Henkel/Cospha; Henkel Canada; Henkel KGaA/Cospha] Cetearyl alcohol, PEG-40 castor oil, and sodium cetearyl sulfate; anionic; SE raw material for cosmetic creams and fluid emulsions; emulsifier for cosmetics, pharmaceuticals; wh. to sl. yel. gran.; sapon. no. 10-15; hyd. no. 160-175; pH 6.5-8.0 (1%); 95% fatty matter.

Emulgade® SE. [Henkel KGaA/Cospha] Glyceryl stearate, ceteareth-20, ceteareth-12, cetearyl alcohol, and cetyl palmitate; self-emulsifying wax mixt. with nonionic emulsifiers for mfg. of heat- and visc.-stable cosmetic and pharmaceutical o/w emulsions; acid no. 1 max.; sapon. no. 90-100; hyd. no. 145-160.

Emulgateur SO. [Witco/H-I-P] Formulated emulsifier; nonionic; emulsifier for min. and veg. oils, solvs.; for personal care prods.; liq.

Emulgator B-6. [Cosmetochem] Ceteareth-6; CAS 68439-49-6; cosmetic ingred.

Emulgator BTO. [Goldschmidt] Laureth-4, glyceryl oleate, and PEG-25 glyceryl trioleate.

Emulgator BTO 2. [Goldschmidt] Oleth-10 and PEG-20 glyceryl oleate.

Emulgator DMR. [Hoechst Celanese/Spec. Chem.] PEG-45 stearate phosphate; thickener for cosmetics and toiletries; 100% act.

Emulgator E 2149. [Goldschmidt; Goldschmidt AG] Steareth-7, stearyl alcohol; nonionic; self-emulsifying emulsifier and stabilizer for cosmetic and pharmaceutical o/w emulsions; resist. to acid and alkaline substances; wh.-ivory waxy solid; sol. warm in veg. and min. oils; disp. warm in water; m.p. 41-47 C; HLB 11.0; acid no. 2 max.; iodine no. 2 max.; sapon. no. 3 max.; 100% conc.

Emulgator E 2155. [Goldschmidt; Goldschmidt AG] Stearyl alcohol, steareth-7, steareth-10; nonionic; self-emulsifying emulsifier and stabilizer for cosmetic and pharmaceutical o/w emulsions; resist. to alkaline and acid substances; wh.-ivory waxy solid; sol. warm in veg. oils, sol. warm with sl. turbidity in min. oil; disp. warm in water; m.p. 49-55 C; HLB 11.0; acid no. 2 max.; iodine no. 2 max.; sapon. no. 3 max.; 100% conc.

Emulgator E 2209. [Goldschmidt] Cetyl alcohol and ceteareth-30; cosmetic ingred.

Emulgator E 2568. [Goldschmidt; Goldschmidt AG] Ceteareth-25; CAS 68439-49-6; nonionic; emulsifier and stabilizer for cosmetic and pharmaceutical o/w emulsions; resist. to alkaline and acid substances; wh.-ivory waxy solid; sol. warm in water; disp. warm in veg. and min. oils; m.p. 43-49 C; HLB 16.0; acid no. 2 max.; iodine no. 1 max.; sapon. no. 3 max.; 100% conc.

Emulmetik™ 100. [Lucas Meyer] Lecithin; CAS 8002-43-5; EINECS 232-307-2; resorbable refatting agent, solubilizer, coemulsifier, and wetting agent for skin care prods., cleansing preps.

Emulmetik™ 110. [Lucas Meyer] Lecithin, oleamide DEA, and soybean oil; resorbable refatting agent, solubilizer, coemulsifier, and wetting agent for cleansing preps., hair care prods., men's toiletries.

Emulmetik™ 120. [Lucas Meyer] Lysolecithin; resorbable refatting agent, solubilizer, coemulsifier, and wetting agent for cleansing preps., lotions, creams, foam baths; vehicle for perfumes; softening agent for skin; stabilizer for emulsions and suspensions; wets hydrophobic substances; antisettling agent for pigmented suspensions; brn. visc. liq.; sol. @ 2% in paraffin oil; partly sol. in alcohols; disp. in water; visc. 13 Pa·s; pH 6-7; usage level: 0.5-2%; 1% max. moisture.

Emulmetik™ 135. [Lucas Meyer] Spray-dried lecithin conc.; CAS 8002-43-5; EINECS 232-307-2; refatting agent providing protection and nourishment for the skin; improves foam stability; stabilizes emulsions and suspensions; for soaps, hand cleansing preps., bath shampoos, hair toiletries, creams and lotions; lt. yel. powd.; usage level: 2-8%; 4.5% moisture.

Emulmetik™ 300. [Lucas Meyer] Lecithin; CAS 8002-43-5; EINECS 232-307-2; resorbable refatting agent, solubilizer, coemulsifier, and wetting agent for skin care prods., skin protectives, liposome preps., sun care prods., face and hand creams, bath and body oils, baby oils, soaps, lipsticks; stabilizes emulsions and suspension; vehicle for perfumes; ylsh. brn. powd.; sol. @ 2% in paraffin, org.

solvs.; partly sol. in alcohol, ketones; disp. in water; usage level: 1-3%; 99% min. solids.

Emulmetik™ 310. [Lucas Meyer] Propylene glycol, lecithin, sodium lauryl sulfate, disodium laureth sulfosuccinate, cocamidopropyl hydroxysultaine, and isopropyl alcohol; resorbable refatting agent, solubilizer, coemulsifier, and wetting agent for cleansing preps., hair care prods.

Emulmetik 320. [Lucas Meyer] Hydrog. lecithin; CAS 92128-87-5; EINECS 295-786-7; resorbable refatting agent, solubilizer, coemulsifier, conditioner, gellant, and wetting agent for skin care prods., skin protectives, liposome preps., sun care prods., decorative cosmetics, nourishing preps.; ylsh.-wh. lt. powd., nearly odorless; partly sol. in alcohol @ 50 C; disp. in water, paraffin oil; iodine no. 10-15; pH 6.0-7.5; usage level: 1-5%.

Emulmetik™ 900. [Lucas Meyer] Phosphatidyl choline-enriched fraction of isolated soybean phospholipids; conditioner, skin protectant; imparts gloss and smoothness; used in hair sprays, setting lotions, face and hair lotions, pre- and aftershave lotions; brn. wax; sol. in alcohol, sol. @ 50 C in paraffin oil; disp. in water; pH 5.5-6.5; usage level: 0.2-1.5%; 1% max. moisture.

Emulmetik 910. [Lucas Meyer] Polysorbate 80, isopropyl alcohol, and lecithin; resorbable refatting agent, nourishing agent, solubilizer, coemulsifier, softener, conditioner, and wetting agent for skin and hair care prods., clear shampoos, cleansing lotions, hair sprays, liq. handwash, preshave and aftershaves, men's toiletries; lt. yel. liq.; sol. opaque in water; sol. clear in alcohol; disp. in paraffin oil; pH 5-6; usage level: 1-3%; 50% solids, 21.4% IPA.

Emulmetik 920. [Lucas Meyer] Isopropyl alcohol, lecithin, hydrolyzed collagen, and ethyl alcohol; resorbable refatting agent, solubilizer, coemulsifier, and wetting agent for hair care prods.; improves pliability and strength of hair, imparts gloss and flexibility; conditions and softens skin; for shampoos, hair sprays, wave preps., day, night, and cleansing creams; lt. yel. liq.; sol. opaque in water; sol. clear in alcohols; disp. in paraffin oil; pH 8-9; usage level: 0.3-2%; 18% solids, 37% IPA, 13% ethanol.

Emulmetik 930. [Lucas Meyer] Phosphatidylcholine; resorbable refatting agent, solubilizer, coemulsifier, gellant, and wetting agent for liposome preps., skin creams/lotions, nourishing preps.; skin conditioner; lt. yel. wax, nearly odorless; sol. @ 60 C in fat, paraffin; sol. @ 20 C in ethanol, hydrocarbons, chlorinated hydrocarbons; disp. in water; iodine no. 95-105; usage level: 0.5-3%.

Emulmetik 950. [Lucas Meyer] Hydrog. lecithin; CAS 92128-87-5; EINECS 295-786-7; resorbable refatting agent, solubilizer, gellant, coemulsifier, and wetting agent for liposome preps., skin creams/lotions, nourishing preps.; skin conditioner; wh. powd., nearly odorless; sol. @ 50 C in ethanol, hydrocarbons, chlorinated hydrocarbons; disp. in water; iodine no. 3 max.; usage level: 0.5-3%.

Emulmetik 970. [Lucas Meyer] Egg lecithin; CAS 8002-43-5; EINECS 232-307-2; resorbable refatting agent, solubilizer, coemulsifier, nourishing and wetting agent for hair and skin care prods., creams, lotions, pharmaceutical preps.; prevents sedimentation; regulates water-binding capacity of the skin; yel.-brn. paste; sol. in ether, ethanol, chlorinated hydrocarbons; sol. @ 50 C in fat, paraffin oil; disp. in water; acid no. 25 max.; iodine no. 80 max.

Emulmin 862. [Sanyo Chem. Industries] PEG distearate; CAS 9005-08-7; nonionic; thickener for cosmetics and textile printing pastes; solid.

Emulpon A. [Witco/H-I-P] Ethoxylated fatty acid; nonionic; emulsifier for sol. min. oil; for personal care prods.; liq.; 100% conc.

Emulpon EL 18. [Witco/H-I-P] Ethoxylated castor oil; nonionic; emulsifier for min. oil; for personal care prods.; liq.; 100% conc.

Emulpon EL 20. [Witco/H-I-P] Ethoxylated castor oil; CAS 61731-12-6; nonionic; emulsifier for waxes, olein; for personal care prods.; liq.; HLB 2.7; 100% conc.

Emulpon EL 33. [Witco/H-I-P] PEG-33 castor oil; CAS 61791-12-6; nonionic; cosmetic ingred.; textile wetting agent; yel. liq.; HLB 12.2; 100% conc.

Emulpon EL 40. [Witco/H-I-P] PEG-40 castor oil; CAS 61731-12-6; nonionic; cosmetic ingred.; textile wetting agent used in dyeing; fluid paste; 100% conc.

Emulsifier 2/014160. [Dragoco] PEG-40 hydrog. castor oil and trideceth-9.

Emulsifier 17 P. [Grau Aromatics] PEG-40 hydrog. castor oil; CAS 61788-85-0; personal care surfactant.

Emulsifier 227 G. [Grau Aromatics] Nonoxynol-4 and non-oxynol-9.

Emulsion 2153. [Siltech] cationic; nonfoaming conditioner for personal care prods.; water-disp.; 40% act.

Emulsion 2170. [Siltech] nonionic; durable conditioner for personal care prods.; disp. in water; 60% act.

Emulsogen EL. [Hoechst Celanese/Spec. Chem.] PEG-36 castor oil; CAS 61791-12-6; emulsifier for w/o cosmetics and toiletries; 100% act.

Emulsogen ELN. [Hoechst Celanese/Colorants & Surf.] Nonoxynol-23; CAS 9016-45-9; cosmetic and personal care surfactant.

Emulsogen LP. [Hoechst Celanese/Spec. Chem.] Oleth-5; CAS 9004-98-2; emulsifier for w/o cosmetics and toiletries; 100% act.

Emulsogen OG. [Hoechst AG] Fatty acid ester; nonionic; emulsifier for prep. of paste-like w/o emulsions from petroleum jelly of from mixts. of petroleum jelly and paraffin wax or oil; also for stearic acid emulsions; wetting agent for water-insol. substances; facilitates pigment grinding; dissolves numerous dyestuffs and chemicals or disperses them very finely; golden yel. clear visc. oil; sol. in hydrocarbons, triglycerides, wool fat, beeswax; insol. in water; 100% act.

Emulsynt® 1055. [ISP Van Dyk] Polyglyceryl-4 oleate, PEG-8 propylene glycol cocoate; nonionic; fragrance solubilizer; emulsifier for w/o cosmetic creams and lotions, hairdressings, pharmaceutical ointments; stabilizer and aux. emulsifier for o/w systems; lt. amber liq.; sol. @ 5% in peanut and min. oils, 95% ethanol, IPM, oleyl alcohol; gels in glycerin; insol. in water; sp.gr. 0.960-0.980; acid no. 5 max.; iodine no. 58-68; sapon. no. 142-152; 100% conc.

Emulsynt® GDL. [ISP Van Dyk] Glyceryl dilaurate; CAS 27638-00-2; EINECS 248-586-9; emollient for creams and lotions; easily emulsified; coupler for more lipophilic materials; melts sl. below body temp.; wh. to off-wh. solid; sol. @ 5% in peanut and min. oil, 95% ethanol, IPM, oleyl alcohol, castor oil; disp. in hot water; HLB 10-12; acid no. 5 max.; sapon. no. 219-229; ref. index 1.4520-1.4560 (35 C); toxicology: LD50 (oral, rat) > 5 g/kg; nonirritating to eyes and skin; nonsensitizing.

Emultex SMS. [Auschem SpA] Sorbitan monostearate; CAS 1338-41-6; EINECS 215-664-9; nonionic; plasticizer, antifoamer, softener, textile lubricant, emulsifier in cosmetics; flakes; HLB 4.5; 100% conc.

Emultex WS. [Auschem SpA] Ester of a polyglycerol deriv.; nonionic; emulsifier for aq. insecticides, deodorant aerosols; liq.; HLB 4.0; 100% conc.

Emulvis®. [C.P. Hall] PEG-150 distearate; CAS 9005-08-7; nonionic; visc. builder in cosmetics, sol. retarder for gums and resins; antiblock agent for decals; thickener in pet shampoos; melt pt. control in suppositories; wh. to cream flake; bland odor; 50% sol. in 70% IPA; 3% sol. in water; m.p. 53–58 C; pH 4–6 (3% aq.); 100% act.

Emulzome. [Exsymol; Biosil Tech.] Hydrog. polyisobutene, stearyl heptanoate, min. oil.; for cosmetic creams and milks; wh. opaque liq.; misc. with water and glycols; sp.gr. 0.9; pH 6.0; usage level: 6-30%; toxicology: nontoxic.

Em-U-Taine. [Emulan] Minkamidopropyl betaine; cosmetic ingred.

Emvelop®. [Mendell] Hydrogenated veg. oil NF; CAS 68334-00-9; EINECS 269-804-9; for prod. of sustained-release tablet formulations; fine powd.; 25% max. -200 mesh; dens. (tapped) 0.57 g/ml; m.p. 61-66 C; iodine no. 5 max.; sapon. no. 188-198.

Enagicol C-30B. [Lion] Cocamidopropyl betaine; CAS 70851-07-9; anionic; mild detergent, visc. builder for shampoos and bubble baths; liq.; 30% conc.

Enagicol C-40H. [Lion] Coconut imidazolinium betaine; amphoteric; nonirritating shampoos, skin cleaners; liq.; 40% conc.

Enagicol CNS. [Lion] Coconut imidazolinium betaine; amphoteric; nonirritating shampoos, skin cleaners; salt-free type; liq.; 40% conc.

Enagicol L-30AN. [Lion] Sodium N-lauroyl-N-methyl-β-aminopropionate; anionic; mild detergent for shampoos and face cleansers; liq.; 30% conc.

Endomine NMF. [Laboratoires Sérobiologiques] Hydrolyzed collagen, glycerin, sodium PCA, sodium lactate, urea.

Endonucleine®. [Laboratoires Sérobiologiques] Polynucleotides, amino acids, polyoside, and oligopeptides; complex providing cutaneous moisturizing action, emollience, anti-free radicals, and enrichment of DNA in human epidermis; used for prods. for anti-aging, antiwrinkle, skin protection and repair; amber limpid liq.; water-sol.; usage level: 3-5%.

Endonucleine LS 2143. [Laboratoires Sérobiologiques] Glycerin, water, propylene glycol, hydrolyzed actin, DNA, glycogen, arginine, RNA.

Enduragloss™. [U.S. Cosmetics] Purified rosin ester gum/2-octyldodecyl myristate; neutral oil improving adhesion, gloss, conditioning in lipsticks, foundation, eye shadow stick, hair creams; liq.

Energisome. [Sederma] Liposome containing L-carnitine and ubiquinone; cell energizer for face and body care prods.; for ageing prevention prods., free scavenger treatments; yel.-orange opalescent liq., char. odor; sp.gr. 1.000-1.050; pH 5.0-6.0; usage level: 5-30%.

Enzyami No. 1. [Alban Muller] Phytoenzymatic complex; Phytoenzymatic complex, anti-free radical protector with anti-solar and anti-bacterial activity; helps prevent skin from aging; usage level: 1-3%.

Enzyami No. 1A. [Alban Muller; Tri-K Industries] Enzymes and herbal extract complex; free radical scavenger; provides solar protection, bactericidal props. for cosmetics; powd.

Enzyami No. 5. [Alban Muller] Phytoenzymatic complex; provides cell stimulation, antisolar and anti-free radical activity for skin care prods.; usage level: 1-3%.

Enzyami No. 5A. [Alban Muller; Tri-K Industries] Enzymes and herbal extract complex; provides stimulation and solar protection in cosmetics; powd.

Enzyami No. 6. [Alban Muller; Tri-K Industries] Enzymes and herbal extract complex; free radical scavenger; provides bactericidal and stimulating props. for cosmetics; powd.

Enzyami No. 7. [Alban Muller; Tri-K Industries] Enzymes and herbal extract complex; deodorant for cosmetics use; powd.

E.O.D. [U.S. Cosmetics] 2-Octyldodecyl erucate; CAS 88103-59-7; neutral oil imparting pleasant, nongreasy "cooling" feel to cosmetic makeup, sunscreens, hair and skin care prods.

Epal® 12. [Ethyl] Dodecanol; CAS 112-53-8; EINECS 203-982-0; detergent and emulsifier intermediate for household prods., industrial and institutional cleaning, emulsion polymerization, and personal care prods.; water-wh. mobile liq., mild char. odor; m.w. 186; sp.gr. 0.830 g/ml; dens. 6.93 lb/gal; f.p. 24 C; b.p. 258-264 C (1 atm); flash pt. (PMCC) 132 C; hyd. no. 301; toxicology: temporary irritation on direct skin or eye contact; 100% conc.

Epal® 12/70. [Ethyl] Dodecanol (70%), tetradecanol (29%); CAS 67762-41-8; EINECS 267-019-6; detergent and emulsifier intermediate for household prods., industrial and institutional cleaning, emulsion polymerization, and personal care prods.; biodeg.; clear liq., mild char. odor; m.w. 195; sp.gr. 0.832 g/ml; dens. 6.94 lb/gal; f.p. 18 C; b.p. 126-129 C (760 mm); flash pt. (PMCC) 135 C; hyd. no. 288; toxicology: temporary irritation on direct skin or eye contact; 100% conc.

Epal® 12/85. [Ethyl] Dodecanol (86%), tetradecanol (14%); CAS 67762-41-8; EINECS 267-019-6; detergent and emulsifier intermediate for household prods., industrial and institutional cleaning, emulsion polymerization, and personal care prods.; biodeg.; clear liq., mild char. odor; m.w. 190; sp.gr. 0.830 g/ml; dens. 6.93 lb/gal; f.p. 20 C; b.p. 126-129 C (760 mm); flash pt. (PMCC) 138 C; hyd. no. 297; toxicology: temporary irritation on direct skin or eye contact; 100% conc.

Epal® 14. [Ethyl] Tetradecanol; CAS 112-72-1; EINECS 204-000-3; detergent and emulsifier intermediate for household prods., industrial and institutional cleaning, emulsion polymerization, and personal care prods.; biodeg.; wh. waxy solid, mild char. odor; m.w. 215; sp.gr. 0.822 g/ml; dens. 6.86 lb/gal; f.p. 35 C; flash pt. (PMCC) 149 C; hyd. no. 261; toxicology: temporary irritation on direct skin or eye contact; 100% conc.

Epal® 16NF. [Ethyl] Hexadecanol NF; CAS 36653-82-4; EINECS 253-149-0; USP grade biodeg. detergent and emulsifier intermediate for household prods., industrial and institutional cleaning, emulsion polymerization, and cosmetic/personal care prods.; wh. waxy solid, mild char. odor; m.w. 242; sp.gr. 0.818 g/ml; dens. 6.83 lb/gal; f.p. 44 C; flash pt. (PMCC) 175 C; hyd. no. 232; toxicology: temporary irritation on direct skin or eye contact; 100% conc.

Epal® 18NF. [Ethyl] Octadecanol NF; CAS 112-92-5; EINECS 204-017-6; USP grade biodeg. detergent and emulsifier intermediate for household prods., cosmetics, deodorants; wh. waxy solid, mild char. odor; m.w. 270; sp.gr. 0.812 g/ml; dens. 6.78 lb/gal; f.p. 54 C; flash pt. (PMCC) 191 C; hyd. no. 207; toxicology: temporary irritation on direct skin or eye contact; 100% conc.

Epal® 20+. [Ethyl] C18-C32 linear and branched alcohols (66%), C24-C40 hydrocarbons (40%); CAS 68911-61-5; EINECS 272-778-1; biodeg. detergent and emulsifier intermediate for household prods., cosmetics, deodorants; off-wh. waxy solid; sp.gr. 0.83 g/ml; dens. 6.9 lb/gal; f.p. 41 C; flash pt. (PMCC) 177 C; hyd. no. 105; toxicology: temporary irritation on direct skin or eye contact; 100% conc.

Epal® 1214. [Ethyl] Dodecanol (66%), tetradecanol (27%), hexadecanol (6%); CAS 67762-41-8; EINECS 267-019-6; biodeg. detergent and emulsifier intermediate for household prods., industrial and institutional cleaners, emulsion polymerization, personal care prods.; clear sl. visc. liq., mild char. odor; m.w. 197; sp.gr. 0.830 g/ml; dens. 6.93 lb/gal; f.p. 22 C; b.p. 233-299 C (1 atm); flash pt. (PMCC) 138 C; hyd. no. 284; toxicology: temporary irritation on direct skin or eye contact; 100% conc.

Epal® 1218. [Ethyl] Dodecanol (48%), tetradecanol (20%), hexadecanol (17%), octadecanol (14%); CAS 67762-25-8; EINECS 267-006-5; biodeg. detergent/emulsifier intermediate for household and personal care prods.; water-wh. mobile liq. at sl. above R.T., mild char. odor; m.w. 214; sp.gr. 0.825 g/ml; dens. 6.89 lb/gal; f.p. 25 C; flash pt. (PMCC) 139 C; hyd. no. 266; toxicology: temporary irrita-

tion on direct skin or eye contact; 100% conc.

Epal® 1412. [Ethyl] Tetradecanol (58%), dodecanol (40%); CAS 67762-41-8; EINECS 267-019-6; intermediate for surfactants, plasticizers, lubricant additives, thioesters, specialty chems., personal care prods.; clear sl. visc. liq., mild char. odor; m.w. 204; sp.gr. 0.820 g/ml; dens. 6.84 lb/gal; f.p. 26 C; b.p. 2 C (1 atm); flash pt. (PMCC) 137 C; hyd. no. 275; toxicology: temporary irritation on direct skin or eye contact; 100% conc.

Epal® 1416. [Ethyl] Tetradecanol (58%), dodecanol (40%); CAS 68333-80-2; EINECS 269-790-4; biodeg. detergent/emulsifier intermediate for household and personal care prods.; wh. waxy solid, mild char. odor; m.w. 224; sp.gr. 0.825 g/ml; dens. 6.88 lb/gal; f.p. 36 C; flash pt. (CC) 143 C; hyd. no. 250; toxicology: temporary irritation on direct skin or eye contact; 100% conc.

Epal® 1416-LD. [Ethox] Tetradecanol (63.5%), hexadecanol (35.6%), low-diol blend; CAS 68333-80-2; EINECS 2679-790-4; detergent/emulsifier intermediate for household and personal care prods.; wh. waxy solid, mild char. odor; m.w. 224; sp.gr. 0.825 g/ml; dens. 6.88 lb/gal; f.p. 38 C; flash pt. (PMCC) 143 C; toxicology: temporary irritation on direct skin or eye contact; 100% conc.

Epal® 1418. [Ethyl] Tetradecanol (35%), hexadecanol (40%), octadecanol (23%); CAS 67762-30-5; EINECS 267-009-1; biodeg. detergent/emulsifier intermediate for household and personal care prods.; wh. waxy solid, mild char. odor; m.w. 239; sp.gr. 0.825 g/ml; dens. 6.89 lb/gal; f.p. 42 C; b.p. 300-315 C (1 atm); flash pt. (PMCC) 149 C; hyd. no. 235; toxicology: temporary irritation on direct skin or eye contact; 100% conc.

Epal® 1618. [Ethyl] Hexadecanol (47%), octadecanol (50%); CAS 67762-27-0; EINECS 267-008-6; biodeg. detergent/emulsifier intermediate for household and personal care prods.; wh. waxy solid, mild char. odor; m.w. 256; sp.gr. 0.819 g/ml; dens. 6.83 lb/gal; f.p. 46 C; flash pt. (PMCC) 202 C; hyd. no. 219; toxicology: temporary irritation on direct skin or eye contact; 100% conc.

Epal® 1618RT. [Ethyl] Hexadecanol (66%), octadecanol (32%), eicosanol (1%); CAS 67762-27-0; EINECS 267-008-6; biodeg. detergent/emulsifier intermediate for household and personal care prods.; wh. waxy solid, mild char. odor; m.w. 250; sp.gr. 0.827 g/ml; dens. 6.90 lb/gal; f.p. 46 C; flash pt. (PMCC) > 149 C; hyd. no. 223; toxicology: temporary irritation on direct skin or eye contact; 100% conc.

Epal® 1618T. [Ethyl] Hexadecanol (32%), octadecanol (65%); CAS 67762-27-0; EINECS 267-008-6; intermediate for surfactants, plasticizers, lubricant additives, thioesters, specialty chems., personal care prods.; wh. waxy solid, mild char. odor; m.w. 260; sp.gr. 0.821 g/ml; dens. 6.86 lb/gal; f.p. 41 C; flash pt. (PMCC) 177 C; hyd. no. 216; toxicology: temporary irritation on direct skin or eye contact; 100% conc.

EPCH. [Vevy] Hydrolyzed casein; CAS 65072-00-6; EINECS 265-363-1; cosmetic protein.

EPC-K. [Senju Pharmaceutical] Potassium ascorbyl tocopheryl phosphate.

Epiderm-Complex O. [Cosmetochem] Olive oil, oleyl erucate, aorta extract, calf skin extract, placental protein, retinyl palmitate, cholecalciferol, and tocopheryl acetate; cosmetic ingred.

Epiderm-Complex W. [Cosmetochem] Water, calf skin extract, spleen extract, udder extract, and placental protein; cosmetic ingred.

Epidermin in Oil. [Dr. Kurt Richter; Henkel/Cospha] Sesame oil, thymus extract, testicular extract, mammary extract, ovarian extract, placental lipids, and pigskin extract; polyvalent tissue complex in oil medium; prod. for aging and sensitive skin; yel. oil.

Epidermin Water-Soluble. [Dr. Kurt Richter; Henkel/ Cospha] Polysorbate 20, balm mint extract, thymus extract, testicular extract, mammary extract, ovarian extract, placental lipids, and pigskin extract; polyvalent tissue complex, hydro-alcohol solubilized; prod. for aging and sensitive skin; yel. liq.

Epikuron 145. [Lucas Meyer] Phosphatidylcholine enriched fraction of soya phospholipids; carrier, wetting agent, stabilizer, emulsifier, and choline enrichment for pharmaceutical applics.; 45% conc.

Epikuron 170. [Lucas Meyer] Conc. phosphatidylcholine from soya; carrier, emulsifier, choline enrichment for pharmaceuticals; 70% conc.

Epikuron 200. [Lucas Meyer] Isolated phosphatidylcholine from soya; carrier, emulsifier, choline enrichment for pharmaceuticals and liposomes; 95% conc.

Epikuron H. [Lucas Meyer] Range of soya phospholipids; hydrophilic emulsifier, dispersant for pharmaceuticals and liposomes; powd.

E.P.O. [Nisshin Oil Mills] Evening primrose oil.

Epomin P-1000. [Aceto] PEI-1750; CAS 9002-98-6; cosmetic ingred.

Epomin SP-006. [Aceto] PEI-15; CAS 9002-98-6; cosmetic ingred.

Epomin SP-012. [Aceto] PEI-30; CAS 9002-98-6; cosmetic ingred.

Epomin SP-018. [Aceto] PEI-45; CAS 9002-98-6; cosmetic ingred.

Epoxyweichmacher LSB. [Bärlocher GmbH] Epoxidized soybean oil; CAS 8013-07-8; EINECS 232-391-0.

Ervol®. [Witco/Petroleum Spec.] Wh. min. oil NF; emulsifier, lubricant, emollient; for cosmetics, food contact; FDA §172.878, 178.3620a; water-wh., odorless, tasteless; sp.gr. 0.849-0.865; visc. 24-26 cSt (40 C); pour pt. -7 C; flash pt. 185 C.

Escalol® 507. [ISP Van Dyk] Octyl dimethyl PABA; CAS 21245-02-3; EINECS 244-289-3; nonstaining uv-B absorber for topical sunscreens; pale yel. mobile liq., very mild char. odor; sol. in min. and peanut oil, ethanol, IPA; insol. in water; m.w. 277; sp.gr. 0.990-1.000; HLB 10-12; acid no. 1 max.; sapon. no. 195-215; ref. index 1.5390-1.5430; usage level: 1.8-8.0%; toxicology: LD50 (oral, rat) 14.9 g/kg; pract. nonirritating to eyes; nonirritating, nonsensitizing to skin; 98% min. purity.

Escalol® 557. [ISP Van Dyk] Octyl methoxycinnamate; CAS 5466-77-3; EINECS 226-775-7; nonstaining uv-B absorber for sunscreens, esp. waterproof formulations; imparts emolliency to emulsions without being tacky or oily; pale yel. liq. with slight odor; sol. in peanut oil, min. oil, ethanol (95%, 100%), oleyl alcohol, castor oil, IPM, cyclomethicone; m.w. 290.4; sp.gr. 1.005-1.013; HLB 6-8; acid no. 1 max.; sapon. no. 189 min.; ref. index 1.542-1.548; toxicology: minimally irritating to eyes; mildly irritating to skin; 98% min. purity.

Escalol® 567. [ISP Van Dyk] Benzophenone-3; CAS 131-57-7; EINECS 205-031-5; uv-A absorber for formulation of high-SPF sunscreens; slightly ylsh. fine cryst. powd.; sol. in peanut oil, ethanol, oleyl alcohol, castor oil; m.w. 228.25; m.p. 62 C min.; usage level: 2-6%; 97% min. assay.

Escalol® 587. [ISP Van Dyk] Octyl salicylate; CAS 118-60-5; EINECS 204-263-4; uv-B sunscreen for high-SPF formulations; boosts efficacy of other sunscreen actives; solubilizer for benzophenone-3; colorless to pale yel. liq., typ. bland odor; sol. in IPA, ethanol, min. oil, dimethicone, cyclomethicone, IPM, octyl palmitate; m.w. 250.34; sp.gr. 1.013-1.022; acid no. 2 max.; sapon. no. 200-230; ref. index 1.495-1.505; usage level: 3-5%; toxicology: LD50 (oral, rat) < 5 g/kg; minimally irritating to eyes; mildly irritating to skin; nonsensitizing.

Escalol® 597. [ISP Van Dyk] Octocrylene; CAS 6197-30-4; EINECS 228-250-8; uv-B sunscreen used when high SPF values are required; esp. for water-resistant formulations; yel. clear visc. liq., bland odor; sol. @ 5% in ethanol, castor oil, IPM, hexylene glycol, IPA; disp. in min. oil, dimethicone; insol. in water; m.w. 361; f.p. -10 C; usage level: 7-10%; toxicology: LD50 (oral, rat) > 64 ml/kg; nonirritating to eyes; minimally irritating to skin; 98% min. assay.

Escin/β-Sitosterol Phytosome®. [Indena SpA; Lipo] Complex of escin, β-sitosterol, and soybean phospholipids; skin lightener, astringent, soothing/moisturizing agent, coadjuvant in external treatment of cellulitis, after-sun, after-depilation, and after-shave prods., dentifrices for swollen gums, prods. for oral cavity; lt. brn. amorphous powd.; water-disp.; usage level: to 3%.

Escorez 1271 U. [Exxon Japan] Polypentene.

ESH-C. [Ethyl] C20-40 isoparaffin.

Esi-Cryl 11. [Emulsion Systems] Styrene/acrylates copolymer.

Esi-Cryl 12. [Emulsion Systems] Styrene/acrylamide copolymer.

Esi-Det CDA. [Emulsion Systems] 1:1 Cocamide DEA; CAS 61791-31-9; EINECS 263-163-9; nonionic; detergent, foam stabilizer, thickener for personal care prods., lt. duty dishwash and household cleaners, industrial prods.; 100% biodeg.; straw color; sp.gr. 0.98; dens. 8.16 lb/gal; pH 9.0-11.0; 99% min. solids.

Esi-Terge 10. [Emulsion Systems] Cocamide DEA; CAS 61791-31-9; EINECS 263-163-9; nonionic; foam stabilizer, thickener for household, cosmetic, industrial prods.; liq.; 100% conc.

Esi-Terge S-10. [Emulsion Systems] 1:1 Cocamide DEA; CAS 61791-31-9; EINECS 263-163-9; nonionic; detergent, emulsifier, foam stabilizer, thickener, for liq. dishwashing and car washing detergents, household, industrial, and cosmetic prods.; lt. straw liq.; sp.gr. 0.98; dens. 8.16 lb/gal; pH 9-10; biodeg.; 100% act.

Eskar Wax R-25, R-35, R-40, R-45, R-50. [Amoco Lubricants] Paraffin; CAS 8002-74-2; EINECS 232-315-6; cosmetic wax.

Espermaceti A. [Fabriquimica] Cetyl esters; regreasing agent for cosmetic emulsions; acid no. < 1; iodine no. < 1; sapon. no. 90-105.

Espermaceti C. [Fabriquimica] Cetyl esters; regreasing agent for cosmetic emulsions; acid no. < 6; iodine no. < 1; sapon. no. 105-120.

Espholip. [Lucas Meyer] Semisyn. phosphatidylcholine; emulsifier, encapsulation aid for pharmaceuticals and liposomes.

Essentiaderm n.1. [CGI-Universal Flavors] Bergamot oil, lavender oil, peppermint oil, thyme oil, lemon oil, and eucalyptus oil.

Essentiaderm n.2. [CGI-Universal Flavors] Rosemary oil, lavender oil, myrtle extract, sweet marjoram oil, lemon oil, and pine oil.

Essentiaderm n.3. [CGI-Universal Flavors] Lavender oil, bergamot oil, cypress oil, clary oil, and chamomile oil.

Essentiaderm n.4. [CGI-Universal Flavors] Clary oil, coriander oil, balm mint oil, and matricaria oil.

Essentiaderm n.4. [CGI-Universal Flavors] Bergamot oil, cypress oil, lemon oil, bitter orange oil, and lavender oil.

Essentiaderm n.6. [CGI-Universal Flavors] Lavender oil, balm mint oil, peppermint oil, coriander oil, bitter orange oil, and matricaria oil.

Essentiaderm n.7. [CGI-Universal Flavors] Lavender oil, camphor, rosemary oil, pine oil, sweet marjoram oil, and thyme oil.

Essentiaderm n.8. [CGI-Universal Flavors] Lavender oil, peppermint oil, coriander oil, balm mint oil.

Essentiaderm n.9. [CGI-Universal Flavors] Rosemary oil,

Estalan 12

lavender oil, sweet marjoram oil, lemon oil, and pine oil.

Estalan 12. [Lanaetex Prods.] Laureth-2 octanoate; nonionic; emollient, lubricant, and skin conditioner for cosmetic creams and lotions; reduces oiliness and greasiness of min. oil and petrolatum-based formulations producing dry skinfeel; lt. color, low odor; sol. in oil and alcohol blends.

Estalan 38. [Lanaetex Prods.] Laureth-2 acetate.

Estalan 42. [Lanaetex Prods.] Laureth-2 acetate; emollient, coupler for use in hydro-alcoholic sol'ns.; blooming agent for bath preps.; also for liq. hand soaps; water-wh., odorless; sol. in alcohol.

Estalan 126. [Lanaetex Prods.] Laureth-2 benzoate; emollient with wetting and mild emulsification props.; blooming agent for bath oils, bath gels; prewetting agent for Carbopol resins and collagen derivs.; alcohol/water coupler for use in hydro-alcoholic systems; leaves soft, conditioned feel on skin and hair.

Estalan 334. [Lanaetex Prods.] Isodecyl octanoate, octyl isononanoate, PEG-2 diisononanoate, and PEG-2 dioctanoate; provides elegant, luxurious, light, dry feel; offsets heavy, greasy feel of oil and petrolatum-based prods. in cosmetic creams and lotions; reduces tackiness; suggested as replacement for volatile silicones.

Estalan 430. [Lanaetex Prods.] Diethylene glycol dioctanoate/diisononanoate; emollient, penetrant, spreading agent, perfume solv. in antiperspirants, deodorants, preshave lotions, and other liqs.

Estalan 560. [Lanaetex Prods.] Diethylene glycol dioctanoate/diisononanoate and octyl isononanoate; provides luxurious, soft, dry feel to cosmetic creams, lotions, makeup, sunscreen formulations.

Estalan 635. [Lanaetex Prods.] Octyl isononanoate, diethylene glycol dioctanoate, laureth-2 benzoate, diethylene glycol diisononanoate; emollient with dry, nonoily skinfeel; reduces tack and drag in formulations; prewetting agent/dispersant for Carbopol powds.; for antiperspirants, lipsticks, creams, lotions, sunscreens, makeup; resin plasticizer in hairsprays.

Estalan 718. [Lanaetex Prods.] Octyl hydroxystearate; CAS 29383-26-4; cosmetic ingred.

Estalan 816. [Lanaetex Prods.] Octyl palmitate; CAS 29806-73-3; EINECS 249-862-1; cosmetic ingred.

Estalan DIA. [Lanaetex Prods.] Diisopropyl adipate; CAS 6938-94-9; EINECS 248-299-9; cosmetic ingred.

Estalan DISD. [Lanaetex Prods.] Diisostearyl dimerate; cosmetic ingred.

Estalan DNPA. [Lanaetex Prods.] Di-n-propyl adipate; CAS 106-19-4; EINECS 203-371-9; emollient giving velvety feel to skin and hair; water-wh., odorless.

Estalan DO. [Lanaetex Prods.] Decyl oleate; CAS 3687-46-5; EINECS 222-981-6; cosmetic ingred.

Estalan DOM. [Lanaetex Prods.] Dioctyl maleate; cosmetic ingred.

Estalan JB. [Lanaetex Prods.] Cetearyl octanoate; cosmetic ingred.

Estalan L-45. [Lanaetex Prods.] Glycereth-4.5 lactate; CAS 125804-13-9; nonionic; emollient, humectant for hydro/alcoholic formulations, aftershave, body-splash prods.; provides extremely soft skinfeel.

Estalan LL. [Lanaetex Prods.] Lauryl lactate; CAS 6283-92-7; EINECS 228-504-8; cosmetic ingred.

Estalan MA. [Lanaetex Prods.] Menthyl anthranilate; CAS 134-09-8; EINECS 205-129-8; uv-A sunscreen.

Estalan ML. [Lanaetex Prods.] Myristyl lactate; CAS 1323-03-1; EINECS 215-350-1; cosmetic ingred.

Estalan OV. [Lanaetex Prods.] Octyl oxystearate; CAS 29710-25-6; cosmetic ingred.

Estalan TC. [Lanaetex Prods.] Trioctyl citrate; cosmetic ingred.

Estamol TR 8-60. [DS Industries] Trimethylolpropane tricaprylate/tricaprate.

Estaram. [Unichema] Suppository bases for pharmaceuticals.

Estasan 3575. See Estasan GT 8-60 3575 [Unichema]

Estasan 3577. See Estasan GT 8-65 3577 [Unichema]

Estasan 3578. See Estasan GT 8-40 3578 [Unichema]

Estasan GT 8-40 3578. [Unichema] Caprylic/capric triglyceride (40% C8 + 60% C10); CAS 65381-09-1; solv. and carrier for drugs, capsules, flavors, fragrances, food ingreds.; lubricant, mold release for food applics.; fat source in dietetic prods.; spreading/penetrating aid, solv. for cosmetics and toiletries; Japan approval; Lovibond 5Y/0.5R color, odorless, bland taste; visc. 29 mPa·s; acid no. 0.1 max.; iodine no. 2 max.; sapon. no. 300-315; hyd. no. 5 max.; cloud pt. 10 C.

Estasan GT 8-60 3575. [Unichema] Caprylic/capric triglyceride (60% C8 + 40% C10); CAS 65381-09-1; EINECS 265-724-3; solv. and carrier for drugs, capsules, flavors, fragrances, food ingreds.; lubricant, mold release for food applics.; fat source in dietetic prods.; spreading/penetrating aid, solv. for cosmetics and toiletries; Japan approval; Lovibond 5Y/0.5R color, odorless, bland taste; visc. 23 mPa·s; acid no. 0.1 max.; iodine no. 0.5 max.; sapon. no. 325-345; hyd. no. 5 max.; cloud pt. -8 C.

Estasan GT 8-60 3580. [Unichema] Caprylic/capric triglyceride (60% C8 + 40% C10), kosher grade; CAS 65381-09-1; solv. and carrier for drugs, capsules, flavors, fragrances, food ingreds.; lubricant, mold release for food applics.; fat source in dietetic prods.; spreading/penetrating aid, solv. for cosmetics and toiletries; Lovibond 5Y/0.5R color, odorless, bland taste; visc. 23 mPa·s; acid no. 0.1 max.; iodine no. 0.5 max.; sapon. no. 325-345; hyd. no. 5 max.; cloud pt. -8 C.

Estasan GT 8-65 3577. [Unichema] Caprylic/capric triglyceride (65% C8 + 35% C10); CAS 65381-09-1; solv. and carrier for drugs, capsules, flavors, fragrances, food ingreds.; lubricant, mold release for food applics.; fat source in dietetic prods.; spreading/penetrating aid, solv. for cosmetics and toiletries; Japan approval; Lovibond 5Y/0.5R color, odorless, bland taste; visc. 23 mPa·s; acid no. 0.1 max.; iodine no. 0.5 max.; sapon. no. 325-360; hyd. no. 5 max.; cloud pt. -5 C.

Estasan GT 8-65 3581. [Unichema] Caprylic/capric triglyceride (65% C8 + 35% C10), kosher grade; CAS 65381-09-1; solv. and carrier for drugs, capsules, flavors, fragrances, food ingreds.; lubricant, mold release for food applics.; fat source in dietetic prods.; spreading/penetrating aid, solv. for cosmetics and toiletries; Lovibond 5Y/0.5R color; visc. 23 mPa·s; acid no. 0.1 max.; iodine no. 0.5 max.; sapon. no. 335-360; hyd. no. 5 max.; cloud pt. -5 C.

Estemol CHS. [Nisshin Oil Mills] Cholesteryl hydroxystearate; CAS 40445-72-5.

Estemol N-01. [Nisshin Oil Mills] Neopentyl glycol dicaprate; CAS 27841-06-1.

Esterlan SN. [Fabriquimica] Acetylated and ethoxylated lanolin alcohol; multifunctional cosmetic ingred.; cloud pt. 8-15 C; acid no. < 3; sapon. no. 65-75.

Estol 1407. [Unichema] Glyceryl oleate; antistat for polyethylene and polypropylene; antifog agent for LDPE and PP; for lubricants, cosmetic emollients.

Estol 1461. [Unichema] Glyceryl monostearate SE; emulsifier for cosmetics.

Estol 1467. [Unichema] Glyceryl stearate; emulsifier for cosmetics; Japan approval; 90% mono.

Estol 1474. [Unichema] Glyceryl stearate; personal care ingred.; Japan approval.

Estol 1476. [Unichema] Isobutyl stearate; CAS 646-13-9; EINECS 211-466-1; lubricant for PVC processing; cos-

156

metic emollients.

Estol 1481. [Unichema] Cetostearyl stearate; CAS 93820-97-4; lubricant for PVC processing; cosmetic emollients.

Estol 1512. [Unichema] Isopropyl myristate (98%); CAS 110-27-0; EINECS 203-751-4; personal care emollient; Japan approval.

Estol 1514. [Unichema] Isopropyl myristate (90%); CAS 110-27-0; EINECS 203-751-4; personal care emollient; Japan approval.

Estol 1517. [Unichema] Isopropyl palmitate; CAS 142-91-6; EINECS 205-571-1; personal care ingred.; Japan approval.

Estol 1526. [Unichema] Propylene glycol dicaprylate/dicaprate; personal care ingred.; Japan approval.

Estol 1527. See Estol GTCC 1527 [Unichema]

Estol 1543. [Unichema] Octyl palmitate; CAS 29806-73-3; EINECS 249-862-1; personal care ingred.; Japan approval.

Estol 3604. See Estol GTCC 60 3604 [Unichema]

Estol 3751. [Unichema] PEG-6 beeswax; cosmetics ingred.

Estol 3752. [Unichema] PEG-8 beeswax; personal care ingred.

Estol 3753. [Unichema] PEG-12 beeswax; cosmetics ingred.

Estol 3754. [Unichema] PEG-20 beeswax; cosmetics ingred.

Estol BUS 1550. [Unichema] Butyl stearate based on triple-pressed stearic acid; CAS 123-95-5; EINECS 204-666-5; emollient ester for cosmetics; APHA 30 max. color; acid no. 0.2 max.; iodine no. 1 max.; sapon. no. 170-180; hyd. no. 1 max.; cloud pt. 23 C.

Estol BWB 3640. [Unichema] Behenyl beeswax.

Estol CEP 3694. [Unichema] Cetyl palmitate; CAS 540-10-3; EINECS 208-736-6; cosmetics ingred.; APHA 50 max. color; m.p. 52 C; acid no. 1 max.; iodine no. 1 max.; sapon. no. 111-122; hyd. no. 5 max.

Estol CEP-b 3653. [Unichema] Cetyl palmitate; CAS 540-10-3; EINECS 208-736-6; emollient.

Estol CES 3705. [Unichema] Cetyl stearate; CAS 1190-63-2; EINECS 214-724-1; emollient.

Estol CSS 3709. [Unichema] Cetearyl stearate; CAS 93820-97-4.

Estol DCO 3662. [Unichema] Decyl oleate; CAS 3687-46-5; EINECS 222-981-6; emollient ester for cosmetics; APHA 200 max. color; acid no. 1.0 max.; iodine no. 55-65; sapon. no. 132-142; hyd. no. 5 max.; cloud pt. 3 C.

Estol DCO-b 3655. [Unichema] Decyl oleate; CAS 3687-46-5; EINECS 222-981-6; emollient ester for cosmetics produced by biosynthesis; APHA 50 max. color; acid no. 0.5 max.; iodine no. 55-65; sapon. no. 132-142; hyd. no. 1 max.; cloud pt. 3 C.

Estol DEMS 3710. [Unichema] PEG-2 stearate; CAS 106-11-6; EINECS 203-363-5; emulsifier.

Estol DEMS-se 3711. [Unichema] PEG-2 stearate SE; CAS 9004-99-3; emulsifier.

Estol DEP 3075. [Unichema] Diethyl phthalate, perfumery grade; CAS 84-66-2; EINECS 201-550-6; cosmetics ingred.; APHA 50 max. color; acid no. 0.07 max.; sapon. no. 501-509; cloud pt. 23 C.

Estol E10DS 3728. [Unichema] PEG-20 distearate; CAS 9005-08-7; personal care surfactant.

Estol E10MS 3727. [Unichema] PEG-20 stearate; CAS 9004-99-3; emulsifier for cosmetics; APHA 100 max. color; m.p. 40 C; acid no. 5 max.; iodine no. 2 max.; sapon. no. 38-50; hyd. no. 45-55.

Estol E60DS 3734. [Unichema] PEG-150 distearate; CAS 9005-08-7; personal care surfactant.

Estol E60MS 3733. [Unichema] PEG-150 stearate; CAS 9004-99-3; emulsifier.

Estol EGDS 3750. [Unichema] Glycol distearate; CAS 627-83-8; EINECS 211-014-3; cosmetic ingred.

Estol EGMS 3749. [Unichema] Glycol stearate; CAS 111-60-

4; EINECS 203-886-9; emulsifier, opacifier, pearlescent for cosmetics.

Estol EHC 1540. [Unichema] Octyl cocoate; CAS 92044-87-6; EINECS 295-366-3; emollient ester for cosmetics; APHA 20 max. color; acid no. 0.2 max.; iodine no. 1 max.; sapon. no. 170-178; hyd. no. 1 max.; cloud pt. < 0 C.

Estol EHL 3613. [Unichema] Octyl laurate; 20292-08-4; EINECS 243-697-9.

Estol EHP 1543. [Unichema] Octyl palmitate; CAS 29806-73-3; EINECS 249-862-1; emollient ester for cosmetics; APHA 30 max. color; acid no. 0.2 max.; iodine no. 1 max.; sapon. no. 150-155; hyd. no. 1 max.; cloud pt. 2 C.

Estol EHP-b 3652. [Unichema] Octyl palmitate; CAS 29806-73-3; EINECS 249-862-1; emollient ester for cosmetics produced by biosynthesis; APHA 30 max. color; acid no. 0.2 max.; iodine no. 1.0 max.; sapon. no. 150-155; cloud pt. 2 C.

Estol EHS 1545. [Unichema] Octyl stearate; emollient ester for cosmetics; APHA 30 max. color; acid no. 0.2 max.; iodine no. 1 max.; sapon. no. 144-152; hyd. no. 1 max.; cloud pt. 10 C.

Estol EHS-b 3654. [Unichema] Octyl stearate; emollient.

Estol EO3BW 3751. [Unichema] PEG-6 beeswax.

Estol EO3GC 3606. [Unichema] PEG-7 glyceryl cocoate; emulsifier for cosmetics; APHA 100 max. color; acid no. 5 max.; iodine no. 4 max.; sapon. no. 90-100; hyd. no. 170-190; cloud pt. 0 C.

Estol EO4BW 3752. [Unichema] PEG-8 beeswax; emulsifier for cosmetics; free of ethylene oxide/p-dioxane; m.p. 64-70 C; acid no. 2 max.; iodine no. 6-12; sapon. no. 72-84; hyd. no. 18-28.

Estol EO4DO 3673. [Unichema] PEG-8 dioleate; CAS 9005-07-6; personal care surfactant.

Estol EO4DS 3724. [Unichema] PEG-8 distearate; CAS 9005-08-7; personal care surfactant.

Estol EO4MO 3672. [Unichema] PEG-8 oleate; CAS 9004-96-0; emulsifier.

Estol EO4MS 3723. [Unichema] PEG-8 stearate; CAS 9004-99-3; emulsifier for cosmetics; APHA 200 max. color; m.p. 31 C; acid no. 2 max.; iodine no. 2 max.; sapon. no. 76-96; hyd. no. 65-85.

Estol EO6BW 3753. [Unichema] PEG-12 beeswax.

Estol EO6DO 3675. [Unichema] PEG-12 dioleate; CAS 9005-07-6; personal care surfactant.

Estol EO6DS 3726. [Unichema] PEG-12 distearate; CAS 9005-08-7; personal care surfactant.

Estol EO6MO 3674. [Unichema] PEG-12 oleate; CAS 9004-96-0; personal care surfactant.

Estol EO6MS 3725. [Unichema] PEG-12 stearate; CAS 9004-99-3; emulsifier.

Estol ETO 3659. [Unichema] Ethyl oleate; CAS 111-62-6; EINECS 203-889-5; emollient ester for cosmetics; APHA 70 max. color; acid no. 0.5 max.; iodine no. 78-90; sapon. no. 180-190; cloud pt. -24 C.

Estol GDS 3748. [Unichema] Glyceryl distearate; CAS 1323-83-7; EINECS 215-359-0; emulsifier, emollient.

Estol GMCC 3602. [Unichema] Glyceryl caprylate/caprate.

Estol GML 3614. [Unichema] Glyceryl laurate; CAS 142-18-7; EINECS 205-526-6; cosmetic emulsifier.

Estol GMS90 1468. [Unichema] Glyceryl stearate, molecular distilled grade; antistat for polyethylene and polypropylene; antifog agent for LDPE; for lubricants; cosmetics emollient and emulsifier; Lovibond 3Y/1R color; m.p. 70 C; acid no. 3 max.; iodine no. 3 max.; > 90% monoglyceride.

Estol GMS 1473. [Unichema] Glyceryl stearate; lubricant for PVC processing; cosmetic emollient and emulsifier; Lovibond 3Y/1R color; m.p. 60 C; acid no. 3 max.; iodine no. 3 max.; sapon. no. 168-184.

Estol GMSse 1462. [Unichema] Glyceryl stearate SE; emulsifier for personal care applics.; Lovibond 7.0Y/1.5R color; m.p. 60 C; acid no. 3 max.; iodine no. 3 max.; sapon. no. 156-170.

Estol GMSveg 1474. [Unichema] Glyceryl stearate, vegetable grade; emulsifier for cosmetics; Lovibond 3Y/1R color; m.p. 60 C; acid no. 3 max.; iodine no. 3 max.; sapon. no. 168-184.

Estol GTC 1803. [Unichema] Tricaprylin; CAS 538-23-8; EINECS 208-686-5; personal care ingred.; APHA 50 max. color; visc. 22 mPa·s; acid no. 0.2 max.; iodine no. 0.5 max.

Estol GTC 3599. [Unichema] Caprylic-capric triglyceride; CAS 65381-09-1; personal care ingred.; APHA 150 max. color; visc. 17 mPa·s (40 C); acid no. 0.1 max.; iodine no. 1 max.

Estol GTCC 60 3604. [Unichema] Caprylic-capric triglyceride; CAS 65381-09-1; personal care ingred.; Japan approval; APHA 50 max. color; visc. 28 mPa·s; acid no. 0.3 max.; iodine no. 1 max.

Estol GTCC 1527. [Unichema] Glyceryl tricaprylate/caprate; for plastics, lubricants, cosmetic emollients; APHA 50 max. color; visc. 24 mPa·s; acid no. 0.1 max.; iodine no. 1 max.; sapon. no. 335-360; hyd. no. 5 max.; cloud pt. -12 C.

Estol GTEH 3609. [Unichema] Trioctanoin; CAS 538-23-8; EINECS 208-686-5; emollient ester for cosmetics; APHA 20 max. color; acid no. 0.1 max.; iodine no. 2 max.; hyd. no. 3 max.; cloud pt. -53 C.

Estol GTOveg 3665. [Unichema] Glyceryl oleate.

Estol IBUS 1552. [Unichema] Isobutyl stearate; CAS 646-13-9; EINECS 211-466-1; emollient, lubricant.

Estol IDCO 3667. [Unichema] Isodecyl oleate; CAS 59231-34-4; EINECS 261-673-6; emollient.

Estol IPL 1511. [Unichema] Isopropyl laurate; CAS 10233-13-3; EINECS 233-560-1; emollient.

Estol IPM 1508. [Unichema] Isopropyl myristate; CAS 110-27-0; EINECS 203-751-4; emollient.

Estol IPM 1509 (BIO-IPM). [Unichema] Isopropyl myristate, veg. derived; CAS 110-27-0; EINECS 203-751-4; penetrating emollient, solv. for cosmetics and topical medicinals with unique spreading props.; reduces heaviness and oiliness of prods. containing triglycerides, liq. waxes, and min. oils; provides gloss and conditioning in hair sprays; for skin creams, sun care preps., aerosols, bath oils, preshave lotions; colorless low-visc. liq., odorless; sp.gr. 0.850-0.855; acid no. 0.1 max.; iodine no. 0.5 max.; sapon. no. 206-211; cloud pt. 0 C max.; 98% min. act.

Estol IPM 1512. [Unichema] Isopropyl myristate; CAS 110-27-0; EINECS 203-751-4; cosmetic emollient ester; APHA 20 max. color; acid no. 0.1 max.; iodine no. 0.5 max.; sapon. no. 206-211; cloud pt. 0 C; 98% min. purity.

Estol IPM 1514. [Unichema] Isopropyl myristate; CAS 110-27-0; EINECS 203-751-4; for plastics, lubricants, cosmetic emollients; APHA 30 max. color; acid no. 0.5 max.; iodine no. 1 max.; sapon. no. 206-211; cloud pt. 0 C; 92% min. purity.

Estol IPM-b 1509. [Unichema] Isopropyl myristate; CAS 110-27-0; EINECS 203-751-4; emollient ester for cosmetics produced by biosynthesis; APHA 20 max. color; acid no. 0.1 max.; iodine no. 0.5 max.; sapon. no. 206-211; cloud pt. 0 C; 98% min. purity.

Estol IPP 1517. [Unichema] Isopropyl palmitate; CAS 142-91-6; EINECS 205-571-1; for plastics, lubricants, cosmetic emollients; APHA 20 max. color; acid no. 0.5 max.; iodine no. 1 max.; sapon. no. 185-191; cloud pt. 12 C; 90% min. purity.

Estol IPP-b 3651. [Unichema] Isopropyl palmitate; CAS 142-91-6; EINECS 205-571-1; emollient ester for cosmetics produced by biosynthesis; APHA 20 max. color; acid no. 0.1 max.; iodine no. 1 max.; sapon. no. 185-191; cloud pt.

12 C.

Estol IPS 3702. [Unichema] Isopropyl stearate based on triple-pressed stearic acid; CAS 112-10-7; EINECS 203-934-9; emollient ester for cosmetics; APHA 30 max. color; acid no. 1.0 max.; iodine no. 2 max.; sapon. no. 176-186; cloud pt. 16-20 C.

Estol MEL 1502. [Unichema] Methyl laurate; CAS 111-82-0; EINECS 203-911-3; detergent intermediate.

Estol MEL 1507. [Unichema] Methyl laurate; CAS 111-82-0; EINECS 203-911-3; detergent intermediate.

Estol MEM 1518. [Unichema] Methyl myristate; CAS 124-10-7; EINECS 204-680-1; detergent intermediate.

Estol MEP 1503. [Unichema] Methyl palmitate; CAS 112-39-0; EINECS 203-966-3; chemical intermediate.

Estol ML/M 1519. [Unichema] Methyl laurate and methyl myristate.

Estol MYM 3645. [Unichema] Myristyl myristate; CAS 124-10-7; EINECS 204-680-1; detergent intermediate.

Estol PDCC 1526. [Unichema] Propylene glycol dicaprylate/dicaprate; emollient ester for cosmetics; APHA 50 max. color; acid no. 0.1 max.; iodine no. 1 max.; sapon. no. 315-335; hyd. no. 10 max.; cloud pt. -40 C.

Estol PDP 3601. [Unichema] Propylene glycol dipelargonate; CAS 41395-83-9; EINECS 255-350-9; emollient.

Estol PMS 3737. [Unichema] Propylene glycol stearate; CAS 1323-39-3; EINECS 215-354-3; personal care surfactant.

Estol SML20 3618. [Unichema] Polysorbate 20; CAS 9005-64-5; emulsifier, solubilizer.

Estol SML 3617. [Unichema] Sorbitan laurate; emulsifier.

Estol SMO20 3686. [Unichema] Polysorbate 80; CAS 9005-65-6; emulsifier.

Estol SMO 3685. [Unichema] Sorbitan oleate; CAS 1338-43-8; EINECS 215-665-4; emulsifier.

Estol SMS 3715. [Unichema] Sorbitan stearate; CAS 1338-41-6; EINECS 215-664-9; emulsifier.

Estol SMS20 3716. [Unichema] Polysorbate 60; CAS 9005-67-8; emulsifier.

Estol STST 3706. [Unichema] Stearyl stearate; CAS 2778-96-3; EINECS 220-476-5; emollient.

Estran™. [Desert King Jojoba] Jojoba oil; CAS 61789-91-1; natural ingred. for hair and skin care formulations; avail. in various grades from single-pressed (golden) to refined (colorless and odorless).

Estran™-Lite. [Desert King Jojoba] Jojoba oil, single-pressed, bleached, and deodorized; CAS 61789-91-1; for skin/hair care cosmetic applics. (moisturizers, creams/lotions, sunscreens, lip care, bath/massage oils, hair/scalp care, makeup, soaps, nail treatments, polishes, and polish removers); emollient, skin softener; base/carrier for active ingreds.; prevents moisture loss from skin without being occlusive; features rapid skin penetration, thermal and oxidative stability; colorless oil, odorless; m.w. 606; sp.gr. 0.863; visc. 58.4 cSt; f.p. 7.0-10.6 C; m.p. 6.8-7.0 C; b.p. 398 C; acid no. < 0.4; iodine no. 82; sapon. no. 92; flash pt. 295 C; ref. index 1.4650; dielec. const. 2.680; toxicology: nonirritating, nontoxic, noncomedogenic.

Estran™-Pure. [Desert King Jojoba] Jojoba oil, single-pressed, filtered; CAS 61789-91-1; for skin/hair care cosmetic applics. (moisturizers, creams/lotions, sunscreens, lip care, bath/massage oils, hair/scalp care, makeup, soaps, nail treatments, polishes, and polish removers); emollient, skin softener; base/carrier for active ingreds.; prevents moisture loss from skin without being occlusive; features rapid skin penetration, high thermal and oxidative stability; golden yel. oil, sl. fatty odor; m.w. 606; sp.gr. 0.863; visc. 58.4 cSt; f.p. 7.0-10.6 C; m.p. 6.8-7.0 C; b.p. 398 C; acid no. < 0.4; iodine no. 82; sapon. no. 92; flash pt. 295 C; ref. index 1.4650; dielec. const. 2.680; toxicology: nonirritating, nontoxic, noncomedogenic.

Estran™-Xtra. [Desert King Jojoba] Jojoba oil, refined,

bleached, deodorized; CAS 61789-91-1; for skin/hair care cosmetic applics. (moisturizers, creams/lotions, sunscreens, lip care, bath/massage oils, hair/scalp care, makeup, soaps, nail treatments, polishes, and polish removers); emollient, skin softener; base/carrier for active ingreds.; prevents moisture loss from skin without being occlusive; features rapid skin penetration, thermal and oxidative stability; lt. yel. oil, odorless; m.w. 606; sp.gr. 0.863; visc. 58.4 cSt; f.p. 7.0-10.6 C; m.p. 6.8-7.0 C; b.p. 398 C; acid no. <<0.03; iodine no. 82; sapon. no. 92; flash pt. 295 C; ref. index 1.4650; dielec. const. 2.680; toxicology: nonirritating, nontoxic, noncomedogenic.

Esuronammina. [Esperis] Hydrolyzed glycosaminoglycans; moisturizer.

Etaphen. [Vevy] Phenethyl alcohol; CAS 60-12-8; EINECS 200-456-2; antiseptic for topical cosmetics; primarily effective against Gram-negative bacteria; USA and Japan approvals; usage level: 1% max.

Etha-Coll 210-20. [Brooks Industries] Myristoyl hydrolyzed collagen; CAS 72319-06-3; film-forming protein.

Etha-Coll AAS-20. [Brooks Industries] Ethyl ester of hydrolyzed collagen; cosmetic ingred.

Etha-Coll ISO. [Brooks Industries] AMP-isostearoyl hydrolyzed collagen; CAS 95032-84-1; raw material for cosmetic and personal care prods.

Etha-Keratin™ ISO. [Brooks Industries] AMP-isostearoyl hydrolyzed keratin; raw material for cosmetic and personal care prods.; alcohol-sol.; 25% alcoholic liq.

Etha-Soy™ ISO. [Brooks Industries] AMP-isostearoyl hydrolyzed soy protein; cosmetic ingredient for skin and hair care prods.; 25% alcoholic liq.

Ethlana 12. [Lanaetex Prods.] Isosteareth-12; CAS 52292-17-8; emulsifier.

Ethlana 22. [Lanaetex Prods.] Isosteareth-22; CAS 52292-17-8; emulsifier.

Ethlana 50. [Lanaetex Prods.] Isosteareth-50; CAS 52292-17-8; emulsifier.

Ethlana 50-M. [Lanaetex Prods.] Isosteareth-50; CAS 52292-17-8; emulsifier.

Ethocel Medium Premium. [Dow] Ethylcellulose NF; CAS 9004-57-3; used for pharmaceutical tablet coating, granulation, controlled release applics.; visc. avail. 50, 70, and 100 cps.

Ethocel Standard Premium. [Dow] Ethylcellulose NF; CAS 9004-57-3; binders for pharmaceutical tableting; visc. avail. 4, 7, 10, 20, 45, and 100 cps.

Ethoduomeen® T/13. [Akzo; Akzo BV] PEG-3 tallow aminopropylamine; CAS 61790-85-0; cationic; emulsifier used in making of bitumen emulsions; dispersant for waxes; for cosmetics, textiles, asphalt, agric. emulsions; wetting agent, corrosion inhibitor; Gardner 18 max. liq.; sp.gr. 0.95; f.p. -20 C; m.p. 17 C; b.p. 150 C; flash pt. (PMCC) > 204 C; surf. tens. 34.5 dynes/cm (0.1%); 100% conc.

Ethoduomeen® T/20. [Akzo; Akzo BV] PEG-10 tallow aminopropylamine; CAS 61790-85-0; cationic; emulsifier, dispersant, wetting agent used in coating preparation on paperboard; corrosion inhibitor; also for cosmetics; Gardner 18 max. liq.; sp.gr. 0.99; f.p. < 25 C; b.p. 150 C; flash pt. 90 C (PMCC); surf. tens. 38.2 dynes/cm (0.1%); 95% min. act.

Ethoduomeen® T/25. [Akzo; Akzo BV] PEG-15 tallow aminopropylamine; CAS 61790-85-0; cationic; corrosion inhibitor in water treatment chemicals in sec. oil recovery; also for cosmetics; Gardner 18 min. liq.; sp.gr. 1.02; f.p. > 25 C; flash pt. 238 C (COC); surf. tens. 43.0 dynes/cm (0.1%); 95% act.

Ethoduomeen® TD/13. [Akzo] Ethoxylated diamine from tallow fatty acid; emulsifier for bitumen emulsions, dispersing waxes; also for cosmetics; Gardner 4 max. clear

liq.; sp.gr. 0.95; surf. tens. 34.2 dynes/cm (0.1%).

Ethofat® 18/14. [Akzo] PEG-4 stearate; CAS 9004-99-3; EINECS 203-358-8; nonionic; industrial surfactant; Gardner 4 max. solid; sp.gr. 0.98; acid no. 3 max.; sapon. no. 121-131; flash pt. (PMCC) 274 C; surf. tens. 39 dynes/cm (0.1%).

Ethofat® 60/15. [Akzo] PEG-5 stearate; CAS 9004-99-3; nonionic; emulsifier, detergent, wetting agent, dispersant, suspending agent, for textile, cosmetic, agric., metal and leather treating; Gardner 8 soft paste; sol. in acetone, IPA, CCl$_4$, benzene, disp. in water; sp.gr. 1.01; acid no. 1 max.; sapon. no. 110–120; surf. tens. 39 dynes/cm (0.1%); pH 6–7.5 (10% aq.).

Ethofat® 60/20. [Akzo] PEG-10 stearate; CAS 9004-99-3; nonionic; emulsifier, detergent, wetting agent, dispersant, suspending agent, for textile, cosmetic, agric., metal and leather treating; Gardner 8 clear liq.; sol. in acetone, IPA, CCl$_4$, benzene, disp. in water; sp.gr. 1.02; acid no. 1 max.; sapon. no. 70–80; surf. tens. 36 dynes/cm (0.1%); pH 6–7.5 (10% aq.).

Ethofat® 242/25. [Akzo] PEG-15 tallate; CAS 61791-00-2; 65071-95-6; nonionic; emulsifier, detergent, dispersant; Gardner 12 clear liq.; sol. in acetone, IPA, CCl$_4$, dioxane, benzene, water; sp.gr. 1.08; acid no. 1 max.; sapon no. 55–65; pH 6–7.5 (10% aq.); flash pt. (PMCC) 274 C; surf. tens. 42 dynes/cm (0.1%); 100% conc.

Ethofat® 433. [Akzo] PEG-15 tallate; CAS 61791-00-2; 65071-95-6; nonionic; personal care surfactant; Gardner 12 max. liq.; acid no. 1.2 max.; sapon. no. 46-54; 9.5-10.5% moisture.

Ethofat® C/15. [Akzo] PEG-5 cocoate; CAS 61791-29-5; nonionic; emulsifier, detergent, dispersant; Gardner 9 clear liq.; sol. in acetone, IPA, CCl$_4$, benzene, disp. in water; sp.gr. 1.00; HLB 10.6; acid no. 1 max.; sapon. no. 120–130; surf. tens. 33 dynes/cm (0.1%); pH 6–7.5 (10% aq.); 100% conc.

Ethofat® C/25. [Akzo] PEG-15 cocoate; CAS 61791-29-5; nonionic; emulsifier, detergent, wetting agent, dispersant, suspending agent, for textile, cosmetic, agric., metal and leather treating; Gardner 8 paste; sol. see Ethofat 60/15; acid no. 1 max.; sapon. no. 60–70; pH 6–7.5 (10% aq.); flash pt. (PM) > 400 F.

Ethofat® O/15. [Akzo] PEG-5 oleate; CAS 9004-96-0; nonionic; emulsifier, detergent, dispersant; Gardner 9 max. clear liq.; sol. in acetone, IPA, CCl$_4$, benzene, disp. in water; sp.gr. 0.99; HLB 8.6; acid no. 1 max.; sapon. no. 110–120; surf. tens. 35 dynes/cm (0.1%); pH 6–7.5 (10% aq.); flash pt. (PM) > 400 F; 100% conc.

Ethofat® O/20. [Akzo] PEG-10 oleate; CAS 9004-96-0; nonionic; emulsifier, detergent, dispersant; Gardner 9 max. clear liq.; sol. in acetone, IPA, CCl$_4$, benzene, disp. in water; sp.gr. 1.028; acid no. 1 max.; sapon. no. 75–85; pH 6–7.5 (10% aq.); flash pt. (PM) 485 F; surf. tens. 41 dynes/cm (0.1%); 100% conc.

Ethomeen® 18/12. [Akzo] PEG-2 stearamine; CAS 10213-78-2; EINECS 233-520-3; cationic; emulsifier, dispersant for textile processing, cosmetics; Gardner 7 solid; sol. in acetone, IPA, CCl$_4$, benzene; sp.gr. 0.96; flash pt. (COC) 400 F; 100% conc.

Ethomeen® 18/15. [Akzo] PEG-5 stearamine; CAS 26635-92-7; cationic; emulsifier, dispersant for textile processing, cosmetics; Gardner 8 solid; sol. in acetone, IPA, CCl$_4$, benzene; sp.gr. 0.98; surf. tens. 34 dynes/cm (0.1%); flash pt. (COC) 500 F; 100% conc.

Ethomeen® 18/20. [Akzo] PEG-10 stearamine; CAS 26635-92-7; cationic; emulsifier, dispersant for textile processing, cosmetics; Gardner 8 clear liq. to paste; sp.gr. 1.02; flash pt. (COC) 540 F; surf. tens. 40 dynes/cm (0.1%).

Ethomeen® 18/25. [Akzo] PEG-15 stearamine; CAS 26635-92-7; cationic; emulsifier, dispersant for textile processing, cosmetics; Gardner 8 clear liq.; sp.gr. 1.04; flash pt. (COC) 560 F; surf. tens. 43 dynes/cm (0.1%).

Ethomeen® 18/60. [Akzo] PEG-50 stearamine; CAS 26635-92-7; cationic; emulsifier, dispersant used in textile processing, cosmetics; prevents premature coagulation of latex rubber; wh. solid; sol. in acetone, IPA, CCl₄, benzene, water; sp.gr. 1.12; flash pt. (COC) 579 F; surf. tens. 49 dynes/cm (0.1%).

Ethomeen® C/12. [Akzo; Akzo BV] PEG-2 cocamine; CAS 61791-14-8; 61791-31-9; cationic; emulsifier, dispersant for textile processing, cosmetics; Gardner 6 max. clear liq.; sol. in acetone, IPA, CCl₄, Stod., benzene; forms gel in water; sp.gr. 0.87; HLB 6.4; flash pt. (COC) 380 F; 100% conc.

Ethomeen® C/15. [Akzo; Akzo BV] PEG-5 cocamine; CAS 61791-14-8; cationic; emulsifier, dispersant for textile processing, dyeing assistant, desizing assistant, softener, antistat; also for cosmetics; Gardner 6 max. clear liq.; sol. in acetone, IPA, CCl₄, Stod., benzene, water (cloudy); sp.gr. 0.98; HLB 13.9; flash pt. (TOC) 460 F; surf. tens. 33 dynes/cm (0.1%); Draves wetting 3.5 s (0.5%); 100% conc.

Ethomeen® C/20. [Akzo] PEG-10 cocamine; CAS 61791-14-8; cationic; emulsifier, dispersant for textile processing, cosmetics; Gardner 11 max. clear liq.; sol. in acetone, IPA, CCl₄, Stod., benzene, water (cloudy); sp.gr. 1.02; flash pt. (COC) 560 F; surf. tens. 39 dynes/cm (0.1%); Draves wetting 14 s (0.5%).

Ethomeen® C/25. [Akzo; Akzo BV] PEG-15 cocamine; CAS 61791-14-8; cationic; emulsifier, dispersant for textile processing, cosmetics; Gardner 12 max. clear liq.; sol. in acetone, IPA, CCl₄, Stod., benzene, water; sp.gr. 1.04; HLB 19.3; flash pt. (COC) 500 F; surf. tens. 41 dynes/cm (0.1%); 100% conc.

Ethomeen® O/12. [Akzo] PEG-2 oleamine; cationic; emulsifier, dispersant for textile processing, cosmetics; Gardner 8 max. clear liq.; sp.gr. 0.90; flash pt. (COC) 470 F; surf tens. 31.5 dynes/cm (0.1%); 100% conc.

Ethomeen® O/15. [Akzo] PEG-5 oleamine; cationic; emulsifier, dispersant for textile processing, cosmetics; Gardner 8 max. clear liq.; sp.gr. 0.96; flash pt. (COC) 540 F; surf tens. 35.3 dynes/cm (0.1%); 100% conc.

Ethomeen® O/25. [Akzo] PEG-15 oleamine; emulsifier, dispersant used in cosmetics, textile processing; Gardner 8 max. paste; sp.gr. 1.04; flash pt. (PM) 380 F.

Ethomeen® S/12. [Akzo; Akzo BV] PEG-2 soyamine; CAS 61791-24-0; cationic; emulsifier, dispersant for textile processing, cosmetics; Gardner 14 max. clear heavy liq; sol. in acetone, IPA, CCl₄, Stod., benzene; insol. water; sp.gr. 0.91; HLB 14.6; flash pt. (TOC) 440 F; surf. tens. 31.4 dynes/cm (0.1%); 100% conc.

Ethomeen® S/15. [Akzo; Akzo BV] PEG-5 soyamine; CAS 61791-24-0; cationic; emulsifier, dispersant for textile processing, cosmetics; Gardner 14 max. clear heavy liq; sol. in acetone, IPA, CCl₄, Stod., benzene; forms gel or disp. in water; sp.gr. 0.95; HLB 19.0; flash pt. (TOC) 460 F; surf. tens. 33 dynes/cm (0.1%); Draves wetting 28 s (0.5%); 100% conc.

Ethomeen® S/20. [Akzo] PEG-10 soyamine; CAS 61791-24-0; cationic; emulsifier, dispersant used in textile processing, cosmetics; Gardner 14 max. clear heavy liq; sol. in acetone (cloudy), IPA, CCl₄, Stod., benzene, water; sp.gr. 1.02; flash pt. (COC) 540 F; surf. tens. 40 dynes/cm (0.1%); Draves wetting 29 s (0.5%).

Ethomeen® S/25. [Akzo; Akzo BV] PEG-15 soyamine; CAS 61791-24-0; cationic; emulsifier, dispersant used in textile processing, cosmetics; Gardner 14–18 max. clear heavy liq; sol. in acetone (cloudy), IPA, CCl₄, Stod., benzene, water; sp.gr. 1.04; HLB 9.8; flash pt. (COC) 540 F; surf. tens. 43 dynes/cm (0.1%); 100% conc.

Ethomeen® T/12. [Akzo; Akzo BV] PEG-2 hydrog. tallow amine; CAS 61791-26-2; cationic; emulsifier, dispersant used in textile processing, cosmetics; Gardner 8 paste; sol. in acetone, IPA, CCl₄, Stod., benzene, water; sp.gr. 0.92; HLB 4.5; flash pt. (COC) 410 F; 100% conc.

Ethomeen® T/15. [Akzo; Akzo BV] PEG-5 hydrog. tallow amine; CAS 61791-26-2; cationic; emulsifier, dispersant for textile processing, cosmetics; Gardner 8 max. paste; sol. cloudy in acetone, IPA, CCl₄, Stod., Benzene; forms gel in water; sp.gr. 0.97; flash pt. (PM) > 400 F; surf. tens. 34 dynes/cm (0.1%); Draves wetting 23 s (0.5%); 100% conc.

Ethomeen® T/25. [Akzo; Akzo BV] PEG-15 hydrog. tallow amine; CAS 61791-26-2; cationic; emulsifier, dispersant used in textile processing, cosmetics; Gardner 8 max. clear liq.; sol. cloudy in acetone, IPA, CCl₄, benzene, water; sp.gr. 1.03; HLB 19.3; flash pt. (COC) > 500 F; surf. tens. 41 dynes/cm (0.1%); Draves wetting 53 s (0.5%); 100% conc.

Ethomeen® T/60. [Akzo] PEG-50 tallow amine; emulsifier, dispersant used in textile processing, cosmetics; Gardner 10 max. paste to solid; m.w. 2362–2562; sp.gr. 1.115; flash pt. > 400 F (PM).

Ethomeen® TD/15. [Akzo] Ethoxylated tert. amine from tallow fatty acid; emulsifier, dispersant used in textile processing, cosmetics; Gardner 4 max. clear liq.; sp.gr. 0.97; surf. tens. 35.8 dynes/cm (0.1%).

Ethomeen® TD/25. [Akzo] Ethoxylated tert. amine from tallow fatty acid; emulsifier, dispersant used in textile processing, cosmetics; Gardner 4 max. clear liq.; sp.gr. 1.03; surf. tens. 43.5 dynes/cm (0.1%).

Ethomid® HT/15. [Akzo BV] Ethoxylated hydrog. tallow amide; nonionic; emulsifier, dispersant, detergent for cosmetics and industrial use; Gardner 10 max. solid; sol. in IPA; disp. in acetone, CCl₄, Stod., benzene, water; sp.gr. 1.03; HLB 13.5; surf. tens. 37 dynes/cm (0.1%); 100% conc.

Ethomid® HT/23. [Akzo] PEG-13 hydrog. tallow amide; CAS 68155-24-8; nonionic; emulsifier, dispersant, detergent, and dye leveling agen used for silicone finishing agents, sizing lubricants; also for cosmetics; Gardner 8 max. solid; sp.gr. 1.028; cloud pt. 130–170 F (1%); flash pt. (PM) > 400 F; hyd. no. 105; surf. tens. 37 dynes/cm (0.1%); 100% conc.

Ethomid® HT/60. [Akzo; Akzo BV] PEG-50 hydrog. tallow amide; CAS 68155-24-8; nonionic; surfactant, emulsifier, sec. stabilizer for emulsion systems; dispersant, detergent; also for cosmetics; Gardner 11 max. hard solid; sol. in IPA, CCl₄, benzene, water; sp.gr. 1.14; HLB 19.0; hyd. no. 45; flash pt. (PMCC) 540 C; surf. tens. 47 dynes/cm (0.1%); 100% conc.

Ethomid® O/15. [Akzo BV] PEG-5 oleamide; CAS 31799-71-0; nonionic; emulsifier, dispersant, detergent; lubricant for syn. and natural fibers; also for cosmetics; Gardner 12 max. liq.; sol. in IPA, CCl₄, gels in water @ 50–80 C; sp.gr. 1.0; HLB 14.0; flash pt. (PM) 225 F; surf. tens. 35 dynes/cm (0.1%); 100% conc.

Ethomid® O/17. [Akzo] PEG-7 oleamide; CAS 26027-37-2; nonionic; emulsifier, dispersant, detergent for cosmetics and industrial use; Gardner 8 max. liq.; sp.gr. 1.00; hyd. no. 110; flash pt. (PMCC) 107 C; surf. tens. 35 dynes/cm (0.1%); 100% conc.

Ethoquad® 18/12. [Akzo] PEG-2 stearmonium chloride and IPA; CAS 3010-24-0; 28724-32-5; cationic; antistat, emulsifier, dyeing assistant, leveling agent, antifoam used in textile industry, as electroplating bath additives; also for cosmetics; Gardner 6 max. paste; sol. in acetone, IPA, benzene, water; sp.gr. 0.919; flash pt. 71 F; surf. tens. 40.2 dynes/cm (0.1%); pH 7–8 (10% aq.); 75% act. in IPA.

Ethoquad® 18/25. [Akzo] PEG-15 stearmonium chloride;

7CAS 28724-32-5; cationic; antistat, emulsifier, dyeing assistant, leveling agent, antifoam used in textile industry, as electroplating bath additives; also for cosmetics; Gardner 11 max. clear liq.; sol. in acetone, IPA, benzene, water, CCl₄; sp.gr. 1.058; flash pt. (PM) 146 F; surf. tens. 50.1 dynes/cm (0.1%); pH 6–9 (10% aq.); 95% act.

Ethoquad® C/12. [Akzo] PEG-2 cocomonium chloride and IPA; CAS 70750-47-9; cationic; antistat, emulsifier, dyeing assistant, electroplating bath additive; also for cosmetics; Gardner 9 max. clear liq.; sol. in acetone, IPA, benzene, water, CCl₄; sp.gr. 0.969; flash pt. (PMCC) 20 C; surf. tens. 35.4 dynes/cm (0.1%); pH 7–8 (10% aq.); 75% act. in IPA.

Ethoquad® C/12B. [Akzo] PEG-2 cocobenzyl ammonium chloride; CAS 61789-68-2; surfactant for cosmetics and industrial use; Gardner 12 max. liq.; pH 6.0-9.0; flash (Seta) 26 C; 73% quat.

Ethoquad® C/12 Nitrate. [Akzo] PEG-2 cocomethyl ammonium nitrate, IPA; CAS 71487-00-8; cationic; industrial surfactant for cosmetics, agric., textiles, protective coatings, inks, pigment dispersions, acid pickling baths, metalworking, electroplating, plastics mfg.; Gardner 8 max. liq.; sol. in water, alcohols, acetone, benzene, CCl₄, hexylene glycol; sp.gr. 0.975 (20 C); pH 6-7.8; flash pt. (PMCC) 20 C; 59-62% quat. in IPA.

Ethoquad® C/25. [Akzo] PEG-15 cocomonium chloride; CAS 61791-10-4; cationic; antistat, emulsifier, dyeing assistant, leveling agent, antifoam used in textile industry, as electroplating bath additives; also for cosmetics; Gardner 11 max. clear liq.; sol. in acetone, IPA, benzene, water, CCl₄; sp.gr. 1.071; flash pt. (PM) 196 F; pH 7–8 (10% aq.); surf. tens. 43.4 dynes/cm (0.1%); 95% act.

Ethoquad® CB/12. [Akzo] PEG-2 cocobenzonium chloride, IPA; CAS 61789-68-2; cationic; industrial surfactant for cosmetics, agric., textiles, protective coatings, inks, pigment dispersions, acid pickling baths, metalworking, electroplating, plastics mfg.; Gardner 12 max. liq.; sol. in water, alcohols, acetone, benzene, CCl₄, hexylene glycol; sp.gr. 0.970; flash pt. (PMCC) 26 C; pH 6-9; 73-77% solids in IPA.

Ethoquad® O/12. [Akzo] PEG-2 oleamonium chloride and IPA; CAS 18448-65-2; cationic; antistat, emulsifier, dyeing assistant, electroplating bath additive; also for cosmetics; Gardner 9 max. clear liq.; sol. in acetone, IPA, benzene, water, CCl₄; sp.gr. 0.932; flash pt. (PM) < 80 F; surf. tens. 40.3 dynes/cm (0.1%); pH 7–8 (10% aq.); 75% act. in IPA.

Ethoquad® O/12H. [Akzo] PEG-2 oleamonium chloride, IPA; CAS 18448-65-2; used for shampoos, hand creams.

Ethoquad® O/25. [Akzo] PEG-15 oleamonium chloride; cationic; antistat, emulsifier, dyeing assistant, leveling agent, antifoam used in textile industry, as electroplating bath additives, in cosmetics; Gardner 11 max. clear liq.; sol. in acetone, IPA, benzene, water, CCl₄; sp.gr. 1.062; flash pt. (PM) 200 F; surf. tens. 40.8 dynes/cm (0.1%); pH 7–9 (10% aq.); 95% act.

Ethoquad® T/12. [Akzo] PEG-2 tallowalkyl methyl ammonium chloride, ethanol; CAS 67784-77-4; cationic; industrial surfactant for cosmetics, agric., textiles, protective coatings, inks, pigment dispersions, acid pickling baths, metalworking, electroplating, plastics mfg.; Gardner 7 max. liq. to paste; sol. in water, alcohols, acetone, benzene, CCl₄, hexylene glycol; pH 7.0-9.0; flash (Seta) 23 C; 74% quat. in ethanol.

Ethoquad® T/13-50. [Akzo] PEG-3 tallow alkyl ammonium acetate, aq. IPA; industrial surfactant for cosmetics, agric., textiles, protective coatings, inks, pigment dispersions, acid pickling baths, metalworking, electroplating, plastics mfg.; EPA listed; Gardner 8 max. liq.; sol. in water, alcohols, acetone, benzene, CCl₄, hexylene glycol; sp.gr.

0.952 (20 C); flash pt. (PMCC) 18 C; 48-52% solids in aq. IPA.

Ethosperse® CA-2. [Lonza] Ceteth-2; CAS 9004-95-9; nonionic; o/w emulsifier, thickener, stabilizer for cosmetics (hair care prods., antiperspirants), household waxes, polishes, and cleaning formulations; wh. soft solid; sol. in ethanol; disp. hot in water; m.p. 29-33 C; HLB 6.0; acid no. 0.5 max.; hyd. no. 160-180; pH 7 (5%); 100% conc.

Ethosperse® CA-20. [Lonza] Ceteth-20; CAS 9004-95-9; nonionic; surfactant, emulsifier, and visc. modifier for hair care prods., lotions, creams; adds body and texture; wh. soft cream, mild odor; HLB 16; acid no. 0.07; hyd. no. 54.6; 100% act.

Ethosperse® G-26. [Lonza] Glycereth-26; CAS 31694-55-0; nonionic; emulsifier, sheen additive, and humectant for cosmetics (hair care prods., skin care prods., makeup), pharmaceutical and industrial uses; tackifier and humectant for hot-melt adhesives; pale straw clear liq.; sol. in water, methanol, ethanol, acetone, toluol; sp.gr. 1.12 (38 C); visc. 150 cps (38 C); HLB 18.0; acid no. 0.5 max.; hyd. no. 128-138; pH 6.0 (5%); 100% conc.

Ethosperse® LA-4. [Lonza] Laureth-4; CAS 9002-92-0; EINECS 226-097-1; nonionic; emulsifier for cosmetic, pharmaceutical and industrial uses (hair and skin care prods., antiperspirants, household waxes, polishes, and cleaners, silicone-based lubricants); water-wh. liq.; sol. in methanol, ethanol, acetone, toluol, min. oil, misc. with water, veg. oils; sp.gr. 0.95; visc. 30 cps; HLB 10.0; acid no. 0.3 max.; hyd. no. 145-160; 100% act.

Ethosperse® LA-12. [Lonza] Laureth-12; CAS 9002-92-0; EINECS 221-286-5; nonionic; emulsifier for cosmetic, pharmaceutical and industrial uses (hair and skin care prods., anti-irritant in deodorants and antiperspirants, household waxes, polishes, and cleaning formulations); Gardner 1 max. turbid liq.; sol. in methanol, ethanol, acetone, toluol, min. oil, misc. with water, veg. oils; sp.gr. 1.10; visc. 1000 cps; HLB 15.0; acid no. 2 max.; hyd. no. 72-82; pH 7 (5%); 100% act.

Ethosperse® LA-23. [Lonza] Laureth-23; CAS 9002-92-0; nonionic; o/w emulsifier, thickener, stabilizer for hair and skin care prods., pharmaceuticals, household waxes, polishes, and cleaning formulations; anti-irritant in deodorants and antiperspirants; wh. waxy solid; sol. in water, hot ethanol; m.p. 30-45 C; HLB 17.0; acid no. 0.3 max.; hyd. no. 45-52; 100% conc.

Ethosperse® OA-2. [Lonza] Oleth-2; CAS 9004-98-2; nonionic; o/w emulsifier, thickener, stabilizer for hair care prods., antiperspirants; as spreading agent and emollient in bath oils; colorless liq.; sol. in ethanol, min. oil; disp. hot in water; visc. 30 cps; HLB 4 ± 1.

Ethosperse® OA-20. [Lonza] Oleth-20; CAS 9004-98-2; emulsifier.

Ethosperse® SL-20. [Lonza] Sorbeth-20; CAS 53694-15-8; nonionic; emulsifier, humectant for in cosmetics (hair and skin care prods., makeup), pharmaceuticals, and industrial uses; tackifier and humectant in hot-melt adhesives; lt. yel. clear liq.; sol. in water, methanol, ethanol, acetone; sp.gr. 1.16; visc. 460 cps; HLB 17; acid no. 0.5 max.; hyd. no. 385-430; pH 7 (5%); 100% act.

Ethoxol 3. [Lanaetex Prods.] Oleth-3; CAS 9004-98-2; cosmetics ingred.

Ethoxol 5. [Lanaetex Prods.] Oleth-5; CAS 9004-98-2; cosmetics ingred.

Ethoxol 10. [Lanaetex Prods.] Oleth-10; CAS 9004-98-2; cosmetics ingred.

Ethoxol 12. [Lanaetex Prods.] Oleth-12.; CAS 9004-98-2; emulsifier.

Ethoxol 20. [Lanaetex Prods.] Oleth-20; CAS 9004-98-2; cosmetics ingred.

Ethoxol 44. [Lanaetex Prods.] Oleth-44.; CAS 9004-98-2;

emulsifier.

Ethoxol 44M. [Lanaetex Prods.] Propylene glycol, oleth-44.

Ethoxol-CO. [Lanaetex Prods.] Oleth-10, PEG-10 coconut oil esters.

Ethoxychol-24. [Lanaetex Prods.] Choleth-24; CAS 27321-96-6; cosmetic ingred.

Ethoxylan® 1685. [Henkel/Cospha; Henkel/Textiles; Henkel Canada] PEG-75 lanolin; CAS 61790-81-6; emollient, emulsifier, dispersant, foam stabilizer, resin plasticizer for cosmetics (antiperspirants, creams, lotions, makeup, hair prods.), pharmaceutical vehicles, textile processing; dk. amber to brn. waxy solid; sol. @ 5% in water, IPA; dens. 9.6 lb/gal; m.p. 39 C; cloud pt. 85 C; flash pt. 530 F.

Ethoxylan® 1686. [Henkel/Cospha; Henkel/Textiles; Henkel Canada] PEG-75 lanolin; CAS 61790-81-6; emollient, emulsifier, dispersant, foam stabilizer, resin plasticizer for cosmetics (antiperspirants, creams, lotions, makeup, hair prods.), pharmaceutical vehicles, textile processing; yel. to lt. amber liq.; sol. @ 5% in water, IPA; dens. 8.9 lb/gal; visc. 1767 cSt (100 F); pour pt. 1 C; cloud pt. 86 C; 50% aq. sol'n.

Ethoxyol® 1707. [Henkel/Cospha; Henkel Canada] Polysorbate 80, cetyl acetate, acetylated lanolin alcohol; nonionic; SE emollient with lubricating and penetrating properties; aux. emulsifier, solubilizer, pigment wetting agent for cosmetics, liq. soaps; Gardner < 8 liq.; sol. @ 5% in water, IPA, IPM, glycerin; dens. 8.7 lb/gal; visc. 132 cSt (100 F); pour pt. 1; cloud pt. –1 C; flash pt. 340 F.

Ethylan® 172. [Harcros UK] Cetoleth-3; nonionic; emulsifier and solubilizer for min. oils, hydrophobic waxes, essential oils, and perfumes for toiletries; lt. amber liq., mild fatty odor; oil-sol.; sp.gr. 0.920; visc. 57 cs; HLB 7.0; pour pt. 16 C; flash pt. (COC) > 175 C; pH 7.0 (1% aq.); 100% act.

Ethylan® CDP2. [Harcros UK] Linear middle fraction fatty alcohol ethoxylate (2 EO); nonionic; surfactant, intermediate for toiletry grade sulfates and other specialty surfactants; coemulsifier for min. oils, waxes, alkyd resins, paraffinic hydrocarbons; colorless clear liq., faint odor; insol. in water; sp.gr. 0.907; HLB 6.2; pour pt. 4 C; flash pt. (COC) > 150 C; 100% act.

Ethylan® CDP3. [Harcros UK] Linear middle fraction fatty alcohol ethoxylate (3 EO); nonionic; surfactant, intermediate for toiletry grade sulfates and other specialty surfactants; coemulsifier for min. oils, waxes, alkyd resins, paraffinic hydrocarbons; colorless clear liq., faint odor; insol. in water; sp.gr. 0.902; HLB 8.0; pour pt. 3 C; flash pt. (COC) > 150 C; 100% act.

Ethylan® CF71. [Harcros UK] Coconut fatty ester; nonionic; emulsifier for cosmetics, pharmaceuticals, fiber lubricant; pale straw liq., mild fatty odor; sol. in water; sp.gr. 1.050; visc. 55 cs (40 C); HLB 14; pour pt. 14 C; cloud pt. 57 C (1% aq.); flash pt. (COC) > 175 C; pH 7.0 (1% aq.); 100% act.

Ethylan® CH. [Harcros UK] Ethoxylated coconut fatty acid alkylolamide; nonionic; foam stabilizer in liq. detergents, general purpose or hard surf. cleaners, shampoos, coemulsifier; amber clear liq.; mild odor; water sol.; sp.gr. 1.033; visc. 250 cs; pour pt. 14 C; cloud pt. 80 C (1% aq.); flash pt. (COC) > 150 C; pH 8.0 (1% aq.); 100% act.

Ethylan® CRS. [Harcros UK] Ethoxylated coconut fatty acid alkylolamide; nonionic; foam stabilizer in liq. detergent, general purpose, or hard surface cleaners and shampoos, coemulsifier; amber clear liq.; mild odor; water sol.; sp.gr. 1.042; visc. 270 cs; pour pt. 10 C; flash pt. (COC) > 150 C; pH 8.0 (1% aq.); 100% act.

Ethylan® GEL2. [Harcros UK] Polysorbate 20; CAS 9005-64-5; nonionic; w/o emulsifier, solubilizer esp. with sorbitan esters; used in cosmetics, agric., perfumes, fiber and textile lubricants, textile antistats, polymer additives, suspension and emulsion polymerization; amber clear liq., mild odor; sol. in water, alcohols, hydrocarbons; sp.gr.

1.10; visc. 350 cs; ; HLB 16.5; pour pt. -10 C; flash pt. (PMCC) > 150 C; 97% act.

Ethylan® GEO8. [Harcros UK] Polysorbate 80; CAS 9005-65-6; nonionic; emulsifier for cosmetics, pharmaceuticals, agrochem. formulations, textile lubricants, plastic additives, emulsion and suspension polymerization; solubilizer for perfume, flavors, essential oils; amber clear liq., mild fatty odor; sol. in water, alcohols, hydrocarbons; sp.gr. 1.10; visc. 720 cs; HLB 15.0; pour pt. -20 C; flash pt. (PMCC) > 150 C; 97% act.

Ethylan® GEO81. [Harcros UK] Polysorbate 81; CAS 9005-65-6; nonionic; emulsifier for cosmetics, agric., plastic additives, textile fiber lubricants and softeners, suspension and emulsion polymerization; solubilizer for perfume, flavors, essential oils; amber clear liq., mild fatty odor; sol. in alcohols, hydrocarbons; disp. in water; sp.gr. 1.15; visc. 465 cs; HLB 10.0; pour pt. -10 C; flash pt. (PMCC) > 150 C; 100% act.

Ethylan® GES6. [Harcros UK] Polysorbate 60; CAS 9005-67-8; nonionic; general purpose, low toxicity emulsifier for cosmetics and agrochem.; textile lubricant; plastics additive; emulsion and suspension polymerization; solubilizer for perfume, flavors, essential oils; pale brn. liq./paste; sol. in water, alcohols, hydrocarbons; sp.gr. 1.07; visc. 190 cs (40 C); HLB 15.0; pour pt. 22 C; flash pt. (PMCC) > 150 C; 97% act.

Ethylan® GL20. [Harcros UK] Sorbitan laurate; CAS 1338-39-2; nonionic; emulsifier for cosmetics, pharmaceuticals, agric., plastic antifog, textile fiber lubricant/softener, suspension and emulsion polymerization; amber visc. liq., mild odor; sol. in alcohols, hydrocarbons, natural and paraffinic oils; sp.gr. 1.04; visc. 5250 cs; HLB 8.0; pour pt. 15 C; flash pt. (PMCC) > 150 C; 100% act.

Ethylan® GO80. [Harcros UK] Sorbitan oleate; CAS 1338-43-8; EINECS 215-665-4; nonionic; emulsifier for cosmetics, pharmaceuticals, agric., plastic antifog, textile fiber lubricant/softener, suspension and emulsion polymerization; amber visc. liq., mild fatty odor; sol. in alcohols, hydrocarbons, natural and paraffinic oils; sp.gr. 1.00; visc. 1100 cs; HLB 4.3; pour pt. -20 C; flash pt. (PMCC) -5 C; 100% act.

Ethylan® GPS85. [Harcros UK] Polysorbate 85; CAS 9005-70-3; nonionic; emulsifier for cosmetics, agric., plastic additives, textile fiber lubricants and softeners, suspension and emulsion polymerization; solubilizer for perfume, flavors, essential oils; amber clear liq., mild fatty odor; sol. in alcohols, hydrocarbons; disp. in water; sp.gr. 1.15; visc. 270 cs; HLB 11.0; pour pt. -20 C; flash pt. (PMCC) > 150 C; 100% act.

Ethylan® GS60. [Harcros UK] Sorbitan stearate; CAS 1338-41-8; EINECS 215-664-9; nonionic; emulsifier for cosmetics, pharmaceuticals, agric., plastic antifog, textile fiber lubricant/softener, suspension and emulsion polymerization; tan waxy solid, mild odor; sol. in alcohols, hydrocarbons, natural and paraffinic oils; sp.gr. 0.98; HLB 4.7; pour pt. 50 C; flash pt. (PMCC) > 150 C; 100% act.

Ethylan® GT85. [Harcros UK] Sorbitan trioleate; CAS 26266-58-0; EINECS 247-569-3; nonionic; emulsifier for cosmetics, pharmaceuticals, agric., plastic antifog, textile fiber lubricant/softener, suspension and emulsion polymerization; amber visc. liq., mild odor; sol. in alcohols, hydrocarbons, natural and paraffinic oils; sp.gr. 1.00; visc. 230 cs; HLB 1.5; pour pt. -10 C; flash pt. (PMCC) -10 C; 100% act.

Ethylan® KEO. [Harcros UK] Nonoxynol-9 (9.5 EO); CAS 9016-45-9; nonionic; detergent, wetting agent, emulsifier, foam stabilizer, solubilizer, used in pesticides, perfumes, emulsion polymerization; EPA approved; clear colorless liq.; negligible odor; water sol.; sp.gr. 1.060; visc. 331 cs; HLB 13; pour pt. 3 C; cloud pt. 54 C (1% aq.); flash pt.

(COC) > 200 C; pH 6–8 (1% aq.); surf. tens. 34 dynes/cm (0.1%); 100% act.

Ethylan® LD. [Harcros UK] Cocamide DEA; CAS 61791-31-9; EINECS 263-163-9; nonionic; foam stabilizer, emulsifier for hand cleaning gels, hard surf. cleaners, shampoos; plastics antistat; clear straw liq.; mild odor; disp. in water; sp.gr. 0.981; visc. 1408 cs; flash pt. (COC) > 350 F; pour pt. 15 C; flash pt. (COC) > 175 C; pH 9.5 (1% aq.); 90% act.

Ethylan® LDA-48. [Harcros] Cocamide DEA; CAS 61791-31-9; EINECS 263-163-9; nonionic; foam stabilizer in liq. detergents, general purpose or hard surf. cleaners, shampoos; amber clear liq., mild odor; water-sol.; sp.gr. 1.008; visc. 1342 cs; pour pt. 5 C; flash pt. (COC) > 175 C; pH 9.5 (1% aq.).

Ethylan® LDG. [Harcros UK] Cocamide DEA; CAS 61791-31-9; EINECS 263-163-9; nonionic; foam stabilizer for liq. detergents, general purpose and hard surf. cleaners, shampoos; amber clear liq., mild odor; disp. in water; sp.gr. 1.007; visc. 1303 cs; pour pt. 5 C; flash pt. (COC) > 175 C; 82% conc.

Ethylan® LM2. [Harcros UK] Ethoxylated coconut fatty acid alkylolamide; nonionic; foam booster/stabilizer, visc. modifier, and emulsifier for detergent and personal care formulations; off-wh. soft paste; mild odor; water sol.; sp.gr. 0.963 (40 C); visc. 108 cs (40 C); flash pt. > 300 F (COC); pour pt. 2 C; pH 7–9 (1% aq.); 100% act.

Ethylan® ME. [Harcros UK] Cetoleth-5.5; nonionic; emulsifier and solubilizer for org. solv., veg. oils, paraffin waxes, essential oils, perfumes for toiletries and cosmetics; plastics antistat; straw liq./soft paste, mild fatty odor; disp. in water; sp.gr. 0.970; visc. 81 cs; HLB 10.0; pour pt. 19 C; flash pt. (COC) > 175 C; pH 7.0 (1% aq.); 100% act.

Ethylan® MLD. [Harcros UK] Lauramide DEA; CAS 120-40-1; EINECS 204-393-1; nonionic; foam booster and stabilizer in toiletries and detergent formulations, antistat for plastics; pale cream waxy flake; negligible odor; disp. in water; visc. 107 cs (60 C); pour pt. 40 C; flash pt. (COC) > 150 C; pH 8.5 (1% aq.); 95% act.

Ethylan® OE. [Harcros UK] Cetoleth-13; nonionic; emulsifier for fatty acids, alcohols, and waxes, oil and latex stabilizer, dye leveling agent; emulsifier/solubilizer for essential oils, perfumes, and waxes for toiletries; mfg. of polishes; emulsion polymerization; cream waxy solid; negligible odor; water sol.; sp.gr. 1.009 (40 C); visc. 55 cs (40 C); HLB 14; pour pt. 31 C; cloud pt. 90 C (1% aq.); flash pt. (COC) > 175 C; pH 7.0 (1% aq.); 100% act.

Ethylan® R. [Harcros UK] Cetoleth-19; nonionic; biodeg. emulsifier for fatty acids, waxes; solubilizer for essential oils, perfumes, and waxes for toiletries; latex stabilizer; polish mfg.; emulsion polymerization; dye leveling agent; cream waxy solid; negligible odor; water sol.; sp.gr. 1.023 (40 C); visc. 141 cs (40 C); HLB 17.5; pour pt. 36 C; cloud pt. > 100 C (1% aq.); flash pt. (COC) > 175 C; pH 7.0 (1% aq.); surf. tens. 40 dynes/cm (0.1%); 100% act.

Ethylan® TC. [Harcros UK] PEG-15 cocamine; CAS 61791-14-8; nonionic; wetting agent for metal cleaning and stripping of surface coatings, textiles, paints, agric., polishes, fiber antistat, used in cosmetics; dk. amber liq.; mild fatty amine odor; water sol.; sp.gr. 1.040; visc. 140 cs; HLB 15; flash pt. (COC) > 150 C; pour pt. < 0 C; pH 9.5 (1% aq.); 100% act.

Ethylan® TN-10. [Harcros UK] PEG-10 cocamine; CAS 61791-14-8; nonionic; wetting agent for acid or alkaline metal cleaners, stripping of surf. coatings; oil emulsifier with anticorrosive properties, antistat for syn. fibers with PS; for cosmetics mfg.; dk. amber liq.; mild fatty amine odor; water sol.; sp.gr. 1.015; visc. 174 cs; HLB 14; pour pt. < 0 C; flash pt. (COC) > 150 C; pH 9.5 (1% aq.); 100% act.

Ethylan® TT-15. [Harcros UK] PEG-15 tallow amine; non-

ionic; wetting agent for metal cleaning and stripping of surface coatings, fiber antistat, used in cosmetics; pale brn. paste; mild fatty amine odor; sp.gr. 1.030; visc. 252 cs; HLB 14; flash pt. (COC) > 150 C; pour pt. 0 C; pH 9.5 (1% aq.); 100% act.

Ethyl Butene-1. [Ethyl] Butene-1 (C4); CAS 106-98-9; intermediate for polyethylene comonomer, oxo alcohols, butylene oxide, household detergents, hard surface and industrial hand cleaners, shampoos, bubble baths; liquified gas; sp.gr. 0.595 (liq.); b.p. -6.1 C; flamm. gas.

Ethyl Decene-1. [Ethyl] Decene-1 (C10); intermediate for oligomers, amines, oxo alcohols, household detergents, hard surface and industrial hand cleaners, shampoos, bubble baths; colorless clear liq.; sp.gr. 0.734; b.p. 170-171 C (5-95%); pour pt. -66 C; flash pt. (CC) 45 C.

Ethyl Dodecene-1. [Ethyl] Dodecene-1 (C12); intermediate for oxo alcohols, alkylated aromatics, mercaptans, sulfonates, fatty amines, ASA, household detergents, hard surface and industrial hand cleaners, shampoos, bubble baths; colorless clear liq.; sp.gr. 0.755; b.p. 213-216 C (5-95%); pour pt. -37 C; flash pt. (CC) 77 C.

Ethyl Dodecene-1/Tetradecene-1 Blend. [Ethyl] Dodecene-1/tetradecene-1 (2:1 ratio); intermediate for oxo alcohols, alkylated aromatics, mercaptans, sulfonates, fatty amines, ASA, household detergents, hard surface and industrial hand cleaners, shampoos, bubble baths; colorless clear liq.; sp.gr. 0.760; b.p. 216-250 C (5-95%); pour pt. -35 C; flash pt. (CC) 81 C.

Ethylene Bodecanedioate. [Henkel/Cospha] Fragrance raw material for cosmetic, personal care, detergent, and cleaning prods.; liq., musk odor; flash pt. 185 C.

Ethylene Brassylate. [Henkel/Cospha] Fragrance raw material for cosmetic, personal care, detergent, and cleaning prods.; liq., musk odor; flash pt. 188 C.

Ethylene Glycol Distearate VA. [Goldschmidt] Glycol distearate; CAS 627-83-8; EINECS 211-014-3; opacifier and pearling agent for hair care.

Ethylene Glycol Monostearate VA. [Goldschmidt] Glycol stearate; CAS 111-60-4; EINECS 203-886-9; stabilizer and thickener for creams and lotions; pearlizing and opacifying agent.

Ethylflo® 162. [Ethyl] Polyalphaolefin; syn. lubricant for automotive crankcase oils, hydraulic fluids, gear and transmission fluids, compressor lubricants, metalworking lubricants, and personal care items.

Ethylflo® 180. [Ethyl] Polyalphaolefin; syn. lubricant for automotive crankcase oils, hydraulic fluids, gear and transmission fluids, compressor lubricants, metalworking lubricants, and personal care items.

Ethylflo® 362 NF. [Ethyl] Didecene; nonoily, non-comedogenic hydrocarbon liq. for use in creams, lotions, cleansers, sunscreens, pigmented cosmetics, conditioners, moisturizers, antiperspirants, deodorants; colorless liq., odorless, tasteless; sp.gr. 0.797 (15.56 C); visc. 5.5 cSt (40 C); acid no. < 0.01; pour pt. < -55 C; flash pt. > 145 C; ref. index 1.4451.

Ethylflo® 364 NF. [Ethyl] Polydecene; CAS 37309-58-3; nonoily, noncomedogenic hydrocarbon liq. for use in creams, lotions, cleansers, sunscreens, pigmented cosmetics, conditioners, moisturizers, antiperspirants, deodorants; colorless liq., odorless, tasteless; sp.gr. 0.818 (15.56 C); visc. 17 cSt (40 C); acid no. < 0.01; pour pt. < -65 C; flash pt. > 204 C; ref. index 1.4555.

Ethylflo® 366 NF. [Ethyl] Polydecene; CAS 37309-58-3; nonoily, noncomedogenic hydrocarbon liq. for use in creams, lotions, cleansers, sunscreens, pigmented cosmetics, conditioners, moisturizers, antiperspirants, deodorants; colorless liq., odorless, tasteless; sp.gr. 0.827 (15.56 C); visc. 31 cSt (40 C); acid no. < 0.01; pour pt. < -60 C; flash pt. > 255 C; ref. index 1.4592.

Ethyl Hexadecene-1/Octadecene-1. [Ethyl] Hexadecene-1/octadecene-1 blend; intermediate for ASA, fuel and lube oil additives, sulfates, olefins for leather tanning, fatty amines, household detergents, hard surface and industrial hand cleaners, shampoos, bubble baths; colorless clear liq.; sp.gr. 0.782; b.p. 285-316 C (5-95%); pour pt. -2 C; flash pt. (CC) 135 C.

Ethyl Hexene-1. [Ethyl] Hexene-1 (C6); CAS 592-41-6; intermediate for polyethylene comonomer, oxo alcohols, syn. fatty acids, household detergents, hard surface and industrial hand cleaners, shampoos, bubble baths; colorless clear liq.; sp.gr. 0.678; b.p. 63-64 C (5 -95%); pour pt. -140 C; flash pt. (CC) -26 C.

Ethyl Octene-1. [Ethyl] Octene-1 (C8); CAS 111-66-0; EINECS 203-893-7; intermediate for polyethylene comonomer, oxo alcohols, syn. fatty acids, oligomers, fatty amines, household detergents, hard surface and industrial hand cleaners, shampoos, bubble baths; colorless clear liq.; sp.gr. 0.711; b.p. 121-123 C (5% -95%); pour pt. -102 C; flash pt. (CC) 10 C.

Ethyl Panthenol No. 26100. [Roche] Ethyl panthenol; deep penetrating moisturizer for hair and skin care prods.

Ethyl Tetradecene-1. [Ethyl] Tetradecene-1 (C14); intermediate for oxo alcohols, alkylated aromatics, mercaptans, sulfonates, fatty amines, ASA, household detergents, hard surface and industrial hand cleaners, shampoos, bubble baths; colorless clear liq.; sp.gr. 0.769; b.p. 245-250 C (5% -95%); pour pt. -18 C; flash pt. (CC) 107 C.

Ethyl Tetradecene-1/Hexadecene-1. [Ethyl] Tetradecene-1/hexadecene-1 (5:3 ratio); intermediate for alpha olefin sulfonates, fatty amines, household detergents, hard surface and industrial hand cleaners, shampoos, bubble baths; colorless clear liq.; sp.gr. 0.773; b.p. 245-279 C (5% -95%); pour pt. -14 C; flash pt. (CC) 113 C.

ETIZM. [Syntex] Corn oil unsaponifiables.

Etocas 5. [Croda Inc.; Croda Chem. Ltd.] PEG-5 castor oil; CAS 61791-12-6; w/o emulsifier, dispersant, solubilizer for cosmetics; pale yel. liq.; HLB 3.9.

Etocas 10. [Croda Chem. Ltd.] PEG-10 castor oil; CAS 61791-12-6; nonionic; cosmetic and essential oil solubilizer, emulsifier, lubricant, softener, leveling agent, emollient, superfatting agent, antistat, softener, detergent; used in personal care prods., fiber processing, metalworking fluids, emulsion polymerization, insecticides; pale yel. liq.; sol. in ethanol, naphtha, MEK, trichlorethylene, disp. in water; HLB 6.3; cloud pt. < 20 C; acid no. 1.0 max.; sapon. no. 120–130; pH 6–7.5; 97% act.

Etocas 15. [Croda Inc.] PEG-15 castor oil; CAS 61791-12-6; o/w emulsifier, dispersant, solubilizer for cosmetics; pale yel. liq.; HLB 12.5.

Etocas 20. [Croda Chem. Ltd.] PEG-20 castor oil.; CAS 61791-12-6; nonionic; emulsifier, wetting agent, dispersant for personal care prods., textile and metal processing; liq.; HLB 9.6; 97% conc.

Etocas 29. [Croda Inc.] PEG-29 castor oil; CAS 61791-12-6; o/w emulsifier, dispersant, solubilizer for cosmetics; pale yel. liq.; HLB 11.7.

Etocas 30. [Croda Chem. Ltd.] PEG-30 castor oil; CAS 61791-12-6; humectant, o/w emulsifier, skin cleanser, conditioner, emollient, solubilizer; liq.; sol. in oil; waterdisp.; HLB 11.7; 97% conc.

Etocas 35. [Croda Chem. Ltd.] PEG-35 castor oil; CAS 61791-12-6; nonionic; cosmetic and essential oil solubilizer, emulsifier, lubricant, emollient, superfatting agent, antistat, softener, detergent; pale yel. liq.; sol. in water, alcohol, naphtha, MEK, oleic acid, trichloroethylene; HLB 12.5; cloud pt. 35–40 C; acid no. 1.0 max.; sapon. no. 62–72; surf. tens. 41.5 dynes/cm (0.1% aq.); pH 6–7.5; 97% act.

Etocas 40. [Croda Inc.; Croda Chem. Ltd.] PEG-40 castor oil;

CAS 61791-12-6; nonionic; o/w emulsifier, wetting agent, dispersant, solubilizer for personal care prods., textile and metal processing; pale yel. liq.; sol. in water, alcohol, naphtha, MEK, oleic acid, trichloroethylene; HLB 13; cloud pt. 50 C; acid no. 1.0 max.; sapon. no. 60–65; pH 6–7.5; 97% act.

Etocas 50. [Croda Chem. Ltd.] PEG-50 castor oil; CAS 61791-12-6; nonionic; emulsifier, wetting agent, dispersant for personal care prods., textile and metal processing; liq.; 97% conc.

Etocas 60. [Croda Inc.; Croda Chem. Ltd.] PEG-60 castor oil; CAS 61791-12-6; nonionic; cosmetic and essential oil solubilizer, o/w emulsifier, lubricant, emollient, superfatting agent, antistat, softener, detergent; pale yel. soft paste; sol. in water, alcohol, naphtha, MEK, oleic acid, trichloroethylene; HLB 14.7; cloud pt. 60 C; acid no. 1.0 max.; sapon. no. 45–50; surf. tens. 43.2 dynes/cm (0.1% aq.); pH 6–7.5.

Ethocas 75. [Croda Chem. Ltd.] PEG-75 castor oil; CAS 61791-12-6; personal care surfactant.

Etocas 100. [Croda Chem. Ltd.] PEG-100 castor oil; CAS 61791-12-6; nonionic; emulsifier, wetting agent, dispersant for personal care prods., textile and metal processing; humectant; pale yel. waxy solid; sol. in water, alcohol, naphtha, MEK, oleic acid, trichloroethylene; HLB 16.5; cloud pt. 66 C; acid no. 1.0 max.; sapon. no. 25–35; surf. tens. 41.6 dynes/cm (0.1% aq.); pH 6–7.5; 97% act.

Etocas 200. [Croda Chem. Ltd.] PEG-200 castor oil.; CAS 61791-12-6; nonionic; antistat for textile processing; hair care prods.; solid; HLB 18.0; 97% conc.

Eucalyptus HS. [Alban Muller] Propylene glycol and eucalyptus extract; botanical extract.

Eucalyptus LS. [Alban Muller] Sunflower seed oil and eucalpytus extract.

Eucalyptus-Extract, Water soluble 4786. [Novarom GmbH] Eucalyptus oil and polysorbate 20.

Eucalyptus Leaves Extract HS 2646 G. [Grau Aromatics] Propylene glycol and eucalyptus extract; botanical extract.

Eucarol B/D. [Auschem SpA] Dilaureth-7 citrate; anionic; nonirritating detergent for cosmetic industry; liq./paste; 100% conc.

Eucarol B/TA. [Auschem SpA] Laureth-7 citrate, acid form; anionic; nonirritating detergent for cosmetic industry; liq./paste; 100% conc.

Eucarol D. [Auschem SpA] Sodium dilaureth-7 citrate; anionic; nonirritating detergent for cosmetic industry; liq./paste; 25% conc.

Eucarol IAS. [Auschem SpA] Disodium hydroxydecyl sorbitol citrate.

Eucarol LS. [Auschem SpA] Sodium dilaureth-7 citrate and sodium lauryl sulfate; anionic; nonirritating detergent for cosmetic industry; liq.; 25% conc.

Eucarol M. [Auschem SpA] Disodium laureth-7 citrate.

Eucarol T. [Auschem SpA] Trilaureth-8 citrate; nonionic; emulsifier, nonirritating detergent for cosmetic industry; liq.; 80% conc.

Eucarol TA. [Auschem SpA] Sodium laureth-7 tartrate; nonionic; nonirritating detergent for cosmetic industry; liq.; 25% conc.

Eucoriol. [Stockhausen] Sodium bischlorophenyl sulfamine.

Eudispert. [Rohm GmbH] Acrylates copolymer; thickener, stabilizer for cosmetics.

Eumulgin® B1. [Henkel/Cospha; Henkel Canada; Henkel KGaA/Cospha] Ceteareth-12; CAS 68439-49-6; nonionic; wetting agent and dispersant for paint systems; emulsifier, emollient, bodying agent, conditioner for ointments, creams, low visc. emulsions, cosmetics, pharmaceuticals; waxy solid; sol. in alcohols, hydrocarbons, and most org. solvs.; sp.gr. 0.95; solid. pt. 50–68 F; HLB 12.0;

100% conc.

Eumulgin® B2. [Henkel/Cospha; Henkel Canada; Henkel KGaA/Cospha; Pulcra SA] Ceteareth-20; CAS 68439-49-6; nonionic; emulsifier, emollient, bodying agent, conditioner for ointments, creams, low visc. emulsions, cosmetics, pharmaceuticals; waxy flakes; sol. in alcohols, hydrocarbons, and most org. solvs.; sp.gr. 0.95; solid. pt. 50–68 F; HLB 15.5; hyd. no. 48-54; pH 6.0-7.5 (1%); 100% conc.

Eumulgin® B3. [Henkel Canada; Henkel KGaA/Cospha; Pulcra SA] Ceteareth-30; CAS 68439-49-6; nonionic; emulsifier for transparent gels and creams, cosmetics, pharmaceuticals; waxy solid; sp.gr. 0.95; solid. pt. 50–68 F; HLB 16.7; hyd. no. 35-40; pH 6.0-7.5 (1%); 100% conc.

Eumulgin® C4. [Henkel; Henkel KGaA/Cospha] PEG-5 cocamide; CAS 61791-08-0; nonionic; foaming agent for detergents; emulsifier; liq.; HLB 8.5; 100% conc.

Eumulgin E-24. [Henkel] PEG-20 glyceryl stearate; emulsifier, solubilizer.

Eumulgin® EO-33. [Pulcra SA] POE distearate; nonionic; thickener, conditioner for shampoos and lotions; flakes; 100% conc.

Eumulgin® EP 5L. [Henkel KGaA/Cospha] Ethoxylated oleyl/cetyl alcohol; nonionic; emulsifier component of pronounced cold behavior; liq.; 100% conc.

Eumulgin® HRE 40. [Henkel KGaA/Cospha] PEG-40 hydrog. castor oil; CAS 61788-85-0; nonionic; solubilizer and o/w emulsifier for cosmetic and pharmaceutical preps.; wh. wax; HLB 14-16; acid no. 1 max.; sapon. no. 50-60; hyd. no. 55-75; pH 6-7 (1%); 100% conc.

Eumulgin® HRE 60. [Henkel KGaA/Cospha] PEG-60 hydrog. castor oil; CAS 61788-85-0; nonionic; solubilizer and o/w emulsifier for cosmetic and pharmaceutical preps.; wax; HLB 15-17; acid no. < 1; sapon. no. 40-50; hyd. no. 50-70; pH 6-7 (1%); 100% conc.

Eumulgin® L. [Henkel/Cospha; Henkel KGaA/Cospha] PPG-2-ceteareth-9; nonionic; emulsifier, solubilizer for aq. or hydroalcoholic media; emollient, bodying agent, conditioner for skin and hair care preps.; lt. yel. clear freeflowing liq., faint char. odor; sol. in alcohols, hydrocarbons, and most org. solvs.; acid no. 1 max.; hyd. no. 145-155; pH 6.0-7.5 (1%); 100% conc.

Eumulgin® M8. [Henkel KGaA/Cospha] Oleth-10 and oleth-5; CAS 9004-98-2; nonionic; emulsifier, solubilizer for pesticides and cosmetics; bright yel. gel-like paste; HLB 11.0; pH 6.5-7.5 (1%); 80% conc.

Eumulgin® O5. [Henkel/Cospha; Henkel Canada; Henkel KGaA/Cospha] Oleth-5; CAS 9004-98-2; nonionic; emulsifier, solubilizer for pesticides, perfumes, cosmetics, floor polishes, hair dressings, creams, lotions, min. oil, terpenes; dispersant improving color acceptance of emulsion paints; bright yel. clear liq.; water-sol.; sp.gr. 0.912-0.9145 (70 C); HLB 12.0; hyd. no. 115-125; cloud pt. 16-22 C; pH 6.5-75 (1%); 100% conc.

Eumulgin® O10. [Henkel/Cospha; Henkel Canada; Henkel KGaA/Cospha] Oleth-10; CAS 9004-98-2; nonionic; wetting agent and dispersant for paint systems; emulsifier for creams, lotions, hair care prods.; used with min. oils and terpenes; ylsh. wh. soft waxy solid; sp.gr. 0.959-0.9615 (70 C); solid. pt. 50–68 F; HLB 12.0; hyd. no. 79-84; cloud pt. 26-30 C; pH 6.5-7.5 (1%); 100% conc.

Eumulgin® PRT 36. [Pulcra SA] PEG-36 castor oil; CAS 61791-12-6; nonionic; detergent, emulsifier, dispersant, solubilizer for conc. pesticides, metal, leather, cosmetics, toiletries, pharmaceuticals, textile, and polymer industries; liq.; HLB 12.7; sapon. no. 59-69; pH 6.0-7.5 (1%); 100% conc.

Eumulgin® PRT 40. [Pulcra SA] PEG-40 castor oil; CAS 61791-12-6; nonionic; detergent, emulsifier, dispersant, solubilizer for conc. pesticides, metal, leather, cosmetics, toiletries, pharmaceuticals, textile, and polymer indus-

tries; liq.; HLB 13.1; sapon. no. 55-65; pH 6.0-7.5 (1%); 100% conc.

Eumulgin® PRT 56. [Pulcra SA] PEG-56 castor oil; CAS 61791-12-6; nonionic; detergent, emulsifier, dispersant, solubilizer for conc. pesticides, metal, leather, cosmetics, toiletries, pharmaceuticals, textile, and polymer industries; paste; HLB 14.5; sapon. no. 45-55; pH 6.0-7.5 (1%); 100% conc.

Eumulgin® PRT 200. [Pulcra SA] PEG-200 castor oil; CAS 61791-12-6; nonionic; detergent, emulsifier, dispersant, solubilizer for conc. pesticides, metal, leather, cosmetics, toiletries, pharmaceuticals, textile, and polymer industries; solid; HLB 18.1; sapon. no. 16-18; pH 5.0-6.5 (10%); 100% conc.

Eumulgin® PWM2. [Pulcra SA] Oleth-2; CAS 9004-98-2; nonionic; w/o emulsifier, dispersant, lipophilic cosolv.; fragrance grade; broad pH and electrolyte tolerance; liq.; HLB 5.0; hyd. no. 155-165; pH 6.0-7.5 (1%); 100% conc.

Eumulgin® PWM5. [Pulcra SA] Oleth-5; CAS 9004-98-2; nonionic; o/w emulsifier, solubilizer; stable over wide pH range; liq.; HLB 9.1; 100% conc.

Eumulgin® PWM10. [Pulcra SA] Oleth-10; CAS 9004-98-2; nonionic; emulsifier for pesticides, cosmetics, floor polishes and detergents; solid; HLB 12.6; hyd. no. 77-83; pH 6.0-7.5 (1%); 100% conc.

Eumulgin® PWM17. [Pulcra SA] Oleth-18; CAS 9004-98-2; nonionic; hydrophilic emulsifier, dispersant, solubilizer, detergent; dyeing assistant for wool/acrylic blends; paste; HLB 14.8; hyd. no. 54-59; pH 6.0-7.5 (1%); 100% conc.

Eumulgin® RO 35. [Henkel KGaA/Cospha] PEG-35 castor oil; CAS 61791-12-6; nonionic; emulsifier and solubilizer for fat-sol. vitamins and essential oils; yields o/w emulsions or clear to sl. opalescent liqs.; ylsh. liq., weak intrinsic odor; sp.gr. 1.014-1.018 (70 C); acid no. 2 max.; iodine no. 25-35; sapon. no. 63-73; hyd. no. 65-80; pH 6.5-7.5 (1%).

Eumulgin® RO 40. [Henkel/Cospha; Henkel Canada; Henkel KGaA/Cospha] PEG-40 castor oil; CAS 61791-12-6; nonionic; o/w emulsifier, solubilizer for perfume oils; for personal care creams and lotions; lt. yel. cloudy visc. liq., faint char. odor; sp.gr. 1.022-1.028 (70 C); sapon. no. 58-62; hyd. no. 74-83; pH 7-8 (1%); 100% conc.

Eumulgin® SML 20. [Henkel KGaA/Cospha; Pulcra SA] Polysorbate 20; CAS 9005-64-5; nonionic; solubilizer and emulsifier for cosmetics and pharmaceuticals; lt. yel. liq.; HLB 16.7; acid no. 2 max.; iodine no. 5 max.; sapon. no. 40-50; hyd. no. 96-108; pH 7.5-8.0 (10%); 100% conc.

Eumulgin® SMO 20. [Henkel KGaA/Cospha] Polysorbate 80 BP, German pharmacopoeia; CAS 9005-65-6; nonionic; solubilizer and emulsifier for cosmetics and pharmaceuticals; ylsh. brn. visc. liq. to paste; acid no. 2 max.; iodine no. 18-24; sapon. no. 45-55; hyd. no. 65-80.

Eumulgin® SMS 20. [Henkel KGaA/Cospha] Polysorbate 60 BP, NF, German pharmacopoeia; CAS 9005-67-8; nonionic; solubilizer and emulsifier for cosmetics and pharmaceuticals; cloudy med.-visc. to pasty wax; acid no. 2 max.; iodine no. 5 max.; sapon. no. 45-55; hyd. no. 81-96.

Eumulgin® ST-8. [Henkel Canada] PEG-8 stearate; CAS 9004-99-3; nonionic; emulsifier for o/w liq. emulsions and creams; waxy solid.

Euperlan® MPK 850. [Henkel/Cospha; Henkel Canada] Sodium laureth sulfate, magnesium laureth sulfate, sodium laureth-8 sulfate, magnesium laureth-8 sulfate, sodium oleth sulfate, magnesium oleth sulfate, glycol stearate, PEG-3 distearate, cocamide MEA, laureth-10; anionic/nonionic; fatty alcohol ether sulfates with pearlescents for use as a pearly gloss conc. for baby shampoos, bath prods.; liq.; 25% conc.

Euperlan® PK 771. [Henkel/Cospha; Henkel Canada; Henkel KGaA/Cospha] Glycol distearate, sodium laureth sulfate, cocamide MEA, and laureth-10; anionic/nonionic; cold-processable pearlescent base for shampoos and bath prods.; refatting props.; very dense, fine silk gloss; wh. high visc. emulsion with pearly gloss, weak intrinsic odor; pH 6.5-7.5 (10%); 44-48% dry residue.

Euperlan® PK 771 BENZ. [Henkel KGaA/Cospha] Glycol distearate, sodium laureth sulfate, cocamide MEA, and laureth-10; cold-processable pearlescent conc. for dense, brilliant surfactant preps. with silky shine; paste, weak intrinsic odor; pH 3.0-4.0 (10%); 44-48% dry residue.

Euperlan® PK 776. [Henkel Canada] Sodium laureth sulfate, glycol distearate, and cocamide MEA; anionic/nonionic; pearlescent base for shampoos and bath prods.; liq.; 41% conc.

Euperlan® PK 789. [Henkel Canada] Sodium laureth sulfate, glycol distearate, and cocamide MEA; anionic; pearl conc. for emulsion-type cosmetics; wh. high-visc. emulsion; 35% conc.

Euperlan® PK 810. [Henkel/Cospha; Henkel Canada] Glycol distearate, sodium laureth sulfate, cocamide MEA, laureth-10; anionic/nonionic; pearlescent base for lotion shampoos and bath prods.; fine, sl. coarse pearly gloss with high density; pumpable wh. liq. disp. with pearly sheen; 37% conc.

Euperlan® PK 810 AM. [Henkel KGaA/Cospha] Glycol distearate, sodium laureth sulfate, cocamide MEA, and laureth-10; cold-processable pumpable pearlescent shine conc. for dense, brilliant surfactant preps.; pumpable, weak intrinsic odor; sp.gr. 1.00; visc. 1000-4000 mPa·s; pH 3-4 (10%); 36-40% dry residue.

Euperlan® PK 900. [Henkel/Cospha; Henkel Canada] PEG-3 distearate, sodium laureth sulfate; anionic/nonionic; pearlescent base for lotion shampoos, bath prods., personal cleansing prods.; opaque gloss effect with very fine structure; wh. liq. disp. with silky gloss; 40% act.

Euperlan® PK 900 BENZ. [Henkel KGaA/Cospha] PEG-3 distearate and sodium laureth sulfate; cold-processable pumpable pearlescent conc. for very dense, fine-structured shining surfactant preps.; pumpable, weak intrinsic odor; sp.gr. 0.95; visc. 500-2000 mPa·s; pH 3-4 (10%); 35-39% dry residue.

Euperlan® PK 3000. [Henkel/Cospha; Henkel Canada] Glycol distearate, laureth-4, cocamidopropyl betaine; surfactant for pearlescent shampoos, bubble bath creams; brilliant, dense pearly gloss; pearly liq.; 45% act.

Euperlan® PK 3000 AM. [Henkel KGaA/Cospha] Glycol distearate, laureth-4, and cocamidopropyl betaine; cold-processable pumpable pearlescent shine concentrate for very dense, brilliant surfactant preps. with silky shine; pumpable, weak intrinsic odor; sp.gr. 0.95; visc. 4000-10,000 mPa·s; pH 3.0-3.5 (10%); 41-45% dry residue.

Euperlan® PK 3000 OK. [Henkel; Henkel KGaA/Cospha] Glycol distearate, glycerin, laureth-4, and cocamidopropyl betaine; cold-processable pumpable pearlescent shine conc. for very dense, brilliant surfactant preps. with silky shine; pumpable, weak intrinsic odor; sp.gr. 0.95; visc. 4000-10,000 mPa·s; pH 3.0-3.5 (10%); 60-64% dry residue.

Euperlan® PL 1000. [Henkel] Glycol distearate, lauryl polyglucose, cocamidopropyl betaine, and propylene glycol; pearlescent surfactant for pearlescent shampoos, bath prods., and liq. soaps; wh. liq. disp. with a pearly luster; 45% act.

European Elastin 10. [Maybrook] Hydrolyzed elastin; CAS 73049-73-7; substantive protein adding to skin elasticity; protective colloid effect; film-former; moisturizer; for skin nourishing creams, shave creams, sun tan prods., hair care and treatment prods.; yel. clear to sl. hazy liq., sl. char. odor; pH 4.5-7.5; 10% min. act.

European Elastin 30. [Maybrook] Hydrolyzed elastin; CAS 73049-73-7; substantive protein contributing to skin elasticity; protective colloid effect; film-former; for skin care (nourishing creams, body lotions, shave creams, suntan products), hair care and treatment prods.; light amber clear to sl. hazy liq., sl. char. odor; pH 4.5-7.5; 30% min. solids.

European Elastin SD. [Maybrook] Hydrolyzed elastin; CAS 73049-73-7; substantive protein adding to skin elasticity; protective colloid effect; film-former; for skin care (nourishing creams, body lotions, shave creams, suntan prods.), hair care and treatment prods.; pale cream free-flowing powd., very sl. char. odor; pH 4.5-7.5 (10% aq.); 92% min. solids.

Eusolex® 232. [Rona; E. Merck] 2-Phenylbenzimidazole-5-sulfonic acid; CAS 27503-81-7; uv-B filter for cosmetics; wh. powd., odorless; water-sol. in salt form; m.w. 274.30; usage level: 0.5-5%; toxicology: LD50 (oral, mouse) > 5 g/kg (free acid); > 98% assay.

Eusolex® 4360. [Rona; E. Merck] Benzophenone-3; CAS 131-57-7; EINECS 205-031-5; uv-A and B filter for cosmetic and dermatological light-screening, skin-protection, and skin-care prods.; greenish-yel. powd., almost odorless; sol. in oil, acetone, chloroform; m.w. 228.25; m.p. 61-63 C; usage level: 1-4%; toxicology: LD50 (oral, rat) > 12.8 g/kg; > 99% assay.

Eusolex® 6007. [Rona; E. Merck] Octyl dimethyl PABA; CAS 21245-02-3; EINECS 244-289-3; uv-B filter for cosmetic light-screen oils and emulsions; not applic. to USA market; ylsh. or pale yel. liq., typ. odor; sol. in paraffin oil, IPM, IPA, ethanol 96%; m.w. 277.41; sp.gr. 0.9952; ref. index 1.5421; usage level: 0.5-5%; toxicology: LD50 (oral, rat) 14.9 g/kg (in corn oil); nonirritating to skin or mucous membranes; > 98.5% assay.

Eusolex® 6300. [Rona; E. Merck] Methylbenzylidene camphor; CAS 38102-62-4; uv-B filter for cosmetics, sun-screens, aerosols, and o/w and w/o oils and emulsions; not applic. to USA market; wh. powd., sl. char. odor; oil-sol.; m.w. 254.37; m.p. 66-68 C; usage level: 0.5-5%; toxicology: LD50 (oral, rat) > 5 g/kg (in oil); 99.5% min. assay.

Eusolex® 8020. [Rona; E. Merck] 4-Isopropyl-dibenzoylmethane; CAS 63250-25-9; EINECS 264-043-9; uv-A filter for cosmetics; not applic. to USA market; ylsh. cryst. powd., sl. char. odor; oil-sol.; m.w. 266.34; m.p. 44-47 C; usage level: 0.5-1.5%; toxicology: LD50 (oral, rat) 6 g/kg (in oil); nonirritating to skin and mucous membranes; > 99% assay.

Eutanol® G. [Henkel/Cospha; Henkel Canada; Henkel KGaA/Cospha] Octyldodecanol; CAS 5333-42-6; EINECS 226-242-9; lubricant, emollient with good spreadability for cosmetics and pharmaceuticals (creams, lotions, depilatories, antiperspirants); carrier for oil-sol. active ingreds.; pigment dispersant; stable to hydrolysis; lt. yel. clear oily liq., pract. odorless and tasteless; sol. in alcohols, esters, cosmetic oils, glycols, ketones, aromatics; insol. in water; m.w. 300; sp.gr. 0.835-0.845; visc. 58-64 mPa·s; acid no. 0.5 max.; iodine no. 8 max.; sapon. no. 5.0; hyd. no. 175-190; cloud pt. < -20 C; ref. index 1.4540-1.4560; 90% min. conc.

Eutanol® G16. [Henkel/Cospha; Henkel Canada; Henkel KGaA/Cospha] Isocetyl alcohol; CAS 36311-34-9; EINECS 252-964-9; emollient for personal care prods.; carrier for oil-sol. active ingreds.; dispersant for pigments; spreading agent; stable to hydrolysis; lt. yel. clear oily liq.; m.w. 250; sp.gr. 0.835-0.840; visc. 40-45 mPa·s; acid no. 0.5 max.; iodine no. 10 max.; sapon. no. 10 max.; hyd. no. 200-225; cloud pt. < -40 C; ref. index 1.4400-1.4600; 85% min. conc.

Eutanol® G 32/36. [Henkel/Cospha] Myristyl eicosanol.

Euxyl K 100. [Schülke & Mayr] Benzyl alcohol, methylchloroisothiazolinone, and methylisothiazolinone; cosmetic preservative; USA and Europe approvals; usage level: 0.03-0.15%.

Euxyl K 400. [Schülke & Mayr] Methyldibromoglutaronitrile and phenoxyethanol; cosmetic preservative; USA and Europe approvals; usage level: 0.03-0.3%.

Euxyl K 702. [Schülke & Mayr] Phenoxyethanol, benzoic acid, and dehydroacetic acid.

Evanol™. [Evans Chemetics] Fatty alcohol mixt.; cosmetic cream base for depilatories, hair relaxing creams, and curl kits; wh. waxy flake; m.p. 50-54 C; acid no. 0.5 max.; iodine no. 3 max.; sapon. no. 0.5 max.; hyd. no. 160-200.

Evanstab® 12. [Evans Chemetics] Dilauryl thiodipropionate; CAS 123-28-4; EINECS 204-614-1; antioxidant for polyethylene, PP, and polyolefins, ABS; stabilizer for polyolefins, oils and fats, food applic.; plasticizer for rubber prods.; lubricating oil additive; syn. lubricant; chemical preservative in fats and oils; wh. cryst. flakes or powd.; m.w. 514; f.p. 40.0 C min.; sol. in acetone, MEK, n-heptane, toluene, ethyl acetate, ethanol; acid no. 1.0 max.; 99.0% min. assay.

Evosina IP 7. [Variati] Isopropyl myristate and iceland moss extract.

Evosina NA 2. [Variati] Alcohol and iceland moss extract; botanical extract.

Exaltex. [Firmenich] Pentadecalactone.

Exaltolide. [Firmenich] Pentadecalactone.

Exceparl DG-MI. [Kao Corp. SA] Isostearic/myristic glycerides.

Exceparl HO. [Kao Corp. SA] Cetyl octanoate; CAS 59130-69-7; EINECS 261-619-1; emollient for cosmetics; liq.

EXP-61. [Genesee Polymers] Stearyl/aminopropyl methicone copolymer.

Explotab®. [Mendell] Sodium starch glycolate NF/BP; CAS 9063-38-1; tablet disintegrant for formulations prepared by direct compression or wet granulation techniques; FDA registered; avg. particle size 42 μ; 100% -140 mesh; insol. in org. solvs.; at 2% disp. in cold water; m.w. 500,000-1,000,000; visc. 200 cps max. (4% disp.); m.p. chars at 200 C; pH 5.5-7.5.

Exsycobalt. [Exsymol] Cobalt acetylmethionate; CAS 105883-52-1; catalyst for oxidoreduction; also for detoxification, transpeptidization, and to promote formation of keratin, enzymes, and hormones; skin moisturizer; m.w. 441.

Exsycuivre. [Exsymol] Copper acetylmethionate; CAS 105883-51-0; catalyst for oxidoreduction; also for detoxification, transpeptidization, and to promote formation of keratin, enzymes, and hormones; skin moisturizer.

Exsyfibroblastes. [Exsymol; Biosil Tech.] Derived from vitro fibroblast cultures; promotes cutaneous cell regeneration and dermal connective tissue in cosmetic formulations; translucent fluid gel; sol. in water; pH 6.0; usage level: 2-10%; toxicology: nontoxic.

Exsymagnesium. [Exsymol] Magnesium acetylmethionate; CAS 105883-49-6.

Exsymanganese. [Exsymol] Manganese acetylmethionate; CAS 105883-50-9.

Exsymol Chromoprotuline. [Exsymol; Biosil Tech.] Hydrolyzed vegetable protein extracted from Spirulina algae; CAS 100209-45-8; pigmented moisturizing agent for oily skin cosmetics, regeneration and skin treatment, anti-aging and antiwrinkle creams; dk. blue liq., algal odor; sol. in water; pH 6.0-6.5; toxicology: nontoxic.

Exsymol Cobalt Acetylmethionate. [Exsymol; Biosil Tech.] Cobalt acetylmethionate; CAS 105883-52-1; detoxification, transpeptidisation element, and keratin, enzyme, and hormone formation promoters; dermal moisturizers for cosmetics; m.w. 441.0.

Exsymol Cupric Acetylmethionate. [Exsymol; Biosil Tech.] Cupric acetylmethionate; CAS 105883-51-0; detoxification, transpeptidisation element, and keratin, enzyme, and hormone formation promoters, dermal moisturizers for cosmetics; m.w. 445.5.

Exsymol Gold Acetylmethionate. [Exsymol; Biosil Tech.] Gold acetylmethionate; CAS 105883-47-4; detoxification, transpeptidisation element, and keratin, enzyme, and hormone formation promoters, dermal moisturizers for cosmetics; m.w. 770.0.

Exsymol Hydrumines. [Exsymol] Total plant extracts incl. liposoluble and hydrosoluble active principles; avail. plants: arnica, calendula, horsetail, hops, liquorice, sage, witch hazel, etc.; cosmetic ingreds.; brn. limpid liqs.; sol. in water; pH 6; usage level: 0.5-2%.

Exsymol Magnesium Acetylmethionate. [Exsymol; Biosil Tech.] Magnesium acetylmethionate; CAS 105883-49-6; detoxification, transpeptidisation element, and keratin, enzyme, and hormone formation promoters, dermal moisturizers for cosmetics; m.w. 406.0.

Exsymol Manganese Acetylmethionate. [Exsymol; Biosil Tech.] Manganese acetylmethionate; CAS 105883-50-9; detoxification, transpeptidisation element, and keratin, enzyme, and hormone formation promoters, dermal moisturizers for cosmetics; m.w. 437.0.

Exsymol Nickel Acetylmethionate. [Exsymol; Biosil Tech.] Nickel acetylmethionate; CAS 105883-48-5; detoxification, transpeptidisation element, and keratin, enzyme, and hormone formation promoters, dermal moisturizers for cosmetics; m.w. 440.7.

Exsymol Oleosterines. [Exsymol; Biosil Tech.] Plant extracts containing liposoluble active principles; avail. plants: arnica, calendula, horsetail, hops, liquorice, sage, witch hazel, etc.; cosmetic ingreds.; for antiwrinkle prods., day and night creams, dry skin treatments; brn. oily liq.; sol. in oils; usage level: 0.5-2%.

Exsymol Parahydroxycinnamic Acid. [Exsymol; Biosil Tech.] Parahydroxycinnamic acid; bactericide extracted from Aloe vera; effective for Gram-positive germs; used in dermal creams, lotions, mouth washes, shaving creams, cosmetic prods. for sensitive skin; wh. to sl. beige cryst. powd.; sol. in alkaline sol'ns., ether, boiling ethylic alcohol, water at 100 C; barely sol. in benzene, cold water; m.w. 164; m.p. 215-220 C; pH 3.3-3.5 (0.1%); usage level: 1-2%.

Exsymol Plant Extracts. [Exsymol; Biosil Tech.] Plant extracts from arnica, chamomile, elder, honeysuckle, hops, horsetail, ivy, marigold, meadowsweet, rosemary, sage, St. John's wort, etc.; cosmetic ingreds.; limpid liqs.; sp.gr. 1.05; pH 5-6; ref. index 1.40.

Exsymol Protuline. [Exsymol; Biosil Tech.] Hydrolyzed vegetable protein extracted from Spirulina algae; CAS 100209-45-8; moisturizing agent for oily skin cosmetics, regeneration and skin treatment, anti-aging and antiwrinkle creams; brn. opalescent, sl. visc. aq. liq., algal odor; misc. with water; pH 6.0-6.5; toxicology: nontoxic.

Exsymol Silver Acetylmethionate. [Exsymol; Biosil Tech.] Gold acetylmethionate; CAS 105883-46-3; detoxification, transpeptidisation element, and keratin, enzyme, and hormone formation promoters, dermal moisturizers for cosmetics; m.w. 297.86.

Exsymol Zinc Acetylmethionate. [Exsymol; Biosil Tech.] Zinc acetylmethionate; CAS 102868-96-2; detoxification, transpeptidisation element, and keratin, enzyme, and hormone formation promoters, dermal moisturizers for cosmetics; m.w. 447.4.

Exsynickel. [Exsymol] Nickel acetylmethionate; CAS 105883-48-5.

Exsyor. [Exsymol] Gold acetylmethionate; CAS 105883-46-3; detoxification, transpeptidisation element, and keratin, enzyme, and hormone formation promoters, dermal moisturizers for cosmetics.

Exsyproteines 2%, 4%. [Exsymol; Biosil Tech.] Hydrolyzed elastin; CAS 9007-58-3; cosmetic ingred. for moisturizers, oily skin treatments, anti-aging creams; yel. sl. visc., opalescent aq. liq.; misc. with water, alcohols, glycols; pH 6.0; usage level: 2-15%; toxicology: nontoxic.

Exsyzinc. [Exsymol] Zinc acetylmethionate; CAS 102868-96-2.

Extan G-7. [Lanaetex Prods.] Glycereth-7; CAS 31694-55-0; cosmetic ingred.

Extan G-26. [Lanaetex Prods.] Glycereth-26; CAS 31694-55-0; cosmetic ingred.

Extan-GMS. [Lanaetex Prods.] Glyceryl stearate, PEG-100 stearate; cosmetics ingred.

Extan-GO. [Lanaetex Prods.] Glyceryl oleate, propylene glycol.

Extan-LT. [Lanaetex Prods.] Sorbitan laurate; cosmetics ingred.

Extan-OT. [Lanaetex Prods.] Sorbitan oleate; CAS 1338-43-8; EINECS 215-665-4; cosmetics ingred.

Extan-PGC. [Lanaetex Prods.] PEG-7 glyceryl cocoate; cosmetic ingred.

Extan-PT. [Lanaetex Prods.] Sorbitan palmitate; CAS 26266-57-9; EINECS 247-568-8; cosmetic ingred.

Extan-SOT. [Lanaetex Prods.] Sorbitan sesquioleate; CAS 8007-43-0; EINECS 232-360-1; emulsifier.

Extan-ST. [Lanaetex Prods.] Sorbitan stearate; CAS 1338-41-6; EINECS 215-664-9; emulsifier.

Extender W. [Rona] Titanium dioxide/mica pigment; nonpearlescent pigment developed by combining the effects of light reflection and light scattering; offers improved skin adhesion, better compressibility, lack of luster.

Extracellular Matrix CLR. [Dr. Kurt Richter] Water and connective tissue extract.

Extract GLM No. 1. [Sederma] Water and mammary extract.

Extract Arnica Special. [Novarom GmbH] Propylene glycol, ethoxydiglycol, and arnica extract; botanical extract.

Extract From Bovine Foetal Skin Cells. [Solabia] Calf skin hydrolysate.

Extrait No. 30. [C.E.P.] Glycerin, mushroom extract, horse chestnut extract, and esculin.

Ectrait Hamamelis LC 452. [Gattefosse] Water, gallic acid, and witch hazel extract.

Extrakt 52. [Zschimmer & Schwarz] Surfactant blend; anionic/nonionic/amphoteric; for bath additives, hair shampoos, baby cosmetics, liq. body cleaners; liq.; 50% act.

Extrapone Arnica Special 2/032591. [Dragoco] Water, ethoxydiglycol, propylene glycol, butylene glycol, and arnica extract.

Extrapone Bio-Tamin Special 2/2032671. [Dragoco] Retinyl palmitate, water, PEG-40 castor oil, ethoxydiglycol, propylene glycol, butylene glycol, menadione, and thiamine HCl.

Extrapone Chamomile Special 2/033021. [Dragoco] Water, ethoxydiglycol, propylene glycol, matricaria extract, butylene glycol, glucose, and bisabolol.

Extrapone Coco-Nut Special 2/033055. [Dragoco] Propylene glycol, water, coconut extract, PEG-60 hydrog. castor oil; botanical extract.

Extrapone Hamamelis Super 2/500010. [Dragoco] Water, ethoxydiglycol, propylene glycol, glucose, butylene glycol, and witch hazel extract.

Extrapone Neo-H-Special 2/032441. [Dragoco] Water, ethoxydiglycol, butylene glycol, calcium pantothenate, colloidal sulfur, and inositol.

Extrapone Poly H Special 2/032451. [Dragoco] Water, ethoxydiglycol, propylene glycol, butylene glycol, coltsfoot extract, horsetail extract, calcium pantothenate, and inositol.

Extrapone Witch Hazel 2/032893. [Dragoco] Water, witch hazel extract, SD alcohol 39-C, and butylene glycol.

Extra Super English Terra Alba. [Charles B. Chrystal] Calcium sulfate; CAS 7778-18-9; EINECS 231-900-3.

Exxal® 16. [Exxon] Hexyldecanol; CAS 36311-34-9; extender and solv. for dyes and fragrances.

Exxal® 18. [Exxon] Octyldecanol; CAS 2745-8-931; cosmetic raw material.

Exxal® 20. [Exxon] Octyldodecanol; CAS 5333-42-6; EINECS 226-242-9; carrier, lubricant, emollient.

Exxal® 26. [Exxon] Undecylpentadecanol; CAS 70693-05-9; cosmetic ingred.

F

F-5W-0 100 cs. [Shin-Etsu Silicones] Diphenyl dimethicone.
F-5W-0 300 cs. [Shin-Etsu Silicones] Diphenyl dimethicone.
F-5W-0 1000 cs. [Shin-Etsu Silicones] Diphenyl dimethicone.
F-5W-0 3000 cs. [Shin-Etsu Silicones] Diphenyl dimethicone.
Facilan. [Lanaetex Prods.] Lanolin acid; CAS 68424-43-1; EINECS 270-302-7; emollient.
Facteur ARL. [Les Colorants Wackherr] Tocopheryl acetate, ascorbyl palmitate, retinyl palmitate, bioflavonoids, and ivy extract; free radical scavenging additive for cosmetics.
Facteur Hydratant PH. [Prod'Hyg] Sodium lactate, lactic acid, glycerin, serine, sorbitol, lauryl aminopropylglycine, lauryl diethylenediaminoglycine, urea, allantoin, and TEA-lactate.
Falba®. [Aceto] cosmetic ingred.
Falba Absorption Base. [Pfaltz & Bauer] Min. oil, lanolin, paraffin, lanolin alcohol, and beeswax.
Famodan SMO. [Grindsted Prods. Denmark] Sorbitan oleate; CAS 1338-43-8; EINECS 215-665-4; emulsifier.
Famous. [Karlshamns] Partially hydrog. soybean oil, stabilized; CAS 8016-70-4; EINECS 232-410-2; emollient, lubricant; iodine no. 88-93.
Fancol 707. [Fanning] PPG-30 cetyl ether; CAS 9035-85-2; skin conditioner, emollient for permanent waves, shampoos, blushers, indoor tanning preps.; lt. yel. liq.; acid no. 1 max.; iodine no. 3 max.
Fancol Acel. [Fanning] Acetylated lanolin; CAS 61788-48-5; EINECS 262-979-2; emollient, superfatting agent, lipophilic spreading agent for oils, creams, lotions, hair grooms, ointments, pharmaceuticals; Gardner 12 max. color; m.p. 30-40 C; acid no. 3 max.; sapon. no. 130 max.; hyd. no. 10 max.
Fancol ALA. [Fanning] Cetyl acetate and acetylated lanolin alcohol; cosmetic, toiletry conditioner, emollient, pigment binder, spreading agent, oil coupler, solv. for skin care prods., hand and body lotions, suntan and bath oils; glossing and plasticizing agent for hairsprays; clear lt. oily liq.; acid no. 1 max.; iodine no. 12 max.; sapon. no. 200 max.; hyd. no. 8 max.
Fancol ALA-10. [Fanning] Polysorbate 80, cetyl acetate, acetylated lanolin alcohol; skin/hair conditioner, sec. emulsifier, pigment wetter, solubilizer, emollient, humectant, superfatting agent for antiperspirants, lotions and creams, sunscreens; amber to yel. liq., pract. odorless; acid no. 2 max.; sapon. no. 60-80; hyd. no. 55-70.
Fancol ALA-15. [Fanning] Polysorbate 80, cetyl acetate, acetylated lanolin alcohol.
Fancol C. [Fanning] Petrolatum, lanolin, lanolin alcohol; w/o emulsifier, moisturizing lubricant, emollient, fatting agent, water absorbent; pale yel.-ivory soft solid, faint char. sterol odor; m.p. 40-46 C; acid no. 1 max.
Fancol CA. [Fanning] Cetyl alcohol; CAS 36653-82-4; EINECS 253-149-0; surfactant, emulsifier, emulsion stabilizer, opacifier, skin conditioner/emollient, visc. booster, foam booster; for makeup, hair conditioners, cleansers,

moisturizing creams and lotions; APHA 40 max. color; m.p. 45-50 C; acid no. 2 max.; iodine no. 0.6 max.; sapon. no. 1 max.; hyd. no. 225-235.
Fancol CAB. [Fanning] Petrolatum, lanolin, lanolin alcohol; w/o emulsifier, moisturizing lubricant, emollient, fatting agent, water absorbent; pale yel.-ivory soft solid, faint char. sterol odor; m.p. 40-46 C; acid no. 1 max.; sapon. no. 10-20.
Fancol CB. [Fanning] Cocoa butter obtained from roasted seeds of *Theobroma cacao*; CAS 8002-31-1; skin conditioner, occlusive solv., skin protectant for OTC drug prods., makeup, moisturizing creams and lotions, suntan preps.; ylsh. wh. solid; iodine no. 35-40; sapon. no. 192-197; ref. index 1.4560-1.4580.
Fancol CB Extra. [Fanning] Cocoa butter USP obtained from roasted seeds of *Theobroma cacao*; CAS 8002-31-1; skin conditioner, occlusive solv., skin protectant for OTC drug prods., makeup, moisturizing creams and lotions, suntan preps.; ylsh. wh. solid; iodine no. 35-43; sapon. no. 188-195; ref. index 1.4560-1.4580.
Fancol CH. [Fanning] Cholesterol NF; CAS 57-88-5; EINECS 200-353-2; film-former with lubricating, protective and anti-irritant props., aids cell regeneration, emulsifier for w/o formulations, precursor for prod. of vitamin D; for cosmetics, pharmaceuticals, hair/skin care prods.; wh. gran.; sol. in acetone, chloroform, dioxane, ether, ethyl acetae, hexane, veg. oils; sl. sol. in alcohol; insol. in water; m.p. 147-150 C.
Fancol CH-24. [Fanning] Choleth-24; CAS 27321-96-6, 9004-95-9; surfactant, emulsifier for hair dyes, bubble bath, moisturizing creams and lotions, cleansing prods.; yel. wax-like solid, faint odor; acid no. 1.5 max.; iodine no. 12-19; hyd. no. 35-45; cloud pt. 88-95 C; pH 4.5-7.5 (10%); 99.5% min. nonvolatiles.
Fancol CO-30. [Fanning] PEG-30 castor oil; CAS 61791-12-6; surfactant, emulsifier for cleansing prods., hair conditioners, wave sets, face, body and hand creams and lotions; amber clear liq.; acid no. 2 max.; sapon. no. 70-80; hyd. no. 70-80.
Fancol DL. [Fanning] DL-Panthenol; CAS 16485-10-2; conditioning agent for hair care prods., makeup, moisturizing creams and lotions; off-wh. to cream cryst. powd., sl. char. odor; sol. in water, acetone, ethanol, and propylene glycol; m.p. 65-69 C; 97% min. assay.
Fancol Gingko Extract. [Fanning] Propylene glycol and ginko extract; biological extract for use in lotions, milks, creams, shampoos, bubble baths, soaps, gels; amber liq.; sol. in water and alcohol.
Fancol HCO-25. [Fanning] PEG-25 hydrog. castor oil; CAS 61788-85-0; surfactant, emulsifier for bath oils, tablets and salts, aftershave lotions, skin fresheners; HLB 10.8; acid no. 2 max.; sapon. no. 80-90; pour pt. 4-8 C.
Fancol HL. [Fanning] Hydrog. lanolin; CAS 8031-44-5; EINECS 232-452-1; emollient, moisturizer, lubricant,

plasticizer, chemical intermediate, humectant, mold release agent for pharmaceuticals, cosmetics, industrial applications; wh. solid, trace odor; sol. in IPM, min. oil, castor oil, ethyl acetate, acetone (@ 75 C); insol. water; sp.gr. 0.855–0.865; m.p. 48–53 C; iodine no. 15 max.; sapon. no. 6 max.; ref. index 1.460–1.469 (50 C).

Fancol HL-20. [Fanning] PEG-20 hydrog. lanolin; CAS 68648-27-1; solubilizer, superfatting agent, gelling agent for cosmetics, pharmaceuticals, makeup, nail polish, night creams, microemulsions; pale cream soft waxy solid, very sl. odor; m.p. 40-50 C; sapon. no. 7 max.; hyd. no. 55 max.

Fancol HL-24. [Fanning] PEG-24 hydrog. lanolin; CAS 68648-27-1; solubilizer, superfatting agent for cosmetic/ pharmaceutical creams and lotions, makeup, nail polish, lipstick, night creams, microemulsions; gelling agent for transparent gels; pale cream soft waxy solid, very sl. odor; m.p. 40-50 C; sapon. no. 7 max.; hyd. no. 55 max.

Fancol HON. [Fanning] Honey; CAS 8028-66-8; biological additive, flavoring, skin conditioner, humectant for shampoos, face, body and hand creams and lotions, bath prods., hair conditioners, cleansing prods., moisturizing creams and lotions; clear; pH 3.0-4.9; 80% min. solids.

Fancol IPL. [Fanning] Isopropyl lanolate; CAS 63393-93-1; EINECS 264-119-1; emollient.

Fancol ISO. [Fanning] Isopropyl myristate, lanolin oil, oleyl alcohol; cosmetic ingred.

Fancol Karite Butter. [Fanning] Shea butter; CAS 68424-60-2; ointment base, anti-irritant for skin, skin conditioner, occlusive agent, solv. for suntan preps., body lotions, winter sports prods., wrinkle creams, soaps, shave foams, shampoos, balsams; Gardner 4 max. color; m.p. 32-45 C; acid no. 0.5 max.; iodine no. 60-70; sapon. no. 178-190; hyd. no. 5.

Fancol Karite Extract. [Fanning] Shea butter extract; CAS 68424-59-9; emollient with exc. spreadability for suntan preps., skin toners, lipsticks, eye liners, ointments, suppositories; Gardner 3 max. color; sol. in castor oil; sl. sol. in min. oil, propylene glycol, glycerin, ethyl acetate, isopropyl lanolate; insol. in water; iodine no. 63-70.

Fancol LA. [Fanning] Lanolin alcohol; CAS 8027-33-6; EINECS 232-430-1; nonionic; emollient, thickener, emulsifier, stabilizer, plasticizer, superfatting agent, dye dispersant, chemical intermediate, lubricant, humectant, mold release agent, conditioner for cosmetics, pharmaceuticals, soaps, industrial applics.; lt. amber to yel. wax-like solid, faint char. odor; sol. in CCl₄, chloroform, IPM (@ 75 C), min. oil (@ 75 C), oleyl alcohol; insol. water; m.p. 56 C; acid no. 3 max.; sapon. no. 12 max.; 100% act.

Fancol LA-5. [Fanning] Laneth-5; CAS 61791-20-6; emollient, emulsifier, moisturizer, spreading agent, coupler for shampoos, skin care prods., cosmetics; yel. solid; acid no. 5 max.; hyd. no. 120-135; 100% act.

Fancol LA-15. [Fanning] Laneth-15; CAS 61791-20-6; nonionic; emollient, emulsifier for stable o/w cosmetics/ pharmaceutical emulsions and microemulsions; coupling agent for lanolin oil into shampoos; yel. solid; HLB 12.7; acid no. 5 max.; hyd. no. 85; 100% act.

Fancol LAO. [Fanning] Min. oil and lanolin alcohol; CAS 8012-95-1, 9027-33-6; nonionic; conditioner, surfactant, stabilizer, moisturizer, humectant, penetrant, emollient, plasticizer, and primary emulsifier for use in cosmetics and pharmaceuticals; plasticizer in aerosol formulas; yel. clear oily liq.; odorless; sol. in oils; insol. in water; sp.gr. 0.84–0.86; acid no. 1 max.; iodine no. 12 max.; sapon. no. 3.0 max.; hyd. no. 16 max.; 100% conc.

Fancol Menthol. [Fanning] Menthol; CAS 89-78-1; EINECS 201-939-0; denaturant, flavoring agent, fragrance component for mouthwashes, aftershaves, cleansing prods., face, body and hand creams/lotions, skin care prods.;

m.p. 41-44 C.

Fancol OA-95. [Fanning] Oleyl alcohol; CAS 143-28-2; EINECS 205-597-3; nonionic; plasticizer, emulsion stabilizer, antifoam and coupling agent, aerosol lubricant, petrol. additive, pigment dispersant; rust preventive; detergent, release agent, cosolvent, softener, tackifier, spreading agent used for metalworking, petrochemicals, pulp and paper, paints and coatings, plastics and polymers, inks, food applics., pharmaceuticals, cosmetics; chemical intermediate; liq.; sol. in IPA, acetone, lt. min. oil, trichloroethylene, kerosene, VMP naphtha, benzene, turpentine; acid no. 0.05 max.; iodine no. 90-96; sapon no. 1 max.; hyd. no. 200-212; cloud pt. 5 C max.

Fancol SA. [Fanning] Stearyl alcohol; CAS 112-92-5; EINECS 204-017-6; emulsion stabilizer, opacifier, skin conditioner, emollient, visc. booster, foam booster for makeup, hair conditioners, moisturizing creams and lotions, cleansers; m.p. 55-60 C; acid no. 2 max.; iodine no. 1 max.; sapon. no. 1.5 max.; hyd. no. 200-220; 98% act.

Fancol SA-15. [Fanning] PPG-15 stearyl ether; CAS 25231-21-4; skin conditioner, emollient for bath oils, tablets and salts, fragrance prods., lipsticks, deodorants, cleansers; APHA 150 color; acid no. 1.5 max.; iodine no. 2 max.; sapon. no. 3 max.; hyd. no. 60-75.

Fancol SORB. [Fanning] Sorbitol; CAS 50-70-4; EINECS 200-061-5; cosmetic/pharmaceutical ingred.

Fancol TOIN. [Fanning] Allantoin; CAS 97-59-6; EINECS 202-592-8; skin conditioner for makeup, cleansers, face, body and hand creams and lotions, moisturizing creams, skin care prods.; wh. cryst.; pH 4.5-6.0 (0.5%).

Fancor IPL. [Fanning] Isopropyl lanolate; CAS 63393-93-1; EINECS 264-119-1; hydrophilic emollient, moisturizer, w/ o aux. emulsifier, stabilizer and opacifier, wetting and dispersing agent for pigments and talc, aids slip and gloss of stick cosmetics, plasticizes wax systems, mold release, superfatting agent; binder for pressed powds.; buttery yel. solid; sol. @ 75 C in IPM, min. oil, castor oil; acid no. 18 max.; iodine no. 20 max.; sapon. no. 165 max.; hyd. no. 68 max.

Fancor ISO Cholesterol. [Fanning] used for cosmetic, pharmaceutical, hair and skin prods.; m.p. 138-145 C; acid no. 0.5 max.

Fancor LFA. [Fanning] Lanolin fatty acids; CAS 68424-43-1; EINECS 270-302-7; nonionic; emollient, stabilizer, emulsifier, corrosion inhibitor for personal care and pharmaceutical prods.; used in industrial leather treating, coatings, polishes, corrosion inhibitors, lubricants; wax-like solid; sol. in ethyl acetate; sl. sol. in IPM, min. oil; sol. @ 75 C in IPM, min. and castor oil, acetone, ethyl acetate, ethyl alcohol; m.p. 57–65 C; acid no. 135–170; iodine no. 10 max.; sapon. no. 158–175; hyd. no. 50 max.; 100% conc.

Fancor Lansil. [Fanning] Dimethicone copolyol adipate.

Fancor Lanwax. [Fanning] Natural lanolin wax ester; CAS 68201-49-0; EINECS 269-220-4; plasticizer in wax crayons; water repellent, humectant, conditioner, corrosion inhibitor, emollient, lubricant for cosmetics, toiletries, pharmaceuticals, industrial applics.; extender and crystallization inhibitor for natural waxes in industrial applics.; emulsifier; semisolid; m.p. 48–52 C; iodine no. 36 max.; sapon. no. 90–110; hyd. no. 35 max.

Fancorsil A. [Fanning] Cyclomethicone and dimethicone; CAS 69430-24-6, 9006-65-9; hair/skin conditioner, emollient, solv.; used in hair conditioners, makeup, moisturizing creams and lotions; provides lubricity, long lasting gloss; clear visc. liq.; sp.gr. 0.960; visc. 5000 cps min.; 100% solids.

Fancorsil P. [Fanning] Modified silicone hydrocarbon; skin/ hair conditioning agent, emollient; exc. afterfeel and lubricity; long lasting high gloss; clear liq.; sol. in ethyl acetate, IPM; sl. sol. in castor and min. oils, propylene glycol, glycerin; insol. in water; iodine no. 40-50; sapon. no. 80-90.

Fancorsil SLA. [Fanning] Dimethicone copolyol adipate; skin/hair conditioning agent, emollient; provides soft and velvety afterfeel; good shine; amber hazy liq.; sol. in min. oil, ethyl acetate, IPM; sl. sol. in castor oil, propylene glycol, glycerin, ethanol, water; acid no. 12 max.; pH 4-6 (1%).

Fancorsil SLA-LT. [Fanning] Dimethicone copolyol adipate; skin/hair conditioning agent, emollient; provides good shine, exc. soft and velvety afterfeel; yel. to brn. paste; sol. in min. oil, ethyl acetae, IPM; sl. sol. in castor oil, propylene glycol, glycerin, ethanol, water; acid no. 12 max.; pH 4-6 (1%).

Fanwax G. [Fanning] Stearyl alcohol, ceteareth-20; CAS 112-92-5, 977054-66-2; nonionic; o/w self-emulsifying wax for cosmetics and toiletries, skin/hair lotions, antiperspirants, depilatories, creme rinses, opacified hair dyes, bleaches; wh. to off-wh. waxy solid or flakes, bland char. odor; m.p. 55-63 C; acid no. 1 max.; sapon. no. 1 max.

Fanwax P. [Fanning] Cetearyl alcohol, polysorbate 60; CAS 8005-44-5, 9005-67-8; nonionic; o/w self-emulsifying wax for lotions, creams, hair and skin care prods., creme rinses, antiperspirants; creamy wh. waxy solid or flake, bland char. odor; m.p. 48-52 C; iodine no. 3.5 max.; sapon. no. 14 max.; hyd. no. 178-192; pH 5.5-7.0 (3% aq.).

Fibrastil. [Sederma] Hydrolyzed spinal protein, glycerin, spleen extract, and thymus hydrolysate.

Fibronex. [Tri-K Industries] Fibronectin.

Fibro-Silk™ Powd. [Brooks Industries] Silk; CAS 9009-99-8; silk protein pigment; powd.

Fibrostimuline P. [Sederma] Glycerin and calf skin extract.

Fibrostimuline S. [Sederma] Serum protein.

Filagrinol®. [Vevy; Vevy Europe] Pollen extract, soybean oil unsaponifiables, olive oil unsaponifiables, and wheat germ oil unsaponifiables; basic active ingred. for cosmetics; filament aggregating protein enhancer; improves skin hydration; usage level: 8-10%.

Filter-Cel. [Celite] Diatomaceous earth; CAS 7631-86-9; EINECS 231-545-4; carrier, filler for cosmetics.

Filtered Verajuice-Cold Processed. [Apree] Aloe vera gel; moisturizer, soothing/healing aid for personal care.

Finamine CO. [Finetex] Cocamidopropylamine oxide; CAS 68155-09-9; EINECS 268-938-5; cosmetic surfactant.

Finecat MOGL. [Finetex] Methyl hydroxycetyl glucaminium lactate.

Fine Oxocol. [Nissan Chem. Ind.] Heptylundecanol.

Finester EH-25. [Finetex] C12-15 alkyl octanoate; emollient, solubilizer.

Finex-25. [Presperse] Micronized zinc oxide; CAS 1314-13-2; EINECS 215-222-5; provide exc. feel, covering power and skin adherance; uv absorber, SPF booster for sun care prods.; JSCI/JCID approved; wh. fine powd.; particle size 0.1μ; sp.gr. 5.6; oil absorp. 18 ml/100 g; ref. index 1.2-2.0.

Finquat CT. [Finetex] Quaternium-75; cationic; hair and skin conditioner used in thioglycolate permanent waving sol'ns. to reduce processing time and condition hair; also in depilatories; liq.; water-sol.

Finsoft HCM-100. [Finetex] Quaternium-77, quaternium-78; hair conditioner, non-eye irritating cream rinses; solid.

Finsolv® 116. [Finetex] Stearyl benzoate; CAS 10578-34-4; EINECS 234-169-9; emollient, solubilizer.

Finsolv® BOD. [Finetex] Octyldodecyl benzoate; emollient, solubilizer, foam modifier for syn. detergents.

Finsolv® EMG-20. [Finetex] Methyl gluceth-20 benzoate; emollient, solubilizer.

Finsolv® P. [Finetex] PPG-15 stearyl ether benzoate; emollient, solubilizer, foam modifier for soap and soap/syndet systems.

Finsolv® PL-62. [Finetex] Poloxamer 182 benzoate; emollient, solubilizer.

Finsolv® PL-355. [Finetex] Poloxamer 105 benzoate; emollient, solubilizer.

Finsolv® SB. [Finetex] Isostearyl benzoate; nongreasy emollient, noncomedogenic; for cosmetics, sunscreen, antiperspirants, deodorants; lubricant; plasticizer for hair resins, in anhyd. systems; perfume solubilizer; liq.; sol. in org. solvs. and oils.

Finsolv® TN. [Finetex; Witco SA] C12-15 alkyl benzoate; CAS 68411-27-8; emollient, solubilizer, conditioner, sunscreen vehicle, deoiler for cosmetic creams and oils; binder in pressed powds.; noncomedogenic; liq.; 100% act.

Firmogen®. [Laboratoires Sérobiologiques] Hydrolyzed wheat protein, barley extract, and arnica extract; phytocomplex providing cutaneous tensor power, strengthening of cutaneous elasticity and firmness; for facial and body care, anti-aging formulations; amber limpid liq.; water-sol.; usage level: 5-10%.

Fishlan LS. [Laboratoires Sérobiologiques] Glycerin, hydrolyzed actin.

Fitoderm. [Hispano Quimica] Squalane; CAS 111-01-3; EINECS 203-825-6; emollient, lubricant.

Fitoestesina. [Vevy] Zedoary oil, ginger oil, cinnamon oil, and thyme oil.

Fitoxantina. [Vevy] Xanthophyll; CAS 11138-66-2; EINECS 234-394-2; gum for cosmetics.

Fizul MD-318C. [Finetex] Disodium oleamido MIPA sulfosuccinate; CAS 43154-85-4; EINECS 256-120-0; anionic; cosmetic grade detergent, conditioner for shampoos, bath prods.; high foam, low toxicology; liq.; 35% conc.

FK 500LS. [Degussa] Precipitated silica; thickener for cosmetic creams and lotions; also in thermal insulation, paper, films, pesticides, pharmaceuticals; FDA approved; tapped dens 80 g/l; surf. area 475 m²/g; pH 6.7; 99% SiO₂.

Flamenco®. [Mearl] Titanium dioxide coated mica; pearl and color pigments of exceptional brilliance displaying twin colors; for cosmetics, frosted nail enamels; grades avail.: Ultra Fine, Velvet, Satina, Pearl, Gold, Orange, Red, Violet, Blue, Green, Twilight Gold, Twilight Red, Twilight Blue, Twilight Green, Superpearl, Super Gold, Super Red, Super Blue, Super Green.

Flamenco® Gold. [Mearl] Mica and titanium dioxide.

Flamenco® Gold CC. [Mearl] Castor oil, mica, titanium dioxide, oleyl alcohol, and carnauba.

Flamenco® Pearl. [Mearl] Mica and titanium dioxide.

Flamenco® Pearl CC. [Mearl] Castor oil, mica, titanium dioxide, oleyl alcohol, and carnauba.

Flamenco® Twilight Blue. [Mearl] Mica, titanium dioxide, and iron oxides.

Flamenco® Ultra Fine. [Mearl] Mica and titanium dioxide.

Flexan® 130. [Nat'l. Starch] Sodium polystyrene sulfonate; CAS 9003-59-2; hair fixative for setting lotions, conditioners, blow drying aid; gloss and antistatic chars.; liq.; sol. in water, glycerin, low m.w. glycols, and ethanol/water blends; visc. 100 cps; pH 6.0; 30% aq. sol'n.

Flexiquat. [Brooks Industries] Gelatin/keratin amino acids/lysine hydroxypropyltrimonium chloride; cosmetic ingred.

Flexiquat AAS-15. [Brooks Industries] AMP-isostearoyl gelatin/keratin amino acids/lysine hydroxypropyltrimonium chloride; raw material for cosmetic and personal care prods.

Flexiqua B. [Brooks Industries] Gelatin/lysine/polyacrylamide hydroxypropyltrimonium chloride; cosmetic ingred.

Flexricin® 9. [CasChem] Propylene glycol ricinoleate; CAS 26402-31-3; EINECS 247-669-7; nonionic; wetting agent, dye solv., wax plasticizer, stabilizer for textile, household, and cosmetic applics., rewetting dried skins; FDA approval; Gardner 2+ liq.; sol. in toluene, butyl acetate, MEK, ethanol; sp.gr. 0.96; visc. 3 stokes; pour pt. -15 F; acid no. 2; iodine no. 77; sapon. no. 159; hyd. no. 288; 100% act.

Flexricin® 13. [CasChem] Glyceryl ricinoleate; CAS 141-08-2; EINECS 205-455-0; nonionic; wetting agent, wax plasticizer, and mold release agent for rubber polymers, antifoam agent, household and cosmetic applics., rewetting dried skins; FDA approval; Gardner 2 min. liq.; sol. in toluene, butyl acetate, MEK, ethanol; sp.gr. 0.985; visc. 8.8 stokes; pour pt. 20 F; acid no. 5; iodine no. 77; sapon. no. 160; hyd. no. 345; 100% act.

Flexricin® 15. [CasChem] Glycol ricinoleate; CAS 106-17-2; EINECS 203-369-8; nonionic; wetting agent, plasticizer, textile, household, and cosmetic applics., rewetting dried skins; chemical intermediate; FDA approval; Gardner 4 liq.; sol. in toluene, butyl acetate, MEK, ethanol; sp.gr. 0.965; visc. 3.9 stokes; 100% act.

Flo-Mo® AJ-85. [Witco/H-I-P] Trideceth-7 (7.5 EO); CAS 24938-91-8; nonionic; detergent, wetting agent for personal care prods.; USDA-MID approved for cleaning food handling equipment; liq.; cloud pt. 102–109 F; 85% act.

Flo-Mo® AJ-85. [Witco/H-I-P] Trideceth-7 (7.5 EO); CAS 24938-91-8; nonionic; detergent, wetting agent for personal care prods.; USDA-MID approved for cleaning food handling equipment; liq.; cloud pt. 102–109 F; 85% act.

Flo-Mo® AJ-100. [Witco/H-I-P] Trideceth-7 (7.5 EO); CAS 24938-91-8; nonionic; detergent, wetting agent for personal care prods.; USDA-MID approved for cleaning food handling equip.; paste; 100% act.

Flonac ME 10 C. [Presperse] Mica, titanium dioxide; silver pearl pigment for cosmetics use; particle size 5-45 µ; 30% TiO_2.

Flonac MG 30 C. [Presperse] Mica, titanium dioxide, and iron oxide; gold pearl pigment for cosmetics use; particle size 15-70 µ; 17% TiO_2.

Flonac MI 10 C. [Presperse] Mica, titanium dioxide; silver pearl pigment for cosmetics use; particle size 10-50 µ; 29% TiO_2.

Flonac ML 10 C. [Presperse] Mica, titanium dioxide; silver pearl pigment for cosmetics use; particle size 30-120 µ; 16% TiO_2.

Flonac MS 5 C. [Presperse] Mica, titanium dioxide; interference pearl pigment for cosmetics use; violet; particle size 15-70 µ; 35% TiO_2.

Flonac MS 10 C. [Presperse] Mica, titanium dioxide; silver pearl pigment for cosmetics use; particle size 15-70 µ; 22% TiO_2.

Flonac MS 20 C. [Presperse] Mica, titanium dioxide; interference pearl pigment for cosmetics use; gold; particle size 15-70 µ; 30% TiO_2.

Flonac MS 30 C. [Presperse] Mica, titanium dioxide, and iron oxide; gold pearl pigment for cosmetics use; particle size 15-70 µ; 30% TiO_2.

Flonac MS 33 C. [Presperse] Mica, titanium dioxide, and iron oxide; gold pearl pigment for cosmetics use; particle size 15-70 µ; 29% TiO_2.

Flonac MS 40 C. [Presperse] Mica, titanium dioxide; interference pearl pigment for cosmetics use; red; particle size 15-70 µ; 34% TiO_2.

Flonac MS 60 C. [Presperse] Mica, titanium dioxide; interference pearl pigment for cosmetics use; blue; particle size 15-70 µ; 36% TiO_2.

Flonac MS 70 C. [Presperse] Mica, titanium dioxide; interference pearl pigment for cosmetics use; green; particle size 15-70 µ; 44% TiO_2.

Flonac MX 10 C. [Presperse] Mica, titanium dioxide; silver pearl pigment for cosmetics use; particle size 40-230 µ; 14% TiO_2.

Flonac MX 30 C. [Kemira Oy] Mica, titanium dioxide, and iron oxides.

Florabeads. [Int'l. Flora Tech.] Jojoba wax; CAS 66625-78-3; exfolient for cosmetic use; hard microspheres in the form of free-flowing beads; particle size 85% 250-420 µ; m.p. 69 C.

Florabeads 28/60 Jade. [Int'l. Flora Tech.] Hard microspheres of microcrystalline wax colored with chromium oxide; exfolient for cosmetic use; jade green free-flowing beads; 85% 250-600 µ particle size; m.p. 88 C.

Florabeads JM 28/60. [Int'l. Flora Tech.] Microspheres containing jojoba seed powd. coated with jojoba wax; exfolient for cosmetic use; free-flowing beads; particle size 80% 250-600 µ.

Florabeads Micro 28/60 Gypsy Rose. [Int'l. Flora Tech.] Hard microspheres of microcrystalline wax colored with D&C Red No. 30; exfolient for cosmetic use; red free-flowing beads; 85% 250-600 µ particle size; m.p. 88 C.

Florabeads Micro 28/60 Lapis. [Int'l. Flora Tech.] Hard microspheres of microcrystalline wax colored with ultramarine blue; exfolient for cosmetic use; deep blue free-flowing beads; 85% 250-600 µ particle size; m.p. 88 C.

Florabeads Micro 28/60 White. [Int'l. Flora Tech.] Hard microspheres of microcrystalline wax; CAS 63231-60-7; EINECS 264-038-1; exfolient for cosmetic use; wh. free-flowing beads; 85% 250-600 µ particle size; m.p. 88 C.

Floraesters. [Int'l. Flora Tech.] Transesterified jojoba oil and wax; for cosmetic use.

Floramat. [Henkel/Cospha] Ethyl-2-t-butylcyclohexylcarbonate; fragrance raw material for personal care and detergent applics.; colorless liq., woody odor; b.p. 73 C; flash pt. 120 C.

Florasun™-90. [Int'l. Flora Tech.] Pure cold-pressed sunflower seed oil; CAS 8001-21-6; EINECS 232-273-9; lipid for cosmetics; water clear oil, trace odor; sp.gr. 0.916; m.p. 1 C; acid no. 0.1; iodine no. 81.5; sapon. no. 190.4.

Flowtone R. [Southern Clay Prods.] Trihydroxystearin; CAS 8001-78-3; thixotrope.

Fluid AP. [Amerchol] PPG-14 butyl ether; CAS 9003-13-8; cosmetic ingred.

Fluidamid DF 12. [Roquette] Aluminum starch octenylsuccinate; CAS 9087-61-0; ingred. for body powds.

Fluilan. [Croda Inc.; Croda Chem. Ltd.] Lanolin oil; CAS 8006-54-0; nonionic; w/o emulsifier; dispersant for pigments; conditioning agent; emollient, penetrant, superfatting agent for lipsticks, baby oils, brilliantines, cleansing lotions, pharmaceutical ointments, creams, and lotions; plasticizer for hair spray resins; moisturizer in w/o emulsions; also for soaps, shampoos, dishwashing liqs., germicidal skin cleansers; pale yel. visc. liq.; pleasant, char. odor; sol. in min. oils, IPA, fatty alcohol, hydrocarbons, and aerosol propellents; cloud pt. 18 C max.; pour pt. 8 C max.; acid no. 2 max.; iodine no. 24-40; sapon. no. 80–100; usage level: 2-10%; toxicology: LD50 (oral, rat) > 20 g/kg; mild skin and eye irritant; 100% act.

Fluilan AWS. [Croda Inc.] PPG-12-PEG-65 lanolin oil; CAS 68458-58-8; emollient, cleanser, and solubilizer for pharmaceuticals, cleansing wipe formulations, moisturizing creams and lotions; plasticizer and film modifier for hair sprays; amber visc. liq., nearly odorless; sol. in water and alcohol; disp. in propylene glycol; acid no. 3 max.; iodine no. 7–15; sapon. no. 10–25; pH 5–7 (10%); usage level: 0.1-2%; toxicology: LD50 (oral, rat) > 5 g/kg; moderate skin irritant, minimal eye irritant.

FMB 128 T. [Crystal] Cocamide DEA; CAS 61791-31-9; EINECS 263-163-9; cosmetic surfactant.

FMB 451-8 Quat. [Crystal] Myristalkonium chloride; CAS 139-08-2; EINECS 205-352-0; for formulation of disinfectants, sanitizers, fungicides, water treatment microbicides, swimming pool algicides, mildewcides; 80% act.

FMB 500-15 Quat U.S.P. [Crystal] Benzalkonium chloride;

preservative in OTC drug prods.; 50% act.

FMB 551-5 Quat. [Crystal] Myristalkonium chloride; CAS 139-08-2; EINECS 205-352-0; antimicrobial.

FMB BT. [Crystal] Cocamide DEA; CAS 61791-31-9; EINECS 263-163-9; cosmetic surfactant.

FMB CAP B. [Crystal] Cocamidopropyl betaine; foaming agent for hair and baby shampoos, industrial applics. in strongly alkaline and acid systems; golden clear visc. liq.; limited sol. in water, lower alcohols, and most polar solvs.; sp.gr. 1.047; dens. 8.732 lb/gal; visc. 30-60 cps; pH 4.5-5.5 (5%); 30% act., 35% total solids.

FMB Cocamide DEA. [Crystal] Cocamide DEA; CAS 61791-31-9; EINECS 263-163-9; cosmetic surfactant.

FMB Coco Condensate. [Crystal] Cocamide DEA; CAS 61791-31-9; EINECS 263-163-9; cosmetic surfactant.

FM Extract. [Ichimaru Pharcos] Alcohol and yogurt filtrate.

Foamamino 40CT. [Brooks Industries] TEA-lauroyl collagen amino acids; cosmetic ingred.

Foam Base F. [Lowenstein] anionic; foaming surfactant for prod. of dry powd. colors.; 100% act.

Foam Base G. [Lowenstein] anionic; surfactant for prod. of dry powd. colors.; gel/lotion base; gel; 100% act.

Foam Blast 5, 7. [Ross Chem.] Silicone antifoam compd.; food-grade antifoam for foam control in nonaq. systems; applics. incl. edible oil processing, meat processing, fat rendering, and synthesis of pharmaceuticals; 100% act.

Foam Blast 10. [Ross Chem.] Silicone antifoam compd.; food-grade antifoam for foam control in nonaq. systems; applics. incl. edible oil processing, meat processing, fat rendering, and synthesis of pharmaceuticals; more compat. and dispersible than Foam Blast 5, but less defoaming efficiency.

Foam Blast 100 Kosher. [Ross Chem.] Silicone defoamer; nonionic; food-grade defoamer for starch and proteinaceous systems requiring an acid or alkaline tolerant defoamer; for yeast fermentations, sugar beet processing, caustic potato peeling, vegetable processing, soups, gravies, fruit juices, jellies/jams, freeze-dried coffee, clam processing, distillations, pharmaceuticals, animal feeds; FDA §173.340, USDA, kosher compliance; wh. emulsion; disp. in water; dens. 8.50 lb/gal; visc. 1200-1600 cps; flash pt. (PMCC) none; pH 6.5-7.5; 10% act.

Foam Blast 150 Kosher. [Ross Chem.] Silicone defoamer; nonionic; food-grade defoamer for starch and proteinaceous systems requiring an acid or alkaline tolerant defoamer; for yeast fermentations, sugar beet processing, caustic potato peeling, seafood/vegetable processing, soups, gravies, fruit juices, jellies/jams, freeze-dried coffee, pharmaceuticals, animal feeds; FDA §173.340, kosher compliance; wh. emulsion; disp. in water; dens. 8.30 lb/gal; visc. 2100 cps; flash pt. (PMCC) none; pH 7.0; 30% act.

Foam-Coll™ 4C. [Brooks Industries] Potassium coco-hydrolyzed collagen; CAS 68920-65-0; foaming protein, cosmetic ingred.; mild surfactant; liq.; 35% act.

Foam-Coll™ 4CT. [Brooks Industries] TEA coco-hydrolyzed collagen; CAS 68952-16-9; foaming protein, cosmetic ingred.; mild surfactant; liq.; 40% act.

Foam-Coll™ 5. [Brooks Industries] Potassium coco-hydrolyzed collagen and sorbitol; foaming protein, mild surfactant for cosmetics use; liq.; 70% act.

Foam-Coll™ 5W. [Brooks Industries] Sorbitol, sodium cocoyl collagen amino acids, cocoyl sarcosine, wheat germ acid, and wheat germ oil; cosmetic ingred.

Foam-Coll™ SK. [Brooks Industries] Sodium cocoyl hydrolyzed collagen; CAS 68188-38-5; substantive cosmetic protein.

foamid 24. [Alzo] Lauramide DEA and diethanolamine.

Foamid 117. [Alzo] Cocamidopropyl dimethylamine propionate, water; CAS 68425-43-4; surfactant, softener,

emollient for creams, lotions, fingernail polish removers; pale to med. yel. clear to sl. hazy liq., sl. mild char. odor; sol. in water; sp.gr. 1.01; b.p. 212 F; flash pt. (COC) 350 F; pH 6-7; toxicology: nonhazardous; 37-44% solids.

Foamid AME-70. [Alzo] Acetamide MEA; CAS 142-26-7; EINECS 205-530-8; nonionic; wetting agent with broad solv. power for org. and inorg. materials and high b.p.; for cosmetic and health prods.; Gardner 2 clear liq., mild organoleptic odor; sol. in most alcohols, glycols, diols, polyols, glycol ethers, ketones, and water; sp.gr. 1.100; dens. 9.2 lb/gal; acid no. 15 max.; alkali no. 15 max.; flash pt. (OC) > 180 C; ref. index 1.4400; pH 6.0-8.5 (50% aq.); toxicology: low toxicity.; 70% min. act. in water.

Foamid AME-75. [Alzo] Acetamide MEA; CAS 142-26-7; EINECS 205-530-8; nonionic; wetting agent with broad solv. power for org. and inorg. materials and high b.p.; for cosmetic and health prods.; Gardner 2 clear liq., mild organoleptic odor; sol. in most alcohols, glycols, diols, polyols, glycol ethers, ketones, and water; sp.gr. 1.100; dens. 9.2 lb/gal; acid no. 15 max.; alkali no. 15 max.; flash pt. (OC) > 180 C; ref. index 1.4410; pH 6.0-8.5 (50% aq.); toxicology: low toxicity.; 75% min. act. in water.

Foamid AME-100. [Alzo] Acetamide MEA; CAS 142-26-7; EINECS 205-530-8; nonionic; wetting agent with broad solv. power for org. and inorg. materials and high b.p.; for cosmetic and health prods.; Gardner 2 clear liq., mild organoleptic odor; sol. in most alcohols, glycols, diols, polyols, glycol ethers, ketones, and water; sp.gr. 1.120; dens. 9.3 lb/gal; acid no. 15 max.; alkali no. 15 max.; flash pt. (OC) > 180 C; ref. index 1.4700; pH 6.0-8.5 (50% aq.); toxicology: low toxicity.; 95% min. act.

Foamid C. [Alzo] Cocamide DEA; CAS 68603-42-9; EINECS 263-163-9; nonionic; thickener, foam builder/stabilizer for shampoos, bubble bath, liq. body and hand soaps, bath gels, laundry detergents, floor cleaners, dishwash; emulsifier for aliphatic, aromatic, and chlorinated hydrocarbons and in waterless hand cleaners, engine shampoos, wax strippers, and tar removers; lt. amber clear liq., mild odor; sol. in water and most org. solvs. (alchols, glycols, polyols, glycol ethers, lower aliphatic, aromatic, and chlorinated hydrocarbons, natural fats); disp. in min. oil; sp.gr. 0.99; dens. 8.25 lb/gal; congeal pt. 10 C max.; acid no. 2 max.; alkali no. 30 max.; flash pt. (OC) > 180 C; 100% act.

Foamid LM2E. [Alzo] Lactamide DGA; nonionic; humectant, emollient, o/w emulsifier, and cosolv. for skin and hair creams and lotions; imparts light, smooth, nongreasy feel to the skin, and sheen, conditioning, moisture balancing, and antistatic props. to overtreated hair; solv., freeze pt. depressant, coupling and wetting agent in "oil-free" pigmented prods.; straw to lt. yel. clear liq., mild organoleptic odor; sol. in most low m.w. alcohols, diols, triols, polyols, glycol ethers, and water; sp.gr. 1.150; dens. 9.58 lb/gal; acid no. 30 max.; alkali no. 35 max.; flash pt. (OC) > 180 C; ref. index 1.4350; 80% min. act. in water.

Foamid LME-75. [Alzo] Lactamide MEA and lactamide DGA; nonionic; humectant for skin and hair applics.; "oil-free" emollient for o/w emulsions; imparts light, smooth, nongreasy feel to the skin; wetting agent in pigmented prods.; adds sheen and conditioning to overtreated hair; lt. yel. clear liq., mild organoleptic odor; sol. in most low m.w. alcohols, diols, triols, polyols, glycol ethers, and water; sp.gr. 1.160; dens. 9.65 lb/gal; acid no. 30 max.; alkali no. 45 max.; flash pt. (OC) > 180 C; ref. index 1.445; 74% min. act. in water.

Foamid PK. [Alzo] Lauramide DEA; CAS 120-40-1; EINECS 204-393-1; nonionic; visc. builder and copious foamer for shampoos, facial scrubs, bubble baths, liq. hand soaps, etc.; wh. cryst. solid, mild odor; sol. in most org. solvs. (alcohols, glycols, glycol ethers, polyols, lower aliphatic, aromatic, and chlorinated hydrocarbons, natural fats and oils); disp. in water and min. oil; sp.gr. 0.97; dens. 8.1 lb/gal; congeal pt. 36 ± 3 C; acid no. 1 max.; alkali no. 25 max.; flash pt. (OC) > 170 C; 100% act.

Foamid SCE. [Alzo] Cocamide DEA; CAS 68603-42-9; EINECS 263-163-9; nonionic; visc. builder, foam booster/stabilizer for mild gel and regular shampoos, shampoo concs., bubble bath, mild liq. hand soaps, syn. detergent formulations; high amide content with exceptionally low free amine level; lt. amber clear visc. liq., mild odor; sol. in most org. solvs. (alcohols, glycols, glycol ethers, polyols, lower aliphatic, aromatic, and chlorinated hydrocarbons, natural fats and oils); partly sol. in water; disp. in min. oil; sp.gr. 0.99; dens. 8.1 lb/gal; congeal pt. 10-15 C; acid no. 1 max.; alkali no. 25 max.; flash pt. (OC) > 170 C; 100% act.

Foamid SL-Extra. [Alzo] Lauramide DEA; CAS 120-40-1; EINECS 204-393-1; nonionic; visc. builder, foam booster/stabilizer for mild gel and regular shampoos, shampoo concs., bubble bath, mild liq. hand soaps, syn. detergent formulations; high amide content with exceptionally low free amine level; off-wh. waxy solid, mild odor; sol. in most org. solvs. (alcohols, glycols, glycol ethers, polyols, lower aliphatic, aromatic, and chlorinated hydrocarbons, natural fats and oils); partly sol. in water; disp. in min. oil; sp.gr. 0.97; dens. 8.1 lb/gal; congeal pt. 40 ± 3 C; acid no. 1 max.; alkali no. 25 max.; flash pt. (OC) > 170 C; 100% act.

Foamid SLM. [Alzo] Luaramide/myristamide DEA; CAS 120-40-1, 7545-23-5; nonionic; visc. builder, foam booster/stabilizer for mild gel and regular shampoos, shampoo concs., bubble bath, mild liq. hand soaps, syn. detergent formulations; high amide content with exceptionally low free amine level; off-wh. waxy solid, mild odor; sol. in most org. solvs. (alcohols, glycols, glycol ethers, polyols, lower aliphatic, aromatic, and chlorinated hydrocarbons, natural fats and oils); partly sol. in water; disp. in min. oil; sp.gr. 0.97; dens. 8.1 lb/gal; congeal pt. 36 ± 3 C; acid no. 1 max.; alkali no. 25 max.; flash pt. (OC) > 170 C; 100% act.

Foamine O-80. [Alzo] Linoleamidopropyl dimethylamine; CAS 81613-56-1; cosmetic emulsifier, softener.

Foam-Keratin LK. [Brooks Industries] Sodium/TEA-lauroyl hydrolyzed collagen; cosmetic protein.

Foamkill® 8G. [Crucible] Silicone compd.; defoamer for food applics. incl. general nonaq. systems, drug extraction and separation, drug processing, starch extractions and processing, anaerobic fermentations, vitamins, coatings, adhesives, polishes, textile processing, detergents, inks, fermentation, insecticides, cutting oils, monomer stripping, cosmetics; FDA §173.340; gray sl. hazy liq., bland odor; insol. in water; sp.gr. 1.020; b.p. > 300 F; flash pt. (TOC) > 300 F; toxicology: may cause eye irritation, mild skin irritation on prolonged/repeated contact; 100% act.

Foamkill® 634C. [Crucible] Nonsilicone; nonionic; alkaline and acid-stable defoamer for food and cosmetic applics., starch and proteinous systems, yeast processing, soya slurries, sugar beet refining, caustic potato peeling, canning trade, pasteurizer defoaming, juice and wine making, fermentations; FDA §173.340, 173.315; pale straw med. visc. liq., mild fatty odor; disp. in water; dens. 7.4 lb/gal; b.p. > 400 F; flash pt. (TOC) 370 F; pH 7.4 (2%); 100% act.

Foamkill® 639J-F. [Crucible] Organo-silicone; nonionic; alkaline and acid-stable defoamer for latex monomer stripping formulations, food and cosmetic applics., warm starch and proteinous systems, soya slurries, sugar beet refining, caustic potato peeling, yeast fermentations, canning, paper coatings; FDA §172.340, 172.315; wh. semitransparent liq., bland odor; sp.gr. 0.895; dens. 7.45 lb/gal; b.p. 390 F; flash pt. (TOC) 160 F; pH 6.6 (2%); usage level: 333 ppm max.; toxicology: skin and eye irritant; may cause harmful effects on ingestion; 100% act.

Foamkill® 810F. [Crucible] Dimethicone emulsion; nonionic;

defoamer for food/pharmaceutical/cosmetic applics. incl. general aq. systems, paper coatings and adhesives in contact with food, egg washing, cleaning/sanitizing sol'ns., pulp/paper applics., soft drink and wine making, vegetable processing, yeast processing, jam/jellies, starch sol'ns., protein processing, water-based inks, detergents; FDA §173.340, 176.210, 175.105, 175.320, 176.200; wh. pourable visc. liq., bland odor; disp. in water; sp.gr. 1.000; dens. 8.3 lb/gal; visc. 300 cps; b.p. 212 F; flash pt. (TOC) > 212 F; pH 7.0; usage level: 100 ppm max.; toxicology: may cause eye irritation, mild skin irritation on prolonged/repeated contact; 10% act.

Foamkill® 830F. [Crucible] Dimethicone; nonionic; defoamer for food/pharmaceutical/cosmetic applics. incl. general aq. systems, paper coatings and adhesives in contact with food, soft drink mfg., cleaning/sanitizing sol'ns., cosmetics, fermentation, bottle filling operations, vegetable washing, sugar beet processing, jams/jellies, coatings, starch and protein processing, pharmaceuticals; FDA §172.340, 173.340, 176.210, 175.105, 175.300, 176.200; wh. pourable visc. liq., bland odor; disp. in water; sp.gr. 0.993; dens. 8.3 lb/gal; visc. 3500 cps; b.p. 212 F; flash pt. (TOC) > 212 F; pH 7.0; usage level: to 33 ppm; toxicology: may cause eye irritation, mild skin irritation on prolonged/repeated contact; 30% act.

Foamkill® MSF Conc. [Crucible] Organo-silicone; nonionic; conc. for formulating defoamers for wide variety of high and low temp. applics., esp. food applics. (fruit and veg. washing, egg washing, soft drinks, wine making, yeast processing, jam/jellies, sugar refining, water-based inks and coatings, detergents, rendering of oils and fats, cosmetics, starch sol'ns., adhesives; FDA §173.340, 176.210, 175.105, 175.300, 176.200; wh. visc. liq., mild pleasant odor; readily disp. in water; sp.gr. 1.084; dens. 9.02 lb/gal; visc. 20,000 cps; b.p. 212 F; flash pt. > 212 F; pH 9.02 (1%); usage level: 66 ppm max.; toxicology: may cause eye irritation, mild skin irritation on prolonged/repeated skin contact; 15% dimethylpolysiloxane.

Foamole A. [ISP Van Dyk] Linoleamide DEA (1:1); CAS 56863-02-6; EINECS 260-410-2; hair conditioner for shampoos, hair dyes; visc. booster, foam stabilizer for shampoos, liq. soaps; amber liq.; sol. in 70% ethanol, propylene glycol, peanut oil; gels in water; sp.gr. 0.972-0.982; acid no. 5 max.; alkali no. 21-35.

Foamole B. [ISP Van Dyk] Minkamidopropyl dimethylamine; CAS 68953-11-7; EINECS 273-187-1; superfatting agent, conditioner for hair care prods.; sol. in propylene glycol; disp. in water.

Foamole M. [ISP Van Dyk] Cocamide MEA (1:1); CAS 68140-00-1; EINECS 268-770-2; foam booster/stabilizer, thickener, emulsifier for creams and lotions, shampoos, bubble baths, other detergents; cream colored flake; sol. in 70% ethanol, propylene glycol, oleyl alcohol; m.p. 70-74 C; acid no. 2 max.; alkali no. 12 max.; 100% conc.

Foamox CDO. [Alzo] Cocamidopropyl amine oxide; CAS 68155-09-9; EINECS 268-938-5; nonionic/catinic; foam booster/stabilizer, detergent, wetting agent, conditioner for shampoos, rinses, shaving creams, lt.-duty dishwash; enhances emolliency and lubricity on skin; antistat for hair care prods.; fully biodeg.; Gardner 2 max. clear to sl. hazy liq.; sol. in water and most hydrophilic solvs. (alcohols, glycols, triols, polyols, glycol ethers); m.w. 320; sp.gr. 0.995; pH 6-8; Ross-Miles foam 245 mm (initial, 0.1%); 35% min. amine oxide in water.

Foamquat 2IAE. [Alzo] Bisisostearamidopropyl ethoxyethyl dimonium chloride; CAS 111381-08-9; cationic; conditioner, thickener, foaming agent, and antistat for hair and skin care prods., industrial applics.; amber clear visc. liq., sl. mild odor; sol. in most alcohols, glycols, glycol ethers, esters, aliphatic, aromatic, and chlorinated hydrocarbons, water, veg. oil; partly sol. in min. oil; m.w. 932; sp.gr. 1.00; dens. 8.3 lb/gal; flash pt. (OC) 115 C; pH 5-7 (5% aq.); 85% min. NV, 65% min. act.

Foamquat BAS. [Alzo] Behenamidopropyl ethyldimonium ethosulfate; CAS 68797-65-9; EINECS 258-377-8; cationic; conditioner with increased substantivity, silkiness, luster, body, and smooth afterfeel for hair care formulations; cream-colored soft waxy solid, mild typ. odor; water-sol.; m.w. 578; sp.gr. 0.98; dens. 8.16 lb/gal; congeal pt. 45 C; flash pt. (OC) 160 C min.; pH 4-7 (5% aq.); 80% min. NV, 70% min. quat.

Foamquat CAS. [Alzo] Cocamidopropyl ethyldimonium ethosulfate; CAS 113492-03-8; cationic; surfactant, detergent, antistat for cosmetic, laundry, and industrial applics. incl. shampoos, liq. detergents, degreasers, hard surf. cleaners, liq. dishwash; perfume solubilizer; o/w emulsifier for glycols, aliphatic, aromatic, and chlorinated hydrocarbons, alcohols; visc. liq., mild amine odor; water-sol.; m.w. 445; sp.gr. 1.04; dens. 8.7 lb/gal; pH 4-7 (5% aq.); 98% min. NV, 80% min. quat.

Foamquat CHP. [Alzo] Propylene glycol, linoleamidopropyl ethyldimonium ethosulfate.

Foamquat COAS. [Alzo] Canolamidopropyl ethyldimonium ethosulfate; cationic; substantive quat. for skin and hair care prods., clear oil-free hair conditioners; dk. amber clear sl. visc. liq., mild typ. odor; water-sol.; m.w. 530; sp.gr. 0.990; dens. 8.2 lb/gal; flash pt. (OC) 160 C min.; pH 4-7 (5% aq.); 90% min. NV, 75% min. quat.

Foamquat IAES. [Alzo] Isostearyl dimethylamidopropyl ethonium ethosulfate; CAS 67633-63-0; EINECS 266-778-0; conditioner.

Foamquat IALA. [Alzo] Isostearamidopropyl lauryl-acetodimonium chloride; CAS 134112-42-8; cationic; w/o and o/w emulsifier for oleic acid, vegetable oil, min. oil, and a variety of solvs.; dk. amber liq., mild odor; m.w. 642; sp.gr. 0.97; dens. 8.1 lb/gal; pH 3.5-6.5 (5% aq.); 80% min. NV, 65% min. quat.

Foamquat ODES. [Alzo] Oleamidopropyl ethyldimonium ethosulfate.

Foamquat SAQ-90. [Alzo] Linoleamidopropyl ethyldimonium ethosulfate; CAS 99542-23-1; conditioner, bodying agent.

Foamquat SOAS. [Alzo] Soyamidopropyl ethyldimonium ethosulfate; CAS 90529-57-0; EINECS 291-990-5; cationic; substantive conditioner for hair and skin prods., clear hair rinses, skin lotions; antistat; emulsifier for min. oil, veg. oil, esters, aromatic, aliphatic, and chlorinated hydrocarbons; amber clear visc. liq., sl. mild odor; sol. in most alcohols, glycols, glycol ethers, aliphatic, aromatic, and chlorinated hydrdocarbons, water; partly sol. in min. oil, esters, and veg. oil; m.w. 516; sp.gr. 1.03; dens. 8.6 lb/gal; flash pt. (COC) 160 C; pH 4-7 (5% aq.); 90% min. NV, 75% min. quat.

Foamquat SOAS-MOD. [Alzo] Oleamidopropyl ethyldimonium ethosulfate, oleamidopropyl dimethylamino glycolate; CAS 90529-57-0; cationic; yel. clear visc. liq., mild odor; sp.gr. 1.00; dens. 8.33 lb/gal; pH 4-7 (5% aq.); 23% min. NV.

Foamquat VG. [Alzo] Linoleamidopropyl dimethylamine lactate; cationic; conditioner, humectant enhancing wet and dry combing props. of hair, detangling props.; antistat for fly-away hair; emulsifier, emollient for creams and lotions; emulsifier for aliphatic, aromatic, and chlorinated hydrocarbons and in waterless hand cleaners, engine shampoos, wax strippers, and tar removers; yel. to lt. amber clear visc. liq., typ. clean odor; sp.gr. 1.015; dens. 8.45 lb/gal; acid no. 25-35; alkali no. 25-35; pH 4-6 (5%); 25% min. solids.

Foam-Soy™ C. [Brooks Industries] Sodium cocoyl hydrolyzed soy protein; foaming cosmetic ingredient for skin

and hair care prods.; mild surfactant; 30% act.

Foamtaine CAB-A. [Alzo] Cocamidopropyl betaine and ammonium chloride; CAS 140203-35-6; amphoteric; mild detergent, foamer, wetting agent, emulsifier, fragrance solubilizer, cloud pt. depressant for low-irritation shampoos, mild acid shampoos, skin cleansers, bath prods.; softener for skin and hair; antistat in shampoos; completely biodeg.; yel. clear liq., sl. char. odor; m.w. 380; sp.gr. 1.052; dens. 8.76 lb/gal; visc. 50 cps; cloud pt. -10 C; pH 5-7; Ross-Miles foam 250 mm (initial, 0.1%); 45% min. solids, 39% min. act.

Foamtaine CAB-G. [Alzo] Cocamidopropyl betaine; CAS 61789-40-0; EINECS 263-058-8; amphoteric; mild detergent, foamer, wetting agent, emulsifier, fragrance solubilizer, cloud pt. depressant for low-irritation shampoos, skin cleansers, bath prods., acid or alkaline detergents; softener for skin and hair; antistat in shampoos; completely biodeg.; Gardner 5 max. clear liq., sl. char. odor; m.w. 372; sp.gr. 1.067; dens. 8.9 lb/gal; visc. 50 cps; cloud pt. -5 C; pH 5-7; Ross-Miles foam 235 mm (initial, 0.1%); 45% min. solids, 39% min. act.

Foamtaine SCAB-K. [Alzo] Cocamidopropyl hydroxysultaine and potassium.

Foam-Wheat C. [Brooks Industries] Sodium cocoyl hydrolyzed wheat protein; mild foaming protein for use in shampoos; gentle cleanser in facial makeup removers; yel. liq.; low odor; 30% act.

Fomblin® HC/04, HC/25, HC/R. [Ausimont; Brooks Industries; ICI Surf. Am.; ICI Surf. UK] Perfluoropolymethylisopropyl ether; emollients for cosmetic formulations; three visc. grades; Japan approval; colorless liq.

Fomblin® HC/P-04, HC/P-25, HC/P-R. [Ausimont] Perfluoropolymethylisopropyl ether and PTFE.

Fondix G Bis. [Gattefosse SA] Propylene glycol, sodium methylparaben, sodium dehydroacetate, sorbic acid, tetrasodium EDTA; cosmetic preservative system; USA, Japan, and Europe approvals; usage level: 1-2%.

Fongasel. [Gattefosse] Sodium dehydroacetate; CAS 4418-26-2; EINECS 224-580-1; cosmetics preservative.

Fonoline® White. [Witco/Petroleum Spec.] Petrolatum USP; CAS 8027-32-5; EINECS 232-373-2; soft, low m.p. for consumer use as petrol. jelly, ointments, industrial applics.; as emollient, protective coating, binder, carrier, lubricant, moisture barrier, plasticizer, protective agent, softener; FDA §172.880 clearance; wh., odorless; visc. 9-14 cSt (100 C); m.p. 53-58 C; pour pt. 20 F.

Fonoline® Yellow. [Witco/Petroleum Spec.] Petrolatum USP; CAS 8027-32-5; EINECS 232-373-2; soft, low m.p. for consumer use as petrol. jelly, ointments, industrial applics.; as emollient, protective coating, binder, carrier, lubricant, moisture barrier, plasticizer, protective agent, softener; yel., odorless; visc. 9-14 cSt (100 C); m.p. 53-58 C; pour pt. 20 F; 99% solids.

Forestall. [ICI Am.] Soyaethyl morpholinium ethosulfate aq. sol'n.; CAS 61791-34-2; EINECS 263-167-0; conditioner and deodorizer for odor control in household cleaners and cosmetic permanent wave preps.; red-brn. liq.; HLB 25-30; 35% act. in water.

Forlan. [R.I.T.A.] Petrolatum, lanolin alcohol, lanolin; absorp. base, emollient for personal care prods.; yel. paste.

Forlan 200. [R.I.T.A.] Petrolatum, lanolin alcohol; absorp. base for personal care prods.; enhances stability of emulsions, dispersions and suspensions; epidermal emollient, moisturizer, lubricant; yel. paste.

Forlan 300. [R.I.T.A.] Petrolatum, lanolin, lanolin alcohol; absorp. base for personal care prods.; enhances stability of emulsions, dispersions and suspensions; epidermal emollient, moisturizer, lubricant; yel. paste.

Forlan 500. [R.I.T.A.] Petrolatum, lanolin, and lanolin alcohol; absorp. base for personal care prods.; enhances stability of emulsions, dispersions and suspensions; epidermal emollient, moisturizer, lubricant; emulsifier for creams and lotions; yel. paste.

Forlan C-24. [R.I.T.A.] Choleth-24 and ceteth-24; nonionic; emulsifier, emulsion stabilizer, emollient, moisturizer, solubilizer, visc. modifier, pigment dispersant, plasticizer for cosmetics, pharmaceuticals; wh. flakes; sol. in alcohol, water; 100% conc.

Forlan L. [R.I.T.A.] Petrolatum, lanolin, hydrog. coconut oil, sorbitan sesquioleate, stearyl alcohol, cetyl alcohol; nonionic; lanolin replacement; as emulsifier, emulsion stabilizer, skin lubricant and emollient in creams and lotions; aids in wetting and dispersion of pigments in facial makeup, lipstick and eye shadows; yel. paste; sparingly water-sol.; 100% conc.

Forlan L Conc. [R.I.T.A.] Petrolatum, lanolin, hydrog. coconut oil, sorbitan sesquioleate, stearyl alcohol, and cetyl alcohol.

Forlan LM. [R.I.T.A.] Petrolatum, hydrog. lanolin, hydrog. coconut oil, sorbitan sesquioleate, stearyl alcohol, and cetyl alcohol; absorption base enhancing stability of emulsions, dispersions, and suspensions; epidermal emollient, moisturizer, and lubricant; yel. paste.

Forlanit® E. [Henkel KGaA/Cospha] Hydroxycetyl phosphate; o/w emulsifier for cosmetic and pharmaceutical emulsions; flakes; 99% conc.

Fortex®. [Petrolite] Hard microcryst. wax consisting of n-paraffinic, branched paraffinic, and naphthenic hydrocarbons; CAS 63231-60-7; EINECS 264-038-1; used in hot-melt coatings and adhesives, paper coatings, printing inks, plastic modification (as lubricant and processing aid), lacquers, paints, and varnishes, as binder in ceramics, for potting, filling, and impregnating elec./electronic components, in investment casting, rubber and elastomers (plasticizer, antisunchecking, antiozonant), as emulsion wax size, as fabric softener ingred., in emulsion and latex coatings, and in cosmetic hand creams and lipsticks; wax; very low sol. in org. solvs.; sp.gr. 0.93; visc. 40 cps (99 C); m.p. 95 C.

Fo-Ti 5:1 PG. [Lipo] Propylene glycol and polygonum extract; botanical extract.

Fractalite 499. [Fractal Labs] Diethylene glycol diisononanoate; CAS 106-01-4; EINECS 203-353-0.

Fractalite IDS. [Fractal Labs] Isodecyl stearate; CAS 31565-38-5; EINECS 250-704-9; lubricant.

Fractalite ISB. [Fractal Labs] Isostearyl behenate.

Fractalite ISL. [Fractal Labs] Isostearyl lactate; CAS 42131-28-2; EINECS 255-674-0; emollient.

Fractein HCP. [Fractal Labs] Hydrolyzed corn protein.

Fractein HWP. [Fractal Labs] Hydrolyzed wheat protein; CAS 70084-87-6; cosmetic protein.

Freederm. [Advanced Polymer Systems] Acrylates copolymer; thickener, stabilizer for cosmetics.

Frescolat, Type ML. [Haarmann & Reimer GmbH] Menthyl lactate; CAS 59259-38-0; EINECS 261-678-3; cooling agent for body care prods. and cosmetics, e.g., facial masks; good skin and mucous membrane compat.; mild cooling flavor in powd. drink mixes, chewing gums, sweets, and tobacco; colorless liq. or solid, faintly minty odor, pract. tasteless; sol. in ethanol (50 vol. %), diethyl phthalate, min. oil, 1,2-propanediol; m.w. 228.4; acid no. 1 max.; flash pt. > 100 C; pH 4-8; avoid combustible substances.

Frigydil. [Prod'Hyg] Menthyl lactate; CAS 59259-38-0;

EINECS 261-678-3; cooling agent for cosmetics.

FRS-Diffuser Microreservoir. [Sederma] Water, glycerin, butylene glycol, lecithin, lactoferrin, thioxanthine, and uric acid.

Frutalone. [Hercules/PFW] 2-Heptylcyclopentanone.

FSP Liq. [Ichimaru Pharcos] Natto gum.

Ftalato 2/46. [Industrial Quimica Lasem] Diethyl phthalate; CAS 84-66-2; EINECS 201-550-6; plasticizer for nail polish.

Fungal Lactase 100,000. [Solvay Enzymes] Fungal lactase derived from *Aspergillus oryzae*; enzyme for hydrolyzing lactose in dairy prods. (milk, whey, cheese, yogurt), pharmaceuticals (digestive aids, lactose intolerance); lt tan amorphous dry powd., free of offensive odor and taste; water-sol.; usage level: 0.2%.

Fungal Protease 31,000. [Solvay Enzymes] Protease derived from *Aspergillus oryzae var.*, maltodextrin diluent; enzyme for hydrolysis of peptide bonds; for baking (improves grain, texture, loaf volume), meat tenderizer formulations; hydrolyzes and modifies plant and animal protein under acid conditions; brewing, fermentation; pharmaceuticals (digestive aid); animal feed supplement; waste treatment; cleaning protein processing equip.; lt. tan to wh. powd., free of offensive odor and taste; water-sol.; usage level: 0.01-0.1%.

Fungal Protease 60,000. [Solvay Enzymes] Protease derived from *Aspergillus oryzae var.*, maltodextrin diluent; enzyme for hydrolysis of peptide bonds; for baking (improves grain, texture, loaf volume), meat tenderizer formulations; hydrolyzes and modifies plant and animal protein under acid conditions; brewing, fermentation; pharmaceuticals (digestive aid); animal feed supplement; waste treatment; cleaning protein processing equip.; lt. tan to wh. powd., free of offensive odor and taste; water-sol.; usage level: 0.01-0.1%.

Fungal Protease 500,000. [Solvay Enzymes] Protease derived from *Aspergillus oryzae var.*, maltodextrin diluent; enzyme for hydrolysis of peptide bonds; for baking (improves grain, texture, loaf volume), meat tenderizer formulations; hydrolyzes and modifies plant and animal protein under acid conditions; brewing, fermentation; pharmaceuticals (digestive aid); animal feed supplement; waste treatment; cleaning protein processing equip.; lt. tan to wh. powd., free of offensive odor and taste; water-sol.; usage level: 0.01-0.1%.

Fungal Protease Conc. [Solvay Enzymes] Protease derived from *Aspergillus oryzae var.*; enzyme for hydrolysis of peptide bonds; for baking (improves grain, texture, loaf volume), meat tenderizer formulations; hydrolyzes and modifies plant and animal protein under acid conditions; brewing, fermentation; pharmaceuticals (digestive aid); animal feed supplement; waste treatment; cleaning protein processing equip.; lt. tan to wh. dry powd., free of offensive odor and taste; water-sol.; usage level: 0.01-0.1%.

Fungicide DA 2/938070. [Dragoco] Undecylenamide DEA; CAS 60239-68-1; EINECS 246-914-5; personal care surfactant.

Fungicide UMA 2/938080. [Dragoco] Undecylenamide MEA; CAS 20545-92-0; EINECS 243-870-9; personal care surfactant.

Fungitex R. [Ciba-Geigy] Domiphen bromide; CAS 538-71-6; EINECS 208-702-0; antimicrobial, fungicide for use in mouthwashes, antiseptics, cold sterilization; water-sol.

G

G-1096. [ICI Surf. Am.; ICI Surf. Belgium] PEG-50 sorbitol hexaoleate; CAS 57171-56-9; nonionic; emulsifier and coupling agent for personal care prods., textiles, hydraulic and metalworking fluids, polymerization; pale yel. liq.; sol. in veg. oils, acetone, cellosolve, lower alcohols, some aromatic solv., tetrachloride; sp.gr. 1.0; visc. 220 cps; HLB 11.4; flash pt. > 300 F; 100% act.; formerly Atlas G-1096.

G-1144. [ICI Am.] PEG-30 sorbitol tetraoleate laurate; formerly Atlas G-1144.

G-1292. [ICI Am.; ICI Surf. Belgium] PEG-25 hyrog. castor oil; CAS 61788-85-0; nonionic; emulsifier for agric., emulsions, textile formulations; solubilizer for creams and lotions; pale yel. liq. to soft paste; sol. in water, ethanol, IPA; sp.gr. 1.0; HLB 10.8; flash pt. > 300 F; 100% conc.

G-1425. [ICI Surf. Belgium] PEG-20 sorbitol lanolin deriv.; nonionic; emulsifier for cosmetic waxes; paste; HLB 8.0; 100% conc.; formerly Atlas G-1425.

G-1441. [ICI Am.; ICI Surf. UK] PEG-40 sorbitan lanolate; nonionic; emulsifier for cosmetic waxes, surfactant for personal care prods., pharmaceuticals; amber paste; sol. in water (hazy), IPA; sp.gr. 1; HLB 14; flash pt. > 300 F; pour pt. 33 C; 100% conc.; formerly Atlas G-1441.

G-1471. [ICI Am.] PEG-75 sorbitol lanolin deriv.; nonionic; surfactant, emulsifier, cosmetic use; amber, soft paste; sol. in IPA, ethylene glycol; HLB 16; flash pt. > 300 F; 100% conc.; formerly Atlas G-1471.

G-1702. [ICI Am.; ICI Spec. Chem.; ICI Surf. Belgium] PEG-6 sorbitan beeswax; CAS 8051-15-8; nonionic; emulsifier in cosmetic creams; tan waxy solid; slight sol. in veg. oils; HLB 5; flash pt. > 300 F; 100% conc.; formerly Atlas G-1702.

G-1726. [ICI Surf. Am.; ICI Surf. Belgium] PEG-20 sorbitan beeswax; CAS 8051-73-8; nonionic; cosmetic emulsifier; yel. brn. solid; HLB 5; 100% conc.; formerly Atlas G-1726.

G-1790. [ICI Am.; ICI Surf. UK] Laneth-20; CAS 61791-20-6; nonionic; emulsifier for cosmetic use; brn. waxy solid; water-sol.; HLB 11; flash pt. > 300 F.; formerly Atlas G-1790.

G-1821. [ICI Surf. Am.; ICI Surf. Belgium] PEG-150 distearate; CAS 9005-08-7; nonionic; thickener, rheology control agent for shampoos, paints; wh. flakes; 100% conc.; formerly Atlas G-1821.

G-2151. [ICI Am.] PEG-30 stearate; CAS 9004-99-3; nonionic; surfactant; ivory, waxy solid; sol. in propylene glycol, ethylene glycol, water; HLB 16; flash pt. > 300 F.; formerly Atlas G-2151.

G-2153. [ICI Am.] PEG-50 stearate; CAS 9004-99-3; emulsifier; formerly Atlas G-2153.

G-2162. [ICI Am.; ICI Surf. UK] PEG-25 propylene glycol stearate; nonionic; emulsifier for personal care prods.; cream-colored semisolid; sol. in water, methanol, ethanol; HLB 16; pour pt. 23 C; flash pt. > 300 F; 100% act.; formerly Atlas G-2162.

G-2162. [ICI Am.; ICI Spec. Chem.] PEG-25 propylene glycol stearate; nonionic; surfactant; cream-colored semisolid; sol. in water, methanol, ethanol; HLB 16; pour pt. 23 C; flash pt. > 300 F; 100% act.

G-2240. [ICI Am.] Sorbeth-6; formerly Atlas G-2240.

G-2320. [ICI Am.] Sorbeth-20; formerly Atlas G-2320.

G-2330. [ICI Surf. Am.] PEG-30 sorbitol; surfactant, humectant in creams and lotions; colorless liq.

G-3707. [ICI Surf. Belgium] POE lauryl alcohol; nonionic; o/w emulsifiers used in topical cosmetic applics.; liq.; HLB 12.8; water-sol./disp.; 100% conc.; formerly Atlas G-3707.

G-3780-A. [ICI Spec. Chem.] PEG-20 hydrog. tallow amine; CAS 61791-26-2; nonionic; antistat, emulsifier; liq.; HLB 15.5.

G-3816. [ICI Surf. Belgium] Ceteth-16; CAS 9004-95-9; nonionic; general purpose emulsifier, lubricant used in cosmetic formulas; wh. solid; HLB 14.9; 100% conc.; formerly Atlas G-3816.

G-3820. [ICI Surf. UK] PEG-20 cetyl alcohol; CAS 9004-95-9; emulsifier for personal care prods.; wh. waxy solid; HLB 15.7; formerly Atlas G-3820.

G-3887. [ICI Surf. UK] Alkoxylated alcohol; emulsifier for personal care prods.; colorless liq.; formerly Atlas G-3887.

G-3904. [ICI Surf. UK] PEG-4 oleylcetyl alcohol; emulsifier for personal care prods.; straw-colored waxy liq.; HLB 8.0; formerly Atlas G-3904.

G-3908S. [ICI Am.] Oleth-8; CAS 9004-98-2; emulsifier, emollient; formerly Atlas G-3908S.

G-3910. [ICI Surf. UK] Oleth-10; CAS 9004-98-2; emulsifier for personal care prods.; yel. oily liq.; HLB 12.4; formerly Atlas G-3910.

G-4252. [ICI Surf. UK] PEG-80 sorbitan palmitate; CAS 9005-66-7; surfactant for baby shampoos; yel. liq.; HLB 18.9.

G-4280. [ICI Spec. Chem.] PEG-80 sorbitan laurate; CAS 9005-64-5; nonionic; surfactant; yel. liq.; sol. in water, alcohol; disp. in propylene glycol; visc. 1000 cps; HLB 19.1.

G-4822. [ICI Surf. Belgium] Ceteareth-12, self-emulsifying; CAS 68439-49-6; nonionic; surfactant for personal care applics.; wh. waxy solid; HLB 13.9; 100% conc.; formerly Atlas G-4822.

G-4829. [ICI Surf. Belgium] Laureth-9; CAS 3055-99-0; EINECS 221-284-4; nonionic; topical anaesthetic; coloress to pale yel. liq.; HLB 14.3; 100% conc.; formerly Atlas G-4829.

G-4909. [ICI Surf. Belgium] Glycerol sorbitan fatty acid ester; nonionic; lanolin absorp. base substitute; amber waxy solid; 100% conc.; formerly Atlas G-4909.

G-4929. [ICI Surf. UK] PEG-9 ricinoleate; CAS 9004-97-1; surfactant, emulsifier for cosmetic creams; yel. liq.; HLB 11.7.

G-4933. [ICI Surf. UK] POE stearyl alcohol; emulsifier for personal care prods.; wh. to amber waxy solid; HLB 7.8;

formerly Atlas G-4933.

G-4935. [ICI Surf. UK] POE stearyl alcohol; emulsifier for personal care prods.; wh. waxy solid; HLB 12.4; formerly Atlas G-4935.

G-4936. [ICI Surf. UK] Ceteareth-10; CAS 68439-49-6; emulsifier for personal care prods.; wh. waxy solid; HLB 12.5; formerly Atlas G-4936.

G-4938. [ICI Surf. UK] Ceteareth-20; CAS 68439-49-6; emulsifier for personal care prods.; wh. waxy solid; HLB 15.3; formerly Atlas G-4938.

G-4940. [ICI Surf. UK] Ceteareth-30; CAS 68439-49-6; emulsifier for personal care prods.; wh. waxy solid; HLB 16.6; formerly Atlas G-4940.

G-4964. [ICI Surf. UK] Myreth-2 myristate; surfactant; wh. solid; HLB 3.5; formerly Atlas G-4964.

G-4972. [ICI Am.] PEG-15 hydroxystearate; solv. for injection sol'ns.; formerly Atlas G-4972.

G-5507. [ICI Surf. Am.; ICI Surf. UK] PEG-7 oleate; CAS 9004-96-0; surfactant; red brn. liq.; HLB 10.4; formerly Atlas G-5507.

G-5511. [ICI Am.] PEG-11 oleate; CAS 9004-96-0; personal care surfactant; formerly Atlas G-5511.

G-70147. [ICI Am.; ICI Surf. UK] Ceteareth-17; CAS 68439-49-6; surfactant; wh. solid; HLB 14.9; formerly Atlas G-70147.

Gadeneel Liq. [Ichimaru Pharcos] Water, alcohol, butylene glycol, and gardenia extract; botanical extract.

Gaffix® VC-713. [ISP] Vinylcaprolactam/PVP/dimethylaminoethyl methacrylate copolymer, ethanol; cationic; film-forming, fixative resin for use in mousses, gels, glazes, lotions, and hairsprays; APHA 100 max. clear visc. liq., ethanolic odor; sol. in water and alcohol; b.p. 173 F; cloud pt. 44 C (1% aq.); flash pt. (CC) 55 F; 37% solids in ethanol.

Gafquat® 734. [ISP] Polyquaternium-11; CAS 53633-54-8; film-forming substantive polymer, conditioner for formulation of hair conditioners, rinses, sprays, shampoos, dyes, semipermanents, deodorants, antiperspirants, shaving preparations, antiseptics, toilet soaps, skin creams, sunburn remedies; 50% alcoholic sol'n.

Gafquat® 755. [ISP] Polyquaternium-11; CAS 53633-54-8; high m.w. film-forming polymer for superior hair and skin care prods., deodorants, antiperspirants, shaving preparations, antiseptics, toilet soaps, skin creams, sunburn remedies; sol'n.; 20% aq. sol'n.

Gafquat® 755N. [ISP] Polyquaternium-11; CAS 53633-54-8; film-forming substantive polymer, conditioner for formulation of hair conditioners, rinses, sprays, shampoos, dyes, semipermanents, deodorants, antiperspirants, shaving preparations, antiseptics, toilet soaps, skin creams, sunburn remedies; liq.; high m.w.; 20% aq. sol'n.

Gafquat® HS-100. [ISP] Polyquaternium-28; cationic; conditioning polymer for personal care prods.; substantive, film-forming props.; for shampoos, conditioners, permanent waves, glazes, moisturizing creams, gels, mousses; lt. pink to straw hazy, highly visc. liq.; visc. 50,000-125,000 cps; pH 5-8; 19-21% solids.

Gafquat® HSi. [ISP] Polymer-silicone encapsulate (dimethicone with polyquaternium-28 shell); delivery vehicle providing silicone and film-forming polymer benefits to hair and skin care applics.; offers conditioning for dry or damaged hair, moisturization for skin care applics.

Galactene. [Vevy] PEG-2 milk solids; cosmetic ingred.

Galenol® 1618 AE. [Condea Chemie GmbH] Cetearyl alcohol (80%) and ceteareth-20 (20%); self-emulsifying cosmetic and pharmaceutical raw material, o/w emulsion base for creams, ointments, liniments, and lotions; flakes.

Galenol® 1618 CS. [Condea Chemie GmbH] Cetearyl alcohol (90%) and sodium cetearyl sulfate (10%); self-emulsifying cosmetic and pharmaceutical raw material,

o/w emulsion base for creams, ointments, liniments, and lotions; flakes or pellets.

Galenol® 1618 DSN. [Condea Chemie GmbH] Cetearyl alcohol (90%) and sodium lauryl sulfate (10%); self-emulsifying cosmetic and pharmaceutical raw material, o/w emulsion base for creams, ointments, liniments, and lotions; flakes or pellets.

Galenol® 1618 KS. [Condea Chemie GmbH] Cetearyl alcohol (90%) and sodium C12-C18 alkyl sulfate (10%); self-emulsifying cosmetic and pharmaceutical raw material, o/w emulsion base for creams, ointments, liniments, and lotions; flakes or pellets.

Gamma W8. [Wacker-Chemie GmbH] γ-Cyclodextrin; CAS 7585-39-9; EINECS 231-493-2; complex hosting guest molecules; increases the sol. and bioavailability of other substances; masks flavor, odor, or coloration; stabilizes against light, oxidation, heat, and hydrolysis; turns liqs. or volatiles into stable solid powds.; for use in pharmaceuticals, cosmetics, toiletries, foods, tobacco, pesticides, textiles, paints, plastics, synthesis, polymers; wh. cryst. powd.; sol. 23.2 g/100 ml in water; m.w. 1297.

Gamma Oryzanol. [Tri-K Industries] Rice bran extract; cosmetic ingred.

Gamma Oryzanol. [Ikeda] Oryzanol; CAS 11042-64-1; uv absorbent and antioxidant for drugs, foods, feeds, and cosmetics (skin creams, moisturizing creams, milk lotions, sunscreen creams and sticks); wh. or pale yel. cryst. powd., odorless; toxicology: LD50 (oral, mice) > 10,000 mg/kg; 98% min. assay.

Ganex® Et-201. [ISP] PVP/decene copolymer.

Ganex® P-904. [ISP] Butylated PVP; used in cosmetics and toiletries as moisture barrier, adhesive, protective colloid, and microencapsulating resin; as dispersant for pigments; as solubilizer for dyes; in petroleum industry as sludge and detergent dispersant; protective colloid in coatings; suspending aid in polymerization; dyeing assistant; antiredeposition agent in drycleaning; esp. as dispersant in aq. agric. chemicals or pigmented skin care prods.; sol'n.; sol. in water; m.w. 16,000; 45% solids in IPA, M-Pyrol, or water.

Ganex® V-216. [ISP] PVP/hexadecene copolymer; CAS 32440-50-9; used in cosmetics, toiletries, and OTC prods. as moisture barrier, adhesive, protective colloid, and microencapsulating resin; as dispersant for pigments; as solubilizer for dyes; in petroleum industry as sludge and detergent dispersant; pale yel. visc. liq.; sol. in min. oil, kerosnee, castor oil, org. solvs., and other polymers; partly sol. in ethanol; m.w. 7300; HLB 10.0; toxicology: LD (oral, rat) > 64 ml/kg; sl. irritating to skin, minimal eye irritation; 100% act.

Ganex® V-220. [ISP] PVP/eicosene copolymer; CAS 28211-18-9; used in cosmetics, toiletries, and OTC prods. as moisture barrier, adhesive, protective colloid, and microencapsulating resin; as dispersant for pigments; as solubilizer for dyes; in petroleum industry as sludge and detergent dispersant; off-wh. waxy solid; sol. in min. oil, kerosene, org. solvs., and other polymers; m.w. 8600; solid. pt. 35-40 C; HLB 8.0; toxicology: LD (oral, rat) > 17.1 g/kg; nonirritating to skin; 100% act.

Ganex® WP-660. [ISP] Tricontanyl PVP; waterproofing polymer for personal care prods.; for sunscreens, skin care prods., cosmetics, makeup, baby care prods.; off-wh. flakes; sol. in min. oil; insol. in water, ethanol; m.p. 60 C; HLB 6.0; toxicology: LD50 (oral, rat) > 5 g/kg; mild eye and skin irritant; 100% act.

Gantrez® AN. [ISP] PVM/MA copolymer; CAS 9011-16-9; anionic; dispersant, coupling, stabilizing agent, thickener, emulsifier, solubilizer, corrosion inhibitor, film former, antistat, used in agric., paper and textile industries, chemical processing, industrial products, detergents, cosmetics;

wh. fluffy powd.; sol. in water, acid, and several org. solvs.; dens. 0.32 g/cc; sp.gr. 1.37; soften. pt. 200–225 C; pH 2 (free acid, 5% aq.); 100% conc.

Gantrez® ES-225. [ISP] Ethyl ester of PVM/MA copolymer, ethanol; anionic; copolymer forming clear, glossy films with substantivity and moisture resistance; used in hairsprays, mousses, gels and lotions, coatings, polishes; emulsion stabilizer in creams and lotions; clear, visc. sol'n.; sol. [1 g resin (100% solids) in 9 g solv.] in ethanol, IPA, diethylene glycol, tetrahydrofuran, ethylene glycol monomethyl ether, butyl Carbitol, acetone, cyclohexanone, dioxane, water; sp.gr. 0.983; dens. 8.18 lb/gal; acid no. 275–300 (100% solids); 50% in ethanol.

Gantrez® ES-335. [ISP] Isopropyl ester of PVM/MA copolymer, IPA; anionic; copolymer forming clear, glossy films with substantivity and moisture resistance; used in hairsprays, mousses, gels and lotions, coatings, polishes; emulsion stabilizer in creams and lotions; clear, visc. sol'n.; sol. in alcohols, alkali, esters, ketones, and glycol ethers; sp.gr. 0.957; dens. 7.98 lg/gal; acid no. 250–280 (100% solids); 50% in IPA.

Gantrez® ES-425. [ISP] n-Butyl ester of PVM/MA copolymer, ethanol; anionic; copolymer forming clear, glossy films with substantivity and moisture resistance; used in hairsprays, mousses, gels and lotions, coatings, polishes; emulsion stabilizer in creams and lotions; clear, visc. sol'n.; sol. [1 g resin (100% solids) in 9 g solv.] in ethanol, IPA, diethylene glycol, tetrahydrofuran, ethylene glycol monomethyl ether, butyl Carbitol, ethyl acetate, acetone, cyclohexanone, dioxane, water; sp.gr. 0.977; dens. 8.13 lb/gal; acid no. 235–265 (100% solids); 50% solids in ethanol.

Gantrez® ES-435. [ISP] n-Butyl ester of PVM/MA copolymer, IPA; anionic; copolymer forming clear, glossy films with substantivity and moisture resistance; used in hairsprays, mousses, gels and lotions, coatings, polishes; emulsion stabilizer in creams and lotions; clear, visc. sol'n.; sol. in alcohols, alkali, esters, ketones, and glycol ethers; sp.gr. 0.962; dens. 8.02 lb/gal; acid no. 245–275 (100% solids); 50% in IPA.

Gantrez® MS-955. [ISP] Calcium/sodium PVM/MA copolymer.

Gantrez® SP-215. [ISP] Ethyl ester of PVM/MA copolymer; hair fixative for stiffer, harder holding prods.; up to 10% can be formulated in pump hair sprays; lt. yel. to straw clear visc. liq.; toxicology: LD50 (oral, rat) > 25.6 g/kg; nonirritating to skin and eyes; 48–52% solids.

Gantrez® V-215. [ISP] Methylvinyl ether/maleic anhydride copolymer, ethyl ester, ethanol SDA-40B; forms tough, clear, glossy, tack-free films with exc. substantivity, hair-holding props., and moisture resist.; for hairsprays, mousses, gels, and lotions; emulsion stabilizer for creams and lotions; clear visc. sol'n.; sol. in alcohols, esters, ketones, glycol ethers.

Gantrez® V-225. [ISP] Methylvinyl ether/maleic anhydride copolymer, ethyl ester, ethanol SDA-40B; forms tough, clear, glossy, tack-free films with exc. substantivity, hair-holding props., and moisture resist.; for hairsprays, mousses, gels and lotions; emulsion stabilizer for creams and lotions; clear visc. sol'n.; sol. in alcohols, esters, ketones, glycol ethers.

Gantrez® V-425. [ISP] Methylvinyl ether/maleic anhydride copolymer, monobutyl ester, ethanol SDA-40B; forms tough, clear, glossy, tack-free films with exc. substantivity, hair-holding props., and moisture resist.; for hairsprays, mousses, gels and lotions; emulsion stabilizer for creams and lotions; clear visc. sol'n.; sol. in alcohols, esters, ketones, glycol ethers.

Gantrez® XL-80. [ISP] PVM/MA decadiene crosspolymer.

Gardinol WA Paste. [Ronsheim & Moore] Sodium lauryl sulfate; CAS 151-21-3; EINECS 205-788-1; anionic; detergent for shampoos, fabrics; emulsifier for cosmetics; wh. to cream stiff paste; 40% conc.

Garionzet. [Ichimaru Pharcos] Water, alcohol, and garlic extract; botanical extract.

Garlic Extract HS 2710 G. [Grau Aromatics] Propylene glycol and garlic extract; botanical extract.

Gatarol M 30 M. [Chem-Y GmbH] Myreth-3 myristate; CAS 59686-68-9; nonionic; cosmetics surfactant; co-emulsifier and stabilizer for creams and lotions mfg.; solid; 99% conc.

Gatuline® A. [Gattefosse SA] Purified saponins extracted from lesser celandine; active ingred. for treatment of sensitive skin; sooths skin and reduces red blotchiness; for cosmetic gels, lotions, and emulsions, makeup, aftersun prods., aftershave preps.; beige powd.; sol. cloudy in water, propylene glycol, glycerin, alcohol; pH 5 ± 0.5 (5% aq.); usage level: 0.1-2%; toxicology: nonirritating to skin.

Gatuline® R. [Gattefosse SA] Water and fagus silvatica extract; amino acids, flavonoids, and peptides of plant origin (from fresh young tissues of beech trees); active ingred. producing anti-aging effects in skin (regeneration, invigoration); used in cosmetic emulsions, gels, shampoos, clear lotions, day creams, eye gels; brn.-amber liq.; sol. in water, propylene glycol, glycerin, alcohol; pH 5.0 ± 0.5; toxicology: nonirritating to skin; very sl. irritating to eyes.

GBL. [Arco] γ-Butyrolactone; CAS 96-48-0; EINECS 202-509-5; spinning and coagulating solv. for textiles, in nail polish removers, detergents, sunscreens, household cleaners, paint removers, agric. use, polymers, petrol. industry.

Geahlene. [Penreco] Min. oil, hydrog. butylene/ethylene/styrene copolymer, and hydrog. ethylene/propylene/styrene copolymer.

Gelcarin LA. [Marine Colloids] Carrageenan; CAS 9000-07-1; EINECS 232-524-2; gellant and stabilizer for cosmetics.

Geleol. [Gattefosse; Gattefosse SA] Glyceryl stearate; CAS 31566-31-1; nonionic; emulsifier; solid; drop pt. 54.5-58.5 C; HLB 3.0; acid no. < 3; iodine no. < 3; sapon. no. 160-180; toxicology: sl. irritating to eyes, nonirritating to skin; 100% conc.

Geliderm 3000 P. [DGF Stoess] Sodium cocoyl hydrolyzed collagen; CAS 68188-38-5; substantive cosmetic protein.

Geliderm 3000 S. [DGF Stoess] Sodium cocoyl hydrolyzed collagen; CAS 68188-38-5; substantive cosmetic protein.

Gelling Agent GP-1. [Ajinomoto] Dibutyl lauroyl glutamide; CAS 63663-21-8; EINECS 264-391-1.

Gelot 64®. [Gattefosse; Gattefosse SA] Glyceryl stearate and PEG-75 stearate; nonionic; SE base for o/w cosmetic and pharmaceutical emulsions; Gardner < 5 waxy solid; weak odor; HLB 10; m.p. 59–65 C; acid no. < 6; iodine no. < 3; sapon. no. 105–125; usage level: 15-25%; toxicology: LD50 (oral, rat) > 5 g/kg; nonirritating to skin and eyes; 100% conc.

Gelot WL 3122. [Gattefosse] PEG-6 stearate, glyceryl stearate.

Geltone. [Cimbar Perf. Minerals] Organophilic sodium bentonite; temp.-stable thickening and suspending agent for coatings, agric., adhesives, caulks, sealants, greases, inks, cosmetics and personal care prods.; lt. cream-colored powd.; 98% thru 200 mesh; mean particle size 20 μ; sp.gr. 1.7; bulk dens. 39 lb/ft³; oil absorp. 34; 3% moisture.

Geltone 1665. [Cimbar Perf. Minerals] Organophilic sodium bentonite; temp.-stable thickening and suspending agent for coatings, agric., adhesives, caulks, sealants, greases, inks, cosmetics and personal care prods.; lt. cream-colored powd.; 100% thru 200 mesh; mean particle size 3 μ; sp.gr. 1.7; bulk dens. 29 lb/ft³; oil absorp. 56; 3% moisture.

Geltone II. [Cimbar Perf. Minerals] Organophilic sodium bentonite; temp.-stable thickening and suspending agent for coatings, agric., adhesives, caulks, sealants, greases, inks, cosmetics and personal care prods.; lt. cream-colored powd.; 98% thru 200 mesh; mean particle size 20 μ; sp.gr. 1.7; bulk dens. 39 lb/ft³; oil absorp. 37; 3% moisture.

Gelucire 33/01. [Gattefosse SA] Hemisynthetic glycerides; excipient for hard gelatin capsules; drop pt. 33-38 C; HLB 1.0; acid no. < 2; iodine no. ≤ 3; sapon. no. 240-260; toxicology: LD50 (oral, rat) > 20 g/kg.

Gelucire 35/10. [Gattefosse SA] Saturated polyglycolized glycerides; excipient for hard gelatin capsules; drop pt. 29-34 C; HLB 10.0; acid no. < 2; iodine no. < 2; sapon. no. 120-135; toxicology: LD50 (oral, rat) > 20 g/kg.

Gelucire 37/02. [Gattefosse SA] Saturated polyglycolized glycerides; excipient for hard gelatin capsules; drop pt. 34.5-39.5 C; HLB 2.0; acid no. < 2; iodine no. < 2; sapon. no. 200-215; toxicology: LD50 (oral, rat) > 20 g/kg.

Gelucire 42/12. [Gattefosse SA] Saturated polyglycolized glycerides; excipient for hard gelatin capsules; drop pt. 41.5-46.5 C; HLB 12.0; acid no. < 2; iodine no. < 2; sapon. no. 95-115; toxicology: LD50 (oral, rat) > 20 g/kg.

Gelucire 44/14. [Gattefosse SA] Saturated polyglycolized glycerides; excipient for hard gelatin capsules; drop pt. 42.5-47.5 C; HLB 14.0; acid no. < 2; iodine no. < 2; sapon. no. 75-95; toxicology: LD50 (oral, rat) > 20 g/kg.

Gelucire 46/07. [Gattefosse SA] Saturated polyglycolized glycerides; excipient for hard gelatin capsules; drop pt. 47-52 C; HLB 7.0; acid no. < 2; iodine no. < 2; sapon. no. 125-140; toxicology: LD50 (oral, rat) > 20 g/kg.

Gelucire 48/09. [Gattefosse SA] Saturated polyglycolized glycerides; excipient for hard gelatin capsules; drop pt. 46-51 C; HLB 9.0; acid no. < 2; iodine no. < 2; sapon. no. 105-125; toxicology: LD50 (oral, rat) > 20 g/kg.

Gelucire 50/02. [Gattefosse SA] Saturated polyglycolized glycerides; excipient for hard gelatin capsules; drop pt. 46.5-51.5 C; HLB 2.0; acid no. < 2; iodine no. < 2; sapon. no. 180-195; toxicology: LD50 (oral, rat) > 18 ml/kg.

Gelucire 50/13. [Gattefosse SA] Saturated polyglycolized glycerides; excipient for hard gelatin capsules; drop pt. 46-51 C; HLB 13.0; acid no. < 2; iodine no. < 2; sapon. no. 65-80; toxicology: LD50 (oral, rat) > 20 g/kg.

Gelucire 53/10. [Gattefosse SA] Saturated polyglycolized glycerides; excipient for hard gelatin capsules; drop pt. 47.5-52.5 C; HLB 10.0; acid no. < 2; iodine no. < 2; sapon. no. 95-115; toxicology: LD50 (oral, rat) > 20 g/kg.

Gelucire 62/05. [Gattefosse SA] Polyglycolized natural wax; excipient for hard gelatin capsules; drop pt. 59-70 C; HLB 5.0; acid no. < 5; iodine no. < 10; sapon. no. 70-90; toxicology: LD50 (oral, rat) > 8.5 g/kg; sl. irritating to skin and eyes.

Gelwhite GP, H. [Southern Clay Prods.] Montmorillonite; CAS 1318-93-0; EINECS 215-288-5; thickener for cosmetics.

Gelwhite L. [Southern Clay Prods.] Montmorillonite; CAS 1318-93-0; EINECS 215-288-5; thickener for cosmetics.

Gelwhite MAS-H, MAS-L. [Southern Clay Prods.] Magnesium aluminum silicate; CAS 12199-37-0; EINECS 235-374-6; emulsifier, thickener, stabilizer.

Gemstone Sunstone CC. [Mearl] Castor oil, mica, titanium dioxide, oleyl alcohol, carnauba, iron oxides, and carmine.

Gemtex PA-70. [Finetex] Dioctyl sodium sulfosuccinate; CAS 577-11-7; EINECS 209-406-4; surfactant.

Gemtex PA-70P. [Finetex] Dioctyl sodium sulfosuccinate, propylene glycol.; CAS 577-11-7; EINECS 209-406-4;

anionic; wetting agent, penetrant; liq.; 70% conc.

Gemtex PA-75. [Finetex] Dioctyl sodium sulfosuccinate, isopropyl alcohol; CAS 577-11-7; EINECS 209-406-4; anionic; wetting agent, penetrant for textile uses and emulsion polymerization; dye leveler; bubble baths, bath oils; liq.; 75% conc.

Gemtex PA-75E. [Finetex] Dioctyl sodium sulfosuccinate; CAS 577-11-7; EINECS 209-406-4; anionic; wetting agent, penetrant.

Gemtex PA-85P. [Finetex] Dioctyl sodium sulfosuccinate, propylene glycol; CAS 577-11-7; EINECS 209-406-4; anionic; wetting agent, penetrant for textiles, emulsion polymerization; dye leveler; bubble baths, bath oils; liq.; 85% conc.

Gemtex PAX-60. [Finetex] Dioctyl sodium sulfosuccinate, anhyd.; CAS 577-11-7; EINECS 209-406-4; anionic; wetting agent for textile uses and emulsion polymerization; dye leveler; bubble baths, bath oils; liq.; 60% conc.

Gemtex SC-75E, SC Powd. [Finetex] Dioctyl sodium sulfosuccinate; CAS 577-11-7; EINECS 209-406-4; anionic; wetting agent for textile uses and emulsion polymerization; dye leveler; bubble baths, bath oils; liq. and powd. resp.; 75 and 83% conc. resp.

Gemtone®. [Mearl] Titanium dioxide-coated mica with iron oxides, iron blue, carmine, or chromium oxide; rich, lustrous pigments deriving color from both light interference and light absorption; for cosmetics and personal care prods. (lipsticks, nail enamels, liq. makeup, lotions, pressed powds.); grades incl. Aquamarine, Azurite, Copperstone, Goldstone, Mauve Quartz, Sunstone, Sapphire, Turquoise, etc.; powd.; avg. particle size 25 μ; sp.gr. 3.0.

Gemtone® Amber. [Mearl] Mica, titanium dioxide, and iron oxides.

Gemtone® Amethyst. [Mearl] Mica, titanium dioxide, ferric ferrocyanide, and carmine.

Gemtone® Emerald. [Mearl] Mica, titanium dioxide, chromium oxide greens, and ferric ferrocyanide.

Gemtone® Mauve Quartz. [Mearl] Mica, titanium dioxide, carmine, and ferric ferrocyanide.

Gemtone® Sunstone. [Mearl] Mica, titanium dioxide, iron oxides, and carmine.

Gemtone® Tan Opal CC. [Mearl] Castor oil, mica, iron oxides, titanium dioxide, oleyl alcohol, and carnauba.

Genagen BPMS. [Hoechst Celanese/Spec. Chem.] 1,4-Butanediol polyglycol ether monostearate; quaternary for cosmetics and toiletries; 90% act.

Genagen CA-050. [Hoechst Celanese/Colorants & Surf.; Hoechst AG] PEG-5 cocamide; CAS 61791-08-0; nonionic; cleansing skin protective component for detergents and cleaning agents; cosmetic emulsifier; 100% conc.

Genagen CAB. [Hoechst Celanese/Colorants & Surf.] Cocamidopropyl betaine; base detergent for cosmetics, toiletries; 30% act.

Genamin CTAC. [Hoechst Celanese/Colorants & Surf.] Cetrimonium chloride; CAS 112-02-7; EINECS 203-928-6; cationic; cosmetic raw material for hair treatment preps.; antistat; pale ylsh. liq.; 29% act.

Genamin DSAC. [Hoechst Celanese/Colorants & Surf.] Distearyldimonium chloride; CAS 107-64-2; EINECS 203-508-2; cationic; cosmetic raw material for hair and skin treatment preps.; good wet combing, skin softening props.; ylsh. wh. powd.; 97% act.

Genamin KDB. [Hoechst AG] Behenalkonium chloride; CAS 16841-14-8; EINECS 240-865-3.

Genamin KDM. [Hoechst AG] Behentrimonium chloride; CAS 17301-53-0; EINECS 241-327-0; cationic; conditioner and antistat in hair care prods.; yel. paste; water-sol.; pH 6–7 (1%); 80% act.

Genamin KDM-F. [Hoechst Celanese/Colorants & Surf.]

Behentrimonium chloride; CAS 17301-53-0; EINECS 241-327-0; cationic; base, antistat, emulsifier for preparation of hair care prods.; conditioner; wh. waxy flake; sol. in water with use of alcohol; 80% act.

Genamin KS 5. [Hoechst AG] PEG-5 stearyl ammonium chloride; cationic; cosmetic raw material, conditioner for hair care prods.; yel.-brn. aq. sol'n.; pleasant odor; water-misc.; pH 6.5 ± 0.3 (1%); 20% act.

Genamin KSE. [Hoechst Celanese/Colorants & Surf.] Distearyldimonium chloride, cetyl alcohol, ceteareth-15, ceteareth-3, PEG-3 distearate; cationic; SE base material, surfactant, conditioner for hair treatment preps.; ylsh. wh. powd.; 100% act.

Genamin KSL. [Hoechst Celanese/Colorants & Surf.; Hoechst AG] PEG-5 stearyl ammonium lactate; cationic; gloss aid for hair care prods.; clear ylsh.; 30% act.

Genamin PDAC. [Hoechst Celanese/Spec. Chem.] Polyquaternium-6; CAS 26062-79-3; quaternary for cosmetics and toiletries; 40% act.

Genamin STAC. [Hoechst Celanese/Spec. Chem.; Hoechst AG] Steartrimonium chloride; CAS 112-03-8; EINECS 203-929-1; cationic; quaternary for cosmetics and toiletries; 80% act.

Genamine C-020. [Hoechst Celanese] Coconut fatty amine oxethylate; cationic; raw material for min. oil additives, insecticides, pesticides, cosmetic bases, adhesives; clear liq.; sol. in min. oil, turbid in water (10 g/l); sp.gr. 0.895 (50 C); visc. 28.8 cps (50 C); flash pt. 188 C (Marcusson); surf. tens. 26 dynes/cm; pH 9–10; 100% act.

Genaminox CS. [Hoechst AG] Coco dimethyl amine oxide; CAS 61788-90-7; EINECS 263-016-9; nonionic; foaming agent and stabilizer, thickener for personal care prods.; hair conditioner; liq.; 30% conc.

Genaminox CST. [Hoechst AG] Alkyl dimethylamine oxide; nonionic; hair conditioner, surfactant; liq.; 30% conc.

Genaminox KC. [Hoechst Celanese/Colorants & Surf.; Hoechst AG] Cocamine oxide; CAS 61788-90-7; EINECS 263-016-9; nonionic; foam booster/stabilizer over wide pH range, thickener for shampoos, bath prods.; surfactant for textile processing; yel. clear liq.; pH 7; 30% act.

Genapol® 24-L-3. [Hoechst Celanese/Colorants & Surf.] C12-14 pareth-2.9; CAS 68439-50-9; nonionic; biodeg. detergent intermediate for sulfation for use in cosmetics, shampoos, lt. duty detergents; emulsifier, prewash spotter, agric. adjuvant, hydrocarbon-based cleaning systems; APHA 10 liq.; oil-sol.; m.w. 331; sp.gr. 0.93; visc. 25 cst; HLB 8.0; hyd. no. 170; pour pt. 7 C; flash pt. (FTCOC) 157 C; pH 6.5 (1% aq.); 100% conc.

Genapol® 26-L-1. [Hoechst Celanese/Colorants & Surf.] C12-16 pareth-1; CAS 68551-12-2; nonionic; biodeg. detergent intermediate for sulfation for use in cosmetics, shampoos, lt. duty detergents; emulsifier, prewash spotter, agric. adjuvant, hydrocarbon-based cleaning systems; APHA 10 liq.; oil-sol.; m.w. 238; sp.gr. 0.87; HLB 3.7; hyd. no. 235; pour pt. 8 C; flash pt. (FTCOC) 149 C; pH 6.5 (1% aq.); 100% conc.

Genapol® 26-L-1.6. [Hoechst Celanese/Colorants & Surf.] C12-16 pareth-1.6; nonionic; biodeg. detergent intermediate for sulfation for use in cosmetics, shampoos, lt. duty detergents; emulsifier, prewash spotter, agric. adjuvant, hydrocarbon-based cleaning systems; FDA compliance; APHA 10 liq.; oil-sol.; m.w. 264; sp.gr. 0.9; visc. 22 cst; HLB 5.0; hyd. no. 213; pour pt. 10 C; flash pt. (FTCOC) 143 C; pH 6.6 (1% aq.); 100% conc.

Genapol® 26-L-2. [Hoechst Celanese/Colorants & Surf.] C12-16 pareth-2; nonionic; biodeg. detergent intermediate for sulfation for use in cosmetics, shampoos, lt. duty detergents; emulsifier, prewash spotter, agric. adjuvant, hydrocarbon-based cleaning systems; APHA 10 liq.; oil-

sol.; m.w. 281; sp.gr. 0.91; visc. 24 cst; HLB 6.0; hyd. no. 200; pour pt. 10 C; flash pt. (FTCOC) 143 C; pH 6.4 (1% aq.); 100% conc.

Genapol® 26-L-3. [Hoechst Celanese/Colorants & Surf.] C12-16 pareth-3; nonionic; biodeg. detergent intermediate for sulfation for use in cosmetics, shampoos, lt. duty detergents; emulsifier, prewash spotter, agric. adjuvant, hydrocarbon-based cleaning systems; FDA compliance; APHA 15 liq.; oil-sol.; m.w. 328; sp.gr. 0.93; visc. 27 cst; HLB 8.0; hyd. no. 171; pour pt. 8 C; flash pt. (FTCOC) 154 C; pH 6.6 (1% aq.); 100% conc.

Genapol® 26-L-5. [Hoechst Celanese/Colorants & Surf.] C12-16 pareth-5; nonionic; biodeg. detergent intermediate for sulfation for use in cosmetics, shampoos, lt. duty detergents; emulsifier, prewash spotter, agric. adjuvant, hydrocarbon-based cleaning systems; FDA compliance; APHA 10 liq.; oil-sol.; m.w. 419; sp.gr. 0.97; visc. 29 cst; HLB 10.6; hyd. no. 134; pour pt. 8 C; flash pt. (FTCOC) 160 C; pH 6.6 (1% aq.); 100% conc.

Genapol® 26-L-45. [Hoechst Celanese/Colorants & Surf.] C12-16 pareth-6; nonionic; biodeg. detergent intermediate for sulfation for use in cosmetics, shampoos, lt. duty detergents; emulsifier, prewash spotter, agric. adjuvant, hydrocarbon-based cleaning systems; APHA 20 liq.; oil-sol.; m.w. 479; sp.gr. 0.96; visc. 49.5 cst; HLB 11.6; hyd. no. 117; pour pt. 6 C; cloud pt. 45 C (1% aq.); flash pt. (FTCOC) 216 C; pH 7.0 (1% aq.); 100% conc.

Genapol® 42-L-3. [Hoechst Celanese/Colorants & Surf.] C12-14 pareth-3; CAS 68439-50-9; nonionic; biodeg. detergent intermediate for sulfation for use in cosmetics, shampoos, lt. duty detergents; emulsifier, prewash spotter, agric. adjuvant, hydrocarbon-based cleaning systems; liq.; oil-sol.; HLB 7.7; 100% conc.

Genapol® AMG. [Hoechst AG] Magnesium PEG-3 cocamide sulfate; nonionic; basic material for cosmetics and toiletries; 30% conc.

Genapol® AMS. [Hoechst Celanese/Colorants & Surf.; Hoechst AG] TEA-PEG-3 cocamide sulfate; anionic; detergent, foaming agent used in top-grade cosmetics cleansers; lime soap dispersant; biodeg.; clear yel. low-visc. liq.; weak odor; dens. 1.0 g/cm³; visc. 200 cps max.; pH 6.5–8.0 (1%); 40% act.

Genapol® ARO Paste. [Hoechst Celanese/Colorants & Surf.; Hoechst AG] Sodium laureth sulfate; CAS 9004-82-4; anionic; raw material for cosmetics, detergents, and cleaning agents; paste.

Genapol® C-050. [Hoechst Celanese/Colorants & Surf.] Coceth-5; CAS 61791-13-7; nonionic; raw material for mfg. of textile, leather, paper auxs., detergents, emulsifiers, cosmetics, agric.; turbid liq.; sol. in min. oil, benzene, turbid in water; sp. gr. 0.952 (50 C); visc. 17.6 cps (50 C); flash pt. 201 C (Marcusson); surf. tens. 32 dynes/cm; 100% act.

Genapol® C-080. [Hoechst Celanese/Colorants & Surf.] Coceth-8; CAS 61791-13-7; nonionic; raw material for mfg. of textile, leather, paper auxs., detergents, emulsifiers, cosmetics, agric.; paste; sol. in water, benzene, turbid in min. oil; sp. gr. 0.979 (50 C); visc. 25.4 cps (50 C); flash pt. 246 C (Marcusson); surf. tens. 36 dynes/cm; 100% act.

Genapol® C-100. [Hoechst Celanese/Colorants & Surf.] Coceth-10; CAS 61791-13-7; nonionic; raw material for mfg. of textile, leather, paper auxs., detergents, emulsifiers, cosmetics, agric.; paste; sol. in water, benzene, turbid in min. oil; sp. gr. 0.990 (50 C); visc. 30.4 cps (50 C); flash pt. 251 C (Marcusson); surf. tens. 38 dynes/cm; 100% act.

Genapol® C-150. [Hoechst Celanese/Colorants & Surf.] Coceth-15; CAS 61791-13-7; nonionic; raw material for mfg. of textile, leather, paper auxs., detergents, emulsifiers, cosmetics, agric.; wax; sol. in water, benzene; sp. gr. 1.027 (50 C); visc. 45.8 cps (50 C); flash pt. 260 C

(Marcusson); surf. tens. 43 dynes/cm; 100% act.

Genapol® C-200. [Hoechst Celanese/Colorants & Surf.] Coceth-20; CAS 61791-13-7; nonionic; raw material for mfg. of textile, leather, paper auxs., detergents, emulsifiers, cosmetics, agric.; wax; sol. in water, benzene; sp. gr. 1.032 (50 C); visc. 61.5 cps (50 C); flash pt. 264 C (Marcusson); surf. tens. 44 dynes/cm; 100% act.

Genapol® CRT 40. [Hoechst Celanese/Colorants & Surf.; Hoechst AG] TEA-lauryl sulfate; CAS 139-96-8; EINECS 205-388-7; anionic; detergent raw material for cosmetics, shampoos, body cleansing agents, detergents; biodeg.; pale yel. clear liq.; slight odor; m.w. 422; sol. in water; dens. 1.0–1.05 g/ cm³; visc. 100 cps max.; pH 6.5–7.5 (1%); 40% conc.

Genapol® L-3. [Hoechst Celanese/Spec. Chem.] Laureth-3; CAS 3055-94-5; EINECS 221-280-2; thickener for cosmetics and toiletries; 100% act.

Genapol® LRO Liq., Paste. [Hoechst Celanese/Colorants & Surf.; Hoechst AG] Sodium laureth sulfate; CAS 9004-82-4; anionic; detergent, foaming agent used in cosmetic prods., personal care prods., agric., lime soap dispersant; biodeg.; pale yel. clear liq., mobile paste resp.; slight odor; misc. with water; dens. 1.05 and 1.0 g/ cm³ resp.; visc. 100 cps max. (liq.); pH 6.5–8.0 (1% aq., liq.), 7.2±0.6 (1% aq., paste); 27 and 68% conc.

Genapol® LRT 40. [Hoechst Celanese/Colorants & Surf.] TEA-lauryl sulfate; CAS 139-96-8; EINECS 205-388-7; personal care surfactant.

Genapol® O-020. [Hoechst Celanese/Colorants & Surf.] Oleth-2; CAS 9004-98-2; nonionic; raw material for mfg. of textile, leather, paper auxs., detergents, emulsifiers, cosmetics, agric.; clear liq.; sol. in min. oil, benzene, turbid in water; sp.gr. 0.894 (50 C); visc. 12.4 cps (50 C); flash pt. 186 C (Marcusson); 100% act.

Genapol® O-050. [Hoechst Celanese/Colorants & Surf.] Oleth-5; CAS 9004-98-2; nonionic; raw material for mfg. of textile, leather, paper auxs., detergents, emulsifiers, cosmetics, agric.; turbid liq.; sol. in benzene, turbid in water, min. oil; sp.gr. 0.936 (50 C); visc. 18.4 cps (50 C); flash pt. 225 C (Marcusson); surf. tens. 54 dynes/cm; 100% act.

Genapol® O-080. [Hoechst Celanese/Colorants & Surf.] Oleth-8; CAS 9004-98-2; nonionic; raw material for mfg. of textile, leather, paper auxs., detergents, emulsifiers, cosmetics, agric.; turbid liq.; sol. in water, benzene, turbid in min. oil; sp.gr. 0.960 (50 C); visc. 25.1 cps (50 C); flash pt. 246 C (Marcusson); surf. tens. 44 dynes/cm; 100% act.

Genapol® O-090. [Hoechst Celanese/Colorants & Surf.] Oleth-9; CAS 9004-98-2; nonionic; raw material for mfg. of textile, leather, paper auxs., detergents, emulsifiers, cosmetics, agric.; yel. liq.; visc. 45 cps; hyd. no. 90; pH 7 (1% aq.); 99% conc.

Genapol® O-100. [Hoechst Celanese/Colorants & Surf.] Oleth-10; CAS 9004-98-2; nonionic; raw material for mfg. of textile, leather, paper auxs., detergents, emulsifiers, cosmetics, agric.; paste; sol. in water, benzene, turbid in min. oil; sp.gr. 0.989 (50 C); visc. 33 cps (50 C); flash pt. 260 C (Marcusson); surf. tens. 41 dynes/cm; 100% act.

Genapol® O-120. [Hoechst Celanese/Colorants & Surf.] Oleth-12; CAS 9004-98-2; nonionic; raw material for mfg. of textile, leather, paper auxs., detergents, emulsifiers, cosmetics, agric.; paste; sol. in water, benzene, turbid in min. oil; sp.gr. 1.0 (50 C); visc. 42.5 cps (50 C); flash pt. 265 C (Marcusson); surf. tens. 42 dynes/cm; 100% act.

Genapol® O-150. [Hoechst Celanese/Colorants & Surf.] Oleth-15; CAS 9004-98-2; nonionic; raw material for mfg. of textile, leather, paper auxs., detergents, emulsifiers, cosmetics, agric.; wax; sol. in water, benzene, turbid in min. oil; sp.gr. 1.02 (50 C); visc. 49.1 cps (50 C); flash pt. 271 C (Marcusson); surf. tens. 45 dynes/cm; 100% act.

Genapol® O-200. [Hoechst Celanese/Colorants & Surf.]

Oleth-20; CAS 9004-98-2; nonionic; raw material for mfg. of textile, leather, paper auxs., detergents, emulsifiers, cosmetics, agric.; wh. waxy solid; sol. in water, benzene, turbid in min. oil; sp.gr. 1.037 (50 C); visc. 65.9 cps (50 C); hyd. no. 50; flash pt. 278 C (Marcusson); pH 7 (1% aq.); surf. tens. 47 dynes/cm; 100% act.

Genapol® O-230. [Hoechst Celanese/Colorants & Surf.] Oleth-23; CAS 9004-98-2; nonionic; raw material for mfg. of textile, leather, paper auxs., detergents, emulsifiers, cosmetics, agric.; wh. waxy solid; sol. in water, benzene, turbid in min. oil; sp.gr. 1.042 (50 C); visc. 79.5 cps (50 C); hyd. no. 44; flash pt. 279 C (Marcusson); pH 7 (1% aq.); surf. tens. 47 dynes/cm; 100% act.

Genapol® PGC. [Hoechst Celanese/Spec. Chem.] Glycol distearate, laureth-4, and cocamidopropyl betaine; pearlescent for cosmetics and toiletries; 45% act.

Genapol® PGM Conc. [Hoechst Celanese/Colorants & Surf.; Hoechst AG] Sodium laureth sulfate, glycol distearate, and cocamide MEA; anionic; pearl-luster conc. used in shampoos, bubble baths, cosmetics, liq. soaps, detergents; biodeg.; wh. fluid paste; slight odor; misc. with water; dens. 1.0 g/ cm³; pH 7.2 ± 0.8 (1% act.); 40.0 ± 1.0% act.

Genapol® PGM Liq. [Hoechst Celanese/Colorants & Surf.; Hoechst AG] Sodium laureth sulfate, glycol distearate, and cocamide MEA; pearl-luster conc. for cosmetics, toiletries; 39% act.

Genapol® PL 120. [Hoechst AG] EO/PO fatty alcohol adduct; nonionic; low foaming surfactant.

Genapol® PMS. [Hoechst Celanese/Colorants & Surf.; Hoechst AG] Glycol distearate; CAS 627-83-8; EINECS 211-014-3; nonionic; pearlescent agent for cosmetic washing agents and shampoo; powd.; 100% act.

Genapol® SBE. [Hoechst Celanese/Spec. Chem.] Disodium laureth sulfosuccinate; basic material for cosmetics and toiletries; 35% conc.

Genapol® T Grades. [Hoechst Celanese/Colorants & Surf.; Hoechst AG] Tallow alcohol polyglycol ether (8–25 EO); nonionic; detergent base and basic material for cosmetic and specialty chemical industries, agric. formulations; biodeg.; liq., paste, wax; 100% conc.

Genapol® T-500. [Hoechst AG] C16-18 fatty alcohol polyalkoxylate; auxiliary for detergent bases; powd.

Genapol® TSM. [Hoechst Celanese/Colorants & Surf.; Hoechst AG] PEG-3 distearate and sodium laureth sulfate; detergent, opacifier, silk luster agent for shampoos, bubble baths, shower preps.; wh. med.-visc. disp.; 36% act.

Genapol® TS Powd. [Hoechst Celanese/Colorants & Surf.; Hoechst AG] PEG-3 distearate; CAS 9005-08-7; detergent, pearlescent, opacifier for shampoos, bubble baths, shower preps.; wh. powd.; 100% act.

Genapol® ZRO Liq., Paste. [Hoechst Celanese/Colorants & Surf.; Hoechst AG] Sodium laureth sulfate; CAS 9004-82-4; anionic; raw material with good foaming and cleansing for cosmetics, detergents, cleaning agents; 28% pale yel. clear liq., 70% sl. yel. mobile paste.

Generol® 122. [Henkel/Cospha; Henkel Canada; Henkel KGaA/Cospha] Soya sterol; nonionic; emollient, aux. or primary w/o emulsifier, emulsion stabilizer, visc. modifier, solubilizer for cosmetics; ylsh. waxy flakes; sol. in abs. alcohol, min. and veg. oils; insol. in water; m.p. 135-141 C; HLB 2.0; acid no. 0.1; sapon. no. 2.0; hyd. no. 110-147; usage level: 2-8%; 90% conc.

Generol® 122E5. [Henkel/Cospha; Henkel Canada; Henkel KGaA/Cospha] PEG-5 soya sterol; nonionic; emollient, primary and sec. emulsifier, conditioner, stabilizer and consistency modifier in o/w emulsions; substantive to hair and in shampoo; ylsh. soft, waxy, amorphous solid; faint odor; sol. in ethanol, isopropyl esters; water-disp.; m.p.

70-90 C; HLB 5.0; hyd. no. 90-110; pH 7 (1% aq.); usage level: 2-8%; 100% conc.

Generol® 122E10. [Henkel/Cospha; Henkel KGaA/Cospha] PEG-10 soya sterol; nonionic; emollient, aux. emulsifier, appearance modifier, gloss enhancer, solubilizer; less substantivity in hair care formulations; emulsion stabilizer; modifies consistency of a firm cream to a pourable lotion in high solids o/w emulsions; lt. amber soft wax; faint odor; sol. in ethanol, isopropyl esters; water-disp. (translucent); m.p. 50-70 C; HLB 12; hyd. no. 70-85; pH 7 (1% aq.); usage level: 2-8%; 100% conc.

Generol® 122E16. [Henkel/Cospha; Henkel Canada; Henkel KGaA/Cospha] PEG-16 soya sterol; nonionic; emollient, primary or aux. emulsifier, solubilizer, stabilizer and consistency modifier in o/w emulsions, makeup formulations; improves pigment disp.; ivory hard wax; faint odor; sol. in water, isopropyl esters, veg. oils, and ethanol; m.p. 45-55 C; HLB 15; hyd. no. 55-70; pH 7 (1% aq.); usage level: 2-8%; 100% conc.

Generol® 122E25. [Henkel/Cospha; Henkel Canada; Henkel KGaA/Cospha] PEG-25 soya sterol; nonionic; emulsifier, emollient, pigment dispersant and wetter, deflocculating agent in cosmetics; solubilizer for perfumes or preservatives; ivory hard wax; faint odor; sol. in water and ethanol; at 80 C, sol. in isopropyl esters and veg. oils; m.p. 40-50 C; HLB 17; hyd. no. 45-55; pH 7 (1% aq.); usage level: 2-8%; 100% conc.

Genetron® 152a. [FMC] Hydrofluorocarbon 152a; CAS 75-37-6; EINECS 200-866-1.

Genu Carrageenan. [Hercules] Refined carrageenan; CAS 9000-07-1; EINECS 232-524-2; emulsifier, stabilizer, thickener, or gelling agent in foods, pharmaceuticals, and cosmetics; powd.

Genugel. [Hercules] Carrageenan; CAS 9000-07-1; EINECS 232-524-2; gellant, thickener, stabilizer, and suspender used in foods, pharmaceuticals, and cosmetics; water binder; imparts desirable body and mouthfeel.

Genulacta Series. [Hercules] Carrageenan; CAS 9000-07-1; EINECS 232-524-2; gellant, thickener, stabilizer, and suspender used in foods, pharmaceuticals, and cosmetics; water binder; imparts desirable body and mouthfeel.

Genu Pectins. [Hercules] Pectin; high-methoxy and low-methoxy purified natural hydrocolloid derived from citrus peels; CAS 9000-69-5; EINECS 232-553-0; consists chiefly of partially methoxylated polygalacturonic acid; used as gelling agent for jellies, and as a visc. builder, protective colloid, and stabilizer for food systems, pharmaceutical, and cosmetic industries; lt. cream to grayish powd.; no odor and flavor.

Genurol 122 E-5. [Universal Preserv-A-Chem] PEG-5 soya sterol; emollient, emulsifier.

Genurol 122 E-10. [Universal Preserv-A-Chem] PEG-10 soya sterol; emollient, emulsifier.

Genurol 122 E-25. [Universal Preserv-A-Chem] PEG-25 soya sterol; emollient, emulsifier.

Genuvisco. [Hercules] Carageenan; CAS 9000-07-1; EINECS 232-524-2; gellant, thickener, stabilizer, and suspender used in foods, pharmaceuticals, and cosmetics; water binder; imparts desirable body and mouthfeel.

George's Aloe Vera. [Warren Labs] Aloe vera gel; moisturizer, soothing/healing aid for personal care.

Geranonitril. [Henkel/Cospha] Fragrance raw material for cosmetic, personal care, detergent, and cleaning prods.; colorless to sl. yel. liq., lemon odor; b.p. 86-89 C; flash pt. 99 C.

Gerbavert. [Henkel/Cospha] Fragrance raw material for cosmetic, personal care, detergent, and cleaning prods.; colorless liq., fruity odor; b.p. 108 C; flash pt. 51 C.

Germaben® II. [Sutton Labs] Diazolidinyl urea (30%), propylene glycol (56%), methylparaben (11%), and propylparaben (3%); broad-spectrum antimicrobial preservative for cosmetic prods.; USA and Europe approvals; pale to lt. yel. clear visc. liq.; char. mild odor; sol. @ 1% in aq. sol'n. and oil-water emulsions; sp.gr. 1.1731-1.1839; b.p. 369 F; flash pt. (TCC) > 200 F; usage level: 1% max.; toxicology: LD50 (oral, rat) > 2000 mg/kg; moderate skin irritant; severe eye irritant at full strength; 42.5-45.5% total solids; 5.8-6.4% N.

Germaben® II-E. [Sutton Labs] Diazolidinyl urea (20%), propylene glycol (60%), methylparaben (10%), and propylparaben (10%); broad-spectrum antimicrobial preservative system for cosmetic creams and lotions; effective against Gram-positive and Gram-negative bacteria, yeast, and mold; pale yel. clear visc. liq., char. mild odor; sol. 0.5 g/100 g water; sp.gr. 1.1353-1.1438; b.p. 369 F; flash pt. (TCC) > 200 F; 38.5-41.5% total solids; 3.8-4.4% N.

Germall® 115. [Sutton Labs] Imidazolidinyl urea; CAS 39236-46-9; EINECS 254-372-6; antimicrobial preservative for cosmetics, esp. cold mix formulations; effective against Gram-negative bacteria; active over wide pH range; synergistic with other preservatives; EC approved; wh. free-flowing fine powd., char. mild odor or odorless; sol. (g/100 g): 200 g in water, 50 g in propylene glycol, 16 g in glycerin; m.w. 406.33; pH 6.0-7.5 (1% aq.); usage level: 0.2-0.6%; toxicology: LD50 (oral, rat) 5200 mg/kg; nonirritating to skin and eyes as aq. so'n.; mild transient eye irritant (powd.); 26-28% N.

Germall® II. [Sutton Labs] Diazolidinyl urea; CAS 78491-02-8; EINECS 278-928-2; broad-spectrum antimicrobial preservative for cosmetics and toiletries (creams, lotions, shampoos, liq. makeup, eye area prods.); effective against Gram-negative and house isolate bacteria; synergistic with other preservatives; EC approved; wh. free-flowing fine powd. char. mild odor or odorless; m.w. 278.23; sol. in water, propylene glycol, glycerin; usage level: up to 0.5%; toxicology: LD50 (oral, rat) 2570 mg/kg; nonirritating to skin and eyes @ 5% aq. sol'n.; 19-21% N.

Geronol ACR/4. [Rhone-Poulenc Surf. & Spec.] Disodium laurethsulfosuccinate; anionic; emulsifier for emulsion polymerization of acrylate, polyvinyl acetate; detergent base, foamer, foam stabilizer, dispersant; liq.; insol. in org. solv.; 30% conc.

Geronol ACR/9. [Rhone-Poulenc Surf. & Spec.] Disodium nonoxynol-10 sulfosuccinate; CAS 67999-57-9; anionic; emulsifier for emulsion polymerization of acrylate, polyvinyl acetate; detergent base, foamer, foam stabilizer, dispersant; liq.; insol. in org. solv.; 30% conc.

Geropon® 99. [Rhone-Poulenc Surf. & Spec.] Dioctyl sodium sulfosuccinate and propylene glycol; CAS 577-11-7; EINECS 209-406-4; anionic; detergent; textile scouring and dispersant for dyes; paper rewetting and felt washing surfactant; wetting agent in cosmetics; detergent additive in dry cleaning fluids; dishwashing compds.; wallpaper removers; agric. sprays; emulsion polymerization; water-based paint formulations; antifog; EPA compliance; clear liq.; water-sol.; sp.gr. 1.08–1.13 (70 F); visc. 500–1000 cps (70 F); pour pt. 40 F; 70% act.; formerly Pentex® 99.

Geropon® AB/20. [Rhone-Poulenc Surf. & Spec.] Ammonium laureth-9 sulfate; anionic; emulsifier for emulsion polymerization and min. oils; detergent, dispersant, foam stabilizer; stable to pH and temp.; liq.; 30% conc.

Geropon® ACR/4. [Rhone-Poulenc Surf. & Spec.] Disodium laureth-4 sulfosuccinate; amphoteric; emulsifier for emulsion polymerization, detergent base, foamer, foam stabilizer, dispersant; mild detergent, emulsifier, foaming agent for shampoos, liq. soaps, facial cleansers, bath gels, and bubble baths; liq.; 30% conc.; formerly Geronol ACR/4.

Geropon® ACR/9. [Rhone-Poulenc Surf. & Spec.] Disodium nonoxynol-10 sulfosuccinate; CAS 67999-57-9; anionic; emulsifier for emulsion polymerization, detergent base, foamer, foam stabilizer, dispersant; liq.; 30% conc.; formerly Geronol ACR/9.

Geropon® AS-200. [Rhone-Poulenc Surf. & Spec.] Sodium cocoyl isethionate, coconut acid, stearic acid; anionic; detergent, emulsifier, foam booster/stabilizer, visc. builder, wetting agent, dispersant, suspending agent for textile wet processing, industrial/household detergents, cosmetics (shampoos, liq. soaps, bar soaps, facial cleansers, bath gels, bubble baths), agric. pesticides, leather, rubber, etc.; readily biodeg.; APHA 100 max. color.

Geropon® AS-250. [Rhone-Poulenc Surf. & Spec.] Sodium cocoyl isethionate, coconut acid, stearic acid; 50% active form of Geropon AS-200; 50% act.

Geropon® LSS. [Rhone-Poulenc Surf. & Spec.] Disodium lauryl sulfosuccinate; CAS 36409-57-1; anionic; low-irritant detergent for shampoos and bubble baths; wh. creamy solid; pH 7.0 (10%); 35% act.; formerly Miranate® LSS.

Geropon® SB-5. [Rhone-Poulenc Surf. & Spec.] Disodium laneth-5 sulfosuccinate.

Geropon® SBDO. [Rhone-Poulenc Surf. & Spec.] Dioctyl sodium sulfosuccinate; CAS 577-11-7; EINECS 209-406-4; surfactant.

Geropon® SBF-12. [Rhone-Poulenc Surf. & Spec.] Disodium lauryl sulfosuccinate.

Geropon® SBFA-30. [Rhone-Poulenc Surf. & Spec.] Disodium laureth sulfosuccinate; CAS 68815-56-5; anionic; skin protecting anti-irritant surfactant; liq.; 40% conc.; formerly Alconate® SBFA 30.

Geropon® SBG-280. [Rhone-Poulenc Surf. & Spec.] Disodium oleamido PEG-2 sulfosuccinate; CAS 56388-43-3; EINECS 260-143-1; cosmetic surfactant.

Geropon® SBL-203. [Rhone-Poulenc Surf. & Spec.] Disodium lauramido MEA-sulfosuccinate; CAS 25882-44-4; EINECS 247-310-4; improves flash foam of anionic systems; produces brittle, tack-free residue for carpet shampoos; liq.; 40% conc.; formerly Alconate® SBL-203.

Geropon® SBR-3. [Rhone-Poulenc Surf. & Spec.] Disodium ricinoleamido MEA-sulfosuccinate; CAS 40754-60-7; anionic; skin protecting anti-irritant surfactant; liq.; 40% conc.; formerly Alconate® SBR-3.

Geropon® SBU-185. [Rhone-Poulenc Surf. & Spec.] Disodium undecylenamido MEA-sulfosuccinate.

Geropon® SS-L9ME. [Rhone-Poulenc Surf. & Spec.] Sodium lauramido MEA sulfosuccinate; anionic; high foaming and non-irritating surfactant for toiletry and carpet shampoo formulations; liq.; 40% conc.; formerly Alkasurf® SS-L9ME.

Geropon® SS-LA-3. [Rhone-Poulenc Surf. & Spec.] Disodium laureth sulfosuccinate; cosmetic surfactant.

Geropon® T-77. [Rhone-Poulenc Surf. & Spec.] Sodium N-methyl-N-oleoyl taurate; CAS 137-20-2; EINECS 205-285-7; anionic; foamer, wetting agent, emulsifier, dispersant for textile and general-purpose applics.; dye assistant; kier boiling; in industrial detergents, rug shampoos, bottle washing compds., metal cleaners, paper industry; foaming agent, conditioner, detergent, emulsifier, foam booster/stabilizer, visc. builder for shampoos, liq. soaps, facial cleansers, bath gels, and bubble baths; cream flakes, fatty odor; m.w. 425; water sol.; pH 6.5–8.0 (5%); 67% act.; formerly Igepon® T-77.

Geropon® TBS. [Rhone-Poulenc Surf. & Spec.] Alkyl polyglycolic ether, modified; anionic; detergent for fibers, cosmetics, leather, paper, and metal industry; liq.

Geropon® TC-42. [Rhone-Poulenc Surf. & Spec.] Sodium N-methyl-N-cocoyl taurate; CAS 61791-42-2; anionic; foamer, foam stabilizer, dispersant, detergent, emulsifier, visc. builder for detergent bars, shampoos, bath gels, bubble baths, liq. soaps, facial cleansers, cosmetics, and toiletries; chemically stable; wh. soft, smooth paste; m.w. 363; pH 7.0–8.5 (10%); 24% act.; formerly Igepon® TC-42.

Gilugel ALM. [Giulini] Sweet almond oil, 20% aluminum/magnesium hydroxide stearate; stabilizer and visc. control agent imparting smooth, nongreasy feel to cosmetic creams, lotions, and stick formulations; soft brn. gel.

Gilugel CAO. [Giulini] Castor oil, 20% aluminum/magnesium hydroxide stearate; stabilizer and visc. control agent imparting smooth, nongreasy feel to lipsticks, lip glosses, lip balms, and lip pencils; tan sl. tacky gel.

Gilugel EUG. [Giulini] Octyldodecanol, 20% aluminum/magnesium hydroxide stearate; emollient, stabilizer, and visc. control agent imparting smooth, nongreasy feel to skin conditioners, eyeliners, lipsticks, creams, and lotions; off-wh. soft gel.

Gilugel IPM. [Giulini] Isopropyl myristate, aluminum/magnesium hydroxide stearate; stabilizer and visc. control agent imparting smooth, nongreasy feel to cosmetics.

Gilugel IPP. [Giulini] Isopropyl palmitate, aluminum/magnesium hydroxide stearate; stabilizer and visc. control agent imparting smooth, nongreasy feel to cosmetic .

Gilugel MIG. [Giulini] Caprylic/capric triglyceride, 20% aluminum/magnesium hydroxide stearate; occlusive solv., stabilizer, and visc. control agent imparting smooth, nongreasy feel to eye shadows, foundations, lipsticks, and creams and lotions; off-wh. soft gel.

Gilugel MIN. [Giulini] Min. oil, 20% aluminum/magnesium hydroxide stearate; emollient, occlusive solv., stabilizer, and visc. control agent imparting smooth, nongreasy feel to makeup, creams, lotions, and sunscreens; moderately stiff translucent gel.

Gilugel OS. [Giulini] Octyl stearate and 20% aluminum/magnesium hydroxide stearate; emollient, stabilizer and visc. control agent imparting smooth, nongreasy feel to cosmetic creams, lotions, and sunscreens; quick rub-in; sl. tan moderately soft gel.

Gilugel R. [Giulini] Soybean oil, aluminum hydroxide, glyceryl isostearate, and microcryst. wax; stabilizer and visc. control agent imparting smooth, nongreasy feel to cosmetics.

Gilugel SIL5. [Giulini] Cyclomethicone and 20% aluminum/magnesium hydroxide stearate; emollient, solv., stabilizer, and visc. control agent imparting smooth, nongreasy feel to eyeliners, eye shadows, makeup bases, creams, lotions, sunscreens; hair conditioning agent.

Gilugels. [Giulini] Thickeners and stabilizers for w/o and anhydrous cosmetic formulations (skin care prods., sunscreens, lip, eye, or face makeup, antiperspirants, hair care prods.).

Ginkgo Biloba Dimeric Flavonoids Phytosome®. [Indena SpA; Lipo] Complex of ginkgo biloba dimeric flavonoids and soybean phospholipids; free-radical scavenger, skin toning/microcirculation stimulant, soothing/moisturizing agent for preps. for aging, dry, and chapped skin, prods. for oily comedonic skin, sun care prods., treatments for cellulitis, prods. for tonic massage; brn. amorphous powd.; water-disp.; usage level: to 3%.

Ginkgo Biloba Phytosome®. [Indena SpA; Lipo] Complex of ginkgo biloba flavonoids and soybean phospholipids; free-radical scavenger, skin toning stimulant, soothing/moisturizing agent for preps. for aging, dry and chapped skin, sun care prods., anti-aging treatments, prods. for oily comedonic skin, treatment of cellulitis, prods. for tonic massage; lt. brn. amorphous powd.; water-disp.; usage level: to 3%.

Ginseng HS. [Alban Muller] Propylene glycol and ginseng

extract; botanical extract.

Ginseng LS. [Alban Muller] Sunflower seed oil and ginseng extract.

Ginseng Extract HS 2457 G. [Grau Aromatics] Propylene glycol and ginseng extract; botanical extract.

Ginseng Glycolysat. [C.E.P.] Propylene glycol, water, and ginseng extract; botanical extract.

Ginseng Oleat M. [C.E.P.] Propylene glycol dicaprylate/dicaprate and ginseng extract.

Ginseng Phytosome® . [Indena SpA; Lipo] Complex of ginseng saponins and soybean phospholipids; soothing, moisturizing, toning, stimulant, eutrophic, firming, elasticizing conditioner for preps. for skin toning, anti-aging treatments, preps. for prevention of wrinkles and stretch marks, hair prods.; lt. brn.-yel. amorphous powd.; water-disp.; usage level: to 2%.

Ginseng Vegebios. [C.E.P.] Water and ginseng extract; CAS 90045-38-8.

Glicoceride OCS. [Vevy] Cetyl oleate; CAS 22393-86-8; EINECS 244-950-6.

Glicolene. [Vevy] Laureth-3; CAS 3055-94-5; EINECS 221-280-2; emulsifier.

Glicosterina DPG. [Vevy] PEG-2 stearate; CAS 106-11-6; EINECS 203-363-5; emulsifier.

Gloria® . [Witco/Petroleum Spec.] Wh. min. oil USP; emollient, lubricant for food, drug, and cosmetic industries; FDA §172.878, 178.3620a; water-wh., odorless, tasteless; sp.gr. 0.859-0.880; visc. 39-42 cSt (40 C); pour pt. -12 C; flash pt. 193 C.

Gluadin® AGP. [Henkel/Cospha; Henkel Canada; Henkel KGaA/Cospha] Hydrolyzed wheat protein; CAS 100684-25-1; EINECS 309-696-3; proteinaecous protective film-former providing pleasant skin feel for cosmetic emulsions and surfactant preps.; lt. colored powd., weak intrinsic odor; sol. in water; sl. sol. in 40% ethanol and IPA; m.w. 2000-25,000; pH 4.5-5.0 (10% aq.); usage level: 1-6%; 94% min. total solids.

Gluadin® Almond. [Henkel/Cospha; Henkel KGaA/Cospha] Hydrolyzed almond protein; CAS 100209-19-6; EINECS 309-327-6; veg. protein for personal care prods.; substantive to skin and hair; anti-irritancy props.; protective film-former; moisturizer; for skin care creams and lotions, facial cleansers, bath prods., skin tonics, liq. soap; for use in o/w and w/o emulsions, surfactant preps., and clear alcoholic/aq. formulations; amber clear liq., char. odor; pH 4.0-5.0 (30%); usage level: 1-5%; 24% act.

Gluadin® Wheat. [Henkel/Cospha] Hydrolyzed wheat protein; CAS 100684-25-1; veg. protein for personal care prods.; substantive to skin and hair; anti-irritancy props.; protective film-former; moisturizer; for skin care creams and lotions, mild cleansers, bath foam, body talc, liq. soap, dental care prods., shave creams; wh. hydrophilic powd., faint char. natural wheat odor; sol. in water, sl. sol. in ethanol; pH 4.5-5.0 (10%); usage level: 0.5-5%; 94% act.

Glucam® E-10. [Amerchol] Methyl gluceth-10; CAS 68239-42-9; nonionic; humectant for personal care prods.; freezing pt. depressant; emollient in aq. and hydroalcoholic prods.; moisturizer; foam modifier in detergent and shampoo systems; solv. and solubilizer for topical pharmaceuticals; film plasticizer; adds gloss, conditioning; used in emulsions, toilet articles, shampoos, shaving creams, shower gels, eye gels, facial cleansers; pale yel. med. visc. syrup; pract. odorless; sol. in water, alcohol, hydroalcoholic systems; acid no. 1.5 max.; iodine no. 1 max.; sapon. no. 1.5 max; hyd. no. 350-370; toxicology: LD50 (acute oral) > 5 ml/kg; nonirritating to eyes and skin; 100% conc.

Glucam® E-20. [Amerchol] Methyl gluceth-20; CAS 68239-43-0; humectant for personal care prods.; freezing pt. depressant; emollient in aq. and hydroalcoholic prods.;

moisturizer; foam modifier in detergent and shampoo systems; solv. and solubilizer for topical pharmaceuticals; for sunscreens, soap bars, dry skin creams, shampoos, liq. soaps; pale yel. thin syrup; pract. odorless; sol. in water, alcohol, hydroalcoholic systems; acid no. 1.0 max.; iodine no. 1 max.; sapon. no. 1.0 max.; hyd. no. 205-225; toxicology: LD50 (acute oral) > 5 ml/kg; nonirritating to eyes and skin; 100% conc.

Glucam® E-20 Distearate. [Amerchol] Methyl gluceth-20 distearate; CAS 98073-10-0; nonionic; aux. o/w emulsifier, moisturizer, emollient, conditioner, and lubricant for cosmetics and pharmaceuticals, aerosol shave creams, nonaerosol styling sprays, deodorant sticks, lip balms, creams, conditioning soaps; yel. semisolid; HLB 12.5; toxicology: LD50 (acute oral) > 5 g/kg; pract. nonirritating to eyes; not a primary skin irritant; 100% conc.

Glucam® P-10. [Amerchol] PPG-10 methyl glucose ether; nonionic; humectant for personal care prods.; freezing pt. depressant; emollient in aq. and hydroalcoholic prods.; moisturizer; foam modifier in detergent and shampoo systems; solv. and solubilizer for topical pharmaceuticals; for eye makeup removers, hair conditioners, styling prods., makeups, moisturizing creams; pale yel. heavy visc. syrups; pract. odorless; sol. in water, alcohol, hydroalcoholic systems, castor oil, IPM, IPP; visc. 8500 cps; acid no. 1.0 max.; iodine no. 1 max.; sapon. no. 1.0 max.; hyd. no. 285-305; toxicology: LD50 (acute oral) > 5 ml/kg; nonirritating to skin; mild transient irritation to eyes; 100% conc.

Glucam® P-20. [Amerchol] PPG-20 methyl glucose ether; nonionic; humectant for personal care prods.; freezing pt. depressant; emollient in aq. and hydroalcoholic prods.; moisturizer; foam modifier in detergent and shampoo systems; solv. and solubilizer for topical pharmaceuticals; for face cleansing toners, nail conditioners, fragrances, aftershaves; pale yel. med. visc. syrup; pract. odorless; sol. in water, alcohol, and hydroalcoholic systems, castor oil, IPM, IPP; visc. 1700 cps; acid no. 1.0 max.; iodine no. 1 max.; sapon. no. 1.0 max.; hyd. no. 160-180; toxicology: LD50 (acute oral) > 3 ml/kg; nonirritating to skin; mild transient irritation to eyes; 100% conc.

Glucam® P-20 Distearate. [Amerchol] PPG-20 methyl glucose ether distearate; skin moisturizer, conditioner, slip agent, and emollient for cosmetics and pharmaceuticals (dry skin creams, cream makeup, moisturizing lotions); binder and plasticizer for pressed powds.; barrier to reduce water loss from stratum corneum; pale amber liq.; sol. in IPM, castor oil, corn oil, ethanol, hot min. oil; insol. in water, propylene glycol, aq. ethanol; acid no. 2.5 max.; sapon. no. 58-72; hyd. no. 50-70; flash pt. (COC) 545 F; toxicology: LD50 (acute oral) > 5 g/kg; not a primary skin irritant; pract. nonirritating to eyes.

Glucamate® DOE-120. [Amerchol] PEG-120 methyl glucoside dioleate; nonionic; thickener, emulsifier, solubilizer for shampoos, baby shampoos, liq. hand soaps; reduces irritation of surfactants; lt. yel. waxy solid, faint char. odor; water-sol.; flash pt. (COC) 695 F; acid no. 1 max.; iodine no. 5-15; hyd. no. 14-26; sapon. no. 14-26; pH 4.5-7.5 (10% aq.); toxicology: LD50 (acute oral) > 5 g/kg; not a primary skin irritant; nonirritating to eyes; 100% conc.

Glucamate® MLE-80. [Amerchol] PEG-80 methyl glucose laurate.

Glucamate® SSE-20. [Amerchol; Amerchol Europe] PEG-20 methyl glucose sesquistearate; CAS 68389-70-8; nonionic; o/w emulsifier, solubilizer used with Glucate SS; cleanser, stabilizer for pigmented makeup suspensions; for hand/body lotions, skin care prods., mild facial creams, eye makeup removers; effective at low concs.; pale yel. soft solid; sol. in water, IPA, ethanol, castor oil, corn oil; HLB 15.0; cloud pt. 74 C (1% in 5% NaCl); flash pt. 570 F

(OC); sapon. no. 47; pH 6.5 (10% aq.); toxicology: LD50 (acute oral) > 5 g/kg; mild transient eye irritant; not a primary skin irritant; 100% conc.

Glucate® DO. [Amerchol; Amerchol Europe] Methyl glucose dioleate; CAS 83933-91-3; nonionic; w/o emulsifier, aux. emulsifier for o/w systems; conditioner, emollient, lubricant, plasticizer, and pigment dispersant; lubricant for molded stick prods.; for dry skin and night creams, sunscreens, lipstick, makeup, pressed powds., skin gels; amber visc. liq.; HLB 5.0; toxicology: LD50 (acute oral) > 5 g/kg; nonirritating to eyes; not a primary skin irritant; 100% conc.

Glucate® IS. [Amerchol] Methyl glucose sesquiisostearate; nonionic; primary w/o emulsifier adding lubricious/satiny feel to personal care prods.; for skin creams, lotions, and mousses, makeup, dry skin and night creams, sunscreen lotions; pale amber syrup, sl. char. odor; sol. in min. oil, IPM; disp. in castor oil, corn oil, glycerin; insol. in water, ethanol, IPA; HLB 6.0; toxicology: LD50 (acute oral) > 5 g/kg; moderate skin irritation, minimal eye irritation; 100% act.

Glucate® ML. [Amerchol] Methyl glucose laurate.

Glucate® SS. [Amerchol; Amerchol Europe] Methyl glucose sesquistearate; CAS 68936-95-8; EINECS 273-049-0; nonionic; w/o emulsifier used with Glucamate SSE-20 to provide visc. stability, mildness; mild barrier supplement for moisture retention in topicals; for hand/body lotions, skin care prods., mild lotions, emulsion makeups; off wh. flakes; sol. in IPA, misc. with common oil phase ingred., water insol.; m.p. 51 C; HLB 6.0; flash pt. 530 F (OC); sapon. no. 136; pH 5.5 (10% in 1:1 IPA:water); toxicology: LD50 (acute oral) > 5 g/kg; nonirritating to eyes; not a primary skin irritant; 100% conc.

Gluconal® CA A. [Akzo Chemie] Calcium gluconate anhydrous; CAS 299-28-5; EINECS 206-075-8; pharmaceutical/food grade mineral source for human and veterinary pharmaceutical preps., dietary supplements, fortified foods and animal feed; wh. powd.; sol. 30 g/l water; m.w. 430.4; bulk dens. 250-350 kg/m³; pH 7.4 (1%); toxicology: LD50 (oral, rat) > 5000 mg/kg; 95-100% act.

Gluconal® CA M. [Akzo Chemie] Calcium gluconate monohydrate; CAS 299-28-5; EINECS 206-075-8; pharmaceutical/food grade mineral source for human and veterinary pharmaceutical preps., dietary supplements, fortified foods and animal feed; wh. powd./gran.; sol. 40 g/l water; m.w. 448.4; bulk dens. 300-650 kg/m³; pH 7.5 (1%); toxicology: LD50 (oral, rat) > 5000 mg/kg; 98.5-100% act.

Gluconal® CA M B. [Akzo Chemie] Calcium borogluconate; pharmaceutical/food grade mineral source for human and veterinary pharmaceutical preps., dietary supplements, fortified foods and animal feed; wh. powd.; sol. 200 g/l water; m.w. 448.4 + 61.8; bulk dens. 550-650 kg/m³; pH 5.1 (1%); toxicology: LD50 (oral, rat) > 2000 mg/kg; 82-89% act.

Gluconal® CO. [Akzo Chemie] Cobalt gluconate; pharmaceutical/food grade mineral source for human and veterinary pharmaceutical preps., dietary supplements, fortified foods and animal feed; pink powd.; sol. 200 g/l water; m.w. 449.3; bulk dens. 450-550 kg/m³; pH 6.5 (1%); toxicology: LD50 (oral, rat) 1420 mg/kg; 88-100% act.

Gluconal® CU. [Akzo Chemie] Copper gluconate; CAS 527-09-3; EINECS 208-408-2; pharmaceutical/food grade mineral source for human and veterinary pharmaceutical preps., dietary supplements, fortified foods and animal feed; lt. blue powd.; sol. 500 g/l water; m.w. 453.8; bulk dens. 450-550 kg/m³; pH 4.6 (1%); toxicology: LD50 (oral, rat) 1710 mg/kg; 98-100% act.

Gluconal® FE. [Akzo Chemie] Ferrous gluconate; CAS 299-29-6; pharmaceutical/food grade mineral source for human and veterinary pharmaceutical preps., dietary

supplements, fortified foods and animal feed; yel.-gray powd./gran.; sol. 100 g/l water; m.w. 446.1; bulk dens. 650-850 kg/m³; pH 4.5 (1%); toxicology: LD50 (oral, rat) 4600 mg/kg; 87.5-95% act.

Gluconal® K. [Akzo Chemie] Potassium gluconate; CAS 299-27-4; EINECS 206-074-2; pharmaceutical/food grade mineral source for human and veterinary pharmaceutical preps., dietary supplements, fortified foods and animal feed; wh. powd./gran.; sol. 1000 g/l water; m.w. 234.3; bulk dens. 500-650 kg/m³; pH 7.1 (1%); toxicology: LD50 (oral, rat) 6060 mg/kg; 95-100% act.

Gluconal® MG. [Akzo Chemie] Magnesium gluconate; CAS 3632-91-5; EINECS 222-848-2; pharmaceutical/food grade mineral source for human and veterinary pharmaceutical preps., dietary supplements, fortified foods and animal feed; wh. powd./gran.; sol. 160 g/l water; m.w. 414.6; bulk dens. 500-750 kg/m³; pH 7.3 (1%); toxicology: LD50 (oral, rat) 9100 mg/kg; 86-99% act.

Gluconal® MN. [Akzo Chemie] Manganese gluconate; CAS 6485-39-8; EINECS 229-350-4; pharmaceutical/food grade mineral source for human and veterinary pharmaceutical preps., dietary supplements, fortified foods and animal feed; off-wh. powd.; sol. 110 g/l water; m.w. 445.2; bulk dens. 700-800 kg/m³; pH 6.4 (1%); toxicology: LD50 (oral, rat) 5850 mg/kg; 90.5-100% act.

Gluconal® NA. [Akzo Chemie] Sodium gluconate; CAS 527-07-1; EINECS 208-407-7; pharmaceutical/food grade mineral source for human and veterinary pharmaceutical preps., dietary supplements, fortified foods and animal feed; wh. powd./gran.; sol. 600 g/l water; m.w. 218.1; bulk dens. 600-780 kg/m³; pH 6.9 (1%); toxicology: LD50 (oral, rat) > 5000 mg/kg; 98-100% act.

Gluconal® ZN. [Akzo Chemie] Zinc gluconate; CAS 4468-02-4; pharmaceutical/food grade mineral source for human and veterinary pharmaceutical preps., dietary supplements, fortified foods and animal feed; wh. powd./gran.; sol. 100 g/l water; m.w. 455.7; bulk dens. 600-800 kg/m³; pH 6.5 (1%); toxicology: LD50 (oral, rat) > 5000 mg/kg; 85.5-100% act.

Glucquat® 100. [Amerchol] Lauryl methyl gluceth-10 hydroxypropyl dimonium chloride.

Glucquat® 125. [Amerchol] Lauryl methyl gluceth-10 hydroxypropyldimonium chloride; substantive conditioner, humectant, and moisturizer for hair and skin care prods.; for hand lotions, shampoos, dry skin creams, conditioning cream rinses, hair styling prods., soap bars and liqs.; pale yel. med. visc. liq., sl. char. odor; sol. in water, ethanol, glycerin; insol. in min. oil, IPP; visc. < 10 cps; pH 5.5-6.5 (10% aq.); surf. tens. 33.8 dynes/cm (0.25% aq.); toxicology: LD50 (acute oral) > 2.4 ml/kg; mild transient eye irritation, not a primary skin irritant; 25% solids max.

Glucuron. [Ursa-Chemie] Urea-d-glucuronic acid.

Gluplex® AC. [Kelisema Srl] Native wheat protein/cocoyl carboxylate complex; protein contributing mild detergency to cosmetics and low-irritation bar soaps and medicinal soaps; protects against surfactant irritancy; yel. clear to hazy liq, sl. char. odor; sol. in water @ pH 9-11; pH 9-10; usage level: 2-10%.

Gluplex® LES. [Kelisema Srl] Native wheat protein/lauryl ether sulfate complex; protein contributing mild detergency to cosmetics and low-irritation hygiene prods. (cleansing creams, bubble baths, soaps/syndets, emollient baths, hair conditioners, shampoos, baby prods., shave creams), toothpastes, skin-friendly dishwash; protects against surfactant irritancy; yel. clear liq, sl. char. odor; sol. in water; pH 5-6; usage level: 1-10%.

Gluplex® LS. [Kelisema Srl] Native wheat protein/lauryl sulfate complex; protein contributing mild detergency to cosmetics and low-irritation hygiene prods. (cleansing bars, bubble baths, soaps/syndets, emollient baths, hair conditioners, shampoos, baby prods., shave creams), toothpastes, skin-friendly dishwash; protects against surfactant irritancy; yel. clear liq, sl. char. odor; sol. in water; pH 5-6; usage level: 1-10%.

Gluplex® OS. [Kelisema Srl] Native wheat protein/C14-16 olefin sulfonate complex; protein contributing mild detergency to cosmetics and low-irritation hygiene prods. (cleansing creams, bubble baths, soaps/syndets, emollient baths, hair conditioners, shampoos, baby prods., shave creams), toothpastes, skin-friendly dishwash; protects against surfactant irritancy; yel. clear liq, sl. char. odor; sol. in water; pH 5-6; usage level: 1-10%.

Glusol. [Kelisema Srl] Hydrolyzed wheat gluten; substantivity agent, moisturizer skin protective emulsions, hair restoring and protective treatments, shampoos, conditioners, cleansers; reduces irritation of surfactants; yel. transparent liq. or wh. odorless powd.; water-sol.; pH 4-6; toxicology: nontoxic.

Glycacil L, S. [Lonza] Iodopropynyl butylcarbamate; CAS 55406-53-6; EINECS 259-627-5; preservative for cosmetics; effective fungicide; temp. stable to 105 C; stable at pH 3-10; USA, Japan, Europe approved; liq.; sol. in oil, water, polar org. compds.; usage level: 0.1-1.0%.

Glycerox HE. [Croda Chem. Ltd.] PEG-7 glyceryl cocoate; emulsifier, solubilizer, emollient for cosmetics; liq.; HLB 11.0.

Glycerox L8. [Croda Chem. Ltd.] PEG-8 glyceryl laurate; nonionic; emulsifier for cosmetic preparation; liq.; HLB 11.0; 100% conc.

Glycerox L15. [Croda Chem. Ltd.] PEG-15 glyceryl laurate; CAS 59070-56-3; nonionic; solubilizer and emulsifier for cosmetics; liq.; HLB 14.0; 100% conc.

Glycerox L30. [Croda Chem. Ltd.] PEG-30 glyceryl laurate; CAS 59070-56-3; emulsifier.

Glycerox L40. [Croda Chem. Ltd.] PEG-40 glyceryl laurate; nonionic; emulsifier for cosmetics; soft paste; HLB 17.0; 100% conc.

Glyceryl Behenate WL 251. [Gattefosse] Glyceryl behenate.

Glyceryl Myristate WL 2130. [Gattefosse] Glyceryl myristate; CAS 589-68-4; cosmetic emulsifier.

Glyco/Cer. [Intergen; Tri-K Industries] Sphingolipids and phospholipids; contains BHT; CAS 85116-74-1; a naturally occurring glycoceramide; incorporated in skin care prods., allows hydrophilic and hydrophobic materials to traverse the stratum corneum; helps replenish intercorneal lipids lost due to environmental stress; wh. to cream-colored powd., char. odor; usage level: 0.025-0.075%; toxicology: nonirritating to eyes; nonprimary irritant to skin; orally nontoxic; 40% glycoceramides.

Glyco/Cer HA. [Intergen; Tri-K Industries] 1% Glyco/Cer (sphingolipids, phospholipids) in 0.5% hyaluronic acid emulsion with preservatives; forms hydrated viscoealstic film for moisturizing and protecting skin against aggressive agents; results in smooth, nongreasy feel on skin; imparts softness; for aq. creams and lotions; wh. to off-wh. visc. liq., char. odor; sp.gr. 0.98-1.01; pH 6.5±0.5; usage level: 2.5-7.5%; 0.40% glycoceramides.

Glyco/Cer HALA. [Intergen; Tri-K Industries] Linoleic acid (1%), hyaluronic acid (0.5%), sphingolipids, and phospholipids emulsion with preservatives; repairs barrier function in detergent-treated skin; for cosmetic creams and lotions; wh. visc. liq., char. odor; sp.gr. 0.99-1.02; pH 6.0±0.5; usage level: 2.5-7.5%; 0.40% glycoceramides.

Glycoderm. [Dr. Kurt Richter; Henkel/Cospha] Sphingolipid liposomes with glycosaminoglycans and phospholipids; prep. for dry and cracked skin; for restoration of the lipid barrier of the stratum corneum; ivory nontransparent suspension.

Glycol 1000 Succinate. [Eastman] d-α Tocopheryl polyeth-

ylene; CAS 9002-96-4; natural vitamin E source for cosmetics.

Glycoliv. [Pentapharm Ltd; Centerchem] Water and liver extract.

Glycolysat de Camomille. [C.E.P.] Propylene glycol, water, and chamomile extract; botanical extract.

Glycolysat de Ginseng. [C.E.P.] Propylene glycol, water, and ginseng extract; botanical extract.

Glycolysat de Houblon. [C.E.P.] Propylene glycol, water, and hops extract; botanical extract.

Glycolysat de Placenta bovin. [C.E.P.] Propylene glycol and placental protein; cosmetic ingred.

Glycomul® L. [Lonza] Sorbitan laurate; CAS 1338-39-2; nonionic; emulsifier for edible, cosmetic, industrial, pharmaceutical uses; antistat, antifog for PVC; amber liq.; sol. in methanol, ethanol, naphtha; sp.gr. 1.0; visc. 4500 cps; HLB 8.6; acid no. 5; sapon. no. 157-171; 100% conc.

Glycomul® O. [Lonza] Sorbitan oleate; CAS 1338-43-8; EINECS 215-665-4; nonionic; emulsifier for cosmetic, pharmaceutical, and industrial applics.; amber liq.; sol. in ethyl acetate, min. and veg. oils, disp. in water; sp.gr. 1.0; visc. 1000 cps.; HLB 4.3; sapon. no. 148-161; 100% conc.

Glycomul® P. [Lonza] Sorbitan palmitate; CAS 26266-57-9; EINECS 247-568-8; nonionic; emulsifier for cosmetic, pharmaceutical, and industrial applics.; cream beads; sol. in veg. and min. oil, ethyl acetate, ethanol, acetone, toluol; HLB 6.7; sapon. no. 139-150; 100% conc.

Glycomul® S. [Lonza] Sorbitan stearate (also avail. in veg. and kosher grade); CAS 1338-41-6; EINECS 215-664-9; nonionic; emulsifier for cosmetic, pharmaceutical, and industrial applics.; antistat for PVC; cream beads; sol. in veg. oil; HLB 5.0; sapon. no. 146-158; 100% conc.

Glycomul® S FG. [Lonza] Sorbitan stearate; CAS 1338-41-6; EINECS 215-664-9; nonionic; emulsifier for food, cosmetic, household and industrial use; Gardner 5 beads; m.p. 53 C; HLB 5; acid no. 5.

Glycomul® S KFG. [Lonza] Sorbitan stearate; CAS 1338-41-6; EINECS 215-664-9; nonionic; emulsifier for food, cosmetic, household and industrial prods.; Gardner 5 beads; m.p. 53 C; HLB 5; acid no. 5.

Glycomul® SOC. [Lonza] Sorbitan sesquioleate; CAS 8007-43-0; EINECS 232-360-1; nonionic; emulsifier for cosmetic, pharmaceutical, and industrial applics.; cream beads; sol. in methanol, ethanol, ethyl acetate; sp.gr. 1.0; visc. 1000 cps; HLB 4.0; sapon. no. 149-166; 100% conc.

Glycomul® TO. [Lonza] Sorbitan trioleate; CAS 26266-58-0; EINECS 247-569-3; nonionic; emulsifier for cosmetic, pharmaceutical, and industrial applics.; amber, oily liq.; sol. in ethyl acetate, toluol, naphtha, min. and veg. oils, disp. in water; sp.gr. 0.95; visc. 200 cps; HLB 1.8; sapon. no. 171-185; 100% conc.

Glycomul® TS. [Lonza] Sorbitan tristearate; CAS 26658-19-5; EINECS 247-891-4; nonionic; emulsifier for cosmetic, pharmaceutical, and industrial applics.; lt. tan beads; poorly sol. in ethyl acetate, toluol, disp. in acetone, naphtha, min. and veg. oils; HLB 2.1; sapon. no. 175-190; 100% conc.

Glycomul® TS KFG. [Lonza] Sorbitan tristearate; CAS 26658-19-5; EINECS 247-891-4; nonionic; emulsifier for food, cosmetic, household and industrial applics.; Gardner 2 beads; m.p. 55 C; HLB 2; acid no. 14.

Glycon® G 100. [Lonza] Glycerin; CAS 56-81-5; EINECS 200-289-5; humectant, bodying agent, moisture control agent for toothpaste, cosmetics, sugarless confections, controlled moisture foods and industrial applics.; sp.gr. 1.2607; 99.5% act.

Glycon® G-300. [Lonza] Glycerin; CAS 56-81-5; EINECS 200-289-5; humectant, bodying agent, moisture control agent for toothpaste, cosmetics, sugarless confections, controlled moisture foods and industrial applics.; sp.gr. 1.2517; 96% act.

Glycoproteins from Milk. [Sederma] Hydrolyzed casein; CAS 65072-00-6; EINECS 265-363-1; cosmetic protein.

Glycosome. [Pentapharm Ltd; Centerchem] Water, phospholipids, sphingolipids, and cholesterol; cosmetic ingred.

Glycosperse® HTO-40. [Lonza] PEG-40 sorbitan hexatallate; emulsifier for food, cosmetic, household or industrial applics.; Gardner 7 liq.; HLB 10; acid no. 10.

Glycosperse® L-10. [Lonza] PEG-10 sorbitan laurate; CAS 9005-64-5; emulsifier for food, cosmetic, household or industrial applics.; Gardner 5 liq.; HLB 8; acid no. 2.

Glycosperse® L-20. [Lonza] Polysorbate 20; CAS 9005-64-5; 9062-73-1; nonionic; emulsifier for food, cosmetic, pharmaceutical, and industrial uses; flavor solubilizer and dispersant; yel. liq.; sol. in water, alcohol, acetone; sp.gr. 1.1; visc. 400 cps; HLB 16.7; sapon. no. 39–52; 100% conc.

Glycosperse® O-5. [Lonza] Polysorbate 81; CAS 9005-65-6; nonionic; flavor solubilizer and dispersant; emulsifier for cosmetic, pharmaceutical, and industrial use; amber liq.; sol. in alcohol, ethyl acetate, min. oil; disp. in water; sp.gr. 1.0; visc. 450 cps; HLB 10.0; sapon. no. 95–105; 100% conc.

Glycosperse® O-20. [Lonza] Polysorbate 80; CAS 9005-65-6; nonionic; emulsifier for food, cosmetic, pharmaceutical, and industrial uses; flavor solubilizer and dispersant; also antifog for PVC; yel. liq.; sol. in water, alcohol, ethyl acetate, toluol, veg. oil; sp.gr. 1.0; visc. 400 cps; HLB 15; sapon. no. 44–56; 100% conc.

Glycosperse® P-20. [Lonza] Polysorbate 40; CAS 9005-66-7; nonionic; emulsifier for food, cosmetic, pharmaceutical, and industrial uses; flavor solubilizer and dispersant; yel. liq.; sol. in water, methanol, ethanol, acetone, ethyl acetate; sp.gr. 1.0; visc. 550 cps; HLB 15.6; sapon. no. 40–53; 100% conc.

Glycosperse® S-20. [Lonza] Polysorbate 60; CAS 9005-67-8; nonionic; emulsifier for food, cosmetic, pharmaceutical, and industrial uses; flavor solubilizer and dispersant; yel. liq.; sol. in water, ethyl acetate, toluol; sp.gr. 1.1; HLB 15.0; sapon. no. 44–56; 100% conc.

Glycosperse® TO-20. [Lonza] Polysorbate 85; CAS 9005-70-3; nonionic; emulsifier for food, cosmetic, pharmaceutical, and industrial uses; flavor solubilizer and dispersant; yel. liq., gels on standing; sol. in ethanol, methanol, ethyl acetate; water disp.; sp.gr. 1.0; visc. 300 cps; HLB 11.0; sapon. no. 82–95; 100% conc.

Glycosperse® TS-20. [Lonza] Polysorbate 65; CAS 9005-71-4; nonionic; emulsifier for food, cosmetic, pharmaceutical, and industrial uses; flavor solubilizer and dispersant; tan waxy solid; sol. in ethanol, methanol, acetone, ethyl acetate, naphtha, min. and veg. oils; disp. water, toluol; sp.gr. 1.05; HLB 11.0; sapon. no. 88–98; 100% conc.

Glycyrrhetinic Acid Phytosome® . [Indena SpA; Lipo] Complex of 18β-glycyrrhetinic acid and soybean phospholipids; skin protectant with smoothing, soothing, moisturizing props.; coadjuvant in treatment of wrinkles and stretch marks, treatment of sensitive, chapped, irritated skin, after-sun, after-depilation, and after-shave prods.; baby toiletries, dentifrices for sensitive gums, prods. for oral cavity and lip protection; lt. yel. amorphous powd.; water-disp.; usage level: to 3%.

Glydant®. [Lonza] DMDM hydantoin in water; CAS 6440-58-0; EINECS 229-222-8; preservative, broad spectrum antimicrobial for cosmetics and toiletries; effective against Gram-positive and Gram-negative bacteria, fungi, and yeast; water-wh. liq., sl. formaldehyde odor; sol. in water and ethanol; sp.gr. 1.1579 ± 0.0026; f.p. -11 ± 0.6 C; pH 6.5–7.5.; contains 2% max. formaldehyde; usage level:

0.05-0.5%; toxicology: LD50 (oral, rat) 3300 mg/kg; mild skin, eye, and mucous membrane irritant.

Glydant® Plus. [Lonza] DMDM hydantoin, iodopropynyl butylcarbamate; high performance, broad-spectrum personal care preservative; heat stable at 80 C for 6 h; stable at pH 3-10; USA, Japan, and Europe approvals; powd.; m.p. 93 C; usage level: 0.03-0.3%; 100% act.

Glydant® XL-1000. [Lonza] DMDM hydantoin; CAS 6440-58-0; EINECS 229-222-8; preservative for personal care prods.; powd.; m.p. 95 C; usage level: 0.05-0.5%; 100% act.

Glyprosol™ 20. [Brooks Industries] Yeast glycoproteins; natural skin smoothing protein; m.w. 30,000.

Glyprosol™ SD. [Brooks Industries] Yeast glycoproteins; natural skin smoothing protein; powd.; 30% conc.

Golden Dawn Grade 1, 2. [Westbrook Lanolin] Anhyd. lanolin; CAS 8006-54-0; EINECS 232-348-6; nonionic; emollient, w/o emulsifier, ointment base, hair conditioner, wax crystal inhibitor, lipstick binder; soft wax, Grade 2 slightly darker color.

Golden-Pea-Pro™ EN-15. [Brooks Industries] Hydrolyzed golden-pea protein; cosmetic ingredient for skin and hair care prods.; m.w. 1000; 15% act.

Gomme Xanthane. [Laserson SA] Xanthan gum; CAS 11138-66-2; EINECS 234-394-2; thickener, stabilizer, and suspending agent for cosmetics; JCID, USA, and Europe approvals; creamy wh. powd.; sol. in water; insol. in oils and most org. solvs.; usage level: 0.1-0.5%.

GP-4 Silicone Fluid. [Genesee Polymers] Amodimethicone; intermediate for synthesis of silicone/org. copolymers used in textiles, coatings car polishes; also in lubricant, coating and mold release formulations; cosmetic and personal care applics. incl. hair care.

GP-71-SS Mercapto Modified Silicone Fluid. [Genesee Polymers] Dimethicone/mercaptopropyl methicone copolymer; plastic and rubber release agent; internal lubricant and release agent for sulfur and peroxide cure rubber; coreactant in vinyl polymerization; synthesis of org./silicone copolymers; heat stabilizer; in corrosion inhibitor coatings, inks; cosmetic and personal care applics. incl. hair care.

GP-209 Silicone Polyol Copolymer. [Genesee Polymers] Dimethicone copolyol; nonionic; emulsifier, wetting agent, pigment dispersant, leveling agent, profoaming additive for PU foams, hard surf. cleaners, polishes, cosmetic formulations; inverse sol. suggests use as defoamer for hot aq. surfactant sol'ns.; lt. straw clear liq.; sol. in water; m.w. 7800; sp.gr. 1.03; dens. 8.5 lb/gal; visc. 2600 cst; f.p. -50 F; flash pt. (PMCC) > 300 F; 100% act., 15% silicone.

GP-215 Silicone Polyol Copolymer. [Genesee Polymers] Dimethicone copolyol; emulsifier, wetting agent, pigment dispersant, leveling agent, profoaming additive for PU foams, hard surf. cleaners, polishes, cosmetics; inverse sol. suggests use as defoamer for hot aq. surfactant sol'ns.; cosmetic and personal care applics. incl. hair care; lt. straw clear liq.; sol. in water; m.w. 9800; sp.gr. 1.03; dens. 8.5 lb/gal; visc. 2000 cst; f.p. -50 F; flash pt. (PMCC) > 300 F; 100% act., 18% silicone.

GP-217 Silicone Polyol Copolymer. [Genesee Polymers] Dimethicone copolyol; wetting agent, emulsifier for water-based coatings, inks, polishes, hard surf. cleaners; dispersant for clays, pigments; thread lubricant; leveling and flow control agent; profoaming additive in aq. systems; cosmetic and personal care applics. incl. hair care; lt. straw clear liq.; sol. in water; m.w. 3800; sp.gr. 1.05; dens. 8.75 lb/gal; visc. 240 cst; f.p. 65 F; flash pt. (PMCC) > 300 F; 100% act., 33% silicone.

GP-218. [Genesee Polymers] Dimethylpolysiloxane PO block copolymer; wetting, leveling, flow control agent, lubricant for solv.-based coatings, industrial finishes; profoamer additive in PU foams; textile and thread lubricants; internal lubricant for plastics; base for aq. defoamers; pigment dispersant; release agent; cosmetic and personal care applics. incl. hair care; colorless clear liq.; sol. in aliphatic, aromatic, and chlorinated hydrocarbons, alcohols; insol. in water; m.w. 11,000; sp.gr. 0.98; dens. 8.0 lb/gal; visc. 1500 cst; f.p. 65 F; flash pt. (CC) > 300 F; 100% act., 32% silicone.

GP-226. [Genesee Polymers] Dimethicone copolyol; wetting agent, emulsifier for water-based coatings, inks, polishes, hard surf. cleaners; pigment/clay dispersant; thread lubricant; leveling and flow control agent; profoaming additive for aq. systems; cosmetic and personal care applics. incl. hair care; lt. straw clear liq.; disp. in water; m.w. 4340; sp.gr. 1.03; dens. 8.5 lb/gal; visc. 150 cst; f.p. 32 F; flash pt. (PMCC) > 300 F; 100% act., 42% silicone.

GPC. [Rhone-Poulenc Rorer] sn-Glycero(3)phosphocholine; CAS 28319-77-9; natural raw material for pharmaceuticals; cryst.

GP-RA-157 Amine Functional Silicone Fluid. [Genesee Polymers] Dimethoxysilyl ethylenediaminopropyl dimethicone; CAS 71750-80-6.

Granamine S3A. [Grant Industries] Marine plant and animal extracts; complex for cosmetic preps.; nutrient, moisturizer, revitalizer, softener for skin and hair care prods., moisturizing creams, nutrient creams/lotions, anticellulitis prods., face mask, aftershaves, sunburn creams/lotions; protects skin and hair from harmful environmental effects; amber transparent liq., sl. char. odor; sol. in water; sp.gr. 1.128-1.133; pH 7.0 ± 0.3 (10% aq.); usage level: 1.0-5.0%; 36% min. total solids, 6.1% min. act. protein.

Grancol SP-01. [Grant Industries] Soluble collagen; CAS 9007-34-5; EINECS 232-697-4; protein for cosmetic creams, lotions, tonics, masks, etc.; water-wh. sl. opaque visc. liq., typ. odor; pH 3.5 ± 0.3; toxicology: nonirritating/ nonsensitizing to skin and eyes; 1.0-1.4% total solids, 0.8% min. act. collagen.

Granlastin 10%. [Grant Industries] Soluble elastin; protein for cosmetic creams, lotions, tonics, masks, etc.; lt. yel. liq., sl. char. odor; pH 6 ± 0.5; toxicology: nonirritating/ nonsensitizing to skin and eyes; 9.5% min. solids, 7.3% min. act. elastin.

Granoliq. Wheat Germ Extract, Water soluble. [Novarom GmbH] Propylene glycol and wheat germ extract; botanical extract.

Granosol 25. [Variati] Hydrolyzed wheat protein; CAS 70084-87-6; cosmetic protein.

Granosol 100. [Variati] Hydrolyzed wheat protein; CAS 70084-87-6; cosmetic protein.

Granpro-5. [Grant Industries] Hydrolyzed collagen; CAS 9015-54-7; cosmetic protein.

Granpro-10. [Grant Industries] TEA-coco-hydrolyzed collagen; CAS 68952-16-9.

Granpro-40, -50, -55, -100. [Grant Industries] Hydrolyzed collagen; CAS 9015-54-7; cosmetic protein.

Granquat S. [Grant Industries] Steartrimonium hydrolyzed animal protein; CAS 111174-62-0; cationic; provides lubricity, smoothness, manageability, and substantivity to hair and skin conditioners, skin creams and lotions, cream rinses, shampoos, liq. soaps; lt. amber liq., sl. char. odor; pH 6.0 ± 0.5 (10%); 40 ± 2% total solids.

Gransil DM-100. [Grant Industries] Trifluoromethyl C1-4 alkyl dimethicone.

Gransil DMG-6. [Grant Industries] Dimethicone and organopolysiloxane; colorless translucent paste; 93 ± 2% NV.

Gransil FL-D 55. [Grant Industries] Silicone fluid containing trifluoroalkyl groups; provides water resistance and lubricity to cosmetic protective creams (liq. glove), suntan

creams/lotions, and body lotions; liq.; sp.gr. 0.98-1.02; visc. 100 cs; ref. index 1.398-1.402; 97% NV.

Gransil GCM. [Grant Industries] Octamethylcyclotetrasiloxane and organopolysiloxane; emollient; colorless to transparent paste; 10% max. NV.

Gransurf 71. [Grant Industries] Dimethicone copolyol; surfactant with exc. wettability, foam chars., and after-feel on skin and hair; for high quality hair and skin care cosmetics; pale ylsh. liq., nearly odorless; sp.gr. 1.06; visc. 100 cs; HLB 14.5; cloud pt. 65 C; ref. index 1.456.

Gransurf 72. [Grant Industries] Dimethicone copolyol; surfactant with exc. wettability, foam chars., and after-feel on skin and hair; for high quality hair and skin care cosmetics; pale ylsh. liq., nearly odorless; sp.gr. 1.03; visc. 1600 cs; HLB 7.0; cloud pt. 35 C; ref. index 1.446.

Gransurf 73. [Grant Industries] Dimethicone copolyol; surfactant with exc. wettability, foam chars., and after-feel on skin and hair; for high quality hair and skin care cosmetics; pale ylsh. liq., nearly odorless; sp.gr. 1.03; visc. 400 cs; HLB 10.0; ref. index 1.436.

Gransurf 75. [Grant Industries] Dimethicone copolyol; surfactant with exc. wettability, foam chars., and after-feel on skin and hair; for high quality hair and skin care cosmetics; pale ylsh. liq., nearly odorless; sp.gr. 1.00; visc. 220 cs; HLB 4.5; ref. index 1.420.

Gransurf 76. [Grant Industries] Dimethicone copolyol; surfactant with exc. wettability, foam chars., and after-feel on skin and hair; for high quality hair and skin care cosmetics; pale ylsh. liq., nearly odorless; sp.gr. 1.01; visc. 150 cs; HLB 4.5; ref. index 1.417.

Gransurf 77. [Grant Industries] Dimethicone copolyol; surfactant with exc. wettability, foam chars., and after-feel on skin and hair; for high quality hair and skin care cosmetics; pale ylsh. liq., nearly odorless; sp.gr. 1.01; visc. 600 cs; HLB 4.5; ref. index 1.420.

Granular Hennegg Albumen Type G-1. [Henningsen Foods] Albumen; CAS 9006-50-2.

Green Clay. [Alban Muller] Montmorillonite; CAS 1318-93-0; EINECS 215-288-5; thickener for cosmetics.

Grhetinol-O. [Maruzen Fine Chems.] Glycyrrhetinyl stearate.

Grillocam E10. [Grillo-Werke AG; R.I.T.A.] Methyl gluceth-10; CAS 68239-42-9; emulsifier, skin moisturizer and emollient imparting a smooth and gentle skin feel to cosmetic formulations; improves lather consistency of bar soaps and surfactants; reduces f.p. and enhances stability; used for creams, lotions, aftershaves, eau de toilet and bar soaps; extremely milkd to skin and eyes; pale yel. visc. liq.; sol. in water and alcohol; acid no. 1 max.; iodine no. 1 max.; sapon. no. 3 max.; hyd. no. 350-370; usage level: 1-5%; toxicology: LD50 (oral, rat) > 2000 mg/kg; nonirritating to skin and eyes.

Grillocam E20. [Grillo-Werke AG; R.I.T.A.] Methyl gluceth-20; CAS 68239-43-0; emulsifier, skin moisturizer and emollient imparting a smooth and gentle skin feel to cosmetic formulations; improves lather consistency of bar soaps and surfactants; used for creams, lotions, aftershaves, eau de toilet and bar soaps; extremely mild to skin and eyes; pale yel. visc. liq.; sol. in water and alcohol; acid no. 1 max.; iodine no. 1 max.; sapon. no. 3 max.; hyd. no. 205-225; usage level: 1-5%; toxicology: LD50 (oral, rat) > 2000 mg/kg; nonirritating to skin and eyes.

Grillocin® AT Basis. [Grillo-Werke AG; R.I.T.A.] Zinc ricinoleate, propylene glycol, disodium PEG-8 ricinosuccinate, PEG-7 glyceryl cocoate, glycerin, triethanolamine; raw material for personal care prods.; absorbent for malodorous materials; deodorant for antiperspirants, esp. those containing aluminum chlorhydrate; ivory solid; dens. 1.04 g/cc; iodine no. 55 ± 7; sapon. no. 133 ± 7;

iodine no. 55 ± 5; pH 7.0 ± 0.5 (1% in ethanol); usage level: 1.5-3.0%; toxicology: LD50 (oral, rat) > 5000 mg/kg; sl. skin irritant; moderate eye irritant; nonsensitizing; 98% act.; 6.1 ± 0.2% zinc.

Grillocin® CW 90. [Grillo-Werke AG; R.I.T.A.] Zinc ricinoleate, tetrahydroxypropyl ethylenediamine, laureth-3, propylene glycol; raw material for personal care prods.; deodorant for aerosols, creams, pump sprays, roll-ons, soaps, and sticks; cleansing agent for liq. and bar soaps; 96% biodeg.; amber visc. liq.; dens. 1.01 ± 0.05 g/cc; iodine no. 55 ± 10; pH 8.0 ± 0.5 (1% in ethanol); do not store below 5 C; usage level: 1.5-3.0%; toxicology: LD50 (oral, rat) > 2000 mg/kg; eye irritant; nonirritating to skin; nonmutagenic; 98% act.; 5 ± 0.2% zinc.

Grillocin® HY 77. [Grillo-Werke AG] Zinc ricinoleate, triethanolamine, dipropylene glycol, and lactic acid; deodorant for aerosols, creams, pump sprays, roll-ons, soaps, and sticks; cleansing agent for liq. and bar soaps; 74% biodeg.; amber liq.; dens. 1.10 ± 0.05 g/cc; iodine no. 70 ± 8; pH 8.0 ± 0.5 (1% in ethanol); do not store below 5 C; usage level: 1.5-3.0%; toxicology: LD50 (oral, rat) > 2000 mg/kg; sl. irritating to skin; nonirritating to eyes; nonmutagenic; 98% act.; 6.6 ± 0.2% zinc.

Grillocin HY-77. [R.I.T.A.] Zinc ricinoleate, triethanolamine, zinc rosinate, isostearic acid, dipropylene glycol, sodium lactate, abietic acid, tocopherol; absorbs malodors from sol'ns. and surfs.; brn. visc. liq.; sol. in ethanol, IPA, dipropylene glycol; sp.gr. 1.09; iodine no. 58 ± 5; pH 7.30 (1% in ethanol); toxicology: LD50 (oral, rat) > 20 g/kg; nonsensitizing.

Grillocin® P 176. [Grillo-Werke AG; R.I.T.A.] Zinc ricinoleate and talc; raw material for personal care prods.; absorbent for malodorous materials; deodorant for powders; 99% biodeg.; wh. powd.; bulk dens. 500 kg/m³; iodine no. 48 ± 5; pH 6.5 ± 0.5 (1% in ethanol); usage level: 1.5-3.0%; toxicology: (tested without talc): LD50 (oral, rat) > 2000 mg/kg; nonirritating to skin and eyes; nonmutagenic; 99% act.; 6.1 ± 0.2% zinc.

Grillocin® PY 88 Pellets. [Grillo-Werke AG; R.I.T.A.] Zinc ricinoleate; CAS 13040-19-2; EINECS 235-911-4; raw material for personal care prods.; deodorant for creams, soaps; cleanser for bar soaps; 99% biodeg.; ivory pellets; bulk dens. 1.10 g/cc; iodine no. 78 ± 6; pH 6.6 (1% in ethanol); usage level: 1.5-3.0%; toxicology: LD50 (oral, rat) > 2000 mg/kg; nonirritating to skin and eyes; nonmutagenic; 98% act.; 9.5 ± 0.7% zinc.

Grillocin® PY 88 Pulver/Powd. [Grillo-Werke AG; R.I.T.A.] Zinc ricinoleate; CAS 13040-19-2; EINECS 235-911-4; raw material for personal care prods.; deodorant for powders, soaps; cleanser for bar soaps; 99% biodeg.; wh. powd.; bulk dens. 500 kg/m³; iodine no. 78 ± 6; pH 6.6 (1% in ethanol); usage level: 1.5-3.0%; toxicology: LD50 (oral, rat) > 2000 mg/kg; nonirritating to skin and eyes; nonmutagenic; 98% act.; 9.5 ± 0.7% zinc.

Grillocin® S 803/7. [Grillo-Werke AG; R.I.T.A.] Zinc rincinoleate with solubilizers; CAS 13040-19-2; EINECS 235-911-4; raw material for personal care prods.; deodorant for deodorant soap formulations; readily biodeg.; yel. paste; dens. 1.05 ± 1.15 g/cc; iodine no. 65 ± 5; pH 7.5 ± 0.5 (1% in ethanol); usage level: 1.5-3.0%; 5.4 ± 0.3% zinc.

Grillocin S-803/12. [R.I.T.A.] Zinc ricinoleate with synergists; CAS 13040-19-2; EINECS 235-911-4; absorbent for malodorous materials; paste; sp.gr. 1.09; iodine no. 58 ± 5; pH 7.3 (1% in ethanol); toxicology: LD50 (oral, rat) > 9.33 g/kg; nonsensitizing.

Grillocin WE-106. [R.I.T.A.] Zinc ricinoleate, castor oil, ricinoleic acid, PEG-7 ricinoleate, glyceryl stearate, isostearic acid, succinic acid; absorbent for malodorous materials; sp.gr. 1.02; iodine no. 55 ± 5; pH 5.35 ± 0.15

(1% in ethanol); toxicology: LD50 (oral, rat) > 25 ml/kg.

Grillocose® DO. [Grillo-Werke AG; R.I.T.A.] Methyl glucose dioleate; CAS 83933-91-3; w/o emulsifier for skin care prods. (baby creams/lotions, night creams, sunscreens, emulsions); skin moisturizer; extremely mild to skin and eyes; pale yel. liq.; usage level: 2.0-5.0%; 95% act.

Grillocose® IS. [Grillo-Werke AG; R.I.T.A.] Methyl glucose isostearate; w/o emulsifier and moisturizer for skin care prods. (baby creams/lotions, night creams, sunscreens, emulsions); extremely mild to skin and eyes; 75% biodeg.; pale yel. liq.; dens. 1.00 ± 0.05 g/cc; acid no. 18 ± 5; iodine no. 5 max.; sapon. no. 143 ± 5; pH 7.5 ± 0.5 (5% in methanol/water); usage level: 2.0-5.0%; toxicology: LD50 (oral, rats) > 2000 mg/kg; nonirritating to skin and eyes; nonmutagenic; 95% act.

Grillocose® PS. [Grillo-Werke AG] Methyl glucose stearate; o/w emulsifier, moisturizer for skin care prods. (baby creams/lotions, makeup, shaving prods., sunscreens, day creams, emulsions); deodorant for creams and soaps; skin cleanser for bar soaps, lotions; 85% biodeg.; lt. yel. pellets; bulk dens. 600 kg/m³; acid no. 20 ± 5; iodine no. 5 max.; sapon. no. 132 ± 5; pH 8.0 ± 0.5 (5% in methanol/water); usage level: 2.0-5.0%; toxicology: LD50 (oral, rats) > 2000 mg/kg; nonirritating to skin and eyes; nonmutagenic; 95% act.

Grillocose PS. [R.I.T.A.] Methyl glucose sesquistearate; CAS 68936-95-8; EINECS 273-049-0; emulsifier, skin moisturizer; extremely mild to skin and eyes; off-wh. pellets.

Grillocose PSE-20. [Grillo-Werke AG] PEG-20 methyl glucose sesquistearate; CAS 68389-70-8; emulsifier, solubilizer.

Grilloderm L 60. [R.I.T.A.] Zinc pentadecene tricarboxylate; wh. powd.; iodine no. 80 ± 2; pH 5.5 ± 0.2; toxicology: LD50 (oral, rat) > 16 g/kg; nonsensitizing; 14-15% zinc; 0.5% moisture.

Grillomuls L90. [Grillo-Werke AG] Glyceryl laurate; CAS 142-18-7; EINECS 205-526-6; o/w coemulsifiers and stabilizers for cosmetic emulsions; thickener for surfactant sol'ns.; wh.-ivory powd.; bulk dens. 600 kg/m³; drop pt. 56 C; acid no. 3 max.; iodine no. 1 max.; sapon. no. 200-210; usage level: 1-5%; 90% min. monoester.

Grillomuls O60. [Grillo-Werke AG] Glyceryl oleate; w/o emulsifier for cosmetics; wh.-ivory paste; bulk dens. 600 kg/m³; drop pt. 47 C; acid no. 3 max.; iodine no. 63-77; sapon. no. 160-180; usage level: 1-5%; 60% min. monoester.

Grillomuls O90. [Grillo-Werke AG] Glyceryl oleate; w/o emulsifier for cosmetics; thickener for surfactant sol'ns.; wh.-ivory paste; bulk dens. 600 kg/m³; acid no. 2 max.; iodine no. 105; sapon. no. 155-170; usage level: 1-5%; 90% min. monoester.

Grillomuls S40. [Grillo-Werke AG] Glyceryl stearate; o/w coemulsifier and stabilizer for cosmetic emulsions; wh.-ivory powd.; bulk dens. 600 kg/m³; drop pt. 60 C; acid no. 2 max.; iodine no. 2 max.; sapon. no. 160-180; usage level: 1-10%; 40% min. monoester.

Grillomuls S60. [Grillo-Werke AG] Glyceryl stearate; o/w coemulsifier and stabilizer for cosmetic emulsions; wh.-ivory powd.; bulk dens. 600 kg/m³; drop pt. 65 C; acid no. 2 max.; iodine no. 2 max.; sapon. no. 155-175; usage level: 1-10%; 60% min. monoester.

Grillomuls S90. [Grillo-Werke AG] Glyceryl stearate; o/w coemulsifier and stabilizer for cosmetic emulsions; wh.-ivory powd.; bulk dens. 600 kg/m³; drop pt. 70 C; acid no. 2 max.; iodine no. 1 max.; sapon. no. 150-165; usage level: 1-10%; 90% min. monoester.

Grillosan DS 7911. [R.I.T.A.] Disodium dihydroxyethyl sulfosuccinylundecylenate; yel. clear liq.; sp.gr. 1.140-1.24; pH 6.5 ± 0.5 (1% aq.); toxicology: LD50 (oral, rat) >

5.6 g/kg; nonsensitizing; 58-60% act.

Grillosol 8C. [R.I.T.A.] Sodium bisglycol ricinosulfosuccinate; anionic; detergent; solubilizer for Grilloten in water and alcohol-based systems; yel. clear liq.; sp.gr. 1.14; pH 6.5 ± 0.5 (1% aq.); toxicology: LD50 (oral, rat) > 16 g/kg; nonsensitizing; 22% moisture.

Grillosol 8C12. [R.I.T.A.] Disodium PEG-8 ricinosuccinate; anionic; detergent; solubilizer for Grilloten in water and alcohol-based systems; soft paste; sp.gr. 1.10; pH 6.5 ± 0.5 (1% aq.); toxicology: LD50 (oral, rat) > 16 g/kg; nonsensitizing; 1% moisture.

Grillosol SB3/12. [R.I.T.A.] Disodium laureth sulfosuccinate; raw material for personal care prods.; pale yel. liq.

Grilloten LSE 65. [R.I.T.A.] Sucrose laurate; CAS 25339-99-5; EINECS 246-873-3; nonionic; anti-irritant, emulsifier, emollient, moisturizer, and conditioner for skin and hair care preps.; wh. creamy soft prod.; HLB 14-15; iodine no. 5 max.; sapon. no. 65 ± 7.0; pH 7.5 ± 0.5 (5% in 1/1 methanol/water); toxicology: LD50 (oral, rat) > 16 g/kg; nontoxic; nonirritating; nonsensitizing; 8.5% moisture.

Grilloten® LSE 65 K. [R.I.T.A.; Grillo-Werke AG] Sucrose cocoate; CAS 91031-88-8; nonionic; mild cosurfactant for skin and hair care prods., esp. transparent prods. (baby shampoos, conditioners, shampoos, shower gels, baby baths, foam baths, liq. and bar soaps, cleansing gels and lotions, shaving prods.); deodorant for soaps; increases visc., improves foam consistency, has moisturizing and refatting props., reduces irritancy of other raw materials; 94% biodeg.; lt. yel. solid; dens. 1.21 g/cc; HLB 14-15; iodine no. 10 max.; sapon. no. 68 ± 5; pH 7.5 ± 1.5 (5% in 1/1 methanol/water); usage level: 1.5-4.0%; toxicology: LD50 (oral, rats) > 2000 mg/kg; sl. irritant to skin; nonirritating to eyes; nonmutagenic; 93% act.

Grilloten® LSE 65 K Soft. [R.I.T.A.; Grillo-Werke AG] Sucrose cocoate; CAS 91031-88-8; nonionic; cosurfactant for skin and hair care prods., esp. transparent prods. and cold processing (baby shampoos, conditioners, shampoos, shower gels, baby baths, foam baths, liq. soaps, cleansing gels and lotions, shaving prods.); reduces irritancy of other raw materials; increases visc.; has moisturizing and refatting props.; improves foam consistency; 94% biodeg.; wh. to cream-colored paste; dens. 1.07 g/cc; HLB 14-15; iodine no. 5 max.; sapon. no. 52 ± 5; pH 7.0 ± 0.5 (5% in 1/1 methanol/water); usage level: 2.0-5.0%; toxicology: LD50 (oral, rats) > 2000 mg/kg; sl. irritating to skin; nonirritating to eyes; nonmutagenic; 65% act. in water.

Grilloten LSE 65 Soft. [R.I.T.A.] Sucrose laurate; CAS 25339-99-5; EINECS 246-873-3; nonionic; anti-irritant, emulsifier, emollient, moisturizer, and conditioner for skin and hair care preps.; lower actives for ease of handling; wh. to cream-colored paste.

Grilloten LSE 87. [R.I.T.A.] Sucrose laurate; CAS 25339-99-5; EINECS 246-873-3; nonionic; o/w emulsifier, solubilizer, foam booster, counter-irritant, emollient, moisturizer, and conditioner for skin and hair care preps.; stable over wide pH range; wh. creamy soft prod.; HLB 12.5; iodine no. 5 max.; sapon. no. 85 ± 5.0; pH 7.3 ± 0.5 (5% in 1/1 methanol/water); toxicology: LD50 (oral, rat) > 16 g/kg; nontoxic, nonirritating, nonsensitizing; 6.5% moisture.

Grilloten® LSE 87 K. [Grillo-Werke AG; R.I.T.A.] Sucrose cocoate; CAS 91031-88-8; nonionic; o/w emulsifier, solubilizer, foam booster, counter-irritant, emollient, moisturizer, conditioner, and cosurfactant for skin and hair care prods. (baby shampoos, conditioners, shampoos, shower gels, baby baths, foam baths, liq. and bar soaps, cleansing gels and lotions, shaving prods.); deodorant for soaps; reduces irritancy of other raw materials; increases visc., improves foam consistency; moisturizing and refatting props.; stable over wide pH range; 100% biodeg.; lt. yel.

solid; dens. 1.16 g/cc; iodine no. 10 max.; sapon. no. 87 ± 7; pH 7.3 ± 0.6 (5% in 1/1 methanol/water); usage level: 1.5-4.0%; toxicology: LD50 (oral, rats) > 2000 mg/kg; sl. irritating to skin; nonirritating to eyes; nonmutagenic; 93% act.

Grilloten® LSE 87 K Soft. [Grillo-Werke AG; R.I.T.A.] Sucrose cocoate; CAS 91031-88-8; nonionic; anti-irritant, emulsifier, emollient, moisturizer, conditioner, and cosurfactant for skin and hair care prods., esp. cold processing (baby shampoos, conditioners, shampoos, shower gels, baby baths, foam baths, liq. soaps, cleansing gels and lotions, shaving prods.); reduces irritancy of other raw materials; increases visc., improves foam consistency; moisturizing and refatting props.; 100% biodeg.; lt. yel. paste; dens. 1.04 g/cc; iodine no. 5 max.; sapon. no. 45 ± 5; pH 7.5 ± 0.5 (5% in 1/1 methanol/water); usage level: 3.0-8.0%; toxicology: LD50 (oral, rats) > 2000 mg/kg; sl. irritating to skin; nonirritating to eyes; nonmutagenic; 47% act.

Grilloten LSE 87 Soft. [R.I.T.A.] Sucrose laurate; CAS 25339-99-5; EINECS 246-873-3; nonionic; anti-irritant, emulsifier, emollient, moisturizer, and conditioner for skin and hair care preps.; lower actives for ease of handling; wh. to cream-colored paste; HLB 12-13; iodine no. 5 max.; sapon. no. 45 ± 5.0; pH 7.3 ± 0.5 (5% in 1/1 methanol/water); 55% moisture.

Grilloten® PSE 141 G Pellets. [Grillo-Werke AG; R.I.T.A.] Sucrose stearate; CAS 37318-31-3; EINECS 246-705-9; nonionic; o/w emulsifier, solubilizer, emollient, moisturizer, conditioner, and cosurfactant for skin care prods. (bar soaps, cleansing lotions, baby and skin creams and lotions, day creams); deodorant for creams and soaps; reduces irritancy of other raw materials; moisturizing and refatting props.; > 95% biodeg.; lt. yel. pellets; dens. 1.13 g/cc; iodine no. 10 max.; sapon. no. 90 ± 6; pH 9.0 ± 0.5 (5% in methanol/water); usage level: 2.0-5.0%; toxicology: LD50 (oral, rats) > 2000 mg/kg; nonirritating to skin and eyes; nonmutagenic; 97% act.

Grindox Ascorbyl Palmitate. [Grindsted Prods. Denmark] Ascorbyl palmitate; CAS 137-66-6; EINECS 205-305-4.

Grit-O'Cobs®. [Andersons] Corn cob meal; chemically inert plastic extender and filler; replaces wood flour in wood particle molding with phenolic resins, in profile and sheet stock prod.; filler in glue, asphalt, caulking compds., and rubber; also used in industrial abrasives, as industrial absorbent, as agric. chemical carriers, livestock feed roughage; fine grades used in soaps and cosmetics; tan gran.; essentially odorless; 20.9% sol. in 1% sodium hydroxide, 9.5% in hot water, 5.6% in alcohol, 2.5% in acetone and in 10% sulfuric acid; sp.gr. 1.2; bulk dens. 20–30 lb/ft³; oil absorp. 100%; water absorp. 133.0%; pH 7.4 (surface); flash pt. (OC) 350 F; hardness (Mohs) 4.5; 47.1% cellulose.

Growthphyllin. [Ichimaru Pharcos] Hematin.

GU-61-A. [Cosmetochem] Propylene glycol, lichen extract, licorice extract, and comfrey extract; botanical extract.

Gu-61-Standard. [Cosmetochem] Propylene glycol, lichen extract, licorice extract, and comfrey extract; botanical extract.

Guerbo. [Nova Molecular Tech.] Trioctyldodecyl borate.

Guineshing-LV. [Ichimaru Pharcos] Alcohol, water, and ginseng extract; botanical extract.

Gulftene® 4. [Chevron] 1-Butene (C4 alpha olefins); CAS 106-98-9; intermediate for biodeg. surfactants for personal care and laundry, and specialty industrial chemicals (polyethylene and other polymers; plasticizers; syn. lubricants; gasoline additives; paper sizing; PVC lubricants); gas; sp.gr. 0.602 (60/60 F); dens. 5.01 lb/gal (60 F); flamm. gas; 100% conc.

Gulftene® 6. [Chevron] 1-Hexene (C6 alpha olefins); CAS

592-41-6; intermediate for biodeg. surfactants for personal care and laundry, and specialty industrial chemicals (polyethylene and other polymers; plasticizers; syn. lubricants; gasoline additives; paper sizing; PVC lubricants); water-wh. bright, clear liq., char. olefinic odor; ; m.w. 84; sp.gr. 0.677 (60/60 F); dens. 5.64 lb/gal (60 F); b.p. 147 F; flash pt. (TOC) < 20 F; flamm. liq.; toxicology: LD50 (oral, rat) > 10 g/kg (nontoxic); minimal skin and eye irritation.

Gulftene® 8. [Chevron] 1-Octene (C8 alpha olefins); CAS 111-66-0; intermediate for biodeg. surfactants for personal care and laundry, and specialty industrial chemicals (polyethylene and other polymers; plasticizers; syn. lubricants; gasoline additives; paper sizing; PVC lubricants); water-wh. bright, clear liq., char. olefinic odor; ; sp.gr. 0.719 (60/60 F); dens. 6.00 lb/gal (60 F); b.p. 240 F; flash pt. (TCC) 55 F; flamm. liq.

Gulftene® 10. [Chevron] 1-Decene (C10 alpha olefins); CAS 872-05-9; intermediate for biodeg. surfactants for personal care and laundry, and specialty industrial chemicals (polyethylene and other polymers; plasticizers; syn. lubricants; gasoline additives; paper sizing; PVC lubricants); water-wh. bright, clear liq., char. olefinic odor; ; m.w. 140; sp.gr. 0.745 (60/60 F); dens. 6.21 lb/gal (60 F); b.p. 338 F; flash pt. (TOC) 128 F; combustible liq.; toxicology: LD50 (oral, rat) > 10 g/kg (nontoxic); minimal skin and eye irritation.

Gulftene® 12. [Chevron] 1-Dodecene (C12 alpha olefins); CAS 112-41-4; intermediate for biodeg. surfactants for personal care and laundry, and specialty industrial chemicals (polyethylene and other polymers; plasticizers; syn. lubricants; gasoline additives; paper sizing; PVC lubricants); water-wh. bright, clear liq., char. olefinic odor; ; sp.gr. 0.762 (60/60 F); dens. 6.36 lb/gal (60 F); f.p. -31 F; b.p. 400 F; pour pt. -33 F; flash pt. (TCC) 171 F; combustible liq.

Gulftene® 14. [Chevron] 1-Tetradecene (C14 alpha olefins); CAS 1120-36-1; intermediate for biodeg. surfactants for personal care and laundry, and specialty industrial chemicals (polyethylene and other polymers; plasticizers; syn. lubricants; gasoline additives; paper sizing; PVC lubricants); water-wh. bright, clear liq., char. olefinic odor; ; sp.gr. 0.775 (60/60 F); dens. 6.46 lb/gal (60 F); f.p. 9 F; b.p. 440 F; pour pt. 10 F; flash pt. (PM) 225 F; combustible liq.

Gulftene® 16. [Chevron] 1-Hexadecene (C16 alpha olefins);

CAS 629-73-2; intermediate for biodeg. surfactants for personal care and laundry, and specialty industrial chemicals (polyethylene and other polymers; plasticizers; syn. lubricants; gasoline additives; paper sizing; PVC lubricants); water-wh. bright, clear liq., char. olefinic odor; m.w. 224; sp.gr. .785 (60/60 F); dens. 6.54 lb/gal (60 F); f.p. 39 F; b.p. 539 F; pour pt. 45 F; flash pt. (TOC) > 200 F; combustible liq.; toxicology: LD50 (oral, rat) > 10 g/kg (nontoxic); minimal skin and eye irritation.

Gulftene® 18. [Chevron] 1-Octadecene (C18 alpha olefins); CAS 112-88-9; intermediate for biodeg. surfactants for personal care and laundry, and specialty industrial chemicals (polyethylene and other polymers; plasticizers; syn. lubricants; gasoline additives; paper sizing; PVC lubricants); water-wh. bright, clear liq., char. olefinic odor; sp.gr. 0.793 (60/60 F); dens. 6.60 lb/gal (60 F); f.p. 64 F; b.p. 165 F; pour pt. 65 F; flash pt. (PM) 310 F.

Gulftene® 20-24. [Chevron] C20-24 alpha olefins; intermediate for biodeg. surfactants for personal care and laundry, and specialty industrial chemicals (polyethylene and other polymers; plasticizers; syn. lubricants; gasoline additives; paper sizing; PVC lubricants); wh. bright, clear waxy solid; sp.gr. 0.856 (60/60 F); dens. 6.67 lb/gal (60 F); visc. 2.1 cSt (99 C); flash pt. (PM) 362 F; toxicology: LD50 (oral, rat) > 5 g/kg.

Gulftene® 24-28. [Chevron] C24-28 alpha olefins; intermediate for biodeg. surfactants for personal care and laundry, and specialty industrial chemicals (polyethylene and other polymers; plasticizers; syn. lubricants; gasoline additives; paper sizing; PVC lubricants); wh. bright, clear waxy solid; sp.gr. 0.891 (60/60 F); dens. 6.83 lb/gal (60 F); visc. 2.5 cSt (99 C); m.p. 143 F; congeal pt. 126 F; b.p. 190 F; flash pt. (PM) 425 F.

Gulftene® 30+. [Chevron] C30 alpha olefin; intermediate for biodeg. surfactants for personal care and laundry, and specialty industrial chemicals (polyethylene and other polymers; plasticizers; syn. lubricants; gasoline additives; paper sizing; PVC lubricants); wh. bright, clear waxy solid; sp.gr. 0.919 (60/60 F); dens. 6.95 lb/gal (60 F); visc. 8.0 cSt (99 C); drop m.p. 163 F; congeal pt. 155 F; b.p. 204 F; flash pt. (PM) 485 F; toxicology: LD50 (oral, rat) > 2 g/kg.

Gunther Pro-Tein 1550. [A.E. Staley Mfg.] Hydrolyzed veg. protein; CAS 100209-45-8; cosmetic moisturizer.

H

H-40. [U.S. Cosmetics] Hollow nonporous silica microballoons; impart light and fluffy ball bearing props. to cosmetic anhyd. makeup prods.; spherical beads.

Hair Complex 20/70n. [Dr. Kurt Richter; Henkel/Cospha] Placental protein, inositol, calcium pantothenate, PABA, methionine, cysteine, and tryptophan; aq.-alcoholic lotions for regenerative hair care, oily scalps and dandruff; water-wh. to lt. yel. liq.

Haircomplex AKS. [Novarom GmbH] Propylene glycol, matricaria extract, arnica extract, and horsetail extract.

Hair Complex Aquosum. [Dr. Kurt Richter; Henkel/Cospha] Water, alcohol, horsetail extract, nettle extract, coltsfoot extract, PEG-8, panthenol, and inositol; herbs and B vitamins in water-alcohol medium for treatment of scalps with dandruff or greasiness; general hair protection; dk. brn. liq.

Hair-cure 2/011500. [Dragoco] Cetyl alcohol, behentrimonium chloride, and wheat bran lipids; cosmetic ingred.

Hair Gloss Polymer. [Cosmetochem] A blend of resins with special gloss-imparting additives.

Hair Saccharides. [Provital; Centerchem] Hydrolyzed glycosaminoglycans; moisturizer.

Hairspray Additive S. [BASF; BASF AG] Rosin acrylate; improves setting strength and reduces tack in hairspray formulations; powd.

Hairwax 7686 o.E. [Kahl] Cetyl palmitate, beeswax, and microcryst. wax.

Halpasol 190/240. [Haltermann GmbH] C10-13 alkane.

Halpasol 230 W. [Haltermann GmbH] Petroleum distillates.

Halpasol 240/270. [Haltermann GmbH] C14-17 alkane.

Hamamelis Extract HS 2456 G. [Grau Aromatics] Propylene glycol and witch hazel extract; botanical extract.

Hamamelis Liq. [Ichimaru Pharcos] Water, butylene glyocl, and witch hazel extract.

Hamamelitannin Conc. 250A. [E.E. Dickinson] Witch hazel extract.

Hamamelitannin Conc. 250M. [E.E. Dickinson] Witch hazel extract.

Hamp-Ene® 100. [Hampshire] Tetrasodium EDTA; CAS 64-02-8; EINECS 200-573-9; general purpose chelating agent; pale straw clear liq.; m.w. 380.2; water-misc.; sp.gr. 1.26–1.28; dens. 10.6 lb/gal; chel. value 100 mg CaCO$_3$/g min. (@ pH 11); pH 11–12 (1%); 38% min. act.

Hamp-Ene® 220. [Hampshire] Tetrasodium EDTA, tech.; CAS 64-02-8; EINECS 200-573-9; chelating agent; wh. cryst. powd.; m.w. 452.3; sol. 50% in water; dens. 6.5 lb/gal; chel. value 219 mg CaCO$_3$/g min (@ pH 11); pH 10.5–11.5 (1%); 99% min. act.

Hamp-Ene® Acid. [Hampshire] EDTA; CAS 60-00-4; EINECS 200-449-4; chelating agent; used where sodium ion is undesirable; synergizes the preservative system toward gram-negative bacteria in personal care prods.; protects fragrance components; stabilizes color and org. thickeners; protects against rancidity in cosmetic creams and lotions; wh. cryst. powd.; m.w. 292.3; dens. 6.0 lb/gal; chel. value 340 mg CaCO$_3$/g min.; pH 2.6–3.1; 99.3% min. act.

Hampene® CaNa$_2$ Pure Crystals. [Hampshire] Calcium disodium EDTA; CAS 62-33-9; EINECS 200-529-9; preservative for cosmetics.

Hampene® Na$_2$ Pure Crystals. [Hampshire] Disodium EDTA; CAS 139-33-3; EINECS 205-358-3; chelating agent; preservative for cosmetics; usage level: 0.1-0.5%.

Hamp-Ene® Na$_3$T. [Hampshire] Trisodium EDTA (trihydrate); chelating agent; wh. cryst. powd.; m.w. 412.3; sol. 40% in water; dens. 6.0 lb/gal; chel. value 242 mg CaCO$_3$/g min.; pH 8.3–8.7 (1%); 99% min. act.

Hamp-Ene® Na$_4$. [Hampshire] Tetrasodium EDTA (dihydrate); CAS 64-02-8; EINECS 200-573-9; chelating agent; wh. cryst. powd.; m.w. 416.2; sol. 48% in water; dens. 6.5 lb/gal; chel. value 240 mg CaCO$_3$/g min. (@ pH 11); pH 10.7–11.7 (1%); 99.5% min. act.

Hamp-Ene® OH Powd. [Hampshire] TEA hydrochloride, disodium EDTA; chelating agent for iron in alkaline conditions; off-wh. to tan cryst. powd.; sol. 30% in water; dens. 6.4 lb/gal; chel. value 115 mg CaCO$_3$/g min.; pH 4.3–5.1 (15%); 100% act.

Hamp-Ex® 80. [Hampshire] Pentasodium pentetate; CAS 140-01-2; EINECS 205-391-3; chelating agent for alkaline earth and heavy metal ions; peroxide bleaching; pale straw clear liq.; m.w. 503.3; water-misc.; sp.gr. 1.29–1.31; dens. 10.8 lb/gal; chel. value 80 mg CaCO$_3$/g min.; pH 11–12 (1%); 40.2% min. act.

Hamp-Ex® Acid. [Hampshire] Pentetic acid; CAS 67-43-6; EINECS 200-652-8; chelating agent; wh. cryst. powd.; m.w. 393.4; dens. 7.0 lb/gal; chel. value 253 mg CaCO$_3$/g min.; pH 2.1–2.5; 99% min. act.

Hamplex DPS. [Hampshire] Sodium polydimethylglycinophenolsulfonate.

Hamp-Ol® 120. [Hampshire] Trisodium HEDTA; CAS 139-89-9; EINECS 205-381-9; general purpose chelating agent for control of iron at pH 6.5–9.5 as well as Ca and Mg; pale straw clear liq.; m.w. 344.2; water-misc.; sp.gr. 1.28–1.31; dens. 10.8 lb/gal; chel. value 120 mg CaCO$_3$/g min.; pH 11–12 (1%); 41.3% min. act.

Hamp-Ol® Acid. [Hampshire] HEDTA; CAS 150-39-0; EINECS 205-759-3; chelating agent; wh. cryst. powd.; m.w. 278.3; dens. 6.0 lb/gal; chel. value 353 mg CaCO$_3$/g min.; pH 2.1–2.4; 98% min. act.

Hamp-Ol® Crystals. [Hampshire] Trisodium HEDTA (dihydrate); CAS 139-89-9; EINECS 205-381-9; chelating agent; wh. cryst. powd.; m.w. 389.3; sol. 59% in water; dens. 6.0 lb/gal; chel. value 255 mg CaCO$_3$/g min.; pH 11–12 (1%); 99.0% min. act.

Hamposyl® AC-30. [Hampshire] Ammonium cocoyl sarcosinate; anionic; surfactant.

Hamposyl® AL-30. [Hampshire] Ammonium lauroyl sarcosinate; CAS 68003-46-3; EINECS 268-130-2; anionic;

surfactant for shampoos, skin cleansers, bath gels; sec. emulsifier for emulsion polymerization; liq.; HLB 29.0; 30% conc.

Hamposyl® C. [Hampshire; Chemplex Chems.] Cocoyl sarcosine; CAS 68411-97-2; EINECS 270-156-4; anionic; detergent, wetting and foaming agent, foam stabilizer, emulsifier, anticorrosive agent, conditioner for hair and rug shampoos, cosmetics, skin cleansers; biodeg.; pale yel. liq.; sol. in most org. solv.; m.w. 280; sp.gr. 0.97–0.99; m.p. 23–26 C; soften. pt. 18-22 C; HLB 10.0; 100% conc.

Hamposyl® C-30. [Hampshire; Chemplex Chems.] Sodium cocoyl sarcosinate; CAS 61791-59-1; EINECS 263-193-2; anionic; detergent, wetting and foaming agent, foam stabilizer, emulsifier, anticorrosive agent, conditioner for hair and rug shampoos, cosmetics, skin cleansers; biodeg.; colorless to very pale yel. liq.; misc. in water; m.w. 301; sp.gr. 1.02–1.03; visc. 30 cps; f.p. –1 C; HLB 27.0; pH 7.5-8.5 (10%); surf. tens. 30 dynes/cm; 30% act.

Hamposyl® CZ. [Hampshire; Chemplex Chems.] Cocoyl sarcosine; CAS 68411-97-2; EINECS 270-156-4; surfactant for industrial and personal care prods.; pale yel. liq.; sp.gr. 0.97-0.99; m.w. 280; m.p. 18-22 C; 95.5% min. act.

Hamposyl® L. [Hampshire; Chemplex Chems.] Lauroyl sarcosine; CAS 97-78-9; EINECS 202-608-3; anionic; detergent, wetting and foaming agent, foam stabilizer, emulsifier, anticorrosive agent, conditioner for hair and rug shampoos, cosmetics, skin cleansers; biodeg.; wh. waxy solid; sol. in most org. solvs.; m.w. 270; sp.gr. 0.97-0.99; m.p. 34–37 C; HLB 13.0; 94% act.

Hamposyl® L-30. [Hampshire; Chemplex Chems.] Sodium lauroyl sarcosinate; CAS 137-16-6; EINECS 205-281-5; anionic; detergent, wetting and foaming agent, foam stabilizer, emulsifier, anticorrosive agent, conditioner for hair and rug shampoos, cosmetics, skin cleansers; biodeg.; colorless liq.; misc. in water; m.w. 292; sp.gr. 1.02–1.03; visc. 30 cps; f.p. –1 C; HLB 30.0; pH 7.5-8.5 (10%); surf. tens. 30 dynes/cm; 30% act.

Hamposyl® L-95. [Hampshire; Chemplex Chems.] Sodium lauroyl sarcosinate; CAS 137-16-6; EINECS 205-281-5; anionic; detergent, wetting and foaming agent, foam stabilizer, emulsifier, anticorrosive agent, conditioner for hair and rug shampoos, cosmetics, skin cleansers; biodeg.; wh. powd.; sol. in water; m.w. 292; dens. 25 lb/ft³; HLB 30.0; pH 7.5-8.5 (10%); 94% act.

Hamposyl® M. [Hampshire; Chemplex Chems.] Myristoyl sarcosine; CAS 52558-73-3; EINECS 258-007-1; anionic; detergent, wetting and foaming agent, foam stabilizer, emulsifier, anticorrosive agent, conditioner for hair and rug shampoos, cosmetics, skin cleansers; biodeg.; wh. waxy solid; sol. in most org. solv.; m.w. 298; sp.gr. 0.97–0.99; m.p. 48–53 C; 94% act.

Hamposyl® M-30. [Hampshire] Sodium myristoyl sarcosinate; CAS 30364-51-3; EINECS 250-151-3; anionic; detergent, wetting and foaming agent, foam stabilizer, emulsifier, anticorrosive agent, conditioner for hair and rug shampoos, cosmetics, skin cleansers; biodeg.; colorless liq.; misc. in water; m.w. 320; sp.gr. 1.02–1.03; visc. 30 cps; f.p. –1 C; pH 7.5-8.5 (10%); surf. tens. 30 dynes/cm; 30% act.

Hamposyl® O. [Hampshire; Chemplex Chems.] Oleoyl sarcosine; CAS 110-25-8; EINECS 203-749-3; anionic; detergent, wetting and foaming agent, foam stabilizer, emulsifier, corrosion inhibitor, mold release agent, conditioner for hair and rug shampoos, cosmetics, skin cleansers; ceramic dispersant; biodeg.; yel. liq.; sol. in most org. solv.; m.w. 349; sp.gr. 0.95–0.97; visc. 250 cps; HLB 10.0; 94% act.

Hamposyl® S. [Hampshire] Stearoyl sarcosine; CAS 142-48-3; EINECS 205-539-7; anionic; detergent, wetting and

foaming agent, foam stabilizer, emulsifier, anticorrosive agent, conditioner for hair and rug shampoos, cosmetics, skin cleansers; biodeg.; wh. waxy solid; sol. in most org. solv.; m.w. 338; sp.gr. 0.96–0.98; m.p. 53–58 C; 94% act.

Hamposyl® TL-40. [Hampshire] TEA lauroyl sarcosinate; CAS 16693-53-1; EINECS 240-736-1; anionic; provides mild, high lathering props. to skin cleansers; liq.; HLB 30.0; 40% conc.

Hamposyl® TOC-30. [Hampshire] TEA-oleoyl sarcosinate, TEA-cocoyl sarcosinate.; anionic; biodeg. surfactant for hair and rug shampoos; liq.; 30% act.

Hampshire® DEG. [Hampshire] Sodium dihydroxyethylglycinate; CAS 139-41-3; EINECS 205-360-4; chelating agent used for for control of iron only in alkaline sol'ns.; pale straw clear liq.; m.w. 185.2; water-misc.; sp.gr. 1.19–1.23; dens. 10 lb/gal; chel. value 50 mg Fe/g min. (@ pH 10); pH 11–12 (1%); 41% act.

Hampshire® Glycine. [Hampshire] Glycine; CAS 56-40-6; EINECS 200-272-2.

Haro® Chem ALMD-2. [Harcros] Aluminum distearate; CAS 300-92-5; EINECS 206-101-8; metal soap stabilizer for cosmetics, oils, fats, lubricants, pharmaceuticals, paints, and printing inks; solid.

Haroil SCO-50. [Graden] Sulfated castor oil; CAS 8002-33-3; EINECS 232-306-7; anionic; emulsifier, superfatting agent for cosmetic creams, soaps, etc.; liq.; 50% conc.

Hartamide LDA. [Hart Chem. Ltd.] Lauramide DEA; CAS 120-40-1; EINECS 204-393-1; nonionic; detergent, foam stabilizer and thickener for liq. and powd. detergent systems, shampoos, bubble baths; wh. solid; 100% act.

Hartamide LMEA. [Hart Chem. Ltd.] Lauramide MEA; CAS 142-78-9; EINECS 205-560-1; anionic; foam stabilizer for spray-dried powd. detergents and bubble bath preparations; visc. modifier for detergents, shampoos, bubble baths; wh. solid; 95% amide.

Hartamide OD. [Hart Chem. Ltd.] Cocamide DEA; CAS 61791-31-9; EINECS 263-163-9; nonionic; detergent, foam stabilizer and visc. regulator for liq. and powd. detergent systems, shampoos, bubble baths; yel. liq.; dens. 1.02 lb/gal; visc. 900 cps; 100% act.

Hartofol 40. [Hart Prods. Corp.] Sodium dodecylbenzene sulfonate; CAS 25155-30-0; EINECS 246-680-4; anionic; high foaming biodeg. surfactant for heavy-duty liq. detergents, textile processing, industrial cleaners, shampoos, automotive cleaners, cold water cleaners; lt. amber liq.; sp.gr. 1.102; dens. 9.2 lb/gal; pH 6.5-7.5 (1%); 40% act.

Hartofol 60T. [Hart Prods. Corp.] TEA dodecylbenzene sulfonate; CAS 27323-41-7; EINECS 248-406-9; anionic; surfactant for cosmetics, shampoos, liq. detergents, wool wash formulations; biodeg.; mild, high purity; lt. amber visc. liq.; sp.gr. 1.087; dens. 9.0 lb/gal; pH 6.5-7.5 (1%); 60% act.

Hartolan. [Croda Inc.; Croda Chem. Ltd.] Lanolin alcohols; CAS 8027-33-6; EINECS 232-430-1; nonionic; spreading agent, dispersant, stabilizer, plasticizer, w/o emulsifier, conditioner, superfatting agent, moisturizer, and emollient for cosmetic and pharmaceutical systems; brn. solid wax; sol. in oils, esters; m.p. 58 C; acid no. 2 max.; sapon. no. 5 mg max; usage level: 0.5-3%; 100% conc.

Hartolite. [Croda Chem. Ltd.] Lanolin alcohols fraction; CAS 8027-33-6; EINECS 232-430-1; nonionic; w/o emulsifier, emollient, skin conditioner, moisturizing agent; pale yel. soft waxy solid; 100% act.

Hawthorn Extract Code 9033. [Brooks Industries] Hawthorn (*Crataegus oxycantha*) extract; rich in natural antioxidants and org. acids for skin care prods. to control erythema and acne; amber clear liq.

HD-Eutanol® . [Henkel/Cospha; Henkel Canada; Henkel KGaA/Cospha] Oleyl alcohol; CAS 143-28-2; EINECS 205-597-3; ultra pure grade used as as solubilizer for dyes and waxes; superfatting agent, emollient in cosmetic emulsions, creams, alcoholic lotions; colorless clear oily liq., bland odor; sp.gr. 0.848-0.851; acid no. 0.1 max.; iodine no. 94-100; sapon. no. 1 max.; hyd. no. 202-212; cloud pt. < 5 C; flash pt. > 150 C; ref. index 1.461-1.463.

HD-Ocenol® 90/95. [Henkel/Emery] Oleyl alcohol (2-10% C16, 87-95% C18); CAS 143-28-2; EINECS 205-597-3; emollient, superfatting agent, carrier for cosmetics; intermediate for surfactant mfg.; APHA 100 clear liq.; oil-sol.; sp.gr. 0.830-0.840 g/cc (40 C); solid. pt. 2-12 C; b.p. 330-360 C; acid no. < 0.2; iodine no. 90-97; sapon. no. < 1.0; hyd. no. 205-215; flash pt. 190 C; 100% conc.

HD-Ocenol® 92/96. [Henkel/Emery] Oleyl alcohol (2-8% C16, 87-93% C18); CAS 143-28-2; EINECS 205-597-3; emollient, superfatting agent for alcohol preparations and emulsions; intermediate for surfactant mfg.; clear oily liq.; sp.gr. 0.830-0.840 g/cc (40 C); solid. pt. 2-6 C; b.p. 330-360 C; acid no. < 0.2; iodine no. 95-105; sapon. no. < 1.0; hyd. no. 205-220; flash pt. 190 C; 100% conc.

HD Oleyl Alcohol 70/75. [Henkel] Oleyl alcohol; CAS 143-28-2; EINECS 205-597-3; emollient.

HD Oleyl Alcohol 80/85. [Henkel] Oleyl alcohol; CAS 143-28-2; EINECS 205-597-3; emollient.

HD Oleyl Alcohol 90/95. [Henkel] Oleyl alcohol; CAS 143-28-2; EINECS 205-597-3; emollient.

HD Oleyl Alcohol CG. [Henkel] Oleyl alcohol; CAS 143-28-2; EINECS 205-597-3; emollient.

Hectabrite® AW. [Am. Colloid] Hectorite USP/NF; CAS 12173-47-6; EINECS 235-340-0; emulsifier, thickener, suspension agent in pharmaceutical, cosmetic and personal care prods.; effective at low solids levels; wh. soft flakes, 20-100 mesh particle size; pH 8.5-10.5 (2% disp.); dry brightness (GE) 78-85; 5-8% moisture.

Hectabrite® DP. [Am. Colloid] Hectorite USP/NF; CAS 12173-47-6; EINECS 235-340-0; very high visc., stabilizing and suspending agent for household and industrial specialties; emulsifier and thickener for low solids formulations; wh. powd.; 90% min. thru 200 mesh; visc. 3000 cps (4% disp.); pH 9.5-10.5 (2% disp.); dry brightness (GE) 82-86; 10% max. moisture.

Hectalite® 200. [Am. Colloid] Sodium hectorite USP/NF; viscosifier, suspension agent, binder for pharmaceutical, cosmetic and personal care prods. where color is important; wh. fine powd.; 90% min. thru 200 mesh; visc. 2000 cps (5% disp.); pH 9.5-10.5 (2% disp.); 10% max. moisture.

Hedione. [Firmenich] Methyldihydrojasmonate; CAS 37172-53-5; EINECS 253-379-1.

Hefti AMS-33. [Hefti Ltd.] Ethyl stearate; CAS 111-61-5; EINECS 203-887-4; emollient, solubilizer for cosmetics.

Hefti DMS-33. [Hefti Ltd.] PEG-2 stearate; CAS 106-11-6; EINECS 203-363-5; emulsifier.

Hefti DO-33-F. [Hefti Ltd.] Sorbitan dioleate; CAS 29116-98-1; EINECS 249-448-0; personal care surfactant.

Hefti GMM-33. [Hefti Ltd.] Glyceryl myristate; CAS 67701-33-1; nonionic; emulsifier for cosmetics and pharmaceutical creams and bases; flakes; HLB 5.5; 100% conc.

Hefti GMS-33. [Hefti Ltd.] Glyceryl stearate; nonionic; emulsifier for cosmetics, pharmaceuticals, emollient and sunscreen creams; base for suppositories; lubricant for tablets; thickener for emulsions; food emulsifier; flakes; HLB 3.5; 100% conc.

Hefti GMS-33-SEN. [Hefti Ltd.] Glyceryl stearate and POE stearate, SE; nonionic; emulsifier for creams; flakes; HLB 11.0; 100% conc.

Hefti GMS-33-SES. [Hefti Ltd.] Glyceryl stearate SE; anionic; emulsifier for cosmetics, foods; flakes; HLB 5.0; 100% conc.

Hefti GMS-99. [Hefti Ltd.] Glyceryl stearate; nonionic; emulsifier for cosmetics, pharmaceuticals, foods; powd.; HLB

5.0; 100% conc.

Hefti GMS-233. [Hefti Ltd.] Polyglyceryl stearate; CAS 61790-95-2; nonionic; emulsifier for cosmetics, pharmaceuticals, foods; flakes; HLB 7.5; 100% conc.

Hefti GMS-333. [Hefti Ltd.] Polyglyceryl-3 stearate; CAS 61790-95-2; EINECS 248-403-2; nonionic; emulsifier for cosmetics, pharmaceuticals, foods; solid; HLB 7.5; 100% conc.

Hefti ML-33-F. [Hefti Ltd.] Sorbitan laurate; CAS 1338-39-2; nonionic; emulsifier for creams, sun lotions, ointments; coemulsifier for latex stabilization; lubricant; liq.; HLB 8.0; 100% conc.

Hefti ML-55-F. [Hefti Ltd.] Polysorbate 20; CAS 9005-64-5; nonionic; solubilizer for essential oils, fragrances, vitamins; emulsifier for cosmetics, pharmaceuticals, stabilizer in syrups; liq.; HLB 16.5; 100% conc.

Hefti ML-55-F-4. [Hefti Ltd.] Polysorbate 21; CAS 9005-64-5; nonionic; coemulsifier with ML-55-F for creams and ointments, pigment dispersions, color pastes, fiber preps., polishes, hydraulic fluids; liq.; HLB 12.0; 100% conc.

Hefti MO-33-F. [Hefti Ltd.] Sorbitan oleate; CAS 1338-43-8; EINECS 215-665-4; nonionic; emulsifier for w/o creams, lotions, shampoos, ointments, biocides, paints, varnishes, anticorrosion oils, polishes, cutting oils; liq.; HLB 4.4; 100% conc.

Hefti MO-55-F. [Hefti Ltd.] Polysorbate 80; CAS 61790-86-1; nonionic; emulsifier for foods and cosmetics applics.; liq.; HLB 15.0; 100% conc.

Hefti MP-33-F. [Hefti Ltd.] Sorbitan palmitate; CAS 26266-57-9; EINECS 247-568-8; nonionic; surfactant for w/o emulsions based on min. oils and triglycerides, cosmetic creams, sun lotions, deodorant sticks, gels, ointments; softener and lubricant for polymers; flakes; HLB 6.5; 100% conc.

Hefti MS-33-F. [Hefti Ltd.] Sorbitan stearate; CAS 1338-41-6; EINECS 215-664-9; nonionic; surfactant for w/o emulsions based on min. oils and saponifiable fats and oils, cosmetic and pharmaceutical creams, emulsifier for milk replacers; coemulsifier in latex stabilization; flakes; HLB 5.0; 100% conc.

Hefti MS-55-F. [Hefti Ltd.] Polysorbate 60; CAS 9005-67-8; nonionic; o/w emulsifier for cosmetics, pharmaceuticals, tech. applics.; latex stabilizer for emulsion polymerization; antistatic agent; liq./paste; HLB 15.0; 100% conc.

Hefti MYM-33. [Hefti Ltd.] Myristyl myristate; CAS 3234-85-3; EINECS 221-787-9; emollient.

Hefti NP-55-60. [Hefti Ltd.] Nonoxynol-6; CAS 9016-45-9; personal care surfactant.

Hefti NP-55-80. [Hefti Ltd.] Nonoxynol-8; CAS 9016-45-9; personal care surfactant.

Hefti NP-55-90. [Hefti Ltd.] Nonoxynol-9; CAS 9016-45-9; personal care surfactant.

Hefti PGE-400-DS. [Hefti Ltd.] PEG-8 distearate; CAS 9005-08-7; nonionic; surfactant for pharmaceuticals, cosmetics, to incorporate fats and ester waxes in creams; homogenizer for suppository bases; plasticizer for plastics; solid; HLB 8.0; 100% conc.

Hefti PGE-400-MS. [Hefti Ltd.] PEG-8 stearate; CAS 9004-99-3; nonionic; o/w emulsifier for cosmetic creams, pharmaceutical ointments, active ingreds.; paper industry deinking; solid; HLB 11.5; 100% conc.

Hefti PGE-600-DS. [Hefti Ltd.] PEG-12 distearate; CAS 9005-08-7; nonionic; o/w emulsifier for cosmetics, pharmaceuticals; plasticizer for plastics, various tech. applics.; flakes; HLB 11.5; 100% conc.

Hefti PGE-600-ML. [Hefti Ltd.] PEG-12 laurate; CAS 9004-81-3; nonionic; emulsifier, solubilizer for pharmaceuticals, cosmetics, textile oils, insecticides, pesticides; antistat for plastics; liq.; HLB 15.0; 100% conc.

Hefti PGE-600-MO. [Hefti Ltd.] PEG-12 oleate; CAS 9004-96-0; personal care surfactant.

Hefti PGE-600-MS. [Hefti Ltd.] PEG-12 stearate; CAS 9004-99-3; nonionic; emulsifier, solubilizer for pharmaceuticals, cosmetics, textile oils, insecticides, pesticides; solid; HLB 13.5; 100% conc.

Hefti PMS-33. [Hefti Ltd.] Propylene glycol stearate; CAS 1323-39-3; EINECS 215-354-3; nonionic; emulsifier, consistency regulator for shampoos, lotions, makeup, cosmetics; solubilizer for lipstick colorants; food emulsiifer; solid; HLB 3.5; 100% conc.

Hefti QO-33-F. [Hefti Ltd.] Sorbitan sesquioleate; CAS 8007-43-0; EINECS 232-360-1; nonionic; emulsifier for cosmetic w/o emulsions; liq.; HLB 4.0; 100% conc.

Hefti RS-55-40. [Hefti Ltd.] PEG-40 stearate; CAS 9004-99-3; 31791-00-2; nonionic; o/w emulsifier for cosmetic creams, lotions, pharmaceutical ointments; glass surface finishing agent; for silicone oil, cooling emulsions; solid; HLB 17.0; 100% conc.

Hefti RS-55-100. [Hefti Ltd.] PEG-100 stearate; CAS 9004-99-3; emulsifier.

Hefti Sorbex-R. [Hefti Ltd.] Sorbitol; CAS 50-70-4; EINECS 200-061-5; cosmetic/pharmaceutical ingred.

Hefti Sorbex-RP. [Hefti Ltd.] Sorbitol; CAS 50-70-4; EINECS 200-061-5; cosmetic/pharmaceutical ingred.

Hefti TO-33-F. [Hefti Ltd.] Sorbitan trioleate; CAS 26266-58-0; EINECS 247-569-3; nonionic; w/o emulsifier for cosmetics, pharmaceuticals; antifoamer, solubilizer; for various tech. applics.; liq.; HLB 2.5; 100% conc.

Hefti TO-55-E. [Hefti Ltd.] PEG-18 sorbitan trioleate; CAS 9005-70-3; nonionic; o/w and w/o emulsifier for min. oils, veg. oils, train oils, waxes, etc.; for cattle feed, textiles, biocides, paints, varnishes, plastics, leather, fur, tech. applics., cosmetics, pharmaceuticals; liq.; HLB 10.5; 100% conc.

Hefti TO-55-EL. [Hefti Ltd.] PEG-17 sorbitan trioleate; CAS 9005-70-3; nonionic; o/w and w/o emulsifier for min. oils, veg. oils, train oils, waxes, etc.; for cattle feed, textiles, biocides, paints, varnishes, plastics, leather, fur, tech. applics., cosmetics, pharmaceuticals; liq.; HLB 10.0; 100% conc.

Hefti TO-55-F. [Hefti Ltd.] Polysorbate 85; CAS 9005-70-3; nonionic; o/w and w/o emulsifier cosmetics, pharmaceuticals, tech. emulsions (wood preservation, pigment stabilization, furniture polishes); liq.; HLB 11.0; 100% conc.

Hefti TS-33-F. [Hefti Ltd.] Sorbitan tristearate; CAS 26658-19-5; EINECS 247-891-4; nonionic; w/o emulsifier for cosmetics, pharmaceuticals; stabilizer for textile printing inks; for silicone antifoams, polish mfg., wax working; flakes; HLB 2.0; 100% conc.

Heparinoid HpDl. [Bioiberica] Sodium dermatan sulfate, heparin, sodium heparin, and sodium chondroitin sulfate.

Herbalcomplex 1 Special. [Novarom GmbH] Propylene glycol, matricaria extract, coltsfoot extract, hypericum extract, sage extract, yarrow extract, and pansy extract.

Herbalcomplex 2 Special. [Novarom GmbH] Propylene glycol, witch hazel extract, tormentil extract, sage extract, and wild thyme extract.

Herbaliquid Alpine Herbs Special. [Novarom GmbH] Propylene glycol, horsetail extract, arnica extract, juniper extract, gentian extract, and pine needle extract; botanical extract.

Herbaliquid Camomile Special. [Novarom GmbH] Propylene glycol and matricaria extract; botanical extract.

Herbaliquid Hops Special. [Novarom GmbH] Propylene glycol and hops extract; botanical extract.

Herbaliquid Rosemary Special. [Novarom GmbH] Propylene glycol and rosemary extract; botanical extract.

Herbaliquid Watercress Special. [Novarom GmbH] Propylene glycol, polysorbate 20, and watercress extract.

Herbasol 7 Herb Complex. [Cosmetochem] Birch, stinging nettle, horsetail, coltsfoot, yarrow, rosemary, and mother of thyme extracts in propylene glycol/water; botanical extract for bath preps. and hair cosmetics; brn. clear sol'n.; sol. in water, water/ethanol mixts. to 60% alcohol content, anionic, cationic, and nonionic surfactants.

Herbasol Alpine Herbs Complex. [Cosmetochem] Gentian root, arnica montana, balm mint, sage, mother of thyme, and rosemary extracts in propylene glycol/water; botanical extract for bath preps.; brn. clear sol'n.; sol. in water, water/ethanol mixts. to 60% alcohol content, anionic, cationic, and nonionic surfactants.

Herbasol Complexes. [Cosmetochem] Water and alcohol-sol. natural plant extracts; cosmetic specialties.

Herbasol Complex A. [Cosmetochem] Yarrow, balm mint, sage, camomile, and arnica extracts in propylene glycol/water; botanical extract for use in skin cosmetics, esp. for sensitive and delicate skin, in creams, lotions, face masks, suntan and after-sun preps.; brn. clear sol'n.; sol. in water, water/ethanol mixts. to 60% alcohol content, anionic, cationic, and nonionic surfactants.

Herbasol Complex B. [Cosmetochem] Camomile and arnica extracts in propylene glycol/water; botanical extract for use in skin cosmetics, esp. suntan lotions and after-sun preps. to soothe the skin; brn. clear sol'n.; sol. in water, water/ethanol mixts. to 60% alcohol content, anionic, cationic, and nonionic surfactants.

Herbasol Complex C. [Cosmetochem] Balm mint and sage extracts in propylene glycol/water; botanical extract for invigorating bath and massage preps., face masks, etc.; brn. clear sol'n.; sol. in water, water/ethanol mixts. to 60% alcohol content, anionic, cationic, and nonionic surfactants.

Herbasol Complex D. [Cosmetochem] Horsetail, witch hazel, St. John's wort, yarrow, and balm mint extracts in propylene glycol/water; botanical extract for after-shave lotions and facial cleansers; brn. clear sol'n.; sol. in water, water/ethanol mixts. to 60% alcohol content, anionic, cationic, and nonionic surfactants.

Herbasol Complex E. [Cosmetochem] Stinging nettle, birch, horsetail, and camomile extracts in propylene glycol/water; botanical extract for hair treatment preps. (hair tonics, anti-dandruff preps., shampoos); brn. clear sol'n.; sol. in water, water/ethanol mixts. to 60% alcohol content, anionic, cationic, and nonionic surfactants.

Herbasol Complex GU-61. [Cosmetochem] A glycolic extract from alpine lichen and liquorice root; botanical extract with bactericidal, fungicidal, antipholigistic, and anti-inflammatory props. used in skin care preps., after-shave prods., massage emulsions, and facial tonics.

Herbasol Distillates. [Cosmetochem] Steam-distilled botanical extracts; cosmetic specialties.; colorless.

Herbasol Dry Extracts. [Cosmetochem] Spray-dried powd. botanical extracts; cosmetic specialties.

Herbasol-Extract Algae. [Cosmetochem] Water, propylene glycol, and algae extract; botanical extract for cosmetics.

Herbasol-Extract Almond. [Cosmetochem] Water, propylene glycol, and sweet almond extract; botanical extract for cosmetics.

Herbasol-Extract Aloe. [Cosmetochem] Water, propylene glycol, and aloe extract; botanical extract for cosmetics.

Herbasol-Extract Arnica. [Cosmetochem] Water, propylene glycol, and arnica extract; botanical extract for cosmetics.

Herbasol-Extract Balm Mint. [Cosmetochem] Water, propylene glycol, and balm mint extract; botanical extract for cosmetics.

Herbasol-Extract Calendula. [Cosmetochem] Water, propylene glycol, and calendula extract; botanical extract for cosmetics.

Herbasol-Extract Eucalyptus. [Cosmetochem] Water, propylene glycol, and eucalyptus extract; botanical extract for cosmetics.

Herbasol-Extract Ginseng. [Cosmetochem] Water, propylene glycol, and ginseng extract; botanical extract for cosmetics.

Herbasol-Extract Hamemelis. [Cosmetochem] Water, propylene glycol, and witch hazel extract; botanical extract for cosmetics.

Herbasol-Extract Ivy. [Cosmetochem] Water, propylene glycol, and ivy extract; botanical extract for cosmetics.

Herbasol-Extract Marigold. [Cosmetochem] Water, propylene glycol, and calendula extract; botanical extract for cosmetics.

Herbasol-Extract Peppermint. [Cosmetochem] Water, propylene glycol, and peppermint extract; botanical extract for cosmetics.

Herbasol-Extract St. John's Wort. [Cosmetochem] Water, propylene glycol, and hypericum extract; botanical extract for cosmetics.

Herbasol Extract Walnut Shell Oil-Sol. [Cosmetochem] Green walnut shells extract in sunflower oil; oily botanical extract for use as a tanning component in suntan oils.

Herbasol Extract Walnut Shell Water-Sol. [Cosmetochem] A propylene glycol/water extract from green walnut shells; botanical extract for use as a tanning agent in suntan preps.

Herbasol-Extract Yarrow. [Cosmetochem] Water, propylene glycol, and yarrow extract; botanical extract for cosmetics.

Herbasol Forte Extracts. [Cosmetochem] Aromatic botanical extracts in anhyd. dipropylene glycol; cosmetic specialties.

Herbasol Herbes de Provence Complex. [Cosmetochem] Sage, rosemary, lavender, laurel, juniper, and mother of thyme extracts in propylene glycol/water; botanical extract for bath and skin preps.; brn. clear sol'n.; sol. in water, water/ethanol mixts. to 60% alcohol content, anionic, cationic, and nonionic surfactants.

Herbasol HP Extracts. [Cosmetochem] High performance, conc. botanical extracts; cosmetic specialties.

Herbasol IPA Extracts. [Cosmetochem] Alcohol-sol. botanical extracts in isopropyl alcohol; avail. extracts incl. birch, yarrow, arnica, calendula, ginseng, witch hazel, camomile, walnut, etc.; for use in hair sprays, deodorant sprays, foot sprays, dry powd. shampoos, nail varnish removers, sun protection sprays, bath preps.; sol. in alcohols, chlorinated hydrocarbons, aerosol propellants, esters, and ketones.

Herbasol O/S Extracts. [Cosmetochem] Oil-sol. botanical extracts in IPM or veg. oil; cosmetic specialties.

Herbasol Sedative Complex. [Cosmetochem] Camomile, balm mint, and valerian extracts in propylene glycol/water; botanical extract for relaxing bath preps.; brn. clear sol'n.; sol. in water, water/ethanol mixts. to 60% alcohol content, anionic, cationic, and nonionic surfactants.

Herbasol Stimulant Complex. [Cosmetochem] Rosemary, sage, arnica, and St. John's wort extracts in propylene glycol/water; botanical extract for stimulating and invigorating bath preps.; brn. clear sol'n.; sol. in water, water/ethanol mixts. to 60% alcohol content, anionic, cationic, and nonionic surfactants.

Herbasol W/S Extracts. [Cosmetochem] Water-sol. botanical extracts in propylene glycol and water; cosmetic specialties.

Hercolyn® D. [Hercules] Methyl hydrog. rosinate; resinous plasticizer or tackifier in finished prods. such as lacquers, inks, adhesives, floor tiles, vinyl plastisols, artificial leather, and antifouling paints; fixative and carrier in perfumes and cosmetic preps.; lt. amber visc. liq.; low odor; sol. in ester, ketones, alcohols, ethers, coal tar, petrol. hydrocarbons, and veg. and min. oils; insol. in water; dens. 1.02 kg/l; visc. (G-H) Z2–Z3; b.p. 360–364 C; acid no. 7; sapon. no. 155; ref. index 1.52; flash pt. 183 C (COC).

Hest CSO. [Heterene] Cetearyl octanoate; cosmetic ingred. for moisturizing creams, night creams, replenishing creams.

Hest E.G.D.S. [Heterene] Glycol distearate; CAS 627-83-8; EINECS 211-014-3; cosmetic ingred. for conditioning shampoos, liq. soap, shower gels.

Hest MS. [Heterene] Myristyl stearate; CAS 17661-50-6; EINECS 241-640-2; bodying agent, emollient for creams and lotions; pearlescent in anionic systems; spermaceti replacement; wh. to off-wh. flake; m.p. 43-47 C; acid no. 5 max.; iodine no. 1 max.; sapon. no. 109-120.

Hetaine CLA. [Heterene] Canolamidopropyl betaine; cosmetic ingred. for shampoos, conditioning shampoos, low-irritation shampoos, liq. soap, pearlescent shower gels.

Hetamide 1069. [Heterene] Capramide DEA; CAS 136-26-5; EINECS 205-234-9; cosmetic ingred.; pale yel. liq.; acid no. 0.5 max.

Hetamide CMA. [Heterene] Modified cocamide MEA; CAS 68140-00-1; EINECS 268-770-2; thickener, foam booster, foam stabilizer, emulsifier for cosmetics; Gardner 8 max. flake; m.p. 68-74 C; acid no. 5.0 max.; 99% conc.

Hetamide CME. [Heterene] Cocamide MEA; CAS 68140-00-1; EINECS 268-770-2; thickener, foam booster, foam stabilizer, emulsifier for cosmetics; tan flake; pH 7.5-9.0 (5%); 99% conc.

Hetamide CME-CO. [Heterene] Cocamide MEA; CAS 68140-00-1; EINECS 268-770-2; thickener, foam booster/stabilizer, emulsifier; Gardner 5 max. flake; acid no. 1.0 max.; pH 9.5-10.5 (5%).

Hetamide DO. [Heterene] Oleamide DEA, diethanolamine; Gardner 7 liq.; acid no. 12-16; pH 9.0-10.5 (5%).

Hetamide DS. [Heterene] Stearamide DEA; CAS 93-82-3; EINECS 202-280-1; thickener, foam booster, foam stabilizer, emulsifier for cosmetics; tan flake; acid no. 5 max.; pH 9.0-10.5 (5%); 99% conc.

Hetamide DSUC. [Heterene] Modified cocamide DEA; CAS 61791-31-9; EINECS 263-163-9; cosmetic ingred.; yel. to lt. amber clear liq.; acid no. 18-22.

Hetamide DT. [Heterene] Tallamide DEA; CAS 68155-20-4; EINECS 268-949-5; emulsifier.

Hetamide IS. [Heterene] Isostearamide DEA; CAS 52794-79-3; EINECS 258-193-4; conditioner.

Hetamide LL. [Heterene] Lauramide DEA; CAS 120-40-1; EINECS 204-393-1; thickener, foam booster, foam stabilizer, emulsifier for cosmetics; Gardner 2 max. solid; acid no. 2.0 max.; pH 9.5-10.5 (5%); 99% conc.

Hetamide LML. [Heterene] Lauramide/linoleamide DEA; thickener, foam booster, foam stabilizer, emulsifier; Gardner 8 max. liq.; 99% conc.

Hetamide LN. [Heterene] Linoleamide DEA; CAS 56863-02-6; EINECS 260-410-2; thickener, foam booster, foam stabilizer, emulsifier for cosmetics; Gardner 8 max. liq.; acid no. 2 max.; pH 9.5-11.0 (5%); 99% conc.

Hetamide LNO. [Heterene] Linoleamide DEA; CAS 56863-02-6; EINECS 260-410-2; foam builder, thickener; Gardner 9 max. liq.; acid no. 1.0 max.

Hetamide M. [Heterene] Myristamide DEA; CAS 7545-23-5; EINECS 231-426-7; thickener, foam booster, foam stabilizer, emulsifier for cosmetics; Gardner 2 max. solid; acid no. 2 max.; pH 9.5-10.5 (5%); 99% conc.

Hetamide MA. [Heterene] Acetamide MEA; CAS 142-26-7; EINECS 205-530-8; thickener, foam booster, foam stabilizer, emulsifier for cosmetics; Gardner 1 max. liq.; acid no. 15 max.

Hetamide MC. [Heterene] Cocamide DEA; CAS 61791-31-9; EINECS 263-163-9; nonionic; thickener, foam booster, foam stabilizer, emulsifier for cosmetics; Gardner 5 max. liq.; sp.gr. 0.98; pH 9.5–11.0 (5%); 100% act.

Hetamide MCS. [Heterene] Cocamide DEA; CAS 61791-31-9; EINECS 263-163-9; thickener, foam booster, foam stabilizer, emulsifier; liq.

Hetamide ML. [Heterene] Lauramide/myristamide DEA; CAS 120-40-1; EINECS 204-393-1; nonionic; thickener, foam booster, foam stabilizer, emulsifier for cosmetics; Gardner 5 max. solid; sp.gr. 0.96; m.p. 35 C; acid no. 1 max.; pH 9.5-11.0 (5%); 100% act.

Hetamide MM. [Heterene] Myristamide MEA; CAS 142-58-5; EINECS 205-546-5; cosmetic emulsifer, pearlescent.

Hetamide MML. [Heterene] Lauramide MEA; CAS 142-78-9; EINECS 205-560-1; personal care surfactant.

Hetamide MO. [Heterene] Oleamide MEA; CAS 111-58-0; EINECS 203-884-8; foam stabilizer, thickener.

Hetamide MOC. [Heterene] Lauramide DEA; CAS 120-40-1; EINECS 204-393-1; thickener, foam booster, foam stabilizer, emulsifier for cosmetics; Gardner 5 max. liq.; acid no. 2 max.; pH 9.5-10.5 (5%); 99% conc.

Hetamide MS. [Heterene] Stearamide MEA; CAS 111-57-9; EINECS 203-883-2; personal care surfactant, thickener, pearlescent.

Hetamide OC. [Heterene] Oleamide DEA; CAS 93-83-4; EINECS 202-281-7; thickener, foam booster, foam stabilizer, emulsifier; liq.

Hetamide RC. [Heterene] Cocamide DEA; CAS 61791-31-9; EINECS 263-163-9; nonionic; thickener, foam booster, foam stabilizer, emulsifier for shampoos, liq. soap; Gardner 8 max. liq.; sp.gr. 1.01; pH 9.5-11.0 (5%); 100% act.

Hetamine 5L-25. [Heterene] Stearamidopropyl dimethylamine lactate; CAS 55819-53-9; EINECS 259-837-7; cationic; antistat, conditioner for hair; compat. with most anionic surfactants; Gardner 4 max. stratified liq. to paste; pH 4.0–5.0; 19-21% solids.

Hetan SL. [Heterene] Sorbitan laurate; CAS 1338-39-2; nonionic; lipophilic emulsifier for cosmetics; flake.

Hetan SO. [Heterene] Sorbitan oleate; CAS 1338-43-8; EINECS 215-665-4; nonionic; lipophilic emulsifier for cosmetics; flake.

Hetan SS. [Heterene] Sorbitan stearate; CAS 1338-41-6; EINECS 215-664-9; nonionic; lipophilic emulsifier for cosmetics, moisturizing creams, replenishing creams; ivory flake; acid no. 11 max.; sapon. no. 140-154; hyd. no. 230-260; 99% conc.

Hetester 412. [Heterene; Bernel] Stearyl stearate; CAS 2778-96-3; EINECS 220-476-5; emollient for stick cosmetics; FDA, EEC, and Japanese compliances; wh. to off-wh. flake; sol. in oil; m.p. 52-56 C; acid no. 2 max.; iodine no. 1 max.; sapon. no. 100-115; usage level: 2-10%.

Hetester 3236S. [Heterene; Bernel] Myristyleicosyl stearate.

Hetester FAO. [Heterene; Bernel] C12–15 alcohols octanoate; unique skin feel ingred., wetting agent; used in personal care prods., hair and skin care prods., makeup, antiperspirants; emollient IPM replacement; FDA, EEC compliances; yel. clear liq.; sol. @ 5% in corn, safflower, and min. oils, octyl palmitate, oleyl alcohol, ethanol; insol. in water; acid no. 0.5 max.; sapon. no. 138–152; hyd. no. 20 max.; pH 6.5–7.5.; usage level: 2-10%.

Hetester HCA. [Heterene; Bernel] Glyceryl triacetyl hydroxystearate.; CAS 27233-00-7; EINECS 248-351-0; gloss agent, film-former for lip oils, skin oils, lipsticks, eye makeup; high visc. and adherence; FDA, EEC compliance; yel. clear to hazy visc. liq.; sol. @ 5% in castor oil, min. oil, octyl palmitate, SD-40 alcohol; iodine no. 3.0 max.; sapon. no. 270-305; pH 5.0 ± 1.5 (3% in IPA/water 1:1); usage level: 10-30%.

Hetester HCP. [Heterene; Bernel] PPG-3 hydrog. castor oil; emollient for lip and cosmetic prods.; FDA, EEC compliance; yel. clear visc. liq.; sol. @ 5% in castor oil, min. oil, octyl palmitate, SD-40 alcohol; disp. in water; acid no. 5 max.; iodine no. 3 max.; sapon. no. 140-150; hyd. no. 130-145; pH 7.0 ± 1.5 (3%); usage level: 3-15%.

Hetester HSS. [Heterene; Bernel] Isocetyl stearoyl stearate; CAS 97338-28-8; emollient with unusual skin feel, pigment dispersant for stick prods., emulsion systems; binding oil for pressed powds.; FDA, EEC, and Japanese compliances; yel. liq.; sol. in most cosmetic oils; partly sol. in 95% ethanol; insol. in water; acid no. 5 max.; sapon. no. 130-150; hyd. no. 15 max.; usage level: 1-6%.

Hetester ISS. [Heterene; Bernel] Isostearyl stearoyl stearate; CAS 134017-12-2; emollient for use in stick prods., pigmented emulsion-type systems; binding oil for use in pressed powds.; FDA, EEC compliance; yel. liq.; sol. @ 5% in most cosmetic oils; partly sol. in 95% ethanol; insol. in water; acid no. 4.0 max.; sapon. no. 115–135; hyd. no. 20 max.; usage level: 1-6%.

Hetester MS. [Heterene; Bernel] Myristyl stearate; CAS 17661-50-6; EINECS 241-640-2; bodying agent in creams and lotions; in certain anionic systems, imparts pearling effects; replacement for spermaceti; wh. to off-wh. flake; m.p. 43–47 C; acid no. 5.0 max.; iodine no. 1.0 max.; sapon. no. 109–120.

Hetester PCA. [Heterene; Bernel] Propylene glycol ceteth-3 acetate; CAS 93385-03-6; nonionic; emulsifier, pigment wetter, antichalking agent, emollient used in personal care prods., antiperspirants; FDA, EEC, and Japanese compliances; colorless clear liq.; sol. @ 5% in water, 95% ethanol, most cosmetic oils; cloud pt. 15 C; acid no. 2 max.; sapon. no. 110–130; hyd. no. 10 max.; pH 6.0–7.0; usage level: 5-15%; 100% conc.

Hetester PCP. [Heterene; Bernel] Propylene glycol ceteth-3 propionate.

Hetester PHA. [Heterene; Bernel] Propylene glycol isoceteth-3 acetate; CAS 93385-13-8; nonionic; emulsifier, pigment wetter, antichalking agent, emollient used in personal care prods., antiperspirants; FDA, EEC, and Japanese compliances; wh. to pale yel. clear liq.; self-emulsifying in water; sol. in 95% ethanol, most cosmetic oils; acid no. 2 max.; sapon. no. 110–130; hyd. no. 10 max.; pH 6.0–7.0; usage level: 2-15%; 100% conc.

Hetester PMA. [Heterene; Bernel] Propylene glycol myristyl ether acetate; emollient, solv., and plasticizer for anhyd. oil systems, emulsions; FDA, EEC, and Japanese compliances; colorless clear liq.; sol. @ 5% in most cosmetic oils; insol. in water, glycols, 70% ethanol; acid no. 2.0 max.; sapon. no. 140–160; hyd. no. 10.0 max.; pH 6.0–7.0 (5% in 50/50 IPA/water); cloud pt. ≈ 0 C.; usage level: 2-10%.

Hetester SSS. [Heterene; Bernel] Stearyl stearoyl stearate; emollient used in cosmetic stick formulations, emulsion systems; FDA, EEC compliance; cream to lt. tan cryst. solid; sol. @ 5% and 45 C in most cosmetic oils; partly sol. in 95% ethanol; insol. in water; acid no. 4.0 max.; sapon. no. 130–140; hyd. no. 20 max.; usage level: 1-12%.

Hetester TICC. [Heterene; Bernel] Triisocetyl citrate; oily liq. emollient useful in stick and pigmented emulsion-type prods., skin care prods., cleansing creams, makeup; pigment dispersing properties; yel. clear liq.; sol. @ 5% in castor oil, min. oil, safflower oil, octyl palmitate, oleyl alcohol, SD-40 ethyl alcohol (95%); insol. in water and propylene glycol; acid no. 4.0 max.; sapon. no. 165–180.

Hetlan AC. [Heterene] Acetylated lanolin alcohols; CAS 61788-49-6; EINECS 262-980-8; emollient for creams and lotions; pale yel. liq., faint char. odor; acid no. 1.0 max.; sapon. no. 180–200; hyd. no. 8.0 max.; 99% conc.

Hetlan AWS. [Heterene] PPG-12 PEG-50 lanolin; CAS 68458-88-8; cosmetics ingred.; Gardner 10 max. liq.; acid no. 2 max.; iodine no. 10 max.; hyd. no. 33-50; pH 5-7 (10% aq.).

Hetlan OH. [Heterene] Hydroxylated lanolin; CAS 68424-66-8; EINECS 270-315-8; cosmetic ingred.; Gardner 10 soft sticky solid; m.p. 39-46 C; acid no. 10 max.; iodine no. 15-23; sapon. no. 95-110; 99% conc.

Hetol CA. [Heterene] Cetyl alcohol; CAS 36653-82-4; EINECS 253-149-0; cosmetic ingred. for night creams.

Hetol CS. [Heterene] Cetearyl alcohol; cosmetic ingred. for moisturizing creams.

Hetoxalan 75. [Heterene] PEG-75 lanolin; CAS 61790-81-6; emulsifier, emollient; Gardner 11 max. solid; m.p. 48-52 C; acid no. 2 max.; sapon. no. 20 max.; hyd. no. 55 max.; pH 5.5-7.0 (10% aq.); 99% conc.

Hetoxalan 75-50%. [Heterene] PEG-75 lanolin; CAS 61790-81-6; emulsifier, emollient; Gardner 11 max. liq.; acid no. 2 max.; sapon. no. 10 max.; pH 5.5-7.0 (10% aq.); 50% conc.

Hetoxalan 100. [Heterene] PEG-100 lanolin; CAS 61790-81-6; emollient; Gardner 10 max. flake; m.p. 46-54 C; acid no. 2 max.; iodine no. 10 max.; sapon. no. 8-16; 99% conc.

Hetoxamate 100S. [Heterene] PEG-100 stearate; CAS 9004-99-3; cosmetic ingred. for moisturizing creams.

Hetoxamate 150 DSA. [Heterene] PEG-150 distearate; CAS 9005-08-7; cosmetics ingred.

Hetoxamate 200 DL. [Heterene] PEG-4 dilaurate; CAS 9005-02-1; nonionic; thickener, foam booster, foam stabilizer, emulsifier for cosmetics; Gardner 4 max. liq.; sol. in IPA, min. oil; acid no. 10 max.; sapon. no. 165-180.

Hetoxamate 400 DL. [Heterene] PEG-8 dilaurate; CAS 9005-02-1; personal care surfactant.

Hetoxamate 400 DS. [Heterene] PEG-8 distearate; CAS 9005-08-7; thickener, foam booster, foam stabilizer, emulsifier for cosmetics; Gardner 3 max. solid; disp. in water, min. oil; sol. in IPA; acid no. 10 max.; sapon. no. 120-130.

Hetoxamate 600 DS. [Heterene] PEG-12 distearate; CAS 9005-08-7; cosmetics ingred.

Hetoxamate 600 DT. [Heterene] PEG-12 ditallate; CAS 61791-01-3; cosmetics ingred.

Hetoxamate FA 2-5. [Heterene] PEG-4 tallate; CAS 61791-00-2; personal care surfactant.

Hetoxamate FA-5. [Heterene] PEG-5 tallate; CAS 61791-00-2; nonionic; detergent, emulsifier, lubricant, softener, coupling agent for cosmetics, textiles, leather, metal cleaning; Gardner 7 max. liq.; sol. in IPA, min. oil, disp. in water; HLB 8.8; acid no. 2.0 max.; sapon. no. 100–120; 99% conc.

Hetoxamate FA-20. [Heterene] PEG-20 tallate; CAS 61791-00-2; nonionic; detergent, emulsifier, lubricant, softener, coupling agent for cosmetics, textiles, leather, metal cleaning; semisolid; sol. in water, IPA; disp. min. oil; HLB 14.9; acid no. 2.0; sapon. no. 50–60.

Hetoxamate LA-4. [Heterene] PEG-4 laurate; CAS 9004-81-3; emulsifier.

Hetoxamate LA-5. [Heterene] PEG-5 laurate; CAS 9004-81-3; nonionic; detergent, emulsifier, lubricant, softener, coupling agent for cosmetics, textiles, leather, metal cleaning; Gardner 1 max. liq.; sol. in IPA; disp. in water; HLB 10.5; acid no. 2.0 max. ; sapon. no. 125–145; 99% conc.

Hetoxamate LA-9. [Heterene] PEG-9 laurate; CAS 9004-81-3; nonionic; detergent, emulsifier, lubricant, softener, coupling agent for cosmetics, textiles, leather, metal cleaning; Gardner 1 max. liq.; sol. in water, IPA; HLB 13.3; acid no. 2.0 max.; sapon. no. 90-100; 99% conc.

Hetoxamate MO-2. [Heterene] PEG-2 oleate; CAS 106-12-7; EINECS 203-364-0; detergent, emulsifier for personal care prods.; softener for leather; Gardner 2 max. liq.; sol. in IPA, min. oil; insol. in water; HLB 5.3; acid no. 1 max.; sapon. no. 145–160; 99% conc.

Hetoxamate MO-4. [Heterene] PEG-4 oleate; CAS 9004-96-0; EINECS 233-293-0; softener, emulsifier, coupling agent, lubricant.

Hetoxamate MO-5. [Heterene] PEG-5 oleate; CAS 9004-96-0; nonionic; detergent, emulsifier, lubricant, softener, coupling agent for cosmetics, textiles, leather, metal cleaning; Gardner 3 max. liq.; sol. in IPA; disp. water; HLB 8.8; acid no. 2.0 max. ; sapon. no. 115–125.

Hetoxamate MO-9. [Heterene] PEG-9 oleate; CAS 9004-96-0; nonionic; detergent, emulsifier, lubricant, softener, coupling agent for cosmetics, textiles, leather, metal cleaning; Gardner 4 max. liq.; sol. in IPA; disp. water; HLB 11.7; acid no. 2.0 max.; sapon. no. 80–88; 99% conc.

Hetoxamate MO-14. [Heterene] PEG-14 oleate; CAS 9004-96-0; personal care surfactant.

Hetoxamate SA-5. [Heterene] PEG-5 stearate; CAS 9004-99-3; nonionic; detergent, emulsifier, lubricant, softener, coupling agent for cosmetics, textiles, leather, metal cleaning; Gardner 2 max. solid; sol. in IPA; disp. hot water, min. oil; HLB 8.8; acid no. 2.0 max. ; sapon. no. 105-120.

Hetoxamate SA-6. [Heterene] PEG-6 stearate; CAS 9004-99-3; cosmetics ingred.

Hetoxamate SA-7. [Heterene] PEG-7 stearate; CAS 9004-99-3; nonionic; detergent, emulsifier for personal care prods.; softener for leather; Gardner 1 max. solid; sol. in IPA; disp. in water; HLB 10.5; acid no. 2 max.; sapon. no. 90–100.

Hetoxamate SA-8. [Heterene] PEG-8 stearate; CAS 9004-99-3; cosmetics ingred.

Hetoxamate SA-9. [Heterene] PEG-9 stearate; CAS 9004-99-3; EINECS 226-312-9; nonionic; detergent, emulsifier, lubricant, softener, coupling agent for cosmetics, textiles, leather, metal cleaning; Gardner 1 max. solid; sol. in IPA; disp. hot water; HLB 11.5; acid no. 2.0 max.; sapon. no. 80-90.

Hetoxamate SA-12. [Heterene] PEG-12 stearate; CAS 9004-99-3; cosmetics ingred.

Hetoxamate SA-13. [Heterene] PEG-12 stearate; CAS 9004-99-3; detergent, emulsifier for personal care prods.; softener for leather; Gardner 2 max. liq.; sol. in water, IPA; HLB 13.4; acid no. 2 max.; sapon. no. 60–70.

Hetoxamate SA-20. [Heterene] PEG-20 stearate; CAS 9004-99-3; cosmetics ingred.

Hetoxamate SA-23. [Heterene] PEG-20 stearate; CAS 9004-99-3; detergent, emulsifier for personal care prods.; softener for leather; Gardner 2 max. solid; sol. in water, IPA; HLB 15.6; acid no. 2 max.; sapon. no. 39–49.

Hetoxamate SA-25. [Heterene] PEG-25 stearate; CAS 9004-99-3; cosmetics ingred.

Hetoxamate SA-35. [Heterene] PEG-35 stearate, dioxane-free; CAS 9004-99-3; nonionic; detergent, emulsifier, lubricant, softener, coupling agent for cosmetics, textiles, leather, metal cleaning; Gardner 2 max. flake; sol. in water, IPA; HLB 16.9; acid no. 2.0 max.; sapon. no. 24–34; hyd. no. 33-43.

Hetoxamate SA-40. [Heterene] PEG-40 stearate; CAS 9004-99-3; nonionic; detergent, emulsifier for personal care prods., moisturizing creams, night creams; softener for leather; Gardner 2 max. flake; sol. in water, IPA; HLB 17.2; sapon. no. 24–34.

Hetoxamate SA-90. [Heterene] PEG-90 stearate; CAS 9004-99-3; nonionic; detergent, emulsifier, lubricant, softener, coupling agent for cosmetics, textiles, leather, metal cleaning; Gardner 3 max. solid; sol. in water IPA; HLB 18.6; sapon. no. 9-20; hyd. no. 11-18.

Hetoxamate SA-90F. [Heterene] PEG-90 stearate; CAS 9004-99-3; nonionic; detergent, emulsifier, lubricant, softener, coupling agent for cosmetics, textiles, leather, metal cleaning; off-wh. to tan flakes; sol. in water, IPA; acid no. 2 max.; sapon. no. 9-20; hyd. no. 11-18.

Hetoxamate SA-100. [Heterene] PEG-100 stearate; CAS

9004-99-3; cosmetic ingred. for night creams, replenishing creams.

Hetoxamide C-4. [Heterene] PEG-5 cocamide; CAS 61791-08-0; cosmetics ingred.; dk. brn. liq.; hyd. no. 180-210; pH 8.5-9.5 (10%); 99% conc.

Hetoxamide CD-4. [Heterene] PEG-3 cocamide; CAS 61791-08-0; personal care surfactant.

Hetoxamide CD-6. [Heterene] PEG-6 cocamide; CAS 61791-08-0; personal care surfactant.

Hetoxamine C-2. [Heterene] PEG-2 cocamine; CAS 61791-14-8; cationic; emulsifier, softener, antistat, water repellent, desizing agent in cosmetics, agriculture, waxes, oils, textile/leather, metal cleaning; Gardner 8 max. liq.; sol. in IPA, min. oil; gels in water; m.w. 285; 95% tert. amine.

Hetoxamine C-5. [Heterene] PEG-5 cocamine; CAS 61791-14-8; cationic; emulsifier, softener, antistat, water repellent, desizing agent in cosmetics, agriculture, waxes, oils, textile/leather, metal cleaning; Gardner 8 max. liq.; sol. in water, IPA, min. oil; m.w. 425; 95% tert. amine.

Hetoxamine C-15. [Heterene] PEG-15 cocamine; CAS 61791-14-8; cationic; emulsifier, softener, antistat, water repellent, desizing agent in cosmetics, agriculture, waxes, oils, textile/leather, metal cleaning; Gardner 12 max. liq.; sol. in water, IPA; m.w. 860; 95% tert. amine.

Hetoxamine O-2. [Heterene] PEG-2 oleamine; nonionic; emulsifier, softener, antistat, water repellent, desizing agent in agriculture, waxes, oils, textile/leather, metal cleaning; liq.; m.w. 350; sol. in IPA, min. oil; 99% conc.

Hetoxamine O-5. [Heterene] PEG-5 oleamine; nonionic; emulsifier, softener, antistat, water repellent, desizing agent in agriculture, waxes, oils, textile/leather, metal cleaning; liq.; m.w. 492; sol. in IPA, min. oil; 99% conc.

Hetoxamine O-15. [Heterene] PEG-15 oleamine; nonionic; emulsifier, softener, antistat, water repellent, desizing agent in agriculture, waxes, oils, textile/leather, metal cleaning; liq.; m.w. 930; sol. in water, IPA.

Hetoxamine S-2. [Heterene] PEG-2 soyamine; CAS 61791-24-0; cationic; emulsifier, softener, antistat, water repellent, desizing agent in agriculture, waxes, oils, textile/leather, metal cleaning, cosmetics; liq.; m.w. 350; sol. in IPA, min. oil.

Hetoxamine S-5. [Heterene] PEG-5 soyamine; CAS 61791-24-0; cationic; emulsifier, softener, antistat, water repellent, desizing agent in agriculture, waxes, oils, textile/leather, metal cleaning, cosmetics; liq.; m.w. 480; sol. in IPA; partly sol. in min. oil; gel in water.

Hetoxamine S-15. [Heterene] PEG-15 soyamine; CAS 61791-24-0; cationic; desizing agent, antistat; emulsifier in cosmetics, agriculture, waxes and oils, leather processing, and metal cleaning industries; water repellent and wet spinning assistant in textile industries; Gardner 12 max. liq., solid; sol. see Hetoxamate SA-13; 95.0% min. tert. amine.

Hetoxamine ST-2. [Heterene] PEG-2 stearamine; CAS 10213-78-2; EINECS 233-520-3; nonionic; emulsifier, softener, antistat, water repellent, desizing agent in cosmetics, agriculture, waxes, oils, textile/leather, metal cleaning; Gardner 7 max. solid; sol. in IPA, min. oil; m.w. 388; 95% tert. amine.

Hetoxamine ST-5. [Heterene] PEG-5 stearamine; CAS 26635-92-7; nonionic; emulsifier, softener, antistat, water repellent, desizing agent in agriculture, waxes, oils, textile/leather, metal cleaning; Gardner 8 max. solid; sol. in IPA, min. oil; insol. in water; m.w. 520; 95% tert. amine.

Hetoxamine ST-15. [Heterene] PEG-15 stearamine; CAS 26635-92-7; nonionic; desizing agent, antistat; emulsifier in cosmetics, agriculture, waxes and oils, leather processing, and metal cleaning industries; water repellent and wet spinning assistant in textile industries; Gardner 8 max. solid; sol. in water, IPA; 95% min. tert. amine.

Hetoxamine ST-50. [Heterene] PEG-50 stearamine; CAS 26635-92-7; nonionic; desizing agent, antistat; emulsifier in cosmetics, agriculture, waxes and oils, leather processing, and metal cleaning industries; water repellent and wet spinning assistant in textile industries; Gardner 8 max. semisolid; sol. in water, IPA.

Hetoxamine T-2. [Heterene] PEG-2 hydrog. tallowamine; CAS 61791-26-2; cationic; emulsifier, softener, antistat, water repellent, desizing agent in cosmetics, agriculture, waxes, oils, textile/leather, metal cleaning; Gardner 10 max. liq.; sol. in IPA, min. oil; insol. in water; m.w. 350; 95% tert. amine.

Hetoxamine T-5. [Heterene] PEG-5 hydrog. tallow amine; CAS 61791-26-2; cationic; emulsifier, softener, antistat, water repellent, desizing agent in cosmetics, agriculture, waxes, oils, textile/leather, metal cleaning; Gardner 10 max. semisolid; sol. in water, IPA, min. oil; m.w. 490; 95% tert. amine.

Hetoxamine T-15. [Heterene] PEG-15 hydrog. tallowamine; CAS 61791-26-2; nonionic; emulsifier, softener, antistat, water repellent, desizing agent in cosmetics, agriculture, waxes, oils, textile/leather, metal cleaning; Gardner 10 max. semisolid; sol. in water, IPA; m.w. 925; 95% tert. amine.

Hetoxamine T-20. [Heterene] PEG-20 hydrog. tallow amine; CAS 61791-26-2; nonionic; emulsifier, softener, antistat, water repellent, desizing agent in cosmetics, agriculture, waxes, oils, textile/leather, metal cleaning; Gardner 10 max. semisolid; sol. in water, IPA; m.w. 1150; 95% tert. amine.

Hetoxamine T-30. [Heterene] PEG-30 hydrog. tallow amine; CAS 61791-26-2; nonionic; emulsifier, softener, antistat, water repellent, desizing agent in cosmetics, agriculture, waxes, oils, textile/leather, metal cleaning; Gardner 10 max. semisolid; sol. in water, IPA; 90% tert. amine.

Hetoxamine T-50. [Heterene] PEG-50 tallowamine; emulsifier, antistat, dyeing assistant, softener, detergent for cosmetics; Gardner 10 max. solid; sol. in water, IPA; 90% tert. amine.

Hetoxamine T-50-70%. [Heterene] PEG-50 tallowamine; emulsifier, softener, antistat, water repellent, desizing agent in cosmetics, agriculture, waxes, oils, textile/leather, metal cleaning; Gardner 10 max. liq.; sol. in water, IPA; 70% act.

Hetoxide BN-13. [Heterene] PEG-13 β-naphthol ether; CAS 35545-57-4; nonionic; emollient, emulsifier, visc. control agent, lubricant, pigment dispersant, perfume solubilizer, used in cosmetics, household, textile industry, metal treating and plating; intermediate; Gardner 8 max. paste; sol. in water, IPA, min. oil; HLB 16.0; acid no. 1.0; hyd. no. 73-83; 99% conc.

Hetoxide C-2. [Heterene] PEG-2 castor oil; CAS 61791-12-6; nonionic; emollient, emulsifier, solubilizer, pigment dispersant, detergent used in cosmetics, household, textile industry; Gardner 6 max. liq.; sol. in IPA, min. oil; insol. in water; HLB 1.7; acid no. 2 max.; sapon. no. 155–170; 99% conc.

Hetoxide C-9. [Heterene] PEG-9 castor oil; CAS 61791-12-6; nonionic; emollient, emulsifier, solubilizer, pigment dispersant, detergent used in cosmetics, household, textile industry; Gardner 5 max. liq.; sol. in IPA, min. oil; disp. in water; HLB 6.0; acid no. 2 max.; sapon. no. 120–136.

Hetoxide C-15. [Heterene] PEG-15 castor oil; CAS 61791-12-6; nonionic; emollient, emulsifier, solubilizer, pigment dispersant, detergent, lubricant used in cosmetics, household, textile industry; Gardner 5 max. liq.; sol. in IPA, min. oil; disp. in water; HLB 8.3; acid no. 2 max.; sapon. no. 95–105.

Hetoxide C-25. [Heterene] PEG-25 castor oil; CAS 61791-12-6; nonionic; emollient, emulsifier, lubricant, solubilizer, pigment dispersant, detergent used in cosmetics, household, textile industry; Gardner 5 max. liq.; sol. in IPA; disp. in water, min. oil; HLB 10.8; acid no. 2 max.; sapon. no. 74–82.

Hetoxide C-30. [Heterene] PEG-30 castor oil; CAS 61791-12-6; nonionic; perfume solubilizer, emollient, emulsifier, visc. control and scouring agent, lubricant, dispersant for cosmetic formulations; dyeing assistant, dye carrier for textiles; used in household cleaning comps., metal treatment, metal plating, chemical intermediate; Gardner 5 max. liq.; sol. in IPA; disp. in water, min. oil; HLB 11.7; acid no. 2 max.; sapon. no. 65–75.

Hetoxide C-40. [Heterene] PEG-40 castor oil; CAS 61791-12-6; nonionic; emollient, emulsifier, lubricant, solubilizer, pigment dispersant, detergent used in cosmetics, household, textile industry; Gardner 4 max. paste; sol. in water, IPA; HLB 13.1; acid no. 1 max.; sapon. no. 55–65; 99% conc.

Hetoxide C-52. [Heterene] PEG-52 castor oil; CAS 61791-12-6; nonionic; cosmetics ingred.

Hetoxide C-60. [Heterene] PEG-60 castor oil; CAS 61791-12-6; nonionic; emollient, emulsifier, solubilizer, pigment dispersant, detergent used in cosmetics, household, textile industry; Gardner 4 max. soft solid; sol. in water, IPA; HLB 14.8; acid no. 2 max.; sapon. no. 41-51; pH 6-8 (3%).

Hetoxide C-200. [Heterene] PEG-200 castor oil; CAS 61791-12-6; nonionic; emollient, emulsifier, lubricant, wetting agent, solubilizer, pigment dispersant, detergent used in cosmetics, household, textile industry; Gardner 4 max. solid; sol. in water, IPA; acid no. 1 max.; sapon. no. 16–18.

Hetoxide C-200-50%. [Heterene] PEG-200 castor oil; CAS 61791-12-6; lubricant, emulsifier, solubilizer for cosmetics; Gardner 4 max. liq.; sol. in water, acid no. 1 max.; sapon no. 7–10; 50% conc.

Hetoxide DNP-4. [Heterene] Nonyl nonoxynol-4; CAS 9014-93-1; nonionic; intermediate, emulsifier for cosmetics; Gardner 4 max. liq.; sol. in IPA, min. oil; disp. in water; HLB 6.7; hyd. no. 120-140; 99% conc.

Hetoxide DNP-5. [Heterene] Nonyl nonoxynol-5; CAS 9014-93-1; nonionic; emollient, emulsifier, solubilizer, pigment dispersant, detergent used in cosmetics, household, textile industry; liq.; sol. in IPA, min. oil, disp. in water.

Hetoxide DNP-9.6. [Heterene] Nonyl nonoxynol-9.6; CAS 9014-93-1; nonionic; intermediate, emulsifier, surfactant for cosmetics; Gardner 5 max. liq.; sol. in IPA, min. oil; disp. in water; HLB 11.0; hyd. no. 65-75; 99% conc.

Hetoxide DNP-10. [Heterene] Nonyl nonoxynol-10; CAS 9014-93-1; nonionic; emollient, emulsifier, solubilizer, pigment dispersant, detergent used in cosmetics, household, textile industry; liq.; sol. in IPA, min. oil, disp. in water.

Hetoxide G-7. [Heterene] Glycereth-7; CAS 31694-55-0; nonionic; emulsifier for cosmetics; Gardner 2 max. liq.; sol. in IPA, water; acid no. 1.0 max.; hyd. no. 412-428; 99% conc.

Hetoxide G-26. [Heterene] Glycereth-26; CAS 31694-55-0; nonionic; humectant for pressure-sensitive adhesives; emulsifier for cosmetics, night creams; Gardner 2 max. liq.; sol. in water, IPA; acid no. 2.0 max.; hyd. no. 127-137; 99% conc.

Hetoxide HC-16. [Heterene] PEG-16 hydrog. castor oil; CAS 61788-85-0; nonionic; emollient, emulsifier, solubilizer, pigment dispersant, detergent used in cosmetics, household, textile industry; Gardner 4 max. liq.; sol. in IPA, min. oil; HLB 8.6; acid no. 1.5 max.; sapon. no. 85–95; 99% conc.

Hetoxide HC-25. [Heterene] PEG-25 hydrog. castor oil; CAS 61788-85-0; nonionic; cosmetics ingred.; Gardner 4 max. semisolid; sol. in water, IPA; HLB 10.8; acid no. 1.5 max.; sapon. no. 67-77; 99% conc.

Hetoxide HC-40. [Heterene] PEG-40 hydrog. castor oil; CAS

61788-85-0; nonionic; emulsifier, lubricant for cosmetics, moisturizing creams; Gardner 4 max. semisolid; sol. in water, IPA; HLB 13.1; acid no. 1.5 max.; sapon. no. 50–60; 99% conc.

Hetoxide HC-60. [Heterene] PEG-60 hydrog. castor oil; CAS 61788-85-0; emulsifier, lubricant for cosmetics; Gardner 4 max. solid; sol. in water, IPA; HLB 14.8; acid no. 1.5 max.; sapon. no. 41–51; hyd. no. 39-49; 99% conc.

Hetoxide NP-4. [Heterene] Nonoxynol-4; CAS 9016-45-9; nonionic; detergent and emulsifier for cosmetics; Gardner 1 max. liq.; sol. in IPA, min. oil; insol. in water; HLB 8.7; hyd. no. 135-139; 99% conc.

Hetoxide NP-6. [Heterene] Nonoxynol-6; CAS 9016-45-9; nonionic; cosmetics ingred.; Gardner 1 max. liq.; sol. in IPA; disp. in water, min. oil; HLB 10.7; hyd. no. 113-119.

Hetoxide NP-9. [Heterene] Nonoxynol-9; CAS 9016-45-9; nonionic; cosmetics ingred.; Gardner 1 max. liq.; sol. in water, IPA; HLB 12.7; hyd. no. 88-93; 99% conc.

Hetoxide NP-10. [Heterene] Nonoxynol-10; CAS 9016-45-9; EINECS 248-294-1; nonionic; cosmetics ingred.; Gardner 1 max. liq.; sol. in water, IPA; acid no. 1 max.; hyd. no. 81-95.

Hetoxide NP-12. [Heterene] Nonoxynol-12; CAS 9016-45-9; nonionic; cosmetics ingred.; Gardner 1 max. semisolid; sol. in water, IPA; HLB 15.7; hyd. no. 72-78; 99% conc.

Hetoxide NP-15. [Heterene] Nonoxynol-15; CAS 9016-45-9; nonionic; cosmetics ingred.; Gardner 1 max. liq.; sol. in water, IPA; HLB 16.4; 85% conc.

Hetoxide NP-30. [Heterene] Nonoxynol-30; CAS 9016-45-9; nonionic; emulsifier for cosmetics, emulsion polymerization; Gardner 4 max. solid; sol. in water, IPA; HLB 17.0; hyd. no. 35-45; 99% conc.

Hetoxide NP-40. [Heterene] Nonoxynol-40; CAS 9016-45-9; nonionic; cosmetics ingred.; Gardner 2 max. solid; sol. in water, IPA; HLB 17.7; 99% conc.

Hetoxide NP-50. [Heterene] Nonoxynol-50; CAS 9016-45-9; nonionic; cosmetics ingred.; Gardner 2 max. solid; sol. in water, IPA; 99% conc.

Hetoxide PEG-200. [Heterene] PEG-4; CAS 25322-68-3; EINECS 203-989-9; cosmetic ingred.

Hetoxide PEG-300. [Heterene] PEG-6; CAS 25322-68-3; EINECS 220-045-1; cosmetic ingred.

Hetoxol 15 CSA. [Heterene] Ceteareth-15; CAS 68439-49-6; detergent, emulsifier, leveling agent, intermediate for cosmetics, textiles, scouring agents, dyes, silicone prods., silicone emulsification, surfactants; Gardner 1 max. solid; sol. in IPA, water; acid no. 1 max.; hyd. no. 59-69; 99% conc.

Hetoxol CA-2. [Heterene] Ceteth-2; CAS 9004-95-9; nonionic; detergent, emulsifier, leveling agent, intermediate, used for cosmetics, household formulations, silicone emulsification, textile processing; Gardner 1 max. solid; sol. in IPA, min. oil; insol. in water; HLB 5.1; acid no. 1 max.; hyd. no. 160–180; 99% conc.

Hetoxol CA-10. [Heterene] Ceteth-10; CAS 9004-95-9; nonionic; detergent, emulsifier, leveling agent, intermediate, used for cosmetics, household formulations, silicone emulsification, textile processing; Gardner 1 max. solid; sol. in water, IPA; HLB 12.7; acid no. 1 max.; hyd. no. 75-90; 99% conc.

Hetoxol CA-20. [Heterene] Ceteth-20; CAS 9004-95-9; nonionic; detergent, emulsifier, leveling agent, intermediate, used for cosmetics, household formulations, silicone emulsification, textile processing; Gardner 1 max. solid; sol. in water; HLB 15.5; acid no. 1 max.; hyd. no. 45–60; 97% conc.

Hetoxol CAWS. [Heterene] PPG-5, ceteth-20; nonionic; intermediate, emulsifier, wetting agent, solubilizer, coupling agent for cosmetics; Gardner 1 max. liq.; sol. in water, IPA; disp. in min. oil; HLB 14.4; acid no. 1 max.; hyd.

no. 40-60.

Hetoxol CD-3. [Heterene] PEG-3 2-ethylhexyl ether; intermediate, emulsifier, wetting agent, solubilizer, coupling agent; liq.; HLB 11.5; 99% conc.

Hetoxol CD-4. [Heterene] PEG-4 2-ethyl hexyl ether; nonionic; intermediate, emulsifier, wetting agent, solubilizer, coupling agent for cosmetics; APHA 100 max. liq.; sol. in water, IPA; disp. in min. oil; HLB 11.5; hyd. no. 160-172; 99% conc.

Hetoxol CS. [Heterene] Cetearyl alcohol; cosmetics ingred.; Gardner 1 max. flake; acid no. 1 max.; iodine no. 2 max.; sapon. no. 2 max.; hyd. no. 204-218; 99% conc.

Hetoxol CS-4. [Heterene] Ceteareth-4; CAS 68439-49-6; detergent, emulsifier, leveling agent, intermediate for personal care prods., wax, oils, textiles, scouring agents, dyes, household prods., silicone emulsification, surfactdants; Gardner 1 max. solid; sol. in IPA; disp. in water, min. oil; HLB 8.2; acid no. 1 max.; hyd. no. 130-150; 99% conc.

Hetoxol CS-5. [Heterene] Ceteareth-5; CAS 68439-49-6; detergent, emulsifier, leveling agent, intermediate for personal care prods., wax, oils, textiles, scouring agents, dyes, household prods., silicone emulsification, surfactants; Gardner 1 max. solid; sol. in IPA; disp. in water, min. oil; HLB 9.2; acid no. 1 max.; hyd. no. 115-130; 99% conc.

Hetoxol CS-9. [Heterene] Ceteareth-9; CAS 68439-49-6; nonionic; detergent, emulsifier, leveling agent, intermediate, used for cosmetics, household formulations, silicone emulsification, textile processing; Gardner 1 max. solid; sol. in water, IPA; HLB 12.2; acid no. 1 max.; hyd. no. 85–90; 99% conc.

Hetoxol CS-15. [Heterene] Ceteareth-15; CAS 68439-49-6; nonionic; detergent, emulsifier, leveling agent, intermediate used for cosmetics, household formulations, silicone emulsification, textile processing; Gardner 1 max. solid; sol. water, IPA; HLB 14.2; acid no. 2 max.; hyd. no. 65-73; 98.5% conc.

Hetoxol CS-20. [Heterene] Ceteareth-20; CAS 68439-49-6; nonionic; detergent, emulsifier, leveling agent, intermediate, used for cosmetics, household formulations, silicone emulsification, textile processing; Gardner 2 max. solid; sol. in water, IPA; HLB 15.4; acid no. 2 max.; hyd. no. 50–70; 99% conc.

Hetoxol CS-30. [Heterene] Ceteareth-30; CAS 68439-49-6; nonionic; detergent, emulsifier, leveling agent, intermediate, used for cosmetics, household formulations, silicone emulsification, textile processing; Gardner 2 max. solid; sol. in water, IPA; HLB 16.7; acid no. 2 max.; hyd. no. 40–52; 99% conc.

Hetoxol CS-40. [Heterene] Ceteareth-40; CAS 68439-49-6; cosmetic ingred.

Hetoxol CS-40W. [Heterene] Ceteareth-40; CAS 68439-49-6; cosmetic ingred.; Gardner 1 max. solid; sol. in IPA; gels in water; acid no. 1 max.; hyd. no. 25-30; 99% conc.

Hetoxol CS-50. [Heterene] Ceteareth-50; CAS 68439-49-6; nonionic; detergent, emulsifier, leveling agent, intermediate, used for cosmetics, household formulations, silicone emulsification, textile processing; Gardner 2 max. flake; sol. in water, IPA; acid no. 2 max.; hyd. no. 20-40; 99% conc.

Hetoxol CS-50 Special. [Heterene] Ceteareth-50; CAS 68439-49-6; detergent, emulsifier, leveling agent, intermediate, used for cosmetics, household formulations, silicone emulsification, textile processing; Gardner 2 max. flake; sol. in IPA; gels in water; set pt. 44-48 C; hyd. no. 18-24; 99% conc.

Hetoxol CSA-15. [Heterene] Ceteareth-15; CAS 68439-49-6; nonionic; detergent, emulsifier, leveling agent, intermediate; used in personal care prods., wax, oil and textiles, scouring agents, dyes, household formulations, silicone

emulsification, surfactants; Gardner 1 max. solid; HLB 14.2.

Hetoxol D. [Heterene] Ceteareth alcohol and ceteareth-20; nonionic; intermediate, emulsifier, wetting agent, solubilizer, coupling agent; for cosmetics, paper, textile industries; flake; m.p. 47-55 C; acid no. 1 max.; iodine no. 2 max.; sapon. no. 2 max.; 99% conc.

Hetoxol G. [Heterene] Stearyl alcohol and ceteareth-20; nonionic; intermediate, emulsifier, wetting agent, solubilizer, coupling agent for cosmetics, moisturizing creams, replenishing creams; flake; acid no. 1 max.; sapon. no. 2 max.; 99% conc.

Hetoxol IS-2. [Heterene] Isosteareth-2; CAS 52292-17-8; emulsifier; Gardner 1 max. solid (clear on remelt); acid no. 1 max.; hyd. no. 140-150; pH 5.5-7.5 (3% aq.).

Hetoxol IS-3. [Heterene] Isosteareth-3; CAS 52292-17-8; emulsifier.

Hetoxol IS-10. [Heterene] Isosteareth-10; CAS 52292-17-8; emulsifier.

Hetoxol IS-20. [Heterene] Isosteareth-20; CAS 52292-17-8; emulsifier.

Hetoxol J. [Heterene] Cetearyl alcohol and ceteareth-20; nonionic; intermediate, emulsifier, wetting agent, solubilizer, coupling agent for cosmetics; flake; m.p. 47-55 C; acid no. 1 max.; iodine no. 2 max.; sapon. no. 2 max.; hyd. no. 166-178; 99% conc.

Hetoxol L. [Heterene] Cetearyl alcohol and ceteareth-30; nonionic; intermediate, emulsifier, wetting agent, solubilizer, coupling agent for cosmetics; flake; acid no. 1 max.; iodine no. 2 max.; sapon. no. 2 max.; hyd. no. 178-192; 99% conc.

Hetoxol L-1. [Heterene] Laureth-1; CAS 4536-30-5; EINECS 224-886-5; emulsifier; Gardner 1 max. liq.; sol. in IPA, min. oil; insol. in water; HLB 3.6; hyd. no. 231-238; 99% conc.

Hetoxol L-2. [Heterene] Laureth-2; CAS 3055-93-4; EINECS 221-279-7; cosmetic ingred. for shower gels; Gardner 1 max. liq.; sol. in IPA, min. oil; insol. in water; HLB 6.1; hyd. no. 191-201; 99% conc.

Hetoxol L-3N. [Heterene] Laureth-3; CAS 3055-94-5; EINECS 221-280-2; nonionic; detergent, emulsifier, leveling agent, intermediate, used for cosmetics, household formulations, silicone emulsification, textile processing; liq.; sol. in IPA, min. oil; HLB 7.9; hyd. no. 170–176.

Hetoxol L-4. [Heterene] Laureth-4; CAS 5274-68-0; EINECS 226-097-1; intermediate, emulsifier, wetting agent, solubilizer, coupling agent for cosmetics, shower gels, night creams; Gardner 1 max. liq.; sol. in IPA, min. oil; disp. in water; HLB 9.4; acid no. 2 max.; hyd. no. 145-160; 99% conc.

Hetoxol L-9. [Heterene] Laureth-9; CAS 3055-99-0; EINECS 221-284-4; intermediate, emulsifier, wetting agent, solubilizer, coupling agent for cosmetics; Gardner 1 max. liq.; sol. in water, IPA; HLB 13.3; acid no. 1 max.; hyd. no. 95-105; 99% conc.

Hetoxol L-12. [Heterene] Laureth-12; CAS 3056-00-6; EINECS 221-286-5; emulsifier for personal care prods.; Gardner 1 max. semisolid; sol. in water, IPA; HLB 14.6; acid no. 1 max.; hyd. no. 74-82; 99% conc.

Hetoxol L-23. [Heterene] Laureth-23; CAS 9002-92-0; nonionic; detergent, emulsifier, leveling agent, intermediate, used for cosmetics, household formulations, silicone emulsification, textile processing; Gardner 1 max. solid; sol. in water, IPA; HLB 16.7; acid no. 0.5 max.; hyd. no. 42-52.

Hetoxol LS-9. [Heterene] Laureth-9, steareth-9; nonionic; detergent, emulsifier, leveling agent, intermediate, used for cosmetics, household formulations, silicone emulsification, textile processing; APHA 75 max. semisolid; sol. in water, IPA; HLB 12.6; hyd. no. 94-104; cloud pt. 64-69 C

(1% aq.); pH 4.5-7.5 (1% aq.); 99% conc.

Hetoxol M-3. [Heterene] Myreth-3; CAS 27306-79-2; EINECS 248-016-9; emulsifier and pigment dispersant in makeup; intermediate, wetting agent, solubilizer, coupling agent; Gardner 1 max. clear thin liq.; sol. in IPA; disp. in water, min. oil; HLB 7.6; acid no. 0.2 max.; hyd. no. 150-162; pH 5.5–7.0 (5% in IPA/water 1:1); 97% conc.

Hetoxol MP-3. [Heterene] PPG-3 myristyl ether; CAS 63793-60-2; emollient; Gardner 1 max. liq.; sol. in IPA, min. oil; insol. in water; acid no. 1.5 max.; sapon. no. 2 max.; hyd. no. 135-155; 99% conc.

Hetoxol OA-3 Special. [Heterene] Oleth-3; CAS 9004-98-2; nonionic; emulsifier and pigment dispersant for cosmetic applics.; pale yel. liq., low odor; sol. in IPA, min. oil; insol. in water; HLB 6.4; acid no. 2 max.; iodine no. 57-62; hyd. no. 135-150.

Hetoxol OA-5 Special. [Heterene] Oleth-5; CAS 9004-98-2; nonionic; intermediate, emulsifier, wetting agent, solubilizer, coupling agent for cosmetics; pale yel. liq.; sol. in IPA, min. oil; disp. in water; HLB 9.0; acid no. 2 max.; iodine no. 40-52; hyd. no. 120-135; 99% conc.

Hetoxol OA-10 Special. [Heterene] Oleth-10; CAS 9004-98-2; nonionic; emulsifier and pigment dispersant for cosmetic applics.; wh. semisolid, low odor; sol. in water, IPA; HLB 12.4; acid no. 2 max.; iodine no. 31-37; hyd. no. 79-91.

Hetoxol OA-20 Special. [Heterene] Oleth-20; CAS 9004-98-2; nonionic; emulsifier and pigment dispersant for cosmetic applics.; wh. solid; sol. in water, IPA; HLB 15.3; acid no. 2 max.; iodine no. 18-25; hyd. no. 50-58.

Hetoxol OCS. [Heterene] Oleth-15; CAS 9004-98-2; cosmetics ingred.

Hetoxol OL-2. [Heterene] Oleth-2; CAS 9004-92-2; nonionic; intermediate, emulsifier, wetting agent, solubilizer, coupling agent for cosmetics; Gardner 2 max. liq.; sol. in IPA, min. oil; insol. in water; HLB 4.9; acid no. 1 max.; hyd. no. 160-180; 99% conc.

Hetoxol OL-3. [Heterene] Oleth-3; CAS 9004-98-2; intermediate, emulsifier, wetting agent, solubilizer, coupling agent for cosmetics.

Hetoxol OL-4. [Heterene] Oleth-4; CAS 9004-98-2; nonionic; intermediate, emulsifier, wetting agent, solubilizer, coupling agent for cosmetics; Gardner 4 max. liq.; sol. in IPA, min. oil; insol. in water; HLB 7.9; hyd. no. 123-133; 99% conc.

Hetoxol OL-5. [Heterene] Oleth-5; CAS 9004-98-2; nonionic; intermediate, emulsifier, wetting agent, solubilizer, coupling agent for cosmetics; Gardner 4 max. liq.; sol. in IPA; disp. in water, min. oil; HLB 9.0; hyd. no. 110–121; 99% conc.

Hetoxol OL-10. [Heterene] Oleth-10; CAS 9004-98-2; nonionic; surfactant for cosmetic formulations; intermediate, emulsifier, wetting agent, solubilizer, coupling agent; Gardner 3 semisolid; sol. in water, IPA; HLB 12.4; hyd. no. 77-83; 99% conc.

Hetoxol OL-10H. [Heterene] Oleth-10; CAS 9004-98-2; nonionic; surfactant for cosmetic formulations; intermediate, emulsifier, wetting agent, solubilizer, coupling agent; Gardner 1 max. semisolid; sol. in water, IPA; HLB 12.8; acid no. 0.5 max.; iodine no. 25-37; hyd. no. 75-88; cloud pt. 71–77 C (1% aq.).; 99% conc.

Hetoxol OL-20. [Heterene] Oleth-20; CAS 9004-98-2; nonionic; surfactant for cosmetic formulations; intermediate, emulsifier, wetting agent, solubilizer, coupling agent; Gardner 2 max. solid; sol. in water, IPA; HLB 15.3; acid no. 2 max.; hyd. no. 50-58; 99% conc.

Hetoxol OL-23. [Heterene] Oleth-23; CAS 9004-98-2; nonionic; intermediate, emulsifier, wetting agent, solubilizer, coupling agent, lubricant for cosmetics; Gardner 2 max. semisolid; sol. in water, IPA; HLB 15.8; acid no. 2 max.;

hyd. no. 47–62; 99% conc.

Hetoxol OL-40. [Heterene] Oleth-40; CAS 9004-98-2; nonionic; intermediate, emulsifier, wetting agent, solubilizer, coupling agent for cosmetics; Gardner 2 max. solid; sol. in water, IPA; HLB 17.4; hyd. no. 28-38; 99% conc.

Hetoxol P. [Heterene] Emulsifying wax NF; emulsion base for cosmetics, replenishing creams; flake; acid no. 2 max.; sapon. no. 14.0 max.; hyd. no. 178-192; 99% conc.

Hetoxol PLA. [Heterene] PPG-30 lanolin ether; CAS 68439-53-2; nonionic; oily emollient, intermediate, emulsifier, wetting agent, solubilizer, coupling agent for cosmetics; liq.; sol. in min. oil, IPA; insol. in water; acid no. 1.0 max.

Hetoxol SA. [Heterene] Stearyl alcohol; CAS 112-92-5; EINECS 204-017-6; cosmetics ingred.

Hetoxol SP-15. [Heterene] PPG-15 stearyl ether; CAS 25231-21-4; nonionic; oily emollient material in cosmetics; ASTM 100 max. liq.; sol. in IPA, min. oil; insol. in water; acid no. 1.5 max.; sapon. no. 2.0 max.; hyd. no. 62–70; 99% conc.

Hetoxol STA-2. [Heterene] Steareth-2; CAS 9005-00-9; nonionic; intermediate, emulsifier, wetting agent, solubilizer, coupling agent for cosmetics; Gardner 1 max. solid; sol. in IPA, min. oil; disp. in water; HLB 4.9; acid no. 2 max.; hyd. no. 155–165; 99% conc.

Hetoxol STA-10. [Heterene] Steareth-10; CAS 9005-00-9; nonionic; intermediate, emulsifier, wetting agent, solubilizer, coupling agent for cosmetics; Gardner 1 max. solid; sol. in water, IPA; HLB 12.4; acid no. 1 max.; hyd. no. 75-90; 99% conc.

Hetoxol STA-20. [Heterene] Steareth-20; CAS 9005-00-9; nonionic; intermediate, emulsifier, wetting agent, solubilizer, coupling agent for cosmetics; Gardner 1 max. solid; sol. in water, IPA; insol. in min. oil; HLB 15.3; acid no. 2 max.; hyd. no. 45-60 C; 99% conc.

Hetoxol STA-30. [Heterene] Steareth-30; CAS 9005-00-9; nonionic; intermediate, emulsifier, wetting agent, solubilizer, coupling agent for cosmetics; Gardner 2 max. flake; sol. in water, IPA; HLB 16.6; m.p. 46–50 C; acid no. 2 max.; hyd. no. 35-45; 99% conc.

Hetoxol TA-6. [Heterene] Talloweth-6; CAS 61791-28-4; emulsifier.

Hetoxol TD-3. [Heterene] Trideceth-3; CAS 4403-12-7; EINECS 224-540-3; nonionic; detergent, emulsifier, leveling agent, intermediate, used for cosmetics, household formulations, silicone emulsification, textile processing; Gardner 1 max. liq.; sol. in IPA, min. oil; insol. in water; HLB 7.9; acid no. 2 max.; hyd. no. 165–175; 99% conc.

Hetoxol TD-6. [Heterene] Trideceth-6; CAS 24938-91-8; nonionic; detergent, emulsifier, leveling agent, intermediate, used for cosmetics, household formulations, silicone emulsification, textile processing; Gardner 1 max. liq.; sol. in IPA, water; HLB 11.3; acid no. 2 max.; hyd. no. 115-1205; 99% conc.

Hetoxol TD-9. [Heterene] Trideceth-9; CAS 24938-91-8; nonionic; wetting agent, industrial surfactant, solubilizer for cosmetics; Gardner 1 max. liq.; sol. in water, IPA; HLB 13.2; acid no. 2 max.; hyd. no. 90-100; 99% conc.

Hetoxol TD-12. [Heterene] Trideceth-12; CAS 24938-91-8; nonionic; detergent, emulsifier, leveling agent, intermediate, used for cosmetics, household formulations, silicone emulsification, textile processing; Gardner 1 max. liq.; sol. in IPA, water; HLB 14.5; acid no. 2 max.; hyd. no. 72–87; 99% conc.

Hetoxol TD-18. [Heterene] Trideceth-18; CAS 24938-91-8; nonionic; leveling agent, solubilizer for cosmetics; Gardner 1 max. solid; sol. in water, IPA; HLB 15.7; hyd. no. 54-62; 99% conc.

Hetoxol TD-25. [Heterene] Trideceth-25; CAS 24938-91-8; nonionic; wetting agent, surfactant, solubilizer for cosmetics and industrial use; Gardner 2 max. semisolid; sol. in water, IPA; HLB 16.9; acid no. 2 max.; hyd. no. 40-60; 99% conc.

Hetoxol TDEP-15. [Heterene] PEG-10 PPG-15 tridecyl ether; nonionic; surfactant for cosmetics, industrial use, automatic dishwashing formulations; Gardner 2 max. liq.; sol. in water, IPA; acid no. 2 max.; hyd. no. 40-60; cloud pt. 21–23 C (1% aq.).; 99% conc.

Hetoxol TDEP-63. [Heterene] PEG-6 PPG-3 tridecyl ether; nonionic; surfactant for cosmetics, industrial use, automatic dishwashing formulations; Gardner 2 max. liq.; sol. in water, IPA; hyd. no. 80-115; cloud pt. 27–33 C (1% aq.).

Hetoxolan 75. [Heterene] PEG-75 lanolin; CAS 61790-81-6; cosmetics ingred.

Hetoxolan 75-50% [Heterene] PEG-75 lanolin; CAS 61790-81-6; cosmetics ingred.; 50% conc.

Hetoxolan 100. [Heterene] PEG-100 lanolin; CAS 61790-81-6; cosmetics ingred.

Hetphos OA-3. [Heterene] Oleth-3 phosphate; CAS 39464-69-2; cosmetics ingred.; Gardner 8 max. liq.; acid no. 90-110; iodine no. 35-50; sapon. no. 105-120; pH 6-7 (2% aq.).

Hetphos SG. [Heterene] PPG-5 ceteth-10 phosphate; CAS 50643-20-4; cosmetics ingred.; Gardner 4 max. color; acid no. 85-105; iodine no. 5 max.; sapon. no. 90-110; pH 1-3 (3%).

Hetquat S-20. [Heterene] Stearalkonium chloride; CAS 122-19-0; EINECS 204-527-9; cationic; cosmetics ingred.; paste; pH 3-4 (10%); 16-19% act. quat.

Hetsorb L-4. [Heterene] Polysorbate 21; CAS 9005-64-5; nonionic; emulsifier, lubricant, thickener, corrosion inhibitor for cosmetics; Gardner 8 max. liq.; sol. in IPA; disp. in water, min. oil; HLB 13.3; acid no. 3 max.; sapon. no. 100–115; hyd. no. 225-255; 99% conc.

Hetsorb L-10. [Heterene] PEG-10 sorbitan laurate; CAS 9005-64-5; nonionic; detergent, emulsifier, lubricant for cosmetics; corrosion inhibitor; Gardner 7 max. liq.; sol. in water, IPA; HLB 8.4; acid no. 2 max.; sapon. no. 66–76; hyd. no. 150-170; 97% conc.

Hetsorb L-20. [Heterene] Polysorbate 20; CAS 9005-64-5; nonionic; detergent, emulsifier, lubricant for cosmetics; corrosion inhibitor; Gardner 6 max. liq.; sol. in water, IPA; HLB 16.7; acid no. 2 max.; sapon. no. 41-50; hyd. no. 97-108; 97% conc.

Hetsorb L-44. [Heterene] PEG-44 sorbitan laurate; CAS 9005-64-5; cosmetics ingred.

Hetsorb L-80-72%. [Heterene] PEG-80 sorbitan laurate; CAS 9005-64-5; surfactant for shampoos; used as counterirritant; Gardner 5 max. clear liq.; sol. in water, IPA; acid no. 3 max.; sapon. no. 8-18; hyd. no. 22-35; 70–74% solids.

Hetsorb O-5. [Heterene] Polysorbate 81; CAS 9005-65-6; emulsifier for food, cosmetics; Gardner 8 max. liq.; sol. in IPA; disp. in water; HLB 10.0; acid no. 2 max.; sapon. no. 96–104; hyd. no. 134-150; 97% conc.

Hetsorb O-20. [Heterene] Polysorbate 80; CAS 9005-65-6; nonionic; emulsifier, lubricant for cosmetics; corrosion inhibitor; Gardner 7 max. liq.; sol. in water, IPA; HLB 15.0; acid no. 2 max.; sapon. no. 45–55; hyd. no. 65-80; 97% conc.

Hetsorb P-20. [Heterene] Polysorbate 40; CAS 9005-66-7; nonionic; general purpose emulsifier; Gardner 6 max. liq. to semisolid; sol. in water, IPA; disp. in min. oil; HLB 15.6; acid no. 2 max.; sapon. no. 40–53; hyd. no. 91-107; 97% conc.

Hetsorb S-4. [Heterene] Polysorbate 61; CAS 9005-67-8; nonionic; emulsifier for cosmetics; amber semisolid; sol. in IPA; disp. in water, min. oil; acid no. 3 max.; sapon. no. 95–115; hyd. no. 165-200; 97% conc.

Hetsorb S-20. [Heterene] Polysorbate 60; CAS 9005-67-8; emulsifier for vitamins; Gardner 6 max. liq. to gel; sol. in

water, misc. in IPA; HLB 14.9; acid no. 2 max.; sapon. no. 45–55; hyd. no. 81-96; 97% conc.

Hetsorb TO-20. [Heterene] Polysorbate 85; CAS 9005-70-3; nonionic; general purpose emulsifier, thickener, lubricant, corrosion inhibitor; Gardner 8 max. liq.; sol. in IPA, min. oil; disp. in water; HLB 11.0; acid no. 2 max.; sapon. no. 82–95; hyd. no. 39-52; 95% conc.

Hetsorb TS-20. [Heterene] Polysorbate 65; CAS 9005-71-4; nonionic; general purpose emulsifier, thickener, lubricant for cosmetics; corrosion inhibitor; Gardner 7 max. solid; sol. in IPA, hot min. oil; disp. in water; HLB 10.5; acid no. 2 max.; sapon. no. 88–98; hyd. no. 44-60; 97% conc.

Hetsulf Acid. [Heterene] Sodium dodecylbenzene sulfonate; CAS 25155-30-0; EINECS 246-680-4; anionic; wetting agent, emulsifier, dispersant, intermediate, base for neutralized surfactant; liq.; dens. 1.05; biodeg.; 97% act.

Hetsulf IPA. [Heterene] MIPA-dodecylbenzenesulfonate; CAS 42504-46-1; EINECS 255-854-9; anionic; wetting agent, emulsifier, dispersant; liq.; pH 5.0–6.5 (5% aq.); biodeg.

Hexaplant Richter. [Dr. Kurt Richter; Henkel/Cospha] Water, alcohol, fennel extract, hops extract, balm mint extract, mistletoe extract, matricaria extract, yarrow extract; polyvalent herbal extract in aq. alcohol; emollient for aq. and hydroalcoholic herbal cosmetics, skin and hair prods., emulsified preparations; dk. brn. liq.; herbal odor.

Hexaryl D 60 L. [Witco/H-I-P] TEA-dodecylbenzenesulfonate; CAS 27323-41-7; EINECS 248-406-9; anionic; multipurpose detergent for personal care use; liq.

Hexetidine 90, 99. [Angus] Hexetidine; CAS 141-94-6; EINECS 205-513-5; antimicrobial, antifungal agent for pharmaceuticals, oral hygiene, body cavity, and skin care prods. (ointments, vaginal gels, dentifrice, mouthwash); EEC approved; clear ylsh. oily liq.; sol. in glycols, nonpolar solvs.; sparingly sol. in water; m.w. 339.6; sp.gr. 0.866; b.p. 172-176 C (1 mm Hg); ref. index 1.462-1.466 and 1.463-1.467 resp.; toxicology: LD50 (oral, rat) 0.61 g/kg; toxic by intravenous route; corrosive to eyes, irritating to skin; 90 and 97% act. min.

Hexyl Jasmat®. [BASF AG] Acetyl ethyl octanoate; floral, herbal, green, jasmine-like fragrance.

HGC 5000. [Siltech] nonionic; gloss agent for hair care prods.; insol. in water; 100% act.

Hi-Care® 1000. [Rhone-Poulenc Surf. & Spec.] Guar hydroxypropyltrimonium chloride; CAS 65497-29-2; conditioner providing silky soft feel and mildness to skin care prods., bar soaps, creams, and facial cleansers.

Hidrolisado de Colageno. [Fabriquimica] Hydrolyzed collagen; CAS 9015-54-7; protein for cosmetics use; pH 6.5; 5.2% solids.

Hidrolisado de Elastina. [Fabriquimica] Hydrolyzed elastin; CAS 100085-10-7; protein for cosmetics use; pH 6.5; 4.9% solids.

Hidrolisado de Placenta. [Fabriquimica] Hydrolyzed placental protein; protein for cosmetics use; pH 6.5; 5.2% solids.

Hidrolisado de Queratina. [Fabriquimica] Hydrolyzed keratin; CAS 69430-36-0; EINECS 274-001-1; protein for cosmetics use; pH 6.5; 5.0% solids.

Hidroxilan. [Fabriquimica] Hydroxylated lanolin; CAS 68424-66-8; EINECS 270-315-8; multifunctional cosmetic ingred.; drop pt. 39-46 C; acid no. < 10; iodine no. 15-23; sapon. no. 90-105.

HiPure Liq. Gelatin, Cosmetic Grade. [Norland Prods.] Gelatin; CAS 9000-70-8; EINECS 232-554-6; cosmetics ingred.

Hispagel® 100. [Hispano Quimica; Centerchem] Glycerin and glyceryl polyacrylate; thickener, stabilizer, lubricant, and humectant for personal care prods. for skin and hair care, aftershave lotions, sun care prods.; base for moisturizing aq. gels; exc. moisture retention; forms permeable film on skin that is easily washed away; suspending agent for insoluble components; vehicle for topical dermatological prods.; provides max. slip and lubricity; colorless transparent visc. gel, odorless; sol. in water; sp.gr. 1.15; visc. < 200,000 cps; b.p. > 250 F; pH 5-6; 43% water.

Hispagel® 200. [Hispano Quimica; Centerchem] Glycerin and glyceryl polyacrylate; thickener, stabilizer, lubricant, and humectant for personal care prods. for skin and hair care, aftershave lotions, sun care prods.; base for moisturizing aq. gels; exc. moisture retention; forms permeable film on skin that is easily washed away; suspending agent for insoluble components; vehicle for topical dermatological prods.; for use where higher visc. is desired; colorless transparent visc. gel, odorless; sol. in water; sp.gr. 1.15; visc. > 250,000 cps; pH 5-6; 48% water.

Hodag 20-L. [Calgene] PEG-4 laurate; CAS 9004-81-3; nonionic; emulsifier, wetting agent, plasticizer for cosmetic, pharmaceutical and other uses; liq.; HLB 10.0; 100% conc.

Hodag 20-O. [Calgene] PEG-4 oleate; CAS 9004-96-0; EINECS 233-293-0; for personal care applics.; yel. liq.; disp. in water; sp.gr. 0.99; dens. 8.24 lb/gal; m.p. < 5 C.

Hodag 20-S. [Calgene] PEG-4 stearate; CAS 9004-99-3; EINECS 203-358-8; for personal care prods.

Hodag 22-L. [Calgene] PEG-4 dilaurate; CAS 9005-02-1; nonionic; emulsifier, wetting agent, plasticizer for cosmetic, pharmaceutical and other uses; liq.; HLB 6.6; 100% conc.

Hodag 22-O. [Calgene] PEG-4 dioleate; CAS 9005-07-6; for personal care use.

Hodag 22-S. [Calgene] PEG-4 distearate; CAS 9005-08-7; for personal care industry; wh. to cream soft solid; disp. in hot water; sp.gr. 0.9067 (45 C); m.p. 34 C; acid no. 10 max.; pH 4-7 (3% aq.).

Hodag 32-O. [Calgene] PEG-6 dioeate; CAS 9005-07-6; personal care surfactant; lt. amber clear, oily liq.; sol. in acetone, IPA, toluene, min. and veg. oils; disp. in water; sp.gr. 0.960-0.967; solid. pt. 5 C; pH 4-6.

Hodag 40-L. [Calgene] PEG-8 laurate; CAS 9004-81-3; nonionic; emulsifier, wetting agent, plasticizer for cosmetic, pharmaceutical and other uses; liq.; HLB 12.8; 100% conc.

Hodag 40-O. [Calgene] PEG-8 oleate; CAS 9004-96-0; nonionic; emulsifier, wetting agent, plasticizer for cosmetics, pharmaceuticals, other uses; liq.; HLB 11.4; 100% conc.

Hodag 40-R. [Calgene] PEG-8 ricinoleate; CAS 9004-97-1; nonionic; emulsifier, wetting agent, plasticizer for general cosmetic, pharmaceutical and other uses; liq.; HLB 11.6; 100% conc.

Hodag 40-S. [Calgene] PEG-8 stearate; CAS 9004-99-3; nonionic; emulsifier, wetting agent, plasticizer for cosmetic, pharmaceutical and other uses; paste; HLB 11.1; 100% conc.

Hodag 40-T (redesignated Hodag WA-56). [Calgene] PEG-8 tallate; CAS 61791-00-2; personal care surfactant.

Hodag 42-L. [Calgene] PEG-8 dilaurate; CAS 9005-02-1; nonionic; emulsifier, wetting agent, plasticizer for cosmetic, pharmaceutical and other uses; liq.; HLB 10.0; 100% conc.

Hodag 42-O. [Calgene] PEG-8 dioleate; CAS 9005-07-6; nonionic; emulsifier, wetting agent, plasticizer for cosmetic, pharmaceutical and other uses; liq.; HLB 8.4; 100% conc.

Hodag 42-S. [Calgene] PEG-8 distearate; CAS 9005-08-7; nonionic; emulsifier, wetting agent, plasticizer for cosmetic, pharmaceutical and other uses; paste; HLB 8.2; 100% conc.

Hodag 60-L. [Calgene] PEG-12 laurate; CAS 9004-81-3;

nonionic; emulsifier, wetting agent, plasticizer for cosmetic, pharmaceutical and other uses; liq.; HLB 14.8; 100% conc.

Hodag 60-O. [Calgene] PEG-12 oleate; CAS 9004-96-0; for personal care applics.

Hodag 60-S. [Calgene] PEG-12 stearate; CAS 9004-99-3; nonionic; emulsifier, wetting agent, plasticizer for cosmetic, pharmaceutical and other uses; solid; HLB 13.6; 100% conc.

Hodag 62-O. [Calgene] PEG-12 dioleate; CAS 9005-07-6; nonionic; emulsifier, wetting agent, plasticizer for cosmetic, pharmaceutical and other uses; liq.; HLB 10.0; 100% conc.

Hodag 62-S. [Calgene] PEG-12 disearate; CAS 9005-08-7; for personal care applics.

Hodag 100-S. [Calgene] PEG-20 stearate; CAS 9004-99-3; nonionic; emulsifier, wetting agent, plasticizer for cosmetic, pharmaceutical and other uses; solid; HLB 15.6; 100% conc.

Hodag 102-S. [Calgene] PEG-20 disearate; CAS 9005-08-7; for personal care applics.

Hodag 150-S. [Calgene] PEG-6-32 stearate; CAS 9004-99-3; nonionic; emulsifier, wetting agent, plasticizer for cosmetic, pharmaceutical and other uses; solid; HLB 16.8; 100% conc.

Hodag 154-S. [Calgene] PEG-32 stearate; CAS 9004-99-3; for personal care applics.

Hodag 600-L. [Calgene] PEG-150 laurate; CAS 9004-81-3; for personal care applics.

Hodag 600-S. [Calgene] PEG-150 stearate; CAS 9004-99-3; for personal care applics.; wh. flake; sol. in water; sp.gr. 1.080; m.p. 61 C; HLB 19.0; acid no. 5 max.; sapon. no. 7-13; cloud pt. > 100 C (1% aq.).

Hodag 602-S. [Calgene] PEG-150 disearate; CAS 9005-08-7; nonionic; thickener and aux. emulsifier for creams and lotions, esp. amphoteric type shampoos; wh. flakes; sol. in water, IPA; insol. in min. and veg. oils; sp.gr. 1.075; m.p. 53.5-57.5 C; HLB 18.4; acid no. 9 max.; iodine no. 0.1 max.; sapon.no. 14-20.

Hodag CC-22. [Calgene] Propylene glycol dicaprylate/dicaprate; nonionic; surfactant for food, cosmetics, and pharmaceutical industries; vehicle/diluent/carrier for vitamins, drugs, flavors, color, fragrance; emollient for makeup, bath and skin oils; FDA compliance as food additive; clear, almost colorless, tasteless, odorless liq.; sol. in ethanol, min. oil, acetone; sp.gr. 0.916; set pt. -20 C; iodine no. 0.5; sapon. no. 325; 100% conc.

Hodag CC-22-S. [Calgene] Propylene glycol dicaprylate/dicaprate; nonionic; surfactant for food, cosmetics, and pharmaceutical industries; vehicle/diluent/carrier for vitamins, drugs, flavors, color, fragrance; emollient for makeup, bath and skin oils; FDA compliance as food additive; clear, almost colorless, tasteless, odorless liq.; sol. in ethanol, min. oil acetone; sp.gr. 0.919; set pt. -20 C; iodine no. 0.5; sapon. no. 325; 100% conc.

Hodag CC-33. [Calgene] Caprylic/capric triglyceride; CAS 65381-09-1; nonionic; surfactant for food, cosmetics, and pharmaceutical industries; vehicle/diluent/carrier for vitamins, drugs, flavors, color, fragrance; emollient for makeup, bath and skin oils; GRAS; clear, almost colorless, tasteless, odorless liq.; sol. in ethanol, min. oil, acetone; sp.gr. 0.945; set pt. -2 C; iodine no. 0.5; sapon. no. 340; 100% conc.

Hodag CC-33-F. [Calgene] Caprylic/capric triglyceride; CAS 65381-09-1; nonionic; surfactant for food, cosmetics, and pharmaceutical industries; vehicle/diluent/carrier for vitamins, drugs, flavors, color, fragrance; emollient for makeup, bath and skin oils; GRAS; clear, almost colorless, tasteless, odorless liq.; sol. in min. oil, acetone; sp.gr. 0.935; set pt. 5 C; iodine no. 8; sapon. no. 305;

100% conc.

Hodag CC-33-L. [Calgene] Caprylic/capric triglyceride; CAS 65381-09-1; nonionic; surfactant for food, cosmetics, and pharmaceutical industries; vehicle/diluent/carrier for vitamins, drugs, flavors, color, fragrance; emollient for makeup, bath and skin oils; GRAS; clear, almost colorless, tasteless, odorless liq.; sol. in min. oil, acetone; sp.gr. 0.938; set pt. 0 C; iodine no. 8; sapon. no. 308; 100% conc.

Hodag CC-33-S. [Calgene] Caprylic/capric triglyceride; CAS 65381-09-1; nonionic; surfactant for food, cosmetics, and pharmaceutical industries; vehicle/diluent/carrier for vitamins, drugs, flavors, color, fragrance; emollient for makeup, bath and skin oils; GRAS; clear, almost colorless, tasteless, odorless liq.; sol. in ethanol, min. oil, acetone; sp.gr. 0.945; set pt. -5 C; iodine no. 0.5; sapon. no. 347; 100% conc.

Hodag CSA-70. [Calgene] PPG-11 stearyl ether; CAS 25231-21-4; for personal care applics.

Hodag CSA-75. [Calgene] PPG-15 stearyl ether; CAS 25231-21-4; for personal care applics.

Hodag CSA-80. [Calgene] PPG-26 oleate; CAS 31394-71-5; nonionic; nongreasy spreading agent, skin moisturizer, emollient, vehicle for skin and hair care prods., bath oils; carrier and dispersant for additives (hormones, vitamins, essnetial oils, germicides, etc.); foam depressing props.; cleary oily fluid; sol. in min. oil, veg. oil, isopropyl esters, alcohol, hydroalcohol blends, lanolin derivs.; insol. in water; sp.gr. 0.985-0.990; acid no. 1; sapon. no. 20-35.

Hodag CSA-86. [Calgene] PEG-2 tallow amine; CAS 61791-44-4; for personal care applics.

Hodag CSA-91. [Calgene] PPG-10 oleyl ether; CAS 52581-71-2; for personal care applics.

Hodag CSA-101. [Calgene] Ceteary alcohol, ceteth-20, glycol stearate; for personal care applics.

Hodag CSA-102. [Calgene] Cetearyl alcohol, polysorbate 60, PEG-150 stearate, steareth-20; for personal care applics.

Hodag CSA-103. [Calgene] Cetearyl alcohol, cetear eth-20; for personal care applics.

Hodag DCA. [Calgene] Dicapryl adipate; CAS 105-97-5; EINECS 203-349-9; cosmetic ester.

Hodag DGL. [Calgene] PEG-2 laurate; CAS 9004-81-3; nonionic; emulsifier for industrial and cosmetic applics.; yel. liq.; nondisp. in water; sp.gr. 0.95; HLB 6.5; pour pt. 1 C; 100% conc.

Hodag DGO. [Calgene] PEG-2 oleate; CAS 106-12-7; EINECS 203-364-0; nonionic; lubricant; yel. liq.; nondisp. in water; sp.gr. 0.95; HLB 4.7; 100% conc.

Hodag DGS. [Calgene] PEG-2 stearate; CAS 9004-99-3; EINECS 203-363-5; nonionic; emulsifier, opacifier, thickener for cosmetics, o/w emulsions; lubricant for stamping and drawing; protective coating for hygroscopic materials (tablets); opacifier/lubricant for paper industry; antitack agent; wh. flake; insol. in water; m.p. 44-48 C; HLB 4.7; acid no. 5 max.; sapon. no. 153-165; pour pt. 46 C; pH 4.5-6.5 (3% disp.); 100% conc.

Hodag DGS-C. [Calgene] PEG-2 stearate SE; CAS 9004-99-3; self-emulsifying emulsifier, opacifier, thickener for cosmetics, o/w emulsions; lubricant for stamping and drawing; protective coating for hygroscopic materials (tablets); opacifier/lubricant for paper industry; antitack agent; wh. flake; disp. in water; m.p. 47-53 C; acid no. 95-105; sapon. no. 160-170; pH 6.5-7.5 (3% disp.).

Hodag DGS-N. [Calgene] PEG-2 stearate; CAS 106-11-6; EINECS 203-363-5; emulsifier, opacifier, thickener for cosmetics, o/w emulsions; lubricant for stamping and drawing; protective coating for hygroscopic materials (tablets); opacifier/lubricant for paper industry; antitack agent; wh. flake; insol. in water; m.p. 43-50 C; acid no. 95-

105; sapon. no. 175-185; pH 4.5-6.5 (3% disp.).

Hodag DOSS-70. [Calgene] Dioctyl sodium sulfosuccinate; CAS 577-11-7; EINECS 209-406-4; anionic; surfactant, wetting agent, surface tension reducer used in emulsion and suspension polymerization, dry cleaning, cleaning compds., industrial compds., paints, textiles, and cosmetics; colorless liq.; sol. in polar and nonpolar org. solvs.; water-disp.; sp.gr. 1.08; dens. 9.0 lb/gal; flash pt. (OC) 85 C; surf. tens. 26 dynes/cm (1% aq.); 70% act.

Hodag DOSS-75. [Calgene] Dioctyl sodium sulfosuccinate; CAS 577-11-7; EINECS 209-406-4; anionic; surfactant, wetting agent, surface tension reducer used in emulsion and suspension polymerization, dry cleaning, cleaning compds., industrial compds., paints, textiles, and cosmetics; colorless liq.; sol. in polar and nonpolar org. solvs.; disp. in water; sp.gr. 1.08; dens. 9.0 lb/gal; flash pt. (OC) 85 C; surf. tens. 26 dynes/cm (1% aq.); 75% act.

Hodag DTSS-70. [Calgene] Sodium ditridecyl sulfosuccinate; CAS 2673-22-5; EINECS 220-219-7; anionic; surfactant, wetting agent, surface tension reducer used in emulsion and suspension polymerization, dry cleaning, cleaning compds., industrial compds., paints, textiles, and cosmetics; pale liq.; sol. in polar and nonpolar org. solvs.; water-disp.; sp.gr. 1.02; dens. 8.5 lb/gal; flash pt. (OC) 91 C; surf. tens. 29 dynes/cm (1% aq.); 70% act.

Hodag EGDS. [Calgene] Glycol distearate; CAS 627-83-8; EINECS 211-014-3; nonionic; surfactant for industrial and cosmetic applics.; cream solid; nondisp. in water; sp.gr. 0.95; HLB 1.5; pour pt. 56 C.

Hodag EGMS. [Calgene] Glycol stearate; CAS 111-60-4; EINECS 203-886-9; nonionic; pearlescent, opacifier for shampoos, lotions, creams, hand dishwash detergents; contributes to thickening; wh. waxy flakes; sol. in aliphatic and aromatic hydrocarbons, veg. oils, alcohols, glycols; insol. in water; m.p. 55-58 C; HLB 3.5; acid no. 2 max.; sapon. no. 174-185; pH 4.5-6.0 (5% aq.); 100% conc.

Hodag EGS. [Calgene] Ethylene glycol monostearate; CAS 111-60-4; EINECS 203-886-9; nonionic; surfactant for industrial and cosmetic applics.; wh. solid; nondisp. in water; sp.gr. 0.96; HLB 3.5; pour pt. 57 C.

Hodag GML. [Calgene] Glyceryl laurate; CAS 142-18-7; EINECS 205-526-6; nonionic; emulsifier, opacifier, stabilizer for food, drug, and cosmetic industries; paste; HLB 3.0; 100% conc.

Hodag GMO. [Calgene] Glyceryl oleate; nonionic; emulsifier, opacifier, stabilizer for food, drug, and cosmetic industries; liq.; HLB 2.7; 100% conc.

Hodag GMO-D. [Calgene] Glyceryl oleate; anionic; emulsifier, opacifier, stabilizer for food, drug, and cosmetic industries; liq.; HLB 2.7; 100% conc.

Hodag GMP. [Calgene] Glyceryl palmitate; nonionic; surfactant.

Hodag GMR. [Calgene] Glyceryl ricinoleate; CAS 141-08-2; EINECS 205-455-0; nonionic; emulsifier, opacifier, stabilizer for food, drug, and cosmetic industries; amber liq.; nondispersible in water; sp.gr. 0.99; dens. 8.25 lb/gal; 100% conc.

Hodag GMR-D. [Calgene] Glyceryl ricinoleate; CAS 141-08-2; EINECS 205-455-0; anionic; emulsifier, opacifier, stabilizer for food, drug, and cosmetic industries; amber liq.; disp. in water; sp.gr. 1.00; dens. 8.25 lb/gal; 100% conc.

Hodag GMS. [Calgene] Glyceryl stearate; nonionic; emulsifier, opacifier, stabilizer for food, drug, and cosmetic industries; solid; sp.gr. 0.97; m.p. 58 C; HLB 2.7; acid no. 5 max.; iodine no. 0.5; sapon. no. 160-175; pH 5.3 (5% in 25% IPA); 100% conc.

Hodag GMS-A. [Calgene] Glyceryl stearate, PEG-100 stearate; nonionic; self-emulsifying, acid-stable prod. for use in neutral or sl. acidic cosmetic and pharmaceutical lotions or cream emulsions; wh. flake; m.p. 50-60 C; acid no. 1

max.; sapon. no. 90-105; pH 6.0-8.5 (1% disp.).

Hodag GMS-D. [Calgene] Glyceryl stearate SE; for personal care applics.; wh. waxy solid; acid no. 10 max.; sapon. no. 135-145.

Hodag GTO. [Calgene] Glyceryl trioleate; CAS 122-32-7; EINECS 204-534-7; nonionic; emulsifier, opacifier, stabilizer for food, drug, and cosmetic industries; liq.; HLB 1.0; 100% conc.

Hodag PB-285. [Calgene] PPG-15 butyl ether; CAS 9003-13-8; for personal care applics.

Hodag PB-300. [Calgene] PPG-16 butyl ether; CAS 9003-13-8; for personal care applics.

Hodag PB-625. [Calgene] PPG-24 butyl ether; CAS 9003-13-8; functional fluid as replacement for animal, veg. and min. oils; for personal care applics.; insol. in water; sp.gr. 1.000; dens. 8.35 lb/gal; pour pt. -32 C.

Hodag PB-1715. [Calgene] PPG-40 butyl ether; CAS 9003-13-8; functional fluid as replacement for animal, veg. and min. oils; for personal care applics.; insol. in water; sp.gr. 1.003; dens. 8.38 lb/gal; pour pt. -23 C.

Hodag PE-004. [Calgene] Phosphate ester; anionic; emulsifier, lubricant, antistat, corrosion inhibitor for pesticides, industrial alkaline detergents, drycleaning, textile wet processing, syn. fiber lubricants, emulsion polymerization, cosmetics; lt. amber clear visc. liq.; sol. in water, aromatic solvs.; sp.gr. 1.18-1.22; acid no. 140-165; pH 1.5-2.5 (10% aq.).

Hodag PE-104. [Calgene] Alkylaryl phosphate ester; anionic; emulsifier, EP lube additive, antistat, corrosion inhibitor, surfactant; for pesticides, industrial detergents, drycleaning, textile wet processing, lubricants, emulsion polymerization, cosmetics; lt. amber clear visc. liq.; sol. in aromatic and aliphatic solvs., disp. in water; sp.gr. 0.98-1.02; acid no. 110-130; pH 1.5-2.5 (10% aq.); 100% conc.

Hodag PE-106. [Calgene] Alkylaryl phosphate ester; anionic; emulsifier, EP lube additive, antistat, corrosion inhibitor, surfactant; for pesticides, industrial detergents, drycleaning, textile wet processing, lubricants, emulsion polymerization, cosmetics; lt. amber clear visc. liq.; sol. in aromatic and aliphatic solvs., disp. in water; sp.gr. 1.09-1.13; acid no. 100-115; pH 1.5-2.5 (10% aq.); 100% conc.

Hodag PE-109. [Calgene] Alkylaryl phosphate ester; anionic; emulsifier, EP lube additive, antistat, corrosion inhibitor, surfactant; for pesticides, industrial detergents, drycleaning, textile wet processing, lubricants, emulsion polymerization, cosmetics; lt. amber clear visc. liq.; sol. in water, aromatic and aliphatic solvs.; sp.gr. 1.07-1.11; acid no. 75-90; pH 1.5-2.5 (10% aq.); 100% conc.

Hodag PE-206. [Calgene] Alkylaryl phosphate ester; anionic; emulsifier, EP lube additive, antistat, corrosion inhibitor, surfactant; for pesticides, industrial detergents, drycleaning, textile wet processing, lubricants, emulsion polymerization, cosmetics; lt. amber sl. hazy visc. liq.; disp. in water; sol. in aromatic and aliphatic solvs.; sp.gr. 1.03-1.08; acid no. 85-100; pH 1.5-2.5 (10% aq.); 100% conc.

Hodag PE-209. [Calgene] Alkylaryl phosphate ester; anionic; emulsifier, EP lube additive, antistat, corrosion inhibitor, surfactant; for pesticides, industrial detergents, drycleaning, textile wet processing, lubricants, emulsion polymerization, cosmetics; lt. amber sl. hazy visc. liq.; disp. in water; sol. in aromatic and aliphatic solvs.; sp.gr. 1.04-1.08; acid no. 70-90; pH 1.5-2.5 (10% aq.); 100% conc.

Hodag PE-1203. [Calgene] Laureth-3 phosphate; CAS 39464-66-9; for personal care applics.

Hodag PE-1803. [Calgene] Oleth-3 phosphate; CAS 39464-69-2; emulsifier for cosmetics, pharmaceuticals, and industrial use; anticorrosion agent; lt. amber liq.; acid no. 125-145; toxicology: relatively low skin irritation; 50% conc.

Hodag PE-1810. [Calgene] Oleth-10 phosphate; CAS 39464-69-2; emulsifier for cosmetics, esp. highly stable o/w emulsions, pharmaceuticals, industrial use; anticorrosion agent; cream paste; sol. in water, alcohol, fatty alcohols, min. oil, IPM, IPP; acid no. 80-100; toxicology: relatively low skin irritation; 70% conc.

Hodag PE-1820. [Calgene] Oleth-20 phosphate; CAS 39464-69-2; surfactant for cosmetic, pharmaceutical, and industrial use; corrosion inhibitor; waxy solid; acid no. 60-80; toxicology: relatively low skin irritation.

Hodag PEG 200. [Calgene] PEG-4; CAS 25322-68-3; EINECS 203-989-9; cosmetics and pharmaceuticals formulation; plasticizer for adhesives; inks; resins and coatings; clear liq.; water-sol.; m.w. 190-210; pH 4.5-7.5 (5%).

Hodag PEG 300. [Calgene] PEG-6; CAS 25322-68-3; EINECS 220-045-1; cosmetics and pharmaceutical formulation; latex coagulating bath; plasticizer for adhesives, spray-on bandages; resins and coatings; clear liq.; water-sol.; m.w. 285-315; visc. 5.4-6.4 cSt (210 F); pH 4.5-7.5 (5%).

Hodag PEG 400. [Calgene] PEG-8; CAS 25322-68-3; EINECS 225-856-4; cosmetic and pharmaceutical formulation; humectant, coupler for lotions; release agent for rubber; latex coagulating bath; in PVAc paints; clear liq.; water-sol.; m.w. 380-420; visc. 6.8-8.0 cSt (210 F); pH 4.5-7.5 (5%).

Hodag PEG 540. [Calgene] PEG-6, PEG-32 (50/50 mixt.); cosmetic, pharmaceutical, and suppository formulation; humectant, plasticizer in adhesives; base for metal polishes; lubricant for paper sizes; inks; in alkyd resins and coatings; wh. waxy solid; water-sol.; m.w. 500-600; visc. 26-33 cSt (210 F); f.p. 38-41 C; pH 4.5-7.5 (5%).

Hodag PEG 600. [Calgene] PEG-12; CAS 25322-68-3; EINECS 229-859-1; cosmetic and pharmaceutical formulation; resins and coatings; liq.; water-sol.; m.w. 570-630; visc. 9.9-11.3 cSt (210 F); pH 4.5-7.5 (5%).

Hodag PEG 1000. [Calgene] PEG-20; CAS 25322-68-3; cosmetic and pharmaceutical formulation; resins and coatings; imparts dimensional stability to paper wet str. resins, improves coatings gloss; wh. waxy solid; water-sol.; m.w. 950-1050; visc. 16-19 cSt (210 F); f.p. 37-40 C; pH 4.5-7.5 (5%).

Hodag PEG 1450. [Calgene] PEG-32; CAS 25322-68-3; cosmetic and pharmaceutical formulation; resins and coatings; wh. waxy solid; water-sol.; m.w. 1300-1600; visc. 25-32 cSt (210 F); f.p. 43-46 C; pH 4.5-7.5 (5%).

Hodag PEG 3350. [Calgene] PEG-75; CAS 25322-68-3; cosmetic and pharmaceutical formulation; resins and coatings; humectant, plasticizer for adhesives; antistat for rubber conveyor belt; in shoe polish; lubricant for paper sizing; printing inks; tablet binder, lubricant; wh. waxy solid; water-sol.; m.w. 3015-3685; visc. 76-110 cSt (210 F); f.p. 53-56 C; pH 4.5-7.5 (5%).

Hodag PEG 8000. [Calgene] PEG-150; CAS 25322-68-3; cosmetic and pharmaceutical formulation; resins and coatings; antistat for rubber conveyor belting; in shoe polish; lubricant for paper size; printing inks; release agent for rubber; tablet binder/lubricant; wh. waxy solid; water-sol.; m.w. 7000-9000; visc. 470-900 cSt (210 F); f.p. 60-63 C; pH 4.5-7.5 (5%).

Hodag PGML. [Calgene] Propylene glycol laurate; CAS 142-55-2; EINECS 205-542-3; nonionic; surfactant for food, industrial, and cosmetic uses; wh. liq.; disp. in water; sp.gr. 0.92; HLB 4.0; pour pt. -4 C; 100% conc.

Hodag PGMP. [Calgene] Propylene glycol palmitate; nonionic; surfactant for industrial and cosmetic applics.; wh. solid; nondisp. in water; sp.gr. 0.95; HLB 3.6; pour pt. 36 C.

Hodag PGMS. [Calgene] Propylene glycol stearate; CAS 1323-39-3; EINECS 215-354-3; nonionic; surfactant for food, industrial, and cosmetic applics.; waxy solid;

nondisp. in water; sp.gr. 0.95; HLB 3.4; pour pt. 38 C; 100% conc.

Hodag PGO-1010. [Calgene] Decaglycerol decaoleate; CAS 11094-60-3; EINECS 234-316-7; nonionic; for personal care applics.; amber liq.; sol. in flavoring oils, brominated veg. oils, ethanol, glycerin, propylene glycol; disp. in water; sp.gr. 0.93-0.97; HLB 2.5; acid no. 15 max.; iodine no. 85 max.; sapon. no. 160-180; pH 7-8; formerly Hodag SVO-10107.

Hodag POE (7) GML. [Calgene] PEG-7 glyceryl laurate; for personal care applics.; yel. liq.; HLB 10.4; acid no. 1; sapon. no. 100.

Hodag POE (12) Glycerine. [Calgene] Glycereth-12; CAS 31694-55-0; for personal care applics.; Gardner 1 max. clear liq.; sp.gr. 1.2; hyd. no. 265-280; flash pt. (COC) > 350 F; pH 5-7 (5% aq.).

Hodag POE (20) GMS. [Calgene] PEG-20 glyceryl stearate; emulsifier for cakes, icings, whipped toppings and personal care prods.; pale yel. semisolid; sol. in ethanol, partly sol. in veg. oil, disp. in propylene glycol, insol. in water; acid no. 2 max.; iodine no. 2 max.; sapon. no. 65-75.

Hodag POE (26) Glycerine. [Calgene] Glycereth-26; CAS 31694-55-0; for personal care applics.

Hodag POE (40) MS. [Calgene] PEG-40 stearate; CAS 9004-99-3; for personal care applics.

Hodag PPG-150. [Calgene] PPG (150); used for lubricants, metalworking compds., cosmetics, paints, urethane foams, hydraulic fluids, plasticizers, release agents, surfactant intermediates, textile lubricants, antifoam agents; straw clear liq.; water-sol.; m.w. 150; pour pt. -42 C; flash pt. (COC) 250 F.

Hodag PPG-400. [Calgene] PPG-9; CAS 25322-69-4; used for lubricants, metalworking compds., cosmetics, paints, urethane foams, hydraulic fluids, plasticizers, release agents, surfactant intermediates, textile lubricants, antifoam agents; straw clear liq.; water-sol.; m.w. 400; pour pt. -45 C; flash pt. (COC) 420 F.

Hodag PPG-1200. [Calgene] PPG-20; CAS 25322-69-4; used for lubricants, metalworking compds., cosmetics, paints, urethane foams, hydraulic fluids, plasticizers, release agents, surfactant intermediates, textile lubricants, antifoam agents; straw clear liq.; sol. 2% in water; m.w. 1200; pour pt. -40 C; flash pt. (COC) 450 F.

Hodag PPG-2000. [Calgene] PPG-26; CAS 25322-69-4; used for lubricants, metalworking compds., cosmetics, paints, urethane foams, hydraulic fluids, plasticizers, release agents, surfactant intermediates, textile lubricants, antifoam agents; straw clear liq.; sol. 0.2% in water; m.w. 2000; pour pt. -35 C; flash pt. (COC) 450 F.

Hodag PPG-4000. [Calgene] PPG-30; CAS 25322-69-4; used for lubricants, metalworking compds., cosmetics, paints, urethane foams, hydraulic fluids, plasticizers, release agents, surfactant intermediates, textile lubricants, antifoam agents; straw clear liq.; sol. 0.1% in water; m.w. 4000; pour pt. -29 C; flash pt. (COC) 440 F.

Hodag PSML-4. [Calgene] Polysorbate 21; CAS 9005-64-5; nonionic; for personal care applics.

Hodag PSML-20. [Calgene] Polysorbate 20; CAS 9005-64-5; nonionic; food-grade emulsifier; also for personal care applics.; yel. liq.; sol. in water; sp.gr. 1.1; HLB 16.7; acid no. 2 max.; sapon. no. 40-50; hyd. no. 96-108; 100% conc.

Hodag PSML-80. [Calgene] PEG-80 sorbitan laurate; CAS 9005-64-5; nonionic; food-grade emulsifier; also for personal care applics.; yel. liq.; water-sol.; sp.gr. 1.1; HLB 19.4; acid no. 3 max.; sapon. no. 7-15; hyd. no. 25-40; 27-29% moisture.

Hodag PSMO-5. [Calgene] Polysorbate 81; CAS 9005-65-6; nonionic; food-grade emulsifier; also for personal care applics.; yel. liq. (may gel on standing); disp. in water;

sp.gr. 1.0; HLB 10.0; acid no. 2 max.; sapon. no. 95-105; hyd. no. 136-152.

Hodag PSMO-20. [Calgene] Polysorbate 80; CAS 9005-65-6; nonionic; emulsifier for food processing, personal care, and industrial applics.; yel. liq.; water-sol.; sp.gr. 1.1; HLB 15.0; acid no. 2 max.; sapon. no. 45-55; hyd. no. 65-80; 100% conc.

Hodag PSMP-20. [Calgene] Polysorbate 40; CAS 9005-66-7; nonionic; emulsifier for food processing, personal care, and industrial applics.; yel. liq. (may gel on standing); sol. in water; sp.gr. 1.1; HLB 15.6; acid no. 2 max.; sapon. no. 43-49; hyd. no. 89-105; 100% conc.

Hodag PSMS-4. [Calgene] Polysorbate 61; CAS 9005-67-8; nonionic; for personal care applics.

Hodag PSMS-20. [Calgene] Polysorbate 60; CAS 9005-67-8; nonionic; emulsifier for food processing, personal care, and industrial applics.; yel. liq. (may gel on standing); water-sol.; sp.gr. 1.1; HLB 14.9; acid no. 2 max.; sapon. no. 45-55; hyd. no. 81-96; 100% conc.

Hodag PSTO-20. [Calgene] Polysorbate 85; CAS 9005-70-3; nonionic; food-grade emulsifier; also for personal care prods.; yel. liq. (may gel on standing); disp. in water; sp.gr. 1.0; HLB 11.0; acid no. 2 max.; sapon. no. 82-95; hyd. no. 39-52.

Hodag PSTS-20. [Calgene] Polysorbate 65; CAS 9005-71-4; nonionic; emulsifier for food processing, personal care, and industrial applics.; tan solid; disp. in water; sp.gr. 1.1; HLB 10.5; acid no. 2 max.; sapon. no. 88-98; hyd. no. 42-60; 100% conc.

Hodag SML. [Calgene] Sorbitan laurate; CAS 1338-39-2; nonionic; emulsifier, oil additive, corrosion inhibitor; food-grade emulsifier; yel. liq.; water-disp.; oil-sol.; sp.gr. 1.0; HLB 8.6; acid no. 7 max.; sapon. no. 158-170; hyd. no. 330-358; 100% conc.

Hodag SMO. [Calgene] Sorbitan oleate; CAS 1338-43-8; EINECS 215-665-4; nonionic; emulsifier, oil additive, corrosion inhibitor; food-grade emulsifier; also for personal care prods.; amber liq.; oil-sol.; sp.gr. 1.0; HLB 4.3; acid no. 7.5; sapon. no. 149-160; hyd. no. 193-209; 100% conc.

Hodag SMP. [Calgene] Sorbitan palmitate; CAS 26266-57-9; EINECS 247-568-8; nonionic; emulsifier, oil additive, corrosion inhibitor; food-grade emulsifier; tan solid; oil-sol.; sp.gr. 1.0; HLB 6.7; acid no. 7.5 max.; sapon. no. 140-150; hyd. no. 275-305; 100% conc.

Hodag SMS. [Calgene] Sorbitan stearate; CAS 1338-41-6; EINECS 215-664-9; nonionic; emulsifier for food processing and personal care prods.; cream solid; nondisp. in water; sp.gr. 1.0; HLB 4.7; acid no. 10 max.; sapon. no. 147-157; hyd. no. 235-260; 100% conc.

Hodag SSO. [Calgene] Sorbitan sesquioleate; CAS 8007-43-0; EINECS 232-360-1; nonionic; for personal care applics.; yel. liq.; sol. in min. oil, IPA; insol. in water; dens. 8.2 lb/gal; visc. 400-500 cSt (100 F); m.p. < 0 C; HLB 3.75; acid no. 10; hyd. no. 195.

Hodag STO. [Calgene] Sorbitan trioleate; CAS 26266-58-0; EINECS 247-569-3; nonionic; emulsifier, oil additive, corrosion inhibitor; food-grade emulsifier; also for personal care prods.; amber liq.; oil-sol.; sp.gr. 1.0; HLB 1.8; acid no. 13.5 max.; sapon. no. 171-185; hyd. no. 58-69; 100% conc.

Hodag STS. [Calgene] Sorbitan tristearate; CAS 26658-19-5; EINECS 247-891-4; nonionic; emulsifier, oil additive, corrosion inhibitor; food-grade emulsifier; cream solid; oil-sol.; sp.gr. 1.0; HLB 2.1; acid no. 15 max.; sapon. no. 175-190; hyd. no. 65-80; 100% conc.

Hodag Antifoam F-1. [Calgene] Simethicone; antifoam for aq. and nonaq. systems; for fermentation, chem. processing, food, cosmetics, pharmaceutical, paint, adhesives, paper coatings, metalworking, lubricants, textile processing, petroleum, pulp and paper, cleaning compds.

Hodag Nonionic 1017-R. [Calgene] Meroxapol 171; CAS 9003-11-6; nonionic; surfactant for personal care applics.; liq.; m.w. 1900; sp.gr. 1.02; visc. 300 cP; HLB 2.5; cloud pt. 33 C (1%); 100% conc.

Hodag Nonionic 1031-L. [Calgene] Poloxamer 101; CAS 9003-11-6; for personal care applics.

Hodag Nonionic 1035-L. [Calgene] Poloxamer 105; CAS 9003-11-6; nonionic; detergent, antifoam, wetting agent, emulsifier, antistat, demulsifier, visc. modifier, deduster, gelation aid, metalworking lubricants, dispersants; also for personal care prods.; liq.; m.w. 1900; sp.gr. 1.06; visc. 375 cP; HLB 18.5; pour pt. 7 C; cloud pt. 77 C (1% aq.); 100% conc.

Hodag Nonionic 1038-F. [Calgene] Poloxamer 108; CAS 9003-11-6; for personal care applics.

Hodag Nonionic 1042-L. [Calgene] Poloxamer 122; CAS 9003-11-6; for personal care applics.; clear liq.; m.w. 1630; sp.gr. 1.03; visc. 250 cps; cloud pt. 37 C (1% aq.).

Hodag Nonionic 1043-L. [Calgene] Poloxamer 123; CAS 9003-11-6; for personal care applics.

Hodag Nonionic 1044-L. [Calgene] Poloxamer 124; CAS 9003-11-6; nonionic; detergent, antifoam, wetting agent, emulsifier, antistat, demulsifier, visc. modifier, deduster, gelation aid, metalworking lubricants, dispersants; also for personal care applics.; liq.; m.w. 2200; sp.gr. 1.05; visc. 400 cP; HLB 16.0; pour pt. 16 C; cloud pt. 67 C (1% aq.); 100% conc.

Hodag Nonionic 1061-L. [Calgene] Poloxamer 181; CAS 9003-11-6; nonionic; detergent, antifoam, wetting agent, emulsifier, antistat, demulsifier, visc. modifier, deduster, gelation aid, metalworking lubricants, dispersants; also for personal care applics.; liq.; m.w. 2000; sp.gr. 1.02; visc. 300 cP; HLB 3.0; pour pt. -29 C; cloud pt. 24 C (1% aq.); 100% conc.

Hodag Nonionic 1062-L. [Calgene] Poloxamer 182; CAS 9003-11-6; nonionic; detergent, antifoam, wetting agent, emulsifier, antistat, demulsifier, visc. modifier, deduster, gelation aid, metalworking lubricants, dispersants; also for personal care applics.; liq.; m.w. 2500; sp.gr. 1.03; visc. 450 cP; HLB 7.0; pour pt. -4 C; cloud pt. 32 C (1% aq.); 100% conc.

Hodag Nonionic 1063-L. [Calgene] Poloxamer 183; CAS 9003-11-6; for personal care applics.; clear liq.; m.w. 2650; sp.gr. 1.04; visc. 490 cps; cloud pt. 34 C (1% aq.).

Hodag Nonionic 1064-L. [Calgene] Poloxamer 184; CAS 9003-11-6; nonionic; detergent, antifoam, wetting agent, emulsifier, antistat, demulsifier, visc. modifier, deduster, gelation aid, metalworking lubricants, dispersants; also for personal care applics.; liq.; m.w. 2900; sp.gr. 1.05; visc. 700 cP; HLB 15.0; pour pt. 16 C; cloud pt. 58 C (1% aq.); 100% conc.

Hodag Nonionic 1065-P. [Calgene] Poloxamer 185; CAS 9003-11-6; for personal care applics.

Hodag Nonionic 1068-F. [Calgene] Poloxamer 188; CAS 9003-11-6; nonionic; detergent, antifoam, wetting agent, emulsifier, antistat, demulsifier, visc. modifier, deduster, gelation aid, metalworking lubricants, dispersants; also for personal care applics.; flake; m.w. 8400; visc. 1000 cP (77 C); HLB 29.0; pour pt. 52 C; cloud pt. > 100 C (1% aq.); 100% conc.

Hodag Nonionic 1072-L. [Calgene] Poloxamer 212; CAS 9003-11-6; for personal care applics.

Hodag Nonionic 1075-P. [Calgene] Poloxamer 215; CAS 9003-11-6; for personal care applics.

Hodag Nonionic 1077-F. [Calgene] Poloxamer 217; CAS 9003-11-6; surfactant for personal care applics.; flake; m.w. 6600; visc. 480 cP (77 C); HLB 24.5; pour pt. 48 C; cloud pt. > 100 C (1% aq.).

Hodag Nonionic 1081-L. [Calgene] Poloxamer 231; CAS 9003-11-6; for personal care applics.

Hodag Nonionic 1084-P. [Calgene] Poloxamer 234; CAS 9003-11-6; for personal care applics.

Hodag Nonionic 1085-P. [Calgene] Poloxamer 235; CAS 9003-11-6; for personal care applics.

Hodag Nonionic 1087-F. [Calgene] Poloxamer 237; CAS 9003-11-6; nonionic; surfactant for personal care applics.; flake; m.w. 7700; visc. 700 cP (77 C); HLB 24.0; pour pt. 49 C; cloud pt. > 100 C (1% aq.).

Hodag Nonionic 1088-F. [Calgene] Poloxamer 238; CAS 9003-11-6; nonionic; detergent, antifoam, wetting agent, emulsifier, antistat, demulsifier, visc. modifier, deduster, gelation aid, metalworking lubricants, dispersants; also for personal care applics.; flake; m.w. 11,400; visc. 2300 cP (77 C); HLB 28.0; pour pt. 54 C; cloud pt. > 100 C (1% aq.); 100% conc.

Hodag Nonionic 1092-L. [Calgene] Poloxamer 282; CAS 9003-11-6; for personal care applics.

Hodag Nonionic 1094-P. [Calgene] Poloxamer 284; CAS 9003-11-6; for personal care applics.

Hodag Nonionic 1098-F. [Calgene] Poloxamer 288; CAS 9003-11-6; for personal care applics.

Hodag Nonionic 1101-L. [Calgene] Poloxamer 331; CAS 9003-11-6; for personal care applics.

Hodag Nonionic 1103-P. [Calgene] Poloxamer 333; CAS 9003-11-6; for personal care applics.

Hodag Nonionic 1104-P. [Calgene] Poloxamer 334; CAS 9003-11-6; for personal care applics.

Hodag Nonionic 1105-P. [Calgene] Poloxamer 335; CAS 9003-11-6; for personal care applics.

Hodag Nonionic 1108-F. [Calgene] Poloxamer 338; CAS 9003-11-6; nonionic; surfactant for personal care applics.; flake; m.w. 14,600; visc. 2800 cP (77 C); HLB 27.0; pour pt. 57 C; cloud pt. > 100 C (1% aq.).

Hodag Nonionic 1121-L. [Calgene] Poloxamer 401; CAS 9003-11-6; for personal care applics.

Hodag Nonionic 1122-L. [Calgene] Poloxamer 402; CAS 9003-11-6; for personal care applics.

Hodag Nonionic 1123-P. [Calgene] Poloxamer 403; CAS 9003-11-6; for personal care applics.

Hodag Nonionic 1127-F. [Calgene] Poloxamer 407; CAS 9003-11-6; nonionic; surfactant for personal care applics.; flake; m.w. 12,600; visc. 3100 cP (77 C); HLB 22.0; pour pt. 56 C; cloud pt. > 100 C (1% aq.).

Hodag Nonionic 1802. [Calgene] Oleth-2; CAS 9004-98-2; for personal care applics.; clear liq.; visc. 30 cps; acid no. 1 max.; hyd. no. 160-180; pH 5-7 (5% aq.).

Hodag Nonionic 1804. [Calgene] Oleth-4; CAS 9004-98-2; for personal care applics.; Gardner 2 turbid liq.; visc. 35 cps; acid no. 2 max.; hyd. no. 118-140; pH 5-7 (5% aq.).

Hodag Nonionic 1809. [Calgene] Oleth-9; CAS 9004-98-2; for personal care applics.

Hodag Nonionic 1810. [Calgene] Oleth-10; CAS 9004-98-2; for personal care applics.; turbid liq.; visc. 40 cps; acid no. 2 max.; hyd. no. 78-85; pH 5-7 (5% aq.).

Hodag Nonionic 1820. [Calgene] Oleth-20; CAS 9004-98-2; for personal care applics.; Gardner 1 solid; visc. 55 cps; acid no. 2 max.; hyd. no. 47-60; pH 5-7 (5% aq.).

Hodag Nonionic 2017-R. [Calgene] Meroxapol 172; CAS 9003-11-6; nonionic; detergent, antifoam, dispersant, demulsifier, dishwashing rinse visc. control agent for personal care prods.; liq.; m.w. 2150; sp.gr. 1.03; visc. 400 cP; HLB 4.1; cloud pt. 38 C (1%); 100% conc.

Hodag Nonionic 5010-R. [Calgene] Meroxapol 105; CAS 9003-11-6; for personal care applics.

Hodag Nonionic 8017R. [Calgene] EO/PO block polymer; nonionic; surfactant; flake; m.w. 7000; sp.gr. 1.06 (77 C); HLB 13.4; cloud pt. 81 C (1%).

Hodag Nonionic 8025R. [Calgene] EO/PO block polymer; nonionic; surfactant; flake; m.w. 8000; sp.gr. 1.06; cloud pt. 45 C (1%).

Hodag Nonionic C-2. [Calgene] Ceteth-2; CAS 9004-95-9; for personal care applics.

Hodag Nonionic C-4. [Calgene] Ceteth-4; CAS 9004-95-9; for personal care applics.

Hodag Nonionic C-10. [Calgene] Ceteth-10; CAS 9004-95-9; for personal care applics.

Hodag Nonionic C-20. [Calgene] Ceteth-20; CAS 9004-95-9; for personal care applics.

Hodag Nonionic CS-2. [Calgene] Ceteareth-2; CAS 68439-49-6; for personal care applics.

Hodag Nonionic CS-5. [Calgene] Ceteareth-5; CAS 68439-49-6; for personal care applics.

Hodag Nonionic CS-10. [Calgene] Ceteareth-10; CAS 68439-49-6; for personal care applics.

Hodag Nonionic CS-15. [Calgene] Ceteareth-15; CAS 68439-49-6; for personal care applics.

Hodag Nonionic CS-20. [Calgene] Ceteareth-20; CAS 68439-49-6; for personal care applics.

Hodag Nonionic CS-40. [Calgene] Ceteareth-40; CAS 68439-49-6; for personal care applics.

Hodag Nonionic E-2. [Calgene] Nonoxynol-2; EINECS 248-291-5; for personal care applics.

Hodag Nonionic E-4. [Calgene] Nonoxynol-4; CAS 9016-45-9; for personal care applics.

Hodag Nonionic E-5. [Calgene] Nonoxynol-5; CAS 9016-45-9; nonionic; detergent and wetting agent for cosmetics, insecticides and other formulations; liq.; 100% conc.

Hodag Nonionic E-6. [Calgene] Nonoxynol-6; CAS 9016-45-9; nonionic; detergent and wetting agent for cosmetics, insecticides and other formulations; liq.; HLB 10.6; 100% conc.

Hodag Nonionic E-7. [Calgene] Nonoxynol-7; CAS 9016-45-9; EINECS 248-292-0; nonionic; detergent and wetting agent for cosmetics, insecticides and other formulations; liq.; 100% conc.

Hodag Nonionic E-8. [Calgene] Nonoxynol-8; CAS 9016-45-9; for personal care applics.

Hodag Nonionic E-9. [Calgene] Nonoxynol-9; CAS 9016-45-9; for personal care applics.

Hodag Nonionic E-10. [Calgene] Nonoxynol-10; CAS 9016-45-9; EINECS 248-294-1; nonionic; detergent and wetting agent for cosmetics, insecticides and other formulations; liq.; HLB 12.6; 100% conc.

Hodag Nonionic E-12. [Calgene] POE alkylaryl ether; nonionic; detergent and wetting agent for cosmetics, insecticides and other formulations; liq.; HLB 14.0; 100% conc.

Hodag Nonionic E-20. [Calgene] Nonoxynol-20; CAS 9016-45-9; nonionic; detergent and wetting agent for cosmetics, insecticides and other formulations; solid; HLB 17.0; 100% conc.

Hodag Nonionic E-30. [Calgene] Nonoxynol-30; CAS 9016-45-9; nonionic; detergent and wetting agent for cosmetics, insecticides and other formulations; solid; HLB 17.5; 100% conc.

Hodag Nonionic E-40. [Calgene] Nonoxynol-40; CAS 9016-45-9; nonionic; for personal care applics.

Hodag Nonionic E-50. [Calgene] Nonoxynol-50; CAS 9016-45-9; nonionic; for personal care applics.

Hodag Nonionic E-100. [Calgene] Nonoxynol-100; CAS 9016-45-9; nonionic; emulsifier, stabilizer, surfactant effective at high temps.; for personal care prods.; wh. waxy flake; water-sol.; visc. 150 cps (100 C); m.p. 52 C; HLB 19.0; cloud pt. > 100 C (1% aq.).

Hodag Nonionic GR-8. [Calgene] PEG-8 castor oil; CAS 61791-12-6; nonionic; surfactant for personal care applics.

Hodag Nonionic GR-25. [Calgene] PEG-25 castor oil; CAS 61791-12-6; nonionic; surfactant for industrial and cos-

metic applics.; sol. hazy in water; sp.gr. 1.05; dens. 8.6 lb/gal; HLB 13.0; pour pt. 5 C.

Hodag Nonionic GR-36. [Calgene] PEG-36 castor oil; CAS 61791-12-6; nonionic; surfactant for personal care applics.

Hodag Nonionic GR-40. [Calgene] PEG-40 castor oil; CAS 61791-12-6; nonionic; surfactant for industrial and cosmetic applics.; sol. in water; sp.gr. 1.05; dens. 8.7 lb/gal; HLB 14.5; pour pt. 14 C; cloud pt. 59-64 C (1%).

Hodag Nonionic GR-52. [Calgene] PEG-52 castor oil; CAS 61791-12-6; surfactant for industrial and cosmetic applics.; sol. in water; sp.gr. 1.07; dens. 8.9 lb/gal; HLB 16.0; pour pt. 18 C; cloud pt. 72-76 C (1%).

Hodag Nonionic GR-200. [Calgene] PEG-200 castor oil; CAS 61791-12-6; nonionic; surfactant for personal care applics.

Hodag Nonionic GRH-25. [Calgene] PEG-25 hydrog. castor oil; CAS 61788-85-0; nonionic; surfactant for personal care applics.

Hodag Nonionic GRH-40. [Calgene] PEG-40 hydrog. castor oil; CAS 61788-85-0; nonionic; surfactant for personal care applics.

Hodag Nonionic ID-5. [Calgene] Isodeceth-5; nonionic; surfactant for personal care applics.

Hodag Nonionic L-4. [Calgene] Laureth-4; CAS 5274-68-0; EINECS 226-097-1; nonionic; surfactant for industrial and cosmetic applics.; disp. in water; sp.gr. 0.94; dens. 7.9 lb/gal; HLB 9.7; pour pt. 12 C.

Hodag Nonionic L-9. [Calgene] Laureth-9; CAS 3055-99-0; EINECS 221-284-4; nonionic; surfactant for personal care applics.

Hodag Nonionic L-12. [Calgene] Laureth-12; CAS 3056-00-6; EINECS 221-286-5; nonionic; surfactant for industrial and cosmetic applics.; sol. in water; sp.gr. 1.00; dens. 8.3 lb/gal; HLB 14.7; pour pt. 29 C; cloud pt. 65-68 C (1% in 10% NaCl).

Hodag Nonionic L-23. [Calgene] Laureth-23; CAS 9002-92-0; nonionic; surfactant for industrial and cosmetic applics.; sol. in water; sp.gr. 1.05; dens. 8.7 lb/gal; HLB 16.9; pour pt. 33 C; cloud pt. 75-78 C (1% in 10% NaCl).

Hodag Nonionic S-2. [Calgene] Steareth-2; CAS 9005-00-9; nonionic; surfactant for industrial and cosmetic applics.; nondisp. in water; sp.gr. 0.98; dens. 8.1 lb/gal; HLB 4.9; pour pt. 43 C; cloud pt. 55 C (1%).

Hodag Nonionic S-10. [Calgene] Steareth-10; CAS 9005-00-9; nonionic; surfactant for industrial and cosmetic applics.; disp. in water; sp.gr. 1.02; dens. 8.5 lb/gal; HLB 12.4; pour pt. 38 C; cloud pt. 44 C (1%).

Hodag Nonionic S-13. [Calgene] Steareth-13; CAS 9005-00-9; nonionic; surfactant for industrial and cosmetic applics.

Hodag Nonionic S-20. [Calgene] Steareth-20; CAS 9005-00-9; nonionic; surfactant for industrial and cosmetic applics.; sol. hot in water; sp.gr. 1.04; dens. 8.7 lb/gal; HLB 15.3; pour pt. 38 C; cloud pt. 47 C (1%).

Hodag Nonionic S-40. [Calgene] Steareth-40; CAS 9005-00-9; nonionic; surfactant for personal care applics.; wh. waxy solid; sol. in water; visc. 100-130 cps (60 C); m.p. 47 C; HLB 17.3; cloud pt. > 100 C (1%); pH 5.0-7.5 (5% aq.).

Hodag Nonionic TD-6. [Calgene] Trideceth-6; CAS 24938-91-8; surfactant for industrial and cosmetic applics.; disp. in water; sp.gr. 0.99; dens. 8.1 lb/gal; HLB 11.4; pour pt. 16 C.

Hodag Nonionic TD-12. [Calgene] Trideceth-12; CAS 24938-91-8; surfactant for industrial and cosmetic applics.; sol. in water; sp.gr. 1.02; dens. 8.5 lb/gal; HLB 14.5; pour pt. 13 C; cloud pt. 53-60 C (1% in 10% NaCl).

Hodag Nonionic TD-15. [Calgene] Trideceth-15; CAS 24938-91-8; nonionic; surfactant for industrial and cosmetic applics.; sol. in water; sp.gr. 1.04; dens. 8.7 lb/gal;

HLB 15.4; pour pt. 16 C; cloud pt. 65-70 C (1%).

Hodag Polyglycol 5035. [Calgene] PPG-28-buteth-35; for personal care applics.

Hodag Polyglycol 5051. [Calgene] PPG-33-buteth-45; for personal care applics.

Hodag Polyglycol 5055. [Calgene] PPG-2-buteth-3; for personal care applics.

Hodag Polyglycol 5066. [Calgene] PPG-12-buteth-16; for personal care applics.

Hoe S 2650. [Hoechst Celanese/Colorants & Surf.] Dilaureth-4 dimonium chloride; cationic; surfactant for clear conditioners, shampoos; lt. colored soft paste; 90% act.

Hoe S 2721. [Hoechst Celanese/Colorants & Surf.] Polyglyceryl-2 sesquiisostearate; nonionic; w/o emulsifier for personal care prods.; for prods. with high temp. stability; pale yel. clear, low-visc. liq.; HLB 3.5; 100% act.

Hoe S 3121. [Hoechst AG] Dioleoyl EDTHP-monium methosulfate.

Hoechst Wax E Pharma. [Hoechst AG] Montan acid wax; CAS 68476-03-9; EINECS 270-664-6; retarding agent for pharmaceutical use; pale ylsh. fine powd. (< 125 μm); dens. 1.01-1.03 g/cc; visc. ≈ 30 mm²/s (100 C); drop pt. 79-85 C; acid no. 15-20; sapon. no. 130-160.

Hoechst Wax PP 690. [Hoechst Celanese] Polypropylene; CAS 9003-07-0.

Hoechst Wax SW. [Hoechst Celanese; Hoechst AG] Montan acid wax; CAS 68476-03-9; EINECS 270-664-6; wax for beauty cosmetic pastes, gels, lipstick; lubricant for plastics; almost wh. flakes; dens. 1.00-1.02 g/cc; visc. ≈ 30 mm²/s (100 C); drop pt. 81-87 C; acid no. 115-135; sapon. no. 145-165.

H₂old™ EP-1. [ISP] Vinylpyrrolidone terpolymer; CAS 9003-39-8; EINECS 201-800-4; alcohol-free environmentally friendly hair spray polymer featuring faster drying times and superior holding; for water-based hair sprays, fragrance-free prods.; nontacky; odorless; water-sol.

Homosalate®. [Aceto] Homomenthyl salicylate; CAS 118-56-9; EINECS 204-260-8; sunscreen agent.

Homulgator 920 G. [Grau Aromatics] Myristyl alcohol, cetyl alcohol, stearyl alcohol, myreth-4, ceteareth-15, and ceteareth-5.

Hops HS. [Alban Muller] Propylene glycol and hops extract; botanical extract.

Hops LS. [Alban Muller] Sunflower seed oil and hops extract.

Hops Extract HS 2367 G. [Grau Aromatics] Propylene glycol and hops extract; botanical extract.

Hops Malt Extract HS 2518 G. [Grau Aromatics] Propylene glycol and hops extract; botanical extract.

Hops Oleat M. [C.E.P.] Propylene glycol dicaprylate/dicaprate and hops extract.

Hormo Fruit Apricot. [Esperis] Apricot extract and glycerin.

Hormo Fruit Pineapple. [Esperis] Pineapple juice and glycerin.

Hostacerin CG. [Hoechst Celanese/Colorants & Surf.; Hoechst AG] Cetearyl alcohol, triceteareth-4 phosphate, PEG-6 oleamide, and sodium C14-17 alkyl sec sulfonate; anionic; self-emulsifying base material for mfg. of o/w creams; ylsh. to wh. waxy flakes; 100% act.

Hostacerin DGI. [Hoechst Celanese/Spec. Chem.; Hoechst AG] Polyglyceryl-2 sesquiisostearate; emulsifier for cosmetic w/o emulsions; liq.; 100% act.

Hostacerin DGL. [Hoechst Celanese/Spec. Chem.] PEG-10 polyglyceryl-2 laurate; emulsifier for cosmetics and toiletries; 100% act.

Hostacerin DGS. [Hoechst Celanese/Colorants & Surf.; Hoechst AG] Polyglyceryl-2-PEG-4 stearate; nonionic; coemulsifier and thickener for cosmetic o/w emulsions; flake; HLB 7.5; 100% conc.

Hostacerin DGSB. [Hoechst Celanese/Spec. Chem.] Polyglycerol-2 PEG-4 stearate; emulsifier for cosmetics

and toiletries; 100% act.

Hostacerin O-20. [Hoechst Celanese/Colorants & Surf.] Oleth-20; CAS 9004-98-2; nonionic; surfactant; wax; 100% conc.

Hostacerin PN 73. [Hoechst Celanese/Colorants & Surf.] Acrylamide/sodium acrylate copolymer; CAS 25085-02-3; preneutralized thickener for cosmetic use; wh. powd.; water-sol.

Hostacerin T-3. [Hoechst Celanese/Colorants & Surf.; Hoechst AG] Ceteareth-3; CAS 68439-49-6; nonionic; emulsifier, superfatting agent, base for ointments, creams, liq. emulsions, shampoo additive; wh. soft, wax-like substance; sol. warm in all hydrocarbons, fatty alcohols; sp.gr. 0.905 (50 C); visc. 15 ± 3 cps (50 C); HLB 7-8; cloud pt. 54 C (in butyl diglycol); flash pt. 220 C; sapon. no. 1 max.; 100% act.

Hostacerin WO. [Hoechst Celanese/Colorants & Surf.; Hoechst AG] Polyglyceryl-2 sesquiisostearate, beeswax, microcryst. wax, min. oil, magnesium stearate, and aluminum stearate; anionic; emulsifier conc. for cosmetic w/o emulsions; ylsh. to wh. soft wax; HLB 4.5; 100% conc.

Hostacerin WOL. [Hoechst Celanese/Spec. Chem.] Polyglyceryl-2 sesquiisostearate, min. oil, magnesium stearate, and aluminum stearate; emulsifier for w/o cosmetics and toiletries; 100% act.

Hostaphat K Grades. [Hoechst AG] Organic phosphoric acid esters; emulsifiers; liq. to paste.

Hostaphat KL 240. [Hoechst Celanese/Colorants & Surf.] Dilaureth-4-phosphate.

Hostaphat KL 340N. [Hoechst Celanese/Colorants & Surf.; Hoechst AG] Trilaureth-4 phosphate; anionic; o/w emulsifier for cosmetic purposes; clear pale ylsh. liq.; disp. in water; HLB 11.5; 100% act.

Hostaphat KO 300. [Hoechst Celanese/Colorants & Surf.; Hoechst AG] Trioleyl phosphate; nonionic; emulsifier for cosmetic w/o emulsions; liq.; insol. in water; 100% conc.

Hostaphat KO 380. [Hoechst Celanese/Colorants & Surf.; Hoechst AG] Trioleth-8 phosphate; nonionic; emulsifier for o/w emulsions for cosmetics industry; liq.; 100% conc.

Hostaphat KW 340 N. [Hoechst Celanese/Colorants & Surf.; Hoechst AG] Triceteareth-4 phosphate; nonionic; emulsifier for creamy cosmetic emulsions based on hydrocarbons, fatty alcohols and fatty acids; wh. wax; HLB 10.5; 100% act.

Hostaphat LPKN158. [Hoechst Celanese/Colorants & Surf.] Phosphate ester; nonionic; surfactant; wh. wax; 100% conc.

Hostapon CT Paste. [Hoechst Celanese/Colorants & Surf.; Hoechst AG] Sodium methyl cocoyl taurate; anionic; base detergent used in shampoos; good foaming, skin compat.; wh. paste; 30% act.

Hostapon KA Powd. [Hoechst Celanese/Colorants & Surf.; Hoechst AG] Sodium cocoyl isethionate; EINECS 263-052-5; anionic; detergent base for cosmetic industry, detergent bars; foamer, dispersant; for syn. soaps with unique lather feel; wh. powd.; 78% conc.

Hostapon KCG. [Hoechst AG] Sodium cocoyl glutamate; CAS 68187-32-6; EINECS 269-087-2; base detergent for cosmetics and toiletries; 25% act.

Hostapon KTW. [Hoechst Celanese/Colorants & Surf.; Hoechst AG] Sodium lauroyl taurate; CAS 70609-66-4; EINECS 274-695-6; anionic; detergent base for cosmetics, toothpastes; powd.; 50% act.

Hostapon LEC. [Hoechst Celanese/Spec. Chem.] Laureth carboxylic acid; base detergent for cosmetics and toiletries; 92% act.

Hostapon SCHC. [Hoechst Celanese/Spec. Chem.] Sodium coco hydrolyzed collagen; CAS 68188-38-5; base detergent for cosmetics and toiletries; 30% act.

Hostapon SCHC-Powd. [Hoechst Celanese/Spec. Chem.]

Sodium coco hydrolyzed collagen; CAS 68188-38-5; base detergent for cosmetics and toiletries; powd.; 85% act.

Hostapon SCI. [Hoechst Celanese/Spec. Chem.] Sodium cocoyl isethionate; EINECS 263-052-5; base detergent for cosmetics and toiletries; 87% act.

Hostapon SCID. [Hoechst Celanese/Spec. Chem.] Sodium cocoyl isethionate; EINECS 263-052-5; base detergent for cosmetics and toiletries; 66% act.

Hostapon SO. [Hoechst Celanese/Colorants & Surf.] Sodium methyl oleoyl tauride; CAS 137-20-2; EINECS 205-285-7; anionic; detergent, foamer, dispersant for cosmetic industry; paste; 33% conc.

Hostapon STT Paste. [Hoechst Celanese/Colorants & Surf.; Hoechst AG] Sodium methyl stearoyl taurate; CAS 149-39-3; anionic; detergent for high quality cream shampoos; paste; 30% conc.

Hostapon T Paste 33. [Hoechst Celanese/Colorants & Surf.] Sodium methyl oleoyl tauride; CAS 137-20-2; EINECS 205-285-7; anionic; detergent, foamer, dispersant for cosmetic industry; paste; 33% conc.

Hostapon T Powd. Highly Conc. [Hoechst Celanese/Colorants & Surf.; Hoechst AG] Sodium methyl oleoyl taurate; CAS 137-20-2; EINECS 205-285-7; anionic; base detergent, cleaner for textile, leather, household prods., agric., cosmetics, etc.; powd.; 63% act.

Hostapur SAS 30. [Hoechst Celanese/Colorants & Surf.] Sodium C14-17 alkyl sec sulfonate; CAS 68037-49-0; EINECS 268-213-3; basic material for cosmetics and toiletries; 30% act.

Hostapur SAS 60. [Hoechst Celanese/Colorants & Surf.; Hoechst AG] Sodium C14–17 alkyl sec sulfonate; CAS 68037-49-0; EINECS 268-213-3; detergent base for mfg. of washing-up liq., detergent, shampoo, wetting agent; surfactant for textile processing; biodeg.; colorless to weakly yel. clear liq., yel. soft paste, flake; virtually odorless; m.w. 328; sp.gr. 1.048–1.087; visc. 26–6500 cps; 60% act.

Hostapur SAS 93. [Hoechst Celanese/Colorants & Surf.] Sodium C14-17 alkyl sec sulfonate; CAS 68037-49-0; EINECS 268-213-3; basic material for cosmetics and toiletries; 93% act.

HPCH Liq. [U.S. Cosmetics] Hydroxypropyl chitosan sol'n.; CAS 84069-44-3; film-forming agent and hair protectant for hair care, styling and setting prods.; provides strong, natural-feeling hold; helps prevent split ends; liq.; m.w. 800,000; 4% act.

HPCH Liq. [Ichimaru Pharcos] Hydroxypropyl chitosan; CAS 84069-44-3; film-former for hair care.

HSA. [CasChem] Hydroxystearic acid.; CAS 106-14-9; EINECS 203-366-1.

Hubersorb®. [J.M. Huber] Calcium silicate; CAS 1344-95-2; EINECS 215-710-8.

Hyala-Dew. [Dasco] Sodium hyaluronate; CAS 9067-32-7; moisturizer.

Hyalase. [Seporga] A stabilized enzymatic complex which contains a range of mucopolysaccharides; cosmetics ingred.

Hyalo-Mucopolysaccharides. [Sederma] Glycosaminoglycans.

Hyaluronic Acid. [Solabia] Hyaluronic acid; CAS 9004-61-9; EINECS 232-678-0; cosmetics moisturizer.

Hyaluronic Acid. [Pentapharm Ltd; Centerchem] Sodium hyaluronate; CAS 9067-32-7; moisturizer.

Hyaluronic Acid AH-602. [Bioiberica] Sodium hyaluronate; CAS 9067-32-7; moisturizer.

Hyaluronic Acid-BT. [Pentapharm Ltd; Centerchem] Sodium hyaluronate; CAS 9067-32-7; moisturizer.

Hyaluronic Acid (Na). [Ichimaru Pharcos] Sodium hyaluronate; CAS 9067-32-7; moisturizer.

Hyamide 1:1. [Hysan] Cocamide DEA; CAS 61791-31-9; EINECS 263-163-9; cosmetic surfactant.

Hyamine® 10X. [Lonza] Methylbenzethonium chloride; CAS 25155-18-4; EINECS 246-675-7; cationic; germicide, disinfectant, sanitizer in restaurant, veterinary, and pharmaceutical uses; wh. cryst.; dens. 27.5 lb/ ft³; surf. tens. 40 dynes/cm (0.01% aq.); 100% act.

Hyamine® 1622 50%. [Lonza] Benzethonium chloride; CAS 121-54-0; EINECS 204-479-9; cationic; germicide, disinfectant for restaurant, veterinary, surgical, pharmaceutical topicals, industrial/household sanitizers; antistat, bacteriostat on fabrics; preservative for starch, glue, casein; cocatalyst for curing polyesters; deodorant; swimming pool algicide; lt. amber liq.; sol. in water, lower alcohols, glycols, ethoxyethanol, tetrachloroethane; misc. with ethylene dichloride, CCl₄; sp.gr. 1.03; dens. 8.56 lb/gal; pour pt. 25 F; flash pt. (Seta) 110 F; pH 8-10 (5%); surf. tens. 30 dynes/cm (0.1%); toxicology: LD50 (oral, rat) 420 mg/kg, (dermal, rabbit) > 3 g/kg; may cause eye and skin irritation; 50% act.

Hyamine® 1622 Crystals. [Lonza] Benzethonium chloride; CAS 121-54-0; EINECS 204-479-9; bactericide, deodorant, preservative for veterinary and pharmaceutical prods.; APHA 40 max. powd.; sol. in water, lower alcohols, glycols, ethoxyethanol, tetrachloroethane; misc. with ethylene dichloride, CCl₄; sp.gr. 0.44 g/cc; dens. 27.5 lb/ft³; 100% act.

Hyamine® 3500 50%. [Lonza] Benzalkonium chloride [n-Alkyl = 50% C14, 40% C12, 10% C16]; CAS 68424-85-1; cationic; bactericide, disinfectant in restaurant and pharmaceutical uses, sanitizers for homes, farms, hospitals, dairies, food processing; antistat, bacteriostat on fabrics, sanitized paper; deodorant, preservative; algicide and slimicide for swimming pools, industrial water treatment, cooling towers; FDA approved: sanitizer for food processing equip.; pale yel. clear liq., mild odor; misc. with water, lower alcohols, ketones; m.w. 359.6; sp.gr. 0.96; dens. 8.0 lb/gal; visc. 42 cps; pour pt. 15 F; flash pt. (PM) 105 F; pH 7-9 (5%); surf. tens. 34 dynes/cm (0.1%); do not mix with oxidizing/reducing agents; toxicology: LD50 (oral, rat) 894 mg/kg; toxic to fish; 50% act.

Hyasol. [Pentapharm Ltd; Centerchem] Sodium hyaluronate; CAS 9067-32-7; moisturizer.

Hyasol-BT. [Pentapharm Ltd; Centerchem] Sodium hyaluronate; CAS 9067-32-7; moisturizer.

Hy Case SF. [Sheffield Prods.] Hydrolyzed casein; CAS 65072-00-6; EINECS 265-363-1; cosmetic protein.

Hy Case Amino. [Sheffield Prods.] Hydrolyzed casein; CAS 65072-00-6; EINECS 265-363-1; cosmetic protein.

Hycollan. [Pentapharm Ltd; Centerchem] Collagen amino acids; CAS 9105-54-7; moisturizer.

Hydagen® B. [Henkel/Cospha; Henkel Canada] α-Bisabolol; CAS 515-69-5; EINECS 208-205-9; antiphlogistic active agent for emulsions, oils, lotions, and oral hygiene preps.; liq.; sp.gr. 0.922-0.928; ref. index 1.492-1.498; usage level: 0.1-1%; 85% min. act.

Hydagen® C.A.T. [Henkel/Cospha; Henkel Canada; Henkel KGaA/Cospha] Triethyl citrate USP/NF; CAS 77-93-0; EINECS 201-070-7; nonmicrobiocidal deodorant active agent; stable in acid and neutral ranges; pale yel. oily clear liq., pract. odorless; sp.gr. 1.135-1.139; acid no. 0.2 max.; sapon. no. 603-609; ref. index 1.439-1.441; usage level: 1-5%; 99% act.

Hydagen® DEO. [Henkel/Cospha; Henkel Canada] Triethyl citrate and BHT; nonmicrobiocidal act. ingred. for deodorant systems and personal care prods.; pale yel. clear oily liq.; sol. in hydroalcoholic sol'ns.; sp.gr. 1.112–1.122; acid no. 0.2 max.; usage level: 1-3%; 99% act.

Hydagen® P. [Henkel/Cospha; Henkel Canada] Diethylene tricaseinamide; softening agent, conditioner for emulsion-type shampoos, hair care preparations; brightening agent for shampoos; improves feel and gloss of hair, esp. damaged hair; paste; m.w. 3000; pH 9.0 (5% aq.); usage level: 0.2-5%.

Hydex® 100 Gran. 206. [Lonza] Sorbitol; CAS 50-70-4; EINECS 200-061-5; humectant, bodying agent, moisture control agent for toothpaste, cosmetics, sugarless confections, controlled moisture foods, industrial applics.; wh. powd., 90% max. on 80 mesh screen; 100% act.

Hydex® Coarse Powd. [Lonza] Sorbitol; CAS 50-70-4; EINECS 200-061-5; humectant, bodying agent, moisture control agent for toothpaste, cosmetics, sugarless confections, controlled moisture foods, industrial applics.; wh. powd., 90% max. on 200 mesh screen; 100% act.

Hydex® Powd. 60. [Lonza] Sorbitol; CAS 50-70-4; EINECS 200-061-5; humectant, bodying agent, moisture control agent for toothpaste, cosmetics, sugarless confections, controlled moisture foods, industrial applics.; wh. powd., 1% max. on 60 mesh screen; 100% act.

Hydex® Tablet Grade. [Lonza] Sorbitol; CAS 50-70-4; EINECS 200-061-5; humectant, bodying agent, moisture control agent for toothpaste, cosmetics, sugarless confections, controlled moisture foods, industrial applics.; wh. powd., 75% max. on 200 mesh screen; 100% act.

Hydracol®. [Gattefosse] Soluble collagen; CAS 9007-34-5; EINECS 232-697-4; biological active providing skin soothing, moisturizing, elasticity, and tonicity improvement; used for skin care prods. incl. moisturizers, body lotions, solar creams; powd., odorless; water-sol.; 90% min. act.

Hydral® 710. [Alcoa] Hydrated alumina; fire retardant, smoke suppressant improving arc track resist. in thermosets, thermoplastics, elastomerics; in fillers and coating pigments in fine printing papers for increased brightness; for vinyl compding.; as reinforcing pigment in adhesives; fine mild abrasive in waxes and polishes; filler for cosmetic powds., lotions; polishing agent in dentifrices.

Hydrane L. [Alban Muller] Hydrolyzed lupine protein.

Hydrane R. [Alban Muller] Hydrolyzed rice protein; CAS 97759-33-8.

Hydrane S. [Alban Muller] Hydrolyzed soy protein; CAS 68607-88-5; cosmetic protein.

Hydrane W. [Alban Muller] Hydrolyzed wheat protein; CAS 70084-87-6; cosmetic protein.

Hydraprotectol-SM. [Sederma] Glycosaminoglycans; 2-in-1 moisturizer providing direct hydration of the superficial layers of the epidermis and in-depth, long-term hydration by reinforcement of the cutaneous barrier, limiting transepidermal water loss.

Hydratherm CGI Glycolic. [CGI-Universal Flavors] Propylene glycol, water, and algae extract; botanical extract.

Hydratherm CGI Hydroalcoholic. [CGI-Universal Flavors] Water, alcohol, and algae extract; botanical extract.

Hydratherm CGI Lyophilized. [CGI-Universal Flavors] Lactose and algae extract.

Hydrenol® D. [Henkel/Cospha; Henkel KGaA/Cospha] Hydrog. tallow alcohol (25-35% C16, 60-67% C18); wetting agent, emulsifier, emollient, consistency giving agent for skin creams and lotions; intermediate for surfactant mfg.; wh. fused/flakes; sp.gr. 0.805-0.815 g/cc (60 C); solid. pt. 48-52 C; b.p. 300-360 C; acid no. < 0.1; iodine no. < 1.0; sapon. no. < 1.2; hyd. no. 210-220; flash pt. 180 C; 100% conc.

Hydrenol® DD. [Henkel/Emery; Henkel KGaA] Hydrog. tallow alcohol; intermediate for surfactant mfg.; APHA 20 fused/flakes; sp.gr. 0.805-0.815 g/cc (60 C); solid. pt. 48-52 C; b.p. 310-360 C; acid no. < 0.1; iodine no. < 1.0; sapon. no. < 0.5; hyd. no. 210-220; flash pt. 180 C; 100% conc.

Hydrine. [Gattefosse; Gattefosse SA] PEG-2 stearate; CAS

9004-99-3; 106-11-6; EINECS 203-363-5; consistency stabilizer for ointments, cream lotions, opacifier in shampoos, liq. soaps; solid; drop pt. 45.5-48.5 C; HLB 5.0; acid no. < 6; iodine no. < 3; sapon. no. 150-160; toxicology: nonirritating to skin and eyes; 100% conc.

Hydrobase 32/34. [Prod'Hyg] Hydrog. coconut oil.

Hydrocell™ AYP-30. [Brooks Industries] Autolyzed yeast protein extract; CAS 100684-36-4; cosmetic ingred.; 30% conc.

Hydrocell™ YP-30. [Brooks Industries] Hydrolyzed yeast protein; CAS 100684-36-4; cosmetic ingredient for skin and hair care prods.; m.w. 1000; 30% act.

Hydrocell YP-30-P. [Brooks Industries] Hydrolyzed yeast protein; CAS 100684-36-4; cosmetic protein.

Hydrocell YP-SD. [Brooks Industries] Hydrolyzed yeast protein; CAS 100684-36-4; cosmetic protein.

Hydrocoll™ AC-30. [Brooks Industries] Acid hydrolyzed collagen; CAS 9015-54-7; cationic; film-forming and moisture retentive substantive protein for hair and skin care prods.; provides hair setting props., builds body and bounce into the hair; protective colloid, counter-irritant for skin protection; amber, very sl. odor; sol. in water; m.w. 6000; 30% conc.

Hydrocoll AG-SD. [Brooks Industries] Gelatin; CAS 9000-70-8; EINECS 232-554-6; cosmetics ingred.

Hydrocoll AL-50, AL-55, EN-40, EN-55-X, EN-SD-1M, EN-SD-10M. [Brooks Industries] Hydrolyzed collagen; CAS 9015-54-7; cosmetic protein.

Hydrocoll™ EN-55. [Brooks Industries] Enzyme hydrolyzed collagen; CAS 9015-54-7; film-forming and moisture-retentive substantive protein with exc. light color, very low odor, controlled m.w.; for hair and skin care prods., shampoos, conditioners; protective colloid, counter-irritant for skin protection; low salt; lt. amber liq., very sl. odor; water-sol.; m.w. 2000; 55% act.

Hydrocoll™ EN-SD. [Brooks Industries] Enzyme hydrolyzed collagen; CAS 9015-54-7; film-forming and moisture-retentive substantive protein with exc. light color, very low odor, controlled m.w.; for hair and skin care prods., shampoos, conditioners; protective colloid, counter-irritant for skin protection; low salt; wh. powd., very sl. odor; water-sol.; m.w. 2000; 100% conc.

Hydrocoll™ G-40. [Brooks Industries] Gelatin; CAS 9000-70-8; EINECS 232-554-6; cosmetics ingred.; liq.; m.w. 100,000.

Hydrocoll™ G-55. [Brooks Industries] Hydrolyzed gelatin; CAS 9000-70-8; EINECS 232-554-6; cosmetic ingred.; liq.; m.w. 2500.

Hydrocoll™ HE-35. [Brooks Industries] Acid hydrolyzed collagen; CAS 9015-54-7; film-forming and moisture retentive substantive protein for hair and skin care prods.; used in Europe for mildness in shampoos, permanent waves; protective colloid, counter-irritant for skin protection; low iron grade compat. with alkaline thioglycolic acid sol'ns.; wh., very sl. odor; water-sol.; m.w. 1000; 40% conc.

Hydrocoll™ LE-35. [Brooks Industries] Acid hydrolyzed collagen; CAS 9015-54-7; film-forming and moisture retentive substantive protein for hair and skin care prods.; used in Europe for mildness in shampoos, permanent waves; lt. amber, very sl. odor; water-sol.; m.w. 1000; 40% conc.

Hydrocoll PGA, PGB. [Brooks Industries] Gelatin; CAS 9000-70-8; EINECS 232-554-6; cosmetics ingred.

Hydrocoll SS-40, SS-55, T-37, T-55, T-LSN, T-LSN-SD, T-P52. [Brooks Industries] Hydrolyzed collagen; CAS 9015-54-7; cosmetic protein.

Hydrocoll™ T-LSN. [Brooks Industries] Alkaline hydrolyzed collagen; CAS 9015-54-7; film-forming and moisture retentive substantive protein for hair and skin care prods., esp. intensive hair treatments to repair and seal damaged hair; provides hard lustrous smooth finish to hair; dk. amber, sl. odor; water-sol.; m.w. 1000; 30% conc.

Hydrocolloid 219. [Brooks Industries] Hydrolyzed collagen; CAS 9015-54-7; cosmetic protein.

Hydrocos. [Cosmetochem] Sodium lactate, urea, hydrolyzed collagen, sorbitol, PEG-40 hydrog. castor oil, phosphoric acid, and allantoin; cosmetic ingred.

Hydrocotyl HS. [Alban Muller] Propylene glycol and hydrocotyl extract; botanical extract.

Hydrocotyl Glycolysat. [C.E.P.] Propylene glycol, water, and hydrocotyl extract; botanical extract.

Hydrocotyl Oleat M. [C.E.P.] Propylene glycol dicaprylate/dicaprate and hydrocotylextract.

Hydrocotyl Vegebios. [C.E.P.] Water and hydrocotyl extract.

Hydro-Diffuser Microreservoir. [Sederma] Water, glycerin, butylene glycol, lecithin, serine, PCA, gycine, proline, ornithine, alanine, citrulline, and glutamic acid.

Hydroessential Jasminum. [Vevy] Jasmine extract.

Hydroessential Matricaria. [Vevy] Matricaria extract.

Hydroessential Thymus. [Vevy] Thyme extract.

Hydrofacteur LC. [Les Colorants Wackherr] A blend of moisturizing substances for cosmetics.

Hydrokeratin™ 100M. [Brooks Industries] Hydrolyzed keratin; CAS 69430-36-0; EINECS 274-001-1; cosmetic ingred.

Hydrokeratin™ AL-30. [Brooks Industries] Hydrolyzed keratin; CAS 69430-36-0; EINECS 274-001-1; cosmetics ingred.; liq.; m.w. 1000; 30% act.

Hydrokeratin™ AL-SD. [Brooks Industries] Hydrolyzed keratin; CAS 69430-36-0; EINECS 274-001-1; cosmetics ingred.; powd.; m.w. 1000.

Hydrokeratin™ WKP. [Brooks Industries] Hydrolyzed keratin (wool keratin with cysteine); CAS 69430-36-0; EINECS 274-001-1; cosmetics ingred.; liq.; m.w. 1000; 20% act.

Hydrokote® 95. [Karlshamns] Hydrog. veg. oil; CAS 68334-28-1; EINECS 269-820-6; specialty base used as replacement for cocoa butter in cosmetic and pharmaceutical applics. (lipsticks, glosses, solid fragrances, antiperspirant sticks, emollient creams and lotions); FDA compliance; m.p. 35.6-36.7 C; iodine no. 5 max.; sapon. no. 240-255.

Hydrokote® 97. [Karlshamns] Hydrog. veg. oil; CAS 68334-28-1; EINECS 269-820-6; specialty base used as replacement for cocoa butter in cosmetic and pharmaceutical applics. (lipsticks, glosses, solid fragrances, antiperspirant sticks, emollient creams and lotions); FDA compliance; m.p. 36.1-37.2 C; iodine no. 5 max.; sapon. no. 238-255.

Hydrokote® 102. [Karlshamns] Hydrog. veg. oil; CAS 68334-28-1; EINECS 269-820-6; specialty base used as replacement for cocoa butter in cosmetic and pharmaceutical applics. (lipsticks, glosses, solid fragrances, antiperspirant sticks, emollient creams and lotions); FDA compliance; m.p. 38.3-39.4 C; iodine no. 5 max.; sapon. no. 230-250.

Hydrokote® 108. [Karlshamns] Hydrog. veg. oil; CAS 68334-28-1; EINECS 269-820-6; specialty base used as replacement for cocoa butter in cosmetic and pharmaceutical applics. (lipsticks, glosses, solid fragrances, antiperspirant sticks, emollient creams and lotions); FDA compliance; m.p. 41.1-42.8 C; iodine no. 5 max.; sapon. no. 230-250.

Hydrokote® 112. [Karlshamns] Hydrog. veg. oil; CAS 68334-28-1; EINECS 269-820-6; specialty base used as replacement for cocoa butter in cosmetic and pharmaceutical applics. (lipsticks, glosses, solid fragrances, antiperspirant sticks, emollient creams and lotions); FDA compliance; m.p. 45.6-47.8 C; iodine no. 5 max.; sapon. no. 225-245.

Hydrokote® 118. [Karlshamns] Hydrog. veg. oil; CAS 68334-28-1; EINECS 269-820-6; specialty base used as replacement for cocoa butter in cosmetic and pharmaceutical applics. (lipsticks, glosses, solid fragrances, antiperspirant sticks, emollient creams and lotions); FDA compliance; m.p. 47.2-48.9 C; iodine no. 5 max.; sapon. no. 230-250.

Hydrokote® AR, HL. [Karlshamns] Hydrog. veg. oil.; CAS 68334-28-1; EINECS 269-820-6; emollient, emulsifier.

Hydrokote® RM. [Karlshamns] Hydrog. veg oil; CAS 68334-28-1; EINECS 269-820-6; emollient, emulsifier.

Hydrolactin 2500. [Croda Inc.] Hydrolyzed milk protein; CAS 92797-39-2; substantive skin and hair care conditioner, moisturizer; for shampoos, conditioner rinses, setting and waving lotions, moisturizing creams and lotions, night creams and lotions; cream colored powd., sl. char. odor; sol. in water; partly sol. in water/ethanol mixts.; m.w. 2500; pH 5.0-7.0; usage level: 0.2-2%; 85% act.

Hydrolactol 70. [Gattefosse] Glyceryl stearate, propylene glycol stearate, glyceryl isostearate, propylene glycol isostearate, oleth-25, ceteth-25.; nonionic; self-emulsifying base for fluid, semifluid lotions and o/w creams, min. pigment formulations (sun filters); Gardner < 6 waxy solid, faint odor; sol. in chloroform, methylene chloride; disp. in water; insol. in ethanol, min. oils; drop pt. 36-45 C; HLB 10.0; acid no. < 3; iodine no. < 5; sapon. no. 125-145; toxicology: sl. irritating to skin, nonirritating to eyes.

Hydrolactol 93. [Gattefosse] Glyceryl stearate, propylene glycol stearate, glyceryl isostearate, propylene glycol isostearate, oleth-25, and ceteth-25.

Hydrolan. [Lanaetex Prods.] Hydrolyzed collagen; CAS 9015-54-7; cosmetic protein.

Hydrolastan. [Pentapharm Ltd; Centerchem] Hydrolyzed elastin; CAS 100085-10-7; cosmetic protein.

Hydrolyzed NMF. [Proalan SA] Hydrolyzed collagen, sodium PCA, lactic acid, allantoin, and glucose.

Hydrolyzed Animal Protein-55. [ChemMark Development] Hydrolyzed collagen; CAS 9015-54-7; cosmetic protein.

Hydrolyzed Animal Protein SD. [ChemMark Development] Hydrolyzed collagen; CAS 9015-54-7; cosmetic protein.

Hydrolyzed Elastin RE-10 No. 26202. [Roche] Hydrolyzed elastin; CAS 100085-10-7; substantive hair and skin care moisturizer; improves elasticity of skin.

Hydrolyzed Elastin RE-30 No. 26203. [Roche] Hydrolyzed elastin; CAS 100085-10-7; substantive hair and skin care moisturizer; improves elasticity of skin.

Hydrolyzed Mucopolysaccharides SD. [Brooks Industries] Hydrolyzed glycosaminoglycans; moisturizer for skin care cosmetics; lt. tan powd., char. bland odor; sol. @ 1% in water, propylene glycol, glycerin, 60% ethanol, ammonium laureth sulfate; insol. in min. oil; pH 6-8 (10%); 93% min. NV.

Hydro-Magma. [Marine Magnesium] Water and magnesium hydroxide; CAS 1309-42-8; EINECS 215-170-3; used in mfg. of milk of magnesia and liq. antacids; paste; 30% act.

Hydromarine. [Sederma] Glycerin, water, propylene glycol, and sodium chondroitin sulfate; moisturizer and restructurer of epidermis for skin, face, and body care prods.; colorless, sl. opalescent visc. liq., char. odor; sp.gr. 1.08-1.10; visc. 350-550 cps; ref. index 1.385 ± 0.005; pH 5.5-6.5; usage level: 5-10%.

Hydromilk™ EN-20. [Brooks Industries] Hydrolyzed casein; CAS 65072-00-6; EINECS 265-363-1; complete food containing all essential amino acids; m.w. 4000; 20% act.

Hydromilk ENL-SD. [Brooks Industries] Lactose, hydrolyzed milk protein; cosmetic ingred.

Hydro Myristenol 2/014082. [Dragoco] Ceteareth-6, isopropyl myristate.

Hydrophilol ISO. [Gattefosse SA] Propylene glycol isostearate; CAS 68171-38-0; EINECS 269-027-5; superfatting agent for cosmetic/pharmaceutical emulsions and microemulsions; liq.; HLB 3-4; acid no. < 6; iodine no. < 15; sapon. no. 150-170; toxicology: sl. irritating to eyes, nonirritating to skin.

Hydrophore 312. [Prod'Hyg] PEG-6 laurate/tartarate.

Hydroplastidine Achillea. [Vevy] Water and yarrow extract; CAS 84082-83-7; botanical extract.

Hydroplastidine Calendula. [Vevy] Water and calendula extract; CAS 84776-23-8.

Hydroplastidine Foeniculum. [Vevy] Water and fennel extract; botanical extract.

Hydroplastidine Matricaria. [Vevy] Water and matricaria extract.

Hydrosoy 2000. [Croda Inc.] Hydrolyzed veg. protein; CAS 100209-45-8; conditioner for cosmetic prods.; liq.

Hydrosoy 2000/SF. [Croda Inc.; Croda Chem. Ltd.] Hydrolyzed soy protein; CAS 68607-88-5; substantive protein moisturizer for personal care prods.; amber clear liq.;m.w. 4000; usage level: 0.2-3%; 20% act.

Hydrotriticum™. [Croda Inc.] Hydrolyzed wheat protein; CAS 70084-87-6; amphoteric; substantive conditioning agent, moisturizer for hair waving systems, shampoos, cream rinses, skin care prods.; pale yel. liq., mild char. odor; sol. in water, water/alcohol (50:50), glycerin, propylene glycol; m.w. 3000; sp.gr. 1.0; b.p. 212 F; pH 4-6; usage level: 1-5%; toxicology: nontoxic, nonirritating to skin and eyes; 20% solids.

Hydrotriticum™ QL. [Croda Inc.] Laurdimonium hydroxypropyl hydrolyzed wheat protein; cationic; film-forming conditioner for hair and skin care prods., e.g., waving systems, activated conditioner treatments, shampoos, styling mousses, hair coloring, wrinkle remover creams and lotions, liq. soap, facial scrubs, skin cleansers, bath prods.; lt. amber clear liq., mild char. odor; sol. @ 10% in water, water/ethanol, glycerin, propylene glycol, surfactants; m.w. 3500; sp.gr. 1.05; b.p. > 300 F; pH 4.0-5.0; toxicology: may be a skin and eye irritant; 26% act.

Hydrotriticum™ QM. [Croda Inc.] Cocodimonium hydroxypropyl hydrolyzed wheat protein; cationic; film-forming conditioner for hair and skin care prods., e.g., waving systems, activated conditioner treatments, shampoos, styling mousses, hair coloring, wrinkle remover creams and lotions, liq. soap, facial scrubs, skin cleansers, bath prods.; lt. amber clear liq., mild char. odor; sol. in water, water/ethanol, glycerin, propylene glycol, surfactants; m.w. 3500; sp.gr. 1.05; b.p. > 300 F; pH 4.0-5.0; toxicology: may be a skin and eye irritant; 26% act.

Hydrotriticum™ QS. [Croda Inc.] Steardimonium hydroxypropyl hydrolyzed wheat protein; cationic; film-forming conditioner for hair and skin care prods., e.g., waving systems, activated conditioner treatments, shampoos, styling mousses, hair coloring, wrinkle remover creams and lotions, liq. soap, facial scrubs, skin cleansers, bath prods.; lt. amber opaque paste, mild char. odor; sol. in water, water/ethanol, glycerin, propylene glycol; m.w. 3500; sp.gr. 1.05; b.p. > 300 F; pH 4.0-5.0; toxicology: may be a skin and eye irritant; 26% act.

Hydrotriticum™ WAA. [Croda Inc.] Wheat amino acids; amphoteric; substantive moisturizer, humectant for hair and skin care prods., cleansers, antiwrinkle preps., sun screens; leaves soft and conditioned afterfeel; amber clear liq., char. odor; sol. in water, glycerin, propylene glycol; m.w. 150; pH 4.0-5.5; 16% act.

Hydrotriticum™ WQ. [Croda Chem. Ltd.] Hydroxypropyltrimonium hydrolyzed wheat protein.

Hydroviton 2/059353. [Dragoco] Water, sodium lactate, lactic acid, glycerin, serine, sorbitol, TEA-lactate, triethanolamine, urea, sodium chloride, lauryl diethylenediaminoglycine, allantoin, lauryl aminopropylglycine, and

SD alcohol 39-C; cosmetic ingred.

Hydroxylan. [Fanning] Hydroxylated lanolin; CAS 68424-66-8; EINECS 270-315-8; nonionic; emulsifier for w/o systems, stabilizer for o/w systems, wetting and dispersing agent, conditioner, emollient, tackifier; for pharmaceutical ointments; yel. to lt. tan solid; m.p. 39-46 C; acid no. 10 max.; iodine no. 12-20; sapon. no. 95-110; hyd. no. 60-85; 100% conc.

Hydroxyprolisilane C. [Exsymol; Biosil Tech.] Methylsilanol aspartate hydroxyprolinate; provides collagen restructuring for cosmetic and health prods. incl. stretch mark prevention creams, anti-aging formulations, acne preventives, eye contour creams, etc.; pale pink sl. opalescent liq.; misc. with water, alcohols, glycols; sp.gr. 1.0; pH 5.5; usage level: 2-5%; toxicology: nontoxic.

Hydrumine Calendula. [Exsymol; Biosil Tech.] Propylene glycol, water, and calendula extract with 0.5% phenonip as preservative; plant extract for cosmetic use, restructuring, antiwrinkle prods., day and night creams; brn. liq.; sol. in water, and alcoholic sol'ns.; usage level: 0.5-2%.

Hydrumine Witchazel. [Exsymol; Biosil Tech.] Propylene glycol, water, and witch hazel extract with 0.5% phenonip as preservative; plant extract for cosmetic use, restructuring, antiwrinkle prods., day and night creams; brn. liq.; sol. in water and alcoholic sol'ns.; usage level: 0.5-2%.

Hyfatol 16-95. [Aarhus Oliefabrik A/S] Cetyl alcohol; CAS 36653-82-4; EINECS 253-149-0; cosmetic ingred.

Hyfatol 16-98. [Aarhus Oliefabrik A/S] Cetyl alcohol; CAS 36653-82-4; EINECS 253-149-0; cosmetic ingred.

Hyfatol 18-95. [Aarhus Oliefabrik A/S] Stearyl alcohol; CAS 112-92-5; EINECS 204-017-6; emollient, cosmetic/pharmaceutical raw material.

Hyfatol 18-98. [Aarhus Oliefabrik A/S] Stearyl alcohol; CAS 112-92-5; EINECS 204-017-6; emollient, cosmetic/pharmaceutical raw material.

Hyfatol CS. [Aarhus Oliefabrik A/S] Cetearyl alcohol.

Hyflo Super-Cel. [Celite] Diatomaceous earth; CAS 7631-86-9; EINECS 231-545-4; filter aids for industrial use (beer, dry cleaning, pharmaceuticals, chems., water, industrial waste); wh. powd.; 5% 150 mesh residue; sp.gr. 2.3; dens. 10 lb/ft³ (dry); pH 10.

Hyglyol S-26. [Nikko Chem. Co. Ltd.] Glycerin/oxybutylene copolymer stearyl ether.

Hygroplex HHG. [Dr. Kurt Richter; Henkel/Cospha] Hexylene glycol, fructose, glucose, sucrose, urea, dextrin, alanine, glutamic acid, aspartic acid, and hexyl nicotinate; natural moisturizing factor in hydrophilic medium for emulsified aq. and hydroalcoholic skin and hair moisturizing cosmetics; lt. yel. liq.; faint char. odor.

Hyladerm®. [Biomatrix; Amerchol] Hyaluronic acid; CAS 9004-61-9; EINECS 232-678-0; cosmetics moisturizer; clear to opalescent visc. liq., low char. odor; pH 5-7.

Hylucare™. [Genzyme Fine Chem.; Lipo] Hyaluronic acid; CAS 9004-61-9; EINECS 232-678-0; high purity, high m.w. cosmetic grade for protection and lubrication of cells, fluid retention and regulation, maintenance of structural integrity of tissues; forms hydrated viscoelastic films on skin; moisturizer imparting smooth, silky texture to skin care prods.; wh. powd. or 1% sol'n.; usage level: 0.01-1%; toxicology: nontoxic; nonsensitizing; nonirritating to skin; ≥ 95% purity.

Hypan® C-100. [Kingston Tech.] DMAPA acrylates/acrylic acid/acrylonitrogens copolymer.

Hypan® QT100. [Kingston Tech.; Lipo] Polyquaternium-31; hydrogel polymer substantive to skin and hair; thickener; carrier for active substances; provides protective coating; primary emulsifier; for cosmetic and personal care prods.; ylsh. powd., 50-200 mesh size, sl. musty odor; visc. > 200,000 cps (0.75% , 0.5 rpm); pH 4.5-5.5 (0.25-1%); toxicology: nontoxic, nonirritating.

Hypan® SA100H. [Kingston Tech.; Lipo] Acrylic acid/ acrylonitrogens copolymer; CAS 61788-40-7; emulsifier and gellant for neutral pH; film-former; able to form thixotropic gels, stable water-dilutable emulsions, conjugates with certain drugs for controlled delivery formulations, continuous oil film on drying; semicryst. polymer.

Hypan® SR150H. [Kingston Tech.; Lipo] Acrylic acid/ acrylonitrogens copolymer; CAS 136505-00-5; thickener and gellant for aq. formulations, esp. highly conc. salt sol'ns., surfactants and drugs; emulsifier of various oils to form stable multiple phase emulsions.

Hypan® SS201. [Kingston Tech.; Lipo] Ammonium acrylates/acrylonitrogens copolymer; CAS 123754-28-9; gellant, emulsifier for cosmetics and related applics.

Hypan® SS500V. [Kingston Tech.] Tromethamine acrylates/ acrylonitrogens copolymer; gellant, emulsifier for cosmetics and related applics.

Hypan® SS500W. [Kingston Tech.] TEA-acrylates/ acrylonitrogens copolymer; gellant, emulsifier for cosmetics and related applics.

Hypan® TC-200. [Kingston Tech.] Sodium tauride acrylates/ acrylic acid/acrylonitrogens copolymer.

Hypericum Oil CLR. [Dr. Kurt Richter] Olive oil, hypericum extract, and tocopherol.

Hy-Phi 1055. [Darling] Oleic acid; CAS 112-80-1; EINECS 204-007-1; surfactant intermediate.

Hy-Phi 1088. [Darling] Oleic acid; CAS 112-80-1; EINECS 204-007-1; surfactant intermediate.

Hy-Phi 1199. [Darling] Stearic acid; CAS 57-11-4; EINECS 200-313-4; surfactant intermediate, emulsifier, emollient.

Hy-Phi 1303. [Darling] Stearic acid; CAS 57-11-4; EINECS 200-313-4; surfactant intermediate, emulsifier, emollient.

Hy-Phi 1401. [Darling] Stearic acid; CAS 57-11-4; EINECS 200-313-4; surfactant intermediate, emulsifier, emollient.

Hy-Phi 2066. [Darling] Oleic acid; CAS 112-80-1; EINECS 204-007-1; surfactant intermediate.

Hy-Phi 2088. [Darling] Oleic acid; CAS 112-80-1; EINECS 204-007-1; surfactant intermediate.

Hy-Phi 2102. [Darling] Oleic acid; CAS 112-80-1; EINECS 204-007-1; surfactant intermediate.

Hy-Phi 4204. [Darling] Tallow acid; CAS 61790-37-2; EINECS 263-129-3; surfactant intermediate.

Hy-Phi 6001. [Darling] Hydrog. tallow acid; CAS 61790-38-3; EINECS 263-130-9; used in bar soaps, cosmetics.

Hypol® 2000. [W.R. Grace/Organics] PU prepolymer derived from TDI; foamable hydrophilic prepolymer offering water activation, high additive loading, controllable flexibility and texture, high water absorbence, low temp. exotherms, inherent flame retardancy; absorbent foam, carrier for functional additives, cosmetic pads, bath sponges, foam toys, air fresheners; yel. to amber liq.; sp.gr. 1.19; visc. 18,500 cps; flash pt. (COC) 435 F; 5% free TDI.

Hypol® 2002. [W.R. Grace/Organics] PU prepolymer; foamable hydrophilic prepolymer for medical, dental, health care, and cosmetic applics. (wound dressings, biocompatible coatings, drug delivery vehicles); produces foams with no extractable TDA, TDI, or other primary aromatic amines; yel. to amber; dens. 1.19 g/ml; visc. 20,000 cps; 95.5% min. act.

Hypol® 3000. [W.R. Grace/Organics] PU prepolymer derived from TDI; foamable hydrophilic prepolymer offering water activation, high additive loading, controllable flexibility and texture, high water absorbence, low temp. exotherms, inherent flame retardancy; can be loaded with flame retardants, reinforcers, aux. blowing agents, fragrances, colorants, cleaners, abrasives, medicaments, and pharmaceutical additives; yel. to amber liq.; sp.gr. 1.15; visc. 20,500 cps; flash pt. (COC) 415 F; 13% free TDI.

Hypol® 4000. [W.R. Grace/Organics] PU prepolymer derived from MDI; foamable hydrophilic prepolymer offering water activation, high purity, high additive loading, improved steam autoclave cycling, hydrolysis resist., thermal/oxidative stability; applics. incl. medical and surgical aids, health and personal care prods.; can produce soft to rigid foams; sp.gr. 1.17; visc. 20,000 cps; flash pt. (COC) > 500 F; 16% free MDI.

Hypol® 5000. [W.R. Grace/Organics] PU prepolymer derived from MDI; foamabile hydrophilic prepolymer offering water activation, high purity, high additive loading, improved steam autoclave cycling, hydrolysis resist., thermal/oxidative stability; applics. incl. medical and surgical aids, health and personal care prods.; can produce soft to rigid foams; sp.gr. 1.17; visc. 18,000 cps; flash pt. (COC) 464 F; 20% free MDI.

Hy-SES. [Vitamins, Inc.] Sesame oil; CAS 8008-74-0; EINECS 232-370-6; emollient oil.

Hystar® 3375. [Lonza] Hydrog. starch hydrolysate; CAS 68425-17-2; humectant, bodying agent, moisture control agent for toothpaste, cosmetics, sugarless confections, controlled moisture foods and industrial applics. where sweet taste and low hygroscopicity are required; Kosher certification; water-wh. clear liq.; sp.gr. 1.32; visc. 1500 cps (40 C); pH neutral; 75% act.

Hystar® 4075. [Lonza] Hydrog. starch hydrolysate; CAS 68425-17-2; humectant, bodying agent, moisture control agent for toothpaste, cosmetics, sugarless confections, controlled moisture foods and industrial applics. where sweet taste and low hygroscopicity are required; Kosher certification; water-wh. clear liq.; sp.gr. 1.33; visc. 1000 cps (40 C); pH neutral; 75% act.

Hystar® 5875. [Lonza] Hydrog. starch hydrolysate; CAS 68425-17-2; humectant, bodying agent, moisture control agent for toothpaste, cosmetics, sugarless confections, controlled moisture foods and industrial applics. where texture and taste are important; water-wh. clear liq.; sp.gr. 1.35; visc. 500 cps (40 C); pH neutral; 75% act.

Hystar® 6075. [Lonza] Hydrog. starch hydrolysate; CAS 68425-17-2; humectant, bodying agent, moisture control agent for toothpaste, cosmetics, sugarless confections, controlled moisture foods and industrial applics. where very low hygroscopicity is required; Kosher certification; water-wh. clear liq., bland taste; sp.gr. 1.35; visc. 2000 cps (40 C); pH neutral; 75% act.

Hystar® 7000. [Lonza] Hydrog. starch hydrolysate; CAS 68425-17-2; humectant, bodying agent, moisture control agent for cosmetics, consumer prods., and industrial applics.; plasticizer, softener, and lubricant; water-wh. clear liq.; sp.gr. 1.32; visc. 385 cps; ref. index 1.460-1.468; pH neutral; 70% act.

Hystar® CG. [Lonza] Hydrog. starch hydrolysate; CAS 68425-17-2; lubricant, humectant for toiletries, dentifrices; water-wh. clear liq.; sp.gr. 1.30; visc. 380 cps; ref. index 1.46; pH neutral; 70% act.

Hystar® HM-75. [Lonza] Hydrog. starch hydrolysate; CAS 68425-17-2; humectant, bodying agent, moisture control agent for toothpaste, cosmetics, sugarless confections, controlled moisture foods and industrial applics. where taste and texture is important; Kosher certification; water-wh. clear liq.; sp.gr. 1.48; visc. 500 cps (40 C); pH neutral; 75% act.

Hystar® TPF. [Lonza] Hydrog. starch hydrolysate; CAS 68425-17-2; lubricant; maintains optimal moisture control in industrial, pet food, tobacco, teat dip, oral hygiene prods.; Kosher certification; water-wh. clear liq.; sp.gr. 1.30; visc. 380 cps; pH neutral; 75% act. in water.

Hystrene® 1835. [Witco/H-I-P] Mixt. tallow/coconut acid (CTFA); CAS 67701-05-7; chemical intermediate, emulsifier; used for personal care prods., soaps, waxes, textile aux., pharmaceuticals; paste; solid. pt. 40 C max.; acid no. 214-222; iodine no. 36-42; sapon. no. 211-220.

Hystrene® 3022. [Witco/H-I-P] Hydrog. menhaden acid; chemical intermediate, emulsifier; used for personal care prods., waxes, greases, textile aux., pharmaceuticals; solid; solid. pt. 50-54 C; acid no. 193-202; iodine no. 5; sapon. no. 193-202; 100% conc.

Hystrene® 4516. [Witco/H-I-P] Stearic acid; CAS 57-11-4; EINECS 200-313-4; lubricant, textile aux., emulsifier, plasticizer, intermediate, used in cosmetics, shampoos, pharmaceuticals; solid; acid no. 203-209; iodine no. 1 max.; sapon. no. 204-210; 100% conc.

Hystrene® 5012. [Witco/H-I-P] Hydrog. stripped coconut acid; CAS 68938-15-8; chemical intermediate, emulsifier; used for personal care prods., soaps, lubricants, waxes, textile aux., pharmaceuticals; liq.; solid. pt. 24–33 C; acid no. 250-266; iodine no. 2 max.; sapon. no. 250-266; 100% conc.

Hystrene® 5016 NF. [Witco/H-I-P] Stearic acid NF, triple pressed; CAS 57-11-4; EINECS 200-313-4; stabilizer, lubricant, textile aux., emulsifier, plasticizer, intermediate, used in cosmetics, shampoos, pharmaceuticals; solid; acid no. 206-210; iodine no. 0.5 max.; sapon. no. 206-211; 100% conc.

Hystrene® 7016. [Witco/H-I-P] Palmitic acid; CAS 57-10-3; EINECS 200-312-9; surfactant intermediate; soap and cosmetic formulations.

Hystrene® 7022. [Witco/H-I-P] Behenic fatty acid; CAS 112-85-6; EINECS 204-010-8; lubricant, textile aux., emulsifier, plasticizer, intermediate, used in cosmetics, shampoos, pharmaceuticals; solid; acid no. 170-180; iodine no. 3.5; sapon. no. 170-181; 100% conc.

Hystrene® 9016. [Witco/H-I-P] Palmitic acid (90%); CAS 57-10-3; EINECS 200-312-9; lubricant, textile aux., emulsifier, plasticizer, intermediate, used in cosmetics, shampoos, pharmaceuticals; solid; acid no. 216-220; iodine no. 0.5 max.; sapon. no. 216-221; 100% conc.

Hystrene® 9022. [Witco/H-I-P] Behenic acid (90%); CAS 112-85-6; EINECS 204-010-8; lubricant, textile aux., emulsifier, plasticizer, intermediate, used in cosmetics, shampoos, pharmaceuticals; solid; acid no. 165-175; iodine no. 3; sapon. no. 165-176; 100% conc.

Hystrene® 9512. [Witco/H-I-P] Lauric acid (95%); CAS 143-07-7; EINECS 205-582-1; lubricant, textile aux., emulsifier, plasticizer, intermediate, used in cosmetics, shampoos, pharmaceuticals; solid; acid no. 276-281; iodine no. 0.5 max.; sapon. no. 276-282; 100% conc.

Hystrene® 9718 NF. [Witco/H-I-P] Stearic acid NF(92%); CAS 57-11-4; EINECS 200-313-4; lubricant, textile aux., emulsifier, plasticizer, intermediate, used in cosmetics, shampoos, pharmaceuticals; solid; acid no. 196-201; iodine no. 0.8 max.; sapon. no. 196-202; 100% conc.

Ialuramina. [Vevy] Hydrolyzed glycosaminoglycans; moisturizer.

Ialuramina 10. [Vevy] Hydrolyzed glycosaminoglycans; moisturizer.

Ibbal. [Mitsubishi Gas] p-Isobutylbenzaldehyde; intermediate for pharmaceuticals; fragrance; colorless liq., aromatic odor; sol. in ethanol, ether, toluene; insol. in water; m.w. 162.2; sp.gr. 0.960; b.p. 240 C; acid no. 0.3; flash pt. (COC) 122 C; toxicology: LD50 (oral, rat) 1000-5000 mg/kg; eye and skin irritant; 98.5% purity.

Ibulate. [Lanaetex Prods.] Isobutyl stearate; CAS 646-13-9; EINECS 211-466-1; cosmetic ingred.

Ichou Liq. [Ichimaru Pharcos] Water, butylene glycol, and ginkgo extract.

Ichtyocollagene. [Sederma] Water, propylene glycol, and hydrolyzed gadidae protein; filmogenic and moisturizing; marine source of collagen for hair, skin, face, and body care prods.; sl. opalescent liq., char. odor; sp.gr. 1.00-1.02; ref. index 1.34-1.35; pH 7.0-8.5; usage level: 2-6%.

Ichtyoelastin. [Sederma] Hydrolyzed elastin; CAS 100085-10-7; moisturizing and firming agent for face, body, and hair care prods.; clear liq., char. odor; sp.gr. 1.02-1.04; ref. index 1.35-1.36; pH 5.5-7.0; usage level: 3-8%.

Idrolizzato Della Seta. [Variati] Hydrolyzed silk; CAS 96690-41-4; cosmetic protein.

Idroramnosan. [Vevy] Hydroxyethylcellulose; CAS 9004-62-0; thickener.

Igepal® CA-630. [Rhone-Poulenc Surf. & Spec.] Octoxynol-9; CAS 9002-93-1; nonionic; detergent, wetting agent, emulsifier for personal care prods., metal processing, emulsion cleaners, agric. formulations; as wetting agent with min. acids and corrosion inhibitors; FDA, EPA compliance; pale yel. liq.; aromatic odor; sol. in xylene, butyl Cellosolve, perchloroethylene, ethanol, water; sp.gr. 1.06; visc. 230–260 cps; HLB 13.0; cloud pt. 63-67 C (1% aq.); flash pt. > 200 F (PMCC); pour pt. 45 ± 2 F; surf. tens. 31 dynes/cm (0.01%); 100% act.

Igepal® CO-430. [Rhone-Poulenc Surf. & Spec.] Nonoxynol-4; CAS 9016-45-9; nonionic; coemulsifier, plasticizer, stabilizer, antistat, detergent, dispersant; for plastics, latex emulsions, petrol. oils, agric., personal care prods.; intermediate for anionic surfactants; biodeg.; FDA, EPA compliance; pale yel. liq., aromatic odor; sol. in kerosene, Stod., naphtha, xylene, butyl Cellosolve, perchloroethylene, ethanol; sp.gr. 1.02; visc. 160-260 cps; solid. pt. -21 F; HLB 8.8; flash pt. > 200 F (PMCC); pour pt. −16 ± 2 F; toxicology: severe eye irritant; LD50 (oral, rat) 7.4 g/kg; 100% act.

Igepal® CO-630 Special. [Rhone-Poulenc Surf. & Spec.] Nonoxynol-9 USP-NF; CAS 9016-45-9; nonionic; GMP grade; used as spermicide, microbicide; detergent, emulsifier, solubilizer; liq.; HLB 13.0; 100% act.

Igepal® DM-970 FLK. [Rhone-Poulenc Surf. & Spec.] Nonyl nonoxynol-150; CAS 9014-93-1; nonionic; detergent, dispersant, wetter, stabilizer for laundry, household, textile, hard-surface detergents, cosmetics, insecticides, paper, petrol., paints; EPA compliance; wh. flakes; sol. in water, aromatic solv., methanol, ethanol; sp.gr. 1.05 (80 C); HLB 19; cloud pt. > 100 C (1%); 100% act.

Igepal® NP-4. [Rhone-Poulenc Surf. & Spec.] Nonoxynol-4; CAS 9016-45-9; nonionic; lipophilic coemulsifier for min. oil and solv. emulsions; intermediate for ethoxy sulfates; detergent, emulsifier, and solubilizer for cosmetics.; liq.; HLB 8.8; 100% conc.; formerly Rhodiasurf NP-4.

Igepal® NP-9. [Rhone-Poulenc Surf. & Spec.] Nonoxynol-9; CAS 9016-45-9; nonionic; emulsifier, wetting agent, dispersant for textile scouring, dyeing and finishing, household/industrial cleaners, alkaline degreasers, acid pickling in metalworking; emulsifier/stabilizer for emulsion polymerization; pitch dispersant in pulp prod.; detergent, emulsifier, and solubilizer for cosmetic prods.; liq.; HLB 13.0; 100% conc.; formerly Rhodiasurf NP-9.

Igepal® OP-9. [Rhone-Poulenc Surf. & Spec.] Octoxynol-9; CAS 9002-93-1; nonionic; detergent, emulsifier, and solubilizer for cosmetics; 100% conc.

Imexine BD. [Chimex] Hydroxyanthraquinoneaminopropyl methyl morpholinium methosulfate; CAS 38866-20-5; EINECS 254-161-9.

Imexine FB. [Chimex] N-Methyl-3-nitro-p-phenylenediamine; CAS 2973-21-9; EINECS 221-014-5.

Imexine FD. [Chimex] N,N´-Dimethyl-N-hydroxyethyl-3-nitro-p-phenylenediamine; CAS 10228-03-2; EINECS 233-549-1.

Imexine FE. [Chimex] 2-Nitro-N-hydroxyethyl-p-anisidine; CAS 57524-53-5.

Imexine FH. [Chimex] 3-Nitro-p-hydroxyethylaminophenol; CAS 65235-31-6; EINECS 265-648-0.

Imexine FM. [Chimex] 2-Hydroxyethylamino-t-nitroanisole; CAS 66095-81-6; EINECS 266-138-0.

Imexine FN. [Chimex] 4-Amino-3-nitrophenol; CAS 610-81-1; EINECS 210-236-8.

Imexine FO. [Chimex] 2-Amino-3-nitrophenol; CAS 603-85-0; EINECS 210-060-1.

Imexine FP. [Chimex] 6-Nitro-o-toluidine; CAS 570-24-1; EINECS 209-329-6.

Imexine FR. [Chimex] 3-Methylamino-4-nitrophenoxyethanol.

Imexine FT. [Chimex] 2-Nitro-5-glyceryl methylaniline; CAS 80062-31-3; EINECS 279-383-3.

Imexine OAG. [Chimex] 2-Methyl-5-hydroxyethylaminophenol.

Imexine OAH. [Chimex] N-Methoxyethyl-p-phenylenediamine HCl.

Imexine OAJ. [Chimex] 2,4-Diaminophenoxyethanol HCl; CAS 66422-95-5; EINECS 266-357-1.

Imexine OAM. [Chimex] 1,2,4-Trihydroxybenzene; CAS 533-73-3; EINECS 208-575-1.

Imexine OAY. [Chimex] Dihydroxyindole; CAS 3131-52-0.

Imexine OG. [Chimex] Lawsone.

Imwitor® 191. [Hüls Am.; Hüls AG] Glyceryl stearate; CAS 31566-31-1; 68308-54-3; nonionic; coemulsifier, dispersant for personal care prods.; emulsifier in o/w and w/o emulsions; lubricants and binders used in the pharmaceutical industry; suspending agent, stabilizer, thickener; food emulsifier; ylsh. powd.; sol. in oils, molten fats, acetone, ether; m.p. 66-71 C; solid. pt. 63–68 C; HLB 4.4; acid no. 3 max.; iodine no. 2 max.; sapon. no. 155–170; 90% monoglycerides.

Imwitor® 308. [Hüls Am.] Glyceryl caprylate; CAS 26402-26-6; EINECS 247-668-1; nonionic; solubilizer for pharmaceutical drugs; carrier/vehicle for drugs in capsules; coemulsifier for lipophilic materials; surfactant and bacteriostatic props.; wh. cryst. solid, char. odor, bitter taste; sol. in ethanol, methylene chloride, acetone, ether, heptane; misc. with oils and fats; m.p. 30-34 C; HLB 6.0; acid no. 3 max.; iodine no. 1 max.; sapon. no. 245-265; 80% monoglycerides.

Imwitor® 310. [Hüls Am.; Hüls AG] Glyceryl caprate; CAS 26402-22-2; EINECS 247-667-6; solubilizer for pharmaceutical drugs; carrier/vehicle for drugs in capsules; coemulsifier for lipophilic materials; surfactant and bacteriostatic props.; wh. cryst. solid; m.p. 40-44 C; HLB 5.0; acid no. 2 max.; iodine no. 1 max.; sapon. no. 210-230; 90% min. monoglycerides.

Imwitor® 312. [Hüls Am.; Hüls AG] Glyceryl laurate; CAS 142-18-7; EINECS 205-526-6; nonionic; coemulsifier for o/w emulsions; solubilizer, carrier for lipophilic drugs; superfatting agent for bath prods.; bacteriostatic effect; wh. cryst. solid; sol. in water/ethanol (50/50), acetone, ether, heptane; m.p. 56-60 C; HLB 4.0; acid no. 3 max.; iodine no. 2 max.; sapon. no. 195-205; 90% min. monoglycerides.

Imwitor® 370. [Hüls Am.; Hüls AG] Glyceryl stearate citrate; CAS 91744-38-6; anionic; food emulsifier; o/w emulsifier for highly polar oils, fats and liq. wax esters in cosmetics; ylsh. flakes; m.p. 59-63 C; HLB 10-12; acid no. 10-25; iodine no. 3 max.; sapon. no. 240-260; 100% conc.

Imwitor® 375. [Hüls Am.; Hüls AG] Glyceryl citrate/lactate/linoleate/oleate; nonionic; o/w emulsifier for highly polar oils and fats; for oil baths, cream baths; ylsh. highly visc. liq.; HLB 11.0; acid no. 5-15; iodine no. 90; sapon. no. 230-250; 10-20% monoglcyerides.

Imwitor® 408. [Hüls Am.] Propylene glycol caprylate; CAS 31565-12-5; coemulsifier, solubilizer, absorp. promoter for cosmetics, topical and rectal pharmaceuticals; solvent for lipophilic drugs; sl. yel. liq.; acid no. 2 max.; iodine no. 1 max.; sapon. no. 250-275; 50% monoglycerides.

Imwitor® 412. [Hüls Am.] Propylene glycol laurate; CAS 142-55-2; EINECS 205-542-3; coemulsifier, solubilizer, absorp. promoter for cosmetics, topical and rectal pharmaceuticals; solv. for lipophilic drugs; sl. yel. solid; acid no. 2 max.; iodine no. 1 max.; sapon. no. 220-235; 50% monoglycerides.

Imwitor® 440. [Hüls Am.] Natural oil monodiglyceride; nonionic; emulsifier for cosmetics and food industries; powd.; HLB 3.7; 100% conc.

Imwitor® 708. [Hüls Am.] Diglyceryl caprylate; solubilizer, absorp. promoter for cosmetics; yel. visc. liq.; acid no. 1 max.; iodine no. 0.5 max.; sapon. no. 180-195; 35% min. monoglycerides.

Imwitor® 742. [Hüls Am.] Caprylic/capric glycerides; CAS 26402-26-6; nonionic; plasticizer for hard fats; solv. for lipophilic ingreds., active substances; cosmetic emollient; coemulsifier, solubilizer, carrier for lipophilic drugs; dispersant, absorp. promoter; bacteriostatic effect; German pharmacopoeia compliance; wh-ylsh. cryst. solid, sl. coconut odor, fatty bitter taste; sol. in ethanol, actone, ether, heptane, hexane; misc. with oils and fats;

m.p. 25 C; HLB 3-4; acid no. 2 max.; iodine no. 1 max.; sapon. no. 250-280; toxicology: LD50 (oral, rat) > 5 g/kg; moderate skin irritant (undiluted); 45% min. monoglycerides.

Imwitor® 780 K. [Hüls Am.; Hüls AG] Isostearyl diglyceryl succinate; CAS 66085-00-5; nonionic; w/o emulsifier for highly polar oils and fats, cosmetic and pharmaceutical preparations; produces very heat-stable emulsions with Miglyol Gel; yel., med. visc. liq.; slight char. odor; sol. in chloroform, benzene, ethanol, oils; insol. in water; m.w. 580; sp.gr. 0.96–0.98; visc. 700–900 cps; HLB 3.7; acid no. 3 max.; iodine no. 10 max.; sapon. no. 240–260; usage level: 3-5%; toxicology: LD50 (oral, rat) > 5 g/kg (nontoxic); nonirritating to skin and eyes; 100% conc.

Imwitor® 900. [Hüls Am.; Hüls AG] Glyceryl stearate; nonionic; coemulsifier, consistency regulator, and dispersant for personal care prods.; emulsifier in o/w and w/o emulsions; lubricants and binders used in the pharmaceutical industry; suspending agent, stabilizer, thickener; ylsh. powd.; sol. in fats, oils, waxes; m.p. 56–61 C; HLB 3.0; acid no. 3 max.; iodine no. 3 max.; sapon. no. 160–175; 100% conc., 40–50% 1-monoglyceride.

Imwitor® 908. [Hüls Am.; Hüls AG] Glyceryl caprylate; CAS 26402-26-6; EINECS 247-668-1; nonionic; coemulsifier for o/w emulsions, lipophilic materials; solv., solubilizer for active substances, surfactant, absorp. promoter; carrier of drugs; bacteriostatic effect; cosmetics ingred.; ylsh. oily liq., char. coconut odor, fatty sl. bitter taste; sol. in ether, n-hexane, alcohol; disp. in water; m.p. 20-25 C; HLB 3.0; acid no. 2 max.; iodine no. 1 max.; sapon. no. 250-275; 45% min. monoglycerides.

Imwitor® 910. [Hüls Am.; Hüls AG] Glyceryl caprate; CAS 26402-22-2; EINECS 247-667-6; nonionic; food emulsifier; coemulsifier for o/w emulsions, lipophilic materials in cosmetics; solubilizer for actives, surfactant, absorp. promoter; promotes penetration; bacteriostatic effect; wh. powd.; m.p. 38-41 C; HLB 3.0; acid no. 2 max.; iodine no. 1 max.; sapon. no. 240-260; 40% min. monoglycerides.

Imwitor® 914. [Hüls Am.; Hüls AG] Glyceryl myristate; CAS 589-68-4; nonionic; coemulsifier for o/w emulsions; solubilizer, carrier for lipophilic drugs; dispersant, consistency regulator in creams, lotions, anhyd. formulations; ylsh. cryst. mass which liquefies at 60 C to a brn.-ylsh. clear oily liq., nearly tasteless and odorless; sol. in acetone, ether, ethanol, n-hexane, chloroform; m.p. 60 C; acid no. 2 max.; iodine no. 1 max.; sapon. no. 180-200; 45-55% 1-monoglycerides.

Imwitor® 928. [Hüls AG] Glyceryl cocoate; CAS 61789-05-7; EINECS 263-027-9; surfactant for pharmaceutical, cosmetic and nutritional fields; as emulsifier, solubilizer, dispersion aid, plasticizer, lubricant, consistency regulator, skin and mucous membrane protectant, refatting agent, penetrant, carrier, adsorp. promoter; soft wh. substance; sol. in acetone, ether, water/ethanol; m.p. 33-37 C; acid no. 2 max.; iodine no. 3 max.; sapon. no. 200-220.

Imwitor® 940. [Hüls Am.] Palm oil glycerides; nonionic; coemulsifier, consistency regulator, stabilizer for cosmetic creams; dispersant for clay systems; sec. emulsifier and stabilizer for asphalt emulsions; binder, lubricant; ylsh. flakes, powd., sl. fatty odor; sol. in fats, oils, waxes; partly sol. in chloroform, benzene, ether; m.p. 54-60 C; HLB 3.0; acid no. 3 max.; iodine no. 3 max.; sapon. no. 165-180; 40-50% 1-monoglyceride.

Imwitor® 940 K. [Hüls Am.] Glyceryl stearate/palmitate Ph. Eur.; nonionic; coemulsifier, dispersant for personal care prods.; emulsifier in o/w and w/o emulsions; lubricants and binders used in the pharmaceutical industry; suspending agent, stabilizer, thickener; food emulsifier; Gardner 4 max. powd.; m.p. 53–57 C; solid. pt. 54–60; sapon. no. 165–178; 42–48% 1-monoglyceride.

Imwitor® 945. [Hüls Am.; Hüls AG] Glyceryl palmitate/stearate; nonionic; stabilizer for cosmetics; powd.; HLB 3.8; 100 conc.

Imwitor® 960. [Hüls Am.; Hüls AG] Glyceryl stearate SE; anionic; emulsion base for cosmetics; suspending agent in creams, lotions, emulsions, cosmetics; imparts pleasant skin feel; ylsh. flakes; sol. in fats, oils, waxes; m.p. 56–61 C; HLB 12.0; acid no. 6 max.; iodine no. 3 max.; sapon. no. 150-175; 30–40% 1-monoglyceride.

Imwitor® 960 K. [Hüls Am.; Hüls AG] Glyceryl stearate SE; anionic; emulsifier and ointment base for pharmaceutical and cosmetic creams of the o/w type; ylsh. flakes; typical odor; sol. in all fats, oils, waxes, in chloroform, benzene, ether, ethanol; m.p. 56–61 C; HLB 12.0; acid no. 6 max.; iodine no. 3 max.; sapon. no. 150-175; 30% min. monoglycerides; 100% conc.

Imwitor® 965. [Hüls Am.; Hüls AG] Palm oil glycerides and potassium stearate; anionic; o/w emulsifier, cream base, suspending agent in creams, lotions, emulsions, cosmetics, pharmaceuticals; wh. flakes, powd., faint fatty odor; sol. in fats, oils, waxes; disp. in hot water; m.p. 56-61 C; HLB 13.0; acid no. 6 max.; iodine no. 3 max.; sapon. no. 155-175; toxicology: nontoxic; 30% min. monoglycerides, 100% conc.

Imwitor® 988. [Hüls AG] Glyceryl caprylate; CAS 26402-26-6; EINECS 247-668-1; surfactant for pharmaceutical, cosmetic and nutritional fields; as emulsifier, solubilizer, dispersion aid, plasticizer, lubricant, consistency regulator, skin and mucous membrane protectant, refatting agent, penetrant, carrier, adsorp. promoter; almost colorless liq./semisolid; sol. in water/ethanol (25/75), acetone, ether, heptane; acid no. 2 max.; iodine no. 1 max.; sapon. no. 275-300.

Incense EA. [Alban Muller] Olibanum; CAS 8050-07-5; EINECS 232-474-1; cosmetic gum.

Incense H. [Alban Muller] Olibanum; CAS 8050-07-5; EINECS 232-474-1; cosmetic gum.

Incense HS. [Alban Muller] Propylene glycol and olibanum.

Incense LS. [Alban Muller] Sunflower seed oil and olibanum.

Incrocas 30. [Croda Inc.] PEG-30 castor oil; CAS 61791-12-6; nonionic; emulsifier, solubilizer, emollient, superfatting agent, lubricant for personal care prods., detergents, metalworking fluids, insecticides, herbicides, household prods.; lubricant, antistat, softener, dye leveling agent for textiles; also lime soap dispersant in alkaline scouring systems; pale yel. liq.; sol. in water, ethanol, oleyl alcohol, naphtha, MEK, oleic acid, trichloroethylene; HLB 11.7; cloud pt. 35–40 C (1% in 10% brine); sapon. no. 72–82; pH 6.0–7.5 (3% aq.); surf. tens. 41.5 dynes/cm (0.1% DW); usage level: 0.5-5%; 100% act.

Incrocas 40. [Croda Inc.] PEG-40 castor oil; CAS 61791-12-6; nonionic; emulsifier, solubilizer, emollient, superfatting agent, lubricant for personal care prods., detergents, metalworking fluids, insecticides, herbicides, household prods.; lubricant, antistat, softener, dye leveling agent for textiles; pale yel. liq.; sol. @ 10% see Incrocas 30; HLB 13.0; cloud pt. 50 C (1% in 10% brine); sapon. no. 60–65; pH 6.0–7.5 (3% aq.); surf. tens. 40.90 dynes/cm (0.1% DW); usage level: 0.5-5%; 100% act.

Incrodet TD7-C. [Croda Inc.] Trideceth-7 carboxylic acid; anionic; mild surfactant for shampoos, bath gels, cleansers; neutralizer for trace caustic or thioglycolate residues present after hair permanents or relaxers; in neutralizing shampoos which follow ethnic hair straighteners; lime soap dispersant; emulsifier; stable at low and high pH; pale yel. clear liq.; sol. in water/alcohol, ethanol, propylene glycol; disp. in water, glycerin; acid no. 45-52; cloud pt. 67-80 C; usage level: 1-12%; 98% act.

Incromate CDP. [Croda Inc.] Cocamidopropyl dimethylamine propionate; CAS 68425-43-4; cationic; moderate foaming conditioner for clear rinses and shampoos; good detangling; Gardner 4 max. liq.; pH 6.0–7.0; usage level: 1-10%; 40% act.

Incromate ISML. [Croda Inc.] Isostearamidopropyl morpholine lactate; cationic; substantive surfactant, conditioner, visc. builder for personal care prods. and cationic emulsions; improves slip, wet comb, and manageability in hair, feel in hand creams and lotions; Gardner 6 max. liq.; sol. in water; pH 4–5 (5%); usage level: 1-10%; 25% min. act.

Incromate OLL. [Croda Inc.] Olivamidopropyl dimethylamine lactate; CAS 124046-31-7; cationic; conditioner and foamer for hair and skin care prods.; amber visc. liq.; usage level: 0.5-5%; 75% act.

Incromate SDL. [Croda Inc.; Croda Surf. Ltd.] Stearamidopropyl dimethylamine lactate; CAS 55819-53-9; EINECS 259-837-7; cationic; visc. builder, opacifier, softener for hair shampoos, conditioners, fabrics; emulsifier for hand creams, cleansers, lotions; raw material; Gardner 3 max. slurry; pH 4–5 (10%); usage level: 1-5%; 70% min. act.

Incromate WGL. [Croda Inc.] Wheat germamidopropyl dimethylamine lactate; CAS 124046-40-8; cationic; conditioner with exc. slip, wet comb, and dry feel; amber visc. liq.; sol. in alcohol; usage level: 0.5-5%; 75% act.

Incromectant AMEA-70. [Croda Inc.] Acetamide MEA; CAS 142-26-7; EINECS 205-530-8; solv., humectant for cosmetics; clarifying agent for shampoos; conditioner for creme rinses; sol'n.; sp.gr. 1.07–1.17; dens. 9.3 lb/gal; pH 6.0–8.5; usage level: 0.5-15%; 70% min. act.

Incromectant AMEA-100. [Croda Inc.; Croda Surf. Ltd.] Acetamide MEA; CAS 142-26-7; EINECS 205-530-8; clarifying detangling agent for shampoos, conditioners, cream rinses; humectant in creams and lotions; liq.; usage level: 0.5-15%; 100% act.

Incromectant AQ. [Croda Inc.] Acetamidopropyl trimonium chloride; cationic; antistat for shampoos and conditioners; humectant; plasticizer for hair conditioning/setting polymers; liq.; usage level: 0.5-3%; 75% act.

Incromectant LAMEA. [Croda Inc.] Acetamide MEA and lactamide MEA; humectant, moisturizing agent for hair and skin care prods.; Gardner 4 max. liq.; acid no. 15 max.; pH 5–8 (10%); usage level: 0.5-15%; 100% act.

Incromectant LMEA. [Croda Inc.; Croda Surf. Ltd.] Lactamide MEA; CAS 5422-34-4; EINECS 226-546-1; clarifying detangling agent for shampoos, conditioners, and cream rinses; humectant in creams and lotions; liq.; usage level: 0.5-15%; 100% act.

Incromectant LQ. [Croda Inc.] Lactamidopropyl trimonium chloride; cationic; antistat for shampoos and conditioners; humectant; plasticizer for hair conditioning/setting polymers; liq.; usage level: 0.5-35; 75% act.

Incromide ALD. [Croda Inc.] Almondamide DEA (1:1); nonionic; conditioner, visc. builder, foam stabilizer; for shampoos, bubble baths, soaps, bath prods.; clear liq.; usage level: 1-10%; 100% conc.

Incromide BAD. [Croda Inc.] Babassuamide DEA (1:1); nonionic; visc. builder, foam stabilizer, emulsifier; for shampoos, bubble baths, soaps, bath prods.; clear liq.; usage level: 1-10%; 100% conc.

Incromide CA. [Croda Inc.] Cocamide DEA; CAS 61791-31-9; EINECS 263-163-9; nonionic; surfactant, foam stabilizer, emulsifier and thickener used in household, cosmetic, and industrial formulations; clear liq.; usage level: 1-10%; 100% act.

Incromide CAC. [Croda Inc.] 1:1 Cocamide DEA and cocoyl sarcosinate; anionic; low irritation foamer, clarifying agent for clear soap and shampoo bar preps.; Gardner 4 max. clear liq., bland odor; water-sol.; pH 8.6–9.2 (3%); usage level: 1-10%; 100% conc.

Incromide CME. [Croda Inc.] Cocamide MEA; CAS 68140-

00-1; EINECS 268-770-2; cosmetic surfactant.

Incromide CPM. [Croda Inc.] Cocamidopropyl morpholine.

Incromide L90. [Croda Inc.] Lauramide DEA; CAS 120-40-1; EINECS 204-393-1; nonionic; foam stabilizer, thickener, detergent, and foaming agent in household, industrial and institutional cleaning compds., car washes, rug and upholstery cleaners, and personal care prods.; Gardner 2 max. solid; mild fatty odor; sol. in alcohol, chlorinated and aromatic hydrocarbons; disp. in water; usage level: 1-10%; 100% act.

Incromide LA. [Croda Inc.] Linoleamide DEA; CAS 56863-02-6; EINECS 260-410-2; nonionic; superfatting agent and thickener for personal care and household prods.; useful in increasing visc. of various sulfate and ether sulfate dilutions; conditioner and lubricant; Gardner 5 max. clear liq.; bland odor; usage level: 1-10%; 100% act.

Incromide LI. [Croda Inc.] Lauramide MIPA; CAS 142-54-1; EINECS 205-541-8; foam stabilizer for cosmetics.

Incromide LL. [Croda Inc.] Lauramide DEA; CAS 120-40-1; EINECS 204-393-1; personal care surfactant.

Incromide LLA. [Croda Inc.] Lauramide DEA and linoleamide DEA.

Incromide LMI. [Croda Inc.] Lauramide MIPA; CAS 142-54-1; EINECS 205-541-8; foam stabilizer for cosmetics.

Incromide LR. [Croda Inc.] Lauramide DEA; CAS 120-40-1; EINECS 204-393-1; nonionic; thickener, foam stabilizer used in personal care prods., dishwash detergents and industrial cleaners; Gardner 5 max. liq.; bland odor; usage level: 1-10%; 100% act.

Incromide OLD. [Croda Inc.] Olivamide DEA (1:1); nonionic; visc. builder, foam stabilizer; for shampoos, bubble baths, soaps, bath prods.; clear liq.; usage level: 0.5-10%; 100% conc.

Incromide OPM. [Croda Inc.] Oleamide MEA; CAS 111-58-0; EINECS 203-884-8; foam stabilizer, thickener.

Incromide SED. [Croda Inc.] Sesamide DEA (1:1); CAS 124046-35-1; nonionic; visc. builder and foam stabilizer; for shampoos, bubble baths, soaps, bath prods.; clear liq.; usage level: 0.5-5%; 100% conc.

Incromide SM. [Croda Surf. Ltd.] Stearamide MEA; CAS 111-57-9; EINECS 203-883-2; personal care surfactant, thickener, pearlescent.

Incromide UM. [Croda Inc.] Undecylenamide MEA; CAS 20545-92-0; EINECS 243-870-9; personal care surfactant.

Incromide WGD. [Croda Inc.] Wheat germamide DEA (1:1); CAS 124046-39-5; nonionic; visc. builder and foam stabilizer; for shampoos, bubble baths, soaps, bath prods.; clear liq.; usage level: 1-10%; 100% conc.

Incromine ALB. [Croda Inc.] Almondamidopropyl dimethylamine.

Incromine AVB-CG. [Croda Inc.] Avocadamidopropyl dimethylamine.

Incromine BAB. [Croda Inc.] Babassuamidopropyl dimethylamine.

Incromine BB. [Croda Inc.] Behenamidopropyl dimethylamine; CAS 60270-33-9; EINECS 262-134-8; nonionic/cationic; emollient conditioner, lubricant, visc. builder, and moisturizer for hair care prods.; intermediate for hair conditioning agent; yel. flakes; sol. in alcohol; m.w. 420-450; m.p. 70-72; usage level: 1-5%; 100% act.

Incromine Mink B. [Croda Inc.] Minkamidopropyl dimethylamine; CAS 68953-11-7; EINECS 273-187-1; superfatting agent for cosmetics.

Incromine OLB. [Croda Inc.] Olivamidopropyl dimethylamine.

Incromine OPM. [Croda Inc.] Oleamidopropyl dimethylamine; CAS 109-28-4; EINECS 203-661-5; emollient, emulsifier.

Incromine SB. [Croda Inc.] Stearamidopropyl dimethylamine; CAS 7651-02-7; EINECS 231-609-1; nonionic/cationic; visc. builder, conditioner for hair care prods.; intermediate for hair conditioning agent for shampoo rinses; cream waxy flakes; sol. in alcohol; faint char. odor; m.p. 63 C; usage level: 1-5%; 100% act.

Incromine SEB. [Croda Inc.] Sesamidopropyl dimethylamine.

Incromine Oxide B. [Croda Inc.; Croda Surf. Ltd.] Behenamine oxide; CAS 26483-35-2; EINECS 247-730-8; nonionic; surfactant, lubricant, emollient for creams and lotions; emulsifier, foam booster/stabilizer, wetting agent.

Incromine Oxide B-30P. [Croda Inc.; Croda Surf. Ltd.] Behenamine oxide; CAS 26483-35-2; EINECS 247-730-8; nonionic; softener and conditioner for hair care prods.; visc. builder, emulsifier, lubricant, wetting, and foam stabilizer used in personal care prods.; wh. paste; pH 6.5–8.0 (3%); usage level: 0.5-105; 29–31% act.

Incromine Oxide B50. [Croda Inc.; Croda Surf. Ltd.] Behenamine oxide; CAS 26483-35-2; EINECS 247-730-8; nonionic; surfactant, lubricant, emollient for creams and lotions.

Incromine Oxide BA. [Croda Inc.] Babassuamidopropylamine oxide; nonionic; foamer, foam stabilizer; for hair care prods.; facial cleaners; pale yel. liq.; usage level: 0.5-10%; 30% act.

Incromine Oxide C. [Croda Inc.; Croda Surf. Ltd.] Cocamidopropylamine oxide, aq. sol'n.; CAS 68155-09-9; EINECS 268-938-5; nonionic; emulsifier, visc. builder, foam booster/stabilizer, wetting agent, conditioner used in personal care prods.; lt. straw liq.; pH 6.5–7.5 (5%); usage level: 0.5-20%; 29.5–31.5% act.

Incromine Oxide C-35. [Croda Surf. Ltd.] Cocamidopropylamine oxide; CAS 68155-09-9; EINECS 268-938-5; nonionic; stabilizer, visc. building surfactant for shampoos, hair conditioners, bath prods.; liq.; 35% conc.

Incromine Oxide L. [Croda Inc.; Croda Surf. Ltd.] Lauramine oxide; CAS 1643-20-5; EINECS 216-700-6; nonionic; foam booster/stabilizer, degreaser for dishwashing comps., household prods., hair conditioner used in personal care prods.; essentially colorless clear liq.; pH 7.0–8.0 (5% aq.); usage level: 0.5-20%; 29.0–31.0% amine oxide.

Incromine Oxide M. [Croda Inc.; Croda Surf. Ltd.] Myristamine oxide; CAS 3332-27-2; EINECS 222-059-3; nonionic; surfactant, emulsifier, emollient, conditioner, visc. builder, foam booster/stabilizer, wetting agent used in personal care prods.; essentially colorless liq.; pH 7.0–8.0 (5%); usage level: 0.5-20%; 29.5–30.5% amine oxide.

Incromine Oxide OL. [Croda Inc.] Olivamidopropylamine oxide; nonionic; thickener for clear systems; yel. gel; usage level: 0.5-10%; 25% act.

Incromine Oxide S. [Croda Inc.; Croda Surf. Ltd.] Stearamine oxide; CAS 2571-88-2; EINECS 219-919-5; nonionic; conditioner, emulsifier, visc. builder, foam booster/stabilizer for personal care prods.; wh. paste; usage level: 0.5-10%; 24.5–26.5% amine oxide.

Incromine Oxide WG. [Croda Inc.] Wheat germamidopropylamine oxide; nonionic; visc. builder, conditioner for hair care prods.; yel. gel; usage level: 0.5-10%; 25% act.

Incronam 30. [Croda Inc.; Croda Surf. Ltd.] Cocamidopropyl betaine; CAS 61789-40-0; amphoteric; surfactant, emulsifier, coupling agent, visc. builder, foam detergent for personal care prods., chemical specialities, rug and upholstery shampoos, dishwashing compds.; Gardner 5 max. clear liq.; sol. in water, alcohol; pH 5.5–7.5 (10% aq.); usage level: 2-20%; 30% act.

Incronam AL-30. [Croda Inc.] Almondamidopropyl betaine; amphoteric; foam booster/stabilizer for skin prods.; yel. liq.; sol. in water, alcohol; usage level: 2-20%; 30% act.

Incronam B-40. [Croda Inc.; Croda Surf. Ltd.] Behenyl

betaine; CAS 84082-44-0; amphoteric; foaming surfactant, conditioner, lubricant used in personal care prods.; exc. slip, conditioning; good wetting and rinse aid; wh. paste; pH 5.5–7.0 (3%); usage level: 2-20%; 40% act.

Incronam BA-30. [Croda Inc.] Babassamidopropyl betaine; amphoteric; foam booster/stabilizer for shampoos; yel. liq.; sol. in alcohol, water; usage level: 2-20%; 30% act.

Incronam CD-30. [Croda Surf. Ltd.] Coco betaine; CAS 68424-94-2; EINECS 270-329-4; amphoteric; mild, high foaming surfactant for detergent systems; liq.; 30% conc.

Incronam ISM 30. [Croda Inc.] Carboxymethyl isostearamidopropyl morpholine.

Incronam OD-50. [Croda Surf. Ltd.] Oleyl betaine; CAS 871-37-4; EINECS 212-806-1; amphoteric; high foaming surfactant, visc. builder for conditioning shampoos, clear rinses, cleansing creams and cosmetic lotions; gel; 50% conc.

Incronam OL-30. [Croda Inc.] Olivamidopropyl betaine; amphoteric; foam booster/stabilizer for skin care prods.; amber liq.; sol. in water, alcohol; usage level: 2-20%; 30% act.

Incronam OLB. [Croda Inc.] Olivamidopropyl betaine.

Incronam OP-30. [Croda Inc.; Croda Surf. Ltd.] Oleamidopropyl betaine; CAS 25054-76-6; EINECS 246-584-2; amphoteric; visc. builder, high foaming surfactant for shampoos, bubble baths, cleansing lotions, hand cleaners, skin care; yel. visc. liq.; 30% conc.

Incronam SE-30. [Croda Inc.] Sesamidopropyl betaine; amphoteric; foam booster/stabilizer, conditioner with good slip; yel. liq.; forms clear sol'ns. in alcohol, clear gels in water; usage level: 2-20%; 30% act.

Incronam WG-30. [Croda Inc.] Wheat germamidopropyl betaine; CAS 133934-09-5; amphoteric; foam booster/stabilizer; yel. liq.; forms clear sol'ns. in water and hot alcohol; usage level: 2-20%; 30% act.

Incropol CS-12. [Croda Inc.] Ceteareth-12; CAS 68439-49-6.

Incropol CS-20. [Croda Inc.] Ceteareth-20; CAS 68439-49-6; nonionic; surfactant, emulsifier, lubricant, detergent for industrial and household prods.; coupling agent, antistat, fiber lubricant and solubilizer for personal care prods.; Gardner 1 max. solid; water-sol.; pH 5.5–7.5 (3%); HLB 15.5; usage level: 0.5-10%; 100% conc.

Incropol CS-40. [Croda Inc.] Ceteareth-40; CAS 68439-49-6.

Incropol CS-60. [Croda Inc.] Ceteareth-60; CAS 68439-49-6.

Incroquat 26. [Croda Inc.] Quaternium-26; CAS 68953-64-0; EINECS 273-222-0; hair conditioner.

Incroquat B65C. [Croda Inc.] Behenalkonium chloride, cetyl alcohol; cationic; substantive conditioner for hair care prods.; wh. flake; usage level: 1-5%; 65% act.

Incroquat BA-85. [Croda Inc.] Babassamidopropalkonium chloride; CAS 124046-05-5; cationic; conditioner, foamer, antistat for hair care prods.; amber liq.; usage level: 0.5-5%; 85% act.

Incroquat BES-35 S. [Croda Inc.] Behenamidopropyl ethyldimonium ethosulfate and stearyl alcohol; exc. wet comb and detangling props., good manageability, and setting/styling props. for hair care prods. esp. for dry hair; pale yel. flake; usage level: 2-10%; 36% act.

Incroquat CR Conc. [Croda Inc.] Cetearyl alcohol, PEG-40 castor oil, stearalkonium chloride; cationic; self-emulsifying wax, conditioner, softener, emollient, o/w emulsifier used in cream rinses, conditioners; wh. flake; mild fatty odor; m.p. 58-62 C; pH 6.3 (5% disp.); usage level: 5-7%; 96% min. act.

Incroquat CTC-30. [Croda Inc.; Croda Surf. Ltd.] Cetrimonium chloride; CAS 112-02-7; EINECS 203-928-6; cationic; conditioner, antistat for hair care prods.; Gardner 2

max. liq.; pH 3.5–4.0 (5%); usage level: 0.5-5%; 29% act.

Incroquat CTC-50. [Croda Surf. Ltd.] Cetrimonium chloride; CAS 112-02-7; EINECS 203-928-6; quat. for personal care prods.

Incroquat DBM-90. [Croda Inc.] Dibehenyldimonium methosulfate; cationic; conditioner with good wetting and slip for hair care prods.; wh. flake; sol. in hot alcohol; insol. in water, cold alcohol; usage level: 0.5-5%; 90% act.

Incroquat LI-85. [Croda Inc.] Linoleamidopropalkonium chloride.

Incroquat O-50. [Croda Inc.] Olealkonium chloride; CAS 37139-99-4; EINECS 253-363-4; cationic; conditioner with good slip for hair care prods.; pale yel. liq.; usage level: 0.5-5%; 50% act.

Incroquat S-85. [Croda Inc.] Stearalkonium chloride; CAS 122-19-0; EINECS 204-527-9; cationic; conditioner, softener, foamer, wetting agent, good rinsing, slip, wet comb, antistatic props.; wh. waxy flake; m.p. 140 F; pH 5–7 (0.5%); usage level: 0.5-5%; 85.0% min. act.

Incroquat SBQ 75P. [Croda Inc.] Stearamidopropalkonium chloride; CAS 65694-10-2; EINECS 265-880-2; hair conditioner.

Incroquat SDQ-25. [Croda Inc.; Croda Universal Ltd.] Stearalkonium chloride; CAS 122-19-0; EINECS 204-527-9; cationic; surfactant used as ingred. in personal care prods., textile and paper; dispersant for pigments and dyestuffs; antistat for fibers and synthetics; hair conditioner; wh. paste; m.p. 140 F; pH 3.0–4.0 (1%); usage level: 2-10%; 25% conc.

Incroquat TMC-80. [Croda Inc.] Behentrimonium chloride; CAS 17301-53-0; EINECS 241-327-0; base, antistat, emulsifier, conditioner for hair care prods.

Incroquat TMC-95. [Croda Inc.] Behentrimonium chloride; CAS 17301-53-0; EINECS 241-327-0; base, antistat, emulsifier, conditioner for hair care prods.

Incroquat WG-85. [Croda Inc.] Wheat germamidopropalkonium chloride; CAS 124046-09-9; cationic; conditioner with good foam and slip for hair prods.; amber liq.; sol. in alcohol and water; usage level: 0.5-5%; 85% act.

Incroquat Behenyl BDQ/P. [Croda Inc.; Croda Surf. Ltd.] Propylene glycol and behenalkonium chloride; cationic; o/w emulsifier and conditioner; paste; 25% conc.

Incroquat Behenyl TMC/P. [Croda Inc.; Croda Surf. Ltd.] Propylene glycol and behenalkonium chloride; cationic; o/w emulsifier and conditioner; paste; 25% conc.

Incroquat Behenyl TMS. [Croda Inc.; Croda Surf. Ltd.] Behenalkonium methosulfate, cetearyl alcohol; cationic; self-emulsifying wax, conditioner, softener, emollient, o/w emulsifier used in hair and skin care prods.; wh. flake, char. odor; m.p. 56-62 C; pH 6.0-7.0 (1%); usage level: 1-10%; 25% act.

Incrosoft S-90. [Croda Inc.] Quaternium-27; CAS 86088-85-9; softener base, lubricant, antistat and rewetting agent for fabrics and syns.; also used in textile maintenance and finishing; in personal care for hair conditioners; yel. semisolid; disp. in water; pH 5.0–7.0 (5% in DW); usage level: 5-10%; 85–88% act.

Incrosoft T-90. [Croda Inc.] Quaternium-53; CAS 130124-24-2; fabric softener, lubricant and antistat for home and commercial laundry prods.; good rewetting; hair conditioner; Gardner 7 max. visc. liq., alcoholic odor; disp. in water; pH 4–7 (3%); usage level: 5-10%; 88–90% act.

Incrosorb O-80. [Croda Inc.] Polysorbate 80; CAS 9005-65-6; emulsifier.

Incrosul LAFS. [Croda Inc.] Disodium laneth-5 sulfosuccinate; anionic; mild, low foaming, conditioning surfactant with good emulsifying props. used in personal care prods.; yel. slurry/liq.; usage level: 5-50%; 50% act.

Incrosul OTS. [Croda Inc.] Disodium oleth-3 sulfosuccinate; anionic; mild, conditioning surfactant, foamer for shampoos, baby shampoos, bath gels, mild skin cleansers; anti-irritant for anionic surfactants; Gardner 2 max. clear liq., mild char. odor; sol. @ 10% in water, water/alcohol, glycerin; pH 6.0-7.0; 37% act.

Inducos. [Induchem AG] A range of plastic powds. incl. polyamide, HD and LD polyethylene in particle sizes to 800 μ; abrasives for cosmetics industry.

Industrene® 20. [Witco/H-I-P] Linseed acid; CAS 68424-45-3; EINECS 270-304-8.

Industrene® 105. [Witco/H-I-P] Oleic acid; CAS 112-80-1; EINECS 204-007-1; intermediate used in alkyd resins, rubber compding., water repellents, polishes, soaps, abrasives, cutting oils, candles, crayons, emulsifiers, personal care prods.; Gardner 6 liq.; solid. pt. 145 C max.; acid no. 195-204; iodine no. 85-95; sapon. no. 195-205; 100% conc.

Industrene® 106. [Witco/H-I-P] Oleic acid NF, low titer; CAS 112-80-1; EINECS 204-007-1; chemical intermediate; personal care prods.; solid. pt. 6 C max.; acid no. 198-204; iodine no. 95 max.; sapon. no. 199-205.

Industrene® 206. [Witco/H-I-P] Oleic acid NF; CAS 112-80-1; EINECS 204-007-1; intermediate used in alkyd resins, rubber compding., water repellents, polishes, soaps, abrasives, cutting oils, candles, crayons, emulsifiers, personal care prods.; liq.; solid. pt. 6 C max.; acid no. 199-204; iodine no. 95 max.; sapon. no. 200-205; 100% conc.

Industrene® 223. [Witco/H-I-P] Hydrog. coconut acid; CAS 68938-15-8; chemical intermediate, emulsifier; used for personal care prods., waxes, textile aux., pharmaceuticals; solid. pt. 23–26 C; acid no. 266-274; iodine no. 3 max.; sapon. no. 267-276.

Industrene® 325. [Witco/H-I-P] Dist. coconut acid; CAS 61788-47-4; EINECS 262-978-7; intermediate used in alkyd resins, rubber compding., water repellents, polishes, soaps, abrasives, cutting oils, candles, crayons, emulsifiers, personal care prods.; paste; acid no. 265-277; iodine no. 6-15; sapon. no. 265-278; 100% conc.

Industrene® 328. [Witco/H-I-P] Stripped coconut acid; CAS 61788-47-4; EINECS 262-978-7; intermediate used in alkyd resins, rubber compding., water repellents, polishes, soaps, abrasives, cutting oils, candles, crayons, emulsifiers, personal care prods.; paste; acid no. 253-260; iodine no. 5-14; sapon. no. 253-260; 100% conc.

Industrene® 9018. [Witco/H-I-P] Stearic acid (90%); CAS 57-11-4; EINECS 200-313-4; intermediate used in alkyd resins, rubber compding., water repellents, polishes, soaps, abrasives, cutting oils, candles, crayons, emulsifiers, personal care prods.; solid; acid no. 196-201; iodine no. 2 max.; sapon. no. 196-202; 100% conc.

Infrasome. [Sederma] Lamellar nano vesicle; epidermal restructurer and moisturizer for face and body care prods.; pale yel. sl. opalescent liq., char. odor; sp.gr. 1.05-1.07; ref. index 1.375-1.385; pH 6.0-7.5; usage level: 3-15%.

Iniferine. [Sederma] Water, lactoferrin, thioxanthine, and uric acid; free radical scavenger for face and sun care protection; pink-ylsh. clear liq., char. odor; sp.gr. 1.02 ± 0.001; ref. index 1.340 ± 0.005; pH 7-8; usage level: 5%.

Inositol. [R.I.T.A.] Inositol; CAS 87-89-8; EINECS 201-781-2; emollient, humectant, pigment, conditioner, lubricant with skin soothing props. for personal care prods.; wh. cryst.

Insect repellent 3535, No. 11887. [E. Merck] Ethyl butylacetylaminopropionate; CAS 52304-36-6; EINECS 257-835-0.

Instabronze. [Alban Muller; Tri-K Industries] Glucose tyrosinate; amino acid/enzyme complex for use as suntan facilitator.

Instant Egg White Solids Type P-600. [Henningsen Foods] Albumen; CAS 9006-50-2.

Instapearl. [Lonza] Glycol stearate; CAS 111-60-4; EINECS

203-886-9; opacifier for creams, lotions, shampoos.

Intex Scour Base 706. [Intex] Alkanolamide; nonionic; foam additive, scour, pulling soap, shampoo base; liq.; 100% conc.

Intravon® JU. [Crompton & Knowles] EO condensate; nonionic; detergent, emulsifier, dispersant, wetting agent, penetrant for textile, household and cosmetic applics.; antiprecipitant for dyeing acrylic blends with anionic/cationic dyes in a one-bath method; colorless to pale yel. visc. liq.; water-sol.; sp.gr. 1.02; dens. 8.5 lb/gal; pH 7.0 ± 0.5 (1%).

Iodamicid. [Vevy] MEA-iodine.

Iodobio 45. [Alban Muller] TEA-hydroiodide; slenderizing prod. for cosmetics.

Iodogene. [Esperis] Hydroxypropyl bistrimonium diiodide; EINECS 204-630-9.

Iodorga. [C.E.P.] Ethiodized oil; CAS 8008-53-5.

Iodotrat. [Vevy] TEA-hydroiodide.

Ionet DL-200. [Sanyo Chem. Industries] POE dilaurate; CAS 9005-02-1; nonionic; emulsifier for emulsion polymerization, metal processing lubricant and personal care prods.; liq.; HLB 6.6; 100% conc.

Ionet DO-200. [Sanyo Chem. Industries] POE dioleate; CAS 9005-07-6; nonionic; emulsifier for emulsion polymerization of vinyl resins, for metal processing lubricants, cosmetics; liq.; HLB 5.3; 100% conc.

Ionet DO-400. [Sanyo Chem. Industries] POE dioleate; CAS 9005-07-6; nonionic; emulsifier for emulsion polymerization of vinyl resins, for metal processing lubricants, cosmetics; liq.; HLB 8.4; 100% conc.

Ionet DO-600. [Sanyo Chem. Industries] POE dioleate; CAS 9005-07-6; nonionic; emulsifier for emulsion polymerization of vinyl resins, for metal processing lubricants, cosmetics; liq.; HLB 10.4; 100% conc.

Ionet DO-1000. [Sanyo Chem. Industries] POE dioleate; CAS 9005-07-6; nonionic; emulsifier for emulsion polymerization of vinyl resins, for metal processing lubricants, cosmetics; solid; HLB 12.9; 100% conc.

Ionet DS-300. [Sanyo Chem. Industries] POE distearate; CAS 9005-08-7; nonionic; emulsifier for emulsion polymerization of vinyl resins, for metal processing lubricants, cosmetics; solid; HLB 7.3; 100% conc.

Ionet DS-400. [Sanyo Chem. Industries] POE distearate; CAS 9005-08-7; nonionic; emulsifier for emulsion polymerization of vinyl resins, for metal processing lubricants, cosmetics; solid; HLB 8.5; 100% conc.

Ionet S-20. [Sanyo Chem. Industries] Sorbitan laurate; CAS 1338-39-2; nonionic; emulsifier for personal care prods.; lubricant, rust inhibitor; pigment dispersant; spreading agent for agric. pesticides; base for textile lubricants; liq.; HLB 8.6; 100% conc.

Ionet S-60 C. [Sanyo Chem. Industries] Sorbitan stearate; CAS 1338-41-6; EINECS 215-664-9; nonionic; emulsifier for personal care prods.; lubricant, rust inhibitor; pigment dispersant; spreading agent for agric. pesticides; base for textile lubricants; solid; HLB 4.7; 100% conc.

Ionet S-80. [Sanyo Chem. Industries] Sorbitan oleate; CAS 1338-43-8; EINECS 215-665-4; nonionic; emulsifier for personal care prods.; lubricant, rust inhibitor; pigment dispersant; spreading agent for agric. pesticides; base for textile lubricants; liq.; HLB 4.3; 100% conc.

Ionet S-85. [Sanyo Chem. Industries] Sorbitan trioleate; CAS 26266-58-0; EINECS 247-569-3; nonionic; emulsifier for personal care prods.; lubricant, rust inhibitor; pigment dispersant; spreading agent for agric. pesticides; base for textile lubricants; liq.; HLB 1.8; 100% conc.

Ionet T-20 C. [Sanyo Chem. Industries] Polysorbate 20; CAS 9005-64-5; nonionic; base and emulsifier for personal care prods., metal processing, lubricant and rust inhibitor; pigment dispersant; spreader sticker for agric. pesticides;

base for textile lubricants; liq.; HLB 16.7; 100% conc.

Ionet T-60 C. [Sanyo Chem. Industries] POE sorbitan monostearate; CAS 9005-67-8; nonionic; base and emulsifier for personal care prods., metal processing, lubricant and rust inhibitor; pigment dispersant; spreader sticker for agric. pesticides; base for textile lubricants; liq.; HLB 14.9; 100% conc.

Ionet T-80 C. [Sanyo Chem. Industries] POE sorbitan monooleate; CAS 9005-65-6; nonionic; base and emulsifier for personal care prods., metal processing, lubricant and rust inhibitor; pigment dispersant; spreader sticker for agric. pesticides; base for textile lubricants; liq.; HLB 15.0; 100% conc.

Ionol CP. [Shell] BHT; CAS 128-37-0; EINECS 204-881-4; antioxidant for rubber, paraffin, and plastic used in food and drug prods.; paper pkg.; Pt-Co 15 max.; solid. pt. 69.4 C min.; 99.0% min. purity.

Ionpure Type A. [U.S. Cosmetics] Silver borosilicate; amorphous water-sol. inorg. preservative for cosmetics and plastic pkg.; stable to 500 C; resist. to light; USA approved; usage level: 0.5-1%; toxicology: nontoxic, nonsensitizing, nonmutagenic.

Ionpure Type B. [U.S. Cosmetics] Silver aluminum magnesium phosphate; amorphous water-sol. inorg. preservative for cosmetics and plastic pkg.; stable to 500 C; resist. to light; USA approved; usage level: 0.5-1%; toxicology: nontoxic, nonsensitizing, nonmutagenic.

IPF Meadowsweet. [Solabia] Water, alcohol, and meadowsweet extract; botanical extract.

IPG. [Kuraray] Isopentyldiol; CAS 2568-33-4.

Iramine. [Janssen Research Foundation] Diphenylmethyl piperazinylbenzimidazole; CAS 65215-54-5.

Irgasan DP300. [Ciba-Geigy] Triclosan; CAS 3380-34-5; EINECS 222-182-2; broad spectrum bacteriostat for deodorant prods., e.g., bar soaps, fabric sanitization, institutional fabric softeners; 99% min. act.

Irotyl. [Henkel/Cospha] Fragrance raw material for cosmetic, personal care, detergent, and cleaning prods.; colorless liq., pungent odor; b.p. 81 C; flash pt. 67 C.

IS-CE. [Kao Corp.] Cholesteryl isostearate; CAS 83615-24-1.

Iso-Adipate 2/043700. [Dragoco] Diisopropyl adipate; CAS 6938-94-9; EINECS 248-299-9; cosmetic ester.

Isobeeswax SP 154. [Strahl & Pitsch] Beeswax, candelilla wax, hydrog. soy glyceride, paraffin, carnauba, and stearic acid.

Isocet. [Vevy] Ceteareth-20 and isostearyl alcohol.

Isocholesterol EX. [Nikko Chem. Co. Ltd.] Dihydrolanosterol and lanosterol.

Isodon Extract. [Maruzen Fine Chems.] Alcohol, water, butylene glycol, and isodonis extract; botanical extract.

Isodragol 2/050300. [Dragoco] Triisononanoin.

Isofol® 12. [Condea Chemie GmbH; Vista] Butyl octanol; CAS 3913-02-8; EINECS 223-470-0; for cosmetic/pharmaceutical creams, ointments, emulsions, sticks, body oils; solubilizer for lipid-sol. actives; biodeg.; clear oily liq.; m.w. 186; sp.gr. 0.833; visc. 23 mPa·s; m.p. < -30 C; b.p. 145-149 C (33 mbar); acid no. 0.1 max.; iodine no. 1.0 max.; sapon. no. 1.0 max.; hyd. no. 296-305; flash pt. 120 C; ref. index 1.443; surf. tens. 28 mN/m; toxicology: nontoxic; nonirritating to skin; 95% min. act.

Isofol® 14T. [Condea Chemie GmbH; Vista] C12-C16 Guerbet alcohol; for cosmetic/pharmaceutical creams, ointments, emulsions, sticks, body oils; solubilizer for lipid-sol. actives; biodeg.; clear oily liq.; m.w. 212-223; sp.gr. 0.835; visc. 32 mPa·s; m.p. < -25 C; b.p. 160-195 C (33 mbar); acid no. 0.1 max.; iodine no. 1.0 max.; sapon. no. 1.0 max.; hyd. no. 252-265; flash pt. 139 C; ref. index 1.447; surf. tens. 30 mN/m; toxicology: nontoxic; nonirritating to skin; 95% min. act.

Isofol® 16. [Condea Chemie GmbH; Vista] Hexyl decanol; CAS 2425-77-6; EINECS 219-370-1; for cosmetic/pharmaceutical creams, ointments, emulsions, sticks, body oils; solubilizer for lipid-sol. actives; biodeg.; clear oily liq.; m.w. 242; sp.gr. 0.836; visc. 38 mPa·s; m.p. -21 to -15 C; b.p. 193-197 C (33 mbar); acid no. 0.1 max.; iodine no. 1.0 max.; sapon. no. 1.0 max.; hyd. no. 225-235; flash pt. 156 C; ref. index 1.450; surf. tens. 30 mN/m; toxicology: nontoxic; nonirritating to skin; 97% min. act.

Isofol® 16 Caprylat. [Condea Chemie GmbH] CAS 92777-70-9; EINECS 298-104-6; oily components in cosmetic/pharmaceutical formulations incl. creams, lotions, deodorants, hair conditioners, aerosol and foam prods.; clear oily liq.; m.w. 370; sp.gr. 0.855; visc. 11 mPa·s; solid. pt. -48 C; acid no. 0.1 max.; iodine no. 0.5 max.; sapon. no. 148-155; hyd. no. 0.1 max.; flash pt. 213 C; ref. index 1.446.

Isofol® 16 Laurat. [Condea Chemie GmbH] CAS 34362-27-1; EINECS 251-959-9; oily components in cosmetic/pharmaceutical formulations incl. creams, lotions, deodorants, hair conditioners, aerosol and foam prods.; clear oily liq.; m.w. 426; sp.gr. 0.853; visc. 16 mPa·s; solid. pt. -29 C; acid no. 0.1 max.; iodine no. 0.5 max.; sapon. no. 129-136; hyd. no. 0.1 max.; flash pt. 225 C; ref. index 1.450.

Isofol® 16 Oleat. [Condea Chemie GmbH] CAS 94278-07-6; EINECS 304-693-3; oily components in cosmetic/pharmaceutical formulations incl. creams, lotions, deodorants, hair conditioners, aerosol and foam prods.; clear oily liq.; m.w. 509; sp.gr. 0.861; visc. 26 mPa·s; solid. pt. -40 C; acid no. 0.1 max.; iodine no. 50-54; sapon. no. 108-114; hyd. no. 0.1 max.; flash pt. 260 C; ref. index 1.459.

Isofol® 16 Palmitat. [Condea Chemie GmbH] CAS 69275-02-1; EINECS 273-942-5; oily components in cosmetic/pharmaceutical formulations incl. creams, lotions, deodorants, hair conditioners, aerosol and foam prods.; clear oily liq.; m.w. 482; sp.gr. 0.852; visc. 24 mPa·s; solid. pt. -10 C; acid no. 0.1 max.; iodine no. 0.5 max.; sapon. no. 114-120; hyd. no. 0.1 max.; flash pt. 237 C; ref. index 1.453.

Isofol® 18E. [Condea Chemie GmbH; Vista] C16-C20 Guerbet alcohol; for cosmetic/pharmaceutical creams, ointments, emulsions, sticks, body oils; solubilizer for lipid-sol. actives; biodeg.; clear oily liq.; m.w. 269-279; sp.gr. 0.837; visc. 50 mPa·s; m.p. -10 to -6 C; b.p. 211-218 C (33 mbar); acid no. 0.1 max.; iodine no. 1.0 max.; sapon. no. 1.0 max.; hyd. no. 201-209; flash pt. 170 C; ref. index 1.452; surf. tens. 30 mN/m; toxicology: nontoxic; nonirritating to skin; 95% min. act.

Isofol® 18T. [Condea Chemie GmbH; Vista] C16-C20 Guerbet alcohol; for cosmetic/pharmaceutical creams, ointments, emulsions, sticks, body oils; solubilizer for lipid-sol. actives; biodeg.; clear oily liq.; m.w. 267-285; sp.gr. 0.837; visc. 50 mPa·s; m.p. -10 to -6 C; b.p. 207-236 C (33 mbar); acid no. 0.1 max.; iodine no. 1.0 max.; sapon. no. 1.0 max.; hyd. no. 197-210; flash pt. 170 C; ref. index 1.452; surf. tens. 30 mN/m; toxicology: nontoxic; nonirritating to skin; 95% min. act.

Isofol® 20. [Condea Chemie GmbH; Vista] Octyl dodecanol; CAS 5333-42-6; EINECS 226-242-9; for cosmetic/pharmaceutical creams, ointments, emulsions, sticks, body oils; solubilizer for lipid-sol. actives; biodeg.; clear oily liq.; m.w. 298; sp.gr. 0.838; visc. 60 mPa·s; m.p. -1 to +1 C; b.p. 234-238 C (33 mbar); acid no. 0.1 max.; iodine no. 1.0 max.; sapon. no. 1.0 max.; hyd. no. 184-190; flash pt. 180 C; ref. index 1.454; surf. tens. 31 mN/m; toxicology: nontoxic; nonirritating to skin; 97% min. act.

Isofol® 20 Myristat. [Condea Chemie GmbH] CAS 22766-83-2; EINECS 245-205-8; oily components in cosmetic/pharmaceutical formulations incl. creams, lotions, deodorants, hair conditioners, aerosol and foam prods.;

clear oily liq.; m.w. 510; sp.gr. 0.851; visc. 27 mPa·s; solid. pt. -2 C; acid no. 0.1 max.; iodine no. 0.5 max.; sapon. no. 106-112; hyd. no. 0.1 max.; flash pt. 244 C; ref. index 1.457.

Isofol® 20 Oleat. [Condea Chemie GmbH] CAS 22801-45-2; EINECS 245-228-3; oily components in cosmetic/pharmaceutical formulations incl. creams, lotions, deodorants, hair conditioners, aerosol and foam prods.; clear oily liq.; m.w. 565; sp.gr. 0.860; visc. 32 mPa·s; solid. pt. -24 C; acid no. 0.1 max.; iodine no. 44-48; sapon. no. 92-98; hyd. no. 0.1 max.; flash pt. 272 C; ref. index 1.460.

Isofol®24. [Condea Chemie GmbH; Vista] Decyl dodecanol; for cosmetic/pharmaceutical creams, ointments, emulsions, sticks, body oils; solubilizer for lipid-sol. actives; biodeg.; clear oily liq.; m.w. 354; sp.gr. 0.842; visc. 86 mPa·s; m.p. 17-20 C; b.p. 271-175 C (33 mbar); acid no. 0.1 max.; iodine no. 1.0 max.; sapon. no. 1.0 max.; hyd. no. 154-160; flash pt. 230 C; ref. index 1.457; surf. tens. 32 mN/m; toxicology: nontoxic; nonirritating to skin; 97% min. act.

Isofol® 28. [Condea Chemie GmbH] 2-Dodecyl-hexadecanol; CAS 72388-18-2; EINECS 276-627-0; wax substitute; skin softener in stick formulations, e.g., deodorant sticks, lip salves; wh. waxy substance; m.w. 415; sp.gr. 0.83; visc. 40 mPa·s; m.p. 29-31 C; b.p. 240 C max. (33 mbar); acid no. 2 max.; iodine no. 1.5 max.; sapon. no. 5 max.; hyd. no. 130-140; flash pt. 254 C; ref. index 1.4516; surf. tens. 31 mN/m (50 C); 90% conc.

Isofol® 32. [Condea Chemie GmbH] 2-Tetradecyl octadecanol; CAS 32582-32-4; EINECS 251-110-2; wax substitute; skin softener in stick formulations, e.g., deodorant sticks, lip salves; wh. waxy substance; m.w. 470; sp.gr. 0.83; visc. 53 mPa·s; m.p. 35-37 C; b.p. 240 C max. (33 mbar); acid no. 2 max.; iodine no. 1.5 max.; sapon. no. 5 max.; hyd. no. 116-126; flash pt. 266 C; ref. index 1.4527; surf. tens. 30 mN/m (50 C); 90% conc.

Isofol® 34T. [Condea Chemie GmbH] 2-Tetradecyl octadecanol (19-25%), 2-tetradecyleicosanol/2-hexadecyloctadecanol (43-51%), 2-hexadecyleicosanol (25-31%); CAS 68187-86-0; EINECS 269-131-0; wax substitute; skin softener in stick formulations, e.g., deodorant sticks, lip salves; wh. waxy substance; m.w. 491; sp.gr. 0.83; visc. 63 mPa·s; m.p. 34-36 C; b.p. 240 C max. (33 mbar); acid no. 2 max.; iodine no. 1.5 max.; sapon. no. 5 max.; hyd. no. 110-120; flash pt. 278 C; ref. index 1.4537; surf. tens. 29 mN/m (50 C); 90% conc.

Isofol®36. [Condea Chemie GmbH] 2-Hexadecyleicosanol; CAS 17658-36-8; EINECS 241-637-6; wax substitute; skin softener in stick formulations, e.g., deodorant sticks, lip salves; wh. waxy substance; m.w. 510; sp.gr. 0.83; visc. 65 mPa·s; m.p. 46-48 C; b.p. 240 C max. (33 mbar); acid no. 2 max.; iodine no. 1.5 max.; sapon. no. 5 max.; hyd. no. 105-115; flash pt. 279 C; ref. index 1.4547; surf. tens. 28 mN/m (50 C); 90% conc.

Iso Isotearyle WL 3196. [Gattefosse SA] Isostearyl isostearate; CAS 41669-30-1; EINECS 255-485-3; superfatting agent for cosmetic/pharmaceutical emulsions and microemulsions; liq.; HLB 1-2; acid no. < 6; iodine no. < 8; sapon. no. 90-110; toxicology: LD50 (oral, rat) > 2 g/kg; sl. irritating to skin and eyes.

Isoixol 6. [Vevy] PEG-20 sorbitan isostearate; CAS 66794-58-9; emulsifier.

Isolan® GI 34. [Goldschmidt] Polyglyceryl-3 isostearate; CAS 127512-63-4; w/o emulsifier for veg. oils; low odor, easy to use; forms very stable emulsions; good oxidative stability; for personal care industry; yel. liq.; sol. @ 10% in veg. and paraffin oils; insol. in water; HLB 5 ± 1; acid no. 10 max.; iodine no. 5 max.; sapon. no. 150-190; hyd. no. 60-110; usage level: 2.5-4.0%.

Isolan® GO 33. [Goldschmidt] Polyglyceryl-3 oleate; CAS

9007-48-1; w/o emulsifier for veg. oils and natural triglycerides; for personal care industry w/o creams; yel. liq.; sol. @ 10% in veg. and paraffin oils; insol. in water; HLB 5.5 ± 1; acid no. 3 max.; iodine no. 65-80; sapon. no. 150-170; hyd. no. 80-130; usage level: 2.5-4.0%.

Isolanoate. [Lanaetex Prods.] Octyl isononanoate; CAS 71566-49-9; EINECS 275-637-2; cosmetics ingred.

Isolanoate-BS. [Lanaetex Prods.] Isobutyl stearate, octyl isononanoate.

Isolene. [Vevy] Glyceryl dipalmitate, glyceryl distearate, glyceryl dimyristate, and glyceryl dilaurate.

Isopar® G. [Exxon] C10–11 isoparaffin; CAS 64742-48-9; solvent, diluent, carrier for personal care prods. for sprays.

Isopar® H. [Exxon] C11–12 isoparaffin; CAS 64742-48-9; solvent, diluent, carrier for personal care prods. for sprays.

Isopar® K. [Exxon] C11–12 isoparaffin; CAS 64742-48-9; solvent, diluent, carrier for personal care prods. for sprays.

Isopar® L. [Exxon] C11–13 isoparaffin; CAS 64742-48-9; solvent for skin care formulations.

Isopar® M. [Exxon] C13–14 isoparaffin; CAS 64742-47-8; solvent for hair prods.

Isopropylan® 33. [Amerchol] Isopropyl palmitate, lanolin oil; binder in talc and pearl powd. systems; plasticizer, emollient, and moisturizer; lt. yel. clear oily liq.; slight char. odor; sapon. no. 145–165.

Isopropylmyristat. [Henkel KGaA/Cospha] Isopropyl myristate BP/NF; CAS 110-27-0; EINECS 203-751-4; spreading agent, dermatological carrier for cosmetic/pharmaceutical skin care preps.; good dissolution power for lipid-sol. actives; almost colorless oil, almost odorless; m.w. 270; sp.gr. 0.850-0.855; visc. 5-6 mPa·s; acid no. 0.2 max.; sapon. no. 205-211; cloud pt. 2 C max.; ref. index 1.434-1.436; 41-45% dry residue.

Isopropyl Palmitate. [Henkel KGaA/Cospha] Isopropyl palmitate; CAS 142-91-6; EINECS 205-571-1; carrier, solubilizer for lipid-sol. actives for cosmetic creams, emulsions, and ointments; transparent fluid, odorless; misc. with oily components; sp.gr. 0.852-0.854; acid no. 0.5 max.; iodine no. 1 max.; sapon. no. 186-191; hyd. no. 2 max.; cloud pt. 12-15 C; flash pt. 170 C min.; ref. index 1.438-1.439; 41-45% dry residue.

Isostearene. [Vevy] Isodecyl laurate; CAS 14779-93-2.

Isostearene L. [Vevy] Lauryl isostearate.

Isoxal 5. [Vevy] Ceteth-3, steareth-3, myreth-3, laureth-3.

Isoxal 11. [Vevy] Ceteth-10, steareth-10, myreth-10, laureth-10.

Isoxal 12. [Vevy] Ceteth-5, laureth-5, steareth-5, myreth-5.

Isoxal E. [Vevy] Isoceteareth-8 stearate.

Isoxal H. [Vevy] Isoceteth-10 stearate, isosteareth-10 stearate.

Ivarbase™ 98. [Brooks Industries] Polysorbate 80, cetyl acetate, acetylated lanolin alcohol; nonionic; surface-active emollient, primary emulsifier, plasticizer, superfatting agent for shampoos, cleansers, foaming bath preps.; amber clear liq.; sol. in water and alcohol; 100% act.

Ivarbase™ 101. [Brooks Industries] Min. oil, lanolin alcohol.; easy-to-use o/w emulsifier for cosmetics applics.; enhances cleansing efficiency and imparts a smooth fine texture; pigment dispersant; very pale straw-colored clear liq.; 100% act.

Ivarbase™ 3210. [Brooks Industries] Cetyl acetate, acetylated lanolin alcohol; light greaseless emollient for skin and hair care prods.; penetrates skin leaving soft, silky, emollient feel; forms fine glossy film on hair; glossing and plasticizing agent for hairsprays and cream curl moisturizers.

Ivarbase™ 3230. [Brooks Industries] Min. oil, PEG-30

lanolin, cetyl alcohol; nonionic; self-emulsifying absorb. base for cosmetics; makes very stable milks and creams; compat. with thioglycollates and oxidizing agents, making it ideal for use in cold wave creams, lotions, depilatories, and creamy neutralizers; pale yel. pearly unctuous solid, almost odorless; 100% act.

Ivarbase™ 3231. [Brooks Industries] PEG-30 soya sterol and cetyl alcohol; cosmetic ingred.

Ivarbase™ 3240. [Brooks Industries] Isopropyl lanolate, lanolin oil, oleyl alcohol; absorp. base, cosmetics ingred.

Ivarbase™ 3250. [Brooks Industries] Isopropyl palmitate, lanolin oil; rich light emollient, absorp. base for cosmetics use; forms emulsion prods. with exc. tactile prop. on skin and good stability and shelf-life; pale yel. oily liq., almost odorless; 100% act.

Ivarbase™ T. [Brooks Industries] Petrolatum, lanolin, lanolin alcohol; cosmetic ingred.

Ivarlan™ 3000. [Brooks Industries] Lanolin; CAS 8006-54-0; EINECS 232-348-6; emollient.

Ivarlan™ 3001. [Brooks Industries] Lanolin; CAS 8006-54-0; EINECS 232-348-6; emollient.

Ivarlan™ 3006 Light. [Brooks Industries] Lanolin; CAS 8006-54-0; EINECS 232-348-6; emollient.

Ivarlan™ 3100. [Brooks Industries] Lanolin oil; moisturizer and emollient readily absorbed by the skin; lt. amber clear visc. liq., very sl. char. odor; 100% act.

Ivarlan™ 3300. [Brooks Industries] Acetylated lanolin; CAS 61788-48-5; EINECS 262-979-2; emollient, superfatting agent.

Ivarlan™ 3310. [Brooks Industries] Lanolin alcohol; CAS 8027-33-6; EINECS 232-430-1; distilled grade; primary or coemulsifier for cosmetic creams and lotions; skin moisturizer; hars yel. wax; 99.5% act.

Ivarlan™ 3350. [Brooks Industries] Isopropyl lanolate; CAS 63393-93-1; EINECS 264-119-1; emollient.

Ivarlan™ 3360. [Brooks Industries] Glyceryl lanolate; CAS 97404-50-7; emollient, moisturizer, emulsifier.

Ivarlan™ 3400. [Brooks Industries] PEG-75 lanolin; CAS 61790-81-6; nonionic; emollient and superfatting agent for soaps, skin and hair care formulations; emulsifier with exc. stability and visc. control props.; amber waxy solid, sl. char. odor; water-sol.; 100% act.

Ivarlan™ 3401. [Brooks Industries] PEG-75 lanolin; CAS 61790-81-6; cosmetic ingred.; 50% act.

Ivarlan™ 3405-L30. [Brooks Industries] PEG-30 lanolin; CAS 61790-81-6; emollient, emulsifier.

Ivarlan™ 3406. [Brooks Industries] PEG-60 lanolin; CAS 61790-81-6; cosmetics ingred.; water-sol.; 100% act.

Ivarlan™ 3407-E. [Brooks Industries] PEG-75 lanolin; CAS 61790-81-6; emulsifier, emollient.

Ivarlan™ 3408W. [Brooks Industries] PEG-75 lanolin; CAS 61790-81-6; emulsifier, emollient.

Ivarlan™ 3409-60. [Brooks Industries] PEG-60 lanolin; CAS 61790-81-6; moisturizer, lubricant.

Ivarlan™ 3410. [Brooks Industries] PEG-85 lanolin.; CAS 61790-81-6; emollient.

Ivarlan™ 3420. [Brooks Industries] PPG-12-PEG-50 lanolin; CAS 68458-88-8; emollient and superfatting agent forming tack-free glossy films, providing spreading and glossing props. in ethnic curl activator sprays and creams; amber cloudy visc. liq., sl. char. odor; completely sol. in water and alcohols; 100% act.

Ivarlan™ 3442. [Brooks Industries] Laneth-15; CAS 61791-20-6; cosmetic ingred.

Ivarlan™ 3450. [Brooks Industries] PEG-20 hydrog. lanolin; CAS 68648-27-1; cosmetics ingred.; wh.; water-sol.

Ivarlan™ 3452. [Brooks Industries] PEG-24 hydrog. lanolin; CAS 68648-27-1; emollient, emulsifier.

Ivarlan™ AWS. [Brooks Industries] PPG-12-PEG-65 lanolin oil; CAS 68458-58-8; emollient for aq. and aq./alcoholic cosmetic systems; emulsifier for controlling visc. of an emulsion; amber hazy visc. liq., almost odorless; sol. in alcohol/water; 100% act.

Ivarlan™ C-24. [Brooks Industries] Choleth-24, ceteth-24; cosmetics ingred.

Ivarlan™ HL. [Brooks Industries] Hydrog. lanolin; CAS 8031-44-5; EINECS 232-452-1; cosmetics ingred.

Ivarlan™ HL-20. [Brooks Industries] PEG-20 hydrog. lanolin; CAS 68648-27-1; emollient, emulsifier.

Ivarlan™ L575. [Brooks Industries] PEG-75 lanolin; CAS 61790-81-6; emulsifier, emollient.

Ivarlan™ Light. [Brooks Industries] Lanolin USP; CAS 8006-54-0; EINECS 232-348-6; cosmetic ingred. providing shine and flexibility to the hair while combatting drying, brittleness, and scaling of scalp; pigment binder and dispersant; lt. yel. unctuous soft solid, sl. char. odor; m.p. 40 C; 100% conc.

Ivarlan™ OH. [Brooks Industries] Hydroxylated lanolin; CAS 68424-66-8; EINECS 270-315-8; cosmetic ingred.

Ivex® 10. [CasChem] Zinc undecylenate and undecylenic acid; antifungal powds. for foot care and personal hygiene prods.; wh. powd.; 100 mesh; visc. 1.25 stokes; 99.9% act.

Ivory Beads. [Procter & Gamble] Sodium tallowate and sodium cocoate.

Ixol 2. [Vevy] Polysorbate 20; CAS 9005-64-5; emulsifier, solubilizer.

Ixol 4. [Vevy] Polysorbate 40; CAS 9005-66-7; emulsifier.

Ixol 6. [Vevy] Polysorbate 60; CAS 9005-67-8; emulsifier.

Ixol 8. [Vevy] Polysorbate 80; CAS 9005-65-6; emulsifier.

Ixolene 2. [Vevy] Sorbitan laurate; emulsifier.

Ixolene 4. [Vevy] Sorbitan palmitate; CAS 26266-57-9; EINECS 247-568-8; emulsifier.

Ixolene 6. [Vevy] Sorbitan stearate; CAS 1338-41-6; EINECS 215-664-9; emulsifier.

Ixolene 8. [Vevy] Sorbitan oleate; CAS 1338-43-8; EINECS 215-665-4; emulsifier.

J

J-13. [U.S. Cosmetics] Jet-milled talc; CAS 14807-96-6; EINECS 238-877-9; premium cosmetic raw material for mfg. of eye shadows, face powds., dusting and talcum powds., foundations, and blushers; avg. particle size 1-3 μ; pH 8.5-9.5.

J-24. [U.S. Cosmetics] Jet-milled talc; CAS 14807-96-6; EINECS 238-877-9; premium cosmetic raw material for mfg. of eye shadows, face powds., dusting and talcum powds., foundations, and blushers; avg. particle size 2-4 μ; pH 8.5-9.5.

J-46. [U.S. Cosmetics] Jet-milled talc; CAS 14807-96-6; EINECS 238-877-9; premium cosmetic raw material for mfg. of eye shadows, face powds., dusting and talcum powds., foundations, and blushers; avg. particle size 4-6 μ; pH 8.5-9.5.

J-68. [U.S. Cosmetics] Jet-milled talc; CAS 14807-96-6; EINECS 238-877-9; premium cosmetic raw material for mfg. of eye shadows, face powds., dusting and talcum powds., foundations, and blushers; avg. particle size 6-8 μ; pH 8.5-9.5.

J-80. [U.S. Cosmetics] Jet-milled talc; CAS 14807-96-6; EINECS 238-877-9; premium cosmetic raw material for mfg. of eye shadows, face powds., dusting and talcum powds., foundations, and blushers; avg. particle size 8-10 μ.

Jafaester 14-96. [Pronova Olechems.] Isopropyl myristate; CAS 110-27-0; EINECS 203-751-4; emollient.

Jafaester 14 NF. [Pronova Olechems.] Isopropyl myristate; CAS 110-27-0; EINECS 203-751-4; emollient.

Jafaester 16 NF. [Pronova Olechems.] Isopropyl palmitate; CAS 142-91-6; EINECS 205-571-1; emollient.

Jafaester 2022. [Pronova Olechems.] Isopropyl behenate and isopropyl arachidate.

Jaguar® C. [Rhone-Poulenc/Water Soluble Polymers] Guar gum; CAS 9000-30-0; EINECS 232-536-8; cosmetic thickener.

Jaguar® C-13S. [Rhone-Poulenc Surf. & Spec.] Guar hydroxypropyltrimonium chloride; CAS 65497-29-2; cationic; thickener and conditioner for hair and skin care prods., liq. soaps, shower gels, facial cleansers, toiletries, shampoos, conditioning rinses, lotions, and creams; particle size 90% min. thru 150 mesh; visc. 3500 ± 500 cps (1% aq.); pH 5-7 (1% aq.); 12% max. moisture.

Jaguar® C-14-S. [Rhone-Poulenc Surf. & Spec.] Guar hydroxypropyl trimonium chloride; CAS 65497-29-2; cationic; thickener, conditioner, and antistat for shampoos, liq. soaps, shower gels, creams and lotions, facial cleansers, bath gels, bubble baths, toiletries, and conditioning rinses; particle size 90% min. thru 150 mesh; visc. 3500 ± 500 cps (1% aq.); pH 9-11 (1% aq.); 13% max. moisture.

Jaguar® C-17. [Rhone-Poulenc Surf. & Spec.] Guar hydroxypropyltrimonium chloride; CAS 65497-29-2; cationic; thickener, antistat, and conditioner for hair and skin care prods., shampoos, creme rinses, lotions, creams, liq.

soaps, shower gels, facial cleansers, bath gels, bubble baths, toiletries; particle size 90% thru 150 mesh; visc. 2000-4000 cps (1% aq.); pH 8.5-10.5 (1% aq.); 12% max. moisture.

Jaguar® C-162. [Rhone-Poulenc Surf. & Spec.] Hydroxypropyl guar hydroxypropyltrimonium chloride; CAS 71329-50-5; cationic; conditioner, thickener, and antistat providing gloss and surfactant compat. for hair and skin care prods., conditioning shampoos, bath gels, liq. soaps, creams and lotions, bar soaps; particle size 90% min. thru 150 mesh; visc. 300-1000 cps (1% aq.); pH 8.5-10.5 (1% aq.); 13% max. moisture.

Jaguar® HP 8. [Rhone-Poulenc Surf. & Spec.] Hydroxypropyl guar; CAS 39421-75-5; nonionic; polymer providing thickening, lubricating props., visc., suspension, mildness, and slip to aq. or hydroalcoholic cosmetic systems (shampoos, creme rinses, lotions, creams, toiletries); particle size 90% min. thru 150 mesh; visc. 4100 ± 500 cps (1% aq.); pH 8.5-11.0 (1% aq.); 12% max. moisture.

Jaguar® HP-11. [Rhone-Poulenc Surf. & Spec.] Hydroxypropyl guar; CAS 39421-75-5; nonionic; polymer providing thickening and compat. with electrolytes and surfactants for shampoos, creme rinse conditioners, lotions, creams, and other personal care prods.; pale yel. free-flowing powd.; particle size 90% min. thru 150 mesh; bulk dens. 40 ± 5 lb/ft³; visc. 3500 ± 400 cps; pH 6.0-7.5 (1% aq.); 12% max. moisture.

Jaguar® HP 60. [Rhone-Poulenc/Water Soluble Polymers] Hydroxypropyl guar; CAS 39421-75-5; nonionic; polymer providing thickening, lubricating props., enhanced foam stabilization, visc., suspension, mildness, and slip to aq. or hydroalcoholic cosmetic systems (shampoos, creme rinses, lotions, creams, toiletries); particle size 90% min. thru 150 mesh; visc. 3400 ± 600 cps (1% aq.); pH 9.5-10.5 (1% aq.); 13% max. moisture.

Jaguar® HP 120. [Rhone-Poulenc/Water Soluble Polymers] Hydroxypropyl guar; CAS 39421-75-5; nonionic; polymer providing thickening, lubricating props., visc., suspension, mildness, emolliency, and slip to aq. or hydroalcoholic cosmetic systems (shampoos, creme rinses, lotions, creams, toiletries); particle size 90% min. thru 150 mesh; visc. 1100 cps (1% aq.); pH 8.5-11.0 (1% aq.); 9% max. moisture.

Jaguar® HP-200. [Rhone-Poulenc/Water Soluble Polymers] Hydroxypropyl guar; CAS 39421-75-5.

Jaluronid. [Esperis] Sodium hyaluronate; CAS 9067-32-7; moisturizer.

Japan Wax NJ-9002. [Ikeda] Japan wax; CAS 8001-39-6; cosmetic wax imparting good feel to the skin; for pomades, eyebrow pencils, lipsticks, creams; ylsh. block; m.p. 50-60 C; acid no. 18-25; iodine no. 10-20; sapon. no. 190-220.

Japan Wax Stralpitz. [Strahl & Pitsch] Japan wax; CAS 8001-39-6; cosmetic wax.

JAQ Powdered Quat. [Crystal] Myristalkonium chloride; CAS 139-08-2; EINECS 205-352-0; for formulation of disinfectants, sanitizers, and swimming pool algicides; 95% act.

Jasmacyclat. [Henkel/Cospha] Methylcyclooctylcarbonate; fragrance raw material for personal care and detergent applics.; colorless liq., herbal odor; b.p. 47 C; flash pt. 119 C.

Jasmin Floral Wax. [Biosil Tech.] Fraction of jasmine floral material not sol. in alcohol when the essential oils are distilled off; cosmetics ingred.; m.p. 73-78 C; acid no. 1.2.

Jasmonan. [Henkel/Cospha] Fragrance raw material for cosmetic, personal care, detergent, and cleaning prods.; colorless liq., jasmine odor; b.p. 95 C; flash pt. 95 C.

Jasmorange® . [BASF AG] 2-Methyl-3(4-methylphenyl) propanal; fragrance (fruity, balsamic, green, floral, aldehydic).

Jaune Covasop W 1771. [Les Colorants Wackherr] Iron oxides and propylene glycol.

Jaune Extra W 1800. [Les Colorants Wackherr] Iron oxides.

Jeffersol DE-75. [Texaco] Glycol; CAS 107-21-1; EINECS 203-473-3.

Jeffox PPG-2000. [Texaco] PPG-26; CAS 25322-69-4; cosmetic ingred.

Jeltex. [Lanaetex Prods.] Polyglycerylmethacrylate and propylene glycol; cosmetic ingred.

Jet Amine DMCD. [Jetco] Dimethyl coco amine; CAS 61788-93-0; EINECS 263-020-0; cationic; intermediate for quats., surfactants, agric., detergent formulations for industrial, home, and personal care prods.; Gardner 2 max. liq.; iodine no. 12 max.; 95% min. tert. amine.

Jet Amine DMOD. [Jetco] Dimethyl oleyl amine; CAS 14727-68-5; cationic; intermediate for quats., surfactants, agric., and detergent formulations in industrial, home, and personal care prods.; Gardner 2 max. liq.; iodine no. 70 min.; 95% min. tert. amine.

Jet Amine DMSD. [Jetco] Dimethyl soya amine; CAS 61788-91-8; EINECS 263-017-4; cationic; intermediate for quats., surfactants, agric., and detergent formulations for industrial, home, and personal care prods.; Gardner 2 max. liq.; iodine no. 80 min.; 95% min. tert. amine.

Jet Amine DMTD. [Jetco] Dimethyl tallow amine; CAS 68814-69-7; cationic; intermediate for quats., surfactants, agric., and detergent formulations for industrial, home, and personal care prods.; Gardner 2 max. liq.; iodine no. 31 min.; 95% min. tert. amine.

Jet Amine M2C. [Jetco] Methyl dicocamine; CAS 61788-62-3; cationic; intermediate for quats., surfactants, agric., and detergent formulations for industrial, home, and personal care prods.; Gardner 2 max. solid; iodine no. 5 max.; 95% min. tert. amine.

Jet Quat 2C-75. [Jetco] Dicoco dimethyl ammonium chloride; CAS 61789-77-3; EINECS 263-087-6; cationic; bactericide, textile softener, asphalt emulsifier, petrol. processing; also for home and personal care prods.; Gardner 5 max. liq.; pH 6-9; 75% conc. in IPA/water.

Jet Quat C-50. [Jetco] Coco trimethyl ammonium chloride; CAS 61789-18-2; EINECS 263-038-9; cationic; bactericide, textile softener, asphalt emulsifier, petrol. processing; home and personal care prods.; Gardner 5 max. liq.; pH 6-9; 50% conc. in IPA/water.

Jet Quat DT-50. [Jetco] Methyl quat. of tallow diamine; CAS 68607-29-4; cationic; bactericide, textile softener, asphalt emulsifier, petrol. processing; home and personal care prods.; Gardner 8 max. liq.; pH 6-9; 50% conc. in IPA/water.

Jet Quat S-2C-50. [Jetco] Soya and dicocoammonium chlorides blend; cationic; textile softener, corrosion inhibitor, petrol. processing emulsifier, antistat, hair conditoner, home laundry softener; liq.; 50% conc.

Jet Quat S-50. [Jetco] Soya trimethyl ammonium chloride; CAS 61790-41-8; EINECS 263-134-0; cationic; bactericide, textile softener, asphalt emulsifier, petrol. processing; home and personal care prods.; Gardner 6 max. liq.; pH 6-9; 50% conc. in IPA/water.

Jet Quat 'i-27W. [Jetco] Tallow trimethyl ammonium chloride; CAS 8030-78-2; EINECS 232-447-4; cationic; bactericide, textile softener, asphalt emulsifier, petrol. processing; home and personal care prods.; Gardner 4 max. liq.; pH 6-9; 27% conc. in IPA/water.

Jet Quat T-50. [Jetco] Tallow trimethyl ammonium chloride; CAS 8030-78-2; EINECS 232-447-4; cationic; bactericide, textile softener, asphalt emulsifier, petrol. processing; home and personal care prods.; Gardner 6 max. liq.; pH 6-9; 50% conc. in IPA/water.

Jewelweed Extract Code 9034. [Brooks Industries] Jewelweed (*Impatiens balsamifera*) extract; treatment for poison ivy and other topical irritants; colorless clear liq.

Jodoprolamina. [Variati] Propylene glycol and iodized corn protein; cosmetic ingred.

Jojoba 28/60 Gypsy Rose. [Int'l. Flora Tech.] Hard microspheres containing jojoba wax; CAS 66625-78-3; exfoliant for cosmetics; biodeg., sterile, stable; CTFA & FDA compliance; red free-flowing beads, trace odor; particle size 85% between 250-600 µ; m.p. 69 C; iodine no. 2.0.

Jojoba 28/60 Jade. [Int'l. Flora Tech.] Hard microspheres containing jojoba wax; CAS 66625-78-3; exfoliant for cosmetics; biodeg., sterile, stable; CTFA & FDA compliance; jade green free-flowing beads, trace odor; particle size 85% between 250-600 µ; m.p. 69 C; iodine no. 2.0.

Jojoba 28/60 White. [Int'l. Flora Tech.] Hard microspheres containing jojoba wax; CAS 66625-78-3; exfoliant for cosmetics; biodeg., sterile, stable; CTFA & FDA compliance; wh. free-flowing beads, trace odor; particle size 85% between 250-600 µ; m.p. 69 C; iodine no. 2.0.

Jojoba 40/60 Mandarin. [Int'l. Flora Tech.] Hard microspheres containing jojoba wax; CAS 66625-78-3; exfoliant for cosmetics; biodeg., sterile, stable; CTFA & FDA compliance; orange free-flowing beads, trace odor; particle size 85% between 250-420 µ; m.p. 69 C; iodine no. 2.0.

Jojoba 40/60 White. [Int'l. Flora Tech.] Hard microspheres containing jojoba wax; CAS 66625-78-3; exfoliant for cosmetics; biodeg., sterile, stable; CTFA & FDA compliance; wh. free-flowing beads, trace odor; particle size 85% between 250-420 µ; m.p. 69 C; iodine no. 2.0.

Jojoba 60/100 White. [Int'l. Flora Tech.] Hard microspheres containing jojoba wax; CAS 66625-78-3; exfoliant for cosmetics; biodeg., sterile, stable; CTFA & FDA compliance; wh. free-flowing beads, trace odor; particle size 85% between 150-250 µ; m.p. 69 C; iodine no. 2.0.

Jojoba PEG-80. [Int'l. Flora Tech.] PEG-80 jojoba acids and PEG-80 jojoba alcohols; nonionic; surfactant, emulsifier for cosmetics; off-wh. waxy solid, typ. fatty odor; water-sol.; acid no. 3; iodine no. 14; sapon. no. 15; pH 6-7 (3%); 0.8% moisture.

Jojoba PEG-120. [Int'l. Flora Tech.] PEG-120 jojoba acids and PEG-120 jojoba alcohols; nonionic; surfactant, emulsifier for cosmetics; off-wh. waxy flake, typ. fatty odor; water-sol.; acid no. 3; iodine no. 10; sapon. no. 8; pH 6-7 (3%); 0.8% moisture.

Jojoba Meal 24/60. [Int'l. Flora Tech.] Milled cold pressed jojoba seeds containing about 9% jojoba oil; exfoliant for cosmetic use; lt. brn. powd., earthy sl. fatty odor; particle size 75% between 250-750 µ; pH 5-6 (10% aq.); 8% moisture.

Jojoba Meal 40. [Int'l. Flora Tech.] Milled cold-pressed jojoba seeds containing 9% jojoba oil; exfoliant for cosmetics; lt. brn. powd., earthy sl. fatty odor; particle size 95% < 370 µ;

pH 5-6 (10% aq.); 8% moisture.

Jojoba Meal 60. [Int'l. Flora Tech.] Milled cold-pressed jojoba seeds containing 9% jojoba oil; exfoliant for cosmetics; lt. brn. powd., earthy sl. fatty odor; particle size 95% < 250 μ; pH 5-6 (10% aq.); 8% moisture.

Jojoba Oil. [Goldschmidt AG] Jojoba oil; CAS 61789-91-1; natural liq. wax ester for high quality cosmetics; yel. liq.; sol. in veg. and min. oils; insol. in water.

Jojoba Oil Cosmetic Grade. [Frank B. Ross] Jojoba oil; CAS 61789-91-1; liq. wax ester for use as emollient, lubricant, and conditioner; provides spreadability and rub-in chars. with nonoily afterfeel; lt. yel. clear liq., mild pleasant odor; sol. in benzene, petrol. ether, chloroform, CCl₄, carbon disulfide, hexane; sp.gr. 0.86-0.89; visc. 56-59 cs; pour pt. 10 C; solid. pt. 7 C; acid no. 0.23-0.57; iodine no. 80 min.; sapon. no. 90 min.; ref. index 1.464 ± 0.004.

Jojoba Oil Pure Grade. [Int'l. Flora Tech.] Pure cold-pressed jojoba oil; CAS 61789-91-1; emollient for cosmetics; dk. golden liq. wax, typ. fatty odor; m.w. 606; sp.gr. 0.863; m.p. 7 C; acid no. 1; iodine no. 80; sapon. no. 93; ref. index 1.4587 (40 C).

Jojoba Oil Refined Grade. [Int'l. Flora Tech.] Pure cold-pressed jojoba oil; CAS 61789-91-1; emollient for cosmetics; very pale yel. liq. wax, trace odor; m.w. 606; sp.gr. 0.863; m.p. 7 C; acid no. 1; iodine no. 82; sapon. no. 90; ref. index 1.4587 (40 C).

Jojobead Gypsy Rose 40/60. [Int'l. Flora Tech.] Jojoba wax colored with D&C Red No. 30; CAS 66625-78-3; exfoliant for cosmetic use; hard microspheres in the form of free-flowing red beads; particle size 85% 250-420 μ; m.p. 69 C.

Jojobead Jade 40/60. [Int'l. Flora Tech.] Jojoba wax colored with chromium hydroxide; CAS 66625-78-3; exfoliant for cosmetic use; hard microspheres in the form of free-flowing green beads; particle size 85% 250-420 μ; m.p. 69 C.

Jojobead Lapis 40/60. [Int'l. Flora Tech.] Jojoba wax colored with ultramarine blue; CAS 66625-78-3; exfoliant for cosmetic use; hard microspheres in the form of free-flowing deep blue beads; particle size 85% 250-420 μ; m.p. 69 C.

Jojobead White 28/60. [Int'l. Flora Tech.] Jojoba wax; CAS 66625-78-3; exfoliant for cosmetic use; wh. free-flowing beads, trace odor; particle size 85% 250-600 μ; m.p. 69 C; iodine no. 2.0.

Jordapon® ACI-30. [PPG/Specialty Chem.] Ammonium cocoyl isethionate; surfactant, wetting agent with exc. foaming, mildness for skin and eyes; imparts soft afterfeel to skin; completely biodeg.; Gardner 3 clear liq.; water-sol.; visc. 50 cps; pH 6.8; surf. tens. 32 dynes/cm (0.1%); Ross-Miles foam 235 mm (initial, 0.2%, 50 C); toxicology: LD50 (oral) 4.33 g/kg; low toxicity; sl. irritating to skin; 27% act. in water.

Jordapon® CI-60. [PPG/Specialty Chem.] Sodium cocoyl isethionate and 40% stearic acid; anionic; mild, high foaming surfactant for syn. detergent soap bars, facial cleansers, aerosol shave creams; lime soap dispersant; biodeg.; wh. sm. flowable, nondusting flake, mild odor; pH 5.0 (10%); 50% act.

Jordapon® CI 60. [PPG/Specialty Chem.] Sodium cocoyl isethionate and stearic acid.

Jordapon® CI 65. [PPG/Specialty Chem.] Sodium cocoyl isethionate and stearic acid.

Jordapon® CI 75. [PPG/Specialty Chem.] Sodium cocoyl isethionate and 25% stearic acid; surfactant with exc. foaming, mildness for skin and eyes; imparts soft afterfeel to skin; for syndet bars, facial cleansers, aerosol shave creams; completely biodeg.; wh. nondusting sm. flowable flakes, mild odor; pH 5.5 (10%); 65% act.

Jordapon® CI Disp. [PPG/Specialty Chem.] Sodium cocoyl isethionate; EINECS 263-052-5; anionic; mild foaming surfactant for shampoos, bubble baths, creams and lotions; firm paste @ R.T., pumpable fluid @ 140 F; 50% act.

Jordapon® CI Powd. [PPG/Specialty Chem.] Sodium cocoyl isethionate; EINECS 263-052-5; anionic; mild high foaming detergent; lime soap dispersant; for syn. detergent soap bars, liq. soaps, facial cleansers; wh. fine powd.; pH 5.8 (10%); surf. tens. 27 dynes/cm (0.1%); Ross-Miles foam 220 mm (initial, 0.2%, 50 C); toxicology: LD50 (oral) > 5 g/kg; low toxicity; nonirritating to skin; 85% act.

Jordapon® CI Prill. [PPG/Specialty Chem.] Sodium cocoyl isethionate; EINECS 263-052-5; anionic; super-mild, high-foaming surfactant for liq. soaps, facial cleansers, liq. and lotion formulations; provides lather with char. lubricity; APHA < 75 clear fluid; sol. in cyclomethicone, almond oil, benzyl laurate, IPM, SD alcohol 40B; disp. in min. oil, propylene glycol; insol. in water; sp.gr. 0.960; visc. < 75 cps; m.p. < -25 C; b.p. > 150 C; flash pt. (CC) > 95 C; ref. index 1.443; toxicology: mild dermal and eye irritation; essentially nontoxic by oral ingestion.

Jordapon® CI-UP. [PPG/Specialty Chem.] Sodium cocoyl isethionate; EINECS 263-052-5; surfactant with exc. foaming, mildness for skin and eyes; imparts soft afterfeel to skin; for shampoos, bath and shower gels, liq. soaps; completely biodeg.; wh. irregular gran.; pH 5.8 (10%); 85% act.

Jox 3. [Int'l. Flora Tech.] Ozonized jojoba oil.

Junipal. [Henkel/Cospha] Fragrance raw material for cosmetic, personal care, detergent, and cleaning prods.; colorless liq., juniper odor; b.p. 84-88 C; flash pt. > 100 C.

Junlon PW-110. [Nihon Junyaku] Carbomer; emulsifier, thickener, stabilizer, suspending agent used in cosmetics.

Junlon PW-111. [Nihon Junyaku] Carbomer; emulsifier, thickener, stabilizer, suspending agent used in cosmetics.

Jurymer. [Les Colorants Wackherr] Microfine poly-methylmethacrylate beads; CAS 9011-14-7; provides lubricant film in cosmetics; beads; 90% between 5-10 μ.

Jurymer MB-1. [Nihon Junyaku] Polymethyl methacrylate; CAS 9011-14-7; provides lubricant film in cosmetics.

K

Kalidone®. [UCIB; Barnet Prods.] Potassium PCA aq. sol'n.; CAS 4810-50-8; EINECS 225-373-9; moisturizing agent for dermatological soap, shampoo, after-sun lotion, shower gel, nutritive and regenerative creams, hair comb-out balm; liq., odorless; very water-sol.; m.w. 167.2; usage level: 0.5-5%; toxicology: nontoxic; nonirritating to skin; very sl. irritating to eyes; 50% act. in water.

Kalixide AS. [Vevy] Talc, kaolin, silica.

Kalixide CT. [Vevy] Titanium dioxide, bismuth subnitrate, magnesium oxide.

Kalixide DPG. [Vevy] Zinc oxide, calcium titanate, bismuth subnitrate.

Kalixide Grassa. [Vevy] Talc, coconut oil, lecithin.

Kalixide Idrata. [Vevy] Talc, PEG-8.

Kalixide LT. [Vevy] Calcium carbonate, magnesium silicate.

Kallikrein. [Waitaki Int'l. Biosciences; Tri-K Industries] Serine protease extracted from pancreas and urine; skin rectifier; antihypertensive promoting vasodilation, cell re-newal, wound healing, increased nutrient and oxygen uptake, and radiation protection in skin care prods., cos-metics, and pharmaceuticals; powd. and sol'n.

Kalokiros HS 263. [Alban Muller] Propylene glycol, horsetail extract, sunflower seed extract, olibanum, wheat germ extract, and arnica extract; soothing prod. for hand creams.

Kalokiros LS 663. [Alban Muller] Sunflower seed oil, horse-tail extract, sunflower seed extract, olibanum, wheat germ extract, arnica extract; soothing prod. for hand creams.

Kamitsure Liq. [Ichimaru Pharcos] Water, alcohol, butylene glycol, and matricaria extract; botanical extract.

Kankoh SO 201. [Japanese Research Institute] Quaternium-73.

Kaopaque 10, 20. [Kaopolite] Kaolin; CAS 1332-58-7; EINECS 296-473-8; cosmetic ingred.

Kaopolite® SF. [Kaopolite] Aluminum silicate, anhyd.; CAS 1327-36-2; EINECS 215-475-1; gentle abrasive for auto polish, metals, plastics, household, dentifrices, cosmet-ics; antiblocking agent in plastic film.

Karajel. [Guardian Labs] Glyceryl alginate.

Karamide 121. [Clark] Cocamide DEA (1:1); CAS 61791-31-9; EINECS 263-163-9; heavy-duty detergent, thickener, foam stabilizer in cleaning compds., shampoos, textile scours; as lubricant, antistat.

Karamide 363. [Clark] Cocamide DEA (1:1); CAS 61791-31-9; EINECS 263-163-9; heavy-duty detergent, thickener, foam stabilizer in cleaning compds., shampoos, textile scours; as lubricant, antistat.

Karamide HTDA. [Clark] Fatty alkanolamide; coemulsifier, thickener for emulsions of oils and waxes; thickener for cleaners, shampoos; as textile softener base.

Karapeg 400-ML. [Clark] PEG-8 laurate; CAS 9004-81-3; emulsifier, coemulsifier for toiletry prep.; defoamer and leveling agent for latex paints; yel. liq.

Karapeg 600-ML. [Clark] PEG-12 laurate; CAS 9004-81-3;

emulsifier and coemulsifier for toiletry preps.; defoamer and leveling agent for latex paints; yel. liq.

Karapeg DEG-MS. [Clark] PEG-2 stearate; CAS 9004-99-3; EINECS 203-363-5; opacifier, pearlescent for liq. cos-metic and detergent compds.; wh. solid.

Karite Butter. [Sederma] Shea butter; CAS 68424-60-2; emollient oil.

Karite Nonsaponifiable. [Sederma] Shea butter unsaponifiables; skin protectant.

Kartacid 1299. [Akzo BV] Lauric acid; CAS 143-07-7; EINECS 205-582-1; surfactant.

Kartacid 1495. [Akzo BV] Myristic acid; CAS 544-63-8; EINECS 208-875-2; surfactant intermediate.

Kartacid 1498. [Akzo BV] Myristic acid; CAS 544-63-8; EINECS 208-875-2; surfactant intermediate.

Kartacid 1692. [Akzo BV] Palmitic acid; CAS 57-10-3; EINECS 200-312-9; surfactant intermediate; soap and cosmetic formulations.

Kartacid 1890. [Akzo BV] Stearic acid; CAS 57-11-4; EINECS 200-313-4; surfactant intermediate, emulsifier, emollient.

Kartacid C 60. [Akzo BV] Coconut acid; intermediate.

Kartacid C 70. [Akzo BV] Coconut acid; intermediate.

Katemul IG-70. [Scher] Isostearamidopropyl dimethylamine glycolate in propylene glycol; CAS 118777-77-8; cationic; emulsifier, conditioner and softener for skin and hair prods.; dk. yel. slight visc. liq., mild typ. odor; water-sol.; sp.gr. 0.99; visc. 600; pH 7.0 (as is), 5.5 (5.0%); 70% NV; 30% propylene glycol.

Katemul IGU-70. [Scher] Isostearamidopropyl dimethyl-amine gluconate; CAS 129541-36-2; emulsifier, condi-tioner and softener for skin and hair prods.; dk. amber visc. liq.; sp.gr. 1.06; visc. 7500; pH 7.0 (as is); 5.5 (5.0%); 70% conc.

Katemul MP. [Scher] Myristamidopropyl dimethylamine phosphate.

Kathon® CG. [Rohm & Haas] 1.15% Methylchloro-isothiazolinone and 0.35% methylisothiazolinone; antimi-crobial, preservative for cosmetics and toiletries; EEC, FDA, and Japan approved; lt. amber clear liq.; mild odor; misc. in water, lower alcohols and glycols; low sol. in hydrocarbons; sp.gr. 1.21; pH 3.5–5.0; 1.5% act. in water and magnesium salts.

Kathon® CG II Biocide. [Rohm & Haas] Methylchloro-isothiazolinone and methylisothiazolinone.

Kaydol® . [Witco/Petroleum Spec.] Wh. min. oil USP; emollient and lubricant in cosmetics and pharmaceuti-cals; also for food processing, agric., chemicals, pkg., plastics, textiles; FDA §172.878, §178.3620a; water-wh., odorless, tasteless; sp.gr. 0.869-0.885; visc. 64-70 cSt (40 C); pour pt. -23 C; flash pt. 216 C.

Kelacid® . [Kelco] Alginic acid; CAS 9005-32-7; EINECS 232-680-1; used as gelling agent, emulsifier and stabilizer in food, pharmaceutical, and industrial applics.; stabilizer in paper and textile industry; wh. fibrous particles; sol. in alkaline sol'n.; swells in water; pH 2.9 (1% aq.); surf. tens. 53 dynes/cm; 7% moisture.

Kelate 220. [Hickson Danchem; Tri-K Industries] Tetrasodium EDTA; CAS 64-02-8; EINECS 200-573-9; chelating agent; wh. spray-dried powd., odorless; sol. 50% in water; sp.gr. 0.6; flash pt. (PMCC) > 200 F; pH 10.5-11.5 (1%); toxicology: dust may irritate nasal/respiratory tract; skin/ temporary eye irritant; ingestion of large amts. may be fatal; 99% min. act.

Kelate Acid. [Tri-K Industries] EDTA; CAS 60-00-4; EINECS 200-449-4; chelating agent.

Kelate CDS. [Tri-K Industries] Calcium disodium EDTA; CAS 62-33-9; EINECS 200-529-9; cosmetic preservative.

Kelate Cu Liq. [Hickson Danchem; Tri-K Industries] Disodium EDTA-copper; CAS 14025-15-1; chelating agent; turquoise blue liq., odorless; completely sol. in water; sp.gr. 1.20; flash pt. (PMCC) > 200 F; pH 5.5-6.5; toxicology: ingestion may cause copper poisoning; temporary eye irritant; 25.5-28.5% EDTA, 5.5-6.1% Cu.

Kelco® HV. [Kelco] Low-calcium sodium alginates; CAS 9005-38-3; used as gelling agent, emulsifier and stabilizer in food, pharmaceutical, and industrial applics.; stabilizer in paper and textile industry; cream fibrous particles; sp.gr. 1.64; dens. 43.38 lb/ft³; visc. 400 cps; ref. index 1.3342; pH 7.2; 9% moisture.

Kelco® LV. [Kelco] Low-calcium sodium alginates; CAS 9005-38-3; used as gelling agent, emulsifier and stabilizer in food, pharmaceutical, and industrial applics.; stabilizer in paper and textile industry; cream fibrous particles; sp.gr. 1.64; dens. 43.38 lb/ft³; visc. 50 cps; ref. index 1.3342; pH 7.2; 9% moisture.

Kelco-Gel® Gellan Gum. [Kelco] Purified gellan gum; high m.w. anionic polysaccharide; gelling agent for use in foods, pet foods, personal care prods., industrial applics.; cream to wh. dry free-flowing powd.; 100% thru 28 mesh.

Kelcoloid® D. [Kelco] Propylene glycol alginate; used as gelling agent, emulsifier and stabilizer in food, pharmaceutical, and industrial applics.; stabilizer in paper and textile industry; cream fibrous particles; sp.gr. 1.46; dens. 33.71 lb/ ft³; visc. 170 cps; ref. index 1.3343; pH 4.4; surf. tens. 58 dynes/cm; 13% max. moisture.

Kelcoloid® DH, DO, DSF. [Kelco] Propylene glycol alginate; used as gelling agent, emulsifier and stabilizer in food, pharmaceutical, and industrial applics.; stabilizer in paper and textile industry; cream agglomerated; sp.gr. 1.46; dens. 33.71 lb/ ft³; visc. 400, 25, 20 cps resp.; ref. index 1.3343; pH 4.0, 4.3, 4.0 resp.; surf. tens. 58 dynes/cm.

Kelcoloid® HVF, LVF, O, S. [Kelco] Propylene glycol alginate; used as gelling agent, emulsifier and stabilizer in food, pharmaceutical, and industrial applics.; stabilizer in paper and textile industry; cream fibrous particles; sp.gr. 1.46; dens. 33.71 lb/ft³; visc. 400, 120, 25, 20 cps resp.; ref. index 1.3343; pH 4.0, 4.0, 4.3, 4.0 resp.; surf. tens. 58 dynes/cm.

Kelcosol® . [Kelco] Algin; CAS 9005-38-3; used as gelling agent, emulsifier and stabilizer in food, pharmaceutical, and industrial applics.; stabilizer in paper and textile industry; cream fibrous particles; water-sol.; sp.gr. 1.64; dens. 43.38 lb/ ft³; visc. 1300 cps; pH 7.2; surf. tens. 70 dynes/cm; 9% moisture.

Kelene 77. [Lowenstein] Sodium dihydroxyethylglycinate and trisodium HEDTA; chelating agent for cosmetics prods. (shampoos, bleaches, colorants, lotions, creams); slight yel. clear liq.; pH 9.5 min.; 41% min. act.

Kelgin® F. [Kelco] Algin, refined; CAS 9005-38-3; used as gelling agent, emulsifier and stabilizer in food, pharmaceutical, and industrial applics.; stabilizer in paper and textile industry; ivory gran. particles; sp.gr. 1.59; dens. 54.62 lb/ ft³; visc. 300 cps; ref. index 1.3343; surf. tens. 62

dynes/cm; 13% moisture.

Kelgin® HV. [Kelco] Algin; CAS 9005-38-3; used as gelling agent, emulsifier and stabilizer in food, pharmaceutical, and industrial applics.; stabilizer in paper and textile industry; ivory gran. particles; sp.gr. 1.59; dens. 54.62 lb/ ft³; visc. 800 cps; ref. index 1.3343; pH 7.5; surf. tens. 62 dynes/cm; 13% moisture.

Kelgin® LV, MV. [Kelco] Algin; CAS 9005-38-3; used as gelling agent, emulsifier and stabilizer in food, pharmaceutical, and industrial applics.; stabilizer in paper and textile industry; ivory gran. particles; sp.gr. 1.59; dens. 54.62 lb/ft³; visc. 60 and 400 cps resp.; ref. index 1.3343; pH 7.5; surf. tens. 62 dynes/cm; 13% moisture.

Kelgin® QL. [Kelco] Treated sodium alginate; CAS 9005-38-3; used as gelling agent, emulsifier and stabilizer in food, pharmaceutical, and industrial applics.; stabilizer in paper and textile industry; improved disp.; ivory gran. particles; visc. 30 cps; pH neutral.

Kelgin® XL. [Kelco] Refined sodium alginate; CAS 9005-38-3; used as gelling agent, emulsifier and stabilizer in food, pharmaceutical, and industrial applics.; stabilizer in paper and textile industry; ivory gran. particles; sp.gr. 1.59; dens. 54.62 lb/ ft³; visc. 30 cps; ref. index 1.3343; pH 7.5; surf. tens. 62 dynes/cm; 13% moisture.

Kelgum CG. [Calgon] Xanthan gum; CAS 11138-66-2; EINECS 234-394-2; gum for cosmetics.

Kelisema Bovine Natural Insoluble Elastin. [Kelisema Srl] Elastin; natural ingred. for cosmetics/pharmaceuticals (soaps, medicinal soaps, dry shampoos, skin masks, skin care foundations, eye shadows); straw-yel. powd., particle size < 0.1 mm; insol. in water.

Kelisema Collagen-CCK Complex. [Kelisema Srl] Macromolecular soluble collagen and potassium cocoate; mild ingred. for medicinal soaps, hand cleansers, detergents for dishwash and laundry soaps.

Kelisema Collagen-IMZ Complex. [Kelisema Srl] Macromolecular soluble collagen and cocoamphoacetate; very mild detergent for sensitive skin, personal hygiene prods., shampoos for damaged hair, detergent tissues.

Kelisema Collagen-LSS Complex. [Kelisema Srl] Macromolecular soluble collagen and sodium lauryl sulfate; mild surfactant, high foam builder for bubble baths, shampoos, liq. soaps.

Kelisema Natural Pure Shea Butter. [Kelisema Srl] Shea butter; CAS 68424-60-2; natural ingred. for skin-protecting treatments and in preps. against dry skin, dermatitis, dermatosis, eczema, solar erythema, burns, and gingivitis.

Kelisema Sodium Hyaluronate Bio. [Kelisema Srl] Sodium hyaluronate; CAS 9067-32-7; natural ingred. for cosmetics/pharmaceuticals.

Kelmar® . [Kelco] Potassium alginate; CAS 9005-36-1; gellant, emulsifier, and stabilizer in food and indust. applic.; gum, bodying agent for creams and lotions, dental impression materials; used for water holding in foods and industry; cream gran. and fibrous particles resp.; watersol.; visc. 270 and 400 cps resp.; pH neutral.

Kelmar® Improved. [Kelco] Potassium alginate; CAS 9005-36-1; gellant, emulsifier, and stabilizer in food and indust. applic.; used for water holding in foods and industry; cream granular particles; visc. 400 cps; pH neutral.

Kelset® . [Kelco] Alginate; used as gelling agent, emulsifier and stabilizer in food, pharmaceutical, and industrial applics.; stabilizer in paper and textile industry; selfgelling gum; lt. ivory fibrous particles; water-sol.; pH neutral.

Keltone. [Kelco] Algin; CAS 9005-38-3; gelling agent, emulsifier and stabilizer in food, pharmaceutical, and industrial applics.

Keltose® . [Kelco] Calcium alginate and ammonium alginate;

gellant, binder, emulsifier, and stabilizer in food and indust. applic.; ivory gran. particles; water-sol.; visc. 250 cps; pH neutral.

Keltrol®. [Kelco] Food-grade xanthan gum; CAS 11138-66-2; EINECS 234-394-2; stabilizer for foods; thickener and emulsion stabilizer in creams and lotions; binder in toothpaste; suspending agent for fruit pulp; cream dry powd.; 80 mesh; water-sol.; swells in glycerin and propylene glycol; sp.gr. 1.5; bulk dens. 52.2 lb/ft³; visc.1400 cps (1% visc. with 1% electrolyte added, LVF, 60 rpm); surf. tens. 75 dynes/cm; pH 7.0; 11% moisture.

Keltrol CG. [Calgon] Xanthan gum; CAS 11138-66-2; EINECS 234-394-2; gum for cosmetics.

Keltrol CG 1000. [Calgon] Xanthan gum; CAS 11138-66-2; EINECS 234-394-2; gum for cosmetics.

Keltrol CG BT. [Calgon] Xanthan gum; CAS 11138-66-2; EINECS 234-394-2; gum for cosmetics.

Keltrol CG F. [Calgon] Xanthan gum; CAS 11138-66-2; EINECS 234-394-2; gum for cosmetics.

Keltrol CG GM. [Calgon] Xanthan gum; CAS 11138-66-2; EINECS 234-394-2; gum for cosmetics.

Keltrol CG RD. [Calgon] Xanthan gum; CAS 11138-66-2; EINECS 234-394-2; gum for cosmetics.

Keltrol CG SF. [Calgon] Xanthan gum; CAS 11138-66-2; EINECS 234-394-2; gum for cosmetics.

Keltrol CG T. [Calgon] Xanthan gum; CAS 11138-66-2; EINECS 234-394-2; gum for cosmetics.

Keltrol CG TF. [Calgon] Xanthan gum; CAS 11138-66-2; EINECS 234-394-2; gum for cosmetics.

Keltrol® F. [Kelco] Food-grade xanthan gum; CAS 11138-66-2; EINECS 234-394-2; stabilizer for foods; thickener and emulsion stabilizer in creams and lotions; binder in toothpaste; suspending agent for fruit pulp; cream dry powd.; 200 mesh size; water-sol.; swells in glycerin and propylene glycol; sp.gr. 1.5; bulk dens. 52.2 lb/ft³; visc.1400 cps (1% visc. with 1% electrolyte added, LVF, 60 rpm); surf. tens. 75 dynes/cm; pH 7.0; 11% moisture.

Kemamide® S-65. [Witco/H-I-P] Tallow amide.

Kemamide® W-35. [Witco/H-I-P] Ethylene distearamide; CAS 110-30-5; EINECS 203-755-6; emollient, solubilizer for cosmetics.

Kemamide® W-42. [Witco/H-I-P] Ethylene distearamide; CAS 110-30-5; EINECS 203-755-6; emollient, solubilizer for cosmetics.

Kemamine® BQ-2982B. [Witco/H-I-P] Erucalkonium chloride; CAS 90730-68-0.

Kemamine® BQ-6502C. [Witco/H-I-P] Benzalkonium chloride.

Kemamine® BQ-9701C. [Witco/H-I-P] Dihydrog. tallow benzylmonium chloride.

Kemamine® P-650. [Witco/H-I-P] Cocamine; CAS 61788-46-3; EINECS 262-977-1; emulsifier.

Kemamine® P-690. [Witco/H-I-P] Lauramine; CAS 124-22-1; EINECS 204-690-6; personal care surfactant.

Kemamine® P-890. [Witco/H-I-P] Palmitamine; CAS 143-27-1; EINECS 205-596-8; emulsifier.

Kemamine® P-974. [Witco/H-I-P] Tallow amine; CAS 61790-33-8; EINECS 263-125-1; emulsifier.

Kemamine® P-989. [Witco/H-I-P] Oleamine; CAS 112-90-3; EINECS 204-015-5; emulsifier.

Kemamine® P-997. [Witco/H-I-P] Soyamine; CAS 61790-18-9; EINECS 263-112-0; emulsifier.

Kemamine® Q-1902C. [Witco/H-I-P] Dibehenyl/diarachidyl dimonium chloride; cationic; germicide, sanitizer, slimicide, antistat, textile softening agent, dyeing aid, corrosion inhibitor, emulsifier; Gardner 4 max. solid; m.w. 680; disp. in water; pH 9 max (5%); 75% act.

Kemamine® Q-1902X. [Witco/H-I-P] Dibehenyl/diarachidyl dimonium chloride.

Kemamine® Q-6503B. [Witco/H-I-P] Cocotrimonium chloride; CAS 61789-18-2; EINECS 263-038-9; surfactant.

Kemamine® Q-6902C. [Witco/H-I-P] Dilauryldimonium chloride; CAS 3401-74-9; EINECS 222-274-2.

Kemamine® Q-6903B. [Witco/H-I-P] Laurtrimonium chloride; CAS 112-00-5; EINECS 203-927-0; emulsifier.

Kemamine® Q-7903B. [Witco/H-I-P] Myristalkonium chloride; CAS 139-08-2; EINECS 205-352-0; antimicrobial.

Kemamine® Q-9703B. [Witco/H-I-P] Tallowtrimonium chloride; CAS 8030-78-2; EINECS 232-447-4; cosmetic ingred.

Kemamine® Q-9902C. [Witco/H-I-P] Distearyldimonium chloride; CAS 107-64-2; EINECS 203-508-2; conditioner for cosmetics.

Kemamine® Q-9903B. [Witco/H-I-P] Steartrimonium chloride; CAS 112-03-8; EINECS 203-929-1; hair conditioner base.

Kemamine® Q-9973B. [Witco/H-I-P] Soytrimonium chloride; CAS 61790-41-8; EINECS 263-134-0; emulsifier.

Kemamine® T-2801. [Witco/H-I-P] Dibehenyl methylamine; CAS 61372-91-6; EINECS 262-740-2.

Kemamine® T-2802D. [Witco/H-I-P] Dimethyl behenamine; CAS 215-42-9; emulsifier, conditioner for cosmetics.

Kemamine® T-6502. [Witco/H-I-P] Dimethyl cocamine; CAS 61788-93-0; EINECS 263-020-0; surfactant intermediate.

Kemamine® T-6902. [Witco/H-I-P] Dimethyl lauramine; CAS 112-18-5; EINECS 203-943-8; surfactant intermediate.

Kemamine® T-7902. [Witco/H-I-P] Dimethyl myristamine; CAS 112-75-4; EINECS 204-002-4; surfactant intermediate.

Kemamine® T-8902. [Witco/H-I-P] Dimethyl palmitamine; CAS 112-69-6; EINECS 203-997-2; surfactant intermediate.

Kemamine® T-9701. [Witco/H-I-P] Dihydrog. tallow methylamine; CAS 61788-63-4; EINECS 262-991-8; cationic; chemical intermediate for quat. ammonium derivs. used for cosmetics and textiles; acid scavenger in petrol. prods.; epoxy hardener, catalyst in mfg. of flexible PU foams; corrosion inhibitor; gasoline additive; Gardner 3 max. liq.; 95% conc.

Kemamine® T-9702. [Witco/H-I-P] Dimethyl hydrog. tallowamine; CAS 61788-95-2; EINECS 263-022-1; cosmetic raw material.

Kemamine® T-9742. [Witco/H-I-P] Dimethyl tallowamine; CAS 68814-69-7.

Kemamine® T-9902. [Witco/H-I-P] Dimethyl stearamine; CAS 124-28-7; EINECS 204-694-8; intermediate for quats. used in cosmetics and textiles; acid scavenger in petrol. prods.; Gardner 1 max. color; 95% min. tert. amine.

Kemamine® T-9972. [Witco/H-I-P] Dimethyl soyamine; CAS 61788-91-8; EINECS 263-017-4; surfactant intermediate.

Kemester® 115. [Witco/H-I-P] Methyl oleate; CAS 112-62-9; EINECS 203-992-5; detergent intermediate.

Kemester® 1000. [Witco/H-I-P] Triolein; CAS 122-32-7; EINECS 204-534-7; nonionic; emollient used in cosmetics, textiles, leather, metalworking lubricants; base for sulfation; Gardner 6 max. liq.; m.p. -8 C; acid no. 5 max.; iodine no. 85-90; sapon. no. 190–198; 100% conc.

Kemester® 1418. [Witco/H-I-P] Myristyl stearate; CAS 17661-50-6; EINECS 241-640-2; emollient for cosmetics/pharmaceuticals.

Kemester® 2000. [Witco/H-I-P] Glycerol oleate; CAS 111-03-5; nonionic; emollient, emulsifier, stabilizer, wetting agent for textiles, personal care prods.; Gardner 6 max. liq.; m.p. 25 C; acid no. 3 max.; iodine no. 73-83; sapon. no. 160–175; 100% conc.

Kemester® 3681. [Witco/H-I-P] Dioctyl dimer dilinoleate; lubricant for crankcase, turbine, compressor, gear, and metalworking formulations; also cosmetic emollient, pearling and bodying agent; Gardner 10 max.; visc. 12.5 cSt (100 C); pour pt. –40 C; acid no. 3.0 max.; flash pt.

(COC) 310 C .

Kemester® 3684. [Witco/H-I-P] Ditridecyl dimer dilinoleate; CAS 16958-92-2; EINECS 241-029-0; cosmetic emollient.

Kemester® 4000. [Witco/H-I-P] Butyl oleate; CAS 142-77-8; EINECS 205-559-6; nonionic; emollient, wetting agent; plasticizer for textiles, leathers, elastomers, personal care prods.; Gardner 2 max. liq.; m.p. 2 C; acid no. 2 max.; iodine no. 72-81; sapon. no. 164–172; 100% conc.

Kemester® 5220. [Witco/H-I-P] Glycol stearate; CAS 111-60-4; EINECS 203-886-9; emulsifier, opacifier, pearlescent for cosmetics.

Kemester® 5221. [Witco/H-I-P] PEG-2 stearate; CAS 106-11-6; EINECS 203-363-5; emulsifier.

Kemester® 5221SE. [Witco/H-I-P] PEG-2 stearate SE; CAS 9004-99-3; anionic; emollient, emulsifier, plasticizer, lubricant for cosmetics, rubber, textiles; Gardner 3 max. flake; m.p. 46–56 C; acid no. 95–105; iodine no. 3 max.; sapon. no. 163–178; 100% conc.

Kemester® 5410. [Witco/H-I-P] Butyl stearate; CAS 123-95-5; EINECS 204-666-5; emollient.

Kemester® 5415. [Witco/H-I-P] Isobutyl stearate; CAS 646-13-9; EINECS 211-466-1; emollient, lubricant for textiles, metalworking fluids, personal care prods.; Gardner < 1 liq.; m.p. 21 C; acid no. 4 max.; iodine no. 1 max.; sapon. no. 170–176.

Kemester® 5500. [Witco/H-I-P] Glyceryl stearate; nonionic; emollient, emulsifier; stabilizer, plasticizer, lubricant for cosmetic, paper, textile, and industrial uses; Gardner 3 max. bead, flake; m.p. 56–60 C; acid no. 3 max.; iodine no. 0.5 max.; sapon. no. 164–177; 100% conc.

Kemester® 5510. [Witco/H-I-P] Butyl stearate; CAS 123-95-5; EINECS 204-666-5; emollient for cosmetics; lubricant, plasticizer; Gardner < 1 max. color; m.p. 23 C; acid no. 2 max.; iodine no. 1 max.; sapon. no. 170–176.

Kemester® 5654. [Witco/H-I-P] Ditridecyl adipate; lubricant for crankcase, turbine, compressor, gear, and metalworking formulations; also cosmetic emollient, pearling and bodying agent; Gardner 2 liq.; f.p. –50 C; acid no. 0.1 max.

Kemester® 5721. [Witco/H-I-P] Tridecyl stearate; CAS 31556-45-3; EINECS 250-696-7; emollient, dye carrier, textile lubricant, cosmetics/pharmaceuticals; Gardner 1 max. color; m.p. 8 C; acid no. 2 max.; iodine no. 4 max.; sapon. no. 117–126.

Kemester® 5822. [Witco/H-I-P] Isocetyl stearate; CAS 25339-09-7; EINECS 246-868-6; emollient, plasticizer for cosmetics; Gardner 1 max. color; m.p. 0 C; acid no. 2 max.; iodine no. 4 max.; sapon. no. 102–114.

Kemester® 6000. [Witco/H-I-P] Glyceryl stearate; nonionic; cosmetic and industrial emulsifier, emollient; plasticizer for elastomers; Gardner 3 max. bead; m.p. 57–60 C; acid no. 3 max.; iodine no. 2 max.; sapon. no. 162–176; 100% conc.

Kemester® 6000SE. [Witco/H-I-P] Glyceryl stearate SE; anionic; emulsifier, emollient, lubricant, plasticizer for cosmetic, paper and textiles; Gardner 3 max. beads; m.p. 56–61 C; acid no. 10 max.; iodine no. 3 max.; sapon. no. 140–156; 100% conc.

Kemester® 7018. [Witco/H-I-P] Methyl stearate; CAS 112-61-8; EINECS 203-990-4; detergent intermediate.

Kemester® 8002. [Witco/H-I-P] Methyl oleate; CAS 112-62-9; EINECS 203-992-5; detergent intermediate.

Kemester® 9012. [Witco/H-I-P] Methyl laurate; CAS 111-82-0; EINECS 203-911-3; detergent intermediate.

Kemester® 9014. [Witco/H-I-P] Methyl myristate; CAS 124-10-7; EINECS 204-680-1; detergent intermediate.

Kemester® 9016. [Witco/H-I-P] Methyl palmitate; CAS 112-39-0; EINECS 203-966-3; chemical intermediate.

Kemester® 9718. [Witco/H-I-P] Methyl stearate; CAS 112-61-8; EINECS 203-990-4; detergent intermediate.

Kemester® BE. [Witco/H-I-P] Behenyl erucate; CAS 18312-32-8; EINECS 242-201-8; industrial lubricant, cosmetic emollient; Gardner 1 solid; m.p. 40–44 C; acid no. 1; iodine no. 50 max.; sapon. no. 80–95.

Kemester® CP. [Witco/H-I-P] Cetyl palmitate; CAS 540-10-3; EINECS 208-736-6; industrial lubricant, cosmetic emollient; wh. solid; m.p. 46-53 C; acid no. 1.

Kemester® DMP. [Witco/H-I-P] Dimethyl phthalate; CAS 131-11-3; EINECS 205-011-6; emollient used in cosmetics; textiles, metalworking lubricants; APHA 10 max. color; m.p. 1 C; acid no. 0.1 max.

Kemester® EE. [Witco/H-I-P] Erucyl erucate; CAS 27640-89-7; EINECS 248-587-4; industrial lubricant, cosmetic emollient; Gardner 2 liq. (@ ambient temp.); acid no. 1.

Kemester® EGDL. [Witco/H-I-P] Glycol dilaurate; CAS 624-04-4; EINECS 210-827-0; emollient for cosmetics/pharmaceuticals.

Kemester® EGDS. [Witco/H-I-P] Glycol distearate; CAS 627-83-8; EINECS 211-014-3; intermediate in prod. of superamides, in metalworking lubricants, specialized solv.; industrial lubricant; opacifier, pearling additive, thickener for cosmetics and pharmaceuticals; Gardner 2 max. solid; m.p. 60-63 C; acid no. 6 max.; iodine no. 1 max.; sapon. no. 190-200; 100% conc.

Kemester® EGMS. [Witco/H-I-P] Glycol stearate; CAS 111-60-4; EINECS 203-886-9; intermediate in prod. of superamides, in metalworking lubricants, specialized solv.; industrial lubricant; opacifier, pearling additive, thickener for cosmetics and pharmaceuticals; Gardner 1 solid; m.p. 56–60 C; acid no. 1; iodine no. 1 max.; sapon. no. 179-195.

Kemester® GDL. [Witco/H-I-P] Glyceryl dilaurate; CAS 27638-00-2; EINECS 248-586-9; emollient for cosmetics/ pharmaceuticals.

Kemester® HMS. [Witco/H-I-P] Homosalate; CAS 118-56-9; EINECS 204-260-8; uv absorber; sunscreen agent; used in cosmetic skin preps.; clear liq.; sp.gr. 1.049-1.053; ref. index 1.516-1.519; 99% min. purity.

Kemester® MM. [Witco/H-I-P] Myristyl myristate; CAS 3234-85-3; EINECS 221-787-9; lubricant for crankcase, turbine, compressor, gear, and metalworking formulations; also cosmetic emollient, pearling and bodying agent; wh. m.p. 38-40 C; acid no. 1.

Kemester® S20. [Witco/H-I-P] Sorbitan laurate; for cosmetics/pharmaceuticals.

Kemester® S40. [Witco/H-I-P] Sorbitan palmitate; CAS 26266-57-9; EINECS 247-568-8; for cosmetics/pharmaceuticals.

Kemester® S60. [Witco/H-I-P] Sorbitan stearate; CAS 1338-41-6; EINECS 215-664-9; for cosmetics/pharmaceuticals.

Kemester® S65. [Witco/H-I-P] Sorbitan tristearate; CAS 26658-19-5; EINECS 247-891-4; for cosmetics/pharmaceuticals.

Kemester® S80. [Witco/H-I-P] Sorbitan oleate; CAS 1338-43-8; EINECS 215-665-4; for cosmetics/pharmaceuticals.

Kemester® S85. [Witco/H-I-P] Sorbitan trioleate; CAS 26266-58-0; EINECS 247-569-3; for cosmetics/pharmaceuticals.

Kemstrene® 96.0% USP. [Witco/H-I-P] Refined glycerin USP; CAS 56-81-5; EINECS 200-289-5; humectant, solv.; used in cosmetics, liq. soaps, confections, inks, and lubricants; intermediate used in polyester and PU formulations; sp.gr. 1.25165 min; 96.0% purity.

Kemstrene® 99.7% USP. [Witco/H-I-P] Refined glycerin USP; CAS 56-81-5; EINECS 200-289-5; humectant, solv.; used in cosmetics, liq. soaps, confections, inks, and lubricants; intermediate used in polyester and PU formulations; sp.gr. 1.26124; 99.7% purity.

Ken-React® KR TTS. [Kenrich Petrochemicals] Isopropyl titanium triisostearate; CAS 61417-49-0; EINECS 262-774-8.

Kerabiol. [Laserson SA] Keratin amino acids; CAS 68238-35-7; improves appearance and stimulates hair growth; amber clear liq.; water-sol.; usage level: 15%.

Kerafix 620. [Variati] Ethoxydiglycol, hydrolyzed corn protein, and PVP.

Keramino™ 20. [Brooks Industries] Keratin amino acids; CAS 68238-35-7; protein conditioner.

Keramino™ 25. [Brooks Industries] Keratin amino acids; CAS 68238-35-7; cosmetics ingred.; liq.; m.w. 200; 25% act.

Keramino™ SD. [Brooks Industries] Keratin amino acids and sodium chloride; protein for cosmetics formulations; powd.; m.w. 200; 50% act.

Keramois L. [Ikeda] Hydrolyzed keratin; CAS 69430-36-0; EINECS 274-001-1; protects and restores hair from damage during permanent wave treatment, bleaching, and dyeing; also for hair shampoos; amber clear liq.; sp.gr. 1.030-1.130; pH 6.5-8.5.

Kerapro S. [Proalan SA] Hydrolyzed keratin; CAS 69430-36-0; EINECS 274-001-1; cosmetic protein.

Keraquat HK. [Innovachem; Tri-K Industries] Cocodimonium hydroxypropyl hydrolyzed hair keratin; CAS 68915-25-3; cationic; substantive quaternary conditioner for hair care prods.; amber clear liq.; misc. with water; sp.gr. 1.1; b.p. 215 F; pH 6.0-7.5 (10% aq.); toxicology: LD50 (rat) > 2 g/ kg; ingestion may cause abdominal upset; mild ocular irritant; not a primary skin irritant; 22-28% NV.

Kera-Quat WKP. [Maybrook] Cocodimonium hydroxypropyl hydrolyzed keratin; CAS 68915-25-3; substantive protein, moisturizer for hair and skin care prods. (shampoos, conditioners, styling prods., liq. hand soaps, creams, lotions); amber clear liq., char. odor; pH 5.0-6.0 (10% aq.); 30-36% nonvolatiles.

Kerasol. [Croda Inc.] Hydrolyzed keratin and sodium chloride; proteinic conditioner for hair and nail care prods.; slightly hazy amber liq., char. odor; m.w. 125,000; sol. in water; pH 5–7; usage level: 1-10%; 15% act. aq. sol'n.

Kera-Tein 1000. [Maybrook] Hydrolyzed keratin; CAS 69430-36-0; EINECS 274-001-1; moisturizer for skin and hair care prods.; protective colloid effect; provides cystine to hair, minimizing damage from harsh treatments; low ash, low odor; amber clear liq., char. odor; pH 5.5-7.0; 30% min. solids.

Kera-Tein 1000 AS. [Maybrook] Hydrolyzed keratin, ethyl ester; cationic; substantive protein forming moisture-retentive films; anti-irritant; plasticizer for hair styling resins; used for hair care (conditioners, mousses), skin care (skin and shave balms, toners, masks); amber clear liq., char. ethanolic odor; sol. in alcohol; pH 3.0-5.0 (5% aq.); 20% min. solids in ethanol.

Kera-Tein 1000 RM/50. [Maybrook] Hydrolyzed keratin; CAS 69430-36-0; EINECS 274-001-1; moisture-binding protein reducing irritancy, increasing tens. str. and protecting hair, and resulting in a more hydrated and elastic skin surface; for hair care (shampoos, conditioners, mousses, bleaches, permanent waves) and skin care (moisturizers, creams, lotions, bath preps.); dark clear to sl. hazy liq., char. odor; pH 5.0-7.0; 48-52% solids.

Kera-Tein 1000 RM SD. [Maybrook] Hydrolyzed keratin; CAS 69430-36-0; EINECS 274-001-1; moisture-binding protein reducing irritancy, increasing tens. str. and protecting hair, and resulting in a more hydrated and elastic skin surface; for hair care (shampoos, conditioners, mousses, bleaches, permanent waves) and skin care (moisturizers, creams, lotions, bath preps.); pale cream powd., sl. char. odor; pH 5.0-7.0 (10% aq.); 8% max. moisture.

Kera-Tein 1000 SD. [Maybrook] Hydrolyzed keratin; CAS 69430-36-0; EINECS 274-001-1; substantive protein with protective colloid and anti-irritant effect; moisturizer for skin and hair care prods. (shampoos, conditioners, mousses, waving preps., creams and lotions); pale cream free-flowing powd., sl. char. odor; pH 5.0-7.0 (10% aq.); 8% max. moisture.

Kera-Tein AA. [Maybrook] Keratin amino acids; CAS 68238-35-7; substantive/protective protein, penetrant, moisturizer for skin and hair care prods.; source of cystine; dark amber clear to sl. hazy liq., char. amino acid odor; pH 5.0-7.0; 25% min. solids.

Kera-Tein AA-SD. [Maybrook] Keratin amino acids; CAS 68238-35-1; moisturizer for skin and hair care prods. (shampoos, conditioners, styling prods., skin care creams/lotions, liq. soaps, bubble baths); esp. suitable for treating hair damaged due to permanent waving and bleaching; pale cream powd., char. odor; pH 3.5-5.5 (10% aq.); very hygroscopic; 93% min. solids.

Kera-Tein H. [Maybrook] Keratin amino acids and sodium chloride; cosmetics ingred.

Kera-Tein V. [Maybrook] Hydrolyzed keratin derived from wool; CAS 69430-36-0; EINECS 274-001-1; substantive protein, film-former, moisture-binder for hair and skin care prods.; reduces split ends, increases flexibility and tens. str., improves shine, and provides protective colloid effect on hair; esp. suitable for perming processes; amber clear to sl. hazy liq., char. odor; pH 6.0-7.5; 20% min. solids.

Kera-Tein W. [Maybrook] Keratin amino acids and hydrolyzed keratin derived from wool; substantive protein for skin and hair care prods.

Keratin P. [Provital; Centerchem] Hydrolyzed keratin; CAS 69430-36-0; EINECS 274-001-1; cosmetic protein.

Keratin S. [Provital; Centerchem] Hydrolyzed keratin; CAS 69430-36-0; EINECS 274-001-1; cosmetic protein.

Keratine Hydrolysate H.T.K. [Solabia] Hydrolyzed keratin; CAS 69430-36-0; EINECS 274-001-1; cosmetic protein.

Keratin Hydrolysate. [Shin-Etsu Silicones] Hydrolyzed keratin; CAS 69430-36-0; EINECS 274-001-1; cosmetic protein.

Keratolan. [Laboratoires Sérobiologiques] Hydrolyzed keratin and glycerin.

Keratoplast. [Vevy] Isodecyl salicylate.

Kessco® 653. [Stepan; Stepan Canada] Cetyl palmitate; CAS 540-10-3; EINECS 208-736-6; nonionic; syn. spermaceti wax, emollient, thickener, visc. booster for pharmaceutical and cosmetic creams and lotions; base material for cosmetic stick prods.; w/o emulsifier, lubricant for metalworking fluids; wh. flakes; sol. in boiling alcohol, ether, chloroform, other waxes, oils, hydrocarbons; insol. in water; m.p. 51–55 C; acid no. 2.0 max.; sapon. no. 109–117.

Kessco® 3283. [Stepan] Propylene glycol soyate; CAS 67784-79-6; EINECS 267-054-7.

Kessco BE. [Akzo BV] Behenyl erucate; CAS 18312-32-8; EINECS 242-201-8; emollient.

Kessco CP. [Akzo BV] Cetyl palmitate; CAS 540-10-3; EINECS 208-736-6; nonionic; replaces native spermaceti in cosmetics and pharmaceuticals; flakes.

Kessco® DCA. [Stepan] Dicapryl adipate; CAS 105-97-5; EINECS 203-349-9; cosmetic ester.

Kessco DEHS. [Akzo BV] Dioctyl sebacate; CAS 122-62-3; EINECS 204-558-8; emollient.

Kessco DHS. [Akzo BV] Octyl hydroxystearate; CAS 29383-26-4; emollient.

Kessco DO. [Akzo BV] Decyl oleate; CAS 3687-46-5; EINECS 222-981-6; emollient.

Kessco® EGAS. [Stepan; Stepan Canada] Glyceryl stearate, stearamide AMP; nonionic; pearlescent, bodying agent, emulsion stabilizer for shampoos, liq. hand soaps;

imparts soft, smooth skin feel to formulations; wh. to cream flakes; m.p. 56-59 C; acid no. 5.0 max.; iodine no. 0.5 max.; sapon. no. 174-184.

Kessco EGMS. [Akzo BV] Glycol stearate; CAS 111-60-4; EINECS 203-886-9; emulsifier, opacifier, pearlescent for cosmetics.

Kessco EHP. [Akzo BV] Octyl palmitate; CAS 29806-73-3; EINECS 249-862-1; emollient.

Kessco EO. [Akzo BV] Ethyl oleate; CAS 111-62-6; EINECS 203-889-5; emollient.

Kessco® GDS 386F. [Stepan; Stepan Canada] Glyceryl distearate; CAS 1323-83-7; EINECS 215-359-0; emulsifier, opacifier, bodying agent; waxy flake; 100% conc.

Kessco GMN. [Akzo BV] Glyceryl myristate; CAS 589-68-4; cosmetic emulsifier.

Kessco GMO. [Akzo BV] Glyceryl oleate.

Kessco GMS. [Akzo BV] Glyceryl stearate; nonionic; bodying agent, emulsifier, and thickener in o/w emulsions; flakes.

Kessco GTM. [Akzo BV] Triheptanoin.

Kessco ICS. [Akzo BV] Isocetyl stearate; CAS 25339-09-7; EINECS 246-868-6; emollient for makeup formulations.

Kessco IPS. [Akzo BV] Isopropyl stearate; CAS 112-10-7; EINECS 203-934-9; emollient.

Kessco OE. [Akzo BV] Oleyl erucate; CAS 17673-56-2; EINECS 241-654-9; emollient.

Kessco® PEG 200 DL. [Stepan; Stepan Canada] PEG-4 dilaurate; CAS 9005-02-1; emulsifier, thickener, solubilizer, emollient, opacifier, spreading agent, wetting agent, dispersant for cosmetics (creams/lotions, makeup, bath oils, shampoos, conditioners, sunscreens), pharmaceuticals (ointments, suppositories), food, agric., plastics, etc.; lubricant, emollient, softener for textile and metalworking applics.; lt. yel. liq.; sol. in IPA, acetone, CCl_4, ethyl acetate, toluol, IPM, wh. oil; water-disp.; sp.gr. 0.951; dens. 7.9 lb/gal; f.p. < 9C; HLB 5.9; acid no. 10.0 max.; iodine no. 9.0; sapon. no. 176–186; flash pt. (COC) 460 F; fire pt. 510 F; 100% act.

Kessco® PEG 200 DO. [Stepan; Stepan Canada] PEG-4 dioleate; CAS 9005-07-6; nonionic; emulsifier, thickener, solubilizer, emollient, opacifier, spreading agent, wetting agent, dispersant for cosmetics (creams/lotions, makeup, bath oils, shampoos, conditioners, sunscreens), pharmaceuticals (ointments, suppositories), food, agric., plastics, etc.; lt. amber liq.; f.p. < –15 C; sol. in naptha, kerosene, IPA, acetone, CCl_4, ethyl acetate, toluol, IPM, peanut oil, wh. oil; water-disp.; sp.gr. 0.942; dens. 7.9 lb/gal; HLB 6.0; acid no. 10.0 max; sapon. no. 148–158; pH 5.0 (3%); flash pt. (COC) 545 F.

Kessco® PEG 200 DS. [Stepan; Stepan Canada] PEG-4 distearate; CAS 9005-08-7; nonionic; emulsifier, thickener, solubilizer, emollient, opacifier, spreading agent, wetting agent, dispersant for cosmetics (creams/lotions, makeup, bath oils, shampoos, conditioners, sunscreens), pharmaceuticals (ointments, suppositories), food, agric., plastics, etc.; wh. to cream soft solid; sol. in naptha, kerosene, IPA, acetone, CCl_4, ethyl acetate, toluol, IPM, peanut oil, wh. oil; water-disp.; sp.gr. 0.9060 (65 C); HLB 5.0; m.p. 34 C; acid no. 10.0 max.; sapon. no. 153–162; pH 5.0 (3%); flash pt. (COC) 475 F.

Kessco® PEG 200 ML. [Stepan; Stepan Canada] PEG-4 laurate; CAS 9004-81-3; nonionic; emulsifier, thickener, solubilizer, emollient, opacifier, spreading agent, wetting agent, dispersant for cosmetics (creams/lotions, makeup, bath oils, shampoos, conditioners, sunscreens), pharmaceuticals (ointments, suppositories), food, agric., plastics, etc.; lt. yel. liq.; f.p. < 5 C; sol. in IPA, acetone, CCl_4, ethyl acetate, toluol, IPM, water-disp.; sp.gr. 0.985; dens. 8.2 lb/gal; HLB 9.8; acid no. 5.0 max.; sapon. no. 132–142; pH 4.5; flash pt. (COC) 385 F.

Kessco® PEG 200 MO. [Stepan; Stepan Canada] PEG-4

oleate; CAS 9004-96-0; EINECS 233-293-0; nonionic; emulsifier, thickener, solubilizer, emollient, opacifier, spreading agent, wetting agent, dispersant for cosmetics (creams/lotions, makeup, bath oils, shampoos, conditioners, sunscreens), pharmaceuticals (ointments, suppositories), food, agric., plastics, etc.; lt. amber liq.; f.p. < –15 C; sol. in IPA, acetone, CCl_4, ethyl acetate, toluol, water-disp.; sp.gr. 0.973; dens. 8.1 lb/gal; HLB 8.0; acid no. 5.0 max.; sapon. no. 115–124; pH 5.0; flash pt. (COC) 395 F.

Kessco® PEG 200 MS. [Stepan; Stepan Canada] PEG-4 stearate; CAS 9004-99-3; EINECS 203-358-8; nonionic; emulsifier, thickener, solubilizer, emollient, opacifier, spreading agent, wetting agent, dispersant for cosmetics (creams/lotions, makeup, bath oils, shampoos, conditioners, sunscreens), pharmaceuticals (ointments, suppositories), food, agric., plastics, etc.; wh. to cream soft solid; sol. in IPA, acetone, CCl_4, ethyl acetate, toluol, IPM, peanut oil; water-disp.; sp.gr. 0.9360 (65 C); HLB 7.9; m.p. 31 C; acid no. 5.0 max.; sapon. no. 120–129; flash pt. (COC) 410 F.

Kessco® PEG 300 DL. [Stepan; Stepan Canada] PEG-6 dilaurate; CAS 9005-02-1; nonionic; emulsifier, thickener, solubilizer, emollient, opacifier, spreading agent, wetting agent, dispersant for cosmetics (creams/lotions, makeup, bath oils, shampoos, conditioners, sunscreens), pharmaceuticals (ointments, suppositories), food, agric., plastics, etc.; lt. yel. liq.; f.p. < 13 C; sol. in naptha, IPA, acetone, toluol, IPM; water-disp.; sp.gr. 0.975; dens. 8.1 lb/gal; HLB 9.8; acid no. 10.0 max.; sapon. no. 148–158; flash pt. (COC) 475 F.

Kessco® PEG 300 DO. [Stepan; Stepan Canada] PEG-6 dioleate; CAS 9005-07-6; nonionic; emulsifier, thickener, solubilizer, emollient, opacifier, spreading agent, wetting agent, dispersant for cosmetics (creams/lotions, makeup, bath oils, shampoos, conditioners, sunscreens), pharmaceuticals (ointments, suppositories), food, agric., plastics, etc.; lt. amber liq.; f.p. < –5 C; sol. in IPA, acetone, CCl_4, ethyl acetate, toluol, IPM, peanut oil; water-disp.; sp.gr. 0.962; dens. 8.0 lb/gal; HLB 7.2; acid no. 10.0 max.; sapon. no. 128–137; pH 5.0; flash pt. (COC) 510 F.

Kessco® PEG 300 DS. [Stepan; Stepan Canada] PEG-6 distearate; CAS 9005-08-7; nonionic; emulsifier, thickener, solubilizer, emollient, opacifier, spreading agent, wetting agent, dispersant for cosmetics (creams/lotions, makeup, bath oils, shampoos, conditioners, sunscreens), pharmaceuticals (ointments, suppositories), food, agric., plastics, etc.; wh. to cream soft solid; sol. in naptha, kerosene, IPA, acetone, CCl_4, ethyl acetate, toluol, IPM, peanut oil, wh. oil; water-disp.; HLB 6.5; m.p. 32 C; acid no. 10.0 max.; sapon. no. 130–139; pH 5.0.

Kessco® PEG 300 ML. [Stepan; Stepan Canada] PEG-6 laurate; CAS 9004-81-3; EINECS 219-136-9; nonionic; emulsifier, thickener, solubilizer, emollient, opacifier, spreading agent, wetting agent, dispersant for cosmetics (creams/lotions, makeup, bath oils, shampoos, conditioners, sunscreens), pharmaceuticals (ointments, suppositories), food, agric., plastics, etc.; lt. yel. liq.; f.p. < 8C; sol. in IPA, acetone, CCl_4, ethyl acetate, toluol; water-disp.; sp.gr. 1.011; dens. 8.4 lb/gal; HLB 11.4; acid no. 5.0 max.; sapon. no. 104–114; pH 4.5; flash pt. (COC) 445 F.

Kessco® PEG 300 MO. [Stepan; Stepan Canada] PEG-6 oleate; CAS 9004-96-0; nonionic; emulsifier, thickener, solubilizer, emollient, opacifier, spreading agent, wetting agent, dispersant for cosmetics (creams/lotions, makeup, bath oils, shampoos, conditioners, sunscreens), pharmaceuticals (ointments, suppositories), food, agric., plastics, etc.; lt. amber liq.; f.p. < –5 C; sol. in IPA, acetone, CCl_4, ethyl acetate, toluol; water-disp.; sp.gr. 0.998; dens. 8.3 lb/gal; HLB 9.6; acid no. 5.0 max.; sapon. no. 94–102; pH 5.0 (3% disp.); flash pt. (COC) 450 F.

Kessco® PEG 300 MS. [Stepan; Stepan Canada] PEG-6 stearate; CAS 9004-99-3; nonionic; emulsifier, thickener, solubilizer, emollient, opacifier, spreading agent, wetting agent, dispersant for cosmetics (creams/lotions, makeup, bath oils, shampoos, conditioners, sunscreens), pharmaceuticals (ointments, suppositories), food, agric., plastics, etc.; wh. to cream soft solid; sol. in IPA, acetone, CCl₄, ethyl acetate, toluol, IPM, peanut oil; water-disp.; sp.gr. 0.9660 (65 C); HLB 9.7; m.p. 28 C; acid no. 5.0 max.; sapon. no. 97–105; pH 5.0 (3% disp.); flash pt. (COC) 475 F.

Kessco® PEG 400 DL. [Stepan; Stepan Canada] PEG-8 dilaurate; CAS 9005-02-1; nonionic; emulsifier, thickener, solubilizer, emollient, opacifier, spreading agent, wetting agent, dispersant for cosmetics (creams/lotions, makeup, bath oils, shampoos, conditioners, sunscreens), pharmaceuticals (ointments, suppositories), food, agric., plastics, etc.; lt. yel. liq.; f.p. 18 C; sol. in naptha, IPA, acetone, CCl₄, ethyl acetate, toluol, IPM, peanut oil; water-disp.; sp.gr. 0.990; dens. 8.3 lb/gal; HLB 9.8; acid no. 10.0 max.; sapon. no. 127–137; flash pt. (COC) 480 F.

Kessco® PEG 400 DO. [Stepan; Stepan Canada] PEG-8 dioleate; CAS 9005-07-6; nonionic; emulsifier, thickener, solubilizer, emollient, opacifier, spreading agent, wetting agent, dispersant for cosmetics (creams/lotions, makeup, bath oils, shampoos, conditioners, sunscreens), pharmaceuticals (ointments, suppositories), food, agric., plastics, etc.; lt. amber liq.; f.p. < 7 C; sol. in naptha, IPA, acetone, CCl₄, ethyl acetate, toluol, IPM, peanut oil; water-disp.; sp.gr. 0.977; dens. 8.1 lb/gal; HLB 8.5; acid no. 10.0 max.; sapon. no. 113–122; pH 5.0; flash pt. (COC) 520 F.

Kessco PEG-400 DS-356. [Stepan] PEG-8 distearate; CAS 9005-08-7; personal care surfactant.

Kessco® PEG 400 DS. [Stepan; Stepan Canada] PEG-8 distearate; CAS 9005-08-7; emulsifier, thickener, solubilizer, emollient, opacifier, spreading agent, wetting agent, dispersant for cosmetics (creams/lotions, makeup, bath oils, shampoos, conditioners, sunscreens), pharmaceuticals (ointments, suppositories), food, agric., plastics, etc.; lubricant, emulsifier, softener for textile and metalworking applics.; wh. to cream soft solid; sol. in naptha, IPA, acetone, CCl₄, ethyl acetate, toluol, IPM, peanut oil, wh. oil; water-disp; sp.gr. 0.9390 (65 C); HLB 8.5; m.p. 36 C; acid no. 10.0 max.; sapon. no. 115–124; pH 5.0 (3% disp.); flash pt. (COC) 500 F; 100% act.

Kessco® PEG 400 ML. [Stepan; Stepan Canada] PEG-8 laurate; CAS 9004-81-3; nonionic; emulsifier, thickener, solubilizer, emollient, opacifier, spreading agent, wetting agent, dispersant for cosmetics (creams/lotions, makeup, bath oils, shampoos, conditioners, sunscreens), pharmaceuticals (ointments, suppositories), food, agric., plastics, etc.; lt. yel. liq.; f.p. 12 C; sol. in water, IPA, acetone, CCl₄, ethyl acetate, toluol; sp.gr. 1.028; dens. 8.6 lb/gal; HLB 13.1; acid no. 5.0 max.; sapon. no. 86–96; flash pt. (COC) 475 F.

Kessco® PEG 400 MO. [Stepan; Stepan Canada] PEG-8 oleate; CAS 9004-96-0; nonionic; emulsifier, thickener, solubilizer, emollient, opacifier, spreading agent, wetting agent, dispersant for cosmetics (creams/lotions, makeup, bath oils, shampoos, conditioners, sunscreens), pharmaceuticals (ointments, suppositories), food, agric., plastics, etc.; lt. amber liq.; f.p. < 10 C; sol. in IPA, acetone, CCl₄, ethyl acetate, toluol; water-disp.; sp.gr. 1.013; dens. 8.4 lb/gal; HLB 11.4; acid no. 5.0 max.; sapon. no. 80–89; pH 5.0 (3% disp.); flash pt. (COC) 510 F.

Kessco® PEG 400 MS. [Stepan; Stepan Canada] PEG-8 stearate; CAS 9004-99-3; nonionic; emulsifier, thickener, solubilizer, emollient, opacifier, spreading agent, wetting agent, dispersant for cosmetics (creams/lotions, makeup, bath oils, shampoos, conditioners, pharma-

ceuticals (ointments, suppositories), food, agric., plastics, etc.; wh. to cream soft solid; sol. in IPA, acetone, CCl₄, ethyl acetate, toluol; water-disp.; sp.gr. 0.9780 (65 C); HLB 11.6; m.p. 32 C; acid no. 5.0 max.; sapon. no. 83–92; pH 5.0 (3% disp.); flash pt. (COC) 480 F.

Kessco® PEG 600 DL. [Stepan; Stepan Canada] PEG-12 dilaurate; CAS 9005-02-1; emulsifier, thickener, solubilizer, emollient, opacifier, spreading agent, wetting agent, dispersant for cosmetics (creams/lotions, makeup, bath oils, shampoos, conditioners, sunscreens), pharmaceuticals (ointments, suppositories), food, agric., plastics, etc.; lubricant, emulsifier, softener for textile and metalworking applics.; liq.; sol. in IPA, acetone, CCl₄, ethyl acetate, toluol, IPM; water-disp.; sp.gr. 0.9820 (65 C); f.p. 24 C; HLB 11.7; acid no. 10.0 max.; sapon. no. 102–112; flash pt. (COC) 465 F; 100% act.

Kessco® PEG 600 DO. [Stepan; Stepan Canada] PEG-12 dioleate; CAS 9005-07-6; nonionic; emulsifier, thickener, solubilizer, emollient, opacifier, spreading agent, wetting agent, dispersant for cosmetics (creams/lotions, makeup, bath oils, shampoos, conditioners, sunscreens), pharmaceuticals (ointments, suppositories), food, agric., plastics, etc.; lt. amber liq.; f.p. 19 C; sol. in IPA, acetone, CCl₄, ethyl acetate, toluol, IPM, peanut oil; water-disp.; sp.gr. 1.001; dens. 8.3 lb/gal; HLB 10.5; acid no. 10.0 max.; sapon. no. 92–102; pH 5.0 (3% disp.); flash pt. (COC) 495 F.

Kessco® PEG 600 DS. [Stepan; Stepan Canada] PEG-12 distearate; CAS 9005-08-7; emulsifier, thickener, solubilizer, emollient, opacifier, spreading agent, wetting agent, dispersant for cosmetics (creams/lotions, makeup, bath oils, shampoos, conditioners, sunscreens), pharmaceuticals (ointments, suppositories), food, agric., plastics, etc.; lubricant, emulsifier, softener for textile and metalworking applics.; wh. to cream soft solid; sol. in IPA, acetone, CCl₄, ethyl acetate, toluol, IPM, peanut oil; water-disp.; sp.gr. 0.9670 (65 C); HLB 10.7; m.p. 39 C; acid no. 10.0 max.; sapon. no. 93–102; pH 5.0 (3% disp.); flash pt. (COC) 490 F; 100% act.

Kessco® PEG 600 ML. [Stepan; Stepan Canada] PEG-12 laurate; CAS 9004-81-3; emulsifier, thickener, solubilizer, emollient, opacifier, spreading agent, wetting agent, dispersant for cosmetics (creams/lotions, makeup, bath oils, shampoos, conditioners, sunscreens), pharmaceuticals (ointments, suppositories), food, agric., plastics, etc.; lubricant, emulsifier, softener for textile and metalworking applics.; lt. yel. liq.; sol. in water, Na₂SO₄, IPA, acetone, CCl₄, ethyl acetate, toluol; sp.gr. 1.050; dens. 8.8 lb/gal; f.p. 23 C; HLB 14.6; acid no. 5.0 max.; sapon. no. 64–74; flash pt. (COC) 475 F; 100% act.

Kessco® PEG 600 MO. [Stepan; Stepan Canada] PEG-12 oleate; CAS 9004-96-0; nonionic; emulsifier, thickener, solubilizer, emollient, opacifier, spreading agent, wetting agent, dispersant for cosmetics (creams/lotions, makeup, bath oils, shampoos, conditioners, sunscreens), pharmaceuticals (ointments, suppositories), food, agric., plastics, etc.; lt. amber liq.; f.p. 23 C; sol. in water, IPA, acetone, CCl₄, ethyl acetate, toluol; sp.gr. 1.037; dens. 8.7 lb/gal; HLB 13.5; acid no. 5.0 max.; sapon. no. 60–69; pH 5.0 (3% disp.); flash pt. (COC) 525 F.

Kessco® PEG 600 MS. [Stepan; Stepan Canada] PEG-12 stearate; CAS 9004-99-3; nonionic; emulsifier, thickener, solubilizer, emollient, opacifier, spreading agent, wetting agent, dispersant for cosmetics (creams/lotions, makeup, bath oils, shampoos, conditioners, sunscreens), pharmaceuticals (ointments, suppositories), food, agric., plastics, etc.; wh. to cream soft solid; sol. in water, IPA, acetone, CCl₄, ethyl acetate, toluol; sp.gr. 1.000 (65 C); HLB 13.6; m.p. 37 C; acid no. 5.0 max.; sapon. no. 61–70; pH 5.0 (3% disp.); flash pt. (COC) 480 F.

Kessco® PEG 1000 DL. [Stepan; Stepan Canada] PEG-20 dilaurate; CAS 9005-02-1; nonionic; emulsifier, thickener, solubilizer, emollient, opacifier, spreading agent, wetting agent, dispersant for cosmetics (creams/lotions, makeup, bath oils, shampoos, conditioners, sunscreens), pharmaceuticals (ointments, suppositories), food, agric., plastics, etc.; cream soft solid; f.p. 38 C; sol. in water, IPA, acetone, CCl_4, ethyl acetate; toluol, IPM; sp.gr. 1.015 (65 C); HLB 14.5; acid no. 10.0 max.; sapon. no. 68–78; flash pt. 475 (COC).

Kessco® PEG 1000 DO. [Stepan; Stepan Canada] PEG-20 dioleate; CAS 9005-07-6; nonionic; emulsifier, thickener, solubilizer, emollient, opacifier, spreading agent, wetting agent, dispersant for cosmetics (creams/lotions, makeup, bath oils, shampoos, conditioners, sunscreens), pharmaceuticals (ointments, suppositories), food, agric., plastics, etc.; cream soft solid; f.p. 37 C; sol. in water, IPA, acetone, CCl_4, ethyl acetate, toluol; sp.gr. 1.005 (65 C); HLB 13.1; acid no. 10.0 max.; sapon. no. 64–74; pH 5.0 (3% disp.); flash pt. (COC) 505 F.

Kessco® PEG 1000 DS. [Stepan; Stepan Canada] PEG-20 distearate; CAS 9005-08-7; nonionic; emulsifier, thickener, solubilizer, emollient, opacifier, spreading agent, wetting agent, dispersant for cosmetics (creams/lotions, makeup, bath oils, shampoos, conditioners, sunscreens), pharmaceuticals (ointments, suppositories), food, agric., plastics, etc.; cream wax; sol. in water, IPA, acetone, CCl_4, ethyl acetate, toluol; sp.gr. 1.005 (65 C); HLB 12.3; m.p. 40 C; acid no. 10.0 max.; sapon. no. 65–74; pH 5.0 (3% disp.); flash pt. (COC) 485 F.

Kessco® PEG 1000 ML. [Stepan; Stepan Canada] PEG-20 laurate; CAS 9004-81-3; nonionic; emulsifier, thickener, solubilizer, emollient, opacifier, spreading agent, wetting agent, dispersant for cosmetics (creams/lotions, makeup, bath oils, shampoos, conditioners, sunscreens), pharmaceuticals (ointments, suppositories), food, agric., plastics, etc.; cream soft solid; f.p. 40 C; sol. in water, propylene glycol (hot), Na_2SO_4, IPA, acetone, CCl_4, ethyl acetate, toluol; sp.gr. 1.035 (65 C); HLB 16.5; acid no. 5.0 max.; sapon. no. 41–51; flash pt. (COC) 490.

Kessco® PEG 1000 MO. [Stepan; Stepan Canada] PEG-20 oleate; CAS 9004-96-0; nonionic; emulsifier, thickener, solubilizer, emollient, opacifier, spreading agent, wetting agent, dispersant for cosmetics (creams/lotions, makeup, bath oils, shampoos, conditioners, sunscreens), pharmaceuticals (ointments, suppositories), food, agric., plastics, etc.; cream soft solid; f.p. 39 C; sol. in water, Na_2SO_4 (5%), IPA, acetone, CCl_4, ethyl acetate, toluol; sp.gr. 1.035 (65 C); HLB 15.4; acid no. 5.0 max.; sapon. no. 40–49; pH 5.0; flash pt. (COC) 515 F.

Kessco® PEG 1000 MS. [Stepan; Stepan Canada] PEG-20 stearate; CAS 9004-99-3; nonionic; emulsifier, thickener, solubilizer, emollient, opacifier, spreading agent, wetting agent, dispersant for cosmetics (creams/lotions, makeup, bath oils, shampoos, conditioners, sunscreens), pharmaceuticals (ointments, suppositories), food, agric., plastics, etc.; cream wax; sol. in water, Na_2SO_4 (5%), IPA, acetone, CCl_4, ethyl acetate, toluol; sp.gr. 1.030 (65 C); HLB 15.6; m.p. 41 C; acid no. 5.0 max.; sapon. no. 40–48; pH 5.0 (3% disp.); flash pt. (COC) 475 F.

Kessco® PEG 1540 DL. [Stepan; Stepan Canada] PEG-32 dilaurate; CAS 9005-02-1; nonionic; emulsifier, thickener, solubilizer, emollient, opacifier, spreading agent, wetting agent, dispersant for cosmetics (creams/lotions, makeup, bath oils, shampoos, conditioners, sunscreens), pharmaceuticals (ointments, suppositories), food, agric., plastics, etc.; cream wax; f.p. 42 C; sol. in water, Na_2SO_4 (5%); hot in propylene glycol, IPA, acetone, CCl_4, ethyl acetate, toluol; sp.gr. 1.04 (65 C); HLB 15.7; acid no. 10.0 max.; sapon. no. 48–56; pH 4.5 (3% disp.); flash pt. (COC)

450 F.

Kessco® PEG 1540 DO. [Stepan; Stepan Canada] PEG-32 dioleate; CAS 9005-07-6; nonionic; emulsifier, thickener, solubilizer, emollient, opacifier, spreading agent, wetting agent, dispersant for cosmetics (creams/lotions, makeup, bath oils, shampoos, conditioners, sunscreens), pharmaceuticals (ointments, suppositories), food, agric., plastics, etc.; cream wax; f.p. 44 C; sol. in water, propylene glycol, Na_2SO_4; hot in IPA, acetone, CCl_4, ethyl acetate, toluol; sp.gr. 1.025 (65 C); HLB 15.0; acid no. 10.0 max.; sapon. no. 45–55; pH 5.0 (3% disp.); flash pt. (COC) 480 F.

Kessco® PEG 1540 DS. [Stepan; Stepan Canada] PEG-32 distearate; CAS 9005-08-7; nonionic; emulsifier, thickener, solubilizer, emollient, opacifier, spreading agent, wetting agent, dispersant for cosmetics (creams/lotions, makeup, bath oils, shampoos, conditioners, sunscreens), pharmaceuticals (ointments, suppositories), food, agric., plastics, etc.; cream wax; sol. in water, IPA, acetone, CCl_4, ethyl acetate, toluol; sp.gr. 1.015 (65 C); HLB 14,8; m.p. 45 C; acid no. 10.0 max.; sapon. no. 49–58; pH 5.0; flash pt. (COC) 490 F.

Kessco® PEG 1540 ML. [Stepan; Stepan Canada] PEG-32 laurate; CAS 9004-81-3; nonionic; emulsifier, thickener, solubilizer, emollient, opacifier, spreading agent, wetting agent, dispersant for cosmetics (creams/lotions, makeup, bath oils, shampoos, conditioners, sunscreens), pharmaceuticals (ointments, suppositories), food, agric., plastics, etc.; cream wax; f.p. 46 C; sol. in water, Na_2SO_4 (5%); sol. hot in propylene glycol, IPA, acetone, CCl_4, ethyl acetate, toluol; sp.gr. 1.06 (65 C); HLB 17.6; acid no. 5.0 max.; sapon. no. 26–36; pH 4.5 (3% disp.); flash pt. (COC) 445 F.

Kessco® PEG 1540 MO. [Stepan; Stepan Canada] PEG-32 oleate; CAS 9004-96-0; nonionic; emulsifier, thickener, solubilizer, emollient, opacifier, spreading agent, wetting agent, dispersant for cosmetics (creams/lotions, makeup, bath oils, shampoos, conditioners, sunscreens), pharmaceuticals (ointments, suppositories), food, agric., plastics, etc.; cream wax; f.p. 45 C; sol. in water, propylene glycol, Na_2SO_4; sol. hot in IPA, acetone, CCl_4, ethyl acetate, toluol; sp.gr. 1.050 (65 C); HLB 17.0; f.p. 47 C; acid no. 5.0 max.; sapon. no. 28–37; pH 5.0 (3% disp.); flash pt. (COC) 520 F.

Kessco® PEG 1540 MS. [Stepan; Stepan Canada] PEG-32 stearate; CAS 9004-99-3; nonionic; emulsifier, thickener, solubilizer, emollient, opacifier, spreading agent, wetting agent, dispersant for cosmetics (creams/lotions, makeup, bath oils, shampoos, conditioners, sunscreens), pharmaceuticals (ointments, suppositories), food, agric., plastics, etc.; cream wax; sol. in water, Na_2SO_4 (5%), IPA, acetone, CCl_4, ethyl acetate, toluol; sp.gr. 1.050 (65 C); HLB 17.3; m.p. 47 C; acid no. 5.0 max.; sapon. no. 27–36; pH 5.0; flash pt. (COC) 485 F.

Kessco® PEG 4000 DL. [Stepan; Stepan Canada] PEG-75 dilaurate; CAS 9005-02-1; nonionic; emulsifier, thickener, solubilizer, emollient, opacifier, spreading agent, wetting agent, dispersant for cosmetics (creams/lotions, makeup, bath oils, shampoos, conditioners, sunscreens), pharmaceuticals (ointments, suppositories), food, agric., plastics, etc.; cream wax; f.p. 52 C; sol. in water, Na_2SO_4 (5%); sol. hot in propylene glycol, IPA, acetone, CCl_4, ethyl acetate, toluol; sp.gr. 1.065 (65 C); HLB 17.6; acid no. 5.0 max.; sapon. no. 20–30; pH 4.5 (3% disp.); flash pt. (COC) 495 F.

Kessco® PEG 4000 DO. [Stepan; Stepan Canada] PEG-75 dioleate; CAS 9005-07-6; nonionic; emulsifier, thickener, solubilizer, emollient, opacifier, spreading agent, wetting agent, dispersant for cosmetics (creams/lotions, makeup, bath oils, shampoos, conditioners, sunscreens), pharmaceuticals (ointments, suppositories), food, agric., plastics, etc.; cream wax; f.p. 49 C; sol. in water, propylene glycol, Na_2SO_4; sol. hot in IPA, acetone, CCl_4, ethyl acetate, toluol; sp.gr. 1.060 (65 C); HLB 17.8; acid no. 5.0 max.; sapon. no. 19–27; pH 5.0; flash pt. (COC) 500 F.

Kessco® PEG 4000 DS. [Stepan; Stepan Canada] PEG-75 distearate; CAS 9005-08-7; nonionic; emulsifier, thickener, solubilizer, emollient, opacifier, spreading agent, wetting agent, dispersant for cosmetics (creams/lotions, makeup, bath oils, shampoos, conditioners, sunscreens), pharmaceuticals (ointments, suppositories), food, agric., plastics, etc.; cream wax; sol. in water, Na_2SO_4 (5%), IPA, acetone, CCl_4, ethyl acetate, toluol; sp.gr. 1.060 (65 C); HLB 17.3; m.p. 51 C; acid no. 5.0 max.; sapon. no. 19–27; pH 5.0 (3% disp.); flash pt. (COC) 515 F.

Kessco® PEG 4000 ML. [Stepan; Stepan Canada] PEG-75 laurate; CAS 9004-81-3; nonionic; emulsifier, thickener, solubilizer, emollient, opacifier, spreading agent, wetting agent, dispersant for cosmetics (creams/lotions, makeup, bath oils, shampoos, conditioners, sunscreens), pharmaceuticals (ointments, suppositories), food, agric., plastics, etc.; cream wax; f.p. 55 C; sol. in water, Na_2SO_4 (5%); sol. hot in propylene glycol, IPA, acetone, CCl_4, ethyl acetate, toluol; sp.gr. 1.075 (65 C); HLB 18.8; acid no. 5.0 max.; sapon. no. 9–18; pH 4.5; flash pt. (COC) 515 F.

Kessco® PEG 4000 MO. [Stepan; Stepan Canada] PEG-75 oleate; CAS 9004-96-0; nonionic; emulsifier, thickener, solubilizer, emollient, opacifier, spreading agent, wetting agent, dispersant for cosmetics (creams/lotions, makeup, bath oils, shampoos, conditioners, sunscreens), pharmaceuticals (ointments, suppositories), food, agric., plastics, etc.; cream wax; f.p. 55 C; sol. in water, propylene glycol, Na_2SO_4; sol. hot in IPA, acetone, CCl_4, ethyl acetate, toluol; sp.gr. 1.075 (65 C); HLB 18.3; acid no. 5.0 max.; sapon. no. 10–18; pH 5.0; flash pt. (COC) 495 F.

Kessco® PEG 4000 MS. [Stepan; Stepan Canada] PEG-75 stearate; CAS 9004-99-3; nonionic; emulsifier, thickener, solubilizer, emollient, opacifier, spreading agent, wetting agent, dispersant for cosmetics (creams/lotions, makeup, bath oils, shampoos, conditioners, sunscreens), pharmaceuticals (ointments, suppositories), food, agric., plastics, etc.; cream wax; sol. in water, Na_2SO_4 (5%), IPA, acetone, CCl_4, ethyl acetate, toluol; sp.gr. 1.075 (64 C); HLB 18.6; m.p. 56 C; acid no. 5.0 max.; sapon. no. 10–18; pH 5.0; flash pt. (COC) 465 F.

Kessco® PEG 6000 DL. [Stepan; Stepan Canada] PEG-150 dilaurate; CAS 9005-02-1; nonionic; emulsifier, thickener, solubilizer, emollient, opacifier, spreading agent, wetting agent, dispersant for cosmetics (creams/lotions, makeup, bath oils, shampoos, conditioners, sunscreens), pharmaceuticals (ointments, suppositories), food, agric., plastics, etc.; cream wax; f.p. 57 C; sol. in water, Na_2SO_4 (5%); sol. hot in propylene glycol, IPA, acetone, CCl_4, ethyl acetate, toluol; sp.gr. 1.077 (65 C); HLB 18.7; m.p. 56 C; acid no. 9.0 max.; sapon. no. 12–20; pH 4.5 (3% disp.); flash pt. (COC) 435 F.

Kessco® PEG 6000 DO. [Stepan; Stepan Canada] PEG-150 dioleate; CAS 9005-07-6; nonionic; emulsifier, thickener, solubilizer, emollient, opacifier, spreading agent, wetting agent, dispersant for cosmetics (creams/lotions, makeup, bath oils, shampoos, conditioners, sunscreens), pharmaceuticals (ointments, suppositories), food, agric., plastics, etc.; cream wax; f.p. 56 C; sol. in water, propylene glycol, Na_2SO_4 (5%); sol. hot in IPA, acetone, CCl_4, ethyl acetate, toluol; sp.gr. 1.070 (65 C); HLB 18.3; acid no. 9.0 max.; sapon. no. 13–21; pH 5.0 (3% disp.); flash pt. 500 F.

Kessco PEG 6000DS. [Akzo BV] PEG-150 distearate; CAS 9005-08-7; nonionic; thickener for mild shampoos; flakes.

Kessco® PEG 6000 DS. [Stepan; Stepan Canada] PEG-150 distearate; CAS 9005-08-7; emulsifier, thickener, solubilizer, emollient, opacifier, spreading agent, wetting agent,

dispersant for cosmetics (creams/lotions, makeup, bath oils, shampoos, conditioners, sunscreens), pharmaceuticals (ointments, suppositories), food, agric., plastics, etc.; lubricant, emulsifier, softener for textile and metalworking applics.; cream wax; sol. in propylene glycol, Na_2SO_4 (5%), IPA, acetone, CCl_4, ethyl acetate, toluol; sp.gr. 1.075 (65 C); HLB 18.4; m.p. 55 C; acid no. 9.0 max.; sapon. no. 14–20; pH 5.0 (3% disp.); flash pt. (COC) 475 F; 100% act.

Kessco® PEG 6000 ML. [Stepan; Stepan Canada] PEG-150 laurate; CAS 9004-81-3; nonionic; emulsifier, thickener, solubilizer, emollient, opacifier, spreading agent, wetting agent, dispersant for cosmetics (creams/lotions, makeup, bath oils, shampoos, conditioners, sunscreens), pharmaceuticals (ointments, suppositories), food, agric., plastics, etc.; cream wax; f.p. 61 C; sol. in water, Na_2SO_4 (5%); sol. hot in propylene glycol, IPA, acetone, CCl_4, ethyl acetate, toluol; sp.gr. 1.085 (65 C); HLB 19.2; acid no. 5.0 max.; sapon. no. 7–13; pH 4.5.

Kessco® PEG 6000 MO. [Stepan; Stepan Canada] PEG-150 oleate; CAS 9004-96-0; nonionic; emulsifier, thickener, solubilizer, emollient, opacifier, spreading agent, wetting agent, dispersant for cosmetics (creams/lotions, makeup, bath oils, shampoos, conditioners, sunscreens), pharmaceuticals (ointments, suppositories), food, agric., plastics, etc.; cream wax; f.p. 59 C; sol. in water, propylene glycol, Na_2SO_4 (5%); sol. hot in IPA, acetone, CCl_4, ethyl acetate, toluol; sp.gr. 1.085 (65 C); HLB 19.0; acid no. 5.0 max.; sapon. no. 7–13; pH 5.0; flash pt. 470 F.

Kessco® PEG 6000 MS. [Stepan; Stepan Canada] PEG-150 stearate; CAS 9004-99-3; nonionic; emulsifier, thickener, solubilizer, emollient, opacifier, spreading agent, wetting agent, dispersant for cosmetics (creams/lotions, makeup, bath oils, shampoos, conditioners, sunscreens), pharmaceuticals (ointments, suppositories), food, agric., plastics, etc.; cream wax; sol. in water, propylene glycol, Na_2SO_4 (5%), IPA, acetone, CCl_4, ethyl acetate, toluol; sp.gr. 1.080 (65 C); HLB 18.8; m.p. 61 C; acid no. 5.0 max.; sapon. no. 7–13; pH 5.0 (3% disp.); flash pt. (COC) 480 F.

Kessco® PGML-X533. [Stepan] Propylene glycol laurate; CAS 142-55-2; EINECS 205-542-3; emollient, emulsifier.

Kessco PGMS. [Akzo BV] Propylene glycol stearate; CAS 1323-39-3; EINECS 215-354-3; nonionic; solubilizer for Eosin dyes in lipsticks; bodying agent in emulsions; flakes.

Kessco PGMS-8615. [Stepan] Propylene glycol stearate SE.

Kessco PGMS-R. [Stepan] Propylene glycol stearate; CAS 1323-39-3; EINECS 215-354-3; personal care surfactant.

Kessco PGMS-X174. [Stepan] Propylene glycol stearate SE.

Kessco PGMS-X534F. [Stepan] Propylene glycol stearate; CAS 1323-39-3; EINECS 215-354-3; personal care surfactant.

Kessco PGNM. [Akzo BV] Propylene glycol myristate; CAS 29059-24-3; EINECS 249-395-3; personal care surfactant.

Kessco PTIS. [Akzo BV] Pentaerythrityl tetraisostearate.

Kessco PTS. [Akzo BV] Pentaerythrityl tetrastearate; CAS 115-83-3; EINECS 204-110-1; emollient, lubricant.

Kessco® Butyl Stearate. [Stepan] Butyl stearate; CAS 123-95-5; EINECS 204-666-5; emollient.

Kessco® Diethylene Glycol Monostearate. [Stepan] PEG-2 stearate; CAS 106-11-6; EINECS 203-363-5; emulsifier.

Kessco® Diglycol Laurate A Neutral. [Stepan] PEG-2 laurate; CAS 141-20-8; EINECS 205-468-1; emulsifier.

Kessco® Diglycol Laurate ASE. [Stepan] PEG-2 laurate; CAS 141-20-8; EINECS 205-468-1; emulsifier.

Kessco® Diglycol Laurate N. [Stepan] PEG-2 laurate; CAS

141-20-8; EINECS 205-468-1; emulsifier.

Kessco® Diglycol Laurate N-Syn. [Stepan] PEG-2 laurate; CAS 141-20-8; EINECS 205-468-1; emulsifier.

Kessco® Diglycol Laurate SE. [Stepan] PEG-2 laurate SE; emulsifier.

Kessco® Diglycol Oleate L-SE. [Stepan] PEG-2 oleate SE; personal care surfactant.

Kessco® Diglycol Stearate. [Stepan] PEG-2 stearate and stearic acid.

Kessco® Diglycol Stearate Neutral. [Stepan] PEG-2 stearate; CAS 106-11-6; EINECS 203-363-5; emulsifier.

Kessco® Diglycol Stearate SE [Stepan] PEG-2 stearate SE and stearic acid.

Kessco® Ethylene Glycol Distearate. [Stepan; Stepan Canada] Glycol distearate; CAS 627-83-8; EINECS 211-014-3; pearlescent, emollient, emulsifier for personal care prods.; wh. to off-wh. flakes, typ. mild fatty odor; insol. in water; sol. in IPA, min. oil, peanut oil; m.p. 60-63 C; HLB 1.5; acid no. 15 max.; iodine no. 0.5 max.; sapon. no. 191-199; flash pt. (COC) 390 F; 100% conc.

Kessco® Ethylene Glycol Monostearate. [Stepan; Stepan Canada] Glycol stearate; CAS 111-60-4; EINECS 203-886-9; pearlescent, bodying agent, emulsion stabilizer for shampoos, liq. hand soaps; wh. flakes, typ. mild fatty odor; insol. in water; sol. in IPA, min. oil, peanut oil; m.p. 56-60 C; HLB 2.9; acid no. 2 max.; iodine no. 0.5 max.; sapon. no. 180-188; 100% conc.

Kessco® Glycerol Dilaurate. [Stepan; Stepan Canada] Glyceryl dilaurate; CAS 27638-00-2; EINECS 248-586-9; nonionic; emulsifier, emollient for free-flowing cosmetic lotions and creams; cream-colored solid, typ. mild fatty odor; insol. in water; partly sol. in peanut oil; sol. in IPA, min. oil; m.p. 28-32 C; HLB 4.0; acid no. 5 max.; iodine no. 6 max.; sapon. no. 219-229; flash pt. (COC) 480 F; 100% conc.

Kessco® Glycerol Dioleate. [Stepan] Glyceryl dioleate; CAS 25637-84-7; EINECS 247-144-2; emulsifier, emollient.

Kessco® Glycerol Distearate 386F. [Stepan; Stepan Canada] Glyceryl distearate; CAS 1323-83-7; EINECS 215-359-0; food-grade emulsifier for pharmaceutical use; wh. to off-wh. waxy flake, typ. mild fatty odor; insol. in water; sol. in IPA, min. oil; partly sol. in peanut oil; m.p. 56-59 C; HLB 2.4; acid no. 5.0 max.; sapon. no. 182-188; flash pt. (COC) 450 F; 100% conc.

Kessco® Glycerol Monolaurate. [Stepan] Glyceryl laurate; CAS 142-18-7; EINECS 205-526-6; cosmetic emulsifier.

Kessco® Glycerol Monoleate. [Stepan; Stepan Canada] Glyceryl oleate; CAS 111-03-5; w/o emulsifier, emollient, slip aid, spreading agent, pigment dispersant for bath oil, makeup, vanishing and moisturizing creams; lubricant for textiles, metalworking compds.; sperm oil replacement; dk. amber liq., typ. mild fatty odor; insol. in water; sol. in IPA, min. oil, peanut oil; m.p. 20 C; HLB 3.8; acid no. 3.0 max.; sapon. no. 166-174; flash pt. (COC) 435 F; 100% act.

Kessco® Glycerol Monostearate SE. [Stepan; Stepan Canada] Glyceryl stearate SE; anionic; primary emulsifier for use in o/w emulsions at pH 5-9; anionic modified for broader emulsification props.; cream flakes, typ. mild fatty odor; disp. in water; sol. in min. oil, peanut oil; partly sol. in IPA; m.p. 56.5-59.5 C; acid no. 20 max.; iodine no. 1 max.; sapon. no. 152-162; flash pt. (COC) 400 F; 100% conc.

Kessco® Glycerol Monostearate SE, Acid Stable [Stepan; Stepan Canada] Glyceryl stearate, PEG-100 stearate; nonionic; emulsifier, self-emulsifying cream base, hair and skin conditioner; for use at pH 3-5; nonionic modified for broader emulsification props.; provides good electrolyte stability in creme rinses and antiperspirants; wh. to

cream flakes, typ. mild fatty odor; sol. in IPA, min. oil; partly sol. in peanut oil; disp. in water; m.p. 54-58 C; HLB 11.2; acid no. 3.0 max.; sapon. no. 95-103; flash pt. (COC) 460 F; 100% conc.

Kessco® Glyceryl Monostearate Pure. [Stepan; Stepan Canada] Glyceryl stearate; emollient, emulsifier, opacifier, bodying agent for cosmetic creams, lotions, antiperspirants, hair care prods., and sunscreens and pharmaceutical topical creams, lotions, and ointments; lubricant for textiles, metalworking compds.; wh. flakes, typ. mild fatty odor; insol. in water; sol. in IPA, min. oil; partly sol. in peanut oil; m.p. 56.5-58.5 C; HLB 3.8; acid no. 3.0; iodine no. 0.5 max.; sapon. no. 168-176; flash pt. (COC) 410 F; 100% act.

Kessco® Isobutyl Stearate. [Stepan; Stepan Canada] Isobutyl stearate; CAS 646-13-9; EINECS 211-466-1; lubricant for textiles, metalworking compds.; slip aid, wetting agent for pigments; emollient used in lipsticks, bath oils, nail polish and removers, skin cleaners, creams, lotions; APHA 35 max. clear liq., typ. mild fatty odor; insol. in water; sol. in IPA, min. oil, peanut oil; sp.gr. 0.850-0.854; f.p. 15 C; b.p. 200 C (4 mm); acid no. 1 max.; iodine no. 1 max.; sapon. no. 170-180; flash pt. (COC) 360 F; ref. index 1.441; 100% act.

Kessco® Isocetyl Stearate. [Stepan; Stepan Canada] Isocetyl stearate; CAS 25339-09-7; EINECS 246-868-6; emollient with very dry, velvety feel for makeup formulations; industrial fiber lubricant; APHA 100 max. clear liq., typ. mild fatty odor; insol. in water; sol. in IPA, min. oil, peanut oil; sp.gr. 0.853-0.859; f.p. 0 C; acid no. 2 max.; iodine no. 2 max.; sapon. no. 110-118; flash pt. (COC) 450 F; ref. index 1.452; 100% act.

Kessco® Isopropyl Myristate. [Stepan; Stepan Canada] Isopropyl myristate; CAS 110-27-0; EINECS 203-751-4; biodeg. replacement for min. oil; used as lubricants in textile spin finish, coning oils, carding, dye bath; emollient, solubilizer, vehicle, solv. for makeup, shaving preps., bath oils, hair preps., highly pigmented prods.; APHA 20 max. clear liq., pract. odorless; insol. in water; sol. in IPA, min. oil, peanut oil; f.p. -3 C; m.p. -3 C; b.p. 162.5 C; acid no. 1 max.; iodine no. 1 max.; sapon. no. 204-212; flash pt. (COC) 305 F; ref. index 1.433; 100% act.

Kessco® Isopropyl Myristate NF. [Stepan] Isopropyl myristate; CAS 110-27-0; EINECS 203-751-4; emollient.

Kessco® Isopropyl Palmitate. [Stepan; Stepan Canada] Isopropyl palmitate; CAS 142-91-6; EINECS 205-571-1; biodeg. replacement for min. oil; used as lubricants in textile spin finish, coning oils, carding, dye bath; emollient, solubilizer, vehicle, solv. for makeup, shaving preps., bath oils, hair preps., highly pigmented prods.; APHA 20 max. clear liq., pract. odorless; insol. in water; sol. in IPA, min. oil, peanut oil; sp.gr. 0.849-0.855; f.p. 13 C; b.p. 172 C (4 mm); acid no. 1 max.; iodine no. 1 max.; sapon. no. 185-191; flash pt. (COC) 323 F; ref. index 1.437; 100% act.

Kessco® Octyl Isononanoate. [Stepan] Octyl isononanoate; CAS 71566-49-9; EINECS 275-637-2; emollient with dry, nonoily skin feel for creams, lotions, makeup, lipsticks; antitack agent in antiperspirants; plasticizer for hair spray resins; APHA 20 max. clear liq., typ. mild fatty odor; insol. in water; sol. in IPA, min. oil, peanut oil; sp.gr. 0.853-0.859; f.p. -30 C; acid no. 1 max.; iodine no. 1 max.; sapon. no. 202-210; flash pt. (COC) 260 F; ref. index 1.434.

Kessco® Octyl Palmitate. [Stepan; Stepan Canada] Octyl palmitate; CAS 29806-73-3; EINECS 249-862-1; biodeg. replacement for min. oil; used as lubricants in textile spin finish, coning oils, carding, dye bath; gloss aid, emollient for stick makeup, hair grooms, creams, lotions, suntan preps., bath oils; binder for pressed powds.; APHA 25 max. clear liq., typ. mild fatty odor; insol. in water; sol. in

IPA, min. oil, peanut oil; sp.gr. 0.850-0.858; ; f.p. 0 C; acid no. 3 max.; iodine no. 1 max.; sapon. no. 146-156; flash pt. (COC) 395 F; ref. index 1.4453; 100% act.

Kessco® Propylene Glycol Monolaurate E. [Stepan; Stepan Canada] Propylene glycol laurate; CAS 142-55-2; EINECS 205-542-3; emollient and aux. emulsifier imparting soft, velvety skin feel to cosmetic prods.; off-wh. clear liq., typ. mild fatty odor; insol. in water; sol. in IPA, min. oil, peanut oil; m.p. 8-12 C; HLB 3.2; acid no. 3.0 max.; iodine no. 1.0 max.; sapon. no. 231-241; flash pt. (COC) 370 F; 100% conc.

Kessco® Propylene Glycol Monostearate Pure. [Stepan; Stepan Canada] Propylene glycol stearate; CAS 1323-39-3; EINECS 215-354-3; aux. emulsifier and opacifier with m.p. near body temp.; used in suppositories, lipsticks, and sunscreens; wh. to off-wh. flakes, typ. mild fatty odor; insol. in water; sol. in IPa, min. oil, peanut oil; m.p. 33.5-38.5 C; HLB 3.4; acid no. 3.0 max.; iodine no. 0.5 max.; sapon. no. 180-188; flash pt. (COC) 392 F; 100% conc.

Kester Wax® 48. [Koster Keunen] Syn. spermaceti (cetyl esters); CAS 136097-97-7; moisturizer, thickener, emollient, gellant, ointment base; pearlescent for hair care prods.; cosmetic creams/lotions, sun care, hair care, shampoos, conditioners, shaving creams, makeup, leather tanning; pastilles; m.w. 478; m.p. 47-49 C; acid no. < 2.

Kester Wax® 56. [Koster Keunen] Cetearyl stearate; CAS 136097-82-0; moisturizer, thickener, emollient, and gellant for cosmetic creams, lotions, sun care preps., shampoos, conditioners, makeup, stick formulations; substitute for animal-based prods.; pastilles; m.w. 538; m.p. 54-56 C; acid no. < 2.

Kester Wax® 59. [Koster Keunen] Coco rapeseedate; CAS 136097-94-4; moisturizer, thickener, emollient, and gellant for cosmetic creams, lotions, sun care preps., shampoos, conditioners, makeup, and stick formulations; substitute for animal-based prods.; pastilles; m.w. 553; m.p. 57-79 C; acid no. < 2.

Kester Wax® 62. [Koster Keunen] Cetearyl behenate; CAS 136097-81-9; moisturizer, thickener, emollient, and gellant for cosmetic creams, lotions, sun care, shampoos, hair conditoners, makeup; pastilles; m.w. 580; m.p. 61-63 C; acid no. < 2.

Kester Wax® 72. [Koster Keunen] Behenyl behenate; CAS 17671-27-1; EINECS 241-646-5; emollient, moisturizer, thickener, and gellant for cosmetic creams, lotions, sun care preps., lipsticks, and makeup; pastilles.

Kester Wax® 82. [Koster Keunen] Octacosanyl stearate; CAS 136097-96-6; emollient, moisturizer, thickener, and gellant for cosmetic creams, lotions, sun care preps., lipsticks, and makeup; pastilles.

Kester Wax® 85. [Koster Keunen] Ester wax; CAS 136097-96-6; moisturizers, thickener, emollient, gellant for cosmetic creams, lotions, sun care, hair conditoners, makeup; m.w. 709; m.p. 83-86 C; acid no. < 2.

Kester Wax® 105. [Koster Keunen] Ester wax; emollient, moisturizer, thickener, and gellant for cosmetic creams, lotions, sun care preps., lipsticks, and makeup; pastilles.

Ketjenflex® MH. [Akzo] Toluenesulfonamide/formaldehyde resin; used for nail lacquer preps.

Ketjenflex® MS-80. [Akzo] Toluenesulfonamide/formaldehyde resin; used for nail lacquer preps.

Ketosesquine. [Hercules/PFW] Isolongifolene ketone exo; CAS 29461-14-1; EINECS 249-649-3.

KF54. [Shin-Etsu Silicones] Diphenyl dimethicone.

KF56, KF58. [Shin-Etsu Silicones] Phenyl trimethicone; CAS 2116-84-9; EINECS 218-320-6; emollient, conditioner.

KF351A. [Shin-Etsu Silicones] Dimethicone copolyol methyl ether; CAS 68951-97-3.

KF351AS. [Shin-Etsu Silicones] Dimethicone copolyol meth-

yl ether; CAS 68951-97-3.

KF352A. [Shin-Etsu Silicones] Dimethicone copolyol butyl ether.

KF353A. [Shin-Etsu Silicones] Dimethicone copolyol.

KF354A, KF355A, KF615A. [Shin-Etsu Silicones] Dimethicone copolyol butyl ether.

KF625A, KF945A. [Shin-Etsu Silicones] Dimethicone copolyol.

KF994. [Shin-Etsu Silicones] Cyclomethicone; CAS 69430-24-6; cosmetic ingred.

KF9937. [Shin-Etsu Silicones] Diphenyl dimethicone.

KF9945. [Shin-Etsu Silicones] Cyclomethicone; CAS 69430-24-6; cosmetic ingred.

K2 Glycyrrhizinate. [Ichimaru Pharcos] Dipotassium glycyrrhizate; CAS 68797-35-3; EINECS 272-296-1; cosmetic ingred.

Killitol. [Collaborative Labs] Butylene glycol, glycerin, chlorphenesin, and methylparaben; cosmetic preservative system; USA, Japan, and Europe approvals; usage level: 3.5% max.

Klearol®. [Witco/Petroleum Spec.] Wh. min. oil NF; emollient in cosmetics; FDA §172.878, 178.3620a; water-wh., odorless, tasteless; sp.gr. 0.822-0.833; visc. 7-10 cSt (40 C); pour pt. -7 C; flash pt. 138 C.

Klensoft. [Guardian Labs] Disodium cocoamphodiacetate, sodium lauryl sulfate, and hexylene glycol; cosmetic surfactant.

Kleptose. [Roquette] Cyclodextrin; CAS 7585-39-9; EINECS 231-493-2; encapsulant.

Klucel® EF. [Aqualon] Hydroxypropylcellulose, premium grade; CAS 9004-64-2; nonionic; stabilizer, film-former, suspending agent, protective colloid; esp. for nonaerosol hairspray formulations; off-wh. powd., tasteless; 99% thru 20 mesh; sol. in water and many polar org. solvs.; m.w. 80,000; visc. 150–700 cps (10% aq.); bulk dens. 0.5 g/ml; soften. pt. 100-150 C.

Klucel® ELF, GF, HF, JF, LF, MF. [Aqualon] Hydroxypropylcellulose, premium grades; CAS 9004-64-2; nonionic; surface active thickener, stabilizer, film-former, suspending agent, protective colloid for food, cosmetics, pharmaceuticals; FCC clearance; off-wh. powd., tasteless; 99% thru 20 mesh; sol. in water and many polar org. solvs.; m.w. 80,000; visc. 150–700 cps (10% aq.); bulk dens. 0.5 g/ml; soften. pt. 100-150 C.

Kodaflex® DBP. [Eastman] Dibutyl phthalate; CAS 84-74-2; EINECS 201-557-4; plasticizer used in coatings industry as primary plasticizer-solv. for nitrocellulose lacquers; for rubbers and CAB, ethyl cellulose, PVAc, and syn. resins; solv. for oil-sol. dyes, insecticides, peroxides, and org. compds.; antifoamer and fiber lubricant in textile mfg.; cosmetics plasticizer; Pt-Co 15 ppm liq.; m.w. 278; f.p. –35 C; b.p. 340 C; sp.gr. 1.048; dens. 1.04 kg/l; visc. 15 cP; ref. index 1.4920; flash pt. 190 C (COC); fire pt. 202 C (COC); vol. resist. 3.0 x 10⁹ ohm cm; 99.0% min. assay.

Kodaflex® DEP. [Eastman] Diethyl phthalate; CAS 84-66-2; EINECS 201-550-6; plasticizer; wetting agent in grinding pigments; pigment-disp. medium in cellulose acetate sol'ns. and plastics, and solv. for natural resins and polymers; PVC prods. due to relatively high volatility; also for cosmetics; Pt-Co 10 ppm liq.; m.w. 222; f.p. < –50 C; b.p. 298 C; sol. 0.12 g/l in water; sp.gr. 1.120; dens. 1.12 kg/l; visc. 9.5 cP; ref. index 1.4990; flash pt. 161 C (COC); fire pt. 171 C (COC); vol. resist. 1.45 x 10⁹ ohm cm; 99.0% min. assay.

Kodaflex® DMP. [Eastman] Dimethyl phthalate; CAS 131-11-3; EINECS 205-011-6; plasticizer with high solv. power for cellulose acetate extrusion compds.; compatible with ethyl cellulose, CAB, PS, PVAc, polyvinyl butyral, and PVC; used in NC-based printing inks; also for cosmetics and personal care prods.; Pt-Co 5 ppm liq.; m.w. 194;

f.p. –1 C; b.p. 284 C; sol. 0.45 g/l in water; sp.gr. 1.192; dens. 1.19 kg/l; visc. 11.0 cP; ref. index 1.513; flash pt. 157 C (COC); fire pt. 168 C (COC); vol. resist. 1.07 x 10^9 ohm cm; 99.0% min. assay.

Kodaflex® DOA. [Eastman] Dioctyl adipate; CAS 103-23-1; EINECS 203-090-1; plasticizer providing flexibility at low temps. to vinyl prods.; used in unfilled garden hose, clear sheeting, elec. insulation; also for cosmetics and personal care prods.; Pt-Co 20 ppm liq.; m.w. 370; f.p. < –70 C; b.p. 417 C; sol. < 0.1 g/l in water; sp.gr. 0.927; dens. 0.924 kg/l; visc. 12 cP; ref. index 1.4472; flash pt. 206 C (COC); fire pt. 229 C (COC); vol. resist. 9.3 x 10^{11} ohm cm; 99.0% min. assay.

Kodaflex® DOTP. [Eastman] Dioctyl terephthalate; CAS 422-86-2; primary plasticizer used with PVC resins, in PVC plastisols, rubber; applic. incl. wire coatings, automotive and furniture upholstery; compatible with acrylics, CAB, cellulose nitrate, polyvinyl butyral, styrene, oxidizing alkyds, nitrile rubber; also for cosmetics; Pt-Co 15 ppm liq.; m.w. 390.57; f.p. 48 C; b.p. 400 C; sol. 0.004 g/l in water; sp.gr. 0.9835; dens. 0.980 kg/l; visc. 63 cP; ref. index 1.4867; flash pt. 238 C (COC); fire pt. 266 C (COC); vol. resist. 3.9 x 10^{12} ohm-cm.

Kodaflex® TOTM. [Eastman] Trioctyl trimellitate; CAS 3319-31-1; primary plasticizer used in vinyl film and vinyl-coated fabrics; also for cosmetics; Pt-Co 100 ppm liq.; m.w. 547; f.p. –38 C; b.p. 414 C; sol. 0.006 g/l in water; sp.gr. 0.989; dens. 0.984 kg/l; visc. 194 cP; ref. index 1.4832; flash pt. 263 C (COC); fire pt. 297 C (COC); 99.0% min. assay.

Kodaflex® TXIB. [Eastman] 2,2,4-Trimethyl-1,3-pentanediol diisobutyrate; CAS 6846-50-0; primary plasticizer used in surf. coatings, vinyl floorings, moldings, and vinyl prods.; compatible with film-forming vehicles used in lacquers for wood, paper, and metals; primary plasticizer for PVC plastisols for rotocasting and slush molding; used in PVC organosols processed by extrusion and inj. molding; also for cosmetics and personal care prods.; clear liq.; slightly fruity odor; m.w. 286.4; f.p. –70 C; b.p. 280 C; sol. 0.42 g/l in water; sp.gr. 0.945; dens. 0.941 kg/l; visc. 9 cP; ref. index 1.4300; flash pt. 143 C (COC); fire pt. 152 C (COC); vol. resist. 1.5 ¥ 1011 ohm-cm.

Kohacool L-400. [Toho Chem. Industry] Alkylether sulfosuccinate; anionic; wetting and foaming agent, base material for nonirritating hair shampoos, bubble baths, hair conditioners, lotions, and detergents; liq.; 40% conc.

Kojic Acid. [Ikeda] Lightener for skin creams; inhibits activation of tyrosinase which causes skin flecks and dark spots; wh. to sl. ylsh. crystal or cryst. powd., odorless; m.p. 154-158 C; 98-102% assay.

Kollagen KD. [Herstellung von Naturextrakten GmbH; Lipo] Soluble collagen; CAS 9007-34-5; EINECS 232-697-4; water-binding film-former, moisture regulator used in face creams, collagen ampoules, body lotions, after-sun lotions, hair conditioning treatments, skin care prods.; visc. opalescent sol'n., weak intrinsic odor; acid no. 5.5-6.5; pH 3.5-4.0.

Kollagen S. [Herstellung von Naturextrakten GmbH; Lipo] Soluble collagen; CAS 9007-34-5; EINECS 232-697-4; water-binding film-former, moisture regulator used in face creams/masks, collagen ampoules, body lotions, after-sun lotions, hair conditioning treatments; visc. opalescent sol'n., weak intrinsic odor; acid no. 5.5-6.5; pH 3.5-4.0; 1% sol'n.

Kollaplex 0.3. [Herstellung von Naturextrakten GmbH; Lipo] Soluble collagen; CAS 9007-34-5; EINECS 232-697-4; water-binding film-former, moisture regulator used in face creams, collagen ampoules, body lotions, after-sun lotions, hair conditioning treatments, skin care prods.; sl. visc. clear sol'n., weak odor; acid no. 20-23; pH 3.5-4.0.

Kollaplex 1.0. [Herstellung von Naturextrakten GmbH; Lipo]

Soluble collagen; CAS 9007-34-5; EINECS 232-697-4; water-binding film-former, moisture regulator used in face creams, collagen ampoules, body lotions, after-sun lotions, hair conditioning treatments, skin care prods.; visc. opalescent sol'n., weak intrinsic odor; acid no. 5.5-6.5; pH 3.5-4.0.

Kollaron. [Herstellung von Naturextrakten GmbH; Lipo] Soluble collagen; CAS 9007-34-5; EINECS 232-697-4; skin softener, water-binder, film-former, moisture regulator used in face creams/masks, ampoules, body lotions, after-sun lotions, and hair conditioning treatments; visc. milky sol'n., weak intrinsic odor; acid no. 5.5-6.5; pH 3.4-4.0; 1% sol'n.

Kollidon®. [BASF AG] PVP; CAS 9003-39-8; EINECS 201-800-4; solubilizers, crystallization retarders, stabilizers for antibiotic suspensions, etc.; binders for tablets, dispersants; for improving catgut; as thickeners, hydrophilic agents.

Kollidon® 12PF, 17PF. [BASF] Polymeric stabilizer for pharmaceutical injectables.

Kollidon® 25, 30, 90. [BASF] Tablet coatings, binders, suspension stabilizers, thickening agents, and excipients for pharmaceutical use.

Kollidon® CL. [BASF; BASF AG] Crospovidone; tablet-disintegrating agent, suspension stabilizer, excipient for pharmaceuticals.; insol. but swells in water.

Kollidon® CLM. [BASF] Excipient and tablet disintegrant for pharmaceuticals.

Kortacid 1295. [Akzo; Akzo BV] Lauric acid; CAS 143-07-7; EINECS 205-582-1; surfactant.

Korthix H-NF. [Kaopolite] Bentonite; CAS 1302-78-9; EINECS 215-108-5; bacteria-controlled grade for cosmetics and pharmaceuticals.

Koster Keunen Auto-Oxidized Beeswax. [Koster Keunen] Oxidized beeswax; esp. designed for depilatories, polishes, etc.; wax; sp.gr. 0.950-0.980; m.p. 61-67 C; acid no. 25-35; iodine no. 1-10; sapon. no. 90-120; flash pt. > 250 C.

Koster Keunen Beeswax. [Koster Keunen] Beeswax, white and yel.; emulsifier, thickener, emollient, opacifier, oil gellant used in creams, lotions, lipstick, makeup; depilatories; ointments, salves; sustained release pharmaceuticals; furniture, wood, and leather polishes; leather, textile, wood, and paper finishes; candles; molding; lithography; emulsions other than cosmetics; FDA §184.1973, 184.1975; wax; sol. 24.2 g/100 ml in benzene; sp.gr. 0.950-0.960; m.p. 61-65 C; acid no. 17-24; iodine no. 8-11; cloud pt. < 65 C; flash pt. 242-250 C; ref. index 1.4398-1.4451; dielec. const. 3.1-3.3.

Koster Keunen Beeswax AO2535. [Koster Keunen] Oxidized beeswax; CAS 138724-55-7; plasticizer, thickener, and wetting agent for depilatories, makeup; slabs.

Koster Keunen Beeswax, Filtered. [Koster Keunen] Beeswax; CAS 8012-89-3; antioxidant, uv-A and uv-B absorber with mild antimicrobial activity; for creams, lotions, sun care, makeup, lipsticks, soaps, fragrances; slabs.

Koster Keunen Beeswax, S&P ISOW. [Koster Keunen] Beeswax, candelilla wax, hydrog. soy glyceride, paraffin, carnauba, stearic acid; oil gellant for creams, lotions, sun care, makeup, and lipsticks; slabs and pastilles.

Koster Keunen Behenyl-Beeswaxate. [Koster Keunen] Behenyl beeswaxate; beeswax deriv. for cosmetic applics.; wh. to lt. yel. amorphous solid, char. odor; insol. in water; sp.gr. 0.92-0.98; m.p. 66-71 C; b.p. > 250 C; acid no. < 2; sapon. no. 80-90; flash pt. (COC) 240-250 C; toxicology: nontoxic, nonirritating; molten wax may cause skin burns, fumes may cause mild upper respiratory irritation.

Koster Keunen Candelilla. [Koster Keunen] Candelilla wax; CAS 8006-44-8; EINECS 232-347-0; gellant, emollient used for lipsticks, creams, lotions, gel prods.; leather dressings; furniture and other polish; cements; varnishes; sealing wax; elec. insulating compositions; phonograph records; paper sizing; rubber; waterproofing and insectproofing; paint removers; soft wax stiffeners; lubricants; adhesives; candy and gum; FDA §172.615, 175.105, 175.320, 176.180; wax; sol. hot in alcohol, benzene, petrleum ether; sp.gr. 0.9820-0.9930; m.p. 68.5-72.5 C; acid no. 11-19; iodine no. 19-44; sapon. no. 44-66; ref. index 1.4555; dielec. const. 2.50-2.63.

Koster Keunen Candelilla Ester. [Koster Keunen] Cetearyl candelillate; CAS 138724-54-6; gellant, emollient, and stabilizer for makeup, lipsticks, gels; pastilles.

Koster Keunen Carnauba. [Koster Keunen] Carnauba; CAS 8015-86-9; EINECS 232-399-4; used for lipsticks, salves, creams, ointments; pill coatings; shoe, furniture, and car polishes; lacquers, varnishes; phonograph records; hardener for candles; leather finishes; elec.-insulating composition; waterproofing textiles, wood; inks; mold lubricant; candies; paper glazing; FDA §182.1978; wax; sol. (g/100 cc): 1.690 g chloroform, 0.610 g xylene, 0.518 g benzene, 0.440 g turpentine, 0.324 g acetone; sp.gr. 0.996-0.998; m.p. 82.5-86 C; acid no. 2-6; iodine no. 7-14; sapon. no. 78-88; flash pt. > 300 C; ref. index 1.463; dielec. const. 2.67-4.20.

Koster Keunen Carnauba, Micro Granulated. [Koster Keunen] Carnauba; CAS 8015-86-9; EINECS 232-399-4; exfoliating agent for creams, lotions, aq. gels; gran.; 20-60 mesh.

Koster Keunen Carnauba No. 1. [Koster Keunen] Carnauba; CAS 8015-86-9; EINECS 232-399-4; barrier, emollient, and stabilizer for lipsticks, gels; flakes and pastilles.

Koster Keunen Carnauba, Powd. [Koster Keunen] Carnauba; CAS 8015-86-9; EINECS 232-399-4; used for tablets, coatings; powd.; 120 mesh.

Koster Keunen Carnauba T-2. [Koster Keunen] Carnauba; CAS 8015-86-9; EINECS 232-399-4; barrier, emollient, and stabilizer for lipsticks, gels; flakes and pastilles.

Koster Keunen Carnauba T-3. [Koster Keunen] Carnauba; CAS 8015-86-9; EINECS 232-399-4; barrier, emollient, and stabilizer for cosmetic gels; flakes and pastilles.

Koster Keunen Ceresine. [Koster Keunen] Ceresine; CAS 8001-75-0; EINECS 232-290-1; used for cosmetics, creams, lotions, ointments, salves, pharmaceuticals; candles; shoe, floor, and leather polishes; antifouling paints; wood polishes/filler; incandescent gas mantles; paper sizing; waxed paper; lubricants; wax figures; toys; elec. insulation; impregnating/preserving agent; crayons; perfume pastes; pomades; rubber mixtures; waterproofing textiles; adhesives; FDA §175.105; wax; sp.gr. 0.88-0.92; m.p. various grades from 133-163 F; acid no. 0; sapon. no. < 1; ref. index 1.4416-1.4465; dielec. const. 2.15-2.33.

Koster Keunen Ceresine 130/135. [Koster Keunen] Ceresin; CAS 8001-75-0; EINECS 232-290-1; gellant, thickener, and stabilizer for creams, lotions, makeup, lipsticks, sun care prods., gels; slabs and pastilles.

Koster Keunen Ceresine 140/145. [Koster Keunen] Ceresin; CAS 8001-75-0; EINECS 232-290-1; gellant, thickener, and stabilizer for creams, lotions, makeup, lipsticks, sun care prods., gels; slabs and pastilles.

Koster Keunen Ceresine 155. [Koster Keunen] Ceresin; CAS 8001-75-0; EINECS 232-290-1; gellant, thickener, and stabilizer for creams, lotions, makeup, lipsticks, sun care prods., gels; slabs and pastilles.

Koster Keunen Ceresine 192. [Koster Keunen] Ceresin; CAS 8001-75-0; EINECS 232-290-1; gellant, thickener, and stabilizer for creams, lotions, makeup, lipsticks, sun care prods., gels; slabs and pastilles.

Koster Keunen Fatty Alcohol 1618. [Koster Keunen] Cetearyl alcohol; CAS 8005-44-5; emollient, emulsifier, thickener, and opacifier for creams, lotions, shampoos, conditioners, soaps, deodorants; flakes.

Koster Keunen Hydroxy-Hexanyl-Behenyl-Beeswaxate. [Koster Keunen] Hexanediol beeswax; CAS 144514-54-5; gellant for silicone oils, moisturizer, emollient; for creams, lotions, shampoos, conditioners, silicone oil gels, lipsticks, makeup, and powds.; lt. yel. to wh. solid amorphous slabs and pastilles, char. odor; insol. in water; sp.gr. 0.92-0.98; m.p. 62-68 C; b.p. > 250 C; acid no. < 2; sapon. no. 80-90; flash pt. (COC) 240-250 C.

Koster Keunen Hydroxy-Polyester. [Koster Keunen] Beeswax substitute; plasticizer, stabilizer, gellant, thickener, emollient, dispersant, and wetting agent for cosmetic creams/lotions, lipsticks, sun care preps.; FDA compliance for food contact; slabs; m.p. 70-80 C; HLB 2.17; acid no. < 10; sapon. no. 50-70; hyd. no. 38-48; flash pt. > 350 F.

Koster Keunen Isostearyl-Behenyl Beeswaxate. [Koster Keunen] Isostearyl behenyl beeswaxate; beeswax deriv. for cosmetic applics.; wh. to lt. yel. amorphous solid, char. odor; insol. in water; sp.gr. 0.92-0.98; m.p. 66-72 C; b.p. > 250 C; acid no. < 2; sapon. no. 80-90; flash pt. (COC) 240-250 C.

Koster Keunen Japan Wax, Synthetic. [Koster Keunen] Syn. Japan wax; CAS 67701-27-3; gellant, thickener, and emulsifier for stick pencils, makeup; pastilles.

Koster Keunen Microcrystalline Waxes. [Koster Keunen] Microcrystalline wax; CAS 64742-42-3; used for cosmetics, pharmaceuticals; laminating of paper, cloth; waterproofing paper, fiberboard, textiles, wood; potting ocmpds. for condensers; polishes for floor, furniture, skis, leather; rust prevention compding. of rubber; patternmaking; printing inks; lubricants; records; FDA §172.886, 178.3710; wh. to amber wax; sp.gr. 0.90-0.94; visc. 50-100 (210 F); m.p. 140-190 F; acid no. 0-0.2; iodine no. 0.-1.5; sapon. no. 0-2; flash pt. > 425 F; fire pt. > 550 F.

Koster Keunen Microcrystalline Wax 170/180. [Koster Keunen] Microcrystalline wax; CAS 63231-60-7; EINECS 264-038-1; stabilizer, emollient, and thickener for cosmetic creams, lotions, sun care preps., lipsticks, makeup, powds., gels; slabs.

Koster Keunen Microcrystalline Wax 193/198. [Koster Keunen] Microcrystalline wax; CAS 64742-42-3; stabilizer, emollient, and thickener for sun care, lipsticks, gels; pastilles.

Koster Keunen Ozokerite. [Koster Keunen] Ozokerite; CAS 8021-55-4; used for cosmetics, creams, lotions, pomades; paints, varnishes; polishes for leather, automobile, floor; printing inks; pharmaceutical ointments; crayons; waxed paper; linen/cotton sizing; elec. insulating; lubricants and sealing wax compositions; process engraving, lithography; rubber filler; FDA approved; wax; sol. (g/100 g): 12.99 carbon bisulfide, 11.83 g petrol. ether (75 C), 6.06 g turpentine (160 C), 3.95 g xylene (137 C), 2.83 g toluene (109 C), 2.42 g chloroform; sp.gr. 0.85-0.95; m.p. various grades from 149-190 F; acid no. 0; iodine no. 7-9; sapon. no. 0; ref. index 1.440 (60 C); dielec. const. 2.37-2.55.

Koster Keunen Ozokerite 153/160. [Koster Keunen] Ozokerite; CAS 8021-55-4; gellant, thickener, and emollient for cosmetic creams, lotions, sun care, lipsticks, and gels; slabs and pastilles.

Koster Keunen Ozokerite 158/160. [Koster Keunen] Ozokerite; CAS 8021-55-4; gellant, thickener, and emollient for cosmetic creams, lotions, sun care, lipsticks, and gels; slabs.

Koster Keunen Ozokerite 160/164. [Koster Keunen] Ozokerite; CAS 8021-55-4; gellant, thickener, and emollient for cosmetic creams, lotions, sun care, lipsticks, and gels; slabs.

Koster Keunen Ozokerite 164/170. [Koster Keunen] Ozokerite; CAS 8021-55-4; gellant, thickener, and emollient for cosmetic creams, lotions, sun care, lipsticks, and gels; slabs and pastilles.

Koster Keunen Ozokerite 170. [Koster Keunen] Ozokerite; CAS 8021-55-4; gellant, thickener, and emollient for cosmetic creams, lotions, sun care, lipsticks, and gels; slabs and pastilles.

Koster Keunen Ozokerite 190. [Koster Keunen] Ozokerite; CAS 8021-55-4; gellant, thickener, and emollient for cosmetic creams, lotions, sun care, lipsticks, and gels; pastilles.

Koster Keunen Paraffin Wax. [Koster Keunen] Paraffin; CAS 8002-74-2; EINECS 232-315-6; wax used for cosmetics, pharmaceutical ointments and salves; candles; waterproofing, sealing; lubricating; protection of food, plants, fruits, cheese, and vegetables; paper; polishes; crayons; electronic insulation; hot-melt adhesives; FDA §172.615, 175.250, 175.300; wax; sol. (g/100 cc): 40 g benzene, 9 g min. oil, 3 g dichloroethane, 0.4 g IPA; m.p. various grades from 118-165 F; ref. index 1.4219-1.4357.

Koster Keunen Paraffin Wax 122/128. [Koster Keunen] Paraffin; CAS 8002-74-2; EINECS 232-315-6; moisturizer and stabilizer for cosmetic creams, lotions, sun care, makeup, hair care, and shaving creams; slabs, gran., and pastilles.

Koster Keunen Paraffin Wax 130/135. [Koster Keunen] Paraffin; CAS 8002-74-2; EINECS 232-315-6; moisturizer and stabilizer for cosmetic creams, lotions, sun care, makeup, hair care, and shaving creams; slabs, gran., and pastilles.

Koster Keunen Paraffin Wax 140/145. [Koster Keunen] Paraffin; CAS 8002-74-2; EINECS 232-315-6; moisturizer and stabilizer for sun care, lipsticks, creams; slabs, gran., and pastilles.

Koster Keunen Paraffin Wax 150/155. [Koster Keunen] Paraffin; CAS 8002-74-2; EINECS 232-315-6; moisturizer and stabilizer for sun care, lipsticks, gels; slabs and pastilles.

Koster Keunen Stearic Acid XXX. [Koster Keunen] Stearic acid; CAS 57-11-4; EINECS 200-313-4; emulsifier and emollient for cosmetic creams, lotions, sun care, makeup, shampoos, conditioners, shaving creams, and soaps; flakes.

Koster Keunen Substitute Beeswax. [Koster Keunen] Syn. beeswax; CAS 97026-94-0; used where pure beeswax not required; for creams, lotions, lipstick, makeup; depilatories; ointments, salves; sustained release pharmaceuticals; furniture, wood, and leather polishes; leather, textile, wood, and paper finishes; candles; molding; lithography; wax; m.p. 62-65 C; acid no. 17-24.

Koster Keunen Synthetic Beeswax. [Koster Keunen] Syn. beeswax; CAS 97026-94-0; gellant, emulsifier, and thickener for cosmetic creams, lotions, sun care, lipsticks, and gels; pastilles.

Koster Keunen Synthetic Candelilla. [Koster Keunen] Syn. candelilla wax; CAS 136097-95-5; gellant, thickener, stabilizer, and moisturizer used for lipsticks, creams, lotions, gel prods.; leather dressings; furniture and other polish; cements; varnishes; sealing wax; elec. insulating compositions; phonograph records; paper sizing; rubber; waterproofing and insectproofing; paint removers; soft wax stiffeners; lubricants; adhesives; candy and gum; wax; sol. hot in alcohol, benzene, petrleum ether; m.p. 68.5-

72.5 C; acid no. 11-20; sapon. no. 44-66.

Koster Keunen Synthetic Candelilla R-4. [Koster Keunen] Syn. candelilla; CAS 136097-95-5; gellant, thickener, stabilizer, and moisturizer for lipsticks and gels; pastilles.

Koster Keunen Synthetic Candelilla R-8. [Koster Keunen] Syn. candelilla; CAS 136097-95-5; gellant, thickener, stabilizer, and moisturizer for lipsticks and gels; pastilles.

Koster Keunen Synthetic Carnauba. [Koster Keunen] Syn. carnauba; CAS 136097-96-6; stabilizer used for lipsticks, salves, creams, ointments; pill coatings; shoe, furniture, and car polishes; lacquers, varnishes; phonograph records; hardener for candles; leather finishes; elec.-insulating composition; waterproofing textiles; wood; inks; pastilles; sol. in chloroform, xylene, benzene, turpentine, acetone; m.p. 80-83 C; acid no. 2-6; ref. index 1.463; dielec. const. 2.67-4.20.

Koster Keunen Synthetic Japan Wax. [Koster Keunen] Syn. Japan wax; CAS 67701-27-3; used for cosmetics, pharmaceuticals; metal buffing compds.; candles; crayons and pencils; textile and leather finishes; lubricants; wax; sol. in hot alcohol, carbon disulfide, chloroform, ether, benzene, petrol. ether, isopropyl ether, naphtha, pyridine, toluene, xylene, turpentine; insol. in water; sp.gr. 0.975-0.984; m.p. 50-56 C; acid no. 6-20; iodine no. 4-15; sapon. no. 210-237; flash pt. > 200 C; ref. index 1.450-1.4560 (60 C); dielec. const. 3.1-3.2.

Koster Keunen Synthetic Spermaceti. [Koster Keunen] Syn. spermaceti (cetyl palmitate and other esters); CAS 136097-97-7; wax for mfg. of emulsions, candles, soaps, sweetmeats, candies, confectionery; cosmetics, ointments, pomades, toiletries; textile finishes; pharmaceuticals; FDA approved; wax; sol. in boiling alcohol, chloroform, carbon disulfide, volatile oils; sp.gr. 0.940-0.946; visc. 6.7-7.4 (100 C); m.p. 45-49 C; acid no. 0-0.5; iodine no. < 3; sapon. no. 116-125; flash pt. > 240 C; ref. index 1.440 (60 C).

Koster Keunen Tallow Glyceride. [Koster Keunen] Tallow glycerides; CAS 67701-27-3; emulsifier and emollient for cosmetic creams, lotions, and shaving creams; gran.

Koucha Liq. [Ichimaru Pharcos] Water, alcohol, butylene glycol, thea sinensis extract; botanical extract.

Kowet Titanium Dioxide. [HK Color Group] Titanium dioxide; CAS 13463-67-7; EINECS 236-675-5; mineral sunscreen.

K-Preserve Liq. [Kraft] Phenoxyethanol; CAS 122-99-6; EINECS 204-589-7; cosmetic preservative; broad activity, esp. against Gram-negative bacteria; USA, Japan, Europe approvals; liq., sl. aromatic odor; usage level: up to 1%.

Krim 32. [Fabriquimica] Self-emulsifying wax; nonionic; emulsifier and thickener for cosmetic emulsions; acid no. < 4; iodine no. < 2; sapon. no. 95-105.

Krim 400. [Fabriquimica] Cetearyl alcohol, cetrimonium chloride; cationic; self-emulsifying wax; emulsifier and thickener for cosmetic emulsions; acid no. < 1; iodine no. < 1; sapon. no. 12-18.

Krim CH 25. [Fabriquimica] Glycol stearate, cocamide DEA, sodium laureth sulfate.

Kronos® 1025. [Kronos] Titanium dioxide; CAS 13463-67-7; EINECS 236-675-5; mineral sunscreen.

Kytamer® KC. [Amerchol] Polyquaternium-29.

Kytamer® L. [Amerchol] Chitosan lactate.

Kytamer® PC. [Amerchol] Chitosan PCA; water-sol. polymer for cosmetics applics.; tan powd., mild char. odor; water-sol.; pH 3.5 min. (1% aq.).

L

L-310. [Procter & Gamble] Linseed acid; CAS 68424-45-3; EINECS 270-304-8.

Labrafac® Hydro WL 1219. [Gattefosse; Gattefosse SA] Caprylic/capric triglycerides PEG-4 esters; nonionic; hydrophilic oil for pharmaceutical and cosmetic formulations; liq.; HLB 4.0; acid no. < 2; iodine no. < 2; sapon. no. 265-285; toxicology: LD50 (oral, rat) > 20 ml/kg; sl. irritating to skin and eyes; 100% conc.

Labrafac® Lipophile WL 1349. [Gattefosse] Caprylic/capric triglyceride; CAS 65381-09-1; superfatting agent for cosmetic/pharmaceutical emulsions and microemulsions; liq.; toxicology: LD50 (oral, rat) > 10 ml/kg; sl. irritating to eyes; nonirritating to skin.

Labrafil® ISO. [Gattefosse SA] Isostearic ethoxylated glycerides; nonionic; hydrophilic oil; liq.; HLB 4.0; acid no. < 2; iodine no. < 15; sapon. no. 145-165; toxicology: LD50 (oral, rat) > 20 ml/kg; nonirritating to skin and eyes; 100% conc.

Labrafil® Isostearique. [Gattefosse] Triisostearin PEG-6 esters; amphiphilic agent for improving drug delivery; liq.; HLB 3-4; toxicology: LD50 (oral, rat) > 20 ml/kg; nonirritating to skin and eyes.

Labrafil® M 1944 CS. [Gattefosse; Gattefosse SA] Apricot kernel oil PEG-6 esters; CAS 97488-91-0; nonionic; hydrophilic oil for pharmaceutical and cosmetic formulations; excipient, solubilizer, dispersion vehicle; cosurfactant of Tefose 63; for drinkable sol'ns., nasal sol'ns., sprays, emulsions, hard shell capsules, softgel capsules, microemulsions; French pharmacopeia compliance; Gardner < 5 liq. (40 C), faint odor; very sol. in chloroform, methylene chloride, min. oils; sol. in n-hexane; disp. in water; sp.gr. 0.935-0.955; visc. 75-95 mPa·s; HLB 4.0; acid no. ≤ 2; iodine no. 79-89; sapon. no. 155-169; hyd. no. 45-65; pH 4.5-6.0 (10% aq.); toxicology: LD50 (oral, rat) > 20 ml/kg; nonirritating to skin; 100% conc.

Labrafil® M 1966 CS. [Gattefosse] Almond oil PEG-6 esters.

Labrafil® M 1969 CS. [Gattefosse; Gattefosse SA] Peanut oil PEG-6 esters; nonionic; hydrophilic oil for pharmaceutical and cosmetic formulations; amphiphilic agent for improving drug delivery; liq.; HLB 4.0; acid no. ≤ 2; iodine no. 70-90; sapon. no. 150-165; toxicology: LD50 (oral, rat) > 5 g/kg; 100% conc.

Labrafil® M 1980 CS. [Gattefosse; Gattefosse SA] Olive oil PEG-6 esters; CAS 103819-46-1; nonionic; hydrophilic oil for pharmaceutical and cosmetic formulations; amphiphilic agent improving drug delivery; liq.; HLB 4.0; acid no. ≤ 2; iodine no. 60-80; sapon. no. 50-170; toxicology: LD50 (oral, rat) > 20 ml/kg; 100% conc.

Labrafil® M 2125 CS. [Gattefosse; Gattefosse SA] Corn oil PEG-6 esters; CAS 85536-08-9; nonionic; hydrophilic oil for pharmaceutical and cosmetic formulations; solubilizer, cosurfactant, oily dispersions vehicle; for formulation of drinkable sol'ns., nasal sol'ns., emulsions, softgel capsules, hard shell capsules; French pharmacopeia compliance; Gardner < 5 liq. (45 C), faint odor; sol. in chloroform, methylene chloride, min. oils; disp. in water; insol. in ethanol; sp.gr. 0.935-0.955; visc. 70-90 mPa·s; HLB 4.0; acid no. < 2; iodine no. 100-110; sapon. no. 156-170; hyd. no. 45-65; ref. index 1.465-1.475; toxicology: LD50 (oral, rat) > 20 ml/kg; 100% conc.

Labrafil® M 2130 BS. [Gattefosse; Gattefosse SA] Hydrog. palm/palm kernel oil PEG-6 esters; nonionic; hydrophilic wax for pharmaceutical and cosmetic formulations; amphiphilic agent for improving drug delivery; solid; drop pt. 30.5-35.5 C; HLB 4.0; acid no. < 2; iodine no. < 2; sapon. no. 162-176; toxicology: LD50 (oral, rat) > 20 ml/kg; 100% conc.

Labrafil® M 2130 CS. [Gattefosse; Gattefosse SA] Palm kernel oil, palm oil, PEG-6, and hydrog. palm/palm kernel oil PEG-6 esters; nonionic; hydrophilic wax for pharmaceutical and cosmetic formulations; bioavailability enhancer for oral use (hard shell capsule); cutaneous absorption enhancer for penetration of active drugs through the skin (lotions, creams); French pharmacopeia compliance; Gardner < 5 doughy solid, faint odor; sol. in chloroform, methylene chloride; partly sol. in ethanol; disp. in water; insol. in min. oils; drop pt. 33-38 C; HLB 4.0; acid no. < 2; iodine no. < 2; sapon. no. 190-204; hyd. no. 65-85; toxicology: LD50 (oral, rat) > 2 g/kg; nonirritating to skin and eyes; 100% conc.

Labrafil® M 2735 CS. [Gattefosse; Gattefosse SA] Triolein PEG-6 esters; nonionic; hydrophilic hydrog. oil; excipient for pharmaceutical and cosmetic formulations; liq.; HLB 4.0; acid no. ≤ 2; iodine no. 70-85; sapon. no. 150-170; toxicology: LD50 (oral, rat) > 20 ml/kg; sl. irritating to skin and eyes; 100% conc.

Labrafil® WL 1958 CS. [Gattefosse SA] Ricinoleic ethoxylated glycerides; nonionic; hydrophilic wax; emulsion stabilizer; liq.; 100% conc.

Labrafil® WL 2609 BS. [Gattefosse] Corn oil PEG-8 esters.

Labrasol. [Gattefosse; Gattefosse SA] PEG-8 caprylic/capric glycerides; CAS 85536-07-8; nonionic; hydrophilic oil; excipient, solubilizer for pharmaceutical and cosmetic formulations; surfactant for microemulsions; wetting agent; penetration enhancer; Gardner < 5 oily liq., faint odor; sol. in water; very sol. in ethanol, chloroform, methylene chloride; sp.gr. 1.060-1.070; visc. 80-110 mPa·s; HLB 14.0; acid no. < 1; iodine no. < 2; sapon. no. 85-105; ref. index 1.450-1.470; toxicology: LD50 (oral, rat) > 20 ml/kg; sl. ocular irritant at 0.1 ml; nonirritating to skin; 100% conc.

Lacol. [Lanaetex Prods.] Isobutyl tallowate, trilinolein, laureth-2 acetate.

Lactabase C14. [Prod'Hyg] Myristyl lactate; CAS 1323-03-1; EINECS 215-350-1; emollient.

Lactabase C16. [Prod'Hyg] Cetyl lactate; CAS 35274-05-6; EINECS 252-478-7; emollient.

Lactabase C18. [Prod'Hyg] Stearyl lactate.

Lactacet. [Vevy] Cetyl lactate; CAS 35274-05-6; EINECS 252-478-7; emollient.

Lactil® . [Goldschmidt; Goldschmidt AG] Sodium lactate, sodium PCA, hydrolyzed animal protein, fructose, urea, niacinamide, inositol, sodium benzoate, lactic acid; nonionic; humectant, moisturizing agent for creams and lotions, anti-aging preps., after-swim prods.; yel. liq.; sp.gr. 1.27; pH 6.7-7.6; 50% conc.

Lactobiol. [Biodev] Milk protein; CAS 9000-71-9; cosmetic protein.

Lactodan F 15. [Grindsted Prods.] Glyceryl palmitate lactate; aerator prod.; hair mousse, facial prods.

Lactodan P 22. [Grindsted Prods.] Lactylated monoglyceride; food emulsifier and functional additive for cosmetics/toiletries; sm. beads; drop pt. 45 C; sapon. no. 270-300.

Lactofil. [Gattefosse] Lactose and milk protein.

Lactolan®. [Laboratoires Sérobiologiques] Hydrolyzed milk protein (oligopeptides, amino acids, lactose, lactate, min. salts, and biocatalyzers); CAS 92797-39-2; moisturizer, conditioner, elasticity strengthener, cutaneous softener, regenerator of epidermal keratinocytes with photo-protecting effect; for nutritive care, prods. for dry, rough skin, babies, facial care, body care, bathing, hair care; yel. limpid liq.; water-sol.; usage level: 2.5-10%.

Lactomul 466. [Henkel/Functional Prods.] Blended glyceride; nonionic; for animal milk replacer prods.; emulsion stability; liq.; 100% conc.

Lactomul 468. [Henkel/Functional Prods.] Blended glyceride; nonionic; for animal milk replacer prods.; suitable for wet process concs.; soft solid; 100% conc.

Lactomul CN-28. [Henkel/Functional Prods.] Blended glyceride; nonionic; for milk replacer prods. with spray drying processes; waxy solid; 100% conc.

LactoPro CLP Code 1580. [Brooks Industries] Skin nourishing complex containing carbohydrates, lipids, and proteins.

Lafil WL 3254. [Gattefosse SA] Polyglyceryl isostearostearate; superfatting agent for cosmetic/pharmaceutical emulsions; drop pt. 35.5-40.5 C; HLB 3.0; acid no. < 1; iodine no. ≤6; sapon. no. 155-175; toxicology: LD50 (oral, rat) > 2 g/kg; sl. irritating to skin and eyes.

Lamacit® GML 20. [Henkel Canada; Henkel KGaA/Cospha; Grünau] PEG-20 glyceryl laurate; CAS 51248-32-9; nonionic; o/w emulsifier for creams and lotions; solubilizer for essential oils in aq./alcoholic systems; used for essential oil baths and water-based skin cleansing preps. containing large quantities of essential oils; lt. yel. clear liq., neutral odor; visc. 500 mPa·s max.; HLB 17.0; acid no. 2 max.; sapon. no. 45-55; pH 6.5-7.5 (10%); usage level: 10-15%; 100% conc.

Lamecreme® AOM. [Grünau] Hydrog. palm oil glycerides, PEG-20 hydrog. palm oil glycerides, cetyl alcohol, steareth-7.

Lamecreme® DGE-18. [Henkel KGaA/Cospha; Grünau] PEG-4 polyglyceryl-2 stearate; o/w emulsifier and consistency agent; at high use levels, forms transparent skin care gels; wh. to ylsh. waxy solid; sol. in most cosmetic oils and emollients; acid no. 2 max.; iodine no. 1 max.; sapon. no. 115-135.

Lamecreme® KSM. [Grünau] Glyceryl stearate SE.

Lamecreme® LPM. [Henkel/Cospha; Henkel Canada; Grünau] Hydrog. palm oil glycerides, cetyl alcohol, TEA-isostearyl hydrolyzed collagen; self-emulsifying raw material for o/w emulsions, hair conditioners, creams, lotions; pale ylsh. pellets; acid no. 12 max.; iodine no. 2 max.; sapon. no. 120-135.

Lameform® TGI. [Henkel/Cospha; Henkel KGaA/Cospha; Grünau] Polyglyceryl-3 diisostearate; CAS 66082-42-6; nonionic; emulsifier, emollient for cosmetic/pharmaceutical w/o emulsions with good stability; yel. visc. liq.; HLB

6.0; acid no. 3 max.; sapon. no. 140-160; hyd. no. 190-220; 100% conc.

Lamegin® EE. [Grünau] Acetylated hydrog. tallow glyceride; CAS 68990-58-9; EINECS 273-612-0; nonionic; emulsifier and plasticizer for cosmetic, food, and edible coatings; solid; 100% conc.

Lamegin® GLP 10, 20. [Grünau] Hydrog. tallow glyceride lactate; CAS 68990-06-7; EINECS 273-576-6; nonionic; emulsifier and plasticizer for cosmetics, foods, and drugs; solid; 100% conc.

Lamegin® ZE 30, 60. [Grünau] Hydrog. tallow glyceride citrate; CAS 68990-59-0; EINECS 273-613-6; anionic; emulsifier for cosmetic, margarine and meat industry; solid; 100% conc.

Lamepon® 4SK. [Henkel/Cospha; Henkel Canada] Potassium coco-hydrolyzed animal protein; CAS 68920-65-0; anionic; surfactant, anti-irritant, foaming and cleansing agent for personal care prods.; skin compatible; lt. yel. clear liq.; 34-38% act.

Lamepon® LPO. [Grünau] Oleoyl hydrolyzed collagen; CAS 68458-51-5.

Lamepon® LPO 30. [Grünau] Isopropyl alcohol, oleoyl hydrolyzed collagen.

Lamepon® PA-K. [Henkel KGaA/Cospha; Grünau] Potassium abietoyl hydrolyzed collagen; CAS 68918-77-4; anionic; additive for anti-fat shampoos; skin compatible; amber clear liq., faint intrinsic odor; sp.gr. 1.05-1.08; visc. 500 mPa·s max.; pH 6.5-7.0 (10%); 30-32% conc.

Lamepon® PA-K/NP. [Henkel KGaA/Cospha] Potassium abietoyl hydrolyzed collagen; CAS 68918-77-4; protein with high substantivity to hair; retards refatting in anti-grease shampoos and hair treatments; amber clear low-visc. liq., char. odor; pH 6.5-7.0; 30-32% dry solids.

Lamepon® PA-TR. [Henkel Canada; Henkel KGaA/Cospha; Grünau] TEA-abietoyl hydrolyzed collagen; CAS 68918-77-4; anionic; mild detergent for shampoos, cleansers; skin compatible; amber clear low-visc. liq., char. intrinsic odor; sp.gr. 1.05-1.09; visc. 150 mPa·s; pH 6.2-7.0; 30-32% act.

Lamepon® PA-TR/NP. [Henkel KGaA/Cospha] TEA-abietoyl hydrolyzed collagen; CAS 68918-77-4; protein with high substantivity to hair; retards refatting in anti-grease shampoos and hair treatments; amber clear low-visc. liq., char. inherent odor; pH 6.2-7.0; 30-32% dry solids.

Lamepon® S. [Henkel/Cospha; Henkel Canada; Henkel KGaA/Cospha; Grünau] Potassium coco-hydrolyzed collagen; CAS 68920-65-0; anionic; mild detergent with good foaming and good foam stability; for shampoos, bath and shower preps., dermatological skin cleansers; lt. yel. clear liq., weak intrinsic odor; sp.gr. 1.04-1.09; visc. 800 mPa·s max.; pH 6.6-7.0; 32% act.

Lamepon® S/NP. [Henkel KGaA/Cospha] Potassium cocoyl hydrolyzed collagen; CAS 68920-65-0; protein, cosurfactant for mild shower and foam baths, shampoos, body cleaners; improves skin and eye mucosa compatibility of surfactants; lt. yel. clear sl. visc. liq., mild inherent odor; visc. 1000 mPa·s max.; pH 6.6-7.0; 31.5-32.5% dry solids.

Lamepon® ST 40/NP. [Henkel KGaA/Cospha] TEA-cocoyl hydrolyzed collagen; CAS 68952-16-9; protein, cosurfactant for prep. of body cleansing preps., foam baths, oily foam baths; improves skin and eye mucosa compatibility of surfactants; lt. yel. clear sl. visc. liq., mild inherent odor; pH 6.5-7.0; 40-41% dry solids.

Lamepon® S-TR/NP. [Henkel KGaA/Cospha] TEA-cocoyl hydrolyzed collagen preserved with methylparaben, ethylparaben, and phenoxyethanol; CAS 68952-16-9; protein, cosurfactant for prep. of mild body cleansing preps.; improves skin and eye mucosa compatibility of surfactants; lt. yel. clear low-visc. liq., mild inherent odor;

pH 6.5-7.0; 31.5-32.5% dry solids.

Lamepon® UD/NP. [Henkel KGaA/Cospha] Potassium undecylenoyl hydrolyzed collagen; CAS 68951-92-8; protein with exc. skin and eye mucosa compatibility and anti-dandruff effect; for anti-dandruff shampoos; lt. amber clear liq., char. odor; pH 6.2-7.0; 31.5-32.5% dry solids.

Lamequat® L. [Henkel/Cospha; Henkel Canada; Henkel KGaA/Cospha; Grünau] Lauryldimonium hydroxypropyl hydrolyzed collagen; CAS 118441-80-8; cationic; proteinaceous conditioning component for hair and body care preps., hair conditioners, shampoos, shower and bath prods.; improves sheen, antistatic props., feel of dry hair; yel. clear low visc. liq., weak intrinsic odor; visc. 800 mPa·s max.; pH 4-5; 35% act.

Lamequat® L/NP. [Henkel KGaA/Cospha] Lauryldimonium hydroxypropyl hydrolyzed collagen; CAS 118441-80-8; cationic; protein for use in shampoos and mild shower gels and foam baths; yel. clear sl. visc. liq., mild inherent odor; pH 5.0-6.5; 34-36% dry solids.

Lamesoft® 156. [Henkel/Cospha; Henkel KGaA/Cospha; Grünau] Hydrog. tallow glycerides, potassium cocoyl hydrolyzed collagen preserved with benzoic acid and pHB esters; anionic; visc. builder, consistency agent, conditioner, opacifier, pearlizing agent, and antistat for personal care prods.; produces very dense, finely structured wh. surfactant preps.; pearly liq.; visc. < 1500 mPa·s; pH 5.0-5.5; 23.5-25.0% dry residue.

Lamesoft® 156/NP. [Henkel KGaA/Cospha] Hydrog. tallow glycerides and potassium cocoyl hydrolyzed collagen; opacifier for very compact, fine-structured cosmetic surfactant preps.; wh. pumpable prod.; visc. ≤ 1500 mPa·s; pH 5.0-5.5; 23.5-25.0% dry residue.

Lamesoft® LMG. [Henkel/Cospha; Henkel Canada; Henkel KGaA/Cospha; Grünau] Glyceryl laurate, potassium cocoyl hydrolyzed collagen preserved with benzoic acid and pHB esters; anionic; refatting agent and thickener for foam baths, shower gels, and shampoos; wh. microcryst. pumpable dispersion; visc. < 1500 mPa·s; pH 5.0-5.5; 25% conc.

Lamesoft® LMG/NP. [Henkel KGaA/Cospha] Glyceryl laurate and potassium cocoyl hydrolyzed collagen; refatting agent for cosmetic surfactant preps.; wh. microcryst. pumpable disp.; visc. ≤ 1500 mPa·s; pH 5.0-5.5; 23.5-25.0% dry residue.

Laminarina. [Vevy] Propylene glycol and algae extract; botanical extract.

Lanacet® 1705. [Henkel/Organic Prods.] Acetylated lanolin USP; CAS 61788-48-5; EINECS 262-979-2; nonionic; emollient, superfatting agent; used in personal care prods.; solid; sol. in IPM, min. oil; 100% conc.

Lanaetex-75. [Lanaetex Prods.] Cetyl acetate and acetylated lanolin alcohols; cosmetic ingred.

Lanaetex A-15. [Lanaetex Prods.] Laneth-15; CAS 61791-20-6; cosmetic ingred.

Lanaetex-A16. [Lanaetex Prods.] Laneth-16; CAS 61791-20-6.

Lanaetex C-40. [Lanaetex Prods.] PEG-40 castor oil; CAS 61791-12-6; cosmetic ingred.

Lanaetex CLC. [Lanaetex Prods.] Petrolatum, lanolin, lanolin alcohol.

Lanaetex CO. [Lanaetex Prods.] Castor oil USP; CAS 8001-79-4; EINECS 232-293-8; cosmetics ingred.

Lanaetex CO-25. [Lanaetex Prods.] PEG-25 hydrog. castor oil; CAS 61788-85-0; cosmetics ingred.

Lanaetex CO-40. [Lanaetex Prods.] PEG-40 castor oil; CAS 61791-12-6; personal care surfactant.

Lanaetex CPS. [Lanaetex Prods.] PEG-15 cocamine phosphate oleate; easily solubilized in water to acheive long lasting emolliency and conditioning; for whirlpool baths, foaming bubble baths, after-bath splashes, pre-electric

shaves, conditioning after-shaves, shampoos, conditioners, liq. soaps; sol. in water and alcohol.

Lanaetex FB. [Lanaetex Prods.] Min. oil, lanolin, paraffin, lanolin alcohol, beeswax.

Lanaetex H. [Lanaetex Prods.] Petrolatum, lanolin, lanolin alcohol, sorbitan sesquioleate, beeswax.

Lanaetex-HG. [Lanaetex Prods.] Hydrog. lanolin; CAS 8031-44-5; EINECS 232-452-1; cosmetics ingred.

Lanaetex L-15. [Lanaetex Prods.] Petrolatum, lanolin, lanolin alcohol.

Lanaetex-LO. [Lanaetex Prods.] Dimethyl lauramine oleate; cosmetic ingred.

Lanaetex-OS. [Lanaetex Prods.] Octyl salicylate; CAS 118-60-5; EINECS 204-263-4; cosmetic sunscreen.

Lanaetex Aloe Vera Gel. [Lanaetex Prods.] Aloe vera gel; moisturizer, soothing/healing aid for personal care.

Lanaetex Jojoba Oil. [Lanaetex Prods.] Jojoba oil; CAS 61789-91-1; cosmetic emollient.

Lanafos-N3. [Lanaetex Prods.] DEA oleth-3 phosphate; cosmetic ingred.

Lanafos-N10. [Lanaetex Prods.] DEA oleth-10 phosphate; cosmetic ingred.

Lanagen-50, -55, -SD. [Lanaetex Prods.] Hydrolyzed collagen; CAS 9015-54-7; cosmetic protein.

Lanalan. [Lanaetex Prods.] Lanolin, lanolin alcohol.

Lanalol. [Lanaetex Prods.] Petrolatum, lanolin, lanolin alcohol.

Lanalox L 30. [Maybrook] PEG-30 lanolin; CAS 61790-81-6; emollient, emulsifier.

Lanamine®. [Amerchol] Mixed isopropanolamines myristate; anionic; high foaming mild detergent for shampoos, shaving soaps; pale yel. gel, sl. char. odor; pH 7.8-8.8 (10% aq.); 50% conc.

Lanapeg-15. [Lanaetex Prods.] Octoxynol-9; CAS 9002-93-1; cosmetic ingred.

Lanapene. [Lanaetex Prods.] Isopropyl palmitate, lecithin.

Lanapol CT. [Seppic] Isopropanolamine lanolate; anionic; cosmetic assistant; 50% conc.

Lan-Aqua-Sol 50. [Fanning] PEG-75 lanolin; CAS 8039-09-6; anionic; emulsifier for cosmetic and pharmaceutical emulsions; emollient, superfatting agent, conditioner for skin and hair care prods., household detergents; solubilizer, wetting agent, dispersing aid.; Gardner 10 max. color, faint odor; sol. in ethanol, water; sl. sol. in glycerin, ethyl acetate; sp.gr. 1.00-1.04 (50/4 C); acid no. 3 max.; sapon. no. 9 max.; pH 5.5-7.0 (4% aq.).

Lan-Aqua-Sol 100. [Fanning] PEG-75 lanolin; CAS 8039-09-6; anionic; emulsifier for cosmetic and pharmaceutical emulsions; emollient, superfatting agent, conditioner for skin and hair care prods., household detergents; solubilizer, wetting agent, dispersing aid.; Gardner 12 max. color, faint odor; sol. in ethanol, water; sl. sol. in ethyl acetate, glycerin; sp.gr. 1.02-1.07 (50/4 C); m.p. 45-51 C; acid no. 5 max.; sapon. no. 18 max.; pH 5.5-7.0 (4% aq.).

Lanatein-25. [Lanaetex Prods.] PEG-75 lanolin, hydrolyzed collagen; cosmetics ingred.

Lanbritol Wax N21. [Ronsheim & Moore] Cetearyl alcohol, ceteth-12, and oleth-12; nonionic; SE wax, emulsifier for pharmaceuticals, cosmetics and hair care preparations; wh. waxy solid; m.p. 45-53 C; biodeg.; 100% conc.

Lancol. [Lanaetex Prods.] Oleyl alcohol; CAS 143-28-2; EINECS 205-597-3; cosmetics ingred.

Landrox. [Lanaetex Prods.] Hydroxylated lanolin; CAS 68424-66-8; EINECS 270-315-8; cosmetic ingred.

Lanesta 10. [Lanaetex Prods.] Isopropyl isostearate; EINECS 250-651-1; emollient.

Lanesta 23. [Lanaetex Prods.] Isopropyl palmitate; CAS 142-91-6; EINECS 205-571-1; cosmetics ingred.

Lanesta 24. [Lanaetex Prods.] Glyceryl stearate; cosmetics ingred.

Lanesta 31. [Lanaetex Prods.] Isopropyl myristate; CAS 110-27-0; EINECS 203-751-4; cosmetics ingred.

Lanesta 35. [Lanaetex Prods.] Glycol stearate; CAS 111-60-4; EINECS 203-886-9; cosmetics ingred.

Lanesta 40. [Lanaetex Prods.] Glyceryl stearate SE; cosmetics ingred.

Lanesta EGD. [Lanaetex Prods.] Glycol distearate; CAS 627-83-8; EINECS 211-014-3; cosmetics ingred.

Lanesta-EO. [Lanaetex Prods.] Glycol distearate and other ingreds.; CAS 627-83-8; EINECS 211-014-3; cosmetic ingred.

Lanesta G. [Westbrook Lanolin] Glyceryl lanolate; CAS 97404-50-7; nonionic; emollient, moisturizer, emulsifier for baby creams/lotions, day/night creams, sunscreen preps.; forms stable w/o emulsions; pale yel. soft wax; m.p. 42-50 C; HLB 4.5; acid no. 3 max.; sapon. no. 140-160; hyd. no. 165 min.; 100% conc.

Lanesta L. [Westbrook Lanolin] Isopropyl lanolate; CAS 63393-93-1; EINECS 264-119-1; nonsticky emollient with lubricant properties; for baby oils, cleansers, foam baths/gels, sunscreens; liq.; sp.gr. 0.850-0.870; acid no. 7 max.; sapon. no. 160-190; pour pt. 10 C.

Lanesta P. [Westbrook Lanolin] Isopropyl lanolate; CAS 63393-93-1; EINECS 264-119-1; emollient, moisturizer, lubricant, glossing agent for baby creams, cleansers, eye preps., lipsticks, toilet soaps; m.p. 28-38 C; acid no. 4 max.; iodine no. 6-20; sapon. no. 125-155.

Lanesta S. [Westbrook Lanolin] Isopropyl lanolate; CAS 63393-93-1; EINECS 264-119-1; nonsticky emollient rapidly absorbed by skin; lubricant; for lipsticks, nailcare, sunscreen preps., toilet soap; binder for pressed powds.; soft wax; m.p. 30-39 C; acid no. 5 max.; iodine no. 6-20; sapon. no. 115-145.

Lanesta SA-30. [Westbrook Lanolin] Isopropyl lanolate; CAS 63393-93-1; EINECS 264-119-1; emollient, moisturizer, lubricant for baby creams/lotions, day/night creams, toilet soaps; binder for pressed powds.; m.p. 30-40 C; acid no. 18 max.; sapon. no. 140-160; hyd. no. 48-68.

Laneto 40. [R.I.T.A.] PEG-40 lanolin; CAS 61790-81-6; nonionic; moisturizer, lubricant, emulsifier, and solubilizer surfactant for soap and detergent systems; emollient, resin modifier and solubilizer for personal care prods.; glossing agent for hair; plasticizer; Gardner 12 max.; char. odor; sol. in alcohol; slightly sol. in water; 50 ± 1% water.

Laneto 50. [R.I.T.A.] PEG-75 lanolin; CAS 8039-09-6; nonionic; moisturizer, lubricant, emulsifier, emollient, plasticizer, solubilizer for soap and detergent systems, personal care prods., fragrances; glossing agent for hair; amber liq., char. odor; water-sol.; sp.gr. 1.00–1.10; acid no. 1 max.; sapon. no. 10 max.; 50 ± 1% water.

Laneto 60. [R.I.T.A.] PEG-60 lanolin; CAS 61790-81-6; moisturizer, lubricant, emulsifier, and solubilizer surfactant for soap and detergent systems; emollient, resin modifier and solubilizer for personal care prods.; glossing agent for hair; plasticizer; amber liq.; m.p. 48–52 C; sapon. no. 10–16.

Laneto 100. [R.I.T.A.] PEG-75 lanolin; CAS 61790-81-6; nonionic; emulsifier, emollient, conditioner, moisturizer, stabilizer, and solubilizer in makeup, lipsticks, skin care prods., bath preps., shampoos, soaps, shave creams, ointments, sun preps., veterinary prods.; amber solid.

Laneto 100-Flaked. [R.I.T.A.] PEG-75 lanolin; CAS 61790-81-6; nonionic; emollient, lubricant, solubilizer, emulsifier, plasticizer for cosmetics and pharmaceuticals; promotes emolliency and surface activity in aq. and hydroalcoholic systems; conditioner for shampoos; superfatting agent for hand soaps and waterless cleaners; imparts soft, nonsticky feel in creams and ointments; solubilizer for pharmaceuticals; yel. flakes, char. odor; water sol.; m.p. 45 C min.; acid no. 2 max.; iodine no. 8 max.; sapon. no.

20 max.; 100% conc.

Laneto AWS. [R.I.T.A.] PPG-12-PEG-50 lanolin; CAS 68458-88-8; nonionic; aux. emulsifier, moisturizer, emollient for personal care prods.; plasticizer for hair spray, resins; amber liq.; sol. in water and alcohol; HLB 16.0; 100% conc.

Lanette® 14. [Henkel/Cospha; Henkel Canada; Henkel KGaA/Cospha] Myristyl alcohol; CAS 112-72-1; EINECS 204-000-3; nonionic; emollient, consistency agent for cosmetic and pharmaceutical o/w and w/o creams, emulsions, sticks; wh. flakes; sp.gr. 0.82-0.83 (40 C); m.p. 35-38 C; acid no. < 0.1; iodine no. < 0.3; sapon. no. < 0.3; hyd. no. 255-262; flash pt. 148 C; 100% conc.

Lanette® 16. [Henkel/Cospha; Henkel Canada; Henkel KGaA/Cospha] Cetyl alcohol; CAS 36653-82-4; EINECS 253-149-0; nonionic; emollient, consistency agent for cosmetic and pharmaceutical o/w and w/o creams, emulsions, sticks; wh. flakes; sp.gr. 0.815-0.830 (40 C); m.p. 46-49 C; acid no. 0.1 max.; iodine no. < 0.5; sapon. no. < 0.5; hyd. no. 225-235; flash pt. 157 C; 100% conc.

Lanette® 18. [Henkel/Cospha; Henkel KGaA/Cospha] Stearyl alcohol USP; CAS 112-92-5; EINECS 204-017-6; nonionic; emollient, consistency agent for cosmetic and pharmaceutical o/w and w/o creams, emulsions, sticks; colorless flakes; m.p. 55-57.5 C; acid no. 0.1 max.; iodine no. 1 max.; sapon. no. 0.5 max.; hyd. no. 203-210; usage level: 1-10%; 100% conc.

Lanette® 18 DEO. [Henkel/Cospha; Henkel Canada] Stearyl alcohol; CAS 112-92-5; EINECS 204-017-6; emollient, consistency agent for cosmetic and pharmaceutical o/w and w/o creams, emulsions, sticks; flakes; acid no. < 0.1; iodine no. < 1.0; sapon. no. < 0.5.

Lanette® 22 Flakes. [Henkel KGaA/Cospha] Behenyl alcohol; CAS 97552-91-5; EINECS 211-546-6; nonionic; emollient, consistency agent for cosmetic and pharmaceutical o/w and w/o creams, emulsions, sticks; wh. to pale ylsh. hydrophilic waxy fused flakes; solid. pt. 64-67 C; acid no. 0.2 max.; iodine no. 1 max.; sapon. no. 0.5 max.; hyd. no. 170-180; 100% conc.

Lanette® E. [Henkel/Cospha; Henkel/Functional Prods; Henkel Canada; Henkel KGaA/Cospha] Sodium cetearyl sulfate; CAS 68955-20-4; anionic; emulsifier and wetting agent for o/w emulsions, creams, and ointments; wh. to lt. yel. powd., almost odorless; dens. 150-250 g/l; pH 6.5-7.5; 90% min. act.

Lanette® N. [Henkel/Cospha; Henkel Canada; Henkel KGaA/Cospha] Cetearyl alcohol (90%) and sodium cetearyl sulfate (10%); anionic; self-emulsifying raw material for o/w creams, ointments, and liq. liniments; wh. gran., faint char. odor; pH 6.5-8.0 (1%); 100% conc.

Lanette® O. [Henkel/Cospha; Henkel KGaA/Cospha] Cetearyl alcohol; CAS 67762-27-0; nonionic; emollient, base, consistency factor for cosmetic/pharmaceutical ointments, creams, o/w emulsions; wh. gran. flakes; insol. in water; m.p. 48-52 C; acid no. 0.1 max.; iodine no. 0.5 max.; sapon. no. 1 max.; hyd. no. 215-225; 100% conc.

Lanette® SX. [Henkel/Cospha; Henkel Canada] Cetearyl alcohol (90%) and sodium lauryl sulfate (10%); anionic; emulsifier; SE base for mfg. of o/w ointment, creams, and emulsions; wh. gran.

Lanette® W. [Henkel] Cetearyl alcohol and sodium lauryl sulfate; anionic; SE base for mfg. of ointments, creams and liniments; gran.; 100% conc.

Lanette® Wax SX, SXBP. [Henkel] Cetearyl alcohol and sodium C12–15 alcohols sulfate (SXBP complies to B.P. specifications); anionic; o/w emulsifier, SE wax for use in toiletry, pharmaceutical preparations, creams, ointments and lotions; cream to pale yel. waxy flakes; faint char. odor; partially sol. in alcohol, almost insol. in water; m.p. 50 C; biodeg.; 100% conc.

Lanette Wax SX. [Ronsheim & Moore] Cetearyl alcohol and sodium C12-15 alkyl sulfate.

Lanexol AWS. [Croda Inc.] PPG-12-PEG-50 lanolin; CAS 68458-88-8; nonionic; emollient, conditioner, cleanser, superfatting agent, foam stabilizer, and lubricant for alcoholic and aq. compositions, pharmaceuticals, plasticizer for hair sprays, o/w emulsifier, solubilizer; amber visc. liq.; sol. in oil, water, ethanol and mixts.; disp. in propylene glycol; cloud pt. 65–80 C (1% aq.); pour pt. 13 C max.; acid no. 2 max.; iodine no. 10 max.; sapon. no. 10–20; pH 6.0–7.0 (1% aq.); usage level: 1-5%; toxicology: LD50 (oral, rat) 32 g/kg; moderate skin irritant, minimal eye irritant; 97% conc.

Lanfrax® . [Henkel/Organic Prods.] Lanolin wax; CAS 68201-49-0; EINECS 269-220-4; nonionic; cosmetic emulsion stabilizer, w/o emulsifier and waxing agent, o/w aux. emulsifier; slip reducing agent; for floor finishing prods., polishes; wax; 100% conc.

Lanfrax® 1776. [Henkel/Cospha; Henkel Canada] USP lanolin wax fraction; CAS 68201-49-0; EINECS 269-220-4; nonionic; w/o emulsifier, emollient, crystallization inhibitor, and film-former for personal care prods. (creams, lotions, makeup, lip prods., suntan preps.); waxing agent, o/w aux. emulsifier; slip reducing agent in floor finishing compds.; emulsion stabilizer and thickener; lt. yel. waxy solid; 100% conc.

Lanfrax® 1779. [Henkel/Cospha; Henkel Canada] Lanolin wax; CAS 68201-49-0; EINECS 269-220-4; w/o emulsifier, emollient, conditioner, moisturizer, film-former, stabilizer, crystallization inhibitor, pigment dispersant for cosmetics, pharmaceuticals (creams, lotions, makeup, lip prods., suntan preps.); lt. yel. waxy solid, low odor; m.p. 49-52 C.

Lanidox-5. [Lanaetex Prods.] PEG-6 lauramide; CAS 26635-75-6; emulsifier, detergent.

Lanidrol. [Esperis] PEG-20 hydrog. lanolin; CAS 68648-27-1; emollient, emulsifier.

Lanion-27. [Lanaetex Prods.] PEG-75 lanolin, stearalkonium chloride.

Lanion-28. [Lanaetex Prods.] Lanolin alcohol, stearalkonium chloride.

Lanisolate. [Lanaetex Prods.] Isopropyl lanolate; CAS 63393-93-1; EINECS 264-119-1; emollient.

Lankropol® KNB22. [Harcros UK] Monoalkyl sulfosuccinate; anionic; foaming agent for personal care prods.; primary emulsifier for latex prod.; cement foaming agent; liq.; 29% conc.

Lankropol® KSG72. [Harcros UK] Monoester sulfosuccinate; anionic; mild foaming agent for toiletries; primary emulsifier for latex prod.; cement foaming agents; liq.; 35% conc.

Lanobase SE. [Lanaetex Prods.] PEG-6-32 and PEG-75 lanolin.

Lanocerin® . [Amerchol] Lanolin wax; CAS 68201-49-0; EINECS 269-220-4; w/o emulsifier, emollient, conditioner used in cosmetics; yel.-tan waxy solid; faint pleasant odor; insol. in water; m.p. 41–51 C; acid no. 2.5 max.; sapon. no. 85–115.

Lanocerina. [Esperis] Hydrog. lanolin; CAS 8031-44-5; EINECS 232-452-1; emollient.

Lanogel® 21. [Amerchol] PEG-27 lanolin; CAS 61790-81-6; nonionic; emollient, emulsifier, dispersant, wetting agent, solubilizer, foam stabilizer, used in cosmetics, personal care prods., pharmaceuticals, facial tissues, antiperspirants, germicidal hand soaps; ASTM 3 max. gel; HLB 15.0; 50% act.

Lanogel® 31. [Amerchol] PEG–40 lanolin; CAS 61790-81-6; nonionic; emollient, emulsifier, dispersant, wetting agent, solubilizer, foam stabilizer, used in cosmetics, personal care prods., pharmaceuticals, facial tissues,

antiperspirants, germicidal hand soaps; ASTM 3 max. gel; 50% act.

Lanogel® 41. [Amerchol] PEG-75 lanolin; CAS 61790-81-6; nonionic; emollient, emulsifier, dispersant, wetting agent, solubilizer, foam stabilizer, used in cosmetics, personal care prods., pharmaceuticals, facial tissues, antiperspirants, germicidal hand soaps; ASTM 3 max. gel; HLB 15.0; 50% act.

Lanogel® 61. [Amerchol] PEG-85 lanolin; CAS 61790-81-6; nonionic; emollient, emulsifier, dispersant, wetting agent, solubilizer, foam stabilizer, used in cosmetics, personal care prods., pharmaceuticals, facial tissues, antiperspirants, germicidal hand soaps; ASTM 3 max. gel; 50% act.

Lanogene® . [Amerchol] Lanolin oil; emollient, moisturizer, and emulsifier which imparts oil sol. and spreading properties; yel.-amber liq.; slight char. odor; sol. in oils, esters, hydrocarbons, and IPA; acid no. 2 max.; sapon. no. 85–105.

Lanoil. [Lanaetex Prods.] Lanolin oil; cosmetics ingred.

Lanoil AWS. [Lanaetex Prods.] PPG-12-PEG-50 lanolin; CAS 68458-88-8; cosmetics ingred.

Lanoil Water/Alcohol Soluble Lanolin. [Lanaetex Prods.] PEG-75 lanolin oil; CAS 68648-38-4; superfatting agent.

Lanol 14 M. [Seppic] Myreth-3 myristate; CAS 59686-68-9; cosmetic emulsifier; paste; 100% act.

Lanol 1688. [Seppic] Cetearyl octanoate; cosmetic emulsifier; liq.; 100% act.

Lanol C. [Seppic] Cetyl alcohol; CAS 36653-82-4; EINECS 253-149-0; nonionic; emollient, cosmetic assistant; wax; 100% conc.

Lanol CS. [Seppic] Cetearyl alcohol; nonionic; emollient, cosmetic assistant; wax; 100% conc.

Lanol P. [Seppic] Glycol palmitate; CAS 4219-49-2; EINECS 224-160-8; cosmetic emulsifier; wax; 100% act.

Lanol S. [Seppic] Stearyl alcohol; CAS 112-92-5; EINECS 204-017-6; nonionic; emollient, cosmetic assistant; wax; 100% conc.

Lanola 90. [Lanaetex Prods.] Lanolin and PEG-8 stearate; cosmetic ingred.

Lanolex L-40. [Nihon Emulsion] PEG-50 lanolin; CAS 61790-81-6; reforming agent, emollient for shampoos, hair conditioners; JSCI compliance; pale yel. visc. liq.; HLB 18.

Lanolide. [Vevy] PEG-5 pentaerythritol ether, PPG-5 pentaerythritol ether, soy sterol.

Lanolin A.C. [Lanaetex Prods.] Acetylated lanolin; CAS 61788-48-5; EINECS 262-979-2; cosmetics ingred.

Lanolin Anhydrous USP. [Lanaetex Prods.] Lanolin; CAS 8006-54-0; EINECS 232-348-6; emollient.

Lanolin Anhydrous USP. [ChemMark Development] Lanolin; CAS 8006-54-0; EINECS 232-348-6; emollient.

Lanolin Cosmetic. [R.I.T.A.] Lanolin; CAS 8006-54-0; EINECS 232-348-6; epidermal moisturizer, lubricant, and emollient for personal care; stabilizer for emulsions, dispersions, and suspensions; yel. grease.

Lanolin Extra-Deodorized. [R.I.T.A.] Lanolin; CAS 8006-54-0; EINECS 232-348-6; epidermal moisturizer, lubricant, and emollient for personal care; stabilizer for emulsions, dispersions, and suspensions; yel. grease.

Lanolin Pharmaceutical. [R.I.T.A.] Lanolin; CAS 8006-54-0; EINECS 232-348-6; epidermal moisturizer, lubricant, and emollient for personal care; stabilizer for emulsions, dispersions, and suspensions; yel. grease.

Lanolin Tech. [Amerchol] Lanolin, tech.; CAS 8006-54-0; EINECS 232-348-6; cosmetic emollient.

Lanolin Tech. Grade. [R.I.T.A.] Lanolin; CAS 8006-54-0; EINECS 232-348-6; emollient.

Lanolin U.S.P. [Amerchol] Lanolin USP; CAS 8006-54-0; EINECS 232-348-6; cosmetic emollient.

Lanolin USP. [R.I.T.A.] Lanolin USP; CAS 8006-54-0;

EINECS 232-348-6; epidermal moisturizer, lubricant, and emollient for personal care; stabilizer for emulsions, dispersions, and suspensions; yel. grease.

Lanoquat® 1751A. [Henkel/Cospha] Lanolin quat.; o/w emulsifier, emollient, and conditioner for liq. soaps, creams, lotions, shaving preps., and hair care prods.; amber clear visc. liq.

Lanoquat® 1756. [Henkel/Cospha; Henkel Canada] Quaternium-33, ethyl hexanediol; cationic; conditioner; emulsifier for skin moisturizers; substantive to hair; provides lubricating, conditioning, antistatic properties; Gardner < 12 visc. liq.; sol. in water, ethanol, glycols; 50% conc.

Lanoquat® 1757. [Henkel/Cospha; Henkel Canada] Quaternium-33, ethyl hexanediol; emollient, conditioner, emulsifier in creams, lotions, makeup, shampoos; Gardner < 12 liq.; sol. in water, IPA, IPM; disp. in triolein, glycerin; dens. 8.2 lb/gal; visc. 226 cSt (100 F); pour pt. < 1 C; flash pt. 270 F.

Lanosil. [Lanaetex Prods.] Isopropyl palmitate and lanolin oil; cosmetics ingred.

Lanosoluble A. [Prod'Hyg] Peanut oil, lanolin, and cholesterol; cosmetic ingred.

Lanosterol. [Solvay Duphar BV] Lanolin deriv.; CAS 79-63-0; EINECS 201-214-9; nonionic; gelling agent for cosmetic preps. such as lipstick, creams, nail polish; crystal powd.; 90+% conc.

Lanotein AWS 30. [Fanning] Propylene glycol, hydrolyzed animal protein, PPG-12-PEG-65 lanolin oil; conditioner, film former, lubricant, humectant, and emollient used in hair prods., shave creams, soaps, conditioning creams and lotions; lt. amber liq.; bland odor; sol. in water; sl. sol. in glycerin @ 75 C; sp.gr. 1.05–1.08; pH 5.0–6.0.

Lanowax. [Lanaetex Prods.] Lanolin wax; CAS 68201-49-0; EINECS 269-220-4; emulsifier, emollient.

Lanoxal 75. [Seppic] PEG-75 lanolin; CAS 61790-81-6; nonionic; cosmetic assistant; wax; 100% conc.

Lanoxide-52. [Lanaetex Prods.] PEG-40 stearate; CAS 9004-99-3; cosmetics ingred.

Lanoxide-53. [Lanaetex Prods.] PEG-50 stearate; CAS 9004-99-3; cosmetics ingred.

Lanoxide-59. [Lanaetex Prods.] PEG-100 stearate; CAS 9004-99-3; cosmetics ingred.

Lanoxide-6000DS. [Lanaetex Prods.] PEG-6000 distearate; CAS 9005-08-7; cosmetic ingred.

Lanpol 5. [Croda Chem. Ltd.] PEG-5 lanolin acids, dist.; CAS 68459-50-7; nonionic; o/w emulsifier, solv. for bromo acid dyes in lipsticks, skin care and makeup prods., solubilizer, wetting agent, dispersant; pale yel. pasty solid; sol. in oil, disp. in water; HLB 7.5; sapon. no. 105–120; pH 4–7 (3%); 97% conc.

Lanpol 10. [Croda Chem. Ltd.] PEG-10 lanolin acids, dist.; CAS 68459-50-7; nonionic; see Lanpol 5; pale yel. pasty solid; HLB 10.9; sapon. no. 60–80; pH 4–7 (3%); 97% conc.

Lanpol 20. [Croda Chem. Ltd.] PEG-20 lanolin acids, dist.; CAS 68459-50-7; nonionic; see Lanpol 5; solid; HLB 14.1; 97% conc.

Lanpro-1. [Lanaetex Prods.] Cocoyl hydrolyzed collagen, min. oil, hydrog. lanolin, ceteareth-5, and myristyl myristate.

Lanpro-2. [Lanaetex Prods.] Lecithin, butyl stearate, cocoyl hydrolyzed collagen, oleoyl sarcosine, sesame oil, and lanolin alcohol.

Lanpro-10. [Lanaetex Prods.] Hydrolyzed collagen, PEG-75 lanolin, propylene glycol, ceteth-16, and lanolin oil.

Lantox 55, 110. [Lanaetex Prods.] PEG-75 lanolin; CAS 61790-81-6; cosmetics ingred.

Lantrol® 1673. [Henkel/Cospha; Henkel Canada] Lanolin oil; emollient and moisturizer for makeup, creams, lotions, hair care prods., bath oils, medicinal preps.; pigment dispersant; amber visc. liq.; sol. in min. oil, triolein, IPM; disp. in IPA; dens. 7.8 lb/gal; visc. 948 cSt (100 F); pour pt. 6 C; cloud pt. 18 C; flash pt. 525 F.

Lantrol® 1674. [Henkel/Cospha; Henkel Canada] Lanolin oil; low odor version of Lantrol 1673; dispersant, vehicle for pigment grinds in makeups; amber visc. liq.; sol. in min. oil, castor oil, triolein, IPM; disp. in IPA; dens. 7.8 lb/gal; visc. 835 cSt (100 F); pour pt. 9 C; cloud pt. 20 C; flash pt. 525 F.

Lantrol® 1675. [Henkel/Cospha; Henkel Canada] Lanolin oil; premium grade for lt. colored or delicate fragrance applics., lip preps., pigment dispersion; Gardner < 7 liq.; sol. in min. oil, triolein, IPM; disp. in IPA; dens. 7.8 lb/gal; visc. 820 cSt (100 F); pour pt. 9 C; cloud pt. < 10 C; flash pt. 525 F.

Lantrol® AWS 1692. [Henkel/Cospha; Henkel Canada] PPG-12-PEG-65 lanolin oil; CAS 68458-58-8; emollient, plasticizer, solubilizer, and conditioner for hair prods., shaving lotions, antiperspirants, body colognes; lt. amber visc. liq.; sol. in water, IPA; disp. in triolein, glycerin; dens. 8.9 lb/gal; visc. 788 cSt (100 F); HLB 18.0; pour pt. 8 C; cloud pt. 57 C; flash pt. 545 F; 100% conc.

Lantrol® HP-2073. [Henkel/Cospha; Henkel Canada] Lanolin oil; CAS 8006-54-0; emulsifier, emollient, conditioner, moisturizer, pigment dispersant for personal care prods., pharmaceuticals; provides hair and skin lubrication; amber visc. liq.; sol. in min. oil, IPM; disp. in IPA; insol. in water; iodine no. 18-36; sapon. no. 90-110; cloud pt. 18 C.

Lantrol® HP-2074. [Henkel/Cospha; Henkel Canada] Lanolin oil; emulsifier, emollient, conditioner, moisturizer, pigment dispersant for personal care prods., pharmaceuticals; Gardner 9 liq.; cloud pt. 20 C.

Lantrol® PLN. [Pulcra SA] Ethoxylated lanolin; CAS 8039-09-6; nonionic; cleaning and wetting agent; solubilizer for perfumes and germicides; conditioner for shampoos; superfatting agent for soaps; o/w emulsifier for nonfatty preps.; plasticizer for aerosols and hair sprays; solid; HLB 17.0; sapon. no. 10-15; pH 6.0-7.5 (1%); 100% conc.

Lantrol® PLN/50. [Pulcra SA] Ethoxylated lanolin; nonionic; cleaning and wetting agent; solubilizer for perfumes and germicides; conditioner for shampoos; superfatting agent for soaps; o/w emulsifier for nonfatty preps.; plasticizer for aerosols and hair sprays; paste; sapon. no. 4-10; pH 6.0-7.5 (1%); 50% conc.

Lanycol-30. [Lanaetex Prods.] Laureth-30; CAS 9002-92-0; cosmetics ingred.

Lanycol-35. [Lanaetex Prods.] Laureth-35; CAS 9002-92-0; cosmetics ingred.

Lanycol-52. [Lanaetex Prods.] Ceteth-2; CAS 9004-95-9; cosmetics ingred.

Lanycol-58. [Lanaetex Prods.] Ceteth-20; CAS 9004-95-9; cosmetics ingred.

Lanycol-72. [Lanaetex Prods.] Steareth-2; CAS 9005-00-9; cosmetics ingred.

Lanycol-78. [Lanaetex Prods.] Steareth-20; CAS 9005-00-9; cosmetics ingred.

Lanycol-79. [Lanaetex Prods.] Steareth-21; CAS 9005-00-9; cosmetic ingred.

Lanycol-92. [Lanaetex Prods.] Oleth-2; CAS 9004-98-2; cosmetics ingred.

Lanycol-96. [Lanaetex Prods.] Oleth-10; CAS 9004-98-2; cosmetic ingred.

Lanycol-97. [Lanaetex Prods.] Oleth-10; CAS 9004-98-2; cosmetic ingred.

Lanycol-98. [Lanaetex Prods.] Oleth-20; CAS 9004-98-2; cosmetics ingred.

Lanycol-99. [Lanaetex Prods.] Oleth-20; CAS 9004-98-2; cosmetics ingred.

Lanycol-700. [Lanaetex Prods.] Steareth-100; CAS 9005-00-9; personal care surfactant.

Lapomer. [Southern Clay Prods.] Sodium magnesium silicate and cellulose gum.

Laponite® D. [Laporte/Southern Clay] Sodium magnesium silicate; CAS 53320-86-8; EINECS 258-476-2; used in conjunction with other thickeners for imparting a shear sensitive structure to clear gel and conventional toothpastes; wh. free-flowing powd.; insol. in water but hydrates and swells to give clear and colorless colloidal disp. in water or aq. alcohol sol'ns.; bulk dens. 1000 kg/m³; surf. area 370 m²/g; pH 9.8 (2% susp.).

Laponite® XLG. [Laporte/Southern Clay] Sodium magnesium silicate; CAS 53320-86-8; EINECS 258-476-2; inert base/carrier for act. ingreds.; suspending agent; promotes thixotropy giving stable suspensions; thickens cosmetic, toiletry creams, lotions, toothpaste prods.; wh. free-flowing powd.; insol. in water but hydrates and swells to give clear, colorless colloidal disps. in water or aq. alocholic sol'ns.; bulk dens. 1000 kg/m³; surf. area 370 m²/g; pH 9.8 (2% susp.).

Laponite® XLS. [Laporte/Southern Clay] Sodium magnesium silicate, tetrasodium pyrophosphate; inert base/carrier for act. ingreds.; suspending agent; promotes thixotropy giving stable suspensions; thickens cosmetic, toiletry creams, lotions, toothpaste prods.; clarification aid, adsorbent; wh. free-flowing powd.; hydrates and swells in water to give clear, colorless colloidal disps. of low visc.; bulk dens. 1000 kg/m³; surf. area 330 m²/g; pH 9.7 (2% susp.).

L.A.S. [Gattefosse SA] PEG-8 caprylic/capric glycerides; CAS 85536-07-8; nonionic; nontoxic excipient for creams, lotions; surfactant for microemulsions; Gardner < 5 oily liq., faint odor; sol. in water; very sol. in ethanol, chloroform, methylene chloride; sp.gr. 1.060-1.070; visc. 80-110 mPa·s; HLB 14.0; acid no. < 1; iodine no. < 2; sapon. no. 85-105; ref. index 1.450-1.470; toxicology: LD50 (oral, rat) > 20 ml/kg; sl. ocular irritant at 0.1 ml.

Lasemul 60. [Industrial Quimica Lasem] Isopropyl stearate; CAS 112-10-7; EINECS 203-934-9; emollient.

Lasemul 62 E. [Industrial Quimica Lasem] Glycol stearate; CAS 111-60-4; EINECS 203-886-9; emulsifier, opacifier, pearlescent for cosmetics.

Lasemul 74 NP. [Industrial Quimica Lasem] Butyl stearate; CAS 123-95-5; EINECS 204-666-5; emollient.

Lasemul 92 AE. [Industrial Quimica Lasem] Glyceryl stearate.

Lasemul 92 AE/A. [Industrial Quimica Lasem] Glyceryl stearate.

Lasemul 92 N 40. [Industrial Quimica Lasem] Glyceryl stearate.

Lasemul 130. [Industrial Quimica Lasem] Octyl stearate; emollient.

Lasemul 400 E. [Industrial Quimica Lasem] PEG-8 stearate; CAS 9004-99-3; emulsifier.

Lasilium [Exsymol] Sodium lactate methylsilanol.

Lasilium C. [Exsymol; Biosil Tech.] Lactoyl methylsilanol elastinate; provides hydrating, anti-inflammatory action, tissue regeneration, slimming action for hand creams, slimming prods., toothpastes, cosmetic and health prods.; colorless to pale yel. sl. opalescent liq.; misc. with water, alcohols, glycols; sp.gr. 1.0; pH 5.5; usage level: 3-4%; toxicology: nontoxic.

Lathanol® LAL. [Stepan; Stepan Canada; Stepan Europe] Sodium lauryl sulfoacetate; CAS 1847-58-1; EINECS 217-431-7; anionic; emulsifier, wetting agent, detergent, foaming agent, thickener used in cosmetics and personal care prods. (powd. bubble baths, shampoos, cleansing creams, cream and paste shampoos, syndet bars); wh. flake, powd.; faint lauryl alcohol odor; slightly acrid taste; water sol. 3.5 g/100 ml; surf. tens. 30.1 dynes/cm (0.1%) pH 5.0-7.5 (5% conc.); 65% act.

Laural D. [Ceca SA] TEA lauryl sulfate; CAS 139-96-8; EINECS 205-388-7; anionic; base for shampoos and foams baths; detergent for wool and syn. fibers; yel. liq.; visc. < 100 mPa·s; pH 6.0-7.5 (10% aq.); ≥ 40% act.

Laural EC. [Ceca SA] Ammonium laureth sulfate; CAS 32612-48-9; anionic; emulsifier, degreaser, foaming shampoo; liq.; 28% conc.

Laural LS. [Ceca SA] Sodium laureth sulfate; CAS 9004-82-4; anionic; base for shampoo and foaming baths; detergent for household prods.; emulsifier for emulsion polymerization; APHA < 500 gel; pH 4-7 (10%); surf. tens. 32 dynes/cm; ≥ 22% act.

Lauramide 11. [Zohar Detergent Factory] Cocamide DEA; CAS 61791-31-9; EINECS 263-163-9; nonionic; foam booster, thickener, superfatting agent for cosmetics; liq.; 80% conc.

Lauramide EG. [Zohar Detergent Factory] Ethylene glycol stearate; CAS 111-60-4; EINECS 203-886-9; nonionic; opacifying agent for cosmetics; paste; 50% conc.

Lauramide ME. [Zohar Detergent Factory] Cocamide DEA; CAS 61791-31-9; EINECS 263-163-9; nonionic; foam booster, thickener, superfatting agent for cosmetics; liq. to paste; 90% conc.

Lauramide R. [Zohar Detergent Factory] Fatty acid DEA; nonionic; foam booster, thickener, superfatting agent for cosmetics; liq.; 85% conc.

Lauramina. [Vevy] Lauramide DEA; CAS 120-40-1; EINECS 204-393-1; personal care surfactant.

Laurate de Cetyle. [Prod'Hyg] Cetyl laurate; CAS 20834-06-4; EINECS 244-071-8; refatting agent for cosmetics.

Laurate de PEG 400. [Prod'Hyg] PEG-8 laurate; CAS 9004-81-3; emulsifier.

Laurate de Propylene Glycol. [Prod'Hyg] Propylene glycol laurate.

Laurel R-50. [Reilly-Whiteman] Sulfated castor oil; CAS 8002-33-3; EINECS 232-306-7; anionic; penetrant, lubricant, emulsifier used in detergent cleaners, metalworking lubricants, paint, textile lubricants, low-irritation and ethnic hair preps. and dyes, skin cleaners and lotions; liq.; 50% conc.

Laurel SD-900M. [Reilly-Whiteman] Cocamide DEA (1:1); CAS 61791-31-9; EINECS 263-163-9; nonionic; surfactant, visc. builder, foam stabilizer for lt. duty liqs., dishwash, shampoos; lt. amber liq.; 100% act.

Laurel SD-1500. [Reilly-Whiteman] Coconut superamide (1:1); thickener, w/o emulsifier, visc. bulder for shampoos, lt. duty liqs.; corrosion inhibitor for sol. oils; liq.; 100% conc.

Laurene. [Vevy] Laurtrimonium chloride; CAS 112-00-5; EINECS 203-927-0; preservative for cosmetics; USA, Japan, Europe approvals; usage level: up to 0.1%.

Laurex® 4550 [Albright & Wilson Am.] Cetearyl alcohol; for mfg. of surfactants; wh. waxy flakes; dens. 0.4 g/cc (20 C); m.p. 48-53 C; acid no. 0.5 max.; sapon. no. 2.0 max; 100% act.

Laurex® CS [Albright & Wilson Am.; Albright & Wilson UK] Cetearyl alcohol BP; nonionic; mfg. of surfactants; raw material for ethoxylation, sulfation, etc.; stabilizer in emulsion polymerization; lubricant in rigid PVC, also for pharmaceutical creams, hand lotions, bath oils, shaving creams; wh. waxy flake; dens. 0.4 g/cc; m.p. 48–53 C; acid no. 0.5 max.; sapon. no. 2.0 max.; flash pt. 150 C; 100% act.

Laurex® CS/D. [Albright & Wilson UK] Cetearyl alcohol BP; nonionic; raw material for ethoxylation, sulfation, etc.; also for pharmaceutical creams, hand lotions, bath oils, shaving creams; wh. waxy flake; dens. 0.4 g/cc; m.p. 48–53 C; acid no. 0.28 max.; sapon. no. 2.0 max.; flash pt. 150 C; 100% conc.

Laurex® CS/W. [Albright & Wilson UK] Cetearyl alcohol;

nonionic; surfactant; liq.; 100% conc.

Laurex® L1. [Albright & Wilson UK] Lauryl alcohol; CAS 112-53-8; EINECS 203-982-0; raw material for ethoxylation, sulfation, etc.; superfatting agent for shampoos; wh. soft solid; dens. 0.84 g/cc; m.p. 20–25 C; acid no. 0.2 max.; sapon. no. 1.0 max.; flash pt. 130 C.

Laurex® NC. [Albright & Wilson UK] Lauryl alcohol; CAS 112-53-8; EINECS 203-982-0; raw material for ethoxylation, sulfation, etc.; stabilizer in emulsion polymerization; foam stabilizer for fire-fighting foams; superfatting agent for shampoos; wh. soft solid; dens. 0.84 g/cc; m.p. 20–25 C; acid no. 0.2 max.; sapon. no. 1.0 max.; flash pt. 132 C.

Laurex® PKH. [Albright & Wilson UK] Palm kernel alcohol; superfatting agent in shampoos, raw material for sulfation, ethoxylation; wh. soft solid; m.p. 18–23 C; sapon. no. 1.5.

Lauricidin 802, 812, 1012, E. [Lauricidin] Glyceryl laurate; CAS 142-18-7; EINECS 205-526-6; cosmetic preservative; usage level: 0.1-1.0%.

Lauridit® KD. [Akzo BV] Cocamide DEA; CAS 61791-31-9; EINECS 263-163-9; nonionic; detergent, emulsifier for cosmetic and household applics., visc. increasing additive; yel. liq.; water sol. 40 g/l; sp.gr. 1.02; flash pt. (PMCC) 104 C; pH 9.0–9.5; 90% act.

Lauridit® KDG. [Akzo BV] Cocamide DEA; CAS 61791-31-9; EINECS 263-163-9; nonionic; detergent, emulsifier for cosmetic and household applics., visc. increasing additive; yel. liq.; water sol. 800 g/l; sp.gr. 1.02; flash pt. (PMCC) 114 C; pH 9.0–9.5; 85% act.

Lauridit® KM. [Akzo BV] Cocamide MEA; CAS 68140-00-1; EINECS 268-770-2; nonionic; detergent for textile, household and cosmetic applics., foam stabilizer for detergents, shampoos, bubble baths; yel. flakes; poor water sol.; sp.gr. 0.97; m.p. 65–70 C; sapon. no. 14 max.; 93% act.

Lauridit® LM. [Akzo BV] Lauramide MEA; CAS 142-78-9; EINECS 205-560-1; nonionic; detergent for textile, household and cosmetic applics., foam stabilizer for detergents, shampoos, bubble baths; ylsh. flakes; poor water sol.; sp.gr. 1.01 (80 C); m.p. 80–84 C; sapon. no. 20 max; pH 9; 93% act.

Lauridit® OD. [Akzo BV] Oleamide DEA; CAS 93-83-4; EINECS 202-281-7; nonionic; detergent, emulsifier for cosmetic and household applics., visc. increasing additive; yel. liq.; water sol. 100 g/l; sp.gr. 0.97; f.p. 0 C; flash pt. 100 C (PMCC); pH 9; 85% act.

Lauroglycol. [Gattefosse] Propylene glycol laurate.; CAS 142-55-2; EINECS 205-542-3; emulsifier.

Lauropal 2. [Witco/H-I-P] Laureth-2; CAS 3055-93-4; EINECS 221-279-7; nonionic; base for liq. detergents and shampoos; liq.; HLB 6.2; 100% act.

Lauropal 3. [Witco/H-I-P] Laureth-3; CAS 3055-94-5; EINECS 221-280-2; viscosifier for shampoos and bath prods.; liq.; 100% act.

Lauropal 4. [Witco/H-I-P] Laureth-4; CAS 9002-92-0; EINECS 226-097-1; nonionic; emulsifier for min. oils and cosmetics; liq.; HLB 9.5; 100% conc.

Lauropal 0207L. [Witco/H-I-P] Ethoxylated fatty alcohol; nonionic; biodeg. detergent for personal care use; liq.; HLB 13.0; 80% conc.

Lauropal X 1003. [Witco/H-I-P] Ethoxylated alcohol; nonionic; wetting agent, detergent, emulsifier for personal care applics.; liq.; HLB 9.1; 100% conc.

Lauropal X 1005. [Witco/H-I-P] Ethoxylated alcohol; nonionic; wetting agent, detergent, emulsifier for personal care applics.; liq.; HLB 11.6; 100% conc.

Lauropal X 1007. [Witco/H-I-P] Ethoxylated alcohol; nonionic; wetting agent, detergent, emulsifier for personal care applics.; liq.; HLB 13.2; 100% conc.

Lauropal X 1103. [Witco/H-I-P] Ethoxylated alcohol; non-

ionic; wetting agent, detergent, emulsifier for personal care applics.; liq.; HLB 8.7; 100% conc.

Lauropal X 1105. [Witco/H-I-P] Ethoxylated branched fatty alcohol; nonionic; wetting agent, detergent for personal care applics.; liq.; HLB 11.0; 100% conc.

Lauropal X 1107. [Witco/H-I-P] Ethoxylated branched fatty alcohol; nonionic; wetting agent, detergent for personal care applics.; liq.; HLB 12.8; 100% conc.

Lauropal X 1203. [Witco/H-I-P] Ethoxylated alcohol; nonionic; wetting agent, detergent, emulsifier for personal care applics.; liq.; HLB 8.3; 100% conc.

Lauropal X 1207. [Witco/H-I-P] Ethoxylated branched fatty alcohol; nonionic; wetting agent, detergent for personal care applics.; liq.; HLB 12.5; 100% conc.

Laurydone® . [UCIB; Barnet Prods.] Lauryl PCA; CAS 30657-38-6; emulsifier in oily or aq. continuous phase; lipophilic moisturizer for skin care prods., hair care prods., pigmented cosmetics, toiletries, makeup; exceptionally soft touch; wh. or creamy-wh. powd. with oily touch; sol. in propylene glycol, ethanol; insol. in water; m.w. 297.4; m.p. 42 C; HLB 8.6; usage level: 0.5-3%; toxicology: sl. irritating to skin; very sl. irritating to eyes.

Laxan-ESE. [Lanaetex Prods.] Polysorbate 61; CAS 9005-67-8; emulsifier.

Laxan-ESL. [Lanaetex Prods.] Polysorbate 20; CAS 9005-64-5; cosmetics ingred.

Laxan-ESM. [Lanaetex Prods.] Polysorbate 81; CAS 9005-65-6; emulsifier.

Laxan-ESO. [Lanaetex Prods.] Polysorbate 80; CAS 9005-65-6; cosmetics ingred.

Laxan-ESP. [Lanaetex Prods.] Polysorbate 40; CAS 9005-66-7; cosmetics ingred.

Laxan-ESR. [Lanaetex Prods.] Polysorbate 65; CAS 9005-71-4; emulsifier.

Laxan-ESS. [Lanaetex Prods.] Polysorbate 60; CAS 9005-67-8; cosmetics ingred.

Laxan-EST. [Lanaetex Prods.] Polysorbate 85; CAS 9005-70-3; emulsifier.

Laxan-S. [Lanaetex Prods.] PEG-80 sorbitan laurate; CAS 9005-64-5; personal care surfactant.

L.C.R.E. [Kolmar Labs] Erucyl oleate, squalane, wheat germ oil, avocado oil, C10-30 cholesterol/lanosterol esters, tocopheryl acetate, retinyl palmitate.

Lebon 101H, 105. [Sanyo Chem. Industries] Alkylimidazoline type surfactant; amphoteric; nontoxic and nonirritating shampoo base; lt.-duty detergents; good foam and foam stability; stable to acids, alkalies, and hard water; liq.; 36 and 35% conc. resp.

Lebon 2000. [Sanyo Chem. Industries] Cocoamidopropyl betaine; amphoteric; low irritation surfactant for shampoos and lt. duty detergents; liq.; 30% conc.

Lebon A-5000. [Sanyo Chem. Industries] Disodium lauroyl ethanolamine POE sulfosuccinate; anionic; raw material for mild shampoos, bubble baths, cleansing agents; liq.; 30% conc.

Lecithin Ex Ovo. [Novarom GmbH] Egg yolk extract and ethoxydiglycol.

Lecithin Extract Kosmaflor, Water-Disp. [Novarom GmbH] Lecithin; CAS 8002-43-5; EINECS 232-307-2; emulsifier.

Lecithin Water Dispersible CLR. [Dr. Kurt Richter; Henkel/Cospha] TEA-dodecylbenzenesulfonate, lecithin, and PEG-40 castor oil; mild refatting agent, emollient for aq. skin and hair care preparations, face cleansers, shampoos; brn. turbid visc. prod.; char. odor.

Lecsoy E. [Fabriquimica] Soya lecithin; CAS 8002-43-5; EINECS 232-307-2; emulsifier; acid no. 18-30; iodine no. 90-100; sapon. no. 190-200.

Lecsoy S. [Fabriquimica] Soya lecithin, emulsifiable; CAS 8002-43-5; EINECS 232-307-2; cosmetic emulsifier; acid no. 16-27; iodine no. 80-90; sapon. no. 175-185.

Lemon HS. [Alban Muller] Propylene glycol and lemon extract; botanical extract.

Lemon Extract HS 2364 G. [Grau Aromatics] Propylene glycol and lemon extract; botanical extract.

Lemon Liq. [Alban Muller] Water, butylene glycol, and lemon extract.

Lencoll. [Lensfield Prods. Ltd.] Collagen; CAS 9007-34-5; EINECS 232-697-4; moisturizing protein.

Leniplex. [Laboratoires Sérobiologiques] Hydroxylated lanolin, petrolatum, glycerin, barley extract, arnica extract, castor oil, serum protein, phenyl salicylate, yarrow extract, ceteth-20, and menthol.

Lensol. [Lensfield Prods. Ltd.] Hydrolyzed collagen; CAS 9015-54-7; cosmetic protein.

Leogard GP. [Akzo BV] Polyquaternium-10; conditioner.

Letocil LP 80, SP 1000. [Chem-Y GmbH] Fatty acid polyglycol ester; nonionic; emulsifier for cosmetic industry; liq., solid resp.; 100% conc.

Leucocyanidins. [Indena SpA] Grapeseed extract.

Leucocyanidins Phytosome®. [Indena SpA; Lipo] Complex of leucocyanidins and soybean phospholipids; free-radical scavenger, elasticizer, anti-aging, soothing, and moisturizing agent for anti-aging skin prods., preps. for prevention of stretch marks, pre-sun prods.; lt. brn. amorphous powd.; water-disp.; usage level: to 2%.

Lexaine® C. [Inolex] Cocamidopropyl betaine; amphoteric; visc. builder, foam booster, thickener in conditioners, specialty shampoos, personal care prods., dishwash, sanitizers; Gardner 4 max. clear liq.; sp.gr. 1.044; f.p. -4 C; pH 4.5–5.5; 30% act.

Lexaine® CG-30. [Inolex] Cocamidopropyl betaine; amphoteric; surfactant, foam and visc. modifier, lime soap dispersant, thickener used in light duty liq. detergent systems, personal care prods.; straw to lt. amber clear nonvisc. liq.; bland odor; sp.gr. 1.06; f.p. -6 C; pH 6.5–8.0; 29% act.

Lexaine® CS. [Inolex] Cocamidopropyl betaine; amphoteric; mild surfactant for shampoo, bubble bath, dishwash, conditioners, sanitizers, creams and lotions; stable in acid and alkaline systems; clear liq.; sp.gr. 1.044; f.p. -4 C; pH 4.5-5.5; 30% conc.

Lexaine® CSB-50. [Inolex] Cocamidopropylhydroxysultaine; CAS 68139-30-0; EINECS 268-761-3; amphoteric; surfactant, foaming and wetting agent used in personal care prods. (shampoos, conditioners, bath prods.), industrial (heavy-duty alkaline cleaners, paint strippers, metal cleaners); stable in systems containing acids, alkali, and electrolytes; lime soap dispersant; clear liq.; sp.gr. 1.10; f.p. -11 C; pH 7-9; 48% conc.

Lexaine® IS. [Inolex] Isostearamidopropyl betaine; amphoteric; mild surfactant, foam booster and thickener for shampoos, bubble baths, foaming conditioners; stable in acid and alkaline systems; liq.; 25% conc.

Lexaine® LM. [Inolex] Lauramidopropyl betaine; CAS 4292-10-8; EINECS 224-292-6; amphoteric; mild surfactant, foam booster for bath prods., shampoos, liq. soaps, dishwash liqs.; pale yel. clear liq.; sp.gr. 1.045; pH 4.5-8.0; 30% conc.

Lexaine® O. [Inolex] Oleamidopropyl betaine; CAS 25054-76-6; EINECS 246-584-2; amphoteric; mild surfactant, foam booster, and thickener used in personal care prods. (shampoos, bubble baths, foaming conditioners); stable in acid and alkaline systems; liq.; 30% conc.

Lexamine 22. [Inolex] Stearamidoethyl diethylamine; CAS 16889-14-8; EINECS 240-924-3; cationic; conditioner, emulsifier for hair and skin care prods.; lt. tan waxy flakes, faint char. amine odor; water-sol. when neutralized with water-sol. acids; m.p. 50 C; acid no. 1.5; pH 9.5 (3%); 100% conc.

Lexamine C-13. [Inolex] Cocamidopropyl dimethylamine;

CAS 68140-01-2; EINECS 268-771-8; cationic; emulsifier for creams and lotions; when neutralized as conditioners for hair care prods.; soft waxy solid; m.p. 30 C; HLB 10.2; acid no. 4 max.; pH 9.5 (3%); toxicology: strong skin and severe eye irritant; moderately corrosive to skin; 100% conc.

Lexamine L-13. [Inolex] Lauramidopropyl dimethylamine; CAS 3179-80-4; EINECS 221-661-3; cationic; conditioner, emulsifier for hair and skin care prods.; lt. tan waxy solid, faint char. amine odor; m.p. 37 C; acid no. 4 max.; pH 9.5 (3%); 100% conc.

Lexamine O-13. [Inolex] Oleamidopropyl dimethylamine; CAS 109-28-4; EINECS 203-661-5; cationic; emulsifier for creams and lotions; when neutralized as conditioners for hair care prods.; golden clear visc. liq.; m.p. 4 C; HLB 7.8; acid no. 4 max.; pH 9.5 (3%); toxicology: strong skin and severe eye irritant; moderately corrosive to skin; 100% conc.

Lexamine S-13. [Inolex] Stearamidopropyl dimethylamine; CAS 7651-02-7; EINECS 231-609-1; cationic; emulsifier for creams and lotions; when neutralized as conditioners for hair care prods.; lt. tan waxy flakes; m.p. 67 C; HLB 7.8; acid no. 4 max.; pH 9.5 (3%); 100% conc.

Lexamine S-13 Lactate. [Inolex] Stearamidopropyl dimethylamine lactate; CAS 55819-53-9; EINECS 259-837-7; cationic; conditioner for shampoos and hair rinses; free rinsing, compat. with lauryl sulfates; fluid slurry, mild char. char. odor; sp.gr. 0.997; f.p. 17 C; pH 4-5; 25% solids.

Lexate® BPQ. [Inolex] Lauramidopropyl betaine, TEA-cocoyl hydrolyzed collagen, oleamidopropyl PG dimonium chloride; blended detergent, conditioner, and protein used as economical base for shampoo, bath gel, liq. soaps, dishwash, bubble baths, cleansers; lt. amber liq., char. odor; pH 5.5-6.5; 35% solids; 4% protein.

Lexate® CRC. [Inolex] Stearamidopropyl dimethylamine, glycol stearate, and ceteth-2; cationic; economical cream rinse conc. and conditioner, emulsifier; cream to tan hard waxy flake, mild fatty amino odor; easily melted and dispersed in water; m.p. 49–53 C; acid no. 2.0; sapon. no. 58; amine no. 64-70; 100% act.

Lexate® PX. [Inolex] Petrolatum, lanolin, and ozokerite; o/w and aux. emulsifier, emollient, surfactant, lanolin cream base, conditioner in soaps, shaving cream, night creams, cleansing creams, hair creams, lipsticks; vehicle in topical pharmaceuticals; faintly yel. semisolid; mild fatty char. odor; sol. in oils, insol. in water; m.p. 36-46 C; acid no. 0.3; sapon. no. 1.0; 100% solids.

Lexate® TA. [Inolex] Glyceryl stearate, IPM, and stearyl stearate; aux. lipophilic emulsifier in w/o emulsions, emollient in cosmetic creams and lotions; provides barrier properties and slip; wh. soft waxy solid; odorless to bland, fatty odor; sol. in oils, insol. in water; m.p. 45–50 C; acid no. 5–9; sapon. no. 159–169; 100% conc.

Lexate® TL. [Inolex] Glyceryl stearate, butyl stearate, and stearyl stearate; superfatting agent in milled bar soap, aux. lipophilic emulsifier in w/o systems, emollient; enhances barrier properties in creams and lotions; wh. waxy solid; mild, fatty odor; sol. in oils, insol. in water; m.p. 50-55 C; acid no. 3 max.; iodine no. 2 max.; sapon. no. 145-152; 100% conc.

Lexein® A-200. [Inolex] Myristoyl hydrolyzed collagen; CAS 72319-06-3; film-forming collagen protein deriv.; resin modifier for hair sprays, makeups, protection skin lotions and creams; wh. to cream fluffy free-flowing powd., mild char. proteinaceous odor; sol. in methanol, ethanol, IPA; insol. in water; pH 3.5-4.5 (5% aq. disp.); 95% min. solids.

Lexein® A-210. [Inolex] Myristoyl hydrolyzed collagen; CAS 72319-06-3; hair fixative, film-former, hair spray resin plasticizer; used in hair preps., lacquers, aftershaves, bath oils, sunscreen prods.; amber clear liq., char. fatty ethanolic odor; sol. in anhyd. ethanol and IPA, propylene glycol, hexylene glycol, water/ethanol 30/70; insol. in water; pH 3.5-45. (5% aq. disp.); 20% conc.

Lexein® A-220. [Inolex] TEA-myristoyl hydrolyzed collagen; film-former for face makeups, shampoos, hair conditioners, skin care prods., creams, lotions, shave creams, bar and liq. soaps; aq. sol'ns. above pH 6.0.; amber sl. hazy to clear liq., mild char. proteinaceous odor; sol. in aq. sol'ns. ≥ pH 6.0; pH 6.8-8.0 (50% aq.); 20% conc.

Lexein® A-240. [Inolex] Isopropyl myristate, sorbitan oleate, myristoyl hydrolyzed collagen; cosmetic protein, emollient, film-former for oil-based personal care prods. (bath oils, lipsticks, suntan oils, hair care prods.); golden brn. clear to hazy liq., neutral odor; sol. in min. oil, isopropyl esters, alcohols; misc. in petrolatum; pH 2.0-3.0 (10% in 50/50 ethanol/water); 20% conc.

Lexein® A-520. [Inolex] TEA-abietoyl hydrolyzed collagen; CAS 68918-77-4; sebum control additive for oily hair and skin care prods.; causes delay in refatting of the scalp when used in shampoos; substantive to skin and hair; amber clear liq., char. proteinaceous odor; water-sol.; pH 6-7 (10%); toxicology: nonirritating to skin and eyes; 30% conc.

Lexein® CP-125. [Inolex] Oleamidopropyl dimethylamine hydrolyzed collagen; cationic; protein for shampoos, cream rinses, hair conditioners; imparts improvement in combing, luster, and body without buildup on hair; amber clear liq., mild char. proteinaceous odor; disp. in water; easily solubilized in aq. systems; pH 5.5-6.5; 50% conc.

Lexein® QX-3000. [Inolex] Quaternium-76 hydrolyzed collagen; cationic; protein providing substantivity, outstanding body, wet and dry combability, renewable skin feel; for cream rinses, conditioners, skin care prods.; amber clear liq., mild char. proteinaceous odor; misc. with water; pH 5.5-7.5; 30% conc.

Lexein® S620S/Superpro 5A. [Inolex] TEA-coco-hydrolyzed animal protein and sorbitol; CAS 68952-16-9, 50-70-4; anionic; mild, high foaming cleansing agent, humectant, moisturizer for skin care prods.; aq. sol'n.; HLB 60.0.

Lexein® S620TA. [Inolex] TEA-coco-hydrolyzed collagen; CAS 68952-16-9; anionic; visc. builder, foam modifier; aq. sol'n.

Lexein® X-250. [Inolex] Hydrolyzed collagen; CAS 9015-54-7; substantive protein for setting lotions, gels, hair groom aids, shampoos, hair conditioners, wave lotions, cream rinses, skin care prods., skin moisturizers; clear aq. sol'n., mild char. proteinaceous odor; sol. in aq. alcoholic sol'ns., water; pH 5.8-6.3; 55% conc.

Lexein® X-250HP. [Inolex] Hydrolyzed collagen; CAS 9015-54-7; low odor and color version of Lexein X250; cosmetic protein exhibiting substantivity for hair and skin care prods. (quality shampoos, conditioners, waving lotions, skin creams and lotions); clear aq. sol'n., char. proteinaceous odor; pH 5.5-6.3; 55% conc.

Lexein® X-300. [Inolex] Hydrolyzed collagen; CAS 9015-54-7; cosmetic protein conditioner with bacterial stability, improved odor, ease of handling and storage; dry powd.; water-sol.; 94% conc.

Lexein® X-350. [Inolex] Hydrolyzed collagen; CAS 9015-54-7; substantive protein for shampoos, hair conditioners, skin creams and lotions, hair color; water sol'n.; sol. in water and hydroalcoholic sol'n.; 55% conc.

Lexemul® 55G. [Inolex] Glyceryl stearate; nonionic; surfactant, emulsifier, opacifier used in cosmetics and topical pharmaceuticals; improves lubricity, gloss in creams and lotions; wh. flakes; mild fatty char. odor; m.p. 55–59 C; HLB 4.1; acid no. 2 max.; iodine no. 1 max.; sapon. no. 160–170; pH 5.5 (3% aq.); 100% conc.

Lexemul® 55SE. [Inolex] Glyceryl stearate SE; anionic; primary emulsifier for o/w emulsion systems, cosmetic

creams, lotions, hair dressing, shave creams; flakes, mild fatty char. odor; sol. @ 60 C in CCl₄, ethyl acetate, IPA, min. oil; disp. in water @ 60 C; m.p. 56 C; HLB 5.4; acid no. 16-20; iodine no. 1 max.; sapon. no. 148-156; pH 8.5.

Lexemul® 200 DL. [Inolex] PEG-4 dilaurate; CAS 9005-02-1; personal care surfactant.

Lexemul® 503. [Inolex] Glyceryl stearate; nonionic; emulsifier, stabilizer, thickener, opacifier in emulsions or surfactant systems, cosmetics, toiletries, pharmaceuticals; flakes, mild fatty char. odor; m.p. 57-60 C; HLB 3.2; acid no. 2 max.; iodine no. 3 max.; sapon. no. 158-168; pH 6.5 (3% aq. disp.); 100% conc.

Lexemul® 515. [Inolex] Glyceryl stearate; nonionic; emulsifier, stabilizer, thickener, opacifier in emulsions or surfactant systems, cosmetics, topical pharmaceuticals; emollient in nonaq. oil and wax-based systems, e.g., lipsticks; flakes, mild fatty char. odor; m.p. 60 C; HLB 3.8; acid no. 16-20; iodine no. 3 max.; sapon. no. 166-176; 100% conc.

Lexemul® 530. [Inolex] Glyceryl stearate SE; anionic; primary emulsifier in o/w systems, cosmetic creams and lotions, hair dressings, shave creams; wh. to cream flakes; low odor; sol. @ 60 C in CCl₄, ethyl acetate, IPA, min. oil; disp. in water; HLB 5.2; m.p. 56 C; acid no. 16-20; iodine no. 1 max.; sapon. no. 146–154; pH 8.5 (3% aq. disp.); 100% conc.

Lexemul® 561. [Inolex] Glyceryl stearate and PEG-100 stearate; nonionic; cosmetic grade emulsifier for o/w cream or lotion systems; wh., brittle flakes; mild fatty char. odor; disp. in water (60 C); m.p. 54 C; HLB 11.1; acid no. 2 max.; iodine no. 1 max.; sapon. no. 90–100; pH 4.3 (3% aq. disp.); 100% conc.

Lexemul® AR. [Inolex] Glyceryl stearate and stearamidoethyl diethylamine; cationic; emulsifier, stabilizer, opacifier, and emollient for cationic systems in cosmetics, toiletries, topical pharmaceuticals, deodorants and antiperspirants; self-emulsifying, acid-stable; wh. to cream flakes; mild fatty odor; disp. in water (60 C); m.p. 60 C; HLB 3.3; acid no. 25–31; iodine no. 3 max.; sapon. no. 166–174; 100% conc.

Lexemul® AS. [Inolex] Glyceryl stearate, sodium lauryl sulfate; anionic; SE, acid-stable emulsifier, stabilizer, opacifier and emollient in cosmetics, toiletries, topical pharmaceuticals; wh to cream flakes; m.p. 60 C; HLB 4.4; acid no. 14–18; iodine no. 3 max.; sapon. no. 153–162; pH 5.5 (3% aq.); 100% conc.

Lexemul® CS-20. [Inolex] Cetearyl alcohol, ceteareth-20; nonionic; emulsifier, emollient used in cosmetics, antiperspirant creams and lotions, ointments, hydroquinone creams, shampoos, topical pharmaceuticals; APHA 50 max. brittle flakes, mild fatty char. odor; m.p. 50 C; HLB 16.6; acid no. 1 max.; iodine no. 2 max.; sapon. no. 2 max.; pH 7.2 (3% aq. disp.); 100% conc.

Lexemul® EGDS. [Inolex] Glycol distearate; CAS 627-83-8; EINECS 211-014-3; nonionic; lubricant, opacifier and pearling agent for cosmetic surfactant systems; liq. hand soaps, lt. duty liqs.; flakes, mild fatty char. odor; m.p. 60 C; HLB 1.5; acid no. 3-6; iodine no. 1 max.; sapon. no. 188-198; hyd. no. 33-43; pH 6.0 (3% aq. susp.); 100% conc.

Lexemul® EGMS. [Inolex] Glycol stearate; CAS 111-60-4; EINECS 203-886-9; nonionic; opacifier and pearling agent for personal care prods., lt. duty liqs.; emulsifier for creams, lotions, topicals; sec. suspending agent in o/w systems; flakes, mild fatty char. odor; sol. in hot min. and veg. oils; water-insol.; m.p. 57 C; HLB 2.3; acid no. 2 max.; iodine no. 1 max.; sapon. no. 180-190; 100% conc.

Lexemul® GDL. [Inolex] Glyceryl dilaurate; CAS 27638-00-2; EINECS 248-586-9; nonionic; lipid for creams and lotions formulated to produce a dry skin feel; melts just below body temp.; emollient; coupling agent for more lipophilic materials; emulsion stabilizer; off-wh. paste,

Lexemul® P

mild odor; water-disp.; m.p. 29.5 C; HLB 2.4; acid no. 5 max.; iodine no. 7; sapon. no. 219-229; ref. index 1.4505-1.4535 (35 C); pH 8.7 (3% aq.); 100% conc.

Lexemul® P. [Inolex] Propylene glycol stearate SE; anionic; emulsifier for low visc. cosmetic creams and lotions; flakes, mild fatty char. odor; m.p. 70 C; HLB 3.8; acid no. 16-20; iodine no. 3 max.; sapon. no. 165-174; pH 9.5 (3% aq. disp.); 100% conc.

Lexemul® PEG-200 DL. [Inolex] PEG-4 dilaurate; CAS 9005-02-1; nonionic; emulsifier, emollient, lubricant for cosmetics, pharmaceuticals, metalworking fluids, paints, polishes and misc. industrial formulations; straw to yel. liq., typ. mild fatty odor; water-disp.; sp.gr. 0.954; m.p. 2-3 C; HLB 5.9; acid no. 5 max.; iodine no. 8 max.; sapon. no. 170-180; 100% conc.

Lexemul® PEG-400 DL. [Inolex] PEG-8 dilaurate; CAS 9005-02-1; nonionic; emulsifier, emollient, lubricant for bath oils, suppositories, creams, lotions for cosmetic, pharmaceutical and industrial formulations; straw to yel. liq., typ. mild fatty odor; water-disp.; sp.gr. 0.988; m.p. 10-11 C; HLB 9.8; acid no. 10 max.; iodine no. 10 max.; sapon. no. 127-137; 100% conc.

Lexemul® PEG-400ML. [Inolex] PEG-8 laurate; CAS 9004-81-3; nonionic; emulsifier, emollient, lubricant, dispersant for creams, lotions, spreading bath oils, cosmetic, pharmaceutical and industrial applics.; pale yel. clear liq., typ. mild fatty odor; water-disp.; sp.gr. 1.024; m.p. 5-6 C; HLB 13.1; acid no. 4 max.; iodine no. 5 max.; sapon. no. 86-96; 100% conc.

Lexemul® T. [Inolex] Glyceryl stearate SE; anionic; for use as emulsifier, opacifier, stabilizer, and emollient in alkaline anionic systems, cosmetics; flakes, mild fatty char. odor; m.p. 60 C; HLB 5.5; acid no. 16-20; iodine no. 3 max.; sapon. no. 146-154; pH 8.5 (3% aq. disp.); 100% conc.

Lexgard® B. [Inolex] Butylparaben; CAS 94-26-8; EINECS 202-318-7; broad spectrum biostatic/biocidal preservative for cosmetics, toiletries, and topical pharmaceuticals; wh. fine powd., odorless, tasteless; sol. in ethanol, propylene glycol; slightly sol. in water; m.p. 68-72 C; usage level: 0.001-0.2%; toxicology: nonirritating to skin, nonsensitizing; 100% conc.

Lexgard® Bronopol. [Inolex] 2-Bromo-2-nitropropane-1,3-diol; CAS 52-51-7; EINECS 200-143-0; broad-spectrum preservative for cosmetics/toiletries, esp. difficult-to-preserve materials and nonionics; effective against bacteria and fungi; primary preservative in neutral or acidic formulas and for initial sterilization at higher pH; wh. to sl. yel. cryst. powd., char. odor; sol. (g/100 ml): 50 g ethanol, 25 g water, IPA, 14.3 g propylene glycol; usage level: < 0.1%; 99% act.

Lexgard® E. [Inolex] Ethyl paraben; CAS 120-47-8; EINECS 204-399-4; broad spectrum biostatic/biocidal preservative for cosmetics, toiletries, and topical pharmaceuticals; wh. fine powd.; sol. in ethanol, propylene glycol; m.p. 115-118 C; usage level: 0.08-1.0%; 100% conc.

Lexgard® M. [Inolex] Methylparaben USP; CAS 99-76-3; EINECS 202-785-7; broad spectrum biostatic/biocidal preservative for cosmetics, toiletries, foods, and topical pharmaceuticals; FDA, Japan, Europe compliance; wh. fine powd.; sol. in ethanol, propylene glycol; sl. sol. in water; m.p. 125-128 C; usage level: 0.1-1.0%; toxicology: nontoxic; 100% conc.

Lexgard® Myacide SP. [Inolex] Dichlorobenzyl alcohol; CAS 1777-82-8; EINECS 217-210-5; cosmetic preservative.

Lexgard® P. [Inolex] Propylparaben USP; CAS 94-13-3; EINECS 202-307-7; broad spectrum biostatic/biocidal preservative for cosmetics, toiletries, and topical pharmaceuticals; FDA, Japan, Europe compliance; wh. fine

powd.; sol. in ethanol, propylene glycol; slightly sol. in water; m.p. 95-98 C; usage level: 0.02-1.0%; 100% conc.

Lexin K. [Am. Lecithin] Lecithin; CAS 8002-43-5; EINECS 232-307-2; nonionic; emulsifier; semisolid, low odor and taste.

Lexol® 60. [Inolex] IPP, IPM, and isopropyl stearate; nonionic; emollient for bath oils, topical pharmaceuticals, personal care prods., preshave lotions, aerosol antiperspirants, creams, and lotions; biodeg.; colorless clear liq., odorless; sol. in acetone, benzene, CCl$_4$, castor oil, chloroform, ethanol, heptane, IPA; insol. in water; sp.gr. 0.848; dens. 7.1 lb/gal; visc. 7 cps; f.p. 8 C; acid no. 1 max.; iodine no. 1 max.; sapon. no. 190–198; flash pt. (PMCC) 165 C; ref. index 1.4358; 100% conc.

Lexol® 3975. [Inolex] Isopropyl palmitate, isopropyl myristate, isopropyl stearate; emollient and solv. for cosmetics and topicals; replacement for IPM; oxidative resist.; colorless liq., odorless; sol. in acetone, benzene, CCl$_4$, castor oil, chloroform, ethanol, heptane, IPA; insol. in water; sp.gr. 0.850-0.858; visc. 7 cps; f.p. 11 C; acid no. 1 max.; iodine no. 1 max.; sapon. no. 184-194; flash pt. (PMCC) 169 C; ref. index 1.4367; 100% conc.

Lexol® EHP. [Inolex] Octyl palmitate; CAS 29806-73-3; EINECS 249-862-1; emollient for nonocclusive creams and lotions, bath oils, antiperspirants, other cosmetic and topical formulations; colorless clear liq., odorless; sol. in acetone, benzene, CCl$_4$, chloroform, ether, heptane, alcohol, veg. and min. oils; insol. in water; sp.gr. 0.858; visc. 13 cps; f.p. -2 C; acid no. 1 max.; iodine no. 1 max.; sapon. no. 145-155; flash pt. (PMCC) 206 C; ref. index 1.4460; 100% conc.

Lexol® GT-855. [Inolex] Caprylic/capric triglyceride; CAS 65381-09-1; emollient with nonoily skin feel; moisturizer; for creams, lotions, bath oils, lipstick, makeup; solv. for perfume and flavor ingreds.; vehicle for medicinals, antibiotics, vitamins; solubilizer; oxidative stability; APHA 100 max. clear liq., odorless; tasteless; alcohol-sol.; sp.gr. 0.943; visc. 27 cps; f.p. -19 C; acid no. 0.1 max.; iodine no. 1 max.; sapon. no. 325-355; flash pt. (PMCC) 224 C; ref. index 1.4479; 100% conc.

Lexol® GT-865. [Inolex] Caprylic/capric triglyceride; CAS 65381-09-1; emollient, emulsion stabilizer, vehicle for cosmetic creams, lotions, bath oils, preshave lotions, lipsticks, makeup; solv. for perfume; carrier for flavors; vehicle for medicinals, antibiotics, vitamins; APHA 100 max. clear liq., odorless; sp.gr. 0.947; visc. 25 cps; f.p. -19 C; acid no. 0.1 max.; iodine no. 1 max.; sapon. no. 335-355; flash pt. (PMCC) 233 C; ref. index 1.4471; 100% conc.

Lexol® IPM. [Inolex] Isopropyl myristate NF; CAS 110-27-0; EINECS 203-751-4; emollient, solv., penetrant, cloud pt. depressant; used in personal care prods.; colorless clear liq.; odorless; sol. in acetone, benzene, CCl$_4$, castor oil, chloroform, ethanol, heptane, IPA; insol. in water; m.w. 270; sp.gr. 0.847–0.854; dens. 7.1 lb/gal; visc. 4.8 cp; f.p. 3 C; b.p. 170 C; acid no. 1 max.; iodine no. 1 max.; sapon. no. 202–212; flash pt. 305 F; ref. index 1.433.

Lexol® IPM-NF. [Inolex] Isopropyl myristate NF; CAS 110-27-0; EINECS 203-751-4; emollient, solv., penetrant for cosmetic applics. (bath oils, elec. preshaves); low visc., low f.p., outstanding spreading, good sol., high oxidative stability; colorless clear liq., odorless; sol. in acetone, benzene, CCl$_4$, castor oil, chloroform, ethanol, heptane, IPA; insol. in water, glycerol, propylene glycol; sp.gr. 0.852; visc. 0.5 cps; f.p. 2 C; acid no. 0.1; iodine no. 0.3; sapon. no. 208; flash pt. (COC) 155 C; ref. index 1.4327; 100% conc.

Lexol® IPP. [Inolex] Isopropyl palmitate; CAS 142-91-6; EINECS 205-571-1; emollient in conditioning cosmetics; solubilizer, carrier for cosmetic and topical pharmaceuticals; colorless clear liq.; odorless; sol. in acetone, benzene, CCl₄, castor oil, chloroform, ethanol, heptane, IPA; insol. in water; m.w. 298; sp.gr. 0.850–0.855; dens. 7.1 lb/gal; visc. 7 cps; f.p. 11 C; acid no. 1 max.; iodine no. 1 max.; sapon. no. 182–191; flash pt. (PMCC) 170 C; ref. index 1.437.

Lexol® IPP-A. [Inolex] Isopropyl palmitate; CAS 142-91-6; EINECS 205-571-1; emollient with exc. spreading and solubilizing props.; carrier for many cosmetic and topical pharmaceuticals; oxidative stability; colorless clear liq., odorless; sol. in acetone, benzene, CCl₄, castor oil, chloroform, ethanol, heptane, IPA, min. oil, dimethicone, cyclomethicone; insol. in water; visc. 7 cps; f.p. 11 C; HLB 13.5; acid no. 1 max.; iodine no. 1 max.; sapon. no. 182-191; flash pt. (PMCC) 170 C; ref. index 1.4370; 100% conc.

Lexol® IPP-NF. [Inolex] Isopropyl palmitate NF; CAS 142-91-6; EINECS 205-571-1; emollient with exc. spreading and solubilizing props.; solubilizer, carrier for many cosmetic and topical pharmaceuticals; APHA 20 max. clear liq., odorless; sol. in acetone, benzene, CCl₄, castor oil, chloroform, ethanol, heptane, IPA; insol. in water; sp.gr. 0.850-0.855; visc. 7 cps; f.p. 11 C; acid no. 1 max.; iodine no. 1 max.; sapon. no. 184-190; flash pt. (PMCC) 170 C; ref. index 1.4350-1.4380; 100% conc.

Lexol® PG-800. [Inolex] Propylene glycol dioctanoate; CAS 56519-71-2; emollient and moisturizer with nonoily feel, oxidation stability; for cosmetic/pharmaceutical creams, lotions, topicals, lipsticks, glossers, makeup bases, bath oils, aftershaves; solv., carrier/vehicle for flavors, fragrance, vitamins, antibiotics, medicinals; colorless clear liq., char. odor; sol. in alcohol, min. oil, acetone; sp.gr. 0.918; visc. 10 cps; f.p. -34 C; acid no. 1 max.; iodine no. 1 max.; sapon. no. 320-340; flash pt. (COC) 272 C; ref. index 1.4350; 100% conc.

Lexol® PG-855. [Inolex] Propylene glycol dicaprylate/dicaprate; nonionic; emollient, solubilizer for cosmetic creams and lotions; carrier/vehicle for flavors, fragrances, pigmented cosmetics, antibiotics; APHA 100 max. clear liq., odorless; sp.gr. 0.919; visc. 10 cps; f.p. -38 C; acid no. 0.1 max.; iodine no. 1 max.; sapon. no. 315-335; flash pt. (PMCC) 196 C; ref. index 1.4397; 100% act.

Lexol® PG-865. [Inolex] Propylene glycol dicaprylate/dicaprate; emollient, moisturizer with lubricity and nonoily skin deposition for creams, lotions, makeup, bath oils, pre-electric shave lotions, aerosol systems; vehicle for flavors, fragrances, pigmented cosmetics, vitamins, antibiotics, medicinals; solubilizer; APHA 100 max. clear liq., odorless; sol. in alcohol, min. and veg. oil, acetone; sp.gr. 0.922; visc. 10 cps; f.p. -38 C; acid no. 0.1 max.; iodine no. 1 max.; sapon. no. 315-335; flash pt. (PMCC) 195 C; ref. index 1.4391; 100% conc.

Lexol® PG-900. [Inolex] Propylene glycol dipelargonate; CAS 41395-83-9; EINECS 255-350-9; emollient for bath oils, preshave lotions, aerosol systems, lipsticks, glosses, makeup bases; carrier for fragrances; colorless clear liq., odorless; sp.gr. 0.918; visc. 11.5 cps; f.p. -36 C; acid no. 0.5 max.; iodine no. 1 max.; sapon. no. 305-320; flash pt. (PMCC) 195 C; ref. index 1.4404; 100% conc.

Lexol® SS. [Inolex] Stearyl stearate; CAS 2778-96-3; EINECS 220-476-5; emollient, lubricant, and opacifier for bath oils, creams, lotions; provides less oily skin feel than min. oil; oxidative stability; Gardner 2 max. flakes; oil sol.; m.p. 56 C; acid no. 4 max.; iodine no. 1 max.; sapon. no. 104-114; flash pt. (PMCC) 230 C; 100% conc.

Lexquat® 2240. [Inolex] Polymethacrylamidopropyl trimonium chloride; CAS 68039-13-4; cationic; polymeric film former, hair fixative, skin protectant, humectant, conditioner, antistat for hair cream rinses, conditioners, bleaches, neutralizers, shampoos, perms, day/night

creams, sun care prods.; pH stable; exceptional low use levels; colorless to buff clear liq.; sp.gr. 1.0380-1.0620; visc. 500 cp; f.p. 32 F; pH 3.5-4.5; ref. index 1.3782; 22-28% solids.

Lexquat® AMG-BEO. [Inolex] Behenamidopropyl PG-dimonium chloride; cationic; mild conditioning surfactant, emollient, and emulsifier for shampoos, bath gels, conditioners, shave prods., esp. for prods. for dry and damaged hair; amber liq., low typ. odor; HLB 8.0; pH 6.0-8.0; 23% min. act., 27-34% solids.

Lexquat® AMG-IS. [Inolex] Isostearamidopropyl PG-dimonium chloride.; cationic; mild conditioning surfactant, emollient, emulsifier for shampoos, bath gels, conditioners, shave prods., skin creams and lotions; amber liq., typ. low odor; HLB 10.0; pH 6.0-8.0; 25% conc.

Lexquat® AMG-M. [Inolex] Lauramidopropyl PG-dimonium chloride; cationic; conditioner, emulsifier for hair and skin prods.; emollient in bath prods., liq. soaps; amber liq., typ. odor; HLB pH 6-8; 33-37% solids, 30% min. act.

Lexquat® AMG-O. [Inolex] Oleamidopropyl PG-dimonium chloride; cationic; conditioner, emulsifier, emollient for hair and skin prods., bath gels; forms clear dilutable gels with other fatty quats; amber liq., typ. odor; HLB 9.7; pH 6-8; 28-32% solids, 25% min. act.

Lexquat® AMG-WC. [Inolex] Cocamidopropyl PG-dimonium chloride; cationic; foaming conditioner, emulsifier for hair and skin prods., bath gels; amber liq.; typ. odor; HLB 12.0; pH 6-8; 33-37% solids, 30% min. act.

Lexquat® CH. [Inolex] Polyquaternium-29; film former, hair fixative, skin protectant, humectant, conditioner, antistat; pH stable; exceptional low use levels; liq.; 7% conc.

Lilaminox M4. [Berol Nobel AB] Tetradecyl dimethylamine oxide; CAS 3332-27-2; EINECS 222-059-3; amphoteric; detergency booster, thickener for household bleaches based on sodium hypochlorite; foaming agent for hair shampoos; clear liq.; sol. in water and polar solvs.; dens. 973 kg/m³; visc. 1500 mPa·s; pour pt. 3 C; pH 7±1 (20%); surf. tens. 32 mN/m (0.1%); Ross-Miles foam 85 ml (initial, 20 ml of 1% aq.); 24-26% act.

Lilaminox M24. [Berol Nobel AB] Lauramine oxide; CAS 1643-20-5; EINECS 216-700-6; amphoteric; foam booster/stabilizer, detergent, thickener, antistat, softener for hair shampoos; thickener for household bleaches based on sodium hypochlorite, hard surf. cleaners; clear liq.; sol. in water and polar solvs.; dens. 969 kg/m³; visc. 30 mPa·s; pour pt. -12 C; pH 6-8 (20%); surf. tens. 32 mN/m (0.1%); Ross-Miles foam 100 ml (initial, 20 ml of 1% aq.); 30-32% act.

Linde A. [Union Carbide Specialty Powds.] Alumina.

Linoleate de Tocopherol. [Prod'Hyg] Tocopheryl linoleate; CAS 36148-84-2; cosmetic ingred.2.

Linoleic Safflower Oil. [Natural Oils Int'l.; Tri-K Industries] Linoleic safflower oil; CAS 8001-23-8; cosmetic ingred.; pale straw clear oil, bland odor and taste; immiscible in water; sp.gr. 0.923-0.928; iodine no. 135-150; sapon. no. 180-195; flash pt. (OC) 640 F; toxicology: nonhazardous; edible; trace moisture.

Linsol ETO. [Lanaetex Prods.] Laneth-10 acetate; cosmetic ingred.

Lion English Kaolin. [Charles B. Chrystal] Kaolin; CAS 1332-58-7; EINECS 296-473-8; cosmetic ingred.

Lipacid LML. [Seppic] Lysine lauroyl methionate.

Lipacid PVB. [Seppic] Palmitoyl hydrolyzed wheat protein.

Lipacid UCO Al. [Seppic] Aluminum undecylenoyl collagen amino acids.

Lipacide C3CO. [Seppic] Propionyl collagen amino acids.

Lipacide C8CO. [Seppic] Capryloyl collagen amino acids.

Lipacide C8CO Al. [Seppic] Aluminum capryloyl hydrolyzed collagen.

Lipacide C8CY. [Seppic] Dicapryloyl cystine; CAS 41760-

23-0; EINECS 255-537-5.

Lipacide C8G. [Seppic] Capryloyl glycine; CAS 14246-53-8.

Lipacide C8K. [Seppic] Capryloyl keratin amino acids.

Lipacide CCO. [Rhone-Poulenc; R.T. Vanderbilt] Capryloyl hydrolyzed collagen; mild surfactant with exc. lathering and wetting props., substantivity to hair and skin; for frequent-use shampoos, bath gels, soaps, shaving creams.

Lipacide DPHP. [Rhone-Poulenc; R.T. Vanderbilt; Seppic] Dipalmitoyl hydroxyproline; CAS 41672-81-5; EINECS 255-490-0; mild surfactant with exc. lathering and wetting props., substantivity to hair and skin; for frequent-use shampoos, bath gels, soaps, shaving creams; used in cosmetic preps. for maintenance of skin's physiological balance; wh. powd.; 100% conc.

Lipacide LCO. [Seppic] Lauroyl collagen amino acids.

Lipacide PCA. [Seppic] Palmitoyl hydrolyzed milk protein.

Lipacide PCO. [Rhone-Poulenc; R.T. Vanderbilt] Palmitoyl animal collagen amino acids; mild surfactant with exc. lathering and wetting props., substantivity to hair and skin; for frequent-use shampoos, bath gels, soaps, shaving creams; for first aid creams, sunburn lotions; beige wax; 100% conc.

Lipacide PK. [Rhone-Poulenc; R.T. Vanderbilt; Seppic] Palmitoyl keratin amino acids; mild surfactant with exc. lathering and wetting props., substantivity to hair and skin; for frequent-use shampoos, bath gels, soaps, shaving creams.

Lipacide SH-CO. [Seppic] Lipoaminoacid complex; shampoo additive for control of dandruff.

Lipacide SH-K. [Seppic] Lipoaminoacid complex; shampoo additive for normal hair.

Lipacide UCO. [Rhone-Poulenc; R.T. Vanderbilt; Seppic] Undecylenoyl collagen amino acids; mild surfactant with exc. lathering and wetting props., substantivity to hair and skin; for frequent-use shampoos, bath gels, soaps, shaving creams.

Lipal 400 DS. [Aquatec Quimica SA] PEG-8 distearate; CAS 977053-29-4; nonionic; emulsifier for o/w and w/o systems; for cosmetics and pharmaceuticals; solid; HLB 7.2; 100% conc.

Lipal 400 S. [Aquatec Quimica SA] PEG-8 stearate; CAS 977055-39-2; nonionic; emulsifier for o/w and w/o systems; for cosmetics and pharmaceuticals; solid; HLB 11.6; 100% conc.

Lipal 6000 DS. [Aquatec Quimica SA] PEG-150 distearate; CAS 977055-48-3; nonionic; emulsifier, visc. builder, superfatting agent for lotions, creams, shampoos; flakes; 100% conc.

Lipal DGMS. [Aquatec Quimica SA] PEG-2 stearate; CAS 9004-99-3; 106-11-6; EINECS 203-363-5; nonionic; emulsifier for lotions and creams; flakes; 100% conc.

Lipal EGDS. [Aquatec Quimica SA] Glycol distearate; CAS 627-83-8; EINECS 211-014-3; nonionic; emulsifier, opacifier, pearlescent, thickener for lotions, creams, shampoos; flakes; 100% conc.

Lipal EGMS. [Aquatec Quimica SA] Glycol stearate; CAS 111-60-4; EINECS 203-886-9; nonionic; thickener, emulsifier, pearlescent for lotions, creams, shampoos; flakes; 100% conc.

Lipal GMS. [Aquatec Quimica SA] Glyceryl stearate; CAS #31566-31-1; nonionic; emulsifier for cosmetic and food prods.; flakes; 100% conc.

Lipal GMS AE. [Aquatec Quimica SA] Glyceryl stearate SE; CAS 977053-96-5; anionic/nonionic; emulsifier for cosmetic prods.; flakes; 100% conc.

Lipal MMDG. [Aquatec Quimica SA] Glycol stearate and glycol distearate; nonionic; emulsifier, opacifier, thickener for creams, lotions, shampoos; flakes; 100% conc.

Lipal PGMS. [Aquatec Quimica SA] Propylene glycol stear-

ate; CAS 1323-39-3; EINECS 215-354-3; nonionic; emulsifier for food and cosmetic prods.; flakes; 100% conc.

Lipamide LMEA. [Lipo] Lactamide MEA; CAS 5422-34-4; EINECS 226-546-1; humectant for cosmetic creams, lotions, antiperspirants, beauty masks, depilatories, and hair care prods.

Lipamide LMWC. [Lipo] Lauramide DEA; CAS 120-40-1; EINECS 204-393-1; cosmetic surfactant.

Lipamide MEAA. [Lipo] Acetamide MEA; CAS 142-26-7; EINECS 205-530-8; nonionic; lubricating humectant for used in personal care prods.; hair conditioner for shampoos, rinses, conditioners; antistat, foam modifier; nontacky liq.; sol. in water, ethanol, IPA, glycols; 75% conc.

Lipamide S. [Lipo] Stearamide DEA; CAS 93-82-3; EINECS 202-280-1; nonionic; emulsifier, opacifier, thickener, emulsion and foam stabilizer, lubricant, used in skin and hair care prods.; off-wh. wax; mild, waxy odor; misc. hot with common oil phase ingred. and most org. solv., disp. in hot water; m.p. 41–46 C; pH 9–10.5 (1% aq.); 100% act.

Lipamine SPA. [Lipo] Stearamidopropyl dimethylamine; CAS 7651-02-7; EINECS 231-609-1; raw material for cosmetics, toiletries, pharmaceuticals.

Lipcare Wax 7782. [Kahl] Microcrystalline wax, polyethylene.

Lipex 20 E-70. [Karlshamns] PEG-70 mango glycerides.

Lipex 101. [Karlshamns] Peanut oil; CAS 8002-03-7; EINECS 232-296-4; emollient.

Lipex 102. [Karlshamns] Shea butter; CAS 68424-60-2; natural oils for pharmaceutical, cosmetic, and personal care prods. (lipsticks, emollient bases, creams and lotions); Lovibond R2.0 max.; m.p. 90-113 F; iodine no. 53-56; sapon. no. 178-190.

Lipex 102 E-75. [Karlshamns] PEG-75 shea butter glycerides.

Lipex 103. [Karlshamns] Sunflower seed oil; CAS 8001-21-6; EINECS 232-273-9; natural oils for pharmaceutical, cosmetic, and personal care prods. (lipsticks, emollient bases, creams and lotions); Gardner 2 max. liq.; acid no. 0.5 max.; iodine no. 125-140; sapon. no. 186-194; hyd. no. 0.5; cloud pt. -7 C.

Lipex 104. [Karlshamns] Corn oil; CAS 8001-30-7; EINECS 232-281-2; natural oils for pharmaceutical, cosmetic, and personal care prods. (lipsticks, emollient bases, creams and lotions); Gardner 2 max. liq.; acid no. 0.5 max.; iodine no. 115-130; sapon. no. 190; hyd. no. 3; cloud pt. -2 C.

Lipex 106. [Karlshamns] Illipe butter; oil of *Shorea stenoptera*; natural oils for pharmaceutical, cosmetic, and personal care prods. (lipsticks, emollient bases, creams and lotions); Gardner 2 max. color; m.p. 81-95 F; acid no. 0.5 max.; iodine no. 30-35; sapon. no. 188-198; hyd. no. 6.

Lipex 106 E-75. [Karlshamns] PEG-75 shorea butter glycerides.

Lipex 109. [Karlshamns] Hydrog. cottonseed oil; CAS 68334-00-9; EINECS 269-804-9; lubricant for pharmaceutical tablets.

Lipex 201. [Karlshamns] Rapeseedoil (canola); natural oils for pharmaceutical, cosmetic, and personal care prods. (lipsticks, emollient bases, creams and lotions); Gardner 1.5 max. liq.; acid no. 0.5 max.; iodine no. 80-90; sapon. no. 185-195; hyd. no. 5; cloud pt. 6 C.

Lipex 202. [Karlshamns] Shea butter liq. fraction; CAS 68424-60-2; natural oils for pharmaceutical, cosmetic, and personal care prods. (lipsticks, emollient bases, creams and lotions); Lovibond R2.5 max.; iodine no. 63-67; sapon. no. 180-185.

Lipex 203. [Karlshamns] Fractionated mango kernel oil; natural oils for pharmaceutical, cosmetic, and personal care prods. (lipsticks, emollient bases, creams and lotions); Gardner 4 max. liq.; acid no. 0.5 max.; iodine no. 55-65; sapon. no. 190; hyd. no. 9; cloud pt. 14 C.

Lipex 203 E-70. [Karlshamns] PEG-70 mango glycerides.

Lipex 205. [Karlshamns] Shea butter; CAS 68424-60-2; emollient oil.

Lipex 401. [Karlshamns] Hydrog. coconut oil; natural oils for pharmaceutical, cosmetic, and personal care prods. (lipsticks, emollient bases, creams and lotions); Gardner 1.5 max. liq.; acid no. 0.5 max.; iodine no. < 3; sapon. no. 245-265; hyd. no. 2; cloud pt. 28 C.

Lipex 402. [Karlshamns] Palm kernel wax and sorbitan tristearate.

Lipex 407. [Karlshamns] Hydrog. soybean oil; CAS 8016-70-4; EINECS 232-410-2; emollient, lubricant.

Lipo 320. [Lipo] Trilaurin; CAS 538-24-9; EINECS 208-687-0; emollient for cosmetics, toiletries, pharmaceuticals.

Lipo AM. [Lipo] Almond meal.; natural abrasive for personal care prods.

Lipo AMS. [Lipo] Almond meal; natural abrasive for facial scrubs, abrasive body scrubs and foot prods.

Lipo APS 40/60. [Lipo] Apricot seed powd.; natural abrasive for facial scrubs, body scrubs, foot prods.

Lipo DGLS. [Lipo] PEG-2 laurate SE; CAS 9004-81-3; nonionic; spreading agent, emulsifier, dispersant, lubricant, opacifier, emulsion stabilizer, emollient, visc. builder used in bath oils, creams, lotions; defoamer for process applics.; yel. liq.; water-disp.; HLB 8.3 ± 1; acid no. 4 max.; sapon. no. 160–170; 100% act.

Lipo EGDS. [Lipo] Glycol distearate; CAS 627-83-8; EINECS 211-014-3; spreading agent, emulsifier, dispersant, lubricant, opacifier, emulsion stabilizer, emollient, visc. builder used in bath oils, creams, lotions; defoamer for process applics.; wh./off wh. beads, flakes; HLB 1.0 ± 1; acid no. 7 max.; sapon. no. 190–205.

Lipo EGMS. [Lipo] Glycol stearate; CAS 111-60-4; EINECS 203-886-9; nonionic; opacifier, pearlizer for shampoos, detergents, w/o emulsifier; stabilizer for o/w systems; wh./off wh. beads, flakes; HLB 2.0 ± 1; acid no. 6 max.; sapon. no. 175–190.; 100% conc.

Lipo GMS 450. [Lipo] Glyceryl stearate; nonionic; general purpose emulsifier, emulsion stabilizer, emollient, opacifier and visc. builder in creams and lotions; food emulsifier; wh. bead or flake; HLB 3.6 ± 1; acid no. 5 max.; sapon. no. 165–182; 100% act.

Lipo GMS 470. [Lipo] Glyceryl stearate SE; nonionic; general purpose emulsifier, emulsion stabilizer, emollient, opacifier and visc. builder in creams and lotions; food emulsifier; wh. bead or flake; HLB 5.8 ± 1; acid no. 5 max.; sapon. no. 138–152; 100% act.

Lipo GMS 600. [Lipo] Glyceryl stearate.

Lipo PE 810. [Lipo] Pentaerythrityl tetracaprylate/caprate; CAS 68441-68-9; EINECS 270-474-3; nonionic; surfactant for creams, lotion, makeup; imparts gloss, leaving skin soft and smooth.

Lipo PE Base G-55. [Lipo] Glycerin, diglycol/cyclohexane-dimethanol/isophthalates/sulfoisophthalates copolymer; raw material for cosmetics, toiletries, pharmaceuticals.

Lipo PE Base GP-55. [Lipo] Glycerin, diglycol/cyclohexanedimethanol/isophthalates/sulfoisophthalates copolymer, propylene glycol; raw material for cosmetics, toiletries, pharmaceuticals.

Lipo PGMS. [Lipo] Propylene glycol stearate; CAS 1323-39-3; EINECS 215-354-3; nonionic; emulsifier, stabilizer for o/w lotions, soft creams; wh. solid wax; HLB 3.0 ± 1; acid no. 6 max.; sapon. no. 180–192; 100% conc.

Lipo PP. [Lipo] Peach pit powd.

Lipo SS. [Lipo] Hydrog. veg. oil; CAS 68334-28-1; EINECS 269-820-6; emollient for skin, sunscreens, lipsticks, balms; enhances gloss, reduces blooming; wh. to tan waxy flake; acid no. 0.1 max.; iodine no. 5 max.; sapon.

no. 230-250.

Lipo WSF 35/60, 60/100. [Lipo] Walnut shell flour; natural abrasive for facial scrubs, abrasive body scrubs and foot prods.

Lipobee 102. [Lipo] Syn. beeswax; raw material for cosmetics, pharmaceuticals, toiletries; oil-misc.; water-insol.

Lipo Buttermilk Powd. [Lipo] Buttermilk powd.

Lipocare HA/EC. [Lipo] Hyaluronic acid and echinacin; raw material for cosmetics, pharmaceuticals, toiletries.

Lipocerina. [Esperis] Acetylated hydrog. lanolin; CAS 91053-41-7; EINECS 293-306-0.

Lipocerite. [Vevy] Hydrog. C12-18 triglycerides.

Lipocerite Standard. [Vevy] Cetyl palmitate, isostearyl palmitate, cetyl stearate, stearyl stearate.

Lipocire A. [Gattefosse] Hydrog. palm glycerides, hydrog. palm kernel glycerides; lipstick base; drop pt. 35-36.5 C; acid no. < 0.5; iodine no. < 2; sapon. no. 225-245.

Lipocire CM. [Gattefosse SA] Hydrog. palm glycerides, hydrog. palm kernel glycerides; lipstick base; drop pt. 38-40 C; acid no. < 0.5; iodine no. < 2; sapon. no. 225-245; toxicology: nonirritating to skin.

Lipocire DM. [Gattefosse SA] Hydrog. palm glycerides, hydrog. palm kernel glycerides; lipstick base; drop pt. 43-45 C; acid no. < 0.5; iodine no. < 2; sapon. no. 215-235.

Lipocol B. [Lipo] PEG-9 stearate, PEG-9 laurate, and PEG-2 laurate SE; nonionic; spreading agent, emulsifier, dispersant, opacifier, lubricant, used in bath oils, creams, lotions; wh. to off-wh., solid wax; water-disp.; HLB 11.0 ± 1; sapon. no. 94–104; 100% act.

Lipocol C. [Lipo] Cetyl alcohol; CAS 36653-82-4; EINECS 253-149-0; emollient, consistency builder for creams, lotions, molded stick prods.; oil-misc.; water-insol.

Lipocol C-2. [Lipo] Ceteth-2; CAS 9004-95-9; nonionic; emulsifier, defoamer, wetting agent, solubilizer, conditioning agent for personal care prods. and pigment disp.; wh. solid wax; HLB 5.3; acid no. 1; hyd. no. 160-180; 100% act.

Lipocol C-4. [Lipo] Ceteth-4; CAS 9004-95-9; emulsifier.

Lipocol C-10. [Lipo] Ceteth-10; CAS 9004-95-9; nonionic; emulsifier, defoamer, wetting agent, solubilizer, conditioning agent for personal care prods. and pigment disp.; wh. solid wax; HLB 12.9; acid no. 1; hyd. no. 75-90; 100% act.

Lipocol C-20. [Lipo] Ceteth-20; CAS 9004-95-9; nonionic; emulsifier, defoamer, wetting agent, solubilizer, conditioning agent for personal care prods. and pigment disp.; wh. solid wax; HLB 15.7; acid no. 2 max; hyd. no. 50-58; 100% act.

Lipocol C-30. [Lipo] Ceteth-30; CAS 9004-95-9; emulsifier.

Lipocol F-33B. [Lipo] Ceteareth-50, ceteth-2, trideceth-12.

Lipocol HCO-40. [Lipo] PEG-40 hydrog. castor oil; CAS 61788-85-0; nonionic; surfactant, emulsifier, defoamer, wetting agent, solubilizer, and conditioner in antiperspirants, depilatories, creams, lotions, pigment dispersions, shampoos, detergents, bleaches, and dyes; wh. waxy paste; HLB 15.0 ± 1; acid no. 1.5 max.; hyd. no. 50-70.

Lipocol HCO-60. [Lipo] PEG-60 hydrog. castor oil; CAS 61788-85-0; nonionic; surfactant, emulsifier, defoamer, wetting agent, solubilizer, and conditioner for antiperspirants, depilatories, creams, lotions, pigment dispersions, shampoos, detergents, bleaches, and dyes; wh. waxy paste; HLB 16.0 ± 1; acid no. 1.0 max.; hyd. no. 60-80.

Lipocol HCO-66. [Lipo] PEG-66 trihydroxystearin; CAS 61788-85-0; emulsifier.

Lipocol IS-20. [Lipo] Isosteareth-20; CAS 52292-17-8; emulsifier.

Lipocol L. [Lipo] Lauryl alcohol; CAS 112-53-8; EINECS 203-982-0; nonoily afterfeel emollient for creams, lotions, makeup; oil-misc.; water-insol.

Lipocol L-1. [Lipo] Laureth-1; CAS 4536-30-5; EINECS 224-

886-5; nonionic; emulsifier, defoamer, wetting agent, solubilizer, conditioning agent for personal care prods. and pigment disp.; HLB 3.6; acid no. 2 max; 100% act.

Lipocol L-4. [Lipo] Laureth-4; CAS 5274-68-0; EINECS 226-097-1; nonionic; surfactant for pigment dispersions, antiperspirants, depilatories, creams, lotions; antistat, emulsifier, defoamer, wetting agent, solubilizer, and conditioning agent in shampoos, detergents, bleaches, and dyes; colorless liq.; HLB 9.7; acid no. 2 max; hyd. no. 145-160; 100% act.

Lipocol L-12. [Lipo] Laureth-12; CAS 3056-00-6; EINECS 221-286-5; nonionic; surfactant for pigment dispersions, antiperspirants, depilatories, creams, lotions; antistat, emulsifier, defoamer, wetting agent, solubilizer, and conditioning agent in shampoos, detergents, bleaches, and dyes; wh. waxy solid; HLB 14.5; acid no. 1 max; hyd. no. 72-87; 100% act.

Lipocol L-23. [Lipo] Laureth-23; CAS 9002-92-0; nonionic; surfactant for pigment dispersions, antiperspirants, depilatories, creams, lotions; antistat, emulsifier, defoamer, wetting agent, solubilizer, and conditioning agent in shampoos, detergents, bleaches, and dyes; wh. waxy solid; HLB 16.9; acid no. 2 max; hyd. no. 42-52; 100% act.

Lipocol M-4. [Lipo] Myreth-4; CAS 27306-79-2; nonionic; emulsifier, defoamer, wetting agent, solubilizer, conditioning agent for personal care prods. and pigment disp.; liq.; HLB 8.8; 100% conc.

Lipocol O. [Lipo] Oleyl alcohol; CAS 143-28-2; EINECS 205-597-3; nontacky afterfeel emollient for bath oils, creams, lotions, makeup; oil-misc.; water-insol.

Lipocol O-2 Special. [Lipo] Oleth-2; CAS 9004-98-2; nonionic; surfactant for pigment dispersions, antiperspirants, depilatories, creams, lotions; antistat, emulsifier, defoamer, wetting agent, solubilizer, and conditioning agent in shampoos, detergents, bleaches, and dyes; yel. liq.; HLB 4.9; acid no. 1 max; hyd. no. 155-175; 100% act.

Lipocol O-3 Special. [Lipo] Oleth-3; CAS 9004-98-2; nonionic; surfactant, emulsifier, defoamer, wetting agent, solubilizer, and conditioner in antiperspirants, depilatories, creams, lotions, pigment dispersions, shampoos, detergents, bleaches, and dyes; yel. liq.; HLB 6.6 ± 1; acid no. 1 max.; hyd. no. 135-150.

Lipocol O-5 Special. [Lipo] Oleth-5; CAS 9004-98-2; nonionic; w/o emulsifier for cold waves, bleaches, dyes, depilatories; yel. liq.; HLB 8.8; acid no. 1 max.; hyd. no. 120-135.

Lipocol O-10. [Lipo] Oleth-10; CAS 9004-98-2; nonionic; surfactant for pigment dispersions, antiperspirants, depilatories, creams, lotions; antistat, emulsifier, defoamer, wetting agent, solubilizer, and conditioning agent in shampoos, detergents, bleaches, and dyes; yel. liq.; HLB 12.4; acid no. 2 max; hyd. no. 74-84; 100% act.

Lipocol O-20. [Lipo] Oleth-20; CAS 9004-98-2; nonionic; surfactant for pigment dispersions, antiperspirants, depilatories, creams, lotions; antistat, emulsifier, defoamer, wetting agent, solubilizer, and conditioning agent in shampoos, detergents, bleaches, and dyes; wh. waxy solid; HLB 15.3; acid no. 2 max; hyd. no. 45-65; 100% act.

Lipocol O-25. [Lipo] Oleth-25.; CAS 9004-98-2; emulsifier.

Lipocol O-80. [Lipo] Oleyl alcohol.; CAS 143-28-2; EINECS 205-597-3; emollient.

Lipocol O/95. [Lipo] Oleyl alcohol; CAS 143-28-2; EINECS 205-597-3; emollient.

Lipocol PT-400. [Lipo] Trideceth-12; CAS 24938-91-8; personal care surfactant.

Lipocol S. [Lipo] Stearyl alcohol; CAS 112-92-5; EINECS 204-017-6; waxy afterfeel emollient, consistency builder for creams, lotions, molded sticks; oil-misc.; water-insol.

Lipocol S-2. [Lipo] Steareth-2; CAS 9005-00-9; nonionic; surfactant for pigment dispersions, antiperspirants, de-

pilatories, creams, lotions; antistat, emulsifier, defoamer, wetting agent, solubilizer, and conditioning agent in shampoos, detergents, bleaches, and dyes; wh. solid wax; HLB 4.9; acid no. 1 max; hyd. no. 155-165; 100% act.

Lipocol S-10. [Lipo] Steareth-10; CAS 9005-00-9; nonionic; surfactant for pigment dispersions, antiperspirants, depilatories, creams, lotions; antistat, emulsifier, defoamer, wetting agent, solubilizer, and conditioning agent in shampoos, detergents, bleaches, and dyes; wh. solid wax; HLB 12.4; acid no. 1 max; hyd. no. 75-90; 100% act.

Lipocol S-20. [Lipo] Steareth-20; CAS 9005-00-9; nonionic; surfactant for pigment dispersions, antiperspirants, depilatories, creams, lotions; antistat, emulsifier, defoamer, wetting agent, solubilizer, and conditioning agent in shampoos, detergents, bleaches, and dyes; wh. solid wax; HLB 15.3; acid no. 1 max; hyd. no. 45-60; 100% act.

Lipocol SC-4. [Lipo] Ceteareth-4; CAS 68439-49-6; nonionic; surfactant for pigment dispersions, antiperspirants, depilatories, creams, lotions; antistat, emulsifier, defoamer, wetting agent, solubilizer, and conditioning agent in shampoos, detergents, bleaches, and dyes; wh. waxy solid; HLB 8.0; acid no. 1 max.; hyd. no. 120-140; 100% conc.

Lipocol SC-6. [Lipo] Ceteareth-6.; CAS 68439-49-6.

Lipocol SC-8. [Lipo] Ceteareth-8; CAS 68439-49-6.

Lipocol SC-10. [Lipo] Ceteareth-10; CAS 68439-49-6; nonionic; emulsifier, defoamer, wetting agent, solubilizer, conditioning agent for personal care prods. and pigment disp.; solid; HLB 12.5; 100% conc.

Lipocol SC-12. [Lipo] Ceteareth-12; CAS 68439-49-6.

Lipocol SC-15. [Lipo] Ceteareth-15; CAS 68439-49-6; nonionic; surfactant for pigment dispersions, antiperspirants, depilatories, creams, lotions; antistat, emulsifier, defoamer, wetting agent, solubilizer, and conditioning agent in shampoos, detergents, bleaches, and dyes; wh. waxy solid; HLB 14.3; acid no. 2 max.; hyd. no. 50-65; 100% conc.

Lipocol SC-20. [Lipo] Ceteareth-20; CAS 68439-49-6; nonionic; surfactant for pigment dispersions, antiperspirants, depilatories, creams, lotions; antistat, emulsifier, defoamer, wetting agent, solubilizer, and conditioning agent in shampoos, detergents, bleaches, and dyes; wh. waxy solid; HLB 15.4; acid no. 1 max.; hyd. no. 45-60; 100% conc.

Lipocol SC-30. [Lipo] Ceteareth-30; CAS 68439-49-6.

Lipocol SC-50. [Lipo] Ceteareth-50.

Lipocol TD-3. [Lipo] Trideceth-3; CAS 4403-12-7; EINECS 224-540-3; nonionic; emulsifier, wetting and scouring agent, dispersant for essential oils; raw material for sulfation and phosphation; liq.; 100% act.

Lipocol TD-6. [Lipo] Trideceth-6; CAS 24938-91-8; nonionic; emulsifier, wetting and scouring agent, dispersant for essential oils; raw material for sulfation and phosphation; liq.; 100% act.

Lipocol TD-12. [Lipo] Trideceth-12; CAS 24938-91-8; nonionic; emulsifier, wetting and scouring agent, dispersant for essential oils; raw material for sulfation and phosphation; solubilizer; wh. paste; HLB 14.6; acid no. 1 max.; hyd. no. 70-85; 100% act.

Lipocutin®. [Henkel KGaA/Cospha; Henkel Canada] Water, lecithin, cholesterol, dicetyl phosphate; liposome; lipid film-forming agent with moisture-retaining props., carrier of encapsulated active agents, esp. for aq. systems such as gels; grades avail.: AQ with Aquadearm moisturizing factor, EP with elastin hydrolysate, RB with calendula extract, and VE with vitamin E; wh. milky cloudy liq., weak intrinsic odor; misc. with water and alcoholic sol'ns.; pH 6.3-6.7; usage level: 5-40%.

Lipodermol®. [Laboratoires Sérobiologiques] Octyldodecanol, phospholipids, glycosphingolipids, retinol, tocopherol, cholesterol, arachidonic acid, linoleic acid, and linolenic acid; substantive lipidic biofilmogen, moisturizer, softener, lubricant with soothing action; structuring agent for epidermis; used for prods. for old and atonic skin, dry or damaged skin, rough and scaly skin; golden yel. limpid liq.; lipo-sol.; usage level: 1-3%.

Lipofacteur Vitentiel. [Les Colorants Wackherr] Vitamin complex rich in essential fatty acids; promotes skin adhesion, hydration, and acts as a free radical scavenger in cosmetic prods.

Lipofilter ODP. [Lipo] Padimate O; CAS 21245-02-3; EINECS 244-289-3; sunscreen.

Lipofirm LCW. [Les Colorants Wackherr] A multifunctional slimming treatment for cosmetics use.

Lipofruit R. [Lipo] Water, lemon juice, pineapple juice, and grapefruit juice.

Lipoid S 75-3. [Lipoid KG] Hydrog. lecithin; CAS 92128-87-5; EINECS 295-786-7; moisturizer.

Lipoid S 100. [Lipoid KG] Lecithin; CAS 8002-43-5; EINECS 232-307-2; emulsifier.

Lipolan. [Lipo] Hydrog. lanolin; CAS 8031-44-5; EINECS 232-452-1; nonionic; aux. w/o emulsifier; emollient; conditioner; lubricant; wh. to off-wh. paste; mild char. odor; water-insol.; m.p. 37–45; acid no. 1 max.; sapon. no. 5 max.; 100% conc.

Lipolan 31. [Lipo] PEG-24 hydrog. lanolin; CAS 68648-27-1; nonionic; o/w emulsifiers, solubilizer, emollient, conditioner used in cosmetics, toiletries and topical pharmaceuticals; cream waxy solid; bland, char. odor; sol. in water and ethanol; acid no. 2 max.; sapon. no. 8; 100% act.

Lipolan 31-20. [Lipo] PEG-20 hydrog. lanolin; CAS 68648-27-1; emollient, emulsifier, solubilizer, stabilizer, conditioner, and moisturizer for cosmetics, toiletries, pharmaceuticals, skin care prods., makeup, lipstick, shampoos/rinses, soap, bath specialties, shaving preps., sun care, ointments, acne preps., veterinary prods.

Lipolan 98. [Lipo] Laneth-10 acetate.

Lipolan Distilled. [Lipo] Dist. hydrog. lanolin; CAS 8031-44-5; EINECS 232-452-1; emollient, emulsifier, solubilizer, stabilizer, conditioner, and moisturizer for cosmetics, pharmaceuticals, skin care prods., makeup, lipstick, shampoos, rinses, soap/bath prods., shaving preps., sun prods., ointments, acne preps., veterinary prods.

Lipolan LB-440. [Lion] α-Olefin sulfonate; anionic; detergent base; emulsifier for cosmetics and emulsion polymerization; liq.; 37% conc.

Lipolan LB-840. [Lion] α-Olefin sulfonate; anionic; detergent base; paste; 37% conc.

Lipolan PJ-400. [Lion] α-Olefin sulfonate; anionic; emulsifier for cosmetics; dispersant for emulsion polymerization; powd.; 100% conc.

Lipolan R. [Lipo] Lanolin oil; emollient, spreading agent, conditioner, cosolv., plasticizer, and lubricant for personal care prods.; dispersant for pigments; yel., amber liq.; mild char. odor; sol. in min. and veg. oils, isopropyl esters, and anhyd. IPA; insol. in water; sapon. no. 85–110; cloud pt. 18 C max.

Lipoliv. [Pentapharm Ltd; Centerchem] Squalane, heart extract, and tocopheryl acetate.

Lipo Lufa 30/100. [Lipo] Luffa.

Lipo LUFFA 30/100. [Lipo] Luffa; natural abrasive for facial scrubs, abrasive body scrubs and foot prods.

Lipomectant AL. [Lipo] Acetamide MEA and lactamide MEA; humectant for cosmetic creams, lotions, antiperspirants, beauty masks, depilatories, and hair care prods.

Lipo Melanin. [Lipo] Melanin; raw material for cosmetics, pharmaceuticals, toiletries.

Lipomicron N.S.L.E. [Sederma] Biomimetic encapsulation of a "natural skin lipid equivalent"; mimics the natural lipidic composition of the epidermis; reinforces structure of cutaneous barrier; provides slow release of the lipid constituent of the upper skin layers; contributes to skin regeneration; makes skin more resist. to exposure; for face, body, sun, and makeup care prods.; milky wh. opalescent liq., char. odor; sp.gr. 1.035-1.055; pH 5.0-6.5; usage level: 5-10%.

Lipomicron Vitamin A Palmitate. [Sederma] Vitamin A palmitate biomimetically encapsulated in lipid spherules containing phospholipids, cholesterol, and fatty acids; provides slow release and protection against denaturization of actives; revitalizes skin, restoring suppleness and youthfulness; alleviates cutaneous dryness and roughness; for face, body, sun, and makeup care prods.; off-wh. opalescent liq., char. odor; sp.gr. 1.04-1.06; pH 6.0-8.0; usage level: 5-10%.

Lipomicron Vitamin E Acetate. [Sederma] Vitamin E acetate biomimetically encapsulated in lipid spherules containing phospholipids, cholesterol, and fatty acids; provides slow release of vitamin E acetate; free radical scavenger, antioxidant for skin care applics.; for face, body, sun, and makeup care prods.; off-wh. liq., char. odor; sp.gr. 1.04-1.06; pH 6.0-8.0; usage level: 5-10%.

Lipomulse 165. [Lipo] Glyceryl stearate and PEG-100 stearate; nonionic; general purpose emulsifier, emulsion stabilizer, emollient, opacifier and visc. builder in creams and lotions; wh. bead or flake; HLB 11.0 ± 1; acid no. 2 max.; sapon. no. 90–100; 100% act.

Liponate 2-DH. [Lipo] PEG-4 diheptanoate; emollient for adjusting rub-in and afterfeel of cosmetic creams, lotions, bath preps.; thickener, visc. control agent; colorless liq.; acid no. 0.5 max.; sapon. no. 249-269.

Liponate 143M. [Lipo] Myreth-3 myristate; CAS 59686-68-9; emollient ester for adjusting rub-in and afterfeel of personal care prods.; thickener and visc. controller; wh./yel. liq./paste; acid no. 6 max.; sapon. no. 90–100.

Liponate CL. [Lipo] Cetyl lactate; CAS 35274-05-6; EINECS 252-478-7; emollient for desired feel and penetration in personal care prods.; thickener and visc. controller; wh. soft solid to liq.; sol. in min. oil, veg. oil, ethanol; partly sol. in water; acid no. 3 max.; sapon. no. 174–195.

Liponate CRM. [Lipo] Cetyl ricinoleate; CAS 10401-55-5; EINECS 233-864-4; glosser, emollient with dry afterfeel; oil-sol., water-disp.; 100% act.

Liponate DPC-6. [Lipo] Dipentaerythrityl hexacaprylate/hexacaprate; CAS 68130-24-5; nontacky emollient for personal care treatment prods.; colorless visc. liq.; acid no. 0.5 max.; sapon. no. 320-340; 100% act.

Liponate EM. [Lipo] Ethyl morrhuate.

Liponate GC. [Lipo] Caprylic/capric triglyceride; CAS 65381-09-1; emollient ester for adjusting rub-in and afterfeel of personal care prods.; thickener and visc. controller; colorless liq.; sol. in anhyd. alcohol, min. and veg. oils; insol. in water; acid no. 0.1 max.; sapon. no. 325–355.

Liponate GDL. [Lipo] Glyceryl dilaurate.; CAS 27638-00-2; EINECS 248-586-9; emulsifier, emollient.

Liponate IPM. [Lipo] IPM; CAS 110-27-0; EINECS 203-751-4; emollient ester for adjusting rub-in and afterfeel of personal care prods.; thickener and visc. controller; colorless liq.; sol. in ethanol, min. and veg. oils; insol. in water; acid no. 2 max.; sapon. no. 202–211.

Liponate IPP. [Lipo] IPP; CAS 142-91-6; EINECS 205-571-1; emollient ester for adjusting rub-in and afterfeel of personal care prods.; thickener and visc. controller; colorless liq.; sol. see Liponate IPM; acid no. 2 max.; sapon. no. 183–190.

Liponate ISA Special. [Lipo] Isostearic acid; CAS 2724-58-5; EINECS 220-336-3; emollient.

Liponate L. [Lipo] Propylene glycol diisononanoate.

Liponate ML. [Lipo] Myristyl lactate; CAS 1323-03-1;

EINECS 215-350-1; nongreasy, soft afterfeel emollient for bath/body oils, hydroalcoholic systems, creams, lotions, anhyd. and emulsified makeups; sol. in min. oil, veg. oil, ethanol, propylene glycol; insol. in water.

Liponate MM. [Lipo] Myristyl myristate; CAS 3234-85-3; EINECS 221-787-9; emollient ester for adjusting rub-in and afterfeel of personal care prods.; thickener and visc. controller; wh. solid wax.; sol. in oils; insol. in water; acid no. 5 max.; sapon. no. 120–135.

Liponate NPG-891. [Lipo] Neopentyl glycol dicaprylate/dipelargonate/dicaprate.

Liponate NPGC-2. [Lipo] Neopentyl glycol dicaprylate/dicaprate; CAS 70693-32-2; dry feel emollient for creams, lotions, cleansers, antiperspirants; colorless liq.; oil-sol.; water-insol.; acid no. 0.5 max.; sapon. no. 292-312; 100% act.

Liponate PB-4. [Lipo] Pentaerythrityl tetrabehenate; CAS 61682-73-3; EINECS 262-895-6; emollient ester for adjusting rub-in and afterfeel of personal care prods.; thickener and visc. controller; off-wh. flakes; oil-misc., water-insol.; acid no. 10 max.; sapon. no. 150-165.

Liponate PC. [Lipo] Propylene glycol dicaprylate/dicaprate; emollient ester for adjusting rub-in and afterfeel of personal care prods.; thickener and visc. controller; colorless liq.; sol. in min. and veg. oils, ethanol; water-insol.; acid no. 0.1 max.; sapon. no. 315–335.

Liponate PE-810. [Lipo] Pentaerythrityl tetracaprylate/tetracaprate; CAS 68441-68-9; EINECS 270-474-3; emollient for adjusting rub-in and afterfeel of cosmetic creams, lotions, bath preps.; thickener, visc. control agent; colorless liq.; acid no. 1 max.; sapon. no. 315-335.

Liponate PO-4. [Lipo] Pentaerythrityl tetraoleate; CAS 19321-40-5; EINECS 242-960-5; emollient ester for adjusting rub-in and afterfeel of personal care prods.; thickener and visc. controller; yel. liq.; sol. in min. and veg. oils, IPA; water-insol.; acid no. 10 max.; sapon. no. 185-195.

Liponate PS-4. [Lipo] Pentaerythrityl tetrastearate; CAS 115-83-3; EINECS 204-110-1; emollient ester for adjusting rub-in and afterfeel of personal care prods.; thickener and visc. controller; wh. flakes; oil-misc., water-insol.; acid no. 10 max.; sapon. no. 183-198.

Liponate SPS. [Lipo] Cetyl esters (syn. spermaceti); emollient ester for adjusting rub-in and afterfeel of personal care prods.; thickener and visc. controller; cream/wh. flakes; oil-misc., water-insol.; acid no. 5 max.; sapon. no. 109-120.

Liponate SS. [Lipo] Stearyl stearate; CAS 2778-96-3; EINECS 220-476-5; emollient ester for adjusting rub-in and afterfeel of personal care prods.; thickener and visc. controller; off-wh. flakes; oil-misc., water-insol.; acid no. 5 max.; sapon. no. 103-117.

Liponate TDS. [Lipo] Tridecyl stearate; CAS 31556-45-3; EINECS 250-696-7; emollient for creams and lotions; colorless liq.; acid no. 1 max.; sapon. no. 110-130; 100% act.

Liponate TDTM. [Lipo] Tridecyl trimellitate; CAS 70225-05-7; nontacky emollient for treatment prods., hair care prods.; pale yel. visc. liq.; acid no. 0.5 max.; sapon. no. 238-258; 100% act.

Liponic 70-NC. [Lipo] Sorbitol; CAS 50-70-4; EINECS 200-061-5; humectant, plasticizer, softener, and lubricant; adds sweet taste and pleasant mouthfeel to oral hygiene prods. such as dentifrices and mouthwashes; oral dosage pharmaceutical, also for adhesives, leather, and paper coatings; clear colorless sol'n.; water-sol.; sp.gr. 1.29–1.32; ref. index 1.455–1.470; pH neutral.

Liponic 76-NC. [Lipo] Sorbitol; CAS 50-70-4; EINECS 200-061-5; humectant, plasticizer, softener, and lubricant; adds sweet taste and pleasant mouthfeel to oral hygiene prods. such as dentifrices and mouthwashes; oral dosage

pharmaceutical, also for adhesives, leather, and paper coatings; colorless to pale wh. clear syrup; odorless; sp.gr. 1.32–1.35; ref. index. 1.468–1.475; 25% max. water.

Liponic 83-NC. [Lipo] Sorbitol; CAS 50-70-4; EINECS 200-061-5; humectant, plasticizer, softener, and lubricant; adds sweet taste and pleasant mouthfeel to oral hygiene prods. such as dentifrices and mouthwashes; oral dosage pharmaceutical, also for adhesives, leather, and paper coatings.

Liponic EG-1. [Lipo] Glycereth-26; CAS 31694-55-0; nonionic; humectant in creams and lotions, lubricant, plasticizer for hair resins, foam stabilizer, pigment dispersant, hair conditioner, foam modifier, antistat; used in personal care prods.; colorless, clear to slightly hazy visc. liq.; sol. in water, alcohol, acetone and ethyl acetate; acid no. 0.5 max.; 100% act.

Liponic EG-7. [Lipo] Glycereth-7; CAS 31694-55-0; humectant, hair conditioner, lubricant, and foam modifier for cosmetics and toiletries; adds lubricity and nongreasy luxurious feel to personal care prods.; colorless to pale yel. liq.; odorless; sol. in water, alcohol; 100% act.

Liponic SO-20. [Lipo] Sorbeth-20; humectant and plasticizer for cosmetics and toiletries; nongreasy rich afterfeel with moderate lubricity; yel. visc. liq.; bland char. odor; sol. in water, alcohol; acid no. 1 max.; 1% max. moisture.

Lipopeg 1-L. [Lipo] PEG-2 laurate; CAS 141-20-8; EINECS 205-468-1; emulsifier.

Lipopeg 1-O. [Lipo] PEG-2 oleate; CAS 106-12-7; EINECS 203-364-0; personal care surfactant.

Lipopeg 1-S. [Lipo] PEG-2 stearate; CAS 106-11-6; EINECS 203-363-5; emulsifier.

Lipopeg 2-DL. [Lipo] PEG-4 dilaurate; CAS 9005-02-1; nonionic; dispersant, emulsifier, spreading agent and lubricant in personal care prods., bath oils; yel. liq.; HLB 6.0 ± 1; acid no. 10 max.; sapon. no. 170–185; 100% conc.

Lipopeg 2-L. [Lipo] PEG-4 laurate; CAS 9004-81-3; mild solubilizer, spreading agent, emulsifier, dispersant, and lubricant for bath oils, creams, and lotions; yel. liq.; HLB 9.0 ± 1; acid no. 5 max.; sapon. no. 140-160.

Lipopeg 2-S. [Lipo] PEG-4 stearate; CAS 9004-99-3; EINECS 203-358-8; emulsifier.

Lipopeg 3-DL. [Lipo] PEG-6 dilaurate.; CAS 9005-02-1; personal care surfactant.

Lipopeg 3-O. [Lipo] PEG-6 oleate; CAS 9004-96-0; emulsifier.

Lipopeg 3-S. [Lipo] PEG-6 stearate; CAS 9004-99-3; emulsifier.

Lipopeg 4-DL. [Lipo] PEG-8 dilaurate; CAS 9005-02-1; nonionic; dispersant, emulsifier, spreading agent and lubricant in personal care prods., bath oils; yel. liq.; HLB 10.0 ± 1; acid no. 10 max.; sapon. no. 125–142; 100% conc.

Lipopeg 4-DO. [Lipo] PEG-8 dioleate; CAS 9005-07-6; dispersant, emulsifier, spreading agent and lubricant in personal care prods., bath oils; amber liq.; HLB 7.2 ± 1; acid no. 10 max.; sapon. no. 113–128.

Lipopeg 4-DS. [Lipo] PEG-8 distearate; CAS 9005-08-7; dispersant, emulsifier, spreading agent and lubricant in personal care prods., bath oils; cream soft wax; HLB 8.0 ± 1; acid no. 10 max.; sapon. no. 113–128.

Lipopeg 4-L. [Lipo] PEG-8 laurate; CAS 9004-81-3; nonionic; spreading agent, emulsifier, dispersant, lubricant for bath oils, creams and lotions; yel. liq.; HLB 13.0 ± 1; acid no. 5 max.; sapon. no. 100; 100% act.

Lipopeg 4-O. [Lipo] PEG-8 oleate; CAS 9004-96-0; nonionic; emulsifier; liq.; HLB 11.0; 100% conc.

Lipopeg 4-S. [Lipo] PEG-8 stearate; CAS 9004-99-3; nonionic; spreading agent, emulsifier, dispersant, lubricant for bath oils, creams and lotions; cream paste; HLB 11.2 ± 1; acid no. 5 max.; sapon. no. 80–90; 100% act.

Lipopeg 6-L. [Lipo] PEG-12 laurate; CAS 9004-81-3; nonionic; spreading agent, emulsifier, dispersant, lubricant for bath oils, creams and lotions; yel. liq.; HLB 14.6 ± 1; acid no. 5 max.; sapon. no. 65–76; 100% act.

Lipopeg 6-O. [Lipo] PEG-12 oleate; CAS 9004-96-0; personal care surfactant.

Lipopeg 6-S. [Lipo] PEG-12 stearate; CAS 9004-99-3; emulsifier.

Lipopeg 10-DS. [Lipo] PEG-20 distearate; CAS 9005-08-7; personal care surfactant.

Lipopeg 10-S. [Lipo] PEG-20 stearate; CAS 9004-99-3; nonionic; spreading agent, emulsifier, dispersant, and lubricant for personal care prods.; wh. solid wax; HLB 15.2; acid no. 5 max.; sapon. no. 39-49; 100% conc.

Lipopeg 15-S. [Lipo] PEG-6-32 stearate; CAS 9004-99-3; nonionic; spreading agent, emulsifier, dispersant, lubricant for bath oils, creams and lotions; solid; HLB 13.8; 100% conc.

Lipopeg 16-S. [Lipo] PEG-35 stearate; CAS 9004-99-3; emulsifier.

Lipopeg 20-S. [Lipo] PEG-45 stearate.; CAS 9004-99-3; emulsifier.

Lipopeg 39-S. [Lipo] PEG-40 stearate; CAS 9004-99-3; nonionic; emulsifier for o/w creams and lotions; wh. solid wax; HLB 16.9 ± 1; acid no. 2 max.; sapon. no. 23–35; 100% act.

Lipopeg 100-S. [Lipo] PEG-100 stearate; CAS 9004-99-3; nonionic; dispersant, emulsifier, spreading agent and lubricant in personal care prods., bath oils; tan flake or bead; HLB 18.8 ± 1; acid no. 1 max.; sapon. no. 9–20; 100% act.

Lipopeg 6000-DL. [Lipo] PEG-150 dilaurate; CAS 9005-02-1; personal care surfactant.

Lipopeg 6000-DS. [Lipo] PEG-150 distearate; CAS 9005-08-7; nonionic; dispersant, emulsifier, spreading agent and lubricant in personal care prods., bath oils; off-wh. flake; HLB 18.4 ± 1; acid no. 10 max.; sapon. no. 12–20; 100% act.

Lipo-Peptide AME 30. [Maybrook] Acetamide MEA, lauroyl hydrolyzed collagen, glycerin; moisturizer, humectant, emollient, softener, aux. emulsifier for skin prods.; conditioner, bodying agent, antistat for hair prods.; foam booster in shampoos, mousses, liq. hand soaps; amber clear to sl. hazy liq., char. sl. acetic odor; pH 4.5-5.5; 60% min. solids.

Lipophos. [Vevy] Soybean oil, lecithin.

Lipophos LMP. [Lipo] Lauryl phosphate; CAS 12751-23-4; EINECS 235-798-1; detergent, emollient.

Lipoplastidine Achillea. [Vevy] Coconut oil and yarrow extract.

Lipoplastidine Aesculus. [Vevy] Coconut oil and horse chestnut extract.

Lipoplastidine Aloe. [Vevy] Coconut oil and aloe extract.

Lipoplastidine Calendula. [Vevy] Min. oil and calendula extract.

Lipoplastidine Laminaria. [Vevy] Coconut oil and algae extract.

Lipoplastidine Pappa Regalis. [Vevy] Min. oil and royal jelly extract.

Lipoplastidine Soja. [Vevy] Soybean oil and soy germ extract.

Lipo Polyglycol 200. [Lipo] PEG-4; CAS 25322-68-3; EINECS 203-989-9; nonirritating neutral polymer functioning as humectant, solubilizer, lubricant, fixative, and visc. regulator for cosmetics and toiletries; odorless; water-sol.

Lipo Polyglycol 300. [Lipo] PEG-6; CAS 25322-68-3; EINECS 220-045-1; nonirritating neutral polymer func-

tioning as humectant, solubilizer, lubricant, fixative, and visc. regulator for cosmetics and toiletries; odorless; water-sol.

Lipo Polyglycol 400. [Lipo] PEG-8; CAS 25322-68-3; EINECS 225-856-4; nonirritating neutral polymer functioning as humectant, solubilizer, lubricant, fixative, and visc. regulator for cosmetics and toiletries; odorless; water-sol.

Lipo Polyglycol 600. [Lipo] PEG-12; CAS 25322-68-3; EINECS 229-859-1; nonirritating neutral polymer functioning as humectant, solubilizer, lubricant, fixative, and visc. regulator for cosmetics and toiletries; odorless; water-sol.

Lipo Polyglycol 1000. [Lipo] PEG-20; CAS 25322-68-3; nonirritating neutral polymer functioning as humectant, solubilizer, lubricant, fixative, and visc. regulator for cosmetics and toiletries; odorless; water-sol.

Lipo Polyglycol 3350. [Lipo] PEG-75; CAS 25322-68-3; nonirritating neutral polymer functioning as humectant, solubilizer, lubricant, fixative, and visc. regulator for cosmetics and toiletries; odorless; water-sol.

Lipo Polyol NC. [Lipo] Hydrog. starch hydrolysate; CAS 68425-17-2; humectant for creams, lotions, antiperspirants, depilatories, wavesets.

Lipoproteol LCO. [Rhone-Poulenc; R.T. Vanderbilt] Sodium/TEA-lauroyl hydrolyzed collagen amino acid; nonionic; mild additive with good foaming props. for rich lather shampoos, facial cleaners, infant shampoos, detergents; liq.; 22% conc.

Lipoproteol LCOK. [Seppic] Lipoaminoacid salt; anionic; shampoo base and detergent; liq.; 22–25% conc.

Lipoproteol LK. [Rhone-Poulenc; R.T. Vanderbilt] Sodium/TEA-lauroyl hydrolyzed keratin amino acids; anionic; shampoo base; liq.; 25% conc.

Lipoproteol UCO. [Seppic] Sodium/TEA-undecylenoyl animal collagen amino acids; anionic; shampoo base for oily hair; antiseborrheic; liq.; 23% conc.

Lipoquat R. [Lipo] Ricinoleamidopropyl ethyldimonium ethosulfate; CAS 112324-16-0; cationic; conditioner, antistat, emollient, glosser, softener for personal care prods. and anhyd. systems; amber visc. liq.; char. odor; water-sol.; pH 6.5–7.5 (3% aq.); 95% act.

Liporamnosan. [Vevy] Hydroxyethylcellulose; CAS 9004-62-0; thickener.

Liporez NEP-Special. [Lipo] Trimethylpentanediol/isophthalic acid/trimellitic anhydride copolymer.

Liposiliol C. [Exsymol; Biosil Tech.] Dioleyl tocopheryl methylsilanol; aids tissue regeneration; for anti-aging formulations, oily cosmetics and sticks; sl. yel. oily limpid liq., sl. aromatic odor; misc. with most fatty substances; nonmisc. with water; sp.gr. 0.85; sapon. no. < 2; ref. index 1.45; usage level: 3-6%; toxicology: nontoxic.

Liposoluble Placental Extract E.M.L. [Solabia] Human placental lipids.

Liposome Anti-Age LS. [Laboratoires Sérobiologiques] Water, serum protein, honey extract, collagen, lecithin, and cholesterol.

Liposome Centella. [Sederma] Water, glycerin, propylene glycol, lecithin, and hydrocotyl extract; cutaneous collagen renewal vector for face and body care prods.; beige sl. visc. opalescent liq., char. odor; sp.gr. 1.00-1.10; pH 5.0-6.0; usage level: 5-30%.

Liposome Conc. E-10. [Cosmetochem] A lecithin-based liposome conc.; CAS 8002-43-5; EINECS 232-307-2; cosmetic specialty for use in skin care preps.

Liposomes CLR. [Dr. Kurt Richter] Water, sphingolipids, and phospholipids.

Liposomes Anti-Age LS. [Laboratoires Sérobiologiques] Water, serum protein, honey extract, collagen, lecithin, and cholesterol; liposomed biocomplex; moisturizer, antiwrinkle action for skin care; beige-ivory opalescent suspension; disp. in water; usage level: 5-15%.

Liposomes Slimmigen® . [Laboratoires Sérobiologiques] Xanthic bases, amino acids, vegetable extracts, and phospholipids; complex providing lipolytic effect, tonifying effect on the veins, local slimming effect, antistasis effect; ivory yel. liq.; disp. in water; usage level: 5-7%.

Liposome Unsapo KM. [Sederma] Water, propylene glycol, glycerin, lecithin, shea butter unsaponifiables, and corn oil unsaponifiables; protective and soothing liposome for sensitive skin protection prods. for face, body, and sun care; prevents erythema caused by long sun exposure; anti-inflammatory; beige sl. visc. opalescent liq., char. odor; sp.gr. 1.00-1.10; pH 4.8-5.8; usage level: 5-30%.

Liposorb 70. [Lipo] Sorbitol.; CAS 50-70-4; EINECS 200-061-5; cosmetic/pharmaceutical ingred.

Liposorb L. [Lipo] Sorbitan laurate; CAS 1338-39-2; nonionic; emulsifier, thickener, lubricant, antistat, all-purpose lipophilic surfactant used with POE Liposorb series; also used in defoamers, aerosol w/o emulsions, corrosion inhibition; amber liq.; HLB 8.6 ± 1; sapon. no. 158–170; hyd. no. 330-360; 100% act.

Liposorb L-10. [Lipo] PEG-10 sorbitan laurate; CAS 9005-64-5; nonionic; o/w emulsifier, lubricant, antistat, all-purpose hydrophilic surfactant used for solubilizing oils and in conjunction with Liposorb esters; for cosmetics/toiletries; yel. liq.; HLB 14.9 ± 1; sapon. no. 66–76; hyd. no. 150-170; 100% act.

Liposorb L-20. [Lipo] Polysorbate 20; CAS 9005-64-5; nonionic; o/w emulsifier, lubricant, antistat, all-purpose hydrophilic surfactant used for solubilizing oils and in conjunction with Liposorb esters; for cosmetics/toiletries; yel. liq.; HLB 16.7 ± 1; sapon. no. 40–50; hyd. no. 96-108; 100% act.

Liposorb O. [Lipo] Sorbitan oleate; CAS 1338-43-8; EINECS 215-665-4; nonionic; emulsifier, thickener, lubricant, antistat, all-purpose lipophilic surfactant used with POE Liposorb series for cosmetics/toiletries; also used in defoamers, aerosol w/o emulsions, corrosion inhibition; yel./amber liq.; HLB 4.3 ± 1; sapon. no. 145–160; hyd. no. 193-210; 100% act.

Liposorb O-5. [Lipo] Polysorbate 81; CAS 9005-65-6; nonionic; hydrophilic surfactant used for solubilizing oils; emulsifier, lubricant, antistat; liq.; HLB 10.0; 100% conc.

Liposorb O-20. [Lipo] Polysorbate 80; CAS 9005-65-6; nonionic; surfactant for food processing; flavor and color dispersant for pickles; defoamer for beet sugar, yeast processing; wetting agent for poultry defeathering; crystal control agent for salt; emulsifier, lubricant, and antistat for cosmetics and toiletries; yel. liq.; HLB 15.0 ± 1; sapon. no. 45–55; hyd. no. 65-80; 100% act.

Liposorb P. [Lipo] Sorbitan palmitate; CAS 26266-57-9; EINECS 247-568-8; nonionic; lipophilic surfactant, emulsifier, thickener, lubricant, antistat for cosmetics and toiletries; also in defoamers, aerosol w/o emulsions, corrosion inhibition; tan beads or flakes; HLB 6.7 ± 1; sapon. no. 139–151; hyd. no. 272-306; 100% act.

Liposorb P-20. [Lipo] Polysorbate 40; CAS 9005-66-7; nonionic; hydrophilic surfactant, solubilizer for oils, emulsifier, lubricant, antistat for cosmetics and toiletries; yel. liq.; HLB 15.6 ± 1; sapon. no. 40–53; hyd. no. 90-107; 100% act.

Liposorb S. [Lipo] Sorbitan stearate; CAS 1338-41-6; EINECS 215-664-9; nonionic; emulsifier, thickener, lubricant, antistat, all-purpose lipophilic surfactant used with POE Liposorb series for cosmetics/toiletries; also for defoamers, aerosol w/o emulsions, corrosion inhibition; cream beads or flakes; HLB 4.7 ± 1; sapon. no. 147–157; hyd. no. 235-260; 100% act.

Liposorb S-4. [Lipo] Polysorbate 61; CAS 9005-67-8;

nonionic; hydrophilic surfactant used for solubilizing oils and in conjunction with Liposorb sorbitan esters for emulsification, lubrication, and antistatic props. in cosmetics and toiletries; tan waxy solid; HLB 9.6 ± 1; sapon. no. 95-115; hyd. no. 170-200.

Liposorb S-20. [Lipo] Polysorbate 60; CAS 9005-67-8; nonionic; hydrophilic surfactant for solubilizing oils and in conjunction with Liposorb sorbitan esters for emulsification, lubrication and antistatic props. in cosmetics and toiletries; food emulsifier, defoamer; yel. paste; HLB 14.9 ± 1; sapon. no. 45–55; hyd. no. 81-96; 100% act.

Liposorb SC. [Lipo] Sorbitan stearate; CAS 1338-41-6; EINECS 215-664-9; emulsifier.

Liposorb SQO. [Lipo] Sorbitan sesquioleate; CAS 8007-43-0; EINECS 232-360-1; nonionic; emulsifier, thickener, lubricant, antistat, all-purpose lipophilic surfactant used with POE Liposorb series for cosmetics/toiletries; amber liq.; HLB 3.7 ± 1; sapon. no. 149–160; hyd. no. 185-215; 100% act.

Liposorb TO. [Lipo] Sorbitan trioleate; CAS 26266-58-0; EINECS 247-569-3; nonionic; emulsifier, thickener, lubricant, antistat, all-purpose lipophilic surfactant used with POE Liposorb series for cosmetics/toiletries; amber liq.; HLB 1.8 ± 1; sapon. no. 171–185; hyd. no. 58-69; 100% act.

Liposorb TO-20. [Lipo] Polysorbate 85; CAS 9005-70-3; nonionic; o/w emulsifier, lubricant, antistat, all-purpose hydrophilic surfactant used for solubilizing oils and in conjunction with Liposorb esters for cosmetics and toiletries; yel. liq.; HLB 11.0 ± 1; sapon. no. 82–95; hyd. no. 39-52; 100% act.

Liposorb TS. [Lipo] Sorbitan tristearate; CAS 26658-19-5; EINECS 247-891-4; nonionic; emulsifier, thickener, lubricant, antistat, all-purpose lipophilic surfactant used with POE Liposorb series for cosmetics/toiletries; cream flakes or beads; HLB 2.1 ± 1; sapon. no. 175–190; hyd. no. 65-80; 100% act.

Liposorb TS-20. [Lipo] Polysorbate 65; CAS 9005-71-4; nonionic; hydrophilic surfactant for solubilizing oils and in conjunction with Liposorb sorbitan esters for emulsification, lubrication and antistatic props. in cosmetics and toiletries; food emulsifier, defoamer; tan solid wax; HLB 10.5 ± 1; sapon. no. 88–98; hyd. no. 44-60; 100% act.

Lipostim. [Sederma] Water, glycerin, propylene glycol, hydrolyzed soy protein, and lecithin; cell stimulator and regulator for face and body care prods.; provides cutaneous firming, seborrheic regulation; yel. opalescent liq., char. odor; pH 6.5-7.5; usage level: 5-15%.

Liposurf EST-30. [Lipo] Sodium trideceth sulfate; personal care surfactant.

Liposurf TD-7C. [Lipo] Trideceth-7 carboxylic acid.

Lipotrofina A. [Vevy] Linoleic acid, linolenic acid, arachidonic acid, lecithin, soy sterol, soybean oil, and tocopherol.

Lipotrofina M. [Vevy] Muscle extract, calf skin extract, placental lipids, embryo extract, soybean oil, and lauryl isostearate.

Lipotrofina Placentare. [Vevy] Placental lipids.

Lipovol A. [Lipo] Avocado oil; CAS 8024-32-6; EINECS 232-428-0; conditioner, glosser, emollient imparting a lt., nongreasy, silky afterfeel to skin and hair prods.; high film gloss and rapid spread; used in personal care prods.; yel. to green visc. oil.; bland char. odor; sol. in oils; sp.gr. 0.908–0.925; acid no. 3 max.; iodine no. 65-95; sapon. no. 177–198; ref. index 1.460–1.470.

Lipovol ALM. [Lipo] Sweet almond oil; conditioner, glosser, emollient imparting a lt., nongreasy, silky afterfeel to skin and hair prods.; high film gloss and rapid spread; used in personal care prods.; pale yel. clear oily liq.; bland, odorless; sol. in min. oil, isopropyl esters, ether, chloroform, benzene, and solv. hexane; water-insol.; acid no. 2 max.; iodine no. 95-115; sapon. no. 185–200.

Lipovol C-76. [Lipo] Coconut oil; CAS 8001-31-8; EINECS 232-282-8; natural emollient, lubricant, conditioner for luxury skin prods., hair care prods., makeup, fine soaps, bath oils, and anhyd. systems; soft solid/liq.; acid no. 0.5 max.; iodine no. 12 max.; sapon. no. 250-265.

Lipovol CAN. [Lipo] Canola oil; natural emollient, lubricant, conditioner for luxury skin prods., hair care prods., makeup, fine soaps, bath oils, and anhyd. systems; yel. oil; acid no. 0.5 max.; iodine no. 94-126; sapon. no. 186-198.

Lipovol CO. [Lipo] Castor oil; CAS 8001-79-4; EINECS 232-293-8; natural emollient, lubricant, conditioner for luxury skin prods., hair care prods., makeup, fine soaps, bath oils, and anhyd. systems; yel. oil; acid no. 0.5 max.; iodine no. 83-88; sapon. no. 186-198.

Lipovol CP. [Lipo] Cherry pit oil; CAS 8022-29-5; conditioner, glosser, emollient imparting a lt., nongreasy, silky afterfeel to skin and hair prods.; high film gloss and rapid spread; used in personal care prods.; lt. amber oil; sapon. no. 182-202.

Lipovol G. [Lipo] Grape seed oil; CAS 8024-22-4; conditioner, glosser, emollient imparting a lt., nongreasy, silky afterfeel to skin and hair prods.; high film gloss and rapid spread; used in personal care prods.; yel. amber oil; oil-sol.; acid no. 5 max.; iodine no. 132-152; sapon. no. 183–205.

Lipovol GTB. [Lipo] Glyceryl tribehenate; CAS 18641-57-1; EINECS 242-471-7; emulsifier, emulsion stabilizer, emollient, visc. builder, opacifier, pearlescent for cosmetic creams and lotions; wh. flakes; HLB 1.0 ± 1; acid no. 10 max.; sapon. no. 160-180.

Lipovol HS. [Lipo] Hydrog. soybean oil; CAS 8016-70-4; EINECS 232-410-2; emollient, lubricant, conditioner for luxury skin prods., hair care prods., makeup, fine soaps, bath oils, and anhyd. systems; yel. oil; acid no. 0.5 max.; iodine no. 101-114; sapon. no. 186-197.

Lipovol J. [Lipo] Jojoba oil, refined; CAS 61789-91-1; emollient, conditioner, and lubricant for cosmetics and toiletries; rapid spread and soft, nontacky afterfeel; used in skin and personal care prods. and oils, anhyd. and emulsified makeups; yel. oil; char. nut-like odor; sol. in min. and veg. oils; insol. in water; acid no. 5 max.; iodine no. 75-95; sapon. no. 85–110.

Lipovol J Lite. [Lipo] Jojoba oil; CAS 61789-91-1; natural emollient, lubricant, conditioner for luxury skin prods., hair care prods., makeup, fine soaps, bath oils, and anhyd. systems; colorless liq.; acid no. 5 max.; iodine no. 75-95; sapon. no. 85-110.

Lipovol MAC. [Lipo] Macadamia nut oil; natural emollient, lubricant, conditioner for luxury skin prods., hair care prods., makeup, fine soaps, bath oils, and anhyd. systems; yel. oil; acid no. 1 max.; iodine no. 73-80; sapon. no. 193-198.

Lipovol MOS-70. [Lipo] Tridecyl stearate, neopentyl glycol dicaprylate/dicaprate, tridecyl trimellitate; specialty ester exhibiting tactile props. of min. oil; used in cosmetics and toiletries; colorless liq.; acid no. 0.5 max.; sapon. no. 206-226.

Lipovol MOS-130. [Lipo] Tridecyl stearate, tridecyl trimellitate, dipentaerythrityl hexacaprylate/hexacaprate; specialty ester exhibiting tactile props. of min. oil for cosmetics and toiletries; colorless liq.; acid no. 0.5 max.; sapon. no. 187-207.

Lipovol MOS-350. [Lipo] Dipentaerythrityl hexacaprylate/hexacaprate, tridecyl trimellitate, tridecyl stearate, neopentyl glycol dicaprylate/dicaprate; specialty ester exhibiting tactile props. of min. oil for cosmetics and toiletries; colorless to straw liq.; acid no. 0.5 max.; sapon.

no. 268-288.

Lipovol M-SYN. [Lipo] Oleic/palmitoleic/linoleic glycerides; natural emollient, lubricant, conditioner for luxury skin prods., hair care prods., makeup, fine soaps, bath oils, and anhyd. systems; yel. oil; acid no. 1 max.; iodine no. 85-98; sapon. no. 190-198.

Lipovol O. [Lipo] Olive oil; CAS 8001-25-0; EINECS 232-277-0; natural emollient, lubricant, conditioner for luxury skin prods., hair care prods., makeup, fine soaps, bath oils, and anhyd. systems; yel. oil; acid no. 3 max.; iodine no. 77-88; sapon. no. 188-195.

Lipovol P. [Lipo] Apricot kernel oil; CAS 72869-69-3; emollient used in cosmetics and pharmaceuticals; soft, nontacky afterfeel and high film gloss; straw oily liq.; bland char. fatty odor; sol. in min. oil and isopropyl esters; insol. in water; acid no. 1 max.; iodine no. 90-115; sapon. no. 185–195.

Lipovol PAL. [Lipo] Palm oil; CAS 8002-75-3; EINECS 232-316-1; emollient, lubricant, conditioner for luxury skin prods., hair care prods., makeup, fine soaps, bath oils, and anhyd. systems; off-wh. paste; acid no. 1 max.; iodine no. 44-59; sapon. no. 195-205.

Lipovol SAF. [Lipo] Safflower oil; CAS 8001-23-8; EINECS 232-276-5; conditioner, glosser, emollient imparting a lt., nongreasy, silky afterfeel to skin and hair prods.; high film gloss and rapid spread; used in personal care prods.; yel. oil; acid no. 2 max.; iodine no. 135-155; sapon. no. 182–202.

Lipovol SES. [Lipo] Sesame oil; CAS 8008-74-0; EINECS 232-370-6; emollient, solv., and vehicle used in cosmetics, toiletries, and pharmaceuticals; offers lt., nontacky feel and enhances gloss and spread of pigmented sticks and pot prods.; yel. clear liq.; bland char. odor; sol. in isopropyl esters and min. oil; insol. in water; acid no. 0.2 max.; iodine no. 103-116; sapon. no. 188–195.

Lipovol SES-S. [Lipo] Veg. oil, sesame oil; emollient, solv., and vehicle used in cosmetics, toiletries, and pharmaceuticals; offers lt., nontacky feel and enhances gloss and spread of pigmented sticks and pot prods.; economical replacement for natural sesame oil; yel. clear liq.; bland char. odor; acid no. 1.0 max.; sapon. no. 188–195.

Lipovol SO. [Lipo] Hybrid safflower oil; conditioner, glosser, emollient imparting a lt., nongreasy, silky afterfeel to skin and hair prods.; high film gloss and rapid spread; used in personal care prods.; yel. oil; oil-sol.; acid no. 1 max.; iodine no. 90-105; sapon. no. 184-196.

Lipovol SOY. [Lipo] Soybean oil; CAS 8001-22-7; EINECS 232-274-4; natural emollient oil, lubricant, conditioner for luxury skin prods., hair care prods., makeup, fine soaps, bath oils, anhyd. systems; yel. oil; acid no. 1 max.; iodine no. 120-145; sapon. no. 180-200.

Lipovol SUN. [Lipo] Sunflower seed oil; CAS 8001-21-6; EINECS 232-273-9; emollient imparting a pleasant, nongreasy feel to skin and hair care prods. and makeups; adds conditioning, spread, and sheen to personal care prods.; used in preparation of margarine; lt. yel. oily liq.; bland, char. fatty odor; sol. in min. oil and isopropyl esters; insol. in water; acid no. 2 max.; iodine no. 120-140; sapon. no. 185–195; 0.05% max. moisture.

Lipovol W. [Lipo] Walnut oil; emollient for makeup, skin, and hair care prods. where a rich, nontacky, persistent afterfeel is desired; rapid spread; yel./amber oil; bland char. odor; sol. in min. oil and isopropyl esters; acid no. 0.5 max.; sapon. no. 185–202.

Lipovol WGO. [Lipo] Wheat germ oil; CAS 8006-95-9; emollient imparting perceptible afterfeel to skin and hair care prods., gloss to anhyd. and emulsified makeups; yel./brn. oil; char. fatty odor; sol. in oils; insol. in water; acid no. 5 max.; iodine no. 120-140; sapon. no. 175–195.

Lipowax. [Lipo] Cetearyl alcohol, cetyl esters, myristyl alcohol; nonionic; wax used for building visc. in personal care prods.; solid; 100% conc.

Lipowax 6138G. [Lipo] Syn. beeswax; cosmetics ingred.

Lipowax D. [Lipo] Cetearyl alcohol, ceteareth-20; nonionic; o/w SE wax, used in skin and hair creams and lotions, personal care prods.; wh. to off-wh. waxy solid; bland, char. odor; sol. in alcohol, misc. warm with most oil phase ingredients, disp. in warm water; m.p. 46–55 C; HLB 11; sapon. no. 2; 100% act.

Lipowax G. [Lipo] Stearyl alcohol and ceteareth-20; non-ionic; emulsifier for personal care prods.; solid; water-disp.; 100% conc.

Lipowax NI. [Lipo] Cetearyl alcohol and ceteth-20; nonionic; o/w SE wax, used in skin and hair creams and lotions, personal care prods.; solid; water-disp.; 100% conc.

Lipowax P. [Lipo] Cetearyl alcohol, polysorbate 60; nonionic; o/w self-emulsifying wax for neutral and mildly acidic and alkaline pH systems; creamy, waxy solid; bland, char. odor; sol. in alcohol, misc. warm with most oil phase ingred., disp. in warm water; m.p. 48–52 C; HLB 9; sapon. no. 14; 100% act.

Lipowax P-31. [Lipo] Emulsifying wax; for formulation of creams, lotions, and ointments.

Lipowax PR. [Lipo] Cetearyl alcohol, polysorbate 60, PEG-150 stearate, steareth-20; emulsifying wax for formulation of creams, lotions, and ointments.

Lipowax P-SPEC. [Lipo] Cetearyl alcohol, polysorbate 60; emulsifying wax for formulation of creams, lotions, and ointments.

Lipoxol® 200 MED. [Hüls Am.; Hüls AG] PEG-4; CAS 25322-68-3; EINECS 203-989-9; moisture and consistency regulators in creams, lotions, shaving preps., tooth-pastes, and hair care prods. (m.w. < 2000), lipstick, deodorant stick, soap bars, powd. bases, and makeup pastes (m.w. > 2000); German pharmacopoeia compli-ance; colorless clear liq.; water-sol.; visc. 60-70 mPa·s; solid. pt. -40 to -55 C; acid no. 0.2 max.; pH 4-7 (10% aq.).

Lipoxol® 300 MED. [Hüls Am.; Hüls AG] PEG-6; CAS 25322-68-3; EINECS 220-045-1; moisture and consistency regulators in creams, lotions, shaving preps., tooth-pastes, and hair care prods. (m.w. < 2000), lipstick, deodorant stick, soap bars, powd. bases, and makeup pastes (m.w. > 2000); German pharmacopoeia compli-ance; colorless clear liq.; water-sol.; visc. 85-95 mPa·s; solid. pt. -10 to -20 C; acid no. 0.2 max.; pH 4-7 (10% aq.).

Lipoxol® 400 MED. [Hüls Am.; Hüls AG] PEG-8; CAS 25322-68-3; EINECS 225-856-4; moisture and consistency regulators in creams, lotions, shaving preps., tooth-pastes, and hair care prods. (m.w. < 2000), lipstick, deodorant stick, soap bars, powd. bases, and makeup pastes (m.w. > 2000); German pharmacopoeia compli-ance; colorless clear liq.; water-sol.; visc. 105-140 mPa·s; solid. pt. 4-8 C; acid no. 0.2 max.; pH 4-7 (10% aq.).

Lipoxol® 550 MED. [Hüls Am.; Hüls AG] PEG-6 and PEG-32; moisture and consistency regulators in creams, lo-tions, shaving preps., toothpastes, and hair care prods. (m.w. < 2000), lipstick, deodorant stick, soap bars, powd. bases, and makeup pastes (m.w. > 2000); German pharmacopoeia compliance; wh. paste; water-sol.; visc. 22-26 mPa·s (50% aq.); solid. pt. 37-40 C; acid no. 0.2 max.; pH 4-7 (10% aq.).

Lipoxol® 600 MED. [Hüls Am.; Hüls AG] PEG-12; CAS 25322-68-3; EINECS 229-859-1; moisture and consis-tency regulators in creams, lotions, shaving preps., tooth-pastes, and hair care prods. (m.w. < 2000), lipstick, deodorant stick, soap bars, powd. bases, and makeup pastes (m.w. > 2000); German pharmacopoeia compli-ance; colorless to wh. liq./solid; water-sol.; visc. 15-20 mPa·s (50% aq.); solid. pt. 15-25 C; acid no. 0.2 max.; pH 4-7 (10% aq.).

Lipoxol® 800 MED. [Hüls Am.; Hüls AG] PEG-16; CAS 25322-68-3; moisture and consistency regulators in creams, lotions, shaving preps., toothpastes, and hair care prods. (m.w. < 2000), lipstick, deodorant stick, soap bars, powd. bases, and makeup pastes (m.w. > 2000); German pharmacopoeia compliance; wh. solid; water-sol.; visc. 20-25 mPa·s (50% aq.); solid. pt. 25-35 C; acid no. 0.2 max.; pH 4-7 (10% aq.).

Lipoxol® 1000 MED. [Hüls Am.; Hüls AG] PEG-20; CAS 25322-68-3; moisture and consistency regulators in creams, lotions, shaving preps., toothpastes, and hair care prods. (m.w. < 2000), lipstick, deodorant stick, soap bars, powd. bases, and makeup pastes (m.w. > 2000); German pharmacopoeia compliance; wh. solid; water-sol.; visc. 24-29 mPa·s (50% aq.); solid. pt. 30-40 C; acid no. 0.2 max.; pH 4-7 (10% aq.).

Lipoxol® 1550 MED. [Hüls Am.; Hüls AG] PEG-32; CAS 25322-68-3; moisture and consistency regulators in creams, lotions, shaving preps., toothpastes, and hair care prods. (m.w. < 2000), lipstick, deodorant stick, soap bars, powd. bases, and makeup pastes (m.w. > 2000); German pharmacopoeia compliance; wh. flakes; water-sol.; visc. 35-50 mPa·s (50% aq.); solid. pt. 40-50 C; acid no. 0.2 max.; pH 4-7 (10% aq.).

Lipoxol® 2000 MED. [Hüls Am.; Hüls AG] PEG-40; CAS 25322-68-3; moisture and consistency regulators in creams, lotions, shaving preps., toothpastes, and hair care prods. (m.w. < 2000), lipstick, deodorant stick, soap bars, powd. bases, and makeup pastes (m.w. > 2000); German pharmacopoeia compliance; wh. flakes; water-sol.; visc. 47-60 mPa·s (50% aq.); solid. pt. 47-52 C; acid no. 0.2 max.; pH 4-7 (10% aq.).

Lipoxol® 3000 MED. [Hüls Am.; Hüls AG] PEG-60; CAS 25322-68-3; moisture and consistency regulators in creams, lotions, shaving preps., toothpastes, and hair care prods. (m.w. < 2000), lipstick, deodorant stick, soap bars, powd. bases, and makeup pastes (m.w. > 2000); German pharmacopoeia compliance; wh. flakes; water-sol.; visc. 70-110 mPa·s (50% aq.); solid. pt. 50-56 C; acid no. 0.2 max.; pH 4-7 (10% aq.).

Lipoxol® 4000 MED. [Hüls Am.; Hüls AG] PEG-75; CAS 25322-68-3; moisture and consistency regulators in creams, lotions, shaving preps., toothpastes, and hair care prods. (m.w. < 2000), lipstick, deodorant stick, soap bars, powd. bases, and makeup pastes (m.w. > 2000); German pharmacopoeia compliance; wh. flakes/powd.; water-sol.; visc. 115-170 mPa·s (50% aq.); solid. pt. 50-58 C; acid no. 0.2 max.; pH 4-7 (10% aq.).

Lipoxol® 6000 MED. [Hüls Am.; Hüls AG] PEG-150; CAS 25322-68-3; moisture and consistency regulators in creams, lotions, shaving preps., toothpastes, and hair care prods. (m.w. < 2000), lipstick, deodorant stick, soap bars, powd. bases, and makeup pastes (m.w. > 2000); German pharmacopoeia compliance; wh. flakes/powd.; water-sol.; visc. 205-350 mPa·s (50% aq.); solid. pt. 55-62 C; acid no. 0.2 max.; pH 4-7 (10% aq.).

Lipoxol® 12000. [Hüls Am.; Hüls AG] PEG-240; CAS 25322-68-3; cosmetic ingred. for lipsticks, deodorant sticks, soap bars, powd. bases, creams, and pastes; wh. flakes/powd.; water-sol.; visc. 1000-2000 mPa·s (50% aq.); solid. pt. 57-60 C; acid no. 0.2 max.; pH 4-7 (10% aq.).

Lipoxol® 20000. [Hüls Am.; Hüls AG] PEG-350; cosmetic ingred. for lipsticks, deodorant sticks, soap bars, powd. bases, creams, pastes; wh. flakes; water-sol.; visc. 2000-3500 mPa·s (50% aq.); solid. pt. 57-60 C; acid no. 0.2 max.; pH 4-7 (10% aq.).

Liprot CK. [Fabriquimica] Potassium cocoyl hydrolyzed collagen; CAS 68920-65-0; protein for cosmetics use; pH 7.0-8.5 (10%); 30-32% solids.

Liprot CT. [Fabriquimica] TEA-cocoyl hydrolyzed collagen;

CAS 68952-16-9; protein for cosmetics use; pH 7.0-8.5 (10%); 30-32% solids.

Liprot CTS. [Fabriquimica] TEA-cocoyl hydrolyzed collagen and sorbitol; CAS 68952-16-9, 50-70-4.

Liprot UK. [Fabriquimica] Potassium undecylenoyl hydrolyzed collagen; CAS 68951-92-8; protein for cosmetics use; pH 7.0-8.5 (10%); 30-32% solids.

Liprot UT. [Fabriquimica] TEA-undecylenoyl hydrolyzed collagen; CAS 68951-91-7; protein for cosmetics use; pH 7.0-8.5 (10%); 30-32% solids.

LiquaPar® Oil. [Sutton Labs] Isopropylparaben, isobutylparaben, n-butylparaben; broad-spectrum preservative for cosmetics and topical pharmaceuticals; effective against Gram-positive and Gram-negative bacteria, yeast, and mold even at low concs.; USA, Japan, and Europe approvals; yel. clear visc. liq., mild char. odor; sol. in alcohol, propylene glycol; slightly sol. in water; sp.gr. 1.103; visc. 6450 cps; b.p. 268 C; sapon. no. 292-296; cloud pt. -12 C; ref. index 1.53; pH 5-8; usage level: up to 0.5%; toxicology: LD50 (oral, rat) > 5000 mg/kg (pract. nontoxic); moderately irritating to skin; severe eye irritant; 100% act.

Liquid Absorption Base. [ChemMark Development] Min. oil and lanolin alcohol.

Liquid Absorption Base Type A, T. [Croda Inc.] Min. oil, lanolin alcohol; mild surfactant, emollient for liq. make-up to improve dispersion and applic. properties of pigments; primary oil phase ingred. in o/w emulsions; type T is better solv. for oil-sol. dyes; also for facial cleansers, surgical scrubs, baby wipes; solubilizer for oil-sol. actives in pharmaceuticals; clear yel. liqs.; sol. in min. oil, IPA (Type A); usage level: 2-10%.

Liquid Animal Collagen. [Phillip Rockley] Soluble collagen; CAS 9007-34-5; EINECS 232-697-4; cosmetic protein.

Liquid Crystal CN/9. [Presperse] Cholesteric esters; CAS 57-88-5; EINECS 200-353-2; carriers for nutrients in skin care prods.; provides decorative, functional and aesthetic effects to cosmetics; iridescent free-flowing oily visc. liq.; avail. colors: red, orange, green, blue, violet, silver; f.p. < 0 C; clearing pt. > 40 C.

Liquid Vegetal Tan DH. [Les Colorants Wackherr] Self-tanning agent of vegetable origin.

Liquiritina. [Vevy] Alcohol, water, and licorice extract; botanical extract.

Liquiwax™ DC-EFA/SS. [Brooks Industries] Dicetyl dilinoleate; emollient to soften the skin without greasiness and oiliness; liq. wax; 100% act.

Liquiwax™ DIADD. [Brooks Industries] Diisoarachidyl dodecanedioate; emollient to soften the skin without greasiness and oiliness; liq. wax; 100% act.

Liquiwax™ DIADD/TiO₂ Disp. [Brooks Industries] Diisoarachidyl dodecanedioate, titanium dioxide; emollient for formulation of high SPF natural sunscreen prods. which do not whiten up on the skin and have a pleasant afterfeel.

Liquiwax™ DICDD. [Brooks Industries] Diisocetyl dodecanedioate; emollient to soften the skin without greasiness and oiliness; liq. wax; 100% act.

Liquiwax™ DIEFA. [Brooks Industries] Diisoarachidyl dilinoleate; emollient to soften the skin without greasiness and oiliness; liq. wax; 100% act.

Lisato RNA. [Variati] Hydrolyzed RNA.

Lithol. [Rhone-Poulenc] Ichthammol.

LMB. [Vevy] Lauryl betaine; CAS 683-10-3; EINECS 211-669-5; detergent.

Lobra. [Karlshamns] Partially hydrog. canola oil; m.p. 66-72 F; iodine no. 88-93; sapon. no. 178-195.

Locron Extra, Flakes, L, P, P Extra, Powd., S, Sol'n. [Hoechst Celanese/Colorants & Surf.] Aluminum chlorohydrate; CAS 1327-41-9; EINECS 215-477-2; anti-

perspirant active.

Lo-Micron Black Extender B.C. 34-3062-1. [Hilton-Davis] Iron oxides and talc.

Lo-Micron Talc 1. [Whittaker, Clark & Daniels] Talc; CAS 14807-96-6; EINECS 238-877-9; cosmetic ingred.

Lonzabac-12.100. [Lonza Ltd.] Laurylamine dipropylenediamine; CAS 2372-82-9; EINECS 219-145-8.

Lonzaine® 12C. [Lonza] Coco betaine; CAS 68424-94-2; EINECS 270-329-4; amphoteric; conditioner, foaming agent, visc. modifier, irritation mitigant used in personal care prods. and industrial applics.; biodeg.; liq.; visc. 14 cps; pour pt. 3 C; pH 7.5 (3%); surf. tens. 34.4 dynes/cm (0.1%); Draves wetting 11 s; 35% conc.

Lonzaine® 14. [Lonza] Lauryl betaine.; CAS 683-10-3; EINECS 211-669-5; mild detergent for shampoos.

Lonzaine® 16S. [Lonza] Cetyl betaine; CAS 693-33-4; EINECS 211-748-4; cosmetic surfactant.

Lonzaine® 16SP. [Lonza] Cetyl betaine; CAS 693-33-4; EINECS 211-748-4; surfactant; solid; visc. 720 cps; surf. tens. 32 dynes/cm (0.1%); Draves wetting 11 s; 35% solids.

Lonzaine® 18S. [Lonza] Stearyl betaine; CAS 820-66-6; EINECS 212-470-6; surfactant.

Lonzaine® C. [Lonza] Cocamidopropyl betaine; amphoteric; foaming agent, conditioner, visc. booster, wetting agent, used in cosmetics, toiletries, detergents, metal finishing, textile finishing, etc.; biodeg.; Gardner 2 nonvisc. liq.; char. odor; visc. 29 cps; pour pt. 3 C; pH 4.5–5.5 (10%); surf. tens. 33.6 dynes/cm (0.1%); Draves wetting 28 s; 30% act.

Lonzaine® CO. [Lonza] Cocamidopropyl betaine; amphoteric; foaming agent, conditioner, visc. booster, wetting agent, used in cosmetics, toiletries, detergents, metal finishing, textile finishing, etc.; biodeg.; Gardner 2 nonvisc. liq.; char. odor; visc. 28 cps; pour pt. 3 C; pH 6–8 (10%); surf. tens. 33.9 dynes/cm (0.1%); Draves wetting 16 s; 35% solids.

Lonzaine® CS. [Lonza] Cocoamidopropylhydroxysultaine; CAS 68139-30-0; EINECS 268-761-3; amphoteric; conditioner used in personal care prods. and industrial applics.; liq.; water-sol.; visc. 189 cps; pour pt. 9 C; pH 8.0 (10%); surf. tens. 35.2 dynes/cm (0.1%); Draves wetting > 2 min; 50% conc.

Lonzaine® JS. [Lonza] Cocamidopropylhydroxysultaine; CAS 68139-30-0; EINECS 268-761-3; amphoteric; foaming agent, visc. modifier, irritation mitigant for personal care and industrial applics.; liq.; 50% solids.

Lonza Insta-Pearl®. [Lonza] Proprietary blend; high intensity pearlescent, opacifier for hair and skin care prods.

Lonzest® 143-S. [Lonza] Myristyl propionate; CAS 6221-95-0; EINECS 226-300-9; nonionic; emollient, penetrant, and spreading agent in hair and skin cosmetics; perfume solv. in bath oils, antiperspirants, preshave lotions, sunburn lotions; solv./emollient in lipsticks, waterless hand cleaners, makeup, facial cleaners; humectant; APHA 10 clear liq., odorless; sol. in acetone, CCl₄, castor, lanolin, peanut, silicone, and cottonseed oils, ethanol, ethyl acetate, heptane, IPA, toluene; sp.gr. 0.852; visc. 5 cps; f.p. -5 C; acid no. 0.5 max.; sapon. no. 195-210; ref. index 1.433; pH 6-8 (10% aq. disp.); toxicology: LD50 (oral) > 39 g/kg; not a primary skin or eye irritant; noncomedogenic; 100% act.

Lonzest® 153-S. [Lonza] Trimethylol propane tricaprate/caprylate; CAS 4826-87-3; emollient and solubilizer for bath oils, antiperspirants, preshave lotions, tanning prods., body lotions; offers barrier and lubricating props.; APHA 100 color, low odor; solvent soluble; sp.gr. 0.94; visc. 34 cts; HLB 1; acid no. 0.5; iodine no. 0.2; sapon. no. 310; 100% conc.

Lonzest® 163-S. [Lonza] Pentaerythrityl tetracaprate/caprylate; CAS 3008-50-2; emollient and solubilizer with lubricating and barrier props.; for bath oils, preshave lotions, tanning prods., and body lotions; imparts pleasant feel; APHA 80 color, low odor; solvent soluble; sp.gr. 0.96; visc. 59 cts; HLB 1; acid no. 0.5; sapon. no. 327; hyd. no. 4; 100% conc.

Lonzest® EGMS. [Lonza] Glycol stearate; CAS 111-60-4; EINECS 203-886-9; pearlescent and opacifier for cosmetics, personal care and household prods.; modifies feel/cosmetic appeal in creams and lotions; wh. free-flowing flakes; water-insol.; m.p. 50-60 C; acid no. 4 max.; sapon. no. 180-190; 100% act.

Lonzest® SML-20. [Lonza] Polysorbate 20; CAS 9005-64-5; nonionic; emulsifier used where o/w and w/o emulsions are required; solubilizer; liq.; HLB 17.0; 100% conc.

Lonzest® SMO-20. [Lonza] Polysorbate 80; CAS 9005-65-6; nonionic; emulsifier, solubilizer and stabilizer used in foods, personal care prods. and industrial applics.; liq.; HLB 15.0; 100% conc.

Lonzest® SMP-20. [Lonza] Polysorbate 40; CAS 9005-66-7; nonionic; emulsifier, solubilizer and stabilizer used in foods, personal care prods. and industrial applics.; liq.; HLB 16.0; 100% conc.

Lonzest® SMS-20. [Lonza] Polysorbate 60; CAS 9005-67-8; nonionic; emulsifier, solubilizer and stabilizer used in foods, personal care prods. and industrial applics.; liq.; HLB 15.0; 100% conc.

Lonzest® STO-20. [Lonza] Polysorbate 85; CAS 9005-70-3; nonionic; emulsifier, solubilizer and stabilizer used in foods, personal care prods. and industrial applics.; liq.; HLB 11.0; 100% conc.

Lonzest® STS-20. [Lonza] Polysorbate 65; CAS 9005-71-4; nonionic; emulsifier, solubilizer and stabilizer used in foods, personal care prods. and industrial applics.; solid; HLB 11.0; 100% conc.

Loofah Extract. [Koshiro] Luffa extract.

Loralan-CH. [Lanaetex Prods.] Cholesterol USP; CAS 57-88-5; EINECS 200-353-2; cosmetics ingred.

Loropan CME. [Triantaphyllou] Cocamide MEA; CAS 68140-00-1; EINECS 268-770-2; nonionic; foam stabilizer and thickening agent for shampoos and detergents; bead; 92–96% conc.

Loropan KD. [Triantaphyllou] Cocamide DEA; CAS 61791-31-9; EINECS 263-163-9; nonionic; emulsifier, stabilizer, thickener for shampoos and bubble baths; liq., paste; 85–90% conc.

Loropan KM. [Triantaphyllou] Cocamide MEA; CAS 68140-00-1; EINECS 268-770-2; nonionic; foam stabilizer, thickener for shampoos and bubble baths; paste; 30% conc.

Loropan LD. [Triantaphyllou] Lauramide DEA; CAS 120-40-1; EINECS 204-393-1; nonionic; foam stabilizer for shampoos, detergents, fortifier for perfumes in soap; solid; 90% conc.

Loropan LM. [Triantaphyllou] Lauramide MEA; CAS 142-78-9; EINECS 205-560-1; nonionic; foam stabilizer and thickening agent for shampoos and detergents; bead; 92–96% conc.

Loropan LMD. [Triantaphyllou] Lauric/myristic DEA; nonionic; foam stabilizer; superfatting and thickening agent for shampoos; fortifier for perfume in soaps; paste; 90% conc.

Loropan OD. [Triantaphyllou] Oleamide DEA; CAS 93-83-4; EINECS 202-281-7; nonionic; foam stabilizer, thickener, and superfatting agent for shampoos and bubble bath prods.; liq.; 90% conc.

Louryl T-50. [Triantaphyllou] TEA-alkylbenzene sulfonate; anionic; detergent base for shampoos and bubble bath prods.; liq.; 50% conc.

Lowenol 710. [Lowenstein] anionic; dispersant for semipermanent hair color systems utilizing basic/disperse solv. dyes.

Lowenol 915. [Lowenstein] Phenylether-based solv. for hair color systems.

Lowenol 1957. [Lowenstein] Coco-based; cationic; surfactant for semipermanent hair color systems.

Lowenol 1985. [Lowenstein] PEG-8 tallow amine; weakly cationic; surfactant for semipermanent hair color systems.

Lowenol 3238. [Lowenstein] Surfactant; anionic; for prep. of semipermanent/temporary color systems based on certified and Lowalan dyes.

Lowenol C-243. [Lowenstein] PEG-3 cocamine; CAS 61791-14-8; nonionic; lubricant, foam stabilizer, dispersant, visc. control agent for shampoos and hair colors.

Lowenol C-279. [Lowenstein] Ceteareth-2; CAS 68439-49-6; emulsifier/opacifier for oxidation color systems (creams).

Lowenol C-420. [Lowenstein] Coco-based; mildly cationic; dye leveling and visc. control agent for hair color systems.

Lowenol C-11034. [Lowenstein] Cocamidopropyl betaine.

Lowenol C Acid. [Lowenstein] Coco-based; anionic; substantive surfactant, foam modifier, lubricant for shampoos, foaming color systems, skin care prods.; reactive coupling agent for cationic/anionic systems.

Lowenol L Acid. [Lowenstein] Lauroyl-based; anionic; substantive surfactant, foam modifier, lubricant for shampoos, foaming color systems, skin care prods.; reactive coupling agent for cationic/anionic systems.

Lowenol M Acid. [Lowenstein] Myristoyl-based; anionic; substantive surfactant, foam modifier, lubricant for shampoos, foaming color systems, and skin care prods.; reactive coupling agent for cationic/anionic systems.

Lowenol O Acid. [Lowenstein] Oleoyl-based; anionic; substantive surfactant, foam modifier, lubricant for shampoos, foaming color systems, and skin care prods.; reactive coupling agent for cationic/anionic systems.

Lowenol OT-216. [Lowenstein] PEG-5 oleamide dioleate.

Lowenol P-1030. [Lowenstein] Polyacrylic acid copolymer; visc. control agent for cream, semipermanent, oxidation hair color systems.

Lowenol P Acid. [Lowenstein] Palmitic-based; anionic; substantive surfactant, foam modifier, lubricant for shampoos, foaming color systems, and skin care prods.; reactive coupling agent for cationic/anionic systems.

Lowenol S-216. [Lowenstein] Dihydroxyethyl soyamine dioleate; mildly cationic; dye leveling and visc. control agent for oxidation hair color systems.

Lowenol T-1106-A. [Lowenstein] Surfactant; anionic; for prep. of temporary hair color systems.

Lubrajel® CG, DV, MS, TW. [Guardian Labs; Amerchol] Polyglycerylmethacrylate and propylene glycol; autoclavable nondrying water-sol. lubricant for medical and surgical use; clear, colorless visc. gel; sp.gr. 1.3 g/ml; visc. 300,000–400,000 cps; pH 5.0–6.0.

Lubrajel® NP. [Guardian Labs; Amerchol] Polyglycerylmethacrylate; CAS 9003-01-4; cosmetic and personal care applics.

Lubrajel® Oil. [Guardian Labs; Amerchol] Polyglycerylmethacrylate; CAS 9003-01-4; cosmetics and personal care applics.

Lubrajel® WA. [Guardian Labs; Amerhcol] Polyglycerylmethacrylate; CAS 9003-01-4; cosmetics and personal care applics.

Lubritab®. [Mendell] Hydrogenated veg. oil NF; CAS 68334-00-9; EINECS 269-804-9; lubricant for pharmaceutical tablets; aux. dry binder when tablets tend to cap or laminate; fine powd.; avg. particle size 104 μ; 25% -200 mesh; dens. (tapped) 0.57 g/ml; m.p. 61-66 C; acid no. 2 max.; sapon. no. 188-198.

Ludipress®. [BASF AG] Based on lactose and Kollidon®; direct tableting auxiliary for pharmaceuticals.

Luminex. [Ikeda] Quaternium-45; CAS 21034-17-3; EINECS 244-158-0; active ingred. improving skin function and esp. useful for treating dry and chapped skin; for hair lotions, body oils, moisturizing lotions/creams, emollient creams, skin fresheners; faint yel. cryst. powd.; m.p. 227-232 C; pH neutral; 97% max. assay.

Lumorol K 28. [Zschimmer & Schwarz] Disodium laurethsulfosuccinate, cocamidopropyl betaine, magnesium lauryl sulfate; anionic; detergent for cosmetics, shampoos, bath preps.; liq.; 28% conc.

Lumorol K 5019. [Zschimmer & Schwarz] Disodium laurethsulfosuccinate, sodium lauryl sulfoacetate; anionic; detergent for cosmetics, shampoos, bath preps.; liq.; 40% conc.

Lumorol RK. [Zschimmer & Schwarz] Surfactant blend; anionic/amphoteric; detergent for cosmetics, shampoos, bath preps., household cleaners; liq.; 28% conc.

Lumosäure A. [Zschimmer & Schwarz] Dodecylbenzene sulfonic acid; CAS 27176-87-0; EINECS 248-289-4; anionic; for low pH cleansing agents; liq.; 100% act.

Lustrabrite® S. [Telechemische] Toluene sulfonamide/epoxy resin; patented formaldehyde-free nail enamel resin providing superior clarity, brilliance, high gloss, adhesion; plasticizer for nitrocellulose.

Lustra-Pearl® . [ISP Van Dyk] Mica, titanium dioxide; pearlescent pigments for cosmetic eye, face, lip, and body makeup; nail lacquers; imparts wide range of luster effects (silk, satin, gloss, glimmer, gold, and amethyst); powd.

Lutrol® E 300. [BASF AG] PEG-6; CAS 25322-68-3; EINECS 220-045-1; emulsifier, emollient, lubricant, and solv. for liq. preps.; liq.; 100% conc.

Lutrol® E 400. [BASF AG] PEG-8; CAS 25322-68-3; EINECS 225-856-4; emulsifier, emollient, lubricant, and solv. for liq. preps.; liq.; 100% conc.

Lutrol® E1450 NF. [BASF] PEG-32; CAS 25322-68-3; cosmetic ingred.; prill.

Lutrol® E 1500. [BASF AG] PEG-32; CAS 25322-68-3; nonionic; emulsifier, binder, solubilizer, resorption promoter for substances insol. or sparingly sol. in water; microbeads; 100% conc.

Lutrol® E 4000. [BASF AG] PEG-75; CAS 25322-68-3; nonionic; emulsifier, binder, solubilizer, resorption promoter for substances insol. or sparingly sol. in water; microbeads; 100% conc.

Lutrol® E 6000. [BASF AG] PEG-150; CAS 25322-68-3; nonionic; emulsifier, binder, solubilizer, resorption promoter for substances insol. or sparingly sol. in water; microbeads; 100% conc.

Lutrol® F 127. [BASF AG] EO/PO block copolymer; CAS 106392-12-5; nonionic; thickening and gelling agent for pharmaceuticals; microbeads; 100% conc.

Lutrol® OP 2000. [BASF] PPG-26 oleate; CAS 31394-71-5; cosmetic emollient, lubricant, defoamer, visc. control agent, dispersant, spreading agent for personal care prods.; biodeg.; pale yel. liq., mild, pleasant odor; m.w. 2000; sol. in IPM, IPA; insol. water; sp.gr. 0.986; dens. 8.3 lb/gal; visc. 267 cps; pour pt. –20 F; acid no. < 1.0; sapon no. 23.

Luviflex® VBM 35. [BASF; BASF AG] Acrylates/PVP copolymer; CAS 26589-26-4; hair fixative, film former with exc. hydrocarbon compatibility for weatherproof hairstyles; sol'n.

Luviform® FA 119. [BASF AG] PVM/MA copolymer; CAS 9011-16-9; stabilizing and binding agent for toothpastes, denture retaining agents, shampoos, etc.

Luviquat® FC 370. [BASF; BASF AG] Polyquaternium-16 (methylvinylimidazolium chloride/vinylpyrrolidone copolymer (30:70 ratio) aq. sol'n.); CAS 29297-55-0; cationic; substantive polymer used as conditioner in prods. for hair and skin care; film former; foam stabilizing, lubri-

cating, and bactericidal effects; ylsh. clear visc. liq., faint char. odor; sol. in water, ethanol, water/IPA mixts., anionic surfactants; m.w. 100,000; pH 5-8 (10% aq.); 40 ± 2% solids.

Luviquat® FC 550. [BASF; BASF AG] Polyquaternium-16 (methylvinylimidazolium chloride/vinylpyrrolidone copolymer (50:50 ratio) aq. sol'n.); CAS 29297-55-0; cationic; substantive polymer used as conditioner in prods. for hair and skin care; film former; foam stabilizing, lubricating, bactericidal effects; ylsh. clear visc. liq., faint char. odor; sol. in water, ethanol, water/IPA mixts., anionic surfactants; m.w. 80,000; pH 5-8 (10% aq.); 40 ± 2% solids.

Luviquat® FC 905. [BASF; BASF AG] Polyquaternium-16 (vinylimidazolium methochloride/vinylpyrrolidone copolymer (95:5 ratio) aq. sol'n.); CAS 29297-55-0; cationic; conditioner and film-former for hair conditioners, rinses, shampoos, bleaches, dyes, liq. soaps, bath preps., skin care prods., coatings; bactericidal effects; ylsh. clear visc. liq., faint char. odor; misc. with water, ethanol; m.w. 4,000; pH 5-8 (10% aq.); 40% act. in water.

Luviquat® HM 552. [BASF; BASF AG] Polyquaternium-16 (vinylimidazolium methochloride/vinylpyrrolidone copolymer (50:50 ratio) aq. sol'n.); CAS 29297-55-0; cationic; substantive film-former, conditioner, and setting resin for hair and skin care prods.; ylsh. clear visc. liq., faint char. odor; misc. with water and ethanol; m.w. 800,000; pH 4.5-7.5 (10% aq.); 19-21% solids.

Luviquat® Mono CP. [BASF] Hydroxyethyl cetyldimonium phosphate; film-former, conditioner for hair cosmetics, esp. cold waves; sol'n.

Luviset® CA66. [BASF AG] Vinyl acetate/crotonic acid copolymer; CAS 25609-89-6; film-former, hair fixative for aerosols, hair sprays, setting lotions, conditioners; colorless powd.; when neutralized, sol. in water, water/alcohol and hydrocarbon/alcohol blends; acid no. 66 ± 4.

Luviset® CAP. [BASF AG] Vinyl acetate/crotonic acid/vinyl propionate copolymer; film-forming agent, fixative for hair-sprays and fixing lotions; compatible in aerosols with propane/butane; powd.; acid no. 66 ± 4.

Luviskol® K17. [BASF; BASF AG] PVP; CAS 9003-39-8; EINECS 201-800-4; film-forming agent, hair fixative, thickener, protective colloid, suspending agent, and dispersant for cosmetics, adhesives, paints, coatings, paper, detergents, glass fibers, inks, ceramics, nonpharmaceutical tableting, photographic films; powd. or liq.; > 99% > 250 µm particle size (powd.); sol. in alcohols, esters, ether alcohols, ketones, lactams, chlorinated hydrocarbons, nitroparaffins, acids, amines; bulk dens. 0.4-0.5 g/cc (powd.); visc. 5.4 cps (5% in methanol); pH 3-7 (10% , powd.), 7-10 (10% , sol'n.); > 92% solids (powd.), 50% solids in water (sol'n.).

Luviskol® K30. [BASF; BASF AG] PVP; CAS 9003-39-8; EINECS 201-800-4; film-forming agent, hair fixative, thickener, protective colloid, suspending agent, and dispersant for cosmetics, adhesives, paints, coatings, paper, detergents, glass fibers, inks, ceramics, nonpharmaceutical tableting, photographic films; powd. or liq.; particle size > 99% > 250 µm (powd.); sol. in alcohols, esters, ether alcohols, ketones, lactams, chlorinated hydrocarbons, nitroparaffins, acids, amines; bulk dens. 0.4-0.5 g/cc; visc. 7.0 cps (5% in methanol); pH 3-7 (10% , powd.), 7-10 (10% , sol'n.); > 95% solids (powd.), 30% solids in water (sol'n.).

Luviskol® K60. [BASF; BASF AG] PVP; CAS 9003-39-8; EINECS 201-800-4; film-forming agent, hair fixative, thickener, protective colloid, suspending agent, and dispersant for cosmetics, adhesives, paints, coatings, paper, detergents, glass fibers, inks, ceramics, nonpharmaceutical tableting, photographic films; liq.; sol. in alcohols, esters, ether alcohols, ketones, lactams, chlorinated hydrocarbons, nitroparaffins, acids, amines; pH 7-10 (10%); 45% solids in water.

Luviskol® K80. [BASF; BASF AG] PVP; CAS 9003-39-8; EINECS 201-800-4; film-forming agent, hair fixative, thickener, protective colloid, suspending agent, and dispersant for cosmetics, adhesives, paints, coatings, paper, detergents, glass fibers, inks, ceramics, nonpharmaceutical tableting, photographic films; powd. or liq.; particle size > 99% > 250 µm (powd.); sol. in alcohols, esters, ether alcohols, ketones, lactams, chlorinated hydrocarbons, nitroparaffins, acids, amines; bulk dens. 0.3-0.4 g/cc (powd.); visc. 27 cps (5% in methanol); pH 5-8 (10% , powd.), 7-10.5 (10% , sol'n.); > 95% solids (powd.), 20% solids in water (sol'n.).

Luviskol® K90. [BASF; BASF AG] PVP; CAS 9003-39-8; EINECS 201-800-4; film-forming agent, hair fixative, thickener, protective colloid, suspending agent, and dispersant for cosmetics, adhesives, paints, coatings, paper, detergents, glass fibers, inks, ceramics, nonpharmaceutical tabletting, photographic films; powd. or liq.; particle size > 99% > 250 µm (powd.); sol. in alcohols, esters, ether alcohols, ketones, lactams, chlorinated hydrocarbons, nitroparaffins, acids, amines; bulk dens. 0.3-0.4 g/cc (powd.); visc. 30.8 cps (5% in methanol); pH 5-9 (10%, powd.), 7-10.5 (10% , sol'n.); > 95% solids (powd.), 15% or 20% solids in water (sol'n.).

Luviskol® LD-9025. [BASF] PVP aq. sol'n.; CAS 9003-39-8; EINECS 201-800-4; film-forming agent, hair fixative, thickener, protective colloid, suspending agent, and dispersant for cosmetics, adhesives, inks, ceramics, nonpharmaceutical tabletting, photographic films; liq.

Luviskol® VA28E. [BASF; BASF AG] PVP/VA copolymer (20:80 ratio) ethanol sol'n.; CAS 25086-89-9; film-forming agents for hair-sprays and fixing lotions; suspending agent, dispersant, thickener, stabilizer, adhesion promoter, coatings; liq.; sol. in alcohols, aromatic hydrocarbons, chlorinated hydrocarbons, esters, ethers, ether alcohols, ketones, lactones; m.w. 58,000; sp.gr. 0.95; visc. 600 cps; 50 ± 2% conc. in ethanol.

Luviskol® VA28I. [BASF; BASF AG] PVP/VA copolymer (20:80 ratio) isopropanol sol'n.; CAS 25086-89-9; film-forming agents for hair-sprays and fixing lotions; suspending agent, dispersant, thickener, stabilizer, adhesion promoter, coatings; liq.; sol. in alcohols, aromatic hydrocarbons, chlorinated hydrocarbons, esters, ethers, ether alcohols, ketones, lactones; m.w. 53,000; sp.gr. 0.95; visc. 300 cps; 50 ± 2% conc. in IPA.

Luviskol® VA37E. [BASF; BASF AG] PVP/VA copolymer (30:70 ratio) ethanol sol'n.; CAS 25086-89-9; film-forming agents for hair-sprays and fixing lotions; suspending agent, dispersant, thickener, stabilizer, adhesion promoter, coatings; liq.; sol. in alcohols, aromatic hydrocarbons, chlorinated hydrocarbons, esters, ethers, ether alcohols, ketones, lactones; m.w. 45,000; sp.gr. 0.95; visc. 1600 cps; 50 ± 2% in ethanol.

Luviskol® VA37I. [BASF; BASF AG] PVP/VA copolymer (30:70 ratio) isopropanol sol'n.; CAS 25086-89-9; film-forming agents for hair-sprays and fixing lotions; suspending agent, dispersant, thickener, stabilizer, adhesion promoter, coatings; liq.; sol. in alcohols, aromatic hydrocarbons, chlorinated hydrocarbons, esters, ethers, ether alcohols, ketones, lactones; m.w. 40,000; sp.gr. 0.95; visc. 2300 cps; 50 ± 2% in IPA.

Luviskol® VA55E. [BASF; BASF AG] PVP/VA copolymer (50:50 ratio) ethanol sol'n.; CAS 25086-89-9; film-forming agents for hair-sprays and fixing lotions; suspending agent, dispersant, thickener, stabilizer, adhesion promoter, coatings; liq.; sol. in alcohols, aromatic hydrocar-

bons, chlorinated hydrocarbons, esters, ethers, ether alcohols, ketones, lactones; 50 ± 2% in ethanol.

Luviskol® VA55I. [BASF; BASF AG] PVP/VA copolymer (50:50 ratio) isopropanol sol'n.; CAS 25086-89-9; film-forming agents for hair-sprays and fixing lotions; suspending agent, dispersant, thickener, stabilizer, adhesion promoter, coatings; liq.; sol. in alcohols, aromatic hydrocarbons, chlorinated hydrocarbons, esters, ethers, ether alcohols, ketones, lactones; 50 ± 2% in IPA.

Luviskol® VA64. [BASF; BASF AG] PVP/VA copolymer (60:40 ratio); CAS 25086-89-9; film-forming agents for hair-sprays and fixing lotions; powd.; sol. in alcohols, aromatic hydrocarbons, chlorinated hydrocarbons, esters, ethers, ether alcohols, ketones, lactones; m.w. 44,000; > 95% solids.

Luviskol® VA64E. [BASF; BASF AG] PVP/VA copolymer (60:40 ratio) ethanol sol'n.; CAS 25086-89-9; film-forming agent for hair sprays and fixing lotions; suspending agent, dispersant, thickener, stabilizer, adhesion promoter, coatings; liq.; sol. in alcohols, aromatic hydrocarbons, chlorinated hydrocarbons, esters, ethers, ether alcohols, ketones, lactones; m.w. 38,000; sp.gr. 0.95; visc. 1700 cps; 50 ± 2% solids in ethanol.

Luviskol® VA64W. [BASF] PVP/VA copolymer (60:40 ratio) aq. sol'n.; CAS 25086-89-9; film-forming agent for hair sprays and fixing lotions; suspending agent, dispersant, thickener, stabilizer, adhesion promoter, coatings; liq.; sol. in water, alcohols, aromatic hydrocarbons, chlorinated hydrocarbons, esters, ethers, ether alcohols, ketones, lactones; m.w. 34,000; sp.gr. 1.22; visc. 1600 cps; 50 ± 2% solids in water.

Luviskol® VA73E. [BASF; BASF AG] PVP/VA copolymer (70:30 ratio) ethanol sol'n.; CAS 25086-89-9; film-forming agents for hair-sprays and fixing lotions; suspending agent, dispersant, thickener, stabilizer, adhesion promoter, coatings; liq.; sol. in alcohols, aromatic hydrocarbons, chlorinated hydrocarbons, esters, ethers, ether alcohols, ketones, lactones; m.w. 55,000; sp.gr. 0.95; visc. 2300 cps; 50 ± 2% conc. in ethanol.

Luviskol® VA73I [BASF; BASF AG] PVP/VA copolymer (70:30 ratio) isopropanol sol'n.; CAS 25086-89-9; film-forming agents for hair-sprays and fixing lotions; suspending agent, dispersant, thickener, stabilizer, adhesion promoter, coatings; liq.; sol. in alcohols, aromatic hydrocarbons, chlorinated hydrocarbons, esters, ethers, ether alcohols, ketones, lactones; m.w. 30,000; sp.gr. 0.95; visc. 2100 cps; 50 ± 2% conc. in IPA.

Luviskol® VA73W. [BASF] PVP/VA copolymer (70:30 ratio) aq. sol'n.; CAS 25086-89-9; film-forming agent for hair sprays and fixing lotions; suspending agent, dispersant, thickener, stabilizer, adhesion promoter, coatings; liq.; sol. in water, alcohols, aromatic hydrocarbons, chlorinated hydrocarbons, esters, ethers, ether alcohols, ketones, lactones; m.w. 33,000; sp.gr. 1.22; visc. 1400 cps; 50 ± 2% solids in water.

Luviskol® VAP 343 E. [BASF AG] PVP/VA/vinyl propionate copolymer (30:40:30 ratio) ethanol sol'n.; film-forming agent, fixative for hair-sprays and fixing lotions; compatible in aerosols with propane/butane; 50% in ethanol.

Luviskol® VAP 343 I. [BASF AG] PVP/VA/vinyl propionate copolymer (30:40:30 ratio) isopropanol sol'n.; film-forming agent, fixative for hair-sprays and fixing lotions; compatible in aerosols with propane/butane; 50% in IPA.

Luvitol® EHO. [BASF; BASF AG] Cetearyl octanoate; nonionic; emollient oil component for cosmetics and pharmaceuticals; liq.; 100% conc.

Luxelen® D. [Presperse] Anatase titanium dioxide; CAS 13463-67-7; EINECS 236-675-5; inorganic SPF for personal care and sun care prods.; JSCI/JCID approved.

Luxelen® SS. [Presperse] Titanium dioxide (77-87%), silica

(13-23%); CAS 13463-67-7, 7631-86-9; makeup ingred. providing blend of transparency, gloss with coverage power, uv absorp., good skin adherence, spreadability; JSCI/JCID approved; wh. free-flowing cryst. powd.; particle size 5-10 μ; pH 5.0-7.5.

Luxelen® SS-020. [Presperse] Titanium dioxide (75-87%), silica (11-23%), methicone (2%); makeup ingred. providing transparency, gloss, coverage power, uv absorp., good skin adherence, spreadability; JSCI/JCID approved; wh. free-flowing cryst. powd.; particle size 5-10 μ.

Lysidone®. [UCIB; Barnet Prods.] Lysine PCA; CAS 30657-38-6; moisturizer, cellular regenerative agent, antioxidant and free radical scavenger for cosmetic/pharmaceuticals, facial skin care (day and night creams, anti-age serum), body skin care (body milk, sun creams, after-sun milks); stable in aq. and hydroalcoholic phases; yel. liq., odorless; sol. in water; pract. insol. in ethanol, ether, chloroform; m.w. 275.3; sp.gr. 1.10-1.14; visc. 16-20 cps; pH 6.5-8.0; usage level: 1-5%; toxicology: LD50 (oral, rat) > 2000 mg/kg; nonirritating to skin, very sl. irritating to eyes; 40% aq. sol'n.

Lysmeral®. [BASF AG] 2-Methyl-3-(4-t-butylphenyl) propanol; fragrance (floral, powdery, fresh, lily-of-the-valley-like).

Lytron 284. [Morton Int'l.] DEA-styrene/acrylates/divinylbenzene copolymer, ammonium nonoxynol-4 sulfate; opacifier for cosmetics, shampoos, aq. ammonia, dishwash liqs., lt. duty and industrial detergents; emulsion; misc. with water; sp.gr. 1.032; dens. 8.6 lb/gal; pH 9.5; 40% solids.

Lytron 288. [Morton Int'l.] DEA-styrene/acrylates/divinylbenzene copolymer, ammonium nonoxynol-4 sulfate, diethanolamine; opacifier for cosmetics, shampoos, aq. ammonia, dishwash liqs., lt. duty and industrial detergents; emulsion; misc. with water; sp.gr. 1.032; dens. 8.6 lb/gal; pH 9.6; 40% solids.

Lytron 295. [Morton Int'l.] Sodium styrene/acrylates/divinylbenzene copolymer, ammonium nonoxynol-4 sulfate; opacifier for cosmetics, shampoos, aq. ammonia, dishwash liqs., lt. duty and industrial detergents; emulsion; misc. with water; sp.gr. 1.032; dens. 8.6 lg/bal; pH 10.0; 40% solids.

Lytron 300. [Morton Int'l.] Sodium styrene/acrylate/PEG-10 dimaleate copolymer, ammonium nonoxynol-4 sulfate; opacifier for cosmetics, shampoos, aq. ammonia, dishwash liqs., lt. duty and industrial detergents; emulsion; misc. with water; sp.gr. 1.059; dens. 8.82 lb/gal; pH 7.3; 40% solids.

Lytron 305. [Morton Int'l.] Sodium styrene/PEG-10 maleate/nonoxynol-10 maleate/acrylate copolymer, ammonium nonoxynol-4 sulfate; opacifier for cosmetics, shampoos, aq. ammonia, dishwash liqs., lt. duty and industrial detergents; emulsion; misc. with water; sp.gr. 1.024; dens. 8.53 lb/gal; pH 6.8; 40% solids.

Lytron 308. [Morton Int'l.] Styrene/acrylamide copolymer, ammonium nonoxynol-4 sulfate; opacifier for cosmetics, shampoos, aq. ammonia, dishwash liqs., lt. duty and industrial detergents; emulsion; misc. with water; sp.gr. 1.026; dens. 8.55 lb/gal; pH 8.0; 40% solids.

Lytron 614 Latex. [Morton Int'l.] Modified PS latex; CAS 9003-53-6; anionic; opacifier for liq. detergents, personal care prods.; wh. low-visc. liq.; sp.gr. 1.032; dens. 8.60 lb/gal; visc. 100 cps max.; pH 5.5 ± 0.3; 40% act.

Lytron 621. [Morton Int'l.] Styrene/acrylates copolymer, sodium lauryl sulfate, and octoxynol-9; opacifier for cosmetics, shampoos, aq. ammonia, dishwash liqs., lt. duty and industrial detergents; emulsion; misc. with water; sp.gr. 1.032; dens. 8.6 lb/gal; pH 5.5; 40% solids.

M

M-102. [U.S. Cosmetics] Mica; CAS 12001-26-2; cosmetic raw material; avg. particle size 1-20 μ.

M-302. [U.S. Cosmetics] Mica; CAS 12001-26-2; cosmetic raw material; avg. particle size 1-20 μ.

Macadamia Nut Oil. [Int'l. Flora Tech.] Refined macadamia nut oil; lipid for cosmetics; lt. yel. clear oil, trace odor, sl. nutty flavor; sp.gr. 0.913; acid no. 0.1; iodine no. 74; sapon. no. 192; ref. index 1.4604 (40 C).

Mackadet™ 40K. [McIntyre] Potassium coconate; CAS 61789-30-8; EINECS 263-049-9; anionic; liq. hand soap; liq.; pH 9.0; 38% conc.

Mackadet™ BBC. [McIntyre] Blend; very mild childrens bubble bath conc.; liq.; pH 6.5; 35% conc.

Mackadet™ BGC. [McIntyre] Blend; bath gel conc.; flowable gel; pH 6.5; 57% conc.

Mackadet™ BSC. [McIntyre] Blend; very mild baby shampoo conc.; liq.; pH 7.0; 45% conc.

Mackadet™ CA. [McIntyre] Blend; high foaming shampoo conc. providing high visc. at low conc.; liq.; pH 7.0; 42% conc.

Mackadet™ CBC. [McIntyre] Blend; conditioner conc. for visc. cream consistency; flakes; pH 4.0; 100% conc.

Mackadet™ INC. [McIntyre] Blend; leave-on conditioner conc.; liq.; pH 4.5; 16.5% conc.

Mackadet™ LCB. [McIntyre] Blend; liq. conditioner conc. that can be cold-blended; liq.; pH 3.0; 30% conc.

Mackadet™ SBC-8. [McIntyre] Blend; surfactant for multi-purpose shampoo, hand soap, bubble bath conc.; liq.; pH 6.5; 46% conc.

Mackadet™ WGS. [McIntyre] Mixed wheat germ oil, coconut oil soap; surfactant for "animal-free" shampoo or skin cleanser; liq.; pH 9.0; 40% conc.

Mackadet™ WHC. [McIntyre] Blend; waterless hand cleaner conc.; liq.; pH 8.0; 100% conc.

Mackalene™ 116. [McIntyre] Cocamidopropyl dimethyl-amine lactate; CAS 68425-42-3; cationic; softener and hair conditioner for cream rinses; liq.; pH 5.0; 25% conc.

Mackalene™ 117. [McIntyre] Cocamidopropyl dimethyl-amine propionate; CAS 68425-43-4; cationic; conditioner for skin and hair care prods.; liq.; pH 6.5; 40% conc.

Mackalene™ 216. [McIntyre] Ricinoleamidopropyl dimethyl-amine lactate; CAS 977012-91-1; cationic; conditioner for skin and hair care prods.; liq.; pH 6.0; 95% conc.

Mackalene™ 316. [McIntyre] Stearamidopropyl dimethyl-amine lactate; CAS 55819-53-9; EINECS 259-837-7; cationic; conditioner for skin and hair care prods.; liq.; pH 4.5; 25% conc.

Mackalene™ 326. [McIntyre] Stearamidopropyl morpholine lactate; CAS 55852-14-7; EINECS 259-860-2; cationic; conditioner for skin and hair care prods.; nonirritating; recommended for applics. requiring extra mildness, e.g., baby shampoos and leave-on conditioners; liq.; pH 4.5; toxicology: mild to eyes; 25% conc.

Mackalene™ 416. [McIntyre] Isostearamidopropyl dimethyl-amine lactate; CAS 55852-15-8; cationic; conditioner for skin and hair care prods.; liq.; pH 6.0; 25% conc.

Mackalene™ 426. [McIntyre] Isostearamidopropyl morpholine lactate; cationic; conditioner for skin and hair care prods.; nonirritating; recommended for applics. requiring extra mildness, e.g., baby shampoos and leave-on conditioners; readily biodeg.; liq.; pH 4.0; toxicology: mild to eyes; 25% conc.

Mackalene™ 616. [McIntyre] Behenamidopropyl dimethyl-amine lactate; cationic; conditioner for skin and hair care prods.; liq.; pH 4.5; 25% conc.

Mackalene™ 716. [McIntyre] Wheat germamidopropyl di-methylamine lactate; CAS 124046-40-8; cationic; condi-tioner for skin and hair care prods.; paste; pH 6.0; 95% conc.

Mackam™ 1C. [McIntyre] Sodium cocoamphoacetate; am-photeric; surfactant for high alkaline cleansers, sham-poos, baby shampoos; liq.; pH 11; 45% conc.

Mackam™ 1CY. [McIntyre] Sodium caproamphoacetate; personal care surfactant.

Mackam™ 1L. [McIntyre] Sodium lauramphoacetate; am-photeric; surfactant for nonirritant shampoos, cleaners; liq.; pH 10.0; 38% conc.

Mackam™ 1L-30. [McIntyre] Sodium lauroamphoacetate; amphoteric; surfactant for high alkaline cleansers, sham-poos, baby shampoos; liq.; 36% conc.

Mackam™ 1W. [McIntyre] Sodium wheat germam-phoacetate.

Mackam™ 2C. [McIntyre] Disodium cocoamphodiacetate; CAS 68650-39-5; EINECS 272-043-5; amphoteric; sur-factant for baby shampoo, high alkaline cleaners; liq.; pH 8.5; 50% conc.

Mackam™ 2CA. [McIntyre] Disodium cocoamphodiacetate, sodium lauryl sulfate.; cosmetic surfactant.

Mackam™ 2CAS. [McIntyre] Disodium cocoamphodiac-etate, sodium laureth sulfate, sodium lauryl sulfate.; cos-metic surfactant.

Mackam™ 2CSF. [McIntyre] Disodium cocoamphodipropio-nate; amphoteric; salt-free surfactant for shampoos, cleaners, dishwash formulations; emulsifier for aerosol and emulsion systems; liq.; pH 10.0; 39% conc.

Mackam™ 2CSF-70. [McIntyre] Disodium cocoamphodipro-pionate and propylene glycol; amphoteric; mild surfactant for cosmetic and industrial use; liq.; pH 6.0; 70% conc.

Mackam™ 2CT. [McIntyre] Disodium cocoamphodiacetate, sodium trideceth sulfate, and hexylene glycol; ampho-teric; nonirritating shampoo; liq.; pH 6.5; 50% conc.

Mackam™ 2CY. [McIntyre] Disodium capryloamphodiace-tate; CAS 7702-01-4; EINECS 231-721-0; amphoteric; low-foaming alkaline cleaner; liq.; pH 11; 50% conc.

Mackam™ 2CYSF. [McIntyre] Disodium capryloamphodi-propionate; amphoteric; surfactant for cosmetics, heavy duty, all-purpose and metal cleaners; emulsifier for aero-sol and emulsion systems; liq.; pH 10.0; 50% conc.

Mackam™ 2L. [McIntyre] Disodium lauroamphodiacetate; CAS 14350-97-1; EINECS 238-306-3; amphoteric; surfactant for nonirritating shampoos, cleaners; liq.; pH 9.0; 38% conc.

Mackam™ 2LES. [McIntyre] Disodium lauroamphodiacetate, sodium trideceth sulfate, hexylene glycol.

Mackam™ 2LSF. [McIntyre] Disodium lauroamphodipropionate; amphoteric; surfactant for heavy duty cleaners, metal and all-purpose cleaners, nonirritating shampoos; emulsifier for aerosol and emulsion systems; liq.; pH 10.0; 39% conc.

Mackam™ 2MCA. [McIntyre] Disodium cocoamphodiacetate, sodium lauryl sulfate, hexylene glycol; amphoteric; mild surfactant for cosmetic and industrial use; liq.; pH 8.0; 47% conc.

Mackam™ 2MCAS. [McIntyre] Disodium cocoamphodiacetate, sodium lauryl sulfate, sodium laureth sulfate, and propylene glycol; amphoteric; mild surfactant for cosmetic and industrial use; liq.; pH 7.5; 47% conc.

Mackam™ 2MHT. [McIntyre] Disodium lauroamphodiacetate, sodium trideceth sulfate, and hexylene glycol; amphoteric; mild surfactant for cosmetic and industrial use; liq.; pH 8.0; 50% conc.

Mackam™ 2W. [McIntyre] Disodium wheat germamphodiacetate; amphoteric; mild surfactant for baby shampoos; wetting agent in caustic cleaners; liq.; pH 9.5; 35% conc.

Mackam™ 35. [McIntyre] Cocamidopropyl betaine; amphoteric; foamer for shampoos, bubble baths, dishwash; liq.; pH 6.0; 35% conc.

Mackam™ 35 HP. [McIntyre] Cocamidopropyl betaine; amphoteric; foamer, visc. builder for shampoos, bubble baths, dishwash; liq.; pH 6.0; 35% conc.

Mackam™ 151C. [McIntyre] Cocaminopropionic acid; CAS 84812-94-2; EINECS 284-219-9; amphoteric; mild surfactant, conditioner for shampoos; liq.; pH 5.0; 40% conc.

Mackam™ 151L. [McIntyre] Lauraminopropionic acid; CAS 1462-54-0; EINECS 215-968-1; amphoteric; mild surfactant, conditioner for shampoos; liq.; pH 5.0; 40% conc.

Mackam™ 160C-30. [McIntyre] Sodium lauriminodipropionate; CAS 14960-06-6; EINECS 239-032-7; amphoteric; surfactants for personal care and industrial applics.; liq.; pH 7.0; 30% conc.

Mackam™ BA. [McIntyre] Behenamidopropyl betaine; amphoteric; conditioner, visc. builder; liq.; 25% act.

Mackam™ CAP. [McIntyre] Cocamidopropyl dimethylamine propionate; CAS 68425-43-4; anionic; surfactant for industrial cleaners and personal care prods.; liq.; 30% conc.

Mackam™ CB-35. [McIntyre] Coco-betaine; CAS 68424-94-2; EINECS 270-329-4; amphoteric; surfactant, conditioner, visc. builder, foam booster for shampoos, skin cleansers, bath prods., heavy duty cleaners; liq.; pH 8.0; 35% conc.

Mackam™ CBS-50. [McIntyre] Cocamidopropyl hydroxysultaine; CAS 68139-30-0; EINECS 268-761-3; thickener and foam booster for cosmetic and industrial applics.; liq.; pH 8.0; 50% conc.

Mackam™ CBS-50G. [McIntyre] Cocamidopropyl hydroxysultaine; CAS 68139-30-0; EINECS 268-761-3; thickener and foam booster for cosmetic and industrial applics.; liq.; pH 8.0; 50% conc.

Mackam™ CET. [McIntyre] Cetyl betaine; CAS 693-33-4; EINECS 211-748-4; surfactant, conditioner, visc. builder, foam booster for shampoos, skin cleansers, bath prods., heavy duty cleaners; gel; pH 7.0; 33% conc.

Mackam™ CM-100. [McIntyre] Disodium cocamido MEA-sulfosuccinate; cosmetic surfactant.

Mackam™ CS. [McIntyre] Sodium cocoamphohydroxypropylsulfonate; CAS 68604-73-9; EINECS 271-705-0; amphoteric; mild surfactant for cosmetic and industrial use;

liq.; pH 8.0; 45% conc.

Mackam™ CSF. [McIntyre] Sodium cocoamphopropionate; CAS 68919-41-5; amphoteric; surfactant for heavy duty cleanser, metal and all-purpose cleaner, nonirritating shampoos; liq.; pH 10.0; 39% conc.

Mackam™ HV. [McIntyre] Oleamidopropyl betaine; CAS 25054-76-6; EINECS 246-584-2; amphoteric; hair conditioner, foamer, emollient, visc. builder; liq.; pH 6.5; 35% conc.

Mackam™ ISA. [McIntyre] Isostearamidopropyl betaine; amphoteric; surfactant, conditioner, visc. builder, foam booster for shampoos, skin cleansers, bath prods., heavy duty cleaners; liq.; water-sol.; pH 7.5; 33% conc.

Mackam™ J. [McIntyre] Cocamidopropyl betaine; surfactant, conditioner, visc. builder, foam booster for shampoos, skin cleansers, bath prods., heavy duty cleaners; liq.; pH 6.0; 35% conc.

Mackam™ JS. [McIntyre] Sodium capryloamphohydroxypropylsulfonate; CAS 68610-39-9; amphoteric; mild surfactant for cosmetic and industrial use; liq.; pH 8.0; 49% conc.

Mackam™ L. [McIntyre] Cocamidopropyl betaine; thickener and foam booster for cosmetic and industrial applics.; liq.; pH 5.0; 35% conc.

Mackam™ LA. [McIntyre] Lauramidopropyl betaine.; EINECS 224-292-6; cosmetic surfactant.

Mackam™ LAP. [McIntyre] Lauramidopropyl dimethylamine propionate; anionic; surfactant for industrial cleaners and personal care prods.; liq.; 30% conc.

Mackam™ LMB. [McIntyre] Lauramidopropyl betaine; EINECS 224-292-6; amphoteric; surfactant for shampoos, bubble baths, dishwash formulations; liq.; pH 6.0; 35% conc.

Mackam™ LMB-LS. [McIntyre] Lauramidopropyl betaine; EINECS 224-292-6; amphoteric; visc. builder and foam booster; amber liq.; 35% conc.

Mackam™ LOS. [McIntyre] Disodium lauroamphodiacetate, sodium C14–16 olefin sulfonate.

Mackam™ LT. [McIntyre] Disodium lauroamphodiacetate and sodium trideceth sulfate; amphoteric; shampoos, cleaners, detergents; liq.; 38 and 35% conc. resp.

Mackam™ MEJ. [McIntyre] Mixed alkylamphocarboxylate; amphoteric; surfactants for personal care and industrial applics.; liq.; pH 10.0; 34% conc.

Mackam™ MLT. [McIntyre] Sodium lauroamphoacetate and sodium trideceth sulfate; amphoteric; surfactant for shampoos, cleaners, detergents; liq.; pH 10.0; 35% conc.

Mackam™ NLB. [McIntyre] Oleamidopropyl dimethylamine propionate, palmitamidopropyl dimethylamine propionate, palmitoleamidopropyl dimethylamine propionate; liq.; pH 7.0; 30% conc.

Mackam™ OB-30. [McIntyre] Oleyl betaine; CAS 871-37-4; EINECS 212-806-1; amphoteric; visc. builder for alkaline cleanser; cosmetic and industrial applics.; amber liq.; pH 7.0; 30% conc.

Mackam™ OS. [McIntyre] Sodium oleamphohydroxypropylsulfonate; CAS 68610-38-8; amphoteric; mild surfactant for cosmetic and industrial use; visc. liq.; pH 8.0; 78% conc.

Mackam™ TM. [McIntyre] Dihydroxyethyl tallow glycinate; amphoteric; surfactant, conditioner for shampoos; thickener for alkaline oven cleaners, acid bowl cleaners; liq.; water-sol.; pH 5.0; 40% conc.

Mackam™ WGB. [McIntyre] Wheat germamidopropyl betaine; CAS 133934-09-5; surfactant, conditioner, visc. builder, foam booster for shampoos, skin cleansers, bath prods., heavy duty cleaners; liq.; pH 6.5; 34% conc.

Mackamide™ AME-75, AME-100. [McIntyre] Acetamide MEA; CAS 142-26-7; EINECS 205-530-8; nonionic; humectant; surfactant, thickener, foam booster/stabilizer for personal care and industrial applics.; liq.; pH 7.0; 75 and

100% conc.

Mackamide™ C. [McIntyre] Cocamide DEA (1:1); CAS 61791-31-9; EINECS 263-163-9; nonionic; foam stabilizer and thickener for shampoos, industrial applics.; liq.; pH 10.0; 100% conc.

Mackamide™ CD. [McIntyre] Cocamide DEA (2:1); CAS 61791-31-9; EINECS 263-163-9; nonionic; surfactant, thickener, foam booster/stabilizer for personal care and industrial applics.; liq.; pH 10.0; 100% conc.

Mackamide™ CD-10. [McIntyre] Capramide DEA; CAS 136-26-5; EINECS 205-234-9; nonionic; surfactant, thickener, foam booster/stabilizer for personal care and industrial applics.; liq.; pH 10.0; 100% conc.

Mackamide™ CDS-80. [McIntyre] Cocamide DEA, DEA dodecylbenzene sulfonate; nonionic; surfactant, thickener, foam booster/stabilizer for personal care and industrial applics.; liq.; pH 9.0; 80% conc.

Mackamide™ CMA. [McIntyre] Cocamide MEA; CAS 68140-00-1; EINECS 268-770-2; nonionic; surfactant, thickener, foam booster/stabilizer for personal care and industrial applics.; flake; pH 10.0; 100% conc.

Mackamide™ CS. [McIntyre] Cocamide DEA (1:1); CAS 61791-31-9; EINECS 263-163-9; nonionic; surfactant, thickener, foam booster/stabilizer for personal care and industrial applics.; liq.; pH 10.0; 100% conc.

Mackamide™ ISA. [McIntyre] Isotearamide DEA; CAS 52794-79-3; EINECS 258-193-4; nonionic; lubricant, surfactant, thickener, foam booster/stabilizer for personal care and industrial applics.; liq.; pH 10.0; 100% conc.

Mackamide™ L-10. [McIntyre] Lauramide DEA; CAS 120-40-1; EINECS 204-393-1; nonionic; surfactant, thickener, foam booster/stabilizer for personal care and industrial applics.; liq.; pH 10.0; 100% conc.

Mackamide™ L95. [McIntyre] Lauramide DEA (95% lauric); CAS 120-40-1; EINECS 204-393-1; nonionic; surfactant, thickener, foam booster/stabilizer for personal care and industrial applics.; solid; pH 10.0; 100% conc.

Mackamide™ LLM. [McIntyre] Lauramide DEA; CAS 120-40-1; EINECS 204-393-1; nonionic; surfactant, thickener, foam booster/stabilizer for personal care and industrial applics.; liq.; pH 10.0; 100% conc.

Mackamide™ LMD. [McIntyre] Lauramide DEA (70% lauric); CAS 120-40-1; EINECS 204-393-1; nonionic; surfactant, thickener, foam booster/stabilizer for personal care and industrial applics.; solid; pH 10.0; 100% conc.

Mackamide™ LME. [McIntyre] Lactamide MEA; CAS 5422-34-4; EINECS 226-546-1; nonionic; conditioner for shampoos; surfactant, thickener, foam booster/stabilizer for personal care and industrial applics.; liq.; water-sol.; pH 5.0; 100% conc.

Mackamide™ LM-Flake. [McIntyre] Cocamide MEA.; CAS 68140-00-1; EINECS 268-770-2; nonionic; cosmetic surfactant.

Mackamide™ LMM. [McIntyre] Lauramide MEA; CAS 142-78-9; EINECS 205-560-1; nonionic; surfactant, thickener, foam booster/stabilizer for personal care and industrial applics.; flake; pH 10.0; 100% conc.

Mackamide™ LOL. [McIntyre] Linoleamide DEA; CAS 56863-02-6; EINECS 260-410-2; nonionic; surfactant, thickener, foam booster/stabilizer for personal care and industrial applics.; liq.; pH 10.0; 100% conc.

Mackamide™ MC. [McIntyre] Cocamide DEA (1:1); CAS 61791-31-9; EINECS 263-163-9; nonionic; surfactant, thickener, foam booster/stabilizer for personal care and industrial applics.; liq.; pH 10.0; 100% conc.

Mackamide™ MO. [McIntyre] Oleamide DEA (1:1); CAS 93-83-4; EINECS 202-281-7; nonionic; surfactant, thickener, foam booster/stabilizer for personal care and industrial applics.; liq.; pH 10.0; 100% conc.

Mackamide™ NOA. [McIntyre] Oleamide DEA (1:1); CAS 93-83-4; EINECS 202-281-7; nonionic; surfactant, thickener, foam booster/stabilizer for personal care and industrial applics.; liq.; pH 10.0; 100% conc.

Mackamide™ O. [McIntyre] Oleamide DEA (2:1); CAS 93-83-4; EINECS 202-281-7; nonionic; surfactant, thickener, foam booster/stabilizer for personal care and industrial applics.; solv. degreaser; liq.; pH 10.0; 100% conc.

Mackamide™ ODM. [McIntyre] Oleamide DEA, DEA oleate; nonionic; surfactant, thickener, foam booster/stabilizer for personal care and industrial applics.; gel; pH 9.0; 100% conc.

Mackamide™ PK. [McIntyre] Palm kernelamide DEA; CAS 73807-15-5; nonionic; surfactant, thickener, foam booster/stabilizer for personal care and industrial applics.; liq.; pH 10.0; 100% conc.

Mackamide™ PKM. [McIntyre] Palm kernelamide MEA; nonionic; surfactant, thickener, foam booster/stabilizer for personal care and industrial applics.; flake; pH 10.0; 100% conc.

Mackamide™ R. [McIntyre] Ricinoleamide DEA; CAS 40716-42-5; EINECS 255-051-3; nonionic; emulsifier; softener; surfactant, thickener, foam booster/stabilizer for personal care and industrial applics.; liq.; pH 10.0; 100% conc.

Mackamide™ S. [McIntyre] Soyamide DEA (1:1); CAS 68425-47-8; EINECS 270-355-6; nonionic; surfactant, thickener, foam booster/stabilizer for personal care and industrial applics.; hair conditioner; liq.; pH 10.0; 100% conc.

Mackamide™ SD. [McIntyre] Soyamide DEA (2:1); CAS 68425-47-8; EINECS 270-355-6; nonionic; surfactant, thickener, foam booster/stabilizer for personal care and industrial applics.; liq.; pH 10.0; 100% conc.

Mackamide™ SMA. [McIntyre] Stearamide MEA; CAS 111-57-9; EINECS 203-883-2; nonionic; surfactant, thickener, foam booster/stabilizer for personal care and industrial applics.; flake; pH 10.0; 100% conc.

Mackamine™ CAO. [McIntyre] Cocamidopropylamine oxide; CAS 68155-09-9; EINECS 268-938-5; cationic; detergent, wetting agent for heavy-duty cleaners; hair conditioner, visc. builder, foam booster for personal care prods.; liq.; pH 7.0; 30% conc.

Mackamine™ CO. [McIntyre] Cocamine oxide; CAS 61788-90-7; EINECS 263-016-9; amphoteric; detergent, wetting agent for heavy-duty cleaners; hair conditioner, visc. builder, foam booster/stabilizer for personal care prods.; liq.; pH 7.0; 30% conc.

Mackamine™ LAO. [McIntyre] Lauramidopropylamine oxide; CAS 61792-31-2; EINECS 263-218-7; nonionic; detergent, wetting agent for heavy-duty cleaners; hair conditioner, visc. builder, foam booster for personal care prods.; water-wh. liq.; pH 7.0; 30% conc.

Mackamine™ LO. [McIntyre] Lauramine oxide; CAS 1643-20-5; EINECS 216-700-6; nonionic; detergent, wetting agent for heavy-duty cleaners; hair conditioner, visc. builder, foam booster for personal care prods.; water-wh. liq.; pH 7.0; 30% conc.

Mackamine™ O2. [McIntyre] Oleamine oxide; CAS 14351-50-9; EINECS 238-311-0; nonionic; detergent, wetting agent for heavy-duty cleaners; hair conditioner, visc. builder, foam booster for personal care prods.; amber liq.; pH 7.5; 35% conc.

Mackamine™ OAO. [McIntyre] Oleamidopropylamine oxide; CAS 25159-40-4; EINECS 246-684-6; nonionic; detergent, wetting agent for heavy-duty cleaners; hair conditioner, visc. builder, foam booster for personal care prods.; amber gel; pH 7.0; 50% conc.

Mackamine™ SO. [McIntyre] Stearamine oxide; CAS 2571-88-2; EINECS 219-919-5; detergent, wetting agent for heavy-duty cleaners; hair conditioner, visc. builder, foam booster for personal care prods.; paste; pH 7.0; 25% conc.

Mackamine™ TAO. [McIntyre] Tallow amine oxide.

Mackamine™ WGO. [McIntyre] Wheat germamido-propylamine oxide; detergent, wetting agent for heavy-duty cleaners; hair conditioner, visc. builder, foam booster for personal care prods.; amber gel; pH 7.0; 30% conc.

Mackanate™ A-102. [McIntyre] Disodium deceth-6 sulfosuccinate; CAS 68311-03-5; mild surfactant, anti-irritant for personal care prods.; liq.; pH 6.0; 30% conc.

Mackanate™ A-103. [McIntyre] Disodium nonoxynol-10 sulfosuccinate; CAS 67999-57-9; mild surfactant, anti-irritant for personal care prods.; liq.; pH 6.0; 35% conc.

Mackanate™ CM. [McIntyre] Disodium cocamido MEA-sulfosuccinate; anionic; mild surfactant, anti-irritant for personal care prods.; base for rug cleaners; liq.; pH 6.0; 40% conc.

Mackanate™ CM-100. [McIntyre] Disodium cocamido MEA-sulfosuccinate; anionic; mild surfactant, anti-irritant for personal care prods.; base for rug cleaners; powd.; pH 6.0; 100% conc.

Mackanate™ CP. [McIntyre] Disodium cocamido MIPA-sulfosuccinate; CAS 68515-65-1; EINECS 271-102-2; anionic; mild surfactant, anti-irritant for personal care prods.; liq; pH 6.0; 40% conc.

Mackanate™ DC-30. [McIntyre] Disodium dimethicone copolyol sulfosuccinate; mild surfactant, anti-irritant for personal care prods.; liq.; pH 5.0; 30% conc.

Mackanate™ DC-30A. [McIntyre] Diammonium dimethicone copolyol sulfosuccinate; mild surfactant, anti-irritant for personal care prods.; liq.; pH 5.0; 30% conc.

Mackanate™ DC-50. [McIntyre] Disodium dimethicone copolyol sulfosuccinate; mild surfactant for personal care prods.; reduces irritation of anionics; for baby shampoos, facial cleansers, mild bath prods., mild liq. hand soaps, syndet bars; liq.; pH 5.0; 50% conc.

Mackanate™ EL. [McIntyre] Disodium laureth sulfosuccinate; anionic; mild surfactant, anti-irritant for personal care prods., shampoos, bubble baths; liq.; pH 6.0; 40% conc.

Mackanate™ ISP. [McIntyre] Disodium isostearamido MIPA-sulfosuccinate.

Mackanate™ LA. [McIntyre] Diammonium lauryl sulfosuccinate; anionic; mild surfactant, anti-irritant for personal care prods., hand cleaners; liq.; pH 6.0; 40% conc.

Mackanate™ LM-40. [McIntyre] Disodium lauramido MEA-sulfosuccinate; CAS 25882-44-4; EINECS 247-310-4; anionic; high foaming mild surfactant, anti-irritant for personal care prods.; lt. colored liq.; pH 6.0; 40% conc.

Mackanate™ LO. [McIntyre] Disodium lauryl sulfosuccinate; anionic; mild surfactant, anti-irritant for hand and skin cleaners, shampoos, bubble baths; paste; pH 6.0; 40% conc.

Mackanate™ LO-100. [McIntyre] Disodium lauryl sulfosuccinate; anionic; mild surfactant, anti-irritant for hand and skin cleaners, shampoos, bubble baths; powd.; pH 6.0; 100% conc.

Mackanate™ LO-Special. [McIntyre] Disodium lauryl sulfosuccinate; anionic; mild surfactant, anti-irritant for prods. with a cream consistency, e.g., hand and skin cleansers, shampoos, bubble baths; paste; pH 6.0; 40% conc.

Mackanate™ NLD. [McIntyre] Disodium oleamido PEG-2 sulfosuccinate, disodium palmitamido PEG-2 sulfosuccinate, disodium palmitoleamido PEG-2 sulfosuccinate.; cosmetic surfactant.

Mackanate NLP. [McIntyre] Oleamidopropyl dimethylamine propionate, palmitamidopropyl dimethylamine propionate, palmitoleamidopropyl dimethylamine propionate.

Mackanate™ OD-35. [McIntyre] Disodium oleamido PEG-2 sulfosuccinate; CAS 56388-43-3; EINECS 260-143-1; anionic; mild surfactant, anti-irritant for personal care

prods., mild conditioning shampoo; liq.; pH 6.0; 35% act.

Mackanate™ OM. [McIntyre] Disodium oleamido MEA-sulfosuccinate; anionic; nonirritating high foaming surfactant for shampoos; liq.; pH 6.0; 35% conc.

Mackanate™ OP. [McIntyre] Disodium oleamido MIPA-sulfosuccinate; CAS 43154-85-4; EINECS 256-120-0; anionic; mild, skin-protective surfactant for personal care prods.; liq.; pH 6.0; 38% conc.

Mackanate™ RM. [McIntyre] Disodium ricinoleamido MEA-sulfosuccinate; anionic; mild, skin-protective surfactant for personal care prods.; liq.; pH 6.0; 40% conc.

Mackanate™ TDS. [McIntyre] Disodium tridecyl sulfosuccinate; anionic; surfactant; liq.; 40% conc.

Mackanate™ UM-50. [McIntyre] Disodium undecylenamido MEA-sulfosuccinate; mild surfactant, anti-irritant for personal care prods.; liq.; pH 6.0; 50% conc.

Mackanate™ WGD. [McIntyre] Disodium wheat germamido PEG-2 sulfosuccinate; anionic; nonirritating emollient surfactant, mild conditioner for personal care prods.; liq.; pH 6.0; 35% conc.

Mackanate™ WGO. [McIntyre] Wheat germamido-propylamine oxide.

Mackernium™ 006. [McIntyre] Polyquaternium-6; CAS 26062-79-3; slip agent for liq. hand soaps, conditioner for shampoos without buildup; liq.; pH 7.0; 40% conc.

Mackernium™ 007. [McIntyre] Polyquaternium-7; CAS 26590-05-6; slip agent for liq. hand soaps; conditioner for shampoos without buildup; liq.; pH 7.0; 9% conc.

Mackernium™ CTC-30. [McIntyre] Cetrimonium chloride; CAS 112-02-7; EINECS 203-928-6; conditioner, lubricant, and antistat for personal care prods.; liq.; pH 4.0; 30% conc.

Mackernium™ KP. [McIntyre] Oleakonium chloride; CAS 37139-99-4; EINECS 253-363-4; conditioner, lubricant, antistat for personal care prods.; liq.; pH 5.0; 50% conc.

Mackernium™ NLE. [McIntyre] Quaternium-84; conditioner, lubricant, antistat for personal care prods.; liq.; pH 7.0; 100% conc.

Mackernium™ SDC-25. [McIntyre] Stearalkonium chloride; CAS 122-19-0; EINECS 204-527-9; conditioner, lubricant, antistat for personal care prods.; wh. paste; pH 4.0; 25% conc.

Mackernium™ SDC-85. [McIntyre] Stearalkonium chloride; CAS 122-19-0; EINECS 204-527-9; conditioner, lubricant, antistat for personal care prods.; wh. flake; pH 6.0; 100% conc.

Mackernium™ WLE. [McIntyre] Wheat lipid epoxide; conditioner, lubricant, and antistat for personal care prods.; liq.; pH 5.0; 100% conc.

Mackester™ EGDS. [McIntyre] Glycol distearate; CAS 627-83-8; EINECS 211-014-3; emulsifier, lubricant, antistat, defoamer for metalworking, textile lubricants, plastics, paper; emulsifier, pearlescent, emollient for cosmetics; flake; 100% conc.

Mackester™ EGMS. [McIntyre] Glycol stearate; CAS 111-60-4; EINECS 203-886-9; emulsifier, lubricant, antistat, defoamer for metalworking, textile lubricants, plastics, paper; emulsifier, pearlescent, emollient for cosmetics; flake; 100% conc.

Mackester™ IP. [McIntyre] Glycol stearate, other ingreds.; CAS 111-60-4; EINECS 203-886-9; emulsifier, lubricant, antistat, defoamer for metalworking, textile lubricants, plastics, paper; emulsifier, pearlescent, emollient for cosmetics; flake; 100% conc.

Mackester™ SP. [McIntyre] Glycol stearate and stearamide MEA; emulsifier, lubricant, antistat, defoamer for metalworking, textile lubricants, plastics, paper; emulsifier, pearlescent, emollient for cosmetics; flake; 100% conc.

Mackine™ 101. [McIntyre] Cocamidopropyl dimethylamine; CAS 68140-01-2; EINECS 268-771-8; cationic; intermediate for cationic surfactants, chemical specialties, hair conditioners, mild cleansers; corrosion inhibitor; salts as emulsifier for acid systems; liq.; 100% act.

Mackine™ 201. [McIntyre] Ricinoleamidopropyl dimethylamine; CAS 20457-75-4; EINECS 243-835-8; cationic; intermediate for cationic surfactants, chemical specialties, hair conditioners, mild cleansers; corrosion inhibitor; salts as emulsifier for acid systems; liq.; 100% act.

Mackine™ 301. [McIntyre] Stearamidopropyl dimethylamine; CAS 7651-02-7; EINECS 231-609-1; cationic; intermediate for cationic surfactants, chemical specialties, hair conditioners, mild cleansers; corrosion inhibitor; salts as emulsifier for acid systems; flake; 100% act.

Mackine™ 321. [McIntyre] Stearamidopropyl morpholine; CAS 55852-13-6; cationic; intermediate for cationic surfactants, chemical specialties, hair conditioners, mild cleansers; corrosion inhibitor; salts as emulsifier for acid systems; flake; 100% act.

Mackine™ 401. [McIntyre] Isostearamidopropyl dimethylamine; CAS 67799-04-6; EINECS 267-101-1; cationic; intermediate for cationic surfactants, chemical specialties, hair conditioners, mild cleansers; corrosion inhibitor; salts as emulsifier for acid systems; liq.; 100% act.

Mackine™ 421. [McIntyre] Isostearamidopropyl morpholine; cationic; intermediate for cationic surfactants, chemical specialties, hair conditioners, mild cleansers; corrosion inhibitor; salts as emulsifier for acid systems; liq.; 100% act.

Mackine™ 501. [McIntyre] Oleamidopropyl dimethylamine; CAS 109-28-4; EINECS 203-661-5; cationic; intermediate for cationic surfactants, chemical specialties, hair conditioners, mild cleansers; corrosion inhibitor; salts as emulsifier for acid systems; amber liq.; 100% conc.

Mackine™ 601. [McIntyre] Behenamidopropyl dimethylamine; CAS 60270-33-9; EINECS 262-134-8; nonionic; intermediate for cationic surfactants, chemical specialties, hair conditioners, mild cleansers; corrosion inhibitor; salts as emulsifier for acid systems; flake; 100% act.

Mackine™ 701. [McIntyre] Wheat germamidopropyl dimethylamine; intermediate for cationic surfactants, chemical specialties, hair conditioners, mild cleansers; corrosion inhibitor; salts as emulsifier for acid systems; amber paste; 100% conc.

Mackine™ 801. [McIntyre] Lauramidopropyl dimethylamine; CAS 3179-80-4; EINECS 221-661-3; intermediate for cationic surfactants, chemical specialties, hair conditioners, mild cleansers; corrosion inhibitor; salts as emulsifier for acid systems; amber solid; 100% conc.

Mackine™ 901. [McIntyre] Soyamidopropyl dimethylamine; CAS 68188-30-7; intermediate for cationic surfactants, chemical specialties, hair conditioners, mild cleansers; corrosion inhibitor; salts as emulsifier for acid systems; amber paste; 100% conc.

Mackol 16. [McIntyre] Cetyl alcohol.; CAS 36653-82-4; EINECS 253-149-0; cosmetic ingred.

Mackol 18. [McIntyre] Stearyl alcohol.; CAS 112-92-5; EINECS 204-017-6; emollient, cosmetic/pharmaceutical raw material.

Mackol 1618. [McIntyre] Cetearyl alcohol.

Mackpro™ CHP. [McIntyre] Cocamidopropyl dimethylamine hydrolyzed animal protein.

Mackpro™ FC. [McIntyre] Cocamidopropyl dimethylamine hydrolyzed animal protein.

Mackpro™ FP. [McIntyre] Cocamidopropyl dimethylamine hydrolyzed animal protein, wheatgermamidopropyl dimethylamine hydrolyzed animal protein.

Mackpro™ KLP. [McIntyre] Quaternium-79 hydrolyzed keratin; protective conditioner for hair and skin care prods.; liq.; pH 5.0; 35% conc.

Mackpro™ MLP. [McIntyre] Quaternium-79 hydrolyzed milk

protein; protective conditioner for hair and skin care prods.; liq.; pH 5.0; 35% conc.

Mackpro™ NLP. [McIntyre] Quaternium-79 hydrolyzed collagen; protective conditioner for hair and skin care prods.; liq.; pH 5.0; 40% conc.

Mackpro™ NLW. [McIntyre] Quaternium-79 hydrolyzed wheat protein; protective conditioner for hair and skin care prods.; liq.; pH 5.0; 35% conc.

Mackpro™ NSP. [McIntyre] Quaternium-79 hydrolyzed silk; protective conditioner for hair and skin care prods.; liq.; pH 5.0; 33% conc.

Mackpro™ OLP. [McIntyre] Oleamidopropyldimonium hydroxypropyl hydrolyzed collagen.

Mackpro™ SLP. [McIntyre] Quaternium-79 hydrolyzed soy protein; protective conditioner for hair and skin care prods.; liq.; pH 5.0; 35% conc.

Mackpro™ WLW. [McIntyre] Wheatgermamidopropyldimonium hydroxypropyl hydrolyzed wheat protein; protective conditioner for hair and skin care prods.; liq.; pH 5.0; 37% conc.

Mackpro™ WWP. [McIntyre] Wheatgermamidopropyl dimethylamine hydrolyzed wheat protein; conditioner for hair and skin care prods.; liq.; pH 5.0; 35% conc.

Mackstat® DM. [McIntyre] DMDM hydantoin; CAS 6440-58-0; EINECS 229-222-8; broad spectrum cosmetic preservative effective against gram negative and positive bacteria, yeast, mold, and fungi; for shampoos, skin cleansers, bath prods., lotions and creams; colorless clear liq., mild odor; sol. in water; pH 7.0; usage level: 0.05-0.5%; 55% conc.

Mackstat® DM-PG. [McIntyre] DMDM hydantoin, propylene glycol; broad spectrum cosmetic preservative for shampoos, skin cleansers, bath prods., lotions and creams; the propylene glycol acts as an antifreeze to prevent crystallization at low temp. storage; pale to lt. yel. clear liq., mild odor; pH 7.0; 55% act.

Macol® 1. [PPG/Specialty Chem.] Poloxamer 181; CAS 9003-11-6; nonionic; defoamer, deduster, emulsifier, detergent, dispersant, dye leveler, gellant, antistat, solubilizer, dispersant, wetting agent, lubricant base for metalworking and textile lubricants, cosmetics, medical, paper, pharmaceutical, chemical intermediates; APHA < 100 liq.; water-sol.; m.w. 2000; sp.gr. 1.015; dens. 8.5 lb/gal; visc. 285 cps; HLB 3.0; pour pt. –29 C; flash pt. (PMCC) 455 F; cloud pt. 24 C (1% aq.); ref. index 1.4520; Ross-Miles foam 10 mm (0.1%); 100% conc.

Macol® 2. [PPG/Specialty Chem.] Poloxamer 182; CAS 9003-11-6; nonionic; detergent, emulsifier, wetting agent, dispersant, antistat, defoamer, gellant, solubilizer, lubricant base for cosmetic, medical, paper, metalworking, pharmaceutical and textile industries; liq.; sol. in aromatic solvs.; m.w. 2500; sp.gr. 1.03; visc. 415 cps; HLB 7.0; pour pt. -4 C; cloud pt. 32 C (1% aq.); surf. tens. 42.8 dynes/cm (0.1%); Ross-Miles foam 35 mm (0.1%); 100% conc.

Macol® 2D. [PPG/Specialty Chem.] EO/PO block copolymer; nonionic; wetting agent, dispersant, antistat, defoamer, gellant, solubilizer, lubricant base for cosmetic, medical, paper, metalworking, pharmaceutical and textile industries; liq.; sol. in aromatic solvs.; m.w. 2360; sp.gr. 1.03; visc. 400 cps; HLB 7.6; pour pt. -1 C; cloud pt. 35 C (1% aq.); surf. tens. 43.0 dynes/cm (0.1%); Ross-Miles foam 15 mm (0.1%); 100% conc.

Macol® 2LF. [PPG/Specialty Chem.] Block polymer; nonionic; detergent, wetting agent, dispersant, antistat, defoamer, gellant, solubilizer, lubricant base for cosmetic, medical, paper, metalworking, pharmaceutical and textile industries; liq.; sol. in aromatic solvs.; m.w. 2300; sp.gr. 1.02; visc. 400 cps; HLB 6.6; pour pt. -7 C; cloud pt. 28 C (1% aq.); surf. tens. 41.2 dynes/cm (0.1%); Ross-Miles foam 26 mm (0.1%); 100% conc.

Macol® 4. [PPG/Specialty Chem.] Poloxamer 184; CAS 9003-11-6; nonionic; detergent, foaming agent, emulsifier, wetting agent, dispersant, antistat, defoamer, gellant, solubilizer, lubricant base for cosmetic, medical, paper, pharmaceutical and textile industries; liq.; sol. in aromatic solvs.; m.w. 2900; sp.gr. 1.05; visc. 800 cps; HLB 15.0; pour pt. 16 C; cloud pt. 60 C (1% aq.); surf. tens. 43.2 dynes/cm (0.1%); Ross-Miles foam > 600 mm (0.1%); 100% conc.

Macol® 8. [PPG/Specialty Chem.] Poloxamer 188; CAS 9003-11-6; nonionic; detergent, foaming agent, wetting agent, dispersant, antistat, gellant, solubilizer, lubricant base for cosmetic, medical, paper, pharmaceutical and textile industries; flake; sol. in aromatic solvs.; m.w. 8500; sp.gr. 1.06; visc. 1100 cps; HLB 29.0; pour pt. 52 C; cloud pt. > 100 C (1% aq.); surf. tens. 50.3 dynes/cm (0.1%); Ross-Miles foam > 600 mm (0.1%); 100% conc.

Macol® 10. [PPG/Specialty Chem.] PO-EO block copolymers; nonionic; wetting agent, dispersant, antistat, defoamer, gellant, solubilizer, lubricant base for cosmetic, medical, paper, pharmaceutical and textile industries; liq.; sol. in aromatic solvs.; m.w. 3200; sp.gr. 1.04; visc. 660 cps; HLB 4.5; pour pt. -5 C; cloud pt. 32 C (1% aq.); surf. tens. 40.6 dynes/cm (0.1%); Ross-Miles foam 90 mm (0.1%); 100% conc.

Macol® 16. [PPG/Specialty Chem.] Meroxapol 108; CAS 9003-11-6; slip agent and solubilizer for fragrances and emollients; humectant for skin care lotions; defoamer, deduster, detergent, emulsifier, dispersant, dye leveler, gellant, antistat; flake; sol. in water, aromatic solvs.; m.w. 4600; sp.gr. 1.06; visc. 400 cps; m.p. 46 C; cloud pt. 95 C (1% aq.); surf. tens. 54.1 dynes/cm (0.1%); Ross-Miles foam 120 mm (0.1%); 100% conc.

Macol® 22. [PPG/Specialty Chem.] Block polymer; nonionic; wetting agent, dispersant, antistat, defoamer, gellant, solubilizer, lubricant base for cosmetic, medical, paper, metalworking, pharmaceutical and textile industries; liq.; sol. in aromatic solvs.; m.w. 2000; sp.gr. 1.01; visc. 520 cps; pour pt. -10 C; cloud pt. 17 C (1% aq.); 100% conc.

Macol® 23. [PPG/Specialty Chem.] Poloxamer 403; CAS 9003-11-6; nonionic; foaming agent, emulsifier, wetting agent, dispersant, antistat, gellant, solubilizer, lubricant base for cosmetic, medical, paper, pharmaceutical and textile industries; paste; sol. in aromatic solvs.; m.w. 5600; sp.gr. 1.01 (60 C); visc. 350 cps (60 C); pour pt. 31 C; cloud pt. 90 C (1% aq.); surf. tens. 34.1 dynes/cm (0.1%); Ross-Miles foam 360 mm (0.1%).

Macol® 27. [PPG/Specialty Chem.] Poloxamer 407; CAS 9003-11-6; nonionic; emulsifier, wetting agent, foamer, dispersant, antistat, defoamer, gellant, solubilizer, lubricant base for cosmetic, medical, paper, pharmaceutical and textile industries, mouthwashes, mild cleansers, baby shampoos; flake; sol. in aromatic solvs.; m.w. 12,500; sp.gr. 1.05 (77 C); visc. 3100 cps (77 C); HLB 2.2; m.p. 56 C; cloud pt. > 100 C (1% aq.); surf. tens. 40.7 dynes/cm (0.1%); Ross-Miles foam > 600 mm (0.1%); 100% conc.

Macol® 31. [PPG/Specialty Chem.] EO-PO block copolymer; nonionic; wetting agent, dispersant, antistat, defoamer, gellant, solubilizer, lubricant base for cosmetic, medical, paper, pharmaceutical and textile industries; APHA < 100 liq.; sol. in water, aromatic solvs.; m.w. 3300; sp.gr. 1.05; dens. 8.5 lb/gal; visc. 950 cps; HLB 6.3; pour pt. 24 C; cloud pt. 40 C (1% aq.); flash pt. (PMCC) 439 F; ref. index 1.4515.

Macol® 32. [PPG/Specialty Chem.] Meroxapol 251; CAS 9003-11-6; nonionic; wetting agent, dispersant, antistat, defoamer, gellant, solubilizer, lubricant base for cosmetic, medical, paper, pharmaceutical and textile industries; APHA < 100 liq.; sol. in water, aromatic solvs.; m.w. 2700; sp.gr. 1.017; dens. 8.5 lb/gal; visc. 460 cps; HLB 4.0; pour pt. -27 C; cloud pt. 26 C (1% aq.); flash pt. (PMCC) < 450 F; ref. index 1.4521; surf. tens. 36.3 dynes/cm (0.1%); Ross-Miles foam < 5 mm (0.1%).

Macol® 33. [PPG/Specialty Chem.] Meroxapol 311; CAS 9003-11-6; nonionic; wetting agent, dispersant, antistat, defoamer, gellant, solubilizer, lubricant base for cosmetic, medical, paper, metalworking, pharmaceutical and textile industries; APHA < 100 liq.; sol. in water, aromatic solvs.; m.w. 3200; sp.gr. 1.018; dens. 8.5 lb/gal; visc. 578 cps; HLB 4.0; pour pt. -25 C; cloud pt. 25 C (1% aq.); flash pt. (PMCC) < 450 F; ref. index 1.4522; surf. tens. 34.1 dynes/cm (0.1%); Ross-Miles foam < 5 mm (0.1%); 100% conc.

Macol® 34. [PPG/Specialty Chem.] Meroxapol 254; CAS 9003-11-6; nonionic; wetting agent, dispersant, antistat, defoamer, gellant, solubilizer, lubricant base for cosmetic, medical, paper, pharmaceutical and textile industries; paste; sol. in aromatic solvs.; m.w. 3600; sp.gr. 1.05 (60 C); visc. 1100 cps (60 C); HLB 10.0; pour pt. 25 C; cloud pt. 40 C (1% aq.); surf. tens. 41.0 dynes/cm (0.1%); Ross-Miles foam 70 mm (0.1%); 100% conc.

Macol® 35. [PPG/Specialty Chem.] Poloxamer 105; CAS 9003-11-6; nonionic; wetting agent, dispersant, antistat, defoamer, gellant, solubilizer, lubricant base for cosmetic, medical, paper, pharmaceutical and textile industries; liq.; sol. in aromatic solvs.; m.w. 1900; sp.gr. 1.06; visc. 375 cps; HLB 8.0; pour pt. 7 C; cloud pt. 78 C (1% aq.); surf. tens. 48.8 dynes/cm (0.1%); Ross-Miles foam 145 mm (0.1%); 100% conc.

Macol® 40. [PPG/Specialty Chem.] Meroxapol 252; CAS 9003-11-6; nonionic; wetting agent, dispersant, antistat, defoamer, gellant, solubilizer, lubricant base for cosmetic, medical, paper, metalworking, pharmaceutical and textile industries; liq.; sol. in aromatic solvs.; m.w. 3100; sp.gr. 1.03; visc. 700 cps; pour pt. -5 C; cloud pt. 29 C (1% aq.); surf. tens. 37.5 dynes/cm (0.1%); Ross-Miles foam < 5 mm (0.1%); 100% conc.

Macol® 42. [PPG/Specialty Chem.] Poloxamer 122; CAS 9003-11-6; nonionic; wetting agent, dispersant, antistat, defoamer, gellant, solubilizer, lubricant base for cosmetic, medical, paper, pharmaceutical and textile industries; APHA < 100 liq.; sol. in water, aromatic solvs.; m.w. 1600; sp.gr. 1.03; dens. 8.5 lb/gal; visc. 250 cps; HLB 12.0; pour pt. -26 C; cloud pt. 37 C (1% aq.); flash pt. (PMCC) 450 F; ref. index 1.4541; surf. tens. 46.5 dynes/cm (0.1%); Ross-Miles foam 10 mm (0.1%); 100% conc.

Macol® 44. [PPG/Specialty Chem.] Poloxamer 124; CAS 9003-11-6; nonionic; wetting agent, dispersant, antistat, defoamer, gellant, solubilizer, lubricant base for cosmetic, medical, paper, pharmaceutical and textile industries; liq.; sol. in aromatic solvs.; m.w. 2200; sp.gr. 1.05; visc. 450 cps; HLB 3.0; pour pt. 15 C; cloud pt. 68 C (1% aq.); surf. tens. 45.4 dynes/cm (0.1%); Ross-Miles foam 360 mm (0.1%); 100% conc.

Macol® 46. [PPG/Specialty Chem.] Poloxamer 101; CAS 9003-11-6; nonionic; wetting agent, dispersant, antistat, defoamer, gellant, solubilizer, lubricant base for cosmetic, medical, paper, pharmaceutical and textile industries; liq.; sol. in aromatic solvs.; m.w. 1100; sp.gr. 1.02; visc. 180 cps; HLB 18.5; pour pt. -32 C; cloud pt. 36 C (1% aq.); surf. tens. 47.1 dynes/cm (0.1%); Ross-Miles foam 18 mm (0.1%); 100% conc.

Macol® 57. [PPG/Specialty Chem.] PPG-10 butanediol; nongreasy emollient and nonwhitening aid for colognes, aftershaves, skin fresheners, antiperspirants, nail enamel removers; high ref. index, good spreading props.; glossing agent for nail; good solv. for many sunscreen actives; crystal growth inhibitor; water-wh. clear liq., mild char. odor; sol. in water, SD alcohol 40B, butylene glycol, IPM, benzyl laurate, almond oil; disp. in cyclomethicone, min. and jojoba oils; insol. in glycerin; sp.gr. 1.005; visc. < 100 cps; m.p. < -25 C; b.p. > 150 C; cloud pt. 42 C; flash pt. (CC) > 95 C; ref. index 1.450; pH 6.0; toxicology: LD50 (oral) < 5 g/kg; nontoxic inhalation hazard; safe for external use.

Macol® 65. [PPG/Specialty Chem.] Functional fluid with lubricating, antiwear props. for hydraulic systems, cosmetics; chemical intermediate for prep. of resins, plasticizers, modifiers, and surfactants; in ink and dye solvs.; liq.; sol. @ 5% in alcohols, ketones, kerosene, min. oil; disp. in water; sp.gr. 0.960; visc. 12 cst (100 F); pour pt. -58 C; flash pt. (PMCC) 245 F; ref. index 1.440.

Macol® 72. [PPG/Specialty Chem.] Poloxamer 212; CAS 9003-11-6; nonionic; wetting agent, dispersant, antistat, defoamer, gellant, solubilizer, lubricant base for cosmetic, medical, paper, pharmaceutical and textile industries; liq.; sol. in aromatic solvs.; m.w. 2750; sp.gr. 1.03; visc. 500 cps; HLB 2.0; pour pt. -7 C; cloud pt. 25 C (1% aq.); surf. tens. 39 dynes/cm (0.1%); Ross-Miles foam 20 mm (0.1%); 100% conc.

Macol® 77. [PPG/Specialty Chem.] Poloxamer 217; CAS 9003-11-6; nonionic; wetting agent, dispersant, antistat, defoamer, gellant, solubilizer, lubricant base for cosmetic, medical, paper, pharmaceutical and textile industries; flake; sol. in aromatic solvs.; m.w. 6600; sp.gr. 1.04; visc. 475 cps; HLB 24.5; pour pt. 48 C; cloud pt. > 100 C (1% aq.); surf. tens. 47.0 dynes/cm (0.1%); Ross-Miles foam > 600 mm (0.1%); 100% conc.

Macol® 85. [PPG/Specialty Chem.] Poloxamer 235; CAS 9003-11-6; nonionic; wetting agent, dispersant, antistat, defoamer, gellant, solubilizer, lubricant base for cosmetic, medical, paper, pharmaceutical and textile industries; paste; sol. in aromatic solvs.; m.w. 4600; sp.gr. 1.04 (60 C); visc. 320 cps (60 C); HLB 16.0; pour pt. 29 C; cloud pt. 85 C (1% aq.); surf. tens. 42.5 dynes/cm (0.1%); Ross-Miles foam > 600 mm (0.1%); 100% conc.

Macol® 88. [PPG/Specialty Chem.] Block polymer; nonionic; wetting agent, dispersant, antistat, defoamer, gellant, solubilizer, lubricant base for cosmetic, medical, paper, pharmaceutical and textile industries; flake; sol. in aromatic solvs.; m.w. 11,500; sp.gr. 1.06 (77 C); visc. 2300 cps (77 C); pour pt. 54 C; cloud pt. > 100 C (1% aq.); surf. tens. 48.5 dynes/cm (0.1%); Ross-Miles foam > 600 mm (0.1%).

Macol® 90. [PPG/Specialty Chem.] Functional fluid with lubricating, antiwear props. for hydraulic systems, cosmetics; chemical intermediate for prep. of resins, plasticizers, modifiers, and surfactants; in ink and dye solvs.; liq.; sol. @ 5% in water, alcohols, ketones; disp. in min. oil; sp.gr. 1.097; visc. 19,500 cst (100 F); pour pt. 5 C; flash pt. (PMCC) 350 F; ref. index 1.465; 100% act.

Macol® 90(70). [PPG/Specialty Chem.] Functional fluid with lubricating, antiwear props. for hydraulic systems, cosmetics; chemical intermediate for prep. of resins, plasticizers, modifiers, and surfactants; in ink and dye solvs.; liq.; sol. @ 5% in water, alcohols, ketones; disp. in min. oil; sp.gr. 1.049; visc. 1700 cst (100 F); pour pt. 1 C; flash pt. none; ref. index 1.418; 70% act.

Macol® 101. [PPG/Specialty Chem.] Poloxamer 331; CAS 9003-11-6; nonionic; wetting agent, dispersant, antistat, defoamer, gellant, solubilizer, lubricant base for cosmetic, medical, paper, pharmaceutical and textile industries; APHA < 100 liq.; sol. in water, aromatic solvs.; sp.gr. 1.020; dens. 8.5 lb/gal; visc. 800 cps; HLB 1.0; pour pt. – 23 C; cloud pt. 15 C (1% aq.); flash pt. (PMCC) < 450 F; ref. index 1.4524; Ross-Miles foam 10 mm (0.1%); 100% conc.

Macol® 108. [PPG/Specialty Chem.] Poloxamer 338; CAS 9003-11-6; nonionic; wetting agent, dispersant, antistat, defoamer, gellant, solubilizer, lubricant base for cosmetic, medical, paper, pharmaceutical and textile industries;

flake; sol. in aromatic solvs.; m.w. 14,600; sp.gr. 1.06 (77 C); visc. 3000 cps (77 C); HLB 17.5; pour pt. 57 C; cloud pt. > 100 C (1% aq.); surf. tens. 41.2 dynes/cm (0.1%); Ross-Miles foam > 600 mm (0.1%); 100% conc.

Macol® 123. [PPG/Specialty Chem.] Ceteareth alcohol, ceteareth-20, ceteareth-10; nonionic; emulsifier for cosmetic and pharmaceutical applics.; flake; m.p. 52 C; acid no. 0.5; iodine no. 0.7; sapon. no. 2; flash pt. (PMCC) > 350 F; usage level: 6-12%.

Macol® 124. [PPG/Specialty Chem.] Cetearyl alcohol, ceteareth-20; nonionic; emulsifier for cosmetic and pharmaceutical applics.; recommended for very mild and hypo-allergenic skin care prods.; flake; m.p. 52 C; acid no. 0.5; iodine no. 0.5; sapon. no. 2; flash pt. (PMCC) > 350 F.

Macol® 125. [PPG/Specialty Chem.] Stearyl alcohol, ceteareth-20; nonionic; emulsifier for cosmetic and pharmaceutical applics.; recommended for very mild and hypo-allergenic skin care prods.; flake; m.p. 60 C; acid no. 1; iodine no. 2.0; sapon. no. 2; flash pt. (PMCC) > 350 F.

Macol® 625. [PPG/Specialty Chem.] Functional fluid with lubricating, antiwear props. for hydraulic systems, cosmetics; chemical intermediate for prep. of resins, plasticizers, modifiers, and surfactants; in ink and dye solvs.; liq.; sol. @ 5% in alcohols, ketones, kerosene, min. oil; disp. in water; sp.gr. 1.000; visc. 135 cst (100 F); pour pt. -31 C; flash pt. (PMCC) 360 F; ref. index 1.450.

Macol® 626. [PPG/Specialty Chem.] Functional fluid with lubricating, antiwear props. for hydraulic systems, cosmetics; chemical intermediate for prep. of resins, plasticizers, modifiers, and surfactants; in ink and dye solvs.; liq.; sol. @ 5% in alcohols, ketones, kerosene, min. oil; disp. in water; sp.gr. 1.002; visc. 300 cst (100 F); pour pt. -27 C; flash pt. (PMCC) 360 F; ref. index 1.451.

Macol® 627. [PPG/Specialty Chem.] Functional fluid with lubricating, antiwear props. for hydraulic systems, cosmetics; chemical intermediate for prep. of resins, plasticizers, modifiers, and surfactants; in ink and dye solvs.; liq.; sol. @ 5% in alcohols, ketones, kerosene, min. oil; disp. in water; sp.gr. 1.002; visc. 370 cst (100 F); pour pt. -23 C; flash pt. (PMCC) 360 F; ref. index 1.452.

Macol® CA-2. [PPG/Specialty Chem.] Ceteth-2; CAS 9004-95-9; nonionic; emulsifier, detergent, wetting agent, dispersant, solubilizer, coupling agent for cosmetics, textile, metalworking, household, industrial and other applics.; solid; sol. @ 5% in IPA; insol. in water; m.p. 38 C; HLB 4.9; iodine no. 0.5; hyd. no. 170; flash pt. (PMCC) > 350 F.

Macol® CA-10. [PPG/Specialty Chem.] Ceteth-10; CAS 9004-95-9; nonionic; emulsifier, detergent, wetting agent, dispersant, solubilizer, coupling agent for cosmetics, textile, metalworking, household, industrial and other applics.; solid; sol. @ 5% in IPA; disp. in water, min. spirits; m.p. 41 C; HLB 12.3; iodine no. 0.5; hyd. no. 95; flash pt. (PMCC) > 350 F.

Macol® CA 30P. [PPG/Specialty Chem.] PPG-30 cetyl ether; CAS 9035-85-2; light, easily emulsified emollient for cosmetic creams, lotions, permanent waves, skin care prods.; lt. yel. liq.; acid no. 1 max.; iodine no. 3 max.; hyd. no. 35-45; 0.5% max. water.

Macol® CPS. [PPG/Specialty Chem.] Cetearyl alcohol, polysorbate 60, PEG-150 stearate, steareth-20; nonionic; emulsifier for cosmetic and pharmaceutical applics.; recommended for very mild and hypo-allergenic skin care prods.; flake; m.p. 51 C; acid no. 1.5; iodine no. 2; sapon. no. 12; flash pt. (PMCC) > 350 F.

Macol® CSA-2. [PPG/Specialty Chem.] Ceteareth-2; CAS 68439-49-6; nonionic; detergent, wetting agent, emulsifier, dispersant, solubilizer, and coupling agent for cosmetics, textiles, metalworking lubricants, household prods., and industrial applics.; wh. solid; sol. @ 5% in IPA;

insol. in water; m.p. 39 C; HLB 5.1; iodine no. 0.5; hyd. no. 160; flash pt. (PMCC) > 350 F.

Macol® CSA-4. [PPG/Specialty Chem.] Ceteareth-4; CAS 68439-49-6; nonionic; detergent, wetting agent, emulsifier, dispersant, solubilizer, and coupling agent for cosmetics, textiles, metalworking lubricants, household prods., and industrial applics.; wh. solid; sol. @ 5% in IPA; insol. water and min. oil; m.p. 38 C; HLB 7.9; iodine no. 0.5; hyd. no. 128; flash pt. (PMCC) > 350 F.

Macol® CSA-10. [PPG/Specialty Chem.] Ceteareth-10; CAS 68439-49-6; nonionic; detergent, wetting agent, emulsifier, dispersant, solubilizer, and coupling agent for cosmetics, textiles, metalworking lubricants, household prods., and industrial applics.; wh. solid; sol. @ 5% in IPA; disp. in water, min. spirits; m.p. 38 C; HLB 12.3; iodine no. 0.5; hyd. no. 80; flash pt. (PMCC) > 350 F.

Macol® CSA-15. [PPG/Specialty Chem.] Ceteareth-15; CAS 68439-49-6; nonionic; detergent, wetting agent, emulsifier, dispersant, solubilizer, and coupling agent for cosmetics, textiles, metalworking lubricants, household prods., and industrial applics.; wh. solid; sol. @ 5% in water, IPA; disp. in min. spirits; insol. min. oil; m.p. 38 C; HLB 14.2; iodine no. 0.5; hyd. no. 65; flash pt. (PMCC) > 350 F.

Macol® CSA-20. [PPG/Specialty Chem.] Ceteareth-20; CAS 68439-49-6; nonionic; detergent, wetting agent, emulsifier, dispersant, solubilizer, and coupling agent for cosmetics, mascara, hair rinses, hand/body lotions, foundations, textiles, metalworking lubricants, household prods., and industrial applics.; wh. solid; sol. @ 5% in water, IPA; insol. min. oil; m.p. 40 C; HLB 15.2; iodine no. 0.5; hyd. no. 52; flash pt. (PMCC) > 350 F; 100% conc.

Macol® CSA-40. [PPG/Specialty Chem.] Ceteareth-40; CAS 68439-49-6; nonionic; detergent, wetting agent, emulsifier, dispersant, solubilizer, and coupling agent for cosmetics, textiles, metalworking lubricants, household prods., and industrial applics.; solid; sol. @ 5% in water, IPA; m.p. 40 C; HLB 16.8; iodine no. 0.5; hyd. no. 30; flash pt. (PMCC) > 350 F.

Macol® DNP-5. [PPG/Specialty Chem.] Nonyl nonoxynol-5; CAS 9014-93-1; nonionic; emulsifier, detergent, wetting agent, dispersant, solubilizer, coupling agent for cosmetics, textile, metalworking, household, industrial and other applics.; liq.; sol. @ 5% in toluene, perchloroethylene; disp. in water, min. oil, min. spirits; sp.gr. 0.97; visc. 385 cps; HLB 8.2; pour pt. -10 C; flash pt. (PMCC) > 350 F.

Macol® DNP-10. [PPG/Specialty Chem.] Nonyl nonoxynol-10; CAS 9014-93-1; nonionic; emulsifier, detergent, wetting agent, dispersant, solubilizer, coupling agent for cosmetics, textile, metalworking, household, industrial and other applics.; liq.; sol. @ 5% in toluene, perchloroethylene; disp. in water, min. oil, min. spirits; sp.gr. 1.00; visc. 390 cps; HLB 11.3; pour pt. 0 C; flash pt. (PMCC) > 350 F; 100% conc.

Macol® DNP-15. [PPG/Specialty Chem.] Nonyl nonoxynol-15; CAS 9014-93-1; nonionic; emulsifier, detergent, wetting agent, dispersant, solubilizer, coupling agent for cosmetics, textile, metalworking, household, industrial and other applics.; paste; sol. @ 5% in toluene, perchloroethylene; disp. in water, min. oil, min. spirits; sp.gr. 1.02; HLB 13.0; pour pt. 30 C; flash pt. (PMCC) > 350 F.

Macol® DNP-21. [PPG/Specialty Chem.] Nonyl nonoxynol-21; CAS 9014-93-1; nonionic; emulsifier, detergent, wetting agent, dispersant, solubilizer, coupling agent for cosmetics, textile, metalworking, household, industrial and other applics.; solid; HLB 14.8; cloud pt. 91 C (1% aq.).

Macol® E-200. [PPG/Specialty Chem.] PEG-4; CAS 25322-68-3; EINECS 203-989-9; chemical intermediate for fatty acid esters, lubricant bases in textile and metalworking, as

components in pharmaceutical and cosmetic preps.; nonirritating humectant for moisturizing creams/lotions, eyeshadows, blushers, skin fresheners; improves freeze-thaw stability of hair conditioners, aftershave lotions; liq.; sol. @ 5% in water; m.w. 200; visc. 3 cst (210 F); flash pt. (PMCC) 300 F.

Macol® E-300. [PPG/Specialty Chem.] PEG-6; CAS 25322-68-3; EINECS 220-045-1; chemical intermediate for fatty acid esters, lubricant bases in textile and metalworking, as components in pharmaceutical and cosmetic preps.; nonirritating humectant for moisturizing creams/lotions, eyeshadows, blushers, skin fresheners; improves freeze-thaw stability of hair conditioners, aftershave lotions; liq.; water-sol.; visc. 6 cst (210 F).

Macol® E-400. [PPG/Specialty Chem.] PEG-8; CAS 25322-68-3; EINECS 225-856-4; chemical intermediate for fatty acid esters, lubricant bases in textile and metalworking, as components in pharmaceutical and cosmetic preps.; nonirritating humectant for moisturizing creams/lotions, eyeshadows, blushers, skin fresheners; improves freeze-thaw stability of hair conditioners, aftershave lotions; liq.; water-sol.; visc. 7.5 cst (210 F).

Macol® E-600. [PPG/Specialty Chem.] PEG-12; CAS 25322-68-3; EINECS 229-859-1; chemical intermediate for fatty acid esters, lubricant bases in textile and metal-working, as components in pharmaceutical and cosmetic preps.; nonirritating humectant for moisturizing creams/lotions, eyeshadows, blushers, skin fresheners; improves freeze-thaw stability of hair conditioners, aftershave lotions; solid; water-sol.; visc. 10.5 cSt (210 F).

Macol® E-1000. [PPG/Specialty Chem.] PEG-20; CAS 25322-68-3; chemical intermediate for fatty acid esters, lubricant bases in textile and metalworking, as components in pharmaceutical and cosmetic preps.; nonirritating humectant for moisturizing creams/lotions, eyeshadows, blushers, skin fresheners; improves freeze-thaw stability of hair conditioners, aftershave lotions; solid; water-sol.; visc. 17.5 cSt (210 F).

Macol® E-1450. [PPG/Specialty Chem.] PEG-32; CAS 25322-68-3; chemical intermediate for fatty acid esters, lubricant bases in textile and metalworking, as components in pharmaceutical and cosmetic preps.; water-sol.

Macol® E-3350. [PPG/Specialty Chem.] PEG-75; CAS 25322-68-3; chemical intermediate for fatty acid esters, lubricant bases in textile and metalworking, as components in pharmaceutical and cosmetic preps.; nonirritating humectant for moisturizing creams/lotions, eyeshadows, blushers, skin fresheners; improves freeze-thaw stability of hair conditioners, aftershave lotions; flake; water-sol.; visc. 90 cSt (210 F).

Macol® E-5000. [PPG/Specialty Chem.] PEG (5000); chemical intermediate for fatty acid esters, lubricant bases in textile and metalworking, as components in pharmaceutical and cosmetic preps.

Macol® E-8000. [PPG/Specialty Chem.] PEG-150; CAS 25322-68-3; chemical intermediate for fatty acid esters, lubricant bases in textile and metalworking, as components in pharmaceutical and cosmetic preps.; water-sol.

Macol® LA-4. [PPG/Specialty Chem.] Laureth-4; CAS 5274-68-0; EINECS 226-097-1; nonionic; detergent, wetting agent, emulsifier, dispersant, solubilizer, stabilizer, coupling agent for cosmetics, eye makeup, roll-on deodorants, reactive hair care prods., textiles, metalworking lubricants, household prods., industrial uses; colorless liq.; sol. @ 5% in IPA, min. oil; disp. in min. spirits; m.p. 12 C; HLB 9.5; iodine no. 0.1; hyd. no. 155; flash pt. (PMCC) > 350 F; 100% conc.

Macol® LA-9. [PPG/Specialty Chem.] Laureth-9; CAS 3055-99-0; EINECS 221-284-4; nonionic; detergent, wetting agent, emulsifier, dispersant, solubilizer, stabilizer, coupling agent for cosmetics, textiles, metalworking lubricants, household prods., industrial uses; colorless paste; sol. @ 5% in water; disp. in min. spirits; HLB 13.3; pour pt. 26 C; iodine no. 0.1; hyd. no. 95; flash pt. (PMCC) > 350 F; 100% conc.

Macol® LA-12. [PPG/Specialty Chem.] Laureth-12; CAS 3056-00-6; EINECS 221-286-5; nonionic; detergent, wetting agent, emulsifier, dispersant, solubilizer, stabilizer, coupling agent for cosmetics, eye makeup, deodorants, permanent waves, textiles, metalworking lubricants, household prods., industrial uses; wh. solid; sol. @ 5% in water; disp. in min. spirits; m.p. 30 C; HLB 14.6; iodine no. 0.1; hyd. no. 75; flash pt. (PMCC) > 350 F; 100% conc.

Macol® LA-23. [PPG/Specialty Chem.] Laureth-23; CAS 9002-92-0; nonionic; detergent, wetting agent, emulsifier, dispersant, solubilizer, stabilizer, coupling agent for cosmetics, eye makeup, deodorants, permanent waves, textiles, metalworking lubricants, household prods., industrial uses; wh. solid; sol. @ 5% in water; disp. in min. spirits; m.p. 40 C; HLB 16.4; iodine no. 0.1; hyd. no. 47; flash pt. (PMCC) > 350 F; 100% conc.

Macol® LA-790. [PPG/Specialty Chem.] Laureth-7; CAS 3055-97-8; EINECS 221-283-9; nonionic; detergent, wetting agent, emulsifier, dispersant, and coupling agent for cosmetics, textiles, metalworking lubricants, household prods., and industrial applics.; solubilizer for fragrance and emollients in bubble baths and shower gels; colorless liq.; sol. @ 5% in water, IPA; disp. in min. spirits; insol. min. oil; HLB 10.8; pour pt. 5 C; iodine no. 0.1; flash pt. (PMCC) > 350 F; 90% act. in water.

Macol® NP-4. [PPG/Specialty Chem.] Nonoxynol-4; CAS 9016-45-9; nonionic; emulsifier, detergent, wetting agent, dispersant, solubilizer, coupling agent for cosmetics, textile, metalworking, household, industrial and other applics.; liq.; sol. @ 5% in min. oil, min. spirits, toluene, perchloroethylene; sp.gr. 1.02; visc. 350 cps; HLB 8.9; pour pt. -27 C; flash pt. (PMCC) > 350 F; 100% conc.

Macol® NP-5. [PPG/Specialty Chem.] Nonoxynol-5; CAS 9016-45-9; nonionic; emulsifier, detergent, wetting agent, dispersant, solubilizer, coupling agent for cosmetics, textile, metalworking, household, industrial and other applics.; liq.; sol. @ 5% in min. oil, min. spirits, toluene, perchloroethylene; sp.gr. 1.03; visc. 320 cps; HLB 10.0; pour pt. -27 C; flash pt. (PMCC) > 350 F.

Macol® NP-6. [PPG/Specialty Chem.] Nonoxynol-6; CAS 9016-45-9; nonionic; emulsifier, detergent, wetting agent, dispersant, solubilizer, coupling agent for cosmetics, textile, metalworking, household, industrial and other applics.; liq.; sol. @ 5% in min. spirits, toluene, perchloroethylene; disp. in water, min. oil; sp.gr. 1.04; visc. 300 cps; HLB 10.9; pour pt. -28 C; flash pt. (PMCC) > 350 F; 100% conc.

Macol® NP-8. [PPG/Specialty Chem.] Nonoxynol-8; CAS 9016-45-9; nonionic; emulsifier, detergent, wetting agent, dispersant, solubilizer, coupling agent for cosmetics, textile, metalworking, household, industrial and other applics.; liq.; sol. @ 5% in water, min. spirits, toluene, perchloroethylene; sp.gr. 1.05; visc. 260 cps; HLB 12.3; pour pt. 5 C; cloud pt. 25 C (1% aq.); flash pt. (PMCC) > 350 F.

Macol® NP-11. [PPG/Specialty Chem.] Nonoxynol-11; CAS 9016-45-9; nonionic; emulsifier, detergent, wetting agent, dispersant, solubilizer, coupling agent for cosmetics, textile, metalworking, household, industrial and other applics.; liq.; sol. @ 5% in water, toluene, perchloroethylene; sp.gr. 1.06; visc. 275 cps; HLB 13.7; pour pt. 14 C; cloud pt. 74 C (1% aq.); flash pt. (PMCC) > 350 F; 100% conc.

Macol® NP-12. [PPG/Specialty Chem.] Nonoxynol-12; CAS 9016-45-9; nonionic; emulsifier, detergent, wetting agent,

dispersant, solubilizer, coupling agent for cosmetics, textile, metalworking, household, industrial and other applics.; liq.; sol. @ 5% in water, toluene, perchloroethylene; sp.gr. 1.06; visc. 325 cps; HLB 14.0; pour pt. 17 C; cloud pt. 81 C (1% aq.); flash pt. (PMCC) > 350 F; 100% conc.

Macol® NP-15. [PPG/Specialty Chem.] Nonoxynol-15; CAS 9016-45-9; nonionic; emulsifier, detergent, wetting agent, dispersant, solubilizer, coupling agent for cosmetics, textile, metalworking, household, industrial and other applics.; paste; sol. @ 5% in water; disp. in toluene, perchloroethylene; sp.gr. 1.07; HLB 15.0; pour pt. 26 C; cloud pt. 65 C (1% in 10% NaCl); flash pt. (PMCC) > 350 F.

Macol® NP-20. [PPG/Specialty Chem.] Nonoxynol–20; CAS 9016-45-9; nonionic; emulsifier, detergent, wetting agent, dispersant, solubilizer, coupling agent for cosmetics, textile, metalworking, household, industrial and other applics.; solid; sol. @ 5% in water; sp.gr. 1.08; HLB 16.0; pour pt. 30 C; cloud pt. 70 C (1% in 10% NaCl); flash pt. (PMCC) > 350 F; 100% conc.

Macol® NP-20(70). [PPG/Specialty Chem.] Nonoxynol-20; CAS 9016-45-9; nonionic; emulsifier, detergent, wetting agent, dispersant, solubilizer, coupling agent for cosmetics, textile, metalworking, household, industrial and other applics.; liq.; sol. @ 5% in water; sp.gr. 1.06; visc. 900 cps; HLB 16.0; pour pt. 0 C; cloud pt. 70 C (1% in 10% NaCl); flash pt. (PMCC) > 350 F; 70% act. in water.

Macol® NP-30(70). [PPG/Specialty Chem.] Nonoxynol-30; CAS 9016-45-9; nonionic; emulsifier, detergent, wetting agent, dispersant, solubilizer, coupling agent for cosmetics, textile, metalworking, household, industrial and other applics.; liq.; sol. @ 5% in water; sp.gr. 1.06; visc. 1100 cps; HLB 17.2; pour pt. 4 C; cloud pt. 75 C (1% in 10% NaCl); flash pt. (PMCC) > 350 F; 70% act. in water.

Macol® NP-100. [PPG/Specialty Chem.] Nonoxynol–100; CAS 9016-45-9; nonionic; emulsifier, detergent, wetting agent, dispersant, solubilizer, coupling agent for cosmetics, textile, metalworking, household, industrial and other applics.; flake; sol. @ 5% in water; sp.gr. 1.11; HLB 19.0; pour pt. 54 C; cloud pt. > 100 C (1% aq.); flash pt. (PMCC) > 350 F; 100% conc.

Macol® OA-2. [PPG/Specialty Chem.] Oleth-2; CAS 9004-98-2; nonionic; detergent, wetting agent, emulsifier, dispersant, solubilizer, stabilizer, coupling agent for cosmetics, hair conditioners, skin cleansers, textiles, metalworking lubricants, household prods., industrial uses; coupler for emollients and alcohol in bath oils and salts; colorless liq.; sol. @ 5% in IPA, min. oil; HLB 3.8; pour pt. < 0 C; iodine no. 70; hyd. no. 170; flash pt. (PMCC) > 350 F; 100% conc.

Macol® OA-4. [PPG/Specialty Chem.] Oleth-4; CAS 9004-98-2; nonionic; detergent, wetting agent, emulsifier, dispersant, solubilizer, stabilizer, coupling agent for cosmetics, textiles, metalworking lubricants, household prods., industrial uses; colorless liq.; sol. @ 5% in IPA, min. oil; disp. in min. spirits; HLB 8.0; pour pt. < 0 C; iodine no. 53; hyd. no. 128; flash pt. (PMCC) > 350 F; 100% conc.

Macol® OA-5. [PPG/Specialty Chem.] Oleth-5; CAS 9004-98-2; nonionic; detergent, wetting agent, emulsifier, dispersant, solubilizer, stabilizer, coupling agent for cosmetics, aftershave lotions, suntan gels, hair coloring prods., textiles, metalworking lubricants, household prods., industrial uses; colorless liq.; sol. @ 5% in IPA, min. oil; disp. in min. spirits; insol. in water; HLB 8.2; pour pt. 5 C; iodine no. 53; hyd. no. 125; flash pt. (PMCC) > 350 F; 100% conc.

Macol® OA-10. [PPG/Specialty Chem.] Oleth-10; CAS 9004-98-2; nonionic; detergent, wetting agent, emulsifier, dispersant, solubilizer, stabilizer, coupling agent for cosmetics, hair tonics/grooms, colognes, skin fresheners, facial masks, moisturizing creams and lotions, textiles, metalworking lubricants, household prods., industrial uses; liq.; sol. @ 5% in water, IPA; disp. min. oil, min. spirits; HLB 12.5; pour pt. 16 C; iodine no. 33; hyd. no. 80; flash pt. (PMCC) > 350 F; 100% conc.

Macol® OA-20. [PPG/Specialty Chem.] Oleth-20; CAS 9004-98-2; nonionic; detergent, wetting agent, emulsifier, dispersant, solubilizer, stabilizer, coupling agent for cosmetics, hair tonics, colognes, skin fresheners, facial masks, moisturizing creams, textiles, metalworking lubricants, household prods., industrial uses; cream solid; sol. @ 5% in water, IPA; m.p. 30 C; HLB 14.7; iodine no. 23; hyd. no. 58; flash pt. (PMCC) > 350 F; 100% conc.

Macol® OP-3. [PPG/Specialty Chem.] Octoxynol-3; CAS 9002-93-1; nonionic; emulsifier, detergent, wetting agent, dispersant, solubilizer, coupling agent for cosmetics, textile, metalworking, household, industrial and other applics.; liq.; sol. @ 5% in min. oil, min. spirits, toluene, perchloroethylene; sp.gr. 1.02; visc. 350 cps; HLB 7.8; pour pt. -23 C; flash pt. (PMCC) > 350 F; 100% conc.

Macol® OP-5. [PPG/Specialty Chem.] Octoxynol-5; CAS 9002-93-1; nonionic; emulsifier, detergent, wetting agent, dispersant, solubilizer, coupling agent for cosmetics, textile, metalworking, household, industrial and other applics.; liq.; sol. @ 5% in min. spirits, toluene, perchloroethylene; disp. in min. oil; sp.gr. 1.04; visc. 300 cps; HLB 10.4; pour pt. -26 C; flash pt. (PMCC) > 350 F; 100% conc.

Macol® OP-8. [PPG/Specialty Chem.] Octoxynol-8; CAS 9002-93-1; nonionic; emulsifier, detergent, wetting agent, dispersant, solubilizer, coupling agent for cosmetics, textile, metalworking, household, industrial and other applics.; liq.; sol. @ 5% in water, toluene, perchloroethylene; sp.gr. 1.05; visc. 275 cps; HLB 12.3; pour pt. 5 C; cloud pt. 23 C (1% aq.); flash pt. (PMCC) > 350 F.

Macol® OP-10. [PPG/Specialty Chem.] Octoxynol-10; CAS 9002-93-1; nonionic; emulsifier, detergent, wetting agent, dispersant, solubilizer, coupling agent for cosmetics, textile, metalworking, household, industrial and other applics.; liq.; sol. @ 5% in toluene, perchloroethylene; disp. in water; sp.gr. 1.06; visc. 250 cps; HLB 13.4; pour pt. 8 C; cloud pt. 65 C (1% aq.); flash pt. (PMCC) > 350 F; 100% conc.

Macol® OP-10 SP. [PPG/Specialty Chem.] Modified octoxynol-10; CAS 9002-93-1; nonionic; emulsifier, detergent, wetting agent, dispersant, solubilizer, coupling agent for cosmetics, textile, metalworking, household, industrial and other applics.; visc. 250 cps; HLB 13.4; cloud pt. 65 C (1% aq.).

Macol® OP-12. [PPG/Specialty Chem.] Octoxynol-12; CAS 9002-93-1; nonionic; emulsifier, detergent, wetting agent, dispersant, solubilizer, coupling agent for cosmetics, textile, metalworking, household, industrial and other applics.; liq.; sol. @ 5% in water, toluene, perchloroethylene; sp.gr. 1.07; visc. 335 cps; HLB 14.6; pour pt.16 C; cloud pt. 88 C (1% aq.); flash pt. (PMCC) > 350 F; 100% conc.

Macol® OP-16(75). [PPG/Specialty Chem.] Octoxynol-16; CAS 9002-93-1; nonionic; emulsifier, detergent, wetting agent, dispersant, solubilizer, coupling agent for cosmetics, textile, metalworking, household, industrial and other applics.; liq.; sol. @ 5% in water; sp.gr. 1.08; visc. 540 cps; HLB 15.8; pour pt. 13 C; cloud pt. > 100 C (1% aq.); flash pt. (PMCC) > 350 F; 75% act. in water.

Macol® OP-30(70). [PPG/Specialty Chem.] Octoxynol-30; CAS 9002-93-1; nonionic; emulsifier, detergent, wetting agent, dispersant, solubilizer, coupling agent for cosmetics, textile, metalworking, household, industrial and other applics.; liq.; sol. @ 5% in water; sp.gr. 1.10; visc. 470 cps; HLB 17.3; pour pt. 2 C; cloud pt. > 100 C (1% aq.); flash pt. (PMCC) > 350 F; 70% act. in water.

Macol® OP-40(70). [PPG/Specialty Chem.] Octoxynol-40; CAS 9002-93-1; nonionic; emulsifier, detergent, wetting agent, dispersant, solubilizer, coupling agent for cosmetics, textile, metalworking, household, industrial and other applics.; emulsifier for vinyl acetate and acrylate polymerization; liq.; sol. @ 5% in water; sp.gr. 1.10; visc. 490 cps; HLB 17.9; pour pt. 4 C; cloud pt. > 100 C (1% aq.); flash pt. (PMCC) > 350 F; 70% act. in water.

Macol® P-1200. [PPG/Specialty Chem.] PPG-20; CAS 25322-69-4; nonionic; skin softener, nonoily emollient for cosmetic creams/lotions, bath oils, blushers, skin fresheners, aftershaves, nail enamel removers; defoamer for aq. systems, in mold release applics., lubricant bases for textile, paper, metalworking formulations, chemical intermediates for fatty acid esters, components for urethane resins; liq.; sol. @ 5% in min. oil, perchloroethylene; m.w. 1200; sp.gr. 1.007; visc. 160 cps; pour pt. -40 C; flash pt. (PMCC) > 350 F; ref. index 1.449.

Macol® P-2000. [PPG/Specialty Chem.] PPG-26; CAS 25322-69-4; nonionic; skin softener, nonoily emollient for cosmetic creams/lotions, bath oils, blushers, skin fresheners, aftershaves, nail enamel removers; defoamer for aq. systems, in mold release applics., lubricant bases for textile, paper, metalworking formulations, chemical intermediates for fatty acid esters, components for urethane resins; liq.; sol. @ 5% in min. oils, min. spirits, aromatic solvs., perchloroethylene; m.w. 2000; sp.gr. 1.002; visc. 230 cps; pour pt. -31 C; flash pt. (PMCC) > 350 F; ref. index 1.450.

Macol® P-4000. [PPG/Specialty Chem.] PPG-30; CAS 25322-69-4; nonionic; cosmetic ingred.; defoamer for aq. systems, in mold release applics., lubricant bases for textile, paper, metalworking formulations, chemical intermediates for fatty acid esters, components for urethane resins; liq.; sol. @ 5% in min. oils, min. spirits, perchloroethylene; m.w. 4000; sp.gr. 1.002; visc. 1150 cps; pour pt. -20 C; flash pt. (PMCC) > 350 F; ref. index 1.450.

Macol® SA-2. [PPG/Specialty Chem.] Steareth-2; CAS 9005-00-9; nonionic; detergent, wetting agent, emulsifier, dispersant, solubilizer, stabilizer, coupling agent for cosmetics, makeup, moisturizing creams/lotions, hair dressings, textiles, metalworking lubricants, household prods., industrial uses; wh. solid; sol. @ 5% in IPA; m.p. 43 C; HLB 4.7; iodine no. 0.1; hyd. no. 158; flash pt. (PMCC) > 350 F; 100% conc.

Macol® SA-5. [PPG/Specialty Chem.] Steareth-5; CAS 9005-00-9; nonionic; detergent, wetting agent, emulsifier, dispersant, solubilizer, stabilizer, coupling agent for cosmetics, textiles, metalworking lubricants, household prods., industrial uses; wh. solid; sol. @ 5% in IPA; m.p. 41 C; HLB 9.0; iodine no. 0.1; hyd. no. 116; flash pt. (PMCC) > 350 F; 100% conc.

Macol® SA-10. [PPG/Specialty Chem.] Steareth-10; CAS 9005-00-9; nonionic; detergent, wetting agent, emulsifier, dispersant, solubilizer, stabilizer, coupling agent for cosmetics, textiles, metalworking lubricants, household prods., industrial uses; wh. solid; sol. @ 5% in IPA; disp. in water, min. spirits; m.p. 40 C; HLB 12.3; iodine no. 0.1; hyd. no. 80; flash pt. (PMCC) > 350 F; 100% conc.

Macol® SA-15. [PPG/Specialty Chem.] Steareth-15; CAS 9005-00-9; nonionic; detergent, wetting agent, emulsifier, dispersant, solubilizer, stabilizer, coupling agent for cosmetics, textiles, metalworking lubricants, household prods., industrial uses; wh. solid; sol. @ 5% in water, IPA; disp. in min. spirits; m.p. 38 C; HLB 14.3; iodine no. 0.1; hyd. no. 64; flash pt. (PMCC) > 350 F; 100% conc.

Macol® SA-20. [PPG/Specialty Chem.] Steareth-20; CAS 9005-00-9; nonionic; detergent, wetting agent, emulsifier, dispersant, solubilizer, stabilizer, coupling agent for cosmetics, textiles, metalworking lubricants, household prods., industrial uses; wh. solid; sol. @ 5% in water, IPA; m.p. 39 C; HLB 15.4; iodine no. 0.1; hyd. no. 52; flash pt. (PMCC) > 350 F; 100% conc.

Macol® SA-40. [PPG/Specialty Chem.] Steareth-40; CAS 9005-00-9; nonionic; detergent, wetting agent, emulsifier, dispersant, solubilizer, stabilizer, coupling agent for cosmetics, textiles, metalworking lubricants, household prods., industrial uses; wh. solid; sol. @ 5% in water, IPA; m.p. 40 C; HLB 17.4; iodine no. 0.1; hyd. no. 32; flash pt. (PMCC) > 350 F; 100% conc.

Macol® TD-3. [PPG/Specialty Chem.] Trideceth-3; CAS 4403-12-7; EINECS 224-540-3; nonionic; detergent, wetting agent, emulsifier, dispersant, solubilizer, stabilizer, coupling agent for cosmetics, textiles, metalworking lubricants, household prods., industrial uses; liq.; sol. @ 5% in min. spirits, toluene, perchloroethylene; disp. in water, min. oil; sp.gr. 0.96; visc. 17 cps; HLB 8.0; pour pt. -32 C; flash pt. (PMCC) > 250 F; 100% conc.

Macol® TD-8. [PPG/Specialty Chem.] Trideceth-8; CAS 24938-91-8; nonionic; detergent, wetting agent, emulsifier, dispersant, solubilizer, stabilizer, coupling agent for cosmetics, textiles, metalworking lubricants, household prods., industrial uses; liq.; sol. @ 5% in water, min. oil, min. spirits, toluene, perchloroethylene; sp.gr. 1.02; visc. 50 cps; HLB 12.4; pour pt. 8 C; cloud pt. 55 C (1% aq.); flash pt. (PMCC) > 275 F; 100% conc.

Macol® TD-10. [PPG/Specialty Chem.] Trideceth-10; CAS 24938-91-8; nonionic; detergent, wetting agent, emulsifier, dispersant, solubilizer, stabilizer, coupling agent for cosmetics, textiles, metalworking lubricants, household prods., industrial uses; liq.; sol. @ 5% in water, min. spirits, toluene, perchloroethylene; disp. in min. oil; sp.gr. 1.02; visc. 60 cps; HLB 13.6; pour pt. 10 C; cloud pt. 76 C (1% aq.); flash pt. (PMCC) > 300 F; 100% conc.

Macol® TD-12. [PPG/Specialty Chem.] Trideceth-12; CAS 24938-91-8; nonionic; detergent, wetting agent, emulsifier, dispersant, solubilizer, stabilizer, coupling agent for cosmetics, textiles, metalworking lubricants, household prods., industrial uses; liq.; sol. @ 5% in water, toluene, perchloroethylene; disp. in min. spirits; sp.gr. 1.03; visc. 540 cps; HLB 14.1; pour pt. 14 C; cloud pt. 91 C (1% aq.); flash pt. (PMCC) > 300 F; 100% conc.

Macol® TD-15. [PPG/Specialty Chem.] Trideceth-15; CAS 24938-91-8; nonionic; detergent, wetting agent, emulsifier, dispersant, solubilizer, stabilizer, coupling agent for cosmetics, textiles, metalworking lubricants, household prods., industrial uses.

Macol® TD-100. [PPG/Specialty Chem.] Trideceth-100; CAS 24938-91-8; nonionic; detergent, wetting agent, emulsifier, dispersant, solubilizer, stabilizer, coupling agent for cosmetics, textiles, metalworking lubricants, household prods., industrial uses; solid; sol. @ 5% in water; sp.gr. 1.06; HLB 18.9; pour pt. 55 C; cloud pt. > 100 C (1% aq.); flash pt. (PMCC) > 300 F; 100% conc.

Macol® TD-610. [PPG/Specialty Chem.] Trideceth-6; CAS 24938-91-8; nonionic; detergent, wetting agent, emulsifier, dispersant, solubilizer, stabilizer, coupling agent for cosmetics, textiles, metalworking lubricants, household prods., industrial uses; liq.; sol. @ 5% in min. spirits, toluene, perchloroethylene; disp. in water, min. oil; sp.gr. 0.98; visc. 115 cps; HLB 11.2; pour pt. 6 C; cloud pt. 41 C (1% aq.); flash pt. (PMCC) > 275 F; 86% conc.

Macromelt. [Henkel] Dilinoleic acid/ethylene diamine copolymer.

Macrospherical® 95. [Reheis] Aluminum chlorohydrate; CAS 1327-41-9; EINECS 215-477-2; antiperspirant active for aerosols with controlled particle size; spray-dried to a relatively thick walled hollow sphere; spherical powd., 90% min. > 10 μ; 47% Al$_2$O$_3$, 16.3% Cl.

Mafo® C. [PPG/Specialty Chem.] Cocamidopropyl betaine; amphoteric; biodeg. solubilizer, emollient, coupling agent, emulsifier, foam booster for shampoos; sp.gr. 1.010; 35% solids in water.

Mafo® CAB. [PPG/Specialty Chem.] Cocamidopropyl betaine; amphoteric; detergent, dispersant, surfactant, conditioner, foam and visc. stabilizer, chelating agent, wetting agent, solubilizer, lubricant, emulsifier; used in personal care, shampoos, liq. soaps, bath gels, dishwashing, rug and carpet cleaning, metalworking applics.; liq.; watersol.; sp.gr. 1.010; 35% solids in water.

Mafo® CAB 425. [PPG/Specialty Chem.] Cocamidopropyl betaine; amphoteric; biodeg. solubilizer, wetting agent, emollient, coupling agent, emulsifier, foam booster for shampoos; liq.; sp.gr. 1.040; 42.5% solids in water.

Mafo® CAB SP. [PPG/Specialty Chem.] Cocamidopropyl betaine; amphoteric; biodeg. solubilizer, emollient, coupling agent, emulsifier, foam booster for shampoos, metalworking formulations; sp.gr. 1.050; 43% solids in water.

Mafo® CB 40. [PPG/Specialty Chem.] Coco betaine; CAS 68424-94-2; EINECS 270-329-4; amphoteric; biodeg. foam booster, visc. builder, emollient, coupling agent, emulsifier for shampoos; oil and fragrance solubilizer; liq.; sp.gr. 1.040; 40% solids in water.

Mafo® CFA 35. [PPG/Specialty Chem.] Cocamidopropyl betaine; amphoteric; biodeg. solubilizer, emollient, coupling agent, emulsifier, foam booster for shampoos; sp.gr. 1.040; 35% solids in water.

Mafo® CSB. [PPG/Specialty Chem.] Cocamidopropyl hydroxysultaine; CAS 68139-30-0; EINECS 268-761-3; amphoteric; biodeg. solubilizer, emollient, coupling agent, emulsifier, foam booster for shampoos; sp.gr. 1.094; 35% solids in water.

Mafo® CSB 50. [PPG/Specialty Chem.] Cocamidopropyl hydroxysultaine; CAS 68139-30-0; EINECS 268-761-3; amphoteric; biodeg. solubilizer, emollient, coupling agent, emulsifier, foam booster, visc. builder for shampoos; reduces irritation of anionics; liq.; sp.gr. 1.100; 50% solids in water.

Mafo® CSB W. [PPG/Specialty Chem.] Cocamidopropyl hydroxysultaine; CAS 68139-30-0; EINECS 268-761-3; amphoteric; biodeg. solubilizer, emollient, coupling agent, emulsifier, foam booster for shampoos; sp.gr. 1.100; 50% solids in water.

Mafo® KCOSB 50. [PPG/Specialty Chem.] Cocamidopropyl hydroxysultaine; CAS 68139-30-0; EINECS 268-761-3; amphoteric; biodeg. solubilizer, emollient, coupling agent, emulsifier, foam booster for shampoos; sp.gr. 1.100; 50% solids in water.

Mafo® LMAB. [PPG/Specialty Chem.] Lauramidopropyl betaine; EINECS 224-292-6; amphoteric; biodeg. solubilizer, emollient, coupling agent, emulsifier, visc. and foam booster for shampoos; sp.gr. 1.100; 35% solids in water.

Mafo® OB. [PPG/Specialty Chem.] Oleyl betaine; CAS 871-37-4; EINECS 212-806-1; amphoteric; biodeg. solubilizer, emollient, coupling agent, emulsifier, foam booster for shampoos; sp.gr. 1.020; 50% solids in water.

Mafo® SBAO 110. [PPG/Specialty Chem.] amphoteric; biodeg. solubilizer, emollient, coupling agent, emulsifier, foam booster for shampoos; lime soap dispersant; sp.gr. 1.049; 42% solids in water.

Magnabrite® F. [Am. Colloid] Magnesium aluminum silicate USP/NF; CAS 12199-37-0; EINECS 235-374-6; disintegrant, binder, stabilizing and suspending agent for cosmetic and pharmaceutical tablets, ointments, and pastes where dry blending is essential; wh. fine powd.; 100% thru 325 mesh; insol. in water or alcohol; surf. area > 750 m^2/g; visc. 150-450 cps (5% solids); pH 9–10 (5% disp.); dry brightness (GE) 83-87; 8% max. moisture.

Magnabrite® FS. [Am. Colloid] Magnesium aluminum silicate USP/NF; CAS 12199-37-0; EINECS 235-374-6;

disintegrant, binder, and suspension agent for tablets, ointments, and pastes where dry incorporation is essential; wh. micronized powd.; 100% thru 325 mesh; insol. in water and alcohol; surf. area > 750 m²/g; visc. 150-450 cps (5% solids); pH 9.0-10.0 (5% disp.); dry brightness (GE) 83-87; 8% max. moisture.

Magnabrite® HS. [Am. Colloid] Magnesium aluminum silicate USP/NF; CAS 12199-37-0; EINECS 235-374-6; suspending agent, gellant, and binder for use in cosmetic, personal care, and pharmaceutical applics. where stability in acidic systems is essential; wh. soft flakes, 20-100 mesh particle size; insol. in water and alcohol; surf. area > 750 m²/g; visc. 40-200 cps (5% solids); pH 9.0-10.0 (5% disp.); dry brightness (GE) 70 min.; 8% max. moisture.

Magnabrite® HV. [Am. Colloid] Magnesium aluminum silicate USP/NF; CAS 12199-37-0; EINECS 235-374-6; emulsifying, thickening, stabilizing, and suspending agent for cosmetic, toiletry, and pharmaceutical formulations at low solids; wh. soft flakes, 20-100 mesh particle size; insol. in water and alcohol; surf. area > 750 m²/g; visc. 800-2200 cps (5% solids); pH 9-10 (5% disp.); dry brightness (GE) 83-87; 8% max. moisture.

Magnabrite® K. [Am. Colloid] Magnesium aluminum silicate USP/NF, acid-stable; CAS 12199-37-0; EINECS 235-374-6; stabilizing and suspending agent for acidic personal care prods., cosmetics, and pharmaceuticals; controls flocculation; wh. soft flakes.; 20-100 mesh particle size; insol. in water and alcohol; surf. area > 750 m²/g; visc. 100-300 cps (5% solids); pH 9-10 (5% disp.); dry brightness (GE) 83-87; 8% max. moisture.

Magnabrite® S. [Am. Colloid] Magnesium aluminum silicate USP/NF; CAS 12199-37-0; EINECS 235-374-6; stabilizing and suspending agent for cosmetics, toiletries, and pharmaceuticals; used where good dispersibility, high visc., and wh. color are essential; wh. soft flakes; 20-100 mesh particle size; insol. in water and alcohol; surf. area > 750 m²/g; visc. 225-600 cps (5% solids); pH 9-10 (5% disp.); dry brightness (GE) 83-87; 8% max. moisture.

Makon® 4. [Stepan; Stepan Canada; Stepan Europe] Nonoxynol-4; CAS 9016-45-9; nonionic; detergent, emulsifier used in chemical specialties, cosmetic, agric., industrial and metal cleaners, textile, paper and petrol. industries; lt. straw liq.; oil-sol.; dens. 8.5 lb/gal; visc. 260 cps; pour pt. –20 C; pH 7.7 (1%); 100% act.

Makon® 6. [Stepan; Stepan Canada; Stepan Europe] Nonoxynol-6; CAS 9016-45-9; nonionic; detergent, emulsifier used in chemical specialties, cosmetic, agric., industrial and metal cleaners, textile, paper and petrol. industries; lt. straw liq.; disp. in water; dens. 8.67 lb/gal; visc. 255 cps; pour pt. –29 C; pH 7.9 (1%); 100% act.

Makon® 8. [Stepan; Stepan Canada; Stepan Europe] Nonoxynol-8; CAS 9016-45-9; nonionic; detergent, emulsifier used in chemical specialties, cosmetic, agric., industrial and metal cleaners, textile, paper and petrol. industries; lt. straw liq.; sol. in water; dens. 8.76 lb/gal; visc. 205 cps; cloud pt. 24 C (1%); pour pt. –5 C; pH 7.0 (1%); 100% act.

Makon® 10. [Stepan; Stepan Canada; Stepan Europe] Nonoxynol-10; CAS 9016-45-9; EINECS 248-294-1; nonionic; detergent, emulsifier used in chemical specialties, cosmetic, agric., industrial and metal cleaners, textile, paper and petrol. industries; lt. straw liq.; sol. in water; dens. 8.85 lb/gal; visc. 235 cps; cloud pt. 54 C (1%); pour pt. 2.8 C; pH 8.2 (1%); 100% act.

Makon® 12. [Stepan; Stepan Canada; Stepan Europe] Nonoxynol-12; CAS 9016-45-9; nonionic; detergent, emulsifier used in chemical specialties, cosmetic, agric., industrial and metal cleaners, textile, paper and petrol. industries; lt. straw liq.; sol. in water; dens. 8.9 lb/gal; visc. 300 cps; cloud pt. 81 C (1%); pour pt. 12.2 C; pH 7.2 (1%); 100% act.

Makon® 14. [Stepan; Stepan Canada; Stepan Europe] Nonoxynol-14; CAS 9016-45-9; nonionic; detergent, emulsifier used in chemical specialties, cosmetic, agric., industrial and metal cleaners, textile, paper and petrol. industries; lt. straw liq.; sol. in water; dens. 8.9 lb/gal; visc. 520 cps; cloud pt. 94 C (1%); pour pt. 18.9 C; pH 7.2 (1%); 100% act.

Makon® 30. [Stepan; Stepan Canada; Stepan Europe] Nonoxynol-30; CAS 9016-45-9; nonionic; detergent, emulsifier used in chemical specialties, cosmetic, agric., industrial and metal cleaners, textile, paper and petrol. industries; off-wh. waxy solid; sol. in water; dens. 9.0 lb/gal; pour pt. 40 C; pH 8.5 (1%); 100% act.

Maltrin® M040. [Grain Processing] Maltodextrin; CAS 9050-36-6; EINECS 232-940-4; nonsweet, nutritive polymer useful for wet binding and anticaking; adds sol'n. visc., good mouthfeel; for pharmaceuticals, foods; DE 4–7; bulk dens. 0.51 g/cc (packed); pH 4–5.

Maltrin® M050. [Grain Processing] Maltodextrin; CAS 9050-36-6; EINECS 232-940-4; nonsweet, nutritive polymer useful for adding visc. and mouthfeel; for pharmaceuticals, foods; DE 4–7; bulk dens. 0.56 g/cc (packed); pH 4–5.

Maltrin® M100. [Grain Processing] Maltodextrin; CAS 9050-36-6; EINECS 232-940-4; nonsweet, nutritive polymer useful as carrier and bulking agent; provides exc. mouthfeel for chewable tablets; functions in binding, coating, and spray drying; for pharmaceuticals, foods; DE 9–12; bulk dens. 0.56 g/cc (packed); pH 4.0–4.7.

Maltrin® M150. [Grain Processing] Maltodextrin; CAS 9050-36-6; EINECS 232-940-4; very slightly sweet, nutritive polymer useful for binding properties; directly compressible; for pharmaceuticals, foods; DE 13–17; bulk dens. 0.61 g/cc (packed); pH 4.0–4.7.

Maltrin® M180. [Grain Processing] Maltodextrin; CAS 9050-36-6; EINECS 232-940-4; slightly sweet, nutritive polymer; directly compressible; binding properties; for pharmaceuticals, foods; DE 16.5–19.5; bulk dens. 0.63 g/cc (packed); pH 4.0–4.7.

Maltrin® M200. [Grain Processing] Corn syrup solids; CAS 68131-37-3; dried glucose syrup with very good coating and binding properties; directly compressible; for pharmaceutical use; DE 20–23; bulk dens. 0.64 g/cc (packed); pH 4.0–4.7.

Maltrin® M250. [Grain Processing] Corn syrup solids; CAS 68131-37-3; dried glucose syrup with good binding properties; directly compressible; for pharmaceutical use; DE 23–27; bulk dens. 0.67 g/cc (packed); pH 4.5–5.5.

Maltrin® M365. [Grain Processing] High maltose corn syrup solids; CAS 68131-37-3; dried glucose syrup with noticeable sweetness; for pharmaceutical use; DE 34–38; bulk dens. 0.67 g/cc (packed); pH 4.5–5.2.

Maltrin® M510. [Grain Processing] Agglomerated maltodextrin; CAS 9050-36-6; EINECS 232-940-4; flowable form of Maltrin M100; exhibits exc. dispersibility and dissolution; directly compressible binder and diluent; for pharmaceutical use; free-flowing gran.; DE 9–12; bulk dens. 0.56 g/cc (packed); pH 4.0–4.7.

Maltrin® M700. [Grain Processing] Agglomerated maltodextrin; CAS 9050-36-6; EINECS 232-940-4; agglomerated form of Maltrin M100; exhibits exc. dissolution; very good carrier when low bulk dens. is required; for pharmaceutical use; free-flowing gran.; DE 9–12; bulk dens. 0.13 g/cc (packed); pH 6.0–7.0.

Maltrin® QD M440. [Grain Processing] Agglomerated maltodextrin; CAS 9050-36-6; EINECS 232-940-4; agglomerated form of Maltrin M040; exhibits exc. dispersibility and dissolution; for pharmaceutical use; free-flowing gran.; DE 4–7; bulk dens. 0.30 g/cc (packed); pH 4.0–5.1.

Maltrin® QD M500. [Grain Processing] Agglomerated maltodextrin; CAS 9050-36-6; EINECS 232-940-4; agglomerated form of Maltrin M100; exhibits exc. dispersibility and dissolution; directly compressible binder and good carrier; for pharmaceutical use; free-flowing gran.; DE 9–12; bulk dens. 0.34 g/cc (packed); pH 4.0–5.1.

Maltrin® QD M550. [Grain Processing] Agglomerated maltodextrin; CAS 9050-36-6; EINECS 232-940-4; agglomerated form of Maltrin M150; exhibits exc. dispersibility and dissolution; directly compressible binder and good carrier; for pharmaceutical use; free-flowing gran.; DE 13–17; bulk dens. 0.37 g/cc (packed); pH 4.0–5.1.

Maltrin® QD M580. [Grain Processing] Maltodextrin; CAS 9050-36-6; EINECS 232-940-4; for pharmaceutical use; DE 16.5–19.5; bulk dens. 0.40 g/cc (packed); pH 4.0–5.1.

Maltrin® QD M600. [Grain Processing] Agglomerated corn syrup solids; CAS 68131-37-3; agglomerated form of Maltrin M200; directly compresible binder and good carrier; for pharmaceutical use; free-flowing gran.; DE 20–23; bulk dens. 0.40 g/cc (packed); pH 4.0–5.1.

N,L-Malyl-L-Tyrosine. [Sederma] Disodium malyl tyrosinate; photoprevention care for pre-tan, sun tan and sun protective prods., and skin and makeup care prods.; wh. to cream hygroscopic lyophilized powd., char. odor; sol. > 300g/l in water; pH 6.0-7.5 (5%); usage level: 0.2-1%; > 80% act.

Manro ALEC 25. [Hickson Manro Ltd.] Ammonium laureth sulfate (3 mole), natural based; CAS 32612-48-9; surfactant for hair care and bath prods., household detergents; liq.; 25% act.

Manro ALEC 27. [Hickson Manro Ltd.] Ammonium laureth sulfate (3 mole), natural based; CAS 32612-48-9; surfactant for hair care prods., bath prods., household detergents; liq.; 27% act.

Manro ALES 60. [Hickson Manro Ltd.] Ammonium laureth sulfate (3 mole); CAS 32612-48-9; anionic; surfactant used in liq. detergents, cleaning prods., fire fighting foams, hair care prods.; biodeg.; amber, slightly hazy, mobile gel; slight alcoholic odor; sp.gr. 1.033; pH 7–8 (10% aq.); 60% act.

Manro ALS 25. [Hickson Manro Ltd.] Ammonium lauryl sulfate; CAS 2235-54-3; EINECS 218-793-9; anionic; biodeg. surfactant for cosmetics and toiletries; liq.; 25% conc.

Manro ALS 27/30. [Hickson Manro Ltd.] Ammonium alkyl sulfate; surfactant for hair care and bath prods., and household detergents; liq.; 27-30% act.

Manro ALS 30. [Hickson Manro Ltd.] Ammonium lauryl sulfate; CAS 2235-54-3; EINECS 218-793-9; anionic; used in cosmetics and toiletries, esp. shampoos, and household detergents; biodeg.; pale yel. clear to slightly hazy, visc. liq.; mild odor; sp.gr. 1.02; visc. 5000 cps; pH 6–7 (10% aq.); 28% min. act.

Manro AO 25M. [Hickson Manro Ltd.] Myristyl dimethylamine oxide; CAS 3332-27-2; EINECS 222-059-3; surfactant for hair care and bath prods., household detergents, and industrial cleaning; liq.; 25% act.

Manro AO 3OC. [Hickson Manro Ltd.] N-Alkyl dimethyl amine oxide; amphoteric; foam booster, detergent for toiletries, household and industrial cleaners; thickener for bleaches; liq.; 30% act.

Manro BEC 28. [Hickson Manro Ltd.] Sodium laureth sulfate (3 mole); anionic; foaming and wetting in shampoos and toiletry prods.; liq.; 28% conc.

Manro BEC 70. [Hickson Manro Ltd.] Sodium laureth sulfate (3 mole), natural based; surfactant for hair care and bath prods.; mobile gel; 68% act.

Manro BES 27. [Hickson Manro Ltd.] Sodium laureth sulfate (3 mole); CAS 9004-82-4; anionic; foaming agent, emulsifier used in cosmetics, toiletries, household detergent and industrial prods.; biodeg.; pale yel., mobile liq.; mild odor; sp.gr. 1.04; visc. 200 cps; pH 6.5–7.5 (10% aq.); 26.5% min. act.

Manro BES 60. [Hickson Manro Ltd.] Sodium laureth sulfate (3 mole); CAS 9004-82-4; anionic; high foaming surfactant used in liq. detergents, cleaning prods., fire fighting foams, personal care prods.; biodeg.; amber, slightly hazy, mobile gel; slight alcoholic odor; sp.gr. 1.090; pH 7–8 (10% aq.); 60% act.

Manro BES 70. [Hickson Manro Ltd.] Sodium laureth sulfate (3 mole); CAS 9004-82-4; anionic; foaming agent, emulsifier for chlorinated solvs., lime soap dispersant, intermediate used in cosmetics, household cleaning prods. and fire fighting foams; biodeg.; pale yel., mobile gel; mild odor; sp.gr. 1.05; pH 7–9 (10% aq.); 67.5% min. act.

Manro CD. [Hickson Manro Ltd.] Cocamide DEA; CAS 61791-31-9; EINECS 263-163-9; anionic; solubilizer, foam stabilizer, detergent for shampoos, liq. detergents, hand cleaners; liq.; 90% conc.

Manro CD/G. [Hickson Manro Ltd.] Cocamide DEA, up to 10% glycerin; anionic; foam stabilizer and solubilizer for liq. detergents, shampoos, bubble baths; liq.; 78% conc.

Manro CDS. [Hickson Manro Ltd.] Cocamide DEA; CAS 61791-31-9; EINECS 263-163-9; anionic; biodeg. foam stabilizer and solubilizer for liq. detergents, shampoos, bubble baths; liq.; 85% conc.

Manro CDX. [Hickson Manro Ltd.] Cocamide DEA, 25% free amine; CAS 61791-31-9; EINECS 263-163-9; anionic; foam stabilizer and solubilizer; liq.; 70% conc.

Manro CMEA. [Hickson Manro Ltd.] Cocamide MEA; CAS 68140-00-1; EINECS 268-770-2; anionic; foam booster/stabilizer for powd. and liq. detergents, hair shampoos; flake; 94% conc.

Manro ML 33. [Hickson Manro Ltd.] MEA-lauryl sulfate; CAS 4722-98-9; EINECS 225-214-3; anionic; foaming and wetting agent used in cosmetics and toiletries; biodeg.; pale yel. clear to slightly hazy visc. liq.; mild odor; sp.gr. 1.03; visc. 7500 cps; pH 6.3–7.3 (10% aq.); 32% act.

Manro NEC 28. [Hickson Manro Ltd.] Sodium laureth sulfate (2 mole), natural based; surfactant for hair care and bath prods.; liq.; 28% act.

Manro NEC 28H. [Hickson Manro Ltd.] Sodium laureth sulfate (2 mole), natural based; anionic; foaming agent, detergent for liq. and lotion hair shampoos; visc. liq.; 28% conc.

Manro NEC 28L. [Hickson Manro Ltd.] Sodium laureth sulfate (2 mole), natural based; anionic; foaming agent, detergent for liq. and lotion hair shampoos; liq.; 28% conc.

Manro NEC 70. [Hickson Manro Ltd.] Sodium laureth sulfate; anionic; foaming agent used in shampoos, bubble baths; biodeg.; pale yel. mobile gel; mild odor; sp.gr. 1.05; pH 6–7 (10% aq.); 68% act.

Manro NES 70. [Hickson Manro Ltd.] Sodium alkyl ether sulfate; anionic; surfactant for shampoos, bubble baths; liq.; 70% conc.

Manro PSC. [Hickson Manro Ltd.] Formulated blend; pearlized shampoo conc.; wh. opaque gel; 35% act.

Manro PSC 40. [Hickson Manro Ltd.] Formulated blend; pearlizing agent for hair care and bath prods.; wh. opaque gel; 40% act.

Manro SLS 28. [Hickson Manro Ltd.] Sodium lauryl sulfate; CAS 151-21-3; EINECS 205-788-1; anionic; foaming and wetting agent used in cosmetics, toiletries, emulsion polymerization, plastics, rubber, foam rubber, carpet and upholstery shampoos, industrial cleaning; biodeg.; very pale yel. clear liq.; mild odor; sp.gr. 1.04; visc. 200–7000 cps; pH 7–8 (10% aq.); 28% min. act.

Manro TDBS 60. [Hickson Manro Ltd.] TEA dodecylbenzene

sulfonate; CAS 27323-41-7; EINECS 248-406-9; anionic; mild detergent used in car shampoos, bubble baths, emulsion polymerization, household and industrial cleaners; amber clear visc. liq.; slight, alcoholic odor; sp.gr. 1.06; visc. 400 cps; pH 6.5–7.5 (10% aq.); 60% act.

Manro TL 40. [Hickson Manro Ltd.] TEA lauryl sulfate; CAS 139-96-8; EINECS 205-388-7; anionic; foaming and wetting agent used in shampoos, bubble baths, household detergents; biodeg.; pale yel. clear liq.; mild odor; sp.gr. 1.025; visc. 100 cps; pH 6.5–7.0 (10% aq.); 40% act.

Manro TMA 23. [Hickson Manro Ltd.] Mixed amine alkyl sulfate; anionic; surfactant for shampoos, bubble baths; liq.; 23% act.

Manromate LEO40. [Hickson Manro Ltd.] Sulfosuccinate half ester; surfactant for hair care and bath prods.; liq.; 40% act.

Manromate LNT40. [Hickson Manro Ltd.] Ammonium lauryl sulfosuccinate; anionic; high foaming, low irritating surfactant for shampoos, toiletries; liq.; 40% conc.

Manromid 150-ADY. [Hickson Manro Ltd.] Soyamide DEA (1:1); CAS 68425-47-8; EINECS 270-355-6; nonionic; thickener, emulsifier, corrosion inhibitor; for personal care prods., household and industrial cleaning, metalworking; liq.; 78% act.

Manromid 1224. [Hickson Manro Ltd.] Lauramide DEA; CAS 120-40-1; EINECS 204-393-1; nonionic; foam booster/ stabilizer for cosmetics and toiletries, household and industrial cleaning; liq.; 82% act.

Manromid AV150. [Hickson Manro Ltd.] Avocadamide DEA, avocado oil; nonionic; foam stabilizer, visc. builder, natural oil replacement for shampoos, creams, and lotions; liq.; 100% conc.

Manromid CD. [Hickson Manro Ltd.] Cocamide DEA (1:1); CAS 61791-31-9; EINECS 263-163-9; surfactant for personal care prods., household and industrial cleaning, metalworking; liq.; 92% act.

Manromid CDG. [Hickson Manro Ltd.] Cocamide DEA (1:1); CAS 61791-31-9; EINECS 263-163-9; surfactant for personal care prods., household and industrial cleaning; liq.; 78% act.

Manromid CDS. [Hickson Manro Ltd.] Cocamide DEA (1:1); CAS 61791-31-9; EINECS 263-163-9; surfactant for personal care prods., household and industrial cleaning; liq.; 85% act.

Manromid CMEA. [Hickson Manro Ltd.] Cocamide MEA (1:1); CAS 68140-00-1; EINECS 268-770-2; surfactant for hair care and bath prods., household and industrial cleaning; flake; 95% act.

Manromid LMA. [Hickson Manro Ltd.] Lauramide MEA (1:1); CAS 142-78-9; EINECS 205-560-1; nonionic; foam booster/stabilizer for solid or powd. detergents for household and industrial cleaning, hair care and bath prods.; flake; 95% act.

Manrosol AXS40. [Hickson Manro Ltd.] Ammonium xylene sulfonate; CAS 26447-10-9; EINECS 247-710-9; surfactant for hair care and bath prods., household detergents, and industrial cleaning; liq.; 40% act.

Manrosol SXS30. [Hickson Manro Ltd.] Sodium xylene sulfonate; CAS 1300-72-7; EINECS 215-090-9; anionic; hydrotrope for personal care prods., household and industrial cleaning; liq.; 30% act.

Manrosol SXS40. [Hickson Manro Ltd.] Sodium xylene sulfonate; CAS 1300-72-7; EINECS 215-090-9; anionic; hydrotrope for personal care prods., household and industrial cleaning; liq.; 40% act.

Manroteric 1202. [Hickson Manro Ltd.] Bis-2-hydroxyethyl tallow glycinate; amphoteric; conditioning agent for hair care prods.; visc. liq.; 40% act.

Manroteric CAB. [Hickson Manro Ltd.] Cocamidopropylbetaine; amphoteric; mild high foaming base surfactant for shampoos, bubble baths, household and industrial cleaning; liq.; 30% act.

Manroteric CDX38. [Hickson Manro Ltd.] Cocoamphocarboxy glycinate; CAS 68650-39-5; EINECS 272-043-5; amphoteric; mild detergent for personal care prods., household detergents; visc. liq.; 39% act.

Manroteric NAB. [Hickson Manro Ltd.] N-Alkyl dimethyl betaine; amphoteric; mild surfactant, foam booster for shampoos, household and industrial cleaners; liq.; 30% act.

Manroteric SAB. [Hickson Manro Ltd.] N-Alkyl dimethyl betaine; amphoteric; surfactant for personal care prods., household and industrial cleaners; liq.; 30% act.

Mapeg® 200 DL. [PPG/Specialty Chem.] PEG-4 dilaurate; CAS 9005-02-1; nonionic; emulsifier, spreading agent, and dispersant used in cosmetics, bath oils/salts, hair conditioners, skin care emulsions, pharmaceuticals, metalworking and fiber lubricants, etc.; yel. clear liq.; sol. in IPA, toluol, soybean and min. oil, water disp.; sp.gr. 0.95; m.p. 10 C; HLB 7.6; acid no. 10 max.; sapon. no. 176–192; flash pt. (PMCC) > 350 F; 100% conc.

Mapeg® 200 DO. [PPG/Specialty Chem.] PEG-4 dioleate; CAS 9005-07-6; nonionic; emulsifier, emollient, and dispersant used in cosmetics, bath oils, skin care emulsions, w/o formulations, pharmaceuticals, metalworking and fiber lubricants, etc.; yel. clear liq.; sol. in IPA, toluol, soybean and min. oil, water disp.; sp.gr. 0.95; m.p. < –10 C; HLB 6.0; acid no. 10 max.; sapon. no. 148–158; flash pt. (PMCC) > 350 F; 100% conc.

Mapeg® 200 DOT. [PPG/Specialty Chem.] PEG-4 ditallate; CAS 61791-01-3; nonionic; surfactant, emulsifier for metalworking lubricants; emollient for hair preps., creams and lotions; solubilizer for bath oils and fragrances; liq.; sol. in IPA, min. spirits, toluene, min. oil; disp. in water; sp.gr. 0.95; HLB 6.0; pour pt. –18 C; acid no. 10 max.; sapon. no. 150; flash pt. (PMCC) > 350 F.

Mapeg® 200 DS. [PPG/Specialty Chem.] PEG-4 distearate; CAS 9005-08-7; nonionic; emulsifier, dispersant used in cosmetics, pharmaceuticals, metalworking and fiber lubricants, etc.; wh. solid; sol. in IPA, toluol, soybean and min. oil; disp. in hot water; m.p. 34 C; HLB 4.7; acid no. 10 max.; sapon. no. 155–165; flash pt. (PMCC) > 350 F; 100% conc.

Mapeg® 200 ML. [PPG/Specialty Chem.] PEG-4 laurate; CAS 9004-81-3; nonionic; emulsifier, emollient, pigment dispersant used in cosmetics, creams, lotions, cuticle softeners, eye shadows, blushes, pharmaceuticals, metalworking and fiber lubricants, etc.; yel. clear liq.; sol. in IPA, toluol, soybean and min. oil, water disp.; sp.gr. 0.991; m.p. 5 C; HLB 9.3; acid no. 5 max.; sapon. no. 139–159; flash pt. (PMCC) > 350 F; 100% conc.

Mapeg® 200 MO. [PPG/Specialty Chem.] PEG-4 oleate; CAS 9004-96-0; EINECS 233-293-0; nonionic; emulsifier, dispersant used in cosmetics, pharmaceuticals, metalworking and fiber lubricants, etc.; yel. clear liq.; sol. in IPA, toluol, soybean oil; disp. hot in water; sp.gr. 0.97; m.p. < –10 C; HLB 8.3; acid no. 5 max.; sapon. no. 115–125; flash pt. (PMCC) > 350 F; 100% conc.

Mapeg® 200 MOT. [PPG/Specialty Chem.] PEG-4 tallate; CAS 61791-00-2; nonionic; emulsifier, dispersant used in cosmetics, pharmaceuticals, metalworking and fiber lubricants, etc.; liq.; sol. @ 5% in IPA, toluene; disp. in water, min. oil, min. spirits; sp.gr. 0.98; HLB 8.3; acid no. 5 max.; sapon. no. 120; pour pt. -22 C; flash pt. (PMCC) > 350 F; 100% conc.

Mapeg® 200 MS. [PPG/Specialty Chem.] PEG-4 stearate; CAS 9004-99-3; EINECS 203-358-8; nonionic; emulsifier, dispersant used in cosmetics, pharmaceuticals, metalworking and fiber lubricants, etc.; wh. solid; sol. in IPA, toluol, soybean oil; disp. hot in water; m.p. 33 C; HLB 8.0;

acid no. 5 max.; sapon. no. 120–130; flash pt. (PMCC) > 350 F; 100% conc.

Mapeg® 400 DL. [PPG/Specialty Chem.] PEG-8 dilaurate; CAS 9005-02-1; nonionic; emulsifier, dispersant used in cosmetics, hair grooms, conditioners, cleansing prods., bath oils, nail enamels, pharmaceuticals, metalworking and fiber lubricants, etc.; lt. yel. liq.; sol. in IPA, toluol, soybean oil, water disp.; sp.gr. 0.98; m.p. 18 C; HLB 10.8; acid no. 10 max.; sapon. no. 130–140; flash pt. (PMCC) > 350 F; 100% conc.

Mapeg® 400 DO. [PPG/Specialty Chem.] PEG-8 dioleate; CAS 9005-07-6; nonionic; emulsifier, emollient, and dispersant used in cosmetics, bubble baths, bath oils/salts, night creams, pharmaceuticals, metalworking and fiber lubricants, etc.; plasticizer for hairspray resins; yel. liq.; sol. in IPA, toluol, soybean and min. oil, water disp.; sp.gr. 0.98; m.p. < 7 C; HLB 8.8; acid no. 10 max.; sapon. no. 114–122; flash pt. (PMCC) > 350 F; 100% conc.

Mapeg® 400 DOT. [PPG/Specialty Chem.] PEG-8 ditallate; CAS 61791-01-3; nonionic; emulsifier, dispersant used in cosmetics, pharmaceuticals, metalworking and fiber lubricants, etc.; liq.; sol. @ 5% in IPA, min. spirits, toluene, min. oil; disp. in water; sp.gr. 0.98; HLB 8.8; acid no. 10 max.; sapon. no. 118; pour pt. 6 C; flash pt. (PMCC) > 350 F; 100% conc.

Mapeg® 400 DS. [PPG/Specialty Chem.] PEG-8 distearate; CAS 9005-08-7; nonionic; emulsifier, dispersant used in cosmetics, hair conditioners, hair coloring prods., skin lotions, cleansing prods., pharmaceuticals, metalworking and fiber lubricants, etc.; provides high visc. and opacity; wh. solid; sol. in IPA, toluol, soybean and min. oil, hot water disp.; m.p. 36 C; HLB 8.1; acid no. 10 max.; sapon. no. 116–125; flash pt. (PMCC) > 350 F; 100% conc.

Mapeg® 400 ML. [PPG/Specialty Chem.] PEG-8 laurate; CAS 9004-81-3; nonionic; emulsifier and dispersant used in cosmetics, hair grooms, conditioners, cleansing prods., bath oils, nail enamels, pharmaceuticals, metalworking and fiber lubricants, etc.; lt. yel., liq.; sol. in IPA, toluol, water; disp. in min. spirits; sp.gr. 1.01; m.p. 12 C; HLB 13.2; acid no. 5 max.; sapon. no. 89–96; flash pt. (PMCC) > 350 F; 100% conc.

Mapeg® 400 MO. [PPG/Specialty Chem.] PEG-8 oleate; CAS 9004-96-0; nonionic; emulsifier, spreading agent, dispersant used in cosmetics, bath oils, cleansing prods., creams, lotions, pharmaceuticals, metalworking and fiber lubricants, etc.; yel. liq.; sol. in IPA, toluol, soybean oil, water disp.; sp.gr. 1.01; m.p. < 10 C; HLB 11.8; acid no. 5 max.; sapon. no. 80–88; flash pt. (PMCC) > 350 F; 100% conc.

Mapeg® 400 MOT. [PPG/Specialty Chem.] PEG-8 tallate; CAS 61791-00-2; nonionic; emulsifier, dispersant used in cosmetics, pharmaceuticals, metalworking and fiber lubricants, etc.; liq.; sol. @ 5% in IPA, toluene; disp. in water, min. spirits, min. oil; sp.gr. 1.01; HLB 11.8; acid no. 5 max.; sapon. no. 84; pour pt. 5 C; flash pt. (PMCC) > 350 F; 100% conc.

Mapeg® 400 MS. [PPG/Specialty Chem.] PEG-8 stearate; CAS 9004-99-3; nonionic; emulsifier, dispersant used in cosmetics, hair conditioners, hair coloring prods., skin lotions, cleansing prods., pharmaceuticals, metalworking and fiber lubricants, etc.; provides high visc. and opacity; wh. solid; sol. in IPA, toluol, soybean oil, hot water disp.; m.p. 33 C; HLB 11.5; acid no. 5 max.; sapon. no. 84–93; flash pt. (PMCC) > 350 F; 100% conc.

Mapeg® 600 DL. [PPG/Specialty Chem.] PEG-12 dilaurate; CAS 9005-02-1; nonionic; dispersant and emulsifier for metalworking lubricants, fiber lubricants and softeners, solubilizers, defoamers, antistats, cosmetics, pharmaceuticals, and chemical intermediates; lt. yel. semisolid; sol. in IPA, toluol, soybean oil; partly sol. min. oil; disp.

water; sp.gr. 0.99; HLB 12.2; m.p. 24 C; acid no. 10 max.; sapon. no. 102–112; flash pt. (PMCC) > 350 F.

Mapeg® 600 DO. [PPG/Specialty Chem.] PEG-12 dioleate; CAS 9005-07-6; nonionic; emulsifier, dispersant used in cosmetics, pharmaceuticals, metalworking and fiber lubricants, etc.; yel. liq.; sol. in IPA, toluol, soybean oil, water disp.; sp.gr. 1.00; m.p. 20 C; HLB 10.3; acid no. 10 max.; sapon. no. 92–102; flash pt. (PMCC) > 350 F; 100% conc.

Mapeg® 600 DOT. [PPG/Specialty Chem.] PEG-12 ditallate; CAS 61791-01-3; nonionic; dispersant and emulsifier for metalworking lubricants, fiber lubricants and softeners, solubilizers, defoamers, antistats, cosmetics, pharmaceuticals, and chemical intermediates; amber liq.; sol. IPA, toluol, soybean oil; disp. water; sp.gr. 1.00; HLB 10.3; m.p. 15 C; acid no. 10 max.; sapon. no. 85–95; flash pt. (PMCC) > 350 F; 100% conc.

Mapeg® 600 DS. [PPG/Specialty Chem.] PEG-12 distearate; CAS 9005-08-7; nonionic; emulsifier, dispersant used in cosmetics, hair conditioners, cleansing prods., shaving creams, makeup bases, pharmaceuticals, metalworking and fiber lubricants, etc.; wh. solid or flake; sol. in IPA, toluol, soybean oil, hot water disp.; m.p. 41 C; HLB 10.6; acid no. 10 max.; sapon. no. 94–104; flash pt. (PMCC) > 350 F; 100% conc.

Mapeg® 600 ML. [PPG/Specialty Chem.] PEG-12 laurate; CAS 9004-81-3; nonionic; dispersant and emulsifier for metalworking lubricants, fiber lubricants and softeners, solubilizers, defoamers, antistats, cosmetics, pharmaceuticals, and chemical intermediates; lt. yel. liq.; sol. in water, IPA, toluol; sp.gr. 1.02; HLB 14.8; m.p. 23 C; acid no. 5 max.; sapon. no. 64–74; flash pt. (PMCC) > 350 F.

Mapeg® 600 MO. [PPG/Specialty Chem.] PEG-12 oleate; CAS 9004-96-0; nonionic; emulsifier, dispersant used in cosmetics, pharmaceuticals, metalworking and fiber lubricants, etc.; yel. liq.; sol. in IPA, toluol, soybean oil, water; sp.gr. 1.03; m.p. 25 C; HLB 13.6; acid no. 5 max.; sapon. no. 60–70; flash pt. (PMCC) > 350 F; 100% conc.

Mapeg® 600 MOT. [PPG/Specialty Chem.] PEG-12 tallate; CAS 61791-00-2; nonionic; emulsifier, dispersant used in cosmetics, pharmaceuticals, metalworking and fiber lubricants, etc.; visc. 175 cps; HLB 13.6.

Mapeg® 600 MS. [PPG/Specialty Chem.] PEG-12 stearate; CAS 9004-99-3; nonionic; emulsifier, dispersant used in cosmetics, hair conditioners, cleansing prods., shaving creams, makeup bases, pharmaceuticals, metalworking and fiber lubricants, etc.; wh. solid; sol. in IPA, toluol, soybean oil, water, propylene glycol; disp. hot in min. oil; m.p. 36 C; HLB 13.6; acid no. 5 max.; sapon. no. 62–70; flash pt. (PMCC) > 350 F; 100% conc.

Mapeg® 1000 MS. [PPG/Specialty Chem.] PEG-20 stearate; CAS 9004-99-3; nonionic; emulsifier, dispersant used in cosmetics, pharmaceuticals, metalworking and fiber lubricants, etc.; wh. solid or flake; sol. in IPA, toluol, propylene glycol, water; m.p. 42 C; HLB 15.7; acid no. 5; sapon. no. 41–49; flash pt. (PMCC) > 350 F; 100% conc.

Mapeg® 1500 MS. [PPG/Specialty Chem.] PEG-6-32 stearate; CAS 9004-99-3; nonionic; emulsifier, dispersant used in cosmetics, pharmaceuticals, metalworking and fiber lubricants, etc.; solid; sol. @ 5% in water, IPA, toluene, propylene glycol; disp. in min. spirits; HLB 16.1; pour pt. 37 C; acid no. 5 max.; sapon. no. 62; flash pt. (PMCC) > 350 F; 100% conc.

Mapeg® 1540 DS. [PPG/Specialty Chem.] PEG-32 distearate; CAS 9005-08-7; nonionic; emulsifier, dispersant used in cosmetics, pharmaceuticals, metalworking and fiber lubricants, etc.; wh. solid or flake; sol. in IPA, toluol, soybean oil, propylene glycol, water; m.p. 45 C; HLB 14.8; acid no. 10 max.; sapon. no. 49–58; flash pt. (PMCC) > 350 F; 100% conc.

Mapeg® 6000 DS. [PPG/Specialty Chem.] PEG-150 distearate; CAS 9005-08-7; nonionic; emulsifier, thickener, dispersant used in mild cosmetics, baby shampoos, bubble baths, shower gels, pharmaceuticals, metalworking and fiber lubricants, etc.; wh. solid or flake; sol. in IPA, toluol, propylene glycol, water; m.p. 55 C; HLB 18.4; acid no. 9 max.; sapon. no. 14–20; flash pt. (PMCC) > 350 F; 100% conc.

Mapeg® CO-16H. [PPG/Specialty Chem.] PEG-16 hydrog. castor oil; CAS 61788-85-0; nonionic; surfactant, emulsifier, dispersant, wetting agent, emollient for hair preps., creams and lotions; solubilizer for bath oils and fragrances; liq.; sol. in toluene, min. oil; disp. in water, IPA, min. spirits; sp.gr. 1.010; HLB 8.6; pour pt. 7 C; acid no. 2 max.; sapon. no. 105; flash pt. (PMCC) > 350 F; 100% conc.

Mapeg® CO-25. [PPG/Specialty Chem.] PEG-25 castor oil; CAS 61791-12-6; nonionic; surfactant; solubilizer, coupling agent for oils, solvs., waxes; for cosmetic, paper, metalworking fluid, and emulsion polymerization; liq.; sol. @ 5% in IPA; disp. in water, min. spirits, toluene; sp.gr. 1.040; HLB 10.8; acid no. 2 max.; sapon. no. 83; pour pt. 5 C; flash pt. (PMCC) > 350 F.

Mapeg® CO-25H. [PPG/Specialty Chem.] PEG-25 hydrog. castor oil; CAS 61788-85-0; nonionic; surfactant for formulation of gels; solubilizer, coupling agent; for cosmetic, paper, metalworking fluids, and emulsion polymerization; liq.; sol. @ 5% in IPA, toluene, min. oil; disp. in water, min. spirits; sp.gr. 1.040; HLB 10.8; acid no. 2 max.; sapon. no. 82; pour pt. 5 C; flash pt. (PMCC) > 350 F; 100% conc.

Mapeg® CO-30. [PPG/Specialty Chem.] PEG-30 castor oil; CAS 61791-12-6; nonionic; surfactant, emulsifier, emollient for hair preps., creams and lotions; solubilizer for bath oils and fragrances; liq.; sol. in water, IPA, toluene; sp.gr. 1.046; HLB 11.8; pour pt. 9 C; acid no. 2 max.; sapon. no. 75; flash pt. (PMCC) > 350 F.

Mapeg® CO-36. [PPG/Specialty Chem.] PEG-36 castor oil; CAS 61791-12-6; nonionic; surfactant, emulsifier, emollient for hair preps., creams and lotions; solubilizer for bath oils and fragrances; liq.; sol. in water, IPA, toluene; sp.gr. 1.055; HLB 12.6; pour pt. 12 C; acid no. 2 max.; sapon. no. 73; flash pt. (PMCC) > 350 F.

Mapeg® CO-200. [PPG/Specialty Chem.] PEG-200 castor oil; CAS 61791-12-6; nonionic; surfactant, emulsifier, emollient for hair preps., creams and lotions; solubilizer for bath oils and fragrances; solid; sol. in water, IPA; HLB 18.1; pour pt. 50 C; acid no. 2 max.; sapon. no. 17.5; flash pt. (PMCC) > 350 F.

Mapeg® EGDS. [PPG/Specialty Chem.] Glycol distearate; CAS 627-83-8; EINECS 211-014-3; nonionic; emulsifier, thickener, opacifier, pearling additive, and dispersant used in cosmetics, shampoos, bubble baths, hair conditioners, pharmaceuticals, metalworking and fiber lubricants, etc.; wh. solid or flake; sol. in IPA, toluol, soybean and min. oil; disp. in min. spirits; m.p. 63 C; HLB 1.4; acid no. 6 max.; sapon. no. 190–199; flash pt. (PMCC) > 350 F; 100% conc.

Mapeg® EGMS. [PPG/Specialty Chem.] Glycol stearate; CAS 111-60-4; EINECS 203-886-9; nonionic; emulsifier, thickener, opacifier, pearling additive, and dispersant used in cosmetics, shampoos, bubble baths, hair conditioners, pharmaceuticals, metalworking and fiber lubricants, etc.; wh. to cream solid or flake; sol. @ 5% in IPA, toluol, soybean and min. oil; disp. in min. spirits; m.p. 56 C; HLB 2.9; acid no. 4 max.; sapon. no. 180–188; flash pt. (PMCC) > 350 F; 100% conc.

Mapeg® EGMS-K. [PPG/Specialty Chem.] Ethylene glycol monostearate; CAS 111-60-4; EINECS 203-886-9; emulsifier, dispersant; flake; 100% conc.

Mapeg® S-40. [PPG/Specialty Chem.] PEG-40 stearate; CAS 9004-99-3; nonionic; emulsifier, dispersant used in cosmetics, pharmaceuticals, metalworking and fiber lubricants, etc.; wh. solid or flake; sol. in IPA, toluol, propylene glycol, water; m.p. 48 C; HLB 17.2; acid no. 1 max.; sapon. no. 25–35; flash pt. (PMCC) > 350 F; 100% conc.

Mapeg® S-40K. [PPG/Specialty Chem.] PEG-40 stearate, kosher; CAS 9004-99-3; nonionic; hydrophilic emulsifier for skin care emulsions and hair grooms; emulsifier for defoamer formulations; Gardner 2 max. flake; congeal pt. 37-47 C; HLB 17.2; acid no. 1 max.; sapon. no. 25-35; hyd. no. 27-40; 100% conc.

Mapeg® S-100. [PPG/Specialty Chem.] PEG-100 stearate; CAS 9004-99-3; nonionic; surfactant, emulsifier, emollient for hair preps., creams and lotions; solubilizer for bath oils and fragrances; flake; sol. in water, IPA, toluene, propylene glycol; disp. in min. spirits; HLB 18.7; pour pt. 50 C; acid no. 1 max.; sapon. no. 16; flash pt. (PMCC) > 350 F.

Mapeg® S-150. [PPG/Specialty Chem.] PEG-150 stearate; CAS 9004-99-3; nonionic; surfactant, emulsifier, emollient for hair preps., creams and lotions; solubilizer for bath oils and fragrances; flake; sol. @ 5% in water, IPA, toluene, propylene glycol; disp. in min. spirits; HLB 19.0; pour pt. 51 C; acid no. 1 max.; sapon. no. 9.5; flash pt. (PMCC) > 350 F.

Mapeg® TAO-15. [PPG/Specialty Chem.] PEG-660 tallate; CAS 61791-00-2; nonionic; emulsifier, dispersant used in cosmetics, pharmaceuticals, metalworking and fiber lubricants, etc.; clear amber liq.; sol. in IPA, toluol, water; sp.gr. 1.03; m.p. 20 C; HLB 13.8; acid no. 5 max.; sapon. no. 55–65; flash pt. (PMCC) > 350 F; 100% conc.

Maprosyl® 30. [Stepan; Stepan Canada] Sodium n-lauroyl sarcosinate; CAS 137-16-6; EINECS 205-281-5; anionic; detergent, wetting and foaming agent used in personal care and household detergent prods.; anticorrosive props.; liq.; sp.gr. 1.03; flash pt. > 200 F; 30% act.

Maquat 4450-E. [Mason] Didecyl dimonium chloride; CAS 7173-51-5; EINECS 230-525-2; disinfectants, algicides, sanitizers, deodorant; 50% quat.

Maquat LC-12S-50%. [Mason] Benzalkonium chloride; antimicrobial; sol. in water, polar solvs.; 50% act.

Maquat SC-18. [Mason] Stearalkonium chloride; CAS 122-19-0; EINECS 204-527-9; germicide with good wetting and penetration; paste, flake, or powd.; 25% , 85% and 94% act. resp.

Maquat SC-1632. [Mason] Cetearyl alcohol, PEG-40 castor oil, stearalkonium chloride; germicide with good wetting and penetration; sol. in water, polar solvs

Maricol CLR. [Dr. Kurt Richter] Soluble collagen; CAS 9007-34-5; EINECS 232-697-4; moisturizing protein forming skin protective film for treatment of dry or aging skin or skin damaged by light or environmental influences; colorless to sl. ylsh. visc. liq., faint char. odor; sol. in water or water-alcohol mixts.; dens. 1.010 g/ml; ref. index 1.337; pH 3.8; usage level 3-10%; toxicology: LD50 (oral, rat) > 2000 mg/kg; nonirritating to eyes; low skin irritation.

Marinco H-USP. [Marine Magnesium] Magnesium hydroxide USP, FCC; CAS 1309-42-8; EINECS 215-170-3; antacid and alkaline buffer for milk of magnesia tablets and for making magnesium citrate; wh. free-flowing powd.; 99% min. thru 325 mesh; bulk dens. 25-33 lb/ft^3.

Marinco OH. [Marine Magnesium] Magnesium oxide USP, FCC; CAS 1309-48-4; EINECS 215-171-9; antacid, alkaline buffer, and mineral supplement; wh. free-flowing powd.; 99.5% min. thru 325 mesh; bulk dens. (loose) 18-26 lb/ft^3.

Marinco OL. [Marine Magnesium] Magnesium oxide; CAS 1309-48-4; EINECS 215-171-9; antacid and alkaline buffer; lt. powd.

Marine Dew. [Ajinomoto; Ajinomoto USA] Partially deacetylated chitin, derived from marine sources; CAS

1398-61-4; EINECS 215-744-3; cationic; high m.w. humectant for skin care creams and lotions, hair treatment and styling prods.; visc. builder, film-former; prevents water evaporation.

Marine Native Collagen. [Seporga] A soluble collagen derived from fish skins, containing 18 amino acids; cosmetics ingred.

Marine Plasma Extract. [Brooks Industries] Hydrolyzed marine protein, brown algae extract, marine plasma fluid, iodine, silicon, iron, sodium, potassium, magnesium, calcium, ascorbic acid, niacinamide; sea plasma extract containing essential elements for development of ocean life.

Marine Plasma Extract I. [Brooks Industries] Hydrolyzed marine protein, brown algae extract, marine plasma fluid, iodine, silicon, iron, sodium, potassium, magnesium, calcium, ascorbic acid, niacinamide; cosmetic ingred.; 10% act.

Mark® 5095. [Witco/Argus] Lauryl/stearyl thiodipropionate; antioxidant for polyolefins and other polymeric systems incl. syn. rubber; also for pharmaceuticals, cosmetics, industrial oils, greases, lubricants; FDA regulated; wh. free-flowing powd.

Marlamid® D 1218. [Hüls Am.; Hüls AG] Cocamide DEA; CAS 61791-31-9; EINECS 263-163-9; nonionic; foam stabilizer, thickener, superfatting agent for liq. detergents, shampoos; increases soil suspending power in felting auxiliaries; liq.; 100% conc.

Marlamid® D 1885. [Hüls Am.; Hüls AG] Oleamide DEA; CAS 93-83-4; EINECS 202-281-7; nonionic; foam stabilizer, thickener, superfatting agent for liq. detergents, shampoos; liq.; water-sol.; 100% act.

Marlamid® DF 1218. [Hüls Am.; Hüls AG] Cocamide DEA; CAS 61790-63-4; EINECS 263-163-9; nonionic; foam stabilizer, thickener, superfatting agent for hair shampoos, foam baths, shower foams, liq. soaps; yel. clear liq.; water-sol; visc. 450 mPa·s; clear pt. 10 C max.; acid no. 5 max.; pH 10 (1% aq.); 100% act.

Marlamid® DF 1818. [Hüls Am.; Hüls AG] Soyamide DEA; CAS 68425-47-8; EINECS 270-355-6; nonionic; foam stabilizer, thickener, superfatting agent for liq. soaps, hair shampoos, foam baths; yel. clear liq.; visc. 1000 mPa·s; clear pt. 10 C max.; acid no. 5 max.; pH 10 (1% aq.); 100% act.

Marlamid® KL. [Hüls Am.; Hüls AG] Cocamidopropyl lauryl ether; nonionic; pearlescent surfactant, silk luster agent, foam stabilizer, thickener, opacifier for liq. and paste detergents, hair shampoos, foam baths, liq. soaps; ylsh. flakes; insol. in water; solid. pt. 55 C; 100% conc.

Marlamid® KLA. [Hüls Am.] Fatty acid alkylolamide and fatty alcohol ether sulfate; nonionic; pearlescent surfactant for personal care prods.; liq.; 40% conc.

Marlamid® KLP. [Hüls Am.; Hüls AG] Cocamidopropyl lauryl ether, sodium laureth sulfate; anionic/nonionic; pumpable pearlescent base for shampoos, bubble baths, liq. soaps; mother-of-pearl wh. free-flowing paste; visc. 1500 mPa·s max. (30 C); solid. pt. 0 C; pH 6.5-7.5 (1% aq.); 30-31% act.

Marlamid® M 1218. [Hüls Am.; Hüls AG] Cocamide MEA; CAS 68140-00-1; EINECS 268-770-2; nonionic; foam stabilizer, superfatting agent, and thickener in household, personal care, and industrial detergents; ylsh. flake; water-insol.; acid no. 6 max.; pH 9 (1% aq.); 100% act.

Marlamid® M 1618. [Hüls Am.; Hüls AG] Tallowamide MEA; CAS 68153-63-9; nonionic; foam stabilizer, thickener for household, personal, and industrial detergents; consistency-providing component for cosmetics sticks (lipsticks); pale yel. flakes; acid no. 5 max.; pH 8 (1% aq.); 100% act.

Marlamid® PG 20. [Hüls Am.; Hüls AG] Cocamide MEA,

glycol ditallowate; nonionic; pumpable pearlescent base for shampoos, bubble baths, liq. soaps; mother-of-pearl luster wh. free-flowing paste; visc. 3000 mPa8s (30 C); pH 6-7 (1% aq.); 21-23% act.

Marlazin® KC 21/50. [Hüls Am.; Hüls AG] Cocoalkonium chloride; CAS 61789-71-7; EINECS 263-080-8; cationic; bactericide, conditioner for hair care prods. with good antistatic props.; improves wet and dry combability; prod. of disinfectant cleaning agents; clear liq.; visc. 20 mPa·s; pH 6-8 (1% aq.); 47-48% act.

Marlazin® KC 30/50. [Hüls Am.; Hüls AG] Cocotrimonium chloride; CAS 61789-18-2; EINECS 263-038-9; cationic; surfactant, conditioner, antistat for hair care prods.; improves wet and dry combability and of hair; clear liq.; visc. 20 mPa·s; pH 6-8 (1% aq.); 47-48% act.

Marlinat® 24/28. [Hüls AG] Anionic; surfactant for detergents, cleaners, cosmetics.

Marlinat® 24/70. [Hüls AG] Anionic; surfactant for detergents, cleaners, cosmetics.

Marlinat® 242/28. [Hüls Am.; Hüls AG] Sodium laureth (2) sulfate; CAS 9004-82-4; anionic; strongly foaming base surfactant for detergents, shampoos, liq. soaps, foam baths; colorless clear liq.; visc. 25 mPa·s; clear pt. 20 C max.; pH 7-8 (1% aq.); 27-28% act.

Marlinat® 242/70. [Hüls Am.; Hüls AG] Sodium laureth (2 EO) sulfate; CAS 9004-82-4; anionic; strongly foaming base surfactant for detergents, shampoos, liq. soaps, foam baths; pale yel. free-flowing paste; pH 7-9 (1% aq.); 68-70% act.

Marlinat® 242/70 S. [Hüls AG] Sodium laureth (2 EO) sulfate; CAS 9004-82-4; anionic; strongly foaming base surfactant for detergents, shampoos, liq. soaps; dioxane content < 10 ppm; liq./paste; 70% act.

Marlinat® 243/28. [Hüls Am.; Hüls AG] Sodium laureth (3) sulfate; CAS 9004-82-4; anionic; strong foaming base surfactant for detergents, shampoos, foam baths, liq. soaps, cleaners; pale yel. clear liq.; visc. 100-300 mPa·s; clear pt. 20 C max.; pH 6.5-7.5 (1% aq.); 27-28% act.

Marlinat® 243/70. [Hüls Am.; Hüls AG] Sodium laureth (3) sulfate; CAS 9004-82-4; anionic; strongly foaming base surfactant for detergents, shampoos, foam baths, liq. soaps, cleaners; pale yel. free-flowing paste; pH 6-8 (1% aq.); 68-70% act.

Marlinat® CM 20. [Hüls Am.; Hüls AG] Laureth-3 carboxylic acid; anionic; surfactant for mild detergents, shampoos, cleaners; liq.; 90% act.

Marlinat® CM 40. [Hüls Am.; Hüls AG] Laureth-5 carboxylic acid; anionic; surfactant for mild detergents, shampoos, foam baths, liq. soaps, cleaners; good emulsifying and foaming props.; insensitive to water hardness; pale yel. clear to sl. cloudy liq.; visc. 200 mPa·s; clear pt. 18 C; pH 2.5-3 (1% aq.); 88-90% act.

Marlinat® CM 45. [Hüls Am.; Hüls AG] Sodium laureth-5 carboxylate; CAS 33939-64-9; anionic; surfactant for prod. of very mild detergents, hair shampoos, foam baths, liq. soaps; good emulsifying and foaming props.; insensitive to water hardness; colorless clear liq.; visc. 30 mPa·s; clear pt. 10 C max.; pH 6-7 (1% aq.); 21-23% act.

Marlinat® CM 100. [Hüls Am.; Hüls AG] Laureth-11 carboxylic acid; CAS 27306-90-7; anionic; surfactant for mild detergents, shampoos, foam baths, shower foams, liq. soaps, cleaners; good emulsifying and foaming props.; insensitive to water hardness; colorless clear to sl. cloudy liq.; visc. 300 mPa·s; clear pt. 11 C; pH 2.5-3 (1% aq.); 85-90% act.

Marlinat® CM 105. [Hüls Am.; Hüls AG] Sodium laureth-11 carboxylate; CAS 33939-64-9; anionic; surfactant for prod. of very mild detergents, hair shampoos, foam baths, liq. soaps, baby prods., sensitive skin formulations; good emulsifying and foaming props.; insensitive to water hardness; colorless clear liq.; visc. 100 mPa·s; clear pt. 4 C max.; pH 6-7 (1% aq.); 21-23% act.

Marlinat® DF 8. [Hüls Am.; Hüls AG] Dioctyl sodium sulfosuccinate; CAS 577-11-7; EINECS 209-406-4; anionic; highly act. wetting agent for textile, paint and paper industries; used in cleaners, cosmetic preparations; liq.; 65% act.

Marlinat® DFK 30. [Hüls Am.; Hüls AG] Sodium lauryl sulfate; CAS 151-21-3; EINECS 205-788-1; anionic; base surfactant for hair shampoos, foam baths, shower foams, liq. soaps; good foam and detergent props.; pale yel. pasty liq.; pH 7-8 (1% aq.); 29-31% act.

Marlinat® DFL 40. [Hüls AG] TEA-lauryl sulfate; CAS 139-96-8; EINECS 205-388-7; anionic; finely porous foaming base surfactant for prod. of hair shampoos, foam baths, shower foams, and liq. soaps; ≈ 90% biodeg.; ylsh. clear liq.; dens. 1.05 g/ml; visc. 50 mPa·s; set pt. < 0 C; clear pt. 13 C; pH 6-7 (1% aq.); 39-41% act.

Marlinat® DFN 30. [Hüls Am.; Hüls AG] Ammonium lauryl sulfate; CAS 2235-54-3; EINECS 218-793-9; anionic; base surfactant for hair shampoos, foam baths, shower foams, liq. soaps; ylsh. clear liq.; visc. 800 mPa·s; clear pt. 15 C; 26-27% act.

Marlinat® KT 50. [Hüls Am.; Hüls AG] Sodium tallow sulfate, sodium coco-sulfate; anionic; surfactant for prod. of handwashing pastes; paste; 50% act.

Marlinat® SL 3/40. [Hüls Am.; Hüls AG] Disodium laureth sulfosuccinate; anionic; base surfactant for hair shampoos, foam baths, shower foams, liq. soaps, baby and child care prods.; colorless clear liq.; visc. 500 mPa·s; clear pt. 12 C; pH 6.5-7.5 (1% aq.); 32-34% act.

Marlinat® SRN 30. [Hüls Am.; Hüls AG] Disodium lauramido MEA-sulfosuccinate, sodium C12-14 olefin sulfonate; anionic; mild base surfactant for prod. of strongly foaming hair shampoos, foam baths, liq. soaps, carpet and upholstery cleaners; good stability in hard water; ylsh. clear to sl. cloudy liq.; visc. 50 mPa·s max.; clear pt. 2 C max.; pH 5.5-7.0 (1% aq.); 30-33% act.

Marlipal® 24/300. [Hüls Am.; Hüls AG] Laureth-30; CAS 9002-92-0; nonionic; dispersant, wetting agent, emulsifier, detergent for washing, cleaning, soil suspension, textiles; waxy solid; HLB 17.4; cloud pt. 76 C (2% in 10% NaCl); 100% act.

Marlipal® 124. [Hüls Am.; Hüls AG] Laureth-4; CAS 9002-92-0; EINECS 226-097-1; nonionic; surfactant for cosmetics, textile aux. agents; solubilizer for oils and perfumes; liq.; HLB 9.7; cloud pt. 68 C (10% in 25% BDG); 100% act.

Marlipal® 129. [Hüls Am.; Hüls AG] Laureth-9; CAS 3055-99-0; EINECS 221-284-4; nonionic; surfactant; solubilizer for oils and perfumes; paste; sol. in oil and water; cloud pt. 71 C (2% aq.); 100% act.

Marlipal® 1012/4. [Hüls Am.] Deceth-4; nonionic; wetting surfactant, esp. for hard surf. cleaning; liq.; cloud pt. 66 C (2% in 10% NaCl); 100% act.

Marlipal® 1618/11. [Hüls Am.; Hüls AG] Ceteareth-11; CAS 68439-49-6; nonionic; dispersant; prod. of powd. detergents; binding agent and base material for solid cleaning agents (toilet sticks); coating material for foam suppressant, enzymes, etc.; dyeing auxiliaries; waxy solid; HLB 13.1; cloud pt. 87 C (2% aq.); 100% act.

Marlipal® 1885/2. [Hüls Am.] Oleth-2; CAS 9004-98-2; emulsifier, emollient.

Marlipal® FS. [Hüls Am.] PEG-12 dioleate; CAS 9005-07-6; nonionic; surfactant used for liq. and paste detergents, esp. hair shampoos, cosmetic preparations; liq.; 100% act.

Marlipal® MG. [Hüls Am.; Hüls AG] Laureth-7; CAS 9002-92-0; EINECS 221-283-9; nonionic; solubilizer for act. ingreds. and oils in cosmetics; liq.; cloud pt. 62 C (2% aq.); 100% act.

Marlon® AFR. [Hüls Am.] Sodium dodecylbenzene sulfonate, modified with urea; CAS 25155-30-0; EINECS 246-680-4; anionic; base material for dishwashing agents, cosmetic detergents, car shampoos; liq.; 30% act.

Marlon® AS3. [Hüls Am.; Hüls AG] Dodecylbenzene sulfonic acid; CAS 85536-14-7; anionic; intermediate for mfg. of anionic surfactants, detergents, sulfonates, textile auxiliaries; biodeg.; liq.; 98% act.

Marlon® PF 40. [Hüls Am.; Hüls AG] Sodium C13-17 alkane sulfonate, sodium laureth sulfate; anionic/nonionic; mild, high foaming detergent for domestic and industrial applics. and personal care prods.; substantially insensitive to hard water; biodeg.; pale yel. clear liq.; visc. 2000 mPa·s max.; clear pt. 15 C max.; pH 7-8 (1% aq.); 39-40% act.

Marlon® PS 30. [Hüls Am.; Hüls AG] Sodium C13-17 alkane sulfonate; anionic; surfactant for prod. of liq., conc., mild cleaning agents, hair shampoos, foam baths, liq. soaps, and textile auxiliaries; sl. ylsh. clear liq.; visc. 300 mPa·s max.; clear pt. 26 C max.; pH 7-8 (1% aq.); 29.5-30.5% act.

Marlon® PS 60. [Hüls Am.; Hüls AG] Sodium C13-17 alkane sulfonate; anionic; base for detergents, cleaners, hair shampoos, foam baths, liq. soaps, textile auxiliaries; pale yel. free-flowing paste; pH 7-8 (1% aq.); 59.5-60.5% act.

Marlon® PS 65. [Hüls Am.; Hüls AG] Sodium C13-17 alkane sulfonate; anionic; mfg. of liq. conc. cleaners, hair shampoos, foam baths, liq. soaps, textile auxiliaries; pale yel. free-flowing paste; pH 7-8 (1% aq.); 64.5-65.5% act.

Marlophor® LN-Acid. [Hüls Am.; Hüls AG] Trilauryl phosphate; anionic; wetting agent, antistat, conditioning base for textile, paper, and personal care industries; improves dry combability of hair; drycleaning detergent; pale yel. pasty wax; solid. pt. 30-35 C; acid no. 215-235; pH 1.5-2.0 (1% aq.); 100% conc.

Marlophor® MO 3-Acid. [Hüls Am.; Hüls AG] Laureth-3 phosphate; CAS 39464-66-9; anionic; surfactant for prod. of textile and dyeing auxiliaries, antistats, drycleaning detergents; conditioning base for hair shampoos and hair care preps.; improves dry combability of hair; antistat; pale yel. clear liq.; solid. pt. 18 C; acid no. 150-170; pH 2.5-3.0 (1% aq.); 100% act.

Marlophor® T10-Acid. [Hüls Am.; Hüls AG] Diceteareth-10 phospate; anionic; special liq. formulation for prod. of drycleaning detergents with antistatic props., textile and dyeing auxiliaries; o/w emulsifier for cosmetic creams, lotions, and gels; pale yel. solid; solid pt. 35 C; acid no. 65-70; pH 1.5-2.0 (1% aq.); 100% act.

Marlophor® T10-Sodium Salt. [Hüls Am.; Hüls AG] Sodium diceteareth-10 phosphate; anionic; special liq. formulation for prod. of drycleaning detergents; o/w emulsifier for cosmetic creams, lotions, and gels; pale yel. solid; solid. pt. 30-40 C; pH 6.5-7.5 (1% aq.); 100% act.

Marlopon® AMS 60. [Hüls Am.; Hüls AG] Amine dodecylbenzene sulfonate/nonionic blend; anionic/nonionic; surfactant used for detergents, dishwashing agents, industrial cleaners, car shampoos, hand cleaners; fluid paste; 60% act.

Marlopon® AT. [Hüls Am.] TEA-dodecylbenzene sulfonate.; CAS 29381-93-9; surfactant for mfg. of cosmetic detergents, dishwashing agents.

Marlopon® AT 50. [Hüls Am.; Hüls AG] TEA-dodecylbenzene sulfonate; CAS 68411-31-4; anionic; surfactant with fine-bubble foam used as neutral detergent base; for hair and bath shampoos, dishwashes, car shampoos, toilet preps.; biodeg.; ylsh. clear liq.; visc. 1800-2500 mPa·s; clear pt. 5 C max.; pH 7-8 (1% aq.); 51-53% act.

Marlopon® CA. [Hüls Am.; Hüls AG] TEA-dodecylbenzene sulfonate, modified; CAS 27323-41-7; EINECS 248-406-9; anionic; detergent; superfatting and dishwashing agent; personal care prods.; liq.; 60% act.

Marlosol® 183. [Hüls Am.; Hüls AG] PEG-3 stearate; CAS 9004-99-3; EINECS 233-562-2; nonionic; raw material for finishing agents in the syn. fiber industry; w/o emulsifier and o/w coemulsifier for cosmetic creams and lotions; superfatting agent for shaving preps. and foam baths; pale yel. waxy solid; water-insol.; visc. 20 mPa·s (50 C); solid. pt. 40 C; HLB 6.4; acid no. 2; cloud pt. 65 C (2% in 60% BDG); pH 5-7 (1% aq.); 100% act.

Marlosol® 188. [Hüls Am.; Hüls AG] PEG-8 stearate; CAS 9004-99-3; nonionic; raw material for processing agents for syn. fiber industry; w/o emulsifier and o/w coemulsifier for cosmetic creams and lotions; superfatting agent for shaving preps. and foam baths; pale yel. waxy paste; water-insol.; visc. 35 mPa·s (50 C); solid. pt. 26-30 C; HLB 11.1; acid no. 2; cloud pt. 65 C (10% in 25% BDG); pH 5-7 (1% aq.); 100% act.

Marlosol® 1820. [Hüls Am.; Hüls AG] PEG-20 stearate; CAS 9004-99-3; nonionic; raw material for finishing agents in the syn. fiber industry, fabric softeners; o/w emulsifier for cosmetic creams and lotions; pale yel. waxy solid; water-sol.; visc. 75 mPa·s; solid. pt. 40 C; HLB 15.1; acid no. 2; cloud pt. 80 C (2% aq.); pH 5-7 (1% aq.); 100% act.

Marlosol® BS. [Hüls Am.; Hüls AG] PEG-12 distearate; CAS 9005-08-7; nonionic; superfatting agent and thickener for hair shampoos, foam baths, shower foams, liq. soaps, cosmetic preps., fabric softeners, syn. fiber finishing; pale yel. waxy solid; visc. 100 mPa·s (50 C); solid. pt. 35-39 C; acid no. < 25; pH 4-6 (1% aq.); 100% act.

Marlosol® F08. [Hüls AG] PEG-12 dioleate/olein polyglycol ester blend; nonionic; refatting and thickening agent for shampoos; raw materials for prep. agents for syn. fibers, fabric softeners; liq.; 100% act.

Marlosol® FS. [Hüls Am.; Hüls AG] PEG-12 dioleate; CAS 9005-07-6; 52668-97-0; nonionic; superfatting agent and thickener for hair shampoos, foam baths, liq. soaps, cosmetic preps., fabric softeners, syn. fiber finishing; yel. clear liq.; visc. 100 mPa·s (50 C); solid. pt. 16 C; acid no. < 18; pH 6 (1% aq.); 100% act.

Marlosol® OL7. [Hüls Am.; Hüls AG] PEG-7 oleate; CAS 9004-96-0; nonionic; raw material for finishing agents in the syn. fiber industry; o/w coemulsifier, superfatting agent for hair shampoos, foam baths, shower foams, and liq. soaps; yel. clear liq.; visc. 35 mPa·s (50 C); solid. pt. -5 C; HLB 10.4; acid no. 2; cloud pt. 62 C (10% in 25% BDG); pH 6.5-7.5 (1% aq.); 100% act.

Marlosol® OL15. [Hüls Am.; Hüls AG] PEG-15 oleate; CAS 9004-96-0; nonionic; raw material for finishing agents in the syn. fiber industry; o/w emulsifier for cosmetic creams and lotions; yel. paste; solid. pt. 30 C; HLB 14.0; cloud pt. 46 C (2% in 5% NaCl); pH 9-11 (1% aq.); 100% act.

Marlosol® R70. [Hüls Am.; Hüls AG] PEG-70 castor oil; CAS 61791-12-6; nonionic; thickener, conditioner for toilet sticks; flakes; 100% act.

Marlowet® 5001. [Hüls Am.; Hüls AG] C18 alcohol polyalkylene glycol ether; nonionic; emulsifier for min. oils, wh. oils, textile aux., cosmetics, textile lubricants and finishes; liq.; cloud pt. 61 C (10% in 25% BDG); 100% act.

Marlowet® CA 5. [Hüls Am.; Hüls AG] Coceth-5; CAS 61791-13-7; o/w emulsifier for cosmetic creams and lotions; colorless clear to sl. cloudy liq.; visc. 60 mPa·s; HLB 10.4; pH 5-7 (1% aq.).

Marlowet® CA 10. [Hüls Am.; Hüls AG] Coceth-10; CAS 61791-13-7; o/w coemulsifier for cosmetic creams and lotions; pale yel. solid; HLB 13.7; pH 5-7 (1% aq.).

Marlowet® EF. [Hüls Am.] Mixt. of carboxylic acid polyglycol esters; nonionic; emulsifier for textile lubricants, pest control, cosmetic preparations; paste; 100% act.

Marlowet® G 12 DO. [Hüls Am.; Hüls AG] PEG-12 glyceryl dioleate; w/o and o/w coemulsifier for cosmetic creams

and lotions; codispersant for bath oils; conditioner for hair care prods. imparting silky luster; yel. clear liq.; visc. 220 mPa·s; HLB 8.9; pH 5-7 (1% aq.).

Marlowet® GDO 4. [Hüls Am.; Hüls AG] PEG-5 glyceryl dioleate; w/o and o/w coemulsifier for cosmetic creams and lotions; codispersant for bath oils; conditioner for hair care prods. imparting silky luster; yel. liq.; visc. 150 mPa·s; HLB 5.5; pH 7-8 (1% aq.).

Marlowet® LA 4. [Hüls Am.; Hüls AG] Laureth-4; CAS 5274-68-0; EINECS 226-097-1; solubilizer for bath oils, active substances, and perfume oils; colorless clear to cloudy liq.; visc. 50 mPa·s; HLB 9.7; pH 5-7 (1% aq.).

Marlowet® LA 7. [Hüls Am.; Hüls AG] Laureth-7; CAS 3055-97-8; EINECS 221-283-9; solubilizer for bath oils, active substances, and perfume oils; colorless clear to cloudy liq.; visc. 500 mPa·s; HLB 12.5; pH 5-7 (1% aq.).

Marlowet® LMA 2. [Hüls Am.; Hüls AG] Laureth-2; CAS 3055-93-4; EINECS 221-279-7; o/w emulsifier for cosmetic creams and lotions, solubilizer for bath oils; colorless clear to cloudy liq.; visc. 25 mPa·s; HLB 6.2; pH 5-7 (1% aq.).

Marlowet® LMA 4. [Hüls Am.; Hüls AG] Laureth-4; CAS 5274-68-0; EINECS 226-097-1; o/w coemulsifier for cosmetic creams and lotions, solubilizer for bath oils; colorless clear to cloudy liq.; visc. 35 mPa·s; HLB 9.5; pH 5-7 (1% aq.).

Marlowet® LMA 5. [Hüls AG] Laureth-5; CAS 3055-95-6; EINECS 221-281-8; o/w coemulsifier for cosmetic creams and lotions, solubilizer for bath oils; colorless clear to cloudy liq.; visc. 44 mPa·s; HLB 10.6; pH 5-7 (1% aq.).

Marlowet® LMA 10. [Hüls Am.; Hüls AG] Laureth-10; CAS 6540-99-4; o/w coemulsifier for cosmetic creams and lotions; colorless pasty wax; HLB 13.9; pH 5-7 (1% aq.).

Marlowet® LMA 20. [Hüls Am.; Hüls AG] Laureth-20; CAS 9002-92-0; o/w coemulsifier for cosmetic creams and lotions; wh. solid; HLB 16.4; pH 5-7 (1% aq.).

Marlowet® LVS/K. [Hüls Am.; Hüls AG] PEG-18 castor oil dioleate; w/o emulsifier for creams, lotions, bath oils, massage oils; esp. suitable for animal and veg. oils; ylsh. clear liq.; visc. 500 mPa·s; pH 7-8 (1% aq.).

Marlowet® LVX/K. [Hüls Am.; Hüls AG] PEG-18 castor oil dioleate, PEG-12 dioleate; emulsifier for bath oils, massage oils; esp. suitable for animal and veg. oils; ylsh. clear liq.; visc. 270 mPa·s; pH 5-7 (1% aq.).

Marlowet® OA 4/1. [Hüls Am.; Hüls AG] Propylene glycol oleth-5; o/w emulsifier for cosmetic creams and lotions, bath and massage oils; emulsifier for liq. paraffin; colorless clear liq.; visc. 61 mPa·s; pH 5-7 (1% aq.).

Marlowet® OA 5. [Hüls Am.; Hüls AG] Oleth-5; CAS 9004-98-2; nonionic; o/w emulsifier for cosmetic creams and lotions; pale yel. cloudy liq.; visc. 78 mPa·s; HLB 9.2; pH 5-7 (1% aq.).

Marlowet® OA 10. [Hüls Am.; Hüls AG] Oleth-10; CAS 9004-98-2; nonionic; o/w emulsifier for cosmetic creams and lotions; pale yel. pasty wax; HLB 12.6; pH 5-7 (1% aq.).

Marlowet® OA 30. [Hüls Am.; Hüls AG] Oleth-30; CAS 9004-98-2; nonionic; o/w coemulsifier for cosmetic creams and lotions; wh. solid; HLB 16.8; pH 5-7 (1% aq.).

Marlowet® R 11/K. [Hüls Am.; Hüls AG] PEG-11 castor oil; CAS 61791-12-6; w/o emulsifier for creams and lotions, bath and massage oils, esp. for animal and veg. oils; ylsh. clear liq.; visc. 1000 mPa·s; HLB 6.8; pH 5-7 (1% aq.).

Marlowet® R 20. [Hüls AG] Ethoxylated castor oil; emulsifier for fatty acids, solvs., cosmetic oils; textile lubricants, dyeing auxiliaries, pesticides, creams; liq.; 100% act.

Marlowet® R 22. [Hüls AG] Ethoxylated castor oil; emulsifier for fatty acids, solvs., cosmetic oils; textile lubricants, dyeing auxiliaries, pesticides, creams; liq.; 100% act.

Marlowet® R 25. [Hüls AG] Ethoxylated castor oil; emulsifier for fatty acids, solvs., cosmetic oils; textile lubricants, dyeing auxiliaries, pesticides, creams; liq.; 100% act.

Marlowet® R 25/K. [Hüls AG] PEG-25 castor oil; CAS 61791-12-6; w/o emulsifier for cosmetic creams and lotions; ylsh. clear liq.; visc. 820 mPa·s; HLB 10.8; pH 5-7 (1% aq.).

Marlowet® R 32. [Hüls AG] Ethoxylated castor oil; emulsifier for fatty acids, solvs., cosmetic oils; textile lubricants, dyeing auxiliaries, pesticides, creams; liq.; 100% act.

Marlowet® R 36. [Hüls AG] Ethoxylated castor oil; emulsifier for fatty acids, solvs., cosmetic oils; textile lubricants, dyeing auxiliaries, pesticides, creams; liq.; 100% act.

Marlowet® R 40. [Hüls Am.; Hüls AG] PEG-40 castor oil; CAS 61791-12-6; nonionic; emulsifier for fatty acids, solvs., cosmetic oils; textile lubricants, dyeing auxiliaries, pesticides, creams; biodeg.; liq.; cloud pt. 50 C (2% in 10% NaCl); 100% act.

Marlowet® R 40/K. [Hüls Am.; Hüls AG] PEG-40 castor oil; CAS 61791-12-6; w/o coemulsifier for cosmetic creams and lotions; solubilizer for perfume and bath oils; ylsh. cloudy, highly visc. liq.; visc. 1000 mPa·s; HLB 13.1; pH 5-7 (1% aq.).

Marlowet® R 54. [Hüls AG] Ethoxylated castor oil; emulsifier for fatty acids, solvs., cosmetic oils; textile lubricants, dyeing auxiliaries, pesticides, creams; liq.; 100% act.

Marlowet® RA. [Hüls Am.; Hüls AG] Mixt. of n-alkylbenzene sulfonate and carboxylic acid polyglycol esters; anionic/nonionic; emulsifier for essential oils, cosmetic preparations; biodeg.; liq.; 70% act.

Marlowet® RNP. [Hüls Am.; Hüls AG] Mixt. of carboxylic acid polyglycol ether and a glycol deriv.; nonionic; emulsifier for essential oils; liq.; cloud pt. 68 C (2% aq.); 100% act.

Marlowet® RNP/K. [Hüls Am.; Hüls AG] Octoxynol-9, PEG-40 castor oil, ethoxydiglycol; nonionic; emulsifier for perfume oils for cosmetics; ylsh. clear liq.; visc. 160 mPa·s; pH 5-7 (1% aq.).

Marlowet® SAF/K. [Hüls Am.; Hüls AG] Oleth-5, laureth-4; CAS 9004-98-2; nonionic; o/w emulsifier for cosmetics, hand washing gels; colorless clear liq.; visc. 50 mPa·s; pH 5-7 (1% aq.).

Marlowet® TA 6. [Hüls Am.; Hüls AG] Ceteareth-6; CAS 68439-49-6; o/w emulsifier for highly stable cosmetic creams and lotions; wh. solid; HLB 10.1; pH 5-7 (1% aq.).

Marlowet® TA 8. [Hüls Am.; Hüls AG] Ceteareth-8; CAS 68439-49-6; o/w emulsifier for highly stable cosmetic creams and lotions; wh. solid; HLB 11.5; pH 5-7 (1% aq.).

Marlowet® TA 10. [Hüls Am.; Hüls AG] Ceteareth-10; CAS 68439-49-6; o/w emulsifier for highly stable cosmetic creams and lotions; wh. solid; HLB 12.5; pH 5-7 (1% aq.).

Marlowet® TA 25. [Hüls Am.; Hüls AG] Ceteareth-25; CAS 68439-49-6; o/w coemulsifier for highly stable cosmetic creams and lotions; wh. flake; HLB 16.1; pH 4.5-6.0 (1% aq.).

Marsorb 24. [Aceto] Benzophenone-3; CAS 131-57-7; EINECS 205-031-5.

Masil® 280. [PPG/Specialty Chem.] Dimethicone copolyol; antistat, wetting agent for personal care prods., shampoos; improves wet and dry combing; coupling, spreading, and fixative props. for fragrance prods.; paste; sol. in water; sp.gr. 1.065; cloud pt. 75 C (1% aq.); flash pt. (PMCC) > 300 F; pour pt. –35 C; surf. tens. 27.2 dynes/cm (1% aq.).

Masil® 280LP. [PPG/Specialty Chem.] Dimethicone copolyol; antistat, wetting agent for personal care prods., shampoos; improves wet and dry combing; coupling, spreading, and fixative props. for fragrance prods.; liq.; sp.gr. 1.065; visc. 500 cSt; cloud pt. 76 C (1% aq.); PMCC flash pt. > 300 F; pour pt. –16 C; surf. tens. 26.3 dynes/cm (1% aq.).

Masil® 556. [PPG/Specialty Chem.] Phenyl trimethicone; CAS 2116-84-9; EINECS 218-320-6; hair conditioner, glossing agent, and skin emollient with water barrier props.; used in hair grooms, nail care prods., skin care creams and lotions; sol. in alcohol; visc. 25 cSt.

Masil® 756. [PPG/Specialty Chem.] Tetrabutoxypropyl methicone; high ref. index, nonoily emollient with improved lubricity and organic emollient compatibility for skin care and to provide high gloss to hair care prods.; features water barrier props., elegant nongreasy feel; APHA < 75 clear fluid; sol. in cyclomethicone, almond oil, benzyl laurate, IPM, SD alcohol 40B; disp. in min. oil, propylene glycol; insol. in water; sp.gr. 0.960; visc. < 75 cps; m.p. < -25 C; b.p. > 150 C; flash pt. (CC) > 95 C; ref. index 1.443; toxicology: mild dermal and eye irritation; essentially nontoxic by oral ingestion.

Masil® 1066C. [PPG/Specialty Chem.] Dimethicone copolyol; provides lubricity and soft feel to cosmetic creams and lotions, hair conditioners; resin plasticizer for hair sprays and mousses; lubricant and antistat for plastics, textiles, metal processing; wetting and leveling char.; antifog for glass cleaners; liq.; water-sol.; sp.gr. 1.02; visc. 1800 cSt; cloud pt. 42 C (1% aq.); flash pt. (PMCC) > 300 F; pour pt. –50 C; surf. tens. 25.9 dynes/cm (1% aq.).

Masil® 1066D. [PPG/Specialty Chem.] Dimethicone copolyol; provides lubricity and soft feel to cosmetic creams and lotions, hair conditioners; resin plasticizer for hair sprays and mousses; lubricant and antistat for plastics, textiles, and metal processing; wetting props.; liq.; water-sol.; sp.gr. 1.03; visc. 1050 cSt; cloud pt. 39 C (1% aq.); flash pt. (PMCC) > 300 F; pour pt. –33 C; surf. tens. 25.2 dynes/cm (1% aq.).

Masil® 2132. [PPG/Specialty Chem.] Silicone glycol; antistat and wetting agent for personal care prods., textile, plastics, lubricants and formulations; solv. based coating, dispersant, and antifoam; liq.; sp.gr. 1.03; visc. 2000 cSt; cloud pt. 38 C (1% aq.); flash pt. (PMCC) > 300 F; pour pt. –40 C; surf. tens. 26.5 dynes/cm (1% aq.); 100% conc.

Masil® 2133. [PPG/Specialty Chem.] Silicone glycol; antistat and wetting agent for personal care prods., textile, plastics, lubricants and formulations; solv. based coating, dispersant, and antifoam; liq.; sp.gr. 1.03; visc. 1050 cSt; cloud pt. 37 C (1% aq.); flash pt. (PMCC) > 300 F; pour pt. -33 C; surf. tens. 25.8 dynes/cm (1% aq.).

Masil® 2134. [PPG/Specialty Chem.] Silicone glycol; antistat and wetting agent for personal care prods., textile, plastics, lubricants and formulations; solv. based coating, dispersant, and antifoam; liq.; sp.gr. 1.02; visc. 1800 cSt; cloud pt. 39 C (1% aq.); flash pt. (PMCC) > 300 F; pour pt. -50 C; surf. tens. 32.0 dynes/cm (1% aq.).

Masil® SF 5. [PPG/Specialty Chem.] Dimethicone; release aid, defoamer for nonaq. processes, esp. in the petrol., foods, and printing inks industries; internal lubricant for plastics, rubber, and metal; also in furniture and auto-wax polishes, household and personal care prods.; textile lubricant; lower visc. fluids recommended as emollients and antiwhitening agents for cosmetic applications (antiperspirants, creams and lotions); water-wh. oily, clear liq.; odorless, tasteless; sp.gr. 0.916; visc. 5 cSt; pour pt. -65 C; flash pt. (PMCC) 280 F; ref. index 1.3970.

Masil® SF 10. [PPG/Specialty Chem.] Dimethicone; release aid, defoamer for nonaq. processes, esp. in the petrol., foods, and printing inks industries; internal lubricant for plastics, rubber, and metal; also in furniture and auto-wax polishes, household and personal care prods.; lower visc. fluids recommended as emollients and antiwhitening agents for cosmetic applications (antiperspirants, creams and lotions); sp.gr. 0.940; pour pt. -65 C; flash pt. (PMCC) 320 F; ref. index 1.3990.

Masil® SF 20. [PPG/Specialty Chem.] Dimethicone; release aid, defoamer for nonaq. processes, esp. in the petrol., foods, and printing inks industries; internal lubricant for plastics, rubber, and metal; also in furniture and auto-wax polishes, household and personal care prods.; lower visc. fluids recommended as emollients and antiwhitening agents for cosmetic applications (antiperspirants, creams and lotions); water-wh. oily, clear liq.; odorless, tasteless; sp.gr. 0.953; visc. 20 cSt; pour pt. –65 C; flash pt. (PMCC) 395 F; ref. index 1.4010.

Masil® SF 50. [PPG/Specialty Chem.] Dimethicone; release aid, defoamer for nonaq. processes, esp. in the petrol., foods, and printing inks industries; internal lubricant for plastics, rubber, and metal; also in furniture and auto-wax polishes, household and personal care prods.; elegant, nongreasy emollient for skin care props.; provides nontacky water barrier props. to eyeliners and eyeshadows; water-wh. oily, clear liq.; odorless, tasteless; sp.gr. 0.963; visc. 50 cps; pour pt. –55 C; flash pt. (PMCC) 460 F; ref. index 1.4020.

Masil® SF 100. [PPG/Specialty Chem.] Dimethicone; release aid, defoamer for nonaq. processes, esp. in the petrol., foods, and printing inks industries; internal lubricant for plastics, rubber, and metal; also in furniture and auto-wax polishes, household and personal care prods.; elegant, nongreasy emollient for skin care props.; provides nontacky water barrier props. to eyeliners and eyeshadows; water-wh. oily, clear liq.; odorless, tasteless; sp.gr. 0.968; visc. 100 cps; pour pt. –55 C; flash pt. (PMCC) 461 C; ref. index 1.4030.

Masil® SF 200. [PPG/Specialty Chem.] Dimethicone; release aid, defoamer for nonaq. processes, esp. in the petrol., foods, and printing inks industries; internal lubricant for plastics, rubber, and metal; also in furniture and auto-wax polishes, household and personal care prods.; water-wh. oily, clear liq.; odorless, tasteless; sp.gr. 0.972; visc. 200 cSt; pour pt. –50 C; flash pt. (PMCC) 460 F; ref. index 1.4031.

Masil® SF 350. [PPG/Specialty Chem.] Dimethicone; release aid, defoamer for nonaq. processes, esp. in the petrol., foods, and printing inks industries; internal lubricant for plastics, rubber, and metal; also in furniture and auto-wax polishes, household and personal care prods.; elegant, nongreasy emollient for skin care props.; provides nontacky water barrier props. to eyeliners and eyeshadows; water-wh. oily, clear liq.; odorless, tasteless; sp.gr. 0.973; visc. 350 cSt; pour pt. –50 C; flash pt. (PMCC) 500 F; ref. index 1.4032.

Masil® SF 350 FG. [PPG/Specialty Chem.] Dimethicone; release aid, defoamer for nonaq. processes, esp. in the petrol., foods, and printing inks industries; internal lubricant for plastics, rubber, and metal; also in furniture and auto-wax polishes, household and personal care prods.; sp.gr. 0.973; pour pt. –50 C; flash pt. (PMCC) 500 F; ref. index 1.4032.

Masil® SF 500. [PPG/Specialty Chem.] Dimethicone; release aid, defoamer for nonaq. processes, esp. in the petrol., foods, and printing inks industries; internal lubricant for plastics, rubber, and metal; also in furniture and auto-wax polishes, household and personal care prods.; elegant, nongreasy emollient for skin care props.; provides nontacky water barrier props. to eyeliners and eyeshadows; water-wh. oily, clear liq.; odorless, tasteless; sp.gr. 0.973; visc. 500 cSt; pour pt. –50 C; flash pt. (PMCC) 500 F; ref. index 1.4033.

Masil® SF 1000. [PPG/Specialty Chem.] Dimethicone; release aid, defoamer for nonaq. processes, esp. in the petrol., foods, and printing inks industries; internal lubricant for plastics, rubber, and metal; also in furniture and auto-wax polishes, household and personal care prods.; nonoily gloss and lubricity aid for hair conditioners, skin protectants, water-barrier props. in creams, lotions, foundations, and blushers; water-wh. oily, clear liq.; odorless, tasteless; sp.gr. 0.974; visc. 1000 cSt; pour pt. –50 C;

flash pt. (PMCC) 500 F; ref. index 1.4035; CC flash pt. 260 C.

Masil® SF 5000. [PPG/Specialty Chem.] Dimethicone; release aid, defoamer for nonaq. processes, esp. in the petrol., foods, and printing inks industries; internal lubricant for plastics, rubber, and metal; also in furniture and auto-wax polishes, household and personal care prods.; water-wh. oily, clear liq.; odorless, tasteless; sp.gr. 0.975; visc. 5000 cSt; pour pt. –49 C; flash pt. (PMCC) 500 F; ref. index 1.4035.

Masil® SF 10,000. [PPG/Specialty Chem.] Dimethicone; release aid, defoamer for nonaq. processes, esp. in the petrol., foods, and printing inks industries; internal lubricant for plastics, rubber, and metal; also in furniture and auto-wax polishes, household and personal care prods.; nonoily gloss and lubricity aid for hair conditioners, skin protectants, water-barrier props. in creams, lotions, foundations, and blushers; water-wh. oily, clear liq.; odorless, tasteless; sp.gr. 0.975; visc. 10,000 cSt; pour pt. –47 C; flash pt. (PMCC) 500 F; ref. index 1.4035.

Masil® SF 12,500. [PPG/Specialty Chem.] Dimethicone; release aid, defoamer for nonaq. processes, esp. in the petrol., foods, and printing inks industries; internal lubricant for plastics, rubber, and metal; also in furniture and auto-wax polishes, household and personal care prods.; skin protectant, water repellent, emollient, softener for cuticle care prods., hair care prods.; water-wh. oily, clear liq.; odorless, tasteless; sp.gr. 0.975; visc. 12,500 cSt; pour pt. –47 C; flash pt. (PMCC) 500 F; ref. index 1.4035.

Masil® SF 30,000. [PPG/Specialty Chem.] Dimethicone; release aid, defoamer for nonaq. processes, esp. in the petrol., foods, and printing inks industries; internal lubricant for plastics, rubber, and metal; also in furniture and auto-wax polishes, household and personal care prods.; skin protectant, water repellent, emollient, softener for cuticle care prods., hair care prods.; water-wh. oily, clear liq.; odorless, tasteless; sp.gr. 0.976; visc. 30,000 cSt; pour pt. –46 C; flash pt. (PMCC) 500 F; ref. index 1.4035.

Masil® SF 60,000. [PPG/Specialty Chem.] Dimethicone; release aid, defoamer for nonaq. processes, esp. in the petrol., foods, and printing inks industries; internal lubricant for plastics, rubber, and metal; also in furniture and auto-wax polishes, household and personal care prods.; skin protectant, water repellent, emollient, softener for cuticle care prods., hair care prods.; water-wh. oily, clear liq.; odorless, tasteless; sp.gr. 0.977; visc. 60,000 cSt; pour pt. –44 C; flash pt. (PMCC) 500 F; ref. index 1.4035.

Masil® SF 100,000. [PPG/Specialty Chem.] Dimethicone; release aid, defoamer for nonaq. processes, esp. in the petrol., foods, and printing inks industries; internal lubricant for plastics, rubber, and metal; also in furniture and auto-wax polishes, household and personal care prods.; water-wh. oily, clear liq.; odorless, tasteless; sp.gr. 0.978; visc. 100,000 cSt; pour pt. –40 C; flash pt. (PMCC) 500 F; ref. index 1.4035.

Masil® SF 300,000. [PPG/Specialty Chem.] Dimethicone; release aid, defoamer for nonaq. processes, esp. in the petrol., foods, and printing inks industries; internal lubricant for plastics, rubber, and metal; also in furniture and auto-wax polishes, household and personal care prods.; water-wh. oily, clear liq.; odorless, tasteless; sp.gr. 0.978; visc. 300,000 cSt; pour pt. –40 C; flash pt. (PMCC) 500 F; ref. index 1.4035.

Masil® SF 500,000. [PPG/Specialty Chem.] Dimethicone; release aid, defoamer for nonaq. processes, esp. in the petrol., foods, and printing inks industries; internal lubricant for plastics, rubber, and metal; also in furniture and auto-wax polishes, household and personal care prods.; sp.gr. 0.978; pour pt. -40 C; flash pt. (PMCC) 500 F; ref. index 1.4035.

Masil® SF 600,000. [PPG/Specialty Chem.] Dimethicone; release aid, defoamer for nonaq. processes, esp. in the petrol., foods, and printing inks industries; internal lubricant for plastics, rubber, and metal; also in furniture and auto-wax polishes, household and personal care prods.; water-wh. oily, clear liq.; odorless, tasteless; sp.gr. 0.979; visc. 600,000 cSt; pour pt. –34 C; flash pt. (PMCC) 500 F; ref. index 1.4035.

Masil® SF 1,000,000. [PPG/Specialty Chem.] Dimethicone; release aid, defoamer for nonaq. processes, esp. in the petrol., foods, and printing inks industries; internal lubricant for plastics, rubber, and metal; also in furniture and auto-wax polishes, household and personal care prods.; sp.gr. 0.979; pour pt. -25 C; flash pt. (PMCC) 500 F; ref. index 1.4035.

Masil® SFR 70. [PPG/Specialty Chem.] Dimethiconol; CAS 31692-79-2; spreading agent and emollient in antiperspirant formulations; offers humidity resist. to hair spray formulas; reactive fluid; raw material in compding. silicone RTV systems, textile and paper coatings, plasticizer/processing aid for silicone elastomers, hydrophobizing silica, in water repellent formulations; water-wh. clear liq.; visc. 55-90 cst; 92.5% mi. solids.

Mazol® SFR 100. [PPG/Specialty Chem.] Dimethiconol; CAS 31692-79-2; spreading agent and emollient in antiperspirant formulations; offers humidity resist. to hair spray formulas; water-wh. clear liq.; visc. 90-150 cSt; acid no. 0.05 max.

Mazol® SFR 750. [PPG/Specialty Chem.] Dimethiconol; CAS 31692-79-2; uniform spreading agent, softener, and nongreasy emollient for skin and nail care prods.; water-wh. clear liq.; visc. 675-825 cps.

Mazol® SFR 2000. [PPG/Specialty Chem.] Dimethiconol; CAS 31692-79-2; uniform spreading agent, softener, and nongreasy emollient for skin and nail care prods.; water-wh. clear liq.; visc. 1800-2200 cps.

Mazol® SFR 3500. [PPG/Specialty Chem.] Dimethiconol; CAS 31692-79-2; uniform spreading agent, softener, and nongreasy emollient for skin and nail care prods.; water-wh. clear liq.; visc. 3150-3850 cSt.

Mazol® SFR 18,000. [PPG/Specialty Chem.] Dimethiconol; CAS 31692-79-2; very high m.w. for highest substantivity, softening, and lubricity for hair, skin, and nail care prods.; water-wh. clear liq.; visc. 16,000-20,000 cps.

Mazol® SFR 50,000. [PPG/Specialty Chem.] Dimethiconol; CAS 31692-79-2; very high m.w. for highest substantivity, softening, and lubricity for hair, skin, and nail care prods.; water-wh. clear liq.; visc. 45,000-55,000 cSt.

Mazol® SFR 150,000. [PPG/Specialty Chem.] Dimethiconol; CAS 31692-79-2; very high m.w. for highest substantivity, softening, and lubricity for hair, skin, and nail care prods.; water-wh. clear liq.; sp.gr. 0.980; visc. 150,000 cSt; acid no. 0.03; flash pt. (PMCC) > 300 F; 1% volatiles.

Masil® SFV. [PPG/Specialty Chem.] Cyclomethicone; CAS 69430-24-6; volatile silicone fluid imparting silky light feel and spreadability to cosmetics (hair care prods., skin creams and lotions, antiperspirants, deodorants, suntan preps.); carrier for fragrances and emollients; liq.; sp.gr. 0.952; f.p. 7 C; flash pt. (PMCC) 140 F; ref. index 1.394.

Masil® SF-V (4). [PPG/Specialty Chem.] Cyclomethicone; CAS 69430-24-6; volatile silicone fluid imparting silky light feel and spreadability to cosmetics (hair care prods., skin creams and lotions, antiperspirants, deodorants, suntan preps.); liq.; sp.gr. 0.950; f.p. 12 C; flash pt. (PMCC) 140 F; ref. index 1.394.

Masil® SF-V (5). [PPG/Specialty Chem.] Cyclomethicone; CAS 69430-24-6; volatile silicone fluid imparting silky light feel and spreadability to cosmetics (hair care prods., skin creams and lotions, antiperspirants, deodorants, suntan preps.); liq.; sp.gr. 0.962; f.p. -40 C; flash pt. (PMCC) 170 F; ref. index 1.399.

Masil® SF-VL. [PPG/Specialty Chem.] Cyclomethicone; CAS 69430-24-6; volatile silicone fluid imparting silky light feel and spreadability to cosmetics (hair care prods., skin creams and lotions, antiperspirants, deodorants, suntan preps.); liq.; sp.gr. 0.957; f.p. -17 C; flash pt. (PMCC) 170 F; ref. index 1.398.

Masil® SF-VV. [PPG/Specialty Chem.] Cyclomethicone; CAS 69430-24-6; volatile silicone fluid imparting silky light feel and spreadability to cosmetics (hair care prods., skin creams and lotions, antiperspirants, deodorants, suntan preps.); carrier for fragrances and emollients; liq.; sp.gr. 0.950; f.p. 10 C; flash pt. (PMCC) 140 F; ref. index 1.394.

Masilwax 135. [PPG/Specialty Chem.] Stearoxymethicone/dimethicone copolymer; wax melting at body temp.; offers emollient, water-barrier props. and gloss to skin and hair care prods.; compat. with organic waxes and antiperspirant stick materials; solid.

Masque Poudre No. 2. [Laserson SA] Calcium alginate, calcium sulfate, tetrasodium pyrophosphate, and diatomaceous earth; quick-setting gel providing a cosmetic mask base for addition of hydrosoluble actives; greyish-wh. to beige powd.; misc. with water; insol. in oils; usage level: 25%.

Massa Estarinum® 299. [Hüls AG] Suppository bases for pharmaceuticals; m.p. 33.5-35.5 C; solid. pt. 32-34.5 C; acid no. 0.3 max.; iodine no. 3 max.; sapon. no. 240-255; hyd. no. 2 max.

Massa Estarinum® A. [Hüls AG] Suppository bases for pharmaceuticals; m.p. 33-35 C; solid. pt. 29-31 C; acid no. 0.5 max.; iodine no. 3 max.; sapon. no. 225-240; hyd. no. 35-45.

Massa Estarinum® AB. [Hüls AG] Suppository bases for pharmaceuticals; m.p. 29-31 C; solid. pt. 26.5-28.5 C; acid no. 0.3 max.; iodine no. 3 max.; sapon. no. 235-245; hyd. no. 25-40.

Massa Estarinum® AM. [Hüls Am.] Trilaurin; CAS 538-24-9; EINECS 208-687-0; raw material for cosmetics, pharmaceutical, and food industries; wh. to ivory solid, natural odor; sol. in ether, sl. sol. in ethanol, pract. insol. in water; m.p. 33.5-35.5 C; solid. pt. 31-34 C; acid no. 0.5 max.; iodine no. 3 max.; sapon. no. 235-245; hyd. no. 3 max.

Massa Estarinum® B. [Hüls AG] Suppository bases for pharmaceuticals; m.p. 33.5-35.5 C; solid. pt. 31-33 C; acid no. 0.3 max.; iodine no. 3 max.; sapon. no. 225-240; hyd. no. 20-30.

Massa Estarinum® BB. [Hüls AG] Suppository bases for pharmaceuticals; m.p. 33.5-35.5 C; solid. pt. 31.5-33.5 C; acid no. 0.3 max.; iodine no. 3 max.; sapon. no. 225-240; hyd. no. 18.5-28.5.

Massa Estarinum® BC. [Hüls AG] Suppository bases for pharmaceuticals; m.p. 33.5-35.5 C; solid. pt. 30.5-32.5 C; acid no. 0.3 max.; iodine no. 3 max.; sapon. no. 225-240; hyd. no. 30-40.

Massa Estarinum® BCF. [Hüls AG] Suppository bases for pharmaceuticals; m.p. 35-36.5 C; solid. pt. 33.5-35 C; acid no. 0.3 max.; iodine no. 3 max.; sapon. no. 225-240; hyd. no. 25-30.

Massa Estarinum® BD. [Hüls AG] Suppository bases for pharmaceuticals; m.p. 33.5-35.5 C; solid. pt. 32-34 C; acid no. 0.3 max.; iodine no. 3 max.; sapon. no. 225-240; hyd. no. 15 max.

Massa Estarinum® C. [Hüls AG] Suppository bases for pharmaceuticals; m.p. 36-38 C; solid. pt. 33-35 C; acid no. 0.3 max.; iodine no. 3 max.; sapon. no. 225-235; hyd. no. 20-30.

Massa Estarinum® CM. [Hüls Am.] Hydrog. palm glycerides, hydrog. palm kernel glycerides; consistency regulator for decorative cosmetics, sticks, pencils, powds., glosses, and eye shadows; wh. to ivory solid; m.p. 33.5-

35.5 C; acid no. 0.5 max.; iodine no. 3 max.; sapon. no. 230-240; hyd. no. 10 max.

Massa Estarinum® D. [Hüls AG] Suppository bases for pharmaceuticals; m.p. 40-42 C; solid. pt. 38-40 C; acid no. 0.3 max.; iodine no. 3 max.; sapon. no. 220-230; hyd. no. 30-40.

Massa Estarinum® E. [Hüls AG] Suppository bases for pharmaceuticals; m.p. 34-36 C; solid. pt. 29-31 C; acid no. 1 max.; iodine no. 3 max.; sapon. no. 215-230; hyd. no. 45-60.

Mattina®. [Mearl] Fine particle size mica coated with titanium dioxide and carmine or iron blue; matte pigments displaying intense color with subtle pearlescent glow for soft luster or matte effects; recommended for pressed powd. makeups; avail. violet, red, or blue; particle size 4-32 μ; bulk dens. 14-17 lb/ft³.

Mayoquest 300. [Mayo] Pentasodium pentetate; CAS 140-01-2; EINECS 205-391-3; chelating agent.

Mayoquest 1530. [Mayo] Tetrasodium etidronate; CAS 3794-83-0; EINECS 223-267-7; chelating agent.

Mayoquest 1545M. [Mayo] Pentasodium pentetate, tetrasodium etidronate; chelating agent.

Mayphos 5C10. [Maybrook] PPG-5-ceteth-10 phosphate; CAS 50643-20-4; cosmetic ingred.

Mayphos OL 3N. [Maybrook] DEA-oleth-3 phosphate; CAS 977060-94-8; o/w emulsifier, coupling agent; shampoo additive and buffer providing wet combability, after-shampoo manageability; amber very visc. semisolid, sl. char. odor; acid no. 80-120; pH 5.0-7.0 (2% aq.); 2.5% max.moisture.

Maypon 4C. [Inolex] Potassium coco-hydrolyzed collagen; CAS 68920-65-0; anionic; low-irritation, high foaming protein surfactant used in personal care prods. (baby shampoos, shower gels, bubble baths, facial cleansers), general purpose cleansers; clear to slightly hazy amber liq.; misc. with water; visc. 500 cps max; pH 6.7–7.3; 34-36% solids.

Maypon 4CT. [Inolex] TEA-coco-hydrolyzed collagen; CAS 68952-16-9; protein surfactant, visc. builder, foam modifier for personal care prods., conditioning shampoos, mild liq. hand cleansers, bubble bath, protective agent in permanent waves, anti-irritant with high foaming surfactants; clear to slightly hazy amber liq., mild char. proteinaceous odor; misc. with water; visc. 150 cps max; pH 6.7–7.3; 38–40% solids.

Maypon UD. [Inolex] Potassium undecylenoyl hydrolyzed collagen; CAS 68951-92-8; anionic; substantive skin conditioner, foaming agent, cleanser with antimycotic and antibacterial props.; used in personal care prods.; dk. amber clear liq.; sol. in alcohol, glycerin, glycols, other polyols, misc. with water; sp.gr. 1.06–1.09; visc. 100 cps max.; pH 6.3–6.8; 34–38% solids.

May-Tein C. [Maybrook] Potassium cocoyl hydrolyzed collagen; CAS 68920-65-0; anionic; mild surfactant, conditioner, softener, moisturizer, lubricant, antistat, anti-irritant for hair relaxers, shampoos, conditioners, liq. soaps, depilatories; biodeg.; lt. amber clear to sl. hazy liq., mild char. odor; pH 6.7-7.3; 34-36% solids.

May-Tein CT. [Maybrook] TEA-cocoyl hydrolyzed collagen; CAS 68952-16-9; anionic; mild surfactant, conditioner, anti-irritant for shampoos, conditioners, baby prods., mousses, makeup removers, shave creams, liq. soaps; biodeg.; lt. amber clear to sl. hazy liq., mild char. odor; pH 6.7-7.3; 38-42% solids.

May-Tein KK. [Maybrook] Potassium cocoyl hydrolyzed keratin; mild biodeg. surfactant providing protection and gentle cleaning to skin and hair prods., hand, body and face soaps, bath prods.; substantive, foaming protein, softener, conditioner, antistat; anti-irritant in depilatories and hair relaxers; amber clear to sl. hazy liq., char. odor;

pH 6.5-7.5; 28-32% solids.

May-Tein KT. [Maybrook] Sodium cocoyl hydrolyzed keratin; mild biodeg. surfactant providing gentle cleansing to skin and hair; source of cystine for damaged hair; substantive, foaming protein, lubricant, antistat; anti-irritant for harsh ingreds.; amber hazy liq., char. odor; pH 8.0-9.0; 30-35% solids.

May-Tein KTS. [Maybrook] Sodium/TEA lauryl hydrolyzed keratin; mild, biodeg. substantive protein foaming surfactant, lubricant, conditioner, moisturizer, counter-irritant for hair, skin, and nail care prods. (shampoos, conditioners, foaming mousses, face/body cleansers, makeup removers); aux. emulsifier in creams and lotions; amber clear to sl. hazy liq., char. odor; pH 7.0-8.0; 30% min. solids.

May-Tein SK. [Maybrook] Sodium cocoyl hydrolyzed collagen; CAS 68188-38-5; anionic; mild substantive protein surfactant, detergent, foaming agent, moisturizer, conditioner, antistat, anti-irritant, hair dye leveling, aux. emulsifier for hair and skin care, dish detergents; textile softener for fine woolen, silk, and hand washables; biodeg.; amber clear to sl. hazy visc. liq., mild char. odor; sol. in cold water; pH 8.0-9.0; 43-45% solids.

May-Tein SY. [Maybrook] TEA-cocoyl hydrolyzed soy protein; mild surfactant, substantive foaming lipoprotein, conditioner, lubricant, antistat providing gentle cleansing to hair and skin, anti-irritancy props.; aux. emulsifier; for shampoos, conditioners, mousses, styling prods., skin care mousses, makeup removers, facial soaps; biodeg.; amber clear to sl. hazy liq.; pH 7.0-8.0; 35-40% solids.

Maywax D. [Maybrook] Cetearyl alcohol and ceteareth-20; cosmetic ingred.

Maywax P. [Maybrook] Emulsifying wax NF; cosmetic ingred.

Mazamide® 65. [PPG/Specialty Chem.] 2:1 mixed fatty acid DEA; nonionic/anionic; detergent, thickener for liq. detergent systems and shampoos, emulsifier, foam booster, rust inhibitor; used in hard surf. cleaners, metalworking fluids/syn. coolants, waterless hand cleaners, automotive specialties; also solubilizer; biodeg.; liq.; sp.gr. 0.99–1.02; flash pt. (PMCC) > 300 F; pH 9.0–10.0; 100% conc.

Mazamide® 68. [PPG/Specialty Chem.] Cocamide DEA (2:1); CAS 61791-31-9; EINECS 263-163-9; nonionic; biodeg. thickener, emulsifier, foam builder; for hard surf. cleaners, dishwash, shampoos, metalworking fluids, waterless hand cleaners, automotive specialties; liq.; sp.gr. 0.99; flash pt. (PMCC) > 300 F; 100% conc.

Mazamide® 80. [PPG/Specialty Chem.] 1:1 Cocamide DEA; CAS 61791-31-9; EINECS 263-163-9; nonionic; thickener, foam stabilizer, solubilizer for emollients and fragrances, emulsifier used in cosmetic and toiletry formulations, hard surface wetters and cleaners, household and industrial detergents; biodeg.; liq.; sp.gr. 0.98–1.00; pH 9–10.5; flash pt. (PMCC) > 300 F; 100% conc.

Mazamide® 124. [PPG/Specialty Chem.] Lauramide DEA (1:1); CAS 120-40-1; EINECS 204-393-1; biodeg. foam booster, stabilizer, thickener, emulsifier for cosmetics and pharmaceuticals; liq.; sp.gr. 0.98; flash pt. (PMCC) > 300 F.

Mazamide® 524. [PPG/Specialty Chem.] Cocamide DEA (2:1); CAS 61791-31-9; EINECS 263-163-9; biodeg. thickener, emulsifier, foam builder; for hard surf. cleaners, dishwash, shampoos, metalworking fluids, waterless hand cleaners, automotive specialties; liq.; sp.gr. 1.01; flash pt. (PMCC) > 300 F; 100% conc.

Mazamide® 1214. [PPG/Specialty Chem.] Lauramide DEA (2:1); CAS 120-40-1; EINECS 204-393-1; biodeg. thickener, emulsifier, foam builder; for hard surf. cleaners, dishwash, shampoos, metalworking fluids, waterless hand cleaners, automotive specialties; liq.; sp.gr. 1.02; flash pt. (PMCC) > 300 F.

Mazamide® 1281. [PPG/Specialty Chem.] Cocamide DEA

(2:1); CAS 61791-31-9; EINECS 263-163-9; nonionic; biodeg. foam booster/stabilizer, visc. builder, detergent, emulsifier; for hard surf. cleaners, dishwash, shampoos, metalworking fluids, waterless hand cleaners, automotive specialties; liq.; sp.gr. 0.99; flash pt. (PMCC) > 300 F; 100% conc.

Mazamide® C-2. [PPG/Specialty Chem.] PEG-3 cocamide MEA; biodeg. foam builder/stabilizer for cosmetic and pharmaceutical shampoos; solubilizer for coupling emollients and fragrances into high-foaming surfactant systems; liq.; sp.gr. 0.95; flash pt. (PMCC) > 300 F.

Mazamide® C-5. [PPG/Specialty Chem.] PEG-6 cocamide MEA; nonionic; emulsifier, lubricant, rust inhibitor, buffing compd., thickener, foam booster, detergent, solubilizer for coupling emollients and fragrances into high-foaming surfactant systems, cosmetics; biodeg.; liq.; sp.gr. 1.05; flash pt. (PMCC) > 300 F; pH 9.5–10.5; 100% conc.

Mazamide® CCO. [PPG/Specialty Chem.] Cocamide DEA (2:1); CAS 61791-31-9; EINECS 263-163-9; nonionic; biodeg. emulsifier, wetting agent for heavy and lt. duty cleansing applics., hard surf. cleaners, dishwash, shampoos, metalworking fluids, waterless hand cleaners, automotive specialties; good visc. at low concs.; liq.; sp.gr. 1.02; flash pt. (PMCC) > 300 F; 100% conc.

Mazamide® CFAM. [PPG/Specialty Chem.] Cocamide MEA (1:1); CAS 68140-00-1; EINECS 268-770-2; nonionic; biodeg. foam stabilizer, visc. builder for cosmetic and pharmaceutical shampoos; flake; sp.gr. 0.93; solid. pt. 70 C; flash pt. (PMCC) > 300 F; 100% conc.

Mazamide® CMEA. [PPG/Specialty Chem.] Cocamide MEA (1:1); CAS 68140-00-1; EINECS 268-770-2; biodeg. foam booster/stabilizer, thickener, emulsifier for cosmetic and pharmaceutical shampoos; flake; sp.gr. 0.93; flash pt. (PMCC) > 300 F.

Mazamide® CMEA Extra. [PPG/Specialty Chem.] Cocamide MEA (1:1); CAS 68140-00-1; EINECS 268-770-2; nonionic; biodeg. foam stabilizer, thickener, emulsifier for shampoos, bubble bath, dishwash, household and cosmetic preps.; flake; sp.gr. 0.93; solid. pt. 61 C; flash pt. (PMCC) > 300 F; 100% conc., 85% amide.

Mazamide® CS 148. [PPG/Specialty Chem.] 1:1 Cocamide DEA; CAS 61791-31-9; EINECS 263-163-9; thickener, foam stabilizer, emulsifier, solubilizer used in cosmetic and toiletry formulations, industrial and household detergents; biodeg.; liq.; sp.gr. 0.98–1.00; flash pt. (PMCC) > 300 F; pH 9.0–10.5; 100% conc.

Mazamide® J 10. [PPG/Specialty Chem.] Mixed alkanolamide (2:1); biodeg. thickener, emulsifier, foam builder; for hard surf. cleaners, dishwash, shampoos, metalworking fluids, waterless hand cleaners, automotive specialties; liq.; sp.gr. 1.01; flash pt. (PMCC) > 300 F.

Mazamide® JR 300. [PPG/Specialty Chem.] Mixed alkanolamide (2:1); biodeg. thickener, emulsifier, foam builder; for hard surf. cleaners, dishwash, shampoos, metalworking fluids, waterless hand cleaners, automotive specialties; liq.; sp.gr. 1.01; flash pt. (PMCC) > 300 F.

Mazamide® JR 400. [PPG/Specialty Chem.] Mixed alkanolamide (2:1); biodeg. thickener, emulsifier, foam builder; for hard surf. cleaners, dishwash, shampoos, metalworking fluids, waterless hand cleaners, automotive specialties; liq.; sp.gr. 1.00; flash pt. (PMCC) > 300 F.

Mazamide® JT 128. [PPG/Specialty Chem.] Cocamide DEA (2:1); CAS 61791-31-9; EINECS 263-163-9; nonionic; biodeg. foam stabilizer, thickener, emulsifier for shampoos, bubble bath, dishwash, household and cosmetic preps.; liq.; sp.gr. 0.99; flash pt. (PMCC) > 300 F; 100% conc.

Mazamide® L-5. [PPG/Specialty Chem.] PEG-6 lauramide DEA; nonionic; emulsifier, lubricant, rust inhibitor, buffing compd., detergent, foam builder, stabilizer for cosmetic

and pharmaceutical creams, lotions, bath oils, shampoos; solubilizer for coupling emollients and fragrances into high-foaming systems; biodeg.; solid; sp.gr. 1.05; flash pt. (PMCC) > 300 F; pH 9.5– 10.5; 100% conc.

Mazamide® L-298. [PPG/Specialty Chem.] 2:1 Lauramide DEA; CAS 120-40-1; EINECS 204-393-1; nonionic/anionic; foam builder and stabilizer, emulsifier, dispersant, visc. builder, solubilizer for hard surface cleaners, dishwashing, shampoos, metalworking fluids, automotive specialties, fiber and hair conditioners, dry cleaning, agric. sprays, leather/fur preparations, emulsifiable waxes, rust inhibitors, polishes, paint removers, rug shampoos, fuel oil additives, textile detergents; biodeg.; solid; water sol.; sp.gr. 1.00; flash pt. (PMCC) > 300 F; pH 9.4 (5% aq.).

Mazamide® LLD. [PPG/Specialty Chem.] Linoleamide DEA (2:1); CAS 56863-02-6; EINECS 260-410-2; biodeg. thickener, emulsifier, foam builder; for hard surf. cleaners, dishwash, shampoos, metalworking fluids, waterless hand cleaners, automotive specialties; liq.; sp.gr. 0.97; flash pt. (PMCC) > 300 F.

Mazamide® LM. [PPG/Specialty Chem.] Lauramide DEA (2:1); CAS 120-40-1; EINECS 204-393-1; biodeg. thickener, emulsifier, foam builder; for hard surf. cleaners, dishwash, shampoos, metalworking fluids, waterless hand cleaners, automotive specialties; liq.; sp.gr. 1.00; flash pt. (PMCC) > 300 F.

Mazamide® LM 20. [PPG/Specialty Chem.] 2:1 Lauramide DEA; CAS 120-40-1; EINECS 204-393-1; nonionic/anionic; biodeg. thickener, emulsifier, foam builder; for hard surf. cleaners, dishwash, shampoos, metalworking fluids, waterless hand cleaners, automotive specialties; liq.; sp.gr. 0.99–1.01; flash pt. (PMCC) > 300 F; pH 9.2–10.0; 100% conc.

Mazamide® LS 196. [PPG/Specialty Chem.] 1:1 Lauramide DEA; CAS 120-40-1; EINECS 204-393-1; nonionic; biodeg. thickener, foam stabilizer, emulsifier used in cosmetic and toiletry formulations; liq.; sp.gr. 0.98–1.00; flash pt. (PMCC) > 300 F; pH 9.0–10.5.

Mazamide® O 20. [PPG/Specialty Chem.] 2:1 Oleamide DEA; CAS 93-83-4; EINECS 202-281-7; nonionic; biodeg. thickener, emulsifier, foam builder, corrosion inhibitor, dispersant; for hard surf. cleaners, dishwash, shampoos, metalworking fluids, waterless hand cleaners, automotive specialties; liq.; sp.gr. 0.99–1.01; flash pt. (PMCC) > 300 F; pH 9–10; 100% conc.

Mazamide® PCS. [PPG/Specialty Chem.] Mixed alkanolamide (2:1); biodeg. thickener, emulsifier, foam builder; for hard surf. cleaners, dishwash, shampoos, metalworking fluids, waterless hand cleaners, automotive specialties; liq.; sp.gr. 0.99; flash pt. (PMCC) > 300 F.

Mazamide® RO. [PPG/Specialty Chem.] Mixed alkanolamide (2:1); biodeg. thickener, emulsifier, foam builder; for hard surf. cleaners, dishwash, shampoos, metalworking fluids, waterless hand cleaners, automotive specialties; liq.; sp.gr. 0.99; flash pt. (PMCC) > 300 F.

Mazamide® SCD. [PPG/Specialty Chem.] Mixed alkanolamide (1:1); biodeg. foam booster/stabilizer, thickener, emulsifier for cosmetic and pharmaceutical shampoos; liq.; sp.gr. 1.00; flash pt. (PMCC) > 300 F.

Mazamide® SMEA. [PPG/Specialty Chem.] Stearamide MEA (1:1); CAS 111-57-9; EINECS 203-883-2; biodeg. emulsifier, pearlescent for syndet soap bars; improves appearance and stability of glycol stearate-pearlized systems; flake; sp.gr. 0.89; flash pt. (PMCC) > 300 F.

Mazamide® SS-10. [PPG/Specialty Chem.] 1:1 Linoleamide DEA; CAS 56863-02-6; EINECS 260-410-2; nonionic; emulsifier, lubricant, thickener, solubilizer, visc. booster for shampoos, liq. soaps, shower gels; corrosion inhibitor, buffing compd., metalworking; biodeg.; liq.; sp.gr. 0.98–

1.00; flash pt. (PMCC) > 300 F; pH 9.0–10.5; 100% conc.

Mazamide® SS 20. [PPG/Specialty Chem.] 2:1 Linoleamide DEA; CAS 56863-02-6; EINECS 260-410-2; nonionic/ anionic; biodeg. thickener, emulsifier, foam builder, corrosion inhibitor; for hard surf. cleaners, dishwash, shampoos, metalworking fluids, waterless hand cleaners, automotive specialties; liq.; water sol.; sp.gr. 1.01; flash pt. (PMCC) > 300 F; pH 9.8 (5% aq.); 100% conc.

Mazamide® T 20. [PPG/Specialty Chem.] 2:1 tall oil alkanolamide; nonionic/anionic; thickener for aq. systems; w/o emulsifier, corrosion inhibitor for sol. oils; metalworking; biodeg.; liq.; water sol.; sp.gr. 1.00; flash pt. (PMCC) > 300 F; pH 9.5 (5% aq.); 100% conc.

Mazamide® TC. [PPG/Specialty Chem.] Lauric alkanolamide (2:1); biodeg. thickener, emulsifier, foam builder; for hard surf. cleaners, dishwash, shampoos, metalworking fluids, waterless hand cleaners, automotive specialties; liq.; sp.gr. 1.01; flash pt. (PMCC) > 300 F.

Mazamide® WC Conc. [PPG/Specialty Chem.] Cocamide DEA (1:1); CAS 61791-31-9; EINECS 263-163-9; nonionic; biodeg. foam stabilizer, thickener, emulsifier for shampoos, bubble baths, dishwash, household and cosmetic preps.; liq.; sp.gr. 0.99; flash pt. (PMCC) > 300 F; 100% conc.

Mazawax® 163R. [PPG/Specialty Chem.] Cetearyl alcohol and polysorbate 60; nonionic; emulsifier for pharmaceutical and cosmetic applics.; base; emolliency and thickening properties; wh. flake; m.p. 51 C; acid no. 1; iodine no. 0.5; sapon. no. 12; flash pt. (PMCC) > 350 F; 100% conc.

Mazawax® 163SS. [PPG/Specialty Chem.] Cetearyl alcohol and polysorbate 60; nonionic; emulsifying wax for pharmaceutical and cosmetic creams; recommended for very mild and hypo-allergenic skin care prods.; flake; m.p. 51 C; 100% conc.

Mazeen® 173. [PPG/Specialty Chem.] Tetrahydroxypropyl ethylenediamine; CAS 102-60-3; EINECS 203-041-4; insecticide and herbicide emulsifier, antistat and rewetting agent, grease additive, textile lubricant; emulsifier for lubricants, inks, and cosmetics; chelant in electroless deposition formulations for electronics industry; crosslinker for rigid polyurethane; Gardner 2 liq.; sol. in water, benzene, acetone, IPA, min. spirits, toluene; m.w. 292; sp.gr. 1.01; flash pt. (PMCC) > 350 F; surf. tens. 51.4 dynes/cm (0.1%).

Mazeen® 174. [PPG/Specialty Chem.] Tetrahydroxypropyl ethylenediamine; CAS 102-60-3; EINECS 203-041-4; cationic; insecticide and herbicide emulsifier, antistat and rewetting agent, grease additive, textile lubricant; emulsifier for lubricants, inks, and cosmetics; chelant in electroless deposition formulations for electronics industry; crosslinker for rigid polyurethane; Gardner < 1 liq.; sol. in water, acetone, IPA, min. spirits, toluene; m.w. 292; sp.gr. 1.00; flash pt. (PMCC) > 350 F; surf. tens. 54.2 dynes/cm (0.1%).

Mazeen® 174-75. [PPG/Specialty Chem.] Tetrahydroxypropyl ethylenediamine; CAS 102-60-3; EINECS 203-041-4; cationic; insecticide and herbicide emulsifier, antistat and rewetting agent, grease additive, textile lubricant; emulsifier for lubricants, inks, and cosmetics; in electroless deposition formulations for electronics industry; Gardner < 1 liq.; sol. in water, acetone, IPA, min. spirits, toluene; m.w. 292; sp.gr. 1.00; flash pt. (PMCC) > 350 F; surf. tens. 54.2 dynes/cm (0.1%).

Mazeen® C-2. [PPG/Specialty Chem.] PEG-2 cocamine; CAS 61791-14-8; cationic; emulsifier, rewetting agent, lubricant, coupler used in insecticides and herbicides, grease additives, textile lubricants, water-based inks, cosmetics; plastics antistat; visc. modifier and rust inhibitor in acid media for metalworking; Gardner 10 liq.; sol. in benzene, acetone, IPA, min. oil, toluene, min. spirits,

forms gel in water; m.w. 285; sp.gr. 0.874; flash pt. (PMCC) > 350 F; surf. tens. 28 dynes/cm (0.1%); 100% conc.

Mazeen® C-5. [PPG/Specialty Chem.] PEG-5 cocamine; CAS 61791-14-8; cationic; emulsifier, rewetting agent, lubricant, coupler used in insecticides and herbicides, grease additives, textile lubricants, water-based inks, cosmetics; plastics antistat; rust inhibitor in acid media for metalworking; Gardner 10 liq.; sol. in water, benzene, acetone, IPA, min. oil, toluene; disp. in min. spirits; m.w. 425; sp.gr. 0.976; flash pt. (PMCC) > 350 F; surf. tens. 33 dynes/cm (0.1%); 100% conc.

Mazeen® C-10. [PPG/Specialty Chem.] PEG-10 cocamine; CAS 61791-14-8; cationic; emulsifier, rewetting agent, lubricant, coupler used in insecticides and herbicides, grease additives, textile lubricants, water-based inks, cosmetics; plastics antistat; Gardner 11 liq.; sol. in water, benzene, acetone, IPA, toluene; m.w. 645; sp.gr. 1.017; flash pt. (PMCC) > 350 F; surf. tens. 39 dynes/cm (0.1%); 100% conc.

Mazeen® C-15. [PPG/Specialty Chem.] PEG-15 cocamine; CAS 61791-14-8; cationic; emulsifier, rewetting agent, lubricant, coupler used in metalworking, insecticides and herbicides, grease additives, textile lubricants, water-based inks, cosmetics; plastics antistat; Gardner 9 liq.; sol. in water, benzene, acetone, IPA, toluene; m.w. 860; sp.gr. 1.042; flash pt. (PMCC) > 350 F; surf. tens. 41 dynes/cm (0.1%); 100% conc.

Mazeen® S-2. [PPG/Specialty Chem.] PEG-2 soyamine; CAS 61791-24-0; cationic; emulsifier, rewetting agent, lubricant, coupler used in insecticides and herbicides, grease additives, textile lubricants, water-based inks, cosmetics; plastics antistat; Gardner 14 liq.; sol. in benzene, acetone, IPA, min. oil; disp. in min. spirits, toluene; m.w. 350; sp.gr. 0.911; flash pt. (PMCC) > 350 F; surf. tens. 26 dynes/cm (0.1%); 100% conc.

Mazeen® S-5. [PPG/Specialty Chem.] PEG-5 soyamine; CAS 61791-24-0; cationic; emulsifier, rewetting agent, lubricant, coupler used in insecticides and herbicides, grease additives, textile lubricants, water-based inks, cosmetics; plastics antistat; Gardner 14 liq.; sol. in benzene, IPA; partly sol. acetone, min. oil; m.w. 480; sp.gr. 0.951; flash pt. (PMCC) > 350 F; surf. tens. 33 dynes/cm (0.1%); 100% conc.

Mazeen® S-10. [PPG/Specialty Chem.] PEG-10 soyamine; CAS 61791-24-0; cationic; emulsifier, rewetting agent, lubricant, coupler used in insecticides and herbicides, grease additives, textile lubricants, water-based inks, cosmetics; plastics antistat; Gardner 14 liq.; sol. in water, benzene, acetone, IPA, toluene; m.w. 710; sp.gr. 1.020; flash pt. (PMCC) > 350 F; surf. tens. 40 dynes/cm (0.1%); 100% conc.

Mazeen® S-15. [PPG/Specialty Chem.] PEG-15 soyamine; CAS 61791-24-0; cationic; emulsifier, rewetting agent, lubricant, coupler used in insecticides and herbicides, grease additives, textile lubricants, water-based inks, cosmetics; plastics antistat; Gardner 18 liq.; sol. in water, benzene, acetone, IPA, toluene; m.w. 930; sp.gr. 1.040; flash pt. (PMCC) > 350 F; surf. tens. 43 dynes/cm (0.1%); 100% conc.

Mazeen® T-2. [PPG/Specialty Chem.] PEG-2 tallow amine; CAS 61791-44-4; cationic; emulsifier, rewetting agent, lubricant, coupler used in insecticides and herbicides, grease additives, textile lubricants, water-based inks, cosmetics, metalworking; plastics antistat; visc. modifier, rust inhibitor in acid media; Gardner 11 liq.; sol. in benzene, acetone, IPA, min. oil; m.w. 350; sp.gr. 0.916; flash pt. (PMCC) > 350 F; surf. tens. 29 dynes/cm (0.1%); 100% conc.

Mazeen® T-5. [PPG/Specialty Chem.] PEG-5 tallow amine;

CAS 61791-44-4; cationic; emulsifier, rewetting agent, lubricant, coupler used in insecticides and herbicides, grease additives, textile lubricants, water-based inks, cosmetics, metalworking; plastics antistat; Gardner 12 liq.; sol. in benzene, acetone, IPA, min. oil; gels in water; m.w. 480; sp.gr. 0.966; flash pt. (PMCC) > 350 F; surf. tens. 34 dynes/cm (0.1%); 100% conc.

Mazeen® T-10. [PPG/Specialty Chem.] PEG-10 tallow amine; cationic; emulsifier, rewetting agent, lubricant, coupler used in insecticides and herbicides, grease additives, textile lubricants, water-based inks, cosmetics; plastics antistat.

Mazeen® T-15. [PPG/Specialty Chem.] PEG-15 tallow amine; cationic; emulsifier, rewetting agent, lubricant, coupler used in insecticides and herbicides, grease additives, textile lubricants, water-based inks, cosmetics; plastics antistat; Gardner 18 liq.; sol. in water, benzene, acetone, IPA; m.w. 925; sp.gr. 1.028; flash pt. (PMCC) > 350 F; surf. tens. 41 dynes/cm (0.1%); 100% conc.

Mazol® 80 MGK. [PPG/Specialty Chem.] PEG-20 glyceryl stearate; nonionic; emulsifier for natural triglycerides in personal care prods.; emulsifier, dough conditioner for cakes, icings, whipped toppings; yel. liq.; sol. in ethanol, water; partly sol. in soybean oil, disp. in propylene glycol; m.p. 25–27 C; HLB 13.5; acid no. 2 max.; sapon. no. 65–75; flash pt. (PMCC) > 350 F; 100% conc.

Mazol® 159. [PPG/Specialty Chem.] PEG-7 glyceryl cocoate; emulsifier for food prods.; emollient and solubilizer used in cosmetics, toiletries, pharmaceuticals, cleansing prods., bath oils, shower gels, skin fresheners, lubricants, mold release compds.; plasticizer in syn. fabrics and plastics; amber liq.; sol. in water, min. oil; disp. in min. spirits, toluene, IPA; HLB 13.0; acid no. 5 max.; sapon. no. 82-98; flash pt. (PMCC) > 350 F.

Mazol® 165C. [PPG/Specialty Chem.] Glyceryl stearate and PEG-100 stearate; nonionic; emulsifier blend, thickener, and opacifier for cosmetic and pharmaceutical o/w emulsions; acid-stable; tan flake; sol. in IPA; disp. in water; sol. hot in min. oil, toluene; HLB 11.2; acid no. 2 max.; sapon. no. 90-100; flash pt. (PMCC) > 350 F; 100% conc.

Mazol® 300 K. [PPG/Specialty Chem.] Glyceryl oleate, kosher; CAS 111-03-5; nonionic; GRAS dispersant for oil or solv. systems; antifoam for sugar and protein processing; coemulsifier with T-Maz 60 or 80; amber liq.; sol. in min. oil, toluene, IPA; disp. in min. spirits; insol. in water; HLB 3.8; acid no. 2 max.; flash pt. (PMCC) > 350 F; 100% conc.

Mazol® 1400. [PPG/Specialty Chem.] Caprylic/capric triglyceride; CAS 65381-09-1; carrier for flavors, fragrances, vitamins, antibiotics, pigmented cosmetics, medicinals; Gardner 1 clear liq.; sol. in min. oil, min. spirits, toluene, IPA; insol. in water; HLB 1.0; acid no. 0.5 max.; sapon. no. 335–360; flash pt. (PMCC) > 350 F.

Mazol® GMO. [PPG/Specialty Chem.] Glyceryl oleate; CAS 111-03-5; nonionic; GRAS dispersant for oil or solv. systems; antifoam for food processing; base for cosmetic creams, lotions, ointments; w/o emulsifier with emolliency, thickening properties; plasticizer; lubricant; antifog for PVC; emulsifier, coupling agent for metalworking applics.; yel. liq.; sol. in soybean oil, min. oil, toluene, IPA; disp. in ethanol, propylene glycol; HLB 3.8; acid no. 2 max.; sapon. no. 150-170; flash pt. (PMCC) > 350 F; 100% conc.

Mazol® GMO K. [PPG/Specialty Chem.] Glyceryl oleate, kosher; CAS 111-03-5; GRAS-type antistat for plastic fibers in contact with food; dispersant for oil or solv. systems; antifoam for sugar and protein processing; co-emulsifier with T-Maz 60 or 80; emollient ester for lipsticks and pigmented makeup; emulsifier and emollient for cosmetic creams and lotions; amber liq./paste; sol. in min. oil,

toluene, IPA; disp. in min. spirits; HLB 3.8; acid no. 2 max.; flash pt. (PMCC) > 350 F; 100% act.

Mazol® GMR. [PPG/Specialty Chem.] Glyceryl ricinoleate; CAS 141-08-2; EINECS 205-455-0; base for cosmetic creams, lotions, ointments; w/o emulsifier with emolliency, thickening properties; plasticizer; dk. liq.; sol. in toluene, IPA; disp. in min. spirits; HLB 6.0; acid no. 7 max.; sapon. no. 138–145; flash pt. (PMCC) > 350 F.

Mazol® GMS. [PPG/Specialty Chem.] Glyceryl stearate; lubricant, emulsifier, plasticizer, and thickener for foods, drugs, and cosmetics; tan flake; sol. in IPA; sol. hot in min. oil, toluene; HLB 3.9; acid no. 5 max.; sapon. no. 172; flash pt. (PMCC) > 350 F.

Mazol® GMS-90. [PPG/Specialty Chem.] Glyceryl stearate; emulsifier for food prods., cosmetics, toiletries, pharmaceuticals, lubricants, mold release compds., in plasticizers for syn. fabrics and plastics; tan flake; sol. in IPA; sol. hot in min. oil, toluene; HLB 3.9; acid no. 2 max.

Mazol® GMS-D. [PPG/Specialty Chem.] Glyceryl stearate SE; emulsifier for food prods.; emollient; used in cosmetics, toiletries, pharmaceuticals, lubricants, mold release compds., metalworking applics.; plasticizer in syn. fabrics and plastics; tan flake; sol. in IPA; sol. hot in min. oil, toluene; disp. in water; HLB 6.0; acid no. 3.5 max.; sapon. no. 145-160; flash pt. (PMCC) > 350 F.

Mazol® GMSDK. [PPG/Specialty Chem.] Glyceryl stearate SE; nonionic; provides opacity and visc. to cosmetic creams and lotions; tan flake; HLB 6.0.

Mazol® GMS-K. [PPG/Specialty Chem.] Glyceryl stearate, kosher; nonionic; w/o emulsifier, low-HLB component of o/w cosmetic emulsions; provides opacity and visc. to creams and lotions; emulsifier for frozen desserts, ice cream, custard, nondairy creamers; used in combination with T-Maz 80 and 65; tan flake; sol. in IPA; sol. hot in min. oil, toluene; HLB 3.9; acid no. 3 max.; flash pt. (PMCC) > 350 F; 100% conc.

Mazol® PGMSK. [PPG/Specialty Chem.] Propylene glycol stearate, kosher; CAS 1323-39-3; EINECS 215-354-3; nonionic; aux. emulsifier/opacifier and pearlizing agent for personal care prods.; coemulsifier for edible oil and shortenings; dispersant for nondairy creamers; tan solid; sol. in min. oil, min. spirits, toluene, IPA; HLB 3.4; acid no. 3 max.; sapon. no. 170-190; flash pt. (PMCC) > 350 F; 100% conc.

Mazol® PGO-31 K. [PPG/Specialty Chem.] Triglyceryl oleate, kosher; CAS 9007-48-1; nonionic; emulsifier for food prods., in cosmetics, toiletries, pharmaceuticals, lubricants, mold release compds., plasticizers; solubilizer for essential oils and flavors; Gardner 8 max. liq.; sol. in min. oil, toluene, IPA; disp. in min. spirits; HLB 6.2; acid no. 2 max.; sapon. no. 140-150; 100% conc.

Mazol® PGO-104. [PPG/Specialty Chem.] Decaglyceryl tetraoleate; CAS 34424-98-1; EINECS 252-011-7; emulsifier for food prods., cosmetics, toiletries, pharmaceuticals, lubricants, mold release compds., in plasticizers for syn. fabrics and plastics; dk. liq.; sol. in IPA, min. oil, toluene; disp. in min. spirits; HLB 6.2; acid no. 8 max.; sapon. no. 125-145; flash pt. (PMCC) > 350 F.

Mazon® 60T. [PPG/Specialty Chem.] TEA dodecylbenzene sulfonate; CAS 27323-41-7; EINECS 248-406-9; anionic; high foaming formulated detergent, emulsifier for shampoos, dishwashing, car wash, textile, hard surf. cleaners, metal cleaners and other formulations; liq.; sp.gr. 1.08; flash pt. (PMCC) > 350 F; 60% act.

Mazon® EE-1. [PPG/Specialty Chem.] Benzyl laurate; CAS 140-25-0; EINECS 204-405-8; nonoily emollient, lubricant for skin care, bath, and hair care formulations; readily emulsified; spreads easily; solv. and degreaser in sunscreens; APHA < 150 clear liq., mild odor; sol. in min. oil, jojoba oil, almond oil, IPM, cyclomethicone, SD alcohol

40-B; misc. with sunscreens; insol. in water; sp.gr. 0.920; visc. < 50 cps; m.p. -5 C; b.p. 95 C; flash pt. (CC) 95 C; toxicology: nontoxic, nonirritating, nonsensitizing.

Mazox® CAPA. [PPG/Specialty Chem.] Cocamidopropylamine oxide; CAS 68155-09-9; EINECS 268-938-5; nonionic/cationic; surfactant, conditioner, emollient, emulsifier, foam booster, visc. builder, lime soap dispersant for cosmetics, toiletries, household and industrial uses; low color for water-wh. or pastel-tinted formulations; low color liq.; sp.gr. 1.02; flash pt. > 200 F; 30% amine oxide.

Mazox® CAPA-37. [PPG/Specialty Chem.] Cocamidopropylamine oxide; CAS 68155-09-9; EINECS 268-938-5; nonionic/cationic; surfactant, conditioner, emollient, emulsifier, foam booster, visc. builder for cosmetics, toiletries, household and industrial uses.

Mazox® CDA. [PPG/Specialty Chem.] Palmitamine oxide; CAS 7128-91-8; EINECS 230-429-0; nonionic/cationic; surfactant, conditioner, emollient, emulsifier, foam booster, visc. builder for cosmetics, toiletries, household and industrial uses; textile softener; good hair conditioning and wet-comb improvement; liq.; sp.gr. 0.96; flash pt. > 200 F; 30% amine oxide.

Mazox® LDA. [PPG/Specialty Chem.] Lauramine oxide; CAS 1643-20-5; EINECS 216-700-6; nonionic/cationic; surfactant, conditioner, emollient, emulsifier, foam booster, visc. builder for cosmetics, toiletries, household and industrial uses; low color for water-wh. or pastel-tinted formulations; liq.; sp.gr. 0.96; flash pt. > 200 F; 30% amine oxide.

Mazox® MDA. [PPG/Specialty Chem.] Myristamine oxide; CAS 3332-27-2; EINECS 222-059-3; nonionic/cationic; surfactant, conditioner, emollient, emulsifier, foam booster, visc. builder for cosmetics, toiletries, household and industrial uses; liq.; sp.gr. 0.96; flash pt. > 200 F; 30% amine oxide.

Mazox® ODA-30. [PPG/Specialty Chem.] Oleamine oxide; CAS 14351-50-9; EINECS 238-311-0; nonionic/cationic; surfactant, conditioner, emollient, emulsifier, foam booster, visc. builder for cosmetics, toiletries, household and industrial uses; textile softener; good hair conditioning and wet-comb improvement; liq.; 30% amine oxide.

Mazox® SDA. [PPG/Specialty Chem.] Stearamine oxide; CAS 2571-88-2; EINECS 219-919-5; nonionic/cationic; surfactant, conditioner, emollient, emulsifier, foam booster, visc. builder for cosmetics, toiletries, household and industrial uses; textile softener; hair conditioner, slip agent; low foaming; paste; sp.gr. 0.99; flash pt. > 200 F; 25% amine oxide.

Mazu® DF 200SP. [PPG/Specialty Chem.] Simethicone; food grade defoamer for fermentation, veg. oils; also is formulated to meet the specific needs of pharmaceutical industry; FDA compliance; liq.; sp.gr. 0.99; dens. 8.3 lb/gal; visc. 1720 cSt; flash pt. (PMCC) > 350 F; 100% silicone.

MEA Commercial Grade. [Dow] Monoethanolamine; used in surfactants, cosmetics/toiletries, pharmaceuticals, metalworking fluids, textile chemicals, gas conditioning chemicals, agric. intermediates, adhesives, coatings, petroleum, rubber, wood pulping, and cement grinding aids; sp.gr. 1.0113 (25/4 C); dens. 8.45 lb/gal; visc. 18.9 cps; f.p. 10 C; b.p. 171 C (760 mm Hg); flash pt. (Seta CC) 201 F; fire pt. 200 F; ref. index 1.4525.

MEA Electronics Grade. [Dow] Monoethanolamine; high purity prod. essentially free of iron, chloride, calcium, lithium, potassium, sodium; used in surfactants, cosmetics/toiletries, metalworking fluids, textile chemicals, gas conditioning chemicals, agric. intermediates, and cement grinding aids; sp.gr. 1.0113 (25/4 C); dens. 8.45 lb/gal; visc. 18.9 cps; f.p. 10 C; b.p. 171 C (760 mm Hg); flash pt. (Seta CC) 201 F; fire pt. 200 F; ref. index 1.4525.

MEA Low Freeze Grade. [Dow] Monoethanolamine; used in surfactants, cosmetics/toiletries, pharmaceuticals, metalworking fluids, textile chemicals, gas conditioning chemicals, agric. intermediates, adhesives, coatings, petroleum, rubber, wood pulping, and cement grinding aids; sp.gr. 1.0113 (25/4 C); dens. 8.45 lb/gal; visc. 18.9 cps; f.p. 10 C; b.p. 171 C (760 mm Hg); flash pt. (Seta CC) 201 F; fire pt. 200 F; ref. index 1.4525.

MEA Low Iron Grade. [Dow] Monoethanolamine; used in surfactants, cosmetics/toiletries, pharmaceuticals, metalworking fluids, textile chemicals, gas conditioning chemicals, agric. intermediates, adhesives, coatings, petroleum, rubber, wood pulping, and cement grinding aids; sp.gr. 1.0113 (25/4 C); dens. 8.45 lb/gal; visc. 18.9 cps; f.p. 10 C; b.p. 171 C (760 mm Hg); flash pt. (Seta CC) 201 F; fire pt. 200 F; ref. index 1.4525.

MEA Low Iron-Low Freeze Grade. [Dow] Monoethanolamine; used in surfactants, cosmetics/toiletries, pharmaceuticals, metalworking fluids, textile chemicals, gas conditioning chemicals, agric. intermediates, adhesives, coatings, petroleum, rubber, wood pulping, and cement grinding aids; sp.gr. 1.0113 (25/4 C); dens. 8.45 lb/gal; visc. 18.9 cps; f.p. 10 C; b.p. 171 C (760 mm Hg); flash pt. (Seta CC) 201 F; fire pt. 200 F; ref. index 1.4525.

MEA NF Grade. [Dow] Monoethanolamine NF; used in surfactants, cosmetics/toiletries, pharmaceuticals, metalworking fluids, textile chemicals, gas conditioning chemicals, agric. intermediates, adhesives, coatings, petroleum, rubber, wood pulping, and cement grinding aids; sp.gr. 1.0113 (25/4 C); dens. 8.45 lb/gal; visc. 18.9 cps; f.p. 10 C; b.p. 171 C (760 mm Hg); flash pt. (Seta CC) 201 F; fire pt. 200 F; ref. index 1.4525.

Mearlite® GBU. [Mearl] Bismuth oxychloride; CAS 7787-59-9; EINECS 232-122-7; pearl pigments and pastes used for high opacitiy and smooth luster providing frosted effects in makeups, lipsticks, blushers, etc.; powd.; avg. particle size 8 μ; 100% act.

Mearlite® GEH. [Mearl] Bismuth oxychloride, castor oil; pearl pigment for cosmetics and personal care prods. (lipsticks, blushers); paste; 70% act.

Mearlite® GEJ. [Mearl] Bismuth oxychloride, min. oil; pearl pigment for cosmetics and personal care prods. (cream eye shadows, other oil-based makeups); paste; 70% act.

Mearlite® GGH. [Mearl] Bismuth oxychloride, water; CAS 7787-59-9; EINECS 232-122-7; pearl pigment for cosmetics and personal care prods. (eye shadows, water-based makeups); paste; 70% act.

Mearlite® LBU. [Mearl] Bismuth oxychloride; CAS 7787-59-9; EINECS 232-122-7; pearl pigment for cosmetics and personal care prods.; powd.; avg. particle size 20 μ; 100% act.

Mearlite® LEM. [Mearl] Bismuth oxychloride, castor oil; pearl pigment for cosmetics and personal care prods. (lipsticks, blushers); paste; 70% act.

Mearlmaid® AA. [Mearl] Water, guanine, isopropyl alcohol, methylcellulose; pearl colors for nail enamels, makeup, lotions, creams, shampoos, hair care prods., natural cosmetics, soap, aq. systems; paste.

Mearlmaid® CKD. [Mearl] Butyl acetate, guanine, isopropyl alcohol, nitrocellulose; pigment for frosted nail enamels of highest brilliance; avg. particle size 30 μ; sp.gr. 1.6.

Mearlmaid® CP. [Mearl] Butyl acetate, guanine, nitrocellulose, isopropyl alcohol; natural pearl colorant for nail enamels of highest brilliance; paste.

Mearlmaid® KND. [Mearl] Butyl acetate, isopropyl alcohol, guanine, nitrocellulose; pigment for frosted nail enamels; avg. particle size 30 μ; sp.gr. 1.6.

Mearlmaid® OL. [Mearl] Isopropyl alcohol, guanine, polysorbate 80; natural pearl colorant for lotions, nail enamel removers, and liqs. based on alcohol-water mixts.; paste.

Mearlmaid® PLN. [Mearl] Water, carbomer, guanine, diisopropanolamine, methylcellulose; natural pearl colorant for lotions, gels, shave balms; paste.

Mearlmaid® TR. [Mearl] Water, guanine, TEA-lauryl sulfate, isopropyl alcohol, methylcellulose; natural pearl colorant for shampoos, lotions, and liq. hand soaps; paste.

Mearlmica® MMCF. [Mearl] Mica; CAS 12001-26-2; extender in loose powds.; increased slip in pressed powds.; binder and reinforcement in lipsticks and other lanolin and wax-based make-ups; 26 μ avg.

Mearlmica® MMSV. [Mearl] Mica; CAS 12001-26-2; extender in loose powds.; increased slip in pressed powds.; binder and reinforcement in lipsticks and other lanolin and wax-based make-ups; 7–8 μ avg.

Mearlmica® SVA. [Mearl] Mica (95.5-97.5%), lauroyl lysine (2.5-4.5%); imparts smooth texture, soft feel, soft luster or matte effect to cosmetics (pressed powd. makeup, eye shadows); nearly wh. platy particles; particle size 400 mesh; sp.gr. 2.7; bulk dens. 16 g/100 cm³; ref. index 1.58.

Medialan Brands. [Hoechst Celanese/Colorants & Surf.; Hoechst AG] Fatty acid sarcosides, sodium salt; anionic; basic material for cosmetic industry; detergent for textile industry; paste; 50% conc.

Medialan KA. [Hoechst Celanese/Colorants & Surf.] Sodium cocoyl sarcosinate; CAS 61791-59-1; EINECS 263-193-2; anionic; detergent used in cream shampoos, foaming agent, mild toiletries, hair shampoos; features mildness, skin compat.; yel. soft paste; weak odor; m.w. 310 ± 5; misc. with water; biodeg.; 53% act.

Medialan KF. [Hoechst Celanese/Colorants & Surf.] TEA-palm kernel sarcosinate; anionic; base detergent used in preparation of clear, liq. shampoos and body lotions; clear yel. low-visc. liq.; misc. with water; 40% act.

Medialan LD. [Hoechst Celanese/Colorants & Surf.; Hoechst AG] Sodium lauroyl sarcosinate; CAS 137-16-6; EINECS 205-281-5; base detergent for dental care prods.; clear ylsh. liq.; 30% act.

Medical Fluid 360. [Dow Corning] Dimethicone.

Mekon® White. [Petrolite] Hard microcryst. wax; CAS 63231-60-7; EINECS 264-038-1; release agent; used in hot-melt coatings and adhesives, paper coatings, printing inks, plastic modification (as lubricant and processing aid), lacquers, paints, varnishes, as binder in ceramics, for potting/filling in elec./electronic components, in investment casting, rubber and elastomers (plasticizer, antisunchecking, antiozonant), as emulsion wax size in papermaking, as fabric softener ingred., in emulsion and latex coatings, and in cosmetic hand creams and lipsticks; chewing gum base; incl. FDA §172.230, 172.615, 175.105, 175.300, 176.170, 176.180, 176.200, 177.1200, 178.3710, 179.45; wh. wax; very low sol. in org. solvs.; dens. 0.78 g/cc (99 C); visc. 15 cps (99 C); m.p. 94 C.

Melanol LP 1. [Seppic] MIPA-lauryl sulfate; CAS 21142-28-9; EINECS 244-238-5; anionic; detergent base for shampoos; gel; 60% conc.

Melhydran®. [Laboratoires Sérobiologiques] Honey extract; CAS 91052-92-5; EINECS 293-255-4; substantive hydroregulator for facial and body moisturizers, sun care, after shave prods., makeup, hair care prods.; pale yel. limpid liq.; water-sol.; usage level: 3-7%.

Melusat. [Henkel/Cospha] Fragrance raw material for cosmetic, personal care, detergent, and cleaning prods.; colorless liq., fruity odor; b.p. 83-85 C; flash pt. 76 C.

Merezan® 8. [Meer] Xanthan gum from *Xanthomonas campestris*; CAS 11138-66-2; EINECS 234-394-2; high m.w. polysaccharide for the food and pharmaceutical industries; cream-colored powd., ≥ 97% thru 80 mesh; readily sol. in hot and cold water; visc. ≥ 1200 cps (1%); pH 6.1-8.1.

Merezan® 20. [Meer] Xanthan gum from *Xanthomonas*

campestris; CAS 11138-66-2; EINECS 234-394-2; high m.w. polysaccharide for the food and pharmaceutical industries; meets FCC specs.; cream-colored powd., ≥ 97% thru 200 mesh; readily sol. in hot and cold water; visc. ≥ 1200 cps (1%); pH 6.1-8.1.

Merguard 1190. [Calgon; Chemviron SA] Methyldibromo glutaronitrile and dipropylene glycol; cosmetic preservative system; USA and Europe approvals; usage level: 0.04-0.4%.

Merguard 1200. [Calgon; Chemviron SA] Methyldibromo glutaronitrile and phenoxyethanol; cosmetic preservative system; USA and Europe approvals; usage level: 0.02-0.2%.

Meristami. [Alban Muller; Tri-K Industries] Oak meristem extract; soothing prod. for sun prods.; water-sol.

Merpol® A. [DuPont] Ethoxylated phosphate; nonionic; low foaming wetting agent, surf. tens. reducer for chemical mfg., cosmetics, metal processing, paper, petrol., inks, plastics, soaps, syn. fibers, textiles; stable to acids, bases, heat to 100 C, freezing; colorless to pale yel. liq., mild odor; sol. in polar solvs., 0.1-1% in nonpolar solvs.; disp. in water to 1%; sp.gr. 1.07 g/mL; dens. 8.9 lb/gal; visc. 104 cP; HLB 6.7; cloud pt. < 25 C (upper, 1%); flash pt. (TCC) 138 C; pH 5-7 (1% emulsion); surf. tens. 26 dynes/cm (0.1%); 100% act.

Merpol® HCS. [DuPont] Alcohol ethoxylate; nonionic; wetting agent, detergent, emulsifier, penetrant, antistat, leveling agent, dyeing assistant, stabilizer used in textiles, leather, paper, metal processing, rubber, emulsion polymerization, paints, inks, medicinal ointments, antiperspirants, cutting oils, polishes, cosmetics; pigment dispersant; lt. yel. clear, visc. liq.; mild fatty odor; 40% sol. in water, sol. in org. solvs. that are misc. with water; sp.gr. 1.03 g/mL; dens. 8.63 lb/gal; HLB 15.3; cloud pt. > 100 C (upper, 1%); flash pt. > 235 F; pH 6–8 (10%); surf. tens. 42.9 dynes/cm (0.1%); 60% act.

Merquat® 100. [Calgon] Polyquaternium-6; CAS 26062-79-3; cationic; conditioner, antistat for hair shampoos, conditioners, rinses, moisturizing creams, lotions, bath prods., skin care; sol. in water, propylene glycol; limited sol. in alcohol.; 40% act.

Merquat® 280. [Calgon; Chemviron SA] Polyquaternium-22; CAS 53694-17-0; cationic; conditioner contributing softness, slip, lubricity to hair and skin prods., baby prods.; improves clarity of bath gels and shampoos; 35% act.

Merquat® 550. [Calgon; Chemviron SA] Polyquaternium-7; CAS 26590-05-6; cationic; foam stabilizing film former for pearlized/opaque systems; used in soaps, skin care, and hair care prods.; 8% act.

Merquat® 2200. [Calgon; Chemviron SA] Methyldibromo glutaronitrile, phenoxyethanol, polyquaternium-7.

Merquat® S. [Calgon; Chemviron SA] Polyquaternium-7; CAS 26590-05-6; foam stabilizing film formers for hair shampoos, rinses, conditioners, bath and skin care prods.; sol. see Merquat 100; 8% act.

Mersolat H 30. [Miles/Organic Prods.] Sodium alkane sulfonates based on n-paraffin; anionic; biodeg. detergent base, wetting agent for mfg. electrolyte-resistant textile and leather auxiliaries, alkaline and acid detergents, floor cleaners, bubble baths, disinfectants, car shampoos; colorless clear sol'n.; m.w. 310-320; visc. 15 mPa·s; cloud pt. < 10 C; pH alkaline; surf. tens. 34.9 dynes/cm (0.1%); 30% act.

Mersolat H 40. [Miles/Organic Prods.] Sodium alkane sulfonates based on n-paraffin; anionic; biodeg. detergent base, wetting agent for mfg. electrolyte-resistant textile and leather auxiliaries, alkaline and acid detergents, floor cleaners, bubble baths, disinfectants, car shampoos; colorless clear sol'n.; m.w. 310-320; visc. 80-160 mPa·s; cloud pt. < 20 C; pH alkaline; surf. tens. 34.9 dynes/cm

(0.1%); 40% act.

Mersolat H 68. [Miles/Organic Prods.] Sodium alkane sulfonates based on n-paraffin; anionic; biodeg. detergent base, wetting agent for mfg. electrolyte-resistant textile and leather auxiliaries, alkaline and acid detergents, floor cleaners, bubble baths, disinfectants, car shampoos; colorless-ylsh. pumpable paste; m.w. 310-320; pH alkaline; surf. tens. 34.9 dynes/cm (0.1%); 68% act.

Mersolat H 76. [Miles/Organic Prods.] Sodium alkane sulfonates based on n-paraffin; anionic; biodeg. detergent base, wetting agent for mfg. electrolyte-resistant textile and leather auxiliaries, alkaline and acid detergents, floor cleaners, bubble baths, disinfectants, car shampoos; wh.-ylsh. stiff paste, virtually odorless; m.w. 310-320; pH alkaline; surf. tens. 34.9 dynes/cm (0.1%); 76% act.

Mersolat H 95. [Bayer AG; Miles/Organic Prods.] Sodium C9-22 alkyl sec sulfonate; CAS 68188-18-1; anionic; biodeg. detergent base, wetting agent for mfg. electrolyte-resistant textile and leather auxiliaries, alkaline and acid detergents, floor cleaners, bubble baths, disinfectants, car shampoos; wh.-ylsh. flakes; m.w. 310-320; pH alkaline; surf. tens. 34.9 dynes/cm (0.1%); toxicology: LD50 (oral, rats) 2100 mg/kg; 95% act.

Mersolat W 40. [Miles/Organic Prods.] Sodium alkane sulfonates based on n-paraffin; anionic; biodeg. detergent base, wetting agent for mfg. electrolyte-resistant textile and leather auxiliaries, alkaline and acid detergents, floor cleaners, bubble baths, disinfectants, car shampoos; colorless clear sol'n.; m.w. 290; visc. 50 mPa·s; cloud pt. < 10 C; surf. tens. 35.0 dynes/cm (0.1%); 40% % act.

Mersolat W 68. [Miles/Organic Prods.] Sodium alkane sulfonates based on n-paraffin; anionic; biodeg. detergent base, wetting agent for mfg. electrolyte-resistant textile and leather auxiliaries, alkaline and acid detergents, floor cleaners, bubble baths, disinfectants, car shampoos; colorless-ylsh. pumpable paste; m.w. 290; surf. tens. 35.0 dynes/cm (0.1%); 68% act.

Mersolat W 76. [Miles/Organic Prods.] Sodium alkane sulfonates based on n-paraffin; anionic; biodeg. detergent base, wetting agent for mfg. electrolyte-resistant textile and leather auxiliaries, alkaline and acid detergents, floor cleaners, bubble baths, disinfectants, car shampoos; wh.-ylsh. stiff paste, virtually odorless; m.w. 290; pH alkaline; surf. tens. 35.0 dynes/cm (0.1%); 76% act.

Mersolat W 93. [Miles/Organic Prods.] Sodium alkane sulfonates based on n-paraffin; anionic; biodeg. detergent base, wetting agent for mfg. electrolyte-resistant textile and leather auxiliaries, alkaline and acid detergents, floor cleaners, bubble baths, disinfectants, car shampoos; wh.-ylsh. flakes; m.w. 290; surf. tens. 35.0 dynes/cm (0.1%); toxicology: LD50 (oral, rats) 2000 mg/kg; 93% act.

Methocel® 40-100. [Dow] Hydroxypropyl methylcellulose; CAS 9004-65-3; visc. control agent, gellant, lather enhancer/stabilizer, film-former, dispersant, lubricant, binder, emulsion stabilizer, and suspending agent for personal care prods., shampoos, facial masks, shave gel, sun care, bubble bath; disp. in cold water; visc. 12,000 mPa·s.

Methocel® 40-101. [Dow] Hydroxypropyl methylcellulose; CAS 9004-65-3; visc. control agent, gellant, lather enhancer/stabilizer, film-former, dispersant, lubricant, binder, emulsion stabilizer, and suspending agent for personal care prods., shampoos, hand/body soaps, facial mask, shave gels, sun care, bubble bath; disp. in cold water; visc. 75,000 mPa·s.

Methocel® 40-202. [Dow] Hydroxypropyl methylcellulose; CAS 9004-65-3; visc. control agent, gellant, lather enhancer/stabilizer, film-former, dispersant, lubricant, binder, emulsion stabilizer, and suspending agent for personal care prods., shampoo, hand/body soaps, condi-

tioners, clear cleansers, skin toners; sun care, bubble bath, makeup; disp. in cold water; visc. 400 mPa·s.

Methocel® A4CP. [Dow] Methylcellulose; CAS 9004-67-5; visc. control agent, gellant, lather enhancer/stabilizer, film-former, dispersant, lubricant, binder, emulsion stabilizer, and suspending agent for personal care prods.; visc. 400 mPa·s.

Methocel® A4MP. [Dow] Methylcellulose; CAS 9004-67-5; visc. control agent, gellant, lather enhancer/stabilizer, film-former, dispersant, lubricant, binder, emulsion stabilizer, and suspending agent for personal care prods.; visc. 4000 mPa·s.

Methocel® A15-LV. [Dow] Methylcellulose; CAS 9004-67-5; food gums used as thickener, stabilizer, emulsifier, adhesive, and gellant; also for tablet coating applics.

Methocel® A15LVP. [Dow] Methylcellulose; CAS 9004-67-5; visc. control agent, gellant, lather enhancer/stabilizer, film-former, dispersant, lubricant, binder, emulsion stabilizer, and suspending agent for personal care prods., pharmaceutical tablet coating; wh./off-wh. powd.; visc. 15 mPa·s.

Methocel® A Premium. [Dow] Methylcellulose USP; 9004-67-5; used for pharmaceutical tablet coating, granulation, controlled release applics.; visc. avail. 15, 400, 1500, and 4000 cps.

Methocel® E3P. [Dow] Hydroxypropyl methylcellulose; CAS 9004-65-3; visc. control agent, gellant, lather enhancer/stabilizer, film-former, dispersant, lubricant, binder, emulsion stabilizer, and suspending agent for personal care prods., pharmaceutical tablet coating; wh./off-wh. powd.; visc. 3 mPa·s.

Methocel® E4MP. [Dow] Hydroxypropyl methylcellulose; CAS 9004-65-3; visc. control agent, gellant, lather enhancer/stabilizer, film-former, dispersant, lubricant, binder, emulsion stabilizer, suspending agent for personal care prods., shampoos, facial mask, shave gels, sun care, bubble bath, controlled drug release; wh./off-wh. powd.; visc. 4000 mPa·s.

Methocel® E5P. [Dow] Hydroxypropylmethylcellulose; CAS 9004-65-3; used for pharmaceutical tablet coating; wh./off-wh. powd.; visc. 4-6 mPa·s.

Methocel® E6P. [Dow] Hydroxypropyl methylcellulose; CAS 9004-65-3; visc. control agent, gellant, lather enhancer/stabilizer, film-former, dispersant, lubricant, binder, emulsion stabilizer, and suspending agent for personal care prods., pharmaceutical tablet coating; wh./off-wh. powd.; visc. 6 mPa·s.

Methocel® E10MP CR. [Dow] Hydroxypropylmethylcellulose; CAS 9004-65-3; controlled-release grade for pharmaceutical release formulations; wh./off-wh. powd.; visc. 10,000 mPa·s.

Methocel® E15LVP. [Dow] Hydroxypropyl methylcellulose; CAS 9004-65-3; visc. control agent, gellant, lather enhancer/stabilizer, film-former, dispersant, lubricant, binder, emulsion stabilizer, and suspending agent for personal care prods., pharmaceutical tablet coating; wh./off-wh. powd.; visc. 15 mPa·s.

Methocel® E50LVP. [Dow] Hydroxypropyl methylcellulose; CAS 9004-65-3; visc. control agent, gellant, lather enhancer/stabilizer, film-former, dispersant, lubricant, binder, emulsion stabilizer, and suspending agent for personal care prods.; visc. 50 mPa·s.

Methocel® E50P. [Dow] Hydroxypropyl methylcellulose; CAS 9004-65-3; visc. control agent, gellant, lather enhancer/stabilizer, film-former, dispersant, lubricant, binder, emulsion stabilizer, and suspending agent for personal care prods., pharmaceutical tablet coating, mouthwashes; wh./off-wh. powd.; visc. 40-60 mPa·s.

Methocel® E Premium. [Dow] Hydroxypropyl methylcellulose USP; CAS 9004-65-3; used for pharmaceutical tablet coating, granulation, controlled release applics.; visc. avail. 3, 5, 6, 15, 50, 4000, and 10,000 cps.

Methocel® F Premium. [Dow] Hydroxypropylmethyl-cellulose USP; CAS 9004-65-3; used for pharmaceutical tablet coating, granulation, controlled release applics.; visc. avail. 50 and 4000 cps.

Methocel® J Premium. [Dow] Hydroxypropylmethyl-cellulose USP; CAS 9004-65-3; used for pharmaceutical tablet coating, granulation, controlled release applics., water-sol. thermoplastics; visc. avail. 5, 15, 100, 4000, 15,000, and 100,000 cps.

Methocel® K3P. [Dow] Hydroxypropylmethylcellulose; CAS 9004-65-3; used for pharmaceutical tablet coating; wh./off-wh. powd.; visc. 3 mPa·s.

Methocel® K4MP. [Dow] Hydroxypropyl methylcellulose; CAS 9004-65-3; visc. control agent, gellant, lather enhancer/stabilizer, film-former, dispersant, lubricant, binder, emulsion stabilizer, and suspending agent for personal care prods., shampoos, facial mask, sun care, creams and lotions, and controlled drug release; visc. 4000 mPa·s.

Methocel® K4MS. [Dow] Hydroxypropyl methylcellulose; CAS 9004-65-3; visc. control agent, gellant, lather enhancer/stabilizer, film-former, dispersant, lubricant, binder, emulsion stabilizer, and suspending agent for personal care prods.; disp. in cold water; visc. 4000 mPa·s.

Methocel® K15MP. [Dow] Hydroxypropyl methylcellulose; CAS 9004-65-3; visc. control agent, gellant, lather enhancer/stabilizer, film-former, dispersant, lubricant, binder, emulsion stabilizer, and suspending agent for personal care prods., emulsion conditioners, and controlled drug release; wh./off-wh. powd.; visc. 15,000 mPa·s.

Methocel® K15MS. [Dow] Hydroxypropyl methylcellulose; CAS 9004-65-3; visc. control agent, gellant, lather enhancer/stabilizer, film-former, dispersant, lubricant, binder, emulsion stabilizer, and suspending agent for personal care prods., emulsion conditioners; disp. in cold water; visc. 15,000 mPa·s.

Methocel® K35. [Dow] Hydroxypropyl methylcellulose; CAS 9004-65-3; food gums used as thickener, stabilizer, emulsifier, adhesive, and gellant.

Methocel® K100LVP. [Dow] Hydroxypropyl methylcellulose; CAS 9004-65-3; visc. control agent, gellant, lather enhancer/stabilizer, film-former, dispersant, lubricant, binder, emulsion stabilizer, and suspending agent for personal care prods. and controlled drug release; wh./off-wh. powd.; visc. 100 mPa·s.

Methocel® K100MP. [Dow] Hydroxypropyl methylcellulose; CAS 9004-65-3; visc. control agent, gellant, lather enhancer/stabilizer, film-former, dispersant, lubricant, binder, emulsion stabilizer, and suspending agent for personal care prods., styling gels, toothpaste, and controlled drug release; wh./off-wh. powd.; visc. 100,000 mPa·s.

Methocel® K Premium. [Dow] Hydroxypropylmethyl-cellulose USP; CAS 9004-65-3; used for pharmaceutical tablet coating, granulation, controlled release applics.; visc. avail. 3, 100, 4000, 15,000, and 100,000 cps.

Methomid 60. [Scher] PEG-50 tallow amide.

Methyl-Steriline. [Zimmerli] Methylparaben; CAS 99-76-3; EINECS 202-785-7; preservative for cosmetics; colorless; usage level: 0.1-1.0%; toxicology: nontoxic.

Mexanyl GQ. [Chimex] Octoxyglyceryl behenate.

Mexanyl GR. [Chimex] C14-16 glycol palmitate.

Mexanyl GU. [Chimex] Lauryl glycol; CAS 1119-87-5; EINECS 214-289-8.

Mexomere PL. [Chimex] Diethylene glycolamine/epichloro-hydrin/piperizine copolymer.

Mexomere PO. [Chimex] Hexadimethrine chloride.

Mexomere PP. [Chimex] Polyvinyl laurate.

Mexpectin LA 100 Range. [Grindsted Prods.] Amidated low-ester pectin; CAS 9000-69-5; EINECS 232-553-0; gellant and mouthfeel modifier for fruit-based prods.; protein stabilizer for cultured milk prods.; also for cosmetics, toiletries, and pharmaceuticals.

Mexpectin LC 700 Range. [Grindsted Prods.] Low-ester pectin; CAS 9000-69-5; EINECS 232-553-0; gellant and mouthfeel modifier for fruit-based prods.; protein stabilizer for cultured milk prods.; also for cosmetics, toiletries, and pharmaceuticals.

Mexpectin XSS 100 Range. [Grindsted Prods.] Pectin; CAS 9000-69-5; EINECS 232-553-0; gellant and mouthfeel modifier for fruit-based prods., confectionery; protein stabilizer for cultured milk prods.; also for cosmetics, toiletries, and pharmaceuticals.

MFA™ Complex. [Barnet Prods.] Sugar cane extract, citrus extract, apple extract, green tea extract; (mixed fruit acid); provides retexturization action on the skin, cell renewal, anti-irritancy props.; liq.; pH ≤ 2; usage level: 3-7.5%; toxicology: caustic to eyes; skin exfoliant.

MFF Series. [Siltech] Dimethicone copolyol; nonionic; high foaming gloss additive, mild conditioner for personal care prods.; water-sol.; 50% act.

Mibiron® N-50. [Rona; E. Merck] Bismuth oxychloride-coated mica; pearlescent pigment for lipsticks, pressed powds., eye makeups, for frosted effects; offers slip, soft skin feel, and good skin adhesion.

Mica PGM-3. [Presperse] Mica; CAS 12001-26-2; natural powd. for pressed powds., pigmented cosmetics; JSCI/JCID approved; powd.; oil absorp. 48-55%; sp.gr. 2.84; bulk dens. 1.85-3.30 g/in.³; m.p. 2800 F; ref. index 1.58; pH 7-9; Moh hardness 2.5.

Mica PGM-4. [Presperse] Mica; CAS 12001-26-2; natural powd. for pressed powds., pigmented cosmetics; JSCI/JCID approved; powd.; oil absorp. 48-55%; sp.gr. 2.84; bulk dens. 1.85-3.30 g/in.³; m.p. 2800 F; ref. index 1.58; pH 7-9; Moh hardness 2.5.

Mica PGM-5. [Presperse] Mica; CAS 12001-26-2; natural powd. for pressed powds., pigmented cosmetics; JSCI/JCID approved; powd.; oil absorp. 48-55%; sp.gr. 2.84; bulk dens. 1.85-3.30 g/in.³; m.p. 2800 F; ref. index 1.58; pH 7-9; Moh hardness 2.5.

Michel XO-150-16. [M. Michel] Isocetyl alcohol; CAS 36311-34-9; EINECS 252-964-9; emollient; Hazen 20 color; m.w. 242; sp.gr. 0.836; visc. 38 cps; m.p. -21 to -15 C; b.p. 285 C; acid no. 0.1 max.; iodine no. 1 max.; sapon. no. 1 max.; hyd. no. 229-235; flash pt. (COC) 156 C; ref. index 1.446-1.451; surf. tens. 29.6 dynes/cm; 100% conc.

Michel XO-150-20. [M. Michel] Octyldodecanol; CAS 5333-42-6; EINECS 226-242-9; carrier, lubricant, emollient; Hazen 20 max. color; m.w. 298; sp.gr. 0.838; visc. 60 cps; m.p. -1 to 1 C; b.p. 324 C; acid no. 0.1 max.; iodine no. 1 max.; sapon. no. 1 max.; hyd. no. 184-190; flash pt. (COC) 180 C; ref. index 1.451-1.456; surf. tens. 30.6 dynes/cm; 100% conc.

Michel XO-150-1620. [M. Michel] Isostearyl alcohol; CAS 70693-04-8; cosmetic ingred.; Hazen 20 color; m.w. 267-285; sp.gr. 0.837; visc. 50 cps; m.p. -10 to -6 C; b.p. 290 C; acid no. 0.1 max.; iodine no. 1 max.; sapon. no. 1 max.; hyd. no. 197-210; flash pt. (COC) 170 C; ref. index 1.449-1.454; surf. tens. 30.3 dynes/cm; 100% conc.

Microat™ E. [Nurture] Oat protein; emulsifier, thickener, film-former, gelling agent, and protein source; wh. fine powd., mild oat flavor; 100% thru 200 mesh; 11% protein, 80% starch, 5% moisture.

Micro-Cel® C. [Celite] Syn. calcium silicate; CAS 1344-95-2; EINECS 215-710-8; functional filler used to convert sticky, visc. liqs. to dry liqs. for use in rubber, agric., chemical, plastics, food processing, animal feed, and pharmaceutical industries; wh. fine powd.; 3.3% 325-mesh residue; sp.gr. 2.40; dens. 8.6 lb/ft³; oil absorp. 380%; surf. area 175 m²/g; ref. index 1.55; pH 10.

Micro-Dry®. [Reheis] Aluminum chlorohydrate; CAS 1327-41-9; EINECS 215-477-2; antiperspirant active used where particle size and surface area are important factors; widely used for aerosols; powd.; 97% min. thru 325 mesh; 47% Al₂O₃, 16.3% Cl.

Micro-Dry® Superultrafine. [Reheis] Aluminum chlorohydrate; CAS 1327-41-9; EINECS 215-477-2; antiperspirant active with finer particle size; used in suspensoid type sticks, suspension and powder roll-ons; powd.; 85% min. thru 10 μ; 47% Al₂O₃, 16.3% Cl.

Micro-Dry® Ultrafine. [Reheis] Aluminum chlorohydrate; CAS 1327-41-9; EINECS 215-477-2; antiperspirant active for use in suspensoid type sticks, suspension and powder roll-ons; powd.; 99% min. thru 400 mesh; 47% Al₂O₃, 16.3% Cl.

Microduct®. [CasChem] Maltodextrin; CAS 9050-36-6; EINECS 232-940-4; carrier for fragrances; emollient oils, bath prods.; food additive; powd.; 100% act.

Microfine 2, 2F, 2FS, 8, 8F. [Astor Wax] Syn. wax.; CAS 8002-74-2; cosmetic wax.

Microma-100. [Ikeda] Polymethylmethacrylate; CAS 9011-14-7; filler, lubricant, and adsorbent with exc. fluidity for pressed and loose powds., eyeshadow, liq. foundations; wh. transparent spherical powd., sl. char. odor, tasteless; 2-16 μm particle size.

Micronasphere™ M. [Rona; E. Merck] Fine mica coated with submicron silica spheres; provides exceptional skin feel to cosmetic formulations.

Micropearl M100. [Seppic] Polymethylmethacrylate; CAS 9011-14-7; provides very soft touch to skin; used in loose and pressed powds., creams and lotions, lipsticks and other makeup prods.; fine spherical powd.

Micropoly 520. [Presperse] Polyethylene; CAS 9002-88-4; EINECS 200-815-3; improves body, texture, visual attributes (luster, coverage, opacity) for wide variety of prod. formulations, pressed powds., pigmented cosmetics; JSCI/JCID approved; off-wh. opaque powd.; particle size 7 μ; sp.gr. 0.95; m.p. 230-237 F.

Micropoly 524. [Presperse] Polyethylene; CAS 9002-88-4; EINECS 200-815-3; improves body, texture, visual attributes (luster, coverage, opacity) for wide variety of prod. formulations, pressed powds., pigmented cosmetics; JSCI/JCID approved; off-wh. opaque powd.; particle size 4 μ (16 max.); sp.gr. 0.96; m.p. 253-257 F.

Micropoly 524-XF. [Presperse] Polyethylene; CAS 9002-88-4; EINECS 200-815-3; improves body, texture, visual attributes (luster, coverage, opacity) for wide variety of prod. formulations, pressed powds., pigmented cosmetics; JSCI/JCID approved; off-wh. opaque powd.; particle size 3 μ (12 max.); sp.gr. 0.50; m.p. 253-257 F.

Micropoly 2001. [Presperse] Polyethylene, syn. wax, and PTFE; improves body, texture, visual attributes (luster, coverage, opacity) for wide variety of prod. formulations, pigmented cosmetics; enhances compressability of pressed powds.; JSCI/JCID approved; off-wh. opaque powd.; particle size 9 μ; sp.gr. 0.99; m.p. 250-270 F.

MicroReservoir FRS-Diffuser. [Sederma] 8-Hydroxy-xanthine, lactoferrine, and vitamin E in encapsulated form; slow-release free radical scavenger for face, body, and sun care prods.; pink opalescent liq., char. odor; sp.gr. 1.040-1.070; ref. index 1.360-1.380; pH 6.0-8.0; usage level: 3-8%.

MicroReservoir Hydro-Diffuser. [Sederma] Natural moisturizing factor of the skin in encapsulated form; slow-release moisturizer for skin, face, body, and sun care prods.; beige liq., char. odor; sp.gr. 1.065-1.085; ref. index

1.380-1.390; pH 6.0-8.0; usage level: 3-8%.

MicroReservoir Nutri-Diffuser. [Sederma] Bacterian filtrate rich in peptides, mineral salts, and vitamin B₃ in encapsulated form; slow-release nutrient system for skin, face, body, and sun care prods.; beige liq., char. odor; sp.gr. 1.050-1.070; ref. index 1.370-1.380; pH 6.0-8.0; usage level: 3-8%.

Microsphere M-100. [Matsumoto Yushi-Seiyaku] Polymethyl methacrylate; CAS 9011-14-7; cosmetic ingred.

Microsphere M-305. [Tomen Am.] Methyl methyacrylate crosspolymer.

Microsponge®. [Advanced Polymer Systems] Styrene/DVB copolymer.

Microsponge® 5640. [Dow Corning; Advanced Polymer Systems] Acrylates copolymer; patented adsorbent for skin secretions; reduces shine and feathering, minimizes syneresis, provides elegant skin feel; for pigmented makeup, loose and compressed powds., facial cleansers, underarm prods., sticks, and oil-control treatments; wh. free-flowing spherical powd.; particle size 25 ± 10 μ; apparent dens. 0.34 g/cc; surf. area 150-260 m²/g; severe explosive hazard.

Microsponge® 5647. [Dow Corning; Advanced Polymer Systems] Acrylates copolymer and glycerin; improves feel of high-glycerin content cosmetic formulations, prolongs humectant props. of glycerin, improves moisture retention; for cleansers, foundations, lipsticks, facial treatments, hand and body moisturizers; patented; wh. to off-wh. free-flowing spherical powd.; particle size 25 ± 10 μ; apparent dens. 0.57 g/cc; 50% glycerin.

Microsponge® 5650. [Dow Corning; Advanced Polymer Systems] Acrylates copolymer, retinyl palmitate (25%), and corn oil (15%); improves stability of vitamin A palmitate formulations; for facial treatments, sun care prods., moisturizers, foundations, and powds.; patented; straw-yel. to yel. free-flowing spherical powd.; mean particle size 25 ± 10 μ; apparent dens. 0.29 g/cc; 60% act.

Microthene® MN-714, MN-722. [Quantum/USI] Polyethylene; CAS 9002-88-4; EINECS 200-815-3; cosmetic wax.

Midecol ACS. [Microbial Systems Int'l.; Ellis & Everard Personal Care; Tri-K Industries] Natural elemental sulfur complexed with fatty acid ethoxylates; cosmetic preservative; anti-dandruff, anti-sebhorrheic, and anti-parasitic agent, hair and skin conditioner.

Midecol CF. [Microbial Systems Int'l.; Ellis & Everard Personal Care; Tri-K Industries] Natural preservative extracted from seeds of *Azadirachta indica*; CAS 84696-25-3; EINECS 283-644-7; broad-spectrum antimicrobial preservative for cosmetic prods.

Midpol 97. [Microbial Systems Int'l.; Ellis & Everard Personal Care; Tri-K Industries] 2-Bromo-2-nitropropane-1,3-diol; CAS 52-51-7; EINECS 200-143-0; water-sol. antibacterial preservative for cosmetics applics.

Midpol 100. [Microbial Systems Int'l.; Ellis & Everard Personal Care; Tri-K Industries] 2-Bromo-2-nitropropane-1,3-diol; CAS 52-51-7; EINECS 200-143-0; water-sol. antibacterial preservative for cosmetics applics.

Midpol 2000. [Microbial Systems Int'l.; Tri-K Industries] Stabilized 2-bromo-2-nitropropane-1,3-diol (< 25%) with trishydroxy nitromethane (< 15%), dioctyl sodium sulfosuccinate (> 20%), α-tocopherol acetate, ethanol (< 10%), water; versatile, cost-effective, broad spectrum preservative for cosmetics and toiletries (shampoos, bath preps., sunscreens, skin care prods., colored cosmetics, creams, cleansers); effective against Gram-positive and Gram-negative bacteria, yeast, and molds; stable to 60 C and at pH 4-8.5; stable to light; biodeg.; USA and Europe approvals; pale straw-colored transparent liq., light pleasant odor; sol. in water, ethanol, IPA; forms emulsions with benzyl alcohol, propylene glycol, veg. oils; sp.gr. ≈ 1.0; pH

4.5; usage level: 200-500 ppm; toxicology: poisonous if swallowed; skin and eye irritant.

Midpol PHN. [Microbial Systems Int'l.; Ellis & Everard Personal Care; Tri-K Industries] 2-Bromo-2-nitropropane-1,3-diol and phenoxyethanol; water-sol. preservative for cosmetics applics. where bacteria is major hazard but yeast and mold contamination is present; USA and Europe approvals; water-sol.; usage level: 0.04-0.16%.

Midtect TF-60. [Microbial Systems Int'l.; Ellis & Everard Personal Care; Tri-K Industries] Potentiated dichlorobenzyl alcohol; CAS 1777-82-8; EINECS 217-210-5; broad-spectrum preservative for cosmetics applics.; effective against molds, yeast, Gram-positive and Gram-negative bacteria incl. *Pseudomonas*; USA and Europe approvals; usage level: 1000-5000 ppm.

Midtect TFP. [Microbial Systems Int'l.; Ellis & Everard Personal Care; Tri-K Industries] Dichlorobenzyl alcohol and phenoxyethanol; preservative for cosmetics applics. esp. highly alkaline formulations such as hair preps., toothpastes, and hard-surf. cleaners; gives broad-spectrum protection at pH > 10.5; USA and Europe approvals; usage level: 0.1-0.3%.

Miglyol® 808. [Hüls Am.] Tricaprylin; CAS 538-23-8; EINECS 208-686-5; emollient with good skin spreading/penetrating props. for cosmetics prods.; colorless to sl. yel. liq.; visc. 25-30 mPa·s; acid no. 0.1 max.; iodine no. 0.5 max.; sapon. no. 350-360.

Miglyol® 810. [Hüls Am.; Hüls AG] Caprylic/capric triglyceride; CAS 65381-09-1; nonionic; emollient, dispersant, lubricant, suspending agent, solubilizer; act. ingred. for cosmetics and pharmaceuticals; carrier/vehicle and solv. for inj. prods., topical ointments, creams, lotions, suppositories; dietetic prods.; penetrating and spreading props. on skin; colorless liq.; neutral odor; sol. in diethyl ether, petrol. ether, chloroform, IPA, toluene, alcohol, min. oil, acetone; sp.gr. 0.94-0.95; visc. 25-35 mPa·s; acid no. 0.1 max.; iodine no. 0.5 max.; sapon. no. 335-355; pH neutral; cloud pt. 0 C.

Miglyol® 812. [Hüls Am.; Hüls AG] Caprylic/capric triglyceride; CAS 65381-09-1; nonionic; dispersant, lubricant, anticaking agent, carrier, solv., solubilizer, suspending agent for cosmetics, pharmaceuticals (oral, external, suppositories), dietetic prods.; spreading and penetrating props. on skin; stable to oxidation; colorless liq.; sol. in alcohol, min. oil, acetone; visc. 25-35 mPa·s; acid no. 0.1 max.; iodine no. 0.5 max.; sapon. no. 325-345; cloud pt. 10 C; 100% conc.

Miglyol® 818. [Hüls Am.; Hüls AG] Caprylic/capric/linoleic triglyceride; CAS 67701-28-4; emollient for topical creams, lotions, and oil formulations for cosmetics and pharmaceuticals; spreading and penetrating props. on skin; virtually colorless liq.; visc. 30-35 mPa·s; acid no. 0.2 max.; iodine no. 10 max.; sapon. no. 315-335; cloud pt. 10 C.

Miglyol® 829. [Hüls Am.; Hüls AG] Caprylic/capric/diglyceryl succinate; emollient, suspending agent for cosmetic and pharmaceutical topicals, cream and liq. emulsions, oral suspensions, and capsules; ylsh. visc. liq.; sp.gr. 1.01; visc. 230-260 mPa·s; acid no. 1 max.; iodine no. 1 max.; sapon. no. 400-430; cloud pt. -30 C; toxicology: nontoxic.

Miglyol® 840. [Hüls Am.; Hüls AG] Propylene glycol dicaprylate/dicaprate; emollient, dispersant, lubricant, suspending agent, solubilizer; act. ingred. for cosmetics and pharmaceuticals; carrier/vehicle and solv. for inj. prods., topical ointments, creams, lotions, suppositories; dietetic prods.; flavor fixative; oxidation-stable; colorless liq.; sol. in alcohol, min. oil, acetone; visc. 8-14 mPa·s; acid no. 0.1 max.; iodine no. 0.5 max.; sapon. no. 320-340; cloud pt. -30 C.

Miglyol® 840 Gel B. [Hüls Am.; Hüls AG] Propylene glycol dicaprylate/dicaprate, stearalkonium hectorite, propylene carbonate; consistency regulator for creams; high temp. stabilizer esp. for w/o emulsions and anhyd. skin care and decorative formulations, pharmaceuticals; cream-colored paste; acid no. 0.5 max.; iodine no. 1 max.; sapon. no. 290-315.

Miglyol® 840 Gel T. [Hüls Am.; Hüls AG] Propylene glycol dicaprylate/dicaprate, stearalkonium bentonite, propylene carbonate; consistency regulator for creams; high temp. stabilizer esp. for w/o emulsions and anhyd. skin care and decorative formulations, pharmaceuticals; greenish paste; acid no. 0.5 max.; iodine no. 1 max.; sapon. no. 290-315.

Miglyol® Gel B. [Hüls Am.; Hüls AG] Caprylic/capric triglyceride, stearalkonium hectorite, propylene carbonate; pale oily gel with neutral props. for anhyd. formulations (ointments, makeup, lip gloss); consistency regulator in anhyd. and aq. cosmetics, pharmaceuticals; stabilizer for emulsions; flesh-colored hard paste; acid no. 0.5 max.; iodine no. 1 max.; sapon. no. 290-320.

Miglyol® Gel T. [Hüls Am.; Hüls AG] Caprylic/capric triglyceride, stearalkonium bentonite, propylene carbonate; consistency regulator for creams; high temp. stabilizer esp. for w/o emulsions and anhyd. skin care and decorative formulations; pharmaceutical ointments; greenish hard paste; acid no. 0.5 max.; iodine no. 1 max.; sapon. no. 290-315.

Mikrokill 2. [Brooks Industries] Polyaminopropyl biguanide, chloroxylenol; cosmetic preservative system; USA and Europe approvals; usage level: 0.2%.

Mikrokill 20. [Brooks Industries] Polyaminopropyl biguanide; CAS 27083-27-8; cosmetic preservative; usage level: 0.2-1.0% , 20% sol'n.

Milkamino™ 20. [Brooks Industries] Milk amino acids; CAS 65072-00-6; substantive moisturizer for cosmetics field; low salt; m.w. 200; 20% act.

Milkpro. [Ikeda] Hydrolyzed casein; CAS 65072-00-6; EINECS 265-363-1; emollient providing protective colloidal effect, chelating function, affinity to skin, and substantivity to hair; for body and hair shampoos, hair conditioners; emulsion stabilizer; ylsh. liq., char. odor; pH 4.0-7.0.

Milkpro-Q. [Ikeda] N-(3-Trimethylammonio-2-hydroxypropyl) hydrolyzed casein; soft film-former with exc. water retention; provides exc. adsorption, glossiness, and fine touch to the skin; for body and hair shampoos, hair conditioners; lt. amber clear liq., char. odor; pH 4.0-7.0; 10.5-12.5% solids.

Millithix® 925. [Milliken] Dibenzylidene sorbitol; CAS 32647-67-9; EINECS 251-136-4; thixotrope and gellant for use in unsat. polyester and vinyl ester resins; also as clear antiperspirant; solid wh. powd.

Mimosoie® . [Alban Muller] Silk worm extract and tepescohuite extract; Cell stimulating complex derived from *Bombyx mori* and *Mimosa tenuiflora* for dermocosmetological applics. incl. anti-aging, delicate, or protective skin creams, gels, and emulsions; brn. liq., odorless; water-sol.; sp.gr. 1.025 ± 0.010; b.p. > 100 C; flash pt. (OC) > 107 C; pH 6.0-8.0; ref. index 1.3650-1.3750; usage level: 3-5%; 60-75% water, 25-35% propylene glycol.

Mineral Jelly No. 5. [Penreco] Petrolatum; CAS 8009-03-8; EINECS 232-373-2; preblended base for cosmetic mfg., hair prods., makeup, creams and lotions; Lovibond 2Y color; odorless; tasteless; misc. with cosmetic ingred. used in oil-base formulations; visc. 38-43 SUS (210 F); pour pt. 75-90 F.

Mineral Jelly No. 10. [Penreco] Petrolatum; CAS 8009-03-8; EINECS 232-373-2; preblended base for cosmetic mfg. (hair prods., makeup, creams and lotions); Lovibond 1Y color; odorless; tasteless; misc. with cosmetic ingred.

used in oil-base formulations; visc. 40-43 SUS (210 F); m.p. (Saybolt) 97-105 F; pour pt. 95-105 F.

Mineral Jelly No. 10. [Witco/Petroleum Spec.] Petrolatum; EINECS 232-373-2; cosmetic ingred.; Lovibond 1.0Y color; visc. 2.6-5.7 cSt (100 C); m.p. 38-43 C.

Mineral Jelly No. 14. [Witco/Petroleum Spec.] Petrolatum; CAS 8009-03-8; EINECS 232-373-2; cosmetics ingred.; Lovibond 1.0Y color; visc. 2.6-5.7 cSt (100 C); m.p. 38-52 C.

Mineral Jelly No. 15. [Penreco] Petrolatum; CAS 8009-03-8; EINECS 232-373-2; preblended base for cosmetic mfg. (hair prods., makeup, creams and lotions); Lovibond 0.5Y color; odorless; tasteless; misc. with cosmetic ingred. used in oil-base formulations; visc. 40-44 SUS (210 F); m.p. (Saybolt) 97-108 F; pour pt. 95-105 F.

Mineral Jelly No. 17. [Witco/Petroleum Spec.] Petrolatum; CAS 8009-03-8; EINECS 232-373-2; cosmetics ingred.; Lovibond 1.0Y color; visc. 2.6-5.7 cSt (100 C); m.p. 36-49 C.

Mineral Jelly No. 20. [Penreco] Petrolatum; CAS 8009-03-8; EINECS 232-373-2; preblended base for cosmetic mfg. (hair prods., makeup, creams and lotions); Lovibond 0.5Y color; odorless; tasteless; misc. with cosmetic ingred. used in oil-base formulations; visc. 37-40 SUS (210 F); m.p. (Saybolt) 111-116 F; pour pt. 110-120 F.

Mineral Jelly No. 25. [Penreco] Petrolatum; CAS 8009-03-8; EINECS 232-373-2; preblended base for cosmetic mfg. (hair prods., makeup, creams and lotions); Lovibond 0.5Y color; odorless; tasteless; misc. with cosmetic ingred. used in oil-base formulations; visc. 38-40 SUS (210 F); m.p. (Saybolt) 103-108 F; pour pt. 100-110 F.

Mink Oil W. [Cosmetochem] PEG-13 mink glycerides; cosmetic ingred.

MIPA. [Dow] Monoisopropanolamine; used to produce soaps with good hard surf. detergency, shampoos, emulsifiers, textile specialties, agric. and polymer curing chemicals, adhesives, coatings, metalworking, petroleum, rubber processing, gas conditioning chemicals; sp.gr. 0.960 (20/4 C); dens. 7.95 lb/gal; visc. 23 cps; f.p. 3 C; b.p. 159 C (760 mm Hg); flash pt. (TCC) 173 F; ref. index 1.4456.

Miracare® 2MCA. [Rhone-Poulenc Surf. & Spec.] Disodium cocoamphodiacetate, sodium lauryl sulfate, and hexylene glycol; mild base used in formulating nonirritating and baby shampoos; lt. amber clear liq.; water sol.; pH 8.0–8.5 (20% aq.); 46–48% solids.; formerly Miranol® 2MCA MOD.

Miracare® 2MCAS. [Rhone-Poulenc Surf. & Spec.] Disodium cocoamphodiacetate, sodium lauryl sulfate, sodium laureth sulfate, and propylene glycol; amphoteric; surfactant for nonirritating and non-eye-sting shampoos, bath gels; lt. yel. clear liq.; water sol.; pH 7.5–8.0; 45.5–48.0% solids.; formerly Miranol® 2MCAS MOD.

Miracare® 2MCA-SF. [Rhone-Poulenc Surf. & Spec.] Disodium cocoamphodipropionate, sodium lauryl sulfate, hexylene glycol; amphoteric; surfactant for nonirritating and non-eye-sting shampoos; visc. liq.; 41% conc.; formerly Miranol® 2MCA-SF MOD.

Miracare® 2MCT. [Rhone-Poulenc Surf. & Spec.] Disodium cocoamphodiacetate, sodium trideceth sulfate, hexylene glycol; amphoteric; surfactant for nonirritating and non-eye-sting shampoos, make-up removers; lt. amber clear liq.; water-sol.; pH 7.5-8.0; 48.5-51.5% solids.; formerly Miranol® 2MCT MOD.

Miracare® 2MHT. [Rhone-Poulenc Surf. & Spec.] Disodium lauroamphodiacetate, sodium trideceth sulfate, and hexylene glycol; amphoteric; detergent base; surfactant for nonirritating and non-eye-sting shampoos and liq. hand soaps; liq.; 42% conc.; formerly Miranol® 2MHT MOD.

Miracare® ANL. [Rhone-Poulenc Surf. & Spec.] Sodium C14-16 olefin sulfonate, sodium laureth sulfate, lauramide DEA; anionic/nonionic; high foaming surfactant conc. for high-performance shampoos and skin cleansers; liq.; 50% conc.; formerly Cycloryl ANL.

Miracare® BC-10. [Rhone-Poulenc Surf. & Spec.] PEG-80 sorbitan laurate, cocamidopropyl betaine, sodium trideceth sulfate, sodium lauroamphoacetate, PEG-150 distearate, sodium laureth-13 carboxylate; conc. for prep. of baby shampoo, bubble bath, bath gel and liq. hand soap prods. requiring mildness.

Miracare® BC-20. [Rhone-Poulenc Surf. & Spec.] PEG-80 sorbitan laurate, cocamidopropyl betaine, sodium trideceth sulfate, glycerin, sodium lauroamphoacetate, PEG-150 distearate, sodium laureth-13 carboxylate; conc. for prep. of baby shampoo, bubble bath, bath gel, and liq. hand soap prods. where mildness is primary concern.

Miracare® BT. [Rhone-Poulenc Surf. & Spec.] Disodium lauroamphodiacetate and sodium trideceth sulfate; amphoteric; surfactant for nonirritating and non-eye-sting shampoos; liq.; 33% conc.; formerly Miranol® BT.

Miracare® CT100. [Rhone-Poulenc Surf. & Spec.] Stearyl alcohol and cetrimonium bromide; cationic; emulsifier for creme rinse/conditioner; base for permanent wave foam neutralizers; wh. flakes; m.p. 76–77 C.; formerly Cycloton® CT100.

Miracare® M1. [Rhone-Poulenc Surf. & Spec.] Sodium lauryl sulfate, stearamide MEA, glycol stearate and cocamide MEA; anionic; built pearlized base for cream shampoos having high flash foam; wh. creamy liq.; 34–36% act.; formerly Cycloryl M1.

Miracare® MHT. [Rhone-Poulenc Surf. & Spec.] Sodium lauroamphoacetate and sodium trideceth sulfate; amphoteric; surfactant for nonirritating and non-eye-sting shampoos, foaming skin cleansing prods.;; lt. amber clear liq.; water sol.; pH 9.4–10.2; 33.5-36.5% solids.; formerly Miranol® MHT.

Miracare® MS-1. [Rhone-Poulenc Surf. & Spec.] PEG-80 sorbitan laurate, sodium trideceth sulfate, PEG-150 distearate, disodium lauraminopropionate, cocamidopropyl hydroxysultaine, sodium laureth-13 carboxylate; anionic/nonionic; conc. for prep. of baby shampoo, bubble bath, bath gel and liq. hand soap prods. requiring mildness; liq.; formerly Compound MS-1.

Miracare® MS-2. [Rhone-Poulenc Surf. & Spec.] PEG-80 sorbitan laurate, sodium trideceth sulfate, PEG-150 distearate, disodium lauraminopropionate, cocamidopropyl hydroxysultaine, sodium laureth-13 carboxylate; anionic/nonionic; conc. for prep. of baby shampoo, bubble bath, bath gel and liq. hand soap prods. requiring mildness; liq.; formerly Compound MS-2.

Miracare® MS-4. [Rhone-Poulenc Surf. & Spec.] PEG-80 sorbitan laurate, sodium trideceth sulfate, PEG-150 distearate, disodium lauraminopropionate, cocamidopropyl hydroxysultaine, sodium laureth-13 carboxylate; anionic/nonionic; conc. for prep. of baby shampoo, bubble bath, bath gel and liq. hand soap prods. requiring mildness; liq.; formerly Compound MS-4.

Miracare® NWC. [Rhone-Poulenc Surf. & Spec.] Sodium laureth sulfate, cocamide DEA, TEA-lauryl sulfate; anionic; biodeg. base for shampoos and bubble baths; amber liq.; 62-64% act.; formerly Cycloryl NWC.

Miracare® SCS. [Rhone-Poulenc Surf. & Spec.] Stearalkonium chloride in compatible emulsifier base; CAS 122-19-0; EINECS 204-527-9; formulated base for simplified prod. of cream rinse conditioners.; formerly Cycloton SCS.

Miracare® XL. [Rhone-Poulenc Surf. & Spec.] DEA-lauryl sulfate, DEA-lauraminopropionate, sodium lauraminopropionate, propylene glycol; anionic/amphoteric; high foaming base for prep. of hair and body shampoos; liq.;

35% conc.; formerly Mirataine® XL.

Miramine® SODI. [Rhone-Poulenc Surf. & Spec.] Stearamidopropyl dimethylamine; CAS 7651-02-7; EINECS 231-609-1; emulsifier, conditioner, foam booster/stabilizer, visc. builder for shampoos, liq. soaps, facial cleansers, bath preps., toiletries, hair conditioners; produces cationic emulsions; off-wh. solid; 100% act., 98% amide.; formerly Cyclomide SODI.

Miranate® LEC. [Rhone-Poulenc Surf. & Spec.] Sodium laureth-13 carboxylate; CAS 70632-06-3; anionic; aux. detergent, foaming agent, emulsifier for shampoo systems, liq. soaps, facial cleansers, bath gels, and bubble baths; lime soap dispersant; emulsifier, lubricant for metalworking fluids; hazy gel; water-sol.; dens. 8.996 lb/gal; flash pt. > 200 C; pH 8.0 (10%); 70% act.

Miranol® 2CIB. [Rhone-Poulenc Surf. & Spec.] Disodium cocoamphodiacetate; CAS 68647-53-0; amphoteric; detergent for high foaming, nonirritating shampoos, skin cleansers, cosmetics, industrial detergents; emulsifier, solubilizer, coupling agent for heavy-duty liq. cleaners; amber clear liq.; sol. in water; dens. 1.18 g/ml; pH 8-9.5; 49.5-50.5% solids.; formerly Alkateric® 2CIB.

Miranol® BM Conc. [Rhone-Poulenc Surf. & Spec.] Disodium lauroamphodiacetate; CAS 68608-66-2; amphoteric; foaming agent, conditioner, detergent, emulsifier, foam stabilizer for nonirritating shampoos, skin cleansers, liq. soaps, bath gels, and bubble baths; liq.; 38% conc.

Miranol® C2M Conc. NP. [Rhone-Poulenc Surf. & Spec.] Disodium cocoamphodiacetate; CAS 68650-39-5; EINECS 272-043-5; amphoteric; detergent, foaming agent, emulsifier, solubilizer, foam stabilizer used in nonirritating shampoos, skin cleansers, make-up removers, liq. soaps, bath gels, bubble baths; emulsifier, solubilizer, and stabilizer in pharmaceuticals, household and industrial cleaners; clear, visc. liq.; sol. in water; pH 8.0–8.5 (20% aq.); 38% act.

Miranol® C2M Conc. NP-PG. [Rhone-Poulenc Surf. & Spec.] Disodium cocoamphodiacetate, propylene glycol; CAS 68650-39-5; surfactant.

Miranol® C2M Conc. OP. [Rhone-Poulenc Surf. & Spec.] Disodium cocoamphodiacetate; CAS 68650-39-5; EINECS 272-043-5; amphoteric; surfactant for nonirritating shampoos, skin cleansers, medicated cosmetics, medium-duty liq. cleaners; liq.; 50% conc.

Miranol® C2M-SF 70%. [Rhone-Poulenc Surf. & Spec.] Disodium cocoamphodipropionate; CAS 68604-71-7; amphoteric; detergent used for heavy-duty liq. cleaning compds., steam cleaners, nonirritating shampoos, medicated cosmetics; paste at R.T., pumps and pours at 50 C; pH 9–10 (10% aq.); 70% act.

Miranol® C2M-SF Conc. [Rhone-Poulenc Surf. & Spec.] Disodium cocoamphodipropionate; CAS 68604-71-7; amphoteric; detergent for extra heavy duty cleaners, steam, pressure, metal, all-purpose cleaners, shampoos, medicated cosmetics; also coupling agent, solubilizer, wetting agent; biodeg.; amber clear liq., fruity odor; sol. in water and alcohol; sp.gr. 1.07; f.p. < 0 C; b.p. 98 C; flash pt. 144 F; pH 9.4–9.8; toxicology: minimally irritating to skin and eyes; LD50 (oral, mouse) > 5 ml/kg; 39% act.

Miranol® CM Conc. NP. [Rhone-Poulenc Surf. & Spec.] Sodium cocoamphoacetate; CAS 68608-65-1; amphoteric; detergent, wetting and foaming agent, sequestrant, emulsifier, dispersant, germicidal, visc. builder; for extra heavy duty cleaners, steam, pressure, metal, all-purpose cleaners; conditioner, detergent, emulsifier, foam booster/stabilizer for shampoos, liq. soaps, facial cleansers, bath gels, bubble baths; biodeg.; lt. amber visc. liq.; pH 9.0–13.0; 44% conc.

Miranol® CM-SF Conc. [Rhone-Poulenc Surf. & Spec.] Sodium cocoamphopropionate; CAS 68919-41-5; amphoteric; mild foaming agent, conditioner, detergent, emulsifier, foam booster/stabilizer for shampoos, liq. soaps, facial cleansers, bath gels, bubble baths; coemulsifier for emulsion polymerization; emulsifier, wetting agent for industrial, institutional and household cleaners; biodeg.; lt. amber clear liq.; sol. in water and alcohol; pH 9.5–10.5; 36–38% solids.

Miranol® CS Conc. [Rhone-Poulenc Surf. & Spec.] Sodium cocoamphohydroxypropylsulfonate; CAS 68604-73-9; EINECS 271-705-0; amphoteric; detergent, wetting agent, corrosion inhibitor, emulsifier, sequestrant, foaming agent for shampoos, cold water fabrics, household and industrial cleaners; biodeg.; yel. visc. liq., fruity odor; water-sol.; sp.gr. 1.16; f.p. < 0 C; b.p. 102 C; pH 8.0; toxicology: minimally irritating to skin and eyes; LD50 (oral, mouse) > 5 ml/kg; 38% conc.

Miranol® DM. [Rhone-Poulenc Surf. & Spec.] Sodium stearoamphoacetate; CAS 68608-63-9; amphoteric; antistat, household softener, lubricant, dispersant used in textile industry, hair conditioners; biodeg.; wh. creamy paste, readily pourable @ 60 C; pH 5.4–6.0 (65 C); 25–27% solids.

Miranol® DM Conc. 45%. [Rhone-Poulenc Surf. & Spec.] Sodium stearoamphoacetate; CAS 68608-63-9; amphoteric; viscosifier, lubricant, softener, conditioner for cosmetics, textiles, industrial, institutional and household cleaners; paste; water-disp.; 45% conc.

Miranol® FB-NP. [Rhone-Poulenc Surf. & Spec.] Disodium cocoamphodiacetate; CAS 68650-39-5; EINECS 272-043-5; amphoteric; surfactant for nonirritating shampoos, skin cleansers, medicated cosmetics, med.-duty liq. cleaners; liq.; 50% conc.; formerly Mirapon FB-NP.

Miranol® H2M Conc. [Rhone-Poulenc Surf. & Spec.] Disodium lauroamphodiacetate; CAS 68608-66-2; amphoteric; conditioner, detergent, emulsifier, foam booster/stabilizer for nonirritating shampoos, skin cleaners, liq. soaps, bath gels, and bubble baths; biodeg.; lt. amber visc. liq.; water sol.; pH 8.0–8.5 (20% aq.); 49–51% solids.

Miranol® H2M-SF Conc. [Rhone-Poulenc Surf. & Spec.] Disodium lauroamphodipropionate; CAS 68610-43-5; amphoteric; surfactant for nonirritating shampoos and skin cleaners, esp. aerosols; biodeg.; lt. amber clear liq.; sol. in water, alcohol; pH 9.2–9.8; 38–40% solids.

Miranol® HM Conc. [Rhone-Poulenc Surf. & Spec.] Sodium lauroamphoacetate; CAS 68608-66-2; amphoteric; detergent, wetting agent, foam booster/stabilizer, sequestrant, emulsifier, dispersant, and germicidal for shampoos, liq. soaps, facial cleansers, dishwashing, and paints; biodeg.; lt. amber, visc. liq.; pH 9.0–9.5; 43–45% solids.

Miranol® JBS. [Rhone-Poulenc Surf. & Spec.] Disodium capryloamphodipropionate; CAS 68815-55-4; amphoteric; low foaming surfactant for medicated shampoos and skin cleansers; emulsifier, wetting agent for industrial cleaners; liq.; 38% conc.; formerly Mirapon JBS.

Miranol® SM Conc. [Rhone-Poulenc Surf. & Spec.] Sodium caproamphoacetate; CAS 68608-61-7; amphoteric; wetting agent, foaming agent, detergent used in medicated and germicidal shampoos and hand soaps, rug and upholstery shampoos, in emulsion polymerization; biodeg.; clear liq.; pH 9.0–9.5; 40–42% solids.

Miranol® TBS. [Rhone-Poulenc Surf. & Spec.] Sodium tallamphodipropionate; CAS 68991-88-8.

Mirapol® 550. [Rhone-Poulenc Surf. & Spec.] Polyquaternium-7; CAS 26590-05-6; cationic; conditioning polymer used in hair and skin care prods. to impart lubricity, slip, detangling, and luster to hair and a smooth, soft feel to skin; used for shampoos, creams and lotions, bath gels, bubble baths, and toiletries.

Mirapol® A-15. [Rhone-Poulenc Surf. & Spec.] Polyquaternium-2; CAS 68555-36-2; cationic; softening, conditioning, lubricant, antistat, surface modifying agent used in cream rinses, conditioning-type shampoos, toiletries, creams and lotions, and textile processing; amber visc. liq.; m.w. 2260; dissolves readily in water; pH 8.5; 64% act. in water.

Mirapol® AD-1. [Rhone-Poulenc Surf. & Spec.] Polyquaternium-17; CAS 90624-75-2; cationic; conditioner and antistat for personal care prods.; amber visc. liq.; m.w. 50,000; water-sol.; pH 8.0 (10%); 62% act. in water.

Mirapol® CP40. [Rhone-Poulenc Surf. & Spec.] Polyquarternium-6; CAS 26062-79-3; cationic; conditioner for shampoos, creams and lotions, and toiletries.

Mirasheen® 202. [Rhone-Poulenc Surf. & Spec.] Glycol stearate, lauramide DEA, cocamidopropyl betaine, glycerin; pearl conc. for cold blend cosmetic formulations; liq. soaps; contains visc. building, foam boosting, and mild conditioning agents; lotion/paste; 42% conc.; formerly Cyclosheen 202.

Mirasoft™ CO 11. [Rhone-Poulenc Surf. & Spec.] Castor oil sucroglyceride; nonionic; mild moisturizer and stabilizer for creams and facial cleansers.

Mirasoft™ LMO. [Rhone-Poulenc Surf. & Spec.] Coconut oil sucroglyceride; nonionic; mild moisturizer and stabilizer for creams and facial cleansers.

Mirasoft™ MSPO 11. [Rhone-Poulenc Surf. & Spec.] Palm oil sucroglyceride; nonionic; mild moisturizer and stabilizer for creams and facial cleansers.

Mirataine® BB. [Rhone-Poulenc Surf. & Spec.] Lauramidopropyl betaine; CAS 86438-78-0; EINECS 224-292-6; amphoteric; mild substantive surfactant, visc. builder and foam booster, wetting agent for shampoos and dishwashing liqs.; conditioner, antistat, emollient; as solubilizer, visc. builder, foam booster with lauryl sulfates; stable to acid and alkali media; clear liq.; 30% conc.

Mirataine® BD-J. [Rhone-Poulenc Surf. & Spec.] Cocamidopropyl betaine; CAS 70851-07-9; amphoteric; detergent and visc. builder for shampoos, bubble baths; liq.; 30% conc.

Mirataine® BD-R. [Rhone-Poulenc Surf. & Spec.] Cocamidopropyl betaine; CAS 70851-07-9.

Mirataine® BET-C-30. [Rhone-Poulenc Surf. & Spec.] Cocamidopropyl betaine; CAS 70851-07-9; amphoteric; mild foaming agent, conditioner, detergent, emulsifier, foam booster/stabilizer, visc. builder for shampoos, liq. soaps, facial cleansers, bath gels, bubble baths; yel. liq.; pH 4.5-5.5; 29-31% act.; formerly Cycloteric BET-C-30.

Mirataine® BET-O-30. [Rhone-Poulenc Surf. & Spec.] Oleamidopropyl betaine; CAS 25054-76-6; EINECS 246-584-2; amphoteric; conditioner, detergent, emulsifier, foam booster/stabilizer, visc. builder for shampoos, liq. soaps, facial cleansers, bath gels, bubble baths; yel. liq.; pH 5.5-6.5; 29-31% act.; formerly Cycloteric BET-O-30.

Mirataine® BET-W. [Rhone-Poulenc Surf. & Spec.] Cocamidopropyl betaine, tech.; CAS 61789-40-0; foam booster, foaming agent, thickener, conditioner for shampoos, cosmetic, and industrial applics.; irritation mollifying agent for baby shampoos; 30% act.; formerly Cycloteric BET-W.

Mirataine® CAB-A. [Rhone-Poulenc Surf. & Spec.] Cocamidopropyl betaine; CAS 61789-40-0; amphoteric; high foaming, mild, substantive detergent, conditioner for shampoos; solubilizer for lauryl sulfate in conc. shampoos; visc. builder, conditioner, antistat, emollient; clear liq.; 34-36% solids.; formerly Alkateric® CAB-A.

Mirataine® CAB-O. [Rhone-Poulenc Surf. & Spec.] Cocamidopropyl betaine; CAS 61789-40-0; amphoteric; mild substantive surfactant for personal care prods.; conditioner, antistat, emollient; as solubilizer, visc. builder, foam booster with lauryl sulfates; stable to acid and alkali media; clear liq.; 30-32% solids.; formerly Alkateric® CAB-O.

Mirataine® CB. [Rhone-Poulenc Surf. & Spec.] Cocamidopropyl betaine; CAS 70851-07-9; amphoteric; glycerin-free conditioner, detergent, emulsifier, foam booster/stabilizer, visc. builder providing mildness to shampoos, liq. soaps, facial cleansers, bath gels, and bubble baths.

Mirataine® CBC. [Rhone-Poulenc Surf. & Spec.] Cocamidopropyl betaine; CAS 70851-07-9; amphoteric; high foaming visc. builder, foam booster, emulsifier, wetting agent, dispersant for shampoos and dishwashing liqs.; liq.; 30% conc.

Mirataine® CB/M. [Rhone-Poulenc Surf. & Spec.] Cocamidopropyl betaine; amphoteric; mild, high foaming, substantive surfactant, emulsifier, wetting agent, dispersant, visc. builder, foam booster for shampoo formulations, dishwashing liqs.; conditioner, antistat, emollient, solubilizer; stable to acid and alkaline media; pale-colored clear liq.; dens. 8.71 lb/gal; sp.gr. 1.045; pH 8.5; 35% act. in water.

Mirataine® CBR. [Rhone-Poulenc Surf. & Spec.] Cocamidopropyl betaine; CAS 70851-07-9; amphoteric; visc. builder and foam booster for shampoos and dishwashing liqs.; liq.; 30% conc.

Mirataine® CBS, CBS Mod. [Rhone-Poulenc Surf. & Spec.] Cocamidopropyl hydroxysultaine; CAS 70851-08-0; EINECS 268-761-3; amphoteric; mild high foaming surfactant, visc. builder, foam booster, emulsifier, wetting agent for shampoo formulations, liq. bubble baths, industrial cleaners; liq.; water-sol.; dens. 9.1 lb/gal; cloud pt. ≤ −12 C; pH 8.2; 50% act. in water.

Mirataine® CCB. [Rhone-Poulenc Surf. & Spec.] Cocamidopropyl betaine; CAS 70851-07-9.

Mirataine® COB. [Rhone-Poulenc Surf. & Spec.] Coco/oleamidopropyl betaine; CAS 86438-79-1; amphoteric; surfactant and conditioner for use in personal care prods. (shampoos, liq. soaps, facial cleansers, bath gels, bubble baths); oil solubilizer, visc. builder, foam booster, stabilizer; yel. sl. visc. liq., faint fruity odor; water-sol.; sp.gr. 1.05; f.p. < 0 C; b.p. 100 C; pH 7.0; toxicology: minimally irritating to skin and eyes; LD50 (oral, mouse) > 5 ml/kg; 34.0% solids.

Mirataine® H2C-HA. [Rhone-Poulenc Surf. & Spec.] Sodium lauriminodipropionate; CAS 14960-06-6; EINECS 239-032-7; amphoteric; high foaming surfactant, foam booster, wetting agent, dispersant for shampoos and skin cleansers, and hard surface cleaners; liq.; 30% conc.

Mirataine® T2C-30. [Rhone-Poulenc Surf. & Spec.] Disodium tallowiminodipropionate; CAS 61791-56-8; EINECS 263-190-6; amphoteric; detergent, solubilizer, moderate foaming surfactant used in textile, leather, metalworking, industrial and personal care prods.; liq.; sol. in water; dens. 8.746 lb/gal; surf. tens. 31.6 dynes/cm (1% aq.); pH 11.5; biodeg.; 30% act. in water.

Mirataine® TM. [Rhone-Poulenc Surf. & Spec.] Dihydroxyethyl tallow glycinate; CAS 61791-25-1; EINECS 274-845-0; amphoteric; wetting agent, viscosifier for industrial and household cleaners; conditioner for shampoos; HCl thickener; lt. amber slightly hazy visc. liq.; pH 5.1; 35% conc.

Mircoat™ Oil. [Nurture] Oat extract; CAS 84012-26-0; antioxidant and fat-sol. vitamin source; amber clear liq., mild oat flavor.

Miristamina. [Vevy] Myristamide DEA; CAS 7545-23-5; EINECS 231-426-7; thickener, foam booster/stabilizer.

Miristocor. [Roche] Myristamidopropyldimethylamine phosphate.

M.O.D. [U.S. Cosmetics] 2-Octyldodecyl myristate; neutral oil imparting pleasant, nongreasy "cool feeling" to cosmetic makeup, sunscreens, hair care, and skin care prods.

M.O.D. WL 2949. [Gattefosse] Octyldodecyl myristate;

emollient; rancidless additive for cosmetics and pharmaceuticals; oily liq.; HLB 1.0; acid no. ≤ 7; iodine no. ≤ 7; sapon. no. 90-110; toxicology: LD50 (oral, rat) > 2 g/kg; sl. irritating to eyes; nonirritating to skin.

Modulan®. [Amerchol] Acetylated lanolin; CAS 61788-48-5; EINECS 262-979-2; conditioner, emollient, softener, lubricant for cosmetic and pharmaceutical prods.; yel.-amber soft solid; faint, pleasant odor; sol. in min. oil; m.p. 30–40 C; acid no. 2.5 max.; sapon. no. 95–120; hyd. no. 10 max.

Moisturizing Factor L. [Sederma] β-Lactoglobuline rich in essential amino acids and a lactic fermentation filtrate rich in amino acids and L-lactic acid; moisturizer for skin care prods.; rich in disulfide bonds.

Molo-Jel. [Witco/Petroleum Spec.] Petrolatum, min. oil.

Monacet. [Argeville] DEA-cetyl phosphate, isopropyl myristate, cetyl alcohol, glyceryl stearate SE.

Monalux CAO-35. [Mona Industries] Cocamidopropylamine oxide; CAS 68155-09-9; EINECS 268-938-5; foam booster/stabilizer and thickener for personal care prods.; yel. clear liq.; 35% conc.

Monamate C-1142. [Mona Industries] Disodium cocamido MIPA sulfosuccinate; CAS 68515-65-1; EINECS 271-102-2; foaming/cleaning surfactants for personal care and household prods.; liq.; toxicology: low skin and eye irritation; 40% act.

Monamate CPA-40. [Mona Industries] Disodium cocamido MIPA-sulfosuccinate; CAS 68515-65-1; EINECS 271-102-2; anionic; high foaming, nonirritating surfactant for shampooos, bubble baths, body cleansers, and household prods.; imparts talc-like feel to skin and soft feel to hair; biodeg.; yel. clear to hazy liq.; pH 6; Ross-Miles foam 210 mm (1% , 120 F); toxicology: LD50 (oral) > 5 g/kg; low eye and skin irritation; 40% act.

Monamate CPA-100. [Mona Industries] Disodium cocamido MIPA sulfosuccinate; CAS 68515-65-1; EINECS 271-102-2; anionic; foaming/cleaning surfactants for personal care and household prods.; powd.; toxicology: low skin and eye irritation; 100% act.

Monamate LA-100. [Mona Industries] Disodium lauryl sulfosuccinate; anionic; high foaming, low irritation surfactant for syndet and combo soap bars, shampoos, bubble baths, body cleansers, and household prods.; imparts soft talc-like after-feel to skin; wh. fine powd.; pH 6.9 (10%); toxicology: LD50 (oral) > 5 g/kg; low eye irritation, nonirritating to skin; 85% act.

Monamate LNT-40. [Mona Industries] Ammonium lauryl sulfosuccinate; anionic; high foaming, low irritation surfactant used in shampoos, bubble baths, body cleansers; imparts talc-like after-feel to skin and soft feel to hair; 100% biodeg.; water-wh. clear liq.; sp.gr. 1.07; dens. 8.88 lb/gal; pH 5.5; toxicology: not a primary skin irritant; only minimally irritating to eyes; 40 ± 1% solids.

Monamate OPA-30. [Mona Industries] Disodium oleamido PEG-2 sulfosuccinate; CAS 56388-43-3; EINECS 260-143-1; anionic; high foaming, nonirritating surfactant for shampoos, bubble baths, body cleansers, soap bars; imparts talc-like after-feel to skin and soft feel to hair; 100% biodeg.; lt. yel. clear liq.; sp.gr. 1.06; dens. 8.85 lb/gal; pH 5.6; toxicology: nonirritating to eyes and skin @ 15% act.; 30% solids.

Monamate OPA-100. [Mona Industries] Disodium oleamido PEG-2 sulfosuccinate; CAS 56388-43-3; EINECS 260-143-1; anionic; high foaming, nonirritating surfactant for shampoos, bubble baths, soap bars; powd.; toxicology: low skin and eye irritation; 100% conc.

Monamate RMEA-40. [Mona Industries] Disodium ricinoleamido MEA-sulfosuccinate.

Monamid® 15-70W. [Mona Industries] 1:1 Linoleamide DEA; CAS 56863-02-6; EINECS 260-410-2; nonionic; thickener, visc. builder, hair and fiber conditioner; biodeg.; Gvcs-33 11 max. liq.; sol. @ 10% in ethanol, chlorinated and aromatic hydrocarbons, min. spirits, kerosene, natural oils and fats, gels in water; dens. 8.00 lb/gal; sp.gr. 0.96; acid no. 0–1; alkali no. 25-40; pH 10–11 (10%); toxicology: very mild primary skin irritant; 100% act.

Monamid® 15-MW. [Mona Industries] Alkanolamide; thickener, visc. builder in shampoos, bubble baths, other aq. systems; sol. in aromatic hydrocarbons, chlorinated solvs.; sol to disp. in water.

Monamid® 31. [Mona Industries] Lauramide DEA; CAS 120-40-1; EINECS 204-393-1; foam booster/stabilizer, fragrance solubilizer, visc. builder for shampoos, hand soaps, other personal care prods.; component in clear deodorant sticks; clear liq.

Monamid® 150-ADY. [Mona Industries] 1:1 Linoleamide DEA; CAS 56863-02-6; EINECS 260-410-2; nonionic; thickener for aq. systems; conditioner; w/o emulsifier, corrosion inhibitor for sol. oils; for cosmetics; biodeg.; Gvcs-33 10 max. liq.; sol. @ 10% in ethanol, chlorinated and aromatic hydrocarbons, min. spirits, kerosene, gels in water; dens. 8.20 lb/gal; sp.gr. 0.97; acid no. 0–1; alkali no. 30-45; pH 10–11 (10%); toxicology: nontoxic orally; not a primary skin irritant; 100% act.

Monamid® 150-CW. [Mona Industries] 1:1 Capramide DEA; CAS 136-26-5; EINECS 205-234-9; nonionic; flash foamer, foam stabilizer, detergent for cosmetic preps., shampoos, bubble baths, bath oils; also as emulsifier, solubilizer, visc. control agent; biodeg.; amber liq./paste, crystallizes on aging; sol. @ 10% in water, ethanol, chlorinated and aromatic hydrocarbons, natural oils and fats; dens. 8.25 lb/gal; sp.gr. 0.99; acid no. 0; alkali no. 40-55; pH 10.3–11.3 (10%); usage level: 1-3%; 100% act.

Monamid® 150-GLT. [Mona Industries] Lauramide DEA; CAS 120-40-1; EINECS 204-393-1; nonionic; thickener and foam booster/stabilizer for cosmetic and toiletry prods.; fragrance solubilizer; amber clear liq.; sol. @ 10% in ethanol, chlorinated and aromatic hydrocarbons, min. spirits, kerosene; gels in water; sp.gr. 0.96; dens. 8.00 lb/gal; acid no. 0.5; alkali no. 30-45; pH 10.3–11.3 (10%); toxicology: very mild to skin and eyes; 100% act.

Monamid® 150-IS. [Mona Industries] 1:1 Isostearamide DEA; CAS 52794-79-3; EINECS 258-193-4; nonionic; lubricant, slip agent, and conditioner for cosmetic and industrial prods.; used in prep. of invert emulsions; emulsifier, corrosion inhibitor and lubricant in syn. coolants; biodeg.; lt. amber clear liq.; sol. 10% in ethanol, chlorinated and aromatic hydrocarbons, min. spirits, kerosene, wh. min. oil, natural oils and fats, water disp.; dens. 8.00 lb/gal; sp.gr. 0.96; acid no. 5–10; alkali no. 30-60; cloud pt. < -5 C; pH 8.8–9.8 (10%); toxicology: not a primary skin irritant; 100% act.

Monamid® 150-LMWC. [Mona Industries] Lauramide DEA; CAS 120-40-1; EINECS 204-393-1; nonionic; foam booster/stabilizer, fragrance solubilizer, and visc. builder for industrial and household detergents and cosmetics; biodeg.; Gvcs-33 3 max. solid; sol. @ 10% in ethanol, chlorinated and aromatic hydrocarbons, min. spirits, gels in water; dens. 8.20 lb/gal; sp.gr. 0.98 (40 C); acid no. 0–1; alkali no. 30-45; pH 10.2–11.2 (10%); toxicology: not a primary skin irritant; 100% act.

Monamid® 150-LWA. [Mona Industries] Lauramide DEA; CAS 120-40-1; EINECS 204-393-1; nonionic; foam booster/stabilizer, fragrance solubilizer, and visc. builder for personal care prods., industrial and household detergents; biodeg.; solid; sol. @ 10% in water, ethanol, chlorinated and aromatic hydrocarbons, natural oils and fats; sp.gr. 1.00; dens. 8.3 lb/gal; acid no. 0-3; alkali no. 58-68; pH 10-11 (10%); 100% act.

Monamid® 150-MW. [Mona Industries] 1:1 Myristamide

DEA; CAS 7545-23-5; EINECS 231-426-7; nonionic; nonirritating foam stabilizer, emulsifier for aq. or nonaq. cosmetics and toiletries; thickener for systems containing sodium ions; biodeg.; wh. solid wax; sol. @ 10% in ethanol, chlorinated and aromatic hydrocarbons, disp. in water; dens. 8.20 lb/gal; sp.gr. 0.98 (45 C); m.p. 50 C; acid no. 0-3; alkali no. 35-50; pH 9.5-10.5 (10%); toxicology: not a primary skin irritant; 100% act.

Monamid® 664-MC. [Mona Industries] Coconut alkanolamide; nonionic; foam booster, stabilizer and thickener for industrial and household detergents; liq.; 100% conc.

Monamid® 705. [Mona Industries] Cocamide DEA; CAS 61791-31-9; EINECS 263-163-9; foam booster/stabilizer and thickener for personal care prods.; amber clear liq.

Monamid® 716. [Mona Industries] Lauramide DEA; CAS 120-40-1; EINECS 204-393-1; nonionic; detergent, foam booster and stabilizer, visc. builder, solubilizer, coupler, wetting agent, used in shampoos, bubble baths, facial/body cleansers, and household liq. detergent formulations; component in clear deodorant sticks; biodeg.; lt. amber clear liq.; sol. @ 10% in water, ethanol, chlorinated and aromatic hydrocarbons, natural oils and fats; sp.gr. 0.98; dens. 8.2 lb/gal; cloud pt. < 1 C; acid no. 2; alkali no. 55; pH 10.8 (10%); toxicology: not a primary skin irritant; 100% act.

Monamid® 718. [Mona Industries] Stearamide DEA; CAS 93-82-3; EINECS 202-280-1; nonionic; emulsifier, thickener, opacifier for cosmetic creams and lotions; biodeg.; Gvcs-33 4 max. solid; sol. @ 10% in ethanol, aromatic hydrocarbons, gels in water; dens. 8.00 lb/gal; sp.gr. 0.96 (45 C); acid no. 21 ± 3; alkali no. 45-65; pH 9.3–10.3 (10%); toxicology: not a primary skin irritant; 100% act.

Monamid® 759. [Mona Industries] Cocamide DEA; CAS 61791-31-9; EINECS 263-163-9; nonionic; foam booster and stabilizer, visc. builder, and conditioner for personal care prods.; very low irritation props.; amber liq.; alkali no. 35 ± 5; acid no. 1 max.; pH 10.5 ± 0.5 (10%); cloud pt. 0 C; clear pt. 33 C; 100% act.

Monamid® 853. [Mona Industries] Alkanolamide, modified; nonionic; detergent, wetting emulsifier, foam stabilizer used in shampoos, bubble baths, skin cleansers, liq. household and industrial detergents, dairy cleaners, wool scouring, waterless hand cleaners; liq.; 100% conc.

Monamid® 1007. [Mona Industries] 1:1 Lauramide DEA and linoleamide DEA; foam booster/stabilizer, visc. builder, conditioner, and emulsifier used in shampoos, bubble baths, skin cleansers, household and industrial liq. detergents; amber clear liq.; dens. 8.16 lb/gal; acid no. 1; alkali no. 35; iodine no. 40; pH 10.5 (10% aq.); usage level: 4-6%; 100% act.

Monamid® 1034. [Mona Industries] Lauramide DEA; CAS 120-40-1; EINECS 204-393-1; nonionic; foam booster and visc. builder for shampoos; liq.; 100% conc.

Monamid® 1159. [Mona Industries] Cocamide DEA; CAS 61791-31-9; EINECS 263-163-9; foam booster/stabilizer and thickener for personal care prods.; amber clear liq.

Monamid® 1224. [Mona Industries] Lauramide DEA; CAS 120-40-1; EINECS 204-393-1; foam booster/stabilizer, fragrance solubilizer, visc. builder for shampoos, hand soaps, other personal care prods.; component in clear deodorant sticks; clear liq.

Monamid® C-305. [Mona Industries] Cocamide DEA; CAS 61791-31-9; EINECS 263-163-9; foam booster/stabilizer and thickener for personal care prods.; amber clear liq.

Monamid® C-310. [Mona Industries] Cocamide DEA; CAS 61791-31-9; EINECS 263-163-9; foam booster/stabilizer and thickener for personal care prods.; amber clear liq.

Monamid® CMA. [Mona Industries] 1:1 Cocamide MEA; CAS 68140-00-1; EINECS 268-770-2; nonionic; foam booster/stabilizer, thickener for liq. and powd. detergents,

cosmetics, shampoos, hand washes, body cleansers, toilet bowl blocks, syn. soap bars, tablet formulations; biodeg.; tan granular; sol. @ 10% in ethanol, disp. in water, chlorinated and aromatic hydrocarbons, min. spirits, kerosene, wh. min. oil, natural oils and fats; solid. pt. 63 ± 2 C; acid no. 6-12; pH 9.4–10.8 (10%); toxicology: nontoxic orally; not a primary skin irritant; 100% act.

Monamid® CMA-A. [Mona Industries] Cocamide MEA; CAS 68140-00-1; EINECS 268-770-2; nonionic; visc. builder, foam stabilizer for anionic systems (shampoos, hand washes, body cleansers), toilet bowl blocks, syn. soap bars, tablet formulations; gran.; m.p. 70 C.

Monamid® CMA-A/F [Mona Industries] Cocamide MEA; CAS 68140-00-1; EINECS 268-770-2; nonionic; visc. builder, foam stabilizer for anionic systems (shampoos, hand washes, body cleansers), toilet bowl blocks, syn. soap bars, tablet formulations; flakes; m.p. 70 C.

Monamid® CMA-A/M. [Mona Industries] Cocamide MEA; CAS 68140-00-1; EINECS 268-770-2; nonionic; visc. builder, foam stabilizer for anionic systems (shampoos, hand washes, body cleansers), toilet bowl blocks, syn. soap bars, tablet formulations; milled; m.p. 70 C.

Monamid® CMA/F. [Mona Industries] Cocamide MEA; CAS 68140-00-1; EINECS 268-770-2; nonionic; visc. builder, foam stabilizer for anionic systems (shampoos, hand washes, body cleansers), toilet bowl blocks, syn. soap bars, tablet formulations; flakes; m.p. 63 C.

Monamid® CMA/M. [Mona Industries] Cocamide MEA; CAS 68140-00-1; EINECS 268-770-2; nonionic; visc. builder, foam stabilizer for anionic systems (shampoos, hand washes, body cleansers), toilet bowl blocks, syn. soap bars, tablet formulations; milled; m.p. 63 C.

Monamid® CMA-S. [Mona Industries] Cocamide MEA; CAS 68140-00-1; EINECS 268-770-2; nonionic; visc. builder, foam stabilizer for anionic systems (shampoos, hand washes, body cleansers), toilet bowl blocks, syn. soap bars, tablet formulations; gran.; m.p. 73 C.

Monamid® CMA-S/F. [Mona Industries] Cocamide MEA; CAS 68140-00-1; EINECS 268-770-2; nonionic; visc. builder, foam stabilizer for anionic systems (shampoos, hand washes, body cleansers), toilet bowl blocks, syn. soap bars, tablet formulations; flakes; m.p. 73 C.

Monamid® CMA-S/M. [Mona Industries] Cocamide MEA; CAS 68140-00-1; EINECS 268-770-2; nonionic; visc. builder, foam stabilizer for anionic systems (shampoos, hand washes, body cleansers), toilet bowl blocks, syn. soap bars, tablet formulations; milled; m.p. 73 C.

Monamid® CP-205. [Mona Industries] Capramide DEA; CAS 136-26-5; EINECS 205-234-9; produces highest flash foam and detergency for personal care prods.; clear liq.-solid.

Monamid® L-350. [Mona Industries] Lauramide DEA; CAS 120-40-1; EINECS 204-393-1; foam booster/stabilizer, fragrance solubilizer, and thickener for shampoos, hand soaps, other personal care prods.; component in clear deodorant sticks; clear liq.

Monamid® L-355. [Mona Industries] Lauramide DEA; CAS 120-40-1; EINECS 204-393-1; foam booster/stabilizer, fragrance solubilizer, and thickener for shampoos, hand soaps, other personal care prods.; component in clear deodorant sticks; clear liq.

Monamid® L-360. [Mona Industries] Lauramide DEA; CAS 120-40-1; EINECS 204-393-1; foam booster/stabilizer, fragrance solubilizer, and thickener for shampoos, hand soaps, other personal care prods.; component in clear deodorant sticks; clear liq.-solid.

Monamid® L-365. [Mona Industries] Lauramide DEA; CAS 120-40-1; EINECS 204-393-1; foam booster/stabilizer, fragrance solubilizer, and thickener for shampoos, hand soaps, other personal care prods.; component in clear deodorant sticks; solid.

Monamid® LL-370. [Mona Industries] Lauramide DEA; CAS 120-40-1; EINECS 204-393-1; foam booster/stabilizer, fragrance solubilizer, and thickener for shampoos, hand soaps, other personal care prods.; component in clear deodorant sticks; clear liq.

Monamid® LLN-380. [Mona Industries] Lauramide DEA and linoleamide DEA; visc. builder, conditioner, and emulsifier for personal care prods.; amber clear liq.

Monamid® LM-375. [Mona Industries] Lauramide DEA; CAS 120-40-1; EINECS 204-393-1; foam booster/stabilizer, fragrance solubilizer, and thickener for shampoos, hand soaps, other personal care prods.; component in clear deodorant sticks; solid.

Monamid® LMIPA. [Mona Industries] Lauramide MIPA; CAS 142-54-1; EINECS 205-541-8; nonionic; foam booster, thickener used in personal care prods., household, and industrial detergent systems; off-wh. solid; m.p. 61 ± 2 C; acid no. 1 max.; alkali no. 10–25; pH 10.5 ± 0.5 (10% aq.); toxicology: not a primary skin irritant; 100% act.

Monamid® LMMA. [Mona Industries] 1:1 Lauramide MEA; CAS 142-78-9; EINECS 205-560-1; nonionic; foam booster, thickener for cosmetic, household and industrial detergents; biodeg.; tan granular; sol. @ 10% in ethanol, disp. in water, aromatic hydrocarbons, kerosene, wh. min. oil, natural oils and fats; solid. pt. 80 ± 2 C; acid no. 0–1; alkali no. 5-12; pH 9.7–10.7 (10%); 100% act.

Monamid® LN-605. [Mona Industries] Linoleamide DEA; CAS 56863-02-6; EINECS 260-410-2; visc. builder, conditioner, and emulsifier for personal care prods.; clear liq.

Monamid® R31-42. [Mona Industries] Lauramide DEA and propylene glycol; nonionic; foam stabilizer for cosmetic preps.; biodeg.; Gvcs-33 2 max liq.; sol. @ 10% in water, ethanol, chlorinated and aromatic hydrocarbons, disp. in natural oils and fats; dens. 8.25 lb/gal; sp.gr. 0.99; acid no. 0–1; alkali no. 25-35; pH 10–11 (10%); 80% act.

Monamid® S. [Mona Industries] 1:1 Stearamide MEA; CAS 111-57-9; EINECS 203-883-2; nonionic; emulsifier, thickener, m.p. modifier for aq. and solv. systems in cosmetics, deodorant sticks; pearlizing agent; gives uniform visc. and prevents settling in liqs. containing talcs, pigments, and fillers; biodeg.; tan granular; disp. @ 10% in water, chlorinated and aromatic hydrocarbons, min. spirits, kerosene, wh. min. oil, natural oils and fats; m.p. 87 ± 2 C; acid no. 0-1; alkali no. 5-18; pH 9.5-11.0 (10%); toxicology: nontoxic orally; 100% act.

Monamid® S/M. [Mona Industries] Stearamide MEA; CAS 111-57-9; EINECS 203-883-2; nonionic; m.p. modifier for solid formulations, such as deodorant sticks; pearlizing agent; milled; m.p. 87 C.

Monamide. [Zohar Detergent Factory] Cocamide MEA; CAS 68140-00-1; EINECS 268-770-2; nonionic; foam booster, thickener, superfatting agent for cosmetics; flakes; 90% conc.

Monamilk. [Argeville] DEA-cetyl phosphate, oleyl alcohol, isopropyl myristate, PEG-2 stearate.

Monamine 779. [Mona Industries] Cocamide DEA and DEA-laureth sulfate; nonionic/anionic; foaming agent, visc. builder, detergent, soil suspending agent, solubilizer, wetting and penetrating agent used in shampoos, bubble baths, household and industrial cleaners, germicides, uv absorbers; biodeg.; lt. yel. clear to hazy visc. liq.; sol. @ 10% in water, polar solvs., alcohol, glycols, fatty acid esters, chlorinated and aromatic hydrocarbons, dens. 8.75 lb/gal; sp.gr. 1.05 ± 0.1; cloud pt. 2 C; pH 9.25 ± 0.5 (10%); surf. tens. 29 dynes/cm (0.1%); toxicology: very mild primary skin irritant; 100% act.

Monamine AA-100. [Mona Industries] 1:2 Dist. cocamide DEA and diethanolamine; nonionic/anionic; detergent,

emulsifier, thickener; biodeg.; Gvcs-33 7 max. liq.; sol. @ 10% in water, ethanol, chlorinated and aromatic hydrocarbons; dens. 8.30 lb/gal; sp.gr. 1.00; acid no. 28–32; alkali no. 165-185; pH 9.5–10.5 (10%); 100% act.

Monamine AC-100. [Mona Industries] Cocamide DEA and linoleamide DEA; nonionic/anionic; detergent, emulsifier, thickener; biodeg.; Gvcs-33 13 max. liq.; sol. @ 10% in ethanol, chlorinated and aromatic hydrocarbons, gels in water; dens. 8.30 lb/gal; sp.gr. 1.00; acid no. 22–32; alkali no. 170-190; pH 9.5–10.5 (10%); 100% act.

Monamine ACO-100. [Mona Industries] Lauramide DEA and diethanolamine; nonionic/anionic; detergent, emulsifier, thickener; biodeg.; Gvcs-33 5 max. paste; sol. @ 10% in water, ethanol, chlorinated and aromatic hydrocarbons; dens. 8.40 lb/gal; sp.gr. 1.01; acid no. 10–14; alkali no. 180-200; pH 9.5–10.5 (10%); 100% act.

Monamine ADD-100. [Mona Industries] Cocamide DEA (1:2); CAS 61791-31-9; EINECS 263-163-9; nonionic; detergent, emulsifier, thickener; biodeg.; Gardner 3 liq.; sol. @ 10% in water, ethanol, chlorinated hydrocarbons; disp. in aromatic hydrocarbons; sp.gr. 1.02; dens. 8.5 lb/gal; acid no. 2-6; alkali no. 105-125; pH 9.5-10.5; 100% act.

Monamine ADY-100. [Mona Industries] Linoleamide DEA and diethanolamine; nonionic; detergent, emulsifier, thickener; biodeg.; Gvcs-33 9 max. liq.; sol. @ 10% in ethanol, min. spirits, kerosene; disp. in water, chlorinated and aromatic hydrocarbons; dens. 8.20 lb/gal; sp.gr. 0.98; acid no. 0–2; alkali no. 110-130; pH 10.5–11.5 (10%); 100% act.

Monamine C-100. [Mona Industries] Capramide DEA, diethanolamine; CAS 136-26-5; EINECS 205-234-9.

Monamine CF-100 M. [Mona Industries] Cocamide DEA and diethanolamine; nonionic/anionic; detergent, emulsifier, thickener; biodeg.; Gvcs-33 11 max. liq.; sol. @ 10% in water, ethanol, chlorinated and aromatic hydrocarbons; dens. 8.40 lb/gal; sp.gr. 1.01; acid no. 56–64; alkali no. 110-120; pH 8.5–9.5 (10%); 100% act.

Monaquat ISIES. [Mona Industries] Isostearyl ethylimidonium ethosulfate; CAS 67633-57-2; EINECS 266-778-0; cationic; antistat, lubricant, softener, corrosion inhibitor used in hair care prods., industrial and textile applics.; biodeg.; amber visc. liq.; sol. @ 10% in water, ethanol, butyl Cellosolve, aromatic, chlorinated and fluorinated hydrocarbons; sp.gr. 1.03; pH 6.9 (10%); toxicology: very mild primary skin irritant; 100% act.

Monaquat P-TC. *See Phospholipid P-TC* [Mona Industries] Cocamidopropyl PG-dimonium chloride phosphate; patented (U.S., Canada, Japan, Europe) substantive conditioner, antistat, detergent, foaming agent, emulsifier, solubilizer, dispersant, thickener, wetting agent, bactericide for personal care and household prods., topical pharmaceuticals and veterinary prods., paper, photography, agric., mining, and textiles; amber clear liq.; sp.gr. 1.10; dens. 9.1 lb/gal; pH 7.0 (10%); surf. tens. 37.7 dynes/cm (1%); Draves wetting 64 s (1%); foam height 91 mm (1 min, 1%); toxicology: LD50 > 5 ml/kg; low skin and eye irritation; 47% total solids.

Monaquat P-TD. *See Phospholipid P-TD* [Mona Industries] Lauramidopropyl PG-dimonium chloride phosphate; patented (U.S., Canada, Japan, Europe) substantive conditioner, antistat, detergent, foaming agent, emulsifier, solubilizer, dispersant, thickener, wetting agent, bactericide for personal care and household prods., topical pharmaceuticals and veterinary prods., paper, photography, agric., mining, and textiles; amber clear liq.; sp.gr. 1.05; dens. 8.7 lb/gal; pH 7.5 (10%); surf. tens. 43.1 dynes/cm (1%); Draves wetting 91 s (1%); foam height 96 mm (1 min, 1%); toxicology: LD50 > 5 ml/kg; very mild to skin, somewhat irritating to eyes; 41% total solids.

Monaquat P-TL. See Phospholipid P-TL [Mona Industries] Lauroampho PG-glycinate phosphate; patented (U.S., Canada, Japan, Europe) substantive conditioner, anti-stat, detergent, foaming agent, emulsifier, solubilizer, dispersant, thickener, wetting agent, bactericide for personal care and household prods., topical pharmaceuticals and veterinary prods., paper, photography, agric., mining, and textiles; clear visc. liq.; sp.gr. 1.10; dens. 9.1 lb/gal; pH 7.5 (10%); surf. tens. 33.7 dynes/cm (1%); Draves wetting 4 s (1%); foam height 61 mm (1 min, 1%); toxicology: LD50 > 5 ml/kg; very low skin and eye irritation; 38% total solids.

Monaquat P-TS. See Phospholipid P-TS [Mona Industries] Stearamidopropyl PG-dimonium chloride phosphate; patented (U.S., Canada, Japan, Europe) primary emulsifier, substantive skin/hair conditioner providing long-lasting skin smoothing props.; for moisturizing/replenishing creams and lotions, sunscreens, hair conditioners, mousses; fully biodeg.; lt. yel. paste to opaque solid; sp.gr. 1.01; dens. 8.4 lb/gal; m.p. 40-50 C; pH 7.6 (10% in 50/50 IPA/water); toxicology: LD50 (oral, mouse) > 5 g/kg; not a primary skin or eye irritant; 35% total solids, 30% act.

Monaquat P-TZ. See Phospholipid P-TZ. [Mona Industries] Cocohydroxyethyl PG-imidazolinium chloride phosphate; patented (U.S., Canada, Japan, Europe) substantive conditioner, antistat, detergent, foaming agent, emulsifier, solubilizer, dispersant, thickener, wetting agent, bactericide for personal care and household prods., topical pharmaceuticals and veterinary prods., paper, photography, agric., mining, and textiles; amber clear liq.; sp.gr. 1.07; dens. 8.9 lb/gal; pH 7 (10%); surf. tens. 37.6 dynes/cm (1%); Draves wetting 10 s (1%); foam height 67 mm (1 min, 1%); toxicology: LD50 > 5 ml/kg; very low skin and eye irritation; 41% total solids.

Monaquat SL-5. [Mona Industries] POE dihydroxypropyl linoleaminium chloride; cationic; conditioner and shampoo additive providing exc. wet comb and lubrication props.; yel. clear liq.; 40% conc.

Monaquat :G. [Mona Industries] Bishydroxyethyl dihydroxypropyl stearaminium chloride; cationic; surfactant used in personal care prods.; conditioner for hair rinses imparting exc. wet comb props.; antistat and foaming agent used in fabric laundering and softening prods.; thickener for acid bowl cleaners, naval gels; biodeg.; Gardner 3 slightly hazy liq.; sp.gr. 1.011; dens. 8.39 lb/gal; solid. pt. –10 to –12 C; cloud pt. 3 C; pH 5.5 (10%); toxicology: LD50 (oral) > 5 g/kg (10%); moderate skin irritant, nonirritating to eyes @ 3%; 30% act.

Monaterge 779. [Mona Industries] Cocamide DEA and DEA-laureth sulfate; used for shampoos, body cleansers, bubble baths, hand cleansers, other personal care prods.; yel. clear liq.; 100% conc.

Monaterge 1164. [Mona Industries] Sodium lauryl sulfate and disodium lauryl sulfosuccinate; provides high foaming, good detergency, and mildness to personal care systems; yel. clear liq.; 30% conc.

Monateric 949J. [Mona Industries] Disodium lauroamphodiacetate; CAS 14350-97-1; EINECS 238-306-3; amphoteric; counter-irritant for baby care prods., no-eye-sting shampoos, other mild cleansers; clear liq.; 38% conc.

Monateric 985A. [Mona Industries] Sodium lauroamphoacetate, sodium trideceth sulfate; amphoteric; high foaming, mild shampoo base for adult and baby prods.; biodeg.; amber clear liq.; sp.gr. 1.07; dens. 8.9 lb/gal; pH 9.3 (10%); Draves wetting instantaneous (1%); 36% act., 39% total solids.

Monateric 1188M. [Mona Industries] Disodium lauryl β-iminodipropionate; CAS 3655-00-3; EINECS 222-899-0; amphoteric; high foaming surfactant, hydrotrope for household and industrial hard surf. cleaners, shampoos, bubble bath, mild skin cleansers, down hole foamers, air

drilling; textile wetter; biodeg.; stable to acid and alkali; Gardner 3 clear liq.; pH 10; Draves wetting 43 s (0.1% aq.); Ross-Miles foam 165 mm (0.1% , initial); 30% act. in water.

Monateric CA-35. [Mona Industries] Sodium cocoamphopropionate; amphoteric; salt-free detergent, wetting agent, emulsifier, dispersant, foaming agent used in cosmetic, household, and industrial prods.; coupling agent, solubilizer; biodeg.; stable to acid, alkali, electrolytes; amber clear liq.; sol. in high concs. of phosphates, silicates, carbonates; m.w. 360; sp.gr. 1.02; dens. 8.5 lb/gal; pH 5.7 (10%); surf. tens. 29.5 dynes/cm (0.1% conc.); Draves wetting 11 s (1%); Ross-Miles foam 160 mm (0.1% aq., initial); toxicology: low skin and eye irritation; 35% act. in water.

Monateric CAB. [Mona Industries] Cocamidopropyl betaine; amphoteric; mild high foaming base surfactant for shampoos, bubble baths, hair conditioners; lt. yel. clear liq.; sp.gr. 1.04; dens. 8.7 lb/gal; pH 7.1 (10%); Draves wetting 18 s (1%); 30% act., 35% total solids.

Monateric CAB-LC. [Mona Industries] Cocamidopropyl betaine; amphoteric; high foaming surfactant providing mildness and visc. building to anionic systems for personal care; clear liq.; 35% conc.

Monateric CAB-XLC. [Mona Industries] Cocamidopropyl betaine; amphoteric; high foaming surfactant providing mildness and visc. building to anionic systems for personal care; clear liq.; 35% conc.

Monateric CDL. [Mona Industries] Cocoamphodiacetate, sodium laureth sulfate; amphoteric; mild, high foaming shampoo base; yel. clear liq.; sp.gr. 1.11; dens. 9.2 lb/gal; pH 8.5 (10%); Draves wetting 4 s (1%); 31% act., 37% total solids.

Monateric CDX-38. [Mona Industries] Disodium cocoamphodiacetate; CAS 68650-39-5; EINECS 272-043-5; amphoteric; detergent, foaming agent, mild base surfactant for shampoos and skin cleansers; counter-irritant for baby care prods., no-eye-sting shampoos; biodeg.; lt. amber visc. liq.; sp.gr. 1.18; dens. 9.8 lb/gal; pH 8.4 (10%); Draves wetting 18 s (1%); 39% act., 50% total solids.

Monateric CDX-38 Mod. [Mona Industries] Disodium cocoamphodiacetate; CAS 68650-39-5; EINECS 272-043-5; amphoteric; high foaming detergent for nonirritating shampoos, skin cleansers, cosmetics; biodeg.; yel. clear liq.; sp.gr. 1.18; dens. 9.8 lb/gal; pH 8.8 (10%); Draves wetting 20 s (1%); 39% act., 50% total solids.

Monateric CEM-38. [Mona Industries] Disodium cocoamphodipropionate; amphoteric; detergent, wetting agent, emulsifier, dispersant, solubilizer, hydrotrope used in liq. detergent systems, heavy-duty detergents, acid bowl cleaners, cosmetics; anti-irritant for anionics; biodeg.; amber clear to hazy liq.; sp.gr. 1.05; dens. 8.75 lb/gal; pH 8.5 ± 0.5 (10%); surf. tens. 35 dynes/cm (0.1%); Draves wetting 4.5 min (1%); toxicology: not a primary skin irritant; 39% act.

Monateric CLV. [Mona Industries] Disodium cocoamphodiacetate; CAS 68650-39-5; EINECS 272-043-5; amphoteric; counter-irritant for baby care prods., no-eye-sting shampoos, other mild cleansers; yel. clear liq.; 50% conc.

Monateric CM-36S. [Mona Industries] Sodium cocoamphoacetate; amphoteric; foaming agent, emulsifier, high foaming detergent, wetting agent, solubilizer, conditioner, coupling agent, fulling agent used in cosmetic and textile industries; ultra-mild, detoxifies and thickens anionics; biodeg.; clear yel. liq.; water sol.; sp.gr. 1.10; dens. 9.2 lb/gal; pH 11.9 (10%); surf. tens. 32 dynes/cm (0.015%); Draves wetting 5 s (1%); 36% act., 42% total solids.

Monateric CNa-40. [Mona Industries] Coconut monocarboxylic propionate, imidazoline-derived, salt-free; amphoteric; surfactant for nonirritating cosmetics; wetting agent and detergent in high electrolyte systems; amber clear liq.; sp.gr. 1.09; dens. 9.1 lb/gal; pH 10.9 (10%); Draves wetting 6 s (1%); 40% act.

Monateric COAB. [Mona Industries] Cocamidopropyl betaine; amphoteric; high foaming surfactant for personal care prods., industrial detergents, cleaners; hydrotrope, coupling agent, and/or solubilizer; corrosion inhibitor in metalworking systems, oil well flooding, and aerosol pkgs.; yel. clear liq.; sp.gr. 1.04; dens. 8.7 lb/gal; pH 7.9 (10%); Draves wetting 10 s (1%); 32% act., 37% total solids.

Monateric CSH-32. [Mona Industries] Disodium cocoamphodiacetate; CAS 68650-39-5; EINECS 272-043-5; amphoteric; high foaming, nonirritating surfactant for baby shampoos; biodeg.; clear yel. liq.; sp.gr. 1.13; dens. 9.4 lb/gal; visc. 2000 cps; f.p. < 0 C; cloud pt. < 0 C; pH 8.4 (10%); Draves wetting 20 s (1%); 32% act., 40% total solids.

Monateric CyA-50. [Mona Industries] Caprylic dicarboxylic propionate, imadazoline-derived, salt-free; amphoteric; surfactant for industrial detergents, cleaners, cosmetics; hydrotrope, coupling agent, and/or solubilizer; corrosion inhibitor in metalworking systems, oil well flooding, and aerosol pkgs.; dk. br. clear liq.; sp.gr. 1.07; dens. 8.9 lb/gal; pH 5.6 (10%); Draves wetting 9 s (1%); 50% act.

Monateric ISA-35. [Mona Industries] Sodium isostearoamphopropionate; CAS 68630-96-6; EINECS 271-929-9; amphoteric; salt-free surfactant used in cosmetic and industrial prods.; conditioner, lubricant, thickener; biodeg.; amber clear to hazy flowable gel; sol. @ 10% in water, alcohol, glycol ethers and alkanolamines, disp. in min. oil and natural oils and fats; sp.gr. 1.01; dens. 8.4 lb/gal; pH 5–6 (10%); surf. tens. 30 dynes/cm (0.1%); Draves wetting 10 min (1%); toxicology: nontoxic orally; not a primary skin irritant; 35% act.

Monateric LMAB. [Mona Industries] Lauramidopropyl betaine; EINECS 224-292-6; amphoteric; high foaming surfactant providing mildness and visc. building to anionics for personal care; shampoo base; lt. yel. clear liq.; sp.gr. 1.04; dens. 8.7 lb/gal; pH 8.3 (10%); Draves wetting 9 s (1%); 30% act., 35% total solids.

Monateric LMM-30. [Mona Industries] Sodium lauroamphoacetate; amphoteric; high foaming detergent for nonirritating shampoos, skin cleansers, other cosmetics; ultramild; detoxifies and thickens anionics; biodeg.; amber visc. liq.; sp.gr. 1.09; dens. 9.1 lb/gal; pH 9.2 (10%); Draves wetting 5 s (1%); 30% act., 36% total solids.

Monateric MCB. [Mona Industries] Cocamidopropyl betaine; amphoteric; high foaming shampoo base with conditioning props.; lt. yel. clear liq.; sp.gr. 1.02; dens. 8.5 lb/gal; pH 4.8 (10%); Draves wetting 18 s (1%); 30% act., 33% total solids.

Monawet MM-80. [Mona Industries] Dihexyl sodium sulfosuccinate, 15% water, 5% IPA; CAS 3006-15-3; EINECS 221-109-1; anionic; wetting agent, detergent for emulsion and suspension polymerization, rug backing, paper coating, textiles, paint, agric., cosmetic, detergent, mining, water treatment, electroplating baths, and food industries; electrolyte tolerant; EPA and FDA §175.105, 176.170, 177.1210, 178.3400 compliances; colorless clear liq.; sol. 33 g/100 g water, in polar and nonpolar solvs.; m.w. 388; sp.gr. 1.10; dens. 9.2 lb/gal; cloud pt. < 0 C; flash pt. (PMCC) 110 F; pH 6 ± 1 (10%); surf. tens. 46 dynes/cm (0.1%); Ross-Miles foam 60 mm (0.1%); toxicology: not a primary skin irritant; 80% act.

Monawet MO-65-150. [Mona Industries] Dioctyl sodium sulfosuccinate, anhyd.; CAS 577-11-7; EINECS 209-406-4; anionic; wetting, penetrating and spreading agent, emulsifier used in oil well cleaning, drycleaning detergents, solv. cleaners and strippers, lubricants, agric.,

paints, mining, water treatment, cosmetic applics.; APHA 50 colorless clear liq.; sp.gr. 1.05; dens. 8.75 lb/gal; acid no. 0.5; flash pt. (COC) 42–43 C; pH 5.5 (10%); 65% act.

Monawet MO-70. [Mona Industries] Dioctyl sodium sulfosuccinate, 20% water, 10% diethylene glycol butyl ether; CAS 577-11-7; EINECS 209-406-4; anionic; wetting, dispersing, emulsifying, penetrating and solubilizing agent used in emulsion and suspension polymerization, adhesives, paints, textile, fertilizer, mining, water treatment, fire fighting, cosmetic, food industries; EPA and FDA §175.105, 175.300, 175.320, 176.170, 176.210, 177.1200, 177.2800, 178.3400 compliance; colorless clear liq.; sol. in polar and nonpolar solvs.; m.w. 444; sp.gr. 1.08; dens. 9.0 lb/gal; cloud pt. < –5 C; flash pt. (PMCC) 325 F; pH 6.0 (10%); surf. tens. 29 dynes/cm (0.1%); Ross-Miles foam 225 mm (0.1%); 70% act.

Monawet MO-70-150. [Mona Industries] Dioctyl sodium sulfosuccinate; CAS 577-11-7; EINECS 209-406-4; anionic; emulsifier, wetting agent, spreading agent, penetrant for agric., paints, mining, water treatment, cosmetic applics.; liq.; sol. in oils, solvs.; 70% conc.

Monawet MO-70E. [Mona Industries] Dioctyl sodium sulfosuccinate, 19% water, 11% ethanol; CAS 577-11-7; EINECS 209-406-4; anionic; wetting agent for industrial applics., emulsion polymerization, adhesives, paints, textiles, agric., cosmetics, glass cleaners, mining, water treatment, wall paper removal, food pkg. plants; EPA and FDA §175.105, 175.300, 175.320, 176.170, 176.210, 177.1200, 177.2800, 178.3400 compliance; colorless clear liq.; sol. in polar and nonpolar solvs.; m.w. 444; sp.gr. 1.08; dens. 9.0 lb/gal; cloud pt. < –5 C; flash pt. (PMCC) 82 F (10%); surf. tens. 29 dynes/cm (0.1%); Ross-Miles foam 220 mm (0.1%); 70% act.

Monawet MO-70R. [Mona Industries] Dioctyl sodium sulfosuccinate, 15% water, 15% propylene glycol; CAS 577-11-7; EINECS 209-406-4; anionic; wetting, dispersing, emulsifying, penetrating and solubilizing agent for textile, printing, agric., paints, mining, water treatment, fire fighting, cosmetic, food industries; EPA and FDA §175.105, 175.300, 175.320, 176.170, 176.210, 177.1200, 177.2800, 178.3400 compliance; colorless clear liq.; sol. in polar and nonpolar solvs.; m.w. 444; sp.gr. 1.06; dens. 8.8 lb/gal; cloud pt. < –5 C; flash pt. (PMCC) 280 F; pH 6.0 (10%); surf. tens. 29 dynes/cm (0.1%); Ross-Miles foam 210 mm (0.1%); 70% act.

Monawet MO-70RP. [Mona Industries] Dioctyl sodium sulfosuccinate; CAS 577-11-7; EINECS 209-406-4; anionic; wetting agent for pharmaceuticals; liq.; 70% conc.

Monawet MO-70S. [Mona Industries] Dioctyl sodium sulfosuccinate, 30% odorless min. spirits; CAS 577-11-7; EINECS 209-406-4; anionic; wetting agent for dry cleaning soaps, spotting compds; wetting agent and emulsifier; agric., paints, mining, water treatment, cosmetics applics.; EPA and FDA §175.105, 175.300, 175.320, 176.170, 176.210, 177.1200, 177.2800, 178.3400 compliance; APHA 25 clear liq.; oil and solv. sol.; sp.gr. 1.08; dens. 9.0 lb/gal; pH 5.5 (10%); Ross-Miles foam 190 mm (0.1%); 70% conc.

Monawet MO-75E. [Mona Industries] Dioctyl sodium sulfosuccinate, 18% water, 7% ethanol; CAS 577-11-7; EINECS 209-406-4; anionic; wetting agent for industrial, agric., paints, mining, water treatment, cosmetics applics.; EPA and FDA §175.105, 175.300, 175.320, 176.170, 176.210, 177.1200, 177.2800, 178.3400 compliance; colorless clear liq.; sol. in polar and nonpolar solvs.; m.w. 444; sp.gr. 1.08; dens. 9.0 lb/gal; cloud pt. < –5 C; flash pt. (PMCC) 80 F; pH 6.0 (10%); surf. tens. 29 dynes/cm (0.1%); Ross-Miles foam 220 mm (0.1%); 75% act.

Monawet MO-84R2W. [Mona Industries] Dioctyl sodium

sulfosuccinate, 16% propylene glycol; CAS 577-11-7, 57-55-6; anionic; wetting agent for general use, agric., paints, mining, water treatment, cosmetics applics.; EPA and FDA §175.105, 175.300, 175.320, 176.170, 176.210, 177.1200, 177.2800, 178.3400 compliance; lt. yel. clear visc. liq.; m.w. 444; sol. in polar and nonpolar solvs.; sp.gr. 1.10; dens. 9.16 lb/gal; b.p. 298 F; cloud pt. < -10 C; flash pt. (PMCC) 223 F; pH 5.5 (10%); surf. tens. 29 dynes/cm (0.1%); Ross-Miles foam 190 mm (0.1%); toxicology: severe eye and skin irritant on overexposure; 84% act.

Monawet MO-85P. [Mona Industries] Dioctyl sodium sulfosuccinate, 15% sodium benzoate; anionic; wetting for wettable powds., pigments, paints, mining, water treatment, cosmetics; EPA and FDA §175.105, 175.300, 175.320, 176.170, 176.210, 177.1200, 177.2800, 178.3400 compliance; wh. fine powd.; 0.85% sol. in water; pH 5.5 (10%); surf. tens. 26 dynes/cm (0.1%); Ross-Miles foam 200 mm (0.1%); 85% act.

Monawet SNO-35. [Mona Industries] Tetrasodium dicarboxyethyl stearyl sulfosuccinamate; CAS 3401-73-8; EINECS 222-273-7; anionic; wetting agent, solubilizer, emulsifier, dispersant, visc. depressant, mild detergent used in polymerization, paints, coatings, textile, cosmetic, agric. prods.; biodeg.; EPA and FDA §175.105, 176.170, 176.180, 178.3400 compliances; lt. amber clear liq.; m.w. 653; sol. in water, high electrolyte salt sol'ns.; sp.gr. 1.14; dens. 9.5 lb/gal; visc. 16-18 s (#2 Zahn cup); f.p. 45 ± 5 F; acid no. 2.0; iodine no. 0.5; pH 7.5; surf. tens. 43 dynes/cm (0.1%); Draves wetting 232 s (0.25% , 30 C); Ross-Miles foam 185 mm (0.1%); toxicology: very low acute oral toxicity; mild eye irritant; 35% solids.

Monomuls® 90-25. [Henkel; Henkel KGaA/Cospha; Grünau] Dist. hydrog. tallow glyceride; CAS 61789-09-1; EINECS 263-031-0; nonionic; nonself-emulsifying base and aux. material for mfg. of cosmetics and pharmaceuticals; fatting agent, consistency factor, emulsifier for o/w emulsions and stick preps. and foodstuffs; wh. powd., neutral odor; m.p. 64-72 C; HLB 3.8; acid no. < 3; pH 4-5 (1:10 methanol/water 1:1); usage level: 1-5%; 90-96% monoglycerides.

Monomuls® 90-L12. [Henkel/Cospha; Henkel Canada; Grünau] Glyceryl laurate; CAS 142-18-7; EINECS 205-526-6; nonionic; coemulsifier, refatting agent, and thickener for personal care prods., bath additives, shampoos; wh. pellets; 100% conc.

Monomuls® 90-O18. [Henkel/Cospha; Henkel KGaA/Cospha; Grünau] Glyceryl oleate; CAS 111-03-5; nonionic; w/o emulsifier, stabilizer, refatting agent, thickener for cosmetics, food and drugs; almost wh. paste, sl. fatty odor; HLB 3.4; acid no. 3 max.; iodine no. 67-80; sapon. no. 150-160; 100% conc.

Monosiliol. [Exsymol] Methylsilanol PEG-7 glyceryl cocoate.

Monosiliol C. [Exsymol; Biosil Tech.] Methylsilanol tri PEG-8 glyceryl cocoate; aids tissue regeneration; for anti-aging formulations, cosmetic and health emulsions, oils, milks, and soaps; sl. yel. oily limpid liq., sl. aromatic odor; misc. with water, alcohol, various oils; sp.gr. 1.05; sapon. no. 95; ref. index 1.50; usage level: 3-6%; toxicology: nontoxic.

Monosteol. [Gattefosse SA; Gattefosse] Propylene glycol palmitostearate; nonionic; emulsifier; stabilizer for ointments, cream lotions; solid; drop pt. 33-36 C; HLB 4.0; acid no. < 6; iodine no. < 3; sapon. no. 165-175; toxicology: sl. irritating to skin and eyes; 100% conc.

Montane 20. [Seppic] Sorbitan laurate; CAS 1338-39-2; EINECS 215-663-3; nonionic; biodeg. emulsifier for cosmetics use; liq.; sol. in ethanol; disp. in water, min. and veg. oils; visc. 4500 mPa·s; HLB 8.6; acid no. 6 max.; sapon. no. 158-170; hyd. no. 330-358; pH 7; toxicology: nonirritating to skin and eyes; 100% conc.

Montane 40. [Seppic] Sorbitan palmitate; CAS 26266-57-9; EINECS 247-568-8; nonionic; biodeg. emulsifier for cosmetics use; flakes; sol. hot in ethanol, with turbidity in min. and veg. oils; gels in water; m.p. 49 C; HLB 6.7; acid no. 5 max.; sapon. no. 140-150; hyd. no. 275-305; pH 7; toxicology: nonirritating to skin and eyes; 100% conc.

Montane 60. [Seppic] Sorbitan stearate; CAS 1338-41-6; EINECS 215-664-9; nonionic; biodeg. emulsifier for cosmetics use; flakes; sol. hot in ethanol, veg. oil, turbid in min. oil; insol. in water; m.p. 55 C; HLB 4.7; acid no. 5-10; sapon. no. 147-157; hyd. no. 235-260; pH 7; toxicology: nonirritating to eyes, mildly irritating to skin; 100% conc.

Montane 65. [Seppic] Sorbitan tristearate; CAS 26658-19-5; EINECS 247-891-4; nonionic; biodeg. emulsifier for cosmetics use; solid; disp. in min. and veg. oils; insol. in water, ethanol; m.p. 54 C; acid no. 15 max.; sapon. no. 176-188; hyd. no. 66-80; HLB 2.7; pH 7; toxicology: nonirritating to skin and eyes; 100% conc.

Montane 70. [Seppic] Sorbitan isostearate; CAS 71902-01-7; nonionic; biodeg. emulsifier; liq.; 100% conc.

Montane 73. [Seppic] Sorbitan sesquiisostearate; cosmetic ingred.

Montane 80. [Seppic] Sorbitan oleate; CAS 1338-43-8; EINECS 215-665-4; nonionic; biodeg. emulsifier for cosmetics use; liq.; sol. in ethanol, min. and veg. oils; insol. in water; visc. 1000 mPa·s; HLB 4.3; acid no. 6 max.; iodine no. 62-76; sapon. no. 145-160; hyd. no. 193-209; pH 7; toxicology: nonirritating to skin and eyes; 100% conc.

Montane 80 SP. [Seppic] Sorbitan oleate with low peroxide value; CAS 1338-43-8; EINECS 215-665-4; emulsifier.

Montane 83. [Seppic] Sorbitan sesquioleate; CAS 8007-43-0; EINECS 232-360-1; nonionic; biodeg. emulsifier for cosmetics use; liq.; sol. in ethanol, min. and veg. oils; insol. in water; visc. 10,000 mPa·s; HLB 3.7; acid no. 6 max.; iodine no. 68-76; sapon. no. 150-166; hyd. no. 180-205; pH 7; toxicology: nonirritating to eyes; 100% conc.

Montane 85. [Seppic] Sorbitan trioleate; CAS 26266-58-0; EINECS 247-569-3; nonionic; biodeg. emulsifier; liq.; sol. in min. and veg. oils, sol. hot in ethanol; insol. in water; visc. 200 mPa·s; HLB 1.8; acid no. 15 max.; sapon. no. 170-190; hyd. no. 55-70; pH 7; toxicology: nonirritating to eyes, mildly irritating to skin; 100% conc.

Montane 481. [Seppic] Sorbitan oleate, beeswax, and stearic acid; biodeg. cosmetic w/o emulsifier; soft wax; toxicology: nonirritating to skin and eyes; 100% act.

Montanol 68. [Seppic] Cetearyl glucoside; nonionic; emulsifier for cosmetic and dermopharmaceutical prods.; flakes; 100% conc.

Montanox 20. [Seppic] Polysorbate 20; CAS 9005-64-5; nonionic; emulsifier for cosmetics use; liq.; sol. in water, ethanol; insol. in min. and veg. oils; visc. 400 mPa·s; HLB 16.7; acid no. 1 max.; sapon. no. 40-50; hyd. no. 96-108; cloud pt. 85-94 C; pH 6.0-7.5; toxicology: nonirritating to skin and eyes.

Montanox 20 DF. [Seppic] Polysorbate 20, dioxane-free; CAS 9005-64-5; nonionic; emulsifier for cosmetics use; liq.; HLB 16.7; 100% conc.

Montanox 21. [Seppic] PEG-5 sorbitan laurate; nonionic; emulsifier; liq.; HLB 13.3; 100% conc.

Montanox 40. [Seppic] Polysorbate 40; CAS 9005-66-7; nonionic; emulsifier for cosmetics use; liq. to gel; sol. in water, ethanol; insol. in min. and veg. oils; HLB 15.6; acid no. 1 max.; sapon. no. 41-52; hyd. no. 89-105; pH 6.0-7.5; toxicology: nonirritating to skin and eyes.

Montanox 40 DF. [Seppic] Polysorbate 40, dioxane-free; CAS 9005-66-7; nonionic; emulsifier for cosmetics use; gel; HLB 15.6; 100% conc.

Montanox 60. [Seppic] Polysorbate 60; CAS 9005-67-8; nonionic; emulsifier for cosmetics use; liq. to gel; sol. in water, ethanol; sol. hot with turbidity in min. oil; insol. in veg. oils; HLB 14.9; acid no. 1 max.; sapon. no. 45-55; hyd. no. 81-96; cloud pt. 60-76 C; pH 6.0-7.5; toxicology: nonirritating to skin and eyes.

Montanox 60 DF. [Seppic] Polysorbate 60, dioxane-free; CAS 9005-67-8; nonionic; emulsifier for cosmetics use; gel; HLB 14.9; 100% conc.

Montanox 61. [Seppic] PEG-4 sorbitan stearate; CAS 9005-67-8; nonionic; emulsifier; solid; HLB 9.6; 100% conc.

Montanox 65. [Seppic] Polysorbate 65; CAS 9005-71-4; nonionic; emulsifier for cosmetics use; solid; sol. in ethanol, min. oil; disp. in water, veg. oil; HLB 10.5; acid no. 2 max.; sapon. no. 88-98; hyd. no. 44-60; pH 6.0-7.5; toxicology: nonirritating to skin and eyes; 100% conc.

Montanox 70. [Seppic] PEG-20 sorbitan isostearate; CAS 66794-58-9; nonionic; emulsifier; liq.; 100% conc.

Montanox 71. [Seppic] PEG-5 sorbitan isostearate; CAS 66794-58-9.

Montanox 80. [Seppic] Polysorbate 80; CAS 9005-65-6; nonionic; emulsifier for cosmetics use; liq.; sol. in water, ethanol; insol. in min. and veg. oils; visc. 500 mPa·s; HLB 15; acid no. 1 max.; sapon. no. 45-55; hyd. no. 65-80; cloud pt. 57-63 C; pH 6.0-7.5; toxicology: nonirritating to skin and eyes.

Montanox 80 DF. [Seppic] Polysorbate 80, dioxane-free; CAS 9005-65-6; nonionic; emulsifier for cosmetics use, pharmaceutical ointments; solubilizer for oral or injectable pharmaceuticals; liq.; HLB 15.0; 100% conc.

Montanox 81. [Seppic] Polysorbate 81; CAS 9005-65-6; nonionic; emulsifier; liq.; HLB 10.0; 100% conc.

Montanox 85. [Seppic] Polysorbate 85; CAS 9005-70-3; nonionic; emulsifier for cosmetics use; solubilizer; liq.; sol. in ethanol, min. oil; sol. hot in veg. oil; disp. in water; visc. 200 mPa·s; HLB 11.0; acid no. 1 max.; sapon. no. 82-95; hyd. no. 39-52; pH 6.0-7.5; toxicology: nonirritating to skin and eyes; 100% conc.

Montanox 90. [Seppic] PEG-20 sorbitan resinolate.

Monteine CA. [Seppic] Hydrolyzed collagen; CAS 9015-54-7; cosmetic protein.

Monteine KL 150. [Seppic] Keratin amino acids; CAS 68238-35-7; protein conditioner.

Monteine LCK-32. [Seppic] Potassium cocoyl hydrolyzed collagen; CAS 68920-65-0; surfactant for cosmetics; liq.; 40% act.

Monteine LCQ. [Seppic] Cocamidopropyl dimethylaminohydroxypropyl hydrolyzed collagen; raw material for shampoos and hair conditioners; liq.; 32% act.

Monteine LCS 30. [Seppic] Sodium cocoyl hydrolyzed collagen; CAS 68188-38-5; substantive cosmetic protein.

Monteine LCT. [Seppic] TEA-cocoyl hydrolyzed collagen; CAS 68952-16-9; anionic; surfactant for shampoo and general cosmetic use; liq.; 40% act.

Monteine PCO. [Seppic] Palmitoyl collagen amino acids.

Monteine PRO. [Seppic] Glycine, alanine, proline, hydroxyproline.

Monteine V. [Seppic] TEA-cocoyl hydrolyzed collagen, sorbitol; CAS 68952-16-9, 50-70-4.

Montelane LT 4088. [Seppic] TEA-laureth sulfate; CAS 27028-82-6; personal care surfactant.

Monthybase. [Gattefosse] Glycol stearate SE; CAS 86418-55-5.

Monthyle. [Gattefosse; Gattefosse SA] Glycol stearate; CAS 111-60-4; EINECS 203-886-9; nonionic; emulsifier, stabilizer for ointments, cream lotions; solid; drop pt. 55-58 C; HLB 3.0; acid no. < 6; iodine no. < 3; sapon. no. 170-180; toxicology: sl. irritating to eyes; nonirritating to skin; 100% conc.

Morillol®. [BASF AG] 1-Octene-3-ol; fragrance and flavoring.

M-P-A® 14. [Rheox] Attapulgite and quaternium-18 hectorite; antisettling additive; lt. cream powd.; sp.gr. 2.3.

MPG Granular Beads. [U.S. Cosmetics] Irregularly shaped beads which remain in suspension and provide a sensory tactile effect and visual color change when applied to the skin; spherical beads; avail. in five colors.

M-Quat® 40. [PPG/Specialty Chem.] Polyquaternium 6; CAS 26062-79-3; homopolymer quat. for hair and skin prods.; emollient; clear visc. liq.; 39.0–41.0% act.

M-Quat® 522. [PPG/Specialty Chem.] Isostearamidopropyl ethyldimonium ethosulfate; CAS 67633-63-0; EINECS 266-778-0; cationic; conditioner for hair conditioners, clear shampoos, and hot oil treatment formulations; clear visc. liq.; exc. water sol.; 85% act.

M-Quat® 1033. [PPG/Specialty Chem.] Soya ethyldimonium ethosulfate; cationic; conditioner for hair conditioners and shampoos; antistat for cleaners, rug shampoos; low foaming; clear yel. liq.; 58% act.

M-Quat® B-25. [PPG/Specialty Chem.] Stearalkonium chloride; CAS 122-19-0; EINECS 204-527-9; quat. for hair conditioners; paste; 25% act.

M-Quat® JS-25. [PPG/Specialty Chem.] Stearalkonium chloride; CAS 122-19-0; EINECS 204-527-9; cationic; conditioner, softener, emollient for hair care prods.; wh. paste; pH 3.6-4.5 (2% aq.); 24-28% solids.

MTD-25. [Ikeda] Micronized titanium dioxide; CAS 13463-67-7; EINECS 236-675-5; uv absorber providing coverage in 200-320 nm range; for sun care prods.; wh. powd.; 99% min. thru 325 mesh; surf. area 40-45 mm^2/g; oil absorb. 27-34; pH 6.5-8.0; 90% min. purity.

Mulsifan CB. [Zschimmer & Schwarz] Beheneth-10; nonionic; emulsifier for cosmetic creams and lotions; wh. waxlike; sol. in paraffin oils, ethanol, IPA; disp. in water; dens. 0.94 g/cc; setting pt. 48 C; HLB 10.0; pH 5-7 (1%); 100% act.

Mulsifan CPA. [Zschimmer & Schwarz] Laureth-4; CAS 5274-68-0; EINECS 226-097-1; nonionic; o/w emulsifier for cosmetic creams and lotions; colorless liq.; sol. in paraffin oils, soya bean oil, ethanol; disp. in water; dens. 0.94 g/cc; HLB 9.3; cloud pt. 57-62 C (5 g/20 ml butyl diglycol 25%); pH 5-7 (1%); 100% act.

Mulsifan RT 18. [Zschimmer & Schwarz] Alkylaryl polyglycol ether; nonionic; emulsifier for solvs.; solubilizer for perfumes and essential oils; for cleaning of metal, engines, machinery, leather degreasing, drycleaning booster; colorless visc. liq.; sol. in water, ethanol, petrol., benzene, toluene, xylene, acetone, chlorinated hydrocarbons; dens. 1.06 g/cc; HLB 13; pH 4-6 (10%); 100% act.

Mulsifan RT 23. [Zschimmer & Schwarz] Laureth-5; CAS 3055-95-6; EINECS 221-281-8; nonionic; emulsifier for paraffin oils, wh. oils for formulation of lubricating agents, spin finishes, coning oils, emulsions for cosmetics; colorless liq.; sol. in wh. oils, min. oils, petrol., benzene, toluene, CCl$_4$, kerosene, perchloroethylene, turpentine; disp. in water; dens. 0.96 g/cc; HLB 11.0; pH 5-7 (10%); 100% act.

Mulsifan RT 141. [Zschimmer & Schwarz] Polysorbate 20; CAS 9005-64-5; nonionic; solubilizer for perfumes and volatile oils; straw-colored visc. liq.; sol. in water, ethanol, IPA, acetone, benzene, toluene, chlorinated hydrocarbons; sp.gr. 1.09; HLB 15–16; pH 5–7 (10%); 100% act.

Mulsifan RT 146. [Zschimmer & Schwarz] Polysorbate 80; CAS 9005-65-6; nonionic; solubilizer for perfumes and volatile oils; yel. visc. liq.; sp.gr. 1.09; sol. in water, ethanol, IPA, acetone, benzene, toluene, chlorinated hydrocarbons; HLB 15–16; pH 5–7 (10%); 100% act.

Mulsifan RT 203/80. [Zschimmer & Schwarz] C12-15 pareth-12; CAS 68131-39-5; nonionic; solubilizer for perfumes and volatile oils; colorless liq.; sp.gr. 1.04; sol. in water; HLB 14.0; cloud pt. 89–94 C (1% aq.); pH 5–7 (10%); 80% act.

Mulsifan RT 275. [Zschimmer & Schwarz] Abietic acid

polyglycol ester; nonionic; shampoo additive; paste; 100% conc.

Mulsor OC. [Fabriquimica] Self-emulsifying wax; nonionic; emulsifier and thickener for cosmetic emulsions; acid no. 4-8; iodine no. < 2; sapon. no. 130-140.

Multifruit BSC. [Brooks Industries] Mixed fruit extract based on bilberry/citrus fruits and sugar cane extracts which contain lactic, citric, and glycolic acids; used for smoothing and line reduction in skin care prods.

Multifruit BSCY. [Brooks Industries] Mixed fruit extract containing yeast peptides; used for moisturizing and soothing props. in skin care prods.

Multi-Grain Barley Code 1851. [Brooks Industries] Oligosaccharide derived from barley, *Hordeum vulgare*; contains high levels of glucans; deposits protective film on proteinaceous substrates; reduces damage caused by repeated washings to hair; 35% act.

Multilan A. [Fabriquimica] Lanolin deriv.; multifunctional cosmetic ingred.; cloud pt. 12-18 C; acid no. < 1; iodine no. < 12; sapon. no. < 1.

Multilan D. [Fabriquimica] Lanolin deriv.; absorption base; drop pt. 40-46 C; acid no. < 1; iodine no. < 14; sapon. no. < 2.

Multiwax® 180-M. [Witco/Petroleum Spec.] Microcryst. wax NF; CAS 63231-60-7; EINECS 264-038-1; plasticizer or modifier for polymeric coatings and adhesives; hot melt adhesives and coatings, chewing gum base, protective coatings, cosmetics/pharmaceuticals; FDA §172.886, 178.3710; lt. yel.; misc. with petrol. prods., many essential oils, most animal and veg. fats, oils, and waxes; visc. 14.3-18.0 cSt (99 C); m.p. 82-88 C; flash pt. (COC) 277 C min.

Multiwax® 180-W. [Witco/Petroleum Spec.] Microcryst. wax; CAS 63231-60-7; EINECS 264-038-1; cosmetic wax.

Multiwax® ML-445. [Witco/Petroleum Spec.] Microcryst. wax NF; CAS 63231-60-7; EINECS 264-038-1; laminating agent for paper, film, foil; hot-melt adhesives; chewing gum base; elec. insulation; sealants; rustproofing compds.; waterproofing/protective coatings; crayons; dental waxes; candles; paraffin wax modifier; cosmetics and pharmaceuticals; FDA §172.886, 178.3710; lt. yel.; misc. with petrol. prods., many essential oils, most animal and veg. fats, oils, and waxes; visc. 14.3-18.0 cSt (99 C); m.p. 77-82 C; flash pt. (COC) 274 C min.

Multiwax® W-445. [Witco/Petroleum Spec.] Microcryst. wax NF; CAS 63231-60-7; EINECS 264-038-1; wax for hair dressings, medicated creams and unguents, chewing gum base, artificial flowers, dental waxes, lubricants, candles, hot-melt adhesives; FDA §172.886, 178.3710; wh. wax; misc. with petrol. prods., many essential oils, most animal and veg. fats, oils, and waxes; visc. 14.3-18.0 cSt (99 C); m.p.77-82 C; flash pt. (COC) 274 C min.

Multiwax® W-835. [Witco/Petroleum Spec.] Microcryst. wax; CAS 63231-60-7; EINECS 264-038-1; plasticizer or modifier for polymeric coatings and adhesives; used in silk screen printing, cold creams, cleansing creams, hair pomades, pharmaceuticals, crayons, paste-up adhesive; FDA §172.886, 178.3710; wh.; visc. 14.3-18.0 cSt (99 C); m.p. 74-79 C; flash pt. (COC) 246 C min.

Multiwax® X-145A. [Witco/Petroleum Spec.] Microcryst. wax NF; CAS 63231-60-7; EINECS 264-038-1; plasticizer or modifier for polymeric coatings and adhesives; cheese coating, laminating of cellophane and plastic film, waterproofing/protective linings, cosmetics/pharmaceuticals; FDA §172.886, 178.3710; lt. yel.; misc. with petrol. prods., many essential oils, most animal and veg. fats, oils, and waxes; visc. 14.3-18.0 cSt (99 C); m.p. 66-71 C; flash pt. (COC) 260 C min.

Musol™ 20. [Brooks Industries] Glycoproteins; cosmetic ingred. for moisturizing; visc. liq.; m.w. 25,000; 20% act.

Musol™ SD. [Brooks Industries] Maltodextrin and sol. yeast mucins; moisture binding props. for cosmetics; powd.

M Violet 112. [Presperse] Manganese violet (90%), bismuth-oxychloride (10%); CAS 10101-66-3, 7787-59-9; inorg. colorant for pigmented cosmetics; JSCI/JCID approved.

Myacide® BT. [Boots Co plc] 2-Bromo-2-nitropropane-1,3-diol; CAS 52-51-7; EINECS 200-143-0; preservative for cosmetics and toiletries; usage level: 0.01-0.1%.

Myacide® SP. [Inolex; Boots Co. plc] 2,4-Dichlorobenzyl alcohol; CAS 1777-82-8; EINECS 217-210-5; antifungal agent, preservative for pharmaceutical, cosmetic, and toiletry formulations for areas where contamination by spoilage yeasts and molds is the problem; stable at pH 3-10 and to 100 C; wh. to sl. yel. crystal; sol. (g/100 ml): 95 g in acetone, 80 g in methanol, 45 g in propylene glycol, 0.1 g in water; m.w. 177; m.p. 57-60 C; 98.5% min. act.

Myavert C. [Brooks Industries; Boots Microcheck] Glucose, glucose oxidase, lactoperoxidase; enzymatic natural preservative, bactericide for cosmetics.

Myristocor™. [Roche] Myristamidopropyl dimethylamino phosphate; quaternary for hair conditioners and mousses; for use in tin-plated aerosols (chloride and corrosion-free).

Myritol® 312. [Henkel KGaA/Cospha] Caprylic/capric triglyceride; CAS 85409-09-2; med. fatting oil component of o/w and w/o emulsions, skin care oils, and bath oils; almost colorless clear oil, odorless; m.w. 490; sp.gr. 0.943-0.950; visc. 27-33 mPa·s; acid no. 0.2 max.; iodine no. 1 max.; sapon. no. 330-345; ref. index 1.448-1.450.

Myritol® 318. [Henkel/Cospha; Henkel Canada; Henkel KGaA/Cospha] Caprylic/capric triglyceride; CAS 85409-09-2; nonionic; emollient for pharmaceutical and cosmetic preps. in emulsion form (bath oils, lotions, lipsitcks); oily component with solv. capacity; solubilizer; oil binder for pressed powd. cosmetics; exc. oxidative stability; almost colorless clear low-visc. oily liq., odorless; m.w. 490; sp.gr. 0.945-0.949; visc. 27-33 mPa·s; acid no. 0.1 max.; iodine no. 0.5 max.; sapon. no. 335-350; ref. index 1.448-1.450; 100% conc.

Myritol® PC. [Henkel/Cospha; Henkel KGaA/Cospha] Propylene glycol dicaprylate/dicaprate; CAS 68583-51-7; emollient for cosmetics, pharmaceuticals, bath oils, aerosols, and antiperspirants; exc. solv. for active ingreds.; stable vehicle for pigmented cosmetics; yel. low visc. liq., faint char. odor; m.w. 340; sp.gr. 0.91-0.93; visc. 9-12 mPa·s; acid no. 0.2 max.; iodine no. 0.5 max.; sapon. no. 320-340; cloud pt. < -20 C; ref. index 1.440-1.442.

Myrj® 45. [ICI Spec. Chem.; ICI Surf. Am.; ICI Surf. Belgium] PEG-8 stearate; CAS 9004-99-3; nonionic; general purpose o/w emulsifiers for cosmetics, pharmaceuticals, etc.; wh. cream-colored soft waxy solid; sol. in alcohol, disp. in water; sp.gr. 1.0; HLB 11.1; pour pt. 28 C; sapon. no. 82-95; 100% conc.

Myrj® 49. [ICI Spec. Chem.; ICI Surf. Am.; ICI Surf. Belgium] PEG-20 stearate; CAS 9004-99-3; nonionic; o/w emulsifier for cosmetic and pharmaceutical applics.; wh. cream solid; HLB 15.0; 100% conc.

Myrj® 51. [ICI Spec. Chem.; ICI Surf. Am.; ICI Surf. Belgium] PEG-30 stearate; CAS 9004-99-3; nonionic; o/w emulsifier for cosmetic and pharmaceutical applics.; wh. cream solid; HLB 16.0; 100% conc.

Myrj® 52. [ICI Spec. Chem.; ICI Surf. Am.; ICI Surf. Belgium] PEG-40 stearate NF; CAS 9004-99-3; nonionic; o/w emulsifier for cosmetic and pharmaceutical applics.; ivory waxy solid or flake; sol. in water, acetone, ether, alcohol; sp.gr. 1.1; HLB 16.9; pour pt. 38 C; sapon. no. 25-35; 100% conc.

Myrj® 52S. [ICI Spec. Chem.] PEG-40 stearate NF; CAS 9004-99-3; nonionic; o/w emulsifier for cosmetic and pharmaceutical applics.; wh. waxy granular solid; sol. in water, toluol, acetone, ether, Cellosolve, CCl_4, alcohol;

sp.gr. 1.1; HLB 16.9; pour pt. 38 C; sapon. no. 25–35; 100% conc.

Myrj® 53. [ICI Spec. Chem.; ICI Surf. Am.; ICI Surf. Belgium] PEG-50 stearate; CAS 9004-99-3; nonionic; o/w emulsifier for cosmetic and pharmaceutical applics.; wh. cream-colored solid; sol. in water, alcohol; HLB 17.9; pour pt. 42 C; sapon. no. 20–28; 100% conc.

Myrj® 59. [ICI Spec. Chem.; ICI Surf. Am.; ICI Surf. Belgium] PEG-100 stearate; CAS 9004-99-3; nonionic; o/w emulsifier for cosmetic and pharmaceutical applics.; off-wh. to lt. tan solid; sol. in water, alcohol; HLB 18.8; pour pt. 46 C; 100% conc.

Myrlene. [Gattefosse] PEG-8 myristate.

Myrol-S. [Lanaetex Prods.] Isopropyl myristate, diisopropyl sebacate.

Mytab®. [Zeeland] Myrtrimonium bromide; CAS 1119-97-7; EINECS 214-291-9; surfactant used as emulsifier and antistat in hair rinses; antimicrobial for cosmetics, topicals; wh. powd.; characteric odor; sol. in water, alcohols, chloroform; m.w. 336.40; pH 5–8 (1% aq.); 100% act.

Myvacet® 5-07. [Eastman] Acetylated hydrog. cottonseed glyceride; CAS 977055-83-6; nonionic; emulsifier, emollient forming highly flexible films with good moisture-vapor barrier props. for cosmetics; waxy solid; sp.gr. 0.94 (80 C); m.p. 41-46 C; HLB 3.8-4.0; acid no. 3 max.; iodine no. 5 max.; sapon. no. 279-292; hyd. no. 133-152.

Myvacet® 7-07. [Eastman] Acetylated monoglycerides; nonionic; emulsifier, emollient forming highly flexible films with good moisture-vapor barrier props. for cosmetics; waxy solid; sp.gr. 0.94 (80 C); m.p. 37-40 C; HLB 3.8-4.0; acid no. 3 max.; iodine no. 5 max.; sapon. no. 316-331; hyd. no. 80.5-95.0.

Myvacet® 9-08. [Eastman] Acetylated monoglycerides; nonionic; emulsifier, emollient, lubricant, and deaerator for cosmetic systems; liq.; sp.gr. 0.94 (80 C); m.p. -12 to -14 C; HLB 3.8-4.0; acid no. 3 max.; iodine no. 2 max.; sapon. no. 440-455; hyd. no. 20 max.

Myvacet® 9-45. [Eastman] Acetylated vegetable glycerides; emulsifier, emollient, lubricant, and dearating agent for cosmetic systems; liq.; sp.gr. 0.94 (80 C); m.p. 4-12 C; HLB 3.8-4.0; acid no. 3 max.; iodine no. 43-53; sapon. no. 370-382; hyd. no. 0-15.

Myvaplex® 600P. [Eastman] Glyceryl monostearate (from hydrog. soy glycerides); CAS 61789-08-0; emulsifier for cosmetics and personal care prods.

Myvatem® 30. [Eastman] Diacetyl tartaric acid ester of dist. monoglycerides (from edible tallow); emulsifier, dispersant for food, pharmaceutical, and cosmetic applics.; semisolid; m.p. 33 C.

Myvatem® 35K. [Eastman] Diacetyl tartaric acid ester of dist. monoglycerides (from refined palm oil); emulsifier, dispersant for food, pharmaceutical, and cosmetic applics.; semisolid; m.p. 26 C.

Myvatex® 3-50. [Eastman] Dist. monoglycerides and dist. propylene glycol monoesters, soybean oil source; emulsifier for cosmetic applics.; beads; sp.gr. 0.91 (80 C); m.p. 58 C; acid no. < 3; iodine no. 5 max.; 90% min. monoester.

Myvatex® 7-85. [Eastman] Dist. cottonseed oil monoglycerides; CAS 8029-44-5; EINECS 232-438-5; emulsifier for cosmetic applics.; plastic; sp.gr. 0.94 (80 C); m.p. 49 C; acid no. < 3; iodine no. 91-101; 63% min. monoester.

Myvatex® 8-06. [Eastman] Dist. hydrog. soybean oil monoglycerides; emulsifier for cosmetic applics.; beads; sp.gr. 0.93 (80 C); m.p. 67 C; acid no. < 3; iodine no. 24-30; 72% min. monoester.

Myvatex® 8-16. [Eastman] Dist. hydrog. palm oil monoglycerides; CAS 67784-87-6; emulsifier for cosmetic applics.; beads; m.p. 61 C; acid no. < 3; iodine no. 28 max.; 72% min. monoester.

Myvatex® 40-06S. [Eastman] Myvatex 3-50, lactylic stearate, potassium sorbate, and water; nonionic; emulsifier for cosmetics, cakes; soft plastic; HLB 3.8–4.0; acid no. < 13; iodine no. < 2; prod. must not be allowed to freeze; 25% solids.

Myvatex® 60. [Eastman] Dist. acetoglycerides with polysorbate 60; emulsifier for cosmetic applics.; liq.; sp.gr. 0.97 (80 C); m.p. 19 C; acid no. 0.8; iodine no. 24; 45% min. monoester.

Myvatex® MSPS. [Eastman] Soybean oil monoglycerides with 25% polysorbate 80; emulsifier for cosmetic applics.; beads; m.p. 69 C; acid no. < 3; iodine no. 6 max.; 67.5% min. monoester.

Myvatex® SSH. [Eastman] Dist. soybean oil monoglycerides, lecithin, water, and propionic acid; emulsifier for cosmetic applics.; soft plastic; acid no. < 7.3; iodine no. 6 min.; prod. must not be allowed to freeze; 45% solids.

Myvatex® Texture Lite. [Eastman] Glyceryl stearate, propylene glycol stearate, sodium stearoyl lactylate; nonionic; emulsifier for cosmetic applics.; powd.; sp.gr. 0.94 (80 C); m.p. 55 C; acid no. < 13; iodine no. 5 max.; 80% min. monoester.

Myverol® 18-04. [Eastman] Dist. hydrog. palm oil glyceride; CAS 67784-87-6; nonionic; emulsifier for cosmetics, personal care prods., baked goods, confectionery prods., dehydrated potatoes, etc.; small beads; sp.gr. 0.94 (80 C); m.p. 66 C; HLB 3.8-4.0; acid no. 3 max.; iodine no. 5 max.; 90% min. monoester.

Myverol® 18-06. [Eastman] Hydrog. soy glyceride, dist.; CAS 61789-08-0; nonionic; emulsifier for foods, cosmetics; small beads; sp.gr. 0.92 (80 C); m.p. 69 C; HLB 3.8-4.0; acid no. 3 max.; iodine no. 5 max.; 90% min. monoester.

Myverol® 18-07. [Eastman] Hydrog. cottonseed glyceride, dist.; CAS 61789-07-9; nonionic; emulsifier for foods, cosmetics; small beads; sp.gr. 0.92 (80 C); m.p. 68 C; HLB 3.8-4.0; acid no. 3 max.; iodine no. 5 max.; 90% min. monoester.

Myverol® 18-30. [Eastman] Tallow glyceride, dist.; CAS 61789-13-7; EINECS 263-035-2; nonionic; emulsifier for baked goods, confectionery prods., cosmetics, etc.; plastic; sp.gr. 0.92 (80 C); 100% act.

Myverol® 18-35. [Eastman] Palm oil glyceride, dist.; CAS 977013-38-9; nonionic; emulsifier for baked goods, confectionery prods., cosmetics, etc.; plastic; sp.gr. 0.94 (80 C); m.p. 60 C; HLB 3.8-4.0; acid no. 3 max.; iodine no. 36-45; 90% min. monoester.

Myverol® 18-40. [Eastman] Lard glyceride, dist.; CAS 61789-10-4; EINECS 263-032-6; nonionic; emulsifier for baked goods, confectionery prods., cosmetics, etc.; plastic; sp.gr. 0.91 (80 C); 100% act.

Myverol® 18-50. [Eastman] Hydrog. veg. glyceride; CAS 69028-36-0; nonionic; emulsifier for cosmetics and personal care prods.; plastic; sp.gr. 0.94 (80 C); m.p. 54 C; HLB 3.8-4.0; acid no. 3 max.; iodine no. 50-60; 90% min. monoester.

Myverol® 18-85. [Eastman] Cottonseed glyceride, dist.; CAS 8029-44-5; EINECS 232-438-5; nonionic; emulsifier for baked goods, confectionery prods., cosmetics, etc.; soft plastic; sp.gr. 0.95 (80 C); m.p. 46 C; HLB 3.8-4.0; acid no. 3 max.; iodine no. 85-95; 90% min. monoester.

Myverol® 18-92. [Eastman] Sunflower seed oil glyceride; nonionic; emulsifier for cosmetics and personal care prods.; semiplastic; sp.gr. 0.90 (80 C); m.p. 41 C; HLB 3.8-4.0; acid no. 3 max.; iodine no. 105-115; 90% min. monoester.

Myverol® 18-99. [Eastman] Canola oil glyceride; nonionic; emulsifier for cosmetics and personal care prods.; forms cubic phase in presence of water; suitable for sustained release formulations and microspheres, topical permeation enhancement, solubilization; semiplastic; sp.gr. 0.93 (80 C); m.p. 35 C; HLB 3.8-4.0; acid no. 3 max.; iodine no. 90-95; 90% min. monoester.

Myverol® P-06. [Eastman] Propylene glycol stearate; CAS 1323-39-3; EINECS 215-354-3; aerating agent for cosmetics; food emulsifier, stabilizer; small beads; sp.gr. 0.89 (80 C); m.p. 45 C; acid no. 3 max.; iodine no. 5 max.; 90%

min. monoester content.

Myverol® SMG. [Eastman] Dist. succinylated monoglycerides; emulsifier for cosmetics and personal care prods.

MZO-25. [Ikeda] Micronized zinc oxide; CAS 1314-13-2; EINECS 215-222-5; uv absorber providing wide coverage (200-350 nm) for sun care prods.; wh. to pale yel. powd.; 99.5% min. purity.

N

Nacconol® 35SL. [Stepan; Stepan Canada] Sodium dode-cylbenzenesulfonate; CAS 25155-30-0; EINECS 246-680-4; anionic; detergent, wetting agent; pale clear, low visc. liq.; very low haze pt.

Nacol® 4-99. [Condea Chemie GmbH; Vista] 1-Butanol; CAS 71-36-3; EINECS 200-751-6; cosmetic and pharmaceutical raw material; Hazen 5 max. color; m.w. 74; sp.gr. 0.809-0.812 (20/4 C); b.p. 116.5-118 C; acid no. 0.02 max.; iodine no. 0.05 max.; hyd. no. 753-760; flash pt. (Abel-Pensky) 35 C; 99.6% min. act.

Nacol® 6-98. [Condea Chemie GmbH; Vista] 1-Hexanol; CAS 111-27-3; EINECS 203-852-3; cosmetic and pharmaceutical raw material; Hazen 10 max. color; m.w. 101-104; sp.gr. 0.819 (20/4 C); pour pt. -52 C; b.p. 150-170 C; acid no. 0.02 max.; iodine no. 0.1 max.; hyd. no. 540-555; flash pt. 58 C; 98% min. act.

Nacol® 8-97. [Condea Chemie GmbH; Vista] 1-Octanol; CAS 111-87-5; EINECS 203-917-6; cosmetic and pharmaceutical raw material; Hazen 10 max. color; m.w. 129-131; sp.gr. 0.825 (20/4 C); pour pt. -16 C; b.p. 185-200 C; acid no. 0.05 max.; iodine no. 0.15 max.; hyd. no. 428-435; flash pt. 82 C; 97.5% min. act.

Nacol® 8-99. [Condea Chemie GmbH; Vista] 1-Octanol; CAS 111-87-5; EINECS 203-917-6; cosmetic and pharmaceutical raw material; Hazen 10 max. color; m.w. 129-131; sp.gr. 0.825 (20/4 C); pour pt. -14 C; b.p. 188-198 C; acid no. 0.03 max.; iodine no. 0.1 max.; hyd. no. 428-435; flash pt. 82 C; 99.5% min. act.

Nacol® 10-97. [Condea Chemie GmbH; Vista] 1-Decanol; CAS 112-30-1; EINECS 203-956-9; cosmetic and pharmaceutical raw material; Hazen 10 max. color; m.w. 157-160; sp.gr. 0.829 (20/4 C); pour pt. 6 C; b.p. 220-235 C; acid no. 0.05 max.; iodine no. 0.2 max.; hyd. no. 350-357; flash pt. 95 C; 97.5% min. act.

Nacol® 10-99. [Condea Chemie GmbH; Vista] 1-Decanol; CAS 112-30-1; EINECS 203-956-9; cosmetic and pharmaceutical raw material; Hazen 10 max. color; m.w. 157-160; sp.gr. 0.829 (20/4 C); pour pt. 6 C; b.p. 220-235 C; acid no. 0.05 max.; iodine no. 0.1 max.; hyd. no. 350-357; flash pt. 95 C; 99% min. act.

Nacol® 12-96. [Condea Chemie GmbH; Vista] 1-Dodecanol; CAS 112-53-8; EINECS 203-982-0; cosmetic and pharmaceutical raw material; Hazen 10 max. color; m.w. 185-190; sp.gr. 0.822 (40/4 C); solid. pt. 22-24 C; b.p. 255-265 C; acid no. 0.05 max.; iodine no. 0.2 max.; hyd. no. 295-305; flash pt. 116 C; 96.5% min. act.

Nacol® 12-99. [Condea Chemie GmbH; Vista] 1-Dodecanol; CAS 112-53-8; EINECS 203-982-0; cosmetic and pharmaceutical raw material; Hazen 10 max. color; m.w. 185-187; sp.gr. 0.822 (40/4 C); solid. pt. 23-25 C; b.p. 258-265 C; acid no. 0.03 max.; iodine no. 0.15 max.; hyd. no. 299-304; flash pt. 119 C; 99% min. act.

Nacol® 14-95. [Condea Chemie GmbH; Vista] 1-Tetradecanol; CAS 112-72-1; EINECS 204-000-3; cos-metic and pharmaceutical raw material; Hazen 20 max. color; m.w. 212-219; sp.gr. 0.809 (60/4 C); solid. pt. 36-38 C; b.p. 275-290 C; acid no. 0.08 max.; iodine no. 0.3 max.; hyd. no. 256-262; flash pt. 145 C; 95% min. act.

Nacol® 14-98. [Condea Chemie GmbH; Vista] Myristyl alcohol; CAS 112-72-1; EINECS 204-000-3; cosmetic and pharmaceutical raw material; emollient, consistency giving factor for creams, ointments, liniments, lotions, and sticks; Hazen 20 max. color; m.w. 212-216; sp.gr. 0.809 (60/4 C); solid. pt. 37-39 C; b.p. 270-290 C; acid no. 0.05 max.; iodine no. 0.25 max.; hyd. no. 258-262; flash pt. 145 C; 98.5% min. act.

Nacol® 16-95. [Condea Chemie GmbH; Vista] 1-Hexadecanol; CAS 36653-82-4; EINECS 253-149-0; cosmetic and pharmaceutical raw material; Hazen 20 max. color; m.w. 240-244; sp.gr. 0.812 (60/4 C); solid. pt. 45-49 C; b.p. 300-320 C; acid no. 0.1 max.; iodine no. 0.5 max.; hyd. no. 226-235; flash pt. 150 C; 95% min. act.

Nacol® 16-98. [Condea Chemie GmbH; Vista] Cetyl alcohol; CAS 36653-82-4; EINECS 253-149-0; cosmetic and pharmaceutical raw material; emollient, consistency giving factor for creams, ointments, liniments, lotions, and sticks; Hazen 20 max. color; m.w. 240-244; sp.gr. 0.812 (60/4 C); solid. pt. 47-50 C; b.p. 305-320 C; acid no. 0.1 max.; iodine no. 0.4 max.; hyd. no. 226-235; flash pt. 155 C; 98% min. act.

Nacol® 18-94. [Condea Chemie GmbH; Vista] 1-Octadecanol; CAS 112-92-5; EINECS 204-017-6; cos-metic and pharmaceutical raw material; Hazen 40 max. color; m.w. 267-275; sp.gr. 0.815 (60/4 C); solid. pt. 55-58 C; b.p. 320-340 C; acid no. 0.2 max.; iodine no. 0.5 max.; hyd. no. 200-210; flash pt. 174 C; 94.5% min. act.

Nacol® 18-98. [Condea Chemie GmbH; Vista] Stearyl alcohol; CAS 112-92-5; EINECS 204-017-6; cosmetic and pharmaceutical raw material; emollient, consistency giving factor for creams, ointments, liniments, lotions, and sticks; Hazen 30 max. color; m.w. 267-275; sp.gr. 0.815 (60/4 C); solid. pt. 56-59 C; b.p. 325-340 C; acid no. 0.1 max.; iodine no. 0.5 max.; hyd. no. 200-210; flash pt. 174 C; 98% min. act.

Nacol® 20-95. [Condea Chemie GmbH; Vista] Eicosanol; CAS 629-96-9; cosmetic and pharmaceutical raw material; emollient, consistency giving factor for creams, ointments, liniments, lotions, and sticks; Hazen 50 max. color; m.w. 298; sp.gr. 0.802 (80/4 C); solid. pt. 61-64 C; acid no. 0.3 max.; iodine no. 1 max.; hyd. no. 180-185; flash pt. 195 C; 95% min. act.

Nacol® 22-97. [Condea Chemie GmbH; Vista] Docosanol; CAS 661-19-8; EINECS 211-546-6; cosmetic and pharmaceutical raw material; emollient, consistency giving factor for creams, ointments, liniments, lotions, and sticks; Hazen 50 max. color; m.w. 326; sp.gr. 0.807 (80/4 C); solid. pt. 67-70 C; acid no. 0.1 max.; iodine no. 0.5 max.; hyd. no. 168-171; flash pt. 227 C; 97.5% min. act.

Nacolox® . [Condea Chemie GmbH] Fatty alcohol ethoxylates; cosmetic and pharmaceutical raw material; emulsifier and consistency giving factor for creams, ointments, liniments, lotions, and sticks.

Nadex 360. [Nat'l. Starch] Dextrin; CAS 9004-53-9; EINECS 232-675-4.

Naetex-CHP. [Lanaetex Prods.] Oleylamidopropyl dimethylamine ethonium ethosulfate; cationic; provides wetcomb, body, and antistatic props. to hair leaving silky, nongreasy afterfeel and texture; for after-shampoo conditioners, cream rinses, leave-on prods.; usage level: 0.3-5%.

Naetex-L. [Lanaetex Prods.] PEG-2 lactamide; coupling agent, lubricant, emollient, and humectant for personal care prods.; enhances wet combing, imparts softness and antistatic props. to hair; solv. in cosmetic creams and lotions; hygroscopic nature prevents dry skin.

Naetex-LAM. [Lanaetex Prods.] Lactic acid MEA; CAS 5422-34-4; EINECS 226-546-1; cosmetic ingred.

Naetex-LD. [Lanaetex Prods.] Oleyl dimethylamidopropyl ethonium ethosulfate isostearate; cationic; substantivity agent for skin and hair; provides wet and dry combability and antistatic props.

Naetex-LS. [Lanaetex Prods.] Lauramide/lineamide DEA; thickener, conditioner, and emollient for shampoos; synergistic with foaming agents.

Naetex O-20. [Lanaetex Prods.] Oleamide DEA, diethanolamine; thickening agent and conditioner for shampoos, liq. hand soaps; also provides lubricity, corrosion inhibiting props. and enhances w/o emulsions.

Naetex O-80. [Lanaetex Prods.] Linoleamidopropyl-dimethylamine; CAS 81613-56-1; cationic; softener, plasticizer, antistat, combability aid, lubricity agent, emulsifier for hair and skin prods., creams, lotions; provides persistent soft, velvety skinfeel; stable.

Naetex-Q. [Lanaetex Prods.] Linoleamidopropyl ethyldimonium ethosulfate; CAS 99542-23-1; conditioner and bodying agent preventing fly-away and providing combability and antistatic props. in hair care prods.; sol. in water.

Naetex-S. [Lanaetex Prods.] Isostearamidopropyl ethyldimonium ethosulfate; CAS 67633-63-0; EINECS 266-778-0; cosmetics ingred.

Naetex-WS. [Lanaetex Prods.] Linoleylamidopropyl polyoxyethylene ethonium ethosulfate; cationic; provides combability and conditioning and prevents fly-away in hair care prods.; water-sol.

Nafol® 10 D. [Vista] C10 alcohol (90% C10, 10% C8); intermediate for mfg. of toiletries, cosmetics, detergents, laundry softeners, lubricating oil additives, plasticizers, plastics additives, textile/leather additives, disinfectants, agrochem., paper defoamers, flotation agents; Hazen 10 max. color; m.w. 155-162; sp.gr. 0.829 (20/4 C); solid. pt. 3 C; b.p. 215-240 C; acid no. 0.05 max.; iodine no. 0.2 max.; hyd. no. 345-365; flash pt. 95 C; 99% min. act.

Nafol® 20+. [Vista] C20-24 alcohol (50% C20, 29% C22, 14% C24); intermediate for mfg. of toiletries, cosmetics, detergents, laundry softeners, lubricating oil additives, plasticizers, plastics additives, textile/leather additives, disinfectants, agrochem., paper defoamers, flotation agents; Hazen 1800 max. color; sp.gr. 0.804 (80/4 C); solid. pt. 53-58 C; acid no. 1.0 max.; iodine no. 20 max.; hyd. no. 130-150; flash pt. 210 C; 80% act.

Nafol® 810 D. [Vista] C8-10 alcohol (43% C8, 55% C10); intermediate for mfg. of toiletries, cosmetics, detergents, laundry softeners, lubricating oil additives, plasticizers, plastics additives, textile/leather additives, disinfectants, agrochem., paper defoamers, flotation agents; Hazen 10 max. color; m.w. 143-148; sp.gr. 0.827 (20/4 C); b.p. 195-240 C; acid no. 0.05 max.; iodine no. 0.15 max.; hyd. no. 380-390; pour pt. 11 C; flash pt. 85 C; 99% min. act.

Nafol® 1014. [Vista] C10-14 alcohol (15% C10, 47% C12, 38% C14); intermediate for mfg. of toiletries, cosmetics, detergents, laundry softeners, lubricating oil additives, plasticizers, plastics additives, textile/leather additives, disinfectants, agrochem., paper defoamers, flotation agents; Hazen 20 max. color; m.w. 187-193; sp.gr. 0.832 (20/4 C); solid. pt. 14-18 C; b.p. 230-285 C; acid no. 0.05 max.; iodine no. 0.2 max.; hyd. no. 290-300; flash pt. 118 C; 99% min. act.

Nafol® 1218. [Vista] C12-18 alcohol (40% C12, 30% C14, 18% C16, 10% C180; intermediate for mfg. of toiletries, cosmetics, detergents, laundry softeners, lubricating oil additives, plasticizers, plastics additives, textile/leather additives, disinfectants, agrochem., paper defoamers, flotation agents; Hazen 30 max. color; m.w. 204-216; sp.gr. 0.823 (40/4 C); solid. pt. 25-28 C; b.p. 270-335 C; acid no. 0.1 max.; iodine no. 0.4 max.; hyd. no. 260-275; flash pt. 145 C; 98.5% min. act.

Nafol® 1618 H. [Condea Chemie GmbH] Cetearyl alcohol; cosmetic and pharmaceutical raw material.

Nafol® C14-C22. [Condea Chemie GmbH] Fatty alcohol blend; cosmetic and pharmaceutical raw material; emollient, consistency giving factor for creams, ointments, liniments, lotions, and sticks.

Nagellite® 3050. [Telechemische] Toluenesulfonamide/epoxy resin; patented formaldehyde-free nail enamel resin providing superior clarity, brilliance, gloss, adhesion; plasticizer for nitrocellulose.

Nagellite® 3050-80. [Telechemische] Toluenesulfonamide/epoxy resin, butyl acetate; nail enamel resin.

Nailsyn® . [Rona; E. Merck] Dispersions of syn. pearl pigments in thixotropic nitrocellulose lacquer; pearlescent for nail polish.

Nalco® 634. [Nalco] PEI-1400; CAS 9002-98-6; cosmetic ingred.

Nalco® 2395. [Nalco] PEG-50 castor oil; CAS 61791-12-6; personal care surfactant.

Nalidone® . [UCIB; Barnet Prods.] Sodium PCA aq. sol'n.; CAS 28874-51-3; EINECS 249-277-1; moisturizer for dermatological soap, shampoo, after-sun gel, nutritive and regenerative creams and lotions, hair comb-out balm; liq., odorless; sol. in water; m.w. 151.1; usage level: 1-5%; toxicology: nontoxic; nonirritating to skin and eyes; 50% act. in water.

Nalquat 2240. [Nalco] Polymethacrylamidopropyltrimonium chloride; CAS 68039-13-4; film-former, hair fixative.

Nanospheres 100 Conc. in O.M.C. [Exsymol; Biosil Tech.] Porous polymer loaded with octyl methoxy cinnamate; CAS 5466-77-3; EINECS 226-775-7; controlled release system for solar creams or gels, anti-aging prods., cosmetic and health prods. such as milks, emulsions, creams, lotions, solutions; sl. colored opalescent visc. liq.; misc. with ethylic alcohol, oils; toxicology: nontoxic.

Nanospheres 100 Dihydroxyacetone. [Exsymol; Biosil Tech.] Porous polymer loaded with dihydroxyacetone; CAS 96-26-4; EINECS 202-494-5; controlled release system containing a tanning activator for cosmetic and health prods. such as milks, emulsions, creams, lotions, and solutions; pale yel. opaque liq.; misc. with water, ethylic alcohol, glycols; pH 5.0; toxicology: nontoxic.

Nanospheres 100 Lipo Plus. [Exsymol; Biosil Tech.] Porous polymer loaded with theophyllisilane and theophyllin; controlled release system for slimming treatments, cosmetic and health prods. such as milks, emulsions, creams, lotions, solutions; sl. colored very opalescent liq.; misc. with water, ethylic alcohol, glycols; pH 5.5; toxicology: nontoxic.

Nanospheres 100 Menthol. [Exsymol; Biosil Tech.] Porous polymer loaded with menthol; CAS 89-78-1; EINECS 201-939-0; controlled release system for slimming treatments, creams or gels for heavy legs, cosmetic and health prods. such as milks, emulsions, creams, lotions, solutions; whitish opalescent liq.; misc. with ethylic alcohol, oils; toxicology: nontoxic.

Nanospheres 100 Silanol. [Exsymol; Biosil Tech.] Porous polymer loaded with Silanol; controlled release system for cosmetic and health prods. such as milks, emulsions, creams, lotions, solutions; sl. colored opaque liq.; misc. with water, ethylic alcohol, glycols; pH 5.0; toxicology: nontoxic.

Nanospheres 100 Vitamin A Acetate. [Exsymol; Biosil Tech.] Porous polymer loaded with vitamin A acetate; controlled release system for anti-aging prods., hydration, tissue regeneration, skin maintenance, cosmetic and health prods. such as milks, emulsions, creams, lotions, solutions; ylsh. opalescent liq.; misc. with ethylic alcohol, oils; toxicology: nontoxic.

Nanospheres 100 Vitamine E Acetate. [Exsymol; Biosil Tech.] Porous polymer loaded with vitamin E acetate; CAS 7695-91-2; EINECS 231-710-0; controlled release system for anti-aging prods., tissue regeneration, skin maintenance, cosmetic and health prods. such as milks, emulsions, creams, lotions, solutions; liq., translucent in 2-octyl dodecanol, opalescent in ethylic alcohol; misc. with ethylic alcohol, oils; toxicology: nontoxic.

Nasuna® B. [Henkel Canada] PVP/VA copolymer; CAS 25086-89-9; basic material for hair setting lotions, sprays; powd.; sol. in alcohol, water.

National Starch 28-4979. [Nat'l. Starch] Acrylates/octylacrylamide copolymer.; hairspray polymer for aerosol and pump hairsprays, setting lotions.

Natipide 08010A. [Rhone-Poulenc Rorer] Water, lecithin; CAS 8002-43-5; EINECS 232-307-2; moisturizer, liposomes; for skin care, creams and lotions, cleansers, and sunscreens.

Natipide 08010E. [Rhone-Poulenc Rorer] Water, alcohol, lecithin; moisturizer, liposomes; for skin care, creams and lotions, cleansers, and sunscreens.

Natipide® II. [Am. Lecithin; Rhone-Poulenc Rorer] Lecithin/water/ethanol liposome conc. containing 20% purified phospholipid fractions with high phosphatidylcholine content; transparent gel containing empty liposomes ready to be loaded with actives; for dermatology, cosmetics, and personal care prods.; improves skin humidity and penetration; transparent gel; usage level: 10%.

Natipide® II PG. [Am. Lecithin] Water/lecithin/propylene glycol liposome; alcohol-free version of Natipide II; easy loading of actives for cosmetics prods.; moisturizer; reduces skin roughness; transparent gel.

Natoil ALM. [Universal Preserv-A-Chem] Almond oil; cosmetic ingred.

Natoil AVO. [Universal Preserv-A-Chem] Avocado oil; CAS 8024-32-6; EINECS 232-428-0; cosmetic ingred.

Natoil RBO. [Universal Preserv-A-Chem] Rice bran oil; EINECS 271-397-8; cosmetic ingred.

Natoil SAF. [Universal Preserv-A-Chem] Safflower oil; CAS 8001-23-8; EINECS 232-276-5; emollient oil.

Natrosol® 250. [Aqualon] Hydroxyethylcellulose; CAS 9004-62-0; nonionic; thickener, protective colloid, binder, stabilizer, suspending agent; for coatings, cosmetics, pharmaceuticals, textile printing pastes, paints, inks, adhesives, electroplating, ceramics, textile and paper sizing, acid thickening for acidizing oil wells; FDA compliance; wh. to lt. tan gran. powd.; particle size 90% thru 40 mesh; water-sol.; avail. in various visc. grades; pH 6.0-8.5 (2%).

Natrosol® Hydroxyethylcellulose. [Aqualon] Hydroxyethylcellulose; CAS 9004-62-0; thickener for hair care prods., creams and lotions, latex paints; protective colloid in emulsion polymerization; suspending aid in joint and tile cements; binder for welding rods; sol. in hot and cold water, DMSO; tolerates up to 70% polar org. solv. in water.

Natrosol® Plus CS. [Aqualon] Cetyl hydroxyethylcellulose; nonionic; associative thickener and visc. stabilizer for aq. and surfactant systems in personal care field; binder, stabilizer, film-former, suspending agent, moisture barrier; costabilizer in emulsion systems; surf. tens. 62 dynes/cm.

Natrosol® Plus CS, Grade 330. [Aqualon] Cetyl hydroxyethylcellulose; nonionic; associative thickener providing visc. stability to aq. and surfactant cosmetic and pharmaceutical systems; binder, stabilizer, film-former, suspending agent; wh. to off-wh. powd.; water-sol.; bulk dens. 0.75 g/ml; visc. 300 cps (1%); surf. tens. 62 dynes/cm; toxicology: LD50 > 5 g/kg (nontoxic); nonirritating to skin; mild ocular irritant.

Natural Beeswax. [R.I.T.A.] Beeswax; emollient, humectant, pigment, conditioner, lubricant with skin soothing props. for personal care prods.; waxy solid.

Natural Extract AP. [R.I.T.A.] Trimethyl glycine; emollient, humectant, pigment, conditioner, lubricant with skin soothing props. for personal care formulations; wh. gran. solid.

Natural Extract AP. [Rewo GmbH] Betaine; moisturizer, conditioner; reduces skin irritation; cryst.; 99% conc.

Naturechem® CAR. [CasChem] Cetyl acetyl ricinoleate; mild, noncomedogenic, nonoily emollient for skin care prods.; Gardner -1 liq.; m.p. 7 C; acid no. < 1; iodine no. 45; hyd. no. < 5.

Naturechem® CR. [CasChem] Cetyl ricinoleate; CAS 10401-55-5; EINECS 233-864-4; mild, noncomedogenic, nonoily emollient for cosmetics; wh. solid, liquefies on skin; m.p. 27 C; acid no. < 1; iodine no. 45; hyd. no. 100; 100% act.

Naturechem® EGHS. [CasChem] Glycol hydroxystearate; CAS 33907-46-9; EINECS 251-732-4; nonionic; aux. emulsifier, emollient, thickener, opacifier for cosmetics, household prods.; wh. flakes; m.p. 66 C; HLB 2.0; acid no. 3; iodine no. < 5; hyd. no. 266; 100% conc.

Naturechem® GMHS. [CasChem] Glyceryl hydroxystearate; CAS 1323-42-8; EINECS 215-355-9; nonionic; aux. emulsifier, emollient, opacifier, bodying and thickening agent for cosmetics, household prods.; wh. flakes; m.p. 69 C; HLB 3.4; acid no. 6; iodine no. < 5; hyd. no. 320; 100% conc.

Naturechem® GTH. [CasChem] Glyceryl triacetyl hydroxystearate; CAS 27233-00-7; EINECS 248-351-0; mild, noncomedogenic emollient, wetting agent, stabilizer for pigmented prods.; imparts gloss; Gardner -1 color; m.p. - 1 C; acid no. 1; iodine no. < 3; hyd. no. < 3.

Naturechem® GTR. [CasChem] Glyceryl triacetyl ricinoleate; CAS 101-34-8; EINECS 202-935-1; mild emollient, pigment wetter, cosolv.; softener for waxes and resins; Gardner 2+ color; m.p. -40 C; acid no. < 1; iodine no. 76; hyd. no. 5.

Naturechem® MAR. [CasChem] Methyl acetyl ricinoleate; CAS 140-03-4; EINECS 205-392-9; light emollient; reduces greasiness of emollients such as min. oil; cosolv. props.; solubilizer for benzophenone-3; superior freeze/thaw props.; Gardner 1 color; m.p. -25 C; acid no. < 1; iodine no. 77; hyd. no. < 5.

Naturechem® MHS. [CasChem] Methyl hydroxystearate; CAS 141-23-1; EINECS 205-471-8; opacifier, pearlescent, emulsifier, visc. builder for surfactant systems; Gardner 1 color; m.p. 52 C; acid no. 2; iodine no. < 5; hyd. no. 164.

Naturechem® OHS. [CasChem] Octyl hydroxystearate; CAS 29383-26-4; emollient, softener for cosmetics; refatting additive for soaps, cleansers; lt. yel. liq.; m.p. 5 C; acid no. 1; iodine no. < 5; hyd. no. 75; 100% act.

Naturechem® PGHS. [CasChem] Propylene glycol hydroxystearate; CAS 33907-47-0; EINECS 251-734-5; nonionic; aux. emulsifier, dispersant, opacifier, thickener, emollient, stabilizer for cosmetics, household prods.; wh. flakes; m.p. 53 C; HLB 2.6; acid no. 2; iodine no. < 5; hyd. no. 289; 100% conc.

Naturechem® PGR. [CasChem] Propylene glycol ricinoleate; CAS 26402-31-3; EINECS 247-669-7; wetting agent, stabilizer, pigment/dye dispersant providing emolliency, gloss, plasticization to cosmetics, household prods.; pale yel. liq.; m.p. -26 C; acid no. 2.5; iodine no. 76; hyd. no. 296; 100% act.

Naturechem® THS-200. [CasChem] PEG-200 trihydroxystearin; CAS 61788-85-0; nonionic; emulsifier, emollient, thickener, stabilizer for cosmetics, household prods.; stable over broad pH range; wh. wax-like solid; sol. in water and alcohol; m.p. 52 C; HLB 18.0; acid no. 1.2; iodine no. < 5; 100% conc.

Naturol. [Lanaetex Prods.] Mink oil; cosmetics ingred.

Naturon® 2X AQ. [Rona] Water, guanine, methylcellulose; pearlescent pigments for cosmetics and toiletries.

Naturon® 2X IPA. [Rona; E. Merck] Isopropyl alcohol, guanine, polysorbate 80, cetyl acetate, acetylated lanolin alcohol; pearlescent pigments for cosmetics and toiletries.

Naturon® CSN-22. [Rona; E. Merck] Butyl acetate, guanine, nitrocellulose, isopropyl alcohol; pearlescent in nail polish, lotions; 22% conc.

Natwax BEE. [Universal Preserv-A-Chem] Beeswax; wax for personal care prods.

Natwax CAN. [Universal Preserv-A-Chem] Candelilla wax; CAS 8006-44-8; EINECS 232-347-0; wax for cosmetics use.

Natwax CAR. [Universal Preserv-A-Chem] Carnauba wax; CAS 8015-86-9; wax for cosmetics.

Natwax CER. [Universal Preserv-A-Chem] Ceresin wax; CAS 8001-75-0; EINECS 232-290-1; wax for gelling and stabilizing cosmetics.

Natwax RB. [Universal Preserv-A-Chem] Rice bran wax; CAS 8016-60-2; EINECS 232-409-7; cosmetic wax.

Naxchem™ CD-6M. [Ruetgers-Nease] Surfactant blend; detergent, foam booster/stabilizer for cosmetics, carpet shampoos, dishwash, laundry detergents, textile processing, pigment dispersions; lt. amber clear liq.; 100% act.

Naxel™ AAS-40S. [Ruetgers-Nease] Sodium dodecylbenzene sulfonate; CAS 25155-30-0; EINECS 246-680-4; anionic; biodeg. surfactant, foamer, wetting agent, detergent for household and industrial detergents, rug shampoos, textile wet processing, metal cleaners, dairy cleaners, cosmetics; 40% act.

Naxel™ AAS-45S. [Ruetgers-Nease] Sodium dodecylbenzene sulfonate; CAS 25155-30-0; EINECS 246-680-4; anionic; surfactant for household and industrial detergents, dairy cleaners, textile scouring compds., car wash prods., leather prods., cosmetics, rug shampoos, aircraft cleaners; gold liq.; 40-43% act.

Naxel™ AAS-60S. [Ruetgers-Nease] TEA dodecylbenzene sulfonate; CAS 27323-41-7; EINECS 248-406-9; anionic; foaming agent for bubble baths, shampoos, household and industrial detergents, textile dyeing compds., etc.; gold liq.; sol. in water, methanol; dens. 9.3 lb/gal; 60% act.

Naxel ™AAS-98S. [Ruetgers-Nease] Dodecylbenzenesulfonic acid; CAS 27176-87-0; EINECS 248-289-4; anionic; biodeg. detergent intermediate, wetting agent, emulsifier; Klett 70 max. liq.; dens. 8.82 lb/gal; visc. 478 cSt (100 F); 96% act.

Naxide™ 1230. [Ruetgers-Nease] Cocamine oxide; CAS 61788-90-7; EINECS 263-016-9; detergent, foam booster/stabilizer, visc. builder, conditioner for shampoos, hand cleaners, dishwash, lt. duty detergents, tex-

tiles, lubricants, paper coatings; APHA 125 max. color; 30% min. act.

Naxolate™ WA-97. [Ruetgers-Nease] Sodium lauryl sulfate USP, BP; CAS 151-21-3; EINECS 205-788-1; anionic; biodeg. detergent, wetting agent, foamer, emulsifier for cosmetic and household prods. incl. shampoos, bubble baths, rug shampoos, toothpaste, dishwash, laundry detergents; wh. powd.; dens. 200 ± 50 g/l; 96-98% act.

Naxolate™ WAG. [Ruetgers-Nease] Sodium lauryl sulfate USP, BP; CAS 151-21-3; EINECS 205-788-1; anionic; biodeg. detergent, wetting agent, foamer, emulsifier for cosmetic and household prods. incl. shampoos, bubble baths, rug shampoos, toothpaste, dishwash, laundry detergents, textile scouring; ivory wh. needles; dens. 500 ± 50 g/l; pH 7-10 (1% aq.); 89% act.

Naxolate™ WA Special. [Ruetgers-Nease] Sodium lauryl sulfate; CAS 151-21-3; EINECS 205-788-1; anionic; detergent, wetting agent, foamer for cosmetic and household prods. incl. shampoos, bubble baths, rug shampoos, toothpaste, acid soap processing, pigment dispersion, compounded detergents; lt. yel. liq., pleasant odor; visc. 50-300 cps; cloud pt. 22 C max.; 30% act.

Naxonic™ NI-40. [Ruetgers-Nease] Nonoxynol-4; CAS 9016-45-9; nonionic; wetting agent, dispersant, penetrant, emulsifier, detergent, solubilizer for textile wet processing, agric., cosmetic, industrial and household detergents, latex and polymers, wax/polishes; demulsifier for petrol.; clear liq.; oil-sol.; sp.gr. 1.02-1.04.

Naxonic™ NI-60. [Ruetgers-Nease] Nonoxynol-6; CAS 9016-45-9; nonionic; wetting agent, dispersant, penetrant, emulsifier, detergent, solubilizer for textile wet processing, agric., cosmetic, industrial and household detergents, latex and polymers, wax/polishes; demulsifier for petrol.; clear liq.; oil-sol.; sp.gr. 1.03-1.05; cloud pt. 32 F.

Naxonic™ NI-100. [Ruetgers-Nease] Nonoxynol-10; CAS 9016-45-9; EINECS 248-294-1; nonionic; wetting agent, dispersant, penetrant, emulsifier, detergent, solubilizer for textile wet processing, agric., cosmetic, industrial and household detergents, latex and polymers, wax/polishes; demulsifier for petrol.; clear liq.; water-sol.; sp.gr. 1.05-1.07; cloud pt. 52-56 C.

Naxonol™ CO. [Ruetgers-Nease] Cocamide DEA (2:1); CAS 61791-31-9; EINECS 263-163-9; nonionic; detergent, wetting agent, thickener for household and industrial detergents, shampoos, textile wet processing, leather and fur processing, metal cleaning, solv. emulsification; amber liq.; sol. in water; sp.gr. 2.47 g/ml; 97% conc.

Naxonol™ PN 66. [Ruetgers-Nease] Cocamide DEA; CAS 61791-31-9; EINECS 263-163-9; nonionic; wetting agent, foam booster/stabilizer, emulsifier, thickener, detergent for household and heavy-duty cleaners, shampoos, leather and fur processing, car wash, textile wet processing, metal cleaners; amber liq.; 98% act.

Naxonol™ PO. [Ruetgers-Nease] Cocamide DEA (1:1); CAS 61791-31-9; EINECS 263-163-9; nonionic; detergent, emulsifier, wetting agent, foam booster, thickener, lubricant, dispersant for household and industrial cleaners, cosmetics, buffing and polishing compds., textiles; lt. yel. visc. liq.; sp.gr. 2.46 g/ml; 85% conc.

NB. [Angus] 2-Nitro-1-butanol; CAS #609-31-4; CAS 609-31-4; chemical and pharmaceutical intermediate, in tire cord adhesives, as formaldehyde release agents, deodorants, antimicrobials; m.w. 119.1; sol. 54 g/100 ml water; m.p. -48 C; b.p. 105 C; flash pt. > 200 F (TCC); pH 4.5 (0.1 M aq. sol'n.).

Necon 655. [Alzo] Dihydroxyethyl tallowamine oleate.

Necon A. [Alzo] Dimethyl lauramine oleate.

Necon BDB. [Alzo] Behenamidopropyldimethylamine behenate; CAS 125804-04-8.

Necon DLD. [Alzo] Dimethyl lauramine dimer dilinoleate.

Necon LO. [Alzo] Dimethyl lauramine oleate.

Necon LO-80. [Alzo] Linoleamidopropyldimethylamine dimer dilinoleate; CAS 125804-10-6.

Necon SOG. [Alzo] Soyamidopropyl dimethylamino glycolate; CAS 118777-77-8; cationic; surfactant, emulsifier, conditioning agent with exc. hair substantivity, fly-away control, softening props., and enhanced wet and dry combing; emulsifier for paper and pulp industry; dk. yel. sl. visc. liq., mild ammoniacal odor; water-sol.; sp.gr. 0.99; pH 7.0; 70% NV in propylene glycol.

Necon SOGU. [Alzo] Soyamidopropyl dimethylamino gluconate; CAS 129541-36-2; cationic; surfactant, emulsifier, conditioning agent with exc. hair substantivity, fly-away control, softening props., and enhanced wet and dry combing; emulsifier for paper and pulp industry; dk. amber visc. liq., mild ammoniacal odor; water-sol.; sp.gr. 1.06; pH 7.0; 70% NV in propylene glycol.

Necon SOLC. [Alzo] Linoleamido dimethylamino lactate; CAS 81613-56-1; cationic; surfactant, emulsifier, conditioning agent with exc. skin and hair substantivity, fly-away control, softening props., and enhanced wet and dry combing; emulsifier for paper and pulp industry; dk. amber visc. liq., mild ammoniacal odor; water-sol.; sp.gr. 1.00; pH 7.0; 70% NV in propylene glycol.

Neobee® 18. [Stepan/PVO; Stepan Europe] Hybrid safflower oil; CAS 8001-23-8; EINECS 232-276-5; emollient oil for cosmetics and pharmaceuticals, solubilizer, solv., lubricant, nutritional fluid; liq.; bland taste and odor; sol. in alcohol, min. oil, acetone; sp.gr. 0.915; visc. 70 cps; sapon. no. 190–200; surf. tens. 31.6 dynes/cm.

Neobee® 20. [Stepan/PVO] Propylene glycol dicaprylate/dicaprate; emollient oil for cosmetics and pharmaceuticals (bath oils, creams, lotions, lipsticks, makeup bases, shaving preps.), carrier/extender for flavors, fragrances, and colors in foods; vehicle for vitamins, antibiotics, and medicinals; solubilizer, cosolv.; APHA 50 max. liq.; sol. in alcohol, min. oil, acetone; sp.gr. 0.920; visc. 9 cps; acid no. 0.10 max.; sapon. no. 315–335; surf. tens. 31.0 dynes/cm.

Neobee® 1053. [Stepan/PVO] Coconut oil-derived triglycerides; diluent vehicle for flavoring, medicinals, colorings, clouding agent in beverages; liq.; odorless and tasteless; sol. in min. oil, acetone, alcohol; sp.gr. 0.930–0.960; sapon. no. 325–355.

Neobee® 1054. [Stepan/PVO] Propylene glycol diester of coconut fatty acids; cosolv. for cosmetics and pharmaceuticals, carrier for flavors and colors; medicinal diluent; emollient; liq.; sol. in alcohol, min. oil, acetone; sp.gr. 0.910–0.923; sapon. no. 315–335.

Neobee® 1062. [Stepan/PVO] Coconut oil-derived triglycerides; cosolv., carrier for fat-sol. vitamins, medicinals, and ointments in food, cosmetic and pharmaceutical industries; liq.; sol. in min. oil, acetone; sp.gr. 0.925–0.945; sapon. no. 295–315.

Neobee® M-5. [Stepan/PVO; Stepan Europe] Caprylic/capric triglyceride; CAS 65381-09-1; diluent vehicle/carrier for vitamins, antibiotics, nutritional fluids, and medicinals; solubilizer, cosolv. for fragrance/flavoring, medicinals, food colors; clouding agent for beverages; emollient oil for cosmetics and pharmaceuticals (bath oils, creams, lotions, lipsticks, makeup base, shaving preps.); sl. yel. liq., bland odor, tasteless; sol. in alcohol, min. oil, acetone; sp.gr. 0.930-0.960; visc. 23 cps; acid no. 0.10 max.; iodine no. 1; sapon. no. 335–360; hyd. no. 5; surf. tens. 32.3 dynes/cm.; 0.1% moisture.

Neobee® M-20. [Stepan/PVO; Stepan Europe] Propylene glycol dicaprylate/dicaprate; low visc. emollient oil for creams, lotions, and ointments; solubilizer for antibiotics, medicinals; diluent for essential oils, injectables; solv. and lubricating agent; exc. deposition on skin; FDA §172.856; pale yel. liq., bland odor; sol. in alcohol containing up to 20% water; iodine no. 1 max.; sapon. no. 315-335; hyd. no. 10 max.; 100% act.

Neobee® O. [Stepan/PVO] Caprylic/capric triglyceride; CAS 65381-09-1; cosolv., carrier for fat-sol. vitamins, medicinals, and ointments in food, cosmetic and pharmaceutical industries; spreading agent, penetrant, solubilizer; liq.; sol. in min. oil, acetone; sp.gr. 0.938; visc. 30 cps; sapon. no. 300–315; surf. tens. 32 dynes/cm.

NeoCryl B-1000. [ICI Resins] Styrene/acrylates/acrylonitrile copolymer.

Neodol® 1. [Shell] Undecyl alcohol; CAS 112-42-5; nonionic; detergent intermediate; clear liq.; m.w. 173; sp.gr. 0.831; visc. 11 cSt (100 F); m.p. 42–57 F; acid no. < 0.001; sapon. no. < 0.001; hyd. no. 323-327; pour pt. 52 F; flash pt. (PMCC) 250 F; ref. index 1.4379; toxicology: low acute oral toxicity; irritating to skin and eyes in undiluted form; 100% act.

Neodol® 5. [Shell] Pentadecyl alcohol; CAS 629-76-5; detergent intermediate; paste; 100% conc.

Neodol® 23. [Shell] C12-13 alcohols; CAS 75782-86-4; detergent intermediate; surfactant for household, personal care, and industrial applics.; APHA 0-5 liq.; m.w. 194; sp.gr. 0.833; visc. 14 cSt (100 F); m.p. 7-22 C; pour pt. 17 C; acid no. < 0.001; hyd. no. 289; flash pt. (PMCC) 137 C; toxicology: LD50 (oral, rat) 28.2 g/kg; practically nonirritating to eyes, mild skin irritant; 100% act.

Neodol® 23-3. [Shell] C12–13 pareth-3; CAS 66455-14-9; nonionic; detergent intermediate used in preparation of sulfates for high-foaming liq. detergents; emulsifier; for cosmetic, specialty industrial, dishwashing applics.; biodeg.; APHA 50 max., clear to slightly hazy liq.; m.w. 310–342; dens. 7.7 lb/gal; sp.gr. 0.925; visc. 19 cs (100 F); m.p. 5–6 C; HLB 7.9; flash pt. 300 F (PMCC); pour pt. 4 C; 100% act.

Neodol® 23-6.5. [Shell] C12-13 pareth-7; CAS 66455-14-9; nonionic; detergent intermediate used in preparation of sulfates for high-foaming liq. detergents, personal care, household and industrial use; biodeg.; practically colorless liq., mild odor; m.w. 484; sp.gr. 0.984; dens. 8.08 lb/gal (100 F); visc. 29 cSt (100 F); m.p. 11-15 C; HLB 12.1; acid no. < 0.001; hyd. no. 115; pour pt. 16 C; cloud pt. 113 F (1% aq.); flash pt. (PMCC) 334 F; pH 6.0 (1% aq.); surf. tens. 28 dynes/cm (0.1% aq.); Draves wetting 9 s (0.1%); Ross-Miles foam 8 cm (0.1% , initial); toxicology: LD50 (oral, rat) 4.6 g/kg; severe eye irritant, mild skin irritant; 100% act.

Neodol® 25. [Shell] C12-15 alcohols; CAS 63393-82-8; detergent, emulsifier intermediate; for household and personal care applics.; emollient for creams and lotions; APHA 0-5 liq.; m.w. 203; sp.gr. 0.834; visc. 15 cSt (100 F); m.p. 12-25 C; acid no. < 0.001; hyd. no. 276; pour pt. 19 C; flash pt. (PMCC) 141 C; toxicology: LD50 (oral, rat) > 23.1 g/kg; minimal eye irritant; mild skin irritant; 100% act.

Neodol® 25-3. [Shell] C12–15 pareth-3; CAS 68131-39-5; nonionic; detergent intermediate used in preparation of sulfates for high-foaming liq. detergents; emulsifier; for cosmetic, industrial, dishwashing and liq. detergents; biodeg.; colorless, clear to slightly hazy liq., mild odor; m.w. 338; sp.gr. 0.921; dens. 7.70 lb/gal; visc. 19 cst (100 F); m.p. 5-6 C; HLB 7.8; acid no. < 0.001; hyd. no. 166; pour pt. 4 C; cloud pt. 30 F (1% aq.); flash pt. (PMCC) 315 F; pH 7.1 (1% aq.); toxicology: LD50 (oral, rat) 2.5 g/kg; severe eye irritant, extreme skin irritant; 100% act.

Neodol® 25-3A. [Shell] Ammonium C12–15 pareth sulfate; anionic; detergent used in high-foaming liq. detergents, dishwash, personal care applics.; biodeg.; lt. clear visc. liq.; mild ethanol odor; m.w. 434; sp.gr. 1.02; dens. 8.5 lb/gal (60 F); visc. 45 cs (100 F); flash pt. (PMCC) 74 F; pH

7.3; toxicology: LD50 (oral, rat) 10.2 g/kg; severe eye irritant, mild skin irritant; 59% act.

Neodol® 25-3S. [Shell] Sodium C12–15 pareth sulfate; anionic; detergent used in high-foaming liq. detergents, dishwash, personal care applics.; lt., visc. liq., mild ethanol odor; m.w. 439; sp.gr. 1.05; dens. 8.76 lb/gal (60 F); visc. 45 cs (100 F); flash pt. (PMCC) 73 F; pH 7.7; toxicology: LD50 (oral, rat) 10.2 g/kg; severe eye irritant, mild skin irritant; 59% act.

Neodol® 25-7. [Shell] C12-15 pareth-7; CAS 68131-39-5; nonionic; detergent intermediate used in preparation of sulfates for high-foaming liq. detergents; wetting agent, dispersant; for personal care, general industrial and household detergents; biodeg.; APHA 5-10 paste-like, mild odor.; m.w. 524; sp.gr. 0.965 (122/77 F); visc. 34 cSt (100 F); m.p. 36-70 F; HLB 12.3; acid no. < 0.001; hyd. no. 107; pour pt. 66 F; cloud pt. 121 F (1% aq.); flash pt. (PMCC) 367 F; pH 6.0 (1%); surf. tens. 30 dynes/cm (0.1% aq.); Draves wetting 11 s (0.1%); Ross-Miles foam 7 cm (0.1% , initial); toxicology: LD50 (oral, rat) 2.7 g/kg; moderate eye irritant, mild skin irritant; 100% act.

Neodol® 25-9. [Shell] C12-15 pareth-9; CAS 68131-39-5; nonionic; detergent intermediate used in preparation of sulfates for high-foaming liq. detergents; wetting agent, dispersant; for personal care, general industrial, and household detergents; biodeg.; APHA 5-10 paste-like.; m.w. 597; sp.gr. 0.982 (122/77 F); visc. 41 cSt (100 F); m.p. 57-77 F; HLB 13.1; acid no. < 0.001; hyd. no. 94; pour pt. 70 F; cloud pt. 163 F (1% aq.); flash pt. (PMCC) 370 F; pH 6.0 (1% aq.); surf. tens. 30 dynes/cm (0.1% aq.); Draves wetting 14 s (0.1%); Ross-Miles foam 12 cm (0.1% , initial); toxicology: LD50 (oral, rat) 1.6 g/kg; extreme eye irritant, severe skin irritant; 100% act.

Neodol® 25-12. [Shell] C12-15 pareth-12; CAS 68131-39-5; nonionic; detergent intermediate used in preparation of sulfates for high-foaming liq. detergents; wetting agent, dispersant, emulsifier; for personal care, general industrial, and household detergent prods.; perfume solubilizer; biodeg.; APHA 5-10 color.; m.w. 729; sp.gr. 0.999 (122/77 F); visc. 53 cSt (100 F); m.p. 68-86 F; HLB 14.4; acid no. < 0.001; hyd. no. 77; pour pt. 81 F; cloud pt. 173 F (5% aq. NaCl); flash pt. (PMCC) 433 F; pH 6.0 (1% aq.); surf. tens. 34 dynes/cm (0.1% aq.); Draves wetting 35 s (0.1%); Ross-Miles foam 14 cm (0.1% , initial); toxicology: LD50 (oral, rat) 1.8 g/kg; severe eye irritant, minimal skin irritant; 100% act.

Neodol® 45. [Shell] C14-15 alcohol; CAS 75782-87-5; detergent intermediate; for household and personal care applics.; emollient for creams and lotions; APHA 0-5 liq.; m.w. 221; sp.gr. 0.820 (122/77 F); visc. 18 cSt (100 F); m.p. 15-36 C; acid no. < 0.001; hyd. no. 254; pour pt. 29 C; flash pt. (PMCC) 157 C; toxicology: LD50 (oral, rat) 26.4 g/kg; minimal eye irritant; mild skin irritant; 100% act.

Neodol® 45-7. [Shell] C14-15 pareth-7; CAS 68951-67-7; nonionic; detergent, wetting agent, emulsifier for personal care, general industrial and household detergent prods.; biodeg.; APHA 5-10 color; sol. in alcohols, esters, ketones, chlorinated solvs., aromatic and aliphatic hydrocarbons; m.w. 529; sp.gr. 0.959 (122/77 F); dens. 8.20 lb/gal; visc. 35 cSt (38 C); m.p. 21–25 C; HLB 11.8; acid no. < 0.001; hyd. no. 106; pour pt. 66 F; cloud pt. 46 C (1% aq.); flash pt. (PMCC) 204 C; pH 6.0 (1% aq.); surf. tens. 29 dynes/cm (0.1% aq.); Draves wetting 17 s (0.1%); Ross-Miles foam 9 cm (0.1% , initial); 100% act.

Neodol® 45-11. [Shell] C14-15 pareth-11; nonionic; detergent; m.w. 702; sp.gr. 0.993 (50/25 C); visc. 51 cst (38 C); HLB 13.8; hyd. no. 80; pour pt. 29 C; cloud pt. 88 C (1% aq.); flash pt. (PMCC) 232 C; pH 6.0 (1% aq.); 100% act.

Neodol® 45-13. [Shell] C14-15 pareth-13; nonionic; surfactant, detergent, wetting agent, emulsifier for personal

care, general industrial, and household detergent prods.; biodeg.; APHA 5-10 color; sol. in alcohols, esters, ketones, chlorinated solvs., aromatic and aliphatic hydrocarbons; m.w. 790; sp.gr. 1.003 (50/25 C); dens. 8.39 lb/gal (49 C); visc. 59 cSt (38 C); m.p. 31-36 C; HLB 14.5; acid no. < 0.001; hyd. no. 71; pour pt. 86 F; cloud pt. 78 C (5% aq. NaCl); flash pt. (PMCC) 241 C; pH 6.4 (1% aq.); surf. tens. 34 dynes/cm (0.1%); Draves wetting 48 s (0.1%); Ross-Miles foam 13 cm (0.1% , initial); 100% act.

Neodol® 91. [Shell] C9-11 alcohols; CAS 66455-17-2; nonionic; detergent intermediate; clear liq.; m.w. 160; sp.gr. 0.835; dens. 6.95 lb/gal; visc. 9 cSt (100 F); m.p. -9 C; pour pt. 10 F; flash pt. (PMCC) 107 C; acid no. < 0.001; hyd. no. 350; toxicology: LD50 (oral, rat) > 10 g/kg; moderate eye irritant, mild skin irritant; 100% act.

Neo Heliopan, Type 303. [Haarmann & Reimer GmbH] Octocrylene; CAS 6197-30-4; EINECS 228-250-8; uv-B absorber for cosmetics, waterproof sunscreens; provides some absorp. in the shorter wave uv-A II spectrum; max. absorp. 303 nm; FDA approval; yel. clear visc. liq., faint odor; sol. in decyl oleate, IPM, caprylic/capric triglyceride, olive oil, dipropylene glycol, ethanol; insol. in water; m.w. 361.5; sp.gr. 1.045-1.055; flash pt. > 100 C; ref. index 1.461-1.571; usage level: 7-10%; 98% min. assay.

Neo Heliopan, Type AV. [Haarmann & Reimer GmbH] 2-Ethylhexyl p-methoxycinnamate; CAS 5466-77-3; EINECS 226-775-7; uv-B absorber for cosmetic applics., waterproof sunscreens; also provides absorp. in shortwave uv-A spectrum; max. absorp. 308 nm; EEC, FDA approvals; colorless to pale yel. clear liq., pract. odorless; sol. in oils, IPM, decyl oleate, ethanol, IPA; insol. in water; m.w. 290.4; sp.gr. 1.007-1.012; acid no. 1 max.; flash pt. 1 max.; usage level: 2-7.5% (USA); toxicology: LD50 (oral/dermal, rat) > 20 g/kg; 98% min. assay.

Neo Heliopan, Type BB. [Haarmann & Reimer GmbH] Benzophenone-3; CAS 131-57-7; EINECS 205-031-5; uv-A and uv-B broad spectrum absorber for sunscreen formulations; EEC and FDA approvals; pale yel. fine cryst. powd., pract. odorless; partly sol. in oils, IPM, decyl oleate, ethanol, IPA; insol. in water; m.w. 228.3; m.p. 62-64 C; usage level: 2-6% (USA); toxicology: LD50 (oral, rat) 12.8 g/kg; exc. skin and mucous membrane compat.; 98% min. assay.

Neo Heliopan, Type Hydro. [Haarmann & Reimer GmbH] 2-Phenylbenzimidazole-5-sulfonic acid; CAS 27503-81-7; uv-B filter for sunscreen formulations; EEC and FDA approvals; wh. fine cryst. powd., odorless; sol. (as salt) in ethanol, IPA; sol. > 30% in water; insol. in oil, IPM; m.p. > 30 C; usage level: 1-4% (USA); toxicology: LD50 (oral, rat) > 16 g/kg; exc. skin and mucous membrane compat.; 98% min. assay.

Neo Heliopan, Type MA. [Haarmann & Reimer GmbH] Menthyl anthranilate; CAS 134-09-8; EINECS 205-129-8; uv-A absorber for waterproof sunscreen formulations; FDA approved; colorless to pale ylsh. clear, visc. liq., faint sweet odor; sol. in paraffin oil, olive oil, IPM, propanol, ethanol; insol. in water; m.w. 275.0; sp.gr. 1.036-1.041; acid no. 1 max.; flash pt. > 100 C; ref. index 1.540-1.544; usage level: 3.5-5%; toxicology: LD50 (oral, rat) > 5 g/kg; exc. skin and mucous membrane compat.

Neo Heliopan, Type OS. [Haarmann & Reimer GmbH] 2-Ethylhexyl salicylate; CAS 118-60-5; EINECS 204-263-4; uv-B absorber for cosmetic applics., waterproof sunscreens; solubilizer for oxybenzone; EEC and FDA approvals; colorless liq., sl. floral odor; sol. in oil, IPM, propanol, ethanol; insol. in water; m.w. 250.4; sp.gr. 1.011-1.016; acid no. 1 max.; flash pt. > 100 C; ref. index 1.500-1.503; usage level: 3-5% (USA); toxicology: LD50 (oral, rat) 4.8 ± 0.3 g/kg; exc. skin and mucous membrane compat.

Neopon LAM. [Witco/H-I-P] Ammonium lauryl sulfate; CAS 2235-54-3; EINECS 218-793-9; anionic; detergent, base for cosmetics; liq.; 27% conc.

Neopon LOA. [Witco/H-I-P] Ammonium laureth sulfate; CAS 32612-48-9; anionic; detergent, base for shampoos, creams, bubble baths; liq.; 25% conc.

Neopon LOS 2 N 70. [Witco/H-I-P] Sodium laureth sulfate; cosmetic ingred.; paste; 70% act.

Neopon LOS 3 N 70. [Witco/H-I-P] Sodium laureth sulfate; cosmetic ingred.; paste; 70% act.

Neopon LOS 70. [Witco/H-I-P] Sodium laureth sulfate; CAS 1335-72-4; anionic; detergent, base for cosmetics (shampoos, creams); liq.; 70% conc.

Neopon LOS/NF. [Witco/H-I-P] Sodium laureth sulfate; CAS 1335-72-4; anionic; detergent, base for cosmetics (shampoos, creams); liq.; 27% conc.

Neopon LOT/NF. [Witco/H-I-P] TEA-laureth sulfate; CAS 27028-82-6; for special shampoos; 27% conc.

Neopon LS/NF. [Witco/H-I-P] Sodium lauryl sulfate; CAS 151-21-3; EINECS 205-788-1; detergent, base for cosmetic creams, shampoos; liq.; 27% act.

Neopon LT/NF. [Witco/H-I-P] TEA-lauryl sulfate; CAS 139-96-8; EINECS 205-388-7; anionic; for special shampoos; liq.; 40% act.

Neotan L. [Fabriquimica] Octyl salicylate; CAS 118-60-5; EINECS 204-263-4; sunscreen for cosmetics; oil-sol.; sp.gr. 1.010-1.015; acid no. < 5; sapon. no. 200-220.

Neotan W. [Fabriquimica] TEA-salicylate; CAS 2174-16-5; EINECS 218-531-3; sunscreen for cosmetics; water-sol.; iodine no. < 2; sapon. no. 155-165; pH 7 (10%).

NEPD. [Angus] 2-Nitro-2-ethyl-1,3-propanediol; CAS 597-09-1; chemical and pharmaceutical intermediate, in tire cord adhesives, as formaldehyde release agents, deodorants, antimicrobials; m.w. 149.2; sol. 400 g/100 ml water; m.p. 56 C; b.p. decomposes; pH 5.5 (0.1 M aq. sol'n.).

Neptuline® C. [Gattefosse SA] Hydrolyzed collagenic protein of marine origin; CAS 9015-54-7; moisturizing filmformer which increases cutaneous hydration in cosmetic creams, lotions, and gels, e.g., moisturizing body lotion, facial lotion, dry skin cream; opalescent liq.; sol. in water; pH 4.0 ± 0.5; toxicology: nonirritating to skin; very sl. irritating to eyes.

Neral. [BASF AG] Z-3,7-Dimethyl-2,6-octadiene-1-al; fragrance and flavoring; fresh, lemon-like, green, sl. lime-like.

Nerolidol. [BASF AG] Z,E-3,7,11-Trimethyl-1,6,10-dodecatriene-3-ol; fragrance and flavoring; sweetly floral, green, woody, lilly-like.

Nervanaid™ BA2 (BP). [Rhone-Poulenc Surf. & Spec.] Disodium EDTA; CAS 139-33-3; EINECS 205-358-3; sequestrant for personal care prods.

Nesatol. [Vevy] C10-18 triglycerides; CAS 85665-33-4.

Neustrene® 053. [Witco/H-I-P] Hydrog. menhaden oil; CAS 68002-72-2; used in mfg. of alkali metal soaps, monoglycerides, textile auxiliaries, greases, personal care prods.; solid; acid no. 5 max.; iodine no. 5 max.; sapon. no. 186-201; 100% conc.

Neustrene® 060. [Witco/H-I-P] Refined hydrog. tallow glycerides; CAS 67701-27-3; textile lubricant, pharmaceutical intermediate, emulsifier, mold release agent, buffing compd.; solid; acid no. 2.5 max.; iodine no. 1 max.; sapon. no. 193-205; 100% conc.

Neustrene® 064. [Witco/H-I-P] Hydrog. soybean oil; CAS 68002-71-1; textile lubricant, pharmaceutical intermediate, emulsifier, mold release agent, buffing compd.; solid; acid no. 4 max.; iodine no. 2 max.; sapon. no. 188-200; 100% conc.

Neutrol® TE. [BASF; BASF AG] Tetrahydroxypropyl ethylenediamine; CAS 102-60-3; EINECS 203-041-4; neutralizing agent for cosmetics industry; liq.

New Econa 200 CH. [Kao Corp. SA] Hydrog. tallow glycerides, hydrog. coconut oil.

N-Hance® 3000. [Aqualon] Guar hydroxypropyltrimonium chloride; CAS 65497-29-2; cationic; conditioner, viscosifier, substantive polymer for hair and skin care prods., shampoos, lotions, liq. soaps; particle size 80% thru 200 mesh; visc. 2400-3200 mPa·s (1%); pH 8.5-9.5; usage level: 0.2-1.0%.

Niacin USP, FCC No. 69902. [Roche] Nicotinic acid; CAS 59-67-6; rubifacient for cosmetics.

Niacinamide USP, FCC No. 69905. [Roche] Niacinamide; CAS 98-92-0; EINECS 202-713-4; cosmetics ingred.

Niaproof® Anionic Surfactant 4. [Niacet] Sodium tetradecyl sulfate; CAS 139-88-8; anionic; detergent, wetting agent, penetrant, emulsifier used in adhesives and sealants, coatings, photo chemicals, emulsion polymerization, metal processing, electrolytic cleaning, pickling baths, plating, pharmaceuticals, leather, textiles; FDA compliance; colorless liq., mild char. odor; misc. with water; sp.gr. 1.031; dens. 8.58 lb/gal; b.p. 92 C; COC flash pt. none; pH 8.5 (0.1% aq.); surf. tens. 47 dynes/cm (0.1% aq.); Draves wetting 20 s (0.26%); Ross-Miles foam 10 mm; corrosive, slippery; toxicology: moderate oral and skin toxicity; eye irritant; LD50 (oral, rats) 4.95 ml/kg; 27% act. in water.

Niaproof® Anionic Surfactant 08. [Niacet] Sodium 2-ethylhexyl sulfate; CAS 126-92-1; EINECS 204-812-8; anionic; detergent, wetting agent, penetrant, emulsifier used in textile mercerizing, metal cleaning, electroplating, photo chemicals, adhesives, emulsion polymerization, household and industrial cleaners, agric., pharmaceuticals; stable to high concs. of electrolytes; FDA compliance; colorless liq., mild char. odor; misc. with water; sp.gr. 1.109; dens. 9.23 lb/gal; b.p. 95 C; COC flash pt. none; pH 7.3 (0.1% aq.); surf. tens. 63 dynes/cm (0.1% aq.); Ross-Miles foam 10 mm (initial); toxicology: moderate oral and skin toxicity; eye irritant; LD50 (oral, rats) 7.27 ml/kg; 39% act.

Nidaba 3. [Vevy] Lauramide MIPA; CAS 142-54-1; EINECS 205-541-8; foam stabilizer for cosmetics.

Nidaba 318. [Vevy] DEA-hydrolyzed lecithin.

Nihon Polyglyceryl-10 Distearate. [Nihon Surfactant] Polyglyceryl-10 distearate; CAS 12764-60-2.

Nikkol ALS-25. [Nikko Chem. Co. Ltd.] Ammonium lauryl sulfate aq. sol'n.; CAS 2235-54-3; EINECS 218-793-9; foaming and cleansing agent for cosmetics; yel. visc. liq.

Nikkol AM-101. [Nikko Chem. Co. Ltd.] 2-Alkyl-N-carboxymethyl-N-hydroxyethyl imidazolinium betaine aq. sol'n.; foaming and cleansing agent for cosmetics; low irritation; brn. liq.

Nikkol AM-102EX. [Nikko Chem. Co. Ltd.] Cocoamphocarboxypropionate; foaming and cleansing agent for cosmetics; low irritation; brn. liq.

Nikkol AM-103EX. [Nikko Chem. Co. Ltd.] 2-Alkyl-N-sodium carboxymethyl-N-carboxymethyl oxyethyl imidazolinium betaine aq. sol'n.; foaming and cleansing agent for cosmetics; low irritation; brn. liq.

Nikkol AM-301. [Nikko Chem. Co. Ltd.] Lauryl betaine; CAS 683-10-3; EINECS 211-669-5; foaming and cleansing agent for cosmetics; low irritation; colorless liq.

Nikkol AM-3130N. [Nikko Chem. Co. Ltd.] Cocamidopropyl betaine aq. sol'n.; foaming and cleansing agent for cosmetics; low irritation; pale yel. liq.

Nikkol AM-3130T. [Nikko Chem. Co. Ltd.] Cocamidopropyl betaine aq. sol'n.; foaming and cleansing agent for cosmetics; low irritation; pale yel. liq.

Nikkol BB-5. [Nikko Chem. Co. Ltd.] Beheneth-5; nonionic; emulsifier for cosmetics; provides good heat resist.; wh. solid; HLB 7.0; 100% conc.

Nikkol BB-10. [Nikko Chem. Co. Ltd.] Beheneth-10; nonionic; emulsifier for cosmetics; provides good heat resist.; wh. solid; HLB 10.0; 100% conc.

Nikkol BB-20. [Nikko Chem. Co. Ltd.] Beheneth-20; nonionic; emulsifier for cosmetics; provides good heat resist.; wh. solid; HLB 16.5; 100% conc.

Nikkol BB-30. [Nikko Chem. Co. Ltd.] Beheneth-30; nonionic; emulsifier for cosmetics; provides good heat resist.; wh. solid; HLB 18.0; 100% conc.

Nikkol BC-2. [Nikko Chem. Co. Ltd.] Ceteth-2; CAS 9004-95-9; nonionic; emulsifier for o/w type creams and lotions, hair dressings, medicated ointments; wh. solid; HLB 8.0; 100% conc.

Nikkol BC-5.5. [Nikko Chem. Co. Ltd.] Ceteth-6; CAS 9004-95-9; nonionic; emulsifier for cosmetic and pharmaceuticals; wh. solid; HLB 10.5; 100% conc.

Nikkol BC-7. [Nikko Chem. Co. Ltd.] Ceteth-7; CAS 9004-95-9; nonionic; hydrophilic emulsifier for cosmetics and pharmaceuticals; wh. solid; HLB 11.5; 100% conc.

Nikkol BC-10TX. [Nikko Chem. Co. Ltd.] Ceteth-10; CAS 9004-95-9; nonionic; hydrophilic emulsifier for cosmetics and pharmaceuticals; wh. solid; HLB 13.5; 100% conc.

Nikkol BC-15TX. [Nikko Chem. Co. Ltd.] Ceteth-15; CAS 9004-95-9; nonionic; emulsifier for cosmetics and pharmaceuticals; used in refining techniques; wh. solid; HLB 15.5; 100% conc.

Nikkol BC-20TX. [Nikko Chem. Co. Ltd.] Ceteth-20; CAS 9004-95-9; nonionic; hydrophilic emulsifier for cosmetics, pharmaceuticals; wh. solid; HLB 17.0; 100% conc.

Nikkol BC-23. [Nikko Chem. Co. Ltd.] Ceteth-23; CAS 9004-95-9; nonionic; hydrophilic emulsifier, dispersant, solubilizer for o/w creams, lotions, hair dressings, medicated ointments; solid; HLB 18.0; 100% conc.

Nikkol BC-25TX. [Nikko Chem. Co. Ltd.] Ceteth-25; CAS 9004-95-9; nonionic; hydrophilic emulsifier, dispersant, and solubilizer for cosmetics and pharmaceuticals; wh. solid; HLB 18.5; 100% conc.

Nikkol BC-30TX. [Nikko Chem. Co. Ltd.] Ceteth-30; CAS 9004-95-9; nonionic; hydrophilic emulsifier, dispersant, and solubilizer for cosmetics and pharmaceuticals; wh. solid; HLB 19.5; 100% conc.

Nikkol BC-40TX. [Nikko Chem. Co. Ltd.] Ceteth-40; CAS 9004-95-9; nonionic; hydrophilic emulsifier, dispersant, and solubilizer for cosmetics and pharmaceuticals; wh. solid; HLB 20.0; 100% conc.

Nikkol BD-2. [Nikko Chem. Co. Ltd.] C12-15 pareth-2; CAS 68131-39-5; emulsifier, dispersant for cosmetics; colorless liq.

Nikkol BD-4. [Nikko Chem. Co. Ltd.] C12-15 pareth-4; CAS 68131-39-5; emulsifier, dispersant for cosmetics; colorless liq.

Nikkol BD-10. [Nikko Chem. Co. Ltd.] C12-15 pareth-10; CAS 68131-39-5; emulsifier, dispersant for cosmetics; wh. solid.

Nikkol BH-30. [Nikko Chem. Co. Ltd.] Isoceteth-30.

Nikkol BL-2. [Nikko Chem. Co. Ltd.] Laureth-2; CAS 3055-93-4; EINECS 221-279-7; nonionic; for emulsifying prods. requiring abundant liquidity; colorless liq.; HLB 9.5; 100% conc.

Nikkol BL-4.2. [Nikko Chem. Co. Ltd.] Laureth-4 (4.2 EO); CAS 5274-68-0; EINECS 226-097-1; nonionic; for emulsifying prods. requiring abundant liquidity; colorless liq.; HLB 11.5; 100% conc.

Nikkol BL-9EX. [Nikko Chem. Co. Ltd.] Laureth-9; CAS 3055-99-0; EINECS 221-284-4; nonionic; for emulsifying prods. requiring abundant liquidity; analgesic; antipruritic; colorless liq.; HLB 14.5; 100% conc.

Nikkol BL-21. [Nikko Chem. Co. Ltd.] Laureth-21; nonionic; for emulsifying prods. requiring abundant liquidity; solubilizer for cosmetics; wh. solid; HLB 19.0; 100% conc.

Nikkol BL-25. [Nikko Chem. Co. Ltd.] Laureth-25; CAS 9002-

92-0; nonionic; for emulsifying prods. requiring abundant liquidity; solubilizer for cosmetics; wh. solid; HLB 19.5; 100% conc.

Nikkol BM. [Nikko Chem. Co. Ltd.] Butyl myristate; CAS 110-36-1; EINECS 203-759-8; oily cosmetic ingred.; colorless liq.

Nikkol BO-2. [Nikko Chem. Co. Ltd.] Oleth-2; CAS 9004-98-2; nonionic; emulsifier for preparations requiring abundant liquidity; superfatting agent for hair care prods.; pale yel. liq.; HLB 7.5; 100% conc.

Nikkol BO-7. [Nikko Chem. Co. Ltd.] Oleth-7; CAS 9004-98-2; nonionic; emulsifier for preparations requiring abundant liquidity; superfatting agent for hair care prods.; pale yel. liq.; HLB 10.5; 100% conc.

Nikkol BO-10TX. [Nikko Chem. Co. Ltd.] Oleth-10; CAS 9004-98-2; nonionic; emulsifier for preparations requiring abundant liquidity; hydrophilic emulsifier, dispersant for cosmetics; pale yel. liq.; HLB 14.5; 100% conc.

Nikkol BO-15TX. [Nikko Chem. Co. Ltd.] Oleth-15; CAS 9004-98-2; nonionic; emulsifier for preparations requiring abundant liquidity; hydrophilic emulsifier, dispersant for cosmetics; pale yel. liq.; HLB 16.0; 100% conc.

Nikkol BO-20. [Nikko Chem. Co. Ltd.] Oleth-20; CAS 9004-98-2; solubilizer for cosmetics; pale yel. solid.

Nikkol BO-20TX. [Nikko Chem. Co. Ltd.] Oleth-20; CAS 9004-98-2; nonionic; emulsifier for preparations requiring abundant liquidity; solid; HLB 17.0; 100% conc.

Nikkol BO-50. [Nikko Chem. Co. Ltd.] Oleth-50; CAS 9004-98-2; nonionic; emulsifier for preparations requiring abundant liquidity; solubilizer for cosmetics; wh. flake; HLB 18.0; 100% conc.

Nikkol BPS-5. [Nikko Chem. Co. Ltd.] PEG-5 phytosterol; nonionic; emulsifier for o/w and w/o compds., solubilizer, dispersant, emollient, foam stabilizer, visc. modifier, conditioner used in cosmetics, pharmaceuticals; yel. paste; sol. in propylene glycol, ethanol; partly sol. in water; HLB 9.5; acid no. 0.25 max.; pH 4.8 (5%); 100% conc.

Nikkol BPS-10. [Nikko Chem. Co. Ltd.] PEG-10 phytosterol; nonionic; see Nikkol BPS-5; yel. paste or solid; sol. in water, propylene glycol, ethanol; HLB 12.5; acid no. 0.18 max.; pH 5.2 (5%); 100% conc.

Nikkol BPS-20. [Nikko Chem. Co. Ltd.] PEG-20 phytosterol; nonionic; see Nikkol BPS-5; pale yel. wax-like solid; sol. in water, propylene glycol, ethanol; HLB 15.5; acid no. 0.07 max.; pH 5.5 (5%); 100% conc.

Nikkol BPS-30. [Nikko Chem. Co. Ltd.] PEG-30 phytosterol; nonionic; see Nikkol BPS-5; pale yel. wax-like solid; sol. in water, propylene glycol, ethanol; HLB 18.0; acid no. 0.09 max.; pH 5.7 (5%); 100% conc.

Nikkol BPSH-25. [Nikko Chem. Co. Ltd.] PEG-25 phytosterol; emulsifier and dispersant for cosmetics; pale yel. solid.

Nikkol BS. [Nikko Chem. Co. Ltd.] Butyl stearate; CAS 123-95-5; EINECS 204-666-5; oily cosmetic ingred.; low visc.; permeates skin and spreads easily; colorless liq.

Nikkol BS-2. [Nikko Chem. Co. Ltd.] Steareth-2; CAS 9005-00-9; lipophilic emulsifier for cosmetics; wh. solid.

Nikkol BS-4. [Nikko Chem. Co. Ltd.] Steareth-4; CAS 9005-00-9; lipophilic emulsifier for cosmetics; wh. solid.

Nikkol BS-20. [Nikko Chem. Co. Ltd.] Steareth-20; CAS 9005-00-9; hydrophilic emulsifier and dispersant for cosmetics; wh. solid.

Nikkol BWA-5. [Nikko Chem. Co. Ltd.] PEG-5 lanolin alcohol; CAS 61791-20-6; nonionic; emulsifier, solubilizer, and softener for shampoos; provides hydrophilic props. to oil phase; ylsh. brn. paste; HLB 12.5; 100% conc.

Nikkol BWA-10. [Nikko Chem. Co. Ltd.] PEG-10 lanolin alcohol; CAS 61791-20-6; nonionic; emollient for cream, milk lotion; provides hydrophilic props. to oil phase; ylsh. brn. solid.

Nikkol BWA-20. [Nikko Chem. Co. Ltd.] PEG-20 lanolin alcohol; CAS 61791-20-6; nonionic; emulsifier, solubilizer, softener for lotions, creams, milk lotions, shampoos; ylsh. brn. solid; HLB 16.0; 100% conc.

Nikkol BWA-40. [Nikko Chem. Co. Ltd.] PEG-40 lanolin alcohol; CAS 61791-20-6; nonionic; emulsifier, solubilizer, softener for lotions, creams, shampoos; ylsh. brn. solid; HLB 17.0; 100% conc.

Nikkol CA-101. [Nikko Chem. Co. Ltd.] Benzalkonium chloride aq. sol'n.; antimicrobial, disinfectant for cosmetics; colorless liq.

Nikkol CA-1485. [Nikko Chem. Co. Ltd.] Stearalkonium chloride; CAS 122-19-0; EINECS 204-527-9; conditioner, softener for cosmetics; wh. flake.

Nikkol CA-2150. [Nikko Chem. Co. Ltd.] Cocotrimonium chloride; CAS 61789-18-2; EINECS 263-038-9; antimicrobial agent, disinfectant, softener for cosmetics; colorless liq.

Nikkol CA-2330. [Nikko Chem. Co. Ltd.] Cetrimonium chloride; CAS 112-02-7; EINECS 203-928-6; conditioner, antistat, and softener for cosmetics; pale yel. liq.

Nikkol CA-2350. [Nikko Chem. Co. Ltd.] Cetrimonium chloride; CAS 112-02-7; EINECS 203-928-6; conditioner, antistat, and softener for cosmetics; pale yel. liq.

Nikkol CA-2450. [Nikko Chem. Co. Ltd.] Steartrimonium chloride; CAS 112-03-8; EINECS 203-929-1; conditioner, antistat, and softener for cosmetics; pale yel. liq.

Nikkol CA-2450T. [Nikko Chem. Co. Ltd.] Tallowtrimonium chloride; CAS 8030-78-2; EINECS 232-447-4; conditioner, antistat, and softener for cosmetics; yel. liq.

Nikkol CA-2465. [Nikko Chem. Co. Ltd.] Steartrimonium chloride; CAS 112-03-8; EINECS 203-929-1; conditioner, antistat, and softener for cosmetics; wh. paste.

Nikkol CA-2580. [Nikko Chem. Co. Ltd.] Behentrimonium chloride; CAS 17301-53-0; EINECS 241-327-0; conditioner, antistat, and softener for cosmetics; pale yel. solid.

Nikkol CA-3080. [Nikko Chem. Co. Ltd.] Dioctyl trimonium chloride; antimicrobial, disinfectant for cosmetics; pale yel. liq.

Nikkol CA-3080M. [Nikko Chem. Co. Ltd.] Mixture; antimicrobial, disinfectant for cosmetics; pale yel. liq.

Nikkol CA-3475. [Nikko Chem. Co. Ltd.] Distearyldimonium chloride; CAS 107-64-2; EINECS 203-508-2; conditioner, softener for cosmetics; pale yel. paste.

Nikkol CCK-40. [Nikko Chem. Co. Ltd.] Potassium cocohydrolyzed animal protein; CAS 68920-65-0; anionic; foaming and cleansing agent used in shampoos, cleansing cream, kitchen cleaning agents; mild to hair and skin; yel. liq.; 30% conc.

Nikkol CCN-40. [Nikko Chem. Co. Ltd.] Sodium cocohydrolyzed animal protein aq. sol'n.; CAS 68188-38-5; anionic; foaming and cleansing agent for shampoos, cleansing creams, kitchen cleaning agents; mild to hair and skin; yel. liq.; 30% conc.

Nikkol CCP-40. [Nikko Chem. Co. Ltd.] Hydrolyzed animal protein; CAS 9015-54-7; cosmetic ingred. for skin and hair protection; yel. liq.

Nikkol CCP-100. [Nikko Chem. Co. Ltd.] Hydrolyzed collagen; CAS 9015-54-7; cosmetic ingred. for skin and hair protection; yel. liq.

Nikkol CCP-100P. [Nikko Chem. Co. Ltd.] Hydrolyzed animal protein; CAS 9015-54-7; cosmetic ingred. for skin and hair protection; pale yel. powd.

Nikkol CDIS-400. [Nikko Chem. Co. Ltd.] PEG diisostearate; emulsifier for cosmetics; pale yel. liq.

Nikkol CDO-600. [Nikko Chem. Co. Ltd.] PEG dioleate; emulsifier for cosmetics; pale yel. liq.

Nikkol CDS-400. [Nikko Chem. Co. Ltd.] PEG distearate; emulsifier for cosmetics; pale yel. solid.

Nikkol CDS-6000P. [Nikko Chem. Co. Ltd.] PEG distearate;

emulsifier and thickener for cosmetics; pale yel. flake.

Nikkol CIO, CIO-P. [Nikko Chem. Co. Ltd.] Cetyl octanoate; CAS 59130-69-7; EINECS 261-619-1; oily cosmetic ingred. with low f.p.; stable for hydrolysis and oxidation; colorless liq.

Nikkol CMT-30. [Nikko Chem. Co. Ltd.] Sodium methyl cocoyl taurate aq. sol'n.; anionic; shampoo base, foamer and detergent; colorless liq.; 30% conc.

Nikkol CO-3. [Nikko Chem. Co. Ltd.] PEG-3 castor oil; CAS 61791-12-6; nonionic; hydrotrope, w/o emulsifier used in cosmetic and pharmaceutical preparations; pale yel. liq.; HLB 3.0; 100% conc.

Nikkol CO-10. [Nikko Chem. Co. Ltd.] PEG-10 castor oil; CAS 61791-12-6; nonionic; emulsifier for cosmetics; pale yel. liq.; HLB 6.5; 100% conc.

Nikkol CO-20TX. [Nikko Chem. Co. Ltd.] PEG-20 castor oil; CAS 61791-12-6; nonionic; emulsifier for cosmetics; pale yel. liq.; HLB 10.5; 100% conc.

Nikkol CO-40TX. [Nikko Chem. Co. Ltd.] PEG-40 castor oil; CAS 61791-12-6; nonionic; solubilizer for cosmetics; pale yel. liq.; HLB 12.5; 100% conc.

Nikkol CO-50TX. [Nikko Chem. Co. Ltd.] PEG-50 castor oil; CAS 61791-12-6; nonionic; solubilizer for cosmetics; pale yel. liq.

Nikkol CO-60TX. [Nikko Chem. Co. Ltd.] PEG-60 castor oil; CAS 61791-12-6; nonionic; solubilizer for cosmetics; pale yel. liq.; HLB 14.0; 100% conc.

Nikkol CP. [Nikko Chem. Co. Ltd.] Ascorbyl dipalmitate; CAS 28474-90-0; oil-sol. vitamin C deriv.; whitening agent for skin lightening creams; promotes collagen synthesis; wh. cryst. powd.

Nikkol CS. [Nikko Chem. Co. Ltd.] Cholesteryl stearate; CAS 35602-69-8; EINECS 252-637-0; oily cosmetic ingred.; emollient; emulsion stabilizer; wh. cryst. powd.

Nikkol DCIS. [Nikko Chem. Co. Ltd.] Dihydrocholesteryl octyldecanoate.

Nikkol DDP-2. [Nikko Chem. Co. Ltd.] Di-PEG-2 alkyl ether phosphate; anionic; emulsifier, stabilizer, dispersant, anticorrosive agent and detergent used in cosmetics, drugs, agric. chemicals and general industrial use; yel. liq.; HLB 6.5; 100% conc.

Nikkol DDP-4. [Nikko Chem. Co. Ltd.] Di-PEG-4 alkyl ether phosphate; anionic; see Nikkol DDP-2; yel. liq.; HLB 9.0; 100% conc.

Nikkol DDP-6. [Nikko Chem. Co. Ltd.] Di-PEG-6 alkyl ether phosphate; anionic; see Nikkol DDP-2; yel. liq.; HLB 9.0; 100% conc.

Nikkol DDP-8. [Nikko Chem. Co. Ltd.] Di-PEG-8 alkyl ether phosphate; anionic; see Nikkol DDP-2; yel. liq.; HLB 11.5; 100% conc.

Nikkol DDP-10. [Nikko Chem. Co. Ltd.] Di-PEG-10 alkyl ether phosphate; anionic; see Nikkol DDP-2; yel. paste; HLB 13.5; 100% conc.

Nikkol DEGS. [Nikko Chem. Co. Ltd.] PEG-2 stearate; CAS 106-11-6; EINECS 203-363-5; emulsifier for cosmetics; pale yel. solid.

Nikkol DES-SP. [Nikko Chem. Co. Ltd.] Diethyl sebacate; CAS 110-40-7; EINECS 203-764-5; oily cosmetic ingred. which permeates the skin; colorless liq.

Nikkol DGDO. [Nikko Chem. Co. Ltd.] Polyglyceryl-2 dioleate; nonionic; w/o emulsifier for cosmetics and pharmaceuticals; yel. liq.; HLB 7.0; 100% conc.

Nikkol DGMIS. [Nikko Chem. Co. Ltd.] Polyglyceryl-2 isostearate; w/o emulsifier for cosmetics; pale yel. liq.

Nikkol DGMO-90. [Nikko Chem. Co. Ltd.] Polyglyceryl-2 oleate; CAS 9007-48-1; emulsifier for cosmetics; high monoester content (90%); pale yel. liq.

Nikkol DGMO-C. [Nikko Chem. Co. Ltd.] Polyglyceryl-2 oleate; CAS 9007-48-1; nonionic; w/o emulsifier for cosmetics and pharmaceuticals; yel. liq.; HLB 5.5; 100%

conc.

Nikkol DGMS. [Nikko Chem. Co. Ltd.] Polyglyceryl-2 stearate; CAS 12694-22-3; EINECS 235-777-7; nonionic; w/o emulsifier for cosmetics, pharmaceuticals, food applics.; pale yel. solid; HLB 5.0; 100% conc.

Nikkol DGO-80. [Nikko Chem. Co. Ltd.] Glyceryl dioleate; CAS 25637-84-7; EINECS 247-144-2; nonionic; emollient, emulsifier for cosmetics; yel. liq.; 100% conc.

Nikkol DGS-80. [Nikko Chem. Co. Ltd.] Glyceryl distearate; CAS 1323-83-7; EINECS 215-359-0; nonionic; emollient, emulsifier for cosmetics; wh. powd.; 100% conc.

Nikkol DHC-15. [Nikko Chem. Co. Ltd.] Dihydrocholeth-15.

Nikkol DHC-20. [Nikko Chem. Co. Ltd.] Dihydrocholeth-20.

Nikkol DHC-30. [Nikko Chem. Co. Ltd.] Dihydrocholeth-30.

Nikkol DID. [Nikko Chem. Co. Ltd.] Diisopropyl adipate; CAS 6938-94-9; EINECS 248-299-9; oily cosmetic ingred. which permeates the skin; colorless liq.

Nikkol DIS. [Nikko Chem. Co. Ltd.] Diisopropyl sebacate; CAS 7491-92-3; EINECS 231-306-4; oily cosmetic ingred. which permeates the skin; colorless liq.

Nikkol DK. [Nikko Chem. Co. Ltd.] Pyridoxine dicaprylate; CAS 106483-04-9; oil-sol. vitamin B_6 deriv.; effective for pimples, rough skin, dandruff, sunburn; wh. cryst. powd.

Nikkol DL. [Nikko Chem. Co. Ltd.] Pyridoxine dilaurate.

Nikkol DLP-10. [Nikko Chem. Co. Ltd.] Dilaureth-10 phosphate; anionic; emulsifier, dispersant, hydrotrope, surfactant, solubilizer for cosmetics; pale yel. paste; 100% conc.

Nikkol DMI. [Nikko Chem. Co. Ltd.] Dimethyl imidazolidinone; CAS 80-73-9; EINECS 201-304-8.

Nikkol DNPP-4. [Nikko Chem. Co. Ltd.] Dinoxynol-4 phosphate; cosmetics ingred.; yel. liq.

Nikkol DOP-8N. [Nikko Chem. Co. Ltd.] Sodium dioleth-8 phosphate; anionic; solubilizer for cosmetic and pharmaceutical applics.; pale yel. liq.; 100% conc.

Nikkol DP. [Nikko Chem. Co. Ltd.] Pyridoxine dipalmitate; CAS 635-38-1; oil-sol. vitamin B_6 deriv.; effective for pimples, rough skin, dandruff, sunburn; wh. cryst. powd.

Nikkol DPIS. [Nikko Chem. Co. Ltd.] Dihydrophytosteryl octyldecanoate.

Nikkol ECT-3. [Nikko Chem. Co. Ltd.] Trideceth-3 carboxylic acid; foaming and cleansing agent for cosmetics; pale yel. liq.

Nikkol ECT-3NEX, ECTD-3NEX. [Nikko Chem. Co. Ltd.] Sodium trideceth-3 carboxylate; anionic; shampoo base, foamer, detergent, and emulsifier; hard water tolerant; low skin irritation; pale yel. visc. liq.; 85% conc.

Nikkol ECT-7. [Nikko Chem. Co. Ltd.] Trideceth-7 carboxylic acid; foaming and cleansing agent for cosmetics; pale yel. liq.

Nikkol ECTD-6NEX. [Nikko Chem. Co. Ltd.] Sodium trideceth-6 carboxylate; anionic; shampoo base, foamer, detergent and emulsifier; hard water tolerant; low skin irritation; pale yel. visc. liq.; 85% conc.

Nikkol EGDS. [Nikko Chem. Co. Ltd.] Glycol distearate; CAS 627-83-8; EINECS 211-014-3; pearling agent for cosmetics; pale yel. solid.

Nikkol EGMS-70. [Nikko Chem. Co. Ltd.] Glycol stearate; CAS 111-60-4; EINECS 203-886-9; pearling agent for cosmetics, shampoos; pale yel. flake.

Nikkol EOO. [Nikko Chem. Co. Ltd.] Ethyl olive oleate; oily cosmetic ingred.; pale yel. liq.

Nikkol GBW-8. [Nikko Chem. Co. Ltd.] PEG-8 sorbitan beeswax; nonionic; emulsifier for cosmetics and pharmaceuticals.

Nikkol GBW-25. [Nikko Chem. Co. Ltd.] PEG-6 sorbitan beeswax; CAS 8051-15-8; nonionic; emulsifier and emulsion stabilizer for cosmetic and pharmaceutical; yel. solid; HLB 7.5; 100% conc.

Nikkol GBW-125. [Nikko Chem. Co. Ltd.] PEG-20 sorbitan beeswax; CAS 8051-73-8; nonionic; emulsifier and emul-

sion stabilizer for cosmetic and pharmaceuticals; yel. solid; HLB 9.5; 100% conc.

Nikkol GL-1. [Nikko Chem. Co. Ltd.] PEG-6 sorbitan laurate; emulsifier for oils in cosmetic field; colorless liq.

Nikkol GM-18IS. [Nikko Chem. Co. Ltd.] Batyl isostearate; nonionic; emollient, emulsion stabilizer used in cosmetics, medicated ointments; wh. paste; 100% conc.

Nikkol GM-18S. [Nikko Chem. Co. Ltd.] Batyl stearate; CAS 13232-26-3; nonionic; emollient, emulsion stabilizer used in cosmetics, medicated ointments; wh. solid; sol. in warm ethanol, castor oil, olive oil, oleyl alcohol; insol. in water; 100% conc.

Nikkol GO-4. [Nikko Chem. Co. Ltd.] PEG-6 sorbitan tetraoleate; emulsifier for oils in cosmetic field; pale yel. liq.

Nikkol GO-430. [Nikko Chem. Co. Ltd.] PEG-30 sorbitan tetraoleate; nonionic; emulsifier, solubilizer, superfatting agent used in drugs and cosmetics, for emulsion polymerization, agric. chemicals, printing inks; pale yel. liq.; sol. in ethanol, ethyl acetate, xylene; partly sol. in water; sp.gr. 1.048; HLB 11.5; ref. index 1.4727; 100% conc.

Nikkol GO-440. [Nikko Chem. Co. Ltd.] PEG-40 sorbitan tetraoleate; CAS 9003-11-6; nonionic; emulsifier, solubilizer, superfatting agent used in drugs and cosmetics, for emulsion polymerization, agric. chemicals, printing inks; pale yel. liq.; sol. in ethanol, ethyl acetate, xylene; partly sol. in water, propylene glycol; sp.gr. 1.054; HLB 12.5; 100% conc.

Nikkol GO-460. [Nikko Chem. Co. Ltd.] PEG-60 sorbitan tetraoleate; nonionic; emulsifier, solubilizer, superfatting agent used in drugs and cosmetics, for emulsion polymerization, agric. chemicals, printing inks; pale yel. liq.; sol. in water, ethanol, ethyl acetate, xylene; partly sol. in propylene glycol; sp.gr. 1.060; HLB 14.0; 100% conc.

Nikkol GS-6. [Nikko Chem. Co. Ltd.] Sorbeth-6 hexastearate; CAS 66828-20-4; cosmetics emulsifier; wh. waxy solid.

Nikkol GS-460. [Nikko Chem. Co. Ltd.] PEG-60 sorbitan tetrastearate; nonionic; emulsifier for cosmetic creams; pale yel. paste; HLB 13.0; 100% conc.

Nikkol HCO-5. [Nikko Chem. Co. Ltd.] PEG-5 hydrog. castor oil; CAS 61788-85-0; nonionic; hydrotrope, w/o emulsifier used in cosmetics and pharmaceuticals; pale yel. liq.; HLB 6.0; 100% conc.

Nikkol HCO-7.5. [Nikko Chem. Co. Ltd.] PEG-7.5 hydrog. castor oil; CAS 61788-85-0; nonionic; hydrotrope, emulsifier used in cosmetics and pharmaceuticals; liq.; HLB 6.0; 100% conc.

Nikkol HCO-10. [Nikko Chem. Co. Ltd.] PEG-10 hydrog. castor oil; CAS 61788-85-0; nonionic; hydrotrope, emulsifier used in cosmetics and pharmaceuticals; pale yel. liq.; HLB 6.5; 100% conc.

Nikkol HCO-20. [Nikko Chem. Co. Ltd.] PEG-20 hydrog. castor oil; CAS 61788-85-0; nonionic; hydrotrope, emulsifier used in cosmetics and pharmaceuticals; pale yel. liq.; HLB 10.5; 100% conc.

Nikkol HCO-30. [Nikko Chem. Co. Ltd.] PEG-30 hydrog. castor oil; CAS 61788-85-0; nonionic; hydrotrope, emulsifier used in cosmetics and pharmaceuticals; pale yel. liq.; HLB 11.0; 100% conc.

Nikkol HCO-40. [Nikko Chem. Co. Ltd.] PEG-40 hydrog. castor oil; CAS 61788-85-0; nonionic; hydrotrope, emulsifier used in cosmetics and pharmaceuticals; pale yel. liq.; HLB 12.5; 100% conc.

Nikkol HCO-40 Pharm. [Nikko Chem. Co. Ltd.] PEG-40 hydrog. castor oil; CAS 61788-85-0; nonionic; pharmaceutical grade emulsifier; pale yel. liq.; high water sol.

Nikkol HCO-50. [Nikko Chem. Co. Ltd.] PEG-50 hydrog. castor oil; CAS 61788-85-0; nonionic; hydrotrope, emulsifier used in cosmetics and pharmaceuticals; wh. paste; HLB 13.5; 100% conc.

Nikkol HCO-50 Pharm. [Nikko Chem. Co. Ltd.] PEG-50 hydrog. castor oil; CAS 61788-85-0; nonionic; pharmaceutical grade emulsifier; wh. paste; high water sol.

Nikkol HCO-60. [Nikko Chem. Co. Ltd.] PEG-60 hydrog. castor oil; CAS 61788-85-0; nonionic; hydrotrope, emulsifier used in cosmetics and pharmaceuticals; wh. paste; HLB 14.5; 100% conc.

Nikkol HCO-60 Pharm. [Nikko Chem. Co. Ltd.] PEG-60 hydrog. castor oil; CAS 61788-85-0; nonionic; pharmaceutical grade emulsifier; wh. paste; high water sol.

Nikkol HCO-80. [Nikko Chem. Co. Ltd.] PEG-80 hydrog. castor oil; CAS 61788-85-0; nonionic; hydrotrope, emulsifier used in cosmetics and pharmaceuticals; pale yel. liq.; HLB 15.0; 100% conc.

Nikkol HCO-100. [Nikko Chem. Co. Ltd.] PEG-100 hydrog. castor oil; CAS 61788-85-0; nonionic; hydrotrope, emulsifier used in cosmetics and pharmaceuticals; wh. solid; HLB 16.5; 100% conc.

Nikkol ICIS. [Nikko Chem. Co. Ltd.] Isocetyl isostearate; emollient used as oil phase component; low congealing pt.; stable to hydrolysis and oxidation; colorless liq.; 100% conc.

Nikkol ICM-R. [Nikko Chem. Co. Ltd.] Isocetyl myristate; CAS 83708-66-1; oily cosmetic ingred. with low f.p.; stable for hydrolysis and oxidation; colorless liq.

Nikkol ICS-R. [Nikko Chem. Co. Ltd.] Isocetyl stearate; CAS 25339-09-7; EINECS 246-868-6; emollient used as oil phase component; low congealing pt.; stable for hydrolysis and oxidation; colorless liq.; 100% conc.

Nikkol IPIS. [Nikko Chem. Co. Ltd.] Isopropyl isostearate; EINECS 250-651-1; oily cosmetic ingred.; low visc.; permeates skin and spreads easily; refreshing feel; pale yel. liq.

Nikkol IPM-100. [Nikko Chem. Co. Ltd.] Isopropyl myristate; CAS 110-27-0; EINECS 203-751-4; oily cosmetic ingred.; low visc.; permeates skin and spreads easily; refreshing feel; colorless liq.

Nikkol IPM-EX. [Nikko Chem. Co. Ltd.] Isopropyl myristate; CAS 110-27-0; EINECS 203-751-4; oily cosmetic ingred.; low visc.; permeates skin and spreads easily; refreshing feel; colorless liq.

Nikkol IPP. [Nikko Chem. Co. Ltd.] Isopropyl palmitate; CAS 142-91-6; EINECS 205-571-1; oily cosmetic ingred.; low visc.; permeates skin and spreads easily; refreshing feel; colorless liq.

Nikkol IPP-EX. [Nikko Chem. Co. Ltd.] Isopropyl palmitate; CAS 142-91-6; EINECS 205-571-1; oily cosmetic ingred.; low visc.; permeates skin and spreads easily; refreshing feel; colorless liq.

Nikkol ISP. [Nikko Chem. Co. Ltd.] Isostearyl palmitate; CAS 72576-80-8; EINECS 276-719-0; oily cosmetic ingred. with low f.p.; stable for hydrolysis and oxidation; colorless liq.

Nikkol KLS. [Nikko Chem. Co. Ltd.] Potassium lauryl sulfate; CAS 4706-78-9; EINECS 225-190-4; foaming and cleansing agent for cosmetics; wh. cryst. powd.

Nikkol LMT. [Nikko Chem. Co. Ltd.] Sodium N-lauroyl methyl taurate; CAS 4337-75-1; EINECS 224-388-8; anionic; shampoo base, foamer and detergent; wh. cryst. solid; 92% conc.

Nikkol LSA. [Nikko Chem. Co. Ltd.] Sodium lauryl sulfoacetate; CAS 1847-58-1; EINECS 217-431-7; anionic; acid-stable foaming and cleansing agent for cosmetics; wh. cryst. solid; 92.5% conc.

Nikkol MGIS. [Nikko Chem. Co. Ltd.] Glyceryl monoisostearate; emulsifier for cosmetics; pale yel. liq.

Nikkol MGM. [Nikko Chem. Co. Ltd.] Glyceryl myristate; CAS 589-68-4; lipophilic emulsifier for cosmetics; wh. flake.

Nikkol MGO. [Nikko Chem. Co. Ltd.] Glyceryl oleate; nonionic; emulsifier for foods and cosmetics; pale yel. paste;

HLB 3.0; 100% conc.

Nikkol MGS-150. [Nikko Chem. Co. Ltd.] Glyceryl stearate SE; emulsifier for foods and cosmetics; wh. solid.

Nikkol MGS-A. [Nikko Chem. Co. Ltd.] Glyceryl stearate; nonionic; emulsifier, stabilizer for foods and cosmetics; wh. flake; HLB 4.5; 100% conc.

Nikkol MGS-ASE. [Nikko Chem. Co. Ltd.] Glyceryl stearate SE; nonionic; emulsifier, stabilizer for foods and cosmetics; wh. flake; HLB 6.5; 100% conc.

Nikkol MGS-B. [Nikko Chem. Co. Ltd.] Glyceryl stearate; nonionic; lipophilic emulsifier, stabilizer for foods and cosmetics; wh. flake; HLB 5.0; 100% conc.

Nikkol MGS-BSE-C. [Nikko Chem. Co. Ltd.] Glyceryl stearate SE; lipophilic emulsifier for cosmetics; wh. flake.

Nikkol MGS-C. [Nikko Chem. Co. Ltd.] Glyceryl stearate; lipophilic emulsifier for cosmetics; wh. flake.

Nikkol MGS-DEX. [Nikko Chem. Co. Ltd.] Glyceryl stearate SE; nonionic; lipophilic emulsifier, stabilizer used in foods and cosmetics; wh. flake; HLB 6.5; 100% conc.

Nikkol MGS-F20. [Nikko Chem. Co. Ltd.] Glyceryl stearate; nonionic; emulsifier, stabilizer for foods and cosmetics; wh. flake; HLB 7.5; 100% conc.

Nikkol MGS-F40. [Nikko Chem. Co. Ltd.] Glyceryl stearate; nonionic; emulsifier, stabilizer for foods and cosmetics; wh. flake; HLB 4.0; 100% conc.

Nikkol MGS-F50. [Nikko Chem. Co. Ltd.] Glyceryl stearate; nonionic; emulsifier, stabilizer for foods and cosmetics; wh. flake; HLB 3.5; 100% conc.

Nikkol MGS-F50SE. [Nikko Chem. Co. Ltd.] Glyceryl stearate SE; emulsifier for foods and cosmetics; wh. flake.

Nikkol MGS-F75. [Nikko Chem. Co. Ltd.] Glyceryl stearate; nonionic; emulsifier, stabilizer for food and cosmetics; wh. flake; HLB 0.5; 100% conc.

Nikkol MGS-TG. [Nikko Chem. Co. Ltd.] Glyceryl stearate; acid-stable emulsifier for foods and cosmetics; wh. flake.

Nikkol MGS-TGL. [Nikko Chem. Co. Ltd.] Glyceryl stearate; acid-stable emulsifier for foods and cosmetics; wh. flake.

Nikkol MM. [Nikko Chem. Co. Ltd.] Myristyl myristate; CAS 3234-85-3; EINECS 221-787-9; oily cosmetic wax with low m.p.; wh. cryst. solid.

Nikkol MMT. [Nikko Chem. Co. Ltd.] Sodium N-myristoyl methyl taurate; CAS 18469-44-8; EINECS 242-349-3; anionic; shampoo base, foaming agent and detergent; wh. cryst. solid; 92% conc.

Nikkol MYL-10. [Nikko Chem. Co. Ltd.] PEG-10 laurate; CAS 9004-81-3; emulsifier for cosmetics; pale yel. liq.

Nikkol MYO-2. [Nikko Chem. Co. Ltd.] Diethylene glycol oleate; CAS 106-12-7; EINECS 203-364-0; nonionic; w/o or o/w emulsifier for creams, lotions and ointments; pale yel. liq.; HLB 4.5; 100% conc.

Nikkol MYO-6. [Nikko Chem. Co. Ltd.] PEG-6 oleate; CAS 9004-96-0; nonionic; w/o or o/w emulsifier for creams, lotions, ointments; pale yel. liq.; HLB 8.5; 100% conc.

Nikkol MYO-10. [Nikko Chem. Co. Ltd.] PEG-10 oleate; CAS 9004-96-0; solubilizer for lotions, toiletries; pale yel. liq.

Nikkol MYS-1EX. [Nikko Chem. Co. Ltd.] PEG-1 stearate; nonionic; pearling agent, emulsifier, or solubilizer for cosmetics and pharmaceuticals; pale yel. solid; HLB 2.0; 100% conc.

Nikkol MYS-2. [Nikko Chem. Co. Ltd.] PEG-2 stearate; CAS 106-11-6; EINECS 203-363-5; nonionic; emulsifier or solubilizer for cosmetics and pharmaceuticals; pale yel. flake; HLB 4.0; 100% conc.

Nikkol MYS-4. [Nikko Chem. Co. Ltd.] PEG-4 stearate; CAS 9004-99-3; EINECS 203-358-8; nonionic; emulsifier or solubilizer for cosmetics and pharmaceuticals; pale yel. solid; HLB 6.5; 100% conc.

Nikkol MYS-10. [Nikko Chem. Co. Ltd.] PEG-10 stearate; CAS 9004-99-3; nonionic; emulsifier or solubilizer for cosmetics and pharmaceuticals; pale yel. solid; HLB 11.0;

100% conc.

Nikkol MYS-25. [Nikko Chem. Co. Ltd.] PEG-25 stearate; CAS 9004-99-3; nonionic; emulsifier or solubilizer for cosmetics and pharmaceuticals; pale yel. solid; HLB 15.0; 100% conc.

Nikkol MYS-40. [Nikko Chem. Co. Ltd.] PEG-40 stearate; CAS 9004-99-3; nonionic; emulsifier or solubilizer for cosmetics and pharmaceuticals; pale yel. solid; HLB 17.5; 100% conc.

Nikkol MYS-45. [Nikko Chem. Co. Ltd.] PEG-45 stearate; CAS 9004-99-3; nonionic; emulsifier or solubilizer for cosmetics and pharmaceuticals; pale yel. flake; HLB 18.0; 100% conc.

Nikkol MYS-55. [Nikko Chem. Co. Ltd.] PEG-55 stearate; CAS 9004-99-3; nonionic; emulsifier or solubilizer for cosmetics and pharmaceuticals; pale yel. flake; HLB 18.0; 100% conc.

Nikkol N-20. [Nikko Chem. Co. Ltd.] Octyldodecyl neodecanoate; cosmetic ingred.

Nikkol NES-203. [Nikko Chem. Co. Ltd.] POE alkyl ether sulfate, sodium salt; anionic; shampoo base, foamer, emulsifier and detergent; liq.; 20% conc.

Nikkol NES-203-27. [Nikko Chem. Co. Ltd.] Sodium PEG-3 alkyl ether sulfate aq. sol'n.; foaming and cleansing agent for cosmetics; hard water tolerant; sol. at low temp.; colorless liq.

Nikkol NES-303. [Nikko Chem. Co. Ltd.] POE alkyl ether sulfate, TEA salt; anionic; shampoo base, foamer, detergent, emulsifier; liq.; 30% conc.

Nikkol NES-303-36. [Nikko Chem. Co. Ltd.] TEA PEG-3 alkyl ether sulfate aq. sol'n.; foaming and cleansing agent for cosmetics; hard water tolerant; sol. at low temp.; colorless liq.

Nikkol NET-FS. [Nikko Chem. Co. Ltd.] Silicone and oil emulsion blend; conc. emulsion for skin care prods.; wh. visc. liq.

Nikkol NET-HO. [Nikko Chem. Co. Ltd.] Silicone emulsion; conc. emulsion for hair care prods.; wh. visc. liq.

Nikkol NET SG-60A. [Nikko Chem. Co. Ltd.] Silicone emulsion; protective film coating for split ends; colorless visc. liq.

Nikkol NP-2. [Nikko Chem. Co. Ltd.] Nonoxynol-2; EINECS 248-291-5; nonionic; emulsifier for cosmetics; colorless liq.

Nikkol NP-5. [Nikko Chem. Co. Ltd.] Nonoxynol-5; CAS 9016-45-9; nonionic; emulsifier, detergent, solubilizer, and wetting agent used in cosmetics, insecticide, and other industrial applics.; colorless liq.

Nikkol NP-7.5. [Nikko Chem. Co. Ltd.] Nonoxynol-8 (7.5 EO); CAS 9016-45-9; nonionic; emulsifier, detergent, solubilizer, and wetting agent used in cosmetics, insecticide, and other industrial applics.; colorless liq.; HLB 14.0; 100% conc.

Nikkol NP-10. [Nikko Chem. Co. Ltd.] Nonoxynol-10; CAS 9016-45-9; EINECS 248-294-1; nonionic; emulsifier, detergent, solubilizer, and wetting agent used in cosmetics, insecticide, and other industrial applics.; colorless liq.; HLB 16.5; 100% conc.

Nikkol NP-15. [Nikko Chem. Co. Ltd.] Nonoxynol-15; CAS 9016-45-9; nonionic; emulsifier, detergent, solubilizer, and wetting agent used in cosmetics, insecticide, and other industrial applics.; colorless liq.; HLB 18.0; 100% conc.

Nikkol NP-18TX. [Nikko Chem. Co. Ltd.] Nonoxynol-18; CAS 9016-45-9; nonionic; emulsifier, detergent, solubilizer, and wetting agent used in cosmetics, insecticide, and other industrial applics.; colorless liq.; HLB 19.0; 100% conc.

Nikkol NP-20. [Nikko Chem. Co. Ltd.] Nonoxynol-20; CAS 9016-45-9; nonionic; solubilizer for cosmetics; wh. paste.

Nikkol N-SP. [Nikko Chem. Co. Ltd.] Cetyl palmitate; CAS 540-10-3; EINECS 208-736-6; syn. spermaceti; emollient for cosmetics; wh. flake; sol. in warm oils; 100% conc.

Nikkol ODM-100. [Nikko Chem. Co. Ltd.] Octyldodecyl myristate; oily cosmetic ingred. with low f.p.; stable to hydrolysis and oxidation; colorless liq.

Nikkol OP-3. [Nikko Chem. Co. Ltd.] Octoxynol-3; CAS 9002-93-1; nonionic; emulsifier, penetrant, detergent, solubilizer, and wetting agent used in cosmetics, insecticide and other industrial applics.; colorless liq.; HLB 6.0; 100% conc.

Nikkol OP-10. [Nikko Chem. Co. Ltd.] Octoxynol-10; CAS 9002-93-1; nonionic; emulsifier, penetrant, detergent, solubilizer, and wetting agent used in cosmetics, insecticide and other industrial applics.; colorless liq.; HLB 11.5; 100% conc.

Nikkol OP-30. [Nikko Chem. Co. Ltd.] Octoxynol-30; CAS 9002-93-1; nonionic; emulsifier, detergent, solubilizer, and wetting agent used in cosmetics, insecticide and other industrial applics.; wh. solid; HLB 17.0; 100% conc.

Nikkol OR Wax. [Nikko Chem. Co. Ltd.] Hydrog. orange roughy oil.

Nikkol OS-14. [Nikko Chem. Co. Ltd.] Sodium alpha-olefin sulfonate; foaming and cleansing agent for cosmetics; wh. powd.

Nikkol OTP-75. [Nikko Chem. Co. Ltd.] Sodium dioctyl sulfosuccinate; CAS 577-11-7; EINECS 209-406-4; wetting and penetrating agent, dispersant for cosmetics; colorless liq.

Nikkol OTP-100. [Nikko Chem. Co. Ltd.] Sodium dioctyl sulfosuccinate; CAS 577-11-7; EINECS 209-406-4; wetting and penetrating agent, dispersant for cosmetics; wh. sponge.

Nikkol OTP-100S. [Nikko Chem. Co. Ltd.] Sodium dioctyl sulfosuccinate USP; CAS 577-11-7; EINECS 209-406-4; anionic; dispersant, wetting agent; sponge-like solid; 98% conc.

Nikkol PBC-31. [Nikko Chem. Co. Ltd.] PPG-4-ceteth-1; nonionic; emulsifier, solubilizer, dispersant used in cosmetic, pharmaceuticals and other industrial applics.; colorless liq.; HLB 9.4; 100% conc.

Nikkol PBC-33. [Nikko Chem. Co. Ltd.] PPG-4-ceteth-10; nonionic; see Nikkol PBC-31; pale yel. paste; HLB 10.5; 100% conc.

Nikkol PBC-34. [Nikko Chem. Co. Ltd.] PPG-4-ceteth-20; nonionic; see Nikkol PBC-31; wh. solid; HLB 16.5; 100% conc.

Nikkol PBC-41. [Nikko Chem. Co. Ltd.] PPG-8-ceteth-1; nonionic; see Nikkol PBC-31; colorless liq.; HLB 9.5; 100% conc.

Nikkol PBC-44. [Nikko Chem. Co. Ltd.] PPG-8-ceteth-20; nonionic; see Nikkol PBC-31; pale yel. solid; HLB 12.5; 100% conc.

Nikkol PDD. [Nikko Chem. Co. Ltd.] Propylene glycol didecanoate; cosmetic ingred. imparting light feel; low visc.; colorless liq.

Nikkol PEN-4612. [Nikko Chem. Co. Ltd.] PPG-6-decyltetradeceth-12; nonionic; low foaming solubilizer for cosmetic lotions and toiletry prods.; pale yel. solid; HLB 8.5; 100% conc.

Nikkol PEN-4620. [Nikko Chem. Co. Ltd.] PPG-6-decyltetradeceth-20; nonionic; see Nikkol PEN-4612; pale yel. solid; HLB 11.0; 100% conc.

Nikkol PEN-4630. [Nikko Chem. Co. Ltd.] PPG-6 decyltetradeceth-30; nonionic; see Nikkol PEN-4612; pale yel. solid; HLB 12.0; 100% conc.

Nikkol PMEA. [Nikko Chem. Co. Ltd.] Palmitamide MEA; CAS 544-31-0; EINECS 208-867-9; pearling agent for hair rinses; pale yel. powd.

Nikkol PMS-1C. [Nikko Chem. Co. Ltd.] Propylene glycol

stearate; CAS 1323-39-3; EINECS 215-354-3; nonionic; emulsifier, emulsion stabilizer, and dispersant for cosmetics and pharmaceuticals; wh. solid; HLB 3.5; 100% conc.

Nikkol PMS-1CSE. [Nikko Chem. Co. Ltd.] Propylene glycol stearate SE; nonionic; emulsifier, emulsion stabilizer, and dispersant for cosmetics and pharmaceuticals; wh. solid; HLB 4.0; 100% conc.

Nikkol PMS-FR. [Nikko Chem. Co. Ltd.] Propylene glycol stearate; CAS 1323-39-3; EINECS 215-354-3; emulsifier and emulsion stabilizer for cosmetics; wh. solid.

Nikkol PMT. [Nikko Chem. Co. Ltd.] Sodium N-palmitoyl methyl taurate; CAS 3737-55-1; EINECS 223-114-4; anionic; shampoo and cleansing cream base, foamer, detergent, thickener; wh. cryst. solid; 92% conc.

Nikkol SBL-2A-27. [Nikko Chem. Co. Ltd.] Ammonium laureth-2 sulfate aq. sol'n.; CAS 32612-48-9; foaming and cleansing agent for cosmetics; hard water tolerant; sol. at low temp.; pale yel. visc. liq.

Nikkol SBL-2N-27. [Nikko Chem. Co. Ltd.] Sodium laureth-2 sulfate aq. sol'n.; foaming and cleansing agent for cosmetics; hard water tolerant; sol. at low temp.; pale yel. liq.

Nikkol SBL-2T-36. [Nikko Chem. Co. Ltd.] TEA laureth-2 sulfate aq. sol'n.; CAS 27028-82-6; foaming and cleansing agent for cosmetics; hard water tolerant; sol. at low temp.; pale yel. liq.

Nikkol SBL-3N-27. [Nikko Chem. Co. Ltd.] Sodium laureth-3 sulfate aq. sol'n.; foaming and cleansing agent for cosmetics; hard water tolerant; sol. at low temp.; pale yel. liq.

Nikkol SBL-4N. [Nikko Chem. Co. Ltd.] Sodium laureth-4 sulfate aq. sol'n.; foaming and cleansing agent for cosmetics; sol. at low temps.; hard water tolerant; pale yel. liq.

Nikkol SBL-4T. [Nikko Chem. Co. Ltd.] TEA laureth-4 sulfate aq. sol'n.; CAS 27028-82-6; foaming and cleansing agent for cosmetics; hard water tolerant; sol. at low temp.; pale yel. liq.

Nikkol SCS. [Nikko Chem. Co. Ltd.] Sodium cetyl sulfate; CAS 1120-01-0; EINECS 214-292-4; anionic; emulsifier, detergent for cosmetics; sodium chloride-free; wh. powd.; 100% conc.

Nikkol SGC-80N. [Nikko Chem. Co. Ltd.] Sodium hydrog. cocomonoglyceride sulfate; CAS 61789-04-6; EINECS 263-026-3; anionic; foamer and detergent for shampoos, facial cleansers, soap; nonirritating to skin; wh. powd.; 70% conc.

Nikkol SI-10R. [Nikko Chem. Co. Ltd.] Sorbitan isostearate; CAS 54392-26-6; nonionic; w/o emulsifier for cosmetics and pharmaceuticals; refined grade (low color/odor); yel. liq.; HLB 5.0; 100% conc.

Nikkol SI-10T. [Nikko Chem. Co. Ltd.] Sorbitan isostearate; CAS 54392-26-6; nonionic; w/o emulsifier for cosmetics and pharmaceuticals; liq.; HLB 5.0; 100% conc.

Nikkol SI-15R. [Nikko Chem. Co. Ltd.] Sorbitan sesquiisostearate; nonionic; w/o emulsifier for cosmetics and pharmaceuticals; refined grade (low color/odor); pale yel. visc. liq.; HLB 4.5; 100% conc.

Nikkol SI-15T. [Nikko Chem. Co. Ltd.] Sorbitan isostearate; CAS 54392-26-6; nonionic; w/o emulsifier for cosmetics and pharmaceuticals; liq.; HLB 4.5; 100% conc.

Nikkol SL-10. [Nikko Chem. Co. Ltd.] Sorbitan laurate; nonionic; emulsifier for foods and cosmetics; pale yel. liq.; HLB 8.6; 100% conc.

Nikkol SLP-N. [Nikko Chem. Co. Ltd.] Sodium lauryl phosphate; foaming and cleansing agent for cosmetics; wh. cryst. powd.

Nikkol SLS. [Nikko Chem. Co. Ltd.] Sodium lauryl sulfate; CAS 151-21-3; EINECS 205-788-1; anionic; foaming and cleansing agent for cosmetics; sodium chloride-free; wh. cryst. powd.; 97% conc.

Nikkol SLS-30. [Nikko Chem. Co. Ltd.] Sodium lauryl sulfate aq. sol'n.; CAS 151-21-3; EINECS 205-788-1; foaming and cleansing agent for cosmetics; yel. liq.

Nikkol SMS. [Nikko Chem. Co. Ltd.] Sodium myristyl sulfate; CAS 1191-50-0; EINECS 214-737-2; foaming and cleansing agent for cosmetics; effective at high temps.; wh. cryst. powd.

Nikkol SMT. [Nikko Chem. Co. Ltd.] Sodium N-stearoyl methyl taurate; CAS 149-39-3; anionic; shampoo and cleansing cream base, foamer, detergent, thickener; wh. cryst. solid; 92% conc.

Nikkol SNP-4N. [Nikko Chem. Co. Ltd.] Sodium nonoxynol-4 sulfate; CAS 9014-90-8; foaming and cleansing agent for cosmetics; hard water tolerant; sol. at low temp.; pale yel. liq.

Nikkol SNP-4T. [Nikko Chem. Co. Ltd.] TEA nonoxynol-4 sulfate aq. sol'n.; foaming and cleansing agent for cosmetics; hard water tolerant; sol. at low temp.; pale yel. liq.

Nikkol SO-10. [Nikko Chem. Co. Ltd.] Sorbitan oleate; CAS 1338-43-8; EINECS 215-665-4; nonionic; w/o emulsifier for cosmetics; food emulsifier; yel. liq.; HLB 5.0; 100% conc.

Nikkol SO-10R. [Nikko Chem. Co. Ltd.] Sorbitan oleate; CAS 1338-43-8; EINECS 215-665-4; cosmetics emulsifier; refined grade (low color/odor); pale yel. liq.

Nikkol SO-15. [Nikko Chem. Co. Ltd.] Sorbitan sesquioleate; CAS 8007-43-0; EINECS 232-360-1; nonionic; w/o emulsifier for cosmetics, foods; yel. liq.; HLB 4.5; 100% conc.

Nikkol SO-15EX. [Nikko Chem. Co. Ltd.] Sorbitan sesquioleate; CAS 8007-43-0; EINECS 232-360-1; cosmetics emulsifier; refined grade; pale yel. liq.; sol. in polar oils.

Nikkol SO-15R. [Nikko Chem. Co. Ltd.] Sorbitan sesquioleate; CAS 8007-43-0; EINECS 232-360-1; cosmetics emulsifier; refined grade (low color/odor); pale yel. liq.

Nikkol SO-30. [Nikko Chem. Co. Ltd.] Sorbitan trioleate; CAS 26266-58-0; EINECS 247-569-3; nonionic; w/o emulsifier for cosmetics; yel. liq.; HLB 4.0; 100% conc.

Nikkol SO-30R. [Nikko Chem. Co. Ltd.] Sorbitan trioleate; CAS 26266-58-0; EINECS 247-569-3; cosmetics emulsifier; refined grade (low color/odor); pale yel. liq.

Nikkol SP-10. [Nikko Chem. Co. Ltd.] Sorbitan palmitate; CAS 26266-57-9; EINECS 247-568-8; nonionic; emulsifier for foods and cosmetics; pale yel. flake; HLB 6.7; 100% conc.

Nikkol SS-10. [Nikko Chem. Co. Ltd.] Sorbitan stearate; CAS 1338-41-6; EINECS 215-664-9; nonionic; lipophilic emulsifier for cosmetics; wh. to pale yel. flake; HLB 4.7; 100% conc.

Nikkol SS-15. [Nikko Chem. Co. Ltd.] Sorbitan sesquistearate; nonionic; lipophilic emulsifier for foods and cosmetics; wh. to pale yel. flake; HLB 4.2; 100% conc.

Nikkol SS-30. [Nikko Chem. Co. Ltd.] Sorbitan tristearate; CAS 26658-19-5; EINECS 247-891-4; nonionic; lipophilic emulsifier for cosmetics; wh. to pale yel. flake; HLB 2.1; 100% conc.

Nikkol SSS. [Nikko Chem. Co. Ltd.] Sodium stearyl sulfate; CAS 1120-04-3; EINECS 214-295-0; emulsifier for cosmetics; wh. powd.

Nikkol TAMDS-4. [Nikko Chem. Co. Ltd.] PEG-4 stearamide.

Nikkol TCP-5. [Nikko Chem. Co. Ltd.] Triceteth-5 phosphate; emulsifier and dispersant for cosmetics; wh. paste.

Nikkol TDP-2. [Nikko Chem. Co. Ltd.] C12-15 pareth-2 phosphate; anionic; emulsifier and solubilizer for cosmetics, drugs, agric. chemicals, dispersant, anticorrosive agent and detergent for general industrial use; yel. liq.; HLB 7.0; 100% conc.

Nikkol TDP-4. [Nikko Chem. Co. Ltd.] Tri-PEG-4 alkyl ether phosphate; anionic; see Nikkol TDP-2; liq.; HLB 7.0; 100% conc.

Nikkol TDP-6. [Nikko Chem. Co. Ltd.] Tri-PEG-6 alkyl ether phosphate; anionic; see Nikkol TDP-2; yel. liq.; HLB 8.0; 100% conc.

Nikkol TDP-8. [Nikko Chem. Co. Ltd.] Tri-PEG-8 alkyl ether phosphate; anionic; see Nikkol TDP-2; yel. liq.; HLB 11.5; 100% conc.

Nikkol TDP-10. [Nikko Chem. Co. Ltd.] Tri-PEG-10 alkyl ether phosphate; anionic; see Nikkol TDP-2; pale yel. paste; HLB 14.0; 100% conc.

Nikkol TEALS. [Nikko Chem. Co. Ltd.] TEA-lauryl sulfate aq. sol'n.; CAS 139-96-8; EINECS 205-388-7; foaming and cleansing agent for cosmetics; pale yel. liq.

Nikkol TEALS-42. [Nikko Chem. Co. Ltd.] TEA-lauryl sulfate aq. sol'n.; CAS 139-96-8; EINECS 205-388-7; foaming and cleansing agent for cosmetics; yel. liq.

Nikkol TI-10. [Nikko Chem. Co. Ltd.] PEG-20 sorbitan isostearate; CAS 66794-58-9; nonionic; emulsifier, solubilizer, and dispersant for cosmetics; pale yel. liq.; HLB 15.0; 100% conc.

Nikkol TL-10, TL-10EX. [Nikko Chem. Co. Ltd.] Polysorbate 20; CAS 9005-64-5; nonionic; hydrophilic emulsifier, solubilizer, dispersant; used in cosmetics and pharmaceuticals; pale yel. liq.; HLB 16.9; 100% conc.

Nikkol TLP-4. [Nikko Chem. Co. Ltd.] Trilaureth-4 phosphate; emulsifier and dispersant for cosmetics; pale yel. liq.

Nikkol TMGO-5. [Nikko Chem. Co. Ltd.] PEG-5 glyceryl oleate; emulsifier and dispersant for cosmetics; yel. liq.

Nikkol TMGO-10. [Nikko Chem. Co. Ltd.] PEG-10 glyceryl oleate; CAS 68889-49-6; emulsifier.

Nikkol TMGO-15. [Nikko Chem. Co. Ltd.] PEG-15 glyceryl oleate; CAS 68889-49-6; emulsifier and dispersant for cosmetics; yel. liq.

Nikkol TMGS-5. [Nikko Chem. Co. Ltd.] PEG-5 glyceryl stearate; emulsifier and dispersant for cosmetics; pale yel. semisolid.

Nikkol TMGS-15. [Nikko Chem. Co. Ltd.] PEG-15 glyceryl stearate; emulsifier and dispersant for cosmetics; wh. solid.

Nikkol TO-10. [Nikko Chem. Co. Ltd.] Polysorbate 80; CAS 9005-65-6; nonionic; hydrophilic emulsifier, solubilizer, and dispersant; for cosmetics, pharmaceuticals, food; yel. liq.; HLB 15.0; 100% conc.

Nikkol TO-10M. [Nikko Chem. Co. Ltd.] Polysorbate 80; CAS 9005-65-6; emulsifier, solubilizer, and dispersant for cosmetics; yel. liq.

Nikkol TO-30. [Nikko Chem. Co. Ltd.] Polysorbate 85; CAS 9005-70-3; nonionic; hydrophilic emulsifier; for cosmetics, pharmaceuticals; yel. liq.; HLB 11.0; 100% conc.

Nikkol TO-106. [Nikko Chem. Co. Ltd.] PEG-6 sorbitan oleate; nonionic; hydrophilic emulsifier; for cosmetics, pharmaceuticals; yel. liq.; HLB 10.0; 100% conc.

Nikkol TOP-O. [Nikko Chem. Co. Ltd.] Sodium oleyl phosphate; CAS 1847-55-8; EINECS 217-430-1; cosmetic ingred.; pale yel. liq.

Nikkol TP-10. [Nikko Chem. Co. Ltd.] Polysorbate 40; CAS 9005-66-7; emulsifier, solubilizer, and dispersant for cosmetics; yel. liq.

Nikkol TS-10. [Nikko Chem. Co. Ltd.] Polysorbate 60; CAS 9005-67-8; nonionic; emulsifier, solubilizer, and dispersant for o/w prods., cosmetics, pharmaceuticals, foods; yel. visc. liq.; sol. in water, ethanol, ethyl acetate, toluene; HLB 14.9; sapon. no. 43–49; pH 5.7–7.7 (5%); 100% conc.

Nikkol TS-30. [Nikko Chem. Co. Ltd.] Polysorbate 65; CAS 9005-71-4; nonionic; emulsifier, solubilizer for o/w prods., cosmetics, pharmaceuticals; yel. semisolid; HLB 11.0; 100% conc.

Nikkol TS-106. [Nikko Chem. Co. Ltd.] PEG-6 sorbitan stearate; CAS 9005-67-8; nonionic; emulsifier, solubilizer for o/w prods., cosmetics, pharmaceuticals; yel. paste.

Nikkol TW-10. [Nikko Chem. Co. Ltd.] PEG-10 lanolin; CAS 61790-81-6; nonionic; emulsifier, superfatting agent, solubilizer, or bodying agent for soap, cleanser, shampoos, and hair rinses; ylsh. brn. paste; HLB 12.0; 100% conc.

Nikkol TW-20. [Nikko Chem. Co. Ltd.] PEG-20 lanolin; CAS 61790-81-6; nonionic; emulsifier, superfatting agent, solubilizer, or bodying agent for soap, cleanser, shampoos, and hair rinses; ylsh. brn. paste; HLB 13.0; 100% conc.

Nikkol TW-30. [Nikko Chem. Co. Ltd.] PEG-30 lanolin; CAS 61790-81-6; nonionic; emulsifier, superfatting agent, solubilizer, or bodying agent for soap, cleanser, shampoos, and hair rinses; ylsh. brn. paste; HLB 15.0; 100% conc.

Nikkol VC-PMG. [Nikko Chem. Co. Ltd.] Magnesium ascorbyl phosphate; CAS 114040-31-2; water-sol. vitamin C deriv.; whitening agent for skin lightening creams; promotes collagen synthesis; for cosmetics use; wh. cryst. powd.

Nikkol VC-SS. [Nikko Chem. Co. Ltd.] Disodium ascorbate sulfate; water-sol. vitamin C deriv.; whitening agent; promotes collagen synthesis; for cosmetics use; wh. cryst. powd.

Nikkol VF-E. [Nikko Chem. Co. Ltd.] Ethyl linoleate; CAS 544-35-4; EINECS 208-868-4; oily cosmetic ingred. providing stability, absorption, smooth applic. of linoleic acid; pale yel. liq.

Nikkol VF-IP. [Nikko Chem. Co. Ltd.] Isopropyl linoleate; CAS 22882-95-7; EINECS 245-289-6; oily cosmetic ingred. providing stability, absorption, smooth applic. of linoleic acid; colorless liq.

Nikkol Akypo RLM 45 NV. [Nikko Chem. Co. Ltd.] Sodium PEG-4.5 lauryl ether carboxylate aq. sol'n.; CAS 33939-64-9; foaming and cleansing agent for cosmetics; hard water tolerant; low skin irritation; pale yel. liq.

Nikkol Alaninate LN-30. [Nikko Chem. Co. Ltd.] Sodium lauroyl methylamino propionate; anionic; shampoo and facial cleanser base, foaming agent, detergent; colorless liq.; 30% conc.

Nikkol Amidoamine S. [Nikko Chem. Co. Ltd.] Stearamidoethyl diethylamine; CAS 16889-14-8; EINECS 240-924-3; cationic; low irritant cosmetic ingred.; pale yel. powd.

Nikkol Apricot Kernel Oil. [Nikko Chem. Co. Ltd.] Apricot kernel oil; CAS 72869-69-3; oily cosmetic ingred. with oleic acid as main component; pale yel. liq.

Nikkol Aquasome AE. [Nikko Chem. Co. Ltd.] Liposome containing vitamin A, E; cosmetic ingred. stimulating metabolism; slows aging of skin; pale yel. turbid liq.

Nikkol Aquasome BH. [Nikko Chem. Co. Ltd.] Liposome containing polyol; moisturizer for cosmetics; pale yel. translucent liq.

Nikkol Aquasome EC-5. [Nikko Chem. Co. Ltd.] Butylene glycol, hydrog. lecithin, choleth-20 trioctanoin, tocopheryl acetate, PEG-100 hydrog. castor. oil.

Nikkol Aquasome EC-30. [Nikko Chem. Co. Ltd.] Liposome containing vitamin E, C; cosmetic ingred. which restrains lipid peroxide; slows aging of skin; pale yel. turbid liq.

Nikkol Aquasome LA. [Nikko Chem. Co. Ltd.] Water, hydrog. lecithin, maltitol, alanine, sorbitol, dipropylene glycol, glycerin, cholesterol; moisturizer for cosmetics; pale yel. turbid liq.

Nikkol Aquasome VA. [Nikko Chem. Co. Ltd.] Liposome containing vitamin A; cosmetic ingred. stimulating metabolism; slows aging of skin; pale yel. turbid liq.

Nikkol Aquasome VE. [Nikko Chem. Co. Ltd.] Hydrog. lecithin, butylene glycol, tocopheryl acetate, PEG-60 hydrog. castor oil; cosmetic ingred. containing vitamin E; restrains lipid peroxide; slows aging of skin.

Nikkol Avocado Oil. [Nikko Chem. Co. Ltd.] Avocado oil;

CAS 8024-32-6; EINECS 232-428-0; oily cosmetic ingred. with oleic acid as main component; pale yel. liq.

Nikkol Batyl Alcohol 100, EX. [Nikko Chem. Co. Ltd.] Batyl alcohol; CAS 544-62-7; EINECS 208-874-7; nonionic; emollient, emulsifier, hydrotrope, emulsion thickener; cosmetic and pharmaceutical preparations; wh. powd.; 100% conc.

Nikkol Behenyl Alcohol 65, 80. [Nikko Chem. Co. Ltd.] Behenyl alcohol; CAS 661-19-8; EINECS 211-546-6; emollient, emulsion stabilizer for cosmetics and pharmaceuticals; wh. flake; sol. in warm ethanol, min. oil, 2-hexyldecanol, IPM; insol. in water.

Nikkol Bio-Sodium Hyaluronate Powd. and 1% Sol'n. [Nikko Chem. Co. Ltd.] Sodium hyaluronate; CAS 9067-32-7; humectant for cosmetics use.

Nikkol Cetanol 50, 70. [Nikko Chem. Co. Ltd.] Cetanol; fragrance-free fatty alcohol cosmetic base; wh. cryst. solid.

Nikkol Cetyl Lactate. [Nikko Chem. Co. Ltd.] Cetyl lactate.; CAS 35274-05-6; EINECS 252-478-7; emollient.

Nikkol Chimyl Alcohol 100. [Nikko Chem. Co. Ltd.] Cetyl glyceryl ether; nonionic; oily cosmetic ingred.; emulsifier, hydrotrope, emollient, emulsion thickener used for cosmetic and pharmaceutical prods.; wh. powd.; 100% conc.

Nikkol Corn Germ Oil. [Nikko Chem. Co. Ltd.] Corn oil; CAS 8001-30-7; EINECS 232-281-2; oily cosmetic ingred. with oleic and linoleic acids as main components; yel. liq.

Nikkol Decaglyn 1-IS. [Nikko Chem. Co. Ltd.] Polyglyceryl-10 isostearate; CAS 133738-23-5; nonionic; emulsifier, solubilizer, dispersant for cosmetics, pharmaceuticals and foods; pale yel. visc. liq.; HLB 12.5; 100% conc.

Nikkol Decaglyn 1-L. [Nikko Chem. Co. Ltd.] Polyglyceryl-10 laurate; CAS 34406-66-1; nonionic; emulsifier, solubilizer, dispersant for cosmetics, pharmaceuticals and foods; pale yel. visc. liq.; HLB 17.0; 100% conc.

Nikkol Decaglyn 1-LN. [Nikko Chem. Co. Ltd.] Polyglyceryl-10 linoleate; nonionic; emulsifier, solubilizer, dispersant for cosmetics, pharmaceuticals and foods; pale yel. visc. liq.; HLB 12.0; 100% conc.

Nikkol Decaglyn 1-M. [Nikko Chem. Co. Ltd.] Polyglyceryl-10 myristate; nonionic; emulsifier, solubilizer, dispersant for cosmetics, pharmaceuticals and foods; pale yel. visc. liq.; HLB 14.5; 100% conc.

Nikkol Decaglyn 1-O. [Nikko Chem. Co. Ltd.] Polyglyceryl-10 oleate; CAS 9007-48-1; nonionic; emulsifier, solubilizer, dispersant for cosmetics, pharmaceuticals and foods; pale yel. visc. liq.; HLB 13.5; 100% conc.

Nikkol Decaglyn 1-S. [Nikko Chem. Co. Ltd.] Polyglyceryl-10 stearate; CAS 79777-30-3; nonionic; emulsifier, solubilizer, dispersant for cosmetics, pharmaceuticals and foods; pale yel. plate; HLB 12.5; 100% conc.

Nikkol Decaglyn 2-IS. [Nikko Chem. Co. Ltd.] Polyglyceryl-10 diisostearate; CAS 102033-55-6; nonionic; hydrophilic emulsifier and dispersant for cosmetics; lubricant, coating agent and anticrystallization agent; pale yel. visc. liq.

Nikkol Decaglyn 2-O. [Nikko Chem. Co. Ltd.] Polyglyceryl-10 dioleate; CAS 33940-99-7; nonionic; o/w emulsifier for cosmetics, pharmaceuticals and foods; pale yel. visc. liq.; HLB 10.0; 100% conc.

Nikkol Decaglyn 2-S. [Nikko Chem. Co. Ltd.] Polyglyceryl-10 distearate; CAS 12764-60-2; nonionic; o/w emulsifier for cosmetics, pharmaceuticals and foods; pale yel. plate; HLB 12.0; 100% conc.

Nikkol Decaglyn 3-IS. [Nikko Chem. Co. Ltd.] Polyglyceryl-10 triisostearate; lipophilic emulsifier for cosmetics; pale yel. visc. liq.

Nikkol Decaglyn 3-O. [Nikko Chem. Co. Ltd.] Polyglyceryl-10 trioleate; CAS 102051-00-3; nonionic; lipophilic emulsifier for cosmetics; gelling agent for hydrocarbon; pale yel. visc. liq.; HLB 6.5; 100% conc.

Nikkol Decaglyn 3-S. [Nikko Chem. Co. Ltd.] Polyglyceryl-10 tristearate; CAS 12709-64-7; nonionic; lipophilic emulsifier for cosmetics; gelling agent for hydrocarbons; wh. plate; HLB 6.5; 100% conc.

Nikkol Decaglyn 5-IS. [Nikko Chem. Co. Ltd.] Polyglyceryl-10 pentaisostearate; nonionic; w/o emulsifier for cosmetics, lubricant, coating agent and anticrystallization agent; pale yel. visc. liq.; HLB 3.5; 100% conc.

Nikkol Decaglyn 5-O. [Nikko Chem. Co. Ltd.] Polyglyceryl-10 pentaoleate; CAS 86637-84-5; nonionic; w/o emulsifier for cosmetics, lubricant, coating agent and anticrystallization agent; pale yel. visc. liq.; HLB 4.0; 100% conc.

Nikkol Decaglyn 5-S. [Nikko Chem. Co. Ltd.] Polyglyceryl-10 pentastearate; nonionic; w/o emulsifier for cosmetics, lubricant, coating agent and anticrystallization agent; wh. flake; HLB 3.5; 100% conc.

Nikkol Decaglyn 7-IS. [Nikko Chem. Co. Ltd.] Polyglyceryl-10 heptaisostearate; nonionic; w/o emulsifier for cosmetics, lubricant, coating agent and anticrystallization agent; pale yel. visc. liq.; 100% conc.

Nikkol Decaglyn 7-O. [Nikko Chem. Co. Ltd.] Polyglyceryl-10 heptaoleate; CAS 103175-09-3; nonionic; w/o emulsifier for cosmetics, lubricant, coating agent and anticrystallization agent; pale yel. visc. liq.; 100% conc.

Nikkol Decaglyn 7-S. [Nikko Chem. Co. Ltd.] Polyglyceryl-10 heptastearate; CAS 99126-54-2; nonionic; emulsifier for cosmetics, lubricant, coating agent, anticrystallization agent for fats; wh. flake; 100% conc.

Nikkol Decaglyn 10-IS. [Nikko Chem. Co. Ltd.] Polyglyceryl-10 decaisostearate; nonionic; cosmetics emulsifier, superfatting agent, lubricant, coating agent, and anticrystallization agent; pale yel. visc. liq.; 100% conc.

Nikkol Decaglyn 10-O. [Nikko Chem. Co. Ltd.] Polyglyceryl-10 decaoleate; CAS 11094-60-3; EINECS 234-316-7; nonionic; cosmetics emulsifier, superfatting agent, lubricant, coating agent, and anticrystallization agent; pale yel. visc. liq.; 100% conc.

Nikkol Decaglyn 10-S. [Nikko Chem. Co. Ltd.] Polyglyceryl-10 decastearate; CAS 39529-26-5; EINECS 254-495-5; nonionic; cosmetics emulsifier, lubricant, coating agent, anticrystallization agent for fats; wh. flake; 100% conc.

Nikkol Dipotassium Glycyrrhizinate. [Nikko Chem. Co. Ltd.] Dipotassium glycyrrhizinate; CAS 68797-35-3; EINECS 272-296-1; anti-inflammatory, anti-allergenic surfactant for cosmetics and pharmaceuticals; pale yel. cryst. powd.; water-sol.

Nikkol Estepearl 10, 15. [Nikko Chem. Co. Ltd.] Glycol distearate; CAS 627-83-8; EINECS 211-014-3; pearlescent for shampoos, rinse and hair conditioners; heat resist.; wh. flake; large crystals; 100% conc.

Nikkol Estepearl 30. [Nikko Chem. Co. Ltd.] PEG-3 distearate; CAS 9005-08-7; pearlescent for shampoos, rinse and hair conditioners; wh. flake; 100% conc.

Nikkol Glycyrrhetinic Acid. [Nikko Chem. Co. Ltd.] Glycyrrhetinic acid; CAS 471-53-4; EINECS 207-444-6; anti-inflammatory, anti-allergenic for cosmetics and pharmaceuticals; wh. cryst. powd.

Nikkol Glycyrrhizic Acid. [Nikko Chem. Co. Ltd.] Glycyrrhizic acid; CAS 1405-86-3; EINECS 215-785-7; anti-inflammatory, anti-allergenic surfactant for cosmetics and pharmaceuticals; wh. powd.; water-sol.

Nikkol Grapeseed Oil. [Nikko Chem. Co. Ltd.] Grape seed oil; CAS 8024-22-4; oily cosmetic ingred. with linoleic acid as main component; yel. liq.

Nikkol Hazel Nut Oil. [Nikko Chem. Co. Ltd.] Hazel nut oil; oily cosmetic ingred. with high palmitoleic acid content; pale yel. liq.

Nikkol Hexaglyn 1-L. [Nikko Chem. Co. Ltd.] Polyglyceryl-6 laurate; CAS 51033-38-6; nonionic; o/w emulsifier for cosmetics, anticrystallizing agent; pale yel. visc. liq; HLB 13.0; 100% conc.

Nikkol Hexaglyn 1-M. [Nikko Chem. Co. Ltd.] Polyglyceryl-6 myristate; hydrophilic emulsifier for cosmetics; pale yel. visc. liq.

Nikkol Hexaglyn 1-O. [Nikko Chem. Co. Ltd.] Polyglyceryl-6 oleate; CAS 9007-48-1; nonionic; o/w emulsifier for cosmetics, anticrystallizing agent; pale yel. visc. liq.; HLB 9.5; 100% conc.

Nikkol Hexaglyn 1-S. [Nikko Chem. Co. Ltd.] Polyglyceryl-6 stearate; nonionic; hydrophilic emulsifier, dispersant, lubricant for cosmetics; wh. plate; HLB 9.5; 100% conc.

Nikkol Hexaglyn 3-S. [Nikko Chem. Co. Ltd.] Polyglyceryl-6 tristearate; CAS 71185-87-0; nonionic; o/w emulsifier for cosmetics, anticrystallizing agent; wh. flake; HLB 2.5; 100% conc.

Nikkol Hexaglyn 5-O. [Nikko Chem. Co. Ltd.] Polyglyceryl-6 pentaoleate; CAS 104934-17-0; nonionic; w/o emulsifier for cosmetics, anticrystallizing agent; pale yel. liq.; HLB 6.0; 100% conc.

Nikkol Hexaglyn 5-S. [Nikko Chem. Co. Ltd.] Polyglyceryl-6 pentastearate; CAS 99734-30-2; nonionic; o/w emulsifier for cosmetics, anticrystallizing agent for fats; wh. flake; 100% conc.

Nikkol Hexaglyn PR-15. [Nikko Chem. Co. Ltd.] Polyglyceryl-6 polyricinoleate; nonionic; w/o emulsifier for cosmetics, anticrystallizing agent; yel. visc. liq.; 100% conc.

Nikkol Jojoba Oil S. [Nikko Chem. Co. Ltd.] Jojoba oil; CAS 61789-91-1; refined grade; decolored and deodorized emollient; pale yel. liq.; sol. in min. and veg. oils.

Nikkol Jojoba Wax. [Nikko Chem. Co. Ltd.] Jojoba wax; CAS 66625-78-3; oily cosmetic ingred. with high m.p.; wh. solid.

Nikkol Kukui Nut Oil. [Nikko Chem. Co. Ltd.] Kukui nut oil; oily cosmetic ingred. with high linoleic and linolenic acids content; pale yel. liq.

Nikkol Lanoquat DES-50. [Nikko Chem. Co. Ltd.] Lanolin quat. ammonium salt; cationic; cosmetic ingred.; brn. visc. liq.

Nikkol Lecinol LL-20. [Nikko Chem. Co. Ltd.] Hydrog. lysolecithin; emulsifier, emulsion stabilizer for cosmetics; pale yel. powd.

Nikkol Lecinol S-10. [Nikko Chem. Co. Ltd.] Hydrog. soya lecithin; CAS 92128-87-5; EINECS 295-786-7; amphoteric; moisturizer, solubilizer, liposoming agent used in skin and hair care prods.; raises absorption, lessens irritant props.; stable; pale yel. powd.; 100% conc.

Nikkol Lecinol S-10E. [Nikko Chem. Co. Ltd.] Hydrog. lecithin; CAS 92128-87-5; EINECS 295-786-7; moisturizer, solubilizer, liposoming agent for cosmetics; raises absorption, lessens irritant props.; stable; pale yel. powd.

Nikkol Lecinol S-10EX. [Nikko Chem. Co. Ltd.] Hydrog. lecithin; CAS 92128-87-5; EINECS 295-786-7; moisturizer, solubilizer, liposoming agent for cosmetics; raises absorption, lessens irritant props.; stable; pale yel. powd.

Nikkol Lecinol S-10M. [Nikko Chem. Co. Ltd.] Hydrog. lecithin; CAS 92128-87-5; EINECS 295-786-7; moisturizer, solubilizer, liposoming agent for cosmetics; raises absorption, lessens irritant props.; stable; pale yel. powd.

Nikkol Lecinol S-30. [Nikko Chem. Co. Ltd.] Hydrog. lecithin; CAS 92128-87-5; EINECS 295-786-7; moisturizer, solubilizer, liposoming agent for cosmetics; raises absorption, lessens irritant props.; stable; pale yel. powd.

Nikkol Lecinol SH. [Nikko Chem. Co. Ltd.] Hydroxylated lecithin; CAS 8029-76-3; EINECS 232-440-6; emulsifier, moisturizer, and emulsion stabilizer for cosmetics; pale yel. powd.

Nikkol Macadamia Nut Oil. [Nikko Chem. Co. Ltd.] Macadamia nut oil; oily cosmetic ingred. with high palmitoleic acid content; pale yel. liq.

Nikkol Meadowfoam Oil. [Nikko Chem. Co. Ltd.] Meadowfoam seed oil; oily cosmetic ingred. containing > 95% unsat. fatty acids (> C_{20}); pale yel. liq.

Nikkol Myristyl Lactate. [Nikko Chem. Co. Ltd.] Myristyl lactate; CAS 1323-03-1; EINECS 215-350-1; emollient.

Nikkol Naphthenic Acid. [Nikko Chem. Co. Ltd.] Cyclopentane carboxylic acid; CAS 3400-45-1; EINECS 222-269-5.

Nikkol Neodecanoate-20. [Nikko Chem. Co. Ltd.] Octyldodecyl neodecanoate; oily cosmetic ingred. with low f.p.; stable to hydrolysis and oxidation; colorless liq.

Nikkol Olive Oil. [Nikko Chem. Co. Ltd.] Olive oil; CAS 8001-25-0; EINECS 232-277-0; oily cosmetic ingred. with oleic acid as main component; pale yel. liq.

Nikkol Pearl 1218. [Nikko Chem. Co. Ltd.] Glycol stearate; CAS 111-60-4; EINECS 203-886-9; pearling agent for shampoo; wh. flake, fine crystals.

Nikkol Pearl 1222. [Nikko Chem. Co. Ltd.] Glycol distearate; CAS 627-83-8; EINECS 211-014-3; pearling agent for cleansing cream; wh. flake.

Nikkol Pentarate 408. [Nikko Chem. Co. Ltd.] Pentaerythrityl tetraoctanoate; CAS 7299-99-2; EINECS 230-743-8; oily cosmetic ingred. imparting light feel; chemically stable; colorless liq.

Nikkol Phosten HLP. [Nikko Chem. Co. Ltd.] Lauryl phosphate; CAS 12751-23-4; EINECS 235-798-1; foaming and cleansing agent for cosmetics; wh. solid.

Nikkol Phosten HLP-1. [Nikko Chem. Co. Ltd.] Laureth-1 phosphate; anionic; cleansing agent base for facial and body cleansers, shampoos; pale yel. paste; 100% conc.

Nikkol Phosten HLP-N. [Nikko Chem. Co. Ltd.] Sodium lauryl phosphate; cleansing agent base for powd. and paste cosmetic prods.; wh. powd.

Nikkol Plastic Powder FP-SQ. [Nikko Chem. Co. Ltd.] Styrene/DVB copolymer.

Nikkol Pulvsome VE. [Nikko Chem. Co. Ltd.] Liposome containing vitamin E; cosmetic ingred. which restrains lipid peroxide; slows aging of skin; pale yel. powd.

Nikkol Rose Hip Oil. [Nikko Chem. Co. Ltd.] Rose hip oil; oily cosmetic ingred. with high linoleic and linolenic acids content; pale yel. liq.

Nikkol Safflower Oil. [Nikko Chem. Co. Ltd.] Safflower oil; CAS 8001-23-8; EINECS 232-276-5; oily cosmetic ingred. with linoleic acid as main component; pale yel. liq.

Nikkol Sarcosinate CN-30. [Nikko Chem. Co. Ltd.] Sodium cocoyl sarcosinate; CAS 61791-59-1; EINECS 263-193-2; foaming and cleansing agent for shampoo; pale yel. liq.

Nikkol Sarcosinate LH. [Nikko Chem. Co. Ltd.] Lauroyl sarcosine; CAS 97-78-9; EINECS 202-608-3; foaming and cleansing agent for cosmetics; pale yel. cryst. solid.

Nikkol Sarcosinate LK-30. [Nikko Chem. Co. Ltd.] Potassium lauroyl sarcosinate aq. sol'n.; cleansing cream base; raw material for bar soap; pale yel. liq.

Nikkol Sarcosinate LN. [Nikko Chem. Co. Ltd.] Sodium lauroyl sarcosinate; CAS 137-16-6; EINECS 205-281-5; anionic; detergent, cleansing and foaming agent for shampoo and dentifrice; wh. cryst. powd.; 100% conc.

Nikkol Sarcosinate LN-30. [Nikko Chem. Co. Ltd.] Sodium lauroyl sarcosinate aq. sol'n.; CAS 137-16-6; EINECS 205-281-5; foaming and cleansing agent for shampoos; pale yel. liq.

Nikkol Sarcosinate MN. [Nikko Chem. Co. Ltd.] Sodium myristoyl sarcosinate; CAS 30364-51-3; EINECS 250-151-3; anionic; detergent for shampoos, dentifrices; cleansing cream base; raw material for bar soap; wh. cryst. powd.; 100% conc.

Nikkol Sarcosinate OH. [Nikko Chem. Co. Ltd.] Oleoyl sarcosine; CAS 110-25-8; EINECS 203-749-3; foaming and cleansing agent for cosmetics; corrosion inhibitor; yel. liq.

Nikkol Sarcosinate PN. [Nikko Chem. Co. Ltd.] Sodium palmitoyl sarcosinate; cleansing cream base; raw material for bar soap; wh. cryst. powd.

Nikkol Sasanqua Oil. [Nikko Chem. Co. Ltd.] Sasanqua oil; cosmetic ingred. with oleic acid as main component; pale yel. liq.

Nikkol Sefsol 218. [Nikko Chem. Co. Ltd.] Propylene glycol monocaprylate; CAS 31565-12-5; cosmetic solubilizer of sl. sol. ingreds.; colorless liq.

Nikkol Sefsol 228. [Nikko Chem. Co. Ltd.] Propylene glycol dicaprylate; CAS 7384-98-7; EINECS 230-962-9; cosmetic solubilizer of sl. sol. ingreds.; colorless liq.

Nikkol Selachyl Alcohol. [Nikko Chem. Co. Ltd.] Selachyl alcohol; an ether-type lipid which maintains membrane structure of cells and gives exc. emolliency to skin.

Nikkol Sericite. [Nikko Chem. Co. Ltd.] Liposome-treated sericite containing either Nikkol VC-PMG or natural moisturizing factors.; cosmetic ingred.

Nikkol Shiso Extract NA. [Nikko Chem. Co. Ltd.] A glucoside extract with anti-allergenic props. for cosmetic use.

Nikkol Sodium Hyaluronate. [Nikko Chem. Co. Ltd.] Sodium hyaluronate; CAS 9067-32-7; humectant for cosmetics; wh. powd.; m.w. 800,000-1,600,000; also avail. as 1% aq. sol.

Nikkol Sodium Naphthenate. [Nikko Chem. Co. Ltd.] Sodium cyclopentane carboxylate.

Nikkol Squalane. [Nikko Chem. Co. Ltd.] Squalane; CAS 111-01-3; EINECS 203-825-6; oily cosmetic ingred. derived from animals; good skin lubricant; extremely fluid; colorless liq.

Nikkol Squalene EX. [Nikko Chem. Co. Ltd.] Squalene; CAS 111-02-4; EINECS 203-826-1; oily cosmetic ingred. derived from animals; skin lubricant; colorless liq.

Nikkol Stearyl Alcohol. [Nikko Chem. Co. Ltd.] Stearyl alcohol; CAS 112-92-5; EINECS 204-017-6; fragrance-free fatty alcohol cosmetic base; wh. cryst. solid.

Nikkol Stearyl Glycyrrhetinate. [Nikko Chem. Co. Ltd.] Stearyl glycyrrhetinate; CAS 13832-70-7; anti-inflammatory, anti-allergenic for cosmetics and pharmaceuticals; wh. to pale yel. cryst. powd.; oil-sol.

Nikkol Sunflower Oil. [Nikko Chem. Co. Ltd.] Sunflower oil; CAS 8001-21-6; EINECS 232-273-9; oily cosmetic ingred. with linoleic acid as main component; pale yel. liq.

Nikkol Super Mica D. [Nikko Chem. Co. Ltd.] Mica coated with titanium dioxide; cosmetic ingred. giving softer glow to makeup.

Nikkol Sweet Almond Oil. [Nikko Chem. Co. Ltd.] Sweet almond oil; oily cosmetic ingred. with oleic acid as main component; pale yel. liq.

Nikkol Syncelane 30. [Nikko Chem. Co. Ltd.] C6-14 polyolefins; oily cosmetic ingred. with similar feel to squalane; colorless liq.; sol. in olive oil, min. oil, ester, 2-octyl dodecanol.

Nikkol Tetraglyn 1-O. [Nikko Chem. Co. Ltd.] Polyglyceryl-4 oleate; CAS 9007-48-1; nonionic; o/w emulsifier, anticrystallizing agent; food emulsifier; pale yel. visc. liq.; HLB 6.0; 100% conc.

Nikkol Tetraglyn 1-S. [Nikko Chem. Co. Ltd.] Polyglyceryl-4 stearate; nonionic; hydrophilic emulsifier for cosmetics; food emulsifier; wh. flake; HLB 6.0; 100% conc.

Nikkol Tetraglyn 3-S. [Nikko Chem. Co. Ltd.] Polyglyceryl-4 tristearate; nonionic; o/w emulsifier for cosmetics, anticrystallizing agent; food emulsifier; wh. flake; 100% conc.

Nikkol Tetraglyn 5-O. [Nikko Chem. Co. Ltd.] Polyglyceryl-4 pentaoleate; nonionic; o/w emulsifier for cosmetics; anticrystallizing agent; food emulsifier; pale yel. liq.; 100% conc.

Nikkol Tetraglyn 5-S. [Nikko Chem. Co. Ltd.] Polyglyceryl-4 pentastearate; nonionic; o/w emulsifier for cosmetics;

anticrystallizing agent for fats; food emulsifier; wh. flake; 100% conc.

Nikkol Trialan 308. [Nikko Chem. Co. Ltd.] Trimethylolpropane trioctanoate; CAS 4826-87-3; EINECS 225-404-6; oily cosmetic ingred. imparting light feel; chemically stable; colorless liq.

Nikkol Trialan 318. [Nikko Chem. Co. Ltd.] Trimethylolpropane triisostearate; CAS 68541-50-4; EINECS 271-347-5; oily cosmetic ingred. imparting light feel; chemically stable; pale yel. liq.

Nikkol Trifat C-24. [Nikko Chem. Co. Ltd.] Coco fatty acid triglyceride; oily cosmetic ingred. with lauric acid as main component; pale yel. liq.

Nikkol Trifat P-52. [Nikko Chem. Co. Ltd.] Hydrog. palm fatty acid triglyceride; oily cosmetic ingred.; natural wax with low m.p.; pale yel. solid.

Nikkol Trifat S-308. [Nikko Chem. Co. Ltd.] Glyceryl trioctanoate; CAS 538-23-8; EINECS 208-686-5; emollient for creams, lotions, makeups, hair preps.; pale yel. liq.; sol. in ethanol, olive oil, min. oil.

Nikkol Trifat T-42. [Nikko Chem. Co. Ltd.] Tallow fatty acid triglyceride; oily cosmetic ingred. derived from animals; natural wax with low m.p.; wh. soft solid.

Nikkol Trifat T-52. [Nikko Chem. Co. Ltd.] Hydrog. tallow fatty acid triglyceride; oily cosmetic ingred. derived from animals; natural wax with low m.p.; wh. solid.

Nikkol Wax-100. [Nikko Chem. Co. Ltd.] Self-emulsifying wax; anionic; cosmetic ingred.; wh. solid.

Nikkol Wax-110. [Nikko Chem. Co. Ltd.] Self-emulsifying wax; anionic; cosmetic ingred.; wh. solid.

Nikkol Wax-220. [Nikko Chem. Co. Ltd.] Self-emulsifying wax; nonionic; cosmetic ingred.; wh. solid.

Nikkol Wax-230. [Nikko Chem. Co. Ltd.] Self-emulsifying wax; nonionic; cosmetic ingred.; wh. flake.

Nikkol Wax-500. [Nikko Chem. Co. Ltd.] Hydrog. lanolin; CAS 8031-44-5; EINECS 232-452-1; cosmetic ingred.; good water retainer; wh. paste.

Nikkol Wax-600. [Nikko Chem. Co. Ltd.] Tricetyl phosphate; wax with high affinity to the skin; wh. solid.

Nikkol Wheat Peptide 5000. [Nikko Chem. Co. Ltd.] A glucoside extract with anti-allergenic props. for cosmetic use.

Nimcolan® 1740. [Henkel/Emery] Absorp. base of lanolin esters, alcohols, and sterols; nonionic; emollient, w/o emulsifier, aux. o/w emulsifier; soft solid; 100% act.

Nimlesterol® 1732. [Henkel/Organic Prods.] Min. oil, lanolin alcohol; nonionic; hypoallergenic w/o emulsifier, emollient, aux. o/w emulsifier for skin care prods.; base; liq.; 100% act.

Ninol® 30-LL. [Stepan; Stepan Canada] Lauramide DEA; CAS 120-40-1; EINECS 204-393-1; nonionic; foam booster/stabilizer, visc. builder/modifier for liq. detergents, shampoos, hand soaps, bath prods.; amber clear liq.; 100% act.

Ninol® 40-CO. [Stepan; Stepan Canada] Cocamide DEA; CAS 61791-31-9; EINECS 263-163-9; nonionic; foam booster/stabilizer, visc. booster, and conditioner for liq. detergents, textile applics., personal care prods. (shampoos, hand soaps, bath prods.); lt. color liq.; 100% act.

Ninol® 49-CE. [Stepan; Stepan Canada] Cocamide DEA; CAS 61791-31-9; EINECS 263-163-9; nonionic; detergent, foam booster and stabilizer, thickener in detergent formulations, personal care prods.; lt. color liq.; 100% act.; formerly Onyxol SD.

Ninol® 55-LL. [Stepan; Stepan Canada] Lauramide DEA (1:1); CAS 120-40-1; EINECS 204-393-1; surfactant for improved visc. in AOS systems; foam booster/stabilizer for shampoos, hand soaps, bath prods.; Gardner 3 liq.; 100% act.

Ninol® 70-SL. [Stepan; Stepan Canada] Lauramide DEA;

Ninol® 96-SL

CAS 120-40-1; EINECS 204-393-1; nonionic; foam booster/stabilizer, thickener for shampoos, hand soaps, bath prods.; gel; 100% act.

Ninol® 96-SL. [Stepan; Stepan Canada] Lauramide DEA; CAS 120-40-1; EINECS 204-393-1; nonionic; thickener, foam booster/stabilizer for liq. detergents, shampoos, hand soaps, and bath prods.; lt. color wax; 100% act.

Ninol® 201. [Stepan; Stepan Canada] Oleamide DEA; CAS 93-83-4; EINECS 202-281-7; nonionic; emulsifier, corrosion inhibitor in industrial lubricant systems, cutting fluids, drawing compds., metal cleaners; thickener for personal care and liq. detergent prods.; emulsifier, lubricant, antistat for textiles; amber liq.; sol. in oils, disp. in water; dens. 8.23 lb/gal; pH 9.5-10.5; 100% act.

Ninol® CNR. [Stepan Europe] Cocamide MEA; CAS 68140-00-1; EINECS 268-770-2; nonionic; emollient, thickener, foam booster/stabilizer for shampoos, bubble baths, liq. soaps, shower gels, toilet soaps; yel. to ivory colored wax; 98% act.

Ninol® GR. [Stepan; Stepan Canada] Cocamide DEA; CAS 61791-31-9; EINECS 263-163-9; nonionic; foam booster/stabilizer, emulsifier, thickener for general cosmetic use, shampoos, bubble baths; liq.; 100% act.

Ninol® L-9. [Stepan; Stepan Canada] Lauramide DEA; CAS 120-40-1; EINECS 204-393-1; nonionic; foam booster/stabilizer, emulsifier, thickener for general cosmetic use, shampoos, bubble baths; paste; 100% act.

Ninol® LMP. [Stepan; Stepan Canada; Stepan Europe] Lauramide MEA; CAS 142-78-9; EINECS 205-560-1; nonionic; foam booster/stabilizer, thickener, emollient, detergent for dishwash, liq. detergents, detergent blocks or bars, shampoos, hand soaps, bath prods.; wh. beads; 100% act.

Ninol® M10. [Stepan Europe] Monoisopropanolamide; nonionic; thickener, emollient, anticorrosive agent, foam booster/stabilizer for shampoos, bubble baths, liq. soaps, shower gels, toilet soaps; wh. to beige flakes; 96% act.

Ninox® FCA. [Stepan Europe] Cocamidopropylamine oxide; CAS 68155-09-9; EINECS 268-938-5; nonionic; thickener, foam booster/stabilizer, detergent, antistat for scale-removing liqs., liq. soaps, cleaning foams, personal care prods.; water-wh. to pale yel. liq.; 33% act.

Nipabenzyl. [Nipa Labs] Benzylparaben; CAS 94-18-8; EINECS 202-311-9; preservative, bactericide, fungicide for pharmaceuticals, cosmetics, foods, medicinal preps., industrial applics.; chemical intermediate; color developing agent for heat-sensitive recording papers; BP, NF, Euorpean pharmacopoeia, FCC compliance; wh. fine cryst. powd., odorless, tasteless; sol. (g/100 g solv.) 102 g acetone, 79 g methanol, 72 g ethanol, 60 g lanolin, 42 g ether; m.w. 228.25; m.p. 110-112 C; toxicology: LD50 (oral, rat) > 5 g/kg; nonirritating to skin; sl. harmful by ingestion, sl. irritating to eyes; 99% assay.

Nipabutyl. [Nipa Labs] Butylparaben; CAS 94-26-8; EINECS 202-318-7; preservative, bactericide, fungicide for pharmaceuticals, cosmetics, foods, medicinal preps., industrial applics.; BP, NF, Euorpean pharmacopoeia, FCC compliance; wh. cryst. powd., odorless or very faint aromatic odor, tasteless; sol. (g/100 g solv.) 240 g acetone, 220 g methanol, 208 g ethanol, > 200 g IPA, 150 g ether, > 100 g lanolin; m.w. 194.23; m.p. 68-69 C; toxicology: LD50 (oral, mouse) > 5 g/kg; nonirritating to skin; sl. irritating to eyes; > 99% act.

Nipabutyl Potassium. [Nipa Labs] Potassium butylparaben; CAS 38566-94-8; preservative, bactericide, fungicide for pharmaceuticals, cosmetics, foods, medicinal preps., industrial applics.; wh. fine hygroscopic powd.; sol. in cold water; m.w. 232.32; pH 9.5-10.5 (0.1% aq.); toxicology: nonirritating to skin; sl. irritating to eyes and nasal passages; > 99% act.

Nipabutyl Sodium. [Nipa Labs] Sodium butylparaben; CAS 36457-20-2; preservative, bactericide, fungicide for pharmaceuticals, cosmetics, foods, medicinal preps., industrial applics.; wh. fine hygroscopic powd.; sol. in cold water; m.w. 216.21; pH 9.5-10.5 (0.1% aq.); toxicology: LD50 (oral, mouse) > 2 g/kg; pure material irritating to skin; sl. irritating to eyes and nasal passages; > 99% act.

Nipacide® MX. [Nipa Labs] p-Chloro-m-xylenol; CAS 88-04-0; EINECS 201-793-8; antimicrobial, preservative for cosmetics, disinfectant, algicide, slimicide, and water treatment pesticide prods., polymer emulsions, adhesives, latex paints, metalworking cutting fluids.

Nipacide® PX-R. [Nipa Labs] Chloroxylenol; CAS 88-04-0; EINECS 201-793-8; pharmaceutical grade antimicrobial agent used as an antiseptic base for OTC drug prods. incl. medicated powds., soaps, surgical scrubs, and antidandruff shampoos and as preservative in cosmetics and toiletries; usage level: 0.5-3.75%.

Nipacide® Potassium. [Nipa Labs] Preservative for aq. foodstuffs, pharmaceuticals, and cosmetics; sol. in cold water.

Nipacide® Sodium. [Nipa Labs] Preservative for aq. foodstuffs, pharmaceuticals, and cosmetics; sol. in cold water.

Nipacombin PK. [Nipa Labs] Preservative for aq. foodstuffs, pharmaceuticals, and cosmetics; sol. in cold water.

Nipacombin SK. [Nipa Labs] Preservative for liq. antacid suspensions and other alkaline sol'ns.; sol. in cold water.

Nipagin A. [Nipa Labs] Ethylparaben; CAS 120-47-8; EINECS 204-399-4; preservative, bactericide, fungicide for pharmaceuticals, cosmetics, foods, medicinal preps., industrial applics.; BP, NF, Euorpean pharmacopoeia, FCC compliance; wh. fine cryst. powd., odorless or very faint aromatic odor, tasteless; sol. (g/100 g solv.) 84 g acetone, 81 g methanol, 70 g ethanol, 40 g ether, 30 g lanolin; m.w. 166.18; m.p. 115-117 C; toxicology: LD50 (oral, rat) > 8 g/kg; nonirritating to skin; sl. irritating to eyes; > 99% act.

Nipagin A Potassium. [Nipa Labs] Potassium ethylparaben; CAS 36457-19-9; preservative, bactericide, fungicide for pharmaceuticals, cosmetics, foods, medicinal preps., industrial applics.; wh. fine hygroscopic powd., tasteless; sol. in cold water; m.w. 204.27; pH 9.5-10.5 (0.1% aq.); toxicology: nonirritating to skin; sl. irritating to eyes and nasal passages; > 99% act.

Nipagin A Sodium. [Nipa Labs] Sodium ethylparaben; CAS 35285-68-8; EINECS 252-487-6; preservative, bactericide, fungicide for pharmaceuticals, cosmetics, foods, medicinal preps., industrial applics.; wh. fine hygroscopic powd., tasteless; sol. in cold water; m.w. 188.16; pH 9.5-10.5 (0.1% aq.); toxicology: LD50 (oral, mouse) 2.5 g/kg; pure material irritating to skin; sl. irritating to eyes and nasal passages; > 99% act.

Nipagin M. [Nipa Labs] Methylparaben; CAS 99-76-3; EINECS 202-785-7; preservative, bactericide, fungicide for pharmaceuticals, cosmetics, foods, medicinal preps., industrial applics.; BP, NF, Euorpean pharmacopoeia, FCC compliance; wh. fine cryst. powd., odorless or very faint aromatic odor, tasteless; sol. (g/100 g solv.): 64 g acetone, 60 g IPA, 58 g methanol, 48 g ethanol, 35 g propylene glycol, 23 g ether; m.w. 152.15; m.p. 125-128 C; toxicology: LD50 (oral, rat) > 8 g/kg; sl. irritating to eyes; nonirritating to skin; > 99% act.

Nipagin M Potassium. [Nipa Labs] Potassium methylparaben.; CAS 26112-07-2; EINECS 247-464-2; preservative, bactericide, fungicide for pharmaceuticals, cosmetics, foods, medicinal preps., industrial applics.; wh. fine hygroscopic powd., odorless or very faint aromatic odor, tasteless; sol. in cold water; m.w. 190.24; pH 9.5-10.5 (0.1% aq.); toxicology: LD50 (oral, rat) > 8 g/kg; nonirritating to skin; sl. irritating to eyes; > 99% act.

Nipagin M Sodium. [Nipa Labs] Sodium methylparaben; CAS 5026-62-0; EINECS 225-714-1; preservative, bactericide, fungicide for pharmaceuticals, cosmetics, foods, medicinal preps., toothpaste; wh. hygroscopic powd.; sol. in cold water; m.w. 174.1; pH 9.5-10.5 (0.1%); toxicology: LD50 (oral, mouse) 2.0 g/kg; nonirritating to skin; sl. irritating to eyes and nasal passages; > 99% act.

Nipaguard BPA. [Nipa Labs] Liquid preservative for sunscreens.

Nipaguard® BPX. [Nipa Labs] Phenoxyethanol, methylparaben, propylparaben, and bronopol; broad-spectrum cosmetic preservative system for use at pH 4.5-8.5; readily incorporated in aq. phase; used in sunscreens; USA and Europe approvals; usage level: 0.25-0.5%.

Nipaguard® DMDMH. [Nipa Labs] DMDM hydantoin; CAS 6440-58-0; EINECS 229-222-8; broad-spectrum antimicrobial effective against gram-postive bacteria, yeast, and molds for cosmetics and personal care prods.; water-wh. clear liq., sl. formaldehyde odor; sol. in water; m.w. 188.12; sp.gr. 1.15 g/ml; dens. 9.68 lb/gal; f.p. -7.5 C; b.p. 108 C; flash pt. > 150 F; pH 6.7-7.5; usage level: 0.15-0.4%; toxicology: LD50 (oral) 3300 mg/kg (moderately toxic); mild skin and eye irritant; respiratory irritant; > 54% act. in water.

Nipaguard® MPA. [Nipa Labs] Benzyl alcohol, methylparaben, and propylparaben; broad-spectrum cosmetic preservative system for use at pH 4.5-8.5; readily incorporated in aq. phase; USA, Japan, and Europe approvals; usage level: 0.3-0.6%.

Nipaguard® MPS. [Nipa Labs] Propylene glycol, methylparaben, and propylparaben; broad-spectrum cosmetic preservative system for use at pH 4.5-8.5; readily incorporated in aq. phase; USA, Japan, and Europe approvals; usage level: 0.3-0.6%.

Nipaheptyl. [Nipa Labs] n-Heptyl p-hydroxybenzoate; preservative, bactericide, fungicide for pharmaceuticals, cosmetics, foods, medicinal preps., industrial applics.

Nipanox® S-1. [Nipa Labs] Propyl gallate (20%), citric acid (10%) in propylene glycol (70%); antioxidant for veg. oil industry and cosmetics; clear to lt. amber liq., very sl. odor; sol. in animal and veg. fats.

Nipanox® Special. [Nipa Labs] BHA (13%), propyl gallate (13%), citric acid (4%) in propylene glycol (70%); antioxidant for foods and cosmetics; fat and oil stabilizer; clear to lt. straw liq., sl. odor; sol. in animal and veg. fats, fatty acids, glycerides; insol. in water.

Nipasept Potassium. [Nipa Labs] Preservative for aq. foodstuffs, pharmaceuticals, and cosmetics; sol. in cold water.

Nipasept Sodium. [Nipa Labs] Sodium methylparaben, sodium propylparaben, and sodium ethylparaben; preservative for aq. foodstuffs, pharmaceuticals, and cosmetics, oral medicines; sol. in cold water.

Nipasol M. [Nipa Labs] Propylparaben; CAS 94-13-3; EINECS 202-307-7; preservative, bactericide, fungicide for pharmaceuticals, cosmetics, foods, medicinal preps., industrial applics.; BP, NF, Euorpean pharmacopoeia, FCC compliance; wh. fine cryst. powd., odorless or very faint aromatic odor, tasteless; sol. (g/100 g solv.): 105 g acetone, 100 g in methanol, ethanol, 88 g IPA, 80 g lanolin, 50 g ether; m.w. 180.20; m.p. 95-98 C; toxicology: LD50 (oral, rat) > 8 g/kg (pract. nonharmful by ingestion); nonirritant to skin; sl. irritant to eyes; > 99% act.

Nipasol M Potassium. [Nipa Labs] Potassium propylparaben; CAS 84930-16-5; preservative, bactericide, fungicide for pharmaceuticals, cosmetics, foods, medicinal preps., industrial applics.; wh. fine hygroscopic powd., odorless or very faint aromatic odor, tasteless; sol. in cold water; m.w. 218.29; pH 9.5-10.5 (0.1% aq.); toxicology: LD50 (oral, rat) > 8 g/kg (pract. nonharmful by ingestion); nonirritating to skin; sl. irritating to eyes; > 99% act.

Nipasol M Sodium. [Nipa Labs] Sodium propylparaben; CAS 35285-69-9; preservative, bactericide, fungicide for pharmaceuticals, cosmetics, foods, medicinal preps., industrial applics.; wh. hygroscopic powd.; sol. in cold water; m.w. 202.2; pH 9.5-10.5 (0.1%); toxicology: LD50 (oral, mouse) 3.7 g/kg (pract. nonharmful); nonirritating to skin; sl. irritating to eyes, nasal passages; > 99% act.

Nipastat. [Nipa Labs] Methylparaben (> 50%), butylparaben (> 20%), ethylparaben (<15%), and propylparaben (< 10%); preservative, bactericide, fungicide for pharmaceuticals, cosmetics, foods, medicinal preps., industrial applics.; USA and Europe approvals; wh. fine cryst. powd., virtually odorless, tasteless; sol. 0.14% in water; m.p. 60-125 C; pH 7.0 (10% aq.); usage level: 0.05-0.3%; toxicology: pract. nonharmful by ingestion; nonirritating to skin; sl. irritating to eyes.

Nissan Diapon T. [Nippon Oils & Fats] Sodium N-methyl tallow taurate; anionic; dyeing aux. for hair dye detergent, emulsifier; powd.; 30% conc.

Nissan Monogly I. [Nippon Oils & Fats] Glyceryl stearate SE; nonionic; emulsifier for creams and lotions of the o/w type; wh. flake; disp. in water; m.p. 55–63 C; HLB 11.0; 100% conc.

Nissan Monogly M. [Nippon Oils & Fats] Glyceryl stearate; nonionic; emulsifier for cosmetics and pharmaceuticals; wh. flake; m.p. 53–61 C; HLB 3.0; 40% min. monoglyceride content.

Nissan Nonion CP-08R. [Nippon Oils & Fats] Sorbitan caprylate; nonionic; emulsifier for cosmetic, pharmaceutical and food applics.; liq.; oil-sol.; HLB 7.3; 100% conc.

Nissan Nonion DN-202. [Nippon Oils & Fats] POE lauryl ether; nonionic; emulsifier for cosmetic, pharmaceutical and food applics.; liq.; oil-sol.; HLB 6.2; 100% conc.

Nissan Nonion DN-203. [Nippon Oils & Fats] POE lauryl ether; nonionic; emulsifier for cosmetic, pharmaceutical and food applics.; liq.; oil-sol.; HLB 7.9; 100% conc.

Nissan Nonion DN-209. [Nippon Oils & Fats] POE lauryl ether; nonionic; emulsifier for cosmetic, pharmaceutical and food applics.; liq.; oil-sol.; HLB 13.2; 100% conc.

Nissan Nonion DS-60HN. [Nippon Oils & Fats] PEG distearate; nonionic; emulsifier, thickener used in cosmetics, textile, industrial uses; solid; sol. in water, methanol, warm in diethylene glycol; m.p. 54–62 C; HLB 19; acid no. 2 max.; 100% conc.

Nissan Nonion E-205. [Nippon Oils & Fats] POE oleyl ether; nonionic; emulsifier, dispersant, detergent, wetting agent used in textile processing, cosmetics, metalworking, agric. preparations, industrial cleaners; APHA 140 max. liq.; sol. in xylene, kerosene, methanol, disp. in water; HLB 9.0; cloud pt. 0 C (1% aq.); 100% conc.

Nissan Nonion E-206. [Nippon Oils & Fats] POE oleyl ether; nonionic; emulsifier, dispersant, detergent, wetting agent used in textile processing, cosmetics, metalworking, agric. preparations, industrial cleaners; liq.; HLB 9.9; 100% conc.

Nissan Nonion E-208. [Nippon Oils & Fats] POE oleyl ether; nonionic; emulsifier, dispersant, detergent, wetting agent used in textile processing, cosmetics, metalworking, agric. preparations, industrial cleaners; liq.; 100% conc.

Nissan Nonion E-215. [Nippon Oils & Fats] POE oleyl ether; nonionic; emulsifier, dispersant, detergent, wetting agent used in textile processing, cosmetics, metalworking, agric. preparations, industrial cleaners; APHA 140 max. semisolid; sol. in water, methanol, cloudy in xylene; HLB 14.2; cloud pt. 95 C (1% aq.); 100% conc.

Nissan Nonion E-220. [Nippon Oils & Fats] POE oleyl ether; nonionic; emulsifier, dispersant, detergent, wetting agent used in textile processing, cosmetics, metalworking, agric. preparations, industrial cleaners; solid; HLB 15.3; 100% conc.

Nissan Nonion E-230. [Nippon Oils & Fats] POE oleyl ether; nonionic; emulsifier, dispersant, detergent, wetting agent used in textile processing, cosmetics, metalworking, agric. preparations, industrial cleaners; APHA 140 max. solid; sol. in water, methanol, cloudy in xylene; HLB 16.6; cloud pt. 100 C resp. (1% aq.); 100% conc.

Nissan Nonion K-202. [Nippon Oils & Fats] POE lauryl ether; nonionic; emulsifier, dispersant, detergent, wetting agent used in textile processing, cosmetics, metalworking, agric. preparations, industrial cleaners; APHA 200 max. liq.; sol. in xylene, ether, methanol; disp. in kerosene; HLB 6.0; cloud pt. 0 C max. (1% aq.); 100% conc.

Nissan Nonion K-203. [Nippon Oils & Fats] POE lauryl ether; nonionic; emulsifier, dispersant, detergent, wetting agent used in textile processing, cosmetics, metalworking, agric. preparations, industrial cleaners; APHA 200 max. liq.; sol. in xylene, ether, methanol; disp. in kerosene; HLB 8.0; cloud pt. 0 C max. (1% aq.); 100% conc.

Nissan Nonion K-204. [Nippon Oils & Fats] POE lauryl ether; nonionic; emulsifier, dispersant, detergent, wetting agent used in textile processing, cosmetics, metalworking, agric. preparations, industrial cleaners; APHA 200 max. semisolid; sol. in xylene, ether, methanol; sol. warm in kerosene; disp. in water; HLB 9.2; cloud pt. 0 C max. (1% aq.); 100% conc.

Nissan Nonion K-207. [Nippon Oils & Fats] POE lauryl ether; nonionic; emulsifier, dispersant, detergent, wetting agent used in textile processing, cosmetics, metalworking, agric. preparations, industrial cleaners; APHA 50 max. semisolid; sol. in water, xylene, methanol; sol. warm in ether; HLB 12.1; cloud pt. 55–63 C max. (1% aq.); 100% conc.

Nissan Nonion K-211. [Nippon Oils & Fats] POE lauryl ether; nonionic; emulsifier, dispersant, detergent, wetting agent used in textile processing, cosmetics, metalworking, agric. preparations, industrial cleaners; APHA 50 max. semisolid; sol. in water, xylene, methanol; HLB 14.1; cloud pt. 90–98 C max. (1% aq.); 100% conc.

Nissan Nonion K-215. [Nippon Oils & Fats] POE lauryl ether; nonionic; emulsifier, dispersant, detergent, wetting agent used in textile processing, cosmetics, metalworking, agric. preparations, industrial cleaners; APHA 140 max. semisolid; sol. in water, xylene, methanol; HLB 15.2; cloud pt. 100 C min. (1% aq.); 100% conc.

Nissan Nonion K-220. [Nippon Oils & Fats] POE lauryl ether; nonionic; emulsifier, dispersant, detergent, wetting agent used in textile processing, cosmetics, metalworking, agric. preparations, industrial cleaners; APHA 120 max. solid; sol. in water, xylene, methanol; HLB 16.2; cloud pt. 100 C min. (1% aq.); 100% conc.

Nissan Nonion K-230. [Nippon Oils & Fats] POE lauryl ether; nonionic; emulsifier, dispersant, detergent, wetting agent used in textile processing, cosmetics, metalworking, agric. preparations, industrial cleaners; APHA 120 max. semisolid; sol. in water, xylene, methanol; HLB 17.3; cloud pt. 100 C min. (1% aq.); 100% conc.

Nissan Nonion LP-20R, LP-20RS. [Nippon Oils & Fats] Sorbitan laurate; CAS 1338-39-2; nonionic; emulsifier for cosmetic, pharmaceutical and food applics., o/w emulsion stabilizer and thickener, fiber lubricant and softener; Gardner 5 max. oily liq.; sol. in methanol, ethanol, acetone, xylene, ethyl ether, kerosene, disp. in water; HLB 8.6; 100% conc.

Nissan Nonion LT-221. [Nippon Oils & Fats] Polysorbate 20; CAS 9005-64-5; nonionic; emulsifier for cosmetic, pharmaceutical and food applics.; Gardner 6 max. oily liq.; sol. in water, methanol, ethanol, acetone, xylene, ethyl ether, ethylene glycol, HLB 16.7; 100% conc.

Nissan Nonion MP-30R. [Nippon Oils & Fats] Sorbitan myristate; nonionic; emulsifier for cosmetic, pharmaceutical and food applics.; solid; oil-sol.; HLB 6.6; 100% conc.

Nissan Nonion OP-80R. [Nippon Oils & Fats] Sorbitan oleate; CAS 1338-43-8; EINECS 215-665-4; nonionic; emulsifier for cosmetic, pharmaceutical and food applics.; Gardner 9 max. oily liq.; oil-sol.; HLB 4.3; 100% conc.

Nissan Nonion OP-83RAT. [Nippon Oils & Fats] Sorbitan sesquioleate; CAS 8007-43-0; EINECS 232-360-1; nonionic; emulsifier for cosmetic, pharmaceutical and food applics.; Gardner 9 max. oily liq.; sol. in ethanol, acetone, xylene, ethyl ether, kerosene, methanol; warm in water; HLB 3.7; 100% conc.

Nissan Nonion OP-85R. [Nippon Oils & Fats] Sorbitan trioleate; CAS 26266-58-0; EINECS 247-569-3; nonionic; emulsifier for cosmetic, pharmaceutical and food applics.; Gardner 9 max. oily liq.; oil-sol.; HLB 1.8; 100% conc.

Nissan Nonion OT-221. [Nippon Oils & Fats] POE sorbitan monooleate; nonionic; emulsifier for cosmetic, pharmaceutical and food applics.; Gardner 6 max. oily liq.; sol. in water, ethanol, acetone, xylene, disp. in methanol; HLB 15.0; 100% conc.

Nissan Nonion P-6. [Nippon Oils & Fats] PEG monopalmitate; nonionic; emulsifier and thickener for cosmetic applics., textile and other industrial uses; semisolid; HLB 13.8; 100% conc.

Nissan Nonion P-208. [Nippon Oils & Fats] POE cetyl ether; nonionic; emulsifier, dispersant, detergent, wetting agent used in textile processing, cosmetics, metalworking, agric. preparations, industrial cleaners; APHA 120 liq.; sol. in water, xylene, methanol; HLB 11.9; cloud pt. 43–53 C (1% aq.); 100% conc.

Nissan Nonion P-210. [Nippon Oils & Fats] POE cetyl ether; nonionic; emulsifier, dispersant, detergent, wetting agent used in textile processing, cosmetics, metalworking, agric. preparations, industrial cleaners; APHA 120 max. semisolid; sol. in water, xylene, methanol; HLB 12.9; cloud pt. 64–74 C (1% aq.); 100% conc.

Nissan Nonion P-213. [Nippon Oils & Fats] POE cetyl ether; nonionic; emulsifier, dispersant, detergent, wetting agent used in textile processing, cosmetics, metalworking, agric. preparations, industrial cleaners; APHA 120 max. semisolid; sol. in water, kerosene, ether, methanol; HLB 14.1; cloud pt. 87–97 C (1% aq.); 100% conc.

Nissan Nonion PP-40R. [Nippon Oils & Fats] Sorbitan palmitate; CAS 26266-57-9; EINECS 247-568-8; nonionic; emulsifier for cosmetic, pharmaceutical and food applics.; Gardner 7 max. waxy solid; oil-sol.; HLB 6.7; 100% conc.

Nissan Nonion PT-221. [Nippon Oils & Fats] POE sorbitan monopalmitate; nonionic; emulsifier for cosmetic, pharmaceutical and food applics.; Gardner 8 max. oily liq.; sol. in water, methanol, ethanol, acetone, xylene, ethyl ether, ethylene glycol; HLB 15.3; 100% conc.

Nissan Nonion S-2. [Nippon Oils & Fats] PEG monostearate; nonionic; emulsifier, thickener used in cosmetics, textile, industrial uses; Gardner 4 max. semisolid; sol. in methanol, warm in xylene, disp. in water, kerosene, ether; m.p. 33–41 C; HLB 8.0; 100% conc.

Nissan Nonion S-4. [Nippon Oils & Fats] PEG monostearate; nonionic; emulsifier, thickener used in cosmetics, textile, industrial uses; Gardner 4 max. semisolid; sol. in kerosene, ether, methanol, warm in xylene, disp. in water; m.p. 30–40 C; HLB 11.6; 100% conc.

Nissan Nonion S-6. [Nippon Oils & Fats] PEG monostearate; nonionic; emulsifier, thickener used in cosmetics, textile, industrial uses; Gardner 4 max. semisolid; sol. in water, methanol, warm in xylene, ether, cloudy in kerosene; m.p. 35–41 C; HLB 13.6; 100% conc.

Nissan Nonion S-10. [Nippon Oils & Fats] PEG monostearate; nonionic; emulsifier, thickener used in cosmetics, textile, industrial uses; Gardner 4 max. semisolid; sol. in water, xylene, ether, methanol; m.p. 38–44 C; HLB 15.2; 100% conc.

Nissan Nonion S-15. [Nippon Oils & Fats] PEG monostearate; nonionic; emulsifier, thickener used in cosmetics, textile, industrial uses; Gardner 4 max. semisolid; sol. in kerosene, ether, methanol, warm in xylene; disp. in water; m.p. 39–45 C; HLB 12.8; 100% conc.

Nissan Nonion S-15.4. [Nippon Oils & Fats] PEG monostearate; nonionic; emulsifier, thickener used in cosmetics, textile, industrial uses; Gardner 4 max. semisolid; sol. in water, xylene, ether, methanol; m.p. 42–48 C; HLB 16.7; 100% conc.

Nissan Nonion S-40. [Nippon Oils & Fats] PEG monostearate; nonionic; emulsifier, thickener used in cosmetics, textile, industrial uses; Gardner 6 max. semisolid; sol. in water, xylene, ether, methanol; m.p. 49–55 C; HLB 18.2; 100% conc.

Nissan Nonion S-206. [Nippon Oils & Fats] POE stearyl ether; nonionic; emulsifier, dispersant, detergent, wetting agent for textile processing, cosmetics, metalworking, agric., industrial cleaners; solid; HLB 9.9; 100% conc.

Nissan Nonion S-207. [Nippon Oils & Fats] POE stearyl ether; nonionic; emulsifier, dispersant, detergent, wetting agent for textile processing, cosmetics, metalworking, agric., industrial cleaners; APHA 120 max. semisolid; sol. in xylene, kerosene, liq. paraffin, soybean oil, tetrachloromethan, methanol, diethylene glycol; water-disp.; HLB 10.7; cloud pt. 0 C max. (1% aq.); 100% conc.

Nissan Nonion S-215. [Nippon Oils & Fats] POE stearyl ether; nonionic; emulsifier, dispersant, detergent, wetting agent for textile processing, cosmetics, metalworking, agric., industrial cleaners; APHA 120 max. semisolid; sol. in water, xylene, kerosene, soybean oil, ether, tetrachloromethan, methanol, diethylene glycol; HLB 14.2; cloud pt. 100 C min. (1% aq.); 100% conc.

Nissan Nonion S-220. [Nippon Oils & Fats] POE stearyl ether; nonionic; emulsifier, dispersant, detergent, wetting agent for textile processing, cosmetics, metalworking, agric., industrial cleaners; APHA 120 max. semisolid; sol. in water, xylene, kerosene, soybean oil, ether, tetrachloromethan, methanol, diethylene glycol; HLB 15.3; cloud pt. 100 C min. (1% aq.); 100% conc.

Nissan Nonion SP-60R. [Nippon Oils & Fats] Sorbitan stearate; CAS 1338-41-6; EINECS 215-664-9; nonionic; emulsifier for cosmetics, pharmaceutical and food applics.; Gardner 5 max. waxy solid; sol. in methanol, ethanol, xylene, kerosene, ethyl ether, disp. in warm water; HLB 4.7; 100% conc.

Nissan Nonion ST-221. [Nippon Oils & Fats] POE sorbitan monostearate; nonionic; emulsifier for cosmetic, pharmaceutical and food applics.; Gardner 5 max. oily liq.; sol. in water, methanol, ethanol, acetone, xylene, ethyl ether, kerosene; HLB 14.9; 100% conc.

Nissan Nonion T-15. [Nippon Oils & Fats] PEG monotallow acid ester; nonionic; emulsifier and thickener for cosmetics, textiles, industrial uses; liq.; HLB 12.8; 100% conc.

Nissan Panacete 810. [Nippon Oils & Fats] Med. chain triglyceride; nonionic; diluent for perfumes; raw material for pharmaceuticals and special foods; liq.; 100% conc.

Nissan Persoft SK. [Nippon Oils & Fats] Sulfated fatty alcohol, sodium salt; anionic; detergent, emulsifier, dispersant, wetting agent; base for shampoo and liq. detergent; biodeg.; liq.; 30% conc.

Nissan Stafoam DO, DOS. [Nippon Oils & Fats] Oleamide DEA; CAS 93-83-4; EINECS 202-281-7; nonionic; thickener, foam stabilizer for shampoo and liq. detergents; liq.; 100% conc.

Nissan Stafoam MF. [Nippon Oils & Fats] Cocamide MEA;

CAS 68140-00-1; EINECS 268-770-2; nonionic; foam stabilizer for paste shampoos; flake; 100% conc.

Nissan Sunamide C-3, CF-3, CF-10. [Nippon Oils & Fats] Fatty alkylolamide ether sulfate; anionic; base for preparation of low irritation and biodeg. shampoos and dishwashing detergents; liq.; 30, 30 and 35% conc. resp.

Nissan Unilube MB-38. [Nippon Oils & Fats] PPG-3 butyl ether.

NM. [Angus] Nitromethane; CAS 75-52-5; EINECS 200-876-6; intermediate, stabilizer for halogenated solvs., as fuels, explosives, and solvs. for coatings or industrial processes; cosmetic and personal care raw material; m.w. 61.0; dens. 1.14 g/ml; b.p. 101 C; flash pt. 96 F (TCC).

Nonasol N4AS. [Hart Chem. Ltd.] Ammonium laureth sulfate; CAS 32612-48-9; anionic; detergent base for dishwash, hard surf. cleaners, shampoos; wetting agent; biodeg.; yel. liq.; sp.gr. 1.02; 58% act.

Nonasol N4SS. [Hart Chem. Ltd.] Sodium laureth sulfate; CAS 9004-82-4; anionic; detergent base for high foaming liq. detergents, dishwash, hard surf. cleaners, shampoos; wetting agent; biodeg.; yel. liq.; sp.gr. 1.04; 60% act.

Nonionic E-4. [Calgene] POE alkylaryl ethers; nonionic; detergent and wetting agent used in cosmetics, insecticide and other formulations; liq.; HLB 8.6; 100% conc.

Nonisol 100. [Ciba-Geigy] PEG-8 laurate; CAS 9004-81-3; nonionic; emulsifier, solubilizing and wetting agent, thickener, used in textiles, cosmetics, hand cleaners, spreading agents; yel. liq.; water-sol.; 100% conc.

Nonychosine. [Exsymol; Biosil Tech.] Blend of acrylic and methacrylic polyesters with methionin; hardener and normalizer for nail growth; colorless to ocher visc., limpid liq., acid bitter odor; misc. with org. solvs., acetone, ethyl acetate; sp.gr. 1.15; visc. 350 cps; ref. index 1.48; usage level: pure or 5-20%; toxicology: nontoxic.

Nopalcol 1-S. [Henkel/Functional Prods.] Diethylene glycol stearate; CAS 9004-99-3; EINECS 203-363-5; nonionic; emulsifier, plasticizer, lubricant, wetting agent, defoamer, binding and thickening agent, used in cosmetics, dry cleaning, leather, textile industries; solid; HLB 3.8; 98% conc.

Nopalcol 1-TW. [Henkel/Functional Prods.] PEG-2 tallowate; nonionic; emulsifier, plasticizer, lubricant, wetting agent, defoamer, binding and thickening agent, used in cosmetics, dry cleaning, leather, textile industries; solid; HLB 4.1; 99% act.

Nopcocastor. [Henkel/Functional Prods.] Sulfated castor oil; CAS 8002-33-3; EINECS 232-306-7; anionic; emulsifier; superfatting agent for cosmetics; liq.; 75% conc.

Noram DMC. [Ceca SA] N-Coco dimethylamine; CAS 61788-93-0; EINECS 263-020-0; cationic; industrial detergent; synthesis intermediate, anticaking agent, flotation, antistripping for road making, soil stabilization; auxs. for fuel additives, rust inhibition, paint, cosmetics; chemical intermediate for quats., betaines, amine oxides; liq.

Noramium DA.50. [Ceca SA] Benzalkonium chloride aq. sol'n.; CAS 8001-54-5; cationic; bactericide, algicide, fungicide, preservative, disinfectant for cosmetics, household disinfectants, food and drink industry, veterinary prods., masonry, swimming pool and industrial water treatment, wood industry, latex coagulation, flotation, electrostatic paints, demulsification of hydrocarbons; emulsifier for emulsion polymerization of acrylic monomers; Gardner ≤ 2 liq.; sp.gr. 980 kg/m³; solid. pt. -2 to 2 C; pH 6-7; 49-51% act.

Noramium M2C. [Ceca SA] Dicoco dimethyl ammonium chloride in isopropanol sol'n.; CAS 61789-77-3; EINECS 263-087-6; cationic; textile softener; hair conditioner with detangling, softening, and antistatic props.; wetting and dispersing agent for pigments in paint industry; biostat, biocide, mold growth inhibitor, and fungicide; carwash ingred.; emulsifier for lubricants, fatliquoring (leather), waxes and silicone oils in home care prods.; dispersant for car polish compds.; liq.; sol. in ethanol; sp.gr. 855 kg/m³; solid. pt. -10 C; pH 5-7; 74-77% act.

Noramium M2SH. [Ceca SA] Dihydrog. tallow dimethyl ammonium chloride; CAS 61789-80-8; EINECS 263-090-2; cationic; textile softener; hair conditioner; pasty; 75% conc.

Noramium MC 50. [Ceca SA] Coco trimethyl ammonium chloride; CAS 61789-18-2; EINECS 263-038-9; cationic; additive for antibiotics mfg.; liq.; 50% conc.

Noramium MO 50. [Ceca SA] Oleyl trimethyl ammonium chloride; cationic; additive for antibiotics mfg.; liq.

Noramium MS 50. [Ceca SA] Tallow trimethyl ammonium chloride; CAS 8030-78-2; EINECS 232-447-4; cationic; emulsifier; pharmaceuticals; liq.; 50% conc.

Noramium MSH 50. [Ceca SA] Hydrog. tallow trimethyl ammonium chloride; CAS 61788-78-1; EINECS 263-005-9; cationic; additive for antibiotics mfg.; liq.; 75% conc.

Norfox® 165C. [Norman, Fox] Glyceryl stearate, acid-stable; nonionic; cosmetic emulsifier; flake; HLB 3.9; 100% conc.

Norfox® 1101. [Norman, Fox] Potassium cocoate; CAS 61789-30-8; EINECS 263-049-9; anionic; flash foamer, emulsifier for shampoo bases, liq. hand soaps; lubricant for conveyors; coupling agent for heavily built liq. alkali systems such as steam cleaners and whitewall tire cleaners; liq.; HLB 20.0; sapon. no. 250 min.; pH 10 (1%); 40% solids.

Norfox® ALKA. [Harcros UK] Fatty amidoalkyl betaine; amphoteric; substantive surfactant, flash foamer for industrial, household and personal care prods. incl. heavy-duty caustic steam cleaners, baby shampoos, bubble baths; exc. electrolyte tolerance; yel. clear liq.; sp.gr. 1.04; cloud pt. 0 C; pH 6.0-7.5 (1% aq.); 29-32% act., 34-37% total solids.

Norfox® ALPHA XL. [Norman, Fox] Sodium C14-16 alpha olefin sulfonate; CAS 68439-57-6; EINECS 270-407-8; anionic; base for shampoos, hand soaps, bath prods., home and janitorial cleaners, dishwash, and lt. duty liqs.; Klett 100 max. liq.; pH 7-9 (5%); 38-41% act.

Norfox® ALS. [Norman, Fox] Ammonium lauryl sulfate; CAS 2235-54-3; EINECS 218-793-9; anionic; base for woolen carpet shampoo, hair shampoo; liq.; 30% conc.

Norfox® B. [Norman, Fox] Sodium stearate; CAS 822-16-2; EINECS 212-490-5; anionic; gelling agent; stabilizer in cosmetics; lubricant; gran.; 96% conc.

Norfox® B-54. [Norman, Fox] Butyl stearate; CAS 123-95-5; EINECS 204-666-5; cosmetic ester.

Norfox® Coco Betaine. [Norman, Fox] Cocamidopropyl betaine; amphoteric; mild substantive surfactant, flash foamer; base for mild shampoos; reduces irritation of sulfates; used for heavy-duty caustic steam cleaners, baby shampoos, bubble baths; electrolyte tolerance over wide pH range; yel. clear liq.; sp.gr. 1.04; dens. 8.67 lb/gal; pH 6.0-7.5 (1% aq.); 29-32% act., 34-37% total solids.

Norfox® Coco Powder. [Norman, Fox] Sodium cocoate; CAS 61789-31-9; EINECS 263-050-4; anionic; soap base; stabilizer; gelling agent; for powd. hand soaps; gran.; 92% conc.

Norfox® DC. [Norman, Fox] Cocamide DEA and diethanolamine; CAS 61791-31-9; nonionic; intermediate for detergent mfg., liq. dishwash, cosmetics; suds stabilizer and dedusting agent for dry prods.; straw-colored visc. liq.; sp.gr. 1.02; pour pt. -8 C; flash pt. 166 C; pH 9.5 (1%); 100% conc.

Norfox® DCS. [Norman, Fox] Alkylaryl sulfonate modified coconut oil DEA condensate; CAS 61791-31-9; EINECS 263-163-9; anionic/nonionic; biodeg. wetting agent and detergent base for textiles, paper, auto and home care prods.; shampoos, bubble bath, liq. dishwash, hand soap,

car wash; dye dispersant; demulsifier; straw-colored visc. liq., bland odor; sp.gr. 1.05; pour pt. 40 F; pH 9.0 (1-5%); 100% act.

Norfox® DCSA. [Norman, Fox] Cocamide DEA; CAS 61791-31-9; EINECS 263-163-9; nonionic; foam booster/stabilizer, detergent, wetting agent, visc. builder for household/industrial cleaners, drycleaning, cosmetics, lt. duty detergents, dishwash, shampoos, bubble bath; Gardner < 4 liq.; sol. in water, alcohol, chlorinated hydrocarbons, aromatic hydrocarbons, natural fats and oils; disp. in min. oil; sp.gr. 1.0016; dens. 8.3 lb/gal; visc. 11.5 poises; m.p. 0 C; acid no. < 2.0; amine no. < 38; flash pt. (OC) 405 F; fire pt. 415 F; pH 10 (1%); 100% conc.

Norfox® DLSA. [Norman, Fox] Lauramide DEA; CAS 120-40-1; EINECS 204-393-1; nonionic; specialty foam booster and visc. builder for shampoo and bubble baths; waxy solid; 100% conc.

Norfox® DOSA. [Norman, Fox] Cocamide DEA; CAS 61791-31-9; EINECS 263-163-9; nonionic; foam stabilizer, emollient, conditioner, emulsifier, corrosion inhibitor; visc. builder for use at reduced concs.; for shampoos, bubble baths, industrial applics.; lubricant for auto-wash brushes; degreaser for heavy-duty cleaners; lt. yel. oily liq.; amine no. < 2.0; pH 10 (1% aq.); 100% conc.

Norfox® GMS. [Norman, Fox] Glyceryl stearate; nonionic; lotion and cream base in cosmetics; opacifier in liq. shampoos and detergents; emulsion stabilizer; beads; 40-80% alpha mono, 100% org.

Norfox® GMS-FG. [Norman, Fox] Glyceryl stearate; nonionic; cosmetic opacifier, food grade emulsifier; flake; HLB 3.9; 100% conc.

Norfox® KD. [Norman, Fox] Cocamide DEA; CAS 61791-31-9; EINECS 263-163-9; nonionic; visc. enhancer and foam booster/stabilizer for shampoos or cleaners; straw-colored liq.; dens. 8.2 lb/gal; pH 9.4 (1%); 100% conc.

Norfox® KO. [Norman, Fox] Potassium oleate; CAS 143-18-0; EINECS 205-590-5; anionic; liq. soap for hand cleaners, tire mounting lubricant; emulsifier and corrosion control in paint strippers; surfactant in insecticides; liq.; HLB 20.0; 80% conc.

Norfox® NP-1. [Norman, Fox] Nonoxynol-1; EINECS 248-762-5; nonionic; emulsion stabilizer and defoamer; liq.; oil-sol.; HLB 4.5; 100% conc.

Norfox® NP-4. [Norman, Fox] Nonoxynol-4; CAS 9016-45-9; nonionic; emulsifier, detergent and dispersant for petrol. based lubricants; intermediate for sulfonation to produce foaming agent; liq.; oil-sol.; HLB 9.0; 100% conc.

Norfox® NP-6. [Norman, Fox] Nonoxynol-6; CAS 9016-45-9; nonionic; emulsifier; wetting agent for oil-based systems; liq.; HLB 11.0; 100% conc.

Norfox® SLES-02. [Norman, Fox] Sodium laureth sulfate; CAS 9004-82-4; anionic; foaming and wetting agent for household and cosmetic specialties; liq.; 28% conc.

Norfox® SLES-03. [Norman, Fox] Sodium laureth sulfate; CAS 9004-82-4; anionic; foaming agent; liq.; 28% conc.

Norfox® SLES-60. [Norman, Fox] Sodium laureth sulfate, 14% denatured alcohol; CAS 9004-82-4; anionic; base for shampoos and lt. duty liq. formulators; flash foam enhancer for automotive, household, personal care and industrial cleaners; in mfg. of gypsum wallboard, gas drilling of deep wells; APHA 100 liq., mild alcoholic odor; sp.gr. 1.05; pH 7.7 (10%); 59% act.

Norfox® SLS. [Norman, Fox] Sodium lauryl sulfate; CAS 151-21-3; EINECS 205-788-1; anionic; biodeg. foamer and wetting agent for household, industrial and personal care prods., shampoos, hand and body soaps, fabric care prods.; Gardner 1 max. paste; sp.gr. 1.02; dens. 8.5 lb/gal; HLB 20.0; 28-30% act.

Norfox® Sorbo T-20. [Norman, Fox] Polysorbate 20; CAS 9005-64-5; nonionic; flavor and fragrance solubilizer; liq.;

HLB 16.7; 100% act.

Norfox® Sorbo T-80. [Norman, Fox] Polysorbate 80; CAS 9005-65-6; nonionic; solubilizer for fat-sol. actives; emulsifier for shortening; whipped topping stabilizer; liq.; HLB 15.0; 100% act.

Norfox® T-60. [Norman, Fox] TEA dodecylbenzene sulfonate; CAS 27323-41-7; EINECS 248-406-9; anionic; detergent, wetting agent and foamer for agric. and industrial/household use, lt. duty detergents, hard surf. cleaners, shampoos, wool and fine fabric washing; yel. clear visc. liq., mild odor; dens. 9.1 lb/gal; HLB 20.0; pH 5.7; 60% act.

Norfox® TLS. [Norman, Fox] TEA lauryl sulfate; CAS 139-96-8; EINECS 205-388-7; biodeg. mild ingred. for shampoo, lt. duty liqs., fine fabric detergents; Gardner 2 max. liq.; sp.gr. 1.05; dens. 8.8 lb/gal; visc. 100 cps (30 C); HLB 20.0; pH 7.2 (10% aq.); 39-42% act.

Norfox® XXX Granules. [Norman, Fox] Sodium tallowate; CAS 8052-48-0; EINECS 232-491-4.

Norgel. [Sederma] Polymeric gel of acrylic and methacrylic acid complexed with glycerin; stabilizer functioning through physical, nontoxic mechanism; reduces or eliminates need for preservatives or propylene glycol in formulations; high moisturizing props.; thickener, water absorber; for creams, lotions, shampoos.

Novata® 299, A, AB, B, BBC, BC, BCF, BD, C, D, E. [Henkel KGaA/Cospha] Cocoglycerides; nonionic; suppository and vaginal prep. bases; consistency giving agent for pharmaceutical ointments, creams, stick preps.; wh. fatty fused, flakes, or pastille which melt to a colorless to sl. ylsh. liq. when heated; almost odorless and tasteless; 100% conc.

Novel® N2.2-810. [Vista] C8-10 pareth-2.2; intermediate for prod. of nonionic biodeg. surfactants and emulsifiers for use in household laundry detergents, liq. cleaners, hard surf. cleaners, cosmetics, and industrial solvs. and degreasers; APHA 5 color; m.w. 242; HLB 10; hyd. no. 232; pH 6.5 (1% aq.).

Novel® N3.0-1216CO. [Vista] C12-16 pareth-3; intermediate for prod. of nonionic biodeg. surfactants and emulsifiers for use in household laundry detergents, liq. cleaners, hard surf. cleaners, cosmetics, and industrial solvs. and degreasers; APHA 10 color; m.w. 330; HLB 8; hyd. no. 167; pH 7.0 (1% aq.).

Novel® N4.9-810. [Vista] C8-10 pareth-4.9; intermediate for prod. of nonionic biodeg. surfactants and emulsifiers for use in household laundry detergents, liq. cleaners, hard surf. cleaners, cosmetics, and industrial solvs. and degreasers; APHA 10 color; m.w. 361; m.p. -10.4 to -7.9 C; HLB 12; hyd. no. 155; cloud pt. 50 C (1% aq.); pH 7.0 (1% aq.).

Novel® N5.1-1618. [Vista] C16-18 pareth-5.1; intermediate for prod. of nonionic biodeg. surfactants and emulsifiers for use in household laundry detergents, liq. cleaners, hard surf. cleaners, cosmetics, and industrial solvs. and degreasers; APHA 20 color; m.w. 469; m.p. 28.3-30.8 C; HLB 9; hyd. no. 116; pH 7.0 (1% aq.).

Novel® N7.7-810. [Vista] C8-10 pareth-7.7; intermediate for prod. of nonionic biodeg. surfactants and emulsifiers for use in household laundry detergents, liq. cleaners, hard surf. cleaners, cosmetics, and industrial solvs. and degreasers; APHA 10 color; m.w. 484; m.p. 8.0-10.6 C; HLB 14; hyd. no. 115; cloud pt. 84 C (1% aq.); pH 7.0 (1% aq.).

Novogel® ST. [Rhone-Poulenc] Aluminum stearate, min. oil; gellant for toiletries; 55% conc.

Novol. [Croda Inc.; Croda Chem. Ltd.] Super refined oleyl alcohol; CAS 143-28-2; EINECS 205-597-3; emollient, emulsion stabilizer, solubilizer, superfatting agent, penetrant, pigment suspending aid used in cosmetics, personal care prods., pharmaceuticals; lipsticks, sunscreens, antiperspirants, bath oils; Gardner 1 max. liq.; mild odor; sol. in min. oil, IPA, propylene glycol; misc. with fat, oil and wax mixts.; sp.gr. 0.845-0.855 (15 C); visc. 24-32 cps; acid no. 0.1 max.; sapon. no. 0.3 max.; hyd. no. 195-210; usage level: 2-30%; toxicology: mild skin irritant, nonirritating to eyes.

Noxamine CA 30. [Ceca SA] Cocamine oxide; CAS 61788-90-7; EINECS 263-016-9; nonionic; raw material for foaming shampoos; foam stabilizer, base for hair prods.; detergent, wetting, dispersing, emulsifying, foaming and degreasing agent; Gardner ≤ 2 liq.; sp.gr. 950 kg/m³; visc. 20 cst; solid. pt. -2 C; 30% act.

NPG® Glycol. [Eastman] Neopentyl glycol; CAS 126-30-7; EINECS 204-781-0; cosmetic ingred.; resin intermediate.

Nuodex S-1421 Food Grade. [Syn. Prods.] Calcium stearate FCC; CAS 1592-23-0; EINECS 216-472-8; tablet mold release, powder flow aid, plastic additive, direct food additive; wh. free-flowing powd.; 100% thru 325 mesh; apparent dens. 0.20 g/cc; m.p. 154 C; 2.5% moisture.

Nuodex S-1520 Food Grade. [Syn. Prods.] Calcium stearate FCC; CAS 1592-23-0; EINECS 216-472-8; tablet mold release, powder flow aid, plastic additive, direct food additive; wh. free-flowing powd.; 95% thru 200 mesh; apparent dens. 0.35 g/cc; m.p. 154 C; 2.5% moisture.

Nuodex Magnesium Stearate Food Grade. [Syn. Prods.] Magnesium stearate FCC; CAS 557-04-0; EINECS 209-150-3; tablet mold release, powder flow aid, direct food additive; wh. free-flowing powd.; 100% thru 325 mesh; apparent dens. 0.25 g/cc; m.p. 155 C; 1.0% moisture.

Nuosept 101 CG. [Hüls Am.] Dimethyl oxazolidine; CAS 51200-87-4; EINECS 257-048-2; preservative for cosmetics; sol. in water and oil; usage level: 0.05-0.5%.

Nuosept C. [Hüls Am.; Hüls AG; Costec] Polymethoxy bicyclic oxazolidine; CAS 56709-13-8; nonionic; broad spectrum preservative for cosmetics and toiletries; effective against gram-positive and gram-negative bacteria, yeasts, and molds; suitable for indirect food additives for industrial applics.; USA, Europe approvals; colorless clear liq., low char. odor; sol. in water, alcohol, ethylene glycol, propylene glycol, glycerin; limited sol. in min. oil, IPM, hexane; sp.gr. 1.133-1.155; dens. 9.45-9.64 lb/gal; visc. 3.5-4 cts; f.p. -25 C; flash pt. (TCC) 140 F; ref. index 1.404-1.412; pH 6.0-7.5; usage level: 0.1-0.5%; 50-51% solids.

Nutrapon AL 1. [Clough] Ammonium lauryl ether (1) sulfate; CAS 32612-48-9; anionic; surfactant for shampoos, bubble baths, and other cosmetic prods. below pH 7; liq.; 27-29% conc.

Nutrapon AL 2. [Clough] Ammonium lauryl ether (2) sulfate; CAS 32612-48-9; anionic; surfactant for shampoos, bubble baths, dishwashing detergents; liq.; 25% conc.

Nutrapon AL 30. [Clough] Ammonium lauryl ether (3) sulfate; CAS 32612-48-9; anionic; surfactant for shampoos, bubble baths, dishwashing, and lt. duty detergents; liq.; 26-28% conc.

Nutrapon AL 60. [Clough] Ammonium laureth-3 sulfate; CAS 32612-48-9; anionic; surfactant for shampoo concs., bubble baths, dishwashing, and lt. duty detergents; liq.; 57-60% conc.

Nutrapon AN-3 0481. [Clough] Ammonium laureth sulfate; CAS 32612-48-9; for use in formulating shampoos and bubble baths; liq.; 27-29% act.

Nutrapon B 1365. [Clough] Sodium lauryl sulfate and ethylene glycol stearate; anionic/nonionic; shampoo and detergent blend with pearlizing agent for pearlescent formulations; for shampoos, bubble baths, liq. hand soaps; liq.; 26.5-28.5% act.

Nutrapon BM 3960. [Clough] Sodium laureth-3 sulfate; surfactant for clear liq. shampoos, bubble baths, other cosmetics; visc. liq.; 27-29% act.

Nutrapon BSK 0501. [Clough] Proprietary blend; baby shampoo concs. suitable for cold batch processing; liq.; 36-38% act.

Nutrapon DE 3796. [Clough] DEA-lauryl sulfate; CAS 143-00-0; EINECS 205-577-4; anionic; mild bubble bath and shampoo conc.; liq.; 36% min. conc.

Nutrapon DL 3891. [Clough] Sodium lauryl sulfate; CAS 151-21-3; EINECS 205-788-1; high foaming surfactant for personal care and industrial formulations; liq.; 28-30% act.

Nutrapon ES-2 3677. [Clough] Sodium laureth (2) sulfate; anionic; mild surfactant used in personal care prods.; high tolerance to hard water; liq.; low color and odor; low cloud pt.; 25-26% conc.

Nutrapon ES-60 3568. [Clough] Sodium laureth (3) sulfate; CAS 9004-82-4; anionic; mild surfactant for personal care and industrial prods.; flash foam in hard water; liq.; 56-59% conc.

Nutrapon ESY 2299. [Clough] Sodium laureth-1 sulfate; anionic; surfactant for shampoos, bubble baths, cosmetics; high tolerance to hard water; liq.; 24.5-25.5% act.

Nutrapon HA 3841. [Clough] Ammonium lauryl sulfate; CAS 2235-54-3; EINECS 218-793-9; anionic; surfactant for personal care prods. and detergent cleaners; liq.; 27.0-28.5% conc.

Nutrapon KA 0461. [Clough] Proprietary blend; baby shampoo concs. suitable for cold batch processing; visc. liq.; 37-39% act.

Nutrapon KB-1 0366. [Clough] Proprietary blend; conc. for prep. of clear shampoos, liq. hand soaps; liq.; 34-36% act.

Nutrapon KF 3846. [Clough] Sodium laureth-3 sulfate; anionic; buffered sulfate for use in mild shampoos, bubble baths, shower gels; flash foam in hard water; liq.; 27-29% conc.

Nutrapon KPC 0156. [Clough] Sodium laureth-3 sulfate; CAS 9004-82-4; anionic; surfactant for shampoos, bubble bath, dishwashing detergents; liq.; 27-28% act.

Nutrapon PA 0436. [Clough] Proprietary blend; conc. for prep. of pearlescent shampoos, liq. hand soaps; liq.; 37-38% act.

Nutrapon PP 3563. [Clough] Ammonium lauryl sulfate; CAS 2235-54-3; EINECS 218-793-9; used in nonalkaline shampoos, bubble baths, mild detergents and cleaners below pH 7.0; visc. liq.; 27-30% act.

Nutrapon TK 3603. [Clough] Sodium lauryl sulfate, glycol stearate; pearlized base for shampoos and liq. hand soaps.

Nutrapon TLS-500. [Clough] TEA-lauryl sulfate; CAS 139-96-8; EINECS 205-388-7; anionic; mild ingred. in cosmetic and industrial formulations; liq.; 39% min. act.

Nutrapon TW 3987. [Clough] TEA-lauryl sulfate, sodium lauryl sulfate; surfactant for shampoos, bubble baths, liq. hand soaps; liq.; 33-34% act.

Nutrapon W 1367. [Clough] Sodium lauryl sulfate; CAS 151-21-3; EINECS 205-788-1; anionic; high foaming surfactant for personal care and industrial formulations; liq.; 28-30% conc.

Nutrapon WAC 3005. [Clough] Sodium lauryl sulfate; CAS 151-21-3; EINECS 205-788-1; anionic; surfactant for personal care and industrial formulations; visc. liq.; 28-30% conc.

Nutrapon WAQ. [Clough] Sodium lauryl sulfate; CAS 151-21-3; EINECS 205-788-1; anionic; surfactant for personal care prods. and industrial formulations; very visc. liq.; 28-30% conc.

Nutrapon WAQE 2364. [Clough] Sodium lauryl sulfate; CAS 151-21-3; EINECS 205-788-1; high foaming surfactant for personal care and industrial formulations; liq.; 28.5-29.5% act.

Nutrex PG. [Fabriquimica] Glycosaminoglycans; biological additive for emulsions and clear cosmetics; sp.gr. 1.020-1.030; pH 5.5-6.5; 5.0-5.5% solids.

Nutrex PV. [Fabriquimica] Hydrolyzed corn starch; biological additive for emulsions and clear cosmetics; sp.gr. 1.250-1.270; pH 6.0-7.0; 50-55% solids.

Nutrex RT. [Fabriquimica] Water, spleen extract; biological additive for emulsions and clear cosmetics; sp.gr. 1.015-1.045; pH 5.5-6.5; 2.8-3.5% solids.

Nutrex TM. [Fabriquimica] Water, thymus hydrolysate; biological additive for emulsions and clear cosmetics.

Nutriderme HS 210. [Alban Muller] Propylene glycol, carrot seed extract, cucumber extract, watercress extract, and calendula extract; phytocomplex; face care prod. for dry skin.

Nutriderme HS 240. [Alban Muller] Propylene glycol, fenugreek extract, sunflower seed extract, and myrrh extract; phytocomplex; face care prod. for normal skin.

Nutriderme HS 243. [Alban Muller] Propylene glycol, sunflower seed extract, fenugreek extract, hops extract, and watercress extract; phytocomplex; face care prod. for oily skin.

Nutriderme HS 313. [Alban Muller] Propylene glycol, hops extract, sunflower seed extract, faba bean extract, and wheat germ extract; phytocomplex; face care prod. for normal skin.

Nutriderme LS 613. [Alban Muller] Sunflower seed oil, hops extract, sunflower seed extract, faba bean extract, and wheat germ extract; phytocomplex; face care prod. for normal skin.

Nutriderme LS 640. [Alban Muller] Sunflower seed oil, fenugreek extract, sunflower seed extract, and myrrh extract; phytocomplex; face care prod. for normal skin.

Nutrilan® FPK. [Henkel KGaA/Cospha] Hydrolyzed collagen; CAS 9015-54-7; substantive to skin and hair; powd.; m.w. 5000; pH 5.5-6.5; usage level: 1-4%.

Nutrilan® H. [Henkel KGaA/Cospha; Grünau] Hydrolyzed collagen; CAS 9015-54-7; substantive to skin and hair.

Nutrilan® I. [Henkel/Cospha; Henkel Canada; Henkel KGaA/Cospha; Grünau] Hydrolyzed collagen; CAS 9015-54-7; substantive protein for shampoos, conditioning rinses, hair care prods., cold waves, bath and shower preps.; amber low-visc. clear liq., intrinsic odor; sp.gr. 1.10-1.20; pH 4.0-5.0; 38-40% act.

Nutrilan® I-50. [Henkel/Cospha; Henkel Canada; Henkel KGaA/Cospha; Grünau] Hydrolyzed collagen; CAS 9015-54-7; substantive protein for skin cleansers, shampoos, conditioning rinses, hair care prods.; improves dermatological props. of anionics; amber clear liq., intrinsic odor; sp.gr. 1.16-1.24; pH 4.0-5.0; 50-52% act.

Nutrilan® I-50/NP. [Henkel KGaA/Cospha] Hydrolyzed collagen; CAS 9015-54-7; substantive protein for skin and hair care preps.; improves dermatological props. of anionics; amber clear to sl. turbid liq., char. inherent odor; pH 4.0-5.0; 50-52% dry solids.

Nutrilan® I Powd. [Henkel KGaA/Cospha] Hydrolyzed collagen; CAS 9015-54-7; substantive protein for shampoos, hair care preps.; improves dermatological props. of anionics; beige powd., weak intrinsic odor; pH 4.0-5.0; 94% min. act.

Nutrilan® I-Powd./NP. [Henkel KGaA/Cospha] Hydrolyzed collagen; CAS 9015-54-7; substantive protein for skin and hair care preps.; improves dermatological props. of anionics; beige powd., mild inherent odor; pH 4.0-5.0; 92% min. dry solids.

Nutrilan® L. [Henkel/Cospha; Henkel Canada; Grünau] Hydrolyzed collagen; CAS 9015-54-7; protein for shampoos, conditioning rinses, hair care prods., cold waves, bath and shower preps.; sl. visc. clear liq.; 35% act.

Nutrilan® L/NP. [Henkel KGaA/Cospha] Hydrolyzed collagen; CAS 9015-54-7; substantive protein for skin and hair care preps.; improves dermatological props. of anionics; amber low-visc. clear to sl. turbid liq., char. inherent odor; pH 5.5-6.5; 35-36% dry solids.

Nutrilan® M. [Henkel KGaA/Cospha] Hydrolyzed collagen; CAS 9015-54-7; cosmetics ingred. substantive to skin and hair.

Nutrilan® Cashmere W. [Henkel KGaA/Cospha; Henkel Canada] Hydrolyzed keratin; CAS 69430-36-0; EINECS 274-001-1; hair-identical protective protein with good brightening props.; liq.; pH 5.0-5.8; usage level: 2-6%.

Nutrilan® Elastin E20. [Henkel KGaA/Cospha] Hydrolyzed elastin; CAS 91080-18-1; EINECS 293-509-4; protective protein for skin care prods.; helps skin retain moisture and suppleness; protective colloid in hair cosmetics and other surfactants; amber clear liq., char. intrinsic odor; sol. in water and water/alcohol mixts.; pH 4.5-6.5; 20% min. total solids.

Nutrilan® Elastin P. [Henkel KGaA/Cospha] Hydrolyzed elastin; CAS 91080-18-1; EINECS 293-509-4; protective protein for hair and skin care prods.; film-former helping skin retain its moisture and suppleness; lt. colored powd., char. intrinsic odor; pH 4.8-6.5; 93% min. solids.

Nutrilan® Keratin W. [Henkel/Cospha; Henkel Canada; Henkel KGaA/Cospha] Hydrolyzed keratin; CAS 69430-36-0; EINECS 274-001-1; protective protein for hair care prods., shampoos, and skin cleansers; brownish yel. liq.; m.w. 3000-5000; pH 5.0-5.8; usage level: 2-10%; 20% act.

Nutrimarine. [Sederma] Water, propylene glycol, fish extract, algae extract, and mussel extract; nutritive complex for skin, face, body, and hair care prods.; pale yel. clear liq., char. odor; sp.gr. 1.02-1.04; ref. index 1.370 ± 0.005; pH 5.5-6.5; usage level: 3-7%.

Nutrol Betaine MD 3863. [Clough] Cocamidopropyl betaine; amphoteric; surfactant, foaming agent, foam stabilizer, wetting agent for shampoos, bubble baths, liq. hand soaps; liq.; 33-37% conc.

Nylon N-012. [Presperse] Nylon 6/6, methicone; CAS 32131-17-2, 9004-73-3; imparts soft, lubricious feel to pigmented cosmetic formulations, anhyd. systems, emulsions, and pressed powds.; JSCI/JCID approved; wh. fine powd.; m.p. 175-179 C; pH 6.5-7.5 (5% aq. slurry).

Nylon SI-N. [Presperse] Nylon 6/6, methicone, min. oil; imparts soft, lubricious feel to pigmented cosmetic formulations, anhyd. systems, emulsions, and pressed powds.; JSCI/JCID approved; wh. fine powd.; m.p. 175-179 C; pH 6.5-7.5 (5% aq. slurry).

O

Oasis™. [U.S. Cosmetics] Polyacrylate/lecithin; surface treatment to enhance cosmetic prods.; exc. moisturizing props., feel, and spreadability; absorbs 30 times more moisture than silicone-treated prods.; hygroscopic and hydrophobic.

Obazoline 662Y. [Toho Chem. Industry] Imidazoline deriv.; amphoteric; antistat and softener for syn. fibers; base material for shampoos and hair rinse, nonirritating detergents; liq.; 35% conc.

Obazoline LB-40. [Toho Chem. Industry] n-Alkyl betaine; amphoteric; antistat for hair prods.; liq.; 40% conc.

Oceagen®. [Laboratoires Sérobiologiques] Soluble native collagen; CAS 9007-34-5; EINECS 232-697-4; moisturizer, conditioner improving cell adhesion and growth; for repair activity, anti-aging, and hair care prods.; yel. limpid syrupy liq.; water-sol.; usage level: 1-5%.

Octaprotein. [Vevy] Soy protein; CAS 68153-28-6; cosmetic protein.

OHlan®. [Amerchol; Amerchol Europe] Hydroxylated lanolin; CAS 68424-66-8; EINECS 270-315-8; nonionic; primary w/o emulsifier, aux. emulsifier and stabilizer, pigment wetting and dispersing agent, emollient and conditioner in personal care prods., absorp. bases, pharmaceuticals; yel.-amber to lt. tan waxy solid; misc. with common oil phase ingredients, sol. at low levels in castor oil; oil-misc.; m.p. 39–46 C; HLB 4; acid no. 10 max.; sapon. no. 95–110; 100% conc.

Oil-Soluble Vegetols®. [Gattefosse SA] Plant extracts.

Ointment Base No. 3. [Penreco] Wh. petrolatum USP; CAS 8027-32-5; EINECS 232-373-2; ointment base for eye and skin medications; carrier for medical materials; absorption base in cosmetics; visc. 55–65 SUS (210 F); m.p. 118–125 F; congeal pt. 104–115 F.

Ointment Base No. 4. [Penreco] Wh. petrolatum USP; CAS 8027-32-5; EINECS 232-373-2; ointment base for eye and skin medications; carriers for medical materials; absorption base in cosmetics; Lovibond 1.5Y color; visc. 60-70 SUS (210 F); m.p. 118-125 F; congeal pt. 109-119 F.

Ointment Base No. 6. [Penreco] Wh. petrolatum USP; CAS 8027-32-5; EINECS 232-373-2; ointment base for eye and skin medications; carriers for medical materials; absorption base in cosmetics; Lovibond 1.5Y color; visc. 60-70 SUS (210 F); m.p. 122-133 F; congeal pt. 120-130 F.

Olamida. [Fabriquimica] Alkanolamides; foam booster and thickener for shampoos.

Olamida CD. [Fabriquimica] Cocamide DEA (1:1); CAS 61791-31-9; EINECS 263-163-9; foam booster and thickener for shampoos; acid no. < 6; amine no. 25-35; pH 8-10 (5%).

Olamida CM. [Fabriquimica] Cocamide MEA (1:1); CAS 68140-00-1; EINECS 268-770-2; foam booster and thickener for shampoos; acid no. < 3; amine no. 5-12; pH 8-10 (5%).

Olamida ED. [Fabriquimica] Stearamide DEA (1:1); CAS 93-

82-3; EINECS 202-280-1; foam booster and thickener for shampoos; acid no. < 6; amine no. 25-45; pH 8-10 (5%).

Olamida RD. [Fabriquimica] Ricinoleamide DEA (1:1); CAS 40716-42-5; EINECS 255-051-3; foam booster and thickener for shampoos; acid no. < 6; amine no. 25-35; pH 8-10 (5%).

Olamida SM. [Fabriquimica] Stearamide MEA (1:1); CAS 111-57-9; EINECS 203-883-2; foam booster and thickener for shampoos; acid no. < 3; amine no. 5-20; pH 8-10 (5%).

Olamida UD. [Fabriquimica] Undecylenamide DEA (1:1); CAS 60239-68-1; EINECS 246-914-5; foam booster and thickener for shampoos; anti-dandruff agent; acid no. < 10; amine no. 35-55; pH 8-10 (5%).

Olamida UD 21. [Fabriquimica] Undecylenamide DEA (2:1); CAS 60239-68-1; EINECS 246-914-5; foam booster and thickener for shampoos; anti-dandruff agent; acid no. < 10; amine no. 115-125; pH 9-11 (5%).

Olamin® K. [Henkel Canada; Henkel KGaA/Cospha; Grünau] Sodium laureth sulfate, sodium dodecylbenzenesulfonate, hydrolyzed collagen, potassium cocoyl hydrolyzed collagen, and sodium C14-17 alkyl sec sulfonate; anionic; surfactant blend, base for liq. shampoos; wetting agent, protectant for permanent wave lotions and neutralizers; produces stable H_2O_2 foam fixatives for cold waves; liq.; 25% conc.

Olamin® K/NP. [Henkel KGaA/Cospha] Sodium laureth sulfate, sodium dodecylbenzene sulfonate, hydrolyzed collagen, potassium cocoyl hydrolyzed collagen, and sodium C13-17 alkane sulfonate; surfactant with good dermatological props. for prep. of stable hydrogen peroxide fixatives for cold waves; ylsh. clear liq.; mild inherent odor; visc. 1500-6000 mPa·s; pH 8.0-8.5; 35-37% dry solids.

Oleo-A.F.R. [Laboratoires Sérobiologiques] Flavonoides and liposoluble vitamins; complex providing anti-free radical and anti-lipoperoxide activity; for anti-aging and sun care preps.; golden yel. liq.; lipo-sol.; usage level: 2-3%.

Oleo-Coll™ A240. [Brooks Industries] Isopropyl myristate, sorbitan oleate, myristoyl hydrolyzed collagen; cosmetic ingred.

Oleo-Coll™ A240-20. [Brooks Industries] Isopropyl myristate, sorbitan oleate, myristoyl hydrolyzed collagen; cosmetic ingred.

Oleo-Coll™ ISO. [Brooks Industries] Isostearoyl hydrolyzed collagen; cosmetic ingred.

Oleo-Coll™ LP. [Brooks Industries] Lecithin, butyl stearate, coco-hydrolyzed animal protein, oleoyl sarcosine, sesame oil, lanolin alcohol; cosmetics ingred.; oily liq.; oil-sol.; 100% act.

Oleo-Coll™ LP/LF. [Brooks Industries] Lecithin, butyl stearate, coco-hydrolyzed animal protein, oleoyl sarcosine, sesame oil; cosmetic ingred.

Oleo Keratin™ ISO. [Brooks Industries] AMP isostearoyl hydrolyzed keratin, isostearic acid, myristyl myristate, isopropyl palmitate; raw material for cosmetic and personal care prods.; oily liq.; oil-sol.; 100% act.

Oleoplex. [Fabriquimica] A family of oil-sol. botanical extracts; for cosmetics use.

Oleo-Soy™ C. [Brooks Industries] Cocoyl hydrolyzed soy protein; cosmetic ingredient for hair and skin care prods.; oily liq.; oil-sol.; 100% act.

Oleosterine Arnica. [Exsymol; Biosil Tech.] *Arnica montana* extract; CAS 8057-65-6; plant extract for cosmetics, restructuring, anti-wrinkle prods., day and night creams; brn. oily liq.; sol. in oils; usage level: 0.5-2%.

Olepal 1. [Gattefosse] PEG-6 oleate; CAS 9004-96-0; emulsifier.

Olepal ISO. [Gattefosse SA] PEG-6 isostearate; CAS 56002-14-3; solvent and emulsifier for cosmetic/pharmaceutical emulsions and microemulsions; liq.; HLB 12-13; acid no. < 6; iodine no. < 15; sapon. no. 95-125.

Oligoceane. [Sederma] Water, propylene glycol, oyster shell extract, and sea silt extract; oligoelement hair and skin toner; energizing treatments for face, body, and hair care prods.; pale yel. clear liq., char. odor; sp.gr. 1.00-1.02; ref. index 1.345 ± 0.005; pH 6.5-7.5; usage level: 2-4%.

Oligoidyne Magnesium. [Vevy] Magnesium aspartate; CAS 18962-61-3; EINECS 242-703-7.

Oligoidyne Manganese. [Vevy] Manganese aspartate.

Oligoidyne Selenium. [Vevy] Selenium aspartate.

Oligoidyne Zincum. [Vevy] Zinc aspartate.

Olive Oil, Refined. [Natural Oils Int'l.; Tri-K Industries] Olive oil; CAS 8001-25-0; EINECS 232-277-0; cosmetic ingred.; pale straw clear oil, bland odor and taste; immiscible in water; sp.gr. 0.910-0.915; iodine no. 79-88; sapon. no. 190-195; flash pt. 640 F; toxicology: nonhazardous; edible; trace moisture.

Olympic. [Luzenac Am.] Talc; CAS 14807-96-6; EINECS 238-877-9; for cosmetic applics. incl. baby powds., creams and lotions, foot powds., dusting powds.

Omadine® MDS. [Olin] Bispyrithione, magnesium sulfate; antidandruff agent for nonalkaline hair care prods.; antimicrobial agent for gram-negative and gram-positive bacteria; also inhibits the growth of fungi; wh. to off-wh. powd.; 90% < 100 μ; no or slight odor; sol. in water; m.w. 426.7; sp.gr. 1.730; bulk dens. 0.36 g/cm³; m.p. 210 C; pH 5.5–6.9 (1% in neut. dist. water); toxicology: LD50 (oral, rat) 1 g/kg, (dermal, rabbit) > 2 g/kg; primary skin irritant; eye irritant; 90% min. act.

Omega 6 Complex. [Seporga] A powerful cell membrane revitalizer based on long chain polyunsat. fatty acids, sterols, natural lipids, and vitamins A and E.

Omega-CH Activator. [Herstellung von Naturextrakten GmbH; Lipo] Panthenol, mannitol, tromethamine, glycine, glutamic acid, arginine, alanine, aspartic acid, lysine, leucine, valine, phenylalanine, isoleucine, tyrosine, and histidine; scavenger of oxygen and hydroxyl radicals; increases cell metabolism; enhances water retention; used for high quality cosmetics such as face creams/masks, ampoules, body lotions, after-sun and after-shave prods.; clear aq. sol'n., weak intrinsic odor; sol. in water (100%); sp.gr. 1.124; pH 6.0-7.0; usage level: 1-4%; 46-50% water content.

Onymyrrhe. [Alban Muller] Myrrh extract and polysorbate 20; biological nail regenerator.

O.O.D. [U.S. Cosmetics] 2-Octyldodecyl oleate; CAS 22801-45-2; EINECS 245-228-3; neutral oil imparting pleasant, nongreasy "cooling" feel to cosmetic makeup, sunscreens, hair and skin care prods.

Optigel CD, CF, CG, CK, CL. [United Catalysts] Smectite prod.; thixotrope for latex emulsion systems incl. coatings, sealants, and adhesives; emulsion stabilizer for cosmetics and pharmaceuticals.

Optigel WM. [United Catalysts] Bentonite, cellulose gum;

thixotrope for aq. cosmetic/toiletry creams and lotions, putty, caulk, cleaning compds., waxes, polishes; lt. cream powd.; particle size 85% < 125 μm; sp.gr. 2.41 g/cc; dens. 20.13 lb/gal; pH 9-11 (2% aq. disp.); usage level: 0.5-1.0%; 8% max. moisture.

Optim. [Dow] Glycerin; CAS 56-81-5; EINECS 200-289-5; high purity grade for use as a humectant and moisturizer in personal care prods.

Oramide DL 200 AF. [Seppic] Cocamide DEA; CAS 61791-31-9; EINECS 263-163-9; nonionic; cosmetic emulsifier; liq.; 90% act.

Oramide ML 115. [Seppic] Cocamide MEA; CAS 68140-00-1; EINECS 268-770-2; cosmetic surfactant.

Oramide ML 200. [Seppic] Fatty amide; nonionic; cosmetic additive; flakes; 100% conc.

Oramide MLM 02. [Seppic] PEG-3 cocamide; CAS 61791-08-0; personal care surfactant.

Oramide MLM 06. [Seppic] PEG-7 cocamide; CAS 61791-08-0; personal care surfactant.

Oramide MLM 10. [Seppic] PEG-11 cocamide; CAS 61791-08-0; personal care surfactant.

Oramix CG 110-60. [Seppic] Caprylyl/capryl glucoside; CAS 68515-73-1; nonionic; foaming surfactant, solubilizer used in cosmetic and dermopharmaceutical prods.; liq.; 60% conc.

Oramix L. [Seppic] Lauroyl sarcosine; CAS 97-78-9; EINECS 202-608-3; detergent.

Oramix L30. [Seppic] Sodium lauroyl sarcosinate; CAS 137-16-6; EINECS 205-281-5; anionic; mild surfactant for liq. or gel hand cleaners, personal care prods.; liq.; 30% conc.

Oramix NS 10. [Seppic] Decyl glucoside; CAS 54549-25-6; EINECS 259-218-1; nonionic; foaming surfactant used in cosmetic and dermopharmaceutical prods.; maintains natural biological balance; Gardner 5 max. clear liq.; sp.gr. 1.07; visc. 2000 mPa·s; pH 3-5; usage level: 1-20%; toxicology: LD50 (oral, rat) > 35,000 mg/kg; moderate eye irritant; 55% act. sol'n.

Oramix O. [Seppic] Oleoyl sarcosine; CAS 110-25-8; EINECS 203-749-3; surfactant.

Orange Wax. [Koster Keunen] Orange waxes; CAS 144514-51-2; moisturizer, emollient, uv-A and -B absorber, natural antioxidant and fragrance, mild natural antimicrobial, anti-inflammatory, dispersant, and wetting agent for cosmetic creams, lotions, sun care, makeup, powds., shampoos, conditioners, deodorants, lipsticks, shaving creams, soaps, gels, fragrances; analgesic on burns; solubilizer; improves water resist.; lt. brn. to lt. orange semisolid, char. odor; very sl. sol. in water; sp.gr. 0.92-0.97; m.p. 45-57 C; congeal pt. 45-55 C; b.p. > 200 C; acid no. 8-20; sapon. no. 70-110; hyd. no. 20-50; flash pt. > 200 C; usage level: 1-10%; toxicology: virtually no irritation potential; molten wax may burn skin, cause mild upper respiratory irritation.

Orange Wax, Deodorized. [Koster Keunen] Orange waxes; CAS 144514-51-2; moisturizer, emollient, uv-A and -B absorber, antioxidant, mild antimicrobial, anti-inflammatory for cosmetic creams, lotions, sun care, makeup, powds., shampoos, conditioners, deodorants, lipsticks, shaving creams, soaps, gels, fragrances.

Orapol DL 210. [Seppic] Cocamide DEA, diethanolamine.

Orgasol 1002 D NAT COS. [Atochem N. Am.] Nylon 6; CAS 25038-54-4; raw material for cosmetics, toiletries, pharmaceuticals; absorbent, carrier used in face powds., talc, foundations, tinted creams, lipstick, nail lacquers, skin care, perfumery, and personal hygiene prods.; natural uncolored powd.; avg. particle size 20 μ.

Orgasol 1002 D WHITE 5 COS. [Atochem N. Am.] Nylon 6; CAS 25038-54-4; raw material for cosmetics, toiletries, pharmaceuticals; absorbent, carrier used in face powds., talc, foundations, tinted creams, lipstick, nail lacquers, skin care, perfumery, and personal hygiene prods.

Orgasol 1002 EX D WHITE 10 COS. [Atochem N. Am.] Nylon 6, titanium dioxide; raw material for cosmetics, toiletries, pharmaceuticals; absorbent, carrier used in face powds., talc, foundations, tinted creams, lipstick, nail lacquers, skin care, perfumery, and personal hygiene prods.; wh. extra-fine powd.; avg. particle size 10 μ.

Orgasol 2002 D EXTRA NAT COS. [Atochem N. Am.; Lipo] Nylon 12; CAS 25038-74-8; cosmetic raw material.

Orgasol 2002 D NAT COS. [Atochem N. Am.; Lipo] Nylon 12; CAS 25038-74-8; raw material for cosmetics, toiletries, pharmaceuticals; absorbent, carrier used in face powds., talc, foundations, tinted creams, lipstick, nail lacquers, skin care, perfumery, and personal hygiene prods.; natural uncolored powd.; avg. particle size 20 μ.

Orgasol 2002 EX D NAT COS. [Atochem N. Am.] Nylon 12; CAS 25038-74-8; raw material for cosmetics, toiletries, pharmaceuticals; absorbent, carrier used in face powds., talc, foundations, tinted creams, lipstick, nail lacquers, skin care, perfumery, and personal hygiene prods.; absorbs between 15-25% perfume and enables its release over a period of time; natural uncolored extra-fine powd.; avg. particle size 10 μ.

Orgasol 2002 UD NAT COS. [Atochem N. Am.; Lipo] Nylon 12; CAS 25038-74-8; raw material for cosmetics, toiletries, pharmaceuticals; absorbent, carrier used in face powds., talc, foundations, tinted creams, lipstick, nail lacquers, skin care, perfumery, and personal hygiene prods.; can be supplied impregnated with 12.5% vitamin E or other actives; natural uncolored ultra-fine powd.; avg. particle size 5 μ.

Orgasol 20030 White 5 Cos. [Atochem N. Am.] Nylon.

Ormagel AC-400. [Assessa-Industria] Algae extract, alcohol, sorbitol; conditioner.

Ormagel SH. [Assessa-Industria; Int'l. Sourcing] Algae extract, sorbitol; seaweed extract for cosmetic moisturizing applics., nutrient creams, anticellulitis creams, massage creams, face masks, after-shaves, sunburn preps., hair care prods.; protecting, hydrating, softening, and nutrient agent; pale greenish-yel. to pale brownish-yel. gel, very sl. seaweed odor, sweetish saline taste; sol. in hot water (above 50 C); sp.gr. 1.02; m.p. 50 C; b.p. 212 F; pH 6-7; toxicology: nontoxic, nonirritating; 18% total solids.

Ormagel XPU. [Assessa-Industria; Int'l. Sourcing] Algae extract and sorbitol; hydrating agent, antistat for hair toiletries, shampoos, hair vitalizers; softens and increases luster and body of hair; protects hair fibers; also for body shampoos, soaps as protecting, hydrating, softening, and nutrient agent; pale greenish-yel. to brownish-yel. gellified aq. sol'n., very sl. seaweed odor, saline taste; b.p. 212 F; pH 6-7; toxicology: nontoxic, nonirritating to skin and eyes; 14% total solids.

Oronal BLD. [Seppic] Sodium laureth sulfate; mild surfactant for cosmetics use; 33% conc.

Oronal LCG. [Seppic] Sodium coceth sulfate, PEG-40 glyceryl cocoate; mild surfactant for cosmetics; liq.; 50% act.

Orvus K Liq. [Procter & Gamble] Ammonium laureth sulfate, cocamide MEA, SD alcohol 40-B.

Orzol®. [Witco/Petroleum Spec.] Wh. min. oil USP; emollient, lubricant for food, drug, and cosmetic industry; also for agric., chemicals, pkg., plastics, textiles; FDA §172.878, 178.3620a; water-wh.; sp.gr. 0.869-0.885; visc. 61-64 cSt (40 C); pour pt. -20 C; flash pt. 202 C.

O Silicate. [PQ Corp.] Sodium silicate; CAS 1344-09-8; EINECS 215-687-4.

Ovonol. [Lucas Meyer] Unbleached lipid mixture from egg yolk; emulsifier and dispersant for cosmetic creams and lotions.

Ovothin. [Lucas Meyer] Range of native egg yolk phospholipids; emulsifier and refatting agent for cosmetic creams, lotions, shampoos, lipsticks.

Ovothin 160. [Lucas Meyer] Egg yolk, phospholipids conc.; emulsifier for pharmaceuticals.

Ovothin 170. [Lucas Meyer] Complex of egg yolk phospholipids; emulsifier and dispersant for pharmaceuticals and liposomes.

Ovothin 180. [Lucas Meyer] Isolated phosphatidylcholine from egg yolk; emulsifier and dispersant for pharmaceuticals; 80% conc.

Ovothin 200. [Lucas Meyer] Isolated phosphatidylcholine from egg yolk; emulsifier and dispersant for pharmaceuticals and liposomes; 94% conc.

Ovucire WL 2558. [Gattefosse SA] Hemisynthetic glycerides; excipient for pharmaceutical suppositories; drop pt. 31-36 C; acid no. < 0.5; iodine no. ≤ 3; sapon. no. 240-260.

Ovucire WL 2944. [Gattefosse SA] Hemisynthetic glycerides; excipient for pharmaceutical suppositories; drop pt. 32.5-35.5 C; acid no. < 0.5; iodine no. < 3; sapon. no. 215-235; toxicology: nonirritating rectally.

Oxaban®-A. [Angus] Dimethyl oxazolidine; CAS 51200-87-4; EINECS 257-048-2; cosmetic preservative, antimicrobial; alkaline pH buffering agent; corrosion inhibitor for aq. systems; EEC approved; APHA 25 max. liq.; sol. in water, alcohols, glycols, and min. oil; sp.gr. 0.98-0.99; dens. 8.2 lb/gal; visc. ≈ 7.5 cp; f.p. < -20 F; flash pt. (TCC) 120 F; pH 10.5-11.5; combustible liq.; usage level: 500-2000 ppm; toxicology: LD50 (oral, rats) 950 mg/kg, (dermal, rabbits) 1400 mg/kg; can cause severe eye burns; harmful if swallowed; 78% act. in water.

Oxaban®-E. [Angus] 7-Ethyl bicyclooxazolidine; CAS 7747-35-5; EINECS 231-810-4; antibacterial for cosmetics and toiletries; EEC approved; low odor; sol. in water, alcohols, glycols, min. oil, benzene, acetone, chlorinated hydrocarbons; sp.gr. 1.085 (30/20 C); f.p. 0 C; b.p. 71 C (15 mm Hg); flash pt. (TCC) 175 F; pH 8-9; surf. tens. 36.5 dynes/cm; usage level: 500-2000 ppm; toxicology: LD50 (oral, male rat) 5250 mg/kg, (dermal, rabbits) 1948 mg/kg; severely irritating to skin and eyes.

Oxamin LO. [ICI Australia] Lauryl dimethyl amine oxide; CAS 1643-20-5; EINECS 216-700-6; nonionic; detergent, foamer and foam stabilizer for personal care prods. and detergent formulations; biodeg.; liq.; 30% conc.

Oxetal VD 20. [Zschimmer & Schwarz] Laureth-2; CAS 3055-93-4; EINECS 221-279-7; nonionic; washing and cleansing agent; liq.; 100% act.

Oxetal VD 28. [Zschimmer & Schwarz] Laureth-3; CAS 3055-94-5; EINECS 221-280-2; nonionic; washing and cleansing agent; liq.; 100% act.

Oxylastil. [Sederma] Hydrolyzed soy protein and propylene glycol; cell oxygenation and regeneration for face and body care prods.; prevents damage due to cutaneous ageing; pale yel. clear liq., char. odor; sp.gr. 1.01-1.02; ref. index 1.35-1.37; pH 5.8-7.3; usage level: 3-8%.

Oxynex® 2004. [Rona; E. Merck] BHT (20%), ascorbyl palmitate (10%), citric acid (10%), glyceryl stearate, propylene glycol; antioxidant for pharmaceuticals, cosmetics, and essential oils; EC and US GRAS compliance; unctuous mass, almost odorless, pract. tasteless; sol. in many org. solvs.; insol. in water; usage level: 0.01-0.2%.

Oxynex® K. [Rona; E. Merck] PEG-8 (62%), tocopherol (30%), ascorbyl palmitate (5%), ascorbic acid (1%), and citric acid (1%); antioxidant, stabilizer for fats and oils; esp. for protection of sat. and unsat. components of the oil phase and for inhibition of formation of free radicals; used for food, pharmaceuticals, cosmetics, and essential oils; EC, GRAS compliance; yel. to lt. brn. transparent liq., char. faint odor; usage level: 0.05-0.2%.

Oxynex® L. [Rona; E. Merck] Tocopherol (30%), ascorbyl

palmitate (5%), ascorbic acid (1%), citric acid (1%), ethanol (53%), veg. oil (20%); antioxidant for stabilization of high-grade fats, oils and fat-containing foodstuffs (e.g., shortenings), anti-adhesive emulsions, dried soups, instant cake mixes, cosmetic preps., essential oils; yel. to reddish brn. transparent liq., char. odor; highly flamm.; usage level: 0.005-0.2%.

Oxynex® LM. [Rona; E. Merck] Tocopherol (25%), lecithin (25%), ascorbyl palmitate (20%), glyceryl stearate, glyceryl oleate, citric acid (2.5%); antioxidant esp. suitable for high-grade veg. fats and fat-containing foodstuffs (e.g., shortenings), anti-adhesive emulsions, mayonnaises, margarine, cake mixes, fat-containing pharmaceutical and cosmetics preps., essential oils; German, EC, US GRAS compliances; lt. brn. waxy solid; odorless and tasteless in dilution; sol. in oils and fats; usage level: 0.005-0.1%.

Oxypol. [Gattefosse] Octoxynol-11; CAS 9002-93-1; cosmetic surfactant.

Oxypon 288. [Zschimmer & Schwarz] Olive oil PEG-10 esters; emollient, solubilizer and refatting agent for cosmetics, perfumes, essential oils; paste; 100% act.

Oxypon 306. [Zschimmer & Schwarz] Mink oil PEG-13 esters; emollient, solubilizer and refatting agent for cosmetics, perfumes, essential oils; liq.; water-sol.; 100% act.

Oxypon 328. [Zschimmer & Schwarz] PEG-26 jojoba acid, PEG-26 jojoba alcohol; refatting agent for cosmetics; wax; 100% act.

Oxypon 365. [Zschimmer & Schwarz] Avocado oil PEG-11 esters; refatting agent for cosmetics; liq.; 100% act.

Oxypon 2145. [Zschimmer & Schwarz] PEG-15 glyceryl isostearate; nonionic; emollient, superfatting agent for cosmetics, bath preps., hand cleaners; liq.; 100% act.

Oxyvet. [Henkel/Cospha] Fragrance raw material for cosmetic, personal care, detergent, and cleaning prods.; colorless liq., animal odor; b.p. 112 C; flash pt. 68 C.

P

Pacific Sea Kelp Glycolic Extract B-1063. [Bell Flavors & Fragrances] Source of minerals, vitamins, and amino acids; used in hair care cosmetics adding luster to hair and helping to keep scalp healthy; water-wh. clear liq., char. odor; sol. in water; sp.gr. 1.030-1.050; flash pt. (CC) > 200 F; ref. index 1.320-1.520; toxicology: may cause eye irritation, mild skin irritation on prolonged contact; 0.3-1.5% total solids.

Pad-1. [Vevy] Magnesium carbonate, aluminum silicate.

Padimate O. [Lipo] Octyl dimethyl PABA; CAS 21245-02-3; EINECS 244-289-3; sunscreen agent.

Palatinol® A. [BASF AG] Diethyl phthalate; CAS 84-66-2; EINECS 201-550-6; plasticizer for nail polish, deodorants.

Palatinol® M. [BASF AG] Dimethyl phthalate; CAS 131-11-3; EINECS 205-011-6; plasticizer for nail polish, deodorants; supplementary plasticizer for paints and varnishes.

Pamak 4. [Hercules] Tall oil acid; CAS 61790-12-3; EINECS 263-107-3; surfactant.

Panalane® L-14E. [Amoco] Hydrog. polyisobutene; specifically designed for cosmetics applics.; outstanding feel and moisturizing ability.

Pancogene® S. [Gattefosse] Soluble collagen; CAS 9007-34-5; EINECS 232-697-4; humectant for cosmetics; moisturizer for upper layers of the stratum corneum; improves cutaneous elasticity and tonicity; reduces irritation of lauryl sulfates; used for cosmetic gels, emulsions; sl. visc. liq., faint specific odor; pH 3.5-4.5; 0.3% aq. sol'n.

Pancreatic Lipase 250. [Solvay Enzymes] Lipase; enzyme for hydrolysis of triglycerides to glycerol and fatty acids; used for development of flavors; hydrolysis of egg yolk lipids; pet food improvement; fat modification; pharmaceuticals (digestive aids); waste treatment; cream-colored amorphous dry powd., free from offensive odor; water-sol.

DL-Panthenol Cosmetic Grade No. 63920. [Roche] DL-Panthenol; long-lasting moisturizer for hair and skin care prods.

DL-Panthenol USP, FCC No. 63915. [Roche] DL-Panthenol; long-lasting moisturizer for hair and skin care prods.

Panthequat® . [Innovachem; Tri-K Industries] Panthenyl hydroxypropyl steardimonium chloride; CAS 132467-76-6; cationic; patented substantive quat. used in skin and hair conditioning applics.; 30% more substantive than panthenol; yel. clear to stratified visc. liq.; misc. with water; sp.gr. 1.15 (50 C); b.p. 105 C; pH 6-8 (5% aq.); toxicology: may cause skin and eye irritation; ingestion may cause abdominal upset; 40-50% solids.

Papain 16,000. [Solvay Enzymes] Protease; enzyme for hydrolysis of proteins; for brewing (stabilizes and chillproofs beer); meat tenderizers; pharmaceutical (digestion aids); protein modification; animal feed supplement; leather bating; in paper, photographic, and textile processing; tan to lt. brn. amorphous dry powd., free of offensive odors and taste; water-sol.; usage level: 0.01-0.1%.

Papain 30,000. [Solvay Enzymes] Protease; enzyme for hydrolysis of proteins; for brewing (stabilizes and chillproofs beer); meat tenderizers; pharmaceutical (digestion aids); protein modification; animal feed supplement; leather bating; in paper, photographic, and textile processing; tan to lt. brn. amorphous dry powd., free of offensive odors and taste; water-sol.; usage level: 0.01-0.1%.

Papain Conc. [Solvay Enzymes] Protease; enzyme for hydrolysis of proteins; for brewing (stabilizes and chillproofs beer); meat tenderizers; pharmaceutical (digestion aids); protein modification; animal feed supplement; leather bating; in paper, photographic, and textile processing; tan to lt. brn. amorphous dry powd., free of offensive odors and taste; water-sol.; usage level: 0.01-0.1%.

Paragon™. [McIntyre] Propylene glycol, DMDM hydantoin, methylparaben; patented dual action cosmetics preservative with bactericidal and fungicidal props.; disperses readily in cold systems; USA and Europe approvals; pale to lt. yel. clear liq., mild odor; pH 7.5 (10% aq.); usage level: 0.4-0.8%; 50% conc.

Paragon™ II. [McIntyre] Propylene glycol, DMDM hydantoin, methylparaben, propylparaben; patented dual action cosmetics preservative with bactericidal and fungicidal props.; USA and Europe approvals; pale to lt. yel. clear liq., mild odor; pH 7.5 (10% aq.); usage level: 0.4-0.8%; 44% conc.

Paramul® SAS. [Bernel] Stearamide DIBA-stearate; nonionic; emulsifier, pearlizing agent, opacifier; FDA, EEC compliances; yel. solid; sol. in oil; usage level: 1-3%; 100% conc.

Parapel® HC. [Bernel] Linoleamidopropyl ethyldimonium ethosulfate, dimethyl lauramine isostearate; cationic; emulsifier for after-shampoo conditioner; compat. with hydrogen peroxide; FDA, EEC compliances; yel. liq.; sol. in oil, disp. in water; usage level: 0.5-3.0%.

Parapel® HC-85. [Bernel] Linoleamidopropyl ethyldimonium ethosulfate, dimethyl lauramine isostearate; cationic; emulsifier compat. with most anionic surfactants; hair conditioner; FDA, EEC compliances; yel. liq.; sol. in oil, water; usage level: 0.5-3.0%.

Parapel® HC-99. [Bernel] Linoleamidopropyl ethyl dimonium ethosulfate, dimethyl lauramine isostearate; cationic; fragrance solubilizer for clear conditioners and shampoos; FDA, EEC compliances; yel. liq.; sol. in water; usage level: 0.5-3.0% .

Parapel® LAM-100. [Bernel] Lactamide MEA; CAS 5422-34-4; EINECS 226-546-1; hair conditioner, humectant; compatible with thioglycolate; FDA, EEC compliances; colorless liq.; sol. in water, oil; usage level: 1-5%.

Parapel® LIS. [Bernel] Dimethyl lauramine isostearate; CAS

70729-87-2; shampoo and conditioner additive; silky, velvety emollient; FDA, EEC compliance; yel. liq.; sol. in oil; usage level: 0.5-4.0%.

Parasonarl Mark II. [Nippon Chem. Co. Ltd.] Ethyl urocanate; CAS 27538-35-8; EINECS 248-515-1.

Paridol B. [Jan Dekker BV] Butylparaben; CAS 94-26-8; EINECS 202-318-7; preservative for cosmetics; usage level: 0.001-0.2%.

Paridol E. [Jan Dekker BV] Ethylparaben; CAS 120-47-8; EINECS 204-399-4; preservative for cosmetics; usage level: 0.08-1.0%.

Paridol M. [Jan Dekker BV] Methylparaben; CAS 99-76-3; EINECS 202-785-7; preservative for cosmetics; colorless; usage level: 0.1-1.0%; toxicology: nontoxic.

Paridol P. [Jan Dekker BV] Propylparaben; CAS 94-13-3; EINECS 202-307-7; cosmetic preservative; USA, Japan, Europe approvals; colorless; usage level: 0.02-1.0%; toxicology: nontoxic.

Parsol® 1789. [Bernel; Givaudan-Roure] Butyl methoxydibenzoylmethane; CAS 70356-09-1; uv-A absorber (320-400 nm) and uv-B absorber (290-320 nm) photostability of cosmetic creams, lotions, skin care prods., sunscreens; EEC and Japanese compliance; lt. tan cryst. powd., weakly aromatic odor; sol. 6-25% in esters, 2% i ethanol; m.w. 310.4; m.p. 83.5 C; usage level: 0.5-3%; 97.5% purity.

Parsol® 5000. [Givaudan-Roure] Methylbenzylidene camphor; CAS 36861-47-9; EINECS 253-242-6; cosmetic uv-B filter for use with Parsol MCX; can raise the SPF above 15; EEC compliance; wh. to off-wh. powd., sl. aromatic odor; sol. in cosmetic lipids; m.w. 254.4; m.p. 66-70 C; flash pt. (TCC) > 100 C; usage level: 0.5-6%; 99% min. purity.

Parsol® HS. [Givaudan-Roure] Phenylbenzimidazole sulfonic acid; CAS 27503-81-7; hydro-sol. cosmetic uv-B filter used with oil-sol. Parsol prods. to obtain cost-effective high SPF formulations; for aq. sunscreen gels; FDA, EEC compliance; wh. fine cryst. powd., odorless; insol. in water in acid form—neutralize before adding; m.w. 274.30; 98% min. purity.

Parsol® MCX. [Bernel; Givaudan-Roure] Octyl methoxycinnamate; CAS 5466-77-3; EINECS 226-775-7; uv-B absorber, sunscreening agent in the wavelength range of 2900–3200 Å which causes sunburn and skin damage, stimulates tanning; FDA, EEC, and Japanese compliances; pale yel sl. visc. liq., pract. odorless; m.w. 290.4; sol. (g/l 100 g solv.): sol. > 50 g in ethanol, 99% IPA, IPM, sweet almond oil, min. oil, coconut oil, dipropylene glycol; 1 g in propylene glycol; sp.gr. 1.007–1.017; b.p. 198–200 C (3 mm); f.p. < -25 C; acid no. 1.0 max.; ref. index 1.545; usage level: 1-10%; 98% min. purity.

Parvan® 127. [Exxon] Petroleum hydrocarbon wax; fully refined wax with enhanced oxidation resist. for food, health, and cosmetic applics.; suited for barbeque lighter bricks, butcher wrap, candles, cheese coating, corrugated paperboard, lumber end coating; FDA compliance; Saybolt +30 color; dens. 6.78 lb/gal (60 F); kinematic visc. 3.5 cSt (210 F); m.p. 127 F; flash pt. 420 F; trace materials constitute explosive hazard; toxicology: may cause skin irritation on prolonged/repeated contact.

Parvan® 129. [Exxon] Petroleum hydrocarbon wax; fully refined wax with enhanced oxidation resist. for food, health, and cosmetic applics.; FDA compliance; Saybolt +30 color; dens. 6.79 lb/gal (60 F); kinematic visc. 3.6 cSt (210 F); m.p. 129 F; flash pt. 420 F; trace materials constitute explosive hazard; toxicology: may cause skin irritation on prolonged/repeated contact.

Parvan® 131. [Exxon] Petroleum hydrocarbon wax; fully refined wax with enhanced oxidation resist. for food, health, and cosmetic applics.; suited for butcher wrap,

corrugated paperboard, cups, drinking straws, shoe polish, wax paper; FDA compliance; Saybolt +30 color; dens. 6.79 lb/gal (60 F); kinematic visc. 3.7 cSt (210 F); m.p. 131 F; flash pt. 425 F; trace materials constitute explosive hazard; toxicology: may cause skin irritation on prolonged/repeated contact.

Parvan® 137. [Exxon] Petroleum hydrocarbon wax; fully refined wax with enhanced oxidation resist. for food, health, and cosmetic applics.; suited for candles, corrugated paperboard, cups, glassine, paste wax, wax paper; FDA compliance; Saybolt +30 color; dens. 6.81 lb/gal (60 F); kinematic visc. 4.1 cSt (210 F); m.p. 137 F; flash pt. 440 F; trace materials constitute explosive hazard; toxicology: may cause skin irritation on prolonged/repeated contact.

Parvan® 138. [Exxon] Petroleum hydrocarbon wax; fully refined wax with enhanced oxidation resist. for food, health, and cosmetic applics.; FDA compliance; Saybolt +30 color; dens. 6.83 lb/gal (60 F); kinematic visc. 4.2 cSt (210 F); m.p. 138 F; flash pt. 446 F; trace materials constitute explosive hazard; toxicology: may cause skin irritation on prolonged/repeated contact.

Parvan® 142. [Exxon] Petroleum hydrocarbon wax; fully refined wax with enhanced oxidation resist. for food, health, and cosmetic applics.; suited for candles, crayons and industrial markers, paste wax, tires; FDA compliance; Saybolt +30 color; dens. 6.85 lb/gal (60 F); kinematic visc. 5.0 cSt (210 F); m.p. 142 F; flash pt. 450 F; trace materials constitute explosive hazard; toxicology: may cause skin irritation on prolonged/repeated contact.

Parvan® 145. [Exxon] Petroleum hydrocarbon wax; fully refined wax with enhanced oxidation resist. for food, health, and cosmetic applics.; FDA compliance; Saybolt +30 color; dens. 6.85 lb/gal (60 F); kinematic visc. 5.1 cSt (210 F); m.p. 145 F; flash pt. 460 F; trace materials constitute explosive hazard; toxicology: may cause skin irritation on prolonged/repeated contact.

Parvan® 147. [Exxon] Petroleum hydrocarbon wax; fully refined wax with enhanced oxidation resist. for food, health, and cosmetic applics.; FDA compliance; Saybolt +30 color; dens. 6.87 lb/gal (60 F); kinematic visc. 5.4 cSt (210 F); m.p. 147 F; flash pt. 470 F; trace materials constitute explosive hazard; toxicology: may cause skin irritation on prolonged/repeated contact.

Parvan® 154. [Exxon] Petroleum hydrocarbon wax; fully refined wax with enhanced oxidation resist. for food, health, and cosmetic applics.; suited for hot-melt adhesives, candles, paper plates, paste wax, tires; FDA compliance; Saybolt +30 color; dens. 6.91 lb/gal (60 F); kinematic visc. 6.6 cSt (210 F); congeal pt. 154 F; flash pt. 500 F; trace materials constitute explosive hazard; toxicology: may cause skin irritation on prolonged/repeated contact.

Parvan® 158. [Exxon] Petroleum hydrocarbon wax; fully refined wax with enhanced oxidation resist. for food, health, and cosmetic applics.; FDA compliance; Saybolt +28 color; dens. 6.93 lb/gal (60 F); kinematic visc. 7.6 cSt (210 F); congeal pt. 158 F; flash pt. 500 F; trace materials constitute explosive hazard; toxicology: may cause skin irritation on prolonged/repeated contact.

Parvan® 161. [Exxon] Petroleum hydrocarbon wax; fully refined wax with enhanced oxidation resist. for food, health, and cosmetic applics.; FDA compliance; Saybolt +27 color; dens. 6.95 lb/gal (60 F); kinematic visc. 8.6 cSt (210 F); congeal pt. 161 F; flash pt. 500 F; trace materials constitute explosive hazard; toxicology: may cause skin irritation on prolonged/repeated contact.

Pationic® 122A. [R.I.T.A.] Sodium capryl lactylate; anionic; emulsifier/foam booster for facial cleansers and personal care prods.; microbial inhibitor properties; amber clear visc. liq.; sol. in propylene glycol, IPM, IPA, hazy in water; visc. 24 cps (2% aq.); HLB 11.3; acid no. 65-85; sapon. no. 235-265; pH 5.25 (2% aq.); surf. tens. 24.72 dynes/cm (0.1%); toxicology: LD50 (oral, rat) 5.84 g/kg; nontoxic by ingestion; nonirritating to skin, eyes; 100% conc.

Pationic® 138C. [R.I.T.A.] Sodium lauroyl-2-lactylate; CAS 13557-75-0; EINECS 236-942-6; anionic; detergent, conditioner, foam booster, visc. builder, lipophilic emulsifier, cleansing agent used in shampoos, facial cleansers; beige waxy solid; sol. in distilled water; visc. 19 cps; m.p. 55-59 C; HLB 14.4; acid no. 50-70; sapon. no. 175-205; pH 6.90 (2% aq.); surf. tens. 24.30 dynes/cm (0.1%); toxicology: LD50 (oral, rat) 6.81 g/kg; nontoxic by ingestion; nonirritating to skin, eyes; 100% conc.

Pationic® CSL. [R.I.T.A.] Calcium stearoyl-2-lactylate; CAS 5793-94-2; EINECS 227-335-7; anionic; w/o emulsifier and protein complexer for cosmetics; off-wh. to lt. tan powd.; visc. 85 cps; m.p. 45-55 C; HLB 5.1; acid no. 50-65; sapon. no. 195-230; pH 4.90 (2% aq.); surf. tens. 37 dynes/cm (0.1%); toxicology: LD50 (oral, rat) > 25 g/kg; nontoxic by ingestion; not a primary skin irritant; nonirritating to eyes; 100% conc.

Pationic® ISL. [R.I.T.A.] Sodium isostearoyl-2-lactylate; CAS 66988-04-3; EINECS 266-533-8; anionic; surfactant, emulsifier for cosmetics; perfume solubilizer; substantive conditioner for hair and skin; exc. moisture absorp.; straw, honey clear visc. liq.; sol. in min. oil, propylene glycol, IPM, IPA; disp. in water; HLB 5.9; acid no. 60-70; sapon. no. 205-225; pH 6.30 (2% aq.); surf. tens. 26.28 dynes/cm (0.1%); toxicology: LD50 (oral, rat) 6.1 g/kg; nontoxic by ingestion; irritating to eyes; 100% act.

Pationic® SBL. [R.I.T.A.] Sodium behenoyl lactylate; anionic; surfactant, humectant, substantive conditioner for hair care prods.; beige solid.

Pationic® SCL. [R.I.T.A.] Sodium cocoyl lactylate; anionic; surfactant, humectant, substantive conditioner for hair care prods.; beige solid.

Pationic® SSL. [R.I.T.A.] Sodium stearoyl 2-lactylate; CAS 25383-99-7; EINECS 246-929-7; anionic; emulsifier, visc. builder, protein complexer for cosmetics prods.; off-wh. to lt. tan powd.; sol. @ 1% conc. and 25 C; disp. in dist. water and min. oil; visc. 175 cps; HLB 6.5; m.p. 47-53 C; acid no. 60-70; sapon. no. 210-235; pH 5.95 (2% aq.); surf. tens. 32.34 dynes/cm (0.1%); toxicology: LD50 (oral, rat) > 2.5 g/kg; nontoxic by ingestion; not a primary skin irritant; nonirritating to eyes; 100% conc.

Patlac® IL. [Am. Ingredients/Patco; R.I.T.A.] Isostearyl lactate; CAS 42131-28-2; EINECS 255-674-0; nonionic; surfactant, emollient for cosmetics; pale yel. low visc. liq.; sol. in ethanol, propylene glycol, min. oil, IPM; insol. in water; sp.gr. 0.92; HLB 10.3 ± 1.0; acid no. 2 max.; sapon. no. 162-182; pH 4.5 (2% aq.); toxicology: LD50 (oral, rat) 7.5 g/kg; nontoxic and nonirritating; 100% conc.

Patlac® LA. [Am. Ingredients/Patco; R.I.T.A.] Lactic acid; CAS 50-21-5; EINECS 200-018-0; moisture binder, humectant for cosmetics; clear liq.; sp.gr. 1.195-1.20; toxicology: irritant to eyes, skin, and mucous membranes in conc. form; 88% act.

Patlac® NAL. [Am. Ingredients/Patco; R.I.T.A.] Sodium lactate; CAS 72-17-3; EINECS 200-772-0; pH buffer, humectant, stabilizer, component of stratum corneum; for food, pharmaceutical, and cosmetic industries; clear liq.; sp.gr. 1.31-1.34; pH 8-9; toxicology: nontoxic if ingested; nonirritating to skin and eyes; 60% conc.

PCL Liq. 2/066210. [Dragoco] Cetearyl octanoate, isopropyl myristate.

PCL Liq. 100. [Dragoco] Cetearyl octanoate and trace amts. of cetyl octanoate; CAS 59130-70-0; emollient for cosmetics; colorless lt. oily liq., odorless; insol. in water; sp.gr.

0.8500-0.8550; flash pt. (CC) 212 F; ref. index 1.4440-1.4460; toxicology: skin and eye irritant.

PCL Liq. 1002/066240. [Dragoco] Cetearyl octanoate; emollient.

PCL Liq. Watersoluble 2/966213. [Dragoco] PEG-13 octanoate.

PCL SE w/o 2/066255. [Dragoco] Ceresin, lanolin, cetearyl octanoate, sorbitan sesquioleate, stearyl heptanoate, min. oil, trihydroxystearin, isopropyl myristate.

Pea Pro-Tein BK. [Maybrook] Hydrolyzed pea protein; CAS 9008-99-8; substantive protein, film-former, moisturizer for skin and hair car prods. (shampoos, conditioners, creams, lotions, liq. hand soaps); anti-irritant in anionic formulations; amber clear liq., mild char. odor; pH 4.-6.0; 12-17% nonvolatiles.

Pearex® L. [Solvay Enzymes] Fungal pectinase; CAS 9032-75-1; EINECS 232-885-6; enzyme used to prevent haze formation in pear and apple processing; clarification and stabilization of fruit juices; vegetable processing; extraction of flavors and fragrances; clear to amber brn. liq.; misc. with water; sp.gr. 1.05-1.15.

Pearl I. [Presperse] Bismuth oxychloride; CAS 7787-59-9; EINECS 232-122-7; pearl pigment for pigmented cosmetics; JSCI/JCID approved; silvery wh. pearlescent free-flowing powd.; particle size 5-25 μ; 98% BiOCl.

Pearl II. [Presperse] Bismuth oxychloride; CAS 7787-59-9; EINECS 232-122-7; pearl pigment for pigmented cosmetics; JSCI/JCID approved; wh. pearlescent free-flowing powd.; particle size 5-20 μ; 98% BiOCl.

Pearlex GC 0311. [Clough] Proprietary blend; pearlizing/opacifying agent for shampoos, bubble baths, liq. hand soaps at low addition levels; visc. liq.; 37-39% act.

Pearl-Glo®. [ISP Van Dyk] Bismuth oxychloride; CAS 7787-59-9; EINECS 232-122-7; pearlescent pigment powds. and disps. for cosmetic eye, face, lip, and body makeup; exc. binding chars. for pressed powds.; high skin adhesion and covering power; uv-resist.

Pearl Super Supreme. [Presperse] Bismuth oxychloride; CAS 7787-59-9; EINECS 232-122-7; pearlescent pigment for cosmetics; JSCI/JCID approved; speckly silver free-flowing powd.; particle size 25-100 μ; 98% BiOCl.

Pearl Supreme UVS. [Presperse] Bismuth oxychloride; CAS 7787-59-9; EINECS 232-122-7; uv-stable pearlescent pigment for cosmetics use; JSCI/JCID approved; silver pearlescent free-flowing powd.; particle size 10-50 μ.

Peceol. [Gattefosse] Glyceryl oleate.

Peceol Isostearique. [Gattefosse SA] Glyceryl isostearate; CAS 32057-14-0; nonionic; w/o coemulsifier; pigment dispersant; additive for lipsticks; superfatting agent for emulsified preps.; Gardner < 6 semicryst., faint odor; very sol. in min. oils; sol. in ethanol, chloroform, methylene chloride; insol. in water; sp.gr. 0.930-0.970; visc. 0.7-1.2 Pa·s; HLB 3.0; acid no. < 4; iodine no. < 15; sapon. no. 150-170; hyd. no. 240-280; ref. index 1.455-1.475; toxicology: nonirritating to skin; sl. irritating to eyes; 100% conc.

Pecogel A-12. [Phoenix] PVP/polycarbamyl polyglycol ester; hydrogel.

Pecogel GC-310, GC-1110. [Phoenix] PVP/dimethylaminoethylmethacrylate/polycarbamyl polyglycol ester; hydrogel.

Pecogel H-12, H-115, H-1220. [Phoenix] PVP/polycarbamyl polyglycol ester; hydrogel.

Pecogel S-1120. [Phoenix] PVP/dimethiconylacrylate/polycarbamyl polygycol ester; hydrogel.

Pecosil® OS-100B. [Phoenix] Dimethicone propylethylenediamine behenate; CAS 133448-12-1; film-former imparting high sheen to skin and hard surfaces; humectant and protective barrier on skin and hair; used in creams, lotions, mascara, lipstick, hair conditioners and styling prods., eyeliners, shampoos, mousses; very visc. paste; toxicology: nontoxic orally; nonirritating to skin and eyes; noncomedogenic; 100% act.

Pecosil® PS-100. [Phoenix] Dimethicone copolyol phosphate; CAS 132207-31-9; anionic; o/w emulsifier, pigment wetting and dispersing agent; imparts silky feel to aq. formulations, skin creams/lotions, mousses, hair conditioners, shaving prods., bath prods. and gels, shampoos, sunscreens, makeup; clear to sl. hazy visc. liq.; water-sol.; sp.gr. 1.01 g/ml; acid no. 37-47; flash pt. (TCC) > 200 F; pH 2-4 (1%); toxicology: nonirritating to skin and eyes; nontoxic orally; noncomedogenic; 100% act.

Pecosil® PS-100K. [Phoenix] Potassium dimethicone copolyol phosphate; o/w emulsifier exhibiting increased cushion in creams, lotions, hair conditioners, sunscreen prods., after-perm treatments; yel. clear to sl. hazy liq.; pH 6.5; toxicology: orally nontoxic; nonprimary skin irritant; nonirritating to eyes; noncomedogenic; 55% solids in water.

Pegosperse® 50 DS. [Lonza] Glycol distearate; CAS 627-83-8; EINECS 211-014-3; nonionic; emulsifier, opacifier, visc. modifier, and stabilizer for suspensions and dispersions, cosmetic hair and skin care prods., household dishwashing liqs., liq. hand soap; emollient, lubricant and pigment dispersant in pharmaceuticals and cosmetics; thickener, wetting agent and plasticizer in hair prods.; wh. beads; sol. in ethanol, min. and veg. oil; insol. in water; HLB 1; m.p. 59 C; acid no. 6 max.; iodine no. < 1; sapon. no. 190-200; pH 5 (3%); 100% conc.

Pegosperse® 50 MS. [Lonza] Glycol stearate; CAS 111-60-4; EINECS 203-886-9; nonionic; surfactant, opacifier, pearlescent, aux. emulsifier for cosmetics (hair and skin care prods.), bath and shower prods., household formulations; dispersant, emulsifier for o/w emulsions for industrial, textile, plastics, water treatment; wh. beads; sol. in methanol, ethanol, acetone, ethyl acetate, toluol, naphtha, min. and veg. oils; sp.gr. 0.96; m.p. 58 C; HLB 2; acid no. < 5; iodine no. < 1; sapon. no. 170-190; pH 5.0 (3% aq.); 100% conc.

Pegosperse® 100 L. [Lonza] PEG-2 laurate SE; nonionic; self-dispersing surfactant, w/o or o/w emulsifier for cosmetic creams and lotions, textile spin finishes and lubricants, solv. and solventless coatings, paper defoamer formulations; straw clear liq.; sol. in ethanol, toluol, naphtha, min. oil; disp. in water; sp.gr. 0.97; HLB 7; solid. pt. < 13 C; acid no. < 4; sapon. no. 160-170; pH 9 (5% aq.); 100% conc.

Pegosperse® 100 O. [Lonza] PEG-2 oleate SE; CAS 106-12-7; nonionic; self-dispersing surfactant, w/o and aux. o/w emulsifier for latex and aq. paints, solv. and solventless coatings, min. oil-based defoamers, inks, drycleaning soaps; emollient and lubricant in cosmetic creams and lotions; amber clear liq.; sol. in methanol, ethanol, toluol, naphtha; disp. in water; sp.gr. 0.93; f.p. < 0 C; HLB 4; acid no. 80-95; iodine no. 70-80; sapon. no. 160-175; pH 8 (5% aq.); 100% conc.

Pegosperse® 100-S. [Lonza] PEG-2 stearate SE; CAS 106-11-6; nonionic; self-emulsifying surfactant; thickener for cosmetic creams and lotions; dispersant and thickener for household polishes, waxes, pastes; antitack agent in rubber molding lubricants; off-wh. beads; sol. in methanol, ethanol, toluol, naphtha, min. and veg. oils; disp. in water; sp.gr. 0.96; m.p. 52 C; HLB 4; acid no. 95-105; sapon. no. 165-175; pH 7 (5%); 100% conc.

Pegosperse® 200 DL. [Lonza] PEG-4 dilaurate; CAS 9005-02-1; nonionic; surfactant, dispersant, emulsifier for cosmetic bath oils, lotions, household pastes, polishes; emulsifier, dispersant, opacifier, visc. control agent, defoamer for textiles, plastics, water treatment; yel. clear liq.; sol. in ethanol, min. and veg. oil; disp. in water; sp.gr. 0.96; solid.

pt. 3 C; HLB 7 ± 1; acid no. 5 max.; sapon. no. 170-185; 100% conc.

Pegosperse® 200 ML. [Lonza] PEG-4 laurate; CAS 9004-81-3; nonionic; dispersant, emulsifier, emollient, visc. modifier for cosmetics (bath oils, lotions, cream rinses, shampoos); visc. modifier for PVC plastisols; defoamer for aq. coatings; emulsifier for textile spin finish formulations; lt. yel. clear liq.; sol. in methanol, ethanol, acetone, ethyl acetate, toluol; misc. with water, sp.gr. 0.99; HLB 9; solid pt. < 5; acid no. 5 max.; sapon. no. 149-159; pH 5 (5% aq.); 100% conc.

Pegosperse® 200 MO. [Lonza] PEG-4 oleate; CAS 9004-96-0; EINECS 233-293-0; nonionic; emulsifier for creams, dispersant, visc. control agent, defoamer.

Pegosperse® 200 MS. [Lonza] PEG-4 stearate; CAS 9004-99-3; EINECS 203-358-8; nonionic; emulsifier and solubilizer for creams and lotions.

Pegosperse® 300 MO. [Lonza] PEG-6 oleate; CAS 9004-96-0; nonionic; emulsifier and solubilizer for creams and lotions.

Pegosperse® 400 DL. [Lonza] PEG-8 dilaurate; CAS 9005-02-1; nonionic; surfactant, emulsifier for cosmetic lotions, bath oils, formulations requiring clarity; provides low temp. flexibility and visc. modification for PVC plastisols; lubricant in textile spin finishes; yel. clear liq.; sol. in methanol, ethanol, acetone, ethyl acetate, toluol, naphtha, min. and veg. oils; sp.gr. 0.99; solid. pt. 5-12 C; HLB 15; acid no. < 5; iodine no. 7.5; sapon. no. 130-140; pH 4 (5% aq.); 100% conc.

Pegosperse® 400 DO. [Lonza] PEG-8 dioleate; CAS 9005-07-6; nonionic; surfactant for cosmetic lotions, bath oils; visc. modifier for PVC plastisols; yel. clear liq.; sol. in methanol, ethanol, ethyl acetate, toluol, naphtha, min. and veg. oils; disp. in water; sp.gr. 0.97; solid. pt. < 0 C; HLB 8.0 ± 0.5; acid no. < 10; iodine no. 52; sapon. no. 115-125; pH 5.5 (5% aq.); 100% conc.

Pegosperse® 400 DOT. [Lonza] PEG-8 ditallate; CAS 61791-01-3; nonionic; surfactant, emulsifier for paper defoamers, solv. and solventless coatings; emulsifier, dispersant, opacifier, visc. control agent, defoamer for cosmetic, household prods., textiles, paper, water treatment; yel. liq.; HLB 8; acid no. 16 max.; iodine no. 75-85; sapon. no. 115-125; pH 4 (5%).

Pegosperse® 400 DS. [Lonza] PEG-8 distearate; CAS 9005-08-7; nonionic; surfactant, visc. modifier, and thickener in hair care prods., creams and lotions; thickener and binder in deodorant sticks; emulsifier for o/w emulsions; dispersant; for industrial, household, and cosmetic use; cream soft solid; sol. in ethanol, ethyl acetate, toluol, naphtha, min. and veg. oil, methanol; disp. in water; sp.gr. 0.98; m.p. 33 C; HLB 8; acid no. < 10; sapon. no. 115-125; pH 5 (5% aq.); 100% conc.

Pegosperse® 400 ML. [Lonza] PEG-8 laurate; CAS 9004-81-3; nonionic; surfactant, emulsifier, dispersant for cosmetic lotions, hair conditioners, clear bath oils; visc. modifier in PVC plastisols; emulsifier, lubricant in textile spin finishes; emulsifier, leveling agent, pigment dispersant, and wetting agent for coatings; solubilizer for oils and solvs.; straw clear liq.; sol. in methanol, ethanol, acetone, ethyl acetate, toluol, veg. and min. oil; misc. with water; sp.gr. 1.03; HLB 14; solid. pt. < 7 C; acid no. < 3; sapon. no. 90-100; pH 5 (5% aq.); 100% conc.

Pegosperse® 400 MO. [Lonza] PEG-8 oleate; CAS 9004-96-0; nonionic; surfactant, emulsifier for cosmetic lotions, bath oils; emulsifier, processing aid for calf-milk replacer formulations; emulsifier, lubricant, softener, scouring agent for textiles; emulsifier for coatings; emulsifier for cutting oils and solvs. in industrial degreasers; yel. clear liq.; sol. in methanol, ethanol, acetone, ethyl acetate, toluol, naphtha; disp. in water; sp.gr. 1.01; solid. pt. < 0 C;

HLB 11.0 ± 0.5; acid no. 2 max.; iodine no. 34-38; sapon. no. 80-88; pH 5 (5% aq.); 100% conc.

Pegosperse® 400 MS. [Lonza] PEG-8 stearate; CAS 9004-99-3; nonionic; surfactant, o/w emulsifier, thickener, pigment grinding aid in hair, skin, and makeup prods., household polishes, cleaners, silicone-based lubricants; emulsifier, lubricant, and softener for textile processing oils and finishes; component of diamond abrasive pastes; antigel agent in starch sol'ns. for paper industry; wh. soft solid; sol. in methanol, ethanol, acetone, ethyl acetate, toluol, naphtha, min. and veg. oils; disp. in water; ; sp.gr. 1.0; m.p. 30 C min.; HLB 11; acid no. 3 max.; sapon. no. 83-94; pH 5 (5% aq.); 100% conc.

Pegosperse® 600 DOT. [Lonza] PEG-12 ditallate; CAS 61791-01-3; nonionic; emulsifier, dispersant, opacifier, visc. control agent, defoamer for cosmetic, household prods., textiles, paper, water treatment; Gardner 10 liq.; HLB 9; acid no. 15; sapon. no. 101.

Pegosperse® 600 ML. [Lonza] PEG-12 laurate; CAS 9004-81-3; nonionic; surfactant, emulsifier, dispersant for cosmetic lotions, clear bath oils; emulsifier and pigment grinding aid in coatings; emulsifier, lubricant in textile spin finishes; lt. yel. clear liq.; sol. in water, methanol, ethanol, acetone, ethyl acetate, naphtha; sp.gr. 1.01; solid. pt. 16–21 C; HLB 15; acid no. < 1; sapon. no. 65-75; pH 5 (5% aq.); 100% conc.

Pegosperse® 600 MO. [Lonza] PEG-12 oleate; CAS 9004-96-0; nonionic; emulsifier and solubilizer for creams and lotions.

Pegosperse® 1500 DL. [Lonza] PEG-6-32 dilaurate; nonionic; visc. control agent for creams and lotions.

Pegosperse® 1500 MS. [Lonza] PEG-6-32 stearate; CAS 9004-99-3; nonionic; emulsifier for cosmetic creams, skin care prods., silicone-based lubricants; wh. solid; sol. in ethanol, ethyl acetate, toluol, veg. oil, methanol, naphtha; misc. with water; sp.gr. 1.05; m.p. 27-31 C; HLB 14; acid no. 8.5 max.; sapon. no. 57-67; pH 4 (5% aq.); 100% conc.

Pegosperse® 1750 MS. [Lonza] PEG-40 stearate; CAS 9004-99-3; nonionic; emulsifier for o/w emulsions; dispersant for industrial, household, and cosmetic use; wh. flakes; sol. in water, ethanol; HLB 18 ± 1; m.p. 46 C; sapon. no. 25–35; 100% conc.

Pegosperse® 1750 MS K Spec. [Lonza] PEG-40 stearate; CAS 9004-99-3; nonionic; surfactant, emulsifier, visc. modifier for cosmetic creams, skin care prods.; emulsifier for silicone-based lubricants; Kosher certified; wh. flakes; HLB 18; acid no. 1 max.; sapon. no. 25-35.

Pegosperse® PMS CG. [Lonza] Propylene glycol stearate; CAS 1323-39-3; EINECS 215-354-3; nonionic; thickener, whipping agent for cosmetic creams; m.p. modifier for lipsticks, deodorant sticks; w/o emulsifier; Gardner 2 max. flakes, waxy solid; m.p. 51 C; HLB 3; acid no. 3 max.; sapon. no. 180.

Pelemol 88. [Phoenix] Octyl octanoate; CAS 7425-14-1; EINECS 231-057-1; very dry cosmetic ester for use in skin preps. where initial light oiliness and dryness on rub-on are desirable; liq.

Pelemol 89. [Phoenix] Octyl isononanoate; CAS 71566-49-9; EINECS 275-637-2; very dry cosmetic ester useful in skin preps. where initial light oiliness and dryness on rub-in are desirable; liq.

Pelemol 108. [Phoenix] Isodecyl octanoate; CAS 89933-26-6; cosmetic ester; liq.; oil-sol.

Pelemol 300B. [Phoenix] C20-40 alcohols behenate; m.p. modifier for solid sticks, lip and makeup prods.; brittle flake; m.p. 85-90 C.

Pelemol 2022. [Phoenix] Octyldodecyl behenate; cosmetic ester with good cushion; for skin creams and lotions; visc. liq.

Pelemol BB. [Phoenix] Behenyl behenate; CAS 17671-27-1; EINECS 241-646-5; emollient and visc. builder imparting richness to oil phase of creams and lotions; also for stick deodorants; wh. flake; oil-sol.

Pelemol BIS. [Phoenix] Behenyl isostearate; emollient for makeup, lip and skin prods.; solid; oil-sol.; m.p. 41 C.

Pelemol CA. [Phoenix] Cetyl acetate; CAS 629-70-9; EINECS 211-103-7; Acetulan replacement for skin preps.; very lt. liq.

Pelemol CR. [Phoenix] Cetyl ricinoleate; CAS 10401-55-5; EINECS 233-864-4; emollient for lipstick and makeup; cryst. solid; oil-sol.

Pelemol DIA. [Phoenix] Diisopropyl adipate; CAS 6938-94-9; EINECS 248-299-9; cosmetic ingred.; liq.; oil-sol.

Pelemol DIPS. [Phoenix] Diisopropyl sebacate; CAS 7491-92-3; EINECS 231-306-4; ester preventing whitening in stick antiperspirants; liq.; oil-sol.

Pelemol DNPA. [Phoenix] Di-n-propyl adipate; CAS 106-19-4; EINECS 203-371-9; cosmetic ester; liq.; oil-sol.

Pelemol EE. [Phoenix] Eicosyl erucate; emollient for skin creams and lotions, makeup prods.; liq.; oil-sol.

Pelemol G7A. [Phoenix] Glycereth-7 triacetate; CAS 57569-76-3; solv. for sunscreen ingreds.; used in facial cleaners, creams and lotions; lt. oily to dry liq.; completely water-sol.

Pelemol G7B. [Phoenix] Glycereth-7 benzoate; used in bath prods., creams and lotions, and pharmaceutical topicals; blooms heavily in water; visc. liq.; sol. in hydro-alcoholic sol'ns., disp. in water.

Pelemol G45L. [Phoenix] Glycereth-5 lactate; CAS 125804-13-9; source of lactic acid; useful in skin prods. where slow release of lactic acid is desirable; visc. liq.; water-sol.

Pelemol GMU. [Phoenix] Glyceryl monoundecylenate; cosmetic ester; liq.; oil-sol.

Pelemol GTB. [Phoenix] Glyceryl tribehenate; CAS 18641-57-1; EINECS 242-471-7; emollient imparting body and richness to oil phase of creams and lotions, makeup; off-wh. gran.; oil-sol.

Pelemol GTO. [Phoenix] Glyceryl tri-2-ethylhexanoate; CAS 538-23-8; EINECS 208-686-5; cosmetic ester.

Pelemol HAB. [Phoenix] Dihydroabietyl behenate; substantivity agent for skin preps., night creams; binder in lipstick prods.; visc. liq.; oil-sol.

Pelemol ICB. [Phoenix] Isocetyl behenate; emollient for skin and makeup preps.; lt. liq.; oil-sol.

Pelemol ICS. [Phoenix] Isocetyl stearate; CAS 25339-09-7; EINECS 246-868-6; emollient for skin and makeup preps.; lt. liq.; oil-sol.

Pelemol IDO. [Phoenix] Isodecyl oleate; CAS 59231-34-4; EINECS 261-673-6; imparts sheen to hair; also for oil phase of creams and lotions; med. visc. liq.

Pelemol ISB. [Phoenix] Isostearyl behenate; emollient for makeup prods., mascara, lipstick, creams and lotions; melts at skin temp.; solid; oil-sol.

Pelemol ISL. [Phoenix] Isostearyl lactate; CAS 42131-28-2; EINECS 255-674-0; cosmetic ester for skin preps.; liq.; oil-sol.

Pelemol L2A. [Phoenix] Laureth-2 acetate; very lt. emollient for skin preps., body oils, and bath preps.; blooms in water; liq.; sol. in hydro-alcoholic sol'ns.

Pelemol L2O. [Phoenix] Laureth-2 octanoate; cosmetic ester; water-wh. liq.

Pelemol LB. [Phoenix] Lauryl behenate; CAS 42233-07-8; ester for stick deodorants; off-wh. solid; oil-sol.; m.p. 46 C.

Pelemol MAR. [Phoenix] Methyl acetyl ricinoleate; CAS 140-03-4; EINECS 205-392-9; light-feel moisture barrier; cosolubilizer for min. and castor oils; lt. visc. oil.

Pelemol MM. [Phoenix] Myristyl myristate; CAS 3234-85-3; EINECS 221-787-9; cosmetic ester for creams and lotions; solid.

Pelemol MS. [Phoenix] Myristyl stearate; CAS 17661-50-6; EINECS 241-640-2; cosmetic emollient.

Pelemol OE. [Phoenix] Oleyl erucate; CAS 17673-56-2; EINECS 241-654-9; emollient which appears to be nonpenetrating; amber liq.

Pelemol OL. [Phoenix] Oleyl lactate; CAS 42175-36-0; ester which leaves skin very soft and supple on rub-in; for skin creams and lotions; liq.; oil-sol.

Pelemol OP. [Phoenix] Octyl palmitate; CAS 29806-73-3; EINECS 249-862-1; cosmetic ester for creams and lotions; liq.

Pelemol OPG. [Phoenix] Octyl pelargonate; CAS 59587-44-9; EINECS 261-819-9; very dry cosmetic ester for skin preps. where initial light oiliness and dryness on rub-in are desirable; liq.

Pelemol P-49. [Phoenix] Pentaerythrityl tetraisononanoate; CAS 93803-89-5; EINECS 298-364-0; cosmetic ester providing emolliency and cushion in creams and lotions; water-wh. to off-wh. visc. liq.; oil-sol.

Pelemol PTL. [Phoenix] Pentaerythrityl tetralaurate; CAS 13057-50-6; EINECS 235-946-5; cosmetic ester for lipstick and makeup prods.; liq.; oil-sol.

Pelemol PTO. [Phoenix] Pentaerythrityl tetraoleate; CAS 19321-40-5; EINECS 242-960-5; cosmetic ester; liq.; oil-sol.

Pelemol SB. [Phoenix] Stearyl behenate; visc. builder and emollient for stick deodorants, creams, lotions; m.p. modifier in solid makeup preps.; wh. flake; oil-sol.

Pelemol TDE. [Phoenix] Tridecyl erucate; CAS 131154-74-0; very lt. oily feel emollient for skin creams and lotions, makeup prods.

Pelemol TGC. [Phoenix] Trioctyldodecyl citrate; CAS 126121-35-5; useful in skin preps. where cushion is desirable; wetting agent for pigments; visc. liq.; oil-sol.

Pemulen®TR-1, TR-2. [BFGoodrich] Acrylates/C10-30 alkyl acrylate crosspolymer; anionic; o/w emulsifier for virtually all hydrophobic substances; for low-irritancy creams, lotions, waterproof sunscreens, low or no alcohol fragrance prods.; powd.; 100% conc.

Peneteck. [Penreco] Min. oil tech.; CAS 8042-47-5; emollient; FDA compliance; sp.gr. 0.802-0.811; dens. 6.73-6.81 lb/gal; visc. 3.4-4.7 cSt (40 C); pour pt. -1 C; flash pt. 129 C; ref. index 1.4517.

Penreco 2251 Oil. [Penreco] Petroleum distillates; CAS 64742-14-9; high purity hydrocarbon processing solv., foam control agent, in waterless hand cleaners, agric. sprays, polishes, fruit and veg. processing, cleaning oils; sp.gr. 0.779–0.797 (60 F); dens. 6.56 lb/gal (60 F); visc. 30.5 SUS (100 F); b.p. 375 F min.; flash pt. (COC) 165 F; pour pt. –40 F.

Penreco 2263 Oil. [Penreco] Petroleum distillates; CAS 64742-47-8; high purity hydrocarbon processing solv., foam control agent, in waterless hand cleaners, agric. sprays, polishes, fruit and veg. processing, cleaning oils; sp.gr. 0.779–0.797 (60 F); dens. 6.56 lb/gal (60 F); visc. 30.5 SUS (100 F); b.p. 375 F min.; flash pt. (COC) 165 F; pour pt. –40 F.

Penreco Amber. [Penreco] Petrolatum USP; CAS 8027-32-5; EINECS 232-373-2; emollient, base for cosmetic and pharmaceutical preparations; waterproofing agent for butcher paper; lubricant, water repellent, moisture barrier for textile and paper; carrier for modeling clays, soldering paste and flux; pigment carrier for carbon paper; binder and conditioner for crayons; animal feed supplements; fruit/veg. coatings; food pkg. materials; FDA compliance; visc. 68–82 SUS (210 F); m.p. 122–135 F; congeal pt. 123 F; solid. pt. 122 F.

Penreco Blond. [Penreco] Petrolatum USP; CAS 8027-32-5; EINECS 232-373-2; emollient, base for cosmetic and pharmaceutical preparations; lubricant, water repellent, moisture barrier for textile and paper; FDA compliance; visc. 68–82 SUS (210 F); m.p. 122–135 F; congeal pt. 123

F; solid. pt. 122 F.

Penreco Cream. [Penreco] Wh. petrolatum USP; CAS 8027-32-5; EINECS 232-373-2; emollient, base, and carrier for cosmetic and pharmaceutical preparations; lubricant for textile and paper; FDA compliance; visc. 64–75 SUS (210 F); m.p. 122–135 F; congeal pt. 125 F; solid. pt. 122 F.

Penreco Lily. [Penreco] Wh. petrolatum USP; CAS 8027-32-5; EINECS 232-373-2; emollient, base, and carrier for cosmetic and pharmaceutical preparations; lubricant for textile and paper; FDA compliance; visc. 64–75 SUS (210 F); m.p. 122–135 F; congeal pt. 124 F; solid. pt. 123 F.

Penreco Regent. [Penreco] Wh. petrolatum USP; CAS 8027-32-5; EINECS 232-373-2; emollient, base, and carrier for cosmetic and pharmaceutical preparations (creams, lotions, petrol. jellies, makeup, absorp. base, ophthalmic and topical ointments, dental adhesives); water repellent, moisture barrier, lubricant for textile and paper; plasticizer and softener for putty; shoe polishes; FDA compliance; visc. 57–70 SUS (210 F); m.p. 118–130 F; congeal pt. 120 F; solid. pt. 119 F.

Penreco Royal. [Penreco] Petrolatum USP; CAS 8027-32-5; EINECS 232-373-2; emollient, base, and carrier for cosmetic and pharmaceutical preparations; lubricant for textile and paper; FDA compliance; visc. 57–70 SUS (210 F); m.p. 118–130 F; congeal pt. 118 F; solid. pt. 115 F.

Penreco Snow. [Penreco] Wh. petrolatum USP; CAS 8027-32-5; EINECS 232-373-2; emollient, base, solv., and carrier for cosmetic and pharmaceutical preparations (creams, lotions, petrol. jellies, ointments, dental adhesives); foods (animal feed supplement, fruit/veg. coatings, food pkg.); sanitary lubricant in food prod. machinery; rust-preventive coating in food processing equipment; carrier in adhesive tapes and compds.; lubricant for textile and paper; shoe polishes; FDA compliance; visc. 64–75 SUS (210 F); m.p. 122–135 F; congeal pt. 123 F; solid. pt. 121 F.

Penreco Super. [Penreco] Wh. petrolatum USP; CAS 8027-32-5; EINECS 232-373-2; emollient, base, and carrier for cosmetic and pharmaceutical preparations; lubricant for textile and paper; FDA compliance; visc. 60–75 SUS (210 F); m.p. 122–135 F; congeal pt. 125 F; solid. pt. 124 F.

Penreco Ultima. [Penreco] Wh. petrolatum USP; CAS 8027-32-5; EINECS 232-373-2; emollient, base, and carrier for cosmetic and pharmaceutical preparations (creams, lotions, hair prods., lip balms, makeup, absorp. bases, ophthalmic and topical ointments, dental adhesives); foods (fruit/veg. coatings, food pkg.); lubricant for textile and paper; FDA compliance; visc. 60–70 SUS (210 F); m.p. 130–140 F; congeal pt. 130 F; solid. pt. 128 F.

Pentacare-HP. [Pentapharm Ltd; Centerchem] Proprietary formulation incorporating plant polysaccharides and a selective casein hydrolysate; cosmetic active ingred., film-former imparting pleasant, soft skinfeel and skin tightening effect; for facial care prods. esp. treatments for mature or sun-damaged skin.

Pentagen. [Pentapharm Ltd] Glycogen; CAS 9005-79-2; EINECS 232-683-8; used in biochemical research.

Pentavitin® . [Pentapharm Ltd; Centerchem] Saccharide isomerate; patented, highly effective moisture magnet for formulation of superior moisturizing creams and lotions; provides long-lasting water-retention in the skin; sl. yel. to amber clear, sl. visc. sol'n.; odorless to sl. caramel-like odor; m.w. 120-400; sp.gr. 1.240-1.255; ref. index 1.422-1.430; pH 4-5; usage level: 3-6%; toxicology: nontoxic, nonirritating, nonsensitizing; 50-55% solids in water.

Pepsobiol. [Laserson SA] Hydrolyzed soy protein preserved with methylparaben and phenoxyethanol in 0.3% butylene glycol sol'n.; CAS 68607-88-5; nourishing and hydrating agent for cosmetics; stimulates metabolic action of fibroblasts; pale yel. clear liq.; water-sol.; usage level:

5-10%.

Peptein® 2000®. [Hormel] Hydrolyzed collagen; CAS 9015-54-7; conditioner for cosmetic applics.; esp. substantive to hair; enhances shine, gloss, and body in shampoos, conditioners, and styling aids; clear amber liq. or lt. tan powd., bland odor; m.w. 1500–2500; sp.gr. 1.15; visc. 100 cps max.; pH 5.8–6.3; toxicology: LD50 (oral, rat) 5 g/kg; nonirritating to eyes and skin; 55% min. solids.

Peptein® 2000XL. [Hormel] Hydrolyzed collagen; CAS 9015-54-7; enhances shine, gloss, and body in hair care prods. (shampoos, conditioners, styling aids); lt. amber clear liq.; m.w. 2000.

Peptein® CAA. [Hormel] Collagen amino acids; CAS 9105-54-7; natural humectant with efficient moisture binding props.; for cosmetic formulations where low inorganic salt is critical; lt. amber clear liq.; m.w. 500; sp.gr. 1.15; pH 5.0-6.5 (diluted 2:1); toxicology: LD50 (oral) > 5 g/kg; sl. irritating to eyes, mildly irritating to skin; 50% min. solids.

Peptein® KC. [Hormel] Potassium cocoyl hydrolyzed collagen; CAS 68920-65-0; protein-based surfactant producing enhanced foam and rich lather for shampoos, foaming conditioners, facial cleansers; improves spreadability, reduces irritation in shaving systems; clear amber liq.; m.w. 650.

Peptein® Qs. [Hormel] Hydroxypropyl trimonium hydrolyzed soy protein; cationic; substantive protein, moisture-binding agent for personal care prods.; clear amber liq., bland char. odor; m.w. 2500-3500; pH 5.5-6.5; 23-27% total solids.

Peptein® Qw. [Hormel] Hydroxypropyl trimonium hydrolyzed wheat protein; cationic; substantive protein and humectant for personal care prods.; clear amber liq., bland char. odor; m.w. 2500-3000; pH 5.5-6.5; 23-27% total solids.

Peptein® TEAC. [Hormel] TEA-coco hydrolyzed collagen; CAS 68952-16-9; protein-based surfactant producing enhanced foam and rich lather for shampoos, foaming conditioners, facial cleansers; improves spreadability, reduces irritation in shaving systems; clear amber liq.; m.w. 650.

Peptein® VgS. [Hormel] Hydrolyzed soy protein; CAS 68607-88-5; film-forming and moisture binding props. for cosmetic hair and skin care prods. (shampoos, conditioners, styling prods., creams and lotions); natural humectant; lt. amber clear liq., bland char. odor; water-sol.; m.w. 2500; pH 4.0-4.5; usage level: 1-5%; 23-27% total solids.

Peptein® VgW. [Hormel] Hydrolyzed wheat protein; CAS 70084-87-6; film-forming and moisture binding props. for hair and skin care prods. (shampoos, conditioners, styling prods.); biodeg.; amber to nearly clear liq., lt. char. proteinaceous odor; water-sol.; m.w. 2500-3000; sp.gr. 1.1; b.p. 215-230 F; pH 4.0-4.5; toxicology: nontoxic; very low skin irritation; 23-27% total solids.

Peptidyl. [Laboratories Sérobiologiques] Glycerin, water, serum protein, glycogen.

Peranat. [Henkel/Cospha] Fragrance raw material for cosmetic, personal care, detergent, and cleaning prods.; colorless liq., fruity, pear-like odor; b.p. 113 C; flash pt. 95 C.

Perfecta® USP. [Witco/Petroleum Spec.] Petrolatum USP; CAS 8027-32-5; EINECS 232-373-2; cosmetic/pharmaceutical grade with lightest color, med. consistency, high m.p.; as carrier, lubricant, moisture barrier, protective agent, softener; FDA §172.880 clearance; Lovibond 0.3Y color; visc. 9–14 cSt (100 C); m.p. 57–60 C.

Perlankrol® ADP3. [Harcros UK] Sodium laureth (3) sulfate; anionic; biodeg. surfactant; base for preparation of high foaming shampoos and toiletries; clear water-wh. liq.; mild odor; water-sol.; sp.gr. l.048; visc. 28 cs.; flash pt. (PMCC) > 100 C; pour pt. < O C; pH 7.0 (1% aq.); 27% act.

Perlankrol® ASC2. [Harcros UK] Sodium laureth (2) sulfate; anionic; biodeg. surfactant for prep. of high foaming shampoos and toiletries; water-wh. clear liq.; mild odor; water-sol.; sp.gr. 1.047; visc. 600 cs; pour pt. < 0 C; flash pt. (PMCC) > 100 C; pH 7.0 (1% aq.); 27.5% act.

Perlankrol® ASC38. [Harcros UK] Sodium laureth (2) sulfate; anionic; toiletry intermediate; water-wh. clear liq., mild odor; water-sol.; sp.gr. 1.047; visc. 1000 cs; pour pt. < 0 C; flash pt. (COC) > 95 C; pH 7.0 (1% aq.); 27.5% act.

Perlankrol® ASC49. [Harcros] Sodium laureth (2) sulfate; anionic; surfactant for toiletries; water-wh. clear liq., mild odor; water-sol.; sp.gr. 1.047; visc. 2500 cs; pour pt. < 0 C; flash pt. (COC) > 95 C; pH 7.0 (1% aq.); 27.5% act.

Perlankrol® ASC82. [Harcros UK] Sodium laureth (2) sulfate; anionic; surfactant for cosmetics and toiletries; clear water-wh. liq., mild odor; sol. in water; sp.gr. 1.047; visc. 2100 cs; pour pt. < 0 C; flash pt. (PMCC) > 100 C; pH 6.5-7.5 (1% aq.); 27.5% act.

Perlankrol® ATL40. [Harcros UK] TEA lauryl sulfate; CAS 139-96-8; EINECS 205-388-7; anionic; biodeg. surfactant for prep. of high foaming shampoos and toiletries; emulsifier for emulsion polymerization; pale straw clear liq.; mild odor; water-sol.; sp.gr. 1.048; visc. 60 cs.; pour pt. < 0 C; flash pt. (COC) > 95 C; pH 7.5 (1% aq.); surf. tens. 32 dynes/cm (0.1%); 40% act.

Perlankrol® DAF25. [Harcros UK] Ammonium lauryl sulfate; CAS 2235-54-3; EINECS 218-793-9; anionic; foaming agent, base; formulation of toiletries and carpet shampoos; pale yel. mobile gel, mild nonammoniacal odor; water-sol.; sp.gr. 1.007; visc. 1600 cs; pour pt. 5 C; flash pt. (COC) > 95 C; pH 6.4 (1% aq.); 25% act.

Perlankrol® DSA. [Harcros UK] Sodium lauryl sulfate; CAS 151-21-3; EINECS 205-788-1; anionic; foaming agent for syn. latexes, emulsion polymerization aid; base for prep. of high foaming shampoos and toiletries; wetting agent; industrial detergent additive; wh. slurry; faint fatty alcohol odor; water-sol.; sp.gr. 1.041; visc. 220 cs (40 C); pour pt. 12 C; flash pt. (COC) > 95 C; pH 8.0 (1% aq.); surf. tens. 30 dynes/cm (0.1%); 28% act.

Perlankrol® TM1. [Harcros UK] Fatty amide ether sulfate, sodium salt; anionic; biodeg. surfactant; base for preparation of high foaming shampoos and toiletries; clear pale yel. liq.; mild odor; water-sol.; sp.gr. 1.045; visc. 715 cs; flash pt. > 200 F (COC); pour pt. < 0 C; pH 7–8 (1% aq.); 30% act.

Perlex B.67, B.70. [Rhone-Poulenc] Bismuth compd.; pearlescent for use in lipsticks, emulsion systems; paste; 67 and 70% resp. in castor oil.

Perlex B.67M. [Rhone-Poulenc] Bismuth compd.; pearlescent for use in lipsticks, emulsion systems; 67% in min. oil.

Perlex BU. [Rhone-Poulenc] Bismuth compd.; pearlescent for dry applics. such as face powd., eye shadow or rouge; solid.

Perlex BUA.35. [Rhone-Poulenc] Bismuth compd.; pearlescent for aq.-based emulsions or lotions; 35% disp. in aq. base.

Perlextra B.70. [Rhone-Poulenc] Bismuth compd.; pearlsecent for lipsticks, other wax-based prods., emulsion systems; insol. in water, alcohol; 70% in castor oil.

Perlextra BU. [Rhone-Poulenc] Bismuth compd.; pearlescent for use in eye shadows and powd. prods. or fluid creams and lotions; dry powd.; insol. in water, alcohol.

Perlextra BUA.70. [Rhone-Poulenc] Bismuth compd.; pearlescent for aq. formulations; 70% aq. disp.

Perlglanzmittel GM 4006. [Zschimmer & Schwarz] Sodium laureth sulfate, glycol stearate, cocamide MEA, cocamidopropyl lauryl ether; pearlescent for hair shampoos and bath additives; fluid; 30% act.

Perlglanzmittel GM 4055. [Zschimmer & Schwarz] Glycol stearate, MIPA C12-15 pareth sulfate; opacifier and pearlescent for cosmetics; fluid; 38% act.

Perlglanzmittel GM 4175. [Zschimmer & Schwarz] Sodium laureth sulfate, cocamide DEA, cocamide MEA, glycol stearate, propylene glycol; pearlescent for hair shampoos and bath additives; fluid; 42% act.

Permethyl® 99A. [Presperse] Isododecane; CAS 13475-82-6; cosolubilizer for nonhydrocarbon materials; for mascara, eyeliner, antiperspirant and where residual film is not desirable; solv. for debris on skin; clean feel, very little residual; JSCI/JCID approved; colorless clear liq.; sol. in cyclomethicone, hydrocarbons, isoparaffins, min. spirits; m.w. 170; sp.gr. 0.747; visc. 1 cps (20 C); ref. index 1.424; toxicology: actue oral > 5 g/kg; pract. nonirritating to eyes; mild skin irritant; noncomedogenic.

Permethyl® 101A. [Presperse] Isohexadecane; CAS 4390-04-9; EINECS 224-506-8; cosolubilizer for non-hydrocarbon materials; in eyeliners, mascaras, sun care and skin prods.; cleanser for eye and face makeup; light silky texture; JSCI/JCID approved; colorless clear liq.; sol. in cyclomethicone, hydrocarbons, isoparaffins, min. spirits; m.w. 226; sp.gr. 0.790; visc. 4 cps; ref. index 1.440; toxicology: acute oral > 5 g/kg; nonirritating to eyes; mildly irritating to skin; noncomedogenic.

Permethyl® 102A. [Presperse] Isoeicosane; CAS 93685-79-1; cosolubilizer for nonhydrocarbon materials; for skin care and sun care prods.; plasticizer for mascara; satiny texture; JSCI/JCID approved; colorless clear liq.; sol. in cyclomethicone, hydrocarbons, isoparaffins, min. spirits; m.w. 282; sp.gr. 0.830; visc. 16 cps; ref. index 1.460; toxicology: acute oral > 5 g/kg; minimal eye irritant; mild skin irritant; noncomedogenic.

Permethyl® 104A. [Presperse] Polyisobutene (iso-octahexacontane); CAS 9003-29-6; cosolubilizer for nonhydrocarbon materials; for lipsticks and glossers to improve wear and impart sheen; in skin care and sun care prods.; luxurious liq. waxy feel combined with Permethyl 102A; colorless clear visc. liq.; sol. in cyclomethicone, hydrocarbons, isoparaffins, min. spirits; m.w. 954; sp.gr. 0.890; visc. 7600 cps (40 C); ref. index 1.505; toxicology: acute oral > 5 g/kg; minimal eye irritant, mild skin irritant; noncomedogenic.

Permethyl® 106A. [Presperse] Polyisobutene (iso-hexapentacontahectane); CAS 9003-29-6; cosolubilizer for nonhydrocarbon materials; for skin care and sun care prods.; luxurious liq. waxy feel combined with Permethyl 102A; JSCI/JCID approved; colorless clear very visc. liq.; sol. in cyclomethicone, hydrocarbons, isoparaffins, min. spirits; m.w. 2186; sp.gr. 0.910; visc. 3200 cps (100 C); ref. index 1.510; toxicology: acute oral > 5 g/kg; minimal eye irritant, mild skin irritant; noncomedogenic.

Permethyl® 108A. [Presperse] Polyisobutene (iso-pentacontaoctactane); CAS 9003-27-4; cosolubilizer for nonhydrocarbon materials; for skin care and sun care prods.; rich emollient feel on skin in combination with Permethyl 102A; pale yel. clear tacky semiliq.; sol. in cyclomethicone, hydrocarbons, isoparaffins, min. spirits; m.w. 12,000; sp.gr. 0.914; visc. 58,000 cps (177 C); ref. index 1.505.

Permethyl® 1082. [Presperse] Polyisobutene (50%), isoeicosane (50%); CAS 9003-27-4, 93685-79-1; used for pigmented cosmetics, personal care prods., skin care prods.; visc. 250,000 cps (22 C).

Permulgin 835. [Koster Keunen] Microcrystalline wax; CAS 63231-60-7; EINECS 264-038-1; stabilizer, emollient, and thickener for cosmetic creams, lotions, sun care, lipsticks, makeups, powds., gels; slabs.

Permulgin CSB. [Koster Keunen] Syn. beeswax; CAS 71243-51-1; gellant, emulsifier, and thickener for cosmetic creams, lotions, sun care, lipsticks, and gels; slabs and pastilles.

Permulgin RWB. [Koster Keunen] Syn. beeswax; CAS 71243-51-1; gellant, emulsifier, and thickener for cosmetic creams, lotions, sun care, lipsticks, and gels; slabs and pastilles.

Petro® 11. [Witco/H-I-P] Sodium alkyl naphthalene sulfonate; CAS 9084-06-4; anionic; hydrotrope, surfactant, germicidal agent, liquid hand soaps, personal care prods., wetting agent in plating and electrolytic baths; 50% act. liq., 95% act. powd.; water-sol.

Petrolite® C-700. [Petrolite] Hard microcryst. wax consisting of n-paraffinic, branched paraffinic, and naphthenic hydrocarbons; CAS 63231-60-7; EINECS 264-038-1; used in hot-melt coatings and adhesives, paper coatings, printing inks, plastic modification (as lubricant and processing aid), lacquers, paints, varnishes, as binder in ceramics, for potting, filling in elec./electronic components; in investment castings, as emulsion wax size in papermaking, as fabric softener ingred. in permanent-press fabrics, in emulsion and latex coatings, and in cosmetic hand creams and lipsticks; color 1.5 (D1500) wax; very low sol. in org. solvs.; sp.gr. 0.93; visc. 16 cps (99 C); m.p. 93 C.

Petrolite® C-1035. [Petrolite] Hard microcryst. wax consisting of n-paraffinic, branched paraffinic, and naphthenic hydrocarbons; CAS 63231-60-7; EINECS 264-038-1; used in hot-melt coatings and adhesives, paper coatings, printing inks, plastic modification (as lubricant and processing aid), lacquers, paints, varnishes, as binder in ceramics, for potting, filling in elec./electronic components; in investment castings, as emulsion wax size in papermaking, as fabric softener ingred. in permanent-press fabrics, in emulsion and latex coatings, and in cosmetic hand creams and lipsticks; incl. FDA §172.230, 172.615, 175.105, 175.300, 176.170, 176.180, 176.200, 177.1200, 178.3710, 179.45; color 0.5 (D1500) wax; very low sol. in org. solvs.; sp.gr. 0.93; visc. 15 cps (99 C); m.p. 94 C.

Petrolite® CP-7. [Petrolite] Ethylene/propylene compd.; CAS 9010-79-1; component for solv.-based PU mold release agents; additives for adhesives, cosmetics, paraffin modification, printing inks, investment casting; FDA §175.105; m.w. 650; dens. 0.94 g/cc; visc. 12 cps (99 C); m.p. 96 C.

Petrolite® CP-11. [Petrolite] Syn. copolymer; component for PU mold release, laminating and hot-melt adhesives, printing inks, cosmetics, investment casting wax; m.w. 1100; dens. 0.94 g/cc; visc. 13 cs (149 C); m.p. 110 C.

Petrolite® CP-12. [Petrolite] Syn. copolymer; component for PU mold release, laminating and hot-melt adhesives, printing inks, cosmetics, investment casting wax; m.w. 1200; dens. 0.94 g/cc; visc. 16 cs (149 C); m.p. 112 C.

PF. [Siltech] nonionic; gloss agent for hair care prods.; insol. in water; 100% act.

PF-6®. [Hormel] Hydrolyzed collagen; CAS 9015-54-7; all-purpose protein for use in shampoos, conditioners, and maintenance prods.; lt. tan liq. or powd.; m.w. 2000; 55% (liq.).

P-Flakes [Karlshamns] Hydrogenated palm oil; Lovibond R4.0 max.; m.p. 138–141 F; iodine no. 5 max.; sapon. no. 196–202.

Pharmaceutical Lanolin USP. [Croda Inc.] Lanolin; CAS 8006-54-0; EINECS 232-348-6; superfatting emollient, emulsifier for pharmaceutical ointments, dressing creams, diaper rash and hemorrhoidal preps.; amber soft solid; partly sol. in min. oil; m.p. 38-44 C.

Pharmasorb Colloidal Pharmaceutical Grade. [Engelhard] Attapulgite clay; CAS 1337-76-4; adsorbent for pharmaceuticals featuring superior adsorptive properties with effective acid adsorp.; powd.; particle size 2.9 and 0.14 μ resp., 0.10 and 0.30% resp.; cream and lt. cream resp.; sp.gr. 2.47 and 2.36 resp.; pH 7.5–9.5 resp.

Phenonip. [Nipa Labs] Phenoxyethanol (> 70%), methylparaben > (15%), ethylparaben (< 5%), propylparaben (< 5%), butylparaben (< 10%); fully active liq. preservative system with low toxicity and wide spectrum activity, esp. against pseudomonads; for cosmetics and pharmaceuticals (shampoos, foam baths, liq. detergents, proteinaceous prods., emulsions, skin antiseptics, deodorants); USA, Japan, and Europe approvals; pract. colorless visc. liq., faint aromatic odor; sol. 0.5% in water; misc. with ethanol, IPA, acetone, propylene glycol, IPM, ethyl acetate; sp.gr. 1.124; m.p. 13 C; b.p. 224-250 C (1013 m.bar); flash pt. (OC) 130 C; ref. index 1.5415; pH 7 (20 g/l water); usage level: 0.25-0.75%; toxicology: LD50 (oral, rat) 1.5 g/kg (sl. harmful); pure material irritating to skin, moderately irritating to eyes; 100% conc.

Phenosept. [Nipa Labs] Phenoxyisopropanol and p-chloro-m-xylenol; antiseptic for skin care prods.

Phenoxen. [Vevy] Phenoxyethanol; CAS 122-99-6; EINECS 204-589-7; cosmetic preservative; broad activity, esp. against Gram-negative bacteria; USA, Japan, Europe approvals; liq., sl. aromatic odor; usage level: up to 1%.

Phenoxetol. [Nipa Labs] Phenoxyethanol; CAS 122-99-6; EINECS 204-589-7; broad-spectrum antimicrobial preservative for cosmetics and pharmaceuticals (antiseptic creams, bath preps., ethnic prods., hair and skin care prods.); colorless sl. visc. liq., faint or pleasant odor; sol. 2.3% in water; misc. with acetone, ethanol, benzene, ether, propylene glycol, glycerin; m.w. 138.2; sp.gr. 1.1 (20/4 C); f.p. 11 C; b.p. 245.6 C; flash pt. (OC) 121 C; toxicology: LD50 (oral, rat) 1.3 g/kg (sl. harmful); moderate eye irritant; pure material sl. irritating to skin; 99% min. assay.

Phenoxyethanol O. [Hüls AG] Phenoxyethanol; CAS 122-99-6; EINECS 204-589-7; fragrance material used for perfume compositions and as a fixative; antistatic props.; liq., mild rose-like odor; dens. 1.10 kg/l; solid. pt. 5-10 C; flash pt. 130 C; ≥ 91% purity.

Philcohol 1600. [United Coconut Chem.] C16 alcohols; CAS 36653-82-4; EINECS 253-149-0; intermediate for surfactant mfg.; cosmetic ingred.; APHA 10 max. flakes; acid no. 0.2 max.; iodine no. 0.3 max.; sapon. no. 0.5 max.; hyd. no. 230-233.

Philcohol 1618. [United Coconut Chem.] C18-18 alcohols; intermediate for surfactant mfg.; cosmetic ingred.; APHA 10 max. flakes; acid no. 0.2 max.; iodine no. 0.3 max.; sapon. no. 2 max.; hyd. no. 211-220.

Philcohol 1800. [United Coconut Chem.] C18 alcohols; CAS 112-92-5; EINECS 204-017-6; intermediate for surfactant mfg.; cosmetic ingred.; APHA 10 max. flakes; acid no. 0.2 max.; iodine no. 0.3 max.; sapon. no. 1.5 max.; hyd. no. 206-209.

Phoenamid CMA, CMA-70. [Phoenix] Cocamide MEA; CAS 68140-00-1; EINECS 268-770-2; foam builder and stabilizer; CMA-70 offers higher m.p.; off-wh. gran. powd.

Phoenamid LD, LD Special. [Phoenix] Lauramide DEA; CAS 120-40-1; EINECS 204-393-1; foam stabilizer; LD Special has low iodine value; solid (LD).

Phoenamid LMM. [Phoenix] Lauramide MEA; CAS 142-78-9; EINECS 205-560-1; personal care surfactant.

Phoenamid SM. [Phoenix] Stearamide MEA; CAS 111-57-9; EINECS 203-883-2; personal care surfactant, thickener, pearlescent.

Phoenate 3 DSA. [Phoenix] PEG-3 distearate; CAS 9005-08-7; pearlizer and emulsifier for shampoos; off-wh. flake.

Phoenoxol J. [Phoenix] Cetearyl alcohol, ceteareth-10; emulsifier.

Phoenoxol T. [Phoenix] Cetearyl alcohol, ceteareth-20; emulsifier.

Phosal 12WD. [Rhone-Poulenc Rorer] Soybean oil, coceth-3, lecithin.

Phosal 15. [Rhone-Poulenc Rorer] Lecithin; CAS 8002-43-5; EINECS 232-307-2; emulsifier.

Phosal 25 PG. [Rhone-Poulenc Rorer] Propylene glycol, lecithin; cosmetic ingred.

Phosal 25 SB. [Seppic] Phosphatidylcholine; natural emulsifying aid, hair conditioner, oil restorer, source of essential fatty acids for cosmetics (shampoos, creams, oil baths, soap additive, hair rinses); so-called vitamin F.

Phosal 25 SB. [Rhone-Poulenc Rorer] Phosphatidylcholine; natural emulsifying aid, hair conditioner, oil restorer, source of essential fatty acids for cosmetics (shampoos, creams, oil baths, soap additive, hair rinses); so-called vitamin F; golden brn. clear to milky liq., nut-like taste; sol. in ethanol; visc. 15,000 mPa·s max.; 100% conc.

Phosal 35SB. [Rhone-Poulenc Rorer] Sunflower seed oil, lecithin.

Phosal® 50 PG. [Am. Lecithin] A preliposome system containing 50% phosphatidylcholine in a propylene glycol/ethanol carrier; dispersant, coemulsifier, and solubilizer for cosmetics, personal care prods., pharmaceuticals, lotions, creams, oil baths; honey yel. fluid, nut-like taste; visc. 5000 mPa·s max.; iodine no. ≈ 50.

Phosal® 50 SA. [Am. Lecithin; Rhone-Poulenc Rorer] Safflower oil and lecithin; improves skin humidity and penetration for dermatology, cosmetics, and personal care prods.; solubilizer for lipophilic substances; phosphatidylcholine source for nutritional supplements; honey yel. fluid; visc. 5000 mPa·s max.; usage level: 5-15%.

Phosal® 53 MCT. [Am. Lecithin; Rhone-Poulenc Rorer] Lecithin, caprylic/capric triglyceride, and alcohol; improves skin humidity and penetration for dermatology, cosmetics, and personal care prods.; solubilizer for lipophilic substances; phosphatidylcholine source for dietetics, esp. as filling mass for soft gelatin capsules; honey yel. fluid; visc. 5000 mPa·s max.; usage level: 5-15%.

Phosal® 60 PG. [Am. Lecithin; Rhone-Poulenc Rorer] A preliposome system containing 60% lecithin in propylene glycol; moisturizer, emulsifier for dermatology, cosmetics, and personal care prods.; controls skin humidity, penetration, roughness; honey yel. liq.; usage level: 2-5%; 60% act.

Phosal® 75 SA. [Am. Lecithin; Rhone-Poulenc Rorer] Lecithin, alcohol, and safflower oil; moisturizer, emollient, emulsifier for skin care, creams and lotions, cleansers, bath and toiletry prods.; improves skin humidity and penetration in dermatology, cosmetics, and personal care prods.; solubilizer for lipophilic substances; phosphatidylcholine source for nutritional supplements, esp. as capsule filling mass; honey yel. fluid; visc. 5500 mPa·s max.; pH 6 ± 2; usage level: 3-10%.

Phosal® NAT-50-PG. [Am. Lecithin; Rhone-Poulenc Rorer] Lecithin, propylene glycol; an alcohol-free phospholipid system for mfg. of perfumes/fragrances in water disps.; emollient, emulsifier, stabilizer for skin and hair care, pharmaceuticals, soap/syndets, creams and lotions, cleansing prods., sunscreens, bath and toiletries.; brn. liq., acetic acid smell possible.

Phosfetal 201 K. [Zschimmer & Schwarz] Calcium alkyl polyglycol ether phosphate; cosmetics surfactant; liq.; 90% act.

Phosphanol Series. [Toho Chem. Industry] Phosphate ester surfactants; emulsifier for textile spinning oils, polymerization; antistat; anticorrosive agent; cosmetics solubilizer and emulsifier; liq., paste, solid.

PhosPho 642. [Fanning] Hydroxylated lecithin; CAS 8029-76-3; EINECS 232-440-6; surfactant, suspending agent for nail polish, hair/skin conditioner; Gardenr 13 max. liq.; sol. @ 5% in water, IPM, castor oil, propylene glycol, ethyl acetate, min. oil, glycerol; visc. 50-125 poises; HLB 9.0; acid no. 34 max.; pH 4-6 (10% aq.).

PhosPho E-100. [Fanning] Lecithin; CAS 8002-43-5; EINECS 232-307-2; emulsifier, suspending agent, solubilizer, superfatting agent for face and hand creams; ylsh. brn. paste; sol. in paraffin, alcohol; disp. in water; acid no. 25 max.; iodine no. 70 max.

PhosPho F-97. [Fanning] Lecithin; CAS 8002-43-5; EINECS 232-307-2; for makeup, cleansers, body creams and lotions, shampoos, moisturizing creams; lt. golden gran.; sol. in IPM, ethyl acetate, water; insol. in castor oil, propylene glycol, ethanol, min. oil, glycerol; HLB 7.0; acid no. 35 max.

PhosPho H-00. [Fanning] Hydrogenated soya lecithin; CAS 92128-87-5; EINECS 295-786-7; for liposome applics.; ylsh.-wh. powd.; iodine no. 8-15; pH 7.0 max.

PhosPho H-150. [Fanning] Hydrog. lecithin; CAS 92128-87-5; EINECS 295-786-7; for liposome applics.; wh. powd.; sol. in alcohol, hydrocarbons; disp. in water; iodine no. 1 mqx.

PhosPho LCN-TS. [Fanning] Lecithin; CAS 8002-43-5; EINECS 232-307-2; phospholipid used as surfactant/ emulsifier and skin conditioning agent for makeup, cleansers, body creams, shampoos, moisturizing creams, face creams, cosmetics, pharmaceuticals; opaque appearance; sol. in IPM, castor oil, propylene glycol, ethyl acetate, min. oil, glycerol; insol. in water, ethanol; dens. 8.48 lb/gal (60 F); visc. 75 poises; HLB 4.0; acid no. 24; pH 5-7 (10% aq.).

PhosPho PL-50. [Fanning] Phospholipids; emulsifier, refatting agent, source of vitamin F; for soft gelatin capsules, lotions, creams, oil baths, natural cosmetics; golden brn. clear-milky fluid; acid no. 10 max.

PhosPho S-85. [Fanning] Phospholipids; CAS 8002-43-5; wetting agent for makeup, cleansers, body creams and lotions, shampoos, moisturizing creams; translucent; sol. @ 5% in water, IPM, castor oil, ethyl acetate, ethanol, min. oil, glycerol; sl. sol. in propylene glycol; visc. 15 poises; HLB 6.0; acid no. 25 max.; pH 5-7 (10% aq.).

PhosPho T-20. [Fanning] Phospholipids; CAS 8002-43-5; hydrophilic cosmetic ingred. for makeup, cleansers, body creams and lotions, shampoos, moisturizing creams; Gardner 14 max. translucent; sol. in IPM, castor oil, propylene glycol, ethyl acetate, water, min. oil, glycerol; insol. in ethanol; visc. 200 poises; HLB 12-13; acid no. 36 max.; pH 4-6 (10% aq.).

Phospholipid EFA. [Mona Industries] Linoleamidopropyl PG-dimonium chloride phosphate; cationic; patented (U.S., Canada, Japan, Europe) component of skin and hair formulations esp. hypoallergenic prods., medicated prods.; emulsifier, antimicrobial, moisturizer; solubilizer and fixative for fragrances; amber clear liq.; sp.gr. 1.04; dens. 8.7 lb/gal; HLB 17-19; pH 7.6 (10% in 50/50 IPA/ water); toxicology: nontoxic, nonirritating to skin, minimal eye irritation; 30% total solids, 45% moisture, 25% propylene glycol.

Phospholipid PTC. [Mona Industries] Cocamidopropyl PG-dimonium chloride phosphate; cationic; patented (U.S., Canada, Japan, Europe) biodeg. substantive, mild foamer, hydrotrope, visc. builder, wetter, surf. tension reducer, bactericide for personal care prods., baby prods., feminine washes, ophthalmic preps., disinfectant cleansers; yel. clear liq.; sp.gr. 1.01; dens. 8.4 lb/gal; HLB 17-19; pH 7.0 (10% in 50/50 IPA/water); toxicology: non-irritating to skin, minimal eye irritant; 47% solids.

Phospholipid PTD. [Mona Industries] Lauramidopropyl PEG-dimonium chloride phosphate; CAS 83682-78-4; cationic; bactericidal, conditioner, antistat, detergent, foamer, emulsifier, solubilizer, dispersant, thickener and wetting agent for personal care, household, pharmaceutical, veterinary prods., fire fighting foams, petrol. prod., photographic processes, agric., mining, textiles; amber

clear liq.; sp.gr. 1.05; dens. 8.7 lb/gal; pH 7.5 (10%); surf. tens. 43.1 dynes/cm (1%); 34% act.

Phospholipid PTL. [Mona Industries] Laurampho PEG-glycinate phosphate; cationic; bactericidal, conditioner, antistat, detergent, foamer, emulsifier, solubilizer, dispersant, thickener and wetting agent for personal care, household, pharmaceutical, veterinary prods., fire fighting foams, petrol. prod., photographic processes, agric., mining, textiles; clear to opaque visc. liq.; sp.gr. 1.10; dens. 9.1 lb/gal; pH 7.5 (10%); surf. tens. 33.7 dynes/cm (1%); 30% act.

Phospholipid PTS. [Mona Industries] Stearamidopropyl PG-dimonium chloride phosphate; cationic; patented mild substantivity agent, skin conditioner, thickener for personal care prods.; forms stable, low pH, smooth and elegant cosmetic emulsions; lt. yel. paste; sp.gr. 1.01; dens. 8.4 lb/gal; HLB 14; m.p. 40 C; pH 7.6 (10% in 50/50 IPA/water); toxicology: extremely mild to skin and eyes; 35% solids.

Phospholipid PTZ. [Mona Industries] Cocohydroxyethyl PEG-imidazolinium chloride phosphate; cationic; bactericidal, conditioner, antistat, detergent, foamer, emulsifier, solubilizer, dispersant, thickener and wetting agent for personal care, household, pharmaceutical, veterinary prods., fire fighting foams, petrol. prod., photographic processes, agric., mining, textiles; amber clear liq.; sp.gr. 1.07; dens. 8.9 lb/gal; pH 7.0 (10%); surf. tens. 37.6 dynes/cm (1%); 30% act.

Phospholipid SV. [Mona Industries] Stearamidopropyl PG-dimonium chloride phosphate and cetyl alcohol; patented substantive emulsifier, skin conditioner for skin and personal care prods.; moisturizer; wh. waxy solid; sp.gr. 1.02; dens. 8.5 lb/gal; m.p. 50 C; HLB 15; pH 7.0 (10% in 50/50 IPA/water); toxicology: nonirritating to skin, minimal eye irritant; 41.5% solids in water/propylene glycol.

Phospholipon® 25G, 25P, 50. [Rhone-Poulenc Rorer] Lecithin; CAS 8002-43-5; EINECS 232-307-2; emulsifier.

Phospholipon® 80. [Am. Lecithin; Rhone-Poulenc Rorer] Lecithin (soya 3-sn-phosphatidylcholine); CAS 8002-43-5; EINECS 232-307-2; moisturizer, emulsifier for skin care, creams and lotions; min. 73% phosphatidylcholine for the mfg. of liposomes; yel.-brn. solid plastic; acid no. 10 max.; usage level: 1-3%; 80% conc.

Phospholipon® 90/90 G. [Am. Lecithin; Rhone-Poulenc Rorer] Min. 90% soya 3-sn-phosphatidylcholine; CAS 97281-47-5; raw material for liposomes; moisturizer, emulsifier for dermatology, cosmetics, and personal care prods.; solubilizer for parenteralia; phosphatidylcholine source for drugs and dietetics; yel. solid or gran.; acid no. 0.5 max.; usage level: 1-3% topical use; 95% conc.

Phospholipon® 90/90G. [Seppic] Phosphatidylcholine; emulsifier for dermatology and cosmetics, solubilizer for parenteralia, raw material for liposomes; source for drugs and dietetics.

Phospholipon® 90 H. [Am. Lecithin; Rhone-Poulenc Rorer] Hydrog. lecithin; CAS 97281-48-6; moisturizer, emulsifier, and stabilizer for skin care, sunscreens, creams, and lotions; min. 90% phosphatidylcholine for the mfg. of liposomes for drugs and cosmetics; wh. cryst. powd.; acid no. 0.5 max.; iodine no. 1 max.; usage level: 1-3% topical use; 94% conc.

Phospholipon® 100. [Rhone-Poulenc Rorer] Soya 3-sn-Phosphatidylcholine; CAS 97281-47-5; natural active ingred. for pharmaceuticals; gran.

Phospholipon® 100 H. [Rhone-Poulenc Rorer] Hydrog. soya 3-sn-phosphatidylcholine; CAS 97281-48-6; natural active ingred. for pharmaceuticals; powd.

Phospholipon® CC. [Seppic] 1,2-Dicaproyl-sn-glycero(3) phosphatidylcholine; CAS 3436-44-0.

Phospholipon® CC. [Rhone-Poulenc Rorer] 1,2-Dicaproyl-sn-glycero(3)phosphatidylcholine; CAS 3436-44-0; emulsifier, solubilizer for dermatology and cosmetics; wh. cryst.; ≥ 99% act.

Phospholipon® G. [Rhone-Poulenc Rorer] Soya 3-(3-sn-phosphatidyl) glycerol; natural raw material for pharmaceuticals; cryst.

Phospholipon® GH. [Rhone-Poulenc Rorer] Hydrog. soya 3-(3-sn-phosphatidyl) glycerol; natural raw material for pharmaceuticals; cryst.

Phospholipon® LC. [Rhone-Poulenc Rorer] 1,2-Dilauroyl-sn-glycero(3) phosphocholine; CAS 18285-71-7; emulsifier, solubilizer for dermatology and cosmetics; powd.

Phospholipon® MC. [Seppic] 1,2-Dimyristoyl-sn-glycero(3) phosphatidylcholine; CAS 18194-24-6.

Phospholipon® MC. [Rhone-Poulenc Rorer] 1,2-Dimyristoyl-sn-glycero(3)phosphatidylcholine; CAS 18194-24-6; emulsifier, solubilizer for dermatology and cosmetics; wh. cryst.; ≥ 99% act.

Phospholipon® MG Na. [Rhone-Poulenc Rorer] 1,2-Dimyristoyl-sn-glycero(3)phosphatidylcholine sodium salt; CAS 116870-30-5; emulsifier, solubilizer for dermatology and cosmetics; wh. cryst.; ≥ 97% act.

Phospholipon® PC. [Seppic] 1,2-Dipalmitoyl-sn-glycero(3) phosphatidylcholine; CAS 2644-64-6.

Phospholipon® PC. [Rhone-Poulenc Rorer] 1,2-Dipalmitoyl-sn-glycero(3)phosphatidylcholine; CAS 2644-64-6; emulsifier, solubilizer for dermatology and cosmetics; wh. cryst.; ≥ 99% act.

Phospholipon® PG Na. [Rhone-Poulenc Rorer] 1,2-Dipalmitoyl-sn-glycero(3)phosphatidylcholine sodium salt; CAS 116870-31-6; emulsifier, solubilizer for dermatology and cosmetics; wh. cryst.; ≥ 97% act.

Phospholipon® SC. [Seppic] 1,2-Distearoyl-sn-glycero(3) phosphatidylcholine; CAS 816-94-4.

Phospholipon® SC. [Rhone-Poulenc Rorer] 1,2-Distearoyl-sn-glycero(3)phosphatidylcholine; CAS 816-94-4; emulsifier, solubilizer for dermatology and cosmetics; wh. cryst.; ≥ 99% act.

Phospholipon® SG Na. [Rhone-Poulenc Rorer] 1,2-Distearoyl-sn-glycero(3)phosphatidylcholine sodium salt; emulsifier, solubilizer for dermatology and cosmetics; wh. cryst.; ≥ 97% act.

Phosphoteric® QL38. [Mona Industries] Trisodium lauroampho PG-acetate phosphate chloride; amphoteric; offers mildness, high foam, and detergency for mild cleansers and baby care prods.; amber visc. liq.; 38% conc.

Phosphoteric® T-C6. [Mona Industries] Sodium dicarboxyethylcoco phosphoethyl imidazoline; amphoteric; patented surfactant, hydrotrope; synergizes detergency with ethoxylated nonionics; improves wetting, penetrating, and detergency; for high electrolyte industrial cleaners; provides mildness, high foam, and detergency to mild cleansers and baby care prods.; clear thin amber liq.; sp.gr. 1.09; dens. 9.1 lb/gal; pH 7.0 (10%); Draves wetting 40 s (1% in 100 ppm hard water); toxicology: very low eye irritation, low to moderate skin irritation; acute oral > 5.0 ml/kg; 35% act.

Phylderm® Filatov. [Gattefosse SA] Human placental protein; biological additive.

Phylderm Vegetal. [Gattefosse] Hydrolyzed soy protein; CAS 68607-88-5; raw material for cosmetics; brn. clear liq., char. odor; sol. in water; pH 5.0-6.0.

Phytantriol No. 63926. [Roche] Nonvitamin moisturizer for hair and skin care prods.

Phyt'iod. [Alban Muller] Ethylic esters of the iodized fatty acid of poppy seed oil (ethiodized oil); slenderizing prod. for cosmetics.

Phyto/Cer. [Intergen; Tri-K Industries] Steryl glycosides (90%); plant-derived glycoceramide which enhances and restores barrier function, regulates skin's ability to bind and retain moisture, restores intercellular regulatory balance; for high quality skin care prods.; off-wh. to cream-colored powd., char. odor; misc. in water.

Phyto/Cer rHA. [Intergen; Tri-K Industries] Plant-derived glycoceramide and hyaluronic acid; moisturizer for high quality skin care prods.

Phytoderm Complex G. [Cosmetochem] Propylene glycol and licorice root extract; cosmetic specialty with anti-inflammatory and soothing effect on damaged skin, due to the content of glycyrrhetinic acid.

Phytoderm Complex U. [Cosmetochem] Usnic acid complex; antimicrobial activity against Gram-negative and - positive bacteria, molds, and yeasts; for use as a natural active ingred. in deodorants, footcare preps., special skin and scalp care prods., and toothpastes.

Phytotan. [Laboratoires Sérobiologiques] Amino acids complex; tanning accelerator reinforcing the auto-photoprotection of the skin; for sun care prods.; fights premature aging of the skin; wh. powd.; water-sol.; usage level: 2-5%.

Phytotec Anti Stress. [Sederma] Shea butter extract in 15% "cell nutrient system"; provides enhanced efficacy of the plant extracts.

Phytotec Astringent. [Sederma] Witch hazel, hops, and crataegus extracts in 25% "cell nutrient system"; provides enhanced efficacy of the plant extracts.

Phytotec Hair Tonic. [Sederma] Ivy, horse chestnut, and red vine extracts in 25% "cell nutrient system"; provides enhanced efficacy of the plant extracts.

Phytotec Moisturizer. [Sederma] Aloe vera and linden extracts in 25% "cell nutrient system"; provides enhanced efficacy of the plant extracts.

Phytotec Remineralizer. [Sederma] Horsetail extract in 25% "cell nutrient system"; provides enhanced efficacy of the plant extracts.

Phytotec Repair Factor. [Sederma] Centella asiatica, ginseng, and horsetail extracts in 25% "cell nutrient system"; provides enhanced efficacy of the plant extracts.

Phytotec Slimming Factor. [Sederma] Bladder wrack, ivy, and horse chestnut extracts in 25% "cell nutrient system"; provides enhanced efficacy of the plant extracts.

Phytotec Softening. [Sederma] Matricaria extract in 25% "cell nutrient system"; provides enhanced efficacy of the plant extracts.

Pidolidone® . [UCIB; Barnet Prods.] PCA; CAS 98-79-3; EINECS 202-700-3; amino acid, moisturizing agent, cellular penetration vector for amino acids or min. salts; used in aq. phases of skin and hair care formulations; wh. cryst. powd., odorless; water-sol.; m.w. 129.11; usage level: 1-3%; toxicology: nontoxic; sl. irritating to skin; very sl. irritating to eyes.

Placentaliquid Oil-Soluble. [Dr. Kurt Richter; Henkel/Cospha] Extract of unborn bovine placentas; prods. for aging skin; brnsh.-yel. oil.

Placentaliquid Water-Soluble. [Dr. Kurt Richter; Henkel/Cospha] Extract of unborn bovine placentas; improves skin tone, protects against hair loss; wh. to lt. yel. clear liq.

Planell™ Oil. [Brooks Industries] Squalene, squalane, glycolipids, phytosterol, tocopherol; natural plant lipid extract for use as cosmetic emollient; maintains normal skin function by augmenting skin's own naturally occurring lipid membrane.

Plantaren® 1200. [Henkel/Cospha; Henkel Canada] Lauryl polyglucose; CAS 110615-47-9; nonionic; mild surfactant, foamer, cleanser for low-irritation personal care prods., hair shampoos, bath and shower gels, foam baths, facial cleansers; biodeg.; tan paste; 50% act.

Plantaren® 1200 CS/UP. [Henkel KGaA/Cospha] Lauryl polyglucose with traces of boron; CAS 110615-47-9;

nonionic; surfactant with good dermatological compat. and visc. enhancing effects; additive for cosmetic cleansers; cloudy visc. liq.; sp.gr. 1.07-1.08 (40 C); visc. 2000-4000 mPa·s; pH 11.5-12.5 (20% in 15% IPA); 50-53% act.

Plantaren® 1200 UP. [Henkel KGaA/Cospha] Lauryl polyglucose, unpreserved; CAS 110615-47-9; nonionic; surfactant with good dermatological compat. and visc. enhancing effects; additive for cosmetic cleansers; cloudy visc. liq.; sp.gr. 1.07-1.08 (40 C); visc. 2000-4000 mPa·s; pH 11.5-12.5 (20% in 15% IPA); 50-53% act.

Plantaren® 1300. [Henkel/Cospha; Henkel Canada] Lauryl polyglucose; CAS 110615-47-9; nonionic; mild surfactant, foamer, cleanser for low-irritation personal care prods., hair shampoos, bath and shower gels, foam baths, facial cleansers; biodeg.; tan paste; 50% act.

Plantaren® 2000. [Henkel/Cospha; Henkel Canada] Decyl polyglucose; nonionic; mild surfactant, foamer, cleanser for low-irritation personal care prods., hair shampoos, bath and shower gels, foam baths, facial cleansers; biodeg.; pale yel. clear visc. liq.; water-sol.; pH 7 (20%); toxicology: orally nontoxic; very mild to skin and eyes; 50% act.

Plantaren® 2000 CS/UP. [Henkel KGaA/Cospha] Decyl polyglucose with traces of boron; CAS 141464-42-8; nonionic; surfactant with exc. foaming props. and good dermatological compat.; base for cosmetic cleansers; cloudy visc. liq.; visc. 1000-6000 mPa·s; pH 11.5-12.5 (20% in 15% IPA); 51-55% act.

Plantaren® 2000 UP. [Henkel KGaA/Cospha] Decyl polyglucose, unpreserved; CAS 141464-42-8; nonionic; surfactant with exc. foaming props. and good dermatological compat.; base for cosmetic cleansers; cloudy visc. liq.; visc. 1000-6000 mPa·s; pH 11.5-12.5 (20% in 15% IPA); 51-55% act.

Plantaren® PS-100. [Henkel/Cospha; Henkel Canada] Decyl polyglucose and ammonium laureth sulfate; anionic/nonionic; surfactant base providing optimal foam, foam stability, and less irritation for personal care prods., shampoos, shower gels, bubble baths, facial cleansers; biodeg.; pale yel. visc. liq.; water-sol.; visc. 6000 cps; pH 6.5 (20%); 50% act.

Plantaren® PS-200. [Henkel/Cospha] Lauryl polyglucose and sodium laureth sulfate; surfactant base providing optimal foaming, foam stability, and less irritation potential than typical anionics; for shampoos, shower gels, bubble baths, facial cleansers, liq. soaps; biodeg.; pale yel. visc. liq.; easily disp. in water; visc. 7000 cps; pH 6.5 (20%); 50% act.

Plantaren® PS-300. [Henkel/Cospha] Decyl polyglucose and ammonium lauryl sulfate; surfactant for shampoos, bath and shower prods., other personal care cleansers; provides optimal foaming with less irritation than typical anionic surfactants; clear visc. liq.; 50% act.

Plant Ceramides. [Herstellung von Naturextrakten GmbH; Lipo] Wheat germ extract, corn germ extract; used for treatment of dry, aging, and/or damaged skin; lt. yel. to amber fine powd., weak intrinsic odor; usage level: 5%.

Plant Exsyliposomes. [Exsymol; Biosil Tech.] Arnica, calendula, centella saiatica, and licorice liposomes for skin care prods.; sl. colored opalescent liq.; usage level: 2-6%; toxicology: nontoxic.

Plantsol. [Brooks Industries] Yeast cytosol extract; cytoskeletol elements provide cellular support and structure and high m.w. sugars provide moisture-binding capability; leaves a soft, moisture-retentive film on the skin; low color and odor; 4% sol'n.

Plascize L-53. [Goo Chem.] Acrylates/diacetoneacrylamide copolymer.

Plascize L-53D. [Goo Chem.] AMPD acrylates/diacetoneacrylamide copolymer; raw material for cos-

metic and personal care prods.

Plascize L-53P. [Goo Chem.] AMP-acrylates/diacetoneacrylamide copolymer; raw material for cosmetic and personal care prods.

Plasdone® C-15. [ISP] PVP (pyrogen-free Povidone USP K-17); CAS 9003-39-8; EINECS 201-800-4; low m.w. excipient used primarily for veterinary pharmaceuticals; for parenteral applics.; solubilizer, stabilizer, protective colloid; powd.

Plasdone® C-30. [ISP] PVP; USP grade; CAS 9003-39-8; EINECS 201-800-4; for parenteral applics.; solubilizer, stabilizer, protective colloid; minimizes toxic side effects and reduces irritation at site of inj.; accepted blood plasma expander for emergency use; suitable for stock piling; powd.

Plasdone® K-25, K-90. [ISP] PVP (Povidone USP); CAS 9003-39-8; EINECS 201-800-4; pharmaceutical excipient used as tablet binder and coating agent; promotes dye and pigment disp.; as cohesive agent, stabilizer, and protective colloid; detoxicant; drug vehicle and retardant; solubilizer and suspending agent in liq. prods.; for topical applics., liq. pharmaceuticals; film-forming agent in medicinal aerosols; powd.

Plasdone® K-26/28, K-29/32. [ISP] PVP USP; CAS 9003-39-8; EINECS 201-800-4; used as tablet binder and coating agent; promotes dye and pigment disp. in tablets; used as cohesive agent, stabilizer, and protective colloid, as detoxicant for poisons and irritants, as drug vehicle and retardant; minimizes toxic side effects of some drugs; as solubilizer and suspending agent in liq. prods.; as detoxicant and demulcent lubricant in ophthalmic and pharmaceutical topicals.; as film-forming agent in medicinal aerosols; powd.

Plasvita® TSM. [Hüls AG] Methylene casein; tablet disintegration agent for pharmaceuticals; high capillary activity, low swelling effect; wh. powd., odorless, tasteless; insol. in water.

Pluracare® F68. [BASF] Poloxamer 188; CAS 9003-11-6; nonionic; surfactant for cosmetic use; prill.

Pluracare® F77. [BASF] Poloxamer 217; CAS 9003-11-6; nonionic; surfactant for cosmetic use; prill.

Pluracare® F108. [BASF] Poloxamer 338; CAS 9003-11-6; nonionic; surfactant for cosmetic use; prill.

Pluracare® F127. [BASF] Poloxamer 407; CAS 9003-11-6; nonionic; surfactant for cosmetic use; prill.

Pluracare® L64. [BASF] Poloxamer 184; CAS 9003-11-6; nonionic; surfactant for cosmetic use; liq.

Pluracare® P65. [BASF] Poloxamer 185; CAS 9003-11-6; nonionic; surfactant for cosmetic use; paste.

Pluracol® E200. [BASF] PEG-4; CAS 25322-68-3; EINECS 203-989-9; intermediate for preparation of nonionic surfactants; binder, base, coating, stabilizer, solv., vehicle, extender, and coupling agent for pharmaceutical, cosmetic, and toiletries; lubricant for metal applics., rubber industry; wood treatment; textile conditioning, antistat, and sizing agent, softener; colorless clear liq.; m.w. 200; sol. in water and org. solvs. except aliphatic hydrocarbons; dens. 9.4 lb/gal; sp.gr. 1.12; visc. 4.36 cs (210 F); flash pt. 360 F; surf. tens. 57.2 dynes/cm (1%); pH 6.5 (5% aq.).

Pluracol® E300. [BASF] PEG-6; CAS 25322-68-3; EINECS 220-045-1; see Pluracol E200; also dispersant in food tablets and preparations; plasticizer; colorless clear liq.; m.w. 300; sol. in water and org. solvs. except aliphatic hydrocarbons; dens. 9.4 lb/gal; sp.gr. 1.12; visc. 5.9 cs (99 C); flash pt. (COC) 210 C; pour pt. -13 C; surf. tens. 62.9 dynes/cm (1%); pH 5.7 (5% aq.).

Pluracol® E400. [BASF] PEG-8; CAS 25322-68-3; EINECS 225-856-4; see Pluracol E300; colorless clear liq.; sol. in water and org. solvs. except aliphatic hydrocarbons;

dens. 9.4 lb/gal; sp.gr. 1.12; visc. 7.39 cs (210 F); flash pt. 460 F; surf. tens. 66.6 dynes/cm (1%); pH 6.2 (5% aq.).

Pluracol® E400 NF. [BASF] PEG-8; CAS 25322-68-3; EINECS 225-856-4; chemical intermediate, base, coupler, thickener, lubricant, mold release agent, defoamer, softener, conditioner, antistat, sizing agent, dispersant for pharmaceutical, cosmetic, and oral care preparations, in metal polishing and cleaning formulations, rubber prods., paper and wood prods., textile processing, ink formulations; liq.; m.w. 400; visc. 7.4 cs (99 C); pour pt. 5 C; flash pt. (COC) 182 C.

Pluracol® E600. [BASF] PEG-12; CAS 25322-68-3; EINECS 229-859-1; see Pluracol E300; colorless clear liq.; sol. in water and org. solvs. except aliphatic hydrocarbons; dens. 9.4 lb/gal; sp.gr. 1.12; visc. 10.83 cs (210 F); flash pt. 480 F; surf. tens. 65.2 dynes/cm (1%); pH 5.3 (5% aq.).

Pluracol® E600 NF. [BASF] PEG-12; CAS 25322-68-3; EINECS 229-859-1; see Pluracol E400 NF; liq.; m.w. 600; visc. 10.8 cs (99 C); pour pt. 20 C; flash pt. (COC) 249 C.

Pluracol® E1000. [BASF] PEG-20; CAS 25322-68-3; see Pluracol E400 NF; solid; m.w. 1000; visc. 17.5 cs (99 C); m.p. 38 C; flash pt. (COC) 255 C.

Pluracol® E1450. [BASF] PEG-32; CAS 25322-68-3; see Pluracol E400 NF; solid; m.w. 1450; visc. 28.5 cs (99 C); m.p. 45 C; flash pt. (COC) 255 C.

Pluracol® E1450 NF. [BASF] PEG-32; CAS 25322-68-3; see Pluracol E400 NF; solid; m.w. 600; visc. 28.5 cs (99 C); m.p. 45 C; flash pt. (COC) 255 C.

Pluracol® E2000. [BASF] PEG-40; CAS 25322-68-3; see Pluracol E400 NF; solid; m.w. 2000; visc. 43.5 cs (99 C); m.p. 52 C; flash pt. (COC) > 260 C.

Pluracol® E4000. [BASF] PEG-75; CAS 25322-68-3; see Pluracol E300; wh. waxy solid; sol. in water and org. solvs. except aliphatic hydrocarbons; dens. 10.0 lb/gal; sp.gr. 1.20; m.p. 59.5 C; flash pt. > 490 F; surf. tens. 61.9 dynes/cm (1%); pH 6.7 (5% aq.).

Pluracol® E4000 NF. [BASF] PEG-75; CAS 25322-68-3; see Pluracol E400 NF; solid; m.w. 4000; visc. 134 cs (99 C); m.p. 59 C; flash pt. (COC) > 260 C.

Pluracol® E8000. [BASF] PEG-150; CAS 25322-68-3; see Pluracol E400 NF; solid; m.w. 8000; visc. 750 cs (99 C); m.p. 61 C; flash pt. (COC) > 260 C.

Pluracol® E8000 NF. [BASF] PEG-150 NF; CAS 25322-68-3; see Pluracol E400 NF; solid; m.w. 8000; visc. 750 cs (99 C); m.p. 61 C; flash pt (COC) > 260 C.

Pluracol® W3520N. [BASF] PPG-28-buteth-35; CAS 9038-95-3; component in demulsifying and wetting formulations; brake and metalworking fluids; rubber and fiber lubricant; textile applics.; defoamer for hot and cold applics., food and chemical processing; cosmetic formulations; APHA 40 max. visc. liq.; sol. in water, alcohols, ketones, esters, benzene, toluene, glycol ethers, chlorinated solvs.; dens. 8.83 lb/gal; sp.gr. 1.06; visc. 3520 SUS (100 F); cloud pt. 57 C (1%); flash pt. (OC) 437 F (OC); pour pt. –20 F; pH 6.0–7.5 (10% aq.).

Pluracol® W5100N. [BASF] PPG-33-buteth-45; CAS 74623-31-7; component in demulsifying and wetting formulations; brake and metalworking fluids; rubber and fiber lubricant; textile applics.; defoamer for hot and cold applics., food and chemical processing; cosmetic formulations; APHA 40 max. visc. liq.; sol. in water, alcohols, ketones, esters, benzene, toluene, glycol ethers, chlorinated solvs.; dens. 8.83 lb/gal; sp.gr. 1.06; visc. 5100 SUS (100 F); cloud pt. 55 C (1%); flash pt. (OC) 437 F; pour pt. –20 F; pH 5.5–7.0 (10% aq.).

Plurol Isostearique. [Gattefosse SA] Polyglyceryl-6 isostearate; CAS 126928-07-2; nonionic; emulsifier; cosurfactant for microemulsions; Gardner < 10 visc. liq., char. odor; sol. in chloroform, methylene chloride, veg. oils,

ethanol; disp. in water; HLB 10.0; acid no. < 6; iodine no. < 10; sapon. no. 115-135; ref. index 1.470-1.480; toxicology: nonirritating to skin and eyes; 100% conc.

Plurol Oleique WL 1173. [Gattefosse SA] Polyglyceryl-6 dioleate; CAS 76009-37-5; nonionic; emulsifier; cosurfactant for microemulsions; Gardner < 10 visc. liq., char. odor; sol. in ethanol, chloroform, methylene chloride, veg. and min. oils; disp. in water; visc. 8-20 Pa·s; HLB 10.0; acid no. < 6; iodine no. 50-70; sapon. no. 110-140; pH 7.0-9.5 (10% aq.); ref. index 1.470-1.490; toxicology: sl. irritating to skin and eyes; 100% conc.

Plurol Stearique WL 1009. [Gattefosse SA] Polyglyceryl-6 distearate; CAS 34424-97-0; nonionic; consistency agent and stabilizer for heated o/w emulsions; food emulsifier; FCC listed; Gardner < 10 waxy solid, faint odor; sol. in chloroform, methylene chloride; partly sol. in ethanol; disp. in water; HLB 9.0; drop pt. 48-53 C; acid no. < 5; iodine no. < 3; sapon. no. 120-140; pH 7.0-9.5 (10% aq.); toxicology: nonirritating to eyes; 100% conc.

Pluronic® 10R5. [BASF] Meroxapol 105; CAS 9003-11-6; nonionic; emulsifier, wetting agent, binder, stabilizer, plasticizer, lubricant, solubilizer, dispersant, visc. control agent, defoamer, intermediate for hard surface detergents, rinse aids, automatic dishwashing, textile processing; cosmetics; pharmaceuticals, pulp, paper, and petrol. industries, agric. prods., in iodophors, water treating systems, fermentation, cutting and grinding fluids; liq.; m.w. 1970; ref. index. 1.4587; sol. in water, propylene glycol, xylene, IPA, ethyl acetate, perchloroethylene, IPM; sp.gr. 1.058; visc. 400 cps; HLB 21.0; cloud pt. 69 C (1% aq.); flash pt. (COC) > 450 F; pour pt. 15 C; surf. tens. 50.9 dynes/cm; toxicology: minimal to mild eye and skin irritation; 100% act.

Pluronic® 17R2. [BASF] Meroxapol 172; CAS 9003-11-6; nonionic; see Pluronic 10R5; liq.; m.w. 2100; ref. index 1.4535; sol. in water, xylene, IPA; ethyl acetate, perchloroethylene, IPM, trichlorotrifluoroethane; sp.gr. 1.030; visc. 350 cps; HLB 8.0; cloud pt. 39 C (1% aq.); flash pt. (COC) > 450 F; pour pt. –25 C; surf. tens. 41.9 dynes/cm (0.1%); toxicology: minimal to mild eye and skin irritation; 100% act.

Pluronic® 17R4. [BASF] Meroxapol 174; CAS 9003-11-6; nonionic; see Pluronic 10R5; liq.; m.w. 2700; ref. index. 1.4572; sol. in water, propylene glycol, xylene, IPA, ethyl acetate, perchloroethylene, IPM, trichlorotrifluoroethane; sp.gr. 1.048; visc. 560 cps; HLB 16.0; cloud pt. 47 C (1% aq.); flash pt. (COC) > 450 F; pour pt. 18 C; surf. tens. 44.1 dynes/cm (0.1%); toxicology: minimal to mild eye and skin irritation; 100% act.

Pluronic® 25R2. [BASF] Meroxapol 252; CAS 9003-11-6; nonionic; see Pluronic 10R5; also wetting and rinse aid; lubricant and leveling agent for paper coating; liq.; m.w. 3120; ref. index 1.4541; sol. see Pluronic 25R1; sp.gr. 1.039; visc. 680 cps; HLB 6.3; cloud pt. 33 C (1% aq.); flash pt. (COC) > 450 F; pour pt. –5 C; surf. tens. 37.5 dynes/cm (0.1%); toxicology: minimal to mild eye and skin irritation; 100% act.

Pluronic® 25R4. [BASF] Meroxapol 254; CAS 9003-11-6; nonionic; see Pluronic 10R5; liq.; m.w. 3800; ref. index 1.4574; sol. in water, propylene glycol, ethyl acetate, perchloroethylene, IPM, trichlorotrifluoroethane; sp.gr. 1.046; visc. 1110 cps; HLB 14.3; cloud pt. 40 C (1% aq.); flash pt. (COC) > 450 F; pour pt. 25 C; surf. tens. 40.9 dynes/cm (0.1%); toxicology: minimal to mild eye and skin irritation; 100% act.

Pluronic® 25R8. [BASF] Meroxapol 258; CAS 9003-11-6; nonionic; see Pluronic 10R5; also dry toilet bowl cleaners, dye levelers for fabrics; solubilizer for drugs; thickener for cosmetics; deinking operations; felt washing operations; flakable solid; m.w. 9000; sol. in water; sp.gr. 1.062; m.p.

56 C; HLB 30.3; cloud pt. 80 C (1% aq.); flash pt. (COC) > 450 F; surf. tens. 46.1 dynes/cm (0.1%); toxicology: minimal to mild eye and skin irritation; 100% act.

Pluronic® 31R1. [BASF] Meroxapol 311; CAS 9003-11-6; nonionic; see Pluronic 10R5; also floating bath oils; foam control in antifreeze; liq.; m.w. 3200; ref. index 1.4522; sol. Pluronic® 25R1; sp.gr. 1.018; visc. 578 cps; HLB 1.7; cloud pt. 25 C (1% aq.); flash pt. (COC) > 450 F; pour pt. –25 C; surf. tens. 34.1 dynes/cm (0.1%); toxicology: minimal to mild eye and skin irritation; 100% act.

Pluronic® F38. [BASF] Poloxamer 108; CAS 9003-11-6; nonionic; wetting agent, emulsifier, demulsifier, foam and visc. control agent, dispersant, antistat, gelling agent, dyeing assistant, leveler, lubricant for agric., cosmetics, pharmaceuticals, metal cleaning, pulp/paper, textile scouring, water treatment; prilled; m.w. 5000; sol. in ethanol, propylene glycol, water, toluene, dens. 8.9 lb/gal (77 C); sp.gr. 1.07 (77 C); visc. 260 cps (77 C); m.p. 48 C; HLB 30.5; cloud pt. > 100 C (1% aq.); flash pt. (COC) 505 F; surf. tens. 52.2 dynes/cm (0.1% conc.); toxicology: non to sl. eye and skin irritation; 100% act.

Pluronic® F68. [BASF] Poloxamer 188; CAS 9003-11-6; nonionic; wetting agent, emulsifier, demulsifier, foam and visc. control agent, dispersant, antistat, gelling agent, dyeing assistant, leveler, lubricant for agric., cosmetics, pharmaceuticals, metal cleaning, pulp/paper, textile scouring, water treatment; prilled; m.w. 8350; sol. in ethanol, water; dens. 8.8 lb/gal (77 C); sp.gr. 1.06 (77 C); visc. 1000 cps (77 C); m.p. 52 C; HLB 29.0; cloud pt. > 100 C (1% aq.); flash pt. (COC) 500 F; surf. tens. 50.3 dynes/cm (0.1%); toxicology: non to sl. eye and skin irritation; 100% act.

Pluronic® F77. [BASF] Poloxamer 217; CAS 9003-11-6; nonionic; wetting agent, emulsifier, demulsifier, foam and visc. control agent, dispersant, antistat, gelling agent, dyeing assistant, leveler, lubricant for agric., cosmetics, pharmaceuticals, metal cleaning, pulp/paper, textile scouring, water treatment; prilled; m.w. 6600; sol. in ethanol, water, toluene; dens. 8.7 lb/gal (77 C); sp.gr. 1.04 (77 C); m.p. 48 C; HLB 24.5; cloud pt. > 100 C (1% aq.); flash pt. (COC) 485 F; surf. tens. 47.0 dynes/cm (0.1%); toxicology: non to sl. eye and skin irritation; 100% act.

Pluronic® F87. [BASF] Poloxamer 237; CAS 9003-11-6; nonionic; wetting agent, emulsifier, demulsifier, foam and visc. control agent, dispersant, antistat, gelling agent, dyeing assistant, leveler, lubricant for agric., cosmetics, pharmaceuticals, metal cleaning, pulp/paper, textile scouring, water treatment; prilled; m.w. 7700; sol. see Pluronic F77; dens. 8.7 lb/gal (77 C); sp.gr. 1.04 (77 C); visc. 700 cps. (77 C); m.p. 49 C; HLB 24.0; cloud pt. > 100 C (1% aq.); flash pt. (COC) 472 F; surf. tens. 44.0 dynes/cm (0.1%); toxicology: non to sl. eye and skin irritation; 100% act.

Pluronic® F88. [BASF] Poloxamer 238; CAS 9003-11-6; nonionic; wetting agent, emulsifier, demulsifier, foam and visc. control agent, dispersant, antistat, gelling agent, dyeing assistant, leveler, lubricant for agric., cosmetics, pharmaceuticals, metal cleaning, pulp/paper, textile scouring, water treatment; prilled; m.w. 10,800; sol. in ethanol and water; dens. 8.8 lb/gal (77 C); sp.gr. 1.06 (77 C); visc. 2300 cps (77 C); m.p. 54 C; HLB 28.0; cloud pt. > 100 C (1% aq.); surf. tens. 48.5 dynes/cm (0.1%); toxicology: non to sl. eye and skin irritation; 100% act.

Pluronic® F98. [BASF] Poloxamer 288; CAS 9003-11-6; nonionic; wetting agent, emulsifier, demulsifier, foam and visc. control agent, dispersant, antistat, gelling agent, dyeing assistant, leveler, lubricant for agric., cosmetics, pharmaceuticals, metal cleaning, pulp/paper, textile scouring, water treatment; prilled; m.w. 13,000; sol. in ethanol, water, perchoroethylene; dens. 8.8 lb/gal (77 C);

sp.gr. 1.06 (77 C); visc. 2700 cps (77 C); m.p. 55 C; HLB 27.5; cloud pt. > 100 C (1% aq.); flash pt. (COC) 491 F; surf. tens. 43.0 dynes/cm (0.1%); toxicology: non to sl. eye and skin irritation; 100% act.

Pluronic® F108. [BASF] Poloxamer 338; CAS 9003-11-6; nonionic; see Pluronic F38; prilled; m.w. 14,000; sol. in ethanol, water; dens. 8.8 lb/gal (77 C); sp.gr. 1.06 (77 C); visc. 8000 cps (77 C); m.p. 57 C; HLB 27.0; cloud pt. > 100 C (1% aq.); flash pt. (COC) 495 F; surf. tens. 41.2 dynes/cm (0.1%); toxicology: non to sl. eye and skin irritation; 100% act.

Pluronic® F127. [BASF] Poloxamer 407; CAS 9003-11-6; nonionic; see Pluronic F38; prilled; m.w. 12,500; sol. in ethanol, water, toluene, perchloroethylene; dens. 8.8 lb/gal (77 C); sp.gr. 1.05 (77 C); visc. 3100 cps (77 C); m.p. 56 C; HLB 22.0; cloud pt. > 100 C (1% aq.); surf. tens. 40.6 dynes/cm (0.1%); toxicology: non to sl. eye and skin irritation; 100% act.

Pluronic® L35. [BASF] Poloxamer 105; CAS 9003-11-6; nonionic; wetting agent, emulsifier, demulsifier, foam and visc. control agent, dispersant, antistat, gelling agent, dyeing assistant, leveler, lubricant for agric., cosmetics, pharmaceuticals, metal cleaning, pulp/paper, textile scouring, water treatment; liq.; m.w. 1900; sol. in ethanol, propylene glycol, water, toluene, xylene, perchloroethylene; dens. 8.8 lb/gal; sp.gr. 1.06; visc. 340 cps; HLB 18.5; cloud pt. 77 C (1% aq.); pour pt. 7 C; surf. tens. 48.8 dynes/cm (0.1%); toxicology: non to sl. eye and skin irritation; 100% act.

Pluronic® L43. [BASF] Poloxamer 123; CAS 9003-11-6; nonionic; wetting agent, emulsifier, demulsifier, foam and visc. control agent, dispersant, antistat, gelling agent, dyeing assistant, leveler, lubricant for agric., cosmetics, pharmaceuticals, metal cleaning, pulp/paper, textile scouring, water treatment; liq.; m.w. 1850; ref. index 1.4563; sol. in ethanol, propylene glycol, water, toluene, xylene, perchloroethylene; dens. 8.7 lb/gal; sp.gr. 1.04; visc. 310 cps; HLB 12.0; cloud pt. 42 C (1% aq.); pour pt. –1 C; surf. tens. 47.3 dynes/cm (0.1%); toxicology: non to sl. eye and skin irritation; 100% act.

Pluronic® L44. [BASF] Poloxamer 124; CAS 9003-11-6; nonionic; wetting agent, emulsifier, demulsifier, foam and visc. control agent, dispersant, antistat, gelling agent, dyeing assistant, leveler, lubricant for agric., cosmetics, pharmaceuticals, metal cleaning, pulp/paper, textile scouring, water treatment; liq.; m.w. 2200; ref. index 1.4580; dens. 8.8 lb/gal; sp.gr. 1.05; visc. 440 cps; HLB 16.0; cloud pt. 65 C (1% aq.); flash pt. (COC) 464 F; pour pt. 16 C; surf. tens. 45.3 dynes/cm (0.1%); toxicology: non to sl. eye and skin irritation; 100% act.

Pluronic® L61. [BASF] Poloxamer 181; CAS 9003-11-6; nonionic; wetting agent, emulsifier, demulsifier, foam and visc. control agent, dispersant, antistat, gelling agent, dyeing assistant, leveler, lubricant for agric., cosmetics, pharmaceuticals, metal cleaning, pulp/paper, textile scouring, water treatment; liq.; m.w. 2000; ref. index 1.4520; sol. in ethanol, toluene, xylene, perchloroethylene; dens. 8.4 lb/gal; sp.gr. 1.01; visc. 285 cps; HLB 3.0; cloud pt. 24 C (1% aq.); flash pt. (COC) 455 F; pour pt. –29 C; toxicology: non to sl. eye and skin irritation; 100% act.

Pluronic® L62. [BASF] Poloxamer 182; CAS 9003-11-6; nonionic; wetting agent, emulsifier, demulsifier, foam and visc. control agent, dispersant, antistat, gelling agent, dyeing assistant, leveler, lubricant for agric., cosmetics, pharmaceuticals, metal cleaning, pulp/paper, textile scouring, water treatment; liq.; m.w. 2500; sol. in ethanol, propylene glycol, water, toluene, xylene, perchloroethylene; dens. 8.6 lb/gal; sp.gr. 1.03; visc. 400 cps; HLB 7.0; cloud pt. 32 C (1% aq.); flash pt. (COC) 466 F; pour pt. –

4 C; surf. tens. 42.8 dynes/cm (0.1%); toxicology: non to sl. eye and skin irritation; 100% act.

Pluronic® L64. [BASF] Poloxamer 184; CAS 9003-11-6; nonionic; wetting agent, emulsifier, demulsifier, foam and visc. control agent, dispersant, antistat, gelling agent, dyeing assistant, leveler, lubricant for agric., cosmetics, pharmaceuticals, metal cleaning, pulp/paper, textile scouring, water treatment; liq.; m.w. 2900; ref. index 1.4575; sol. in ethanol, propylene glycol, water, toluene, xylene, perchloroethylene; dens. 8.8 lb/gal; sp.gr. 1.05; visc. 550 cps; HLB 15.0; cloud pt. 61 C (1% aq.); flash pt. (COC) 485 F; pour pt. 16 C; surf. tens. 43.2 dynes/cm (0.1%); toxicology: non to sl. eye and skin irritation; 100% act.

Pluronic® L81. [BASF] Poloxamer 231; CAS 9003-11-6; nonionic; wetting agent, emulsifier, demulsifier, foam and visc. control agent, dispersant, antistat, gelling agent, dyeing assistant, leveler, lubricant for agric., cosmetics, pharmaceuticals, metal cleaning, pulp/paper, textile scouring, water treatment; liq.; m.w. 2750; ref. index 1.4526; sol. in ethanol, toluene, xylene, perchloroethylene; dens. 8.5 lb/gal; sp.gr. 1.02; visc. 475 cps; HLB 2.0; cloud pt. 20 C (1% aq.); pour pt. −37 C; toxicology: non to sl. eye and skin irritation; 100% act.

Pluronic® L92. [BASF] Poloxamer 282; CAS 9003-11-6; nonionic; wetting agent, emulsifier, demulsifier, foam and visc. control agent, dispersant, antistat, gelling agent, dyeing assistant, leveler, lubricant for agric., cosmetics, pharmaceuticals, metal cleaning, pulp/paper, textile scouring, water treatment; liq.; m.w. 3650; ref. index 1.4547; sol. in ethanol, toluene, xylene, perchloroethylene; dens. 8.6 lb/gal; sp.gr. 1.03; visc. 700 cps; HLB 5.5; cloud pt. 26 C (1% aq.); flash pt. (COC) 445 F; pour pt. 7 C; surf. tens. 35.9 dynes/cm (0.1%); toxicology: non to sl. eye and skin irritation; 100% act.

Pluronic® L101. [BASF] Poloxamer 331; CAS 9003-11-6; nonionic; wetting agent, emulsifier, demulsifier, foam and visc. control agent, dispersant, antistat, gelling agent, dyeing assistant, leveler, lubricant for agric., cosmetics, pharmaceuticals, metal cleaning, pulp/paper, textile scouring, water treatment; liq.; m.w. 3800; ref. index 1.4524; sol. in ethanol, toluene, xylene, perchloroethylene; dens. 8.5 lb/gal; sp.gr. 1.02; visc. 800 cps; HLB 1.0; cloud pt. 15 C (1% aq.); pour pt. −23 C; toxicology: non to sl. eye and skin irritation; 100% act.

Pluronic® L121. [BASF] Poloxamer 401; CAS 9003-11-6; nonionic; wetting agent, emulsifier, demulsifier, foam and visc. control agent, dispersant, antistat, gelling agent, dyeing assistant, leveler, lubricant for agric., cosmetics, pharmaceuticals, metal cleaning, pulp/paper, textile scouring, water treatment; liq.; m.w. 4400; ref. index 1.4527; sol. in ethanol, toluene, xylene, perchloroethylene; dens. 8.4 lb/gal; sp.gr. 1.01; visc. 1200 cps; HLB 5.0; cloud pt. 14 C (1% aq.); pour pt. 5 C; surf. tens. 33.0 dynes/cm (0.1%); toxicology: non to sl. eye and skin irritation; 100% act.

Pluronic® L122. [BASF] Poloxamer 402; CAS 9003-11-6; nonionic; wetting agent, emulsifier, demulsifier, foam and visc. control agent, dispersant, antistat, gelling agent, dyeing assistant, leveler, lubricant for agric., cosmetics, pharmaceuticals, metal cleaning, pulp/paper, textile scouring, water treatment; liq.; m.w. 5000; ref. index 1.4558; sol. in ethanol, toluene, xylene, perchloroethylene; dens. 8.6 lb/gal; sp.gr. 1.03; visc. 1750 cps; HLB 4.0; cloud pt. 19 C (1% aq.); flash pt. (COC) 490 F; pour pt. 20 C; surf. tens. 33.0 dynes/cm (0.1%); toxicology: non to sl. eye and skin irritation; 100% act.

Pluronic® P65. [BASF] Poloxamer 185; CAS 9003-11-6; nonionic; wetting agent, emulsifier, demulsifier, foam and visc. control agent, dispersant, antistat, gelling agent,

dyeing assistant, leveler, lubricant for agric., cosmetics, pharmaceuticals, metal cleaning, pulp/paper, textile scouring, water treatment; paste; sol. > 10 g/100 ml in 95% ethanol, propylene glycol, water, toluene, xylene, perchloroethylene; m.w. 3400; dens. 8.8 lb/gal (60 C); sp.gr. 1.06 (60 C); visc. 180 cps (60 C); m.p. 30 C; HLB 17.0; cloud pt. 82 C (1% aq.); pour pt. 27 C; surf. tens. 46.3 dynes/cm (0.1%); toxicology: non to sl. eye and skin irritation; 100% act.

Pluronic® P84. [BASF] Poloxamer 234; CAS 9003-11-6; nonionic; wetting agent, emulsifier, demulsifier, foam and visc. control agent, dispersant, antistat, gelling agent, dyeing assistant, leveler, lubricant for agric., cosmetics, pharmaceuticals, metal cleaning, pulp/paper, textile scouring, water treatment; paste; m.w. 4200; dens. 8.6 lb/gal (60 C); sp.gr. 1.03 (60 C); visc. 265 cps (60 C); m.p. 34 C; HLB 14.0; cloud pt. 74 C (1% aq.); flash pt. (COC) 442 F; pour pt. 18 C; surf. tens. 42.0 dynes/cm (0.1%); toxicology: non to sl. eye and skin irritation; 100% act.

Pluronic® P85. [BASF] Poloxamer 235; CAS 9003-11-6; nonionic; wetting agent, emulsifier, demulsifier, foam and visc. control agent, dispersant, antistat, gelling agent, dyeing assistant, leveler, lubricant for agric., cosmetics, pharmaceuticals, metal cleaning, pulp/paper, textile scouring, water treatment; paste; m.w. 4600; sol. in ethanol, propylene glycol, water, toluene, xylene, perchloroethylene; dens. 8.7 lb/gal (60 C); sp.gr. 1.04 (60 C); visc. 310 cps (60 C); m.p. 40 C; HLB 16.0; cloud pt. 85 C (1% aq.); pour pt. 29 C; surf. tens. 42.5 dynes/cm (0.1%); toxicology: non to sl. eye and skin irritation; 100% act.

Pluronic® P103. [BASF] Poloxamer 333; CAS 9003-11-6; nonionic; wetting agent, emulsifier, demulsifier, foam and visc. control agent, dispersant, antistat, gelling agent, dyeing assistant, leveler, lubricant for agric., cosmetics, pharmaceuticals, metal cleaning, pulp/paper, textile scouring, water treatment; paste; m.w. 4950; sol. in ethanol, toluene, xylene, perchloroethylene; dens. 8.7 lb/gal (60 C); sp.gr. 1.04 (60 C); visc. 285 cps (60 C); m.p. 30 C; HLB 9.0; cloud pt. 86 C (1% aq.); pour pt. 21 C; surf. tens. 34.4 dynes/cm (0.1%); toxicology: non to sl. eye and skin irritation; 100% act.

Pluronic® P104. [BASF] Poloxamer 334; CAS 9003-11-6; nonionic; wetting agent, emulsifier, demulsifier, foam and visc. control agent, dispersant, antistat, gelling agent, dyeing assistant, leveler, lubricant for agric., cosmetics, pharmaceuticals, metal cleaning, pulp/paper, textile scouring, water treatment; paste; m.w. 5850; sol. in ethanol, toluene, xylene, perchloroethylene; dens. 8.7 lb/gal (60 C); sp.gr. 1.04 (60 C); visc. 550 cps (60 C); m.p. 37.5; HLB 13.0; cloud pt. 81 C (1% aq.); flash pt. (COC) 448 F; pour pt. 32 C; surf. tens. 33.1 dynes/cm (0.1%); toxicology: non to sl. eye and skin irritation; 100% act.

Pluronic® P105. [BASF] Poloxamer 335; CAS 9003-11-6; nonionic; wetting agent, emulsifier, demulsifier, foam and visc. control agent, dispersant, antistat, gelling agent, dyeing assistant, leveler, lubricant for agric., cosmetics, pharmaceuticals, metal cleaning, pulp/paper, textile scouring, water treatment; paste; m.w. 6500; sol. in ethanol, toluene, xylene, perchloroethylene; dens. 8.8 lb/gal (60 C); sp.gr. 1.05 (60 C); visc. 800 cps (60 C); m.p. 42 C; HLB 15.0; cloud pt. 91 C (1% aq.); pour pt. 35 C; surf. tens. 39.1 dynes/cm (0.1%); toxicology: non to sl. eye and skin irritation; 100% act.

Pluronic® P123. [BASF] Poloxamer 403; CAS 9003-11-6; nonionic; wetting agent, emulsifier, demulsifier, foam and visc. control agent, dispersant, antistat, gelling agent, dyeing assistant, leveler, lubricant for agric., cosmetics, pharmaceuticals, metal cleaning, pulp/paper, textile scouring, water treatment; paste; m.w. 5750; sol. in ethanol, toluene, xylene, perchloroethylene; dens. 8.5 lb/gal

(60 C); sp.gr. 1.02 (60 C); visc. 350 cps (60 C); m.p. 31 C; HLB 8.0; cloud pt. 90 C (1% aq.); pour pt. 31 C; surf. tens. 34.1 dynes/cm (0.1%); toxicology: non to sl. eye and skin irritation; 100% act.

PME. [Vevy] PPG-5 pentaerythritol ether.

PMMA Beads. [U.S. Cosmetics] Polymethylmethacrylate beads; CAS 9011-14-7; provides a smooth feel or glide to aid in applic. of makeup and skin care prods.; avail. in gelling and nongelling types; spherical beads.

Poem-LS-90. [Riken Vitamin Oil] Sodium cocomonoglyceride sulfate; CAS 61789-04-6; EINECS 263-026-3; detergent, foamer.

Poem-S-105. [Riken Vitamin Oil] PEG-5 glyceryl stearate; emulsifier.

Pogol 200. [Hart Chem. Ltd.] PEG; nonionic; intermediate for fatty acid esters; solubilizer, antistat, softener, humectant, fiber and metal lubricant, plasticizer, tablet binder; for pharmaceuticals, cosmetics; clear liq.; m.w. 190-210; sp.gr. 1.14; 100% act.

Pogol 400 NF. [Hart Chem. Ltd.] PEG, NF grade; nonionic; solubilizer, solv. for pharmaceuticals; mold release agent and lubricant for both natural and syn. prods.; dye carrier; clear liq.; m.w. 380-420; sp.gr. 1.12; visc; 92 cps; 100% act.

Polargel® HV. [Am. Colloid] Bentonite USP/NF; CAS 1302-78-9; EINECS 215-108-5; high visc. wh. montmorilonite used as viscosifier, disintegrant, binder, suspension agent for pharmaceutical, cosmetic, and personal care prods.; wh. microfine powd.; 99% min. thru 200 mesh; vic. 800 cps min. (5% solids); pH 9.5-10.5 (2% disp.); dry brightness (GE) 83-87; 5-8% moisture.

Polargel® NF. [Am. Colloid] Purified wh. bentonite USP/NF; CAS 1302-78-9; EINECS 215-108-5; gellant, thickener, and suspending agent for cosmetics, pharmaceuticals, and personal care prods.; wh. fine powd.; 99% thru 200 mesh; visc. 40-200 cps (5% solids); pH 9.0-10.0 (5% disp.); dry brightness (GE) 85-90; 8% max. moisture.

Polargel® T. [Am. Colloid] Bentonite USP/NF; CAS 1302-78-9; EINECS 215-108-5; thickener, suspension agent, and binder for pharmaceutical, cosmetic, and personal care prods.; wh. fine powd.; 99% min. thru 200 mesh; visc. 200-500 cps (5% solids); pH 9.5-10.5 (2% disp.); dry brightness (GE) 83-87; 5-8% moisture.

Polawax®. [Croda Inc.; Croda Surf. Ltd.] Emulsifying wax NF; nonionic; emulsifier, thickener, opacifier, suspending agent; stabilizer for o/w emulsions; for cosmetics, pharmaceuticals, hair straighteners, moisturizers, nail preps., sunscreens, antibiotic creams and lotions, acne preps., analgesic rubs; creamy wh. flaked waxy solid, mild char. odor; sol. in alcohol; disp. in water, propylene glycol; m.p. 48-52 C; iodine no. 3.5 max.; sapon. no. 14 max.; hyd. no. 178-192; pH 5.5-7.0 (3% aq.); usage level: 2-15%; toxicology: LD50 (oral, rat) 16 g/kg; nonirritating to skin and eyes; 100% conc.

Polawax® A31. [Croda Inc.; Croda Surf. Ltd.] Emulsifying wax NF; nonionic; o/w emulsifier and foaming agent used in quick-breaking foams and mousses, cosmetics, pharmaceuticals; creamy wh. waxy solid, mild char. odor; sol. in alcohol and aerosol propellant, disp. in water, propylene glycol; m.p. 48-52 C; iodine no. 3.5 max.; sapon. no. 14 max.; hyd. no. 178-192; pH 5.5-7.0 (3% aq.); usage level: 1-8%; toxicology: LD50 (oral, rat) > 5 g/kg; nonirritating to skin and eyes; 100% conc.

Polawax® GP200. [Croda Inc.; Croda Surf. Ltd.] Self-emulsifying wax; nonionic; self-bodying emulsifier producing stable w/o emulsions for cosmetics, pharmaceuticals, lotions, creams, ointments; effective at high levels of electrolytes and active ingreds.; heat-stable; wh. waxy solid; 97% conc.

Polectron® 430. [ISP] Styrene/PVP copolymer; binder and adhesive for wood, cotton, paper, glass fiber, flour, concrete; stabilizer and opacifier; laundry processing; stabilizer for detergents; surf., textile, and paper coatings, latex rug backings, floor wax emulsions; opacifier for shampoos, conditioners, acid rinses, permanent waves, setting lotions; dye acceptor in hair color preps.; milky-wh. fluid emulsion; particle size < 0.5 μ; 40% solids.

Poliglicoleum. [Vevy] Ricinoleth-40.

Polyaminon-3. [Nippon Chem. Co. Ltd.] Ethyl glutamate, ethyl aspartate.

Polyaminon-5. [Nippon Chem. Co. Ltd.] Diethyl aspartate, diethyl glutamate.

Polyaminon-15. [Nippon Chem. Co. Ltd.] Diethyl glutamate, ethyl serinate, diethyl aspartate.

Polycare® 133. [Rhone-Poulenc Surf. & Spec.] Polymethacrylamidopropyltrimonium chloride; CAS 68039-13-4; cationic; hair fixative, conditioner providing gloss and mildness to shampoos, liq. soaps, shower gels, creams and lotions, facial cleansers, bath gels, bubble baths, toiletries, conditioning rinses.

Polycare® 509. [Rhone-Poulenc Surf. & Spec.] Vinyl acetate, isobutyl maleate, vinylneodecanoate copolymer; hair styling fixative resin providing superior hold and curl retention even under extremely humid conditions; fine wh. transparent beads, practically odorless; sol. 100% in abs. ethanol; acid no. 60-66; formerly Meyprofix 509.

Polychol 5. [Croda Inc.; Croda Chem. Ltd.] Laneth-5; CAS 61791-20-6; nonionic; o/w emulsifier, dispersant, gellant, emollient, solubilizer for personal care prods., hair straighteners, pharmaceuticals; bromo dye solv.; soft yel. wax; sol. in IPA, disp. in water, propylene glycol, min. oil; m.p. 35-48 C; HLB 7.5; acid no. 5 max.; hyd. no. 120-135; pH 4.5–6.0 (10% aq.); usage level: 1-10%; toxicology: LD50 (oral, rat) 7.7 g/kg; mild skin irritant, nonirritating to eyes; 100% conc.

Polychol 15. [Croda Inc.; Croda Chem. Ltd.] Laneth-15; CAS 61791-20-6; nonionic; o/w emulsifier, dispersant, solubilizer, emollient, thickener, and gelling agent for cosmetics and pharmaceuticals; yel. semihard wax; sol. in water, IPA, propylene glycol; disp. in min. oil; m.p. 38-46 C; HLB 12.7; acid no. 5 max.; hyd. no. 82-92; pH 3.5–5.5 (10% aq.); usage level: 1-10%; toxicology: nonirritating to skin and eyes; 100% conc.

Polychol 16. [Croda Inc.] Laneth-16; CAS 61791-20-6; nonionic; emulsifier, dispersant, solubilizer, emollient and gelling agent for cosmetics and pharmaceuticals.

Polyethylene 1000 HE. [Koster Keunen] Polyethylene; CAS 9002-88-4; EINECS 200-815-3; gellant, thickener, and stabilizer for lipsticks, gels; pastilles.

Poly-G® 200. [Olin] PEG 200; CAS 25322-68-3; EINECS 203-989-9; chemical intermediate for prod. of surfactants for cleaners, textiles, paper, cosmetics; carrier for pharmaceuticals; also in cosmetics and personal care prods., textiles, rubber mold releases, printing inks and dyes, metalworking fluids, foods, paints, paper, wood prods., adhesives, agric. prods., ceramics, elec. equipment, petrol. prods., photographic prods., resins; APHA 25 max. liq.; m.w. 200; sol. in water, acetone, ethanol, ethyl acetate, toluene; sp.gr. 1.125; dens. 9.38 lb/gal; visc. 4.3 cs (99 C); flash pt. 171 C (COC).

Poly-G® 300. [Olin] PEG 300; CAS 25322-68-3; EINECS 220-045-1; see Poly-G 200; APHA 25 max. liq.; m.w. 300; sol. in water, acetone, ethanol, ethyl acetate, toluene; sp.gr. 1.125; dens. 9.38 lb/gal; visc. 5.8 cs (99 C); f.p. –15 to –8 C; flash pt. 196 C (COC).

Poly-G® 400. [Olin] PEG 400; CAS 25322-68-3; EINECS 225-856-4; see Poly-G 200; APHA 25 max. liq.; m.w. 400; sol. in water, acetone, ethanol, ethyl acetate, toluene; sp.gr. 1.127; dens. 9.4 lb/gal; visc. 7.3 cs (99 C); f.p. 4–10 C; flash pt. 224 C (COC); pour pt. 3–10 C.

Poly-G® 600. [Olin] PEG 600; CAS 25322-68-3; EINECS 229-859-1; see Poly-G 200; APHA 25 max. liq.; m.w. 600; sol. in water, acetone, ethanol, ethyl acetate, toluene; sp.gr. 1.127; dens. 9.4 lb/gal; visc. 10.5 cs (99 C); f.p. 20–25 C; flash pt. 246 C (COC); pour pt. 19–24 C.

Poly-G® 1000. [Olin] PEG 1000; CAS 25322-68-3; see Poly-G 200; wh. waxy solid; m.w. 1000; somewhat less sol. in water than liq. glycols; sp.gr. 1.104 (50/20 C); dens. 9.20 lb/gal (50/20 C); visc. 17.4 cs (99 C); f.p. 38–41 C; flash pt. 260 C (COC); pour pt. 40 C.

Poly-G® 1500. [Olin] PEG 1500; see Poly-G 200; wh. waxy solid; m.w. 1500; somewhat less sol. in water than liq. glycols; sp.gr. 1.104 (50/20 C); dens. 9.20 lb/gal (50/20 C); visc. 28 cs (99 C); f.p. 43–46 C; flash pt. 266 C (COC); pour pt. 45 C.

Poly-G® 2000. [Olin] PEG 2000; CAS 25322-68-3; see Poly-G 200; APHA 25 max. liq.; m.w. 2000; somewhat less sol. in water than lower m.w. glycols; sp.gr. 1.113; dens. 9.26 lb/gal; visc. 11.7 cs (99 C); f.p. –20 C; 60% aq. sol'n.

Poly-G® B1530. [Olin] PEG 500-600; see Poly-G 200; wh. waxy solid; m.w. 900; somewhat less sol. in water than liq. glycols; sp.gr. 1.104 (50/20 C); dens. 9.20 lb/gal (50/20 C); visc. 15 cs (99 C); f.p. 38–41 C; flash pt. 254 C (COC); pour pt. 38 C.

Polyglucadyne™. [Brooks Industries] 1-3 and 1-6 β-glucans copolymer; patented material for protection of skin in cosmetics; macrophage stimulating factor; high m.w. hollow spheres of submicron size.

Polymer SBOCP. [Brooks Industries] Cocamidopropyl dimethylammonium C8-16 isoalkylsuccinyl lactoglobulin sulfonate; cosmetic ingred.

Polymer T-1172. [Lowenstein] Film-former and setting agent for temporary hair color systems.

Polymin® FG SG. [BASF] PEI-10; CAS 25987-06-8; cosmetic ingred. with affinity for skin and hair (hair conditioners, hair fixatives, waving prods., antidandruff prods., hair dyes, skin softener/protectant/conditioner); surface modifier for cosmetic powds.; complexing agent for heavy metal ions (antiperspirants); used in paper, food pkg., medical diagnostics, adhesives; FDA approval; liq.; sol. in water and other poalr solvs.; m.w. 700-800; visc. 17,000-28,000 cps; toxicology: sl. or moderately toxic by oral dose; nonirritating to sl. irritating to skin and eyes; 99% conc.

Polymin® G-35 SG. [BASF] PEI-35; CAS 9002-98-6; cosmetic ingred. with affinity for skin and hair (hair conditioners, hair fixatives, waving prods., antidandruff prods., hair dyes, skin softener/protectant/conditioner); surface modifier for cosmetic powds.; complexing agent for heavy metal ions (antiperspirants); used in paper, food pkg., medical diagnostics, adhesives; liq.; m.w. 1700-2000; visc. ≈ 450 cps; 50% conc.

Polymin® P SG. [BASF] PEI-1500; CAS 68130-97-2; cosmetic ingred. with affinity for skin and hair (hair conditioners, hair fixatives, waving prods., antidandruff prods., hair dyes, skin softener/protectant/conditioner); surface modifier for cosmetic powds.; complexing agent for heavy metal ions (antiperspirants); used in paper, food pkg., medical diagnostics, adhesives; liq.; m.w. 70,000-750,000; visc. 17,000-40,000 cps; 50% conc.

Polymin® PS SG. [BASF] PEI-1500; CAS 68130-97-2; cosmetic ingred. with affinity for skin and hair (hair conditioners, hair fixatives, waving prods., antidandruff prods., hair dyes, skin softener/protectant/conditioner); surface modifier for cosmetic powds.; complexing agent for heavy metal ions (antiperspirants); used in paper, food pkg., medical diagnostics, adhesives; liq.; m.w. 70,000-750,000; visc. 1200-1700 cps; 33% conc.

Polymin® Waterfree SG. [BASF] PEI-250; CAS 9002-98-6; cosmetic ingred. with affinity for skin and hair (hair condi-

tioners, hair fixatives, waving prods., antidandruff prods., hair dyes, skin softener/protectant/conditioner); surface modifier for cosmetic powds.; complexing agent for heavy metal ions (antiperspirants); used in paper, food pkg., medical diagnostics, adhesives; liq.; m.w. 10,000-25,000; visc. 100,000-200,000 cps; 99% conc.

Polymoist® Mask. [Henkel/Cospha; Henkel Canada] Collagen fiber material; CAS 9007-34-5; EINECS 232-697-4; network of insol. collagen fibers for topical short-term applic. as a moisturizer and vehicle for cosmetic active agents; nonwoven fabric.

Polyolprepolymer-2. [Penederm; Barnet Prods.] PPG-12/SMDI copolymer; CAS 9042-82-4; deposition and delivery system for cosmetic formulations; binds to skin forming noninvasive, water-resist. film which remains in the upper layers of the skin and is resist. to washoff; enhances release of actives; provides moisturizing and spreading props.; for sunscreens, pigmented cosmetics, hair and personal care formulas; clear visc. liq., odorless; sol. < 1% in water; m.w. ≈ 4000; visc. 2500-4500 cps (35 C); f.p. < 0 C; b.p. dec.; toxicology: LD50 (acute oral) > 5 g/kg; noncomedogenic, nonirritating to eyes or skin, nonsensitizing.

Polyox® WSR 35. [Union Carbide] PEG-5M; CAS 25322-68-3; reduces friction in shave prods.; feel modifier providing soft feel; film-former, thickener for aq. systems.

Polyox® WSR 205. [Amerchol] PEG-14M; CAS 25322-68-3; nonionic; thickener; wh. powd., mild ammoniacal odor; 100% thru 10 mesh, 96% min. thru 20 mesh; sol. in water, some chlorinated solvs., alcohols, aromatic hydrocarbons, ketones; visc. 4500-8800 cps (5% aq.); pH 8-10 (5% aq.).

Polyox® WSR 301. [Amerchol] PEG-90M; CAS 25322-68-3; nonionic; thickener; wh. powd., mild ammoniacal odor; 100% thru 10 mesh, 96% min. thru 20 mesh; sol. in water, some chlorinated solvs., alcohols, aromatic hydrocarbons, ketones; visc. 1650-5500 cps (1% aq.); pH 8-10 (1% aq.).

Polyox® WSR 1105. [Amerchol] PEG-20M; CAS 25322-68-3; nonionic; thickener; wh. powd., mild ammoniacal odor; 100% thru 10 mesh, 96% min. thru 20 mesh; sol. in water, some chlorinated solvs., alcohols, aromatic hydrocarbons, ketones; viscs. 8800-17,600 cps (5% aq.); pH 8-10 (5% aq.).

Polyox® WSR 3333. [Amerchol] PEG-9M; CAS 25322-68-3; nonionic; water-sol. polymer, thickener; wh. powd., mild ammoniacal odor; 100% thru 10 mesh, 96% min. thru 20 mesh; visc. 2250-3350 cps (5% aq.); pH 8-10 (5% aq.).

Polyox® WSR N-10. [Amerchol] PEG-2M; CAS 25322-68-3; nonionic; thickener; wh. powd., mild ammoniacal odor; 100% thru 10 mesh, 96% min. 20 mesh; sol. in water, some chlorinated solvs., alcohols, aromatic hydrocarbons, ketones; visc. 30-50 cps (5% aq.); pH 8-10 (5% aq.).

Polyox® WSR N-12K. [Amerchol] PEG-23M; CAS 25322-68-3; nonionic; thickener; wh. powd., mild ammoniacal odor; 100% thru 10 mesh, 96% min. thru 20 mesh; sol. in water, some chlorinated solvs., alcohols, aromatic hydrocarbons, ketones; visc. 400-800 cps (2% aq.); pH 8-10 (2% aq.).

Polyox® WSR N-60K. [Amerchol] PEG-45M; CAS 25322-68-3; nonionic; thickener; wh. powd., mild ammoniacal odor; 100% thru 10 mesh, 96% min. thru 20 mesh; sol. in water, some chlorinated solvs., alcohols, aromatic hydrocarbons, ketones; visc. 2000-4000 cps (2% aq.); pH 8-10 (2% aq.).

Polyox® WSR N-80. [Amerchol] PEG-5M; CAS 25322-68-3; nonionic; thickener; wh. powd., mild ammoniacal odor; 100% thru 10 mesh, 96% min. thru 20 mesh; sol. in water, some chlorinated solvs., alcohols, aromatic hydrocarbons, ketones; visc. 65-115 cps (5% aq.); pH 8-10 (5%

aq.).

Polyox® WSR N-750. [Amerchol] PEG-7M; CAS 25322-68-3; nonionic; thickener; wh. powd., mild ammoniacal odor; 100% thru 10 mesh, 96% min. thru 20 mesh; sol. in water, some chlorinated solvs., alcohols, aromatic hydrocarbons, ketones; visc. 600-1200 cps (5% aq.); pH 8-10 (5% aq.).

Polyox® WSR N-3000. [Amerchol] PEG-14M; CAS 25322-68-3; nonionic; thickener; wh. powd., mild ammoniacal odor; 100% thru 10 mesh, 96% min. thru 20 mesh; sol. in water, some chlorinated solvs., alcohols, aromatic hydrocarbons, ketones; visc. 2250-4500 cps (5% aq.); pH 8-10 (5% aq.).

Polyox® Coagulant. [Amerchol] PEG-115M; reduces friction in shave prods.; feel modifier providing soft feel; film-former, thickener for aq. systems.

Polypeptide 10. [Maybrook] Hydrolyzed collagen; CAS 9015-54-7; protective colloid, anti-irritant, substantivity agent, moisturizer for hair and skin care prods., dish detergents; dye leveler and fiber protectant in textile industry; amber clear liq., char. odor; pH 6.7-7.3; 48-52% solids.

Polypeptide 12. [Maybrook] Hydrolyzed collagen; CAS 9015-54-7; substantive protein with protective colloid effect, anti-irritancy benefits; moisturizer; for hair care (styling prods., shampoos, conditioners), skin care (creams, lotions, shave creams), liq. detergents, dish detergents; amber clear liq., char. odor; pH 6.7-7.4; 40-43% solids.

Polypeptide 37. [Inolex] Hydrolyzed collagen; CAS 9015-54-7; anionic; substantive protein for use in personal care prods. not sensitive to electrolytes, e.g., shampoos and conditioners; dk. amber clear liq., mild char. proteinaceous odor; misc. with water; sp.gr. 1.20–1.23; visc. 75 cps max.; pH 6.5-7.5; 48–50% solids.

Polypeptide LSN Anhydrous. [Inolex] Hydrolyzed collagen; CAS 9015-54-7; anionic; protein for aerosols, soaps, syndet bars, anhyd. shampoos; wh. to cream fluffy dry powd., mild char. proteinaceous odor; misc. with water; dens. 20–21 lb/ft³; pH 5.0-6.5 (10% aq.); 94% min. solids.

Polypeptide SF. [Inolex] Hydrolyzed collagen; CAS 9015-54-7; anionic; protein for use in personal care prods. sensitive to electrolytes; greater emulsion stability; amber clear liq.; misc. with water; pH 6.5–7.0; 56–58% solids.

Polypro® 5000. [Hormel] Hydrolyzed collagen; CAS 9015-54-7; food-grade protein with exc. film-forming and moisturizing props.; ivory powd.; m.w. 5000.

Polypro® 15000. [Hormel] Hydrolyzed collagen; CAS 9015-54-7; food-grade protein with exc. film forming and moisturizing props.; ivory powd.; m.w. 15,000.

Polyquart® H. [Henkel/Cospha; Henkel Canada] PEG-15 cocopolyamine; cationic; surfactant, conditioner used in hair and skin care prods.; antistat; leaves hair manageable, glossy, easy to comb; amber clear liq.; sol. in water, alcohol; visc. 1500–4000 cps; pH 5.0–6.0 (1%); 50% act.

Polyquart® H 81. [Henkel/Emery] PEG-15 cocopolyamine; antistatic and softening agent for shampoos and hair care preps.; 49–51% conc.

Polyquart® H 7102. [Henkel/Cospha; Henkel Canada] PEG-15 cocopolyamine and stearalkonium chloride; cationic; surfactant used in personal care prods.; hair conditioner, antistat; hair fixative; Gardner 6.0 max. liq.; sol. in water, alcohol; visc. 1500–4000 cps; pH 5.5–6.5 (1%); 49–52% solids.

Polyspend™. [U.S. Cosmetics] Polyethylene; CAS 9002-88-4; EINECS 200-815-3; inert surface treatment to enhance cosmetic prods.; imparts smoothness, good adhesion; less settling, color striation/separation in nail enamels; good misc. and disp. into oil phase.

Polystate C. [Gattefosse; Gattefosse SA] PEG-6 stearate; CAS 9004-99-3; nonionic; base for cosmetic lotions; solid;

drop pt. 26.5-30.5 C; HLB 9.0-10.0; acid no. < 6; iodine no. < 3; sapon. no. 90-110; toxicology: sl. skin irritant, nonirritating to eyes; 100% conc.

PolySurf. [Aqualon] Cetyl hydroxyethylcellulose; hydrophobically modified hydroxyethylcellulose; thickener and visc. stabilizer for aq. and surfactant systems in personal care applics.

Polysynlane. [Nippon Oils & Fats] Hydrog. polyisobutene; patented (U.S., Germany, France, Japan) base oil for cosmetics.

Polytex 10M. [Lipo] Glycol stearate and stearamide AMP; emulsifier, emulsion stabilizer, emollient, visc. builder, opacifier, pearlescent for cosmetic creams and lotions; wh. flakes; HLB 2.0 ± 1; acid no. 5 max.; sapon. no. 174-184.

Polytrap® 6035. [Dow Corning; Advanced Polymer Systems] Cyclomethicone (80%) and acrylates copolymer; provides elegant skin feel and adsorbs secreted skin oils in pigmented makeups, loose and compressed powds., facial cleaners, sticks, foundations, and oil-control treatments; patented; wh. free-flowing amorphous powd.; particle size 100 μ; apparent dens. 0.4-0.5 g/cc; surf. area 0.32 m²/m³; dust is severe explosive hazard; combustible.

Polytrap® 6603. [Dow Corning; Advanced Polymer Systems] Acrylates copolymer; adsorbs secreted skin oils, converts liqs. to solid powd. form, reduces feathering, minimizes syneresis, provides an elegant skin feel; for pigmented makeup, loose and compressed powds., facial cleansers, sticks, and oil-control treatments; patented; wh. free-flowing amorphous powd.; particle size 200-1200 μ; apparent dens. 0.06 g/cc; surf. area 0.32 m²/g; surf. tens. 39.6 mNm⁻¹; dust is severe explosive hazard.

Polytrap® Q5-6035. [Dow Corning] Cyclomethicone and acrylates copolymer; delivers volatile silicone fluid in powd. form; provides lubricious skin feel for skin care and cosmetics formulations, facial cleansers, foundations; wh. free-flowing powd.; particle size 100 μ max.; apparent dens. 0.4-0.5 g/cc; surf. area 0.32 m²/cm³; combustible.

Polytrap® Q5-6038 Polymer Beads. [Dow Corning] Acrylates copolymer and min. oil; beaded and abrasive form to aid in the gentle sloughing off of outer layers of epidermis; for use in facial scrubs, sloughing lotions, facial cleansers, and skin polishers; low chem. reactivity; wh. free-flowing powd.; 200-800 μ particle size; sp.gr. 0.837-0.853; apparent dens. 0.5 g/cc; visc. 11-14 cst.

Polytrap® Q5-6603. [Dow Corning] Acrylates copolymer; adsorbs high levels of lipopholic and certain hydrophilic liqs.; for skin care, sun care, and cosmetic formulations; low chem. reactivity; wh. free-flowing powd.; 200-1200 μ particle size; apparent dens. 0.06 g/cc; surf. area 0.32 m²/cm³; decomp. temp. > 200 C; dust is severe explosive hazard; toxicology: LD50 (acute oral) > 5 g/kg (virtually nontoxic); moderate eye irritant; nonirritating to skin.

Polytrix™. [Biomatrix; Amerchol] PEG-115M and hyaluronic acid.

Polywax® 500. [Petrolite] Polyethylene homopolymer; CAS 9002-88-4; EINECS 200-815-3; lubricant, flow modifier, release agent, antiblock for plastics processing; nucleating agent for expandable PS; slip aid for printing inks; leveling/slip agent for powd. coatings; visc. modifier for hot-melt adhesives; cosmetic ingreds.; wax modifier; chewing gum base; incl. FDA §172.888, 175.105, 175.300, 176.170, 176.180, 176.200, 177.1200, 178.3720, 179.45; prilled; low sol. in org. solvs., esp. at R.T.; sol. in CCl₄, benzene, xylene, toluene, turpentine; m.w. 500; melt index > 5000 g/10 min; dens. 0.93 g/cc; visc. 6.6 cps (99 C); m.p. 88 C; soften. pt. (R&B) 88 C.

Polywax® 655. [Petrolite] Polyethylene homopolymer; CAS 9002-88-4; EINECS 200-815-3; lubricant, flow modifier, release agent, antiblock for plastics processing; nucleating agent for expandable PS; slip aid for printing inks; leveling/slip agent for powd. coatings; visc. modifier for hot-melt adhesives; cosmetic ingreds.; wax modifier; chewing gum base; incl. FDA §172.888, 175.105, 175.300, 176.170, 176.180, 176.200, 177.1200, 178.3720, 179.45; prilled; low sol. in org. solvs., esp. at R.T.; sol. in CCl₄, benzene, xylene, toluene, turpentine; m.w. 655; melt index > 5000 g/10 min; dens. 0.94 g/cc; visc. 5 cps (149 C); m.p. 99 C; soften. pt. (R&B) 99 C.

Polywax® 850. [Petrolite] Polyethylene homopolymer; CAS 9002-88-4; EINECS 200-815-3; lubricant, flow modifier, release agent, antiblock for plastics processing; nucleating agent for expandable PS; slip aid for printing inks; leveling/slip agent for powd. coatings; visc. modifier for hot-melt adhesives; cosmetic ingreds.; wax modifier; incl. FDA §172.888, 175.105, 175.300, 176.170, 176.180, 176.200, 177.1200, 178.3720, 179.45; m.w. 850; melt index > 5000 g/10 min; dens. 0.96 g/cc; visc. 8.5 cs (149 C); m.p. 107 C; soften. pt (R&B) 107 C.

Polywax® 1000. [Petrolite] HDPE; CAS 9002-88-4; EINECS 200-815-3; lubricant, flow modifier, release agent, antiblock for plastics processing; nucleating agent for expandable PS; slip aid for printing inks; leveling/slip agent for powd. coatings; visc. modifier for hot-melt adhesives; cosmetic ingreds.; wax modifier; incl. FDA §172.888, 175.105, 175.300, 176.170, 176.180, 176.200, 177.1200, 178.3720, 179.45; prilled; low sol. in org. solvs., esp. at R.T.; sol. in CCl₄, benzene, xylene, toluene, turpentine; m.w. 1000; melt index > 5000 g/10 min; dens. 0.96 g/cc; visc. 12 cps (149 C); m.p. 113 C; soften. pt. (R&B) 113 C.

Polywax® 2000. [Petrolite] HDPE; CAS 9002-88-4; EINECS 200-815-3; lubricant, flow modifier, release agent, antiblock for plastics processing; nucleating agent for expandable PS; slip aid for printing inks; leveling/slip agent for powd. coatings; visc. modifier for hot-melt adhesives; cosmetic ingreds.; wax modifier; incl. FDA §173.20, 175.105, 175.300, 176.170, 176.180, 177.1520(c) (2.1)-(2.3), 178.3570, 179.45; prilled; low sol. in org. solvs., esp. at R.T.; sol. in CCl₄, benzene, xylene, toluene, turpentine; m.w. 2000; melt index > 5000 g/10 min; dens. 0.97 g/cc; visc. 48 cps (149 C); m.p. 126 C; soften. pt. (R&B) 126 C.

Polywax® 3000. [Petrolite] Polyethylene homopolymer; CAS 9002-88-4; EINECS 200-815-3; lubricant, flow modifier, release agent, antiblock for plastics processing; nucleating agent for expandable PS; slip aid for printing inks; leveling/slip agent for powd. coatings; visc. modifier for hot-melt adhesives; cosmetic ingreds.; wax modifier; incl. FDA §173.20, 175.105, 175.300, 176.170, 176.180, 177.1520(c) (2.1)-(2.3), 178.3570, 179.45; m.w. 3000; melt index > 5000 g/10 min; dens. 0.98 g/cc; visc. 130 cps (149 C); m.p. 129 C; soften. pt. (R&B) 129 C.

Porosponge. [Advanced Polymer Systems] Acrylates copolymer; thickener, stabilizer for cosmetics.

Potato-Pro™ EN-15. [Brooks Industries] Hydrolyzed potato protein; cosmetic ingredient for skin and hair care prods.; m.w. 10,000; 15% act.

Pot Marigold AMI. [Alban Muller] Natural ingred. with soothing props. for sun prods.; oil-sol.

Powdered Aloe Vera (1:200) Food Grade. [Tri-K Industries] Aloe vera gel; for personal care prods., suntan, sun treatment, burn gels, first aid creams, soaps, hair care, cosmetics, weight control, oral hygiene.

Pran H. [Fabriquimica] Hydrolyzed collagen; CAS 9015-54-7; cosmetic protein.

Pran LIQ. [Fabriquimica] Hydrolyzed collagen; CAS 9015-54-7; protein for cosmetics use; pH 5.0-7.0 (10%); 30-32% solids.

Pran QC. [Fabriquimica] Steartrimonium hydrolyzed collagen; CAS 111174-62-0; protein for cosmetics use; pH

5.5-6.5 (10%); > 30% solids.

Precifac ATO. [Gattefosse SA] Cetyl palmitate; CAS 540-10-3; EINECS 208-736-6; tableting agent and lipophilic matrix for pharmaceuticals/cosmetics; drop pt. 48-52 C; HLB 2.0; acid no. < 6; iodine no. < 3; sapon. no. 95-120; toxicology: LD50 (oral, rat) > 5 mg/kg.

Precirol ATO 5. [Gattefosse SA] Tripalmitin and tristearin; CAS 8067-32-1; nonionic; additive for tablets, binder, lubricant, sustained release; solid; drop pt. 53-57 C; HLB 2.0; acid no. < 6; iodine no. < 3; sapon. no. 175-195; toxicology: LD50 (oral, rat) > 6 g/kg; 100% conc.

Precirol WL 2155 ATO. [Gattefosse; Gattefosse SA] Glyceryl ditristearate; CAS 8067-32-1; nonionic; additive for tablets mfg.; solid; drop pt. 63.5-67.5 C; HLB 2.0; acid no. < 6; iodine no. < 3; sapon. no. 180-190; toxicology: LD50 (oral, rat) > 6 g/kg; 100% conc.

Prenol. [BASF AG] 3-Methyl-2-butene-1-ol; fragrance and flavoring (fresh, herbal, green, fruity, sl. lavender-like).

Preserval B. [Laserson SA] Butylparaben; CAS 94-26-8; EINECS 202-318-7; preservative for cosmetics.

Preserval E. [Laserson SA] Ethylparaben; CAS 120-47-8; EINECS 204-399-4; preservative for cosmetics.

Preserval M. [Laserson SA] Methylparaben; CAS 99-76-3; EINECS 202-785-7; preservative for cosmetics; colorless; usage level: 0.1-1.0%; toxicology: nontoxic.

Preserval P. [Laserson SA] Propylparaben; CAS 94-13-3; EINECS 202-307-7; cosmetic preservative; USA, Japan, Europe approvals; colorless; usage level: 0.02-1.0%; toxicology: nontoxic.

Preserval Butylique. [Laserson SA] Butylparaben; CAS 94-26-8; EINECS 202-318-7; preservative for cosmetics.

Presome Type I. [Ikeda] Phospholipids and cholesterol; lipid compound for easy prep. of liposomes for skin care prods.; wh. to off-wh. powd., char. odor.

Press-Aid™. [Presperse] Synthetic wax, corn gluten protein; CAS 8002-74-2, 9010-66-6; binder for pressed powds.; provides high adhesion, transparency, exc. powd. compressibility; wh. opaque powd.; particle size 7.5 μ; congeal pt. 94 C min.

Press-Aid™ SP. [Presperse] Synthetic wax; CAS 8002-74-2; binder for pressed powds.; JSCI/JCID approved; wh. opaque spherical powd.; particle size 7.5 μ; bulk dens. 290 kg/m³; congeal pt. 94 C min.

Press-Aid™ XF. [Presperse] Synthetic wax, corn gluten protein; CAS 8002-74-2, 9010-66-6; binder for pressed powds.; wh. opaque powd.; particle size 3.0 μ; congeal pt. 91 C min.

Press-Aid™ XP. [Presperse] Synthetic wax; CAS 8002-74-2; binder for pressed powds.

Preventol BP. [Bayer AG] Chlorophene; CAS 120-32-1; EINECS 204-385-8.

Preventol D2. [Bayer AG] Benzylhemiformal; CAS 14548-60-8; EINECS 238-588-8.

Preventol GD. [Bayer AG] Dichlorophene; CAS 97-23-4; EINECS 202-567-1; fungicide, bactericide.

Priacetin. [Unichema] Glyceryl triacetate; CAS 102-76-1; EINECS 203-051-9; cosmetics ingred.

Prifac 7920. [Unichema] Tallow acid; CAS 61790-37-2; EINECS 263-129-3; raw material for surfactants, soaps, nitrogen derivs., buffing formulations; low melting solid; acid no. 200-206; iodine no. 50-62; sapon. no. 201-207.

Prifac 7935. [Unichema] Dist. tallow fatty acid; CAS 61790-37-2; EINECS 263-129-3; raw material for surfactants, soaps, nitrogen derivs., buffing formulations; low melting solid; acid no. 198-204; iodine no. 52-62; sapon. no. 200-208.

Prifrac 2901. [Unichema] Caprylic acid; CAS 124-07-2; EINECS 204-677-5; intermediate for ester prod., syn. lubes, latex stabilizers, substituted glycerides used as skin protectors; liq.; acid no. 385-390; iodine no. 0.5 max.;

98% conc.

Prifrac 2910. [Unichema] Caprylic acid; CAS 124-07-2; EINECS 204-677-5; intermediate for ester prod., syn. lubes, and substituted glycerides used as skin protectors; liq.; 98% conc.

Prifrac 2940. [Unichema] Myristic acid; CAS 544-63-8; EINECS 208-875-2; intermediate for ester, detergent, and surfactant prods.; solid; acid no. 243-248; iodine no. 0.5 max.; 92-94% conc.

Prifrac 2960. [Unichema] Palmitic acid; CAS 57-10-3; EINECS 200-312-9; intermediate for surfactants, soap and cosmetic formulations; cryst. solid; acid no. 216-220; iodine no. 1 max.; 92% min. conc.

Prifrac 2980. [Unichema] Stearic acid; CAS 57-11-4; EINECS 200-313-4; intermediate for surfactants, soap and cosmetic formulations; cryst. solid; acid no. 195-199; iodine no. 2 max.; 93% min. conc.

Prifrac 2981. [Unichema] Stearic acid; CAS 57-11-4; EINECS 200-313-4; intermediate for surfactants, soap and cosmetic formulations; cryst. solid; acid no. 194-198; iodine no. 2 max.; 98-100% conc.

Prifrac 2989. [Unichema] Behenic acid; CAS 112-85-6; EINECS 204-010-8; intermediate for surfactants, soap and cosmetic formulations; solid; acid no. 160-166; iodine no. 2 max.; 85-90% conc.

Prifrac 5901, 7901. [Unichema] Coconut acid.; hardened fatty acid used in toilet soaps.

Prifrac 7948. [Unichema] Tallow acid, coconut acid.; hardened fatty acid used in toilet soaps.

Priolene 6900. [Unichema] Oleic acid; CAS 112-80-1; EINECS 204-007-1; intermediate for ethoxylates, esters, nitrogen derivs., surfactants; used in soaps, personal care prods., lubricant and metalworking fluids, for NR latex stabilization; liq.; acid no. 196-204; iodine no. 89-97; sapon. no. 197-205.

Priolene 6905. [Unichema] Oleic acid; CAS 112-80-1; EINECS 204-007-1; intermediate for ethoxylates, esters, nitrogen derivs., surfactants; used in soaps, personal care prods., lubricant and metalworking fluids; liq.; acid no. 199-204; iodine no. 95 max.; sapon. no. 201-206.

Priolene 6906. [Unichema] Oleic acid; CAS 112-80-1; EINECS 204-007-1; intermediate for ethoxylates, esters, nitrogen derivs., surfactants; used in soaps, personal care prods., lubricant and metalworking fluids; liq.; acid no. 199-204; iodine no. 95 max.; sapon. no. 201-206.

Priolene 6910. [Unichema] Oleic acid; CAS 112-80-1; EINECS 204-007-1; intermediate for ethoxylates, esters, nitrogen derivs., surfactants; used in soaps, personal care prods., lubricant and metalworking fluids; liq.; acid no. 196-204; iodine no. 89-97; sapon. no. 197-205.

Priolene 6933. [Unichema] Oleic acid; CAS 112-80-1; EINECS 204-007-1; intermediate for ethoxylates, esters, nitrogen derivs., surfactants; used in soaps, personal care prods., lubricant and metalworking fluids; liq.; acid no. 197-203; iodine no. 89-95; sapon. no. 199-205.

Pripol 2033. [Unichema] Dimer diol; cosmetics ingred.

Pripure 3785. [Unichema] Diisostearyl dimer dilinoleate; personal care ingred.

Pripure 3786. [Unichema] Diisopropyl dimerate (diisopropyl dilinoleate); emollient ester for cosmetics; Japan approval; APHA 150 max. color; acid no. 1 max.; iodine no. 10 max.; sapon. no. 165-175; hyd. no. 2 max.; cloud pt. -35 C.

Prisorine 2021. *See Prisorine IPIS 2021*

Prisorine 2039. *See Prisorine ISIS 2039*

Prisorine 2040. *See Prisorine GMIS 2040*

Prisorine 3501. [Unichema] Isostearic acid, std. grade; CAS 2724-58-5; EINECS 220-336-3; emollient ester for cosmetics.

Prisorine 3505. [Unichema] Isostearic acid; CAS 2724-58-

5; EINECS 220-336-3; personal care ingred.; Japan approval.

Prisorine 3515. [Unichema] Isostearyl alcohol; CAS 27458-93-1; EINECS 248-470-8; personal care ingred.; Japan approval.

Prisorine EHIS 2036. [Unichema] 2-Ethylhexyl isostearate; very light, nonfatting penetrant, emollient for sunscreens, daytime cosmetic preps., baby toiletries, and cosmetics for sensitive skin; APHA 50 max. color; acid no. 0.2 max.; iodine no. 2 max.; sapon. no. 140-145; cloud pt. -25 C.

Prisorine GMIS 2040. [Unichema] Glyceryl isostearate; emollient ester for protective cosmetics; coemulsifier for w/o emulsions; Japan approval; APHA 150 max. color; HLB 5.2; acid no. 1.0 max.; iodine no. 2 max.; sapon. no. 150-180; hyd. no. 176-196; cloud pt. 4 C; 40-50% monoglycerides.

Prisorine GTIS 2041. [Unichema] Glyceryl triisostearate; fat oil, emollient, skin protectant for cosmetics, esp. for sensitive skin; Japan approval; APHA 150 max. color; acid no. 2 max.; iodine no. 2 max.; sapon. no. 180-190; cloud pt. -13 C.

Prisorine IPIS 2021. [Unichema] Isopropyl isostearate; EINECS 250-651-1; emollient ester for cosmetics; spreading agent, penetrant, skin softener; Japan approval; APHA 100 max. color; acid no. 1.0 max.; iodine no. 3 max.; sapon. no. 170-180; cloud pt. -20 C.

Prisorine ISAC 3505. [Unichema] Isostearic acid, cosmetic grade; CAS 2724-58-5; EINECS 220-336-3; cosmetic emollient for creams and lotions, leaving rich afterfeel; intermediate for prod. of isostearyl alcohol and other derivs.; in neutralized form, emulsifier for thixotropic o/w emulsions; Japan approval; APHA 100 max. color; sp.gr. 0.89; visc. 45 mPa·s; acid no. 190-197; iodine no. 2 max.; sapon. no. 193-200; cloud pt. 8 C; flash pt. 175 C; ref. index 1.452.

Prisorine ISIS 2039. [Unichema] Isostearyl isostearate; CAS 41669-30-1; EINECS 255-485-3; rich emollient ester for cosmetic skin care prods.; forms lipid films on the skin which are highly permeable to oxygen and water vapor; refatting agent in hair care prods.; Japan approval; APHA 100 max. liq.; acid no. 0.5 max.; iodine no. 3 max.; sapon. no. 95-110; hyd. no. 10 max.; cloud pt. 15 C.

Prisorine ISOH 3515. [Unichema] Isostearyl alcohol; CAS 27458-93-1; EINECS 248-470-8; emollient ester for decorative cosmetics, skin care emulsions, sunscreen prods., hair dyeing, perming, and bleaching prods.; forms nongreasy, highly substantive, water-resist. lipid films on the skin without exhibiting occlusivity; Japan approval; APHA 20 max. liq.; acid no. 0.1 max.; iodine no. 1 max.; sapon. no. 1.0; hyd. no. 205 min.; cloud pt. 0 C.

Prisorine MIS 3760. [Unichema] Methyl isostearate; CAS 68517-10-2; personal care ingred.; intermediate for producing derivs. where color and odor are critical; APHA 100 max. color; acid no. 0.2 max.; iodine no. 2 max.; sapon. no. 180 min.; cloud pt. -20 C max.

Prisorine PDIS 2035. [Unichema] Propylene glycol diisostearate; substantive emollient covering skin with a wax-like layer leaving an oily feeling; for night creams, afterbath oils, sunscreen formulations where formation of a barrier film is important; Japan approval; APHA 100 max. color; acid no. 1 max.; iodine no. 2 max.; sapon. no. 176-186; hyd. no. 34 max.

Prisorine PMIS 2034. [Unichema] Propylene glycol isostearate; CAS 68171-38-0; EINECS 269-027-5; personal care ingred. providing emolliency and thixotropic behavior to emulsions; lipid film-former for protective cosmetics; coemulsifier for w/o emulsions; Japan approval; APHA 50 mnax. color; HLB 3.0; acid no. 1 max.; iodine no. 2 max.; sapon. no. 160-164; hyd. no. 160-175; > 90% monoester.

Prisorine SQS 3758. [Unichema] Syn. squalane; CAS 111-

01-3; EINECS 203-825-6; personal care ingred.

Pristerene 4904. [Unichema] Stearic acid; CAS 57-11-4; EINECS 200-313-4; intermediate for ethoxylates, esters, nitrogen derivs., personal prod. formulations; heat-stable; wh. cryst. solid; acid no. 206-212; iodine no. 0.5 max.; sapon.no. 208-214.

Pristerene 4905. [Unichema] Stearic acid, triple pressed; CAS 57-11-4; EINECS 200-313-4; intermediate for ethoxylates, esters, nitrogen derivs., personal prod. formulations; wh. cryst. solid; acid no. 206-212; iodine no. 0.5 max.; sapon. no. 208-214.

Pristerene 4910. [Unichema] Stearic acid; CAS 57-11-4; EINECS 200-313-4; intermediate for ethoxylates, esters, nitrogen derivs., personal prod. formulations; wh. solid; acid no. 200-208; iodine no. 2 max.; sapon. no. 201-209.

Pristerene 4911. [Unichema] Stearic acid, triple pressed; CAS 57-11-4; EINECS 200-313-4; intermediate for ethoxylates, esters, nitrogen derivs., personal prod. formulations; wh. solid; acid no. 206-210; iodine no. 0.5 max.; sapon. no. 207-211.

Pristerene 4915. [Unichema] Stearic acid, triple pressed; CAS 57-11-4; EINECS 200-313-4; intermediate for ethoxylates, esters, nitrogen derivs., personal prod. formulations; heat-stable; wh. solid; acid no. 206-210; iodine no. 0.5 max.; sapon. no. 207-211.

Pristerene 4921. [Unichema] Stearic acid, double pressed; CAS 57-11-4; EINECS 200-313-4; intermediate for ethoxylates, esters, nitrogen derivs., personal prod. formulations; heat-stable; wh. solid; acid no. 203-208; iodine no. 7 max.; sapon. no. 205-210.

Probiol™ L/N. [Rhone-Poulenc Surf. & Spec.] Water, lecithin, and custom active; CAS 8002-43-5; EINECS 232-307-2; moisturizer, stabilizer, liposomes; for skin and hair care, creams and lotions, cleansers, and sunscreens.

Probutyl 14. [Croda Inc.] PPG-14 butyl ether; CAS 9003-13-8; facilitates dispersion in antiperspirant sticks to help release the active and provide uniformity; nonstaining; clear liq.; sol. in oil, alcohol, lanolin oil; usage level: 2-25%.

Probutyl DB-10. [Croda Inc.] PPG-10 butanediol; imparts light, nonoily feel to skin; used in antiperspirant sticks, makeup removers, lotions, and foundations; clear liq.; sol. in water, alcohol; usage level: 2-25%.

Proceramide L. [Sederma] A natural ceramide precursor to native ceramides; contains sphingomyelin; replenishes native ceramides for skin function.

Procetyl 10. [Croda Inc.; Croda Chem. Ltd.] PPG-10 cetyl ether; CAS 9035-85-2; nonionic; emollient, coupler, cosolvent, plasticizer, superfatting, wetting and spreading agent, penetrant; lubricant in cosmetics and personal care prods.; alcoholic and aq. alcoholic compositions; APHA 150 max. clear liq.; faint, char. sweet odor; sol. in min. oil, acetone, IPM, lanolin oil, alcohol; acid no. 1 max.; hyd. no. 80-100; pH 6.0–7.5 (3% disp.); usage level: 5-30%; toxicology: nontoxic; 100% act.

Procetyl 30. [Croda Inc.; Croda Chem. Ltd.] PPG-30 cetyl ether; CAS 9035-85-2; emollient, coupler, cosolvent, plasticizer, superfatting, wetting and spreading agent, penetrant; lubricant in cosmetics and personal care prods.; alcoholic and aq. alcoholic compositions; APHA 150 max. clear liq.; faint, char. sweet odor; pH 6.0–7.5 (3% disp.); 100% act.

Procetyl 50. [Croda Inc.; Croda Chem. Ltd.] PPG-50 cetyl ether; CAS 9035-85-2; emollient, coupler, cosolvent, plasticizer, superfatting, wetting and spreading agent, penetrant; lubricant in cosmetics and personal care prods.; alcoholic and aq. alcoholic compositions; APHA 150 max. clear liq.; faint, char. sweet odor; sol. in PEG-200, lanolin oil, alcohol; acid no. 1 max.; hyd. no. 30-50; pH 6–7.5 (3% disp); usage level: 5-30%; toxicology: nontoxic; 100% act.

Procetyl AWS. [Croda Inc.; Croda Chem. Ltd.] PPG-5 ceteth-20; CAS 9087-53-0; nonionic; emulsifier, plasticizer, coupler, humectant, dispersant, emollient, and fragrance solubilizer in aq. and aq. alcoholic systems, personal care prods., antiperspirants, bath oils; water-wh. turbid oily liq.; char. sweet odor; sol. in water, alcohol, IPM, PEG-200, glycerin, propylene glycol, lanolin oil; acid no. 1 max.; hyd. no. 35-50; HLB 16.0; pH 6.0–7.5 (30% aq.); usage level: 0.5-5%; 100% act.

Prochem 12K. [Protameen] Hydrolyzed collagen; CAS 9015-54-7; cosmetic protein.

Prochem 35. [Protameen] Butyl stearate, lecithin, oleic acid, peach kernel oil.

Prochem 35A. [Protameen] Butyl stearate, lecithin, oleic acid, peach kernel oil, hydrolyzed collagen.

Prochem 100-CG Powd. [Protameen] Hydrolyzed collagen; CAS 9015-54-7; cosmetic protein.

Prochem SPA. [Protameen] Hydrolyzed collagen; CAS 9015-54-7; cosmetic protein.

Procol CA-2. [Protameen] Ceteth-2; CAS 9004-95-9; emulsifier.

Procol CA-4. [Protameen] Ceteth-4; CAS 9004-95-9; emulsifier.

Procol CA-6. [Protameen] Ceteth-6; CAS 9004-95-9; emulsifier.

Procol CA-10. [Protameen] Ceteth-10; CAS 9004-95-9; emulsifier.

Procol CA-20. [Protameen] Ceteth-20; CAS 9004-95-9; emulsifier.

Procol CA-30. [Protameen] Ceteth-30; CAS 9004-95-9; emulsifier.

Procol CS-3. [Protameen] Ceteareth-3; CAS 68439-49-6.

Procol CS-4. [Protameen] Ceteareth-4; CAS 68439-49-6.

Procol CS-5. [Protameen] Ceteareth-5; CAS 68439-49-6.

Procol CS-6. [Protameen] Ceteareth-6; CAS 68439-49-6.

Procol CS-8. [Protameen] Ceteareth-8; CAS 68439-49-6.

Procol CS-10. [Protameen] Ceteareth-10; CAS 68439-49-6.

Procol CS-12. [Protameen] Ceteareth-12; CAS 68439-49-6.

Procol CS-15. [Protameen] Ceteareth-15; CAS 68439-49-6.

Procol CS-17. [Protameen] Ceteareth-17; CAS 68439-49-6.

Procol CS-20. [Protameen] Ceteareth-20; CAS 68439-49-6.

Procol CS-20-D. [Protameen] Ceteareth-20, cetearyl alcohol.

Procol CS-27. [Protameen] Ceteareth-27; CAS 68439-49-6.

Procol CS-30. [Protameen] Ceteareth-30; CAS 68439-49-6.

Procol LA-2. [Protameen] Laureth-2; CAS 3055-93-4; EINECS 221-279-7; surfactant.

Procol LA-3. [Protameen] Laureth-3; CAS 3055-94-5; EINECS 221-280-2; emulsifier.

Procol LA-4. [Protameen] Laureth-4; CAS 5274-68-0; EINECS 226-097-1; emulsifier.

Procol LA-7. [Protameen] Laureth-7; CAS 3055-97-8; EINECS 221-283-9; cosmetic surfactant.

Procol LA-9. [Protameen] Laureth-9; CAS 3055-99-0; EINECS 221-284-4; personal care surfactant.

Procol LA-10. [Protameen] Laureth-10; CAS 6540-99-4; personal care emulsifier.

Procol LA-12. [Protameen] Laureth-12; CAS 3056-00-6; EINECS 221-286-5; emulsifier.

Procol LA-15. [Protameen] Laureth-15; CAS 9002-92-0; emulsifier.

Procol LA-20. [Protameen] Laureth-20; CAS 9002-92-0; emulsifier.

Procol LA-23. [Protameen] Laureth-23; CAS 9002-92-0; emulsifier.

Procol LA-30. [Protameen] Laureth-30; CAS 9002-92-0; cosmetics surfactant.

Procol LA-40 [Protameen] Laureth-40; CAS 9002-92-0; cosmetics surfactant.

Procol MA-4. [Protameen] Myreth-4; CAS 27306-79-2;

personal care ingred.

Procol NIN. [Protameen] Cetearyl alcohol, ceteth-20.

Procol OA-2. [Protameen] Oleth-2; CAS 9004-98-2; emulsifier, emollient.

Procol OA-3. [Protameen] Oleth-3; CAS 9004-98-2; emulsifier, emollient.

Procol OA-4. [Protameen] Oleth-4; CAS 9004-98-2; emulsifier, emollient.

Procol OA-5. [Protameen] Oleth-5; CAS 9004-98-2; emulsifier, emollient.

Procol OA-10. [Protameen] Oleth-10; CAS 9004-98-2; emulsifier, emollient.

Procol OA-20. [Protameen] Oleth-20; CAS 9004-98-2; emulsifier.

Procol OA-23. [Protameen] Oleth-23; CAS 9004-98-2; emulsifier.

Procol OA-25. [Protameen] Oleth-25; CAS 9004-98-2; emulsifier.

Procol P. [Protameen] Cetearyl alcohol, polysorbate 60, PEG-150 stearate, steareth-20.

Procol PMA-3. [Protameen] PPG-3 myristyl ether; CAS 63793-60-2; emollient.

Procol PSA-11. [Protameen] PPG-11 stearyl ether; CAS 25231-21-4; emollient.

Procol PSA-15. [Protameen] PPG-15 stearyl ether; CAS 25231-21-4; emollient.

Procol SA-2. [Protameen] Steareth-2; CAS 9005-00-9; personal care surfactant.

Procol SA-4. [Protameen] Steareth-4; CAS 9005-00-9; personal care surfactant.

Procol SA-10. [Protameen] Steareth-10; CAS 9005-00-9; personal care surfactant.

Procol SA-20. [Protameen] Steareth-20; CAS 9005-00-9; personal care surfactant.

Procol ST-20-G. [Protameen] Ceteareth-20, stearyl alcohol.

Procol TDA-3. [Protameen] Trideceth-3; CAS 4403-12-7; EINECS 224-540-3; surfactant.

Procol TDA-6. [Protameen] Trideceth-6; CAS 24938-91-8; personal care surfactant.

Procol TDA-12. [Protameen] Trideceth-12; CAS 24938-91-8; personal care surfactant.

Procol TDA-15. [Protameen] Trideceth-15; CAS 24938-91-8; personal care surfactant.

Prodew 100. [Ajinomoto] Sorbitol, sodium lactate, proline, sodium PCA, and hydrolyzed collagen; formulated moisturizer for cosmetics, soaps, hair care prods.; humectant; lt. yel. and transparent sol'n.; sp.gr. 1.20-1.24; pH 6.3-7.5; 50% aq. sol'n.

Prodew 200. [Ajinomoto] Sodium lactate, sodium PCA, sorbitol, hydrolyzed collagen, proline; formulated moisturizer for cosmetics, soaps, hair care prods.; humectant; lt. yel. transparent sol'n.; sp.gr. 1.15-1.19; pH 6.5-7.7.

Produkt W 37194. [Stockhausen] Acrylamidopropyltrimonium chloride/acrylates copolymer.

Profan 24 Extra, 128 Extra. [Sanyo Chem. Industries] Cocamide DEA (1:1); CAS 61791-31-9; EINECS 263-163-9; nonionic; foam stabilizer and thickener for shampoo; resistant to antifoaming action of oily soils; liq.; 100% conc.

Profan 2012E. [Sanyo Chem. Industries] Cocamide DEA (1:2); CAS 61791-31-9; EINECS 263-163-9; nonionic; foam stabilizer and thickener for shampoo; resistant to antifoaming action of oily soils; liq.; 100% conc.

Profan AA62. [Sanyo Chem. Industries] 1:1 Lauramide DEA; CAS 120-40-1; EINECS 204-393-1; nonionic; foam stabilizer, thickener for shampoos; resistant to antifoaming action of oily soils; solid; 100% conc.

Profan AB20. [Sanyo Chem. Industries] Coconut MEA; CAS 68140-00-1; EINECS 268-770-2; nonionic; foam stabilizer and thickener for shampoos; resistant to antifoaming

action of oily soils; solid; 100% conc.

Profan AD31. [Sanyo Chem. Industries] Lauramide MIPA; CAS 142-54-1; EINECS 205-541-8; nonionic; foam stabilizer, thickener for shampoos; resistant to antifoaming action of oily soils; solid; 100% conc.

Profan ME-20. [Sanyo Chem. Industries] POE coconut fatty acid amide; nonionic; used in pH balanced shampoos, dishwashing detergents and acid cleansers; stable in acid or alkali media; liq.; 97% conc.

Progallin® LA. [Nipa Labs] Dodecyl gallate; CAS 1166-52-5; EINECS 214-620-6; antioxidant for cosmetics (creams, ointments, emulsions, lipsticks, soaps, suntan preps., and dental preps.); wh. to creamy-wh. powd., odorless; insol. in ethanol, acetone, and veg. oils; m.p. 97 C; toxicology: LD50 (oral, rat) 6.5 g/kg (pract. nonharmful); sl. irritant to eyes and mucous membranes.

Progallin® P. [Nipa Labs] Propyl gallate; CAS 121-79-9; EINECS 204-498-2; antioxidant for cosmetics; wh. to creamy-wh. fine powd., odorless; sol. 0.1% in water; m.w. 212.21; m.p. 148-151 C; toxicology: LD50 (oral, rat) 3.7 g/kg (pract. nonharmful); local sensitization or irritation on skin contact or inhalation; > 98% act.

Prolagen C. [Proalan SA] Hydrolyzed collagen; CAS 9015-54-7; cosmetic protein.

Pro-Lan V. [Lanaetex Prods.] Sorbitol, TEA-cocoyl hydrolyzed collagen.

Prolastine. [Proalan SA] Hydrolyzed elastin; CAS 100085-10-7; cosmetic protein.

Promarine. [Sederma] Water, propylene glycol, and hydrolyzed gadus protein; nourishing, regenerating, and cell stimulating factor for face, body, and hair care prods.; treatment of cutaneous ageing; pale yel. clear liq., char. odor; sp.gr. 1.010-1.030; ref. index 1.345-1.355; pH 7-8; usage level: 3-8%.

Promodan SPV. [Grindsted Prods.] Dist. propylene glycol ester; functional additive for cosmetics/toiletries.

Promois E118D. [Seiwa Kasei; R.I.T.A.] AMPD isostearoyl hydrolyzed collagen; protein for skin and hair care prods.; 50% alcohol sol'n.

Promois ECP. [Seiwa Kasei; R.I.T.A.] Potassium cocoyl hydrolyzed collagen; CAS 68920-65-0; protein for skin and hair care prods.; water sol'n.; m.w. 450.

Promois® ECP-C. [Seiwa Kasei; R.I.T.A.] Potassium coco-hydrolyzed collagen; CAS 68920-65-0; protein for skin and hair care prods.; water sol'n.; m.w. 350.

Promois ECP-P. [Seiwa Kasei; R.I.T.A.] Potassium coco-hydrolyzed collagen; CAS 68920-65-0; protein for skin and hair care prods.; powd.; m.w. 450.

Promois ECS. [Seiwa Kasei; R.I.T.A.] Sodium cocoyl hydrolyzed collagen; CAS 68188-38-5; protein for skin and hair care prods.; aq. sol'n.; m.w. 450.

Promois ECT. [Seiwa Kasei; R.I.T.A.] TEA-cocoyl hydrolyzed collagen; CAS 68952-16-9; protein for skin and hair care prods.; aq. sol'n.; m.w. 450.

Promois ECT-C. [Seiwa Kasei; R.I.T.A.] TEA-cocoyl hydrolyzed collagen; CAS 68952-16-9; protein for skin and hair care prods.; aq. sol'n.; m.w. 350.

Promois EFLS. [Seiwa Kasei; R.I.T.A.] Lauroyl hydrolyzed silk sodium salt; protein for skin and hair care prods.; liq.

Promois EUP. [Seiwa Kasei; R.I.T.A.] Potassium undecylenoyl hydrolyzed collagen; CAS 68951-92-8; protein for skin and hair care prods.; aq. sol'n.

Promois EUT. [Seiwa Kasei; R.I.T.A.] TEA undecylenoyl hydrolyzed collagen; CAS 68951-91-7; protein for skin and hair care prods.; aq. sol'n.

Promois S-CAQ. [Seiwa Kasei; R.I.T.A.] Cocodimonium hydroxypropyl hydrolyzed silk; protein for skin and hair care prods.; liq.

Promois S-LAQ. [Seiwa Kasei; R.I.T.A.] Lauryldimonium hydroxypropyl hydrolyzed silk; protein for skin and hair care prods.; liq.

Promois S-SAQ. [Seiwa Kasei; R.I.T.A.] Stearyldimonium hydroxypropyl hydrolyzed silk; protein for skin and hair care prods.; liq.

Promois W-32. [Seiwa Kasei; R.I.T.A.] Hydrolyzed collagen; CAS 9015-54-7; protein for skin and hair care prods.; aq. sol'n.; m.w. 400.

Promois W-32LS. [Seiwa Kasei; R.I.T.A.] Hydrolyzed collagen; CAS 9015-54-7; protein for skin and hair care prods.; aq. sol'n.; m.w. 400.

Promois W-32R. [Seiwa Kasei; R.I.T.A.] Hydrolyzed collagen; CAS 9015-54-7; protein for skin and hair care prods.; aq. sol'n.; m.w. 400.

Promois W-42. [Seiwa Kasei; R.I.T.A.] Hydrolyzed collagen; CAS 9015-54-7; protein for skin and hair care prods.; aq. sol'n.; m.w. 1000.

Promois W-42 CAQ. [Seiwa Kasei; R.I.T.A.] Cocodimonium hydroxypropyl hydrolyzed collagen; protein for skin and hair care prods.; liq.

Promois W-42CP. [Seiwa Kasei; R.I.T.A.] Hydrolyzed collagen; CAS 9015-54-7; protein for skin and hair care prods.; aq. sol'n.; m.w. 1000.

Promois W-42K. [Seiwa Kasei; R.I.T.A.] Hydrolyzed collagen; CAS 9015-54-7; protein for skin and hair care prods.; aq. sol'n.; m.w. 1000.

Promois W-42 LAQ. [Seiwa Kasei; R.I.T.A.] Lauryldimonium hydroxypropyl hydrolyzed collagen; protein for skin and hair care prods.; liq.

Promois W-42LS. [Seiwa Kasei; R.I.T.A.] Hydrolyzed collagen; CAS 9015-54-7; protein for skin and hair care prods.; aq. sol'n.; m.w. 1000.

Promois W-42Q. [Seiwa Kasei; R.I.T.A.] Hydroxypropyltrimonium hydrolyzed collagen; CAS 11308-59-1; protein for skin and hair care prods.; aq. sol'n.; m.w. 1000.

Promois W-42QP. [Seiwa Kasei; R.I.T.A.] Hydroxypropyltrimonium hydrolyzed collagen; CAS 11308-59-1; protein for skin and hair care prods.; powd.; m.w. 1000.

Promois W-42R. [Seiwa Kasei; R.I.T.A.] Hydrolyzed collagen; CAS 9015-54-7; protein for skin and hair care prods.; aq. sol'n.; m.w. 1000.

Promois W-42 SAQ. [Seiwa Kasei; R.I.T.A.] Stearyldimonium hydroxypropyl hydrolyzed collagen; protein for skin and hair care prods.; liq.

Promois W-52. [Seiwa Kasei; R.I.T.A.] Hydrolyzed collagen; CAS 9015-54-7; protein for skin and hair care prods.; aq. sol'n.; m.w. 2000.

Promois W-52P. [Seiwa Kasei; R.I.T.A.] Hydrolyzed collagen; CAS 9015-54-7; protein for skin and hair care prods.; powd.; m.w. 2000.

Promois W-52Q. [Seiwa Kasei; R.I.T.A.] Hydroxypropyltrimonium hydrolyzed collagen; CAS 11308-59-1; protein for skin and hair care prods.; aq. sol'n.; m.w. 2000.

Promois W-52QP. [Seiwa Kasei; R.I.T.A.] Hydroxypropyltrimonium hydrolyzed collagen; CAS 11308-59-1; protein for skin and hair care prods.; powd.; m.w. 2000.

Promois WG. [Seiwa Kasei; R.I.T.A.] Hydrolyzed wheat protein; CAS 70084-87-6; protein for skin and hair care prods.; aq. sol'n.

Promois WG-Q. [Seiwa Kasei; R.I.T.A.] Hydroxypropyl trimonium chloride hydrolyzed wheat protein; protein for skin and hair care prods.; liq.

Promois WK. [Seiwa Kasei; R.I.T.A.] Hydrolyzed keratin; CAS 69430-36-0; EINECS 274-001-1; protein for skin and hair care prods.; aq. sol'n.; m.w. 400.

Promois WK-H. [Seiwa Kasei; R.I.T.A.] Hydrolyzed keratin; CAS 69430-36-0; EINECS 274-001-1; protein for skin and hair care prods.; aq. sol'n.; m.w. 1000.

Promois WK-HQ. [Seiwa Kasei; R.I.T.A.] Hydroxypropyltrimonium hydrolyzed keratin; protein for skin and hair care prods.; aq. sol'n.

Promois WS. [Seiwa Kasei; R.I.T.A.] Hydrolyzed soy protein; CAS 68607-88-5; protein for skin and hair care prods.; aq. sol'n.

Promois WS-Q. [Seiwa Kasei; R.I.T.A.] Hydroxypropyl trimonium chloride hydrolyzed soy protein; protein for skin and hair care prods.; liq.

Promois Milk. [Seiwa Kasei; R.I.T.A.] Hydrolyzed casein; CAS 65072-00-6; EINECS 265-363-1; protein for skin and hair care prods.; aq. sol'n.

Promois Milk CAQ. [Seiwa Kasei; R.I.T.A.] Cocodimonium hydroxypropyl hydrolyzed collagen; protein for skin and hair care prods.; liq.

Promois Milk LAQ. [Seiwa Kasei; R.I.T.A.] Lauryldimonium hydroxypropyl hydrolyzed collagen; protein for skin and hair care prods.; liq.

Promois Milk Q. [Seiwa Kasei; R.I.T.A.] Hydroxypropyltrimonium hydrolyzed casein; protein for skin and hair care prods.; aq. sol'n.

Promois Milk SAQ. [Seiwa Kasei; R.I.T.A.] Stearyldimonium hydroxypropyl hydrolyzed collagen; protein for skin and hair care prods.; liq.

Promois Pearl P. [Seiwa Kasei; R.I.T.A.] Hydrolyzed conchiorin protein; protein for skin and hair care prods.; aq. sol'n.

Promois Silk 700 QSP. [Seiwa Kasei; R.I.T.A.] Hydroxypropyl trimonium hydrolyzed silk; protein for skin and hair care prods.; powd.; m.w. 500.

Promois Silk 700 SP. [Seiwa Kasei; R.I.T.A.] Hydrolyzed silk; CAS 96690-41-4; protein for skin and hair care prods.; powd.; m.w. 350.

Promois Silk-1000. [Seiwa Kasei; R.I.T.A.] Hydrolyzed silk; CAS 96690-41-4; protein for skin and hair care prods.; aq. sol'n.

Promois Silk-1000 Q. [Seiwa Kasei; R.I.T.A.] Hydroxypropyltrimonium hydrolyzed silk; protein for skin and hair care prods.; aq. sol'n.

Promois Silk-1000 QP. [Seiwa Kasei; R.I.T.A.] Hydroxypropyltrimonium hydrolyzed silk; protein for skin and hair care prods.; powd.

Promois Silk A. [Seiwa Kasei; R.I.T.A.] Ethyl ester of hydrolyzed silk; protein for skin and hair care prods.; alcohol sol'n.

Promulgen® D. [Amerchol] Cetearyl alcohol and ceteareth-20; nonionic; gelling agent; o/w emulsifier, emollient, and stabilizer for cosmetics and pharmaceuticals; highly resistant to acidic and alkaline conditions; wh. waxy solid; odorless; m.p. 47–55 C; acid no. 1 max.; sapon. no. 2 max.; 100% conc.

Promulgen® G. [Amerchol] Stearyl alcohol and ceteareth-20; nonionic; gelling agent; o/w emulsifier, emollient, and stabilizer for cosmetics and pharmaceuticals; highly resistant to acidic and alkaline conditions; yel. liq.; sp.gr. 0.848; visc. 35 cps; m.p. 55–63 C; acid no. 1 max.; sapon. no. 2 max.; 100% act.

Promyr. [Amerchol] Isopropyl myristate; CAS 110-27-0; EINECS 203-751-4; emollient and solv. for cosmetics, toiletries, makeups; nongreasing rub in; water-wh. low visc. liq.; odorless; oil-sol.; acid no. 1.0 max.; sapon. no. 202–211.

Promyristyl PM-3. [Croda Inc.; Croda Chem. Ltd.] PPG-3 myristyl ether; CAS 63793-60-2; low-visc. emollient for clear analgesic, deodorant, and fragrance sticks; Gardner 1 max. clear liq.; sol. in oil, alcohol, lanolin oil; acid no. 1 max.; usage level: 5-15% .

Pronova™. [Protan Biopolymer A/S] Sodium hyaluronate; CAS 9067-32-7; polysaccharides used for medical, pharmaceutical, veterinary, botanical, microbiological, and cosmetic uses, as well as for bioreactor processes.

Propal. [Amerchol] Isopropyl palmitate; CAS 142-91-6; EINECS 205-571-1; emollient and solv. for cosmetics, toiletries, makeups; nongreasing rub in; water-wh. liq.; odorless; acid no. 1.0 max.; sapon. no. 182–191.

Propoxyol® 1695. [Henkel/Cospha; Henkel Canada] PPG-5 lanolin wax glyceride; nonionic; emollient, stabilizer, and pigment dispersant for anhyd. makeups; cosmetic additive; imparts glossy finish to skin care prods.; produces lipsticks with low drag; amber waxy solid; sol. in most cosmetic oils and waxes; m.p. 50-55 C; 100% conc.

Propylene Phenoxetol. [Nipa Labs] Phenoxyisopropanol; CAS 4169-04-4; EINECS 2240-27-4; antiseptic for skin care prods.

Propyl-Steriline. [Zimmerli] Propylparaben; CAS 94-13-3; EINECS 202-307-7; cosmetic preservative; USA, Japan, Europe approvals; colorless; usage level: 0.02-1.0%; toxicology: nontoxic.

Pro Soy AMP. [Lanaetex Prods.] AMP-coco hydrolyzed soy protein; cosmetic ingred.

Pro Soy CO. [Lanaetex Prods.] Sodium-coco hydrolyzed soy protein; cosmetic ingred.

Protachem 26. [Protameen] Glyceryl stearate.

Protachem 35A. [Protameen] Butyl stearate, lecithin, oleic acid, peach kernel oil, hydrolyzed collagen.

Protachem 100. [Protameen] Polyglyceryl-4 oleate; CAS 9007-48-1; emulsifier.

Protachem 1450 NF. [Protameen] PEG-32; CAS 25322-68-3; cosmetic ingred.

Protachem CA-9. [Protameen] PEG-9 castor oil; CAS 61791-12-6; personal care surfactant.

Protachem CA-25. [Protameen] PEG-25 castor oil; CAS 61791-12-6; personal care surfactant.

Protachem CA-30. [Protameen] PEG-30 castor oil; CAS 61791-12-6; personal care surfactant.

Protachem CA-40. [Protameen] PEG-40 castor oil; CAS 61791-12-6; personal care surfactant.

Protachem CA-100. [Protameen] PEG-100 castor oil; CAS 61791-12-6; personal care surfactant.

Protachem CA-200. [Protameen] PEG-200 castor oil; CAS 61791-12-6; personal care surfactant.

Protachem CAH-16. [Protameen] PEG-16 hydrog. castor oil; CAS 61788-85-0; emulsifier.

Protachem CAH-25. [Protameen] PEG-25 hydrog. castor oil; CAS 61788-85-0; personal care surfactant.

Protachem CAH-40. [Protameen] PEG-40 hydrog. castor oil; CAS 61788-85-0; personal care surfactant.

Protachem CAH-60. [Protameen] PEG-60 hydrog. castor oil; CAS 61788-85-0; personal care surfactant.

Protachem CAH-100. [Protameen] PEG-100 hydrog. castor oil; CAS 61788-85-0; emulsifier.

Protachem CAH-200. [Protameen] PEG-200 hydrog. castor oil; CAS 61788-85-0; emulsifier.

Protachem CB 45. [Protameen] Coco-betaine; CAS 68424-94-2; EINECS 270-329-4; cosmetic surfactant.

Protachem CER. [Protameen] Cetyl ricinoleate; CAS 10401-55-5; EINECS 233-864-4; emollient.

Protachem CTG. [Protameen] Caprylic/capric triglyceride; CAS 65381-09-1.

Protachem DGS. [Protameen] PEG-2 stearate; CAS 106-11-6; EINECS 203-363-5; emulsifier.

Protachem DGS-C. [Protameen] PEG-2 stearate; CAS 106-11-6; EINECS 203-363-5; emulsifier.

Protachem EGMS. [Protameen] Glycol stearate; CAS 111-60-4; EINECS 203-886-9; emulsifier, opacifier, pearlescent for cosmetics.

Protachem G 5509, G 5566. [Protameen] Glyceryl stearate.

Protachem GL-7. [Protameen] Glycereth-7; CAS 31694-55-0; cosmetic ingred.

Protachem GL-26. [Protameen] Glycereth-26; CAS 31694-55-0; cosmetic ingred.

Protachem GMS-165. [Protameen] Glyceryl stearate, PEG-100 stearate.

Protachem GMS-450. [Protameen] Glyceryl stearate.

Protachem HMS. [Protameen] Glyceryl stearate.

Protachem IPM. [Protameen] Isopropyl myristate; CAS 110-27-0; EINECS 203-751-4'; emollient.

Protachem IPP. [Protameen] Isopropyl palmitate; CAS 142-91-6; EINECS 205-571-1; emollient.

Protachem ISP. [Protameen] Isostearyl palmitate; CAS 72576-80-8; EINECS 276-719-0; cosmetic ingred.

Protachem JS. [Protameen] Cocamidopropyl hydroxysultaine; CAS 68139-30-0; EINECS 268-761-3; cosmetic surfactant.

Protachem LP-40. [Protameen] Potassium cocoate; CAS 61789-30-8; EINECS 263-049-9; personal care surfactant.

Protachem MLD. [Protameen] Glyceryl laurate; CAS 142-18-7; EINECS 205-526-6; cosmetic emulsifier.

Protachem MST. [Protameen] Cetyl esters; raw material for personal care prods.

Protachem NP-4. [Protameen] Nonoxynol-4; CAS 9016-45-9; personal care surfactant.

Protachem NP-6. [Protameen] Nonoxynol-6; CAS 9016-45-9; personal care surfactant.

Protachem NP-9. [Protameen] Nonoxynol-9; CAS 9016-45-9; personal care surfactant.

Protachem SDM. [Protameen] Stearamidopropyl dimethylamine lactate; CAS 55819-53-9; EINECS 259-837-7; conditioner.

Protachem SML. [Protameen] Sorbitan laurate.

Protachem SMO. [Protameen] Sorbitan oleate; CAS 1338-43-8; EINECS 215-665-4; emulsifier.

Protachem SMP. [Protameen] Sorbitan palmitate; CAS 26266-57-9; EINECS 247-568-8; emulsifier.

Protachem SMS. [Protameen] Sorbitan stearate; CAS 1338-41-6; EINECS 215-664-9; emulsifier.

Protachem SOC. [Protameen] Sorbitan sesquioleate; CAS 8007-43-0; EINECS 232-360-1; emulsifier.

Protachem SQI. [Protameen] Sorbitan sesquiisostearate; cosmetic ingred.

Protachem STO. [Protameen] Sorbitan trioleate; CAS 26266-58-0; EINECS 247-569-3; emulsifier.

Protachem STS. [Protameen] Sorbitan tristearate; CAS 26658-19-5; EINECS 247-891-4; emulsifier.

Protalan 85. [Protameen] PEG-85 lanolin; CAS 61790-81-6.

Protalan 98. [Protameen] Polysorbate 80, cetyl acetate, acetylated lanolin alcohol.

Protalan AC. [Protameen] Cetyl acetate, acetylated lanolin alcohol.

Protalan H. [Protameen] Hydroxylated lanolin; CAS 68424-66-8; EINECS 270-315-8; cosmetic emulsifier.

Protalan L-30. [Protameen] PEG-30 lanolin; CAS 61790-81-6; emollient, emulsifier.

Protalan L-60. [Protameen] PEG-60 lanolin; CAS 61790-81-6; moisturizer, lubricant.

Protalan L-75. [Protameen] PEG-75 lanolin; CAS 61790-81-6; emulsifier, emollient.

Protalan M-16, M-26. [Protameen] Min. oil, lanolin alcohol.

Protalan MOD. [Protameen] Acetylated lanolin alcohol; CAS 61788-49-6; EINECS 262-980-8; emollient.

Protalan Oil. [Protameen] Lanolin oil; emollient, moisturizer.

Protalan SS-100. [Protameen] Petrolatum, lanolin, lanolin alcohol.

Protalan Wax. [Protameen] Lanolin wax; CAS 68201-49-0; EINECS 269-220-4; emulsifier, emollient.

Protamate 200 DL. [Protameen] PEG-2 dilaurate; CAS 9005-02-1; EINECS 228-486-1; oil-phase cosmetic ingred.

Protamate 200 DPS. [Protameen] PEG-4 stearate; CAS 9004-99-3; EINECS 203-358-8; emulsifier.

Protamate 200 ML. [Protameen] PEG-4 laurate; CAS 9004-81-3; emulsifier.

Protamate 200 OC. [Protameen] PEG-4 oleate; CAS 9004-96-0; EINECS 233-293-0; personal care surfactant.

Protamate 200 T. [Protameen] PEG-4 tallate; CAS 61791-00-2; personal care surfactant.

Protamate 300 DPS. [Protameen] PEG-6 stearate; CAS 9004-99-3; emulsifier.

Protamate 300 OC. [Protameen] PEG-6 oleate; CAS 9004-96-0; emulsifier.

Protamate 400 DL. [Protameen] PEG-4 dilaurate; CAS 9005-02-1; personal care surfactant.

Protamate 400 DO. [Protameen] PEG-8 dioleate; CAS 9005-07-6; personal care surfactant.

Protamate 400 DPS. [Protameen] PEG-8 stearate; CAS 9004-99-3; emulsifier.

Protamate 400 DS. [Protameen] PEG-8 distearate; CAS 9005-08-7; personal care surfactant.

Protamate 400 ML. [Protameen] PEG-8 laurate; CAS 9004-81-3; emulsifier.

Protamate 400 OC. [Protameen] PEG-8 oleate; CAS 9004-96-0; emulsifier.

Protamate 400 T. [Protameen] PEG-8 tallate; CAS 61791-00-2; personal care surfactant.

Protamate 600 DPS. [Protameen] PEG-12 stearate; CAS 9004-99-3; emulsifier.

Protamate 600 DS. [Protameen] PEG-12 distearate; CAS 9005-08-7; personal care surfactant.

Protamate 600 OC. [Protameen] PEG-10 oleate; CAS 9004-96-0; personal care surfactant.

Protamate 600 T. [Protameen] PEG-12 tallate; CAS 61791-00-2; personal care surfactant.

Protamate 1000 DPS. [Protameen] PEG-20 stearate; CAS 9004-99-3; emulsifier.

Protamate 1000 OC. [Protameen] PEG-20 oleate; CAS 9004-96-0; personal care surfactant.

Protamate 1000 T. [Protameen] PEG-20 tallate; CAS 61791-00-2; personal care surfactant.

Protamate 1500 DPS. [Protameen] PEG-6-32 stearate; CAS 9004-99-3; emulsifier.

Protamate 1540 DPS. [Protameen] PEG-32 stearate; CAS 9004-99-3; emulsifier.

Protamate 2000 DPS. [Protameen] PEG-40 stearate; CAS 9004-99-3; emulsifier.

Protamate 4000 DPS. [Protameen] PEG-75 stearate; CAS 9004-99-3; emulsifier.

Protamate 4400 DPS. [Protameen] PEG-100 stearate; CAS 9004-99-3; emulsifier.

Protamate 6000 DS. [Protameen] PEG-150 distearate; CAS 9005-08-7; personal care surfactant.

Protamide 15W. [Protameen] Linoleamide DEA; CAS 56863-02-6; EINECS 260-410-2; foam builder, thickener.

Protamide CA. [Protameen] Ricinoleamide DEA; CAS 40716-42-5; EINECS 255-051-3; personal care surfactant.

Protamide CKD. [Protameen] Cocamide DEA; CAS 61791-31-9; EINECS 263-163-9; cosmetic surfactant.

Protamide CME. [Protameen] Cocamide MEA; CAS 68140-00-1; EINECS 268-770-2; cosmetic surfactant.

Protamide DCA. [Protameen] Cocamide DEA; CAS 61791-31-9; EINECS 263-163-9; cosmetic surfactant.

Protamide DCAW. [Protameen] Cocamide DEA; CAS 61791-31-9; EINECS 263-163-9; cosmetic surfactant.

Protamide HCA. [Protameen] Cocamide DEA; CAS 61791-31-9; EINECS 263-163-9; cosmetic surfactant.

Protamide L-80M, L90, L90A, LM 73, LM 73-L, LM-73 PG, LMAV. [Protameen] Lauramide DEA; CAS 120-40-1; EINECS 204-393-1; cosmetic surfactant.

Protamide LNO. [Protameen] Linoleamide DEA; CAS 56863-02-6; EINECS 260-410-2; foam builder, thickener.

Protamide MRCA. [Protameen] Myristamide DEA; CAS 7545-23-5; EINECS 231-426-7; thickener, foam booster/stabilizer.

Protamide N-1918. [Protameen] Stearamide DEA, diethanolamine.

Protamide OFO. [Protameen] Oleamide DEA, diethanolamine.

Protamide SA. [Protameen] Stearamide DEA; CAS 93-82-3; EINECS 202-280-1; thickener, emulsifier.

Protamide T. [Protameen] Oleamide DEA, diethanolamine.

Protaphos 400-A. [Protameen] Oleth-4 phosphate; CAS 39464-69-2; personal care surfactant.

Protaphos P-610. [Protameen] Nonoxynol-10 phosphate; CAS 51609-41-7.

Protaphos SDA. [Protameen] Laureth-8 phosphate; CAS 39464-66-9; surfactant.

Protapon 24A. [Protameen] Sodium methyl cocoyl taurate; personal care surfactant.

Protapon 33. [Protameen] Sodium methyl oleoyl taurate; CAS 137-20-2; EINECS 205-285-7; personal care surfactant.

Protaquat 2HT-75. [Protameen] Distearyldimonium chloride; CAS 107-64-2; EINECS 203-508-2; conditioner for cosmetics.

Protasorb L-5. [Protameen] Polysorbate 21; CAS 9005-64-5; emulsifier.

Protasorb L-20. [Protameen] Polysorbate 20; CAS 9005-64-5; emulsifier, solubilizer.

Protasorb O-5. [Protameen] Polysorbate 81; CAS 9005-65-6; emulsifier.

Protasorb O-20. [Protameen] Polysorbate 80; CAS 9005-65-6; emulsifier.

Protasorb P-20. [Protameen] Polysorbate 40; CAS 9005-66-7; emulsifier.

Protasorb S-20. [Protameen] Polysorbate 60; CAS 9005-67-8; emulsifier.

Protasorb TO-20. [Protameen] Polysorbate 85; CAS 9005-70-3; emulsifier.

Protastat P-211. [Protameen] Methylparaben, propylparaben, potassium sorbate; cosmetic preservative.

Protectein™. [Hormel] Propyltrimonium hydrolyzed collagen; cationic; substantive quaternary protein reducing irritation potential of surfactants; antistat; used for skin and hair prods. (shampoos, conditioners where mildness is important); amber clear liq., bland char. odor; m.w. 2000; pH 6–7 (diluted 2:1); 54-56% solids.

Protegin®. [Goldschmidt; Goldschmidt AG] Min. oil, petrolatum, ozokerite, glyceryl oleate, lanolin alcohol; nonionic; emollient, emulsifier; absorption base for w/o cosmetic/pharmaceutical emulsions; iovry soft waxy solid; sol. warm in min. oil, sol. warm with sl. turbidity in veg. oils; insol. in water; m.p. 58-65 C; HLB 3.0; acid no. 1 max.; sapon. no. 8-12; hyd. no. 18-30; 100% conc.

Protegin® W. [Goldschmidt; Goldschmidt AG] Petrolatum, ozokerite, hydrog. castor oil, glyceryl isostearate, polyglyceryl-3 oleate; nonionic; SE w/o emulsifier, emollient, absorp. base for cosmetics and pharmaceuticals; ivory waxy solid; sol. warm in veg. and min. oils; disp. warm in water; m.p. 75-82 C; HLB 3.0; acid no. 1 max.; sapon. no. 18-28; hyd. no. 18-28; 100% conc.

Protegin® WX. [Goldschmidt; Goldschmidt AG] Petrolatum, ozokerite, hydrog. castor oil, glyceryl isostearate, polyglyceryl-3 oleate; nonionic; SE w/o emulsifier, emollient, absorp. base for cosmetics and pharmaceuticals; ivory waxy solid; sol. warm in veg. and min. oils; disp. warm in water; m.p. 76-83 C; HLB 3.5; acid no. 1 max.; sapon. no. 27-37; hyd. no. 32-42; 100% conc.

Protegin® X. [Goldschmidt; Goldschmidt AG] Min. oil, petrolatum, ozokerite, glyceryl oleate, lanolin alcohol; nonionic; SE w/o emulsifier, emollient, absorp. base for cosmetics and pharmaceuticals; ivory waxy paste; sol. warm in min. oil, sol. warm with sl. turbidity in veg. oils;

insol. in water; m.p. 58-65 C; HLB 3.5; acid no. 1 max.; sapon. no. 10-16; hyd. no. 25-38; 100% conc.

Pro-Tein ES-20. [Maybrook] Hydrolyzed collagen, ethyl ester; CAS 68951-89-3; cationic; substantive to hair; plasticizer for styling resins; improves film props. and gloss in cream rinses, hair conditioners, mousses; anti-irritant and protectant in facial toners, antiperspirants; lt. amber clear liq., char. sweet ethanolic odor; sp.gr. 0.930-0.980; pH 3.5-4.5 (5% aq.); 20% min. solids. in ethanol.

Pro-Tein SA-20. [Maybrook] Lauroyl hyrolyzed collagen in ethanol; CAS 68952-15-8; adds body, mitigates drying effects of alcohol in skin and hair care prods. (hair sprays, aftershaves, facial toners, antiperspirants); plasticizer for hair styling resins; lt. amber clear liq., char. ethanolic odor; insol. in water; sp.gr. 0.800-0.900; pH 3.5-4.5 (5% aq.); 20% min. solids. in ethanol.

Protein SC. [Lowenstein] Hydrolyzed animal protein; CAS 9015-54-7; protein for shampoo and hair color systems; solid.

Pro-Tein SM-20. [Maybrook] Myristoyl hydrolyzed collagen; CAS 72319-06-3; cosmetic ingred.

Protein TC. [Lowenstein] Hydrolyzed protein; CAS 9015-54-7; protein for shampoo and hair color systems; liq.

Proteodermin CLR. [Dr. Kurt Richter; Henkel/Cospha] Sol. proteoglycans; for skin care preps. for aging or sun damaged skin; wh.-gray, optically dense, sl. visc. liq.

Proteol VS22. [Seppic] Sodium cocoyl hydrolyzed soya protein; foaming surfactant for cosmetics use.

Proteolene H. [Vevy] Hydrolyzed collagen; CAS 9015-54-7; cosmetic protein.

Proteosilane C. [Exsymol; Biosil Tech.] Methylsilanol elastinate; aids tissue regeneration; for regenerative creams, anti-aging formulations, stretch mark preventives, other cosmetic and health emulsions, creams, alcoholic lotions; pale yel. opalescent liq.; misc. with water, alcohols, glycols; pH 5.5; usage level: 2-6%; toxicology: nontoxic.

Proteric CAB. [Protameen] Cocamidopropyl betaine.

Proteric CDL. [Protameen] Disodium cocoamphodiacetate, sodium lauryl sulfate, sodium laureth sulfate; cosmetic surfactant.

Proteric CDTD. [Protameen] Disodium cocoamphodiacetate, sodium trideceth sulfate; cosmetic surfactant.

Proteric CDX-38. [Protameen] Disodium cocoamphodiacetate; CAS 68650-39-5; EINECS 272-043-5; cosmetic surfactant.

Proteric CM-36 S. [Protameen] Sodium cocoamphoacetate; personal care surfactant.

Prote-sorb SML. [Protex] Sorbitan laurate; CAS 1338-39-2; nonionic; emulsifier for food, cosmetic, household and industrial, agric., leather, metalworking, and textile industries; liq.; HLB 8.6; sapon. no. 162.

Prote-sorb SMO. [Protex] Sorbitan oleate; CAS 1338-43-8; EINECS 215-665-4; nonionic; emulsifier for food, cosmetic, household and industrial, agric., leather, metalworking, and textile industries; liq.; HLB 4.3; sapon. no. 153.

Prote-sorb SMP. [Protex] Sorbitan palmitate; CAS 26266-57-9; EINECS 247-568-8; nonionic; emulsifier for food, cosmetic, household and industrial, agric., leather, metalworking, and textile industries; solid; HLB 6.7; sapon. no. 155.

Prote-sorb SMS. [Protex] Sorbitan stearate; CAS 1338-41-6; EINECS 215-664-9; nonionic; emulsifier for food, cosmetic, household and industrial, agric., leather, metalworking, and textile industries; solid; HLB 4.7; sapon. no. 152.

Prote-sorb STO. [Protex] Sorbitan trioleate; CAS 26266-58-0; EINECS 247-569-3; nonionic; emulsifier for food, cosmetic, household and industrial, agric., leather, metal-working, and textile industries; liq.; HLB 1.8; sapon. no. 180.

Prote-sorb STS. [Protex] Sorbitan tristearate; CAS 26658-19-5; EINECS 247-891-4; emulsifier for food, cosmetic, household and industrial, agric., leather, metalworking, and textile industries; solid; HLB 2.1; sapon. no. 182.

Prothera™. [ICN Pharmaceuticals] Cleanser and protectant for dry, itchy skin and skin assaulted by wind, cold, sun, and cosmetics; provides protective moisturizing layer.

Protol® . [Witco/Petroleum Spec.] Wh. min. oil USP; emollient, lubricant in cosmetic creams and lotions, pharmaceuticals, food processing; FDA §172.878, 178.3620a; water-wh., odorless, tasteless; sp.gr. 0.859-0.875; visc. 35-37 cSt (40 C); pour pt. -12 C; flash pt. 188 C.

Proto-Lan 4R. [Maybrook] Min. oil, coco-hydrolyzed collagen, cetyl alcohol, myristyl myristate, ceteth-16, hydrog. lanolin; emollient, moisturizer, aux. emulsifier, antistat, conditioner, base for skin and hair care prods. (hair conditioners, creams, lotions, lipsticks); provides lubricious film, water emulsifying/binding props.; pale amber soft solid, char. sl. fatty odor; pH 3.5-5.0; 95% min. solids.

Proto-Lan 8. [Maybrook] Lecithin, butyl stearate, coco-hydrolyzed animal protein, oleoyl sarcosine, sesame oil, lanolin alcohol.; nongreasy emollient, moisturizer, emulsifier, conditioner, antistat, lubricant for creams, lotions, ethnic formulations, conditioners, baby oils, bath oils, suntan prods., shave creams, makeup, face soaps; amber clear to sl. hazy liq., char. sl. fatty odor; sp.gr. 0.940-0.970; 95% min. solids.

Proto-Lan 20. [Maybrook] Hydrolyzed animal protein, PEG-75 lanolin, propylene glycol, ceteth-16, lanolin oil; substantive emollient, softener, conditioner, moisturizer, lubricant, base for skin and hair prods. (shampoos, conditioners, ethnic prods., creams, lotions, face masks, bath prods.); lt. amber clear liq., char. mild odor; pH 6.0-7.5; 28-32% solids.

Proto-Lan 30. [Maybrook] Propylene glycol, PPG-12-PEG-65 lanolin oil, hydrolyzed animal protein; substantive emollient, moisturizer, adjunct emulsifier for skin and hair care prods. (shampoos, conditioners, creams, lotions, bath prods., antiperspirants, facial toners); lt. amber clear liq., char. mild odor; pH 5.0-6.0; 28-34% solids.

Proto-Lan IP. [Maybrook] Isostearic acid, isostearoyl hydrolyzed collagen; CAS 2724-58-5, 977066-20-8; nongreasy emollient, moisturizer for ethnic formulations, conditioners, hair treatments, lip care, skin care, nail polish, soap bars, antiperspirants; yel. clear to sl. hazy liq., char. fatty odor; acid no. 180-200; pH 5.5-6.0 (10% aq.).

Proto-Lan KT. [Maybrook] Isostearic acid, sorbitan oleate, cocoyl hydrolyzed keratin; cosmetic ingred.

Protopet® Alba. [Witco/Petroleum Spec.] Petrolatum USP; CAS 8027-32-5; EINECS 232-373-2; med. consistency and m.p. petrolatum functioning as carrier, lubricant, emollient, moisture barrier, protective agent, softener for cosmetics, pharmaceutical ointment, food processing, industrial applics.; FDA §172.880 approved; Lovibond 1.0Y color, odorless; visc. 10-16 cSt (100 C); m.p. 54-60 C.

Protopet® White 1S. [Witco/Petroleum Spec.] Petrolatum USP; CAS 8027-32-5; EINECS 232-373-2; med. consistency and m.p. petrolatum functioning as carrier, lubricant, emollient, moisture barrier, protective agent, softener for cosmetics, pharmaceutical ointment, food processing, industrial applics.; FDA §172.880 clearance; Lovibond 1.5Y color, odorless; visc. 10–16 cSt (100 C); m.p. 54–60 C.

Protopet® White 2L. [Witco/Petroleum Spec.] Petrolatum USP; CAS 8027-32-5; EINECS 232-373-2; med. consistency and m.p. petrolatum functioning as carrier, lubricant, emollient, moisture barrier, protective agent, softener for cosmetics, pharmaceutical ointment, food processing, industrial applics.; FDA §172.880 clearance; Lovibond 8Y0.6R color, odorless; visc. 10–16 cSt (100 C); m.p. 54–60 C.

Protopet® White 3C. [Witco/Petroleum Spec.] Petrolatum USP; CAS 8027-32-5; EINECS 232-373-2; med. consistency and m.p. petrolatum functioning as carrier, lubricant, emollient, moisture barrier, protective agent, softener for cosmetics, pharmaceutical ointment, food processing, industrial applics.; FDA §172.880 clearance; Lovibond 25Y1.0R color, odorless; visc. 10–16 cSt (100 C); m.p. 54–60 C.

Protopet® Yellow 2A. [Witco/Petroleum Spec.] Petrolatum USP; CAS 8027-32-5; EINECS 232-373-2; med. consistency and m.p. petrolatum functioning as carrier, lubricant, emollient, moisture barrier, protective agent, softener for cosmetics, pharmaceutical ointment, food processing, industrial applics.; FDA §172.880 clearance; Lovibond 30Y/2.5R color, odorless; visc. 10–16 cSt (100 C); m.p. 54–60 C.

Protox C-2. [Protameen] PEG-2 cocamine; CAS 61791-14-8; emulsifier.

Protox C-5. [Protameen] PEG-5 cocamine; CAS 61791-14-8; emulsifier.

Protox C-10. [Protameen] PEG-10 cocamine; CAS 61791-14-8; emulsifier.

Protox C-15. [Protameen] PEG-15 cocamine; CAS 61791-14-8; emulsifier.

Protox HTA-2. [Protameen] PEG-2 stearamine; CAS 10213-78-2; EINECS 233-520-3; emulsifier.

Protox HTA-10. [Protameen] PEG-10 stearamine; CAS 26635-92-7; emulsifier.

Protox HTA-15. [Protameen] PEG-15 stearamine; CAS 26635-92-7; emulsifier.

Protox HTA-50. [Protameen] PEG-50 stearamine; CAS 26635-92-7; emulsifier.

Protox O-2. [Protameen] PEG-2 oleamine; emulsifier.

Protox O-5. [Protameen] PEG-5 oleamine; emulsifier.

Protox O-15. [Protameen] PEG-15 oleamine; emulsifier.

Protox S-2. [Protameen] PEG-2 soyamine; CAS 61791-24-0; personal care surfactant.

Protox S-5. [Protameen] PEG-5 soyamine; CAS 61791-24-0; personal care surfactant.

Protox S-10. [Protameen] PEG-10 soyamine; CAS 61791-24-0; personal care surfactant.

Protox S-15. [Protameen] PEG-15 soyamine; CAS 61791-24-0; personal care surfactant.

Protox T-2. [Protameen] PEG-2 hydrog. tallowamine; CAS 61791-26-2; emulsifier.

Protox T-5. [Protameen] PEG-5 hydrog. tallowamine; CAS 61791-26-2; emulsifier.

Protox T-15. [Protameen] PEG-15 hydrog. tallowamine; CAS 61791-26-2; emulsifier.

Protox T-20. [Protameen] PEG-20 hydrog. tallowamine; CAS 61791-26-2; emulsifier.

Protox T-40. [Protameen] PEG-40 hydrog. tallowamine; CAS 61791-26-2; emulsifier.

Protox T-50. [Protameen] PEG-50 hydrog. tallowamine; CAS 61791-26-2; emulsifier.

Protulines. [Exsymol; Biosil Tech.] Hydrolyzed vegetable protein; CAS 100209-45-8; moisturizer for cosmetics, oily skin care, regeneration and skin treatment, anti-ageing and anti-wrinkle creams; brn. opalescent sl. visc. liq., algal odor; misc. in water; pH 6.0-6.5; usage level: 2-10% of a 4% sol'n.; toxicology: nontoxic.

Prove HM. [Fabriquimica] Hydrolyzed corn protein.

Prove HS. [Fabriquimica] Hydrolyzed soy protein; CAS 68607-88-5; cosmetic protein.

Prove HT. [Fabriquimica] Hydrolyzed wheat protein; CAS 70084-87-6; cosmetic protein.

Provol 50. [Croda Inc.] PPG-50 oleyl ether; CAS 52581-71-2; emollient, superfatting agent, lubricant, pigment dispersant, and coupler for personal care prods., ethnic hair prods.; aids spreading and pigment dispersion in makeup systems; Gardner 10 max. liq.; sol. in acetone, IPM, lanolin oil; sol. hazy in min. oil; insol. in water; acid no. 1 max.; iodine no. 12 max.; pH 5.5–7.5 (3% aq.).; usage level: 5-20% .

Pro Wheat CO. [Lanaetex Prods.] Sodium-coco hydrolyzed wheat protein; cosmetic ingred.

Prox-onic CC-05. [Protex] PEG-5 cocoate; CAS 61791-29-5; emulsifier, lubricant additive for metalworking, textiles, cosmetics, defoamers; visc. control agent in plastisols; liq.; sapon. no. 135.

Prox-onic CC-09. [Protex] PEG-9 cocoate; CAS 61791-29-5; emulsifier, lubricant additive for metalworking, textiles, cosmetics, defoamers; visc. control agent in plastisols; liq.; sapon. no. 90.

Prox-onic CC-014. [Protex] PEG-14 cocoate; CAS 61791-29-5; emulsifier, lubricant additive for metalworking, textiles, cosmetics, defoamers; visc. control agent in plastisols; liq.; sapon. no. 68.

Prox-onic CSA-1/04. [Protex] Ceteareth-4; CAS 68439-49-6; emulsifier, emulsion stabilizer, detergent, wetting agent, dispersant, solubilizer, defoamer, dye assistant, leveling agent for cosmetics, textiles, metal cleaners, industrial, institutional and household cleaners, emulsion polymerization; solid; HLB 8.0.

Prox-onic CSA-1/06. [Protex] Ceteareth-6; CAS 68439-49-6; see Prox-onic CSA-1/04; solid; HLB 10.1.

Prox-onic CSA-1/010. [Protex] Ceteareth-10; CAS 68439-49-6; see Prox-onic CSA-1/04; solid; HLB 12.4; cloud pt. 73 C (1% aq.).

Prox-onic CSA-1/015. [Protex] Ceteareth-15; CAS 68439-49-6; see Prox-onic CSA-1/04; paste; HLB 14.3; cloud pt. 95-100 C (1% aq.).

Prox-onic CSA-1/020. [Protex] Ceteareth-20; CAS 68439-49-6; see Prox-onic CSA-1/04; solid; cloud pt. > 100 C (1% aq.).

Prox-onic CSA-1/030. [Protex] Ceteareth-30; CAS 68439-49-6; see Prox-onic CSA-1/04; solid; cloud pt. > 100 C (1% aq.).

Prox-onic CSA-1/050. [Protex] Ceteareth-50; CAS 68439-49-6; see Prox-onic CSA-1/04; solid; HLB 16.9; cloud pt. < 100 C (1% aq.).

Prox-onic EP 1090-1. [Protex] Difunctional block polymer ending in primary hydroxyl groups; nonionic; defoamer for metalworking, cosmetic, pharmaceuticals, paper, textiles; base for low foaming surfactants, antifoams, dishwash, dispersing and wetting agents for paints, drilling muds, emulsifiers, petrol. demulsifiers, emulsion polymerization; liq.; m.w. 2000; HLB 3.0; cloud pt. 24 C (1% aq.); 100% act.

Prox-onic EP 1090-2. [Protex] Difunctional block polymer ending in primary hydroxyl groups; nonionic; defoamer for metalworking, cosmetic, paper, textiles; base for low foaming surfactants, antifoams, dishwash, dispersing and wetting agents for paints, drilling muds, emulsifiers, petrol. demulsifiers, emulsion polymerization; liq.; m.w. 2600; HLB 6.5; cloud pt. 28 C (1% aq.); 100% act.

Prox-onic EP 2080-1. [Protex] Difunctional block polymer ending in primary hydroxyl groups; nonionic; defoamer for metalworking, cosmetic, paper, textiles; base for low foaming surfactants, antifoams, dishwash, dispersing and wetting agents for paints, drilling muds, emulsifiers, petrol. demulsifiers, emulsion polymerization; liq.; m.w. 2500; HLB 7.0; cloud pt. 30 C (1% aq.); 100% act.

Prox-onic EP 4060-1. [Protex] Difunctional block polymer ending in primary hydroxyl groups; nonionic; defoamer for metalworking, cosmetic, paper, textiles; base for low foaming surfactants, antifoams, dishwash, dispersing and wetting agents for paints, drilling muds, emulsifiers, petrol. demulsifiers, emulsion polymerization; liq.; m.w. 3000; HLB 1.0; cloud pt. 16 C (1% aq.); 100% act.

Prox-onic HR-05. [Protex] PEG-5 castor oil; CAS 61791-12-6; nonionic; emulsifier, pigment dispersant, leveling agent, softener, rewetting agent, degreaser, antistat, emulsion stabilizer, lubricant for leather, paint, paper, plastics, textile, and cosmetics industries; solubilizer for perfumes; liq.; HLB 3.8; sapon. no. 145.

Prox-onic HR-016. [Protex] PEG-16 castor oil; CAS 61791-12-6; nonionic; see Prox-onic HR-05; liq.; HLB 8.6; sapon. no. 100.

Prox-onic HR-025. [Protex] PEG-25 castor oil; CAS 61791-12-6; nonionic; see Prox-onic HR-05; liq.; HLB 10.8; sapon. no. 80.

Prox-onic HR-030. [Protex] PEG-30 castor oil; CAS 61791-12-6; nonionic; see Prox-onic HR-05; liq.; HLB 11.7; sapon. no. 73.

Prox-onic HR-036. [Protex] PEG-36 castor oil; CAS 61791-12-6; nonionic; see Prox-onic HR-05; liq.; HLB 12.6; sapon. no. 68.

Prox-onic HR-040. [Protex] PEG-40 castor oil; CAS 61791-12-6; nonionic; see Prox-onic HR-05; liq.; HLB 12.9; sapon. no. 61.

Prox-onic HR-080. [Protex] PEG-80 castor oil; CAS 61791-12-6; nonionic; see Prox-onic HR-05; solid; HLB 15.8; sapon. no. 34.

Prox-onic HR-0200. [Protex] PEG-200 castor oil; CAS 61791-12-6; nonionic; see Prox-onic HR-05; liq.; HLB 18.1; sapon. no. 16.

Prox-onic HR-0200/50. [Protex] PEG-200 castor oil; CAS 61791-12-6; nonionic; see Prox-onic HR-05; liq.; HLB 18.1; sapon. no. 16; 50% act.

Prox-onic HRH-05. [Protex] PEG-5 hydrogenated castor oil; CAS 61788-85-0; nonionic; emulsifier, pigment dispersant, leveling agent, softener, rewetting agent, degreaser, antistat, emulsion stabilizer, lubricant for leather, paint, paper, plastics, textile, and cosmetics industries; solubilizer for perfumes; liq.; HLB 3.8; sapon. no. 142.

Prox-onic HRH-016. [Protex] PEG-16 hydrogenated castor oil; CAS 61788-85-0; nonionic; see Prox-onic HRH-05; liq.; HLB 8.6; sapon. no. 100.

Prox-onic HRH-025. [Protex] PEG-25 hydrogenated castor oil; CAS 61788-85-0; nonionic; see Prox-onic HRH-05; liq.; HLB 10.8; sapon. no. 80.

Prox-onic HRH-0200. [Protex] PEG-200 hydrogenated castor oil; CAS 61788-85-0; nonionic; see Prox-onic HRH-05; liq.; HLB 18.1; sapon. no. 17.

Prox-onic HRH-0200/50. [Protex] PEG-200 hydrogenated castor oil; CAS 61788-85-0; nonionic; see Prox-onic HRH-05; liq.; HLB 18.1; sapon. no. 17; 50% act.

Prox-onic L 081-05. [Protex] POE (5) linear alcohol ether; biodeg. low foam detergent, wetting agent, emulsifier for household, agric. and industrial cleaners; coupling agent and solubilizer for perfumes and org. additives; cosmetic and pharmaceutical emulsions, shampoos, gels, shaving creams, antiperspirant.

Prox-onic L 101-05. [Protex] POE (5) linear alcohol ether; biodeg. low foam detergent, wetting agent, emulsifier for household, agric. and industrial cleaners; coupling agent and solubilizer for perfumes and org. additives; cosmetic and pharmaceutical emulsions, shampoos, gels, shaving creams, antiperspirant.

Prox-onic L 102-02. [Protex] POE (2) linear alcohol ether; biodeg. low foam detergent, wetting agent, emulsifier for household, agric. and industrial cleaners; coupling agent and solubilizer for perfumes and org. additives; cosmetic and pharmaceutical emulsions, shampoos, gels, shaving creams, antiperspirant.

Prox-onic L 121-09. [Protex] POE (9) linear alcohol ether; biodeg. low foam detergent, wetting agent, emulsifier for household, agric. and industrial cleaners; coupling agent and solubilizer for perfumes and org. additives; cosmetic and pharmaceutical emulsions, shampoos, gels, shaving creams, antiperspirant.

Prox-onic L 161-05. [Protex] POE (5) linear alcohol ether; biodeg. low foam detergent, wetting agent, emulsifier for household, agric. and industrial cleaners; coupling agent and solubilizer for perfumes and org. additives; cosmetic and pharmaceutical emulsions, shampoos, gels, shaving creams, antiperspirant.

Prox-onic L 181-05. [Protex] POE (5) linear alcohol ether; biodeg. low foam detergent, wetting agent, emulsifier for household, agric. and industrial cleaners; coupling agent and solubilizer for perfumes and org. additives; cosmetic and pharmaceutical emulsions, shampoos, gels, shaving creams, antiperspirant.

Prox-onic L 201-02. [Protex] POE (2.5) linear alcohol ether; biodeg. low foam detergent, wetting agent, emulsifier for household, agric. and industrial cleaners; coupling agent and solubilizer for perfumes and org. additives; cosmetic and pharmaceutical emulsions, shampoos, gels, shaving creams, antiperspirant.

Prox-onic LA-1/02. [Protex] Laureth-2; CAS 3055-93-4; EINECS 221-279-7; coupling agent, solubilizer, emulsion stabilizer for cosmetic and hair care prods.; with anionic surfactants for emulsion polymerization; in coning and textile spin finishes; liq.; HLB 6.4.

Prox-onic LA-1/04. [Protex] Laureth-4; CAS 5274-68-0; EINECS 226-097-1; see Prox-onic LA-1/02; liq.; HLB 9.2; cloud pt. 52 C (1% aq.).

Prox-onic LA-1/09. [Protex] Laureth-9; CAS 3055-99-0; EINECS 221-284-4; see Prox-onic LA-1/02; liq.; HLB 13.3; cloud pt. 73-76 C (1% aq.).

Prox-onic LA-1/012. [Protex] Laureth-12; CAS 3056-00-6; EINECS 221-286-5; see Prox-onic LA-1/02; solid; HLB 14.5; cloud pt. < 100 C (1% aq.).

Prox-onic LA-1/023. [Protex] Laureth-23; CAS 9002-92-0; see Prox-onic LA-1/02; solid; HLB 16.7.

Prox-onic MG-010. [Protex] POE (10) methyl glucoside; CAS 68239-42-9; emollient; liq.

Prox-onic MG-020. [Protex] POE (20) methyl glucoside; CAS 68239-43-0; emollient; liq.

Prox-onic MG-020 P. [Protex] POP (20) methyl glucoside; cosolv., perfume fixative; liq.

Prox-onic NP-1.5. [Protex] Nonoxynol-1; EINECS 248-762-5; nonionic; emulsifier, detergent, wetting agent, dispersant, solubilizer, coupling agent, defoamer for textiles, metalworking, household, industrial, agric., paper, paint, and cosmetics industries; liq.; oil-sol.; HLB 4.6.

Prox-onic NP-04. [Protex] Nonoxynol-4; CAS 9016-45-9; nonionic; emulsifier, detergent, wetting agent, dispersant, solubilizer, defoamer, coupling agent for textiles, metalworking, household, industrial, agric., paper, paint, and cosmetics industries; liq.; HLB 8.9.

Prox-onic NP-06. [Protex] Nonoxynol-6; CAS 9016-45-9; nonionic; emulsifier, detergent, wetting agent, dispersant, solubilizer, coupling agent for textiles, metalworking, household, industrial, agric., paper, paint, and cosmetics industries; liq.; HLB 10.9; cloud pt. < 25 C (1% aq.).

Prox-onic NP-09. [Protex] Nonoxynol-9; CAS 9016-45-9; nonionic; emulsifier, detergent, wetting agent, dispersant, solubilizer, coupling agent for textiles, metalworking, household, industrial, agric., paper, paint, and cosmetics industries; liq.; HLB 13.0; cloud pt. 54 C (1% aq.).

Prox-onic NP-010. [Protex] Nonoxynol-10; CAS 9016-45-9; EINECS 248-294-1; nonionic; emulsifier, detergent, wetting agent, dispersant, solubilizer, coupling agent for textiles, metalworking, household, industrial, agric., paper, paint, and cosmetics industries; liq.; HLB 13.5; cloud pt. 72 C (1% aq.).

Prox-onic NP-015. [Protex] Nonoxynol-15; CAS 9016-45-9; nonionic; emulsifier, detergent, wetting agent, dispersant, solubilizer, coupling agent for textiles, metalworking, household, industrial, agric., paper, paint, and cosmetics industries; detergent, wetting agent at elevated temps. and electrolyte; paste; HLB 15.0; cloud pt. 96 C (1% aq.).

Prox-onic NP-020. [Protex] Nonoxynol-20; CAS 9016-45-9; nonionic; emulsifier, detergent, wetting agent, dispersant, solubilizer, coupling agent for textiles, metalworking, household, industrial, agric., paper, paint, and cosmetics industries; detergent, wetting agent at elevated temps. and electrolyte; solid; HLB 16.0; cloud pt. > 100 C (1% aq.).

Prox-onic NP-030. [Protex] Nonoxynol-30; CAS 9016-45-9; nonionic; emulsifier for fats, oils, and waxes; detergent, wetting agent, dispersant, solubilizer, coupling agent for textiles, metalworking, household, industrial, agric., paper, paint, and cosmetics industries; solid; HLB 17.1; cloud pt. > 100 C (1% aq.).

Prox-onic NP-030/70. [Protex] Nonoxynol-30; CAS 9016-45-9; nonionic; emulsifier for fats, oils, and waxes; detergent, wetting agent, dispersant, solubilizer, coupling agent for textiles, metalworking, household, industrial, agric., paper, paint, and cosmetics industries; liq.; HLB 17.1; cloud pt. > 100 C (1% aq.); 70% act.

Prox-onic NP-040. [Protex] Nonoxynol-40; CAS 9016-45-9; nonionic; emulsifier, detergent, wetting agent, dispersant, solubilizer, coupling agent for textiles, metalworking, household, industrial, agric., paper, paint, and cosmetics industries; for high temps. and electrolyte use; solid; HLB 17.8; cloud pt. > 100 C (1% aq.).

Prox-onic NP-040/70. [Protex] Nonoxynol-40; CAS 9016-45-9; nonionic; emulsifier, detergent, wetting agent, dispersant, solubilizer, coupling agent for textiles, metalworking, household, industrial, agric., paper, paint, and cosmetics industries; for high temps. and electrolytes; liq.; HLB 17.8; cloud pt. > 100 C (1% aq.); 70% act.

Prox-onic NP-050. [Protex] Nonoxynol-50; CAS 9016-45-9; nonionic; emulsifier, detergent, wetting agent, dispersant, solubilizer, coupling agent for textiles, metalworking, household, industrial, agric., paper, paint, and cosmetics industries; for high temps. and electrolyte; emulsifier for waxes and polishes; solid; HLB 18.2; cloud pt. > 100 C (1% aq.).

Prox-onic NP-050/70. [Protex] Nonoxynol-50; CAS 9016-45-9; nonionic; emulsifier, detergent, wetting agent, dispersant, solubilizer, coupling agent for textiles, metalworking, household, industrial, agric., paper, paint, and cosmetics industries; for high temps. and electrolyte; emulsifier for waxes and polishes; liq.; HLB 18.2; cloud pt. > 100 C (1% aq.); 70% act.

Prox-onic NP-0100. [Protex] Nonoxynol-100; CAS 9016-45-9; nonionic; emulsifier, detergent, wetting agent, dispersant, coupling agent for textiles, metalworking, household, industrial, agric., paper, paint, and cosmetics industries; for high temps. and electrolyte; emulsifier for waxes and polishes; solid; HLB 19.0; cloud pt. > 100 C (1% aq.).

Prox-onic NP-0100/70. [Protex] Nonoxynol-100; CAS 9016-45-9; nonionic; emulsifier, detergent, wetting agent, dispersant, solubilizer, coupling agent for textiles, metalworking, household, industrial, agric., paper, paint, and cosmetics industries; for high temps. and electrolyte; emulsifier for waxes and polishes; liq.; HLB 19.0; cloud pt. > 100 C (1% aq.); 70% act.

Prox-onic OA-1/04. [Protex] Oleth-4; CAS 9004-98-2; nonionic; coupling agent, solubilizer, emulsion stabilizer for cosmetic and hair care prods.; with anionic surfactants for

emulsion polymerization; in coning and textile spin finishes; liq.; HLB 7.9.

Prox-onic OA-1/09. [Protex] Oleth-9; CAS 9004-98-2; nonionic; see Prox-onic OA-1/04; liq.; HLB 11.9; cloud pt. 52 C (1% aq.).

Prox-onic OA-1/020. [Protex] Oleth-20; CAS 9004-98-2; nonionic; emulsifier for min. oils, fatty acids, waxes; for polishes, cosmetics, polyethylene aq. disps.; stabilizer for rubber latex; solubilizer/emulsifier for essential oils, pharmaceuticals; wetting agent in metal cleaners; dyeing assistant; dyestuff dispersant for leather; solid; HLB 15.3; cloud pt. > 100 C (1% aq.).

Prox-onic OA-2/020. [Protex] Oleth-20; CAS 9004-98-2; nonionic; emulsifier for min. oils, fatty acids, waxes; for polishes, cosmetics, polyethylene aq. disps.; stabilizer for rubber latex; solubilizer/emulsifier for essential oils, pharmaceuticals; wetting agent in metal cleaners; dyeing assistant; dyestuff dispersant for leather; liq.; HLB 15.3; cloud pt. > 100 C (1% aq.).

Prox-onic OL-1/05. [Protex] PEG-5 oleate; CAS 9004-96-0; surfactant for cutting oils, degreasing solvs., metal cleaners, textiles, leather, cosmetics; dyeing assistant; emulsifier for min. oils, fatty oils; liq.; sapon. no. 118.

Prox-onic OL-1/09. [Protex] PEG-9 oleate; CAS 9004-96-0; see Prox-onic OL-1/05; liq.; sapon. no. 85.

Prox-onic OL-1/014. [Protex] PEG-14 oleate; CAS 9004-96-0; see Prox-onic OL-1/05; liq.; sapon. no. 65.

Prox-onic PEG-2000. [Protex] PEG-2M; CAS 25322-68-3; low foam wetting in paper pulping; emulsifier for metal degreasing; bottle cleaner defoamer; binder for tobacco; polyurethane mfg.; mold release agent; agric.; cosmetic/pharmaceutical emulsions; m.w. 2000; solid. pt. 48-52 C; hyd. no. 51-62.

Prox-onic PEG-4000. [Protex] PEG-4M; low foam wetting in paper pulping; emulsifier for metal degreasing; bottle cleaner defoamer; binder for ceramics, tobacco; in depilatories; agric.; m.w. 4000; solid. pt. 53-58 C; hyd. no. 25-30.

Prox-onic PEG-6000. [Protex] PEG-6M; CAS 25322-68-3; low foam wetting in paper pulping; emulsifier for metal degreasing; bottle cleaner defoamer; dispersant, binder for ceramics; plasticizer for cement; anticaking agent for fertilizer; soap molding; in depilatories; agric.; m.w. 6000; solid. pt. 55-60 C; hyd. no. 16-20.

Prox-onic PEG-10,000. [Protex] PEG-10M; low foam wetting in paper pulping; emulsifier for metal degreasing; plasticizer for cement; ceramics binder; bottle cleaning defoamer; agric.; cosmetic/pharmaceutical emulsions; m.w. 10,000; solid. pt. 55-60 C; hyd. no. 9-12.

Prox-onic PEG-20,000. [Protex] PEG-20M; CAS 25322-68-3; low foam wetting in paper pulping; emulsifier for metal degreasing; bottle cleaner defoamer; plasticizer for cement; ceramics binder; mold release for rubber; agric.; cosmetic/pharmaceutical emulsions; m.w. 20,000; solid. pt. 60 C; hyd. no. 7-11.

Prox-onic PEG-35,000. [Protex] PEG-35M; low foam wetting in paper pulping; emulsifier for metal degreasing; bottle cleaner defoamer; plasticizer for cement; ceramics binder; agric.; cosmetic/pharmaceutical emulsions; m.w. 35,000; solid. pt. 60 C; hyd. no. < 7.

Prox-onic SML-020. [Protex] Polysorbate 20; CAS 9005-64-5; nonionic; emulsifier, solubilizer for petrol. oils, solvs., veg. oils, waxes, silicones, etc.; for agric., cosmetic, leather, metalworking and textile industries; liq.; HLB 16.7; sapon. no. 45.

Prox-onic SMO-05. [Protex] Polysorbate 81; CAS 9005-65-6; emulsifier, solubilizer for petrol. oils, solvs., veg. oils, waxes, silicones, etc.; for agric., cosmetic, leather, metalworking and textile industries; liq.; HLB 10.0; sapon. no. 100.

Prox-onic SMO-020. [Protex] Polysorbate 80; CAS 9005-65-

6; emulsifier, solubilizer for petrol. oils, solvs., veg. oils, waxes, silicones, etc.; for agric., cosmetic, leather, metalworking and textile industries; liq.; HLB 15.0; sapon. no. 50.

Prox-onic SMP-020. [Protex] Polysorbate 40; CAS 9005-66-7; nonionic; emulsifier, solubilizer for petrol. oils, solvs., veg. oils, waxes, silicones, etc.; for agric., cosmetic, leather, metalworking and textile industries; liq.; HLB 15.6; sapon. no. 46.

Prox-onic SMS-020. [Protex] Polysorbate 60; CAS 9005-67-8; emulsifier, solubilizer for petrol. oils, solvs., veg. oils, waxes, silicones, etc.; for agric., cosmetic, leather, metalworking and textile industries; soft paste; HLB 14.9; sapon. no. 50.

Prox-onic ST-05. [Protex] PEG-5 stearate; CAS 9004-99-3; emulsifier, lubricant additive for metalworking, textiles, cosmetics, defoamers; visc. control agent in plastisols; paste; sapon. no. 112.

Prox-onic ST-09. [Protex] PEG-9 stearate; CAS 9004-99-3; EINECS 226-312-9; emulsifier, lubricant additive for metalworking, textiles, cosmetics, defoamers; visc. control agent in plastisols; paste; sapon. no. 87.

Prox-onic ST-014. [Protex] PEG-14 stearate; CAS 9004-99-3; EINECS 233-641-1; emulsifier, lubricant additive for metalworking, textiles, cosmetics, defoamers; visc. control agent in plastisols; paste; sapon. no. 62.

Prox-onic ST-023. [Protex] PEG-23 stearate; CAS 9004-99-3; emulsifier, lubricant additive for metalworking, textiles, cosmetics, defoamers; visc. control agent in plastisols; solid; sapon. no. 43.

Prox-onic STO-020. [Protex] Polysorbate 85; CAS 9005-70-3; nonionic; emulsifier, solubilizer for petrol. oils, solvs., veg. oils, waxes, silicones, etc.; for agric., cosmetic, leather, metalworking and textile industries; soft paste; HLB 11.0; sapon. no. 88.

Prox-onic STS-020. [Protex] Polysorbate 65; CAS 9005-71-4; nonionic; emulsifier, solubilizer for petrol. oils, solvs., veg. oils, waxes, silicones, etc.; for agric., cosmetic, leather, metalworking and textile industries; solid; HLB 10.5; sapon. no. 93.

Pruv™. [Mendell] Sodium stearyl fumarate NF/FCC; CAS 4070-80-8; lubricant for pharmaceutical tablets; wh. fine powd. with agglomerates of flat, circular shaped particles ≤ 8 μm; sol. 20 g/100 ml of water (90 C); dens. (tapped) 0.3-0.5 g/cm; m.p. 224-245 C with decomp.; sapon. no. 142-146; 100% conc.

Pseudocollagen™. [Brooks Industries] High m.w. matric oligosaccharides and sol. proteins; cosmetic ingredient forming moisture-retentive films on skin, leaving skin soft and supple; thermally stable; visc. sol'n., pract. colorless and odorless; 5% conc.

PT-46. [U.S. Cosmetics] Platy talc; CAS 14807-96-6; EINECS 238-877-9; premier talc for cosmetic makeup and skin care formulations; yields smoothness, transparency, and exc. skin adhesion; avg. particle size 4-7 μ; surf. area 7-10 m²/g.

PT-0602. [Astor Wax] Syn. wax; CAS 8002-74-2; narrow fraction syn. paraffin obtained from a F-T wax; filler/binder in cosmetic stick prods.; ivory slabs; m.p. 77–78 C; penetration 10–11; acid no. nil; sapon. no. nil.

PTAL. [Mitsubishi Gas] p-Tolualdehyde; CAS 140-87-0; EINECS 203-246-9; additive for resins; intermediate for pharmaceuticals; fragrance; 86% biodeg.; colorless liq., aromatic odor; sol. 0.27% in water @ 40 C; m.w. 120.2; b.p. 205.9 C; m.p. -5.6 C; acid no. 0.2; flash pt. (COC) 88 C; toxicology: LD50 (oral, rat) 1000 mg/kg; eye and skin irritant; 96.4% purity.

PTFE-20. [Presperse] PTFE; CAS 9002-84-0; binder for pressed powds.; exc. thermal and chem. resist., good skin adhesion; imparts luxurious, lubricious feel; off-wh.

opaque free-flowing powd.; particle size 2 μ (9 max.); sp.gr. 2.2; soften. pt. > 600 F.

Pulvi-Lan. [Lanaetex Prods.] Lanolin oil, calcium silicate; cosmetics ingred.

Punctilious® Ethyl Alcohol. [Quantum/USI] Ethanol; solv. and extraction medium; sol. in methanol; misc. in ether, water, chloroform.

Pur-Cellin Oil. [Dragoco] Cetearyl octanoate (90%) and isopropyl myristate; CAS 59130-70-0; emollient for cosmetics; colorless lt. oily liq., odorless; insol. in water; sp.gr. 0.8500-0.8550; flash pt. (CC) 212 F; ref. index 1.4440-1.4460; toxicology: skin and eye irritant.

Pur-Cellin Wax. [Dragoco] Stearyl heptanoate and stearyl caprylate; CAS 66009-41-4, 18312-31-7; emollient for cosmetics; colorless soft oily solid, odorless; insol. in water; flash pt. (CC) 212 F; toxicology: skin and eye irritant; skin sensitizer.

Pureco® 76. [Karlshamns] Coconut oil; CAS 8001-31-8; EINECS 232-282-8; used in hand soaps, liq. soaps, beauty bars; Lovibond R1.0 max.; m.p. 76–80 F; iodine no. 12 max.; sapon. no. 248–264.

Pureco® 92. [Karlshamns] Partially hydrog. coconut oil; used in hand soaps, liq. soaps, beauty bars; Lovibond R1.0 max.; m.p. 100–104 F; iodine no. 4 max.; sapon. no. 248–264.

Pureco® 110. [Karlshamns] Partially hydrog. coconut and palm oils; used in hand soaps, liq. soaps, beauty bars; Lovibond R1.0 max.; m.p. 112–115 F; iodine no. 4 max.; sapon. no. 246–262.

Pure-Dent® B700. [Grain Processing] Corn starch USP, NF; CAS 9005-25-8; EINECS 232-679-6; binder and diluent for granulations and tablets when used wet or dry; disintegrant; for pharmaceutical use; wh. powd.; no odor, bland flavor; pH 5.5–7.0; 9–12.5% moisture.

Pure-Dent® B810. [Grain Processing] Corn starch NF; CAS 9005-25-8; EINECS 232-679-6; binder, diluent, absorbent, and disintegrant for pharmaceutical applics.; wh. powd., no odor, bland flavor; pH 4.5–7.0; 8–11% moisture.

Purity® 21. [Nat'l. Starch] Corn starch NF; CAS 9005-25-8; EINECS 232-679-6; binder, filler and disintegrant for cosmetic and pharmaceutical formulations, body powds., foot powds., dry shampoos, makeup, eye liner, mascara; wh. free-flowing powd.; disp. in water; 12% volatiles.

Pur-Oba® . [Goldschmidt AG] Natural wax ester; for high-quality cosmetics; nearly colorless liq.; sol. in veg. and min. oils; insol. in water.

Purtalc USP. [Charles B. Chrystal] Talc; CAS 14807-96-6; EINECS 238-877-9; cosmetic ingred.

Purton CFD. [Zschimmer & Schwarz] Cocamide DEA; CAS 61791-31-9; EINECS 263-163-9; nonionic; foam stabilizer, emollient, thickener and superfatting agent for cosmetics, shampoos, cleaners; liq.; 100% conc.

Purton SFD. [Zschimmer & Schwarz] Linoleamide DEA; CAS 56863-02-6; EINECS 260-410-2; nonionic; foam stabilizer, emollient, thickener and superfatting agent for cosmetics, shampoos, cleaners; liq.; 100% conc.

PVP-Iodine 17/12, 30/06. [BASF; BASF AG] PVP-iodine; CAS 25655-41-8; broad spectrum microbicide for pharmaceuticals.

PVP K-15. [ISP] PVP; CAS 9003-39-8; EINECS 201-800-4; binder, stabilizer, protective colloid, carrier, film-former, emollient, moisturizer; detoxifier for poison and irritants; visc. modifier for aq. systems; used in cosmetics, adhesives, detergents, coatings, paper, ink, textiles, printing, antifreeze, agric. and specialty formulations; powd.; m.w. 10,000; sol. in water and org. solv.; dens. (bulk) 36 lb/ft³; 95% min. active.

PVP K-30. [ISP] PVP; CAS 9003-39-8; EINECS 201-800-4; film-former, protective colloid, detoxicant, emollient,

373

emulsifier, emulsion/foam stabilizer in hair prods, cream, lotions, makeup, lipsticks, toothpaste, etc.; dispersant for hair colorants; off wh. powd.; m.w. 40,000; sol. in water and many organic solvs., incl. alcohols, some chlorinated compds., nitroparaffins, and amines; dens. (bulk) 28 lb/ft^3; 95% min. active.

PVP/Si-10. [ISP] Polymer-silicone encapsulate (dimethicone with PVP shell); cationic; delivery vehicle providing silicone and film-forming polymer benefits to hair and skin care applics.; imparts conditioning, body, and manageability to hair, moisturization for skin care applics.

PVP/VA E-335, E-535, E-635. [ISP] PVP/VA copolymer with mole ratios of 30/70, 50/50, and 60/40 resp., ethanol; CAS 25086-89-9; film-formers for hairsprays, gels, mousses, lotions, hair thickeners, tints, and dyes; sol'n; 50% ethanol sol'ns.

PVP/VA E-735. [ISP] PVP/VA copolymer (mole ratio 70/30), ethanol; forms adhesive, glossy, water-removable films; wide compatibility permits various degrees of hygroscopicity, flexibility, and abrasion resistance; used in cosmetics, e.g., hair grooming aids, protective masks and bandages, spray-or rub-on protective gloves, etc.; sol'n.; 50% ethanol sol'n.

PVP/VA S-630. [ISP] PVP/VA copolymer (60/40 mole ratio); CAS 25086-89-9; solv.-sol. prod. used where absence of water or alcohol is desirable; forms stable emulsions when dispersed in water by stirring; solid.

Pyridoxine Hydrochloride USP. [Roche] Vitamin B$_6$; oil control agent in skin and makeup prods.

Pyroter CPI-30. [Nihon Emulsion] PEG-30 hydrog. castor oil pyroglutamate isostearate; nonionic; surfactant, emulsifier, solubilizer, thickener, superfatting agent, emulsion stabilizer for shampoos, cleansing foams, and soaps; JCID compliance; pale yel. oil; HLB 10.

Pyroter CPI-40. [Ajinomoto; Nihon Emulsion] PEG-40 hydrog. castor oil PCA isostearate; nonionic; emulsifier, solubilizer and thickener used in personal care prods. and detergents; low irritation, nontoxic; JCID compliance; pale yel. soft paste; water-sol.; HLB 11; 100% conc.

Pyroter CPI-60. [Nihon Emulsion] PEG-60 hydrog. castor oil pyroglutamate isostearate; nonionic; surfactant, emulsifier, solubilizer, thickener, superfatting agent, emulsion stabilizer for shampoos, cleansing foams, and soaps; JCID compliance; pale yel. soft wax; HLB 13.

Pyroter GPI-25. [Ajinomoto; Nihon Emulsion] Glycereth-25 PCA isostearate; nonionic; moisturizer, emulsifier, solubilizer, dispersant, reforming agent, and emollient for hair conditioners, hair liqs. and lotions; JCID compliance; pale yel. oily liq.; water-sol.; HLB 15.

Q

Quamectant™ AM-50. [Brooks Industries] 6-(N-Acetylamino)-4-oxahexyltrimonium chloride; substantive humectant with emollient feel; nonoily and nongreasy; skin moisturizer; hair care prods.; 50% act.

Quat-Coll™ CDMA-30QX. [Brooks Industries] Cocamidopropyldimonium hydroxypropyl hydrolyzed collagen; cosmetic ingred.

Quat-Coll™ CDMA 40. [Brooks Industries] Cocodimonium hydroxypropyl hydrolyzed animal protein.; cosmetics ingred.; liq.; m.w. 2000; 40% act.

Quat-Coll™ IP10-30. [Brooks Industries] Hydroxypropyltrimonium gelatin; cosmetics ingred.; liq.; m.w. 25,000; 30% act.

Quat-Coll™ QS. [Brooks Industries] Steartrimonium hydroxyethyl hydrolyzed collagen; CAS 111174-62-0; cosmetics ingred.; powd.; m.w. 10,000.

Quatex S. [Lanaetex Prods.] Steartrimonium hydrolyzed animal protein; CAS 111174-62-0; cosmetic protein.

Quat Keratin™ QTM-30. [Brooks Industries] Hydroxypropyltrimonium hydrolyzed keratin; cosmetic ingred.

Quat Keratin™ WKP. [Brooks Industries] Cocodimonium hydroxypropyl hydrolyzed keratin; CAS 68915-25-3; cosmetics ingred.; 35% act.

Quat-Pro E. [Maybrook] Triethonium hydrolyzed collagen ethosulfate; CAS 111174-64-2; substantive protein for hair and skin care prods. (shampoos, leave-on conditioners, mousses, creams, lotions, face tonics, liq. soaps); lt. amber clear to sl. hazy, visc. liq., char. odor; pH 4.5-5.5; 28% min. solids.

Quat-Pro S. [Maybrook] Steartrimonium hydroxyethyl hydrolyzed collagen; CAS 111174-62-0; cationic; substantive film-former, moisturizer, conditioner, protectant for hair and skin care prods. (shampoos, conditioners, creams, lotions, liq. hand soaps, bath prods.); wh. to sl. off-wh. powd., char. odor; pH 5.5-6.5 (10% aq.); 92% min. solids.

Quat-Pro S 30. [Maybrook] Steartrimonium hydroxyethyl hydrolyzed collagen; CAS 111174-62-0; cationic; substantive film-former, moisturizer, conditioner, protectant for hair and skin care prods. (shampoos, conditioners, creams, lotions, liq. hand soaps, bath prods.); clear to sl. hazy liq., char. odor; pH 5.5-6.5 (10% aq.); 28-32% solids.

Quatrex CRC. [Chemron] Cetearyl alcohol, stearalkonium chloride, PEG-40 castor oil; conc. surfactant for cream rinses; fully compat. with esters, fatty alcohols, and proteins; waxy flakes.

Quatrex CT-100. [Chemron] Stearyl alcohol, cetrimonium chloride; cream rinse conc., conditioner for quality salon and professional hair care prods.; wh. flakes.

Quatrex CTAC. [Chemron] Cetrimonium chloride; CAS 112-02-7; EINECS 203-928-6; surfactant, conditioner for hair treatment applics.; liq.; cold water disp.; 29% act.

Quatrex S. [Chemron] Soyamidopropalkonium chloride; cationic; substantivity and conditioning agent for conditioning shampoos, sprays, mousses, setting gels, conditioners; amber liq.; 25% act.

Quatrex STC-25. [Chemron] Stearalkonium chloride; CAS 122-19-0; EINECS 204-527-9; personal care surfactant for after-shampoo cream rinses; wh. paste; 18% act.

Quatrex STC-85. [Chemron] Stearalkonium chloride; CAS 122-19-0; EINECS 204-527-9; personal care surfactant, hair conditioner, softener for conditioners, protein packs, mousses; waxy flakes; 85% act.

Quatrisoft® Polymer LM-200. [Amerchol] Polyquaternium-24; CAS 107987-23-5; stabilizer for emulsions; thickener for surfactant systems; substantive conditioner for hair and skin care prods.; tan powd.

Quat-Silk™ QTM-10. [Brooks Industries] Hydroxypropyltrimonium hydrolyzed silk; cosmetics ingred.; liq.; 10% act.

Quat-Soy™ CDMA-25. [Brooks Industries] Cocodimonium hydroxypropyl hydrolyzed soy protein; cosmetic ingredient for hair and skin care prods.; 25% act.

Quat-Soy™ LDMA-30. [Brooks Industries] Lauryldimonium hydroxypropyl hydrolyzed soy protein; cosmetic ingredient for skin and hair care prods.; 35% act.

Quat-Soy™ QTM-30. [Brooks Industries] Hydroxypropyltrimonium hydrolyzed soy protein; cosmetic ingred.

Quat-Veg™ Q-30. [Brooks Industries] Hydroxypropyltrimonium hydrolyzed vegetable protein; cosmetic ingredient for skin and hair care prods.; 30% act.

Quat-Wheat™ CDMA-30. [Brooks Industries] Cocodimonium hydroxypropyl hydrolyzed wheat protein; cosmetic ingred. for skin and hair care prods.; 25% act.

Quat-Wheat™ QTM-20. [Brooks Industries] Hydroxypropyltrimonium hydrolyzed wheat protein.; cosmetic ingred. for hair and skin care prods.; 20% act.

Quat-Wheat™ SDMA-25. [Brooks Industries] Soya dimonium hydrolyzed wheat protein; substantivity agent for hair care prods.; enhances combability, softness, conditioning; esp. as pre-wrap before chemical treatment or as post-perm treatment; amber liq.; low odor; 25% act.

Queen of the Prairie Extract Code 9031. [Brooks Industries] Queen of the Prairie (*Filipendula rubra*) extract; provides cell renewal and stimulatory props. for poultices; amber clear liq.

Querton 16Cl-29. [Berol Nobel AB] Cetrimonium chloride; CAS 112-02-7; EINECS 203-928-6; cationic; emulsifier, dispersant, antistat for hair conditiners, shampoos, detergent sanitizers; clear liq.; sol. in water, alcohols, other polar solvs.; dens. 964 kg/m³; visc. 30 mPa·s; pour pt. 2 C; pH 6.5 ± 1 (20%); surf. tens. 41 mN/m (0.1%); 29% act., 3% ethanol.

Querton 16Cl-50. [Berol Nobel AB] Cetrimonium chloride; CAS 112-02-7; EINECS 302-928-6; cationic; emulsifier, dispersant, antistat, and substantivity agent for hair conditiners, shampoos, detergent sanitizers; clear liq.; sol. in water, alcohols, other polar solvs.; dens. 899 kg/m³; visc. 30 mPa·s; pour pt. 6 C; pH 6.5 ± 1 (20%); surf. tens. 42 mN/m (0.1%); 50% act., 30-35% ethanol.

Querton 442. [Berol Nobel AB] Dihydrog. tallow dimethyl ammonium chloride; CAS 61789-80-8; EINECS 263-090-2; imparts soft feel and antistatic props. to textile softeners for commercial laundry and textile mfg. applics.; also for hair conditioners, paper chemicals, mfg. of organoclays.

Querton 442-11 [Berol Nobel AB] Dihydrog. tallow dimethyl ammonium chloride; CAS 61789-80-8; EINECS 263-090-2; imparts soft feel and antistatic props. to textile softeners for commercial laundry and textile mfg. applics.; also for hair conditioners, paper chemicals, mfg. of organoclays; off-wh. paste; sol. in warm ethanol, IPA, or similar solvs.; disp. in hot water; dens. 860 kg/m³; visc. 90 mPa·s; solid. pt. 35-40 C; pH 6-8 (5% in IPA/water 50/50); 76-78.5% act.

Querton 442-82. [Berol Nobel AB] Dihydrog. tallow dimethyl ammonium chloride; CAS 61789-80-8; EINECS 263-090-2; imparts soft feel and antistatic props. to textile softeners for consumer rinse cycle softeners, commercial laundry, textile mfg. applics.; also for hair conditioners, paper chemicals, mfg. of organoclays; off-wh. paste; sol. in warm ethanol, IPA, similar solvs.; disp. in hot water; dens. 860 kg/m³; visc. 150 mPa·s; solid. pt. 35-40 C; pH 6-8 (5% in IPA/water 50/50); 81-83% act.

Querton 442E. [Berol Nobel AB] Dihydrog. tallow dimethyl ammonium chloride; CAS 61789-80-8; EINECS 263-090-2; imparts soft feel and antistatic props. to textile softeners for consumer rinse cycle softeners, commercial laundry, textile mfg. applics.; also for hair conditioners, paper chemicals, mfg. of organoclays; off-wh. paste; sol. in warm ethanol, IPA, similar solvs.; disp. in hot water; dens. 860 kg/m³; visc. 50 mPa·s; solid. pt. 30 C; pH 6-9 (5% in IPA/water 50/50); 75-77% act.

Querton 442H. [Berol Nobel AB] Dihydrog. tallow dimethyl ammonium chloride; CAS 61789-80-8; EINECS 263-090-2; imparts soft feel and antistatic props. to textile softeners for consumer rinse cycle softeners, commercial laundry, textile mfg. applics.; also for hair conditioners, paper chemicals, mfg. of organoclays; off-wh. paste; sol. in warm ethanol, IPA, similar solvs.; disp. in hot water; dens. 860 kg/m³; visc. 50 mPa·s; solid. pt. 30 C; pH 6-9 (5% in IPA/water 50/50); 75-77% act.

Querton 442P. [Berol Nobel AB] Di(C12-20 alkyl) dimethyl-ammonium chloride; CAS 68514-95-4; EINECS 271-064-7; imparts soft feel and antistatic props. to textile softeners for consumer rinse cycle softeners, commercial laundry, textile mfg. applics.; also for hair conditioners, paper chemicals, mfg. of organoclays; off-wh. paste; sol. in warm ethanol, IPA, similar solvs.; disp. in hot water; dens. 860 kg/m³; visc. 50 mPa·s; solid. pt. 30 C; pH 6-9 (5% in IPA/water 50/50).

Querton 442P-11. [Berol Nobel AB] Di(C12-20 alkyl) di-methylammonium chloride; CAS 68514-95-4; EINECS 271-064-7; imparts soft feel and antistatic props. to textile softeners for consumer rinse cycle softeners, commercial laundry, textile mfg. applics.; also for hair conditioners, paper chemicals, mfg. of organoclays; off-wh. paste; sol. in warm ethanol, IPA, similar solvs.; disp. in hot water; dens. 860 kg/m³; visc. 90 mPa·s; solid. pt. 35-40 C; pH 6-8 (5% in IPA/water 50/50); 76-78.5% act.

Quimipol EA 2512. [Quimigal-Quimica] Syn. primary alcohol ethoxylate; nonionic; wetting agent at elevated temps.; cosmetic emulsifier; solid; HLB 14.2; 100% conc.

Quimipol ENF 65. [Quimigal-Quimica] Nonylphenol ethoxylate; nonionic; acid wool scouring, drycleaning and emulsifier for oils, hydrocarbon solvs. and waxes; liq.; HLB 10.9; 100% conc.

Quso® G27, G29, G35, G38, WR55, WR83. [Degussa] Precipitated silica; thickener for pastes, creams, lotions in cosmetics and toiletries; suspending agent; improves free-flowing chars. of fine powds.; for pulp and paper defoaming; microfine; sol. in hot, strong alkaline sol'ns.

Quso® WR55-FG. [Degussa] Precipitated silica; thickener for pastes, creams, lotions in cosmetics and toiletries; suspending agent; improves free-flowing chars. of fine powds.; for food grade defoamers; FDA approved.

R

Radia® 7051. [Fina Chemicals] Butyl stearate; CAS 85408-76-0; EINECS 287-039-9; chemical intermediate, lubricant, plasticizer; chemical synthesis; lubricant in min., cutting, lamination, and textile oils, rust inhibitors; textile and leather applic.; cosmetics and pharmaceuticals; APHA 65 liq.; m.w. 325; insol. in water; sol. in hexane, benzene, IPA, trichlorethylene, min. and veg. oils; sp.gr. 0.844 (37.8 C); visc. 6.10 cps (37.8 C); acid no. 0.5 max.; iodine no. < 1; pour pt. 20 C; cloud pt. 23 C; flash pt. (COC) 200 C; ref. index 1.4432.

Radia® 7060. [Fina Chemicals] Methyl oleate; CAS 67762-38-3; EINECS 267-015-4; chemical intermediate, lubricant; chemical synthesis; lubricity improvers in min. oils; formulation of cutting, lamination, and textile oils; rust inhibitors; textile and leather industry; cosmetics and pharmaceuticals; Lovibond 10Y-1.5R liq.; insol. in water, sol. in hexane, benzene, IPA, trichlorethylene, min. and veg. oils; m.w. 286; sp.gr. 0.862 (37.8 C); visc. 4.10 cps (37.8 C); acid no. 1 max.; iodine no. 83-91; pour pt. -26 C; cloud pt. < -10 C; flash pt. (COC) 180 C; ref. index 1.4513.

Radia® 7106. [Fina Chemicals] Caprylic-capric triglyceride; CAS 65381-09-1; nongreasy emollient with spreading props. and skin penetration; for makeup, skin care prods., bath oils; diluents for active ingreds. and carriers of fragrances; min. oil substitute in creams, lotions, oil formulations, and other cosmetics; APHA 120 liq., odorless; acid no. 0.5 max.; iodine no. 1 max.; cloud pt. < -10 C.

Radia® 7108. [Fina Chemicals] Glyceryl C8-10 triester; CAS 85409-09-2; EINECS 287-075-5; chemical intermediate, chemical synthesis; lubricant in min., cutting, lamination, textile oils, and rust inhibitors; textile and leather applic.; also as emollient, plasticizer, solubilizer of act. components in cosmetics and pharmaceuticals; Lovibond 5Y-1R liq.; insol. in water; sol. in hexane, benzene, IPA, trichlorethylene, min. and veg. oils; sp.gr. 944 kg/m³; acid no. 1 max.; iodine no. < 1; pour pt. < -35 C; cloud pt. < -10 C; flash pt. (COC) 240 C.

Radia® 7110. [Fina Chemicals] Methyl stearate; CAS 85586-21-6; EINECS 287-824-6; chemical intermediate, chemical synthesis; lubricant in min., cutting, lamination, textile oils, and rust inhibitors; textile and leather applic.; cosmetics and pharmaceuticals; APHA 65 paste; insol. in water, sol. in hexane, benzene, IPA, trichlorethylene, min. and veg. oils; m.w. 285; sp.gr. 811 kg/m³ (100 C); m.p. 28 C; acid no. 1 max.; iodine no. < 2; flash pt. (COC) 165 C.

Radia® 7117. [Fina Chemicals] Methyl cocoate; CAS 61788-59-8; EINECS 262-988-1; emollient, plasticizer, lubricant for cosmetics, pharmaceuticals, plastics, lubricating oils, textile and leather additives, cutting oils for metallurgy; chemical intermediate; Lovibond 5Y-1R liq.; insol. in water, sol. in hexane, benzene, IPA, trichlorethylene, min. and veg. oils; sp.gr. 865 kg/m³; pour pt. -3 C; cloud pt. < 0 C; flash pt. (COC) 128 C; acid no. 1; iodine no. < 12.

Radia® 7120. [Fina Chemicals] Methyl palmitate; CAS 112-

39-0; EINECS 203-966-3; chemical intermediate, chemical synthesis; lubricant in min., cutting, lamination, textile oils, and rust inhibitors; textile and leather applic.; cosmetics and pharmaceuticals; Lovibond 5Y-1R paste; insol. in water, sol. in hexane, benzene, IPA, trichlorethylene, min. and veg. oils; m.w. 267; sp.gr. 0.855 (37.8 C); visc. 4.30 cps (37.8 C); m.p. 27.5 C; acid no. 1 max.; iodine no. < 1; flash pt. (COC) 149 C.

Radia® 7131. [Fina Chemicals] Isooctyl stearate; CAS 91031-48-0; EINECS 292-951-5; cosmetics emollient, solv.; plasticizer for PVC; lubricant for PS; APHA 100 liq.; insol. in water; sol. in hexane, benzene, IPA, trichlorethylene, min. and veg. oils; sp.gr. 854 kg/m³; acid no. 1 max.; iodine no. < 1; pour pt. 7 C; cloud pt. < 10 C; flash pt. (COC) 215 C.

Radia® 7171. [Fina Chemicals] Pentaerythritol tetraoleate; CAS 68604-44-4; EINECS 271-694-2; lubricant, chemical intermediate; formulation of cutting, lamination, and textile oils; corrosion inhibitors; chemical synthesis; cosmetics and pharmaceuticals; Lovibond 10Y-2.5R liq.; sol. (@ 10%) in trichloroethylene, min. and veg. oil, hexane, benzene, IPA; m.w. 1160; sp.gr. 0.913 (37.8 C); visc. 70.80 cps (37.8 C); acid no. 3 max.; iodine no. 85-95; pour pt. -19 C; cloud pt. < -3 C; flash pt. (COC) 300 C; ref. index 1.4733.

Radia® 7176. [Fina Chemicals] Pentaerythritol tetrastearate; CAS 91050-82-7; EINECS 293-029-5; lubricant, chemical intermediate; formulation of cutting, lamination, and textile oils; corrosion inhibitors; chemical synthesis; cosmetics and pharmaceuticals; Lovibond 5Y-1R flakes; sol. (@ 10%) in trichlorethylene; m.w. 1140; sp.gr. 0.868 (98.9 C); visc. 14.50 cps (98.9 C); m.p. 61 C; acid no. 3 max.; iodine no. < 1; flash pt. (COC) 290 C.

Radia® 7178. [Fina Chemicals] Caprylic-capric pentaerythrtol tetraester; CAS 68441-68-9; EINECS 270-474-3; nongreasy emollient with spreading props. and skin penetration; for makeup, skin care prods., bath oils; diluents for active ingreds. and carriers of fragrances; min. oil substitute in creams, lotions, oil formulations, and other cosmetics; APHA 100 liq., odorless; acid no. 0.5 max.; iodine no. 2 max.; cloud pt. -11 C.

Radia® 7185. [Fina Chemicals] Ethyl stearate; CAS 91031-43-5; EINECS 292-945-2; chemical intermediate, chemical synthesis; lubricant in min., cutting, lamination, textile oils, and rust inhibitors; textile and leather applic.; also as emollient, plasticizer, solubilizer of act. components in cosmetics and pharmaceuticals; Lovibond 4Y-0.4R paste; insol. in water; sol. in hexane, benzene, IPA, trichlorethylene, min. and veg. oils; sp.gr. 857 kg/m³; m.p. 27 C; acid no. 1 max.; iodine no. < 1; flash pt. (COC) 190 C.

Radia® 7187. [Fina Chemicals] Ethyl oleate; CAS 85049-36-1; EINECS 285-206-0; chemical intermediate, chemical synthesis; lubricant in min., cutting, lamination, textile oils, and rust inhibitors; textile and leather applic.; also as emollient, plasticizer, solubilizer of act. components in cosmetics and pharmaceuticals; Lovibond 5Y-0.5R liq.; insol. in water; sol. in hexane, benzene, IPA, trichlorethylene, min. and veg. oils; sp.gr. 865 kg/m³; acid no. 5 max.; iodine no. 74-84; pour pt. -10 C; cloud pt. < 0 C; flash pt. (COC) 195 C.

Radia® 7190. [Fina Chemicals] Isopropyl myristate; CAS 110-27-0; EINECS 203-751-4; chemical intermediate, chemical synthesis; lubricant in min., cutting, lamination, textile oils, and rust inhibitors; textile and leather applic.; also as emollient, plasticizer, solubilizer of act. components in cosmetics and pharmaceuticals; APHA 35 liq.; insol. in water; sol. in hexane, benzene, IPA, trichlorethylene, min. and veg. oils; m.w. 271; sp.gr. 0.840 (37.8 C); visc. 3.50 cps (37.8 C); acid no. 0.5 max.; iodine no. < 1; pour pt. -3 C; cloud pt. -4 C; flash pt. (COC) 155 C; ref. index 1.4345.

Radia® 7200. [Fina Chemicals] Isopropyl palmitate; CAS 142-91-6; EINECS 205-571-1; chemical intermediate, chemical synthesis; lubricant in min., cutting, lamination, textile oils, and rust inhibitors; textile and leather applic.; also as emollient, plasticizer, solubilizer of act. components in cosmetics and pharmaceuticals; m.w. 300; insol. in water; sol. in hexane, benzene, IPA, trichlorethylene, min. and veg. oils; sp.gr. 0.843 (37.8 C); visc. 5.05 cps (37.8 C); acid no. 0.5 max.; iodine no. < 1; pour pt. < 12 C; cloud pt. < 12 C; flash pt. (COC) 165 C; ref. index 1.4373.

Radia® 7204. [Fina Chemicals] Propylene glycol dioleate; CAS 85049-34-9; EINECS 285-203-4; chemical intermediate, chemical synthesis; lubricant in min., cutting, lamination, textile oils, and rust inhibitors; textile and leather applic.; also as emollient, plasticizer, solubilizer of act. components in cosmetics and pharmaceuticals; Lovibond 15Y-2.5R liq.; sol. in hexane, benzene, IPA, trichlorethylene, min. and veg. oils; insol. in water; sp.gr. 902 kg/m³; acid no. 2 max.; iodine no. 82-92; pour pt. < -5 C; cloud pt. < 0 C; flash pt. (COC) 250 C.

Radia® 7230. [Fina Chemicals] Isobutyl oleate; CAS 84988-79-4; EINECS 284-868-8; chemical intermediate, lubricant; chemical synthesis; carbon source in antibiotic culture broths; lubricity improvers in min. oils; formulation of cutting, lamination, and textile oils, rust inhibitors; textile and leather industry; emollient in cosmetics and pharmaceuticals; m.w. 327; insol. in water; sol. in hexane, benzene, IPA, trichlorethylene, min. and veg. oils; sp.gr. 0.854 (37.8 C); visc. 5.60 cps (37.8 C); acid no. 1 max.; iodine no. 66-74; pour pt. -18 C; cloud pt. < -8 C; flash pt. (COC) 190 C; ref. index 1.4499; surf. tens. 31.50 dynes/cm.

Radia® 7231. [Fina Chemicals] Isopropyl oleate; CAS 85116-87-6; EINECS 285-540-7; chemical intermediate, lubricant; chemical synthesis; lubricity improvers in min. oils; formulation of cutting, lamination, and textile oils; rust inhibitors; textile and leather industry; cosmetics and pharmaceuticals; Lovibond 10Y-1.5 liq.; m.w. 313; insol. in water; sol. in hexane, benzene, IPA, trichlorethylene, min. and veg. oils; sp.gr 0.853 (37.8 C); visc. 5.05 cps (37.8 C); acid no. 0.5 max.; iodine no. 73-83; pour pt. -15 C; cloud pt. < -8 C; flash pt. (COC) 170 C; ref. index 1.4479.

Radia® 7241. [Fina Chemicals] Isobutyl stearate; CAS 85865-69-6; EINECS 288-668-1; cosmetics emollient, solv.; plasticizer for PVC; lubricant for PS; APHA 65 liq.; insol. in water; sol. in hexane, benzene, IPA, trichlorethylene, min. and veg. oils; sp.gr. 853 kg/m³; acid no. 0.5 max.; iodine no. < 1; pour pt. 18 C; cloud pt. < 20 C; flash pt. (COC) 180 C.

Radia® 7266. [Fina Chemicals] Ethylene glycol distearate; CAS 91031-31-1; EINECS 292-932-1; chemical interme-

diate, chemical synthesis; lubricant in min., cutting, lamination, textile oils, and rust inhibitors; textile and leather applic.; also as emollient, plasticizer, solubilizer of act. components in cosmetics and pharmaceuticals; Lovibond 15Y-3R flakes; sol. (@ 75 C) in trichlorethylene, sol. cloudy in hexane, benzene, IPA, min. and veg. oils; sp.gr. 837 kg/m³ (100 C); m.p. 69 C; acid no. 3 max.; iodine no. < 1; flash pt. (COC) 240 C.

Radia® 7331. [Fina Chemicals] Ethylhexyl oleate; CAS 85049-37-2; EINECS 285-207-6; chemical intermediate, lubricant; chemical synthesis; lubricity improvers in min. oils; formulation of cutting, lamination, and textile oils; rust inhibitors; textile and leather industry; cosmetics and pharmaceuticals; Lovibond 10Y-1R liq.; insol. in water; sol. in hexane, benzene, IPA, trichlorethylene, min. and veg. oils; m.w. 373; sp.gr. 0.857 (37.8 C); visc. 7.50 cps (37.8 C); acid no. 0.5 max.; iodine no. 60-70; pour pt. -30 C; cloud pt. < -15 C; flash pt. (COC) 195 C; ref. index 1.4538.

Radia® 7345. [Fina Chemicals] Sorbitan tristearate; CAS 72869-62-6; EINECS 276-951-2; chemical intermediate, chemical synthesis; lubricant in min., cutting, lamination, textile oils, and rust inhibitors; textile and leather applic.; also as emollient, plasticizer, solubilizer of act. components in cosmetics and pharmaceuticals; Gardner 6 flakes; sol. (@ 75 C) in trichlorethylene, min. and veg. oils; sol. cloudy in hexane, IPA; sp.gr. 893 kg/m³ (100 C); m.p. 55 C; acid no. 15 max.; iodine no. < 1; flash pt. (COC) 255 C.

Radia® 7355. [Fina Chemicals] Sorbitan trioleate; CAS 85186-88-5; EINECS 286-074-7; chemical intermediate, chemical synthesis; lubricant in min., cutting, lamination, textile oils, and rust inhibitors; textile and leather applic.; also as emollient, plasticizer, solubilizer of act. components in cosmetics and pharmaceuticals; Gardner 10 liq.; insol. in water; sol. in hexane, benzene, IPA, trichlorethylene, min. and veg. oils; sp.gr. 940 kg/m³; acid no. 15 max.; iodine no. 75-90; pour pt. -14 C; cloud pt. < -11 C; flash pt. (COC) 230 C.

Radia® 7363. [Fina Chemicals] Glyceryl trioleate; CAS 67701-30-8; EINECS 266-948-4; lubricant, chemical intermediate; formulation of cutting, lamination, and textile oils; corrosion inhibitors; chemical synthesis; as carbon source in antibiotic culture broths; cosmetics and pharmaceuticals; Lovibond 10Y-2.5R liq.; sol. in hexane, benzene, IPA, trichlorethylene, veg. and min. oils; insol. in water; m.w. 880; sp.gr. 0.906 (37.8 C); visc. 41.20 cps (37.8 C); acid no. 2 max.; iodine no. 86-96; pour pt. -18 C; cloud pt. < -10 C; flash pt. (COC) 290 C; ref. index 1.4691.

Radia® 7370. [Fina Chemicals] Trimethylpropane trioleate; CAS 68002-79-9; EINECS 268-093-2; lubricant, chemical intermediate; formulation of cutting, lamination, and textile oils; corrosion inhibitors; chemical synthesis; cosmetics and pharmaceuticals; Gardner 8 liq.; insol. in water; sol. in hexane, benzene, IPA, trichlorethylene, min. and veg. oils; m.w. 900; sp.gr. 0.904 (37.8 C); visc. 45.90 cps (37.8 C); acid no. 2 max.; iodine no. 95-105; pour pt. -37 C; cloud pt. < -10 C; flash pt. (COC) 305 C; ref. index 1.4712.

Radia® 7371. [Fina Chemicals] Trimethylol propane triester, unsat.; CAS 68002-79-9; EINECS 268-093-2; chemical intermediate, chemical synthesis; lubricant in min., cutting, lamination, textile oils, and rust inhibitors; textile and leather applic.; also as emollient, plasticizer, solubilizer of act. components in cosmetics and pharmaceuticals; Gardner 8 liq.; insol. in water; sol. in hexane, benzene, trichlorethylene, min. and veg. oils; sol. cloudy in IPA; sp.gr. 930 kg/m³; acid no. 2 max.; iodine no. 90-100; cloud pt. < -10 C; flash pt. (COC) 305 C.

Radia® 7500. [Fina Chemicals] Cetyl palmitate; CAS 97404-

33-6; EINECS 306-797-4; chemical intermediate, chemical synthesis; lubricant in min., cutting, lamination, textile oils, and rust inhibitors; textile and leather applic.; also used for wax formulation due to its high m.p.; emollient, film-former, consistency factor, texture promoter, binder for emulsions, skin preps., lipsticks, mascaras, compact powds.; Lovibond 5Y-0.6R flakes; sol. (@ 10%) in benzene and trichlorethylene; m.w. 484; sp.gr. 0.805 (98.9 C); visc. 4.30 cps (98.9 C); m.p. 54 C; acid no. 1.5 max.; iodine no. 2 max.; flash pt. (COC) 215 C.

Radia® 7501. [Fina Chemicals] Stearyl stearate; CAS 85536-04-5; EINECS 287-484-9; chemical intermediate, chemical synthesis; lubricant in min., cutting, lamination, textile oils, and rust inhibitors; textile and leather applic.; also used for wax formulation due to its high m.p.; emollient, film-former, consistency factor, texture promoter, binder for emulsions, skin preps., lipsticks, mascaras, compact powds.; Lovibond 5Y-1R flake; sol. (@ 10%) in trichlorethylene; m.w. 534; sp.gr. 0.807 (98.9 C); visc. 4.60 cps (98.9 C); m.p. 57 C; acid no. 1.5 max.; iodine no. 2 max.; flash pt. (COC) 215 C.

Radia® 7505. [Fina Chemicals] Distearyl phthalate; CAS 90193-76-3; EINECS 290-580-3; chemical intermediate, chemical synthesis; lubricant in min., cutting, lamination, textile oils, and rust inhibitors; textile and leather applic.; also as emollient, plasticizer, solubilizer of act. components in cosmetics and pharmaceuticals; Lovibond 5Y-1R flakes; sol. cloudy in hexane, benzene, trichlorethylene; sp.gr. 864 kg/m³ (100 C); m.p. 44 C; acid no. 3 max.; iodine no. < 1; flash pt. (COC) 240 C.

Radia® 7506. [Fina Chemicals] Ethylene bis-stearamide; CAS 68955-45-3; EINECS 273-277-0; chemical intermediate, chemical synthesis; lubricant in min., cutting, lamination, textile oils, and rust inhibitors; textile and leather applic.; also as emollient, plasticizer, solubilizer of act. components in cosmetics and pharmaceuticals; flakes; sol. @ 75 C in trichlorethylene; gels @ 75 C in benzene, min. and veg. oil; m.p. 141 C; acid no. 8 max.; iodine no. < 2; flash pt. (COC) 280 C.

Radia® 7510. [Fina Chemicals] Isononyl stearate; CAS 91031-57-1; EINECS 292-960-4; chemical intermediate, chemical synthesis; lubricant in min., cutting, lamination, textile oils, and rust inhibitors; textile and leather applic.; cosmetics and pharmaceuticals; APHA 100 liq.; insol. in water; sol. in hexane, benzene, IPA, trichlorethylene, min. and veg. oils; m.w. 380; sp.gr. 0.851 (37.8 C); visc. 11.30 cps (37.8 C); acid no. 1 max.; iodine no. < 1; pour pt. 9 C; cloud pt. 10 C; flash pt. (COC) 200 C; ref. index 1.4493.

Radia® 7514. [Fina Chemicals] Pentaerythritol tetrabehenate; CAS 84539-90-2; EINECS 283-078-0; lubricant, chemical intermediate; formulation of cutting, lamination, and textile oils; corrosion inhibitors; chemical synthesis; cosmetics and pharmaceuticals; Lovibond 5Y-1R flakes; sol. in trichlorethylene, min. oil; m.w. 1300; sp.gr. 0.860 (98.9 C); visc. 17.20 cps (98.9 C); m.p. 62 C; acid no. 3 max.; iodine no. < 3; flash pt. (COC) 290 C.

Radia® 7730. [Fina Chemicals] Isopropyl myristate; CAS 110-27-0; EINECS 203-751-4; emollient, solvent for cosmetic creams and lotions, bath oils, sun oils, hair conditioners, shaving creams, aerosol hair sprays, decorative cosmetics; APHA 35 liq., odorless; acid no. 0.5 max.; iodine no. 1 max.; cloud pt. -4 C.

Radia® 7732. [Fina Chemicals] Isopropyl palmitate; CAS 142-91-6; EINECS 205-571-1; emollient, solvent for cosmetic creams and lotions, bath oils, sun oils, hair conditioners, shaving creams, aerosol hair sprays, decorative cosmetics; APHA 35 liq., odorless; acid no. 0.5 max.; iodine no. 1 max.; cloud pt. < 12 C.

Radia® 7752. [Fina Chemicals] n-Butyl stearate; CAS 123-95-5; EINECS 204-666-5; emollient, solvent for cosmetic

creams and lotions, bath oils, sun oils, hair conditioners, shaving creams, aerosol hair sprays, decorative cosmetics; gloss agent for nail polish; slip agent for lipsticks; APHA 65 liq., odorless; acid no. 0.5 max.; iodine no. 1 max.; cloud pt. 23 C.

Radia® 7761. [Fina Chemicals] Isobutyl stearate; CAS 646-13-9; EINECS 211-466-1; emollient, solvent for cosmetic creams and lotions, bath oils, sun oils, hair conditioners, shaving creams, aerosol hair sprays, decorative cosmetics; APHA 65 liq., odorless; acid no. 0.5 max.; iodine no. 1 max.; cloud pt. < 20 C.

Radia® 7770. [Fina Chemicals] Octyl stearate; emollient, solvent for cosmetic creams and lotions, bath oils, sun oils, hair conditioners, shaving creams, aerosol hair sprays, decorative cosmetics; APHA 100 liq., odorless; acid no. 1 max.; iodine no. 1 max.; cloud pt. < 10 C.

Radiacid® 152. [Fina Chemicals] Stearic acid; CAS 57-11-4; EINECS 200-313-4; emollient, binder, bodying agent, stabilizer for cosmetics, esp. soaps; acid no. 195-201; iodine no. < 2.

Radiacid® 212. [Fina Chemicals] Oleic acid; CAS 112-80-1; EINECS 204-007-1; emollient, binder, bodying agent, stabilizer for cosmetics, esp. liq. pump soaps; acid no. 198-205; iodine no. 88-95; cloud pt. < 6 C.

Radiacid® 416. [Fina Chemicals] Stearic acid; CAS 57-11-4; EINECS 200-313-4; emollient, binder, bodying agent, stabilizer for cosmetics, esp. soaps; acid no. 202-209; iodine no. < 0.5.

Radiacid® 423. [Fina Chemicals] Stearic acid; CAS 57-11-4; EINECS 200-313-4; emollient, binder, bodying agent, stabilizer for cosmetics, esp. soaps and shaving sticks; acid no. 208-212; iodine no. < 1.

Radiacid® 427. [Fina Chemicals] Stearic acid; CAS 57-11-4; EINECS 200-313-4; extra heat-stable emollient, binder, bodying agent, stabilizer for cosmetics, esp. soaps and shaving sticks; acid no. 208-212; iodine no. < 0.5.

Radiacid® 428. [Fina Chemicals] Stearic acid; CAS 57-11-4; EINECS 200-313-4; heat-stable emollient, binder, bodying agent, stabilizer for cosmetics, esp. soaps and shaving sticks; acid no. 208-212; iodine no. < 1.

Radiacid® 464. [Fina Chemicals] Stearic acid; CAS 57-11-4; EINECS 200-313-4; emollient, binder, bodying agent, stabilizer for cosmetics, esp. soaps; acid no. 210-214; iodine no. < 1.

Radiacid® 631. [Fina Chemicals] Coconut fatty acid; emollient, binder, bodying agent, stabilizer for cosmetics, esp. high foaming shaving foams, aerosols, and soaps; acid no. 260-276; iodine no. < 1.

Radiamine 6140. [Fina Chemicals] Hydrog. tallow amine; CAS 61788-45-2; EINECS 262-976-6; cationic; min. flotation, corrosion inhibitor, pigment dispersant; cosmetics; lubricant and mold release for hard rubber, textile chemical, chemical synthesis; antistat and antifog additive for plastic foils; Gardner 3 max. solid; m.p. 46 C; amine no. 210; iodine no. < 3; 100% conc.

Radiamine 6141. [Fina Chemicals] Hydrog. tallow amine, distilled; CAS 61788-45-2; EINECS 262-976-6; cationic; min. flotation, corrosion inhibitor, pigment dispersant; cosmetics; lubricant and mold release for hard rubber, textile chemical, chemical synthesis; antistat and antifog additive for plastic foils; Gardner 1 max. solid; m.p. 48 C; amine no. 212; iodine no. < 3; 98% amine.

Radiamine 6160. [Fina Chemicals] Coconut oil amine; CAS 61788-46-3; EINECS 262-977-1; cationic; min. flotation, corrosion inhibitor, pigment dispersant; cosmetics; lubricant and mold release for hard rubber, textile chemical, chemical synthesis; antistat and antifog additive for plastic foils; Gardner 3 max. liq.; m.p. 16 C; amine no. 275; iodine no. < 13; 100% conc.

Radiamine 6161. [Fina Chemicals] Coconut oil amine, distilled; CAS 61788-46-3; EINECS 262-977-1; cationic; min. flotation, corrosion inhibitor, pigment dispersant; cosmetics; lubricant and mold release for hard rubber, textile chemical, chemical synthesis; antistat and antifog additive for plastic foils; Gardner 1 max. liq.; m.p. 15 C; amine no. 282; iodine no. < 12; 98% amine.

Radiamine 6163. [Fina Chemicals] Lauramine; CAS 124-22-1; EINECS 204-690-6; cationic; min. flotation, corrosion inhibitor, pigment dispersant; cosmetics; lubricant and mold release for hard rubber, textile chemical, chemical synthesis; antistat and antifog additive for plastic foils; liq.; 100% conc.

Radiamine 6164. [Fina Chemicals] Lauramine, distilled; CAS 124-22-1; EINECS 204-690-6; min. flotation, corrosion inhibitor, pigment dispersant; cosmetics; lubricant and mold release for hard rubber, textile chemical, chemical synthesis; antistat and antifog additive for plastic foils.

Radiamine 6170. [Fina Chemicals] Tallow amine; CAS 61790-33-8; EINECS 263-125-1; cationic; min. flotation, corrosion inhibitor, pigment dispersant; cosmetics; lubricant and mold release for hard rubber, textile chemical, chemical synthesis; antistat and antifog additive for plastic foils; Gardner 3 max. paste; m.p. 32 C; amine no. 210; iodine no. 40; 100% conc.

Radiamine 6171. [Fina Chemicals] Tallow amine, distilled; CAS 61790-33-8; EINECS 263-125-1; cationic; min. flotation, corrosion inhibitor, pigment dispersant; cosmetics; lubricant and mold release for hard rubber, textile chemical, chemical synthesis; antistat and antifog additive for plastic foils; Gardner 1 max. liq.; m.p. 30 C; amine no. 212; iodine no. 40; 98% amine.

Radiamine 6172. [Fina Chemicals] Oleyl amine; CAS 112-90-3; EINECS 204-015-5; cationic; min. flotation, corrosion inhibitor, pigment dispersant; cosmetics; lubricant and mold release for hard rubber, textile chemical, chemical synthesis; antistat and antifog additive for plastic foils; Gardner 2 max. liq.; cloud pt. < 20 C; amine no. 207; iodine no. 82; 95% amine.

Radiamine 6173. [Fina Chemicals] Oleamine, distilled; CAS 112-90-3; EINECS 204-015-5; cationic; min. flotation, corrosion inhibitor, pigment dispersant; cosmetics; lubricant and mold release for hard rubber, textile chemical, chemical synthesis; antistat and antifog additive for plastic foils; Gardner 2 max. liq.; cloud pt. < 20 C; amine no. 209; iodine no. 80; 97% amine.

Radiamox® 6800. [Fina Chemicals] Cocamine oxide; CAS 61788-90-7; EINECS 263-016-9; cationic/nonionic; substantive hair conditioner, antistat, foam booster for nonirritating and coloring shampoos, antidandruff prods., foam baths, cream rinses; good viscosifiers with anionics; Gardner 1 color; pH 7-8 (10% aq.); 30±1% act.

Radiamox® 6804. [Fina Chemicals] Lauramine oxide; CAS 1643-20-5; EINECS 216-700-6; cationic/nonionic; substantive hair conditioner, antistat, foam booster for nonirritating and coloring shampoos, antidandruff prods., foam baths, cream rinses; good viscosifiers with anionics; Gardner 1 color; pH 7-8 (10% aq.); 30±1% act.

Radianol® 1712. [Fina Chemicals] Lauryl alcohol; CAS 112-53-8; EINECS 203-982-0; emollient, bodying agent, stabilizer for skin care prods. incl. creams, lotions, cleansing milks, shave creams, depilatories, makeup, hair care, and foam prods.; also for synthesis of perfume materials and surfactants; acid no. 0.1; iodine no. 0.2; sapon. no. 1; hyd. no. 296-302; solid. pt. 23 C.

Radianol® 1724. [Fina Chemicals] C12-14 alcohol; emollient, bodying agent, stabilizer for skin care prods. incl. creams, lotions, cleansing milks, shave creams, depilatories, makeup, hair care, and foam prods.; also for synthesis of perfume materials and surfactants; acid no. 0.1;

iodine no. 0.2; sapon. no. 0.5; hyd. no. 285-294; solid. pt. 17-23 C.

Radianol® 1726. [Fina Chemicals] C12-16 alcohol; CAS 68855-56-1; emollient, bodying agent, stabilizer for skin care prods. incl. creams, lotions, cleansing milks, shave creams, depilatories, makeup, hair care, and foam prods.; also for synthesis of perfume materials and surfactants; acid no. 0.1; iodine no. 0.2; sapon. no. 1; hyd. no. 280-292; solid. pt. 18-22 C.

Radianol® 1728. [Fina Chemicals] Coconut alcohol; CAS 68425-37-6; EINECS 270-351-4; emollient, bodying agent, stabilizer for skin care prods. incl. creams, lotions, cleansing milks, shave creams, depilatories, makeup, hair care, and foam prods.; also for synthesis of perfume materials and surfactants; acid no. 0.1; iodine no. 0.2; sapon. no. 1; hyd. no. 265-275; solid. pt. 25-28 C.

Radianol® 1763. [Fina Chemicals] Cetearyl alcohol; emollient, bodying agent, stabilizer for skin care prods. incl. creams, lotions, cleansing milks, shave creams, depilatories, makeup, hair care, and foam prods.; also for synthesis of perfume materials and surfactants; flake; acid no. 0.2; iodine no. 0.2; sapon. no. 1; hyd. no. 210-225; solid. pt. 48-52 C.

Radianol® 1765. [Fina Chemicals] Cetearyl alcohol; emollient, bodying agent, stabilizer for skin care prods. incl. creams, lotions, cleansing milks, shave creams, depilatories, makeup, hair care, and foam prods.; also for synthesis of perfume materials and surfactants; flake; acid no. 0.2; iodine no. 0.2; sapon. no. 1; hyd. no. 215-225; solid. pt. 48-52 C.

Radianol® 1768. [Fina Chemicals] Cetearyl alcohol; emollient, bodying agent, stabilizer for skin care prods. incl. creams, lotions, cleansing milks, shave creams, depilatories, makeup, hair care, and foam prods.; also for synthesis of perfume materials and surfactants; acid no. 0.2; iodine no. 0.2; sapon. no. 1; hyd. no. 210-225; solid. pt. 48-52 C.

Radianol® 1769. [Fina Chemicals] Cetearyl alcohol; emollient, bodying agent, stabilizer for skin care prods. incl. creams, lotions, cleansing milks, shave creams, depilatories, makeup, hair care, and foam prods.; also for synthesis of perfume materials and surfactants; flake; acid no. 0.2; iodine no. 0.2; sapon. no. 1; hyd. no. 210-225; solid. pt. 48-52 C.

Radianol® 1898. [Fina Chemicals] Stearyl alcohol; CAS 112-92-5; EINECS 204-017-6; emollient, bodying agent, stabilizer for skin care prods. incl. creams, lotions, cleansing milks, shave creams, depilatories, makeup, hair care, and foam prods.; also for synthesis of perfume materials and surfactants; acid no. 0.2; iodine no. 0.2; sapon. no. 0.7; hyd. no. 200-215; solid. pt. 56-60 C.

Radiaquat® 6442. [Fina Chemicals] Dihydrog. tallow dimethyl ammonium chloride; CAS 61789-80-8; EINECS 263-090-2; cationic; surfactant, softener for laundry applics.; substantive conditioner for hair care prods.; bacteriostat for personal hygiene prods., deodorants, antidandruff prods.; Gardner 3 max. paste; 74% conc.

Radiaquat® 6444. [Fina Chemicals] Palmityl trimethyl ammonium chloride; CAS 112-02-7; EINECS 203-928-6; cationic; softener, antistat, detergent for textile, leather, detergent, and cosmetic industries; clay modifier; substantive conditioner for hair care prods.; bacteriostat in personal hygiene prods., deodorants, antidandruff prods.; Gardner 3 max. liq.; 50% conc.

Radiaquat® 6445. [Fina Chemicals] Cetrimonium chloride; CAS 112-02-7; EINECS 203-928-6; cationic; substantive conditioner for hair care prods.; bacteriostat for personal hygiene prods., deodorants, antidandruff prods.; Gardner 3 max. color; 30% conc.

Radiaquat® 6460. [Fina Chemicals] Cocotrimonium chloride; CAS 61789-18-2; EINECS 263-038-9; cationic; surfactant, substantive conditioner for hair care prods.; bacteriostat for personal hygiene prods., deodorants, antidandruff prods.; Gardner 5 max. color; 32-35% conc.

Radiaquat® 6462. [Fina Chemicals] Dicoco dimethyl ammonium chloride; CAS 61789-77-3; EINECS 263-087-6; cationic; detergent, antistat, softener, bactericide for detergents, textiles, fabric softeners, cosmetics; substantive hair conditioner; bacteriostat for personal hygiene prods., deodorants, antidandruff prods.; Gardner 4 max. paste; 75% conc.

Radiaquat® 6471. [Fina Chemicals] Tallow trimethyl ammonium chloride; CAS 68002-61-9; cationic; detergent, antistat, softener for textile, leather, detergent and cosmetic prods.; Gardner 5 max. liq.; 50% conc.

Radiastar® 1060. [Fina Chemicals] Calcium stearate; CAS 1592-23-0; EINECS 216-472-8; emulsifier for cleansing and night creams; opacifiers, dry binders for body powds., eye shadows, cream shampoos (pearlescent effect); anticking agent for powd. food prods.; wh. fluffy powd.; 99%—300 mesh fineness; m.p. 150-160 C.

Radiastar® 1100. [Fina Chemicals] Magnesium stearate; CAS 557-04-0; EINECS 209-150-3; emulsifier for cleansing and night creams; opacifiers, dry binders for body powds., eye shadows, cream shampoos (pearlescent effect); anticaking agent for powd. food prods.; wh. fluffy powd.; 98%—200 mesh fineness; m.p. 130-150 C.

Radiastar® 1170. [Fina Chemicals] Zinc stearate; CAS 557-05-1; EINECS 209-151-9; emulsifier for cleansing and night creams; opacifier, dry binder for body powds., eye shadows, cream shampoos (pearlescent effect); powd.; 99%-200 mesh fineness; m.p. 118-122 C.

Radiastar® 1200. [Fina Chemicals] Aluminum stearate; emulsifier for cleansing and night creams; opacifier, dry binder for body powds., eye shadows; thickener and gelling agent for oil-type cosmetics, e.g., waterproof mascaras; powd.; 75%-100 mesh fineness; m.p. 150-160 C.

Radiastar® 1208. [Fina Chemicals] Aluminum stearate, high gel; emulsifier for cleansing and night creams; opacifier, dry binder for body powds., eye shadows; thickener and gelling agent for oil-type cosmetics, e.g., waterproof mascaras; powd.; 85%-100 mesh fineness; m.p. 190-205 C.

Radiasurf® 7125. [Fina Chemicals] Sorbitan laurate; CAS 68154-36-9; EINECS 268-910-2; nonionic; emulsifier, descouring aid, antistat; anticorrosive agent for pipelines; cleaner for metallic surfaces; superfatting, bodying and antifog aid; pigment dispersant; detergent; emulsion of solv.; cutting oils; textile lubricant additive; concrete and paper additives; leather aux.; cosmetics and pharmaceuticals; plastics; pesticides; dry cleaning formulations; amber liq.; sol. in hexane, trichlorethylene, min. and veg. oil, benzene, IPA; disp. in water; m.w. 450; sp.gr. 1.025; visc. 1193.0 cps (37.8 C); acid no. 7 max.; iodine no. < 10; sapon. no. 155–175; cloud pt. 23 C.; flash pt. (COC) 198 C; ref. index 1.4718.

Radiasurf® 7141. [Fina Chemicals] Glyceryl stearate SE; nonionic; emulsifier, wetting agent, defoamer, rust inhibitor, pigment grinding, antistat; primary emulsifier for cosmetics; powd., flakes; m.p. 58 C; acid no. 3 max.; iodine no. < 3; 35% alpha monoester content.

Radiasurf® 7146. [Fina Chemicals] Glyceryl mono-12-hydroxystearate; nonionic; chemical intermediate, emulsifier, detergent, wetting agent, lubricant; chemical synthesis; cosmetics and pharmaceuticals; pearlescent shampoo formulations; detergency and cleaning prods.; cutting, lamination, and textile oils; rust inhibitor; pigment wetting, grinding, and improved gloss in paints, lacquers, printing inks; paper industry; lubricant and mold release in plastics; textile and leather processing; m.w. 550; sol. (@ 10%); @ 75 C in benzene, IPA, trichlorethylene; sp.gr.

0.925 (98.9 C); visc. 25.80 cps (98.9 C); HLB 1.9; m.p. 70 C; flash pt. 260 C (COC).

Radiasurf® 7150. [Fina Chemicals] Glyceryl oleate; CAS 68424-61-3; EINECS 270-312-1; internal lubricant for PVC; biodeg. surfactant, wetting agent, emulsifier for cosmetics, pharmaceuticals, agric., chem. synthesis, explosives, polymers, glass fibers, surface coatings, textiles and leather; Lovibond 15Y-3R liq.; sol. in hexane, benzene, IPA, min. oil; sol. cloudy in trichlorethylene, veg. oil; sp.gr. 934 kg/m³; HLB 2.7; acid no. 3 max.; iodine no. 75-85; pour pt. 3 C; cloud pt. < 10 C; flash pt. (COC) 230 C; 40% alpha monoglycerides.

Radiasurf® 7151. [Fina Chemicals] Glyceryl oleate, SE; nonionic; chemical intermediate, emulsifier, detergent, wetting agent, lubricant; chemical synthesis; cosmetic and pharmaceuticals; detergency and cleaning prods.; cutting, lamination, and textile oils; rust inhibitors; pigment wetting, grinding, and improved gloss in paints, lacquers, and printing inks; paper industry; lubricant and mold release in plastics; textile and leather processing; Lovibond 15Y-3R liq.; m.w. 515; sol. in IPA, min. and veg. oil, hexane, benzene, trichlorethylene; sp.gr. 0.947 (37.8 C); visc. 137.70 cps (37.8 C); HLB 3.3; acid no. 3 max.; iodine no. 75-85; cloud pt. 12.0 C.; flash pt. 208 C (COC); ref. index 1.4696.

Radiasurf® 7152. [Fina Chemicals] Glyceryl oleate; CAS 111-03-5; nonionic; chemical intermediate, emulsifier, detergent, wetting agent, lubricant; chemical synthesis; cosmetic and pharmaceuticals; detergency and cleaning prods.; cutting, lamination, and textile oils; rust inhibitors; pigment wetting; liq.; m.w. 521; sol. in IPA, min. and veg. oil, hexane, benzene, trichlorethylene; sp.gr. 0.934 (37.8 C); visc. 77.10 cps (37.8 C); HLB 2.8; ref. index 1.4697; flash pt. 232 C (COC); cloud pt. 7.5 C.

Radiasurf® 7153. [Fina Chemicals] Glyceryl ricinoleate; CAS 141-08-2; EINECS 205-455-0; nonionic; chemical intermediate, emulsifier, detergent, wetting agent, lubricant; cosmetic and pharmaceuticals; detergency and cleaning prods.; cutting, lamination, and textile oils; rust inhibitors; pigment wetting; antistat/antifog in plastics; m.w. 554; sol. (@ 10%); in benzene, IPA, trichlorethylene, min. and veg. oils; sp.gr. 0.982 (37.8 C); visc. 356.20 cps (37.8 C); HLB 2.5; ref. index 1.4774; flash pt. 229 C (COC); cloud pt. −16.0 C; 40% conc.

Radiasurf® 7156. [Fina Chemicals] Pentaerythritol oleate; CAS 85711-45-1; EINECS 288-305-7; nonionic; corrosion inhibitor for lubricating oils and greases; biodeg. surfactant, wetting agent, emulsifier for cosmetics, pharmaceuticals, agric., chem. synthesis, explosives, polymers, glass fibers, surface coatings, textiles and leather; Lovibond 15Y-3R liq.; sol. in bezene, IPA, trichlorethylene, min. and veg. oils; sol. cloudy in hexane; sp.gr. 938 kg/m³; HLB 2.1; acid no. 3 max.; iodine no. 80-90; cloud pt. < 0 C; flash pt. (COC) 280 C.

Radiasurf® 7175. [Fina Chemicals] Pentaerythritol stearate; CAS 85116-93-4; EINECS 285-547-5; nonionic; chemical intermediate, emulsifier, detergent, wetting agent, lubricant; chemical synthesis; cosmetics and pharmaceuticals; pearlescent shampoo formulations; detergency and cleaning prods.; cutting, lamination, and textile oils; rust inhibitor; pigment wetting, grinding, and improved gloss in paints, lacquers, printing inks; paper industry; lubricant and mold release in plastics; textile and leather processing; Lovibond 5Y-1R flakes; sol. in trichlorethylene; m.w. 675; sp.gr. 0.886 (98.9 C); visc. 17.60 cps (98.9 C); HLB 2.3; m.p. 52 C; acid no. 2 max.; iodine no. < 1; flash pt. (COC) 260 C.

Radiasurf® 7196. [Fina Chemicals] Propylene glycol myristate; CAS 29059-24-3; EINECS 249-395-3; nonionic; wetting aid, lubricant, opacifier, antistat, dispersant, w/o emulgent, scouring and detergent aid, defoamer, plasticizer, rust inhibitor; cosmetics and pharmaceuticals, lubricating and cutting oils, textile and leather aids, pigment grinding; in paints and printing inks, latex and emulsion paints, plastics, waxes, and maintenance prods., insecticides; wh. to amber liq.; m.w. 378; sol. in trichlorethylene, hexane, benzene, IPA, min. and veg. oils; disp. in water; sp.gr. 0.902 (37.8 C); visc. 17.30 cps (37.8 C); HLB 3.9; acid no. 5 max.; sapon. no. 190–205; ref. index 1.4379; flash pt. 145 C (COC).

Radiasurf® 7201. [Fina Chemicals] Propylene glycol stearate; CAS 1323-39-3; EINECS 215-354-3; nonionic; wetting aid, lubricant, opacifier, antistat, dispersant, w/o emulgent, scouring and detergent aid, defoamer, plasticizer, rust inhibitor; lubricating and cutting oils, textile and leather aids, pigment grinding; aux. emulsifier, visc. modifier for cosmetics and pharmaceuticals, cream shampoos, shower and bath prods.; wh. to cream solid; m.w. 457; sol. (@ 10%) in hexane, trichlorethylene, min. oil; sp.gr. 0.849 (98.9 C); visc. 4.50 cps (98.9 C); m.p. 40 C; HLB 3.0; acid no. 2 max.; iodine no. < 3; sapon. no. 177; flash pt. 206 C (COC).

Radiasurf® 7206. [Fina Chemicals] Propylene glycol oleate; CAS 1330-80-9; EINECS 215-549-3; nonionic; wetting aid, lubricant, opacifier, antistat, dispersant, w/o emulgent, scouring and detergent aid, defoamer, plasticizer, rust inhibitor; cosmetics and pharmaceuticals, lubricating and cutting oils, textile and leather aids, pigment grinding; amber liq.; m.w. 460; sol. in benzene, IPA, trichlorethylene, veg. and min. oil, hexane; sp.gr. 0.900 (37.8 C); visc. 18.80 cps (37.8 C); HLB 2.3; acid no. 2 max.; sapon. no. 172–180; ref. index. 1.4606; flash pt. 157 C (COC); cloud pt. –9 C.

Radiasurf® 7269. [Fina Chemicals] Ethylene glycol distearate; CAS 627-83-8; EINECS 211-014-3; nonionic; wetting aid, lubricant, opacifier, antistat, dispersant, w/o emulgent, scouring and detergent aid, defoamer, plasticizer, rust inhibitor; cosmetics and pharmaceuticals, lubricating and cutting oils, textile and leather aids, pigment grinding; wh. solid; sol. in trichlorethylene, hexane, benzene, IPA, min. and veg. oils; HLB 1.5; m.p. 65 C; acid no. 3 max.; sapon. no. 190–200.

Radiasurf® 7270. [Fina Chemicals] Ethylene glycol stearate; CAS 97281-23-7; EINECS 306-522-8; nonionic; wetting aid, lubricant, opacifier, antistat, dispersant, w/o emulgent, scouring and detergent aid, defoamer, plasticizer, rust inhibitor; lubricating and cutting oils, textile and leather aids, pigment grinding; weak emulsifier; bodying agent, opacifier, thickener, pearlescent for cosmetic creams and lotions, cream shampoos, and pharmaceuticals; adds body, hardness, slip, and opacity to lipsticks and makeup; wh. flakes; m.w. 445; sol. (@ 10% and 75 C) in benzene, IPA, trichlorethylene, veg. oil; sp.gr. 0.851 (98.9 C); visc. 4.80 cps (98.9 C); HLB 2.1; m.p. 57 C; acid no. 2 max.; iodine no. < 1; sapon. no. 180–190; flash pt. (COC) 214 C.

Radiasurf® 7400. [Fina Chemicals] Diethylene glycol oleate; CAS 93455-78-8; EINECS 297-364-8; nonionic; emulsifier, wetting agent, defoamer, rust inhibitor, pigment grinder, antistat; for agric., chem. synthesis, cosmetics/pharmaceuticals, explosives, polymers, surf. coatings, textile and leather; amber liq.; m.w. 478; sol. in trichlorethylene, hexane, benzene, IPA, min. and veg. oil; disp. in water; sp.gr. 0.929 (37.8 C); visc. 58.50 cps (37.8 C); HLB 3.8; pour pt. -12 C; cloud pt. < -2 C;acid no. 4 max.; iodine no. 75-85; sapon. no. 155–168; ref. index 1.4642; flash pt. (COC) 180 C.

Radiasurf® 7402. [Fina Chemicals] PEG-4 oleate; CAS 85736-49-8; EINECS 288-459-5; nonionic; wetting aid, lubricant, opacifier, antistat, dispersant, o/w emulgent,

scouring and detergent aid, defoamer, plasticizer, rust inhibitor, visc. modifier, antifog aid; cosmetics and pharmaceuticals; lubricating and cutting oils; textile and leather aids; pigment grinding aids in paints and printing inks; latex and emulsion paints; plastics; waxes and maintenance prods.; glass fiber; insecticides; silicones; amber liq.; sol. (@ 10%) in benzene, isopropyl, trichlorethylene, hexane, min. and veg. oils; water-disp.; sp.gr. 0.962 (37.8 C); visc. 34.00 cps (37.8 C); HLB 7.4; acid no. < 3; sapon. no. 105–125; iodine no. 55-65; ref. index 1.4645; flash pt. (COC) 218 C; cloud pt. –10 C.

Radiasurf® 7403. [Fina Chemicals] PEG-8 oleate; CAS 85736-49-8; EINECS 288-459-5; nonionic; wetting aid, lubricant, opacifier, antistat, dispersant, o/w emulgent, scouring and detergent aid, defoamer, plasticizer, rust inhibitor, visc. modifier, antifog aid; cosmetics and pharmaceuticals; lubricating and cutting oils; amber liq.; sol. in trichlorethylene, hexane, benzene, IPA, min. and veg. oil; disp. in water; m.w. 728; sp.gr. 1.007 (37.8 C); visc. 49.50 cps (37.8 C); HLB 11.5; acid no. < 3; sapon. no. 75–90; ref. index 1.4672; flash pt. (COC) 261 C; cloud pt. –1 C.

Radiasurf® 7404. [Fina Chemicals] PEG-12 oleate; CAS 85736-49-8; EINECS 288-459-5; nonionic; wetting aid, lubricant, opacifier, antistat, dispersant, o/w emulgent, scouring and detergent aid, defoamer, plasticizer, rust inhibitor, visc. modifier, antifog aid; cosmetics and pharmaceuticals; lubricating and cutting oils; amber liq.; sol. (@ 10%) in water, benzene, IPA, trichlorethylene, hexane, min. and veg. oils; m.w. 920; sp.gr. 1.030 (37.8 C); visc. 66.30 cps (37.8 C); HLB 13.2; acid no. < 3; sapon. no. 60–75; cloud pt. 19 C; flash pt. (COC) 254 C; ref. index 1.4669.

Radiasurf® 7410. [Fina Chemicals] Diethylene glycol stearate; CAS 85116-97-8; EINECS 285-550-1; nonionic; wetter, lubricant, opacifier, antistat, dispersant, detergent, defoamer, plasticizer, rust inhibitor; for textiles, leather, paints, inks, plastic, waxes, maintenance prods., insecticides; aux. emulsifier, thickener, opacifier for for cosmetic shampoos and creams, vanishing creams, pharmaceuticals; wh. paste; sol. in trichlorethylene, hexane, benzene, IPA, min. and veg. oils; disp. in water; m.w. 475; sp.gr. 0.873 (100 C); visc. 5.95 cps (98.9 C); HLB 3.5; m.p. 49 C; acid no. 3 max.; iodine no. < 1; sapon. no. 160–175; flash pt. (COC) 191 C.

Radiasurf® 7411. [Fina Chemicals] Diethylene glycol stearate, SE; CAS 9004-99-3; nonionic; wetter, lubricant, opacifier, antistat, dispersant, detergent, defoamer, plasticizer, rust inhibitor; for cosmetics, pharmaceuticals, textiles, leather, paints, inks, plastic, waxes, maintenance prods., insecticides; wh. solid; m.w. 470; sol. in trichlorethylene, hexane, benzene, IPA, min. and veg. oils; disp. in water; sp.gr. 0.878 (98.9 C); visc. 5.90 cps (98.9 C); HLB 4.1; m.p. 52 C; acid no. 3 max.; sapon. no. 160–170; flash pt. 176 C (COC).

Radiasurf® 7413. [Fina Chemicals] PEG-8 stearate; CAS 9004-99-3; nonionic; wetting aid, lubricant, opacifier, antistat, dispersant, o/w emulgent, scouring and detergent aid, defoamer, plasticizer, rust inhibitor, visc. modifier, antifog aid; cosmetics and pharmaceuticals; lubricating and cutting oils; wh. paste; m.w. 722; sol. (@ 10%) in benzene, trichlorethylene, min. oil, hexane; sp.gr. 0.951 (98.9 C); visc. 9.45 cps (98.9 C); HLB 11.9; m.p. 34 C; acid no. < 3; sapon. no. 75–90; flash pt. 248 C (COC).

Radiasurf® 7414. [Fina Chemicals] PEG-12 stearate; CAS 97281-23-7; EINECS 306-522-8; nonionic; wetting aid, lubricant, opacifier, antistat, dispersant, o/w emulgent, scouring and detergent aid, defoamer, plasticizer, rust inhibitor, visc. modifier, antifog aid; cosmetics and pharmaceuticals; lubricating and cutting oils; wh. paste; sol. in benzene, IPA, hexane, min. and veg. oil, trichlorethylene;

m.w. 906; sp.gr. 0.981 (98.9 C); visc. 12.60 cps (98.9 C); m.p. 38 C; HLB 13.5; acid no. < 3; sapon. no. 60–75; flash pt. (COC) 241 C.

Radiasurf® 7417. [Fina Chemicals] PEG-1500 stearate; CAS 97281-23-7; EINECS 306-522-8; nonionic; wetting aid, lubricant, opacifier, antistat, dispersant, o/w emulgent, scouring and detergent aid, defoamer, plasticizer, rust inhibitor, visc. modifier, antifog aid; cosmetics and pharmaceuticals; lubricating and cutting oils; wh. flakes; sol. in benzene, trichlorethylene; m.w. 1812; sp.gr. 1.023 (98.9 C); visc. 28.40 cps (98.9 C); m.p. 47 C; HLB 15.5; acid no. < 3; sapon. no. 30–40; flash pt. (COC) 248 C.

Radiasurf® 7420. [Fina Chemicals] Diethylene glycol laurate; CAS 9004-81-3; nonionic; wetting aid, lubricant, opacifier, antistat, dispersant, w/o emulgent, scouring and detergent aid, defoamer, plasticizer, rust inhibitor; cosmetics and pharmaceuticals, lubricating and cutting oils, textile and leather aids, pigment grinding; wh. paste; m.w. 352; sol. in IPA, trichlorethylene, hexane, min. and veg. oil; sp.gr. 0.942 (37.8 C); visc. 15.20 cps (37.8 C); HLB 5.7; acid no. 3 max.; sapon. no. 195–205; flash pt. 164 C (COC); cloud pt. 28.5 C.

Radiasurf® 7422. [Fina Chemicals] PEG-4 laurate; CAS 9004-81-3; nonionic; wetting aid, lubricant, opacifier, antistat, dispersant, o/w emulgent, scouring and detergent aid, defoamer, plasticizer, rust inhibitor, visc. modifier, antifog aid; cosmetics and pharmaceuticals; lubricating and cutting oils; wh. liq.; m.w. 379; sol. in trichlorethylene, hexane, benzene, IPA, min. and veg. oil; disp. in water; sp.gr. 0.983 (37.8 C); visc. 23.40 cps (37.8 C); HLB 9.6; acid no. < 3; sapon. no. 140–150; ref. index 1.4542; flash pt. 188 C (COC); cloud pt. –3 C.

Radiasurf® 7423. [Fina Chemicals] PEG-8 laurate; CAS 37318-14-2; EINECS 253-458-0; nonionic; wetting aid, lubricant, opacifier, antistat, dispersant, o/w emulgent, scouring and detergent aid, defoamer, plasticizer, rust inhibitor, visc. modifier, antifog aid; cosmetics and pharmaceuticals; lubricating and cutting oils; wh. liq.; sol. in benzene, IPA, trichlorethylene, water, hexane, min. and veg. oil; m.w. 610; sp.gr. 1.023 (37.8 C); visc. 41.70 cps (37.8 C); HLB 12.8; acid no. < 3; sapon. no. 90–100; ref. index 1.4596; flash pt. (COC) 238 C; cloud pt. 4 C.

Radiasurf® 7431. [Fina Chemicals] PEG-6 oleate; CAS 9004-96-0; nonionic; wetting aid, lubricant, opacifier, antistat, dispersant, o/w emulgent, scouring and detergent aid, defoamer, plasticizer, rust inhibitor, visc. modifier, antifog aid; cosmetics and pharmaceuticals; lubricating and cutting oils; amber liq.; sol. in trichlorethylene, hexane, benzene, IPA, min. and veg. oil; disp. in water; HLB 9.5; acid no. < 3; sapon. no. 95–115; cloud pt. –8 C.

Radiasurf® 7432. [Fina Chemicals] PEG-6 stearate; CAS 9004-99-3; nonionic; wetting aid, lubricant, opacifier, antistat, dispersant, o/w emulgent, scouring and detergent aid, defoamer, plasticizer, rust inhibitor, visc. modifier, antifog aid; cosmetics and pharmaceuticals; lubricating and cutting oils; wh. paste; sol. in benzene, IPA, trichlorethylene, min. oil, hexane; HLB 9.7; m.p. 28–35 C; acid no. < 3; sapon. no. 95–115.

Radiasurf® 7443. [Fina Chemicals] PEG-8 dioleate; CAS 85736-49-8; EINECS 288-459-5; nonionic; wetting aid, lubricant, opacifier, antistat, dispersant, o/w emulgent, scouring and detergent aid, defoamer, plasticizer, rust inhibitor, visc. modifier, antifog aid; cosmetics and pharmaceuticals; lubricating and cutting oils; amber liq.; sol. in trichlorethylene, hexane, benzene, IPA, min. and veg. oil; disp. in water; m.w. 911; sp.gr. 0.962 (37.8 C); visc. 47.00 cps (37.8 C); HLB 7.4; acid no. < 5; sapon. no. 120–130; cloud pt. –3 C; flash pt. (COC) 248 C; ref. index 1.4655.

Radiasurf® 7444. [Fina Chemicals] PEG-12 dioleate; CAS

85736-49-8; EINECS 288-459-5; nonionic; biodeg. surfactant, wetting agent, emulsifier for cosmetics, pharmaceuticals, agric., chem. synthesis, explosives, polymers, glass fibers, surface coatings, textiles and leather; Lovibond 10Y-1.5R liq.; sol. cloudy in water, min. oil; sol. clear in hexane, benzene, IPA, trichlorethylene, veg. oil; sp.gr. 992 kg/m³; HLB 9.9; acid no. 5 max.; iodine no. 45-55; pour pt. 2 C; cloud pt. < 15 C; flash pt. (COC) 275 C.

Radiasurf® 7453. [Fina Chemicals] PEG-8 distearate; CAS 97281-23-7; EINECS 306-522-8; nonionic; wetting aid, lubricant, opacifier, antistat, dispersant, o/w emulgent, scouring and detergent aid, defoamer, plasticizer, rust inhibitor, visc. modifier, antifog aid; cosmetics and pharmaceuticals; lubricating and cutting oils; wh. paste; sol. (@ 10%) in benzene, IPA, trichlorethylene; m.w. 901; sp.gr. 0.920 (98.9 C); visc. 9.85 cps (98.9 C); HLB 7.8; m.p. 39 C; acid no. < 5; sapon. no. 120–130; flash pt. (COC) 242 C.

Radiasurf® 7454. [Fina Chemicals] PEG-12 distearate; CAS 97281-23-7; EINECS 306-522-8; nonionic; wetting aid, lubricant, opacifier, antistat, dispersant, o/w emulgent, scouring and detergent aid, defoamer, plasticizer, rust inhibitor, visc. modifier, antifog aid; cosmetics and pharmaceuticals; lubricating and cutting oils; wh. paste; sol. in benzene, trichlorethylene, hexane, IPA, min. oil; m.w. 1101; sp.gr. 0.940 (98.9 C); visc. 12.20 cps (98.9 C); m.p. 41 C; HLB 10.6; acid no. < 5; sapon. no. 100–110; flash pt. (COC) 249 C.

Radiasurf® 7473. [Fina Chemicals] PEG-8 stearate; CAS 97281-23-7; EINECS 306-522-8; nonionic; biodeg. surfactant, wetting agent, emulsifier for cosmetics, pharmaceuticals, agric., chem. synthesis, explosives, polymers, glass fibers, surface coatings, textiles and leather; Lovibond 5R-0.6Y paste; sol. cloudy in water, min. and veg. oil; sol. clear in hexane, benzene, IPA, trichlorethylene; sp.gr. 945 kg/m³ (100 C); m.p. 27 C; HLB 11.1; acid no. 3 max.; iodine no. < 1; flash pt. (COC) 260 C.

Radiasurf® 7600. [Fina Chemicals] Glyceryl stearate; CAS 85251-77-0; EINECS 286-490-9; nonionic; wetter, defoamer, rust inhibitor, pigment grinder, emulsifier, antistat; aux. emulsifier for cosmetic creams and lotions, imparting body, opacity, and smoothness; flakes, powd.; sol. (@ 75 C) in hexane, benzene, IPA, trichlorethylene, min. and veg. oils; sp.gr. 893 kg/m³ (100 C); HLB 3.3; m.p. 58 C; acid no. 3 max.; iodine no. < 1; flash pt. (COC) 225 C; 60% conc.

Radiasurf® 7900. [Fina Chemicals] Glyceryl stearate; CAS 91052-47-0; EINECS 293-208-8; nonionic; biodeg. surfactant, wetting agent, emulsifier for cosmetics, pharmaceuticals, agric., chem. synthesis, explosives, polymers, glass fibers, surface coatings, textiles and leather; Lovibond 5Y-1R powd.; sol. (@ 75 C) in hexane, benzene, IPA, trichlorethylene, min. and veg. oils; sp.gr. 902 kg/m³; HLB 4.8; m.p. 68 C; acid no. 3 max.; iodine no. < 2; flash pt. (COC) 220 C; 90% alpha monoglycerides.

Radiateric® 6860. [Fina Chemicals] Coco-betaine; CAS 68424-94-2; EINECS 270-329-4; amphoteric; high foaming detergent with antistatic, bacteriostatic, and substantive props. for nonirritating shampoos, conditioners, cream rinses, bubble baths, liq. soaps, shaving prods.; Gardner 2 color; pH 5-8 (10% aq.); 30% act.

Radiateric® 6864. [Fina Chemicals] Lauryl betaine; CAS 683-10-3; EINECS 211-669-5; amphoteric; high foaming detergent with antistatic, bacteriostatic, and substantive props. for nonirritating shampoos, conditioners, cream rinses, bubble baths, liq. soaps, shaving prods.; Gardner 2 color; pH 5-8 (10% aq.); 30% act.

Reach® 101, 201, 501. [Reheis] Aluminum chlorohydrate; CAS 1327-41-9; EINECS 215-477-2; antiperspirant for increased wetness protection, esp. for aerosols; powd.;

97% thru 325 mesh; pH 4.0–4.4 (15% aq.); 46–48.5, 46–48.5, and 46–48% Al$_2$O$_3$ resp., 15.8–17.5, 15.8–17.5, and 15.8–16.8% Cl.

Reach® AZP-701, AZP-703. [Reheis] Aluminum zirconium tetrachlorohydrex glycine; enhanced efficacy antiperspirant for nonaq. systems, sticks, roll-ons; 15% Al, 14% Zr, 12% Gly.

Reach® AZZ-902. [Reheis] Aluminum zirconium trichlorohydrex GLY; antiperspirant.

Red 119. [Presperse] D&C Red #7 calcium lake and bismuth oxychloride; organic colorant for pigmented cosmetics.

Red 139. [Presperse] Iron oxides (90%), bismuthoxychloride (10%); CAS 1309-37-1; inorg. colorant for pigmented cosmetics; JSCI/JCID approved.

Red 150. [Presperse] D&C red #30 aluminum lake and bismuth oxychloride; organic colorant for pigmented cosmetics.

Red 219. [Presperse] D&C red #36 and bismuth oxychloride; organic colorant for pigmented cosmetics; Japanese approval.

Regederme HS 236. [Alban Muller] Propylene glycol, olibanum extract, horsetail extract, hops extract, arnica extract; face care prod. for elderly skin.

Regederme HS 330. [Alban Muller] Propylene glycol, myrrh extract, horsetail extract, wheat germ extract, hops extract; face care prod. for elderly skin.

Regederme LS 630. [Alban Muller] Sunflower seed oil, horsetail extract, hops extract, wheat germ extract, and myrrh extract; face care prod. for elderly skin.

Regederme LS 636. [Alban Muller] Sunflower seed oil, olibanum extract, horsetail extract, hops extract, and arnica extract; face care prod. for elderly skin.

Rehydragel® Compressed Gel. [Reheis] Aluminum hydroxide; CAS 21645-51-2; EINECS 244-492-7; adsorbent gel for pharmaceuticals (enhances suspensions, builds visc.); carrier for toxins in veterinary vaccines; translucent gel; 9% Al$_2$O$_3$.

Rehydragel® Low Visc. Gel. [Reheis] Aluminum hydroxide; CAS 21645-51-2; EINECS 244-492-7; adsorbent gel and protein binder for use as a fluid adjuvant in the prep. of parenteral sol'ns.; low visc. gel; 2% Al$_2$O$_3$.

Rehydragel® Thixotropic Gel. [Reheis] Aluminum hydroxide; CAS 21645-51-2; EINECS 244-492-7; adsorbent, protein binder for biological materials; wh. opaque thixotropic gel; 2% Al$_2$O$_3$.

Rehydrol® II. [Reheis] Aluminum chlorohydrex PG; antiperspirant active for pumps, roll-ons and alcoholic sticks; solid; sol. 50% max. in alcohol and water; 36% min. Al$_2$O$_3$, 12.5% min. Cl, 22% min. propylene glycol.

Relaxant HS 278. [Alban Muller] Propylene glycol, spiraea extract, hops extract, matricaria extract, and laurel extract; phytocomplex; relaxing prod. for bubble baths.

Relaxant LS 678. [Alban Muller] Sunflower seed oil, spiraea extract, hops extract, matricaria extract, and laurel extract; phytocomplex; relaxing prod. for bubble baths.

Relaxer Conc. No. 2. [Brooks Industries] Cetearyl alcohol, cetyl alcohol, polysorbate 60, laneth-15, PEG-60 lanolin, steareth-20, TEA-coco-hydrolyzed collagen, PEG-150 stearate.; an emulsion conc. to which is added min. oil, petrolatum, a base, and water to form a stable hair relaxer; emulsifier; flakes; 100% act.

Remcopal 40 S3. [Ceca SA] PEG-40 castor oil; CAS 61791-12-6; nonionic; emulsifier for vitamins and essential oils; cosmetic base; liq., pleasant odor; sp.gr. 1.03-1.04; sol. in water, aromatic, chlorinated, and terpene solvs., veg. oil; disp. in min. oil, kerosene; HLB 12.9; acid no. ≤ 2; iodine no. 30 ± 5; sapon. no. 75 ± 8; hyd. no. 75 ± 10; pH 6-7 (10%); surf. tens. 44 dynes/cm; 97% conc.

Remcopal 207. [Ceca SA] PEG-4.5 oleate; CAS 9004-96-0; EINECS 233-293-0; nonionic; emulsifier for vitamins; liq.;

HLB 8.0; 100% act.

Remcopal 334. [Ceca SA] Nonoxynol-4; CAS 9016-45-9; nonionic; emulsifier, dispersant for pigments, paints, cosmetics, industrial emulsions; emulsive base for hair dyes, oxidative coloring; liq., faint odor; sol. in terpene solvs., kerosene, veg. and min. oils; disp. in water, aromatic solvs.; HLB 8.5; surf. tens. 28.1 dynes/cm; 100% conc.

Remcopal 21411. [Ceca SA] Laureth-11; CAS 9002-92-0; nonionic; emulsifier for lt. hydrocarbons, raw material shampoos; paste; HLB 13.5; 100% conc.

Remcopal HC 7. [Ceca SA] PEG-7 hydrog. castor oil; CAS 61788-85-0; nonionic; surfactant, solubilizer for essential oils and liposoluble vitamins; visc. liq., very faint odor; insol. in water; HLB 5.0; iodine no. 0.16; pH 6.5 — 0.5 (101%); 100% conc.

Remcopal HC 33. [Ceca SA] PEG-33 hydrog. castor oil; CAS 61788-85-0; nonionic; surfactant, solubilizer for essential oils and liposoluble vitamins; paste, very fait odor; HLB 12.0; iodine no. 0.16; pH 6.5 ± 0.5 (10%); surf. tens. 42 dynes/cm); 100% conc.

Remcopal HC 40. [Ceca SA] PEG-40 hydrog. castor oil; CAS 61788-85-0; nonionic; surfactant, solubilizer for essential oils and vitamins; Gardner < 4 paste, very faint odor; sol. in water, ethyl acetate, aromatic and chlorinated solvs., alcohols, veg. oil; disp. in min. oil, aliphatic solvs.; HLB 13.0; acid no. 1.5; iodine no. 0.2; sapon. no. 64; hyd. no. 65; ref. index 1.467; pH 6.5 ± 0.5 (10%); surf. tens. 42 dynes/cm; 100% conc.

Remcopal HC 60. [Ceca SA] PEG-60 hydrog. castor oil; CAS 61788-85-0; nonionic; surfactant, solubilizer for essential oils and vitamins; paste, very faint odor; HLB 15.0; iodine no. 0.21; pH 6.5 ± 0.5 (10%); surf. tens. 42.5 dynes/cm; 100% conc.

Remcopal O9. [Ceca SA] Octoxynol-9; CAS 9002-93-1; nonionic; solubilizer for essential oils; emulsifier; liq.; HLB 13.0; 100% conc.

Remcopal O11. [Ceca SA] Octoxynol-10; CAS 9002-93-1; nonionic; solubilizer for essential oils; emulsifier; liq.; HLB 13.4; 100% conc.

Remcopal O12. [Ceca SA] Octoxynol-11; CAS 9002-93-1; nonionic; solubilizer for essential oils; emulsifier; paste; HLB 14.1; 100% conc.

Renex® 20. [ICI Am.; ICI Surf. Belgium] PEG-16 tallate; CAS 61791-00-2; nonionic; detergent for personal care, home laundry, textile scouring, spotting agent, rug shampoos; emulsifier, dispersant; yel. amber clear liq.; sol. in water, lower alcohols, toluene, acetone, diethyl ether, dioxane, Cellosolve, ethyl acetate, aniline; sp.gr. 1.1; visc. 350 cps; HLB 13.8; cloud pt. 126 F (1% aq.); flash pt. > 300 F; pour pt. 55 F; surf. tens. 41 dynes/cm (0.01%); 100% act.

Renex® 22. [ICI Am.; ICI Surf. UK] Mixed fatty and resin acids POE ester (12 EO); detergent for personal care, home laundry, textile scouring, rug shampoos, mechanical dishwashing, metal cleaning; amber liq.; sol. in acetone, ethyl acetate, dioxane, Cellosolve, aniline, ethyl alcohol; disp. in water; sp.gr. 1.1; visc. 300 cps; HLB 12.2; cloud pt. 32 F (1% aq.); flash pt. > 300 F; pour pt. 35 F; surf. tens. 39 dynes/cm (0.01%).

Renex® 30. [ICI Am.; ICI Surf. Belgium] Trideceth-12; CAS 24938-91-8; nonionic; detergent, emulsifier, and wetting agent used for raw wool scouring and carbonizing, metal cleaning, bottle washing, home laundry, personal care prods.; colorless clear-hazy liq.; sol. in water, lower alcohols, xylene, butyl Cellosolve, carbon tetrachloride, ethylene glycol, propylene glycol; sp.gr. 1.0; visc. 60 cps; HLB 14.5; cloud pt. 183 F (1% aq.); flash pt. > 300 F; pour pt. 55 F; surf. tens. 28 dynes/cm (0.01%); pH 6 (1%); 100% conc.

Renex® 36. [ICI Am.; ICI Surf. Belgium] Trideceth-6; CAS 24938-91-8; nonionic; detergent, wetting agent, emulsifier, dye leveling agent used in personal care prods., alkaline cleaners, dishwashing, textiles, dairy cleaners, sanitizers; dispersant for solids and paint pigments; colorless clear-cloudy thin oily liq.; sol. in acetone, CCl_4, ethyl acetate, Cellosolve, ethanol, toluene, aniline; disp. in water; sp.gr. 1.0; visc. 80 cps.; HLB 11.4; cloud pt. < 32 F (1% aq.); flash pt. > 300 F; surf. tens. 27 dynes/cm (0.01%); pH 6 (1%); 100% conc.

Renex® 647. [ICI Am.; ICI Surf. Belgium] Nonoxynol-4; CAS 9016-45-9; nonionic; emulsifier, detergent for personal care, industrial, and agrochem. industries; pale yel. liq.; HLB 8.9; 100% conc.

Renex® 648. [ICI Am.; ICI Surf. Belgium] Nonoxynol-5; CAS 9016-45-9; nonionic; detergent, solv. and emulsion cleaning applications; metal cleaning; personal care applics.; yel. clear liq.; sol. in propylene glycol, perchlorethylene, IPA, cottonseed oil; sp.gr. 1.03; visc. 223 cps; HLB 10.5; flash pt. > 200 F; pour pt. –20 F; 100% act.

Renex® 649. [ICI Am.; ICI Surf. Belgium] Nonoxynol-20; CAS 9016-45-9; nonionic; emulsifier, detergent for personal care, industrial, and agrochem. industries; cream-colored solid; HLB 16.0; 100% conc.

Renex® 650. [ICI Am.; ICI Surf. Belgium] Nonoxynol-30; CAS 9016-45-9; nonionic; detergent, emulsifier, stabilizer; surfactant for detergent use, personal care, industrial, and agrochem. applics.; latex stabilizer; cream-colored solid; sol. in water, propylene glycol, IPA glycol, IPA, xylene; sp.gr. 1.15; HLB 17.1; cloud pt. 212 F; flash pt. > 300 F; pour pt. 91 F; surf. tens. 42 dynes/cm (0.01%); 100% act.

Renex® 670. [ICI Surf. UK] Nonoxynol-11; CAS 9016-45-9; surfactant for personal care, industrial, and agrochem. applics.; colorless to pale yel. liq.; HLB 13.6.

Renex® 678. [ICI Am.; ICI Surf. Belgium] Nonoxynol-15; CAS 9016-45-9; nonionic; detergent, wetting agent used in dishwashing, personal care, industrial, agrochem. applics.; colorless to pale yel. clear liq.; sol. in water, propylene glycol, perchloroethylene, IPA, xylene; sp.gr 1.08; visc. 319 cps; HLB 15; cloud pt. 211 F (1%); flash pt. > 300 F; pour pt. 69 F; surf. tens. 33 dynes/cm (0.01%); 100% act.

Renex® 679. [ICI Am.; ICI Surf. Belgium] Nonoxynol-13; CAS 9016-45-9; nonionic; emulsifier, detergent for personal care, industrial, and agrochem. applics.; colorless to pale liq.; HLB 14.4; 100% conc.

Renex® 682. [ICI Am.; ICI Surf. Belgium] Nonoxynol-12; CAS 9016-45-9; nonionic; emulsifier and detergent for personal care, industrial, and agrochem. applics.; colorless to pale yel. liq.; HLB 13.9; 100% conc.

Renex® 688. [ICI Am.; ICI Surf. Belgium] Nonoxynol-8; CAS 9016-45-9; nonionic; detergent, wetting agent; surfactant for dishwashing, textile scouring, personal care, industrial, agrochem. applics.; colorless to pale yel. liq.; sol. in propylene glycol, perchloroethylene, IPA, xylene, water and cottonseed oil; sp.gr. 1.05; visc. 240 cps; HLB 12.3; cloud pt. 87 F (1%); flash pt. > 300 F; pour pt. 12 F; surf. tens. 30 dynes/cm (0.01%); 100% act.

Renex® 690. [ICI Am.; ICI Surf. Belgium] Nonoxynol-10; CAS 9016-45-9; EINECS 248-294-1; nonionic; wetting agent, detergent for home and commercial laundry products, textile scouring, dyeing and desizing, acid metal cleaner, sanitizer, hard surface cleaning, personal care prods.; colorless to pale yel. liq.; sol. in propylene glycol, perchloroethylene, IPA, xylene, water and cottonseed oil; sp.gr. 1.06; visc. 260 cps; HLB 13.3; cloud pt. 150 F (1%); flash pt. > 300 F; pour pt. 33 F; surf. tens. 31 dynes/cm (0.01%); 100% act.

Renex® 697. [ICI Am.; ICI Surf. Belgium] Nonoxynol-6; CAS 9016-45-9; nonionic; emulsifier, detergent for personal care, industrial, and agrochem. applics.; colorless to pale yel. clear liq.; sol. in propylene glycol, perchloroethylene,

IPA, xylene, cottonseed oil; sp.gr. 1.04; visc. 250 cps; HLB 10.9; cloud pt. < 32 F (1%); flash pt. > 300 F; pour pt. –21 F; surf. tens. 30 dynes/cm (0.01%); 100% act.

Renex® 698. [ICI Am.; ICI Surf. Belgium] Nonoxynol-9 (9–9.5 EO); CAS 9016-45-9; nonionic; emulsifier, detergent for personal care, industrial, and agrochem. applics.; colorless to pale yel. clear liq.; sol. in propylene glycol, perchloroethylene, IPA, xylene, water, cottonseed oil; sp.gr. 1.06; visc. 245 cps; HLB 13; cloud pt. 129 F (1%); flash pt. > 300 F; pour pt. 28 F; surf. tens. 30 dynes/cm (0.01%); 100% act.

Renex® 702. [ICI Am.; ICI Surf. Belgium] PEG-2 syn. primary C13–15 alcohol; nonionic; biodeg. general purpose detergent, emulsifier for personal care, industrial, and agrochem. applics.; colorless liq.; HLB 5.9; 100% conc.

Renex® 703. [ICI Am.; ICI Surf. Belgium] PEG-3 syn. primary C13–15 alcohol; nonionic; biodeg. general purpose detergent, emulsifier for personal care, industrial, and agrochem. applics.; colorless liq.; HLB 7.8; 100% conc.

Renex® 707. [ICI Am.; ICI Surf. Belgium] PEG-7 syn. primary C13–15 alcohol; nonionic; biodeg. general purpose detergent, emulsifier for personal care, industrial, and agrochem. applics.; colorless liq.; HLB 12.2; 100% conc.

Renex® 709. [ICI Surf. UK] PEG-9 syn. primary C13-15 alcohol; surfactant for personal care, industrial, and agrochem. applics.; wh. paste; HLB 12.5.

Renex® 711. [ICI Am.; ICI Surf. Belgium] PEG-11 syn. primary C13–15 alcohol; nonionic; biodeg. general detergent, emulsifier for personal care, industrial, and agrochem. applics.; wh. paste; HLB 13.9; 100% conc.

Renex® 720. [ICI Am.; ICI Surf. Belgium] PEG-20 syn. primary C13–15 alcohol; nonionic; biodeg. general detergent, emulsifier for personal care, industrial, and agrochem. applics.; wh. solid; HLB 16.2; 100% conc.

Renex® 750. [ICI Am.; ICI Surf. Belgium] Octoxynol-10; CAS 9002-93-1; nonionic; biodeg. emulsifier, detergent for personal care, industrial, and agrochem. applics.; pale yel. liq.; HLB 13.6; 100% conc.

Renex® 759. [ICI Surf. UK] Octoxynol-9 USP/NF; CAS 9002-93-1; surfactant for personal care, industrial, and agrochem. applics.; pale yel. liq.; HLB 13.0.

Renex® PEG 200. [ICI Surf. Am.] PEG; surfactant; colorless liq.

Renex® PEG 300. [ICI Surf. Am.; ICI Surf. UK] PEG-6 USP/NF; CAS 25322-68-3; EINECS 220-045-1; surfactant for personal care, industrial, and agrochem. applics.; colorless liq.

Renex® PEG 300. [ICI Surf. Am.; ICI Surf. UK] PEG USP/NF; surfactant for personal care, industrial, and agrochem. applics.; colorless liq.

Renex® PEG 400. [ICI Surf. Am.; ICI Surf. UK] PEG-8 USP/NF; CAS 25322-68-3; EINECS 225-856-4; surfactant for personal care, industrial, and agrochem. applics.; colorless liq.

Renex® PEG 600. [ICI Surf. Am.; ICI Surf. UK] PEG-12 USP/NF; CAS 25322-68-3; EINECS 229-859-1; surfactant for personal care, industrial, and agrochem. applics.; wh. paste.

Renex® PEG 1000. [ICI Surf. Am.; ICI Surf. UK] PEG-20 USP/NF; CAS 25322-68-3; surfactant for personal care, industrial, and agrochem. applics.; wh. solid.

Renex® PEG 1500FL. [ICI Surf. UK] PEG-32 USP/NF; CAS 25322-68-3; surfactant for personal care, industrial, and agrochem. applics.; wh. solid.

Renex® PEG 4000FL. [ICI Surf. UK] PEG-75 USP/NF; CAS 25322-68-3; surfactant for personal care, industrial, and agrochem. applics.; wh. solid.

Renex® PEG 6000FL. [ICI Surf. UK] PEG-150 USP/NF; CAS 25322-68-3; surfactant for personal care, industrial, and agrochem. applics.; wh. solid.

Renex® PEG 8000FL. [ICI Surf. UK] PEG USP/NF; surfactant for personal care, industrial, and agrochem. applics.; wh. solid.

Resyn® 28-1310. [Nat'l. Starch] Vinyl acetate/crotonic acid copolymer; CAS 25609-89-6; hair fixative; for hair sprays, setting lotions, conditioners, skin applics., cosmetics; dry beads; when neutralized sol. in water, water/alcohol and hydrocarbon/ethanol blends.; 2% volatiles.

Resyn® 28-2913. [Nat'l. Starch] Vinyl acetate/crotonic acid/ vinyl neodecanoate copolymer.; CAS 55353-21-4; hair fixative providing exc. holding power, manageability, gloss; for aerosol and pump hairsprays, setting lotions, spritzes, cosmetics; translucent beads; sol. in low m.w. alcohols (ethanol, IPA); sol. in water when neutralized; 2% volatiles.

Resyn® 28-2930. [Nat'l. Starch] Vinyl acetate/crotonic acid/ vinyl neodecanoate copolymer; CAS 55353-21-4; hair fixative; for aerosol and pump hair sprays, setting lotions, conditioners, spritzes, and cosmetics; fine translucent beads; sol. in anhyd. ethanol and IPA; when neutralized sol. in water; 2% volatiles.

Resyn® 28-3307. [Nat'l. Starch] Carboxylated polyvinyl acetate; uv absorber for hair and skin prods., protective coatings; when neutralized, sol. in water, alcohol/water mixts.

Reticusol. [Croda Inc.; Croda Chem. Ltd.] Hydrolyzed reticulin; moisturizer, conditioner for skin care prods.; pale straw liq.; m.w. 3000; usage level: 0.5-2%; 20% act. in water.

Rewocid® DU 185. [Rewo GmbH] Undecylenamide DEA and diethanolamine; nonionic; detergent, emulsifier used as bacteriocide, thickener, foam stabilizer in shampoos; fungicide, antimycotic agent; yel. visc. liq.; sol. in water, oil, alcohols, glycols; sp.gr. 1.0; high visc.; 100% act.

Rewocid® SBU 185. [Rewo GmbH] Disodium undecylenamido MEA-sulfosuccinate; anionic; fungicide, detergent, foamer used in antidandruff shampoos; pale yel. liq., sl. odor; sol. in alcohol, glycol; sp.gr. 1.0; pH 6.5–7.5 (5% solids); 50% act.

Rewocid® SBU 185 P. [Rewo GmbH] Disodium undecylenamido MEA-sulfosuccinate; anionic; antidandruff shampoo surfactant, fungicide; powd.; 95% conc.

Rewocid® U 185. [Rewo GmbH] Undecylenamide MEA; CAS 20545-92-0; EINECS 243-870-9; nonionic; fungicide, anti-mycotic agent; detergent; improves foam quality, stability, superfatting, increases visc.; yel. flakes; strong odor; sol. in alcohol, glycol, disp. in water; m.p. 50 C; 100% act.

Rewocid® UTM 185. [Rewo GmbH] Undecylenamidopropyltrimonium methosulfate; cationic; bacteri-cide, fungicide for toiletries; conditioner for shampoos, antistat; low visc. liq.; 47% conc.

Rewoderm® ES 90. [Rewo GmbH] PEG-7 glyceryl cocoate; nonionic; emulsifier for cosmetics, superfatting agent, solubilizer; visc. liq.; 100% conc.

Rewoderm® LI 48. [Rewo GmbH] PEG-80 glyceryl tallowate; nonionic; mild surfactant, thickener and super-fatting agent for shampoos, foam baths, baby shampoos; wh. paste; 100% conc.

Rewoderm® LI 48-50. [Rewo GmbH] PEG-80 glyceryl tallowate; nonionic; mild surfactant, thickener for shampoos, foam baths, baby shampoos; gel; 50% conc.

Rewoderm® LI 63. [Rewo GmbH] PEG-30 glyceryl cocoate; nonionic; mild surfactant, thickener, solubilizer and super-fatting agent for shampoos, foam baths, and baby shampoos; soft paste; 100% conc.

Rewoderm® LI 67. [Rewo GmbH] PEG-78 glyceryl cocoate; nonionic; mild surfactant with thickening props. for use in shampoos, foam baths, baby shampoos; wax; 100% conc.

Rewoderm® LI 67-75. [Rewo GmbH] PEG-78 glyceryl cocoate; nonionic; mild surfactant, thickener, solubilizer and superfatting agent for shampoos, foam baths, baby shampoos; med.-visc. liq.; 75% conc.

Rewoderm® LI 420. [Rewo GmbH] PEG-200 glyceryl tallowate; nonionic; mild surfactant with thickening props. for use in shampoos, foam baths, baby shampoos; wax; 100% conc.

Rewoderm® LI 420-70. [Rewo GmbH] PEG-200 glyceryl tallowate; nonionic; mild surfactant, thickener for shampoos, foam baths, baby shampoos; gel; 70% conc.

Rewoderm® LIS 75. [Rewo GmbH] PEG-200 glyceryl tallowate and PEG-7 glyceryl cocoate; nonionic; mild surfactant, thickener, and superfatting agent for cosmetics (shampoos, foam baths, baby shampoos, shower gels); gel; 75% conc.

Rewoderm® LIS 80. [Rewo GmbH] PEG-200 hydrog. glyceryl palmate and PEG-7 glyceryl cocoate; cold-processable mild thickening agent for shampoos, foam baths, baby shampoos, shower gels; liq.; 70% conc.

Rewoderm® S 1333. [Rewo GmbH] PEG-78 glyceryl MEA-sulfosuccinate; anionic; detergent for very mild and skin-friendly shampoos, intimate preps., dermatological lotions, skin protection prods., washing up liqs.; decreases irritancy of alkylbenzene sulfonate and other surfactants; emulsifier for emulsion polymerization; amber liq.; pH 6.5–7.5 (5%); surf. tens. 28 mN/m; 40% act.

Rewoderm® SPS. [Rewo GmbH] Disodium sitosteareth-14 sulfosuccinate; anionic; surfactant for shampoos, shower and foam baths, mild skin cleaners, baby shampoos, skin care prods.; liq.; 35% conc.

Rewolan® 5. [Rewo GmbH] Disodium laneth-5 sulfosuccinate; anionic; detergent, moisturizer, superfatting agent for personal care prods.; skin protective agent; liq.; pH 6.5–7.5 (5% solids); 50% act.

Rewolan® AWS. [Rewo GmbH] PEG-75 lanolin oil; CAS 68648-38-4; nonionic; superfatting agent for shower and foam baths, shampoos, hair sprays, hair lotions; visc. liq.; 100% conc.

Rewolan® E 50, E 100. [Rewo GmbH] PEG-75 lanolin; CAS 61790-81-6; nonionic; superfatting agent for shower and foam baths, shampoos, liq. soaps; visc. liq. and hard wax resp.; 50 and 100% conc. resp.

Rewolan® LP. [Rewo GmbH] Isopropyl lanolate and lanolin; nonionic; emollient for skin care, toiletries; liq.; 100% conc.

Rewomid® C 212. [Rewo GmbH] Cocamide MEA; CAS 68140-00-1; EINECS 268-770-2; nonionic; detergent, thickener, foam booster/stabilizer, superfatting agent used in detergent products; stabilizer for emulsions; off-wh. flakes; amidic slight odor; m.p. 73 C; 100% act.

Rewomid® DC 212 LS. [Rewo GmbH] Cocamide DEA; CAS 61791-31-9; EINECS 263-163-9; cosmetic surfactant.

Rewomid® DC 212 S. [Rewo GmbH] Cocamide DEA; CAS 61791-31-9; EINECS 263-163-9; nonionic; detergent, foam stabilizer and visc. modifier used for shampoos, foam baths, and all-purpose detergents; lt. yel. visc. liq.; slight odor; dens. 0.99 g/cm³; 100% act.

Rewomid® DC 212 SE. [Rewo GmbH] Cocamide DEA; CAS 61791-31-9; EINECS 263-163-9; nonionic; foam booster/ stabilizer, detergent, detergent builder, thickener for toiletries; med. visc. liq.; 100% conc.

Rewomid® DC 220 SE. [Rewo GmbH] Cocamide DEA; CAS 61791-31-9; EINECS 263-163-9; nonionic; detergent, thickener, foam stabilizer and superfatting agent; soft paste; 100% act.

Rewomid® DL 203 S. [Rewo GmbH] Lauramide DEA and diethanolamine; nonionic; foam booster/stabilizer, super-fatting agent, and thickener for personal care prods., floor cleaners, general purpose cleaners, textile lubricants;

wax; 100% conc.

Rewomid® DL 240. [Rewo GmbH] Cocamide DEA (2:1) and diethanolamine; nonionic; detergent, thickener added to cosmetic preparations and household cleaning and washing agents; stabilizer of emulsions; superfatting agent; yel. liq.; faint odor; visc. med.; 100% act.

Rewomid® DO 280. [Rewo GmbH] Oleamide DEA and diethanolamine; nonionic; detergent, thickener, and superfatting agent for cosmetic and household prods.; amber liq.; slight odor; sp.gr. 1.0; 100% act.

Rewomid® DO 280 S. [Rewo GmbH] Mixed fatty acid DEA; nonionic; emulsifier; superfatter; aerosol anticorrosive agent; hair cosmetic specialty; cream bath additive; dye and perfume solubilizer; paste; 100% conc.

Rewomid® DO 280 SE. [Rewo GmbH] Oleamide DEA (1:1); CAS 93-83-4; EINECS 202-281-7; nonionic; detergent, thickener, foam booster/stabilizer, superfatting agent for cosmetic products; conditioner for shampoos, bath oils; honey liq.; dens. 0.96 g/cm³; 100% act.

Rewomid® F. [Rewo GmbH] Linoleamide DEA and diethanolamine; nonionic; foam booster, superfatting agent and thickener for shampoos; med. visc. liq.; 100% conc.

Rewomid® IPE 280. [Rewo GmbH] Oleamide MIPA; CAS 111-05-7; EINECS 203-828-2; nonionic; detergent, emulsifier, foam stabilizer, thickener, superfatting agent; additive for skin protecting products; yel. paste; slight odor; 100% act.

Rewomid® IPL 203. [Rewo GmbH] Lauramide MIPA; CAS 142-54-1; EINECS 205-541-8; nonionic; foam stabilizer, thickener, detergent for shampoos, shaving foams, and dishwashing liqs.; additive for solid and paste end prods.; improved washing power; stabilizer of emulsions; wh. flakes; slight odor; m.p. 55 C; 100% act.

Rewomid® IPP 240. [Rewo GmbH] Cocamide MIPA; CAS 68333-82-4; EINECS 269-793-0; nonionic; detergent, foam stabilizer, thickener, additive for solid and paste end prods.; improved washing power; emulsion stabilizer; wh. flakes; slight odor; m.p. 50 C; 100% act.

Rewomid® L 203. [Rewo GmbH] Lauramide MEA; CAS 142-78-9; EINECS 205-560-1; nonionic; detergent, thickener, foam booster/stabilizer, superfatting agent for detergent preparations; fixation of perfumes; stabilizer of emulsions; wh. flakes; slight odor; m.p. 84 C; 100% act.

Rewomid® R 280. [Rewo GmbH] Ricinoleamide MEA; CAS 106-16-1; EINECS 203-368-2; nonionic; surfactant for syn. soap bars; foam stabilizer, thickener; wax; 100% conc.

Rewomid® S 280. [Rewo GmbH] Stearamide MEA; CAS 111-57-9; EINECS 203-883-2; nonionic; detergent, thickener, foam booster, superfatting agent; stabilizer of emulsions; syn. soap bars; anti-inflammatory agent; wh. flakes; slight odor; m.p. 92 C; 100% act.

Rewominox B 204. [Rewo GmbH] Cocamidopropylamine oxide; CAS 68155-09-9; EINECS 268-938-5; nonionic; foam booster, thickener for shampoos, foam baths; antistat; hair conditioner; skin compatible; liq.; 35% conc.

Rewominox L 408. [Rewo GmbH] Lauramine oxide; CAS 1643-20-5; EINECS 216-700-6; nonionic; foam booster, thickener for shampoos, foam baths; hair conditioner; antistat; liq.; 30% conc.

Rewominox S 300. [Rewo GmbH] Stearamine oxide; CAS 2571-88-2; EINECS 219-919-5; nonionic; foam booster, antistat, hair conditioning agent; liq.; 25% conc.

Rewomul HL. [Rewo GmbH] Hexyl laurate; CAS 34316-64-8; EINECS 251-932-1; emollient, vehicle for cosmetics.

Rewomul IS. [Rewo GmbH] Isostearyl isostearate; CAS 41669-30-1; EINECS 255-485-3; emollient.

Rewomul MG. [Rewo GmbH] Glyceryl stearate; nonionic; emulsifier for cosmetics; flake; 100% conc.

Rewomul MG SE. [Rewo GmbH] Glyceryl stearate SE; CAS

977053-96-5; nonionic; emulsifier for cosmetic creams and lotions; waxy flakes; HLB 5.5; 100% conc.

Rewopal® C 6. [Rewo GmbH] PEG-6 cocamide; CAS 61791-08-0; nonionic; dispersant, emulsifier, foam booster, wetting agent for calcium soap, personal care prods.; solubilizer for perfume oils; amber liq.; cloud pt. 80–90 C (2%); pH 8–10 (1% solids); 100% act.

Rewopal® LA 3. [Rewo GmbH] Laureth-3; CAS 3055-94-5; EINECS 221-280-2; nonionic; emulsifier for solvs. (cold water detergents), cosmetic oils (bath oils), min. oils (textile aux., metalworking); intermediate, coupler, raw material for the prod. of ether sulfates and sulfosuccinates; clear liq.; sol. in min. and org. solvs.; pH 5–7 (1% solids); biodeg.; 100% conc.

Rewopal® LA 6. [Rewo GmbH] Laureth-6; CAS 3055-96-7; EINECS 221-282-3; nonionic; detergent; liq.; 100% conc.

Rewopal® MPG 10. [Rewo GmbH] Phenoxyethanol; CAS 122-99-6; EINECS 204-589-7; nonionic; solv., solubilizer, preservative; liq.; 100% conc.

Rewopal® PEG 6000 DS. [Rewo GmbH] PEG-150 distearate; CAS 9005-08-7; nonionic; thickener for personal care prods.; flake; 100% conc.

Rewopal® PG 280. [Rewo GmbH] Glycol distearate; CAS 627-83-8; EINECS 211-014-3; anionic; pearlizing agent for cosmetics; flake; 100% conc.

Rewopal® PG 340. [Rewo GmbH] Glycol dibehenate; CAS 79416-55-0; nonionic; pearlizing agent for cosmetics and detergents; flake; 100% conc.

Rewopol® ALS 30. [Rewo GmbH] Ammonium lauryl sulfate; CAS 2235-54-3; EINECS 218-793-9; anionic; surfactant for shampoos, foam baths; liq.; 28% conc.

Rewopol® CL 30. [Rewo GmbH] Laureth-3 carboxylic acid; anionic; surfactant for household cleaners and toiletries; liq.; 90% conc.

Rewopol® CLN 100. [Rewo GmbH] Sodium laureth-11 carboxylate; CAS 33939-64-9; anionic; surfactant for toiletries (shampoo, shower gel, liq. soap); liq.; 23% conc.

Rewopol® CT 65. [Rewo GmbH] Trideceth-7 carboxylic acid; anionic; acid-stable cleaner for household and industrial use, textile auxiliaries, min. oil emulsions, tert. oil recovery; emulsifier, wetting agent for personal care products; opaque liq.; 90% conc.

Rewopol® HM 14. [Rewo GmbH] Surfactant blend; anionic; mild shampoos, bath preps.; liq.; 28% conc.

Rewopol® HM 30. [Rewo GmbH] Surfactant blend; for mild shampoos and bath preps.; liq.; 28% solids.

Rewopol® MLS 30. [Rewo GmbH] MEA-lauryl sulfate; CAS 4722-98-9; EINECS 225-214-3; anionic; surfactant for personal care products, foam baths, shampoos, liq. detergents; detergent raw material; visc. liq.; 30% conc.

Rewopol® NL 2-28. [Rewo GmbH] Sodium laureth sulfate; CAS 9004-82-4; anionic; surfactant for shampoos, shower gels, foam baths, liq. soaps, dishwashing liqs., emulsion polymerization, air entrainment agent, textile auxiliaries; liq.; 28% conc.

Rewopol® NL 3. [Rewo GmbH] Sodium laureth sulfate; CAS 9004-82-4; anionic; detergent, foamer; cleaning formulations; personal care products; emulsifier for emulsion polymerization; BGA compliance; colorless clear liq.; low odor; visc. 50–150 cps; pH 6.5-7.5 (1%); surf. tens. 38 mN/m; 28% act.

Rewopol® NL 3-28. [Rewo GmbH] Sodium laureth sulfate; CAS 9004-82-4; anionic; surfactant for shampoos, shower gels, foam baths, liq. soaps, dishwashing liqs., emulsion polymerization, air entrainment agent, textile auxiliaries; liq.; 28% conc.

Rewopol® NL 3-70. [Rewo GmbH] Sodium laureth sulfate; CAS 9004-82-4; anionic; surfactant for shampoos, shower gels, foam baths, liq. soaps, dishwashing liqs., emulsion polymerization, air entrainment agent, textile auxiliaries; paste; HLB 18.0; 70% conc.

Rewopol® NLS 28. [Rewo GmbH] Sodium lauryl sulfate; CAS 151-21-3; EINECS 205-788-1; anionic; detergent, emulsifier in emulsion polymerization; raw material for lt. duty detergents, body cleaning agents, shampoos, detergent pastes, cosmetics; air entrainment agents; BGA and FDA compliance; lt. yel. low visc. liq.; water-sol.; m.w. 300; pH 7–8 (1%); surf. tens. 30 mN/m; 28% act.

Rewopol® NLS 90. [Rewo GmbH] Sodium lauryl sulfate; CAS 151-21-3; EINECS 205-788-1; anionic; raw material for mild detergents, syndet soaps, shampoos in powd. form; wh.-lt. yel. powd.; m.w. 300; pH 7–9 (1% solids); 95% conc.

Rewopol® PGK 2000. [Rewo GmbH] Surfactant blend with pearlizing agent; anionic; pearlizing agent for shampoos, foam baths, household cleaners; liq.; 35% conc.

Rewopol® SBC 212. [Rewo GmbH] Disodium cocamido MEA-sulfosuccinate; anionic; surfactant for foam cleaners, lt. duty detergents, shampoos, foam baths; low visc. liq.; 40% conc.

Rewopol® SBC 212 G. [Rewo GmbH] Disodium cocamido MEA-sulfosuccinate; anionic; surfactant for foam cleaners, lt. duty detergents, and personal care products; granules; 95% conc.

Rewopol® SBC 212 P. [Rewo GmbH] Disodium cocamido MEA-sulfosuccinate; surfactant for foam cleaners, lt. duty detergents, shampoos; powd.; 95% solids.

Rewopol® SBCS 50. [Rewo GmbH] Disodium PEG-10 laurylcitrate sulfosuccinate; surfactant for mild, skin-friendly shampoos, shower and foam baths, baby shampoos, skin cleansers; liq.; 40% solids.

Rewopol® SBDO 75. [Rewo GmbH] Dioctyl sodium sulfosuccinate; CAS 577-11-7; EINECS 209-406-4; anionic; wetting agent, solubilizer; emulsion polymerization; BGA and FDA compliance; visc. liq.; sol. 10 g/1000 ml water; very sol. in org. solvs.; pH 5-7 (1%); surf. tens. 27 dynes/cm; 75% conc.

Rewopol® SBE 280. [Rewo GmbH] Disodium oleamido MEA-sulfosuccinate.

Rewopol® SBF 12. [Rewo GmbH] Disodium lauryl sulfosuccinate; anionic; detergent raw material for personal care products, soaps; spray drying additive; carpet and upholstery shampoos; toilet and syndet soaps; wh. paste; pH 6.5–7.5 (5% solids); 40% solids.

Rewopol® SBF 18. [Rewo GmbH] Disodium stearyl sulfosuccinamate; CAS 14481-60-8; EINECS 238-479-5; anionic; raw material for detergents; additive to syndet soap; flakes; 95% conc.

Rewopol® SBFA 30. [Rewo GmbH] Disodium laureth sulfosuccinate; anionic; detergent raw material for personal care products, mild shampoos, skin-friendly foam baths, liq. soaps, cleansing agents; colorless clear liq.; visc. 100–299 cps; pH 6.5–7.5 (5% solids); 40% solids.

Rewopol® SBL 203. [Rewo GmbH] Disodium lauramido MEA-sulfosuccinate; CAS 25882-44-4; EINECS 247-310-4; anionic; detergent for mild detergents, syndet bar soaps, shampoos; aids spray-drying; carpet and upholstery shampoos; yel. turbid paste; pH 6.5–7.5 (5% solids); 40% solids.

Rewopol® SBLC, SBLC G. [Rewo GmbH] Fatty acid alkylolamide sulfosuccinate; anionic; surfactant for foam cleaners, lt. duty detergents, shampoos; paste, granules resp.; 40 and 95% conc.

Rewopol® SBV. [Rewo GmbH] Disodium laureth sulfosuccinate, sodium laureth sulfate, cocamide DEA; anionic; raw material for mild and skin-friendly bubble baths, shampoos, dishwashing and lt. duty detergents; lt. yel. clear liq.; visc. 2500 cps; pH 6.5–7.5 (1% solids); 28% min. solids.

Rewopol® SBZ. [Rewo GmbH] Disodium PEG-4 cocamido

MIPA-sulfosuccinate; anionic; surfactant for mild and skin-friendly foam baths, shampoos, lt. duty detergents; low visc. liq.; 50% conc.

Rewopol® TLS 40. [Rewo GmbH] TEA-lauryl sulfate; CAS 139-96-8; EINECS 205-388-7; anionic; surfactant raw material for shampoos, foam baths, liq. detergents; liq.; 40% conc.

Rewopol® TLS 90 L. [Rewo GmbH] TIPA-lauryl sulfate; CAS 66161-60-2; anionic; raw material for high active ingred. cosmetic prods., foaming bath oils; med. visc. liq.; 75% conc.

Rewoquat CPEM. [Rewo GmbH] PEG-5 cocomonium methosulfate; CAS 68989-03-7; cationic; conditioner for antistatic hair care prods., emulsifier in emulsion polymerization; visc. liq.; 100% conc.

Rewoquat DQ 35. [Rewo GmbH] PEG-3 tallow propylenedimonium dimethosulfate; CAS 93572-63-5; EINECS 297-495-0; cationic; antistat and wetting agent; liq.; 35% conc.

Rewoquat RTM 50. [Rewo GmbH] Ricinoleamidopropyltrimonium methosulfate; CAS 85508-38-9; EINECS 287-462-9; cationic; conditioner for shampoos, liq. soaps; antistat; low visc. liq.; 40% conc.

Rewoquat W 75. [Rewo GmbH] Quaternium-27; cationic; fabric softener, hair care prods.; liq.; 75% conc.

Rewoquat W 75 PG. [Rewo GmbH] Quaternium-27, free of isopropanol; cationic; fabric softener, hair care prods.; liq.; 75% conc.

Rewoquat W 222 PG. [Rewo GmbH] Quaternium-53; CAS 68410-69-5; hair conditioner.

Rewoquat WE 16. [Rewo GmbH] Quaternary dialkyl ester; fabric softener, hair care prods.; paste; 90% conc.

Rewoquat WE 18. [Rewo GmbH] Quaternary dialkyl ester; fabric softener, hair care prods.; paste; 90% conc.

Rewoquat WE 18-85. [Rewo GmbH] Quaternary dialkyl ester; fabric softener, hair care prods.; paste; 85% conc.

Rewoquat WE 20. [Rewo GmbH] Quaternary dialkyl ester; fabric softener, hair care prods.; paste; 90% conc.

Rewoquat WE 28. [Rewo GmbH] Quaternary dipalm ester; fabric softener, hair care prods.; paste; 90% conc.

Reworyl® K. [Rewo GmbH] Dodecylbenzene sulfonic acid; CAS 27176-87-0; EINECS 248-289-4; anionic; biodeg. raw material for anionic detergent systems; liq.; 97% conc.

Rewotein CPK. [Rewo GmbH] Potassium cocoyl hydrolyzed collagen; CAS 68920-65-0; for very mild and skin-friendly shampoos, foam baths, shower gels, skin cleansers for sensitive skin; liq.; 32% conc.

Rewotein CPT. [Rewo GmbH] TEA-cocoyl hydrolyzed collagen; CAS 68952-16-9; for very mild and skin-friendly shampoos, foam baths, shower gels, skin cleansers for sensitive skin; liq.; 32% conc.

Rewoteric® AM 2C NM. [Rewo GmbH] Disodium cocoamphodiacetate; CAS 61791-32-0; amphoteric; mild nonirritating raw material for foam baths, shampoos, intimate hygiene and baby prods.; visc. liq.; pH 8.0-8.6 (12.5%); wetting 1 min 10 s; Ross-Miles foam 180/170 mm; 50% conc.

Rewoteric® AM 2C SF. [Rewo GmbH] Disodium cocoamphodipropionate; high-foaming surfactant for baby and intimate hygiene prods.; exc. for high pH systems; coupler and detergent in high electrolyte formulations; liq.; 40% solids.

Rewoteric® AM 2C W. [Witco/H-I-P] Disodium cocoamphodiacetate; CAS 68650-39-5; EINECS 272-043-5; amphoteric; high-foaming surfactant for low-irritation shampoos, foam baths, skin cleansers, medicated cosmetics; conditioning agent; visc. liq.; 50% conc.; formerly Varion 2C.

Rewoteric® AM 2L-40. [Witco/H-I-P] Disodium lauroamphodiacetate; CAS 14350-97-1; EINECS 238-306-3; amphoteric; mild nonirritating raw material for baby shampoos, mild shampoos, foam baths, intimate hygiene prods.; liq.; 40% conc.; formerly Varion 2L.

Rewoteric® AM 2T. [Rewo GmbH] Disodium tallow-amphodiacetate.

Rewoteric® AM B 13. [Rewo GmbH] Cocamidopropyl betaine; amphoteric; foam booster for foam baths, shower gels, shampoos, liq. soaps, all-purpose cleaners; liq.; 35% conc.

Rewoteric® AM B-13. [Witco/H-I-P] Cocamidopropyl betaine; CAS 61789-40-0; amphoteric; mild raw material, foam booster, visc. builder for personal care products (shampoos, skin cleansers), liq. soaps, all-purpose cleaners; lime soap dispersant; coemulsifier; low visc. liq.; pH 5-6 (10%); wetting 1 min 34 s; Ross-Miles foam 200/185 mm; 35% conc.

Rewoteric® AM B-14. [Witco/H-I-P] Cocamidopropyl betaine; CAS 61789-40-0; amphoteric; mild raw material, foam booster, visc. builder for shampoos, bubble baths, liq. soaps, all-purpose cleaners; lime soap dispersant; liq.; 35% conc.; formerly Varion AM B-14, Varion CADG-W.

Rewoteric® AM B 14 [Rewo GmbH] Cocamidopropyl betaine; amphoteric; foam booster for foam baths, shower gels, shampoos, liq. soaps, all-purpose cleaners; liq.; 35% conc.

Rewoteric® AM B-14 LS. [Witco/H-I-P] Cocamidopropyl betaine; low-salt surfactant for personal care prods.; liq.; 35% solids.; formerly Varion CADG-LS.

Rewoteric® AM B-15. [Witco/H-I-P] Cocamidopropyl betaine; foam booster for shampoos, visc. builder, low-irritation skin cleanser, lime soap dispersant; aids in deposition of protein and cationic polymers on hair; coemulsifier; liq.; 35% solids.; formerly Varion CADG-HS.

Rewoteric® AM CA. [Rewo GmbH] Disodium lauroamphodiacetate and sodium laureth sulfate; amphoteric; raw material for mild foam baths, hair shampoos, baby preps.; med. visc. liq.; pH 8.0-8.5 (10%); 30% conc.

Rewoteric® AM CAS. [Witco/H-I-P] Cocamidopropyl hydroxysultaine; CAS 68139-30-0; EINECS 268-761-3; amphoteric; high-foaming mild detergent for shampoos, bubble bath; coemulsifier; liq.; 50% solids.; formerly Varion CAS-W.

Rewoteric® AM CAS. [Rewo GmbH] Cocamidopropyl hydroxysultaine; CAS 68139-30-0; EINECS 268-761-3; amphoteric; surfactant for shampoos, baby prods., foam baths, shower gels, acidic and alkaline cleaners; liq.; 50% conc.

Rewoteric® AM CAS-15. [Witco/H-I-P] Cocamidopropyl hydroxysultaine; CAS 68139-30-0; EINECS 268-761-3; amphoteric; high-foaming mild detergent used in shampoos, bubble baths, and acid and alkaline cleaners; coemulsifier; better response to salt than regular betaines; low visc. liq.; pH 7-8 (10%); wetting 1 min 34 s; Ross-Miles foam 170/165 mm; 50% conc.; formerly Varion CAS.

Rewoteric® AM DML. [Rewo GmbH] Lauryl betaine; CAS 683-10-3; EINECS 211-669-5; amphoteric; surfactant for shampoos, foam baths, hard surf. cleaners; liq.; 40% conc.

Rewoteric® AM DML-35. [Witco/H-I-P] Lauryl betaine; CAS 11140-78-6; amphoteric; high-foaming mild surfactant for baby shampoos, hard surf. cleaners, steam jet cleaners, and pickling baths; Gardner 1 max. liq.; pH 7-8 (10%); 35% conc.

Rewoteric® AM G 30. [Rewo GmbH] Sodium lauroamphoacetate, sodium lauryl sulfate and hexylene glycol; amphoteric; surfactant for baby and child care cosmetic formulations, shower baths, shampoos; low visc. liq.; pH 7.5-8.5 (10%); 38% conc.

Rewoteric® AM HC. [Witco/H-I-P] Lauryl hydroxysultaine; CAS 13197-76-7; EINECS 236-164-7; amphoteric; mild

detergent, foam booster, skin conditioning agent; hydrotrope; exc. for high pH systems; liq.; 50% conc.; formerly Varion HC.

Rewoteric® AM KSF-40. [Rewo GmbH] Sodium cocoamphopropionate, salt-free; CAS 93820-52-1; amphoteric; raw material, high-foaming surfactant, wetting agent used in personal care products (baby and intimate hygiene prods.) and industrial cleaners; exc. for high pH systems; visc. liq.; pH 9-10 (10%); wetting 1 min 12 s; Ross-Miles foam 175/165 mm; 40% conc.; formerly Varion AM KSF-40.

Rewoteric® AM LP. [Witco/H-I-P] Sodium lauryliminodipropionate; CAS 14960-06-6; EINECS 239-032-7; high-foaming surfactant for baby and intimate hygiene prods.; exc. for high pH systems; liq.; 40% solids.; formerly Varion LP.

Rewoteric® AM R40. [Rewo GmbH] Ricinoleamidopropyl betaine; CAS 86089-12-5; amphoteric; mild cosmetic and medicated cleaning agents; baby shampoos; med. visc. liq.; pH 5.5-6.0 (10%); 40% conc.

Rewoteric® AM TEG. [Rewo GmbH] Dihydroxyethyl tallow glycinate; CAS 61791-25-1; EINECS 274-845-0; cationic; high-foaming mild surfactant for acidic and alkaline cleaning products, conditioning shampoos, bubble baths; conditioner, thickener; amber hazy liq.; pH 4.5-5.5 (10%); wetting 2 min 30 s; Ross-Miles foam 145/135 mm; 40% solids.; formerly Varion TEG.

Rewoteric® QAM 50. [Rewo GmbH] Cocobetainamido amphopropionate; CAS 100085-64-1; EINECS 309-206-8; cationic/amphoteric; surfactant for hard surf. disinfectants, skin disinfectants, deodorants, cleaning and bacteriocidal prods. for use in industrial catering, hotels, hospitals, and households; biodeg.; straw clear liq.; pH 8-9 (10% aq.); Draves wetting 1 min 4 s; Ross-Miles foam 180/0; toxicology: LD50 (acute oral, rat) 5100 mg/kg; 50% conc.

Rewowax CG. [Rewo GmbH] Cetyl palmitate; CAS 540-10-3; EINECS 208-736-6; nonionic; spermaceti wax replacement; emulsifier for cosmetic creams and lotions; flakes; 100% conc.

Rexol AE-1. [Hart Chem. Ltd.] Linear alcohol ethoxylate; nonionic; intermediate for shampoo and detergent mfg.; liq.; HLB 4.2; cloud pt. 36–39 C (1% in 25% diethylene glycol butyl ether); 100% act.

Rexol AE-2. [Hart Chem. Ltd.] Linear alcohol ethoxylate; nonionic; intermediate for shampoo and detergent mfg.; liq.; HLB 6.1; cloud pt. 50-52 C (1% in 25% diethylene glycol butyl ether); 100% act.

Rexol AE-23. [Hart Chem. Ltd.] Linear alcohol ethoxylate; nonionic; dispersant, emulsifier in cosmetic applications; solid; HLB 17.0; cloud pt. 90–95 C (1% in 5% NaCl); 100% act.

Rexonic N91-6. [Hart Chem. Ltd.] Alcohol ethoxylate; nonionic; detergent for industrial use; emulsifier; shampoo intermediate, dispersant; biodeg.; liq.; water-sol.; HLB 12.5; cloud pt. 51–53 C (1% aq.); 100% act.

Rexonic N91-8. [Hart Chem. Ltd.] Alcohol ethoxylate; nonionic; detergent, emulsifier, dispersant for general industrial usage, hard surf. cleaners, liq. detergents; shampoo intermediate; biodeg.; liq.; water-sol.; HLB 14.1; cloud pt. 80-82 C (1% aq.); 100% act.

Rezal® 36. [Reheis] Aluminum zirconium tetrachlorohydrex-glycine; antiperspirant active for high alcohol content antiperspirants; liq.; 45% total solids.

Rezal® 36G. [Reheis] Aluminum zirconium tetra-chlorohydrex-glycine; antiperspirant active for aq. nonaerosol systems, roll-ons, creams; liq.; 35% act.

Rezal® 36G Conc. [Reheis] Aluminum zirconium tetrachlorohydrex-glycine; antiperspirant active for nonaerosol systems; liq.; 46% act.

Rezal® 36GP. [Reheis] Aluminum zirconium tetrachlorohydrex-glycine; antiperspirant active for suspension roll-ons and suspensoid type sticks; powd.; 98.5% min. thru 325 mesh.

Rezal® 36GP Superultrafine. [Reheis] Aluminum zirconium tetrachlorohydrex-glycine; antiperspirant active for suspension roll-ons and suspensoid sticks; fine particle size results in improved aesthetics; powd.; 85% min. thru 10 μ.

Rezal® 67. [Reheis] Aluminum zirconium pentachlorohydrate; antiperspirant active for hydroalcoholic and aq. systems such as clear and emulsified roll-ons and creams; liq.; 40% act.

Rezal® 67P. [Reheis] Aluminum zirconium pentachlorohydrate; antiperspirant active for use in suspensoid sticks and suspension roll-ons; powd., 97% thru 325 mesh.

Rhaballgum CG-M. [Ikeda] Guar hydroxypropyltrimonium chloride; CAS 65497-29-2; stabilizer, thickener, emulsifier, dispersant, suspending agent, gellant for cosmetics; wh. to sl. ylsh. powd., faint char. odor; sol. in water; visc. 1500-3000 cps (1%); pH 5.0-7.5.

Rheodol 440. [Kao Corp. SA] PEG-40 sorbitan tetraoleate; CAS 9003-11-6; nonionic; emulsifier for cosmetics; liq.; HLB 11.8; 100% conc.

Rheodol 460. [Kao Corp. SA] PEG-60 sorbitan tetraoleate; emulsifier, solubilizer.

Rheopearl KL. [Chiba Flour Milling] Dextrin palmitate; CAS 83271-10-7.

Rhodacal® 301-10F. [Rhone-Poulenc Surf. & Spec.] Sodium C14-16 olefin sulfonate; CAS 68439-57-6; EINECS 270-407-8; anionic; detergent, foam booster, emulsifier, wetting agent, dispersant for dry bubble baths, powd. hand soaps, lt. duty and fine fabric detergents, metal soak cleaners, aerosol rug and upholstery cleaners; flake; 90% conc.; formerly Siponate® 301-10F.

Rhodacal® 330. [Rhone-Poulenc Surf. & Spec.] Isopropylamine dodecylbenzene sulfonate; CAS 26264-05-1; EINECS 247-556-2; anionic; emulsifier, wetting agent, grease/pigment dispersant, lubricant, solubilizer, solv., penetrant, high foaming base for shampoos and cleaners, metalworking fluids, agric. pesticides, emulsion polymerization, drycleaning, latex paints, metal cleaning; amber liq.; oil-sol.; sp.gr. 1.03; dens. 8.497 lb/gal; visc. 6500 cps; HLB 11.7; flash pt. > 200 C; pH 3-6 (5%); 90% act.; formerly Siponate® 330.

Rhodacal® A-246L. [Rhone-Poulenc Surf. & Spec.] Sodium C14-16 olefin sulfonate; CAS 68439-57-6; EINECS 270-407-8; anionic; detergent, foaming agent, emulsifier, wetting agent, dispersant for hair shampoos, liq. soaps, skin cleansers, industrial cleaners, emulsion polymerization; liq.; surf. tens. 29 dynes/cm (@ CMC); 40% act.; formerly Siponate® A-246L.

Rhodacal® A-246 LX. [Rhone-Poulenc Surf. & Spec.] Sodium C14-16 olefin sulfonate; CAS 68439-57-6; EINECS 270-407-8; detergent, visc. builder; liq.; 40% act.; formerly Siponate® A-246 LX.

Rhodacal® DDB 60T. [Rhone-Poulenc Surf. & Spec.] TEA-dodecylbenzenesulfonate; CAS 27323-41-7; EINECS 248-406-9; personal care surfactant; formerly Siponate® DDB 60T.

Rhodafac® MC-470. [Rhone-Poulenc Surf. & Spec.] Sodium laureth-4 phosphate; CAS 42612-52-2; anionic; detergent, emulsifier, visc. builder for creams and lotions, facial cleansers, polymerization and stabilization of latexes; fatliquoring of leathers; metalworking fluids; textile antistat, lubricant, softener; emulsifier for min. oils; clear visc. liq.; sol. in min. oil, kerosene, xylene, perchloroethylene, disp. in water; sp.gr. 1.02-1.04; dens. 8.580 lb/gal; pour pt. 0 C; flash pt. > 200 C; pH 5.0-6.5 (10%); 95% act.; formerly Gafac® RM-470.

Rhodafac® RD-510. [Rhone-Poulenc Surf. & Spec.] Laureth-4 phosphate; CAS 39464-66-9; anionic; emulsifier, antistat, lubricant, solubilizer for fibers, metals, cosmetics, agric. formulations; FDA, EPA compliance; clear visc. liq.; sol. in min. oil, kerosene, xylene, butyl Cellosolve, perchloroethylene, ethanol; disp. in water; sp.gr. 1.05-1.06; dens. 8.8 lb/gal; pour pt. 13 C; pH < 2.5 (10%); 98% act.; formerly Gafac® RD-510.

Rhodafac® RM-510. [Rhone-Poulenc Surf. & Spec.] Nonyl nonoxynol-10 phosphate; CAS 39464-64-7; anionic; emulsifier for chlorinated and phosphated pesticide concs., polyethylene; wetting agent, emulsifier for industrial cleaners, drycleaning, cosmetics; EPA compliance; hazy, visc. liq.; sol. in kerosene, Stod., xylene, butyl Cellosolve, perchloroethylene, ethanol; disp. in water; sp.gr. 1.05-1.07; dens. 8.8 lb/gal; pour pt. 5 C; pH < 2.5 (10%); 100% act.; formerly Gafac® RM-510.

Rhodafac® RM-710. [Rhone-Poulenc Surf. & Spec.] Nonyl nonoxynol-15 phosphate; CAS 39464-64-7; anionic; emulsifier for chlorinated and phosphated pesticide concs. and polyethylene; wetting agent, emulsifier for industrial cleaners, drycleaning, cosmetics; EPA compliance; hazy, visc. liq.; sol. in xylene, butyl Cellosolve, perchloroethylene, ethanol, water; sp.gr. 1.06-1.08; dens. 8.9 lb/gal; pour pt. 15 C; acid no. 33-41; pH < 3 (10%); 100% conc.; formerly Gafac® RM-710.

Rhodameen® OS-12. [Rhone-Poulenc Surf. & Spec.] PEG-2 oleyl/stearyl amine; cationic; coemulsifier and antistat for cosmetics, textile and plastic processing; flowable paste; 99% conc.; formerly Rhodiasurf OS-12.

Rhodamox® CAPO. [Rhone-Poulenc Surf. & Spec.] Cocamidopropyl dimethylamine oxide; CAS 68155-09-9; EINECS 268-938-5; nonionic/cationic; foaming agent/stabilizer, thickener, emollient for shampoos, bath prods., dishwash, rug shampoos, fine fabric detergents, shaving creams, lotions, foam rubber, electroplating, paper coatings; used in toiletries for mildness; colorless clear liq.; faint odor; water sol.; disp. in min. oil; dens. 1.0 g/ml; f.p. < 0 C; 30% conc.; formerly Alkamox® CAPO.

Rhodamox® LO. [Rhone-Poulenc Surf. & Spec.] Lauryl dimethylamine oxide; CAS 1643-20-5; EINECS 216-700-6; cationic; foaming agent/stabilizer, thickener, emollient for shampoos, bath prods., dishwash, fine fabric detergents, shaving creams, lotions, textile softeners, foam rubber, in electroplating, paper coatings; used in toiletries for mildness; colorless clear liq.; faint odor; water sol.; disp. in min. oil; dens. 1.0 g/ml; f.p. < 0 C; 30% conc.; formerly Alkamox® LO, Cyclomox® L.

Rhodapex® 674/C. [Rhone-Poulenc Surf. & Spec.] Sodium trideceth sulfate; CAS 25446-78-0.

Rhodapex® CO-433. [Rhone-Poulenc Surf. & Spec.] Sodium nonoxynol-4 sulfate; CAS 68891-39-4; anionic; high foaming detergent, wetting agent, dispersant for dishwashing, scrub soaps, car washes, rug and hair shampoos; emulsifier for emulsion polymerization, petrol. waxes; antistat for plastics and syn. fibers; lime soap dispersant; FDA compliance; Varnish 4 max. clear liq.; mild aromatic odor; water-sol.; sp.gr. 1.065; dens. 8.9 lb/gal; visc. 2500 cps; surf. tens. 32 dynes/cm (1%); 28% act.; formerly Alipal® CO-433.

Rhodapex® CO-436. [Rhone-Poulenc Surf. & Spec.] Ammonium nonoxynol-4 sulfate; CAS 9051-57-4; anionic; high foaming detergent, wetting agent, dispersant for dishwashing, scrub soaps, car washes, rug and hair shampoos; emulsifier for emulsion polymerization, petrol. waxes; antistat for plastics and syn. fibers; lime soap dispersant; FDA, EPA compliance; Varnish 5 max clear liq.; alcoholic odor; water-sol.; sp.gr. 1.065; dens. 8.9 lb/gal; visc. 100 cps; surf. tens. 34 dynes/cm (1%); 58% act.; formerly Alipal® CO-436.

Rhodapex® EA-2. [Rhone-Poulenc Surf. & Spec.] Ammonium laureth sulfate; CAS 67762-19-0; anionic; detergent used in personal care prods.; liq.; 26% conc.; formerly Sipon EA-2.

Rhodapex® ES. [Rhone-Poulenc Surf. & Spec.] Sodium laureth (3) sulfate; CAS 9004-82-4; anionic; emulsifier, high foaming base for shampoos, lt. duty detergents, bubble baths; polymerization surfactant; liq.; 27% conc.; formerly Sipon® ES.

Rhodapex® ES-2. [Rhone-Poulenc Surf. & Spec.] Sodium laureth (2) sulfate; CAS 68585-34-2; anionic; detergent for shampoos, bubble baths; liq.; 26% act.; formerly Sipon® ES-2.

Rhodapex® ES-12. [Rhone-Poulenc Surf. & Spec.] Sodium laureth sulfate (12 EO); surfactant for personal care prods.; liq.; 60% act.

Rhodapex® EST-30. [Rhone-Poulenc Surf. & Spec.] Sodium trideth sulfate; CAS 25446-78-0; anionic; emulsifier, wetting agent, dispersant for baby shampoo, other personal care prods., household, industrial, institutional and industrial formulations, emulsion polymerization of styrene systems, textile scouring, dishwash; FDA compliance; Gardner 2 max. liq.; cloud pt. 14 C max.; pH 7.5–8.5 (10%); surf. tens. 33 dynes/cm (@ CMC); 29-30% act.; formerly Sipex® EST-30.

Rhodapex® ESY. [Rhone-Poulenc Surf. & Spec.] Sodium laureth (1) sulfate; CAS 68585-34-2; anionic; base, cosurfactant, emulsifier for shampoos, lt. duty detergents; liq.; 30% conc.; formerly Sipon® ESY.

Rhodapex® HF-433. [Rhone-Poulenc Surf. & Spec.] Ammonium nonoxynol-4 sulfate; anionic; high foaming surfactant base for shampoos, bubble baths; mild to skin; FDA compliance; liq.; 27% act.; formerly Alipal® HF-433.

Rhodapon® EC111. [Rhone-Poulenc Surf. & Spec.] Sodium cetyl/stearyl sulfate; CAS 59186-41-3; anionic; emulsifier, detergent, flotation agent; collector in ore flotation; softener/lubricant for textiles; cosmetics and toiletries; wh. thick paste; pH 8 (10%); 25% act.; formerly Sipex® EC111.

Rhodapon® L-22, L-22/C. [Rhone-Poulenc Surf. & Spec.] Ammonium lauryl sulfate; CAS 2235-54-3; EINECS 218-793-9; anionic; high foaming detergent, emulsifier for shampoo, bubble bath, pet shampoos, industrial and institutional cleaners, wool scouring, fire fighting foams, assistant for pigment dispersion; emulsion polymerization aid; clear visc. liq.; visc. 1000 cps; HLB 31.0; cloud pt. 14 C; pH 6.8 (10%); 28% act.; formerly Sipon® L-22.

Rhodapon® L-22HNC. [Rhone-Poulenc Surf. & Spec.] Ammonium lauryl sulfate; CAS 2235-54-3; EINECS 218-793-9; surfactant for personal care prods. and SBR latex froth applics.; liq.; 30% act.; formerly Sipon® L-22HNC.

Rhodapon® LM. [Rhone-Poulenc Surf. & Spec.] Magnesium lauryl sulfate; CAS 3097-08-3; EINECS 221-450-6; anionic; high-foaming emulsifier, wetting agent, dispersant, detergent for rug and upholstery shampoos, bubble baths, shampoos; food pkg. applics.; clear liq.; visc. 50 cps; cloud pt. 2 C; pH 6.5 (10%); 27% act.; formerly Sipon® LM.

Rhodapon® LSB, LSB/CT. [Rhone-Poulenc Surf. & Spec.] Sodium lauryl sulfate; CAS 151-21-3; EINECS 205-788-1; anionic; high foaming detergent, emulsifier for hair shampoo, lotion, pastes, industrial, institutional and household cleaners; pale clear liq.; visc. 150 cps; HLB 40; cloud pt. 20 C; pH 8 (10%); 29% act.; formerly Sipon® LSB.

Rhodapon® LT-6. [Rhone-Poulenc Surf. & Spec.] TEA lauryl sulfate; CAS 139-96-8; EINECS 205-388-7; anionic; emulsifier and high foaming base for industrial and household detergents, shampoos, bubble baths; obtains creamy, mild lather; pale yel. clear liq.; visc. 50 cps; HLB 34.0; cloud pt. 2 C; pH 7 (10%); 40% act.; formerly Sipon®

LT-6.

Rhodapon® SB-8208/S. [Rhone-Poulenc Surf. & Spec.] Sodium lauryl sulfate; CAS 151-21-3; EINECS 205-788-1; detergent/emulsifier and foaming agent for shampoos, liq. soaps, bath gels, bubble baths; 30% conc.; formerly Sipon® 21LS.

Rhodapon® SM Special. [Rhone-Poulenc Surf. & Spec.] Sodium lauryl sulfate; CAS 151-21-3; EINECS 205-788-1; anionic; cosurfactant for household, institutional and industrial cleaner formulations, personal care prods.; liq.; 35% conc.; formerly Sipon® SM Spec.

Rhodapon® TDS. [Rhone-Poulenc Surf. & Spec.] Sodium tridecyl sulfate; CAS 3026-63-9; EINECS 221-188-2; anionic; emulsifier, wetting agent, emulsion polymerization of vinyl chloride, styrene, and styrene/acrylic monomers; detergent formulations; base for shampoos, foaming bath oils, cosmetic emulsions; FDA compliance; colorless liq.; visc. 100 cps; cloud pt. 10 C; pH 8.5 (10%); surf. tens. 34 dynes/cm (@ CMC); 25% act.; formerly Sipex® TDS.

Rhodaquat® M214B/99. [Rhone-Poulenc Surf. & Spec.] Myrtrimonium bromide; CAS 1119-97-7; EINECS 214-291-9; cationic; conditioner with superior antistatic properties and lt. feel; flake; 99% act.; formerly Cycloton® M214B/99.

Rhodaquat® M242B/99. [Rhone-Poulenc Surf. & Spec.] Cetrimonium bromide; CAS 57-09-0; EINECS 200-311-3; cationic; quat. ammonium compd. used in conditioners to increase antistatic and comb out effects; 100% act.; formerly Cycloton® M242B/99.

Rhodaquat® M242C/29. [Rhone-Poulenc Surf. & Spec.] Cetrimonium chloride; CAS 112-02-7; EINECS 203-928-6; cationic; surfactant with conditioning and emolliency effect on hair; liq.; 29% act.; formerly Cycloton® M242C/29.

Rhodaquat® M270C/18. [Rhone-Poulenc Surf. & Spec.] Stearalkonium chloride; CAS 122-19-0; EINECS 204-527-9; high stability surfactant base for cream rinse and conditioners; formerly Cycloton® M270C/18.

Rhodasurf® C-20. [Rhone-Poulenc Surf. & Spec.] Ceteareth-20; CAS 68439-49-6; nonionic; emollient, detergent, emulsifier for creams and lotions; HLB 5.3; 100% act.; formerly Siponic® C-20.

Rhodasurf® E 400. [Rhone-Poulenc Surf. & Spec.] PEG-8; CAS 25322-68-3; EINECS 225-856-4; nonionic; surfactant intermediate; binder and lubricant in compressed tablets; softener for paper, plasticizer for starch pastes and polyethylene films; coupling agent for skin care lotions; liq.; pour pt. 6 C; 100% conc.; formerly Pegol® E-400.

Rhodasurf® E 600. [Rhone-Poulenc Surf. & Spec.] PEG-14; CAS 25322-68-3; nonionic; surfactant intermediate; binder and lubricant in compressed tablets; color stabilizer for fuel oils; liq.; pour pt. 22 C; 100% conc.; formerly Pegol® E-600.

Rhodasurf® L-4. [Rhone-Poulenc Surf. & Spec.] Laureth-4; CAS 68002-97-1; EINECS 226-097-1; nonionic; emulsifier, thickener, wetting agent, pigment dispersant, lubricant, solubilizer for cosmetic and industrial emulsions; textile scouring agent, emulsion polymerization, metal cleaning, monomer systems, floor waxes, paper finishes, rubber; emollient for pharmaceuticals; liq.; HLB 9.7; pH 6.5 (1%); 100% conc.; formerly Siponic® L-4.

Rhodasurf® L-25. [Rhone-Poulenc Surf. & Spec.] Laureth-23; CAS 9002-92-0; nonionic; surfactant for cosmetic and industrial emulsions; wetting agent, pigment dispersant, lubricant, solubilizer, textile scouring agent, emulsion polymerization, metal cleaning, rubber and monomer systems; stabilizer for emulsion polymers; floor waxes, paper finishes, emollient for pharmaceuticals; wax; HLB 16.9; cloud pt. > 95 C (1%); pH 6.5 (1%); 100% act.;

formerly Siponic® L-25.

Rhodasurf® L-790. [Rhone-Poulenc Surf. & Spec.] Laureth-7; CAS 9002-92-0; EINECS 221-283-9; nonionic; surfactant for cosmetic and industrial emulsions; wetting agent, pigment dispersant, lubricant, solubilizer, textile scouring agent, emulsion polymerization, metal cleaning; liq.; HLB 12.1; 90% act.; formerly Siponic® L-790.

Rhodasurf® LA-3. [Rhone-Poulenc Surf. & Spec.] C12-15 pareth-3; CAS 68131-39-5; nonionic; detergent base and emulsifier for dishwash, personal care prods., industrial applics.; textile lubricant; translucent to opaque liq.; sol. in min. oil, aromatic solv, perchloroethylene; sp.gr. 0.93; visc. 19 cps (100 F); HLB 7.8; cloud pt. 58-62 C; 100% act.; formerly Alkasurf® LA-3.

Rhodasurf® LA-30. [Rhone-Poulenc Surf. & Spec.] Linear syn. alcohol ethoxylate; nonionic; coemulsifier for pesticides, cosmetics, min. oil emulsions for metalworking, textile processing, degreasers; intermediate for biodeg. ether sulfate prod.; liq.; HLB 8.0; 99% conc.; formerly Rhodiasurf LA-30.

Rhodasurf® LA-90. [Rhone-Poulenc Surf. & Spec.] Linear syn. alcohol ethoxylate; nonionic; wetting agent for textile wet processing, cosmetic preps.; solid; HLB 13.5; 99% conc.; formerly Rhodiasurf LA-90.

Rhodasurf® ON-870. [Rhone-Poulenc Surf. & Spec.] Oleth-20; CAS 9004-98-2; nonionic; high foaming emulsifier, stabilizer, dispersant, wetting agent, solubilizer for min. oils, fatty acids, waxes; for industrial cleaners, metal cleaners, agric., paints, adhesives, textile, leather, cosmetic, pharmaceutical industries; FDA, EPA compliance; wh. solid wax; sol. in water, xylene, ethanol, ethylene glycol, butyl Cellosolve; sp.gr. 1.04; HLB 15.4; pour pt. 46 C; cloud pt. > 100 C; flash pt. (PMCC) 93 C; surf. tens. 37 dynes/cm (0.1%); 100% act.; formerly Emulphor® ON-870.

Rhodasurf® ON-877. [Rhone-Poulenc Surf. & Spec.] Oleth-20; CAS 9004-98-2; nonionic; stabilizer for natural and syn. rubber latex emulsions; acid degreaser, dyeing assistant for textiles; dyestuff dispersant, tanning assistant, fat liquor, degreaser for leathers; solubilizer and emulsifier for essential oils and pharmaceuticals; emulsifier for aq. dispersions of polyethylene; liq.; 70% conc.; formerly Emulphor® ON-877.

Rhodasurf® PEG 400. [Rhone-Poulenc Surf. & Spec.] PEG-9; CAS 25322-68-3; EINECS 222-206-1; intermediate, plasticizer, solv., lubricant, coupler in cosmetic lotions; wh. liq.; water-sol.; m.w. 380-420; sp.gr. 1.13; f.p. 4-8 C; pH 5-8; 100% conc.; formerly Alkapol PEG 400.

Rhodasurf® PEG 600. [Rhone-Poulenc Surf. & Spec.] PEG-14; CAS 25322-68-3; plasticizer, solv.; lubricant, binder for pharmaceuticals; color stabilizer for fuel oils; intermediate for processing surfactants; wh. liq.; m.w. 570–630; water sol.; sp.gr. 1.13 (30/15.5 C); f.p. 20-25 C; pH 5–8; 100% conc.; formerly Alkapol PEG 600.

Rhodasurf® S-2. [Rhone-Poulenc Surf. & Spec.] Steareth-2; CAS 9005-00-9; nonionic; emollient, detergent, emulsifier for creams and lotions, facial cleansers, bath and toiletries; solid; HLB 4.9; 100% conc.; formerly Siponic® S-2.

Rhodasurf® S-20. [Rhone-Poulenc Surf. & Spec.] Steareth-20; CAS 9005-00-9; nonionic; emollient, detergent, emulsifier for creams and lotions, facial cleansers, bath and toiletries; solid; HLB 15.2; 100% conc.; formerly Siponic® S-20.

Rhodasurf® TD-9 [Rhone-Poulenc Surf. & Spec.] Trideceth-9; CAS 24938-91-8; nonionic; emulsifier, emollient and lubricant for skin creams and lotions; solubilizer for fragrance and oils; liq.; water-sol.; HLB 12.9; 90% conc.; formerly Siponic® TD-9.

Rhodaterge® SSB. [Rhone-Poulenc Surf. & Spec.] Sodium lauryl sulfate, disodium lauryl sulfosuccinate, propylene glycol; surfactant; formerly Miranate® SSB.

Rhodicare™ D. [Rhone-Poulenc Surf. & Spec.] Xanthan gum; CAS 11138-66-2; EINECS 234-394-2; polymer which imparts visc. building and thickening, and suspends insol. additives in cosmetic formulations (shampoos, creams and lotions, toiletries, tooth paste, mouthwash).

Rhodicare™ H. [Rhone-Poulenc Surf. & Spec.] Xanthan gum; CAS 11138-66-2; EINECS 234-394-2; polymer which imparts visc. and suspends insol. additives in cosmetic formulations (shampoos, creams and lotions, toiletries, tooth paste, mouthwash).

Rhodicare™ S. [Rhone-Poulenc Surf. & Spec.] Xanthan gum; CAS 11138-66-2; EINECS 234-394-2; polymer which imparts visc. and suspends insol. additives in cosmetic formulations (shampoos, creams and lotions, toiletries, tooth paste, mouthwash).

Rhodicare™ SC-225. [Rhone-Poulenc Surf. & Spec.] Guar gum and xanthan gum; polymer providing visc. building and suspension props. to tooth paste, and mouth wash.

Rhodicare™ XC. [Rhone-Poulenc Surf. & Spec.] Xanthan gum; CAS 11138-66-2; EINECS 234-394-2; thickening and stabilizing hydrocholloid; emulsion/foam stabilizer; imparts visc. and suspends insol. additives in cosmetics and toiletry formulations (shampoos, creams and lotions, tooth paste, mouthwash).

Rhodigel®. [Rhone-Poulenc Food Ingreds.; R.T. Vanderbilt] Xanthan gum; CAS 11138-66-2; EINECS 234-394-2; emulsion stabilizer, suspending agent, thickener for cosmetic and pharmaceutical applics.; water-sol.

Rhodigel® 23. [Rhone-Poulenc Surf. & Spec.; R.T. Vanderbilt] Xanthan gum; CAS 11138-66-2; EINECS 234-394-2; cosmetic/pharmaceutical grade thickener, stabilizer, and suspending agent.

Rhodigel® 200. [Rhone-Poulenc Food Ingreds.; R.T. Vanderbilt] Xanthan gum; CAS 11138-66-2; EINECS 234-394-2; used in pharmaceuticals, cosmetic applics. to suspend insol. additives; exc. pseudo plastic props.; in baking, cereal, meat, poultry, dairy/cheese, processed foods, beverages, confections.

Rhodigel® EZ. [Rhone-Poulenc Food Ingreds.] Xanthan gum; CAS 11138-66-2; EINECS 234-394-2; used in cosmetic applics. to suspend insol. additives; exc. pseudo plastic props.; in baking, cereals, meat, poultry, dairy/cheese, processed foods, beverages, and confections.

Rhodocap-A, G, N. [Rhone-Poulenc] Cyclodextrin; CAS 7585-39-9; EINECS 231-493-2; encapsulant.

Rhodopol® SC. [Rhone-Poulenc/Water Soluble Polymers] Xanthan gum; CAS 11138-66-2; EINECS 234-394-2; gum for cosmetics.

Rhodorsil® AF 70414, 70416, 70426 R, 70452. [Rhone-Poulenc Silicones] Simethicone; foam control agent.

Rhodorsil® Oils 70041 VO.65. [Rhone-Poulenc Silicones] Hexamethyldisiloxane; CAS 107-46-0; EINECS 203-492-7.

Rhodorsil® Oils 70045. [Rhone-Poulenc Silicones] Cyclomethicone; CAS 69430-24-6; cosmetic ingred.

Rhodorsil® Oils 70045 V2, 70045 V3, 70045 V5. [Rhone-Poulenc Surf. & Spec.] Cyclomethicone; CAS 69430-24-6; conditioner and emollient providing silky soft feel to cosmetic creams, facial cleansers, and deodorants.; formerly Silbione 70045 V2, V3, V5.

Rhodorsil® Oils 70047 V2, V5. [Rhone-Poulenc Silicones] Dimethicone; conditioner and emollient providing silky soft feel to cosmetic creams.; formerly Silbione 70047.

Rhodorsil® Oils 70633 V30. [Rhone-Poulenc Silicones] Bisphenylhexamethicone; CAS 18758-91-3; conditioner and emollient providing silky soft feel to cosmetic creams, facial cleansers, and deodorants.; formerly Silbione 70633 V30.

Rhodorsil® Oils 70641 V 200. [Rhone-Poulenc Silicones] Phenyl trimethicone; CAS 2116-84-9; EINECS 218-320-6; emollient, conditioner.

Rhodorsil® Oils 70646. [Rhone-Poulenc Silicones] Dimethicone copolyol; conditioner, detergent, emulsifier, foam booster/stabilizer for shampoos, liq. soaps, creams and lotons, facial cleansers, and toiletries; 100% conc.; formerly Silbione 70646.

Rhodorsil® Oils 71631. [Rhone-Poulenc Surf. & Spec.] Cyclomethicone/dimethicone; emollient, conditioner, and antistat for shampoos, creams, and facial cleansers.; formerly Silbione 71631.

Rhodorsil® Oils 71634. [Rhone-Poulenc Surf. & Spec.] Cyclomethicone/phenyl dimethicone; conditioner, emollient, antistat, and gloss agent for shampoos, liq. soaps, shower gels, creams and lotions, facial cleansers, and conditioning rinses.; formerly Silbione 71634.

Rhumacalm HS 328. [Alban Muller] Propylene glycol, harpagophytum extract, spiraea extract, and juniper extract; for articular pains.

Riboflavin-5′-Phosphate Sodium USP, FCC. [Roche] Vitamin B2; catalyst in tan-accelerating formulations.

Riboflavin USP, FCC Type S. [Roche] Vitamin B2; colorant for cosmetics use.

Rice Bran Oil. [Ikeda] Rice bran oil; EINECS 271-397-8; nutritive oil providing cholesterol control; for skin care prods., foods; acid no. 0.1 max.; iodine no. 102-110; sapon. no. 185-195; cloud pt. -4 C max.

Rice Bran Oil SO. [Tsuno Rice Fine Chems.; Tri-K Industries] Rice bran oil; EINECS 271-397-8; cosmetic ingred.; also suitable for food use; lt. yel. liq.; insol. in water; sp.gr. 0.916-0.922; b.p. 310 C; acid no. 0.1 max.; iodine no. 92-115; sapon. no. 180-195; cloud pt. -7 C max.; ref. index 1.470-1.473; toxicology: nonhazardous; edible; trace moisture.

Rice-Pro™ EN-20. [Brooks Industries] Hydrolyzed rice protein; CAS 97759-33-8; cosmetic ingredient for skin and hair care prods.; m.w. 1000; 20% act.

Rice Pro-Tein BK. [Maybrook] Hydrolyzed rice protein; CAS 97759-33-8; bland substantive protein with oil binding, film forming, moisturizing props.; anti-irritant; ingred. in oil-absorbent formulations, hair and skin care prods. (shampoos, makeup bases, moisturizers for sensitive skin, cleansing masks); amber clear liq., mild char. odor; pH 4.0-6.0; 17-23% nonvolatiles.

Rice Wax No. 1. [Ikeda] Rice bran wax from deoiling and decoloring process; CAS 8016-60-2; EINECS 232-409-7; natural prod. for use in lipsticks; m.p. 78-82 C; acid no. 13 max.; iodine no. 10 max.; sapon. no. 75-90.

Rice Wax RX-100. [Ikeda] Hydrog. rice bran wax, decolorized; natural prod. for use in lipsticks; m.p. 70-77 C; acid no. 10 max.; iodine no. 10 max.; sapon. no. 120-150.

Ricinion. [Gattefosse] PEG-33 castor oil; CAS 61791-12-6; solv., emulsifier for cosmetic/pharmaceutical emulsions; liq.; HLB 12-13; acid no. 30-40; sapon. no. 60-80; toxicology: LD50 (oral, rat) > 10 ml/kg; nonirritating to skin and eyes.

Ricino Viscoil. [Vevy] PEG-25 castor oil; CAS 61791-12-6; personal care surfactant.

Ringdex-A, B. [Mercian; Ringdex] Cyclodextrin; CAS 7585-39-9; EINECS 231-493-2; encapsulant.

RITA CA. [R.I.T.A.] Cetyl alcohol NF; CAS 36653-82-4; EINECS 253-149-0; thickener, opacifier, emollient for cosmetic formulations; wh. waxy flakes; m.p. 45-50 C; acid no. 2 max.; iodine no. 5 max.; hyd. no. 218-238.

RITA EDGS. [R.I.T.A.] Glycol distearate; CAS 627-83-8; EINECS 211-014-3; emulsifier, emulsion stabilizer, emollient, pearlescent, opacifier, visc. builder for cosmetic systems; wh. flakes.

RITA EGMS. [R.I.T.A.] Glycol stearate; CAS 111-60-4; EINECS 203-886-9; emulsifier, emulsion stabilizer, emollient, pearlescent, opacifier, visc. builder for cosmetic systems; wh. flakes.

RITA GMS. [R.I.T.A.] Glyceryl stearate; emulsifier, emulsion stabilizer, emollient, pearlescent, opacifier, visc. builder for cosmetic systems; wh. flakes.

RITA HA C-1-C. [R.I.T.A.] Sodium hyaluronate; CAS 9067-32-7; protein for use in skin and hair care preps.; 1% aq. sol'n.

RITA SA. [R.I.T.A.] Stearyl alcohol NF; CAS 112-92-5; EINECS 204-017-6; thickener, opacifier, emollient for cosmetic formulations; m.p. 56-60 C; iodine no. 2 max.; sapon. no. 3 max.; hyd. no. 200-212.

Ritabate 20. [R.I.T.A.] Polysorbate 20; CAS 9005-64-5; nonionic; surfactant, emulsifier for personal care prods.; yel. liq.

Ritabate 40. [R.I.T.A.] Polysorbate 40; CAS 9005-66-7; nonionic; surfactant, emulsifier for personal care prods.; yel. liq.

Ritabate 60. [R.I.T.A.] Polysorbate 60; CAS 9005-67-8; nonionic; surfactant, emulsifier for personal care prods.; yel. liq.

Ritabate 80. [R.I.T.A.] Polysorbate 80; CAS 9005-65-6; nonionic; surfactant, emulsifier for personal care prods.; yel. liq.

Ritacet-20. [R.I.T.A.] Ceteareth-20; CAS 68439-49-6; nonionic; surfactant, emulsifier for personal care prods.; wh. solid wax.

Ritaceti. [R.I.T.A.] Cetyl esters; raw material for personal care prods.; wh. flakes.

Ritacetyl®. [R.I.T.A.] Acetylated lanolin; CAS 61788-48-5; EINECS 262-979-2; nonionic; superfatting agent, emollient, spreading agent, foam stabilizer for soaps, shampoos; moisture barrier, film-former for creams and lotions, water resistant films; provides sheen and conditioning to hair prods.; suitable for baby prods., bath preps., makeup, colognes, hair/skin care prods., shaving preps.; yel./amber soft waxy semisolid, bland odor; oil-sol.; m.p. 30-40 C; acid no. 3 max.; sapon. no. 125 max.; hyd. no. 10 max.; usage level: 0.1-50%; 100% conc.

Ritachlor 50%. [R.I.T.A.] Aluminum chlorohydrate; CAS 1327-41-9; EINECS 215-477-2; raw material for personal care prods.; aq. sol'n.

Ritachol®. [R.I.T.A.] Min. oil and lanolin alcohol; nonionic; absorp. base, primary or aux. emulsifier used in cosmetics, toiletries, pharmacueticals, household specialties; stabilizer for emulsions, dispersions, and suspensions; epidermal moisturizer, lubricant, and emollient; plasticizer for hair spray resins and aerosol bandage films; reduces stickiness and tackiness; pale straw liq.; faint sterol-type odor; misc. with min. oil, esters, and glycerides; sp.gr. 0.84-0.86; HLB 8; acid no. 1 max.; iodine no. 12 max.; sapon. no. 2 max.; toxicology: nontoxic; nonirritating to skin and eyes; nonsensitizing; 100% act.

Ritachol® 1000. [R.I.T.A.] Cetearyl alcohol, polysorbate 60, PEG-150 stearate, steareth-20; nonionic; emulsifer for cosmetics, pharmaceuticals, and household specialties (skin treatment creams/lotions, hair treatments such as conditioners, straighteners, perms, and dyes, antiperspirants); wh. waxy flakes, low odor; m.p. 48-52 C; acid no. 1.5 max.; iodine no. 3.5 max.; sapon. no. 9–14; hyd. no. 178-192; pH 5.5-7.0 (3% aq.); toxicology: nonirritating; 100% conc.

Ritachol® 2000. [R.I.T.A.] Cetearyl alcohol and polysorbate 60; nonionic; emulsifier, conditioner for cosmetics and pharmaceuticals; used in powd. suspension formulas; stable over wide pH and temp. range; wh. waxy flakes; m.p. 48-52 C; acid no. 0.1-1.0; iodine no. 3.5 max.; sapon. no. 9-14; hyd. no. 178-192; pH 5.5-7.0 (3% aq.); toxicology: nonirritating; 100% conc.

Ritachol® 3000. [R.I.T.A.] Cetearyl alcohol, polysorbate 60, PEG-150 stearate, steareth-20, cetyl alcohol, laneth-16, PEG-60 lanolin; nonionic; emulsifying wax for cosmetic, pharmaceutical, and industrial prods.; exc. for curl relaxer systems, perms, color treatments, depilatories, antiperspirants, germicides; high electrolyte tolerance; ylsh. waxy flake; acid no. 2 max.; iodine no. 6 max.; sapon. no. 14 max.; hyd. no. 168-186; pH 5.3-6.8 (3% aq.); toxicology: nonirritating; 100% conc.

Ritachol® 4000. [R.I.T.A.] Cetyl alcohol, steareth-20, PEG-60 lanolin; nonionic; emulsifying wax, emollient, and thickener for cosmetics, pharmaceuticals, industrial use; exc. for curl relaxer systems; ylsh. waxy flake; acid no. 1 max.; sapon. no. 5 max.; hyd. no. 160-180; toxicology: nonirritating; 100% conc.

Ritachol 5000. [R.I.T.A.] Cetearyl alcohol, polysorbate 60, PEG-150 stearate, cetyl alcohol, ceteareth-20, PEG-20 hydrog. lanolin, and PEG-40 stearate; nonionic; emulsifier, hair conditioner; wh. flakes.

Ritachol SS. [R.I.T.A.] Stearyl stearate; CAS 2778-96-3; EINECS 220-476-5; raw material for personal care prods.; wh. flakes.

Ritacollagen BA-1. [R.I.T.A.] Soluble collagen; CAS 9007-34-5; EINECS 232-697-4; protein for use in skin and hair care preps.; 1% aq. sol'n.

Ritacollagen S-1. [R.I.T.A.] Soluble collagen; CAS 9007-34-5; EINECS 232-697-4; protein for skin and hair care prods.; 1% aq. sol'n.

Ritacomplex DF 10. [R.I.T.A.] Soluble animal elastin and soluble animal collagen; protein for skin and hair care prods.; amber liq.

Ritacomplex DF 11. [R.I.T.A.] Hydrolyzed animal elastin and soluble animal collagen; protein for skin and hair care prods.; amber liq.

Ritacomplex DF 12, DF 13. [R.I.T.A.] Soluble animal collage and sodium hyaluronate; protein for skin and hair care prods.; amber liq.

Ritacomplex DF 14. [R.I.T.A.] Hydrolyzed animal elastin, sodium hyaluronate, and soluble animal collagen; protein for skin and hair care prods.; amber liq.

Ritacomplex DF 15. [R.I.T.A.] Sodium hyaluronate, hydrolyzed wheat protein, and aloe vera gel; protein for skin and hair care prods.; amber liq.

Ritacomplex DF 26. [R.I.T.A.] Pineapple extract and sodium hyaluronate; protein for skin and hair care prods.; amber liq.

Ritaderm® . [R.I.T.A.] Petrolatum, lanolin, sodium PCA, polysorbate 85; nonionic; emollient, moisturizer, and lubricant used in cosmetics; off-wh. paste; sol. in oil, alcohol; m.p. 42–48 C; 100% act.

Ritahydrox. [R.I.T.A.] Hydroxylated lanolin; CAS 68424-66-8; EINECS 270-315-8; nonionic; w/o emulsifier, hypoallergenic emollient, superfatting agent, pigment dispersant, emulsion stabilizer, thickener with high water absorp., skin wetting; for skin care prods., emulsions, soap and cleansing systems; yel. paste; HLB 4.0; m.p. 39-46 C; acid no. 10 max.; iodine no. 15-23; sapon. no. 95-110; hyd. no. 60-85; 100% conc.

Ritalafa® . [R.I.T.A.] Lanolin acid; CAS 68424-43-1; EINECS 270-302-7; nonionic; film-former, emollient, wetting agent, dispersant; gellant for oils and detergents; solubilizer for propellants; rewetting of makeup preparations; prevents defatting; for eye makeup, hair/skin care prods., shaving preps.; yel.-tan hard waxy solid, mild waxy odor; oil-sol.; m.p. 50-65 C; acid no. 135 min.; iodine no. 10 max.; sapon. no. 155 min.; hyd. no. 40-60; usage level: 0.1-10%; 100% conc.

Ritalan® . [R.I.T.A.] Lanolin oil USP; nonionic; moisturizer, plasticizer, penetrant, emollient with high spreading coefficient; hypoallergenic nonsensitizing skin lubricant; pre-

vents defatting; for baby prods., bath preps., makeup, hair/skin preps., cleansers, shaving preps., sunscreens; amber clear liq., sl. odor; sol. in lipids, min. oil; insol. in water; acid no. 2 max.; iodine no. 18-36; cloud pt. 18 C; usage level: 0.1-50%; 100% conc.

Ritalan® AWS. [R.I.T.A.] PPG-12-PEG-65 lanolin oil; CAS 68458-58-8; nonionic; aux. emulsifier, moisturizer, emollient for cosmetic formulations; plasticizer for hair sprays; lt. amber liq., odorless; sol. in water and alcohol; HLB 18.0; acid no. 3 max.; iodine no. 10 max.; sapon. no. 10-25; hyd. no. 50 max.; pH 5-7 (10%); 100% act.

Ritalan® C. [R.I.T.A.] Isopropyl palmitate and lanolin oil; nonionic; blending agent, emollient, epidermal penetrant, rewetting agent, and solubilizer for waxes and other oil-sol. or disp. materials; personal care prods.; yel. liq., bland odor; sol. in min. oil; 100% act.

RITA Lanolin. [R.I.T.A.] Lanolin; CAS 8006-54-0; EINECS 232-348-6; emollient, emulsifier, penetrant, moisturizer with good skin feel, adhesive/cohesive and tackifying props. for cosmetic and pharmaceutical formulations (baby prods., bath preps., makeup, colognes, hair/skin care prods., shaving preps., suntans); ointment-like material, sl. char. odor; sol. in chloroform, ether; partly sol. in alcohol; insol. in water, min. oil; usage level: 0.1-50%.

R.I.T.A. Lanolin Wax. [R.I.T.A.] Lanolin wax; CAS 68201-49-0; EINECS 269-220-4; w/o emulsifier, thickener, bodying agent, hardener for wax systems (lipsticks, makeup); improves visc. stability in creams and lotions; for suntans, colognes, shaving preps., skin care prods., hair preps.; Gardner 7 max. waxy solid, odorless, tasteless; m.p. 49-52 C; sapon. no. 90-110; hyd. no. 20-35; usage level: 0.1-50%.

Ritalastin EL-10. [R.I.T.A.] Hydrolyzed elastin; CAS 100085-10-7; protein for use in skin and hair care preps.; 10% aq. sol'n.

Ritalastin EL-30. [R.I.T.A.] Hydrolyzed elastin; CAS 100085-10-7; protein for skin and hair care prods.; 30% aq. sol'n.

Ritaloe 1X, 10X, 20X, 40X. [R.I.T.A.] Aloe vera; emollient, humectant, pigment, conditioner, lubricant with skin soothing props. for personal care formulations; clear liq.

Ritaloe 200M. [R.I.T.A.] Aloe vera gel; emollient, humectant, pigment, conditioner, lubricant with skin soothing props. for personal care prods.; wh. powd.

Ritamectant K2. [R.I.T.A.] Dipotassium glycyrrhizinate; CAS 68797-35-3; EINECS 272-296-1; humectant for personal care prods.; wh. powd.

Ritamectant PCA. [R.I.T.A.] Sodium PCA; CAS 28874-51-3; EINECS 249-277-1; humectant for personal care prods.; clear liq.

Ritamide C. [R.I.T.A.] Cocamide DEA; CAS 61791-31-9; EINECS 263-163-9; raw material for personal care prods.; clear liq.

Ritapan D. [R.I.T.A.] D-panthenol; CAS 81-13-0; nutrient, humectant for hair and skin care formulations; hair repair agent; soothing to skin; clear visc. liq.

Ritapan DL. [R.I.T.A.] DL-panthenol; nutrient, humectant for hair and skin care formulations; hair repair agent; soothing to skin; wh. powd.

Ritapan TA. [R.I.T.A.] Panthenyl triacetate; CAS 98133-47-2; nutrient, humectant for hair and skin care formulations; hair repair agent; soothing to skin; clear visc. liq.

R.I.T.A. d-Panthenol. [R.I.T.A.] d-Panthenol; CAS 81-13-0; penetrant, humectant for restoring/maintaining natural skin moisture; stimulates cell proliferation and soothes irritated skin; repairs and strengthens damaged hair; colorless clear visc. liq., char. odor, sl. bitter taste; sol. in water and ethanol; m.w. 205.25; visc. 105,000 mPa·s (30 C); ref. index 1.495-1.502; toxicology: nontoxic, nonirritating; 100% conc.

R.I.T.A. dl-Panthenol. [R.I.T.A.] dl-Panthenol; penetrant, humectant for restoring/maintaining natural skin moisture; stimulates cell proliferation and soothes irritated skin; thickens, moisturizes, repairs, and strengthens damaged hair; wh. to creamy wh. cryst. hygroscopic powd., char. odor; sl. bitter taste; sol. in water, ethanol, propylene glycol, chloroform, ether; sl. sol. in glycerin; m.w. 205.25; m.p. 64.5-68.5 C; toxicology: nontoxic, nonirritating; 100% conc.

Ritapeg 150 DS. [R.I.T.A.] PEG-150 stearate; CAS 9004-99-3; nonionic; surfactant, emulsifier for personal care prods.; off-wh. flakes.

Ritaplast. [R.I.T.A.] Min. oil and polyethylene; raw material for personal care prods.; gelled oil.

Ritapro 100. [R.I.T.A.] Cetearyl alcohol, steareth-20, and steareth-10; nonionic; o/w emulsifier for personal care prods.; hair conditioner; wh. flakes; 100% conc.

Ritapro 165. [R.I.T.A.] Glyceryl stearate and PEG-2 stearate; nonionic; o/w emulsifier for creams, lotions; wh. flakes; 100% conc.

Ritapro 200. [R.I.T.A.] Stearyl alcohol, ceteareth-20; nonionic; o/w emulsifier for creams, lotions, hair conditoners; wh. flake; 100% conc.

Ritapro 300. [R.I.T.A.] Cetearyl alcohol, ceteareth-20; nonionic; o/w emulsifier for personal care prods.; wh. flake; 100% conc.

Ritasol. [R.I.T.A.] Isopropyl lanolate; CAS 63393-93-1; EINECS 264-119-1; nonionic; emollient, spreading agent, water-resistant film former for lip preparations; yel. paste; 100% conc.

Ritasynt IP. [R.I.T.A.] Glycol stearate and other ingreds.; CAS 111-60-4; EINECS 203-886-9; nonionic; foam booster, thickener, opacifier for cosmetics; wh. flakes; 100% conc.

Ritavena™ 5. [R.I.T.A.] Hydrolyzed oat flour and [gb]-glucan; suspending agent, emulsion stabilizer, and synergistic thickener; conditioning agent for 2 in 1 shampoos; suspending agent for liq. makeup, abrasive cleaners, antidandruff shampos, sunscreens; provides lubricious feel in aq. systems; slip aid in soaps and shave creams, stick prods.; additive for foaming bath prods.; off-wh. powd., char. odor; sol. hazy in water, glycerin to 2%; dens. 25.05 lb/ft³; pH 5.5-6.5 (10%); toxicology: nonirritating to skin and eyes; nonsensitizing; 4-8% moisture.

Ritawax. [R.I.T.A.] Lanolin alcohol; CAS 8027-33-6; EINECS 232-430-1; nonionic; emulsifier, emollient, stabilizer, and thickener for cosmetics/pharmaceuticals; hardener for wax systems; strong water absorp. props.; for baby prods., bath preps., makeup, colognes, hair/skin care prods., sunscreens, shaving preps.; amber firm waxy solid, char. odor; sol. in alcohol, IPM, other oils; m.p. 53-61 C; acid no. 2 max.; sapon. no. 10 max.; hyd. no. 118-160; usage level: 0.1-50%; 100% conc.

Ritawax 5. [R.I.T.A.] Laneth-5; CAS 61791-20-6; nonionic; emulsifier, solubilizer, emollient for creams and lotions; solid; 100% conc.

Ritawax 10. [R.I.T.A.] Laneth-10; CAS 61791-20-6; nonionic; emulsifier, solubilizer, emollient for creams and lotions; solid; 100% conc.

Ritawax 20. [R.I.T.A.] Laneth-20; CAS 61791-20-6; nonionic; emulsifier, solubilizer, emollient for creams and lotions; solid; 100% conc.

Ritawax AEO. [R.I.T.A.] Polysorbate 80, acetylated lanolin alcohol, cetyl acetate; nonionic; emollient, lubricant, moisturizer, penetrant, solubilizer, dispersant, plasticizer, cosolv., emulsifier for personal care prods.; hair and skin softening and conditioning; vehicle for medicaments; degreases and detackifies emulsion systems; lemon yel. to straw-colored clear oily liq., char. bland odor; sol. in water, IPA, castor oil, min. oil, veg. oil; acid no. 2 max.; sapon. no. 65-80; hyd. no. 60-70; 100% conc.

Ritawax ALA. [R.I.T.A.] Cetyl acetate and acetylated lanolin alcohol; nonionic; emollient, lubricant, moisturizer, penetrant, plasticizer, cosolv., solubilizer, emulsifier; hair and skin softening and conditioning; vehicle for medicaments; degreases and detackifies emulsion systems; lemon yel. to straw-colored oily liq., char. bland odor; sol. in min. oil, castor oil, veg. oil, alcohol; acid no. 1 max.; iodine no. 10 max.; sapon. no. 180-200; hyd. no. 8 max.; 100% conc.

Ritawax Super. [R.I.T.A.] Lanolin alcohol; CAS 8027-33-6; EINECS 232-430-1; emulsifier, emollient, conditioner, moisturizer, stabilizer, and solubilizer in makeup, lipsticks, skin care prods., bath preps., shampoos, soaps, shave creams, ointments, sun preps., veterinary prods.; amber solid.

Ritoleth 2. [R.I.T.A.] Oleth-2; CAS 9004-98-2; nonionic; o/w emulsifier, solubilizer; stable over wide pH range; clear liq.; HLB 4.9; 100% conc.

Ritoleth 5. [R.I.T.A.] Oleth-5; CAS 9004-98-2; nonionic; o/w emulsifier, solubilizer; stable over wide pH range; clear liq.; HLB 9.6; 100% conc.

Ritoleth 10. [R.I.T.A.] Oleth-10; CAS 9004-98-2; nonionic; o/w emulsifier, solubilizer; stable over wide pH range; wh. paste; HLB 12.4; 100% conc.

Ritoleth 20. [R.I.T.A.] Oleth-20; CAS 9004-98-2; nonionic; o/w emulsifier, solubilizer; stable over wide pH range; wh. solid wax; HLB 15.1; 100% conc.

Ritox 35. [R.I.T.A.] Laureth-23; CAS 9002-92-0; nonionic; surfactant, emulsifier for personal care prods.; wh. solid wax.

Ritox 52. [R.I.T.A.] PEG-40 stearate; CAS 9004-99-3; nonionic; surfactant, emulsifier for personal care prods.; wh. solid wax or flakes.

Ritox 53. [R.I.T.A.] PEG-50 stearate; CAS 9004-99-3; nonionic; surfactant, emulsifier for personal care prods.; wh. solid wax.

Ritox 59. [R.I.T.A.] PEG-100 stearate; CAS 9004-99-3; nonionic; surfactant, emulsifier for personal care prods.; wh. waxy flakes.

Robane®. [Robeco] Squalane NF; CAS 111-01-3; EINECS 203-825-6; liq. vehicle natural to skin and sebum; moisturizer, emollient, lubricant, humectant; aids spread of topical agents over the skin, increases skin respiration, prevents insensible water loss, imparts suppleness to skin without greasy feel; cosmetics and pharmaceuticals; colorless liq. oil, odorless, tasteless; misc. with veg. and min. oils, org. solvs., lipophilic substances, and human sebum; m.w. 422.83; sp.gr. 0.807-0.810; visc. 32-34 cps; f.p. -38 C; b.p. 350 C; acid no. 0.2 max.; iodine no. 4 max.; sapon. no. 2 max.; flash pt. 230 C; ref. index 1.4510-1.4525; toxicology: nontoxic, nonirritating.

Robeco-DNA. [Robeco] DNA; CAS 9007-49-2; cosmetic ingred.

Robeco-DNA-K. [Robeco] Potassium DNA.

Robeco-DNA-Na. [Robeco] Sodium DNA.

Rocou AMI. [Alban Muller] Natural ingred. with soothing props. for sun prods.; oil-sol.

R.O.D. [U.S. Cosmetics] 2-Octyldodecyl ricinoleate; neutral oil imparting pleasant, nongreasy "cooling" feel to cosmetic makeup, sunscreens, hair and skin care prods.

Rodol 2A3PYR. [Lowenstein] 2-Amino-3-hydroxypyridine; CAS 16867-03-1; EINECS 240-886-8; intermediate for prep. of oxidation color systems.

Rodol 2G. [Lowenstein] o-Aminophenol; CAS 95-55-6; EINECS 202-431-1; intermediate for prep. of oxidation color systems.

Rodol 4GP. [Lowenstein] 4-Nitro-o-phenylenediamine HCl; CAS 6219-77-8; EINECS 228-293-2; intermediate for prep. of oxidation color systems.

Rodol 4J. [Lowenstein] 4-Nitro-o-phenylenediamine; CAS 99-56-9; EINECS 202-766-3; intermediate for prep. of oxidation color systems.

Rodol 15N. [Lowenstein] 1,6-Naphthalenediol; CAS 575-44-6; EINECS 209-386-7; intermediate for prep. of oxidation color systems.

Rodol 23N. [Lowenstein] 2,3-Naphthalenediol; CAS 92-44-4; EINECS 202-156-7; intermediate for prep. of oxidation color systems.

Rodol 26PYR. [Lowenstein] 2,6-Diaminopyridine; CAS 141-86-6; EINECS 205-507-2; intermediate for prep. of oxidation color systems.

Rodol 27N. [Lowenstein] 2,7-Naphthalenediol; CAS 582-17-2; EINECS 209-478-7; intermediate for prep. of oxidation color systems.

Rodol BA. [Lowenstein] 4-Methoxy-m-phenylenediamine; CAS 615-05-4; intermediate for prep. of oxidation color systems.

Rodol BLFX. [Lowenstein] Toluene-2,5-diamine sulfate; CAS 615-50-9; EINECS 210-431-8; intermediate for prep. of oxidation color systems.

Rodol Brown 2R. [Lowenstein] 2-Nitro-p-phenylenediamine; intermediate for prep. of oxidation color systems.

Rodol Brown SO. [Lowenstein] 2-Chloro-p-phenylenediamine sulfate; CAS 6219-71-2; EINECS 228-291-1; intermediate for prep. of oxidation color systems.

Rodol C. [Lowenstein] Pyrocatechol; CAS 120-80-9; EINECS 204-427-5; intermediate for prep. of oxidation color systems.

Rodol CRS. [Lowenstein] 4-Chlororesorcinol; CAS 95-88-5; EINECS 202-462-0; intermediate for prep. of oxidation color systems.

Rodol D. [Lowenstein] p-Phenylenediamine; CAS 106-50-3; EINECS 203-404-7; intermediate for prep. of oxidation color systems.

Rodol DEMAP. [Lowenstein] N,N-Diethyl-m-aminophenol; CAS 91-68-9; EINECS 202-090-9; intermediate for prep. of oxidation color systems.

Rodol DEMAPS. [Lowenstein] N,N-Diethyl-m-aminophenol sulfate; CAS 68239-84-9; EINECS 269-478-8; intermediate for prep. of oxidation color systems.

Rodol DS. [Lowenstein] p-Phenylenediamine sulfate; CAS 16245-77-5; EINECS 240-357-1; intermediate for prep. of oxidation color systems.

Rodol EACS. [Lowenstein] N-Hydroxyethyl-2-amino-4-hydroxytoluene sulfate; intermediate for prep. of oxidation color systems.

Rodol EG. [Lowenstein] m-Aminophenol; CAS 591-27-5; EINECS 209-711-2; intermediate for prep. of oxidation color systems.

Rodol EGC. [Lowenstein] m-Aminophenol HCl; CAS 51-81-0; EINECS 200-125-2; intermediate for prep. of oxidation color systems.

Rodol EGS. [Lowenstein] m-Aminophenol sulfate; CAS 68239-81-6; EINECS 269-475-1; intermediate for prep. of oxidation color systems.

Rodol EOX. [Lowenstein] 4-Ethoxy-m-phenylenediamine sulfate; CAS 68015-98-5; EINECS 268-164-8; intermediate for prep. of oxidation color systems.

Rodol ERN. [Lowenstein] 1-Naphthol; intermediate for prep. of oxidation color systems.

Rodol Gray B Base. [Lowenstein] N-Phenyl-p-phenylenediamine; CAS 101-54-2; EINECS 202-951-9; intermediate for prep. of oxidation color systems.

Rodol Gray BS. [Lowenstein] N-Phenyl-p-phenylenediamine sulfate; CAS 4698-29-7; EINECS 225-173-1; intermediate for prep. of oxidation color systems.

Rodol Gray DMS. [Lowenstein] N,N-Dimethyl-p-phenylenediamine sulfate; CAS 6219-73-4; EINECS 228-292-7; intermediate for prep. of oxidation color systems.

Rodol HQ. [Lowenstein] Hydroquinone; CAS 123-31-9; EINECS 204-617-8; intermediate for prep. of oxidation

color systems.

Rodol LY. [Lowenstein] 4-Nitro-m-phenylenediamine; intermediate for prep. of oxidation color systems.

Rodol MPD. [Lowenstein] m-Phenylenediamine; intermediate for prep. of oxidation color systems.

Rodol MPDS. [Lowenstein] m-Phenylenediamine sulfate; CAS 541-70-8; EINECS 208-791-6; intermediate for prep. of oxidation color systems.

Rodol P Base. [Lowenstein] p-Aminophenol; CAS 123-30-8; EINECS 204-616-2; intermediate for prep. of oxidation color systems.

Rodol PAOC. [Lowenstein] 4-Amino-2-hydroxytoluene; CAS 2835-95-2; EINECS 220-618-6; intermediate for prep. of oxidation color systems.

Rodol PDAS. [Lowenstein] 2-Methoxy-p-phenylenediamine sulfate; CAS 42909-29-5; EINECS 255-999-8; intermediate for prep. of oxidation color systems.

Rodol PG. [Lowenstein] Pyrogallol; CAS 87-66-1; EINECS 201-762-9; intermediate for prep. of oxidation color systems.

Rodol PM. [Lowenstein] p-Methylaminophenol sulfate; CAS 55-55-0; EINECS 200-237-1; intermediate for prep. of oxidation color systems.

Rodol PS. [Lowenstein] p-Aminophenol sulfate; CAS 63084-98-0; EINECS 263-847-7; intermediate for prep. of oxidation color systems.

Rodol RS. [Lowenstein] Resorcinol; CAS 108-46-3; EINECS 203-585-2; intermediate for prep. of oxidation color systems.

Rodol YBA. [Lowenstein] 2-Amino-5-nitrophenol; CAS 121-88-0; EINECS 204-503-8; intermediate for prep. of oxidation color systems.

Rohadon® M-449. [Rohm Tech] Polymethyl methacrylate; CAS 9011-14-7; dental grade polymer for prostheses and bridges with superior shape and color matching qualities; also for nail care formulations; bead in powd. form.

Rohadon® M-527. [Rohm Tech] Polymethyl methacrylate; CAS 9011-14-7; dental grade polymer for prostheses and bridges with superior shape and color matching qualities; also for nail care formulations; ground bulk form.

Rohadon® MW-235. [Rohm Tech] Polymethyl methacrylate; CAS 9011-14-7; dental grade polymer for prostheses and bridges with superior shape and color matching qualities; also for nail care formulations; bead in powd. form.

Rohadon® MW-332. [Rohm Tech] Polymethyl methacrylate; CAS 9011-14-7; dental grade polymer for prostheses and bridges with superior shape and color matching qualities; also for nail care formulations; bead in powd. form.

Rohadon® MW-422. [Rohm Tech] Polymethyl methacrylate; CAS 9011-14-7; dental grade polymer for prostheses and bridges with superior shape and color matching qualities; also for nail care formulations; bead in powd. form.

Rohagit® S, SD 15. [Rohm GmbH] Acrylates copolymer; thickener, stabilizer for cosmetics.

Rohagum® M-335. [Rohm Tech] Methyl methacrylate and modified PVC; heat sealing raw material for pkg. of foods and pharmaceuticals; bead in powd. form.

Rohagum® M-345. [Rohm Tech] Methyl methacrylate; heat sealing raw material for pkg. of foods and pharmaceuticals; bead in powd. form.

Rohagum® M-825. [Rohm Tech] Methyl methacrylate; heat sealing raw material for pkg. of foods and pharmaceuticals; ground bulk form.

Rohagum® M-890. [Rohm Tech] Methyl methacrylate; heat sealing raw material for pkg. of foods and pharmaceuticals; ground bulk form.

Rohagum® M-914. [Rohm Tech] Polymethyl methacrylate; CAS 9011-14-7; heat sealing raw material for pkg. of foods and pharmaceuticals.

Rohagum® M-920. [Rohm Tech] Methyl methacrylate; heat

sealing raw material for pkg. of foods and pharmaceuticals; bead in powd. form.

Rohagum® MB-319. [Rohm Tech] Methyl methacrylate and ethyl acrylate; heat sealing raw material for pkg. of foods and pharmaceuticals; bead in powd. form.

Rohagum® N-80. [Rohm Tech] Ethyl methacrylate and methyl acrylate; heat sealing raw material for pkg. of foods and pharmaceuticals; pelletized bulk form.

Rohagum® N-742. [Rohm Tech] Ethyl methacrylate; CAS 97-63-2; EINECS 202-597-5; heat sealing raw material for pkg. of foods and pharmaceuticals; ground bulk form.

Rohagum® P-24. [Rohm Tech] n-Butyl methacrylate; CAS 97-88-1; EINECS 202-615-1; heat sealing raw material for pkg. of foods and pharmaceuticals; bead in powd. form.

Rohagum® P-26. [Rohm Tech] Isobutyl methacrylate; CAS 97-86-9; heat sealing raw material for pkg. of foods and pharmaceuticals; bead in powd. form.

Rohagum® P-28. [Rohm Tech] Isobutyl methacrylate; CAS 97-86-9; heat sealing raw material for pkg. of foods and pharmaceuticals; ground bulk form.

Rohagum® P-675. [Rohm Tech] Isobutyl methacrylate; CAS 97-86-9; heat sealing raw material for pkg. of foods and pharmaceuticals; bead in powd. form.

Rohagum® PM-381. [Rohm Tech] Butyl and methyl methacrylate; heat sealing raw material for pkg. of foods and pharmaceuticals; ground bulk form.

Rohagum® PM-685. [Rohm Tech] n-Butyl methacrylate, methyl methacrylate; heat sealing raw material for pkg. of foods and pharmaceuticals; bead in powd. form.

Rohagum® PQ-610. [Rohm Tech] Isobutyl methacrylate; CAS 97-86-9; heat sealing raw material for pkg. of foods and pharmaceuticals; ground bulk form.

Rohamere® 4885F. [Rohm Tech] Methyl and isobutyl methacrylate emulsion; high quality, nonyel. thickener for hair care prods. (perms, colorants); powd.

Rohamere® 4899F. [Rohm Tech] Methyl methacrylate copolymer; high quality, nonyel. thickener for hair care prods. (perms, colorants).

Rohamere® 4944F. [Rohm Tech] Methyl methacrylate with carboxylic groups; high quality, nonyel. thickener for hair care prods. (perms, colorants).

Rohamere® 6639F. [Rohm Tech] Acrylic copolymer with carboxylic groups; high quality, nonyel. thickener for hair care prods. (perms, colorants); ground form.

Rohamere® 7525L. [Rohm Tech] Methacrylic acid polyelectrolyte aq. sol'n.; cationic; high quality, nonyel. thickener for hair care prods. (perms, colorants); liq.

Rohamere® 8744F. [Rohm Tech] Polymethyl methacrylate; CAS 9011-14-7; high quality, nonyel. thickener for hair care prods. (perms, colorants); bead in powd. form.

Rohasol® P-550. [Rohm Tech] n-Butyl methacrylate/min. spirits sol'n.; CAS 97-88-1; EINECS 202-615-1; heat sealing raw material for pkg. of foods and pharmaceuticals; liq.

Rohasol® PM-555. [Rohm Tech] Methacrylic esters and olefins in org. emulsion; heat sealing raw material for pkg. of foods and pharmaceuticals; liq.

Rohasol® PM-560. [Rohm Tech] n-Butyl and methyl methacrylate in Shellsol A sol'n.; heat sealing raw material for pkg. of foods and pharmaceuticals; liq.

Rohasol® PM-709. [Rohm Tech] n-Butyl and methyl methacrylate in xylene sol'n.; heat sealing raw material for pkg. of foods and pharmaceuticals; liq.

Rol 52. [Fabriquimica] PEG-40 stearate; CAS 9004-99-3; thickener, emulsifier, coemulsifier, and emollient for cosmetics; acid no. < 3; iodine no. < 1; sapon. no. 25-40.

Rol 53. [Fabriquimica] PEG-50 stearate; CAS 9004-99-3; thickener, emulsifier, coemulsifier, and emollient for cosmetics; acid no. < 3; iodine no. < 1; sapon. no. 20-35.

Rol 59. [Fabriquimica] PEG-100 stearate; CAS 9004-99-3; thickener, emulsifier, coemulsifier, and emollient for cosmetics; acid no. < 3; iodine no. < 1; sapon. no. 10-25.

Rol 400. [Fabriquimica] PEG-8 stearate; CAS 9004-99-3; thickener, emulsifier, coemulsifier, and emollient for cosmetics; acid no. < 2; iodine no. < 2; sapon. no. 75-85.

Rol AG. [Fabriquimica] PEG-8 oleate; CAS 9004-96-0; thickener, emulsifier, coemulsifier, and emollient for cosmetics; acid no. < 1; iodine no. 50-60; sapon. no. 80-95.

Rol D 600. [Fabriquimica] PEG-150 disterate; CAS 9005-08-7; thickener for shampoos; acid no. < 1; iodine no. 0.5 max.; sapon. no. 14-20.

Rol DGE. [Fabriquimica] PEG-2 stearate; CAS 106-11-6; EINECS 203-363-5; thickener, emulsifier, coemulsifier, and emollient for cosmetics; acid no. < 2; iodine no. < 1; sapon. no. 145-160.

Rol DL 40. [Fabriquimica] PEG-8 dilaurate; CAS 9005-02-1; thickener, emulsifier, coemulsifier, and emollient for cosmetics; acid no. < 1; iodine no. 10-20; sapon. no. 120-135.

Rol DO 40. [Fabriquimica] PEG-8 dioleate; CAS 9005-07-6; thickener, emulsifier, coemulsifier, and emollient for cosmetics; acid no. < 1; iodine no. 65-80; sapon. no. 100-115.

Rol GE. [Fabriquimica] Glycol stearate; CAS 111-60-4; EINECS 203-886-9; thickener, emulsifier, coemulsifier, and emollient for cosmetics; acid no. < 8; iodine no. < 1; sapon. no. 180-190.

Rol L 40. [Fabriquimica] PEG-8 laurate; CAS 9004-81-3; thickener, emulsifier, coemulsifier, and emollient for cosmetics; acid no. < 1; idoine no. < 12; sapon. no. 75-95.

Rol LP. [Fabriquimica] Propylene glycol laurate; CAS 142-55-2; EINECS 205-542-3; thickener, emulsifier, coemulsifier, and emollient for cosmetics; acid no. < 1; iodine no. 20-30; sapon. no. 175-195.

Rol MOG. [Fabriquimica] Glyceryl oleate; thickener, emulsifier, coemulsifier, and emollient for cosmetics; acid no. < 2; iodine no. 80-100; sapon. no. 155-165.

Rol RP. [Fabriquimica] Propylene glycol ricinoleate; CAS 26402-31-3; EINECS 247-669-7; thickener, emulsifier, coemulsifier, and emollient for cosmetics; acid no. < 1; iodine no. 60-75; sapon. no. 140-150.

Rol TR. [Fabriquimica] Glyceryl trihydroxystearate; CAS 8001-78-3; thickener, emulsifier, coemulsifier, and emollient for cosmetics; acid no. < 4; iodine no. < 5; sapon. no. 170-190.

Rolamid CD. [Auschem SpA] Cocamide DEA; CAS 61791-31-9; EINECS 263-163-9; nonionic; thickener, foam booster, superfatting agent for toiletries; liq.; 100% conc.

Rolpon 24/230. [Auschem SpA] Sodium laureth-2 sulfate; CAS 9004-82-4; 15826-16-1; anionic; raw material for use in detergent toiletry preps.; liq.; 27% conc.

Rolpon 24/270. [Auschem SpA] Sodium laureth-2 sulfate; CAS 9004-82-4; 15826-16-1; anionic; raw material for use in detergent toiletry preps.; paste; 70% conc.

Rolpon 24/330. [Auschem SpA] Sodium alkyl ether sulfate; CAS 91648-56-5; anionic; detergent; liq.; 27% conc.

Rolpon 24/330 N. [Auschem SpA] Sodium laureth-3 sulfate; CAS 9004-82-4; 15826-16-1; anionic; raw material for detergent toiletry preps.; liq.; 27% conc.

Rolpon 24/370. [Auschem SpA] Sodium alkyl ether sulfate; CAS 91648-56-5; anionic; detergent; paste; 70% conc.

Rolpon C 200. [Auschem SpA] Sodium trideceth-7 carboxylate; anionic; raw material for use in detergent toiletry preps.; liq.; 30% conc.

Rolpon LSX. [Auschem SpA] Sodium lauryl sulfate; CAS 151-21-3; EINECS 205-788-1; anionic; raw material for use in detergent toiletry preps.; liq./paste; 28% conc.

Rolpon SE 138. [Auschem SpA] Disodium laureth sulfosuccinate; CAS 39354-45-5; anionic; raw material for use in detergent toiletry preps.; liq.; 40% conc.

Romilat. [Henkel/Cospha] Fragrance raw material for cosmetic, personal care, detergent, and cleaning prods.; colorless liq., herbal odor; b.p. 64 C; flash pt. 58 C.

Rose Ether Phenoxyethanol. [Henkel/Cospha] Fragrance raw material for cosmetic, personal care, detergent, and cleaning prods.; liq., rose odor; flash pt. 121 C.

Rose Hip Seed Oil. [Les Colorants Wackherr] Source of essential fatty acids.

Rose Talc. [Presperse] Talc; CAS 14807-96-6; EINECS 238-877-9; elegant, silky smooth, creamy natural powd. for pressed powds. and pigmented cosmetics; large particle size renders it virtually transparent on skin; platy particle shape provides unsurpassed compressibility and high skin adhesion.

Ross Bayberry Wax. [Frank B. Ross] Bayberry wax; CAS 8038-77-5; avail. as crude and refined wh. bleached grades; for use in buffing compds., candles, cosmetics, crayons, laundry wax, textile sizing; grayish-green wax-like fat, aromatic odor; sp.gr. 0.977-0.982; m.p. 38-49 C; acid no. 5-24; sapon. no. 210-239; flash pt. 470 F min.; ref. index 1.4360.

Ross Bayberry Wax Substitute. [Frank B. Ross] Bayberry wax substitute; film-forming wax for use in buffing compds., candles, cosmetics, crayons, laundry wax, and textile sizing; m.p. 125-135 F; acid no. 3-10; iodine no. 5 max.; sapon. no. 170-185; flash pt. (COC) 450 F min.

Ross Beeswax. [Frank B. Ross] Beeswax; avail. as crude, yel. refined, and wh. bleached grades; for use in polishes, cosmetics, medicinal ointments/salves, candles, leather/textile/wood/paper finishes, confectionery, modeling, engraving, acid etching, lithography, emulsions; FDA §184.1973, 184.1975; lt. taffy to deep brn. wax, char. honey odor; m.p. 62-65 C; acid no. 17-24; cloud pt. -65 C max.

Ross Beeswax Substitute. [Frank B. Ross] Beeswax substitutes; various grades (Yel. No. 11, 30, 662, 909, 1595, White No. 145, 1776, 1623, 628/5, 1892); for use where pure beeswax is not required in polishes, cosmetics, medicinals (ointments, salves), candles, textile, leather, wood, and paper finishes, confectionary, modeling, engraving, acid etching, lithography, and emulsions; avail. in various grades: yel. or wh.; m.p. from 130-160 F; acid no. from nil to 27; sapon. no. from nil to 103.

Ross Beeswax Substitute 628/5. [Frank B. Ross] Paraffin, candelilla wax, hydrog. tallow glycerides, stearic acid, and cetyl alcohol; for use where pure beeswax is not required in polishes, cosmetics, medicinals (ointments, salves), candles, textile, leather, wood, and paper finishes, confectionary, modeling, engraving, acid etching, lithography, and emulsions.

Ross Beeswax Synthetic. [Frank B. Ross] Synthetic beeswax.

Ross Beeswax Synthetic Cosmetic Grade. [Frank B. Ross] Synthetic beeswax.

Ross Bleached Montan Wax. [Frank B. Ross] Montan wax; CAS 8002-53-7; EINECS 232-313-5; cosmetic wax.

Ross Bleached Montan Wax Cosmetic. [Frank B. Ross] Montan wax; CAS 8002-53-7; EINECS 232-313-5; cosmetic wax.

Ross Bleached Refined Shellac Wax. [Frank B. Ross] Shellac wax.

Ross Bleached Refined Shellac Wax Cosmetic Grade. [Frank B. Ross] Shellac wax.

Ross Brazil Wax. [Frank B. Ross] Carnauba; CAS 8015-86-9; EINECS 232-399-4; wax for cosmetics use.

Ross Candelilla Wax. [Frank B. Ross] Candelilla wax; CAS 8006-44-8; EINECS 232-347-0; avail. as crude and refined grades; used in polishes, leather/textile finishes, cosmetics (lipstick), casting, lubricants/greases, adhesives, chewing gum, paper size, paper coatings; FDA §172.615, 175.105, 175.320, 176.180; grayish-green

wax-like fat, aromatic odor; sp.gr. 0.977-0.982; m.p. 38-49 C; acid no. 5-24; iodine no. 2-10; sapon. no. 210-239; flash pt. 470 F min.; ref. index 1.4360.

Ross Carnauba Wax. [Frank B. Ross] Carnauba wax; CAS 8015-86-9; avail. as Prime or No. 1 Yel., Med. or No. 2 Yel., No. 2 or No. 3 North Country grades; used for polishes, leather finishes, cosmetic creams and lipsticks, casting, lubricants, buffing compds., glazing of candies, gum, pills, and paper, inks, protective coatings, candles, medicinal ointments and salves; FDA §182.1978; flakes or powd.; sp.gr. 0.996-0.998; m.p. 181.4 F min.; acid no. 2-10; iodine no. 7-14; sapon. no. 78-88; flash pt. 570 F min.; ref. index 1.4540.

Ross Castor Wax. [Frank B. Ross] Hydrog. castor oil; CAS 8001-78-3; EINECS 232-292-2; wax for cosmetics, pharmaceuticals.

Ross Ceresine Wax. [Frank B. Ross] Ceresine wax; CAS 8001-75-0; EINECS 232-290-1; avail. in various grades; used for adhesives, textile waterproofing/mildewproofing, polishes, sunchecking in rubbers, cosmetic pomades and perfumes, crayons, medicinal ointments and slaves, lubricants, mold releases, paper impregnants/sizes, paints, casting; FDA §175.105; wh., yel., tan, or orange grades; sp.gr. 0.880-0.935; m.p. 53.3-87.8 C; acid no. nil; sapon. no. 2 max.; ref. index 1.425-1.435.

Ross Crude Scale Wax. [Frank B. Ross] Paraffin; CAS 8002-74-2; EINECS 232-315-6; cosmetic wax.

Ross Japan Wax. [Frank B. Ross] Japan wax; CAS 8001-39-6; wax used in package coatings, textile finishes, cosmetics, lubricants for textile, metal, and rope, pencils, crayons, wax modeling, buffing compds., pharmaceuticals, anticorrosion agent for metal; FDA §175.105, 175.300, 175.350, 176.170, 182.10; pale cream colored wax, gummy feel; sp.gr. 0.975-0.984; m.p. 46.5-51.5 C; acid no. 6-30; iodine no. 4-15; sapon. no. 200-225; flash pt. 385 F min.; ref. index 1.4550.

Ross Japan Wax Substitute 473. [Frank B. Ross] Microcryst. wax, fish glycerides, tallow glycerides, oleostearine.

Ross Japan Wax Substitute 525. [Frank B. Ross] Fish glycerides, tallow glycerides, oleostearine, microcryst. wax; for coatings, textile finishes, cosmetics, lubricants, crayons, wax modeling, buffing compds., pharmaceuticals; m.p. 53-56 C; acid no. 4; sapon. no. 185-195.

Ross Japan Wax Substitute 930. [Frank B. Ross] Microcryst. wax, hydrog. tallow glycerides.

Ross Japan Wax Substitute 966. [Frank B. Ross] Hydrog. soybean oil, paraffin; for coatings, textile finishes, cosmetics, lubricants, crayons, wax modeling, buffing compds., pharmaceuticals; m.w. 51-55 C; acid no. 5; sapon. no. 185-195.

Ross Ozokerite Wax. [Frank B. Ross] Ozokerite; CAS 8021-55-4; waxes used in adhesives, cosmetic creams and pomades, paints, varnishes, leather, auto, and floor polishes, and printing inks; FDA §175.105; avail. in various grades: wh. or yel.; m.p. from 145 to 198 F.

Ross Rice Bran Wax. [Frank B. Ross] Rice bran wax, refined grade; CAS 8016-60-2; EINECS 232-409-7; wax for use in confectionery, chewing gum, leather/textile/cordage finishes, cosmetics, and coatings for fruit and vegetables; FDA §172.615, 172.890; tan to lt. brn. flake or powd.; m.p. 76-82 C; acid no. 5-15; iodine no. 10 max.; sapon. no. 70-105; flash pt. 520 F min.

Ross Spermaceti Wax Substitute 573. [Frank B. Ross] Cetyl esters; for adhesives, cosmetic creams, lotions, and soaps, medicinals (ointments, salves), candles, textiles, coatings; sp.gr. 0.940-0.946; m.p. 42-50 C; acid no. 2-8; iodine no. 3 max.; sapon. no. 117-148; flash pt. 470 F min.

Ross Synthetic Candelilla Wax. [Frank B. Ross] Paraffin, myristyl lignocerate, stearic acid, hydrog. tallow glyceride;

hard lustrous wax for use in furniture, leather, auto, and floor polishes, leather and textile finishes, cosmetics (lipsticks), casting, lubricants/greases, adhesives, chewing gum, paper size and coatings; pale yel. hard wax, faint aromatic odor; m.p. 155-165 F; acid no. 12-22; sapon. no. 43-65; flash pt. 435 F min.

Rudol® . [Witco/Petroleum Spec.] Lt. min. oil NF; white oil functioning as binder, carrier, conditioner, defoamer, dispersant, extender, heat transfer agent, lubricant, moisture barrier, plasticizer, protective agent, and/or softener in adhesives, agric., chemicals, cleaning, cosmetics, food, pkg., plastics, and textiles industries; FDA §172.878, 178.3620a; water-wh., odorless, tasteless; sp.gr. 0.852–0.870; visc. 28-30 cSt (40 C); pour pt. -7 C; flash pt. 188 C.

Rueterg SA. [Finetex] Dodecylbenzene sulfonic acid; CAS 27176-87-0; EINECS 248-289-4; anionic; intermediate for detergents and emulsifiers; liq.; 97% conc.

Ruscogenins Phytosome® . [Indena SpA; Lipo] Complex of butcher's broom sapogenins and soybean phospholipids; astringent, skin lightener, soothing, moisturizing agent; coadjuvant in external treatment of cellulitis and for heavy legs; after-sun, after-depilation, and after-shave prods., personal hygiene prods.; lt. brn. amorphous powd.; water-disp.; usage level: to 2%.

Ryoto Sugar Ester B-370. [Mitsubishi Kasei Foods] Sucrose tribehenate; biodeg. emulsifier with antibacterial, wetting, and dispersing effect for foods, drugs, and cosmetics industries; powd.; partly sol. in propylene glycol, glycerin, liq. paraffin, soybean oil, cottonseed oil, water; m.p. 53-63 C; decomp. pt. 241 C; HLB 3.

Ryoto Sugar Ester L-195. [Mitsubishi Kasei Foods] Sucrose polylaurate; emulsifier for foods, drugs, and cosmetics applics.

Ryoto Sugar Ester L-595. [Mitsubishi Kasei Foods] Sucrose dilaurate; emulsifier with antibacterial, wetting, and dispersing effect for foods, drugs, cosmetics industries; pellet; sol. in water, ethanol; partly sol. in glycerin; HLB 5.

Ryoto Sugar Ester L-1570. [Mitsubishi Kasei Foods] Sucrose laurate; CAS 25339-99-5; EINECS 246-873-3; emulsifier with antibacterial, wetting, and dispersing effect for foods, drugs, cosmetics industries; surf. tens. 31.7 dynes/cm (0.1% aq.); Ross-Miles foam 177 mm (0.25% aq., initial).

Ryoto Sugar Ester L-1695. [Mitsubishi Kasei Foods] Sucrose laurate; CAS 25339-99-5; EINECS 246-873-3; emulsifier with antibacterial, wetting, and dispersing effect for foods, drugs, cosmetics industries; pellet; sol. in water, ethanol; partly sol. in glycerin; m.p. 35-47 C; decomp. pt. 235 C; HLB 16; surf. tens. 31.6 dynes/cm (0.1% aq.).

Ryoto Sugar Ester LN-195. [Mitsubishi Kasei Foods] Sucrose polylinoleate; emulsifier for foods, drugs, and cosmetics.

Ryoto Sugar Ester M-1695. [Mitsubishi Kasei Foods] Sucrose myristate; emulsifier with antibacterial, wetting, and dispersing effect for foods, drugs, cosmetics industries; pellet; sol. in water, propylene glycol, ethanol; partly sol. in glycerin; m.p. 27-40 C; decomp. pt. 243 C; HLB 16.

Ryoto Sugar Ester O-170. [Mitsubishi Kasei Foods] Sucrose polyoleate; emulsifier for foods, drugs, and cosmetics.

Ryoto Sugar Ester O-1570. [Mitsubishi Kasei Foods] Sucrose oleate; emulsifier with antibacterial, wetting, and dispersing effect for foods, drugs, cosmetics industries; vegetable/fruit scrubbing, baby bottle cleaning, demulsification; pellet; sol. in water, ethanol; partly sol. in glycerin; m.p. 27-43 C; decomp. pt. 227 C; HLB 15; surf. tens. 34.5 dynes/cm (0.1% aq.); Ross-Miles foam 14 mm (0.25% aq., initial).

Ryoto Sugar Ester OWA-1570. [Mitsubishi Kasei Foods] Sucrose oleate; nonionic; emulsifier, conditioner, soft-

ener, detergent for foods, drugs, cosmetics; tablet lubricant; vegetable/fruit scrubbing; baby bottle cleaning; demulsification; paste; HLB 15.0; 40% conc.

Ryoto Sugar Ester P-1570. [Mitsubishi Kasei Foods] Sucrose palmitate; CAS 26446-38-8; EINECS 247-706-7; nonionic; emulsifier, conditioner, softener, detergent for foods, drugs, cosmetics; tablet lubricant; polymerization emulsifier for food pkg. film; demulsifier; solubilizer, dispersant for flavors and preservatives; powd.; partly sol. in water, propylene glycol, glycerin, liq. paraffin, soybean and cottonseed oils; m.p. 47-54 C; decomp. pt. 237 C; HLB 15.0; surf. tens. 35.4 dynes/cm (0.1% aq.); Ross-Miles foam 15 mm (0.25% aq., initial); 100% conc.

Ryoto Sugar Ester P-1570S. [Mitsubishi Kasei Foods] Sucrose palmitate; CAS 26446-38-8; EINECS 247-706-7; nonionic; emulsifier, conditioner, softener, detergent for foods, drugs, cosmetics; tablet lubricant; demulsifier; for use with high ignition residue; powd.; sol. in water; partly sol. in propylene glycol, glycerin, liq. paraffin, soybean and cottonseed oils; HLB 15.

Ryoto Sugar Ester P-1670. [Mitsubishi Kasei Foods] Sucrose palmitate; CAS 26446-38-8; EINECS 247-706-7; nonionic; emulsifier, conditioner, softener, detergent for foods, drugs, cosmetics; tablet lubricant; demulsifier; solubilizer, dispersant for flavors and preservatives; powd.; sol. in water; partly sol. in propylene glycol, glycerin, liq. paraffin, soybean and cottonseed oils; m.p. 40-48 C; decomp. pt. 235 C; HLB 16; surf. tens. 34.5 dynes/cm (0.1% aq.); Ross-Miles foam 24 mm (0.25% aq., initial).

Ryoto Sugar Ester S-070. [Mitsubishi Kasei Foods] Sucrose polystearate; nonionic; o/w and w/o emulsifier, softener, conditioner, and aerating agent in foods; also for cosmetics/pharmaceticals; powd.; 100% conc.

Ryoto Sugar Ester S-170. [Mitsubishi Kasei Foods] Sucrose di, tristearate; nonionic; emulsifier, conditioner, softener, detergent for foods, drugs, cosmetics; tablet lubricant; powd.; partly sol. in propylene glycol, glycerin, liq. paraffin, soybean and cottonseed oils; insol. in water; m.p. 51-61 C; decomp. pt. 260 C; HLB 1.0; 100% conc.

Ryoto Sugar Ester S-170 Ac. [Mitsubishi Kasei] Sucrose tetrastearate triacetate; emulsifier for foods, drugs, and cosmetics.

Ryoto Sugar Ester S-270. [Mitsubishi Kasei Foods] Sucrose di, tristearate; nonionic; emulsifier, conditioner, softener, detergent for foods, drugs, cosmetics; tablet lubricant; powd.; partly sol. in propylene glycol, glycerin, liq. paraffin, soybean and cottonseed oils; insol. in water; m.p. 52-61 C; decomp. pt. 253 C; HLB 2.0; 100% conc.

Ryoto Sugar Ester S-370. [Mitsubishi Kasei Foods] Sucrose tristearate; nonionic; emulsifier, conditioner, softener, detergent for foods, drugs, cosmetics; tablet lubricant; powd.; partly sol. in propylene glycol, glycerin, liq. paraffin, soybean and cottonseed oils; insol. in water; m.p. 51-58 C; decomp. pt. 238 C; HLB 3; 100% conc.

Ryoto Sugar Ester S-370F. [Mitsubishi Kasei Foods] Sucrose tristearate; nonionic; emulsifier, conditioner, softener, detergent for foods, drugs, cosmetics; tablet lubricant; ultrafine version of S-370; powd.; HLB 3.

Ryoto Sugar Ester S-570. [Mitsubishi Kasei Foods] Sucrose distearate; CAS 27195-16-0; EINECS 248-317-5; nonionic; emulsifier, conditioner, softener, detergent for foods, drugs, cosmetics; tablet lubricant; polymerization emulsifier for food pkg. film; powd.; partly sol. in propylene glycol, glycerin, liq. paraffin, soybean and cottonseed oils; insol. in water; m.p. 50-57 C; decomp. pt. 231 C; HLB 5.0; surf. tens. 38.1 dynes/cm (0.1% aq.); 100% conc.

Ryoto Sugar Ester S-770. [Mitsubishi Kasei Foods] Sucrose distearate; CAS 27195-16-0; EINECS 248-317-5; emulsifier, conditioner, softener, detergent for foods, drugs, cosmetics; tablet lubricant; polymerization emulsifier for food pkg. film; powd.; partly sol. in propylene glycol, glycerin, liq. paraffin, soybean and cottonseed oils, water; m.p. 49-60 C; decomp. pt. 233 C; HLB 7.0; surf. tens. 37.4 dynes/cm (0.1% aq.).

Ryoto Sugar Ester S-970. [Mitsubishi Kasei Foods] Sucrose mono, distearate; CAS 27195-16-0; EINECS 248-317-5; nonionic; emulsifier, conditioner, softener, detergent for foods, drugs, cosmetics; powd.; partly sol. in propylene glycol, glycerin, liq. paraffin, soybean and cottonseed oils, water; m.p. 49-56 C; decomp. pt. 234 C; HLB 9.0; surf. tens. 35.8 dynes/cm (0.1% aq.); 100% conc.

Ryoto Sugar Ester S-1170. [Mitsubishi Kasei Foods] Sucrose stearate; CAS 25168-73-4; EINECS 246-705-9; nonionic; emulsifier, conditioner, detergent for foods, drugs, cosmetics; softener, antistat for textiles; solubilizer, dispersant for flavors and preservatives; powd.; partly sol. in propylene glycol, glycerin, liq. paraffin, soybean and cottonseed oils, water; m.p. 49-55 C; decomp. pt. 234 C; HLB 11; surf. tens. 34.8 dynes/cm (0.1% aq.); 100% conc.

Ryoto Sugar Ester S-1170S. [Mitsubishi Kasei Foods] Sucrose stearate; CAS 25168-73-4; EINECS 246-705-9; nonionic; emulsifier, conditioner, detergent for foods, drugs, cosmetics; softener, antistat for textiles; solubilizer, dispersant for flavors and preservatives; for use with high ignition residue; powd.; sol. in water; partly sol. in propylene glycol, glycerin, liq. paraffinn, soybean and cottonseed oils; HLB 11.

Ryoto Sugar Ester S-1570. [Mitsubishi Kasei Foods] Sucrose stearate; CAS 25168-73-4; EINECS 246-705-9; nonionic; emulsifier, conditioner, detergent for foods, drugs, cosmetics; softener, antistat for textiles; solubilizer, dispersant for flavors and preservatives; powd.; sol. in water; partly sol. in propylene glycol, glycerin, liq. paraffin, soybean and cottonseed oils; m.p. 49-55 C; decomp. pt. 234 C; HLB 15.0; surf. tens. 34.7 dynes/cm (0.1% aq.); Ross-Miles foam 11 mm (0.25% aq., initial); 100% conc.

Ryoto Sugar Ester S-1670. [Mitsubishi Kasei Foods] Sucrose stearate; CAS 25168-73-4; EINECS 246-705-9; nonionic; emulsifier, conditioner, detergent for foods, drugs, cosmetics; softener, antistat for textiles; solubilizer, dispersant for flavors and preservatives; powd.; sol. in water; partly sol. in propylene glycol, glycerin, liq. paraffin, soybean and cottonseed oils; m.p. 49-56 C; decomp. pt. 237 C; HLB 16; surf. tens. 34.7 dynes/cm (0.1% aq.); Ross-Miles foam 12 mm (0.25% aq., initial).

Ryoto Sugar Ester S-1670S. [Mitsubishi Kasei Foods] Sucrose stearate; CAS 25168-73-4; EINECS 246-705-9; nonionic; emulsifier, conditioner, softener, detergent for foods, drugs, cosmetics; for use with high ignition residue; powd.; sol. in water; partly sol. in propylene glycol, glycerin, liq. paraffin, soybean and cottonseed oils; HLB 16.

S

S-100. [U.S. Cosmetics] Sericite; cosmetic raw material; avg. particle size 1-15 μ.

S-152. [U.S. Cosmetics] Sericite; cosmetic raw material; avg. particle size 1-20 μ.

S-210. [Procter & Gamble] Soya fatty acid; CAS 67701-08-0; intermediate for mfg. of soaps, amides, esters, alcoholamides; raw material for non-surfactant applics.; Gardner 2 max. liq.; m.w. 279; acid no. 197-203; iodine no. 133 min.; sapon. no. 199-205; 100% conc.

S.A.B. [Gattefosse SA] Bovine albumin serum; biological additive.

Saccaluronate CC. [Les Colorants Wackherr] Fermentation grade of sodium hyaluronate; CAS 9067-32-7; cosmetics ingred.; 1% sol'n. of lower m.w. material.

Saccaluronate CW. [Les Colorants Wackherr] Fermentation grade of sodium hyaluronate; CAS 9067-32-7; cosmetics ingred.; high m.w. powd.

Saccaluronate LC. [Les Colorants Wackherr] Fermentation grade of sodium hyaluronate; CAS 9067-32-7; cosmetics ingred.; 1% sol'n. of high m.w. material.

Safester A-75. [Induchem AG; Lipo] Ethyl linoleate; CAS 544-35-4; EINECS 208-868-4; vitamin deriv. for cosmetics, toiletries, pharmaceuticals.

Safester A 75 WS. [Induchem AG] Solubilized ethyl linoleate with PEG-12 glyceryl laurate and PEG-36 castor oil; vitamin deriv. for cosmetics and pharmaceuticals.

SAG-710, -730. [Union Carbide] Dimethicone and silica; antifoams.

Salacos 99. [Nisshin Oil Mills] Isononyl isononanoate; CAS 42131-25-9.

Salacos 618. [Nisshin Oil Mills] Diisostearyl adipate.

Salacos 913. [Nisshin Oil Mills] Isotridecyl isononanoate.

Salacos 6318. [Nisshin Oil Mills] Trimethylolpropane triisostearate; CAS 68541-50-4; EINECS 271-347-5; lipid for cosmetics.

Salcare SC10. [Allied Colloids] Polyquaternium-7 aq. sol'n.; CAS 26590-05-6; cationic; conditioner, antistat, film-former for hair care formulas (shampoo, conditioner, setting lotions, styling gels and mousses), foam baths, suntan lotions, lip preps.; clear to pale yel. liq., mild aldehydic odor; sp.gr. 1.010-1.015; visc. 7500-15,000 cps; pH 6.5-7.5; 8.1-9.1% solids.

Salcare SC30. [Allied Colloids] Polyquaternium-6 aq. sol'n.; CAS 26062-79-3; cationic; alkaline-stable conditioner, antistat, film-former for hair care formulas (shampoo, conditioner, setting lotion, styling gel and mousse), foam baths, suntan lotions, lip preps.; clear visc. liq., mild odor; sp.gr. 1.085; visc. 10,000 cps; pH 6.0-7.0; 40% solids.

Salcare SC90. [Allied Colloids] Steareth-10 allyl ether/ acrylates copolymer aq. emulsion; anionic; thickener, gellant, stabilizer, and suspending agent producing consistent, clear gels on addition of alkali; for hair and skin care prods. incl. shampoos, setting gels, permanent waves, styling gels, hand and body lotions; wh. liq.; pH 3.0; 30% solids.

Salcare SC91. [Allied Colloids] Sodium polyacrylate copolymer, min. oil, and PPG-1 trideceth-6; anionic; base, gellant, moisturizer, thickener, suspending agent, stabilizer, conditioner, softener for cosmetics, hand and body lotions, suntan lotions/creams, foundation, makeup remover, facial washing creams, hair care prods.; wh. to cream mobile liq., very sl. acrylic odor; sp.gr. 1.10-1.25; visc. 250 cps; pH 6.0-8.0 (2%); 48-52% solids.

Salcare SC92. [Allied Colloids] Polyquaternium 32 and min. oil; cationic; conditioner, thickener, gellant, emulsion stabilizer, suspending agent, opacifier, moisturizer for hair conditioners and shampoos; wh. to cream mobile liq., sl. paraffinic odor; sp.gr. 0.950-1.050; visc. 100-500 cps; pH 3.0-5.0 (2% aq.); 48-52% act.

Salcare SC95. [Allied Colloids] Polyquaternium 37, min. oil, and PPG-1 trideceth-6; cationic; conditioner, thickener, gellant, emulsion stabilizer, suspending agent, and opacifier for hair conditioners; cosmetic base, gellant, moisturizer, spread enhancer, substantivity aid for skin care, hand and body lotions, suntan preps.; off-wh. to cream mobile liq., very sl. acrylic odor; 48-52% act.

Salfax 77. [Chem-Y GmbH] Veg. and animal fats, aliphatic alcohols, fatty acids and cationics; cationic; hair conditioner; base for cream rinses; opaque paste; visc. 3000 mPa·s; acid no. 5; pH 2.6-3.4; 22% act.

Sandet EN. [Sanyo Chem. Industries] Sodium laureth sulfate; CAS 9004-82-4; anionic; shampoo base; liq.; 31.5% conc.

Sandet END, ENN. [Sanyo Chem. Industries] Sodium alkyl ether sulfate; anionic; shampoo base; liq.; 26.5% conc.

Sandobet SC. [Sandoz] Cocoamidopropylhydroxy sultaine; CAS 68139-30-0; EINECS 268-761-3; amphoteric; high foaming, mild surfactant for cosmetic and toiletry applics.; acid and alkali stable; liq.; 50% conc.

Sandogen NH. [Sandoz] PEG-105 behenyl propylenediamine; leveling agent used in mfg. hair dyes.

Sandopan® DTC. [Sandoz] Sodium trideceth-7 carboxylate; anionic; detergent, emulsifier, wetting agent, solubilizer; cosmetics, household, specialty, industrial and institutional cleaner; dishwashing detergent; lime soap dispersant; clear gel; water-sol.; sp.gr. 1.06; visc. 5000 cps; b.p. 220 F; HLB 16.0 (@ pH 8); pH 6.5 (10%); Ross-Miles foam 150 mm (0.1%, 40 C, initial); 68% act.

Sandopan® DTC-100. [Sandoz] Sodium trideceth-7 carboxylate; anionic; detergent, emulsifier, wetting agent for liq. detergents, solv. cleaners, all-purpose cleaners, germicidal cleaners, shampoos, bubble baths; oil solubilizer for aq. systems, acid bowl cleaners; yel. clear liq.; HLB 15.0 (@ pH 8); pH 7.0 (10%); Ross-Miles foam 150 mm (0.1%, 40 C, initial); 70 ± 2% solids.

Sandopan® DTC-Acid. [Sandoz] Trideceth-7 carboxylic acid; anionic; detergent, emulsifier, wetting agent for industrial and personal care, conditioning shampoos, liq.

soaps, household and industrial cleaners; clear liq.; sol. in oils, solvs.; HLB 13.0 (@ pH 2.5); pH 2.5 (10%); surf. tens. 31.6 dynes/cm (0.01%); Ross-Miles foam 145 mm (0.1%, 40 C, initial); 90% conc.

Sandopan® DTC Linear P. [Sandoz] Sodium C12-15 pareth-6 carboxylate; CAS 70632-06-3; anionic; detergent, emulsifier, wetting agent, solubilizer, visc. booster for industrial, personal care, and household prods.; stable in alkali high temps.; wh. opaque paste; HLB 15.0 (pH 8); pH 8.5 (10%); Ross-Miles foam 130 mm (0.1%, 40 C, initial); 70% conc.

Sandopan® DTC Linear P Acid. [Sandoz] C12–15 pareth-7 carboxylic acid; CAS 88497-58-9; anionic; detergent, emulsifier, wetting agent for industrial, personal care, and household use; oil solubilizer; clear liq.; HLB 10 (pH 2.5); pH 3.5 (10%); Ross-Miles foam 120 mm (0.1%, 40 C, initial); 90% conc.

Sandopan® JA-36. [Sandoz] Trideceth-19 carboxylic acid; anionic; moderate foaming mild surfactant, oil solubilizer, wetting agent cosmetics/toiletries, laundry prods., cleaners, industrial specialties; clear to sl. hazy liq.; HLB 16 (pH 2.5); pH 2.5 (10% aq.); surf. tens. 43.7 dynes/cm (0.01%); Ross-Miles foam 130 mm (0.1%, 40 C, initial); 90 ± 2% solids.

Sandopan® KST-A. [Sandoz] Sodium ceteth-13 carboxylate; CAS 33939-65-0; anionic; mild emulsifier, detergent, lime soap dispersant for use in sticks, bar soaps, antiperspirants, other personal care prods., industrial specialties, laundry prods.; inhibits sodium stearate crystal formation; off-wh. waxy solid; HLB 11 (pH 8); pH 6.5 (10% aq.); surf. tens. 42.9 dynes/cm (0.01%); Ross-Miles 70 mm (0.1%, 40 C, initial); 97 ± 2% solids.

Sandopan® LA-8. [Sandoz] Laureth-5 carboxylic acid; anionic; surfactant for cosmetics/toiletries, laundry prods., cleaners, industrial specialties.

Sandopan® LA-8-HC. [Sandoz] Sodium laureth-5 carboxylic acid; CAS 33939-64-9; anionic; mild surfactant for cosmetic and personal care prods., household and industrial applics.; clear liq.; pH 2.5 (10%); surf. tens. 38.6 dynes/cm (0.01%); Ross-Miles foam 155 mm (initial); 91% act.

Sandopan® LS-24. [Sandoz] Sodium laureth-13 carboxylate; CAS 33939-64-9; anionic; mild detergent, emulsifier, solubilizer for baby shampoos and personal care prods.; clear to sl. hazy gel; HLB 16 (pH 8); pH 7.8 (10%); surf. tens. 36.5 dynes/cm (0.01%); Ross-Miles foam 125 mm (0.1%, 40 C, initial); 69 ± 2% solids.

Sandopan® TA-10. [Sandoz] Isosteareth-6 carboxylic acid; anionic; surfactant for cosmetics/toiletries.

Sandopan® TA-20. [Sandoz] Isosteareth-11 carboxylic acid; anionic; surfactant for cosmetics/toiletries.

Sandopan® TFL Conc. [Sandoz] Sodium oleoamphohydroxypropylsulfonate; CAS 68610-38-8; amphoteric; detergent, cosmetic and toiletries prods.; leather industry; amber gel; mild fatty odor; water-sol.; sp.gr. 1.14; b.p. 220 F; 48% conc.

Sandopan® TS-10. [Sandoz] Sodium isosteareth-6 carboxylate; anionic; surfactant for cosmetics/toiletries.

Sandopan® TS-20. [Sandoz] Sodium isosteareth-11 carboxylate; anionic; used for conditioning shampoos.

Sandoperm FE. [Sandoz] Dimethiconol and amodimethicone; cationic; gloss agent, lubricant, and conditioner for hair prods.

Sandoteric CFL. [Sandoz] Cocamphohydroxypropyl sulfonate; CAS 68604-73-9; EINECS 271-705-0; extremely mild surfactant producing synergistic visc. increase with alkyl sulfates; weak ampholyte.

Sandoteric TFL Conc. [Sandoz] Sodium oleoamphohydroxypropyl sulfonate; CAS 68610-38-8; extremely mild surfactant producing synergistic visc. increase with alkyl

sulfates; weak ampholyte; toxicology: zero skin and eye irritation in rabbits.

Sandotex A. [Sandoz] Stearamidoethyl ethanolamine phosphate, cetoleth-24; antistatic agent for hair care; provides light conditioning props.

Sandoz Sulfate 216. [Sandoz] Ammonium laureth sulfate (3 EO); CAS 32612-48-9; anionic; foamer and visc. modifier for personal care prods.; basic ingred. in shampoos and liq. dishwashing prods.; textile scouring; emulsifier and suspending agent in fabrics; pale yel. liq.; visc. 1000 cps max.; cloud pt. 15 C; pH 6.5–7.5 (10%); 58.5–60% act.

Sandoz Sulfate 219. [Sandoz] Sodium laureth sulfate (3 EO); CAS 9004-82-4; anionic; foamer and visc. modifier in personal care prods.; textile scouring; pale yel. liq.; visc. 1000 cps max.; cloud pt. 15 C; pH 7.5–8.5 (15%); 58.5–60% act.

Sandoz Sulfate 219 Special. [Sandoz] Sodium laureth sulfate; anionic; surfactant used in personal and cosmetic prods.; liq.; 30% conc.

Sandoz Sulfate TL. [Sandoz] TEA-lauryl sulfate; CAS 139-96-8; EINECS 205-388-7; anionic; low cloud pt. surfactant for shampoos, other personal care prods.; biodeg.; lt. yel. liq.; visc. 225 cps; cloud pt. 2.5 C; pH 6.4–7.7 (10%); 38.5–42.5% act.

SanSurf™. [Collaborative Labs] Colloidal suspension of nano-sized particles, stabilized by high charge density; provides high levels of immiscible materials dispersed in water, incl. silicones, sunscreens, and oils; devoid of surfactants, liposome-compat. with low irritation potential.

Santone® 10-10-O. [Van Den Bergh Foods] Polyglycerol-10-decaoleate; CAS 11094-60-3; EINECS 234-316-7; nonionic; food emulsifier; solubilizer; emulsion stabilizer; dispersant aid in flavors; liq.; HLB 2.0; sapon. no. 165–180; 100% conc.

Sanwet® COS-905. [Sanyo Chem. Industries; Hoechst Celanese] Sodium polyacrylate starch; cosmetic grade superabsorbent polymer, thickener, gellant for personal care prods.; reduces tack, enhances smoothness and feel; suitable for clear gels, hydro-alcoholic gels, lotions, abrasive mixts.

Sanwet® COS-915. [Sanyo Chem. Industries; Hoechst Celanese] Sodium polyacrylate starch; cosmetic grade superabsorbent polymer, thickener, gellant for personal care prods.; reduces tack, enhances smoothness and feel; suitable for clear gels, hydro-alcoholic gels, lotions, powd. mixts.; wh. gran. powd.; sl. sol. in water; bulk dens. 25-31 lb/ft³; toxicology: LD50 (oral, rat) > 5000 mg/kg (sl. toxic); sl. to moderate eye irritant; pract. nonirritating to skin; > 99% act.

Sanwet® COS-960. [Sanyo Chem. Industries; Hoechst Celanese] Sodium polyacrylate starch; cosmetic grade superabsorbent polymer, thickener, gellant for personal care prods.; reduces tack, enhances smoothness and feel; suitable for clear gels, hydro-alcoholic gels, creams, powd. mixts., as suspension agent.; wh. gran. powd.; sl. sol. in water; bulk dens. 25-31 lb/ft³; toxicology: LD50 (oral, rat) > 5000 mg/kg (sl. toxic); sl. to moderate eye irritant; pract. nonirritating to skin; > 99% act.

Sanwet® COS-965. [Sanyo Chem. Industries; Hoechst Celanese] Sodium polyacrylate starch; cosmetic grade superabsorbent polymer, thickener, gellant for personal care prods.; reduces tack, enhances smoothness and feel; suitable for clear gels, hydro-alcoholic gels, creams, abrasive mixts., as suspension agent.

Sarkosyl® L. [Ciba-Geigy AG] Lauroyl sarcosine; CAS 97-78-9; EINECS 202-608-3; anionic; detergent, corrosion inhibitor, foam booster and stabilizer, wetting agent, lubricant, emulsifier used dentifrices, personal care, and household cleaning prods.; pharmaceuticals, metal processing and finishing, metalworking and cutting oils;

powd.; m.w. 264–285; sol. in org. solvs.; insol. in water; sp.gr. 0.969; m.p. 35–37 C; 94% min. purity.

Satialgine™ H8. [Mendell] Alginic acid NF/FCC; CAS 9005-32-7; EINECS 232-680-1; tablet disintegrant for compressed tablets in wet or dry granulations; wh. to ylsh. wh. fibrous powd.; 75% max. -325 mesh; acid no. ≥ 230; pH 1.5-3.5 (3% aq.).

SB-150. [U.S. Cosmetics] Silica beads; carriers for actives, fragrances, excess oils, and other ingreds. in cosmetic formulations; spherical porous beads; avg. particle size 4 µ; surf. area 150 m²/g.

SB-700. [U.S. Cosmetics] Silica beads; carriers for active ingreds. such as vitamins, sunscreens, moisturizers, fragrances, esters, etc. for cosmetic use; spherical porous beads; surf. area 700 m²/g.

ScentCap. [M-CAP Tech. Int'l.] Microencapsulated fragrance oils for use in soap, clothing, personal care prods., cosmetics, emollients in skin creams/powds.; avail. prods.: min. oil, strawberry oil, rose oil, wintergreen oil, odor masking oils; capsule avg. size 10-30 µ.

Schercamox C-AA. [Scher] Cocamidopropylamine oxide; CAS 68155-09-9; EINECS 268-938-5; nonionic; conditioner, detergent, wetting agent, antistat used in personal care prods. and lt. dishwashing detergents; biodeg.; Gardner 4.0 max. clear to slightly hazy liq.; sol. in water and hydrophilic solvs.; m.w. 320; sp.gr. 0.986 ± 0.01; pH 7.0 ± 0.5; 30% min. act.

Schercamox CMA. [Scher] Dihydroxyethyl cocamine oxide; CAS 61791-47-7; EINECS 263-180-1; nonionic; softener, and wetting agent for cosmetics; builds visc. and stabilizes foam in personal care prods.; soft emollient feel on the skin; emolliency, lubricity, and slip to shave creams; conditions and prevents fly-away in hair shampoos; Gardner 3.0 max. clear liq.; mild odor; m.w. 301; sol. in water and hydrophilic solvs.; sp.gr. 0.99 ± 0.05; pH 7.0 ± 0.5 (1.0%); 39% min. conc.

Schercamox DMA. [Scher] Myristamine oxide; CAS 3332-27-2; EINECS 222-059-3; nonionic; wetting and foaming agent; foam booster for shampoos, bubble baths, dishwashing compds.; visc. liq.; 30% conc.

Schercamox DMC. [Scher] Cocamine oxide; CAS 61788-90-7; EINECS 263-016-9; wetting agent, foam stabilizer, visc. enhancer; yel. clear liq.; 29% amine oxide.

Schercamox DML. [Scher] Lauramine oxide; CAS 1643-20-5; EINECS 216-700-6; nonionic; antistat; emulsifier, emulsion stabilizer for used in cosmetics industry; wetting agent, foam booster/stabilizer, and visc. builder for shampoos, bath preps., shave creams; Gardner 1.0 max. clear liq., mild odor; sol. in water and hydrophilic solvs.; m.w. 235; sp.gr. 0.99±0.01; pH 7.0±1.0 (1%); 30% min. conc.

Schercamox DMM. [Scher] Myristamine oxide; CAS 3332-27-2; EINECS 222-059-3; nonionic; wetting and foaming agent, surfactant for lt. duty dishwashing compds., shampoos; emulsifier and emulsion stabilizer for min. oils; Gardner 1.0 max. clear liq.; mild odor; m.w. 263; sol. in water and hydrophilic solvs.; sp.gr. 0.98; pH 7.0 ± 1.0 (1%); 29% min. conc.

Schercamox DMS. [Scher] Stearamine oxide; CAS 2571-88-2; EINECS 219-919-5; nonionic/cationic; skin emollient, softener, visc. controller, foam stabilizer, and hair conditioner in personal care prods.; wh. to off-wh. paste, typ. odor; sol. in alcohols, glycols, triols, polyols, and glycol ethers; slightly sol. in water; m.w. 326; sp.gr. 0.90; pH 7.0 ± 1.0 (1.0%); 25% min. amine oxide.

Schercemol 65. [Scher] Isohexyl neopentanoate; CAS 5434-57-1; penetrating emollient with good sol. in hydroalcoholic systems; constituent in aroma chemicals.; clear liq.; f.p. < -15 C; acid no. 2 max.; iodine no. nil; sapon. no. 290-305.

Schercemol 105. [Scher] Isodecyl neopentanoate; CAS

60209-82-7; EINECS 262-108-6; emollient; Gardner 1 max. clear liq., sl. typ. odor; sol. in esters, veg. oils, min. oils, aliphatic, aromatic, and chlorinated hydrocarbons; partly sol. in glycols; insol. in water; m.w. 242; sp.gr. 0.850-0.855; dens. 7.1 lb/gal; f.p. < -5 C; acid no. 2 max.; iodine no. nil; sapon. no. 220-240; flash pt. (OC) > 170 C; ref. index 1.4270-1.4290.

Schercemol 145. [Scher] Myristyl neopentanoate; CAS 116518-82-2; light emollient; reduces tackiness in skin and hair preps.; clear liq.; f.p. 4 C; acid no. 2 max.; iodine no. nil; sapon. no. 180-200.

Schercemol 185. [Scher] Isostearyl neopentanoate; CAS 58958-60-4; EINECS 261-521-9; substantive emollient with low cloud pt.; aids as cloud and freeze point depressant, emulsion and freeze-thaw stabilizer; cosmetic preparations for skin care esp. near eyes; low level of skin and eye irritation; binder for pigmented makeup; Gardner 2.0 max. clear liq.; slight typ. odor; sol. in many solvs.; m.w. 368; sp.gr. 0.865; dens. 7.2 lb/gal; acid no. 2.0 max.; iodine no. 12 max.; sapon. no. 135-155; cloud pt. -10 C; flash pt. (OC) > 180 C; ref. index 1.450 ± 0.002.

Schercemol 318. [Scher] Isopropyl isostearate; CAS 68171-33-5; EINECS 250-651-1; emollient for bath oils, creams, lotions, and lipsticks; lubricity without oiliness; lt. lemon yel. clear liq.; bland odor; m.w. 326; sp.gr. 0.855 ± 0.01; dens. 7.12 lb/gal; f.p. -28 C; acid no. 1.0 max.; iodine no. 3 max.; sapon. no. 170 ± 10; flash pt. > 170 C; ref. index 1.422 ± 0.001; 99.0% min. conc.

Schercemol 1688. [Scher] Cetearyl octanoate; CAS 59130-69-7, 59130-70-7; EINECS 261-619-1; moisturizing emollient for bath and skin preps.; spreads evenly on skin imparting velvety softness; functions as waterproofing agent due to adhesion properties; colorless clear liq., sl. char. odor; sol. in org. solvs., insol. in water; m.w. 388; sp.gr. 0.852; dens. 7.1 lb/gal; acid no. 1.0 max.; iodine no. nil; sapon. no. 135-150; cloud pt. 4.0 C; flash pt. (OC) 170 C; ref. index 1.4448.

Schercemol 1818. [Scher] Isostearyl isostearate; CAS 41669-30-1; EINECS 255-485-3; substantive emollient imparting luxurious softness to skin; used in cosmetics imparting slip and lubricity, luster, and sheen; cosolv. and solubilizer in perfumes; yel. clear liq., slight typ. odor; sol. in org. solvs., insol. in water; m.w. 536; sp.gr. 0.865-0.875; f.p. -5 C; acid no. 2.0 max.; iodine no. 13 max.; sapon. no. 95-110; cloud pt. 17 C; flash pt. (OC) > 180 C; ref. index 1.4610.

Schercemol BE. [Scher] Behenyl erucate; CAS 18312-32-8; EINECS 242-201-8; emollient base for lip care cosmetics, skin creams and lotions; chemically comparable to one of main constituents of jojoba oil; melts close to body temp.; nontoxic; cream-colored soft solid, slight typ. odor; sol. in hydrophobic solvs.; insol. in water; m.w. 631; sp.gr. 0.840; dens. 7.0 lb/gal; m.p. 45 C; acid no. 2 max.; iodine no. 55 max.; sapon. no. 80-95; flash pt. (OC) > 170 C.

Schercemol CO. [Scher] Cetyl octanoate; CAS 59130-69-7; EINECS 261-619-1; solvency properties for use in make-up removers; clear liq.; f.p. 10 C; acid no. 3 max.; iodine no. nil; sapon. no. 140-155.

Schercemol DIA. [Scher] Diisopropyl adipate; CAS 6938-94-9; EINECS 248-299-9; nonoily penetrating emollient, lubricant, and solv. with mild drying effects used in hydroalcoholic cosmetic formulations; water-wh. clear liq., faint ester odor; sol. in alcohols, higher glycols, ketones, ester, aromatic, chlorinated, and aliphatic hydrocarbons; insol. in water; m.w. 230; sp.gr. 0.960 ± 0.01; dens. 8.0 lb/gal; f.p. -1 C; b.p. 87-89 C; acid no. 2 max.; iodine no. nil; sapon. no. 480-500; flash pt. > 170 C; ref. index 1.423 ± 0.001.

Schercemol DID. [Scher] Diisopropyl dimer dilinoleate; CAS 103213-20-3; nonoily, glossy emollient producing a cushiony feel and body to skin and makeup preparations; improves disp. and spreading of pigments; binder for pressed powd.; offers sheen, emolliency in lip preparations; highly substantive; suitable for sun tan preparations requiring some water repellency; yel. clear to slightly hazy liq., slight char. odor; sol. in org. solvs., insol. in water; m.w. 650; sp.gr. 0.895–0.905; dens. 7.5 lb/gal; f.p. -9 C; acid no. 3.0 max.; iodine no. 15 max.; sapon. no. 165-185; flash pt. (OC) > 170 C; ref. index 1.4600–1.4650.

Schercemol DIS. [Scher] Diisopropyl sebacate; CAS 7491-02-3; EINECS 231-306-4; nonoily emollient, lubricant, solubilizer with mild drying effects used in hydro-alcoholic personal care prods.; solv. and coupling properties; fast spreading action; colorless clear liq., bland odor; sol. in alcohols, higher glycols, ketones, esters, aromatic, aliphatic, and chlorinated hydrocarbons, min. and natural oils; insol. in water; m.w. 286; sp.gr. 0.932 ± 0.01; dens. 7.8 lb/gal; f.p. 0 C; acid no. 1.0 max.; iodine no. nil; sapon. no. 380-400; flash pt. > 170 C; ref. index 1.4320; 99% min. ester conc.

Schercemol DISD. [Scher] Diisostearyl dimer dilinoleate; CAS 103213-19-0; heavy moisturizing emollient offering lingering effect retained on skin after washing; binder for pigmented prods.; for rich night creams, lipsticks, makeup; yel. to amber clear to slightly hazy liq., slight char. odor; sol. in org. solvs., insol. in water; m.w. 1078; sp.gr. 0.895; f.p. -3 C; acid no. 5 max.; iodine no. 20 max.; sapon. no. 90-110; flash pt. (OC) 170 C max.; ref. index 1.4720; 96% conc.

Schercemol DISF. [Scher] Diisostearyl fumarate; CAS 113431-53-1; lubricant, conditioner; colorless liq.; f.p. -5 C; acid no. 2 max.; iodine no. nil; sapon. no. 160-175.

Schercemol DO. [Scher] Decyl oleate; CAS 3687-46-5; EINECS 222-981-6; high m.w. low freeze pt. nonoily lubricant, emollient, penetrant, and moisturizer for cosmetic and personal care prods.; yel. clear liq., bland char. odor; sol. in hydrophobic solvs.; insol. in water; m.w. 422; sp.gr. 0.86 ± 0.02; f.p. –10 C; acid no. 3 max.; iodine no. 65 max.; sapon. no. 130-140; ref. index 1.4540; 87.0% conc.

Schercemol EGMS. [Scher] Glycol stearate; CAS 111-60-4; EINECS 203-886-9; nonionic; emulsifier, opacifier, thickener, visc. controller, and pearlescent for hair and skin preps.; wh. to cream-colored flakes; sol. in most org. solvs.; insol. in water; m.w. 312; m.p. 58 C; acid no. 5 max.; iodine no. 1 max.; sapon. no. 170-190; 100% conc.

Schercemol GMIS. [Scher] Glyceryl isostearate; CAS 66085-00-5; EINECS 266-124-4; nonionic; emulsifier and emollient for creams and lotions; straw-colored clear liq. to soft solid, slight typ. odor; sol. in org. solvs., insol. in water; m.w. 385; sp.gr. 0.960; dens. 8.0 lb/gal; f.p. 5 C; acid no. 5 max.; iodine no. 10 max.; sapon. no. 160-180; flash pt. (OC) > 170 C; ref. index 1.4715; 100% conc.

Schercemol GMS. [Scher] Glyceryl stearate; nonionic; emulsifier, opacifier, stabilizer, and thickener for cosmetic and personal care prods.; wh. to cream flakes; m.w. 342; sol. in most org. solvs.; insol. in water; m.p. 55–60 C; acid no. 3.0 max.; sapon. no. 160–176; 40% conc.

Schercemol ICS. [Scher] Isocetyl stearate; CAS 25339-09-7; EINECS 246-868-6; nongreasy emollient used in creams; imparts elegant feel to makeup, lotions, bath preps.; remains liq. even @ low temps.; straw-colored clear liq., slight typ. odor; sol. in hydrophobic solvs.; insol. in water; m.w. 494; sp.gr. 0.850; dens. 7.1 lb/gal; f.p. –5 C; acid no. 2 max.; iodine no. nil; sapon. no. 105-120; flash pt. > 180 C.

Schercemol IDO. [Scher] Isodecyl oleate; CAS 59231-34-4; EINECS 261-673-6; emollient, lubricant, penetrant with pigment dispersing props.; for makeup and makeup removers; clear liq.; f.p. 10 C; acid no. 5 max.; iodine no. 65

max.; sapon. no. 130-140.

Schercemol MEL-3. [Scher] Myreth-3 laurate; CAS 84605-13-0; EINECS 283-390-7; nonoily rich penetrating emollient for cosmetic and personal care prods.; dispersibility and spreadability in bath oils; coupler in hydro-alcoholic systems; emulsifier and solubilizer in lotions; straw-colored clear liq., mild typ. odor; sol. in hydrophobic solvs.; water-disp.; m.w. 528; sp.gr. 0.907; f.p. 15 C; acid no. 3.0 max.; iodine no. nil; sapon. no. 100-120; flash pt. (OC) 160 C; ref. index 1.4510; 98% ester conc.

Schercemol MEM-3. [Scher] Myreth-3 myristate; CAS 59686-68-9; nonoily rich penetrating emollient for cosmetic and personal care prods.; dispersibility and spreadability in bath oils; coupler in hydro-alcoholic systems; emulsifier and solubilizer in lotions; straw-colored clear liq., slight typ. odor; sol. in hydrophobic solvs.; water-disp.; m.w. 556; sp.gr. 0.901; f.p. 23 C; acid no. 3.0 max.; iodine no. nil; sapon. no. 95-115; flash pt. (OC) 160 C; ref. index 1.4525; 98% conc.

Schercemol MEP-3. [Scher] Myreth-3 palmitate; CAS 84605-14-1; EINECS 293-391-2; nonoily rich penetrating emollient for cosmetic and personal care prods.; dispersibility and spreadability in bath oils; coupler in hydro-alcoholic systems; emulsifier and solubilizer in lotions; cream-colored soft wax, mild typ. odor; sol. in hydrophobic solvs.; water-disp.; m.w. 584; sp.gr. 0.890; m.p. 26 C; HLB 4.5; acid no. 3.0 max.; iodine no. nil; sapon. no. 85-100; flash pt. (OC) 160 C; 95% ester conc.

Schercemol ML. [Scher] Myristyl lactate; CAS 1323-03-1; EINECS 215-350-1; nonoily soft waxy emollient with low m.p.; conditioner; used in creams and body lotions giving velvety feel to skin; imparts luster and body to hair in shampoos and cream rinses; reduces tackiness; lubricant and plasticizer for polymer resins in aerosol hair spray formulations and antiperspirants; Gardner 2.0 max. liq. to soft solid, typ. sl. odor; sol. in org. solvs., alcohols, glycols, glycol ethers, esters, min. oils, insol. in water; m.w. 286; sp.gr. 0.90 (30 C); dens. 7.5 lb/gal; m.p. 28–34 C; acid no. 10 max.; iodine no. 1 max.; sapon. no. 165-185; flash pt. (OC) > 160 C.

Schercemol MM. [Scher] Myristyl myristate; CAS 3234-85-3; EINECS 221-787-9; soft, waxy emollient that melts near body temp.; visc. builder; imparts substantivity to personal care prods.; ease of combing of hair preparations; velvety feel on skin; wh. to pale yel. waxy solid; mild char odor; sol. in hydrophobic solvs.; m.w. 424; sp.gr. 0.839 (45 C); dens. 7.0 lb/gal (45 C); m.p. 36–40 C; acid no. 2.0 max.; iodine no. nil; sapon. no. 120-135; flash pt. (OC) > 170 C.

Schercemol MP. [Scher] Myristyl propionate; CAS 6221-95-0; EINECS 226-300-9; emollient for antiperspirants, body oils, creams, and lotions; straw-colored clear liq.; acid no. 2 max.; iodine no. nil; sapon. no. 190-210.

Schercemol NGDC. [Scher] Neopentyl glycol dicaprate; CAS 27841-06-1; solvency properties for use in make-up removers; clear liq.; f.p. 2 C; acid no. 3 max.; iodine no. nil; sapon. no. 255–270.

Schercemol NGDL. [Scher] Neopentyl glycol dilaurate; emollient and skin conditioner for creams and lotions; yel. clear liq.; f.p. 6 C; acid no. 3 max.; iodine no. nil; sapon. no. 230-250.

Schercemol NGDO. [Scher] Neopentyl glycol dioctanoate; CAS 28510-23-8; low freeze pt. emollient; solv. for makeup remover; clear liq.; f.p. < -12 C; acid no. 3 max.; iodine no. nil; sapon. no. 290-310.

Schercemol OHS. [Scher] Octyl hydroxystearate; CAS 29383-26-4; emollient producing slip, lubricity and tackiness reduction in skin preps.; clear liq.; f.p. 20 C; acid no. 1 max.; iodine no. 3 max.; sapon. no. 140-160.

Schercemol OLO. [Scher] Oleyl oleate; CAS 3687-45-4;

EINECS 222-980-4; nonoily emollient for cosmetic formulations contributing luster, softness, and high degree of lubricity in skin and hair preparations; cosolv. and solubilizer in perfumes; lubricant for metal working and wire drawing; amber clear liq., mild oleic odor; sol. in org. solvs., insol. in water; m.w. 332; sp.gr. 0.860 ± 0.01; dens. 7.2 lb/gal; acid no. 2 max.; iodine no. 95 max.; sapon. no. 95-110; cloud pt. 13 C; flash pt. (OC) > 180 C; ref. index 1.4630 ± 0.001.

Schercemol OP. [Scher] Octyl palmitate; CAS 29806-73-3; EINECS 249-862-1; nonoily emollient ester for cosmetic and personal care prods. giving sheen without greasiness; anticlogging and suspending agent in antiperspirants; soft velvety feel in skin creams, lotions, and aftershaves; straw-colored clear liq., bland odor; sol. in hydrophobic solvs.; m.w. 368; sp.gr. 0.855 ± 0.01; dens. 7.12 lb/gal; f.p. 0 C max.; acid no. 3.0 max.; iodine no. nil; sapon. no. 145-160; flash pt. (OC) > 170 C; ref. index 1.4460.

Schercemol OPG. [Scher] Octyl pelargonate; CAS 59587-44-9; EINECS 261-819-9; dry, nonoily rich penetrating emollient for cosmetic and personal care prods.; anticlogging agent in antiperspirants; soft, luxurious feel in skin creams and aftershaves; straw-colored clear liq., mild odor; sol. in hydrophobic solvs.; m.w. 270; sp.gr. 0.857 ± 0.01; dens. 7.13 lb/gal; f.p. < -10. 0 C; acid no. 1.0 max.; iodine no. nil; sapon. no. 200-215; flash pt. (OC) > 170 C; ref. index 1.4363 ± 0.001.

Schercemol PGDP. [Scher] Propylene glycol dipelargonate; CAS 41395-83-9; EINECS 255-350-9; nonionic; emollient offering low f.p.; cosolv. for perfumed bath oils, creams, and lotions; straw-colored clear liq., slight typ. odor; sol. in org. solvs., insol. in water; m.w. 360; sp.gr. 0.917; dens. 7.6 lb/gal; f.p. −25 C; acid no. 5 max.; iodine no. nil; sapon. no. 300-320; flash pt. (OC) > 170 C; ref. index 1.440.

Schercemol PGML. [Scher] Propylene glycol laurate; CAS 27194-74-7; EINECS 205-542-3; nonionic; emollient and solv.; stable base for cosmetics; emulsion stabilizer; solubilizes and couples ingred. such as perfumes, coloring and flavoring agents, sunscreen compds. into natural fatty veg. or min. oils; solv. for org. pesticides for spray applic.; produces sprayable oils which spread well, have good adherence, and are not readily removed by rainfall; plasticizer and stabilizer in vinyl copolymers made from PVAc and PVC; defoaming agent in PVAc emulsions; yel. clear liq., mild odor; sol. in most org. solvs. such as alcohols, ketones, esters, glycol ethers, veg. oil, min. oil, aliphatic, aromatic, chlorinated hydrocarbons; disp. in glycols, triols, polyols; m.w. 258 (theoret.); sp.gr. 0.905 ± 0.01; dens. 7.45 lb/gal; f.p. 10 C; acid no. 5 max.; iodine no. 1 max.; sapon no. 225-240; flash pt. (OC) 160 C min.; pH 7.0 (10% disp.).

Schercemol PGMS. [Scher] Propylene glycol stearate; CAS 1323-39-3; EINECS 215-354-3; nonionic; emulsifier for creams and lotions; wh. to cream-colored solid, slight typ. odor; sol. in org. solvs.; insol. in water; m.w. 326; m.p. 35 C; acid no. 4 max.; iodine no. 1 max.; sapon. no. 175-190; flash pt. (OC) > 170 C; 100% conc.

Schercemol TISC. [Scher] Triisostearyl citrate; CAS 113431-54-2; high visc. ester imparting gloss to lipsticks and lip gloss preps.; colorless liq.; f.p. -5 C; acid no. 3 max.; iodine no. 3 max.; sapon. no. 150-165.

Schercemol TIST. [Scher] Triisostearyl trilinoleate; CAS 103213-22-5; emollient; provides superior gloss, moisturizing, shine, visc., and good binding chars.; dk. amber slightly hazy, syrupy liq., slight typ. odor; sol. in hydrophobic solvs.; insol. in water; m.w. 1656; sp.gr. 0.92; dens. 7.7 lb/gal; f.p. −10 C; acid no. 5 max.; iodine no. 30 max.; sapon. no. 90-110; flash pt. (OC) > 170 C; ref. index

1.4760.

Schercodine B. [Scher] Behenamidopropyl dimethylamine; CAS 60270-33-9; EINECS 262-134-8; cationic; emulsifier with conditioning properties for hair and skin preparations; tan hard waxy flakes; m.w. 394; m.p. 63-68 C; alkali value 135-145; 98% min. amide.

Schercodine C. [Scher] Cocamidopropyl dimethylamine; CAS 68140-01-2; EINECS 268-771-8; cationic; good foaming surfactant for hair and bath preps.; emulsifier, intermediate for betaine amphoterics; tan soft solid; m.w. 304; alkali no. 177-187; 100% conc.

Schercodine I. [Scher] Isostearamidopropyl dimethylamine; CAS 67799-04-6; EINECS 267-101-1; cationic; versatile liq. o/w emulsifier for creams and lotions; lubricant for hair rinses and conditioners; lt. amber liq., ammoniacal odor; m.w. 394; acid no. 4.0 max.; alkali no. 150-160; flash pt. (OC) > 160 C; 98% min. amide.

Schercodine L. [Scher] Lauramidopropyl dimethylamine; CAS 3179-80-4; EINECS 221-661-3; cationic; emulsifier; surfactant, intermediate for betaine amphoterics; lt. tan solid; m.w. 284; m.p. 35-40 C; alkali value 196-206; 98% min. amide.

Schercodine M. [Scher] Myristamidopropyl dimethylamine; CAS 45267-19-4; EINECS 256-214-1; cationic; o/w emulsifier, conditioner, visc. builder; lt. tan wax; m.w. 312; sol. in org. solvs.; m.p. 45-50 C; alkali value 180-190; 98% min. amide.

Schercodine O. [Scher] Oleamidopropyl dimethylamine; CAS 109-28-4; EINECS 203-661-5; cationic; o/w emulsifier; emollient conditioner for hair and skin preparations; amber liq.; m.w. 366; alkali value 150-160; 98% min. amide.

Schercodine P. [Scher] Palmitamidopropyl dimethylamine; CAS 39669-97-1; EINECS 254-585-4; cationic; substantive conditioner and emulsifier in creams, lotions, rinses; tan hard wax; m.w. 340; sol. in org. solvs.; m.p. 55-60 C; alkali value 160-170; 98% min. amide.

Schercodine S. [Scher] Stearamidopropyl dimethylamine; CAS 7651-02-7; EINECS 231-609-1; cationic; softener, emulsifier, and conditioner in hair and skin preparations; tan hard waxy flakes; sol. in org. solvs.; m.w. 368; m.p. 65-70 C; alkali value 145-155; 98% min. amide.

Schercodine T. [Scher] Tallamidopropyl dimethylamine; CAS 68650-79-3; conditioner for cationic emulsions; substantivity and thickening properties; amber liq.; m.w. 366; alkali value 150-160; 98% min. amide.

Schercomid 1214. [Scher] Lauramide DEA and diethanolamine; CAS 120-40-1, 7545-23-5; nonionic; foam booster/stabilizer for detergent compositions; good detergency by itself and works synergistically with other surfactants; thickening agent and visc. builder; used in personal care items and cleaners for hard surfaces; lt. amber clear liq., sl. typ. odor; sol. in water and in most org. solvs.; disp. in aliphatic hydrocarbons, min. oil, and natural fats; sp.gr. 1.01; dens. 8.4 lb/gal; acid no. 12–16; alkali no. 150-170; flash pt. (OC) > 170 C; 100% act.; 60% min. amide content.

Schercomid AME. [Scher] Acetamide MEA; CAS 142-26-7; EINECS 205-530-8; nonionic; solubilizer, humectant, skin and hair conditioner, intermediate, coupling agent, pigment dispersant; straw-colored clear liq., mild organoleptic odor; sol. in most alcohols, glycols, diols, polyols, glycol ethers, ketones, and water; sp.gr. 1.120; dens. 9.3 lb/gal; acid no. 10.0 max.; alkali no. 15.0 max.; flash pt. (OC) > 180 C; ref. index 1.4700; pH 6.0–8.5 (50% aq.); 100% conc.

Schercomid CCD. [Scher] Cocamide DEA and diethanolamine; CAS 68603-42-9; EINECS 263-163-9; nonionic; emulsifier, thickener, detergent, soil dispersing and suspending agent; for floor cleaners, liq. hand dishwashing, car waxes, liq. hand soaps, all-purpose industrial and household cleaners, lubricants, emulsifiable oils, agric. sprays, cosmetics; dk. amber visc. liq.; sol. in water, alcohols, diols, triols, glycol ethers, polyols, aromatic and chlorinated hydrocarbons; sp.gr. 0.99±0.01; dens. 8.3 lb/gal; acid no. 15-20; alkali no. 140-160; flash pt. (OC) > 170 C; pH 9.9 ± 0.5 (10%); 100% act., 60% min. amide.

Schercomid CDA. [Scher] Cocamide DEA and diethanolamine; CAS 68603-42-9; nonionic/anionic; foam stabilizer, soil suspender, lime soap dispersant, and detergency booster for industrial and household cleaners and cosmetics; lt. amber clear liq.; sol. in water, alcohols, diols, triols, glycol ethers, polyols, aromatic and chlorinated hydrocarbons; sp.gr. 1.01 ± 0.01; dens. 8.33 lb/gal; visc. 1000 cps min.; acid no. 40-50; alkali value 150-170; flash pt. (OC) > 170 C; pH 9.6±0.5 (10%); 100% act., 60% min. amide.

Schercomid CDO-Extra. [Scher] Cocoamide DEA and diethanolamine; CAS 68603-42-9; EINECS 263-163-9; nonionic/anionic; detergent, wetting agent, foam stabilizer, visc. builder; shampoos, household cleaners, industrial cleaners with builders, liq. dishwashing compds., floor cleaners, personal care formulations; visc. yel. liq.; sl. odor; sol. in water, alcohols, diols, triols, glycol ethers, polyols, aromatic and chlorinated hydrocarbons; sp.gr. 1.00±0.01; visc. 950 cps min.; acid no. 5; alkali no. 110-140; flash pt. (OC) > 170 C; pH 10±0.5 (10% sol'n.); 100% act., 65% min. amide.

Schercomid CME. [Scher] Cocamide MEA; CAS 68140-00-1; EINECS 268-770-2; nonionic; foam booster and visc. builder for shampoos, bubble baths, and powded. detergent compositions; emulsifier for creams and lotions, esp. in cream hair dye formulations; tan wax; ammoniacal odor; sol. in alcohols, glycols, glycol ethers, aliphatic, aromatic, and chlorinated hydrocarbons; disp. in water; m.p. 63 ± 3 C; flash pt. (OC) > 180 C; acid no. 1.0 max.; 100% active; 85% min. amide content.

Schercomid HT-60. [Scher] PEG-50 hydrog. tallow amide; CAS 68783-22-2; nonionic; thickener, detergent, emulsifier, dispersant with foam char.; tan hard waxy solid, ammoniacal odor; sol. in alcohols, glycols, triols, polyols, glycol ethers, water, in some aromatic and chlorinated hydrocarbons; sp.gr. 1.064 (60 C); dens. 9.6 lb/gal; m.p. 50-55 C; acid no. 2 max.; alkali no. 10; flash pt. (OC) > 180 C; pH 9.0–10.0 (10% aq.); 100% act.

Schercomid LME. [Scher] Lactamide MEA; CAS 5422-34-4; EINECS 226-546-1; nonionic; humectant, skin and hair conditioner, coupling agent, emollient; yel. clear liq.; acid no. 20 max.; alkali no. 20 max.; 90% min. amide.

Schercomid ODA. [Scher] Oleamide DEA and diethanolamine; CAS 93-83-4; EINECS 202-281-7; nonionic/anionic; w/o emulsifier, pigment dispersant, conditioner, corrosion inhibitor, and visc. builder; emulsifier for aromatic and aliphatic hydrocarbon solv.; used in gel-type pine cleaners, shampoo formulations, hair conditioning agent; lt. amber clear liq., mild char. odor; sol. in alcohols, glycols, glycol ethers, aliphatic and chlorinated hydrocarbons; water-disp.; sp.gr. 0.950 ± 0.01; dens. 7.9 lb/gal; visc. 1200 cps min.; acid no. 12-16; alkali no. 120-140; flash pt. (OC) > 170 C; pH 9.9 ± 0.5 (10% disp.); 100% active; 60% min. amide content.

Schercomid OME. [Scher] Oleamide MEA; CAS 111-58-0; EINECS 203-884-8; w/o emulsifier, conditioner, and thickener; tan wax; acid no. 10 max.; alkali no. 20 max.; 85% min. amide.

Schercomid OMI. [Scher] Oleamide MIPA; CAS 111-05-7; EINECS 203-828-2; nonionic; thickener, foam stabilizer for shampoos; hair conditioning agent; emulsifier for min. oil, IPP, IPM, butyl stearate, creams and lotions; imparts slip, lubrication, some emolliency, and softening effects upon the skin; amber clear liq. to soft solid, mild ammoniacal odor; sol. in alcohols, esters, glycol ethers, min. and veg. oils, aliphatic, aromatic, and chlorinated hydrocarbons; sp.gr. 0.90 ± 0.01; dens. 7.5 lb/gal; acid no. 5-15; alkali no. 7-17; flash pt. (OC) 180 C; 100% active; 85% min. amide.

Schercomid SAP. [Scher] Apricotamide DEA; nonionic; thickener, foam stabilizer for natural and herbal shampoos; amber clear liq.; acid no. 3 max.; alkali no. 20-40; 80% min. amide.

Schercomid SCE. [Scher] Cocamide DEA (1:1); CAS 68603-42-9; EINECS 263-163-9; nonionic; detergent, visc. builder and foam stabilizer for cosmetic formulations, bubble baths, liq. dishwash detergents, and rug shampoos; lt. amber clear visc. liq., mild odor; sol. in alcohols, diols, triols, polyols, glycol ethers, aliphatic, aromatic, and chlorinated hydrocarbons; water-disp.; sp.gr. 0.97; dens. 8.1 lb/gal; acid no. 2.0 max.; alkali no. 20-40; flash pt. (OC) > 180 C; 100% active; 87% min. amide content.

Schercomid SCO-Extra. [Scher] Cocamide DEA (1:1); CAS 68603-42-9; EINECS 263-163-9; nonionic; thickener, foam builder, foam stabilizer, and detergency booster for alkylaryl sulfonates and lauryl sulfates; used in shampoos, bubble baths, floor cleaners and liq. and powd. dishwashing detergents; for making self-emulsifiable solv. from aliphatic, aromatic, or chlorinated hydrocarbons, used in waterless hand cleaners, engine shampoos, concrete floor cleaners, wax strippers, and tar removers; lt. amber clear liq., mild odor; sol. in water, alcohols, glycols, polyols, glycol ethers, aliphatic (lower members), aromatic, chlorinated hydrocarbons, and natural fats; disp. in min. oil; sp.gr. 0.99; dens. 8.25 lb/gal; acid no. 3.0 max.; alkali no. 20-40; flash pt. (OC) > 180 C; 100% active; 77% min. amide content.

Schercomid SLE. [Scher] Linoleamide DEA (1:1); CAS 56863-02-6; EINECS 260-410-2; nonionic; solubilizer, thickener, w/o emulsifier, conditioner, and emollient for personal care prods.; emulsion stabilizer for o/w emulsions; dk. amber clear liq., mild, typical odor; sol. in most org. solvs., min. and veg. oil; disp. in water; sp.gr. 0.965; dens. 8.0 lb/gal; acid no. 1.0 max.; alkali no. 20-40; flash pt. (OC) > 180 C; 100% act., 87% min. amide.

Schercomid SL-Extra. [Scher] Lauramide DEA (1:1); CAS 120-40-1; EINECS 204-393-1; nonionic; thickener, foam booster/stabilizer for hair shampoos, soaps, syn. detergent formulations; bubble bath applics.; industrial applics. incl. manual dishwashing formulations, liq. heavy-duty laundry detergents, all-purpose cleaning prods.; emulsifier for aliphatic, aromatic hydrocarbons and oils for o/w emulsions; off-wh. cryst. solid; mild odor; sol. in alcohols, glycols, glycol ethers, polyols, aliphatic (lower members); aromatic, and chlorinated hydrocarbons, and natural fats and oils; disp. in water and min. oils; sp.gr. 0.97 (45 C); dens. 8.1 lb/gal (45 C); m.p. 42 C; acid no. 1.0 max.; alkali no. 20-40; flash pt. (OC) > 170 C; 100% active; 87% min. amide content.

Schercomid SL-ML. [Scher] Lauramide DEA, myristamide DEA; CAS 120-40-1, 7545-23-5; nonionic; detergent, aux, skin and hair conditioner, visc. builder which generates thick, copious foam; for mild shampoos, bubble baths, aerosol shave creams, and other detergent compositions; o/w and w/o emulsifier in creams and lotions; lt. amber clear liq., mild odor; sol. in alcohols, glycols, glycol ethers, polyols, aliphatic, aromatic, and chlorinated hydrocarbons, natural fats and oils; disp. in min. oil and water; sp.gr. 0.97; dens. 8.0 lb/gal; acid no. 1 max.; alkali no. 20-40; flash pt. (OC) > 180 C; 100% act.; 87% min. amide content.

Schercomid SLM-LC. [Scher] Lauramide DEA, myristamide DEA; CAS 120-40-1, 7545-23-5; nonionic; wetting agent, thickener, and foam stabilizer; amber clear liq.; acid no. 1 max.; alkali no. 30-50; 85% min. amide.

Schercomid SLM-S. [Scher] Lauramide DEA, myristamide DEA; CAS 120-40-1, 7545-23-5; EINECS 204-393-1; nonionic; visc. builder for the cosmetic industry; thick, copious foam in shampoos, facial scrubs, bubble baths, hand soaps, etc.; lt. yel. liq. when fresh (cryst. on aging), mild odor; sol. in alcohols, glycols, glycol ethers, polyols, aliphatic, aromatic, and chlorinated hydrocarbons, natural fats and oils; disp. in min. oil and water; sp.gr. 0.97 ± 0.01 (45 C); dens. 8.1 lb/gal; acid no. 1.0 max.; alkali no. 20-40; flash pt. (OC) > 170 C; 100% act.; 88% min. amide content.

Schercomid SLS. [Scher] Soyamide DEA (1:1); CAS 68425-47-8; EINECS 270-355-6; nonionic; conditioner and emollient for personal care prods.; emulsifier for w/o systems and hydrocarbons; dispersant for pigments and min. clays; visc. builder; emulsion stabilizer; amber clear liq., mild fruity odor; sol. in most org. solvs., min. and veg. oil; disp. in water; sp.gr. 0.980; dens. 8.0 lb/gal; acid no. 2.0 max.; alkali no. 20-40; flash pt. (OC) > 180 C; 100% conc., 82% min. amide.

Schercomid SO-A. [Scher] Oleamide DEA (1:1); CAS 93-83-4; EINECS 202-281-7; nonionic/anionic; w/o emulsifier, lubricant, conditioner; lt. amber clear liq., slight typ. oleic odor; sol. in most org. solvs.; water-disp.; sp.gr. 0.95 ± 0.01; dens. 7.9 lb/gal; visc. 450 cps min.; acid no. 5 max.; alkali no. 40-60; flash pt. (OC) > 180 C; 100% act., 85% min. amide.

Schercomid SO-T. [Scher] Tallamide DEA (1:1); CAS 68155-20-4; EINECS 268-949-5; anionic/nonionic; w/o emulsifier; amber clear liq.; acid no. 15 max.; alkali no. 40-50; 100% conc., 85% min. amide.

Schercomid SWG. [Scher] Wheatgermamide DEA; CAS 124046-39-5; nonionic; thickener, foam stabilizer for natural and herbal shampoos; amber clear liq.; acid no. 3 max.; alkali no. 20-40; 80% min. amide.

Schercomid TO-2. [Scher] Tallamide DEA and diethanolamine; CAS 68155-20-4; EINECS 268-949-5; nonionic/anionic; w/o emulsifier, visc. builder, pigment and min. clay dispersant, corrosion inhibitor; emulsifier for aromatic and aliphatic hydrocarbon solv.; used in shampoos where it generates a creamy, luxurious foam; stabilizes foam when used with surfactants and detergents; hair conditioning agent; dk. amber clear liq., mild char. odor; sol. in alcohols, glycols, glycol ethers, aliphatic and chlorinated hydrocarbons; disp. in water; sp.gr. 0.990; dens. 8.25 lb/gal; acid no. 16-19; alkali no. 130-150; flash pt. (OC) > 170 C; 100% act.; 65% min. amide.

Schercopol CMA-Na. [Scher] Disodium cocamido-MEA sulfosuccinate; surfactant for cosmetic use; 29% conc.

Schercopol CMS-Na. [Scher] Disodium cocamido MEA-sulfosuccinate; CAS 68784-08-7; EINECS 272-219-1; anionic; nonirritating surfactant, foam-stabilizer, solubilizer, softener for personal care prods.; home and industrial detergent cleaning formulations; anti-irritant for other surfactants; biodeg.; m.w. 477; sol. in water; partly sol. in most org. solvs.; sp.gr. 1.12; dens. 9.3 lb/gal; visc. 100 cps max.; pH 5-7; cloud pt. 5.0 C; 30% solids.

Schercopol DOS-70. [Scher] Dioctyl sodium sulfosuccinate and propylene glycol; CAS 577-11-7; EINECS 209-406-4; anionic; wetting agent, surf. tens. depressant; straw-colored clear visc. liq., mild char. odor; m.w. 446; sp.gr. 1.10; dens. 9.16 lb/gal; acid no. 2.5 max.; flash pt. (OC) 140 C min.; pH 4-6 (1%); Draves wetting 25 s; 70% act.

Schercopol DOS-PG-70. [Scher] Dioctyl sodium sulfosuccinate, propylene glycol; CAS 577-11-7; EINECS 209-406-4; wetting agent, surf. tens. depressant; visc. liq.; pH 6-8; 70% min. dry solids.

Schercopol DOS-PG-85. [Scher] Dioctyl sodium sulfosucci-

nate; CAS 577-11-7; EINECS 209-406-4; anionic; wetting agent, surf. tens. depressant; visc. liq.; 85% min. dry solids.

Schercopol LPS. [Scher] Disodium laureth sulfosuccinate; CAS 39354-45-5; EINECS 255-062-3; mild high foaming surfactant; visc. enhancer; yel. clear liq.; pH 5-7; 39% min. dry solids.

Schercopol OMS-Na. [Scher] Disodium oleamido MEA-sulfosuccinate; CAS 68479-64-1; EINECS 270-864-3; anionic; solubilizer; nonirritating surfactant imparting soft, emollient feel on skin and conditioning effect on hair; foamer in toiletries, hand dishwashing detergents, and personal care prods.; yel. clear liq.; mild char. odor; sol. in water; partly sol. in most org. solvs.; sp.gr. 1.10 ± 0.05; dens. 9.16 lb/gal; visc. 1000 cps max.; pH 6.0 ± 1.0; cloud pt. 5.0 C max.; 34% min. solids conc.

Schercoquat 2IAE. [Scher] Hydroxypropyl bis-isostear-amidopropyldimonium chloride; cationic; w/o and o/w emulsifier; conditioner for hair and skin care prods.; antistat; liq.; 85% conc.

Schercoquat 2IAP. [Scher] Hydroxypropyl bis-isostear-amidopropyldimonium chloride; cationic; o/w and o/w emulsifier; conditioner for hair and skin care prods.; liq.; 85% conc.

Schercoquat ALA. [Scher] Dilauryl acetyl dimonium chloride; CAS 90283-04-8; cationic; w/o and o/w emulsifier; conditioner for hair and skin care prods.; lt. yel. liq. (30 C); m.w. 504; 70% min. dry solids.

Schercoquat APAS. [Scher] Apricotamidopropyl ethyldimonium ethosulfate; CAS 115340-78-8; natural, mild conditioner; imparts good slip and shine; amber visc. liq.; m.w. 515; 90% min. dry solids.

Schercoquat BAS. [Scher] Behenamidopropyl ethyl-dimonium ethosulfate; CAS 68797-65-9; EINECS 258-377-8; conditioner for dry and over-processed hair; amber liq.; m.w. 548; 50% min. dry solids.

Schercoquat CAS. [Scher] Cocamidopropyl ethyl dimonium ethosulfate; CAS 113492-03-8; cationic; w/o and o/w emulsifier, conditioner, antistat for hair care prods.; amber visc. liq.; m.w. 445; 98% min. solids.

Schercoquat COAS. [Scher] Canola oil amidopropyl ethyldimonium ethosulfate; natural, mild hair and skin conditioner; imparts good slip and velvety feel; amber visc. liq.; m.w. 529.

Schercoquat DAS. [Scher] Quaternium-61; CAS 111905-55-6; cationic; conditioner for skin and hair care prods., esp. low irritation cosmetics; amber visc. liq., sl. mild odor; water-sol.; m.w. 1050; sp.gr. 1.01; dens. 8.4 lb/gal; flash pt. (OC) 90 C; pH 4-7 (5% aq.); 90% min. NV.

Schercoquat FOAS. [Scher] Saffloweramidopropyl ethyldimonium ethosulfate; CAS 113492-04-9; quat. effective in hair conditioners; good slip, shine, and combability; amber visc. liq.; water-sol.; m.w. 520; 90% min. dry solids.

Schercoquat IALA. [Scher] Isostearamidopropyl laurylacetodimonium chloride; CAS 134112-42-8; cationic; w/o and o/w emulsifier; conditioner for hair and skin care prods. with high lubricity and substantivity; amber visc. liq.; m.w. 670; 80% min. dry solids.

Schercoquat IAS. [Scher] Isostearamidopropyl ethyldimonium ethosulfate; CAS 67633-63-0; EINECS 266-778-0; cationic; conditioner for clear conditioning shampoos where it contributes body, combability, and antistatic props.; amber clear visc. liq., slight mild odor; water-sol.; m.w. 522; sp.gr. 0.99 ± 0.01; dens. 8.2 lb/gal; pH 5-7 (5.0% aq.); 90% min. act.

Schercoquat IEP. [Scher] Quaternium-62; CAS 84605-15-2; conditioning quat. offering good compat. with many anionic surfactants; amber visc. liq.; water-sol.; m.w. 486; 80% min. dry solids.

Schercoquat IIS. [Scher] Isostearyl ethylimidonium ethosulfate; CAS 67633-57-2; EINECS 266-778-0; cationic; conditioner for skin and hair care prods. where it contributes softness to skin, fullness and body to hair; dk. amber clear to slighty hazy visc. liq., slight mild odor; m.w. 532; sp.gr. 1.036 ± 0.01; dens. 8.6 lb/gal; pH 4–7 (5.0% aq.); 98% min. dry solids.

Schercoquat ROAS. [Scher] Rapeseedamidopropyl ethyldimonium ethosulfate; CAS 94552-41-7; cationic; conditioner for personal care prods., esp. for dry and overprocessed hair care prods.; visc. builder in anionic systems; dk. amber clear to hazy visc. liq., mild amine odor; m.w. 560; sp.gr. 0.990; dens. 8.2 lb/gal; flash pt. (OC) 90 C; pH 4–7 (5.0% aq.); 90% min. NV; 80% min. quat.

Schercoquat ROEP. [Scher] Rapeseedamidopropyl epoxypropyl dimonium chloride; CAS 112324-11-5; conditioner for conditioning shampoos and hair sprays; dk. amber visc. liq.; water-sol.; m.w. 533; 80% min. dry solids.

Schercoquat SAS. [Scher] Stearamidopropyl ethyl dimonium ethosulfate; CAS 67846-16-6; EINECS 267-360-0; conditioner for hair rinses providing body and bounce and improving shine; yel. liq.; m.w. 508; water-sol.; 80% min. dry solids.

Schercoquat SOAS. [Scher] Soyamidopropyl ethyldimonium ethosulfate; CAS 90529-57-0; EINECS 291-990-5; cationic; conditioner for personal care prods.; offers slip, shine, and combability to hair conditioners; amber clear visc. liq., mild amine odor; water-sol.; m.w. 516; sp.gr. 1.04; dens. 8.6 lb/gal; pH 4–7 (5.0% aq.); 90% min. dry solids.

Schercoquat WOAS. [Scher] Wheatgermamidopropyl ethyldimonium ethosulfate; CAS 115340-80-2; cationic; surfactant, mild conditioner imparting body, bounce, antistatic properties, shine to hair; amber visc. liq.; m.w. 528; 90% act.

Schercotaine APAB. [Scher] Apricotamidopropyl betaine; CAS 133934-08-4; amphoteric; mild detergent, conditioner, emollient, visc. enhancer; amber clear liq.; pH 5-7; 35% min. dry solids.

Schercotaine CAB. [Scher] Cocamidopropyl betaine; CAS 61789-40-0; EINECS 263-058-8; amphoteric; detergent, wetting agent, foamer, cloud pt. depressant, antistat and softener in nonirritating shampoos and bubble baths; pale yel. clear liq., slight char. odor; water-sol.; m.w. 386; sp.gr. 1.05 ± 0.01; dens. 8.75 lb/gal; visc. 100 cps max.; cloud pt. –2.0 C max.; pH 5.5 ± 1.0; 45% min. dry solids.

Schercotaine CAB-A. [Scher] Cocamidopropyl betaine, ammonium chloride; amphoteric; mild surfactant with higher foam than the sodium counterpart, decreased defatting properties; lt. yel. clear liq.; pH 5-7; 45% solids.

Schercotaine CAB-K. [Scher] Cocamidopropyl betaine, potassium chloride; amphoteric; mild detergent, surfactant, foamer with decreased defatting props.; visc. stabilizer in natural soap systems; lt. yel. clear liq.; pH 5-7; 45% min. dry solids.

Schercotaine CAB-KG. [Scher] N-[3-(cocoamido)-propyl]-N,N-dimethyl betaine, potassium salt; amphoteric; surfactant with increased solubility and lower cloud pt.; visc. stabilizer for natural soap systems; yel. clear liq.; typ. odor; m.w. 401; sp.gr. 1.06; dens. 8.8 lb/gal; pH 5.0–7.0; 40% min. act.

Schercotaine CAB-Mg. [Scher] Coconut amido betaine; amphoteric; mild surfactant with moderate foam; used in hair care prods.; liq.; 35% conc.

Schercotaine IAB. [Scher] Isostearamidopropyl betaine; CAS 6179-44-8; EINECS 228-227-2; amphoteric; conditioner and detergent for shampoos and emollient body treatments; visc. control agent; textile softener; amber visc. liq., soft opaque gel, slight char. odor; sol. in aq.

alcohol, glycols; m.w. 477; sp.gr. 1.05; dens. 8.75 lb/gal; pH 5.5 ± 1.0; 35% min. dry solids.

Schercotaine MAB. [Scher] Myristamidopropyl betaine; CAS 59272-84-3; EINECS 261-684-6; amphoteric; detergent, thickener, wetting agent with antistatic properties for cosmetic and toiletry preps.; yel. clear to hazy liq., sl. char. odor; m.w. 393; sp.gr. 1.030; dens. 8.58 lb/gal; visc. 90 cps; cloud pt. -1 C; pH 5.5 ± 1.0; 30.0% min. solids; 25% min. act.

Schercotaine MKAB. [Scher] Minkamidopropyl betaine and sodium chloride; amphoteric; surfactant, conditioner imparting sheen to hair; softens skin; emulsification properties; liq.; 35% conc.

Schercotaine PAB. [Scher] Palmitamidopropyl betaine; CAS 32954-43-1; EINECS 251-306-8; amphoteric; thickening agent, good hair and skin conditioner for lotions and cream rinses; lt. yel. soft gel; sol. in aq. alcohol, glycols; pH 5–7; 35% min. dry solids.

Schercotaine SCAB. [Scher] Cocamidopropyl hydroxysultaine; CAS 68139-30-0; EINECS 268-761-3; amphoteric; detergent, wetting agent and foamer, cloud pt. depressant used in personal care prods.; lt. lemon clear liq., typ. odor; water-sol.; m.w. 500; sp.gr. 1.07 ± 0.01; dens. 8.9 lb/gal; visc. 100 cps max.; cloud pt. –7 C; pH 6.0 ± 1.0; 50% min. dry solids.

Schercotaine SCAB-A. [Scher] Cocamidopropylhydroxysultaine, ammonium chloride; amphoteric; low cloud pt. surfactant with higher foam and decreased defatting properties; lt. yel. clear liq.; pH 5-7; 50% min. dry solids.

Schercotaine SCAB-K. [Scher] Cocamidopropyl hydroxysultaine, potassium salt; amphoteric; low cloud pt. surfactant, visc. stabilizer in natural soap systems; lt. yel. clear liq.; pH 5-7; 50% min. dry solids.

Schercotaine SCAB-KG. [Scher] Cocamidopropylhydroxysultaine, potassium chloride; visc. stabilizer in natural soap systems; low cloud pt. surfactant; lt. yel. clear liq.; typ. odor; m.w. 480; sp.gr. 1.10; dens. 9.1 lb/gal; pH 5–7; 50% min. dry solids.

Schercotaine UAB. [Scher] Undecylenamidopropyl betaine; CAS 133798-12-6; amphoteric; surfactant with germicidal/bactericidal activity; for shampoos; amber clear liq.; pH 5-7; 35% min. dry solids.

Schercotaine WOAB. [Scher] Wheat germamidopropyl betaine; CAS 133934-09-5; amphoteric; detergent with emulsification properties, conditioner, surfactant with vitamin E; imparts good body to hair; amber clear liq.; pH 5-7; 35% min. dry solids.

Schercoteric CY-2. [Scher] Disodium capryloamphodiacetate; CAS 7702-01-4; EINECS 231-721-0; amphoteric; low foaming surfactant for household and industrial cleaning prods., cosmetics; amber clear liq.; 50% min. dry solids.

Schercoteric I-AA. [Scher] Sodium isostearoamphopropionate; CAS 68630-96-6; EINECS 271-929-9; amphoteric; surfactant for cosmetic and industrial cleaners; amber visc. liq.; 34% min. dry solids.

Schercoteric MS. [Scher] Sodium cocoamphoacetate; CAS 68334-21-4; EINECS 269-819-0; amphoteric; foamer, mild detergent, conditioner used in shampoos and industrial cleaners; amber clear visc. liq.; 45% min. dry solids.

Schercoteric MS-2. [Scher] Disodium cocoamphodiacetate; CAS 68650-39-5; EINECS 272-043-5; amphoteric; mild detergent used in shampoos and industrial cleaners; amber clear visc. liq.; 50% min. dry solids.

Schercoteric MS-EP. [Scher] Sodium cocoamphohydroxypropylsulfonate; CAS 68604-73-9; EINECS 271-705-0; amphoteric; surfactant for personal care prods.; low skin irritation, low cloud pt.; amber clear liq.; 45% min. dry solids.

Schercozoline C. [Scher] Cocoyl hydroxyethyl imidazoline;

CAS 61791-38-6; EINECS 263-170-7; cationic; antistat, dispersant, wetting agent, emulsifier, microbicide, detergent, intermediate for quat. ammonium compds., primer paints, emulsion cleaning, cleaners, polishes, surf. treatment, textile and leather processing, agriculture and cosmetic; tan semisolid; m.w. 278; alkali no. 200-214; 90% min. imidazoline.

Schercozoline I. [Scher] Isostearyl hydroxyethyl imidazoline; CAS 68966-38-1; EINECS 273-429-6; cationic; surfactant, softener, antistat, dye assistant for textiles, paper, cutting oils, metal lubricants, polishes, cosmetics, agric., corrosion inhibitors, building materials; amber clear liq.; m.w. 378; alkali no. 150-160; 90% min. imidazoline.

Schercozoline L. [Scher] Lauryl hydroxyethyl imidazoline; CAS 136-99-2; EINECS 205-271-0; cationic; surfactant, softener, dye assistant, antistat for textiles, paper, cutting oils, metal lubricants, polishes, cosmetics, corrosion inhibitors, building materials; intermediate for quats.; cream solid; m.w. 268; m.p. 38-42 C; alkali no. 204-214; 90% min. imidazoline.

Schercozoline O. [Scher] Oleyl hydroxyethyl imidazoline; CAS 95-38-5; EINECS 248-248-0; cationic; surfactant, softener, dye assistant, antistat, w/o emulsifier, corrosion inhibitor, intermediate for quat. ammonium compds., textiles, paper, cutting oils, metal lubricants, polishes, cosmetics, agric., building materials; dk. amber liq.; m.w. 350; alkali no. 160-170; 90% min. imidazoline.

SCS 40. [Witco/H-I-P] Sodium cumenesulfonate; CAS 32073-22-6; EINECS 250-913-5; hydrotrope, solubilizer.

Seagel L. [Marine Colloids] Locust bean gum; CAS 9000-40-2; EINECS 232-541-5; stabilizer, thickener, emulsifier for cosmetics, pharmaceuticals, foods.

Seakem 3, LCM. [Marine Colloids] Carrageenan; CAS 9000-07-1; EINECS 232-524-2; gellant and stabilizer for cosmetics.

Seanami MY. [Laboratoires Sérobiologiques] Ostreosidic complex of oses, peptides, and amino acids; metabolic activator with cytophilic power, survival maintenance of living cutaneous cells; for facial care, skin freshness, and hair and nail care prods.; yel. opalescent liq.; water-sol.; usage level: 5-8%.

Seanamin AT. [Laboratoires Sérobiologiques] Biomolecules extracted from structural and protective marine tissues; water, sorbitol, hydrolyzed actin, glycosaminoglycans, glycogen, and sodium gluconate; provides stimulation of cellular vitality, structuring effect on skin; used as nutrient, energizer, hydro-regulator in cosmetics; amber liq.; water-sol.; usage level: 5-10%.

Seanamin BD. [Laboratoires Sérobiologiques] Carrageenan, sorbitol, mannitol, sodium chloride, hydrolyzed actin, glucosamine, sodium glucuronate, and calcium gluconate; marine complex containing electrolytes, heteropolysaccharides, and peptides; visc. enhancer; skin detoxifier providing mobilization of interstitial water; used for face/body detoxification, astringent and hemostatic care, slimming and strengthening local effect; wh. powd.; water-sol.; usage level: 0.5-3%.

Seanamin FP. [Laboratoires Sérobiologiques] Water, hydrolyzed actin, glycerin, and bladderwrack extract; biopeptides providng stimulation and protection of bulbar hair cells, conditioning of capillary fibers, protection/photo-protection/repair of hair altered by light, permanent waving, or coloring; also for nail and eyelash care; amber syrupy limpid liq.; water-sol.; usage level: 2-5%.

Seanamin SU. [Laboratoires Sérobiologiques] Whole deodorized seaweeds and seaweed extracts; water, sorbitol, and algae extract; skin softener, moisturizer, and conditioner for facial hydration and softness, body care prods.; amber unctuous gel; disp. in water; usage level: 5-8%.

Seanamin TH. [Laboratoires Sérobiologiques] Sorbitol, glycine, glucosamine, and glycogen; hydro-regulator for prods. for dry, rough skin, enrichment of dermis and epidermis, anti-aging and protection prods.; wh. powd., odorless; water-sol.; usage level: 3-5%.

Seaspen PF. [Marine Colloids] Carrageenan; CAS 9000-07-1; EINECS 232-524-2; gellant and stabilizer for cosmetics.

Sebase. [Westbrook Lanolin] PEG-30 lanolin, cetearyl alcohol, min. oil, and p-chloro-m-cresol; nonionic; complete self-emulsifying cosmetic base, emollient, moisturizer, emulsifier, lubricant, visc. stabilizer for o/w cosmetic emulsions, cleansers, day/night creams, face masks, nailcare, sunscreens; binder for pressed powds.; carrier for foundations; paste; m.p. 30-38 C; HLB 8.0; acid no. 1.5 max.; sapon. no. 6-24; hyd. no. 9-16; 100% conc.

Sebomine SB12. [Sederma] Water, potassium thiocyanate, lactoferrin, lactoperoxidase, and glucose oxidase; prod. for treatment of oily skin with acne tendency and dandruff; brownish clear liq., char. odor; sp.gr. 1.025 ± 0.005; ref. index 1.345 ± 0.005; pH 6.0-7.5; usage level: 4%.

Sebopessina. [Vevy] Polyisoprene, soy sterol.

Seboregular HS 312. [Alban Muller] Watercress, ivy, and rocket phytocomplex; prod. for treatment of oily hair and scalp, oily skin.

Seboside. [Vevy] Soy sterol, PPG-5 pentaerythritol ether, PEG-5 pentaerythritol ether.

Sebum Control COS-218/2-A. [Cosmetochem] PEG-6 isolauryl thioether; a synergistic blend of ingreds. with effectively reduce the rate of sebum production; cosmetic specialty for use in shampoos, hair tonics, and skin care preps.

Secosol® AL 959. [Stepan Europe] Sodium lauryl sulfosuccinate; anionic; mild foamer for shampoos, bubble baths, liq. soaps, shower gels, bath salts; paste; 25% conc.

Secosol® ALL40. [Stepan Europe] Sodium laureth sulfosuccinate; anionic; mild foamer for shampoos, bubble baths, liq. soaps, shower gels, bath salts; emulsifier for emulsion polymerization; water-wh. to pale yel. liq.; 31% act.

Secoster® DMS. [Stepan Europe] Glycol distearate; CAS 627-83-8; EINECS 211-014-3; nonionic; emollient, pearl-escent, emulsifier, opacifier for creams, cleansing milks, shampoos; wh. to beige solid; 100% act.

Secoster® EMS. [Stepan Europe] Glycol stearate; CAS 111-60-4; EINECS 203-886-9; nonionic; emulsifier for creams and cleansing milks; emollient, pearlescent, opacifier; wh. solid; 100% act.

Secosyl. [Stepan Europe] Sodium N-lauroyl sarcosinate; CAS 137-16-6; EINECS 205-281-5; anionic; detergent, foaming agent, base, anticorrosion additive for rug shampoos, mild dishwash, household cleaners, personal care prods.; stable in hard water; water-wh. to pale yel. liq.; 30% act.

Sedamon. [Henkel/Cospha] Fragrance raw material for cosmetic, personal care, detergent, and cleaning prods.; sl. yel. liq., jasmine odor; b.p. 55-58 C; flash pt. 87 C.

Sedaplant Richter. [Dr. Kurt Richter; Henkel/Cospha] Polyvalent herbal extract plus anti-irritants (fennel, hops, balm mint, mistletoe, matricaria, and yarrow extracts, urea, and allantoin) in water-alcohol medium; emollient for aq. and hydroalcoholic herbal cosmetics, skin and hair protection prods.; emulsified preparations; dk. brn. liq.; herbal odor.

Sedefos 75®. [Gattefosse; Gattefosse SA] Glycol stearate, PEG-2 stearate, and trilaneth-4 phosphate; anionic; SE base for cosmetics and pharmaceuticals; Gardner < 5 waxy solid; weak odor; HLB 10-11; m.p. 43-48 C; acid no. < 6; iodine no. < 3; sapon. no. 105-120; usage level: 15-20%; toxicology: sl. irritating to skin, nonirritating to eyes; 100% conc.

Sedermasome. [Sederma] Water, glycerin, propylene glycol, and lecithin; liposome moisturizer for face and body care prods.; reconstitutes cutaneous film and increases intercellular cohesion; beige sl. visc. opalescent liq., char. odor; sp.gr. 1.00-1.10; pH 4.8-5.8; usage level: 5-30%.

Sellig LA 1150. [Ceca SA] Laureth-20; CAS 9002-92-0; nonionic; surfactant for shampoos, degreaser, textile applics.; liq.; sp.gr. 1.0 ± 0.2; HLB 14.5; pH 7 ± 0.5 (10% aq.); 50% conc.

Sellig Lano 30. [Ceca SA] PEG-30 lanolin; CAS 61790-81-6; nonionic; emollient for cosmetic preps., shampoos, liq. or gel soaps, ointments; brown clear wax; sp.gr. 1.01 ± 0.2; HLB 13; pH 8 ± 0.5 (10% aq.); 49-52% act.

Sellig LET 630. [Ceca SA] Alkylamine laureth sulfate; base for shampoos, hair lotions, foam baths; detergents for wool, fine lingerie, syn. fibers; pale yel. liq.; sp.gr. 1.03 ± 0.2; pH 7 ± 0.5 (10% aq.); 30 ± 1 act.

Sellig R 3395. [Ceca SA] PEG-33 castor oil; CAS 61791-12-6; nonionic; surfactant, emulsifier for pharmaceuticals, veterinary, and cosmetic applics.; solubilizer for essential oils; pale yel. visc. liq.; sp.gr. 1.08±0.06; HLB 12.0; iodine no. 33±4; sapon. no. 67±4; pH 7±0.5 (10%); 95% conc.

Sellig T 14 100. [Ceca SA] PEG-14 tallate; CAS 61791-00-2; nonionic; detergent base with controlled foam; solubilizer for essential oils; Gardner < 6 liq., char. odor; sp.gr. 1.05; HLB 13.4; pH 7-9 (10%); 100% active.

Selligor DC 100. [Ceca SA] DEA-coprah oil; surfactant and foam stabilizer for shampoo, foam baths, liq. soaps; greasing agent for creams; yel. liq.; sp.gr. 1.02 ± 0.1; > 99% act.

Semburi Extract BG. [Ikeda] Swertia herb extract, 1,3-butyleneglycol; bitter component claimed to stimulate hair growth and prevent hair loss in hair care prods.; yel. brn. clear visc. liq., char. odor; sp.gr. 1.030-1.065; pH 3.0-5.0.

Semburi Extract Ethanol. [Ikeda] Swertia herb extract, ethanol; bitter component claimed to stimulate hair growth and prevent hair loss in hair care prods.; yel. brn. clear visc. liq., char. odor; sp.gr. 0.800-1.000; pH 5.5-6.5.

Seodol E-2016. [Nihon Emulsion] Octyldodeceth-16; cosmetic emulsifier.

Seodol E-2020. [Nihon Emulsion] Octyldodeceth-20; cosmetic emulsifier.

Seodol E-2025. [Nihon Emulsion] Octyldodeceth-25; cosmetic emulsifier.

Sepicide CI. [Seppic] Imidazolidinyl urea; CAS 39236-46-9; EINECS 254-372-6; preservative for cosmetics; effective against Gram-negative bacteria; active over wide pH range; water-sol.; usage level: 0.2-0.6%.

Sepicide HB. [Seppic] Phenoxyethanol, methylparaben, ethylparaben, propylparaben, butylparaben; cosmetic preservative; liq.; 100% act.

Sepicide LD. [Seppic] Phenoxyethanol; CAS 122-99-6; EINECS 204-589-7; cosmetics preservative; esp. effective against Gram-negative bacteria; USA, Japan, Europe approvals; liq., al. aromatic odor; usage level: up to 1%.

Sepicide MB. [Seppic] Phenoxyethanol, methylparaben, ethylparaben, propylparaben, and butylparaben; cosmetic preservative system; USA and Europe approvals; usage level: 0.6-1.4%.

Sepigel 305. [Seppic] Polyacrylamide, C13-14 isoparaffin, laureth-7; thickener for cosmetics; supplied as dispersion; thickens instantly on addition of water; liq.; 50% act.

Sequestrene® 220. [Ciba-Geigy/Dyestuffs] Tetrasodium EDTA dihydrate; CAS 64-02-8; EINECS 200-573-9; chelating agent used in powd. cleaning compds.; scale removal, hair rinses; processing of syn. fibers and textiles, and industrial cleaning preparations; wh. cryst. powd.; water-sol.

Sequestrene® AA. [Ciba-Geigy/Dyestuffs] EDTA; CAS 60-00-4; EINECS 200-449-4; chelating agent for photographic developer baths, shampoos, cosmetics, electro-

plating, rare earth separations, metal determinations, liq. soaps, germicides, herbicide sprays; wh. powd.; insol. in water.

Sequestrene® NA2. [Ciba-Geigy/Dyestuffs] Disodium EDTA dihydrate; CAS 139-33-3; EINECS 205-358-3; chelating agent for control of trace metal contamination in pharmaceutical and cosmetic prods.; wh. cryst. powd.; odorless; water-sol.; pH 6.0 (5%); 99% act.

Sequestrene® NA3. [Ciba-Geigy/Dyestuffs] Trisodium EDTA trihydrate; chelating agent used in personal care prods.; processing of syn. fibers and textiles; stabilizer for resin systems; photographic baths, electrolytic and electroless plating; foam stabilizer, water treatment; powd.; water-sol.; pH 8.5 (10%).

Serdox NSG 400. [Servo Delden BV] PEG-9 stearate; CAS 9004-99-3; EINECS 226-312-9; nonionic; biodeg. surfactant for textile processing and cosmetic emulsions; antistat for plastics; solid; water-disp.; 100% conc.

Sericite 5, 300S. [Les Colorants Wackherr] Mica (aluminum potassium silicate); CAS 12001-26-2; lubricity agent giving exceptional smoothness and soft feel to cosmetic powds., lotions, and creams.

Sericite DNN. [Ikeda] Refined mica; CAS 12001-26-2; cosmetic grade with exc. color shade and remarkable shape; provides longer lasting activity and pleasant finish in makeup, pressed powd.; wh. fine powd.; 99% min. thru 325 mesh.

Sericite DNN-2SH. [Ikeda] Mica and dimethicone; cosmetic grade with exc. color shade and remarkable shape; provides longer lasting activity and pleasant finish in makeup, pressed powd.; wh. fine powd.; 99% min. thru 325 mesh.

Sericite FSE. [Presperse] Mica; CAS 12001-26-2; filler imparting softness, smooth feel, skin adhesion, and spreadability to pigmented cosmetics; JSCI/JCID approved; wh. fine powd.; particle size 3.3 µ; 95% min. thru 325 mesh.

Sericite SL. [Presperse] Mica; CAS 12001-26-2; filler imparting softness, smooth feel, skin adhesion, and spreadability to pigmented cosmetics; JSCI/JCID approved; wh. fine powd.; particle size 4.7 µ; 95% min. thru 325 mesh.

Sericite SL-012. [Presperse] Mica, methicone; CAS 12001-26-2, 9004-73-3; surf.-treated powd. providing creamier, more lubricious feel, improved spreadability and skin adhesion; ideal for wet and dry applics., pressed powds., pigmented cosmetics; JSCI/JCID approved; wh. fine powd.; 95% thru 325 mesh.

Sericite SL-012P. [Presperse] Mica, methicone, min. oil; surf.-treated powd. providing creamier, more lubricious feel, improved spreadability and skin adhesion; ideal for wet and dry applics., pressed powds., pigmented cosmetics; JSCI/JCID approved; wh. fine powd.; 95% thru 325 mesh.

Sericite SLZ. [Presperse] Mica; CAS 12001-26-2; cosmetic raw material, colorant.

Sericite SLZ-012P. [Presperse] Mica, methicone, min. oil; surf.-treated powd. providing creamier, more lubricious feel, improved spreadability and skin adhesion; ideal for wet and dry applics., pressed powds., pigmented cosmetics; JSCI/JCID approved; wh. fine powd.; 95% thru 325 mesh.

Sericite SP. [Presperse] Mica; CAS 12001-26-2; cosmetic raw material, colorant.

Sericite WL. [Ikeda] Mica, lauroyl lysine, lecithin; provides good dispersion and compatibility with oils, good water repellency, and good affinity to the skin; for use in pressed powd. prods. such as eyeshadow, or oil-based liq. foundations; sl. ylsh. fine powd., char. odor.

Sericoside Phytosome®. [Indena SpA; Lipo] *Terminalia sericea* extract; elasticizing, eutrophic, firming, soothing, moisturizing agent, skin protectant; coadjuvant in external treatment of cellulitis and for heavy legs; after-sun, after-depilation, and after-shave prods.; preps. for prevention of wrinkles and stretch marks; eye contour prods.; preps. for sensitive and chapped skin; lt. brn. amorphous powd.; water-disp.; usage level: to 3%.

Seromarine. [Sederma] Water and hemolymph extract; skin oxygenation stimulator for face care prods.; colorless to sl. bluish clear liq., char. odor; sp.gr. 1.020-1.040; ref. index 1.360 ± 0.005; pH 7.5-8.5; usage level: 3-7%.

Serumpro™ EN-10. [Brooks Industries] Hydrolyzed serum protein; cosmetics ingred.; contains all essential amino acids; m.w. 7000; 10% act.

Servirox OEG 45. [Servo Delden BV] PEG-17 castor oil; CAS 61791-12-6; nonionic; used in textile, phytopharmaceutical, leather, paper and cosmetic industries; liq.; 100% conc.

Servirox OEG 55. [Servo Delden BV] PEG-26 castor oil; CAS 61791-12-6; nonionic; used in textile, phytopharmaceutical, leather, paper and cosmetic industries; liq.; 100% conc.

Servirox OEG 65. [Servo Delden BV] PEG-32 castor oil; CAS 61791-12-6; nonionic; used in textile, phytopharmaceutical, leather, paper and cosmetic industries; liq.; 100% conc.

Servirox OEG 90/50. [Servo Delden BV] PEG-180 castor oil; CAS 61791-12-6; nonionic; used in textile, phytopharmaceutical, leather, paper and cosmetic industries; liq.; 50% conc.

Sesame Oil USP/NF 16. [Natural Oils Int'l.; Tri-K Industries] Sesame oil; CAS 8008-74-0; EINECS 232-370-6; cosmetic ingred.; pale straw clear oil, bland odor and taste; insol. in water; sp.gr. 0.916-0.921; iodine no. 103-116; sapon. no. 188-195; flash pt. (OC) 640 F; toxicology: nonhazardous.

Setacin 103 Spezial. [Zschimmer & Schwarz] Disodium laurethsulfosuccinate; anionic; detergent for personal care prods.; cleaning agent; liq.; 40% conc.

Setacin F Spezial Paste. [Zschimmer & Schwarz] Disodium lauryl sulfosuccinate; anionic; detergent, cosmetics, washing and cleaning agent; paste; 40% conc.

Setacin M. [Zschimmer & Schwarz] Semisulfosuccinate of ethoxylated fatty alcohols/fatty acid derivs., neutralized; anionic; detergent, personal care prods. and cleaning agents; yel. liq.; sol. in water, alcohol; pH 6-7; 42% act. in water.

Sexadecyl Alcohol, Cosmetic Grade. [Lanaetex Prods.] Isostearyl alcohol, min. oil; cosmetics ingred.

SF81-50. [GE Silicones] Dimethyl silicone; defoamers, release agents, in cosmetics, polishes, paint additives, and mechanical devices; lubricant in rubber or plastic-to-metal applics.; for damping and heat transfer in mechanical/elec. applics.; water-wh. clear, oily fluid; sp.gr. 0.972; visc. 50 cstk; pour pt. –120 F; ref. index 1.4030; flash pt. 460 F; surf. tens. 21.0 dynes/cm; conduct. 0.087 Btu/h-°F ft²/ft; sp. heat 0.36 Btu/lb/°F; dissip. factor 0.0001; dielec. str. 35.0 kV; dielec. const. 2.74; vol. resist. 1 x 10¹⁴ ohm-cm.

SF96® (5 cst). [GE Silicones] Dimethicone; emollient for hair spray, suntan lotion, antiperspirants; thread and fiber lubricants for textiles; fluid; sol. in lower alcohols, aliphatic, aromatic, and chlorinated hydrocarbons; sp.gr. 0.916; visc. 5 cSt; pour pt. –120 F; ref. index 1.397; surf. tens. 19.7 dynes/cm; sp. heat 0.36 Btu/lb °F; dissip. factor 0.0001; dielec. str. 35 kV; dielec. const. 2.60; vol. resist. 1 x 10¹⁵ ohm-cm; 100% act.

SF96® (100 cst) [GE Silicones] Dimethicone; used for damping, heat transfer, hydraulic fluids, rubber/plastic, base fluid for grease, polishes, cosmetics/toiletries, mold release for tires, rubber, plastics, aq. defoaming prods., thread/fiber lubricants; paint additives for flow control, mar

resist., gloss; sp.gr. 0.968; visc. 100 cSt; pour pt. -67 F; flash pt. (PMCC) 575 F; ref. index 1.4030; surf. tens. 20.9 dynes/cm; sp. heat 0.36 Btu/lb F; dissip. factor 0.0001; dielec. str. 35 kV; dielec. const. 2.74; vol. resist. 1 x 10¹⁴ ohm-cm.

SF96® (350 cst) [GE Silicones] Dimethicone; used for damping, heat transfer, hydraulic fluids, rubber/plastic, base fluid for grease, polishes, cosmetics/toiletries, mold release for tires, rubber, plastics, aq. defoaming prods., thread/fiber lubricants; paint additives for flow control, mar resist., gloss; sp.gr. 0.973; visc. 350 cSt; pour pt. -58 F; flash pt. (PMCC) 637 F; ref. index 1.4032; surf. tens. 21.1 dynes/cm; sp. heat 0.36 Btu/lb F; dissip. factor 0.0001; dielec. str. 35 kV; dielec. const. 2.75; vol. resist. 1 x 10¹⁴ ohm-cm.

SF96® (500 cst) [GE Silicones] Dimethicone; used for damping, heat transfer, hydraulic fluids, rubber/plastic, base fluid for grease, polishes, cosmetics/toiletries, mold release for tires, rubber, plastics, aq. defoaming prods., thread/fiber lubricants; paint additives for flow control, mar resist., gloss; sp.gr. 0.973; visc. 350 cSt; pour pt. -58 F; flash pt. (PMCC) 662 F; ref. index 1.4033; surf. tens. 21.1 dynes/cm; sp. heat 0.36 Btu/lb F; dissip. factor 0.0001; dielec. str. 35 kV; dielec. const. 2.76; vol. resist. 1 x 10¹⁴ ohm-cm.

SF96® (1000 cst) [GE Silicones] Dimethicone; used for damping, heat transfer, hydraulic fluids, rubber/plastic, base fluid for grease, polishes, cosmetics/toiletries, mold release for tires, rubber, plastics, aq. defoaming prods., thread/fiber lubricants; paint additives for flow control, mar resist., gloss; sp.gr. 0.974; visc. 350 cSt; pour pt. -58 F; flash pt. (PMCC) 658 F; ref. index 1.4035; surf. tens. 21.1 dynes/cm; sp. heat 0.36 Btu/lb F; dissip. factor 0.0001; dielec. str. 35 kV; dielec. const. 2.77; vol. resist. 1 x 10¹⁴ ohm-cm.

SF1080. [GE Silicones] Methyl alkyl polysiloxane silicone fluid; nonionic; mold release agent, lubricant; used in rubber, plastic, and metal industries, hair care prods.; internal mold release agent in vinyl slush molding; aluminum die cast mold release agent; lt. yel. liq.; sol. in aliphatic, aromatic, and chlorinated hydrocarbons, higher alcohols, and higher ketones; sp.gr. 1.035; visc. 1500 cs; pour pt. –50 F; ref. index 1.4930; flash pt. 400 F (CC); 100% act.

SF1173. [GE Silicones] Cyclomethicone; CAS 69430-24-6; emollient, lubricant used in antiperspirants, skin care prods., sunscreen prods., hair conditioners, facial makeup, particle treatment; liq.; insol. in water; misc. in the lower alcohols and in typ. aliphatic, aromatic, and halogenated hydrocarbon solvs.; sp.gr. 0.960; visc. 2.4 ctks; f.p. 17 C; b.p. 175 C; m.p. 63 F; flash pt. (PMCC) 130 F; ref. index 1.3935; surf. tens. 17.4 dynes/cm; sp. heat 0.36 Btu/lb F.

SF1188. [GE Silicones] Dimethicone copolyol; emollient, lubricant, and release agent for cosmetics and toiletries, paint, plastic mold release, and rubber lubricants; textile softener/modifier and thread/fiber lubricants; amber clear fluid; sol. in water below 43 C; sol. in acetone, toluene, lower alcohols, and some hydrocarbons; sp.gr. 1.04; dens. 8.65 lb/gal; visc. 1000 cps; flash pt. (PMCC) 200 F; ref. index 1.4470; surf. tens. 25.5 dynes/cm; 100% silicone.

SF1202. [GE Silicones] Cyclomethicone; CAS 69430-24-6; emollient, lubricant used in antiperspirants, skin care prods., sunscreen prods., hair conditioners, facial makeup, particle treatment; liq.; insol. in water; misc. in the lower alcohols and in typ. aliphatic, aromatic, and halogenated hydrocarbon solvs.; sp.gr. 0.950; visc. 3.8 ctks; f.p. –40 C; b.p. 190–210 C; m.p. -40 F; flash pt. (PMCC) 170 F; ref. index 1.3982; surf. tens. 17.4 dynes/

cm; sp. heat 0.36 Btu/lb F.

SF1204. [GE Silicones] Cyclomethicone (85% SF 1173 and 15% SF 1202); CAS 69430-24-6; emollient, lubricant used in antiperspirants, skin care prods., sunscreen prods., hair conditioners, facial makeup, particle treatment; liq.; insol. in water; misc. in the lower alcohols and in typ. aliphatic, aromatic, and halogenated hydrocarbon solvs.; sp.gr. 0.960; visc. 2.6 ctks; f.p. 11 C; b.p. 175–210 C; m.p. 53 F; flash pt. (PMCC) 140 F; ref. index 1.3939; surf. tens. 17.4 dynes/cm; sp. heat 0.36 Btu/lb F.

SF1706. [GE Silicones] Amine functional silicone fluid; for durable car polishes and cosmetics/toiletries; liq.; sol. in aromatic, aliphatic solvs, IPA; sp.gr. 0.986; visc. 15-40 ctks; flash pt. (PMCC) 150 F; 100% act.

S-Flakes. [Karlshamns] Hydrog. soybean oil; CAS 8016-70-4; EINECS 232-410-2; emollient, lubricant; Lovibond R2.0 max.; m.p. 153–157 F; iodine no. 5 max.; sapon. no. 189–197.

Shampoo Base 733A. [Mona Industries] Fully compounded shampoo conc. which can be diluted either 1:8 or 1:15 with water for the professional beauty salon market.

Shea Butter. [Sederma] Shea butter; CAS 68424-60-2; skin protective and healing agent for the skin against climatic, mechanical, and chemical agressions; treatment for dry and sensitive skin, body and hand care, hair care, presun, sun, and after-sun care; pale yel. fatty matter, char. odor; sp.gr. 0.91-0.98; iodine no. 50-80; usage level: 2-10%.

Shea Unsaponifiable Conc. [Sederma] Shea butter unsaponifiables; treatment for sensitive or dry skin, lip care, sun protection; for face, sun, and makeup care prods.; green-brownish fatty matter, char. odor; sp.gr. 0.92-0.98; usage level: 0.2-2%.

Shebu® WS. [R.I.T.A.] PEG-50 shea butter; emollient, humectant, pigment, conditioner, lubricant for personal care formulations; solubilizer and emulsifier of other fatty components; superfatting agent for cleansing prods.; suggested for aq. systems, shampoos, hand soaps, conditioners, creams, lotions, after-sun moisturizers; amber clear very visc. liq.; sol. in water, min. oil; toxicology: nontoxic; 50% conc.

Shebu® Refined. [R.I.T.A.] Shea butter; CAS 68424-60-2; emollient, humectant, moisturizer, pigment, conditioner, lubricant for personal care formulations; unique unsaponifiable fraction; alleviates dryness, reduces erythema, provides sun protection props. to skin; reduces sunlight damage to hair; fast penetration; melts at body temp.; suggested for sun care prods., antiwrinkle creams, lip care, baby prods., soaps, cleansers, pomades and hair dressings; off-wh. paste, char. nutty odor; sp.gr. 0.91-0.98; m.p. 30-39 C; acid no. 48-60; iodine no. 48-60; sapon. no. 160-180; ref. index 1.46 (40 C); toxicology: nontoxic.

Shinju® White 100T. [Mearl] Fine particle size mica (50%) coated with bismuth oxychloride; pearl pigment with increased opacity and better light stability for cosmetics (face powds., pressed powds.); powd.; particle size 2-20 μ; sp.gr. 4.0; bulk dens. 16 lb/ft³.

Sicomet®. [BASF AG] Anionic dyes, cationic dyes, fat-sol. dyes, org. pigments, inorg. pigments, pigment concs.; colorants for cosmetics.

Sicopharm®. [BASF AG] Sol. dyes and pigments for coloring pharmaceuticals.

Sident® 15. [Degussa] Silica; abrasiveness and thickening agent for toothpastes.

Sident® 22LS. [Degussa] Silica; nonabrasive thickening agent for toothpastes.

Sident® 22S. [Degussa] Syn. amorphous precipitated silica; CAS 112926-00-8; nonabrasive thickening agent for toothpastes; FDA compliance; wh. loose powd.; tapped

dens. 90 g/l; surf. area 190 m²/g; pH 6.2 (5%); 100% act.

Silagen AA. [Hormel] Collagen amino-polysilocane hydrolysate; cosmetic protein; 40% conc.

Silagen HC. [Hormel] Collagen amino-polysilocane hydrolysate; cosmetic protein; 40% conc.

Silagen MP. [Hormel] Collagen amino-polysilocane hydrolysate; cosmetic protein; 40% conc.

Silamide DCA-100. [Siltech] nonionic; moderate foaming conditioner for personal care prods.; water-sol.; 100% act.

Silamine 50. [Siltech] cationic; low foaming softener and gloss agent for personal care prods.; water-insol.; 100% act.

Silamine 65. [Siltech] Dimethicone copolyolamine; cationic; moderate foaming gloss and conditioning agent for personal care prods.; water-sol.; 100% act.

Silanol Exsyliposomes. [Exsymol; Biosil Tech.] Liposomes for skin care prods.; sl. colored opalescent liq.; usage level: 2-6%; toxicology: nontoxic.

Silatex SF-50. [Lanaetex Prods.] Dimethicone; cosmetic ingred.

Silatex SF-280. [Lanaetex Prods.] Dimethicone copolyol; cosmetic ingred.

Silatex SF-300. [Lanaetex Prods.] Dimethicone; cosmetic ingred.

Silatex SF-V. [Lanaetex Prods.] Cyclomethicone; CAS 69430-24-6; cosmetic ingred.

Silflex A22. [Rhone-Poulenc] Sodium/TEA-lauroyl animal collagen amino acids.; shampoo base.

Silhydrate C. [Exsymol; Biosil Tech.] Copper PCA methylsilanol; provides skin moisturization, skin restructuring for anti-aging formulations, skin treatments, cosmetic and toiletry emulsions, creams, lotions; pale blue, limpid liq., without any particular odor; misc. with water, alcohol, glycols; sp.gr. 1.1; pH 5.5; usage level: 5-10%; toxicology: nontoxic.

Silicone L-31. [Union Carbide] Methicone; CAS 9004-73-3.

Silicone L-45. [Union Carbide] Dimethicone.

Silicone Emulsion E-130. [Wacker-Chemie GmbH] Silicone emulsion; used for auto/furniture polish emulsions, cosmetics, textile lubricants and release aids, and aerosol window cleaners; wh. liq.; dens. 8.3 lb/gal; visc. 100 cSt; 60% solids in water.

Silicone Emulsion E-131. [Wacker Silicones] Silicone emulsion; used for mold release, auto/furniture polish emulsions, aerosol window cleaners, cosmetics, textile thread lubricants; wh. liq.; dens. 8.3 lb/gal; visc. 350 cSt6; 60% solids in water.

Silicone Emulsion E-133. [Wacker Silicones] Silicone emulsion; used for mold release, auto/furniture polish emulsions, cosmetics, textile lubricants and softeners; wh. liq.; dens. 8.3 lb/gal; visc. 1000 cSt6; 60% solids in water.

Silkall 100. [Ikeda] Silk; protein improving humectancy, flexibility, and anticracking props.; for use in powdery makeup, pressed powd., eyeshadow, lipstick, liq. foundation; moisturizing function on skin; ivory to sl. grayish powd., faint pleasant odor; particle size thru 200 mesh; pH 4.5-7.5; 99% min. protein.

Silkall CA. [Ikeda] Calcium carbonate and silk; silk-coated inorg. pigment offering good moisturizing effect, good adhesion to the skin, pleasant feel, elegance, and gloss; used in pressed powds.; ivory to sl. grayish powd., faint pleasant odor; particle size thru 500 mesh; pH 6.5-8.7 (10% aq. susp.); 38-43% protein.

Silkall TI. [Ikeda] Titanium dioxide and silk; silk-coated inorg. pigment offering good moisturizing effect, good adhesion to the skin, pleasant feel, elegance, and gloss; used in pressed powds.; ivory to sl. grayish powd., faint pleasant odor; particle size thru 200 mesh; pH 4.5-7.5 (10% aq. susp.); 15-20% protein.

Silkall TL. [Ikeda] Talc and silk; silk-coated inorg. pigment offering good moisturizing effect, good adhesion to the skin, pleasant feel, elegance, and gloss; used in pressed powds.; ivory to sl. grayish powd., faint pleasant odor; particle size thru 500 mesh; pH 4.5-7.5 (10% aq. susp.); 17.5-22.5% protein.

Silkall ZN. [Ikeda] Zinc oxide and silk; silk-coated inorg. pigment offering good moisturizing effect, good adhesion to the skin, pleasant feel, elegance, and gloss; used in pressed powds.; ivory to sl. grayish powd., faint pleasant odor; particle size thru 200 mesh; pH 4.5-7.5 (10% aq. susp.); 15-20% protein.

Silkies. [Int'l. Flora Tech.] Semisolid microspheres containing jojoba esters, hydrog. sunflower oil and wax; exfoliant for cosmetics; biodeg., sterile, stable; CTFA & FDA compliance; semisolid beads, sl. fatty odor; m.p. 55-65 C.

Silkpro. [Ikeda] Hydrolyzed silk; CAS 96690-41-4; cosmetic ingred. in skin creams/lotions, soft liq. soaps, cleansing foams, conditioning shampoos, hair moisturizers; imparts gentle and glossy feel to hair due to effective absorption and film-forming props.; amber clear liq., char. odor; m.w. 400; pH 5.0-7.0; 9-13% protein.

Silkpro AS. [Ikeda] Ethyl ester of hydrolyzed silk; protein providing glossy films, pleasant touch; sol. in alcohol makes it ideal for hair sprays, hair treatments, styling mousses, nail enamels, etc.; lt. ylsh. clear liq.; sol. in ethanol; sp.gr. 0.820-0.950; pH 3.0-6.5; 34% min. Ca, 1.5% min Mg.

Silkpro CM-1000. [Ikeda] Hydrolyzed silk; CAS 96690-41-4; water-retaining film-former imparting gentle touch to hair shampoos and treatments, skin creams and lotions; lt. amber clear liq., char. odor; m.w. 1000; pH 6.0-8.0; 5-8% solids.

Silkpro CM-2000. [Ikeda] Hydrolyzed silk; CAS 96690-41-4; water-retaining film-former imparting gentle touch to hair shampoos and treatments, skin creams and lotions; amber clear liq., char. odor; m.w. 2000; pH 5.5-7.5; 10.5-12.5% solids.

Silkpro-Q. [Ikeda] N-(3-Trimethylammonio-2-hydroxypropyl) hydrolyzed silk; soft film-former with exc. water holding capacity; provides exc. adsorption on skin, gloss, fine touch; for hair shampoos, treatments, rinses; lt. amber clear liq., char. odor; pH 5.5-7.5.

Silk Pro-Tein. [Maybrook] Hydrolyzed silk; CAS 96690-41-4; moisturizer, substantive protein, protective barrier for elegant skin and hair preps. (lotions, creams, bath gels, shampoos, conditioners, treatment prods., shave preps., soap bars); amber clear liq., mild char. odor; pH 5.0-7.0; 8-14% solids.

Silquat AD. [Siltech] cationic; moderate foaming softener and emulsifier for personal care prods.; anionic-compat.; water-sol.; 40% act.

Silquat AM. [Siltech] Silicone quaternium-2; cationic; moderate foaming softener for personal care prods.; anionic-compat.; water-sol.; 40% act.

Silquat Q-100. [Siltech] Quaternium-80; CAS 134737-05-6; cationic; low foaming, nonrewetting conditioner and softener for personal care prods.; water-disp.; 70% act.

Silquat Q-200. [Siltech] cationic; moderate foaming, mild conditioner for personal care prods.; water-sol.; 50% act.

Silquat Q-300. [Siltech] cationic; low foaming conditioner and softener for personal care prods.; water-disp.; 70% act.

Siltek® GR. [Petrolite] Polyethylene; CAS 9002-88-4; EINECS 200-815-3; polymer for use in cosmetics applics.; visc. 80 SUS (300 F); m.p. 235 F.

Siltek® L. [Petrolite] Ethylene/propylene copolymer; CAS 9010-79-1; polymer for use in cosmetic stick formulations; offers compat., improved oil retention and better stick structure; visc. 70 SUS (210 F); m.p. 202 F.

Siltek® M. [Petrolite] Polyethylene; CAS 9002-88-4; EINECS

200-815-3; binder for pressed powds. in eyeshadows and blushers; eliminates "bleeding" of pigments during processing; visc. 47 SUS (300 F); m.p. 210 F.

Siltek® M Super. [Petrolite] Polyethylene; CAS 9002-88-4; EINECS 200-815-3; binder for pressed powds. in eyeshadows and blushers; eliminates "bleeding" of pigments during processing; smaller particle size prod. than Siltek M; visc. 47 SUS (300 F); m.p. 210 F.

Siltek® PL. [Petrolite] Polyethylene; CAS 9002-88-4; EINECS 200-815-3; cosmetic ingred. improving dimensional stability, binding oil in stick applics., controlling visc. over wide temp. range in oil-based systems; visc. 52 SUS (210 F); m.p. 187 F.

Silwax® C. [Siltech] Dimethiconol hydroxystearate; patented, highly lubricious wax for personal care applics., polishes, textile lubrication and softening, laundry prods., dryer sheet softeners, syn. lubricants, plastics lubricants; buff wax; sol. @ 5% in IPA; disp. in silicone fluid; insol. in water.

Silwax® F. [Siltech] Dimethiconol fluoroalcohol dilinoleic acid; patented prod. forming films which are hydrophobic, nonocclusive, and resist. to many chemical agents; additive for barrier creams and other skin care prods.; yel. opaque liq.; water-insol.; sp.gr. 1.00 g/ml; b.p. 212 F; flash pt. (TCC) > 200 F; pH 5-7 (10%); toxicology: skin exposure can cause irritation; ingestion may cause nausea; 100% solids, 8% F.

Silwax® F-D. [Siltech] Fluorine-containing silicone polymers; patented prod. forming films which are hydrophobic, nonocclusive, and resist. to many chemical agents; additive for barrier creams and other skin care prods.; wh. solid; water-insol.; sp.gr. 1.00 g/ml; b.p. 212 F; flash pt. (TCC) > 200 F; pH 5-7 (10%); toxicology: skin exposure can cause irritation; ingestion may cause nausea; 100% solids, 8% F.

Silwax® S. [Siltech] Silicone wax; nonionic; patented, highly lubricious wax for personal care applics., polishes, textile lubrication and softening, laundry prods., dryer sheet softeners, syn. lubricants, plastics lubricants; wh. paste-like wax; sol. @ 5% in IPA, min. spirits; disp. in min. oil, oleic acid; insol. in water; 100% act.

Silwax® WD-IS. [Siltech] Dimethicone copolyol isostearate; CAS 133448-16-5; nonionic; patented, highly lubricious wax for personal care conditioning, polishes, textile lubrication and softening, laundry prods., dryer sheet softeners, syn. lubricants, plastics lubricants; forms microemulsions in water without added surfactants; wax; sol. @ 5% in IPA, glyceryl trioleate, oleic acid; disp. in water; 100% act.

Silwax® WD-S. [Siltech] Silicone wax; patented, highly lubricious wax for personal care applics., polishes, textile lubrication and softening, laundry prods., dryer sheet softeners, syn. lubricants, plastics lubricants; more dispersible than Silwax S, more substantive than WD-IS; wax; sol. @ 5% in IPA, glyceryl trioleate, oleic acid; initially disp. in water, but creams upon standing.

Silwax® WS. [Siltech] Silicone wax; nonionic; patented, highly lubricious wax for personal care applics., polishes, textile lubrication and softening, laundry prods., dryer sheet softeners, syn. lubricants, plastics lubricants; produces high gloss on a variety of substrates; wax; sol. @ 5% in water, IPA, PEG 400, glyceryl trioleate, oleic acid; insol. in min. oil; 100% act.

Silwet® L-77. [OSi Specialties] Polyalkylene oxide-modified polymethylsiloxane; CAS 27306-78-1; nonionic; surfactant, flow/leveling agent, antistat, antifog, dispersant, wetting agent, flotation agent, spreading agent for coatings, printing inks, adhesives, agric., automotive, cleaners, antifogging agent, mining, paper, pharmaceutical applics.; pale amber clear liq.; m.w. 600; sol. in methanol,

IPA, acetone, xylene, methylene chloride; disp. in water; sp.gr. 1.007; dens. 8.37 lb/gal; visc. 20 cSt; HLB 5–8; cloud pt. < 10 C (0.1%); flash pt. (PMCC) 116 C; pour pt. 2 C; surf. tens. 20.5 dyne/cm (0.1% aq.); Draves wetting 8 s (0.1%); Ross-Miles foam 33 mm (0.1%, initial); 100% act.

Silwet® L-711. [OSi Specialties] Dimethicone copolyol.

Silwet® L-720. [OSi Specialties] Dimethicone copolyol; CAS 68554-65-4; nonionic; surfactant; anticaking agent; slip additive for paper; also for pharmaceutical use, printing inks; FDA approved; colorless clear liq.; m.w. 12,000; sol. in water, methanol, IPA, acetone, xylene, methylene chloride; sp.gr. 1.036; dens. 8.61 lb/gal; visc. 1100 cSt; HLB 9-12; cloud pt. 42 C (1%); flash pt. (PMCC) 96 C; pour pt. -34 C; surf. tens. 29.3 dyne/cm (0.1% aq.); Draves wetting > 300 s (0.1%); Ross-Miles foam 43 mm (0.1%, initial); 50% act.

Silwet® L-721. [OSi Specialties] Dimethicone copolyol.

Silwet® L-7000. [OSi Specialties] Dimethicone copolyol.

Silwet® L-7001. [OSi Specialties] Dimethicone copolyol; CAS 67762-85-0; nonionic; surfactant, dispersant, emulsifier, leveling/flow control agent, antifog, lubricant, antiblock, slip additive for adhesives, agric., automotive, coatings, printing inks, textiles, household specialties, cutting fluids, petrol. extraction, paper, personal care prods., plastics and rubber; pale yel. clear liq.; m.w. 20,000; sol. in water, methanol, IPA, acetone, xylene, methylene chloride; sp.gr. 1.023; dens. 8.50 lb/gal; visc. 1700 cSt; HLB 9–12; cloud pt. 39 C (1%); flash pt. (PMCC) 97 C; pour pt. -48 C; surf. tens. 30.5 dyne/cm (0.1% aq.); Draves wetting > 300 s (0.25%); Ross-Miles foam 46 mm (0.1%, initial); 75% act.

Silwet® L-7002. [OSi Specialties] Dimethicone copolyol; CAS 67762-87-2; nonionic; low surf. tension, high wetting surfactant, lubricant, antistat, dispersant, emulsifier; lt. amber clear liq.; sol. in water, methanol, IPA, acetone, xylene, methylene chloride; m.w. 8000; sp.gr. 1.028; dens. 8.54 lb/gal; visc. 900 cSt; HLB 5-8; pour pt. -40 C; cloud pt. 39 C (1% aq.); flash pt. (PMCC) 88 C; surf. tens. 30.5 dynes/cm (1.1% aq.); Ross-Miles foam 64 mm (0.1%, initial); 100% act.

Silwet® L-7004. [OSi Specialties] Dimethicone copolyol; nonionic.

Silwet® L-7500. [OSi Specialties] Dimethicone copolyol; CAS 68440-66-4; nonionic; surfactant, antifoam, dispersant, emulsifier, leveling and flow control agent, lubricant, slip additive for adhesives, automotive, chemical processing, coatings, petrol. extraction, paper, personal care prods., plastics and rubber, pharmaceutical, textile applics.; lt. yel. clear liq.; sol. in methanol, IPA, acetone, xylene, hexanes, methylene chloride; insol. in water; m.w. 3000; sp.gr. 0.982; dens. 8.16 lb/gal; visc. 140 cSt; HLB 5-8; pour pt. -43 C; flash pt. (PMCC) 121 C; 100% act.

Silwet® L-7600. [OSi Specialties] Dimethicone copolyol; CAS 68938-54-5; nonionic; surfactant, wetting agent for adhesives, window cleaners, textiles, personal care prods.; internal lubricant for plastics and rubber; lt. amber clear liq.; sol. in water, methanol, IPA, acetone, xylene, methylene chloride; m.w. 4000; sp.gr. 1.066; dens. 8.86 lb/gal; visc. 110 cSt; HLB 13-17; pour pt. 2 C; cloud pt. 64 C (1% aq.); flash pt. (PMCC) 74 C; surf. tens. 25.1 dyne/cm (1.1% aq.); Draves wetting 131 s (0.1%); Ross-Miles foam 94 mm (0.1%, initial); 100% act.

Silwet® L-7602. [OSi Specialties] Dimethicone copolyol; CAS 68938-54-5; nonionic; surfactant, defoamer, dispersant, emulsifier, leveling and flow control agent, gloss agent, lubricant, release agent, antiblock and slip additive, wetting agent for adhesives, agric., automotive specialties, chemical processing, coatings, petrol. extraction, skin care prods., urethane bubble release, pharmaceuti-

cal, printing inks, textiles; pale yel. clear liq.; sol. in methanol, IPA, acetone, xylene, methylene chloride; disp. in water; m.w. 3000; sp.gr. 1.027; dens. 8.54 lb/gal; visc. 100 cSt; HLB 5-8; flash pt. (PMCC) 127 C; pour pt. -15 C; surf. tens. 26.6 dyne/cm (1.1% aq.); 100% act.

Silwet® L-7604. [OSi Specialties] Dimethicone copolyol; CAS 68937-54-2; nonionic; surfactant, dispersant, emulsifier, wetting agent, flotation agent, spreading agent for automotive specialties, coatings, window cleaners, mining, personal care prods., textiles; pale yel. clear liq.; sol. in water, methanol, IPA, acetone, xylene, methylene chloride; m.w. 4000; sp.gr. 1.074; dens. 8.93 lb/gal; visc. 420 cSt; HLB 13-17; pour pt. -1 C; cloud pt. 50 C (1% aq.); flash pt. (PMCC) 79 C; surf. tens. 25.4 dyne/cm (1.1% aq.); Draves wetting 210 s (0.1%); Ross-Miles foam 71 mm (0.1%, initial); 100% act.

Silwet® L-7610. [OSi Specialties] Dimethicone copolyol.

Silwet® L-7614. [OSi Specialties] Dimethicone copolyol; nonionic; low surf. tension and high wetting surfactant, lubricant, antistat, dispersant, emulsifier; for personal care prods.; pale yel. clear liq.; sol. in water, methanol, IPA, acetone, xylene, methylene chloride; m.w. 5000; sp.gr. 1.084; dens. 9.03 lb/ga; visc. 480 cSt; HLB 5-8; pour pt. 55 F; cloud pt. 88 C (1% aq.); flash pt. (PMCC) 174 F; surf. tens. 27.6 dynes/cm (0.1% aq.); Draves wetting > 300 s (0.1%); Ross-Miles foam 84 mm (0.1%, initial); 100% act.

Silymarin Phytosome® . [Indena SpA; Lipo] Complex of silymarin and soybean phospholipids; free-radical scavenger, dermopurifier, skin protectant, soothing/moisturizing agent; for prods. for aging skin, sun preps., prods. for oily, comedonic skin; yel. to lt. yel.-brn. amorphous powd.; water-disp.; usage level: to 3%.

Simchin® WS. [R.I.T.A.] PEG-40 jojoba oil; superfatting agent, emollient, humectant, pigment, conditioner, foam stabilizer, plasticizer, moisturizer, and lubricant for personal care formulations (soaps, hair preps., creams, lotions, antiperspirants); yel. clear visc. liq.; water-sol.; acid no. 2 max.; sapon. no. 30 max.; hyd. no. 60 max.; pH 5-8 (3%); toxicology: nontoxic; 45-52% moisture.

Simchin® Natural. [R.I.T.A.] Jojoba oil; CAS 61789-91-1; moisturizer, emollient, conditioner, spreading agent for skin and hair care prods.; coating material and carrier for pharmaceuticals and topicals; yel. liq.; sp.gr. 0.863-0.864; f.p. 7-10.6 C; m.p. 6.8-7 C; acid no. 2 max.; iodine no. 82-93; sapon. no. 92-95.6; ref. index 1.4650-1.4665; toxicology: nontoxic.

Simchin® Refined. [R.I.T.A.] Jojoba oil; CAS 61789-91-1; highest quality jojoba oil for use when low odor and color is important; moisturizer, emollient, conditioner, spreading agent for skin and hair care prods.; coating material and carrier for pharmaceuticals and topicals; Gardner 1 liq. wax, almost odorless; sp.gr. 0.863-0.864; f.p. 7-10.6 C; m.p. 6.8-7 C; acid no. 2 max.; iodine no. 82-93; sapon. no. 92-95.6; ref. index 1.4650-1.4665; toxicology: nontoxic, nonirritating; 100% conc.

Simulsol 7. [Seppic] Steareth-20; CAS 9005-00-9; cosmetics emulsifier.

Simulsol 52. [Seppic] Ceteth-2; CAS 9004-95-9; nonionic; emulsifier; solid; HLB 5.3; 100% conc.

Simulsol 56. [Seppic] Ceteth-10; CAS 9004-95-9; nonionic; emulsifier; solid; HLB 12.9; 100% conc.

Simulsol 58. [Seppic] Ceteth-20; CAS 9004-95-9; nonionic; cosmetics emulsifier; solid; HLB 15.7; 100% conc.

Simulsol 72. [Seppic] Steareth-2; CAS 9005-00-9; nonionic; emulsifier; solid; HLB 4.9; 100% conc.

Simulsol 76. [Seppic] Steareth-10; CAS 9005-00-9; nonionic; emulsifier; solid; HLB 12.4; 100% conc.

Simulsol 78. [Seppic] Steareth-20; CAS 9005-00-9; nonionic; emulsifier; solid; HLB 15.3; 100% conc.

Simulsol 92. [Seppic] Oleth-2; CAS 9004-98-2; nonionic; emulsifier; liq.; HLB 4.9; 100% conc.

Simulsol 96. [Seppic] Oleth-10; CAS 9004-98-2; nonionic; emulsifier; liq.; HLB 12.4; 100% conc.

Simulsol 98. [Seppic] Oleth-20; CAS 9004-98-2; nonionic; cosmetic emulsifier; solid; HLB 15.3; 100% conc.

Simulsol 165. [Seppic] PEG-100 stearate, glyceryl stearate; acid-stable cosmetics emulsifier; flakes; 100% act.

Simulsol 220 TM. [Seppic] PEG-200 glyceryl stearate; thickening agent for cosmetic surfactant systems.

Simulsol 989. [Seppic] PEG-7 hydrog. castor oil; CAS 61788-85-0; cosmetic w/o emulsifier; paste; 100% act.

Simulsol 1030 NP. [Seppic] Nonoxynol-10; CAS 9016-45-9; EINECS 248-294-1; nonionic; personal care surfactant.

Simulsol 1285. [Seppic] PEG-60 castor oil; CAS 61791-12-6; solubilizer; liq.

Simulsol 1292. [Seppic] PEG-25 hydrog. castor oil; CAS 61788-85-0; solubilizer, emulsifier for cosmetics; liq.; 100% act.

Simulsol 1293. [Seppic] PEG-40 hydrog. castor oil; CAS 61788-85-0; cosmetic emulsifier and solubilizer; paste; 100% act.

Simulsol 1294. [Seppic] PEG-60 hydrog. castor oil; CAS 61788-85-0; cosmetic emulsifier and solubilizer; paste; 100% act.

Simulsol 5719. [Seppic] Ethoxydiglycol, ceteareth-16, nonoxynol-8; cosmetic emulsifier and solubilizer; liq.; 100% act.

Simulsol 5817. [Seppic] PEG-35 castor oil; CAS 61791-12-6; solubilizer for cosmetics.

Simulsol CG. [Seppic] PEG-78 glyceryl cocoate; personal care surfactant.

Simulsol CS. [Seppic] Ceteareth-33; CAS 68439-49-6; cosmetics emulsifier; flakes; 100% act.

Simulsol M 45. [Seppic] PEG-8 stearate; CAS 9004-99-3; nonionic; cosmetics emulsifier; solid; HLB 11.1; 100% conc.

Simulsol M 49. [Seppic] PEG-20 stearate; CAS 9004-99-3; nonionic; cosmetics emulsifier; solid; HLB 15.0; 100% conc.

Simulsol M 51. [Seppic] PEG-30 stearate; CAS 9004-99-3; nonionic; emulsifier; solid; HLB 16.0; 100% conc.

Simulsol M 52. [Seppic] PEG-40 stearate; CAS 9004-99-3; nonionic; cosmetics emulsifier; solid; HLB 16.9; 100% conc.

Simulsol M 53. [Seppic] PEG-50 stearate; CAS 9004-99-3; nonionic; cosmetics emulsifier; solid; HLB 17.9; 100% conc.

Simulsol M 59. [Seppic] PEG-100 stearate; CAS 9004-99-3; nonionic; cosmetics emulsifier; solid; HLB 18.8; 100% conc.

Simulsol NP 575. [Seppic] Alkylphenyl polyethoxy ether; nonionic; emulsifier; liq.; 100% conc.

Simulsol O. [Seppic] Alkyl polyethoxy ether; nonionic; emulsifier; paste; 100% conc.

Simulsol OL 50. [Seppic] PEG-40 castor oil; CAS 61791-12-6; solubilizer for cosmetics use.

Simulsol P4. [Seppic] Laureth-4; CAS 5274-68-0; EINECS 226-097-1; nonionic; cosmetics emulsifier; liq.; HLB 9.7; 100% conc.

Simulsol P23. [Seppic] Laureth-23; CAS 9002-92-0; cosmetics emulsifier; liq.; 100% act.

Simulsol PS20. [Seppic] PEG-25 propylene glycol stearate.

Sinochem GMS. [Sino-Japan] Glyceryl monostearate; nonionic; emulsifier; flake; HLB 4.2; 99.5% conc.

Sinopol 1100H. [Sino-Japan] POE lauryl ether; nonionic; emulsifier for silicone, min. oil; liq.; HLB 12.9; 100% conc.

Sipernat® 22. [Degussa] Hydrated silica; CAS 112926-00-8; adsorbent, anticaking and free-flow agents; used as aid to convert liqs. into powds.; processing aid; hydrophilic;

for adhesives, sealants, detergents, food, cosmetics industries; FDA approved; wh. fluffy powd., particle size 18 nanometer; tapped dens. 260 g/l; surf. area 190 m²/g; pH 6.2 (5%); 98% SiO₂.

Sipernat® 22LS. [Degussa] Precipitated silica; thickening agent for cosmetics, pharmaceuticals, elec., insulation, paper, film, pesticides, plastics industries; FDA approved; tapped dens. 80 g/l; surf. area 190 m²/g; pH 6.2; 98% SiO₂.

Sipernat® 22S. [Degussa] Hydrated silica; CAS 112926-00-8; free-flow/anticaking agent for powd. detergents, sealants, foodstuffs, pharmaceuticals, fire extinguishers; FDA approved; loose wh. powd.; tapped dens. 90 g/l; surf. are 190 m²/g; pH 6.2 (5%); 98% SiO₂.

Sipernat® 50. [Degussa] Hydrated silica; CAS 112926-00-8; carrier, free-flow agent, anticaking agent for cosmetics, detergents, food industries; FDA approved; loose wh. powd.; pH 6.0-7.4 (5%).

Sipernat® 50S. [Degussa] Precipitated silica; CAS 112926-00-8; free-flow agent for uniform packing of metal powds. in elec. industry; also for cosmetics, detergents, food, pharmaceuticals industries; FDA approved; loose wh. powd.; tapped dens. 100 g/l; surf. area 480 m²/g; pH 6.7 (5%).

Sitostene. [Vevy] Soy sterol.

Skinotan S 10. [Zschimmer & Schwarz] Polysiloxane polyglycol ether; nonionic; shampoo additive; liq.; 100% conc.

SM 2112. [GE Silicones] Dimethiconol and PEG-15 cocomonium chloride; 35% silicone emulsion used in textiles as softener; also for hair mousse; disp. in water.

S-Maz® 20. [PPG/Specialty Chem.] Sorbitan laurate; CAS 1338-39-2; nonionic; lubricant, antistat, textile softener, process defoamer, opacifier, coemulsifier, solubilizer, dispersant, suspending agent, coupler; prepares exc. w/o emulsions; with T-Maz Series used as o/w emulsifiers in cosmetics, lipstick, makeup, skin care prods., food formulations, industrial oils, and household prods.; lipophilic; amber liq.; sol. in ethanol, naphtha, min. oils, toluene, veg. oil; water-disp.; sp.gr. 1.0; visc. 4500 cps; HLB 8.0; acid no. 7 max.; sapon. no. 158–170; hyd. no. 330-358; flash pt. (PMCC) > 55 F; 100% conc.

S-Maz® 40. [PPG/Specialty Chem.] Sorbitan palmitate; CAS 26266-57-9; EINECS 247-568-8; nonionic; lubricant, antistat, textile softener, process defoamer, opacifier, coemulsifier, solubilizer, dispersant, suspending agent, coupler; prepares exc. w/o emulsions; tan flakes; partly sol. in hot ethanol, acetone, toluol, min. and veg. oils; m.p. 45–46 C; HLB 6.5; acid no. 7.5 max.; sapon. no. 140–150; hyd. no. 275-305; flash pt. (PMCC) > 55 F; 100% conc.

S-Maz® 60. [PPG/Specialty Chem.] Sorbitan stearate; CAS 1338-41-6; EINECS 215-664-9; nonionic; lubricant, antistat, textile softener, process defoamer, opacifier, coemulsifier, solubilizer, dispersant, suspending agent, coupler; prepares exc. w/o emulsions; cream flakes; insol. in water, min. oils; m.p. 50–53 C; HLB 4.7; acid no. 10 max.; sapon. no. 147–157; hyd. no. 235-260; flash pt. (PMCC) > 350 F; 100% conc.

S-Maz® 60K. [PPG/Specialty Chem.] Sorbitan stearate; CAS 1338-41-6; EINECS 215-664-9; nonionic; emulsifier for cosmetic creams and lotions; food emulsifier for veg. and dairy prods., cakes; gloss aid in chocolate, nondairy creamers; tan flake; insol. in water, min. oils; HLB 4.7; acid no. 10 max.; sapon. no. 147-157; hyd. no. 235-260; flash pt. (PMCC) > 350 F.

S-Maz® 60KHM. [PPG/Specialty Chem.] Sorbitan stearate; CAS 1338-41-6; EINECS 215-664-9; nonionic; lubricant, antistat, textile softener, process defoamer, opacifier, coemulsifier, solubilizer, dispersant, suspending agent, coupler; prepares exc. w/o emulsions; kosher high melt grade; Gardner 3 flake; insol. in water, min. oils; HLB 4.7;

acid no. 10 max.; sapon. no. 147-157; hyd. no. 235-260; flash pt. (PMCC) > 350 F.

S-Maz® 65K. [PPG/Specialty Chem.] Sorbitan tristearate; CAS 26658-19-5; EINECS 247-891-4; nonionic; lubricant, antistat, textile softener, process defoamer, opacifier, coemulsifier, solubilizer, dispersant, suspending agent, coupler; prepares exc. w/o emulsions; Gardner 3 flake; sol. in min. spirits, toluene; disp. in min. and veg. oils; HLB 2.2; acid no. 15 max.; sapon. no. 176-188; hyd. no. 66-80; flash pt. (PMCC) > 350 F; 100% conc.

S-Maz® 80. [PPG/Specialty Chem.] Sorbitan oleate; CAS 1338-43-8; EINECS 215-665-4; nonionic; lubricant, antistat, textile softener, process defoamer, opacifier, coemulsifier, solubilizer, dispersant, suspending agent, coupler; prepares exc. w/o emulsions; binder in eye shadow, pressed powd. makeup; emulsifier for cleansing and night creams; lubricant, rust inhibitor, penetrant in metalworking formulations; amber liq.; sol. in ethanol, naphtha, min. oils, min. spirits, toluene, veg. oil; disp. in water; sp.gr. 1.0; visc. 1000 cps; HLB 4.6; acid no. 7.5 max.; sapon. no. 149–160; hyd. no. 193-209; flash pt. (PMCC) > 350 F; 100% conc.

S-Maz® 80K. [PPG/Specialty Chem.] Sorbitan oleate; CAS 1338-43-8; EINECS 215-665-4; nonionic; lubricant, antistat, textile softener, process defoamer, opacifier, coemulsifier, solubilizer, dispersant, suspending agent, coupler; prepares exc. w/o emulsions; kosher grade; Gardner 6 liq.; sol. in min. oils, min. spirits, toluene, veg. oil; insol. in water; HLB 4.6; acid no. 8 max.; sapon. no. 149-160; hyd. no. 193-209; flash pt. (PMCC) > 350 F.

S-Maz® 83R. [PPG/Specialty Chem.] Sorbitan sesquioleate; CAS 8007-43-0; EINECS 232-360-1; nonionic; solubilizer, emulsifier and dispersant; Gardner 5 liq.; sol. in oils and solvs.; HLB 4.6; acid no. 12 max.; sapon. no. 145-160; hyd. no. 185-215; flash pt. (PMCC) > 350 F; 100% conc.

S-Maz® 85. [PPG/Specialty Chem.] Sorbitan trioleate; CAS 26266-58-0; EINECS 247-569-3; nonionic; lubricant, antistat, textile softener, process defoamer, opacifier, coemulsifier, solubilizer, dispersant, suspending agent, coupler; prepares exc. w/o emulsions; binder in eye shadow, pressed powd. makeup; emulsifier for cleansing and night creams; lubricant, rust inhibitor, penetrant in metalworking formulations; amber liq.; sol. in toluol, naphtha, min. and veg. oils; water-disp.; sp.gr. 1.0; visc. 200 cps; HLB 2.1; acid no. 14 max.; sapon. no. 172–186; hyd. no. 56-68; flash pt. (PMCC) > 350 F; 100% conc.

S-Maz® 85K. [PPG/Specialty Chem.] Sorbitan trioleate; CAS 26266-58-0; EINECS 247-569-3; nonionic; lubricant, antistat, textile softener, process defoamer, opacifier, coemulsifier, solubilizer, dispersant, suspending agent, coupler; prepares exc. w/o emulsions;kosher grade; Gardner 6 liq.; sol. in min. oils, min. spirits, toluene, veg. oil; insol. in water; HLB 2.1; acid no. 14 max.; sapon. no. 172-186; hyd. no. 56-68; flash pt. (PMCC) > 350 F.

S-Maz® 90. [PPG/Specialty Chem.] Sorbitan tallate; nonionic; lubricant, antistat, textile softener, process defoamer, opacifier, coemulsifier, solubilizer, dispersant, suspending agent, coupler; prepares exc. w/o emulsions; also as lubricant, rust inhibitor, penetrant in metalworking formulations; amber liq.; sol. in min. and veg. oils; water-disp.; sp.gr. 1.0; visc. 800 cps; HLB 4.3; acid no. 10 max.; sapon. no. 145–160; hyd. no. 180-210; flash pt. (PMCC) > 350 F; 100% conc.

S-Maz® 95. [PPG/Specialty Chem.] Sorbitan tritallate; nonionic; antistat, textile softener, lubricant, process defoamer, opacifier, coemulsifier; prepares w/o emulsions; together with T-Maz series, as o/w emulsifier in metalworking fluids and coolants, semi-syn. and oil-based metalworking lubricants; and coolants, cosmetics, food formulations, industrial oils, and household prods.; amber liq.; sol. in toluol, naphtha, min. oil, veg. oil; misc. with ethanol, acetone; disp. in water; sp.gr. 0.9; visc. 200 cps; HLB 1.9; acid no. 15 max.; sapon. no. 168–186; hyd. no. 55-85; flash pt. (PMCC) 350 F.

Snow Fine. [Allied-Signal] Sodium sesquicarbonate; CAS 533-96-0; EINECS 208-580-9; used for creams and lotions.

Snow Flake. [Allied-Signal] Sodium sesquicarbonate; CAS 533-96-0; EINECS 208-580-9; used for creams and lotions.

Snow White Petrolatum. [Stevenson Bros.] Petrolatum; EINECS 232-373-2; emollient, ointment base.

Soapearl®. [Mearl] Pearlescent pigments for incorporation into extruded soap bars where they exhibit luxurious color effects.

Sobalg FD 100 Series. [Grindsted Prods.] Sodium alginate; food stabilizer, gellant, film-former for dairy prods., desserts, beverages, fruits and vegetables; also for cosmetics/toiletries; FDA, EEC compliance.

Sobalg FD 200 Series. [Grindsted Prods.] Potassium alginate; CAS 9005-36-1; gellant for foods and cosmetics; FDA, EEC compliance.

Sobalg FD 300 Series. [Grindsted Prods.] Ammonium alginate; CAS 9005-34-9; gellant for foods and cosmetics; FDA, EEC compliance.

Sobalg FD 460. [Grindsted Prods.] Calcium alginate; CAS 9005-35-0; gellant for foods and cosmetics; FDA, EEC compliance.

Sochamine A 755. [Witco/H-I-P] Monocarboxylate coconut deriv., sodium salt; amphoteric; detergent, wetting agent; base for shampoos; liq.; 40% conc.

Sochamine A 7525. [Witco/H-I-P] Disodium cocoamphodiacetate; CAS 68650-39-5; EINECS 272-043-5; amphoteric; detergent, wetting agent, base for nonirritating shampoos; liq.; 40% act.

Sochamine A 7527. [Witco/H-I-P] Sodium cocoamphopropionate; amphoteric; detergent; wetting agent; base for shampoos; liq.; 40% act.

Sochamine A 8955. [Witco/H-I-P] Disodium caproamphodiacetate; CAS 7702-01-4; EINECS 231-721-0; amphoteric; low foaming and wetting agent in alkaline formulations; for personal care applics.; liq.; 38% conc.

Sodium Ascorbate USP, FCC Fine Powd. No. 6047708. [Roche] Sodium ascorbate USP, FCC; CAS 134-03-2; EINECS 205-126-1; cosmetic ingred.

Sodium Citrate USP, FCC (Dihydrate) Fine Gran. No. 69975. [Roche] Sodium citrate; CAS 68-04-2; EINECS 200-675-3; pH adjustor for cosmetic prods.; buffering agent.

Sodium Hyaluronate RCC-1 No. 26228. [Roche] Sodium hyaluronate; CAS 9067-32-7; provides exc. water retention props. in hair, skin, and lipstick prods.

Sodium Omadine®, 40% Aq. Sol'n. [Olin] Sodium 2-pyridinethione in water; CAS 3811-73-2; EINECS 223-296-5; industrial microbiostat, preservative; chelating agent; used in cosmetics, aq. metal coolant and cutting fluids, vinyl acetate latex emulsions, inks, fiber lubricants, laundry rinse aids; amber liq.; mild odor; m.w. 149.2 (solid); sol. 53% in neut. water; 19% in 40A ethanol; 17% in dimethylsulfoxide; 13% in propylene glycol; sp.gr. 1.22; dens. 10.2 lb/gal; m.p. 250 C (dec.); pH 8.3 (10% in water); 40% min. act.

Sodium Stéarate C7L. [Witco/H-I-P] Sodium stearate; CAS 822-16-2; EINECS 212-490-5; gelling agent for cosmetics.

Softigen® 701. [Hüls Am./ Hüls AG] Glyceryl ricinoleate; CAS 141-08-2; EINECS 205-455-0; nonionic; emollient; refatting and skin protecting agent; emulsifier; for personal care prods. (skin protection cream, cleansers, sunscreens, bath and shaving preps., soaps) and pharmaceuticals (creams, suppositories); good adhesion to mucosae; ylsh.-wh. paste/clear oily liq. @ 30-35 C, char. odor; sol. in ether, benzene, toluene, xylene, chloroform, and dichlorethylene; misc. with fats, oils; sp.gr. 0.979-0.981; visc. 550-610 mPa·s (30 C); HLB 4.5; acid no. 3 max.; iodine no. 70-80; sapon. no. 155-170; usage level: 5-10%; 100% conc.

Softigen® 767. [Hüls Am.; Hüls AG] PEG-6 caprylic/capric glycerides; CAS 52504-24-2; nonionic; superfatting base wetting agent, perfume solubilizer, emollient used in cosmetics (shave preps., bath preps, hair fixative), pharmaceuticals, liq. soaps; ylsh. visc. oily liq., char. odor; sol. in water @ 1.3%; sol. in acetone, ethyl and butyl acetate, castor oil, IPA; dens. 1.080 g/ml; visc. 160 mPa·s; HLB 19; acid no. 1 max.; iodine no. 1 max.; sapon. no. 90-110; surf. tens. 29.7 dynes/cm (1%); toxicology: LD50 (oral, rat) > 5 g/kg (pract. nontoxic); nonirritating to skin and eyes; 100% act.

Softisan® 100. [Hüls Am.; Hüls AG] Hydrog. coco-glycerides; CAS 977056-87-3; nonionic; consistency regulator, emollient, ointment base for cosmetic creams, ointments, and sticks, makeup, lip gloss, and pharmaceutical industry; cocoa butter substitute; wh. pastilles; neutral odor and taste; sol. in benzene, ether, xylene, toluene, chloroform, CCl₄, dioxane; sp.gr. 0.950-0.980; visc. 30 cps (40 C); m.p. 33-36 C; solid. pt. 29-33 C; acid no. 0.2 max.; iodine no. 3 max.; sapon. no. 230-250; hyd. no. 15 max.; ref. index 1.4490-1.4510 (40 C).

Softisan® 133. [Hüls Am.; Hüls AG] Hydrog. coco-glycerides; CAS 977056-87-3; hard wax used in cosmetic and pharmaceutical preparations (creams, ointments, sticks, makeup, lip gloss); wh. pastilles; neutral odor and taste; sol. in benzene, toluene, acetone, chloroform, petrol. spirit; insol. in water; m.p. 32-34 C; solid. pt. 29-32 C; acid no. 0.2 max.; iodine no. 3 max.; sapon. no. 235-255; hyd. no. 15 max.; ref. index 1.445-1.449 (50 C).

Softisan® 134. [Hüls Am.; Hüls AG] Hydrog. coco-glycerides; CAS 977056-87-3; fat component and consistency regulator in cosmetic/pharmaceutical creams, ointments, sticks, makeup, lip gloss; wh. pastilles; neutral odor and taste; sol. in benzene, toluene, acetone, chloroform, petrol. spirit; insol. in water; m.p. 33-36 C; solid. pt. 27-32 C; acid no. 0.3 max.; iodine no. 3 max.; sapon. no. 220-235; hyd. no. 40-50; ref. index 1.445-1.449 (50 C).

Softisan® 138. [Hüls Am.; Hüls AG] Hydrog. coco-glycerides; CAS 977056-87-3; fat component and consistency regulator in cosmetic/pharmaceutical creams, ointments, sticks, makeup, lip gloss; wh. blocks; neutral odor and taste; sol. in benzene, toluene, acetone, chloroform, petrol. spirit; insol. in water; m.p. 37-40 C; solid. pt. 32-36 C; acid no. 1.5 max.; iodine no. 3 max.; sapon. no. 215-235; hyd. no. 15 max.; ref. index 1.445-1.449 (50 C).

Softisan® 142. [Hüls Am.; Hüls AG] Hydrog. coco-glycerides; CAS 977056-87-3; fat component and consistency regulator in cosmetic/pharmaceutical creams, ointments, sticks, makeup, lip gloss; wh. pastilles; neutral odor and taste; sol. in benzene, toluene, acetone, chloroform, petrol. spirit; insol. in water; m.p. 42-44 C; solid. pt. 37-42 C; acid no. 0.3 max.; iodine no. 3 max.; sapon. no. 215-235; hyd. no. 15 max.; ref. index 1.445-1.449 (50 C).

Softisan® 154. [Hüls Am.; Hüls AG] Hydrog. palm oil; fat component and consistency regulator in cosmetic/pharmaceutical creams, ointments, sticks, makeup, lip gloss; wh. flakes; neutral odor and taste; sol. in benzene, toluene, acetone, chloroform, petrol. spirit; insol. in water; m.p. 55-60 C; solid. pt. 48-53 C; acid no. 1 max.; iodine no. 3 max.; sapon. no. 195-210; hyd. no. 10 max.; ref. index 1.445-1.460 (50 C).

Softisan® 378. [Hüls Am.] Caprylic/capric/stearic triglyceride; nonionic; absorption-promoting fat base for cosmetic/

pharmaceutical creams and ointments, emollient, moisturizer, stabilizer; good skin compatibility and resorption chars. for the prep. of nonaq. ointments and creams; off-wh. to ylsh. pasty wax; m.p. 37-40 C; acid no. 1 max.; iodine no. 1 max.; sapon no. 245-260; hyd. no. 20 max.; 100% act.

Softisan® 601. [Hüls Am.; Hüls AG] Glyceryl cocoate, hydrog. coconut oil, and ceteareth-25; nonionic; emollient; cosmetic and pharmaceutical self-emulsifying base for o/w or anhyd. prods.; water absorption to 65%; wh.-ylsh. pellets; sp.gr. 0.97 (60 C); m.p. 40-45 C; acid no. 1 max.; iodine no. 5 max.; sapon. no. 120-140; hyd. no. 230-270; 100% conc.

Softisan® 645. [Hüls Am.; Hüls AG] Bis-diglyceryl caprylate/caprate/isostearate/hydroxystearate adipate; adhesion-promoting oil for creams, lotions, and decorative cosmetics; high water-binding capacity, good heat stability; lanolin oil substitute; ylsh. liq.; acid no. 3 max.; iodine no. 5 max.; sapon. no. 260-285; hyd. no. 60-100.

Softisan® 649. [Hüls Am.; Hüls AG] Bis diglyceryl caprylate/caprate/isostearate/stearate/hydroxystearate adipate; emollient, ointment base for creams, lipsticks, other decorative cosmetics, pharmaceuticals; lanolin substitute; good adhesion to skin, high waterbinding power; ylsh. paste; almost odorless; sol. in ether, chloroform; misc. with fats, oils; acid no. 2 max.; iodine no. 3 max.; sapon. no. 270-290; hyd. no. 60-80.

Softisan® Gel. [Hüls Am.] Bis diglyceryl caprylate/caprate/isostearate/hydroxystearate adipate, propylene glycol dicaprylate/dicaprate, stearalkonium hectorite, propylene carbonate; consistency regulator for creams; high temp. stabilizer for w/o emulsions and anhyd. skin care and decorative formulations; flesh-colored hard paste; acid no. 1 max.; iodine no. 3 max.; sapon. no. 250-280.

Sohakuhi Extract BG-100. [Ikeda] Mulberry root extract, 1,3-Butyleneglycol; whitening agent for skin care prods.; anti-inflammatory and moisturizing agent; ylsh. brn. transparent color, faint char. odor; sp.gr. 1.000-1.030; pH 4.3-5.3.

Sohakuhi Extract Ethanol. [Ikeda] Mulberry root extract, Ethanol; whitening agent for skin care prods.; anti-inflammatory and moisturizing agent; lt. ylsh. brn. transparent color, faint char. odor; sp.gr. 0.940-0.960; pH 4.0-5.0.

Solan. [Croda Inc.] PEG-60 lanolin; CAS 61790-81-6; nonionic; surfactant, emollient, conditioner, superfatting agent, emulsifier, solubilizer, foam stabilizer, plasticizer, humectant for soaps, detergent bars, shampoos, skin cleansers, hair sprays, deodorants, chemical specialties, pharmaceuticals; yel. wax; sol. in water, propylene glycol; sol. warm in IPA; m.p. 46-54 C; acid no. 2 max.; iodine no. 10 max.; sapon. no. 8-16; pH 5.5-7.0 (1% aq.); usage level: 1-10%; toxicology: LD50 (oral, rat) > 5 g/kg; nonirritating to skin; 100% act.

Solan 50. [Croda Inc.] PEG-60 lanolin; CAS 61790-81-6; nonionic; hydrophilic surfactant, emollient, conditioner, thickener, superfatting agent, foam stabilizer, plasticizer, humectant for personal care prods., soaps, pharmaceuticals, chemical specialties; fragrance solubilizer; Gardner 11 max. visc. liq.; water-sol.; acid no. 2 max.; iodine no. 6 max.; sapon. no. 8 max.; pH 5.5-7.0 (1% aq.); usage level: 1-10%; 50% act.

Solan E. [Croda Inc.; Croda Chem. Ltd.] PEG-55 lanolin; CAS 61790-81-6; nonionic; emollient and emulsifier; solid; water-sol.; HLB 16.2; 100% conc.

Solarchem® O. [CasChem] Octyl dimethyl PABA; CAS 21245-02-3; EINECS 244-289-3; selective uv absorber for suncare and cosmetic prods.; clear liq.; odorless; sp.gr. 0.99-1.00; acid no. 1 max.; sapon. no. 195-215; ref. index 1.5390-1.5430; 99% min. purity.

Solarium HS 268, LS 668. [Alban Muller] St. John's wort, myrrh, rathany, pot marigold phytocomplex; soothing solar prod.

Solarium HS 269. [Alban Muller] Hypericum extract, propylene glycol, calendula extract, and wheat germ extract; phytocomplex; soothing solar prod.

Solarium HS 270. [Alban Muller] Propylene glycol, myrrh extract, hypericum extract, and laurel extract; phytocomplex; soothing solar prod.

Solarium LS 669. [Alban Muller] Sunflower seed oil, hypericum extract, calendula extract, and wheat germ extract; phytocomplex; soothing solar prod.

Solarium LS 670. [Alban Muller] Sunflower seed oil, myrrh extract, hypericum extract, and laurel extract; phytocomplex; soothing solar prod.

Solarium Special HS 271, LS 671. [Alban Muller] Aloe, buckthorn, German chamomile, everlasting phytocomplex; soothing solar prod.

Solar Shield™. [U.S. Cosmetics] Ultrafine rutile titanium dioxide; CAS 13463-67-7; EINECS 236-675-5; transparent sunscreen agent imparting minimal skin whitening; particle size 0.02-0.05 µ.

Sole Terge 8. [Calgene] Disodium oleamido MIPA-sulfosuccinate; CAS 43154-85-4; EINECS 256-120-0; high foaming base for bubble baths, shampoos, etc.; frother in specialized ore flotation; emulsifier and stabilizer in emulsion polymerization; stable at all concs. at pH 4-7; amber liq.; sol. in water, ethanol, glycols, acetone; sp.gr. 1.09-1.12; dens. 9.1 lb/gal; pH 6-7 (1% aq.); surf. tens. 35 dynes/cm (0.1%); toxicology: mild eye irritant; 32-35% act.

Solka-Floc® BW-40. [James River] Cellulose NF; CAS 9004-34-6; EINECS 232-674-9; binder, diluent, disintegrant, stabilizer, absorption aid, stabilizer, tablet filler for pharmaceutical formulations; moisture absorp. and retention props.; avg. particle size 60 µ; 82-95% thru 100 mesh; dens. (tapped) 0.35 g/ml; pH 5.0-7.5.

Solka-Floc® BW-100. [James River] Cellulose NF; CAS 9004-34-6; EINECS 232-674-9; binder, diluent, disintegrant, stabilizer, absorption aid, stabilizer, tablet filler for pharmaceutical formulations; recommended for direct compression and wet granulations; avg. particle size 40 µ; 95% min. thru 60 mesh; dens. (tapped) 0.46 g/ml; pH 5.0-7.5.

Solka-Floc® BW-200. [James River] Cellulose NF; CAS 9004-34-6; EINECS 232-674-9; binder, diluent, disintegrant, stabilizer, absorption aid, tablet filler for pharmaceutical formulations; avg. particle size 35 µ; 98% min. thru 60 mesh; dens. (tapped) 0.46 g/ml; pH 5.0-7.5.

Solka-Floc® BW-2030. [James River] Cellulose NF; CAS 9004-34-6; EINECS 232-674-9; binder, diluent, disintegrant, stabilizer, absorption aid, tablet filler for pharmaceutical formulations; avg. particle size 35 µ; 80% min. thru 100 mesh; dens. (tapped) 0.45 g/ml; pH 5.0-7.5.

Solka-Floc® Fine Granular. [Mendell] Cellulose NF; CAS 9004-34-6; EINECS 232-674-9; binder, diluent, disintegrant, stabilizer, absorption aid, tablet filler for pharmaceutical formulations; exc. flow and improved compressibility; 15% max. thru 200 mesh; dens. (tapped) 0.68 g/ml; pH 5.0-7.5.

Sollagen® EC. [Hormel] Soluble collagen; CAS 9007-34-5; EINECS 232-697-4; strong moisture-binding props.; provides elegant silky feel in skin care prods.; clear sl. visc. liq.; m.w. 300,000.

Sollagen® LA. [Hormel] Soluble collagen; CAS 9007-34-5; EINECS 232-697-4; natural humectant for cosmetic applics. incl. skin care and body lotions, and hair care prods.; elegant silky feel; translucent sl. visc. liq.; m.w. 300,000.

Soloron-R-Gold. [Rona] Mica, titanium dioxide, tin oxide; pearlescent for pressed powds., eye makeup, frosted pearl effects in cosmetics.

Soloron Silver. [Rona] Mica, titanium dioxide, tin oxide; pearlescent pigment for cosmetics and toiletries.

Soloron Silver CO. [Rona] Castor oil, mica, titanium dioxide, tin oxide; pearlescent pigment for cosmetics and toiletries.

Soloron Silver Fine. [Rona] Mica, titanium dioxide, tin oxide; pearlescent pigment for cosmetics and toiletries.

Soloron Silver Fine CO. [Rona] Castor oil, mica, titanium dioxide, tin oxide; pearlescent pigment for cosmetics and toiletries.

Soloron Silver Sparkle. [Rona] Mica, titanium dioxide, tin oxide; pearlescent pigment for cosmetics and toiletries.

Soloron Silver Sparkle CO. [Rona] Castor oil, mica, titanium dioxide, tin oxide, carnauba; pearlescent pigment for cosmetics and toiletries.

Solubilisant γ 2420. [Gattefosse] Octoxynol-11, polysorbate 20; nonionic; surfactant blend.

Solubilisant γ 2428. [Gattefosse] PEG-40 hydrog. castor oil, polysorbate 20, octoxynol-11; nonionic; surfactant blend.

Solubiliser LRI. [Les Colorants Wackherr] PPG-26-buteth-26 and PEG-40 hydrog. castor oil; cosmetics solubilizer.

Solubilizer L-76. [Lipo] Trideceth-12, laureth-12; cosmetics solubilizer.

Soluble Native Collagen RA-1 No. 26206. [Roche] Soluble collagen; CAS 9007-34-5; EINECS 232-697-4; provides increased water absorption and improved elasticity of skin in cosmetics.

Soluble Native Collagen RS-1 No. 26205. [Roche] Soluble collagen; CAS 9007-34-5; EINECS 232-697-4; provides improved moisture retention props. and elasticity of skin.

Solu-Coll™. [Brooks Industries] Soluble collagen; CAS 9007-34-5; EINECS 232-697-4; protein providing skin elasticity and moisturizing props. to skin care cosmetics; hazy visc. liq., lt. bland odor; m.w. 300,000; pH 3.2-5.0; 1.0-2.0% NV.

Solu-Coll™ C, CLR. [Brooks Industries] Soluble collagen; CAS 9007-34-5; EINECS 232-697-4; cosmetic protein.

Solu-Coll™ D. [Brooks Industries] Desamido collagen; protein providing skin elasticity and moisturizing props. to skin care cosmetics; hazy visc. liq., sl. bland odor; pH 3.5-5.0; 2.1-2.5% NV.

Solu-Coll™ P. [Brooks Industries] Procollagen; protein providing skin elasticity and moisturizing props. to skin care cosmetics; opalescent liq., almost odorless; m.w. 360,000; pH 3.5-4.0; 1-2% NV.

Solu-Coll™ Complex. [Brooks Industries] Soluble collagen, collagen amino acids; cosmetic ingred.

Solu-Coll™ Complex VY. [Brooks Industries] Soluble collagen; CAS 9007-34-5; EINECS 232-697-4; cosmetic protein.

Solu-Coll™ Native. [Brooks Industries] Soluble animal collagen; CAS 9007-34-5; EINECS 232-697-4; protein providing skin elasticity and moisturizing effect in skin cosmetics formulations; clear to hazy liq., l.amost odorless; pH 3.5-4.0; 1.8-2.3% NV.

Solu Kera-Tein M. [Maybrook] Sol. keratin; cosmetics ingred.

Solulan® 5. [Amerchol; Amerchol Europe] Laneth-5, ceteth-5, oleth-5 and steareth-5; nonionic; emulsifier, wetting agent, dispersant, lubricant, solv., conditioner, plasticizer, emollient used in personal care and dermatology prods.; foam stabilizer for detergent systems; amber semisolid; faint pleasant odor; sol. @ 5% in anhyd. ethanol; disp. in water; HLB 8.0; acid no. 3 max.; sapon. no. 14 max.; pH 4.5-7.0 (10% aq.); 100% conc.

Solulan® 16. [Amerchol; Amerchol Europe] Laneth-16, ceteth-16, oleth-16 and steareth-16; nonionic; emulsifier, wetting agent, dispersant, lubricant, solv., conditioner, plasticizer, emollient used in personal care and dermatology prods.; foam stabilizer for detergent systems; lt. tan waxy solid; sol. @ 5% in water, 30% ethanol; HLB 15; cloud pt. 64–70 C; acid no. 3 max.; sapon. no. 8 max.; pH 4.5–7.5 (10% aq.); 100% conc.

Solulan® 25. [Amerchol; Amerchol Europe] Laneth-25, ceteth-25, oleth-25 and steareth-25; nonionic; o/w emulsifier, dispersant, lubricant, solubilizer for cosmetics and pharmaceuticals; yel. waxy solid; faint pleasant odor; sol. see Solulan 16; HLB 16; cloud pt. 85–92 C; acid no. 3 max.; sapon. no. 8 max.; pH 4.5–7.5 (10% aq.); 100% conc.

Solulan® 75. [Amerchol; Amerchol Europe] PEG-75 lanolin; CAS 61790-81-6; nonionic; emulsifier, wetting agent, dispersant, lubricant, solv., conditioner, plasticizer, emollient used in personal care and dermatology prods.; foam stabilizer for detergent systems; lt. yel.-amber waxy solid; faint pleasant odor; sol. see Solulan 16; HLB 15; cloud pt. 80–87 C; acid no. 3 max.; sapon. no. 10–20; pH 4.5–7.5 (10% aq.); 100% conc.

Solulan® 97. [Amerchol; Amerchol Europe] Polysorbate 80 acetate, cetyl acetate and acetylated lanolin alcohol; nonionic; dispersant, lubricant, emollient, conditioner for cosmetics and pharmaceuticals; lt. amber visc. liq.; faint pleasant odor; sol. @ 5% in water, ethanol; HLB 15; acid no. 3 max.; sapon. no. 110–130; pH 4.5–7.5 (10% aq.); 100% conc.

Solulan® 98. [Amerchol; Amerchol Europe] Polysorbate 80, cetyl acetate, acetylated lanolin alcohol; nonionic; dispersant, lubricant, emollient, conditioner for cosmetics and pharmaceuticals; also aids pearling of stearic acid emulsions; lt. amber visc. liq.; faint pleasant odor; sol. @ 5% in water, ethanol; HLB 13; acid no. 3 max.; sapon. no. 65–75; pH 4.5–7.5 (10% aq.); 100% conc.

Solulan® C-24. [Amerchol; Amerchol Europe] Choleth-24 and ceteth-24; nonionic; emulsifier, wetting agent, dispersant, lubricant, solv., conditioner, plasticizer, emollient used in personal care and dermatology prods.; foam stabilizer for detergent systems; off-wh. to pale yel. waxy solid; faint pleasant odor; sol. @ 5% in water; HLB 14; cloud pt. 88–95 C; acid no. 1; sapon. no. 3 max.; 100% conc.

Solulan® L-575. [Amerchol; Amerchol Europe] PEG-75 lanolin; CAS 61790-81-6; nonionic; emulsifier, wetting agent, dispersant, lubricant, solv., conditioner, plasticizer, emollient used in personal care and dermatology prods.; foam stabilizer for detergent systems; lt. yel.-amber visc. liq.; faint pleasant odor; sol. @ 5% in water, 30% ethanol; HLB 15; cloud pt. 80–87 C; acid no. 1 max.; sapon. no. 10 max.; 50% conc.

Solulan® PB-2. [Amerchol; Amerchol Europe] PPG-2 lanolin alcohol ether; CAS 68439-53-2; nonionic; spreading agent, dispersant, plasticizer; emollient and conditioner for personal care prods., detergents, pharmaceuticals, waxes, polishes, leather treatment; amber semisolid, liq.; sol. in castor oil, IPM, IPP, anhyd. ethanol; HLB 8.0; acid no. 3 max.; sapon. no. 7 max.; 100% conc.

Solulan® PB-5. [Amerchol; Amerchol Europe] PPG-5 lanolin alcohol ether; CAS 68439-53-2; nonionic; spreading agent, dispersant, plasticizer; emollient and conditioner for personal care prods., detergents, pharmaceuticals, waxes, polishes, leather treatment; lt. amber clear visc. liq.; sol. see Solulan PB-2; HLB 10.0; acid no. 2 max.; sapon. no. 6 max.; 100% conc.

Solulan® PB-10. [Amerchol; Amerchol Europe] PPG-10 lanolin alcohol ether; CAS 68439-53-2; nonionic; spreading agent, dispersant, plasticizer; emollient and conditioner for personal care prods., detergents, pharmaceuticals, waxes, polishes, leather treatment; straw clear heavy-visc. liq.; sol. see Solulan PB-2; HLB 12.0; acid no. 1 max.; sapon. no. 4 max.; 100% conc.

Solulan® PB-20. [Amerchol; Amerchol Europe] PPG-20 lanolin alcohol ether; CAS 68439-53-2; nonionic; spreading agent, dispersant, plasticizer; emollient and conditioner for personal care prods., detergents, pharmaceuticals, waxes, polishes, leather treatment; lt. straw clear med-visc. liq.; sol. see Solulan PB-2; HLB 14.0; acid no. 0.75 max.; sapon. no. 3 max.; 100% conc.

Solu-Lastin™ 10. [Brooks Industries] Hydrolyzed animal elastin.; CAS 100085-10-7; structural protein giving flexibility and elasticity to tissues; for cosmetics use; low odor; m.w. 4000; 10% act.

Solu-Lastin™ 30. [Brooks Industries] Hydrolyzed elastin; CAS 100085-10-7; structural protein giving flexibility and elasticity to the tissues; for cosmetics use; m.w. 4000; 30% act.

Solu-Mar™ EN-30. [Brooks Industries] Hydrolyzed marine protein; film-former and moisturizer for skin and hair cosmetics; substantive protein; yel. liq., low odor; m.w. > 2000; 30% act.

Solu-Mar™ Native. [Brooks Industries] Soluble marine protein; film-former and moisturizer for skin cosmetics; visc. sol'n., low odor; m.w. 300,000+; 1% act.

Solumin F Range. [Rhone-Poulenc Surf. & Spec.] Ether sulfate; anionic; surfactant for aq. systems; liq.; 25% conc.

Soluphor® P. [BASF; BASF AG] Pyrrolidone-2; solv. for pharmaceutical injectables, veterinary medicine.

Solu-Silk™ 25. [Brooks Industries] Silk amino acids; CAS 977077-71-6; cosmetics ingred.; liq.; m.w. 1000; 30% act., 15% protein.

Solu-Silk™ SF. [Brooks Industries] Silk amino acids; CAS 977077-71-6; protein for cosmetics formulations; low salt; m.w. 100; 15% act.

Solu-Silk™ Protein. [Brooks Industries] Hydrolyzed silk; CAS 96690-41-4; protein; liq.; m.w. 1000; 10% act.

Solusol® 75%. [Am. Cyanamid] Dioctyl sodium sulfosuccinate; CAS 577-11-7; EINECS 209-406-4; anionic; emulsifier, wetting agent for cosmetic formulations; liq.; sp.gr. 1.09; 75% act.

Solusol® 85%. [Am. Cyanamid] Dioctyl sodium sulfosuccinate, sodium benzoate; anionic; emulsifier, wetting agent for cosmetic formulations; wh. solid; sp.gr. 1.1; m.p. < 300 C; 85% act.

Solusol® 100%. [Am. Cyanamid] Dioctyl sodium sulfosuccinate; CAS 577-11-7; EINECS 209-406-4; anionic; emulsifier, wetting agent for cosmetic formulations; wh. solid; sp.gr. 1.1; m.p. 153–157 C; surf. tens. 28.7 dynes/cm (0.1%); 100% act.

Solu-Soy™ EN-25. [Brooks Industries] Hydrolyzed soy protein; CAS 68607-88-5; cosmetic ingred. for skin and hair care prods.; low salt; m.w. 1000; 25% act.

Sol-U-Tein 6861. [Fanning] Hydrolyzed soy protein; CAS 68607-88-5; skin/hair conditioner for permanent waves, rinses, shampoos, tonics, dressings, cleansers, face, body and hand creams and lotions, moisturizing creams; off-wh. to lt. cream powd.; sol. in hot or cold water under acid, alkaline, or neutral conditions; pH 4.5-5.0; 83% total protein.

Sol-U-Tein EA. [Fanning] Albumen; CAS 977000-98-8; binder, coagulant, film-former, skin conditioning agent; used in pharmaceuticals and personal care prods.; dye mordant in textiles, adhesives, veneers, sizing and making papers; gilding leather; book binding; food applic.; yel. powd.; 100% thru 80 mesh; 90% thru 100 mesh; bland odor; pH 6.5–8.0; 75% ovalbumin, ovoconalbumin, ovomucoid, ovomucin, ovoglobulin, lysozyme, and avidin.

Sol-U-Tein FS-1000. [Fanning] Hydrolyzed soy protein; CAS 68607-88-5; skin/hair conditioner for permanent waves, rinses, shampoos, tonics, dressings, cleansers, face, body and hand creams/lotions, moisturizing creams; lt.

cream powd.; pH 4.0-6.0 (5%).

Sol-U-Tein PS-1000. [Fanning] Hydrolyzed soy protein; CAS 68607-88-5; skin/hair conditioner for permanent waves, rinses, shampoos, tonics, dressings, cleansers, face, body and hand creams/lotions, moisturizing creams; lt. cream powd.; pH 4.5-5.5 (5%).

Sol-U-Tein VG. [Fanning] Hydrolyzed soy protein; CAS 68607-88-5; skin/hair conditioner for permanent waves, rinses, shampoos, tonics, dressings, cleansers, face, body and hand creams/lotions, moisturizing creams; off-wh.; sol. in water; pH 4.0-5.5 (5%); 74% min. total protein.

Solu-Tofu EN-10. [Brooks Industries] Hydrolyzed soy protein; CAS 68607-88-5; cosmetic protein.

Solutol® HS 15. [BASF AG] PEG-660 hydroxystearate; nonionic; solv. for injection sol'ns.

Solu-Veg™ EN-35. [Brooks Industries] Hydrolyzed vegetable protein; CAS 100209-45-8; cosmetic ingred. for skin and hair care prods.; low salt; m.w. 2000; 35% act.

Solu-Veg™ Complex #4. [Brooks Industries] Hydrolyzed soy protein, hydrolyzed wheat protein, hydrolyzed keratin; cosmetic ingred.

Soluvit Richter. [Dr. Kurt Richter; Henkel/Cospha] Water, alcohol, PEG-35 castor oil, polysorbate 20, horse chestnut extract, retinyl palmitate, tocopherol, PABA, inositol, calcium pantothenate, linoleic acid, and biotin; mutlivitamin herbal complex, hydro-alcohol solubilized; broad spectrum vitamin treatment for skin and hair protection; reddish-yel. to red liq.

Solvent 111. [Vulcan Materials] Trichloroethane; CAS 71-55-6; EINECS 200-756-3.

Solvent APV Spec. [Hüls AG] Ethoxydiglycol; CAS 111-90-0; EINECS 203-919-7; high boiling solv. for fragrance materials, essential oils, terpene oils for cosmetics use; colorless liq.; dens. 0.986-0.990 kg/l; b.p. 198-203 C; acid no. ≤0.05; hyd. no. 420-490.

Solvent PM. [BASF AG] 1- Methoxypropan-2-ol; solv. for cosmetic industry.

Somepon T25. [Seppic] Sodium methyl cocoyl taurate; surfactant for cosmetics; paste; 25% act.

Sono Jell® No. 4. [Witco/Petroleum Spec.] Petrolatum; EINECS 232-373-2; emollient base for cleansing creams, cosmetics, pharmaceuticals; Lovibond 0.5Y color; visc. 2.6-5.7 cSt (100 C); m.p. 38-52 C.

Sono Jell® No. 9. [Witco/Petroleum Spec.] Petrolatum; EINECS 232-373-2; emollient base for cleansing creams, cosmetics, pharmaceuticals; Lovibond color 0.5Y; visc. 2.6-5.7 Cst (100 C); m.p. 42-49 C.

Soprol VR.50. [Rhone-Poulenc] PEG-200 glyceryl stearate; thickener.

Sorban AO. [Witco/H-I-P] Sorbitan oleate; CAS 1338-43-8; EINECS 215-665-4; nonionic; emulsifier for personal care applics.; liq.; HLB 4.5; 100% conc.

Sorban AST. [Witco/H-I-P] Sorbitan stearate; CAS 1338-41-6; EINECS 215-664-9; nonionic; emulsifier for oils and greases; antifoamer, corrosion inhibitor; cosmetic applics.; flakes; 100% conc.

Sorbanox AOM. [Witco/H-I-P] Ethoxylated sorbitan ester; CAS 9005-65-6; nonionic; emulsifier; solubilizer of vitamins; liq.; HLB 15.0; 100% conc.

Sorbanox AST. [Witco/H-I-P] Ethoxylated sorbitan ester; CAS 9005-67-8; nonionic; emulsifier for paraffin and min. oil; insecticides, cosmetic applics.; liq.; 100% conc.

Sorbanox CO. [Witco/H-I-P] Polysorbate 85; CAS 9005-70-3; nonionic; emulsifier for min. oil; for personal care applics.; liq.; HLB 11.0; 100% conc.

Sorbax PML-20. [Chemax] Polysorbate 20; CAS 9005-64-5; nonionic; o/w emulsifier, solubilizer for perfumes, flavors; for agric., cosmetic, leather, metalworking, and textile industries; liq.; water-sol.; sapon. no. 45; HLB 16.7; 100% conc.

Sorbax PMO-5. [Chemax] Polysorbate 81; CAS 9005-65-6; nonionic; o/w emulsifier, solubilizer for perfumes and flavors; emulsifier for petrol. oils, solvs., veg. oils, waxes, silicones in agric., cosmetic, leather, metalworking, and textile industries; liq.; water-sol.; sapon. no. 100; HLB 10.0; 100% conc.

Sorbax PMO-20. [Chemax] Polysorbate 80; CAS 9005-65-6; nonionic; o/w emulsifier, solubilizer for perfumes and flavors; emulsifier for petrol. oils, solvs., veg. oils, waxes, silicones in agric., cosmetic, leather, metalworking, and textile industries; liq.; water-sol.; sapon. no. 50; HLB 15.0; 100% conc.

Sorbax PMP-20. [Chemax] Polysorbate 40; CAS 9005-66-7; nonionic; o/w emulsifier, solubilizer for perfumes and flavors; emulsifier for petrol. oils, solvs., veg. oils, waxes, silicones in agric., cosmetic, leather, metalworking, and textile industries; liq.; water-sol.; sapon. no. 46; HLB 15.6; 100% conc.

Sorbax PMS-20. [Chemax] Polysorbate 60; CAS 9005-67-8; nonionic; o/w emulsifier, solubilizer for perfumes and flavors; emulsifier for petrol. oils, solvs., veg. oils, waxes, silicones in agric., cosmetic, leather, metalworking, and textile industries; soft paste; water-sol.; sapon. no. 50; HLB 14.9; 100% conc.

Sorbax PTO-20. [Chemax] Polysorbate 85; CAS 9005-70-3; nonionic; o/w emulsifier, solubilizer for perfumes and flavors; emulsifier for petrol. oils, solvs., veg. oils, waxes, silicones in agric., cosmetic, leather, metalworking, and textile industries; liq., gel; water-sol.; sapon. no. 88; HLB 11.0; 100% conc.

Sorbax PTS-20. [Chemax] Polysorbate 65; CAS 9005-71-4; nonionic; o/w emulsifier, solubilizer for perfumes and flavors; emulsifier for petrol. oils, solvs., veg. oils, waxes, silicones in agric., cosmetic, leather, metalworking, and textile industries; solid; water-sol.; sapon. no. 93; HLB 10.5; 100% conc.

Sorbax SML. [Chemax] Sorbitan laurate; CAS 1338-39-2; nonionic; emulsifier for petrol. oils, solvs., veg. oils, waxes, silicones in agric., cosmetic, leather, metalworking, and textile industries; liq.; oil-sol.; sapon. no. 162; HLB 8.6.

Sorbax SMO. [Chemax] Sorbitan oleate; CAS 1338-43-8; EINECS 215-665-4; nonionic; emulsifier, surfactant for o/w emulsion stabilizers and thickeners in cosmetic, agric., metalworking, leather, and textile industries; liq.; oil-sol.; sapon. no. 153; HLB 4.3; 100% conc.

Sorbax SMP. [Chemax] Sorbitan palmitate; CAS 26266-57-9; EINECS 247-568-8; nonionic; emulsifier, surfactant for o/w emulsion stabilizers and thickeners used in cosmetic, agric., leather, metalworking, and textile industries; solid; oil-sol.; sapon. no. 155; HLB 6.7; 100% conc.

Sorbax SMS. [Chemax] Sorbitan stearate; CAS 1338-41-6; EINECS 215-664-9; nonionic; emulsifier; surfactant for o/w emulsion stabilizers and thickeners used in cosmetic, agric., leather, metalworking, and textile industries; solid; oil-sol.; sapon. no. 152; HLB 4.7; 100% conc.

Sorbax STO. [Chemax] Sorbitan trioleate; CAS 26266-58-0; EINECS 247-569-3; nonionic; emulsifier, surfactant for o/w emulsion stabilizers and thickeners used in cosmetic, agric., metalworking, leather, and textile industries; liq.; oil-sol.; sapon. no. 180; HLB 1.8; 100% conc.

Sorbax STS. [Chemax] Sorbitan tristearate; CAS 26658-19-5; EINECS 247-891-4; nonionic; emulsifier, surfactant for o/w emulsion stabilizers and thickeners used in cosmetic, agric., leather, metalworking, and textile industries; solid; oil-sol.; sapon. no. 182; HLB 2.1; 100% conc.

Sorbelite™ C. [Mendell] Crystalline sorbitol NF; CAS 50-70-4; EINECS 200-061-5; provides sweetness and cooling mouthfeel to direct compression tablet mfg.; improved flowability, exc. cohesion; avg. particle size 403 μ; 5%

-100 mesh; dens. (tapped) 0.64 g/ml max.; 91-100.5% assay.

Sorbelite™ FG. [Mendell] Crystalline γ-sorbitol NF; CAS 50-70-4; EINECS 200-061-5; for direct compression of pharmaceutical tablets where added sweetness and cooling mouthfeel are desired; wh. fine gran.; avg. particle size 124 μ; 65% -100 mesh; dens. (tapped) 0.85 g/ml; 91-100.5% assay.

Sorbilene ISM. [Auschem SpA] PEG-20 sorbitan isostearate; CAS 66794-58-9; nonionic; emulsifier for cosmetics and pharmaceuticals; liq.; HLB 15.0; 100% conc.

Sorbilene L. [Auschem SpA] Polysorbate 20; CAS 9005-64-5; nonionic; emulsifier and solubilizer for cosmetics and pharmaceuticals; liq.; HLB 16.7; 100% conc.

Sorbilene L 4. [Auschem SpA] Polysorbate 21; CAS 9005-64-5; nonionic; emulsifier for cosmetics and pharmaceuticals; liq.; HLB 13.3; 100% conc.

Sorbilene LH. [Auschem SpA] Polysorbate 20, low dioxane; CAS 9005-64-5; nonionic; emulsifier for cosmetics and pharmaceuticals; liq.; HLB 16.7; 100% conc.

Sorbilene O. [Auschem SpA] Polysorbate 80; CAS 9005-65-6; nonionic; emulsifier and solubilizer for cosmetics and pharmaceuticals, emulsifiable concs.; liq.; HLB 15.0; 100% conc.

Sorbilene O 5. [Auschem SpA] Polysorbate 81; CAS 9005-65-6; nonionic; emulsifier for cosmetics and pharmaceuticals; liq.; HLB 10.0; 100% conc.

Sorbilene P. [Auschem SpA] Polysorbate 40; CAS 9005-66-7; nonionic; emulsifier for cosmetics and pharmaceuticals; liq./paste; HLB 15.7; 100% conc.

Sorbilene S. [Auschem SpA] Polysorbate 60; CAS 9005-67-8; nonionic; emulsifier for cosmetics and pharmaceuticals; liq./paste; HLB 14.8; 100% conc.

Sorbilene S 4. [Auschem SpA] Polysorbate 61; CAS 9005-67-8; nonionic; emulsifier for cosmetics and pharmaceuticals; solid; HLB 9.6; 100% conc.

Sorbilene TO. [Auschem SpA] Polysorbate 85; CAS 9005-70-3; nonionic; emulsifier for cosmetics and pharmaceuticals; liq.; HLB 11.0; 100% conc.

Sorbilene TS. [Auschem SpA] Polysorbate 65; CAS 9005-71-4; nonionic; emulsifier for cosmetics and pharmaceuticals; solid; HLB 10.5; 100% conc.

Sorbirol ISM. [Auschem SpA] Sorbitan isostearate; CAS 54392-26-6; nonionic; emulsifier for cosmetics and pharmaceuticals; liq.; HLB 4.3; 100% conc.

Sorbirol O. [Auschem SpA] Sorbitan oleate; CAS 1338-43-8; EINECS 215-665-4; nonionic; emulsifier for cosmetics and pharmaceuticals, emulsifiable concs. in agric. preps.; liq.; HLB 4.3; 100% conc.

Sorbirol P. [Auschem SpA] Sorbitan palmitate; CAS 26266-57-9; EINECS 247-568-8; nonionic; emulsifier for cosmetics and pharmaceuticals; solid; HLB 6.7; 100% conc.

Sorbirol S. [Auschem SpA] Sorbitan stearate; CAS 1338-41-6; EINECS 215-664-9; nonionic; emulsifier for cosmetics and pharmaceuticals; flakes; HLB 4.7; 100% conc.

Sorbirol SQ. [Auschem SpA] Sorbitan sesquioleate; CAS 8007-43-0; EINECS 232-360-1; nonionic; emulsifier for cosmetics and pharmaceuticals; liq.; HLB 3.7; 100% conc.

Sorbirol TO. [Auschem SpA] Sorbitan trioleate; CAS 26266-58-0; EINECS 247-569-3; nonionic; emulsifier for cosmetics and pharmaceuticals; liq.; HLB 1.8; 100% conc.

Sorbirol TS. [Auschem SpA] Sorbitan tristearate; CAS 26658-19-5; EINECS 247-891-4; nonionic; emulsifier for cosmetics and pharmaceuticals; solid; HLB 2.1; 100% conc.

Sorbitol L. [Auschem SpA] Sorbitan laurate; CAS 1338-39-2; nonionic; emulsifier for cosmetics and pharmaceuticals; liq.; HLB 8.6; 100% conc.

Sorbo®. [ICI Am.] Sorbitol; CAS 50-70-4; EINECS 200-061-5; cosmetics ingred.

Sorbon S-20. [Toho Chem. Industry] Sorbitan laurate; CAS 1338-39-2; nonionic; emulsifier, dispersant for w/o cosmetic emulsion; liq.; 100% conc.

Sorbon S-40. [Toho Chem. Industry] Sorbitan palmitate; CAS 26266-57-9; EINECS 247-568-8; nonionic; emulsifier, dispersant for w/o cosmetic emulsions; solid; 100% conc.

Sorbon S-60. [Toho Chem. Industry] Sorbitan stearate; CAS 1338-41-6; EINECS 215-664-9; nonionic; emulsifier, dispersant for w/o cosmetic emulsions; solid; 100% conc.

Sorbon S-66. [Toho Chem. Industry] Sorbitan distearate; CAS 36521-89-8; emulsifier, dispersant for w/o cosmetic emulsions.

Sorbon S-80. [Toho Chem. Industry] Sorbitan oleate; CAS 1338-43-8; EINECS 215-665-4; nonionic; emulsifier, dispersant for w/o cosmetic emulsions; liq.; 100% conc.

Sorbon T-20. [Toho Chem. Industry] PEG-20 sorbitan laurate; CAS 9005-64-5; nonionic; emulsifier, dispersant, solubilizer for o/w cosmetic emulsion; liq.; HLB 16.7; 100% conc.

Sorbon T-40. [Toho Chem. Industry] POE sorbitan palmitate; nonionic; emulsifier, dispersant for o/w cosmetic emulsions; liq.; HLB 15.7; 100% conc.

Sorbon T-60. [Toho Chem. Industry] POE sorbitan stearate; nonionic; emulsifier, dispersant for o/w cosmetic emulsions; liq.; HLB 15.3; 100% conc.

Sorbon T-80. [Toho Chem. Industry] POE sorbitan oleate; nonionic; emulsifier, dispersant for o/w cosmetic emulsions; liq.; 100% conc.

Sorbon TR 814. [Toho Chem. Industry] POE sorbitol oleate; nonionic; detergent, emulsifier for cosmetics; liq.; HLB 17.5; 100% conc.

Sorbon TR 843. [Toho Chem. Industry] POE sorbitol oleate; nonionic; detergent, emulsifier for cosmetics; liq.; HLB 11.2; 100% conc.

Sorgen 30. [Dai-ichi Kogyo Seiyaku] Sorbitan sesquioleate; CAS 8007-43-0; EINECS 232-360-1; nonionic; antifoamer and emulsifier for foods, cosmetics, and pharmaceutical prods.; liq.; HLB 3.7; 100% conc.

Sorgen 40. [Dai-ichi Kogyo Seiyaku] Sorbitan oleate; CAS 1338-43-8; EINECS 215-665-4; nonionic; antifoamer and emulsifier for foods, cosmetics, and pharmaceutical prods.; liq.; HLB 4.3; 100% conc.

Sorgen 50. [Dai-ichi Kogyo Seiyaku] Sorbitan stearate; CAS 1338-41-6; EINECS 215-664-9; nonionic; antifoamer and emulsifier for foods, cosmetics, and pharmaceutical prods.; flake; HLB 4.7; 100% conc.

Sorgen 90. [Dai-ichi Kogyo Seiyaku] Sorbitan laurate; nonionic; antifoamer and emulsifier for foods, cosmetics, and pharmaceutical prods.; liq.; HLB 8.6; 100% conc.

Sorgen S-30-H. [Dai-ichi Kogyo Seiyaku] Sorbitan sesquioleate; CAS 8007-43-0; EINECS 232-360-1; nonionic; antifoamer and emulsifier for foods, cosmetics, and pharmaceutical prods.; liq.; HLB 3.7; 100% conc.

Sorgen S-40-H. [Dai-ichi Kogyo Seiyaku] Sorbitan oleate; CAS 1338-43-8; EINECS 215-665-4; nonionic; antifoamer and emulsifier for foods, cosmetics, and pharmaceutical prods.; liq.; HLB 4.3; 100% conc.

Soy-Amino Quat L/O. [Brooks Industries] Lauryloleylmethylamine soy amino acids; cationic; cosmetic ingredient for skin and hair care prods.; conditioning agent; gives exc. gloss in hairsprays; highly compat. with popular resins; 90% act.

Soypro 25. [Tri-K Industries] Hydrolyzed soya protein; CAS 68607-88-5; cosmetic protein.

Soyquat 30. [Tri-K Industries] A quaternary hydrolyzed soya protein; cosmetic ingred.

Soy-Quat C. [Maybrook] Cocodimonium hydroxypropyl hydrolyzed soy protein; CAS 977039-11-4; substantive conditioner, moisturizer for hair and skin care prods. (shampoos, conditioners, creams, lotions, bath prods., face and body cleansers); amber clear to sl. hazy liq., char. odor; pH 4.0-6.0; 26-32% nonvolatiles.

Soy-Tein NL. [Maybrook] Hydrolyzed soy protein; CAS 70084-94-5; protein providing moisture retentive, protective and sealing films, substantivity to hair and skin care prods. (shampoos, conditioners, treatment prods., lotions, creams, bath prods.); mitigates damage due to bleaching, perming, etc.; yel. to lt. amber clear liq., char. odor; pH 4.0-6.0; 20% min. solids.

SP-500. [Kobo] Nylon 12.; CAS 25038-74-8; cosmetic raw material.

Span® 20. [ICI Spec. Chem.; ICI Surf. Am.; ICI Surf. Belgium] Sorbitan laurate NF; CAS 1338-39-2; nonionic; emulsifier, stabilizer, thickener, lubricant, softener, antistatic agent; foods, pharmaceuticals, cosmetics, cleaning compds.; textiles; amber liq.; sol. (@ 1%) in IPA, perchloroethylene, xylene, cottonseed oil, min. oil; sol. (hazy) in propylene glycol; visc. 4250 cps; HLB 8.6; 100% act.

Span® 40. [ICI Spec. Chem.; ICI Surf. Am.; ICI Surf. Belgium] Sorbitan palmitate NF; CAS 26266-57-9; EINECS 247-568-8; nonionic; emulsifier, stabilizer, thickener, lubricant, softener, antistatic agent; foods, pharmaceuticals, cosmetics, cleaning compds., textiles; tan solid; sol. (@ 1%) in IPA, xylene; sol. (hazy) in perchloroethylene; HLB 6.7; pour pt. 48 C; 100% act.

Span® 60, 60K. [ICI Spec. Chem.; ICI Surf. Am.; ICI Surf. Belgium] Sorbitan stearate NF; CAS 1338-41-6; EINECS 215-664-9; nonionic; emulsifier, stabilizer, solubilizer, thickener, lubricant, softener, antistatic agent; foods, pharmaceuticals, cosmetics, household prods., cleaning compds., textiles; also dispersant for inorg. pigments in thermoplastics; pale cream solid; sol. (@1%): sol. in IPA; sol. (hazy) in perchloroethylene, xylene; HLB 4.7; pour pt. 53 C; 100% act.

Span® 60 VS. [ICI Spec. Chem.] Sorbitan stearate; CAS 1338-41-6; EINECS 215-664-9; vegetable source used in foods; emulsifier, solubilizer for pharmaceuticals and cosmetics; beads; HLB 4.7; 100% conc.

Span® 65. [ICI Spec. Chem.; ICI Surf. Am.; ICI Surf. Belgium] Sorbitan tristearate; CAS 26658-19-5; EINECS 247-891-4; nonionic; emulsifier, stabilizer, thickener, lubricant, softener, antistatic agent; foods, pharmaceuticals, cosmetics, cleaning compds., textiles; cream solid; sol. (@ 1%) in IPA, perchloroethylene, xylene; HLB 2.1; pour pt. 53 C; 100% act.

Span® 80. [ICI Spec. Chem.; ICI Surf. Am.; ICI Surf. Belgium] Sorbitan oleate NF; CAS 1338-43-8; EINECS 215-665-4; nonionic; w/o emulsifier for personal care, industrial, and textile applics; oil additive for corrosion inhibition; fiber lubricant and softener; amber liq.; sol. (@ 1%) in IPA, perchloroethylene, xylene, cottonseed and min. oils; visc. 1000 cps; HLB 4.3.; 100% act.

Span® 85. [ICI Spec. Chem.; ICI Surf. Am.; ICI Surf. Belgium] Sorbitan trioleate; CAS 26266-58-0; EINECS 247-569-3; nonionic; emulsifier, stabilizer, thickener, lubricant, softener, antistatic agent; foods, pharmaceuticals, cosmetics, cleaning compds., textiles; amber liq.; sol. (@ 1%) in IPA, perchloroethylene, xylene, cottonseed and min. oils; visc. 210 cps; HLB 1.8; 100% act.

Special Fat 42/44. [Hüls Am.] Hydrog. coconut oil; raw material for cosmetics, pharmaceuticals, and food industries.

Special Fat 168T. [Hüls Am.] Hydrog. tallow; CAS 8030-12-4; EINECS 232-442-7; raw material for food, pharmaceutical and personal care industries.

Special Oil 619. [Hüls Am.; Hüls AG] Triisostearin; lubricant in emulsions, ointments, lipsticks, hair care prods.; adds fine sheen to skin; pigment dispersant in sticks and liners;

stable to oxidation; ylsh. high visc. oil, sl. fatty odor, bland fatty taste; sol. in chloroform, n-hexane, ether; insol. in water; sp.gr. 0.912; visc. 155 mPa·s; acid no. 1 max.; iodine no. 10 max.; sapon. no. 180-200; hyd. no. 10 max.; ref. index 1.456.

Special Oil 888. [Hüls Am.; Hüls AG] Oleic/linoleic triglyceride; release agent and conditioning oil for cast and compression molded cosmetic formulations; stable to oxidation; ylsh. paste; acid no. 0.2 max.; iodine no. 65 max.; sapon. no. 90-210; cloud pt. 15 C.

Spectradyne® G. [Lonza] Chlorhexidine gluconate BP; CAS 18472-51-0; EINECS 242-354-0; antimicrobial for pharmaceuticals, hospital disinfectants, veterinary prods., anti-plaque dental prods.; liq.; 20% act.

Spectra-Pearl®. [ISP Van Dyk] Colored pigments/titanium dioxide on mica; patented pearlescent giving sparkle, luster, and color to cosmetic eye, face, lip, and body makeup, pressed powds., pencil formulations; optimum color intensity, uv light stability, skin adhesion, and flow chars.; free-flowing powds.

Spectra-Sorb® UV 9. [Am. Cyanamid] Benzophenone-3; CAS 131-57-7; EINECS 205-031-5; uv lt. absorber; used in sunscreen, cosmetic, and pharmaceutical formulations; pale cream to off-wh. powd.; m.w. 228.25; sol. (g/100 ml solv.): 100 g propylene glycol monostearate, 57 g in ethoxyethyl alcohol, 47 g in diglycol stearate, 15 g in IPM, 11.3 g in soybean oil, 0 g in water; sp.gr. 1.324; m.p. 63.0-64.5 C; 100% assay.

Spectra-Sorb® UV 24. [Am. Cyanamid] Benzophenone-8; CAS 131-53-3; EINECS 205-026-8; uv lt. absorber for cosmetics, sunscreens; stabilizes formulations; yel. free-flowing powd.; m.w. 244.25; sol. (g/100 ml solv.): 38 g in propylene glycol stearate, 34 g in diglycol stearate, 21.8 g in 95% ethanol, 17 g in IPA, 10 g in IPM; sp.gr. 1.382; m.p. 68-70 C; 100% assay.

Spectra-Sorb® UV 5411. [Am. Cyanamid] Octrizole; CAS 3147-75-9; EINECS 221-573-5; uv lt. absorber for cosmetics; stabilizes formulations, protects colors; off-wh. free-flowing powd.; m.w. 323.44; sol. (g/100 ml solv.): 65 g in benzene, 27.2 g in ethyl acetate, 0 g in water; sp.gr. 1.18; m.p. 101-105 C.

Spermwax®. [Robeco] Cetyl esters wax NF; CAS 17661-50-6; EINECS 241-640-2; syn. spermaceti used in toiletries, cosmetics, dermatologicals as stiffening agent, slip and visc. aid; provides smoothness and rigidity; solid; m.p. 43-47 C; HLB 8.4-9.4; acid no. 5 max.; iodine no. 1 max.; sapon. no. 109-120.

Spherica. [Ikeda] Silica; provides slip and improves smoothness of makeup, eye shadow, mascara, antiperspirants, body powd., loose and pressed powds.; can be modified to increase or decrease absorption of water, oil, or fragrances and hold them within its pores; provides vehicle and slow release for other active ingreds.; wh. spherical powd.; 2-15 μm particle size; 99% min. SiO_2.

Spherica HA. [Ikeda] Silica, 0.2% hyaluronic acid; imparts smoothness and fine touch to powdery cosmetics while providing high moisturizing effect; for lipsticks, foundations, skin lotions and creams; wh. spherical powd., char. odor; 2-15 μm particle size.

Spherititan. [Ikeda] Titanium dioxide; CAS 13463-67-7; EINECS 236-675-5; provides good coverage but with lighter touch due to spherical shape; for liq. foundations, pressed and loose powds., eyeshadow; wh. spherical powd.; 2.0-15.0 μm particle size; pH 3.0-5.0; 95% min. purity.

Spheron L-1500. [Presperse] Silica; CAS 7631-86-9; spherical hollow microbeads as carriers for sunscreens, fragrances, emollients; imparts lubricity; JSCI/JCID approved; wh. fine free-flowing spherical powd.; particle size 3-15 μ; surf. area 200 m²/g.

Spheron P-1000. [Presperse] Silica; CAS 7631-86-9; spherical hollow microbeads as carriers for sunscreens, fragrances, emollients; imparts lubricity; JSCI/JCID approved; wh. fine free-flowing spherical powd.; particle size 3-10 μ; surf. area 150 m²/g.

Spheron P-1500. [Presperse] Silica; CAS 7631-86-9; spherical hollow microbeads as carriers for sunscreens, fragrances, emollients; imparts lubricity; JSCI/JCID approved; wh. fine free-flowing spherical powd.; particle size 3-15 μ; surf. area 150 m²/g.

Spheron P-1500-030. [Presperse] Silica, methicone; CAS 7631-86-9, 9004-73-7; spherical hollow microbeads as carriers for sunscreens, fragrances, emollients; imparts lubricity; JSCI/JCID approved; wh. fine free-flowing spherical powd.; particle size 3-15 μ; surf. area 150 m²/g.

Sphingoceryl® Fluid, Wax, Powd. [Laboratoires Sérobiologiques] Glycosphingolipids, phospholipids, and cholesterol; epidermal structuring agent used in prods. for dry, rough, sensitive, and stressed skin, anti-aging, sun care, and protection/repair of skin and lips; liq., wax, and powd.; lipo-disp.; usage level: 2-5%.

Sphingoceryl® LS. [Laboratoires Sérobiologiques] Octyldodecanol, phospholipids, cholesterol, glycosphingolipids; epidermal structuring agent used in prods. for dry, rough, sensitive, and stressed skin, anti-aging, sun care, and protection/repair of skin and lips.

Sphingoceryl® Powd. LS. [Laboratoires Sérobiologiques] Octyldodecanol, silica, nylon-12, phospholipids, cholesterol, glycosphingolipids; epidermal structuring agent used in prods. for dry, rough, sensitive, and stressed skin, anti-aging, sun care, and protection/repair of skin and lips.

Sphingoceryl® Wax LS 2958 B. [Laboratoires Sérobiologiques] Octyldodecanol, microcryst. wax, petrolatum, phospholipids, cholesterol, castor oil, glyceryl ricinoleate, carnauba, candelilla wax, cetyl alcohol, beeswax, min. oil, and glycosphingolipids; epidermal structuring agent used in prods. for dry, rough, sensitive, and stressed skin, anti-aging, sun care, and protection/repair of skin and lips.

Sphingolipid CB-1. [Nikko Chem. Co. Ltd.; Barnet Prods.] Sphingolipids; humectant for cosmetics.

Sphingosomes® AL. [Laboratoires Sérobiologiques] Water, glycerin, lecithin, glycosphingolipids, allantoin, and cholesterol; liposome for epicutaneous hydration, bioprotection and strengthening of cutaneous barrier functioning; used for prods. for dry, rough, and sensitive skin, sun care, and hair care; wh. ivory liq.; disp. in water; usage level: 3-10%.

Spiroflor. [Henkel/Cospha] 3-Ethyl-2,4-dioxaspiro (5.5) undec-8-ene; complex, natural odor fragrance raw material for personal care and detergent formulations; colorless liq., sweet odor; b.p. 86 C; flash pt. 103 C.

Spirulina Extract COS. [Cosmetochem] An extract of Spirulina algae; cosmetic specialty high in proteins and containing well balanced compositions of minerals and vitamins.

Spotted Geranium Extract Code 9032. [Brooks Industries] Geranium (Geranium maculatum) extract; infusion rich in tannins for use in topicals; yel. clear liq.

Spray Dried Gum Arabic NF Type CSP. [Meer] Gum arabic from Acacia senegal CAS 9000-01-5; EINECS 232-519-5; used in the food, beverage, and pharmaceutical tableting industries; creamy wh. powd., 98% thru 120 mesh; sol. 1 g/2 ml of water yielding lt. amber sol'n.

Spreading Agent ET0672. [Croda Inc.; Croda Chem. Ltd.] Complex alkoxylate; nonionic; o/w emulsifier, surface spreading agent, dispersant for min. oils used for mosquito control, in bath oils; pale straw clear liq.; HLB 7.5; 100% conc.

Squatol S. [Les Colorants Wackherr] Syn. squalene; CAS

111-02-4; EINECS 203-826-1; cosmetics ingred.

SS-88. [U.S. Cosmetics] Sericite; mineral having silky shine, transparency, spreadability, and an oily feel; provides creamy feel when incorporated into cosmetic powd. formulations.

SS-4267. [GE Silicones] Dimethicone and trimethylsiloxysilicate; emollient for water-resistant cosmetics and suntan prods.; sol. in aliphatic, aromatic solvs., IPP, IPM, some lt. min. oils; 100% act.

S-Safe 2010. [Nippon Oils & Fats] PPG-20-decyltetradeceth-10.

S-SM. [U.S. Cosmetics] Sericite; cosmetic raw material; avg. particle size 1-20 μ.

Stabileze™ 06. [ISP] PVM/MA decadiene crosspolymer; thickener and stabilizer for use in pigmented cosmetics, skin creams, lotions, sunscreens, moisturizers, barrier creams, hair styling gels, shampoos, nail polish removers; imparts nontacky emollience; film-former; for aq. and nonaq. systems; wh. powd.; disp. in water; visc. 50,000-70,000 (5% aq. gel).

Stabland®. [Karlshamns] Fractionated partially hydrog. soybean oil; CAS 8016-70-4; EINECS 232-410-2; specialty oil; Lovibond R1.5 max.; m.p. < 40 F; iodine no. 107-115; sapon. no. 189-195.

Stabolec C. [Lucas Meyer] Lecithin, propylene glycol, citric acid, t-butyl hydroquinone.

Stamere®. [Meer] Carrageenan; CAS 9000-07-1; EINECS 232-524-2; suspending agent, stabilizer, thickener, gelling agent for food industry; lubricant, emollient for pharmaceutical jellies, laxatives; tablet binder; emulsion stabilizer; pigment suspender in ceramic glazes; also for cosmetics, toothpaste, wire drawing lubricants, electroplating baths.

Stamid HT 3901. [Clough] Cocamide DEA; CAS 61791-31-9; EINECS 263-163-9; nonionic; foam stabilizer, emulsifier and thickener used in a variety of household, industrial and cosmetic formulations; liq.; pH 9.5-10.5; 85% conc.

Stamid LS 5487. [Clough] Soyamide DEA; CAS 68425-47-8; EINECS 270-355-6; nonionic; stabilizer, emulsifier, thickener for shampoos and bubble bath formulations; liq.; pH 8.0-11.0; 100% conc.

Standamid® CD. [Henkel/Cospha; Henkel Canada] Capramide DEA (2:1) and diethanolamine; CAS 136-26-5; EINECS 205-234-9; nonionic; detergent, foam enhancer for anionic systems; solubilizes fragrances into hydroalcoholic systems; sec. emulsifier in o/w systems, perfume stabilizer; personal care prods., industrial cleaners; amber liq.; sol. in water, propylene glycol, PEG-8, SD-40 alcohol; dens. 8.19 lb/gal; visc. 675 cps; acid no. 15-20; cloud pt. 0 C; gel pt. 0 C; 98% conc.

Standamid® ID. [Henkel/Emery] Isotearamide DEA (1:1); CAS 52794-79-3; EINECS 258-193-4; nonionic; visc. builder esp. in sodium lauryl sulfate systems; foam enhancer; hair conditioning agent; lubricant, mold release agent, emulsifier; amber liq.; sol. in SD-40 alcohol; sp.gr. 0.964; dens. 8.04 lb/gal; visc. 1600 cps; cloud pt. < 0 C; gel pt. < 0 C; pH 8-10 (1.0%); 100% act.

Standamid® KD. [Henkel/Cospha; Henkel Canada] Cocamide DEA (1:1); CAS 61791-31-9; EINECS 263-163-9; nonionic; foaming and thickening agent for liq. or gel shampoos and bubble baths, industrial cleaners, etc.; superfatting agent, foam stabilizer, emulsifier, intermediate; detergent and solubilizer for oily components; hair conditioner; visc. amber liq.; sol. in propylene glycol., PEG-8, SD-40 alcohol; insol. in water; dens. 8.13 lb/gal; visc. 1150 cps; m.p. 100 F; acid no. 1.0 max.; cloud pt. 11 C; gel pt. 5 C; pH 9.0-9.5 (10%); 85-90% amide content.

Standamid® KDL. [Henkel/Cospha] Lauramide DEA; CAS 120-40-1; EINECS 204-393-1; cosmetic surfactant.

Standamid® KDO. [Henkel/Cospha; Henkel Canada]

Cocamide DEA (1:1); CAS 61791-31-9; EINECS 263-163-9; nonionic; visc. builder for anionic systems, good foam enhancement, low odor, good color, broad compatibility, and good handling qualities; used in shampoos, bath prods., liq. hand soaps, industrial cleaners; amber visc. liq.; sol. in lower alcohols, propylene glycol, and polyethylene glycols; sp.gr. 0.982; dens. 8.20 lb/gal; visc. 1050 cps; acid no. 2.0 max.; cloud pt. 12 C; gel pt. 4 C; pH 9–11 (1.0%); 100% conc.

Standamid® KDOL. [Henkel/Cospha] Lauramide DEA; CAS 120-40-1; EINECS 204-393-1; cosmetic surfactant.

Standamid® KDS. [Henkel/Cospha; Henkel Canada] Lauramide DEA (1:1); CAS 120-40-1; EINECS 204-393-1; nonionic; detergent, solubilizer for oils; enhances foam dens., lubricity, stability for shampoos, skin cleansers, bath and shower prods.; lt. amber liq.; dens. 8.20 lb/gal; 80% conc.

Standamid® KM. [Henkel] Cocamide MEA (1:1); CAS 68140-00-1; EINECS 268-770-2; visc. builder for anionic systems; produces lubricious foam for shampoo and bath prods., industrial cleaners; waxy flakes, beads; sol. in lower alcohols; sp.gr. 0.884; m.p. 80 C; acid no. 2.0 max.; cloud pt. 64 C; gel pt. 59 C; pH 9–11 (1.0%).

Standamid® LD. [Henkel/Cospha; Henkel Canada] Lauramide DEA (1:1); CAS 120-40-1; EINECS 204-393-1; nonionic; foam booster/stabilizer, wetting agent, superfatting agent, thickening agent, emulsifier for oils and grease, shampoos, bath prods., industrial cleaners, fortifier for perfumes in soaps; waxy solid; sol. in propylene glycol, PEG-8, SD-40 alcohol; insol. in water; dens. 8.20 lb/gal; m.p. 105 F; acid no. 0–1.0; cloud pt. 1 C; gel pt. < 0 C; pH 9.5–10.5 (10% sol'n.); > 90% amide content.

Standamid® LD 80/20. [Henkel/Cospha; Henkel Canada] Luaramide DEA and propylene glycol; nonionic; foam booster/stabilizer, detergency builder, emulsifier, thickener, conditioner; shampoos, bubble baths, dishwashing detergents, creams, and lotions; clear amber liq.; dens. 8.27 lb/gal; cloud pt. 0 C; acid no. 0.5 max.; pH 9.5–10.5 (10% sol'n.); 80% conc.

Standamid® LDO. [Henkel/Cospha; Henkel Canada] Lauramide DEA (1:1); CAS 120-40-1; EINECS 204-393-1; nonionic; detergent, foam and visc. builder for shampoos, bath prods., cleansers, industrial cleaners; amber liq.; sol. in propylene glycol, PEG-8, SD-40 alcohol; insol. in water; sp.gr. 0.985; dens. 8.22 lb/gal; visc. 850 cps; acid no. 2.0 max.; cloud pt. < 0 C; gel pt. < 0 C; pH 9–11 (1.0%); 100% conc.

Standamid® LDS. [Henkel/Cospha; Henkel Canada] Lauramide DEA (1:1); CAS 120-40-1; EINECS 204-393-1; nonionic; foam booster/stabilizer, thickener; solubilizer for liqs., oils, perfumes; used in personal care prods., dishwashing detergents; lt. amber liq.; sol. in lower alcohols, propylene glycol, polyethylene glycol; disp. in water; sp.gr. 0.98; dens. 8.2 lb/gal; visc. 1000 cps; cloud pt. < 0 C; gel pt. < 0 C; pH 9–11 (1.0%); 100% conc.

Standamid® LM. [Henkel] Lauramide MEA (1:1); CAS 142-78-9; EINECS 205-560-1; visc. builder for anionic systems; produces lubricious foam for shampoo and bath prods., and industrial cleaners; waxy flakes, beads; sol. in lower alcohols; insol. in water; sp.gr. 0.915; m.p. 80 C; acid no. 2.0 max.; cloud pt. 83 C; gel pt. 73 C; pH 9–11 (1.0 %).

Standamid® PD. [Henkel/Cospha; Henkel Canada] Cocamide DEA (2:1) and diethanolamine; nonionic; more efficient foam builder, less efficient visc. builder than 1:1 superamides; stabilizer; used in shampoos, bubble baths with anionics, nonionics, and amphoterics; industrial cleaning; solubilizer for oily additives; amber visc. liq.; sol. in water, propylene glycol, PEG-8, SD-40 alcohol; dens. 8.17 lb/gal; visc. 1050 cps; cloud pt. 0 C; gel pt. 0 C; 100% conc.

Standamid® PK-KD. [Henkel/Cospha; Henkel Canada] Cocamide DEA superamide; CAS 61791-31-9; EINECS 263-163-9; nonionic; visc. builder, foamer; lt. amber liq.

Standamid® PK-KDO. [Henkel/Cospha; Henkel Canada] Cocamide DEA superamide; CAS 61791-31-9; EINECS 263-163-9; nonionic; enhances foam for shampoos, liq. hand soaps, etc.; lt. amber liq.

Standamid® PK-KDS. [Henkel/Cospha; Henkel Canada] Cocamide DEA superamide; CAS 61791-31-9; EINECS 263-163-9; nonionic; solubilizer, foam booster; lt. amber liq.

Standamid® PK-SD. [Henkel/Cospha; Henkel Canada] Cocamide DEA superamide; CAS 61791-31-9; EINECS 263-163-9; nonionic; for liq. conditioners, foaming prods.; lt. amber liq.

Standamid® Resin BC-1283. [Henkel/Cospha] Nylon-66; CAS 32131-17-2; gellant for hydrocarbons and Guerbet alcohols; solid, controlled-release fragrance prods.; lt. amber clear solid.

Standamid® SD. [Henkel/Cospha; Henkel Canada] Cocamide DEA (1:1); CAS 61791-31-9; EINECS 263-163-9; nonionic; high foaming detergent and foam stabilizer with pronounced visc. build-up; used in bath gels, liq. bubble baths, shampoos, dishwashing and laundry detergents; derived from whole coconut oil; contains no amide ester; low cost alkanolamide; amber visc. liq.; sol. in propylene glycol, PEG-8, SD-40 alcohol; insol. in water; visc. 1225 cps; m.p. 25 F; cloud pt. < 0 C; gel pt. < 0 C; pH 9.5–10.5 (10% sol'n.); 100% conc.

Standamid® SDO. [Henkel/Cospha; Henkel Canada] Cocamide DEA (1:1); CAS 61791-31-9; EINECS 263-163-9; nonionic; visc. builder and foam enhancer for aq. systems, shampoo, bubble baths, liq. hand soaps, industrial cleaners, offers excellent handling chars.; residual glycerin to enhance humectancy and hair conditioning effects; amber liq.; sol. in lower alcohols, propylene glycol, polyethylene glycols; sp.gr. 0.991; dens. 8.27 lb/gal; visc. 950 cps; acid no. 2.0 max.; cloud pt. < 0 C; gel pt. < 0 C; pH 9–11 (1.0%); 100% conc.

Standamid® SM. [Henkel/Cospha; Henkel Canada] Cocamide MEA (1:1); CAS 68140-00-1; EINECS 268-770-2; visc. builder for anionic systems; wetting agent; produces lubricious foam for shampoo and bath prods., industrial cleaners; flakes, beads; sol. in lower alcohols; insol. in water; sp.gr. 0.934; m.p. 62 C; acid no. 1.0 max.; cloud pt. 63 C; gel pt. 56 C; pH 9–11 (1.0%); 100% conc.

Standamid® SOMD. [Henkel/Cospha] Linoleamide DEA (1:1); CAS 56863-02-6; EINECS 260-410-2; nonionic; visc. builder with foam enhancement chars.; produces esp. high visc. when used with ethoxylated anionics; used in gel shampoos, bubble baths, liq. hand soaps, industrial cleaners, and formulation; where the amt. of electrolyte must be kept to a min.; low-cost shampoo concentrates; waxy solid; sol. in lower alcohols; sp.gr. 0.935; acid no. 2 max.; cloud pt. 38 C; gel pt. 34 C; pH 9–11 (1.0%); 100% conc.

Standamox CAW. [Henkel/Cospha; Henkel Canada] Cocamidopropylamine oxide; CAS 68155-09-9; EINECS 268-938-5; nonionic; wetting agent, foam builder, stabilizer, thickener, lubricant, emollient for low-irritation baby shampoos, bubble baths, skin care preps.; clear liq.; 30% act.

Standamox O1. [Henkel/Cospha; Henkel Canada] Oleamine oxide; CAS 14351-50-9; EINECS 238-311-0; nonionic; biodeg. thickener, bacteriostat, dye assistant, lubricant, softener used in industrial applics., hair prods., plating compds., lube oils; amber clear thixotropic liq.; 50% act.

Standamox PS. [Pulcra SA] Stearyl dimethylamine oxide;

CAS 2571-88-2; EINECS 219-919-5; nonionic; conditioner, softener for cream rinses, lotions, liq. bath prods.; paste; 25% conc.

Standamul® Conc. 1002. [Henkel/Cospha] Cetearyl alcohol, PEG-40 hydrog. castor oil, stearalkonium chloride; cationic; conditioner and softener used in hair conditioners and cream rinses; cost-effective; off-wh. waxy flakes; m.p. 58 C; pH 5.0 (1%); 99% act.

Standapol® 125-E. [Henkel/Cospha] Sodium laureth-12 sulfate; CAS 9004-82-4; detergent, foamer used in personal care prods.; straw yel. clear liq.; sol. in water and hydrophilic solvs.; cloud pt. 10 C max.; pH 7.5–9.0 (10% aq.); 58–60% act.

Standapol® 130-E. [Henkel/Cospha] Sodium laureth-12 sulfate; CAS 9004-82-4; detergent, foamer used in personal care prods.; pale yel. clear liq.; sol. see Standapol 125-E Conc.; pH 7.5–9.0 (10% aq.); 28–30% act.

Standapol® 230-E. [Henkel/Cospha] Ammonium laureth-12 sulfate; detergent, foamer used in personal care prods.; straw-yel. clear liq.; sol. see Standapol 125-E Conc.; cloud pt. 0 C; pH 6.5–7.0 (10% aq.); 28–30% act.

Standapol® 7088. [Henkel/Cospha; Henkel Canada] Ammonium myreth sulfate, cocamide MEA; anionic/nonionic; foaming surfactant base for personal care cleansing and bath prods.; clear liq.; 38% conc.

Standapol® 7092. [Henkel/Cospha; Henkel Canada] Sodium laureth sulfate, glycol stearate; anionic/nonionic; pearlescent surfactant for shampoos and bath prods.; for cold blending; exc. stability over wide temp. ranges; pearly-wh. visc. liq.; 35% act.

Standapol® A. [Henkel/Cospha; Henkel Canada] Ammonium lauryl sulfate; CAS 2235-54-3; EINECS 218-793-9; anionic; detergent, foamer, suspending agent, base for shampoos, cleaning compds. with near neutral pH; water-wh. visc. liq.; visc. 1500–3000 cps; pH 6.5–7.0 (10% aq.); 27.5–28.5% act.

Standapol® A-215. [Henkel/Cospha] Ammonium C12-15 alkyl sulfate; CAS 68815-61-2; EINECS 272-385-5.

Standapol® AA-1. [Henkel/Cospha; Henkel Canada] DEA-lauryl sulfate, DEA-lauraminopropionate, and sodium lauraminopropionate; anionic-amphoteric; low color, low odor surfactant blend used in personal care prods.; amber liq.; cloud pt. 12 C; pH 7.5–8.5; 34.5–38.5% solids.

Standapol® A-HV. [Henkel/Cospha; Henkel Canada] Ammonium lauryl sulfate; CAS 2235-54-3; EINECS 218-793-9; anionic; surfactant, foamer, visc. modifier used in personal care prods.; water-wh. to pale yel. liq.; water-sol.; dens. 1.025 g/ml; visc. < 10,000 cP; pH 6.0–7.0; 27.5–28.5% act.

Standapol® AP-60. [Henkel] Ammonium C12-15 pareth sulfate; surfactant for personal care, household and industrial cleaning prods.; yel. clear visc. liq.; water-sol.; dens. 1.025 g/ml; visc. 100–200 cps; cloud pt. 10 C max.; pH 6.0–7.0 (10%); 58–60% act.

Standapol® AP Blend. [Henkel/Cospha; Henkel Canada] Sodium laureth sulfate, cocamide DEA, cocamidopropyl betaine; conc. for shampoo, bath and cleansing prods., liq. soaps; exc. foaming and visc. response; lt. amber liq.; 35-40% conc.

Standapol® BW. [Henkel/Cospha; Henkel Canada] Sodium lauryl sulfate, cocamide DEA, cocamidopropyl; anionic/nonionic; formulated conc. for personal care cleaning and bath prods.; base for liq. dishwash; liq.; 37% conc.

Standapol® CAT. [Henkel/Cospha; Henkel Canada] Glycol stearate, lauramine oxide, propylene glycol, and ceteareth-20; pearlescent surfactant for personal care prods., shampoos, bubble bath creams, cationic formulations such as conditioners; pearly liq.; 45% act.

Standapol® CIM-40. [Henkel/Cospha] Sodium cocoamphoacetate; amphoteric; surfactant used in personal care

prods.; lt. clear liq.; pleasant mild odor; cloud pt. 0 C; pH 8.0–9.0 (10%); 40–42% act.

Standapol® Conc. 7021. [Henkel/Cospha] DEA-lauryl sulfate and TEA-lauryl sulfate; anionic; detergent, foamer used in personal care prods.; anhyd. slurry; 100% conc.

Standapol® Conc. 7023. [Henkel/Cospha] Cocamide DEA and DEA-myreth sulfate; anionic; detergent, foamer, solubilizer; conc. shampoos and bath prods. where high foaming is required; gelatin capsules bath beads; solubilizer for fatty alcohols, fatty acid esters, and min. oil; straw-yel. clear liq.; visc. 250 cps max.; pH 8.5–9.5 (1% aq.); cloud pt. 10 C max.; 100% conc.

Standapol® CS-50. [Henkel/Cospha] Sodium lauryl sulfate, sodium cetyl sulfate, and laureth-3; personal care surfactant; pearly wh. visc. liq.; mild char. odor; pH 6.5–7.5 (10% aq.); 28.5–30% act.

Standapol® CS Paste. [Henkel/Cospha; Henkel Canada] Sodium lauryl sulfate, sodium cetyl sulfate, and laureth-3; anionic; detergent, foamer; formulated conc. for pearlescent cream shampoos, bubble baths; pearly creamy paste; mild char. odor; pH 6.5–7.5 (10% aq.); 57–60% act.

Standapol® DEA. [Henkel/Cospha; Henkel Canada] DEA-lauryl sulfate; CAS 143-00-0; EINECS 205-577-4; anionic; base, detergent, foamer used in personal care prods.; lt. yel. clear liq.; 37% conc.

Standapol® DLC. [Henkel/Cospha] DEA-laureth sulfate, cocamide DEA.

Standapol® EA-1. [Henkel/Cospha; Henkel Canada] Ammonium laureth sulfate; CAS 32612-48-9; anionic; surfactant for clear liq. shampoos, bubble baths; water-wh. visc. liq.; visc. 2500 cps; cloud pt. 5 C max.; pH 6.5–7.0 (10% aq.); 25.5–26.5% act.

Standapol® EA-2. [Henkel/Cospha; Henkel Canada] Ammonium laureth sulfate; CAS 32612-48-9; anionic; surfactant for clear liq. shampoos, bubble baths; water-wh. visc. liq.; visc. 2500 cps max.; cloud pt. 0 C max.; pH 6.5–7.0 (10% aq.); 24.5–25.5% act.

Standapol® EA-3. [Henkel/Cospha; Henkel Canada] Ammonium laureth sulfate; CAS 32612-48-9; solubilizer used in personal care prods.; water-wh. visc. liq.; water-sol.; dens. 1.020 g/ml; visc. 2500 cps; cloud pt. 5 C; pH 6.0–7.0 (10%); 26–28% act.

Standapol® EA-40. [Henkel/Cospha; Henkel Canada] Ammonium myreth sulfate; CAS 27731-61-9; anionic; detergent, foamer, base for professional shampoo concs., bubble baths; pale-yel. clear liq.; cloud pt. 10 C max.; pH 6.0–7.0 (10% aq.); 58–60% act.

Standapol® EA-K. [Henkel/Cospha; Henkel Canada] Ammonium myreth sulfate, cocamide DEA; base for manual dishwash, pet shampoos, bath prods., lt. duty cleaners, body cleansers; exc. visc. and foam performance; amber clear liq.; misc. in R.T. water; visc. 200 cps; pH 6.3 ± 0.3; 61.0 ± 1.5% solids.

Standapol® ES-1. [Henkel/Cospha; Henkel Canada] Sodium laureth sulfate; anionic; detergent, foamer, base for liq. shampoos and bubble baths; water-wh. visc. liq.; visc. 500–1200 cps; cloud pt. 5 C max.; pH 7.5–8.5 (10% aq.); 24.5–25.5% act.

Standapol® ES-2. [Henkel/Cospha; Henkel Canada] Sodium laureth sulfate; anionic; detergent, foamer, base for liq. shampoos and bubble baths; water-wh. visc. liq.; visc. 4000–5000 cps; cloud pt. 0 C max.; pH 6.5–7.5 (10% aq.); 25–26% act.

Standapol® ES-3. [Henkel/Cospha; Henkel Canada] Sodium laureth sulfate; anionic; detergent, foamer, base for liq. shampoos and bubble baths; water-wh. visc. liq.; visc. 500 cps max.; cloud pt. 0 C; pH 6.5–8.0 (10% aq.); 28–29% act.

Standapol® ES-40. [Henkel/Cospha; Henkel Canada] Sodium myreth sulfate; CAS 25446-80-4; EINECS 246-986-

8; anionic; detergent, foamer, base for liq. shampoos and bubble baths; pale-yel. clear liq.; cloud pt. 10 C max.; pH 7.5–9.0 (10% aq.); 58–60% act.

Standapol® ES-50. [Henkel/Cospha; Henkel Canada] Sodium myreth sulfate; CAS 25446-80-4; EINECS 246-986-8; anionic; surfactant for liq. shampoos, skin cleansers, cleaning prods., foams; cloudy visc. liq.; 50% conc.

Standapol® ES-250. [Henkel/Cospha; Henkel Canada] Sodium laureth sulfate; CAS 9004-82-4; anionic; surfactant for shampoos, cleaning prods.; pale yel. clear liq.; 53% act.

Standapol® ES-350. [Henkel/Cospha; Henkel Canada] Sodium laureth sulfate; CAS 9004-82-4; anionic; surfactant for shampoos, bath prods., detergent cleaning prods.; pale yel. clear liq.; 53% act.

Standapol® LIS. [Henkel/Cospha; Henkel Canada] Mixture of special alkyl ether sulfates, amphoteric, alkanolamide; anionic/nonionic; blend for mild shampoos and bath prods.; clear visc. liq.; 35-40% act.

Standapol® MG. [Henkel/Cospha; Henkel Canada] Magnesium lauryl sulfate; CAS 3097-08-3; EINECS 221-450-6; anionic; foamer with good dermatological props. for personal care prods.; straw yel. liq.; cloud pt. 3 C max.; pH 6–7 (10% aq.); 28–30% act.

Standapol® MLS. [Henkel/Cospha] MEA-lauryl sulfate; CAS 4722-98-9; EINECS 225-214-3; anionic; detergent, foamer for personal care prods.; lt. yel. clear visc. liq.; visc. 3000–5000 cps; cloud pt. 0 C; pH 7–8 (10% aq.); 32–34% act.

Standapol® Pearl Conc. 7130. [Henkel/Cospha; Henkel Canada] Glycol distearate, sodium laureth sulfate, propylene glycol, cocamide MEA, laureth-9; anionic/nonionic; pearlescent surfactant for shampoos, bath and cleansing prods.; for cold blending; wh. pearly liq.; misc. in R.T. water; visc. 5000 cps max.; pH 6.5 ± 1.0% (10%); 41.0 ± 3.0% solids.

Standapol® S. [Henkel/Cospha; Henkel Canada] Sodium lauryl sulfate, sodium laureth sulfate, lauramide MIPA, cocamide MEA, glycol stearate, and coceth-8; anionic/nonionic; pearlescent shampoo and liq. soap base; pearly-wh. visc. liq.; visc. 1200–1700 cps; pH 6.6–7.4 (10% aq.); 36.8–37.3% act.

Standapol® SCO. [Henkel/Cospha; Henkel Canada] Sulfated castor oil; CAS 8002-33-3; EINECS 232-306-7; anionic; emulsifier and dispersant, wetting agent, foam depressant, emollient surfactant and solubilizer used in personal care prods.; amber visc. liq.; 75% conc.

Standapol® SH-100. [Henkel/Cospha; Henkel Canada] Disodium oleamido PEG-2 sulfosuccinate; CAS 56388-43-3; EINECS 260-143-1; anionic; detergent used in personal care prods.; nonirritating shampoo base; anti-irritant for other surfactants; lt. amber liq.; mild pleasant odor; cloud pt. < 0 C; pH 6.0–7.0 (5%); 29–31% act.

Standapol® SH-124-3. [Henkel/Cospha] Disodium laureth sulfosuccinate; low-irritation shampoo base for babies and adults; gentle on skin; anti-irritants in blends with other surfactants; clear liq.; toxicology: nonirritating to skin and eyes; 30% act.

Standapol® SH-135. [Henkel/Cospha; Henkel Canada] Disodium oleamido PEG-2 sulfosuccinate; CAS 56388-43-3; EINECS 260-143-1; anionic; nonirritating surfactant for mild shampoos, foam baths; anti-irritant for other surfactants; lt. amber liq. mild pleasant odor; cloud pt. 10 C max.; pH 6–7 (5%); 34–36% act.

Standapol® SH-300. [Henkel/Cospha] Di-TEA-oleamido PEG-2 sulfosuccinate; detergent for personal care prods.; lt. amber liq.; char. odor; cloud pt. < 0 C; pH 6–7 (5%); 39–41% act.

Standapol® SHC-101. [Henkel/Cospha; Henkel Canada] Disodium oleamido PEG-2 sulfosuccinate and sodium lauryl sulfate; anionic; base for low-irritation shampoos for babies and adults; anti-irritant for other surfactants; lt. amber liq.; mild pleasant odor; visc. 1000 cps max.; cloud pt. 0 C max.; pH 6.5–7.5 (5%); 30% min. solids.

Standapol® SP-60. [Henkel] Sodium C12–15 pareth sulfate; surfactant for personal care, household, and industrial cleansing prods.; yel. clear liq.; dens. 1.050 g/ml; visc. 100–200 cps; cloud pt. 10 C max.; pH 7.0–9.0 (10%); 58–60% act.

Standapol® T. [Henkel/Cospha; Henkel Canada] TEA-lauryl sulfate; CAS 139-96-8; EINECS 205-388-7; anionic; detergent, foamer, base for mild shampoos, aerosols; water-wh. liq.; 39% conc.

Standapol® T-315. [Henkel KGaA/Cospha] TEA-C12-15 alkyl sulfate.

Standapol® WA-AC. [Henkel/Cospha; Henkel Canada] Sodium lauryl sulfate; CAS 151-21-3; EINECS 205-788-1; anionic; detergent, foamer, base for cream and paste shampoos, bubble baths; extremely low salt content; pearly-wh. paste; visc. 20,000 cps min.; cloud pt. 25 C max.; pH 7.5–8.5 (10% aq.); 28–30% conc.

Standapol® WAQ-115. [Henkel/Cospha; Henkel Canada] Sodium C12-15 alcohols sulfate; anionic; surfactant for liq. and cream shampoos, bubble baths; yields fine dense foam; water-wh. visc. liq.; visc. 1000 cps max.; cloud pt. 12 C max.; pH 7.5–8.5 (10% aq.); 29–31% conc.

Standapol® WAQ-LC. [Henkel/Cospha; Henkel Canada] Sodium lauryl sulfate; CAS 151-21-3; EINECS 205-788-1; foaming agent, detergent, suspending agent for personal care prods., liq. cleaners; low salt content for improved corrosion resistance; water-wh. liq.; visc. 100 cps max.; cloud pt. 8 C max.; pH 7–9 (10% aq.); 28.5–31.5% conc.

Standapol® WAQ Special. [Henkel/Cospha; Henkel Canada] Sodium lauryl sulfate; CAS 151-21-3; EINECS 205-788-1; anionic; detergent, foamer, base for cream and paste shampoos, bubble baths; extremely low salt content; water-wh. visc. liq.; visc. 1500 cps max.; cloud pt. 15 C max.; pH 7.5–8.5 (10% aq.); 28–30% conc.

Standard Super-Cel. [Celite] Diatomaceous earth; CAS 7631-86-9; EINECS 231-545-4; filter aid and carrier for cosmetics; buff/pink powd.; 4% 150 mesh residue; sp.gr. 2.2; wet dens. 18 lb/ft³.

Stanol 212F. [Henkel-Nopco] Organic sulfates with nonionics; anionic; scouring and fulling agent for wool; shampoo base; bubble baths; liq.; 40% conc.

Star. [Procter & Gamble] Glycerin USP; CAS 56-81-5; EINECS 200-289-5; humectant; in pharmaceuticals, toiletries, tobacco, alkyds, food prods., explosives, cellophane, urethane foam, other industries; APHA 10 max. color; sp.gr. 1.2517.

Starfol® CP. [Witco/H-I-P] Cetyl palmitate; CAS 540-10-3; EINECS 208-736-6; emollient for cosmetic creams, lotions, and lipstick formulations; opacifier and feel modifier; cream-colored flakes; sol. in min. oil.; 100% solids.

Starfol® OS. [Witco/H-I-P] Octyldodecyl stearate; CAS 22766-82-1; EINECS 245-204-2; emollient and moisturizer for creams and lotions; imparts luxurious, conditioned feel to the skin without greasiness; high-temp. lubricant for textiles; lt. amber liq.; 100% solids.

Starfol® Wax CG. [Witco/H-I-P] Cetyl esters; nonionic; syn. spermaceti wax; emollient, opacifier, and feel modifier for cosmetics, creams, lotions; APHA 100 max. flake; sol. in min. oil; m.p. 46–49 C; sapon. no. 109–117; 100% conc.

Starwax® 100. [Petrolite] Hard microcryst. wax consisting of n-paraffinic, branched paraffinic, and naphthenic hydrocarbons; CAS 63231-60-7; EINECS 264-038-1; wax used in hot-melt coatings and adhesives, paper coatings, printing inks, plastic modification (as lubricant and processing aid), lacquers, paints, and varnishes, as binder in ceramics, for potting/impregnant in elec./electronic components, rubber and elastomers (plasticizer, antisunchecking, antiozonant), as emulsion wax size in papermaking, as fabric softener ingred., in emulsion and latex coatings, and in cosmetic hand creams and lipsticks; incl. FDA §172.230, 172.615, 175.105, 175.300, 176.170, 176.180, 176.200, 177.1200, 178.3710, 179.45; color 1.0 (D1500) wax; very low sol. in org. solvs.; sp.gr. 0.93; visc. 15 cps (99 C); m.p. 88 C.

Stearal. [Amerchol] Stearyl alcohol; CAS 112-92-5; EINECS 204-017-6; emollient, aux. emulsifier, texturizer; nonoily, velvety feel; higher visc. in emulsions; wh. waxy solid; mild char. odor; m.p. 55–60 C; acid no. 1.0 max.; sapon. no. 2.0 max.

Stearalchol. [Lanaetex Prods.] Min. oil, lanolin alcohol.

Stearate 400 WL 817. [Gattefosse SA] PEG-8 palmito-stearate; solvent and emulsifier for cosmetic/pharmaceutical emulsions; drop pt. 29-34 C; HLB 11-12; acid no. < 6; iodine no. < 3; sapon. no. 70-95.

Stearate 1500. [Gattefosse SA] PEG (1500) palmitostearate; solvent and emulsifier for cosmetic/pharmaceutical emulsions; drop pt. 46-50 C; HLB 16; acid no. < 6; iodine no. < 3; sapon. no. 30-45; toxicology: nonirritating to skin and eyes.

Stearate 6000 WL 1644. [Gattefosse SA] PEG-150 palmitostearate; solvent and emulsifier for cosmetic/pharmaceutical emulsions; drop pt. 55-60 C; HLB 18; acid no. ≤ 2; iodine no. < 3; sapon. no. 15-25; toxicology: nonirritating to skin; sl. irritating to eyes.

Stearate PEG 1000. [Ceca SA] PEG-21 stearate; CAS 9004-99-3; nonionic; surfactant; solid; HLB 15.3; 100% conc.

Stedbac®. [Zeeland] Stearalkonium chloride; CAS 122-19-0; EINECS 204-527-9; cationic; hair conditioner, emulsifier imparting softness, antistatic properties to cream rinse formulations; powd.; very sol. in water, alcohol; 100% conc.

Steol® 4N. [Stepan; Stepan Canada] Sodium laureth sulfate; CAS 9004-82-4; anionic; detergent, emulsifier, foamer, wetting agent used in personal care prods.; car wash, dishwash; textile mill applics.; emulsion polymerization; water-wh. liq.; water-sol.; sp.gr. 1.045; visc. 31 cps; cloud pt. –4 C; pH 8.0; 28% act.

Steol® CA-130. [Stepan; Stepan Canada] Ammonium laureth sulfate; CAS 32612-48-9; anionic; surfactant, foamer, visc. modifier for shampoo and bath prods.; for low pH systems; low skin irritation; good for children's prods.; liq.; 26% conc.

Steol® CA-230. [Stepan; Stepan Canada] Ammonium laureth sulfate; CAS 32612-48-9; anionic; surfactant, foamer, visc. modifier for shampoo and bath prods.; for low pH systems; low skin irritation props.; good for children's prods.; liq.; 25% conc.

Steol® CA-330. [Stepan; Stepan Canada] Ammonium laureth sulfate; CAS 32612-48-9; anionic; surfactant, foamer, visc. modifier for shampoo and bath prods.; for low pH systems; mild to skin; good for children's prods.; liq.; 27-29% conc.

Steol® CA-460. [Stepan; Stepan Canada] Ammonium laureth sulfate; CAS 32612-48-9; anionic; detergent, emulsifier, foamer, dispersant, visc. modifier, and wetting agent used in shampoos, bath and cleansing preps., dishwashers, car washers, textile mill applics., emulsion polymerization; pale yel. liq.; water-sol.; sp.gr. 1.016; visc. 67 cps; cloud pt. 19 C; pH 7.0; 60% conc.

Steol® CS-130. [Stepan; Stepan Canada] Sodium laureth sulfate; anionic; foamer for shampoos, bath prods., mild cleansers, baby prods.; low skin irritation props.; pH 7.5–8.5 (10% aq.); 26% act.

Steol® CS-230. [Stepan; Stepan Canada] Sodium laureth sulfate; anionic; foamer for shampoos, bath prods., mild

cleansers, baby prods.; low skin irritation props.; liq.; pH 6.5–8.5 (10% aq.); 25% act.

Steol® CS-330. [Stepan; Stepan Canada] Sodium laureth sulfate; anionic; foamer for shampoos, bath prods., mild cleansers, baby prods.; low skin irritation props.; liq.; pH 6.5–8.5 (10% aq.); 28% act.

Steol® CS-460. [Stepan; Stepan Canada] Sodium laureth sulfate; CAS 9004-82-4; anionic; surfactant, foamer, emulsifier for shampoos, bath prods., liq. detergents, carwash, dishwash liq., laundry, alkaline detergents, textiles; pale yel. liq.; water-sol.; sp.gr. 1.037; visc. 69 cps; cloud pt. 17 C; pH 8.0 (1% aq.); 59.5% act.

Steol® KA-460. [Stepan; Stepan Canada] Ammonium laureth sulfate, modified; CAS 32612-48-9; anionic; detergent, emulsifier, foamer and wetting agent used in liq. detergents, shampoos, carwash, textile detergents; suitable for soft and hard waters; biodeg.; straw liq.; water-sol.; dens. 8.65 lb/gal; cloud pt. 0 C; pH 7.0 (10% aq.); 60% act.

Steol® KS-460. [Stepan; Stepan Canada] Sodium laureth sulfate, modified; anionic; surfactant, foamer, emulsifier for liq. detergents, shampoos, carwash, textile detergent; biodeg.; straw liq.; water-sol.; dens. 8.94 lb/gal; cloud pt. 0 C; pH 8.0 (10% aq.); 60% act.

Stepanhold® Extra. [Stepan; Stepan Canada; Stepan Europe] PVP/ethyl methacrylate/methacrylic acid terpolymer; CAS 26589-26-4; hair care fixative for super-hold formulations; visc. fluid; 40% act.

Stepanhold® R-1. [Stepan; Stepan Canada] Acrylates/PVP copolymer; CAS 26589-26-4; hair fixative for hair sprays, setting lotions, conditioners; liq.; 50% act.

Stepan-Mild® LSB. [Stepan; Stepan Canada; Stepan Europe] Sodium lauryl sulfoacetate, disodium laurethsulfosuccinate; surfactant combining exc. foaming with visc. building and mildness; for shampoos, hand soaps, bubble baths, facial cleansers, baby prods., sensitive skin prods.; clear liq.; 25% act.

Stepan-Mild® SL3. [Stepan; Stepan Canada] Disodium laurethsulfosuccinate; surfactant for low-irritation shampoos, bubble baths, hand soaps, and dishwashing detergents; liq.; 32% act.

Stepanol® 317. [Stepan; Stepan Canada] Lauramide DEA, TEA-dodecylbenzenesulfonate, and TEA-laureth sulfate; anionic; dilutable base for shampoos; liq.; 92% conc.

Stepanol® 360. [Stepan; Stepan Canada] Sodium lauryl sulfate, lauramide DEA; conc. for shampoo and bath prods.; liq.; 40% act.

Stepanol® AEG. [Stepan; Stepan Canada] Ammonium lauryl sulfate, ammonium laureth sulfate, cocamidopropyl betaine, cocamide DEA; anionic; base for liq. hand and body soaps, shampoos, and bath prods.; liq.; 42% act.

Stepanol® AEM. [Stepan; Stepan Canada] Ammonium laureth sulfate, cocamide MEA; anionic; surfactant conc. for shampoo and bath prods.; liq.; 48% act.

Stepanol® AM. [Stepan; Stepan Canada] Ammonium lauryl sulfate; CAS 2235-54-3; EINECS 218-793-9; anionic; detergent, foamer, visc. booster used in shampoos, hand soaps, bath prods.; rug and upholstery shampoos; household, metal, and industrial cleaners; fruit washing; insecticides; textile and leather processing; pharmaceuticals; pale yel. visc. liq.; water-sol.; pH 6–7 (10%); 28% act.

Stepanol® AM-V. [Stepan; Stepan Canada] Ammonium lauryl sulfate; CAS 2235-54-3; EINECS 218-793-9; anionic; detergent, foamer, visc. booster used in shampoos, hand soaps, bath prods.; rug and upholstery shampoos; household, metal, and industrial cleaners; fruit washing; insecticides; textile and leather processing; pharmaceuticals; visc. liq., lt. gel; water-sol.; pH 6–7 (10%); 27–29% act.

Stepanol® BS-2. [Stepan Canada] Surfactant blend; baby

shampoo conc.

Stepanol® DEA. [Stepan; Stepan Canada] DEA-lauryl sulfate; CAS 143-00-0; EINECS 205-577-4; anionic; detergent, foamer used in shampoos, bubble baths, liq. hand soaps, clear prods.; rug and upholstery shampoos; household, metal, and industrial cleaners; fruit washing; insecticides; textile and leather processing; pharmaceuticals; pale yel. clear liq.; water-sol.; pH 7.3–7.7 (10%); 34% act.

Stepanol® LX. [Stepan; Stepan Canada] DEA lauryl sulfate, DEA lauraaminopropionate, sodium lauraminopropionate; anionic; mild blended conc. for shampoos, baby soaps, bubble baths; foaming power; substantive to hair and skin; liq.; 36% act.

Stepanol® ME Dry. [Stepan; Stepan Canada] Sodium lauryl sulfate; CAS 151-21-3; EINECS 205-788-1; anionic; detergent, foamer for personal care (dentifrices, tablets, powd. baths, cleansing preps.); rug and upholstery shampoos; household, metal, and industrial cleaners; fruit washing; insecticides; textile and leather processing; pharmaceuticals; wh. powd.; water-sol.; pH 7.5–1.0 (10%); 93% min. act.

Stepanol® MG. [Stepan; Stepan Canada] Magnesium lauryl sulfate; CAS 3097-08-3; EINECS 221-450-6; anionic; detergent, foamer used in personal care prods.; rug and upholstery shampoos; household, metal, and industrial cleaners; fruit washing; insecticides; textile and leather processing; pharmaceuticals; water-sol.; pH 6.5–7.5 (10%); 28–30% act.

Stepanol® WA-100. [Stepan; Stepan Canada; Stepan Europe] Sodium lauryl sulfate USP/NF; CAS 151-21-3; EINECS 205-788-1; anionic; detergent, foamer, wetting and suspending agent; dentifrice formulations where minimal taste contribution is important; pharmaceuticals; emulsion polymerization; clay dispersions; wh. powd.; water-sol.; pH 7.5–10 (10%); 98.5% min. act.

Stepanol® WAC. [Stepan; Stepan Canada; Stepan Europe] Sodium lauryl sulfate; CAS 151-21-3; EINECS 205-788-1; anionic; detergent, foamer, visc. booster used in shampoos, hand soaps, bath prods., shaving creams, medicated ointments; rug and upholstery shampoos; household, metal, and industrial cleaners; fruit washing; insecticides; textile and leather processing; pharmaceuticals; pale yel. clear liq.; water-sol.; pH 7.5–8.5 (10%); 28–30% act.

Stepanol® WA Extra. [Stepan; Stepan Canada] Sodium lauryl sulfate; CAS 151-21-3; EINECS 205-788-1; anionic; detergent, foamer, visc. booster used in shampoos, hand soaps, bath prods., shaving creams, medicated ointments; rug and upholstery shampoos; household, metal, and industrial cleaners; fruit washing; insecticides; textile and leather processing; pharmaceuticals; clear liq.; water-sol.; pH 7.5–8.5 (10%); 29% act.

Stepanol® WA Paste. [Stepan; Stepan Canada] Sodium lauryl sulfate; CAS 151-21-3; EINECS 205-788-1; anionic; detergent, foamer, visc. booster used in shampoos, hand soaps, bath prods., shaving creams, medicated ointments; rug and upholstery shampoos; household, metal, and industrial cleaners; fruit washing; insecticides; textile and leather processing; pharmaceuticals; water-wh. clear paste; water-sol.; pH 7.5–8.5 (10%); 29% act.

Stepanol® WAQ. [Stepan; Stepan Canada] Sodium lauryl sulfate; CAS 151-21-3; EINECS 205-788-1; anionic; detergent, foamer, visc. booster used in shampoos, hand soaps, bath prods., shaving creams, medicated ointments; rug and upholstery shampoos; household, metal, and industrial cleaners; fruit washing; insecticides; textile and leather processing; pharmaceuticals; water-wh. clear visc. liq.; water-sol.; pH 7.5–8.5 (10%); 29% act.

Stepanol® WA Special. [Stepan; Stepan Canada] Sodium lauryl sulfate; CAS 151-21-3; EINECS 205-788-1; anionic; detergent, foamer, visc. booster used in shampoos, hand soaps, bath prods., shaving creams, medicated ointments; rug and upholstery shampoos; household, metal, and industrial cleaners; fruit washing; insecticides; textile and leather processing; pharmaceuticals; water-wh. clear liq.; water-sol.; pH 7.5–8.5 (10%); 29% act.

Stepanol® WAT. [Stepan; Stepan Canada] TEA-lauryl sulfate; CAS 139-96-8; EINECS 205-388-7; anionic; detergent, foamer used in shampoos, bubble baths, liq. hand soaps, clear prods.; rug and upholstery shampoos; household, metal, and industrial cleaners; fruit washing; insecticides; textile and leather processing; pharmaceuticals; water-wh. clear liq.; water-sol.; pH 7.0–8.5 (10%); 40% act.

Stepan Pearl Series. [Stepan Europe] Surfactant blend; pearlescent, satining or opacifying agent, conditioning agent for shampoos, liq. soaps, bubble baths, shower gels; wh. paste.

Stepanquat® 6585. [Stepan; Stepan Canada] Dipalitmoylethyl hydroxyethylmonium methosulfate; cationic; mild surfactant for cream rinses and conditioners; wh. soft paste; 85% act.

Stepan TAB®-2. [Stepan; Stepan Europe] Dihydrogenated tallow phthalic acid amide; CAS 127733-92-0; emulsifier, suspending agent for silicones, zinc pyrithione, sulfur, selenium sulfide, coal tar, oil extracts; opacifier; esp. for use in conditioning and anti-dandruff shampoos; off-wh. to sl. yel. solid, typ. mild fatty odor; sol. in min. and veg. oils, IPP, IPM; insol. in water; m.p. 45 C; flash pt. > 200 F; toxicology: nontoxic; nonirritating to skin; sl. conjunctival irritant; nonsensitizing; 99.7% solids.

Steraffine. [Laserson SA] Stearyl alcohol; CAS 112-92-5; EINECS 204-017-6; emollient, cosmetic/pharmaceutical raw material.

Steralchol. [Lanaetex Prods.] Min. oil and lanolin alcohol; cosmetic ingred.

SteriLine 200. [Montana Talc] Platy talc USP; CAS 14807-96-6; EINECS 238-877-9; general purpose, coarse talc for use in dusting and baby powds., soaps, antiperspirant sticks, color extensions.

SteriLine 665. [Montana Talc] Platy talc USP; CAS 14807-96-6; EINECS 238-877-9; ultrafine talc for cosmetic applics. requiring high oil absorp., gloss control, and smoothness; visc. control additive in pharmaceutical excipient applics.

Sterol CC 595. [Auschem SpA] PEG-6 caprylic/capric glycerides; CAS 52504-24-2; nonionic; superfatting agent; liq.; 100% conc.

Sterol GMS. [Auschem SpA] Glyceryl stearate; CAS 31566-31-1; nonionic; w/o emulsifier, thickener for o/w emulsions; flakes; HLB 3.2; 100% conc.

Sterol LA 300. [Auschem SpA] Ethoxylated veg. oil; nonionic; solubilizer in cosmetic preps.; liq.; 100% conc.

Sterol LG 491. [Auschem SpA] PEG-8 glyceryl laurate; nonionic; superfatting agent; liq.; water-sol.; HLB 11.0; 100% conc.

Sterol SES. [Auschem SpA] PEG-8 stearyl stearate; nonionic; coemulsifier and thickener for cosmetic emulsions; solid; HLB 12.0; 100% conc.

Sterol ST 1. [Auschem SpA] Glycol stearate; CAS 111-60-4; EINECS 203-886-9; nonionic; pearling agent, w/o emulsifier; flakes; HLB 2.7; 100% conc.

Sterol ST 2. [Auschem SpA] PEG-2 stearate; CAS 9004-99-3; 106-11-6; EINECS 203-363-5; nonionic; pearling agent, w/o emulsifier; solid; HLB 4.7; 100% conc.

Sterol TE 200. [Auschem SpA] Blend of PEG esters; nonionic; self-emulsifying base for o/w creams in cosmetics and pharmaceuticals; paste; 100% conc.

Sterotex®. [Karlshamns] Hydrog. veg. oil; CAS 68334-28-

1; EINECS 269-820-6; binder and internal lubricant for pressed powds., food and pharmaceutical tablets, compacting and compounding processes in the catalyst, ceramic, and powd. metallurgy fields; powd.; m.p. 60-63 C; acid no. 0.4 max.; iodine no. 5 max.; sapon. no. 188-198.

Sterotex® C. [Karlshamns] Hydrog. soybean oil and carnauba wax; CAS 8016-70-4 and 8105-86-9; tablet lubricant for pharmaceuticals, nutrition, lipstick base in cosmetics; carnauba replacement; mold lubricant and binder in powd. metallurgy, catalysts, and ceramics; wh. to lt. tan powd., odorless; insol. in water; sp.gr. 0.9 (100 F); m.p. 79-82 C; b.p. > 500 F; acid no. 2.5 max.; iodine no. 5 max.; sapon. no. 164-174; flash pt. (COC) > 500 F.

Sterotex® HM NF. [Karlshamns] Hydrog. soybean oils; CAS 8016-70-4; EINECS 232-410-2; lubricant in pharmaceutical tableting, nutrition, powd. compression applics; lipstick base in cosmetics; mold lubricant and binder in powd. metallurgy, catalysts, and ceramics; fine wh. powd., yel. oil when melted; insol. in water; sp.gr. 0.9; m.p. 67-70 C; b.p. > 500 F; acid no. 0.4 max.; iodine no. 5 max.; sapon. no. 186-196; flash pt. (COC) > 550 F.

Sterotex® K. [Karlshamns] Hydrog. soybean oil, hydrog. castor oil; CAS 8016-70-4 and 8001-78-3; tablet lubricant for pharmaceuticals; lipstick base in cosmetics; mold lubricant and binder in powd. metallurgy, catalysts, and ceramics; wh. to lt. tan powd., odorless; insol. in water; sp.gr. 0.9; bulk dens. 0.48; m.p. 81-84 C; b.p. > 500 f; acid no. 1 max.; iodine no. 5 max.; sapon. no. 185-195; flash pt. (COC) > 600 F; toxicology: nontoxic.

Sterotex® NF. [Karlshamns] Hydrog. veg. oil; CAS 68334-00-9; EINECS 269-820-6; lubricant for tableting and compaction in pharmaceuticals, nutritional supplements, powd. metallurgy, catalysts, and ceramics; wh. powd. @ R.T., lt. yel. oil when melted; insol. in water; sp.gr. 0.9; b.p. > 500 F; flash pt. (COC) > 640 F.

Stimulant HS 280. [Alban Muller] Propylene glycol, sage extract, rosemary extract, lavender extract, and thyme extract; herbal extract for tonic shower gels.

Stimulant HS 285. [Alban Muller] Propylene glycol, myrrh extract, ivy extract, tormentil extract, wild marjoram extract, olibanum, and gum benzoin; phytocomplex for tonic shower gels.

Stimulant LS 680. [Alban Muller] Sunflower seed oil, sage extract, rosemary extract, lavender extract, and thyme extract; herbal extract for tonic shower gels.

Stimulant LS 685. [Alban Muller] Benzoin, incense, myrrh, ivy, oregano, tormentil phytocomplex; for tonic shower gels.

St. John's Wort Oil CLR. [Dr. Kurt Richter; Henkel/Cospha] Fatty oil extract of St. John's wort blossoms; general skin protection, esp. for sensitive skin; red-brn. oil.

Stokopol LO. [Stockhausen] Sodium C12-18 alkyl sulfate.

Styrene MC Beads. [U.S. Cosmetics] provides mild, scrubbing action when used in skin care prods.; stimulates blood circulation and removes old horny layers, wastes, and dusts on the skin; spherical beads.

Sucro Ester 7. [Gattefosse SA] Saccharose distearate; CAS 25168-73-4; nonionic; food emulsifier; o/w emulsifier wetting agent, crystallization inhibitor for veg. oils and fats; inhibitor of thermal denaturation of proteins; tableting agent and lipophilic matrix for pharmaceuticals/cosmetics; fine powd., faint odor; sol. in water @ 75 C, in ethanol @ 60 C; insol. in veg. and min. oils; HLB 7.0; acid no. < 5; sapon. no. 115-135; toxicology: LD50 (oral, rat) > 5 g/kg; 100% conc.

Sucro Ester 11. [Gattefosse SA] Saccharose mono/distearate; CAS 25168-73-4; nonionic; food emulsifier; o/w emulsifier wetting agent, crystallization inhibitor for veg. oils and fats; inhibitor of thermal denaturation of proteins; tableting agent and lipophilic matrix for pharmaceuticals/

cosmetics; fine powd., faint odor; sol. in water @ 75 C, in ethanol @ 60 C; insol. in min. and veg. oils; HLB 11.0; acid no. < 5; sapon. no. 110-130; toxicology: LD50 (oral, rat) > 5 g/kg; 100% conc.

Sucro Ester 15. [Gattefosse SA] Saccharose palmitate; CAS 25168-73-4; nonionic; food emulsifier; o/w emulsifier wetting agent, crystallization inhibitor for veg. oils and fats; inhibitor of thermal denaturation of proteins; solvent and emulsifier for pharmaceutical/cosmetic emulsions; fine powd., faint odor; sol. in water and ethanol @ 60 C; insol. in min. and veg. oils; HLB 15.0; acid no. < 5; sapon. no. 95-135; toxicology: LD50 (oral, rat) > 8 g/kg; 100% conc.

Sugartab®. [Mendell] Sucrose (90-93%), invert sugar; CAS 57-50-1; EINECS 200-334-9; inert base for directly compressible pharmaceutical tablets; wh. free-flowing powd.; avg. particle size 296 μ; 30% -80 mesh; very sol. in water; sl. sol. in alcohol; dens. (tapped) 0.6-0.9 g/ml.

Sulcoidal. [Universal Preserv-A-Chem] Colloidal sulfur; cosmetic ingred.

Sulfetal CJOT 38. [Zschimmer & Schwarz] MIPA-lauryl sulfate; CAS 21142-28-9; EINECS 244-238-5; anionic; basic material for hair shampoos, bath additives, cosmetics, liq. detergents; straw-colored clear visc. liq.; dens. 1.02 g/cc; visc. 5000-10,000 mPa·s; cloud pt. 8 C; pH 6.5-7.0 (10%); 38% act. in water.

Sulfetal CJOT 60. [Zschimmer & Schwarz] MIPA-lauryl sulfate; CAS 21142-28-9; EINECS 244-238-5; anionic; for hair shampoos, bath additives; liq.; 60% act.

Sulfetal KT 400. [Zschimmer & Schwarz] TEA-lauryl sulfate; CAS 139-96-8; EINECS 205-388-7; anionic; for detergents, cosmetics, hair shampoos; liq.; 40% conc.

Sulfetal MG 30. [Zschimmer & Schwarz] Magnesium lauryl sulfate; CAS 3097-08-3; EINECS 221-450-6; anionic; for detergents, cosmetics; liq.; 30% conc.

Sulfochem AEG. [Chemron] Blend; anionic; base for personal care prods.; liq.; 42% conc.

Sulfochem ALS. [Chemron] Ammonium lauryl sulfate; CAS 2235-54-3; EINECS 218-793-9; anionic; surfactant, mild detergent for use in low pH systems; foaming and suspending agent; for personal care and industrial applics.; water-wh. liq.; 29% conc.

Sulfochem B-209. [Chemron] Blend; anionic; mild shampoo blend conc.; liq.; 39% conc.

Sulfochem B-209OP. [Chemron] Blend; anionic; mild shampoo blend conc.; pearlized version of Sulfochem B-209 allowing cold blending procedures; liq.; 42% conc.

Sulfochem B-221. [Chemron] Blend; anionic; base with dense, long-lasting foam; for shampoo, body soap, liq. hand cleaner formulations; liq.; 34% conc.

Sulfochem B-221OP. [Chemron] Blend; anionic; base with dense, long-lasting foam; for shampoo, body soap, liq. hand cleaner formulations; pearlized version of Sulfochem B-221 permitting cold blend procedures; liq.; 37% conc.

Sulfochem DLS. [Chemron] DEA-lauryl sulfate; CAS 143-00-0; EINECS 205-577-4; anionic; surfactant foamer with soap-like chars.; for shampoos, bubble baths, skin cleaners, syndet bars, shower gels; liq.; 37% conc.

Sulfochem EA-1. [Chemron] Ammonium laureth (1) sulfate; CAS 32612-48-9; anionic; surfactant for low pH shampoo systems; mildness, high flash foam, low cloud pt., visc. response; for shampoos, cleansers, bath prods., gels; water-wh. liq.; 27% conc.

Sulfochem EA-2. [Chemron] Ammonium laureth (2) sulfate; CAS 32612-48-9; anionic; surfactant for low pH shampoo systems; mildness, high flash foam, low cloud pt., visc. response; water-wh. liq.; 27% conc.

Sulfochem EA-3. [Chemron] Ammonium laureth (3) sulfate; CAS 32612-48-9; anionic; surfactant for low pH shampoo systems; mildness, high flash foam, low cloud pt., visc.

response; water-wh. liq.; 27% conc.

Sulfochem EA-60. [Chemron] Ammonium laureth (3) sulfate; CAS 32612-48-9; anionic; surfactant for shampoo systems, bubble baths, cleansers; water-wh. to pale yel. liq.; 59% conc.

Sulfochem EA-70. [Chemron] Ammonium laureth (2) sulfate; CAS 32612-48-9; anionic; surfactant for toiletries and cosmetics; pale yel. flowing gel; 68% conc.

Sulfochem ES-1. [Chemron] Sodium laureth-1 sulfate; anionic; surfactant for personal care cleansers; water-wh. liq.; 27% conc.

Sulfochem ES-2. [Chemron] Sodium laureth-2 sulfate; CAS 9004-82-4; anionic; flash foamer and detergent for personal cleansing prods., specialty cleaning prods.; water-wh. liq.; 27% conc.

Sulfochem ES-3. [Chemron] Sodium laureth-3 sulfate; anionic; surfactant for personal cleansing prods.; water-wh. liq.; 27% conc.

Sulfochem ES-60. [Chemron] Sodium laureth-3 sulfate; anionic; surfactant for shampoo systems, bubble baths, cleansers; water-wh. to pale yel. liq.; 59% conc.

Sulfochem ES-70. [Chemron] Sodium laureth-2 sulfate; CAS 9004-82-4; anionic; surfactant for toiletries, cosmetics, specialty industrial compds.; pale yel. flowing gel; 69% conc.

Sulfochem K. [Chemron] Potassium lauryl sulfate; CAS 4706-78-9; EINECS 225-190-4; anionic; detergent, foamer; liq.; 30% conc.

Sulfochem MG. [Chemron] Magnesium lauryl sulfate; CAS 3097-08-3; EINECS 221-450-6; anionic; mild detergent, foamer for bubblebath, shampoos, cleansing preps., carpet shampoos; liq.; 30% conc.

Sulfochem MLS. [Chemron] MEA-lauryl sulfate; CAS 4722-98-9; EINECS 225-214-3; anionic; surfactant foamer with soap-like chars.; for shampoos, bubble baths, skin cleaners, shower gels, syndet bars; liq.; 33% conc.

Sulfochem SAC. [Chemron] Sodium lauryl sulfate; CAS 151-21-3; EINECS 205-788-1; anionic; foamer for lotion and paste shampoos; detergent base for pearlescent shampoos, bubble baths, shower gels, cleansers; wh. pearlescent paste; 28-30% act.

Sulfochem SBS. [Chemron] Blend; anionic; mild shampoo conc. for baby and premium shampoos; liq.; 55% conc.

Sulfochem SLC. [Chemron] Sodium lauryl sulfate; CAS 151-21-3; EINECS 205-788-1; surfactant for clear shampoos, bath prods., cleaners; water-wh. liq.; 28-30% act.

Sulfochem SLN. [Chemron] Sodium lauryl sulfate; CAS 151-21-3; EINECS 205-788-1; foamer, dispersant, wetting agent, detergent for dry blends used in cleaning compds., carpet shampoos, shampoo concs., bubble baths, cosmetic cleansers; wh. needles; 88% act.

Sulfochem SLP. [Chemron] Sodium lauryl sulfate; CAS 151-21-3; EINECS 205-788-1; foamer, dispersant, wetting agent, detergent for high-act., cleaning concs., dentifrices, bath prods., cleansers; wh. powd.; 90% act.

Sulfochem SLP-95. [Chemron] Sodium lauryl sulfate; CAS 151-21-3; EINECS 205-788-1; foamer, dispersant, wetting agent, detergent for high-act., cleaning concs., dentifrices, high purity cleansers; wh. powd.; 95% act.

Sulfochem SLS. [Chemron] Sodium lauryl sulfate; CAS 151-21-3; EINECS 205-788-1; anionic; detergent, foamer, suspending agent for hard surf. cleaners, carpet shampoos, upholstery cleaners, spot removers, personal care prods.; water-wh. liq.; 29% conc.

Sulfochem TLS. [Chemron] TEA-lauryl sulfate; CAS 139-96-8; EINECS 205-388-7; anionic; surfactant foamer, wetting agent with soap-like chars.; for liq. soaps and shampoos, industrial applics.; good tolerance to hard water; water-wh. liq.; 40% conc.

Sulfocos 2B. [Cosmetochem] PEG-6 isolauryl thioether;

detergent, emulsifier.

Sul-fon-ate AA-10. [Boliden Intertrade] Sodium dodecylbenzene sulfonate; CAS 25155-30-0; EINECS 246-680-4; anionic; wetting agent; air pollution control; cement, food, commercial laundry and industrial industries; cosmetics; fertilizers, insecticides; leather, paper, petrol., and rubber processing; metal cleaning, electroplating, etching, pickling; mining; wh. crisp flake; sol. in water; pH 6–8 (1%); surf. tens. 33.2 dynes/cm (0.05%, 86 F); toxicology: toxic orally; LD50 (male rat, oral) 1-5 g/kg; eye and skin irritant but nontoxic dermally; 96% act.

Sulfopon® 101 Special. [Henkel KGaA/Cospha; Pulcra SA] Sodium lauryl sulfate; CAS 151-21-3; EINECS 205-788-1; anionic; surfactant for shampoos, specialty cleaners, and lt.-duty detergents; emulsifier for emulsion polymerization; low freezing pt.; paste; m.w. 302; pH 7.5-8.5 (101%); 30% conc.

Sulfopon® 103. [Henkel KGaA/Cospha] Sodium lauryl sulfate; CAS 151-21-3; EINECS 205-788-1; anionic; detergent and wetting agent for personal care prods.; wh. pearly paste; pH 7.0-7.5 (10%); 28-30% act.

Sulfopon® P-40. [Pulcra SA] Sodium lauryl sulfate; CAS 151-21-3; EINECS 205-788-1; anionic; dispersant and emulsifier for acrylates, styrene acrylic, vinyl chloride, vinyl acetate copolymers; also for cream shampoos, specialty cleaners, rug shampoos; paste; m.w. 302; pH 6.0-7.0 (10%); 38-42% act.

Sulfopon® WA 3. [Henkel Canada] Sodium lauryl sulfate; CAS 151-21-3; EINECS 205-788-1; anionic; detergent, foamer for cream and paste shampoos, bubble baths; wh. paste; 28–30% act.

Sulfopon® WAQ LCX. [Henkel Canada] Sodium lauryl sulfate; CAS 151-21-3; EINECS 205-788-1; anionic; detergent, foamer; base for shampoos and bubble baths; rug shampoos; liq.; 30% conc.

Sulfopon® WAQ Special. [Henkel Canada] Sodium lauryl sulfate; CAS 151-21-3; EINECS 205-788-1; anionic; surfactant for personal care prods., rug shampoos, lt. duty detergents; water-wh. liq.; 28–30% act.

Sumquat® 2355. [Zeeland] Benzyl triethyl ammonium chloride; CAS 56-37-1; EINECS 200-270-1.

Sumquat® 6020. [Zeeland] Cetethyldimonium bromide; CAS 124-03-8; EINECS 204-672-8; germicide, detergent.

Sumquat® 6030. [Zeeland] Cetrimonium bromide; CAS 57-09-0; EINECS 200-311-3; quat. for personal care prods.

Sumquat® 6045. [Zeeland] Distearyldimonium chloride; CAS 107-64-2; EINECS 203-508-2; conditioner for cosmetics.

Sumquat® 6050. [Zeeland] Cetalkonium chloride; CAS 122-18-9; EINECS 204-526-3; germicide, surfactant.

Sumquat® 6110. [Zeeland] Myrtrimonium bromide; CAS 1119-97-7; EINECS 214-291-9; antimicrobial surfactant.

Sumquat® 6210. [Zeeland] Stearalkonium chloride; CAS 122-19-0; EINECS 204-527-9; conditioner, antistat.

Sun Chemical Colorants. [Sun Chem. Corp./Colors] Organic and inorganic colorants for the cosmetic industry.

Sun Espol G-318. [Taiyo Kagaku] Triisostearin.

Sungen. [Sederma] Hydrolyzed soy protein and shea butter unsaponifiables; antistress, desensibilization factor, SPF booster with erythema soothing effect for sun care prods., day and foundation creams; pale yel. fluid emulsion, char. odor; sp.gr. 0.95-1.05; pH 5.3-6.3; usage level: 3-8%.

Sunnol 710 H. [Lion] POE alkyl ether sulfate; anionic; detergent and personal care prods.; paste; 70% conc.

Sunnol CM-1470. [Lion] POE laureth sulfate; anionic; shampoos, detergents; paste; 70% conc.

Sunnol DL-1430. [Lion] POE alkyl ether sulfate; anionic; shampoos, detergents, bubble baths; liq.; 27% conc.

Sunnol LM-1100. [Lion] Lauryl sulfate; anionic; foaming

agent for shampoo and toothpaste; powd.; 100% conc.

Sunnol LM-1140T. [Lion] TEA lauryl sulfate; CAS 139-96-8; EINECS 205-388-7; anionic; shampoos, detergents, bubble baths; liq.; 39-41% conc.

Sunsoft 601. [Taiyo Kagaku] Diglyceryl stearate malate.

Sun-Tanning Bioactivator AMI, VITAMI. [Alban Muller] Glucose tyrosinate; sun-tan facilitator.

Sunveil. [Ikeda] Titanium dioxide with 0.15% methyl paraben; sunscreening agent forming a very thin transparent layer on skin; wh. or sl. ylsh. translucent liq.; pH 7.0-9.0; 9-11% TiO_2.

Sunveil 6010. [Ikeda] Titanium dioxide; CAS 13463-67-7; EINECS 236-675-5; sunscreening agent forming a very thin transparent layer on skin; wh. or sl. ylsh. liq.; pH 6.0-8.0; 9-11% TiO_2.

Sunveil 6030. [Ikeda] Titanium dioxide; CAS 13463-67-7; EINECS 236-675-5; sunscreening agent forming a very thin transparent layer on skin; wh. or sl. ylsh. liq.; pH 6.0-8.0; 25-26.5% TiO_2.

Sunveil F. [Ikeda] Titanium dioxide and iron oxides; sunscreen agent providing wider range of uv protection (to 400 nm); for colored sun care prods.; dk. red liq.; particle size 5 μm x 60 μm; pH 7-9; 25-26.5% TiO_2.

Supercol® Guar Gum. [Aqualon] Guar gum; CAS 9000-30-0; EINECS 232-536-8; cosmetic thickener.

Super Corona. [Croda Inc.] Refined anhyd. lanolin USP; CAS 8006-54-0; EINECS 232-348-6; superfatting emollient and emulsifier for cosmetics and pharmaceuticals; improves spreading, penetration, and aesthetic properties of these prods.; plasticizer in aerosol hairsprays; stable w/o emulsions; Gardner 8.5 max. soft solid, pract. odorless; partly sol. in min. oil; m.p. 38-44 C; acid no. 1.0 max; iodine no. 18-36; toxicology: LD50 (oral, rat) > 20 g/kg; mild skin and eye irritant.

Superfine Lanolin. *See Anhydrous Lanolin USP Superfine*

Superfine Lanolin Anhydrous USP. [Croda Inc.] Lanolin; CAS 8006-54-0; EINECS 232-348-6; superfatting emollient with some emulsifying properties; used in pharmaceutical ointments, dressing creams, diaper rash and hemorrhoidal preps.; yel./amber soft solid; low odor; partly sol. in min. oil; m.p. 38-44 C; toxicology: LD50 (oral, rat) > 20 g/kg; mild skin and eye irritant.

Super Floss. [Celite] Diatomaceous earth; CAS 7631-86-9; EINECS 231-545-4; carrier and functional filler for cosmetics; wh. fine powd.; 0.2% 325 mesh residue; surf. area 0.7-3.5 m²/g; sp.gr. 2.3; dens. 8.7 lb/ft³ (loose); wet dens. 21 lb/ft³; oil absorp. 120 lb/100 lb; ref. index 1.48; pH 10 max.

Super Hartolan. [Croda Inc.; Croda Chem. Ltd.] Lanolin alcohol NF; CAS 8027-33-6; EINECS 232-430-1; nonionic; spreading agent, dispersant, stabilizer, plasticizer, w/o emulsifier, emulsion stabilizer, thickener, and emollient for cosmetics and pharmaceuticals; pale amber solid wax; sol. in IPA, partly sol. in min. oil, disp. in propylene glycol; m.p. 60 C min.; HLB 1.0; acid no. 1.5 max.; sapon. no. 5 mg max.; usage level: 0.5-3%; toxicology: LD50 (oral, rat) 20 g/kg; mild skin and eye irritant; 100% conc.

Superla® No. 5. [Amoco Lubricants] Wh. min. oil USP; used in pharmaceuticals, cosmetics, food, agric., plastics, textiles, and polishes; FDA, USDA approved; kosher; colorless, odorless, tasteless; sp.gr. 0.844; visc. 8.4 cSt (40 C); pour pt. -12 C; flash pt. 149 C; ref. index 1.4660.

Superla® No. 6. [Amoco Lubricants] Wh. min. oil USP; used in pharmaceuticals, cosmetics, food, agric., plastics, textile, and polishes; FDA, USDA approved; kosher; colorless, odorless, tasteless; sp.gr. 0.847; visc. 10.9 cSt (40 C); pour pt. -15 C; flash pt. 174 C; ref. index 1.4664.

Superla® No. 7. [Amoco Lubricants] Wh. min. oil USP; used in pharmaceuticals, cosmetics, food, agric., plastics, textile, and polishes; FDA, USDA approved; kosher; color-

less, odorless, tasteless; sp.gr. 0.849; visc. 14.0 cSt (40 C); pour pt. -15 C; flash pt. 185 C; ref. index 1.4666.

Superla® No. 9. [Amoco Lubricants] Wh. min. oil USP; used in pharmaceuticals, cosmetics, food, agric., plastics, textile, and polishes; FDA, USDA approved; kosher; colorless, odorless, tasteless; sp.gr. 0.850; visc. 16.0 cSt (40 C); pour pt. -15 C; flash pt. 193 C; ref. index 1.4715.

Superla® No. 10. [Amoco Lubricants] Wh. min. oil USP; used in pharmaceuticals, cosmetics, food, agric., plastics, textile, and polishes; FDA, USDA approved; kosher; colorless, odorless, tasteless; sp.gr. 0.850; visc. 18.4 cSt (40 C); pour pt. -15 C; flash pt. 193 C; ref. index 1.4728.

Superla® No. 13. [Amoco Lubricants] Wh. min. oil USP; used in pharmaceuticals, cosmetics, food, agric., plastics, textile, and polishes; FDA, USDA approved; kosher; colorless, odorless, tasteless; sp.gr. 0.854; visc. 26.2 cSt (40 C); pour pt. -12 C; flash pt. 190 C; ref. index 1.4728.

Superla® No. 18. [Amoco Lubricants] Wh. min. oil USP; used in pharmaceuticals, cosmetics, food, agric., plastics, textile, and polishes; FDA, USDA approved; kosher; colorless, odorless, tasteless; sp.gr. 0.857; visc. 36.3 cSt (40 C); pour pt. -12 C; flash pt. 193 C; ref. index 1.4738.

Superla® No. 21. [Amoco Lubricants] Wh. min. oil USP; used in pharmaceuticals, cosmetics, food, agric., plastics, textile, and polishes; FDA, USDA approved; kosher; colorless, odorless, tasteless; sp.gr. 0.859; visc. 40.2 cSt (40 C); pour pt. -12 C; flash pt. 210 C; ref. index 1.4744.

Superla® No. 31. [Amoco Lubricants] Wh. min. oil USP; used in pharmaceuticals, cosmetics, food, agric., plastics, textile, and polishes; FDA, USDA approved; kosher; colorless, odorless, tasteless; sp.gr. 0.865; visc. 60.5 cSt (40 C); pour pt. -12 C; flash pt. 227 C; ref. index 1.4763.

Superla® No. 35. [Amoco Lubricants] Wh. min. oil USP; used in pharmaceuticals, cosmetics, food, agric., plastics, textile, and polishes; FDA, USDA approved; kosher; colorless, odorless, tasteless; sp.gr. 0.865; visc. 69.3 cSt (40 C); pour pt. -12 C; flash pt. 232 C; ref. index 1.4772.

Superloid® . [Kelco] Refined ammonium alginate; CAS 9005-34-9; gum used as gelling agent, thickener, emulsifier, film-forming agent, suspending agent, and stabilizer in food, pharmaceutical, and industrial applics.; stabilizer in paper and textile industry; tan gran. particles; water-sol.; sp.gr. 1.73; dens. 56.62 lb/ ft³; visc. 1500 cps; ref. index 1.3347; pH 5.5; 13% moisture.

Supermontaline SLT65. [Seppic] Dioctyl sodium sulfosuccinate; CAS 577-11-7; EINECS 209-406-4; anionic; wetting agent and emulsifier; liq.; 65% conc.

Superol. [Procter & Gamble] Glycerin USP; CAS 56-81-5; EINECS 200-289-5; humectant; in pharmaceuticals, toiletries, tobacco, alkyds, food prods., explosives, cellophane, urethane foam, other industries; APHA 10 max. color; sp.gr. 1.2612.

Superpolystate. [Gattefosse SA] PEG-6 stearate SE; CAS 9004-99-3; nonionic; SE gelling base for pharmaceutical and cosmetic lotions; Gardner < 5 doughy solid; very sol. in chloroform, methylene chloride; disp. in water; insol. in ethanol, min. oils; drop pt. 33-37 C; HLB 9.0; acid no. < 6; iodine no. < 3; sapon. no. 90-110; hyd. no. 75-105; toxicology: LD50 (oral, rat) > 2 g/kg; nonirritating to skin and eyes; 100% conc.

Superpro 5A. [Inolex] TEA coco-hydrolyzed collagen, sorbitol; CAS 68952-16-9, 50-70-4; anionic; detergent, conditioner, emulsifier, moisturizer, foamer used in personal care prods.; Gardner 10 max. liq.; sp.gr. 1.15 min.; visc. 400 cps min.; pH 7.0-7.5; 68% act.

Super Refined™ Almond Oil NF. [Croda Inc.; Croda Surf. Ltd.] Almond oil; emollient; provides elegant skin feel and promotes spreading in creams, lotions, bath oils; solv. and vehicle for pharmaceuticals (parenteral formulations for intramuscular administration, nutritional supplements, IV emulsions, liniments, ointments); APHA 40 color; sol. in min. oil, IPA; toxicology: LD50 (oral, rat) > 5 g/kg; nonirritating to skin.

Super Refined™ Apricot Kernel Oil NF. [Croda Inc.; Croda Surf. Ltd.] Apricot kernel oil; CAS 72869-69-3; emollient; lubricant and softener in nail oils; conditioner for hair care prods.; APHA 30.

Super Refined™ Avocado Oil. [Croda Inc.; Croda Surf. Ltd.] Avocado oil; CAS 8024-32-6; EINECS 232-428-0; emollient; provides elegant skin feel and promotes spreading in creams, lotions, bath oils; emollient for hair care prods.; APHA 30.

Super Refined™ Babassu Oil. [Croda Inc.; Croda Surf. Ltd.] Babassu oil; emollient for sunscreen prods.; APHA 20.

Super Refined™ Corn Oil. [Croda Inc.] Corn oil NF; CAS 8001-30-7; EINECS 232-281-2; solv. and vehicle for pharmaceuticals (parenteral formulations for intramuscular administration, nutritional supplements, IV emulsions, liniments, ointments); APHA 40 color; sol. in min. oil, IPA.

Super Refined™ Cottonseed Oil. [Croda Inc.] Cottonseed oil; CAS 8001-29-4; EINECS 232-280-7; solv. and vehicle for pharmaceuticals (parenteral formulations for intramuscular administration, nutritional supplements, IV emulsions, liniments, ointments); APHA 50 color; sol. in min. oil, IPA.

Super Refined™ Crossential EPO. [Croda Inc.; Croda Surf. Ltd.] Evening primrose oil; emollient; contains essential fatty acids vital to health of skin; APHA 20.

Super Refined™ Grapeseed Oil. [Croda Inc.] Grapeseed oil; CAS 8024-22-4; emollient; APHA 50.

Super Refined™ Menhaden Oil. [Croda Inc.] Menhaden oil; CAS 8002-50-4; EINECS 232-311-4; emollient; contains essential fatty acids vital to health of skin; dietary supplement and therapeutic applics.; APHA 100 color, faint char. odor; sol. in min. oil, IPA.

Super Refined™ Mink Oil. [Croda Inc.; Croda Surf. Ltd.] Mink oil; emollient oil for makeup remover systems; APHA 30.

Super Refined™ Olive Oil. [Croda Inc.; Croda Surf. Ltd.] Olive oil; CAS 8001-25-0; EINECS 232-277-0; cosmetic emollient; lubricant for hair care prods.; solv. and vehicle for pharmaceuticals (parenteral formulations for intramuscular administration, nutritional supplements, IV emulsions, liniments, ointments); APHA 30 color; sol. in min. oil, IPA.

Super Refined™ Orange Roughy Oil. [Croda Inc.; Croda Surf. Ltd.] Orange roughy oil; emollient, softener, spreading agent, and solubilizer in skin care prods. and pharmaceuticals; APHA 30 color, faint char. odor; sol. in min. oil, IPA; toxicology: LD50 (oral, rat) > 5 g/kg; minimal skin irritant, nonirritating to eyes.

Super Refined™ Peanut Oil. [Croda Inc.] Peanut oil; CAS 8002-03-7; EINECS 232-296-4; emollient in skin care prods.; solv. and vehicle for pharmaceuticals (parenteral formulations for intramuscular administration, nutritional supplements, IV emulsions, liniments, ointments); APHA 30 color; sol. in min. oil, IPA.

Super Refined™ Safflower Oil USP. [Croda Inc.; Croda Surf. Ltd.] Safflower oil; CAS 8001-23-8; EINECS 232-276-5; emollient; solv. and vehicle for pharmaceuticals (parenteral formulations for intramuscular administration, nutritional supplements, IV emulsions, liniments, ointments); APHA 30 mobile oil; sol. in min. oil, IPA; toxicology: LD50 (oral, rat) > 5 g/kg; minimal eye and skin irritant.

Super Refined™ Sesame Oil. [Croda Inc.; Croda Surf. Ltd.] Sesame oil; CAS 8008-74-0; EINECS 232-370-6; emollient oil used in skin care preps.; solv. and vehicle for pharmaceuticals (parenteral formulations for intramuscular administration, nutritional supplements, IV emulsions, liniments, ointments); APHA 30 color; sol. in min. oil, IPA;

toxicology: LD50 (oral, rat) > 5 g/kg; mild skin irritant, minimal eye irritant.

Super Refined™ Shark Liver Oil. [Croda Inc.; Croda Surf. Ltd.] Shark liver oil; CAS 68990-63-6; EINECS 273-616-2; emollient, moisture repellent for skin protection; protectant that softens and smooths skin tissues for hemorrhoidal preps.; FDA recognized; APHA 40 color, faint char. odor; sol. in min. oil, IPA; usage level: 3% conc.; toxicology: LD50 (oral, rat) > 5 g/kg; moderate skin irritant, minimal eye irritant.

Super Refined™ Soybean Oil USP. [Croda Inc.; Croda Surf. Ltd.] Soybean oil; CAS 8001-22-7; EINECS 232-274-4; emollient oil used in skin care preps.; solv. and vehicle for pharmaceuticals (parenteral formulations for intramuscular administration, nutritional supplements, IV emulsions, liniments, ointments); APHA 60 color; sol. in min. oil, IPA; toxicology: LD50 (oral, rat) > 5 g/kg; mild skin irritant, minimal eye irritant.

Super Refined™ Sunflower Oil. [Croda Inc.; Croda Surf. Ltd.] Sunflower seed oil; CAS 8001-21-6; EINECS 232-273-9; cosmetic ingred.

Super Refined™ Wheat Germ Oil. [Croda Inc.; Croda Surf. Ltd.] Wheat germ oil; CAS 8006-95-9; emollient; contains essential fatty acids vital to health of skin; used in facial creams; moisturizer in hair care prods.; APHA 250.

Super-Sat. [R.I.T.A.] Hydrog. lanolin; CAS 8031-44-5; EINECS 232-452-1; nonionic; plasticizer, emollient, spreading agent for cosmetics and pharmaceuticals (makeups, night creams, shaving creams); high water absorp.; imparts smooth afterfeel to skin; vehicle for actives in skin prods.; hardener for wax systems; wh. to lt. yel. tacky solid; sol. in ethyl ether, chloroform; insol. in water; sp.gr. 0.855-0.865; m.p. 48-53 C; acid no. 2 max.; iodine no. 20 max.; sapon. no. 6 max.; hyd. no. 140-165; usage level: 0.1-25%; 100% act.

Super-Sat AWS-4. [R.I.T.A.] PEG-20 hydrog. lanolin; CAS 977055-17-6; nonionic; emollient, emulsifier, visc. control agent, and plasticizer for emulsion systems; gelling agent for transparent gels; solubilizer for min./veg. oils and perfumes; suggested for aftershaves, hair dressings, facial cleansers, nail polish removers; amber solid, bland odor; slightly water-sol.; acid no. 1 mqx.; iodine no. 10 max.; sapon. no. 8 max.; hyd. no. 32-47; 100% conc.

Super-Sat AWS-24. [R.I.T.A.] PEG-24 hydrog. lanolin; CAS 977055-17-6; nonionic; emollient, plasticizer, emulsifier, visc. control agent; gelling agent for transparent gels; solubilizer for min./veg. oils and perfumes; suggested for aftershaves, hair dressings, facial cleansers, nail polish removers; wh. flakes, bland odor; acid no. 1 max.; iodine no. 10 max.; sapon. no. 8 max.; hyd. no. 32-47; 100% conc.

Super Solan Flaked. [Croda Inc.] PEG-75 lanolin; CAS 61790-81-6; emollient, conditioner, superfatting agent, solubilizer, and plasticizer; used in cleansing wipe formulations; yel. flake; sol. in water, propylene glycol; sol. warm in IPA; m.p. 46-54 C; usage level: 1-10%; toxicology: LD50 (oral, rat) > 5 g/kg; minimal skin irritant, nonirritating to eyes.

Super Sterol Ester. [Croda Inc.; Croda Chem. Ltd.] C10–30 cholesterol/lanosterol esters; emollient, lubricant, and moisturizer for dry skin, cosmetics, pharmaceuticals (ointments, dressing creams); softening agent in transdermal delivery systems due to its hypoallergenicity; soft wh. solid; sol. in min. oil, IPA, esters; m.p. 30-38 C; usage level: 1-10%; toxicology: LD50 (oral, rat) > 5 g/kg; mild skin irritant.

Super White Fonoline®. [Witco/Petroleum Spec.] Wh. petrolatum USP; CAS 8027-32-5; EINECS 232-373-2; low m.p. grade with superior snow white color, exhibiting elegant feel and texture; for premium cosmetic formulations and food related applics.; FDA clearance; visc. 55-65 SUS (210 F); m.p. 122-133 F.

Super White Protopet® . [Witco/Petroleum Spec.] Wh. petrolatum USP; CAS 8027-32-5; EINECS 232-373-2; high purity, med. consistency, med. m.p. grade for premium cosmetic and pharmaceutical formulations where extra whiteness is preferred; also for food applics.; FDA § 172.880; Lovibond 1.0Y max. color; visc. 60-70 SUS (210 F); m.p. 130-140 F.

Supoweiss. [Unichema] Suppository bases for pharmaceuticals.

Suppocire A. [Gattefosse SA] Hemisynthetic glycerides; excipient for pharmaceutical suppositories; drop pt. 35-40 C; toxicology: LD50 (oral, rat) > 20 ml/kg, nonirritating rectally.

Suppocire AI. [Gattefosse SA] Hemisynthetic glycerides; excipient for pharmaceutical suppositories; drop pt. 33-35 C; acid no. < 0.5; iodine no. < 2; sapon. no. 225-245; toxicology: LD50 (oral, rat) > 20 ml/kg; nonirritating rectally.

Suppocire AIM. [Gattefosse SA] Hemisynthetic glycerides; excipient for pharmaceutical suppositories; drop pt. 33.-40 C; acid no. < 0.2; iodine no. < 2; sapon. no. 230-250; toxicology: LD50 (oral, rat) > 20 ml/kg, nonirritating rectally; sl. irritating to eyes.

Suppocire AIML. [Gattefosse SA] Hemisynthetic glycerides; excipient for pharmaceutical suppositories; drop pt. 33-35 C; acid no. < 0.5; iodine no. < 3; sapon. no. 230-250; toxicology: LD50 (oral, rat) > 20 ml/kg, nonirritating rectally.

Suppocire AIP, AP, BP, CP. [Gattefosse SA] Saturated polyglycolized glycerides; excipient for pharmaceutical suppositories; drop pt. 30-39 C; acid no. < 1; iodine no. < 1; sapon. no. 205-225, 200-220, 200-220, and 195-215 resp.; toxicology: LD50 > 20 ml/kg; nonirritating rectally.

Suppocire AIX. [Gattefosse SA] Hemisynthetic glycerides; excipient for pharmaceutical suppositories; drop pt. 33-35 C; acid no. < 0.5; iodine no. < 2; sapon. no. 220-240; toxicology: nonirritating rectally.

Suppocire AM. [Gattefosse SA] Hemisynthetic glycerides; excipient for pharmaceutical suppositories; drop pt. 33-36.5 C; acid no. < 0.2; iodine no. < 2; sapon. no. 225-245; toxicology: LD50 (oral, rat) > 20 ml/kg, nonirritating rectally; sl. irritating to eyes.

Suppocire AML. [Gattefosse SA] Hemisynthetic glycerides; excipient for pharmaceutical suppositories; drop pt. 35-36.5 C; acid no. < 0.5; iodine no. < 3; sapon. no. 225-245; toxicology: LD50 (oral, rat) > 20 ml/kg, nonirritating rectally.

Suppocire AS2. [Gattefosse SA] Hemisynthetic glycerides; excipient for pharmaceutical suppositories; drop pt. 35-36.5 C; acid no. < 0.5; iodine no. < 2; sapon. no. 225-245; toxicology: LD50 (oral, rat) > 20 ml/kg.

Suppocire AS2X. [Gattefosse SA] Hemisynthetic glycerides; excipient for pharmaceutical suppositories; drop pt. 35-36.5 C; acid no. < 0.5; iodine no. < 2; sapon. no. 225-245; toxicology: nonirritating rectally.

Suppocire B. [Gattefosse SA] Hemisynthetic glycerides; excipient for pharmaceutical suppositories; drop pt. 36-37.5 C; acid no. < 0.5; iodine no. < 2; sapon. no. 225-245; toxicology: LD50 (oral, rat) > 20 ml/kg, nonirritating rectally.

Suppocire BM. [Gattefosse SA] Hemisynthetic glycerides; excipient for pharmaceutical suppositories; drop pt. 36-37.5 C; acid no. < 0.2; iodine no. < 2; sapon. no. 225-245; toxicology: LD50 (oral, rat) > 20 ml/kg, nonirritating rectally; sl. irritating to eyes.

Suppocire BML. [Gattefosse SA] Hemisynthetic glycerides; excipient for pharmaceutical suppositories; drop pt. 36-37.5 C; acid no. < 0.5; iodine no. < 3; sapon. no. 225-245;

toxicology: LD50 (oral, rat) > 20 ml/kg, nonirritating rectally.

Suppocire BS2. [Gattefosse SA] Hemisynthetic glycerides; excipient for pharmaceutical suppositories; drop pt. 36-37.5 C; acid no. < 0.5; iodine no. < 2; sapon. no. 225-245; toxicology: LD50 (oral, rat) > 20 ml/kg.

Suppocire BS2X. [Gattefosse SA] Hemisynthetic glycerides; excipient for pharmaceutical suppositories; drop pt. 36-37.5 C; acid no. < 0.5; iodine no. < 2; sapon. no. 220-240.

Suppocire C. [Gattefosse SA] Hemisynthetic glycerides; excipient for pharmaceutical suppositories; drop pt. 38-40 C; acid no. < 0.5; iodine no. < 2; sapon. no. 220-240; toxicology: LD50 (oral, rat) > 20 ml/kg, nonirritating rectally.

Suppocire CM. [Gattefosse] Hydrog. palm glycerides, hydrog. palm kernel glycerides; excipient for pharmaceutical suppositories; drop pt. 38-40 C; acid no. < 0.2; iodine no. < 2; sapon. no. 225-245; toxicology: LD50 (oral, rat) > 20 ml/kg; sl. irritating to eyes, nonirritating to skin.

Suppocire CS2. [Gattefosse SA] Hemisynthetic glycerides; excipient for pharmaceutical suppositories; drop pt. 38-40 C; acid no. < 0.5; iodine no. < 2; sapon. no. 225-245; toxicology: LD50 (oral, rat) > 20 ml/kg.

Suppocire CS2X. [Gattefosse SA] Hemisynthetic glycerides; excipient for pharmaceutical suppositories; drop pt. 38-40 C; acid no. < 0.5; iodine no. < 2; sapon. no. 220-240.

Suppocire DM. [Gattefosse SA] Hemisynthetic glycerides; excipient for pharmaceutical suppositories; drop pt. 42-45 C; acid no. < 0.2; iodine no. < 2; sapon. no. 220-240.

Suppocire NA. [Gattefosse SA] Hemisynthetic glycerides; excipient for pharmaceutical suppositories; drop pt. 34.5-36.5 C; acid no. < 0.5; iodine no. < 2; sapon. no. 225-245.

Suppocire NAI. [Gattefosse SA] Hemisynthetic glycerides; excipient for pharmaceutical suppositories; drop pt. 33.5-40.5 C; acid no. < 0.5; iodine no. < 2; sapon. no. 225-245.

Suppocire NB. [Gattefosse SA] Hemisynthetic glycerides; excipient for pharmaceutical suppositories; drop pt. 36.5-38.5 C; acid no. < 0.5; iodine no. < 2; sapon. no. 225-245; toxicology: LD50 (oral, rat) > 20 ml/kg, nonirritating rectally.

Suppocire NC. [Gattefosse SA] Hemisynthetic glycerides; excipient for pharmaceutical suppositories; drop pt. 38.5-40.5 C; acid no. < 0.5; iodine no. < 2; sapon. no. 220-240.

Supra A. [Luzenac Am.] Platy talc USP; CAS 14807-96-6; EINECS 238-877-9; extremely platy talc with high brightness, exc. slip; recommended for formulations with very sensitive fragrances and pigments; used in dusting and pressed powds., antiperspirants, creams, lotions, bath and loose powds.; powd.; 99% thru 200 mesh; median diam. 12 μ; tapped dens. 62 lb/ft^3; pH 9 (10% slurry).

Supra EF. [Luzenac Am.] Platy talc; CAS 14807-96-6; EINECS 238-877-9; for cosmetic applics. incl. dusting and pressed powds., creams and lotions, antiperspirants, bath and loose powds.

Supra EF A. [Luzenac Am.] Platy talc USP; CAS 14807-96-6; EINECS 238-877-9; extrafine, extremely platy talc with exc. brightness, purity, surface passivity, and slip; used for dusting and pressed powds., antiperspirants, creams, lotions, bath and loose powds. and as detackifying agent for fine rubber prods.; powd.; 99.6% thru 200 mesh; median diam. 8 μ; tapped dens. 59 lb/ft^3; pH 9 (10% slurry).

Supraene® . [Robeco] Purified squalene; CAS 111-02-4; EINECS 203-826-1; patented natural emollient, protective agent, vehicle for dermatological, cosmetic, and medical use, lubricating and finishing oils, printing oils, carriers of perfumes; lt. straw-colored liq. oil, faint char. odor; misc. with veg. and min. oils, org. solvs., lipophilic substances, human sebum; insol. in water; m.w. 410.73;

sp.gr. 0.855-0.865; visc. 15 cps; f.p. -75 C; b.p. 335 C; acid no. 1 max.; iodine no. 360-380; sapon. no. 2 max.; flash pt. 200 C; ref. index 1.4945-1.4960; toxicology: nontoxic; 99% min. purity.

Suprafino A. [Luzenac Am.] Talc USP; CAS 14807-96-6; EINECS 238-877-9; extremely platy talc with high slip, brightness, and purity; for cosmetic applics. incl. antiperspirants, eye shadows, soaps, creams and lotions, nail polish, aerosols; powd.; 99.9% thru 325 mesh; median diam. 5 µ; tapped dens. 44 lb/ft^3; pH 9 (10% slurry).

Suprafino SMD. [Luzenac Am.] Platy talc surface-modified with a triglyceride; CAS 14807-96-6; EINECS 238-877-9; enhanced emulsifying action for binding pressed powds.; exc. texture for longer wearing makeup without greasy effect; recommended for eye shadows, antiperspirants, soaps, creams, lotions, nail polish, aerosols; powd.; 99.9% thru 325 mesh; median diam. 5 µ; tapped dens. 45 lb/ft^3.

Supralate C. [Witco/H-I-P] Sodium lauryl sulfate USP; CAS 151-21-3; EINECS 205-788-1; anionic; emulsifier, dispersant, detergent, wetting agent for cosmetic, dental and medical preps.; wh. spray-dried beads; mild fatty odor; water sol.; dens. 3.3 lb/gal; 90–96% conc.; formerly Duponol® C.

Supralate EP. [DuPont] DEA-lauryl sulfate, tech.; CAS 143-00-0; EINECS 205-577-4; anionic; foaming agent, detergent, wetting agent, emulsifier used for cosmetics, personal care prods.; very pale golden, slightly visc. liq.; bland and clean odor; sol. in water, polar solv. with some electrolyte precipitation; dens. 8.4 lb/gal; visc. 50–150 cps ; cloud pt. 5 C; 33-36% act.; formerly Duponol® EP.

Supralate FAS. [Witco/H-I-P] Ethoxylated alkyl sulfate, nonionic surfactant; anionic; detergent; liq.; formerly Duponol® FAS.

Supralate G. [Witco/H-I-P] Fatty alcohol amine sulfate; anionic; emulsifier, wetting agent; yel. visc. translucent paste; mild fatty penetrating odor; sol. in hydrocarbons, 50% in water; dens. 8.2 lb/gal; surf. tens. 29.6 dynes/cm (0.1%); 92% act.; formerly Duponol® G.

Supralate QC. [Witco/H-I-P] Sodium lauryl sulfate; CAS 151-21-3; EINECS 205-788-1; anionic; detergent, shampoo base; water wh. slightly visc. liq.; bland clean, char. odor; sol. in water, polar solv. with some electrolyte precipitation; visc. < 500 cps; cloud pt. 65 F; 29–30% act.; formerly Duponol® QC.

Supralate WA Paste. [Witco/H-I-P] Sodium lauryl sulfate; CAS 151-21-3; EINECS 205-788-1; anionic; detergent, shampoo base, superior cleansing and foaming, textile scouring; liq.; formerly Duponol® WA Paste.

Supralate XL. [Witco/H-I-P] Alkyl alcohol sulfate; anionic; shampoo surfactant, detergent, conditioner; golden moderately visc. liq.; faintly spicy odor; sol. in water, in polar solv. with some electrolyte precipitation; visc. 2500–4500 cps; cloud pt. 50 F; clear pt. 50–55 F; 36% solids.; formerly Duponol® XL.

Supreme USP. [Luzenac Am.] Talc; CAS 14807-96-6; EINECS 238-877-9; cosmetic ingred.

Supro-Tein S. [Maybrook] Sodium cocoyl hydrolyzed soy protein and sorbitol; mild foaming substantive protein providing soft afterfeel; protects and conditions skin and hair; mild surfactant for bleached and permed hair; aux. thickener and conditioner; for baby shampoos, conditioners, ethnic shampoos, styling prods.; skin care lotions, hand and face cleansers, bath prods., depilatories; biodeg.; amber sl. hazy liq., char. odor; pH 7.0-8.0; 50-60% solids.

Supro-Tein V. [Maybrook] TEA-coco-hydrolyzed animal protein, sorbitol; CAS 68952-16-9, 50-70-4; anionic; mild surfactant with foam stability; emulsifier, solubilizer, moisturizer; for ethnic and mild shampoos, conditioners, lotions, hair and skin mousses, liq. soap, shave creams; lt. amber clear to sl. hazy visc. liq., mild char. odor; pH 7.0-7.5; 68-72% solids.

Surfactol® 13. [CasChem] Castor oil, modified; CAS 1323-38-2; nonionic; wetting agent, emulsifier, solubilizer, dispersant, wax plasticizer, mold release agent, antifoamer for textiles, leather, paints, household, cosmetics, dyeing, tanning, finishing, sizing, making of cutting and sol. oils, oilfield chems.; biodeg.; FDA approval; Gardner 4 liq.; faint odor; water-sol.; sp.gr. 1.005; dens. 8.36 lb/gal; visc. 17 stokes; iodine no. 70; sapon. no. 130; hyd. no. 425; flash pt. 385 F; toxicology: sl. skin or eye irritant; low oral toxicity; 100% conc.

Surfactol® 318. [CasChem] PEG-5 castor oil; CAS 61791-12-6; nonionic; emulsifier for oils, waxes; solubilizer for fragrances; emollient; used in textiles, paints, household, cosmetics, dyeing, tanning, finishing, sizing, insecticides, herbicides, fungicides, kier boiling, making of cutting and sol. oils, dispersing waxes, pigments, resins, rewetting dried skins; FDA approval; Gardner 3 liq.; faint odor; sol. in toluene, butyl acetate, MEK; sp.gr. 0.984; dens. 8.2 lb/gal; visc. 690 cps; pour pt. -25 C; HLB 3.8; acid no. 0.2; iodine no. 70; sapon. no. 148; hyd. no. 141; flash pt. 525 F; toxicology: sl. eye or skin irritant; low oral toxicity; 100% conc.

Surfactol® 340. [CasChem] Ethoxylated castor oil; CAS 61791-12-6; wetting agent, wax plasticizer, mold release agent, antifoam for textiles, leather, paints, household, cosmetics, dyeing, tanning, finishing, sizing, cutting and sol. oils, dispersing waxes, pigments, resins; Gardner 4 color; sp.gr. 1.015; dens. 8.4 lb/gal; visc. 5 stokes; pour pt. -30 F; acid no. 0.3; iodine no. 51; sapon. no. 108; hyd. no. 112; flash pt. 520 F; toxicology: low oral toxicity.

Surfactol® 365. [CasChem] PEG-40 castor oil; CAS 61791-12-6; nonionic; emulsifier for oils, waxes; solubilizer for fragrances; emollient; used in textiles, paints, household, cosmetics, dyeing, tanning, finishing, sizing, insecticides, herbicides, fungicides, kier boiling, making of cutting and sol. oils; FDA approval; clear amber liq., char. odor; sol. in toluene, butyl acetate, MEK, ethanol, and water; sp.gr. 1.054; dens. 8.8 lb/gal; visc. 500 cps; m.p. 10 C; HLB 13.3; acid no. 0.2; iodine no. 36; sapon. no. 68; hyd. no. 80; flash pt. (PMCC) 520 F; toxicology: sl. eye or skin irritation; low oral toxicity; 100% conc.

Surfactol® 380. [CasChem] Ethoxylated castor oil; CAS 61791-12-6; wetting agent, wax plasticizer, mold release agent, antifoam for textiles, leather, paints, household, cosmetics, dyeing, tanning, finishing, sizing, cutting and sol. oils, dispersing waxes, pigments, resins; Gardner 3 paste; water-sol.; sp.gr. 1.076; dens. 9.0 lb/gal; acid no. 0.2; iodine no. 23; sapon. no. 36; hyd. no. 50; toxicology: sl. eye or skin irritant; low oral toxicity.

Surfactol® 575. [CasChem] PEG-66 trihydroxystearin; CAS 61788-85-0; emulsifier for oils, waxes; solubilizer for fragrances; emollient; used in textiles, paints, household, cosmetics, dyeing, tanning, finishing, sizing, insecticides, herbicides, fungicides, kier boiling, making of cutting and sol. oils; wh. solid; water-sol.; alcohol; sp.gr. 1.08; dens. 9.0 lb/gal; m.p. 39 C; HLB 15.; toxicology: skin and eye irritant; inhalation may cause severe choking reaction.

Surfactol® 590. [CasChem] PEG-200 trihydroxystearin; CAS 61788-85-0; nonionic; emulsifier for oils, waxes; solubilizer for fragrances; emollient; used in textiles, paints, household, cosmetics, dyeing, tanning, finishing, sizing, insecticides, herbicides, fungicides, kier boiling, making of cutting and sol. oils; wh. solid; sol. in water, alcohol; sp.gr. 1.18; dens. 9.8 lb/gal; m.p. 53 C; HLB 18; acid no. 1.2; iodine no. 50; sapon. no. 18; hyd. no. 24; 100% conc.

Surfactol® Q1. [CasChem] Ricinoleamidopropyltrimonium

chloride, propylene glycol; CAS 127311-98-2; cationic; surfactant, emollient, refatting agent, antistat, emulsifier for skin and hair care prods., clear shampoos; Gardner 2 clear liq., mild odor; water-sol.; dens. 7.8 lb/gal; pour pt. -15 C; HLB 13.0; flash pt. (PMCC) > 210 F; pH 3.5 (3% aq.); toxicology: mild irritant to skin and eyes; nontoxic orally; 56% act.

Surfactol® Q2. [CasChem] Hydroxystearamidopropyl trimonium chloride, propylene glycol; cationic; surfactant, emollient, emulsifier, refatting agent, antistat for conditioners, liq. hand soaps, shampoos, skin lotions; Gardner 5 color; water-disp.; m.p. 35 C; HLB 8.0; iodine no. < 5; flash pt. (PMCC) > 200 F; pH 3.5 (3% aq.); toxicology: mild eye irritant; nontoxic orally, dermally; 58% act.

Surfactol® Q3. [CasChem] Hydroxystearamidopropyl trimonium methosulfate, propylene glycol; cationic; surfactant, emulsifier, emollient, antistat for aerosols and mousses, liq. hand soaps, shampoos, skin lotions; compat. in aerosol systems without corroding cans; Gardner 5 color; water-disp.; m.p. 45 C; HLB 8.0; iodine no. < 5; flash pt. (PMCC) > 210 F; pH 3.5 (3% aq.); toxicology: minimal eye or skin irritation; nontoxic orally; 54% act.

Surfactol® Q4. [CasChem] Ricinoleamidopropyl ethyldimonium ethosulfate; CAS 112324-16-0; emollient, emulsifier for personal care prods. (shampoos, conditioners, aerosols); Gardner 3+ clear liq., mild odor; water-sol.; dens. 7.8 lb/gal; pour pt. 20 F; flash pt. (PMCC) > 210 F; toxicology: mild eye or skin irritant; nontoxic orally; 95% act.

Surfadone® LP-100. [ISP] Caprylyl pyrrolidone; surfactant for personal care use; specialty solv. for commercial cleaning, textile processing, lithographic printing prods., water-borne coatings; biodeg.; pale yel. low visc., clear to sl. hazy liq.; sol. in polar and nonpolar solvs. incl. ethanol, acetone, xylene, heptane, paraffin oil, Stod., perchloroethylene; sparingly sol. in water; m.w. 192; sp.gr. 0.92; b.p. 100 C (0.3 mm Hg); solid. pt. -25 C; HLB 6; flash pt. (TCC) 119 C; surf. tens. 28 dynes/cm; Draves wetting 3.5 s (0.1%); Ross-Miles foam 25 mm (initial, 0.1%); toxicology: LD50 (oral) 2.05 g/kg; not a primary skin or eye irritant; noncomedogenic; 97% min. act.

Surfadone® LP-300. [ISP] Lauryl pyrrolidone; surfactant for personal care use; provides enhanced body, improved combability, higher sheen, foam boosting/stabilization, visc., and clarity to shampoos; complete replacement for a variety of additives; specialty solv. for commercial cleaning, textile processing, lithographic printing prods., water-borne coatings; biodeg.; pale yel. low visc., clear to sl. hazy liq.; sol. in polar and nonpolar solvs. incl. ethanol, acetone, xylene, heptane, paraffin oil, Stod., perchloroethylene; sparingly sol. in water; m.w. 253; sp.gr. 0.90; b.p. 145 C (0.2 mm Hg); solid. pt. 10 C; HLB 3; flash pt. (TCC) 116 C; surf. tens. 26 dynes/cm; Draves wetting > 300 s (0.1%); Ross-Miles foam 13 mm (initial, 0.1%); usage level: 1-2%; toxicology: LD50 (oral) > 5 g/kg; not a primary skin or eye irritant; noncomedogenic; 97% min. act.

Surfagene FDD 402. [Chem-Y GmbH] Laureth-3 phosphate; CAS 39464-66-9; anionic; emulsifier for cosmetic formulations, oil baths; additive for mineral collectors; liq.; 99% act.

Surfagene S 30. [Chem-Y GmbH] Disodium laureth-3 sulfosuccinate; CAS 39354-45-5; anionic; mild raw material for personal care prods., baby prods., shampoo, foam baths; mild to skin and eyes; biodeg.; Hazen 200 max. clear liq.; sp.gr. 1.1 kg/l; visc. 200 mPa·s; pH 6.0-7.5; toxicology: less eye irritation than sodium laureth sulfates; 40% conc. in water.

Surfax 40. [Aquatec Quimica SA] TEA lauryl sulfate; CAS 139-96-8; EINECS 205-388-7; anionic; detergent, foam-

ing agent for shampoos and bubble baths; liq.; 40% conc.

Surfax 100. [Aquatec Quimica SA] Sodium lauryl sulfate; CAS 151-21-3; EINECS 205-788-1; anionic; detergent, dispersant, wetting agent for toothpaste, shampoos, bubble baths; powd.; 90% conc.

Surfax 100 AG. [Aquatec Quimica SA] Sodium lauryl sulfate; CAS 151-21-3; EINECS 205-788-1; anionic; detergent, dispersant, wetting agent for toothpaste, shampoos, bubble baths; needles; 90% conc.

Surfax AC 50. [Aquatec Quimica SA] Disodium cocoamphodiacetate; CAS 68650-39-5; EINECS 272-043-5; amphoteric; mild detergent, wetting and foaming agent for baby shampoos; liq.; 50% conc.

Surfax AC 55. [Aquatec Quimica SA] Disodium cocoamphodiacetate, sodium lauryl sulfate; anionic; mild detergent, wetting and foaming agent for shampoos; liq.; 34% conc.

Surfax ACB. [Aquatec Quimica SA] Coco betaine; CAS 68424-94-2; EINECS 270-329-4; amphoteric; mild detergent for shampoos, foam baths, other foaming toiletries; liq.; 30% conc.

Surfax ACI. [Aquatec Quimica SA] Disodium cocoamphodiacetate; CAS 68650-39-5; EINECS 272-043-5; amphoteric; mild detergent, wetting and foaming agent for baby shampoos; liq.; 30% conc.

Surfax ACR. [Aquatec Quimica SA] Cocamidopropyl betaine; CAS 61789-40-0; amphoteric; mild detergent for shampoos, bubble baths, and other foaming toiletries; liq.; 30% conc.

Surfax ASD. [Aquatec Quimica SA] Ammonium lauryl sulfate, buffered; CAS 2235-54-3; EINECS 218-793-9; anionic; detergent for shampoos; liq.; 25% conc.

Surfax CJ. [Aquatec Quimica SA] Ammonium laureth sulfate and ammonium lauryl sulfate; anionic; detergent for shampoos, bubble baths, other foaming toiletries; liq.; 25% conc.

Surfax CN. [Aquatec Quimica SA] Sodium lauryl sulfate; CAS 151-21-3; EINECS 205-788-1; anionic; detergent, dispersant, foaming and wetting agent for shampoos, shaving creams; base for rug and household cleaners; liq.; 30% conc.

Surfax EAD. [Aquatec Quimica SA] Sodium laureth sulfate; anionic; detergent for shampoos; liq.; 27% conc.

Surfax ECM. [Aquatec Quimica SA] MEA laureth sulfate; CAS 977067-77-8; anionic; detergent for shampoos; liq.; 29% conc.

Surfax EDT. [Aquatec Quimica SA] TEA laureth sulfate; CAS 27028-82-6; anionic; detergent for shampoos; liq.; 32% conc.

Surfax EKZ. [Aquatec Quimica SA] Ammonium laureth sulfate; CAS 32612-48-9; anionic; detergent for shampoos; liq.; 24% conc.

Surfax EVE. [Aquatec Quimica SA] Sodium laureth sulfate; CAS 3088-31-1; anionic; detergent for shampoos; liq.; 28% conc.

Surfax MEA. [Aquatec Quimica SA] MEA lauryl sulfate; CAS 4722-98-9; EINECS 225-214-3; anionic; detergent and foaming agent for shampoos and bubble baths; liq.; 32% conc.

Surfax MG. [Aquatec Quimica SA] Magnesium lauryl sulfate; CAS 3097-08-3; EINECS 221-450-6; anionic; detergent and foaming agent for shampoos; base for rug and household cleaners; liq.; 29% conc.

Surfax NH. [Aquatec Quimica SA] Ammonium lauryl sulfate; CAS 2235-54-3; EINECS 218-793-9; anionic; detergent for shampoos; liq.; 28% conc.

Surfax SLA. [Aquatec Quimica SA] Disodium laureth sulfosuccinate and sodium laureth sulfate; anionic; detergent, wetting and foaming agent for baby shampoos; liq.; 27% conc.

Surfax SME. [Aquatec Quimica SA] Disodium cocamido

MEA-sulfosuccinate; anionic; mild detergent for shampoos, foam baths, other foaming toiletries; liq.; 28% conc.

Surfine AZI-A. [Finetex] Nonoxynol-10 carboxylic acid; CAS 53610-02-9; nonionic; detergent, wetter, lime soap dispersant, emulsifier, solubilizer, coupler; for liq. detergents, household, personal care, industrial and institutional prods.; liq.; 90% conc.

Surfine T-A. [Finetex] Trideceth-7 carboxylic acid; nonionic; detergent, wetting agent, lime soap dispersant for cosmetic and household formulations; liq.; 90% conc.

Surfine WLG-A. [Finetex] Ethoxylated alcohol carboxylic acid; coupler, solubilizer, lime soap dispersant for hard surf. cleaners, personal care prods.

Surfine WLL. [Finetex] Sodium laureth-13 carboxylate; CAS 33939-64-9; anionic; solubilizer and coupler, lime soap dispersant for mild hair and body shampoos; improves formulation stability; gel; 70% conc.

Surfine WNG-A. [Finetex] C14-15 pareth-8 carboxylic acid; nonionic; detergent, wetting agent, emulsifier, solubilizer and coupler used in detergents; liq.; 90% conc.

Surfine WNT-A. [Finetex] C12-15 pareth-7 carboxylic acid; CAS 88497-58-9; nonionic; detergent, wetting agent, lime soap dispersant used in cosmetic and household formulations; liq.; 90% conc.

Surfine WNT Conc. [Finetex] Carboxylated alcohol ethoxylate; anionic; detergent, wetting agent; dispersant for household and cosmetic formulations; liq.; 85% conc.

Surfine WNT Gel. [Finetex] Sodium C12–15 pareth-7 carboxylic acid; CAS 70632-06-3; anionic; detergent, wetting agent, lime soap dispersant for cosmetic and household formulations; gel; 60% conc.

Surfine WNT LC. [Finetex] Sodium C12–15 pareth-7 carboxylate; CAS 70632-06-3; anionic; detergent, wetting agent, dispersant for cosmetic and household formulations; liq.; 50% conc.

Surfine WNT-LS. [Finetex] Sodium C12-15 pareth-7 carboxylate; CAS 70632-06-3; anionic; detergent, wetting agent, lime soap dispersant for cosmetic and household formulations; liq.; 95% conc.

Surfonic® L12-3. [Texaco] C10-12 pareth-3; nonionic; biodeg. surfactant for detergent, laundry prespotters, hard surf. cleaners, emulsifiers, personal care prods.; agric. pesticides; clear to sl. turbid liq.; water-insol.; m.w. 295; dens. 7.8 lb/gal; HLB 9.0; hyd. no. 190; pour pt. -15 C; flash pt. (PMCC) 280 F; pH 5.5-6.5 (1% in aq. IPA); 100% conc.

Surfonic® L12-6. [Texaco] C10-12 pareth-6; nonionic; biodeg. surfactant for detergent, laundry prespotters, hard surf. cleaners, emulsifiers, personal care prods.; agric. pesticides; clear to sl. turbid liq.; water-sol.; m.w. 428; dens. 8.2 lb/gal; HLB 12.4; hyd. no. 133; pour pt. 10 C; cloud pt. 48-52 C (1% aq.); flash pt. (PMCC) 325 F; pH 5.5-6.5 (1% in aq. IPA); 100% conc.

Surfonic® L12-8. [Texaco] C10-12 pareth-8; nonionic; surfactant for detergent, laundry prespotters, hard surf. cleaners, emulsifiers, personal care prods., agric. pesticides; liq.; HLB 13.7; 100% conc.

Surfonic® L24-1. [Texaco] Ethoxylated alcohol; nonionic; surfactant for detergents, personal care prods.; liq.; HLB 4.5; 100% conc.

Surfonic® L24-2. [Texaco] C12-14 pareth-2; nonionic; biodeg. surfactant for detergents, laundry prespotters, hard surf. cleaners, personal care prods., agric. pesticides; clear to sl. turbid liq.; water-insol.; m.w. 267; dens. 7.5 lb/gal; HLB 5.3; hyd. no. 210; pour pt. 10 C; flash pt. (PMCC) 240 F; pH 5.5-6.5 (1% in aq. IPA); 100% conc.

Surfonic® L24-3. [Texaco] C12-14 pareth-3; CAS 68439-50-9; nonionic; biodeg. surfactant for detergents, laundry prespotters, hard surf. cleaners, personal care prods., agric. pesticides; clear to sl. turbid liq.; water-insol.; m.w.

330; dens. 7.8 lb/gal; HLB 8.0; hyd. no. 170; pour pt. 5 C; flash pt. (PMCC) 305 F; pH 5.5-6.5 (1% in aq. IPA); 100% conc.

Surfonic® L24-7. [Texaco] C12-14 pareth-7; CAS 68439-50-9; nonionic; biodeg. surfactant for detergents, laundry prespotters, hard surf. cleaners, personal care prods.; agric. pesticides; clear to sl. turbid liq.; water-sol.; m.w. 487; dens. 8.1 lb/gal; HLB 11.9; hyd. no. 117; pour pt. 15 C; cloud pt. 48-52 C (1% aq.); flash pt. (PMCC) 375 F; pH 5.5-6.5 (1% in aq. IPA); 100% conc.

Surfonic® L24-9. [Texaco] C12-14 pareth-8.2; nonionic; biodeg. surfactant for detergents, laundry prespotters, hard surf. cleaners, personal care prods., agric. pesticides; clear to sl. turbid semiliq.; water-sol.; m.w. 561; dens. 8.3 lb/gal; HLB 13.0; hyd. no. 100; pour pt. 20 C; cloud pt. 73-77 C (1% aq.); flash pt. (PMCC) 325 F; pH 5.5-6.5 (1% in aq. IPA); 100% conc.

Surfonic® L24-12. [Texaco] C12-14 pareth-10.8; nonionic; biodeg. surfactant for detergents, laundry prespotters, hard surf. cleaners, personal care prods., agric. pesticides; waxy solid; water-sol.; m.w. 703; dens. 8.4 lb/gal; HLB 14.4; hyd. no. 83; pour pt. 28 C; cloud pt. 65-71 C (1% in 10% NaCl); flash pt. (PMCC) 400 F; pH 5.5-6.5 (1% in aq. IPA); 100% conc.

Surfonic® L42-3. [Texaco] Ethoxylated alcohol; nonionic; surfactant for detergents, personal care prods.; liq.; HLB 7.6; 100% conc.

Surfonic® L46-7. [Texaco] C14-16 pareth-7; nonionic; biodeg. surfactant, detergent, emulsifier, foamer, penetrant, intermediate for detergent, laundry prespotters, hard surf. cleaners, personal care prods., agric. pesticides; clear to sl. turbid liq.; water-sol.; m.w. 534; dens. 8.0 lb/gal; HLB 11.6; hyd. no. 107; pour pt. 22 C; cloud pt. 48-52 C (1% aq.); flash pt. (PMCC) 400 F; pH 5.5-6.5 (1% in aq. IPA); 100% conc.

Surfonic® L46-8X. [Texaco] Alkyl polyoxyalkylene ether; nonionic; low pour pt. surfactant; liq.; 100% conc.

Surfonic® N-10. [Texaco] Nonoxynol-1; EINECS 248-762-5; nonionic; biodeg. emulsifier, wetting agent, detergent, penetrant, solubilizer, dispersant for household cleaners, textile, agric., metal cleaning, petrol, cosmetic, latex paint, cutting oil, janitorial supply industries; FDA compliance; clear sl. visc. liq.; water-insol.; oil-sol.; m.w. 264; dens. 8.1 lb/gal; HLB 3.4; flash pt. (PMCC) 340 F; Ross-Miles foam 5 mm (initial, 0.1%, 120 F); 100% act.

Surfonic® N-31.5. [Texaco] Nonoxynol-3; CAS 9016-45-9; nonionic; biodeg. emulsifier, wetting agent, detergent, penetrant, solubilizer, dispersant for household cleaners, textile, agric., metal cleaning, petrol, cosmetic, latex paint, cutting oil, janitorial supply industries; FDA compliance; clear sl. visc. liq.; water-insol., oil-sol.; m.w. 358; sp.gr. 1.01; dens. 8.4 lb/gal; visc. 480 SUS (100 F); HLB 7.7; hyd. no. 157; flash pt. (PMCC) 405 F; ref. index 1.4950; Ross-Miles foam 8 mm (initial, 0.1%, 120 F); 100% act.

Surfonic® N-40. [Texaco] Nonoxynol-4; CAS 9016-45-9; nonionic; biodeg. emulsifier, wetting agent, detergent, penetrant, solubilizer, dispersant for household cleaners, textile, agric., metal cleaning, petrol, cosmetic, latex paint, cutting oil, janitorial supply industries; FDA compliance; clear sl. visc. liq.; sol. in acetone, methanol, xylene, CCl4, Stoddard; m.w. 396; sp.gr. 1.026; dens. 8.5 lb/gal; visc. 445 SUS (100 F); HLB 8.9; hyd. no. 142; flash pt. (PMCC) 360 F; ref. index 1.4979; surf. tens. 27.5 dynes/cm (0.1%); Ross-Miles foam 10 mm (initial, 0.1%, 120 F); 100% act.

Surfonic® N-60. [Texaco] Nonoxynol-6; CAS 9016-45-9; nonionic; biodeg. emulsifier, wetting agent, detergent, penetrant, solubilizer, dispersant for household cleaners, textile, agric., metal cleaning, petrol, cosmetic, latex paint, cutting oil, janitorial supply industries; FDA compliance; clear sl. visc. liq.; sol. in acetone, methanol, xylene, CCl4,

Stoddard solv.; disp. in water; m.w. 484; sp.gr. 1.041; dens. 8.7 lb/gal; visc. 440 SUS (100 F); f.p. < 0 C; HLB 10.9; hyd. no. 116; flash pt. (PMCC) 430 F; ref. index 1.4938; surf. tens. 28.7 dynes/cm (0.1%); Draves wetting 6 s (0.25%); Ross-Miles foam 12 mm (initial, 0.1%, 120 F); 100% act.

Surfonic® N-85. [Texaco] Nonoxynol-8.5; CAS 9016-45-9; nonionic; biodeg. emulsifier, wetting agent, detergent, penetrant, solubilizer, dispersant for household cleaners, textile, agric., metal cleaning, petrol, cosmetic, latex paint, cutting oil, janitorial supply industries; FDA compliance; liq.; sol. in acetone, methanol, xylene, CCl_4, water; m.w. 596; sp.gr. 1.056; dens. 8.8 lb/gal; visc. 485 SUS (100 F); f.p. -1 C; HLB 12.6; hyd. no. 94; cloud pt. 44 C (1% aq.); flash pt. (PMCC) 470 F; ref. index 1.4923; surf. tens. 30.5 dynes/cm (0.1%); Draves wetting 3.5 s (0.25%); Ross-Miles foam 40 mm (initial, 0.1%, 120 F); 100% act.

Surfonic® N-95. [Texaco] Nonoxynol-10; CAS 9016-45-9; EINECS 248-294-1; nonionic; biodeg. emulsifier, wetting agent, detergent, penetrant, solubilizer, dispersant for household cleaners, textile, agric., metal cleaning, petrol, cosmetic, latex paint, cutting oil, janitorial supply industries; FDA compliance; colorless to straw clear sl. visc. liq., sl. odor; sol. in acetone, methanol, xylene, CCl_4, water; m.w. 632; sp.gr. 1.061; dens. 8.8 lb/gal; visc. 510 SUS (100 F); f.p. 5 C; HLB 12.9; hyd. no. 90; cloud pt. 54.2 (1% aq.); flash pt. (PMCC) 460 F; ref. index 1.4893; pH 7.0; surf. tens. 30.8 dynes/cm (0.1%); Draves wetting 3 s (0.25%); Ross-Miles foam 80 mm (initial, 0.1%, 120 F); toxicology: LD50 (oral, rat) 3 g/kg (sl. toxic); eye irritant; sl. to severe skin irritant; 100% act.

Surfonic® N-100. [Texaco] Nonoxynol-10; CAS 9016-45-9; EINECS 248-294-1; nonionic; biodeg. emulsifier, wetting agent, detergent, penetrant, solubilizer, dispersant for household cleaners, textile, agric., metal cleaning, petrol, cosmetic, latex paint, cutting oil, janitorial supply industries; FDA compliance; clear sl. visc. liq.; sol. in acetone, methanol, xylene, CCl_4, water; m.w. 660; sp.gr. 1.064; dens. 8.8 lb/gal;visc. 69 SUS (210 F); f.p. 8 C; HLB 13.2; hyd. no. 85; cloud pt. 65 C (1% aq.); flash pt. (PMCC) 415 F; ref. index 1.4888; surf. tens. 31.0 dynes/cm (0.1%); Draves wetting 4 s (0.25%); Ross-Miles foam 85 mm (initial, 0.1%, 120 F); 100% act.

Surfonic® N-102. [Texaco] Nonoxynol-10; CAS 9016-45-9; EINECS 248-294-1; nonionic; biodeg. emulsifier, wetting agent, detergent, penetrant, solubilizer, dispersant for household cleaners, textile, agric., metal cleaning, petrol, cosmetic, latex paint, cutting oil, janitorial supply industries; clear sl. visc. liq.; sol. in acetone, methanol, xylene, CCl_4, water; m.w. 668; sp.gr. 1.065; dens. 8.8 lb/gal; f.p. 9 C; HLB 13.5; hyd. no. 84; cloud pt. 81 C (1% aq.); flash pt. (PMCC) 500 F; ref. index 1.4884; surf. tens. 31.2 dynes/cm (0.1%); Draves wetting 4.5 s (0.25%); Ross-Miles foam 85 mm (initial, 0.1%, 120 F); 100% act.

Surfonic® N-120. [Texaco] Nonoxynol-12; CAS 9016-45-9; nonionic; biodeg. emulsifier, wetting agent, detergent, penetrant, solubilizer, dispersant for household cleaners, textile, agric., metal cleaning, petrol, cosmetic, latex paint, cutting oil, janitorial supply industries; FDA compliance; clear sl. visc. liq.; sol. in acetone, methanol, xylene, CCl_4, water; m.w. 748; sp.gr. 1.070; dens. 8.9 lb/gal; visc. 560 SUS (100 F); f.p. 14 C; HLB 14.1; hyd. no. 75; cloud pt. 81 C (1% aq.); flash pt. (PMCC) 400 F; ref. index 1.4869; surf. tens. 32.3 dynes/cm (0.1%); Draves wetting 7 s (0.25%); Ross-Miles foam 110 mm (initial, 0.1%, 120 F); 100% act.

Surfonic® N-130. [Texaco] Nonoxynol-13; CAS 9016-45-9; nonionic; biodeg. emulsifier, wetting agent, detergent, penetrant, solubilizer, dispersant for household cleaners, textile, agric., metal cleaning, petrol, cosmetic, latex paint, cutting oil, janitorial supply industries; sl. turbid, sl. visc.

liq.; water-sol.; m.w. 792; dens. 8.9 lb/gal; f.p. 18 C; HLB 14.4; cloud pt. 56-60 C (1% in 10% brine); flash pt. (PMCC) 750 F; 100% act.

Surfonic® N-150. [Texaco] Nonoxynol-15; CAS 9016-45-9; nonionic; biodeg. emulsifier, wetting agent, detergent, penetrant, solubilizer, dispersant for household cleaners, textile, agric., metal cleaning, petrol, cosmetic, latex paint, cutting oil, janitorial supply industries; FDA compliance; wh. waxy solid; sol. in acetone, methanol, xylene, CCl_4, water; m.w. 880; sp.gr. 1.065 (30/4 C); dens. 8.95 lb/gal; visc. 89 SUS (210 F); f.p. 23 C; HLB 15.0; hyd. no. 64; cloud pt. 94 C (1% aq.); flash pt. (PMCC) 355 F; ref. index 1.4815 (30 C); surf. tens. 34.2 dynes/cm (0.1%); Draves wetting 17 s (0.25%); Ross-Miles foam 120 mm (initial, 0.1%, 120 F); 100% act.

Surfonic® N-200. [Texaco] Nonoxynol-20; CAS 9016-45-9; nonionic; biodeg. emulsifier, wetting agent, detergent, penetrant, solubilizer, dispersant for household cleaners, textile, agric., metal cleaning, petrol, cosmetic, latex paint, cutting oil, janitorial supply industries; FDA compliance; waxy solid; water-sol.; m.w. 1100; dens. 9.0 lb/gal; f.p. 34 C; HLB 15.8; cloud pt. 72-73 C (1% in 10% brine); flash pt. (PMCC) 450 F; 100% act.

Surfonic® N-300. [Texaco] Nonoxynol-30; CAS 9016-45-9; nonionic; biodeg. emulsifier, wetting agent, detergent, penetrant, solubilizer, dispersant for household cleaners, textile, agric., metal cleaning, petrol, cosmetic, latex paint, cutting oil, janitorial supply industries; FDA compliance; sol. in water; m.w. 1540; dens. 9.1 lb/gal; visc. 150-170 SUS (210 F); f.p. 44 C; HLB 17.1; cloud pt. > 100 C (1% aq.); flash pt. (PMCC) 385 F; ref. index 1.4690 (50 C); 100% act.

Surfonic® NB-5. [Texaco] Nonoxynol-30; CAS 9016-45-9; nonionic; biodeg. emulsifier, wetting agent, detergent, penetrant, solubilizer, dispersant for household cleaners, textile, agric., metal cleaning, petrol, cosmetic, latex paint, cutting oil, janitorial supply industries; clear liq.; 70% act. in water.

Surfynol® 82. [Air Prods.] 3,6-Dimethyl-4-octyne-3,6-diol; CAS 78-66-0; nonionic; surfactant, defoamer, wetting agent, visc. reducer used in aq. systems, pesticide concs., shampoos, vinyl plastisols, agric., aq. starch sol'ns., flexographic inks, electroplating baths; detergent for radiator cleaners, descaling compds.; EPA compliance; wh. cryst. powd.; very sol. in acetone, benzene, CCl_4, Cellosolve, ethylene glycol, ethyl acetate, ethanol, MEK;sp.gr. 0.933; m.p. 49-51 C; b.p. 222 C; surf. tens. 55.3 (0.1% aq.); toxicology: LD50 (oral, rat) 1400 mg/k, (dermal, rabbit) > 1000 mg/k; not considered toxic; 100% act.

Surfynol® 82S. [Air Prods.] 3,6-Dimethyl-4-octyne-3,6-diol on amorphous silica carrier; nonionic; defoamer/wetting agent in pesticide wettable powds., electroplating baths, cement, plastics, coatings; solubilizer and clarifier in shampoos; EPA compliance; wh. free-flowing powd.; disp. in water; sp.gr. 0.47 g/ml; dens. 3.9 lb/gal; pH 7.6 (5% aq.); Draves wetting 4 s (4.35%); 46% conc.

Suspengel Elite. [Cimbar Perf. Minerals] Purified dry colloidal hydrated aluminum silicate; CAS 1327-36-2; EINECS 215-475-1; thixotropic thickener giving good sag control, leveling, and suspension props.; used for coatings, inks, foods, beverages, pharmaceuticals, cosmetics, industrial use (adhesives, ceramics, lubricants, mastics, polishes, dishwash, household cleaners, metalworking compds., plasters, slurries, agric.); FDA GRAS §184.1155; kosher; lt. cream-colored powd.; odorless, tasteless; avg. particle size 0.5 µ; surf. area 1.2 m^2/cc; visc. 10,000 cps (6% solids); bulk dens. 38 lb/ft³ (loose); oil absorp. 47; pH 9.4; usage level: 0.25-8.0%; 8.7% moisture.

Suspengel Micro. [Cimbar Perf. Minerals] Purified dry colloidal hydrated aluminum silicate; CAS 1327-36-2;

EINECS 215-475-1; thixotropic thickener giving good sag control, leveling, and suspension props.; used for coatings, inks, foods, beverages, pharmaceuticals, cosmetics, industrial use (adhesives, ceramics, lubricants, mastics, polishes, dishwash, household cleaners, metalworking compds., plasters, slurries, agric.); FDA GRAS §184.1155; kosher; lt. cream-colored powd.; odorless, tasteless; avg. particle size 1.0 μ; surf. area 0.9 m²/cc; visc. 10,000 cps (6% solids); bulk dens. 41 lb/ft³ (loose); oil absorp. 36; pH 9.4; usage level: 0.25-8.0%; 8.7% moisture.

Suspengel Ultra. [Cimbar Perf. Minerals] Purified dry colloidal hydrated aluminum silicate; CAS 1327-36-2; EINECS 215-475-1; thixotropic thickener giving good sag control, leveling, and suspension props.; used for coatings, inks, foods, beverages, pharmaceuticals, cosmetics, industrial use (adhesives, ceramics, lubricants, mastics, polishes, dishwash, household cleaners, metalworking compds., plasters, slurries, agric.); FDA GRAS §184.1155; kosher; lt. cream-colored powd.; avg. particle size 0.18 μ; surf. area 1.8 m²/cc; visc. 15,000 cps (6% solids); bulk dens. 29 lb/ft³ (loose); oil absorp. 52; pH 9.4; usage level: 0.25-8.0%; 8.7% moisture.

Suspentone. [Cimbar Perf. Minerals] Organophilic attapulgite; CAS 1337-76-4; thickening and suspending agent for coatings, agric., adhesives, caulks, sealants, greases, inks, cosmetics and personal care prods.; lt. cream-colored powd.; 98% thru 200 mesh; avg. particle size 1.5 μ; sp.gr. 1.7; bulk dens. 39 lb/ft³; oil absorp. 66; 3% moisture.

Suspentone 1265. [Cimbar Perf. Minerals] Organophilic attapulgite; CAS 1337-76-4; thickening and suspending agent for coatings, agric., adhesives, caulks, sealants, greases, inks, cosmetics and personal care prods.; lt. cream-colored powd.; 100% thru 200 mesh; avg. particle size 0.12 μ; sp.gr. 1.7; bulk dens. 26 lb/ft³; oil absorp. 85; 3% moisture.

Sustane® 1-F. [UOP] BHA; CAS 25013-16-5; EINECS 246-563-8; preservative and antioxidant for foods, flavors, cosmetics, vitamins, oils, waxes, essential oils, tallow, sausage, chewing gum base, shortening, lard, food pkg. materials, potatoes, and cereals; inhibits oxidation reaction of oils and fats in presence of air and retards rancidity and off-flavors caused by oxidation; wh. tablets and flakes; sol. > 30 g/100 g in soybean oil, cottonseed oil; > 25 g/100 g in acetone, ether; > 10 g/100 g in methanol; neg. sol. in water; m.w. 180.2; visc. 3.3 cS (99 C); m.p. 57 C; b.p. 270 F (@ 5 mm Hg); flash pt. (OC) 130 C; 98.5% min. conc.

Sustane® 3. [UOP] BHA (20%), propylene glycol (70%), propyl gallate (6%), citric acid (4%); preservative and antioxidant used in snack foods, cosmetics, and spices; pale yel. liq.; sp.gr. 1.066; dens. 8.7 lb/gal; visc. 40.64 cS (38 C); f.p. -23 C; flash pt. (CC) 99 C; ref. index. 1.4636.

Sustane® BHA. [UOP] BHA; CAS 25013-16-5; EINECS 246-563-8; antioxidant, stabilizer for fats, oils, other foods, in cosmetic creams, lotions, hair dressings; FDA and USDA approvals; wh. solid tablets; sol. in propylene glycol, ethanol, glyceryl oleate, soybean and cottonseed oils; insol. in water; m.w. 180.2; sp.gr. 1.020; visc. 3.3 cSt (100 C); m.p. 57 C; b.p. 270 C (760 mm Hg); flash pt. (CC) 130 C; usage level: 0.02% max.; 100% act.

Sustane® BHT. [UOP] BHT; CAS 128-37-0; EINECS 204-881-4; preservative and antioxidant for foods, food pkg. materials, tallow, animal feeds, soaps, cosmetic creams, lotions, and hair dressings, and plastics; inhibits oxidation of fats and oils and retards rancidity and off-flavors caused by oxidation; FDA and USDA approvals; wh. cryst.; sol. (g/100 solv.): 48 g in lard (50 C); 40 g in benzene; 30 g in min. oil; 28 g in linseed oils; 20 g in methanol; nil in water;

m.w. 220.3; sp.gr. 1.01 (20/4 C); dens. 37.5 lb/ft³; visc. 3.5 cSt (80 C); m.p. 70 C; b.p. 265 C (760 mm Hg); flash pt. (CC) 118 C; ref. index 1.486; usage level: 0.02% max.; 100% act.

Suttocide® A. [Sutton Labs] Sodium hydroxymethylglycinate; CAS 70161-44-3; EINECS 274-357-8; broad-spectrum antimicrobial preservative for cosmetics, esp. shampoos, conditioners, alkaline prods.; effective against Gram-positive and Gram-negative bacteria, yeasts, and molds; remains active at alkaline pH; ISO 9002, USA and Europe compliance; colorless to lt. yel. clear liq.; mild char. odor; m.w. 127.10; sol. (g/100 g): > 100 g in water, 112 g in propylene glycol, 119 g glycerin; sp.gr. 1.28-1.30; pH 10-12; usage level: up to 1.0%; toxicology: LD50 (oral, rat) 1070 mg/kg; not a primary skin irritant; moderately irritating to eyes at full strength; 50% act. in water; 5.5-6.1% N.

Swanol AM-301. [Nikko Chem. Co. Ltd.] Lauryl betaine; CAS 683-10-3; EINECS 211-669-5; amphoteric; detergent, wetting, dispersant; liq.; 35% conc.

Swanol CA-101. [Nikko Chem. Co. Ltd.] Benzalkonium chloride; antimicrobial; liq.

Swanol Amidoamine S. [Nikko Chem. Co. Ltd.] Stearamidoethyl diethylamine; CAS 16889-14-8; EINECS 240-924-3; emulsifier.

Sweetrex® . [Mendell] Dextrose, fructose, maltose, isomaltose, other polysaccharides; directly compressible chewable tablet base with high sweetness, coolness and mouthfeel; wh. gran. powd., neutral odor; avg. particle size 210 μ; 25% -100 mesh; very sol. in water; dens. (tapped) 0.6-0.9 g/ml; pH 3.5-6.0 (10% aq.).

SWS-101. [Wacker Silicones] Dimethylpolysiloxane terminated with nonreactive trimethylsiloxy groups; features inertness, heat and oxidative stability, exc. elec. props. for dielec. coolants, brake fluids, lubricants, auto care prods., release, heat transfer, aerosols, damping media, household prods., antifoam agents, cosmetics, shock absorbers; provides lubricity, antitackiness, emolliency, and water barrier props. to skin care formulations; colorless clear liq.; misc. with nonpolar liqs. (hydrocarbons, chlorinated hydrocarbons, ethers); ref. index 1.35-1.41; dielec. str. 350 V/mil; dielec. const. 2.7 (100 cycles); vol. resist. 1 x 10¹⁴ ohm-cm (500 V).

SWS-231. [Wacker Silicones] Silicone emulsion; nonionic; used for car/furniture polish, aerosol window cleaners, hand creams and lotions; wh. liq.; visc. 350 cSt.

SWS-232. [Wacker Silicones] Silicone emulsion; nonionic; used for car/furniture polish, aerosol window cleaners, hand creams and lotions; wh. liq.; visc. 100 cSt.

SWS-03314. [Wacker Silicones] Cyclomethicone; CAS 69430-24-6; slip agent, lubricant, release agent for personal care industry; emollient for skin care prods.; plasticizer for hair spray resins; replacement for IPM in aerosol antiperspirants; low surf. tens. enhances spreadability and wetting; slow and consistent rate of evaporation; reduces tack and stickiness in cosmetic formulations; for deodorants/antiperspirants, eye makeup, hair sprays, conditioners, hand creams/lotions, shave preps.; colorless clear liq., essentially odorless; sol. in alcohols, hydrocarbons, chlorinates solvs., and a variety of cosmetic ingreds.; sp.gr. 0.95; visc. 2.3 cSt; f.p. 18 C; flash pt. (TCC) 126 F; toxicology: extremely low order of toxicity.

SXS 40. [Witco/H-I-P] Sodium xylenesulfonate; CAS 1300-72-7; EINECS 215-090-9; hydrotrope.

Syncrowax AW1-C. [Croda Inc.] C18-36 acid; anionic; emulsifier, emollient, opacifier; pale cream waxy flakes, mild waxy odor; oil-sol.; HLB 2.0; m.p. 69–74 C; acid no. 155–170; iodine no. 3 max.; sapon. no. 165–175; usage level: 1-15%; 100% conc.

Syncrowax BB-4. [Croda Inc.; Croda Surf. Ltd.] Syn.

beeswax; emulsifier, emollient, opacifier; also suspending agent for anhyd. systems, aux. w/o emulsifier, thickener for oils and waxes; used in creams and sticks; pale cream waxy flakes; oil-sol.; m.p. 60–65 C; usage level: 1-5%.

Syncrowax ERL-C. [Croda Inc.; Croda Surf. Ltd.] C18-36 acid glycol ester; emulsifier, emollient, opacifier; also lubricant, stabilizer, suspending agent for anhyd. systems, thickener, reducer of bleeding and sweating; gloss improver; sticks, creams; lt. tan waxy flakes; mild waxy odor; m.p. 70–75 C; acid no. 10–15; iodine no. 3 max.; sapon. no. 155–160; usage level: 1-4%.

Syncrowax HGL-C. [Croda Inc.; Croda Surf. Ltd.] C18-36 acid triglyceride; emulsifier, emollient, opacifier; also lubricant, suspending agent, strength improver, stabilizer, gloss improver; used in cosmetic makeup; lt. tan waxy flakes; mild waxy odor; m.p. 70–75 C; acid no. 6–12; iodine no. 3 max.; sapon. no. 160–175; usage level: 4-12%.

Syncrowax HR-C. [Croda Inc.] Glyceryl tribehenate; CAS 18641-57-1; EINECS 242-471-7; emulsifier, emollient, opacifier; also suspending agent, thickener, gloss improver used in personal care prods.; off-wh. waxy pastilles/powd.; mild waxy odor; m.p. 60–65 C; acid no. 10 max.; iodine no. 3 max.; sapon. no. 170–175; usage level: 4-12%.

Syncrowax HRS-C. [Croda Inc.; Croda Surf. Ltd.] Glyceryl tribehenate, calcium behenate; emulsifier, emollient, opacifier; also suspending agent for anhyd. systems, aux. w/o emulsifier, gellant, thickener for oils and waxes; pale cream flakes; mild waxy odor; oil-sol.; m.p. 105–115 C; acid no. 8–13; iodine no. 3 max.; sapon. no. 115–125; usage level: 2-10%.

Synotol C-30. [Aquatec Quimica SA] Coconut dimethylamine oxide; CAS 61788-90-7; EINECS 263-016-9; nonionic; foam stabilizer for shampoos, bubble baths, other foaming toiletries; liq.; 30% conc.

Synotol CN 60. [Aquatec Quimica SA] Cocamide DEA; CAS 68603-42-9; EINECS 263-163-9; nonionic; foam stabilizer, thickener, superfatting agent for cosmetic and household prods.; liq.; 60% conc.

Synotol CN 80. [Aquatec Quimica SA] Cocamide DEA; CAS 61791-31-9; EINECS 263-163-9; nonionic; foam stabilizer, thickener, superfatting agent for cosmetic and household prods.; liq.; 80% conc.

Synotol CN 90. [Aquatec Quimica SA] Cocamide DEA; CAS 61791-31-9; EINECS 263-163-9; nonionic; foam stabilizer, thickener, superfatting agent for cosmetic and household prods.; liq.; 90% conc.

Synotol ME 90. [Aquatec Quimica SA] Cocamide MEA; CAS 68140-00-1; EINECS 268-770-2; nonionic; foam booster, wetting agent, thickener, foam stabilizer, and superfatting agent for cosmetic and household preparations; flakes; 90% conc.

Synperonic A2. [ICI Am.; ICI plc] Trideceth-2; CAS 678213-23-0; nonionic; detergent, emulsifier, coemulsifier; base for emulsifiers, textile antistats, scouring and wetting agents, and specialty cleaners; intermediate for sulfation used in personal care prods.; colorless liq.; sol. in alcohol, glycol ethers, kerosene, and min. oil; dens. 0.897 g/ml; visc. 25 cps; HLB 5.9; pour pt. 2 C; pH 6–8 (1% aq.); 99% min. act.

Synperonic A3. [ICI Am.; ICI plc] Trideceth-3; CAS 4403-12-7; EINECS 224-540-3; nonionic; detergent, emulsifier, coemulsifier; base for emulsifiers, textile antistats, scouring and wetting agents, and specialty cleaners; intermediate for sulfation used in personal care prods.; colorless liq.; sol. in alcohol, glycol ethers, kerosene, and min. oil; dens. 0.918 g/ml; visc. 29 cps; HLB 7.9; pour pt. 5 C; pH 6–8 (1% aq.); 99% min. act.

Synperonic A4. [ICI Am.; ICI plc] PEG-4 syn. primary C13-15 alcohol; CAS 68213-23-0; nonionic; detergent, emulsifier, coemulsifier; base for emulsifiers, textile antistats, scouring and wetting agents, and specialty cleaners; intermediate for sulfation used in personal care prods.; colorless liq.; sol. in alcohol, glycol ethers, kerosene; sol./disp. in min. oil; dens. 0.937 g/ml; visc. 34 cps; HLB 9.1; pour pt. 9 C; pH 6–8 (1% aq.); 99% min. act.

Synperonic A7. [ICI Am.; ICI plc] Trideceth-7; CAS 24938-91-8; 68213-23-0; nonionic; detergent, emulsifier, coemulsifier; base for emulsifiers, textile antistats, scouring and wetting agents, and specialty cleaners; intermediate for sulfation used in personal care prods.; wh. paste; sol. in water, glycol ethers and alcohol; dens. 0.977 g/ml; visc. 60 cps; HLB 12.2; cloud pt. 44–48 C (1% aq.); pour pt. 21 C; surf. tens. 30.2 dynes/cm (0.1%); pH 6–8 (1% aq.); 99% min. act.

Synperonic A9. [ICI Am.; ICI plc] Trideceth-9; CAS 24938-91-8; 68213-23-0; nonionic; detergent, emulsifier, coemulsifier; base for emulsifiers, textile antistats, scouring and wetting agents, and specialty cleaners; intermediate for sulfation used in personal care prods.; wh. paste; sol. in water, glycol ethers and alcohol; dens. 0.984 g/ml (40 C); visc. 35 cps (40 C); HLB 13.0; cloud pt. 62–68 C (1% aq.); pour pt. 24 C; surf. tens. 31.4 dynes/cm (0.1%); pH 6–8 (1% aq.); 99% min. act.

Synperonic A11. [ICI Am.; ICI plc] Trideceth-11; CAS 24938-91-8; 68213-23-0; nonionic; detergent, emulsifier, coemulsifier; base for emulsifiers, textile antistats, scouring and wetting agents, and specialty cleaners; intermediate for sulfation used in personal care prods.; wh. solid; sol. in water, glycol ethers and alcohol; dens. 0.998 g/ml (40 C); visc. 42 cps (40 C); HLB 13.9; cloud pt. 85–89 C (1% aq.); pour pt. 27 C; surf. tens. 33.2 dynes/cm (0.1%); pH 6–8 (1% aq.); 99% min. act.

Synperonic A20. [ICI Am.; ICI plc] Trideceth-20; CAS 24938-91-8; nonionic; detergent, solubilizer, dispersant, stabilizer for household, industrial, and agrochem. applics.; used for high temp. and alkaline applics.; emulsifier for creams and lotions; solubilizer for fragrances; wh. hard wax; sol. in water, glycol ethers and alcohol; dens. 1.028 g/ml (50 C); visc. 58 cps (50 C); HLB 16.2; cloud pt. > 100 C (1% aq.); pour pt. 37 C; surf. tens. 40.1 dynes/cm (0.1%); pH 6–8 (1% aq.); 99% min. act.

Synperonic A50. [ICI Am.; ICI plc] Trideceth-50; CAS 24938-91-8; nonionic; detergent, solubilizer, dispersant, stabilizer for household, industrial, and agrochem. applics.; used for high temp. and alkaline applics.; emulsifier for creams and lotions; solubilizer for fragrances; wh. solid; water-sol.; HLB 18.3; 100% conc.

Synperonic NP1. [ICI Surf. Am.; ICI Surf. UK] Nonoxynol-1; EINECS 248-762-5; surfactant for industrial, agrochem., and textile applics.; emulsifier for creams, lotions; solubilizer for topical pharmaceuticals and shampoos; pale yel. liq.; HLB 3.3.

Synperonic NP2. [ICI Surf. Am.; ICI Surf. UK] Nonoxynol-2; EINECS 248-291-5; surfactant for industrial, agrochem., and textile applics.; emulsifier for creams, lotions; solubilizer for topical pharmaceuticals and shampoos; pale yel. liq.; HLB 5.7.

Synperonic NP4. [ICI Am.; ICI plc] Nonoxynol-4; CAS 9016-45-9; 68412-54-4; nonionic; detergent, emulsifier, coemulsifier, surfactant for industrial, agrochem., and textile applics.; intermediate for sulfation in mfg. lubricants and antistats; emulsifier for creams, lotions; solubilizer for topical pharmaceuticals and shampoos; pale yel. liq.; sol. in alcohol, glycol ethers, kerosene, and min. oil; dens. 1.022 g/ml; visc. 400 cps; HLB 8.9; pour pt. < 0 C; pH 6–8 (1% aq.); 99% min. act.

Synperonic NP5. [ICI Am.; ICI plc] Nonoxynol-5; CAS 9016-

45-9; nonionic; detergent, emulsifier, coemulsifier, surfactant for industrial, agrochem., and textile applics.; intermediate for sulfation in mfg. lubricants and antistats; emulsifier for creams, lotions; solubilizer for topical pharmaceuticals and shampoos; pale yel. liq.; sol. in alcohol, glycol ethers, kerosene, min. oil; insol./disp. in water; dens. 1.035 g/ml; visc. 350 cps; HLB 10.5; pour pt. < 0 C; pH 6–8 (1% aq.); 99% min. act.

Synperonic NP5.5. [ICI Surf. Am.; ICI Surf. UK] Nonoxynol-5.5; CAS 9016-45-9; surfactant for industrial, agrochem., and textile applics.; emulsifier for creams, lotions; solubilizer for topical pharmaceuticals and shampoos; pale yel. liq.; HLB 10.7.

Synperonic NP6. [ICI Am.; ICI plc] Nonoxynol-6; CAS 9016-45-9; nonionic; detergent, emulsifier, coemulsifier, surfactant for industrial, agrochem., and textile applics.; intermediate for sulfation in mfg. lubricants and antistats; emulsifier for creams, lotions; solubilizer for topical pharmaceuticals and shampoos; pale yel. liq.; sol. in alcohol, glycol ethers, min. oil; disp. in water; dens. 1.041 g/ml; visc. 355 cps; HLB 10.9; pour pt. < 0 C; pH 6–8 (1% aq.); 99% min. act.

Synperonic NP7. [ICI Am.; ICI plc] Nonoxynol-7; CAS 9016-45-9; EINECS 248-292-0; nonionic; detergent, emulsifier for oils, waxes, solvs.; surfactant for industrial, agrochem., and textile applics.; emulsifier for creams, lotions; solubilizer for topical pharmaceuticals and shampoos; pale yel. liq.; oil-sol.; HLB 11.7; 100% conc.

Synperonic NP8. [ICI Am.; ICI plc] Nonoxynol-8; CAS 9016-45-9; nonionic; detergent for textile scouring; wetting agent; emulsifier for med. polarity oils and solvs.; surfactant for industrial, agrochem., and textile applics.; emulsifier for creams, lotions; solubilizer for topical pharmaceuticals and shampoos; pale yel. liq.; sol. in water, alcohol, glycol ethers; dens. 1.053 g/ml; visc. 355 cps; HLB 12.3; cloud pt. 30–34 C (1% aq.); pour pt. < 0 C; surf. tens. 29.4 dynes/cm (0.1%); pH 6–8 (1% aq.); 99% min. act.

Synperonic NP8.5. [ICI plc] Nonoxynol-8.5; CAS 9016-45-9; nonionic; detergent, wetting agent, emulsifier, surfactant for industrial, agrochem., and textile applics.; emulsifier for creams, lotions; solubilizer for topical pharmaceuticals and shampoos; pale yel. liq.; water-sol.; HLB 12.6; 100% conc.

Synperonic NP8.75. [ICI Surf. UK] Nonoxynol-8.75; CAS 9016-45-9; wetting agent, detergent, emulsifier, surfactant for industrial, agrochem., and textile applics.; emulsifier for creams, lotions; solubilizer for topical pharmaceuticals and shampoos; pale yel. liq.; HLB 12.7.

Synperonic NP9. [ICI Am.; ICI plc] Nonoxynol-9; CAS 9016-45-9; nonionic; detergent for textile scouring; wetting agent; emulsifier for med. polarity oils and solvs.; surfactant for industrial, agrochem., and textile applics.; emulsifier for creams, lotions; solubilizer for topical pharmaceuticals and shampoos; pale yel. liq.; sol. in water, alcohol, glycol ethers; dens. 1.058 g/ml; visc. 340 cps; HLB 12.8; cloud pt. 51–56 C (1% aq.); pour pt. 0 C; surf. tens. 30.6 dynes/cm; pH 6–8 (1% aq.); 99% min. act.

Synperonic NP9.5. [ICI Surf. UK] Nonoxynol-9.5; CAS 9016-45-9; surfactant for industrial, agrochem., and textile applics.; emulsifier for creams, lotions; solubilizer for topical pharmaceuticals and shampoos; pale yel. liq.; HLB 13.0.

Synperonic NP9.75. [ICI Surf. UK] Nonoxynol-9.75; CAS 9016-45-9; EINECS 248-294-1; surfactant for industrial, agrochem., and textile applics.; emulsifier for creams, lotions; solubilizer for topical pharmaceuticals and shampoos; pale yel. liq.; HLB 13.2.

Synperonic NP10. [ICI Am.; ICI plc] Nonoxynol-10; CAS 9016-45-9; EINECS 248-294-1; nonionic; detergent, solubilizer, dispersant, stabilizer, surfactant for industrial,

agrochem., and textile applics.; emulsifier for creams, lotions; solubilizer for topical pharmaceuticals and shampoos; pale yel. liq.; sol. in water, alcohol, glycol ethers; dens. 1.061 g/ml; visc. 360 cps; HLB 13.3; cloud pt. 62–67 C (1% aq.); pour pt. 5 C; surf. tens. 30.6 dynes/cm; pH 6–8 (1% aq.); 99% min. act.

Synperonic NP12. [ICI Am.; ICI plc] Nonoxynol-12; CAS 9016-45-9; nonionic; detergent, solubilizer, dispersant, stabilizer, surfactant for industrial, agrochem., and textile applics.; emulsifier for creams, lotions; solubilizer for topical pharmaceuticals and shampoos; pale yel. liq.; sol. in water, alcohol, glycol ethers; dens. 1.062 g/ml; visc. 265 cps; HLB 13.9; cloud pt. 79–84 C (1% aq.); pour pt. 14 C; surf. tens. 35.2 dynes/cm; pH 6–8 (1% aq.); 99% min. act.

Synperonic NP13. [ICI Am.; ICI plc] Nonoxynol-13; CAS 9016-45-9; nonionic; emulsifier and wetting agent for solvs. and agrochemical pesticides and herbicides; detergent additive, solubilizer, and dispersant; emulsifier for creams, lotions; solubilizer for topical pharmaceuticals and shampoos; pale yel. paste; sol. in water, alcohol, glycol ethers; dens. 1.068 g/ml; visc. 280 cps; HLB 14.4; cloud pt. 87–92 C (1% aq.); pour pt. 17 C; surf. tens. 34.8 dynes/cm; pH 6–8 (1% aq.); 99% min. act.

Synperonic NP15. [ICI Surf. Am.; ICI plc] Nonoxynol-15; CAS 9016-45-9; nonionic; emulsifier and wetting agent for agrochem. powds. and solvs.; detergent additive, solubilizer, dispersant; emulsifier for creams, lotions; solubilizer for topical pharmaceuticals and shampoos; pale yel. paste; sol. in water, alcohol, glycol ethers; dens. 1.058 g/ml (40 C); visc. 125 cps (40 C); HLB 15.0; cloud pt. 95–99 C (1% aq.); pour pt. 21 C; surf. tens. 33.4 dynes/cm; pH 6–8 (1% aq.); 99% min. act.

Synperonic NP17. [ICI Surf. Am.; ICI Surf. UK] Nonoxynol-17; CAS 9016-45-9; surfactant for industrial, agrochem., and textile applics.; emulsifier for creams, lotions; solubilizer for topical pharmaceuticals and shampoos; pale yel. solid; HLB 15.4.

Synperonic NP20. [ICI Surf. Am.; ICI plc] Nonoxynol-20; CAS 9016-45-9; nonionic; surfactant for industrial, agrochem., and textile applics.; solubilizer and emulsifier for polar substrates; emulsifier for creams, lotions; solubilizer for topical pharmaceuticals and shampoos; pale yel. solid; sol. in water, alcohol, glycol ethers; dens. 1.073 g/ml (40 C); visc. 168 cps (40 C); HLB 16.0; cloud pt. > 100 C (1% aq.); pour pt. 30 C; surf. tens. 41.7 dynes/cm; pH 6–8 (1% aq.); 99% min. act.

Synperonic NP25. [ICI Surf. Am.; ICI Surf. UK] Nonoxynol-25; CAS 9016-45-9; surfactant for industrial, agrochem., and textile applics.; emulsifier for creams, lotions; solubilizer for topical pharmaceuticals and shampoos; pale yel. solid; HLB 16.7.

Synperonic NP30. [ICI Surf. Am.; ICI plc] Nonoxynol-30; CAS 9016-45-9; nonionic; surfactant for industrial, agrochem., and textile applics.; solubilizer and emulsifier for high polarity materials; emulsifier for creams, lotions; solubilizer for topical pharmaceuticals and shampoos; pale yel. solid; sol. in water, alcohol, glycol ethers; dens. 1.074 g/ml (50 C); visc. 150 cps (50 C); HLB 17.1; cloud pt. > 100 C (1% aq.); pour pt. 40 C; surf. tens. 42.8 dynes/cm; pH 6–8 (1% aq.); 99% min. act.

Synperonic NP30/70. [ICI Am.] Nonoxynol-30; CAS 9016-45-9; nonionic; surfactant for industrial, agrochem., and textile applics.; solubilizer and emulsifier for high polarity materials; emulsifier for creams, lotions; solubilizer for topical pharmaceuticals and shampoos.

Synperonic NP35. [ICI Surf. Am.; ICI plc] Nonoxynol-35; CAS 9016-45-9; nonionic; surfactant for industrial, agrochem., and textile applics.; solubilizer and emulsifier for high polarity materials; emulsifier for creams, lotions; solubilizer for topical pharmaceuticals and shampoos;

pale yel. solid; HLB 17.5; 100% conc.

Synperonic NP40. [ICI Am.; ICI plc] Nonoxynol-40; CAS 9016-45-9; nonionic; surfactant for industrial, agrochem., and textile applics.; solubilizer and emulsifier for high polarity materials; emulsifier for creams, lotions; solubilizer for topical pharmaceuticals and shampoos; pale yel. solid; HLB 17.8; 100% conc.

Synperonic NP50. [ICI Am.; ICI plc] Nonoxynol-50; CAS 9016-45-9; nonionic; surfactant for industrial, agrochem., and textile applics.; solubilizer and emulsifier for high polarity materials; emulsifier for creams, lotions; solubilizer for topical pharmaceuticals and shampoos; pale yel. solid; HLB 18.2; 100% conc.

Synperonic OP3. [ICI Am.; ICI plc] Octoxynol-3; CAS 9002-93-1; 68987-90-6; nonionic; detergent and emulsifier for oils, waxes, and solvs.; for industrial and agrochem. applics.; emulsifier for creams, lotions; solubilizer for topical pharmaceuticals and shampoos; pale yel. liq.; oil-sol.; HLB 7.1; 100% conc.

Synperonic OP4.5. [ICI Am.; ICI plc] Octoxynol-4.5; CAS 9002-93-1; nonionic; detergent and emulsifier for oils, waxes, and solvs.; for industrial and agrochem. applics.; emulsifier for creams, lotions; solubilizer for topical pharmaceuticals and shampoos; pale yel. liq.; oil-sol.; HLB 9.4; 100% conc.

Synperonic OP6. [ICI Surf. Am.; ICI Surf. UK] Octoxynol-6; CAS 9002-93-1; surfactant for industrial and agrochem. applics.; emulsifier for creams, lotions; solubilizer for topical pharmaceuticals and shampoos; pale yel. liq.; HLB 10.5.

Synperonic OP7.5. [ICI Am.; ICI plc] Octoxynol-7.5; CAS 9002-93-1; nonionic; detergent for textile and paper processing; emulsifier for creams, lotions; solubilizer for topical pharmaceuticals and shampoos; pale yel. liq.; HLB 11.7; 100% conc.

Synperonic OP8. [ICI Surf. Am.; ICI plc] Octoxynol-8; CAS 9002-93-1; nonionic; detergent for textile and paper processing; emulsifier for creams, lotions; solubilizer for topical pharmaceuticals and shampoos; pale yel. liq.; HLB 12.6; 100% conc.

Synperonic OP10. [ICI Am.; ICI plc] Octoxynol-10; CAS 9002-93-1; nonionic; detergent, wetting agent, emulsifier; for textile and paper processing; emulsifier for creams, lotions; solubilizer for topical pharmaceuticals and shampoos; pale yel. liq.; sol. in water, alcohol, glycol ethers; dens. 1.062 g/ml; visc. 393 cps; HLB 13.3; cloud pt. 63–67 C (1% aq.); pour pt. 7 C; surf. tens. 31.8 dynes/cm; pH 6–8 (1% aq.); 99% min. act.

Synperonic OP10.5. [ICI Surf. Am.; ICI plc] Octoxynol-10.5; CAS 9002-93-1; nonionic; detergent for textile and paper processing; emulsifier for creams, lotions; solubilizer for topical pharmaceuticals and shampoos; pale yel. liq.; HLB 13.5; 100% conc.

Synperonic OP11. [ICI Am.; ICI plc] Octoxynol-11; CAS 9002-93-1; nonionic; detergent for textile and paper processing; emulsifier for creams, lotions; solubilizer for topical pharmaceuticals and shampoos; pale yel. liq.; sol. in water, alcohol, glycol ethers; dens. 1.067 g/ml; visc. 371 cps; HLB 13.6; cloud pt. 79–82 C (1% aq.); pour pt. 8 C; surf. tens. 31.0 dynes/cm; pH 6–8 (1% aq.); 99% min. act.

Synperonic OP12.5. [ICI Am.; ICI plc] Octoxynol-12.5; CAS 9002-93-1; nonionic; detergent for hard surf. cleaners; emulsifier for creams, lotions; solubilizer for topical pharmaceuticals and shampoos; pale yel. liq.; water-sol.; HLB 14.3; 100% conc.

Synperonic OP16. [ICI Am.] Octoxynol-16; CAS 9002-93-1; nonionic; emulsifier for emulsion polymerization, cosmetic creams, lotions; solubilizer for topical pharmaceuticals and shampoos; liq.; HLB 15.6; 70% conc.

Synperonic OP16.5. [ICI Surf. Am.; ICI plc] Octoxynol-16.5;

CAS 9002-93-1; nonionic; detergent for hard surf. cleaners; emulsifier for creams, lotions; solubilizer for topical pharmaceuticals and shampoos; pale yel. solid; HLB 15.3; 100% conc.

Synperonic OP20. [ICI Am.] Octoxynol-20; CAS 9002-93-1; nonionic; surfactant for industrial and agrochem. applics.; emulsifier for creams, lotions; solubilizer for topical pharmaceuticals and shampoos; pale yel. solid; HLB 16.2.

Synperonic OP25. [ICI Am.] Octoxynol-25; CAS 9002-93-1; nonionic; surfactant for industrial and agrochem. applics.; emulsifier for creams, lotions; solubilizer for topical pharmaceuticals and shampoos; pale yel. solid; HLB 16.7.

Synperonic OP30. [ICI Am.; ICI plc] Octoxynol-30; CAS 9002-93-1; nonionic; surfactant for emulsion polymerization; emulsifier for creams, lotions; solubilizer for topical pharmaceuticals and shampoos; pale yel. solid; HLB 17.2; 100% conc.

Synperonic OP40. [ICI Am.; ICI plc] Octoxynol-40; CAS 9002-93-1; nonionic; solubilizer, dispersant, emulsifier for highly polar substrates; for industrial and agrochem. applics.; emulsifier for creams, lotions; solubilizer for topical pharmaceuticals and shampoos; pale yel. solid; HLB 17.4; 100% conc.

Synperonic OP40/70. [ICI plc] Octoxynol-40; CAS 9002-93-1; nonionic; solubilizer, dispersant, emulsifier for highly polar substrates; for industrial and agrochem. applics.; emulsifier for creams, lotions; solubilizer for topical pharmaceuticals and shampoos; liq.; HLB 17.4; 70% conc.

Synperonic PE/F68. [ICI Am.; ICI plc] Poloxamer 188; CAS 9003-11-6; nonionic; emulsifier, dispersant for household, industrial, and agrochem. applics.; emulsifier for creams and lotions; wh. flake; cloud pt. > 100 C (10% aq.); 100% conc.

Synperonic PE/F87. [ICI Am.; ICI plc] Poloxamer 237; CAS 9003-11-6; nonionic; emulsifier, dispersant for shampoos, household, industrial, and agrochem. applics.; wh. flake; cloud pt. > 100 C (10% aq.); 100% conc.

Synperonic PE/F127. [ICI Am.; ICI plc] Poloxamer 407; CAS 9003-11-6; nonionic; emulsifier, dispersant for household, industrial, and agrochem. applics.; also for pharmaceutical preps. and mouthwashes; wh. flake; cloud pt. > 100 C (10% aq.); 100% conc.

Synperonic PE/L35. [ICI Am.; ICI plc] Poloxamer 105; CAS 9003-11-6; nonionic; emulsifier, dispersant, detergent for cosmetic creams and lotions, household, industrial, and agrochem. applics.; colorless liq.; cloud pt. 80 C (10% aq.); 100% conc.

Synperonic PE/P85. [ICI Am.; ICI plc] Poloxamer 235; CAS 9003-11-6; nonionic; emulsifier, demulsifier for cosmetic creams and lotions, household, industrial, and agrochem. applics.; wh. paste; cloud pt. 86 C (10% aq.); 100% conc.

Synperonic T/1301. [ICI Am.; ICI plc] Poloxamine 1301; CAS 11111-34-5; nonionic; low foaming agent, wetting agent, dispersant, demulsifier for industrial applics. and cosmetic stick deodorants; yel. liq.; cloud pt. 12.5 C (10% aq.); 100% conc.

Synperonic T/1302. [ICI Am.; ICI plc] Poloxamine 1302; CAS 11111-34-5; nonionic; low foaming agent, wetting agent, dispersant, demulsifier for industrial applics. and cosmetic stick deodorants; yel. liq.; cloud pt. 29 C (10% aq.); 100% conc.

Synperonic T/1307. [ICI Am.] Used in cosmetic stick deodorants.

Synpro® Aluminum Stearate USP. [Syn. Prods.] Aluminum stearate; additive for cosmetics.

Synpro® Calcium Stearate USP. [Syn. Prods.] Calcium stearate; CAS 1592-23-0; EINECS 216-472-8; additive for pharmaceuticals; fineness 99% thru 200 mesh; soften. pt. 155 C; 2.5% moisture.

Synprolam 35DM. [ICI plc] Syn. C13-15 dimethyl tert. fatty amine; CAS 68391-04-8; cationic; chemical intermediate for prod. of quat. salts and amine oxides used in cosmetics; catalyst for PU foam; corrosion inhibitor; Hazen 50 clear liq.; sp.gr. 0.79; visc. 3.9 cps; flash pt. 143 C (PMCC); 97% tert. amine.

Synpro® Magnesium Stearate USP. [Syn. Prods.] Magnesium stearate; CAS 557-04-0; EINECS 209-150-3; additive for pharmaceuticals.

Synpro® Zinc Stearate USP. [Syn. Prods.] Zinc stearate; CAS 557-05-1; EINECS 209-151-9; additive for pharmaceuticals; fineness 99% thru 200 mesh; soften. pt. 120 C; 0.5% moisture.

Syntase® 62. [Rhone-Poulenc Surf. & Spec.] Benzophenone-3; CAS 131-57-7; EINECS 205-031-5; uv absorber for sunscreen lotions and for protection of PS, PVC, methacrylate polymers, and polyesters, against uv degradation over prolonged exposure; useful in protecting clear varnishes and lacquers, linseed oil-based alkyds and phenolic coatings intended for use on uv-sensitive surfaces; pale cream powd.; m.w. 228; sol. in alcohols, aliphatic and aromatic hydrocarbons, ketones, and esters; sp.gr. 1.339; m.p. 62 C min.; 98% min. purity.

Syntase® 230. [Rhone-Poulenc Surf. & Spec.] Benzophenone-4; CAS 4065-45-6; EINECS 223-772-2; uv absorber used in water-based cosmetics, incl. suntan lotions, body creams, shampoos, hair sprays, and hair dyes, and in wool fabrics; protects color integrity of personal care formulations; anti photo oxidant; pale yel. powd.; m.w. 308; sol. 59.3% in methanol, 38.2% in water, 12.0% in acetone; sp.gr. 1.262; m.p. 110 C; acid no. 180.0; pH 0.6 (10% aq.); 99.0% min. purity.

Syntesqual. [Vevy] Polyisoprene; CAS 9003-31-0.

Syntopon 8 A. [Witco/H-I-P] Octyl phenol ethoxylate; anionic; wetting agent for textile and leather; detergent; emulsifier; solubilizer for personal care applics.; liq.; HLB 11.2; 100% conc.

Syntopon 8 B. [Witco/H-I-P] Octyl phenol ethoxylate; anionic; detergent for metal cleaning, low temp. applics.; solubilizer for personal care applics.; liq.; HLB 12.3; 100% conc.

Syntopon 8 C. [Witco/H-I-P] Octoxynol-9; CAS 9002-93-1; 9010-43-9; anionic; detergent for wool; solubilizer for personal care applics.; liq.; HLB 13.0; 100% conc.

Syntopon 8 D. [Witco/H-I-P] Octyl phenol ethoxylate; anionic; detergent for degreasing; wetting agent; emulsifier for insecticides; solubilizer for personal care applics.; liq.; 100% conc.

Syntopon 8 D 1. [Witco/H-I-P] Octoxynol-11; CAS 9002-93-1; solubilizer for personal care applics.; clear liq.

Syntopon A. [Witco/H-I-P] Nonoxynol-6; CAS 9016-45-9; 977057-32-1; nonionic; detergent; emulsifier for solvs. and min. oils; wetting agent; solubilizer for personal care applics.; liq.; HLB 10.9; 100% conc.

Syntopon A 100. [Witco/H-I-P] Nonoxynol-4; CAS 9016-45-9; nonionic; detergent, emulsifier for latex; wetting agent; solubilizer for personal care applics.; liq.; HLB 9.0; 100% conc.

Syntopon B. [Witco/H-I-P] Nonoxynol-8; CAS 9016-45-9; 977057-34-3; nonionic; wetting agent, detergent for textiles; emulsifier; solubilizer for personal care applics.; liq.; HLB 12.6; 100% conc.

Syntopon C. [Witco/H-I-P] Nonoxynol-9; CAS 9016-45-9; nonionic; wetting agent and detergent; emulsifier; solubilizer for personal care applics.; liq.; HLB 12.7; 100% conc.

Syntopon D. [Witco/H-I-P] Nonoxynol-10; CAS 9016-45-9; 977057-35-4; EINECS 248-294-1; nonionic; detergent, emulsifier for perfume; solubilizer for personal care applics.; liq.; HLB 13.2; 100% conc.

Syntopon D2. [Witco/H-I-P] Nonoxynol-12; CAS 9016-45-9; solubilizer for personal care applics.

Syntopon E. [Witco/H-I-P] Nonoxynol-13; CAS 9016-45-9; nonionic; detergent, emulsifier for metal cleaning, high temp. applics.; dispersant; solubilizer for personal care applics.; wax; HLB 14.0; 100% conc.

Syntopon F. [Witco/H-I-P] Nonoxynol-15; CAS 9016-45-9; nonionic; detergent, emulsifier, cleaning agent; solubilizer for personal care applics.; wax; HLB 15.0; 100% conc.

Syntopon G. [Witco/H-I-P] Nonoxynol-20; CAS 9016-45-9; nonionic; detergent, emulsifier, cleaning agent; solubilizer for personal care applics.; wax; HLB 16.0; 100% conc.

Syntopon H. [Witco/H-I-P] Nonoxynol-30; CAS 9016-45-9; nonionic; crude oil demulsifier; solubilizer for personal care applics.; wax; HLB 17.0; 100% conc.

Syntran 5002. [Interpolymer] Styrene/acrylates/ammonium methacrylate copolymer, propylene glycol, potassium octoxynol-12 phosphate, nonoxynol-10.; used for mascara binders; sp.gr. 1.065; dens. 8.88 lb/gal; visc. 400 cps max.; pH 7.5-8.8; 38-42% total solids.

Syntran 5130. [Interpolymer] Ammonium acrylates copolymer, propylene glycol, potassium octoxynol-12 phosphate, sodium laureth sulfate, nonoxynol-10.

Syntran 5170. [Interpolymer] Ammonium acrylates copolymer, propylene glycol, potassium octoxynol-12 phosphate, nonoxynol-10; used in mascara binders; sp.gr. 1.057; dens. 8.82 lb/gal; visc. 300 cps max.; pH 7.5 ± 0.5; 40-42% total solids.

T

T-11. [Procter & Gamble] Tallow fatty acid; CAS 67701-06-8; intermediate for mfg. of soaps, amides, esters, alcoholamides; raw material for non-surfactant applics.; paste; m.w. 276; acid no. 200-206; iodine no. 38-45; sapon. no. 200-208; 100% conc.

T-18. [Procter & Gamble] Tallow fatty acid; CAS 67701-06-8; intermediate for mfg. of soaps, amides, esters, alcoholamides; raw material for non-surfactant applics.; Gardner 5 max. paste; m.w. 275; acid no. 200-208; iodine no. 40-55; 100% conc.

T-20. [Procter & Gamble] Tallow fatty acid; CAS 67701-06-8; intermediate for mfg. of soaps, amides, esters, alcoholamides; raw material for non-surfactant applics.; Gardner 7 max. paste; m.w. 274; acid no. 200-210; iodine no. 40-55; sapon. no. 206; 100% conc.

T-22. [Procter & Gamble] Tallow fatty acid; CAS 67701-06-8; intermediate for mfg. of soaps, amides, esters, alcoholamides; raw material for non-surfactant applics.; Gardner 7 max. paste; m.w. 274; acid no. 200-210; iodine no. 45-70; 100% conc.

TA-1618. [Procter & Gamble] Cetearyl alcohol; CAS 67762-30-5; intermediate; wh. waxy solid; sp.gr. 0.810 (65 C); m.p. 50 C; acid no. 1 max.; iodine no. 1 max.; sapon. no. 3 max.; hyd. no. 204-216.

Tagat® L. [Goldschmidt; Goldschmidt AG] PEG-30 glyceryl laurate; CAS 51248-32-9; nonionic; preparation of o/w emulsions; solubilizer for flavors, perfumes, vitamin oils; dispersant and antistat; pale yel. liq.; sol. in water; insol. in veg. and min. oils; HLB 17.0; acid no. 2 max.; iodine no. 4 max.; sapon. no. 35-55; hyd. no. 52-68; 100% conc.

Tagat® L2. [Goldschmidt; Goldschmidt AG] PEG-20 glyceryl laurate; CAS 51248-32-9; nonionic; preparation of o/w emulsions for pharmaceuticals; solubilizer for flavors, perfumes, vitamin oils; dispersant and antistat; ivory liq.; sol. in water; insol. in veg. and min. oils; m.p. 60-80 C; HLB 15.7; acid no. 2 max.; iodine no. 4 max.; sapon. no. 50-70; hyd. no. 60-80; 100% conc.

Tagat® O. [Goldschmidt; Goldschmidt AG] PEG-30 glyceryl oleate; CAS 51192-09-7; nonionic; preparation of o/w emulsions; solubilizer for flavors, perfumes, vitamin oils; dispersant and antistat; yel. liq.; sol. in water; insol. in veg. and min. oils; HLB 16.4; acid no. 2 max.; iodine no. 15-19; sapon. no. 30-45; hyd. no. 50-65; 100% conc.

Tagat® O2. [Goldschmidt; Goldschmidt AG] PEG-20 glyceryl oleate; CAS 51192-09-7; nonionic; preparation of o/w emulsions for pharmaceuticals; solubilizer for flavors, perfumes, vitamin oils; dispersant and antistat; yel. liq.; sol. in water; insol. in veg. and min. oils; m.p. 70-85 C; HLB 15.0; acid no. 2 max.; iodine no. 21-27; sapon. no. 40-55; hyd. no. 70-85; 100% conc.

Tagat® R40. [Goldschmidt; Goldschmidt AG] PEG-40 hydrog. castor oil; CAS 61788-85-0; nonionic; solubilizer for water-insol. substances, e.g., essential oils, perfumes, vitamins, cosmetic/pharmaceutical active ingreds.; co-emulsifier for o/w emulsions; ivory solid; sol. warm in water; sol. warm with sl. turbidity in veg. and min. oils; m.p. 55-75 C; HLB 13.0; acid no. 2 max.; iodine no. 2 max.; sapon. no. 45-65; hyd. no. 55-75; 100% conc.

Tagat® R60. [Goldschmidt; Goldschmidt AG] PEG-60 hydrog. castor oil; CAS 61788-85-0; nonionic; solubilizer for water-insol. substances, e.g., essential oils, perfumes, vitamins, cosmetic/pharmaceutical active ingreds.; co-emulsifier for o/w emulsions; ivory solid; sol. warm in water; sol. warm with sl. turbidity in veg. and min. oils; HLB 15.0; acid no. 2 max.; iodine no. 2 max.; sapon. no. 35-52; hyd. no. 38-58; 100% conc.

Tagat® R63. [Goldschmidt; Goldschmidt AG] PEG-60 hydrog. castor oil and propylene glycol; CAS 61788-85-0; nonionic; solubilizer for water-insol. substances, e.g., essential oils, perfumes, vitamins, cosmetic/pharmaceutical active ingreds.; coemulsifier for o/w emulsions; pale yel. liq.; sol. in water; insol. in veg. and min. oils; HLB 15.0; acid no. 2 max.

Tagat® S. [Goldschmidt; Goldschmidt AG] PEG-30 glyceryl stearate; CAS 51158-08-8; nonionic; preparation of o/w emulsions; solubilizer for flavors, perfumes, vitamin oils; dispersant and antistat; ivory solid, partially liq.; sol. with sl. turbidity in water; insol. in veg. and min. oils; HLB 16.4; acid no. 2 max.; iodine no. 2 max.; sapon. no. 30-47; hyd. no. 53-70; 100% conc.

Tagat® S2. [Goldschmidt; Goldschmidt AG] PEG-20 glyceryl stearate; CAS 51158-08-8; nonionic; preparation of o/w emulsions for pharmaceuticals; solubilizer for flavors, perfumes, vitamin oils; dispersant and antistat; ivory solid, partially liq.; sol. with sl. turbidity in water; insol. in veg. and min. oils; m.p. 65-85 c; HLB 15.0; acid no. 2 max.; iodine no. 2 max.; sapon. no. 40-60; hyd. no. 65-85; 100% conc.

Tagat® TO. [Goldschmidt; Goldschmidt AG] PEG-25 glyceryl trioleate; CAS 68958-64-5; nonionic; preparation of o/w emulsions; solubilizer for flavors, perfumes, vitamin oils; dispersant and antistat; refatting agent for hair/bath preps.; amber liq.; sol. in veg. oils; disp. in water; insol. in min. oil; HLB 11.3; acid no. 12 max.; iodine no. 34-40; sapon. no. 75-90; hyd. no. 18-33; 100% conc.

Takanal. [Ikeda; Tri-K Industries] Quaternium 51; CAS 1463-95-2; EINECS 215-976-5; cationic; ingred. for hair and scalp treatment formulations, anti-itch and dandruff treatments, hair tonic, shampoo, conditioner; activates metabolism, promotes hair growth; Japan approval; yel. cryst. powd., odorless; sol. in methanol, glycerin, propylene glycol, polyethylene glcyol; m.p. 233-238 C; pH neutral; usage level: 0.002% max.; toxicology: LD50 (mouse, subcutaneous inj.) 369 mg/kg; 97% min. assay.

Talc LCW. [Les Colorants Wackherr] Talc; CAS 14807-96-6; EINECS 238-877-9; cosmetics ingred.; particle size < 2 μ.

Talc OOC. [Les Colorants Wackherr] Talc; CAS 14807-96-6; EINECS 238-877-9; cosmetics ingred.; particle size ≈

10 μ.

Talc Micro-Ace P-2. [Presperse] Talc; CAS 14807-96-6; EINECS 238-877-9; cosmetic ingred. contributing soft, smooth feel, skin adhesion, and spreadability; for pressed powds., pigmented cosmetics; JSCI/JCID approved; wh. fine powd., essentially odorless; particle size 2-4 μ; oil absorp. 0.495 ml/g; 100% act.

Talc Micro-Ace P-2-030. [Presperse] Talc (97%), methicone (3%); CAS 14807-96-6, 9004-73-3; cosmetic ingred. contributing soft, smooth feel, skin adhesion, and spreadability; for pressed powds., pigmented cosmetics; JSCI/JCID approved; wh. fine powd., essentially odorless; particle size 2-4 μ.

Talc Micro-Ace P-4. [Presperse] Talc; CAS 14807-96-6; EINECS 238-877-9; cosmetic ingred. contributing soft, smooth feel, skin adhesion, and spreadability; for pressed powds., pigmented cosmetics; JSCI/JCID approved; wh. fine powd., essentially odorless; particle size 0-2 μ; oil absorp. 0.520 ml/g.

Talcoseptic C. [Vevy] Talc, phenoxyethanol, methylparaben, ethylparaben, propylparaben, butylparaben.

T.A.M. [Exsymol; Biosil Tech.] Thenoyl methionine; cosmetic ingred. rich in org. sulfur; contributes to formation of disulfur bridges in skin tissues; for scalp treatments, prevention of hair fallout; wh. microcryst. powd., sl. but distinctive odor; sol. in hot water and alcohol; sol. in water at pH > 7; m.w. 259; m.p. 115 C; usage level: 1-5%; toxicology: nontoxic.

Tamol® 731-25%. [Rohm & Haas] Isobutylene/maleic anhydride copolymer; CAS 26426-80-2; dispersant for dyes, pigments; lt. yel. aq. sol'n.; dens. 9.2 lb/gal; visc. 200 cps; f.p. 28 F; 25% act.

Tauranol I-78. [Finetex] Sodium cocoyl isethionate; EINECS 263-052-5; anionic; mild detergent, foamer, dispersant for soap-syndet, toilet bars, shampoos, bubble baths, mild foaming facial cleansers; imparts conditioning to hair and skin; emulsifier in creams and lotions; powd.; 83% conc.

Tauranol I-78 Flakes. [Finetex] Sodium cocoyl isethionate; EINECS 263-052-5; anionic; mild detergent, foamer, dispersant for soap-syndet, toilet bars, shampoos, bubble baths, mild foaming facial cleansers; imparts conditioning to hair and skin; emulsifier in creams and lotions; flakes; 83% conc.

Tauranol I-78-3. [Finetex] Sodium cocoyl isethionate; EINECS 263-052-5; anionic; mild detergent, foamer, dispersant for soap-syndet, toilet bars, shampoos, bubble baths, mild foaming facial cleansers; imparts conditioning to hair and skin; emulsifier in creams and lotions; paste; 27% conc.

Tauranol I-78-6. [Finetex] Sodium cocoyl isethionate; EINECS 263-052-5; anionic; mild detergent, foamer, dispersant for soap-syndet, toilet bars, shampoos, bubble baths, mild foaming facial cleansers; imparts conditioning to hair and skin; emulsifier in creams and lotions; paste; 50% conc.

Tauranol I-78/80. [Finetex] Sodium cocoyl isethionate, stearic acid; anionic; mild detergent, foamer, dispersant for soap-syndet, toilet bars, shampoos, bubble baths, mild foaming facial cleansers; imparts conditioning to hair and skin; emulsifier in creams and lotions.

Tauranol I-78E, I-78E Flakes. [Finetex] Sodium cocoyl isethionate; EINECS 263-052-5; anionic; mild detergent, foamer, dispersant for soap-syndet, toilet bars, shampoos, bubble baths, mild foaming facial cleansers; imparts conditioning to hair and skin; emulsifier in creams and lotions.

Tauranol M-35. [Finetex] Sodium N-methyl-N oleoyl taurate; CAS 137-20-2; EINECS 205-285-7; anionic; detergent, wetting agent, all-purpose surfactant for textile processes, soaping prints, naphthols and vats, kier boil-off,

bleaching, dyeing, shampoos, bubble baths, household cleaners; liq.; 23% conc.

Tauranol ML. [Finetex] Sodium methyl oleoyl taurate and isopropyl alcohol; CAS 137-20-2; EINECS 205-285-7; anionic; detergent, dispersant for hard surf. cleaners, personal care prods.; lime soap dispersant; liq.; 33% conc.

Tauranol MS. [Finetex] Sodium methyl oleoyl taurate; CAS 137-20-2; EINECS 205-285-7; anionic; wetting agent and detergent scour; for personal care prods., household cleaners; paste; 33% conc.

Tauranol T-Gel. [Finetex] Sodium N-methyl-N oleoyl taurate; CAS 137-20-2; EINECS 205-285-7; anionic; wetting and detergent scour for textiles, personal care prods.; soaping off agent; gel; 14% conc.

Tauranol WS, WS Conc. [Finetex] Sodium methyl cocoyl taurate; anionic; detergent, foamer used in cosmetic preparations, household cleaners; slurry; 24 and 31% conc. resp.

Tauranol WS H.P. [Finetex] Sodium methyl cocoyl taurate; anionic; foamer, detergent for personal care prods., pharmaceuticals; tolerance to electrolytes, hard water; powd.; 95% conc.

Tauranol WSP. [Finetex] Sodium methyl cocoyl taurate; anionic; detergent, foaming agent for cosmetic preps., household cleaners; powd.; 70% conc.

TBAB. [Zeeland] Tetrabutyl ammonium bromide; CAS 1643-19-2; EINECS 216-699-2.

T-Base. [Tri-K Industries] Mineral oil, PEG-30 lanolin, and cetyl alcohol; emulsifer for skin care cosmetics; biodeg.; pale yel. pearly soft waxy solid, faint odor; disp. in water; sp.gr. 0.89; m.p. 32-42 C; b.p. 375 F; acid no. 1.5 max.; sapon. no. 6-24; flash pt. (OC) 425 F; toxicology: LD50 (oral, rat) > 50 ml/kg; nonirritating to skin and eyes.

TBC. [Morflex] Tri-n-butyl citrate; CAS 77-94-1; EINECS 201-071-2; aq. based pharmaceutical coating.

T-Det® O-407. [Harcros] Octoxynol-40; CAS 9002-93-1; nonionic; detergent, emulsifier, stabilizer for various applics.; FDA compliance; APHA 100 max. liq.; water-sol.; sp.gr. 1.10; dens. 9.1 lb/gal; visc. 600 cps; HLB 17.9; cloud pt. > 100 C (1%); flash pt. > 100 C (TOC); pour pt. 30 F; pH 7 (1%); 70 ± 0.5% act.

TEA 85. [Dow] Triethanolamine (85%), diethanolamine (15%); used in surfactants, cosmetics/toiletries, metalworking, textile chemicals, gas conditioning chemicals, agric. intermediates, adhesives, antistats, cotings, corrosion inhibition, electroplating, petroleum, polymers, rubber, cement grinding aids; sp.gr. 1.1179; dens. 9.34 lb/gal; visc. 590.5 cps; f.p. 17 C; b.p. 325 C (760 mm Hg); flash pt. (PMCC) 354 F; fire pt. 410 F; ref. index 1.4836.

TEA 85 Low Freeze Grade. [Dow] Triethanolamine (85%), water (15%); CAS 102-71-6; EINECS 203-049-8; used in surfactants, cosmetics/toiletries, metalworking, textile chemicals, gas conditioning chemicals, agric. intermediates, adhesives, antistats, cotings, corrosion inhibition, electroplating, petroleum, polymers, rubber, cement grinding aids; sp.gr. 1.1179; dens. 9.34 lb/gal; visc. 590.5 cps; f.p. 17 C; b.p. 325 C (760 mm Hg); flash pt. (PMCC) 354 F; fire pt. 410 F; ref. index 1.4836.

TEA 99 Low Freeze Grade [Dow] Triethanolamine; CAS 102-71-6; EINECS 203-049-8; used in surfactants, cosmetics/toiletries, metalworking, textile chemicals, gas conditioning chemicals, agric. intermediates, adhesives, antistats, cotings, corrosion inhibition, electroplating, petroleum, polymers, rubber, cement grinding aids; sp.gr. 1.1205; dens. 9.35 lb/gal; visc. 600.7 cps; f.p. 21 C; b.p. 340 C (760 mm Hg); flash pt. (COC) 350 F; fire pt. 420 F; ref. index 1.4839; 15% water.

TEA 99 Standard Grade. [Dow] Triethanolamine; CAS 102-71-6; EINECS 203-049-8; used in surfactants, cosmetics/

toiletries, metalworking, textile chemicals, gas conditioning chemicals, agric. intermediates, adhesives, antistats, cotings, corrosion inhibition, electroplating, petroleum, polymers, rubber, cement grinding aids; sp.gr. 1.1205; dens. 9.35 lb/gal; visc. 600.7 cps; f.p. 21 C; b.p. 340 C (760 mm Hg); flash pt. (COC) 350 F; fire pt. 420 F; ref. index 1.4839.

TEC. [Morflex] Triethyl citrate; CAS 77-93-0; EINECS 201-070-7; aq. based pharmaceutical coating.

Tecquinol® USP Grade. [Eastman] Hydroquinone; CAS 123-31-9; EINECS 204-617-8; cosmetics ingred.

Tefose® 63. [Gattefosse; Gattefosse SA] PEG-6-32 stearate and glycol stearate; nonionic; SE base for cosmetics, o/w pharmaceutical ointments; exc. skin and mucosal tolerance; esp. for anti-mycotic preps.; Gardner < 5 waxy solid; weak odor; sol. in chloroform, methylene chloride; disp. in water; insol. in ethanol, min. oils; m.p. 40-45 C; drop pt. 46-53 C; HLB 10.0; acid no. < 6; iodine no. < 3; sapon. no. 110–120; usage level: 15-20%; toxicology: nonrritating to skin and eyes; 100% conc.

Tefose® 70. [Gattefosse] PEG-2 stearate, ceteareth-20.

Tefose® 1500. [Gattefosse; Gattefosse SA] PEG-6-32 stearate; CAS 9004-99-3; nonionic; self-emulsifying base for o/w cosmetic or pharmaceutical emulsions (thick lotions and creams); Gardner < 5 pasty solid; weak odor; sol. in ethanol, chloroform, methylene chloride; insol. in water, min. oils; m.p. 39-45 C; drop pt. 42-46 C; HLB 11.0; acid no. < 6; iodine no. < 3; sapon. no. 75–95; usage level: 5-15%; toxicology: nonirritating to skin and eyes; 100% conc.

Tefose® 2000. [Gattefosse; Gattefosse SA] PEG-6 stearate, ceteth-20, steareth-20; nonionic; self-emulsifying base for o/w cosmetic or pharmaceutical emulsions (fluid, semifluid lotions, and creams); Gardner < 5 pasty solid; weak odor; sol. in chloroform, methylene chloride; sparingly sol. in ethanol; disp. in water, n-hexane; insol. in min. oils; m.p. 32-37 C; HLB 11.0; acid no. < 6; iodine no. < 3; sapon. no. 65–85; usage level: 5-15%; toxicology: nonirritating to skin; sl. irritating to eyes; 100% conc.

Tefose® 2561. [Gattefosse; Gattefosse SA] PEG-6 stearate, glyceryl stearate, and ceteth-20; nonionic; base for o/w cosmetic or pharmaceutical emulsions; Gardner < 3 pasty solid; weak odor; HLB 10.0; m.p. 35–40 C; acid no. < 5; iodine no. < 3; sapon. no. 65–105; usage level: 5-15%; toxicology: LD50 (oral, rat) > 2 g/kg; sl. irritating to skin and eyes; 100% conc.

Tegacid® Regular VA. [Goldschmidt] Glyceryl stearate, stearamidoethyldiethylamine; cationic; self-emulsifying; forms stable emulsions for creams and lotions; acid stable; flake; HLB 4.2; 100% conc.

Tegacid® Special. [Goldschmidt] Glyceryl stearate, sodium lauryl sulfate; anionic; forms very stable personal care emulsions, creams, and lotions; acid stable; broad pH range; flake; HLB 4.9; 100% conc.

Tegacid® Special VA. [Goldschmidt] Glyceryl stearate SE; anionic; self-emulsifying, acid stable surfactant; flake; HLB 4.9; 100% conc.

Tegamine® 18. [Goldschmidt] Stearamidopropyl dimethylamine; CAS 7651-02-7; EINECS 231-609-1; cationic; surfactant, conditioner for hair care and bath prods.; aux. emulsifier for creams and lotions; provides skin feel; flake; 100% act.

Tegamine® Oxide WS-35. [Goldschmidt] Cocamidopropylamine oxide; CAS 68155-09-9; EINECS 268-938-5; nonionic; foam builder/stabilizer for shampoos, bath preps., liq. detergents; visc. builder; liq.; 35% conc.

Tegin® . [Goldschmidt] Glyceryl stearate SE; anionic; self-emulsifying emulsifier for cosmetic and pharmaceutical o/w emulsions; powd.; HLB 5.5; 100% conc.

Tegin® 55G VA. [Goldschmidt] Glyceryl stearate; nonionic;

nonself-emulsifying gloss agent and emollient for creams; flake; HLB 3.8; 100% conc.

Tegin® 90 NSE. [Goldschmidt; Goldschmidt AG] Glyceryl stearate; nonionic; stabilizer for creamy and liq. o/w emulsions in cosmetics, pharmaceuticals; wh.-ivory powd.; sol. warm in min. and veg. oils; insol. in water; m.p. 67-72 C; HLB 4.5; acid no. 3 max.; iodine no. 2 max.; sapon. no. 155-170; 100% conc.

Tegin® 515. [Goldschmidt] Glyceryl stearate; nonionic; emulsifier, stabilizer for creams and lotions; powd.; HLB 3.8; 100% conc.

Tegin® 515 VA. [Goldschmidt] Glyceryl stearate; nonionic; emulsifier, stabilizer, opacifier for skin care creams and lotions; improved afterfeel for leave-on conditioners; flake; HLB 3.8; 100% conc.

Tegin® 4011. [Goldschmidt; Goldschmidt AG] Glyceryl stearate; CAS 31566-31-1; nonionic; emulsifier for pharmaceuticals; wh.-ivory powd.; sol. warm in veg. and min. oils; insol. in water; m.p. 54-60 C; HLB 3.8; acid no. 3 max.; iodine no. 3 max.; sapon. no. 162-173; 100% conc.

Tegin® 4100 NSE. [Goldschmidt; Goldschmidt AG] Glyceryl stearate; CAS 31566-31-1; nonionic; emulsifier for cosmetics and pharmaceuticals; wh.-ivory powd.; sol. warm in veg. and min. oils; insol. in water; m.p. 58-63 C; HLB 3.8; acid no. 2 max.; iodine no. 3 max.; sapon. no. 164-180; 100% conc.

Tegin® 4433. [Goldschmidt; Goldschmidt AG] Glyceryl stearate SE; anionic; emulsifier for pharmaceuticals; British Pharmaceutical Codex; wh.-ivory powd.; sol. warm in veg. and min. oils; disp. warm in water; m.p. 54-57 C; HLB 12.0; acid no. 18 max.; iodine no. 8 max.; sapon. no. 148-156; 100% conc.

Tegin® 4480. [Goldschmidt] Glyceryl stearate; nonionic; emulsifier and stabilizer for cosmetics and pharmaceuticals; semisolid; HLB 3.8; 100% conc.

Tegin® 4600 NSE. [Goldschmidt] Glyceryl caprylate/caprate; nonionic; antistat and lubricant for syn. materials; emulsifier for cosmetic and pharmaceutical prods.; liq.; HLB 4.0; 100% conc.

Tegin® D 1102. [Goldschmidt AG] PEG-3 stearate; CAS 9004-99-3; EINECS 233-562-2; sheen additive for cosmetics; pearlizing agent for shampoos, shower, and bath preps.; wh.-ivory powd.; sol. warm in min. and veg. oils; insol. in water; m.p. 47-52 C; HLB 3.8; acid no. 5-7; iodine no. 3 max.; sapon. no. 168-178; ≈ 90% diester.

Tegin® D 6100. [Goldschmidt; Goldschmidt AG] PEG-2 stearate; CAS 9004-99-3; EINECS 203-363-5; nonionic; lipophilic coemulsifier for o/w emulsions; wh.-ivory waxy solid; sol. warm in veg. and min. oils; insol. in water; m.p. 40-46 C; HLB 2.8; acid no. 5 max.; iodine no. 3 max.; sapon. no. 145-160; 100% conc.

Tegin® G. [Goldschmidt; Goldschmidt AG] Glycol stearate SE; CAS 86418-55-5; anionic; self-emulsifying sheen additive, opacifier for cosmetics and pharmaceuticals; o/w emulsions; wh.-ivory waxy powd.; sol. warm in veg. and min. oils; disp. warm in water; m.p. 48-53 C; HLB 12.0; acid no. 36-38; iodine no. 3 max.; sapon. no. 150-165; 100% conc.

Tegin® G 1100. [Goldschmidt AG] Glycol distearate; CAS 627-83-8; EINECS 211-014-3; sheen additive, pearlescent, opacifier for shampoos; non SE; wh.-ivory powd.; sol. warm in min. and veg. oils; insol. in water; m.p. 59-63 C; acid no. 6 max.; iodine no. 3 max.; sapon. no. 192-208; ≈ 90% diester.

Tegin® G 6100. [Goldschmidt; Goldschmidt AG] Glycol stearate; CAS 111-60-4; EINECS 203-886-9; nonionic; lipophilic coemulsifier for o/w emulsions; promotes silky shine in shampoos; wh.-ivory powd.; sol. warm in min. and veg. oils; insol. in water; m.p. 53-58 C; HLB 3.2; acid no. 3 max.; iodine no. 3 max.; sapon. no. 180-195; 100%

conc.

Tegin® ISO NSE. [Goldschmidt; Goldschmidt AG] Glyceryl mono/diisostearate; CAS 68958-48-5; anionic; w/o emulsifier for cosmetic creams; ivory paste; sol. in veg. and min. oils; insol. in water; HLB 3.4; acid no. 2 max.; iodine no. 15 max.; sapon. no. 150-165; 100% conc.

Tegin® M. [Goldschmidt; Goldschmidt AG] Glyceryl stearate; anionic; emulsifier for o/w cosmetic/pharmaceutical systems; wh.-ivory powd.; sol. warm in veg. and min. oils; insol. in water; m.p. 58-63 C; HLB 3.8; acid no. 2 max.; iodine no. 4 max.; sapon. no. 165-180; 100% conc.

Tegin® O. [Goldschmidt; Goldschmidt AG] Glyceryl mono/dioleate; CAS 25496-72-4; nonionic; emulsifier for w/o emulsions for pharmaceuticals; pale yel. paste; sol. in veg. and min. oils; insol. in water; HLB 3.3; acid no. 2 max.; iodine no. 70-76; sapon. no. 158-175; 100% conc.

Tegin® P. [Goldschmidt; Goldschmidt AG] Propylene glycol stearate SE; anionic; emulsifier for o/w lotions and creams for cosmetics and pharmaceuticals; solubilizer for dye-stuffs; wh.-ivory waxy solid; sol. warm in min. and veg. oils; disp. warm in water; m.p. 39-46 C; HLB 12.0; acid no. 16-18; iodine no. 3 max.; sapon. no. 150-170; 100% conc.

Tegin® Spezial. [Goldschmidt; Goldschmidt AG] Glyceryl stearate; anionic; emulsifier for cosmetic and pharmaceutical o/w emulsions; wh.-ivory powd.; sol. warm in veg. and min. oils; disp. warm in water; m.p. 54-60 C; HLB 12.0; acid no. 16-20; iodine no. 3 max.; sapon. no. 148-158; 100% conc.

Tegin® V. [Goldschmidt] Glyceryl stearate SE; self-emulsifying grade forming o/w emulsions for creams and lotions.

Teginacid® . [Goldschmidt; Goldschmidt AG] Glyceryl stearate and ceteareth-20; nonionic; emulsifier for o/w emulsions; powd.; HLB 12.0; 100% conc.

Teginacid® H. [Goldschmidt; Goldschmidt AG] Glyceryl stearate and ceteth-20; nonionic; emulsifier for o/w emulsions, acid and salt resisting emulsions; self-emulsifying; powd.; HLB 11.2; 100% conc.

Teginacid® H-SE. [Goldschmidt; Goldschmidt AG] Glyceryl monodistearate and other nonionics; nonionic; self-emulsifying; for acid and salt resistant o/w emulsions with liq. or creamy consistency; ivory powd.; sol. warm in veg. and min. oils; disp. warm in water; m.p. 45-51 C; HLB 11.2; acid no. 3 max.; iodine no. 3 max.; sapon. no. 55-70; 100% conc.

Teginacid® SE. [Goldschmidt; Goldschmidt AG] Glyceryl monodistearate; nonionic; self-emulsifying; for acid and salt resistant o/w emulsions with liq. or creamy consistency; ivory powd.; sol. warm in veg. and min. oils; disp. warm in water; m.p. 58-63 C; HLB 12.0; acid no. 3 max.; iodine no. 4 max.; sapon. no. 153-165; 100% conc.

Teginacid® Special. [Goldschmidt; Goldschmidt AG] Glyceryl stearate SE; anionic; self-emulsifying acid-stable emulsifier for cosmetic creams and lotions; solid; HLB 4.8; 100% conc.

Teginacid® Spezial SE. [Goldschmidt AG] Glyceryl stearate, sodium lauryl sulfate; anionic; emulsifier for acid and salt-resisting o/w cosmetic emulsions of liq. or creamy consistency; ivory powd.; sol. warm in veg. oils, sol. warm with sl. turbidity in min. oil; disp. warm in water; m.p. 53-59 C; HLB 12.0; acid no. 16-18; iodine no. 3 max.; sapon. no. 160-172; 100% conc.

Teginacid® X SE. [Goldschmidt; Goldschmidt AG] Glyceryl stearate and ceteareth-20; nonionic; self-emulsifying emulsifier for acid and salt resistant o/w emulsions with liq. or creamy consistency; ivory powd.; sol. warm in veg. and min. oils; disp. warm in water; m.p. 55-61 C; HLB 12.0; acid no. 3 max.; iodine no. 4 max.; sapon. no. 145-160; 100% conc.

Tego®-Amid S 18. [Goldschmidt; Goldschmidt AG] Stearamidopropyl dimethylamine; CAS 7651-02-7; EINECS

231-609-1; cationic; emulsifier for creams and lotions; conditioner for hair care prods.; ivory flakes; sol. warm @ 10% in veg. and min. oils; insol. in water; acid no. 4 max.; 100% conc.

Tego®-Betaine C. [Goldschmidt; Goldschmidt AG] Cocamidopropyl betaine; CAS 61789-40-0; amphoteric; surfactant used as foam stabilizer and visc. builder in personal care prods., nonirritating shampoos, bubble baths, body cleansers, dishwash, liq. soap; lt. clear liq.; pH 5.0; 30% act.

Tego®-Betaine F. [Goldschmidt; Goldschmidt AG] Cocamidopropyl betaine; CAS 61789-40-0; amphoteric; surfactant for nonirritating shampoos, bubble baths, hygiene and baby care prods.; yel. liq.; pH 5-7; 30% act.

Tego®-Betaine HS. [Goldschmidt; Goldschmidt AG] Cocamidopropyl betaine and glyceryl laurate; amphoteric; mild surfactant for nonirritating shampoos, conditioners, and baby care prods.; good refatting props.; yel. liq.; pH 6-7; 30% act.

Tego®-Betaine L-7. [Goldschmidt; Goldschmidt AG] Cocamidopropyl betaine; CAS 61789-40-0; amphoteric; surfactant, detergent, emulsifier, foam stabilizer, visc. builder in low-irritation personal care prods., pharmaceuticals; esp. mild for baby care prods.; ivory powd. or yel. liq.; sp.gr. 1.040-1.050 (liq.); pH 5; toxicology: LD50 (acute oral) 8.10 ml/kg; nonirritating to eyes; 78-85% active. (powd.), 30% act. (liq.).

Tego®-Betaine L-10 S. [Goldschmidt AG] Lauramidopropyl betaine; EINECS 224-292-6; amphoteric; surfactant for personal care and pharmaceutical prods. (nonirritating shampoos, bubble baths, body cleansers, baby prods.); lt. clear liq.; pH 5.0; 30% act.

Tego®-Betaine L-5351. [Goldschmidt; Goldschmidt AG] Cocamidopropyl betaine; CAS 61789-40-0; amphoteric; low-salt surfactant for use in salt-critical formulations, e.g., hair dyes, fixatives, reactive prods., aerosols, electrolyte-sensitive formulations; yel. liq.; pH 6; 30% act.

Tego®-Betaine N-192. [Goldschmidt; Goldschmidt AG] Dihydroxyethyl tallow glycinate; CAS 61791-25-1; EINECS 274-845-0; amphoteric; surfactant for acid and alkali-stable formulations; highly visc. liq.; 35% conc.

Tego® Care 150. [Goldschmidt; Goldschmidt AG] Glyceryl stearate, steareth-25, ceteth-20, stearyl alcohol; nonionic; wax-like o/w balanced emulsifier systems for creams and lotions; optimized for ease of formulation; ivory powd.; sol. warm in veg. and min. oils, cosmetic alcohol, 1,2-propylene glycol (sl. turbid); disp. warm in water; m.p. 52-58 C; HLB 12; acid no. 3 max.; sapon. no. 90-106; usage level: 7-10%; 100% conc.

Tego® Care 215. [Goldschmidt] Ceteareth-15 and glyceryl stearate; nonionic; emulsifier for cosmetic o/w lotions, skin care prods.; produces brilliant appearance; good thermal stability; ivory pellets; acid no. 3 max.; iodine no. 3 max.; sapon. no. 64-74; usage level: 2-3%.

Tego® Care 300. [Goldschmidt] Glyceryl stearate, steareth-25, ceteth-20; nonionic; wax-like o/w balanced emulsifier systems for creams and lotions; optimized for ease of formulation; wh./ivory powd.; sol. warm in veg. oil, min. oil, alcohol, propylene glycol; disp. warm in water; m.p. 56-62 C; HLB 12; acid no. 3 max.; sapon. no. 114-130; 100% conc.

Tego® Care 450. [Goldschmidt] Polyglyceryl methyl glucose distearate; nonionic; o/w emulsifier producing stable emulsions with cosmetics oils and waxes; emulsifier for creams, lotions, hair conditioners, sun prods.; for systems with pH of 6-9; ivory pellets; sol. warm in paraffin and veg. oils; disp. warm in water; HLB 11.5 ± 1; acid no. 12 max.; iodine no. 5 max.; sapon. no. 120-140; usage level: 3%.

Tego®-Pearl B-48. [Goldschmidt; Goldschmidt AG] Cocamidopropyl betaine, glycol distearate, cocamide DEA, cocamide MEA; amphoteric; pearlescent and opacifier for hair care prods.; cold mixable; wh. liq.; pH 5-7 (10% aq.); 44% act.

Tegosoft® CI. [Goldschmidt] Cetearyl isononanoate; cosmetic esters for emolliency, skin softening, and moisture retention in hair and skin care prods., creams and lotions, hair conditioners/glossing systems, sunscreen preps., soaps.

Tegosoft® CO. [Goldschmidt] Cetyl octanoate; CAS 59130-69-7; EINECS 261-619-1; cosmetic esters for emolliency, skin softening, and moisture retention in hair and skin care prods., creams and lotions, hair conditioners/glossing systems, sunscreen preps., soaps.

Tegosoft® CT. [Goldschmidt] Caprylic/capric triglycerides; CAS 65381-09-1; cosmetic esters for emolliency, skin softening, and moisture retention in hair and skin care prods., creams and lotions, hair conditioners/glossing systems, sunscreen preps., soaps.

Tegosoft® DO. [Goldschmidt] Decyl oleate; CAS 3687-46-5; EINECS 222-981-6; cosmetic esters for emolliency, skin softening, and moisture retention in hair and skin care prods., creams and lotions, hair conditioners/glossing systems, sunscreen preps., soaps.

Tegosoft® EE. [Goldschmidt] Octyl octanoate; CAS 7425-14-1; EINECS 231-057-1; cosmetic esters for emolliency, skin softening, and moisture retention in hair and skin care prods., creams and lotions, hair conditioners/glossing systems, sunscreen preps., soaps.

Tegosoft® GC. [Goldschmidt] PEG-7 glyceryl cocoate; mild surfactant for shampoos, bath prods. and personal cleansers; refatting and conditioning agent; foam booster/stabilizer; rinses clean; very sol. in water.

Tegosoft® Liquid. [Goldschmidt] Cetearyl octanoate; cosmetic esters for emolliency, skin softening, and moisture retention in hair and skin care prods., creams and lotions, hair conditioners/glossing systems, sunscreen preps., soaps.

Tegosoft® Liquid M. [Goldschmidt] Cetearyl octanoate and isopropyl myristate; cosmetic esters for emolliency, skin softening, and moisture retention in hair and skin care prods., creams and lotions, hair conditioners/glossing systems, sunscreen preps., soaps.

Tegosoft® M. [Goldschmidt] Isopropyl myristate; CAS 110-27-0; EINECS 203-751-4; cosmetic esters for emolliency, skin softening, and moisture retention in hair and skin care prods., creams and lotions, hair conditioners/glossing systems, sunscreen preps., soaps.

Tegosoft® OP. [Goldschmidt] Octyl palmitate; CAS 29806-73-3; EINECS 249-862-1; cosmetic esters for emolliency, skin softening, and moisture retention in hair and skin care prods., creams and lotions, hair conditioners/glossing systems, sunscreen preps., soaps.

Tegosoft® OS. [Goldschmidt] Octyl stearate; cosmetic esters for emolliency, skin softening, and moisture retention in hair and skin care prods., creams and lotions, hair conditioners/glossing systems, sunscreen preps., soaps.

Tegosoft® P. [Goldschmidt] Isopropyl palmitate; CAS 142-91-6; EINECS 205-571-1; cosmetic esters for emolliency, skin softening, and moisture retention in hair and skin care prods., creams and lotions, hair conditioners/glossing systems, sunscreen preps., soaps.

Tegosoft® S. [Goldschmidt] Isopropyl stearate; CAS 112-10-7; EINECS 203-934-9; cosmetic esters for emolliency, skin softening, and moisture retention in hair and skin care prods., creams and lotions, hair conditioners/glossing systems, sunscreen preps., soaps.

Tegosoft® SH. [Goldschmidt] Stearyl heptanoate; CAS 66009-41-4; cosmetic esters for emolliency, skin softening, and moisture retention in hair and skin care prods., creams and lotions, hair conditioners/glossing systems,

sunscreen preps., soaps.

Teinowax. [Lanaetex Prods.] Cetearyl alcohol, polysorbate 60, PEG-150 stearate, steareth-20; cosmetics ingred.

Tektamer® 38. [Calgon] Methyldibromo glutaronitrile; CAS 35691-65-7; EINECS 252-681-0; antimicrobial for preserving cosmetics and personal care prods.

Tektamer® 38 A.D. [Calgon] Methyldibromo glutaronitrile, sodium chloride, xanthan gum, dimethicone; antimicrobial for preserving cosmetics and personal care prods.

Tektamer® 38 L.V. [Calgon] Methyldibromo glutaronitrile, attapulgite, dimethicone, xanthan gum; antimicrobial for preserving cosmetics and personal care prods.

Tenox® 2. [Eastman] Propylene glycol, BHA, propyl gallate, citric acid; food-grade antioxidant; also for cosmetics.

Tenox® 4. [Eastman] Corn oil, BHA, BHT; food-grade antioxidant; also for cosmetics.

Tenox® 4B. [Eastman] Corn oil, BHT; antioxidant for cosmetics and personal care prods.

Tenox® 6. [Eastman] Corn oil, glyceryl oleate, propylene glycol, BHA, BHT, propyl gallate, citric acid; antioxidant for cosmetics and food applics.

Tenox® 20B. [Eastman] Propylene glycol, t-butyl hydroquinone, and citric acid; antioxidant for cosmetics and personal care prods.

Tenox® 22. [Eastman] Propylene glycol, t-butyl hydroquinone, and citric acid; antioxidant for foods and cosmetics.

Tenox® 25. [Eastman] Corn oil, glyceryl oleate, propylene glycol, BHT, TBHQ, citric acid; antioxidant for cosmetics and personal care prods.

Tenox® 26. [Eastman] Corn oil, glyceryl oleate, propylene glycol, BHA, BHT, t-butyl hydroquinone, citric acid; antioxidant for foods and cosmetics.

Tenox® BHA. [Eastman] BHA; CAS 5013-16-5; antioxidant for food applic., food pkg., plastics, rubber, and cosmetics; wh. waxy tablets; slight odor; m.w. 180; b.p. 264–270 C (733 mm); sol. in ethanol, diisobutyl adipate, propylene glycol, glyceryl monooleate, soya oil, lard, yel. grease, and paraffin; insol. in water; m.p. 48–55 C.

Tenox® BHT. [Eastman] BHT; CAS 128-37-0; EINECS 204-881-4; antioxidant for cosmetics and personal care prods.

Tenox® GT-1, GT-2. [Eastman] Tocopherol; food-grade antioxidant; also for cosmetics and personal care prods.

Tenox® PG. [Eastman] Propyl gallate; CAS 121-79-9; EINECS 204-498-2; antioxidant for cosmetics, fats and oils; stabilizer for food applic.; wh. cryst. powd.; slight odor; sol. in ethanol, propylene glycol, and water; m.w. 212; b.p. 148 C; m.p. 146–148 C.

Tenox® TBHQ. [Eastman] t-Butyl hydroquinone; CAS 1948-33-0; EINECS 217-752-2; antioxidant and stabilizer used in cosmetics and in oils and fats for food applic.; wh. to lt. tan cryst., slight odor; sol. in ethanol, ethyl acetate; < 1% in water; m.w. 166.22; m.p. 126.5–128.5 C.

Tensagex DLM 627. [Hickson Manro Ltd.] Sodium trideceth sulfate; anionic; for liq. detergent blends, shampoos, bubble baths, liq. soaps; liq.; 26-28% conc.

Tensagex DLM 670. [Hickson Manro Ltd.] Sodium trideceth sulfate; anionic; for liq. detergent blends, shampoos, bubble baths, liq. soaps; liq.; 68-72% conc.

Tensagex DLM 927. [Hickson Manro Ltd.] Sodium laureth sulfate (3 mole), syn. based; anionic; for liq. detergent blends, shampoos, bubble baths, liq. soaps, household detergents, industrial cleaning; liq.; 27% act.

Tensagex DLM 970. [Hickson Manro Ltd.] Sodium laureth sulfate (3 mole), syn. based; anionic; for liq. detergent blends, shampoos, bubble baths, liq. soaps, household detergents, industrial cleaning; liq.; 68% act.

Tensagex DLS 670. [Hickson Manro Ltd.] Sodium trideceth sulfate; anionic; for liq. detergent blends, shampoos, bubble baths, liq. soaps; liq.; 68-72% conc.

Tensagex DLS 970. [Hickson Manro Ltd.] Sodium trideceth

sulfate; anionic; for liq. detergent blends, shampoos, bubble baths, liq. soaps; liq.; 68-72% conc.

Tensagex EOC 628. [Hickson Manro Ltd.] Sodium laureth sulfate (2 mole), natural based; CAS 68585-34-2; anionic; for liq. detergent blends, shampoos, bubble baths, liq. soaps, hair care prods.; liq.; 28% conc.

Tensagex EOC 670. [Hickson Manro Ltd.] Sodium laureth sulfate (2 mole), natural based; CAS 68585-34-2; anionic; for liq. detergent blends, shampoos, bubble baths, liq. soaps, hair care prods.; liq.; 70% act.

Tensami 1/05. [Alban Muller; Tri-K Industries] Lecithin, xanthan gum; natural emulsifier for cosmetic field.

Tensami 3/06. [Alban Muller; Tri-K Industries] Casein, xanthan gum; natural emulsifier for cosmetic field.

Tensami 4/07. [Alban Muller; Tri-K Industries] Soy protein, xanthan gum; natural emulsifier for cosmetic field.

Tensami 8/09. [Alban Muller; Tri-K Industries] Corn oil, egg yolk extract; natural emulsifier for cosmetic field.

Tensami 10/06. [Alban Muller; Tri-K Industries] Saponins, xanthan gum; natural emulsifier for cosmetic field.

Tensianol 399 ISL. [ICI Surf. Am.; ICI plc] Syndet based on alkyl sulfate and cocoyl isothiohate; anionic; raw material for mfg. of alkali-free soap bars; wh. to ivory flakes; 36-38% conc.

Tensianol 399 KS1. [ICI Surf. Am.; ICI Surf. UK] Syndet based on alkyl sulfate; anionic; raw material for mfg. of alkali-free soap bars; wh. to ivory flakes; 46-48% conc.

Tensianol 399 N1. [ICI Surf. Am.; ICI plc] Syndet based on alkyl sulfate; anionic; raw material for mfg. of alkali-free soap bars; wh. to ivory flakes; 39-41% conc.

Tensianol 399 SCIL. [ICI Surf. Am.; ICI Surf. UK] Syndet based on cocoylisethionate; anionic; raw material for mfg. of alkali-free soap bars; wh. to ivory flakes; 32-34% conc.

Tensiorex BND57. [Hickson Manro Ltd.] Pearlizing agent for hair care and bath prods.; visc. liq.; 40% act.

Tensopol 528LS. [Hickson Manro Ltd.] Sodium alkyl sulfate; surfactant for hair care and bath prods., household detergents, and industrial cleaning; liq.; 28% act.

Tensopol A 79. [Hickson Manro Ltd.] Sodium fatty alcohol sulfate; CAS 73296-89-6; anionic; surfactant for toiletries, hair care and bath prods., household detergents, industrial cleaning, emulsion polymerization, pigment dispersion; needles; 90% act.

Tensopol A 795. [Hickson Manro Ltd.] Sodium fatty alcohol sulfate; CAS 73296-89-6; anionic; surfactant for toiletries, hair care and bath prods., household detergents, industrial cleaning, emulsion polymerization, pigment dispersion; needles; 95% act.

Tensopol ACL 79. [Hickson Manro Ltd.] Broadcut sodium fatty alcohol sulfate; CAS 68955-19-1; anionic; surfactant for toiletries, hair care and bath prods., household detergents, industrial cleaning, emulsion polymerization, pigment dispersion; needles; 90% act.

Tensopol ACL795. [Hickson Manro Ltd.] Broadcut sodium alkyl sulfate; surfactant for hair care and bath prods., household detergents, and industrial cleaning; needles; 95% act.

Tensopol AG. [Hickson Manro Ltd.] Magnesium alkyl sulfate; surfactant for hair care and bath prods., household detergents, and industrial cleaning; needles; 80% act.

Tensopol LTS. [Hickson Manro Ltd.] TEA fatty alcohol sulfate; CAS 68815-25-8; anionic; surfactant for toiletries, hair care and bath prods., household detergents; liq.; 40% act.

Tensopol SPK. [Hickson Manro Ltd.] Sodium/potassium fatty alcohol sulfate; CAS 4706-78-9; anionic; surfactant for syn. toilet bars, hair care and bath preps., household detergents, industrial cleaning; powd.; 96% act.

Tensopol USP 94. [Hickson Manro Ltd.] Sodium fatty alcohol sulfate; CAS 73296-89-6; anionic; for pharmaceuticals, toothpaste, hair care and bath prods., household detergents, industrial cleaning; powd.; 94% act.

Tensopol USP 97. [Hickson Manro Ltd.] Sodium fatty alcohol sulfate; CAS 73296-89-6; anionic; for pharmaceuticals, toothpaste, hair care and bath prods., household detergents, industrial cleaning; powd.; 97% act.

Tensuccin HM 935. [Hickson Manro Ltd.] Sodium hemi-sulfosuccinate of a modified alcohol ethoxylate; anionic; mild surfactant for shampoos, bubble baths, shower gels, dermatological preps.; liq.; 40% act.

Tepescohuite AMI Watersoluble. [Alban Muller] Mimosa bark extract in water and propylene glycol; natural ingred. with soothing props., regenerative agent for skin tissue; for pharmaceuticals, cosmetics, aftersun lotions, baby skin care prods., protection creams; red brn.; sol. in water, alcohol; sp.gr. 1.035; b.p. 106 C; ref. index 1.3880-1.4090; pH 5.10-7.10.

Tepescohuite HG. [Alban Muller] Mimosa bark extract in water and propylene glycol; regenerative agent for skin tissue; for pharmaceuticals, cosmetics, aftersun lotions, baby skin care prods., protection creams; dk. red; sol. in water, alcohol; sp.gr. 1.030; b.p. 100 C; ref. index 1.3880-1.4090; pH 5-7; usage level: 1-5%.

Tepescohuite HS. [Alban Muller] Mimosa bark extract in propylene glycol (> 95%); regenerative agent for skin tissue; for pharmaceuticals, cosmetics, aftersun lotions, baby skin care prods., protection creams; red brn.; sol. in water, alcohol; sp.gr. 1.045; b.p. 188.2 C; flash pt. (OC) 107 C; ref. index 1.4300-1.4360; pH 6-8; usage level: 1-5%.

Tepescohuite LS. [Alban Muller] Mimosa bark extract in edible sunflower oil; regenerative agent for skin tissue; for pharmaceuticals, cosmetics, aftersun lotions, baby skin care prods., protection creams; yel.; sol. in org. solvs.; insol. in water; sp.gr. 0.915; acid no. < 3; iodine no. 105-135; sapon. no. 180-198; ref. index 1.4735-1.4785; usage level: 1-5%.

Tequat BC. [Auschem SpA] Cetrimonium chloride; CAS 112-02-7; EINECS 203-928-6; softener, after-treatment hair prep.; liq.

Tequat PAN. [Auschem SpA] Lauralkonium chloride; CAS 139-07-1; EINECS 205-351-5; germicide, antistat; liq.

Tergitol® 26-L-3. [Union Carbide] C12-16 pareth-3; nonionic; surfactant, emulsifier, intermediate for sulfation; used for prewash spotters, coning oil, hydrocarbon-based cleaners, agric.; as sulfated prod. in cosmetics, hand dishwash, lt. duty detergents; FDA and EPA compliance; APHA 10 clear to slightly hazy liq.; mild char. odor; misc. with ethyl acetate, ethanol, propylene glycol, IPA, toluene, hexane; m.w. 328; sp.gr. 0.917; visc. 19 cSt (37.8 C); HLB 8.0; hyd. no. 168-178; flash pt. (PMCC) 157 C; pour pt. 6 C; pH 6.9 (1% in 10:6 IPA/water).

Tergitol® NP-9. [Union Carbide] Nonoxynol-9; CAS 9016-45-9; nonionic; detergent, wetting agent, dispersant, emulsifier; yel. clear liq.; mild char. odor; m.w. 616; sol. in butyl acetate, butyl Cellosolve, ethylene glycol, anhyd. IPA, toluene, water; sp.gr. 1.057; dens. 8.80 lb/gal; visc. 318 cs; HLB 12.9; solid. pt. 0 C; b.p. > 250 C; flash pt. 540 F (COC); cloud pt. 54 C; pH 5–8 (10% aq.); surf. tens. 30 dynes/cm (0.1% aq.); 100% act.

Teric 9A6. [ICI Australia] C9-11 ethoxylate (6 EO); CAS 68439-46-3; nonionic; emulsifier for agric.; filter cake dewatering; dust supression in coal industry; domestic, laundry, hard surf. and window cleaners; leather; paper deinking; skin care prods.; textile wetting, carbonizing, leveling, scouring; APHA 100 color; sol. in water, aromatics, ethyl acetate, glycol ethers, trichlorethylene, ethanol, ethylene glycol; sp.gr. 0.987; visc. 38 cps; HLB 12.4; pour pt. < 0 C; cloud pt. 50-55 C; pH 6-8; surf. tens. 24.0 dynes/cm (0.1%); 100% act.

Teric 12A3. [ICI Australia] C12-15 pareth-3 (2.6 EO); CAS 68131-39-5; nonionic; wetting agent, dispersant, coemulsifier, detergent, intermediate used in oil and solv.-based systems; horticultural applics.; w/o emulsions; household/industrial cleaners; skin care prods.; mfg. of sulfate and phosphate surfactants; Hazen 80 liq.; sol. in benzene, ethyl acetate, ethyl lcinol, perchlorethylene, ethanol, kerosene, min. and veg. oil, olein; sp.gr. 0.912; visc. 28 cps; m.p. < 0 C; HLB 7.1; hyd. no. 174-178; pH 6-8 (1% aq.); biodeg.; 100% act.

Teric 12A7. [ICI Australia] C12-15 pareth-7; CAS 68131-39-5; nonionic; surfactant for skin care gels; dairy cleaning; laundry prods.; lt. duty detergents; paper processing; fiber lubricant/antistat for textile spinning, cotton dye leveling; APHA 100 color; sol. in water, aromatics, ethyl acetate, glycol ethers, trichlorethylene, ethanol, ethylene glycol; sp.gr. 0.958 (50 C); visc. 26 cps (50 C); HLB 12.1; pour pt. 15 C; cloud pt. 48-52 C; pH 6-8; surf. tens. 30 dynes/cm (0.1%); 100% act.

Teric LAN70. [ICI Australia] PEG-70 lanolin; CAS 61790-81-6; nonionic; emulsifier, dispersant, detergent additive, sanitizer component, textile lubricant, cosmetic ingred.; yel.-amber soft waxy solid; sol. in water, benzene, ethyl lcinol, perchlorethylene, ethanol, olein; sp.gr. 1.13; visc. 246 cps (50 C); m.p. 42 ± 2 C; HLB 16.3; cloud pt. > 100 C; surf. tens. 48.1 dynes/cm; pH 4.5–7.0 (1% aq.); 100% act.

Teric PEG 200. [ICI Australia] PEG 200; CAS 25322-68-3; EINECS 203-989-9; biodeg.; binder for glazing; intermediate for PEG esters, methacrylate resins, PU foams; plasticizer/solv. for cork; toiletries; metalworking lubricants; paints/resins; paper/film; printing inks; textile emulsifier; APHA 25 color; sol. in water and most polar org. solvs.; m.w. 190-210; sp.gr. 1.127; visc. 4.2 cst (99 C); pour pt. -50 C; flash pt. (OC) > 170 C; ref. index 1.459; pH 4.5-7.5; surf. tens. 44.6 dynes/cm; 99% act.

Teric PEG 300. [ICI Australia] PEG 300; CAS 25322-68-3; EINECS 220-045-1; pesticide solubilizer/carrier; visc. modifier for brake fluids; intermediate for PEG esters, PU foams; plasticizer/solv.; cosmetics; metalworking lubricants; paints/resins; paper/film; pharmaceuticals; printing inks; rubber; textile aux.; biodeg.; APHA 25 color; sol. in water and most polar org. solvs.; m.w. 285-315; sp.gr. 1.128; visc. 5.8 cst (99 C); pour pt. -12 C; flash pt. (OC) > 190 C; ref. index 1.463; pH 4.5-7.5; surf. tens. 44.6 dynes/cm; 99% act.

Teric PEG 400. [ICI Australia] PEG 400; CAS 25322-68-3; EINECS 225-856-4; biodeg.; emulsifier, antistat for textiles; rubber; inks; cosmetics; pharmaceuticals; paper/film; pesticide solubilizer/carrier; intermediate for PEG esters, PU foams; plasticizer/solv. for cork; metalworking lubricants; paints/resins; APHA 25 color; sol. in water and most polar org. solvs.; m.w. 380-420; sp.gr. 1.130; visc. 7.3 cst (99 C); pour pt. 6 C; flash pt. (OC) > 215 C; ref. index 1.465; pH 4.5-7.5; surf. tens. 44.6 dynes/cm; 99% act.

Teric PEG 600. [ICI Australia] PEG 600; CAS 25322-68-3; EINECS 229-859-1; biodeg.; emulsifier for textiles; pesticide solubilizer/carrier; binder for ceramics; intermediate for PEG esters, PU foams; cosmetics; pharmaceuticals; metalworking lubricants; resins; paper/film; inks; rubber; APHA 10 color (25% aq.); sol. in water and most polar org. solvs.; m.w. 560-630; sp.gr. 1.127; visc. 10.4 cst (99 C); pour pt. 19 C; flash pt. (OC) > 230 C; ref. index 1.454; pH 4.5-7.5; surf. tens. 44.6 dynes/cm; 99% act.

Teric PEG 800. [ICI Australia] PEG 800; CAS 25322-68-3; biodeg.; textile aux.; pharmaceutical tabletting; pesticide solubilizer/carrier; intermediate for PEG esters; toiletries; metalworking lubricants; APHA 30 color (25% aq.); sol. in water and most polar org. solvs.; m.w. 760-840; sp.gr. 1.184; visc. 13.8 cst (99 C); pour pt. 28 C; flash pt. (OC)

> 235 C; ref. index 1.455; pH 4.5-7.5; 99% act.

Teric PEG 1000. [ICI Australia] PEG 1000; CAS 25322-68-3; biodeg.; intermediate for PEG esters; cosmetics/toiletries/soaps; metalworking lubricants; wood processing; APHA 30 color; sol. in water and most polar org. solvs.; m.w. 950-1050; sp.gr. 1.198; visc. 17.8 cst (99 C); pour pt. 37 C; flash pt. (OC) > 245 C; ref. index 1.455; pH 4.5-7.5; surf. tens. 54.2 dynes/cm (50% aq.); 100% act.

Teric PEG 1500. [ICI Australia] PEG 1500; biodeg.; textile finishing and sizing; wood processing; latex prod.; printing inks; pharmaceuticals; paper/film; APHA 30 color (25% aq.); sol. in water and most polar org. solvs.; m.w. 1430-1570; sp.gr. 1.208; visc. 28.4 cst (99 C); pour pt. 46 C; flash pt. (OC) > 260 C; ref. index 1.456; pH 4.5-7.5; surf. tens. 53.1 dynes/cm (50% aq.); 100% act.

Teric PEG 3350. [ICI Australia] PEG 3350; biodeg.; intermediates for PEG esters; spinning aid for textiles; pharmaceuticals; APHA 30 color (25% aq.); sol. in water and most polar org. solvs.; m.w. 3000-3700; sp.gr. 1.215; visc. 70-120 cst (99 C); pour pt. 53 C; flash pt. (OC) > 260 C; ref. index 1.456; pH 4.5-7.5; surf. tens. 54.0 dynes/cm (50% aq.); 100% act.

Teric PEG 4000. [ICI Australia] PEG 4000; CAS 25322-68-3; biodeg.; binder/plasticizer for ceramics; intermediate for copolymers, PEG esters; cosmetics; pharmaceticals; metalworking lubricants and electropolishes; resins; paper/film; printing inks; rubber antistat, release, compding. aid; textile aux.; APHA 50 color (25% aq.); sol. in water and most polar org. solvs.; m.w. 3300-4000; sp.gr. 1.217; visc. 130-180 cst (99 C); pour pt. 56 C; flash pt. (OC) > 260 C; ref. index 1.456; pH 4.5-7.5; surf. tens. 54.4 dynes/cm (50% aq.); 100% act.

Teric PEG 6000. [ICI Australia] PEG 6000; CAS 25322-68-3; biodeg.; cosmetics; pharmaceuticals; thickener for inks; wood processing; binder/plasticizer for ceramics; intermediate for copolymers, PEG esters; metalworking lubricants; resins; APHA 50 color (25% aq.); sol. in water and most polar org. solvs.; m.w. 6000-7500; sp.gr. 1.217; visc. 330-500 cst (99 C); pour pt. 55-60 C; flash pt. (OC) > 260 C; ref. index 1.456; pH 4.5-7.5; surf. tens. 55.3 dynes/cm (50% aq.); 100% act.

Teric PEG 8000. [ICI Australia] PEG 8000; CAS 25322-68-3; biodeg.; intermediate for copolymers, PEG esters; cosmetics; pharmaceuticals; thickener for inks; release for rubber molding; sol. in water and most polar org. solvs.; m.w. 7000-9000; sp.gr. 1.2; visc. 700-900 cst (99 C); pour pt. 55-60 C; flash pt. (OC) > 260 C; ref. index 1.456; pH 4.5-7.5; 100% act.

Teric PPG 1650. [ICI Australia] PPG 1650; biodeg.; intermediate for surfactants, ethers, esters; antifoam for ceramics, rubber; lubricant/softener for leather; metalworking lubricant; demulsifier for petrol. industry; plasticizer for plastics; solv. for cosmetics; sol. in polar org. solvs.; sp.gr. 1.006; visc. 330 cps; hyd. no. 67-71; pour pt. -32 C; flash pt. (OC) 230 C; ref. index 1.449; pH 5-8 (1% aq. disp.); surf. tens. 31.8 dynes/cm; 99% act.

Teric PPG 2250. [ICI Australia] PPG 2250; biodeg.; intermediate for surfactants, ethers, esters; hydraulic brake fluids; cosmetics; dyeing; lubricant/softener for leather; metalworking lubricant; demulsifier for petrol.; latex coagulant; rubber release agent; solv. for veg. oils; APHA 50 color; sol. in polar org. solvs.; sp.gr. 1.005; visc. 482 cps; hyd. no. 47-54; pour pt. -29 C; flash pt. (OC) 240 C; ref. index 1.449; pH 4.0-7.5 (10% in aq. methanol); surf. tens. 32.1 dynes/cm; 99% act.

Teric PPG 4000. [ICI Australia] PPG 4000; biodeg.; intermediate for surfactants, ethers, esters; cosmetics; lubricant/softener for leather; metalworking lubricants; demulsifier for petrol. industry; mold release for rubber; APHA 250 color; sol. in polar org. solvs.; sp.gr. 1.004; visc. 1232 cps;

hyd. no. 26-30; pour pt. -30 C; flash pt. (OC) 240 C; ref. index 1.450; pH 5-8 (10% in aq. methanol); surf. tens. 32.2 dynes/cm; 99% act.

Tesal. [Gattefosse] Propylene glycol stearate SE; anionic; SE base for cosmetic/pharmaceutical ointments, lotions, creams; drop pt. 37-43 C; acid no. 90-110; iodine no. < 5; sapon. no. 160-180; toxicology: nonirritating to skin and eyes.

Tetronic® 304. [BASF] Poloxamine 304; CAS 11111-34-5; nonionic; emulsifier, thickener, wetting agent, dispersant, solubilizer, stabilizer for cosmetics and pharmaceuticals; demulsifier in petrol. industry; detergent ingred.; antistat for polyethylene and resin molding powds.; metal treatment; emulsion polymerization; used in latex-based paints, aq.-based syn. cutting fluids and vulcanization of rubber; colorless liq.; m.w. 1650; ref. index 1.4649; water-sol.; sp.gr. 1.06; visc. 450 cps; HLB 16; cloud pt. 94 C (1%); pour pt. −11 C; surf. tens. 53.0 dynes/cm (0.1%); toxicology: none to mild eye and minimal to moderate skin irritation; 100% act.

Tetronic® 701. [BASF] Poloxamine 701; CAS 11111-34-5; nonionic; see Tetronic 304; colorless liq.; m.w. 3400; ref. index. 1.4553; sp.gr. 1.02; visc. 575 cps; HLB 3; cloud pt. 22 C (1%); pour pt. −21 C; surf. tens. 36.1 dynes/cm; toxicology: none to mild eye and minimal to moderate skin irritation; 100% act.

Tetronic® 704. [BASF] Poloxamine 704; CAS 11111-34-5; nonionic; see Tetronic 304; colorless liq.; m.w. 5500; ref. index 1.4613; water-sol.; sp.gr. 1.04; visc. 850 cps; HLB 15; cloud pt. 65 C (1%); pour pt. 18 C; surf. tens. 40.3 dynes/cm (0.1%); toxicology: none to mild eye and minimal to moderate skin irritation; 100% act.

Tetronic® 901. [BASF] Poloxamine 901; CAS 11111-34-5; nonionic; see Tetronic 304; colorless liq.; m.w. 4750; ref. index 1.4545; sp.gr. 1.02; visc. 700 cps; HLB 2.5; cloud pt. 20 C (1%); pour pt. −23 C; toxicology: none to mild eye and minimal to moderate skin irritation; 100% act.

Tetronic® 904. [BASF] Poloxamine 904; CAS 11111-34-5; nonionic; see Tetronic 304; colorless liq.; m.w. 7500; ref. index 1.4604; water-sol.; sp.gr. 1.04; visc. 6000 cps; HLB 14.5; cloud pt. 64 C (1%); pour pt. 29 C; surf. tens. 35.4 dynes; toxicology: none to mild eye and minimal to moderate skin irritation; 100% act.

Tetronic® 908. [BASF] Poloxamine 908; CAS 11111-34-5; nonionic; see Tetronic 304; flakes; m.w. 27,000; water-sol.; m.p. 58 C; HLB 30.5; cloud pt. > 100 C (1%); surf. tens. 45.7 dynes/cm (0.1%); toxicology: none to mild eye and minimal to moderate skin irritation; 100% act.

Tetronic® 1307. [BASF] Poloxamine 1307; CAS 11111-34-5; nonionic; see Tetronic 304; solid; m.w. 18,600; water-sol.; m.p. 54 C; HLB 23.5; cloud pt. > 100 C (1%); surf. tens. 43.8 dynes/cm (0.1%); toxicology: none to mild eye and minimal to moderate skin irritation; 100% act.

Tewax TC 1. [Auschem SpA] Hydrog. tallow alcohol and ceteareth-25; nonionic; cosmetics, hair dye preparations; flakes; 100% conc.

Tewax TC 2. [Auschem SpA] Cetyl/stearyl alcohol with nonionic emulsifiers; nonionic; cosmetics, hair dye preparations; flakes; 100% conc.

Tewax TC 10. [Auschem SpA] Ceteareth-9; CAS 68439-49-6; nonionic; emulsifier for cosmetic and pharmaceutical preps.; flakes; HLB 12.0; 100% conc.

Tewax TC 60. [Auschem SpA] Stearyl alcohol and PEG-100 stearate; nonionic; emulsifier for cosmetic creams; flakes; HLB 11.5; 100% conc.

Tewax TC 65. [Auschem SpA] Glyceryl stearate and PEG-100 stearate; nonionic; emulsifier for cosmetic and pharmaceutical preps.; flakes; HLB 11.0; 100% conc.

Tewax TC 72. [Auschem SpA] Steareth-8; CAS 9005-00-9; nonionic; emulsifier for cosmetic and pharmaceutical preps.; solid; HLB 9.0; 100% conc.

Tewax TC 80. [Auschem SpA] Glyceryl sorbitan oleo/stearate; nonionic; w/o emulsifier for cosmetics and pharmaceuticals; solid; HLB 4.6; 100% conc.

Tewax TC 81. [Auschem SpA] Glyceryl sorbitan oleo/stearate, beeswax; nonionic; w/o emulsifier for cosmetics and pharmaceuticals; solid; HLB 4.0; 100% conc.

Tewax TC 82. [Auschem SpA] PEG-1 glyceryl sorbitan isostearate; nonionic; w/o emulsifier for cosmetics and pharmaceuticals; solid; HLB 5.0; 100% conc.

Tewax TC 83. [Auschem SpA] PEG-5 glyceryl stearate; CAS 51158-08-8; nonionic; w/o emulsifier for cosmetics and pharmaceuticals; solid; HLB 5.0; 100% conc.

Tewax TC 840. [Auschem SpA] Cetearyl alcohol, lanolin, ceteareth-25, and glyceryl stearate; nonionic; emulsifier for depilatory creams and hair care prods.; flakes; 100% conc.

Texal-L. [Lanaetex Prods.] Isopropyl myristate, myristyl alcohol.

Texapon® ALS. [Henkel KGaA/Cospha] Ammonium lauryl sulfate; CAS 2235-54-3; EINECS 218-793-9; anionic; base for shampoos, shower baths, bubble baths; faintly yel. sl. visc. liq.; cloud pt. < 15 C; pH 6-7 (10%); 29-31% conc.

Texapon® ASV. [Henkel/Cospha; Henkel Canada; Henkel KGaA/Cospha] Sodium laureth sulfate, magnesium laureth-8 sulfate, sodium laureth-8 sulfate, sodium oleth sulfate, magnesium oleth sulfate; anionic; extremely mild surfactant base for baby shampoos, facial cleansers, foam baths; lt. yel. clear semivisc. liq.; sp.gr. 1.05; visc. 2000-2500 mPa·s; cloud pt. < 0 C; pH 6.5-7.5 (10%); 28-30% act.

Texapon® BSC-1. [Henkel/Cospha; Henkel Canada] Proprietary surfactant blend; anionic; mild conc. for baby shampoo, foam baths; liq.

Texapon® DEA. [Henkel/Cospha; Henkel Canada] DEA-lauryl sulfate; CAS 143-00-0; EINECS 205-577-4; anionic; detergent, foamer for personal care prods.; lt. yel. clear liq.; 36–38% act.

Texapon® EA-1. [Henkel/Cospha; Henkel Canada] Ammonium laureth sulfate; CAS 32612-48-9; anionic; surfactant, visc. builder, solubilizer in personal care prods.; water-wh. visc. liq.; 25–27% act.

Texapon® EA-2. [Henkel/Cospha; Henkel Canada] Ammonium laureth sulfate; CAS 32612-48-9; anionic; surfactant, visc. builder, solubilizer for personal care prods.; water-wh. visc. liq.; 28% act.

Texapon® EA-3. [Henkel/Cospha; Henkel Canada] Ammonium laureth sulfate; CAS 32612-48-9; anionic; surfactant, visc. builder, solubilizer for personal care prods.; water-wh. visc. liq.; 26-28% act.

Texapon® EA-40. [Henkel/Cospha; Henkel Canada] Ammonium myristyl ether sulfate; CAS 27731-61-9; anionic; detergent, foamer for personal care prods.; lt. yel. liq.; 58-60% act.

Texapon® EA-K. [Henkel/Cospha; Henkel Canada] Proprietary blend; anionic; ready-to-dilute conc. for clear shampoos, foam baths, cleansing preps., liq. soaps, dishwash; liq.; 60% conc.

Texapon® ES-1. [Henkel/Cospha; Henkel Canada] Sodium laureth sulfate; anionic; surfactant and solubilizer for personal care prods.; water-wh. visc. liq.; 25% act.

Texapon® ES-2. [Henkel/Cospha; Henkel Canada] Sodium laureth sulfate; anionic; surfactant and solubilizer for personal care prods.; water-wh. visc. liq.; 26% conc.

Texapon® ES-3. [Henkel/Cospha; Henkel Canada] Sodium laureth sulfate; anionic; surfactant and solubilizer for personal care prods.; water-wh. visc. liq.; 28% conc.

Texapon® ES-40. [Henkel/Cospha; Henkel Canada] Sodium laureth sulfate; anionic; detergent for personal care prods.; lt. yel. liq.; 57.5–60.0% act.

Texapon® ES-250. [Henkel Canada] Sodium laureth sulfate; anionic; surfactant with superior visc. response for shampoos, liq. hand soaps, bubble baths; liq.; 53% conc.

Texapon® EVR. [Henkel Canada; Henkel KGaA/Cospha] Sodium lauryl sulfate, sodium laureth sulfate, lauramide MIPA, cocamide MEA, glycol stearate, and laureth-10; anionic; detergent, foamer; base for pearlescent shampoos; liq.; 40% conc.

Texapon® K-12 Needles. [Henkel/Cospha; Henkel KGaA/Cospha] Sodium lauryl sulfate; CAS 151-21-3; EINECS 205-788-1; anionic; foamer for toothpaste, emulsion and cream shampoos, detergents, wettable powds.; wh. to lt. yel. needles, almost odorless; dens. 400-500 g/l; pH 6.5-9.0 (1%); 88% act.

Texapon® K-12 Powd. [Henkel/Cospha; Henkel KGaA/Cospha] Sodium lauryl sulfate; CAS 151-21-3; EINECS 205-788-1; anionic; wetting agent, dispersant and foamer used in emulsion and cream shampoos, dentifrice mfg.; wh. to lt. yel. fine powd., almost odorless; dens. 200-300 g/l; pH 6.5–9.0 (1% aq.); 90% min. act.

Texapon® K-14S 70 Special. [Henkel KGaA/Cospha] Sodium lauryl/myristyl ether sulfate; CAS 68891-38-3; anionic; skin-compatible detergent for shampoos and foam baths; water-wh. to lt. yel. pumpable paste; pH 7.0-9.5 (3%); 70% conc.

Texapon® K-14S Spec. [Henkel Canada; Henkel KGaA/Cospha] Sodium myreth sulfate; CAS 25446-80-4; EINECS 246-986-8; anionic; mild detergent for personal care prods.; pale clear visc. liq.; sp.gr. 1.05; visc. 2500-3000 mPa·s; cloud pt. < 0 C; pH 6-7 (10%); 27-29% act.

Texapon® K-1296. [Henkel/Cospha; Henkel Canada; Henkel KGaA/Cospha] Sodium lauryl sulfate; CAS 151-21-3; EINECS 205-788-1; anionic; dispersant, wetting agent, cleansing agent, disintegrant, foamer for dentifrices, foaming bubble baths, cosmetic cleansers; wh. to ylsh. powd., almost odorless; dens. 2.08 lb/gal; pH 6–9 (1%); 96% act.

Texapon® L-100. [Henkel/Cospha] Sodium lauryl sulfate; CAS 151-21-3; EINECS 205-788-1; wetting and cleansing agent, dispersant used in dentifrice mfg., high-solids cleansers, wettable powds.; wh. powd.; pH 7.0 (1% aq.); 98% act.

Texapon® LS 100 F. [Henkel/Cospha; Henkel Canada] Sodium lauryl sulfate; CAS 151-21-3; EINECS 205-788-1; surfactant for personal care prods., dentifrices and other oral prods. where taste contribution must be minimal; wh. powd.; 98% act.

Texapon® LS Highly Conc. Needles. [Henkel KGaA/Cospha] Sodium lauryl sulfate (C12-C14); CAS 85586-07-8; anionic; detergent, foamer used in personal care prods. and detergents, toothpastes, emulsion and cream shampoos; wh. to lt. yel. needles, almost odorless; dens. 400-500 g/l; pH 6.5-9.0 (1%); 87% min. act.

Texapon® LT-327. [Pulcra SA] Sodium lauryl ether (2.7) sulfate; CAS 9004-82-4; anionic; for shampoos and lt. duty detergents; liq.; 27% conc.

Texapon® MG. [Henkel/Cospha; Henkel KGaA/Cospha] Magnesium laureth sulfate; CAS 62755-21-9; anionic; mild surfactant for liq. shampoo and bath preparation base, baby shampoos; sl. yel. liq.; sp.gr. 1.05; visc. 2700-3200 mPa·s; cloud pt. < 0 C; pH 6.0-6.7 (10%); 30% act.

Texapon® MGLS. [Henkel Canada] Magnesium lauryl sulfate; CAS 3097-08-3; EINECS 221-450-6; anionic; mild foamer for shampoos, bubble baths, cleansing preps., carpet shampoos; liq.; 30% conc.

Texapon® MLS. [Henkel KGaA/Cospha] MEA-lauryl sulfate; CAS 4722-98-9; EINECS 225-214-3; anionic; detergent for liq. shampoos; sl. yel. clear visc. liq.; sp.gr. 1.0; visc. 5000-7000 mPa·s; cloud pt.< 0 C; pH 6-7 (10%); 31-33%

act.

Texapon® N 70. [Henkel/Cospha; Henkel Canada; Henkel KGaA/Cospha; Pulcra SA] Sodium laureth (2) sulfate; CAS 9004-82-4; 1335-72-4; anionic; detergent in shower and foam baths, shampoos, body cleansers, lt. duty detergents; solubilizer for perfumes; water-wh. to ylsh. paste; m.w. 388; visc. < 9000 mPa·s; pH 7-9 (3%); 68-73% act.

Texapon® NC 70. [Henkel/Cospha; Henkel Canada; Henkel KGaA/Cospha; Pulcra SA] Sodium laureth (2) sulfate; CAS 9004-82-4; 1335-72-4; anionic; detergent in personal care prods., lt. duty detergents; solubilizer for perfumes; water-wh. paste; m.w. 388; visc. < 9000 mPa·s; pH 7-9 (3%); 68-73% act.

Texapon® NSO. [Henkel KGaA/Cospha; Pulcra SA] Sodium lauryl ether (2) sulfate; CAS 9004-82-4; anionic; detergent for liq. shampoos, bubble baths, shower gels, mfg. of household detergents; wetting agent and detergent for textile fibers, esp. wool and blends; liq.; m.w. 382; visc. < 200 mPa·s; pH 6.4-7.5 (10%); 26.5-27.5% act.

Texapon® OT Highly Conc. Needles. [Henkel/Functional Prods.; Henkel KGaA/Cospha] Sodium lauryl sulfate C12-C18; CAS 151-21-3; EINECS 205-788-1; anionic; detergent, shampoo base; for bubble bath, soaps; emulsifier for emulsion polymerization, additive for mech. latex foaming, carpet and upholstery cleaners; needles; 91-92% act.

Texapon® PLT-227. [Pulcra SA] Sodium laureth-2 sulfate; CAS 9004-82-4; 1335-72-4; anionic; for shampoos and liq. detergents; liq.; 27% conc.

Texapon® PN-235. [Pulcra SA] Sodium laureth-2.35 sulfate; CAS 9004-82-4; 1335-72-4; anionic; surfactant for mfg. of shampoos, foam baths, personal foam washers, household detergents; solubilizer for perfumes; wetting agent/detergent for textile fibers, esp. wool and blends; liq.; m.w. 403; visc. < 350 mPa·s; pH 6.5-7.5 (10%); 26.5-27.5% act.

Texapon® PN-254. [Pulcra SA] Sodium laureth-2.4 sulfate; CAS 9004-82-4; anionic; surfactant for mfg. of shampoos, foam baths, personal foam washers, household detergents; solubilizer for perfumes; paste; m.w. 388; visc. 5000-8000 mPa·s; pH 6.5-8.0 (1%); 53-55% act.

Texapon® PNA. [Pulcra SA] Ammonium lauryl sulfate; CAS 2235-54-3; EINECS 218-793-9; anionic; base for liq. shampoos, foam baths, in mfg. of household liq. detergents, fire-fighting foams; visc. liq.; m.w. 296; pH 6.3-6.8 (10%); 26-28% act.

Texapon® PNA-127. [Pulcra SA] Ammonium lauryl ether (1) sulfate; CAS 32612-48-9; anionic; wetting agent for acid or gel-like shampoos, lt. duty detergents, window cleaners; stable foam; low eye and skin irritation; liq./paste; m.w. 336; pH 6.5-7.0 (10%); 25-26% act.

Texapon® QLV. [Henkel Canada] Sodium laureth sulfate; anionic; low salt surfactant for shampoos, cleansing preps., lt. duty detergents; liq.; 25% conc.

Texapon® SB-3. [Henkel Canada; Henkel KGaA/Cospha] Disodium laurethsulfosuccinate; anionic; mild surfactant, foamer for bubble baths, baby shampoos, cleansing preps.; pract. colorless clear liq., may become cloudy on storage; acid no. 6 max.; cloud pt. < 0 C; pH 5.5-6.5; 40% conc.

Texapon® SH 100. [Henkel/Cospha; Henkel Canada] Disodium oleamide PEG-2 sulfosuccinate; CAS 56388-43-3; EINECS 260-143-1; anionic; nonirritating detergent base for shampoos and skin cleansers; liq.; 30% conc.

Texapon® SH-135 Special. [Henkel/Cospha; Henkel Canada] Disodium oleamide PEG-2 sulfosuccinate; CAS 56388-43-3; EINECS 260-143-1; anionic; nonirritating surfactant for personal care prods.; liq.; 35% conc.

Texapon® T. [Henkel/Cospha; Henkel Canada] TEA-lauryl sulfate; CAS 139-96-8; EINECS 205-388-7; anionic; detergent, foamer, mild base for personal care prods., aerosols; water-wh. liq.; 39–41% act.

Texapon® T 42. [Henkel KGaA/Cospha; Pulcra SA] TEA lauryl sulfate; CAS 139-96-8; EINECS 205-388-7; anionic; detergent, emulsifier for hair and rug shampoos, bubble baths, shower gels, fire fighting foams; liq.; m.w. 420; visc. < 100 mPa·s; pH 7.2-7.5 (10%); 40-43% act.

Texapon® TW-1. [Henkel/Cospha; Henkel Canada] Proprietary blend; anionic; ready-to-dilute conc. for mild conditioning shampoos, foam baths, cleansing preps.; liq.; 55% conc.

Texapon® VHC Needles. [Henkel/Cospha; Henkel/Functional Prods; Henkel Canada; Henkel KGaA/Cospha] Sodium lauryl sulfate; CAS 151-21-3; EINECS 205-788-1; anionic; wetting agent, foamer, emulsifier, detergent and cosmetic base for personal care prods., scouring agents, pigment dispersions, emulsion polymerization; wh. fine needles; pH 7–8 (1% aq.); 86-90% act.

Texapon® Z. [Henkel KGaA/Cospha] Sodium lauryl sulfate C12-C14; CAS 151-21-3; EINECS 205-788-1; anionic; detergent, wetting agent, foaming agent, dispersant for shampoos, bath preps., pharmaceutical preparations, toothpastes, mouth and dental care prods., pesticides, paint; wh. to pale yel. powd.; sol. in cold water; dens. 100 g/l; pH 6-9 (1%); 60% min. act.

Texapon® ZHC Needles. [Henkel/Cospha; Henkel KGaA/Cospha] Sodium lauryl sulfate; CAS 68955-19-1; anionic; foaming agent, dispersant, wetting agent for foaming bubble baths, cosmetic cleansing creams and emulsions; air entraining agent; wh. to lt. yel. needles; dens. 400-500 g/l; pH 6.5-9.0 (1%); 88% conc.

Texapon® ZHC Powder. [Henkel/Cospha; Henkel/Functional Prods.] Sodium lauryl sulfate C12-C18; CAS 151-21-3; EINECS 205-788-1; foaming dispersion and wetting agent for bubble baths, cosmetic cleansing creams and emulsions, emulsion polymerization, mech. latex foaming, carpet and upholstery cleaners; wh. fine powd.; pH 7.5–8.5 (0.25% aq.); 88% act.

Texatein C. [Lanaetex Prods.] Potassium cocoyl hydrolyzed collagen; CAS 68920-65-0; cosmetics ingred.

Texatein CT. [Lanaetex Prods.] TEA-cocoyl hydrolyzed collagen; CAS 68952-16-9; cosmetics ingred.

Texofor B7. [Rhone-Poulenc Surf. & Spec.] Alcohol ethoxylate; nonionic; wetting agent and emulsifier for cosmetics/toiletries; liq.; HLB 15.8; 100% conc.

Theophyllisilane C. [Exsymol; Biosil Tech.] Methylsilanol carboxymethyl theophylline alginate; ingred. for slimming and anti-aging formulations, cosmetic and health prods.; sl. opalescent liq.; misc. with water, alcohols, glycols; sp.gr. 1.0; pH 5.5; usage level: 5-6%; toxicology: nontoxic.

Thermoplex. [Herstellung von Naturextrakten GmbH; Lipo] Soluble collagen and glycerol; water-binding film-former, moisture regulator used in face creams, collagen ampoules, body lotions, after-sun lotions, hair conditioning treatments, skin care prods.; visc. clear sol'n., weak intrinsic odor; acid no. 3.0-3.5; pH 3.5-4.0.

Thickagent LC. [Les Colorants Wackherr] A blend of thickeners for thixotropic control of creams and makeup prods.

Thiovanic® Acid. [Evans Chemetics] Thioglycolic acid; CAS 68-11-1; EINECS 200-677-4; intermediate for hair waving, depilatories.

Thiovanol®. [Evans Chemetics] Thioglycerin; CAS 96-27-5; EINECS 202-495-0; stabilizer for acrylonitrile polymers; cross-linking agent for hard high-gloss coatings; accelerator for epoxy-amine condensation reactions; reducing agent; used in hair waving and straightening, hair dyes, depilatories, textiles, furs, pharmaceuticals, surfactants, foam stabilizing additives for detergents, shampoos, insecticides, pesticides, fungicides, and dessi-

cants; practically clear and colorless sol'n.; mild char. odor; m.w. 108.2; b.p. 118 C (5 mm, anhyd.); misc. in all proportions with water and alcohol; insol. in ether; 90% aq. sol'n.

Thixcin® R. [Rheox] Trihydroxystearin; CAS 8001-78-3; rheological additive, thixotrope promoting pigment and filler suspension, controlling flow and leveling; for paints, stains, coatings, mastics, inks, textile backings, solv.-free epoxy systems; adds water resist. to eye shadow and mascara; binder/lubricant for tablets and pressed powds.; also for lipsticks, topical ointments, creams and lotions; stiffens stick prods.; for use in aliphatic solv. systems; wh. fine powd.; fineness 99.8% min. thru 200 mesh; sp.gr. 1.023; dens. 8.51 lb/gal; m.p. 86 C; 100% NV.

Ticalose 15, 30, 75, 150R, 1200, 2000R, 2500, 4000, 4500, 5000R. [TIC Gums] Cellulose gum; CAS 9004-32-4; binder, thickener, suspending agent for cosmetics.

Timica®. [Mearl] Mica platelets coated with titanium dioxide or iron oxide; luster pigments for frosted and iridescent effects in lipsticks, cream makeups, nail enamels, pressed powds.; avail. as white pearlescents (Silkwhite, Pearlwhite, Sparkle, Extra Large Sparkle) and metallic/earth colors (Brilliant Gold, Gold Sparkle, Golden Bronze, Copper, Nu-Antique Silver, Nu-Antique Gold, Nu-Antique Bronze, Nu-Antique Copper); wh. and colored powds.; sp.gr. ≈ 3.0.

Timiron®. [Rona] Titanium dioxide-coated mica; pearlescent pigments for lipsticks, pressed powds., eye makeups, for all frosted effects; incl. silver/wh. pearls, gold pearls, and interference pigments.

Tinopal® CBS-X. [Ciba-Geigy] Disodium distyrylbiphenyl disulfonate; highly soluble, low dusting, lightfast, chlorine stable whitener for cotton and other cellulosics; used in anionic and nonionic laundry detergents, dry bleaches, fabric softeners, commercial laundry prods., toilet bar soaps, liq. prods., and prods. for use at low wash temps.

Tiolisina Complex 30. [Sinerga Srl; Trivent] Lysine carboxymethyl cysteinate and lysine thiazolidine carboxylate.

TIPA 99. [Dow] Triisopropanolamine; CAS 122-20-3; EINECS 204-528-4; used to produce soaps with good hard surf. detergency, shampoos, pharmaceuticals, emulsifiers, textile specialties, agric. and polymer curing chemicals, adhesives, antistats, coatings, metalworking, rubber, gas conditioning chemicals; sp.gr. 0.988 (70/4 C); dens. 8.24 lb/gal (70 C); visc. 100 cps (60 C); f.p. 44 C; b.p. 306 C (760 mm Hg); flash pt. (COC) 320 F; ref. index 1.4595 (30 C).

TIPA 101. [Dow] Triisopropanolamine; CAS 122-20-3; EINECS 204-528-4; used to produce soaps with good hard surf. detergency, shampoos, emulsifiers, textile specialties, agric. and polymer curing chemicals, gas conditioning chemicals; sp.gr. 0.988 (70/4 C); dens. 8.24 lb/gal (70 C); visc. 100 cps (60 C); f.p. 44 C; b.p. 306 C (760 mm Hg); flash pt. (COC) 320 F; ref. index 1.4595 (30 C); 10% water.

TIPA Low Freeze Grade. [Dow] Triisopropanolamine; CAS 122-20-3; EINECS 204-528-4; used to produce soaps with good hard surf. detergency, shampoos, emulsifiers, textile specialties, agric. and polymer curing chemicals, gas conditioning chemicals; sp.gr. 0.988 (70/4 C); dens. 8.24 lb/gal (70 C); visc. 100 cps (60 C); f.p. 44 C; b.p. 306 C (760 mm Hg); flash pt. (COC) 320 F; ref. index 1.4595 (30 C); 15% water.

Tisolate-BS. [Lanaetex Prods.] Isobutyl stearate, octyl isononanoate.

Ti-Sphere AA-1512-030. [Presperse] Titanium dioxide, methicone; CAS 13463-67-7, 9004-73-7; spherical titanium dioxide with exc. spreadability and improved feel for cosmetics use.; JSCI/JCID approved.

Ti-Sphere AA-1512-LL. [Presperse] Anatase titanium dioxide; CAS 13463-67-7; EINECS 236-675-5; spherical titanium dioxide with exc. spreadability and improved feel for cosmetics use, suncare prods.; JSCI/JCID approved; wh. free-flowing powd., essentially odorless; particle size 2-15 μ; oil absorp. 57 ml/100 g; bulk dens. 10.5 g/in.[3]; 99% act.

Ti-Sphere AA-1515. [Presperse] Rutile titanium dioxide; CAS 13463-67-7; EINECS 236-675-5; spherical titanium dioxide with exc. spreadability and improved feel for suncare prods.; JSCI/JCID approved; wh. free-flowing powd., essentially odorless; particle size 2-15 μ; bulk dens. 10.9 g/in.[3]; 99% act.

Ti-Sphere AB-15155A. [Presperse] Titanium dioxide (85%), silica (15%); CAS 13463-67-7, 7631-86-9; spherical powd. imparting spreadability and smooth creamy feel to cosmetic powds.; may be used as nonchemical sunscreen; JSCI/JCID approved; wh. free-flowing powd., essentially odorless; particle size 2-15 μ; oil absorp. 70 ml/100 g; bulk dens. 8.0 g/in[3]

Titanium Dioxide 110. [Presperse] Titanium dioxide (90%), bismuthoxychloride (10%); CAS 13463-67-7, 7787-59-9; inorg. colorant for pigmented cosmetics; JSCI/JCID approved.

Titanium Dioxide P25. [Degussa] Titanium dioxide; CAS 13463-67-7; EINECS 236-675-5; catalyst carrier for fixed bed catalyst; heat stabilizer for HCR silicone rubber and flame retardant; uv absorber for sunscreen lotions.

Titanium Dioxide SPA. [Les Colorants Wackherr] Titanium dioxide; CAS 13463-67-7; EINECS 236-675-5; treated with mild surfactants to produce a milky effect in bath prods.

Tixogel FTN. [United Catalysts] C12-15 alcohols benzoate (87%), stearalkonium bentonite (10%), propylene carbonate (3%); rhelogical additive for makeup bases; sp.gr. 0.97; visc. 24-36 cps.

Tixogel IPM. [United Catalysts] Stearalkonium bentonite (10%), isopropyl myristate (87%), propylene carbonate (3%); rheological additive for antiperspirants, creams, lotions; sp.gr. 0.88; visc. 34-60 cps.

Tixogel LAN. [United Catalysts] Stearalkonium bentonite (10%), lanolin oil (65%), isopropyl palmitate (22%), propylene carbonate (3%); rheological additive for lipsticks, suntan prods., creams and lotions; sp.gr. 0.94; visc. 8-22 cps.

Tixogel LG. [United Catalysts] Stearalkonium bentonite; rheological additive for high polarity and oxygenated solv. systems such as nail lacquers.

Tixogel MIO. [United Catalysts] Quaternium-18 bentonite (10%), min. oil (87%), propylene carbonate (3%); rheological additive for lipsticks, creams, lotions, mascara, eyeshadow; sp.gr. 0.85; visc. 40-60 cps.

Tixogel OMS. [United Catalysts] Quaternium-18 bentonite (10%), odorless min. spirits (87%), propylene carbonate (3%); rheological additive for eye makeup, mascara, eyeshadow; sp.gr. 0.79; visc. 22-30 cps; 10% act.

Tixogel VP. [United Catalysts] Quaternium-18 bentonite; CAS 68953-58-2; EINECS 273-219-4; thixotrope for low to med. polarity systems, e.g., antiperspirants; as suspension aid for active ingreds.; for 100% aliphatic to 100% aromatic systems (automotive undercoats, trade sales alkyds, traffic paints, stains, acrylics, chlorinated rubber); lt. cream powd.; particle size < 1 μm; sp.gr. 1.8 g/cc; dens. 14.99 lb/gal; 2.5% max. moisture.

Tixogel VSP. [United Catalysts] Quaternium-18 bentonite (17.5%), cyclomethicone (79.5%), propylene carbonate (2.5%), water (0.5%); rheological additive for suntan prods., creams, lotions; sp.gr. 1.02; visc. 30-50 cps.

Tixogel VZ. [United Catalysts] Stearalkonium bentonite; thixotrope for high polarity and oxygenated solv. systems such as nail lacquers; also for paints/coatings (nitrocellu-

lose lacquers, sol'n. vinyls, epoxies, acrylics, wash primers, inorg. zinc-rich primers, chlorinated rubber, unsat. polyesters); lt. cream powd.; particle size < 1 μm; sp.gr. 1.7 g/cc; dens. 14.16 lb/gal; 3% max. moisture.

Tixosil 38AB, 43, 53, 63, 73, 83, 93. [Rhone-Poulenc] Hydrated silica.

Tixosil 331. [Rhone-Poulenc] Hydrated silica, amorphous; flatting agents providing gloss and sheen control in coatings; rheology control agent for solv. and water-based systems; for coatings, adhesives, plastics, paper, food, cosmetics, toothpaste, and pharmaceutical applics.; wh. powd.; 3 μ avg. particle size; < 0.1% retained 325 mesh; Hegman grind 7; dens. 17.1 lb/gal; surf. area 310 m²/g; oil absorp. 320%; ref. index 1.45; pH 7; 96% SiO₂.

Tixosil 333, 343. [Rhone-Poulenc] Hydrated silica; rheology control agent for solv. and water-based systems; for coatings, adhesives, plastics, paper, food, cosmetics, toothpaste, and pharmaceutical applics.

T-Maz® 20. [PPG/Specialty Chem.] Polysorbate 20; CAS 9005-64-5; nonionic; emulsifier, solubilizer, wetting agent, antistat, stabilizer, dispersant, visc. modifier, suspending agent used in the food, cosmetic, drug, textile and metalworking industries; very mild ingred. for no-tear shampoos, baby baths; solubilizer for emollients and fragrances into bath prods.; emulsifier for cleansing prods., skin care emulsions; yel. liq.; sol. in water, ethanol, acetone, toluene, veg. oil; sp.gr. 1.1; visc. 400 cps; HLB 16.7; sapon. no. 40–50; hyd. no. 96-108; flash pt. (PMCC) > 350 F; 97% act.

T-Maz® 28. [PPG/Specialty Chem.] PEG-80 sorbitan laurate; CAS 9005-64-5; emulsifier and solubilizer of essential oils, wetting agent, visc. modifier, antistat, stabilizer and dispersant used in food, cosmetic, drug, textile and metalworking industries; very mild ingred. for no-tear shampoos, baby baths; solubilizer for emollients and fragrances into bath prods.; emulsifier for cleansing prods. and skin care emulsions; pale yel. liq.; sol. in water; sp.gr. 1.0; visc. 1100 cps; HLB 19.2; acid no. 2 max.; sapon. no. 5–15; hyd. no. 25-40; flash pt. (PMCC) > 350 F; 30% max. water.

T-Maz® 40. [PPG/Specialty Chem.] Polysorbate 40; CAS 9005-66-7; nonionic; emulsifier, solubilizer, wetting agent, antistat, stabilizer, dispersant, visc. modifier, suspending agent used in the food, cosmetic, drug, textile and metalworking industries; yel. liq.; sol. in water; disp. in toluene, veg. oil; sp.gr. 1.0; visc. 600 cps; HLB 15.8; sapon. no. 41-52; hyd. no. 85-105; flash pt. (PMCC) > 350 F; 97% min. act.

T-Maz® 60. [PPG/Specialty Chem.] Polysorbate 60; CAS 9005-67-8; emulsifier, solubilizer, wetting agent, antistat, stabilizer, dispersant, visc. modifier, suspending agent used in the food, cosmetic, drug, textile and metalworking industries; yel. gel; sol. in water, min. spirits, toluol; sp.gr. 1.1; visc. 550 cps; HLB 14.9; pour pt. 23–25 C; sapon. no. 45-55; hyd. no. 81-96; flash pt. (PMCC) > 350 F; 97% min. act.

T-Maz® 60K. [PPG/Specialty Chem.] Polysorbate 60, kosher; CAS 9005-67-8; nonionic; emulsifier for cosmetic creams, lotions, cleansing prods., foundations, foods; binder for pressed powd. makeup; dough conditioner for bakery goods; amber semisolid; sol. in water, min. spirits, toluene; HLB 14.9; sapon. no. 45-55; hyd. no. 81-96; flash pt. (PMCC) > 350 F; 100% conc.

T-Maz® 61. [PPG/Specialty Chem.] Polysorbate 61; CAS 9005-67-8; nonionic; emulsifier, solubilizer, wetting agent, antistat, stabilizer, dispersant, visc. modifier, suspending agent used in the food, cosmetic, drug, textile and metalworking industries; Gardner 5 paste; disp. @ 5% in water, min. oils, toluene, veg. oils; HLB 9.5; sapon. no. 98-113; hyd. no. 170-200; flash pt. (PMCC) > 350 F; 100%

conc.

T-Maz® 65. [PPG/Specialty Chem.] Polysorbate 65; CAS 9005-71-4; nonionic; emulsifier, solubilizer, wetting agent, antistat, stabilizer, dispersant, visc. modifier, suspending agent used in the food, cosmetic, drug, textile and metalworking industries; sol. in ethanol, acetone, naphtha; disp. in water; sp.gr. 1.1; m.p. 30–32 C; HLB 10.5; sapon. no. 88–98; 97% min. act.

T-Maz® 80. [PPG/Specialty Chem.] Polysorbate 80; CAS 9005-65-6; nonionic; emulsifier, solubilizer, wetting agent, antistat, stabilizer, dispersant, visc. modifier, suspending agent used in the food, cosmetic, drug, textile and metalworking industries; pigment dispersant for makeup; mild emulsifier for makeup bases, skin care emulsions, hair conditioners; solubilizer for fragrances and emollients in body splashes; yel. liq.; sol. in water, ethanol, veg. oil, toluol; sp.gr. 1.0; visc. 400 cps; HLB 15.0; sapon. no. 45–55; hyd. no. 65-80; flash pt. (PMCC) > 350 F; 97% min. act.

T-Maz® 80K. [PPG/Specialty Chem.] Polysorbate 80, kosher; CAS 9005-65-6; nonionic; solubilizer and emulsifier for foods, vitamins, edible oils; Gardner 5 liq.; sol. in water, veg. oil; disp. in toluene; HLB 15.0; sapon. no. 45-55; hyd. no. 65-80; flash pt. (PMCC) > 350 F; 100% conc.

T-Maz® 80KLM. [PPG/Specialty Chem.] Polysorbate 80, kosher, low melt pt.; CAS 9005-65-6; emulsifier, solubilizer, wetting agent, antistat, stabilizer, dispersant, visc. modifier, suspending agent used in the food, cosmetic, drug, textile and metalworking industries; Gardner 5 liq.; sol. @ 5% in water, veg. oil; disp. in toluene; HLB 15.0; sapon. no. 45–55; hyd. no. 65-80; flash pt. (PMCC) > 350 F.

T-Maz® 81. [PPG/Specialty Chem.] Polysorbate 81; CAS 9005-65-6; nonionic; emulsifier, solubilizer, wetting agent, antistat, stabilizer, dispersant, visc. modifier, suspending agent used in the food, cosmetic, drug, textile and metalworking industries; Gardner 6 liq.; sol. in min. spirits; disp. in water, min. oils, toluene, veg. oils; HLB 10.0; sapon. no. 96-104; hyd. no. 134-150; flash pt. (PMCC) > 350 F; 100% conc.

T-Maz® 85. [PPG/Specialty Chem.] Polysorbate 85; CAS 9005-70-3; nonionic; emulsifier, solubilizer, wetting agent, antistat, stabilizer, dispersant, visc. modifier, suspending agent used in the food, cosmetic, drug, textile and metalworking industries; pigment dispersant for makeup; mild emulsifier for makeup bases, skin care emulsions, hair conditioners; solubilizer for fragrances and emollients in body splashes; lt. amber liq.; sol. in mineral. spirits; disp. in water; sp.gr. 1.0; visc. 300 cps; HLB 11.1; sapon. no. 83–93; hyd. no. 39-52; flash pt. (PMCC) > 350 F; 95% min. act.

T-Maz® 90. [PPG/Specialty Chem.] PEG-20 sorbitan tallate; nonionic; emulsifier, solubilizer, wetting agent, antistat, stabilizer, dispersant, visc. modifier, suspending agent used in the food, cosmetic, drug, textile and metalworking industries; amber liq.; sol. in water, ethanol, toluol, veg. oil; sp.gr. 1.0; visc. 500 cps; HLB 14.9; sapon. no. 45–55; hyd. no. 65-80; flash pt. (PMCC) > 350 F; 97% min. act.

T-Maz® 95. [PPG/Specialty Chem.] PEG-20 sorbitan tritallate; emulsifier, solubilizer, wetting agent, visc. modifier, antistat, stabilizer, dispersant for food, cosmetic, drug, textile and metalworking industries; amber liq.; sol. in min. spirits; disp. in water, min. oils, toluene, veg. oils; sp.gr. 1.0; visc. 350 cps; HLB 11.0; sapon. no. 83-93; hyd. no. 39-52; flash pt. (PMCC) > 350 F; 3.0% max. water.

TMPD® Glycol. [Eastman] 2,2,4-Trimethyl-1,3-pentanediol; CAS 144-19-4; cosmetic ingred.; resin intermediate.

dl-a-Tocopherol. [BASF] Tocopherol; antioxidant, vitamin E source.

Tocopherol Oil CLR. [Dr. Kurt Richter; Henkel/Cospha] Vitamin E carrier with natural tocopherols in soya oil medium; general skin care prods.; lt. yel. oil.

dl-α-Tocopheryl Acetate, Cosmetic Grade No. 60574. [Roche] Tocopheryl acetate; moisturizer for cosmetic applics.; stable liq. form of vitamin E; liq.

dl-α-Tocopheryl Linoleate No. 26364. [Roche] Tocopheryl linoleate; CAS 36148-84-2; long-lasting moisturizer for cosmetic applics.; source of essential fatty acids; liq.

Tofupro-U. [Ikeda] Soya protein; CAS 68153-28-6; protein providing substantivity and conditioning effects in hair and skin care prods., creamy shampoos, hair treatments, milk lotions; nutritive high-protein, low-calorie food without cholesterol; yel. to amber clear liq.; pH 3.8-6.2.

Toho PEG Series. [Toho Chem. Industry] Polyethylene glycol (m.w. 200, 300, 400, 600, 1000, 1500, 1540, 2000, 4000); base material for surfactants, syn. resin, plasticizer, lubricating industries; wetting, softening, penetrating, lubricating and cleaning agent for textile, paper, ink, pigments, cosmetics and toiletries, etc.; liq./paste/solid.

Tohol N-220. [Toho Chem. Industry] Cocamide DEA; CAS 61791-31-9; EINECS 263-163-9; nonionic; foam booster/stabilizer and thickener for shampoo, detergent, toothpaste; liq.; 100% conc.

Tohol N-220X. [Toho Chem. Industry] Cocamide DEA; CAS 61791-31-9; EINECS 263-163-9; nonionic; foam stabilizer and thickener for shampoo, detergent, toothpaste; solid; 100% conc.

Tohol N-230. [Toho Chem. Industry] Lauramide DEA; CAS 120-40-1; EINECS 204-393-1; nonionic; foam booster/stabilizer and thickener for shampoo, detergent, toothpaste; liq.; 100% conc.

Tohol N-230X. [Toho Chem. Industry] Lauramide DEA; CAS 120-40-1; EINECS 204-393-1; nonionic; foam stabilizer and thickener for shampoo, detergent, and toothpaste; solid; 100% conc.

Tomah AO-14-2. [Exxon/Tomah] Bishydroxyethylisodecyloxypropylamine oxide; cationic; foam stabilizers/boosters in liq. detergents, shampoos, hard surf. cleaners, laundry detergents; grease emulsifier, soil suspension aid; forms synergistic surfactant base for built household, instititional and industrial cleaners with quats. and nonionics; Gardner 2 clear liq.; sp.gr. 0.956 (15 C); pour pt. < 20 F; amine no. 83-89; flamm.; 50% act.

Tomah AO-728 Special. [Exxon/Tomah] Amine oxide; detergent, foam booster/stabilizer for industrial and household detergents, dishwash, personal care prods.; Gardner 3 max. liq.; sp.gr. 0.958; pour pt. < 20 F; amine no. 72-79; flamm.; 50% act.

Tonique HS 216. [Alban Muller] Cypress, witch hazel, St. John's wort, horsetail, and thyme phytocomplex; facial lotion.

Tonique HS 290. [Alban Muller] Propylene glycol, calendula extract, horse chestnut extract, cypress extract, and arnica extract; phytocomplex for facial creams.

Tonique LS 690. [Alban Muller] Sunflower seed oil, calendula extract, horse chestnut extract, cypress extract, and arnica extract; phytocomplex for facial creams.

Transcutol. [Gattefosse SA] Ethoxydiglycol; CAS 111-90-0; EINECS 203-919-7; solv. for active ingreds. in pharmaceutical preps.; cosurfactant for microemulsions; liq.; toxicology: LD50 (oral, rat) 5.9 ml/kg; nonirritating to skin and eyes; 100% conc.

Transjojoba™ 15. [Int'l. Flora Tech.] Jojoba esters; cosmetic ingred.; clear liq.

Transjojoba™ 30. [Int'l. Flora Tech.] Transesterified jojoba oil and wax; cosmetic ingred.; soft wh. to off-wh. cream, typ. fatty odor; m.p. 29 C; acid no. 1.8; iodine no. 60; sapon. no. 90.

Transjojoba™ 60. [Int'l. Flora Tech.] Transesterified jojoba oil and wax; cosmetic ingred.; wh. to off-wh. soft paste, typ. fatty odor; m.p. 58 C; acid no. 2.5; iodine no. 40;

sapon. no. 90.

Transjojoba™ 70. [Int'l. Flora Tech.] Hydrog. jojoba oil; CAS 61789-91-1; extremely hard, nontacky, lustrous cosmetic ingred.; wh. free-flowing powd., trace odor; m.w. 610; m.p. 69 C; acid no. 2; iodine no. 1; sapon. no. 92.

Transparent Titanium Dioxide PW Covafluor. [Les Colorants Wackherr] Titanium dioxide, fluoroalkyl coated; CAS 13463-67-7; EINECS 236-675-5; mineral sunscreen.

Transparent Titanium Dioxide PW Covalim. [Les Colorants Wackherr] Titanium dioxide, 40% disp. in min. oil; mineral sunscreen.

Transparent Titanium Dioxide PW Covasil S. [Les Colorants Wackherr] Titanium dioxide, silane coated; CAS 13463-67-7; EINECS 236-675-5; mineral sunscreen.

Transparent Titanium Dioxide PW Covasop. [Les Colorants Wackherr] 35% Titanium dioxide disp. in propylene glycol; mineral sunscreen.

Transparent Titanium Dioxide PW Powd. [Les Colorants Wackherr] Titanium dioxide; CAS 13463-67-7; EINECS 236-675-5; mineral uv filter with low opacitiy; for sunscreens; microfine powd.

Transparent Titanium Dioxide PW Squatol S. [Les Colorants Wackherr] 40% Titanium dioxide disp. in syn. squalene; mineral sunscreen.

Trichogen. [Laboratoires Sérobiologiques] Placental protein, hydrolyzed serum protein, propylene glycol, glucose, panthenol, yeast extract, niacinamide, pyridoxine, hydrolyzed glycosaminoglycans, and biotin; keratinocytes growth factor; activates synthesis of proteins, stimulates hair growth; improves dandruff and seborrheic conditions; colloidal liq.; water-sol.; usage level: 10%.

Tri-Derm SE. [Tri-K Industries] Water and spleen extract; an additive which helps increase cell renewal in skin treatment prods.; colorless to pale yel. clear liq., bland odor; sp.gr. 1.015-1.025; b.p. 212 F; ref. index 1.340-1.350; pH 5.5-6.5; 4.5-5.5% NV.

Triethanolamine Pure C. [BASF AG] Neutralizing component for the cosmetic industry.

Tri-K Allantoin. [Tri-K Industries] Allantoin; CAS 97-59-6; EINECS 202-592-8; ingred. for skin care prods.

Tri-K Allantoin Acetyl Methionine. [Tri-K Industries] Allantoin acetyl methionine; CAS 4207-40-3; EINECS 224-126-2; ingred. for skin care and sun care prods.

Tri-K CMF Complex. [Tri-K Industries] Cell moisturizing factor containing collagen, hydrolyzed elastin, hydrolyzed mucopolysaccharides, bovine amniotic fluid, tocopheryl acetate, linoleic acid, linolenic acid, arachidonic acid, and oleic acid; skin care complex providing moisturization, conditioning, and nutrition to the skin; also for hair care and cleansing prods., hand and body lotions, moisturizing creams, cleansing lotions, bar soap, hair/scalp conditioner, shampoo, hair tonics; straw to lt. amber sl. visc. clear liq., char. proteinaceous odor; sol. in water; sp.gr. 1.000; b.p. 212 F; pH 3.5-4.25; toxicology: pract. nonirritating.

Tri-K EFA Complex. [Tri-K Industries] A phytosterol complex containing a stabilized blend of essential fatty acids with sterols, egg lecithin, carotene, and tocopherol; cosmetic ingred.

Tri-K KHP. [Tri-K Industries] Hydrolyzed hair keratin; cosmetic ingred.

Tri-K HMF Complex. [Tri-K Industries] A moisturizing complex containing more than 12 ingreds. for complete spectrum of activity; increases moisture in damaged hair.

Tri-K HMP. [Tri-K Industries] Hydrolyzed mucopolysaccharide; cosmetic ingred.; powd.; 99% act.

Tri-K Soypro-25. [Tri-K Industries] Hydrolyzed soy protein; CAS 68607-88-5; cosmetic/food-grade protein providing substantivity, hair manageability, conditioning, skin smoothing, moisture retention, and film formation; com-

pletely biodeg.; amber clear to sl. hazy liq., sl. pleasant odor; completely sol. in water; sp.gr. 1.16; b.p. 215 F; pH 4-6; toxicology: LD50 anticipated to be > 5 g/kg; may cause temporary eye irritation; 25% act. in water.

Tri-K Soyquat-30. [Tri-K Industries] Hydroxypropyltrimonium hydrolyzed soy protein; cosmetic raw material; amber clear liq., mild char. odor; freely sol. in water; sp.gr. 1.2; b.p. 105 C; pH 4.5-6.0; toxicology: LD50 anticipated to be > 5 g/kg; 30% in water.

Tri-K Sunflower Oil. [Tri-K Industries] Sunflower oil; CAS 8001-21-6; EINECS 232-273-9; cosmetic ingred.; pale straw clear oil, bland odor and taste; sp.gr. 0.922-0.996; iodine no. 120-139; sapon. no. 188-195; ref. index 1.4663-1.6840; trace moisture.

Tri-Lastin 10F. [Tri-K Industries] Hydrolyzed elastin; CAS 100085-10-7; film-former providing moisture-retentive films, protective colloid effects, elasticity and resilience in skin care cosmetics; provides gloss, ease of combing, and silky feel in hair care prods.; completely biodeg.; pale yel. clear liq., very sl. char. odor; completely sol. in water; sp.gr. 1.02; b.p. 105 C; pH 4.5-7.5; toxicology: LD50 (oral, rat) > 50 ml/kg; nonirritating to skin and eyes; 10% act. in water.

Trilipidina. [Vevy] Glyceryl palmitate/stearate and glyceryl laurate/oleate.

Trillagene® . [Gattefosse] Soluble collagen; CAS 9007-34-5; EINECS 232-697-4; biological additive for moisturizing and body lotions and mid/high quality cosmetics; liq.; water-sol.; 1% collagen.

Trimol CE 2000. [Tri-K Industries] Trioctyldodecyl citrate; CAS 126121-35-5; high visc. emollient ester with pigment dispersing props.

Tri-Ol ALM. [Tri-K Industries] Sweet almond oil.

Tri-Ol AVO. [Tri-K Industries] Avocado oil; CAS 8024-32-6; EINECS 232-428-0.

Tri-Ol CAM. [Tri-K Industries] Camellia oil.

Tri-Ol OLV. [Tri-K Industries] Olive oil; CAS 8001-25-0; EINECS 232-277-0; emollient.

Tri-Ol RBO. [Tri-K Industries] Rice bran oil; EINECS 271-397-8; cosmetic ingred.

Tri-Ol SAF. [Tri-K Industries] Safflower oil; CAS 8001-23-8; EINECS 232-276-5; emollient oil.

Tri-Ol SES. [Tri-K Industries] Sesame oil; CAS 8008-74-0; EINECS 232-370-6; emollient oil.

Tri-Ol SUN. [Tri-K Industries] Sunflower seed oil; CAS 8001-21-6; EINECS 232-273-9; lipid for cosmetics.

Tri-Ol WG. [Tri-K Industries] Wheat germ oil; CAS 8006-95-9; emollient.

Trioxene A. [Vevy] Glyceryl adipate; CAS 26699-71-8; EINECS 247-911-1.

Trioxene D. [Vevy] Isotridecyl cocoate.

Trioxene E. [Vevy] Octyl cocoate; CAS 92044-87-6; EINECS 295-366-3; emollient.

Trioxene I. [Vevy] Isodecyl cocoate.

Trioxene L. [Vevy] PEG-5 lauryl tricitrate, PEG-5 decyl tricitrate, PEG-5 caprylyl tricitrate.

Trioxene LV. [Vevy] Isodecyl citrate; CAS 90605-17-7; EINECS 292-416-6.

Trioxene S. [Vevy] PEG-5 myristyl tricitrate, PEG-5 stearyl tricitrate, PEG-5 cetyl tricitrate.

Tripro-5. [Tri-K Industries] TEA-cocoyl hydrolyzed collagen and sorbitol; CAS 68952-16-9, 50-70-4; mild protein-based cosmetic ingred.; lt. amber clear to sl. hazy liq., mild pleasant sl. proteinaceous odor; completely sol. in water; sp.gr. 1.25; b.p. 220 F; pH 7.1-7.4; 70% act. in water.

Tri-Pronectin. [Tri-K Industries] Fibronectin and soluble collagen; designed for max. functionality in cosmetic prods.

Tri-Quat-S. [Tri-K Industries] Steartrimonium hydrolyzed animal protein; CAS 111174-62-0; cationic; cosmetic ingred.

Tris Amino®. [Angus] Tris (hydroxymethyl) aminomethane; CAS 77-86-1; EINECS 201-064-4; pigment dispersant, neutralizing amine, corrosion inhibitor, acid-salt catalyst, pH buffer, chemical, personal care, and pharmaceutical intermediate, solubilizer; m.w. 121.1; sol. 80 g/100 ml water; m.p. 171 C; b.p. 219 C; pH 10.4 (0.1M aq. sol'n.).

Trisept B. [Tri-K Industries] Butylparaben NF/tech.; CAS 94-26-8; EINECS 202-318-7; preservative for cosmetics.

Trisept E. [Tri-K Industries] Ethylparaben NF/tech.; CAS 120-47-8; EINECS 204-399-4; preservative for cosmetics.

Trisept M. [Tri-K Industries] Methylparaben NF/FCC/tech.; CAS 99-76-3; EINECS 202-785-7; preservative for cosmetics; colorless; usage level: 0.1-1.0%; toxicology: nontoxic.

Trisept P. [Tri-K Industries] Propylparaben NF/FCC/tech.; CAS 94-13-3; EINECS 202-307-7; cosmetics preservative; USA, Japan, Europe approvals; colorless; usage level: 0.02-1.0%; toxicology: nontoxic.

Trisept SDHA. [Tri-K Industries] Sodium dehydroacetate FCC; CAS 4418-26-2; EINECS 224-580-1; broad spectrum cosmetics preservative; ideal for lipsticks (does not affect taste); heat stable to 120 C; USA, Japan, Europe approvals; usage level: 0.2-0.5%.

Tri-Sil HGC 5000. [Tri-K Industries] Dimethiconol and cyclomethicone; silicone polymer for use where conditioning, substantivity, and lubricity are required, e.g., in hair laminates and gloss sprays.

Tri-Sil MFF 5010. [Tri-K Industries] A multifunctional silicone copolymer; gives softening, antistatic, and conditioning props. to cosmetic formulations; water-disp.

Tri-Sil MFF 5010-70. [Tri-K Industries] A 70% aq. microemulsion of Tri-Sil MFF 5010; gives softening, antistatic, and conditioning props. to cosmetic formulations; water-disp.; 70% conc.

Tri-Sil MFF 5015. [Tri-K Industries] Amino silicone copolyol; self-dispersing, multifunctional polymer with conditioning props. on skin and hair.

Tri-Sil Wax 105. [Tri-K Industries] Dimethylsiloxane wax; achieves the lubricity and solubility of silicone in a solid form; for use in cosmetic stick prods.

Tris Nitro®. [Angus] Tris (hydroxymethyl) nitromethane; CAS 126-11-4; EINECS 204-769-5; antibacterial agent, preservative for cosmetics, water treatment, metalworking fluids, oil prod., deodorizing; formaldehyde releaser; 100% act. solid or 50% aq. sol'n.

Tristat. [Tri-K Industries] Sorbic acid NF/FCC; CAS 110-44-1; EINECS 203-768-7; preservative.

Tristat BNP. [Tri-K Industries] 2-Bromo-2-nitropropane-1,3-diol; CAS 52-51-7; EINECS 200-143-0; preservative for cosmetics; usage level: 0.01-0.1%.

Tristat IU. [Tri-K Industries] Imidazolidinyl urea; CAS 39236-46-9; EINECS 254-372-6; preservative for cosmetics; effective against Gram-negative bacteria; active over wide pH range; water-sol.; usage level: 0.2-0.6%.

Tristat K. [Tri-K Industries] Potassium sorbate NF/FCC; CAS 590-00-1; EINECS 246-376-1; cosmetics and food preservative; antimycotic effective against yeasts and molds; effective only in acid media; USA GRAS, FCC, Japan, Europe approvals; wh. gran. and powd.; sol. 1 g/ml water; pH 8.5-9.8 (5%); usage level: 0.05-0.5%; 99% min. purity.

Tristat SDHA. [Tri-K Industries] Sodium dehydroacetate; CAS 4418-26-2; EINECS 224-580-1; preservative for cosmetics, lipsticks, beverages, butter and other food prods.; inhibits growth of molds, yeast, gram-positive and gram-negative bacteria; FCC approved; wh. to lt. yel. cryst. powd., char. odor; sol. in water; m.w. 208.15; bulk dens. 0.6; m.p. 109-112 C; usage level: 0.2-0.25% food/0.3-0.5% cosmet; toxicology: nontoxic; 98% min. assay.

Trisynlane. [Tri-K Industries] Hydrog. polyisobutene; substitute for natural squalane for cosmetics and pharmaceuticals; provides exc. feel with good spreading and penetrating props. as base oil for cosmetics; good oxidation stability; colorless liq., odorless, tasteless; misc. with veg. and min. oils.

Tritein-40, -50, -100. [Tri-K Industries] Hydrolyzed collagen; CAS 9015-54-7; cosmetic protein.

Tri-Tein 40N. [Tri-K Industries] Hydrolyzed collagen; CAS 9015-54-7; protein for cosmetics applics.; lt. yel. clear to hazy liq., very sl. char. proteinaceous odor; completely sol. in water; sp.gr. 1.0-1.25; b.p. 215 F; pH 4.5-6.5; toxicology: nonhazardous; 40% min. NV.

Tri-Tein 55. [Tri-K Industries] Hydrolyzed collagen; CAS 9015-54-7; protein for cosmetics applics.; biodeg.; lt. amber clear liq., very sl. char. proteinaceous odor; completely sol. in water; sp.gr. 1.2; b.p. 215 C; pH 5.8-6.3; toxicology: LD50 anticipated to be > 5 g/kg; 55% act. in water.

Tri-Tein Milk Polypeptide. [Tri-K Industries] Hydrolyzed milk protein; CAS 92797-39-2; emollient with good affinity for skin, adsorption to hair; stabilizes colloids and emulsions; for body and body shampoos, soaps, hair conditioners, treatments, and rinses; stable in hard water due to chelating ability; biodeg.; yelsh. clear liq., mild hydrolysate odor; sol. in water; insol. in oils, org. solvs.; pH 4-7.

Tri-Tein Silk AA. [Tri-K Industries] Silk amino acids; CAS 977077-71-6; protein with exc. absorption and film-forming props. imparting softness and gloss to hair and smoothness to the skin; component of natural moisturizing factor; biodeg.; amber clear liq., char. mild odor; sol. in water; sp.gr. 1.10; b.p. 215 F; pH 4.5-7.5; toxicology: nonhazardous; nonirritating to skin and eyes; 15% protein, 15% sodium chloride, 70% water.

Tritisol™. [Croda Inc.] Soluble wheat protein; film-forming conditioning, moisturizing protein improving skin firmness; for hair and skin care preps., permanent waves, activated conditioners; binder in mascara formulations; lt. amber clear visc. sol'n., mild char. odor; sol. in water, water/ethanol, glycerol, propylene glycol; m.w. > 100,000; pH 6.5-7.5; 20-25% solids.

Triton® CG-110. [Union Carbide; Union Carbide Europe] Caprylyl/capryl glucoside; CAS 68515-73-1; nonionic; low irritation surfactant, foaming agent for shampoos, skin creams, lotions, bar soaps, industrial cleaners, alkali bottlewashing, food processing; biodeg.; golden clear liq.; sol. in 50% sodium hydroxide sol'n.; sp.gr. 1.15; dens. 8.9 lb/gal (15.5 C); visc. 940 cP; pour pt. -8 C; cloud pt. > 100 C (1% aq.); flash pt. (COC) none; pH 5.7; surf. tens. 28 dynes/cm (0.1%); Draves wetting 102 s (0.1%); Ross-Miles foam 188 mm (initial, 0.1%); 60% act.

Triton® N-42. [Union Carbide; Union Carbide Europe] Nonoxynol-4; CAS 9016-45-9; nonionic; detergent, emulsifier; colorless-yel. clear visc. liq.; m.w. 405; water-disp., oil-sol.; sp.gr. 1.068; dens. 8.5 lb/gal; visc. 250 cps; HLB 9.1; pour pt. -26 C; flash pt. (TOC) 149 C; pH 7.5; surf. tens. 29 dynes/cm (0.01% aq.); 100% conc.

Triton® N-150. [Union Carbide; Union Carbide Europe] Nonoxynol-15; CAS 9016-45-9; nonionic; detergent, emulsifier; APHA 160 liq.; m.w. 880; dens. 9.0 lb/gal; visc. 4350 cps; HLB 15.0; cloud pt. 95 C (1%); pour pt. 65 F; surf. tens. 33 dynes/cm (1%); 100% conc.

Triton® X-100. [Union Carbide; Union Carbide Europe] Octoxynol-9 (9-10 EO); CAS 9002-93-1; nonionic; wetting agent, dispersant, detergent, household and industrial cleaners; metal cleaners; sanitizers; textile processing, wool scouring; emulsifier for insecticides and herbicides; solubilizer of perfumes; FDA, EPA compliance; clear liq.; sol. in water, toluene, xylene, trichlorethylene, ethylene glycol, alcohols; m.w. 628; sp.gr. 1.065; dens.

8.9 lb/gal; visc. 240 cps; HLB 13.5; cloud pt. 65 C (1% aq.); flash pt. > 300 F (TOC); pour pt. 45 F; pH 6 (5% aq.); surf. tens. 30 dynes/cm (1%); Ross-Miles foam 110 mm (0.1%, 120 F); 100% act.

Trivalon. [Henkel/Cospha] Fragrance raw material for cosmetic, personal care, detergent, and cleaning prods.; colorless liq., walnut odor; b.p. 90-92 C; flash pt. 112 C.

Trivent ALA. [Trivent] Acetylated lanolin alcohol, cetyl acetate; emollient; Gardner 2+ color, typ. odor; acid no. 0.91; iodine no. 5.1; sapon. no. 183.4; hyd. no. 0.43.

Trivent BE-13. [Trivent] Tridecyl behenate; cosmetic emollient which liquefies on contact with skin; provides increased lubricity during rub-out; boosts and stabilizes visc. in emulsions; yel. liq. to semisolid, typ. mild odor; sol. @ 10% in min. oil, oxybenzone, DIA, castor oil, volatile silicone, octyl salicylate, isocetyl alcohol; insol. in water, ethanol; m.w. 522; sp.gr. 0.854; m.p. 24 C; acid no. 2 max.; sapon. no. 95-115; toxicology: LD50 (acute oral) > 5 g/kg; nonirritating to skin and eyes; noncomedogenic.

Trivent CP. [Trivent] Cetyl palmitate; CAS 540-10-3; EINECS 208-736-6; emollient; wh. to off-wh. flakes, typ. mild waxy odor; sol. in min. oil, peanut oil, hot IPA; insol. in water; m.w. 480; m.p. 50.5-55.5 C; acid no. 2 max.; sapon. no. 109-117.

Trivent DIA. [Trivent] Diisopropyl adipate; CAS 6938-94-9; EINECS 248-299-9; lubricating dry emollient with strong solv. props.; hydro/alcoholic compat. for aftershave lotions and afterbath splashes; lubricant and detackifier in antiperspirants; drying agent in heavy oily systems; colorless clear liq., faint typ. odor; sol. in min. oils, lower alcohols, ketones, esters, chlorinated hydrocarbons; insol. in water, glycerin; m.w. 230; sp.gr. 0.960; f.p. -2 C; acid no. 1 max.; iodine no. nil; sapon. no. 480-500; flash pt. (COC) > 170 C.

Trivent DOS. [Trivent] Dioctyl sebacate; CAS 122-62-3; EINECS 204-558-8; emollient; APHA 50 max. color, mild typ. odor; sol. @ 10% in min. oil, IPM, dimethicone, castor oil, 95% alcohol, safflower, soybean, and lanolin oils; insol. in water, glycerin, propylene glycol; m.w. 426; sp.gr. 0.913; acid no. 0.10; toxicology: LD50 (acute oral) > 5 g/kg; nonirritating to skin and eyes; noncomedogenic.

Trivent EG-18. [Trivent] Glycol stearate, stearamide AMP; raw material for cosmetic and personal care prods.

Trivent MA. [Trivent] Menthyl anthranilate; CAS 134-09-8; EINECS 205-129-8; sunscreen; pale to dk. yel. visc. liq., faint sweet aromatic odor; sol. in IPA, 65/75 min. oil, ethanol, peanut oil; insol. in water, glycerin; m.w. 275.38; sp.gr. 1.020-1.060; acid no. 1 max.; sapon. no. 180-210; ref. index 1.532-1.552.

Trivent NP-13. [Trivent] Tridecyl neopentanoate; CAS 106436-39-9; very dry emollient for nonoily creams and lotions; SPF booster for sunscreens; binder and pigment dispersant; plasticizer for hair setting polymers; cosolv. for oils and waxes in anhyd. sticks; wetting agent for Carbopol; colorless to pale yel. liq., sl. mild odor; sol. @ 5% in 95% ethanol, min. oil, cyclomethicone, IPM, dimethicone, isocetyl alcohol, hexyelne glycol; insol. in water, glycerin, propylene glycol; m.w. 284; sp.gr. 0.850-0.860; acid no. 2 max.; sapon. no. 185-205; ref. index 1.434-1.437; toxicology: LD50 (acute oral) > 5 g/kg; may cause eye and skin irritation; noncomedogenic.

Trivent OC-13. [Trivent] Tridecyl octanoate; dry emollient for skin and eye care prods., makeup, skin treatment, sun care, lipsticks, lip glosses; water-wh. to pale yel. liq., typ. mild odor; sol. @ 5% in castor oil, min. oil, peanut oil, 95% ethanol, IPM; insol. in dimethicone, glycerin, propylene glycol, water; m.w. 326.56; sp.gr. 0.861 ± 0.01; acid no. 2 max.; sapon. no. 145-175; ref. index 1.445; toxicology: LD50 (acute oral) > 5 g/kg; nonirritating to skin and eyes; noncomedogenic.

Trivent OC-16. [Trivent] Cetyl octanoate; CAS 59130-69-7; EINECS 261-619-1; dry emollient, lubricity, gloss agent for skin treatment, makeup, lip prods., sun care, bath prods., eye makeup removers, hot oil treatments, pressed powds.; water-wh. to pale yel., typ. mild odor; sol. @ 5% in castor oil, min. oil, peanut oil, IPM, dimethicone, 100% ethanol, isopropanol; insol. in water, glycerin, propylene glycol; m.w. 368; acid no. 1 max.; sapon. no. 130-155; hyd. no. 5 max.; ref. index 1.445; toxicology: LD50 (acute oral) > 5 g/kg; nonirritating to eyes; may cause sl. skin irritation; noncomedogenic.

Trivent OC-143. [Trivent] Myreth-3 octanoate; emollient; water-wh. to pale yel. liq., typ. mild odor; sol. in min. oil, peanut oil, dimethicone, IPM; disp. in glycerin, propylene glycol, sorbitol, water; m.w. 472.73; acid no. 2 max.; sapon. no. 60-80; ref. index 1.451; toxicology: LD50 (acute oral) > 5 g/kg; nonirritating to eyes; may cause skin irritation.

Trivent OC-G. [Trivent] Glyceryl trioctanoate; CAS 538-23-8; EINECS 208-686-5; emollient for cosmetics; provides distinct powd.-like feel on dry-down; exc. pigment wetting/dispersing, and binding props. for use in liq. makeup, pressed powds., lip prods; pigment color booster for pressed powds.; lt. yel. clear liq., typ. mild odor; sol. @ 10% in min. oil, IPM, octyl salicylate, oleyl alcohol, castor oil, 95% IPA, 95% ethanol, cyclomethicone; insol. in dimethicone, water, propylene glycol, glycerin; m.w. 470.69; sp.gr. 0.95; acid no. 2 max.; sapon. no. 340-360; ref. index 1.446; toxicology: LD50 (acute oral) > 5 g/kg; nonirritating to skin and eyes; noncomedogenic.

Trivent OL-10. [Trivent] Decyl oleate; CAS 3687-46-5; EINECS 222-981-6; emollient for cosmetics and toiletries, creams, lotions, anhyd. oils; wets out iron oxide pigments for liq. makeup, pressed powds., makeup removers; min. oil replacement; yel. liq., typ. odor; sol. @ 5% in peanut oil, min. oil, 95% ethanol, IPM, oleyl alcohol; insol. in water, glycerin, propylene glycol; acid no. 2 max.; iodine no. 45-60; sapon. no. 130-145; ref. index 1.454.

Trivent OL-10B. [Trivent] Isodecyl oleate; CAS 59231-34-4; EINECS 261-673-6; emollient for creams and lotions providing dry light feel on skin; wetting agent for pigments in makeup and makeup removers; imparts luster, conditioning, and improved foam props. to mousse hair conditioners; pale yel. liq., typ. odor; sol. @ 5% in peanut oil, min. oil, 95% ethanol, IPM, oleyl alcohol; insol. in water, glyceri, propylene glycol; f.p. < 0 C; acid no. 2 max.; iodine no. 45-60; sapon. no. 120-140; ref. index 1.455.

Trivent OP. [Trivent] Octyl palmitate; CAS 29806-73-3; EINECS 249-862-1; emollient; Gardner 2 max. liq.; sol. in peanut oil, min. oil, 95% ethanol, IPM, oleyl alcohol; insol. in water, glycerin, propylene glycol; sp.gr. 0.854-0.858; f.p. 0 C; acid no. 3 max.; iodine no. 1 max.; flash pt. (COC) 395 F; ref. index 1.445; 90% min. purity.

Trivent OS. [Trivent] Octyl salicylate; CAS 118-60-5; EINECS 204-263-4; sunscreen; colorless clear to lt. yel. liq., typ. bland odor; sol. in alcohol, min. oil; insol. in water; m.w. 250; sp.gr. 1.013-1.022; ref. index 1.495-1.505; 95% min. purity.

Trivent PE-48. [Trivent] Pentaerythrityl tetraoctanoate; CAS 7299-99-2; EINECS 221-123-8; emollient contributing wet feel in skin preps.; lubricant and drag reducer lin lip glosses and lipsticks; Gardner 1 max. clear liq., typ. odor; sol. @ 10% in min. oil, anhyd. ethanol, dimethicone, IPM; insol. in water, propylene glycol; m.w. 640; acid no. 1 max.; sapon. no. 338-368; hyd. no. 10 max.; toxicology: LD50 (acute oral) > 5 g/kg; nonirritating to eyes and skin; noncomedogenic.

Trivent SS-13. [Trivent] Tridecyl stearoyl stearate; emollient; golden yel. clear liq., typ. mild odor; sol. in castor oil, min. oil, peanut oil, 95% ethanol, IPM, volatile silicone; insol. in water, glycerin, propylene glycol; m.w. 482.82; acid no. 2 max.; sapon. no. 100-120; toxicology: LD50 (acute oral) > 5 g/kg; nonirritating to skin and eyes; noncomedogenic.

Trivent SS-20. [Trivent] Octyldodecyl stearoyl stearate; CAS 58450-52-5; EINECS 289-991-0; emollient in emulsion systems providing smooth, nongreasy protective film on skin; visc. stabilizer for soap systems; binder in pressed powds.; pigment dispersant in lipsticks; Gardner 5 max. liq., typ. mild odor; sol. in veg. oil, IPM, safflower oil, min. oil, oleyl alcohol, octyl palmitate; partly sol. in 95% ethanol, propylene glycol, glycerin, 70% sorbitol; insol. in water; acid no. 10 max.; sapon. no. 115-135; ref. index 1.447-1.467.

Troenan. [Henkel/Cospha] Fragrance raw material for cosmetic, personal care, detergent, and cleaning prods.; colorless liq., privet blossom odor; b.p. 72 C; flash pt. 126 C.

Trolamine 85 NF Grade. [Dow] Triethanolamine; CAS 102-71-6; EINECS 203-049-8; used in surfactants, cosmetics/toiletries, metalworking fluids, textile chemicals, gas conditioning chemicals, agric. intermediates, and cement grinding aids; sp.gr. 1.1179; dens. 9.34 lb/gal; visc. 590.5 cps; f.p. 17 C; b.p. 325 C (760 mm Hg); flash pt. (PMCC) 354 F; fire pt. 410 F; ref. index 1.4836.

Trolamine 99 NF Grade. [Dow] Triethanolamine; CAS 102-71-6; EINECS 203-049-8; used in surfactants, cosmetics/toiletries, metalworking fluids, textile chemicals, gas conditioning chemicals, agric. intermediates, and cement grinding aids; sp.gr. 1.1205; dens. 9.35 lb/gal; visc. 600.7 cps; f.p. 21 C; b.p. 340 C (760 mm Hg); flash pt. (COC) 350 F; fire pt. 420 F; ref. index 1.4839.

Trycol® 5882. [Henkel/Emery; Henkel/Textiles] Laureth-4; CAS 5274-68-0; EINECS 226-097-1; nonionic; coemulsifier for silicone in polishes, mold release agents; emulsifier in industrial lubricants, agric., textile applics.; intermediate for shampoo bases; biodeg.; EPA-exempt; Gardner 1 liq.; sol. in butyl stearate, glycerol trioleate, xylene; disp. in water, min. oil; dens. 7.7 lb/gal; visc. 20 cSt (100 F); HLB 9.2; cloud pt. < 25 C; flash pt. 325 F; pour pt. 12 C; 100% conc.

Trycol® 5964. [Henkel/Emery; Henkel/Textiles] Laureth-23; CAS 9002-92-0; nonionic; emulsifier, solubilizer, lubricant used in textiles, agric., and detergent shampoo bases, personal care prods.; coemulsifier for silicone in polishes and mold release agents; solv. emulsifier for textile dye carriers; EPA-exempt; Gardner 1 solid; sol. in water, xylene; dens. 8.6 lb/gal (70 C); HLB 16.7; m.p. 40 C; cloud pt. 93 C (5% saline); flash pt. 440 F; 100% conc.

Trycol® 5967. [Henkel/Emery] Laureth-12; CAS 9002-92-0; EINECS 221-286-5; nonionic; biodeg. detergent, emulsifier; intermediate for shampoo base; textile lubricant; agric. formulations; EPA-exempt; Gardner 1 solid; sol. 5% in water, xylene; dens. 8.4 lb/gal; HLB 14.8; m.p. 32 C; cloud pt. 90 C; flash pt. 465 F; 100% conc.

Trycol® 5971. [Henkel/Emery; Henkel/Textiles] Oleth-20; CAS 9004-98-2; nonionic; emulsifier, dispersant, solubilizer; textile lubricant; intermediate for shampoo base; Gardner 1 solid; sol. in water; disp. in butyl stearate, glycerol trioleate, Stod., xylene; dens. 8.5 lb/gal; HLB 15.3; m.p. 39 C; cloud pt. 87 C (5% saline); flash pt. 500 F.

Trycol® 5972. [Henkel/Emery; Henkel/Textiles] Oleth-23; CAS 9004-98-2; nonionic; emulsifier, dispersant, solubilizer, detergent, stabilizer, anticoagulant, dyeing assistant, lubricant used in textiles, cosmetics and processing of animal fibers; Gardner 2 solid; sol. in water, xylene; HLB 15.8; m.p. 47 C; cloud pt. 89 C (5% saline); flash pt. 440 F; 100% conc.

Trylox® 6746. [Henkel/Emery; Henkel/Textiles] PEG-40 sorbitol hexaoleate; CAS 57171-56-9; nonionic; o/w

emulsifier, dispersant, wetting agent, lubricant, plasticizer, solubilizer for household/industrial/institutional prods., metal lubricants, textile and cosmetic use; Gardner 6 liq.; sol. @ 5% in butyl stearate, glycerol trioleate, Stod., xylene; disp. in water, min. oil; dens. 8.4 lb/gal; visc. 120 cSt (100 F); HLB 10.4; cloud pt. < 25 C; pour pt. < −10 C; flash pt. 515 F; 100% conc.

Trylox® 6753. [Henkel/Emery] PEG-20 sorbitol; nonionic; humectant, plasticizer; intermediate; used in surfactant sol'ns.; emulsifier for textile and cosmetic use; Gardner 1 liq.; sol. in water; dens. 9.7 lb/gal; visc. 200 cSt (100 F); HLB 15.4; cloud pt. > 100 C (10% saline); pour pt. 7 C; flash pt. 435 F; 100% conc.

T-Soft® SA-97. [Harcros] Linear alkylbenzene sulfonic acid; anionic; high foaming detergent intermediate; liq.; 97% conc.

T-Tergamide 1CD. [Harcros] Cocamide DEA; CAS 61791-31-9; EINECS 263-163-9; nonionic; foam stabilizer, thickener, visc. modifier for detergents and shampoos; liq.; 100% conc.

T-Tergamide 1PD. [Harcros] Palm kernelamide DEA; CAS 73807-15-5; nonionic; foam stabilizer, thickener, visc. modifier for detergents and shampoos; liq.; 100% conc.

Tullanox HM-250. [Tulco] Hydrophobic precipitated silica, modified by org. silazane compd.; high surf. area, high water repellency; provides reinforcement, rheology control, corrosion resist., anticaking, thickening to silicone sealants, coatings, powds., polyester resins, liq. systems, elastomers, elec. insulation, defoamers; carrier for catalysts; filler/additive for plastics, paints, coatings, inks, pharmaceuticals, cosmetics, fertilizers, metals, adhesives, toners; extremely fine particle size.

Turkey Red Oil 100%. [Zschimmer & Schwarz] Sulfated castor oil; CAS 8002-33-3; EINECS 232-306-7; anionic; solubilizer, refatting agent; liq.; 85% conc.

Türkischrotöl 100%. [Zschimmer & Schwarz] Sulfated castor oil; CAS 8002-33-3; EINECS 232-306-7; solubilizer for cosmetics, perfumes; liq.; 82% act.

Turpinal® 4 NL. [Henkel/Cospha; Henkel KGaA/Cospha] Tetrasodium etidronate; CAS 3794-83-0; EINECS 223-267-7; chelating agent for heavy metal ions; stabilizer for cosmetic/pharmaceutical hair/skin preps. esp. those containing H_2O_2 or mercaptane, e.g., cold waves; colorless to sl. ylsh., neutral inherent odor; pH 10-12; usage level: 0.1-2%; 29–30% conc.

Turpinal® SL. [Henkel/Cospha; Henkel KGaA/Cospha] Etidronic acid; CAS 2809-21-4; EINECS 220-552-8; chelating agent for heavy metal ions; stabilizer, antioxidant for cosmetic/pharmaceutical hair/skin preps. esp. those containing H_2O_2 or mercaptane, e.g., cold waves; colorless to sl. ylsh. liq., neutral inherent odor; sp.gr. 1.445-1.458; corrosive; usage level: 0.1-2%; toxicology: protect skin and eyes from contact; 58–61% conc.

T-Wax. [Tri-K Industries] Emulsifying wax NF; ingred. for skin care prods.

Tween® 20. [ICI Spec. Chem.; ICI Surf. Am.; ICI Surf. Belgium] Polysorbate 20 NF; CAS 9005-64-5; nonionic; solubilizer, o/w emulsifier, wetting agent; detergent for shampoos; antistat and fiber lubricant used in textile industry; flavor emulsifier; pale yel. liq.; sol. in water, methanol, ethanol, IPA, propylene glycol, ethylene glycol, cottonseed oil; sp.gr. 1.1; visc. 400 cps; HLB 16.7; flash pt. > 300 F; sapon. no. 40–50; 100% act.

Tween® 21. [ICI Spec. Chem.; ICI Surf. Am.; ICI Surf. Belgium] Polysorbate 21; CAS 9005-64-5; nonionic; emulsifier, wetting agent, dispersant, solubilizer for personal care, industrial, and textile applics.; antistat, fiber lubricant for textiles; yel. oily liq.; sol. in corn oil, dioxane, Cellosolve, CCl_4, methanol, ethanol, aniline; disp. in water; sp.gr. 1.1; visc. 500 cps; HLB 13.3; flash pt. > 300 F;

sapon. no. 100–115; 100% act.

Tween® 40. [ICI Spec. Chem.; ICI Surf. Am.; ICI Surf. Belgium] Polysorbate 40 NF; CAS 9005-66-7; nonionic; emulsifier, wetting agent, dispersant, solubilizer for personal care, industrial, and textile applics.; textile antistat, fiber lubricant; pale yel. liq.; sol. in water, methanol, ethanol, IPA, ethylene glycol, cottonseed oil; sp.gr. 1.08; HLB 15.6; flash pt. > 300 F; sapon. no. 41–52; 100% act.

Tween® 60. [ICI Surf. Am.; ICI Surf. UK] Polysorbate 60; CAS 9005-67-8; nonionic; emulsifier, wetting agent, and dispersant for personal care, household, and industrial applics.; pale yel. semisolid; HLB 14.9.

Tween® 61. [ICI Spec. Chem.; ICI Surf. Am.; ICI Surf. Belgium] Polysorbate 61; CAS 9005-67-8; nonionic; emulsifier, solubilizer for perfume, flavor, vitamin oils; wetting agent, dispersant; ivory waxy solid; sol. in methanol, ethanol; disp. in water; sp.gr. 1.06; HLB 9.6; flash pt. > 300 F; pour pt. 100 F; sapon. no. 95–115; 100% act.

Tween® 65. [ICI Surf. Am.; ICI Surf. UK] Polysorbate 65; CAS 9005-71-4; nonionic; emulsifier, wetting agent, and dispersant for personal care, household, and industrial applics.; pale yel. solid; HLB 10.5.

Tween® 80. [ICI Surf. Am.; ICI Surf. UK] Polysorbate 80; CAS 9005-65-6; nonionic; emulsifier, wetting agent, and dispersant for personal care, household, and industrial applics.; yel. brn. liq.; HLB 15.0.

Tween® 80K. [ICI Spec. Chem.; ICI Surf. Am.; ICI Surf. Belgium] Polysorbate 80 NF; CAS 9005-65-6; nonionic; emulsifier, solubilizer for food, vitamins, oils; antifoam; wetting agent, detergent for cleaning contact lenses, skin care prods.; deflocculant; yel. brn. liq.; sol. in water, IPA, ethanol; sp.gr. 1.08; visc. 425 cps; HLB 15.0; flash pt. > 300 F; sapon. no. 45–55; 100% act.

Tween® 81. [ICI Spec. Chem.; ICI Surf. Am.; ICI Surf. Belgium] Polysorbate 81; CAS 9005-65-6; nonionic; emulsifier, wetting agent, dispersant, solubilizer for perfume, flavor, vitamin oils; yel. brn. oily liq.; sol. in min. and corn oil, dioxane, Cellosolve, methanol, ethanol, ethyl acetate, aniline; disp. in water; sp.gr. 1; visc. 450 cps; HLB 10.0; flash pt. > 300 F; sapon. no. 96–104; 100% act.

Tween® 85. [ICI Spec. Chem.; ICI Surf. Am.; ICI Surf. Belgium] Polysorbate 85; CAS 9005-70-3; nonionic; emulsifier, wetting agent, dispersant, solubilizer for perfume, flavor, vitamin oils; floating bath oils; yel. brn. liq.; sol. in veg. oil, Cellosolve, lower alcohols, aromatic solvs., ethyl acetate, min. oils and spirits, acetone, dioxane, CCl_4 and ethylene glycol; disp. in water; sp.gr. 1.0; visc. 300 cps; HLB 11.0; flash pt. > 300 F; sapon. no. 80–95; 100% act.

28-1801. [Nat'l. Starch] Corn starch NF; CAS 9005-25-8; EINECS 232-679-6; binder, filler, and disintegrant in cosmetic and pharmaceutical formulations incl. body powds., foot powds., dry shampoos, makeup, eye liner, mascara; wh. powd.; 12% volatiles.

28-1898. [Nat'l. Starch] Distarch phosphate; CAS 55963-33-2; crosslinked corn starch that will not swell in water; adsorber for oils; for body powds., makeup, eye liner, mascara, dry shampoo; wh. powd.; insol. in water and org. solvs.; 12% volatiles.

Tylorol 2S, 2S/25. [Triantaphyllou] Sodium laureth (2) sulfate; anionic; detergent base for personal care prods.; liq.; 28 and 25% conc. resp.

Tylorol 3S. [Triantaphyllou] Sodium laureth (3) sulfate; anionic; detergent base for liq. shampoos and foam baths; liq.; 28% conc.

Tylorol A. [Triantaphyllou] Ammonium lauryl ether (2) sulfate; CAS 32612-48-9; anionic; detergent base for personal care prods.; liq.; 24% conc.

Tylorol BS. [Triantaphyllou] Sodium lauryl ether (2) sulfate; anionic; detergent base for pearly shampoos; liq.; 22% conc.

Tylorol LM. [Triantaphyllou] MEA lauryl ether (1) sulfate; anionic; detergent base for liq. shampoos; liq.; 30% conc.

Tylorol LT50. [Triantaphyllou] TEA lauryl ether (1) sulfate; CAS 27028-82-6; anionic; detergent base for liq. shampoos; liq.; 42% conc.

Tylorol MG. [Triantaphyllou] Magnesium lauryl ether (3) sulfate; CAS 62755-21-9; anionic; detergent base for the cosmetic industry; liq.; 30% conc.

Tylorol S. [Triantaphyllou] Sodium lauryl ether (1) sulfate; anionic; detergent base for shampoos, foam baths; liq.; 25% conc.

Tylose® C, CB Series. [Hoechst Celanese/Colorants & Surf.] Sodium CMC; CAS 9004-32-4; anionic; binder in pencil leads; thickener in batteries, rubber industry, cosmetics, foodstuffs, pharmaceuticals, tobacco and textile industry; dispersant, emulsifier for insecticidal, fungicidal and herbicidal prods.; plasticizer in ceramics; surface sizing in paper industry; press aid and lubricant in welding electrodes; gran., powd.; 100% act.

Tylose® C-p, CB-p. [Hoechst Celanese/Colorants & Surf.] Cellulose gum; CAS 9004-32-4; cosmetic thickener; powd.

Tylose® H Series. [Hoechst Celanese/Colorants & Surf.; Hoechst AG] Hydroxyethylcellulose; CAS 9004-62-0; nonionic; binder, thickener, plasticizer, visc. control agent, protective colloid in ceramics, emulsion polymerization, tobacco and textile industry, agric., cosmetics, soaps, and hand cleaning pastes; gran.; water-sol.; 100% act.

Tylose® H-p. [Hoechst Celanese/Colorants & Surf.] Hydroxyethyl cellulose; CAS 9004-62-0; cosmetic thickener; powd.

Tylose® H-yp. [Hoechst Celanese/Colorants & Surf.] Hydroxyethyl cellulose; CAS 9004-62-0; cosmetic thickener; powd.

Tylose® MH Grades. [Hoechst Celanese/Colorants & Surf.; Hoechst AG] Methyl hydroxyethylcellulose; CAS 9032-42-2; nonionic; binder, thickener, pigment, foam, and filler stabilizer, dispersant, emulsifier, plasticizer, visc. control and sedimenting aid, and protective colloid used in coatings, paints, resins, mining, batteries, insecticides, fungicides, herbicides; rubber, textile, and leather industry; ceramics, suspension polymerization, and pharmaceuticals; gran.; water-sol.; 100% act.

Tylose® MHB. [Hoechst Celanese/Colorants & Surf.] Methyl hydroxyethylcellulose; CAS 9032-42-2; nonionic; binder, thickener, pigment, foam, and filler stabilizer, dispersant, emulsifier, plasticizer, visc. control and sedimenting aid, and protective colloid used in coatings, paints, resins, mining, batteries, insecticides, fungicides, herbicides; rubber, textile, and leather industry; ceramics, suspension polymerization, and pharmaceuticals; gran.; water-sol.

Tylose® MH-p, MHB-p. [Hoechst Celanese/Colorants & Surf.] Methylhydroxyethyl cellulose; CAS 9032-42-2; cosmetic thickener; powd.

Tyr-Ol. [Sederma] Tan accelerator providing anti-free radical activity and photoprotection.

Tyrosilane. [Exsymol] Methylsilanol acetyltyrosine.

Tyrosilane C. [Exsymol; Biosil Tech.] Copper acetyl tyrosinate methylsilanol; tanning activator and anti-aging action for cosmetic and health prods.; lt. brn. limpid liq.; misc. with water, alcohols, glycols; sp.gr. 1.0; pH 5.5; usage level: 3.5-4.5%; toxicology: nontoxic.

U

Uantox 3. [Universal Preserv-A-Chem] Propylene glycol, BHA, propyl gallate, citric acid; preservative and antioxidant.

Uantox 20. [Universal Preserv-A-Chem] Propylene glycol, t-butyl hydroquinone, citric acid; cosmetic ingred.

Uantox 1250. [Universal Preserv-A-Chem] Natural vitamin E acetate; CAS 7695-91-2; EINECS 231-710-0; cosmetic ingred.

Uantox ASCA. [Universal Preserv-A-Chem] Ascorbic acid; CAS 50-81-7; EINECS 200-066-2; acidulant for cosmetic applics.

Uantox BHA. [Universal Preserv-A-Chem] BHA; CAS 25013-16-5; EINECS 246-563-8; antioxidant.

Uantox BHT. [Universal Preserv-A-Chem] BHT; CAS 128-37-0; EINECS 204-881-4; cosmetic ingred.

Uantox EBATE. [Universal Preserv-A-Chem] Erythorbic acid; CAS 89-65-6; EINECS 201-928-0; antioxidant.

Uantox HQ. [Universal Preserv-A-Chem] Hydroquinone; CAS 123-31-9; EINECS 204-617-8; cosmetics ingred.

Uantox HW-4. [Universal Preserv-A-Chem] Corn oil, BHA, BHT; cosmetic ingred.

Uantox PG. [Universal Preserv-A-Chem] Propyl gallate; CAS 121-79-9; EINECS 204-498-2; cosmetic antioxidant.

Uantox PMBS. [Universal Preserv-A-Chem] Potassium metabisulfite; CAS 16731-55-8; EINECS 240-795-3; antiseptic, bleaching agent.

Uantox POMEBIS. [Universal Preserv-A-Chem] Potassium metabisulfite; CAS 16731-55-8; EINECS 240-795-3; antiseptic, bleaching agent.

Uantox ROSM. [Universal Preserv-A-Chem] Rosemary extract; botanical extract.

Uantox SBS. [Universal Preserv-A-Chem] Sodium bisulfite; CAS 7631-90-5; EINECS 231-548-0; cosmetic ingred.

Uantox SEBATE. [Universal Preserv-A-Chem] Sodium erythorbate; CAS 6381-77-7; EINECS 228-973-9; antioxidant, preservative.

Uantox SMBS. [Universal Preserv-A-Chem] Sodium metabisulfite; CAS 7681-57-4; EINECS 231-673-0; preservative.

Uantox SODASC. [Universal Preserv-A-Chem] Sodium ascorbate; CAS 134-03-2; EINECS 205-126-1; cosmetic ingred.

Uantox SODERT. [Universal Preserv-A-Chem] Sodium erythorbate; CAS 6381-77-7; EINECS 228-973-9; antioxidant, preservative.

Uantox TBHQ. [Universal Preserv-A-Chem] t-Butyl hydroquinone; CAS 1948-33-0; EINECS 217-752-2; cosmetic antioxidant and stabilizer.

Uantox W-1. [Universal Preserv-A-Chem] Corn oil, glyceryl oleate, propylene glyco, BHA, BHT, t-butyl hydroquinone, citric acid; cosmetic ingred.

U Blue 104. [Presperse] Ultramarine blue (90%), bismuth-oxychloride (10%); CAS 1317-97-1, 7787-59-9; inorg. colorant for pigmented cosmetics; JSCI/JCID approved.

Ucarcide® 225. [Union Carbide] Glutaral; CAS 111-30-8; EINECS 203-856-5; broad-spectrum preservative, antimicrobial for cosmetic, toiletry, and chemical specialty prods.; effective against bacteria, fungi, and yeast over wide pH range; EPA registered, EC listed; Pt-Co 100 max. color; sol. in water; sp.gr. 1.064; dens. 8.87 lb/gal; visc. 3.2 cps; b.p. 100.5 C (760 mm Hg); f.p. -10 C; flash pt. (TCC) none; ref. index 1.375; pH 3.1-4.5; surf. tens. 48 dynes/cm; usage level: 0.04-0.40%; toxicology: causes mild to moderate skin irritation, severe eye damage at full strength; 25% act. min.

Ucarcide® 250. [Union Carbide] Glutaral; CAS 111-30-8; EINECS 203-856-5; broad-spectrum preservative, antimicrobial for cosmetic, toiletry, and chemical specialty prods.; effective against bacteria, fungi, and yeast over wide pH range; EPA registered, EC listed; Pt-Co 100 max. color; sol. in water; sp.gr. 1.129; dens. 9.41 lb/gal; visc. 21 cps; b.p. 101.5 C (760 mm Hg); f.p. -21 C; flash pt. (TCC) none; ref. index 1.421; pH 3.1-4.4; surf. tens. 47 dynes/cm; corrosive; usage level: 0.02-0.2%; toxicology: causes skin burns, severe eye damage at full strength; 50% act. min.

Ucare® Polymer JR-30M, JR-125, JR-400. [Amerchol] Polyquaternium-10; cationic; conditioner, hair fixative; contributes substantivity, visc., barrier and anti-irritant props. for cosmetics, toiletries, hair and skin care prods.; suppresses allergic response to poison ivy dermatitis, skin dryness in depilatories; sol. in water; visc. 1000-2500, 75-175, and 300-500 cps resp.

Ucare® Polymer LK. [Amerchol] Polyquaternium-10; water-sol. polymer for cosmetic applications; wh. powd., sl. amine odor; visc. 300-500 cps.

Ucare® Polymer LR 30M, LR 400. [Amerchol] Polyquaternium-10; water-sol. polymer for cosmetic applications; visc. 1000-2500 cps and 300-500 cps resp.

Ucare® Polymer SR-10. [Amerchol] Polyquaternium-10; water-sol. polymer for cosmetic applications; wh. powd., sl. amine odor; 95% min. thru 20 mesh; visc. 8000-12,000 cps (2% aq.).

Ucon® 50-HB-55. [Union Carbide] PPG-2-buteth-3; emollient, lubricant; for applics. where fluid is to be removed by a water rinse; sol. in water, alcohol.

Ucon® 50-HB-100. [Union Carbide] PPG-3-buteth-5; emollient, lubricant.

Ucon® 50-HB-170. [Union Carbide] PPG-5-buteth-7; emollient, lubricant.

Ucon® 50-HB-260. [Union Carbide] PPG-7-buteth-10; emollient, lubricant.

Ucon® 50-HB-400. [Amerchol] PPG-9-buteth-12; emollient; clear liq., char. odor; visc. 380-420 SUS (100 F); pH 5.5-7.5 (10% aq.).

Ucon® 50-HB-660. [Amerchol] PPG-12-buteth-16; emollient; clear liq., low char. odor; visc. 630-690 SUS (100 F); pH 5.5-7.5 (10% aq.).

Ucon® 50-HB-2000. [Union Carbide] PPG-20-buteth-30; emollient.

Ucon® 50-HB-3520. [Amerchol] PPG-28-buteth-35; emollient; clear liq., char. odor; visc. 3370-3670 SUS (100 F); pH 4.5-7.5 (10% aq.).

Ucon® 50-HB-5100. [Amerchol; Union Carbide] PPG-33-buteth-45; emollient; clear visc. liq., low char. odor; visc. 4850-5350 SUS (100 F); pH 5.5-7.5 (10% aq.).

Ucon® 75-H-450. [Amerchol] PEG/PPG-17/6 copolymer; CAS 9003-11-6; lubricant for antiperspirants; emollient, solv., bodying agent; clear to cloudy liq., mild char. odor; visc. 425-475 SUS (100 F); pH 5.5-7.5 (10% aq.).

Ucon® 75-H-1400. [Union Carbide] PEG/PPG-35/9 copolymer; CAS 9003-11-6; lubricant, emollient; for applics. where fluid is to be removed by a water rinse; sol. in water, alcohol; visc. in SUS @ 100 F corresponds to numerical value.

Ucon® 75-H-90000. [Union Carbide] PEG/PPG-125/30 copolymer; CAS 9003-11-6; lubricant.

Ucon® Fluid AP. [Amerchol] PPG-14 butyl ether; CAS 9003-13-8; lubricant for antiperspirants; emollient, solv., bodying agent; clear liq., char. odor; visc. 85-105 cps; acid no. 0.5 max.; flash pt. (COC) 400 F min.

Ucon® LB-65. [Union Carbide] PPG-5 butyl ether; CAS 9003-13-8; lubricant.

Ucon® LB-135. [Union Carbide] PPG-9 butyl ether; CAS 9003-13-8; lubricant.

Ucon® LB-285. [Union Carbide] PPG-15 butyl ether; CAS 9003-13-8; lubricant.

Ucon® LB-385. [Union Carbide] PPG-18 butyl ether; CAS 9003-13-8; emollient, lubricant; low color and odor; sol. in alcohol; insol. in water; visc. 385 SUS (100 F).

Ucon® LB-525. [Union Carbide] PPG-22 butyl ether; CAS 9003-13-8; lubricant.

Ucon® LB-625. [Union Carbide] PPG-24 butyl ether; CAS 9003-13-8; emollient, lubricant; cosolv. for most natural oils in aq. alcoholic compositions; low color and odor; sol. in alcohol; visc. 625 SUS (100 F).

Ucon® LB-1145. [Amerchol] PPG-33 butyl ether; CAS 9003-13-8; emollient; cosolv. for most natural oils in aq. alcoholic compositions; low color and odor; sol. in alcohol; visc. 1145 SUS (100 F).

Ucon® LB-1715. [Amerchol] PPG-40 butyl ether; CAS 9003-13-8; emollient; cosolv. for most natural oils in aq. alcoholic compositions; clear liq., low char. odor; sol. in alcohol; visc. 1630-1800 SUS (100 F); pH 5.0-8.5 (10% w/v).

Ucon® LB-3000. [Union Carbide] PPG-53 butyl ether; CAS 9003-13-8; emollient, lubricant; cosolv. for most natural oils in aq. alcoholic compositions; low color and odor; sol. in alcohol; visc. 3000 SUS (100 F).

U-Dagen DEO. [Universal Preserv-A-Chem] Triethyl citrate and BHT; cosmetic ingred.

Ufablend HS-70. [Unger Fabrikker AS] Lauryl ether sulfate, cocamide DEA blend, with bactericide; anionic/nonionic; biodeg. conc. for clear shampoos, bath preps.; lt. yel. paste; pH 6.5-7.0 (15%); 70% act.

Ufablend MPL. [Unger Fabrikker AS] Sodium laureth sulfate, nacreous agent, cocamide DEA blend; anionic; biodeg. pearlized conc. and pearlizing agent for shampoos, bath preps., hand cleaning soaps; wh. pearlized paste; pH 6.5-7.0 (1%); 30% act.

Ufanon K-80. [Unger Fabrikker AS] Cocamide DEA (2:1); CAS 61791-31-9; EINECS 263-163-9; nonionic; biodeg. detergent, foaming agent, wetting agent, thickener, foam stabilizer for liq. detergents, shampoos, cosmetics, leather industry; confers some corrosion protection; brn. visc. liq., char. amine odor; pH 9-10 (1%); 48-56% conc.

Ufanon KD-S. [Unger Fabrikker AS] Cocamide DEA (1:1); CAS 61791-31-9; EINECS 263-163-9; nonionic; biodeg. visc. modifier, foam booster/stabilizer for liq. detergents,

shampoos, cosmetics, leather industry; pale yel. liq.; sp.gr. 0.997; sapon. no. 150; cloud pt. -11 C; pH 9.5-10.0 (1%); usage level: 1-10%; 90% conc.

Ufarol Am 30. [Unger Fabrikker AS] Ammonium lauryl sulfate; CAS 2235-54-3; EINECS 218-793-9; anionic; biodeg. detergent, wetting and foaming agent for shampoos, bath prods., general-purpose detergents, laundry cleaners, carpet shampoos, furniture cleaning, textiles, leather, paints; stable in hard water and alkali, moderately stable in acids; pale yel. liq.; m.w. 289-295; visc. 2000 ± 1000 cp; pH 6-7 (10%); 28-30% act.

Ufarol Am 70. [Unger Fabrikker AS] Ammonium lauryl sulfate; CAS 2235-54-3; EINECS 218-793-9; anionic; biodeg. detergent, wetting and foaming agent for shampoos, bath prods., general-purpose detergents, laundry cleaners, carpet shampoos, furniture cleaning, textiles, leather, paints; stable in hard water and alkali, moderately stable in acids; water-wh. paste; m.w. 289-295; pH 6-7 (10%); 68-72% act.

Ufarol Na-30. [Unger Fabrikker AS] Sodium lauryl sulfate; CAS 151-21-3; EINECS 205-788-1; anionic; biodeg. detergent, wetting and foaming agent for shampoos, bath prods., general-purpose detergents, laundry cleaners, carpet shampoos, furniture cleaning, textiles, leather, paints; stable in hard water and alkali, moderately stable in acids; water-wh. to pale yel. liq.; m.w. 293-299; visc. < 200 cp; pH 7.5-9.0 (2%); 29-31% act.

Ufarol TA-40. [Unger Fabrikker AS] TEA lauryl sulfate; CAS 139-96-8; EINECS 205-388-7; anionic; biodeg. surfactant for shampoos, bath prods., carpet shampoos, furniture cleaning, laundry, textiles; mild to hair and scalp; water-wh. to pale yel. liq.; m.w. 412-418; visc. 100 cps; cloud pt. 0 C; pH 6.5-7.5 (1%); 39-41% act.

Ufasan 35. [Unger Fabrikker AS] Linear sodium dodecylbenzene sulfonate; CAS 25155-30-0; EINECS 246-680-4; anionic; biodeg. detergent, wetting agent, foaming agent for liq. detergents, dishwash, hair and car shampoos and in plastics, metal, agric., polish, textiles, mining, oil and cement industries; stable in hard water and acids; golden visc. liq., weak char. odor; m.w. 343-345; cloud pt. -7 C; pH 7.5-8.5; 34–36% act.

UFZO. [U.S. Cosmetics] Ultra-fine zinc oxide; CAS 1314-13-2; EINECS 215-222-5; physical uv blocking agent for cosmetic applics.; provides greatly reduced skin whitening, better anti-inflammatory props. than normal zinc oxide; submicron (0.005-0.020 µ).

Uhydagen B. [Universal Preserv-A-Chem] α-Bisabolol; CAS 515-69-5; EINECS 208-205-9; cosmetic ingred.

Ultra® . [Mearl] Bismuth-based; highly lustrous pearl pigments avail. in nitrocellulose paste dispersions for use in frosted nail enamels.

Ultrafine Lanolin. See *Anhydrous Lanolin USP Ultrafine*

Ultrafino. [Luzenac Am.] Talc USP/FCC; CAS 14807-96-6; EINECS 238-877-9; highly refined, extra-fine talc with exc. slip and lustrous, translucent appearance; recommended for fine cosmetics, formulations with sensitive fragrances and pigments, eye shadows, antiperpsirants, nail polish, pressed powds., and aerosols; powd.; 99.96% thru 325 mesh; median diam. 4 µ; tapped dens. 35 lb/ft³; pH 9 (10% slurry).

Ultraflex® . [Petrolite] Microcryst. wax; CAS 63231-60-7; EINECS 264-038-1; plastic wax offering high ductility, flexibility at very low temps., provides protective barrier properties against moisture vapor and gases; uses incl. hot-melt laminating adhesives for papers, films, and foils; hot-melt coatings; in antisunchecking agents in rubber goods, elec. insulating agents, leather treating agents, water repellents for textiles, rustproof coatings, cosmetic ingreds., and as plasticizer for waxes used in crayons, dental compds., chewing gum base, candles; incl. FDA

§172.230, 172.615, 175.105, 175.300, 176.170, 176.180, 176.200, 177.1200, 178.3710, 179.45; amber wax; also avail. in wh.; dens. 0.93 g/cc; visc. 13 cps (99 C); m.p. 69 C; flash pt. 293 C.

Ultrahold® 8. [BASF; BASF AG] Acrylates/acrylamide copolymer; hair spray resin with outstanding hold and humidity resistance; hair fixative; film-former; powd.

Ultra Sil™. [U.S. Cosmetics] Adsorbed silicone surface treatment; surface treatment which bonds to the surface of cosmetic raw materials such as talc, mica, sericite, and pigments and provides creamy, elegant, tactile, wet, smooth feel, exc. adhesion, longer wearabilty, strong hydrophobicity; suggested for liq. makeup, mascaras, other aq. systems.

Umordant P. [Cosmetochem] A moisturizing complex similar to the natural moisturizing factor with added plant extracts; free of animal derivs.; cosmetic specialty.

Umulse-E. [Universal Preserv-A-Chem] Sorbitan sesquioleate, beeswax, aluminum stearate; cosmetic ingred.

Unamide® C-5. [Lonza] PEG-6 cocamide; CAS 61791-08-0; nonionic; foam stabilizer, visc. builder, emulsifier for shampoos, lt. and heavy-duty detergents; stable over broad pH range; lt. yel. liq.; sapon. no. 12 max.; pH 9–10 (5%); 100% act.

Unamide® C-72-3. [Lonza] Cocamide DEA (2:1); CAS 61791-31-9; EINECS 263-163-9; nonionic; visc. builder, foam stabilizer; used for lt. duty liqs., industrial, household hard surface cleaners, surfactant, emulsifier, corrosion inhibitor, lubricant and personal care prods.; amber liq.; acid no. 0–10; pH 9–10.5 (5%); 100% act.

Unamide® D-10. [Lonza] 2:1 Coco DEA, modified; CAS 61791-31-9; EINECS 263-163-9; nonionic; detergent, visc. builder, foam stabilizer; used for lt. duty liqs., industrial, household hard surface cleaners, surfactant, emulsifier, corrosion inhibitor, lubricant and personal care prods.; 100% biodeg.; dk. amber liq.; sp.gr. 1.00; dens. 8.34 lb/gal; acid no. 55-75; pH 8.5-9.5 (1%); 100% act.

Unamide® LDL. [Lonza] Cocamide DEA (1:1); CAS 61791-31-9; EINECS 263-163-9; nonionic; visc. builder, foam stabilizer, surfactant, emulsifier, corrosion inhibitor, lubricant; used for lt. duty liqs., industrial/household hard surface cleaners, dishwash, fine fabric detergent, mild liq. hand soap; 100% biodeg; lt. straw liq.; sp.gr. 0.98; dens. 8.2 lb/gal; acid no. 9-10.5; pH 9-10 (1%); 100% act.

Unamine-MORP. [Universal Preserv-A-Chem] Morpholine; CAS 110-91-8; EINECS 203-815-1; cosmetic ingred.

Unamino GLCN. [Universal Preserv-A-Chem] Glycine; CAS 56-40-6; EINECS 200-272-2; cosmetic ingred.

Unamino GLUT. [Universal Preserv-A-Chem] L-Glutamic acid; CAS 56-86-0; EINECS 200-293-7; flavor enhancer, medicine/biochemical research.

Unamino L-CSTE. [Universal Preserv-A-Chem] L-Cysteine; CAS 52-90-4; EINECS 200-158-2; biochemical and nutritive component.

Unamino L-CSTI. [Universal Preserv-A-Chem] L-Cystine; CAS 56-89-3; EINECS 200-296-3; biochemical and nutritive component.

Unatox. [Universal Preserv-A-Chem] Tocopherol; antioxidant, vitamin E source.

Undamide. [Vevy] Undecylenamide DEA; CAS 60239-68-1; EINECS 246-914-5; personal care surfactant.

Undebenzofene. [Vevy] Phenoxyethylparaben and undecylenoyl PEG-5 paraben; cosmetic preservative.

Undebenzofene C. [Vevy] Phenoxyethanol, methylparaben, ethylparaben, propylparaben, and butylparaben; cosmetic preservative system; USA, Japan (JCID/JSCI), and Europe approvals; usage level: up to 1.5%.

Undelene. [Vevy] PEG-6 undecylenate.

Undenat. [Vevy] Sodium undecylenate; CAS 3398-33-2; EINECS 222-264-8; cosmetics preservative; USA and Europe approvals; usage level: up to 0.2% as acid.

Undezin. [Vevy] Zinc undecylenate; CAS 557-08-4; EINECS 209-155-0; fungistat.

Unette-O. [Universal Preserv-A-Chem] Cetearyl alcohol; cosmetic ingred.

Unette-W. [Universal Preserv-A-Chem] Cetearyl alcohol, sodium laureth sulfate; cosmetic ingred.

Unger EST. [Unger Fabrikker AS] Partially sulfated fatty alcohols; anionic; softener and superfatting agent for fibers, skin and hair care prods. (shampoos, bath foams, hand soap); skin protectant; reduces excessive degreasing; light paste; disp. in water; usage level: 0.5-1.5%.

Ungerol AM3-60. [Unger Fabrikker AS] Ammonium lauryl ether sulfate (3 EO); CAS 32612-48-9; anionic; for liq. detergents, shampoos; paste; 58–62% conc.

Ungerol AM3-75. [Unger Fabrikker AS] Ammonium lauryl ether (3 EO) sulfate; CAS 32612-48-9; anionic; biodeg. detergent, wetting and foaming agent, emulsifier used in liq. detergents, car shampoos, bath foams; stable in hard water, moderately stable in acids; pale straw soft paste; m.w. 440-450; sp.gr. 1.05; flash pt. (Abel Pensky) 42 C; pH 7-9 (1%); 72-75% act.

Ungerol LES 2-28. [Unger Fabrikker AS] Sodium laureth sulfate (2 EO); CAS 9004-82-4; anionic; biodeg. detergent, wetting and foaming agent, emulsifier for liq. detergents, shampoos, bath prods., wallboard mfg., textiles, drilling aux.; exc. stability in hard water, alkalis; moderately stable in acids; colorless liq.; m.w. 379-389; visc. 300-600 cps; cloud pt. 0 C; pH 7-8 (1%); 26-28% act.

Ungerol LES 2-70. [Unger Fabrikker AS] Sodium laureth sulfate (2 EO); CAS 9004-82-4; anionic; biodeg. detergent, wetting and foaming agent, emulsifier for liq. detergents, shampoos, bath prods., wallboard mfg., textiles, drilling aux.; exc. stability in hard water, alkalis; moderately stable in acids; pale straw pumpable paste; m.w. 379-389; pH 7-9 (1%); 68-72% act.

Ungerol LES 3-28. [Unger Fabrikker AS] Sodium laureth sulfate (3 EO); CAS 9004-82-4; anionic; biodeg. detergent, wetting and foaming agent, emulsifier for liq. detergents, shampoos, bath prods., wallboard mfg., textiles, drilling aux.; exc. stability in hard water, alkalis; moderately stable in acids; colorless liq.; m.w. 445-455; sp.gr. 1.02; visc. 500-800 cps; pH 7.0-8.5 (1%); 26-28% act.

Ungerol LES 3-70. [Unger Fabrikker AS] Sodium laureth sulfate (3 EO); CAS 9004-82-4; anionic; biodeg. detergent, wetting and foaming agent, emulsifier for liq. detergents, shampoos, bath prods., wallboard mfg., textiles, drilling aux.; exc. stability in hard water, alkalis; moderately stable in acids; pale straw pumpable paste; m.w. 445-455; sp.gr. 1.05; visc. 40,000 cps; pH 7-9 (1%); 68-72% act.

Ungerol N2-28. [Unger Fabrikker AS] Sodium laureth sulfate (2 EO); CAS 9004-82-4; anionic; biodeg. detergent, wetting and foaming agent, emulsifier for liq. detergents, shampoos, bath prods., wallboard mfg., textiles, drilling aux.; exc. stability in hard water, alkalis; moderately stable in acids; colorless to pale straw liq.; m.w. 377-387; sp.gr. 1.02; visc. 200 cps max.; cloud pt. 0 C; pH 7-8 (1%); 27-29% act.

Ungerol N2-70. [Unger Fabrikker AS] Sodium laureth sulfate (2 EO); CAS 9004-82-4; anionic; biodeg. detergent, wetting and foaming agent, emulsifier for liq. detergents, shampoos, bath prods., wallboard mfg., textiles, drilling aux.; exc. stability in hard water, alkalis; moderately stable in acids; pale straw paste; m.w. 377-387; sp.gr. 1.05; pH 7-9 (1%); 68-72% act.

Ungerol N3-28. [Unger Fabrikker AS] Sodium laureth sulfate (3 EO); CAS 9004-82-4; anionic; biodeg. detergent, wetting and foaming agent, emulsifier for liq. detergents, shampoos, bath prods., wallboard mfg., textiles, drilling aux.; exc. stability in hard water, alkalis; moderately stable in acids; colorless liq.; m.w. 420-430; sp.gr. 1.02; visc. 150 cps; pH 7-8 (1%); 27-29% act.

Ungerol N3-70. [Unger Fabrikker AS] Sodium laureth sulfate (3 EO); CAS 9004-82-4; anionic; biodeg. detergent, wetting and foaming agent, emulsifier for liq. detergents, shampoos, bath prods., wallboard mfg., textiles, drilling aux.; exc. stability in hard water, alkalis; moderately stable in acids; pale straw pumpable paste; m.w. 420-430; sp.gr. 1.05; visc. 40,000 cps; pH 7-9 (1%); 68-72% act.

Unibetaine 2C. [Universal Preserv-A-Chem] Disodium coco-amphodiacetate; CAS 68650-39-5; EINECS 272-043-5; cosmetic surfactant.

Unibetaine 160. [Universal Preserv-A-Chem] Sodium lauriminodipropionate; CAS 14960-06-6; EINECS 239-032-7; personal care surfactant.

Unibetaine 160C. [Universal Preserv-A-Chem] Disodium cocoamphodipropionate; cosmetic surfactant.

Unibetaine AB-30, AB-45. [Universal Preserv-A-Chem] Coco-betaine; CAS 68424-94-2; EINECS 270-329-4; cosmetic surfactant.

Unibetaine BA-35, BC-35. [Universal Preserv-A-Chem] Cocamidopropyl betaine; cosmetic ingred.

Unibetaine CDC. [Universal Preserv-A-Chem] Sodium co-coamphoacetate; personal care surfactant.

Unibetaine G-20. [Universal Preserv-A-Chem] Sodium lauroamphoacetate; personal care surfactant.

Unibetaine GC-88. [Universal Preserv-A-Chem] Sodium cocoamphoacetate; personal care surfactant.

Unibetaine K. [Universal Preserv-A-Chem] Cocamidopropyl betaine; cosmetic ingred.

Unibetaine LB. [Universal Preserv-A-Chem] Lauryl betaine; CAS 683-10-3; EINECS 211-669-5; detergent.

Unibetaine OLB-30, OLB-50. [Universal Preserv-A-Chem] Oleyl betaine; CAS 871-37-4; EINECS 212-806-1; emollient, surfactant.

Unibiovit B-33. [Induchem AG] Decyl oleate, farnesol, ethyl linoleate, farnesyl acetate; a bioactive complex for moisturizing and smoothing the skin.

Unibiovit B-332. [Induchem AG] PEG-12 glyceryl laurate, PEG-36 castor oil, farnesol, ethyl linoleate, farnesyl acetate; water-sol. bioactive complex for moisturizing and smoothing the skin.

Unibotan Arnica CLR. [Universal Preserv-A-Chem] Arnica extract; CAS 8057-65-6; botanical extract.

Unibotan CLR. [Universal Preserv-A-Chem] Botanical extracts.

Unibotan Calendula CLR. [Universal Preserv-A-Chem] Calendula extract; CAS 84776-23-8; botanical extract.

Unibotan Carrot Oil CLR. [Universal Preserv-A-Chem] Carrot oil; CAS 8015-88-1; botanical extract.

Unibotan Chamomile. [Universal Preserv-A-Chem] Chamomile extract; CAS 84649-86-5; botanical extract.

Unibotan Haircomplex Aquosum. [Universal Preserv-A-Chem] Hair complex aquosum; hair care prods.

Unibotan Hexaplant CLR. [Universal Preserv-A-Chem] Hexaplant; botanical extract.

Unibotan Sedaplant CLR. [Universal Preserv-A-Chem] Sedaplant-H; cosmetic ingred.

Unibotan SOLUVIT CLR. [Universal Preserv-A-Chem] Soluvit; botanical extract.

Unibotan St. Johns Wort Oil. [Universal Preserv-A-Chem] St. John's wort oil; botanical extract.

Unibotan Vitaplant O CLR. [Universal Preserv-A-Chem] Sesame oil, soybean oil, pigskin extract, calendula extract, tocopherol; cosmetic ingred.; oil-sol.

Unibotan Vitaplant W CLR. [Universal Preserv-A-Chem] Water, alcohol, coneflower extract, and aloe extract; botanical extract; water-sol.

Unibotan Witch Hazel. [Universal Preserv-A-Chem] Witch

hazel extract; botanical extract.

Unicaine-B. [Universal Preserv-A-Chem] Benzocaine; CAS 51-05-8; local anesthetic in medicine and suntan preps.

Unicast CO. [Universal Preserv-A-Chem] Castor oil; CAS 8001-79-4; EINECS 232-293-8; emollient.

Unichem 1-3 BUT-G. [Universal Preserv-A-Chem] 1,3-Butylene glycol; cosmetic ingred.

Unichem ACETA. [Universal Preserv-A-Chem] Acetic acid; CAS 64-19-7; EINECS 200-580-7; intermediate for mfg. of pharmaceuticals, plastics, dyes, insecticides, photographic chemicals, food additives.

Unichem ALSUL. [Universal Preserv-A-Chem] Aluminum sulfate; CAS 10043-01-3; EINECS 233-135-0; cosmetic ingred.

Unichem AMAL. [Universal Preserv-A-Chem] Ammonium alum; CAS 7784-25-0; EINECS 232-055-3; cosmetic ingred.

Unichem AMST. [Universal Preserv-A-Chem] Ammonium stearate; CAS 1002-89-7; EINECS 213-695-2; vanishing creams, brushless shaving creams, other cosmetic prods.

Unichem BICARB-S. [Universal Preserv-A-Chem] Sodium bicarbonate; CAS 144-55-8; EINECS 205-633-8; cosmetic ingred.

Unichem BUTSTE. [Universal Preserv-A-Chem] Butyl stearate; CAS 123-95-5; EINECS 204-666-5; emollient.

Unichem BZAL. [Universal Preserv-A-Chem] Benzyl alcohol; CAS 100-51-6; EINECS 202-859-9; used for perfumes, flavors, cosmetics; intermediate.

Unichem BZBN. [Universal Preserv-A-Chem] Benzyl benzoate; CAS 120-51-4; EINECS 204-402-9; fixative and solvent for musk in perfumes and flavors; external medicine.

Unichem CA HYD. [Universal Preserv-A-Chem] Calcium hydroxide; CAS 1305-62-0; EINECS 215-137-3; cosmetic ingred.

Unichem CALAC. [Universal Preserv-A-Chem] Calcium lactate; cosmetic ingred.

Unichem CALCARB. [Universal Preserv-A-Chem] Calcium carbonate; CAS 471-34-1; EINECS 207-439-9; cosmetic ingred.

Unichem CALCHLOR. [Universal Preserv-A-Chem] Calcium chloride; CAS 10043-52-4; EINECS 233-140-8; cosmetic ingred.

Unichem CAMP. [Universal Preserv-A-Chem] Camphor; CAS 76-22-2; EINECS 207-355-2; cosmetic ingred.

Unichem CAO. [Universal Preserv-A-Chem] Calcium oxide; CAS 1305-78-8; EINECS 215-138-9; cosmetic ingred.

Unichem CIT-A. [Universal Preserv-A-Chem] Citric acid; CAS 77-92-9; EINECS 201-069-1; cosmetic ingred.

Unichem CS. [Universal Preserv-A-Chem] Calcium stearate; CAS 1592-23-0; EINECS 216-472-8; cosmetic ingred.

Unichem CS White. [Universal Preserv-A-Chem] Calcium sulfate; CAS 7778-18-9; EINECS 231-900-3; cosmetic ingred.

Unichem DEA. [Universal Preserv-A-Chem] Diethanolamine; CAS 111-42-2; EINECS 203-868-0; used in surfactants, cosmetics/toiletries.

Unichem DEG. [Universal Preserv-A-Chem] Diethylene glycol; CAS 111-46-6; EINECS 203-872-2; cosmetic ingred.

Unichem DIPA. [Universal Preserv-A-Chem] Diisopropanolamine; CAS 110-97-4; EINECS 203-820-9; cosmetic ingred.

Unichem DPG. [Universal Preserv-A-Chem] Dipropylene glycol; cosmetic ingred.

Unichem EPSAL. [Universal Preserv-A-Chem] Magnesium sulfate heptahydrate; CAS 7487-88-9; EINECS 231-298-2; used in cosmetic lotions.

Unichem GLYC. [Universal Preserv-A-Chem] Glycerin; CAS

56-81-5; cosmetic ingred.

Unichem GUADIC. [Universal Preserv-A-Chem] Guanidine carbonate; cosmetic ingred.

Unichem KCL. [Universal Preserv-A-Chem] Potassium chloride; CAS 7447-40-7; EINECS 231-211-8; cosmetic ingred.

Unichem KI. [Universal Preserv-A-Chem] Potassium iodide; CAS 7681-11-0; EINECS 231-659-4; cosmetic ingred.

Unichem KIO3. [Universal Preserv-A-Chem] Potassium iodate; CAS 7758-05-6; EINECS 231-831-9; topical antiseptic.

Unichem KOHYD. [Universal Preserv-A-Chem] Potassium hydroxide; CAS 1310-58-3; EINECS 215-181-3; used for soap mfg.

Unichem LACA. [Universal Preserv-A-Chem] Lactic acid; CAS 50-21-5; EINECS 200-018-0; humectant.

Unichem Levula. [Universal Preserv-A-Chem] Levulinic acid; CAS 123-76-2; EINECS 204-649-2; pharmaceutical intermediate.

Unichem MC. [Universal Preserv-A-Chem] Magnesium carbonate; CAS 546-93-0; EINECS 208-915-9; used in pharmaceuticals, dentifrices, cosmetics.

Unichem METSAL. [Universal Preserv-A-Chem] Methyl salicylate; CAS 119-36-8; EINECS 204-317-7; uv absorber.

Unichem MGC. [Universal Preserv-A-Chem] Magnesium carbonate; CAS 546-93-0; EINECS 208-915-9; used in pharmaceuticals, dentifrices, cosmetics.

Unichem MGS. [Universal Preserv-A-Chem] Magnesium stearate; CAS 557-04-0; EINECS 209-150-3; personal care emulsifier.

Unichem MS. [Universal Preserv-A-Chem] Magnesium stearate; CAS 557-04-0; EINECS 209-150-3; personal care emulsifier.

Unichem PBA. [Universal Preserv-A-Chem] Lead acetate; CAS 301-04-2; EINECS 206-104-4; cosmetic ingred.

Unichem POCARB. [Universal Preserv-A-Chem] Potassium carbonate; CAS 584-08-7; EINECS 209-529-3; cosmetic ingred.

Unichem POCHLOR. [Universal Preserv-A-Chem] Potassium chloride; CAS 7447-40-7; EINECS 231-211-8; cosmetic ingred.

Unichem PROP-G. [Universal Preserv-A-Chem] Propylene glycol; CAS 57-55-6; EINECS 200-338-0; cosmetic ingred.

Unichem ROSAL. [Universal Preserv-A-Chem] Potassium sodium tartrate; CAS 6381-59-5; EINECS 206-156-8; cosmetic ingred.

Unichem RSC. [Universal Preserv-A-Chem] Resorcinol; CAS 108-46-3; EINECS 203-585-2; cosmetic ingred.

Unichem SALAC. [Universal Preserv-A-Chem] Salicylic acid; CAS 69-72-7; EINECS 200-712-3; preservative.

Unichem SOBOR. [Universal Preserv-A-Chem] Borax; CAS 1303-96-4; cosmetic ingred.

Unichem SODAC. [Universal Preserv-A-Chem] Sodium acetate; CAS 127-09-3; EINECS 204-823-8; dye intermediate, pharmaceuticals, soaps.

Unichem SODCIT. [Universal Preserv-A-Chem] Sodium citrate; CAS 68-04-2; EINECS 200-675-3; pH adjustor for cosmetic prods.

Unichem SODIOD. [Universal Preserv-A-Chem] Sodium iodate; CAS 7681-55-2; EINECS 231-672-5; antiseptic, disinfectant.

Unichem SOHYD. [Universal Preserv-A-Chem] Sodium hydroxide; CAS 1310-73-2; EINECS 215-185-5; cosmetic ingred.

Unichem SOLAC. [Universal Preserv-A-Chem] Sodium lactate; CAS 72-17-3; EINECS 200-772-0; pH buffer, humectant, stabilizer.

Unichem SS. [Universal Preserv-A-Chem] Sodium stearate;

CAS 822-16-2; EINECS 212-490-5; gellant.

Unichem TANAC. [Universal Preserv-A-Chem] Tannic acid; CAS 1401-55-4; EINECS 215-753-2; cosmetic ingred.

Unichem TAR AC. [Universal Preserv-A-Chem] Tartaric acid; cosmetic ingred.

Unichem TEA. [Universal Preserv-A-Chem] Triethanolamine; CAS 102-71-6; EINECS 203-049-8; cosmetic ingred.

Unichem THYMOL. [Universal Preserv-A-Chem] Thymol; CAS 89-83-8; EINECS 201-944-8; antibacterial, perfumery, preservative, antioxidant.

Unichem TIPA. [Universal Preserv-A-Chem] Triisopropanolamine; CAS 122-20-3; EINECS 204-528-4; soap intermediate.

Unichem UREA. [Universal Preserv-A-Chem] Urea; CAS 57-13-6; EINECS 200-315-5; cosmetic ingred.

Unichem UREA-P. [Universal Preserv-A-Chem] Urea peroxide; CAS 124-43-6; EINECS 204-701-4; OTC active ingred.

Unichem ZO. [Universal Preserv-A-Chem] Zinc oxide; CAS 1314-13-2; EINECS 215-222-5; uv sunscreen.

Unichem ZPS. [Universal Preserv-A-Chem] Zinc phenolsulfonate; CAS 127-82-2; EINECS 204-867-8; antiseptic.

Unichem ZS. [Universal Preserv-A-Chem] Zinc stearate; CAS 557-05-1; EINECS 209-151-9; cosmetic ingred.

Unichol. [Universal Preserv-A-Chem] Cholesterol; CAS 57-88-5; EINECS 200-353-2; emulsifier, moisturizer.

Unichol EUM-L. [Universal Preserv-A-Chem] PPG-2 ceteareth-9; cosmetic ingred.

Unicide U-13. [Induchem AG; Lipo] Imidazolidinyl urea; CAS 39236-46-9; EINECS 254-372-6; biocide for cosmetics, toiletries, and pharmaceuticals, esp. for water phase; effective against Gram-negative bacteria; active over wide pH range; wh. powd., odorless; sol. in water, aq. alcohol; sl. sol. in pure alcohol; insol. in lipoids; m.p. 150 C dec.; pH 7 ± 0.5 (2% aq.); usage level: 0.2-0.4%; toxicology: nontoxic.

Unicol 12. [Universal Preserv-A-Chem] Trideceth-12; CAS 24938-91-8; personal care surfactant.

Unicol 15. [Universal Preserv-A-Chem] Trideceth-15; CAS 24938-91-8; personal care surfactant.

Unicol 50. [Universal Preserv-A-Chem] Benzalkonium chloride; cosmetic ingred.

Unicol 123. [Universal Preserv-A-Chem] Cetearyl alcohol, steareth-10; cosmetic ingred.

Unicol 1200. [Universal Preserv-A-Chem] PPG-20; CAS 25322-69-4; cosmetic ingred.

Unicol AETH-8. [Universal Preserv-A-Chem] PPG-5 laureth-5; superfatting agent.

Unicol CA-2. [Universal Preserv-A-Chem] Ceteth-2; CAS 9004-95-9; emulsifier.

Unicol CA-4. [Universal Preserv-A-Chem] Ceteth-4; CAS 9004-95-9; emulsifier.

Unicol CA-10. [Universal Preserv-A-Chem] Ceteth-10; CAS 9004-95-9; emulsifier.

Unicol CA-20. [Universal Preserv-A-Chem] Ceteth-20; CAS 9004-95-9; emulsifier.

Unicol CPS. [Universal Preserv-A-Chem] Cetearyl alcohol, PEG-150 stearate, steareth-20; cosmetic ingred.

Unicol CSA-2. [Universal Preserv-A-Chem] Ceteareth-2; CAS 68439-49-6; cosmetic ingred.

Unicol CSA-4. [Universal Preserv-A-Chem] Ceteareth-4; CAS 68439-49-6; cosmetic ingred.

Unicol CSA-5. [Universal Preserv-A-Chem] Ceteareth-5; CAS 68439-49-6; cosmetic ingred.

Unicol CSA-10. [Universal Preserv-A-Chem] Ceteareth-10; CAS 68439-49-6; cosmetic ingred.

Unicol CSA-15. [Universal Preserv-A-Chem] Ceteareth-15; CAS 68439-49-6; cosmetic ingred.

Unicol CSA-20. [Universal Preserv-A-Chem] Ceteareth-20; CAS 68439-49-6; cosmetic ingred.

Unicol CSA-30. [Universal Preserv-A-Chem] Ceteareth-30; CAS 68439-49-6; cosmetic ingred.

Unicol CSA-40. [Universal Preserv-A-Chem] Ceteareth-40; CAS 68439-49-6; cosmetic ingred.

Unicol LA-4. [Universal Preserv-A-Chem] Laureth-4; CAS 5274-68-0; EINECS 226-097-1; cosmetic ingred.

Unicol LA-9. [Universal Preserv-A-Chem] Laureth-9; CAS 3055-99-0; EINECS 221-284-4; personal care surfactant.

Unicol LA-23. [Universal Preserv-A-Chem] Laureth-23; CAS 9002-92-0; emulsifier.

Unicol NP-2. [Universal Preserv-A-Chem] Nonoxynol-2; EINECS 248-291-5; personal care surfactant.

Unicol NP-4. [Universal Preserv-A-Chem] Nonoxynol-4; CAS 9016-45-9; personal care surfactant.

Unicol NP-5. [Universal Preserv-A-Chem] Nonoxynol-5; CAS 9016-45-9; personal care surfactant.

Unicol NP-6. [Universal Preserv-A-Chem] Nonoxynol-6; CAS 9016-45-9; personal care surfactant.

Unicol NP-7. [Universal Preserv-A-Chem] Nonoxynol-7; CAS 9016-45-9; EINECS 248-292-0; personal care surfactant.

Unicol NP-8. [Universal Preserv-A-Chem] Nonoxynol-8; CAS 9016-45-9; personal care surfactant.

Unicol NP-9. [Universal Preserv-A-Chem] Nonoxynol-9; CAS 9016-45-9; personal care surfactant.

Unicol NP-10. [Universal Preserv-A-Chem] Nonoxynol-10; CAS 9016-45-9; EINECS 248-294-1; personal care surfactant.

Unicol NP-20. [Universal Preserv-A-Chem] Nonoxynol-20; CAS 9016-45-9; personal care surfactant.

Unicol NP-30. [Universal Preserv-A-Chem] Nonoxynol-30; CAS 9016-45-9; personal care surfactant.

Unicol NP-40. [Universal Preserv-A-Chem] Nonoxynol-40; CAS 9016-45-9; personal care surfactant.

Unicol NP-50. [Universal Preserv-A-Chem] Nonoxynol-50; CAS 9016-45-9; personal care surfactant.

Unicol NP-100. [Universal Preserv-A-Chem] Nonoxynol-100; CAS 9016-45-9; personal care surfactant.

Unicol OA-2. [Universal Preserv-A-Chem] Oleth-2; CAS 9004-98-2; emulsifier, emollient.

Unicol OA-4. [Universal Preserv-A-Chem] Oleth-4; CAS 9004-98-2; emulsifier, emollient.

Unicol OA-10. [Universal Preserv-A-Chem] Oleth-10; CAS 9004-98-2; emulsifier, emollient.

Unicol OA-20. [Universal Preserv-A-Chem] Oleth-20; CAS 9004-98-2; emulsifier.

Unicol P-400. [Universal Preserv-A-Chem] PPG-9; CAS 25322-69-4; personal care surfactant.

Unicol P-2000. [Universal Preserv-A-Chem] PPG-26; CAS 25322-69-4; cosmetic ingred.

Unicol P-4000. [Universal Preserv-A-Chem] PPG-30; CAS 25322-69-4; cosmetic ingred.

Unicol Propox 1695. [Universal Preserv-A-Chem] PPG-5 lanolin wax; cosmetic ingred.

Unicol SA-2. [Universal Preserv-A-Chem] Steareth-2; CAS 9005-00-9; personal care surfactant.

Unicol SA-10. [Universal Preserv-A-Chem] Steareth-10; CAS 9005-00-9; personal care surfactant.

Unicol SA-13. [Universal Preserv-A-Chem] Steareth-13; CAS 9005-00-9; personal care surfactant.

Unicol SA-15. [Universal Preserv-A-Chem] Steareth-15; CAS 9005-00-9; personal care surfactant.

Unicol SA-20. [Universal Preserv-A-Chem] Steareth-20; CAS 9005-00-9; personal care surfactant.

Unicol SA-40. [Universal Preserv-A-Chem] Steareth-40; CAS 9005-00-9; personal care surfactant.

Unicol TD-15. [Universal Preserv-A-Chem] Trideceth-15; CAS 24938-91-8; personal care surfactant.

Unicol W-5. [Universal Preserv-A-Chem] Isodeceth-5; cosmetic ingred.

Uniderm A. [Universal Preserv-A-Chem] Allantoin; CAS 97-59-6; EINECS 202-592-8; skin protectant.

Uniderm HOMSAL. [Universal Preserv-A-Chem] Homosalate; CAS 118-56-9; EINECS 204-260-8; sunscreen agent.

Uniderm SILPOW. [Universal Preserv-A-Chem] Silk powd.; CAS 9009-99-8; cosmetic protein.

Uniderm SSME. [Universal Preserv-A-Chem] Sesame oil; CAS 8008-74-0; EINECS 232-370-6; emollient oil.

Uniderm WGO. [Universal Preserv-A-Chem] Wheat germ oil; CAS 8006-95-9; emollient.

Unifat 5L. [Universal Preserv-A-Chem] Oleic acid; CAS 112-80-1; EINECS 204-007-1; surfactant intermediate.

Unifat 6. [Universal Preserv-A-Chem] Caproic acid; CAS 142-62-1; EINECS 205-550-7; chemical intermediate.

Unifat 8. [Universal Preserv-A-Chem] Caprylic acid; CAS 124-07-2; EINECS 204-677-5; intermediate.

Unifat 10. [Universal Preserv-A-Chem] Capric acid; CAS 334-48-5; EINECS 206-376-4; ester for perfumes and flavors; base for wetting agents; intermediate for chemical synthesis.

Unifat 12. [Universal Preserv-A-Chem] Lauric acid; CAS 143-07-7; EINECS 205-582-1; surfactant.

Unifat 16. [Universal Preserv-A-Chem] Palmitic acid; CAS 57-10-3; EINECS 200-312-9; surfactant intermediate; soap and cosmetic formulations.

Unifat 54. [Universal Preserv-A-Chem] Stearic acid; CAS 57-11-4; EINECS 200-313-4; surfactant intermediate, emulsifier, emollient.

Unifat 55L. [Universal Preserv-A-Chem] Stearic acid; CAS 57-11-4; EINECS 200-313-4; surfactant intermediate, emulsifier, emollient.

Unifilter U-41. [Induchem AG] Butyl methoxydibenzoylmethane, octyl methoxycinnamate, 3-benzylidene camphor; a blend of sunscreens offering broad spectrum protection.

Uniflex 9-88. [Universal Preserv-A-Chem] Dipropylene glycol dibenzoate; CAS 94-51-9; EINECS 202-340-7; cosmetic ingred.

Uniflex 50. [Universal Preserv-A-Chem] Dipropylene glycol dibenzoate, diethylene glycol dibenzoate; cosmetic ingred.

Uniflex DBP. [Universal Preserv-A-Chem] Dibutyl phthalate; CAS 84-74-2; EINECS 201-557-4; plasticizer for nail polish.

Uniflex DEP. [Universal Preserv-A-Chem] Diethyl phthalate; CAS 84-66-2; EINECS 201-550-6; plasticizer for nail polish.

Uniflex TBC. [Universal Preserv-A-Chem] Tributyl citrate; CAS 77-94-1; EINECS 201-071-2; cosmetic ingred.

Uniflex TEC. [Universal Preserv-A-Chem] Triethyl citrate; CAS 77-93-0; EINECS 201-070-7; cosmetic ingred.

Unifluorid D 401. [Induchem AG] Complex organofluoride compd.; pharmaceutical ingred. for caries prophylaxis.

Unifluorid H 101. [Induchem AG] Cetylamine hydrofluoride; CAS 3151-59-5; EINECS 221-588-7; pharmaceutical ingred. for caries prophylaxis.

Unigator B 67. [Induchem AG] Laureth-4, lanolin, petrolatum, and poloxamer 188; self-emulsifying base for high quality o/w cosmetic emulsions.

Uniglaudin A. [Universal Preserv-A-Chem] Hydrolyzed almond protein; cosmetic ingred.

Uniglaudin W. [Universal Preserv-A-Chem] Hydrolyzed wheat protein; CAS 70084-87-6; cosmetic protein.

Unigum PGA. [Universal Preserv-A-Chem] Propylene alginate; cosmetic ingred.

Unigum XAN. [Universal Preserv-A-Chem] Xanthan gum; CAS 11138-66-2; EINECS 234-394-2; gum for cosmetics.

Unihydag Wax 12. [Universal Preserv-A-Chem] Lauryl

alcohol; CAS 112-53-8; EINECS 203-982-0; cosmetic and pharmaceutical raw material.

Unihydag Wax-14. [Universal Preserv-A-Chem] Myristyl alcohol; CAS 112-72-1; EINECS 204-000-3; cosmetic/pharmaceutical raw material.

Unihydag Wax 16. [Universal Preserv-A-Chem] Cetyl alcohol; CAS 36653-82-4; EINECS 253-149-0; cosmetic ingred.

Unihydag Wax-18. [Universal Preserv-A-Chem] Stearyl alcohol; CAS 112-92-5; EINECS 204-017-6; emollient, cosmetic/pharmaceutical raw material.

Unihydag Wax 22. [Universal Preserv-A-Chem] Behenyl alcohol; CAS 661-19-8; EINECS 211-546-6; cosmetic/pharmaceutical raw material.

Unihydag Wax E. [Universal Preserv-A-Chem] Sodium cetearyl sulfate; CAS 59186-41-3; emulsifier.

Unihydag Wax-O. [Universal Preserv-A-Chem] Cetearyl alcohol; cosmetic ingred.

Unihydag Wax-SX. [Universal Preserv-A-Chem] Cetearyl alcohol, sodium lauryl sulfate; cosmetic ingred.

Unihydol 100. [Universal Preserv-A-Chem] Laureth-10; CAS 6540-99-4; personal care emulsifier.

Unihydol LS-2. [Universal Preserv-A-Chem] Laureth-2; CAS 3055-93-4; EINECS 221-279-7; surfactant.

Unihydol LS-3. [Universal Preserv-A-Chem] Laureth-3; CAS 3055-94-5; EINECS 221-280-2; emulsifier.

Unihydol LS-4. [Universal Preserv-A-Chem] Laureth-4; CAS 5274-68-0; EINECS 226-097-1; cosmetic ingred.

Unihydol LS 10. [Universal Preserv-A-Chem] Laureth-10; CAS 6540-99-4; personal care emulsifier.

Unihypro GLADIN A. [Universal Preserv-A-Chem] Soluble almond protein; cosmetic protein.

Unihypro GLADIN W. [Universal Preserv-A-Chem] Soluble wheat protein; cosmetic protein.

Unihypro Hygroplex HHG. [Universal Preserv-A-Chem] Hygroplex HHG; cosmetic ingred.

Unihypro LAN. [Universal Preserv-A-Chem] Soluble collagen; CAS 9007-34-5; EINECS 232-697-4; cosmetic protein.

Unikon A-22. [Induchem AG] 2,4-Dichlorobenzyl alcohol; CAS 1777-82-8; EINECS 217-210-5; cosmetic biocide; usage level: 0.05-0.5%.

Unilan. [Universal Preserv-A-Chem] Lanolin; CAS 8006-54-0; EINECS 232-348-6; emollient.

Unilan W. [Universal Preserv-A-Chem] Lanolin wax; CAS 68201-49-0; EINECS 269-220-4; emulsifier, emollient.

Unilan Acetyl. [Universal Preserv-A-Chem] Acetylated lanolin; CAS 61788-48-5; EINECS 262-979-2; emollient, superfatting agent.

Unilanal. [Universal Preserv-A-Chem] Lanolin alcohol; CAS 8027-33-6; EINECS 232-430-1; emollient, emulsifier.

Unilaneth 75. [Universal Preserv-A-Chem] PEG-75 lanolin; CAS 61790-81-6; emulsifier, emollient.

Unilaneth PPG-12-PEG-65. [Universal Preserv-A-Chem] PPG-12-PEG-65 lanolin oil; CAS 68458-58-8; cosmetic ingred.

Unilan Oil. [Universal Preserv-A-Chem] Lanolin oil; emollient, moisturizer.

Unilec S. [Universal Preserv-A-Chem] Lecithin; CAS 8002-43-5; EINECS 232-307-2; emulsifier.

Unilex, DS, S, SH. [Universal Preserv-A-Chem] Lecithin; CAS 8002-43-5; EINECS 232-307-2; emulsifier.

Unilin® 350 Alcohol. [Petrolite] C20-40 alcohols; chemical intermediate for oxidation, ethoxylation, sulfation, amination, esterification; coemulsifier and direct additive in coatings; plastics additive (processing aid, lubricant, dispersant); thickener, moisturizer, pigment dispersant, oil binder, stabilizer in cosmetic creams, lotions, lipsticks, antiperspirants, and soaps; FDA §175.105; slab; sol. in aliphatic and aromatic solvs.; m.w. 375; sp.gr. 0.78 (121

C); dens. 0.985 g/cc; visc. 5.9 cp (99 C); m.p. 78 C; hyd. no. 127.

Unilin® 425 Alcohol. [Petrolite] C20-40 alcohols; functional polymer for modification of PP, PVC, polyethylene, PS, and high-performance engineering resins; acts as antioxidant, heat stabilizer, uv stabilizer, or visc. depressant; promotes emollient protective films onto the skin in cosmetic creams and lotions; used in hot-melt and solv.-based coatings; textile/leather lubricants and finishes; chemical intermediate; defoamer for pulp/paper processing; FDA §175.105; off-wh. prills; sol. in aliphatic and aromatic solvs.; m.w. 460; sp.gr. 0.78 (121 C); dens. 0.985 g/cc; visc. 7.8 cps (99 C); m.p. 91 C; hyd. no. 105.

Unilin® 550 Alcohol. [Petrolite] C30-50 alcohols; chemical intermediate for oxidation, ethoxylation, sulfation, amination, esterification; coemulsifier and direct additive in coatings; plastics additive (processing aid, lubricant, dispersant); thickener, moisturizer, pigment dispersant, oil binder, stabilizer in cosmetic creams, lotions, lipsticks, antiperspirants, and soaps; FDA §175.105; off-wh. prills; sol. in toluene, MIBK, VM&P naphtha, hexane; m.w. 550; sp.gr. 0.78 (121 C); dens. 0.985 g/cc; visc. 5.5 cps (149 C); m.p. 99 C; hyd. no. 83.

Unilin® 700 Alcohol. [Petrolite] C40-60 alcohols; chemical intermediate for oxidation, ethoxylation, sulfation, amination, esterification; coemulsifier and direct additive in coatings; plastics additive (processing aid, lubricant, dispersant); thickener, moisturizer, pigment dispersant, oil binder, stabilizer in cosmetic creams, lotions, lipsticks, antiperspirants, and soaps; FDA §175.105; off-wh. prills; sol. in toluene, MIBK, VM&P naphtha; m.w. 700; sp.gr. 0.79 g/cc (121 C); dens. 0.985 g/cc; visc. 7.9 cps (149 C); m.p. 105 C; hyd. no. 65.

Unilube MB-370. [Nippon Oils & Fats] PPG-40 butyl ether; CAS 9003-13-8; emollient.

Unimer U-15. [Induchem AG] PVP/eicosene copolymer; CAS 28211-18-9; forms water-resist. films for cosmetics applics.; solid.

Unimer U-151. [Induchem AG] PVP/hexadecene copolymer; CAS 32440-50-9; forms water-resist. films for cosmetics applics.; liq.

Unimin KA. [Universal Preserv-A-Chem] Kaolin; CAS 1332-58-7; EINECS 296-473-8; cosmetic ingred.

Unimoist U-125. [Induchem AG] Glycerin, urea, saccharide hydrolysate, magneisum aspartate, glycine, alanine, creatine; a moisturizing complex for cosmetics use.

Unimox CAW. [Universal Preserv-A-Chem] Cocamidopropylamine oxide; CAS 68155-09-9; EINECS 268-938-5; cosmetic surfactant.

Unimox LO. [Universal Preserv-A-Chem] Lauramine oxide; CAS 1643-20-5; EINECS 216-700-6; personal care surfactant.

Unimox OL. [Universal Preserv-A-Chem] Oleamine oxide; CAS 14351-50-9; EINECS 238-311-0; personal care surfactant.

Unimox SO. [Universal Preserv-A-Chem] Stearamine oxide; CAS 2571-88-2; EINECS 219-919-5; conditioner, surfactant.

Unimul-05. [Universal Preserv-A-Chem] Oleth-5; CAS 9004-98-2; emulsifier, emollient.

Unimul-10. [Universal Preserv-A-Chem] Oleth-10; CAS 9004-98-2; emulsifier, emollient.

Unimul 14. [Universal Preserv-A-Chem] Myristyl myristate; CAS 3234-85-3; EINECS 221-787-9; emollient.

Unimul 14E. [Universal Preserv-A-Chem] Myreth-3-myristate; CAS 59686-68-9; emulsifier, emollient, moisturizer, cosmetic base.

Unimul-1002 Conc. [Universal Preserv-A-Chem] Cetearyl alcohol, PEG-40 hydrog. castor oil, stearalkonium chloride; cosmetic ingred.

Unimul-1410. [Universal Preserv-A-Chem] Myreth-3 caprate; cosmetic ingred.

Unimul-1414EW. [Universal Preserv-A-Chem] Myreth-3 myristate; CAS 59686-68-9; emulsifier, emollient, moisturizer, cosmetic base.

Unimul-1616. [Universal Preserv-A-Chem] Cetyl palmitate; CAS 540-10-3; EINECS 208-736-6; emollient.

Unimul 1818. [Universal Preserv-A-Chem] Stearyl stearate; CAS 2778-96-3; EINECS 220-476-5; emollient.

Unimul-7061. [Universal Preserv-A-Chem] Isocetyl stearate; CAS 25339-09-7; EINECS 246-868-6; emollient.

Unimul-7115. [Universal Preserv-A-Chem] Myristyleicosyl stearate; cosmetic ingred.

Unimul-B-1. [Universal Preserv-A-Chem] Ceteareth-12; CAS 68439-49-6; cosmetic ingred.

Unimul-B-2. [Universal Preserv-A-Chem] Ceteareth-20; CAS 68439-49-6; cosmetic ingred.

Unimul-B-3. [Universal Preserv-A-Chem] Ceteareth-30; CAS 68439-49-6; cosmetic ingred.

Unimul-CTA. [Universal Preserv-A-Chem] Hexyl laurate; CAS 34316-64-8; EINECS 251-932-1; emollient, vehicle for cosmetics.

Unimul-CTV. [Universal Preserv-A-Chem] Decyl oleate; CAS 3687-46-5; EINECS 222-981-6; emollient.

Unimul-G. [Universal Preserv-A-Chem] Octyldodecanol; CAS 5333-42-6; EINECS 226-242-9; carrier, lubricant, emollient.

Unimul-G-16. [Universal Preserv-A-Chem] Isocetyl alcohol; CAS 36311-34-9; EINECS 252-964-9; emollient.

Unimul-G-32/36. [Universal Preserv-A-Chem] Myristyl eicosanol; cosmetic ingred.

Unimul-HE. [Universal Preserv-A-Chem] PEG-7 glyceryl cocoate; personal care surfactant.

Unimul ISN. [Universal Preserv-A-Chem] Cetearyl isononanoate; emollient.

Unimul LAM-TGI. [Universal Preserv-A-Chem] Polyglyceryl-3 diisostearate; CAS 66082-42-6; emulsifier.

Unimul-LC. [Universal Preserv-A-Chem] Coco-caprylate/caprate; cosmetic ingred.

Unimul MYRLAC. [Universal Preserv-A-Chem] Myristyl lactate; CAS 1323-03-1; EINECS 215-350-1; emollient.

Unimulgade-1000NI. [Universal Preserv-A-Chem] Cetearyl alcohol, ceteareth-20; cosmetic ingred.

Unimulgade-F. [Universal Preserv-A-Chem] Cetearyl alcohol, PEG-40 castor oil, sodium cetearyl sulfate; cosmetic ingred.

Unimulgade-F Special. [Universal Preserv-A-Chem] Cetearyl alcohol, PEG-40 castor oil; cosmetic ingred.

Unimulse. [Universal Preserv-A-Chem] Shea butter; CAS 68424-60-2; emollient oil.

Unineut SOBROM. [Universal Preserv-A-Chem] Sodium bromate; CAS 7789-38-0; EINECS 232-160-4; cosmetic ingred.

Uninontan U 34. [Induchem AG] Water, propylene glycol, sodium citrate, lemon extract, and cucumber extract; plant extract blend which inhibits tanning and lightens the skin.

Uninox A 287. [Induchem AG] BHT-based antioxidant; CAS 128-37-0; EINECS 204-881-4; for the cosmetics industry; oil-sol.

Unipabol U-17. [Induchem AG; Lipo] PEG-25 PABA; uv-B sunscreen for cosmetics, toiletries, pharmaceuticals.

Unipeg 75 Cocoa Butter. [Universal Preserv-A-Chem] PEG-75 cocoa butter; cosmetic ingred.

Unipeg 150 DS. [Universal Preserv-A-Chem] PEG-3 distearate; CAS 9005-08-7; pearlescent.

Unipeg 200. [Universal Preserv-A-Chem] PEG-4; CAS 25322-68-3; EINECS 203-989-9; cosmetic ingred.

Unipeg-200 ML. [Universal Preserv-A-Chem] PEG-4 laurate; CAS 9004-81-3; emulsifier.

Unipeg-200 MO. [Universal Preserv-A-Chem] PEG-4 oleate; CAS 9004-96-0; EINECS 233-293-0; personal care surfactant.

Unipeg-200 MS. [Universal Preserv-A-Chem] PEG-4 stearate; CAS 9004-99-3; EINECS 203-358-8; emulsifier.

Unipeg-200 X. [Universal Preserv-A-Chem] PEG-4; CAS 25322-68-3; EINECS 203-989-9; cosmetic ingred.

Unipeg 400. [Universal Preserv-A-Chem] PEG-8; CAS 25322-68-3; EINECS 225-856-4; cosmetic ingred.

Unipeg-400 DL. [Universal Preserv-A-Chem] PEG-8 dilaurate; CAS 9005-02-1; personal care surfactant.

Unipeg-400 DO. [Universal Preserv-A-Chem] PEG-8 dioleate; CAS 9005-07-6; personal care surfactant.

Unipeg-400 DS. [Universal Preserv-A-Chem] PEG-8 distearate; CAS 9005-08-7; personal care surfactant.

Unipeg-400 ML. [Universal Preserv-A-Chem] PEG-8 laurate; CAS 9004-81-3; emulsifier.

Unipeg-400 MO. [Universal Preserv-A-Chem] PEG-8 oleate; CAS 9004-96-0; emulsifier.

Unipeg-400 MOT. [Universal Preserv-A-Chem] PEG-8 tallate; CAS 61791-00-2; personal care surfactant.

Unipeg-400 MS. [Universal Preserv-A-Chem] PEG-8 stearate; CAS 9004-99-3; emulsifier.

Unipeg-400 SO. [Universal Preserv-A-Chem] PEG-8 sesquioleate; cosmetic ingred.

Unipeg-400 X. [Universal Preserv-A-Chem] PEG-8; CAS 25322-68-3; EINECS 225-856-4; cosmetic ingred.

Unipeg-600. [Universal Preserv-A-Chem] PEG-12; CAS 25322-68-3; EINECS 229-859-1; cosmetic ingred.

Unipeg-600 DO. [Universal Preserv-A-Chem] PEG-12 dioleate; CAS 9005-07-6; personal care surfactant.

Unipeg-600 DS. [Universal Preserv-A-Chem] PEG-12 distearate; CAS 9005-08-7; personal care surfactant.

Unipeg-600 ML. [Universal Preserv-A-Chem] PEG-12 laurate; CAS 9004-81-3; emulsifier.

Unipeg-600 MO. [Universal Preserv-A-Chem] PEG-12 oleate; CAS 9004-96-0; personal care surfactant.

Unipeg-600 MS. [Universal Preserv-A-Chem] PEG-12 stearate; CAS 9004-99-3; emulsifier.

Unipeg 1000. [Universal Preserv-A-Chem] PEG-20; CAS 25322-68-3; cosmetic ingred.

Unipeg 1000 DS. [Universal Preserv-A-Chem] PEG-20 distearate; CAS 9005-08-7; personal care surfactant.

Unipeg-1000 MS. [Universal Preserv-A-Chem] PEG-20 stearate; CAS 9004-99-3; emulsifier.

Unipeg-1000 X. [Universal Preserv-A-Chem] PEG-20; CAS 25322-68-3; cosmetic ingred.

Unipeg 1500. [Universal Preserv-A-Chem] PEG-6-32; CAS 25322-68-3; cosmetic ingred.

Unipeg-1500 X. [Universal Preserv-A-Chem] PEG-6 and PEG-32; cosmetic ingred.

Unipeg 1540. [Universal Preserv-A-Chem] PEG-32; CAS 25322-68-3; cosmetic ingred.

Unipeg-1540 MS. [Universal Preserv-A-Chem] PEG-32 stearate; CAS 9004-99-3; emulsifier.

Unipeg-1540 X. [Universal Preserv-A-Chem] PEG-32; CAS 25322-68-3; cosmetic ingred.

Unipeg 4000. [Universal Preserv-A-Chem] PEG-75; CAS 25322-68-3; cosmetic ingred.

Unipeg-4000 DS. [Universal Preserv-A-Chem] PEG-75 distearate; CAS 9005-08-7; personal care surfactant.

Unipeg-4000 MS. [Universal Preserv-A-Chem] PEG-75 stearate; CAS 9004-99-3; emulsifier.

Unipeg-4000 X. [Universal Preserv-A-Chem] PEG-75; CAS 25322-68-3; cosmetic ingred.

Unipeg 6000. [Universal Preserv-A-Chem] PEG-150; CAS 25322-68-3; cosmetic ingred.

Unipeg-6000 DS. [Universal Preserv-A-Chem] PEG-150 distearate; CAS 9005-08-7; personal care surfactant.

Unipeg-6000 ML. [Universal Preserv-A-Chem] PEG-150

laurate; CAS 9004-81-3; emulsifier.

Unipeg-6000 MS. [Universal Preserv-A-Chem] PEG-150 stearate; CAS 9004-99-3; emulsifier.

Unipeg-6000 X. [Universal Preserv-A-Chem] PEG-150; CAS 25322-68-3; cosmetic ingred.

Unipeg-CO-8. [Universal Preserv-A-Chem] PEG-8 castor oil; CAS 61791-12-6; personal care surfactant.

Unipeg-CO-25. [Universal Preserv-A-Chem] PEG-25 castor oil; CAS 61791-12-6; personal care surfactant.

Unipeg-CO-25H. [Universal Preserv-A-Chem] PEG-25 hydrog. castor oil; CAS 61788-85-0; personal care surfactant.

Unipeg-CO-36. [Universal Preserv-A-Chem] PEG-36 castor oil; CAS 61791-12-6; personal care surfactant.

Unipeg-CO-40. [Universal Preserv-A-Chem] PEG-40 castor oil; CAS 61791-12-6; personal care surfactant.

Unipeg-CO-40H. [Universal Preserv-A-Chem] PEG-40 hydrog. castor oil; CAS 61788-85-0; personal care surfactant.

Unipeg-CO-200. [Universal Preserv-A-Chem] PEG-200 castor oil; CAS 61791-12-6; cosmetic ingred.

Unipeg-DGL. [Universal Preserv-A-Chem] PEG-2 laurate; CAS 141-20-8; EINECS 205-468-1; emulsifier.

Unipeg-EGDS. [Universal Preserv-A-Chem] Glycol distearate; CAS 627-83-8; EINECS 211-014-3; cosmetic ingred.

Unipeg-EGMS. [Universal Preserv-A-Chem] Glycol stearate; CAS 111-60-4; EINECS 203-886-9; emulsifier, opacifier, pearlescent for cosmetics.

Unipeg-ETG-12. [Universal Preserv-A-Chem] Glycereth-12; CAS 31694-55-0; cosmetic ingred.

Unipeg-ETG-26. [Universal Preserv-A-Chem] Glycereth-26; CAS 31694-55-0; cosmetic ingred.

Unipeg-PGML. [Universal Preserv-A-Chem] Propylene glycol laurate; CAS 142-55-2; EINECS 205-542-3; emulsifier.

Unipeg-PGMS. [Universal Preserv-A-Chem] Propylene glycol stearate; CAS 1323-39-3; EINECS 215-354-3; personal care surfactant.

Unipeg-S-40. [Universal Preserv-A-Chem] PEG-40 stearate; CAS 9004-99-3; emulsifier.

Unipertan P-24. [Induchem AG] Hydrolyzed collagen, tyrosine, riboflavin.

Unipertan P-24. [Lipo] Hydrolyzed collagen, tyrosine, riboflavin; tanning accelerator complex for cosmetics, toiletries, pharmaceuticals.

Unipertan P-242. [Induchem AG; Lipo] Hydrolyzed collagen, acetyl tyrosine, adenosine triphosphate; tanning accelerator complex for cosmetics, toiletries, pharmaceuticals.

Unipertan P-2002. [Induchem AG] Hydrolyzed collagen, acetyl tyrosine, adenosine triphosphate, and riboflavin; tanning accelerator complex with riboflavin and ATP.

Unipertan VEG 24. [Induchem AG] Butylene glycol, acetyl tyrosine, hydrolyzed vegetable protein, and riboflavin; tanning accelerator complex.

Unipertan VEG 242. [Induchem AG] Butylene glycol, acetyl tyrosine, hydrolyzed vegetable protein, and adenosine triphosphate; tanning accelerator complex.

Unipet. [Universal Preserv-A-Chem] Petrolatum; EINECS 232-373-2; emollient, ointment base.

Uniphen P-23. [Induchem AG; Lipo] Phenoxyethanol, methylparaben, ethylparaben, propylparaben, butylparaben; preservative, biocide for cosmetics, toiletries, pharmaceuticals; esp. to preserve the oil phase of emulsions; additive for deodorants; USA, Japan, and Europe approvals; colorless clear sl. visc. liq., faint aromatic odor; sol. in ethanol, aq. ethanol, ethylene glycol, propylene glycol; misc. with acetone, chloroform; sl. sol. in water; sp.gr. 1.120-1.126; ref. index 1.540-1.543; usage level: 0.3-1.0%.

Unipherol U-14. [Induchem AG] Isopropyl myristate, lecithin,

tocopherol; natural antioxidant blend for cosmetics applics.; oil-sol.

Uniphos STPP. [Universal Preserv-A-Chem] Sodium tripolyphosphate; cosmetic ingred.

Uniphyllin SC. [Universal Preserv-A-Chem] Chlorophyllin-copper complex; CAS 11006-34-1; EINECS 234-242-5; cosmetic ingred.

Uniplant PS-100. [Universal Preserv-A-Chem] Ammonium laureth sulfate and decyl polyglucose; cosmetic ingred.

Uniplant PS-200. [Universal Preserv-A-Chem] Lauryl polyglucose and sodium laureth sulfate; cosmetic ingred.

Uniplex 84. [Unitex] Acetyl tributyl citrate; CAS 77-90-7; EINECS 201-067-0; plasticizer for indirect and direct food contact applics.; milling lubricant for aluminum foil or sheet steel for use in cans for beverage and food prods.; in PVC toys, cellulose nitrate films, aerosol hair sprays, dairy prod. cartons.

Uniplex 110. [Unitex] Dimethyl phthalate; CAS 131-11-3; EINECS 205-011-6; solv. and plasticizer for cellulose acetate butyrate compositions; solv. for org. catalysts; plasticizer and solv. for aerosol hair sprays.

Uniplex 150. [Unitex] Dibutyl phthalate; CAS 84-74-2; EINECS 201-557-4; solv./plasticizer in fingernail polish, nail polish remover, hair sprays, org. peroxide catalysts, adhesives, coatings; compat. with cellulosics, methacrylate, PS, PVB, vinyl chloride, urea-formaldehyde, melamine-formaldehye, phenolics.

Uniplex 260. [Unitex] Glyceryl tribenzoate; CAS 614-33-5; polymer modifier; plasticizer; for heat seal applics., lacquers, films, in PVAc-based adhesives, cellophane coatings, nitrocellulose coatings, nail lacquer formulations, printing inks, polishes; extrusion and inj. molding processing aid.

Unipol 125-E, 130-E. [Universal Preserv-A-Chem] Sodium laureth-12 sulfate; CAS 9004-82-4; personal care surfactant.

Unipol 230. [Universal Preserv-A-Chem] Ammonium C12-15 pareth sulfate; personal care surfactant.

Unipol 230-E. [Universal Preserv-A-Chem] Ammonium laureth-12 sulfate; cosmetic ingred.

Unipol 7092. [Universal Preserv-A-Chem] Sodium laureth sulfate, glycol stearate; pearlescent surfactant.

Unipol A. [Universal Preserv-A-Chem] Ammonium lauryl sulfate; CAS 2235-54-3; EINECS 218-793-9; surfactant.

Unipol A-215. [Universal Preserv-A-Chem] Ammonium C12-15 alkyl sulfate; CAS 68815-61-2; EINECS 272-385-5; cosmetic ingred.

Unipol AP-60. [Universal Preserv-A-Chem] Ammonium C12-15 pareth sulfate; personal care surfactant.

Unipol CIM-40. [Universal Preserv-A-Chem] Sodium coco-amphoacetate; personal care surfactant.

Unipol Conc. 7021. [Universal Preserv-A-Chem] DEA-lauryl sulfate and TEA-lauryl sulfate; cosmetic ingred.

Unipol Conc. 7023. [Universal Preserv-A-Chem] Cocamide DEA, DEA-myreth sulfate; cosmetic ingred.

Unipol CS-50. [Universal Preserv-A-Chem] Sodium lauryl sulfate, sodium cetyl sulfate, laureth-3; personal care surfactant.

Unipol CS Paste. [Universal Preserv-A-Chem] Sodium lauryl sulfate, sodium cetyl sulfate, laureth-3; personal care surfactant.

Unipol DEA. [Universal Preserv-A-Chem] DEA-lauryl sulfate; CAS 143-00-0; EINECS 205-577-4; personal care surfactant.

Unipol EA-1, EA-2, EA-3. [Universal Preserv-A-Chem] Ammonium laureth sulfate; CAS 32612-48-9; surfactant.

Unipol EA-40. [Universal Preserv-A-Chem] Ammonium myreth sulfate; CAS 27731-61-9; surfactant.

Unipol ES. [Universal Preserv-A-Chem] Sodium laureth sulfate; personal care surfactant.

Unipol ES-1, ES-2, ES-3. [Universal Preserv-A-Chem] Sodium laureth sulfate; personal care surfactant.
Unipol ES-40. [Universal Preserv-A-Chem] Sodium laureth-12 sulfate; CAS 9004-82-4; personal care surfactant.
Unipol LAUROYLSAR. [Universal Preserv-A-Chem] Sodium lauroyl sarcosinate; CAS 137-16-6; EINECS 205-281-5; personal care surfactant.
Unipol MEA LES. [Universal Preserv-A-Chem] MEA-laureth sulfate; cosmetic ingred.
Unipol MGLES. [Universal Preserv-A-Chem] Magnesium laureth sulfate; CAS 62755-21-9; personal care surfactant.
Unipol MGLS. [Universal Preserv-A-Chem] Magnesium lauryl sulfate; CAS 3097-08-3; EINECS 221-450-6; personal care surfactant.
Unipol MLS. [Universal Preserv-A-Chem] MEA-lauryl sulfate; CAS 4722-98-9; EINECS 225-214-3; detergent.
Unipol SCO. [Universal Preserv-A-Chem] Sulfated castor oil; CAS 8002-33-3; EINECS 232-306-7; emulsifier.
Unipol SH-100, SH-135. [Universal Preserv-A-Chem] Disodium oleamido PEG-2 sulfosuccinate; CAS 56388-43-3; EINECS 260-143-1; cosmetic surfactant.
Unipol SH-300. [Universal Preserv-A-Chem] TEA-oleamido PEG-2 sulfosuccinate; cosmetic ingred.
Unipol SLS. [Universal Preserv-A-Chem] Sodium lauryl sulfate; CAS 151-21-3; EINECS 205-788-1; personal care surfactant.
Unipol SP-60. [Universal Preserv-A-Chem] Sodium C12-15 pareth sulfate; cosmetic ingred.
Unipol T. [Universal Preserv-A-Chem] TEA-lauryl sulfate; CAS 139-96-8; EINECS 205-388-7; personal care surfactant.
Unipol T-315. [Universal Preserv-A-Chem] TEA-C12-15 alcohols sulfate; cosmetic ingred.
Unipol WA-AC. [Universal Preserv-A-Chem] Sodium lauryl sulfate; CAS 151-21-3; EINECS 205-788-1; personal care surfactant.
Unipol WAC Special. [Universal Preserv-A-Chem] Sodium lauryl sulfate; CAS 151-21-3; EINECS 205-788-1; personal care surfactant.
Unipol WAQ-115. [Universal Preserv-A-Chem] Sodium C12-15 alcohols sulfate; cosmetic ingred.
Unipol WAQ-LC. [Universal Preserv-A-Chem] Sodium lauryl sulfate; CAS 151-21-3; EINECS 205-788-1; personal care surfactant.
Unipoly HSP 1180. [Universal Preserv-A-Chem] Polyacrylamidomethyl propane sulfonic acid; cosmetic ingred.
Unipon K12, K1296, L-100, ZHC Needles, ZHC Powd. [Universal Preserv-A-Chem] Sodium lauryl sulfate; CAS 151-21-3; EINECS 205-788-1; personal care surfactant.
Unipon ZHC Needles. [Universal Preserv-A-Chem] Sodium lauryl sulfate; CAS 151-21-3; EINECS 205-788-1; personal care surfactant.
Unipro Aminoderm CLR. [Universal Preserv-A-Chem] Aminodermin; cosmetic ingred.
Unipro CAL-CASE, CO-CASE. [Universal Preserv-A-Chem] Casein; CAS 9000-71-9; EINECS 232-55-1; cosmetic ingred.
Unipro CLR. [Universal Preserv-A-Chem] Collagen; CAS 9007-34-5; EINECS 232-697-4; moisturizing protein.
Unipro ELAST CLR. [Universal Preserv-A-Chem] Elastin; cosmetic ingred.
Unipro Epidermin/Oil Disp. [Universal Preserv-A-Chem] Epidermin; cosmetic ingred.; oil-disp.
Unipro Epidermin/Water Disp. [Universal Preserv-A-Chem] Epidermin; cosmetic ingred.; water-disp.
Unipro Glycoderm. [Universal Preserv-A-Chem] Glycoderm; cosmetic ingred.
Unipro LAN-S. [Universal Preserv-A-Chem] Potassium cocoyl hydrolyzed collagen; CAS 68920-65-0; cosmetic protein.
Unipro Placenta Liq./OS. [Universal Preserv-A-Chem] Placenta liq.; cosmetic ingred.; oil-sol.
Unipro Placenta Liq./WS. [Universal Preserv-A-Chem] Placenta liq.; cosmetic ingred.; water-sol.
Unipro Protoglycan. [Universal Preserv-A-Chem] Proteodermin; cosmetic ingred.
Unipro SO-CASE. [Universal Preserv-A-Chem] Sodium caseinate; CAS 9005-46-3; emulsifier, stabilizer.
Uniprolam PAJR. [Universal Preserv-A-Chem] TEA-abietoyl hydrolyzed collagen; CAS 68918-77-4; cosmetic protein.
Uniprolam ST-40. [Universal Preserv-A-Chem] TEA-cocyl hydrolyzed collagen; cosmetic ingred.
Uniquart 7102. [Universal Preserv-A-Chem] PEG-15 cocopolyamine, stearalkonium chloride; cosmetic ingred.
Uniquart A. [Universal Preserv-A-Chem] Cetrimonium chloride; CAS 112-02-7; EINECS 203-928-6; quat. for personal care prods.
Uniquart ADBAC-50 USP. [Universal Preserv-A-Chem] Benzalkonium chloride; cosmetic ingred.
Uniquart C. [Universal Preserv-A-Chem] Lauryl pyridiniumchloride; CAS 104-74-5; EINECS 203-232-2; surfactant.
Uniquart COSM GUAR. [Universal Preserv-A-Chem] Guar hydroxypropyl trimonium chloride; CAS 65497-29-2; thickener, conditioner for cosmetics.
Uniquart CPC. [Universal Preserv-A-Chem] Cetyl pyridinium chloride; CAS 123-03-5; EINECS 204-593-9; emulsifier; antibacterial, preservative for cosmetics and pharmaceuticals.
Uniquart E. [Universal Preserv-A-Chem] Hydroxycetyl hydroxyethyl dimonium chloride; CAS 84643-53-8; cosmetic ingred.
Uniquart H. [Universal Preserv-A-Chem] PEG-15 tallow polyamine; cosmetic ingred.
Uniquart LMQL. [Universal Preserv-A-Chem] Lauryldimonium hydroxypropyl hydrolyzed collagen; cosmetic ingred.
Uniquart SP. [Universal Preserv-A-Chem] Quaternium-52; CAS 58069-11-7; emulsifier, conditioner.
Unirep U-18. [Induchem AG] Dimethyl phthalate, diethyl toluamide, ethyl hexanediol; blend of insect repellents for personal care prods.
Unisept B. [Universal Preserv-A-Chem] Butylparaben; CAS 94-26-8; EINECS 202-318-7; cosmetics preservative.
Unisept BNA. [Universal Preserv-A-Chem] Sodium butyl paraben; CAS 36457-20-2; cosmetic ingred.
Unisept BZ. [Universal Preserv-A-Chem] Benzylparaben; CAS 94-18-8; EINECS 202-311-9; cosmetics preservative.
Unisept BZA. [Universal Preserv-A-Chem] Benzoic acid; CAS 65-85-0; EINECS 200-618-2; cosmetics preservative.
Unisept Chlorbut. [Universal Preserv-A-Chem] Chlorobutanol; CAS 57-15-8; EINECS 200-317-6; antimicrobial, preservative.
Unisept DHA. [Universal Preserv-A-Chem] Dehydroacetic acid; CAS 520-45-6; EINECS 208-293-9; cosmetics preservative.
Unisept DSA. [Universal Preserv-A-Chem] Sodium dehydroacetate; CAS 4418-26-2; EINECS 224-580-1; cosmetics preservative.
Unisept E. [Universal Preserv-A-Chem] Ethylparaben; CAS 120-47-8; EINECS 204-399-4; cosmetics preservative.
Unisept IMIDU. [Universal Preserv-A-Chem] Imidurea NF; cosmetic ingred.
Unisept M. [Universal Preserv-A-Chem] Methylparaben; CAS 99-76-3; EINECS 202-785-7; cosmetics preservative.

Unisept M NA. [Universal Preserv-A-Chem] Methyl paraben sodium; CAS 5026-62-0; EINECS 225-714-1; preservative.

Unisept P. [Universal Preserv-A-Chem] Propylparaben; CAS 94-13-3; EINECS 202-307-7; cosmetics preservative.

Unisept PNA. [Universal Preserv-A-Chem] Propyl paraben NA; CAS 94-13-3; EINECS 202-307-7; cosmetic preservative.

Unisept POE. [Universal Preserv-A-Chem] Phenoxyethanol; CAS 122-99-6; EINECS 204-589-7; preservative.

Unisept SB. [Universal Preserv-A-Chem] Sodium benzoate; CAS 532-32-1; EINECS 208-534-8; cosmetics preservative.

Unisil DF-200S, DF-200SP. [Universal Preserv-A-Chem] Simethicone; foam control agent.

Unisil SF. [Universal Preserv-A-Chem] Simethicone; foam control agent.

Unisil SF-R. [Universal Preserv-A-Chem] Dimethiconol; CAS 31692-79-2; cosmetic ingred.

Unisil SF-V. [Universal Preserv-A-Chem] Cyclomethicone; CAS 69430-24-6; cosmetic ingred.

Unisoft 475. [Universal Preserv-A-Chem] Quaternium-27; hair conditioner.

Unisoft SAC. [Universal Preserv-A-Chem] Stearalkonium chloride; CAS 122-19-0; EINECS 204-527-9; conditioner, antistat.

Unisol S-22. [Induchem AG] 3-Benzylidene camphor; CAS 15087-24-8; EINECS 239-139-9; uv-B sunscreen.

Unisorb 20. [Universal Preserv-A-Chem] Polysorbate 20; CAS 9005-64-5; emulsifier, solubilizer.

Unisorb 21. [Universal Preserv-A-Chem] Polysorbate 21; CAS 9005-64-5; emulsifier.

Unisorb 40. [Universal Preserv-A-Chem] Polysorbate 40; CAS 9005-66-7; emulsifier.

Unisorb 60. [Universal Preserv-A-Chem] Polysorbate 60; CAS 9005-67-8; emulsifier.

Unisorb 61. [Universal Preserv-A-Chem] Polysorbate 61; CAS 9005-67-8; emulsifier.

Unisorb 65. [Universal Preserv-A-Chem] Polysorbate 65; CAS 9005-71-4; emulsifier.

Unisorb 80. [Universal Preserv-A-Chem] Polysorbate 80; CAS 9005-65-6; emulsifier.

Unisorb 80L. [Universal Preserv-A-Chem] PEG-80 sorbitan laurate; CAS 9005-64-5; personal care surfactant.

Unisorb 85. [Universal Preserv-A-Chem] Polysorbate 85; CAS 9005-70-3; emulsifier.

Unispheres. [Induchem AG] Spherical beads consisting of cellulose derivs. with lactose in blue, red, yellow, and green; abrasives for cosmetics industry.

Unispheres G-503. [Induchem AG] Lactose, cellulose, hydroxypropyl methylcellulose, and chlorophyllin-copper complex; see Unispheres.

Unispheres R-505. [Induchem AG] Lactose, cellulose, hydroxypropyl methylcellulose, and iron oxides; see Unispheres.

Unispheres U-504. [Induchem AG] Lactose, cellulose, hydroxypropyl methylcellulose, and ultramarines; see Unispheres.

Unispheres YE-501. [Induchem AG] Lactose, cellulose, hydroxypropyl methylcellulose, iron oxides, and tocopheryl acetate; see Unispheres.

Unistab S 69. [Induchem AG] Odor neutralizing prod.

Unistat. [Universal Preserv-A-Chem] Sorbic acid; CAS 110-44-1; EINECS 203-768-7; preservative.

Unistat CALBAN. [Universal Preserv-A-Chem] Calcium propionate; CAS 4075-81-4; EINECS 223-795-8; preservative.

Unistat CALPRO. [Universal Preserv-A-Chem] Calcium propionate; CAS 4075-81-4; EINECS 223-795-8; preservative.

Unistat K. [Universal Preserv-A-Chem] Potassium sorbate; CAS 590-00-1; EINECS 246-376-1; cosmetics and food preservative.

Unistat SOBAN. [Universal Preserv-A-Chem] Sodium propionate; CAS 137-40-6; EINECS 205-290-4; preservative.

Unistat SORBA. [Universal Preserv-A-Chem] Sorbic acid; CAS 110-44-1; EINECS 203-768-7; preservative.

Unisulcoidal. [Universal Preserv-A-Chem] Sulfur; CAS 7704-34-9; EINECS 231-722-6; cosmetic ingred.

Unisuprol S-25. [Induchem AG] Phenoxyethanol, triethylene glycol, 2,4-dichlorobenzyl alcohol; biocide for cosmetics use; USA and Europe approvals; usage level: 0.4-0.6%.

Unisweet 70. [Universal Preserv-A-Chem] Sorbitol; CAS 50-70-4; EINECS 200-061-5; cosmetic/pharmaceutical ingred.

Unisweet 70/CONC. [Universal Preserv-A-Chem] Sorbitol; CAS 50-70-4; EINECS 200-061-5; cosmetic/pharmaceutical ingred.

Unisweet CALSAC. [Universal Preserv-A-Chem] Calcium saccharin; CAS 6485-34-3; EINECS 229-349-9; cosmetic ingred.

Unisweet CONC. [Universal Preserv-A-Chem] Sorbitol; CAS 50-70-4; EINECS 200-061-5; cosmetic/pharmaceutical ingred.

Unisweet EVAN. [Universal Preserv-A-Chem] Ethyl vanillin; CAS 121-32-4; EINECS 204-464-7; flavoring agent.

Unisweet L. [Universal Preserv-A-Chem] Lactose; CAS 63-42-3; EINECS 200-599-2; used in pharmaceuticals, foods.

Unisweet Lactose. [Universal Preserv-A-Chem] Lactose; CAS 63-42-3; EINECS 200-599-2; used in pharmaceuticals, foods.

Unisweet MAN. [Universal Preserv-A-Chem] Mannitol; CAS 69-65-8; EINECS 200-711-8; cosmetics ingred.

Unisweet SAC. [Universal Preserv-A-Chem] Saccharin; CAS 81-07-2; EINECS 201-321-0; noncaloric sweetener, pharmaceutic aid.

Unisweet SODGLYCRZ. [Universal Preserv-A-Chem] Sodium glycyrrhizinate; cosmetic ingred.

Unisweet SOSAC. [Universal Preserv-A-Chem] Sodium saccharin; CAS 128-44-9; EINECS 204-886-1; artificial sweetener.

Unisweet VAN. [Universal Preserv-A-Chem] Vanillin; CAS 121-33-5; EINECS 204-465-2; perfume ingred.

Unisyn BEE. [Universal Preserv-A-Chem] Cetyl esters; raw material for personal care prods.

Unitan-L. [Universal Preserv-A-Chem] Sorbitan laurate; emulsifier.

Unitan-O. [Universal Preserv-A-Chem] Sorbitan oleate; CAS 1338-43-8; EINECS 215-665-4; emulsifier.

Unitan-P. [Universal Preserv-A-Chem] Sorbitan palmitate; CAS 26266-57-9; EINECS 247-568-8; emulsifier.

Unitan-S. [Universal Preserv-A-Chem] Sorbitan stearate; CAS 1338-41-6; EINECS 215-664-9; emulsifier.

Unitan-TRIOL. [Universal Preserv-A-Chem] Sorbitan trioleate; CAS 26266-58-0; EINECS 247-569-3; emulsifier.

Unitan-TRIST. [Universal Preserv-A-Chem] Sorbitan tristearate; CAS 26658-19-5; EINECS 247-891-4; emulsifier.

Uniterge NP 2. [Universal Preserv-A-Chem] Nonoxynol-2; EINECS 248-291-5; personal care surfactant.

Uniterge NP 4. [Universal Preserv-A-Chem] Nonoxynol-4; CAS 9016-45-9; personal care surfactant.

Uniterge NP 5. [Universal Preserv-A-Chem] Nonoxynol-5; CAS 9016-45-9; personal care surfactant.

Uniterge NP 6. [Universal Preserv-A-Chem] Nonoxynol-6; CAS 9016-45-9; personal care surfactant.

Uniterge NP 7. [Universal Preserv-A-Chem] Nonoxynol-7;

CAS 9016-45-9; EINECS 248-292-0; personal care surfactant.

Uniterge NP 8. [Universal Preserv-A-Chem] Nonoxynol-8; CAS 9016-45-9; personal care surfactant.

Uniterge NP 9. [Universal Preserv-A-Chem] Nonoxynol-9; CAS 9016-45-9; personal care surfactant.

Uniterge NP-10. [Universal Preserv-A-Chem] Nonoxynol-10; CAS 9016-45-9; EINECS 248-294-1; personal care surfactant.

Uniterge NP-13. [Universal Preserv-A-Chem] Nonoxynol-13; CAS 9016-45-9; personal care surfactant.

Uniterge NP-15. [Universal Preserv-A-Chem] Nonoxynol-15; CAS 9016-45-9; personal care surfactant.

Uniterge NP-20. [Universal Preserv-A-Chem] Nonoxynol-20; CAS 9016-45-9; personal care surfactant.

Uniterge NP 30. [Universal Preserv-A-Chem] Nonoxynol-30; CAS 9016-45-9; personal care surfactant.

Uniterge NP 40. [Universal Preserv-A-Chem] Nonoxynol-40; CAS 9016-45-9; personal care surfactant.

Uniterge NP-44. [Universal Preserv-A-Chem] Nonoxynol-44; CAS 9016-45-9; personal care surfactant.

Uniterge NP 50. [Universal Preserv-A-Chem] Nonoxynol-50; CAS 9016-45-9; personal care surfactant.

Uniterge NP 100. [Universal Preserv-A-Chem] Nonoxynol-100; CAS 9016-45-9; personal care surfactant.

Unitex 610-L. [Universal Preserv-A-Chem] Sodium lauriminodipropionate; CAS 14960-06-6; EINECS 239-032-7; personal care surfactant.

Unitex 710-L. [Universal Preserv-A-Chem] Lauraminopropionic acid; CAS 1462-54-0; EINECS 215-968-1; cosmetic surfactant.

Unitex P. [Universal Preserv-A-Chem] Etidronic acid; CAS 2809-21-4; EINECS 220-552-8; chelating agent.

Unithox® 420. [Petrolite] C20-40 pareth-3; nonionic; o/w emulsifier for cosmetics, vehicle for inert, difficult-to-disperse colorants, oils, and waxes; provides silky lubricating feel, superior film-forming chars.; for coatings, metalworking fluids, pulp/paper processing, textiles, mold releases; sol. in min. oil, butyl Cellosolve, xylene, toluene, MEK, perchloroethylene; sol. hazy in Stod., VM&P naphtha, kerosene; disp. in water, ethanol, IPA; m.w. 560; m.p. 91 C; HLB 4; hyd. no. 85; flash pt. 204 C; Ross-Miles foam 20 mm (initial, 50 C, 0.1%).

Unithox® 450. [Petrolite] C20-40 pareth-10; nonionic; component for water-based PU mold release agents; metalworking additive; o/w emulsifier for cosmetics, vehicle for inert, difficult-to-disperse colorants, oils, and waxes; provides silky lubricating feel, superior film-forming chars.; also for coatings, pulp/paper processing, textiles; solid; sol. in min. oil, cyclohexane, butyl Cellosolve, xylene, toluene, MEK, perchloroethylene; sol. hazy in Stod., VM&P naphtha, kerosene, ethanol, IPA; disp. in water, ethylene glycol; m.w. 900; m.p. 91 C; HLB 10; hyd. no. 55; flash pt. 218 C; surf. tens. 45 dynes/cm (0.01% aq.); Ross-Miles foam 25 mm (initial, 50 C, 0.1%); 50% EO.

Unithox® 480. [Petrolite] C20-40 pareth-40; nonionic; o/w emulsifier for cosmetics, vehicle for inert, difficult-to-disperse colorants, oils, and waxes; provides silky lubricating feel, superior film-forming chars.; also for coatings, metalworking fluids, pulp/paper processing, textiles, mold releases; sol. in min. oil, cyclohexane, ethylene glycol, butyl Cellosolve, xylene, toluene, MEK, perchloroethylene, ethyl acetate; sol. cloudy in Stod., VM&P naphtha, kerosene, ethanol, IPA; m.w. 2250; m.p. 86 C; HLB 16; hyd. no. 22; flash pt. 218 C; surf. tens. 52 dynes/cm (0.01% aq.); Ross-Miles foam 28 mm (initial, 50 C, 0.1%).

Unithox® 520. [Petrolite] C30-50 pareth-3; nonionic; o/w emulsifier for cosmetics, vehicle for inert, difficult-to-disperse colorants, oils, and waxes; provides silky lubricating feel, superior film-forming chars.; also for coatings, metalworking fluids, pulp/paper processing, textiles, mold releases; m.w. 700; m.p. 99 C; HLB 4; hyd. no. 67; flash pt. 232 C; Ross-Miles foam 15 mm (initial, 50 C, 0.1%).

Unithox® 550. [Petrolite] C30-50 pareth-10; nonionic; o/w emulsifier for cosmetics, vehicle for inert, difficult-to-disperse colorants, oils, and waxes; provides silky lubricating feel, superior film-forming chars.; also for coatings, metalworking fluids, pulp/paper processing, textiles, mold releases; m.w. 1100; m.p. 99 C; HLB 10; hyd. no. 41; flash pt. 232 C; surf. tens. 47 dynes/cm (0.01% aq.); Ross-Miles foam 26 mm (initial, 50 C, 0.1%).

Unithox® 720. [Petrolite] C40-60 pareth-3; nonionic; o/w emulsifier for cosmetics, vehicle for inert, difficult-to-disperse colorants, oils, and waxes; provides silky lubricating feel, superior film-forming chars.; also for coatings, metalworking fluids, pulp/paper processing, textiles, mold releases; m.w. 875; m.p. 106 C; HLB 4; hyd. no. 52; flash pt. 232 C; Ross-Miles foam 15 mm (initial, 50 C, 0.1%).

Unithox® 750. [Petrolite] C40-60 pareth-10; nonionic; o/w emulsifier for cosmetics, vehicle for inert, difficult-to-disperse colorants, oils, and waxes; provides silky lubricating feel, superior film-forming chars.; also for coatings, metalworking fluids, pulp/paper processing, textiles, mold releases; m.w. 1400; m.p. 106 C; HLB 10; hyd. no. 33; flash pt. 232 C; surf. tens. 53 dynes/cm (0.01% aq.); Ross-Miles foam 22 mm (initial, 50 C, 0.1%).

Unitina BW. [Universal Preserv-A-Chem] Glyceryl hydroxystearate, cetyl palmitate, microcryst. wax, trihydroxystearin; cosmetic ingred.

Unitina CP. [Universal Preserv-A-Chem] Cetyl palmitate; CAS 540-10-3; EINECS 208-736-6; emollient.

Unitina E-24. [Universal Preserv-A-Chem] PEG-20 glyceryl stearate; emulsifier, solubilizer.

Unitina GMO. [Universal Preserv-A-Chem] Glyceryl oleate; cosmetic ingred.

Unitina GMRO. [Universal Preserv-A-Chem] Glyceryl ricinoleate; CAS 141-08-2; EINECS 205-455-0; emulsifier.

Unitina HR. [Universal Preserv-A-Chem] Hydrog. castor oil; CAS 8001-78-3; EINECS 232-292-2; wax for cosmetics, pharmaceuticals.

Unitina KD-16. [Universal Preserv-A-Chem] Tallow glycerides and glyceryl stearate; cosmetic ingred.

Unitina LM. [Universal Preserv-A-Chem] Castor oil, glyceryl ricinoleate, octyldodecanol, carnauba, candelilla wax, microcryst. wax, cetyl alcohol, beeswax, min. oil.; cosmetic ingred.

Unitina MD, MD-A. [Universal Preserv-A-Chem] Glyceryl stearate; cosmetic ingred.

Unitol ISA. [Universal Preserv-A-Chem] Isostearic acid; CAS 2724-58-5; EINECS 220-336-3; emollient.

Unitolate. [Universal Preserv-A-Chem] Caprylic capric glyceride; cosmetic ingred.

Unitolate 80MG. [Universal Preserv-A-Chem] PEG-20 glyceryl stearate; emulsifier, solubilizer.

Unitolate 160-K. [Universal Preserv-A-Chem] Caprylic/ capric triglyceride; CAS 65381-09-1; cosmetic ingred.

Unitolate 165-C. [Universal Preserv-A-Chem] Glyceryl stearate, PEG-100 stearate; cosmetic ingred.

Unitolate 302. [Universal Preserv-A-Chem] Propylene glycol dicaprylate/dicaprate; emollient.

Unitolate 380. [Universal Preserv-A-Chem] Propylene glycol dicaprylate/dicaprate; emollient.

Unitolate 868. [Universal Preserv-A-Chem] Octyl stearate; emollient.

Unitolate A. [Universal Preserv-A-Chem] Hexyl laurate; CAS 34316-64-8; EINECS 251-932-1; emollient, vehicle for cosmetics.

Unitolate B. [Universal Preserv-A-Chem] Dibutyl adipate; CAS 105-99-7; EINECS 203-350-4; emollient.

Unitolate CSL. [Universal Preserv-A-Chem] Calcium stearoyl lactylate; CAS 5793-94-2; EINECS 227-335-7; emulsifier.

Unitolate GDS. [Universal Preserv-A-Chem] Glyceryl distearate; CAS 1323-83-7; EINECS 215-359-0; emulsifier, emollient.

Unitolate GMS. [Universal Preserv-A-Chem] Glyceryl stearate; cosmetic ingred.

Unitolate GMS-D. [Universal Preserv-A-Chem] Glyceryl stearate SE; cosmetic ingred.

Unitolate GS. [Universal Preserv-A-Chem] Glyceryl stearate; cosmetic ingred.

Unitolate GTA. [Universal Preserv-A-Chem] Triacetin; CAS 102-76-1; EINECS 203-051-9; cosmetics ingred.

Unitolate HE. [Universal Preserv-A-Chem] PEG-7 glyceryl cocoate; personal care surfactant.

Unitolate ISOST. [Universal Preserv-A-Chem] Glyceryl isostearate; cosmetic ingred.

Unitolate J600. [Universal Preserv-A-Chem] Oleyl erucate; CAS 17673-56-2; EINECS 241-654-9; emollient.

Unitolate LC. [Universal Preserv-A-Chem] Coco-caprylate/ caprate; cosmetic ingred.

Unitolate OLOL. [Universal Preserv-A-Chem] Oleyl oleate; CAS 3687-45-4; EINECS 222-980-4; emollient, lubricant.

Unitolate OPG. [Universal Preserv-A-Chem] Octyl pelargonate; CAS 59587-44-9; EINECS 261-819-9; emollient.

Unitolate PG/DPG. [Universal Preserv-A-Chem] Propylene glycol dipelargonate; CAS 41395-83-9; EINECS 255-350-9; emollient.

Unitolate PGIST. [Universal Preserv-A-Chem] Propylene glycol isostearate; CAS 68171-38-0; EINECS 269-027-5; solubilizer, cosmetic ingred.

Unitolate PGMS. [Universal Preserv-A-Chem] Propylene glycol stearate; CAS 1323-39-3; EINECS 215-354-3; personal care surfactant.

Unitolate PGO-1010. [Universal Preserv-A-Chem] Polyglyceryl-10 decaoleate; CAS 11094-60-3; EINECS 234-316-7; personal care emulsifier.

Unitolate PTP. [Universal Preserv-A-Chem] Pentaerythrityl tetrapelargonate; CAS 14450-05-6; EINECS 238-430-8; emollient.

Unitolate SSL. [Universal Preserv-A-Chem] Sodium stearoyl lactylate; CAS 25383-99-7; EINECS 246-929-7; emulsifier.

Unitolate V. [Universal Preserv-A-Chem] Decyl oleate; CAS 3687-46-5; EINECS 222-981-6; emollient.

Unitrienol T-27. [Induchem AG; Lipo] Farnesyl acetate, farnesol, panthenyl triacetate; a bioactive complex with cell regenerating props. for cosmetics, toiletries, pharmaceuticals.

Unitrienol T-272. [Induchem AG] PEG-12 glyceryl laurate, PEG-36 castor oil, farnesyl acetate, farnesol, panthenyl triacetate; a water-sol. bioactive complex with cell regenerating props. for cosmetics.

Univeg CCB. [Universal Preserv-A-Chem] Cocoa butter; CAS 8002-31-1; skin conditioner.

Univeg CS. [Universal Preserv-A-Chem] Corn starch; CAS 9005-25-8; cosmetic ingred.

Univegoil COCO. [Universal Preserv-A-Chem] Coconut oil; CAS 8001-31-8; EINECS 232-282-8; emollient.

Univegoil COTSD. [Universal Preserv-A-Chem] Cottonseed oil; CAS 8001-29-4; EINECS 232-280-7; cosmetic ingred.

Univegoil CRN. [Universal Preserv-A-Chem] Corn oil; CAS 8001-30-7; EINECS 232-281-2; cosmetic ingred.

Univegoil P-O. [Universal Preserv-A-Chem] Peanut oil; CAS 8002-03-7; EINECS 232-296-4; emollient.

Univegoil SUNFL. [Universal Preserv-A-Chem] Sunflower seed oil; CAS 8001-21-6; EINECS 232-273-9; lipid for cosmetics.

Universal MENT. [Universal Preserv-A-Chem] Menthol; CAS 89-78-1; EINECS 201-939-0; denaturant, flavor and fragrance component.

Universal ZPS. [Universal Preserv-A-Chem] Zinc phenolsulfonate; CAS 127-82-2; EINECS 204-867-8; antiseptic.

Universene AC. [Universal Preserv-A-Chem] Tetrasodium etidronate; CAS 3794-83-0; EINECS 223-267-7; chelating agent.

Universene ACID. [Universal Preserv-A-Chem] EDTA; CAS 60-00-4; EINECS 200-449-4; chelating agent.

Universene CaNa2. [Universal Preserv-A-Chem] Calcium disodium EDTA; CAS 62-33-9; EINECS 200-529-9; cosmetic preservative.

Universene Na2. [Universal Preserv-A-Chem] Disodium EDTA; CAS 139-33-3; EINECS 205-358-3; chelating agent.

Universene Na2 Cu. [Universal Preserv-A-Chem] Disodium EDTA-copper; CAS 14025-15-1; cosmetic ingred.

Universene Na3. [Universal Preserv-A-Chem] Trisodium EDTA; cosmetic ingred.

Universene Na4. [Universal Preserv-A-Chem] Tetrasodium EDTA; CAS 64-02-8; EINECS 200-573-9; chelating agent.

Univit-E Acetate. [Universal Preserv-A-Chem] Tocopheryl acetate; vitamin E source, antioxidant.

Univit-F. [Universal Preserv-A-Chem] Linol linolenic acid; cosmetic ingred.

Univit-F ETHES. [Universal Preserv-A-Chem] Ethyl linoleate, ethyl oleate, ethyl linolenate; cosmetic ingred.

Univit-F Forte. [Universal Preserv-A-Chem] Linolenic acid; CAS 463-40-1; EINECS 207-334-8; cosmetic ingred.

Univit-F Forte CLR. [Universal Preserv-A-Chem] Linoleic acid, linolenic acid; cosmetic ingred.

Univit-F Glyest CLR. [Universal Preserv-A-Chem] Glyceryl linoleate and glyceryllinolenate; cosmetic ingred.

Uniwax 1450. [Universal Preserv-A-Chem] PEG-6 and PEG-32; cosmetic ingred.

Uniwax AW-1060. [Astor Wax] Syn. wax; CAS 8002-74-2; cosmetic wax.

Uniwax C. [Universal Preserv-A-Chem] Emulsifying wax NF; cosmetic ingred.

Uniwax PARA. [Universal Preserv-A-Chem] Paraffin; CAS 8002-74-2; EINECS 232-315-6; cosmetic wax.

Uniwhite AO. [Universal Preserv-A-Chem] Titanium dioxide; CAS 13463-67-7; EINECS 236-675-5; mineral sunscreen.

Uniwhite KO. [Universal Preserv-A-Chem] Titanium dioxide; CAS 13463-67-7; EINECS 236-675-5; mineral sunscreen.

Uniwhite Oil 55, 70, 85, 130, 185, 205, 350. [Universal Preserv-A-Chem] Min. oil; emollient, cosmetic raw material.

Unizeen C-2. [Universal Preserv-A-Chem] PEG-2 cocamine; CAS 61791-14-8; emulsifier.

Unizeen C-5. [Universal Preserv-A-Chem] PEG-5 cocamine; CAS 61791-14-8; emulsifier.

Unizeen C-10. [Universal Preserv-A-Chem] PEG-10 cocamine; CAS 61791-14-8; emulsifier.

Unizeen OA. [Universal Preserv-A-Chem] Oleamidopropyl dimethylamine; CAS 109-28-4; EINECS 203-661-5; emollient, emulsifier.

Unizeen S-10. [Universal Preserv-A-Chem] PEG-10 soyamine; CAS 61791-24-0; personal care surfactant.

Unizeen S-15. [Universal Preserv-A-Chem] PEG-15 soyamine; CAS 61791-24-0; personal care surfactant.

Unizeen SA. [Universal Preserv-A-Chem] Stearamidopropyl dimethylamine; CAS 7651-02-7; EINECS 231-609-1; emulsifier.

Unizeen T-2. [Universal Preserv-A-Chem] PEG-2 hydrog. tallow amine; CAS 61791-26-2; emulsifier.

Unizeen T-5. [Universal Preserv-A-Chem] PEG-5 hydrog. tallow amine; CAS 61791-26-2; emulsifier.
Unizeen T-15. [Universal Preserv-A-Chem] PEG-15 hydrog. tallow amine; CAS 61791-26-2; emulsifier.
Unsoft 475. [Universal Preserv-A-Chem] Quaternium-27; hair conditioner.
Upamate DBA. [Universal Preserv-A-Chem] Dibutyl adipate; CAS 105-99-7; EINECS 203-350-4; emollient.
Upamate DIPA. [Universal Preserv-A-Chem] Diisopropyl adipate; CAS 6938-94-9; EINECS 248-299-9; cosmetic ester.
Upamate IPM. [Universal Preserv-A-Chem] Isopropyl myristate; CAS 110-27-0; EINECS 203-751-4; emollient.
Upamate IPP. [Universal Preserv-A-Chem] Isopropyl palmitate; CAS 142-91-6; EINECS 205-571-1; emollient.
Upamide ACMEA. [Universal Preserv-A-Chem] Acetamide MEA; CAS 142-26-7; EINECS 205-530-8; solvent, humectant for cosmetics.
Upamide C-2. [Universal Preserv-A-Chem] PEG-3 cocamide; CAS 61791-08-0; personal care surfactant.
Upamide C-5. [Universal Preserv-A-Chem] PEG-6 cocamide; CAS 61791-08-0; personal care surfactant.
Upamide CA-20. [Universal Preserv-A-Chem] Cocamide DEA; CAS 61791-31-9; EINECS 263-163-9; cosmetic surfactant.
Upamide CD. [Universal Preserv-A-Chem] Capramide DEA and diethanolamine; CAS 136-26-5; EINECS 205-234-9; cosmetic ingred.
Upamide CS-148. [Universal Preserv-A-Chem] Cocamide DEA; CAS 61791-31-9; EINECS 263-163-9; cosmetic surfactant.
Upamide KD. [Universal Preserv-A-Chem] Cocamide DEA; CAS 61791-31-9; EINECS 263-163-9; cosmetic surfactant.
Upamide L-2. [Universal Preserv-A-Chem] PEG-3 lauramide; CAS 26635-75-6; emulsifier, detergent.
Upamide L-5. [Universal Preserv-A-Chem] PEG-6 lauramide; CAS 26635-75-6; emulsifier, detergent.
Upamide LACAMEA. [Universal Preserv-A-Chem] Lactamide MEA; CAS 5422-34-4; EINECS 226-546-1; cosmetic ingred.
Upamide LD. [Universal Preserv-A-Chem] Lauramide DEA; CAS 120-40-1; EINECS 204-393-1; personal care surfactant.
Upamide LDS, LM-20, LS-173, LS-196. [Universal Preserv-A-Chem] Lauramide DEA; CAS 120-40-1; EINECS 204-393-1; cosmetic surfactant.
Upamide MEA. [Universal Preserv-A-Chem] Lauramide MEA; CAS 142-78-9; EINECS 205-560-1; personal care surfactant.
Upamide MIPA. [Universal Preserv-A-Chem] Lauramide MIPA; CAS 142-54-1; EINECS 205-541-8; foam stabilizer for cosmetics.
Upamide O-20. [Universal Preserv-A-Chem] Oleamide DEA; CAS 93-83-4; EINECS 202-281-7; thickener, foam booster/stabilizer.
Upamide OD. [Universal Preserv-A-Chem] Oleamide DEA; CAS 93-83-4; EINECS 202-281-7; thickener, foam booster/stabilizer.
Upamide PD. [Universal Preserv-A-Chem] Cocamide DEA and diethanolamine; cosmetic ingred.
Upamide Resin 1289. [Universal Preserv-A-Chem] Nylon 66; CAS 32131-17-2; cosmetic raw material.
Upamide Resin UPC-1283. [Universal Preserv-A-Chem] Nylon-66; CAS 32131-17-2; cosmetic raw material.
Upamide SD. [Universal Preserv-A-Chem] Stearamide DEA; CAS 93-82-3; EINECS 202-280-1; thickener, emulsifier.
Upamide SM. [Universal Preserv-A-Chem] Cocamide MEA; CAS 68140-00-1; EINECS 268-770-2; cosmetic surfactant.

Upamide SME-M. [Universal Preserv-A-Chem] Stearamide MEA; CAS 111-57-9; EINECS 203-883-2; personal care surfactant, thickener, pearlescent.
Upamide SS-10. [Universal Preserv-A-Chem] Soyamide DEA and diethanolamine; cosmetic ingred.
Uperlans. [Universal Preserv-A-Chem] Pearlescent agents.
U Pink 113. [Presperse] Ultramarine pink (90%), bismuth oxychloride (10%); inorg. colorant for pigmented cosmetics; JSCI/JCID approved.
Upiwax 163. [Universal Preserv-A-Chem] Cetearyl alcohol, PEG-12 stearate; cosmetic ingred.
Upiwax 163R. [Universal Preserv-A-Chem] Cetearyl alcohol, polysorbate 60; cosmetic ingred.
Upiwax 200. [Universal Preserv-A-Chem] PEG-4; CAS 25322-68-3; EINECS 203-989-9; cosmetic ingred.
Upiwax 300. [Universal Preserv-A-Chem] PEG-6; CAS 25322-68-3; EINECS 220-045-1; cosmetic ingred.
Upiwax 350. [Universal Preserv-A-Chem] PEG-6 methyl ether; CAS 9004-74-4; intermediate, solvent.
Upiwax 400. [Universal Preserv-A-Chem] PEG-8; CAS 25322-68-3; EINECS 225-856-4; cosmetic ingred.
Upiwax 600. [Universal Preserv-A-Chem] PEG-12; CAS 25322-68-3; EINECS 229-859-1; cosmetic ingred.
Upiwax 1000. [Universal Preserv-A-Chem] PEG-20; CAS 25322-68-3; cosmetic ingred.
Upiwax 3350. [Universal Preserv-A-Chem] PEG-75; CAS 25322-68-3; cosmetic ingred.
Upiwax 8000. [Universal Preserv-A-Chem] PEG-150; CAS 25322-68-3; cosmetic ingred.
Upiwax 20000. [Universal Preserv-A-Chem] PEG-350; cosmetic ingred.
Upiwax Synbee. [Universal Preserv-A-Chem] Syn. beeswax; cosmetics ingred.
USP-1. [Zinc Corp. of Am.] Zinc oxide USP; CAS 1314-13-2; EINECS 215-222-5; opacifier with mild deodorant props. for face powds., body powds., nursery powds., sunburn preventives, rouge sticks; protective astringent for dermatological ointments and lotions; used in can lacquers for pkg. of foods, in dental cements, and in silver-zinc batteries; FDA §73.1991; powd.; mean particle size 0.12 µ; 99.99% thru 325 mesh; surf. area 9 m^2/g; dens. 30 lb/ft^3.
USP-2. [Zinc Corp. of Am.] Zinc oxide USP; CAS 1314-13-2; EINECS 215-222-5; provides high covering power, opacity to uv light, and mild deodorant props. to face and body powds., sunburn preventives, rouge sticks; protective astringent in dermatological ointments and lotions; also in dental cements and silver-zinc batteries; powd.; mean particle size 0.31 µ; 99.99% thru 325 mesh; surf. area 3.5 m^2/g; sp.gr. 5.6; dens. 40 lb/ft^3; oil absorp. 12.
Utanol. [Universal Preserv-A-Chem] Guerbet alcohols; cosmetic ingred.
U Tanol G. [Universal Preserv-A-Chem] Octyldodecanol; CAS 5333-42-6; EINECS 226-242-9; carrier, lubricant, emollient.
U Tanol GST. [Universal Preserv-A-Chem] Octyldodecanol stearate; cosmetic ingred.
U Tanol HD, HD 70/75, HD 80/85, HD 90/95, HD CG. [Universal Preserv-A-Chem] Oleyl alcohol; CAS 143-28-2; EINECS 205-597-3; emollient.
U Tanol HDL CG. [Universal Preserv-A-Chem] Oleyl alcohol; CAS 143-28-2; EINECS 205-597-3; emollient.
Uvasorb 20H. [3V-Sigma] Benzophenone-1; CAS 131-56-6; EINECS 205-029-4; uv B absorber with max. absorption at wavelengths 290–320; improves lightfastness of dyes used in cosmetics; also protects colored, liq. detergents; pale yel. powd.; m.w. 214; sol. in polar solvs. (> 10% in acetone, 40% in ethanol, 40% in methanol); insol. in water; m.p. 144–146; 99% min. act.
Uvasorb MET. [3V-Sigma] Benzophenone-3; CAS 131-57-7; EINECS 205-031-5; uv B filter with max. absorp. at

wavelengths 280–320; for cosmetic prods., skin creams, sunscreens; pale yel. powd.; m.w. 228; sol. 20% in chloroform, 10% in flax oil, 4% in ethanol, 3% in methanol; insol. in water; m.p. 62–64 C; 99.5% act.

Uvasorb S-5. [3V-Sigma] Benzophenone-4; CAS 4065-45-6; EINECS 223-772-2; uv B filter with max. absorp. at wavelengths 290–320; for sunscreen preps. and prods. with high water or alcohol content (hair gel, lotions, o/w creams); light stabilizer for colored prods.; pale yel. cryst. powd.; m.w. 308; sol. 50% in methanol, 30% in ethanol, 25% in water; pH 1–2 (1% aq.); 97% min. act.

Uvinul® 400. [BASF; BASF AG] Benzophenone-1; CAS 131-56-6; EINECS 205-029-4; uv-A and B absorber; antiphoto-oxidant used for polyester, acrylics, PS, in outdoor paints and coatings, varnishes, colored liq. toiletries and cleaning agents, filters for photographic color films and prints, and rubber-based adhesives; Japan approval; ylsh. powd.; sol. in oils, alcohols, ether alcohols, propylene glycol, cyclic ethers, ketones, and esters; m.w. 214; m.p. ≥ 144 C; absorp. max. 288 nm; > 98% act.

Uvinul® D 49. [BASF] Benzophenone-6; CAS 131-54-4; EINECS 205-027-3; economical uv-A and B absorber for cosmetics, plastics, coatings, textiles; greater heat stability and more sol. (in chlorinated and aromatic solvs.); gives broad protection to PVC, chlorinated polyesters, epoxies, acrylics, urethanes, cellulosics, oil-based paints and varnishes, and cosmetics; Japan approval; yel. powd.; sol. in oils; m.w. 274; m.p. ≥ 130 C; absorp. max. 339 nm; > 98% act.

Uvinul® D 50. [BASF; BASF AG] Benzophenone-2; CAS 131-55-5; EINECS 205-028-9; uv-A and B absorber with the broadest uv absorp. spectrum; retards fading of colorants, pigments, and dyestuffs; improves stability of fragrances to oxidation; prolongs the life of polymeric materials; photostabilizes cosmetic formulations and minimizes discoloration of syn. rubber of plastic latices; Japan approval; yel. powd.; sol. in oils, ethanol, propylene glycol, 8% in IPM; m.w. 246; m.p. 195 C; absorp. max. 345 nm; > 98% act.

Uvinul® DS 49. [BASF; BASF AG] Benzophenone-9; CAS 3121-60-6; EINECS 221-498-8; sulfonated deriv. of Uvinul D 49; uv-A and B absorber in cosmetic formulations to prevent fading of colors and visc. changes caused by uv lt.; in textiles and water-based paints; Japan approval; yel. powd.; sol. in water, 1% in propylene glycol; m.w. 478; absorp. max. 331 nm; 67% act.

Uvinul® M 40. [BASF; BASF AG] Benzophenone-3; CAS 131-57-7; EINECS 205-031-5; uv-A/B absorber for cosmetics, plastics, and coatings, suncare preps., day creams; good weather resistance in resins and plastics; stabilizes PVC and polyesters against uv-lt. degradation; used in NC lacquers, varnishes, oil-based paints; USA (2-6%), EC (10%), and Japan (5%) approvals; lt. yel. powd.; sol. in oils, 12% in IPM, 6% in ethanol; m.w. 228; m.p. ≥ 62 C; absorp. max. 287 nm; > 98% act.

Uvinul® M 493. [BASF; BASF AG] Benzophenone-11; CAS 1341-54-4; uv-A and B absorber for cosmetics; yel. powd.;

sol. in oils, 2.5% in ethanol, propylene glycol, and IPM; m.p. ≥ 80 C; absorp. max. 347 nm.

Uvinul® MS 40. [BASF; BASF AG] Benzophenone-4; CAS 4065-45-6; EINECS 223-772-2; uv-A and B absorber in sunscreen prods. and in hair sprays and shampoos for dyed and tinted hair; for leather and textile fibers; visc. stabilizer for gels based on polyacrylic acid exposed to uv radiation; USA (5-10%), EC (5%), and Japan approvals; lt. yel. powd.; sol. in water, propylene glycol, alcohol; m.w. 308; pH 2 (1%); absorp. max. 285 nm; > 98% act.

Uvinul® N 35. [BASF] Etocrylene; CAS 5232-99-5; EINECS 226-029-0; noncolor contributing uv absorber; does not contain aromatic hydroxyl groups; effective under varying pH conditions; for NC lacquers and PVC; used in alkaline systems such as urea-formal-dehyde and epoxyamine formulations, and in cosmetics; wh. powd.; m.w. 277; m.p. 94–96 C; > 98% act.

Uvinul® N 539. [BASF] Octocrylene; CAS 6197-30-4; EINECS 228-250-8; uv-B absorber for cosmetics esp. water-resist. formulations, plastics, coatings; in flexible and rigid PVC; used in NC lacquers, varnishes, vinyl flooring, and oil-based paints; in aerosol and oil-based suntan lotions; nonreative with metallic driers; USA (7-10%) approval; yel. clear visc. liq.; sol. in nonpolar plastics; misc. with oils, min. spirits, ethanol, IPM; m.w. 361; f.p. –10 C; absorp. max. 302 nm; > 98% act.

Uvinul® P 25. [BASF; BASF AG] PEG-25 PABA; CAS 113010-52-9; nonionic; uv-B absorber for sunscreen prods., skin cosmetics; mild to the skin; EC (10%) approval; pale yel. slightly visc., turbid liq. that becomes clear at 30-40 C; misc. with water, ethanol, propylene glycol; m.w. 1265; absorp. max. 308 nm; 100% conc.; formerly Lusantan 25.

Uvinul® T 150. [BASF; BASF AG] Octyl triazone; CAS 88122-99-0; uv-B filter for cosmetic sun care preps., esp. water-resist. formulations; effective at small concs. to achieve high SPF values; EC (5%) approval; off-wh. to pale yel. powd.; sol. in oils; insol. in water; m.w. 823; m.p. ≥ 119 C; absorp. max. 312 nm; usage level: to 5%; 50% conc.

U Violet 109. [Presperse] Ultramarine violet (90%), bismuth-oxychloride (10%); CAS 12769-96-9, 7787-59-9; inorg. colorant for pigmented cosmetics; JSCI/JCID approved.

UV-Titan M210. [Presperse] Rutile titanium dioxide, alumina, and trimethylolethane; inorganic SPF for sun care prods., cosmetics, skin care prods.; provides protection against uv-B and uv-A radiation; disp. in water.

UV-Titan M212. [Presperse] Titanium dioxide, alumina, and glycerol; inorganic SPF for sun care prods., cosmetics, skin care prods.; disp. in water.

UV-Titan M260. [Presperse] Titanium dioxide, dimethicone, and alumina; inorganic SPF for sun care prods., cosmetics, skin care prods.; disp. in oil.

UV-Titan M262. [Presperse] Titanium dioxide, alumina, and dimethicone; inorganic SPF for sun care prods., cosmetics, skin care prods.; disp. in oil.

V

Valfor® Zeolite Na-A. [PQ Corp.] Sodium silicoaluminate; CAS 1344-00-9; EINECS 215-684-8; conditioner, anti-caking agent.

Vancide® 89 RE. [R.T. Vanderbilt] Captan; CAS 133-06-2; EINECS 205-087-0; antimicrobial and preservative for cosmetics and topical pharmaceuticals, veterinary prods.; wh. to off-wh. fine powd.; sol. (g/100 g solv.): 7.5 g xylene, 5.8 g cyclohexanone, 5.3 g chloroform, 5.2 g tetrachloroethane, 5.0 g ethyl acetate, 4.2 g acetone; dens. 1.7 mg/m³; m.p. 171–176 C; pH 5–6 (1% disp.); 97% assay.

Vanox® PCX. [R.T. Vanderbilt] 2,6-Di-t-butyl-4-methylphenol; CAS 128-37-0; EINECS 204-881-4; food-grade oxidation inhibitor used in soaps and cosmetics.

Vanseal® CS. [R.T. Vanderbilt] Cocoyl sarcosine; CAS 68411-97-2; EINECS 270-156-4; anionic; biodeg. surfactant, foaming and wetting agent, detergent, foam booster for soaps, bath gels, shampoos, shaving creams, denti-frices, rug shampoos, oven cleaners, dishwash, textile/leather processing; offers tolerance to hard water, mild-ness; pale yel. liq.; sol. in most org. solvs. (alcohols, ketones, glycols, ethers, aliphatic and aromatic hydrocarbons); m.w. 280; 94% min. act.

Vanseal® LS. [R.T. Vanderbilt] Lauroyl sarcosine; CAS 97-78-9; EINECS 202-608-3; anionic; biodeg. surfactant, foaming and wetting agent, detergent, foam booster for soaps, bath gels, shampoos, shaving creams, dentifrices, rug shampoos, oven cleaners, dishwash, textile/leather processing; offers tolerance to hard water, mildness; wh. waxy solid; sol. in most org. solvs. (alcohols, ketones, glycols, ethers, aliphatic and aromatic hydrocarbons); m.w. 270; soften. pt. 34-37 C; 94% min. act.

Vanseal® MS. [R.T. Vanderbilt] Myristoyl sarcosine; CAS 52558-73-3; EINECS 258-007-1; anionic; wetting and foaming agent, detergent, substantive to skin and hair, solubilizer, hydrotrope; for shampoos, cleansers, mouth-wash, dentifrice, shaving preps., styling mousses, house-hold and industrial prods. (rug shampoos, dishwash, alkaline cleaners); wh. waxy solid; sol. in most org. solvs. (alcohols, ketones, glycols, ethers, aliphatic and aromatic hydrocarbons); m.w. 298; soften. pt. 48-53 C; 94% min. act.

Vanseal® NACS-30. [R.T. Vanderbilt] Sodium cocoyl sarco-sinate; CAS 61791-59-1; EINECS 263-193-2; anionic; biodeg. surfactant, foaming and wetting agent, detergent, foam booster for soaps, bath gels, shampoos, shaving creams, dentifrices, rug shampoos, oven cleaners, dish-wash, textile/leather processing; offers tolerance to hard water, mildness; pale yel. liq.; water-sol.; pH 7.5-8.5 (10%); 29-31% act. in water.

Vanseal® NALS-30. [R.T. Vanderbilt] Sodium lauroyl sarco-sinate; CAS 137-16-6; EINECS 205-281-5; anionic; biodeg. surfactant, foaming and wetting agent, detergent, foam booster for soaps, bath gels, shampoos, shaving

creams, dentifrices, rug shampoos, oven cleaners, dish-wash, textile/leather processing; offers tolerance to hard water, mildness; colorless liq.; water-sol.; pH 7.5-8.5 (10%); 29-31% act. in water.

Vanseal® NALS-95. [R.T. Vanderbilt] Sodium lauroyl sarco-sinate; CAS 137-16-6; EINECS 205-281-5; anionic; biodeg. surfactant, foaming and wetting agent, detergent, foam booster for soaps, bath gels, shampoos, shaving creams, dentifrices, rug shampoos, oven cleaners, dish-wash, textile/leather processing; offers tolerance to hard water, mildness; wh. powd.; water-sol.; pH 7.5-8.5 (10%); 94% min. act.

Vanseal® NAMS-30. [R.T. Vanderbilt] Sodium myristoyl sarcosinate; CAS 30364-51-3; EINECS 250-151-3; an-ionic; wetting and foaming agent, detergent, substantive to skin and hair, solubilizer, hydrotrope; for shampoos, cleansers, mouthwash, dentifrice, shaving preps., styling mousses, household and industrial prods. (rug sham-poos, dishwash, alkaline cleaners); colorless liq.; water-sol.; pH 7.5-8.5 (10%); 29-31% act. in water.

Vanseal OS. [R.T. Vanderbilt] Oleoyl sarcosine; CAS 110-25-8; EINECS 203-749-3; anionic; biodeg. surfactant, foaming and wetting agent, detergent, foam booster for soaps, bath gels, shampoos, shaving creams, dentifrices, rug shampoos, oven cleaners, dishwash, textile/leather processing; offers tolerance to hard water, mildness; yel. liq.; sol. in most org. solvs. (alcohols, ketones, glycols, ethers, aliphatic and aromatic hydrocarbons); m.w. 349; 94% min. act.

Varamide® A-2. [Witco/H-I-P] Refined cocamide DEA (2:1); CAS 61791-31-9; EINECS 263-163-9; nonionic; thick-ener, foam stabilizer, and detergent for soaps, hand cleaners, bubble baths, textile applics. as a scouring and fulling agent, and in rug and floor cleaners; clear yel. liq.; water-disp.; dens. 8.5 lb/gal; pH 10.2 (1%); 100% act.

Varamide® A-7. [Witco/H-I-P] Oleamide DEA (2:1); CAS 93-83-4; EINECS 202-281-7; nonionic; rust inhibitor and base for o/w emulsifiers, detergents, anticorrosive clean-ers, and thickener for waterless hand cleaners; degreas-ers; emulsifier for oils in fiber and yarn lubricants; foam suppressor in solv. and dye carrier emulsions; personal care applics.; amber clear liq.; dens. 8.2 lb/gal; pH 10.4 (1%); 100% act.

Varamide® A-10. [Witco/H-I-P] Modified cocamide DEA (2:1); CAS 61791-31-9; EINECS 263-163-9; nonionic; thickener, foam stabilizer, detergent, rust inhibitor for floor cleaners and general-purpose cleaners; reduces neces-sary rinsing and increases visc., perfume and dye solubil-ity in anionic base cleaners; suitable for chain belt lubri-cants and metal-lathe working sol'ns.; also for personal care applics.; clear amber liq.; water-sol.; dens. 8.3 lb/gal; pH 8.8 (1%); 100% act.

Varamide® A-12. [Witco/H-I-P] Modified cocamide DEA (2:1); CAS 61791-31-9; EINECS 263-163-9; anionic; see

Varamide A-10; A-12 is a higher salt tolerance version designed for use at phosphate levels as high as 10%; clear amber liq.; dens. 8.2 lb/gal; pH 9 (1%); 100% act.

Varamide® A-80. [Witco/H-I-P] Modified coco DEA (2:1); CAS 61791-31-9; EINECS 263-163-9; general detergent base which solubilizes quickly and rinses easily; for personal care, household, and industrial applics.; liq.; 100% solids.

Varamide® A-83. [Witco/H-I-P] Modified coco DEA (2:1); CAS 61791-31-9; EINECS 263-163-9; anionic; lower cost version of Varamide A-10 used in personal care, industrial, institutional, and household cleaners, wh. sidewall cleaners, wax strippers, degreasers, and for textile scouring and fulling; liq.; dens. 8.3 lb/gal; pH 9 (1%); 100% conc.

Varamide® A-84. [Witco/H-I-P] Modified coco DEA (2:1); CAS 61791-31-9; EINECS 263-163-9; general-purpose detergent base which solubilizes quickly and rinses easily; for personal care and industrial applics.; liq.; 100% solids.

Varamide® AC-28. [Witco/H-I-P] Modified mixed DEA; emulsifier, anticorrosive in cutting oils, grinding oils, and metalworking liqs.; also for personal care applics.; liq.; sol. in hydrocarbons, emulsified in water; 100% solids.

Varamide® C-212. [Witco/H-I-P] Cocamide MEA (1:1); CAS 68140-00-1; EINECS 268-770-2; nonionic; foam booster/stabilizer in anionic systems; degreaser; hair conditioning agent; visc. modifier; for personal care, household, and industrial applics., powder and stick formulations; flake; 100% solids.

Varamide® FBR. [Witco/H-I-P] Surfactant blend; anionic/nonionic; conc. for floor and hard surf. cleaners, truckwash, personal care applics.; liq.; 100% solids.

Varamide® L-203. [Witco/H-I-P] Lauramide MEA (1:1); CAS 142-78-9; EINECS 205-560-1; nonionic; foam booster and stabilizer for aq. systems; degreaser; hair conditioner, visc. modifier; for household and industrial applics.; flake; 100% act.

Varamide® LL-1. [Witco/H-I-P] Lauramide DEA (1:1); CAS 120-40-1; EINECS 204-393-1; foam stabilizer, thickener, and conditioning agent for personal care prods.; clear liq.; water-disp.; 100% solids.

Varamide® LO-1. [Witco/H-I-P] Linoleamide DEA (1:1); CAS 56863-02-6; EINECS 260-410-2; thickener and foam stabilizer for shampoos, baby bath, and hand soap; conditioning agent; clear liq.; 100% solids.

Varamide® MA-1. [Witco/H-I-P] Refined cocamide DEA (1:1); CAS 61791-31-9; EINECS 263-163-9; nonionic; foam stabilizer and booster, thickener, conditioner; basic liq. superamide for shampoos, bubble bath, and dishwashes; low cost equivalent to lauric superamide; does not require melting; gives higher visc. and foam stability than conventional 2:1 alkanolamides in liq. detergent systems; Gardner 3+ max. clear liq.; readily disp. in water; dens. 8.2 lb/gal; pH 9.8 (1%).; 100% act.

Varamide® ML-1. [Witco/H-I-P] Lauramide DEA (1:1); CAS 120-40-1; EINECS 204-393-1; nonionic; thickener, foam stabilizer, and conditioner for shampoo, bubble bath, and hand laundry detergent; gives the highest visc., foam level, and stability of the superamides in series; wh. wax; water-disp.; dens. 8.1 lb/gal; pH 10.2 (1%); 100% conc.

Varamide® ML-4. [Witco/H-I-P] Lauramide DEA (1:1); CAS 120-40-1; EINECS 204-393-1; nonionic; detergent, foam stabilizer, thickener, and conditioner for shampoos, shower gel formulations, industrial cleaning applics.; wh. wax; dens. 8.2 lb/gal; pH 10.2 (1%); 100% conc.

Varamide® T-55. [Witco/H-I-P] Tallow MEA ethoxylate; detergent base for floor and hard-surface cleaners; tolerant to high builder levels and hard water; also for personal care applics.; liq.; 100% conc.

Varifoam® A. [Witco/H-I-P] Blend; anionic; shampoo conc.

for high performance baby shampoos; liq.; 57% conc.

Varifoam® SXC. [Witco/H-I-P] TEA-lauryl sulfate, cocamidopropyl hydroxysultaine, lauramide DEA, methylparaben; anionic; high-foaming, cost-effective shampoo base; liq.; 38% solids.

Varine C. [Witco/H-I-P] Coco hydroxyethyl imidazoline; CAS 61791-38-6; EINECS 263-170-7; cationic; emulsifier, anticorrosive, raw material for surfactant prod.; shampoo base, penetrating oils, antistats, corrosion inhibitors, paints, printing inks, textiles, adhesives; Gardner 9 liq.; m.w. 274; disp. in water; sol. in polar solvs. and hydrocarbons; m.p. 31 C; 100% act.

Varine O®. [Witco/H-I-P] Oleyl hydroxyethyl imidazoline; cationic; emulsifier, anticorrosive for automotive body panels, raw material; shampoo base, penetrating oils, antistats, corrosion inhibitors, paints, printing inks, textiles, adhesives; Gardner 8 liq.; m.w. 352; sol. in polar solvs. and hydrocarbons; m.p. –10 C; 100% act.

Varine O Acetate. [Witco/H-I-P] Oleic imidazoline acetate; anticorrosive; also for personal care applics.; liq.; 100% solids.

Varine T. [Witco/H-I-P] Tall oil hydroxyethyl imidazoline; CAS 61791-39-7; EINECS 263-171-2; cationic; anticorrosive for automobile industry; also for personal care applics.; Gardner 8; m.w. 350; sol. in polar solvs. and hydrocarbons; disp. in water; m.p. –10 C; 100% solids, 85% tert. amine.

Varion® 2C. *See Rewoteric AM 2C-W*

Varion® AM-KSF-40. *See Rewoteric AM KSF-40*

Varion® AM-R40. [Witco/H-I-P] Ricinoleamidopropyl betaine; CAS 71850-81-2; amphoteric; baby and child cosmetic formulations; liq.; 40% conc.

Varion® AM-V. *See Rewoteric AM V*

Varion® CADG-HS. [Witco/H-I-P] Cocamidopropyl betaine; amphoteric; surfactant; detergent; foam booster and visc. modifier for personal care prods., textile aux., heavy-duty detergents; LS is low-salt version; yel. clear liq.; pH 6.5–8.5; 35–37% solids.

Varion® CDG-LS. [Witco/H-I-P] Lauryl betaine; CAS 683-10-3; EINECS 211-669-5; amphoteric; foaming agent in acid systems; low salt version of CDG; also for personal care prods.; liq.; 35% solids.

Varion® CDG. [Witco/H-I-P] Lauryl betaine; CAS 683-10-3; EINECS 211-669-5; amphoteric; foamer, detergent, solubilizer, conditioner used in shampoos, acid cleaners; lime soap dispersant; liq.; sol. in water and electrolytes; 31% act.

Varion® HC. *See Rewoteric AM HC*

Varion® SDG. [Witco/H-I-P] Stearyl betaine; CAS 820-66-6; EINECS 212-470-6; amphoteric; detergent, softener for fabric and hair applics.; liq.; 50% conc.

Varion® TEG-40%. *See Rewoteric AM TEG-40*

Variquat® 50AC. [Witco/H-I-P] Benzalkonium chloride, IPA; germicidal conc. for disinfection and sanitization; hair conditioner; liq.; 50% solids.

Variquat® 50AE. [Witco/H-I-P] Benzalkonium chloride, ethanol; germicidal conc. for disinfection and sanitization; hair conditioner; liq.; 50% solids.

Variquat® 50MC. [Witco/H-I-P] Benzalkonium chloride; cationic; germicide, algicide, disinfectant, sanitizer, deodorant; used in pesticides and mfg. of sanitizers; food processing, dairy, restaurant, industrial and household prods.; hair conditioner; Gardner 2 max. liq.; m.w. 358; flash pt. (PM) 120 F; 50% act.

Variquat® 50ME. [Witco/H-I-P] Dimethyl alkyl (C12–C16) benzyl ammonium chloride (50%), ethyl alcohol (7.5%) in water; specialty quat., germicide used for disinfection and sanitizing for hospitals, beautician instruments, food processing plants; hair conditioner; Gardner 2 max. liq.; m.w. 358; sol. in water or alcohol; sp.gr. 0.96; dens. 8.0 lb/gal; flash pt. 120 F (P-M); pH 5–8; 57.5% act.

Variquat® 60LC. [Witco/H-I-P] Benzalkonium chloride; cationic; swimming pool and water treatment algicide; hair conditioner; Gardner 2 max. liq.; m.w. 351; flash pt. (PM) 130 F; 49.5–51.5% quat.

Variquat® 66. [Witco/H-I-P] Ethyl bis (polyethoxy ethanol) tallow ammonium chloride; antistat and degreaser for aq. cleaning systems; hair conditioner; liq.; 72% solids.

Variquat® 80AC. [Witco/H-I-P] Benzalkonium chloride, IPA; IPA version of Variquat 80MC; hair conditioner; liq.; 80% solids.

Variquat® 80AE. [Witco/H-I-P] Benzalkonium chloride, ethanol; ethanol version of Variquat 80MC; hair conditioner; liq.; 80% solids.

Variquat® 80LC. [Witco/H-I-P] Benzyl chloride quat.; algicide conc. for swimming pools; hair conditioner; liq.; 80% solids.

Variquat® 80MC. [Witco/H-I-P] Dimethyl alkyl (C12–16) benzyl ammonium chloride; cationic; germicide, disinfectant, deodorant used in pesticides and sanitizers; corrosion inhibitor for water inj. systems; hair conditioner; liq.; m.w. 358; flash pt. (PM) 100 F; 80% act.

Variquat® 80ME. [Witco/H-I-P] Dimethyl alkyl (C12–C16) benzyl ammonium chloride; germicidal conc. for disinfection and sanitization; mildewcide, antistat; catalyst for caustic treatment of polyester yarn or fabric; hair conditioner; liq.; Gardner 2 max.; m.w. 358; flash pt. 100 F (P-M); 80% solids.

Variquat® 477. [Witco/H-I-P] N-Tallow pentamethyl propane diammonium dichloride, IPA/water; hair conditioner.

Variquat® 638. [Witco/H-I-P] PEG-2 cocomonium chloride, IPA; cationic; detergent booster, antistat, emulsifier for hard surf. cleaners, other liq. detergents, textiles; plating bath foam blanket; base for hair conditioners, creme rinses, antistats; coemulsifier; Gardner 9 max. liq.; m.w. 353; flash pt. (PM) 56 F; 74-75% solids in IPA.

Variquat® B200. [Witco/H-I-P] Benzyltrimethyl ammonium chloride; cationic; dispersant, dye leveler and retarder, emulsifier used in textile industry; hair conditioner; APHA 50 max. liq.; pH 6.5–8.0; 60% act.

Variquat® B343. [Witco/H-I-P] Dihydrog. tallow methyl benzyl ammonium chloride; specialty quat.; hair conditioner; Gardner 2 max. paste; m.w. 656; flash pt. 84 F (PM); 74–76% quat.

Variquat® B345. [Witco/H-I-P] Dimethyl hydrog. tallow benzyl ammonium chloride; CAS 61789-72-8; EINECS 263-081-3; specialty quat.; hair conditioner; liq.; Gardner 3 max.; m.w. 417; flash pt. 81 F (PM); 75–77% solids.

Variquat® CE 100. [Witco/H-I-P] Alkyl (C12-16) ethyl dimethyl ethyl sulfate; hair conditioner.

Variquat® E290. [Witco/H-I-P] Cetrimonium chloride; CAS 112-02-7; EINECS 203-928-6; cationic; quat. for personal care prods.; Gardner I max. clear liq.; 28.5–30.0% in water.

Variquat® K300. [Witco/H-I-P] Dimethyl dicoco ammonium chloride, IPA; CAS 61789-77-3; EINECS 263-087-6; cationic; low cloud pt. emulsifier, dispersant; hair conditioner; also for laundry detergent-softeners; Gardner 5 max. liq.; m.w. 460; flash pt. 50 F (PM); 75% conc.

Variquat® K375. [Witco/H-I-P] Dicoco dimethyl ammonium chloride in hexylene glycol; CAS 61789-77-3; EINECS 263-087-6; specialty quat.; hair conditioner; liq.; Gardner 5 max.; m.w. 439; flash pt. > 200 F (P-M); 74–77% quat.

Variquat® K-1215. [Witco/H-I-P] PEG-15 cocomonium chloride; CAS 61791-10-4; cationic; emulsifier, antistat for personal care prods., textiles; Gardner 11 max. liq.; m.w. 910; flash pt. (PM) 258 F; 95% quat. min.

Variquat® S-1202. [Witco/H-I-P] Methyl bis (2-hydroxyethyl) stearyl ammonium chloride, IPA; hair conditioner.

Variquat® SDC. [Witco/H-I-P] Stearalkonium chloride, IPA/water; CAS 122-19-0; EINECS 204-527-9; hair conditioner.

Varisoft® 2TD. [Witco/H-I-P] Ditridecyl dimethyl ammonium chloride, aq. ethanol; CAS 68910-56-5; softener, conditioner, base for hair conditioners and creme rinses; esp. for Afro-Amer. hair; amber clear liq.; pH 7 (5% in 50:50 IPA/water); 75% solids in aq. ethanol.

Varisoft® 5TD. [Witco/H-I-P] PEG-5 ditridecylmonium chloride; hair conditioner, antistat, emulsifier, softener for textured hair; good rinseability, exc. manageability and shine; yel. clear liq.; pH 7; 60% quat.

Varisoft® 110. [Witco/H-I-P] Dihydrog. tallowamidoethyl hydroxyethylmonium methosulfate, IPA/water; cationic; nonyellowing fabric softener conc. for home and commercial laundries, textile processing; hair conditioner and lotion component; Gardner 6 max. paste; flash pt. (PMCC) 99 F; 75% solids.

Varisoft® 110 DEG. [Witco/H-I-P] Methyl bis (hydrog. tallow amidoethyl) 2-hydroxyethyl ammonium methosulfate, modified, diethylene glycol; fabric softener; hair conditioner and lotion component; Gardner 6 solid; flash pt. (PMCC) > 200 F; 75% solids.

Varisoft® 110-PG. [Witco/H-I-P] Dihydrog. tallowamidoethyl hydroxyethylmonium methosulfate in aq. propylene glycol; base for hair conditioners and creme rinses; antistat; paste; 75% solids.

Varisoft® 136-100P. [Witco/H-I-P] Proprietary; quat. for fabric softeners; hair conditioner and lotion component; Gardner 4 solid; flash pt. (PMCC) > 200 F; 100% solids.

Varisoft® 137. [Witco/H-I-P] Dihydrog. tallow dimonium methosulfate, IPA; cationic; quat. for home and commercial laundry fabric and tissue softeners, debonding agent and antistat; emulsifier; hair conditioner and lotion component; Gardner 5 solid paste; m.w. 656; disp. in water; dens. 7.4 lb/gal; flash pt. 78 F (PMCC); pH 5–8; 89–91% solids.

Varisoft® 222 (75%). [Witco/H-I-P] Methyl bis (tallowamidoethyl) 2-hydroxyethyl ammonium methyl sulfate, IPA; cationic; fabric softener conc. for home and commercial laundries, textile processing; hair conditioner and lotion component; Gardner 6 max. liq.; flash pt. (PMCC) 72 F; 74–76% solids.

Varisoft® 222 (90%). [Witco/H-I-P] Methyl bis (tallowamidoethyl) 2-hydroxyethyl ammonium methyl sulfate, IPA; specialty quat. for rinse cycle fabric softeners; hair conditioner and lotion component; Gardner 6 max. paste; flash pt. (PMCC) 85 F; 89–91% solids.

Varisoft® 222 HV (90%). [Witco/H-I-P] Methyl bis (tallow amidoethyl) 2-hydroxyethyl ammonium methosulfate, modified, IPA; fabric softener; hair conditioner and lotion component; Gardner 6 paste; flash pt. (PMCC) 85 F; 90% solids.

Varisoft® 222 LM (90%). [Witco/H-I-P] Methylbis (tallow amidoethyl) 2-hydroxy ethyl ammonium methyl sulfate, IPA; softener with exc. handling properties for laundry rinse-cycle softeners; hair conditioner and lotion component; Gardner 6 liq.; flash pt. (PMCC) 85 F; 90% solids.

Varisoft® 222 LT (90%). [Witco/H-I-P] Methyl bis (oleyl amidoethyl) 2-hydroxyethyl ammonium methylsulfate, IPA; cationic; softener conc. for formulation of liq. detergent-softeners or high solids softener prods.; hair conditioner and lotion component; Gardner 8 liq.; flash pt. (PMCC) 75 F; 90% solids.

Varisoft® 222 PG (90%). [Witco/H-I-P] Methyl bis (tallow amidoethyl) 2-hydroxyethyl ammonium methosulfate, modified, propylene glycol; fabric softener; hair conditioner and lotion component; Gardner 6 hazy liq.; flash pt. (PMCC) > 200 F; 90% solids.

Varisoft® 238 (90%). [Witco/H-I-P] Methyl bis (tallowamidoethyl) 2-hydroxypropyl ammonium methyl sulfate; specialty quat.; hair conditioner and lotion component; Gardner 6 max. liq.; flash pt. 85 F (P-M); 89–91% solids.

Varisoft® 250. [Witco/H-I-P] Cetrimonium chloride; CAS 112-02-7; EINECS 203-928-6; base for hair conditioners/ creme rinses; imparts softness and manageability to hair without greasiness; antistat, surfactant, emulsifier; hair grooming aids; Gardner 1 clear liq.; pH 4 (5% in 50:50 IPA/ water); 24-27% solids in water.

Varisoft® 300. [Witco/H-I-P] Cetrimonium chloride; CAS 112-02-7; EINECS 203-928-6; base for hair conditioners and creme rinses; imparts softness and manageability without greasiness; Gardner 1 clear liq.; pH 9 (5% in 50:50 IPA/water); 28-30% solids in water.

Varisoft® 355. [Witco/H-I-P] Cetrimonium chloride; CAS 112-02-7; EINECS 203-928-6; base for hair conditioners and creme rinses; imparts softness and manageability without greasiness; Gardner 4 clear liq.; pH 7 (5% in 50:50 IPA/water); 50% solids in water/IPA.

Varisoft® 432-100. [Witco/H-I-P] Dicetyl dimonium chloride; CAS 1812-53-9; EINECS 217-325-0; coemulsifier; antistat, conditioner for hair care preps., creme rinses; solv.-free; off-wh. paste; pH 8 (5% in 50:50 IPA/water); 91% quat.

Varisoft® 432-CG. [Witco/H-I-P] Dicetyl dimonium chloride, IPA; CAS 68391-05-9; base, conditioner, antistat for hair conditioners and creme rinses; coemulsifier; Gardner 2 clear liq.; dilutable with cold water; flash pt. (PMCC) 70 F; pH 7 (5% in 50:50 IPA/water); 68% quat. in IPA, 10% water.

Varisoft® 432-ET. [Witco/H-I-P] Dicetyl dimonium chloride, ethanol; CAS 68391-05-9; base, conditioner, and antistat for hair conditioners and cream rinses; coemulsifier; Gardner 2 clear liq.; dilutable with cold water; flash pt. (PMCC) 70 F; pH 7 (5% in 50:50 IPA/water); 68% quat. in ethanol, 10% water.

Varisoft® 432-PPG. [Witco/H-I-P] Dicetyldimonium chloride in propylene glycol; CAS 68391-05-9; antistat, conditioner for hair care preps., creme rinses; Gardner 4 clear liq.; flash pt. (PMCC) > 200 F; pH 8 (5% in 50:50 IPA/water); 68% quat. in propylene glycol, 10% water.

Varisoft® 442-100P. [Witco/H-I-P] Quaternium-18; CAS 61789-80-8; EINECS 263-090-2; base for hair conditioners and creme rinses; coemulsifier; powd.; 100% solids.

Varisoft® 445. [Witco/H-I-P] Methyl (1) hydrog. tallow amidoethyl (2) hydrog. tallow imidazolinium methosulfate; fabric softener conc. for home and commercial laundries, textile processing; hair conditioner and lotion component; Gardner 7 paste; flash pt. (PMCC) 72 F; 75% solids.

Varisoft® 461. [Witco/H-I-P] Cocotrimonium chloride, IPA; CAS 61789-18-2; EINECS 263-038-9; base for hair conditioners and creme rinses; used in hot oil treatments; liq.; 50% solids in IPA.

Varisoft® 462. [Witco/H-I-P] Dicocodimonium chloride, aq. IPA; CAS 61789-77-3; EINECS 263-087-6; base for hair conditioners and creme rinses; liq.; 75% solids in aq. IPA.

Varisoft® 470. [Witco/H-I-P] Ditallowdimonium chloride, aq. IPA; base for hair conditioners and creme rinses; softens hair; paste; 75% solids in aq. IPA.

Varisoft® 471. [Witco/H-I-P] Tallowtrimonium chloride, IPA; CAS 8030-78-2; EINECS 232-447-4; base for hair conditioners and cream rinses; liq.; 50% solids in IPA.

Varisoft® 475. [Witco/H-I-P] Quaternium-27, IPA; CAS 86088-85-9; cationic; fabric softener conc. for home and commercial laundries, textile processing; hair conditioner; Gardner 5 max. liq.; flash pt. 72 F (PM); 75–77% solids.

Varisoft® 910. [Witco/H-I-P] Methyl bis (2-hydroxyethyl) coco ammonium chloride, IPA; fabric softener; hair conditioner and lotion component; soft paste; m.w. 335; flash pt.

(PMCC) 66 F; 75% solids.

Varisoft® 920. [Witco/H-I-P] Tallow bis hydroxyethyl methyl ammonium chloride; cationic; softener conc. for anionic/ nonionic based detergent/softeners; hair conditioner and lotion component; Gardner 6 soft paste; m.w. 400; flash pt. (PMCC) 66 F; 75% act.

Varisoft® 950. [Witco/H-I-P] Quat.; for nonionic-based laundry detergent-softeners; hair conditioner and lotion component; soft paste.

Varisoft® 3690. [Witco/H-I-P] Methyl (1) oleylamidoethyl (2) oleyl imidazolinium methosulfate, IPA; cationic; quat. for laundry detergent-softeners; hair conditioner and lotion component; Gardner 7 max. liq.; m.w. 723; flash pt. (PMCC) 66 F; 75% solids.

Varisoft® 3690N (90%). [Witco/H-I-P] Methyl-1 oleyl amidoethyl 2-oleyl-imidazolinium methyl sulfate; fabric softener; hair conditioner and lotion component; Gardner 6 liq.; m.w. 723; flash pt. (PMCC) > 200 F; 98% solids.

Varisoft® BT-85. [Witco/H-I-P] Behentrimonium chloride; CAS 17301-53-0; EINECS 241-327-0; antistat, suspending agent for body and hand creams and lotions; base for hair conditioners and creme rinses; wh. solid flakes; pH 7 (5% in 50:50 IPA/water); 85% solids, 80% quat.

Varisoft® BTMS. [Witco/H-I-P] Cetearyl alcohol, behenyltrimonium methosulfate; cationic; self-emulsifying wax for hair and skin formulations; flakes; 100% solids.

Varisoft® CRC. [Witco/H-I-P] Cetearyl alcohol, dicetyl dimonium chloride, stearamidopropyl dimethylamine; cost-effective creme rinse conc. for formulating creme rinses and conditioners; waxy flake; m.p. 49 C; pH 8.8 (5% in 1:1 IPA/water); 100% solids.

Varisoft® C SAC. [Witco/H-I-P] Cetearyl alcohol, stearalkonium chloride, PEG-40 castor oil; cost-effective conc. for formulating creme rinses and conditioners; based on Varisoft SDAC; waxy flake; 100% solids.

Varisoft® CTB-40. [Witco/H-I-P] Cetrimonium bromide; CAS 57-09-0; EINECS 200-311-3; base for hair conditioners and creme rinses; antistat; conditioner for skin creams and lotions; synergistic with proteins; Gardner 1+ clear liq.; pH 8 (10% aq.); 40% quat. in water/ethanol.

Varisoft® DHT. [Witco/H-I-P] Quaternium-18, IPA; CAS 68002-59-5; cationic; antistat, base for hair conditioners and creme rinse concs.; coemulsifier; off-wh. paste; disp. in water; m.w. 569; dens. 7.12 lb/gal; flash pt. (PMCC) 68 F; pH 7 (5% in 50:50 IPA/water); 74–77% act. in aq. IPA.

Varisoft® DS-100. [Witco/H-I-P] Proprietary; quat. for fabric softeners; hair conditioner and lotion component; Gardner 4 solid; flash pt. (PMCC) > 200 F; 100% solids.

Varisoft® LAC. [Witco/H-I-P] Lauryltrimonium chloride; CAS 112-00-5; EINECS 203-927-0; base for hair conditioners and creme rinses; liq.; 36-38% solids.

Varisoft® OIMS. [Witco/H-I-P] Quaternium-81, aq. IPA; base for hair conditioners, creme rinses, antistats; coemulsifier; exc. antistat and curl retention props.; liq.; 75% solids in aq. IPA.

Varisoft® PIMS. [Witco/H-I-P] Quaternium 27 in propylene glycol; base for hair conditioners and creme rinses; liq.; 75% solids.

Varisoft® SDAC. [Witco/H-I-P] Stearalkonium chloride, IPA; CAS 122-19-0; EINECS 204-527-9; base for hair conditioners and creme rinses; antistat; detangles and conditions hair, easy wet and dry comb-out; imparts softness without making hair limp or oily; wh. paste; pH 4 (2% in 1:1 IPA/water); toxicology: may cause irritation to eyes, skin, and mucous membranes; 25% solids, 17% quat., 5% IPA.

Varisoft® SDAC-W. [Witco/H-I-P] Stearalkonium chloride; CAS 122-19-0; EINECS 204-527-9; base for hair conditioners; imparts softness, manageability, antistatic props. to hair; easy wet and dry comb-out; wh. paste; pH 4 (2% in 1:1 IPA/water); toxicology: may cause irritation to eyes, skin, and mucous membranes; 25% solids, 18% quat., trace IPA.

Varisoft®SDC-85. [Witco/H-I-P] Stearalkonium chloride and stearyl alcohol; antistat, base for hair conditioners; emulsifier for creams and lotions; Gardner 3 waxy flakes; pH 7 (10% in 50:50 IPA/water); 85% quat.

Varisoft® ST-50. [Witco/H-I-P] Steartrimonium chloride aq. alcohol sol'n.; CAS 112-03-8; EINECS 203-929-1; substantive quat. imprating softness and manageability to hair; Gardner 6 clear liq.; pH 7.5 (5% aq.); 50% act. in water.

Varisoft® TA-100. [Witco/H-I-P] Distearyldimonium chloride; CAS 107-64-2; EINECS 203-508-2; cationic; base for hair conditioners and creme rinses; imparts softness, manageability, and antistatic props. to hair; emulsifier for creams and lotions, skin care prods., pigmented cosmetics; wh. to off-wh. free-flowing powd.; disp. in warm water; pH 8 (10% in 50:50 IPA/water); 91% quat., 4% water.

Varisoft® TC-90. [Witco/H-I-P] Tricetylmonium chloride; CAS 52467-63-7; base for hair conditioners, creme rinses, 2-in-1 shampoos; antistat; Gardner 3 sm. gran.; pH 7 (5% in 50:50 IPA/water); 95% solids, 90% quat.

Varisoft® TIMS. [Witco/H-I-P] Quaternium-27; CAS 68122-86-1; base for creme rinses and conditioners; antistat, substantivity agent, conditioner; Gardner 5 liq.; flash pt. (PMCC) 70 F; pH 6 (5% in 50:50 IPA/water); 75% quat.

Varisoft® TS-50. [Witco/H-I-P] Steartrimonium chloride, aq. alcohol; CAS 112-03-8; EINECS 203-929-1; base for hair conditioners; liq.; 75% solids.

Varisoft® TSC. [Witco/H-I-P] Steartrimonium chloride; CAS 112-03-8; EINECS 203-929-1; base for hair conditioners; liq.; 25% solids in water.

Varonic® 32-E20. [Witco/H-I-P] Oleth-20; CAS 9004-98-2; nonionic; emulsion stabilizer, moisturizer, and emollient for creams and lotions; surfactant for hot oil treatments, hair color, and creme rinses; paste; HLB 15.3; 100% solids.

Varonic® 63 E20. [Witco/H-I-P] Ceteareth-20; CAS 68439-49-6; nonionic; emulsion stabilizer, emulsifier, solubilizer, moisturizer, and emollient for creams and lotions; surfactant for stick formulations and hair conditioners; solid; HLB 15.7; 100% solids.

Varonic® 2271. [Witco/H-I-P] PEG-8 tallowamine; dye leveler; improves wettability and reduces dye affinity at the surf., permitting more even migration onto substrates such as hair; coemulsifier and stabilizer for emulsion systems; neutralizer, plasticizer; antistat in acidic systems; liq.; HLB 10.0; 99% solids.

Varonic® BD. [Witco/H-I-P] Cetearyl alcohol, ceteareth-20; nonionic; self-emulsifying wax, visc. modifier for hair conditioners, creams and lotions; emulsifier, solubilizer; waxy flake; 100% solids.

Varonic® BG. [Witco/H-I-P] Stearyl alcohol, ceteareth-20; nonionic; self-emulsifying wax, visc. modifier for hair conditioners, creams and lotions; emulsifier, solubilizer; waxy flake; 100% solids.

Varonic® DM55. [Witco/H-I-P] Methyl capped glycol ether; solv. with low toxicity and exc. grease cutting properties for surf. cleaners; textile scouring; skin and hair care prods.; liq.; water-emulsifiable; 100% solids.

Varonic® K-202. [Witco/H-I-P] PEG-2 cocamine; CAS 61791-14-8; nonionic; dye leveler for hair dyes; coemulsifier and stabilizer for cosmetic emulsions; neutralizer and plasticizer; emulsifier; antistat in acidic systems; corrosion inhibitor in metal finishing (e.g. as cutting oil additives); detergent, antifouling, antistalling, and deicing agent in gasoline; also in textile lubricants, oil field emulsification; Gardner 2 liq.; sol. in IPA, benzene, Stod., CCl$_4$, MEK; insol. in water; sp.gr. 0.916; HLB 6.2; 99% solids.

Varonic® K-202 SF. [Witco/H-I-P] PEG-2 cocamine; CAS

61791-14-8; nonionic; dye leveler; improves wettability and reduces dye affinity at the surf., permitting more even migration onto substrates such as hair; coemulsifier and stabilizer for emulsion systems; neutralizer, plasticizer; antistat in acidic systems; liq.; HLB 6.2; 99% solids.

Varonic® K-205. [Witco/H-I-P] PEG-5 cocamine; CAS 61791-14-8; nonionic; dye leveler; improves wettability and reduces dye affinity at the surf., permitting more even migration onto substrates such as hair; coemulsifier and stabilizer for emulsion systems; neutralizer, plasticizer; antistat in acidic systems; corrosion inhibitor, antifouling agent in gasoline; antistat, lubricant in wool spinning; emulsifier and leveling agent in textile dyeing; insecticide and herbicide systems; metal finishing; Gardner 7 liq.; sol. in IPA, benzene, Stod., CCl$_4$, MEK; sp.gr. 0.977; HLB 11.0; 99% solids.

Varonic® K-205 SF. [Witco/H-I-P] PEG-5 cocamine; CAS 61791-14-8; nonionic; dye leveler; improves wettability and reduces dye affinity at the surf., permitting more even migration onto substrates such as hair; coemulsifier and stabilizer for emulsion systems; neutralizer, plasticizer; antistat in acidic systems; liq.; HLB 11.0; 99% solids.

Varonic® K-210. [Witco/H-I-P] PEG-10 cocamine; CAS 61791-14-8; nonionic; dye leveling agent, dispersant in hair dyes, paper industry; coemulsifier and stabilizer for cosmetic emulsions; neutralizer and plasticizer; antistat for acidic systems; wetting and spreading agent and emulsifier in insecticides and herbicides; tanning of leather and furs; wetting and redeposition aids in fur treating; Gardner 7 liq.; sol. in water, IPA, benzene, CCl$_4$; sp.gr. 0.995; HLB 13.8; 99% solids.

Varonic® K-210 SF. [Witco/H-I-P] PEG-10 cocamine; CAS 61791-14-8; nonionic; dye leveler; improves wettability and reduces dye affinity at the surf., permitting more even migration onto substrates such as hair; coemulsifier and stabilizer for emulsion systems; neutralizer, plasticizer; antistat in acidic systems; liq.; HLB 13.8; 99% solids.

Varonic® K-215. [Witco/H-I-P] PEG-15 cocamine; CAS 61791-14-8; nonionic; dye leveler for hair colors; coemulsifier and stabilizer for cosmetic emulsions; neutralizer; plasticizer; antistat for acidic systems; wetting agent and redeposition aid in fur treatment; textile additive in spinning bath to reduce jet clogging and disperse sulfur/zinc sulfide particles to prevent cratering; in petrol. industry for corrosion resistance; Gardner 7 liq.; sol. in water, IPA, benzene, CCl$_4$, MEK; sp.gr. 1.040; HLB 15.4; 99% solids.

Varonic® K-215 LC. [Witco/H-I-P] PEG-15 cocamine; CAS 61791-14-8; low-color version of Varonic K215; wetting agent during liming stage in tanning of leathers and furs; textile aid reducing jet clogging in spinning bath and dispersing sulfur/zinc sulfide particles preventing cratering; skin and hair care prods.; Gardner 3 liq.; sol. in water, IPA, benzene, CCl$_4$, MEK; sp.gr. 1.040; HLB 15.4; 100% solids.

Varonic® K-215 SF. [Witco/H-I-P] PEG-15 cocamine; CAS 61791-14-8; nonionic; dye leveler; improves wettability and reduces dye affinity at the surf., permitting more even migration onto substrates such as hair; coemulsifier and stabilizer for emulsion systems; neutralizer, plasticizer; antistat in acidic systems; liq.; HLB 15.4; 99% solids.

Varonic® LI-42. [Witco/H-I-P] PEG-20 glyceryl stearate; nonionic; low-irritation detergent, emulsifier, lubricant, solubilizer for household and industrial applics., personal care prods.; Gardner 2 paste; m.p. 27 C; HLB 13; surf. tens. 44 dynes/cm (1%); 100% solids.

Varonic® LI-48. [Witco/H-I-P] PEG-80 glyceryl tallowate; nonionic; emulsifier, solubilizer, thickener, dispersant, antiirritant surfactant used in household and industrial applics., personal care prods.; Gardner 2 hard solid; sol. in water, methanol, ethanol, IPA, acetone, and butyl

Cellosolve; m.p. 41 C; HLB 18.0; pH 7.0; surf. tens. 49.5 dynes/cm; 100% conc.

Varonic® LI-63. [Witco/H-I-P] PEG-30 glyceryl cocoate; nonionic; low-irritation detergent, emulsifier, solubilizer for soaps, specialized lubricants, personal care prods.; Gardner 2 paste; HLB 15.9; m.p. 27 C; surf. tens. 40 dynes/cm (1%); 100% solids.

Varonic® LI-67. [Witco/H-I-P] PEG-80 glyceryl cocoate; nonionic; low-irritation detergent, emulsifier, solubilizer for personal care prods.; liq. soaps gelling agent; Gardner 2 solid; m.p. 42 C; HLB 18; surf. tens. 47 dynes/cm (1%); 100% solids.

Varonic® LI-67 (75%). [Witco/H-I-P] PEG-80 glyceryl cocoate; nonionic; low-irritation detergent, emulsifier, solubilizer for personal care prods., household and industrial applics.; liq.; HLB 18.0; 75% solids in water.

Varonic® LI-420. [Witco/H-I-P] PEG-200 glyceryl tallowate; nonionic; visc. builder and modifier, moisturizer, emulsifier, and stabilizer for creams and lotions, low-irritation shampoos; solid; m.p. 53 C; HLB 19.0; 100% conc.

Varonic® LI-420 (70%). [Witco/H-I-P] PEG-200 glyceryl tallowate; nonionic; visc. builder and modifier, moisturizer, emulsifier, and stabilizer for creams and lotions, low-irritation shampoos; hazy liq.; HLB 19.0; 70% solids.

Varonic® MT 65. [Witco/H-I-P] Methyl capped alkoxylated fatty alcohol; nonionic; low-foam detergent, wetting agent, textile spinning lubricant; skin and hair care prods.; Gardner 2 clear liq.; sol. in polar and nonpolar solvs.; pH 3.5 (10%); surf. tens. 32 dynes/cm; 100% solids.

Varonic® MT 65. [Witco/H-I-P] Methyl capped alkoxylated fatty alcohol; nonionic; low-foam detergent, wetting agent, textile spinning lubricant; skin and hair care prods.; Gardner 2 clear liq.; sol. in polar and nonpolar solvs.; pH 3.5 (10%); surf. tens. 32 dynes/cm; 100% solids.

Varonic® Q-202. [Witco/H-I-P] PEG-2 oleamine; dye leveler for hair colors; coemulsifier and stabilizer for cosmetic emulsions; neutralizer; plasticizer; antistat in acidic systems; anticorrosive emulsifier for metalworking, grinding oils; liq.; HLB 4.7; 99% solids.

Varonic® Q-202 SF. [Witco/H-I-P] PEG-2 oleamine; dye leveler; improves wettability and reduces dye affinity at the surf., permitting more even migration onto substrates such as hair; coemulsifier and stabilizer for emulsion systems; neutralizer, plasticizer; antistat in acidic systems; liq.; HLB 4.7; 99% solids.

Varonic® Q-205. [Witco/H-I-P] PEG-5 oleamine; nonionic; dye leveler for hair colors; coemulsifier and stabilizer for cosmetic emulsions; neutralizer; plasticizer; antistat in acidic systems; liq.; HLB 8.4; 99% solids.

Varonic® Q-205 SF. [Witco/H-I-P] PEG-5 oleamine; dye leveler; improves wettability and reduces dye affinity at the surf., permitting more even migration onto substrates such as hair; coemulsifier and stabilizer for emulsion systems; neutralizer, plasticizer; antistat in acidic systems; liq.; HLB 8.4; 99% solids.

Varonic® Q-230. [Witco/H-I-P] PEG-30 oleamine; nonionic; compatiblizer or antiprecipitant in dye bath of acid and cationic dyes; mild dye leveler and/or stripping agent for acid dyes; hydrophilic emulsifier; skin and hair care prods.; liq.; 100% solids.

Varonic® S-202. [Witco/H-I-P] PEG-2 stearamine; CAS 10213-78-2; EINECS 233-520-3; dye leveler for hair colors; coemulsifier and stabilizer for cosmetic emulsions; neutralizer; plasticizer; antistat in acidic systems; polymer additive and emulsifier; paste; HLB 5.0; 99% solids.

Varonic® S-202 SF. [Witco/H-I-P] PEG-2 stearamine; CAS 10213-78-2; EINECS 233-520-3; dye leveler; improves wettability and reduces dye affinity at the surf., permitting more even migration onto substrates such as hair; coemulsifier and stabilizer for emulsion systems; neutral-

izer, plasticizer; antistat in acidic systems; paste; HLB 5.0; 99% solids.

Varonic® T-202. [Witco/H-I-P] PEG-2 tallowamine; CAS 61791-44-4; nonionic; dye leveler for hair colors; coemulsifier and stabilizer for cosmetic emulsions; neutralizer; plasticizer; antistat in acidic systems; lubricant, softener, scouring aid, dye leveler and antistat for textiles; in syn. latex paints; emulsifier for latex, dyes, and oils; dispersant; acid cleaners; process modifier in polymer industry; raw material for quat. and amphoteric surfactants; Gardner 2 semiliq.; sol. in IPA, benzene, Stod., CCl₄; insol. in water; sp.gr. 0.915; HLB 5.1; 99% solids.

Varonic® T-202 SF. [Witco/H-I-P] PEG-2 tallowamine; CAS 61791-44-4; dye leveler; improves wettability and reduces dye affinity at the surf., permitting more even migration onto substrates such as hair; coemulsifier and stabilizer for emulsion systems; neutralizer, plasticizer; antistat in acidic systems; paste; HLB 5.1; 99% solids.

Varonic® T-202 SR. [Witco/H-I-P] PEG-2 tallowamine; CAS 61791-44-4; surfactant for optimum visc. control in acid cleaners; skin and hair care prods.; paste; HLB 5.1; 100% solids.

Varonic® T-205. [Witco/H-I-P] PEG-5 tallowamine; CAS 61791-44-4; nonionic; dye leveler for hair colors; coemulsifier and stabilizer for cosmetic emulsions; neutralizer; plasticizer; antistat in acidic systems; lubricant, softener, and antistat for syn. fibers; antistat/lubricant in wool spinning; emulsifier/leveling agent in water/oil dye systems; emulsifier and spreading-wetting agent in insecticides and herbicides; process modifier for polymers; Gardner 7 liq.; sol. in IPA, benzene, Stod., CCl₄, MEK; emul. in water; sp.gr. 0.966; HLB 9.2; 99% solids.

Varonic® T-205 SF. [Witco/H-I-P] PEG-5 tallowamine; CAS 61791-44-4; dye leveler; improves wettability and reduces dye affinity at the surf., permitting more even migration onto substrates such as hair; coemulsifier and stabilizer for emulsion systems; neutralizer, plasticizer; antistat in acidic systems; liq.; HLB 9.2; 99% solids.

Varonic® T-210. [Witco/H-I-P] PEG-10 tallowamine; nonionic; dye leveler for hair colors; coemulsifier and stabilizer for cosmetic emulsions; neutralizer; plasticizer; antistat in acidic systems; lubricant, scouring aid, dye leveler for textile industry; process modifier in polymer industry; raw material for quat. and amphoteric surfactants; liq.; HLB 12.6; 99% solids.

Varonic® T-210 SF. [Witco/H-I-P] PEG-10 tallowamine; dye leveler; improves wettability and reduces dye affinity at the surf., permitting more even migration onto substrates such as hair; coemulsifier and stabilizer for emulsion systems; neutralizer, plasticizer; antistat in acidic systems; liq.; HLB 12.6; 99% solids.

Varonic® T-215. [Witco/H-I-P] PEG-15 tallowamine; nonionic; dye leveler for hair colors; coemulsifier and stabilizer for cosmetic emulsions; neutralizer; plasticizer; antistat in acidic systems; lubricant, softener, and antistat for textiles; wetting aid/emulsifier in tanning; in petrol. industry with caustic to break o/w crude oil emulsions and to impart corrosion resistance; raw material for quat. and amphoteric surfactants; Gardner 7 liq.; sol. in water, IPA, benzene, CCl₄, MEK; sp.gr 1.029; HLB 14.4; 99% conc.

Varonic® T-215LC. [Witco/H-I-P] PEG-15 tallowamine; low-color version of Varonic T215; skin and hair care prods.; liq.; HLB 14.4; 100% solids.

Varonic® T-215 SF. [Witco/H-I-P] PEG-15 tallowamine; dye leveler; improves wettability and reduces dye affinity at the surf., permitting more even migration onto substrates such as hair; coemulsifier and stabilizer for emulsion systems; neutralizer, plasticizer; antistat in acidic systems; liq.; HLB 14.4; 99% solids.

Varonic® T-220. [Witco/H-I-P] PEG-20 tallowamine; nonionic; acid dye leveler for nylon; antiprecipitant for mixed dye baths; migrating agent for dispersed dyes; wool lubricant and antistat; antistat for spin finishes; skin and hair care prods.; liq.; 100% solids.

Varonic® T-250. [Witco/H-I-P] PEG-50 tallowamine; non-ionic; acid dye leveler with less effect on lightfastness; dye bath antiprecipitant; leveling agent for cationic and dispersed dyes; emulsifier; skin and hair care prods.; liq.; 100% solids.

Varonic® U-215. [Witco/H-I-P] PEG-15 hydrog. tallowamine; CAS 61791-26-2; nonionic; nylon leveling agent; antiprecipitant for mixed dye baths; migrating agent for dispersed dyes; skin and hair care prods.; solid; 100% solids.

Varox® 185E. [Witco/H-I-P] Dihydroxyethyl C12-15 alkoxypropylamine oxide; nonionic; detergent, foam booster/stabilizer for anionic surfactants used in liq. dishwashing, shampoos and fabric detergents; Gardner 1 liq.; pH 4.5–5.5; surf. tens. 31.5 dynes/cm; 39–43% amine oxide.

Varox® 270. [Witco/H-I-P] Lauramine oxide; CAS 1643-20-5; EINECS 216-700-6; low-irritation emulsifier, foam booster, and stabilizer; visc. builder; conditioner, antistat for hair care prods.; liq.; 30% solids.

Varox® 365. [Witco/H-I-P] Lauramine oxide; CAS 1643-20-5; EINECS 216-700-6; nonionic; low-irritation emulsifier, detergent, foam booster/stabilizer, visc. modifier for anionic surfactants for shampoo and detergent systems, textiles; conditioner and antistat for hair care prods.; hypochlorite-stable; Gardner 1 liq.; 30% solids.

Varox® 375. [Witco/H-I-P] Lauramine oxide; CAS 1643-20-5; EINECS 216-700-6; hypochlorite-stable foam booster/stabilizer for skin care prods., hair conditioners; liq.; 40% solids.

Varox® 743. [Witco/H-I-P] Cocodihydroxyethylamine oxide; nonionic; detergent, foam booster and stabilizer; liq.; 50% conc.

Varox® 1770. [Witco/H-I-P] Cocamidopropylamine oxide; CAS 68155-09-9; EINECS 268-938-5; nonionic; low-irritation emulsifier, mild detergent, foam booster/stabilizer, visc. modifier for liq. soaps, shampoos, textile scouring; conditioner, antistat for hair care prods.; liq.; 35% act.

Varsulf® MS30. [Witco/H-I-P] Surfactant blend; foaming, dry-residue rug and upholstery shampoo conc.; skin care prods., hair conditioners; liq.; 30% solids.

Varsulf® NOS-25. [Witco/H-I-P] Sodium alkylphenol polyglycol ether sulfate; anionic; emulsifier for emulsion polymerization; skin care prods., hair conditioners; lt. yel. clear liq.; pH 7.0 (1%); 35% conc.

Varsulf® S-1333. [Witco/H-I-P] Disodium ricinoleamido MEA-sulfosuccinate aq. disp.; anionic; mild detergent, refatting agent used in dishwash, liq. soaps, and personal care prods.; skin friendly, improved skin feel; anti-irritant for other surfactants; coemulsifier; pale yel. liq.; dens. 9.4 lb/gal; visc. 300 cps; pH 6.5–7.5; surf. tens. 28.8 dynes/cm; 40% solids in water.

Varsulf® SBF-12. [Witco/H-I-P] Disodium lauryl sulfosuccinate; low-irritation foaming agent for shampoos, bubble bath, body cleansers; some conditioning and moisturizing effects; detergent for fine fabric wash systems; paste; 40% solids.

Varsulf® SBFA-30. [Witco/H-I-P] Disodium laureth sulfosuccinate aq. disp.; anionic; detergent, refatting agent used in dishwash, fine fabric wash, liq. soaps; low-irritation foaming agent, conditioner, moisturizer for shampoos, bubble bath, and body cleansers; wh.-pale yel. liq.; dens. 9.2 lb/gal; visc. 200 cps; pH 6.5–7.5; surf. tens. 21.7 dynes/cm; 40% solids in water.

Varsulf® SBL-203. [Witco/H-I-P] Disodium lauramido MEA-sulfosuccinate aq. disp.; CAS 25882-44-4; EINECS 247-310-4; anionic; low-irritation foaming and cleansing

agent, foam stabilizer for personal care prods.; detergent, refatting agent used in dishwash, lt. duty detergents, rug and upholstery shampoos; Gardner 3 max. liq.; dens. 9.5 lb/gal; visc. 100–500 cps; pH 6.5–7.5; surf. tens. 24.3 dynes/cm; 39.0% min. solids in water.

Vaseline 335 G. [Ceca SA] Vaseline meeting European and US pharmacopoeias; excipient in pharmaceutical and cosmetic industries, as ointments for skin where actives must remain on epidermis, base for laxatives, opthalmologic ointments, creams, and salves, makeup, hair prods., veterinary prods.; Mettler drop pt. 45-50 C.

Vaseline 7702. [Ceca SA] Vaseline meeting European and US pharmacopoeias; excipient in pharmaceutical and cosmetic industries, as ointments for skin where actives must remain on epidermis, base for laxatives, opthalmologic ointments, creams, and salves, makeup, hair prods., veterinary prods.; Mettler drop pt. 46-52 C.

Vaseline 8332. [Ceca SA] Vaseline meeting European and US pharmacopoeias; excipient in pharmaceutical and cosmetic industries, as ointments for skin where actives must remain on epidermis, base for laxatives, opthalmologic ointments, creams, and salves, makeup, hair prods., veterinary prods.; Mettler drop pt. 44-49 C.

Vaseline 10049 BL. [Ceca SA] Vaseline BP/USP; excipient in pharmaceutical and cosmetic industries, as ointments for skin where actives must remain on epidermis, base for laxatives, opthalmologic ointments, creams, and salves, makeup, hair prods., veterinary prods.; Mettler drop pt. 55-60 C.

Vaseline A. [Ceca SA] Vaseline meeting European and US pharmacopoeias; excipient in pharmaceutical and cosmetic industries, as ointments for skin where actives must remain on epidermis, base for laxatives, opthalmologic ointments, creams, and salves, makeup, hair prods., veterinary prods.; Mettler drop pt. 51-57 C.

Veegum®. [R.T. Vanderbilt] Complex colloidal magnesium aluminum silicate derived from natural smectite clays; CAS 12199-37-0; EINECS 235-374-6; thickener, visc. modifier, emulsion stabilizer for emulsions, suspensions, sol'ns., liqs., creams and pastes, cosmetics, toiletries, toothpaste, pharmaceuticals, paints, textile finishes, chemical specialties, industrial applics.; suspending agent for powd. and pigments; binder for inorg. powd. and pigments; disintegrating agent in tablets; pigment dispersant; improves spreadability of lotions, creams, and ointments; wh. to tan sm. flakes, odorless, tasteless; insol. in water or alcohol; swells to many times original vol. in water to form colloidal disp; dens. 2.6 mg/m³; visc. 250 cps ± 25% (5% aq. disp.); pH 9.5 (5% aq disp.); 8% moisture.

Veegum® D. [R.T. Vanderbilt] Magnesium aluminum silicate; CAS 12199-37-0; EINECS 235-374-6; see Veegum; fast dispersing, fluoride compat. grade; good for dentifrice binder systems; wh. flakes, odorless, tasteless; visc. 100-300 cps (5% aq. disp.).

Veegum® F. [R.T. Vanderbilt] Magnesium aluminum silicate; CAS 12199-37-0; EINECS 235-374-6; see Veegum; microfine grade used in tablets for dry blending of fine powd.; prep. of ointments and pastes where dry incorporation is essential; wh. microfine powd., odorless, tasteless; insol. in water or alcohol; swells to many times original vol. in water to form colloidal disp.; visc. 187-312 cps (5.5% disp.); pH 9.5 (5% aq disp.); 8% moisture.

Veegum® HS. [R.T. Vanderbilt] Magnesium aluminum silicate; CAS 12199-37-0; EINECS 235-374-6; see Veegum; max. electrolyte stability; wh. flakes, odorless, tasteless; insol. in water or alcohol; swells to many times original vol. in water to form colloidal disp.; visc. 75-225 cps (5.5% disp.); pH 9 (5% aq. disp.); 8% moisture.

Veegum® HV. [R.T. Vanderbilt] Magnesium aluminum silicate; CAS 12199-37-0; EINECS 235-374-6; see

Veegum; high visc. at low solids is desired; emulsification and suspension are obtained at low solids; mostly for cosmetics and pharmaceuticals; wh. flakes, odorless, tasteless; insol. in water or alcohol; swells to many times original vol. in water to form colloidal disp.; visc. 187-312 cps (4% aq. disp.); 8% moisture.

Veegum® K. [R.T. Vanderbilt] Magnesium aluminum silicate; CAS 12199-37-0; EINECS 235-374-6; see Veegum; for pharmaceutical acid suspensions; has low acid demand and high acid compatibility; wh. flakes, odorless, tasteless; insol. in water or alcohol; swells to many times original vol. in water to form colloidal disp.; visc. 165-275 cps (5.5% disp.); pH 9.5 (5% aq.); 8% moisture.

Veegum® PRO. [R.T. Vanderbilt] Tromethamine magnesium aluminum silicate; emulsion stabilizer, suspending agent for cosmetics, pharmaceuticals, veterinary prods., chem. specialties, household prods.; superior soap and surfactant compatibility; hydrates rapidly in cold or hot water to form high visc. disps.; wh. flakes, odorless, tasteless; visc. 300-500 cps (1.5% aq. disp.).

Veegum® Ultra. [R.T. Vanderbilt] Magnesium aluminum silicate; CAS 12199-37-0; EINECS 235-374-6; efficient thickener, stabilizer, and suspending agent for cosmetics and toiletries, esp. skin care prods.; pH balanced, easy to hydrate; whitest and brightest in series; works synergistically with anionic polymers; wh. free-flowing powd.; visc. 325 cps (5% aq. disp.); pH 4.7 (5% aq. disp.); toxicology: nontoxic, nonirritating; 4% moisture.

Veegum® WG. [R.T. Vanderbilt] Magnesium aluminum silicate; CAS 12199-37-0; EINECS 235-374-6; see Veegum; esp. for use as a disintegrator in the dry compounding of tablets and in ointments and pastes where dry incorporation is essential; low acid demand; wh. powd., odorless, tasteless; 50 mesh.

Vegamide. [Les Colorants Wackherr] Ceramides derived from wheat; cosmetic ingred.

Vegamino™ 30-SF. [Brooks Industries] Vegetable amino acids; moisture binding agent substantive to skin and hair; used in perms and for chemically treated hair; yel. liq.; low odor; m.w. 100; 30% act.

Vegebios. [Solabia; Barnet Prods.] Colorless botanical extracts for use in clear prods.

Vegepro W. [Les Colorants Wackherr] Hydrolyzed wheat protein; CAS 70084-87-6; cosmetic protein.

Vegetol®. [Gattefosse SA] Wide range of plant extracts for use in cosmetics.

Velsan® D8P-3. [Sandoz] Isopropyl PPG-2-isodeceth-7-carboxylate; noncomedogenic emollient that helps to solubilize cosmetic actives; provides emulsion visc., wetting, and softer feel for skin care, sun care, hair care, bath, and pigmented prods.; lt. yel. oil; sol. @ 5% in SDA-40 ethanol, propylene glycol; disp. in dist. water, glycerin; sp.gr. 1.02; HLB 14.; toxicology: LD50 (acute oral) > 5 g/kg; pract. nonirritating to skin and eyes.

Velsan® D8P-16. [Sandoz] Cetyl PPG-2 isodeceth-7 carboxylate; emollient for skin care, sun care, hair care, pigmented prods., bath prods.; solubilizer for cosmetic actives; lt. yel. paste/semisolid; disp. in min. oil; sp.gr. 0.97; HLB 12; toxicology: LD50 (acute oral) > 5 g/kg; not a primary skin irritant; pract. nonirritating to eyes.

Velsan® P8-3. [Hercules; Sandoz] Isopropyl C12-15 pareth-9-carboxylate; emollient for cosmetics providing emulsion visc., wetting, and softer feel to skin care, sun care, bath, and pigmented prods.; lt. yel. oil; sol. in water, SDA-40 ethanol; sp.gr. 1.01; HLB 18; toxicology: LD50 (acute oral) > 5 g/kg; mild eye irritant, not a primary skin irritant.

Velsan® P8-16. [Sandoz] Cetyl C12-15-pareth-9-carboxylate; emollient for cosmetics providing emulsion visc., wetting, and softer feel to skin care, sun care, bath, and pigmented prods.; yel. semisolid paste; disp. @ 20% in

hot min. oil, glycerin; sp.gr. 0.95; HLB 9; toxicology: LD50 (acute oral) > 5 g/kg; not a primary skin irritant; nonirritating to eyes.

Velvetex® AB-45. [Henkel/Cospha; Henkel Canada] Cocobetaine; CAS 68424-94-2; EINECS 270-329-4; amphoteric; surfactant, conditioner, emulsifier, solubilizer used in industrial use, liq. detergents, cleansing emulsions, personal care prods.; visc. builder, gelling agent; lime soap dispersant; frothing agent; Gardner 2 clear liq.; water-sol.; sp.gr. 1.03; visc. < 100 cps; cloud pt. < 0 C; pH 6.5–8.5 (10%); 43–45% solids.

Velvetex® BA-35. [Henkel Canada] Cocamidopropyl betaine; amphoteric; surfactant used in foam drilling and blanketing; air-inhibiting agent for cement gypsum board and cleaners for oily surfaces; mild surfactant and conditioner for hair, bath, and skin care prods.; pronounced substantivity, antistatic props.; stable in strong acid and alkaline sol'ns.; good foaming props.; liq.; dens. 8.2 lb/gal.

Velvetex® BK-35. [Henkel/Cospha; Henkel Canada] Cocamidopropyl betaine; amphoteric; nonirritating surfactant and conditioner for hair care prods., skin cleansers, foam baths; visc. builder; pronounced substantivity, antistatic props.; stable in strong acid and alkaline sol'ns.; good foaming props.; yel. clear liq.; water-sol.; sp.gr. 1.039; visc. < 100 cps; pH 4.5–5.5; 34.0–36.0% solids.

Velvetex® CDC. [Henkel/Cospha; Henkel Canada] Disodium cocoamphodiacetate; CAS 68650-39-5; EINECS 272-043-5; amphoteric; mild, high foaming surfactant for low-irritation liq. and gel shampoos, conditioners, body cleansers, bath and shower preps.; lt. amber visc. liq.; 50% act.

Velvetex® GC-88. [Henkel/Cospha] Sodium cocoamphoacetate; personal care surfactant.

Velvetex® LTD. [Henkel/Cospha] Disodium lauroamphodiacetate, sodium trideceth sulfate.

Velvetex® OLB-30. [Henkel/Cospha] Oleyl betaine; CAS 871-37-4; EINECS 212-806-1; conditioner for shampoos and bath preps.

Velvetex® OLB-50. [Henkel/Cospha; Henkel Canada] Oleyl betaine; CAS 871-37-4; EINECS 212-806-1; amphoteric; mild, foaming detergent, visc. builder, conditioner used in conditioning shampoos, bath and cleansing prods., mfg. of fibers and cutting oils; substantive to hair and skin; imparts unique silky feel to surfactant systems; amber translucent gel; water-sol.; sp.gr. 0.953 (60 C); pH 6.0–8.0 (10%); 50% act.

Velvet Veil 310. [Presperse] Mica (90%), silica beads (10%); CAS 12001-26-2, 7631-86-9; provides lubricious feel to skin for pressed and loose powds.; light stable; produces "soft focus" optical blurring of wrinkles and blemishes; JSCI/JCID approved; wh. fine powd.; pH 8.5-10.5 (10% susp.); 45-55% SiO_2.

Velvet Veil A. [Ikeda] Mica coated 10% with spherical silica particle (diam. 0.3 μm); CAS 12001-26-2, 7631-86-9; provides transparency with dispersion of light for pressed and loose powdered cosmetics, liq. foundations; wh. powd.; pH 8.5-10.5 (10% susp.); 45-55% SiO_2.

Velvetveil X. [Ikeda] Mica coated 20% with spherical silica particle (diam. 0.6 μm); CAS 12001-26-2, 7631-86-9; provides transparency with dispersion of light for pressed and loose powdered cosmetics, liq. foundations; wh. powd.; pH 7.3-9.8 (10% susp.); 50-60% TiO_2.

Velvetveil Y. [Ikeda] Mica coated 20% with spherical silica particle (diam. 0.3 μm); CAS 12001-26-2, 7631-86-9; provides transparency with dispersion of light for pressed and loose powdered cosmetics, liq. foundations; wh. powd.; pH 7.3-9.8 (10% susp.); 50-60% TiO_2.

Velvetveil Z. [Ikeda] Mica coated 40% with spherical silica particle (diam. 0.6 μm); CAS 12001-26-2, 7631-86-9; provides transparency with dispersion of light for pressed and loose powdered cosmetics, liq. foundations; wh. powd.; pH 7.3-9.8 (10% susp.); 62-72% TiO$_2$.

Veragel® 200. [Dr. Madis Labs] Aloe vera gel; moisturizer, soothing/healing aid for personal care; powd.

Veragel® Aq. Conc. 1:10. [Dr. Madis Labs] Aloe extract; CAS 85507-69-3; cosmetic ingred.

Veragel® Lipoid. [Dr. Madis Labs] Aloe extract; CAS 85507-69-3; cosmetic ingred.

Veragel® Liq., Liq. 1:1. [Dr. Madis Labs] Aloe vera gel; moisturizer, soothing/healing aid for personal care.

Verdoxan. [Henkel/Cospha] 2,2,5,5-Tetramethyl-4-isopropyl-1,3-dioxane; fragrance raw material with grn. or fruity notes for personal care or detergent formulations; colorless liq., woody odor; b.p. 70 C; flash pt. 54 C.

Versamid® 930. [Henkel/Functional Prods.] Nylon 66; CAS 32131-17-2; used in cosmetic applics.

Versatyl-42. [Nat'l. Starch] Octyl acrylamide/acrylates copolymer; hairspray polymer for systems containing large proportion of hydrocarbon propellant; for aerosol and pump hairsprays, setting lotions, spritzes; wh. fine powd.; sol. in ethanol, IPA; water-sol. when neutralized; 3% volatiles.

Versene 100. [Dow] Tetrasodium EDTA; CAS 64-02-8; EINECS 200-573-9; chelating agent controlling trace metal ions to improve lathering and stability of personal care prods., pharmaceuticals, in water treatment, textiles, soaps/detergents, electroless copperplating, polymer prod., disinfectants, pulp/paper, enhanced oil recovery, metal cleaning and protection; for control of common heavy metal ions to pH 12, iron to pH 8, water hardness ions above pH 6; lt. straw-colored liq.; m.w. 1.290-1.325; dens. 10.9 lb/gal; pH 11.0-11.8 (1% aq.); chel. value 102; 39% act.

Versene 100 EP. [Dow] Tetrasodium EDTA; CAS 64-02-8; EINECS 200-573-9; chelating agent controlling trace metal ions to improve lathering and stability of personal care prods., pharmaceuticals, in water treatment, textiles, soaps/detergents, electroless copperplating, foods, polymer prod., disinfectants, pulp/paper, enhanced oil recovery, metal cleaning and protection; high purity version of Versene 100; liq.

Versene 100 LS. [Dow] Tetrasodium EDTA; CAS 64-02-8; EINECS 200-573-9; chelating agent controlling trace metal ions to improve lathering and stability of personal care prods., pharmaceuticals, in water treatment, textiles, soaps/detergents, electroless copperplating, foods, polymer prod., disinfectants, pulp/paper, enhanced oil recovery, metal cleaning and protection; low solids grade used in aerosols; liq.

Versene 100 SRG. [Dow] Tetrasodium EDTA; CAS 64-02-8; EINECS 200-573-9; chelating agent controlling trace metal ions to improve lathering and stability of personal care prods., pharmaceuticals, in water treatment, textiles, soaps/detergents, electroless copperplating, foods, polymer prod., disinfectants, pulp/paper, enhanced oil recovery, metal cleaning and protection; pH adjusted; liq.

Versene 100 XL. [Dow] Tetrasodium EDTA; CAS 64-02-8; EINECS 200-573-9; chelating agent controlling trace metal ions to improve lathering and stability of personal care prods., pharmaceuticals, in water treatment, textiles, soaps/detergents, electroless copperplating, foods, polymer prod., disinfectants, pulp/paper, enhanced oil recovery, metal cleaning and protection; low NTA version of Versene 100; liq.

Versene 220. [Dow] Tetrasodium EDTA tetrahydrate; CAS 64-02-8; EINECS 200-573-9; chelating agent controlling trace metal ions to improve lathering and stability of personal care prods., pharmaceuticals, in water treatment, textiles, soaps/detergents, electroless copperplating, polymer prod., disinfectants, pulp/paper, en-

hanced oil recovery, metal cleaning and protection; high purity, crystal form of Versene 100; wh. cryst.; m.w. 452; dens. 45 lb/ft^3; pH 10.5-11.5; chel. value 219; 99% act.

Versene Acid. [Dow] EDTA; CAS 60-00-4; EINECS 200-449-4; chelating agent controlling trace metal ions to improve lathering and stability of personal care prods., pharmaceuticals, in water treatment, textiles, soaps/detergents, electroless copperplating, polymer prod., disinfectants, pulp/paper, enhanced oil recovery, metal cleaning and protection; intermediate for prep. of other salt forms of EDTA; wh. powd.; m.w. 292; dens. 54 lb/ft^3; pH 2.5-3.0 (sat. aq. sol'n.); chel. value 339; 99% act.

Versene CA. [Dow] Calcium-disodium EDTA; CAS 62-33-9; EINECS 200-529-9; chelating agent controlling trace metal ions to improve lathering and stability of personal care prods., pharmaceuticals, in water treatment, textiles, soaps/detergents, electroless copperplating, foods, polymer prod., disinfectants, pulp/paper, enhanced oil recovery, metal cleaning and protection; high purity direct food additive preventing metal catalyzed oxidative breakdown; also for medical and pharmaceutical preps.; FCC, USP, and Kosher compliance; wh. powd.; m.w. 410; dens. 40 lb/ft^3; pH 6.5-7.5 (1%); 97-102% act.

Versene Diammonium EDTA. [Dow] Diammonium EDTA; CAS 20824-56-0; EINECS 244-063-4; chelating agent controlling trace metal ions to improve lathering and stability of personal care prods., pharmaceuticals, in water treatment, textiles, soaps/detergents, electroless copperplating, polymer prod., disinfectants, pulp/paper, enhanced oil recovery, metal cleaning and protection; used when very sol. chelates are required or where sodium ions are undesirable; lt. straw-colored liq.; m.w. 326; sp.gr. 1.19-1.22; dens. 10.0 lb/gal; pH 4.6-5.2; chel. value 137; 44.6% act.

Versene NA. [Dow] Disodium EDTA; CAS 139-33-3; EINECS 205-358-3; chelating agent controlling trace metal ions to improve lathering and stability of personal care prods., pharmaceuticals, in water treatment, textiles, soaps/detergents, electroless copperplating, foods, polymer prod., disinfectants, pulp/paper, enhanced oil recovery, metal cleaning and protection; high purity direct food additive preventing metal catalyzed oxidative breakdown; also for medical and pharmaceutical preps.; FCC, USP, and Kosher compliance; wh. cryst.; m.w. 372; dens. 67 lb/ft^3; pH 4.3-4.7 (1%); 99% act.

Versene Na$_2$. [Dow] Na$_2$H$_2$EDTA·2H$_2$O; chelating agent used primarily in cosmetics and toiletries; crystals.

Versene Tetraammonium EDTA. [Dow] Tetraammonium EDTA; chelating agent controlling trace metal ions to improve lathering and stability of personal care prods., pharmaceuticals, in water treatment, textiles, soaps/detergents, electroless copperplating, polymer prod., disinfectants, pulp/paper, enhanced oil recovery, metal cleaning and protection; used when very sol. chelates are required or where sodium ions are undesirable; for chelation of iron to pH 9.5; lt. straw-colored liq.; m.w. 360; sp.gr. 1.16-1.19; dens. 9.7 lb/gal; pH 9.0-9.5; chel. value 130; 46.8% act.

Versenex 80. [Dow] Pentasodium DTPA; CAS 140-01-2; EINECS 205-391-3; chelating agent controlling trace metal ions to improve lathering and stability of personal care prods., pharmaceuticals, in water treatment, textiles, soaps/detergents, electroless copperplating, polymer prod., disinfectants, pulp/paper, enhanced oil recovery, metal cleaning and protection; used when oxidative conditions exist or when chelates of greater stability are required; lt. straw-colored liq.; m.w. 503; sp.gr. 1.28-1.32; dens. 10.8 lb/gal; pH 11.0-11.8 (1% aq.); chel. value 80; 40.2% act.

Versenol 120. [Dow] Trisodium HEDTA; CAS 139-89-9;

EINECS 205-381-9; chelating agent controlling trace metal ions to improve lathering and stability of personal care prods., pharmaceuticals, in water treatment, textiles, soaps/detergents, electroless copperplating, polymer prod., disinfectants, pulp/paper, enhanced oil recovery, metal cleaning and protection; for iron control to pH 10.5; lt. straw-colored liq.; m.w. 344; sp.gr. 1.26-1.31; dens. 10.7 lb/gal; pH 11.0-11.8 (1% aq.); chel. value 120; 41.3% act.

Vertal CO+. [Luzenac Am.] Hydrous magnesium silicate; CAS 14807-96-6; EINECS 238-877-9; very platy talc whose props. are enhanced by a flotation process improving brightness and purity; used for dusting powds., pressed powds., creams, lotions, and soaps; powd.; median diam. 16 µ; sp.gr. 2.8; surf. area 2 m²/g; oil absorp. 35; tapped dens. 65 lb/ft³; pH 9 (10% slurry).

Vexel. [Sederma] Lecithin, caffeine benzoate, and palmitoyl carnitine; slimming/cellulite regulating complex for body care prods.; activates caffeine diffusion, inhibits lipogenesis; pale yel. opalescent liq., char. odor; sp.gr. 1.030-1.040; ref. index 1.37-1.38pH 6.0-7.0; usage level: 5-10%.

Victory® . [Petrolite] Microcryst. wax; CAS 63231-60-7; EINECS 264-038-1; plastic wax offering high ductility, flexibility at very low temps.; provides protective barrier properties against moisture vapor and gases; used in hot-melt adhesives; hot-melt coatings; in antisunchecking agents in rubber goods, elec. insulating agents, leather treating agents, water repellents for textiles, rustproof coatings, cosmetic ingreds., and as plasticizer for other petrol. waxes used in crayons, dental compds., chewing gum base, and candles; incl. FDA §172.230, 172.615, 175.105, 175.300, 176.170, 176.180, 176.200, 177.1200, 178.3710, 179.45; wh., amber wax; dens. 0.93 g/cc; visc. 13 cps (99 C); m.p. 79 C; flash pt. 293 C.

Vigilan. [Fanning] Lanolin oil; CAS 8038-43-5; nonionic; emulsifier; skin and hair substantive emollient, conditioner, and moisturizer; coupling agent for castor and min. oils; o/w and/or w/o emulsions; adds elegance, lubricity, and hydration to makeup and facial preparations; spreads rapidly; superfatting agent in soap, liq. and solid detergents; plasticizer for hair spray resins; Gardner 8 max. liq. (Regular), 6 max. (Superfine), pleasant mild odor; sol. in IPM, castor and min. oils, propylene glycol laurate, ethyl acetate, silicone fluids; insol. in water; acid no. 2.0 max.; iodine no. 36 max.; sapon. no. 95–110; cloud pt. 20 C; 100% conc.

Vigilan AWS. [Fanning] PPG-12-PEG-65 lanolin oil; CAS 68458-58-8; nonionic; o/w emulsifier; plasticizer, emollient, solubilizer, and wetting agent in personal care prods.; disperses to form milky emulsion in water used in bath oils; Gardner 9–11 color; sol. in water, ethanol, castor oil, propylene glycol laurate, acetone, ethyl acetate; HLB 13.5; acid no. 3.0 max.; iodine no. 15 max.; sapon. no. 10–25; pH 7 max. (10%); 100% conc.

Vinac® 880. [Air Prods./Polymers] Polyvinyl acetate.

Vinol 523, 540. [Air Prods.] Polyvinyl alcohol; CAS 9002-89-5.

Viscarin. [Marine Colloids] Sodium carrageenan.

Viscarin XLV. [Marine Colloids] Carrageenan; CAS 9000-07-1; EINECS 232-524-2; gellant and stabilizer for cosmetics.

Viscasil® (10,000 cSt) [GE Silicones] Dimethicone; used for damping, power transmission, rubber/plastic lubrication, base fluid for grease, polishes, cosmetics/toiletries, mold release for tires, rubber, plastics, petrol. antifoam, textile thread/fiber lubricants; sp.gr. 0.975; visc. 10,000 cSt; pour pt. -53 F; flash pt. (PMOC) 601 F; ref. index 1.4035; surf. tens. 21.3 dynes/cm; sp. heat 0.36 Btu/lb F; dissip. factor 0.0001; dielec. str. 35 kV; dielec. const. 2.75; vol. resist. 1 x 10¹⁴ohm-cm.

Viscasil® (12,500 cSt) [GE Silicones] Dimethicone; used for damping, rubber/plastic lubrication, polishes, cosmetics/toiletries, mold release for tires, rubber, plastics, petrol. antifoam, textile thread/fiber lubricants; sp.gr. 0.975; visc. 12,500 cSt; pour pt. -53 F; flash pt. (PMCC) 500 F; ref. index 1.4035; surf. tens. 21.3 dynes/cm; sp. heat 0.36 Btu/lb F; dissip. factor 0.0001; dielec. str. 35 kV; dielec. const. 2.75; vol. resist. 1 x 10¹⁴ ohm-cm.

Viscolene. [Vevy] PEG-150 stearate, PEG-150 distearate.

Viscontran HEC. [Henkel] Hydroxyethylcellulose; CAS 9004-62-0; thickener.

Viscontran MC. [Henkel] Methylcellulose; CAS 9004-67-5.

Viscontran MHPC. [Henkel] Hydroxypropyl methylcellulose; CAS 9004-65-3.

Visonoil. [Vevy] Hydrog. mink oil.

Vitacap. [Les Colorants Wackherr] A vitamin-dimethicone copolyol; for hair conditioning.

Vitacell. [Laboratoires Sérobiologiques] Amino acids and peptides; yeast extract stimulating cells consumption of oxygen and metabolic action; for prods. for tired, dull skin, premature aging, skin subjected to environmental stress; yel. limpid liq.; water-sol.; usage level: 2-5%.

Vitacell LS. [Laboratoires Sérobiologiques] Yeast extract; CAS 8103-01-2; yeast extract stimulating cells consumption of oxygen and metabolic action; for prods. for tired, dull skin, premature aging, skin subjected to environmental stress.

Vita-Cos. [CasChem] Wheat germ glycerides; CAS 68990-07-8; used for pigmented cosmetics, skin care prods.; substantive counter-irritant.

Vitamarine. [Sederma] Min. oil, docosahexenoic acid, eicosapentaenoic acid, algae extract; for sensitive and stressed skin treatments, body and facial care prods.; prevents cutaneous ageing; yel.-orange clear oil, char. odor; sp.gr. 0.85 ± 0.02; acid no. < 2; iodine no. ≈ 15; sapon. no. ≈ 15; ref. index 1.460 ± 0.005; usage level: 3-7%.

Vitamin A Palmitate 1.0 BHT in Peanut Oil. [BASF] Vitamin A palmitate, BHT, peanut oil; cosmetic ingred.; oil.

Vitamin A Palmitate 1.7 BHT. [BASF] Vitamin A palmitate, BHT; cosmetic ingred.; oil.

Vitamin A Palmitate Type P1.7. [Roche] Vitamin A palmitate, 1,650,000-1,800,000 IU/g; antikeratinizing, moisturizing ingred. for skin care and after-sun tanning prods.

Vitamin A Palmitate Type P1.7/BHT. [Roche] Vitamin A palmitate, 1,600,000-1,800,000 IU/g, stabilized with BHT; antikeratinizing, moisturizing ingred. for skin care and after-sun tanning prods.

Vitamin A Palmitate Type PIMO/BH. [Roche] Vitamin A palmitate, 1,000,000 IU/g, stabilized with BHA/BHT; antikeratinizing, moisturizing ingred. for skin care and after-sun tanning prods.

Vitamin A and D-3. [Roche] Vitamin A palmitate in veg. oil with D-3, 1,000,000 IU vitamin A and 200,000 IU of D-3/g (5:1 ratio); antikeratinizing, moisturizing ingred. for skin care and after-sun tanning prods.

Vitamin B Complex CLR. [Dr. Kurt Richter; Henkel/Cospha] Yeast extract with B vitamins in water-alcohol medium; CAS 8103-01-2; prod. for treatment of greasy hair, dandruff and oily skin; dk. brn. liq.

Vitamin E Acetate Cosmetic Oil. [BASF] Vitamin E acetate; cosmetic ingred.; oil.

Vitamin E Acetate USP Oil. [BASF] Vitamin E acetate USP; cosmetic ingred.; oil.

Vitamin E Nicotinate. [BASF] Vitamin E nicotinate; cosmetic ingred.; oil.

Vitamin E USP Tocopherol. [BASF] Vitamin E; cosmetic ingred.; oil.

Vitamin F Alcohol-Soluble CLR. [Dr. Kurt Richter; Henkel/

Cospha] Hydro-alcohol solubilized complex of essential free fatty acids for treatment of dry skin and hair; lt. yel. liq.

Vitamin F Ethyl Ester CLR. [Dr. Kurt Richter; Henkel/ Cospha] Ethyl linoleate, ethyl oleate, and ethyl linolenate; complex of essential esterified fatty acids in lipophilic medium for treatment of dry skin and hair; lt. yel. oily liq.

Vitamin F Forte CLR. [Dr. Kurt Richter; Henkel/Cospha] Linoleic acid and linolenic acid; complex of essential free fatty acids in lipophilic medium for treatment of dry skin and hair; lt. yel. oily liq.

Vitamin F Glyceryl Ester CLR. [Dr. Kurt Richter; Henkel/ Cospha] Glyceryl linoleate and glyceryl linolenate; complex of essential esterified fatty acids in lipophilic medium for treatment of dry skin and hair; lt. yel. oily liq.

Vitamin F Water-Soluble CLR. [Dr. Kurt Richter; Henkel/ Cospha] Polysorbate 20, linoleic acid, and linolenic acid; Hydro-alcohol solubilized complex of essential free fatty acids for treatment of dry skin and hair; yel. liq.

Vitamine A Palmitate Exsyliposomes. [Exsymol; Biosil Tech.] Vitamin A palmitate (340,000 IU), glycerophospholipids (2%); liposome for anti-aging cosmetics, hydration and tissular regeneration, skin maintenance; pale yel. opalescent liq.; usage level: 4-6%; toxicology: nontoxic.

Vitaphyle ACE. [Les Colorants Wackherr] A blend of vitamins and a uv filter in a min. oil base; for use in cosmetic creams and lotions.

Vitaplant CLR Oil-Soluble N. [Dr. Kurt Richter; Henkel/ Cospha] Sesame oil, soybean oil, pigskin extract, calendula extract, and tocopherol; prod. for aging, damaged and sun-burned skin; brnsh.-yel. oil.

Vitaplant CLR Water-Soluble. [Dr. Kurt Richter; Henkel/ Cospha] Water, alcohol, coneflower extract, and aloe extract; prods. for aging, damaged and sun-burned skin; dk. brn. liq.

Vitazyme® A-Plus. [Brooks Industries] Retinyl palmitate polypeptide; natural protein complexed vitamins for cosmetics use; 175,000 IU vitamin A.

Vitazyme® B3. [Brooks Industries] 25% Niacinamide in a natural protein; CAS 98-92-0; EINECS 202-713-4; protein complexed vitamins for cosmetic use.

Vitazyme® B5. [Brooks Industries] 25% Pantothenic acid in a natural protein; protein complexed vitamins for cosmetic use.

Vitazyme® C. [Brooks Industries] 20% Ascorbic acid in a natural protein; CAS 50-81-7; EINECS 200-066-2; protein complexed vitamins for cosmetic use.

Vitazyme® D. [Brooks Industries] 1,000,000 IU/g vitamin D_3 in a natural protein; cholecalciferol polypeptide; protein complexed vitamins for cosmetic use.

Vitazyme® E. [Brooks Industries] 250 IU/g Vitamin E in a natural protein; tocopherol polypeptide; protein complexed vitamins for cosmetic use.

Volatile Silicone 7158, 7207, 7349. [Union Carbide] Cyclomethicone; CAS 69430-24-6; emollient, lubricant for skin creams and lotions, antiperspirants, bath oils, shaving prods., suntan lotions, colognes, hair care prods.; sol. in alcohols, aerosol propellants, fatty esters, min. oil; insol. in water.

Volclay® NF-BC. [Am. Colloid] Sodium bentonite USP/NF; suspending agent, gellant, binder for pharmaceuticals, cosmetics, and personal care prods. where color is not critical; air-floated powd.; 99% thru 200 mesh; pH 9.5–10.5 (2% disp.); 63.02% SiO_2, 21.08% Al_2O_3; 5-8% moisture.

Volclay NF-ID. [Am. Colloid] Sterilized microfine sodium bentonite NF; suspending agent, gellant, binder for use in pharmaceuticals, cosmetics, and personal care prods. where minimal microbial content is essential; powd.; 99% min. thru 200 mesh; pH 9.5-10.5 (2% disp.); 5-8%

moisture.

Volpo 3. [Croda Inc.] Oleth-3; CAS 9004-98-2; 52581-71-2; nonionic; emollient, lubricant, emulsifier, solubilizer for cosmetic and pharmaceutical applics.; emulsifier in astringent creams and lotions; clear gel formation; superfatting in shampoos, foaming bath preparations, and Carbopol gels; used in cold waves, depilatories, and hair straighteners; solubilizer for bromo acids in lipsticks and liq. rouge; spreading agent for bath oils; off-wh. hazy liq.; sol. in alcohols, glycols, ketones, and chlorinated and aromatic solvs., min. oil, and nonpolar oils; insol. in water; HLB 6.6; acid no. 2.0 max.; iodine no. 57-62; hyd. no. 135-150; pH 5–7 (3% aq.).; usage level: 0.5-5%; toxicology: LD50 (oral, rat) 12.2 g/kg; skin irritant; nonirritating to eyes.

Volpo 5. [Croda Inc.] Oleth-5; CAS 9004-98-2; nonionic; emollient, lubricant, emulsifier, solubilizer for cosmetic and pharmaceutical applics.; off-wh. hazy liq.; sol. in alcohols, glycols, ketones, and chlorinated and aromatic solvs., min. oil, and nonpolar oils; insol. in water; HLB 8.8; acid no. 2.0 max.; iodine no. 40-52; pH 5–7 (3% aq.); usage level: 0.5-5%; toxicology: LD50 (oral, rat) 5 g/kg; mild skin irritant, moderate eye irritant; 100% conc.

Volpo 10. [Croda Inc.] Oleth-10; CAS 9004-98-2; nonionic; emollient, lubricant, emulsifier, solubilizer for cosmetic and pharmaceutical applics.; off-wh. semisolid; sol. in alcohols, glycols, ketones, chlorinated and aromatic solvs., and water; HLB 12.4; acid no. 2.0 max.; iodine no. 31-37; hyd. no. 79-91; pH 5–7 (3% aq.); usage level: 0.5-5%; toxicology: LD50 (oral, rat) 4.3 g/kg; skin irritant, nonirritating to eyes; 100% conc.

Volpo 20. [Croda Inc.] Oleth-20; CAS 9004-98-2; nonionic; emollient, lubricant, emulsifier, fragrance solubilizer for cosmetic and pharmaceutical applics.; off-wh. soft solid; sol. in water, IPa, propylene glycol; HLB 15.4; cloud pt. 100 C (1% aq.); acid no. 2.0 max.; iodine no. 18-25; hyd. no. 50-58; pH 5–7 (3% aq.); usage level: 0.5-5%; toxicology: LD50 (oral, rat) 15.1 g/kg; mild skin and eye irritant; 100% conc.

Volpo 25 D 3. [Croda Chem. Ltd.] PEG-3 C12-15 ether; CAS 68131-39-5; nonionic; emulsifier, dispersant, wetting agent, gelling agent, scouring and solubilizing agent for industrial and cosmetic applics.; liq.; 97% conc.

Volpo 25 D 5. [Croda Chem. Ltd.] PEG-5 C12-15 ether; CAS 68131-39-5; nonionic; emulsifier, dispersant, wetting agent, gelling agent, scouring and solubilizing agent for industrial and cosmetic applics.; liq.; 97% conc.

Volpo 25 D 10. [Croda Chem. Ltd.] PEG-10 C12-15 ether; CAS 68131-39-5; nonionic; emulsifier, dispersant, wetting agent, gelling agent, scouring and solubilizing agent for industrial and cosmetic applics.; paste; 97% conc.

Volpo 25 D 15. [Croda Chem. Ltd.] PEG-15 C12-15 ether; CAS 68131-39-5; nonionic; emulsifier, dispersant, wetting agent, gelling agent, scouring and solubilizing agent for industrial and cosmetic applics.; solid; 97% conc.

Volpo 25 D 20. [Croda Chem. Ltd.] PEG-20 C12-15 ether; CAS 68131-39-5; nonionic; emulsifier, dispersant, wetting agent, gelling agent, scouring and solubilizing agent for industrial and cosmetic applics.; solid; 97% conc.

Volpo CS-3. [Croda Inc.; Croda Chem. Ltd.] Ceteareth-3; CAS 68439-49-6; nonionic; emulsifier, dispersant, wetting agent, gellant for industrial and cosmetic skin care applics.; solubilizer for essential oils and perfumes; off-wh. soft waxy solid; sol. in ethanol, kerosene, trichloroethylene, oleic acid, oleyl alcohol; HLB 7.3; pH 6.0-7.5 (3%); 97% conc.

Volpo CS-5. [Croda Inc.; Croda Chem. Ltd.] Ceteareth-5; CAS 68439-49-6; nonionic; emulsifier, dispersant, wetting agent, gellant for industrial and cosmetic skin care applics.; solubilizer for perfumes and essential oils; off wh. soft waxy solid; sol. in ethanol, trichloroethylene, oleic acid; HLB 9.5; surf. tens. 33.0 dynes/cm (0.1% aq.); pH 6.0-7.5 (3%); 97% conc.

Volpo CS-10. [Croda Inc.; Croda Chem. Ltd.] Ceteareth-10; CAS 68439-49-6; nonionic; emulsifier, dispersant, wetting agent, gellant for industrial and cosmetic skin care applics.; solubilizer for perfumes and essential oils; off wh. soft waxy solid; sol. in ethanol, trichloroethylene, oleic acid; HLB 12.9; cloud pt. 68 C (1% aq.); surf. tens. 34.5 dynes/cm (0.1% aq.); pH 6.0-7.5 (3%); 97% conc.

Volpo CS-15. [Croda Inc.; Croda Chem. Ltd.] Ceteareth-15; CAS 68439-49-6; nonionic; emulsifier, dispersant, wetting agent, gellant for industrial and cosmetic skin care applics.; solubilizer for perfumes and essential oils; off wh. waxy solid; sol. in ethanol, trichloroethylene, oleic acid; HLB 14.6; cloud pt. 94 C (1% aq.); surf. tens. 35.5 dynes/cm (0.1% aq.); pH 6.0-7.5 (3%); 97% conc.

Volpo CS-20. [Croda Inc.; Croda Chem. Ltd.] Ceteareth-20; CAS 68439-49-6; nonionic; emulsifier, dispersant, wetting agent, gellant for industrial, cosmetic skin care, and pharmaceutical applics.; solubilizer for perfumes and essential oils; off-wh. hard waxy solid; sol. in water, ethanol, trichloroethylene, oleic acid; HLB 15.6; cloud pt. 78 C (1% aq.); surf. tens. 41.5 dynes/cm (0.1% aq.); pH 6.0-7.5 (3%); toxicology: LD50 (oral, rat) 2.1 g/kg; mild skin irritant, moderate eye irritant; 97% conc.

Volpo L4. [Croda Chem. Ltd.] C12-13 pareth-4; CAS 9002-92-0; nonionic; general purpose emulsifier and dispersant; liq.; 97% conc.

Volpo L23. [Croda Chem. Ltd.] C12-13 pareth-23; CAS 9002-92-0; nonionic; o/w emulsifier and solubilizer for cosmetics, pharmaceuticals, and household prods.; solid; 97% conc.

Volpo N3. [Croda Inc.; Croda Chem. Ltd.] Oleth-3, distilled; CAS 9004-98-2; nonionic; emulsifier, dispersant, wetting agent, gelling agent, scouring agent for industrial and cosmetic skin care applics.; solubilizer for perfumes and essential oils; pale straw liq.; HLB 6.7; 97% conc.

Volpo N5. [Croda Inc.; Croda Chem. Ltd.] Oleth-5, distilled; CAS 9004-98-2; nonionic; emulsifier, dispersant, wetting agent, gelling agent, scouring agent for industrial and cosmetic skin care applics.; solubilizer for perfumes and essential oils; pale straw liq.; HLB 9.0; 97% conc.

Volpo N10. [Croda Inc.; Croda Chem. Ltd.] Oleth-10, distilled; CAS 9004-98-2; nonionic; emulsifier, dispersant, wetting agent, gelling agent, scouring agent for industrial and cosmetic skin care applics.; solubilizer for perfumes and essential oils; pale straw paste; HLB 12.4; 97% conc.

Volpo N15. [Croda Chem. Ltd.] Oleth-15, distilled; CAS 9004-98-2; nonionic; emulsifier, dispersant, wetting agent, gelling agent, scouring and solubilizing agent for industrial and cosmetic applics.; paste; HLB 14.2; 97% conc.

Volpo N20. [Croda Chem. Ltd.] Oleth-20, distilled; CAS 9004-98-2; nonionic; emulsifier, dispersant, wetting agent, gelling agent, scouring and solubilizing agent for industrial and cosmetic applics.; solid; HLB 15.5; 97% conc.

Volpo O3. [Croda Chem. Ltd.] Oleth-3; CAS 9004-98-2; nonionic; emulsifier, dispersant, wetting agent, gelling agent, scouring and solubilizing agent for industrial and cosmetic applics.; liq.; 97% conc.

Volpo O5. [Croda Chem. Ltd.] Oleth-5; CAS 9004-98-2; nonionic; emulsifier, dispersant, wetting agent, gelling agent, scouring and solubilizing agent for industrial and cosmetic applics.; liq.; 97% conc.

Volpo O10. [Croda Chem. Ltd.] Oleth-10; CAS 9004-98-2; nonionic; emulsifier, dispersant, wetting agent, gelling agent, scouring and solubilizing agent for industrial and cosmetic applics.; paste; 97% conc.

Volpo O15. [Croda Chem. Ltd.] Oleth-15; CAS 9004-98-2;

nonionic; emulsifier, dispersant, wetting agent, gelling agent, scouring and solubilizing agent for industrial and cosmetic applics.; paste; 97% conc.

Volpo O20. [Croda Chem. Ltd.] Oleth-20; CAS 9004-98-2; nonionic; emulsifier, dispersant, wetting agent, gelling agent, scouring and solubilizing agent for industrial and cosmetic applics.; solid; 97% conc.

Volpo S-2. [Croda Inc.; Croda Chem. Ltd.] Steareth-2; CAS 9005-00-9; nonionic; emulsifier for o/w systems, cosmetics, pharmaceuticals; stable over wide pH range; wh. soft solid; sol. in alcohol, glycols, ketones, most chlorinated and aromatic solvs., keroesene, min. oil; cloud pt. < 55 C (1% aq.); HLB 4.9; acid no. 1.0 max.; hyd. no. 150-170; pH 6.0-7.0 (3%); usage level: 0.5-5%; 100% conc.

Volpo S-10. [Croda Inc.; Croda Chem. Ltd.] Steareth-10; CAS 9005-00-9; nonionic; emulsifier for cosmetics and pharmaceuticals, hair straighteners and relaxers; stable over wide pH range; wh. soft solid, low odor; sol. in alcohol, glycol, ketone, most chlorinated and aromatic solvs.; insol. in oil; HLB 12.4; cloud pt. 65-75 C (1% aq.); acid no. 1.0 max.; hyd. no. 75-90; pH 6.0-7.0 (3%); usage level: 0.5-5%; toxicology: LD50 (oral, rat) 2.1 g/kg; moderate skin irritant, severe eye irritant; 100% conc.

Volpo S-20. [Croda Inc.; Croda Chem. Ltd.] Steareth-20; CAS 9005-00-9; nonionic; emulsifier for cosmetics and pharmaceuticals, ethic hair straighteners and relaxers; stable over wide pH range; wh. solid; sol. in water, alcohols, glycols, ketones, most chlorinated and aromatic solvs.; insol. in oil; cloud pt. > 100 C (1% aq.); HLB 15.3; acid no. 1.0 max.; hyd. no. 45-60; usage level: 0.5-5%; toxicology: LD50 (oral, rat) 2.07 g/kg; nonirritating to skin; moderate eye irritant; 100% conc.

Volpo T-3. [Croda Chem. Ltd.] Trideceth-3; CAS 4403-12-7; EINECS 224-540-3; nonionic; emulsifier, dispersant, wetting agent, gelling agent, scouring and solubilizing agent for industrial and cosmetic applics.; liq.; 97% conc.

Volpo T-5. [Croda Chem. Ltd.] Trideceth-5; CAS 24938-91-8; nonionic; emulsifier, dispersant, wetting agent, gelling agent, scouring and solubilizing agent for industrial and cosmetic applics.; liq.; 97% conc.

Volpo T-10. [Croda Chem. Ltd.] Trideceth-10; CAS 24938-91-8; nonionic; emulsifier, dispersant, wetting agent, gelling agent, scouring and solubilizing agent for industrial and cosmetic applics.; paste; 97% conc.

Volpo T-15. [Croda Chem. Ltd.] Trideceth-15; CAS 24938-91-8; nonionic; emulsifier, dispersant, wetting agent, gelling agent, scouring and solubilizing agent for industrial and cosmetic applics.; paste; 97% conc.

Volpo T-20. [Croda Chem. Ltd.] Trideceth-20; CAS 24938-91-8; nonionic; emulsifier, dispersant, wetting agent, gelling agent, scouring and solubilizing agent for industrial and cosmetic applics.; solid; 97% conc.

Vybar® 103. [Petrolite] Syn. wax; ethylene-derived hydrocarbon polymer; CAS 8002-74-2; lubricant, anticaking agent, modifier; used in paraffin; used in candles to replace stearic acid; opacifies the candle and imparts resistance to thermal shock; pigment disp. to wet inorg. pigments and fillers at high loading levels; suitable for hot melt inks, mold release compds., plastic lubricants, protective coatings, polishes, slip and antimar additives; emollient, gloss, lubricant for cosmetics; FDA §175.105, 176.170, 176.180, 178.3850; solid; limited sol. in org. solvs.; m.w. 2800; dens. 0.92 g/cc; visc. 310 cps (99 C); m.p. 72 C; iodine no. 14.

Vybar® 260. [Petrolite] Syn. wax; olefin-derived hydrocarbon polymer; CAS 8002-74-2; paraffin wax modifier; hard, low-melting polymer with low melt visc; additive producing blends with paraffin which are harder and more opaque; upgrades properties of lower-grade waxes; useful in polishes, industrial coatings, hot-melt inks, mold-release compds., plastic lubricants, and slip and antimar additives; emollient, gloss, lubricant for cosmetics; FDA §175.105, 176.170, 176.180, 178.3850; solid; sol. in min. spirits, xylene, and trichloroethylene; m.w. 2600; dens. 0.90 g/cc; visc. 330 cps (99 C); m.p. 51 C; iodine no. 15.

Vybar® 825. [Petrolite] Syn. wax; ethylene-derived hydrocarbon polymer; CAS 8002-74-2; plasticizer, lubricant with good slip chars.; additive in specialty lubricants, polishes, cutting oils, ski wax, and release agents; ozone barrier for elastomers; increases gloss, lubricity, and film deposition on skin for cosmetics applics.; liq.; sol. in org. solvs., min. oil, chlorinated solvs., and selected silicones; m.w. 1500; dens. 0.86 g/cc; visc. 52 cps (99 C); pour pt. -34 C; iodine no. 30.

Vybar® 5013. [Petrolite] C18-28 alkyl acetate; syn. wax contributing gloss to lipsticks, emolliency to creams, visc. to mascara, and water resist. to suntan prods.; m.w. 420; visc. 4 cP (99 C); m.p. 135 F; soften. pt. 53 C; acid no. 23; sapon. no. 114.

Vyox. [Vevy] Tocopherol, triethyl citrate, BHA.

W

Wacker HDK® H20. [Wacker-Chemie GmbH] Fumed silica; hydrophobic thickener, thixotrope, excipient, free-flow aid for paints/coatings, pharmaceuticals/cosmetic powds., sealing and jointing compds., printing inks, PVC dry-blending, rubbers; wh. powd.; apparent dens. 40 g/l; surf. area 170 ± 30 m²/g; ref. index 1.45; pH 3.8-4.5 (4% in 1:1 water/methanol disp.).

Wacker HDK® N20. [Wacker-Chemie GmbH] Fumed silica; hydrophilic thickener, thixotrope for paints/coatings, pharmaceuticals/cosmetics (toothpaste, tablets, powds., aerosols, suspensions, ointments, creams), diazo paper, printing inks, PVC plastisols, rubbers, adhesives; wh. powd.; apparent dens. 40 g/l; surf. area 200 ± 30 m²/g; ref. index 1.45; pH 3.6-4.3 (4% aq.).

Wacker HDK® V15. [Wacker-Chemie GmbH] Fumed silica; hydrophilic thickener, thixotrope for pharmaceuticals/cosmetics (suspensions, ointments, creams), silicone rubber, polyurethane and polysulfide elastomers, acrylates; wh. powd.; apparent dens. 50 g/l; surf. area 150 ± 30 m²/g; ref. index 1.45; pH 3.6-4.3 (4% aq.).

Wacker Silicone Antifoam Agent S 184. [Wacker Silicones] Simethicone; foam control agent.

Wacker Silicone Antifoam Emulsion SE 6. [Wacker Silicones] Simethicone; foam control agent.

Wacker Silicone Antifoam Emulsion SE 9. [Wacker-Chemie GmbH; Wacker Silicones] Simethicone; antifoam, processing aid for foods, cosmetics, pharmaceuticals, fermentation, in mfg. of plastics in contact with food, for degassing of monomers (e.g., PVC, latex stripping); FDA §173.340, BGA II, VII; milky wh. med. visc. o/w emulsion; sp.gr. 1.0; pH 6-8; usage level: 0.02-0.5%; 15-16% solids in water.

Wacker Silicone Fluid AKF. [Wacker Silicones] Dimethicone.

Wacker Silicone Fluid VP 1653. [Wacker Silicones] Amodimethicone.

Water Lock® A-100. [Grain Processing] Starch/acrylates/acrylamide copolymer; superabsorbent polymer; able to absorb or immobilize large quantities of aq. fluids, such as alkalies, dilute acids, body fluids.

Water-Soluble Vegetols®. [Gattefosse SA] Plant extracts.

Waxenol® 801. [CasChem] Arachidyl propionate; CAS 65591-14-2; EINECS 265-839-9; binder; emollient, solubilizer, and ingred. in cosmetic and toiletries; lubricant for pressed powds.; metal working lubricant and corrosion inhibitor for metal surf.; Gardner 3+ color; sol. in min. oil, IPM, chloroform, anhyd. ethanol @ 45 C; misc. with lanolin @ 45 C; pour pt. 36 C; acid no. 0.2; iodine no. 12.

Waxenol® 810. [CasChem] Myristyl myristate; CAS 3234-85-3; EINECS 221-787-9; emollient with unusual afterfeel; esp. for stick preps.; Gardner 2+ color; sol. in IPM, min. oil, oleyl alcohol; insol. in water; pour pt. 38 C; acid no. 1.2; iodine no. 1.0 max.

Waxenol® 815. [CasChem] Cetyl palmitate; CAS 540-10-3;

EINECS 208-736-6; emollient additive; internal lubricant and binder in pressed powds.; in metalworking lubricant coatings; Gardner 1+ powd.; pour pt. 51 C; acid no. 0.2; iodine no. 1.0 max.

Waxenol® 816. [CasChem] Cetyl palmitate; CAS 540-10-3; EINECS 208-736-6; nonionic; internal lubricant and binder in pressed binder operations; emollient additive; metalworking lubricant and corrosion inhibitor coating for metal surfs.; Gardner 1+ flakes; pour pt. 51 C; acid no. 0.2; iodine no. 1.0 max.; 100% act.

Waxenol® 821. [CasChem] Syn. beeswax; lipophilic emulsifier, emollient; Gardner 2+ color; pour pt. 58 C; acid no. 22; iodine no. 15 max.

Waxenol® 822. [CasChem] Arachidyl behenate; CAS 42233-14-7; EINECS 255-728-3; emollient for sticks, creams, lotions; barrier props. for enhanced moisturization; gloss and film-forming props.; Gardner 2+ waxy flakes; pour pt. 65 C; acid no. 22; iodine no. 10.

Wayhib® S. [Olin] TEA phosphate ester, sodium salt; anionic; emulsifier, detergent builder, sequestrant, corrosion inhibitor; for pipeline scale inhibition, water circulating systems, air conditioning, boiler treatment compds., pharmaceutical, and metalworking applics.; Gardner 1 liq.; misc. with water; sp.gr. 1.45; dens. 12.07 lb/gal; pH 4.6 (1% aq.); toxicology: irritating to skin and eyes; 70% act.

Wecobee® FS. [Stepan/PVO] Hydrog. veg. oil; CAS 68334-28-1; EINECS 269-820-6; cocoa butter replacement, emollient used for foods (salad dressing, snack dips, confection coatings), pharmaceuticals (suppositories, ointment bases); base for cosmetic/pharmaceutical creams and ointments; exc. mold release; FDA GRAS §170.30; wh. to off-wh. soft solid, bland odor; m.p. 39 C; iodine no. 3; sapon. no. 240; 0-1% moisture.

Wecobee® FW. [Stepan/PVO] Hydrog. veg. oil; CAS 68334-28-1; EINECS 269-820-6; cocoa butter replacement, emollient used for foods (whipped toppings, salad dressing, snack dips, confection coatings) and pharmaceuticals (suppositories, ointment and cream bases); base for cosmetic/pharmacuetical creams and ointments; exc. mold release; FDA GRAS §170.30; wh. to off-wh. soft solid, bland odor; m.p. 38 C; iodine no. 3; sapon. no. 240; 0.1% moisture.

Wecobee® M. [Stepan/PVO; Stepan Europe] Hydrog. veg. oil; CAS 68334-28-1; EINECS 269-820-6; cocoa butter replacment with exc. mold release chars.; used in personal care prods. (lipsticks, pomades, solid fragrances, antiperspirant sticks, suppositories, emollient creams/lotions), pharmaceuticals (suppositories, ointment and cream bases), food industry (coffee whiteners, whipped toppings, salad dressing, snack dips, confection coatings); APHA 400 max. solid, bland odor; visc. 13.5 cps (150 F); m.p. 36 C; acid no. 0.20 max.; sapon. value 238-250.

Wecobee® S. [Stepan/PVO; Stepan Europe] Hydrog. veg. oil; CAS 68334-28-1; EINECS 269-820-6; cocoa butter replacment with exc. mold release chars.; used in personal care prods. (lipsticks, pomades, solid fragrances, antiperspirant sticks, suppositories, emollient creams/lotions), pharmaceuticals (suppositories, ointment and cream bases), food industry (coffee whiteners, whipped toppings, salad dressing, snack dips, confection coatings); APHA 400 max. flakes, bland odor; visc. 14.0 cps (150 F); m.p. 45 C; acid no. 0.20 max.; sapon. value 230–250.

Wecobee® SS. [Stepan/PVO] Hydrog. veg. oil; CAS 68334-28-1; EINECS 269-820-6; cocoa butter replacement, emollient used for foods (confection coatings), pharmaceuticals (suppositories, ointment bases), cosmetics (lipsticks, glossers, pomades, antiperspirant sticks, cream/ointment base); exc. mold release; FDA GRAS §170.30; sl. yel. flakes, bland odor; m.p. 44-49 C; iodine no. 4 max.; sapon. no. 225-250; 0.1% max. moisture.

Wecobee® W. [Stepan/PVO] Hydrog. veg. oil; CAS 68334-28-1; EINECS 269-820-6; cocoa butter replacement, emollient used for foods (coffee whiteners, whipped toppings, salad dressing, snack dips), pharmaceuticals (suppositories), cosmetics (cream/ointment base); FDA GRAS §170.30; wh. to off-wh. soft solid, bland odor; m.p. 33-36 C; iodine no. 4 max.; sapon. no. 240-254; 0.1% max. moisture.

Westchlor® 170. [Westwood] Aluminum sesquichlorhydrate; CAS 11097-68-0; antiperspirant active for aq. roll-ons or hydroalcoholic pump systems; colorless clear liq., odorless; pH 3.9-4.3 (15% aq.); 45% aq., 11% Al, 8.25% Cl.

Westchlor® 170 Powd. [Westwood] Aluminum sesquichloride; antiperspirant active for hydroalcoholic and high basic sesquichlorhydrate systems; off-wh., sl. yel. fine crystals, pract. odorless; sol. in 95% ethanol; pH 3.9-4.3 (15% aq.); 24.25% Al, 18.25% Cl.

Westchlor® 200. [Westwood] Aluminum chlorhydrate; CAS 1327-41-9; EINECS 215-477-2; antiperspirant active for aq. roll-on emulsions or creams; colorless clear liq., odorless; sp.gr. 1.335-1.345; pH 4.0-4.4 (15% aq.); 50% aq., 12.2-12.7% Al, 7.9-8.4% Cl.

Westchlor® 200 Custom Powd. 10. [Westwood] Basic aluminum chloride; antiperspirant active for anhydr. suspension systems and suspensoid sticks where low visc. are encountered; wh. to off-wh. impalpable powd.; 85% min. < 10 µ; pH 4.0-4.4 (15% aq.); 46-48% Al$_2$O$_3$, 15.8-16.8% Cl.

Westchlor® 200 Impalpable. [Westwood] Basic aluminum chloride; antiperspirant active for dry suspension formulas, aerosols, and creams; wh. impalpable powd.; 97% min. thru 325 mesh; pH 4.0-4.4 (15% aq.); 46-48% Al$_2$O$_3$, 15.8-16.8% Cl.

Westchlor® A2Z 8106. [Westwood] Aluminum zirconium pentachlorhydrex-gly, propylene glycol sol'n. with zinc glycinate as adjusting agent; antiperspirant active for use in dibenzyl sorbitol gellant formulations; features high pH, high efficacy, crystal clear solid formulas with no visible residue; sl. yel. clear liq., faint glycolic odor; sp.gr. 1.230 ± 0.01; visc. 550 ± 150 cps; ref. index 1.460 ± 0.01; pH 4.75±0.15 (10%); 30% act.; 5.50% Al, 2.40% Zr, 4.5% Cl.

Westchlor® DM 200 Impalpable. [Westwood] Basic aluminum chloride; antiperspirant active for dry suspension formulas and aerosols; high efficacy; off-wh. free-flowing powd., typ. odor; 60% min. < 10 µ; pH 4.0-4.5 (10% aq.); 25.5-26.4% Al, 16.3-17.9% Cl.

Westchlor® ZR 30B DM Powd. [Westwood] Aluminum zirconium trichlorhydrex-gly; antiperspirant active for anhyd. silicone suspensions and sticks; high efficacy; wh. to off-wh. free-flowing powd., pract. odorless; 100% < 53 µ; pH 3.8-4.4 (25% aq.); 14.0-15.2% Al, 13.3-17.5% Cl, 13.5-16.5% glycine.

Westchlor® ZR 30B. [Westwood] Aluminum zirconium trichlorhydrex-gly; antiperspirant active for anhyd. silicone suspensions and sticks; yields whiter formulations and lower irritancy levels; wh. to off-wh. free-flowing powd., pract. odorless; 99.9% thru 200 mesh; pH 3.8-4.4 (25% aq.); 14.0-15.2% Al, 13.6-16.3% Zr, 13.3-17.5% Cl, 13.5-16.5% glycine.

Westchlor® ZR 35B. [Westwood] Aluminum zirconium tetrachlorhydrex-gly; antiperspirant active for roll-on emulsions and creams; higher efficacy than basic aluminum chlorides; pH 3.7-4.1 (15% aq.); 35% aq., 5.0-5.7% Al, 4.7-5.4% Zr, 5.9-6.5% Cl.

Westchlor® ZR 35B DM Powd. [Westwood] Aluminum zirconium tetrachlorhydrex-gly; antiperspirant active for anhyd. silicone suspensions and sticks; high efficacy; off-wh. impalpable powd., pract. odorless; 98.5% min. thru 325 mesh; pH 3.6-4.0 (15% aq.); 14.5-15.5% Al, 13.0-15.5% Zr, 17-19% Cl, 10.5-13.5% glycine.

Westchlor® ZR 35B Micro Powd. [Westwood] Aluminum zirconium tetrachlorhydrex-gly; antiperspirant active for anhyd. silicone suspensions, sticks, and creams; offers higher efficacy than conventional aluminum chlorhydrate active suspension formulas; wh. to off-wh. impalpable powd., pract. odorless; 98.5% min. < 325 mesh; pH 3.7-4.1 (15% aq.); 14.5-15.5% Al, 13.0-15.5% Zr, 17.0-18.5% Cl, 10.5-13.5% glycine.

Westchlor® ZR 41. [Westwood] Aluminum zirconium tetrachlorhydrex-gly; antiperspirant active allowing formulator greater flexibility in the use of nonaq. ingreds.; pract. odorless; pH 3.70-4.00 (15% aq.); 45% aq., 6.5-7.2% Al, 5.85-6.40% Zr, 7.65-8.40% Cl.

Westchlor® ZR 80B DM Powd. [Westwood] Aluminum zirconium pentachlorhydrex-gly; antiperspirant active for anhyd. silicone suspensions and sticks; wh. to off-wh. free-flowing powd., pract. odorless; 98.5% min. thru 325 mesh; 19-20% Al, 7.8-8.8% Zr, 15-17% Cl, 7-9% glycine.

Westchlor® ZR 82B DM Powd. [Westwood] Aluminum zirconium octachlorhydrex-gly; antiperspirant active for anhyd. silicone suspensions and sticks; wh. to off-wh. free-flowing powd., pract. odorless; 98.5% min. thru 325 mesh; 18.4-19.4% Al, 7.6-8.6% Zr, 18.5-20.5% Cl, 7-9% glycine.

W.G.S. Cetyl Palmitate. [Werner G. Smith] Cetyl palmitate; CAS 540-10-3; EINECS 208-736-6; cosmetic/pharmaceutical ingred.; wh. flake; m.p. 45-55 C; acid no. 1 max.; iodine no. 5 max.; sapon. no. 110-130; toxicology: passes LD50 toxicity and rabbit skin and eye irritation tests; 92% min. act.

W.G.S. Synaceti 116 NF/USP. [Werner G. Smith] Cetyl esters (syn. spermaceti); emollient, bodying agent for cosmetic emulsions, pharmaceuticals; slip aid for inks; gloss/slip aid for varnish; processing aid and lubricant for plastics; in binder formulations for pencils; extremely stable; FDA §175.105, 175.300 compliance; wh. cryst. flakes; sp.gr. 0.82-0.84 (50 C); m.p. 43-47 C; acid no. 2 max.; iodine no. 1 max.; sapon. no. 109-120; toxicology: passes LD50 toxicity and rabbit eye and skin irritation tests.

Wheat Germ Oil. [R.I.T.A.] Wheat germ oil; CAS 8006-95-9; emollient, humectant, pigment, conditioner, lubricant with skin soothing props. for personal care prods.; yel./brn. oil.

Wheat Germ Oil. [Natural Oils Int'l.; Tri-K Industries] Wheat germ oil; CAS 8006-95-9; Unrefined grade for food and cosmetics applics. where natural vitamin E is required; Refined grade for cosmetics, vitamin E and natural antioxidant for formulations and other veg. oils; Expeller grade for gourmet food applics., natural vitamin E; golden-dk. reddish brn. clear oil, sl. nutty odor and taste; insol. in water; sp.gr. 0.93-0.94; iodine no. 115-130; sapon. no. 180-195; flash pt. (OC) 640 F; ref. index 1.469-1.478; toxicology: nonhazardous; 0.2% max. moisture.

Wheat Germ Oil CLR. [Dr. Kurt Richter; Henkel/Cospha] Wheat germ oil; CAS 8006-95-9; natural vitamin E carrier; used for general skin protection; brn. oil.

Wheat-Pro™ EN-20. [Brooks Industries] Hydrolyzed wheat protein; CAS 70084-87-6; cosmetic ingredient for skin and hair care prods.; m.w. 2000; 20% act.

Wheat-Quat C. [Maybrook] Cocodimonium hydroxypropyl hydrolyzed soy protein; CAS 100684-25-7; cationic; mild substantive protein, conditioner, moisture binder for hair and skin care prods. (shampoos, conditioners, styling prods., skin care creams/lotions, bath prods., face/body cleansers); improves wet and dry combing, hair texture, manageability; improves skin hydration and elasticity; amber clear to sl. hazy liq., char. odor; pH 4.0-6.0; 25% min. nonvolatiles.

Wheat-Tein NL. [Maybrook] Hydrolyzed wheat protein; CAS 100864-25-1; substantive protein, film-former, anti-irritant, protectant, moisturizer for skin and hair care prods. (shampoos, conditioners, styling prods., creams, lotions, hand soaps); amber clear liq., mild char. odor; pH 4.0-6.5; 18-23% nonvolatiles.

White Charcoal MB-15153. [Ikeda] Silica, magnesium oxide.

Wickenol® 101. [CasChem] Isopropyl myristate; CAS 110-27-0; EINECS 203-751-4; emollient, solubilizer, and lubricant for use in cosmetic and toilet preparations; Gardner -1 color; sol. in alcohol, animal, veg., and wh. oils; insol. in water; pour pt. -3 C; acid no. 0.1; ref. index 1.433.

Wickenol® 105. [CasChem] Isopropyl myristate, isopropyl palmitate; emollient, solubilizer, and lubricant for use in cosmetic and toilet preparations; Gardner -1 color; sol. in alcohol, animal, veg., and wh. oils; insol. in water; pour pt. 7 C; acid no. 0.2; ref. index 1.433.

Wickenol® 111. [CasChem] Isopropyl palmitate; CAS 142-91-6; EINECS 205-571-1; emollient, solubilizer, and lubricant for use in cosmetic and toilet preparations; Gardner -1 color; sol. in alcohol, animal, veg., and wh. oils; insol. in water; pour pt. 11 C; acid no. 0.1; ref. index 1.436.

Wickenol® 127. [CasChem] Isopropyl stearate; CAS 112-10-7; EINECS 203-934-9; emollient, cosolv., and lubricant; Gardner -1 color; sol. in acetone, min. and veg. oils, ethyl acetate, alcohol; insol. in water; pour pt. 18 C; acid no. 0.1; ref. index 1.438.

Wickenol® 131. [CasChem] Isopropyl isostearate; EINECS 250-651-1; lubricant, emollient, solubilizer; Gardner 2+ color; sol. in acetone, castor oil, corn oil, ethyl acetate, ethanol, min. oil; pour pt. -10 C; acid no. 0.1; ref. index 1.4418.

Wickenol® 136. [CasChem] IPP, IPM, and isopropyl stearate; emollient, conditioner, moisturizer, solubilizer, vehicle, and solv. for cosmetic and toilet preparations; Gardner -1 liq.; sol. in alcohols, ketones, aromatic and aliphatic hydrocarbons; insol. in water; pour pt. 7 C; acidno. 0.1; ref. index 1.435.

Wickenol® 139. [CasChem] Syn. jojoba oil; CAS 61789-91-1; emollient, plasticizer, lubricant, coupler for hair and skin care prods.; replacement for natural jojoba oil; clear liq. wax; sol. in alcohol, animal and veg. oils, wh. oils; pour pt. -38 C; acid no. 0.1; ref. index 1.960.

Wickenol® 141. [CasChem] Butyl myristate; CAS 110-36-1; EINECS 203-759-8; emollient, solubilizer, and lubricant for use in cosmetic and toilet preparations; plasticizer; Gardner -1 color; sol. in alcohol, animal, wh., and veg. oils; insol. in water; pour pt. 0 C; acid no. 0.1; ref. index 1.437.

Wickenol® 142. [CasChem] Octyldodecyl myristate; emollient ingred., plasticizer for cosmetic and pharmaceutical preparations; Gardner 2+ color; sol. in alcohol, animal,

veg., and wh. oils; insol. in water; pour pt. 0 C; acid no. 0.1; ref. index 1.460.

Wickenol® 143. [CasChem] Oleyl oleate; CAS 3687-45-4; EINECS 222-980-4; lubricant used in cosmetic and toilet preparations; replacement for sperm oil in addition to functioning as cosmetic additive; Gardner 2+ color; sol. in alcohol, animal, wh. and veg. oils; insol. in water; pour pt. 14 C; acid no. 0.1; ref. index 1.463.

Wickenol® 144. [CasChem] Isodecyl oleate; CAS 59231-34-4; EINECS 261-673-6; emollient, wetting agent and pigment binder for cosmetics; Gardner 2+ color; pour pt. -20 C; acid no. 0.1; ref. index 1.45.

Wickenol® 151. [CasChem] Isononyl isononanoate; CAS 42131-25-9; emollient, moisturizer, pigment wetter; silky emolliency and solv. chars.; for hair care prods.; Gardner -1 color; sol. in alcohol, animal, veg., and min. oil; insol. in water; pour pt. < -15 C; acid no. 0.10; ref. index 1.435.

Wickenol® 152. [CasChem] Isodecyl isononanoate; CAS 41395-89-5; silky emollience and solv. char. for skin and hair care prods.; pigment wetter; Gardner -1 color; sol. in alcohol, animal, veg., and min. oils; pour pt. < -15 C; acid no. 0.10; ref. index 1.438.

Wickenol® 153. [CasChem] Isotridecyl isononanoate; silky emollience and solv. char. for skin and hair care prods.; pigment wetter, moisturizer; Gardner -1 color; sol. in alcohol, animal, veg., and min. oils; pour pt. < -18 C; acid no. 0.10; ref. index 1.444.

Wickenol® 155. [CasChem] Octyl palmitate; CAS 29806-73-3; EINECS 249-862-1; emollient, moisturizer, pigment wetter/dispersant; increases water vapor porosity of fatty components used in cosmetic and topical pharmaceutical preparations; Gardner -1 color; sol. in alcohol, animal, veg., and min. oils; insol. in water; pour pt. -3 C; acid no. 0.10; ref. index 1.445.

Wickenol® 156. [CasChem] Octyl stearate; emollient, moisturizer, pigment wetter/dispersant; increases water vapor porosity of fatty components used in cosmetic and topical pharmaceutical preparations; Gardner -1 color; sol. in alcohol, animal, veg., and min. oils; pour pt. 5 C; acid no. 0.10; ref. index 1.4465.

Wickenol® 158. [CasChem] Dioctyl adipate; CAS 103-23-1; EINECS 203-090-1; emollient, moisturizer, pigment wetter/dispersant, cosolv.; increases water vapor porosity of fatty components used in cosmetic and topical pharmaceutical preparations; Gardner -1 color; sol. in alcohol, animal, veg., and min. oils; pour pt. -20 C; acid no. 0.10; ref. index 1.445.

Wickenol® 159. [CasChem] Dioctyl succinate; CAS 2915-57-3; EINECS 220-836-1; emollient, moisturizer, pigment wetter/dispersant; increases water vapor porosity of fatty components used in cosmetic and topical pharmaceutical preparations; Gardner -1 color; sol. in alcohol, animal, veg., and min. oils; pour pt. -18 C; acid no. 0.7; ref. index 1.443.

Wickenol® 160. [CasChem] Octyl pelargonate; CAS 59587-44-9; EINECS 261-819-9; emollient, moisturizer, pigment wetter/dispersant; increases water vapor porosity of fatty components used in cosmetic and topical pharmaceutical preparations; improves stick formulations; Gardner 2+ color; sol. in alcohol, animal, veg., and min. oils; pour pt. -18 C; acid no. 0.10; ref. index 1.437.

Wickenol® 161. [CasChem] Dioctyl adipate, octyl stearate, octyl palmitate; emollient, moisturizer, pigment wetter/dispersant; increases water vapor porosity of fatty components used in cosmetic and topical pharmaceutical preparations; Gardner -1 color; sol. in alcohol, animal, veg., and min. oils; pour pt. -12 C; acid no. 0.1; ref. index 1.446.

Wickenol® 163. [CasChem] Dioctyl adipate, octyl stearate, octyl palmitate; emollient, solubilizer; fragrance enhancer; Gardner -1 color; sol. in alcohol, animal, veg., and min. oils; pour pt. 0 C; acid no. 0.1; ref. index 1.446.

Wickenol® 171. [CasChem] Octyl hydroxystearate; CAS 29383-26-4; emollient, moisturizer, pigment wetter/dispersant; increases water vapor porosity of fatty components used in cosmetic and topical pharmaceutical preparations; refatting agent, counter-irritant, cosolv., solubilizer; Gardner 2+ color; sol. in acetone, castor, corn, and min. oil, chloroform, ethyl acetate, ethanol; pour pt. 5 C; acid no. 0.30; ref. index 1.456.

Wickenol® 174. [CasChem] Myristyl octanoate; emollient; provides soft satiny skin afterfeel; Gardner 2+ liq.; pour pt. 14 C; acid no. 0.1; ref. index 1.443.

Wickenol® 506. [CasChem] Myristyl lactate; CAS 1323-03-1; EINECS 215-350-1; emollient with smooth, satiny afterfeel; Gardner 2+ color; sol. in ethanol, min. oil, IPM, propylene glycol; insol. in water; m.p. 9 C; acid no. 0.50; ref. index 1.444.

Wickenol® 535. [CasChem] Wheat germ glycerides; CAS 68990-07-8; hydrophilic/hydrophobic emollient, emulsifier, skin lubricant; anti-irritant; Gardner 2+ liq.; sol. in veg. and min. oils, IPA, acetone, chloroform; insol. in water; acid no. 0.8; iodine no. 118; 100% act.

Wickenol® 545. [CasChem] Glucose glutamate; substantive humectant, skin conditioner, moisturizer, emulsifier, surfactant, thickener used in personal care prods.; enhances lather in surfactant systems; Gardner 2+ color; sol. in water, slightly sol. in alcohol; 55% conc.

Wickenol® 550. [CasChem] Maltodextrin; CAS 9050-36-6; EINECS 232-940-4; absorbent for lipophilic materials for powd. bath applics.; food-grade carrier for flavors; Gardner 2+ powd.; 100% act.

Wickenol® 707. [CasChem] PPG-30 cetyl ether; CAS 9035-85-2; all-purpose fluid, nongreasy emollient with hydroalcoholic compatibility; provides coupling and emulsion stability; foam modifier; enhances sheen and manageability; Gardner 2+ color; sol. in animal and veg. oils, ethanol; insol. in water; acid no. 0.1; iodine no. 1.0 max.

Wickenol® 727. [CasChem] PPG-30 lanolin alcohol ether; CAS 68439-53-2; nongreasy emollient, solubilizer, bodying agent; also low odor derivative; Gardner 4+ color; sol. in animal and veg. oils, ethanol; insol. in water; acid no. 0.7; iodine no. 12.

Witafrol® 7420. [Hüls Am.] Caprylic/capric glycerides; CAS 26402-26-6; surfactant for pharmaceutical, cosmetic, nutritional fields; as emulsifier, solubilizer, dispersant, plasticizer, lubricant, consistency regulator, skin/mucous membrane protectant, refatting agent, penetrant, carrier, adsorp. promoter, antifoam; sl. ylsh. oil; sol. in water/ethanol (50/50), acetone; sol. cloudy in ether, heptane; acid no. 2 max.; iodine no. 1 max.; sapon. no. 240-275; 40-42% monoglycerides.

Witarix® 212. [Hüls Am.] Hydrog. palm kernel oil; CAS 68990-82-9; fats for chocolate and confectionery prods. with soft consistency; also for personal care prods.

Witarix® 250. [Hüls Am.] Cocoglycerides; fats for chocolate and confectionery prods. with soft consistency; also for personal care applics.

Witarix® 440. [Hüls Am.] Hydrog. soybean oil; CAS 8016-70-4; EINECS 232-410-2; fats for chocolate and confectionery prods. with soft consistency; also for personal care applics.

Witarix® 450. [Hüls Am.] Hydrog. peanut oil; CAS 68425-36-5; EINECS 270-350-9; fats for chocolate and confectionery prods. with soft consistency; also for personal care applics.

Witcamide® 61. [Witco/H-I-P] Oleamide MIPA and isopropanolamire; nonionic; hair conditioner, emulsifier, lubricant; cosmetics and toiletries; yel. paste; disp. in oils, water; sp.gr. 0.90; 100% conc.

Witcamide® 70. [Witco/H-I-P] Stearamide MEA; CAS 111-

57-9; EINECS 203-883-2; nonionic; opacifier, conditioner, lubricant, thickener, gelling agent, mold release agent, binder; cosmetics and toiletries; base for antiperspirant and makeup sticks; flake; sol. in oil; sp.gr. 1.0.

Witcamide® 82. [Witco/H-I-P] Cocamide DEA and diethanolamine; nonionic; foam stabilizer, visc. modifier, lubricant, conditioner, emulsifier, wetting agent, penetrant, dye dispersant, scouring aid, antistat; cosmetics and toiletries, base for scrub soap; thickener; industrial and textile surfactant; metal processing; liq.; 100% conc.

Witcamide® 128T. [Witco/H-I-P] Cocamide DEA; CAS 61791-31-9; EINECS 263-163-9; nonionic; detergent, foam booster/stabilizer, visc. modifier, substantive conditioner for personal care prods.; liq.; sol. in water, disp. in oils; sp.gr. 0.99; formerly Witcamide 6515.

Witcamide® 823/10. [Witco/H-I-P] Isostearic alkanolamide; nonionic; hair conditioner, lubricant used in personal care prods.; lt. amber liq.; sol. in aromatic solv., chlorinated hydrocarbons, min. spirits and oil, kerosene, veg. oil, ethanol; disp. in water; cloud pt. –5 C; acid no. 10 max.; pH 9.5 ± 0.5 (10% disp.); 100% act.

Witcamide® 5024. [Witco/H-I-P] Cocamide DEA, diethanolamine; personal care surfactant.

Witcamide® 5085. [Witco/H-I-P] Oleamide DEA; CAS 93-83-4; EINECS 202-281-7; thickener, foam booster/stabilizer.

Witcamide® 5118S. [Witco/H-I-P] Isostearamide DEA; CAS 52794-79-3; EINECS 258-193-4; personal care surfactant.

Witcamide® 5133. [Witco/H-I-P] Cocamide DEA and diethanolamine; nonionic; emulsifier, foam stabilizer, visc. modifier, lubricant, conditioner, wetting agent, penetrant, dye dispersant, scouring aid, antistat for textiles, industrial use, personal care prods., metal processing; liq.; 100% conc.

Witcamide® 5168. [Witco/H-I-P] Diethanolaminooleamide DEA; cationic; surfactant for cosmetics, textiles, detergents, and industrial uses; liq.; 100% conc.

Witcamide® 5195. [Witco/H-I-P] Lauramide DEA; CAS 120-40-1; EINECS 204-393-1; nonionic; visc. modifier, foam stabilizer, lubricant, conditioner, lubricant, emulsifier, wetting agent, thickener, penetrant, dye dispersant, scouring aid, antistat; cosmetics and toiletries; industrial foamer and stabilizer; metal processing; textile surfactant; aerosol formulations; paste; water-sol.; sp.gr. 0.99.

Witcamide® 6310. [Witco/H-I-P] Lauramide DEA, modified; CAS 120-40-1; EINECS 204-393-1; nonionic; conditioner, foam stabilizer, gelling agent, lubricant, and visc. modifier for cosmetics and toiletries; industrial detergent; paste; water-sol.; sp.gr. 0.97; 100% conc.

Witcamide® 6404. [Witco/H-I-P] Cocamide DEA; CAS 61791-31-9; EINECS 263-163-9; personal care surfactant.

Witcamide® 6507. [Witco/H-I-P] Stearamide MEA; CAS 111-57-9; EINECS 203-883-2; personal care surfactant.

Witcamide® 6510. [Witco/H-I-P] Lauramide DEA; CAS 120-40-1; EINECS 204-393-1; nonionic; personal care surfactant.

Witcamide® 6511. [Witco/H-I-P] Lauramide DEA; CAS 120-40-1; EINECS 204-393-1; nonionic; detergent, foam booster/stabilizer, substantive conditioner, visc. modifier for personal care prods.; liq.; water-sol.; sp.gr. 0.99.

Witcamide® 6514. [Witco/H-I-P] Cocamide DEA; CAS 61791-31-9; EINECS 263-163-9; nonionic; detergent, foam booster/stabilizer, visc. modifier, substantive conditioner for personal care prods.; liq.; water-sol.; sp.gr. 0.98.

Witcamide® 6519. [Witco/H-I-P] Lauramide DEA; CAS 120-40-1; EINECS 204-393-1; personal care surfactant.

Witcamide® 6531. [Witco/H-I-P] Cocamide DEA; CAS 61791-31-9; EINECS 263-163-9; nonionic; detergent, foam booster/stabilizer, conditioner for personal care prods.; liq.; water-sol.; sp.gr. 1.01.

Witcamide® 6533. [Witco/H-I-P] Cocamide DEA, diethanolamine; nonionic; detergent, dispersant, o/w emulsifier, lubricant, visc. modifier, conditioner for personal care prods.; liq.; water-sol.; sp.gr. 0.99.

Witcamide® 6534. [Witco/H-I-P] Cocamide DEA, diethanolamine; personal care surfactant.

Witcamide® 6540. [Witco/H-I-P] Linoleamide DEA; CAS 56863-02-6; EINECS 260-410-2; personal care surfactant.

Witcamide® 6544. [Witco/H-I-P] Capramide DEA, diethanolamine; CAS 136-26-5; EINECS 205-234-9; personal care surfactant.

Witcamide® 6546. [Witco/H-I-P] Oleamide DEA, diethanolamine; nonionic; conditioner, coupling agent, detergent, o/w emulsifier, foam stabilizer for personal care applics.; liq.; oil-sol.; sp.gr. 0.98.

Witcamide® 6570. [Witco/H-I-P] Undecylenamide MEA; CAS 20545-92-0; EINECS 243-870-9; personal care surfactant.

Witcamide® 6590. [Witco/H-I-P] Lauramide DEA; CAS 120-40-1; EINECS 204-393-1; personal care surfactant.

Witcamide® 6625. [Witco/H-I-P] Cocamide DEA, modified; CAS 61791-31-9; EINECS 263-163-9; nonionic; detergent, foam booster/stabilizer, visc. modifier, substantive conditioner for personal care applics.; liq.; water-sol.; sp.gr. 0.98.

Witcamide® 6731. [Witco/H-I-P] Cocamide DEA, DEA-lauryl sulfate.; personal care surfactant.

Witcamide® CD. [Witco/H-I-P] Cocamide DEA; CAS 61791-31-9; EINECS 263-163-9; nonionic; detergent, thickener, foam booster/stabilizer, conditioner for personal care applics.; liq.; water-sol.; sp.gr. 1.02; 100% conc.; formerly Witcamide Coco Condensate.

Witcamide® CDA. [Witco/H-I-P] Cocamide DEA, modified; CAS 61791-31-9; EINECS 263-163-9; nonionic; detergent, dispersant, o/w emulsifier, lubricant, visc. modifier, conditioner for personal care prods.; base for scrub soap formulations; liq.; water-sol.; sp.gr. 1.00; 100% conc.

Witcamide® CMEA. [Witco/H-I-P] Acetamide MEA; CAS 142-26-7; EINECS 205-530-8; nonionic; solvent, humectant for cosmetics; liq.; 70-100% conc.; formerly Acetamide MEA.

Witcamide® GR. [Witco/H-I-P] Cocamide DEA; CAS 61791-31-9; EINECS 263-163-9; personal care surfactant.

Witcamide® L-9. [Witco/H-I-P] Lauramide DEA; CAS 120-40-1; EINECS 204-393-1; personal care surfactant.

Witcamide® LDEA. [Witco/H-I-P] Lauramide DEA; CAS 120-40-1; EINECS 204-393-1; nonionic; substantive conditioner, detergent, foam booster/stabilizer, visc. modifier for personal care applics.; liq.; disp. in water; sp.gr. 0.99.

Witcamide® LDTS. [Witco/H-I-P] Cocamide DEA; CAS 61731-31-9; EINECS 263-163-9; nonionic; detergent, foam stabilizer, softener, visc. control for cosmetics, shampoos, bath prods.; yel. liq.; 100% conc.

Witcamide® LL. [Witco/H-I-P] Lauramide DEA; CAS 120-40-1; EINECS 204-393-1; personal care surfactant.

Witcamide® LM, LMT. [Witco/H-I-P] Alkylolamide; nonionic; thickener for personal care prods.; flakes; 100% conc.

Witcamide® M-3. [Witco/H-I-P] Cocamide DEA; CAS 61791-31-9; EINECS 263-163-9; nonionic; cleansing agent, conditioner, lubricant, and visc. modifier; detergent, foamer and stabilizer for industrial detergents; liq.; water-sol.; 100% conc.

Witcamide® MAS. [Witco/H-I-P] Stearamide MEA-stearate; CAS 14351-40-7; EINECS 238-310-5; nonionic; opacifier, conditioner, lubricant, gelling agent for personal care, household, and institutional liq. soaps; used as partial or total replacement for veg. waxes in polishes; coating

agent for paper and textiles; mold release agent for industrial processing; additive for raising melting pts. of petrol. waxes or glyceride waxes and fats; ingred. of insulating coatings or barriers, and of water-repellent compds.; lt. cream waxy flakes; mild char. odor; sol. in aliphatic, aromatic, and chlorinated hydrocarbons, alcohol, ketones, esters; sp.gr. 0.844; m.p. 81 C; acid no. 5.0; 100% conc.

Witcamide® MM. [Witco/H-I-P] Myristamide MEA; CAS 142-58-5; EINECS 205-546-5; nonionic; opacifier, conditioner, binder, lubricant, gelling and mold release agent for cosmetics; wax.

Witcamide® PPA. [Witco/H-I-P] Cocamide MIPA; CAS 68333-82-4; EINECS 269-793-0; viscosifier for shampoos and bath prods.; wax; 100% act.

Witcamide® S771. [Witco/H-I-P] Cocamide DEA, modified; CAS 61791-31-9; EINECS 263-163-9; nonionic; detergent, emulsifier, foamer, stabilizer, lubricant, coupling agent for shampoos, bubble baths, industrial detergents; liq.; water-sol.; sp.gr. 0.98; 100% conc.

Witcamide® S780. [Witco/H-I-P] Cocamide DEA, modified; CAS 61791-31-9; EINECS 263-163-9; nonionic; emulsifier, coupling agent, foamer, stabilizer, lubricant for shampoos, bubble baths, industrial detergents; liq.; water-sol.; sp.gr. 0.97; 100% conc.

Witcamide® SR200. [Witco/H-I-P] Diethanolamine and cocamide DEA; personal care surfactant.

Witcamide® SSA. [Witco/H-I-P] Soyamide DEA; CAS 68425-47-8; EINECS 270-355-6; nonionic; substantive conditioner, detergent, foam booster/stabilizer, visc. modifier for personal care prods.; liq.; water-sol.; sp.gr. 1.00.

Witcamide® STD-HP. [Witco/H-I-P] Lauramide DEA; CAS 120-40-1; EINECS 204-393-1; nonionic; detergent, conditioner, foam stabilizer, lubricant for cosmetics and toiletries; visc. enhancer; solid; water-sol.; 100% conc.

Witcamine® 100. [Witco/H-I-P] Cocamidopropyl dimethylamine; CAS 68140-01-2; EINECS 268-771-8; personal care surfactant.

Witcamine® 6606. [Witco/H-I-P] PEG-15 tallow amine; cationic; antistat, dispersant, o/w emulsifier, lubricant, substantivity and wetting agent for personal care applics.; lt. amber liq.; water-sol.; sp.gr. 1.02; pH 9.5; 99% solids.

Witcamine® 6622. [Witco/H-I-P] PEG-30 oleamine; cationic; antistat, dispersant, o/w emulsifier, lubricant, substantivity and wetting agent for personal care prods.; lt. amber liq.; water-sol.; sp.gr. 1.07; pH 9.5; 80% solids.

Witco® Aluminum Stearate 18. [Witco/H-I-P] Aluminum stearate; thickener for hydrocarbon fluids, personal care applics.; sol. hot with gelation on cooling in aliphatic and aromatic solvs., oils.

Witco® Aluminum Stearate 132. [Witco/H-I-P] Aluminum tristearate; CAS 637-12-7; EINECS 211-279-5; personal care applics.

Witco® Aluminum Stearate EA Food Grade. [Witco/H-I-P] Aluminum distearate; CAS 300-92-5; EINECS 206-101-8; food and personal care applics.

Witco® Calcium Stearate F.P. [Witco/H-I-P] Calcium stearate; CAS 1592-23-0; EINECS 216-472-8; personal care applics.

Witcodet 4680. [Witco/H-I-P] Formulated prod.; detergent conc. base for bubble baths, shampoos; liq.; 55% conc.

Witcodet AE. [Witco/H-I-P] Pearlized blend; anionic/nonionic/amphoteric; detergent conc. for bubble bath, hand and body soaps, shampoo; liq.; water-sol.; sp.gr. 1.02; visc. 4000 cps; pH 5.5; 43% solids.

Witcodet AEG. [Witco/H-I-P] Blend; anionic/nonionic/amphoteric; detergent conc. for bubble bath, hand and body soaps, shampoo; Gardner 3 liq.; water-sol.; sp.gr. 1.02; visc. 3000 cps; pH 5.5; 42% solids.

Witcolate™ 1050. [Witco/H-I-P] Sodium C12-15 pareth sulfate; anionic; detergent, detergent base, emulsifier, foamer, wetting agent for the detergent and personal care industry; liq.; water-sol.; sp.gr. 1.04; 39% act.
Witcolate™ 3570. [Witco/H-I-P] Sodium alkyl ether sulfate; anionic; detergent for shampoos, bubble baths, household and industrial cleansing compositions; paste; 70% conc.
Witcolate™ 6462. [Witco/H-I-P] Sodium alkyl sulfate; anionic; detergent, dispersant, wetting agent for personal care applics.; liq.; water-sol.; sp.gr. 1.08; 38% act.
Witcolate™ 7093. [Witco/H-I-P] Sodium deceth sulfate; anionic; detergent, foamer and wetting agent for personal care and industrial pressure-spray applics.; electrolyte tolerance; liq.; water-sol.; sp.gr. 1.04; 38.5% act.
Witcolate™ 7103. [Witco/H-I-P] Ammonium alcohol ether sulfate; anionic; high foaming detergent, wetting agent in high electrolyte systems such as oil well drilling; also for personal care formulations; liq.; water-sol.; sp.gr. 1.105; 58% act.
Witcolate™ AE-3. [Witco/H-I-P] Ammonium C12-15 pareth sulfate; anionic; detergent, wetting agent, emulsifier, foamer for the detergent and personal care industry; liq.; water-sol.; sp.gr. 1.04; 59% act.; formerly Witcolate AE.
Witcolate™ AE3S. [Witco/H-I-P] Sodium alkyl ether sulfate; anionic; base for liq. detergents; liq.; 27% conc.
Witcolate™ A Powder. [Witco/H-I-P] Sodium lauryl sulfate; CAS 151-21-3; EINECS 205-788-1; anionic; detergent, wetting agent, foamer used in personal care prods., wool detergents; polymerization emulsifier; powd.; water-sol.; sp.gr. 0.35; 93% act.
Witcolate™ C. [Witco/H-I-P] Sodium lauryl sulfate; CAS 151-21-3; EINECS 205-788-1; anionic; detergent, foaming agent, wetting agent for personal care prods.; paste; water-sol.; sp.gr. 1.06; 29% act.
Witcolate™ D51-51. [Witco/H-I-P] Nonoxynol-4 sulfate; anionic; antistat for syn. fibers and polymer prods.; surfactant, wetting agent and dispersant; emulsifier for polymerization of acrylics, vinyl acetate, vinyl acrylics, styrene, SAN, styrene acrylic, vinyl chloride; personal care formulations; FDA compliance; clear liq.; sol. in water, ethanol; sp.gr. 1.06; visc. 2500 cps; pH 8.0 (5% aq.); flash pt. (PMCC) > 93.3 C; surf. tens. 30.0 dynes/cm (1%); Ross-Miles foam 173 mm (initial, 1% , 49 C); 34% solids.
Witcolate™ D51-51EP. [Witco/H-I-P] Sodium nonoxynol-4 sulfate; CAS 9014-90-8; emulsifier for emulsion polymerization of acrylic, vinyl acetate, vinyl acrylic, vinyl chloride; personal care formulations; FDA compliance; Gardner 4 color; visc. 400 cps; pH 8 (10% aq.); surf. tens. 30 dynes/cm (1%); 30% act.
Witcolate™ D51-52. [Witco/H-I-P] Sodium alkylaryl polyether sulfate; anionic; emulsifier for polymerization, personal care formulations; liq.
Witcolate™ D51-53. [Witco/H-I-P] Nonoxynol-10 sulfate; emulsifier for acrylic, vinyl acetate, vinyl acrylic, styrene, SAN, styrene acrylic, and vinyl chloride polymerization; personal care formulations; visc. 250 cps; surf. tens. 40 dynes/cm (1%); Ross-Miles foam 218 mm (initial, 1% , 49 C); 34% solids.
Witcolate™ D51-53HA. [Witco/H-I-P] Nonoxynol-10 sulfate; emulsifier for acrylic, vinyl acetate, vinyl acrylic, styrene, SAN, styrene acrylic, and vinyl chloride polymerization; personal care formulations; visc. 50 cps; surf. tens. 41.2 dynes/cm (1%); Ross-Miles foam 224 mm (initial, 1% , 49 C); 30% solids.
Witcolate™ D51-60. [Witco/H-I-P] Nonoxynol-30 sulfate; emulsifier for acrylic, vinyl acetate, vinyl acrylic, styrene, SAN, styrene acrylic, and vinyl chloride polymerization; personal care formulations; visc. 300 cps; surf. tens. 43.3 dynes/cm (1%); Ross-Miles foam 234 mm (initial, 1% , 49

C); 40% solids.
Witcolate™ D-510. [Witco/H-I-P] Sodium 2-ethylhexyl sulfate; CAS 126-92-1; EINECS 204-812-8; anionic; detergent, wetting agent and penetrant for industrial use and polymerization reactions; dispersant for bleaching powds.; lime soap and grease dispersant; personal care formulations; clear liq.; sol. (5%) in water, IPA; sp.gr. 1.12; pH 10.5 (10% aq.); flash pt. > 93 C; 39% act.; formerly Witcolate 6465.
Witcolate™ DLS-35. [Witco/H-I-P] DEA-lauryl sulfate; CAS 143-00-0; EINECS 205-577-4; personal care applics.
Witcolate™ ES-1. [Witco/H-I-P] Sodium laureth (1) sulfate; detergent, foaming and wetting agent for personal care applics.; liq.; water-sol.; sp.gr. 1.04; 25% act.; formerly Witcolate 6450.
Witcolate™ ES-2. [Witco/H-I-P] Sodium laureth (2) sulfate; CAS 9004-82-4; anionic; detergent, foaming agent, wetting agent for personal care applics.; liq.; water-sol.; sp.gr. 1.05; 26% act.; formerly Witcolate 6455.
Witcolate™ ES-3. [Witco/H-I-P] Sodium laureth (3) sulfate; CAS 9004-82-4; anionic; detergent, foaming agent, wetting agent for personal care applics.; liq.; water-sol.; sp.gr. 1.05; 28% act.; formerly Witcolate 6453.
Witcolate™ LCP. [Witco/H-I-P] Sodium lauryl sulfate; CAS 151-21-3; EINECS 205-788-1; anionic; detergent, foaming agent, wetting agent for personal care applics.; liq.; water-sol.; sp.gr. 1.04; 29% act.
Witcolate™ LES-60A. [Witco/H-I-P] Ammonium laureth sulfate; CAS 32612-48-9; anionic; detergent, foaming agent, wetting agent for personal care applics.; liq.; water-sol.; sp.gr. 1.06; 59% act.
Witcolate™ LES-60C. [Witco/H-I-P] Sodium laureth sulfate; CAS 9004-82-4; anionic; detergent, foaming agent, wetting agent for personal care applics.; liq.; water-sol.; sp.gr. 1.06; 58% act.
Witcolate™ MG-LS. [Witco/H-I-P] Magnesium lauryl sulfate; CAS 3097-08-3; EINECS 221-450-6; personal care applics.
Witcolate™ NH. [Witco/H-I-P] Ammonium lauryl sulfate; CAS 2235-54-3; EINECS 218-793-9; anionic; detergent, foaming agent, wetting agent for personal care applics.; liq.; water-sol.; sp.gr. 1.01; 28.5% act.; formerly Witcolate 6430, 6431, AM.
Witcolate™ OME. [Witco/H-I-P] Sodium laureth sulfate; CAS 9004-82-4; anionic; used in detergents and personal care prods.; liq.; 24% conc.
Witcolate™ S1285C. [Witco/H-I-P] Sodium laureth sulfate; CAS 9004-82-4; anionic; cleansing agent, detergent, wetting agent, detergent base, and foamer for cosmetics, toiletries, industrial detergents, textiles; liq.; water-sol.; 60% conc.
Witcolate™ S1300C. [Witco/H-I-P] Ammonium laureth sulfate; CAS 32612-48-9; anionic; cleansing agent, detergent, wetting agent, detergent base, and foamer for cosmetics, toiletries, industrial detergents, textiles; liq.; water-sol.; 60% conc.
Witcolate™ SE-2. [Witco/H-I-P] Sodium laureth sulfate.; personal care applics.
Witcolate™ SE-5. [Witco/H-I-P] Sodium C12-15 pareth sulfate; anionic; detergent, detergent base, foamer, o/w emulsifier, wetting agent for industrial and household detergents, textiles, personal care prods.; liq.; water-sol.; sp.gr. 1.04; 59% act.; formerly Witcolate SE.
Witcolate™ SL-1. [Witco/H-I-P] Sodium lauryl sulfate; CAS 151-21-3; EINECS 205-788-1; emulsifier for acrylics, acrylonitrile, carboxylated SBR, chloroprene, styrene, vinyl chloride, vinyl acetate; personal care formulations; FDA compliance; visc. 50 cps; HLB 40; surf. tens. 31.8 dynes/cm (1%); Ross-Miles foam 180 mm (initial, 1% , 49 C); 29% solids.

Witcolate™ T

Witcolate™ T. [Witco/H-I-P] TEA-lauryl sulfate; CAS 139-96-8; EINECS 205-388-7; anionic; cleansing agent, and foamer, emulsifier, solubilizer for cosmetics and toiletries; detergent base; wetting agent for industrial detergents; liq.; water-sol.; 40% conc.

Witcolate™ TLS-500. [Witco/H-I-P] TEA-lauryl sulfate; CAS 139-96-8; EINECS 205-388-7; anionic; detergent, foaming agent, wetting agent for personal care applics.; liq.; water-sol.; sp.gr. 1.05; 40% act.; formerly Witcolate 6434.

Witcolate™ WAC. [Witco/H-I-P] Sodium lauryl sulfate; CAS 151-21-3; EINECS 205-788-1; anionic; detergent, foaming agent, wetting agent for personal care applics.

Witcolate™ WAC-GL. [Witco/H-I-P] Sodium lauryl sulfate; CAS 151-21-3; EINECS 205-788-1; anionic; detergent, foaming agent, wetting agent for personal care applics.; liq.; water-sol.; sp.gr. 1.04; 29% act.

Witcolate™ WAC-LA. [Witco/H-I-P] Sodium lauryl sulfate; CAS 151-21-3; EINECS 205-788-1; anionic; detergent, foaming agent, wetting agent for personal care applics.; liq.; water-sol.; sp.gr. 1.04; 29% act.; formerly Witcolate 6400, A, S.

Witco® Lithium Stearate 306. [Witco/H-I-P] Lithium stearate; CAS 4485-12-5; EINECS 224-772-5; personal care applics.

Witco® Magnesium Stearate N.F. [Witco/H-I-P] Magnesium stearate; CAS 557-04-0; EINECS 209-150-3; personal care applics.

Witconate™ 30DS. [Witco/H-I-P] Sodium dodecylbenzene sulfonate; CAS 25155-30-0; EINECS 246-680-4; anionic; detergent, foaming agent, wetting agent for personal care applics.; liq.; sol. in water; sp.gr. 1.07; pH 7.5; 30% act.

Witconate™ 45 Liq. [Witco/H-I-P] Sodium dodecylbenzene-sulfonate, sodium xylenesulfonate; anionic; detergent base, emulsifier, foamer, and wetting agent for personal care, detergent industry, and industrial surfactants; electrolyte tolerant; liq.; water-sol.; sp.gr. 1.08; pH 7.0; 45% act.; formerly Witconate 45DS.

Witconate™ 45BX. [Witco/H-I-P] Sodium dodecylbenzene sulfonate; CAS 25155-30-0; EINECS 246-680-4; anionic; detergent base for personal care applics.; liq.; 42% conc.

Witconate™ 45LX. [Witco/H-I-P] Sodium dodecylbenzene-sulfonate, sodium xylene sulfonate; anionic; detergent, wetting agent, foaming agent, base for personal care, household and industrial specialties; low cloud pt.; liq.; water-sol.; sp.gr. 1.09; pH 7.5; 43% act.

Witconate™ 60B. [Witco/H-I-P] Sodium dodecylbenzene sulfonate; CAS 25155-30-0; EINECS 246-680-4; anionic; cleansing agent, foamer, solubilizer for cosmetics and toiletries; detergent base, foamer and wetting agent, emulsifier for industrial detergents; liq.; water-sol.; 60% conc.

Witconate™ 60T. [Witco/H-I-P] TEA-dodecylbenzenesulfonate; CAS 27323-41-7; EINECS 248-406-9; anionic; detergent, wetter, emulsifier, foaming agent, antistat, lubricant; base for household, industrial, and cosmetic/toiletry specialty compds.; liq.; water-sol.; sp.gr. 1.08; pH 6.5; 58% act.; formerly Sulframin 60T.

Witconate™ 68KN. [Witco/H-I-P] Blend; anionic/nonionic; detergent, foaming agent, wetting agent for personal care applics.; liq.; sol. in water; sp.gr. 1.09; pH 7.0; 67% act.

Witconate™ 79S. [Witco/H-I-P] TEA-dodecylbenzene sulfonate; CAS 27323-41-7; EINECS 248-406-9; anionic; detergent, dispersant, emulsifier, wetting agent; personal care and industrial surfactant; agric. applics.; EPA clearance; liq.; water-sol.; sp.gr. 1.06; pH 7.0; 52% act.

Witconate™ 90F H. [Witco/H-I-P] Branched sodium dodecylbenzene sulfonate; CAS 25155-30-0; EINECS 246-680-4; anionic; detergent, foaming agent, wetting agent for personal care applics.; flake; sol. in water; sp.gr. 0.40; pH 8.0; 91% act.

Witconate™ 93S. [Witco/H-I-P] Amine dodecylbenzene sulfonate; anionic; detergent, detergent base, emulsifier, foamer, wetting agent, dispersant, solubilizer for the personal care and detergent industry; biodeg.; liq.; sol. in oil, IPA, kerosene, xylene; disp. in water; sp.gr. 1.05; dens. 8.5 lb/gal; visc. 800 cps; pour pt. 25 F; pH 4.5; 91% act.

Witconate™ 1238. [Witco/H-I-P] Sodium dodecylbenzene-sulfonate; CAS 25155-30-0; EINECS 246-680-4; personal care surfactant.

Witconate™ 1240. [Witco/H-I-P] Sodium dodecylbenzene-sulfonate; CAS 25155-30-0; EINECS 246-680-4; anionic; detergent base, emulsifier, foamer, and wetting agent for the personal care, household and industrial detergents; slurry; water-sol.; sp.gr. 1.07; pH 7.5; 40% act.

Witconate™ 1250. [Witco/H-I-P] Sodium dodecylbenzene sulfonate; CAS 25155-30-0; EINECS 246-680-4; anionic; detergent, wetting agent, foaming agent, base for personal care, household, and industrial detergents, emulsion polymerization; slurry; water-sol.; sp.gr. 1.08; pH 7.5; 53% act.

Witconate™ 1260. [Witco/H-I-P] Sodium dodecylbenzene-sulfonate, sodium xylenesulfonate; anionic; detergent, wetting agent, foaming agent, base for personal care, household, and industrial compds.; textile surfactant; slurry; water-sol.; sp.gr. 1.10; pH 7.5; 60% act.

Witconate Acide B. [Witco/H-I-P] Straight chain dodecylbenzene sulfonic acid; CAS 27176-87-0; EINECS 248-289-4; anionic; intermediate for prod. of biodeg. sulfonates; liq.; 97% conc.; formerly Sulframin Acide B.

Witconate™ AOK. [Witco/H-I-P] Sodium C14-16 olefin sulfonate; CAS 68439-57-6; EINECS 270-407-8; anionic; detergent, foaming agent, wetting agent for personal care applics.; flake; sol. in water; sp.gr. 0.40; pH 8.5; 90% act.

Witconate™ AOS. [Witco/H-I-P] Sodium C14-16 olefin sulfonate; CAS 68439-57-6; EINECS 270-407-8; anionic; detergent, foamer, wetting agent, solubilizer for cosmetics and toiletries, shampoos, industrial detergents, textiles, petrol. industry; emulsifier for plastics/rubber polymerization; FDA compliance; liq.; sol. in water; disp. in IPA; sp.gr. 1.05; dens. 8.8 lb/gal; visc. 70 cps; HLB 11.8; pour pt. 32 F; pH 7.7; surf. tens. 35.0 dynes/cm (1%); Ross-Miles foam 168 mm (initial, 1% , 49 C); 39% act.; formerly Sulframin AOS.

Witconate™ AOS-EP. [Witco/H-I-P] Sodium a-olefin sulfonate; CAS 68439-57-6; EINECS 270-407-8; emulsifier for emulsion polymerization, latex paints, adhesives, binders, personal care formulations; lt. clear liq.; dens. 8.92 lb/gal; visc. 200 cps; flash pt. (PMCC) > 200 F; pH 7.5-8.5 (5%); 38-40% act.

Witconate™ AOS-PC. [Witco/H-I-P] Sodium C14-16 olefin sulfonate; CAS 68439-57-6; EINECS 270-407-8; anionic; detergent, foaming agent, wetting agent, visc. modifier for personal care formulations; slurry; water-sol.; sp.gr. 1.05; pH 7.7; 39% act.

Witconate™ C50H. [Witco/H-I-P] Sodium dodecylbenzene sulfonate; CAS 25155-30-0; EINECS 246-680-4; anionic; electrolyte-tolerant detergent, foamer and wetting agent for industrial and personal care formulations; liq.; water-sol.; 44% conc.

Witconate™ CHB. [Witco/H-I-P] Alkyaryl sulfonic acid; demulsifier used in the petrol. industry; also for personal care formulations.

Witconate™ DS. [Witco/H-I-P] Sodium decylbenzenesulfonate; CAS 1322-98-1; EINECS 215-347-5; anionic; detergent, foaming agent, wetting agent for personal care applics.; liq.; water-sol.; sp.gr. 0.45; pH 8.0; 91% act.

Witconate™ DS Dense. [Witco/H-I-P] Sodium dodecylbenzene sulfonate; CAS 25155-30-0; EINECS 246-680-4; anionic; detergent, foaming agent, wetting agent for personal care applics.; powd; sol. in water; sp.gr. 0.50; pH

8.0; 91% act.

Witconate™ LX F. [Witco/H-I-P] Sodium dodecylbenzene-sulfonate and sodium xylenesulfonate; anionic; detergent base, emulsifier, foamer, and wetting agent for personal care, detergent industry, and industrial surfactants; flake; water-sol.; sp.gr. 0.48; pH 8.0; 91% act.

Witconate™ LXH. [Witco/H-I-P] Branched TEA-dodecyl-benzene sulfonate; CAS 27323-41-7; EINECS 248-406-9; anionic; detergent, foaming agent, wetting agent, dispersant for personal care applics.; liq.; water-sol.; sp.gr. 1.09; pH 7.2; 53% act.

Witconate™ LX Powd. [Witco/H-I-P] Sodium dodecylben-zenesulfonate and sodium xylenesulfonate; anionic; detergent, wetting agent; base for personal care, household, and industrial specialty compds.; powd.

Witconate™ NAS-8. [Witco/H-I-P] Sodium alkane sulfonate; anionic; low foaming, biodeg. detergent base with hydro-tropic props.; stable to electrolyte, acid, alkaline, and chlorine bleach; for personal care applics.; liq.; 39% act.

Witconate™ NIS. [Witco/H-I-P] Sodium isethionate; CAS 1562-00-1; EINECS 216-343-6; anionic; detergent, foaming agent, wetting agent for personal care applics.; liq.; water-sol.; sp.gr. 1.37; pH 8.5; 56% act.

Witconate™ NXS. [Witco/H-I-P] Ammonium xylenesulfo-nate; CAS 26447-10-9; EINECS 247-710-9; hydrotrope, solubilizer, coupler and processing aid in personal care and detergent mfg. and industrial processes; antiblocking and anticaking agent in powd. prods.; formulates shampoos, aerosols, cutting oils, glue; textile finishing; Klett 30 liq.; dens. 1.1 g/cc; pH 8.0; 40% act.

Witconate™ S-1280. [Witco/H-I-P] TEA-dodecylbenzene-sulfonate; CAS 27323-41-7; EINECS 248-406-9; personal care surfactant.

Witconate™ SCS 45%. [Witco/H-I-P] Sodium cumene sulfonate; CAS 32073-22-6; EINECS 250-913-5; anionic; hydrotrope, solubilizer, coupler and processing aid in detergent mfg. and industrial processes; antiblocking and anticaking agent in powd. prods.; formulates shampoos, aerosols, cutting oils, glue; textile finishing; Klett 50 liq.; sol. in water; sp.gr. 1.16; pH 8.0; 45% act.

Witconate™ SCS 93%. [Witco/H-I-P] Sodium cumene sulfonate; CAS 32073-22-6; EINECS 250-913-5; anionic; hydrotrope, solubilizer, coupler and processing aid in detergent mfg. and industrial processes; antiblocking and anticaking agent in powd. prods.; formulates shampoos, aerosols, cutting oils, glue; textile finishing; powd.; sol. in water; sp.gr. 0.33; pH 8.0; 93% act.

Witconate™ SE-5. [Witco/H-I-P] Sodium alcohol ether sulfate; anionic; oilfield surfactant, foaming agent; also for personal care formulations; liq.; sol. in water; dens. 8.8 lb/gal; visc. 65 cps; pour pt. 22 F; pH 7.5.

Witconate™ SK. [Witco/H-I-P] Sodium dodecylbenzene sulfonate; CAS 25155-30-0; EINECS 246-680-4; anionic; detergent, foaming agent, wetting agent for personal care applics.; flake; sol. in water; sp.gr. 0.55; pH 8.0; 40% act.

Witconate™ STS. [Witco/H-I-P] Sodium toluene sulfonate; CAS 12068-03-0; EINECS 235-088-1; hydrotrope, solu-bilizer, coupler and processing aid in detergent mfg. and industrial processes; antiblocking and anticaking agent in powd. prods.; formulates shampoos, aerosols, cutting oils, glue; textile finishing; Klett 150 liq., powd.; dens. 0.32–1.2 g/cc; pH 9.0–10.0; 40% act. liq., 90% act. powd.

Witconate™ SXS 40%. [Witco/H-I-P] Sodium xylene sul-fonate; CAS 1300-72-7; EINECS 215-090-9; anionic; hydrotrope, solubilizer, coupler and processing aid in detergent mfg. and industrial processes; antiblocking and anticaking agent in powd. prods.; formulates shampoos, aerosols, cutting oils, glue; textile finishing; Klett 40 liq.; sol. in water; sp.gr. 1.18; pH 8.0; 41% act.

Witconate™ SXS 90%. [Witco/H-I-P] Sodium xylene sul-fonate; CAS 1300-72-7; EINECS 215-090-9; anionic; hydrotrope, solubilizer, coupler and processing aid in detergent mfg. and industrial processes; antiblocking and anticaking agent in powd. prods.; formulates shampoos, aerosols, cutting oils, glue; textile finishing; powd.; sol. in water; sp.gr. 0.35; pH 8.0; 93% act.

Witconate™ TAB. [Witco/H-I-P] TEA-dodecylbenzene sul-fonate; CAS 27323-41-7; EINECS 248-406-9; anionic; detergent, foamer, wetting agent, solubilizer, emulsifier in cosmetics/toiletries, industrial surfactants, paints; elec-trolyte tolerant; liq.; water-sol.; 60% conc.

Witconate™ TDB. [Witco/H-I-P] Sodium tridecylbenzene sulfonate; CAS 26248-24-8; EINECS 247-536-3; anionic; detergent base, emulsifier, foamer, and wetting agent for the detergent industry; used in industrial surfactants and personal care formulations; liq.; water-sol.; 44% conc.

Witconate™ TX Acid. [Witco/H-I-P] Modified toluene sul-fonic acid; CAS 104-15-4; EINECS 203-180-0; anionic; wetting agent, hydrotrope, coupler and solubilizer for liq. detergents, personal care formulations; anticaking aid in dry neutralization; catalyst in org. reactions; liq.; sol. in oil; sp.gr. 1.30; 96% act.

Witconate™ YLA. [Witco/H-I-P] Amine dodecylbenzene sulfonate; anionic; detergent base, emulsifier, solubilizer, foaming and wetting agent for detergents, drycleaning charge soaps, solv. cleaners, metal cleaning, and textile industries, and personal care formulations; liq.; oil-sol.; 95% conc.

Witconol™ 18L. [Witco/H-I-P] Polyglyceryl-4 isostearate; CAS 91824-88-3; nonionic; emulisifier, spreader, sticker, antifoaming agent, solubilizer for w/o emulsions, aero-sols, personal care prods.; liq.; oil-sol.; 100% conc.

Witconol™ 2300. [Witco/H-I-P] Octyl isononanoate; CAS 71566-49-9; EINECS 275-637-2; personal care ingred.

Witconol™ 2301. [Witco/H-I-P] Methyl oleate; CAS 112-62-9; EINECS 203-992-5; nonionic; defoamer, lubricant, moisture barrier for personal care prods.; Gardner 5 liq.; sol. in oil; sp.gr. 0.88; pour pt. -16 C.

Witconol™ 2307. [Witco/H-I-P] Octyl pelargonate; CAS 59587-44-9; EINECS 261-819-9; personal care ingred.

Witconol™ 2310. [Witco/H-I-P] Isopropyl isostearate; EINECS 250-651-1; personal care ingred.

Witconol™ 2314. [Witco/H-I-P] Isopropyl myristate; CAS 110-27-0; EINECS 203-751-4; personal care emollient.

Witconol™ 2316. [Witco/H-I-P] Isopropyl palmitate; CAS 142-91-6; EINECS 205-571-1; personal care ingred.

Witconol™ 2325. [Witco/H-I-P] Butyl stearate; personal care ingred.

Witconol™ 2326. [Witco/H-I-P] Butyl stearate; CAS 123-95-5; EINECS 204-666-5; emollient.

Witconol™ 2355. [Witco/H-I-P] Glycol distearate; CAS 627-83-8; EINECS 211-014-3; personal care ingred.

Witconol™ 2380. [Witco/H-I-P] Propylene glycol stearate; CAS 1323-39-3; EINECS 215-354-3; nonionic; o/w emul-sifier, lubricant, opacifier for personal care prods.; Gardner 2 beads; sol. in oil; sp.gr. 0.90; HLB 1.8; m.p. 36 C.

Witconol™ 2381. [Witco/H-I-P] Propylene glycol stearate SE; personal care ingred.

Witconol™ 2384. [Witco/H-I-P] Propylene glycol isostear-ate; CAS 68171-38-0; EINECS 269-027-5; personal care ingred.

Witconol™ 2400. [Witco/H-I-P] Glyceryl stearate; nonionic; o/w emulsifier, lubricant for personal care prods.; beads; disp. in oil; sp.gr. 0.93; HLB 3.9; m.p. 58 C.

Witconol™ 2401. [Witco/H-I-P] Glyceryl stearate; nonionic; o/w emulsifier, lubricant for personal care prods.; beads; disp. in oil; sp.gr. 0.92; HLB 3.9; m.p. 58 C.

Witconol™ 2407. [Witco/H-I-P] Glyceryl stearate SE; non-ionic; o/w emulsifier, lubricant for personal care applics.;

Witconol™ 2410

Gardner 3 beads; disp. in water, oils; sp.gr. 0.93; HLB 5.1; m.p. 58 C.

Witconol™ 2410. [Witco/H-I-P] Glyceryl isostearate; personal care ingred.

Witconol™ 2421. [Witco/H-I-P] Glyceryl oleate; CAS 111-03-5; nonionic; defoamer, o/w emulsifier, lubricant, moisture barrier for personal care applics.; liq.; oil-sol.; sp.gr. 0.95; HLB 3.4; pour pt. 19 C.

Witconol™ 2423. [Witco/H-I-P] Triolein; CAS 122-32-7; EINECS 204-534-7; personal care ingred.

Witconol™ 2500. [Witco/H-I-P] Sorbitan oleate; CAS 1338-43-8; EINECS 215-665-4; nonionic; w/o emulsifier, lubricant, coupling agent for personal care applics.; Gardner 8 liq.; sol. in oil; sp.gr. 1.00; HLB 4.6; pour pt. < 0 C.

Witconol™ 2502. [Witco/H-I-P] Sorbitan sesquioleate; CAS 8007-43-0; EINECS 232-360-1; personal care ingred.

Witconol™ 2503. [Witco/H-I-P] Sorbitan trioleate; CAS 26266-58-0; EINECS 247-569-3; nonionic; w/o emulsifier, lubricant, coupling agent for personal care prods.; Gardner 7 liq.; sol. in oil; sp.gr. 0.95; HLB 2.1; pour pt. < 0 C.

Witconol™ 2505. [Witco/H-I-P] Sorbitan stearate; CAS 1338-41-6; EINECS 215-664-9; personal care ingred.

Witconol™ 2507. [Witco/H-I-P] Sorbitan tristearate; CAS 26658-19-5; EINECS 247-891-4; personal care ingred.

Witconol™ 2510. [Witco/H-I-P] Sorbitan palmitate; CAS 26266-57-9; EINECS 247-568-8; personal care ingred.

Witconol™ 2515. [Witco/H-I-P] Sorbitan laurate; personal care ingred.

Witconol™ 2620. [Witco/H-I-P] PEG-4 laurate; CAS 9004-81-3; nonionic; o/w emulsifier, lubricant for personal care prods.; Gardner 1 liq.; disp. in water, oil; sp.gr. 0.98; HLB 9.3; pour pt. 9 C.

Witconol™ 2622. [Witco/H-I-P] PEG-4 dilaurate; CAS 9005-02-1; nonionic; o/w emulsifier, lubricant for personal care applics.; Gardner 2 liq.; sol. in oil, disp. in water; sp.gr. 0.96; HLB 7.6; pour pt. 0 C.

Witconol™ 2648. [Witco/H-I-P] PEG-8 dioleate; CAS 9005-07-6; nonionic; o/w emulsifier, lubricant, defoamer for personal care applics.; Gardner 4 liq.; disp. in water, sol. in oil; sp.gr. 0.97; HLB 8.8; pour pt. 6 C.

Witconol™ 2711. [Witco/H-I-P] PEG-8 stearate; CAS 9004-99-3; nonionic; o/w emulsifier, lubricant for personal care applics.; Gardner 1 solid; disp. in water, oil; sp.gr. 1.02; m.p. 32 C; HLB 12; formerly Witconol 2640.

Witconol™ 2712. [Witco/H-I-P] PEG-8 distearate; CAS 9005-08-7; nonionic; o/w emulsifier, lubricant for personal care applics.; Gardner 2 solid; sol. in oil, disp. in water; m.p. 36 C; HLB 7.5; formerly Witconol 2642.

Witconol™ 2713. [Witco/H-I-P] PEG-20 stearate; CAS 9004-99-3; personal care ingred.

Witconol™ 2720. [Witco/H-I-P] Polysorbate 20; CAS 9005-64-5; nonionic; o/w emulsifier, dispersant, visc. modifier, coupling agent for personal care applics.; Gardner 6 liq.; water-sol.; sp.gr. 1.10; HLB 16.7; pour pt. -10 C.

Witconol™ 2722. [Witco/H-I-P] Polysorbate 80; CAS 9005-65-6; nonionic; o/w emulsifier, dispersant, visc. modifier, coupling agent for personal care applics.; Gardner 6 liq.; sol. in water; sp.gr. 1.08; HLB 15.0; pour pt. -12 C.

Witconol™ 2728. [Witco/H-I-P] Polysorbate 60; CAS 9005-67-8; personal care ingred.

Witconol™ 2737. [Witco/H-I-P] PEG-16 hydrog. castor oil; CAS 61788-85-0; personal care ingred.

Witconol™ 2738. [Witco/H-I-P] PEG-25 hydrog. castor oil; CAS 61788-85-0; personal care ingred.

Witconol™ 2739. [Witco/H-I-P] PEG-40 hydrog. castor oil; CAS 61788-85-0; personal care ingred.

Witconol™ 5875. [Witco/H-I-P] Laureth-4; CAS 5274-68-0; EINECS 226-097-1; personal care ingred.

Witconol™ 5906. [Witco/H-I-P] PEG-30 castor oil; CAS 61791-12-6; nonionic; dispersant, o/w emulsifier, lubricant for personal care applics.; Gardner 2 liq.; water-sol.; sp.gr. 1.06; HLB 11.8; clear pt. 55 C.

Witconol™ 5907. [Witco/H-I-P] PEG-36 castor oil; CAS 61791-12-6; nonionic; dispersant, o/w emulsifier, lubricant for personal care applics.

Witconol™ 5909. [Witco/H-I-P] PEG-40 castor oil; CAS 61791-12-6; nonionic; dispersant, o/w emulsifier, lubricant for personal care prods.; Gardner 2 liq.; water-sol.; sp.gr. 1.06; HLB 13.0; clear pt. 80 C.

Witconol™ 5964. [Witco/H-I-P] Laureth-23; CAS 9002-92-0; personal care ingred.

Witconol™ 5969. [Witco/H-I-P] Myreth-3; CAS 27306-79-2; EINECS 248-016-9; personal care ingred.

Witconol™ 6903. [Witco/H-I-P] Polysorbate 85; CAS 9005-70-3; nonionic; o/w emulsifier, dispersant, lubricant, coupling agent for personal care applics.; Gardner 7 liq.; disp. in oils, water; sp.gr. 1.03; HLB 11.1; pour pt. -15 C.

Witconol™ 6907. [Witco/H-I-P] Polysorbate 65; CAS 9005-71-4; personal care ingred.

Witconol™ APB. [Witco/H-I-P] PPG-14 butyl ether; CAS 9003-13-8; personal care ingred.

Witconol™ APEB. [Witco/H-I-P] PPG-26-buteth-26; CAS 9065-63-8; emollient, superfatting agent, skin lubricant, emulsifier; perfume solubilizer; vehicle for suntan oils and lotions; wh. wax; 100% conc.

Witconol™ APEM. [Witco/H-I-P] PPG-3-myreth-3; nonionic; lubricant, emulsifier, wetting agent, penetrant, dye dispersant, scouring aid, antistat, solv. coupler; syn. oils for personal care prods.; metal processing; textile surfactant; liq.; sol. in 3A ethanol, min. oil.

Witconol™ APES. [Witco/H-I-P] PPG-9-steareth-3; CAS 9038-43-1; personal care ingred.

Witconol™ APM. [Witco/H-I-P] PPG-3 myristyl ether; CAS 63793-60-2; nonionic; lubricant, emulsifier, wetting agent, penetrant, dye dispersant, scouring aid, antistat, solv. coupler; metal processing; textile surfactant; emollient oil for cosmetics and toiletries; solubilizer for alcohol in oils; Gardner 1 liq.; sol. in oil; sp.gr. 0.90; pH 7.0; 100% act.

Witconol™ APS. [Witco/H-I-P] PPG-11 stearyl ether; CAS 25231-21-4; nonionic; lubricant, emulsifier, wetting agent, penetrant, dye dispersant, scouring aid, antistat, solv. coupler; syn. oils for personal care prods.; metal processing; textile surfactant; emollient oil for cosmetics and toiletries, solubilizer; Gardner 1 liq.; sol. in oil; sp.gr. 0.94; pH 7.0.

Witconol™ CA. [Witco/H-I-P] Glyceryl stearate SE; nonionic; lubricant, bodying agent, emulsifier, opacifier used in industrial, cosmetic and aerosol formulations; wax; 100% conc.

Witconol™ CAD. [Witco/H-I-P] Diethylene glycol monostearate; CAS 106-11-6; EINECS 203-363-5; anionic; bodying agent, lubricant, and opacifier for cosmetics and toiletries; wax; 100% conc.

Witconol™ CC-43. [Witco/H-I-P] PPG-55 glyceryl ether; CAS 25791-96-2; nonionic; lubricant, emulsifier, antistat; for cosmetics.

Witconol™ CD-17. [Witco/H-I-P] PPG-34; CAS 25322-69-4; nonionic; antistat, emulsifier for personal care prods.; syn. lubricant oil and foam modifier for aerosol formulations.

Witconol™ CD-18. [Witco/H-I-P] PPG-27 glyceryl ether; CAS 25791-96-2; EINECS 247-144-2; nonionic; emollient, visc. control agent, spreading agent for personal care prods., cosmetic emulsifier, lubricant, antistat; liq.; sol. in lower hydrocarbon solvs., lower alcohols; 100% act.

Witconol™ DOSS. [Witco/H-I-P] Diethylene glycol monooleate; CAS 106-12-7; EINECS 203-364-0; nonionic; o/w emulsifier for cosmetic and industrial formulations; self-emulsifying; liq.; 100% conc.

Witconol™ DP60. [Witco/H-I-P] Dodoxynol-6; personal care ingred.

Witconol™ EGMS. [Witco/H-I-P] Glycol stearate; CAS 111-60-4; EINECS 203-886-9; nonionic; opacifier, conditioner for personal care formulations; Gardner 2 beads; sol. in oil; sp.gr. 0.88; HLB 2.2; m.p. 50 C.

Witconol™ EST2. [Witco/H-I-P] MEG distearate; opacifier for shampoos, bath prods.; flakes; 100% act.

Witconol™ F2646. [Witco/H-I-P] PPG-36 oleate; CAS 31394-71-5; nonionic; emollient oil, spreading agent and coupler for cosmetic oil systems; conditioner in hair grooms; surfactant with aux. lubricating, dispersing, and coupling properties; dispersant for industrial use; spreading and anticaking agent for aerosol prods.; visc. and flow control agent; APHA 150 clear liq.; sol. in common alcohols, water/alcohol sol'ns., and hydrocarbons; sp.gr. 0.987; visc. 270 cps; acid no. 1.3; sapon. no. 25.0; flash pt. > 93 C; 0.1% moisture.

Witconol™ H31A. [Witco/H-I-P] PEG-8 oleate; CAS 9004-96-0; nonionic; lubricant and plasticizer in oils and polymers; o/w emulsifier for min. and veg. oils, and solvs., cosmetic and industrial applics.; improves flow and leveling of coatings, increases spreadability of personal care prods.; defoamer; lt. amber liq.; sol. in alcohol, xylene, kerosene, perchloroethylene, wh. min. oil; partially sol. in water; sp.gr. 0.99; HLB 12.5; acid no. 7; pH 3.7 (3% aq.); flash pt. > 93 C (PMCC); 100% act.

Witconol™ L3245. [Witco/H-I-P] PEG-150 distearate; CAS 9005-08-7; thickening agent for aq. systems; stabilizer for o/w emulsions; in hair shampoos, bubble bath formulations, cosmetic and toiletry lotions, water-based paints and lubricants, and protective coatings; aux. agent in corrosion inhibitor formulations; off-wh. waxy flakes; m.p. 57 C; acid no. 7; sapon. no. 18; pH 5.0 (3% aq.).; 100% act.

Witconol™ MST. [Witco/H-I-P] Glyceryl stearate; nonionic; emulsifier for cosmetic, pharmaceutical, aerosol formulations; internal lubricant, plasticizer, and emulsifier in industrial applics.; flow control agent for polymerization reactions; dispersant; flake; disp. in oil; sp.gr. 0.93; HLB 3.9; m.p. 58 C; 100% act.

Witconol™ NP-40. [Witco/H-I-P] Nonoxynol-4; CAS 9016-45-9; nonionic; detergent, o/w emulsifier, solubilizer for oils in metal processing, personal care formulations; liq.; sol. in naphthenic and paraffinic oil.

Witconol™ NP-60. [Witco/H-I-P] Nonoxynol-6; CAS 9016-45-9; personal care surfactant.

Witconol™ NP-90. [Witco/H-I-P] Nonoxynol-9; CAS 9016-45-9; personal care surfactant.

Witconol™ NP-110. [Witco/H-I-P] Nonoxynol-11; CAS 9016-45-9; personal care surfactant.

Witconol™ NP-300. [Witco/H-I-P] Nonoxynol-30; CAS 9016-45-9; nonionic; personal care surfactant; paint industry emulsifier for emulsion polymerization; pigment wetting and grinding agent for aq. systems; spreading agent; solid, liq.; water-sol.

Witconol™ NP-307. [Witco/H-I-P] Nonoxynol-30; CAS 9016-45-9; personal care surfactant.

Witconol™ OP-90. [Witco/H-I-P] Octoxynol-9; CAS 9002-93-1; personal care surfactant.

Witconol™ PPG 400. [Witco/H-I-P] PPG-9; CAS 25322-69-4; personal care surfactant.

Witconol™ RDC-D. [Witco/H-I-P] Diglycol coconate; nonionic; surfactant, emulsifier; cosmetic and industrial use; liq.; oil-sol.

Witconol™ RHP. [Witco/H-I-P] Propylene glycol monostearate SE; nonionic; emollient, conditioner, emulsifier, lubricant, opacifier and visc. modifier for cosmetics and toiletries, general industrial use; paste; sol. in oil; 100% conc.

Witconol™ RHT. [Witco/H-I-P] Glyceryl stearate SE; nonionic; lubricant, plasticizer, o/w emulsifier used in per-

sonal care and industrial applics.; Gardner 2 flake; disp. in water, oil; sp.gr. 0.93; HLB 5.1; m.p. 58 C; 100% conc.

Witconol™ SE-40. [Witco/H-I-P] Sorbeth-40; personal care surfactant.

Witconol™ TD-60. [Witco/H-I-P] Trideceth-6; CAS 24938-91-8; personal care surfactant.

Witconol™ TD-100. [Witco/H-I-P] Trideceth-10; CAS 24938-91-8; personal care surfactant.

Witcopearl 15. [Witco/H-I-P] Mixture; anionic; opacifier for shampoos, bath prods.; liq.; 46% act.

Witco® Potassium Stearate. [Witco/H-I-P] Potassium stearate; CAS 593-29-3; EINECS 209-786-1; personal care applics.

Witco® Sodium Stearate C-1. [Witco/H-I-P] Sodium stearate; CAS 822-16-2; EINECS 212-490-5; gelling agent for cosmetic and toiletry stick prods.; sol. hot with gelation on cooling in water, methanol, ethanol, certain lower glycols.

Witco® Sodium Stearate C-7. [Witco/H-I-P] Sodium stearate; CAS 822-16-2; EINECS 212-490-5; gelling agent for cosmetic and toiletry stick prods.; powd.; sol. hot with gelation on cooling in water, methanol, ethanol, certain lower glycols.

Witco® Zinc Stearate U.S.P.-D. [Witco/H-I-P] Zinc stearate; CAS 557-05-1; EINECS 209-151-9; lubricant, mold release agent, w/o emulsifier for cosmetics, toiletries, pharmaceuticals; wh. powd.; 99.9% thru 325 mesh; sol. in hot turpentine, benzene, toluene, xylene, CCl_4, veg. and min. oils, waxes; sp.gr. 1.09; soften. pt. 120 C.

Witepsol® E75. [Hüls Am.; Hüls AG] Hydrog. coco-glycerides; CAS 977056-87-3; suppository bases for pharmaceuticals; pellets; m.p. 37-39 C; solid. pt. 32-36 C; acid no. 1.3 max.; iodine no. 3 max.; sapon. no. 220-230; hyd. no. 15 max.

Witepsol® E76. [Hüls Am.; Hüls AG] Hydrog. coco-glycerides; CAS 977056-87-3; suppository bases for pharmaceuticals; pellets; m.p. 37-39 C; solid. pt. 31-35 C; acid no. 0.3 max.; iodine no. 3 max.; sapon. no. 220-230; hyd. no. 30-40.

Witepsol® E85. [Hüls Am.; Hüls AG] Hydrog. coco-glycerides; CAS 977056-87-3; suppository bases for hydrophilic and lipophilic drugs; pellets; m.p. 42-44 C; solid. pt. 37-42 C; acid no. 0.3 max.; iodine no. 3 max.; sapon. no. 220-230; hyd. no. 15 max.

Witepsol® H5. [Hüls Am.; Hüls AG] Hydrog. coco-glycerides; CAS 977056-87-3; suppository bases for pharmaceuticals; pellets; m.p. 34-36 C; solid. pt. 33-35 C; acid no. 0.2 max.; iodine no. 2 max.; sapon. no. 235-245; hyd. no. 5 max.

Witepsol® H12. [Hüls Am.; Hüls AG] Hydrog. coco-glycerides; CAS 977056-87-3; suppository bases for pharmaceuticals; pellets; m.p. 32-33.5 C; solid. pt. 29-33 C; acid no. 0.2 max.; iodine no. 3 max.; sapon. no. 240-255; hyd. no. 15 max.

Witepsol® H15. [Hüls Am.; Hüls AG] Hydrog. coco-glycerides; CAS 977056-87-3; suppository bases for pharmaceuticals; pellets; m.p. 33.5-35.5 C; solid. pt. 32.5-34.5 C; acid no. 0.2 max.; iodine no. 3 max.; sapon. no. 230-240; hyd. no. 15 max.

Witepsol® H32. [Hüls Am.; Hüls AG] Hydrog. coco-glycerides; CAS 977056-87-3; suppository bases for pharmaceuticals; pellets; m.p. 31-33 C; solid. pt. 30-32.5 C; acid no. 0.2 max.; iodine no. 3 max.; sapon. no. 240-250; hyd. no. 3 max.

Witepsol® H35. [Hüls Am.; Hüls AG] Hydrog. coco-glycerides; CAS 977056-87-3; suppository bases for pharmaceuticals; pellets; m.p. 33.5-35.5 C; solid. pt. 32-35 C; acid no. 0.2 max.; iodine no. 3 max.; sapon. no. 240-250; hyd. no. 3 max.

Witepsol® H37. [Hüls Am.; Hüls AG] Hydrog. coco-glycerides; CAS 977056-87-3; suppository bases for pharmaceuticals; pellets; m.p. 36-38 C; solid. pt. 35-37 C; acid no. 0.2 max.; iodine no. 3 max.; sapon. no. 225-245; hyd. no. 3 max.

Witepsol® H39. [Hüls Am.; Hüls AG] Hydrog. coco-glycerides; CAS 977056-87-3; suppository bases for pharmaceuticals; pellets; m.p. 38-40 C; solid. pt. 37-39.5 C; acid no. 0.2 max.; iodine no. 3 max.; sapon. no. 220-240; hyd. no. 3 max.

Witepsol® H42. [Hüls Am.; Hüls AG] Hydrog. coco-glycerides; CAS 977056-87-3; suppository bases for pharmaceuticals; pellets; m.p. 41-43 C; solid. pt. 40-42.5 C; acid no. 0.2 max.; iodine no. 3 max.; sapon. no. 220-240; hyd. no. 3 max.

Witepsol® H175. [Hüls Am.; Hüls AG] Hydrog. coco-glycerides; CAS 977056-87-3; suppository bases for pharmaceuticals; pellets; m.p. 34.5-36.5 C; solid. pt. 32-34 C; acid no. 0.7 max.; iodine no. 3 max.; sapon. no. 225-245; hyd. no. 15 max.

Witepsol® H185. [Hüls Am.; Hüls AG] Hydrog. coco-glycerides; CAS 977056-87-3; suppository bases for pharmaceuticals; pellets; m.p. 38-39 C; solid. pt. 34-37 C; acid no. 0.2 max.; iodine no. 3 max.; sapon. no. 220-235; hyd. no. 15 max.

Witepsol® S51. [Hüls AG] Hydrog. coco-glycerides; CAS 977056-87-3; suppository bases for pharmaceuticals; pellets; m.p. 30-32 C; solid. pt. 25-27 C; acid no. 0.5 max.; iodine no. 8 max.; sapon. no. 215-230; hyd. no. 55-70.

Witepsol® S55. [Hüls AG] Hydrog. coco-glycerides; CAS 977056-87-3; suppository bases for pharmaceuticals; pellets; m.p. 33.5-35.5 C; solid. pt. 28-33 C; acid no. 1.0 max.; iodine no. 3 max.; sapon. no. 215-230; hyd. no. 50-65.

Witepsol® S58. [Hüls AG] Hydrog. coco-glycerides; CAS 977056-87-3; suppository bases for pharmaceuticals; pellets; m.p. 32-33.5 C; solid. pt. 27-29 C; acid no. 1.0 max.; iodine no. 7 max.; sapon. no. 215-225; hyd. no. 60-70.

Witepsol® W25. [Hüls Am.; Hüls AG] Hydrog. coco-glycerides; CAS 977056-87-3; suppository bases for pharmaceuticals; pellets; m.p. 33.5-35.5 C; solid. pt. 29-33 C; acid no. 0.3 max.; iodine no. 3 max.; sapon. no. 225-240; hyd. no. 20-30.

Witepsol® W31. [Hüls Am.; Hüls AG] Hydrog. coco-glycerides; CAS 977056-87-3; suppository bases for pharmaceuticals; pellets; m.p. 35-37 C; solid. pt. 30-33 C; acid no. 0.3 max.; iodine no. 3 max.; sapon. no. 225-240; hyd. no. 25-35.

Witepsol® W32. [Hüls Am.; Hüls AG] Hydrog. coco-glycerides; CAS 977056-87-3; suppository bases for pharmaceuticals; pellets; m.p. 32-33.5 C; solid. pt. 25-30 C; acid no. 0.5 max.; iodine no. 3 max.; sapon. no. 225-245; hyd. no. 40-50.

Witepsol® W35. [Hüls Am.; Hüls AG] Hydrog. coco-glycerides; CAS 977056-87-3; suppository bases for pharmaceuticals; pellets; m.p. 33.5-35.5 C; solid. pt. 27-32 C; acid no. 0.3 max.; iodine no. 3 max.; sapon. no. 225-235; hyd. no. 40-50.

Witepsol® W45. [Hüls Am.; Hüls AG] Hydrog. coco-glycerides; CAS 977056-87-3; suppository bases for pharmaceuticals; pellets; m.p. 33.5-35.5 C; solid. pt. 29-34 C; acid no. 0.3 max.; iodine no. 3 max.; sapon. no. 225-235; hyd. no. 40-50.

XY

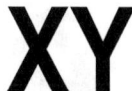

Xalidrene. [Vevy] PEG-20 myristate and PEG-20 palmitate.

Xalifin 15. [Vevy] C12-20 acid PEG-8 ester.

Xanthan XP. [Lowenstein] Xanthan gum; CAS 11138-66-2; EINECS 234-394-2; provides rapid hydration for powd. cosmetic systems.

Yeast Extract SC. [Herstellung von Naturextrakten GmbH; Lipo] Yeast extract; CAS 8103-01-2; activator for cell metabolism; used in high quality cosmetic face creams/masks, ampoules; yel.-brn. clear sol'n., weak intrinsic odor; sol. in water (100%), ethanol (10%); pH 5.0-7.0; usage level: 2-5%; toxicology: LD50 (oral, rat) > 10,000 mg/kg; nonirritating to skin and eyes.

Yeast Lactase L-50,000. [Solvay Enzymes] Yeast lactase; enzyme for hydrolyzing lactose in dairy prods. (milk, whey, cheese, yogurt), pharmaceuticals (digestive aids); lt. amber liq., free from offensive odors and taste.

Yeast Walls. [Sederma] Hydrolyzed yeast; cleansing epidermis care and oily skin treatment; regulates sebaceous secretions; recommended for cleansing masks; ocher atomized powd., char. odor; pH 2.5-4.5 (10% disp.); usage level: 2-10%.

Yellow 134. [Presperse] D&C yellow #5 aluminum lake and bismuth oxychloride; organic colorant for pigmented cosmetics; Japanese approval.

Yellow 201. [Presperse] Iron oxides (85%), bismuthoxychloride (15%); CAS 1309-37-1, 7787-59-9; inorg. colorant for pigmented cosmetics; JSCI/JCID approved.

York Krystal Kleer Castor Oil. [United Catalysts] Castor oil; CAS 8001-79-4; EINECS 232-293-8; high quality oil imparting gloss and emollience and as a dye solv. in personal care prods., e.g., lipsticks.

York USP Castor Oil. [United Catalysts] Castor oil USP; CAS 8001-79-4; EINECS 232-293-8; high quality oil imparting gloss and emollience and as a dye solv. in personal care prods., e.g., lipsticks.

Yucca Extract 50%. [Int'l. Flora Tech.] Mohave yucca/yucca schidigera extract; mild, natural cleansing prod. for cosmetics.; water-misc.

Yucca Glauca Extract Code 9030. [Brooks Industries] Yucca glauca extract; provides moisturization and anti-inflammatory activity for topical treatments for burns and mild abrasions; pale yel. sl. hazy liq.

Z

Z-Cote®. [SunSmart; Trivent] Micronized zinc oxide; CAS 1314-13-2; EINECS 215-222-5; sunscreen providing uv-A and -B protection to cosmetic and healthcare prods. incl. transparent prods.; powd.; avg. particle size 0.1-0.2 μ; ref. index 1.9.

Zeo® 49. [J.M. Huber] Hydrated silica; polishing agent, catalyst support; 9.0 micrometer avg. particle size; surf. area 250 m²/g; oil absorp. 92 cc/100 g; pH 7.0.

Zeodent® 113. [J.M. Huber] Hydrated silica; polishing agent, antiskid agent; 9.0 micrometer avg. particle size; surf. area 200 m²/g; oil absorp. 92 cc/100 g; pH 7.0.

Zeodent® 115, 119, 163, 173, 177. [J.M. Huber] Hydrated silica.

Zeofree® 80. [J.M. Huber] Hydrated silica; defoamer, carrier; anticaking and free-flow aid for powd. detergents; 6.0 μ avg. particle size; surf. area 140 m²/g; oil absorp. 190 cc/100 g; pH 7.0.

Zeofree® 153. [J.M. Huber] Hydrated silica; carrier, filler; 7.0 micrometer avg. particle size; surf. area 120 m²/g; oil absorp. 165 cc/100 g; pH 7.0.

Zeolex® 7. [J.M. Huber] Sodium silicoaluminate; CAS 1344-00-9; EINECS 215-684-8; conditioning and anticaking agent; absorbent carrier; 6 micrometer avg. particle size; surf. area 115 m²/g; oil absorp. 115 cc/100 g; pH 7.0.

Zeolex® 23A. [J.M. Huber] Sodium silicoaluminate; CAS 1344-00-9; EINECS 215-684-8; conditioning and anticaking agent; absorbent carrier; 5 micrometer avg. particle size; surf. 73 m²/g; oil absorp. 115 cc/100 g; pH 10.2.

Zeosyl® 110SD. [J.M. Huber] Hydrated silica; carrier, reinforcing agent; surf. area 140 m²/g; oil absorp. 190 cc/100 g; pH 7.0.

Zeosyl® 200. [J.M. Huber] Hydrated silica; carrier, rheology agent, thickener for liq. detergents; adsorbent that converts liqs. to free flowing powds.; 5.0 micrometer avg. particle size; surf. area 250 m²/g; oil absorp. 200 cc/100 g; pH 7.0.

Zeothix® 95. [J.M. Huber] Hydrated silica; flatting agent; 2.3 μ avg. particle size; surf. area 175 m²/g; oil absorp. 210 cc/100 g; pH 7.0.

Zeothix® 265. [J.M. Huber] Hydrated silica; thickener, thixotrope; anticaking and free-flow agent for hygroscopic powds.; thickener for liq. detergents; adsorbent that converts liqs. to powds.; 1.7 micrometer avg. particle size; surf. area 250 m²/g; oil absorp. 220 cc/100 g; pH 7.0.

Zetesap 813A. [Zschimmer & Schwarz] Disodium lauryl sulfosuccinate, sodium lauryl sulfate, corn starch, cetearyl alcohol, paraffin, titanium dioxide; anionic; basic material for syn. toilet bar soaps; solid; 50% act.

Zetesap 5165. [Zschimmer & Schwarz] Disodium lauryl sulfosuccinate, sodium cocoyl isethionate, cetearyl alcohol, corn starch, glyceryl stearate, paraffin, titanium dioxide.; anionic; basic material for syn. toilet bar soaps; solid; 40% conc.

Zetesol 100. [Zschimmer & Schwarz] MIPA-laureth sulfate,

laureth-4, cocamide DEA; anionic; detergent and emulsifier for personal care prods.; for foam bath preps. with high oil concs.; liq.; 98% conc.

Zetesol 856. [Zschimmer & Schwarz] MIPA-laureth sulfate; anionic; detergent for cosmetics, shampoos, bath preps., liq. syn. soap; liq.; 56% conc.

Zetesol 856 D. [Zschimmer & Schwarz] MIPA C12-15 pareth sulfate; anionic; detergent for cosmetics, shampoos, bath preps., liq. syn. soap; liq.; 58% conc.

Zetesol 856 DT. [Zschimmer & Schwarz] MIPA laureth sulfate with betaine; anionic; detergent for cosmetics, shampoos, bath preps., hand cleaners, liq. syn. soap; liq.; 59% conc.

Zetesol 856 T. [Zschimmer & Schwarz] MIPA-laureth sulfate, cocamidopropyl betaine; anionic; detergent for cosmetics, shampoos, bath preps., liq. syn. soap; liq.; 56% conc.

Zetesol 2056. [Zschimmer & Schwarz] MIPA-laureth sulfate; anionic; detergent for personal care prods., shampoos, household and industrial cleaners; ylsh. clear liq.; misc. with cold water; dens. 1.06 g/cc; visc. 3000 mPa·s; cloud pt. 10 C; pH 6.5-7.0 (10%); 56% act. in water.

Zetesol AP. [Zschimmer & Schwarz] Ammonium C12-15 pareth sulfate, propylene glycol; anionic; detergent for cosmetics, shampoos, bath preps., liq. hand cleaners, dishwash, household cleaners; straw-colored liq.; dens. 1.05 g/cc; pH 6.0-6.8 (10%); 60% act.

Zetesol MS. [Zschimmer & Schwarz] Sodium laureth sulfate, magnesium myreth sulfate; anionic; detergent for baby shampoos, bath preps.; liq.; 28% conc.

Zetesol NL. [Zschimmer & Schwarz] Sodium laureth sulfate; CAS 9004-82-4; 1335-72-4; anionic; detergent for personal care, shampoos, household, hand cleaners, and industrial cleaners; almost colorless clear liq.; dens. 1.04 g/cc; visc. 100 mPa·s; cloud pt. 0 C; pH 6.0-7.0 (10%); 28% act.

Zetesol OM. [Zschimmer & Schwarz] Sodium laureth sulfate, magnesium oleyl ether sulfate; for hair shampoos, baby shampoos, baby bath additives; liq.; 28% act.

Zincidone®. [UCIB; Barnet Prods.] Zinc PCA; CAS 15454-75-8; moisturizing agent, cicatrizing agent, tissue hardening agent, antiseborrhoeic and bacteriostatic agent for skin and hair care, dermatological soap, shampoo, shower gel, spray or stick deodorant, nutritive cream; wh. powd., odorless; m.w. 321.4; usage level: 0.1-1%; toxicology: nonirritating to skin and eyes.

Zinc Omadine® 48% Disp. [Olin] Zinc pyrithione; CAS 13463-41-7; EINECS 236-671-3; antimicrobial inhibiting growth of gram-negative and gram-positive bacterial, fungi, mold and yeast; antidandruff agent for shampoos and hair dressings; preservation of cosmetics, surgical scrubs, acne preps., topical antibacterial prods., metal coolant and cutting fluids, PVC plastics, fabrics; off-wh. disp. (particle size 90% < 5μ), mild odor; m.w. 317.7 (zinc pyrithione); dens. 10 lb/gal; pH 6.5–9.0 (5% active slurry in neut. water); 48–50% act.

Zinc Omadine® Powd. [Olin] Zinc pyrithione; CAS 13463-41-7; EINECS 236-671-3; antidandruff agent for shampoos; inhibits growth of gram-positive and gram-negative bacteria and fungi; preservative for cosmetics, metalworking fluids, fabrics; off-wh. aq. dispersion (particle size: 95% < 7μ; 90% < 5μ); mild odor; insol. in water; m.w. 317.7 (zinc pyrithione); sp.gr. 1.782; dens. 10 lb/gal; m.p. ≈ 240 C (dec.); pH 6.5–8.5 (5% act. slurry in pH 7 water); 48% aq. disp.

Zinc Oxide USP 66. [Whittaker, Clark & Daniels] Zinc oxide; CAS 1314-13-2; EINECS 215-222-5; uv sunscreen.

Zink Pyrion. [Ruetgers-Nease] Zinc pyrithione; CAS 13463-41-7; EINECS 236-671-3; antidandruff agent, preservative, antibacterial, antimicrobial; aq. disp.

Zirkonal L. [Giulini] Aluminum zirconium tetrachlorohydrex GLY; highly effective antiperspirant with a perspiration reduction up to 60% in nonaerosol cosmetic preps.; pale yel. liq.; pH 3.7-4.1 (15%); very hygroscopic; usage level: 20% max.; 35% act.

Zirkonal P. [Giulini] Aluminum zirconium tetrachlorohydrex GLY; highly effective antiperspirant with a perspiration reduction up to 60% in nonaerosol cosmetic preps.; wh. to pale yel. powd.; 100% < 53 μm particle size; pH 3.7-4.1 (15%); very hygroscopic; usage level: 20% max.; 35% act.

Zohar EGDS. [Zohar Detergent Factory] Glycol distearate; CAS 627-83-8; EINECS 211-014-3; nonionic; opacifying agent for cosmetics; flakes; 100% conc.

Zohar EGMS. [Zohar Detergent Factory] Glycol stearate; CAS 111-60-4; EINECS 203-886-9; nonionic; coemulsifier for o/w emulsions; opacifier, pearlescent, emollient, superfatting agent for mfg. of shampoos, liq. toilet soaps, bath prods.; flakes; 100% conc.

Zohar EGMS 771. [Zohar Detergent Factory] Sodium laureth sulfate, ethylene glycol stearate, cocamide MEA; anionic/nonionic; raw material for mfg. of emulsions and pearlescent shampoos in cold processing; paste; 45-47% conc.

Zohar GLST. [Zohar Detergent Factory] Glyceryl stearate; nonionic; emulsifier, thickener, superfatting agent for cosmetics; flakes; 100% conc.

Zohar GLST SE. [Zohar Detergent Factory] Glyceryl stearate and sodium stearate; nonionic/anionic; self-emulsifying emulsifier, coemulsifier, thickener, opacifier, and superfatting agent for cosmetics; flakes; 100% conc.

Zoharconc Bar. [Zohar Detergent Factory] Conc. for syn. bar soap.

Zoharconc BB. [Zohar Detergent Factory] Blend of anionics and mild cationics; anionic/cationic; bubble bath conc.; liq.; 30% conc.

Zoharconc BS. [Zohar Detergent Factory] Blend of anionics, amphoterics, and nonionics; anionic/amphoteric; baby shampoo conc.; liq.

Zoharconc Dead Sea. [Zohar Detergent Factory] Foaming bath conc. (with Dead Sea minerals).

Zoharconc DH. [Zohar Detergent Factory] Alcohol sulfates, nonionics, and mild cationic surfactants; shampoo conc. for dilution with water to ready-to-use shampoo for dry hair; liq.; 29% conc.

Zoharconc H.C.C. [Zohar Detergent Factory] Hair conditioner conc.

Zoharconc NH. [Zohar Detergent Factory] Alcohol sulfates, nonionics, and mild cationic surfactants; anionic/cationic; shampoo conc. for dilution with water to ready-to-use shampoo for normal hair; liq.; 25%.

Zoharconc OH. [Zohar Detergent Factory] Alcohol sulfates, nonionics, and mild cationic surfactants; shampoo conc. for dilution with water to ready-to-use shampoo for oily hair; liq.; 27% conc.

Zoharconc SC. [Zohar Detergent Factory] Blend of anionics, amphoterics, and nonionics; anionic/amphoteric; high active shampoo conc.; liq.; 70% conc.

Zoharconc SPC. [Zohar Detergent Factory] High active pearly shampoo conc.

Zoharlab. [Zohar Detergent Factory] Linear sodium alkylbenzene sulfonate; anionic; raw material for mfg. of detergents; paste; 60% conc.

Zoharpon 3525. [Zohar Detergent Factory] Blend; anionic/nonionic; raw material for pearly shampoos; liq.; 23% conc.

Zoharpon 3560. [Zohar Detergent Factory] Blend; anionic/nonionic; raw material for pearly shampoos; paste; 60% conc.

Zoharpon BB. [Zohar Detergent Factory] Fatty alcohol sulfate/mild cationic surfactant blend; anionic; bubble bath conc. for high quality bubble baths processed at R.T.; gel; 30% conc.

Zoharpon DH. [Zohar Detergent Factory] Alcohol sulfates, nonionics, and mild cationic surfactants; raw material conc. for dilution with water to "ready to use" shampoos; liq.; 29% conc.

Zoharpon DT-80. [Zohar Detergent Factory] Alkanolamine lauryl sulfate; anionic; raw material for shampoo and foam baths; liq.; 80% conc.

Zoharpon EGDS-771. [Zohar Detergent Factory] Sodium laureth sulfate, glycol distearate, and cocamide MEA; nonionic/anionic; pearlizing agent for cold processing of cosmetic formulations; paste; 46-48% conc.

Zoharpon ETA 27. [Zohar Detergent Factory] Sodium laureth (2) sulfate; CAS 9004-82-4; anionic; raw material for liq. shampoos, other cosmetics, lt. duty detergents; liq.; 27% conc.

Zoharpon ETA 35. [Zohar Detergent Factory] Sodium lauryl ether sulfate and nonionic compds.; anionic/nonionic; raw material for mfg. of emulsions, pearlescent shampoos; paste; 35% conc.

Zoharpon ETA 70. [Zohar Detergent Factory] Sodium laureth (2) sulfate; CAS 9004-82-4; anionic; raw material for liq. shampoos and cosmetic preparations; lt.-duty detergents; paste; 70% conc.

Zoharpon ETA 270 (OXO). [Zohar Detergent Factory] Sodium lauryl ether sulfate (3 EO); CAS 9004-82-4; anionic; raw material for shampoos, cosmetics, lt. duty detergents; liq.; 27% conc.

Zoharpon ETA 271. [Zohar Detergent Factory] Sodium lauryl ether sulfate (1 EO); CAS 9004-82-4; anionic; raw material for shampoos, cosmetics, lt. duty detergents; liq.; 25% conc.

Zoharpon ETA 273. [Zohar Detergent Factory] Sodium lauryl ether sulfate (3 EO); CAS 9004-82-4; anionic; raw material for shampoos, cosmetics, lt. duty detergents; liq.; 27% conc.

Zoharpon ETA 603. [Zohar Detergent Factory] Sodium lauryl ether sulfate (3 EO); CAS 9004-82-4; anionic; raw material for shampoos, cosmetics, lt. duty detergents; liq.; 60% conc.

Zoharpon ETA 700 (OXO). [Zohar Detergent Factory] Sodium lauryl ether sulfate (3 EO); CAS 9004-82-4; anionic; raw material for shampoos, cosmetics, lt. duty detergents; paste; 70% conc.

Zoharpon ETA 703. [Zohar Detergent Factory] Sodium lauryl ether sulfate (3 EO); CAS 9004-82-4; anionic; raw material for shampoos, cosmetics, lt. duty detergents; paste; 70% conc.

Zoharpon ETA 3525. [Zohar Detergent Factory] Blend of anionics and nonionics; anionic/nonionic; raw material for pearly shampoos; liq.; 23% conc.

Zoharpon ETA 3560. [Zohar Detergent Factory] Blend of anionics and nonionics; anionic/nonionic; raw material for pearly shampoos; paste; 60% conc.

Zoharpon LAA. [Zohar Detergent Factory] Ammonium lauryl

sulfate; CAS 2235-54-3; EINECS 218-793-9; anionic; raw material for clear body and hair shampoos; liq.; 29% conc.

Zoharpon LAD. [Zohar Detergent Factory] DEA lauryl sulfate; CAS 143-00-0; EINECS 205-577-4; anionic; raw material for shampoos, cosmetics, lt. duty detergents; liq.; 35% conc.

Zoharpon LAEA 253. [Zohar Detergent Factory] Ammonium lauryl ether sulfate (3 EO); CAS 32612-48-9; anionic; raw material for shampoos, cosmetics, lt. duty detergents; liq.; 25% conc.

Zoharpon LAET. [Zohar Detergent Factory] TEA lauryl ether sulfate (2 EO); CAS 27028-82-6; anionic; raw material for shampoos, cosmetics; liq.; 35% conc.

Zoharpon LAM. [Zohar Detergent Factory] MEA-lauryl sulfate; CAS 4722-98-9; EINECS 225-214-3; anionic; raw material for shampoos and foam baths; liq.; 29% conc.

Zoharpon LAS. [Zohar Detergent Factory] Sodium lauryl sulfate USP/BP; CAS 151-21-3; EINECS 205-788-1; anionic; raw material for shampoos, toothpaste, and pharmaceutical prods.; liq. to paste; 30% conc.

Zoharpon LAS 70%. [Zohar Detergent Factory] Sodium lauryl sulfate; CAS 151-21-3; EINECS 205-788-1; anionic; mfg. of toilet soap bar; solid; 70% conc.

Zoharpon LAS Special. [Zohar Detergent Factory] Sodium lauryl sulfate; CAS 151-21-3; EINECS 205-788-1; anionic; raw material for shampoos; liq. to paste; 33% conc.

Zoharpon LAS Spray Dried. [Zohar Detergent Factory] Sodium lauryl sulfate USP/BP; CAS 151-21-3; EINECS 205-788-1; anionic; raw material for mfg. of shampoo, toothpaste, pharmaceutical preparations; powd.; 92% conc.

Zoharpon LAT. [Zohar Detergent Factory] TEA lauryl sulfate; CAS 139-96-8; EINECS 205-388-7; anionic; raw material for mild shampoos and skin care preps.; liq.; 40% conc.

Zoharpon LMT42. [Zohar Detergent Factory] Sodium lauroyl methyl taurate; CAS 4337-75-1; EINECS 224-388-8; anionic; mild detergent, foamer, dispersant used in soap, syndet toilet bars, shampoos, bubble baths; conditioner for skin and hair; paste; 30% conc.

Zoharpon MgES. [Zohar Detergent Factory] Magnesium lauryl ether sulfate (2 EO); CAS 62755-21-9; anionic; raw material for mild, nonirritating shampoos and cosmetic preps.; visc. liq.; 25% conc.

Zoharpon MgS. [Zohar Detergent Factory] Magnesium lauryl sulfate; CAS 3097-08-3; EINECS 221-450-6; anionic; raw material for mild, nonirritating shampoos and cosmetic preps.; liq.; 26% conc.

Zoharpon NH. [Zohar Detergent Factory] Alcohol sulfates, nonionics, and mild cationic surfactants; raw material conc. for dilution with water to "ready to use" shampoos; liq.; 25% conc.

Zoharpon OH. [Zohar Detergent Factory] Alcohol sulfates, nonionics, and mild cationic surfactants; raw material conc. for dilution with water to "ready to use" shampoos; liq.; 27% conc.

Zoharpon SA. [Zohar Detergent Factory] Disodium lauryl sulfosuccinate; anionic; raw material for mild, nonirritating shampoos and cosmetic preps.; paste; 50% conc.

Zoharpon SC. [Zohar Detergent Factory] Blend; amphoteric/anionic/nonionic; shampoo conc. for clear conditioning shampoos processing at R.T.; liq.; 70% conc.

Zoharpon SE. [Zohar Detergent Factory] Disodium laureth sulfosuccinate; anionic; raw material for mild, nonirritating shampoos and cosmetic preps.; liq.; 40% conc.

Zoharpon SM. [Zohar Detergent Factory] Disodium cocamido MEA sulfosuccinate; anionic; raw material for mild shampoos, carpet shampoos; liq. to paste; 40% conc.

Zoharpon ST. [Zohar Detergent Factory] Blend of lauryl ether

sulfate, alkanolamide, and sulfosuccinate; anionic/nonionic; base for mild shampoos, bubble baths, and shower preps.; liq; 28% conc.

Zoharquat 25. [Zohar Detergent Factory] Stearalkonium chloride; CAS 122-19-0; EINECS 204-527-9; cationic; base for hair conditioner; paste; 25% conc.

Zoharquat 75. [Zohar Detergent Factory] Stearalkonium chloride; CAS 122-19-0; EINECS 204-527-9; cationic; base for hair conditioners; paste; 75% conc.

Zoharsyl L-30. [Zohar Detergent Factory] Sodium lauroyl sarcosinate; CAS 137-16-6; EINECS 205-281-5; anionic; raw material for mfg. of hair shampoos, conditioners, toothpastes, carpet and upholstery shampoos; anticorrosive props.; liq.; 30% conc.

Zohartaine AB. [Zohar Detergent Factory] Lauryl betaine; CAS 683-10-3; EINECS 211-669-5; foam booster, mild ingred. for nonirritating shampoos, bubble baths, and detergents; industrial foamer; liq.; 36% conc.

Zohartaine CBS. [Zohar Detergent Factory] Cocamidopropyl hydroxysultaine; CAS 68139-30-0; EINECS 268-761-3; amphoteric; mild detergent for cosmetic applics.; liq.; 50% conc.

Zohartaine TM. [Zohar Detergent Factory] Dihydroxyethyl tallow glycinate; amphoteric; thickener and anticorrosive agent for tech. acid formulations, industrial cleaners; component of mild shampoos based on lauryl sulfates; visc. liq. to paste; 35% conc.

Zoharteric D. [Zohar Detergent Factory] Disodium cocoamphodiacetate; CAS 68650-39-5; EINECS 272-043-5; amphoteric; component for mild, nonirritating conditioning shampoos, bubble baths; detergent for specialty cleaners; liq. to gel; 50% conc.

Zoharteric D-2. [Zohar Detergent Factory] Disodium cocoamphodiacetate, sodium laureth (2) sulfate; amphoteric; component of mild, nonirritating conditioning shampoos, bubble baths, baby prods.; liq.; 38% conc.

Zoharteric D-3. [Zohar Detergent Factory] Disodium cocoamphodiacetate and sodium laureth (3) sulfate; amphoteric; component of mild, nonirritating conditioning shampoos, bubble baths, baby shampoos; liq.; 38 or 50% conc.

Zoharteric DJ. [Zohar Detergent Factory] Disodium lauroamphodiacetate; CAS 14350-97-1; EINECS 238-306-3; amphoteric; component of mild, nonirritating conditioning shampoos, bubble baths; detergent for specialty cleaners; liq.; 35% conc.

Zoharteric D.O. [Zohar Detergent Factory] Disodium cocoamphodiacetate, sodium lauryl sulfate, hexylene glycol; amphoteric; component of extra mild, nonirritating, non-eye-stinging conditioning shampoos, bubble baths, baby shampoos, cleansing materials; liq.; 47% conc.

Zoharteric D.O.T. [Zohar Detergent Factory] Disodium cocoamphodiacetate, sodium laureth (3) sulfate, hexylene glycol; amphoteric; component of extra mild, nonirritating, non-eye-stinging shampoos, cleansing materials; liq.; 50% conc.

Zoharteric D-SF. [Zohar Detergent Factory] Disodiumcocoamphopropionate, salt-free; amphoteric; component of mild, nonirritating shampoos, bubble baths; detergent for heavy-duty household and industrial cleaners with tolerance for alkalies and electrolytes; liq. to paste; 40% conc.

Zoharteric D-SF 70%. [Zohar Detergent Factory] Disodium cocoamphodiacetate, salt-free; CAS 68650-39-5; EINECS 272-043-5; amphoteric; component of mild, nonirritating, conditioning shampoos, bubble baths; detergent for heavy-duty household and industrial cleaners with tolerance for alkalies and electrolytes; liq.; 70% conc.

Zoharteric D-SF/L. [Zohar Detergent Factory] Disodium lauroamphodipropionate, salt-free; amphoteric; component of mild, nonirritating shampoos and bubble baths;

liq.; 40% conc.

Zoharteric M. [Zohar Detergent Factory] Sodium cocoamphoacetate; amphoteric; component for mild, nonirritating conditioning shampoos and bubble baths; detergent for specialty cleaners; liq.; 44% conc.

Zoharteric M-2. [Zohar Detergent Factory] Sodium cocoamphoacetate, sodium laureth (2) sulfate; amphoteric; component of mild, nonirritating conditioning shampoos, bubble baths, baby prods.; liq.; 35% conc.

Zoharteric M-3. [Zohar Detergent Factory] Sodium cocoamphoacetate and sodium laureth (3) sulfate; amphoteric; component of mild, nonirritating, conditioning shampoos and bubble baths; liq.; 35 or 50% conc.

Zoldine® ZT-55. [Angus] Hydroxymethyl dioxoazabicyclo-octane; CAS 6542-37-6; EINECS 229-457-6; cross-linking agent for resorcinol phenol-formaldehyde or protein-based resin systems; raw material for synthesis; used in hair care prods.; m.w. 145.1; water-sol.; m.p. –20 C; b.p. decomposes; flash pt. > 200 F (TCC); pH 7.0 (0.1M aq. sol'n.).

Zoldine® ZT Oxazolidine. [Angus] Hydroxymethyl dioxoazabicyclooctane; CAS 6542-37-6; EINECS 229-457-6.

Zoramide CM. [Zohar Detergent Factory] Cocamide MEA; CAS 68140-00-1; EINECS 268-770-2; nonionic; foam booster, thickener, superfatting agent for cosmetics; flakes; 80% conc.

Zoramox. [Zohar Detergent Factory] Cocamidopropylamine oxide; CAS 68155-09-9; EINECS 268-938-5; amphoteric; wetting agent, foam booster/stabilizer for shampoos, bubble baths; visc. builder for low pH shampoos, other liq. detergents; liq.; 35% conc.

Zoramox E. [Zohar Detergent Factory] Oleamine oxide; CAS 14351-50-9; EINECS 238-311-0; amphoteric; wetting agent, foam booster/stabilizer for shampoos, bubble baths; visc. builder esp. for low pH shampoos; liq.; 48% conc.

Zoramox LO. [Zohar Detergent Factory] Lauramine oxide; CAS 1643-20-5; EINECS 216-700-6; amphoteric; wetting agent, foam booster/stabilizer for shampoos, bubble baths; visc. builder for low pH shampoos, other liq. detergents; liq.; 30% conc.

Part II
Trade Name Functional
Cross-Reference

Trade Name Functional Cross-Reference

Trade name chemicals from the first part of this reference are grouped by broad functional areas derived from manufacturer's specifications. The following trade name products may not be limited to the functional areas represented here.

Absorbents

Aerosil® 200
Aquasorb® A250
Argobase EUC 2
Argobase L1
Argobase L2
Argobase S1
Avicel PH-101
Avicel PH-102
Avicel PH-105
Avicel RC-591
Beeswing 1/16
Beeswing 3/16
Beeswing 3/32
Bio-Pol® OE
Carolane
Celluflow C-25
Celluflow TA-25
Cob Flour #4, 6, 100
Cob Grit #1, 2, 3, 8, 150, 3050
Coral STar

Crosilk Powder
Emery® 1730
Emery® 1732
Emery® 1740
Fancol C
Fancol CAB
Forlan
Forlan 200
Forlan 300
Forlan 500
Forlan LM
G-4909
Hypol® 2000
Imwitor® 408
Imwitor® 412
Imwitor® 708
Imwitor® 742
Imwitor® 908
Imwitor® 910
Imwitor® 928
Imwitor® 988

Ivarbase™ 3230
Ivarbase™ 3240
Ivarbase™ 3250
Labrafil® M 2130 CS
Liquid Absorption Base Type A, T
Nikkol VF-E
Nikkol VF-IP
Norgel
Ointment Base No. 3
Ointment Base No. 4
Ointment Base No. 6
Orgasol 1002 D NAT COS
Orgasol 1002 D WHITE 5 COS
Orgasol 1002 EX D WHITE 10 COS
Orgasol 2002 D NAT COS
Orgasol 2002 EX D NAT COS

Orgasol 2002 UD NAT COS
Protegin® SE
Protegin® W SE
Protegin® WX SE
Protegin® X SE
Ritachol®
Sanwet® COS-905
Sanwet® COS-915
Sanwet® COS-960
Solka-Floc® BW-40
Solka-Floc® BW-100
Solka-Floc® BW-200
Solka-Floc® BW-2030
Solka-Floc® Fine Granular
Water Lock® A-100
Wickenol® 550
Zeolex® 7
Zeolex® 23A
Zeosyl® 200
Zeothix® 265

Analgesics/Anti-Inflammatories/Anti-Irritants

Acylglutamate GS-21
Acylglutamate HS-21
Aldo® PMS
Aloe-Phytogel 199 Powd
Aloe Vera Freeze Dried Powd. 200:1
Aloe Vera Gel
Aloe Vera Gel 1:1
Aloe Vera Gel 1:1 Decolorized
Aloe Vera Gel 1:1 With Pulp
Aloe Vera Gel 1:2
Aloe Vera Gel 1:10
Aloe Vera Gel 1:10 Conc
Aloe Vera Gel 1:50
Aloe Vera Gel 1:50 Conc
Aloe Vera Gel 1:100
Aloe Vera Gel 1:100 Conc
Aloe Vera Gel 10:1 Decolorized
Aloe Vera Gel Conc. 10:1
Aloe Vera Gel Conc. 40:1
Aloe Vera Gel Conc. 40:1 Decolorized
Aloe Vera Gel CS

Aloe Vera Gel CS 10
Aloe Vera Gel CS 40
Aloe Vera Gel DC
Aloe Vera Gel DC 10
Aloe Vera Gel DC 40
Aloe Vera Gel Filtered
Aloe Vera Gel Single Fold
Aloe Vera Gel TEX
Aloe Vera Gel Unfiltered
Aloe Vera Juice
Aloe Vera Powd. A 1-200
Aloe Vera Pulp
Aloe Vera Spray Dried Powd
Alomucin
Alpinamed Chamomile
Alpinamed Ivy
Ami Bioprotector
Ampholak 7CX/C
Ampholak 7TX
Ampholak 7TX/C
Ampholak 7TX-T
Ampholak MDX-1
Ampholak MSX-1
Ampholak XCO-30
Ampholak XO7/C

Ampholak XTP
Anionyx® 12S
Anti-Irritant Complex-1
Aqua-Tein C
Aruba Aloe Vera Gel
Avanel® S-150
Avicel PH-103
Biodynes® TRF
Biodynes® TRF 5% Sol'n
Biophytex®
α-Bisabolol
Brookosome® TRF
CG 10x (Unfiltered and stabilized)
Chembetaine CAS
Clear Filtered Verajuice-Cold Processed
Clintonia Borealis Extract Code 9035
Colla-Gel AC
Collagen Hydrolyzate Cosmetic 50
Collagen Hydrolyzate Cosmetic 55
Collagen Hydrolyzate Cosmetic N-35

Collagen Hydrolyzate Cosmetic N-55
Collagen Hydrolyzate Cosmetic SD
Cosmetic Gelatin
CoVera
Crillon ODE
Crovol A40
Crovol A70
Crovol M40
Crovol M70
Crovol PK40
Crovol PK70
Dermol DISD
Dow Corning® Q2-5220 Resin Modifier
Dow Corning® Q2-5324 Surfactant
Eijitsu Extract BG
Emsorb® 2721
Ethosperse® LA-12
Ethosperse® LA-23
Fancol CH
Fancol Karite Butter
Filtered Verajuice-Cold Processed

507

Analgesics/Anti-Inflammatories/Anti-Irritants *(cont'd.)*

George's Aloe Vera
Geropon® SBFA-30
Geropon® SBR-3
Gluadin® Almond
Gluadin® Wheat
Glucamate® DOE-120
Gluplex® AC
Gluplex® LES
Gluplex® LS
Gluplex® OS
Glusol
Grilloten LSE 65
Grilloten® LSE 65 K
Grilloten® LSE 65 K Soft
Grilloten LSE 65 Soft
Grilloten LSE 87
Grilloten® LSE 87 K
Grilloten® LSE 87 K Soft
Grilloten LSE 87 Soft
Grilloten® PSE 141 G
   Pellets
Grilloten ZT12
Grilloten ZT-40
Grilloten ZT-80
Herbasol Complex GU-61
Hetsorb L-80-72%
Hydagen® B
Hydrocoll™ EN-55
Hydrocoll™ EN-SD
Incrosul OTS
Jewelweed Extract Code
   9034

Kera-Tein 1000 AS
Kera-Tein 1000 RM/50
Kera-Tein 1000 RM SD
Kera-Tein 1000 SD
Lamepon® 4SK
Lanaetex Aloe Vera Gel
Lasilium C
Liposome Unsapo KM
Lonzaine® 12C
Lonzaine® JS
Mackanate™ A-102
Mackanate™ A-103
Mackanate™ CM
Mackanate™ CM-100
Mackanate™ CP
Mackanate™ DC-30
Mackanate™ DC-30A
Mackanate™ DC-50
Mackanate™ EL
Mackanate™ LA
Mackanate™ LM-40
Mackanate™ LO
Mackanate™ LO-100
Mackanate™ LO-Special
Mackanate™ OD-35
Mackanate™ UM-50
Mafo® CSB 50
Maypon 4CT
May-Tein C
May-Tein CT
May-Tein KK
May-Tein KT

May-Tein KTS
May-Tein SK
May-Tein SY
MFA™ Complex
Mirataine® BET-W
Monateric 949J
Monateric CDX-38
Monateric CEM-38
Monateric CLV
Nikkol BL-9EX
Nikkol Dipotassium
   Glycyrrhizinate
Nikkol Glycyrrhetinic Acid
Nikkol Glycyrrhizic Acid
Nikkol Lecinol S-10
Nikkol Lecinol S-10E
Nikkol Lecinol S-10EX
Nikkol Lecinol S-10M
Nikkol Lecinol S-30
Nikkol Stearyl Glycyrrheti-
   nate
Nikkol Wheat Peptide 5000
Norfox® Coco Betaine
Orange Wax
Orange Wax, Deodorized
Pancogene® S
Pea Pro-Tein BK
Peptein® KC
Peptein® TEAC
Phytoderm Complex G
Plasdone® C-30
Plasdone® K-26/28,

K-29/32
Polypeptide 10
Polypeptide 12
Protectein™
Pro-Tein ES-20
PVP K-15
PVP K-30
Rewoderm® S 1333
Rewomid® S 280
Rhumacalm HS 328
Rice Pro-Tein BK
R.I.T.A. d-Panthenol
R.I.T.A. dl-Panthenol
Schercopol CMS-Na
Seanamin BD
Sohakuhi Extract BG-100
Sohakuhi Extract Ethanol
Standapol® SH-100
Standapol® SH-135
Standapol® SHC-101
Sungen
Ucare® Polymer JR-30M,
   JR-125, JR-400
UFZO
Varonic® LI-48
Varsulf® S-1333
Vita-Cos
Wheat-Tein NL
Wickenol® 171
Wickenol® 535
Yucca Glauca Extract Code
   9030

Anticaking Agents/Free-Flow Agents/Flow Improvers

Aerosil® 200
Aerosil® R972
Aluminum Oxide C
Armeen® 18
Armeen® 18D
Armeen® HT
Armeen® HTD
Armeen® T
Avicel PH-101
Avicel PH-102
Avicel PH-103
Avicel PH-105

Cab-O-Sil® L-90
Cab-O-Sil® TS-530
Cecavon AL 11
Cecavon AL 12
Cecavon MG 51
Elcema® F150, G250,
   P100
GP-218
GP-226
Maltrin® M040
Maltrin® M700
Maltrin® QD M550

Maltrin® QD M600
Miglyol® 812
Nuodex Magnesium
   Stearate Food Grade
Nuodex S-1421 Food
   Grade
Nuodex S-1520 Food
   Grade
Quso® G27, G29, G35,
   G38, WR55, WR83
Quso® WR55-FG
Radiastar® 1060

Radiastar® 1100
Silwet® L-720
Sipernat® 22
Sipernat® 22S
Sipernat® 50
Sipernat® 50S
Valfor® Zeolite Na-A
Wacker HDK® H20
Zeofree® 80
Zeolex® 7
Zeolex® 23A
Zeothix® 265

Antifoamers/Defoamers

Ablunol 200ML
Ablunol 200MS
Ablunol 400ML
Ablunol 400MS
Ablunol 600ML
Ablunol 600MS
Adol® 52 NF
Adol® 60
Adol® 80
Adol® 85
Adol® 640
Alcolec® BS
Aldo® MO
Alfol® 1012 HA
Alkamuls® 200-DL
Alkamuls® 200-DO
Alkamuls® CO-15

Amersil® Simethicone EM
Antarox® L-64
Arlacel® 186
Britol® 6NF
Britol® 7NF
Britol® 9NF
Britol® 20USP
Britol® 35USP
Britol® 50USP
Caprol® 3GO
Carbowax® Sentry® PEG
   300
Carbowax® Sentry® PEG
   400
Carbowax® Sentry® PEG
   540 Blend
Carbowax® Sentry® PEG

600
Carbowax® Sentry® PEG
   900
Carbowax® Sentry® PEG
   1000
Carbowax® Sentry® PEG
   1450
Carbowax® Sentry® PEG
   3350
Carbowax® Sentry® PEG
   4600
Carbowax® Sentry® PEG
   8000
Cetodan
Chemal BP-262
Chemal BP-262LF
Chemal BP-2101

Chemal LA-4
Chemal LA-9
Chemal LA-12
Chemal LA-23
Colorin 102, 104, 202
Crill 1
Crill 2
Crill 4
Dehydol® G 202
Dow Corning® Antifoam A
Dow Corning® 200 Fluid
Ethoquad® 18/12
Ethoquad® 18/25
Ethoquad® C/25
Ethoquad® O/25
Fancol OA-95
Flexricin® 13

Antifoamers/Defoamers *(cont'd.)*

Foam Blast 5, 7	Lipocol C-10	Macol® 108	Radiasurf® 7404
Foam Blast 10	Lipocol C-20	Mazol® 300 K	Radiasurf® 7411
Foam Blast 100 Kosher	Lipocol HCO-40	Mazol® GMO K	Radiasurf® 7413
Foam Blast 150 Kosher	Lipocol HCO-60	Mazu® DF 200SP	Radiasurf® 7414
Foamkill® 8G	Lipocol L-1	Nopalcol 1-S	Radiasurf® 7417
Foamkill® 30 Series	Lipocol L-4	Nopalcol 1-TW	Radiasurf® 7420
Foamkill® 80J Series	Lipocol L-12	Norfox® NP-1	Radiasurf® 7422
Foamkill® 618 Series	Lipocol L-23	OP-2000	Radiasurf® 7423
Foamkill® 634 Series	Lipocol M-4	Pegosperse® 400 DOT	Radiasurf® 7431
Foamkill® 634B-HP	Lipocol O-2 Special	Pluracol® E400 NF	Radiasurf® 7432
Foamkill® 634C	Lipocol O-3 Special	Pluracol® E600 NF	Radiasurf® 7443
Foamkill® 634D-HP	Lipocol O-10	Pluracol® E1000	Radiasurf® 7453
Foamkill® 634F-HP	Lipocol O-20	Pluracol® E1450	Radiasurf® 7454
Foamkill® 639J-F	Lipocol S-2	Pluracol® E1450 NF	Rudol®
Foamkill® 644 Series	Lipocol S-10	Pluracol® E2000	Sentry Simethicone NF
Foamkill® 652H	Lipocol S-20	Pluracol® E4000 NF	SF81-50
Foamkill® 652-HF	Lipocol SC-4	Pluracol® E4500	Silwet® L-7602
Foamkill® 684 Series	Lipocol SC-10	Pluracol® E8000	Sorgen 30
Foamkill® 810F	Lipocol SC-15	Pluracol® E8000 NF	Sorgen 40
Foamkill® 830F	Lipocol SC-20	Prox-onic CSA-1/04	Sorgen 50
Foamkill® 836A	Macol® 1	Prox-onic CSA-1/06	Sorgen 90
Foamkill® 1001 Series	Macol® 2LF	Prox-onic CSA-1/010	Sorgen S-30-H
Foamkill® GCP Series	Macol® 4	Prox-onic CSA-1/015	Sorgen S-40-H
Foamkill® MSF Conc	Macol® 16	Prox-onic CSA-1/020	Standapol® SCO
Foamkill® RP	Macol® 22	Prox-onic CSA-1/030	Surfactol® 13
Hodag Antifoam F-1	Macol® 27	Prox-onic CSA-1/050	Surfactol® 340
Hodag CSA-80	Macol® 31	Prox-onic EP 1090-1	Surfactol® 380
Hodag Nonionic 1035-L	Macol® 32	Prox-onic EP 1090-2	Surfynol® 82
Hodag Nonionic 1044-L	Macol® 34	Prox-onic EP 2080-1	Tegosipon®
Hodag Nonionic 1061-L	Macol® 35	Prox-onic EP 4060-1	TO-33-F
Hodag Nonionic 1062-L	Macol® 40	Prox-onic NP-1.5	Tween® 80K
Hodag Nonionic 1064-L	Macol® 42	Prox-onic NP-04	Viscasil®
Hodag Nonionic 1068-F	Macol® 44	Radiasurf® 7196	Viscasil® (10,000 cSt)
Hodag Nonionic 1088-F	Macol® 46	Radiasurf® 7206	Viscasil® (12,500 cSt)
Hodag Nonionic 2017-R	Macol® 72	Radiasurf® 7269	Wacker Silicone Antifoam
Lipo DGLS	Macol® 77	Radiasurf® 7270	Emulsion SE 9
Lipo DGS-SE	Macol® 85	Radiasurf® 7400	Witafrol® 7420
Lipo EGDS	Macol® 88	Radiasurf® 7402	Zeofree® 80
Lipocol C-2	Macol® 101	Radiasurf® 7403	

Antimicrobials/Antiseptics/Disinfectants/Sanitizers

Acetoquat CPC	Amisoft CS-11	Arquad® DM14B-90	Cetrimide™ BP
Acetoquat CTAB	Amisoft CT-12	Arquad® DMMCB-50	CMI 321
Acylglutamate CS-11	Amisoft GS-11	Arquad® S-2C-50	CMI 800
Acylglutamate CS-21	Amisoft HS-11	Arquad® T-2C-50	Comperlan® UDM
Acylglutamate CT-12	Amisoft LS-11	Arquad® T-27W	CPC
Acylglutamate GS-11	Amisoft MS-11	Atomergic Zinc Pyrithione	CPC Sumquat 6060
Acylglutamate HS-11	Amonyl BR 1244	Bactericide MB 2/012582	Crodasinic LS30
Acylglutamate LS-11	Ampholak 7CX/C	Bactiphen 2506 G	Crodasinic LS35
Acylglutamate LT-12	Ampholak 7TX/C	Bardac® 2050	Crodasinic OS35
Acylglutamate MS-11	Ampholak MDX-1	Barquat® MB-50	Cuivridone®
Alberger®	Ampholak MSX-1	Barquat® MB-80	Dehyquart® A
AlcoCare® 2011	Ampholak XO7/C	Barquat® MX-50	Dehyquart® C
AlcoCare® 2012	Amphosol® DM	Barquat® MX-80	Dehyquart® C Crystals
AlcoCare® 2013	Arquad® 2C-75	Biocelose NC-50	Dehyquart® LDB
AlcoCare® 2115	Arquad® 2HT-75	Bretol®	Dehyquart® LT
AlcoCare® 2123	Arquad® 12-33	BTC® 2125	Deo-Usnate
AlcoCare® 2150	Arquad® 12-50	Busan® 1500	Elestab CPN
Alcocare® 3020	Arquad® 16-29	Busan® 1504	Elestab HP 100
Alkaquat® DMB-451-50,	Arquad® 16-50	Busan® 1506	EmCon Tea Tree
DMB-451-80	Arquad® 18-50	Busan® 1507	Empigen® 5073
Alpinamed Burdock	Arquad® B-50	CAE	Empigen® 5089
Aludone®	Arquad® B-90	Cathelios CL 50	Empigen® BAC50
Amical® 48	Arquad® B-100	Catinal HTB-70	Empigen® BAC50/BP
Amical® 50	Arquad® C-33	Catinal MB-50A	Empigen® BAC80
Amical® Flowable	Arquad® C-50	Cetol®	Empigen® BAC90

Antimicrobials/Antiseptics/Disinfectants/Sanitizers *(cont'd.)*

Empigen® CHB
Empigen® CHB40
Enzyami No. 1
Enzyami No. 1A
Enzyami No. 6
ES-1239
Etaphen
Ethylan® HBI-TG
Exsymol Parahydroxy-
cinnamic Acid
FMB 65-15 Quat,
65-28 Quat
FMB 210-8 Quat,
210-15 Quat
FMB 302-8 Quat
FMB 451-5 Quat,
451-8 Quat
FMB 451-8 Quat
FMB 504-5 Quat
FMB 551-5 Quat
FMB 1210-5 Quat,
1210-8 Quat
FMB 3328-5 Quat,
3328-8 Quat
FMB 4500-5 Quat
Fungitex R
Germaben® II
Germaben® II-E
Germall® 115
Germall® II
Glycacil L, S
Glydant®
Herbasol Complex GU-61
Hexetidine 90, 99
Hyamine® 10X
Hyamine® 1622 50%
Hyamine® 1622 Crystals
Hyamine® 2389
Hyamine® 3500 50%
Hyamine® 3500-NF
Igepal® CA-630G
Igepal® CO-630 Special
Irgasan DP300
Ivex® 10
Jet Quat 2C-75
Jet Quat C-50

Jet Quat DT-50
Jet Quat S-50
Jet Quat T-27W
Jet Quat T-50
Kathon® CG
Kemamine® Q-1902C
Kemamine® Q-7903B
Koster Keunen Beeswax,
Filtered
Lexgard B
Lexgard E
Lexgard M
Lexgard P
Lexgard® Bronopol
Luviquat® FC 370
Luviquat® FC 550
Luviquat® FC 905
Maquat 4450-E
Maquat LC-12S
Maquat SC-18
Maquat SC-1632
Marlazin® KC 21/50
Maypon UD
Midecol CF
Midpol 97
Midpol 100
Midpol 2000
Midpol PHN
Midtect TF-60
Miranol® HM Conc
Miranol® OM-SF Conc
Myacide® SP
Myavert C
Mytab®
Nikkol CA-101
Nikkol CA-2150
Nikkol CA-3080
Nikkol CA-3080M
Nipabenzyl
Nipabutyl
Nipabutyl Potassium
Nipabutyl Sodium
Nipacide® MX
Nipacide® PX-R
Nipagin A
Nipagin A Potassium

Nipagin A Sodium
Nipagin M
Nipagin M Potassium
Nipagin M Sodium
Nipaguard® DMDMH
Nipaheptyl
Nipasol M
Nipasol M Potassium
Nipasol M Sodium
Nipastat
Noramium DA.50
Nuosept C
Omadine® MDS
Orange Wax
Orange Wax, Deodorized
Oxaban®-A
Oxaban®-E
Paragon™
Paragon™ II
Pationic® 122A
Phenonip
Phenosept
Phenoxen
Phenoxetol
Phospholipid EFA
Phospholipid PTC
Phospholipid PTD
Phospholipid PTL
Phospholipid PTZ
Phytoderm Complex U
Preventol GD
Propylene Phenoxetol
PVP-Iodine 17/12, 30/06
Radiaquat® 6442
Radiaquat® 6444
Radiaquat® 6445
Radiaquat® 6460
Radiaquat® 6462
Radiateric® 6860
Radiateric® 6864
Rewocid® DU 185
Rewocid® SBU 185
Rewocid® SBU 185 P
Rewocid® U 185
Rewocid® UTM 185
Rewoquat UTM 185

Rewoteric® QAM 50
Ryoto Sugar Ester B-370
Ryoto Sugar Ester L-595
Ryoto Sugar Ester L-1570
Ryoto Sugar Ester L-1695
Ryoto Sugar Ester M-1695
Ryoto Sugar Ester O-1570
Sanisol C
Sanisol CPR, CR, CR-80%
Sanisol HTPR
Sanisol OPR, TPR
Schercoquat IB
Schercotaine UAB
Schercotaine UAB-Z
Schercozoline B
Schercozoline C
Sepicide CI
Sepicide LD
Sodium Omadine®,
40% Aq. Sol'n
Spectradyne® G
Standamox O1
Sumquat® 6020
Sumquat® 6050
Sumquat® 6110
Suttocide® A
Swanol CA-101
Tektamer® 38
Tequat PAN
Tris Nitro®
Tristat IU
Uantox POMEBIS
Ucarcide® 225
Ucarcide® 250
Undezin
Unichem THYMOL
Unicide U-13
Unikon A-22
Uniphen P-23
Unisuprol S-25
Universal ZPS
Vancide® 89 RE
Zincidone®
Zinc Omadine® 48% Disp
Zinc Omadine® Powd
Zink Pyrion

Antioxidants

Alkaterge®-E
Amiox
Antioxidant G-2
Argus DLTDP
Argus DSTDP
Ascorbyl Palmitate No.
60412
Atomergic Propyl Gallate
Beta Carotene 30% in Veg.
Oil No. 65646
CMI 321
CMI 550
CMI 800
Controx® KS
Controx® VP
Copherol® 950LC
Copherol® 1250
Copherol® F 1300

Covi-Ox T-30P
Covi-Ox T-50
Covi-Ox T-70
Covipherol T-75
Covitol 80/20M
Covitol 544
Covitol 700C
Covitol 1100
Covitol 1185
Covitol 1210
Covitol 1360
Covitol F-350M
Covitol F-600
Covitol F-1000
Dascare Orizanol
Evanstab® 12
Gamma Oryzanol
Ionol CP

Koster Keunen Beeswax,
Filtered
Lipomicron Vitamin E
Acetate
Lysidone®
Mark® 5095
Mircoat™ Oil
Nipanox® S-1
Nipanox® Special
Orange Wax
Orange Wax, Deodorized
Oxynex® 2004
Oxynex® K
Oxynex® L
Oxynex® LM
Progallin® LA
Progallin® P
Sustane® 1-F

Sustane® 3
Sustane® BHA
Sustane® BHT
Syntase® 230
Tenox® 2
Tenox® 4
Tenox® 4B
Tenox® 6
Tenox® 20B
Tenox® 22
Tenox® 25
Tenox® 26
Tenox® BHA
Tenox® BHT
Tenox® GT-1, GT-2
Tenox® PG
Tenox® TBHQ
dl-α-Tocopherol

Antioxidants *(cont'd.)*

Turpinal® SL	Uantox EBATE	Uantox TBHQ	Unipherol U-14
Uantox 3	Uantox PG	Unichem THYMOL	Univit-E Acetate
Uantox BHA	Uantox SEBATE		

Antiperspirants/Deodorants

Abscents® Deodorizing Powd.	Dow Corning® ACH-331	Hyamine® 3500-NF	Rezal® 67P
Alchlordrate	Dow Corning® ACH7-308	Hydagen® C.A.T	Unistab S 69
Aloxicoll® L	Dow Corning® ACH7-321	Hydagen® DEO	USP-2
Aloxicoll® PC	Dow Corning® AZG-368	Locron Extra, Flakes, L,	Westchlor® 170
Aloxicoll® PF	Dow Corning® AZG-369	P, P Extra, Powd.,	Westchlor® 170 Powd.
Aloxicoll® PSF	Dow Corning® AZG-370	S, Sol'n	Westchlor® 200
Alpinamed Sage	Dow Corning® Q5-7160	Macrospherical® 95	Westchlor® 200 Custom
Aludone®	AZAG Powd.	Maquat 4450-E	Powd. 10
Aluminum Hydroxychloride 23	Dow Corning® Q5-7171 AACH Powd.	Micro-Dry®	Westchlor® 200 Impalpable
Aluminum Hydroxychloride 47	Emcol® E-607L	Micro-Dry® Superultrafine	Westchlor® A2Z 8106
	Emcol® E-607S	Micro-Dry® Ultrafine	Westchlor® DM 200
Barquat® CME-35	Enzyami No. 7	Microsponge® 5640	Impalpable
Biocelose NC-50	G-271	Millithix® 925	Westchlor® ZR 30B
Carbowax® PEG 600	Grillocin® AT Basis	Polytrap® 6603	Westchlor® ZR 30B DM
Carbowax® PEG 900	Grillocin® CW 90	Reach® 101, 201, 501	Powd.
Carbowax® PEG 1450	Grillocin® HY 77	Reach® AZO-902	Westchlor® ZR 35B
Chloracel® 40% Sol'n	Grillocin® P 176	Reach® AZP-701,	Westchlor® ZR 35B DM
Chloracel® Solid	Grillocin® PY 88 Pellets	AZP-703	Powd.
Chlorhydrol® 50% Sol'n	Grillocin® S 803/7	Reach® AZZ-902	Westchlor® ZR 35B Micro
Chlorhydrol® Granular	Grillocin S-803/12	Rehydrol® II	Powd.
Chlorhydrol, Impalpable	Grillocin WE-106	Rewoteric® QAM 50	Westchlor® ZR 41
Chlorhydrol® Powd.	Grillocose® PS	Rezal® 36	Westchlor® ZR 80B DM
Dehyquart® A	Grilloten® LSE 65 K	Rezal® 36G	Powd.
Dehyquart® LT	Grilloten® LSE 87 K	Rezal® 36G Conc	Westchlor® ZR 82B DM
Deodorant Richter/K	Grilloten® PSE 141 G Pellets	Rezal® 36GP	Powd.
Dow Corning® ACH-303	Hyamine® 1622 Crystals	Rezal® 36GP Super-ultrafine	Zirkonal L
Dow Corning® ACH-323	Hyamine® 3500 50%	Rezal® 67	Zirkonal P

Antistats

Abil®-Quat 3270	Alkamuls® PSMO-5	Carbowax® PEG 600	Chemax E-1000 MS
Abil®-Quat 3272	Alkapol PEG 300	Carbowax® PEG 900	Chemeen 18-2
Ablumine 18	Alkateric® PB	Carbowax® PEG 1000	Chemeen 18-5
Ablumine 280	Aluminum Oxide C	Carbowax® PEG 1450	Chemeen 18-50
Ablumine 1618	Amidex AME	Carbowax® PEG 3350	Chemeen C-2
Ablumine DHT75	Amifat P-21	Carbowax® PEG 4600	Chemeen C-5
Ablumox CAPO	Amifat P-30	Carbowax® PEG 8000	Chemeen C-10
Ablumox LO	Ammonyx® KP	Carsamide® AMEA	Chemeen C-15
Ablunol CO 5	Ammonyx® LKP	Carsonon® 144-P	Chemphos TC-231S
Ablunol CO 15	Antistatique WL 879	Carsonon® 169-P	Chemphos TC-337
Ablunol CO 30	Arlatone® T	Carsoquat® 868	Chemphos TC-341
Accomeen C2	Aromox® C/12	Carsoquat® 868-E	Chemphos TC-349
Accomeen C5	Aromox® C/12-W	Carsoquat® CT-429	Chemphos TR-505
Accomeen C10	Aromox® DMMC-W	Carsoquat® SDQ-25	Chemphos TR-505D
Accomeen C15	Arquad® 2C-75	Cathelios CL 50	Chemphos TR-510
Accomeen S2	Arquad® 2HT-75	Catinal HTB-70	Chemphos TR-510S
Accomeen S10	Arquad® 12-33	Catinal MB-50A	Chemphos TR-515
Accomeen T2	Arquad® 12-50	Celquat® H-100	Chemphos TR-515D
Accomeen T5	Arquad® 16-29	Celquat® L-200	Chemphos TR-541
Accomeen T15	Arquad® 16-50	Celquat® SC-240	Chimin BX
Adogen® S-18 V	Arquad® 18-50	Centrolex® F	Chimin P45
Aerosol® OT-75%	Arquad® C-33	Ceranine PN Base	Chimin P50
Akypoquat 131	Arquad® C-50	Ceraphyl® 60	Chitin Liq
Alkamuls® CO-15	Arquad® DMMCB-50	Ceraphyl® 65	Cithrol 2ML
Alkamuls® EL-620	Arquad® HC	Ceraphyl® 70	Cithrol 4ML
Alkamuls® EL-620L	Arquad® T-2C-50	Ceraphyl® 85	Cithrol 6DS
Alkamuls® GMO	Arquad® T-27W	Cetrimide BP	Cithrol 6ML
Alkamuls® GMO-45LG	Barquat® CME-35	Chemax E-200 MS	Cithrol 10ML
Alkamuls® PSML-20	CAE	Chemax E-600 MS	Cithrol 60ML

Antistats *(cont'd.)*

Cithrol DGMS N/E	Empigen® BS	Incroquat SE-85	Macol® 40
Cithrol DGMS S/E	Empigen® BS/H	Incroquat TMC-80	Macol® 42
Cithrol GDL N/E	Empigen® CM	Incroquat TMC-95	Macol® 44
Cithrol GDL S/E	Empigen® OB	Jaguar® C-14-S	Macol® 46
Cithrol GDO N/E	Empigen® OY	Jaguar® C-17	Macol® 72
Cithrol GDO S/E	Emulgade® CRC	Jaguar® C-162	Macol® 77
Cithrol GDS N/E	ES-1239	Jet Quat S-2C-50	Macol® 85
Cithrol GDS S/E	Ethomeen® C/15	Karamide 121	Macol® 88
Cithrol GML N/E	Ethoquad® 18/12	Karamide 363	Macol® 101
Cithrol GML S/E	Ethoquad® 18/25	Katioran® AF	Macol® 108
Cithrol GMO N/E	Ethoquad® C/12	Lanoquat® 1756	Marlazin® KC 21/50
Cithrol GMO S/E	Ethoquad® C/25	Lexquat® 2240	Marlazin® KC 30/50
Cithrol GMR N/E	Ethoquad® O/12	Lexquat® CH	Marlophor® LN-Acid
Cithrol GMR S/E	Ethoquad® O/25	Lilaminox M24	Marlophor® MO 3-Acid
Cithrol GMS Acid Stable	Etocas 10	Lipamide MEAA	Masil® 280
Cithrol GMS N/E	Etocas 35	Lipocol L-4	Masil® 280LP
Cithrol GMS S/E	Etocas 60	Lipocol L-12	Masil® 2132
Cithrol PGML N/E	Flexan® 130	Lipocol L-23	Masil® 2133
Cithrol PGML S/E	Foamid LM2E	Lipocol O-2 Special	Masil® 2134
Cithrol PGMO N/E	Foamquat 2IAE	Lipocol O-10	May-Tein C
Cithrol PGMO S/E	Foamquat CAS	Lipocol O-20	May-Tein KK
Cithrol PGMR N/E	Foamquat SOAS	Lipocol S-2	May-Tein KT
Cithrol PGMR S/E	Foamquat VG	Lipocol S-10	May-Tein R
Cithrol PGMS N/E	Foamtaine CAB-A	Lipocol S-20	May-Tein SK
Cithrol PGMS S/E	Foamtaine CAB-G	Lipocol SC-4	May-Tein SY
Cosmedia Guar® C-261 N	Gafac® RE-877	Lipocol SC-15	Merpol® HCS
Crafol AP-11	Gantrez® AN	Lipocol SC-20	Merquat® 100
Crapol FU-25	Genamin CTAC	Liponic EG-1	Miramine® CODI
Crill 1	Genamin KDM	Lipo-Peptide AME 30	Miranol® DM
Crill 2	Genamin KDM-F	Lipoquat R	Miranol® Ester PO-LM4
Crill 3	Hetamine 5L-25	Liposorb L	Mirapol® 9, 95, 175
Crill 35	Hetoxamine C-2	Liposorb L-10	Mirapol® A-15
Crillet 4	Hetoxamine C-5	Liposorb L-20	Mirapol® AD-1
Crodafos CAP	Hetoxamine C-15	Liposorb O	Mirapol® AZ-1
Crodafos N-3 Acid	Hetoxamine O-2	Liposorb O-5	Mirataine® BB
Crodasinic LS35	Hetoxamine O-5	Liposorb O-20	Mirataine® CAB-A
Crodasinic OS35	Hetoxamine ST-2	Liposorb P	Mirataine® CAB-O
Croduret 200	Hetoxamine ST-15	Liposorb P-20	Mirataine® CB/M
Crosultaine E-30	Hetoxamine ST-50	Liposorb S	Monaquat ISIES
Dehyquart® A	Hetoxamine T-2	Liposorb S-4	Monolan® PPG440,
Dehyquart® C Crystals	Hetoxamine T-5	Liposorb S-20	PPG1100, PPG2200
Dehyquart® E	Hetoxamine T-15	Liposorb SQO	M-Quat® JO-50
Dehyquart® LT	Hetoxamine T-20	Liposorb TO	Mytab®
Dehyquart® SP	Hetoxamine T-50	Liposorb TO-20	Naetex-CHP
Dehyquart® STC-25	Hetoxamine T-50-70%	Liposorb TS	Naetex-L
Diaformer® Z-301	Hodag Nonionic 1035-L	Liposorb TS-20	Naetex-LD
Diaformer® Z-400	Hodag Nonionic 1044-L	Mackernium™ CTC-30	Naetex O-80
Diaformer® Z-A	Hodag Nonionic 1061-L	Mackernium™ KP	Naetex-Q
Diaformer® Z-AT	Hodag Nonionic 1062-L	Mackernium™ NLE	Nikkol CA-2330
Diaformer® Z-SM	Hodag Nonionic 1064-L	Mackernium™ SDC-25	Nikkol CA-2350
Diaformer® Z-W	Hodag Nonionic 1068-F	Mackernium™ SDC-50	Nikkol CA-2450
Drewmulse® 200K	Hodag Nonionic 1088-F	Mackernium™ SDC-85	Nikkol CA-2450T
Drewpol® 10-4-O	Hodag PE-004	Mackernium™ WLE	Nikkol CA-2465
Elacid Richter	Hodag PE-104	Macol® 1	Nikkol CA-2580
Emcol® 4	Hodag PE-106	Macol® 2	Ninox® FCA
Emcol® CC-9	Hodag PE-109	Macol® 2D	Obazoline LB-40
Emcol® CC-36	Hodag PE-206	Macol® 2LF	Ormagel XPU
Emcol® CC-42	Hodag PE-209	Macol® 4	Phenoxyethanol O
Emcol® CC-55	Igepal® CO-430	Macol® 8	Phospholipid PTD
Emcol® CC-57	Incromectant AQ	Macol® 10	Phospholipid PTL
Emcol® ISML	Incromectant LQ	Macol® 16	Phospholipid PTZ
Emcol® L	Incropol CS-20	Macol® 22	Pluracol® E400 NF
Emcol® M	Incropol CS-50	Macol® 23	Pluracol® E600 NF
Emcol® NA-30	Incropol L-23	Macol® 31	Pluracol® E1000
Emphos™ CS-1361	Incroquat 100	Macol® 32	Pluracol® E1450
Emphos™ D70-30C	Incroquat BA-85	Macol® 33	Pluracol® E1450 NF
Empicol® 0216	Incroquat CTC-30	Macol® 34	Pluracol® E2000
Empigen® 5107	Incroquat S-85	Macol® 35	Pluracol® E4000 NF

Antistats *(cont'd.)*

Pluracol® E4500	Querton 16Cl-50	Schercoquat IB	T-Maz® 81
Pluracol® E8000	Querton 442	Schercoquat WOAS	T-Maz® 85
Pluracol® E8000 NF	Querton 442-11	Schercotaine CAB	T-Maz® 90
Pluronic® F38	Querton 442-82	Schercotaine MAB	T-Maz® 95
Pluronic® F68	Querton 442E	Schercozoline B	Tri-Sil MFF 5010
Pluronic® F68LF	Querton 442H	Schercozoline C	Tri-Sil MFF 5010-70
Pluronic® F77	Querton 442P	Schercozoline I	Unisoft SAC
Pluronic® F87	Querton 442P-11	Schercozoline L	Variquat® K-1215
Pluronic® F88	Radiamox® 6800	Schercozoline O	Varisoft® 5TD
Pluronic® F98	Radiamox® 6804	Schercozoline S	Varisoft® 110-PG
Pluronic® F108	Radiaquat® 6444	Silbione™ 71631	Varisoft® 250
Pluronic® F127	Radiaquat® 6462	Silbione™ 71634	Varisoft® 432-100
Pluronic® L35	Radiaquat® 6471	Silwet® L-77	Varisoft® 432-CG
Pluronic® L42	Radiasurf® 7196	Silwet® L-7002	Varisoft® 432-ET
Pluronic® L43	Radiasurf® 7206	Silwet® L-7614	Varisoft® 432-PPG
Pluronic® L44	Radiasurf® 7269	Span® 20	Varisoft® BT-85
Pluronic® L61	Radiasurf® 7270	Span® 40	Varisoft® CTB-40
Pluronic® L62	Radiasurf® 7400	Span® 60, 60K	Varisoft® DHT
Pluronic® L62D	Radiasurf® 7402	Span® 65	Varisoft® OIMS
Pluronic® L62LF	Radiasurf® 7403	Span® 85	Varisoft® SDAC
Pluronic® L63	Radiasurf® 7404	Stafoam DF-1	Varisoft® SDAC-W
Pluronic® L64	Radiasurf® 7411	Stafoam DF-4	Varisoft® SDC-85
Pluronic® L72	Radiasurf® 7413	Standamul® STC-25	Varisoft® TA-100
Pluronic® L81	Radiasurf® 7414	Standapol® AB-45	Varisoft® TC-90
Pluronic® L92	Radiasurf® 7417	Standapol® BAW	Varisoft® TIMS
Pluronic® L101	Radiasurf® 7420	Stedbac®	Varonic® 2271
Pluronic® L121	Radiasurf® 7422	Sulfostat KNT	Varonic® K-202
Pluronic® L122	Radiasurf® 7423	Sulframin 85	Varonic® K-202 SF
Pluronic® P65	Radiasurf® 7431	Sulframin 90	Varonic® K-205
Pluronic® P75	Radiasurf® 7432	Sulframin 1240, 1245	Varonic® K-205 SF
Pluronic® P84	Radiasurf® 7443	Sulframin 1250, 1260	Varonic® K-210
Pluronic® P85	Radiasurf® 7453	Sulframin 1288	Varonic® K-210 SF
Pluronic® P94	Radiasurf® 7454	Sulframin 1298	Varonic® K-215
Pluronic® P103	Radiateric® 6860	Sulframin 1388	Varonic® K-215 SF
Pluronic® P104	Radiateric® 6864	Sumquat® 6210	Varonic® Q-202
Pluronic® P105	Rewocid® UTM 185	Surfactol® Q1	Varonic® Q-202 SF
Pluronic® P123	Rewominox B 204	Surfactol® Q2	Varonic® Q-205
Polyquart® H	Rewominox L 408	Surfactol® Q3	Varonic® Q-205 SF
Polyquart® H 81	Rewominox S 300	Synoquart P 50	Varonic® S-202
Polyquart® H 7102	Rewominoxid S 300	Tagat® I	Varonic® S-202 SF
Protectein™	Rewoquat CPEM	Tagat® I2	Varonic® T-202
Proto-Lan 4R	Rewoquat DQ 35	Tagat® L	Varonic® T-202 SF
Proto-Lan 8	Rewoquat RTM 50	Tagat® L2	Varonic® T-205
Prox-onic HR-05	Rhodafac® RD-510	Tagat® O	Varonic® T-205 SF
Prox-onic HR-016	Rhodafac® RE-870	Tagat® O2	Varonic® T-210
Prox-onic HR-025	Rhodameen® OS-12	Tagat® RI	Varonic® T-210 SF
Prox-onic HR-030	Rhodaquat® M214B/99	Tagat® S	Varonic® T-215
Prox-onic HR-036	Rhodaquat® M242B/99	Tagat® S2	Varonic® T-215 SF
Prox-onic HR-040	Salcare SC10	Tagat® TO	Varox® 270
Prox-onic HR-080	Salcare SC30	Tequat PAN	Varox® 365
Prox-onic HR-0200	Sandotex A	T-Maz® 20	Varox® 1770
Prox-onic HR-0200/50	Sandoz Amine Oxide XA-C	T-Maz® 28	Velvetex® BA-35
Prox-onic HRH-05	Schercamox C-AA	T-Maz® 40	Velvetex® BC-35
Prox-onic HRH-016	Schercamox DML	T-Maz® 60	Velvetex® BK-35
Prox-onic HRH-025	Schercamox T-12	T-Maz® 61	Witcamide® 82
Prox-onic HRH-0200	Schercoquat 2IAE	T-Maz® 65	Witcamide® 5133
Prox-onic HRH-0200/50	Schercoquat CAS	T-Maz® 80	Witcamide® 5195
Querton 16Cl-29	Schercoquat IAS	T-Maz® 80KLM	Witcamine® 6606
			Witcamine® 6622

Aromatic Extracts/Fragrances/Perfume Fixatives

Abil® AV 8853	Aromaplex™	Bonarox	Cyclamber
Aldehyd 11-11	Arova® N	Carbavert	Cyclohexyl Salicylate
Aldehyd 13-13	Atrinon	Cephene™	Cyclovertal
Ambroxan	Aurantiol®	Corps Celeri	Cypronat
Anthoxan	Boisambrene Forte	Crodamol AB	EmCon Tea Tree

Aromatic Extracts/Fragrances/Perfume Fixatives *(cont'd.)*

Emeressence® 1150
Ethylene Bodecanedioate
Ethylene Brassylate
Fancol Menthol
Floramat
Geranonitril
Gerbavert
Herbavert
Hexyl Jasmat®

Irotyl
Jasmacyclat
Jasmonan
Jasmorange®
Junipal
Lysmeral®
Melusat
Neral
Nerolidol

Orange Wax
Oxyvet
Peranat
Phenoxyethanol O
Prenol
Romilat
Rose Ether Phenoxy-
ethanol
ScentCap

Sedamon
Spiroflor
Trivalon
Troenan
Unichem THYMOL
Unisweet VAN
Universal MENT
Verdoxan

Bases/Ointment Bases/Shampoo Bases

Ablumine 1618
Ablumine DHT75
Ablumine TMC
Ablumine TMS
Abluphat MLP-200
Abluphat MLP-220
Akyporox SAL SAS
Akyposal 23 ST 70
Akyposal ALS 33
Akyposal DS 28
Akyposal DS 56
Akyposal EO 20
Akyposal EO 20 MW
Akyposal EO 2067
Akyposal HF 28
Akyposal MLES 35
Akyposal MLS 30
Akyposal RLM 70
Alscoap LE-240
Alscoap LN-40, LN-90
Alscoap M-3S
Amerchol® BL
Amerchol® C
Amerchol® H-9
Amerchol® L-99
Amiter LGOD-2
Amiter LGOD-5
Amojell Petrolatum Amber,
Dark, Snow White
Amphocerin® K
Amphosol® CA
Amphosol® DM
Apifac
Apifil®
Aquabase
Aremsol MA
Aremsol MR
Aremsol TA
Argobase EU
Argobase EUC 2
Argobase L1
Argobase L2
Argobase S1
Arosurf® 42-E6
Avicel RC-591
Avirol® 300
Base Nacrante 2078
Base Nacrante 6030 CP
Base Nacrante 9578
Beaulight A-5000
Beaulight ECA
Beaulight ESS
Beaulight LCA-30D
Beaulight SSS
Calfoam NLS-30

Calsuds CD-6
Carbowax® PEG 300
Carbowax® PEG 900
Carbowax® PEG 1000
Carbowax® Sentry® PEG
300
Carbowax® Sentry® PEG
400
Carbowax® Sentry® PEG
540 Blend
Carbowax® Sentry® PEG
600
Carbowax® Sentry® PEG
900
Carbowax® Sentry® PEG
1000
Carbowax® Sentry® PEG
1450
Carbowax® Sentry® PEG
3350
Carbowax® Sentry® PEG
4600
Carbowax® Sentry® PEG
8000
Carsofoam® BS-I
Carsoquat® 816-C
Catinal HTB-70
Catinal OB-80E
Cation S
C-Base
Cetax 16
Cetax 18
Cetax 50
Chemical 39 Base
Cithrol GMS A/S ES 0743
Coronet Lanolin
Cosmopon MP
Cosmopon MT
Cutina® CBS
Cutina® GMS
Cutina® KD16
Cutina® LE
Cutina® LM
Cutina® MD-A
Cycloryl ALC
Cycloton® 7LUF
Cycloton® D261C/70
Cycloton® M270C/18
Cycloton® M270C/85
Dehydag® Wax W
Dehydol® LS 2
Dehymuls® K
Dermalcare® 1673
Diadol 18G
Drakeol 6

Drakeol 7
Drakeol 9
Drakeol 13
Dynasan® 110
Dynasan® 112
Dynasan® 114
Dynasan® 116
Dynasan® 118
Elfapur® ML 30 SH
Emal 20C
Emal E-25C, -70C
Emal NC-35
Emalex CC-10
Emalex CC-16
Emalex CC-18
Emalex CC-168
Emalex EG-2854-IS
Emalex EG-2854-O
Emalex EG-2854-S
Emalex HIS-34
Emalex LIP
Emalex LWIS-2
Emalex LWIS-5
Emalex LWS-3
Emalex LWS-5
Emalex LWS-8
Emalex LWS-10
Emalex LWS-15
Emalex PS-1
Emalex PS-1(S)
Emalex PS-2A
Emalex PS-2B
Emcol® ISML
Emery® 1730
Emery® 1732
Emery® 1740
Empicol® AL70
Empicol® EAA70
Empicol® EAB
Empicol® ESB3
Empicol® ESB3/D
Empicol® ESB3/S
Empicol® ESB50
Empicol® ESC70/AU
Empicol® ESC/AU
Empicol® LQ70
Empicol® LS30B
Empicol® LS30P
Empicol® MIPA
Empicol® TA40A
Empicol® TL40/S
Empicol® WAK
Empicol® XC35
Empicol® XC35/S
Empicol® XPA

Empicol® XT 45
Emulgade® 1000 NI
Emulgade® A
Emulgade® CL
Emulgade® CLB
Emulgade® EO-10
Emulgade® F Special
Emulgade® K
Estaram
Estran™-Lite
Estran™-Pure
Estran™-Xtra
Eureka 102-WK
Evanol™
Fancol Karite Butter
Foam Base G
Forlan
Forlan 200
Forlan 300
Forlan 500
Forlan LM
G-4909
Galenol® 1618 AE
Galenol® 1618 CS
Galenol® 1618 DSN
Galenol® 1618 KS
Gelot 64®
Genamin KDM-F
Genamin KSE
Genapol® T Grades
Golden Dawn Grade 1, 2
Golden Dawn Superfine
Golden Fleece DF
Golden Fleece P-80
Golden Fleece P-95
Golden Fleece RA
Hefti GMS-33
Hetoxol P
Hetsulf Acid
Hispagel® 100
Hispagel® 200
Hostacerin CG
Hostacerin T-3
Hostapon KTW New
Hostapur SAS 60
Hydrokote® 25
Hydrokote® 27
Hydrokote® 79
Hydrokote® 95
Hydrokote® 97
Hydrokote® 102
Hydrokote® 108
Hydrokote® 112
Hydrokote® 118
Hydrokote® 711

Bases/Ointment Bases/Shampoo Bases *(cont'd.)*

Hydrokote® S-7
Hydrokote® SP
Hydrolactol 70
Imwitor® 960
Imwitor® 960 K
Imwitor® 965
Imwitor® 965 K
Incromate CDL
Incroquat TMC-80
Incroquat TMC-95
Intex Scour Base 706
Ionet T-20 C
Ionet T-60 C
Ionet T-80 C
Ivarbase™ 3230
Ivarbase™ 3240
Ivarbase™ 3250
Kalcohl 68
Kalcohl 80
Kessco® 653
Kessco® Glycerol
  Monostearate SE,
  Acid Stable
Kester Wax® K 48
Kohacool L-400
Lanette® O
Lanette® SX
Lanette® W
Lanogen 1500
Lauropal 2
Lebon 101H, 105
Lexate® BPQ
Lexate® PX
Lipocire A
Lipocire CM
Lipocire DM
Lipoproteol LCOK
Lipoproteol LK
Lipoproteol UCO
Liquid Absorption Base
  Type A, T
Liquid Base
Louryl T-50
Manroteric CAB
Marlamid® KLP
Marlamid® PG 20
Marlinat® 242/28
Marlinat® 242/70
Marlinat® 242/70 S
Marlinat® 243/28
Marlinat® 243/70
Marlinat® DFK 30
Marlinat® DFL 40
Marlinat® DFN 30
Marlinat® SL 3/40
Marlinat® SRN 30
Marlon® AFR
Marlon® PS 60
Marlophor® LN-Acid
Marlophor® MO 3-Acid
Marlopon® AT 50
Masque Poudre No. 2
Massa Estarinum® 299
Massa Estarinum® A
Massa Estarinum® AB
Massa Estarinum® AM
Massa Estarinum® B
Massa Estarinum® BB

Massa Estarinum® BC
Massa Estarinum® BCF
Massa Estarinum® BD
Massa Estarinum® C
Massa Estarinum® D
Massa Estarinum® E
Mazawax® 163R
Mazol® GMO
Mazol® GMR
Mersolat H 30
Mersolat H 40
Mersolat H 68
Mersolat H 76
Mersolat H 95
Mersolat W 40
Mersolat W 68
Mersolat W 76
Mersolat W 93
Miglyol® 840 Gel
Miglyol® Gel
Mineral Jelly No. 5
Mineral Jelly No. 10
Mineral Jelly No. 14
Mineral Jelly No. 15
Mineral Jelly No. 17
Mineral Jelly No. 20
Mineral Jelly No. 25
Miracare® 2MCA
Miracare® 2MHT
Miracare® CT100
Miracare® M1
Miracare® NWC
Miracare® SCS
Miracare® XL
Miramine® CODI
Monateric 985A
Monateric CAB
Monateric CDL
Monateric CDX-38
Monateric LMAB
Monateric MCB
Multilan D
Nasuna® B
Neopon LAM
Neopon LOA
Neopon LOS 70
Neopon LOS/NF
Neopon LS/NF
Nikkol Alaninate LN-30
Nikkol Cetanol 50, 70
Nikkol CMT-30
Nikkol ECT-3NEX, ECTD-
  3NEX
Nikkol ECTD-6NEX
Nikkol LMT
Nikkol MMT
Nikkol NES-203
Nikkol NES-303
Nikkol Phosten HLP-1
Nikkol Phosten HLP-N
Nikkol PMT
Nikkol Sarcosinate LK-30
Nikkol Sarcosinate MN
Nikkol SMT
Nikkol Stearyl Alcohol
Nimlesterol® 1730
Nimlesterol® 1732
Niox EO-10

Niox EO-26
Niox KS Series
Nissan Persoft SK
Nissan Sunamide C-3,
  CF-3, CF-10
Nonasol N4AS
Nonasol N4SS
Nonisol 300
Norfox® ALPHA XL
Norfox® ALS
Norfox® Coco Betaine
Norfox® Coco Powder
Norfox® DCS
Norfox® GMS
Norfox® SLES-60
Novata® 299, A, AB, B,
  BBC, BC, BCF, BD,
  C, D, E
Nutrapon TK 3603
Obazoline 662Y
Obazoline CS-65
OHlan®
Ointment Base No. 3
Ointment Base No. 4
Ointment Base No. 6
Olamin® K
Penreco Amber
Penreco Blond
Penreco Cream
Penreco Lily
Penreco Regent
Penreco Royal
Penreco Snow
Penreco Super
Penreco Ultima
Perlankrol® ACM2
Perlankrol® ADP3
Perlankrol® DAF25
Perlankrol® DSA
Perlankrol® TM1
Pluracol® E400 NF
Pluracol® E600 NF
Pluracol® E1000
Pluracol® E1450
Pluracol® E1450 NF
Pluracol® E2000
Pluracol® E4000 NF
Pluracol® E4500
Pluracol® E8000
Pluracol® E8000 NF
Polystate C
Polysynlane
Protegin® SE
Protegin® W SE
Protegin® WX SE
Protegin® X SE
Proto-Lan 4R
Proto-Lan 20
Quartamin 86W
Rhodacal® 330
Rhodacal® T
Rhodapex® ES
Rhodapex® ESY
Rhodapex® HF-433
Rhodapon® LT-6
Rhodapon® TDS
Rhodaquat® M270C/18
Ritachol®

Sactol 2 OS 2
Sactol 2 OS 28
Sactol 2 OT
Sactol 2 S 3
Sactol 2 T
Salcare SC91
Salfax 77
Sandet EN
Sandet END, ENN
Sandoz Sulfate 216
Sandoz Sulfate A
Sandoz Sulfate K
Schercemol EE
Schercemol ISE
Schercemol PGML
Schercoteric MS-2ES
  Modified
Schercoteric MS-2 Modified
Schercoteric MS-2TE
  Modified
Schercoteric MS-SF-2
  (38%)
Schercoteric MS-SF-2
  (70%)
Sebase
Secosyl
Sedefos 75®
Sellig LET 630
Sellig T 14 100
Serdet NZ 60
Snow White Petrolatum
Sochamine A 755
Sochamine A 7525
Sochamine A 7527
Softisan® 100
Softisan® 378
Softisan® 601
Softisan® 649
Sole Terge 8
Sono Jell® No. 4
Sono Jell® No. 9
Standamul® 302
Standamul® 318
Standamul® 1414-E
Standamul® 7061
Standamul® 7063
Standamul® 7105
Standamul® CTA
Standamul® CTV
Standamul® G-32/36
  Stearate
Standapol® 7088
Standapol® 7092
Standapol® A
Standapol® DEA
Standapol® EA-40
Standapol® EA-K
Standapol® ES-1
Standapol® ES-2
Standapol® ES-3
Standapol® ES-40
Standapol® ES-7099
Standapol® S
Standapol® SHC-101
Standapol® T
Standapol® WA-AC
Standapol® WAQ Special
Stanol 212F

Bases/Ointment Bases/Shampoo Base *(cont'd.)*

Stepanol® 317
Stepanol® AEG
Sterol TE 200
Sterotex® C
Sterotex® HM NF
Sterotex® K
Sugartab®
Sulfetal CJOT 38
Sulfochem AEG
Sulfochem B-221
Sulfochem B-221OP
Sulfochem SAC
Sulfopon® WAQ LCX
Sulfotex WA
Sulfotex WAT
Sulframin 40RA
Sulframin AOS
Sulphonated 'Lorol' Liquid
　MA, MR
Sulphonated 'Lorol' Liquid
　TA, TN, TNR
Superpolystate
Supoweiss
Swascol L-327
Sweetrex®
Tefose® 63
Tefose® 1500
Tefose® 2000
Tefose® 2561
Tesal
Texapon® A 400
Texapon® ALS
Texapon® ASV
Texapon® EVR
Texapon® N 25

Texapon® N 103
Texapon® OT Highly Conc.
　Needles
Texapon® PNA
Texapon® SBN
Texapon® SH 100
Texapon® T
Texapon® VHC Needles
Texapon® WW 99
Toho PEG Series
Trycol® 5878
Tylorol 2S, 2S/25
Tylorol 3S
Tylorol A
Tylorol BS
Tylorol LM
Tylorol LT50
Tylorol MG
Tylorol S
Ultra Sulfate SE-5
Ultra Sulfate SL-1
Unigator B 67
Unimul-1414EW
Varifoam® SXC
Varine C
Varine O®
Variquat® 638
Varisoft® 2TD
Varisoft® 110-PG
Varisoft® 250
Varisoft® 300
Varisoft® 355
Varisoft® 432-CG
Varisoft® 432-ET
Varisoft® 442-100P

Varisoft® 461
Varisoft® 462
Varisoft® 470
Varisoft® 471
Varisoft® BT-85
Varisoft® CTB-40
Varisoft® DHT
Varisoft® LAC
Varisoft® OIMS
Varisoft® PIMS
Varisoft® SDAC
Varisoft® SDAC-W
Varisoft® SDC-85
Varisoft® TA-100
Varisoft® TC-90
Varisoft® TIMS
Varisoft® TS-50
Varisoft® TSC
Vaseline 335 G
Vaseline 7702
Vaseline 8332
Vaseline 10049 BL
Vaseline A
Wecobee® FS
Wecobee® FW
Wecobee® M
Wecobee® S
Wecobee® SS
Wecobee® W
Witcamide® 70
Witcamide® 82
Witcodet 4680
Witcolate™ 1050
Witcolate™ A
Witcolate™ S1285C

Witcolate™ S1300C
Witcolate™ T
Witconate™ 45 Liq
Witconate™ 60T
Witconate™ 93S
Witconate™ 1240
Witconate™ 1250
Witepsol® E75
Witepsol® E76
Witepsol® E85
Witepsol® H5
Witepsol® H12
Witepsol® H15
Witepsol® H32
Witepsol® H35
Witepsol® H37
Witepsol® H39
Witepsol® H42
Witepsol® H175
Witepsol® H185
Witepsol® S51
Witepsol® S55
Witepsol® S58
Witepsol® W25
Witepsol® W31
Witepsol® W32
Witepsol® W35
Witepsol® W45
Zetesap 5165
Zetesap 813A
Zoharpon ST
Zoharquat 25
Zoharquat 75

Binders

Acetadeps
Acetulan®
ACumist™ B-6
ACumist™ B-12
ACumist™ B-18
ACumist™ C-5
ACumist™ C-9
ACumist™ C-12
ACumist™ C-18
Albalan
Alberger®
Alginic Acid FCC
Alkapol PEG 300
Alumystique™
Anhydrous Lanolin Grade 1
Anhydrous Lanolin Grade 2
Anhydrous Lanolin
　Superfine
Argonol 50
Argonol ACE 5
Argonol ACE 6
Argonol RIC2
Avicel PH-101
Avicel PH-102
Avicel PH-103
Avicel PH-105
BB-1
Benecel® M
Benecel® ME

Benecel® MP
Bernel® Ester NPDC
Blanose 7 Types
Blanose 9 Types
Blanose 12 Types
Britol®
Britol® 6NF
Britol® 7NF
Britol® 9NF
Britol® 20USP
Britol® 35USP
Britol® 50USP
Byco A
Byco C
Byco O
Carbowax® PEG 300
Carbowax® PEG 3350
Carbowax® PEG 4600
Carbowax® PEG 8000
Carbowax® Sentry® PEG
　300
Carbowax® Sentry® PEG
　400
Carbowax® Sentry® PEG
　540 Blend
Carbowax® Sentry® PEG
　600
Carbowax® Sentry® PEG
　900

Carbowax® Sentry® PEG
　1000
Carbowax® Sentry® PEG
　1450
Carbowax® Sentry® PEG
　3350
Carbowax® Sentry® PEG
　4600
Carbowax® Sentry® PEG
　8000
Cellosize® HEC QP
　Grades
Cellosize® HEC QP-3-L
Cellosize® HEC QP-40
Cellosize® HEC QP-100
　M-H
Cellosize® HEC QP-300
Cellosize® HEC QP-4400-
　H
Cellosize® HEC QP-
　15,000-H
Cellosize® HEC QP-
　52,000-H
Cellosize® HEC WP
　Grades
Cellosize® Polymer
　PCG-10
Cellulon
Ceraphyl® 28

Ceraphyl® 31
Ceraphyl®45
Ceraphyl® 55
Ceraphyl® 140
Ceraphyl® 140-A
Ceraphyl® 368
Ceraphyl® 375
Ceraphyl® 847
Ceraphyl® ICA
Chemal BP 261
Chemal BP-262
Chemal BP-262LF
Chemal BP-2101
Crosilk Powder
Crosterene
Dascare MCCP
Dermacryl™ 79
Dermol 185
Dermol OO
Dynasan® 114
Eldew CL-301
Elefac™ I-205
Elvanol® 71-30
Elvanol® 90-50
Emcocel® 50M
Emcocel® 90M
Emcocel® LM
Emerest® 2310
Emery® 6709

Binders *(cont'd.)*

Ethocel Standard Premium	Mearlmica® MMSV	Pluronic® 25R5	Sebase
Fancol ALA	Methocel® 40-100	Pluronic® 25R8	Siltek® M
Fancor IPL	Methocel® 40-101	Pluronic® 31R1	Siltek® M Super
Finsolv® TN	Methocel® 40-202	Pluronic® 31R2	Siltek® PL
Fonoline® White	Methocel® A4CP	Pluronic® 31R4	S-Maz® 80
Fonoline® Yellow	Methocel® A4MP	Pluronic® L10	S-Maz® 85
Glucam® P-20 Distearate	Methocel® A15LVP	Pogol 200	Solka-Floc® BW-40
Golden Dawn Grade 1, 2	Methocel® E3P	Polargel® HV	Solka-Floc® BW-100
Golden Dawn Superfine	Methocel® E4MP	Polargel® T	Solka-Floc® BW-200
Golden Fleece DF	Methocel® E6P	Polysphere 3000 SP	Solka-Floc® BW-2030
Golden Fleece P-80	Methocel® E15LVP	Precirol ATO 5	Solka-Floc® Fine Granular
Golden Fleece P-95	Methocel® E50LVP	Press-Aid™	Sol-U-Tein EA
Golden Fleece RA	Methocel® E50P	Press-Aid™ SP	Stamere®
Hectalite® 200	Methocel® K4MP	Press-Aid™ XF	Standamul® 318
Hetester HSS	Methocel® K4MS	Press-Aid™ XP	Standamul® G-16
Hetester ISS	Methocel® K15MP	PT-0602	Sterotex®
Hodag PEG 3350	Methocel® K15MS	PTFE-19	Thixcin® R
Hodag PEG 8000	Methocel® K100LVP	PTFE-20	Ticalose 15, 30, 75, 150R,
Imwitor® 191	Methocel® K100MP	Pure-Dent® B700	1200, 2000R, 2500,
Imwitor® 900	Natrosol® Plus CS	Pure-Dent® B810	4000, 4500, 5000R
Imwitor® 940	Natrosol® Plus CS, Grade	Purity® 21	T-Maz® 60K
Imwitor® 940 K	330	PVP K-15	Tritisol™
Isopropylan® 33	Nopalcol Series	Radia® 7500	Trivent NP-13
Ivarlan™ Light	Nopalcol 1-S	Radia® 7501	Trivent OC-G
Keltose®	Nopalcol 1-TW	Radiacid® 152	Trivent SS-20
Keltrol®, Keltrol F	Pearl-Glo®	Radiacid® 212	28-1801
Kessco® Octyl Palmitate	Pegosperse® 400 DS	Radiacid® 416	Tylose® H Series
Kollidon®	Plasdone® K-25, K-90	Radiacid® 423	Tylose® MH Grades
Kollidon® 25, 30, 90	Plasdone® K-26/28,	Radiacid® 427	Tylose® MHB
Lanesta S	K-29/32	Radiacid® 428	Tylose® MH-K, MH-xp,
Lanesta SA-30	Pluracol® E200	Radiacid® 464	MHB-y, MHB-yp
Lubritab®	Pluracol® E300	Radiacid® 631	Unilin® 350 Alcohol
Lutrol® E 1500	Pluracol® E400	Radiastar® 1060	Unilin® 550 Alcohol
Lutrol® E 4000	Pluracol® E600	Radiastar® 1100	Unilin® 700 Alcohol
Lutrol® E 6000	Pluracol® E1500	Radiastar® 1170	Veegum®
Luviform® ES 22	Pluracol® E4000	Radiastar® 1200	Veegum® D
Luviform® ES 42	Pluracol® E6000	Radiastar® 1208	Veegum® F
Luviform® FA 119	Pluriol® E 1500	Rehydragel® Low Visc. Gel	Veegum® HS
Magnabrite® F	Pluronic® 10R5	Rehydragel® Thixotropic	Veegum® HV
Magnabrite® FS	Pluronic® 10R8	Gel	Veegum® K
Magnabrite® HS	Pluronic® 12R3	Rhodasurf® E 400	Veegum® WG
Maltrin® M150	Pluronic® 17R1	Rhodasurf® E 600	Volclay® NF-BC
Maltrin® M180	Pluronic® 17R2	Rhodasurf® PEG 600	Volclay NF-ID
Maltrin® M250	Pluronic® 17R4	Rice Pro-Tein BK	Waxenol® 801
Maltrin® M510	Pluronic® 17R8	Rudol®	Waxenol® 815
Maltrin® QD M500	Pluronic® 22R4	Schercemol 185	Waxenol® 816
Maltrin® QD M550	Pluronic® 25R1	Schercemol DID	Wickenol® 144
Maltrin® QD M600	Pluronic® 25R2	Schercemol DISD	Witcamide® 70
Mearlmica® MMCF	Pluronic® 25R4	Schercemol TT	Witcamide® MM

Bleaching Agents/Skin Lighteners

Brookosome® C	Hamp-Ex® 80	Nikkol VC-SS	Tinopal® CBS-X
Empigen® OY	Kojic Acid	Ruscogenins Phytosome®	Uantox POMEBIS
Escin/β-Sitosterol	Nikkol CP	Sohakuhi Extract BG-100	Uninontan U 34
Phytosome®	Nikkol VC-PMG	Sohakuhi Extract Ethanol	

Botanicals and Extracts

Acacia Flower Extract	Actiphyte of Aloe Vera	Actiphyte of Apricot Fruit	Actiphyte of Balm Mint
HS 2744 G	10-Fold	Actiphyte of Apricot Leaves	Actiphyte of Basil
Acacia Glycolysat	Actiphyte of Aloe Vera	Actiphyte of Arbutus	Actiphyte of Bee Pollen
Acerola Extract HS 2855 G	20-Fold	Actiphyte of Arnica	Actiphyte of Black Walnut
Actiphyte of Acacia	Actiphyte of Aloe Vera	Actiphyte of Arrowroot	Actiphyte of Bran
Actiphyte of Alfalfa	40-Fold	Actiphyte of Avocado Fruit	Actiphyte of Calendula
Actiphyte of Almond	Actiphyte of Apple Leaves	Actiphyte of Avocado	Actiphyte of Capsicum
Actiphyte of Aloe Vera	Actiphyte of Apple Pectin	Leaves	Actiphyte of Chamomile

Botanicals and Extracts *(cont'd.)*

Actiphyte of Chaparral
Actiphyte of Chrysanthe-
mum
Actiphyte of Cinnamon
Actiphyte of Coconut
Actiphyte of Comfrey
Actiphyte of Coriander
Actiphyte of Cornsilk
Actiphyte of Eucalyptus
Actiphyte of Flax Seed
Actiphyte of Garlic
Actiphyte of Ginseng
Actiphyte of Goldenseal
Actiphyte of Henna
Actiphyte of Honeysuckle
Actiphyte of Hops
Actiphyte of Irish Moss
Actiphyte of Jojoba Meal
Actiphyte of Lavender
Actiphyte of Lemon Juice
Actiphyte of Lemon Peel
Actiphyte of Malt
Actiphyte of Marigold
Actiphyte of Meadowsweet
Actiphyte of Oat Bran
Actiphyte of Oat Flour
Actiphyte of Olive Leaves
Actiphyte of Orange
Bioflavonoids
Actiphyte of Pennyroyal
Actiphyte of Peppermint
Actiphyte of Rice Bran
Actiphyte of Rose
Actiphyte of Rose Hips
Actiphyte of Royal Jelly
Actiphyte of St. John's Wort
Actiphyte of Tansy
Actiphyte of Wheat
Actiphyte of Wheat Germ
Actiphyte of Wintergreen
Actiphyte of Witch Hazel
Actiplex™ 745
Activegetal™ IPF
Agave Extract HS 2817 G
Alder Buckthorn HS
Alfalfa Herb Extract
HS 2967 G
Aloe Extract HS 2386 G
Aloe Extract Special
Aloe Flower Extract PG
Angelica HS
Anise Seed Extract
HS 2712 G
Apple HS
Apple Extract HS 1806 AT
Apricot Extract HS 2509 G
Apricot Glycolysat
Arnica Extract HS 2397 G
Arnica HS
Aromaphyte of Almond
Aromaphyte of Chamomile
Aromaphyte of Orange
Aromaphyte of Peppermint
Auxina Tricogena
Avocado Extract
HS 2384 G
Awapuhi Extract
Balm Mint HS

Balm Mint Oil Infusion
BBC Mineral Complex
Benibana Liq
Biochelated Extract of
Lemon Grass
Biochelated Sea Kelp
Extract
Bio-Oil GLA-10
Bitter Almond HS
Blend For Bust Cares
HS 201
Blend For Chapped Skins
HS 361
Blend For Deodorant
HS 275
Blend For Elderly Skins
HS 296
Blend For Greasy Hair
HS 312
Blend For Greasy Skin
Imperfections HS 315
Blend For Slenderizing
Prods. HS 255
Broom Glycolysat
Broom HS
Broom Tops Extract HS
2645 G
Carob HS
Carrot Oil Extra
Carrots Extract HS 2597 G
Chamomile CL 2/033026
Chamomile Distillate 2/
380930
Chamomile Extract HS
2382 G
Chamomile Extract HS
2779 G
Chinpi Liq
Cholecithine
Chouji Liq
Eucalyptus Leaves Extract
HS 2646 G
Complex GT
Complex NR
Complex Relax
Complexe AST 1
Complexe AV.a
Coobato Camomilla
Coobato Hamamelis
Coobato Speciale
Corn Silk Extract HS
2969 G
Cremogen AF
Cremogen Aloe Vera
Cremogen Camomile Forte
Cremogen Chamomile
739012
Cremogen Hamamelis
739008
Cremogen M-I 739001
Cremogen Pine Needles
739007
Cremogen Yarrow 739017
Crodarom Avocadin
Crodarom Calendula O
Crodarom Carrot O
Crodarom Chamomile A
Crodarom Chamomile EO

Crodarom Chamomile O
Crodarom Nut O
Crodarom St. John's
Wort O
Cytoplasmine-1
Dandelion HS
Dermascreen
Dragoplant Chamomile
2/034010
Elicrisina
EmCon Eucalyptus
EmCon Ginger
EmCon Hazelnut
EmCon Limnanthes Alba
EmCon Olive
EmCon Orange
EmCon Peanut
EmCon Rice Bran
EmCon Rose
EmCon Soya
EmCon Spearmint
EmCon Tea Tree
EmCon Walnut
Emollient HS 235
Emollient HS 238
Emollient LS 635
Eucalyptus HS
Eucalyptus Leaves Extract
HS 2646 G
Evosina NA 2
Exsymol Hydrumines
Exsymol Oleosterines
Exsymol Plant Extracts
Extract Arnica Special
Extrapone Coco-Nut
Special 2/033055
Fancol Gingko Extract
Fo-Ti 5:1 PG
Gadeneel Liq
Garionzet
Garlic Extract HS 2710 G
Ginseng Extract HS 2457 G
Ginseng Glycolysat
Ginseng HS
Glycolysat de camomille
Glycolysat de ginseng
Glycolysat de Houblon
Granoliq. Wheat Germ
Extract, Water soluble
GU-61-A
Gu-61-Standard
Guineshing-LV
Hamamelis Extract
HS 2456 G
Herbaliquid Alpine Herbs
Special
Herbaliquid Camomile
Special
Herbaliquid Hops Special
Herbaliquid Rosemary
Special
Herbasol HP Extracts
Herbasol IPA Extracts
Herbasol O/S Extracts
Herbasol W/S Extracts
Herbasol Alpine Herbs
Complex
Herbasol Complex A

Herbasol Complex B
Herbasol Complex C
Herbasol Complex D
Herbasol Complex E
Herbasol Complex GU-61
Herbasol Complexes
Herbasol Distillates
Herbasol Dry Extracts
Herbasol-Extract Algae
Herbasol-Extract Almond
Herbasol-Extract Aloe
Herbasol-Extract Arnica
Herbasol-Extract Balm Mint
Herbasol-Extract Calendula
Herbasol-Extract
Eucalyptus
Herbasol-Extract Ginseng
Herbasol-Extract
Hamemelis
Herbasol-Extract Ivy
Herbasol-Extract Marigold
Herbasol-Extract
Peppermint
Herbasol-Extract St. John's
Wort
Herbasol Extract Walnut
Shell Oil-Sol
Herbasol Extract Walnut
Shell Water-Sol
Herbasol-Extract Yarrow
Herbasol Forte Extracts
Herbasol 7 Herb Complex
Herbasol Herbes de
Provence Complex
Herbasol Sedative
Complex
Herbasol Stimulant
Complex
Hexaplant Richter
Hops Extract HS 2367 G
Hops HS
Hops Malt Extract HS
2518 G
Hydratherm CGI Glycolic
Hydratherm CGI
Hydroalcoholic
Hydrocotyl Glycolysat
Hydrocotyl HS
Hydroplastidine Achillea
Hydroplastidine Foeniculum
IPF Meadowsweet
Isodon Extract
Kamitsure Liq
Koucha Liq
Laminarina
Lemon Extract HS 2364 G
Lemon HS
Liquiritina
Marine Plasma Extract
Oleosterine Arnica
Ormagel SH, XPU
Pacific Sea Kelp Glycolic
Extract B-1063
Planell™ Oil
Tonique HS 216
Tonique HS 290, LS 690
Uninontan U 34
Vegebios

Carriers/Vehicles/Excipients/Fillers/Diluents/Extenders

Acticel™ 12
Acticel™ Plus
Aerosil® 130
Aerosil® 300
Alberger®
Aldo® TC
Almond Oil
Altalc 200 USP
Altalc 400 USP
Aqualose SLT
Aqualose SLW
Aqualose W20
Armeen® 3-12
Avicel PH-101
Avicel PH-102
Avicel PH-103
Avicel PH-105
Beeswing 1/16
Beeswing 3/16
Beeswing 3/32
Biron®
Britol®
Britol® 6NF
Britol® 7NF
Britol® 9NF
Britol® 20USP
Britol® 35USP
Britol® 50USP
Byco A
Byco C
Byco O
Cab-O-Sil® TS-530
Candex® Plus
Captex® 200
Captex® 350
Captex® 355
Captex® 800
Captex® 810A
Captex® 810B
Captex® 810C
Captex® 810D
Captex® 910A
Captex® 910B
Captex® 910C
Captex® 910D
Captex® 8000
Captex® 8227
Carbowax® PEG 300
Carbowax® PEG 400
Carbowax® PEG 4600
Carbowax® PEG 8000
Carbowax® Sentry® PEG
    300
Carbowax® Sentry® PEG
    400
Carbowax® Sentry® PEG
    540 Blend
Carbowax® Sentry® PEG
    600
Carbowax® Sentry® PEG
    900
Carbowax® Sentry® PEG
    1000
Carbowax® Sentry® PEG
    1450
Carbowax® Sentry® PEG
    3350
Carbowax® Sentry® PEG

4600
Carbowax® Sentry® PEG
    8000
Celite® 503
Celite® 512
Celite® 521 AW
Celite® 545
Celite® 550
Celite® 560
Celite® 577
Cellulon
Ceraphyl® ICA
Cerasynt® 840
Cetiol®
Cetiol® A
Cetiol® LC
Cetiol® V
Cob Flour #4, 6, 100
Cob Grit #1, 2, 3, 8, 150,
    3050
Coconut Oils® 76, 92, 110
Compactrol®
Compritol HD5 ATO
Crodamol AB
Crodamol DO
Crodamol GTCC
Crodamol IPM
Crodamol IPP
Croderol G7000
Dascare MCCP
Dow Corning® 244 Fluid
Dow Corning® 245 Fluid
Dow Corning® 344 Fluid
Dow Corning® 345 Fluid
Dow Corning® 1401 Fluid
Drakeol 7
Drakeol 9
Edenol 302
Elespher®
Elesponge®
Emcompress®
Emdex®
Emdex® Plus
Emkapol 8000
Emkapol 8500
Emulmetik™ 120
Emulmetik™ 300
Epikuron 145
Epikuron 170
Epikuron 200
Estasan GT 8-40 3578
Estasan GT 8-60 3575
Estasan GT 8-60 3580
Estasan GT 8-65 3577
Estasan GT 8-65 3581
Estran™-Lite
Estran™-Pure
Estran™-Xtra
Eutanol® G
Eutanol® G16
Exxal® 16
Exxal® 20
Filter-Cel
Finsolv® TN
Fonoline® White
Fonoline® Yellow
G-100
Gafquat® HSi

Gelucire 33/01
Gelucire 35/10
Gelucire 37/02
Gelucire 42/12
Gelucire 44/14
Gelucire 46/07
Gelucire 48/09
Gelucire 50/02
Gelucire 50/13
Gelucire 53/10
Gelucire 62/05
Grit-O'Cobs®
HD-Ocenol® 90/95
Hercolyn® D
Hispagel® 100
Hispagel® 200
Hodag CC-22
Hodag CC-22-S
Hodag CC-33
Hodag CC-33-F
Hodag CC-33-L
Hodag CC-33-S
Hodag CSA-80
Hydral® 710
Hypan® QT100
Hypol® 2000
Hypol® 2002
Hypol® 3000
Imwitor® 308
Imwitor® 310
Imwitor® 312
Imwitor® 742
Imwitor® 908
Imwitor® 914
Imwitor® 928
Imwitor® 988
Isopar® G
Isopar® H
Isopar® K
Isopropyl Palmitate
Kessco® Isopropyl
    Myristate
Kessco® Isopropyl
    Palmitate
Kollidon® 25, 30, 90
Kollidon® CL
Kollidon® CLM
Labrafil® M 1944 CS
Labrafil® M 2125 CS
Labrafil® M 2735 CS
Labrasol
Lantrol® 1674 Deodorized
Laponite® XLG
Laponite® XLS
L.A.S
Lexate® PX
Lexol® GT-855
Lexol® GT-865
Lexol® IPP
Lexol® IPP-A
Lexol® IPP-NF
Lexol® PG-800
Lexol® PG-855
Lexol® PG-865
Lexol® PG-900
Lipocutin®
Lipovol SES
Lipovol SES-S

Liquid Crystal CN/9
Liquid Crystal (LC)
    CAPS 122
Maltrin® M100
Maltrin® M510
Maltrin® M700
Maltrin® QD M500
Maltrin® QD M550
Maltrin® QD M600
Masil® SFV
Masil® SF-VV
Mazol® 1400
Mearlmica® MMCF
Mearlmica® MMSV
Michel XO-150-20
Micro-Cel® C
Microduct®
Microma-100
Miglyol® 810
Miglyol® 812
Miglyol® 840
Myritol® PC
Neobee® 20
Neobee® 1053
Neobee® 1054
Neobee® 1062
Neobee® M-5
Neobee® M-20
Neobee® O
Nissan Panacete 810
Ointment Base No. 3
Ointment Base No. 4
Ointment Base No. 6
Onyxol® 42
Orgasol 1002 D NAT COS
Orgasol 1002 D WHITE 5
    COS
Orgasol 1002 EX D WHITE
    10 COS
Orgasol 2002 D NAT COS
Orgasol 2002 EX D NAT
    COS
Orgasol 2002 UD NAT
    COS
Ovucire WL 2558
Ovucire WL 2944
Pegol® P-1000
Pegol® P-2000
Penreco Cream
Penreco Lily
Penreco Regent
Penreco Royal
Penreco Snow
Penreco Super
Penreco Ultima
Perfecta® USP
Phosal® 53 MCT
Phosal® 75 SA
Plasdone® C-15
Plasdone® K-25, K-90
Plasdone® K-26/28,
    K-29/32
Pluracol® E200
Pluracol® E300
Pluracol® E400
Pluracol® E600
Pluracol® E1500
Pluracol® E4000

Carriers/Vehicles/Excipients/Fillers/Diluents/Extenders *(cont'd.)*

Pluracol® E6000
Poly-G® 200
Poly-G® 300
Poly-G® 400
Poly-G® 600
Poly-G® 1000
Poly-G® 1500
Poly-G® 2000
Poly-G® B1530
Polymoist® Mask
Polysphere 3000 SP
Protopet® Alba
Protopet® White 1S
Protopet® White 2L
Protopet® White 3C
Protopet® Yellow 1E
Protopet® Yellow 2A
PT-0602
Pure-Dent® B700
Pure-Dent® B810
Purity® 21
PVP K-15
PVP/Si-10
Radia® 7106
Radia® 7178
Rehydragel® Compressed
    Gel
Rewomul HL
Ritawax AEO
Ritawax ALA
Robane®
Rudol®

SB-150
SB-700
Sebase
Sericite FSE
Sericite SL
Simchin® Natural
Simchin® Refined
Sipernat® 50
Solka-Floc® BW-40
Solka-Floc® BW-100
Solka-Floc® BW-200
Solka-Floc® BW-2030
Solka-Floc® Fine Granular
Spheron L-1500
Spheron P-1000
Spheron P-1500
Spheron P-1500-030
Spheron PL-700
Standamul® 318
Standamul® 1414-E
Standamul® CTA
Standamul® CTV
Standamul® G
Standamul® G-16
Super Floss
Super Refined™ Almond
    Oil NF
Super Refined™ Corn Oil
Super Refined™
    Cottonseed Oil
Super Refined™ Olive Oil

Super Refined™ Peanut Oil
Super Refined™ Safflower
    Oil USP
Super Refined™ Sesame
    Oil
Super Refined™ Soybean
    Oil USP
Super-Sat
Suppocire A
Suppocire AI
Suppocire AIM
Suppocire AIML
Suppocire AIP, AP, BP, CP
Suppocire AIX
Suppocire AM
Suppocire AML
Suppocire AS2
Suppocire AS2X
Suppocire B
Suppocire BM
Suppocire BML
Suppocire BS2
Suppocire BS2X
Suppocire C
Suppocire CM
Suppocire CS2
Suppocire CS2X
Suppocire DM
Suppocire NA
Suppocire NAI
Suppocire NB

Suppocire NC
Supraene®
Tullanox HM-250
28-1801
Unimate® IPM
Unimate® IPP
Unimate® IPPM
Unimul-G
Unithox® 420
Unithox® 450
Unithox® 480
Unithox® 520
Unithox® 550
Unithox® 720
Unithox® 750
U Tanol G
Vaseline 335 G
Vaseline 7702
Vaseline 8332
Vaseline 10049 BL
Vaseline A
Wacker HDK® H20
Wickenol® 136
Wickenol® 550
Witafrol® 7420
Zeofree® 80
Zeofree® 153
Zeolex® 7
Zeolex® 23A
Zeosyl® 110SD
Zeosyl® 200

Colorants/Pigments/Color Fixatives/Dye Stabilizers

Atomergic Carmine
Azulene 50% 2/012990
Azulene 100% 2/912980
Beta Carotene 30% in Veg.
    Oil No. 65646
Bicrona®
Biju® BNT
Biju® BTD, BXD
Biju® BWD, BWS
Biju® BWP
Biju® Ultra UNT
Biju® Ultra UTD, UXD
Biju® Ultra UWD, UWS
Biju® Ultra UWP
Bi-Lite®
Bio-Pol® OE
Biron®
Biron® B-5
Biron® B-50
Biron® ESQ
Biron® Fines
Biron® HB
Biron® NLD-SP
Bismica 46
Bismica 55
Bismica 596
Bital®
Black 103
Bleu De Prusse Pur W 745
Blue 135
Brown 208
Carmine 40

Carmine 224
Carmine 5297
Carmine Ultra-fine
Carmisol-50
Carotene Standard RR
Chrome Green 106
Cloisonné®
Cogilor Amethyst
Cogilor Aquamarine
Cogilor Emerald
Cogilor Jade
Cogilor Jet
Cogilor Ochre
Cogilor Rose
Cogilor Rouge
Cogilor Sapphire
Cogilor Spinel
Colorona®
Cosmetic Micro Blend
    Red Oxide 9268
Cosmica®
Covafluor
Covalac
Covanor
Covasil
Covasol
Coverleaf PC-2035
Coverleaf PC-2055M
Coverleaf PC-2055T
Crystalline Beta Carotene
    No. 65638
Dascolor Carmine

Dichrona®
Duocrome®
Ethomeen® C/15
Ethomid® HT/23
Extender W
Ferric Blue 107
Ferric Blue 114
Fibro-Silk™ Powd
Flamenco®
Flonac ME 10 C
Flonac MG 30 C
Flonac MI 10 C
Flonac ML 10 C
Flonac MS 5 C
Flonac MS 10 C
Flonac MS 20 C
Flonac MS 30 C
Flonac MS 33 C
Flonac MS 40 C
Flonac MS 60 C
Flonac MS 70 C
Flonac MX 10 C
Gemtone®
H Chrome Green 105
Inositol
Lustra-Pearl®
Mattina®
Mearlite® GBU
Mearlite® GEH
Mearlite® GEJ
Mearlite® GGH
Mearlite® LBU

Mearlite® LEM
Mearlmaid® AA
Mearlmaid® CKD
Mearlmaid® CP
Mearlmaid® FL
Mearlmaid® KN
Mearlmaid® KND
Mearlmaid® OL
Mearlmaid® PLN
Mearlmaid® PLO
Mearlmaid® TR
Mibiron® N-50
Microsponge® 5640
M Violet 112
Natural Beeswax
Natural Extract AP
Naturon® 2X AQ
Naturon® 2X IPA
Pearl I
Pearl II
Pearl III
Pearl-Glo®
Pearl Super Supreme
Pearl Supreme
Pearl Supreme UVS
Red 119
Red 139
Red 150
Red 219
Riboflavin USP, FCC
    Type S
Rita AZ

Colorants/Pigments/Color Fixatives/Dye Stabilizers *(cont'd.)*

Rita KA
Ritaloe 1X, 10X, 20X, 40X
Ritaloe 200M
Sericite DNN-2SH
Sericite SLZ
Sericite SP
Shebu® Refined
Shebu® WS
Shinju® White 100T

Sicomet®
Sicopharm®
Silkall CA
Silkall TI
Silkall TL
Silkall ZN
Simchin® WS
Soapearl®

Soloron Silver
Soloron Silver CO
Soloron Silver Fine
Soloron Silver Fine CO
Soloron Silver Sparkle
Soloron Silver Sparkle CO
Timica®
Timiron®

Titanium Dioxide 110
U Blue 104
Ultra®
U Pink 113
U Violet 109
Wheat Germ Oil
Yellow 134
Yellow 201

Depilatories

Koster Keunen Auto-
Oxidized Beeswax

Koster Keunen Beeswax

Thiovanic® Acid

Detergents/Foaming Agents/Foam Boosters/Stabilizers

Abex® LIV/30
Abil® B 8842
Abil® B 8873
Abil® B 9808
Abil® B 88183
Ablumide CDE
Ablumide CDE-G
Ablumide CKD
Ablumide CME
Ablumide LDE
Ablumide LME
Ablumox CAPO
Ablumox LO
Ablunol LA-3
Ablunol LA-5
Ablunol LA-7
Ablunol LA-9
Ablunol LA-12
Ablunol LA-16
Ablunol LA-40
Abluphat MLP-200
Abluphat MLP-220
Ablusol CDE
Ablusol LA
Ablusol LAE
Ablusol LDE
Abluter CPB
Abluter CPS
Abluter DCM-2
Abluter LDB
Accobetaine CL
Accomid 50
Accomid C
Accomid PK
Acconon TGH
Active #4
Acusol® 820
Acylglutamate CS-11
Acylglutamate CS-21
Acylglutamate CT-12
Acylglutamate GS-11
Acylglutamate HS-11
Acylglutamate LS-11
Acylglutamate LT-12
Acylglutamate MS-11
Adinol CT95
Adinol OT16
Admox® 1214
Adogen® 163D
Adogen® MA-102

Adogen® MA-104
Adogen® MA-106
Adogen® MA-108
AE-1214/3
Aerosol® 19
Aerosol® A-102
Aerosol® NPES 458
Afdet™ KCS
Afdet™ WGS
Akypo RLM 38 NV
Akypo RLM 45
Akypo RLM 45 N
Akypo RLM 100 MGV
Akypo RLM 160 N
Akypo RLM 160 NV
Akypogene FP 35 T
Akypogene HM 8
Akypogene HM 12
Akypogene ZA 97 SP
Akyporox SAL SAS
Akyposal 23 ST 70
Akyposal 2010 S
Akyposal ALS 33
Akyposal BA 28
Akyposal DS 28
Akyposal DS 56
Akyposal EO 20 MW
Akyposal MGLS
Akyposal MLES 35
Akyposal MLS 30
Akyposal NLS
Akyposal RLM 56 S
Akyposal RLM 70
Akyposal TLS 42
Akypo®-Soft 100 MgV
Akypo®-Soft 100 NV
Akypo®-Soft 130 NV
Akypo®-Soft 160 NV
AlcoCare® 1000
AlcoCare® 1010
AlcoCare® 2011
AlcoCare® 2012
AlcoCare® 2013
AlcoCare® 6012
Alcodet® 218
Alcodet® SK
Aldo® PMS
Alfol® 610
Alfol® 610 ADE
Alfol® 610 AFC

Alfol® 810
Alfol® 1012 HA
Alfonic® 1012-2.5
Alfonic® 1214-GC-2
Alfonic® 1216-1.5
Alfonic® 1216-CO-2
Alfonic® 1412-3
Algon DS 6000
Algon OL 90
Alkamide® 101 CG
Alkamide® 327
Alkamide® 1002
Alkamide® 1182
Alkamide® 2124
Alkamide® 2204
Alkamide® 2204A
Alkamide® C-5
Alkamide® C-212
Alkamide® CDE
Alkamide® CDM
Alkamide® CDO
Alkamide® CL63
Alkamide® CME
Alkamide® CMO
Alkamide® DC-212
Alkamide® DC-212/S
Alkamide® DC-212/SE
Alkamide® DIN-100
Alkamide® DIN-295/S
Alkamide® DL-203
Alkamide® DL-203/S
Alkamide® DL-207/S
Alkamide® DS-280/S
Alkamide® HTDE
Alkamide® KD
Alkamide® L7DE
Alkamide® L7DE-BT
Alkamide® L7DE-PG
Alkamide® L9DE
Alkamide® LE
Alkamide® SDO
Alkamox® L20
Alkamuls® CO-15
Alkamuls® EGMS
Alkamuls® EL-620
Alkamuls® EL-630
Alkamuls® PEG 400 DS
Alkamuls® PEG 600 DS
Alkasurf® LAN-1
Alkasurf® NP-4

Alkasurf® NP-8
Alkasurf® NP-12
Alkasurf® NP-15
Alkasurf® T
Alkasurf® TDA-12
Alkasurf® TLS
Alkaterge®-E
Alkateric® CIB
Alpha-Step® ML-40
Alscoap LE-240
Alscoap LN-40, LN-90
Alscoap M-3S
Alscoap SS-90
Amfotex FV-10
Amfotex FV-28
Amide CMA-2
Amide RMA-2
Amidex CE
Amidex CME
Amidex CP
Amidex KD
Amidex KDO
Amidex KME
Amidex LD
Amidex LD-8
Amidex LIPA
Amidex LMMEA
Amidex LN
Amidex PK
Amidex S
Amido Betaine C
Amido Betaine C-45
Amido Betaine C Conc
Amido Betaine-L
Amidox® C-2
Amidox® C-5
Amidox® L-2
Amidox® L-5
Aminofoam C
Aminofoam K
Aminol A-15
Aminol CM, CM Flakes,
CM-C Flakes, CM-D
Flakes
Aminol COR-2C
Aminol COR-4C
Aminol HCA
Aminol KDE
Aminol LM-30C,
LM-30C Special

Detergents/Foaming Agents/Foam Boosters/Stabilizers *(cont'd.)*

Aminoxid WS 35
Amisoft CA
Amisoft CS-11
Amisoft CT-12
Amisoft GS-11
Amisoft HA
Amisoft HS-11
Amisoft LS-11
Amisoft MS-11
Ammonyx® CDO
Ammonyx® CO
Ammonyx® DMCD-40
Ammonyx® LO
Ammonyx® MCO
Ammonyx® MO
Ammonyx® OAO
Ammonyx® SO
Amonyl 265 BA
Amonyl 380 BA
Ampho B11-34
Ampho T-35
Ampholak 7CX
Ampholak 7CX/C
Ampholak 7TX
Ampholak 7TX-SD 55
Ampholak 7TX-T
Ampholak BCA-30
Ampholak MSX-1
Ampholak MSX-2
Ampholak XCO-30
Ampholak XCO-40
Ampholak XO7
Ampholak XTP
Ampholak YCE
Ampholan® B-171
Ampholan® D197
Ampholan® E210
Ampholan® U 203
Ampholyt™ JA 140
Ampholyt™ JB 130
Amphoram CP1
Amphosol® CA
Amphosol® CG
Amphoteen 24
Amphoteen BCA-30
Amphotensid 9M
Amphotensid GB 2009
Amphoterge® J-2
Amphoterge® K
Amphoterge® K-2
Amphoterge® KJ-2
Amphoteric L
Amyx CDO 3599
Amyx CO 3764
Amyx LO 3594
Amyx SO 3734
Anionyx® 12S
Annonyx SO
Antaron® FC-34
Antarox® L-64
Antarox® PGP 18-1
Antarox® PGP 18-2
Antarox® PGP 18-2D
Antarox® PGP 18-2LF
Antarox® PGP 18-8
Antarox® PGP 33-8
APG® 300 CS
APG® 325 CS

APG® 600 CS
Arlatone® SCI
Armeen® 2-10
Armeen® 2-18
Armeen® 2S
Armeen® 12
Armeen® 16
Armeen® DM8
Armeen® DM12D
Armeen® DM14D
Armeen® DM16D
Armeen® DM18D
Armeen® DMC
Armeen® DMCD
Armeen® DMHTD
Armeen® DMOD
Armeen® DMSD
Armeen® DMTD
Armeen® M2C
Armeen® Z
Armid® 18
Aromox® C/12
Aromox® C/12-W
Aromox® DM14D-W
Aromox® DM16
Aromox® DMB
Aromox® DMC
Aromox® DMC-W
Aromox® DMCD
Aromox® DMHT
Aromox® DMHTD
Aromox® DMMC-W
Aromox® DMMCD-W
Aromox® T/12
Arquad® 2C-75
Arquad® 2HT-75
Arquad® 12-33
Arquad® 12-50
Arquad® 16-29
Arquad® 16-50
Arquad® 18-50
Arquad® C-33
Arquad® C-50
Arquad® DNHTB-75
Arquad® T-2C-50
Arquad® T-27W
Atmos 150
Atmos 300
Avamid 150
Barlene® 12C
Barlene® 14
Barlox® 10S
Barlox® 12
Barlox® 14
Barlox® 16S
Barlox® 18S
Barlox® C
Base Nacrante 1100 AD
Berol 452
Berol 480
Bio-Soft® D-60
Bio-Soft® E-200
Bio-Soft® E-300
Bio-Soft® E-400
Bio-Soft® EN 600
Bio-Soft® MT 40
Bio-Soft® N-300
Bio-Soft® TD 630

Bio-Surf PBC-460
Bio-Terge® AS-40
Bretol®
Briphos O3D
Britex EMB
Brophos-3
Brophos™ OL-2
Brox HLB-13
Brox S-2
Brox S-20
Brox S-30
C-108
C-110
CAE
Calamide C
Calester
Calfoam ALS-30
Calfoam EA-603
Calfoam ES-30
Calfoam ES-303
Calfoam ES-603
Calfoam NEL-60
Calfoam SEL-60
Calfoam SLS-30
Calfoam TLS-40
Calsoft AOS-40
Calsoft F-90
Calsoft L-40
Calsoft L-60
Calsoft T-60
Calsuds CD-6
Capmul® PGMS
Carbopol® 1706
Carbopol® 1720
Carbowax® PEG 400
Carbowax® PEG 600
Carbowax® PEG 900
Carbowax® PEG 1000
Carbowax® PEG 1450
Carbowax® PEG 3350
Carbowax® PEG 4600
Carbowax® PEG 8000
Carosulf T-60-L
Carroll 40% Coconut
  Hand Soap
Carsamide® CA
Carsamide® CMEA
Carsamide® O
Carsamide® SAC
Carsamide® SAL-7
Carsamide® SAL-9
Carsamide® SAL-82
Carsofoam® DEV
Carsofoam® MS Conc
Carsofoam® MSP
Carsofoam® PS-1, PS-3
Carsofoam® SC
Carsofoam® T-60-L
Carsonol® ALS
Carsonol® ALS-R
Carsonol® ALS-S
Carsonol® ALS Special
Carsonol® ANS
Carsonol® AOS
Carsonol® BD
Carsonol® DLS
Carsonol® ILS
Carsonol® MLS

Carsonol® SES-A
Carsonol® SES-S
Carsonol® SLES
Carsonol® SLES-2
Carsonol® SLES-3
Carsonol® SLES-4
Carsonol® SLS
Carsonol® SLS Paste B
Carsonol® SLS-R
Carsonol® SLS-S
Carsonol® SLS Special
Carsonol® TLS
Carsonon® L-9
Carsonon® N-2
CE-1218
CE-1270
CE-1280
CE-1290
CE-1295
Cedepal TD-403
Cedepal TD-407
Cedepal TD-484
Cedepon LA-30
Cedepon® LS-30PM
Ceraphyl® 140-A
Cerex EL 150
Cetol®
Chemal LA-4
Chemal LA-9
Chemal LA-12
Chemal LA-23
Chemal OA-4
Chemal OA-9
Chemal OA-20G
Chemal TDA-3
Chemal TDA-6
Chemal TDA-9
Chemal TDA-12
Chemal TDA-15
Chemal TDA-18
Chemax/DOSS-75E
Chemax E-200 MO
Chemax E-400 ML
Chemax E-400 MO
Chemax E-400 MT
Chemax E-600 ML
Chemax E-600 MO
Chemax E-1000 MO
Chemax NP-1.5
Chemax NP-4
Chemax NP-6
Chemax NP-9
Chemax NP-10
Chemax NP-15
Chemax NP-20
Chemax NP-30
Chemax NP-30/70
Chemax NP-40
Chemax NP-40/70
Chemax NP-50
Chemax NP-50/70
Chemax OP-3
Chemax OP-5
Chemax OP-7
Chemax OP-9
Chemax OP-40
Chemax PEG 200 DL
Chemax PEG 400 DT

Detergents/Foaming Agents/Foam Boosters/Stabilizers *(cont'd.)*

Chemax PEG 600 DT	Comperlan® LMM	Dehyton® PG	Elfan® A 913
Chembetaine C	Comperlan® LP	Dehyton® PK	Elfan® AT 84
Chembetaine CAS	Comperlan® LS	Dehyton® PLG	Elfan® AT 84 G
Chembetaine CB	Comperlan® OD	Dehyton® W	Elfan® KM 550
Chembetaine CGF	Comperlan® P 100	Demaquillant HS 287,	Elfan® KM 730
Chembetaine L	Comperlan® PD	LS 687	Elfan® KT 550
Chembetaine S	Comperlan® SD	Demaquillant LS 658	Elfan® NS 98 N
Chemoxide CAW	Comperlan® SDO	Demelan CB-28	Elfan® NS 242
Chemoxide L	Comperlan® SM	Demelan FB-12	Elfan® NS 242 A
Chemoxide LM-30	Comperlan® VOD	Depasol AS-26	Elfan® NS 242 Conc
Chemoxide SAO	Cosmopon ME	Deriphat® 151C	Elfan® NS 243 S
Chemoxide ST	Cosmopon MO	Deriphat® 154	Elfan® NS 243 S Conc
Chemoxide T	Cosmopon SES	Deriphat® 154L	Elfan® NS 243 S Mg
Chemoxide TAO	CPH-3-SE	Deriphat® 160	Elfan® NS 252 S
Chemoxide WC	CPH-41-N	Deriphat® 160C	Elfan® NS 252 S Conc
Chemsalan NLS 30	CPH-79-N	Desadipol AX Extra	Elfan® NS 423 SH
Chemsalan RLM 28	CPH-213-N	DeSonate AOS	Elfan® OS
Chemsalan RLM 56	CPH-361-N	DeSonol AES	Elfan® OS 46
Chemsalan RLM 70	CPH-380-N	Detergent CR	Elfan® SG
Chimin AX	Crafol AP-11	Detergent Concentrate 840	Elfan® SP 325
Chimin CMO	Cralane KR-13, -14	Diadol 13	Elfan® SP 400
Chimin IMB	Cralane LR-10	Dionil® OC	Elfan® SP 500
Chimin IMZ	Cralane LR-11	Dionil® OC/K	Elfan® WAT
Chimin L	Crillet 4	Dionil® S 37	Elfanol® 510
Chimin LE 50	Crodacel QL	Dionil® SH 100	Elfanol® 616
Chimin LMO	Crodacel QM	Dionil® W 100	Elfanol® 850
Chimin LX	Crodacel QS	DIPA Commercial Grade	Elfapur® KA 45
Chimin P45	Crodacid PD3160	DIPA Low Freeze Grade 85	Elfapur® LT
Chimipal DCL/M	Crodafos 1214A	DIPA Low Freeze Grade 90	Elfapur® N 50
Chimipal DE 7	Crodafos N2A	DIPA NF Grade	Elfapur® N 70
Chimipal LDA	Crodasinic C	Dow Corning® 190	Elfapur® N 90
Chimipal MC	Crodasinic CS	Surfactant	Elfapur® N 120
Cithrol 2ML	Crodasinic L	Dow Corning® 193	Elfapur® N 150
Cithrol 2MO	Crodasinic LS30	Surfactant	Elfapur® O 80
Cithrol 2MS	Crodasinic LS35	Dow Corning® 2501	Elfapur® O 160
Cithrol 3MS	Crodasinic LT40	Cosmetic Wax	Elfapur® T 110
Cithrol 4DS	Crodasinic MS	Dow Corning® Antifoam	Elfapur® T 250
Cithrol 4ML	Crodasinic OS35	1520-US	Emal 20C
Cithrol 4MO	Crodasinic S	Dow Corning® Medical	Emal E-25C, -70C
Cithrol 4MS	Crodesta F-10	Antifoam A Compound	Emal NC-35
Cithrol 6ML	Crodesta F-50	Dow Corning® Medical	Emalex 102
Cithrol 6MO	Crodesta F-110	Antifoam AF Emulsion	Emalex 103
Cithrol 6MS	Crodesta F-160	Dow Corning® Medical	Emalex 105
Cithrol 10ML	Crodesta SL-40	Antifoam C Emulsion	Emalex 107
Cithrol 10MO	Crodet O23	Drewmulse® POE-SML	Emalex 110
Cithrol 10MS	Crodolene LA1020	Drewmulse® POE-SMO	Emalex 112
Cithrol 15MS	Croduret 10	Drewmulse® POE-SMS	Emalex 115
Cithrol 40MO	Croduret 25	Drewmulse® POE-STS	Emalex 117
Cithrol 40MS	Croduret 30	Drewmulse® SML	Emalex 120
Cithrol 60DS	Croduret 40	Drewmulse® SMO	Emalex 125
Cithrol 60ML	Croduret 60	Drewmulse® SMS	Emalex 130
Cithrol 60MO	Croduret 100	Drewmulse® STS	Emalex 200
Cithrol DEGMO	Cromeen	Duoquad® O-50	Emalex 703
Cithrol PGMM	Crosultaine C-50	Duoquad® T-50	Emalex 705
Closyl 30 2089	Crosultaine T-30	Eccowet® W-50	Emalex 707
Closyl LA 3584	Crotein O	Eccowet® W-88	Emalex 709
Comperlan® 100	Crotein SPA	Edenor L2SM	Emalex 710
Comperlan® CD	Crotein SPC	Elfacos® PEG 400 DS	Emalex 712
Comperlan® COD	Cyclochem® PEG 200DS	Elfacos® PEG 600 DS	Emalex 715
Comperlan® F	Cyclochem® PEG 6000DS	Elfacos® PGMS	Emalex 720
Comperlan® KD	Cyclochem® PEG 600DS	Elfadent SM 514	Emalex 725
Comperlan® KDO	Cyclomox® SO	Elfan® 200	Emalex 730
Comperlan® KM	Cycloryl M1	Elfan® 240T/S	Emalex 750
Comperlan® LD	Cycloteric BET-L31	Elfan® 260 S	Emalex 1605
Comperlan® LD 9	Cycloteric CAPA	Elfan® 280	Emalex 1610
Comperlan® LDO, LDS	Cycloteric SLIP	Elfan® 680	Emalex 1615
Comperlan® LM	Dehyton® AB-30	Elfan® 2240 Mg	Emalex 1620
Comperlan® LMD	Dehyton® PAB-30	Elfan® A 432	Emalex 1625

Detergents/Foaming Agents/Foam Boosters/Stabilizers *(cont'd.)*

Emalex 1805	Emcol® SO	Empicol® LXV	Emthox® 5942
Emalex 1810	Emericide 142	Empicol® LXV/D	Emthox® 5943
Emalex 1815	Emericide 144	Empicol® LZ	Emthox® 6957
Emalex 1820	Emersol® 150	Empicol® LZ/D	Emthox® 6961
Emalex 1825	Emery® 655	Empicol® LZP	Emthox® 6964
Emalex 2405	Emery® 5315	Empicol® LZV	Emthox® 6965
Emalex 2410	Emery® 5412	Empicol® LZV/D	Emthox® 6967
Emalex 2415	Emery® 6744	Empicol® ML 26/F	Emthox® 6968
Emalex 2420	Emery® 6748	Empicol® ML30	Emthox® 6970
Emalex 2425	Emery® 6752	Empicol® ML30	Emthox® 6971
Emalex 2505	Emid® 6500	Empicol® TAS30	Emthox® 6972
Emalex 2510	Emid® 6510	Empicol® TC30/T	Emulsifier 17 P
Emalex 2515	Emid® 6513	Empicol® TC34	Enagicol C-30B
Emalex 2520	Emid® 6515	Empicol® TCR	Enagicol L-30AN
Emalex 2525	Emid® 6518	Empicol® TCR/T	Equex AEM
Emalex N-83	Emid® 6519	Empicol® TL40	Equex S
Emalex NN-5	Emid® 6521	Empicol® TL40/S	Equex STM
Emalex NN-15	Emid® 6531	Empicol® TLP	Equex SW
Emalex NP-2	Emid® 6534	Empicol® TLP/T	Equex T
Emalex NP-3	Emid® 6541	Empicol® TLR	Esi-Det CDA
Emalex NP-5	Emid® 6573	Empicol® TLR/T	Esi-Terge 10
Emalex NP-10	Emid® 6590	Empicol® XDB	Esi-Terge S-10
Emalex NP-11	Emkapol 6000	Empigen® 5083	Espesilor AC-50
Emalex NP-12	Emkapol 8000	Empigen® 5089	Estol E10DS 3728
Emalex NP-13	Emkapol 8500	Empigen® 5107	Estol E60DS 3734
Emalex NP-15	Emphos™ CS-1361	Empigen® 5509	Estol EO4DO 3673
Emalex NP-20	Empicol® 0031/T	Empigen® BB	Estol EO4DS 3724
Emalex NP-25	Empicol® 0045	Empigen® BB-AU	Estol EO6DO 3675
Emalex NP-30	Empicol® 0045V	Empigen® BS	Estol EO6DS 3726
Emalex OD-5	Empicol® 0185	Empigen® BS/AU	Estol EO6MO 3674
Emalex OD-10	Empicol® 0216	Empigen® BS/H	Estol MEL 1502
Emalex OD-16	Empicol® 0251/70	Empigen® BS/P	Estol MEL 1507
Emalex OD-20	Empicol® 0627	Empigen® CDL10	Estol MEM 1518
Emalex OD-25	Empicol® 0919	Empigen® CDL30	Estol MYM 3645
Emalex OP-5	Empicol® 1220/T	Empigen® CDL60	Estol PMS 3737
Emalex OP-8	Empicol® AL30	Empigen® CDR40	Ethofat® 60/15
Emalex OP-10	Empicol® AL30/T	Empigen® CDR60	Ethofat® 60/20
Emalex OP-15	Empicol® AL70	Empigen® OB	Ethofat® 60/25
Emalex OP-20	Empicol® BSD	Empigen® OB/AU	Ethofat® 142/20
Emalex OP-25	Empicol® DLS	Empigen® OH25	Ethofat® 242/25
Emalex OP-30	Empicol® EAA70	Empigen® OS/A	Ethofat® C/15
Emalex OP-40	Empicol® EAB	Empigen® OS/AU	Ethofat® C/25
Emalex OP-50	Empicol® EAB70	Empigen® OY	Ethofat® O/15
Emcol® 1484	Empicol® EAB/T	Empigen® XDR112	Ethofat® O/20
Emcol® 4100M	Empicol® EAC/T	Empilan® 2502	Ethomid® HT/60
Emcol® 4161L	Empicol® EGB	Empilan® CDE	Ethomid® O/15
Emcol® 4300	Empicol® EL	Empilan® CDE/FF	Ethomid® O/17
Emcol® 4400-1	Empicol® EMB	Empilan® CDEY	Ethoquad® C/12B
Emcol® 4403	Empicol® EMD	Empilan® CDX	Ethoquad® C/12 Nitrate
Emcol® 4500	Empicol® ESA	Empilan® CIS	Ethoquad® CB/12
Emcol® 5310	Empicol® ESA70	Empilan® CM	Ethoquad® T/12
Emcol® 5315	Empicol® ESB	Empilan® CM/F	Ethoquad® T/13-50
Emcol® 6748	Empicol® ESB3	Empilan® CME	Ethoxylan® 1685
Emcol® CC-36	Empicol® ESB3/D	Empilan® FD	Ethoxylan® 1686
Emcol® CC-3718	Empicol® ESB3GA	Empilan® FE	Ethylan® CH
Emcol® CDO	Empicol® ESB50	Empilan® KB 2	Ethylan® CL
Emcol® CLA-40	Empicol® ESB70	Empilan® KB 3	Ethylan® CRS
Emcol® CMCD	Empicol® ETB	Empilan® KC 3	Ethylan® KEO
Emcol® Coco Betaine	Empicol® HL25	Empilan® LDE	Ethylan® LD
Emcol® DMCD-40	Empicol® LM	Empilan® LDE/FF	Ethylan® LDA-48
Emcol® E-607L	Empicol® LM45	Empilan® LDX	Ethylan® LDG
Emcol® E-607S	Empicol® LM/T	Empilan® LIS	Ethylan® LDS
Emcol® ISML	Empicol® LMV	Empilan® LME	Ethylan® LM2
Emcol® L	Empicol® LMV/T	Empimin® KSN70	Ethylan® MLD
Emcol® LO	Empicol® LQ70	Empiphos 4KP	Ethylan® TCO
Emcol® M	Empicol® LX	Emsorb® 2721	Etocas 10
Emcol® MO	Empicol® LX28	Emthox® 2738	Etocas 30
Emcol® NA-30	Empicol® LXS95	Emthox® 5941	Etocas 35

Detergents/Foaming Agents/Foam Boosters/Stabilizers *(cont'd.)*

Etocas 60	Geropon® SBR-3	Hetamide CME	Hetoxol LS-9
Ethocas 75	Geropon® SS-L7DE	Hetamide CME-CO	Hetoxol TD-3
Eucarol B/D	Geropon® SS-L9ME	Hetamide DS	Hetoxol TD-6
Eucarol B/TA	Geropon® SS-LA-3	Hetamide LA	Hetoxol TD-12
Eucarol D	Geropon® SS-TA	Hetamide LL	Hetoxol TDEP-15
Eucarol LS	Geropon® T-77	Hetamide LML	Hetsorb L-10
Eucarol T	Geropon® TBS	Hetamide LN	Hetsorb L-20
Eucarol TA	Geropon® TC-42	Hetamide LNO	Hetsorb L-80-72%
Eumulgin® C4	Glo-Mul 4001	Hetamide M	Hexaryl D 60 L
Eumulgin® PRT 36	Glo-Mul 4007	Hetamide MA	Hodag Nonionic 1035-L
Eumulgin® PRT 40	Glucam® E-10	Hetamide MC	Hodag Nonionic 1044-L
Eumulgin® PRT 56	Glucam® E-20	Hetamide MCS	Hodag Nonionic 1061-L
Eumulgin® PRT 200	Glucam® P-10	Hetamide ML	Hodag Nonionic 1062-L
Eumulgin® PWM17	Glucam® P-20	Hetamide MMC, OC	Hodag Nonionic 1064-L
Euperlan® PL 1000	Glucamate® SSE-20	Hetamide MO	Hodag Nonionic 1068-F
Fancol CA	Gluplex® AC	Hetamide MOC	Hodag Nonionic 1088-F
Fancol OA-95	Gluplex® LES	Hetamide MS	Hodag Nonionic 2017-R
Fancol SA	Gluplex® LS	Hetamide OC	Hodag Nonionic E-5
Finsolv® BOD	Gluplex® OS	Hetamide RC	Hodag Nonionic E-6
Finsolv® P	GP-215 Silicone Polyol	Hetoxamate 200 DL	Hodag Nonionic E-7
Fizul MD-318C	Copolymer	Hetoxamate 400 DS	Hodag Nonionic E-10
Fluilan AWS	Gransurf 71	Hetoxamate FA 2-5	Hodag Nonionic E-12
FMB 128 T	Gransurf 72	Hetoxamate FA-5	Hodag Nonionic E-20
Foamid C	Gransurf 73	Hetoxamate FA-20	Hodag Nonionic E-30
Foamid PK	Gransurf 75	Hetoxamate LA-5	Hostapon CT Paste
Foamid SCE	Gransurf 76	Hetoxamate LA-9	Hostapon KA Powd
Foamid SL-Extra	Gransurf 77	Hetoxamate MO-2	Hostapon KCG
Foamid SLM	Grillocin® CW 90	Hetoxamate MO-5	Hostapon KTW New
Foamole A	Grillocin® HY 77	Hetoxamate MO-9	Hostapon LEC
Foamole M	Grillocin® PY 88 Pellets	Hetoxamate MO-15	Hostapon SCHC
Foamox CDO	Grillocin® PY 88 Pulver/	Hetoxamate SA-5	Hostapon SCHC-Powd
Foamquat 2IAE	Powd.	Hetoxamate SA-7	Hostapon SCI
Foamquat CAS	Grillocose® PS	Hetoxamate SA-9	Hostapon SCID
Foam-Soy™ C	Grillosol 8C	Hetoxamate SA-13	Hostapon SO
Foamtaine CAB-A	Grillosol 8C12	Hetoxamate SA-23	Hostapon STT Paste
Foamtaine CAB-G	Grilloten® LSE 65 K	Hetoxamate SA-35	Hostapon T Paste 33
Foam-Wheat C	Grilloten® LSE 65 K Soft	Hetoxamate SA-40	Hostapon T Powd
Fungicide DA 2/938070	Grilloten LSE 87	Hetoxamate SA-90	Hostapur SAS 60
Fungicide UMA 2/938080	Grilloten® LSE 87 K	Hetoxamate SA-90F	Hyamide 1:1
G-2151	Grilloten® LSE 87 K Soft	Hetoxamine T-50	Hydrenol® DD
G-2330	Grilloten ZT12	Hetoxide C-2	Hy-Phi 1055
G-4252	Grilloten ZT-40	Hetoxide C-9	Hy-Phi 1088
G-4280	Hamposyl® C	Hetoxide C-15	Hy-Phi 1199
G-4964	Hamposyl® C-30	Hetoxide C-25	Hy-Phi 1303
G-5507	Hamposyl® L	Hetoxide C-40	Hy-Phi 1401
G-5511	Hamposyl® L-30	Hetoxide C-60	Hy-Phi 2066
G-70147	Hamposyl® L-95	Hetoxide C-200	Hy-Phi 2088
Gafac® RE-877	Hamposyl® M	Hetoxide DNP-5	Hy-Phi 2102
Genaminox CS	Hamposyl® M-30	Hetoxide DNP-10	Hy-Phi 4204
Genaminox KC	Hamposyl® O	Hetoxide HC-16	Hy-Phi 6001
Genapol® AMS	Hamposyl® S	Hetoxide NP-4	Hystrene® 7016
Genapol® CRT 40	Hamposyl® TL-40	Hetoxol 15 CSA	Igepal® CA-630
Genapol® LRO Liq., Paste	Hartamide LDA	Hetoxol CA-2	Igepal® CO-430
Genapol® T Grades	Hartamide LMEA	Hetoxol CA-10	Igepal® CO-630 Special
Genapol® TS Powd	Hartamide OD	Hetoxol CA-20	Igepal® DM-970 FLK
Genapol® TSM	Hartofol 40	Hetoxol CS-4	Igepal® NP-4
Geronol ACR/4	Hartofol 60T	Hetoxol CS-5	Igepal® NP-9
Geronol ACR/9	Hefti DO-33-F	Hetoxol CS-9	Igepal® OP-9
Geropon® AB/20	Hefti NP-55-60	Hetoxol CS-15	Incrodet TD7-C
Geropon® AC-78	Hefti NP-55-80	Hetoxol CS-20	Incromate CDL
Geropon® ACR/4	Hefti NP-55-80	Hetoxol CS-30	Incromate CDP
Geropon® ACR/9	Hefti NP-55-90	Hetoxol CS-50	Incromate Mink L
Geropon® AS-200	Hefti NP-55-90	Hetoxol CS-50 Special	Incromate OLL
Geropon® AS-250	Hefti PGE-400-DS	Hetoxol CSA-15	Incromate SEL
Geropon® LSS	Hefti PGE-600-MO	Hetoxol L-3N	Incromide ALD
Geropon® SBDO	Hefti PMS-33	Hetoxol L-4N	Incromide BAD
Geropon® SBFA-30	Hest E.G.D.S	Hetoxol L-9N	Incromide CA
Geropon® SBG-280	Hetamide CMA	Hetoxol L-23	Incromide CAC

Detergents/Foaming Agents/Foam Boosters/Stabilizers *(cont'd.)*

Incromide CM	Jordapon® CI Prill	Lexaine® C	Mackam™ CBS-50
Incromide CME	Jordapon® CI-UP	Lexaine® CG-30	Mackam™ CBS-50G
Incromide L90	Karamide 121	Lexaine® CS	Mackam™ CET
Incromide LI	Karamide 363	Lexaine® CSB-50	Mackam™ HV
Incromide LL	Kartacid 1299	Lexaine® IS	Mackam™ ISA
Incromide LM-70	Kartacid 1495	Lexaine® LM	Mackam™ J
Incromide LMI	Kartacid 1498	Lexaine® O	Mackam™ L
Incromide LR	Kartacid 1692	Lexate® BPQ	Mackam™ LMB-LS
Incromide Mink D	Kartacid 1890	Lexein® S620S/Superpro	Mackam™ OB
Incromide OLD	Kelisema Collagen-IMZ	5A	Mackam™ RA
Incromide OPM	Complex	Lexein® S620TA	Mackam™ WGB
Incromide SED	Kelisema Collagen-LSS	Lexemul® 200 DL	Mackamide™ 100-A
Incromide SM	Complex	Lilaminox M4	Mackamide™ AME-75,
Incromide UM	Kemamine® P-690	Lilaminox M24	AME-100
Incromide WGD	Kemamine® Q-6503B	Lipacide CCO	Mackamide™ AN55
Incromine CB	Kemamine® T-6502	Lipacide DPHP	Mackamide™ C
Incromine Oxide B	Kemamine® T-6902	Lipacide PCO	Mackamide™ CD
Incromine Oxide B-30P	Kemamine® T-7902	Lipacide PK	Mackamide™ CD-10
Incromine Oxide B50	Kemamine® T-8902	Lipacide UCO	Mackamide™ CDC
Incromine Oxide BA	Kemamine® T-9972	Lipamide MEAA	Mackamide™ CDS-80
Incromine Oxide C	Kemester® 115	Lipamide S	Mackamide™ CMA
Incromine Oxide I	Kemester® 7018	Lipocol PT-400	Mackamide™ CS
Incromine Oxide ISMO	Kemester® 8002	Lipolan LB-440	Mackamide™ EC
Incromine Oxide L	Kemester® 9012	Lipolan LB-840	Mackamide™ ISA
Incromine Oxide L-40	Kemester® 9014	Liponic EG-1	Mackamide™ L-10
Incromine Oxide M	Kemester® 9718	Liponic EG-7	Mackamide™ L95
Incromine Oxide MC	Kessco Diglycol Oleate	Lipo-Peptide AME 30	Mackamide™ LLM
Incromine Oxide Mink	L-SE	Lipophos LMP	Mackamide™ LMD
Incromine Oxide O	Kessco PEG-400 DS-356	Lipoproteol LCO	Mackamide™ LME
Incromine Oxide OD-50	Kessco PGMS-R	Lipoproteol LCOK	Mackamide™ LMM
Incromine Oxide S	Kessco PGMS-X534F	LMB	Mackamide™ LOL
Incronam 30	Kessco PGNM	Lonzaine® 12C	Mackamide™ MC
Incronam AL-30	Klensoft	Lonzaine® 14	Mackamide™ MO
Incronam B-40	Kohacool L-400	Lonzaine® 16S	Mackamide™ NOA
Incronam BA-30	Kortacid 1295	Lonzaine® 16S	Mackamide™ O
Incronam CD-30	Lamepon® 4SK	Lonzaine® C	Mackamide™ ODM
Incronam I-30	Lamepon® PA-TR	Lonzaine® CO	Mackamide™ OP
Incronam Mink 30	Lamepon® S	Lonzaine® JS	Mackamide™ PK
Incronam OD-50	Lamepon® S-TR	Lonzest® PEG 4-O	Mackamide™ PKM
Incronam OL-30	Lamepon® S/NP	Loropan CME	Mackamide™ R
Incronam OP-30	Lamepon® ST40	Loropan KM	Mackamide™ S
Incronam SE-30	Lamepon® ST 40/NP	Loropan LD	Mackamide™ SD
Incronam WG-30	Lamepon® S-TR/NP	Loropan LM	Mackamide™ SMA
Incropol CS-20	Lamepon® UD	Loropan LMD	Mackamine™ BAO
Incropol CS-50	Lanamine®	Loropan OD	Mackamine™ CAO
Incropol L-23	Lanexol AWS	Louryl T-50	Mackamine™ CO
Incroquat AL-85	Lanidox-5	Lowenol C-243	Mackamine™ IAO
Incroquat BA-85	Lankropol® KNB22	Lowenol C Acid	Mackamine™ ISMO
Incroquat Mink-85	Lankropol® KSG72	Lowenol L Acid	Mackamine™ LAO
Incroquat S-85	Lanogel® 21	Lowenol M Acid	Mackamine™ LO
Incrosul LMA	Lanogel® 31	Lowenol O Acid	Mackamine™ O2
Incrosul LMS	Lanogel® 41	Lowenol P Acid	Mackamine™ OAO
Incrosul LS	Lanogel® 61	Lumorol K 28	Mackamine™ SAO
Incrosul LSA	Lantrol® PLN	Lumorol K 5019	Mackamine™ SO
Incrosul LTS	Lantrol® PLN/50	Lumorol RK	Mackamine™ WGO
Incrosul OMS	Lathanol® LAL	Lutensit® AS 2230, 2270	Mackanate™ OD-2
Incrosul OTS	Laural D	Lutensit® AS 3330	Mackanate™ ODT
Incrosul TS	Laural EC	Lutensit® AS 3334	Mackanate™ ODT-2
Intravon® AN	Laural LS	Luviquat® FC 370	Mackanate™ OL
Intravon® JU	Lauramina	Luviquat® FC 550	Mackanate™ OM
Jaguar® HP 60	Laurel SD-900M	Mackadet™ CA	Macol® 2
Jojoba PEG-80	Lauridit® KD, KDG	Mackadet™ SBC-8	Macol® 2LF
Jojoba PEG-120	Lauridit® KM	Mackadet™ TLC-45	Macol® 4
Jordapon® ACI-30	Lauridit® LM	Mackadet™ WGS	Macol® 8
Jordapon® CI-60 Flake	Lauridit® LMI	Mackam™ 35	Macol® 16
Jordapon® CI 75	Lauridit® OD	Mackam™ 35 HP	Macol® 23
Jordapon® CI Disp	Lauridit® PPD	Mackam™ CB-35	Macol® 27
Jordapon® CI-Powd	Lebon 101H, 105	Mackam™ CB-LS	

Detergents/Foaming Agents/Foam Boosters/Stabilizers *(cont'd.)*

Macol® CA-2
Macol® CA-10
Macol® CSA-2
Macol® CSA-4
Macol® CSA-10
Macol® CSA-15
Macol® CSA-20
Macol® CSA-40
Macol® CSA-50
Macol® DNP-5
Macol® DNP-10
Macol® DNP-15
Macol® DNP-21
Macol® LA-4
Macol® LA-9
Macol® LA-12
Macol® LA-23
Macol® LA-790
Macol® NP-4
Macol® NP-5
Macol® NP-6
Macol® NP-8
Macol® NP-11
Macol® NP-12
Macol® NP-15
Macol® NP-20
Macol® NP-20(70)
Macol® NP-30(70)
Macol® NP-100
Macol® OA-2
Macol® OA-4
Macol® OA-5
Macol® OA-10
Macol® OA-20
Macol® OP-3
Macol® OP-5
Macol® OP-8
Macol® OP-10
Macol® OP-10 SP
Macol® OP-12
Macol® OP-16(75)
Macol® OP-30(70)
Macol® OP-40(70)
Macol® SA-2
Macol® SA-5
Macol® SA-10
Macol® SA-15
Macol® SA-20
Macol® SA-40
Macol® TD-3
Macol® TD-8
Macol® TD-10
Macol® TD-12
Macol® TD-15
Macol® TD-100
Macol® TD-610
Mafo® C
Mafo® CAB
Mafo® CAB 425
Mafo® CAB SP
Mafo® CB 40
Mafo® CFA 35
Mafo® CSB
Mafo® CSB 50
Mafo® CSB W
Mafo® KCOSB 50
Mafo® LMAB
Mafo® OB

Mafo® SBAO 110
Makon® 4
Makon® 6
Makon® 8
Makon® 10
Makon® 12
Makon® 14
Makon® 30
Manro AO 3OC
Manro BEC 28
Manro BES 27
Manro BES 60
Manro BES 70
Manro CD
Manro CD/G
Manro CDS
Manro CDX
Manro CMEA
Manro ML 33
Manro NEC 28H
Manro NEC 28L
Manro NEC 70
Manro SLS 28
Manro TDBS 60
Manro TL 40
Manromate LNT40
Manromid 1224
Manromid AV150
Manromid LMA
Manroteric CAB
Manroteric CDX38
Manroteric NAB
Maprosyl® 30
Marlamid® D 1218
Marlamid® D 1885
Marlamid® DF 1218
Marlamid® DF 1818
Marlamid® KL
Marlamid® M 1218
Marlamid® M 1618
Marlinat® 242/28
Marlinat® 242/70
Marlinat® 242/70 S
Marlinat® 243/28
Marlinat® 243/70
Marlinat® CM 40
Marlinat® CM 45
Marlinat® CM 100
Marlinat® CM 105
Marlinat® DFK 30
Marlinat® DFL 40
Marlinat® DFN 30
Marlinat® HA 12
Marlinat® SL 3/40
Marlinat® SRN 30
Marlipal® 24/300
Marlon® AFR
Marlon® PF 40
Marlon® PS 60
Marlopon® AT 50
Marlopon® CA
Maypon 4C
Maypon 4CT
Maypon UD
May-Tein KK
May-Tein KT
May-Tein KTS
May-Tein R

May-Tein SK
May-Tein SY
Mazamide® 65
Mazamide® 68
Mazamide® 124
Mazamide® 524
Mazamide® 1214
Mazamide® 1281
Mazamide® C-2
Mazamide® C-5
Mazamide® CFAM
Mazamide® CMEA
Mazamide® CMEA Extra
Mazamide® CS 148
Mazamide® J 10
Mazamide® JR 300
Mazamide® JR 400
Mazamide® JT 128
Mazamide® L-5
Mazamide® L-298
Mazamide® LLD
Mazamide® LM
Mazamide® LM 20
Mazamide® LS 196
Mazamide® O 20
Mazamide® PCS
Mazamide® RO
Mazamide® SCD
Mazamide® SS 20
Mazamide® TC
Mazamide® WC Conc
Mazon® 60T
Mazox® CAPA
Mazox® CAPA-37
Mazox® CDA
Mazox® LDA
Mazox® MDA
Mazox® ODA
Mazox® SDA
Medialan KA
Medialan KF
Melanol LP 1
Merpol® HCS
Merquat® 550
Merquat® S
Mersolat H 30
Mersolat H 40
Mersolat H 68
Mersolat H 76
Mersolat H 95
Mersolat W 40
Mersolat W 68
Mersolat W 76
Mersolat W 93
Methocel® 40-100
Methocel® 40-101
Methocel® 40-202
Methocel® A4CP
Methocel® A4MP
Methocel® A15LVP
Methocel® E3P
Methocel® E4MP
Methocel® E6P
Methocel® E15LVP
Methocel® E50LVP
Methocel® E50P
Methocel® K4MP
Methocel® K4MS

Methocel® K15MP
Methocel® K15MS
Methocel® K100LVP
Methocel® K100MP
MFF 159-B
Miracare® 2MHT
Miracare® ANL
Miracare® M1
Miracare® XL
Miramine® SODI
Miranate® LEC
Miranol® 2CIB
Miranol® BM Conc
Miranol® C2M Conc. NP
Miranol® C2M-SF 70%
Miranol® C2M-SF Conc
Miranol® CM Conc. NP
Miranol® CM-SF Conc
Miranol® CS Conc
Miranol® H2M Conc
Miranol® HM Conc
Miranol® OM-SF Conc
Miranol® OS-D
Miranol® SM Conc
Mirasheen® 202
Mirataine® AP-C
Mirataine® BB
Mirataine® BD-J
Mirataine® BET-C-30
Mirataine® BET-O-30
Mirataine® BET-P-30
Mirataine® BET-W
Mirataine® CAB-A
Mirataine® CAB-O
Mirataine® CB
Mirataine® CBC
Mirataine® CB/M
Mirataine® CBR
Mirataine® CBS, CBS Mod
Mirataine® COB
Mirataine® H2C-HA
Mirataine® T2C-30
Miristamina
Monalux CAO-35
Monamate C-1142
Monamate CPA-40
Monamate CPA-100
Monamate LA-100
Monamate LNT-40
Monamate OPA-30
Monamate OPA-100
Monamid® 31
Monamid® 150-CW
Monamid® 150-GLT
Monamid® 150-LMWC
Monamid® 150-LWA
Monamid® 150-MW
Monamid® 664-MC
Monamid® 705
Monamid® 716
Monamid® 759
Monamid® 770
Monamid® 853
Monamid® 1007
Monamid® 1034
Monamid® 1159
Monamid® 1224
Monamid® C-305

Detergents/Foaming Agents/Foam Boosters/Stabilizers *(cont'd.)*

Monamid® C-310
Monamid® CMA
Monamid® CMA-A
Monamid® CMA-A/F
Monamid® CMA-A/M
Monamid® CMA/F
Monamid® CMA/M
Monamid® CMA-S
Monamid® CMA-S/F
Monamid® CMA-S/M
Monamid® CP-205
Monamid® L-350
Monamid® L-355
Monamid® L-360
Monamid® L-365
Monamid® LL-370
Monamid® LM-375
Monamid® LMIPA
Monamid® LMMA
Monamid® R31-42
Monamide
Monamine 779
Monamine AA-100
Monamine AC-100
Monamine ACO-100
Monamine ADD-100
Monamine ADY-100
Monamine CF-100 M
Monaterge 1164
Monateric 805
Monateric 951A
Monateric 985A
Monateric 1188M
Monateric 1202
Monateric CA-35
Monateric CAB
Monateric CAB-LC
Monateric CAB-XLC
Monateric CDL
Monateric CDX-38
Monateric CDX-38 Mod
Monateric CEM-38
Monateric CM-36S
Monateric CNa-40
Monateric COAB
Monateric CSH-32
Monateric LMAB
Monateric LMM-30
Monateric MCB
Monawet MM-80
Monawet SNO-35
Monawet TD-30
Montovol GF-15
Montovol RF-13
Mytab®
Nacconol® 35SL
Naxchem™ CD-6M
Naxel™ AAS-40S
Naxel™ AAS-60S
Naxide™ 1230
Naxolate™ WA-97
Naxolate™ WAG
Naxolate™ WA Special
Naxonic™ NI-40
Naxonic™ NI-60
Naxonic™ NI-100
Naxonol™ CO
Naxonol™ PN 66

Naxonol™ PO
Necon SOG
Necon SOGU
Necon SOLC
Neodol® 1
Neodol® 5
Neodol® 23-3
Neodol® 25-3A
Neodol® 25-3S
Neodol® 25-7
Neodol® 25-9
Neodol® 25-12
Neodol® 45-7
Neodol® 45-11
Neodol® 45-13
Neodol® 91
Neopon LAM
Neopon LOA
Neopon LOS 70
Neopon LOS/NF
Neopon LS/NF
Niaproof® Anionic
   Surfactant 4
Niaproof® Anionic
   Surfactant 08
Nidaba 3
Nikkol Akypo RLM 45 NV
Nikkol Alaninate LN-30
Nikkol ALS-25
Nikkol AM-101
Nikkol AM-102EX
Nikkol AM-103EX
Nikkol AM-301
Nikkol AM-3130N
Nikkol AM-3130T
Nikkol BPS-5
Nikkol BPS-10
Nikkol BPS-15
Nikkol BPS-20
Nikkol BPS-25
Nikkol BPS-30
Nikkol CCK-40
Nikkol CCN-40
Nikkol CMT-30
Nikkol DDP-2
Nikkol DDP-4
Nikkol DDP-6
Nikkol DDP-8
Nikkol DDP-10
Nikkol ECT-3
Nikkol ECT-3NEX
Nikkol ECT-7
Nikkol ECTD-3NEX
Nikkol ECTD-6NEX
Nikkol KLS
Nikkol LMT
Nikkol LSA
Nikkol MMT
Nikkol NES-203
Nikkol NES-203-27
Nikkol NES-303
Nikkol NES-303-36
Nikkol NP-5
Nikkol NP-7.5
Nikkol NP-10
Nikkol NP-15
Nikkol NP-18TX
Nikkol OP-3

Nikkol OP-10
Nikkol OP-30
Nikkol OS-14
Nikkol Phosten HLP
Nikkol Phosten HLP-1
Nikkol Phosten HLP-N
Nikkol PMT
Nikkol Sarcosinate CN-30
Nikkol Sarcosinate LH
Nikkol Sarcosinate LN
Nikkol Sarcosinate LN-30
Nikkol Sarcosinate MN
Nikkol Sarcosinate OH
Nikkol Sarcosinate PN
Nikkol SBL-2A-27
Nikkol SBL-2N-27
Nikkol SBL-2T-36
Nikkol SBL-3N-27
Nikkol SBL-4N
Nikkol SBL-4T
Nikkol SCS
Nikkol SGC-80N
Nikkol SLP-N
Nikkol SLS
Nikkol SLS-30
Nikkol SMS
Nikkol SMT
Nikkol SNP-4N
Nikkol SNP-4T
Nikkol TDP-2
Nikkol TDP-4
Nikkol TDP-6
Nikkol TDP-8
Nikkol TDP-10
Nikkol TEALS
Nikkol TEALS-42
Ninol® 30-LL
Ninol® 40-CO
Ninol® 49-CE
Ninol® 55-LL
Ninol® 70-SL
Ninol® 96-SL
Ninol® CNR
Ninol® GR
Ninol® L-9
Ninol® LMP
Ninol® M10
Ninox® FCA
Niox KI Series
Nissan Nonion E-205
Nissan Nonion E-206
Nissan Nonion E-208
Nissan Nonion E-215
Nissan Nonion E-220
Nissan Nonion E-230
Nissan Nonion K-202
Nissan Nonion K-203
Nissan Nonion K-204
Nissan Nonion K-207
Nissan Nonion K-211
Nissan Nonion K-215
Nissan Nonion K-220
Nissan Nonion K-230
Nissan Nonion P-208
Nissan Nonion P-210
Nissan Nonion P-213
Nissan Nonion S-206
Nissan Nonion S-207

Nissan Nonion S-215
Nissan Nonion S-220
Nissan Persoft SK
Nissan Stafoam DO, DOS
Nissan Stafoam MF
Nonasol N4AS
Nonasol N4SS
Nonionic E-4
Norfox® 1101
Norfox® ALKA
Norfox® Coco Betaine
Norfox® DCS
Norfox® DCSA
Norfox® DESA
Norfox® DLSA
Norfox® DOSA
Norfox® KD
Norfox® KO
Norfox® NP-4
Norfox® SLES-02
Norfox® SLES-03
Norfox® SLES-60
Norfox® SLS
Norfox® T-60
Novel® N2.2-810
Novel® N3.0-1216CO
Novel® N4.9-810
Novel® N5.1-1618
Novel® N7.7-810
Noxamine CA 30
Nutrapon DL 3891
Nutrapon KF 3846
Nutrapon W 1367
Nutrapon WAQE 2364
Nutrilan® Elastin E20
Nutrol Betaine MD 3863
Olamida
Olamida CD
Olamida CM
Olamida ED
Olamida RD
Olamida SM
Olamida UD
Olamida UD 21
Olamin® K/NP
Onyxol® 336
Oramix CG 110-60
Oramix L
Oramix NS 10
Oxamin LO
Oxetal VD 20
Oxetal VD 28
Pamak 4
Pationic® 122A
Pationic® 138C
Penreco 2251 Oil
Penreco 2263 Oil
Peptein® KC
Peptein® TEAC
Perlankrol® DAF25
Perlankrol® DSA
Perlglanz-Konzentrat B-48
Permethyl® 101A
P & G Amide No. 27
Phoenamid LMM
Phoenamid SM
Phospholipid PTC
Phospholipid PTD

Detergents/Foaming Agents/Foam Boosters/Stabilizers *(cont'd.)*

Phospholipid PTL	Radiamox® 6800	Rewomid® DL 203	Rhodapon® EC111
Phospholipid PTZ	Radiamox® 6804	Rewomid® DL 203 S	Rhodapon® L-22, L-22/C
Phosphoteric® QL38	Radiaquat® 6444	Rewomid® DL 240	Rhodapon® LM
Phosphoteric® T-C6	Radiaquat® 6462	Rewomid® DLMS	Rhodapon® LSB, LSB/CT
Plantaren™ 1200	Radiaquat® 6471	Rewomid® DO 280	Rhodapon® LT-6
Plantaren® 1200 CS/UP	Radiasurf® 7000	Rewomid® DO 280 SE	Rhodapon® SB-8208/S
Plantaren® 1200 UP	Radiasurf® 7151	Rewomid® F	Rhodasurf® C-20
Plantaren® 1300	Radiasurf® 7152	Rewomid® IPE 280	Rhodasurf® LA-3
Plantaren® 2000	Radiasurf® 7153	Rewomid® IPL 203	Rhodasurf® S-2
Plantaren® 2000 CS/UP	Radiasurf® 7175	Rewomid® IPP 240	Rhodasurf® S-20
Plantaren® 2000 UP	Radiasurf® 7196	Rewomid® L 203	Rhodicare™ XC
Plantaren® PS-100	Radiasurf® 7206	Rewomid® OM 101/G	Rhodorsil® AF 70414,
Plantaren® PS-200	Radiasurf® 7269	Rewomid® OM 101/IG	70416, 70426 R, 70452
Plantaren® PS-300	Radiasurf® 7270	Rewomid® R 280	Ritacetyl®
Pluronic® 12R3	Radiasurf® 7402	Rewomid® S 280	Ritasynt IP
Pluronic® L10	Radiasurf® 7403	Rewomid® SD	Rolamid CD
Poem-LS-90	Radiasurf® 7404	Rewominox B 204	Ryoto Sugar Ester OWA-
Prifac 7920	Radiasurf® 7411	Rewominox L 408	1570
Prifac 7935	Radiasurf® 7413	Rewominox S 300	Ryoto Sugar Ester P-1570
Prifrac 2940	Radiasurf® 7414	Rewominoxid L 408	Ryoto Sugar Ester P-1570S
Priolene 6900	Radiasurf® 7417	Rewominoxid S 300	Ryoto Sugar Ester P-1670
Priolene 6905	Radiasurf® 7420	Rewopal® C 6	Ryoto Sugar Ester S-170
Priolene 6906	Radiasurf® 7422	Rewopal® LA 6	Ryoto Sugar Ester S-370
Priolene 6910	Radiasurf® 7423	Rewopol® HM 30	Ryoto Sugar Ester S-370F
Priolene 6933	Radiasurf® 7431	Rewopol® NL 3	Ryoto Sugar Ester S-570
Profan 24 Extra, 128 Extra	Radiasurf® 7432	Rewopol® NLS 28	Ryoto Sugar Ester S-770
Profan 2012E	Radiasurf® 7443	Rewopol® SBC 212 P	Ryoto Sugar Ester S-970
Profan AA62	Radiasurf® 7453	Rewopol® SBCS 50	Ryoto Sugar Ester S-1170
Profan AB20	Radiasurf® 7454	Rewopol® SBL 203	Ryoto Sugar Ester S-1170S
Profan AD31	Radiateric® 6860	Rewopol® SBR 12-Powder	Ryoto Sugar Ester S-1570
Protamate 200 T	Radiateric® 6864	Rewopon® AM-2C	Ryoto Sugar Ester S-1670
Protamide 15W	Remcopal HC 7	Rewopon® AM-2L	Ryoto Sugar Ester S-1670S
Protamide LNO	Remcopal HC 33	Rewopon® AM-B 13	S-210
Protamide MRCA	Remcopal HC 60	Rewopon® AM-CA	Sandobet SC
Proteol VS22	Renex® 20	Reworyl® K	Sandopan® DTC
Prothera™	Renex® 22	Rewoteric® AM 2C SF	Sandopan® DTC-100
Prox-onic CSA-1/04	Renex® 30	Rewoteric® AM 2C W	Sandopan® DTC-Acid
Prox-onic CSA-1/06	Renex® 36	Rewoteric® AM B 13	Sandopan® DTC Linear P
Prox-onic CSA-1/010	Renex® 647	Rewoteric® AM B 14	Sandopan® DTC Linear P
Prox-onic CSA-1/015	Renex® 648	Rewoteric® AM B-15	Acid
Prox-onic CSA-1/020	Renex® 649	Rewoteric® AM CAS	Sandopan® JA-36
Prox-onic CSA-1/030	Renex® 650	Rewoteric® AM CAS-15	Sandopan® KST
Prox-onic CSA-1/050	Renex® 678	Rewoteric® AM DML	Sandopan® LS-24
Prox-onic L 081-05	Renex® 679	Rewoteric® AM DML-35	Sandopan® TFL Conc
Prox-onic L 101-05	Renex® 682	Rewoteric® AM HC	Sandoz Amide NT
Prox-onic L 102-02	Renex® 688	Rewoteric® AM KSF-40	Sandoz Amide PE
Prox-onic L 121-09	Renex® 690	Rewoteric® AM LP	Sandoz Amide PL
Prox-onic L 161-05	Renex® 697	Rewoteric® AM R40	Sandoz Amide PO
Prox-onic L 181-05	Renex® 698	Rewoteric® AM TEG	Sandoz Amine Oxide XA-C
Prox-onic L 201-02	Renex® 702	Rewoteric® QAM 50	Sandoz Amine Oxide XA-L
Prox-onic NP-1.5	Renex® 703	Rexonic N91-8	Sandoz Amine Oxide XA-M
Prox-onic NP-04	Renex® 707	Rhodacal® 301-10F	Sandoz Sulfate 216
Prox-onic NP-06	Renex® 711	Rhodacal® 330	Sandoz Sulfate 219
Prox-onic NP-09	Renex® 720	Rhodacal® A-246L	Sandoz Sulfate A
Prox-onic NP-010	Renex® 750	Rhodacal® A-246 LX	Sandoz Sulfate EP
Prox-onic NP-015	Renex® PEG 200	Rhodacal® DDB 60T	Sandoz Sulfate ES-3
Prox-onic NP-020	Renex® PEG 300	Rhodacal® LA Acid	Sandoz Sulfate K
Prox-onic NP-030	Rewocid® DU 185	Rhodafac® MC-470	Sandoz Sulfate WA Dry
Prox-onic NP-030/70	Rewocid® SBU 185	Rhodafac® RE-870	Sandoz Sulfate WA Special
Prox-onic NP-040	Rewocid® U 185	Rhodamox® CAPO	Sandoz Sulfate WAG
Prox-onic NP-040/70	Rewoderm® S 1333	Rhodamox® LO	Sandoz Sulfate WAS
Prox-onic NP-050	Rewolan® 5	Rhodapex® CO-433	Sandoz Sulfate WE
Prox-onic NP-050/70	Rewomat B 2003	Rhodapex® CO-436	Sandoz Sulfonate AAS 60S
Prox-onic NP-0100	Rewomid® 203/S	Rhodapex® EA-2	Sarkosyl® L
Prox-onic NP-0100/70	Rewomid® C 212	Rhodapex® EAY	Sarkosyl® LC
Purton CFD	Rewomid® DC 212 S	Rhodapex® ES	Sarkosyl® NL-30
Purton SFD	Rewomid® DC 212 SE	Rhodapex® ES-2	Sarkosyl® O
PVP K-30	Rewomid® DC 220 SE	Rhodapex® HF-433	Schercamox C-AA

Detergents/Foaming Agents/Foam Boosters/Stabilizers *(cont'd.)*

Schercamox CMA
Schercamox DMA
Schercamox DMC
Schercamox DML
Schercamox DMM
Schercamox DMS
Schercamox T-12
Schercodine C
Schercomid 1-102
Schercomid 1214
Schercomid CCD
Schercomid CDA
Schercomid CDA-H
Schercomid CDO-Extra
Schercomid CME
Schercomid CMI
Schercomid HT-60
Schercomid LD
Schercomid MD-Extra
Schercomid MME
Schercomid OMI
Schercomid SAP
Schercomid SCE
Schercomid SCO-Extra
Schercomid SI
Schercomid SLA
Schercomid SL-Extra
Schercomid SLM
Schercomid SLMC-75
Schercomid SL-ML
Schercomid SLM-LC
Schercomid SLM-S
Schercomid SM
Schercomid SME
Schercomid SWG
Schercomid TO-2
Schercopol CMIS-Na
Schercopol CMS-Na
Schercopol LPS
Schercopol OMIS-Na
Schercopol OMS-Na
Schercotaine APAB
Schercotaine CAB
Schercotaine CAB-A
Schercotaine CAB-G
Schercotaine CAB-K
Schercotaine CAB-Mg
Schercotaine IAB
Schercotaine MAB
Schercotaine SCAB
Schercotaine SCAB-A
Schercotaine WOAB
Schercoteric CY-2
Schercoteric LS
Schercoteric LS-2
Schercoteric LS-EP
Schercoteric LS-SF-2
Schercoteric LS-SF-2 Conc
Schercoteric MS
Schercoteric MS-2
Schercoteric MS-2ES
  Modified
Schercoteric MS-2 Modified
Schercoteric MS-2TE
  Modified
Schercoteric MS-SF-2
  (38%)
Schercoteric MS-SF-2

(70%)
Schercozoline C
Secosol® AL 959
Secosol® ALL40
Secosyl
Sellig R 3395
Sellig T 14 100
Selligor DC 100
Serdet DFL 40
Serdet DFM 33
Serdet DFN 30
Serdet DMK 75
Serdolamide POF 61
Serdolamide PYF 77
Setacin 103 Spezial
Setacin F Spezial Paste
Setacin M
Silamine 65
Silbione™ 70646
Silquat AD
Silquat AM
Silwet® L-7002
Simchin® WS
Siponic® NP-7
Sochamine A 755
Sochamine A 7525
Sochamine A 7527
Solan
Solan 50
Sole Terge 8
Solulan® 5
Solulan® 16
Solulan® 75
Solulan® C-24
Solulan® L-575
Solwax L20
Sorbon TR 814
Sorbon TR 843
Stafoam DF-1
Stafoam DF-4
Stafoam DL
Stamid HT 3901
Standamid® 100
Standamid® CD
Standamid® CMG
Standamid® ID
Standamid® KD
Standamid® KDM
Standamid® KDO
Standamid® KDS
Standamid® KM
Standamid® LD
Standamid® LD 80/20
Standamid® LDM
Standamid® LDO
Standamid® LDS
Standamid® LM
Standamid® LP
Standamid® PD
Standamid® PK-KD
Standamid® PK-KDO
Standamid® PK-KDS
Standamid® SD
Standamid® SDO
Standamid® SM
Standamid® SOMD
Standamox C 30
Standamox CAW

Standapol® 125-E Conc
Standapol® 130-E
Standapol® 230-E Conc
Standapol® 7088
Standapol® A
Standapol® AB-45
Standapol® A-HV
Standapol® AMS-100
Standapol® AP Blend
Standapol® BAW
Standapol® Conc. 7021
Standapol® Conc. 7023
Standapol® CS Paste
Standapol® DEA
Standapol® EA-40
Standapol® EA-K
Standapol® ES-1
Standapol® ES-2
Standapol® ES-3
Standapol® ES-40
Standapol® ES-7099
Standapol® MG
Standapol® MLS
Standapol® OLB-30
Standapol® OLB-50
Standapol® SH-100
Standapol® SH-124-3
Standapol® SH-200
Standapol® SH-300
Standapol® SHC-301
Standapol® T
Standapol® TS-100
Standapol® WA-AC
Standapol® WAQ-115
Standapol® WAQ-LC
Standapol® WAQ Special
Standapol® WAS-100
Steol® 4N
Steol® CA-130
Steol® CA-230
Steol® CA-330
Steol® CA-460
Steol® CS-130
Steol® CS-460
Steol® KA-460
Steol® KS-460
Stepan-Mild® LSB
Stepanol® AM
Stepanol® AM-V
Stepanol® DEA
Stepanol® LX
Stepanol® ME Dry
Stepanol® MG
Stepanol® WA-100
Stepanol® WAC
Stepanol® WA Extra
Stepanol® WA Paste
Stepanol® WAQ
Stepanol® WA Special
Stepanol® WAT
Sulfetal CA 30
Sulfochem ALS
Sulfochem B-221
Sulfochem B-221OP
Sulfochem DLS
Sulfochem EA-1
Sulfochem EA-2
Sulfochem EA-3

Sulfochem ES-2
Sulfochem K
Sulfochem MG
Sulfochem MLS
Sulfochem SAC
Sulfochem SLN
Sulfochem SLP
Sulfochem SLP-95
Sulfochem SLS
Sulfochem TLS
Sulfocos 2B
Sulfopon® 103
Sulfopon® WA 3
Sulfopon® WAQ LCX
Sulfotex DOS
Sulfotex WA
Sulfotex WAT
Sulframin 85
Sulframin 90
Sulframin 1240, 1245
Sulframin 1250, 1260
Sulframin 1288
Sulframin 1298
Sulframin 1388
Sulframin AOS
Sumquat® 6020
Sumquat® 6050
Sumquat® 6110
Sunnol LDF-110
Sunnol LL-103
Sunnol LM-1100
Superpro 5A
Supralate C
Supralate EP
Supralate QC
Supralate WA Paste
Supralate XL
Supro-Tein R
Supro-Tein S
Supro-Tein V
Surfadone® LP-300
Surfax 40
Surfax 100
Surfax 100 AG
Surfax AC 50
Surfax AC 55
Surfax ACB
Surfax ACI
Surfax ACR
Surfax ASD
Surfax CJ
Surfax CN
Surfax EAD
Surfax ECM
Surfax EDT
Surfax EKZ
Surfax EVE
Surfax MEA
Surfax MG
Surfax NH
Surfax SLA
Surfax SME
Surfine AZI-A
Surfine T-A
Surfine WNG-A
Surfine WNT-A
Surfine WNT Conc
Surfine WNT Gel

Detergents/Foaming Agents/Foam Boosters/Stabilizers *(cont'd.)*

Surfine WNT LC	Tauranol ML	Tohol N-230X	Vanseal® NALS-95
Surfine WNT-LS	Tauranol MS	Tomah AO-14-2	Vanseal® NAMS-30
Surfonic® L46-7	Tauranol T-Gel	Tomah AO-728 Special	Vanseal OS
Surfonic® N-10	Tauranol WS, WS Conc	Triton® CG-110	Varamide® A-2
Surfonic® N-31.5	Tauranol WS H.P	Triton® N-42	Varamide® C-212
Surfonic® N-40	Tauranol WSP	Triton® N-150	Varamide® L-203
Surfonic® N-60	T-Det® O-407	Triton® X-100	Varamide® LL-1
Surfonic® N-85	Tegamine® Oxide WS-35	Trycol® 5878	Varamide® LO-1
Surfonic® N-95	Tego®-Betaine C	Trycol® 5967	Varamide® MA-1
Surfonic® N-100	Tego®-Betaine L-7	Trycol® 5972	Varamide® ML-1
Surfonic® N-102	Tego®-Betaine L-90	T-Tergamide 1CD	Varamide® ML-4
Surfonic® N-120	Tego®-Betaine S	T-Tergamide 1PD	Varifoam® A
Surfonic® N-130	Tegosoft® GC	Tween® 20	Varifoam® SXC
Surfonic® N-150	Tergelan® 1790	Tween® 20 SD	Varion® CADG-HS
Surfonic® N-200	Tergitol® NP-9	Tween® 80K	Varion® CDG
Surfonic® N-300	Teric 12A3	Tylorol 2S, 2S/25	Varion® SDG
Surfonic® NB-5	Teric LAN70	Tylorol 3S	Varonic® LI-42
Swanol AM-301	Texapon® A	Tylorol A	Varonic® LI-63
Swascol L-327	Texapon® A 400	Tylorol BS	Varonic® LI-67
Synotol 119 N	Texapon® DEA	Tylorol LM	Varonic® LI-67 (75%)
Synotol C-30	Texapon® EA-40	Tylorol LT50	Varox® 185E
Synotol CN 20	Texapon® ES-40	Tylorol MG	Varox® 270
Synotol CN 60	Texapon® EVR	Tylorol S	Varox® 365
Synotol CN 80	Texapon® K-12 Granules	Ufanon K-80	Varox® 743
Synotol CN 90	Texapon® K-12 Needles	Ufanon KD-S	Varox® 1770
Synotol Detergent E	Texapon® K-12 USP	Ufarol Am 30	Varsulf® S-1333
Synotol L 60	Texapon® K-14S 70	Ufarol Am 70	Varsulf® SBF-12
Synotol L 90	Special	Ufarol Na-30	Varsulf® SBFA-30
Synotol LM 60	Texapon® K-14S Spec	Ufasan 35	Varsulf® SBL-203
Synotol LM 90	Texapon® K-1294	Unamide® C-2	Velvetex® BA-35
Synotol ME 90	Texapon® K-1296 USP	Unamide® C-5	Velvetex® BC-35
Synperonic 3S27S	Texapon® L-100	Unamide® C-72-3	Velvetex® BK-35
Synperonic A2	Texapon® LS Highly Conc.	Unamide® CDX	Velvetex® CDC
Synperonic A3	Needles	Unamide® CMX	Velvetex® OLB-50
Synperonic A4	Texapon® MGLS	Unamide® D-10	Vifcoll CCN-40, CCN-40
Synperonic A6	Texapon® MLS	Unamide® J-56	Powd.
Synperonic A7	Texapon® N 40	Unamide® JJ-35	Wacker Silicone Antifoam
Synperonic A9	Texapon® N 70	Unamide® L-2	Agent S 184
Synperonic A11	Texapon® N 70-88	Unamide® L-5	Wacker Silicone Antifoam
Synperonic A20	Texapon® N 70 LS	Unamide® LDL	Emulsion SE 6
Synperonic A50	Texapon® NA	Unamide® LDX	Wickenol® 545
Synperonic NP1	Texapon® N Conc	Unamide® LMDX	Wickenol® 707
Synperonic NP10	Texapon® NSO	Unamide® N-72-3	Witcamide® 82
Synperonic NP12	Texapon® NT	Ungerol AM3-75	Witcamide® 128T
Synperonic NP13	Texapon® OT Highly Conc.	Ungerol LES 2-28	Witcamide® 5085
Synperonic NP15	Needles	Ungerol LES 2-70	Witcamide® 5133
Synperonic PE/L35	Texapon® PN-235	Ungerol LES 3-28	Witcamide® 5195
Synperonic T/1301	Texapon® SB-3	Ungerol LES 3-70	Witcamide® 6310
Synperonic T/1302	Texapon® SBN	Ungerol N2-28	Witcamide® 6511
Synprolam 35DMO	Texapon® SG	Ungerol N2-70	Witcamide® 6514
Synprolam 35MX1/O	Texapon® SH 100	Ungerol N3-28	Witcamide® 6531
Synprolam 35X2/O	Texapon® T	Ungerol N3-70	Witcamide® 6533
Syntopon A	Texapon® T 35	Unibetaine LB	Witcamide® 6546
Syntopon D	Texapon® T 42	Unibetaine OLB-30,	Witcamide® 6625
Syntopon F	Texapon® TH	OLB-50	Witcamide® C
Syntopon G	Texapon® VHC Needles	Unipol 7092	Witcamide® CD
T-11	Texapon® VHC Powd	Unipol MLS	Witcamide® CPA
T-18	Texapon® Z	Unisil DF-200S, DF-200SP	Witcamide® LDEA
T-20	Texapon® Z Granules	Unisil SF	Witcamide® LDTS
T-22	Texapon® ZHC Needles	Upamide L-2	Witcamide® NA
Tauranol I-78	Texapon® ZHC Powder	Upamide L-5	Witcamide® S771
Tauranol I-78-3	Thiovanol®	Upamide O-20	Witcamide® S780
Tauranol I-78-6	TIPA 99	Upamide SME-M	Witcamide® SSA
Tauranol I-78/80	TIPA 101	Vanseal® CS	Witcamide® STD-HP
Tauranol I-78E, I-78E	TIPA Low Freeze Grade	Vanseal® LS	Witco® Acid B
Flakes	Tohol N-220	Vanseal® MS	Witcodet 4680
Tauranol I-78 Flakes	Tohol N-220X	Vanseal® NACS-30	Witcodet AE
Tauranol M-35	Tohol N-230	Vanseal® NALS-30	Witcodet AEG

Detergents/Foaming Agents/Foam Boosters/Stabilizers *(cont'd.)*

Witcolate™ 1050	Witcolate™ LES-60C	Witconate™ 79S	Zetesol NL
Witcolate™ 3570	Witcolate™ NH	Witconate™ 90F H	Zetesol SE 35
Witcolate™ 6400	Witcolate™ S	Witconate™ 93S	Zoharpon LMT42
Witcolate™ 6430	Witcolate™ S1285C	Witconate™ 1240	Zohartaine AB
Witcolate™ 6431	Witcolate™ S1300C	Witconate™ 1250	Zohartaine CBS
Witcolate™ 6462	Witcolate™ T	Yucca Extract 50%	Zoharteric D
Witcolate™ A	Witcolate™ TLS-500	Zetesol 100	Zoharteric D-SF
Witcolate™ A Powder	Witcolate™ WAC	Zetesol 856	Zoharteric D-SF 70%
Witcolate™ AE-3	Witcolate™ WAC-GL	Zetesol 856 D	Zoharteric DJ
Witcolate™ AM	Witcolate™ WAC-LA	Zetesol 856 DT	Zoharteric D-SF/L
Witcolate™ C	Witconate™ 30DS	Zetesol 856 T	Zoharteric M
Witcolate™ ES-1	Witconate™ 45 Liq	Zetesol 2056	Zoramide CM
Witcolate™ ES-2	Witconate™ 45LX	Zetesol 2210	Zoramox
Witcolate™ ES-3	Witconate™ 60B	Zetesol AP	Zoramox E
Witcolate™ LCP	Witconate™ 60T	Zetesol MS	Zoramox LO
Witcolate™ LES-60A	Witconate™ 68KN		

Dispersants/Suspending Agents/Pigment Grinding Aids

Abil® Wax 9814	Acritamer® 941	Amerlate® P	Bentone® Gel LOI
Ablunol 200ML	Active #4	Amerlate® W	Bentone® Gel M20
Ablunol 200MO	ACumist™ B-6	Amerlate® WFA	Bentone® Gel MIO
Ablunol 200MS	ACumist™ B-12	Ameroxol® OE-2	Bentone® Gel MIO A-40
Ablunol 400ML	ACumist™ B-18	Amihope LL-11	Bentone® Gel SS71
Ablunol 400MO	ACumist™ C-5	Aminol CA-2	Bentone® Gel TN
Ablunol 400MS	ACumist™ C-9	AMP	Bentone® Gel TN A-40
Ablunol 600ML	ACumist™ C-12	Ampholan® U 203	Bentone® Gel VS-5
Ablunol 600MO	ACumist™ C-18	Amphoteen 24	Bentone® Gel VS-5 PC
Ablunol 600MS	Adinol OT16	Anhydrous Lanolin USP	Bentone® LT
Ablunol 1000MO	Adogen® 444	Cosmetic Grade	Bentone® MA
Ablunol 1000MS	Aerosil® 300	Anhydrous Lanolin USP	Bentone® SD-3
Ablunol LA-3	Aerosil® R812	Pharmaceutical Grade	Bernel® Ester 2014
Ablunol LA-5	Aerosol® A-102	Anhydrous Lanolin USP	Bio-Pol® NCHAP
Ablunol LA-7	Aerosol® OT-B	Pharmaceutical Light	Bio-Pol® OE
Ablunol LA-9	Ajicoat SPG	Grade	Biosil Basics Fluoro
Ablunol LA-12	Akypo RLM 45	Anhydrous Lanolin USP	Guerbet 1.0%
Ablunol LA-16	Akypo RLMQ 38	X-tra Deodorized	Biosil Basics Fluoro
Ablunol LA-40	Alcolec® BS	Antaron® FC-34	Guerbet 3.5%
Abluter CPB	Alcolec® Z-3	Antaron® WP-660	Biozan
A-C® 8, 8A	Aldosperse® ML-23	Antarox® L-64	Blanose 7 Types
A-C® 9, 9A, 9F	Aldosperse® MS-20	Antarox® PGP 23-7	Blanose 9 Types
A-C® 400A	Alkamide® DC-212	Aqualon® Cellulose Gum	Blanose 12 Types
A-C® 540, 540A	Alkamide® DS-280/S	Armeen® OD	Brij® 93
Accomeen T2	Alkamuls® 200-DL	Armeen® T	Britol® 6NF
Accomeen T5	Alkamuls® 200-DO	Armeen® Z	Britol® 7NF
Accomeen T15	Alkamuls® 400-DL	Armid® 18	Britol® 9NF
Acconon 200-DL	Alkamuls® 400-MO	Arosurf® 66-PE12	Britol® 20USP
Acconon 200-MS	Alkamuls® 400-MS	Arquad® 2C-75	Britol® 35USP
Acconon 400-DO	Alkamuls® 600-DL	Arquad® 2HT-75	Britol® 50USP
Acconon 400-ML	Alkamuls® 600-DO	Arquad® 12-33	Cab-O-Sil® L-90
Acconon 400-MO	Alkamuls® 600-MO	Arquad® 12-50	Cab-O-Sil® TS-530
Acconon 400-MS	Alkamuls® B	Arquad® 16-29	Capmul® GMO
Acconon 1300	Alkamuls® BR	Arquad® 16-50	Caprol® 10G10O
Acconon CA-5	Alkamuls® CO-15	Arquad® 18-50	Carbopol® 907
Acconon CA-8	Alkamuls® EL-620	Arquad® C-33	Carbopol® 910
Acconon CA-9	Alkamuls® EL-620L	Arquad® C-50	Carbopol® 934P
Acconon CA-15	Alkamuls® EL-719	Arquad® T-2C-50	Carbopol® 940
Acconon CA-25	Alkamuls® L-9	Arquad® T-27W	Carbopol® 954
Acconon CON	Alkasurf® L-14	Attasorb RVM Sorbent	Carbopol® 980
Acconon E	Alkasurf® NP-4	Benecel® M	Carbopol® 981
Acconon TGH	Alkasurf® NP-6	Benecel® ME	Carbopol® 1706
Acconon W230	Alkasurf® NP-40, 70%	Benecel® MP	Carbopol® 1720
Acrisint 400, 410, 430	Alkasurf® SA-20	Bentone® 27	Carbopol® 2984
Acritamer® 934	Amerchol L-101®	Bentone® EW	Carbopol® 5984
Acritamer® 934P	Amerchol® RC	Bentone® Gel IPM	Carbowax® Sentry® PEG
Acritamer® 940	Amerlate® LFA	Bentone® Gel ISD	300

Dispersants/Suspending Agents/Pigment Grinding Aids *(cont'd.)*

Carbowax® Sentry® PEG 400	Chemax E-400 MO	Crodesta F-110	Emalex 300 di-O
Carbowax® Sentry® PEG 540 Blend	Chemax E-600 ML	Crodesta F-160	Emalex 400A
Carbowax® Sentry® PEG 600	Chemax E-600 MO	Crodesta SL-40	Emalex 400B
Carbowax® Sentry® PEG 600	Chemax HCO-5	Crodet L4	Emalex 400 di-IS
Carbowax® Sentry® PEG 900	Chemax HCO-16	Crodet L8	Emalex 400 di-O
Carbowax® Sentry® PEG 1000	Chemax NP-1.5	Crodet L12	Emalex 503
Carbowax® Sentry® PEG 1450	Chemax NP-4	Crodet L24	Emalex 506
Carbowax® Sentry® PEG 3350	Chemax NP-6	Crodet L40	Emalex 508
Carbowax® Sentry® PEG 4600	Chemax NP-9	Crodet L100	Emalex 510
Carbowax® Sentry® PEG 8000	Chemax NP-10	Crodet S4	Emalex 512
Carsamide® CA	Chemax OP-5	Crodet S8	Emalex 515
Carsamide® SAC	Chemax OP-30/70	Crodet S12	Emalex 520
Carsoquat® SDQ-25	Chemax OP-40	Crodet S24	Emalex 523
Castorwax® MP-80	Chemeen C-2	Crodet S40	Emalex 550
Cedepon LA-30	Chemeen C-5	Crodet S100	Emalex 600 di-IS
Cedepon® LS-30PM	Chemeen C-10	Crovol A40	Emalex 600 di-O
Cellosize® HEC QP Grades	Chemeen C-15	Crovol M40	Emalex 602
Cellosize® HEC QP-3-L	Chimin BX	Crovol PK40	Emalex 603
Cellosize® HEC QP-40	Cithrol 2DL	Crovol PK70	Emalex 605
Cellosize® HEC QP-100 M-H	Cithrol 2DO	Crystal Crown LP	Emalex 606
Cellosize® HEC QP-300	Cithrol 2ML	Cyclochem® LVL	Emalex 608
Cellosize® HEC QP-4400-H	Cithrol 2MO	Damox® 1010	Emalex 611
Cellosize® HEC QP-15,000-H	Cithrol 4DL	Daxad® 30	Emalex 615
Cellosize® HEC QP-52,000-H	Cithrol 4DO	Daxad® 31	Emalex 620
Cellosize® HEC WP Grades	Cithrol 4ML	Demol EP	Emalex 625
Cellosize® Polymer PCG-10	Cithrol 4MO	Dermacryl™ 79	Emalex 630
Centrolex® P	Cithrol 6DL	Dermol 334	Emalex 640
Centrophase® HR	Cithrol 6DO	Dermol 489	Emalex 703
Ceraphyl® 140	Cithrol 6ML	Detergent CR	Emalex 705
Ceraphyl® 375	Cithrol 6MO	Diaformer® Z-W	Emalex 707
Ceraphyl® 791	Cithrol 10DL	Drewfax® 0007	Emalex 709
Ceraphyl® 847	Cithrol 10DO	Drewmulse® 3-1-O	Emalex 710
Ceraphyl® ICA	Cithrol 10ML	Drewmulse® 3-1-S	Emalex 712
Cerasynt® 303	Cithrol 10MO	Drewmulse® 6-2-S	Emalex 715
Cetiol® HE	Cithrol 40MO	Drewmulse® 10-10-O	Emalex 720
Chemal BP 261	Cithrol 60ML	Drewmulse® 10-10-S	Emalex 725
Chemal BP-262	Cithrol 60MO	Drewmulse® 10-4-O	Emalex 730
Chemal BP-262LF	Cithrol DGMS S/E	Drewmulse® 10-8-O	Emalex 750
Chemal BP-2101	Cithrol GDL N/E	Drewmulse® 900K	Emalex 805
Chemal LA-4	Cithrol GDL S/E	Drewmulse® POE-SML	Emalex 810
Chemal LA-9	Cithrol L, O Range	Drewmulse® POE-SMO	Emalex 820
Chemal LA-12	Cithrol S Range	Drewmulse® POE-SMS	Emalex 830
Chemal LA-23	Citmol™ 316	Drewmulse® POE-STS	Emalex 840
Chemal OA-4	Comperlan® P 100	Drewmulse® SML	Emalex 1605
Chemal OA-9	Corona Lanolin	Drewmulse® SMO	Emalex 1610
Chemal OA-20G	Coronet Lanolin	Drewmulse® SMS	Emalex 1615
Chemal TDA-6	CPH-43-N	Drewmulse® STS	Emalex 1620
Chemal TDA-9	Crill 1	Dulectin	Emalex 1625
Chemal TDA-12	Crill 2	Dur-Em® GMO	Emalex 1805
Chemax CO-16	Crill 4	Eastman® AQ 29D	Emalex 1810
Chemax E-200 ML	Crill 6	Eastman® AQ 35S	Emalex 1815
Chemax E-200 MO	Crill 43	Eastman® AQ 38D	Emalex 1820
Chemax E-400 ML	Crill 45	Eccowet® W-50	Emalex 1825
	Crill 50	Eccowet® W-88	Emalex 2405
	Crillet 1	Eldew CL-301	Emalex 2410
	Crillet 4	Emalex 102	Emalex 2415
	Crodalan AWS	Emalex 103	Emalex 2420
	Crodasinic LT40	Emalex 105	Emalex 2425
	Crodesta A10	Emalex 107	Emalex BHA-5
	Crodesta DKS F10	Emalex 110	Emalex BHA-10
	Crodesta DKS F20	Emalex 112	Emalex BHA-20
	Crodesta DKS F50	Emalex 115	Emalex BHA-30
	Crodesta DKS F70	Emalex 117	Emalex C-20
	Crodesta DKS F110	Emalex 120	Emalex C-30
	Crodesta DKS F140	Emalex 125	Emalex C-40
	Crodesta DKS F160	Emalex 130	Emalex C-50
	Crodesta F-10	Emalex 200 di-O	Emalex CS-5
	Crodesta F-50	Emalex 300 di-IS	Emalex CS-10

Dispersants/Suspending Agents/Pigment Grinding Aids *(cont'd.)*

Emalex CS-15	Emcol® CC-42	Etocas 15	Hetoxide C-40
Emalex CS-20	Emerest® 1723	Etocas 20	Hetoxide C-60
Emalex CS-24	Emerest® 2704	Etocas 29	Hetoxide C-200
Emalex CS-30	Emerest® 11723	Etocas 40	Hetoxide DNP-5
Emalex DEG-di-O	Emery® 1656	Etocas 50	Hetoxide DNP-10
Emalex DEG-m-S	Emery® 1660	Etocas 100	Hetoxide HC-16
Emalex EG-di-O	Emery® HP-2050	Eumulgin® PRT 36	Hetoxol M-3
Emalex EGS-A	Emery® HP-2060	Eumulgin® PRT 40	Hetoxol OA-3 Special
Emalex EGS-B	Emphos™ CS-1361	Eumulgin® PRT 56	Hetoxol OA-10 Special
Emalex GWIS-310	Empicol® 0185	Eumulgin® PRT 200	Hetoxol OA-20 Special
Emalex GWIS-320	Empigen® BB	Eumulgin® PWM2	Hetsulf 60T
Emalex GWIS-330	Empigen® BB-AU	Eumulgin® PWM17	Hetsulf Acid
Emalex GWO-310	Emsorb® 2721	Eutanol® G	Hetsulf IPA
Emalex GWO-320	Emsorb® 2722	Eutanol® G16	Hispagel® 100
Emalex GWO-330	Emthox® 5882	Fancol LA	Hispagel® 200
Emalex HC-5	Emthox® 5940	Fancol OA-95	Hodag CSA-80
Emalex HC-7	Emthox® 5941	Fancor IPL	Hodag Nonionic 2017-R
Emalex HC-10	Emthox® 5942	Fluilan	Hostapon KA Powd
Emalex LWIS-8	Emthox® 5964	Forlan C-24	Hostapon SO
Emalex LWIS-10	Emthox® 6957	Forlan L	Hostapon T Paste 33
Emalex NP-2	Emthox® 6962	Gafac® RE-877	Hydroxylan
Emalex NP-3	Emthox® 6971	Ganex® P-904	Igepal® DM-970 FLK
Emalex NP-5	Emthox® 6972	Ganex® V-216	Imwitor® 191
Emalex NP-10	Emthox® 6984	Ganex® V-220	Imwitor® 742
Emalex NP-11	Emulmetik™ 120	Gantrez® AN	Imwitor® 900
Emalex NP-12	Emulsogen OG	Geltone	Imwitor® 900 K
Emalex NP-13	Epikuron H	Geltone 1665	Imwitor® 914
Emalex NP-15	ES-1239	Geltone II	Imwitor® 928
Emalex NP-20	Estalan 635	Generol® 122E25	Imwitor® 940
Emalex NP-25	Ethoduomeen® T/20	Genugel	Imwitor® 940 K
Emalex NP-30	Ethofat® 60/15	Genulacta Series	Imwitor® 960
Emalex OD-5	Ethofat® 60/20	Genuvisco	Imwitor® 965
Emalex OD-10	Ethofat® 60/25	Geronol ACR/4	Imwitor® 965 K
Emalex OD-16	Ethofat® 142/20	Geronol ACR/9	Imwitor® 988
Emalex OD-20	Ethofat® 242/25	Geropon® AB/20	Incroquat SDQ-25
Emalex OD-25	Ethofat® C/15	Geropon® ACR/9	Intravon® JU
Emalex OP-5	Ethofat® C/25	Geropon® AS-200	Ionet S-20
Emalex OP-8	Ethofat® O/15	Geropon® AS-250	Ionet S-60 C
Emalex OP-10	Ethofat® O/20	Geropon® SS-TA	Ionet S-80
Emalex OP-15	Ethomeen® 18/12	Geropon® TC-42	Ionet S-85
Emalex OP-20	Ethomeen® 18/15	Glo-Mul 4001	Ionet T-20 C
Emalex OP-25	Ethomeen® 18/20	Glo-Mul 4007	Ionet T-60 C
Emalex OP-30	Ethomeen® 18/25	Glucate® DO	Ionet T-80 C
Emalex OP-40	Ethomeen® 18/60	Glycosperse® L-20	Ivarbase™ 101
Emalex OP-50	Ethomeen® C/12	Glycosperse® O-5	Ivarlan™ Light
Emalex PEIS-3	Ethomeen® C/15	Glycosperse® O-20	Jaguar® HP 8
Emalex PEIS-6	Ethomeen® C/20	Glycosperse® O-20 Veg	Jaguar® HP 60
Emalex PEIS-12	Ethomeen® C/25	Glycosperse® O-20X	Jaguar® HP 120
Emalex PEIS-20	Ethomeen® O/12	Glycosperse® P-20	Junlon PW-110
Emalex RWIS-105	Ethomeen® O/15	Glycosperse® S-20	Junlon PW-111
Emalex RWIS-110	Ethomeen® O/25	Glycosperse® TO-20	Keltrol®, Keltrol F
Emalex RWIS-115	Ethomeen® S/12	Glycosperse® TS-20	Kessco® Glycerol
Emalex RWIS-305	Ethomeen® S/15	Gomme Xanthane	Monooleate
Emalex RWIS-310	Ethomeen® S/20	GP-209	Kessco® PEG 200 DL
Emalex RWIS-315	Ethomeen® S/25	GP-218	Kessco® PEG 200 DO
Emalex RWIS-320	Ethomeen® T/12	GP-226	Kessco® PEG 200 DS
Emalex RWL-120	Ethomeen® T/15	Hartolan	Kessco® PEG 200 ML
Emalex RWL-130	Ethomeen® T/25	Hectabrite® AW	Kessco® PEG 200 MO
Emalex SWS-9	Ethomeen® T/60	Hectabrite® DP	Kessco® PEG 200 MS
Emalex SWS-10	Ethomeen® TD/15	Hectalite® 200	Kessco® PEG 300 DL
Emalex SWS-12	Ethomeen® TD/25	Hetester HSS	Kessco® PEG 300 DO
Emalex TEG-di-O	Ethomid® HT/15	Hetester TICC	Kessco® PEG 300 DS
Emcol® 4100M	Ethomid® HT/23	Hetoxide BN-13	Kessco® PEG 300 ML
Emcol® 4161L	Ethomid® O/15	Hetoxide C-2	Kessco® PEG 300 MO
Emcol® 4300	Ethomid® O/17	Hetoxide C-9	Kessco® PEG 300 MS
Emcol® 4500	Ethoxylan® 1685	Hetoxide C-15	Kessco® PEG 400 DL
Emcol® CC-9	Ethoxylan® 1686	Hetoxide C-25	Kessco® PEG 400 DO
Emcol® CC-36	Etocas 5	Hetoxide C-30	Kessco® PEG 400 DS

Dispersants/Suspending Agents/Pigment Grinding Aids *(cont'd.)*

Kessco® PEG 400 ML	Lipopeg 4-DL	Macol® CSA-40	Mapeg® 400 DS
Kessco® PEG 400 MO	Lipopeg 4-DO	Macol® CSA-50	Mapeg® 400 ML
Kessco® PEG 400 MS	Lipopeg 4-DS	Macol® DNP-5	Mapeg® 400 MO
Kessco® PEG 600 DL	Lipopeg 4-L	Macol® DNP-10	Mapeg® 400 MOT
Kessco® PEG 600 DO	Lipopeg 4-S	Macol® DNP-15	Mapeg® 400 MS
Kessco® PEG 600 DS	Lipopeg 6-L	Macol® DNP-21	Mapeg® 600 DL
Kessco® PEG 600 ML	Lipopeg 10-S	Macol® LA-4	Mapeg® 600 DO
Kessco® PEG 600 MO	Lipopeg 15-S	Macol® LA-9	Mapeg® 600 DOT
Kessco® PEG 600 MS	Lipopeg 100-S	Macol® LA-12	Mapeg® 600 DS
Kessco® PEG 1000 DL	Lipopeg 6000-DS	Macol® LA-23	Mapeg® 600 ML
Kessco® PEG 1000 DO	Liquid Absorption Base	Macol® LA-790	Mapeg® 600 MO
Kessco® PEG 1000 DS	Type A, T	Macol® NP-4	Mapeg® 600 MOT
Kessco® PEG 1000 ML	Lonzest® PEG 4-L	Macol® NP-5	Mapeg® 600 MS
Kessco® PEG 1000 MO	Lowenol 710	Macol® NP-6	Mapeg® 1000 MS
Kessco® PEG 1000 MS	Lowenol C-243	Macol® NP-8	Mapeg® 1500 MS
Kessco® PEG 1540 DL	Lutensol® FA 12	Macol® NP-11	Mapeg® 1540 DS
Kessco® PEG 1540 DO	Luviskol® K12	Macol® NP-12	Mapeg® 6000 DS
Kessco® PEG 1540 DS	Luviskol® K17	Macol® NP-15	Mapeg® CO-16
Kessco® PEG 1540 ML	Luviskol® K30	Macol® NP-20	Mapeg® CO-16H
Kessco® PEG 1540 MO	Luviskol® K60	Macol® NP-20(70)	Mapeg® EGDS
Kessco® PEG 1540 MS	Luviskol® K80	Macol® NP-30(70)	Mapeg® EGMS
Kessco® PEG 4000 DL	Luviskol® K90	Macol® NP-100	Mapeg® EGMS-K
Kessco® PEG 4000 DO	Luviskol® LD-9025	Macol® OA-2	Mapeg® S-40
Kessco® PEG 4000 DS	Luviskol® VA28E	Macol® OA-4	Mapeg® TAO-15
Kessco® PEG 4000 ML	Luviskol® VA28I	Macol® OA-5	Marlipal® 24/300
Kessco® PEG 4000 MO	Luviskol® VA37E	Macol® OA-10	Marlipal® 1618/11
Kessco® PEG 4000 MS	Luviskol® VA37I	Macol® OA-20	Marlowet® G 12 DO
Kessco® PEG 6000 DL	Luviskol® VA55E	Macol® OP-3	Marlowet® GDO 4
Kessco® PEG 6000 DO	Luviskol® VA55I	Macol® OP-5	Mazamide® L-298
Kessco® PEG 6000 DS	Luviskol® VA64E	Macol® OP-8	Mazamide® O 20
Kessco® PEG 6000 ML	Luviskol® VA64I	Macol® OP-10	Mazol® 300 K
Kessco® PEG 6000 MO	Luviskol® VA64W	Macol® OP-10 SP	Mazol® GMO
Kessco® PEG 6000 MS	Luviskol® VA73E	Macol® OP-12	Mazol® GMO K
Klucel® EF	Luviskol® VA73I	Macol® OP-16(75)	Merpol® HCS
Klucel® ELF, GF, HF, JF,	Luviskol® VA73W	Macol® OP-30(70)	Methocel® 40-100
LF, MF	Macol® 1	Macol® OP-40(70)	Methocel® 40-101
Koster Keunen Hydroxy-	Macol® 2	Macol® SA-2	Methocel® 40-202
Polyester	Macol® 2D	Macol® SA-5	Methocel® A4CP
Lan-Aqua-Sol 50	Macol® 2LF	Macol® SA-10	Methocel® A4MP
Lan-Aqua-Sol 100	Macol® 4	Macol® SA-15	Methocel® A15LVP
Lanfrax® 1779	Macol® 8	Macol® SA-20	Methocel® E3P
Lanogel® 21	Macol® 10	Macol® SA-40	Methocel® E4MP
Lanogel® 31	Macol® 16	Macol® TD-3	Methocel® E6P
Lanogel® 41	Macol® 22	Macol® TD-8	Methocel® E15LVP
Lanogel® 61	Macol® 23	Macol® TD-10	Methocel® E50LVP
Lanpol 5	Macol® 27	Macol® TD-12	Methocel® E50P
Lanpol 10	Macol® 31	Macol® TD-15	Methocel® K4MP
Lanpol 20	Macol® 32	Macol® TD-100	Methocel® K4MS
Lantrol® 1673	Macol® 33	Macol® TD-610	Methocel® K15MP
Lantrol® 1674	Macol® 34	Mafo® CAB	Methocel® K15MS
Lantrol® 1674 Deodorized	Macol® 35	Magnabrite® F	Methocel® K100LVP
Lantrol® HP-2073	Macol® 40	Magnabrite® FS	Methocel® K100MP
Lantrol® HP-2074	Macol® 42	Magnabrite® HS	Miglyol® 810
Laponite® XLG	Macol® 44	Magnabrite® HV	Miglyol® 812
Laponite® XLS	Macol® 46	Magnabrite® K	Miglyol® 829
Lexemul® EGMS	Macol® 72	Magnabrite® S	Miglyol® 840
Lexemul® PEG-400ML	Macol® 77	Maltrin® M510	Miranol® DM
Lipo DGLS	Macol® 85	Maltrin® QD M550	Miranol® HM Conc
Lipo DGS-SE	Macol® 88	Mapeg® 200 DL	Miranol® OM-SF Conc
Lipo EGDS	Macol® 101	Mapeg® 200 DO	Mirataine® CBC
Lipocol B	Macol® 108	Mapeg® 200 DS	Mirataine® CB/M
Lipocol TD-3	Macol® CA-2	Mapeg® 200 ML	Mirataine® H2C-HA
Lipocol TD-6	Macol® CA-10	Mapeg® 200 MO	Monateric CA-35
Lipocol TD-12	Macol® CSA-2	Mapeg® 200 MOT	Monateric CEM-38
Lipolan R	Macol® CSA-4	Mapeg® 200 MS	Monawet MO-70
Liponic EG-1	Macol® CSA-10	Mapeg® 400 DL	Monawet MO-70R
Lipopeg 2-DL	Macol® CSA-15	Mapeg® 400 DO	Monawet SNO-35
Lipopeg 2-L	Macol® CSA-20	Mapeg® 400 DOT	Monomuls® 60-10

Dispersants/Suspending Agents/Pigment Grinding Aids *(cont'd.)*

Monomuls® 60-15
Monomuls® 60-20
Monomuls® 60-25
Monomuls® 60-25/2
Monomuls® 60-30
Monomuls® 60-35
Monomuls® 60-40
Monomuls® 60-45
Monomuls® 90-10
Monomuls® 90-15
Monomuls® 90-20
Monomuls® 90-25/2,
  90-25/5
Monomuls® 90-30
Monomuls® 90-35
Monomuls® 90-40
Monomuls® 90-45
Montosol PG-17
M-P-A® 14
Myvatem® 06K
Myvatem® 30
Myvatem® 35K
Myvatem® 92K
Natrosol® Plus CS,
  Grade 330
Naturechem® PGHS
Naturechem® PGR
Naxonic™ NI-40
Naxonic™ NI-60
Naxonic™ NI-100
Naxonol™ PO
Neodol® 25-7
Neodol® 25-9
Neodol® 25-12
Nikkol BC-23
Nikkol BC-25TX
Nikkol BC-30TX
Nikkol BC-40TX
Nikkol BD-2
Nikkol BD-4
Nikkol BD-10
Nikkol BO-10TX
Nikkol BO-15TX
Nikkol BPS-5
Nikkol BPS-10
Nikkol BPS-15
Nikkol BPS-20
Nikkol BPS-25
Nikkol BPS-30
Nikkol BPSH-25
Nikkol BS-20
Nikkol DDP-2
Nikkol DDP-4
Nikkol DDP-6
Nikkol DDP-8
Nikkol DDP-10
Nikkol Decaglyn 1-IS
Nikkol Decaglyn 1-L
Nikkol Decaglyn 1-LN
Nikkol Decaglyn 1-M
Nikkol Decaglyn 1-O
Nikkol Decaglyn 1-S
Nikkol Decaglyn 2-IS
Nikkol DLP-10
Nikkol Hexaglyn 1-S
Nikkol OTP-75
Nikkol OTP-100
Nikkol OTP-100S

Nikkol PBC-31
Nikkol PBC-33
Nikkol PBC-34
Nikkol PBC-41
Nikkol PBC-44
Nikkol PMS-1C
Nikkol PMS-1CSE
Nikkol TCP-5
Nikkol TDP-2
Nikkol TDP-4
Nikkol TDP-6
Nikkol TDP-8
Nikkol TDP-10
Nikkol TI-10
Nikkol TL-10, TL-10EX
Nikkol TLP-4
Nikkol TMGO-5
Nikkol TMGO-15
Nikkol TMGS-5
Nikkol TMGS-15
Nikkol TO-10
Nikkol TO-10M
Nikkol TP-10
Nikkol TS-10
Niox KI Series
Niox KJ-10
Nissan Nonion E-205
Nissan Nonion E-206
Nissan Nonion E-208
Nissan Nonion E-215
Nissan Nonion E-220
Nissan Nonion E-230
Nissan Nonion K-202
Nissan Nonion K-203
Nissan Nonion K-204
Nissan Nonion K-207
Nissan Nonion K-211
Nissan Nonion K-215
Nissan Nonion K-220
Nissan Nonion K-230
Nissan Nonion P-208
Nissan Nonion P-210
Nissan Nonion P-213
Nissan Nonion S-206
Nissan Nonion S-207
Nissan Nonion S-215
Nissan Nonion S-220
Nissan Persoft SK
Nopalcol Series
Norfox® NP-4
Novol
Noxamine CA 30
OHlan®
Onyxol® 336
OP-2000
Orange Wax
Ovonol
Ovothin 170
Ovothin 180
Ovothin 200
Peceol Isostearique
Pecosil® PS-100
Pegosperse® 50 DS
Pegosperse® 200 DL
Pegosperse® 200 ML
Pegosperse® 400 DOT
Pegosperse® 400 DS
Pegosperse® 400 ML

Pegosperse® 600 DOT
Pegosperse® 600 ML
Pegosperse® 1750 MS
Pegosperse® 6000 DS
Pegosperse® EGMS-70
Phosal® 50 PG
PhosPho 642
PhosPho E-100
Phospholipid PTD
Phospholipid PTL
Phospholipid PTZ
Phytotec Astringent
Plasdone® K-25, K-90
Plasdone® K-26/28,
  K-29/32
Pluracol® E400
Pluracol® E400 NF
Pluracol® E600
Pluracol® E600 NF
Pluracol® E1000
Pluracol® E1450
Pluracol® E1450 NF
Pluracol® E2000
Pluracol® E4000 NF
Pluracol® E4500
Pluracol® E8000
Pluracol® E8000 NF
Plurio® E 1500
Pluronic® 10R5
Pluronic® 10R8
Pluronic® 12R3
Pluronic® 17R1
Pluronic® 17R2
Pluronic® 17R4
Pluronic® 17R8
Pluronic® 22R4
Pluronic® 25R1
Pluronic® 25R2
Pluronic® 25R4
Pluronic® 25R5
Pluronic® 25R8
Pluronic® 31R1
Pluronic® 31R2
Pluronic® 31R4
Pluronic® F38
Pluronic® F68
Pluronic® F68LF
Pluronic® F77
Pluronic® F87
Pluronic® F88
Pluronic® F98
Pluronic® F108
Pluronic® F127
Pluronic® L10
Pluronic® L35
Pluronic® L42
Pluronic® L43
Pluronic® L44
Pluronic® L61
Pluronic® L62
Pluronic® L62D
Pluronic® L62LF
Pluronic® L63
Pluronic® L64
Pluronic® L72
Pluronic® L81
Pluronic® L92
Pluronic® L101

Pluronic® L121
Pluronic® L122
Pluronic® P65
Pluronic® P75
Pluronic® P84
Pluronic® P85
Pluronic® P94
Pluronic® P103
Pluronic® P104
Pluronic® P105
Pluronic® P123
Polargel® HV
Polargel® NF
Polargel® T
Polawax®
Polychol 5
Polychol 10
Polychol 15
Polychol 16
Polychol 20
Polychol 40
Polylan®
Probutyl 14
Procetyl AWS
Progacyl® COS-10
Propoxyol® 1695
Provol 10
Provol 30
Provol 50
Prox-onic CSA-1/04
Prox-onic CSA-1/06
Prox-onic CSA-1/010
Prox-onic CSA-1/015
Prox-onic CSA-1/020
Prox-onic CSA-1/030
Prox-onic CSA-1/050
Prox-onic HR-05
Prox-onic HR-016
Prox-onic HR-025
Prox-onic HR-030
Prox-onic HR-036
Prox-onic HR-040
Prox-onic HR-080
Prox-onic HR-0200
Prox-onic HR-0200/50
Prox-onic HRH-05
Prox-onic HRH-016
Prox-onic HRH-025
Prox-onic HRH-0200
Prox-onic HRH-0200/50
Prox-onic NP-1.5
Prox-onic NP-04
Prox-onic NP-06
Prox-onic NP-09
Prox-onic NP-010
Prox-onic NP-015
Prox-onic NP-020
Prox-onic NP-030
Prox-onic NP-030/70
Prox-onic NP-040
Prox-onic NP-040/70
Prox-onic NP-050
Prox-onic NP-050/70
Prox-onic NP-0100
Prox-onic NP-0100/70
Puxol CB-22
Pyroter GPI-25
Querton 16Cl-29

Dispersants/Suspending Agents/Pigment Grinding Aids *(cont'd.)*

Querton 16Cl-50
Quso® G27, G29, G35, G38, WR55, WR83
Quso® WR55-FG
Radiasurf® 7196
Radiasurf® 7206
Radiasurf® 7269
Radiasurf® 7270
Radiasurf® 7402
Radiasurf® 7403
Radiasurf® 7404
Radiasurf® 7411
Radiasurf® 7413
Radiasurf® 7414
Radiasurf® 7417
Radiasurf® 7420
Radiasurf® 7422
Radiasurf® 7423
Radiasurf® 7431
Radiasurf® 7432
Radiasurf® 7443
Radiasurf® 7453
Radiasurf® 7454
Rehydragel® Compressed Gel
Remcopal 334
Renex® 20
Renex® 36
Rewomat B 2003
Rewopal® C 6
Rexol AE-23
Rexonic N91-6
Rexonic N91-8
Rhaballgum CG-M
Rhodacal® 301-10F
Rhodacal® 330
Rhodacal® A-246L
Rhodafac® RE-870
Rhodapex® CO-433
Rhodapex® CO-436
Rhodapex® EST-30
Rhodapon® LM
Rhodasurf® L-4
Rhodasurf® ON-870
Rhodicare™ D
Rhodicare™ H
Rhodicare™ S
Rhodicare™ SC-225
Rhodicare™ XC
Rhodigel®
Rhodigel® 23
Rhodigel® 200
Rhodigel® EZ
Ritahydrox
Ritalafa®
Ritavena™ 5
Ritawax AEO
Rudol®
Ryoto Sugar Ester B-370
Ryoto Sugar Ester L-595
Ryoto Sugar Ester L-1570
Ryoto Sugar Ester L-1695
Ryoto Sugar Ester M-1695
Ryoto Sugar Ester O-1570
Ryoto Sugar Ester P-1570
Ryoto Sugar Ester P-1670
Ryoto Sugar Ester S-1170
Ryoto Sugar Ester S-1170S

Ryoto Sugar Ester S-1570
Ryoto Sugar Ester S-1670
Salcare SC90
Salcare SC91
Salcare SC92
Salcare SC95
Santone® 10-10-O
Sanwet® COS-960
Sanwet® COS-965
Schercemol DEIS
Schercemol DID
Schercemol IDO
Schercemol OP
Schercomid AME
Schercomid AME-70
Schercomid CCD
Schercomid HT-60
Schercomid ODA
Schercomid SLS
Schercomid TO-2
Schercozoline B
Schercozoline C
Sericite WL
Silwet® L-77
Silwet® L-7001
Silwet® L-7002
Silwet® L-7500
Silwet® L-7602
Silwet® L-7604
Silwet® L-7614
Siponic® NP-7
S-Maz® 83R
Solulan® 5
Solulan® 16
Solulan® 25
Solulan® 75
Solulan® 97
Solulan® 98
Solulan® C-24
Solulan® L-575
Solulan® PB-2
Solulan® PB-5
Solulan® PB-10
Solulan® PB-20
Sorbon S-20
Sorbon S-40
Sorbon S-60
Sorbon S-66
Sorbon S-80
Sorbon T-20
Sorbon T-40
Sorbon T-60
Sorbon T-80
Special Oil 619
Spinomar NaSS
Spreading Agent ET0672
Stamere®
Standamid® KDM
Standamul® CTA
Standamul® CTV
Standamul® G
Standapol® A
Standapol® SCO
Standapol® WAQ-LC
Steol® CA-460
Stepanol® WA-100
Stepan TAB®-2
Sulfochem ALS

Sulfochem SLN
Sulfochem SLP
Sulfochem SLP-95
Sulfochem SLS
Sulfopon® P-40
Sulframin 1288
Sulframin 1298
Sulframin 1388
Super Hartolan
Superloid®
Supralate C
Surfactol® 13
Surfax 100
Surfax 100 AG
Surfax CN
Surfine WNT Conc
Surfine WNT LC
Surfonic® N-10
Surfonic® N-31.5
Surfonic® N-40
Surfonic® N-60
Surfonic® N-85
Surfonic® N-95
Surfonic® N-100
Surfonic® N-102
Surfonic® N-120
Surfonic® N-130
Surfonic® N-150
Surfonic® N-200
Surfonic® N-300
Surfonic® NB-5
Suspengel Elite
Suspengel Micro
Suspengel Ultra
Suspentone
Suspentone 1265
Swanol AM-301
Syncrowax BB-4
Syncrowax ERL-C
Syncrowax HGL-C
Syncrowax HR-C
Syncrowax HRS-C
Synperonic A20
Synperonic A50
Synperonic NP10
Synperonic NP12
Synperonic NP13
Synperonic NP15
Synperonic PE/F87
Synperonic PE/F127
Synperonic PE/L35
Synperonic T/1301
Synperonic T/1302
Tagat® I
Tagat® I2
Tagat® L
Tagat® L2
Tagat® O
Tagat® O2
Tagat® RI
Tagat® S
Tagat® S2
Tagat® TO
Tamol® 731-25%
Tauranol I-78
Tauranol I-78-3
Tauranol I-78-6
Tauranol I-78/80

Tauranol I-78E, I-78E Flakes
Tauranol I-78 Flakes
Tauranol ML
Tensopol A 79
Tensopol A 795
Tensopol ACL 79
Tergitol® NP-9
Teric 12A3
Teric LAN70
Tetronic® 50R1
Tetronic® 50R4
Tetronic® 50R8
Tetronic® 70R1
Tetronic® 70R2
Tetronic® 70R4
Tetronic® 90R1
Tetronic® 90R4
Tetronic® 90R8
Tetronic® 110R1
Tetronic® 110R2
Tetronic® 110R7
Tetronic® 130R1
Tetronic® 130R2
Tetronic® 150R1
Tetronic® 150R4
Tetronic® 150R8
Tetronic® 304
Tetronic® 504
Tetronic® 701
Tetronic® 702
Tetronic® 704
Tetronic® 707
Tetronic® 901
Tetronic® 904
Tetronic® 908
Tetronic® 909
Tetronic® 1101
Tetronic® 1102
Tetronic® 1104
Tetronic® 1107
Tetronic® 1301
Tetronic® 1302
Tetronic® 1304
Tetronic® 1307
Tetronic® 1501
Tetronic® 1502
Tetronic® 1504
Tetronic® 1508
Texapon® K-12 USP
Texapon® K-1296 USP
Texapon® L-100
Texapon® VHC Powd
Texapon® Z
Texapon® Z Granules
Texapon® ZHC Needles
Ticalose 15, 30, 75, 150R, 1200, 2000R, 2500, 4000, 4500, 5000R
Tixogel VP
T-Maz® 20
T-Maz® 28
T-Maz® 40
T-Maz® 60
T-Maz® 61
T-Maz® 65
T-Maz® 80
T-Maz® 80KLM

Dispersants/Suspending Agents/Pigment Grinding Aids *(cont'd.)*

T-Maz® 81	MHB-y, MHB-yp	Volpo 25 D 15	Volpo T-20
T-Maz® 85	Ultra Lantrol® HP-2074	Volpo 25 D 20	White Swan
T-Maz® 90	Unilin® 350 Alcohol	Volpo CS-3	Wickenol® 155
T-Maz® 95	Unilin® 550 Alcohol	Volpo CS-5	Wickenol® 156
Trimol CE 2000	Unilin® 700 Alcohol	Volpo CS-10	Wickenol® 158
Triton® X-100	Varisoft® BT-85	Volpo CS-15	Wickenol® 159
Trivent NP-13	Varonic® K-210	Volpo CS-20	Wickenol® 160
Trivent OC-G	Varonic® LI-48	Volpo L4	Wickenol® 161
Trivent SS-20	Veegum®	Volpo N3	Wickenol® 171
Trycol® 5972	Veegum® D	Volpo N5	Witafrol® 7420
Trylox® 6746	Veegum® F	Volpo N10	Witcamide® 82
Tween® 21	Veegum® HS	Volpo N15	Witcamide® 5133
Tween® 40	Veegum® HV	Volpo N20	Witcamide® 5195
Tween® 60	Veegum® K	Volpo O3	Witcamide® 6533
Tween® 61	Veegum® PRO	Volpo O5	Witcamine® 6606
Tween® 65	Veegum® Ultra	Volpo O10	Witcamine® 6622
Tween® 80	Veegum® WG	Volpo O15	Witco® Acid B
Tween® 81	Volclay® NF-BC	Volpo O20	Witcolate™ 6462
Tween® 85	Volclay® NF-ID	Volpo T-3	Witconate™ 79S
Tylose® MH Grades	Volpo 25 D 3	Volpo T-5	Witconate™ 93S
Tylose® MHB	Volpo 25 D 5	Volpo T-10	Yeoman
Tylose® MH-K, MH-xp,	Volpo 25 D 10	Volpo T-15	Zoharpon LMT42

Emollients/Conditioners/Softeners/Skin Protectants/ Refatting and Superfatting Agents

AA USP	A-C® 6A	Adol® 66	Alfol® 1618
Abil® 10-10000	A-C® 8, 8A	Adol® 80	Alfol® 1618 CG
Abil® AV 20-1000	A-C® 9, 9A, 9F	Adol® 85	Alfol® 1618 GC
Abil® AV 8853	A-C® 15	Adol® 90	Alkamide® 1188
Abil® B 8	A-C® 16	Adol® 90 NF	Alkamide® 1195
Abil® B 8839	A-C® 143	Adol® 320, 330, 340	Alkamide® DL-203/S
Abil® B 8842	A-C® 400	Adol® 520 NF	Alkamide® DL-207/S
Abil® B 8843	A-C® 430	Adol® 620 NF	Alkamide® DO-280/S
Abil® B 8851	A-C® 540, 540A	Adol® 630	Alkamide® DS-280/S
Abil® B 8852	A-C® 580	Adol® 640	Alkamide® L7DE
Abil® B 8873	A-C® 617, 617A	Aethoxal® B	Alkamide® L7DE-PG
Abil® B 9800, B 9801	A-C® 617G	Afalene™ 117	Alkamide® S-280
Abil® B 9806, B 9808	A-C® 1702	Afalene™ 216	Alkamide® SDO
Abil® B 9808	Acconon CA 10	Afalene™ 416	Alkamox® L20
Abil® B 9905, B 9907, B	Acconon MA3	Afalene™ 716	Alkamuls® EL-620L
9908, B 9909	Acetadeps	Afalene™ AFC	Alkamuls® GMS/C
Abil® B 9950	Acetol® 1706	Akypo RLM 45	Alkamuls® LVL
Abil® B 88183	Acetulan®	Albalan	Alkamuls® MM/M
Abil® EM-90	Actiglow™	Alcolan®	Alkamuls® MST
Abil® K 4	Actiglow™ C	Alcolan® 36W	Alkamuls® SDG
Abil® OSW 12, OSW 13	Actiquat™	Alcolec® BS	Alkamuls® SS
Abil®-Quat 3270	Acylan	Alcolec® PG	Alkateric® PB
Abil®-Quat 3272	Acylglutamate CS-11	Alconate® SBG-280	Almolan HL
Abil®-Wax 2434	Acylglutamate CS-21	Aldo® HMS	Almond Oil
Abil®-Wax 2440	Acylglutamate CT-12	Aldo® MS LG	Almondermin®
Abil®-Wax 9800	Acylglutamate GS-11	Aldo® PMS	Amerchol® 400
Abil®-Wax 9801	Acylglutamate HS-11	Aldo® TC	Amerchol® BL
Abil® Wax 9814	Acylglutamate LS-11	Alfol® 16	Amerchol® C
Ablumide CME	Acylglutamate LT-12	Alfol® 18	Amerchol® CAB
Ablumide LDE	Acylglutamate MS-11	Alfol® 22+	Amerchol® H-9
Ablumine 18	Admox® 1214	Alfol® 1012 HA	Amerchol® L-99
Ablumine 280	Adogen® MA-108 SF	Alfol® 1014 CDC	Amerchol L-101®
Ablumine 1618	Adogen® MA-112 SF	Alfol® 1214	Amerchol® L-500
Ablumine TMC	Adogen® S-18 V	Alfol® 1214 GC	Amerlate® LFA
Ablumox CAPO	Adol® 52 NF	Alfol® 1216	Amerlate® P
Ablumox LO	Adol® 60	Alfol® 1216 CO	Amerlate® W
Ablunol 200MS	Adol® 61	Alfol® 1218 DCBA	Amersil® VS-7158
Ablunol 400MS	Adol® 61 NF	Alfol® 1412	Amersil® VS-7207
Ablunol 600MS	Adol® 62 NF	Alfol® 1416 GC	Amersil® VS-7349
Ablusol LAE	Adol® 63	Alfol® 1418 DDB	Amfotex FV-28
Abluter DCM-2	Adol® 64	Alfol® 1418 GBA	Amidex AME

Emollients/Conditioners/Softeners... *(cont'd.)*

Amidex CIPA
Amidex LN
Amidex O
Amidex RC
Amifat P-21
Amifat P-30
Amino-Collagen-25, -40
Aminodermin CLR
Aminofoam C
Amino Gluten MG
Aminol KDE
Aminoxid WS 35
Amisoft CS-11
Amisoft CT-12
Amisoft GS-11
Amisoft HS-11
Amisoft LS-11
Amisoft MS-11
Amiter LGS-2
Amiter LGS-5
Ammonyx® 4, 4B, 485, 4002
Ammonyx® CA-Special
Ammonyx® CDO
Ammonyx® CETAC, CETAC-30
Ammonyx® KP
Ammonyx® LKP
Ammonyx® LO
Ammonyx® MCO
Ammonyx® MO
Ammonyx® SO
Amojell Petrolatum Amber, Dark, Snow White
Ampholak 7TX
Ampholak 7TX/C
Ampholak 7TX-SD 55
Ampholak 7TX-T
Ampholak XO7
Ampholak XO7/C
Ampholak XTP
Amphosol® CA
Amphosol® DM
Amyx A-25-S 0040
Amyx CDO 3599
Amyx CO 3764
Amyx SO 3734
Anhydrous Lanolin Grade 1
Anhydrous Lanolin Grade 2
Anhydrous Lanolin HP-2050
Anhydrous Lanolin P.80
Anhydrous Lanolin P.95
Anhydrous Lanolin P.95RA
Anhydrous Lanolin Superfine
Anhydrous Lanolin USP Cosmetic
Anhydrous Lanolin USP Cosmetic AA
Anhydrous Lanolin USP Cosmetic Grade
Anhydrous Lanolin USP Deodorized AAA
Anhydrous Lanolin USP Pharmaceutical
Anhydrous Lanolin USP

Pharmaceutical Grade
Anhydrous Lanolin USP Pharmaceutical Light Grade
Anhydrous Lanolin USP Superfine
Anhydrous Lanolin USP Ultrafine
Anhydrous Lanolin USP X-tra Deodorized
Annonyx SO
Antaron® FC-34
Antil® 208
Aqualose L30
Aqualose L75
Aqualose L75/50
Aqualose L100
Aqualose LL100
Aqualose SLT
Aqualose SLW
Aqualose W5
Aqualose W20
Aqualose W20/50
Aquaphil K
Aqua-Tein C
Aqua-Tein S
Argobase 125
Argobase EU
Argobase L1
Argobase L2
Argobase MS 5
Argobase S1
Argonol 1SO
Argonol 40
Argonol 50
Argonol 50 Pharmaceutical
Argonol 50 Super
Argonol 60
Argonol ACE 5
Argonol ACE 6
Argonol LFA Dist
Argonol RIC2
Argowax Cosmetic Super
Argowax Dist
Argowax LFA Distilled
Argowax LFA Standard
Argowax Standard
Arlacel® 989
Arlamol® 801
Arlamol® D4
Arlamol® DOA
Arlamol® E
Arlamol® F
Arlamol® GM
Arlamol® HD
Arlamol® ISML
Arlamol® M812
Arlamol® PAO Series
Arlamol® PC
Arlamol® S3, S7
Arlasolve® DMI
Arlatone® G
Arnica Oil CLR
Arosurf® 66-E2
Arosurf® 66-E10
Arosurf® 66-E20
Arosurf® 66-PE12
Arquad® DM18B-90

Arquad® DMMCB-50
Arquad® HT-50
Atomergic Cocoa Butter
Atomergic Jojoba Oil
Avamid 150
Avocado Oil CLR
Barlox® 10S
Barlox® 12
Barlox® 14
Barlox® 16S
Barlox® 18S
Baysilone Fluid PD 5
Baysilone Fluid PK 20
BBS
Bee's Milk
Belsil ADM 6041 E
Belsil ADM 6042 E
Belsil ADM 6056 E
Belsil ADM 6057 E
Belsil ADM 6059 E
Belsil DMC 6031
Belsil DMC 6032
Belsil DMC 6033
Belsil DMC 6035
Bernel® Ester 168
Bernel® Ester 2014
Bernel® Ester CO
Bernel® Ester DID
Bernel® Ester DISM
Bernel® Ester DOM
Bernel® Ester EHP
Bernel® Ester NPDC
Bernel® Ester TOC
Bernel® OPG
Bina QAT-43
BioCare® Polymer HA-24
BioCare® SA
Biomin® Marine
Biosil Basics A-30
Biosil Basics Amino DL-30
Biosil Basics DL-30
Biosil Basics Fluoro Guerbet 1.0%
Biosil Basics Fluoro Guerbet 3.5%
Biosil Basics Jasmine Wax S
Biosil Basics L-30
Bio-Soft® MT 40
Biosulphur Fluid
Bio-Surf PBC-460
Bovinol 30
Britol®
Britol® 6NF
Britol® 7NF
Britol® 9NF
Britol® 20USP
Britol® 24
Britol® 35USP
Britol® 50USP
Brocose Q
Brookosome® ACEBC
Brookosome® ANE
Brookosome® A-Plus
Brookosome® BC
Brookosome® Biophos
Brookosome® C
Brookosome® CS

Brookosome® CU
Brookosome® DHA
Brookosome® DNA/RNA
Brookosome® E
Brookosome® Elastin
Brookosome® ELL
Brookosome® EPO
Brookosome® F
Brookosome® FIH
Brookosome® GSL
Brookosome® H
Brookosome® Herbal
Brookosome® MT
Brookosome® P
Brookosome® Planell
Brookosome® RJ
Brookosome® RP
Brookosome® S
Brookosome® TA
Brookosome® TE
Brookosome® U
Brookosome® UV
Brookosome® V
Brooksgel 41
Brooks Hydrogenated Lanolin
Brookswax™ D
Brookswax™ G
Brookswax™ P
Brophos™ 5C10
Brophos™ OL-3
Brophos™ OL-3N
Brox OL-2
Brox OL-3
Brox OL-4
Brox OL-5
Brox OL-10
Bumyr
Cachalot® C-50
Cachalot® C-51
Cachalot® M-43
Cachalot® O-3
Cachalot® O-8
Cachalot® O-15
Cachalot® S-54
Cachalot® S-56
Calendula Oil CLR
Camellia Oil
Captex® 200
Captex® 300
Captex® 350
Captex® 810A
Captex® 810B
Captex® 810C
Captex® 810D
Captex® 910A
Captex® 910B
Captex® 910C
Captex® 910D
Captex® 8227
Carbopol® 1706
Carbopol® 1720
Carbowax® Sentry® PEG 300
Carbowax® Sentry® PEG 400
Carbowax® Sentry® PEG 540 Blend

Emollients/Conditioners/Softeners... *(cont'd.)*

Carbowax® Sentry® PEG
  600
Carbowax® Sentry® PEG
  900
Carbowax® Sentry® PEG
  1000
Carbowax® Sentry® PEG
  1450
Carbowax® Sentry® PEG
  3350
Carbowax® Sentry® PEG
  4600
Carbowax® Sentry® PEG
  8000
Carnation®
Carolane
Carrot Oil
Carrot Oil CLR
Carsamide® AMEA
Carsonon® 144-P
Carsonon® 169-P
Carsoquat® 868
Carsoquat® 868-E
Carsoquat® 868P
Carsoquat® CB
Carsoquat® CT-429
Carsoquat® CTM-29
Carsoquat® CTM-429
Carsoquat® SDQ-25
Carsoquat® SDQ-85
Cartaretin F-4
Castor Oil USP
Catigene® ST 70
Catinal HC-100
Cation LQ
Cationic Collagen
  Polypeptides
CE-618
Cegesoft® C 17
Cegesoft® C 19
Cegesoft® C 25
Celquat® H-100
Celquat® L-200
Celquat® SC-230M
Celquat® SC-240
Celquat® SC-240C,
  28-6804
Centella Phytosome®
Centrolex® F
Cera Albalate 101
Cera Albalate 102
Cera Albalate 103
Cera Euphorbia
Ceral 165
Ceral CK
Ceral LE
Ceral MA
Ceral ME
Ceral MET
Ceral MEX
Ceral ML
Ceral MN
Ceral MNT
Ceral MNX
Ceral P
Ceral PA
Ceral TG
Ceral TN

Ceral TP
Ceralan®
Ceranine PN Base
Ceraphyl® 28
Ceraphyl® 31
Ceraphyl® 41
Ceraphyl®45
Ceraphyl® 50
Ceraphyl® 55
Ceraphyl® 60
Ceraphyl® 65
Ceraphyl® 70
Ceraphyl® 85
Ceraphyl® 140
Ceraphyl® 140-A
Ceraphyl® 230
Ceraphyl® 368
Ceraphyl® 375
Ceraphyl® 424
Ceraphyl® 494
Ceraphyl® 791
Ceraphyl® 847
Ceraphyl® GA
Ceraphyl® GA-D
Ceraphyl® ICA
Ceraphyl® IPL
Cerasynt® 840
Cetal
Cetax 16
Cetax 18
Cetax 50
Cetina
Cetiol®
Cetiol® 868
Cetiol® 1414E
Cetiol® A
Cetiol® B
Cetiol® G16S
Cetiol® G20S
Cetiol® HE
Cetiol® J600
Cetiol® LC
Cetiol® MM
Cetiol® OE
Cetiol® R
Cetiol® S
Cetiol® SB45
Cetiol® SN
Cetiol® V
Chemal OA-10
Chemal TDA-12
Chemax E-200 MS
Chemax E-1000 MS
Chemax HCO-5
Chemax HCO-16
Chemax HCO-25
Chembetaine OL
Chembetaine OL-30
Chembetaine S
Chembetaine TG
Chemical 39 Base
Chemical Base 6532
Chemidex B
Chemidex C
Chemidex L
Chemidex M
Chemidex O
Chemidex P

Chemidex R
Chemidex SE
Chemidex SI
Chemidex SO
Chemidex T
Chemidex WC
Chemoxide CAW
Chemoxide SAO
Chemoxide ST
Chemoxide WC
Chemphos TC-231S
Chemphos TC-337
Chemphos TC-341
Chemphos TC-349
Chemphos TR-505
Chemphos TR-505D
Chemphos TR-510
Chemphos TR-510S
Chemphos TR-515
Chemphos TR-515D
Chemphos TR-541
Chemsperse EGDS
Chemsperse GMS-SE
Chesguar C10, C10R
Chesguar C17
Chesguar C20, C20R
Chimin AX
Chimipal FV
Cholesterol NF
Cithrol 2ML
Cithrol 2MO
Cithrol 6ML
Cithrol 6MO
Cithrol 10ML
Cithrol 60MO
Cithrol ES
Cithrol GTO
Citmol™ 316
Citmol 320
Clearcol
Clearlan® 1650
Clearlan® K50
CMI 550
CMI 800
CO-618
CO-1695
CO-1895
Cobee 76
Cobee 92
Cobee 110
Coconut Oils® 76, 92, 110
Cojoba
Colla-Gel AC
Collagen Hydrolyzate
  Cosmetic 50
Collagen Hydrolyzate
  Cosmetic 55
Collagen Hydrolyzate
  Cosmetic N-35
Collagen Hydrolyzate
  Cosmetic N-55
Collagen Hydrolyzate
  Cosmetic SD
Collagen Native Extra 1%
Collamino™ Complex L/O
Collasol
Comperlan® 100
Comperlan® COD

Comperlan® ID
Comperlan® KD
Comperlan® OD
Comperlan® VOD
Compritol 888
Compritol WL 3241
Conditioner P6
Conditioner P7
Copolymer 845
Copolymer 937
Copolymer 958
Corona Lanolin
Corona PNL
Coronet Lanolin
Cosbiol
Cosmedia Guar® C-261 N
Cosmetic Lanolin
Cosmetic Lanolin
  Anhydrous USP
Cosmetol® X
Cosmowax J
Cosmowax K
Cosmowax P
CPH-399-N
Crafol AP-11
Cralane KR-13, -14
Cralane LR-10
Cralane LR-11
Cremba
Cremeol HF-52, HF-62
Cremerol HMG
Crestalans
Crillon LME
Crillon ODE
Crodacel QL
Crodacel QM
Crodacel QS
Crodacol A-10
Crodacol CS-50
Crodacol S-95NF
Crodafos 1214A
Crodafos 25 D2 Acid
Crodafos 25 D5 Acid
Crodafos 25 D10 Acid
Crodafos CAP
Crodafos N-3 Acid
Crodafos O2 Acid
Crodafos O5 Acid
Crodafos O10 Acid
Crodafos T2 Acid
Crodafos T5 Acid
Crodafos T10 Acid
Crodalan 0477
Crodalan AWS
Crodalan LA
Crodamol AB
Crodamol BB
Crodamol BE
Crodamol BM
Crodamol BS
Crodamol CAP
Crodamol CL
Crodamol CP
Crodamol CSS
Crodamol DA
Crodamol DO
Crodamol DOA
Crodamol GHS

Emollients/Conditioners/Softeners... *(cont'd.)*

Crodamol GTCC	Crotein SPA	Dermol MO	Emalex 1000 di-L
Crodamol ICS	Crotein SPC	Dermol OL	Emalex CS-5
Crodamol IPL	Crotein WKP	Dermol OO	Emalex CS-10
Crodamol IPM	Crovol A40	Dermol QE	Emalex CS-15
Crodamol IPP	Crovol A70	Dermol T	Emalex CS-20
Crodamol ISNP	Crovol M40	Dermolan GLH	Emalex CS-24
Crodamol JJ	Crovol M70	Diadol 18G	Emalex CS-30
Crodamol LL	Crovol PK40	Diamond Quality®	Emalex DEG-di-L
Crodamol ML	Crovol PK70	Dionil® OC	Emalex DNP-5
Crodamol MM	Crystal® O	Dionil® OC/K	Emalex EG-di-L
Crodamol MP	Crystal® Crown	Dionil® RS	Emalex GMS-55FD
Crodamol OC	Crystosol NF 70	Dionil® SD	Emalex K.T.G
Crodamol OHS	Crystosol NF 90	Dipsal	Emalex LWIS-2
Crodamol OO	Crystosol USP 200	Distilled Lipolan	Emalex LWIS-5
Crodamol OSU	Crystosol USP 240	Docoil DOS	Emalex LWS-3
Crodamol PC	Crystosol USP 350	Dow Corning® 190	Emalex LWS-5
Crodamol PETS	Cutina® CP-A	Surfactant	Emalex LWS-8
Crodamol PMP	Cutina® KD16	Dow Corning® 193	Emalex LWS-10
Crodamol PTC	Cyclochem® GMO	Surfactant	Emalex LWS-15
Crodamol PTIS	Cyclochem® LVL	Dow Corning® 200 Fluid	Emalex O.T.G
Crodamol SS	Cyclochem® PEG 200DS	Dow Corning® 556 Fluid	Emalex TEG-di-AS
Crodamol W	Cyclochem® PEG 400 DS	Dow Corning® 939	Emalex TEG-di-L
Crodasone W	Cyclochem® PEG 600DS	Dow Corning® 1401 Fluid	Emalex TPS-303
Croderol G7000	Cyclochem® PEG 6000DS	Dow Corning® 1669	Emalex TPS-305
Croderol GA 7000	Cyclomox® SO	Dow Corning® Q2-1403	Emalex TPS-308
Crodesta F-10	Cycloteric BET-L31	Fluid	Emalex TPS-310
Crodesta F-50	Cycloteric CAPA	Dow Corning® Q2-5324	Emcol® 4
Crodesta SL-40	Cycloteric SLIP	Surfactant	Emcol® 3555
Croduret 10	Cycloton® 7LUF	Dow Corning® Q2-7224	Emcol® 4072
Croduret 30	Damox® 1010	Conditioning Additive	Emcol® 4161L
Croduret 40	Dastar	Dow Corning® Q2-8220	Emcol® 6613
Croduret 60	Dehyquart® A	Conditioning Additive	Emcol® CC-9
Croduret 100	Dehyquart® C Crystals	Dow Corning® QF1-3593A	Emcol® CC-42
Crodyne BY-19	Dehyquart® DAM	D.P.P.G	Emcol® CC-55
Crolactil CSL	Dehyquart® E	Dragoxat EH 2/044115	Emcol® CC-57
Crolactil SISL	Dehyquart® LT	Drakeol 5	Emcol® E-607L
Crolactil SSL	Dehyquart® SP	Drakeol 7	Emcol® E-607S
Crolastin	Dehyquart® STC-25	Drakeol 8	Emcol® ISML
Crolastin 10 Powder	Dehyton® AB-30	Drakeol 10	Emcol® L
Crolastin 30 Powder	Dehyton® PK	Drakeol 15	Emcol® M
Crolec 4135	Deltyl® Extra	Drewmulse® 200K	Emcol® NA-30
Cromoist CS	Deltyl® Prime	Drewpol® 10-4-O	Emcol® SML
Cromoist HYA	Dermaffine	Dusoran MD	Emcol® SO
Cronectin	Dermalcare® EGMS/SE	Dynacerin® 660	EmCon CO
Cropepsol	Dermalcare® GTIS	Dynasan® 110	EmCon E
Cropeptide W	Dermalcare® HL	Edenol 302	EmCon E-5
Cropeptone	Dermalcare® LVL	Efevit E	EmCon Limnanthes Alba
Croquat HH	Dermalcare® MST	Efevit S	EmCon Olive
Croquat K	Dermalcare® PGMS	Elacid Richter	EmCon Rice Bran
Croquat L	Dermane	Eldew CL-301	EmCon W
Croquat M	Dermene	Elefac™ I-205	EmCon Walnut
Croquat S	Dermol 89	Eleseryl® SH	Emerest® 1723
Croquat WKP	Dermol 105	Eleseryl® SHT	Emerest® 2310
Crosilk 10,000	Dermol 108	Elfacos® BE	Emerest® 2314
Crosilk Liq	Dermol 109	Elfacos® CP	Emerest® 2316
Crosilkquat	Dermol 126	Elfacos® DEHS	Emerest® 2325
Crosultaine E-30	Dermol 185	Elfacos® DO	Emerest® 2384
Crotein AD Anhyd	Dermol 334	Elfacos® EHP	Emerest® 2388
Crotein ADW	Dermol 489	Elfacos® EO	Emerest® 2410
Crotein ASC	Dermol 2022	Elfacos® IPM	Emerest® 2452
Crotein ASK	Dermol CV	Elfacos® IPP	Emerest® 2486
Crotein BTA	Dermol DISD	Elfacos® ST 9	Emerest® 11723
Crotein HKP Powd	Dermol EB	Elfacos® ST 37	Emery® 912
Crotein HKP/SF	Dermol G-76	Emalex 200 di-L	Emery® 916
Crotein IP	Dermol GL-7A	Emalex 300 di-L	Emery® 917
Crotein K	Dermol ICSA	Emalex 400 di-L	Emery® 918
Crotein O	Dermol Jojoba E	Emalex 600 di-L	Emery® 1650
Crotein Q	Dermol L45	Emalex 800 di-L	Emery® 1656

Emollients/Conditioners/Softeners... *(cont'd.)*

Emery® 1660	Estol 1414	Exxal® 20	HC/R
Emery® 1720	Estol 1427	Facilan	Fonoline® White
Emery® 1730	Estol 1445	Famous	Fonoline® Yellow
Emery® 1732	Estol 1476	Fancol 707	Forestall
Emery® 1740	Estol 1481	Fancol Acel	Forlan
Emery® 1747	Estol 1502	Fancol ALA	Forlan 200
Emery® 1780	Estol 1512	Fancol ALA-10	Forlan 300
Emery® 1781	Estol 1514	Fancol C	Forlan 500
Emery® 1795	Estol 1574	Fancol CA	Forlan C-24
Emery® 2423	Estol 1579	Fancol CAB	Forlan L
Emery® 6748	Estol 1583	Fancol CB	Forlan LM
Emery® HP-2050	Estol 1593	Fancol CB Extra	Fractalite ISL
Emery® HP-2060	Estol BUS 1550	Fancol DL	G-3908S
Emery® HP-2095	Estol CEP-b 3653	Fancol HL	Gafquat® 734
Emid® 6515	Estol CES 3705	Fancol HL-20	Gafquat® 755N
Emphos™ D70-30C	Estol DCO 3662	Fancol HL-24	Gafquat® HS-100
Empicol® 0216	Estol DCO-b 3655	Fancol HON	Gafquat® HSi
Empicol® 0627	Estol EHC 1540	Fancol IPL	Gantrez® ES-225
Empicol® XDB	Estol EHP 1543	Fancol Karite Butter	Gantrez® ES-335
Empigen® 5509	Estol EHP-b 3652	Fancol Karite Extract	Gantrez® ES-425
Empigen® BB	Estol EHS 1545	Fancol LA	Gantrez® ES-435
Empigen® CM	Estol EHS-b 3654	Fancol LA-5	Gantrez® V-215
Empilan® 2125-AU	Estol ETO 3659	Fancol LA-15	Gantrez® V-225
Empilan® EGMS	Estol GDS 3748	Fancol LAO	Gantrez® V-425
Empilan® KB 2	Estol GMS 1473	Fancol OA-95	Geliderm 3000 P
Empilan® KB 3	Estol GMS90 1468	Fancol SA	Geliderm 3000 S
Empilan® KC 3	Estol GTCC 1527	Fancol SA-15	Genamin KDM
Emsorb® 2500	Estol GTEH 3609	Fancol TOIN	Genamin KDM-F
Emsorb® 2503	Estol IBUS 1552	Fancor IPL	Genamin KS 5
Emsorb® 2507	Estol IDCO 3667	Fancor LFA	Genamin KSE
Emsorb® 2729	Estol IPL 1511	Fancor Lanwax	Genaminox CS
Emthox® 2730	Estol IPM 1508	Fancorsil A	Genaminox CST
Emthox® 5964	Estol IPM 1512	Fancorsil P	Generol® 122
Emthox® 5967	Estol IPM 1514	Fancorsil SLA	Generol® 122E5
Emulan®	Estol IPM-b 1509	Fancorsil SLA-LT	Generol® 122E10
Emulgade® CRC	Estol IPP 1517	Finester EH-25	Generol® 122E16
Emulmetik	Estol IPP-b 3651	Finquat CT	Generol® 122E25
Emulmetik™ 100	Estol IPS 3702	Finsoft HCM-100	Geropon® T-77
Emulmetik™ 110	Estol PDCC 1526	Finsolv® 116	Gilugel EUG
Emulmetik™ 120	Estol PDP 3601	Finsolv® BOD	Gilugel MIN
Emulmetik™ 135	Estol STST 3706	Finsolv® EMG-20	Gilugel OS
Emulmetik™ 300	Estran™-Lite	Finsolv® P	Gilugel SIL5
Emulmetik™ 310	Estran™-Pure	Finsolv® PL-62	Ginseng Phytosome®
Emulmetik™ 320	Estran™-Xtra	Finsolv® PL-355	Gloria®
Emulmetik™ 900	Ethosperse® OA-2	Finsolv® SB	Gluadin® AGP
Emulmetik™ 910	Ethoxylan® 1685	Finsolv® TN	Gluadin® Almond
Emulmetik™ 920	Ethoxylan® 1686	Fitoderm	Gluadin® Wheat
Emulmetik™ 930	Ethoxyol® 1707	Fizul MD-318C	Glucam® E-10
Emulmetik™ 950	Etocas 10	Florasun™-90	Glucam® E-20
Emulmetik™ 970	Etocas 30	Fluilan	Glucam® E-20 Distearate
Emulsion 2153	Etocas 35	Fluilan AWS	Glucam® P-10
Emulsion 2170	Etocas 60	Foam-Coll™ SK	Glucam® P-20
Emulsynt® GDL	Eumulgin® B1	Foamid 117	Glucam® P-20 Distearate
Endonucleine®	Eumulgin® B2	Foamid LM2E	Glucate® DO
Enduragloss™	Eumulgin® EO-33	Foamid LME-75	Glucquat® 125
Ervol®	Eumulgin® L	Foamine O-80	Glusol
ES-1239	Euperlan® PK 771	Foamole A	Glycerox HE
Espesilor AC Series	European Elastin 10	Foamole B	GlycoCer HA
Espesilor AC-43	European Elastin 30	Foamox CDO	Golden Dawn Grade 1, 2
Estalan 12	European Elastin SD	Foamquat 2IAE	Golden Dawn Lanolin
Estalan 42	Eutanol® G	Foamquat BAS	Golden Dawn Superfine
Estalan 126	Eutanol® G16	Foamquat COAS	Golden Fleece DF
Estalan 430	Exceparl HO	Foamquat IAES	Golden Fleece Lanolin
Estalan 635	Exceparl IPM	Foamquat SAQ-90	Golden Fleece P-80
Estalan DNPA	Exceparl IPP	Foamquat SOAS	Golden Fleece P-95
Estalan L-45	Exceparl OD-M	Foamquat VG	Golden Fleece RA
Estol 1406	Exceparl OD-OL	Foamtaine CAB-G	Granamine S3A
Estol 1407	Exceparl TGO	Fomblin® HC/04, HC/25,	Gransil GCM

Emollients/Conditioners/Softeners... *(cont'd.)*

Grillocam E10	Hetoxamine C-2	Hydroxylan	Incroquat Behenyl TMC/P
Grillocam E20	Hetoxamine C-5	Hyfatol 18-95	Incroquat Behenyl TMS
Grilloten LSE 65	Hetoxamine C-15	Hyfatol 18-98	Incrosul LAFS
Grilloten® LSE 65 K	Hetoxamine O-2	Hypan® QT100	Incrosul LS
Grilloten® LSE 65 K Soft	Hetoxamine O-5	Hy-Phi 1199	Incrosul OMS
Grilloten LSE 65 Soft	Hetoxamine O-15	Hy-Phi 1303	Incrosul OTS
Grilloten LSE 87	Hetoxamine S-2	Hy-Phi 1401	Inositol
Grilloten® LSE 87 K	Hetoxamine S-5	Hy-SES	Iscolan
Grilloten® LSE 87 K Soft	Hetoxamine ST-2	Hystar® 7000	Isofol® 28
Grilloten LSE 87 Soft	Hetoxamine ST-5	Imwitor® 312	Isofol® 32
Grilloten PSE141G	Hetoxamine T-2	Imwitor® 742	Isofol® 34T
Grilloten® PSE 141 G	Hetoxamine T-5	Imwitor® 928	Isofol® 36
Pellets	Hetoxamine T-15	Imwitor® 988	Iso Isotearyle WL 3196
Grilloten ZT-40	Hetoxamine T-20	Incrocas 30	Isopropylan® 33
Grilloten ZT-80	Hetoxamine T-30	Incrocas 40	Ivarbase™ 98
Hamposyl® C	Hetoxamine T-50	Incromate ALL	Ivarbase™ 3210
Hamposyl® C-30	Hetoxamine T-50-70%	Incromate BAL	Ivarbase™ 3250
Hamposyl® L	Hetoxide BN-13	Incromate CDL	Ivarlan™ 3000
Hamposyl® L-30	Hetoxide BP-3	Incromate CDP	Ivarlan™ 3001
Hamposyl® L-95	Hetoxide BY-3	Incromate IDL	Ivarlan™ 3006 Light
Hamposyl® M	Hetoxide C-2	Incromate ISML	Ivarlan™ 3100
Hamposyl® M-30	Hetoxide C-9	Incromate Mink L	Ivarlan™ 3300
Hamposyl® O	Hetoxide C-15	Incromate OLL	Ivarlan™ 3350
Hamposyl® S	Hetoxide C-25	Incromate SDL	Ivarlan™ 3360
Haroil SCO-50	Hetoxide C-30	Incromate SEL	Ivarlan™ 3400
Haroil SCO-65, -7525	Hetoxide C-40	Incromate WGL	Ivarlan™ 3405-L30
Hartolan	Hetoxide C-60	Incromectant AMEA-70	Ivarlan™ 3407-E
Hartolite	Hetoxide C-200	Incromide ALD	Ivarlan™ 3408W
HD-Eutanol®	Hetoxide DNP-5	Incromide LA	Ivarlan™ 3410
HD-Ocenol® 90/95	Hetoxide DNP-10	Incromine BB	Ivarlan™ 3420
HD-Ocenol® 92/96	Hetoxide HC-16	Incromine CB	Ivarlan™ L575
HD Oleyl Alcohol 70/75	Hetoxol MP-3	Incromine Mink B	Jafaester 14-96
HD Oleyl Alcohol 80/85	Hetoxol PLA	Incromine OPB	Jafaester 14 NF
HD Oleyl Alcohol 90/95	Hetoxol SP-15	Incromine OPM	Jafaester 16 NF
HD Oleyl Alcohol CG	Hexaplant Richter	Incromine PB	Jaguar® C-13S
Hefti AMS-33	Hi-Care® 1000	Incromine SB	Jaguar® C-14-S
Hefti GMS-33	Hodag CC-22	Incromine Oxide AL	Jaguar® C-17
Hefti MYM-33	Hodag CC-22-S	Incromine Oxide B	Jaguar® C-162
Hest MS	Hodag CC-33	Incromine Oxide B-30P	Jaguar® HP 120
Hetamide IS	Hodag CC-33-F	Incromine Oxide B50	Jet Quat S-2C-50
Hetamine 5L-25	Hodag CC-33-L	Incromine Oxide C	Jojoba Oil Cosmetic Grade
Hetester 412	Hodag CC-33-S	Incromine Oxide L	Jojoba Oil Pure Grade
Hetester FAO	Hodag CSA-80	Incromine Oxide M	Jojoba Oil Refined Grade
Hetester HCP	Hostacerin T-3	Incromine Oxide S	Karite Butter
Hetester HSS	Hydagen® P	Incromine Oxide SE	Kartacid 1890
Hetester ISS	Hydrenol® D	Incromine Oxide WG	Katemul IB-70
Hetester PCA	Hydrocoll™ EN-55	Incronam B-40	Katemul IG-70
Hetester PHA	Hydrocoll™ EN-SD	Incronam I-30	Katemul IGU-70
Hetester PMA	Hydrocoll™ HE-35	Incronam Mink 30	Katioran® AF
Hetester SSS	Hydrocoll™ LE-35	Incronam SE-30	Kaydol®
Hetester TICC	Hydrocoll™ T-LSN	Incroquat 100	Kemamide® W-35
Hetlan AC	Hydrokote® AR, HL	Incroquat 248	Kemamide® W-42
Hetoxalan 75	Hydrokote® RM	Incroquat AL-85	Kemamine® Q-9902C
Hetoxalan 75-50%	Hydrolactin 2500	Incroquat B65C	Kemamine® T-2802D
Hetoxalan 100	Hydrolyzed Elastin RE-10	Incroquat BA-85	Kemester® 1000
Hetoxamate FA-5	No. 26202	Incroquat CR Conc	Kemester® 1418
Hetoxamate FA-20	Hydrolyzed Elastin RE-30	Incroquat CTC-30	Kemester® 2000
Hetoxamate LA-5	No. 26203	Incroquat DBM-90	Kemester® 3681
Hetoxamate LA-9	Hydromond	Incroquat I-85	Kemester® 3684
Hetoxamate MO-4	Hydrophilol ISO	Incroquat Mink-85	Kemester® 4000
Hetoxamate MO-5	Hydrosoy 2000	Incroquat O-50	Kemester® 5221SE
Hetoxamate MO-9	Hydrosoy 2000/SF	Incroquat OL-85	Kemester® 5410
Hetoxamate MO-15	Hydrotriticum™	Incroquat S-75CG	Kemester® 5415
Hetoxamate SA-5	Hydrotriticum™ Powd	Incroquat S-85	Kemester® 5500
Hetoxamate SA-9	Hydrotriticum™ QL	Incroquat SDQ-25	Kemester® 5510
Hetoxamate SA-35	Hydrotriticum™ QM	Incroquat SE-85	Kemester® 5654
Hetoxamate SA-90	Hydrotriticum™ QS	Incroquat WG-85	Kemester® 5721
Hetoxamate SA-90F	Hydrotriticum™ WAA	Incroquat Behenyl BDQ/P	Kemester® 5822

Emollients/Conditioners/Softeners... *(cont'd.)*

Kemester® 6000
Kemester® 6000SE
Kemester® BE
Kemester® CP
Kemester® DMP
Kemester® EE
Kemester® EGDL
Kemester® GDL
Kemester® MM
Keraquat HK
Kera-Quat WKP
Kerasol
Kera-Tein 1000 AS
Kera-Tein 1000 SD
Kera-Tein AA
Kera-Tein V
Kessco® 653
Kessco BE
Kessco® Butyl Stearate
Kessco DEHS
Kessco DHS
Kessco DO
Kessco EHP
Kessco EO
Kessco® Ethylene Glycol
  Distearate
Kessco Glycerol Dilaurate
Kessco Glycerol Dioleate
Kessco Glycerol Dioleate
Kessco® Glycerol
  Monooleate
Kessco® Glycerol
  Monostearate Pure
Kessco® Glycerol
  Monostearate SE, Acid
  Stable
Kessco ICS
Kessco IPS
Kessco® Isobutyl Stearate
Kessco® Isocetyl Stearate
Kessco® Isopropyl
  Myristate
Kessco® Isopropyl
  Palmitate
Kessco OE
Kessco Octyl Isononanoate
Kessco® Octyl Palmitate
Kessco® PEG 200 DL
Kessco® PEG 200 DO
Kessco® PEG 200 DS
Kessco® PEG 200 ML
Kessco® PEG 200 MO
Kessco® PEG 200 MS
Kessco® PEG 300 DL
Kessco® PEG 300 DO
Kessco® PEG 300 DS
Kessco® PEG 300 ML
Kessco® PEG 300 MO
Kessco® PEG 300 MS
Kessco® PEG 400 DL
Kessco® PEG 400 DO
Kessco® PEG 400 DS
Kessco® PEG 400 ML
Kessco® PEG 400 MO
Kessco® PEG 400 MS
Kessco® PEG 600 DL
Kessco® PEG 600 DO
Kessco® PEG 600 DS

Kessco® PEG 600 ML
Kessco® PEG 600 MO
Kessco® PEG 600 MS
Kessco® PEG 1000 DL
Kessco® PEG 1000 DO
Kessco® PEG 1000 DS
Kessco® PEG 1000 ML
Kessco® PEG 1000 MO
Kessco® PEG 1000 MS
Kessco® PEG 1540 DL
Kessco® PEG 1540 DO
Kessco® PEG 1540 DS
Kessco® PEG 1540 ML
Kessco® PEG 1540 MO
Kessco® PEG 1540 MS
Kessco® PEG 4000 DL
Kessco® PEG 4000 DO
Kessco® PEG 4000 DS
Kessco® PEG 4000 ML
Kessco® PEG 4000 MO
Kessco® PEG 4000 MS
Kessco® PEG 6000 DL
Kessco® PEG 6000 DO
Kessco® PEG 6000 DS
Kessco® PEG 6000 ML
Kessco® PEG 6000 MO
Kessco® PEG 6000 MS
Kessco® PGML-X533
Kessco® Propylene Glycol
  Monolaurate E
Kessco PTS
Kester Wax® 72
Kester Wax® 82
Kester Wax® 105
Kester Wax® K 48
Kester Wax® K 56
Kester Wax® K 59
Kester Wax® K 62
Kester Wax® K 85
KF56, KF58
Klearol®
Kollaron
Koster Keunen Beeswax
Koster Keunen Candelilla
Koster Keunen Candelilla
  Ester
Koster Keunen Carnauba
  No. 1
Koster Keunen Carnauba
  T-2
Koster Keunen Carnauba
  T-3
Koster Keunen Fatty
  Alcohol 1618
Koster Keunen Hydroxy-
  Hexanyl-Behenyl-
  Beeswaxate
Koster Keunen Hydroxy-
  Polyester
Koster Keunen Microcrys-
  talline Wax 170/180
Koster Keunen Microcrys-
  talline Wax 193/198
Koster Keunen Ozokerite
  153/160
Koster Keunen Ozokerite
  158/160
Koster Keunen Ozokerite

160/164
Koster Keunen Ozokerite
  164/170
Koster Keunen Ozokerite
  170
Koster Keunen Ozokerite
  190
Koster Keunen Stearic Acid
  XXX
Koster Keunen Tallow
  Glyceride
Labrafac® Lipophile WL
  1349
Lactabase C14
Lactabase C16
Lactacet
Lactolan®
Lafil WL 3254
Lamecerin 50-80
Lameform® TGI
Lamequat® L
Lamesoft® LMG
Lamesoft® LMG/NP
Lanacet® 1705
Lanaetex CPS
Lanaetex Jojoba Oil
Lanalox L 30
Lan-Aqua-Sol 50
Lan-Aqua-Sol 100
Lanesta 10
Lanesta G
Lanesta L
Lanesta P
Lanesta S
Lanesta SA-30
Lanethyl
Laneto 20
Laneto 27
Laneto 30
Laneto 49
Laneto 50
Laneto 60
Laneto 85
Laneto 99
Laneto 100
Laneto 100-Flaked
Laneto AWS
Lanette® 14
Lanette® 16
Lanette® 18
Lanette® 18-22
Lanette® 18 DEO
Lanette® 22
Lanette® O
Lanex
Lanexol
Lanexol AWS
Lanfrax® 1776
Lanfrax® 1777 Deodorized
Lanfrax® 1779
Lanidrol
Lanisolate
Lanocerina
Lanocerin®
Lanogel® 21
Lanogel® 31
Lanogel® 41
Lanogel® 61

Lanogene®
Lanoil Water/Alcohol
  Soluble Lanolin
Lanol C
Lanol CS
Lanol S
Lanolex L-40
Lanolic Acid
Lanolin Anhydrous USP
Lanolin Cosmetic
Lanolin Extra-Deodorized
Lanolin Pharmaceutical
Lanolin Tech
Lanolin Tech. Grade
Lanolin USP
Lanoquat® 1751A
Lanoquat® 1756
Lanoquat® 1757
Lanotein AWS 30
Lanotex 730
Lanowax
Lantrol®
Lantrol® 1673
Lantrol® 1674
Lantrol® AWS
Lantrol® AWS 1692
Lantrol® HP-2073
Lantrol® HP-2074
Lantrol® PLN
Lantrol® PLN/50
Lasemul 60
Lasemul 74 NP
Lasemul 130
Laurate de Cetyle
Laurex® CH
Laurex® L1
Laurex® NC
Laurex® PKH
Lecithin Water Dispersible
  CLR
Leogard GP
Leoguard G
Lexamine 22
Lexamine L-13
Lexamine S-13 Lactate
Lexate® BPQ
Lexate® CRC
Lexate® PX
Lexate® TA
Lexate® TL
Lexein® A-240
Lexein® A-520
Lexein® QX-3000
Lexein® X-250
Lexein® X-250HP
Lexein® X-300
Lexein® X-350
Lexemul® 515
Lexemul® AR
Lexemul® AS
Lexemul® CS-20
Lexemul® GDL
Lexemul® PEG-200 DL
Lexemul® PEG-400 DL
Lexemul® PEG-400ML
Lexemul® T
Lexol® 60
Lexol® 3975

Emollients/Conditioners/Softeners... *(cont'd.)*

Lexol® EHP	Lipocol SC-20	Liquid Base	Mackamine™ O2
Lexol® GT-855	Lipodermol®	Liquiwax™ DC-EFA/SS	Mackamine™ OAO
Lexol® GT-865	Lipolan	Liquiwax™ DIADD	Mackamine™ SAO
Lexol® IPM	Lipolan 31	Liquiwax™ DIADD/TiO$_2$	Mackamine™ SO
Lexol® IPM-NF	Lipolan 31-20	Disp	Mackamine™ WGO
Lexol® IPP	Lipolan Distilled	Liquiwax™ DICDD	Mackanate™ DG30
Lexol® IPP-A	Lipolan R	Liquiwax™ DIEFA	Mackanate™ IM
Lexol® IPP-NF	Lipolan S	Lonzaine® 12C	Mackanate™ OP
Lexol® PG-800	Lipomulse 165	Lonzaine® C	Mackanate™ RM
Lexol® PG-855	Liponate 2-DH	Lonzaine® CO	Mackanate™ WG
Lexol® PG-865	Liponate 143M	Lonzaine® CS	Mackanate™ WGD
Lexol® PG-900	Liponate CL	Lonzest® 143-S	Mackernium™ 006
Lexol® SS	Liponate CRM	Lonzest® 153-S	Mackernium™ 007
Lexquat® 2240	Liponate DPC-6	Lonzest® 163-S	Mackernium™ CTC-30
Lexquat® AMG-BEO	Liponate GC	Loropan LMD	Mackernium™ KP
Lexquat® AMG-IS	Liponate GDL	Loropan OD	Mackernium™ NLE
Lexquat® AMG-M	Liponate IPM	Lowenol C Acid	Mackernium™ SDC-25
Lexquat® AMG-O	Liponate IPP	Lowenol L Acid	Mackernium™ SDC-50
Lexquat® AMG-WC	Liponate ISA Special	Lowenol M Acid	Mackernium™ SDC-85
Lexquat® CH	Liponate ML	Lowenol O Acid	Mackernium™ WLE
Lilaminox M24	Liponate MM	Lowenol P Acid	Mackester™ EGDS
Lipacide CCO	Liponate NPGC-2	Lutrol® E 300	Mackester™ EGMS
Lipacide DPHP	Liponate PB-4	Lutrol® E 400	Mackester™ IDO
Lipacide PCO	Liponate PC	Luviquat® FC 370	Mackester™ IP
Lipacide PK	Liponate PE-810	Luviquat® FC 550	Mackester™ SP
Lipacide UCO	Liponate PO-4	Luviquat® FC 905	Mackester™ TD-88
Lipal 6000 DS	Liponate PS-4	Luviquat® HM 552	Mackol 18
Lipal EB	Liponate SPS	Luviquat® Mono CP	Mackpro™ KLP
Lipal LC	Liponate SS	Luvitol® EHO	Mackpro™ MLP
Lipal ST	Liponate TDS	Luvitol® HP	Mackpro™ NLP
Lipamide MEAA	Liponate TDTM	Macadamia Nut Oil	Mackpro™ NLW
Lipex 101	Liponic 70-NC	Mackadet™ CBC	Mackpro™ NSP
Lipex 205	Liponic 76-NC	Mackadet™ INC	Mackpro™ SLP
Lipex 407	Liponic 83-NC	Mackadet™ LCB	Mackpro™ WLW
Lipo 320	Liponic EG-1	Mackalene™ 116	Mackpro™ WWP
Lipo DGLS	Liponic EG-7	Mackalene™ 117	Macol® 57
Lipo DGS-SE	Lipo-Peptide AME 30	Mackalene™ 216	Macol® CA 30P
Lipo EGDS	Lipophos LMP	Mackalene™ 316	Macol® P-1200
Lipo GMS 450	Lipoquat R	Mackalene™ 326	Macol® P-2000
Lipo GMS 470	Lipovol A	Mackalene™ 416	Macol® P-4000
Lipo SS	Lipovol ALM	Mackalene™ 426	Mafo® C
Lipocol	Lipovol ALM-S	Mackalene™ 616	Mafo® CAB
Lipocol C	Lipovol C-76	Mackalene™ 716	Mafo® CAB 425
Lipocol C-2	Lipovol CAN	Mackalene™ NLC	Mafo® CAB SP
Lipocol C-10	Lipovol CO	Mackam™ 151C	Mafo® CB 40
Lipocol C-20	Lipovol CP	Mackam™ 151L	Mafo® CFA 35
Lipocol HCO-40	Lipovol G	Mackam™ BA	Mafo® CSB
Lipocol HCO-60	Lipovol GTB	Mackam™ CB-35	Mafo® CSB 50
Lipocol L	Lipovol HS	Mackam™ CB-LS	Mafo® CSB W
Lipocol L-1	Lipovol J	Mackam™ CET	Mafo® KCOSB 50
Lipocol L-4	Lipovol J Lite	Mackam™ HV	Mafo® LMAB
Lipocol L-12	Lipovol MAC	Mackam™ ISA	Mafo® OB
Lipocol L-23	Lipovol M-SYN	Mackam™ J	Mafo® SBAO 110
Lipocol M-4	Lipovol O	Mackam™ OB	Manroteric 1202
Lipocol O	Lipovol P	Mackam™ RA	Mapeg® 200 DO
Lipocol O-2 Special	Lipovol PAL	Mackam™ TM	Mapeg® 200 DOT
Lipocol O-3 Special	Lipovol P-S	Mackam™ WGB	Mapeg® 200 ML
Lipocol O-10	Lipovol SAF	Mackamate WGD	Mapeg® 400 DO
Lipocol O-20	Lipovol SES	Mackamide™ LME	Mapeg® CO-16
Lipocol O-80	Lipovol SES-S	Mackamide™ R	Mapeg® CO-16H
Lipocol O/95	Lipovol SO	Mackamide™ S	Mapeg® CO-30
Lipocol S	Lipovol SOY	Mackamine™ BAO	Mapeg® CO-36
Lipocol S-2	Lipovol SUN	Mackamine™ CAO	Mapeg® CO-200
Lipocol S-10	Lipovol W	Mackamine™ CO	Mapeg® S-100
Lipocol S-20	Lipovol WGO	Mackamine™ IAO	Mapeg® S-150
Lipocol SC-4	Liquester	Mackamine™ ISMO	Maricol CLR
Lipocol SC-10	Liquid Absorption Base	Mackamine™ LAO	Marlamid® D 1218
Lipocol SC-15	Type A, T	Mackamine™ LO	Marlamid® D 1885

Emollients/Conditioners/Softeners... *(cont'd.)*

Marlamid® DF 1218
Marlamid® DF 1818
Marlamid® M 1218
Marlazin® KC 21/50
Marlazin® KC 30/50
Marlipal® 1885/2
Marlipal® BS
Marlophor® LN-Acid
Marlophor® MO 3-Acid
Marlopon® CA
Marlosol® 183
Marlosol® 188
Marlosol® BS
Marlosol® F08
Marlosol® FS
Marlosol® OL7
Marlosol® R70
Marlowet® G 12 DO
Marlowet® GDO 4
Masil® 556
Masil® 756
Masil® SF 5
Masil® SF 10
Masil® SF 20
Masil® SF 50
Masil® SF 100
Masil® SF 350
Masil® SF 500
Masil® SF 1000
Masil® SF 10,000
Masil® SF 12,500
Masil® SF 30,000
Masil® SF 60,000
Masil® SFR 70
Mazol® SFR 100
Mazol® SFR 750
Mazol® SFR 2000
Mazol® SFR 3500
Mazol® SFR 18,000
Mazol® SFR 50,000
Mazol® SFR 150,000
Masilwax 135
Maypon UD
May-Tein C
May-Tein CT
May-Tein KK
May-Tein KT
May-Tein KTS
May-Tein R
May-Tein SK
May-Tein SY
Mazawax® 163R
Mazol® 159
Mazol® GMO
Mazol® GMO K
Mazol® GMR
Mazol® GMS-D
Mazox® CAPA
Mazox® CAPA-37
Mazox® CDA
Mazox® LDA
Mazox® MDA
Mazox® ODA
Mazox® SDA
Melhydran®
Merquat® 100
Merquat® 280
MFF 159-B

Michel XO-150-16
Michel XO-150-20
Midecol ACS
Miglyol® 808
Miglyol® 810
Miglyol® 818
Miglyol® 829
Miglyol® 840
Miglyol® 840 Gel
Milkamino™ 20
Miramine® CODI
Miramine® SODI
Miranol® BM Conc
Miranol® CM Conc. NP
Miranol® CM-SF Conc
Miranol® DM
Miranol® DM Conc. 45%
Miranol® Ester PO-LM4
Miranol® H2M Conc
Mirapol® 9, 95, 175
Mirapol® 550
Mirapol® A-15
Mirapol® AD-1
Mirapol® AZ-1
Mirapol® CP40
Mirasheen® 202
Mirataine® AP-C
Mirataine® BB
Mirataine® BET-C-30
Mirataine® BET-O-30
Mirataine® BET-P-30
Mirataine® BET-W
Mirataine® CAB-A
Mirataine® CAB-O
Mirataine® CB
Mirataine® CB/M
Mirataine® COB
Mirataine® ODMB-35
Mirataine® TM
M.O.D. WL 2949
Modulan®
Monamid® 15-70W
Monamid® 150-ADY
Monamid® 150-IS
Monamid® 759
Monamid® 1007
Monamid® LLN-380
Monamid® LN-605
Monamide
Monaquat ISIES
Monaquat SL-5
Monaquat TG
Monateric 1202
Monateric 1203
Monateric CM-36S
Monateric ISA-35
Monateric MCB
Monomuls® 90-L12
Monomuls® 90-O18
Monteine LCS 30
M-Quat® 40
M-Quat® 522
M-Quat® 1033
M-Quat® B-25
M-Quat® Dimer 18 PG
M-Quat® Dimer S-50 PG
M-Quat® JB-25
M-Quat® JN

M-Quat® JO-50
M-Quat® JS-25
M-Quat® JS-25 SP
Multi-Grain Barley Code 1851
Myritol® 318
Myritol® PC
Myvacet® 5-07
Myvacet® 7-07
Myvacet® 9-08
Myvacet® 9-45
Nacol® 14-98
Nacol® 16-98
Nacol® 18-98
Nacol® 20-95
Nacol® 22-97
Naetex-L
Naetex-LD
Naetex-LS
Naetex O-20
Naetex O-80
Naetex-Q
Naetex-WS
Nafol® C14-C22
Natural Beeswax
Natural Extract AP
Naturechem® CAR
Naturechem® CR
Naturechem® EGHS
Naturechem® GMHS
Naturechem® GTH
Naturechem® GTR
Naturechem® MAR
Naturechem® OHS
Naturechem® PGHS
Naturechem® PGR
Naturechem® THS-200
Naxide™ 1230
Necon SOG
Necon SOLC
Neobee® 18
Neobee® 20
Neobee® 1054
Neobee® M-5
Neobee® M-20
Neodol® 25
Neodol® 45
N-Hance® 3000
Nikkol Batyl Alcohol 100, EX
Nikkol Behenyl Alcohol 65, 80
Nikkol BO-2
Nikkol BO-7
Nikkol BPS-5
Nikkol BPS-10
Nikkol BPS-15
Nikkol BPS-20
Nikkol BPS-25
Nikkol BPS-30
Nikkol BWA-5
Nikkol BWA-10
Nikkol BWA-20
Nikkol BWA-40
Nikkol CA-1485
Nikkol CA-2150
Nikkol CA-2330
Nikkol CA-2350

Nikkol CA-2450
Nikkol CA-2450T
Nikkol CA-2465
Nikkol CA-2580
Nikkol CA-3475
Nikkol CCP-40
Nikkol CCP-100
Nikkol CCP-100P
Nikkol Cetyl Lactate
Nikkol Chimyl Alcohol 100
Nikkol CS
Nikkol Decaglyn 10-IS
Nikkol Decaglyn 10-O
Nikkol DGO-80
Nikkol DGS-80
Nikkol GM-18IS
Nikkol GM-18S
Nikkol GO-430
Nikkol GO-440
Nikkol GO-460
Nikkol ICIS
Nikkol ICS-R
Nikkol Jojoba Oil N
Nikkol Jojoba Oil S
Nikkol Myristyl Lactate
Nikkol N-SP
Nikkol PEMS
Nikkol Selachyl Alcohol
Nikkol Trifat S-308
Nikkol TW-10
Nikkol TW-20
Nikkol TW-30
Nimco® 1780
Nimco® 1781
Nimcolan® 1740
Nimcolan® 1747
Nimlesterol® 1730
Nimlesterol® 1732
Ninol® 40-CO
Ninol® CNR
Ninol® LMP
Ninol® M10
Niox EO-33
Nopcocastor
Noramium M2C
Noramium M2SH
Norfox® ALKA
Norfox® Coco Betaine
Norfox® DOSA
Novol
Nutrilan® Elastin E20, P
Nutrilan® FPK
Nutrilan® H, M
Nutrilan® I-50
Oceagen®
OHlan®
Onyxol® 42
OP-2000
Orange Wax
Orange Wax, Deodorized
Ormagel AC-400
Ormagel SH, XPU
Orzol®
Ovothin
Oxypon 288
Oxypon 306
Oxypon 328
Oxypon 365

Emollients/Conditioners/Softeners... *(cont'd.)*

Oxypon 2145	Pluracol® E400 NF	Protegin® SE	Radia® 7131
Panthequat®	Pluracol® E400	Protegin® W SE	Radia® 7178
Parapel® HC-85	Pluracol® E600	Protegin® WX SE	Radia® 7185
Parapel® LAM-100	Pluracol® E600 NF	Protegin® X SE	Radia® 7187
Parapel® LIS	Pluracol® E1000	Pro-Tein ES-20	Radia® 7190
Paricin® 9	Pluracol® E1450	Prothera™	Radia® 7200
Paricin® 13	Pluracol® E1450 NF	Protol®	Radia® 7204
Paricin® 15	Pluracol® E2000	Proto-Lan 4R	Radia® 7230
Pationic® 138C	Pluracol® E4000 NF	Proto-Lan 8	Radia® 7241
Pationic® ISL	Pluracol® E4500	Proto-Lan 20	Radia® 7266
Pationic® SBL	Pluracol® E8000	Proto-Lan 30	Radia® 7345
Pationic® SCL	Pluracol® E8000 NF	Proto-Lan IP	Radia® 7355
Patlac® IL	Pogol 200	Protopet® Alba	Radia® 7371
PCL Liq. 100	Polyaldo® DGHO	Protopet® White 1S	Radia® 7500
PCL Liq. 1002/066240	Polycare® 133	Protopet® White 2L	Radia® 7501
Pea Pro-Tein BK	Polychol 5	Protopet® White 3C	Radia® 7505
Peceol Isostearique	Polychol 10	Protopet® Yellow 1E	Radia® 7506
Pegosperse® 50 DS	Polychol 15	Protopet® Yellow 2A	Radia® 7730
Pegosperse® 100 O	Polychol 16	Provol 10	Radia® 7732
Pegosperse® 200 ML	Polychol 20	Provol 30	Radia® 7752
Pegosperse® 6000 DS	Polychol 40	Provol 50	Radia® 7761
Pegosperse® EGMS-70	Polylan®	Prox-onic HR-05	Radia® 7770
Pelemol BB	Polypeptide 10	Prox-onic HR-016	Radiacid® 152
Pelemol BIS	Polypeptide 12	Prox-onic HR-025	Radiacid® 212
Pelemol CR	Polypeptide 37	Prox-onic HR-030	Radiacid® 416
Pelemol EE	Polyquart® H	Prox-onic HR-036	Radiacid® 423
Pelemol GTB	Polyquart® H 81	Prox-onic HR-040	Radiacid® 427
Pelemol HAB	Polyquart® H 7102	Prox-onic HR-080	Radiacid® 428
Pelemol ICB	Polytex 10M	Prox-onic HR-0200	Radiacid® 464
Pelemol ICS	Pripure DIPD 3786	Prox-onic HR-0200/50	Radiacid® 631
Pelemol ISB	Prisorine 3501	Prox-onic HRH-05	Radiamox® 6800
Pelemol MS	Prisorine GMIS 2040	Prox-onic HRH-016	Radiamox® 6804
Pelemol OE	Prisorine IPIS 2021	Prox-onic HRH-025	Radianol® 1712
Pelemol P-49	Prisorine ISAC 3505	Prox-onic HRH-0200	Radianol® 1724
Pelemol TDE	Prisorine ISIS 2039	Prox-onic HRH-0200/50	Radianol® 1726
Peneteck	Prisorine ISOH 3515	Prox-onic MG-010	Radianol® 1728
Penreco Amber	Procetyl 10	Prox-onic MG-020	Radianol® 1763
Penreco Blond	Procetyl 30	Pseudocollagen™	Radianol® 1765
Penreco Cream	Procetyl 50	Pur-Cellin Oil	Radianol® 1768
Penreco Lily	Procetyl AWS	Pur-Cellin Wax	Radianol® 1769
Penreco Regent	Procol OA-2	Purton CFD	Radianol® 1898
Penreco Royal	Procol OA-3	Purton SFD	Radianol® 7106
Penreco Snow	Procol OA-4	PVP K-15	Radiaquat® 6442
Penreco Super	Procol OA-5	PVP K-30	Radiaquat® 6444
Penreco Ultima	Procol OA-10	PVP/Si-10	Radiaquat® 6445
Peptein® 2000®	Procol PMA-3	Pyroter GPI-25	Radiaquat® 6460
Peptein® Qs	Procol PSA-11	Quamectant™ AM-50	Radiaquat® 6462
Peptein® Qw	Procol PSA-15	Quat-Pro E	Radiaquat® 6471
Perfecta® USP	Produkt GS 5001	Quat-Pro S	Radiateric® 6860
Perfecta®	Produkt RT 288	Quat-Pro S 30	Radiateric® 6864
Permethyl® 108A	Promulgen® D	Quatrex CT-100	Reticusol
Permulgin 835	Promulgen® G	Quatrex CTAC	Rewocid® U 185
Pharmaceutical Lanolin	Promyr	Quatrex S	Rewocid® UTM 185
USP	Promyristyl PM-3	Quatrex STC-85	Rewoderm® ES 90
Phosal 25 SB	Propal	Quatrisoft® Polymer LM-	Rewoderm® LI 48
Phosal® 75 SA	Propoxyol® 1695	200	Rewoderm® LI 63
Phosal® NAT-50-PG	Prostearyl 15	Quat-Wheat™ SDMA-25	Rewoderm® LI 67-75
PhosPho 642	Protachem CER	Querton 16Cl-50	Rewoderm® LIS 75
PhosPho E-100	Protachem IPM	Querton 442	Rewolan® 5
PhosPho LCN-TS	Protachem IPP	Querton 442-11	Rewolan® AWS
PhosPho PL-50	Protachem SDM	Querton 442-82	Rewolan® E
Phospholipid PTC	Protalan L-30	Querton 442E	Rewolan® E 50, 100
Phospholipid PTD	Protalan L-75	Querton 442H	Rewolan® LP
Phospholipid PTL	Protalan MOD	Querton 442P	Rewomid® C 212
Phospholipid PTS	Protalan Oil	Querton 442P-11	Rewomid® DC 220 SE
Phospholipid PTZ	Protalan Wax	Radia® 7106	Rewomid® DL 203 S
Phospholipid SV	Protaquat 2HT-75	Radia® 7108	Rewomid® DL 203
Planell™ Oil	Protectein™	Radia® 7117	Rewomid® DL 240

Emollients/Conditioners/Softeners... *(cont'd.)*

Rewomid® DLM SE	Ritawax Super	Schercemol DID	Schercoquat IIB
Rewomid® DO 280 S	Robane®	Schercemol DIS	Schercoquat IIS
Rewomid® DO 280 SE	Robecote	Schercemol DISD	Schercoquat IIS-R
Rewomid® F	Robeyl	Schercemol DISF	Schercoquat IIS-RD
Rewomid® IPE 280	Rol 52	Schercemol DO	Schercoquat MKAS
Rewomid® L 203	Rol 53	Schercemol EE	Schercoquat ROAB
Rewomid® S 280	Rol 59	Schercemol GMIS	Schercoquat ROAS
Rewominox B 204	Rol 400	Schercemol ICS	Schercoquat ROEP
Rewominox L 408	Rol AG	Schercemol IDO	Schercoquat SAB
Rewominox S 300	Rol DGE	Schercemol IPM	Schercoquat SAS
Rewominoxid B 204	Rol DL 40	Schercemol IPO	Schercoquat SOAS
Rewominoxid S 300	Rol DO 40	Schercemol ISE	Schercoquat WOAS
Rewomul HL	Rol GE	Schercemol LL	Schercotaine APAB
Rewomul IS	Rol L 40	Schercemol MEL-3	Schercotaine IAB
Rewoquat CPEM	Rol LP	Schercemol MEM-3	Schercotaine MKAB
Rewoquat RTM 50	Rol MOG	Schercemol MEP-3	Schercotaine OAB
Rewoquat W 7500 H	Rol RP	Schercemol ML	Schercotaine PAB
Rewoquat WE 16	Rol TR	Schercemol MM	Schercotaine WOAB
Rewoteric® AM 2C W	Rolamid CD	Schercemol MP	Schercoteric MS
Rewoteric® AM HC	Rudol®	Schercemol MS	Schercoteric STS
Rewoteric® AM TEG	Ryoto Sugar Ester OWA-	Schercemol NGDL	Schercozoline I
Rhodamox® CAPO	1570	Schercemol NGDO	Schercozoline L
Rhodamox® LO	Ryoto Sugar Ester P-1570	Schercemol OHS	Schercozoline O
Rhodaquat® M214B/99	Ryoto Sugar Ester P-1570S	Schercemol OLO	Schercozoline S
Rhodaquat® M242B/99	Ryoto Sugar Ester P-1670	Schercemol OP	Scheroba Oil
Rhodaquat® M242C/29	Ryoto Sugar Ester S-070	Schercemol OPG	Seanamin FP
Rhodasurf® C-2	Ryoto Sugar Ester S-170	Schercemol PGDP	Seanamin SU
Rhodasurf® C-20	Ryoto Sugar Ester S-270	Schercemol PGML	Sebase
Rhodasurf® L-4	Ryoto Sugar Ester S-370	Schercemol SE	Secoster® DMS
Rhodasurf® L-25	Ryoto Sugar Ester S-370F	Schercemol TIST	Secoster® EMS
Rhodasurf® S-2	Ryoto Sugar Ester S-570	Schercodine B	Sedaplant Richter
Rhodasurf® S-20	Ryoto Sugar Ester S-770	Schercodine M	Sellig Lano 30
Rhodasurf® TD-9	Ryoto Sugar Ester S-970	Schercodine O	Serdolamide POF 61
Rhodorsil® Oils 70641 V	Ryoto Sugar Ester S-1170	Schercodine P	Serdolamide PYF 77
200	Ryoto Sugar Ester S-1170S	Schercodine S	Sericoside Phytosome®
Rice Pro-Tein BK	Ryoto Sugar Ester S-1570	Schercodine T	SF96® (5 cst)
Rita AZ	Ryoto Sugar Ester S-1670	Schercomid AME	SF1173
Rita CA	Ryoto Sugar Ester S-1670S	Schercomid AME-70	SF1188
Rita EDGS	Salcare SC10	Schercomid CMI	SF1202
Rita EGMS	Salcare SC30	Schercomid ID	SF1204
Rita GMS	Salcare SC91	Schercomid IMI	S-Flakes
Rita KA	Salcare SC92	Schercomid LME	Shebu® Refined
Rita SA	Salfax 77	Schercomid M	Shebu® WS
Ritacetyl®	Sandoperm FE	Schercomid ODA	Silamide DCA-100
Ritachol®	Sandotex A	Schercomid OME	Silamine 50
Ritachol® 2000	Sandoz Amine Oxide XA-C	Schercomid OMI	Silamine 65
Ritachol® 4000	Satexlan 20	Schercomid SI	Silbione™ 70045 V2 and
Ritachol 5000	Satulan	Schercomid SLE	V5
Ritaderm®	ScentCap	Schercomid SL-ML	Silbione™ 70047
Ritahydrox	Schercamox C-AA	Schercomid SLS	Silbione™ 70633 V30
Ritalafa®	Schercamox CMA	Schercomid SO-A	Silbione™ 70646
Ritalan®	Schercamox DMS	Schercomid TO-2	Silbione™ 71631
Ritalan® AWS	Schercamox T-12	Schercopol CMS-Na	Silbione™ 71634
Ritalan® C	Schercemol 65	Schercopol OMS-Na	Silk Pro-Tein
RITA Lanolin	Schercemol 105	Schercoquat 2IAE	Silk Protein Complex
Ritaloe 1X, 10X, 20X, 40X	Schercemol 145	Schercoquat 2IAP	Silquat AD
Ritaloe 200M	Schercemol 185	Schercoquat ALA	Silquat AM
Ritapro 100	Schercemol 318	Schercoquat APAS	Silquat Q-100
Ritasol	Schercemol 1688	Schercoquat BAS	Silquat Q-200
Ritavena™ 5	Schercemol 1818	Schercoquat CAS	Silquat Q-300
Ritawax	Schercemol BE	Schercoquat COAS	Simchin® Natural
Ritawax 5	Schercemol CL	Schercoquat DAB	Simchin® Refined
Ritawax 10	Schercemol CM	Schercoquat DAS	Simchin® WS
Ritawax 15	Schercemol CP	Schercoquat IALA	Siponic® E-2
Ritawax 20	Schercemol CS	Schercoquat IAS	Siponic® E-3
Ritawax 40	Schercemol DED	Schercoquat IAS-LC	Siponic® E-5
Ritawax AEO	Schercemol DIA	Schercoquat IB	Siponic® E-7
Ritawax ALA	Schercemol DICA	Schercoquat IEP	Siponic® E-10

Emollients/Conditioners/Softeners... *(cont'd.)*

Siponic® E-15
Siponic® L-1
Skliro Distilled
Snow White Petrolatum
Softigen® 701
Softigen® 767
Softisan® 100
Softisan® 378
Softisan® 601
Softisan® 649
Solan
Solan 50
Solan E
Solidester
Solulan® 5
Solulan® 16
Solulan® 75
Solulan® 97
Solulan® 98
Solulan® C-24
Solulan® PB-2
Solulan® PB-5
Solulan® PB-10
Solulan® PB-20
Solu-Mar™ EN-30
Sol-U-Tein EA
Sol-U-Tein FS-1000
Sol-U-Tein PS-1000
Sol-U-Tein VG
Solwax L20
Solwax LG 35
Sono Jell® No. 4
Sono Jell® No. 9
Sorba
Soy-Amino Quat L/O
Soy-Quat C
Soy-Tein NL
Span® 20
Span® 40
Span® 60, 60K
Span® 65
Span® 85
Special Oil 888
SS 4267
Stabileze™ 06
Stafoam DF-1
Stafoam DF-4
Stafoam DL
Stamere®
Standamid® 100
Standamid® ID
Standamid® KD
Standamid® LD
Standamid® LP
Standamid® SDO
Standamox CAW
Standamox O1
Standamox PS
Standamul® 302
Standamul® 318
Standamul® 1414-E
Standamul® 7061
Standamul® 7063
Standamul® Conc. 1002
Standamul® CTA
Standamul® CTV
Standamul® G-16
Standamul® G-32/36

Standamul® G-32/36
  Stearate
Standamul® HE
Standamul® LC
Standamul® O-5
Standamul® O-10
Standamul® O-20
Standamul® OXL
Standapol® AB-45
Standapol® BAW
Standapol® BC-35
Standapol® OLB-30
Standapol® OLB-50
Standapol® SCO
Starfol® CP
Starfol® OS
Starfol® Wax CG
Stearal
Stedbac®
Stepanol® LX
Stepan Pearl Series
Steraffine
Sterol CC 595
Sterol LG 491
St. John's Wort Oil CLR
Sumquat® 6045
Sumquat® 6210
Super Corona
Superfine Lanolin
  Anhydrous USP
Super Hartolan
Superpro 5A
Super Refined™ Almond
  Oil NF
Super Refined™ Apricot
  Kernel Oil NF
Super Refined™ Avocado
  Oil
Super Refined™ Babassu
  Oil
Super Refined™ Coconut
  Oil
Super Refined™
  Crossential EPO
Super Refined™
  Grapeseed Oil
Super Refined™
  Menhaden Oil
Super Refined™ Mink Oil
Super Refined™ Olive Oil
Super Refined™ Orange
  Roughy Oil
Super Refined™ Peanut Oil
Super Refined™ Safflower
  Oil USP
Super Refined™ Sesame
  Oil
Super Refined™ Shark
  Liver Oil
Super Refined™ Soybean
  Oil USP
Super Refined™ Wheat
  Germ Oil
Super-Sat
Super-Sat AWS-4
Super-Sat AWS-24
Super Solan Flaked
Super Sterol Ester

Supraene®
Supralate XL
Supro-Tein R
Supro-Tein S
Surfactol® 318
Surfactol® 365
Surfactol® 575
Surfactol® 590
Surfactol® Q1
Surfactol® Q2
Surfactol® Q3
Surfactol® Q4
SWS-101
SWS-03314
Syncrowax AW1-C
Syncrowax BB-4
Syncrowax ERL-C
Syncrowax HGL-C
Syncrowax HR-C
Syncrowax HRS-C
Synoquart P 50
Synotol CN 20
Synotol CN 60
Synotol CN 80
Synotol CN 90
Synotol ME 90
Tagat® TO
Tauranol I-78
Tauranol I-78-3
Tauranol I-78-6
Tauranol I-78/80
Tauranol I-78E, I-78E
  Flakes
Tauranol I-78 Flakes
Tegamine® 18
Tegamine® P-7
Tegin® 55G VA
Tegin® E-41
Tegin® E-41 NSE
Tegin® E-61
Tegin® E-61 NSE
Tegin® E-66
Tegin® E-66 NSE
Tegin® L 61, L 62
Tegin® RZ
Tegin® RZ NSE
Tegin® VA 55G
Tego®-Amid D 5040
Tego®-Amid O 18
Tego®-Amid S 18
Tego®-Betaine HS
Tego®-Pearl S-33
Tegosoft® 168
Tegosoft® 189
Tegosoft® CI
Tegosoft® CO
Tegosoft® CT
Tegosoft® DO
Tegosoft® EE
Tegosoft® GC
Tegosoft® Liquid
Tegosoft® Liquid M
Tegosoft® M
Tegosoft® OP
Tegosoft® OS
Tegosoft® P
Tegosoft® S
Tegosoft® SH

Tequat BC
Tofupro-U
Tri-K CMF Complex
Tri-K Soypro-25
Trimol CE 2000
Tri-OI OLV
Tri-OI SAF
Tri-OI SES
Tri-OI WG
Trioxene E
Tri-Sil HGC 5000
Tri-Sil MFF 5010
Tri-Sil MFF 5010-70
Tri-Sil MFF 5015
Trisolan 1720
Tri-Tein Milk Polypeptide
Tri-Tein Silk AA
Tritisol™
Trivent ALA
Trivent BE-13
Trivent CP
Trivent DIA
Trivent DOS
Trivent NP-13
Trivent OC-13
Trivent OC-16
Trivent OC-143
Trivent OC-G
Trivent OL-10
Trivent OL-10B
Trivent OP
Trivent PE-48
Trivent SS-13
Trivent SS-20
Turkey Red Oil 100%
Ucare® Polymer JR-30M,
  JR-125, JR-400
Ucon® 50-HB-55
Ucon® 50-HB-100
Ucon® 50-HB-170
Ucon® 50-HB-260
Ucon® 50-HB-400
Ucon® 50-HB-660
Ucon® 50-HB-1000
Ucon® 50-HB-2000
Ucon® 50-HB-3520
Ucon® 50-HB-5100
Ucon® 75-H-450
Ucon® 75-H-1400
Ucon® Fluid AP
Ucon® LB-385
Ucon® LB-625
Ucon® LB-1145
Ucon® LB-1715
Ucon® LB-3000
Ucon® LO-500
Ucon® LO-1000
Ultra Lantrol® HP-2074
Unger EST
Unibetaine OLB-30,
  OLB-50
Unicast CO
Unicol OA-2
Unicol OA-4
Unicol OA-10
Uniderm SSME
Uniderm WGO
Unifat 54

Emollients/Conditioners/Softeners... *(cont'd.)*

Unilin® 425 Alcohol	Varisoft® 250	Vybar® 103	Wickenol® 535
Unilube MB-370	Varisoft® 300	Vybar® 260	Wickenol® 545
Unimate® BYS	Varisoft® 355	Vybar® 5013	Wickenol® 707
Unimate® DBS	Varisoft® 432-100	Waxenol® 801	Wickenol® 727
Unimate® DIPS	Varisoft® 432-CG	Waxenol® 810	Witafrol® 7420
Unimate® DOS	Varisoft® 432-ET	Waxenol® 815	Witcamide® 61
Unimate® EHP	Varisoft® 432-PPG	Waxenol® 816	Witcamide® 70
Unimate® IPM	Varisoft® 470	Waxenol® 821	Witcamide® 82
Unimate® IPP	Varisoft® 475	Waxenol® 822	Witcamide® 128T
Unimate® IPPM	Varisoft® CTB-40	Wecobee® FS	Witcamide® 823/10
Unimul-05	Varisoft® SDAC	Wecobee® FW	Witcamide® 5133
Unimul-10	Varisoft® ST-50	Wecobee® SS	Witcamide® 5195
Unimul-1414EW	Varisoft® TA-100	Wecobee® W	Witcamide® 6310
Unimul-7061	Varisoft® TIMS	W.G.S. Synaceti 116 NF/	Witcamide® 6511
Unimul-CTV	Varonic® 32-E20	USP	Witcamide® 6514
Unimul-G	Varonic® 63 E20	Wheat Germ Oil	Witcamide® 6531
Unimul-G-16	Varox® 270	Wheat Germ Oil CLR	Witcamide® 6533
Union Carbide® L-45	Varox® 365	Wheat-Quat C	Witcamide® 6546
Series	Varox® 1770	Wheat-Tein NL	Witcamide® 6625
Unisoft SAC	Varsulf® S-1333	White Swan	Witcamide® C
Unitolate 380	Varsulf® SBF-12	Wickenol® 101	Witcamide® CD
Unitolate 868	Varsulf® SBFA-30	Wickenol® 105	Witcamide® CPA
Unitolate B	Varsulf® SBL-203	Wickenol® 111	Witcamide® LDEA
Unitolate V	Vegamino™ 30-SF	Wickenol® 127	Witcamide® LDTS
Uniwhite Oil 55, 70, 85,	Velsan® D8P-3	Wickenol® 131	Witcamide® MAS
130, 185, 205, 350	Velsan® D8P-16	Wickenol® 136	Witcamide® MM
Unizeen OA	Velsan® P8-3	Wickenol® 139	Witcamide® NA
Upamate IPM	Velsan® P8-16	Wickenol® 141	Witcamide® SSA
Upamate IPP	Velvetex® AB-45	Wickenol® 142	Witcamide® STD-HP
U Tanol G	Velvetex® BA-35	Wickenol® 144	Witcamine® 6606
Valfor® Zeolite Na-A	Velvetex® BC-35	Wickenol® 151	Witcamine® 6622
Vanseal® MS	Velvetex® BK-35	Wickenol® 152	Witconol™ 2314
Vanseal® NAMS-30	Velvetex® OLB-30	Wickenol® 153	Yeoman
Varamide® C-212	Velvetex® OLB-50	Wickenol® 155	York Krystal Kleer Castor
Varamide® L-203	Vigilan	Wickenol® 156	Oil
Varamide® LL-1	Vigilan AWS	Wickenol® 158	York USP Castor Oil
Varamide® LO-1	Viscasil®	Wickenol® 159	Zeolex® 23A
Varamide® MA-1	Vita-Cos	Wickenol® 160	Zeolex® 7
Varamide® ML-1	Volatile Silicone 7158,	Wickenol® 161	Zohar EGMS
Varamide® ML-4	7207, 7349	Wickenol® 163	Zohar GLST
Varion® CDG	Volpo 3	Wickenol® 171	Zohar GLST SE
Varion® SDG	Volpo 5	Wickenol® 174	Zoharpon LMT42
Varisoft® 2TD	Volpo 10	Wickenol® 506	Zoramide CM
Varisoft® 5TD	Volpo 20		

Emulsifiers

Abex® LIV/30	Ablunol 1000MS	Ablunol S-85	Accomeen T15
Abil® B 9806, B 9808	Ablunol 6000DS	Ablunol SA-7	Accomid C
Abil® B 9808	Ablunol CO 5	Ablunol T-20	Accomid PK
Abil® EM-90	Ablunol CO 15	Ablunol T-40	Acconon 200-DL
Abil® WE 09	Ablunol CO 30	Ablunol T-60	Acconon 200-MS
Abil® WS 08	Ablunol GMS	Ablunol T-80	Acconon 300-MO
Ablumine DHT75	Ablunol LA-3	Ablusol DBD	Acconon 400-DO
Ablumox CAPO	Ablunol LA-5	Ablusol DBM	Acconon 400-ML
Ablumox LO	Ablunol LA-7	Ablusol DBT	Acconon 400-MO
Ablunol 200ML	Ablunol LA-9	Abluter CPB	Acconon 400-MS
Ablunol 200MO	Ablunol LA-12	Accobetaine CL	Acconon 1300
Ablunol 200MS	Ablunol LA-16	Accomeen C2	Acconon CA-5
Ablunol 400ML	Ablunol LA-40	Accomeen C5	Acconon CA-8
Ablunol 400MO	Ablunol OA-6	Accomeen C10	Acconon CA-9
Ablunol 400MS	Ablunol OA-7	Accomeen C15	Acconon CA-15
Ablunol 600ML	Ablunol S-20	Accomeen S2	Acconon CA-25
Ablunol 600MO	Ablunol S-40	Accomeen S10	Acconon CON
Ablunol 600MS	Ablunol S-60	Accomeen T2	Acconon E
Ablunol 1000MO	Ablunol S-80	Accomeen T5	Acconon TGH

Emulsifiers *(cont'd.)*

Acconon W230
Acrisint 400, 410, 430
Acritamer® 934
Acritamer® 934P
Acritamer® 940
Acritamer® 941
Acrysol® A-1
Adinol CT95
Adinol OT16
Adogen® 160D
Adogen® 170D
Adogen® 444
Adogen® MA-108 SF
Adogen® MA-112 SF
Adogen® S-18 V
Adol® 52 NF
Adol® 80
Adol® 85
Adol® 320, 330, 340
Adol® 630
Adol® 640
AE-1214/3
Aerosol® 19
Aerosol® A-102
Aerosol® A-103
Aerosol® OT-70 PG
Agnosol 3
Agnosol 5
Ajicoat SPG
Akypo NP 70
Akypo RLM 38 NV
Akypo RLM 45
Akypo RLM 100
Akypo RLM 100 MGV
Akypo RLM 130
Akypo RLM 160
Akypo RLM 160 NV
Akypo RLMQ 38
Akypo®-Muls 400
Akyporox CO 400
Akyporox CO 600
Akyporox RLM 22
Akyporox RLM 40
Akyporox RLM 80V
Akyporox RO 90
Akyposal 100 DAL
Akyposal ALS 33
Akypo®-Soft 100 MgV
Akypo®-Soft 100 NV
Akypo®-Soft 130 NV
Akypo®-Soft 160 NV
Alanate 110
Albalan
Alcodet® 218
Alcodet® SK
Alcolan®
Alcolan® 36W
Alcolec® BS
Alcolec® Extra A
Alcolec® F-100
Alcolec® Granules
Alcolec® PG
Alcolec® Powder
Alcolec® S
Alcolec® SFG
Alcolec® Z-3
Alcolec® Z-7
Aldo® DC

Aldo® HMS
Aldo® ML
Aldo® MLD
Aldo® MO
Aldo® MO FG
Aldo® MOD
Aldo® MOD FG
Aldo® MR
Aldo® MS
Aldo® MS-20 FG
Aldo® MSA
Aldo® MSC
Aldo® MSD
Aldo® MS LG
Aldo® MSLG FG
Aldo® PMS
Aldosperse® L L-20
Aldosperse® ML-23
Aldosperse® MS-20
Aldosperse® O-20 FG
Alfonic® 1012-2.5
Alfonic® 1214-GC-2
Alfonic® 1216-1.5
Alfonic® 1216-CO-2
Alfonic® 1412-3
Algon LA 40
Algon LA 80
Algon OL 60
Algon OL 70
Algon ST 50
Algon ST 80
Algon ST 100
Algon ST 200
Algon ST 400
Algon ST 500
Algon ST 1000
Alkamide® 101 CG
Alkamide® 2124
Alkamide® C-5
Alkamide® CDE
Alkamide® CDM
Alkamide® CDO
Alkamide® CL63
Alkamide® DC-212
Alkamide® DC-212/S
Alkamide® DIN-295/S
Alkamide® DO-280
Alkamide® DO-280/S
Alkamide® HTDE
Alkamide® L9DE
Alkamuls® 200-DL
Alkamuls® 200-DO
Alkamuls® 200-DS
Alkamuls® 400-DL
Alkamuls® 400-DO
Alkamuls® 400-DS
Alkamuls® 400-ML
Alkamuls® 400-MO
Alkamuls® 400-MS
Alkamuls® 600-DL
Alkamuls® 600-DO
Alkamuls® 600-DS
Alkamuls® 600-ML
Alkamuls® 600-MO
Alkamuls® 6000-DS
Alkamuls® B
Alkamuls® BR
Alkamuls® CO-15

Alkamuls® EGMS
Alkamuls® EL-620
Alkamuls® EL-620L
Alkamuls® EL-719
Alkamuls® GMO
Alkamuls® GMO-45LG
Alkamuls® GMS/C
Alkamuls® L-9
Alkamuls® PEG 300 DS
Alkamuls® PETS
Alkamuls® PSML-20
Alkamuls® PSMO-5
Alkamuls® PSMO-20
Alkamuls® PSMS-4
Alkamuls® PSMS-20
Alkamuls® PSTO-20
Alkamuls® PSTS-20
Alkamuls® S-6
Alkamuls® SML
Alkamuls® SMO
Alkamuls® SMS
Alkamuls® ST-40
Alkamuls® STS
Alkamuls® T-20
Alkamuls® T-60
Alkamuls® T-65
Alkamuls® T-85
Alkaqua® DMB-451-50,
  DMB-451-80
Alkasurf® L-14
Alkasurf® NP-1
Alkasurf® NP-4
Alkasurf® NP-6
Alkasurf® NP-8
Alkasurf® NP-15
Alkasurf® NP-30, 70%
Alkasurf® NP-40, 70%
Alkasurf® SA-20
Alkasurf® T
Alkasurf® TDA-12
Alkasurf® TLS
Alkaterge®-E
Alrosperse 11P Flake
Amerchol® 400
Amerchol® BL
Amerchol® C
Amerchol® CAB
Amerchol® H-9
Amerchol® L-99
Amerchol® L-500
Amerchol® RC
Amerlate® LFA
Amerlate® P
Amerlate® W
Amerlate® WFA
Ameroxol® LE-4
Ameroxol® LE-23
Ameroxol® OE-2
Ameroxol® OE-5
Ameroxol® OE-10
Ameroxol® OE-20
Amersil® ME-358
Amidex LD
Amidex LN
Amidex O
Amidex RC
Amidex S
Amidex SE

Amidex SME
Amidox® C-2
Amidox® C-5
Amidox® L-2
Amidox® L-5
Amifat P-21
Amifat P-30
Amihope LL-11
Amine 12-98D
Amine 16D
Amine KKD
Aminol CA-2
Aminol COR-2C
Aminol COR-4C
Aminoxid WS 35
Amisoft CT-12
Amisoft GS-11
Amisoft HS-11
Amisoft HT-12
Amisoft LS-11
Amisoft LT-12
Amisol™ MS-12 BA
Amiter LGS-2
Amiter LGS-5
Ammonyx® 4, 4B, 485,
  4002
Ammonyx® CA-Special
Ammonyx® CETAC,
  CETAC-30
Ammonyx® CO
Ammonyx® LO
Ammonyx® SO
AMP
AMPD
Amphisol®
Amphisol® K
Amphocerin® E
Amphoteen 24
AMS-33
Amyx A-25-S 0040
Amyx LO 3594
Amyx SO 3734
Anhydrous Lanolin Grade 1
Anhydrous Lanolin Grade 2
Anhydrous Lanolin HP-
  2050
Anhydrous Lanolin P.80
Anhydrous Lanolin P.95
Anhydrous Lanolin P.95RA
Anhydrous Lanolin
  Superfine
Anhydrous Lanolin USP
  Cosmetic Grade
Anhydrous Lanolin USP
  Pharmaceutical Grade
Anhydrous Lanolin USP
  Pharmaceutical Light
  Grade
Anhydrous Lanolin USP
  X-tra Deodorized
Annonyx SO
Antaron® FC-34
Antaron® MC-44
Antarox® L-64
Antarox® PGP 18-1
Antarox® PGP 18-2
Antarox® PGP 18-2D
Antarox® PGP 18-2LF

Emulsifiers *(cont'd.)*

Antarox® PGP 18-8	Armeen® TD	Biozan	Capmul® POE-O
Antarox® PGP 23-7	Armotan® ML	Brij® 30	Capmul® POE-S
Antarox® PGP 33-8	Armotan® MO	Brij® 30SP	Caprol® 2G4S
Aquabase	Armotan® MP	Brij® 35	Caprol® 3GO
Aquabase N.F	Armotan® MS	Brij® 52	Caprol® 3GS
Aqualose L30	Armotan® NP	Brij® 56	Caprol® 6G2O
Aqualose L75	Armotan® PMD 20	Brij® 58	Caprol® 6G2S
Aqualose L75/50	Armotan® PML 20	Brij® 72	Caprol® 10G2O
Aqualose LL100	Armotan® PMO 20	Brij® 76	Caprol® 10G4O
Aqualose W5	Aromox® C/12	Brij® 78	Caprol® 10G10O
Aqualose W20	Aromox® C/12-W	Brij® 92	Caprol® PGE860
Aqualose W20/50	Aromox® DMMC-W	Brij® 93	Carbopol® 907
Aquaphil K	Arosurf® 42-E6	Brij® 96	Carbopol® 910
Argobase 125	Arosurf® 66-E2	Brij® 97	Carbopol® 934P
Argobase EU	Arosurf® 66-E10	Brij® 98	Carbopol® 940
Argobase L1	Arosurf® 66-E20	Brij® 700	Carbopol® 941
Argobase L2	Arosurf® 66-PE12	Brij® 700S	Carbopol® 954
Argobase MS 5	Arquad® 2C-75	Brij® 721	Carbopol® 980
Argobase S1	Arquad® 2HT-75	Brij® 721S	Carbopol® 981
Argonol 40	Arquad® 12-33	Britex C	Carbopol® 1342
Argonol 60	Arquad® 12-37W	Britex C 20	Carbopol® 1382
Argowax Cosmetic Super	Arquad® 12-50	Britex C 100	Carbopol® 2984
Argowax Dist	Arquad® 16-29	Britex C 200	Carbopol® 5984
Argowax Standard	Arquad® 16-29W	Britex CO 220	Carsamide® CA
Arlacel® 20	Arquad® 16-50	Britex CS 110	Carsamide® SAL-7
Arlacel® 40	Arquad® 18-50	Britex CS 200 B	Carsonol® ALS
Arlacel® 60	Arquad® B-50	Britex CS 250	Carsonol® ALS-R
Arlacel® 80	Arquad® B-90	Britex L 20	Carsonol® ALS-S
Arlacel® 83	Arquad® C-33	Britex L 40	Carsonol® ALS Special
Arlacel® 129	Arquad® C-33W	Britex L 100	Carsonol® DLS
Arlacel® 165	Arquad® C-50	Britex L 230	Carsonol® ILS
Arlacel® 186	Arquad® DM18B-90	Britex O 20	Carsonol® MLS
Arlacel® 481	Arquad® DMMCB-50	Britex O 100	Carsonol® SLES-3
Arlacel® 581	Arquad® HT-50	Britex O 200	Carsonol® SLS
Arlacel® 582	Arquad® S-50	Britex S 20	Carsonol® SLS Paste B
Arlacel® 780	Arquad® T-2C-50	Britex S 100	Carsonol® SLS-R
Arlacel® 986	Arquad® T-27W	Britex S 200	Carsonol® SLS-S
Arlacel® 987	Arquad® T-50	Britex TR 60	Carsonol® SLS Special
Arlacel® 988	Artodan CF 40	Britex TR 120	Carsonol® TLS
Arlacel® 989	Artodan SP 55 Kosher	Brooksgel 41	Carsonon® L-2
Arlacel® 1689	Asol	Brophos™ 5C10	Carsonon® L-3
Arlacel® C	Atmos 150	Brophos™ A	Carsonon® L-5
Arlasolve® 200	Atmos 300	Brophos™ OL-3	Carsonon® L-12
Arlasolve® 200 Liq	Atomergic Cholesterol	Brophos™ OL-3N	Carsonon® N-30
Arlatone® 285	Atsurf 594	Brophos™ OL-3NPG	Carsonon® N-100
Arlatone® 289	Augon 1000	Brox OL-2	Carsoquat® 868P
Arlatone® 983	Avanel® S-30	Brox OL-3	Carsoquat® CB
Arlatone® 983S	Avanel® S-35	Brox OL-4	Cation LQ
Arlatone® 985	Avanel® S-70	Brox OL-5	Cedepon LA-30
Arlatone® 2121	Avanel® S-74	Brox OL-10	Cedepon® LS-30PM
Arlatone® B	Avanel® S-90	Brox OL-20	Centrolene® A, S
Arlatone® T	Avanel® S-150	Brox OL-20 70% Liq	Centrolex® F
Armeen® 2C	Axol® E 61	Brox OL-40	Centrolex® P
Armeen® 2HT	Barlox® 12	Burco Anionic APS	Centromix® E
Armeen® 2T	Barlox® 16S	Calamide C	Cera-E
Armeen® 12D	Barlox® 18S	Calfoam NEL-60	Ceral 10
Armeen® 16D	Basis LP-20	Calfoam NLS-30	Ceral 165
Armeen® 18	Basis LS-60	Calfoam SLS-30	Ceral CK
Armeen® 18D	BBS	Calsoft F-90	Ceral EFN
Armeen® C	Berol 452	Calsoft L-40	Ceral EN 6
Armeen® CD	BFP 640	Calsoft L-60	Ceral G
Armeen® HT	Bina QAT-43	Calsuds CD-6	Ceral LE
Armeen® HTD	Bio-Soft® E-200	Capmul® EMG	Ceral MA
Armeen® OL	Bio-Soft® E-300	Capmul® GDL	Ceral ME
Armeen® OLD	Bio-Soft® E-400	Capmul® GMO	Ceral MET
Armeen® S	Bio-Soft® EN 600	Capmul® MCM	Ceral MEX
Armeen® SD	Bio-Soft® TD 400	Capmul® MCM-90	Ceral ML
Armeen® T	Bio-Soft® TD 630	Capmul® POE-L	Ceral MN

Emulsifiers *(cont'd.)*

Ceral MNT	Chemax CO-200/50	Cithrol 2DL	Cosmowax
Ceral MNX	Chemax/DOSS-75E	Cithrol 2DO	Cosmowax J
Ceral P	Chemax E-200 ML	Cithrol 2ML	Cosmowax K
Ceral PA	Chemax E-200 MO	Cithrol 2MO	CPC
Ceral PW	Chemax E-200 MS	Cithrol 2MS	CPC Sumquat 6060
Ceral TG	Chemax E-400 ML	Cithrol 3MS	CPH-27-N
Ceral TN	Chemax E-400 MO	Cithrol 4DL	CPH-30-N
Ceral TP	Chemax E-400 MS	Cithrol 4DO	CPH-34-N
Ceralan®	Chemax E-600 ML	Cithrol 4ML	CPH-35-N
Ceramol	Chemax E-600 MO	Cithrol 4MO	CPH-37-NA
Ceranine HC Hi Conc	Chemax E-600 MS	Cithrol 4MO	CPH-40-N
Ceranine HCA	Chemax E-1000 ML	Cithrol 4MS	CPH-46-N
Ceranine PN Base	Chemax E-1000 MO	Cithrol 6DL	CPH-50-N
Ceraphyl® 65	Chemax E-1000 MS	Cithrol 6DO	CPH-90-N
Ceraphyl® 70	Chemax HCO-5	Cithrol 6ML	CPH-104-DC-SE
Ceraphyl® 85	Chemax HCO-16	Cithrol 6MO	CPH-104-DG-SE
Cerasynt® 303	Chemax HCO-25	Cithrol 6MS	CPH-233-N
Cerasynt® 840	Chemax HCO-200/50	Cithrol 10DL	Cralane KR-13, -14
Cerasynt® 945	Chemax NP-1.5	Cithrol 10DO	Cralane LR-10
Cerasynt® D	Chemax NP-4	Cithrol 10ML	Cralane LR-11
Cerasynt® GMS	Chemax NP-6	Cithrol 10MO	Cremba
Cerasynt® IP	Chemax NP-9	Cithrol 10MS	Cremeol HF-52, HF-62
Cerasynt® M	Chemax NP-10	Cithrol 15MS	Cremerol HMG
Cerasynt® MN	Chemax NP-15	Cithrol 40MO	Cremophor® A 6
Cerasynt® PA	Chemax NP-20	Cithrol 40MS	Cremophor® A 11
Cerasynt® Q	Chemax NP-30	Cithrol 60ML	Cremophor® A 25
Cerasynt® SD	Chemax NP-30/70	Cithrol 60MO	Cremophor® EL
Cerasynt® WM	Chemax NP-100	Cithrol DGMS N/E	Cremophor® GO32
Cerex ELS 50	Chemax NP-100/70	Cithrol DGMS S/E	Cremophor® GS32
Cerex U 60	Chemax OP-3	Cithrol GDL N/E	Cremophor® RH 40
Cetal	Chemax OP-5	Cithrol GDL S/E	Cremophor® RH 60
Cetax DR	Chemax OP-30/70	Cithrol GDO N/E	Cremophor® RH 410
Cetodan	Chemax OP-40	Cithrol GDO S/E	Cremophor® RH 455
Cetomacrogol 1000 BP	Chemax OP-40/70	Cithrol GDS N/E	Cremophor® S 9
Cetomil	Chemax PEG 400 DO	Cithrol GDS S/E	Cremophor® WO 7
Cetostearyl Alcohol BP	Chemax PEG 600 DO	Cithrol GML N/E	Crill 1
Cetostearyl Alcohol NF	Chemeen 18-2	Cithrol GML S/E	Crill 2
Chemal BP 261	Chemeen 18-5	Cithrol GMM	Crill 3
Chemal BP-262	Chemeen 18-50	Cithrol GMO N/E	Crill 4
Chemal BP-262LF	Chemeen C-2	Cithrol GMO S/E	Crill 6
Chemal BP-2101	Chemeen C-5	Cithrol GMR N/E	Crill 35
Chemal LA-4	Chemeen C-10	Cithrol GMR S/E	Crill 41
Chemal LA-9	Chemeen C-15	Cithrol GMS Acid Stable	Crill 43
Chemal LA-12	Chemical 39 Base	Cithrol GMS A/S ES 0743	Crill 45
Chemal LA-23	Chemical Base 6532	Cithrol GMS N/E	Crill 50
Chemal OA-4	Chemidex S	Cithrol GMS S/E	Crillet 1
Chemal OA-5	Chemoxide SAO	Cithrol PGML N/E	Crillet 2
Chemal OA-9	Chemphos TC-231S	Cithrol PGML S/E	Crillet 3
Chemal OA-10	Chemphos TC-337	Cithrol PGMO N/E	Crillet 4
Chemal OA-20	Chemphos TC-341	Cithrol PGMO S/E	Crillet 6
Chemal OA-20/70CWS	Chemphos TC-349	Cithrol PGMR N/E	Crillet 11
Chemal OA-20G	Chemphos TR-505	Cithrol PGMR S/E	Crillet 31
Chemal OA-23	Chemphos TR-505D	Cithrol PGMS N/E	Crillet 35
Chemal TDA-3	Chemphos TR-510	Cithrol PGMS S/E	Crillet 41
Chemal TDA-6	Chemphos TR-510S	Cithrol PR	Crillet 45
Chemal TDA-9	Chemphos TR-515	Comperlan® COD	Crillon ODE
Chemal TDA-12	Chemphos TR-515D	Comperlan® LD	Crodacol C-70
Chemal TDA-15	Chemphos TR-541	Comperlan® LDO, LDS	Crodacol C-95NF
Chemal TDA-18	Chemsperse GMS	Comperlan® LS	Crodacol S-70
Chema CO-5	Chemsperse GMS-PS	Compritol 888	Crodafos CAP
Chemax CO-16	Chemsperse GMS-SE	Compritol 888 ATO	Crodafos CDP
Chemax CO-25	Ches® 500	Compritol WL 3241	Crodafos CKP
Chemax CO-28	Chimin AX	Corona Lanolin	Crodafos CS2 Acid
Chemax CO-30	Chimin P50	Corona PNL	Crodafos CS5 Acid
Chemax CO-36	Cholesterol	Coronet Lanolin	Crodafos CS10 Acid
Chemax CO-40	Cholesterol BP	Cosmetic Lanolin	Crodafos N-3 Acid
Chemax CO-80	Cholesterol NF	Anhydrous USP	Crodafos N-3 Neutral
Chemax CO-80	Cire De Lanol CTO	Cosmol O-42T	Crodafos N-5 Acid

Emulsifiers *(cont'd.)*

Crodafos N-10 Acid	Dariloid® QH	Drewmulse® TP	Emalex 523
Crodafos N-10 Neutral	Dehydag® Wax E	Drewmulse® V	Emalex 550
Crodafos SG	Dehydol® D 3	Drewmulse® V-SE	Emalex 600 di-AS
Crodalan 0477	Dehydol® LS 2	Drewpol® 3-1-O	Emalex 600 di-IS
Crodalan AWS	Dehydol® PID 6	Drewpol® 6-1-O	Emalex 600 di-L
Crodamol GHS	Dehydol® PLT 6	Drewpol® 10-4-O	Emalex 600 di-O
Crodasinic LT40	Dehymuls® E	Drewpol® 10-10-O	Emalex 600 di-S
Crodesta A10	Dehymuls® F	Dulectin	Emalex 602
Crodesta DKS F10	Dehymuls® FCE	Duoquad® T-50	Emalex 603
Crodesta DKS F20	Dehymuls® HRE 7	Dur-Em® 114	Emalex 605
Crodesta DKS F50	Dehymuls® SML	Dur-Em® 117	Emalex 606
Crodesta DKS F70	Dehymuls® SMO	Dur-Em® 207E	Emalex 608
Crodesta DKS F110	Dehymuls® SMS	Durfax® 20	Emalex 611
Crodesta DKS F140	Dehymuls® SSO	Durfax® 60	Emalex 615
Crodesta DKS F160	Dehyquart® A	Durfax® 80	Emalex 620
Crodesta F-10	Dehyquart® C Crystals	Dusoran MD	Emalex 625
Crodesta F-50	Dehyquart® SP	Eccowet® W-50	Emalex 630
Crodesta F-110	Dehyquart® STC-25	Eccowet® W-88	Emalex 640
Crodesta F-160	Dehyton® G-SF	Elfacos® E200	Emalex 703
Crodesta SL-40	Deltyl® Extra	Elfacos® EGMS	Emalex 705
Crodet L4	Deriphat® 151C	Elfacos® PEG 400 ML	Emalex 707
Crodet L8	Deriphat® 160	Elfacos® PEG 400 MO	Emalex 709
Crodet L12	Dermalcare® C-20	Elfacos® PEG 400 MS	Emalex 710
Crodet L24	Dermalcare® GMS-165	Elfacos® PEG 600 MS	Emalex 712
Crodet L40	Dermalcare® GMS/SE	Elfacos® PEG 1000 MS	Emalex 715
Crodet L100	Dermalcare® NI	Elfan® A	Emalex 720
Crodet O6	Dermalcare® POL	Elfan® OS	Emalex 725
Crodet S4	Dermalcare® SPS	Elfapur® N 50	Emalex 730
Crodet S8	Detergent CR	Elfapur® N 70	Emalex 750
Crodet S12	Dimodan LS Kosher	Elfapur® N 90	Emalex 800 di-L
Crodet S24	Dimodan PM	Elfapur® N 120	Emalex 805
Crodet S40	Dimodan PV	Elfapur® N 150	Emalex 810
Crodet S50	Dow Corning® 190	Emal 20C	Emalex 820
Crodet S100	Surfactant	Emal E-25C, -70C	Emalex 830
Crodex N	Dow Corning® 193	Emal NC-35	Emalex 840
Croduret 7	Surfactant	Emalex 102	Emalex 1000 di-L
Croduret 10	Dow Corning® 3225C	Emalex 103	Emalex 1605
Croduret 30	Formulation Aid	Emalex 105	Emalex 1610
Croduret 40	Dow Corning® Q2-5200	Emalex 107	Emalex 1615
Croduret 50 Special	Dow Corning® Q2-5220	Emalex 110	Emalex 1620
Croduret 60	Resin Modifier	Emalex 112	Emalex 1625
Croduret 100	Dragil 2/027011	Emalex 115	Emalex 1805
Croduret 200	Drewmulse® 3-1-O	Emalex 117	Emalex 1810
Crolactil CSL	Drewmulse® 3-1-S	Emalex 120	Emalex 1815
Crolactil SISL	Drewmulse® 6-2-S	Emalex 125	Emalex 1820
Crolactil SSL	Drewmulse® 10-4-O	Emalex 130	Emalex 1825
Crolec 4135	Drewmulse® 10-8-O	Emalex 200 di-AS	Emalex 2405
Cromeen	Drewmulse® 10-10-O	Emalex 200 di-L	Emalex 2410
Cromul 0685	Drewmulse® 10-10-S	Emalex 200 di-O	Emalex 2415
Cromul 1207	Drewmulse® 85K	Emalex 200 di-S	Emalex 2420
Crothix	Drewmulse® 200K	Emalex 300 di-IS	Emalex 2425
Crovol A40	Drewmulse® 900K	Emalex 300 di-L	Emalex 2505
Crovol A70	Drewmulse® DGMS	Emalex 300 di-O	Emalex 2510
Crovol M40	Drewmulse® EGDS	Emalex 300 di-S	Emalex 2515
Crovol M70	Drewmulse® EGMS	Emalex 400A	Emalex 2520
Crovol PK40	Drewmulse® GMO	Emalex 400B	Emalex 2525
Crovol PK70	Drewmulse® GMRO	Emalex 400 di-AS	Emalex AF-2
CUPL® PIC	Drewmulse® GMS	Emalex 400 di-IS	Emalex AF-4
Cutina® E24	Drewmulse® HM-100	Emalex 400 di-L	Emalex BHA-5
Cutina® FS 25, FS 45	Drewmulse® PGMS	Emalex 400 di-O	Emalex BHA-10
Cutina® FS 45 Flakes	Drewmulse® POE-SML	Emalex 400 di-S	Emalex BHA-20
Cutina® KD16	Drewmulse® POE-SMO	Emalex 503	Emalex BHA-30
Cyclochem® GMO	Drewmulse® POE-SMS	Emalex 506	Emalex C-20
Cyclochem® PEG 200DS	Drewmulse® POE-STS	Emalex 508	Emalex C-30
Cyclochem® PEG 600DS	Drewmulse® SML	Emalex 510	Emalex C-40
Cyclochem® PEG 6000DS	Drewmulse® SMO	Emalex 512	Emalex C-50
Cyclochem® PETS	Drewmulse® SMS	Emalex 515	Emalex CS-5
Damox® 1010	Drewmulse® STS	Emalex 520	Emalex CS-10

Emulsifiers *(cont'd.)*

Emalex CS-15	Emalex MSG-2MA	Emalex TPM-320	Empilan® KB 2
Emalex CS-20	Emalex MSG-2MB	Emalex TPM-325	Empilan® KB 3
Emalex CS-24	Emalex MSG-2ME	Emalex TPM-330	Empilan® KC 3
Emalex CS-30	Emalex MSG-2ML	Emasol L-106	Empilan® KL 6
Emalex CWD-2	Emalex NP-2	Emasol L-120	Empilan® KL 10
Emalex CWD-38	Emalex NP-3	Emasol P-120	Empilan® KL 20
Emalex DEG-di-L	Emalex NP-5	Emcol® 4072	Empiwax SK
Emalex DEG-di-O	Emalex NP-10	Emcol® 4100M	Empiwax SK/BP
Emalex DEG-di-S	Emalex NP-11	Emcol® 4161L	Emsorb® 2500
Emalex DEG-m-S	Emalex NP-12	Emcol® 4300	Emsorb® 2502
Emalex DISG-2	Emalex NP-13	Emcol® 4400-1	Emsorb® 2503
Emalex DISG-3	Emalex NP-15	Emcol® 4500	Emsorb® 2505
Emalex DISG-5	Emalex NP-20	Emcol® CC-9	Emsorb® 2507
Emalex DISG-10	Emalex NP-25	Emcol® CC-36	Emsorb® 2510
Emalex DNP-5	Emalex NP-30	Emcol® CC-42	Emsorb® 2515
Emalex DSG-2	Emalex OD-5	Emcol® CC-55	Emsorb® 2720
Emalex DSG-3	Emalex OD-10	Emcol® CC-57	Emsorb® 2722
Emalex DSG-5	Emalex OD-16	Emcol® E-607L	Emsorb® 2725
Emalex EG-2854-IS	Emalex OD-20	Emcol® E-607S	Emsorb® 2726
Emalex EG-2854-O	Emalex OD-25	Emcon E	Emsorb® 2728
Emalex EG-2854-S	Emalex OP-5	EmCon E-5	Emsorb® 2729
Emalex EG-di-L	Emalex OP-8	Emerest® 2350	Emsorb® 6900
Emalex EG-di-MPS	Emalex OP-10	Emerest® 2355	Emsorb® 6905
Emalex EG-di-O	Emalex OP-15	Emerest® 2380	Emsorb® 6915
Emalex EG-di-S	Emalex OP-20	Emerest® 2400	Emthox® 2730
Emalex EG-di-SE	Emalex OP-25	Emerest® 2401	Emthox® 2737
Emalex EGS-A	Emalex OP-30	Emerest® 2410	Emthox® 5877
Emalex EGS-B	Emalex OP-40	Emerest® 2423	Emthox® 5882
Emalex ET-2020	Emalex OP-50	Emerest® 2452	Emthox® 5885
Emalex ET-8020	Emalex PEIS-3	Emerest® 2642	Emthox® 5940
Emalex ET-8040	Emalex PEIS-6	Emerest® 2662	Emthox® 5943
Emalex FC-1	Emalex PEIS-12	Emerest® 2701	Emthox® 5967
Emalex FC-2	Emalex PEIS-20	Emerest® 2704	Emthox® 6957
Emalex GM-5	Emalex PR-3	Emerest® 2711	Emthox® 6961
Emalex GM-10	Emalex RWIS-105	Emerest® 2712	Emthox® 6962
Emalex GM-15	Emalex RWIS-110	Emerest® 2715	Emthox® 6964
Emalex GM-20	Emalex RWIS-115	Emerest® 2717	Emthox® 6965
Emalex GM-30	Emalex RWIS-120	Emerwax® 1257	Emthox® 6967
Emalex GM-40	Emalex RWIS-130	Emerwax® 1266	Emthox® 6968
Emalex GWIS-110	Emalex RWIS-140	Emery® 1650	Emthox® 6970
Emalex GWIS-115	Emalex RWIS-305	Emery® 1656	Emthox® 6971
Emalex GWIS-115(M)	Emalex RWIS-310	Emery® 1660	Emthox® 6972
Emalex GWIS-120	Emalex RWIS-315	Emery® 1730	Emthox® 6984
Emalex GWIS-125	Emalex RWIS-320	Emery® 1732	Emulgade® 1000 NI
Emalex GWIS-130	Emalex RWL-120	Emery® 1740	Emulgade® CL
Emalex GWIS-140	Emalex RWL-130	Emery® 1747	Emulgade® F
Emalex GWIS-150	Emalex SEF-4	Emery® 1780	Emulgade® SE
Emalex GWIS-160	Emalex SEF-8	Emery® 1795	Emulgator E 2149 SE
Emalex GWIS-160N	Emalex SEF-320(A)	Emery® HP-2050	Emulgator E 2155 SE
Emalex GWIS-310	Emalex SG-37	Emery® HP-2060	Emulgator E 2568 SE
Emalex GWIS-320	Emalex S.T.G	Emery® HP-2095	Emulmetik
Emalex GWIS-330	Emalex S.T.G.-R	Emid® 6515	Emulmetik™ 100
Emalex GWO-310	Emalex SWS-9	Emid® 6531	Emulmetik™ 110
Emalex GWO-320	Emalex SWS-10	Emid® 6534	Emulmetik™ 120
Emalex GWO-330	Emalex SWS-12	Emid® 6541	Emulmetik™ 300
Emalex HC-5	Emalex TEG-di-L	Emphos™ CS-1361	Emulmetik™ 310
Emalex HC-7	Emalex TEG-di-O	Emphos™ D70-30C	Emulmetik™ 320
Emalex HC-10	Emalex TEG-di-S	Empicol® 0185	Emulmetik™ 910
Emalex HC-20	Emalex TISG-2	Empicol® 0919	Emulmetik™ 920
Emalex HC-30	Emalex TPIS-303	Empicol® LXS95	Emulmetik™ 930
Emalex HC-40	Emalex TPIS-320	Empicol® LZ/D	Emulmetik™ 950
Emalex HC-50	Emalex TPIS-325	Empicol® LZV/D	Emulmetik ™970
Emalex HC-60	Emalex TPIS-330	Empigen® BB	Emulphor® VN-430
Emalex HC-80	Emalex TPIS-340	Empigen® BB-AU	Emulsogen EL
Emalex HC-100	Emalex TPIS-350	Empilan® EGMS	Emulsogen LP
Emalex LWIS-8	Emalex TPM-303	Empilan® FD	Emulsogen OG
Emalex LWIS-10	Emalex TPM-305	Empilan® GMS SE32	Emulsynt® 1055
Emalex MSG-2	Emalex TPM-308	Empilan® GMS SE40	Emultex SMS

Emulsifiers *(cont'd.)*

Emultex WS	Ethomeen® T/15	Eucarol T	G-1441
Epikuron 145	Ethomeen® T/25	Eumulgin® B1	G-1471
Epikuron 170	Ethomeen® T/60	Eumulgin® B2	G-1702
Epikuron 200	Ethomeen® TD/15	Eumulgin® B3	G-1726
Epikuron H	Ethomeen® TD/25	Eumulgin® C4	G-1790
Equex S	Ethomid® HT/15	Eumulgin E-24	G-1795
Equex SW	Ethomid® HT/23	Eumulgin® EP 2L	G-2153
Ervol®	Ethomid® HT/60	Eumulgin® EP 5L	G-2162
ES-1239	Ethomid® O/15	Eumulgin® HRE 40	G-3707
Esi-Terge S-10	Ethomid® O/17	Eumulgin® HRE 60	G-3780-A
Espesilor AC-43	Ethoquad® 18/12	Eumulgin® KP92	G-3816
Espholip	Ethoquad® 18/25	Eumulgin® L	G-3820
Estol 1461	Ethoquad® C/12	Eumulgin® M8	G-3887
Estol 1467	Ethoquad® C/25	Eumulgin® O5	G-3904
Estol DEMS 3710	Ethoquad® O/12	Eumulgin® O10	G-3908S
Estol DEMS-se 3711	Ethoquad® O/25	Eumulgin® PRT 36	G-3910
Estol E10MS 3727	Ethosperse® CA-2	Eumulgin® PRT 40	G-4929
Estol E60MS 3733	Ethosperse® CA-20	Eumulgin® PRT 56	G-4935
Estol EGMS 3749	Ethosperse® G-26	Eumulgin® PRT 200	G-4936
Estol EO3GC 3606	Ethosperse® LA-4	Eumulgin® PWM2	G-4938
Estol EO4BW 3752	Ethosperse® LA-12	Eumulgin® PWM5	G-4940
Estol EO4MO 3672	Ethosperse® LA-23	Eumulgin® PWM10	Gafac® RE-877
Estol EO4MS 3723	Ethosperse® OA-2	Eumulgin® PWM17	Gantrez® AN
Estol EO6MS 3725	Ethosperse® OA-20	Eumulgin® RO 35	Gardinol WA Paste
Estol GDS 3748	Ethosperse® SL-20	Eumulgin® RO 40	Gatarol M 30 M
Estol GML 3614	Ethosperse® TDA-6	Eumulgin® SML 20	Geleol
Estol GMS 1473	Ethoxol 12	Eumulgin® SMO 20	Gelwhite MAS-H, MAS-L
Estol GMS90 1468	Ethoxol 44	Eumulgin® SMS 20	Genamin KDM-F
Estol GMSse 1462	Ethoxylan® 1685	Eumulgin® ST-8	Generol® 122
Estol GMSveg 1474	Ethoxylan® 1686	Eumulgin® TI 60	Generol® 122E5
Estol SML20 3618	Ethoxyol® 1707	Eumulgin® TL 30	Generol® 122E10
Estol SML 3617	Ethylan® CF71	Eumulgin® TL 55	Generol® 122E16
Estol SMO20 3686	Ethylan® CH	Extan-SOT	Generol® 122E25
Estol SMO 3685	Ethylan® CL	Extan-ST	Genu Carrageenan
Estol SMS20 3716	Ethylan® CRS	Famodan SMO	Geropon® ACR/4
Estol SMS 3715	Ethylan® GEL2	Fancol ALA-10	Geropon® ACR/9
Ethlana 12	Ethylan® GEO8	Fancol C	Geropon® AS-200
Ethlana 22	Ethylan® GEO81	Fancol CA	Geropon® AS-250
Ethlana 50	Ethylan® GEP4	Fancol CAB	Geropon® SS-TA
Ethlana 50-M	Ethylan® GES6	Fancol CH	Geropon® T-77
Ethoduomeen® T/13	Ethylan® GL20	Fancol CH-24	Geropon® TC-42
Ethoduomeen® T/20	Ethylan® GLE-21	Fancol CO-30	Glicolene
Ethoduomeen® TD/13	Ethylan® GO80	Fancol HCO-25	Glicosterina DPG
Ethofat® 60/15	Ethylan® GOE-21	Fancol LA	Glo-Mul 780
Ethofat® 60/20	Ethylan® GPS85	Fancol LA-5	Glo-Mul 781
Ethofat® 60/25	Ethylan® GS60	Fancol LA-15	Glo-Mul 782
Ethofat® 142/20	Ethylan® GT85	Fancol LAO	Glo-Mul 783
Ethofat® C/15	Ethylan® KEO	Fancor IPL	Glo-Mul 789
Ethofat® C/25	Ethylan® L10	Fancor LFA	Glo-Mul 4001
Ethofat® O/15	Ethylan® LD	Fancor Lanwax	Glo-Mul 4007
Ethofat® O/20	Ethylan® LDS	Fluilan	Glucam® E-20 Distearate
Ethomeen® 18/12	Ethylan® LM2	Foamid C	Glucamate® DOE-120
Ethomeen® 18/15	Ethylan® LM2E	Foamid LM2E	Glucamate® SSE-20
Ethomeen® 18/20	Ethylan® ME	Foamine O-80	Glucate® DO
Ethomeen® 18/25	Ethylan® OE	Foamole M	Glucate® IS
Ethomeen® 18/60	Ethylan® R	Foamquat CAS	Glucate® SS
Ethomeen® C/12	Ethylan® TCO	Foamquat IALA	Glycerox HE
Ethomeen® C/15	Ethylan® TN-10	Foamquat SOAS	Glycerox L8
Ethomeen® C/20	Etocas 5	Foamquat VG	Glycerox L15
Ethomeen® C/25	Etocas 10	Foamtaine CAB-A	Glycerox L30
Ethomeen® O/12	Etocas 15	Foamtaine CAB-G	Glycerox L40
Ethomeen® O/15	Etocas 20	Forlan 500	Glyceryl Myristate WL 2130
Ethomeen® O/25	Etocas 29	Forlan C-24	Glycomul® L
Ethomeen® S/12	Etocas 30	Forlan L	Glycomul® LC
Ethomeen® S/15	Etocas 35	Forlanit® E	Glycomul® MA
Ethomeen® S/20	Etocas 40	G-1096	Glycomul® O
Ethomeen® S/25	Etocas 50	G-1292	Glycomul® P
Ethomeen® T/12	Etocas 60	G-1425	Glycomul® S
	Etocas 100		

Emulsifiers *(cont'd.)*

Glycomul® S FG	Hartolite	Hetoxamate SA-23	Hetoxol IS-10
Glycomul® S KFG	Hectabrite® AW	Hetoxamate SA-35	Hetoxol IS-20
Glycomul® SOC	Hectabrite® DP	Hetoxamate SA-40	Hetoxol J
Glycomul® TAO	Hefti DMS-33	Hetoxamate SA-90	Hetoxol L
Glycomul® TO	Hefti GMM-33	Hetoxamate SA-90F	Hetoxol L-1
Glycomul® TS	Hefti GMS-33	Hetoxamine C-2	Hetoxol L-3N
Glycomul® TS KFG	Hefti GMS-33-SEN	Hetoxamine C-5	Hetoxol L-4
Glycosperse® HTO-40	Hefti GMS-33-SES	Hetoxamine C-15	Hetoxol L-4N
Glycosperse® L-10	Hefti GMS-99	Hetoxamine O-2	Hetoxol L-9
Glycosperse® L-20	Hefti GMS-233	Hetoxamine O-5	Hetoxol L-9N
Glycosperse® O-5	Hefti GMS-333	Hetoxamine O-15	Hetoxol L-12
Glycosperse® O-20	Hefti ML-33-F	Hetoxamine S-2	Hetoxol L-23
Glycosperse® O-20 Veg	Hefti ML-55-F	Hetoxamine S-5	Hetoxol LS-9
Glycosperse® O-20X	Hefti ML-55-F-4	Hetoxamine S-15	Hetoxol M-3
Glycosperse® P-20	Hefti MO-33-F	Hetoxamine ST-2	Hetoxol OA-3 Special
Glycosperse® S-20	Hefti MO-55-F	Hetoxamine ST-5	Hetoxol OA-5 Special
Glycosperse® TO-20	Hefti MP-33-F	Hetoxamine ST-15	Hetoxol OA-10 Special
Glycosperse® TS-20	Hefti MS-33-F	Hetoxamine ST-50	Hetoxol OA-20 Special
Golden Dawn Grade 1, 2	Hefti MS-55-F	Hetoxamine T-2	Hetoxol OL-2
Golden Dawn Lanolin	Hefti PGE-400-MS	Hetoxamine T-5	Hetoxol OL-4
Golden Dawn Superfine	Hefti PGE-600-ML	Hetoxamine T-15	Hetoxol OL-5
Golden Fleece DF	Hefti QO-33-F	Hetoxamine T-20	Hetoxol OL-10
Golden Fleece P-80	Hefti RS-55-40	Hetoxamine T-30	Hetoxol OL-10H
Golden Fleece P-95	Hefti RS-55-100	Hetoxamine T-50	Hetoxol OL-20
Golden Fleece RA	Hefti TO-33-F	Hetoxamine T-50-70%	Hetoxol OL-23
GP-209	Hefti TO-55-F	Hetoxide BN-13	Hetoxol OL-40
GP-215 Silicone Polyol	Hefti TS-33-F	Hetoxide BP-3	Hetoxol PLA
Copolymer	Hetamide CMA	Hetoxide BY-3	Hetoxol STA-2
GP-217 Silicone Polyol	Hetamide CME	Hetoxide C-2	Hetoxol STA-10
Copolymer	Hetamide CME-CO	Hetoxide C-9	Hetoxol STA-20
GP-226	Hetamide DS	Hetoxide C-15	Hetoxol STA-30
Grillocam E10	Hetamide DT	Hetoxide C-25	Hetoxol TA-6
Grillocam E20	Hetamide LA	Hetoxide C-30	Hetoxol TD-3
Grillocose® DO	Hetamide LL	Hetoxide C-40	Hetoxol TD-6
Grillocose DO	Hetamide LML	Hetoxide C-60	Hetoxol TD-12
Grillocose® IS	Hetamide LN	Hetoxide C-200	Hetoxol TDEP-63
Grillocose IS	Hetamide M	Hetoxide C-200-50%	Hetsorb L-4
Grillocose® PS	Hetamide MA	Hetoxide DNP-4	Hetsorb L-10
Grillocose PS	Hetamide MC	Hetoxide DNP-5	Hetsorb L-20
Grillocose PSE-20	Hetamide MCS	Hetoxide DNP-9.6	Hetsorb O-5
Grillomuls L90	Hetamide ML	Hetoxide DNP-10	Hetsorb O-20
Grillomuls O60	Hetamide MM	Hetoxide G-7	Hetsorb P-20
Grillomuls O90	Hetamide MMC, OC	Hetoxide G-26	Hetsorb S-4
Grillomuls S40	Hetamide MOC	Hetoxide HC-16	Hetsorb S-20
Grillomuls S60	Hetamide OC	Hetoxide HC-40	Hetsorb TO-20
Grillomuls S90	Hetamide RC	Hetoxide HC-60	Hetsorb TS-20
Grilloten LSE 65	Hetan SO	Hetoxide NP-4	Hetsulf 60T
Grilloten LSE 65 Soft	Hetan SS	Hetoxide NP-30	Hetsulf Acid
Grilloten LSE 87	Hetester PCA	Hetoxol 15 CSA	Hetsulf IPA
Grilloten LSE87K	Hetester PHA	Hetoxol CA-2	Hodag 20-L
Grilloten LSE 87 K Soft	Hetoxalan 75	Hetoxol CA-10	Hodag 22-L
Grilloten LSE 87 Soft	Hetoxalan 75-50%	Hetoxol CA-20	Hodag 40-L
Grilloten PSE141G	Hetoxamate 200 DL	Hetoxol CAWS	Hodag 40-O
Grilloten ZT12	Hetoxamate 400 DS	Hetoxol CD-3	Hodag 40-R
Grilloten ZT-40	Hetoxamate FA-5	Hetoxol CD-4	Hodag 40-S
Grilloten ZT-80	Hetoxamate FA-20	Hetoxol CS-4	Hodag 42-L
Hamposyl® C	Hetoxamate LA-4	Hetoxol CS-5	Hodag 42-O
Hamposyl® C-30	Hetoxamate LA-5	Hetoxol CS-9	Hodag 42-S
Hamposyl® L	Hetoxamate LA-9	Hetoxol CS-15	Hodag 60-L
Hamposyl® L-30	Hetoxamate MO-2	Hetoxol CS-20	Hodag 60-S
Hamposyl® L-95	Hetoxamate MO-4	Hetoxol CS-30	Hodag 62-O
Hamposyl® M	Hetoxamate MO-5	Hetoxol CS-50	Hodag 100-S
Hamposyl® M-30	Hetoxamate MO-9	Hetoxol CS-50 Special	Hodag 150-S
Hamposyl® O	Hetoxamate MO-15	Hetoxol CSA-15	Hodag 602-S
Hamposyl® S	Hetoxamate SA-5	Hetoxol D	Hodag DGL
Haroil SCO-50	Hetoxamate SA-7	Hetoxol G	Hodag DGS
Haroil SCO-65, -7525	Hetoxamate SA-9	Hetoxol IS-2	Hodag DGS-C
Hartolan	Hetoxamate SA-13	Hetoxol IS-3	Hodag DGS-N

Emulsifiers *(cont'd.)*

Hodag GML
Hodag GMO
Hodag GMO-D
Hodag GMR
Hodag GMR-D
Hodag GMS
Hodag GTO
Hodag Nonionic 1035-L
Hodag Nonionic 1044-L
Hodag Nonionic 1061-L
Hodag Nonionic 1062-L
Hodag Nonionic 1064-L
Hodag Nonionic 1068-F
Hodag Nonionic 1088-F
Hodag Nonionic E-100
Hodag PE-004
Hodag PE-104
Hodag PE-106
Hodag PE-109
Hodag PE-206
Hodag PE-209
Hodag PE-1803
Hodag PE-1810
Hodag POE (20) GMS
Hodag PSML-20
Hodag PSML-80
Hodag PSMO-5
Hodag PSMO-20
Hodag PSMP-20
Hodag PSMS-20
Hodag PSTO-20
Hodag PSTS-20
Hodag SML
Hodag SMO
Hodag SMP
Hodag SMS
Hodag STO
Hodag STS
Hoe S 2721
Hostacerin DGI
Hostacerin DGL
Hostacerin DGO
Hostacerin DGS
Hostacerin DGSB
Hostacerin O-5
Hostacerin T-3
Hostacerin WO
Hostacerin WOL
Hostaphat K Grades
Hostaphat KL 340N
Hostaphat KO 300
Hostaphat KO 380
Hostaphat KW 340 N
Hydrenol® D
Hydrokote® AR, HL
Hydrokote® RM
Hydroxylan
Hypan® QT100
Hypan® SA100H
Hypan® SR150H
Hypan® SS201
Hypan® SS500V
Hypan® SS500W
Hy-Phi 1199
Hy-Phi 1303
Hy-Phi 1401
Hystrene® 1835
Hystrene® 3022

Hystrene® 4516
Hystrene® 5012
Hystrene® 5016 NF
Hystrene® 7022
Hystrene® 9016
Hystrene® 9022
Hystrene® 9512
Hystrene® 9718 NF
Igepal® CA-630
Igepal® CO-430
Igepal® CO-630 Special
Igepal® NP-4
Igepal® NP-9
Igepal® OP-9
Imwitor® 191
Imwitor® 308
Imwitor® 310
Imwitor® 312
Imwitor® 370
Imwitor® 375
Imwitor® 408
Imwitor® 412
Imwitor® 440
Imwitor® 742
Imwitor® 780 K
Imwitor® 900
Imwitor® 900 K
Imwitor® 908
Imwitor® 910
Imwitor® 914
Imwitor® 928
Imwitor® 940
Imwitor® 940 K
Imwitor® 960 K
Imwitor® 965
Imwitor® 988
Incrocas 30
Incrocas 40
Incrodet TD7-C
Incromate SDL
Incromide BAD
Incromide CA
Incromine OPM
Incromine PB
Incromine Oxide B
Incromine Oxide B-30P
Incromine Oxide C
Incromine Oxide I
Incromine Oxide M
Incromine Oxide O
Incromine Oxide OD-50
Incromine Oxide S
Incronam 30
Incropol CS-20
Incropol CS-50
Incropol L-23
Incroquat CR Conc
Incroquat TMC-80
Incroquat TMC-95
Incroquat Behenyl BDQ/P
Incroquat Behenyl TMC/P
Incroquat Behenyl TMS
Incrosorb O-80
Incrosul LAFS
Industrene® 223
Intravon® AN
Intravon® JU
Ionet DL-200

Ionet DO-200
Ionet DO-400
Ionet DO-600
Ionet DO-1000
Ionet DS-300
Ionet DS-400
Ionet S-20
Ionet S-60 C
Ionet S-80
Ionet S-85
Ionet T-20 C
Ionet T-60 C
Ionet T-80 C
Isoixol 6
Isolan® GI 34
Isolan® GO 33
Ivarbase™ 98
Ivarbase™ 101
Ivarlan™ 3310
Ivarlan™ 3360
Ivarlan™ 3400
Ivarlan™ 3405-L30
Ivarlan™ 3407-E
Ivarlan™ 3408W
Ivarlan™ L575
Ixol 2
Ixol 4
Ixol 6
Ixol 8
Ixolene 4
Ixolene 6
Ixolene 8
Jet Quat 2C-75
Jet Quat C-50
Jet Quat DT-50
Jet Quat S-50
Jet Quat T-27W
Jet Quat T-50
Jojoba PEG-80
Jojoba PEG-120
Juniorlan 1664
Junlon PW-110
Junlon PW-111
Karamide HTDA
Karapeg 400-ML
Karapeg 600-ML
Kartacid 1890
Katemul IG-70
Katemul IGU-70
Katioran® AF
Kelacid®
Kelco® HV
Kelco® LV
Kelcoloid® D
Kelcoloid® DH, DO, DSF
Kelcoloid® HVF, LVF, O, S
Kelcosol®
Kelgin® F
Kelgin® HV, LV, MV
Kelgin® QL
Kelgin® XL
Kelmar®
Kelmar® Improved
Kelset®
Keltone
Keltose®
Kemamine® P-650
Kemamine® P-890

Kemamine® P-974
Kemamine® P-989
Kemamine® P-997
Kemamine® Q-1902C
Kemamine® Q-6903B
Kemamine® Q-9973B
Kemamine® T-2802D
Kemester® 2000
Kemester® 5220
Kemester® 5221
Kemester® 5221SE
Kemester® 5500
Kemester® 6000
Kemester® 6000SE
Kessco Diethylene Glycol
  Monostearate
Kessco Diglycol Laurate A
  Neutral
Kessco Diglycol Laurate
  ASE
Kessco Diglycol Laurate N
Kessco Diglycol Laurate
  N-Syn
Kessco Diglycol Laurate SE
Kessco Diglycol Stearate
  Neutral
Kessco EGMS
Kessco® Ethylene Glycol
  Distearate
Kessco® GDS 386F
Kessco® Glycerol
  Distearate 386F
Kessco® Glycerol Dilaurate
Kessco Glycerol Dioleate
Kessco Glycerol
  Monolaurate
Kessco® Glycerol
  Monooleate
Kessco® Glycerol
  Monostearate Pure
Kessco® Glycerol
  Monostearate SE
Kessco® Glycerol
  Monostearate SE,
  Acid Stable
Kessco® GMC-8
Kessco® GML
Kessco GMN
Kessco GMS
Kessco® PEG 200 DL
Kessco® PEG 200 DO
Kessco® PEG 200 DS
Kessco® PEG 200 ML
Kessco® PEG 200 MO
Kessco® PEG 200 MS
Kessco® PEG 300 DL
Kessco® PEG 300 DO
Kessco® PEG 300 DS
Kessco® PEG 300 ML
Kessco® PEG 300 MO
Kessco® PEG 300 MS
Kessco® PEG 400 DL
Kessco® PEG 400 DO
Kessco PEG 400DS
Kessco® PEG 400 DS
Kessco® PEG 400 ML
Kessco® PEG 400 MO
Kessco® PEG 400 MS

Emulsifiers *(cont'd.)*

Kessco® PEG 600 DL
Kessco® PEG 600 DO
Kessco® PEG 600 DS
Kessco® PEG 600 ML
Kessco® PEG 600 MO
Kessco® PEG 600 MS
Kessco® PEG 1000 DL
Kessco® PEG 1000 DO
Kessco® PEG 1000 DS
Kessco® PEG 1000 ML
Kessco® PEG 1000 MO
Kessco® PEG 1000 MS
Kessco® PEG 1540 DL
Kessco® PEG 1540 DO
Kessco® PEG 1540 DS
Kessco® PEG 1540 ML
Kessco® PEG 1540 MO
Kessco® PEG 1540 MS
Kessco® PEG 4000 DL
Kessco® PEG 4000 DO
Kessco® PEG 4000 DS
Kessco® PEG 4000 ML
Kessco® PEG 4000 MO
Kessco® PEG 4000 MS
Kessco® PEG 6000 DL
Kessco® PEG 6000 DO
Kessco® PEG 6000 DS
Kessco® PEG 6000 ML
Kessco® PEG 6000 MO
Kessco® PEG 6000 MS
Kessco® PGML-X533
Kessco® Propylene Glycol
 Monolaurate E
Kessco® Propylene Glycol
 Monostearate Pure
Koster Keunen Beeswax
Koster Keunen Fatty
 Alcohol 1618
Koster Keunen Japan Wax,
 Synthetic
Koster Keunen Stearic Acid
 XXX
Koster Keunen Synthetic
 Beeswax
Koster Keunen Tallow
 Glyceride
Krim 32
Lactodan P 22
Lamacit® ER
Lamacit® GML 12
Lamacit® GML 20
Lamacit® GMO 25
Lamecreme® DGE-18
Lamecreme® SA 7
Lameform® TGI
Lamegin® EE
Lamegin® GLP 10, 20
Lamegin® NSL
Lamegin® ZE 30, 60
Lanalox L 30
Lan-Aqua-Sol 50
Lan-Aqua-Sol 100
Lanbritol Wax N21
Lanesta G
Lanethyl
Laneto 27
Laneto 40
Laneto 60

Laneto 100
Laneto 100-Flaked
Laneto AWS
Lanette® E
Lanette® N
Lanette® SX
Lanette® Wax SX, SXBP
Lanexol AWS
Lanfrax®
Lanfrax® 1776
Lanfrax® 1779
Lanfrax® WS 55
Lanidox-5
Lanidrol
Lanocerin®
Lanogel® 21
Lanogel® 31
Lanogel® 41
Lanogel® 61
Lanogene®
Lanol 14 M
Lanol 1688
Lanol P
Lanoquat® 1751A
Lanoquat® 1756
Lanoquat® 1757
Lanowax
Lanpol 5
Lanpol 10
Lanpol 20
Lanpol 520
Lanpolamide 5
Lantrol® AWS
Lantrol® HP-2073
Lantrol® HP-2074
Lantrol® PLN
Lantrol® PLN/50
Lasemul 62 E
Lasemul 400 E
Lathanol® LAL
Laural EC
Laural LS
Laurate de PEG 400
Laurel R-50
Laurel SD-1500
Lauridit® KD, KDG
Lauridit® OD
Lauroglycol
Lauropal 4
Laurydone®
Laxan-ESE
Laxan-ESM
Laxan-ESR
Laxan-EST
Lecithin Extract Kosmaflor,
 Water-Disp
Lecsoy E
Lecsoy S
Letocil LP 80, SP 1000
Lexamine 22
Lexamine C-13
Lexamine L-13
Lexamine O-13
Lexamine S-13
Lexate® CRC
Lexate® PX
Lexate® TA
Lexate® TL

Lexemul® 55G
Lexemul® 55SE
Lexemul® 503
Lexemul® 515
Lexemul® 530
Lexemul® 561
Lexemul® AR
Lexemul® AS
Lexemul® CS-20
Lexemul® EGMS
Lexemul® P
Lexemul® PEG-200 DL
Lexemul® PEG-400 DL
Lexemul® PEG-400ML
Lexemul® T
Lexin K
Lexquat® AMG-BEO
Lexquat® AMG-IS
Lexquat® AMG-M
Lexquat® AMG-O
Lexquat® AMG-WC
Lipal 400 DS
Lipal 400 S
Lipal 6000 DS
Lipal DGMS
Lipal EGDS
Lipal EGMS
Lipal GMS AE
Lipal GMS
Lipal MMDG
Lipal PGMS
Lipamide S
Lipo DGLS
Lipo DGS-SE
Lipo EGDS
Lipo EGMS
Lipo GMS 450
Lipo GMS 470
Lipo PGMS
Lipocol
Lipocol B
Lipocol C-2
Lipocol C-4
Lipocol C-10
Lipocol C-20
Lipocol C-30
Lipocol HCO-40
Lipocol HCO-60
Lipocol HCO-66
Lipocol IS-20
Lipocol L-1
Lipocol L-4
Lipocol L-12
Lipocol L-23
Lipocol M-4
Lipocol O-2 Special
Lipocol O-3 Special
Lipocol O-5 Special
Lipocol O-10
Lipocol O-20
Lipocol O-25
Lipocol S-2
Lipocol S-10
Lipocol S-20
Lipocol SC-4
Lipocol SC-10
Lipocol SC-15
Lipocol SC-20

Lipocol TD-3
Lipocol TD-6
Lipocol TD-12
Lipoid S 100
Lipolan
Lipolan 31
Lipolan 31-20
Lipolan 1400
Lipolan Distilled
Lipolan LB-440
Lipolan PJ-400
Lipomulse 165
Liponate GDL
Lipopeg 1-L
Lipopeg 1-S
Lipopeg 2-DL
Lipopeg 2-L
Lipopeg 2-S
Lipopeg 3-O
Lipopeg 3-S
Lipopeg 4-DL
Lipopeg 4-DO
Lipopeg 4-DS
Lipopeg 4-L
Lipopeg 4-O
Lipopeg 4-S
Lipopeg 6-L
Lipopeg 6-S
Lipopeg 10-S
Lipopeg 15-S
Lipopeg 16-S
Lipopeg 20-S
Lipopeg 39-S
Lipopeg 100-S
Lipopeg 6000-DS
Lipo-Peptide AME 30
Liposorb L
Liposorb L-10
Liposorb L-20
Liposorb O
Liposorb O-5
Liposorb O-20
Liposorb P
Liposorb P-20
Liposorb S
Liposorb S-4
Liposorb S-20
Liposorb SC
Liposorb SQO
Liposorb TO
Liposorb TO-20
Liposorb TS
Liposorb TS-20
Lipovol GTB
Lipowax G
Lipowax PR
Lipowax P-SPEC
Liquid Base
Lonzest® PEG 4-O
Lonzest® SML-20
Lonzest® SMO-20
Lonzest® SMP-20
Lonzest® SMS-20
Lonzest® STO-20
Lonzest® STS-20
Loropan KD
Lowenol C-279
Lutensol® FA 12

Emulsifiers *(cont'd.)*

Lutrol® E 300	Macol® SA-2	Mapeg® CO-36	Mazamide® 1281
Lutrol® E 400	Macol® SA-5	Mapeg® CO-200	Mazamide® C-5
Lutrol® E 1500	Macol® SA-10	Mapeg® EGDS	Mazamide® CCO
Lutrol® E 4000	Macol® SA-15	Mapeg® EGMS	Mazamide® CMEA
Lutrol® E 6000	Macol® SA-20	Mapeg® EGMS-K	Mazamide® CMEA Extra
Mackam™ 2CSF	Macol® SA-40	Mapeg® S-40	Mazamide® CS 148
Mackam™ 2CYSF	Macol® TD-3	Mapeg® S-40K	Mazamide® J 10
Mackam™ 2LSF	Macol® TD-8	Mapeg® S-100	Mazamide® JR 300
Mackamide™ R	Macol® TD-10	Mapeg® S-150	Mazamide® JR 400
Mackester™ EGDS	Macol® TD-12	Mapeg® TAO-15	Mazamide® JT 128
Mackester™ EGMS	Macol® TD-15	Marlinat® CM 40	Mazamide® L-5
Mackester™ IDO	Macol® TD-100	Marlinat® CM 45	Mazamide® L-298
Mackester™ IP	Macol® TD-610	Marlinat® CM 100	Mazamide® LLD
Mackester™ SP	Mafo® C	Marlinat® CM 105	Mazamide® LM
Mackester™ TD-88	Mafo® CAB	Marlipal® 24/300	Mazamide® LM 20
Macol® 1	Mafo® CAB 425	Marlipal® 1885/2	Mazamide® LS 196
Macol® 2	Mafo® CAB SP	Marlophor® T10-Acid	Mazamide® O 20
Macol® 4	Mafo® CB 40	Marlophor® T10-Sodium	Mazamide® PCS
Macol® 16	Mafo® CFA 35	Salt	Mazamide® RO
Macol® 23	Mafo® CSB	Marlosol® 183	Mazamide® SCD
Macol® 27	Mafo® CSB 50	Marlosol® 188	Mazamide® SMEA
Macol® 123	Mafo® CSB W	Marlosol® 1820	Mazamide® SS-10
Macol® 124	Mafo® KCOSB 50	Marlosol® OL7	Mazamide® SS 20
Macol® 125	Mafo® LMAB	Marlosol® OL15	Mazamide® T 20
Macol® CA-2	Mafo® OB	Marlowet® 5001	Mazamide® TC
Macol® CA-10	Mafo® SBAO 110	Marlowet® CA 5	Mazamide® WC Conc
Macol® CPS	Magnabrite® HV	Marlowet® CA 10	Mazawax® 163R
Macol® CSA-2	Makon® 4	Marlowet® EF	Mazawax® 163SS
Macol® CSA-4	Makon® 6	Marlowet® G 12 DO	Mazeen® 173
Macol® CSA-10	Makon® 8	Marlowet® GDO 4	Mazeen® 174
Macol® CSA-15	Makon® 10	Marlowet® LMA 2	Mazeen® 174-75
Macol® CSA-20	Makon® 12	Marlowet® LMA 4	Mazeen® C-2
Macol® CSA-40	Makon® 14	Marlowet® LMA 5	Mazeen® C-5
Macol® CSA-50	Makon® 30	Marlowet® LMA 10	Mazeen® C-10
Macol® DNP-5	Manro BES 27	Marlowet® LMA 20	Mazeen® C-15
Macol® DNP-10	Manro BES 70	Marlowet® LVS/K	Mazeen® S-2
Macol® DNP-15	Manromid 150-ADY	Marlowet® LVX/K	Mazeen® S-5
Macol® DNP-21	Mapeg® 200 DL	Marlowet® OA 4/1	Mazeen® S-10
Macol® LA-4	Mapeg® 200 DO	Marlowet® OA 5	Mazeen® S-15
Macol® LA-9	Mapeg® 200 DOT	Marlowet® OA 10	Mazeen® T-2
Macol® LA-12	Mapeg® 200 DS	Marlowet® OA 30	Mazeen® T-5
Macol® LA-23	Mapeg® 200 ML	Marlowet® R 11/K	Mazeen® T-10
Macol® LA-790	Mapeg® 200 MO	Marlowet® R 20	Mazeen® T-15
Macol® NP-4	Mapeg® 200 MOT	Marlowet® R 22	Mazol® 80 MGK
Macol® NP-5	Mapeg® 200 MS	Marlowet® R 25	Mazol® 165C
Macol® NP-6	Mapeg® 400 DL	Marlowet® R 25/K	Mazol® 300 K
Macol® NP-8	Mapeg® 400 DO	Marlowet® R 32	Mazol® GMO
Macol® NP-11	Mapeg® 400 DOT	Marlowet® R 36	Mazol® GMO K
Macol® NP-12	Mapeg® 400 DS	Marlowet® R 40	Mazol® GMS
Macol® NP-15	Mapeg® 400 ML	Marlowet® R 40/K	Mazol® GMS-90
Macol® NP-20	Mapeg® 400 MO	Marlowet® R 54	Mazol® GMS-D
Macol® NP-20(70)	Mapeg® 400 MOT	Marlowet® RA	Mazol® GMS-K
Macol® NP-30(70)	Mapeg® 400 MS	Marlowet® RNP	Mazol® PGMSK
Macol® NP-100	Mapeg® 600 DL	Marlowet® RNP/K	Mazol® PGO-31 K
Macol® OA-2	Mapeg® 600 DO	Marlowet® SAF/K	Mazol® PGO-104
Macol® OA-4	Mapeg® 600 DOT	Marlowet® TA 6	Mazon® 60T
Macol® OA-5	Mapeg® 600 DS	Marlowet® TA 8	Mazox® CAPA
Macol® OA-10	Mapeg® 600 ML	Marlowet® TA 10	Mazox® CAPA-37
Macol® OA-20	Mapeg® 600 MO	Marlowet® TA 25	Mazox® CDA
Macol® OP-3	Mapeg® 600 MOT	Mayphos OL 3N	Mazox® LDA
Macol® OP-5	Mapeg® 600 MS	May-Tein KTS	Mazox® MDA
Macol® OP-8	Mapeg® 1000 MS	May-Tein SY	Mazox® ODA
Macol® OP-10	Mapeg® 1500 MS	Mazamide® 65	Mazox® SDA
Macol® OP-10 SP	Mapeg® 1540 DS	Mazamide® 68	Merpol® HCS
Macol® OP-12	Mapeg® 6000 DS	Mazamide® 80	Methocel® A15-LV
Macol® OP-16(75)	Mapeg® CO-16	Mazamide® 124	Methocel® K35
Macol® OP-30(70)	Mapeg® CO-16H	Mazamide® 524	Microat™ E
Macol® OP-40(70)	Mapeg® CO-30	Mazamide® 1214	Miracare® CT100

560

Emulsifiers *(cont'd.)*

Miramine® CODI	Monomuls® 90-O18	Myverol® 18-06	Nikkol BO-10TX
Miramine® SC	Monosteol	Myverol® 18-07	Nikkol BO-15TX
Miramine® SODI	Montane 20	Myverol® 18-30	Nikkol BO-20TX
Miranate® LEC	Montane 40	Myverol® 18-35	Nikkol BO-50
Miranol® 2CIB	Montane 60	Myverol® 18-40	Nikkol BPS-5
Miranol® BM Conc	Montane 65	Myverol® 18-50	Nikkol BPS-10
Miranol® C2M Conc. NP	Montane 70	Myverol® 18-85	Nikkol BPS-15
Miranol® CM Conc. NP	Montane 73	Myverol® 18-92	Nikkol BPS-20
Miranol® CM-SF Conc	Montane 80 SP	Myverol® 18-99	Nikkol BPS-25
Miranol® CS Conc	Montane 80	Myverol® P-06	Nikkol BPS-30
Miranol® Ester PO-LM4	Montane 83	Myverol® SMG	Nikkol BPSH-25
Miranol® H2M Conc	Montane 85	Nacolox®	Nikkol BS-2
Miranol® HM Conc	Montane 481	Naetex O-80	Nikkol BS-4
Miranol® JBS	Montanol 68	Naturechem® EGHS	Nikkol BS-20
Miranol® OM-SF Conc	Montanov 68	Naturechem® GMHS	Nikkol BWA-5
Mirapol® 1941	Montanox 20	Naturechem® MHS	Nikkol BWA-20
Mirataine® BET-C-30	Montanox 20 DF	Naturechem® PGHS	Nikkol BWA-40
Mirataine® BET-O-30	Montanox 21	Naturechem® THS-200	Nikkol CDIS-400
Mirataine® BET-P-30	Montanox 40	Naxel ™AAS-98S	Nikkol CDO-600
Mirataine® CB	Montanox 40 DF	Naxolate™ WA-97	Nikkol CDS-400
Mirataine® CBC	Montanox 60	Naxolate™ WAG	Nikkol CDS-6000P
Mirataine® CB/M	Montanox 60 DF	Naxonic™ NI-40	Nikkol Chimyl Alcohol 100
Mirataine® CBS, CBS Mod	Montanox 61	Naxonic™ NI-60	Nikkol CO-3
Monamid® 150-ADY	Montanox 65	Naxonic™ NI-100	Nikkol CO-10
Monamid® 150-CW	Montanox 70	Naxonol™ PN 66	Nikkol CO-20TX
Monamid® 150-MW	Montanox 71	Naxonol™ PO	Nikkol DDP-2
Monamid® 718	Montanox 80	Necon SOG	Nikkol DDP-4
Monamid® 853	Montanox 80 DF	Necon SOGU	Nikkol DDP-6
Monamid® 1007	Montanox 81	Necon SOLC	Nikkol DDP-8
Monamid® LLN-380	Montanox 85	Neodol® 23-3	Nikkol DDP-10
Monamid® LN-605	Monthyle	Neodol® 25-3	Nikkol Decaglyn 1-IS
Monamid® S	Montovol RF-10	Neodol® 25-12	Nikkol Decaglyn 1-L
Monamine AA-100	M-Quat® Dimer 18 PG	Neodol® 45-7	Nikkol Decaglyn 1-LN
Monamine AC-100	MS-33-F	Neodol® 45-13	Nikkol Decaglyn 1-M
Monamine ACO-100	MS-55-F	Neustrene® 045	Nikkol Decaglyn 1-O
Monamine ADD-100	Mulsifan CB	Neustrene® 060	Nikkol Decaglyn 1-S
Monamine ADY-100	Mulsifan CPA	Neustrene® 064	Nikkol Decaglyn 2-IS
Monamine CF-100 M	Mulsifan RT 18	Niaproof® Anionic	Nikkol Decaglyn 2-O
Monateric CA-35	Mulsifan RT 23	Surfactant 4	Nikkol Decaglyn 2-S
Monateric CEM-38	Mulsifan RT 69	Niaproof® Anionic	Nikkol Decaglyn 3-IS
Monateric CM-36S	Mulsor OC	Surfactant 08	Nikkol Decaglyn 3-O
Monawet MO-65-150	Myrj® 45	Nikkol Batyl Alcohol 100,	Nikkol Decaglyn 3-S
Monawet MO-70	Myrj® 49	EX	Nikkol Decaglyn 5-IS
Monawet MO-70-150	Myrj® 51	Nikkol BB-5	Nikkol Decaglyn 5-O
Monawet MO-70R	Myrj® 52	Nikkol BB-10	Nikkol Decaglyn 5-S
Monawet MO-70S	Myrj® 52S	Nikkol BB-20	Nikkol Decaglyn 7-IS
Monawet SNO-35	Myrj® 53	Nikkol BB-30	Nikkol Decaglyn 7-O
Monawet TD-30	Myrj® 59	Nikkol BC-2	Nikkol Decaglyn 7-S
Monomuls® 60-10	Mytab®	Nikkol BC-5.5	Nikkol Decaglyn 10-IS
Monomuls® 60-15	Myvacet® 5-07	Nikkol BC-7	Nikkol Decaglyn 10-O
Monomuls® 60-20	Myvacet® 7-07	Nikkol BC-10TX	Nikkol Decaglyn 10-S
Monomuls® 60-25	Myvacet® 9-08	Nikkol BC-15TX	Nikkol DEGS
Monomuls® 60-25/2	Myvacet® 9-45	Nikkol BC-20TX	Nikkol DGDO
Monomuls® 60-30	Myvaplex® 600P	Nikkol BC-23	Nikkol DGMIS
Monomuls® 60-35	Myvatem® 06K	Nikkol BC-25TX	Nikkol DGMO-90
Monomuls® 60-40	Myvatem® 30	Nikkol BC-30TX	Nikkol DGMO-C
Monomuls® 60-45	Myvatem® 35K	Nikkol BC-40TX	Nikkol DGMS
Monomuls® 90-10	Myvatem® 92K	Nikkol BD-2	Nikkol DGO-80
Monomuls® 90-15	Myvatex® 3-50	Nikkol BD-4	Nikkol DGS-80
Monomuls® 90-20	Myvatex® 7-85	Nikkol BD-10	Nikkol DLP-10
Monomuls® 90-25	Myvatex® 8-06	Nikkol BEG-1630	Nikkol ECT-3NEX,
Monomuls® 90-25/2,	Myvatex® 8-16	Nikkol BL-2	ECTD-3NEX
90-25/5	Myvatex® 40-06S	Nikkol BL-4.2	Nikkol ECTD-6NEX
Monomuls® 90-30	Myvatex® 60	Nikkol BL-9EX	Nikkol GBW-8
Monomuls® 90-35	Myvatex® MSPS	Nikkol BL-21	Nikkol GBW-25
Monomuls® 90-40	Myvatex® SSH	Nikkol BL-25	Nikkol GBW-125
Monomuls® 90-45	Myvatex® Texture Lite	Nikkol BO-2	Nikkol GL-1
Monomuls® 90-L12	Myverol® 18-04	Nikkol BO-7	Nikkol GO-4

Emulsifiers *(cont'd.)*

Nikkol GO-430	Nikkol PBC-34	Nissan Nonion DN-202	Olepal 1
Nikkol GO-440	Nikkol PBC-41	Nissan Nonion DN-203	Olepal ISO
Nikkol GO-460	Nikkol PBC-44	Nissan Nonion DN-209	Oramide DL 200 AF
Nikkol GS-6	Nikkol PMS-1C	Nissan Nonion DS-60HN	Ovonol
Nikkol GS-460	Nikkol PMS-1CSE	Nissan Nonion E-205	Ovothin
Nikkol HCO-5	Nikkol PMS-FR	Nissan Nonion E-206	Ovothin 160
Nikkol HCO-7.5	Nikkol SCS	Nissan Nonion E-208	Ovothin 170
Nikkol HCO-10	Nikkol SI-10R	Nissan Nonion E-215	Ovothin 180
Nikkol HCO-20	Nikkol SI-10T	Nissan Nonion E-220	Ovothin 200
Nikkol HCO-30	Nikkol SI-15R	Nissan Nonion E-230	Paramul® SAS
Nikkol HCO-40	Nikkol SI-15T	Nissan Nonion K-202	Parapel® HC
Nikkol HCO-40 Pharm	Nikkol SL-10	Nissan Nonion K-203	Parapel® HC-85
Nikkol HCO-50	Nikkol SO-10	Nissan Nonion K-204	Pationic® 122A
Nikkol HCO-50 Pharm	Nikkol SO-10R	Nissan Nonion K-207	Pationic® 138C
Nikkol HCO-60	Nikkol SO-15	Nissan Nonion K-211	Pationic® 145A
Nikkol HCO-60 Pharm	Nikkol SO-15EX	Nissan Nonion K-215	Pationic® CSL
Nikkol HCO-80	Nikkol SO-15R	Nissan Nonion K-220	Pationic® ISL
Nikkol HCO-100	Nikkol SO-30	Nissan Nonion K-230	Pationic® SSL
Nikkol Hexaglyn 1-L	Nikkol SO-30R	Nissan Nonion LP-20R,	Peceol Isostearique
Nikkol Hexaglyn 1-M	Nikkol SP-10	LP-20RS	Pecosil® PS-100
Nikkol Hexaglyn 1-O	Nikkol SS-10	Nissan Nonion LT-221	Pecosil® PS-100K
Nikkol Hexaglyn 1-S	Nikkol SS-15	Nissan Nonion MP-30R	Pegosperse® 50 DS
Nikkol Hexaglyn 3-S	Nikkol SS-30	Nissan Nonion OP-80R	Pegosperse® 50 MS
Nikkol Hexaglyn 5-O	Nikkol SSS	Nissan Nonion OP-83RAT	Pegosperse® 100 L
Nikkol Hexaglyn 5-S	Nikkol TCP-5	Nissan Nonion OP-85R	Pegosperse® 200 DL
Nikkol Hexaglyn PR-15	Nikkol TDP-2	Nissan Nonion OT-221	Pegosperse® 200 ML
Nikkol Lecinol LL-20	Nikkol TDP-4	Nissan Nonion P-6	Pegosperse® 200 MS
Nikkol Lecinol SH	Nikkol TDP-6	Nissan Nonion P-208	Pegosperse® 300 MO
Nikkol MGIS	Nikkol TDP-8	Nissan Nonion P-210	Pegosperse® 400 DL
Nikkol MGM	Nikkol TDP-10	Nissan Nonion P-213	Pegosperse® 400 DOT
Nikkol MGO	Nikkol Tetraglyn 1-O	Nissan Nonion PP-40R	Pegosperse® 400 DS
Nikkol MGS-150	Nikkol Tetraglyn 1-S	Nissan Nonion PT-221	Pegosperse® 400 ML
Nikkol MGS-A	Nikkol Tetraglyn 3-S	Nissan Nonion S-2	Pegosperse® 400 MO
Nikkol MGS-ASE	Nikkol Tetraglyn 5-O	Nissan Nonion S-4	Pegosperse® 400 MS
Nikkol MGS-B	Nikkol Tetraglyn 5-S	Nissan Nonion S-6	Pegosperse® 600 DOT
Nikkol MGS-BSE-C	Nikkol TI-10	Nissan Nonion S-10	Pegosperse® 600 ML
Nikkol MGS-C	Nikkol TL-10, TL-10EX	Nissan Nonion S-15	Pegosperse® 600 MO
Nikkol MGS-DEX	Nikkol TLP-4	Nissan Nonion S-15.4	Pegosperse® 1500 MS
Nikkol MGS-F20	Nikkol TMGO-5	Nissan Nonion S-40	Pegosperse® 1750 MS
Nikkol MGS-F50	Nikkol TMGO-15	Nissan Nonion S-206	Pegosperse® 1750 MS K
Nikkol MGS-F50SE	Nikkol TMGS-5	Nissan Nonion S-207	Spec.
Nikkol MGS-F75	Nikkol TMGS-15	Nissan Nonion S-215	Pegosperse® EGMS-70
Nikkol MGS-TG	Nikkol TO-10	Nissan Nonion S-220	Pegosperse® PMS CG
Nikkol MGS-TGL	Nikkol TO-10M	Nissan Nonion SP-60R	Pemulen® TR-1, TR-2
Nikkol MYL-10	Nikkol TO-30	Nissan Nonion ST-221	Permulgin CSB
Nikkol MYO-2	Nikkol TO-106	Nissan Nonion T-15	Permulgin RWB
Nikkol MYO-6	Nikkol TP-10	Nissan Persoft SK	PGE-400-MS
Nikkol MYS-1EX	Nikkol TS-10	Nonisol 100	PGE-600-DS
Nikkol MYS-2	Nikkol TS-30	Nonisol 300	PGE-600-ML
Nikkol MYS-4	Nikkol TS-106	Nopalcol Series	PGE-600-MS
Nikkol MYS-10	Nikkol TW-10	Nopalcol 1-S	Pharmaceutical Lanolin
Nikkol MYS-25	Nikkol TW-20	Nopalcol 1-TW	USP
Nikkol MYS-40	Nikkol TW-30	Nopcocastor	Phoenate 3 DSA
Nikkol MYS-45	Nimco® 1780	Noramium MS 50	Phosal 15
Nikkol MYS-55	Nimcolan® 1740	Norfox® 165C	Phosal 25 SB
Nikkol NES-203	Nimcolan® 1747	Norfox® 1101	Phosal® 50 PG
Nikkol NES-303	Nimlesterol® 1732	Norfox® DOSA	Phosal® 60 PG
Nikkol NP-2	Ninol® GR	Norfox® EGMS	Phosal® NAT-50-PG
Nikkol NP-5	Ninol® L-9	Norfox® GMS-FG	Phosphanol Series
Nikkol NP-7.5	Niox KG-11	Norfox® NP-4	PhosPho E-100
Nikkol NP-10	Niox KI Series	Norfox® NP-6	PhosPho LCN-TS
Nikkol NP-15	Niox KJ-10	Norfox® Sorbo T-80	PhosPho PL-50
Nikkol NP-18TX	Niox KJ-72	Novel® N3.0-1216CO	Phospholipid EFA
Nikkol OP-3	Niox KP-62, -63, -67	Novel® N4.9-810	Phospholipid PTD
Nikkol OP-10	Nissan Diapon T	Novel® N5.1-1618	Phospholipid PTL
Nikkol OP-30	Nissan Monogly I	Novel® N7.7-810	Phospholipid PTZ
Nikkol PBC-31	Nissan Monogly M	Noxamine CA 30	Phospholipid SV
Nikkol PBC-33	Nissan Nonion CP-08R	OHlan®	Phospholipon® 25G, 25P

Emulsifiers *(cont'd.)*

Phospholipon® 50	Polawax® A31	Protasorb O-20	Prox-onic NP-09
Phospholipon® 80	Polawax® GP200	Protasorb P-20	Prox-onic NP-010
Phospholipon® 90/90 G	Polyaldo® DGHO	Protasorb S-20	Prox-onic NP-015
Phospholipon® 90 H	Polychol 5	Protasorb TO-20	Prox-onic NP-020
Phospholipon® CC	Polychol 10	Protegin® SE	Prox-onic NP-030
Phospholipon® LC	Polychol 15	Protegin® W SE	Prox-onic NP-030/70
Phospholipon® MC	Polychol 16	Protegin® WX SE	Prox-onic NP-040
Phospholipon® MG Na	Polychol 20	Protegin® X SE	Prox-onic NP-040/70
Phospholipon® PC	Polychol 40	Prote-sorb SML	Prox-onic NP-050
Phospholipon® PG Na	Polytex 10M	Prote-sorb SMO	Prox-onic NP-050/70
Phospholipon® SC	Prisorine GMIS 2040	Prote-sorb SMP	Prox-onic NP-0100
Phospholipon® SG Na	Prisorine ISAC 3505	Prote-sorb SMS	Prox-onic NP-0100/70
Plurol Isostearique	Procetyl AWS	Prote-sorb STO	Prox-onic OA-1/020
Plurol Oleique WL 1173	Procol CA-2	Prote-sorb STS	Prox-onic OA-2/020
Pluronic® 10R5	Procol CA-4	Proto-Lan 4R	Prox-onic OL-1/05
Pluronic® 10R8	Procol CA-6	Proto-Lan 8	Prox-onic OL-1/09
Pluronic® 12R3	Procol CA-10	Proto-Lan 30	Prox-onic OL-1/014
Pluronic® 17R1	Procol CA-20	Protox C-2	Prox-onic PEG-2000
Pluronic® 17R2	Procol CA-30	Protox C-5	Prox-onic PEG-4000
Pluronic® 17R4	Procol LA-3	Protox C-10	Prox-onic PEG-6000
Pluronic® 17R8	Procol LA-4	Protox C-15	Prox-onic PEG-10,000
Pluronic® 22R4	Procol LA-10	Protox HTA-2	Prox-onic PEG-20,000
Pluronic® 25R1	Procol LA-12	Protox HTA-10	Prox-onic PEG-35,000
Pluronic® 25R2	Procol LA-15	Protox HTA-15	Prox-onic SML-020
Pluronic® 25R4	Procol LA-20	Protox HTA-50	Prox-onic SMO-05
Pluronic® 25R5	Procol LA-23	Protox O-2	Prox-onic SMO-020
Pluronic® 25R8	Procol OA-2	Protox O-5	Prox-onic SMP-020
Pluronic® 31R1	Procol OA-3	Protox O-15	Prox-onic SMS-020
Pluronic® 31R2	Procol OA-4	Protox T-2	Prox-onic ST-05
Pluronic® 31R4	Procol OA-5	Protox T-5	Prox-onic ST-09
Pluronic® F38	Procol OA-10	Protox T-15	Prox-onic ST-014
Pluronic® F68	Procol OA-20	Protox T-20	Prox-onic ST-023
Pluronic® F68LF	Procol OA-23	Protox T-40	Prox-onic STO-020
Pluronic® F77	Procol OA-25	Protox T-50	Prox-onic STS-020
Pluronic® F87	Promulgen® D	Prox-onic CC-05	PVP K-30
Pluronic® F88	Promulgen® G	Prox-onic CC-09	Pyroter CPI-30
Pluronic® F98	Protachem CAH-100	Prox-onic CC-014	Pyroter CPI-40
Pluronic® F108	Protachem CAH-200	Prox-onic CSA-1/04	Pyroter CPI-60
Pluronic® F127	Protachem DGS	Prox-onic CSA-1/06	Pyroter GPI-25
Pluronic® L10	Protachem DGS-C	Prox-onic CSA-1/010	QO-33-F
Pluronic® L35	Protachem EGMS	Prox-onic CSA-1/015	Querton 16Cl-29
Pluronic® L42	Protachem MLD	Prox-onic CSA-1/020	Querton 16Cl-50
Pluronic® L43	Protachem SMO	Prox-onic CSA-1/030	Quimipol EA 2512
Pluronic® L44	Protachem SMP	Prox-onic CSA-1/050	Radiastar® 1060
Pluronic® L61	Protachem SMS	Prox-onic HR-05	Radiastar® 1100
Pluronic® L62	Protachem SOC	Prox-onic HR-016	Radiastar® 1170
Pluronic® L62D	Protachem STO	Prox-onic HR-025	Radiastar® 1200
Pluronic® L62LF	Protachem STS	Prox-onic HR-030	Radiastar® 1208
Pluronic® L63	Protalan H	Prox-onic HR-036	Radiasurf® 7000
Pluronic® L64	Protalan L-30	Prox-onic HR-040	Radiasurf® 7141
Pluronic® L72	Protalan L-75	Prox-onic HR-080	Radiasurf® 7150
Pluronic® L81	Protalan Wax	Prox-onic HR-0200	Radiasurf® 7151
Pluronic® L92	Protamate 200 DPS	Prox-onic HR-0200/50	Radiasurf® 7152
Pluronic® L101	Protamate 200 ML	Prox-onic HRH-05	Radiasurf® 7153
Pluronic® L121	Protamate 300 DPS	Prox-onic HRH-016	Radiasurf® 7156
Pluronic® L122	Protamate 300 OC	Prox-onic HRH-025	Radiasurf® 7175
Pluronic® P65	Protamate 400 DPS	Prox-onic HRH-0200	Radiasurf® 7196
Pluronic® P75	Protamate 400 ML	Prox-onic HRH-0200/50	Radiasurf® 7201
Pluronic® P84	Protamate 400 OC	Prox-onic L 081-05	Radiasurf® 7206
Pluronic® P85	Protamate 600 DPS	Prox-onic L 101-05	Radiasurf® 7269
Pluronic® P94	Protamate 1000 DPS	Prox-onic L 102-02	Radiasurf® 7270
Pluronic® P103	Protamate 1500 DPS	Prox-onic L 121-09	Radiasurf® 7400
Pluronic® P104	Protamate 1540 DPS	Prox-onic L 161-05	Radiasurf® 7402
Pluronic® P105	Protamate 2000 DPS	Prox-onic L 181-05	Radiasurf® 7403
Pluronic® P123	Protamide SA	Prox-onic L 201-02	Radiasurf® 7404
PMS-33	Protasorb L-5	Prox-onic NP-1.5	Radiasurf® 7410
Pogol 200	Protasorb L-20	Prox-onic NP-04	Radiasurf® 7413
Polawax®	Protasorb O-5	Prox-onic NP-06	Radiasurf® 7414

Emulsifiers *(cont'd.)*

Radiasurf® 7417
Radiasurf® 7420
Radiasurf® 7422
Radiasurf® 7423
Radiasurf® 7431
Radiasurf® 7432
Radiasurf® 7443
Radiasurf® 7444
Radiasurf® 7453
Radiasurf® 7454
Radiasurf® 7473
Radiasurf® 7600
Radiasurf® 7900
Relaxer Conc. No. 2
Remcopal 40 S3
Remcopal 207
Remcopal 334
Remcopal 21411
Remcopal O11
Remcopal O12
Remcopal O9
Renex® 20
Renex® 30
Renex® 36
Renex® 647
Renex® 649
Renex® 650
Renex® 679
Renex® 682
Renex® 697
Renex® 698
Renex® 702
Renex® 703
Renex® 707
Renex® 711
Renex® 720
Renex® 750
Rewocid® DU 185
Rewoderm® ES 90
Rewomat B 2003
Rewomid® DO 280 S
Rewomid® IPE 280
Rewomid® OM 101/G
Rewomid® OM 101/IG
Rewominoxid B 204
Rewomul MG
Rewomul MG SE
Rewopal® C 6
Rewopal® CSF 11
Rewopal® LA 3
Rewopol® CT 65
Rewopol® NLS 28
Rewoquat CPEM
Rewoteric® AM B-15
Rewoteric® AM CAS
Rewoteric® AM CAS-15
Rewowax CG
Rexol AE-23
Rexonic N91-6
Rexonic N91-8
Rhaballgum CG-M
Rheodol 430, 450
Rheodol 440
Rheodol 460
Rheodol AO-10
Rheodol AO-15
Rheodol AS-10
Rheodol MO-60

Rheodol MS-50, MS-60,
    SEM
Rheodol SP-L10
Rheodol SP-P10
Rheodol TW-L106, -L120
Rheodol TW-P120
Rhodacal® 301-10F
Rhodacal® 330
Rhodacal® A-246L
Rhodacal® LA Acid
Rhodafac® MC-470
Rhodafac® RD-510
Rhodafac® RE-870
Rhodafac® RM-510
Rhodafac® RM-710
Rhodameen® OS-12
Rhodapex® ES
Rhodapex® EST-30
Rhodapex® ESY
Rhodapon® EC111
Rhodapon® LM
Rhodapon® LSB, LSB/CT
Rhodapon® LT-6
Rhodapon® SB-8208/S
Rhodasurf® C-20
Rhodasurf® L-4
Rhodasurf® LA-3
Rhodasurf® LA-30
Rhodasurf® LAN-23-75%
Rhodasurf® ON-870
Rhodasurf® ON-877
Rhodasurf® S-2
Rhodasurf® S-20
Rhodasurf® TD-9
Ricinion
Rita EDGS
Rita EGMS
Rita GMS
Ritabate 20
Ritabate 40
Ritabate 60
Ritabate 80
Ritacet-20
Ritachol®
Ritachol® 1000
Ritachol® 2000
Ritachol® 3000
Ritachol® 4000
Ritachol 5000
Ritahydrox
Ritalan® AWS
RITA Lanolin
R.I.T.A. Lanolin Wax
Ritapeg 100 DS
Ritapeg 150 DS
Ritapeg 400 DS
Ritapro 100
Ritapro 165
Ritapro 200
Ritapro 300
Ritapro 300K
Ritapro 300R
Ritawax
Ritawax 5
Ritawax 10
Ritawax 15
Ritawax 20

Ritawax 40
Ritawax AEO
Ritawax ALA
Ritawax Super
Ritoleth 2
Ritoleth 5
Ritoleth 10
Ritoleth 20
Ritox 35
Ritox 52
Ritox 53
Ritox 59
Ritox 721
Rol 52
Rol 53
Rol 59
Rol 400
Rol AG
Rol DGE
Rol DL 40
Rol DO 40
Rol GE
Rol L 40
Rol LP
Rol MOG
Rol RP
Rol TR
RS-55-40
Ryoto Sugar Ester B-370
Ryoto Sugar Ester L-195
Ryoto Sugar Ester L-595
Ryoto Sugar Ester L-1570
Ryoto Sugar Ester L-1695
Ryoto Sugar Ester LN-195
Ryoto Sugar Ester M-1695
Ryoto Sugar Ester O-170
Ryoto Sugar Ester O-1570
Ryoto Sugar Ester OWA-
    1570
Ryoto Sugar Ester P-1570
Ryoto Sugar Ester P-1570S
Ryoto Sugar Ester P-1670
Ryoto Sugar Ester S-070
Ryoto Sugar Ester S-170
Ryoto Sugar Ester S-170
    Ac
Ryoto Sugar Ester S-270
Ryoto Sugar Ester S-370
Ryoto Sugar Ester S-370F
Ryoto Sugar Ester S-570
Ryoto Sugar Ester S-770
Ryoto Sugar Ester S-970
Ryoto Sugar Ester S-1170
Ryoto Sugar Ester S-1170S
Ryoto Sugar Ester S-1570
Ryoto Sugar Ester S-1670
Ryoto Sugar Ester S-1670S
Sandopan® DTC
Sandopan® DTC-100
Sandopan® DTC-Acid
Sandopan® DTC Linear P
Sandopan® DTC Linear P
    Acid
Sandopan® KST
Sandopan® LS-24
Sandoz Amide NT
Santone® 10-10-O
Sarkosyl® L

Sarkosyl® LC
Sarkosyl® NL-30
Sarkosyl® O
Satexlan 20
Satulan
Schercamox DML
Schercamox DMM
Schercemol DEGMS
Schercemol EGMS
Schercemol GMIS
Schercemol GMS
Schercemol MEL-3
Schercemol MEM-3
Schercemol MEP-3
Schercemol PGMS
Schercodine B
Schercodine C
Schercodine I
Schercodine L
Schercodine M
Schercodine O
Schercodine P
Schercodine S
Schercomid 1-102
Schercomid CCD
Schercomid CDA-H
Schercomid CME
Schercomid HT-60
Schercomid ID
Schercomid IMI
Schercomid M
Schercomid MD-Extra
Schercomid MME
Schercomid ODA
Schercomid OME
Schercomid OMI
Schercomid SD-DS
Schercomid SI
Schercomid SLE
Schercomid SL-Extra
Schercomid SLL
Schercomid SL-ML
Schercomid SLS
Schercomid SM
Schercomid SME
Schercomid SME-S
Schercomid SO-A
Schercomid SO-T
Schercomid TO-2
Schercoquat 2IAE
Schercoquat 2IAP
Schercoquat ALA
Schercoquat CAS
Schercoquat IALA
Schercotaine MKAB
Schercotaine WOAB
Schercozoline B
Schercozoline C
Schercozoline O
Seagel L
Sebase
Secoster® DMS
Secoster® EMS
Sellig R 3395
Shebu® WS
Silbione™ 70646
Silquat AD
Silwet® L-7001

Emulsifiers *(cont'd.)*

Silwet® L-7002	Solwax LG 35	Standamul® 1414-E	Surfonic® N-100
Silwet® L-7500	Sorban AST	Standamul® B-1	Surfonic® N-102
Silwet® L-7602	Sorbanox AOM	Standamul® B-2	Surfonic® N-120
Silwet® L-7604	Sorbanox AST	Standamul® B-3	Surfonic® N-130
Silwet® L-7614	Sorbax PML-20	Standamul® HE	Surfonic® N-150
Simulsol 7	Sorbax PMO-5	Standamul® M-8	Surfonic® N-200
Simulsol 52	Sorbax PMO-20	Standamul® O-5	Surfonic® N-300
Simulsol 56	Sorbax PMP-20	Standamul® O-10	Surfonic® NB-5
Simulsol 58	Sorbax PMS-20	Standamul® O-20	Swanol Amidoamine S
Simulsol 72	Sorbax PTO-20	Standapol® SCO	Syncrowax AW1-C
Simulsol 76	Sorbax PTS-20	Stearal	Syncrowax BB-4
Simulsol 78	Sorbax SML	Stearate 400 WL 817	Syncrowax ERL-C
Simulsol 92	Sorbax SMO	Stearate 1500	Syncrowax HGL-C
Simulsol 96	Sorbax SMP	Stearate 6000 WL 1644	Syncrowax HR-C
Simulsol 98	Sorbax SMS	Stedbac®	Syncrowax HRS-C
Simulsol 165	Sorbax STO	Steol® 4N	Synoquart P 50
Simulsol 989	Sorbax STS	Steol® CA-460	Synperonic A2
Simulsol 1292	Sorbilene ISM	Steol® CS-460	Synperonic A3
Simulsol 1293	Sorbilene L	Steol® KA-460	Synperonic A4
Simulsol 1294	Sorbilene L 4	Steol® KS-460	Synperonic A6
Simulsol 5719	Sorbilene LH	Stepan TAB®-2	Synperonic A7
Simulsol CS	Sorbilene O	Sterol GMS	Synperonic A9
Simulsol M 45	Sorbilene O 5	Sterol SES	Synperonic A11
Simulsol M 49	Sorbilene P	Sterol ST 1	Synperonic A50
Simulsol M 51	Sorbilene S	Sterol ST 2	Synperonic NP1
Simulsol M 52	Sorbilene S 4	Sterol TE 200	Synperonic NP2
Simulsol M 53	Sorbilene TO	Sucro Ester 7	Synperonic NP4
Simulsol M 59	Sorbilene TS	Sucro Ester 11	Synperonic NP5
Simulsol NP 575	Sorbirol ISM	Sucro Ester 15	Synperonic NP5.5
Simulsol O	Sorbirol O	Sulfocos 2B	Synperonic NP6
Simulsol P4	Sorbirol P	Sulfopon® P-40	Synperonic NP7
Simulsol P23	Sorbirol S	Sulfotex DOS	Synperonic NP8
Sinochem GMS	Sorbirol SQ	Sulframin 85	Synperonic NP8.5
Siponic® E-2	Sorbirol TO	Sulframin 90	Synperonic NP8.75
Siponic® E-3	Sorbirol TS	Sulframin 1240, 1245	Synperonic NP9
Siponic® E-10	Sorbitol L	Sulframin 1250, 1260	Synperonic NP9.5
Siponic® NP-7	Sorbon S-20	Super Corona	Synperonic NP9.75
Sipothix® H-65	Sorbon S-40	Superfine Lanolin	Synperonic NP10
Skliro Distilled	Sorbon S-60	Anhydrous USP	Synperonic NP12
S-Maz® 20	Sorbon S-66	Super Hartolan	Synperonic NP13
S-Maz® 40	Sorbon S-80	Superloid®	Synperonic NP15
S-Maz® 60	Sorbon T-20	Supermontaline SLT65	Synperonic NP17
S-Maz® 60K	Sorbon T-40	Superpro 5A	Synperonic NP20
S-Maz® 60KHM	Sorbon T-60	Super-Sat AWS-4	Synperonic NP25
S-Maz® 65K	Sorbon T-80	Super-Sat AWS-24	Synperonic NP30
S-Maz® 80	Sorbon TR 814	Suprafino SMD	Synperonic NP30/70
S-Maz® 80K	Sorbon TR 843	Supralate C	Synperonic NP35
S-Maz® 83R	Sorgen 30	Supralate EP	Synperonic NP40
S-Maz® 85	Sorgen 40	Supro-Tein V	Synperonic NP50
S-Maz® 85K	Sorgen 50	Surfactol® 13	Synperonic OP3
S-Maz® 90	Sorgen 90	Surfactol® 318	Synperonic OP4.5
S-Maz® 95	Sorgen S-30-H	Surfactol® 365	Synperonic OP6
Softigen® 701	Sorgen S-40-H	Surfactol® 575	Synperonic OP7.5
Softisan® 601	Span® 20	Surfactol® 590	Synperonic OP8
Solan	Span® 40	Surfactol® Q1	Synperonic OP10
Solan E	Span® 60, 60K	Surfactol® Q2	Synperonic OP10.5
Solangel 401	Span® 60 VS	Surfactol® Q3	Synperonic OP11
Solulan® 5	Span® 65	Surfactol® Q4	Synperonic OP12.5
Solulan® 16	Span® 80	Surfagene FDD 402	Synperonic OP16
Solulan® 25	Span® 85	Surfine AZI-A	Synperonic OP16.5
Solulan® 75	Spreading Agent ET0672	Surfine WNG-A	Synperonic OP20
Solulan® C-24	Stamid HT 3901	Surfonic® L46-7	Synperonic OP25
Solulan® L-575	Stamid LS 5487	Surfonic® N-10	Synperonic OP30
Solusol® 75%	Standamid® CD	Surfonic® N-31.5	Synperonic OP40
Solusol® 85%	Standamid® ID	Surfonic® N-40	Synperonic OP40/70
Solusol® 100%	Standamid® KD	Surfonic® N-60	Synperonic PE/F68
Solwax C-24	Standamid® LD	Surfonic® N-85	Synperonic PE/F87
Solwax L20	Standamid® LD 80/20	Surfonic® N-95	Synperonic PE/F127

Emulsifiers *(cont'd.)*

Synperonic PE/L35
Synperonic PE/P85
Syntofor A03, A04, AB03, AB04, AL3, AL4, B03, B04
Syntopon A
Syntopon D
Syntopon F
Syntopon G
Tagat® R40
Tagat® R60
Tagat® R63
Tauranol I-78
Tauranol I-78-3
Tauranol I-78-6
Tauranol I-78/80
Tauranol I-78E, I-78E Flakes
Tauranol I-78 Flakes
T-Det® O-407
Tegamine® 18
Tegin®
Tegin® 515
Tegin® 515 VA
Tegin® 4011
Tegin® 4433
Tegin® 4480
Tegin® 4600
Tegin® 4600 NSE
Tegin® A-412
Tegin® A-422
Tegin® C-1R
Tegin® C-61
Tegin® C-62 SE
Tegin® C-63
Tegin® C-63 SE
Tegin® D 6100
Tegin® DGS
Tegin® E-41
Tegin® E-41 NSE
Tegin® E-61
Tegin® E-61 NSE
Tegin® E-66
Tegin® E-66 NSE
Tegin® G 6100
Tegin® GO
Tegin® GRB
Tegin® ISO NSE
Tegin® L 61, L 62
Tegin® M
Tegin® O
Tegin® P
Tegin® P-411
Tegin® RZ
Tegin® RZ NSE
Tegin® Spezial SE
Tegin® T 4753
Tegin® VA
Tegin® VA 515
Teginacid®
Teginacid® H
Teginacid® ML
Teginacid® R
Teginacid® R-SE
Teginacid® Special
Teginacid® Spezial SE
Teginacid® X SE
Tego®-Amid D 5040

Tego®-Amid O 18
Tego®-Amid S 18
Tego®-Betaine L-7
Tego® Care 150
Tego® Care 215
Tego® Care 300
Tego® Care 450
Tensami 1/05
Tensami 3/06
Tensami 4/07
Tensami 8/09
Tensami 10/06
Tergitol® 26-L-3
Tergitol® NP-9
Teric 9A6
Teric 12A3
Teric LAN70
Tetronic® 304
Tetronic® 504
Tetronic® 701
Tetronic® 702
Tetronic® 704
Tetronic® 707
Tetronic® 901
Tetronic® 904
Tetronic® 908
Tetronic® 909
Tetronic® 1101
Tetronic® 1102
Tetronic® 1104
Tetronic® 1107
Tetronic® 1301
Tetronic® 1302
Tetronic® 1304
Tetronic® 1307
Tetronic® 1501
Tetronic® 1502
Tetronic® 1504
Tetronic® 1508
Tewax TC 10
Tewax TC 60
Tewax TC 65
Tewax TC 72
Tewax TC 80
Tewax TC 81
Tewax TC 82
Tewax TC 83
Tewax TC 840
Texapon® K-1294
Texapon® T 42
Texapon® VHC Needles
Texapon® WW 99
Texofor B7
T-Maz® 20
T-Maz® 28
T-Maz® 40
T-Maz® 60
T-Maz® 60K
T-Maz® 61
T-Maz® 65
T-Maz® 80
T-Maz® 80K
T-Maz® 80KLM
T-Maz® 81
T-Maz® 85
T-Maz® 90
T-Maz® 95
TO-33-F

TO-55-E
TO-55-EL
TO-55-F
Triton® N-42
Triton® N-150
Triton® X-100
Trycol® 5878
Trycol® 5964
Trycol® 5967
Trycol® 5972
Trydet LA-5
Trydet SA-23
Trydet SA-40
Trylox® 6746
Trylox® 6753
TS-33-F
Tween® 20
Tween® 20 SD
Tween® 21
Tween® 40
Tween® 60
Tween® 61
Tween® 65
Tween® 80
Tween® 80K
Tween® 81
Tween® 85
Tylose® MH Grades
Tylose® MHB
Tylose® MH-K, MH-xp, MHB-y, MHB-yp
Ultra Sulfate SE-5
Ultra Sulfate SL-1
Unamide® C-2
Unamide® C-5
Unamide® L-2
Unamide® L-5
Unamide® LDL
Ungerol AM3-75
Ungerol LES 2-28
Ungerol LES 2-70
Ungerol LES 3-28
Ungerol LES 3-70
Ungerol N2-28
Ungerol N2-70
Ungerol N3-28
Ungerol N3-70
Unichem MS
Unichol
Unicol CA-2
Unicol CA-4
Unicol CA-10
Unicol LA-23
Unicol OA-2
Unicol OA-4
Unicol OA-10
Unicol OA-20
Unifat 54
Unihydol 100
Unihydol LS-3
Unilex, DS, S, SH
Unimul-05
Unimul-10
Unimul-1414EW
Unipeg-200 ML
Unipeg-200 MS
Unipeg-400 ML
Unipeg-400 MO

Unipeg-400 MS
Unipeg-600 ML
Unipeg-600 MS
Unipeg-1000 MS
Unipeg-1540 MS
Unipeg-DGL
Unipeg-EGMS
Unipeg-PGML
Unipeg-S-40
Unipol SCO
Unithox® 420
Unithox® 450
Unithox® 480
Unithox® 520
Unithox® 550
Unithox® 720
Unithox® 750
Unitina E-24
Unitina GMRO
Unitolate 80MG
Unitolate PGO-1010
Unizeen C-2
Unizeen C-5
Unizeen C-10
Unizeen OA
Unizeen SA
Unizeen T-2
Unizeen T-5
Unizeen T-15
Upamide L-2
Upamide L-5
Upamide SD
Variquat® K-1215
Varisoft® 5TD
Varisoft® 250
Varisoft® 432-100
Varisoft® 432-CG
Varisoft® 432-ET
Varisoft® 442-100P
Varisoft® DHT
Varisoft® OIMS
Varisoft® SDC-85
Varisoft® TA-100
Varonic® 63 E20
Varonic® 2271
Varonic® BD
Varonic® BG
Varonic® K-202
Varonic® K-202 SF
Varonic® K-205
Varonic® K-205 SF
Varonic® K-210
Varonic® K-210 SF
Varonic® K-215
Varonic® K-215 SF
Varonic® LI-42
Varonic® LI-48
Varonic® LI-63
Varonic® LI-67
Varonic® LI-67 (75%)
Varonic® LI-420
Varonic® LI-420 (70%)
Varonic® Q-202
Varonic® Q-202 SF
Varonic® Q-205
Varonic® Q-205 SF
Varonic® S-202
Varonic® S-202 SF

Emulsifiers *(cont'd.)*

Varonic® T-202	Volpo 20	Volpo O15	Witcamide® 6533
Varonic® T-202 SF	Volpo 25 D 3	Volpo O20	Witcamide® 6546
Varonic® T-205	Volpo 25 D 5	Volpo S-2	Witcamide® S771
Varonic® T-205 SF	Volpo 25 D 10	Volpo S-10	Witcamide® S780
Varonic® T-210	Volpo 25 D 15	Volpo S-20	Witcamine® 6606
Varonic® T-210 SF	Volpo 25 D 20	Volpo T-3	Witcamine® 6622
Varonic® T-215	Volpo CS-3	Volpo T-5	Witco® Acid B
Varonic® T-215 SF	Volpo CS-5	Volpo T-10	Witcolate™ 1050
Varox® 270	Volpo CS-10	Volpo T-15	Witcolate™ A
Varox® 365	Volpo CS-15	Volpo T-20	Witcolate™ AE-3
Varox® 1770	Volpo CS-20	Waxenol® 821	Witcolate™ T
Varsulf® S-1333	Volpo L4	Wayhib® S	Witconate™ 60T
Velvetex® 610L	Volpo L23	White Swan	Witconate™ 79S
Velvetex® AB-45	Volpo N3	Wickenol® 535	Witconate™ 93S
Vifcoll CCN-40, CCN-40	Volpo N5	Wickenol® 545	Witconate™ 1240
Powd	Volpo N10	Witafrol® 7420	Zetesol 100
Vigilan	Volpo N15	Witcamide® 61	Zinc Stearate USP
Vigilan AWS	Volpo N20	Witcamide® 82	Zohar EGMS
Volpo 3	Volpo O3	Witcamide® 5133	Zohar GLST
Volpo 5	Volpo O5	Witcamide® 5195	Zohar GLST SE
Volpo 10	Volpo O10		

Enzymes

Actibronze	Clarex® 5XL	Fungal Protease 60,000	Papain 16,000
Bromelain 1:10	Clarex® L	Fungal Protease 500,000	Papain 30,000
Bromelain Conc	Dihydroxy-acetone	Fungal Protease Conc	Papain Conc
Brookosome® SOD	Enzyami No. 1	Instabronze	Pearex® L
Cellulase 4000	Fungal Lactase 100,000	Myavert C	Yeast Lactase L-50,000
Cellulase Tr Conc	Fungal Protease 31,000	Pancreatic Lipase 250	

Film Formers

Abil® AV 20-1000	Benecel® ME	Copolymer 937	Elvanol® 71-30
A-C® 6A	Benecel® MP	Copolymer 958	Elvanol® 85-82
A-C® 8, 8A	Bernel® Ester DID	Cosmetic Gelatin	Elvanol® 90-50
A-C® 9, 9A, 9F	Bio-Pol® OE	Crodamol LL	Elvanol® HV
A-C® 15	Blanose 7 Types	Crodasone W	Etha-Coll 210-20
A-C® 16	Blanose 9 Types	Cropeptide W	European Elastin 10
A-C® 143	Blanose 12 Types	Crotein ADW	European Elastin 30
A-C® 400	Brookosome® Elastin	Crotein ASC	European Elastin SD
A-C® 430	Brookosome® SC	Crotein ASK	Fancol CH
A-C® 540, 540A	Byco A	Crotein SPO	Fluilan AWS
A-C® 580	Byco C	Dantoin® DMHF-75	Gaffix® VC-713
A-C® 617, 617A	Byco O	Dantoin® DMHF Refined	Gafquat® 734
A-C® 617G	Carboset 525	Dascare HPCH	Gafquat® 755
A-C® 1702	Cationic Collagen	Desamidocollagen	Gafquat® 755N
Acylan	Polypeptides	Desaron	Gafquat® HS-100
Advantage™ V	Cellow 940	Diaformer® Z-301	Gafquat® HSi
Aloe Vera Whole Leaf	Ceraphyl® 50	Diaformer® Z-400	Gantrez® AN
Dried Powd	Chitin Liq	Diaformer® Z-A	Gantrez® ES-225
Amercell® Polymer HM-	Citmol 320	Diaformer® Z-AT	Gantrez® ES-335
1500	Colla-Gel AC	Diaformer® Z-SM	Gantrez® ES-425
Anhydrous Lanolin USP	Collagen Hydrolyzate	Diaformer® Z-W	Gantrez® ES-435
Cosmetic	Cosmetic 50	Diahold® A-503	Gantrez® V-215
Anhydrous Lanolin USP	Collagen Hydrolyzate	Dow Corning® 580 Wax	Gantrez® V-225
Pharmaceutical	Cosmetic 55	Dow Corning® 939	Gantrez® V-425
Anhydrous Lanolin USP	Collagen Hydrolyzate	Dow Corning® Q2-1403	Gluadin® AGP
Superfine	Cosmetic N-35	Fluid	Gluadin® Almond
Anhydrous Lanolin USP	Collagen Hydrolyzate	Eastman® AQ 29D	Gluadin® Wheat
Ultrafine	Cosmetic N-55	Eastman® AQ 35S	GlycoCer HA
Aquagel	Collagen Hydrolyzate	Eastman® AQ 38D	Hetester HCA
Ateco	Cosmetic SD	Elastein® 5000	Hispagel® 100
Bee's Milk	Collagen Native Extra 1%	Elastinhydrolyzate, Liq	Hispagel® 200
Belsil CM 1000	Collasol	Elastinhydrolyzate, Powd	HPCH Liq
Benecel® M	Copolymer 845	Elastosol	Hydagen® BP1

Film Formers *(cont'd.)*

Hydrocoll™ AC-30
Hydrocoll™ EN-55
Hydrocoll™ EN-SD
Hydrocoll™ HE-35
Hydrocoll™ LE-35
Hydrocoll™ T-LSN
Hydrotriticum™ QL
Hydrotriticum™ QM
Hydrotriticum™ QS
Hypan® SA100H
Ivarbase™ 3210
Ivarlan™ 3420
Jurymer
Kera-Tein 1000 AS
Kera-Tein V
Klucel® EF
Klucel® ELF, GF, HF, JF, LF, MF
Kollagen KD
Kollagen S
Kollaplex 0.3
Kollaplex 1.0
Kollaron
Lanfrax® 1776
Lanfrax® 1779
Lanotein AWS 30
Lexein® A-200
Lexein® A-210
Lexein® A-220
Lexein® A-240
Lexquat® 2240
Lexquat® CH
Lipocutin®
Luviflex® D 430 I, D 455 I
Luviflex® VBM 35
Luviform® ES 22
Luviform® ES 42
Luviquat® FC 370
Luviquat® FC 550
Luviquat® FC 905
Luviquat® HM 552
Luviquat® Mono CP
Luviset® CA66

Luviset® CAP
Luviskol® K12
Luviskol® K17
Luviskol® K30
Luviskol® K60
Luviskol® K80
Luviskol® K90
Luviskol® LD-9025
Luviskol® VA28E
Luviskol® VA28I
Luviskol® VA37E
Luviskol® VA37I
Luviskol® VA55E
Luviskol® VA55I
Luviskol® VA64E
Luviskol® VA64I
Luviskol® VA64 Powd
Luviskol® VA64W
Luviskol® VA73E
Luviskol® VA73I
Luviskol® VA73W
Luviskol® VAP 343 E
Luviskol® VAP 343 I
Maricol CLR
Marine Dew
Merquat® 550
Merquat® S
Methocel® 40-100
Methocel® 40-101
Methocel® 40-202
Methocel® A4CP
Methocel® A4MP
Methocel® A15LVP
Methocel® E3P
Methocel® E4MP
Methocel® E6P
Methocel® E15LVP
Methocel® E50LVP
Methocel® E50P
Methocel® K4MP
Methocel® K4MS
Methocel® K15MP
Methocel® K15MS

Methocel® K100LVP
Methocel® K100MP
Microat™ E
Milkpro-Q
Multi-Grain Barley Code 1851
Myvacet® 5-07
Myvacet® 7-07
Nalquat 2240
Natrosol® Plus CS
Natrosol® Plus CS, Grade 330
Neptuline® C
Nikkol NET SG-60A
Nutrilan® Elastin E20, P
Pea Pro-Tein BK
Pecosil® OS-100B
Pentacare-HP
Peptein® VgS
Peptein® VgW
Plantsol
Plasdone® K-25, K-90
Plasdone® K-26/28, K-29/32
Polymer T-1172
Polyox® Coagulant
Polyox® WSR 35
Polypro® 5000
Polypro® 15000
Prisorine ISIS 2039
Prisorine ISOH 3515
Pro-Tein ES-20
Proto-Lan 4R
Pseudocollagen™
PVP K-15
PVP K-30
PVP/Si-10
PVP/VA E-335, E-535, E-635
PVP/VA E-735
Quat-Pro S
Quat-Pro S 30
Radia® 7500

Radia® 7501
Rice Pro-Tein BK
Ritacetyl®
Ritalafa®
Ritasol
Ritasol Base 100
Ritasol Base 200
Ross Bayberry Wax Substitute
Salcare SC10
Salcare SC30
Schercemol IPM
Silkpro
Silkpro CM-1000
Silkpro CM-2000
Silkpro-Q
Silwax® F
Silwax® F-D
Solu-Mar™ EN-30
Solu-Mar™ Native
Sol-U-Tein EA
Soy-Tein NL
Stabileze™ 06
Superloid®
Thermoplex
Tri-K Soypro-25
Tri-Lastin 10F
Tri-Tein Silk AA
Tritisol™
Trivent SS-20
Ultrahold® 8
Unilin® 425 Alcohol
Unimer U-15
Unimer U-151
Unithox® 420
Unithox® 450
Unithox® 480
Unithox® 520
Unithox® 550
Unithox® 720
Unithox® 750
Waxenol® 822
Wheat-Tein NL

Glossing Agents

Abil® B 88183
Abil® OSW 12, OSW 13
Abil® S201
Abil® S255
Abil®-Wax 9810
A-C® 9, 9A, 9F
Amersil® L-45 Grades
Amersil® L-45/10
Amersil® L-45/20
Amersil® L-45/50
Amersil® L-45/100
Amersil® L-45/200
Amersil® L-45/350
Amersil® L-45/500
Amersil® L-45/1000
Amersil® L-45/12500
Amersil® L-45/60000
Aquarez 7
Argobase 125
Argonol ACE 6
Argonol RIC2

Belsil SDM 6021
Belsil SDM 6022
Bernel® Ester DOM
Caprol® 2G4S
Caprol® 3GO
Caprol® 3GS
Caprol® 6G2O
Caprol® 6G2S
Caprol® 10G2O
Caprol® 10G4O
Caprol® 10G10O
Caprol® 10G10S
Caprol® PGE860
Celquat® H-100
Celquat® L-200
Celquat® SC-240
Ceraphyl® 41
Ceraphyl® 55
Ceraphyl® 368
Ceraphyl® 375
Colla-Gel AC

Comperlan® KM
Crodamol BS
Crodamol ML
Crodamol OSU
Crodasone W
Crosilk 10,000
Crotein Q
Dow Corning® 200 Fluid
Dow Corning® 556 Fluid
Dow Corning® 580 Wax
Dow Corning® 929
Eastman® AQ 38S
Eastman® AQ 55S
Emalex CS-5
Emalex CS-10
Emalex CS-15
Emalex CS-20
Emalex CS-24
Emalex CS-30
Emalex LWIS-8
Emalex LWIS-10

Emery® 1695
Enduragloss™
Ethosperse® G-26
Euperlan® K 771
Euperlan® MPK 850
Euperlan® PK 3000
Fancol ALA
Fancor IPL
Fancorsil A
Fancorsil P
Fancorsil SLA
Fancorsil SLA-LT
Flexan® 130
Gantrez® ES-225
Gantrez® ES-335
Gantrez® ES-425
Gantrez® ES-435
Gantrez® V-215
Gantrez® V-225
Gantrez® V-425
Genamin KSL

TRADE NAME FUNCTIONAL CROSS-REFERENCE

Glossing Agents *(cont'd.)*

Generol® 122E10
Glucam® E-10
Hair Gloss Polymer
Herbalcomplex 2 Special
Hetester HCA
HGC 5000
Hydagen® P
Ivarbase™ 3210
Ivarlan™ 3420
Kera-Tein V
Kessco® Octyl Palmitate
Lanesta P
Laneto 40
Laneto 50
Laneto 60
Lexemul® 55G
Lipo PE 810
Lipo SS
Liponate CRM
Lipoquat R
Lipovol A
Lipovol ALM
Lipovol ALM-S
Lipovol A-S
Lipovol CP
Lipovol G
Lipovol P

Lipovol P-S
Lipovol SAF
Lipovol SES
Lipovol SES-S
Lipovol SO
Lipovol SUN
Lipovol WGO
Lustrabrite® S
Luxelen® Silk D
Luxelen® SS
Luxelen® SS-020
Macol® 57
Masil® 556
Masil® 756
Masil® SF 1000
Masil® SF 10,000
Masilwax 135
MFF 159-B
Mirapol® 550
Nagellite® 3050
Nagellite® 3050-80
Naturechem® GTH
Naturechem® PGR
Pacific Sea Kelp Glycolic
    Extract B-1063
Pecosil® OS-100B
Peptein® 2000®

Peptein® 2000XL
Permethyl® 104A
PF
Polycare® 133
Produkt GM 4055
Pro-Tein ES-20
PVP/VA E-735
Radia® 7752
Resyn® 28-2913
Ritacetyl®
Robeyl
Sandoperm FE
Schercemol 1818
Schercemol CL
Schercemol CP
Schercemol CS
Schercemol DID
Schercemol TISC
Schercemol TIST
Schercoquat SAS
Schercoquat SOAS
Schercoquat WOAS
Schercotaine MKAB
SF96® (500 cst)
SF96® (1000 cst)
Silamine 50
Silamine 65

Silbione™ 71634
Silkpro AS
Silkpro-Q
Silwax® WS
Silwet® L-7602
Soy-Amino Quat L/O
Syncrowax ERL-C
Syncrowax HGL-C
Syncrowax HR-C
Tegin® 55G VA
Tegin® D 1102
Tegin® G
Tegin® G 1100
Tegin® G 6100
Tri-Lastin 10F
Tri-Tein Silk AA
Trivent OL-10B
Vybar® 103
Vybar® 260
Vybar® 825
Vybar® 5013
Waxenol® 822
Wickenol® 707
York Krystal Kleer Castor
    Oil
York USP Castor Oil
Zeodent® 113

Hair Care Additives
(Antidandruff Agents, Hair Fixatives, Dyes, Sets, Waves)

Abil® S201
Abil® S255
Ablumine DHT75
Advantage™ CP
Advantage™ V
Ageflex FM-1
Ageflex mDMDAC
Akypo RLM 45 A
Akypo RLM 45 N
Akypoquat 131
Akyporox NP 30
Alfonic® 1216-1.5
Alfonic® 1216-CO-2
Alfonic® 1412-3
Almond Oil
Alpinamed Burdock
Amphomer® 4910
Amphomer® LV-71
Anti-Dandruff Usnate AO
Aquagel
Aquaron
Aristoflex A
Aristoflex A/60% Sol'n
Arquad® HC
Atomergic Zinc Pyrithione
Barquat® CME-35
Belsil CM 1000
Biodermine
Biosil Basics A-30
Biosil Basics Amino DL-30
Biosil Basics DL-30
Biosil Basics HKP-30
Biosil Basics L-30
Biosil Basics L-Cysteine
Biosulphur Powder

Brookosome® P
D-Calcium Pantothenate
    USP, FCC Type SD
    No. 63924
Camellia Oil
Capigen
Capigen CG
Capigen CS
Capilotonique HS 220
Capilotonique HS 226
Capilotonique HS 245
Capisome
Catinal LQ-75
Cation G-40
Cation S
Centrolene® A, S
Ceraphyl® 65
Ceraphyl® 70
Ceraphyl® 85
Chemsalan NLS 30
Chemsalan RLM 28
Chemsalan RLM 56
Chemsalan RLM 70
Cofix
Coflex
Copolymer 845
Crodasinic L
Crodasinic O
Cryolidone®
Cuivridone®
Dascare HPCH
Delsette
Dexpanthenol USP, FCC
    No. 63909
Diaformer® Z-301

Diaformer® Z-400
Diaformer® Z-A
Diaformer® Z-AT
Diaformer® Z-W
Diahold® A-503
Dow Corning® 225
Dow Corning® 929
Dow Corning® 939
Dow Corning® 1669
Dow Corning® 7224
Dow Corning® Q2-7224
    Conditioning Additive
Dow Corning® Q2-8220
    Conditioning Additive
Dow Corning® X2-1669
Eastman® AQ 29D
Eastman® AQ 35S
Eastman® AQ 38D
Eastman® AQ 38S
Eastman® AQ 55S
Eldew CL-301
Empicol® TAS30
Empigen® OY
Emulmetik™ 110
Emulmetik™ 135
Emulmetik™ 310
Emulmetik™ 900
Emulmetik™ 910
Emulmetik™ 920
Emulmetik™970
Estran™-Lite
Estran™-Pure
Estran™-Xtra
Ethyl Panthenol No. 26100
Etocas 200

Flexan® 130
Foamid LME-75
Foamox CDO
Foamquat 2IAE
Foamquat BAS
Foamquat COAS
Foamquat SOAS
Forestall
Gaffix® VC-713
Gantrez® SP-215
Genamin CTAC
Ginseng Phytosome®
Glusol
GP-4 Silicone Fluid
GP-71-SS Mercapto
    Modified Silicone Fluid
GP-215 Silicone Polyol
    Copolymer
GP-217 Silicone Polyol
    Copolymer
GP-218
GP-226
Granamine S3A
Gransurf 71
Gransurf 72
Gransurf 73
Gransurf 75
Gransurf 76
Gransurf 77
Hair Complex 20/70n
Hair Complex Aquosum
Hair Gloss Polymer
Hairspray Additive S
Herbasol Complex E
Herbasol 7 Herb Complex

569

Hair Care Additives *(cont'd.)*

Hetaine CLA
Hispagel® 100
Hispagel® 200
H₂old™ EP-1
HPCH Liq
Hydrocoll™ AC-30
Hydrocoll™ HE-35
Hydrocoll™ LE-35
Hydrocoll™ T-LSN
Hydrolyzed Elastin RE-10
  No. 26202
Hydrolyzed Elastin RE-30
  No. 26203
Ichtyocollagene
Ichtyoelastin
Incromectant AMEA-100
Incromectant LMEA
Incroquat 26
Incroquat BES-35 S
Incroquat SBQ 75P
Incroquat TMC-80
Incroquat TMC-95
Incrosoft S-90
Incrosoft T-90
Isopar® M
Ivarlan™ Light
Kemamine® Q-9903B
Kerabiol
Keramois L
Kera-Tein 1000
Kessco® PEG 200 DL
Kessco® PEG 400 DS
Kessco® PEG 600 DL
Lamepon® PA-K/NP
Lamepon® PA-TR/NP
Lamepon® UD/NP
Lanoquat® 1751A
Lexein® A-210
Lexein® A-520
Lexein® CP-125
Lexquat® 2240
Lexquat® CH
Lipacide SH-CO
Lipacide SH-K
Lipacide SH-V
Luviflex® D 430 I, D 455 I

Luviflex® VBM 35
Luviset® CA66
Luviset® CAP
Luviset® CAP X
Luviskol® K12
Luviskol® K17
Luviskol® K30
Luviskol® K60
Luviskol® K80
Luviskol® K90
Luviskol® LD-9025
Luviskol® VA28E
Luviskol® VA28I
Luviskol® VAP 343 E
Luviskol® VAP 343 I
Marine Dew
Midecol ACS
Milkpro-Q
Myristocor™
Mytab®
Naetex-CHP
Nalquat 2240
National Starch 28-4979
Necon SOG
Necon SOLC
Noxamine CA 30
Nutrilan® Elastin E20
Nutrilan® I-50/NP
Nutrilan® I Powd
Nutrilan® I-Powd./NP
Nutrilan® L/NP
Nutrimarine
Olamida UD 21
Olamin® K/NP
Oligoceane
Omadine® MDS
Ormagel XPU
DL-Panthenol Cosmetic
  Grade No. 63920
DL-Panthenol USP, FCC
  No. 63915
Pecosil® OS-100B
Pecosil® PS-100K
Pelemol IDO
Phytantriol No. 63926
Phytoderm Complex U

Polycare® 133
Polycare® 509
Polymer T-1172
Polymin® FG SG
Polymin® G-35 SG
Polymin® P SG
Polymin® PS SG
Polymin® Waterfree SG
Polyolprepolymer-2
Polyquart® H 7102
Promarine
Relaxer Conc. No. 2
Remcopal 334
Resyn® 28-1310
Resyn® 28-2913
Resyn® 28-2930
Rewocid® SBU 185 P
Rewomid® DO 280 S
Rewoquat W 75
Rewoquat W 75 PG
Rewoquat W 222 PG
Rewoquat WE 16
Rewoquat WE 18
Rewoquat WE 18-85
Rewoquat WE 20
Rewoquat WE 28
Rhodapon® LM
Rhodaquat® M270C/18
Salcare SC91
Salcare SC92
Salcare SC95
Schercoquat FOAS
Seanamin FP
Seboregular HS 312
Sebum Control COS-218/2-
  A
Sellig LET 630
Semburi Extract BG
Semburi Extract Ethanol
Silkpro
Silkpro AS
Silkpro CM-1000
Silkpro CM-2000
Silkpro-Q
Sodium Hyaluronate RCC-
  1 No. 26228

Softigen® 767
Sol-U-Tein 6861
Spinomar NaSS
Stepanhold® Extra
Stepanhold® R-1
Thiovanic® Acid
Tofupro-U
Trichogen
Trydet LA-5
Ucare® Polymer JR-30M,
  JR-125, JR-400
Ultrahold® 8
Unsoft 475
Uvasorb S-5
Varonic® K-202
Varonic® K-202 SF
Varonic® K-205
Varonic® K-205 SF
Varonic® K-210
Varonic® K-210 SF
Varonic® K-215
Varonic® K-215 SF
Varonic® Q-202
Varonic® Q-202 SF
Varonic® Q-205
Varonic® Q-205 SF
Varonic® S-202
Varonic® S-202 SF
Varonic® T-202
Varonic® T-202 SF
Varonic® T-205
Varonic® T-205 SF
Varonic® T-210
Varonic® T-210 SF
Varonic® T-215
Varonic® T-215 SF
Vaseline 335 G
Vaseline 7702
Vaseline 8332
Vaseline 10049 BL
Vaseline A
Versatyl-42
Zinc Omadine® 48% Disp.
Zinc Omadine® Powd.
Zink Pyrion

Humectants/Moisturizers

A-611
Abil® OSW 12, OSW 13
A-C® 6A
A-C® 8, 8A
A-C® 9, 9A, 9F
A-C® 15
A-C® 16
A-C® 143
A-C® 430
A-C® 540, 540A
A-C® 617, 617A
A-C® 617G
A-C® 1702
Acconon ETG
Acetadeps
Acetamide MEA
Acid Mucopolysaccharides
Actiglide™

Actiglow™
Actimoist™
Actimoist™ Bio-2
Ajidew A-100
Ajidew N-50
Ajidew SP-100
Alcolec® PG
Algisium-C
Alkamuls® MM/M
Alkamuls® SDG
Alkamuls® SS
Alkapol PEG 300
Almond Oil
Almondermin®
Aloe Gel Stabilized
Aloe Phytogel 1:199 Powd.
Aloe-Phytogel 199 Powd.
Aloe Vera Conc. 40 Fold

Aloe Vera Freeze Dried
  Powd. 200:1
Aloe Vera Gel
Aloe Vera Gel 1:1
Aloe Vera Gel 1:1
  Decolorized
Aloe Vera Gel 1:1 With
  Pulp
Aloe Vera Gel 1:2
Aloe Vera Gel 1:10
Aloe Vera Gel 1:10 Conc.
Aloe Vera Gel 1:50
Aloe Vera Gel 1:50 Conc.
Aloe Vera Gel 1:100
Aloe Vera Gel 1:100 Conc.
Aloe Vera Gel 10:1
  Decolorized
Aloe Vera Gel Conc. 10:1

Aloe Vera Gel Conc. 40:1
Aloe Vera Gel Conc. 40:1
  Decolorized
Aloe Vera Gel CS
Aloe Vera Gel CS 10
Aloe Vera Gel CS 40
Aloe Vera Gel DC
Aloe Vera Gel DC 10
Aloe Vera Gel DC 40
Aloe Vera Gel Filtered
Aloe Vera Gel Single Fold
Aloe Vera Gel TEX
Aloe Vera Gel Unfiltered
Aloe Vera Juice
Aloe Vera Powd. A 1-200
Aloe Vera Pulp
Aloe Vera Spray Dried
  Powd.

Humectants/Moisturizers *(cont'd.)*

Aloe Vera Whole Leaf Dried Powd.
Alomucin
Alo-X-11
Aloxe MG-20
Amerchol® 400
Amerchol® BL
Amerchol® C
Amerchol® CAB
Amerchol® L-99
Amerchol L-101®
Amerchol® L-500
Amerchol® RC
Amerlate® P
Amidex AME
Amino-Collagen-25, -40
Amino Gluten MG
Amino-Silk SF
Anhydrous Lanolin Grade 2
Anhydrous Lanolin P.80
Anhydrous Lanolin P.95
Anhydrous Lanolin P.95RA
Aqualose L30
Aqualose L75
Aqualose L100
Aqualose SLT
Aqualose SLW
Aqua-Tein C
Aqua-Tein S
Argidone®
Argobase L2
Argobase MS 5
Argonol 1SO
Argonol 40
Argonol 50
Argonol 50 Super
Argonol 60
Argonol ACE 5
Argonol ACE 6
Argonol RIC2
Argowax Cosmetic Super
Argowax Dist
Argowax LFA Distilled
Argowax Standard
Arosurf® 66-E2
Arosurf® 66-E10
Arosurf® 66-E20
Aruba Aloe Vera Gel
Ateco
Atomergic Cholesterol
Atomergic Hyaluronic Acid
ATP Nucleotides
Avian Sodium Hyaluronate Powd.
Avian Sodium Hyaluronate Sol'n.
Base EAC 20
Basis LS-60H
Belsil DMC 6031
Belsil DMC 6032
Belsil DMC 6033
Belsil DMC 6035
Benecel® M
Benecel® ME
Benecel® MP
BioCare® Polymer HA-24
Biodynes® TRF Ultra-5
Biomatrix®

Biomin® Marine
Biophos 35
Biopol® TE
Brocose Q
Brookosome® ANE
Brookosome® Biophos
Brookosome® CS
Brookosome® DNA/RNA
Brookosome® E
Brookosome® EFA
Brookosome® Elastin
Brookosome® EPO
Brookosome® Fucus
Brookosome® H
Brookosome® MSF
Brookosome® P
Brookosome® SC
Brookosome® U
Brookosome® V
D-Calcium Pantothenate USP, FCC Type SD No. 63924
Caprol® 10G2O
Captex® 300
Carbopol® 1342
Carbopol® 1706
Carbopol® 1720
Carbowax® PEG 300
Carbowax® PEG 400
Carbowax® PEG 600
Carbowax® Sentry® PEG 300
Carbowax® Sentry® PEG 400
Carbowax® Sentry® PEG 540 Blend
Carbowax® Sentry® PEG 600
Carbowax® Sentry® PEG 900
Carbowax® Sentry® PEG 1000
Carbowax® Sentry® PEG 1450
Carbowax® Sentry® PEG 3350
Carbowax® Sentry® PEG 4600
Carbowax® Sentry® PEG 8000
Cartilage Mucopolysaccharides E.M.A.C
Celluflow C-25
Celluflow TA-25
Centella Phytosome®
Cera Albalate 101
Cera Albalate 102
Cera Albalate 103
Ceraphyl® 60
Ceraphyl® GA-D
CG 10x (Unfiltered and stabilized)
Chitin Liq
Cholesterol
Cholesterol BP
Cholesterol NF
Chromoprotulines
Clearcol

Clear Filtered Verajuice-Cold Processed
Colla-Gel AC
Collagen
Collagen 15K
Collagen Amino Acids SF
Collagen Masks
Collagen Native Extra 1%
Collagen S.D
Collagene Lyophilized
Collagen Powd
Collamino™ 40-SF
Collamino™ Complex
Colla-Moist™ CG
Colla-Moist™ WS
Collamoist ZN
Collasol
Copherol® 950LC
Copherol® 1250
Copherol® F 1300
Corona Lanolin
Coronet Lanolin
CoVera
Cremba
Crestalans
Croderol G7000
Croderol GA 7000
Crodyne BY-19
Crolastin
Cromoist CS
Cromoist HYA
Cromoist O-25
Cronectin H
Crosilk 10,000
Crosilk Liq
Crosilkquat
Crotein CAA/SF
Crotein HKP Powd
Crotein K
Cryolidone®
Dermalcare® EGMS/SE
Dermalcare® GTIS
Dermalcare® LVL
Dermalcare® MST
Dermalcare® PGMS
Dermatein® GSL
Dermatein® MPS
Dermidrol
Dermol G-76
Dermol L45
Dermosaccharides® GY
Desamidocollagen
Desamidocollagen K 1.0
Desamidocollagen K 1.5
Desaron
Dexpanthenol USP, FCC No. 63909
DNA Marine
Dow Corning® 190 Surfactant
Dow Corning® 193 Surfactant
Dow Corning® 2501 Cosmetic Wax
D.S.H. C
Elastin PG 2000
Elastinhydrolysate, Liq
Elastinhydrolysate, Powd

Elastosol
Elespher®
Elfacos® E200
EmCon COPA
EmCon E-5
Emery® 912
Emery® 916
Emery® 917
Emery® 918
Emery® 1660
Emery® 1732
Emery® 1740
Emery® 1747
Emery® 6709
Emery® HP-2050
Emery® HP-2060
Emthox® 2730
Endonucleine®
Escin/b-Sitosterol Phytosome®
Estalan L-45
Estran™-Lite
Esuronammina
Ethosperse® G-26
Ethosperse® SL-20
Ethyl Panthenol No. 26100
Etocas 30
Etocas 100
European Elastin 10
Exsycobalt
Exsycuivre
Exsymol Chromoprotuline
Exsymol Cobalt Acetylmethionate
Exsymol Cupric Acetylmethionate
Exsymol Gold Acetylmethionate
Exsymol Magnesium Acetylmethionate
Exsymol Manganese Acetylmethionate
Exsymol Nickel Acetylmethionate
Exsymol Protuline
Exsymol Silver Acetylmethionate
Exsymol Zinc Acetylmethionate
Exsyor
Fancol ALA-10
Fancol C
Fancol CAB
Fancol HL
Fancol HON
Fancol LA
Fancol LA-5
Fancol LAO
Fancor IPL
Fancor Lanwax
Filagrinol®
Filtered Verajuice-Cold Processed
Fluilan
Foamid LM2E
Foamid LME-75
Foamquat VG
Forlan 200

571

Humectants/Moisturizers *(cont'd.)*

Forlan 300
Forlan 500
Forlan C-24
Forlan LM
G-2330
Gafquat® HSi
Gamma Oryzanol
George's Aloe Vera
Ginkgo Biloba Dimeric
   Flavonoids
   Phytosome®
Ginkgo Biloba Phytosome®
Ginseng Phytosome®
Gluadin® Almond
Gluadin® Wheat
Glucam® E-10
Glucam® E-20
Glucam® E-20 Distearate
Glucam® P-10
Glucam® P-20
Glucam® P-20 Distearate
Glucquat® 125
Glusol
GlycoCer HA
Glycon® G 100
Glycon® G-300
Glycyrrhetinic Acid
   Phytosome®
Granamine S3A
Grillocam E10
Grillocam E20
Grillocose DO
Grillocose® IS
Grillocose® PS
Grilloten LSE 65
Grilloten® LSE 65 K
Grilloten® LSE 65 K Soft
Grilloten LSE 65 Soft
Grilloten LSE 87
Grilloten® LSE 87 K
Grilloten® LSE 87 K Soft
Grilloten LSE 87 Soft
Grilloten PSE141G
Grilloten® PSE 141 G
   Pellets
Grilloten ZT-40
Grilloten ZT-80
Gunther Pro-Tein 1550
Hair Saccharides
Hartolan
Hartolite
Hest CSO
Hispagel® 100
Hispagel® 200
Hodag CSA-80
Hodag PEG 400
Hodag PEG 540
Humectant SD-35
Hyala-Dew
Hyaluronic Acid
Hyaluronic Acid AH-602
Hyaluronic Acid-BT
Hyaluronic Acid (Na)
Hyamine® 3500-NF
Hyasol
Hyasol-BT
Hycollan
Hydagen® BP1

Hydagen® F
Hydex® 100 Gran. 206
Hydex® Coarse Powd
Hydex® Powd. 60
Hydex® Tablet Grade
Hydracol®
Hydrocoll™ AC-30
Hydrocoll™ EN-55
Hydrocoll™ EN-SD
Hydrolactin 2500
Hydrolyzed Elastin RE-10
   No. 26202
Hydrolyzed Mucopolysac-
   charides SD
Hydromarine
Hydrosoy 2000/SF
Hydrotriticum™
Hydrotriticum™ Powd
Hydrotriticum™ WAA
Hyladerm®
Hylucare™
Hystar® 3375
Hystar® 4075
Hystar® 5875
Hystar® 6075
Hystar® 7000
Hystar® 7570
Hystar® CG
Hystar® HM-75
Hystar® TPF
Ialuramina
Ialuramina 10
Ichtyocollagene
Ichtyoelastin
Incromectant AMEA-70
Incromectant AMEA-100
Incromectant AQ
Incromectant LAMEA
Incromectant LMEA
Incromectant LQ
Incromine BB
Incromine OPB
Inositol
Isopropylan® 33
Ivarlan™ 3100
Ivarlan™ 3310
Ivarlan™ 3360
Ivarlan™ 3409-60
Jaluronid
Kalidone®
Kemstrene® 96.0%
Kemstrene® 99.7%
Kera-Quat WKP
Kera-Tein 1000
Kera-Tein 1000 RM/50
Kera-Tein 1000 RM SD
Kera-Tein 1000 SD
Kera-Tein AA
Kera-Tein AA-SD
Kera-Tein V
Kester Wax® 72
Kester Wax® 82
Kester Wax® 105
Kester Wax® K 48
Kester Wax® K 56
Kester Wax® K 59
Kester Wax® K 62
Kester Wax® K 85

Kollagen KD
Kollagen S
Kollaplex 0.3
Kollaplex 1.0
Kollaron
Koster Keunen Hydroxy-
   Hexanyl-Behenyl-
   Beeswaxate
Koster Keunen Paraffin
   Wax 122/128
Koster Keunen Paraffin
   Wax 130/135
Koster Keunen Paraffin
   Wax 140/145
Koster Keunen Paraffin
   Wax 150/155
Koster Keunen Synthetic
   Candelilla
Koster Keunen Synthetic
   Candelilla R-4
Koster Keunen Synthetic
   Candelilla R-8
Lactil®
Lactolan®
Lanaetex Aloe Vera Gel
Lanesta G
Lanesta P
Lanesta SA-30
Laneto 27
Laneto 40
Laneto 50
Laneto 60
Laneto 100
Laneto AWS
Lanfrax® 1779
Lanogene®
Lanolin Cosmetic
Lanolin Extra-Deodorized
Lanolin Pharmaceutical
Lanolin USP
Lantrol® 1673
Lantrol® 1674
Lantrol® HP-2073
Lantrol® HP-2074
Laurydone®
Leucocyanidins
   Phytosome®
Lexein® S620S/Superpro
   5A
Lexol® GT-855
Lexol® PG-800
Lexol® PG-865
Lexquat® 2240
Lexquat® CH
Lipamide LMEA
Lipamide MEAA
Lipo Polyol NC
Lipocol
Lipocutin®
Lipodermol®
Lipoid S 75-3
Lipolan 31-20
Lipolan Distilled
Lipomectant AL
Liponic 70-NC
Liponic 76-NC
Liponic 83-NC
Liponic EG-1

Liponic EG-7
Liponic SO-20
Lipo-Peptide AME 30
Lipo Polyglycol 200
Lipo Polyglycol 300
Lipo Polyglycol 400
Lipo Polyglycol 600
Lipo Polyglycol 1000
Lipo Polyglycol 3350
Liposomes Anti-Age
Lipoxol® 200 MED
Lipoxol® 300 MED
Lipoxol® 400 MED
Lipoxol® 550 MED
Lipoxol® 600 MED
Lipoxol® 800 MED
Lipoxol® 1000 MED
Lipoxol® 1550 MED
Lipoxol® 2000 MED
Lipoxol® 3000 MED
Lipoxol® 4000 MED
Lipoxol® 6000 MED
Liquester
Liquid Base
Lonzest® 143-S
Lysidone®
Mackamide™ AME-75,
   AME-100
Macol® E-200
Macol® E-300
Macol® E-400
Macol® E-600
Macol® E-1000
Macol® E-3350
Maricol CLR
Marine Dew
May-Tein C
May-Tein KTS
May-Tein SK
Melhydran®
MicroReservoir Hydro-
   Diffuser
Microsponge® 5647
Microsponge® 5650
Milkamino™ 20
Mirasoft™ CO 11
Mirasoft™ LMO
Mirasoft™ MSPO 11
Moisturizing Factor L
Multifruit BSCY
Musol™ 20
Musol™ SD
Naetex-L
Nalidone®
Natipide®
Natipide® II
Natipide® II PG
Natural Beeswax
Natural Extract AP
Neptuline® C
Nikkol Aquasome BH
Nikkol Aquasome LA
Nikkol Bio-Sodium
   Hyaluronate Powd. and
   1% Sol'n.
Nikkol Lecinol S-10
Nikkol Lecinol S-10E
Nikkol Lecinol S-10EX

Humectants/Moisturizers *(cont'd.)*

Nikkol Lecinol S-10M
Nikkol Lecinol S-30
Nikkol Lecinol SH
Nikkol Sodium Hyaluronate
Niox KS Series
Oasis™
Oceagen®
Optim
Orange Wax
Orange Wax, Deodorized
Ormagel SH, XPU
Panalane® L-14E
Pancogene® S
DL-Panthenol Cosmetic
    Grade No. 63920
DL-Panthenol USP, FCC
    No. 63915
Parapel® LAM-100
Pationic® SBL
Pationic® SCL
Patlac® LA
Patlac® NAL
Pea Pro-Tein BK
Pecosil® OS-100B
Pentavitin®
Peptein® CAA
Peptein® Qs
Peptein® Qw
Peptein® VgS
Peptein® VgW
Phosal® 50 SA
Phosal® 53 MCT
Phosal® 60 PG
Phosal® 75 SA
Phospholipid EFA
Phospholipid SV
Phospholipon® 80
Phospholipon® 90/90 G
Phospholipon® 90 H
Phytantriol No. 63926
Pidolidone®
Plantsol
Pluriol® E 1500
Pogol 200
Polymoist® Mask
Polyolprepolymer-2
Polypeptide 10
Polypeptide 12
Polypro® 5000
Polypro® 15000
Probiol™ L/N
Procetyl AWS
Prodew 100
Prodew 200
Protalan L-60
Protalan Oil
Prothera™
Proto-Lan 4R
Proto-Lan 8

Proto-Lan 20
Proto-Lan 30
Proto-Lan IP
Protulines
PVP K-15
Pyroter GPI-25
Quamectant™ AM-50
Quat-Pro S
Quat-Pro S 30
Reticusol
Rewolan® 5
Rewolan® E
Rice Pro-Tein BK
Rita AZ
Rita KA
Ritacetin
Ritachol®
Ritaderm®
Ritalan®
Ritalan® AWS
RITA Lanolin
Ritaloe 1X, 10X, 20X, 40X
Ritaloe 200M
Ritamectant K2
Ritamectant PCA
Ritapan CAP
Ritapan D
Ritapan DL
Ritapan NAP
Ritapan TA
R.I.T.A. d-Panthenol
R.I.T.A. dl-Panthenol
Ritatin
Ritawax AEO
Ritawax ALA
Ritawax Super
Robane®
Ruscogenins Phytosome®
Salcare SC91
Salcare SC92
Salcare SC95
Schercemol 1688
Schercemol DEIS
Schercemol DO
Schercemol TIST
Schercomid AME
Schercomid AME-70
Schercomid LME
Scheroba Oil
SD-35
Seanamin SU
Seanamin TH
Sebase
Sedermasome
Shebu® Refined
Shebu® WS
Silhydrate C
Silkall 100
Silkall CA

Silkall TI
Silkall TL
Silkall ZN
Silk Pro-Tein
Silymarin Phytosome®
Simchin® Natural
Simchin® Refined
Simchin® WS
Sodium Hyaluronate RCC-
    1 No. 26228
Softisan® 378
Softisan® 645
Sohakuhi Extract BG-100
Sohakuhi Extract Ethanol
Solan
Solan 50
Solangel 401
Solidester
Sollagen® EC
Sollagen® LA
Soluble Native Collagen
    RA-1 No. 26206
Soluble Native Collagen
    RS-1 No. 26205
Solu-Coll™
Solu-Coll™ P
Solu-Mar™ EN-30
Solu-Mar™ Native
Sol-U-Tein 6861
Soy-Quat C
Soy-Tein NL
Standamid® SDO
Standamul® 1414-E
Star
Starfol® OS
Superol
Superpro 5A
Super Refined™ Wheat
    Germ Oil
Super Sterol Ester
Supro-Tein V
Tegosoft® CI
Tegosoft® CO
Tegosoft® CT
Tegosoft® DO
Tegosoft® EE
Tegosoft® Liquid
Tegosoft® Liquid M
Tegosoft® M
Tegosoft® OP
Tegosoft® OS
Tegosoft® P
Tegosoft® S
Tegosoft® SH
Thermoplex
dl-α-Tocopheryl Acetate,
    Cosmetic Grade No.
    60574

dl-α-Tocopheryl Linoleate
    No. 26364
Tri-K CMF Complex
Tri-K HMF Complex
Tri-K Soypro-25
Tri-Lastin 10F
Tritisol™
Ultra Anhydrous Lanolin
    HP-2060
Ultra Lantrol® HP-2074
Umordant P
Unibiovit B-33
Unibiovit B-332
Unichem LACA
Unichol
Unilin® 350 Alcohol
Unilin® 550 Alcohol
Unilin® 700 Alcohol
Unimoist U-125
Unimul-1414EW
Varonic® 32-E20
Varonic® 63 E20
Varonic® LI-420
Varonic® LI-420 (70%)
Varsulf® SBF-12
Varsulf® SBFA-30
Vegamino™ 30-SF
Veragel® 200
Veragel® Liq., Liq. 1:1
Vigilan
Vitamin A Palmitate Type
    P1.7
Vitamin A Palmitate Type
    P1.7/BHT
Vitamin A Palmitate Type
    PIMO/BH
Vitamine A Palmitate
    Exsyliposomes
Waxenol® 822
Wheat Germ Oil
Wheat-Quat C
Wheat-Tein NL
White Swan
Wickenol® 136
Wickenol® 151
Wickenol® 153
Wickenol® 155
Wickenol® 156
Wickenol® 158
Wickenol® 159
Wickenol® 160
Wickenol® 161
Wickenol® 171
Wickenol® 545
Xanthan XP
Yucca Glauca Extract Code
    9030
Zincidone®

Lubricants/Slip Agents/Penetrants/ Spreading Agents/Release Agents

AA USP
Abil® B 8842
Abil® B 8873
Abil® B 88183

Abil®-Wax 2434
Abil®-Wax 2440
Abil®-Wax 9800
Abil® Wax 9814

Ablunol 200ML
Ablunol 200MO
Ablunol 200MS
Ablunol 400ML

Ablunol 400MO
Ablunol 400MS
Ablunol 600ML
Ablunol 600MO

Lubricants/Slip Agents/Penetrants... *(cont'd.)*

Ablunol 600MS
Ablunol 1000MO
Ablunol 1000MS
Ablunol CO 5
Ablunol CO 15
Ablunol CO 30
A-C® 8, 8A
A-C® 9, 9A, 9F
A-C® 540, 540A
Acconon 300-MO
Acconon 400-MO
Acconon CA-9
Acconon CA-15
Acconon CA-25
Acconon ETG
Acconon GTO
Acetol® 1706
Acetulan®
Actiglide™
Adol® 52 NF
Adol® 60
Adol® 80
Adol® 85
Adol® 90 NF
Adol® 640
Alcolec® Granules
Aldo® PMS
Alfol® 610 ADE
Alfol® 1012 HA
Alfol® 1012 HA
Alfol® 1014 CDC
Alfol® 1214
Alfol® 1214 GC
Alfol® 1216
Alfol® 1216 CO
Alfol® 1218 DCBA
Alfol® 1412
Alfol® 1416 GC
Alfol® 1418 DDB
Alfol® 1418 GBA
Alfol® 1618
Alfol® 1618 CG
Alfol® 1618 GC
Alkamuls® 200-DL
Alkamuls® 200-DO
Alkamuls® 400-DO
Alkamuls® 400-MO
Alkamuls® EL-620
Alkamuls® EL-620L
Alkamuls® GMO
Alkamuls® GMO-45LG
Alkamuls® MM/M
Alkamuls® PETS
Alkamuls® PSML-20
Alkamuls® PSMO-5
Alkamuls® SDG
Alkamuls® SS
Alkapol PEG 300
Alkasurf® NP-40, 70%
Almond Oil
Alrosperse 11P Flake
Altalc 200 USP
Altalc 400 USP
Amerchol® 400
Amerchol® H-9
Amerchol L-101®
Amerchol® RC
Amerlate® P

Amerlate® W
Amidex O
Amidex RC
Amidroxy
Amino-Collagen-25, -40
Amino-Silk SF
Anhydrous Lanolin HP-
2050
Argobase 125
Argonol 50
Argonol 50 Pharmaceutical
Argonol ACE 6
Argonol RIC2
Arlatone® T
Armid® O
Arosurf® 66-PE12
Asol
Avamid 150
Axol® E 61
Axol® E 66
Belsil PDM 20
Belsil PDM 200
Belsil PDM 1000
Benol®
BioCare® Polymer HA-24
Biosil Basics Jasmine
Wax S
Blandol®
Britol®
Britol® 6NF
Britol® 7NF
Britol® 9NF
Britol® 20USP
Britol® 35USP
Britol® 50USP
Brookosome® MSF
Cachalot® C-51
Cachalot® O-15
Cachalot® S-54
Capmul® GMS
Caprol® 10G2O
Caprol® 10G10O
Captex® 355
Captex® 800
Captex® 8000
Carbowax® PEG 300
Carbowax® PEG 400
Carbowax® PEG 600
Carbowax® PEG 900
Carbowax® PEG 1000
Carbowax® PEG 1450
Carbowax® PEG 3350
Carbowax® PEG 4600
Carbowax® PEG 8000
Carbowax® Sentry® PEG
300
Carbowax® Sentry® PEG
400
Carbowax® Sentry® PEG
540 Blend
Carbowax® Sentry® PEG
600
Carbowax® Sentry® PEG
900
Carbowax® Sentry® PEG
1000
Carbowax® Sentry® PEG
1450

Carbowax® Sentry® PEG
3350
Carbowax® Sentry® PEG
4600
Carbowax® Sentry® PEG
8000
Carnation®
Carsonon® 144-P
Carsonon® 169-P
Cartaretin F-4
Castorwax® MP-80
Cecavon NA 61
Cecavon ZN 70
Cecavon ZN 71
Cecavon ZN 72
Cecavon ZN 73
Cecavon ZN 735
Celluflow C-25
Celluflow TA-25
Celquat® SC-230M
Cera Albalate 101
Cera Albalate 102
Cera Albalate 103
Ceranine PN Base
Ceraphyl® 28
Ceraphyl® 31
Ceraphyl® 50
Ceraphyl® 55
Ceraphyl® 140
Ceraphyl® 230
Ceraphyl® 375
Ceraphyl® 494
Ceraphyl® 791
Ceraphyl® 847
Cetina
Cetinol 1212
Cetinol EE
Cetinol LA
Cetinol LL
Cetinol LM
Cetinol LU
Cetinol MM
Cetiol® G16S
Cetiol® G20S
Cetiol® LC
Cetiol® V
Cetodan
C-Flakes
Chemal LA-4
Chemal LA-9
Chemal LA-12
Chemal LA-23
Chemal OA-5
Chemal OA-20/70CWS
Chemal TDA-3
Chemal TDA-6
Chemal TDA-9
Chemal TDA-12
Chemal TDA-15
Chemal TDA-18
Chemax E-200 MO
Chemax E-200 MS
Chemax E-400 ML
Chemax E-400 MO
Chemax E-600 ML
Chemax E-600 MO
Chemax E-600 MS
Chemax E-1000 MO

Chemax HCO-5
Chemax HCO-16
Chemax HCO-25
Chemax HCO-200/50
Chemeen C-2
Chemeen C-5
Chemeen C-10
Chemeen C-15
Chemical 39 Base
Chimin P10
Cithrol 2ML
Cithrol 2MO
Cithrol 4ML
Cithrol 4MO
Cithrol 6ML
Cithrol 6MO
Cithrol 10ML
Cithrol 10MO
Cithrol 40MO
Cithrol 60ML
Cithrol 60MO
Cithrol GDO N/E
Cithrol GDO S/E
Cithrol GDS N/E
Cithrol GDS S/E
Cithrol GML N/E
Cithrol GML S/E
Cithrol GMO N/E
Cithrol GMO S/E
Cithrol GMR N/E
Cithrol GMR S/E
Cithrol GMS Acid Stable
Cithrol GMS N/E
Cithrol GMS S/E
Cithrol PGML N/E
Cithrol PGML S/E
Cithrol PGMO N/E
Cithrol PGMO S/E
Cithrol PGMR N/E
Cithrol PGMR S/E
Cithrol PGMS N/E
Cithrol PGMS S/E
Co-Gell® A2/B270
Cosbiol
Cosmetol® X
Covafluor
Cremophor® S 9
Crill 1
Crill 2
Crill 3
Crill 35
Crillet 4
Crillon LME
Crillon ODE
Crodacol CS-50
Crodalan LA
Crodamol CAP
Crodamol DO
Crodamol ICS
Crodamol IPM
Crodamol IPP
Crodamol ISNP
Crodamol JJ
Crodamol OO
Crodamol OP
Crodamol PC
Crodamol PETS
Crodamol PMP

Lubricants/Slip Agents/Penetrants... *(cont'd.)*

Crodamol PTC
Crodamol PTIS
Crodasinic LS35
Crodasinic OS35
Crodasone W
Crodex N
Croduret 200
Crosilk Powder
Crystal® O
Crystal® Crown
Cutina® HR
Cyclochem® GMO
Cyclochem® LVL
Cyclochem® PETS
D-400
D-1000
D-1200
D-1300
D-2000
D-3000
D-4000
Dar Chem-11
Dar Chem-12
Dermalcare® EGMS/SE
Dermalcare® GTIS
Dermalcare® HL
Dermalcare® LVL
Dermalcare® MST
Dermalcare® PGMS
Dermalcare® POL
Dermane
Detergent CR
Diamond Quality®
Distilled Lipolan
Dow Corning® 200 Fluid
Dow Corning® 225
Dow Corning® 244 Fluid
Dow Corning® 245 Fluid
Dow Corning® 344 Fluid
Dow Corning® 345 Fluid
Dow Corning® 556 Fluid
Dow Corning® 580 Wax
Dow Corning® 593 Fluid
Dow Corning® Q2-5220
    Resin Modifier
Dow Corning® Q2-5324
    Surfactant
Drakeol 5
Drakeol 9
Drakeol 19
Drewfax® 0007
Drewmulse® 85K
Dur-Em® GMO
Durfax® 60
Dynasan® 110
Dynasan® 112
Dynasan® 114
Dynasan® 116
Dynasan® 118
Eccowet® W-50
Eccowet® W-88
Emalex 703
Emalex 705
Emalex 707
Emalex 709
Emalex 710
Emalex 712
Emalex 715

Emalex 720
Emalex 725
Emalex 730
Emalex 750
Emcol® CC-9
Emcol® CC-42
Emcol® CC-57
Emcol® L
Emcol® M
Emcol® NA-30
EmCon COPA
EmCon E-5
Emerest® 2310
Emerest® 2325
Emerest® 2381
Emerest® 2388
Emerest® 2410
Emerest® 2423
Emerest® 2704
Emerest® 2715
Emery® 1650
Emery® 1656
Emery® 1660
Emery® 1730
Emsorb® 2500
Emsorb® 2503
Emsorb® 2507
Emsorb® 2729
Emthox® 5940
Emthox® 6964
Emthox® 6965
Ervol®
Espermaceti A
Espermaceti C
Estalan 12
Estalan 430
Estasan GT 8-40 3578
Estasan GT 8-60 3575
Estasan GT 8-60 3580
Estasan GT 8-65 3577
Estasan GT 8-65 3581
Estol IBUS 1552
Ethomid® O/15
Ethosperse® OA-2
Ethoxyol® 1707
Ethylflo® 162
Ethylflo® 180
Etocas 10
Etocas 35
Etocas 60
Eutanol® G
Eutanol® G16
Exxal® 20
Famous
Fancol Acel
Fancol ALA
Fancol C
Fancol CAB
Fancol CH
Fancol HL
Fancol LA
Fancol LA-5
Fancol LAO
Fancol OA-95
Fancor IPL
Fancor Lanwax
Fancorsil A
Fancorsil P

Finsolv® SB
Fitoderm
Flexricin® 13
Fluilan
Foamox CDO
Fonoline® White
Fonoline® Yellow
Forlan 200
Forlan 300
Forlan 500
Forlan L
Forlan LM
Fractalite IDS
G-3816
Gafac® RE-877
Gemtex PA-70P
Gemtex PA-75
Gemtex PA-75E
Gemtex PA-85P
Gloria®
Glucam® E-20 Distearate
Glucam® P-20 Distearate
Glucate® DO
Glucate® IS
Gransil FL-D 55
Hamposyl® O
Hartolan
Hefti GMS-33
Hetoxamate FA-5
Hetoxamate FA-20
Hetoxamate LA-5
Hetoxamate LA-9
Hetoxamate MO-4
Hetoxamate MO-5
Hetoxamate MO-9
Hetoxamate MO-15
Hetoxamate SA-5
Hetoxamate SA-9
Hetoxamate SA-35
Hetoxamate SA-90
Hetoxamate SA-90F
Hetoxide BN-13
Hetoxide C-15
Hetoxide C-25
Hetoxide C-30
Hetoxide C-40
Hetoxide C-200
Hetoxide C-200-50%
Hetoxide HC-40
Hetoxide HC-60
Hetsorb L-4
Hetsorb L-10
Hetsorb L-20
Hetsorb O-20
Hetsorb TO-20
Hetsorb TS-20
Hispagel® 100
Hispagel® 200
Hodag CSA-80
Hodag DGO
Hodag PE-004
Hodag PEG 3350
Hodag PEG 8000
Hylucare™
Hystar® 7000
Hystar® CG
Hystar® TPF
Hystrene® 4516

Hystrene® 5016 NF
Hystrene® 7022
Hystrene® 9016
Hystrene® 9022
Hystrene® 9512
Hystrene® 9718 NF
Imwitor® 900
Imwitor® 928
Imwitor® 940
Imwitor® 940 K
Imwitor® 988
Incrocas 30
Incrocas 40
Incromide LA
Incromine BB
Incromine OPB
Incromine Oxide B
Incromine Oxide B-30P
Incromine Oxide I
Incromine Oxide ISMO
Incromine Oxide O
Incronam B-40
Incronam I-30
Incropol CS-20
Incropol CS-50
Inositol
Intravon® JU
Ionet DL-200
Iscolan
Isopropylmyristate
Ivarbase™ 3210
Ivarlan™ 3409-60
Jaguar® HP 8
Jaguar® HP 60
Jaguar® HP 120
Jojoba Oil Cosmetic Grade
Jurymer
Jurymer MB-1
Karamide 121
Karamide 363
Kaydol®
Kemester® 5221SE
Kemester® 5415
Kemester® 5500
Kemester® 5510
Kemester® 6000SE
Kera-Tein AA
Kessco® Glycerol
    Monooleate
Kessco® Isobutyl Stearate
Kessco® PEG 200 DL
Kessco® PEG 200 DO
Kessco® PEG 200 DS
Kessco® PEG 200 ML
Kessco® PEG 200 MO
Kessco® PEG 200 MS
Kessco® PEG 300 DL
Kessco® PEG 300 DO
Kessco® PEG 300 DS
Kessco® PEG 300 ML
Kessco® PEG 300 MO
Kessco® PEG 300 MS
Kessco® PEG 400 DL
Kessco® PEG 400 DO
Kessco® PEG 400 DS
Kessco® PEG 400 ML
Kessco® PEG 400 MO
Kessco® PEG 400 MS

Lubricants/Slip Agents/Penetrants... *(cont'd.)*

Kessco® PEG 600 DL	Lipocol B	Lutrol® E 300	Mazol® SFR 3500
Kessco® PEG 600 DO	Lipodermol®	Lutrol® E 400	Mazol® SFR 18,000
Kessco® PEG 600 DS	Lipolan	Luviquat® FC 370	Mazol® SFR 50,000
Kessco® PEG 600 ML	Lipolan R	Luviquat® FC 550	Mazol® SFR 150,000
Kessco® PEG 600 MO	Lipolan S	Mackamide™ ISA	Masil® SFV
Kessco® PEG 600 MS	Liponic 70-NC	Mackernium™ 006	Masil® SF-V (4)
Kessco® PEG 1000 DL	Liponic 76-NC	Mackernium™ 007	Masil® SF-V (5)
Kessco® PEG 1000 DO	Liponic 83-NC	Mackernium™ CTC-30	Masil® SF-VL
Kessco® PEG 1000 DS	Liponic EG-1	Mackernium™ KP	Masil® SF-VV
Kessco® PEG 1000 ML	Liponic EG-7	Mackernium™ NLE	May-Tein C
Kessco® PEG 1000 MO	Lipopeg 2-DL	Mackernium™ SDC-25	May-Tein KT
Kessco® PEG 1000 MS	Lipopeg 2-L	Mackernium™ SDC-50	May-Tein KTS
Kessco® PEG 1540 DL	Lipopeg 4-DL	Mackernium™ SDC-85	May-Tein R
Kessco® PEG 1540 DO	Lipopeg 4-DO	Mackernium™ WLE	May-Tein SY
Kessco® PEG 1540 DS	Lipopeg 4-DS	Macol® 22	Mazamide® C-5
Kessco® PEG 1540 ML	Lipopeg 4-L	Macol® 23	Mazamide® L-5
Kessco® PEG 1540 MO	Lipopeg 4-S	Macol® 27	Mazamide® SS-10
Kessco® PEG 1540 MS	Lipopeg 6-L	Macol® 31	Mazeen® C-2
Kessco® PEG 4000 DL	Lipopeg 10-S	Macol® 32	Mazeen® C-5
Kessco® PEG 4000 DO	Lipopeg 15-S	Macol® 33	Mazeen® C-10
Kessco® PEG 4000 DS	Lipopeg 100-S	Macol® 34	Mazeen® C-15
Kessco® PEG 4000 ML	Lipopeg 6000-DS	Macol® 35	Mazeen® S-2
Kessco® PEG 4000 MO	Lipo Polyglycol 200	Macol® 40	Mazeen® S-5
Kessco® PEG 4000 MS	Lipo Polyglycol 300	Macol® 42	Mazeen® S-10
Kessco® PEG 6000 DL	Lipo Polyglycol 400	Macol® 44	Mazeen® S-15
Kessco® PEG 6000 DO	Lipo Polyglycol 600	Macol® 46	Mazeen® T-2
Kessco® PEG 6000 DS	Lipo Polyglycol 1000	Macol® 65	Mazeen® T-5
Kessco® PEG 6000 ML	Lipo Polyglycol 3350	Macol® 72	Mazeen® T-10
Kessco® PEG 6000 MO	Liposorb L	Macol® 77	Mazeen® T-15
Kessco® PEG 6000 MS	Liposorb L-10	Macol® 85	Mazol® GMS
Kessco PTS	Liposorb L-20	Macol® 88	Merpol® HCS
Koster Keunen Synthetic	Liposorb O	Macol® 90	Merquat® 280
Japan Wax	Liposorb O-5	Macol® 90(70)	Methocel® 40-100
Lanesta L	Liposorb O-20	Macol® 101	Methocel® 40-101
Lanesta P	Liposorb P	Macol® 108	Methocel® 40-202
Lanesta S	Liposorb P-20	Macol® 625	Methocel® A4CP
Lanesta SA-30	Liposorb S	Macol® 626	Methocel® A4MP
Laneto 40	Liposorb S-4	Macol® 627	Methocel® A15LVP
Laneto 50	Liposorb S-20	Mafo® CAB	Methocel® E3P
Laneto 60	Liposorb SQO	Mapeg® 200 DL	Methocel® E4MP
Laneto 100-Flaked	Liposorb TO	Mapeg® 400 MO	Methocel® E6P
Lanexol	Liposorb TO-20	Masil® 756	Methocel® E15LVP
Lanexol AWS	Liposorb TS	Masil® 1066C	Methocel® E50LVP
Lanolic Acid	Liposorb TS-20	Masil® 1066D	Methocel® E50P
Lanolin Cosmetic	Lipovol C-76	Masil® SF 5	Methocel® K4MP
Lanolin Extra-Deodorized	Lipovol CAN	Masil® SF 10	Methocel® K4MS
Lanolin Pharmaceutical	Lipovol CO	Masil® SF 20	Methocel® K15MP
Lanolin USP	Lipovol HS	Masil® SF 50	Methocel® K15MS
Lanoquat® 1756	Lipovol J	Masil® SF 100	Methocel® K100LVP
Lanotein AWS 30	Lipovol J Lite	Masil® SF 200	Methocel® K100MP
Lantrol® HP-2073	Lipovol MAC	Masil® SF 350	Michel XO-150-20
Laurel R-50	Lipovol M-SYN	Masil® SF 350 FG	Microma-100
Lexemul® 55G	Lipovol O	Masil® SF 500	Miglyol® 810
Lexemul® EGDS	Lipovol PAL	Masil® SF 1000	Miglyol® 812
Lexemul® PEG-200 DL	Lipovol SOY	Masil® SF 5000	Miglyol® 818
Lexemul® PEG-400 DL	Liquester	Masil® SF 10,000	Miglyol® 840
Lexemul® PEG-400ML	Liquid Base	Masil® SF 12,500	Miranol® DM
Lexol® IPM	Lonzest® 143-S	Masil® SF 30,000	Miranol® DM Conc. 45%
Lexol® IPM-NF	Lonzest® 153-S	Masil® SF 60,000	Mirapol® 550
Lexol® PG-865	Lonzest® 163-S	Masil® SF 100,000	Mirapol® A-15
Lexol® SS	Lowenol C-243	Masil® SF 300,000	Modulan®
Lipamide MEAA	Lowenol C Acid	Masil® SF 500,000	Monamid® 150-IS
Lipamide S	Lowenol L Acid	Masil® SF 600,000	Monamine 779
Lipex 109	Lowenol M Acid	Masil® SF 1,000,000	Monaquat ISIES
Lipex 407	Lowenol O Acid	Masil® SFR 70	Monateric ISA-35
Lipo DGLS	Lowenol P Acid	Mazol® SFR 100	Monawet MO-65-150
Lipo DGS-SE	Lubrajel® CG, DV, MS, TW	Mazol® SFR 750	Monawet MO-70
Lipo EGDS	Lubritab®	Mazol® SFR 2000	Monawet MO-70-150

Lubricants/Slip Agents/Penetrants... *(cont'd.)*

Monawet MO-70R
Monolan® PPG440, PPG1100, PPG2200
Myvacet® 9-08
Myvacet® 9-45
Naetex-L
Naetex O-20
Naetex O-80
Natural Beeswax
Natural Extract AP
Naxonic™ NI-40
Naxonic™ NI-60
Naxonic™ NI-100
Naxonol™ PO
Neobee® 18
Neobee® M-20
Neobee® O
Nikkol Decaglyn 2-IS
Nikkol Decaglyn 5-IS
Nikkol Decaglyn 5-O
Nikkol Decaglyn 5-S
Nikkol Decaglyn 7-IS
Nikkol Decaglyn 7-O
Nikkol Decaglyn 7-S
Nikkol Decaglyn 10-IS
Nikkol Decaglyn 10-O
Nikkol Decaglyn 10-S
Nikkol Hexaglyn 1-S
Nikkol OP-3
Nikkol OP-10
Nikkol OTP-75
Nikkol OTP-100
Nikkol Squalane
Nikkol Squalene EX
Nimlesterol® 1730
Nopalcol Series
Nopalcol 1-S
Nopalcol 1-TW
Norfox® B
Novol
OP-2000
Orzol®
Pegosperse® 50 DS
Pegosperse® 100 O
Pegosperse® 6000 DS
Pegosperse® EGMS-70
Perfecta® USP
Phosal® 50 SA
Phosal® 53 MCT
Phosal® 60 PG
Phosal® 75 SA
Plasdone® K-26/28, K-29/32
Pluracol® E400
Pluracol® E400 NF
Pluracol® E600
Pluracol® E600 NF
Pluracol® E1000
Pluracol® E1450
Pluracol® E1450 NF
Pluracol® E2000
Pluracol® E4000 NF
Pluracol® E4500
Pluracol® E8000
Pluracol® E8000 NF
Pluronic® F38
Pluronic® F68
Pluronic® F68LF

Pluronic® F77
Pluronic® F87
Pluronic® F88
Pluronic® F98
Pluronic® F108
Pluronic® F127
Pluronic® L35
Pluronic® L42
Pluronic® L43
Pluronic® L44
Pluronic® L61
Pluronic® L62
Pluronic® L62D
Pluronic® L62LF
Pluronic® L63
Pluronic® L64
Pluronic® L72
Pluronic® L81
Pluronic® L92
Pluronic® L101
Pluronic® L121
Pluronic® L122
Pluronic® P65
Pluronic® P75
Pluronic® P84
Pluronic® P85
Pluronic® P94
Pluronic® P103
Pluronic® P104
Pluronic® P105
Pluronic® P123
Polyaldo® DGHO
Polylan®
Precirol ATO 5
Prisorine IPIS 2021
Procetyl 10
Procetyl 30
Procetyl 50
Prostearyl 15
Protalan L-60
Protol®
Proto-Lan 8
Proto-Lan 20
Protopet® Alba
Protopet® White 1S
Protopet® White 2L
Protopet® White 3C
Protopet® Yellow 1E
Protopet® Yellow 2A
Provol 10
Provol 30
Provol 50
Prox-onic CC-05
Prox-onic CC-09
Prox-onic CC-014
Prox-onic HR-05
Prox-onic HR-016
Prox-onic HR-025
Prox-onic HR-030
Prox-onic HR-036
Prox-onic HR-040
Prox-onic HR-080
Prox-onic HR-0200
Prox-onic HR-0200/50
Prox-onic HRH-05
Prox-onic HRH-016
Prox-onic HRH-025
Prox-onic HRH-0200

Prox-onic HRH-0200/50
Prox-onic ST-05
Prox-onic ST-09
Prox-onic ST-014
Prox-onic ST-023
Pruv™
PVP/Si-10
Radia® 7106
Radia® 7117
Radia® 7178
Radia® 7752
Radiasurf® 7151
Radiasurf® 7152
Radiasurf® 7153
Radiasurf® 7175
Radiasurf® 7196
Radiasurf® 7206
Radiasurf® 7269
Radiasurf® 7402
Radiasurf® 7403
Radiasurf® 7404
Radiasurf® 7411
Radiasurf® 7413
Radiasurf® 7414
Radiasurf® 7417
Radiasurf® 7420
Radiasurf® 7422
Radiasurf® 7423
Radiasurf® 7431
Radiasurf® 7432
Radiasurf® 7443
Radiasurf® 7453
Radiasurf® 7454
Rhodacal® 330
Rhodacal® LA Acid
Rhodafac® RD-510
Rhodafac® RE-870
Rhodasurf® E 400
Rhodasurf® E 600
Rhodasurf® L-4
Rhodasurf® PEG 400
Rhodasurf® PEG 600
Rhodasurf® TD-9
Rita AZ
Rita KA
Ritacetyl®
Ritachol®
Ritaderm®
Ritalan®
Ritalan® C
RITA Lanolin
Ritaloe 1X, 10X, 20X, 40X
Ritaloe 200M
R.I.T.A. d-Panthenol
R.I.T.A. dl-Panthenol
Ritasol
Ritavena™ 5
Ritawax AEO
Ritawax ALA
Robane®
Rudol®
Ryoto Sugar Ester OWA-1570
Ryoto Sugar Ester P-1570
Ryoto Sugar Ester P-1570S
Ryoto Sugar Ester P-1670
Ryoto Sugar Ester S-170
Ryoto Sugar Ester S-270

Ryoto Sugar Ester S-370
Ryoto Sugar Ester S-370F
Ryoto Sugar Ester S-570
Ryoto Sugar Ester S-770
Salcare SC95
Sandoperm FE
Sarkosyl® L
Sarkosyl® LC
Sarkosyl® NL-30
Sarkosyl® O
Schercamox CMA
Schercemol 65
Schercemol 318
Schercemol 1818
Schercemol DEIS
Schercemol DIA
Schercemol DICA
Schercemol DIS
Schercemol DISF
Schercemol DO
Schercemol IDO
Schercemol IPO
Schercemol LL
Schercemol MEM-3
Schercemol MEP-3
Schercemol ML
Schercemol OHS
Schercemol OLO
Schercemol OPG
Schercodine I
Schercomid ID
Schercomid IMI
Schercomid OMI
Schercomid SM
Schercomid SO-A
Schercoquat IALA
Scheroba Oil
Sebase
Selligor DC 100
Sericite 5, 300S
SF96® (350 cst)
SF1080
SF1173
SF1188
SF1202
SF1204
S-Flakes
Shebu® Refined
Shebu® WS
Silwax® C
Silwax® S
Silwax® WD-IS
Silwax® WD-S
Silwax® WS
Silwet® L-7001
Silwet® L-7002
Silwet® L-7500
Silwet® L-7602
Silwet® L-7614
Simchin® Natural
Simchin® Refined
Simchin® WS
Siponic® E-2
Siponic® E-3
Siponic® E-10
Solidester
Solulan® 5
Solulan® 16

Lubricants/Slip Agents/Penetrants... *(cont'd.)*

Solulan® 25	Sulframin 85	Trivent BE-13	Velvet Veil 640
Solulan® 75	Sulframin 90	Trivent DIA	Vigilan
Solulan® 97	Sulframin 1240, 1245	Trivent PE-48	Viscasil®
Solulan® 98	Sulframin 1250, 1260	Trycol® 5878	Viscasil® (10,000 cSt)
Solulan® C-24	Sulframin 1288	Trycol® 5964	Volatile Silicone 7158,
Solulan® L-575	Sulframin 1298	Trylox® 6746	7207, 7349
Solulan® PB-2	Sulframin 1388	Ucon® 50-HB-55	Volpo 3
Solulan® PB-5	Super Corona	Ucon® 50-HB-100	Volpo 5
Solulan® PB-10	Super Hartolan	Ucon® 50-HB-170	Volpo 10
Solulan® PB-20	Super Refined™ Almond	Ucon® 50-HB-260	Volpo 20
Span® 20	Oil NF	Ucon® 75-H-450	Vybar® 103
Span® 40	Super Refined™ Apricot	Ucon® 75-H-1400	Vybar® 260
Span® 60, 60K	Kernel Oil NF	Ucon® 75-H-90000	Vybar® 825
Span® 65	Super Refined™ Olive Oil	Ucon® Fluid AP	Waxenol® 801
Span® 85	Super Refined™ Orange	Ucon® LB-65	Waxenol® 815
Special Oil 619	Roughy Oil	Ucon® LB-135	Waxenol® 816
Special Oil 888	Super-Sat	Ucon® LB-285	Wheat Germ Oil
Spermwax®	Super Sterol Ester	Ucon® LB-385	Wickenol® 101
Spheron L-1500	Surfactol® 13	Ucon® LB-525	Wickenol® 105
Spheron P-1000	Surfonic® L46-7	Ucon® LB-625	Wickenol® 111
Spheron P-1500	Surfonic® N-10	Ucon® LB-3000	Wickenol® 127
Spheron P-1500-030	Surfonic® N-31.5	Ultra Lantrol® HP-2074	Wickenol® 131
Spheron PL-700	Surfonic® N-40	Ultra Sulfate SE-5	Wickenol® 139
Spreading Agent ET0672	Surfonic® N-60	Ultra Sulfate SL-1	Wickenol® 141
Stamere®	Surfonic® N-85	Unamide® LDL	Wickenol® 143
Standamid® ID	Surfonic® N-95	Unimate® DIPS	Wickenol® 535
Standamid® KDS	Surfonic® N-100	Unimate® IPM	Witafrol® 7420
Standamid® KM	Surfonic® N-102	Unimate® IPP	Witcamide® 61
Standamid® LM	Surfonic® N-120	Unimate® IPPM	Witcamide® 70
Standamid® SM	Surfonic® N-130	Unimul-G	Witcamide® 82
Standamox CAW	Surfonic® N-150	Union Carbide® LE-45	Witcamide® 823/10
Standamox O1	Surfonic® N-200	Unithox® 420	Witcamide® 5133
Standamul® CTA	Surfonic® N-300	Unithox® 450	Witcamide® 5195
Standamul® CTV	Surfonic® NB-5	Unithox® 480	Witcamide® 6310
Standamul® G-32/36	SWS-101	Unithox® 520	Witcamide® 6533
Standamul® G-32/36	SWS-03314	Unithox® 550	Witcamide® MAS
Stearate	Syncrowax ERL-C	Unithox® 720	Witcamide® MM
Standamul® GTO-26	Syncrowax HGL-C	Unithox® 750	Witcamide® S771
Sterotex®	Thixcin® R	U Tanol G	Witcamide® S780
Sterotex® C	Tri-Sil HGC 5000	Varonic® LI-42	Witcamide® STD-HP
Sterotex® HM NF	Tri-Sil Wax 105	Velvet Veil 310	Witcamine® 6606
Sterotex® K	Trisolan 1720	Velvet Veil 320	Witcamine® 6622
Sterotex® NF	Trisynlane	Velvet Veil 620	Zinc Stearate USP

Moisture Barriers/Water Repellents

Abil® AV 8853	Belsil DM 35	Cecavon AL 12	Dow Corning® 556 Fluid
Abil®-Wax 2434	Belsil DM 100	Cecavon NA 61	Dow Corning® 593 Fluid
Abil®-Wax 2440	Belsil DM 350	Cecavon ZN 70	Dow Corning® 2501
Abil®-Wax 9809	Belsil DM 100000	Cecavon ZN 71	Cosmetic Wax
Abil®-Wax 9810	Belsil PDM 20	Cecavon ZN 72	Dow Corning® Q2-1403
A-C® 8, 8A	Belsil PDM 200	Cecavon ZN 73	Fluid
A-C® 9, 9A, 9F	Belsil PDM 1000	Cecavon ZN 735	Dow Corning® Q5-0158A
A-C® 16	Be Square® 175	Cera Albalate 101	Wax
A-C® 143	Biosil Basics Fluoro	Cera Albalate 102	Dow Corning® QF1-3593A
A-C® 400	Guerbet 1.0%	Cera Albalate 103	Emalex SWS-9
A-C® 430	Britol®	Cetodan	Emalex SWS-10
A-C® 540, 540A	Britol® 6NF	Coflex	Emalex SWS-12
A-C® 580	Britol® 7NF	Co-Gell® A2/B270	Emphos™ D70-30C
A-C® 617G	Britol® 9NF	Covafluor	Estran™-Lite
A-C® 1702	Britol® 20USP	Covasil	Estran™-Pure
Acetol® 1706	Britol® 35USP	Crodamol CAP	Fancor Lanwax
Actisea™ 100	Britol® 50USP	Crodamol W	Fonoline® White
Acylan	Brookosome® F	Dermacryl™ 79	Fonoline® Yellow
Antaron® WP-660	Brookosome® GSL	Dow Corning® 200 Fluid	Ganex® P-904
Belsil DM 0.65	Cecavon AL 11	Dow Corning® 225	Ganex® V-216

Moisture Barriers/Water Repellents *(cont'd.)*

Ganex® V-220
Ganex® WP-660
Gantrez® ES-225
Gantrez® ES-335
Gantrez® ES-425
Gantrez® ES-435
Gantrez® V-215
Gantrez® V-225
Gantrez® V-425
Glucam® P-20 Distearate
Glucate® SS
Gransil FL-D 55
Hetoxamine C-2
Hetoxamine C-5
Hetoxamine C-15
Hetoxamine O-2
Hetoxamine O-5

Hetoxamine ST-2
Hetoxamine ST-15
Hetoxamine ST-50
Hetoxamine T-2
Hetoxamine T-5
Hetoxamine T-15
Hetoxamine T-20
Hetoxamine T-50-70%
Hydraprotectol-SM
Hydrocoll™ HE-35
Hydrocoll™ LE-35
Hydrocoll™ T-LSN
Koster Keunen Carnauba
   No. 1
Koster Keunen Carnauba
   T-2
Koster Keunen Carnauba

T-3
Masil® 556
Masil® 756
Masil® SF 50
Masil® SF 350
Masil® SF 500
Masil® SF 1000
Masil® SF 12,500
Masil® SF 30,000
Masil® SF 60,000
Masilwax 135
Myvacet® 5-07
Myvacet® 7-07
Natrosol® Plus CS
Pecosil® OS-100B
Pelemol MAR
Perfecta® USP

Polyolprepolymer-2
Protopet® Alba
Protopet® White 1S
Protopet® White 2L
Protopet® White 3C
Protopet® Yellow 1E
Protopet® Yellow 2A
Ritacetyl®
Rudol®
Schercemol 1688
Sericite WL
Skliro Distilled
Super Refined™ Shark
   Liver Oil
SWS-101
Thixcin® R
Vybar® 5013

Neutralizers

Adogen® MA-108 SF
Adogen® MA-112 SF
Adogen® S-18 V
Alatal
Incrodet TD7-C
Lencoll
Lensol
Monteine CA
Monteine KL 150
Neutrol® TE

Octaprotein
Proteolene H
Silkall 100
Triethanolamine Pure C
Varonic® 2271
Varonic® K-202
Varonic® K-202 SF
Varonic® K-205
Varonic® K-205 SF

Varonic® K-210
Varonic® K-210 SF
Varonic® K-215
Varonic® K-215 SF
Varonic® Q-202
Varonic® Q-202 SF
Varonic® Q-205
Varonic® Q-205 SF
Varonic® S-202

Varonic® S-202 SF
Varonic® T-202
Varonic® T-202 SF
Varonic® T-205
Varonic® T-205 SF
Varonic® T-210
Varonic® T-210 SF
Varonic® T-215
Varonic® T-215 SF

Nutritive Additives (Proteins, Vitamins)

Actigen C
Actigen E
Afpro™ WLP
Afpro™ WWP
Alacen
Alpha-Elastin
Amino-Silk SF
Aquapalm No. 63841
Atelo-Collagen
Atelocollagen M
Atelocollagen MS
Atelocollagen SS
Autolyzed Silk
Autolyzed Silk Protein
Biomin® Acquacinque Liq
Biomin® Ca/P/C
Biomin® Cinque
Biomin® Cu/P/C
Biomin® Cu/P/C Liq
Biomin® F/P/C
Biomin® Fe/P/C
Biomin® Ge/P/C
Biomin® K/P/C
Biomin® Mg/P/C
Biomin® Mn/P/C
Biomin® Se/P/C
Biomin® Si/P/C
Biomin® Z/P/C
Biomin® Z/P/C-20 Liq
Biosil Basics HKP-30
Bovinal-20
Bovinol 30
Brookosome® CU
Brookosome® RJ

Byco A
Byco C
Byco O
Chemodyne Tyrosine
Clearcol
CMP-I
Colladerm Procollagene SC
Colla-Gel AC
Collagen
Collagen BIO-5000
Collagen-CCK-Complex
Collagen Hydrolyzate
   Cosmetic 50
Collagen Hydrolyzate
   Cosmetic N-55
Collagen Hydrolyzate
   Cosmetic SD
Collagen P
Collagen S
Collagen S.D
Collagen-Cocoate-Complex
   V 2037
Collagene SPO
Collagene Lyophilized
Collagen Hydrolysate 30%
Collagen Nativ 1%
Collagenol LS/HC-10
Collagenol LS/HC-50
Collagenon
Collagen Powd
Collagen Protein WN
Colla-Moist™ CG
Colla-Moist™ WS
Collapur®

Collapurol® E 1
Collapuron® DAK
Collapuron N
Crolastin C
Cropepsol 35
Cropepsol 50
Cropepsol SD
Cropeptide W
Cropeptone 35
Cropeptone 50
Croquat HH
Croquat L
Croquat M
Croquat S
Croquat WKP
Crosilk 10,000
Crosilk Liq. Complex
Crosilk Powder
Crossential EPO, Super
   Refined
Crotein A
Crotein AD
Crotein AD Anhyd
Crotein ADW
Crotein ADX
Crotein ASC
Crotein HKP/SF
Crotein IPX
Crotein K
Crotein SPA 55
Crystallin Protein
Cutavit Richter
Cytochrome C
Dascare FSP Liq

Dascare SWP
Dehydrated Keratine
   Hydrolysate
Dermacol
Derma-Vitamincomplex, Oil
   soluble
Eastman® Vitamin E 4-50
Eastman® Vitamin E 4-80
Eastman® Vitamin E 5-40
Eastman® Vitamin E 5-67
Eastman® Vitamin E 6-40
Eastman® Vitamin E 6-81
Eastman® Vitamin E 6-100
Eastman® Vitamin E 700
Eastman® Vitamin E
   Succinate
Eastman® Vitamin E TPGS
Edamin S
Elastin
Elastin 5000
Elastin H.P.M
Elastin Hydrolysate COS
Elastin (Partialhydrolisate)
   NOVA
Elastobiol
Elastolan LS HE 20
Elastosol
Elastovit
Eleseryl® SH
Eleseryl® SHT
Emulmetik™ 135
Emulmetik™ 910
Emulmetik™ 930
Emulmetik™ 950

Nutritive Additives (Proteins, Vitamins) *(cont'd.)*

Emulmetik™ 970
EPCH
Etha-Coll 210-20
European Elastin 10
European Elastin 30
European Elastin SD
Exsyproteines 2%, 4%
Fibro-Silk™ Powd
Foam-Coll™ 4C
Foam-Coll™ 4CT
Foam-Coll™ 5
Foam-Keratin LK
Foam-Wheat C
Fractein HWP
Gluadin® AGP
Gluadin® Almond
Gluadin® Wheat
Gluconal® CA A
Gluconal® CA M
Gluconal® CA M B
Gluconal® CO
Gluconal® CU
Gluconal® FE
Gluconal® K
Gluconal® MG
Gluconal® MN
Gluconal® NA
Gluconal® ZN
Gluplex® AC
Gluplex® LES
Gluplex® LS
Gluplex® OS
Glycol 1000 Succinate
Glycoproteins from Milk
Glyprosol™ 20
Glyprosol™ SD
Granamine S3A
Grancol SP-01
Granlastin 10%
Granosol 25
Granosol 100
Granpro-5
Granpro-40, -50, -55, -100
Hidrolisado de Colageno
Hidrolisado de Elastina
Hidrolisado de Placenta
Hidrolisado de Queratina
HPX
Hy Case Amino
Hy Case SF
Hydrane S
Hydrane W
Hydrocell YP-30-P
Hydrocell YP-SD
Hydrocoll AL-50, AL-55, EN-40, EN-55-X, EN-SD-1M, EN-SD-10M
Hydrocoll™ EN-55
Hydrocoll™ EN-SD
Hydrocoll SS-40, SS-55, T-37, T-55, T-LSN, T-LSN-SD, T-P52
Hydrocolloid 219
Hydrolan
Hydrolastan
Hydrolyzed Animal Protein-55
Hydrolyzed Animal Protein

SD
Hydromilk™ EN-20
Hydrosoy 2000/SF
Idrolizzato Della Seta
Keramino™ 20
Keramino™ SD
Kerapro S
Kera-Quat WKP
Kerasol
Kera-Tein 1000 AS
Kera-Tein 1000 RM/50
Kera-Tein 1000 RM SD
Kera-Tein 1000 SD
Kera-Tein AA
Kera-Tein V
Keratin P
Keratin S
Keratine Hydrolysate H.T.K
Keratin Hydrolysate
Lactobiol
Lactolan®
Lactomul 466
Lactomul 468
Lactomul CN-28
LactoPro CLP Code 1580
Lamepon® PA-K/NP
Lamepon® PA-TR/NP
Lamepon® S/NP
Lamepon® ST 40/NP
Lamepon® S-TR/NP
Lamepon® UD/NP
Lamequat® L/NP
Lanagen-50, -55, -SD
Lexate® BPQ
Lexein® A-240
Lexein® CP-125
Lexein® QX-3000
Lexein® X-250
Lexein® X-250HP
Lexein® X-300
Lexein® X-350
Liprot CK
Liprot CT
Liprot CTS
Liprot UK
Liprot UT
Liquid Animal Collagen
Lutavit® Niacin
Maricol CLR
Maypon 4C
Maypon 4CT
May-Tein KK
May-Tein KT
May-Tein KTS
May-Tein R
May-Tein SK
May-Tein SY
Microat™ E
MicroReservoir Nutri-Diffuser
Neobee® 18
Nikkol Aquasome VE
Nikkol DK
Nikkol DP
Nutrilan® Cashmere W
Nutrilan® Elastin E20, P
Nutrilan® I
Nutrilan® I-50

Nutrilan® I-50/NP
Nutrilan® I Powd
Nutrilan® Keratin W
Nutrilan® L
Nutrilan® L/NP
Nutrimarine
Ormagel SH, XPU
Ormagel XPU
Pacific Sea Kelp Glycolic Extract B-1063
Pea Pro-Tein BK
Pepsobiol
Peptein® KC
Peptein® Qs
Peptein® Qw
Peptein® TEAC
PF-6®
Phosal 25 SB
Phosal® 50 SA
Phosal® 53 MCT
Phosal® 75 SA
PhosPho PL-50
Polypeptide 12
Polypeptide 37
Polypeptide LSN Anhydrous
Polypeptide SF
Polypro® 5000
Polypro® 15000
Pran H
Pran H, LIQ
Pran QC
Prochem 12K
Prochem 100-CG Powd
Prochem SPA
Prolagen C
Prolastine
Promois E118D
Promois ECP
Promois ECP-C
Promois ECP-P
Promois ECS
Promois ECT
Promois ECT-C
Promois EFLS
Promois EUP
Promois EUT
Promois Milk
Promois Milk CAQ
Promois Milk LAQ
Promois Milk Q
Promois Milk SAQ
Promois Pearl P
Promois S-CAQ
Promois Silk 700 QSP
Promois Silk 700 SP
Promois Silk-1000
Promois Silk-1000 Q
Promois Silk-1000 QP
Promois Silk A
Promois S-LAQ
Promois S-SAQ
Promois W-32
Promois W-32LS
Promois W-32R
Promois W-42
Promois W-42 CAQ
Promois W-42CP

Promois W-42K
Promois W-42 LAQ
Promois W-42LS
Promois W-42Q
Promois W-42QP
Promois W-42R
Promois W-42 SAQ
Promois W-52
Promois W-52P
Promois W-52Q
Promois W-52QP
Promois WG
Promois WG-Q
Promois WK
Promois WK-H
Promois WK-HQ
Promois WS
Promois WS-Q
Protectein™
Protein SC
Protein TC
Prove HS
Prove HT
Quatex S
Quat-Pro E
Quinta-Pro Conc
Rice Bran Oil
Rice Pro-Tein BK
Rita HA C-1-C
Ritacetin
Ritacollagen BA-1
Ritacollagen S-1
Ritacomplex DF 10
Ritacomplex DF 11
Ritacomplex DF 12, DF 13
Ritacomplex DF 14
Ritacomplex DF 15
Ritacomplex DF 26
Ritalanine
Ritalastin EL-10
Ritalastin EL-30
Ritapan CAP
Ritapan D
Ritapan DL
Ritapan NAP
Ritapan TA
Ritaquat Q
Ritasilk
Ritasilk Powd
Ritatin
Safester A-75
Safester A 75 WS
Seanamin AT
Silkpro AS
Silk Pro-Tein
Solu-Lastin™ 10
Solu-Lastin™ 30
Solu-Mar™ EN-30
Solu-Silk™ Protein
Solu-Silk™ SF
Solu-Tofu EN-10
Soluvit Richter
Soypro 25
Soy-Tein NL
Spirulina Extract COS
Super Refined™ Menhaden Oil
Super Refined™ Wheat

Nutritive Additives (Proteins, Vitamins) *(cont'd.)*

Germ Oil	Tri-Tein 55	BHT	Vitazyme® B3
Supro-Tein R	Tri-Tein Silk AA	Vitamin E Acetate	Vitazyme® B5
Supro-Tein S	Tritisol™	Cosmetic Oil	Vitazyme® C
Tofupro-U	Univit-E Acetate	Vitamin E Acetate USP Oil	Vitazyme® D
Tri-K CMF Complex	Vitamin A Palmitate 1.0	Vitamin E Nicotinate	Vitazyme® E
Tritein-40, -50, -100	BHT in Peanut Oil	Vitamin E USP Tocopherol	Wheat-Quat C
Tri-Tein 40N	Vitamin A Palmitate 1.7	Vitazyme® A-Plus	Wheat-Tein NL

Opacifiers/Pearlants

Ablucols EDP	Cecavon ZN 735	Emalex EG-di-MPS	Flonac MS 33 C
Ablumide SME	Cerasynt® D	Emalex EG-di-S	Flonac MS 40 C
Ablunol DEGMS	Cerasynt® IP	Emalex EG-di-SE	Flonac MS 60 C
Ablunol EGDS	Cerasynt® LP	Emalex EGS-A	Flonac MS 70 C
Ablunol EGMS	Cerasynt® M	Emalex EGS-B	Flonac MX 10 C
Adol® 61	Cerasynt® MN	Emalex PC-6	Genapol® PGC
Adol® 62 NF	Cerasynt® PA	Emalex PC-7	Genapol® PGM Conc
Adol® 63	Cerasynt® SD	Emalex TEG-di-AS	Genapol® PGM Liq
Adol® 64	Chemsperse EGDS	Emalex TEG-di-S	Genapol® PMS
Adol® 520 NF	Chemsperse EGMS	Emerest® 2350	Genapol® TS Powd
Adol® 620 NF	Chemsperse GMS	Emerest® 2355	Genapol® TSM
Adol® 630	Chemsperse GMS-SE	Emerest® 2380	Hest MS
Akyposal 2010 S	Chroma-Lite®	Emerest® 2381	Hetamide MM
Akyposal 2010 SD	Cithrol GMS A/S ES 0743	Emerest® 2400	Hetamide MS
Alkamide® CME	Colorona®	Emerest® 2401	Hetester MS
Alkamide® CMO	Comperlan® KM	Emerest® 2410	Hodag DGS
Alkamuls® 200-DS	Covamat	Emerest® 2712	Hodag DGS-C
Alkamuls® 400-DS	CPH-37-NA	Emersol® 110	Hodag DGS-N
Alkamuls® 600-DS	CPH-380-N	Emersol® 120	Hodag EGMS
Alkamuls® EGDS	Crodacol C-70	Emersol® 132 NF Lily®	Hodag GML
Alkamuls® EGMS/C	Crodacol C-NF	Emersol® 143	Hodag GMO
Alkamuls® SEG	Crodacol S-70	Empicol® 0384	Hodag GMO-D
Amerlate® P	Crodacol S-USP	Empicol® 0627	Hodag GMR
Ami-Pearl Conc	Crodamol BE	Empicol® 9060X	Hodag GMR-D
Ami-Pearl TS	Crodapearl Liq	Empicol® XC35	Hodag GMS
AMS-33	Crodapearl NI Liquid	Empicol® XPA	Hodag GTO
Arlacel® 165	Cromul 0685	Empilan® EGMS	Hydrine
Avicel RC-591	Crosterene	Estol EGMS 3749	Incromate SDL
Bee's Milk	Cutina® AGS	Ethylene Glycol Distearate	Incromide BED
Bicrona®	Cutina® EGMS	VA	Incromide CM
Biju® BNT	Cutina® TS	Ethylene Glycol	Incromide SM
Biju® BTD, BXD	Cyclochem® GMO	Monostearate VA	Karapeg DEG-MS
Biju® BWD, BWS	Dichrona®	Euperlan® K 771	Kemester® 3681
Biju® BWP	Dragil 2/027011	Euperlan® MPK 850	Kemester® 5220
Biju® Ultra UNT	Drewmulse® 200K	Euperlan® PK 771	Kemester® 5654
Biju® Ultra UTD, UXD	Drewmulse® DGMS	Euperlan® PK 771 BENZ	Kemester® EGDS
Biju® Ultra UWD, UWS	Drewmulse® EGDS	Euperlan® PK 776	Kemester® EGMS
Biju® Ultra UWP	Drewmulse® EGMS	Euperlan® PK 789	Kemester® MM
Bi-Lite®	Drewmulse® GMRO	Euperlan® PK 810	Kessco® EGAS
Biron®	Drewmulse® GMS	Euperlan® PK 810 AM	Kessco EGMS
Biron® B-5	Drewmulse® PGMS	Euperlan® PK 900	Kessco® Ethylene Glycol
Biron® B-50	Drewmulse® TP	Euperlan® PK 900 BENZ	Distearate
Biron® Fines	Drewmulse® V	Euperlan® PK 3000 AM	Kessco® Ethylene Glycol
Biron® HB	Drewmulse® V-SE	Euperlan® PK 3000 OK	Monostearate
Biron® NLD-SP	Drewpol® 10-4-O	Euperlan® PL 1000	Kessco® GDS 386F
Bismica 46	Elfacos® EGMS	Fancol CA	Kessco® Glycerol
Bismica 55	Elfan® L 310	Fancol SA	Monostearate Pure
Bismica 596	Emalex 400A	Fancor IPL	Kessco® PEG 200 DL
Bital®	Emalex 400B	Flonac ME 10 C	Kessco® PEG 200 DO
Brillante	Emalex 805	Flonac MG 30 C	Kessco® PEG 200 DS
Caprol® 2G4S	Emalex 810	Flonac MI 10 C	Kessco® PEG 200 ML
Cecavon NA 61	Emalex 820	Flonac ML 10 C	Kessco® PEG 200 MO
Cecavon ZN 70	Emalex 830	Flonac MS 5 C	Kessco® PEG 200 MS
Cecavon ZN 71	Emalex 840	Flonac MS 10 C	Kessco® PEG 300 DL
Cecavon ZN 72	Emalex DEG-di-S	Flonac MS 20 C	Kessco® PEG 300 DO
Cecavon ZN 73	Emalex DEG-m-S	Flonac MS 30 C	Kessco® PEG 300 DS

Opacifiers/Pearlants *(cont'd.)*

Kessco® PEG 300 ML
Kessco® PEG 300 MO
Kessco® PEG 300 MS
Kessco® PEG 400 DL
Kessco® PEG 400 DO
Kessco® PEG 400 DS
Kessco® PEG 400 ML
Kessco® PEG 400 MO
Kessco® PEG 400 MS
Kessco® PEG 600 DL
Kessco® PEG 600 DO
Kessco® PEG 600 DS
Kessco® PEG 600 MO
Kessco® PEG 600 MS
Kessco® PEG 1000 DL
Kessco® PEG 1000 DO
Kessco® PEG 1000 DS
Kessco® PEG 1000 ML
Kessco® PEG 1000 MO
Kessco® PEG 1000 MS
Kessco® PEG 1540 DL
Kessco® PEG 1540 DO
Kessco® PEG 1540 DS
Kessco® PEG 1540 ML
Kessco® PEG 1540 MO
Kessco® PEG 1540 MS
Kessco® PEG 4000 DL
Kessco® PEG 4000 DO
Kessco® PEG 4000 DS
Kessco® PEG 4000 ML
Kessco® PEG 4000 MO
Kessco® PEG 4000 MS
Kessco® PEG 6000 DL
Kessco® PEG 6000 DO
Kessco® PEG 6000 ML
Kessco® PEG 6000 MO
Kessco® PEG 6000 MS
Kessco® Propylene Glycol
   Monostearate Pure
Kester Wax® K 48
Koster Keunen Beeswax
Koster Keunen Fatty
   Alcohol 1618
Lamesoft® 156/NP
Lankropearl™ T
Lasemul 62 E
Lauramide EG
Lexemul® 55G
Lexemul® 503
Lexemul® 515
Lexemul® AR
Lexemul® AS
Lexemul® EGDS
Lexemul® EGMS
Lexemul® T
Lexol® SS
Lipal EGDS
Lipal EGMS
Lipal MMDG
Lipamide S
Lipo DGLS
Lipo DGS-SE
Lipo EGDS
Lipo EGMS
Lipo GMS 450
Lipo GMS 470
Lipocol B
Lipomulse 165

Lipovol GTB
Lonza Insta-Pearl®
Lonzest® EGMS
Lowenol C-279
Lustra-Pearl®
Lytron 153
Lytron 284
Lytron 288
Lytron 295
Lytron 300
Lytron 305
Lytron 308
Lytron 614 Latex
Lytron 621
Mackester™ EGDS
Mackester™ EGMS
Mackester™ IDO
Mackester™ IP
Mackester™ SP
Mackester™ TD-88
Mackpearl LV
Manro PSC
Manro PSC 40
Mapeg® 400 DS
Mapeg® 400 MS
Mapeg® EGDS
Mapeg® EGMS
Marlamid® KL
Marlamid® KLA
Marlamid® KLP
Marlamid® PG 20
Mattina®
Mazamide® SMEA
Mazol® 165C
Mazol® GMSDK
Mazol® GMS-K
Mazol® PGMSK
Mearlite® GBU
Mearlite® GEH
Mearlite® GEJ
Mearlite® GGH
Mearlite® LBU
Mearlite® LEM
Mearlmaid® AA
Mearlmaid® CP
Mearlmaid® OL
Mearlmaid® PLN
Mearlmaid® TR
Mibiron® N-50
Micropoly 520
Micropoly 524
Micropoly 524-XF
Micropoly 2001
Miracare® M1
Mirasheen® 202
Monamid® 718
Monamid® S
Monamid® S/M
Monomuls® 60-10
Monomuls® 60-15
Monomuls® 60-20
Monomuls® 60-25
Monomuls® 60-25/2
Monomuls® 60-30
Monomuls® 60-35
Monomuls® 60-40
Monomuls® 60-45
Monomuls® 90-10

Monomuls® 90-15
Monomuls® 90-20
Monomuls® 90-25/2, 90-
   25/5
Monomuls® 90-30
Monomuls® 90-35
Monomuls® 90-40
Monomuls® 90-45
Nailsyn®
Naturechem® EGHS
Naturechem® GMHS
Naturechem® MHS
Naturechem® PGHS
Naturon CSN-11
Naturon CSN-22
Naturon® 2X AQ
Naturon® 2X IPA
Nikkol EGDS
Nikkol EGMS-70
Nikkol Estepearl 10, 15
Nikkol Estepearl 30
Nikkol MYS-1EX
Nikkol Pearl 1218
Nikkol Pearl 1222
Nikkol PMEA
Norfox® EGMS
Norfox® GMS
Norfox® GMS-FG
Nutrapon B 1365
Nutrapon TK 3603
Onyxol® 42
Paramul® SAS
Pearl I
Pearl II
Pearl III
Pearlex GC 0311
Pearl-Glo®
Pearl Super Supreme
Pearl Supreme
Pearl Supreme UVS
Pegosperse® 50 DS
Pegosperse® 50 MS
Pegosperse® 400 DOT
Pegosperse® 600 DOT
Pegosperse® 6000 DS
Pegosperse® EGMS-70
Perglanzmittel GM 4006
Perlex B.67, B.70
Perlex B.67M
Perlex BU
Perlex BUA.35
Perlextra B.70
Perlextra BU
Perlextra BUA.70
Perlglanz-Konzentrat B-30
Perlglanz-Konzentrat B-48
Perlglanzmittel GM 4006
Perlglanzmittel GM 4055
Perlglanzmittel GM 4175
Phoenamid SM
Phoenate 3 DSA
Polawax®
Polectron® 430
Polytex 10M
Produkt GM 4055
Protachem EGMS
Radiastar® 1060
Radiastar® 1100

Radiastar® 1170
Radiastar® 1200
Radiastar® 1208
Radiasurf® 7196
Radiasurf® 7206
Radiasurf® 7269
Radiasurf® 7270
Radiasurf® 7402
Radiasurf® 7403
Radiasurf® 7404
Radiasurf® 7410
Radiasurf® 7411
Radiasurf® 7413
Radiasurf® 7414
Radiasurf® 7417
Radiasurf® 7420
Radiasurf® 7422
Radiasurf® 7423
Radiasurf® 7431
Radiasurf® 7432
Radiasurf® 7443
Radiasurf® 7453
Radiasurf® 7454
Radiasurf® 7600
Rewopal® PG 280
Rewopal® PG 340
Rewopal® PGK 2000
Rita CA
Rita EDGS
Rita EGMS
Rita GMS
Rita SA
Ritasynt IP
Salcare SC92
Salcare SC95
Schercemol CP
Schercemol CS
Schercemol EGMS
Schercemol GMS
Schercomid MME
Schercomid SD-DS
Schercomid SME
Schercomid SME-A
Schercomid SME-M
Schercomid SME-S
Schercopearl EA-100
Secoster® DMS
Secoster® EMS
Shinju® White 100T
Soapearl®
Soloron-R-Gold
Soloron Silver
Soloron Silver CO
Soloron Silver Fine
Soloron Silver Fine CO
Soloron Silver Sparkle
Soloron Silver Sparkle CO
Solulan® 98
Spectra-Pearl®
Standamul® G-32/36
Standamul® G-32/36
   Stearate
Standapol® 7092
Standapol® CAT
Standapol® Pearl Conc.
   7130
Standapol® S
Starfol® CP

Opacifiers/Pearlants *(cont'd.)*

Starfol® Wax CG
Stepan Pearl Series
Stepan TAB®-2
Sterol ST 1
Sterol ST 2
Syncrowax AW1-C
Syncrowax BB-4
Syncrowax ERL-C
Syncrowax HGL-C

Syncrowax HR-C
Syncrowax HRS-C
Tegin® 515 VA
Tegin® D 1102
Tegin® G
Tegin® G 1100
Tegin® VA
Tego®-Pearl B-48
Tego®-Pearl S-33

Tensiorex BND57
Texapon® CS Paste
Timiron®
Ufablend MPL
Ultra®
Unamide® S
Unipol 7092
Upamide SME-M
Witcamide® 70

Witcamide® MAS
Witcamide® MM
Witcopearl 15
Zohar EGDS
Zohar EGMS
Zohar GLST SE
Zoharpon EGDS-771

Plasticizers

Acetulan®
Adogen® S-18 V
Adol® 52 NF
Adol® 60
Adol® 80
Adol® 85
Adol® 90 NF
Adol® 640
Aldo® PMS
Alfol® 610
Alfol® 610 ADE
Alfol® 610 AFC
Alfol® 810
Amerchol® CAB
Amerchol® H-9
Amerchol L-101®
Amerlate® LFA
Amerlate® P
Anhydrous Lanolin USP
    Cosmetic
Anhydrous Lanolin USP
    Pharmaceutical
Anhydrous Lanolin USP
    Superfine
Anhydrous Lanolin USP
    Ultrafine
Aqualose L30
Aqualose L75
Aqualose LL100
Aqualose W20
Argonol 1SO
Argonol ACE 6
Argowax Cosmetic Super
Argowax Dist
Argowax Standard
Arosurf® 66-E2
Arosurf® 66-E20
Axol® E 61
Axol® E 66
Belsil DMC 6031
Belsil DMC 6032
Belsil DMC 6033
Belsil DMC 6035
Be Square® 175
Britol® 6NF
Britol® 7NF
Britol® 9NF
Britol® 20USP
Britol® 35USP
Britol® 50USP
Captex® 300
Carbopol® 1706
Carbopol® 1720
Carbowax® PEG 400
Carbowax® PEG 600

Carbowax® PEG 900
Carbowax® PEG 1000
Carbowax® Sentry® PEG
    300
Carbowax® Sentry® PEG
    400
Carbowax® Sentry® PEG
    540 Blend
Carbowax® Sentry® PEG
    600
Carbowax® Sentry® PEG
    900
Carbowax® Sentry® PEG
    1000
Carbowax® Sentry® PEG
    1450
Carbowax® Sentry® PEG
    3350
Carbowax® Sentry® PEG
    4600
Carbowax® Sentry® PEG
    8000
Ceraphyl® 41
Ceraphyl® 230
Cetiol® B
Citroflex A-4
Citroflex A-6
Citroflex B-6
Coflex
Corona Lanolin
Coronet Lanolin
Cralane KR-13, -14
Cralane LR-10
Cralane LR-11
Crestalans
Crodalan AWS
Crodalan LA
Crodamol BS
Crodamol DA
Crodamol IPL
Croderol G7000
Crodet L4
Crodet L8
Crodet L12
Crodet L24
Crodet L40
Crodet L100
Crotein ADW
Crovol A40
Crovol M40
Crovol PK40
Crovol PK70
Dermol 89
Dermol EB
Dow Corning® 190

    Surfactant
Dow Corning® 193
    Surfactant
Dow Corning® 1315
    Surfactant
Dow Corning® 5103
    Surfactant
Dow Corning® Q2-5220
    Resin Modifier
Dow Corning® Q2-5324
    Surfactant
Drakeol 32
Emcol® CC-36
Estalan 635
Ethoxylan® 1685
Ethoxylan® 1686
Fancol ALA
Fancol HL
Fancol LA
Fancol LAO
Fancol OA-95
Fancor IPL
Fancor Lanwax
Finsolv® SB
Flexricin® 9
Flexricin® 13
Flexricin® 15
Fluilan
Fluilan AWS
Fonoline® White
Fonoline® Yellow
Forlan C-24
Ftalato 2/46
Glucam® E-10
Glucam® P-20 Distearate
Glucate® DO
Hartolan
Hetester PMA
Hodag 20-L
Hodag 22-L
Hodag 40-L
Hodag 40-O
Hodag 40-R
Hodag 40-S
Hodag 42-L
Hodag 42-O
Hodag 42-S
Hodag 60-L
Hodag 60-S
Hodag 62-O
Hodag 100-S
Hodag 150-S
Hystar® 7000
Hystrene® 4516
Hystrene® 5016 NF

Hystrene® 7022
Hystrene® 9016
Hystrene® 9022
Hystrene® 9512
Hystrene® 9718 NF
Igepal® CO-430
Imwitor® 742
Imwitor® 928
Imwitor® 988
Incromectant AQ
Incromectant LQ
Isopropylan® 33
Ivarbase™ 98
Ivarbase™ 3210
Kemester® 4000
Kemester® 5221SE
Kemester® 5500
Kemester® 5510
Kemester® 5822
Kemester® 6000
Kemester® 6000SE
Kera-Tein 1000 AS
Ketjenflex® 8
Kodaflex® DBP
Kodaflex® DEP
Kodaflex® DMP
Kodaflex® DOA
Kodaflex® DOTP
Kodaflex® TOTM
Kodaflex® TXIB
Koster Keunen Beeswax
    AO2535
Koster Keunen Hydroxy-
    Polyester
Lamegin® EE
Lamegin® GLP 10, 20
Lanethyl
Laneto 40
Laneto 50
Laneto 60
Laneto 100-Flaked
Laneto AWS
Lanex
Lanexol
Lanexol AWS
Lantrol® AWS 1692
Lantrol® PLN
Lantrol® PLN/50
Lexein® A-200
Lexein® A-210
Lipolan R
Liponic 70-NC
Liponic 76-NC
Liponic 83-NC
Liponic EG-1

Plasticizers *(cont'd.)*

Liponic SO-20	Radia® 7355	Solan	Uniflex DEP
Lustrabrite® S	Radia® 7371	Solan 50	Uniplex 84
Mapeg® 400 DO	Radia® 7505	Solulan® 5	Uniplex 110
Masil® 1066C	Radia® 7506	Solulan® 16	Uniplex 150
Masil® 1066D	Radianol® 7106	Solulan® 75	Uniplex 260
Mazol® GMR	Radiasurf® 7196	Solulan® C-24	Varonic® 2271
Mazol® GMS	Radiasurf® 7206	Solulan® L-575	Varonic® K-202
Monolan® PPG440,	Radiasurf® 7269	Solulan® PB-2	Varonic® K-202 SF
PPG1100, PPG2200	Radiasurf® 7270	Solulan® PB-5	Varonic® K-205
Nagellite® 3050	Radiasurf® 7402	Solulan® PB-10	Varonic® K-205 SF
Naturechem® PGR	Radiasurf® 7403	Solulan® PB-20	Varonic® K-210
Nopalcol Series	Radiasurf® 7404	Super Corona	Varonic® K-210 SF
Nopalcol 1-S	Radiasurf® 7411	Super Hartolan	Varonic® K-215
Nopalcol 1-TW	Radiasurf® 7413	Super-Sat	Varonic® K-215 SF
Palatinol® A	Radiasurf® 7414	Super-Sat AWS-4	Varonic® Q-202
Palatinol® M	Radiasurf® 7417	Super-Sat AWS-24	Varonic® Q-202 SF
Pegosperse® 50 DS	Radiasurf® 7420	Super Solan Flaked	Varonic® Q-205
Pegosperse® 6000 DS	Radiasurf® 7422	Surfactol® 13	Varonic® Q-205 SF
Pegosperse® EGMS-70	Radiasurf® 7423	Surfactol® 340	Varonic® S-202
Permethyl® 102A	Radiasurf® 7431	Surfactol® 380	Varonic® S-202 SF
Pogol 200	Radiasurf® 7432	SWS-03314	Varonic® T-202
Procetyl 10	Radiasurf® 7443	Tegin® E-41	Varonic® T-202 SF
Procetyl 30	Radiasurf® 7453	Tegin® E-41 NSE	Varonic® T-205
Procetyl 50	Radiasurf® 7454	Tegin® E-61	Varonic® T-205 SF
Procetyl AWS	Rhodasurf® PEG 400	Tegin® E-61 NSE	Varonic® T-210
Pro-Tein ES-20	Rhodasurf® PEG 600	Tegin® E-66	Varonic® T-210 SF
Pro-Tein SA-20	Ritachol®	Tegin® E-66 NSE	Varonic® T-215
Radia® 7108	Ritalan®	Tegin® L 61, L 62	Varonic® T-215 SF
Radia® 7117	Ritalan® AWS	Tegin® RZ	Victory®
Radia® 7185	Ritawax AEO	Tegin® RZ NSE	Vigilan
Radia® 7187	Ritawax ALA	Trivent NP-13	Vigilan AWS
Radia® 7190	Rudol®	Trylox® 6746	Wickenol® 139
Radia® 7200	Schercemol DICA	Tylose® H Series	Wickenol® 141
Radia® 7204	Schercemol ML	Ultraflex®	Wickenol® 142
Radia® 7266	Simchin® WS	Uniflex DBP	Witafrol® 7420
Radia® 7345			

Preservatives

Abiol	CoSept BNP	Germall® II	LiquaPar® Oil
Aethyl-Steriline	CoSept E	Glycacil L, S	Mackstat® DM
Amical® Flowable	CoSept M	Glydant®	Mackstat® DM-PG
Ampholak MDX-1	CoSept P	Glydant® Plus	Merguard 1190
Ampholak MSX-1	Cosmocil CQ	Glydant® XL-1000	Merguard 1200
Anti-MB	CPC	Hampene® CaNa$_2$ Pure	Methyl-Steriline
Aseptoform	CPC Sumquat 6060	Crystals	Midcol ACS
Atomergic Imidazolidinyl	Dantoin® MDMH	Hampene® Na$_2$ Pure	Midcol CF
Urea	Dekaben	Crystals	Midpol 97
Bentex E	Dekacymen	Hyamine® 1622 Crystals	Midpol 100
Bentex M	Dekafald	Hyamine® 2389	Midpol 2000
Bentex P	Dowicide 1	Hyamine® 3500 50%	Midpol PHN
Benzoic Acid Powd. No.	Dowicide A	Hyamine® 3500-NF	Midtect TF-60
130	Dowicil® 200	Ionpure Type A	Midtect TFP
Biopure 100	Elestab CPN	Ionpure Type B	Mikrokill 2
Bronidox® L	Elestab HP 100	Kathon® CG	Mikrokill 20
Bronidox® L 5	Emercide® 1199	Kelate CDS	Mikrokill 300
Bronopol	Emeressence® 1160 Rose	Killitol	Myacide® BT
Busan® 1500	Ether	K-Preserve Liq	Myacide® SP
Busan® 1504	Emthox® 6705	Laurene	Myavert C
Busan® 1506	Euxyl K 100	Lauricidin 802, 812, 1012,	Nipabenzyl
Busan® 1507	Euxyl K 400	E	Nipabutyl
Butylparaben NF	FMB 500-15 Quat U.S.P	Lexgard B	Nipabutyl Potassium
Butyl Parasept	Fondix G Bis	Lexgard E	Nipabutyl Sodium
CAE	Fongasel	Lexgard M	Nipacide® MX
Combi-Steriline MP	Germaben® II	Lexgard P	Nipacide® Potassium
CoSept 200	Germaben® II-E	Lexgard® Bronopol	Nipacide® PX-R
CoSept B	Germall® 115	Lexgard® Myacide SP	Nipacide® Sodium

Preservatives *(cont'd.)*

Nipacombin PK	Nuosept C	Sepicide LD	Uantox SEBATE
Nipacombin SK	Oxaban®-A	Sepicide MB	Uantox SMBS
Nipagin A	Paragon™	Sodium Omadine®, 40%	Ucarcide® 225
Nipagin A Potassium	Paragon™ II	Aq. Sol'n	Ucarcide® 250
Nipagin A Sodium	Paridol B	Sustane® 1-F	Undebenzofene C
Nipagin M	Paridol E	Sustane® 3	Undenat
Nipagin M Potassium	Paridol M	Sustane® BHT	Unichem SALAC
Nipagin M Sodium	Paridol P	Suttocide® A	Unichem THYMOL
Nipaguard BPA	Phenonip	Tektamer® 38	Unicide U-13
Nipaguard® BPX	Phenoxen	Trisept B	Unisept BZA
Nipaguard® MPA	Phenoxetol	Trisept E	Unistat
Nipaguard® MPS	Preserval B	Trisept M	Unistat CALBAN
Nipaheptyl	Preserval Butylique	Trisept P	Unistat K
Nipasept Potassium	Preserval E	Trisept SDHA	Unistat SOBAN
Nipasept Sodium	Preserval M	Tris Nitro®	Universene CaNa2
Nipasol M	Preserval P	Tristat	Vancide® 89 RE
Nipasol M Potassium	Propyl-Steriline	Tristat BNP	Zinc Omadine® 48% Disp
Nipasol M Sodium	Rewopal® MPG 10	Tristat IU	Zinc Omadine® Powd
Nipastat	Sepicide CI	Tristat K	Zink Pyrion
Nuosept 101 CG	Sepicide HB	Uantox 3	

Skin Care Additives
(Rejuvinators, Stimulants, Astringents, Tonics)

Actiglow™	Biosil Basics Fluoro	Chemie Linz Allantoin	Dow Corning® Q5-6038
Actimoist™ Bio-2	Guerbet 1.0%	Chromoprotulines	Polymer Beads
Actimulse 250	Biosil Basics Fluoro	Circulatory Blend HS 318	D.S.H. C
Actiplex™ 745	Guerbet 3.5%	Cithrol 6DS	EFA-Liq
A.F.R	Biosil Basics Jasmine	Cithrol 10DS	Eijitsu Extract BG
Alfonic® 1012-2.5	Wax S	Cithrol DGMS N/E	Elacid CLR
Algisium-C	Biosil Basics L-30	Cithrol DGMS S/E	Elastein® 5000
Allantoin	Biosulphur Fluid	CoAxel	Elastin CLR
Allantoin Powd. No. 1015	Biosulphur Powder	Collagen CLR	Elastobiol
Almond Oil	α-Bisabolol	Collapur®	Elastosol
Aloxicoll® L	Blend For Delicate Skins	Collapuron® DAK	Eldew CL-301
Aloxicoll® PC	HS 215	Copherol® 950LC	Eleseryl® SH
Aloxicoll® PF	Brookosome® A	Cosiderm Masks	Eleseryl® SHT
Aloxicoll® PSF	Brookosome® ANE	Cryolidone®	Elfan® NS 423 SH
Alpinamed Balm	Brookosome® Biophos	Cuivridone®	Emulmetik™ 100
Alpinamed Ivy	Brookosome® CU	Cytochrome C	Emulmetik™ 135
Alpinamed Sage	Brookosome® FIH	Cytochrome Marine	Emulmetik™ 300
Alpinamed Witch Hazel	Brookosome® GSL	Dermasome® A	Emulmetik™ 320
Aludone®	Brookosome® Herbal	Dermasome® E	Emulmetik™ 900
Amisoft CA	Brookosome® MPS	Dermasome® EPO	Emulmetik™ 910
Amisoft HA	Brookosome® MSF	Dermasome® H	Emulmetik™ 930
Antiraghades HS 361, LS	Brookosome® P	Dermasome® MPS	Emulmetik™ 950
661	Brookosome® RP	Dermasome® MT	Emulmetik™ 970
Antistretchmarks HS 338	Brookosome® SE	Dermasome® P	Endonucleine®
Aquagel	Brookosome® SOD	Dermasome® RJ	Energisome
Argidone®	Brookosome® TRF	Dermasome® RP	Enzyami No. 1
Ascorbosilane C	Brookosome® TYE	Dermasome® S	Enzyami No. 1A
Asebiol®	D-Calcium Pantothenate	Dermasome® SC	Enzyami No. 5
Ateloglycane	USP, FCC Type SD	Dermasome® SE	Enzyami No. 5A
Atomergic Allantoin	No. 63924	Dermasome® SOD	Enzyami No. 6
Babyderme LS 642	Camellia Oil	Dermasome® TE	Epidermin in Oil
Babyderme LS 665	Carbowax® PEG 400	Dermasome® TRF	Epidermin Water-Soluble
BioCare® SA	Carbowax® PEG 600	Dermasome® U	Escin/β-Sitosterol
Biodermine	Carbowax® PEG 900	Dermasome® V	Phytosome®
Biodynes® TRF	Carbowax® PEG 1000	Dermosaccharides® GY	Estran™-Lite
Biodynes® TRF 5% Sol'n	Carbowax® PEG 1450	Dermosaccharides® HC	Estran™-Pure
BioLac™	Carbowax® PEG 3350	Dermosaccharides® SEA	Estran™-Xtra
Biopeptide CL	Carbowax® PEG 4600	Destressine 2000	Ethyl Panthenol No. 26100
Biopeptide FN	Carbowax® PEG 8000	Dexpanthenol USP, FCC	Exsycobalt
Biophytex®	Cegesoft® C 24	No. 63909	Exsycuivre
Bio-Pol® NCHAP	Centella Phytosome®	Dow Corning® 225	Exsyfibroblastes
Biosil Basics A-30	Ceramide HO3	Dow Corning® Q5-0158A	Exsymol Chromoprotuline
Biosil Basics DL-30	Ceramides	Wax	Exsymol Cobalt

Skin Care Additives *(cont'd.)*

Acetylmethionate
Exsymol Cupric
   Acetylmethionate
Exsymol Gold
   Acetylmethionate
Exsymol Magnesium
   Acetylmethionate
Exsymol Manganese
   Acetylmethionate
Exsymol Nickel
   Acetylmethionate
Exsymol Oleosterines
Exsymol Protuline
Exsymol Silver
   Acetylmethionate
Exsymol Zinc
   Acetylmethionate
Exsyor
Fancol CH
Filagrinol®
Firmogen®
Foamquat 2IAE
Foamquat COAS
Foamquat SOAS
Frigydil
Gamma Oryzanol
Gatuline® A
Gatuline® R
Genagen CA-050
Gilugel EUG
Ginkgo Biloba Dimeric
   Flavonoids
   Phytosome®
Ginkgo Biloba Phytosome®
Ginseng Phytosome®
Gluadin® AGP
GlycoCer
GlycoCer HA
Glyco/Cer HALA
Glycoderm
Glycyrrhetinic Acid
   Phytosome®
Granamine S3A
Grancol SP-01
Granlastin 10%
Gransurf 71
Gransurf 72
Gransurf 73
Gransurf 75
Gransurf 76
Gransurf 77
Hawthorn Extract Code
   9033
Herbasol Complex A
Herbasol Complex B
Herbasol Complex C
Herbasol Complex D
Herbasol Complex GU-61
Herbasol Herbes de
   Provence Complex
Hetol CA
Hetoxamate 100S
Hetoxamate SA-100
Hispagel® 100
Hispagel® 200
Hydagen® BP1
Hydracol®
Hydraprotectol-SM

Hydrocoll™ AC-30
Hydrocoll™ HE-35
Hydrocoll™ LE-35
Hydrolyzed Elastin RE-10
   No. 26202
Hydrolyzed Elastin RE-30
   No. 26203
Hydromarine
Hydroxyprolisilane C
Hydrumine Calendula
Hydrumine Witchazel
Hylucare™
Ichtyocollagene
Ichtyoelastin
Infrasome
Isopropylmyristat
Japan Wax NJ-9002
Jordapon® CI 75
Karite Nonsaponifiable
Kelisema Natural Pure
   Shea Butter
Kojic Acid
Lactolan®
LactoPro CLP Code 1580
Lamecreme® DGE-18
Lanoquat® 1751A
Lasilium C
Leucocyanidins
   Phytosome®
Lipodermol®
Lipofacteur Vitentiel
Lipomicron N.S.L.E
Lipomicron Vitamin A
   Palmitate
Liposiliol C
Liposome Centella
Liposome Unsapo KM
Liposomes Anti-Age
Liposomes Slimmigen®
Lipostim
Lysidone®
N,L-Malyl-L-Tyrosine
Marine Dew
MFA™ Complex
MicroReservoir FRS-
   Diffuser
MicroReservoir Hydro-
   Diffuser
MicroReservoir Nutri-
   Diffuser
Microsponge® 5647
Milkpro-Q
Mimosoie®
Moisturizing Factor L
Monosiliol C
MPG Granular Beads
Multifruit BSC
Multifruit BSCY
Myritol® 312
Natipide® II
Natipide® II PG
Neptuline® C
Nikkol Aquasome AE
Nikkol Aquasome EC-30
Nikkol Aquasome VA
Nikkol Aquasome VE
Nikkol Pulvsome VE
Nikkol Selachyl Alcohol

Nutrilan® Elastin E20
Nutrilan® I-50/NP
Nutrilan® I-Powd./NP
Nutrilan® L/NP
Nutrimarine
Oleo-A.F.R
Oligoceane
Omega-CH Activator
Oxylastil
DL-Panthenol Cosmetic
   Grade No. 63920
DL-Panthenol USP, FCC
   No. 63915
Pecosil® OS-100B
Pelemol 88
Pelemol BIS
Pelemol CA
Pelemol EE
Pelemol ICS
Pelemol OPG
Pelemol TDE
Pelemol TGC
Pentacare-HP
Pepsobiol
Phytantriol No. 63926
Pidolidone®
Placentaliquid Oil-Soluble
Placentaliquid Water-
   Soluble
Planell™ Oil
Plant Ceramides
Plant Exsyliposomes
Plantsol
Polyglucadyne™
Polymin® FG SG
Polymin® G-35 SG
Polymin® P SG
Polymin® PS SG
Polymin® Waterfree SG
Polytrap® Q5-6035
Presome Type I
Proceramide L
Promarine
Proteodermin
Proteosilane C
Protulines
Pyridoxine Hydrochloride
   USP
Queen of the Prairie Extract
   Code 9031
Regederme HS 236,
   LS 636
Regederme HS 330,
   LS 630
Rewoteric® QAM 50
Rice Bran Oil
R.I.T.A. d-Panthenol
R.I.T.A. dl-Panthenol
Ruscogenins Phytosome®
Salcare SC95
Seanami MY
Seanamin AT
Seanamin BD
Seanamin TH
Sebomine SB12
Seboregular HS 312
Sebum Control COS-218/2-
   A

Sedermasome
Sericite WL
Sericoside Phytosome®
Seromarine
Shea Butter
Shea Unsaponifiable Conc
Silanol Exsyliposomes
Silhydrate C
Silkall 100
Silkpro
Silkpro CM-1000
Silkpro CM-2000
Silymarin Phytosome®
Sodium Hyaluronate RCC-
   1 No. 26228
Sohakuhi Extract BG-100
Sohakuhi Extract Ethanol
Soluble Native Collagen
   RA-1 No. 26206
Soluble Native Collagen
   RS-1 No. 26205
Solu-Lastin™ 10
Solu-Lastin™ 30
Sol-U-Tein 6861
Sphingoceryl® Fluid
Sphingoceryl® Wax
Sphingoceryl® Powd
Sphingosomes® AL
Styrene MC Beads
Sungen
Tego® Care 215
Tepescohuite AMI
   Watersoluble
Tepescohuite HG
Tepescohuite HS
Tepescohuite LS
Theophyllisilane C
Tofupro-U
Tonique HS 216
Tonique HS 290, LS 690
Tri-Derm SE
Tri-K CMF Complex
Tri-Lastin 10F
Tyrosilane C
Uniderm A
Unitrienol T-27
Unitrienol T-272
USP-2
Uvasorb MET
Vaseline 335 G
Vaseline 7702
Vaseline 8332
Vaseline 10049 BL
Vaseline A
Vexel
Vitacell
Vitamin A and D-3
Vitamin A Palmitate Type
   P1.7
Vitamin A Palmitate Type
   P1.7/BHT
Vitamin A Palmitate Type
   PIMO/BH
Vitamine A Palmitate
   Exsyliposomes
Vitaplant CLR Oil-Soluble N
Vitaplant CLR Water-
   Soluble

Skin Care Additives *(cont'd.)*

Yeast Extract SC | Yeast Walls | Zincidone® |

Solubilizers/Hydrotropes/Coupling Agents

Abil®-Wax 2440	Ameroxol® OE-10	Caprol® 10G4O	Chemax NP-9
Abil®-Wax 9801	Ameroxol® OE-20	Caprol® 10G10O	Chemax NP-10
Accobetaine CL	Amfotex FV-28	Caprol® 10G10S	Chemax OP-30/70
Acconon 200-DL	Aminol KDE	Caprol® PGE860	Chemax PEG 400 DO
Acconon 200-MS	AMP	Captex® 200	Chemphos TC-231S
Acconon 400-DO	AMPD	Carbowax® PEG 300	Chemphos TC-337
Acconon 400-ML	Ampho B11-34	Carbowax® Sentry® PEG	Chemphos TC-341
Acconon 400-MO	Ampho T-35	300	Chemphos TC-349
Acconon 400-MS	Ampholak YCE	Carbowax® Sentry® PEG	Chemphos TR-505
Acconon 1300	Ampholan® U 203	400	Chemphos TR-505D
Acconon CA-5	Amphoteric N	Carbowax® Sentry® PEG	Chemphos TR-510
Acconon CA-8	Antaron® MC-44	540 Blend	Chemphos TR-510S
Acconon CA-9	Antaron® PC-37	Carbowax® Sentry® PEG	Chemphos TR-515
Acconon CA-15	Antil® 141 Liq	600	Chemphos TR-515D
Acconon CON	Antil® 208	Carbowax® Sentry® PEG	Chemphos TR-541
Acconon E	Aqualose L30	900	Cholesterol NF
Acconon TGH	Aqualose L75	Carbowax® Sentry® PEG	Cithrol 2ML
Acconon W230	Aqualose L100	1000	Cithrol 2MO
ACS 60	Aqualose LL100	Carbowax® Sentry® PEG	Cithrol 2MS
Adol® 90 NF	Aqualose SLT	1450	Cithrol 3MS
Aerosol® A-102	Aqualose SLW	Carbowax® Sentry® PEG	Cithrol 4ML
Aerosol® A-103	Aqualose W20	3350	Cithrol 4MO
Aerosol® MA-80	Argonol 60	Carbowax® Sentry® PEG	Cithrol 4MS
Aerosol® OT-B	Arlasolve® 200	4600	Cithrol 6ML
Akyporox CO 400	Arlasolve® 200 Liq	Carbowax® Sentry® PEG	Cithrol 6MO
Akyporox CO 600	Arlasolve® DMI	8000	Cithrol 6MS
Akyporox OP 250V	Arlatone® 285	Carsonon® 144-P	Cithrol 10ML
Akyporox RC 200	Arlatone® 289	Carsonon® 169-P	Cithrol 10MO
Alcolec® BS	Arlatone® 650	Cegesoft® C 17	Cithrol 10MS
Aldo® DC	Arlatone® 827	Cegesoft® C 19	Cithrol 15MS
Aldo® ML	Arlatone® 970	Cegesoft® C 25	Cithrol 40MO
Aldo® MO FG	Arlatone® 975	Ceraphyl® 45	Cithrol 40MS
Aldo® MOD FG	Arlatone® 980	Ceraphyl® 140-A	Cithrol 60ML
Aldo® MR	Arlatone® G	Ceraphyl® 230	Cithrol 60MO
Aldo® MS-20 FG	Arlatone® T	Ceraphyl® 368	Cithrol ES
Aldo® MSD	Armotan® PML 20	Cerex EL 250	Coconut Oils® 76, 92, 110
Aldo® PMS	Aromaphyte™	Cerex EL 300	CPH-27-N
Aldosperse® ML-23	Arosurf® 66-E2	Cerex EL 360	CPH-43-N
Aldosperse® MS-20	Arosurf® 66-E10	Cerex EL 400	Cralane KR-13, -14
Aldosperse® O-20 FG	Arosurf® 66-E20	Cerex EL 4929	Cralane LR-10
Alkamuls® 400-DL	Arosurf® 66-PE12	Cerex ELS 250	Cralane LR-11
Alkamuls® 400-DO	Axol® E 66	Cerex ELS 400	Cremophor® EL
Alkamuls® 400-MS	Bernel® Ester DOM	Cerex ELS 450	Cremophor® NP 10
Alkamuls® 600-DL	Brij® 56	Cerex U 60	Cremophor® NP 14
Alkamuls® EL-620	Brij® 58	Cetiol® A	Cremophor® RH 40
Alkamuls® EL-620L	Brij® 76	Cetomacrogol 1000 BP	Cremophor® RH 60
Alkamuls® GMS/C	Brij® 78	Chemal LA-4	Cremophor® RH 410
Alkamuls® PSML-20	Brij® 96	Chemal LA-9	Cremophor® RH 455
Alkamuls® PSMO-5	Brij® 98	Chemal LA-12	Crill 4
Alkamuls® SMO	Brij® 700	Chemal LA-23	Crillet 1
Alkamuls® SMS	Brij® 700S	Chemal OA-4	Crillet 2
Alkamuls® T-20	Brij® 721	Chemal OA-5	Crillet 4
Alkamuls® T-60	Brij® 721S	Chemal OA-9	Crillet 6
Alkamuls® T-65	Capmul® MCM	Chemal OA-20/70CWS	Crillet 11
Alkamuls® T-85	Capmul® POE-L	Chemal OA-20G	Crillet 31
Alkasurf® NP-30, 70%	Capmul® POE-O	Chemal TDA-6	Crillet 35
Alkasurf® TDA-12	Capmul® POE-S	Chemal TDA-12	Crillet 41
Alkateric® PB	Caprol® 2G4S	Chemal TDA-15	Crillet 45
Alpha-Step® ML-40	Caprol® 3GO	Chemal TDA-18	Crodafos SG
Ameroxol® LE-4	Caprol® 3GS	Chemax CO-5	Crodalan AWS
Ameroxol® LE-23	Caprol® 6G2O	Chemax NP-1.5	Crodamol BS
Ameroxol® OE-2	Caprol® 6G2S	Chemax NP-4	Crodamol PMP
Ameroxol® OE-5	Caprol® 10G2O	Chemax NP-6	Crodesta F-10

Solubilizers/Hydrotropes/Coupling Agents *(cont'd.)*

Crodesta F-50	Emalex 510	Emalex HC-100	Emery® 918
Crodesta F-110	Emalex 512	Emalex NP-2	Emphos™ CS-1361
Crodesta F-160	Emalex 515	Emalex NP-3	Empigen® 5107
Crodesta SL-40	Emalex 520	Emalex NP-5	Empilan® CDE
Crodet L4	Emalex 523	Emalex NP-10	Empilan® CDX
Crodet L8	Emalex 550	Emalex NP-11	Empilan® LDE
Crodet L12	Emalex 1605	Emalex NP-12	Empilan® LDX
Crodet L24	Emalex 1610	Emalex NP-13	Emsorb® 2500
Crodet L40	Emalex 1615	Emalex NP-15	Emsorb® 2502
Crodet L100	Emalex 1620	Emalex NP-20	Emsorb® 2503
Crodet S4	Emalex 1625	Emalex NP-25	Emsorb® 2505
Crodet S8	Emalex 1805	Emalex NP-30	Emsorb® 2507
Crodet S12	Emalex 1810	Emalex OD-5	Emsorb® 2510
Crodet S24	Emalex 1815	Emalex OD-10	Emsorb® 2515
Crodet S40	Emalex 1820	Emalex OD-16	Emsorb® 2720
Crodet S100	Emalex 1825	Emalex OD-20	Emsorb® 2722
Croduret 10	Emalex 2405	Emalex OD-25	Emsorb® 2726
Croduret 30	Emalex 2410	Emalex OP-5	Emsorb® 6900
Croduret 40	Emalex 2415	Emalex OP-8	Emsorb® 6915
Croduret 50 Special	Emalex 2420	Emalex OP-10	Emthox® 5885
Croduret 60	Emalex 2425	Emalex OP-15	Emthox® 5964
Croduret 100	Emalex 2505	Emalex OP-20	Emulmetik
Croduret 200	Emalex 2510	Emalex OP-25	Emulmetik™ 100
Crovol A40	Emalex 2515	Emalex OP-30	Emulmetik™ 110
Crovol A70	Emalex 2520	Emalex OP-40	Emulmetik™ 300
Crovol M40	Emalex 2525	Emalex OP-50	Emulmetik™ 310
Crovol M70	Emalex AF-2	Emalex PEIS-3	Emulmetik™ 910
Crovol PK40	Emalex AF-4	Emalex PEIS-6	Emulmetik™ 920
Crovol PK70	Emalex BHA-5	Emalex PEIS-12	Emulmetik™ 930
CUPL® PIC	Emalex BHA-10	Emalex PEIS-20	Emulmetik™ 950
Dehydol® D 3	Emalex BHA-20	Emalex RWIS-150	Emulmetik™ 970
Dehydol® LS 2	Emalex BHA-30	Emalex RWIS-160	Emulsynt® 1055
Dehyton® AB-30	Emalex C-20	Emalex RWIS-305	Emulsynt® GDL
Dehyton® PAB-30	Emalex C-30	Emalex RWIS-310	Espesilor AC-43
Dehyton® PK	Emalex C-40	Emalex RWIS-315	Espesilor AC-50
Deriphat® 154	Emalex C-50	Emalex RWIS-320	Estalan 42
Deriphat® 154L	Emalex CS-5	Emalex RWIS-330	Estalan 126
Deriphat® 160	Emalex CS-10	Emalex RWIS-340	Estol SML20 3618
Deriphat® 160C	Emalex CS-15	Emalex RWIS-350	Ethoxyol® 1707
Dermol GL-7A	Emalex CS-20	Emalex RWIS-360	Ethylan® GEL2
Drewmulse® 3-1-O	Emalex CS-24	Emalex RWL-140	Ethylan® GEO8
Drewmulse® 3-1-S	Emalex CS-30	Emalex RWL-150	Ethylan® GEO81
Drewmulse® 6-2-S	Emalex ET-2020	Emalex RWL-160	Ethylan® GEP4
Drewmulse® 10-10-O	Emalex ET-8020	Emalex TPIS-303	Ethylan® GES6
Drewmulse® 10-10-S	Emalex ET-8040	Emalex TPIS-320	Ethylan® GLE-21
Drewmulse® 10-4-O	Emalex GM-20	Emalex TPIS-325	Ethylan® GOE-21
Drewmulse® 10-8-O	Emalex GM-30	Emalex TPIS-330	Ethylan® GPS85
Drewmulse® POE-SML	Emalex GM-40	Emalex TPIS-340	Ethylan® KEO
Drewmulse® POE-SMO	Emalex GWIS-110	Emalex TPIS-350	Ethylan® ME
Drewmulse® POE-SMS	Emalex GWIS-115	Emalex TPM-303	Ethylan® OE
Drewmulse® POE-STS	Emalex GWIS-120	Emalex TPM-305	Ethylan® R
Drewmulse® SML	Emalex GWIS-125	Emalex TPM-308	Etocas 5
Drewmulse® SMO	Emalex GWIS-130	Emalex TPM-320	Etocas 10
Drewmulse® SMS	Emalex GWIS-140	Emalex TPM-325	Etocas 15
Drewmulse® STS	Emalex GWIS-150	Emalex TPM-330	Etocas 29
Drewpol® 10-4-O	Emalex GWIS-160	Emalex TS-8	Etocas 30
Dur-Em® GMO	Emalex GWIS-340	Emalex VS-31	Etocas 35
Eccowet® W-50	Emalex GWIS-350	Emalox CG-4	Etocas 40
Eccowet® W-88	Emalex GWIS-360	Emasol L-106	Etocas 60
Eltesol® ACS 60	Emalex GWO-340	Emasol P-120	Eumulgin E-24
Eltesol® AX 40	Emalex GWO-350	Emcol® NA-30	Eumulgin® HRE 40
Eltesol® ST 34	Emalex GWO-360	Emerest® 2325	Eumulgin® HRE 60
Eltesol® ST 40	Emalex HC-20	Emerest® 2384	Eumulgin® L
Eltesol® SX 30	Emalex HC-30	Emerest® 2389	Eumulgin® M8
Eltesol® SX 93	Emalex HC-40	Emerest® 2452	Eumulgin® O5
Emalex 503	Emalex HC-50	Emery® 912	Eumulgin® PRT 36
Emalex 506	Emalex HC-60	Emery® 916	Eumulgin® PRT 40
Emalex 508	Emalex HC-80	Emery® 917	Eumulgin® PRT 56

Solubilizers/Hydrotropes/Coupling Agents *(cont'd.)*

Eumulgin® PRT 200
Eumulgin® PWM5
Eumulgin® PWM17
Eumulgin® RO 35
Eumulgin® RO 40
Eumulgin® SML 20
Eumulgin® SMO 20
Eumulgin® SMS 20
Fancol ALA
Fancol ALA-10
Fancol HL-20
Fancol HL-24
Fancol LA-5
Fancol LA-15
Fancol OA-95
Finester EH-25
Finsolv® 116
Finsolv® BOD
Finsolv® EMG-20
Finsolv® P
Finsolv® PL-62
Finsolv® PL-355
Finsolv® SB
Finsolv® TN
Fluilan AWS
Foamquat CAS
Foamtaine CAB-A
Foamtaine CAB-G
Forlan C-24
G-1096
G-1292
Gafac® RE-877
Ganex® P-904
Ganex® V-216
Ganex® V-220
Gantrez® AN
Generol® 122
Generol® 122E10
Generol® 122E16
Generol® 122E25
Geropon® SS-TA
Glucam® E-10
Glucam® E-20
Glucam® P-10
Glucam® P-20
Glucamate® DOE-120
Glucamate® SSE-20
Glycerox HE
Glycerox L15
Glycosperse® L-20
Glycosperse® O-5
Glycosperse® O-20
Glycosperse® O-20 Veg
Glycosperse® O-20X
Glycosperse® P-20
Glycosperse® S-20
Glycosperse® TO-20
Glycosperse® TS-20
Grillocose PSE-20
Grillosol 8C
Grillosol 8C12
Grilloten LSE 87
Grilloten LSE87K
Grilloten PSE141G
Grilloten ZT12
Grilloten ZT-40
Grilloten ZT-80
HD-Eutanol®

Hefti AMS-33
Hefti ML-55-F
Hetoxamate FA-5
Hetoxamate FA-20
Hetoxamate LA-5
Hetoxamate LA-9
Hetoxamate MO-4
Hetoxamate MO-5
Hetoxamate MO-9
Hetoxamate MO-15
Hetoxamate SA-5
Hetoxamate SA-9
Hetoxamate SA-35
Hetoxamate SA-90
Hetoxamate SA-90F
Hetoxide BN-13
Hetoxide C-2
Hetoxide C-9
Hetoxide C-15
Hetoxide C-25
Hetoxide C-30
Hetoxide C-40
Hetoxide C-60
Hetoxide C-200
Hetoxide C-200-50%
Hetoxide DNP-5
Hetoxide DNP-10
Hetoxide HC-16
Hetoxol CAWS
Hetoxol CD-3
Hetoxol CD-4
Hetoxol D
Hetoxol G
Hetoxol J
Hetoxol L
Hetoxol L-4
Hetoxol L-9
Hetoxol M-3
Hetoxol OA-5 Special
Hetoxol OL-2
Hetoxol OL-4
Hetoxol OL-5
Hetoxol OL-10
Hetoxol OL-10H
Hetoxol OL-20
Hetoxol OL-23
Hetoxol OL-40
Hetoxol PLA
Hetoxol STA-2
Hetoxol STA-10
Hetoxol STA-20
Hetoxol STA-30
Hetoxol TD-9
Hetoxol TD-18
Hetoxol TD-25
Hodag PEG 400
Igepal® CO-630 Special
Igepal® NP-4
Igepal® NP-9
Igepal® OP-9
Imwitor® 308
Imwitor® 310
Imwitor® 312
Imwitor® 408
Imwitor® 412
Imwitor® 708
Imwitor® 908
Imwitor® 910

Imwitor® 914
Imwitor® 928
Imwitor® 988
Incrocas 30
Incrocas 40
Incronam 30
Incropol CS-20
Incropol CS-50
Incropol L-23
Isofol® 12
Isofol® 14T
Isofol® 16
Isofol® 18E
Isofol® 18T
Isofol® 20
Isofol® 24
Isopropyl Palmitate
Ixol 2
Kemamide® W-35
Kemamide® W-42
Kessco® GMC-8
Kessco® Isopropyl
  Myristate
Kessco® Isopropyl
  Palmitate
Kessco® PEG 200 DL
Kessco® PEG 200 DO
Kessco® PEG 200 DS
Kessco® PEG 200 ML
Kessco® PEG 200 MO
Kessco® PEG 200 MS
Kessco® PEG 300 DL
Kessco® PEG 300 DO
Kessco® PEG 300 DS
Kessco® PEG 300 ML
Kessco® PEG 300 MO
Kessco® PEG 300 MS
Kessco® PEG 400 DL
Kessco® PEG 400 DO
Kessco PEG 400DS
Kessco® PEG 400 DS
Kessco® PEG 400 ML
Kessco® PEG 400 MO
Kessco® PEG 400 MS
Kessco® PEG 600 DL
Kessco® PEG 600 DO
Kessco® PEG 600 DS
Kessco® PEG 600 ML
Kessco® PEG 600 MO
Kessco® PEG 600 MS
Kessco® PEG 1000 DL
Kessco® PEG 1000 DO
Kessco® PEG 1000 DS
Kessco® PEG 1000 ML
Kessco® PEG 1000 MO
Kessco® PEG 1000 MS
Kessco® PEG 1540 DL
Kessco® PEG 1540 DO
Kessco® PEG 1540 DS
Kessco® PEG 1540 ML
Kessco® PEG 1540 MO
Kessco® PEG 1540 MS
Kessco® PEG 4000 DL
Kessco® PEG 4000 DO
Kessco® PEG 4000 DS
Kessco® PEG 4000 ML
Kessco® PEG 4000 MO
Kessco® PEG 4000 MS

Kessco® PEG 6000 DL
Kessco® PEG 6000 DO
Kessco® PEG 6000 DS
Kessco® PEG 6000 ML
Kessco® PEG 6000 MO
Kessco® PEG 6000 MS
Kessco PGMS
Kollidon®
Labrafil® M 1944 CS
Labrafil® M 2125 CS
Labrasol
Lamacit® ER
Lamacit® GML 12
Lamacit® GML 20
Lamacit® GMO 25
Lan-Aqua-Sol 50
Lan-Aqua-Sol 100
Laneto 20
Laneto 27
Laneto 30
Laneto 40
Laneto 49
Laneto 50
Laneto 60
Laneto 85
Laneto 99
Laneto 100
Laneto 100-Flaked
Lanexol AWS
Lanogel® 21
Lanogel® 31
Lanogel® 41
Lanogel® 61
Lanpol 5
Lanpol 10
Lanpol 20
Lanpol 520
Lantrol® AWS 1692
Lantrol® PLN
Lantrol® PLN/50
Lexemul® GDL
Lexol® GT-855
Lexol® IPP
Lexol® IPP-A
Lexol® IPP-NF
Lexol® PG-855
Lexol® PG-865
Lipocol C-2
Lipocol C-10
Lipocol C-20
Lipocol HCO-40
Lipocol HCO-60
Lipocol L-1
Lipocol L-4
Lipocol L-12
Lipocol L-23
Lipocol M-4
Lipocol O-2 Special
Lipocol O-3 Special
Lipocol O-10
Lipocol O-20
Lipocol S-2
Lipocol S-10
Lipocol S-20
Lipocol SC-4
Lipocol SC-10
Lipocol SC-15
Lipocol SC-20

Solubilizers/Hydrotropes/Coupling Agents *(cont'd.)*

Lipocol TD-12	Macol® CSA-20	Manrosol SXS40	Monamid® L-355
Lipolan 31	Macol® CSA-40	Mapeg® 200 DOT	Monamid® L-360
Lipolan Distilled	Macol® CSA-50	Mapeg® 600 DL	Monamid® L-365
Lipopeg 2-L	Macol® DNP-5	Mapeg® 600 DOT	Monamid® LL-370
Lipo Polyglycol 200	Macol® DNP-10	Mapeg® 600 ML	Monamid® LM-375
Lipo Polyglycol 300	Macol® DNP-15	Mapeg® CO-16	Monamine 779
Lipo Polyglycol 400	Macol® DNP-21	Mapeg® CO-16H	Monateric 810-A-50
Lipo Polyglycol 600	Macol® LA-4	Mapeg® CO-25	Monateric 1188M
Lipo Polyglycol 1000	Macol® LA-9	Mapeg® CO-25H	Monateric 1202
Lipo Polyglycol 3350	Macol® LA-12	Mapeg® CO-30	Monateric CA-35
Liposorb L-10	Macol® LA-23	Mapeg® CO-36	Monateric CDTD
Liposorb L-20	Macol® LA-790	Mapeg® CO-200	Monateric CEM-38
Liposorb O-5	Macol® NP-4	Mapeg® S-100	Monateric CEM-38CG
Liposorb P-20	Macol® NP-5	Mapeg® S-150	Monateric CM-36S
Liposorb S-4	Macol® NP-6	Marlipal® 124	Monateric COAB
Liposorb S-20	Macol® NP-8	Marlipal® 129	Monateric CyA-50
Liposorb TO-20	Macol® NP-11	Marlipal® MG	Monateric CyMM-40
Liposorb TS-20	Macol® NP-12	Marlowet® LA 4	Monateric TA-35
Liquid Absorption Base	Macol® NP-15	Marlowet® LA 7	Monawet MO-70
Type A, T	Macol® NP-20	Marlowet® LMA 2	Monawet MO-70R
Lonzest® 153-S	Macol® NP-20(70)	Marlowet® LMA 4	Monawet SNO-35
Lonzest® 163-S	Macol® NP-30(70)	Marlowet® LMA 5	Montanox 80 DF
Lonzest® SML-20	Macol® NP-100	Marlowet® R 40/K	Montanox 85
Lonzest® SMO-20	Macol® OA-2	Masil® 280	Montosol PF-10
Lonzest® SMP-20	Macol® OA-4	Masil® 280LP	Montosol PF-14
Lonzest® SMS-20	Macol® OA-5	Mayphos OL 3N	Montosol PF-26, PG-10
Lonzest® STO-20	Macol® OA-10	Mazamide® 65	Montosol PL-16
Lonzest® STS-20	Macol® OA-20	Mazamide® 80	Montosol PQ-17
Lowenol C Acid	Macol® OP-3	Mazamide® C-2	Mulsifan RT 18
Lowenol L Acid	Macol® OP-5	Mazamide® C-5	Mulsifan RT 69
Lowenol M Acid	Macol® OP-8	Mazamide® CS 148	Mulsifan RT 141
Lowenol O Acid	Macol® OP-10	Mazamide® L-5	Mulsifan RT 146
Lowenol P Acid	Macol® OP-10 SP	Mazamide® L-298	Mulsifan RT 203/80
Lutrol® E 1500	Macol® OP-12	Mazamide® SS-10	Mulsifan RT 302
Lutrol® E 4000	Macol® OP-16(75)	Mazeen® C-2	Myritol® 318
Lutrol® E 6000	Macol® OP-30(70)	Mazeen® C-5	Myverol® 18-99
Macol® 1	Macol® OP-40(70)	Mazeen® C-10	Naetex-L
Macol® 2	Macol® SA-2	Mazeen® C-15	Naturechem® MAR
Macol® 2D	Macol® SA-5	Mazeen® S-2	Naxonic™ NI-40
Macol® 2LF	Macol® SA-10	Mazeen® S-5	Naxonic™ NI-60
Macol® 4	Macol® SA-15	Mazeen® S-10	Naxonic™ NI-100
Macol® 8	Macol® SA-20	Mazeen® S-15	Neobee® 18
Macol® 10	Macol® SA-40	Mazeen® T-2	Neobee® 20
Macol® 16	Macol® TD-3	Mazeen® T-5	Neobee® M-5
Macol® 22	Macol® TD-8	Mazeen® T-10	Neobee® M-20
Macol® 23	Macol® TD-10	Mazeen® T-15	Neobee® O
Macol® 27	Macol® TD-12	Mazol® 159	Neodol® 25-12
Macol® 31	Macol® TD-15	Mazol® PGO-31 K	Neo Heliopan, Type OS
Macol® 32	Macol® TD-100	Miglyol® 810	Nikkol Batyl Alcohol 100,
Macol® 33	Macol® TD-610	Miglyol® 812	EX
Macol® 34	Mafo® C	Miglyol® 840	Nikkol BC-23
Macol® 35	Mafo® CAB	Miranol® 2CIB	Nikkol BC-25TX
Macol® 40	Mafo® CAB 425	Miranol® C2M Conc. NP	Nikkol BC-30TX
Macol® 42	Mafo® CAB SP	Miranol® C2M-SF Conc	Nikkol BC-40TX
Macol® 44	Mafo® CB 40	Mirataine® BB	Nikkol BEG-1630
Macol® 46	Mafo® CFA 35	Mirataine® CAB-A	Nikkol BL-21
Macol® 72	Mafo® CSB	Mirataine® CAB-O	Nikkol BL-25
Macol® 77	Mafo® CSB 50	Mirataine® CB/M	Nikkol BO-20
Macol® 85	Mafo® CSB W	Mirataine® COB	Nikkol BO-50
Macol® 88	Mafo® KCOSB 50	Mirataine® T2C-30	Nikkol BPS-5
Macol® 101	Mafo® LMAB	Monamid® 31	Nikkol BPS-10
Macol® 108	Mafo® OB	Monamid® 150-CW	Nikkol BPS-15
Macol® CA-2	Mafo® SBAO 110	Monamid® 150-GLT	Nikkol BPS-20
Macol® CA-10	Manro CD	Monamid® 150-LMWC	Nikkol BPS-25
Macol® CSA-2	Manro CD/G	Monamid® 150-LWA	Nikkol BPS-30
Macol® CSA-4	Manro CDS	Monamid® 716	Nikkol BWA-5
Macol® CSA-10	Manro CDX	Monamid® 1224	Nikkol BWA-20
Macol® CSA-15	Manrosol SXS30	Monamid® L-350	Nikkol BWA-40

Solubilizers/Hydrotropes/Coupling Agents *(cont'd.)*

Nikkol Chimyl Alcohol 100	Nikkol TP-10	Pluracol® E1450	Prox-onic HRH-0200/50
Nikkol CO-3	Nikkol TS-10	Pluracol® E1450 NF	Prox-onic L 081-05
Nikkol CO-40TX	Nikkol TS-30	Pluracol® E1500	Prox-onic L 101-05
Nikkol CO-50TX	Nikkol TS-106	Pluracol® E2000	Prox-onic L 102-02
Nikkol CO-60TX	Nikkol TW-10	Pluracol® E4000	Prox-onic L 121-09
Nikkol Decaglyn 1-IS	Nikkol TW-20	Pluracol® E4000 NF	Prox-onic L 161-05
Nikkol Decaglyn 1-L	Nikkol TW-30	Pluracol® E4500	Prox-onic L 181-05
Nikkol Decaglyn 1-LN	Niox KI Series	Pluracol® E6000	Prox-onic L 201-02
Nikkol Decaglyn 1-M	Niox KI-29	Pluracol® E8000	Prox-onic LA-1/02
Nikkol Decaglyn 1-O	Niox KJ-10	Pluracol® E8000 NF	Prox-onic LA-1/04
Nikkol Decaglyn 1-S	Noiox KJ-12	Pluriol® E 1500	Prox-onic LA-1/09
Nikkol DLP-10	Noiox KJ-15	Pluronic® 10R5	Prox-onic LA-1/012
Nikkol DOP-8N	Nonisol 100	Pluronic® 10R8	Prox-onic LA-1/023
Nikkol GO-430	Norfox® Sorbo T-20	Pluronic® 12R3	Prox-onic NP-1.5
Nikkol GO-440	Norfox® Sorbo T-80	Pluronic® 17R1	Prox-onic NP-04
Nikkol GO-460	Novol	Pluronic® 17R2	Prox-onic NP-06
Nikkol HCO-5	Oramix CG 110-60	Pluronic® 17R4	Prox-onic NP-09
Nikkol HCO-7.5	Orange Wax	Pluronic® 17R8	Prox-onic NP-010
Nikkol HCO-10	Oxypon 288	Pluronic® 22R4	Prox-onic NP-015
Nikkol HCO-20	Oxypon 306	Pluronic® 25R1	Prox-onic NP-020
Nikkol HCO-30	Parapel® HC-99	Pluronic® 25R2	Prox-onic NP-030
Nikkol HCO-40	Pationic® ISL	Pluronic® 25R4	Prox-onic NP-030/70
Nikkol HCO-50	Pegosperse® 200 MS	Pluronic® 25R5	Prox-onic NP-040
Nikkol HCO-60	Pegosperse® 300 MO	Pluronic® 25R8	Prox-onic NP-040/70
Nikkol HCO-80	Pegosperse® 400 ML	Pluronic® 31R1	Prox-onic NP-050
Nikkol HCO-100	Pegosperse® 600 MO	Pluronic® 31R2	Prox-onic NP-050/70
Nikkol Lecinol S-10	Pelemol MAR	Pluronic® 31R4	Prox-onic NP-0100
Nikkol Lecinol S-10E	Permethyl® 99A	Pluronic® L10	Prox-onic NP-0100/70
Nikkol Lecinol S-10EX	Permethyl® 101A	PMS-33	Prox-onic OA-1/04
Nikkol Lecinol S-10M	Permethyl® 102A	Pogol 200	Prox-onic OA-1/09
Nikkol Lecinol S-30	Permethyl® 104A	Pogol 400 NF	Prox-onic OA-1/020
Nikkol MYO-10	Permethyl® 106A	Polychol 5	Prox-onic OA-2/020
Nikkol MYS-1EX	Permethyl® 108A	Polychol 10	Prox-onic SML-020
Nikkol MYS-2	PGE-600-ML	Polychol 15	Prox-onic SMO-05
Nikkol MYS-4	PGE-600-MS	Polychol 16	Prox-onic SMO-020
Nikkol MYS-10	Phosal® 50 PG	Polychol 20	Prox-onic SMP-020
Nikkol MYS-25	Phosal® 50 SA	Polychol 40	Prox-onic SMS-020
Nikkol MYS-40	Phosal® 53 MCT	Polylan®	Prox-onic STO-020
Nikkol MYS-45	Phosal® 75 SA	Procetyl 10	Prox-onic STS-020
Nikkol MYS-55	Phosphanol Series	Procetyl 30	Pyroter CPI-30
Nikkol NP-5	PhosPho E-100	Procetyl 50	Pyroter CPI-40
Nikkol NP-7.5	Phospholipid EFA	Procetyl AWS	Pyroter CPI-60
Nikkol NP-10	Phospholipid PTC	Produkt RT 288	Pyroter GPI-25
Nikkol NP-15	Phospholipid PTD	Prostearyl 15	Radia® 7108
Nikkol NP-18TX	Phospholipid PTL	Protasorb L-20	Radia® 7185
Nikkol NP-20	Phospholipid PTZ	Provol 10	Radia® 7187
Nikkol OP-3	Phospholipon® 90/90 G	Provol 30	Radia® 7190
Nikkol OP-10	Phospholipon® CC	Provol 50	Radia® 7200
Nikkol OP-30	Phospholipon® LC	Prox-onic CSA-1/04	Radia® 7204
Nikkol PBC-31	Phospholipon® MC	Prox-onic CSA-1/06	Radia® 7266
Nikkol PBC-33	Phospholipon® MG Na	Prox-onic CSA-1/010	Radia® 7345
Nikkol PBC-34	Phospholipon® PC	Prox-onic CSA-1/015	Radia® 7355
Nikkol PBC-41	Phospholipon® PG Na	Prox-onic CSA-1/020	Radia® 7371
Nikkol PBC-44	Phospholipon® SC	Prox-onic CSA-1/030	Radia® 7505
Nikkol PEN-4612	Phospholipon® SG Na	Prox-onic CSA-1/050	Radia® 7506
Nikkol PEN-4620	Phosphoteric® T-C6	Prox-onic HR-05	Radianol® 7106
Nikkol PEN-4630	Plasdone® C-15	Prox-onic HR-016	Remcopal HC 7
Nikkol Sefsol 218	Plasdone® C-30	Prox-onic HR-025	Remcopal HC 33
Nikkol Sefsol 228	Plasdone® K-25, K-90	Prox-onic HR-030	Remcopal HC 40
Nikkol TDP-2	Plasdone® K-26/28,	Prox-onic HR-036	Remcopal HC 60
Nikkol TDP-4	K-29/32	Prox-onic HR-040	Remcopal O9
Nikkol TDP-6	Pluracol® E200	Prox-onic HR-080	Remcopal O11
Nikkol TDP-8	Pluracol® E300	Prox-onic HR-0200	Remcopal O12
Nikkol TDP-10	Pluracol® E400	Prox-onic HR-0200/50	Rewoderm® ES 90
Nikkol TI-10	Pluracol® E400 NF	Prox-onic HRH-05	Rewoderm® LI 63
Nikkol TL-10, TL-10EX	Pluracol® E600	Prox-onic HRH-016	Rewoderm® LI 67-75
Nikkol TO-10	Pluracol® E600 NF	Prox-onic HRH-025	Rewomat B 2003
Nikkol TO-10M	Pluracol® E1000	Prox-onic HRH-0200	Rewomid® DO 280 S

Solubilizers/Hydrotropes/Coupling Agents *(cont'd.)*

Rewopal® C 6	Shebu® WS	Surfonic® N-100	Tagat® S
Rewopal® CSF 11	Simulsol 1285	Surfonic® N-102	Tagat® S2
Rewopal® LA 3	Simulsol 1292	Surfonic® N-120	Tagat® TO
Rewopal® MPG 10	Simulsol 1293	Surfonic® N-130	Tegin® C-1R
Rewopol® SBDO 70	Simulsol 1294	Surfonic® N-150	Tegin® P
Rewopol® SBDO 75	Simulsol 5719	Surfonic® N-200	Tegin® P-411 SE
Reworyl® NCS 40	Simulsol 5817	Surfonic® N-300	Tegin® PL
Reworyl® NTS 40	Simulsol OL 50	Surfonic® NB-5	Tegin® RZ
Rewoteric® AM HC	Siponic® NP-7	Surfynol® 82S	Tegin® RZ NSE
Rheodol 460	Siponic® TD-12	SXS 40	Tetronic® 50R1
Rheodol TW-P120	S-Maz® 83R	Synperonic A20	Tetronic® 50R4
Rhodacal® 330	Softigen® 767	Synperonic A50	Tetronic® 50R8
Rhodafac® RD-510	Solan	Synperonic NP1	Tetronic® 70R1
Rhodasurf® E 400	Solan 50	Synperonic NP2	Tetronic® 70R2
Rhodasurf® L-4	Solubiliser LRI	Synperonic NP4	Tetronic® 70R4
Rhodasurf® LAN-23-75%	Solulan® 25	Synperonic NP5	Tetronic® 90R1
Rhodasurf® ON-870	Solwax C-24	Synperonic NP5.5	Tetronic® 90R4
Rhodasurf® ON-877	Solwax LG 35	Synperonic NP6	Tetronic® 90R8
Rhodasurf® PEG 400	Sorbanox AOM	Synperonic NP7	Tetronic® 110R1
Rhodasurf® TD-9	Sorbax PML-20	Synperonic NP8	Tetronic® 110R2
Ritalafa®	Sorbax PMO-5	Synperonic NP8.5	Tetronic® 110R7
Ritalan® C	Sorbax PMO-20	Synperonic NP8.75	Tetronic® 130R1
Ritawax 5	Sorbax PMP-20	Synperonic NP9	Tetronic® 130R2
Ritawax 10	Sorbax PMS-20	Synperonic NP9.5	Tetronic® 150R1
Ritawax 15	Sorbax PTO-20	Synperonic NP9.75	Tetronic® 150R4
Ritawax 20	Sorbax PTS-20	Synperonic NP10	Tetronic® 150R8
Ritawax 40	Sorbilene L	Synperonic NP12	Tetronic® 304
Ritawax AEO	Sorbilene O	Synperonic NP13	Tetronic® 504
Ritawax ALA	Sorbon T-20	Synperonic NP15	Tetronic® 701
Ritawax Super	Span® 60, 60K	Synperonic NP17	Tetronic® 702
Ritoleth 2	Span® 60 VS	Synperonic NP20	Tetronic® 704
Ritoleth 5	Standamid® CD	Synperonic NP25	Tetronic® 707
Ritoleth 10	Standamid® KD	Synperonic NP30	Tetronic® 901
Ritoleth 20	Standamid® KDS	Synperonic NP30/70	Tetronic® 904
Ryoto Sugar Ester P-1570	Standamid® LDS	Synperonic NP35	Tetronic® 908
Ryoto Sugar Ester P-1670	Standamid® PD	Synperonic NP40	Tetronic® 909
Ryoto Sugar Ester S-1170	Standamid® PK-KDS	Synperonic NP50	Tetronic® 1101
Ryoto Sugar Ester S-1170S	Standamul® 1414-E	Synperonic OP3	Tetronic® 1102
Ryoto Sugar Ester S-1570	Standamul® B-1	Synperonic OP4.5	Tetronic® 1104
Ryoto Sugar Ester S-1670	Standamul® B-2	Synperonic OP6	Tetronic® 1107
Sandopan® DTC	Standamul® B-3	Synperonic OP7.5	Tetronic® 1301
Sandopan® DTC-100	Standamul® G	Synperonic OP8	Tetronic® 1302
Sandopan® DTC Linear P	Standamul® HE	Synperonic OP10	Tetronic® 1304
Sandopan® DTC Linear P	Standapol® Conc. 7023	Synperonic OP10.5	Tetronic® 1307
Acid	Standapol® EA-3	Synperonic OP11	Tetronic® 1501
Sandopan® JA-36	Standapol® SCO	Synperonic OP12.5	Tetronic® 1502
Sandopan® LS-24	Sterol LA 300	Synperonic OP16	Tetronic® 1504
Santone® 10-10-O	Super Refined™ Orange	Synperonic OP16.5	Tetronic® 1508
Satexlan 20	Roughy Oil	Synperonic OP20	Texapon® EA-1
Schercemol 1818	Super-Sat AWS-4	Synperonic OP25	Texapon® EA-2
Schercemol DEIS	Super-Sat AWS-24	Synperonic OP30	Texapon® EA-3
Schercemol DIS	Super Solan Flaked	Synperonic OP40	Texapon® ES-1
Schercemol IPM	Supro-Tein V	Synperonic OP40/70	Texapon® ES-2
Schercemol MEL-3	Surfactol® 13	Syntopon A	Texapon® ES-3
Schercemol MEM-3	Surfactol® 318	Syntopon D	Texapon® N 25
Schercemol MEP-3	Surfactol® 365	Syntopon D2	Texapon® N 70
Schercemol OLO	Surfactol® 575	Syntopon F	Texapon® PN-235
Schercemol PGML	Surfactol® 590	Syntopon G	Texapon® PN-254
Schercomid AME	Surfine AZI-A	Tagat® I	Texapon® T 35
Schercomid AME-70	Surfine WLG-A	Tagat® I2	T-Maz® 20
Schercomid LME	Surfine WLL	Tagat® L	T-Maz® 28
Schercomid SI	Surfine WNG-A	Tagat® L2	T-Maz® 40
Schercomid SLE	Surfonic® N-10	Tagat® O	T-Maz® 60
Schercopol CMS-Na	Surfonic® N-31.5	Tagat® O2	T-Maz® 61
Schercopol OMS-Na	Surfonic® N-40	Tagat® R40	T-Maz® 65
SCS 40	Surfonic® N-60	Tagat® R60	T-Maz® 80
Sellig R 3395	Surfonic® N-85	Tagat® R63	T-Maz® 80K
Sellig T 14 100	Surfonic® N-95	Tagat® RI	T-Maz® 80KLM

Solubilizers/Hydrotropes/Coupling Agents *(cont'd.)*

T-Maz® 81	Vanseal® MS	Volpo 25 D 10	Volpo T-15
T-Maz® 85	Vanseal® NAMS-30	Volpo 25 D 15	Volpo T-20
T-Maz® 90	Varion® CDG	Volpo 25 D 20	Waxenol® 801
T-Maz® 95	Varonic® 63 E20	Volpo CS-3	Wickenol® 101
TO-33-F	Varonic® BD	Volpo CS-5	Wickenol® 105
Triton® X-100	Varonic® BG	Volpo CS-10	Wickenol® 111
Trycol® 5878	Varonic® LI-42	Volpo CS-15	Wickenol® 131
Trycol® 5964	Varonic® LI-48	Volpo CS-20	Wickenol® 136
Trycol® 5972	Varonic® LI-63	Volpo L23	Wickenol® 139
Trylox® 6746	Varonic® LI-67	Volpo N3	Wickenol® 141
Turkey Red Oil 100%	Varonic® LI-67 (75%)	Volpo N5	Wickenol® 163
Türkischrotöl 100%	Velsan® D8P-3	Volpo N10	Wickenol® 171
Tween® 20	Velsan® D8P-16	Volpo N15	Wickenol® 707
Tween® 20 SD	Velvetex® AB-45	Volpo N20	Wickenol® 727
Tween® 21	Vigilan	Volpo O3	Witafrol® 7420
Tween® 40	Vigilan AWS	Volpo O5	Witcamide® 6546
Tween® 61	Volpo 3	Volpo O10	Witcamide® S771
Tween® 80K	Volpo 5	Volpo O15	Witcamide® S780
Tween® 81	Volpo 10	Volpo O20	Witcolate™ A
Tween® 85	Volpo 20	Volpo T-3	Witcolate™ T
Unimate® DIPS	Volpo 25 D 3	Volpo T-5	Witconate™ 60B
Unitina E-24	Volpo 25 D 5	Volpo T-10	Witconate™ 93S
Unitolate 80MG			

Solvents

Acetamide MEA	900	Dow B100-1000	Estasan GT 8-40 3578
Acetol® 1706	Carbowax® Sentry® PEG	Dow B100-2000	Estasan GT 8-60 3575
Acetulan®	1000	Dow B100-4800	Estasan GT 8-60 3580
Adol® 52 NF	Carbowax® Sentry® PEG	Dow EP530	Estasan GT 8-65 3577
Adol® 60	1450	Dow L910	Estasan GT 8-65 3581
Adol® 80	Carbowax® Sentry® PEG	Dow L1150	Eumulgin® PWM2
Adol® 85	3350	Dow MPEG350	Exxal® 16
Adol® 640	Carbowax® Sentry® PEG	Dow MPEG550	Fancol ALA
Agnosol 3	4600	Dow MPEG750	Fancol Karite Butter
Agnosol 5	Carbowax® Sentry® PEG	Dow P425	Fancol OA-95
Alkapol PEG 300	8000	Dow P1000TB	Fancorsil A
Ameroxol® OE-2	Cellosolve®	Dow P1200	Flexricin® 9
Arlamol® E	Cellosolve® Acetate	Dow P2000	Foamid LM2E
Axol® E 61	Ceraphyl® 28	Dow P4000	G-100
Axol® E 66	Ceraphyl® 140	Dow PT250	G-4972
Butyl Carbitol®	Ceraphyl® 140-A	Dow PT700	GBL
Butyl Cellosolve®	Ceraphyl® ICA	Dow PT3000	Gilugel MIG
Capmul® MCM	Cetiol® B	Drakeol 7	Gilugel MIN
Capmul® MCM-90	Chemax E-1000 MO	Edenol 302	Gilugel SIL5
Captex® 200	Cithrol 2DL	Ektasolve® DB	Glucam® E-10
Captex® 300	Cithrol 2DO	Ektasolve® DB Acetate	Glucam® E-20
Captex® 350	Cithrol 4DL	Ektasolve® DE	Glucam® P-10
Captex® 810A	Cithrol 4DO	Ektasolve® DE Acetate	Glucam® P-20
Captex® 810B	Cithrol 6DL	Ektasolve® DM	Hetester PMA
Captex® 810C	Cithrol 6DO	Ektasolve® DP	Imwitor® 408
Captex® 810D	Cithrol 10DL	Ektasolve® EEH	Imwitor® 412
Captex® 910A	Cithrol 10DO	Ektasolve® EP	Imwitor® 742
Captex® 910B	Corona Lanolin	Ektasolve® PM Acetate	Imwitor® 908
Captex® 910C	Coronet Lanolin	Emcol® CC-42	Incromectant AMEA-70
Captex® 910D	Cosmetol® X	Emcol® CC-55	Isopar® G
Captex® 8227	Crill 1	Emcol® CC-57	Isopar® H
Carbitol® Acetate	Crill 2	EmCon CO	Isopar® K
Carbowax® PEG 300	Crodamol DA	EmCon Olive	Isopar® L
Carbowax® Sentry® PEG	Crodamol IPL	EmCon Rice Bran	Isopar® M
300	Crodamol IPM	EmCon W	Kemstrene® 96.0%
Carbowax® Sentry® PEG	Crodamol IPP	EmCon Walnut	Kemstrene® 99.7%
400	Crodamol PMP	Emerest® 2452	Kessco® Isopropyl
Carbowax® Sentry® PEG	Crystal® O	Emery® 912	Myristate
540 Blend	Crystal® Crown	Emery® 916	Kessco® Isopropyl
Carbowax® Sentry® PEG	Dermol ICSA	Emery® 918	Palmitate
600	Dow 15-200	Emery® 6709	Lanpol 5
Carbowax® Sentry® PEG	Dow 112-2	Estalan 430	Lanpol 10

Solvents *(cont'd.)*

Lanpol 20
Lanpol 520
Lexol® 3975
Lexol® GT-855
Lexol® GT-865
Lexol® IPM
Lexol® IPM-NF
Lexol® PG-800
Lipolan R
Lipovol SES
Lipovol SES-S
Liquid Absorption Base
  Type A, T
Lonzest® 143-S
Lowenol 915
Lutrol® E 300
Lutrol® E 400
Macol® 16
Miglyol® 810
Miglyol® 812
Miglyol® 840
Monolan® PPG440,
  PPG1100, PPG2200
Myritol® 318
Myritol® PC
Naetex-L
Naturechem® GTR
Naturechem® MAR
Neobee® 18
Neobee® 20
Neobee® 1054
Neobee® 1062
Neobee® M-5
Neobee® M-20
Neobee® O
Niox KJ-10
Niox KS Series

Olepal ISO
Pegol® P-400
Pegol® P-700
Pegol® P-1000
Pegol® P-2000
Pelemol G7A
Penreco Snow
Permethyl® 99A
Pluracol® E200
Pluracol® E300
Pluracol® E400
Pluracol® E600
Pluracol® E600 NF
Pluracol® E1000
Pluracol® E1450
Pluracol® E1450 NF
Pluracol® E1500
Pluracol® E4000
Pluracol® E6000
Pogol 400 NF
Polychol 5
Polylan®
Procetyl 10
Procetyl 30
Procetyl 50
Promyr
Propal
Prox-onic MG-020 P
Radia® 7131
Radia® 7241
Radia® 7730
Radia® 7732
Radia® 7752
Radia® 7761
Radia® 7770
Rewomid® OM 101/G
Rewomid® OM 101/IG

Rewomid® OM 101/IG/ER
Rewopal® MPG 10
Rhodacal® 330
Rhodasurf® PEG 400
Rhodasurf® PEG 600
Ricinion
Ritawax AEO
Ritawax ALA
Schercemol 1818
Schercemol CO
Schercemol DIA
Schercemol DICA
Schercemol DIS
Schercemol IPM
Schercemol NGDC
Schercemol NGDO
Schercemol OLO
Schercemol PGDP
Schercemol PGML
Solulan® 5
Solulan® 16
Solulan® 75
Solulan® C-24
Solulan® L-575
Soluphor® P
Solutol® HS 15
Solvent APV Spec
Solvent PM
Standamul® G-16
Stearate 400 WL 817
Stearate 1500
Stearate 6000 WL 1644
Super Refined™ Almond
  Oil NF
Super Refined™ Corn Oil
Super Refined™

Cottonseed Oil
Super Refined™ Olive Oil
Super Refined™ Peanut Oil
Super Refined™ Safflower
  Oil USP
Super Refined™ Sesame
  Oil
Super Refined™ Soybean
  Oil USP
Tegosoft® 189
Teric PPG 1650
Transcutol
Trivent NP-13
Ucon® 75-H-450
Ucon® Fluid AP
Ucon® LB-625
Ucon® LB-1145
Ucon® LB-1715
Ucon® LB-3000
Ucon® LO-500
Ucon® LO-1000
Unimate® BYS
Uniplex 110
Uniplex 150
Upiwax 350
Wickenol® 127
Wickenol® 136
Wickenol® 151
Wickenol® 152
Wickenol® 153
Wickenol® 158
Wickenol® 171
York Krystal Kleer Castor
  Oil
York USP Castor Oil

Stabilizers

Ablunol S-20
Ablunol S-40
Ablunol S-60
Ablunol S-80
Ablunol S-85
A-C® 6A
A-C® 15
A-C® 16
A-C® 143
A-C® 430
A-C® 540, 540A
A-C® 580
A-C® 617, 617A
A-C® 617G
Acetulan®
Acrisint 400, 410, 430
Acritamer® 934
Acritamer® 934P
Acritamer® 940
Acritamer® 941
Acrymul AM 123R
Acrysol 22
Acrysol 33
Aculyn™ 22
Aculyn™ 33
Acusol® 820
Adol® 52 NF

Adol® 61
Adol® 62 NF
Adol® 63
Adol® 64
Adol® 80
Adol® 90 NF
Adol® 520 NF
Adol® 620 NF
Adol® 630
Alanate 110
Alcolec® BS
Alcolec® Granules
Alcolec® Powder
Aldo® HMS
Aldo® MS LG
Aldo® PMS
Alkamide® CDE
Alkamuls® EL-620L
Alkamuls® SEG
Alkasurf® NP-4
Alkasurf® NP-40, 70%
Amercell® Polymer HM-
  1500
Amerchol® 400
Amerchol® BL
Amerchol® C
Amerchol® CAB

Amerchol® H-9
Amerchol® L-99
Amerchol L-101®
Amerchol® L-500
Amerchol® RC
Amerlate® LFA
Amerlate® P
Amerlate® WFA
Ameroxol® OE-2
Ameroxol® OE-5
Ameroxol® OE-10
Ameroxol® OE-20
Amidex KME
Amiter LGS-5
AMP
Amphisol®
Amphisol® K
Anhydrous Lanolin USP
  Cosmetic Grade
Anhydrous Lanolin USP
  Pharmaceutical Grade
Anhydrous Lanolin USP
  Pharmaceutical Light
  Grade
Anhydrous Lanolin USP
  X-tra Deodorized
Argobase EU

Argobase L1
Argobase MS 5
Argobase S1
Arlatone® 985
Armeen® Z
Aromox® C/12
Aromox® C/12-W
Arosurf® 66-E2
Arosurf® 66-E10
Arosurf® 66-E20
Aubygel X52
Belsil DMC 6031
Belsil DMC 6032
Belsil DMC 6033
Belsil DMC 6035
Benecel® M
Benecel® ME
Benecel® MP
Bentone® 27
Bentone® Gel CAO
Bentone® Gel IPM
Bentone® Gel ISD
Bentone® Gel LOI
Bentone® Gel M20
Bentone® Gel MIO
Bentone® Gel MIO A-40
Bentone® Gel SS71

Stabilizers *(cont'd.)*

Bentone® Gel TN
Bentone® Gel TN A-40
Bentone® Gel VS-5
Bentone® Gel VS-5 PC
Bentone® LT
Bentone® MA
Biopolymer HI-13DC
Blanose 7 Types
Blanose 9 Types
Blanose 12 Types
Byco A
Byco C
Byco O
Calsoft L-40
Calsoft L-60
Capmul® GMS
Caprol® 3GS
Caprol® 10G4O
Carbopol® 907
Carbopol® 940
Carbopol® 941
Carbopol® 954
Carbopol® 980
Carbopol® 981
Carbopol® 1342
Carbopol® 2984
Carbopol® 5984
Carboset 514
Carboset XL-19X2
Carboset XL-28
Carboset XL-40
Carboset XPD-1616
Carraghenate P, Standard,
   X 2
Carsamide® CMEA
Carsonon® 144-P
Carsonon® 169-P
Carsonon® N-100
Cationic Guar C-261
Cavitron Cyclo-dextrin.™
Cellulon
Cera Bellina®
Cera Euphorbia
Cerasynt® 840
Ceresine Wax Cosmetic
   Stralpitz
Ceresine Wax SP 84
Cetostearyl Alcohol BP
Cetostearyl Alcohol NF
Chel DTPA
Chemal BP 261
Chemal BP-262
Chemal BP-262LF
Chemal BP-2101
Chemax OP-3
Chemax OP-5
Chemsperse GMS
Chemsperse GMS-SE
Chesguar C10, C10R
Chesguar C17
Chesguar C20, C20R
Chesguar HP4
Chesguar HP4R
Chitin Liq
Cholesterol NF
Chronosponge
Cithrol GDO N/E
Cithrol GDO S/E

Cithrol GDS N/E
Cithrol GDS S/E
Cithrol GML N/E
Cithrol GML S/E
Cithrol GMO N/E
Cithrol GMO S/E
Cithrol GMR N/E
Cithrol GMR S/E
Cithrol GMS Acid Stable
Cithrol GMS N/E
Cithrol GMS S/E
Cithrol PGML N/E
Cithrol PGML S/E
Cithrol PGMO N/E
Cithrol PGMO S/E
Cithrol PGMR N/E
Cithrol PGMR S/E
Cithrol PGMS N/E
Cithrol PGMS S/E
Co-Gell® A2/B270
Cosmedia Guar® C-261 N
Cosmedia Guar® U
Cosmowax
Cosmowax J
Cosmowax K
Cosmowax P
Cremophor® S 9
Crillon ODE
Crodacol C-95NF
Crodacol S-95NF
Crodafos CDP
Crodafos CKP
Crodafos CS2 Acid
Crodafos CS5 Acid
Crodafos CS10 Acid
Crodafos N-5 Acid
Crodafos SG
Crodamol BE
Crosilk Powder
Crotein O
Cutina® CBS
Cutina® MD
Cyclomox® SO
Dariloid® QH
Deriphat® 160
Deriphat® 160C
Dermalcare® C-20
Dermalcare® SPS
Dermol 185
Drewmulse® 200K
Drewmulse® GMO
Drewmulse® HM-100
Drewmulse® TP
Drewmulse® V
Drewmulse® V-SE
Drewpol® 10-4-O
Dulectin
Dusoran MD
Dynasan® P60
Elastinhydrolysate, Liq
Elastinhydrolysate, Powd
Elfacos® C26
Elfacos® ST 9
Elfacos® ST 37
Emalex 400A
Emalex 400B
Emalex 805
Emalex 810

Emalex 820
Emalex 830
Emalex 840
Emalex 6300 DI-ST
Emalex DEG-m-S
Emalex EGS-A
Emalex EGS-B
Emalex GMS-55FD
Emalex GWIS-103
Emalex GWIS-105
Emalex GWIS-106
Emalex GWIS-108
Emalex GWS-310
Emalex GWS-320
Emalex LWIS-8
Emalex LWIS-10
Emalex PEIS-3
Emalex PEIS-6
Emalex PGML
Emalex PGMS
Emalex SWS-9
Emalex SWS-10
Emalex SWS-12
Emcol® 4400-1
Emerest® 2350
Emerest® 2355
Emerest® 2715
Emery® 1730
Emery® 1732
Emery® 1780
Emid® 6510
Emid® 6515
Empilan® CME
Empilan® EGMS
Empilan® LME
Emulgator E 2149 SE
Emulgator E 2155 SE
Emulgator E 2568 SE
Emulmetik™ 120
Emulsynt® 1055
Epikuron 145
Ethomid® HT/60
Ethosperse® CA-2
Ethosperse® LA-23
Ethosperse® OA-2
Ethylene Glycol
   Monostearate VA
Eudispert
Fancol CA
Fancol LA
Fancol LAO
Fancol OA-95
Fancol SA
Fancor LFA
Flexricin® 9
Forlan 200
Forlan 300
Forlan 500
Forlan C-24
Forlan L
Forlan LM
Freederm
Gafac® RE-877
Gantrez® AN
Gantrez® ES-225
Gantrez® ES-335
Gantrez® ES-425
Gantrez® ES-435

Gantrez® V-215
Gantrez® V-225
Gantrez® V-425
Gatarol M 30 M
Gelcarin LA
Gelwhite MAS-H, MAS-L
Generol® 122
Generol® 122E5
Generol® 122E10
Generol® 122E16
Genu Carrageenan
Genugel
Genulacta Series
Genu Pectins
Genuvisco
Gilugel ALM
Gilugel CAO
Gilugel EUG
Gilugel IPM
Gilugel IPP
Gilugel MIG
Gilugel MIN
Gilugel R
Gilugel SIL5
Gilugels
Glucamate® SSE-20
Glucate® SS
Gomme Xanthane
Grillocam E10
Grillomuls L90
Grillomuls S40
Grillomuls S60
Grillomuls S90
Hamp-Ene® Acid
Haro® Chem ALMD-2
Hartolan
Hispagel® 100
Hispagel® 200
Hodag GML
Hodag GMO
Hodag GMO-D
Hodag GMR
Hodag GMR-D
Hodag GMS
Hodag GTO
Hodag Nonionic E-100
Hydrine
Hydroxylan
Hystrene® 5016 NF
Igepal® CO-430
Igepal® DM-970 FLK
Imwitor® 191
Imwitor® 900
Imwitor® 900 K
Imwitor® 940
Imwitor® 940 K
Imwitor® 945
Incromine Oxide C-35
Junlon PW-110
Junlon PW-111
Kelacid®
Kelco® HV
Kelco® LV
Kelcoloid® D
Kelcoloid® DH, DO, DSF
Kelcoloid® HVF, LVF, O, S
Kelcosol®
Kelgin® F

Stabilizers *(cont'd.)*

Kelgin® HV, LV, MV
Kelgin® QL
Kelgin® XL
Kelmar®
Kelset®
Keltone
Keltose®
Keltrol®, Keltrol F
Kemester® 2000
Kemester® 5500
Kessco® EGAS
Kessco® Ethylene Glycol
   Monostearate
Klucel® EF
Klucel® ELF, GF, HF, JF,
   LF, MF
Kollidon®
Kollidon® 12PF, 17PF
Kollidon® 25, 30, 90
Kollidon® CL
Koster Keunen Candelilla
   Ester
Koster Keunen Carnauba
   No. 1
Koster Keunen Carnauba
   T-2
Koster Keunen Carnauba
   T-3
Koster Keunen Ceresine
   130/135
Koster Keunen Ceresine
   140/145
Koster Keunen Ceresine
   155
Koster Keunen Ceresine
   192
Koster Keunen Hydroxy-
   Polyester
Koster Keunen Microcrys-
   talline Wax 170/180
Koster Keunen Microcrys-
   talline Wax 193/198
Koster Keunen Paraffin
   Wax 122/128
Koster Keunen Paraffin
   Wax 130/135
Koster Keunen Paraffin
   Wax 140/145
Koster Keunen Paraffin
   Wax 150/155
Koster Keunen Synthetic
   Candelilla
Koster Keunen Synthetic
   Candelilla R-4
Koster Keunen Synthetic
   Candelilla R-8
Koster Keunen Synthetic
   Carnauba
Labrafil® WL 1958 CS
Laneto 27
Laneto 100
Lanfrax®
Lanfrax® 1776
Lanfrax® 1779
Lanolin Cosmetic
Lanolin Extra-Deodorized
Lanolin Pharmaceutical
Lanolin USP

Lanpolamide 5
Lexemul® 503
Lexemul® 515
Lexemul® AR
Lexemul® AS
Lexemul® GDL
Lexemul® T
Lexol® GT-865
Lipamide S
Lipo DGLS
Lipo DGS-SE
Lipo EGDS
Lipo EGMS
Lipo GMS 450
Lipo GMS 470
Lipo PGMS
Lipolan 31-20
Lipolan Distilled
Lipomulse 165
Lipovol GTB
Liquid Base
Lonzest® PEG 4-L
Lonzest® SMO-20
Lonzest® SMP-20
Lonzest® SMS-20
Lonzest® STO-20
Lonzest® STS-20
Loropan KD
Luviform® FA 119
Luviskol® VA28E
Luviskol® VA28I
Luviskol® VA37E
Luviskol® VA37I
Luviskol® VA55E
Luviskol® VA55I
Luviskol® VA64E
Luviskol® VA64I
Luviskol® VA64W
Luviskol® VA73E
Luviskol® VA73I
Luviskol® VA73W
Macol® E-200
Macol® E-300
Macol® E-400
Macol® E-600
Macol® E-1000
Macol® E-3350
Macol® LA-4
Macol® LA-9
Macol® LA-12
Macol® LA-23
Macol® OA-2
Macol® OA-4
Macol® OA-5
Macol® OA-10
Macol® OA-20
Macol® SA-2
Macol® SA-5
Macol® SA-10
Macol® SA-15
Macol® SA-20
Macol® SA-40
Macol® TD-3
Macol® TD-8
Macol® TD-10
Macol® TD-12
Macol® TD-15
Macol® TD-100

Macol® TD-610
Mafo® CAB
Magnabrite® F
Magnabrite® HV
Magnabrite® K
Magnabrite® S
Mazamide® 80
Mazamide® L-5
Mazamide® SMEA
Merpol® HCS
Methocel® 40-100
Methocel® 40-101
Methocel® 40-202
Methocel® A4CP
Methocel® A4MP
Methocel® A15-LV
Methocel® A15LVP
Methocel® E3P
Methocel® E4MP
Methocel® E6P
Methocel® E15LVP
Methocel® E50LVP
Methocel® E50P
Methocel® K4MP
Methocel® K4MS
Methocel® K15MP
Methocel® K15MS
Methocel® K35
Methocel® K100LVP
Methocel® K100MP
Mexpectin LA 100 Range
Mexpectin LC 700 Range
Mexpectin XSS 100 Range
Miglyol® 840 Gel
Miglyol® 840 Gel B
Miglyol® 840 Gel T
Miglyol® Gel
Miglyol® Gel B
Miglyol® Gel T
Miranol® C2M Conc. NP
Mirasoft™ CO 11
Mirasoft™ LMO
Mirasoft™ MSPO 11
Miristamina
Monomuls® 60-10
Monomuls® 60-15
Monomuls® 60-20
Monomuls® 60-25
Monomuls® 60-25/2
Monomuls® 60-30
Monomuls® 60-35
Monomuls® 60-40
Monomuls® 60-45
Monomuls® 90-10
Monomuls® 90-15
Monomuls® 90-20
Monomuls® 90-25/2,
   90-25/5
Monomuls® 90-30
Monomuls® 90-35
Monomuls® 90-40
Monomuls® 90-45
Monomuls® 90-O18
Monosteol
Monthyle
Myverol® P-06
Natrosol® Plus CS
Natrosol® Plus CS,

Grade 330
Naturechem® GTH
Naturechem® PGHS
Naturechem® PGR
Naturechem® THS-200
Nikkol Behenyl Alcohol 65,
   80
Nikkol CS
Nikkol DDP-2
Nikkol DDP-4
Nikkol DDP-6
Nikkol DDP-8
Nikkol DDP-10
Nikkol GBW-25
Nikkol GBW-125
Nikkol GM-18IS
Nikkol GM-18S
Nikkol Lecinol LL-20
Nikkol Lecinol SH
Nikkol MGS-A
Nikkol MGS-ASE
Nikkol MGS-B
Nikkol MGS-DEX
Nikkol MGS-F20
Nikkol MGS-F50
Nikkol MGS-F75
Nikkol PMS-1C
Nikkol PMS-1CSE
Nikkol PMS-FR
Nikkol VF-E
Nikkol VF-IP
Nimco® 1780
Nipanox® Special
Nissan Nonion LP-20R,
   LP-20RS
Norfox® B
Norfox® Coco Powder
Norfox® GMS
Norfox® NP-1
Norgel
Novol
OHlan®
Optigel CD, CF, CG, CK,
   CL
Oxynex® K
Oxynex® L
Patlac® NAL
Pegosperse® 50 DS
Pegosperse® 6000 DS
Pegosperse® EGMS-70
Permulgin 835
Phosal® NAT-50-PG
Phospholipon® 90 H
Plasdone® C-15
Plasdone® C-30
Plasdone® K-25, K-90
Plasdone® K-26/28,
   K-29/32
Pluracol® E200
Pluracol® E300
Pluracol® E400
Pluracol® E600
Pluracol® E600 NF
Pluracol® E1000
Pluracol® E1450
Pluracol® E1450 NF
Pluracol® E1500
Pluracol® E4000

Stabilizers *(cont'd.)*

Pluracol® E6000	Radiacid® 427	Span® 60, 60K	Tetronic® 1504
Plurol Stearique WL 1009	Radiacid® 428	Span® 65	Tetronic® 1508
Pluronic® 10R5	Radiacid® 464	Span® 85	T-Maz® 20
Pluronic® 10R8	Radiacid® 631	Spectra-Sorb® UV 24	T-Maz® 28
Pluronic® 12R3	Radianol® 1712	Spectra-Sorb® UV 5411	T-Maz® 40
Pluronic® 17R1	Radianol® 1724	Stabileze™ 06	T-Maz® 60
Pluronic® 17R2	Radianol® 1726	Stamere®	T-Maz® 61
Pluronic® 17R4	Radianol® 1728	Stamid LS 5487	T-Maz® 65
Pluronic® 17R8	Radianol® 1763	Standamid® CD	T-Maz® 80
Pluronic® 22R4	Radianol® 1765	Standamid® CMG	T-Maz® 80KLM
Pluronic® 25R1	Radianol® 1768	Standamid® KDS	T-Maz® 81
Pluronic® 25R2	Radianol® 1769	Standamul® G-32/36	T-Maz® 85
Pluronic® 25R4	Radianol® 1898	Stearate	T-Maz® 90
Pluronic® 25R5	Renex® 650	Super Hartolan	T-Maz® 95
Pluronic® 25R8	Rewocid® U 185	Superloid®	Tri-Tein Milk Polypeptide
Pluronic® 31R1	Rewomid® DL 203	Sustane® BHA	Trivent BE-13
Pluronic® 31R2	Rewomid® DL 240	Syncrowax ERL-C	Trivent SS-20
Pluronic® 31R4	Rewomid® IPL 203	Syncrowax HGL-C	Trycol® 5972
Pluronic® L10	Rewomid® IPP 240	Synperonic A20	Turpinal® 4 NL
Polawax®	Rewomid® L 203	T-Det® O-407	Turpinal® SL
Polyethylene 1000 HE	Rewomid® S 280	Tegin® 90 NSE	Uantox TBHQ
PolySurf	Rhaballgum CG-M	Tegin® 515	Unilin® 350 Alcohol
Polytex 10M	Rhodasurf® LAN-23-75%	Tegin® 515 VA	Unilin® 550 Alcohol
Porosponge	Rhodasurf® ON-870	Tegin® 4100 NSE	Unilin® 700 Alcohol
Probiol™ L/N	Rhodicare™ XC	Tegin® 4480	Upamide O-20
Promulgen® D	Rhodigel®	Tegin® GO	Uvinul® D 50
Promulgen® G	Rhodigel® 23	Tegin® GRB NSE	Vanate Acid
Propoxyol® 1695	Rita EDGS	Tegin® MAV	Vanate PSPA
Protamide MRCA	Rita EGMS	Tegin® M NSE	Vanate TS
Prox-onic CSA-1/04	Rita GMS	Tenox® PG	Vanate TSD
Prox-onic CSA-1/06	Ritachol®	Tenox® TBHQ	Vanate TSHE
Prox-onic CSA-1/010	Ritahydrox	Tetronic® 50R1	Vanate TS-N
Prox-onic CSA-1/015	R.I.T.A. Lanolin Wax	Tetronic® 50R4	Vanate TST
Prox-onic CSA-1/020	Ritavena™ 5	Tetronic® 50R8	Varonic® 32-E20
Prox-onic CSA-1/030	Ritawax	Tetronic® 70R1	Varonic® 63 E20
Prox-onic CSA-1/050	Ritawax Super	Tetronic® 70R2	Varonic® 2271
Prox-onic HR-05	Rohagit® S, SD 15	Tetronic® 70R4	Varonic® K-202
Prox-onic HR-016	Salcare SC90	Tetronic® 90R1	Varonic® K-202 SF
Prox-onic HR-025	Salcare SC91	Tetronic® 90R4	Varonic® K-205
Prox-onic HR-030	Salcare SC92	Tetronic® 90R8	Varonic® K-205 SF
Prox-onic HR-036	Salcare SC95	Tetronic® 110R1	Varonic® K-210
Prox-onic HR-040	Santone® 10-10-O	Tetronic® 110R2	Varonic® K-210 SF
Prox-onic HR-080	Schercamox DML	Tetronic® 110R7	Varonic® K-215
Prox-onic HR-0200	Schercamox DMM	Tetronic® 130R1	Varonic® K-215 SF
Prox-onic HR-0200/50	Schercemol 185	Tetronic® 130R2	Varonic® LI-420
Prox-onic HRH-05	Schercemol GMS	Tetronic® 150R1	Varonic® LI-420 (70%)
Prox-onic HRH-016	Schercemol PGML	Tetronic® 150R4	Varonic® Q-202
Prox-onic HRH-025	Schercomid SLE	Tetronic® 150R8	Varonic® Q-202 SF
Prox-onic HRH-0200	Schercomid SLS	Tetronic® 304	Varonic® Q-205
Prox-onic HRH-0200/50	Schercotaine CAB-K	Tetronic® 504	Varonic® Q-205 SF
Prox-onic LA-1/02	Schercotaine CAB-KG	Tetronic® 701	Varonic® S-202
Prox-onic LA-1/04	Schercotaine SCAB-K	Tetronic® 702	Varonic® S-202 SF
Prox-onic LA-1/09	Schercotaine SCAB-KG	Tetronic® 704	Varonic® S-202 SF
Prox-onic LA-1/012	Seagel L	Tetronic® 707	Varonic® T-202
Prox-onic LA-1/023	Seakem 3, LCM	Tetronic® 901	Varonic® T-202 SF
Prox-onic OA-1/04	Seaspen PF	Tetronic® 904	Varonic® T-205
Prox-onic OA-1/09	Sebase	Tetronic® 908	Varonic® T-205 SF
PVP K-15	Sobalg FD 100 Series	Tetronic® 909	Varonic® T-210
PVP K-30	Softisan® 378	Tetronic® 1101	Varonic® T-210 SF
PVP/VA S-630	Softisan® Gel	Tetronic® 1102	Varonic® T-215
Pyroter CPI-30	Solka-Floc® BW-40	Tetronic® 1104	Varonic® T-215 SF
Pyroter CPI-60	Solka-Floc® BW-100	Tetronic® 1107	Veegum®
Quatrisoft® Polymer	Solka-Floc® BW-200	Tetronic® 1301	Veegum® D
LM-200	Solka-Floc® BW-2030	Tetronic® 1302	Veegum® F
Radiacid® 152	Solka-Floc® Fine Granular	Tetronic® 1304	Veegum® HS
Radiacid® 212	Solwax C-24	Tetronic® 1307	Veegum® HV
Radiacid® 416	Span® 20	Tetronic® 1501	Veegum® K
Radiacid® 423	Span® 40	Tetronic® 1502	Veegum® PRO
			Veegum® Ultra

Stabilizers *(cont'd.)*

Veegum® WG	Versene 100 XL	EDTA	Versenex 80
Versene 100	Versene 220	Versene NA	Versenol 120
Versene 100 EP	Versene Acid	Versene Tetraammonium	Viscarin XLV
Versene 100 LS	Versene CA	EDTA	Wickenol® 707
Versene 100 SRG	Versene Diammonium		

Suncare Additives (Sunscreens, Tanning Accelerators)

Abil® 10-10000	Escin/β-Sitosterol	190	Solarium HS 270, LS 670
Abil® AV 20-1000	Phytosome®	Koster Keunen Paraffin	Solarium Special HS 271,
Abil® WE 09	Estalan MA	Wax 122/128	LS 671
Actibronze	Estran™-Lite	Koster Keunen Paraffin	Solar Shield™
Activera™ 106 LIPO M	Estran™-Pure	Wax 130/135	Sungen
Alfonic® 1012-2.5	Estran™-Xtra	Koster Keunen Paraffin	Sun-Tanning Bioactivator
Almond Oil	Finex-25	Wax 140/145	AMI, VITAMI
Aloe Vera Gel 1:1	Finex-25-020	Koster Keunen Paraffin	Sunveil 6010
Aloe Vera Gel 1:1, 10:1,	Gamma Oryzanol	Wax 150/155	Sunveil 6030
40:1	Gilugel MIN	Koster Keunen Stearic Acid	Sunveil F
Aloe Vera Oil	Gilugel OS	XXX	Transparent Titanium
Aloe Vera Powd. 200:1	Gilugel SIL5	Koster Keunen Synthetic	Dioxide PW Covafluor
Alpinamed Chamomile	Granamine S3A	Beeswax	Transparent Titanium
Alpinamed Ivy	Gransil FL-D 55	Kowet Titanium Dioxide	Dioxide PW Covalim
Alpinamed Witch Hazel	Herbasol Complex A	Kronos® 1025	Transparent Titanium
Arlatone® 507	Herbasol Complex B	Lanaetex-OS	Dioxide PW Covasil S
Ascorbosilane C	Herbasol Extract Walnut	Lipofilter ODP	Transparent Titanium
Atlas White Titanium	Shell Oil-Sol	Lipomicron N.S.L.E	Dioxide PW Covasop
Dioxide	Herbasol Extract Walnut	Lipomicron Vitamin A	Transparent Titanium
Biophytex®	Shell Water-Sol	Palmitate	Dioxide PW Powd
Bioprotector AMI	Hispagel® 100	Lipomicron Vitamin E	Transparent Titanium
Biosil Basics Fluoro	Hispagel® 200	Acetate	Dioxide PW Squatol S
Guerbet 1.0%	Homosalate®	Liposome Unsapo KM	Trivent MA
Biosil Basics Fluoro	Iniferine	Luxelen® D	Trivent NP-13
Guerbet 3.5%	Instabronze	N,L-Malyl-L-Tyrosine	Trivent OS
Biosil Basics Jasmine	Kemester® HMS	Meristami	Tyr-Ol
Wax S	Kester Wax® 72	MicroReservoir FRS-	Tyrosilane C
α-Bisabolol	Kester Wax® 82	Diffuser	UFZO
Brookosome® TA	Kester Wax® 105	MicroReservoir Hydro-	Uniderm HOMSAL
Brookosome® UV	Koster Keunen Ceresine	Diffuser	Unifilter U-41
Ceramide HO3	130/135	MicroReservoir Nutri-	Uninontan U 34
CMI 321	Koster Keunen Ceresine	Diffuser	Unipertan P-24
CMI 400	140/145	Microsponge® 5650	Unipertan P-242
CMI 551	Koster Keunen Ceresine	MTD-25	Unipertan P-2002
CMI 800	155	Oleo-A.F.R	Unipertan VEG 24
Copherol® 950LC	Koster Keunen Ceresine	Orange Wax, Deodorized	Unipertan VEG 242
Dermoblock MA	192	Padimate O	Uniwhite AO
Dermol 105	Koster Keunen Hydroxy-	Parsol® MCX	Uniwhite KO
Destressine 2000	Polyester	Pecosil® PS-100K	USP-2
Dihydroxyacetone	Koster Keunen Microcrys-	Permulgin 835	Uvasorb MET
Dow Corning® 2501	talline Wax 170/180	Permulgin CSB	Uvasorb S-5
Cosmetic Wax	Koster Keunen Microcrys-	Permulgin RWB	UV-Titan M210
Eastman® AQ 29D	talline Wax 193/198	Phytotan	UV-Titan M212
Eastman® AQ 35S	Koster Keunen Ozokerite	Polyolprepolymer-2	UV-Titan M260
Eastman® AQ 38D	153/160	Pot Marigold AMI	UV-Titan M262
Eijitsu Extract BG	Koster Keunen Ozokerite	Riboflavin-5´-Phosphate	Vitamin A and D-3
Eldew CL-301	158/160	Sodium USP, FCC	Vitamin A Palmitate Type
Elefac™ I-205	Koster Keunen Ozokerite	Rocou AMI	P1.7
Emulmetik™ 300	160/164	Salcare SC91	Vitamin A Palmitate Type
Emulmetik™ 320	Koster Keunen Ozokerite	Salcare SC95	P1.7/BHT
Enzyami No. 1	164/170	Shea Butter	Vitamin A Palmitate Type
Enzyami No. 1A	Koster Keunen Ozokerite	Shea Unsaponifiable Conc	PIMO/BH
Enzyami No. 5	170	Solarium HS 268, LS 668	Z-Cote®
Enzyami No. 5A	Koster Keunen Ozokerite	Solarium HS 269, LS 669	Zinc Oxide USP 66

Thickeners/Gelling Agents/Thixotropes/
Rheological Additives/Viscosity Modifiers

Abil®-Wax 9810
Ablumide CDE
Ablumide CDE-G
Ablumide CKD
Ablumide CME
Ablumide LDE
Ablumide LME
Ablumide SME
Ablumox CAPO
Ablumox LO
Ablunol 200MS
Ablunol 400MS
Ablunol 600MS
Ablunol 6000DS
Ablunol S-20
Ablunol S-40
Ablunol S-60
Ablunol S-80
Ablunol S-85
Abluter CPB
A-C® 6A
A-C® 8, 8A
A-C® 9, 9A, 9F
A-C® 15
A-C® 16
A-C® 143
A-C® 400
A-C® 430
A-C® 540, 540A
A-C® 580
A-C® 617, 617A
A-C® 617G
A-C® 1702
A-C® 5120
Accomid 50
Accomid C
Accomid PK
Acconon 200-DL
Acconon 200-MS
Acconon 400-DO
Acconon 400-ML
Acconon 400-MO
Acconon 400-MS
Acconon 1300
Acconon CA-5
Acconon CA-8
Acconon CA-9
Acconon CA-15
Acconon CON
Acconon E
Acconon TGH
Acconon W230
Acrisint 400, 410, 430
Acritamer® 934
Acritamer® 934P
Acritamer® 940
Acritamer® 941
Acrymul AM 123R
Acrysol 22
Acrysol 33
Acrysol® A-1
Acrysol® ICS-1 Thickener
Aculyn™ 22
Aculyn™ 33
Acusol® 820
Admox® 1214

Adol® 61
Adol® 62 NF
Adol® 63
Adol® 64
Adol® 520 NF
Adol® 620 NF
Adol® 630
Aerosil® 130
Aerosil® 200
Aerosil® 300
Ajidew N-50
Albagel 4446
Albagel Premium USP
  4444
Albagen 4439
Alberger®
Alconate® SBG-280
Alcoramnosan
Aldo® HMS
Aldo® MS LG
Aldo® PMS
Aldosperse® L L-20
Alkamide® 101 CG
Alkamide® 327
Alkamide® 1002
Alkamide® 1182
Alkamide® 1188
Alkamide® 1195
Alkamide® 2124
Alkamide® C-5
Alkamide® C-212
Alkamide® CDE
Alkamide® CDM
Alkamide® CDO
Alkamide® CL63
Alkamide® CME
Alkamide® CMO
Alkamide® DC-212
Alkamide® DC-212/S
Alkamide® DC-212/SE
Alkamide® DIN-100
Alkamide® DIN-295/S
Alkamide® DL-203/S
Alkamide® DL-207/S
Alkamide® DO-280/S
Alkamide® DS-280/S
Alkamide® KD
Alkamide® L7DE
Alkamide® L7DE-BT
Alkamide® L7DE-PG
Alkamide® L9DE
Alkamide® LE
Alkamide® SDO
Alkamuls® 400-DS
Alkamuls® 6000-DS
Alkamuls® EGDS
Alkamuls® EGMS/C
Alkamuls® GMS/C
Alkamuls® MM/M
Alkamuls® PSML-20
Alkamuls® SEG
Alkamuls® SS
Alkamuls® VR/50
Alkateric® PB
Amercell® Polymer
  HM-1500

Amfotex FV-28
Amide CMA-2
Amide RMA-2
Amidex CE
Amidex CME
Amidex KDO
Amidex KME
Amidex LD
Amidex LD-8
Amidex LMMEA
Amidex LN
Amidex O
Amidex PK
Amidex S
Amidex SE
Amidex SME
Amidox® C-2
Amidox® C-5
Amidox® L-5
Amigel
Amino Acid Gelatinization
  Agent
Aminol A-15
Aminol CM, CM Flakes,
  CM-C Flakes,
  CM-D Flakes
Aminol COR-2C
Aminol COR-4C
Aminol N
Aminol OF
Ammonyx® CO
Ammonyx® LO
Ammonyx® MCO
Ammonyx® OAO
Ammonyx® SO
Amphocerin® E
Ampholak BCA-30
Ampholan® E210
Amphosol® CA
Amphosol® CG
Amphosol® DM
Amphoteen BCA-30
Amphoteric N
AMS-33
Annonyx SO
Antarox® PGP 23-7
Antil® 141 Liq
Antil® 171
Antil® 208
APG® 600 CS
APG® 625 CS
Aqualon® Cellulose Gum
Argowax Cosmetic Super
Argowax Dist
Argowax Standard
Arlacel® 165
Arlacel® 186
Arlypon® F
Aromox® DM14D-W
Aromox® DMB
Aromox® DMCD
Aromox® DMMCD-W
Attasorb RVM Sorbent
Aubygel X52
Avamid 150
Barlox® 12

Barlox® 14
Barlox® 16S
Barlox® 18S
Barlox® C
Benecel® M
Benecel® ME
Benecel® MP
Bentolite H
Bentolite H 4430
Bentolite L
Bentolite WH
Bentone® 27
Bentone® 34
Bentone® 38
Bentone® 500
Bentone® EW
Bentone® Gel CAO
Bentone® Gel IPM
Bentone® Gel ISD
Bentone® Gel LOI
Bentone® Gel M20
Bentone® Gel MIO
Bentone® Gel MIO A-40
Bentone® Gel SS71
Bentone® Gel TN
Bentone® Gel TN A-40
Bentone® Gel VS-5
Bentone® Gel VS-5 PC
Bentone® LT
Bentone® MA
Bentone® SD-3
Bentonite USP BC 670
Bio-Pol® NCHAP
Biopolymer HI-13DC
Biosil Basics DL-30
Bio-Surf PBC-460
Biozan
Blanose 7 Types
Blanose 9 Types
Blanose 12 Types
Burtonite V7E
Calamide C
Calsuds CD-6
Caprol® 2G4S
Caprol® 10G4O
Caprol® 10G10S
Carbopol® 907
Carbopol® 910
Carbopol® 934P
Carbopol® 940
Carbopol® 941
Carbopol® 954
Carbopol® 980
Carbopol® 981
Carbopol® 1342
Carbopol® 2984
Carbopol® 5984
Carboset 514
Carboset XL-19X2
Carboset XL-28
Carboset XL-40
Carboset XPD-1616
Carbowax® Sentry® PEG
  300
Carbowax® Sentry® PEG
  400

Thickeners/Gelling Agents/Thixotropes... *(cont'd.)*

Carbowax® Sentry® PEG 540 Blend
Carbowax® Sentry® PEG 600
Carbowax® Sentry® PEG 900
Carbowax® Sentry® PEG 1000
Carbowax® Sentry® PEG 1450
Carbowax® Sentry® PEG 3350
Carbowax® Sentry® PEG 4600
Carbowax® Sentry® PEG 8000
Carraghenate P, Standard, X 2
Carsamide® CA
Carsamide® CMEA
Carsamide® O
Carsamide® SAC
Carsamide® SAL-7
Carsamide® SAL-9
Carsofoam® 1618
Cationic Guar C-261
Cecavon NA 61
Cecavon ZN 70
Cecavon ZN 71
Cecavon ZN 72
Cecavon ZN 73
Cecavon ZN 735
Cellosize® HEC QP Grades
Cellosize® HEC QP-3-L
Cellosize® HEC QP-40
Cellosize® HEC QP-100 M-H
Cellosize® HEC QP-300
Cellosize® HEC QP-4400-H
Cellosize® HEC QP-15,000-H
Cellosize® HEC QP-52,000-H
Cellosize® HEC WP Grades
Cellosize® Polymer PCG-10
Cellow 940
Centrolex® F
Cera-E
Cera Bellina®
Cera Euphorbia
Ceral 10
Ceral EFN
Ceral EN 6
Ceral G
Ceral P
Ceral PA
Ceral PW
Ceral TP
Ceraphyl® 424
Ceraphyl® 847
Cerasynt® 303
Cerasynt® 840
Cerasynt® 945
Cerasynt® D

Cerasynt® GMS
Cerasynt® M
Cerasynt® MN
Cerasynt® SD
Ceresine Wax Cosmetic Stralpitz
Ceresine Wax SP 84
Cetal
Cetax 16
Cetax 18
Cetax 50
Cetiol® SB45
Cetomil
Cetostearyl Alcohol BP
Cetostearyl Alcohol NF
Chembetaine C
Chembetaine CGF
Chembetaine L
Chembetaine OL-30
Chembetaine S
Chemoxide CAW
Chemoxide L
Chemoxide LM-30
Chemoxide O
Chemoxide ST
Chemoxide TAO
Chemoxide WC
Chemsperse EGDS
Chemsperse EGMS
Chemsperse GMS
Chesguar C10, C10R
Chesguar C17
Chesguar C20, C20R
Chesguar HP4
Chesguar HP4R
Chimipal DCL/M
Chimipal LDA
Chimipal MC
Chimipal OLD
Chronosponge
Cirami No. 1
Cithrol 2ML
Cithrol 2MO
Cithrol 2MS
Cithrol 3MS
Cithrol 4ML
Cithrol 4MO
Cithrol 4MS
Cithrol 6ML
Cithrol 6MO
Cithrol 6MS
Cithrol 10ML
Cithrol 10MO
Cithrol 10MS
Cithrol 15MS
Cithrol 40MO
Cithrol 40MS
Cithrol 60ML
Cithrol 60MO
Claytone 34
Claytone 40
Claytone AF
Claytone APA
Claytone XL
Co-Gell® A2/B270
Comperlan® 100
Comperlan® COD
Comperlan® F

Comperlan® HS
Comperlan® KD
Comperlan® KDO
Comperlan® LD
Comperlan® LD 9
Comperlan® LDO, LDS
Comperlan® LM
Comperlan® LMD
Comperlan® LP
Comperlan® LS
Comperlan® OD
Comperlan® P 100
Comperlan® PD
Comperlan® SDO
Comperlan® SM
Comperlan® VOD
Cosmedia Guar® C-261 N
Cosmedia Guar® U
Cosmetic Gelatin
CPH-380-N
Cremophor® S 9
Crodacid B
Crodacol C-70
Crodacol C-95NF
Crodacol C-NF
Crodacol S-70
Crodacol S-95NF
Crodacol S-USP
Crodafos CAP
Crodafos N-3 Acid
Crodafos N-3 Neutral
Crodafos N-10 Acid
Crodafos N-10 Neutral
Crodafos SG
Croda Lanosterol
Crodamol BB
Crodamol BE
Crodamol CSS
Crodamol GHS
Crodamol ICS
Crodamol MM
Crodamol SS
Crodesta F-160
Crodyne BY-19
Crosultaine E-30
Crosultaine T-30
Crothix
Cutina® BW
Cutina® CBS
Cutina® CP
Cutina® EGMS
Cutina® FS 25, FS 45
Cutina® FS 45 Flakes
Cutina® GMS
Cutina® HR
Cutina® MD
Cutina® MD-A
Cyclochem® PEG 200DS
Cyclochem® PEG 600DS
Cyclochem® PEG 6000DS
Cyclomox® SO
Cycloteric BET-OB50
Damox® 1010
Dantoin® MDMH
Dariloid® QH
Dehydag® Wax 14
Dehydag® Wax 16
Dehydag® Wax 18

Dehydag® Wax 22 (Lanette)
Dehydag® Wax O
Dehyton® AB-30
Dehyton® PAB-30
Dehyton® PK
Dermalcare® EGMS/SE
Dermalcare® GTIS
Dermalcare® LVL
Dermalcare® MST
Dermalcare® NI
Dermalcare® PGMS
Dermolan GLH
Detergent CR
Dionil® OC/K
Dow Corning® 580 Wax
Drewmulse® 200K
Drewmulse® GMO
Drewmulse® HM-100
Drewmulse® POE-SML
Drewmulse® POE-SMO
Drewmulse® POE-SMS
Drewmulse® POE-STS
Drewmulse® SML
Drewmulse® SMO
Drewmulse® SMS
Drewmulse® STS
Drewmulse® TP
Drewmulse® V
Drewmulse® V-SE
Drewpol® 10-4-O
Dynasan® 110
Dynasan® 112
Dynasan® 114
Dynasan® 116
Dynasan® 118
Dynasan® P60
EA-209
Edenor GMS
Elfacos® C26
Eltesol® ACS 60
Elvanol® 75-15
Emalex 200 di-AS
Emalex 200 di-L
Emalex 200 di-S
Emalex 300 di-L
Emalex 300 di-S
Emalex 400A
Emalex 400B
Emalex 400 di-AS
Emalex 400 di-L
Emalex 400 di-AS
Emalex 600 di-AS
Emalex 600 di-L
Emalex 600 di-S
Emalex 602
Emalex 603
Emalex 605
Emalex 606
Emalex 608
Emalex 611
Emalex 615
Emalex 620
Emalex 625
Emalex 630
Emalex 640
Emalex 800 di-L
Emalex 805

Thickeners/Gelling Agents/Thixotropes... *(cont'd.)*

Emalex 810
Emalex 820
Emalex 830
Emalex 840
Emalex 1000 di-L
Emalex 2505
Emalex 2510
Emalex 2515
Emalex 2520
Emalex 2525
Emalex 6300 DI-ST
Emalex 6300 M-ST
Emalex CS-5
Emalex CS-10
Emalex CS-15
Emalex CS-20
Emalex CS-24
Emalex CS-30
Emalex DEG-di-L
Emalex DEG-di-S
Emalex DEG-m-S
Emalex EG-di-L
Emalex EG-di-MPS
Emalex EG-di-S
Emalex EG-di-SE
Emalex EGS-A
Emalex EGS-B
Emalex GM-5
Emalex GM-10
Emalex GM-15
Emalex GM-6000
Emalex GWIS-340
Emalex GWIS-350
Emalex GWIS-360
Emalex GWO-340
Emalex GWO-350
Emalex GWO-360
Emalex HC-20
Emalex HC-30
Emalex HC-40
Emalex HC-50
Emalex HC-60
Emalex HC-80
Emalex HC-100
Emalex N-83
Emalex NN-5
Emalex NN-15
Emalex RWIS-150
Emalex RWIS-160
Emalex RWIS-330
Emalex RWIS-340
Emalex RWIS-350
Emalex RWIS-360
Emalex RWL-140
Emalex RWL-150
Emalex RWL-160
Emalex TEG-di-L
Emalex TEG-di-S
Emanon 3199, 3299R
Emanon 4110
Emcol® 6748
Emcol® CC-3718
Emcol® Coco Betaine
Emcol® L
Emcol® LO
Emcol® M
Emcol® NA-30
Emerest® 2350

Emerest® 2355
Emerest® 2452
Emerest® 2642
Emerest® 2662
Emerest® 2704
Emerest® 2711
Emerest® 2712
Emerest® 2717
Emerwax® 1253
Emery® 912
Emery® 916
Emery® 917
Emery® 918
Emery® 1780
Emery® 6709
Emery® 6748
Emery® 6752
Emid® 6500
Emid® 6510
Emid® 6515
Emid® 6518
Emid® 6519
Emid® 6521
Emid® 6531
Emid® 6534
Emid® 6590
Emkapol 6000
Emkapol 8000
Emkapol 8500
Empicol® TLP
Empicol® TLR
Empigen® 5083
Empigen® BB
Empigen® OB
Empigen® OB/AU
Empigen® OH25
Empigen® OS/A
Empigen® OS/AU
Empilan® 2125-AU
Empilan® CDEY
Empilan® CDX
Empilan® CM/F
Empilan® CME
Empilan® FE
Empilan® LDE
Empilan® LDX
Empilan® LIS
Empilan® LME
Emsorb® 2720
Emthox® 5964
Emthox® 5967
Emulgator DMR
Emulmetik 320
Emulmetik 930
Emulmetik 950
Emulmin 862
Emulvis®
Enagicol C-30B
Esi-Det CDA
Esi-Terge 10
Esi-Terge S-10
Espesilor AC Series
Espesilor AC-43
Espesilor AC-50
Ethosperse® CA-2
Ethosperse® CA-20
Ethosperse® LA-23
Ethosperse® OA-2

Ethylan® LM2
Ethylene Glycol
    Monostearate VA
Eudispert
Eumulgin® EO-33
Fancol CA
Fancol HL-20
Fancol HL-24
Fancol LA
Fancol SA
FK 500LS
Flowtone R
Foamid C
Foamid PK
Foamid SCE
Foamid SL-Extra
Foamid SLM
Foamole A
Foamole M
Foamquat 2IAE
Foamquat SAQ-90
Forlan C-24
Freederm
G-1821
Gantrez® AN
Gelcarin LA
Geltone
Geltone 1665
Geltone II
Gelwhite GP, H
Gelwhite L
Gelwhite MAS-H, MAS-L
Genaminox CS
Genaminox KC
Genapol® L-3
Generol® 122
Generol® 122E5
Genu Carrageenan
Genugel
Genulacta Series
Genu Pectins
Genuvisco
Geropon® AS-200
Geropon® AS-250
Geropon® T-77
Geropon® TC-42
Gilugel ALM
Gilugel CAO
Gilugel EUG
Gilugel IPM
Gilugel IPP
Gilugel MIG
Gilugel MIN
Gilugel OS
Gilugel R
Gilugel SIL5
Gilugels
Glucamate® DOE-120
Glycon® G 100
Glycon® G-300
Gomme Xanthane
Green Clay
Grillomuls L90
Grillomuls O90
Grilloten® LSE 65 K
Grilloten® LSE 87 K
Grilloten® LSE 87 K Soft
Hartamide LDA

Hartamide LMEA
Hartamide OD
Hectabrite® AW
Hectabrite® DP
Hectalite® 200
Hefti GMS-33
Hest MS
Hetamide CMA
Hetamide CME
Hetamide CME-CO
Hetamide DS
Hetamide LA
Hetamide LL
Hetamide LML
Hetamide LN
Hetamide LNO
Hetamide M
Hetamide MA
Hetamide MC
Hetamide MCS
Hetamide ML
Hetamide MMC, OC
Hetamide MO
Hetamide MOC
Hetamide MS
Hetamide OC
Hetamide RC
Hetester MS
Hetoxamate 200 DL
Hetoxamate 400 DS
Hetoxide BN-13
Hetoxide C-30
Hetsorb L-4
Hetsorb TO-20
Hetsorb TS-20
Hispagel® 100
Hispagel® 200
Hodag 602-S
Hodag DGS
Hodag DGS-C
Hodag DGS-N
Hodag EGMS
Hodag Nonionic 1035-L
Hodag Nonionic 1044-L
Hodag Nonionic 1061-L
Hodag Nonionic 1062-L
Hodag Nonionic 1064-L
Hodag Nonionic 1068-F
Hodag Nonionic 1088-F
Hodag Nonionic 2017-R
Hostacerin DGS
Hostacerin PN 73
Hydex® 100 Gran. 206
Hydex® Coarse Powd
Hydex® Powd. 60
Hydex® Tablet Grade
Hydrenol® D
Hypan® QT100
Hypan® SA100H
Hypan® SR150H
Hypan® SS201
Hypan® SS500V
Hypan® SS500W
Hystar® 3375
Hystar® 4075
Hystar® 5875
Hystar® 6075
Hystar® 7000

Thickeners/Gelling Agents/Thixotropes... *(cont'd.)*

Hystar® 7570
Hystar® HM-75
Idroramnosan
Imwitor® 191
Imwitor® 900
Imwitor® 900 K
Imwitor® 914
Imwitor® 928
Imwitor® 940
Imwitor® 940 K
Imwitor® 988
Incromate ISML
Incromate SDL
Incromide ALD
Incromide BAD
Incromide CA
Incromide CM
Incromide L90
Incromide LA
Incromide LM-70
Incromide LR
Incromide Mink D
Incromide OD
Incromide OLD
Incromide OPM
Incromide SED
Incromide SM
Incromide WGD
Incromine BB
Incromine PB
Incromine SB
Incromine Oxide AL
Incromine Oxide B-30P
Incromine Oxide C
Incromine Oxide C-35
Incromine Oxide I
Incromine Oxide ISMO
Incromine Oxide M
Incromine Oxide MC
Incromine Oxide Mink
Incromine Oxide O
Incromine Oxide OD-50
Incromine Oxide OL
Incromine Oxide S
Incromine Oxide SE
Incromine Oxide WG
Incronam 30
Incronam I-30
Incronam Mink 30
Incronam OD-50
Incronam OP-30
Incrosul LS
Ivarlan™ 3400
Jaguar® C
Jaguar® C-13S
Jaguar® C-14-S
Jaguar® C-17
Jaguar® C-162
Jaguar® HP 8
Jaguar® HP-11
Jaguar® HP 60
Jaguar® HP 120
Junlon PW-110
Junlon PW-111
Karamide 121
Karamide 363
Karamide HTDA
Katioran® AF

Kelacid®
Kelco® HV
Kelco® LV
Kelco-Gel® Gellan Gum
Kelcoloid® D
Kelcoloid® DH, DO, DSF
Kelcoloid® HVF, LVF, O, S
Kelcosol®
Kelgin® F
Kelgin® HV, LV, MV
Kelgin® QL
Kelgin® XL
Kelmar®
Kelset®
Keltone
Keltose®
Keltrol®, Keltrol F
Kemester® 3681
Kemester® 5654
Kemester® EGDS
Kemester® EGMS
Kemester® MM
Kessco® 653
Kessco® EGAS
Kessco® Ethylene Glycol
    Monostearate
Kessco® GDS 386F
Kessco GMS
Kessco® PEG 200 DL
Kessco® PEG 200 DO
Kessco® PEG 200 DS
Kessco® PEG 200 ML
Kessco® PEG 200 MO
Kessco® PEG 200 MS
Kessco® PEG 300 DL
Kessco® PEG 300 DO
Kessco® PEG 300 DS
Kessco® PEG 300 ML
Kessco® PEG 300 MO
Kessco® PEG 300 MS
Kessco® PEG 400 DL
Kessco® PEG 400 DO
Kessco® PEG 400 DS
Kessco® PEG 400 ML
Kessco® PEG 400 MO
Kessco® PEG 400 MS
Kessco® PEG 600 DO
Kessco® PEG 600 DS
Kessco® PEG 600 ML
Kessco® PEG 600 MO
Kessco® PEG 600 MS
Kessco® PEG 1000 DL
Kessco® PEG 1000 DO
Kessco® PEG 1000 DS
Kessco® PEG 1000 ML
Kessco® PEG 1000 MO
Kessco® PEG 1000 MS
Kessco® PEG 1540 DL
Kessco® PEG 1540 DO
Kessco® PEG 1540 DS
Kessco® PEG 1540 ML
Kessco® PEG 1540 MO
Kessco® PEG 1540 MS
Kessco® PEG 4000 DL
Kessco® PEG 4000 DO
Kessco® PEG 4000 DS
Kessco® PEG 4000 ML
Kessco® PEG 4000 MO

Kessco® PEG 4000 MS
Kessco® PEG 6000 DL
Kessco® PEG 6000 DO
Kessco® PEG 6000 DS
Kessco® PEG 6000 ML
Kessco® PEG 6000 MO
Kessco® PEG 6000 MS
Kessco PGMS
Kester Wax® 72
Kester Wax® 82
Kester Wax® 105
Kester Wax® K 48
Kester Wax® K 56
Kester Wax® K 59
Kester Wax® K 62
Kester Wax® K 85
Klucel® ELF, GF, HF, JF,
    LF, MF
Kollidon®
Kollidon® 25, 30, 90
Koster Keunen Beeswax
Koster Keunen Beeswax
    AO2535
Koster Keunen Beeswax,
    S&P ISOW
Koster Keunen Candelilla
Koster Keunen Candelilla
    Ester
Koster Keunen Carnauba
Koster Keunen Ceresine
    130/135
Koster Keunen Ceresine
    140/145
Koster Keunen Ceresine
    155
Koster Keunen Ceresine
    192
Koster Keunen Fatty
    Alcohol 1618
Koster Keunen Hydroxy-
    Hexanyl-Behenyl-
    Beeswaxate
Koster Keunen Hydroxy-
    Polyester
Koster Keunen Japan Wax,
    Synthetic
Koster Keunen Microcrys-
    talline Wax 170/180
Koster Keunen Microcrys-
    talline Wax 193/198
Koster Keunen Ozokerite
    153/160
Koster Keunen Ozokerite
    158/160
Koster Keunen Ozokerite
    160/164
Koster Keunen Ozokerite
    164/170
Koster Keunen Ozokerite
    170
Koster Keunen Ozokerite
    190
Koster Keunen Synthetic
    Beeswax
Koster Keunen Synthetic
    Candelilla
Koster Keunen Synthetic
    Candelilla R-4

Koster Keunen Synthetic
    Candelilla R-8
Krim 32
Lamecreme® DGE-18
Lamesoft® LMG
Lanette® 14
Lanette® 16
Lanette® 18
Lanette® 18-22
Lanette® 18 DEO
Lanette® 22
Lanette® O
Lanfrax® 1776
Lanogen 1500
Lanosterol
Laponite® D
Laponite® XLG
Laponite® XLS
Lathanol® LAL
Laurel SD-900M
Laurel SD-1500
Lauridit® KD, KDG
Lauridit® OD
Lauropal 3
Lexaine® C
Lexaine® CG-30
Lexaine® IS
Lexaine® O
Lexein® S620TA
Lexemul® 503
Lexemul® 515
Lilaminox M24
Lipal 6000 DS
Lipal EGDS
Lipal EGMS
Lipal MMDG
Lipamide S
Lipo DGLS
Lipo DGS-SE
Lipo EGDS
Lipo GMS 450
Lipo GMS 470
Lipocol C
Lipocol S
Lipomulse 165
Liponate 2-DH
Liponate 143M
Liponate CL
Liponate GC
Liponate IPM
Liponate IPP
Liponate MM
Liponate PB-4
Liponate PC
Liponate PE-810
Liponate PO-4
Liponate PS-4
Liponate SPS
Liponate SS
Lipo-Peptide AME 30
Lipo Polyglycol 200
Lipo Polyglycol 300
Lipo Polyglycol 400
Lipo Polyglycol 600
Lipo Polyglycol 1000
Lipo Polyglycol 3350
Liporamnosan
Liposorb L

Thickeners/Gelling Agents/Thixotropes... *(cont'd.)*

Liposorb O	Mackam™ RA	Mafo® CB 40	Mazox® LDA
Liposorb P	Mackam™ WGB	Mafo® CSB 50	Mazox® MDA
Liposorb S	Mackamide™ 100-A	Mafo® LMAB	Mazox® ODA
Liposorb SQO	Mackamide™ AME-75,	Magnabrite® HS	Mazox® SDA
Liposorb TO	AME-100	Magnabrite® HV	Methocel® 40-100
Liposorb TS	Mackamide™ AN55	Maltrin® M050	Methocel® 40-101
Lipovol GTB	Mackamide™ C	Manromid 150-ADY	Methocel® 40-202
Lipowax	Mackamide™ CD	Manromid AV150	Methocel® A4CP
Lipoxol® 200 MED	Mackamide™ CD-10	Mapeg® 400 DS	Methocel® A4MP
Lipoxol® 300 MED	Mackamide™ CDC	Mapeg® 400 MS	Methocel® A15-LV
Lipoxol® 400 MED	Mackamide™ CDS-80	Mapeg® 6000 DS	Methocel® A15LVP
Lipoxol® 550 MED	Mackamide™ CMA	Mapeg® EGDS	Methocel® E3P
Lipoxol® 600 MED	Mackamide™ CS	Mapeg® EGMS	Methocel® E4MP
Lipoxol® 800 MED	Mackamide™ EC	Marine Dew	Methocel® E6P
Lipoxol® 1000 MED	Mackamide™ ISA	Marlamid® D 1218	Methocel® E15LVP
Lipoxol® 1550 MED	Mackamide™ L-10	Marlamid® D 1885	Methocel® E50LVP
Lipoxol® 2000 MED	Mackamide™ L95	Marlamid® DF 1218	Methocel® E50P
Lipoxol® 3000 MED	Mackamide™ LLM	Marlamid® DF 1818	Methocel® K4MP
Lipoxol® 4000 MED	Mackamide™ LMD	Marlamid® KL	Methocel® K4MS
Lipoxol® 6000 MED	Mackamide™ LME	Marlamid® M 1218	Methocel® K15MP
Lonzaine® 12C	Mackamide™ LMM	Marlamid® M 1618	Methocel® K15MS
Lonzaine® C	Mackamide™ LOL	Marlipal® BS	Methocel® K35
Lonzaine® CO	Mackamide™ MC	Marlosol® BS	Methocel® K100LVP
Lonzaine® JS	Mackamide™ MO	Marlosol® F08	Methocel® K100MP
Loropan CME	Mackamide™ NOA	Marlosol® FS	Mexpectin LA 100 Range
Loropan KD	Mackamide™ O	Marlosol® R70	Mexpectin LC 700 Range
Loropan KM	Mackamide™ ODM	Massa Estarinum® CM	Mexpectin XSS 100 Range
Loropan LM	Mackamide™ OP	Maypon 4CT	Meypro-Guar™ CASA M-
Loropan LMD	Mackamide™ PK	Mazamide® 65	225
Loropan OD	Mackamide™ PKM	Mazamide® 68	Microat™ E
Lowenol C-243	Mackamide™ R	Mazamide® 80	Miglyol® 840 Gel B
Lowenol C-420	Mackamide™ S	Mazamide® 124	Miglyol® 840 Gel T
Lowenol P-1030	Mackamide™ SD	Mazamide® 524	Miglyol® Gel B
Lowenol S-216	Mackamide™ SMA	Mazamide® 1214	Miglyol® Gel T
Lutrol® F 127	Mackamine™ CAO	Mazamide® 1281	Miramine® CODI
Luviskol® K12	Mackamine™ CO	Mazamide® C-5	Miramine® SODI
Luviskol® K17	Mackamine™ IAO	Mazamide® CFAM	Miranol® DM Conc. 45%
Luviskol® K30	Mackamine™ ISMO	Mazamide® CMEA	Mirapol® 9, 95, 175
Luviskol® K60	Mackamine™ LAO	Mazamide® CMEA Extra	Mirapol® 1941
Luviskol® K80	Mackamine™ LO	Mazamide® CS 148	Mirasheen® 202
Luviskol® K90	Mackamine™ O2	Mazamide® J 10	Mirataine® BB
Luviskol® LD-9025	Mackamine™ OAO	Mazamide® JR 300	Mirataine® BD-J
Luviskol® VA28E	Mackamine™ SAO	Mazamide® JR 400	Mirataine® BET-C-30
Luviskol® VA28I	Mackamine™ SO	Mazamide® JT 128	Mirataine® BET-O-30
Luviskol® VA37E	Mackamine™ WGO	Mazamide® L-298	Mirataine® BET-P-30
Luviskol® VA37I	Macol® 2	Mazamide® LLD	Mirataine® BET-W
Luviskol® VA55E	Macol® 2D	Mazamide® LM	Mirataine® CAB-A
Luviskol® VA55I	Macol® 2LF	Mazamide® LM 20	Mirataine® CAB-O
Luviskol® VA64E	Macol® 4	Mazamide® LS 196	Mirataine® CB
Luviskol® VA64I	Macol® 8	Mazamide® O 20	Mirataine® CBC
Luviskol® VA64W	Macol® 10	Mazamide® PCS	Mirataine® CB/M
Luviskol® VA73E	Macol® 16	Mazamide® RO	Mirataine® CBR
Luviskol® VA73I	Macol® 22	Mazamide® SCD	Mirataine® CBS, CBS Mod.
Luviskol® VA73W	Macol® 23	Mazamide® SS-10	Mirataine® COB
Mackam™ 35 HP	Macol® 27	Mazamide® SS 20	Mirataine® ODMB-35
Mackam™ BA	Macol® 31	Mazamide® T 20	Mirataine® TM
Mackam™ CB-35	Macol® 32	Mazamide® TC	Miristamina
Mackam™ CB-LS	Macol® 33	Mazamide® WC Conc	Monalux CAO-35
Mackam™ CBS-50	Macol® 34	Mazawax® 163R	Monamid® 15-70W
Mackam™ CBS-50G	Macol® 40	Mazol® 165C	Monamid® 15-MW
Mackam™ CET	Macol® 42	Mazol® GMO	Monamid® 31
Mackam™ HV	Macol® 46	Mazol® GMR	Monamid® 150-ADY
Mackam™ ISA	Macol® 72	Mazol® GMS	Monamid® 150-CW
Mackam™ J	Macol® 77	Mazol® GMSDK	Monamid® 150-GLT
Mackam™ L	Macol® 85	Mazol® GMS-K	Monamid® 150-LMWC
Mackam™ LMB-LS	Macol® 88	Mazox® CAPA	Monamid® 150-LWA
Mackam™ OB	Macol® 101	Mazox® CAPA-37	Monamid® 150-MW
Mackam™ OB-30	Macol® 108	Mazox® CDA	Monamid® 664-MC

Thickeners/Gelling Agents/Thixotropes... *(cont'd.)*

Monamid® 705
Monamid® 716
Monamid® 718
Monamid® 759
Monamid® 1007
Monamid® 1034
Monamid® 1159
Monamid® 1224
Monamid® C-305
Monamid® C-310
Monamid® CMA
Monamid® CMA-A
Monamid® CMA-A/F
Monamid® CMA-A/M
Monamid® CMA/F
Monamid® CMA/M
Monamid® CMA-S
Monamid® CMA-S/F
Monamid® CMA-S/M
Monamid® L-350
Monamid® L-355
Monamid® L-360
Monamid® L-365
Monamid® LL-370
Monamid® LLN-380
Monamid® LM-375
Monamid® LMIPA
Monamid® LMMA
Monamid® LN-605
Monamid® S
Monamide
Monamine 779
Monamine AA-100
Monamine AC-100
Monamine ACO-100
Monamine ADD-100
Monamine ADY-100
Monamine CF-100 M
Monateric 1202
Monateric CAB-LC
Monateric CAB-XLC
Monateric CM-36S
Monateric ISA-35
Monateric LMAB
Monateric LMM-30
Monomuls® 90-25
Monomuls® 90-L12
Monomuls® 90-O18
Mulsor OC
Nacol® 14-98
Nacol® 16-98
Nacol® 18-98
Nacol® 20-95
Nacol® 22-97
Nacolox®
Naetex-LS
Naetex O-20
Naetex-Q
Nafol® C14-C22
Natrosol® 250
Natrosol® Hydroxyethylcel-
     lulose
Natrosol® Plus CS
Natrosol® Plus CS, Grade
     330
Naturechem® EGHS
Naturechem® GMHS
Naturechem® MHS

Naturechem® PGHS
Naturechem® THS-200
Naxide™ 1230
Naxonol™ CO
Naxonol™ PN 66
Naxonol™ PO
N-Hance® 3000
Nikkol Batyl Alcohol 100,
     EX
Nikkol BPS-5
Nikkol BPS-10
Nikkol BPS-15
Nikkol BPS-20
Nikkol BPS-25
Nikkol BPS-30
Nikkol CDS-6000P
Nikkol Chimyl Alcohol 100
Nikkol Decaglyn 3-O
Nikkol Decaglyn 3-S
Nikkol PMT
Nikkol SMT
Nikkol TW-10
Nikkol TW-20
Ninol® 30-LL
Ninol® 40-CO
Ninol® 49-CE
Ninol® 70-SL
Ninol® 96-SL
Ninol® 201
Ninol® CNR
Ninol® GR
Ninol® L-9
Ninol® LMP
Ninol® M10
Ninox® FCA
Niox EO-33
Nissan Nonion DS-60HN
Nissan Nonion LP-20R,
     LP-20RS
Nissan Nonion P-6
Nissan Nonion S-2
Nissan Nonion S-4
Nissan Nonion S-6
Nissan Nonion S-10
Nissan Nonion S-15
Nissan Nonion S-15.4
Nissan Nonion S-40
Nissan Nonion T-15
Nissan Stafoam DF-1, DF-2
Nissan Stafoam DO, DOS
Nonisol 100
Nopalcol Series
Nopalcol 1-S
Nopalcol 1-TW
Norfox® B
Norfox® Coco Powder
Norfox® DCSA
Norfox® DESA
Norfox® DLSA
Norfox® DOSA
Norfox® EGMS
Norfox® KD
Norgel
Novata® 299, A, AB, B,
     BBC, BC, BCF, BD, C,
     D, E
Novogel® ST
Olamida

Olamida CD
Olamida CM
Olamida ED
Olamida RD
Olamida SM
Olamida UD
Olamida UD 21
Onyxol® 42
OP-2000
Optigel WM
Pationic® 138C
Pationic® SSL
Pegosperse® 50 DS
Pegosperse® 100-S
Pegosperse® 200 ML
Pegosperse® 400 DOT
Pegosperse® 400 DS
Pegosperse® 400 MS
Pegosperse® 600 DOT
Pegosperse® 1750 MS K
     Spec.
Pegosperse® 6000 DS
Pegosperse® EGMS-70
Pegosperse® PMS CG
Pelemol BB
Peptein® 2000®
Peptein® 2000XL
Permulgin 835
Permulgin CSB
Permulgin RWB
P &G Amide No. 27
Phoenamid SM
Phospholipid PTC
Phospholipid PTD
Phospholipid PTL
Phospholipid PTS
Phospholipid PTZ
Pluracol® E400
Pluracol® E400 NF
Pluracol® E600
Pluracol® E600 NF
Pluracol® E1000
Pluracol® E1450
Pluracol® E1450 NF
Pluracol® E2000
Pluracol® E4000 NF
Pluracol® E4500
Pluracol® E8000
Pluracol® E8000 NF
Plurol Stearique WL 1009
Pluronic® 10R5
Pluronic® 10R8
Pluronic® 12R3
Pluronic® 17R1
Pluronic® 17R2
Pluronic® 17R4
Pluronic® 17R8
Pluronic® 22R4
Pluronic® 25R1
Pluronic® 25R2
Pluronic® 25R4
Pluronic® 25R5
Pluronic® 25R8
Pluronic® 31R1
Pluronic® 31R2
Pluronic® 31R4
Pluronic® F38
Pluronic® F68

Pluronic® F68LF
Pluronic® F77
Pluronic® F87
Pluronic® F88
Pluronic® F98
Pluronic® F108
Pluronic® F127
Pluronic® L10
Pluronic® L35
Pluronic® L42
Pluronic® L43
Pluronic® L44
Pluronic® L61
Pluronic® L62
Pluronic® L62D
Pluronic® L62LF
Pluronic® L63
Pluronic® L64
Pluronic® L72
Pluronic® L81
Pluronic® L92
Pluronic® L101
Pluronic® L121
Pluronic® L122
Pluronic® P65
Pluronic® P75
Pluronic® P84
Pluronic® P85
Pluronic® P94
Pluronic® P103
Pluronic® P104
Pluronic® P105
Pluronic® P123
PMS-33
Polargel® HV
Polargel® NF
Polargel® T
Polawax®
Polychol 5
Polychol 10
Polychol 15
Polychol 16
Polychol 20
Polychol 40
Polyethylene 1000 HE
Polyox® Coagulant
Polyox® WSR 35
Polyox® WSR 205
Polyox® WSR 301
Polyox® WSR 1105
Polyox® WSR 3333
Polyox® WSR N-10
Polyox® WSR N-12K
Polyox® WSR N-60K
Polyox® WSR N-80
Polyox® WSR N-750
Polyox® WSR N-3000
PolySurf
Polytex 10M
Porosponge
Profan 24 Extra, 128 Extra
Profan 2012E
Profan AA62
Profan AB20
Profan AD31
Progacyl® COS-1
Progacyl® COS-10
Progacyl® COS-20, -70

Thickeners/Gelling Agents/Thixotropes... *(cont'd.)*

Promulgen® D	Rewoderm® LIS 80	Rol LP	Schercomid SLA
Promulgen® G	Rewomid® 203/S	Rol MOG	Schercomid SLE
Protamide 15W	Rewomid® DC 212 S	Rol RP	Schercomid SL-Extra
Protamide LNO	Rewomid® DC 212 SE	Rol TR	Schercomid SLL
Protamide MRCA	Rewomid® DC 220 SE	Rolamid CD	Schercomid SLM
Protamide SA	Rewomid® DL 203 S	Salcare SC90	Schercomid SLMC-75
Pro-Tein SA-20	Rewomid® DL 240	Salcare SC91	Schercomid SL-ML
Purton CFD	Rewomid® DLM SE	Salcare SC92	Schercomid SLM-LC
Purton SFD	Rewomid® DLMS	Salcare SC95	Schercomid SLM-S
PVP K-15	Rewomid® DO 280 SE	Sandopan® DTC Linear P	Schercomid SLS
PVP/Si-10	Rewomid® F	Sandoteric CFL	Schercomid SM
Pyroter CPI-30	Rewomid® IPE 280	Sandoteric TFL Conc	Schercomid SME
Pyroter CPI-40	Rewomid® IPL 203	Sandoz Amide NT	Schercomid SME-A
Pyroter CPI-60	Rewomid® IPP 240	Sandoz Amide PE	Schercomid SME-M
Quatrisoft® Polymer	Rewomid® L 203	Sandoz Amide PL	Schercomid SME-S
LM-200	Rewomid® R 280	Sandoz Amide PO	Schercomid SWG
Quso® G27, G29, G35,	Rewomid® S 280	Sandoz Amine Oxide XA-C	Schercomid TO-2
G38, WR55, WR83	Rewominox B 204	Sandoz Amine Oxide XA-L	Schercopol LPS
Quso® WR55-FG	Rewominox L 408	Sandoz Amine Oxide XA-M	Schercoquat IAS
Radia® 7500	Rewopal® PEG 6000 DS	Sandoz Sulfate 216	Schercoquat ROAB
Radia® 7501	Rewoteric® AM B 13	Sandoz Sulfate 219	Schercoquat ROAS
Radiacid® 152	Rewoteric® AM B-15	Sandoz Sulfate A	Schercotaine APAB
Radiacid® 212	Rewoteric® AM B-15	Sandoz Sulfate EP	Schercotaine IAB
Radiacid® 416	Rewoteric® AM TEG	Sandoz Sulfate ES-3	Schercotaine MAB
Radiacid® 423	Rhaballgum CG-M	Sandoz Sulfate K	Schercotaine OAB
Radiacid® 427	Rhodacal® A-246 LX	Sandoz Sulfate WA Dry	Schercotaine PAB
Radiacid® 428	Rhodafac® MC-470	Sandoz Sulfate WA Special	Schercotaine WOAB
Radiacid® 464	Rhodamox® CAPO	Sandoz Sulfate WAG	Seagel L
Radiacid® 631	Rhodamox® LO	Sandoz Sulfate WAS	Seakem 3, LCM
Radiamox® 6800	Rhodasurf® L-4	Sandoz Sulfate WE	Seanamin BD
Radiamox® 6804	Rhodicare™ D	Sanwet® COS-905	Seaspen PF
Radianol® 1712	Rhodicare™ H	Sanwet® COS-915	Sepigel 305
Radianol® 1724	Rhodicare™ S	Sanwet® COS-960	Serdolamide POF 61
Radianol® 1726	Rhodicare™ SC-225	Satexlan 20	Serdolamide PYF 77
Radianol® 1728	Rhodicare™ XC	Schercamox CMA	Sident® 15
Radianol® 1763	Rhodigel®	Schercamox DMC	Sident® 22LS
Radianol® 1765	Rhodigel® 23	Schercamox DML	Sident® 22S
Radianol® 1768	Rita CA	Schercamox DMS	Siltek® PL
Radianol® 1769	Rita EDGS	Schercamox T-12	Simulsol 220 TM
Radianol® 1898	Rita EGMS	Schercemol CL	Sipernat® 22LS
Radiastar® 1200	Rita GMS	Schercemol CM	Siponic® L-1
Radiastar® 1208	Rita SA	Schercemol EGMS	Sipothix® H-65
Radiasurf® 7201	Ritachol® 4000	Schercemol GMS	Sobalg FD 100 Series
Radiasurf® 7270	Ritahydrox	Schercemol MM	Sobalg FD 200 Series
Radiasurf® 7404	Ritalafa®	Schercodine M	Sobalg FD 300 Series
Radiasurf® 7410	R.I.T.A. Lanolin Wax	Schercodine T	Sobalg FD 460
Radiasurf® 7413	Ritapeg 100 DS	Schercomid 1-102	Sodium Stéarate C7L
Radiasurf® 7414	Ritasynt IP	Schercomid 1214	Softisan® 100
Radiasurf® 7417	Ritavena™ 5	Schercomid CCD	Softisan® 134
Radiasurf® 7422	Ritawax	Schercomid CDA-H	Softisan® 138
Radiasurf® 7423	Rohagit® S, SD 15	Schercomid CDO-Extra	Softisan® 142
Radiasurf® 7431	Rohamere® 4885F	Schercomid CME	Softisan® 154
Radiasurf® 7432	Rohamere® 4899F	Schercomid HT-60	Softisan® Gel
Radiasurf® 7443	Rohamere® 4944F	Schercomid ID	Solan 50
Radiasurf® 7453	Rohamere® 6639F	Schercomid IMI	Soprol VR.50
Radiasurf® 7454	Rohamere® 7525L	Schercomid LD	Span® 20
Radiasurf® 7600	Rohamere® 8744F	Schercomid M	Span® 40
Rehydragel® Compressed	Rol 52	Schercomid MD-Extra	Span® 60, 60K
Gel	Rol 53	Schercomid MME	Span® 65
Rewocid® DU 185	Rol 59	Schercomid ODA	Span® 85
Rewoderm® LI 48	Rol 400	Schercomid OME	Spermwax®
Rewoderm® LI 48-50	Rol AG	Schercomid OMI	Stabileze™ 06
Rewoderm® LI 63	Rol D 600	Schercomid SAP	Stafoam DL
Rewoderm® LI 67	Rol DGE	Schercomid SCE	Stamere®
Rewoderm® LI 67-75	Rol DL 40	Schercomid SCO-Extra	Stamid HT 3901
Rewoderm® LI 420	Rol DO 40	Schercomid SD-DS	Stamid LS 5487
Rewoderm® LI 420-70	Rol GE	Schercomid SI	Standamid® 100
Rewoderm® LIS 75	Rol L 40	Schercomid SI-M	Standamid® CMG

Thickeners/Gelling Agents/Thixotropes... *(cont'd.)*

Standamid® ID	Synotol Detergent E	T-Maz® 95	Veegum® K
Standamid® KD	Synotol L 60	Tohol N-220	Veegum® Ultra
Standamid® KDM	Synotol L 90	Tohol N-220X	Veegum® WG
Standamid® KDO	Synotol LM 60	Tohol N-230	Velsan® P8-3
Standamid® KM	Synotol LM 90	Tohol N-230X	Velsan® P8-16
Standamid® LD	Synotol ME 90	Trivent BE-13	Velvetex® AB-45
Standamid® LD 80/20	Synprolam 35DMO	Trydet SA-23	Velvetex® BK-35
Standamid® LDM	Synprolam 35MX1/O	T-Tergamide 1CD	Velvetex® OLB-50
Standamid® LDO	Tegamine® Oxide WS-35	T-Tergamide 1PD	Viscarin XLV
Standamid® LDS	Tego®-Betaine C	Tullanox HM-250	Viscontran HEC
Standamid® LM	Tego®-Betaine L-7	Tylose® C, CB Series	Volclay® NF-BC
Standamid® LP	Tego®-Betaine L-90	Tylose® C-p, CB-p	Volclay NF-ID
Standamid® PK-KD	Tego®-Betaine S	Tylose® H Series	Volpo 25 D 3
Standamid® Resin	Tetronic® 304	Tylose® H-p	Volpo 25 D 5
BC-1283	Tetronic® 504	Tylose® H-yp	Volpo 25 D 10
Standamid® SD	Tetronic® 701	Tylose® MH Grades	Volpo 25 D 15
Standamid® SDO	Tetronic® 702	Tylose® MHB	Volpo 25 D 20
Standamid® SM	Tetronic® 704	Tylose® MH-K, MH-xp,	Volpo CS-3
Standamid® SOMD	Tetronic® 707	MHB-y, MHB-yp	Volpo CS-5
Standamox C 30	Tetronic® 901	Tylose® MH-p, MHB-p	Volpo CS-10
Standamox CAW	Tetronic® 904	Ucon® 75-H-450	Volpo CS-15
Standamox O1	Tetronic® 908	Ucon® Fluid AP	Volpo CS-20
Standamul® 1616	Tetronic® 909	Ufanon K-80	Volpo N3
Standamul® O-5	Tetronic® 1101	Ufanon KD-S	Volpo N5
Standamul® O-10	Tetronic® 1102	Unamide® C-2	Volpo N10
Standamul® O-20	Tetronic® 1104	Unamide® C-5	Volpo N15
Standapol® AB-45	Tetronic® 1107	Unamide® C-72-3	Volpo N20
Standapol® A-HV	Tetronic® 1301	Unamide® CDX	Volpo O3
Standapol® BC-35	Tetronic® 1302	Unamide® CMX	Volpo O5
Standapol® EA-K	Tetronic® 1304	Unamide® D-10	Volpo O10
Standapol® OLB-30	Tetronic® 1307	Unamide® J-56	Volpo O15
Standapol® OLB-50	Tetronic® 1501	Unamide® JJ-35	Volpo O20
Steol® CA-130	Tetronic® 1502	Unamide® L-2	Volpo T-3
Steol® CA-230	Tetronic® 1504	Unamide® L-5	Volpo T-5
Steol® CA-330	Tetronic® 1508	Unamide® LDL	Volpo T-10
Steol® CA-460	Texapon® EA-1	Unamide® LDX	Volpo T-15
Stepan-Mild® LSB	Texapon® EA-2	Unamide® LMDX	Volpo T-20
Stepanol® AM	Texapon® EA-3	Unamide® N-72-3	Vybar® 5013
Stepanol® AM-V	Texapon® ES-250	Unamide® S	Wacker HDK® H20
Stepanol® WAC	Thickagent LC	Unichem SS	Wacker HDK® N20
Stepanol® WA Extra	Thixcin® R	Unilin® 350 Alcohol	Wacker HDK® V15
Stepanol® WAQ	Ticalose 15, 30, 75, 150R,	Unilin® 550 Alcohol	W.G.S. Synaceti 116 NF/
Stepanol® WA Special	1200, 2000R, 2500,	Unilin® 700 Alcohol	USP
SteriLine 665	4000, 4500, 5000R	Upamide O-20	Wickenol® 545
Sterol GMS	Tixogel FTN	Upamide SD	Wickenol® 727
Sterol SES	Tixogel IPM	Upamide SME-M	Witafrol® 7420
Supercol® Guar Gum	Tixogel LAN	Varamide® A-2	Witcamide® 70
Super Hartolan	Tixogel LG	Varamide® C-212	Witcamide® 82
Superloid®	Tixogel MIO	Varamide® L-203	Witcamide® 128T
Superpolystate	Tixogel OMS	Varamide® LL-1	Witcamide® 5085
Super-Sat AWS-4	Tixogel VP	Varamide® LO-1	Witcamide® 5133
Super-Sat AWS-24	Tixogel VSP	Varamide® MA-1	Witcamide® 5195
Supro-Tein R	Tixogel VZ	Varamide® ML-1	Witcamide® 6310
Supro-Tein S	Tixosil 38AB, 43, 53, 73, 83	Varamide® ML-4	Witcamide® 6511
Suspengel Elite	Tixosil 311	Varion® CADG-HS	Witcamide® 6514
Suspengel Micro	Tixosil 331	Varonic® BD	Witcamide® 6533
Suspengel Ultra	Tixosil 333, 343	Varonic® BG	Witcamide® 6625
Suspentone	T-Maz® 20	Varonic® LI-48	Witcamide® C
Suspentone 1265	T-Maz® 28	Varonic® LI-420	Witcamide® CD
Syncrowax BB-4	T-Maz® 40	Varonic® LI-420 (70%)	Witcamide® CPA
Syncrowax ERL-C	T-Maz® 60	Varox® 270	Witcamide® LDEA
Syncrowax HR-C	T-Maz® 61	Varox® 365	Witcamide® LDTS
Syncrowax HRS-C	T-Maz® 65	Varox® 1770	Witcamide® LM, LMT
Synotol 119 N	T-Maz® 80	Veegum®	Witcamide® MAS
Synotol CN 20	T-Maz® 80KLM	Veegum® D	Witcamide® MM
Synotol CN 60	T-Maz® 81	Veegum® F	Witcamide® PPA
Synotol CN 80	T-Maz® 85	Veegum® HS	Witcamide® SSA
Synotol CN 90	T-Maz® 90	Veegum® HV	Witcamide® STD-HP

Thickeners/Gelling Agents/Thixotropes... *(cont'd.)*

Witco® Sodium Stearate
  C-1, C-7
Zeosyl® 200

Zeothix® 265
Zohar GLST
Zohar GLST SE

Zoramide CM
Zoramox

Zoramox E
Zoramox LO

UV Absorbers

Arlatone® 507
Arlatone® UVB
BioGir-MBC
BioGir-PISA
Brookosome® BC
Brookosome® UV
CMI 321
CMI 324, 400
CMI 550
CMI 800
Coverleaf PC-2055M
Dascare Orizanol
Dermoblock MA
Dermoblock OS
DHBP Quinsorb 010
Dipsal
Escalol® 507
Escalol® 557
Escalol® 567
Escalol® 587

Escalol® 597
Estalan MA
Eusolex® 232
Eusolex® 4360
Eusolex® 6007
Eusolex® 6300
Eusolex® 8020
Finex-25
Finex-25-020
Kemester® HMS
Koster Keunen Beeswax,
  Filtered
Luxelen® Silk D
Luxelen® SS
Luxelen® SS-020
MTD-25
Neo Heliopan, Type 303
Neo Heliopan, Type AV
Neo Heliopan, Type BB
Neo Heliopan, Type Hydro

Neo Heliopan, Type MA
Neo Heliopan, Type OS
Orange Wax
Orange Wax, Deodorized
Parsol® 1789
Parsol® 5000
Parsol® HS
Parsol® MCX
Resyn® 28-3307
Rhodialux™ A
Rhodialux™ D
Rhodialux™ S
Solarchem® O
Spectra-Sorb® UV 9
Spectra-Sorb® UV 24
Spectra-Sorb® UV 5411
Syntase® 62
Syntase® 230
Titanium Dioxide P25
Unichem METSAL

Unichem ZO
Unipabol U-17
Unisol S-22
Uvasorb 20H
Uvasorb MET
Uvasorb S-5
Uvinul® 400
Uvinul® D 49
Uvinul® D 50
Uvinul® DS 49
Uvinul® M 40
Uvinul® M 493
Uvinul® MS 40
Uvinul® N 35
Uvinul® N 539
Uvinul® P 25
Uvinul® T 150
Z-Cote®
Zinc Oxide USP 66

Waxes

Abil®-Wax 2434
Abil®-Wax 2440
Abil®-Wax 9800
Abil®-Wax 9801
Abil®-Wax 9809
Abil®-Wax 9814
A-C® 6A
A-C® 15
A-C® 316
A-C® 395, 395A
A-C® 400A
A-C® 405M, 405S, 405T
A-C® 430
A-C® 540, 540A
A-C® 617, 617A
A-C® 629
A-C® 655
A-C® 656
ACumist™ B-6
ACumist™ B-9
ACumist™ B-12
ACumist™ B-18
ACumist™ C-5
ACumist™ C-9
ACumist™ C-12
ACumist™ C-18
ACumist™ D-9
Alkamuls® PETS
Beeswax Commercial SP
  1142
Beeswax SP 116
Beeswax SP 125
Beeswax SP 139
Beeswax Synthetic Stralpitz
Beeswax White Refined SP
  44
Beeswax White SP 52

Beeswax White Stralpitz
Beeswax Yellow Refined
  SP 6
Beeswax Yellow SP 57
Be Square® 175
Be Square® 185
Be Square® 195
Biowax 754
Bleached Beeswax
Brookswax™ D
Brookswax™ P
Candelilla Wax Cosmetic
  Grade Stralpitz
Carnauba Wax NC #2
  Stralpitz
Carnauba Wax NC #3
  Stralpitz
Carnauba Wax SP 8
Castorwax® MP-70
Castorwax® MP-80
Castorwax® NF
Ceral EFN
Ceral EN 6
Ceral G
Ceresine Wax Cosmetic
  Stralpitz
Ceresine Wax SP 84
Cetina
Cetomil
Cire De Lanol CTO
Cosmowax
Crodamol GHS
Crodex A
Crodex C
Crodex N
CS-2032
CS-2037

CS-2043
CS-2054
CS-2080W
Cutina® BW
Cutina® EGMS
Cutina® LM
Cyclochem EM 326A
Cyclochem EM 560
Cyclochem® PETS
Cyclogol NI
Cyclol SPS
Dehydag® Wax 14
Dehydag® Wax 16
Dehydag® Wax 18
Dehydag® Wax 22
  (Lanette)
Dehydag® Wax E
Dehydag® Wax O
Dehydag® Wax SX
Dehydag® Wax W
Dermalcare® AC
Dermalcare® HV
Dermalcare® POL
Dow Corning® 2503
  Cosmetic Wax
Emerwax® 1266
Empiwax SK
Empiwax SK/BP
Emulgade® SE
Eskar Wax R-25, R-35, R-
  40, R-45, R-50
Fanwax G
Fanwax P
Glycowax® S 932
Hoechst Wax SW
Incromide BEM
Incroquat CR Conc

Incroquat Behenyl TMS
Japan Wax NJ-9002
Japan Wax Stralpitz
Jojoba Oil
Jojoba Oil Cosmetic Grade
Kessco® 653
Kester Wax® 72
Kester Wax® 82
Kester Wax® 105
Kester Wax® K 48
Kester Wax® K 56
Kester Wax® K 59
Kester Wax® K 62
Kester Wax® K 85
Koster Keunen Auto-
  Oxidized Beeswax
Koster Keunen Beeswax
Koster Keunen Beeswax
  AO2535
Koster Keunen Behenyl-
  Beeswaxate
Koster Keunen Candelilla
Koster Keunen Carnauba
Koster Keunen Carnauba,
  Micro Granulated
Koster Keunen Carnauba,
  Powd
Koster Keunen Ceresine
Koster Keunen Ceresine
  130/135
Koster Keunen Ceresine
  140/145
Koster Keunen Ceresine
  155
Koster Keunen Ceresine
  192
Koster Keunen Isostearyl-

Waxes *(cont'd.)*

Behenyl Beeswaxate
Koster Keunen Japan Wax, Synthetic
Koster Keunen Microcrystalline Waxes
Koster Keunen Microcrystalline Wax 170/180
Koster Keunen Microcrystalline Wax 193/198
Koster Keunen Ozokerite
Koster Keunen Ozokerite 153/160
Koster Keunen Ozokerite 158/160
Koster Keunen Ozokerite 160/164
Koster Keunen Ozokerite 164/170
Koster Keunen Ozokerite 170
Koster Keunen Ozokerite 190
Koster Keunen Paraffin Wax
Koster Keunen Paraffin Wax 122/128
Koster Keunen Paraffin Wax 130/135
Koster Keunen Paraffin Wax 140/145
Koster Keunen Paraffin Wax 150/155
Koster Keunen Substitute Beeswax
Koster Keunen Synthetic Beeswax
Koster Keunen Synthetic Candelilla
Koster Keunen Synthetic Candelilla R-4

Koster Keunen Synthetic Candelilla R-8
Koster Keunen Synthetic Carnauba
Koster Keunen Synthetic Japan Wax
Koster Keunen Synthetic Spermaceti
Labrafil® M 2130 BS
Labrafil® M 2130 CS
Labrafil® WL 1958 CS
Lanbritol Wax N21
Lanette® Wax CAT
Lanette® Wax SX, SXBP
Lipowax
Lipowax D
Lipowax NI
Lipowax P
Lipowax PR
Lipowax P-SPEC
Masilwax 135
Masilwax 148
Mazawax® 163SS
Microfine 2, 2F, 2FS, 8, 8F
Microthene® MN-714, MN-722
Multiwax® 180-M
Multiwax® 180-W
Multiwax® ML-445
Multiwax® W-445
Multiwax® W-835
Multiwax® X-145A
Nikkol MM
Nikkol Trifat P-52
Nikkol Trifat T-42
Nikkol Trifat T-52
Nikkol Wax-100
Nikkol Wax-110
Nikkol Wax-220

Nikkol Wax-230
Nikkol Wax-500
Nikkol Wax-600
Orange Wax
Orange Wax, Deodorized
Paricin® 1
Parvan® 127
Parvan® 129
Parvan® 131
Parvan® 137
Parvan® 138
Parvan® 142
Parvan® 145
Parvan® 147
Parvan® 154
Parvan® 158
Parvan® 161
Permulgin CSB
Ritachol® 3000
Ritachol® 4000
R.I.T.A. Lanolin Wax
Ross Bayberry Wax
Ross Bayberry Wax Substitute
Ross Beeswax
Ross Beeswax Substitute
Ross Beeswax Substitute 628/5
Ross Beeswax Synthetic
Ross Beeswax Synthetic Cosmetic Grade
Ross Bleached Montan Wax
Ross Bleached Montan Wax Cosmetic
Ross Bleached Refined Shellac Wax
Ross Bleached Refined Shellac Wax Cosmetic

Grade
Ross Brazil Wax
Ross Candelilla Wax
Ross Carnauba Wax
Ross Castor Wax
Ross Ceresine Wax
Ross Crude Scale Wax
Ross Japan Wax
Ross Japan Wax Substitute 473
Ross Japan Wax Substitute 525
Ross Japan Wax Substitute 930
Ross Japan Wax Substitute 966
Ross Ozokerite Wax
Rose Rice Bran Wax
Ross Spermaceti Wax Substitute 573
Ross Synthetic Candelilla Wax
Silwax® C
Silwax® S
Silwax® WD-IS
Silwax® WD-S
Silwax® WS
Softisan® 133
Spermwax®
Standamul® G-32/36
Starfol® Wax CG
Starwax® 100
Trivent OC-G
Ultraflex®
Varisoft® BTMS
Varonic® BD
Varonic® BG
Victory®
Vybar® 5013

Wetting Agents

Abex® LIV/30
Abil® B 8842
Abil® B 8863
Ablumox CAPO
Ablunol LA-3
Ablunol LA-5
Ablunol LA-7
Ablunol LA-9
Ablunol LA-12
Ablunol LA-16
Ablunol LA-40
Ablusol DBD
Ablusol DBM
Ablusol DBT
Accobetaine CL
Acconon TGH
Active #4
Acylglutamate CS-11
Adinol OT16
Aerosol® 19
Aerosol® A-102
Aerosol® A-103
Aerosol® OT-70 PG
Aerosol® OT-75%
Aerosol® OT-B

Akypo RLM 38 NV
Akypo RLM 100 MGV
Akypo RLM 160 NV
Akyporox RO 90
Akypo®-Soft 100 MgV
Akypo®-Soft 100 NV
Akypo®-Soft 130 NV
Akypo®-Soft 160 NV
Alcodet® 218
Alcodet® SK
Alcolec® BS
Alcolec® Granules
Alcolec® Z-3
Alkamide® 2124
Alkamide® DL-207/S
Alkamox® L20
Alkamuls® 400-DO
Alkamuls® 400-MO
Alkamuls® CO-15
Alkamuls® EL-620
Alkamuls® GMO
Alkamuls® GMS/C
Alkamuls® PSMO-20
Alkamuls® PSMS-20
Alkamuls® PSTS-20

Alkamuls® SMO
Alkaquat® DMB-451-50, DMB-451-80
Alkasurf® NP-8
Alkasurf® NP-15
Alkasurf® NP-40, 70%
Alkasurf® T
Alkasurf® TLS
Alkateric® CIB
Amerchol L-101®
Amerlate® P
Amerlate® W
Amerlate® WFA
Amfotex FV-10
Amidex CP
Amidex RC
Amidox® C-2
Amidox® C-5
Amidox® L-2
Amidox® L-5
Aminoxid WS 35
Ammonyx® CDO
Ammonyx® CO
Ammonyx® DMCD-40
Ammonyx® LO

Ammonyx® MCO
Ammonyx® MO
Ammonyx® OAO
Ampho B11-34
Ampho T-35
Amphosol® CA
Amphosol® CG
Amphoterge® J-2
Amphoterge® KJ-2
Amphoteric L
Amphoteric N
Amyx CDO 3599
Amyx LO 3594
Annonyx SO
Antaron® FC-34
Antarox® L-64
Armeen® SZ
Armeen® Z
Armotan® PMD 20
Aromox® C/12
Aromox® C/12-W
Aromox® DMMC-W
Arquad® 2C-75
Arquad® 2HT-75
Arquad® 12-33

Wetting Agents *(cont'd.)*

Arquad® 12-50
Arquad® 16-29
Arquad® 16-50
Arquad® 18-50
Arquad® C-33
Arquad® C-50
Arquad® S-2C-50
Arquad® T-2C-50
Arquad® T-27W
Avanel® S-70
Belsil DMC 6031
Belsil DMC 6032
Belsil DMC 6033
Belsil DMC 6035
Bernel® Ester NPDC
Bernel® Ester TOC
Berol 452
Bio-Soft® E-200
Bio-Soft® E-300
Bio-Soft® E-400
Bio-Soft® EN 600
Bio-Soft® N-300
Brij® 30
Brij® 35
Brij® 52
Brij® 56
Brij® 58
Brij® 72
Brij® 76
Brij® 78
Brij® 92
Brij® 93
Brij® 96
Brij® 97
Brij® 98
Brij® 700
Brij® 700S
Brij® 721
Brij® 721S
Calfoam ES-30
Calfoam NEL-60
Calfoam SEL-60
Calsoft F-90
Calsoft L-40
Calsoft L-60
Calsoft T-60
Calsuds CD-6
Capmul® GMO
Caprol® 3GO
Carsamide® CA
Carsamide® SAC
Carsofoam® T-60-L
Carsonol® ALS
Carsonol® ALS-R
Carsonol® ALS-S
Carsonol® ALS Special
Carsonol® DLS
Carsonol® ILS
Carsonol® MLS
Carsonol® SLES-3
Carsonol® SLS
Carsonol® SLS Paste B
Carsonol® SLS-R
Carsonol® SLS-S
Carsonol® SLS Special
Carsonol® TLS
Cedepal TD-403
Cedepal TD-407

Cedepal TD-484
Ceraphyl® 140-A
Cerasynt® 303
Cetomacrogol 1000 BP
Chemal BP 261
Chemal BP-262
Chemal BP-262LF
Chemal BP-2101
Chemal TDA-6
Chemal TDA-9
Chemal TDA-15
Chemal TDA-18
Chemax/DOSS-75E
Chemax E-400 ML
Chemax NP-1.5
Chemax NP-4
Chemax NP-6
Chemax NP-9
Chemax NP-10
Chemax NP-15
Chemax NP-20
Chemax NP-30
Chemax NP-30/70
Chemax OP-3
Chemax OP-5
Chemax OP-30/70
Chemax OP-40
Chemeen C-2
Chemeen C-5
Chemeen C-10
Chemeen C-15
Chemoxide O
Chemoxide SAO
Chemoxide T
Chimin BX
Chimin DOS 70
Chimin P10
Chimin P45
Cithrol 2DL
Cithrol 2DO
Cithrol 2ML
Cithrol 2MO
Cithrol 2MS
Cithrol 3MS
Cithrol 4DL
Cithrol 4DO
Cithrol 4ML
Cithrol 4MO
Cithrol 4MS
Cithrol 6DL
Cithrol 6DO
Cithrol 6ML
Cithrol 6MO
Cithrol 6MS
Cithrol 10DL
Cithrol 10DO
Cithrol 10ML
Cithrol 10MO
Cithrol 10MS
Cithrol 15MS
Cithrol 40MO
Cithrol 40MS
Cithrol 60ML
Cithrol 60MO
Cithrol GDO N/E
Cithrol GDO S/E
Cithrol GDS N/E
Cithrol GDS S/E

Cithrol GML N/E
Cithrol GML S/E
Cithrol GMO N/E
Cithrol GMO S/E
Cithrol GMR N/E
Cithrol GMR S/E
Cithrol GMS Acid Stable
Cithrol GMS N/E
Cithrol GMS S/E
Cithrol PGML N/E
Cithrol PGML S/E
Cithrol PGMO N/E
Cithrol PGMO S/E
Cithrol PGMR N/E
Cithrol PGMR S/E
Cithrol PGMS N/E
Cithrol PGMS S/E
Closyl 30 2089
Corona Lanolin
Coronet Lanolin
Cosmetol® X
Cosmopon SES
Cralane KR-13, -14
Cralane LR-10
Crill 1
Crill 2
Crill 4
Crill 6
Crill 43
Crill 45
Crill 50
Crillet 1
Crillet 2
Crillet 4
Crillet 11
Crillet 31
Crillet 35
Crillet 41
Crillet 45
Crodalan AWS
Crodalan LA
Crodamol CL
Crodasinic LS30
Crodasinic LS35
Crodasinic LT40
Crodasinic OS35
Crodesta A10
Crodesta DKS F10
Crodesta DKS F20
Crodesta DKS F50
Crodesta DKS F70
Crodesta DKS F110
Crodesta DKS F140
Crodesta DKS F160
Crodesta F-10
Crodesta F-50
Crodesta F-110
Crodesta F-160
Crodet L4
Crodet L8
Crodet L12
Crodet L24
Crodet L40
Crodet L100
Crodet S4
Crodet S8
Crodet S12
Crodet S24

Crodet S40
Crodet S100
Crodex N
Croduret 200
Crovol A40
Crovol A70
Crovol M40
Crovol M70
Crovol PK40
Crovol PK70
Crystal® O
Crystal® Crown
Crystal Crown LP
Damox® 1010
Dehydol® PID 6
Dehydol® PLT 6
Dehyquart® C
Dehyquart® LT
Dehyton® PG
Deriphat® 151C
Deriphat® 160
Dermol 126
Detergent CR
Diamond Quality®
Dow Corning® 190
    Surfactant
Dow Corning® 193
    Surfactant
Dow Corning® Q2-5220
    Resin Modifier
Drewfax® 0007
Drewmulse® POE-SML
Drewmulse® POE-SMO
Drewmulse® POE-SMS
Drewmulse® POE-STS
Drewmulse® SML
Drewmulse® SMO
Drewmulse® SMS
Drewmulse® STS
Dur-Em® GMO
Eccowet® W-50
Eccowet® W-88
Elefac™ I-205
Elfan® A
Elfan® NS 242 Conc
Elfan® NS 243 S
Elfan® NS 243 S Conc
Elfan® NS 252 S
Elfan® NS 252 S Conc
Elfan® OS
Elfanol® 883
Emalex 703
Emalex 705
Emalex 707
Emalex 709
Emalex 710
Emalex 712
Emalex 715
Emalex 720
Emalex 725
Emalex 730
Emalex 750
Emalex 1605
Emalex 1610
Emalex 1615
Emalex 1620
Emalex 1625
Emalex 1805

Wetting Agents *(cont'd.)*

Emalex 1810	Emulmetik™ 120	Hamposyl® L-95	Hodag Nonionic E-30
Emalex 1815	Emulmetik™ 300	Hamposyl® M	Hydrenol® D
Emalex 1820	Emulmetik™ 310	Hamposyl® M-30	Hydroxylan
Emalex 1825	Emulmetik™ 320	Hamposyl® O	Igepal® CA-630
Emalex NP-2	Emulmetik™ 910	Hamposyl® S	Igepal® DM-970 FLK
Emalex NP-3	Emulmetik™ 920	Hetester FAO	Incromine Oxide B
Emalex NP-5	Emulmetik™ 930	Hetester PCA	Incromine Oxide B-30P
Emalex NP-10	Emulmetik™ 950	Hetester PHA	Incromine Oxide C
Emalex NP-11	Emulmetik™ 970	Hetoxide C-200	Incromine Oxide I
Emalex NP-12	Epikuron 145	Hetoxol CAWS	Incromine Oxide ISMO
Emalex NP-13	Equex SW	Hetoxol CD-3	Incromine Oxide M
Emalex NP-15	ES-1239	Hetoxol CD-4	Incromine Oxide O
Emalex NP-20	Estalan 126	Hetoxol D	Incromine Oxide OD-50
Emalex NP-25	Estalan 635	Hetoxol G	Incronam B-40
Emalex NP-30	Ethoduomeen® T/13	Hetoxol J	Incropol CS-50
Emalex OD-5	Ethoduomeen® T/20	Hetoxol L	Incropol L-23
Emalex OD-10	Ethofat® 60/20	Hetoxol L-4	Incroquat S-85
Emalex OD-16	Ethofat® 60/25	Hetoxol L-9	Intravon® JU
Emalex OD-20	Ethofat® 142/20	Hetoxol M-3	Iscolan
Emalex OD-25	Ethofat® C/25	Hetoxol OA-5 Special	Kemester® 2000
Emalex OP-5	Ethoxyol® 1707	Hetoxol OL-2	Kemester® 4000
Emalex OP-8	Ethylan® KEO	Hetoxol OL-4	Kessco® Isobutyl Stearate
Emalex OP-10	Ethylan® TC	Hetoxol OL-5	Kessco® PEG 200 DL
Emalex OP-15	Ethylan® TN-10	Hetoxol OL-10	Kessco® PEG 200 DO
Emalex OP-20	Ethylan® TT-15	Hetoxol OL-10H	Kessco® PEG 200 DS
Emalex OP-25	Etocas 20	Hetoxol OL-20	Kessco® PEG 200 ML
Emalex OP-30	Etocas 40	Hetoxol OL-23	Kessco® PEG 200 MO
Emalex OP-40	Etocas 50	Hetoxol OL-40	Kessco® PEG 200 MS
Emalex OP-50	Etocas 100	Hetoxol PLA	Kessco® PEG 300 DL
Emcol® 4100M	Fancol ALA-10	Hetoxol STA-2	Kessco® PEG 300 DO
Emcol® 4161L	Fancor IPL	Hetoxol STA-10	Kessco® PEG 300 DS
Emcol® 4300	Flexricin® 9	Hetoxol STA-20	Kessco® PEG 300 ML
Emcol® 4500	Flexricin® 13	Hetoxol STA-30	Kessco® PEG 300 MO
Emcol® 6748	Flexricin® 15	Hetoxol TD-9	Kessco® PEG 300 MS
Emcol® CC-9	Foamid AME-70	Hetoxol TD-25	Kessco® PEG 400 DL
Emcol® Coco Betaine	Foamid AME-75	Hetsulf 60T	Kessco® PEG 400 DO
Emerest® 1723	Foamid AME-100	Hetsulf Acid	Kessco® PEG 400 DS
Emerest® 2452	Foamid LM2E	Hetsulf IPA	Kessco® PEG 400 ML
Emerest® 11723	Foamid LME-75	Hodag 20-L	Kessco® PEG 400 MO
Emery® 5418	Foamox CDO	Hodag 22-L	Kessco® PEG 400 MS
Empicol® 0185	Foamtaine CAB-A	Hodag 40-L	Kessco® PEG 600 DL
Empicol® 0919	Foamtaine CAB-G	Hodag 40-O	Kessco® PEG 600 DO
Empicol® LZ	Forlan L	Hodag 40-R	Kessco® PEG 600 DS
Empicol® LZ/D	Gafac® RE-877	Hodag 40-S	Kessco® PEG 600 ML
Empicol® LZP	Gemtex PA-70P	Hodag 42-L	Kessco® PEG 600 MO
Empicol® LZV/D	Gemtex PA-75	Hodag 42-O	Kessco® PEG 600 MS
Empigen® BB	Gemtex PA-75E	Hodag 42-S	Kessco® PEG 1000 DL
Empigen® BB-AU	Gemtex PA-85P	Hodag 60-L	Kessco® PEG 1000 DO
Empilan® FD	Gemtex PAX-60	Hodag 60-S	Kessco® PEG 1000 DS
Emsorb® 2721	Gemtex SC-75E, SC Powd	Hodag 62-O	Kessco® PEG 1000 ML
Emthox® 5882	Generol® 122E25	Hodag 100-S	Kessco® PEG 1000 MO
Emthox® 5940	Geropon® 99	Hodag 150-S	Kessco® PEG 1000 MS
Emthox® 5941	Geropon® AC-78	Hodag DOSS-70	Kessco® PEG 1540 DL
Emthox® 5942	Geropon® AS-200	Hodag DOSS-75	Kessco® PEG 1540 DO
Emthox® 5943	Geropon® AS-250	Hodag DTSS-70	Kessco® PEG 1540 DS
Emthox® 6957	Glo-Mul 4001	Hodag Nonionic 1035-L	Kessco® PEG 1540 ML
Emthox® 6962	Glo-Mul 4007	Hodag Nonionic 1044-L	Kessco® PEG 1540 MO
Emthox® 6964	GP-209	Hodag Nonionic 1061-L	Kessco® PEG 1540 MS
Emthox® 6965	GP-215 Silicone Polyol	Hodag Nonionic 1062-L	Kessco® PEG 4000 DL
Emthox® 6967	Copolymer	Hodag Nonionic 1064-L	Kessco® PEG 4000 DO
Emthox® 6968	GP-217 Silicone Polyol	Hodag Nonionic 1068-F	Kessco® PEG 4000 DS
Emthox® 6970	Copolymer	Hodag Nonionic 1088-F	Kessco® PEG 4000 ML
Emthox® 6971	GP-218	Hodag Nonionic E-5	Kessco® PEG 4000 MO
Emthox® 6972	GP-226	Hodag Nonionic E-6	Kessco® PEG 4000 MS
Emthox® 6984	Hamposyl® C	Hodag Nonionic E-7	Kessco® PEG 6000 DL
Emulmetik	Hamposyl® C-30	Hodag Nonionic E-10	Kessco® PEG 6000 DO
Emulmetik™ 100	Hamposyl® L	Hodag Nonionic E-12	Kessco® PEG 6000 DS
Emulmetik™ 110	Hamposyl® L-30	Hodag Nonionic E-20	Kessco® PEG 6000 ML

Wetting Agents *(cont'd.)*

Kessco® PEG 6000 MO
Kessco® PEG 6000 MS
Kodaflex® DEP
Kohacool L-400
Koster Keunen Beeswax
    AO2535
Koster Keunen Hydroxy-
    Polyester
Labrasol
Lan-Aqua-Sol 50
Lan-Aqua-Sol 100
Lanette® E
Lanogel® 21
Lanogel® 31
Lanogel® 41
Lanogel® 61
Lanpol 5
Lanpol 10
Lanpol 20
Lanpol 520
Lantrol® PLN
Lantrol® PLN/50
Lathanol® LAL
Lexaine® CSB-50
Lipacide CCO
Lipacide DPHP
Lipacide PCO
Lipacide PK
Lipacide UCO
Lipocol C-2
Lipocol C-10
Lipocol C-20
Lipocol HCO-40
Lipocol HCO-60
Lipocol L-1
Lipocol L-4
Lipocol L-12
Lipocol L-23
Lipocol M-4
Lipocol O-2 Special
Lipocol O-3 Special
Lipocol O-10
Lipocol O-20
Lipocol S-2
Lipocol S-10
Lipocol S-20
Lipocol SC-4
Lipocol SC-10
Lipocol SC-15
Lipocol SC-20
Lipocol TD-3
Lipocol TD-6
Lipocol TD-12
Lonzaine® C
Lonzaine® CO
Lonzest® PEG 4-L
Lutensol® FA 12
Macol® 1
Macol® 2
Macol® 2D
Macol® 2LF
Macol® 4
Macol® 8
Macol® 10
Macol® 22
Macol® 23
Macol® 27
Macol® 31

Macol® 32
Macol® 33
Macol® 34
Macol® 35
Macol® 40
Macol® 42
Macol® 44
Macol® 46
Macol® 72
Macol® 77
Macol® 85
Macol® 88
Macol® 101
Macol® 108
Macol® CA-2
Macol® CSA-2
Macol® CSA-4
Macol® CSA-10
Macol® CSA-15
Macol® CSA-20
Macol® CSA-40
Macol® CSA-50
Macol® DNP-5
Macol® DNP-10
Macol® DNP-15
Macol® DNP-21
Macol® LA-4
Macol® LA-9
Macol® LA-12
Macol® LA-23
Macol® LA-790
Macol® NP-4
Macol® NP-5
Macol® NP-6
Macol® NP-8
Macol® NP-11
Macol® NP-12
Macol® NP-15
Macol® NP-20
Macol® NP-20(70)
Macol® NP-30(70)
Macol® NP-100
Macol® OA-2
Macol® OA-4
Macol® OA-5
Macol® OA-10
Macol® OA-20
Macol® OP-3
Macol® OP-5
Macol® OP-8
Macol® OP-10
Macol® OP-10 SP
Macol® OP-12
Macol® OP-16(75)
Macol® OP-30(70)
Macol® OP-40(70)
Macol® SA-2
Macol® SA-5
Macol® SA-10
Macol® SA-15
Macol® SA-20
Macol® SA-40
Macol® TD-3
Macol® TD-8
Macol® TD-10
Macol® TD-12
Macol® TD-15
Macol® TD-100

Macol® TD-610
Mafo® CAB
Mafo® CAB 425
Manoxol OT/P
Manro BEC 28
Manro ML 33
Manro SLS 28
Manro TL 40
Mapeg® CO-16
Mapeg® CO-16H
Maprosyl® 30
Maquat SC-18
Maquat SC-1632
Marlinat® DF 8
Marlipal® 24/300
Marlipal® 1012/4
Marlophor® LN-Acid
Masil® 280
Masil® 280LP
Masil® 2132
Masil® 2133
Masil® 2134
Mazamide® CCO
Mazeen® C-2
Mazeen® C-5
Mazeen® C-10
Mazeen® C-15
Mazeen® S-2
Mazeen® S-5
Mazeen® S-10
Mazeen® S-15
Mazeen® T-2
Mazeen® T-5
Mazeen® T-10
Mazeen® T-15
Merpol® A
Merpol® HCS
Mersolat H 30
Mersolat H 40
Mersolat H 68
Mersolat H 76
Mersolat H 95
Mersolat W 40
Mersolat W 68
Mersolat W 76
Mersolat W 93
Miranol® C2M-SF Conc
Miranol® CS Conc
Miranol® HM Conc
Miranol® JBS
Miranol® OM-SF Conc
Miranol® SM Conc
Mirataine® BB
Mirataine® CBC
Mirataine® CB/M
Mirataine® CBS, CBS Mod
Mirataine® H2C-HA
Mirataine® TM
Monamid® 716
Monamid® 853
Monamine 779
Monateric CA-35
Monateric CEM-38
Monateric CM-36S
Monateric CNa-40
Monawet MM-80
Monawet MO-65-150
Monawet MO-65 PEG

Monawet MO-70
Monawet MO-70-150
Monawet MO-70E
Monawet MO-70 PEG
Monawet MO-70R
Monawet MO-70RP
Monawet MO-70S
Monawet MO-75E
Monawet MO-84R2W
Monawet MO-85P
Monawet SNO-35
Montosol PF-16, -18
Montosol PG-12
Montosol PQ-11, -15
Montosol TQ-11
Montovol GF-15
Nacconol 35SL
Naturechem® GTH
Naturechem® GTR
Naturechem® PGR
Naxel™ AAS-40S
Naxel ™AAS-98S
Naxolate™ WA-97
Naxolate™ WAG
Naxolate™ WA Special
Naxonic™ NI-40
Naxonic™ NI-60
Naxonic™ NI-100
Naxonol™ CO
Naxonol™ PN 66
Naxonol™ PO
Neodol® 25-7
Neodol® 25-9
Neodol® 25-12
Neodol® 45-7
Neodol® 45-13
Niaproof® Anionic
    Surfactant 4
Niaproof® Anionic
    Surfactant 08
Nikkol NP-5
Nikkol NP-7.5
Nikkol NP-10
Nikkol NP-15
Nikkol NP-18TX
Nikkol OP-3
Nikkol OP-10
Nikkol OP-30
Nikkol OTP-75
Nikkol OTP-100
Nikkol OTP-100S
Nissan Nonion E-205
Nissan Nonion E-206
Nissan Nonion E-208
Nissan Nonion E-215
Nissan Nonion E-220
Nissan Nonion E-230
Nissan Nonion K-202
Nissan Nonion K-203
Nissan Nonion K-204
Nissan Nonion K-207
Nissan Nonion K-211
Nissan Nonion K-215
Nissan Nonion K-220
Nissan Nonion K-230
Nissan Nonion P-208
Nissan Nonion P-210
Nissan Nonion P-213

Wetting Agents *(cont'd.)*

Nissan Nonion S-206
Nissan Nonion S-207
Nissan Nonion S-215
Nissan Nonion S-220
Nissan Persoft SK
Nonasol N4AS
Nonasol N4SS
Nonionic E-4
Nonisol 100
Nonisol 300
Nopalcol Series
Nopalcol 1-S
Nopalcol 1-TW
Norfox® DCS
Norfox® DCSA
Norfox® NP-6
Norfox® SLES-02
Norfox® SLS
Norfox® T-60
Nutrol Betaine MD 3863
OHlan®
Olamin® K
Onyxol® 336
Orange Wax
Pecosil® PS-100
Pegosperse® 50 DS
Pegosperse® 6000 DS
Pegosperse® EGMS-70
Pelemol TGC
Perlankrol® DSA
PhosPho S-85
Phospholipid PTC
Phospholipid PTD
Phospholipid PTL
Phospholipid PTZ
Pluronic® 10R5
Pluronic® 10R8
Pluronic® 12R3
Pluronic® 17R1
Pluronic® 17R2
Pluronic® 17R4
Pluronic® 17R8
Pluronic® 22R4
Pluronic® 25R1
Pluronic® 25R2
Pluronic® 25R4
Pluronic® 25R5
Pluronic® 25R8
Pluronic® 31R1
Pluronic® 31R2
Pluronic® 31R4
Pluronic® F38
Pluronic® F68
Pluronic® F68LF
Pluronic® F77
Pluronic® F87
Pluronic® F88
Pluronic® F98
Pluronic® F108
Pluronic® F127
Pluronic® L10
Pluronic® L35
Pluronic® L42
Pluronic® L43
Pluronic® L44
Pluronic® L61
Pluronic® L62
Pluronic® L62D

Pluronic® L62LF
Pluronic® L63
Pluronic® L64
Pluronic® L72
Pluronic® L81
Pluronic® L92
Pluronic® L101
Pluronic® L121
Pluronic® L122
Pluronic® P65
Pluronic® P75
Pluronic® P84
Pluronic® P85
Pluronic® P94
Pluronic® P103
Pluronic® P104
Pluronic® P105
Pluronic® P123
Procetyl 10
Procetyl 30
Procetyl 50
Prox-onic HR-05
Prox-onic HR-016
Prox-onic HR-025
Prox-onic HR-030
Prox-onic HR-036
Prox-onic HR-040
Prox-onic HR-080
Prox-onic HR-0200
Prox-onic HR-0200/50
Prox-onic HRH-05
Prox-onic HRH-016
Prox-onic HRH-025
Prox-onic HRH-0200
Prox-onic HRH-0200/50
Prox-onic L 081-05
Prox-onic L 101-05
Prox-onic L 102-02
Prox-onic L 121-09
Prox-onic L 161-05
Prox-onic L 181-05
Prox-onic L 201-02
Prox-onic NP-1.5
Prox-onic NP-04
Prox-onic NP-06
Prox-onic NP-09
Prox-onic NP-010
Prox-onic NP-015
Prox-onic NP-020
Prox-onic NP-030
Prox-onic NP-030/70
Prox-onic NP-040
Prox-onic NP-040/70
Prox-onic NP-050
Prox-onic NP-050/70
Prox-onic NP-0100
Prox-onic NP-0100/70
Prox-onic PEG-2000
Prox-onic PEG-4000
Prox-onic PEG-6000
Prox-onic PEG-10,000
Prox-onic PEG-20,000
Prox-onic PEG-35,000
Radiasurf® 7150
Radiasurf® 7151
Radiasurf® 7152
Radiasurf® 7153
Radiasurf® 7156

Radiasurf® 7175
Radiasurf® 7196
Radiasurf® 7206
Radiasurf® 7269
Radiasurf® 7270
Radiasurf® 7400
Radiasurf® 7402
Radiasurf® 7403
Radiasurf® 7404
Radiasurf® 7411
Radiasurf® 7413
Radiasurf® 7414
Radiasurf® 7417
Radiasurf® 7420
Radiasurf® 7422
Radiasurf® 7423
Radiasurf® 7431
Radiasurf® 7432
Radiasurf® 7443
Radiasurf® 7444
Radiasurf® 7453
Radiasurf® 7454
Radiasurf® 7473
Radiasurf® 7900
Renex® 30
Renex® 36
Renex® 678
Renex® 688
Renex® 690
Rewopal® C 6
Rewopol® CT 65
Rewopol® SBDO 70
Rewopol® SBDO 75
Rewopon® AM-2C
Rewoquat DQ 35
Rewoteric® AM KSF-40
Rhodacal® 301-10F
Rhodacal® 330
Rhodacal® A-246L
Rhodacal® LA Acid
Rhodafac® RE-870
Rhodafac® RM-510
Rhodafac® RM-710
Rhodapex® CO-433
Rhodapex® CO-436
Rhodapex® EST-30
Rhodapon® LM
Rhodasurf® L-4
Rhodasurf® LA-90
Rhodasurf® ON-870
Ritalafa®
Ritalan® C
Ryoto Sugar Ester B-370
Ryoto Sugar Ester L-595
Ryoto Sugar Ester L-1570
Ryoto Sugar Ester L-1695
Ryoto Sugar Ester M-1695
Ryoto Sugar Ester O-1570
Sandopan® DTC
Sandopan® DTC-100
Sandopan® DTC-Acid
Sandopan® DTC Linear P
Sandopan® DTC Linear P
   Acid
Sandopan® JA-36
Sandoz Amide PE
Sandoz Amide PL
Sandoz Amide PO

Sandoz Sulfonate AAS 60S
Sarkosyl® L
Sarkosyl® LC
Sarkosyl® NL-30
Sarkosyl® O
Schercamox C-AA
Schercamox CMA
Schercamox DMA
Schercamox DMC
Schercamox DML
Schercamox DMM
Schercomid CDO-Extra
Schercomid SLM-LC
Schercopol DOS-70
Schercopol DOS-PG-70
Schercopol DOS-PG-85
Schercotaine CAB
Schercotaine CAB-G
Schercotaine MAB
Schercotaine SCAB
Schercozoline B
Schercozoline C
Silwet® L-77
Silwet® L-7002
Silwet® L-7600
Silwet® L-7602
Silwet® L-7604
Silwet® L-7614
Siponic® NP-7
Sochamine A 755
Sochamine A 7525
Sochamine A 7527
Softigen® 767
Solulan® 5
Solulan® 16
Solulan® C-24
Solulan® L-575
Solusol® 75%
Solusol® 85%
Solusol® 100%
Standamid® KDM
Standamid® LD
Standamid® SM
Standamox C 30
Standamox CAW
Standamul® GTO-26
Standapol® SCO
Steol® 4N
Steol® CA-460
Steol® KA-460
Stepanol® WA-100
Sucro Ester 7
Sucro Ester 11
Sucro Ester 15
Sulfochem SLN
Sulfochem SLP
Sulfochem SLP-95
Sulfochem TLS
Sul-fon-ate AA-9
Sul-fon-ate AA-10
Sulfopon® 103
Sulfotex WAT
Sulframin 85
Sulframin 90
Sulframin 1240, 1245
Sulframin 1250, 1260
Supermontaline SLT65
Supralate C

Wetting Agents *(cont'd.)*

Supralate EP	Tetronic® 110R7	Tween® 80	Volpo O10
Surfactol® 13	Tetronic® 130R1	Tween® 80K	Volpo O15
Surfactol® 340	Tetronic® 130R2	Tween® 81	Volpo O20
Surfactol® 380	Tetronic® 150R1	Tween® 85	Volpo T-3
Surfax 100	Tetronic® 150R4	Ufanon K-80	Volpo T-5
Surfax 100 AG	Tetronic® 150R8	Ufarol Am 30	Volpo T-10
Surfax AC 50	Tetronic® 304	Ufarol Am 70	Volpo T-15
Surfax AC 55	Tetronic® 504	Ufarol Na-30	Volpo T-20
Surfax ACI	Tetronic® 701	Ufasan 35	Wickenol® 144
Surfax CN	Tetronic® 702	Ultra Sulfate SE-5	Wickenol® 151
Surfax SLA	Tetronic® 704	Ultra Sulfate SL-1	Wickenol® 152
Surfine AZI-A	Tetronic® 707	Ungerol AM3-75	Wickenol® 153
Surfine T-A	Tetronic® 901	Ungerol LES 2-28	Wickenol® 155
Surfine WNG-A	Tetronic® 904	Ungerol LES 2-70	Wickenol® 156
Surfine WNT-A	Tetronic® 908	Ungerol LES 3-28	Wickenol® 158
Surfine WNT Conc	Tetronic® 909	Ungerol LES 3-70	Wickenol® 159
Surfine WNT Gel	Tetronic® 1101	Ungerol N2-28	Wickenol® 160
Surfine WNT LC	Tetronic® 1102	Ungerol N2-70	Wickenol® 161
Surfine WNT-LS	Tetronic® 1104	Ungerol N3-28	Wickenol® 171
Surfonic® N-10	Tetronic® 1107	Ungerol N3-70	Witcamide® 82
Surfonic® N-31.5	Tetronic® 1301	Vanseal® CS	Witcamide® 5133
Surfonic® N-40	Tetronic® 1302	Vanseal® LS	Witcamide® 5195
Surfonic® N-60	Tetronic® 1304	Vanseal® MS	Witcamine® 6606
Surfonic® N-85	Tetronic® 1307	Vanseal® NACS-30	Witcamine® 6622
Surfonic® N-95	Tetronic® 1501	Vanseal® NALS-30	Witco® Acid B
Surfonic® N-100	Tetronic® 1502	Vanseal® NALS-95	Witcolate™ 1050
Surfonic® N-102	Tetronic® 1504	Vanseal® NAMS-30	Witcolate™ 6400
Surfonic® N-120	Tetronic® 1508	Vanseal OS	Witcolate™ 6430
Surfonic® N-130	Texapon® K-12 USP	Varonic® 2271	Witcolate™ 6431
Surfonic® N-150	Texapon® K-1294	Varonic® K-202 SF	Witcolate™ 6462
Surfonic® N-200	Texapon® K-1296 USP	Varonic® K-205	Witcolate™ A
Surfonic® N-300	Texapon® L-100	Varonic® K-205 SF	Witcolate™ A Powder
Surfonic® NB-5	Texapon® PNA-127	Varonic® K-210 SF	Witcolate™ AE-3
Surfynol® 82	Texapon® VHC Needles	Varonic® K-215 SF	Witcolate™ AM
Swanol AM-301	Texapon® VHC Powd	Varonic® Q-202 SF	Witcolate™ C
Sykanol DKM 45, 80	Texapon® Z	Varonic® Q-205 SF	Witcolate™ ES-1
Synotol 119 N	Texapon® Z Granules	Varonic® S-202 SF	Witcolate™ ES-2
Synotol Detergent E	Texapon® ZHC Needles	Varonic® T-202 SF	Witcolate™ ES-3
Synotol L 60	Texapon® ZHC Powder	Varonic® T-205 SF	Witcolate™ LCP
Synotol L 90	Texofor B7	Varonic® T-210 SF	Witcolate™ LES-60A
Synotol LM 60	T-Maz® 20	Varonic® T-215 SF	Witcolate™ LES-60C
Synotol LM 90	T-Maz® 28	Velsan® D8P-3	Witcolate™ NH
Synotol ME 90	T-Maz® 40	Velsan® P8-3	Witcolate™ S
Synperonic T/1301	T-Maz® 60	Velsan® P8-16	Witcolate™ S1285C
Synperonic T/1302	T-Maz® 61	Vigilan AWS	Witcolate™ S1300C
Syntopon A	T-Maz® 65	Volpo 25 D 3	Witcolate™ TLS-500
Tauranol M-35	T-Maz® 80	Volpo 25 D 5	Witcolate™ WAC
Tauranol MS	T-Maz® 80KLM	Volpo 25 D 10	Witcolate™ WAC-GL
Tauranol T-Gel	T-Maz® 81	Volpo 25 D 15	Witcolate™ WAC-LA
Tergitol® NP-9	T-Maz® 85	Volpo 25 D 20	Witconate™ 30DS
Teric 12A3	T-Maz® 90	Volpo CS-3	Witconate™ 45LX
Tetronic® 50R1	T-Maz® 95	Volpo CS-5	Witconate™ 60T
Tetronic® 50R4	Triton® X-100	Volpo CS-10	Witconate™ 68KN
Tetronic® 50R8	Trivent OL-10	Volpo CS-15	Witconate™ 79S
Tetronic® 70R1	Trivent OL-10B	Volpo CS-20	Witconate™ 90F H
Tetronic® 70R2	Trylox® 6746	Volpo N3	Witconate™ 93S
Tetronic® 70R4	Tween® 20	Volpo N5	Witconate™ 1240
Tetronic® 90R1	Tween® 21	Volpo N10	Witconate™ 1250
Tetronic® 90R4	Tween® 40	Volpo N15	Zoramox
Tetronic® 90R8	Tween® 60	Volpo N20	Zoramox E
Tetronic® 110R1	Tween® 61	Volpo O3	Zoramox LO
Tetronic® 110R2	Tween® 65	Volpo O5	

Part III
Chemical Component
Cross-Reference

Chemical Component Cross-Reference

Abietic acid (INCI)
CAS 514-10-3; EINECS 208-178-3
Synonyms: Abietinic acid; Sylvic acid
Trade names containing: Grillocin HY-77

Acacia (INCI)
CAS 9000-01-5; EINECS 232-519-5
Synonyms: Acacia gum; Gum arabic
Trade names: Spray Dried Gum Arabic NF Type CSP
Trade names containing: Liquid Crystal (LC) CAPS 122

Acacia extract (INCI)
Synonyms: Acacia farnesiana extract; Acacia senegal extract
Trade names containing: Acacia Flower Extract HS 2744 G; Actiphyte of Acacia

Acetamide MEA (INCI)
CAS 142-26-7; EINECS 205-530-8
Synonyms: N-Acetyl ethanolamine; N-(2-Hydroxy-ethyl)acetamide
Trade names: Amidex AME; Carsamide® AMEA; Foamid AME-70; Foamid AME-75; Foamid AME-100; Hetamide MA; Incromectant AMEA-70; Incromectant AMEA-100; Lipamide MEAA; Mackamide™ AME-75, AME-100; Schercomid AME; Upamide ACMEA; Witcamide® CMEA;
Trade names containing: Aqua-Tein C; Aqua-Tein S; Collamino™ Complex ESC; Collamino™ Complex S; Collamino™ Complex SS; Collamino™ Complex; Incromectant LAMEA; Lipo-Peptide AME 30

Acetamidopropyl trimonium chloride (INCI)
CAS 123776-56-7
Trade names: Incromectant AQ

Acetic acid (INCI)
CAS 64-19-7; EINECS 200-580-7
Synonyms: Ethanoic acid; Vinegar acid; Methane-car-boxylic acid
Trade names: Unichem ACETA

6-(N-Acetylamino)-4-oxahexyltrimonium chloride
Trade names: Quamectant™ AM-50

Acetylated glycol stearate
Trade names: Cetacene

Acetylated hydrogenated cottonseed glyceride (INCI)
CAS 977055-83-6
Synonyms: Glycerides, cottonseed-oil, mono-, hydroge-nated, acetates
Trade names: Myvacet® 5-07

Acetylated hydrogenated lanolin (INCI)
CAS 91053-41-7; EINECS 293-306-0
Trade names: Lipocerina

Acetylated hydrogenated tallow glyceride (INCI)
CAS 68990-58-9; EINECS 273-612-0
Synonyms: Glycerides, tallow mono-, hydrogenated, acetates
Trade names: Lamegin® EE

Acetylated lanolin (INCI)
CAS 61788-48-5; EINECS 262-979-2
Trade names: Acelan L; Acetadeps; Acylan; Fancol Acel; Ivarlan™ 3300; Lanacet® 1705; Lanolin A.C; Modulan®; Ritacetyl®; Unilan Acetyl

Acetylated lanolin alcohol (INCI)
CAS 61788-49-6; EINECS 262-980-8
Synonyms: Lanolin, alcohols, acetates
Trade names: Hetlan AC; Protalan MOD
Trade names containing: Acelan A; Acetol® 1706; Acetulan®; Argonol ACE 5; Crodalan AWS; Crodalan LA; Ethoxyol® 1707; Fancol ALA-10; Fancol ALA-15; Fancol ALA; Ivarbase™ 3210; Ivarbase™ 98; Lanalene 97; Lanalene 98; Lanalene AC; Lanaetex-75; Naturon® 2X IPA; Protalan 98; Protalan AC; Ritawax AEO; Ritawax ALA; Solulan® 97; Solulan® 98; Trivent ALA

Acetylated palm kernel glycerides (INCI)
Synonyms: Glycerides, palm kernel oil mono-, di-, and tri, acetates
Trade names: Cetodan® 95 CO

Acetylated vegetable glycerides (INCI)
Trade names: Myvacet® 9-45

Acetyl ethyl octanoate
Synonyms: 2-n-Hexyl-aceto-acetic ethyl ester
Trade names: Hexyl Jasmat®

Acetyl hexamethyl indan (INCI)
CAS 15323-35-0; EINECS 239-360-0
Synonyms: 1-(2,3-Dihydro-1,1,2,3,3,6-hexamethyl-1H-inden-5-yl) ethanone; 6-Acetyl-1,1,2,3,3,5-hexa-methyl indan
Trade names containing: Amtolide

Acetyl hexamethyl tetralin (INCI)
CAS 1506-02-1; EINECS 216-133-4
Synonyms: 6-Acetyl-1,1,2,4,4,7-hexamethyl-1,2,3,4-tetrahydronaphthalene; 1-(5,6,7,8-Tetrahydro-3,5,5,6,8,8-hexamethyl-2-naphthalenyl) ethanone
Trade names containing: Amtolide

Acetyl tributyl citrate (INCI)
CAS 77-90-7; EINECS 201-067-0
Synonyms: 2-(Acetyloxy)-1,2,3-propanetricarboxylic acid, tributyl ester; 1,2,3-Propanetricarboxylic acid, 2-acetyloxy)-, tributyl est
Trade names: ATBC; Citroflex A-4; Uniplex 84

Acetyl triethyl citrate (INCI)
CAS 77-89-4; EINECS 201-066-5
Synonyms: 2-(Acetyloxy)-1,2,3-propanetricarboxylic acid, triethyl ester
Trade names: ATEC

Acetyl tri-n-hexyl citrate (INCI)
CAS 24817-92-3
Trade names: Citroflex A-6

Acetyltyrosine (INCI)
CAS 537-55-3; EINECS 208-671-3
Trade names: Chemodyne N-Acetyltyrosine
Trade names containing: Unipertan P-2002; Unipertan P-242; Unipertan VEG 24; Unipertan VEG 242

Achillea millefolium extract. *See Yarrow extract*

Acrylamide/sodium acrylate copolymer (INCI)
CAS 25085-02-3
Synonyms: 2-Propenamide, polymer with 2-propenoic acid, sodium salt; 2-Propenoic acid, sodium salt, polymer with 2-propenamide
Trade names: Hostacerin PN 73

Acrylamidopropyltrimonium chloride/acrylates copolymer (INCI)
Trade names: Produkt W 37194

Acrylates/acrylamide copolymer (INCI)
Trade names: Ultrahold® 8

Acrylates/C10-30 alkyl acrylate crosspolymer (INCI)
Trade names: Carbopol® 1342; Carbopol® 1382; Pemulen® TR-1, TR-2

Acrylates copolymer (INCI)
Synonyms: Acrylic/acrylate copolymer
Trade name: Acrymul AM 123R; Acrysol® 33 Polymer; Acusol® 820; Acylyn™ 33; Carboset 514; Carboset XL-19X2; Carboset XL-28; Carboset XL-40; Carboset XPD-1616; Chronosponge; Eudispert; Freederm; Microsponge® 5640; Polytrap® 6603; Polytrap® Q5-6603; Porosponge; Rohagit® S, SD 15
Trade names containing: Blanc Covanail W 9737; DHA Melanosponge; Dow Corning® Q5-6038 Polymer Beads; Microsponge® 5647; Microsponge® 5650; Polytrap® 6035; Polytrap® Q5-6035; Polytrap® Q5-6038 Polymer Beads

Acrylates/diacetoneacrylamide copolymer (INCI)
Trade names: Plascize L-53

Acrylates/octylacrylamide copolymer (INCI)
CAS 9002-93-1 (generic); 9036-19-5 (generic); 9004-87-9 (generic)
Synonyms: Acrylates/octylpropenamide copolymer
Trade names: Dermacryl™ 79; National Starch 28-4979

Acrylates/PVP copolymer (INCI)
CAS 26589-26-4
Synonyms: Methacrylic acid, polymer with ethyl methacrylate and 1-vinyl-2-pyrrolidinone
Trade names: Luviflex® VBM 35; Stepanhold® Extra; Stepanhold® R-1

Acrylate/steareth-20 methacrylate copolymer (INCI)
Trade names: Aculyn™ 22; Acrysol® 22 Polymer; Acrysol® ICS-1 Thickener

Acrylic acid/acrylonitrogens copolymer (INCI)
CAS 61788-40-7; 136505-00-5, 136505-01-6
Trade names: Hypan® SA100H; Hypan® SR150H

Acrylic/acrylate copolymer. *See Acrylates copolymer*

Acrylic resin
Synonyms: Acrylic polymer; Acrylic fiber; Nitrile rubber
Trade names: Carboset 525
Trade names containing: Carboset 514A; Carboset 514H; Carboset 531

Actin hydrolysate. *See Hydrolyzed actin*

Adenosine triphosphate (INCI)
CAS 56-65-5; EINECS 200-283-2

Synonyms: ATP; Adenosine, 5´-(tetrahydrogen triphosphate)
Trade names containing: ATP Nucleotides; Unipertan P-242; Unipertan P-2002; Unipertan VEG 242

Adipic acid/dimethylaminohydroxypropyl diethylenetriamine copolymer (INCI)
CAS 61840-27-5
Trade names: Cartaretin F-4; Cartaretin F-23

Adipic acid/epoxypropyl diethylenetriamine copolymer (INCI)
CAS 52932-31-7, 25212-19-5
Trade names: Delsette 101

AEPD. *See 2-Amino-2-ethyl-1,3-propanediol*

Alabaster. *See Calcium sulfate (dihydrate)*

Alanine (INCI)
CAS 56-41-7 (L-form); EINECS 200-273-8
Synonyms: 2-Aminopropionic acid
Trade names containing: Hydro-Diffuser Microreservoir; Hygroplex HHG; Monteine PRO; Nikkol Aquasome LA; Omega-CH Activator; Unimoist U-125

Albumen (INCI)
CAS 9006-50-2
Synonyms: Dried egg white; Egg albumin; Albumin
Trade names: Egg White Solids Type P-20; Granular Hennegg Albumen Type G-1; Instant Egg White Solids Type P-600; Sol-U-Tein EA
Trade names containing: BioCare® SA

Albumin. *See Albumen*

Alcohol (INCI)
CAS 64-17-5; EINECS 200-578-6
Synonyms: EtOH; Ethyl alcohol, undenatured; Ethanol, undenatured; Distilled spirits; Absolute alcohol
Trade names: Punctilious® Ethyl Alcohol
Trade names containing: Advantage™ CP; Advantage™ V; Aloe Extract Vera; Auxina Tricogena; Benibana Liq.; Biochelated Extract of Lemon Grass; Biochelated Sea Kelp Extract; Chinpi Liq.; Cholecithine; Chouji Liq.; Collapurol® E 1; Complex GT; Copolymer 958; Emulmetik 920; Ethoquad® T/12; Evosina NA 2; FM Extract; Gadeneel Liq.; Gaffix® VC-713; Gantrez® ES-225; Gantrez® ES-425; Gantrez® V-215; Gantrez® V-225; Gantrez® V-425; Garionzet; Guineshing-LV; Hair Complex Aquosum; Hexaplant Richter; Hydratherm CGI Hydroalcoholic; IPF Meadowsweet; Isodon Extract; Kamitsure Liq.; Koucha Liq.; Liquiritina; Midpol 2000; Monawet MO-75E; Natipide®; Natipide 08010E; Natipide® II; Oxynex® L; Ormagel AC-400; Phosal® 53 MCT; Phosal® 75 SA; Pro-Tein SA-20; PVP/VA E-735; Sedaplant Richter; Semburi Extract Ethanol; Sohakuhi Extract Ethanol; Soluvit Richter; Unibotan Vitaplant W CLR; Variquat® 50AE; Variquat® 50AE; Variquat® 50ME; Variquat® 50ME; Variquat® 80AE; Variquat® 80AE; Varisoft® 432-ET; Varisoft® TS-50; Vitaplant CLR Water-Soluble

Alcohol C-10. *See n-Decyl alcohol*

Alcohols, C12-13. *See C12-13 alcohols*

Alfalfa extract (INCI)
CAS 84082-36-0
Synonyms: Medicago sativa extract
Trade names containing: Actiphyte of Alfalfa; Alfalfa Herb Extract HS 2967 G; BBC Mineral Complex

Algae extract (INCI)
CAS 68917-51-1, 92128-82-0
Synonyms: Absolute algae; Extract of algae
Trade names containing: Actisea™ 100; Algogen; Blend

For Slenderizing Prods. HS 255; Elespher® Almondermin; Elespher® Dermosaccharides GY; Elespher® Dermosaccharides HC; Elespher® Eleseryl SH; Herbasol-Extract Algae; Hydratherm CGI Glycolic; Hydratherm CGI Hydroalcoholic; Hydratherm CGI Lyophilized; Laminarina; Lipoplastidine Laminaria; Nutrimarine; Ormagel AC-400; Ormagel SH; Ormagel XPU; Seanamin SU; Vitamarine

Algin (INCI)
CAS 9005-38-3
Synonyms: Sodium alginate; Sodium polymannuronate
Trade names: Dariloid® QH; Kelco® HV; Kelco® LV; Kelcosol®; Kelgin® F; Kelgin® HV; Kelgin® LV, MV; Kelgin® QL; Kelgin® XL; Keltone; Sobalg FD 100 Series

Alginic acid (INCI)
CAS 9005-32-7; EINECS 232-680-1
Synonyms: Norgine
Trade names: Alginic Acid FCC; Kelacid®; Satialgine™ H8

Alkanes, C11-12-iso-. *See C11-12 isoparaffin*

Alkanet extract (INCI)
Synonyms: Alkanna tinctoria extract; Spanish bugloss extract
Trade names containing: Alkanet LS

Alkyl C12-16 ethyldimethyl ethosulfate
Trade names: Variquat® CE 100

Alkyl dimethyl benzyl ammonium chloride. *See Benzalkonium chloride*

Alkyl trimethyl ammonium bromide
Trade names: Empigen® CHB40

Allantoin (INCI)
CAS 97-59-6; EINECS 202-592-8
Synonyms: (2,5-Dioxo-4-imidazolidinyl) urea; Glyoxyldiureide; 5-Ureidohydrantoin
Trade names: Allantoin Powd. No. 1015; Atomergic Allantoin; Chemie Linz Allantoin; Fancol TOIN; Tri-K Allantoin; Uniderm A
Trade names containing: Antiphlogistic ARO; Asebiol® LS; Brookosome® A; Dermasome® A; Facteur Hydratant PH; Hydrolyzed NMF; Hydroviton 2/ 059353; Sedaplant Richter; Sphingosomes® AL

Allantoin acetyl methionine (INCI)
CAS 4207-40-3; EINECS 224-126-2
Synonyms: Allantoin N-acetyl-DL-methionine
Trade names: Tri-K Allantoin Acetyl Methionine

Alligator pear oil. *See Avocado oil*

Allium sativum extract. *See Garlic extract*

Almondamide DEA (INCI)
Synonyms: Almond amides, N,N-bis (2-hydroxyethyl)-; Diethanolamine almond fatty acid condensate; Almond diethanolamide
Trade names: Incromide ALD

Almondamidopropyl betaine (INCI)
Synonyms: Almondamidopropyl dimethyl glycine; Almond amide propylbetaine
Trade names: Incronam AL-30

Almondamidopropyl dimethylamine (INCI)
Trade names: Incromine ALB

Almondamidopropyl dimethyl glycine. *See Almondamidopropyl betaine*

Almond meal (INCI)
Trade names: Lipo AM; Lipo AMS

Almond oil
Synonyms: Amygdalin
Trade names: Natoil ALM; Super Refined™ Almond Oil NF

Almond oil PEG-6 esters (INCI)
Trade names: Labrafil® M 1966 CS

Aloe (INCI)
CAS 8001-97-6
Synonyms: Aloe vera
Trade names: Aloe Vera Whole Leaf Dried Powd

Aloe barbadensis extract. *See Aloe extract*

Aloe extract (INCI)
CAS 85507-69-3
Synonyms: Aloe barbadensis extract; Extract of aloe; Curacao aloe extract
Trade names: Activera™ 106 LIPO M; Activera™ 107 LIPO C; Aloe Extract #101; Aloe Vera Aqueous Extract Conc; Aloe Vera Lipo-Quinone Extract; Aloe Vera Polysaccharide #0179121B01; Veragel® Aq. Conc. 1:10; Veragel® Lipoid
Trade names containing: Actiphyte of Aloe Vera 10-Fold; Actiphyte of Aloe Vera 20-Fold; Actiphyte of Aloe Vera 40-Fold; Actiphyte of Aloe Vera; Aloe Extract #102; Aloe Extract #103; Aloe Extract #104; Aloe Extract #105; Aloe Extract HS 2386 G; Aloe Extract Special; Aloe Extract Vera; Aloe HS; Aloe Vera Oil 0030X; Aloe Vera Oil 0040X; Alowcape Liq. B-7; Cremogen Aloe Vera; Dermascreen; Herbasol-Extract Aloe; Lipoplastidine Aloe; Unibotan Vitaplant W CLR; Vitaplant CLR Water-Soluble

Aloe flower extract (INCI)
Trade names containing: Aloe Flower Extract PG

Aloe vera. *See Aloe*

Aloe vera gel (INCI)
Trade names: Activera™; Activera™ 1-1FA (Filtered); Activera™ 1-10; Activera™ 1-20; Activera™ 1-200 A; Activera™ 104; Aloe Con UP 10; Aloe Con UP 40; Aloe-Con UP-200; Aloe Con WG 10; Aloe Con WG 40; Aloe Con WG 200; Aloe Con WLG 10; Aloe Con WLG 200; Aloe Gel Stabilized; Aloe Phytogel 1:199 Powd.; Aloe-Phytogel 199 Powd.; Aloe Vera Conc. 40 Fold; Aloe Vera Freeze Dried Powd. 200:1; Aloe Vera Gel; Aloe Vera Gel 1:1; Aloe Vera Gel 1:1; Aloe Vera Gel 1:1 Decolorized; Aloe Vera Gel 1:1 With Pulp; Aloe Vera Gel 1:2; Aloe Vera Gel 1:2; Aloe Vera Gel 1:10; Aloe Vera Gel 1:10 Conc.; Aloe Vera Gel 1:50; Aloe Vera Gel 1:50 Conc.; Aloe Vera Gel 1:100; Aloe Vera Gel 1:100 Conc.; Aloe Vera Gel 10:1 Decolorized; Aloe Vera Gel 10:1, 40:1; Aloe Vera Gel Conc. 10:1; Aloe Vera Gel Conc. 40:1; Aloe Vera Gel Conc. 40:1 Decolorized; Aloe Vera Gel CS; Aloe Vera Gel CS 10; Aloe Vera Gel CS 40; Aloe Vera Gel DC; Aloe Vera Gel DC 10; Aloe Vera Gel DC 40; Aloe Vera Gel Filtered; Aloe Vera Gel Single Fold; Aloe Vera Gel TEX; Aloe Vera Gel Unfiltered; Aloe Vera Juice; Aloe Vera Oil; Aloe Vera Powd. 200:1; Aloe Vera Powd. 200XXX Extract-Microfine; Aloe Vera Powd. A 1-200; Aloe Vera Pulp; Aloe Vera Spray Dried Powd.; Alomucin; Alo-X-11; Aruba Aloe Vera Gel; Cal-O-Vera 1:1; Cal-O-Vera 10:1; Cal-O-Vera 40:1; Cal-O-Vera 200XXX Powd.; CG 10x (Unfiltered and stabilized); Clear Filtered Verajuice-Cold Processed; CoVera; CoVera Dry; Filtered Verajuice-Cold Processed; George's Aloe Vera; Lanaetex Aloe Vera Gel; Powdered Aloe Vera (1:200) Food Grade; Ritaloe 1X, 10X, 20X, 40X; Ritaloe 200M; Veragel® 200; Veragel® Liq., Liq. 1:1

Trade names containing: Actisea™ 100; Brookosome®
V; Dermasome® V; Ritacomplex DF 15

Althea extract (INCI)
CAS 97676-24-9
Synonyms: Althea officinalis extract; Marshmallow root
extract
Trade names containing: Almondermin® LS; Althea Liq.;
BBC Moisture Trol; Bio-Chelated Sauna-Derm I;
Elespher® Almondermin

Alum. *See Aluminum sulfate*

Alumina
CAS 1344-28-1; EINECS 215-691-6
Synonyms: Aluminum oxide; Calcined alumina; Alumite
Trade names: Alumina, Activated 4082; Alumina, Cal-
cined 612; Alumina, Tabular 635; Alumina Trihydrate
617; Aluminum Oxide C; Cosmetic Alumina Hydrate;
Dispal; Linde A
Trade names containing: UV-Titan M210; UV-Titan
M212; UV-Titan M260; UV-Titan M262

Alumina, hydrate (INCI)
CAS 1333-84-2; 21645-51-2
Synonyms: Alumina trihydrate; Aluminum hydroxide;
Aluminum trihydroxide
Trade names: Hydral® 710

Alumina trihydrate. *See Alumina, hydrate*

Aluminum ammonium sulfate. *See Ammonium alum*

Aluminum capryloyl hydrolyzed collagen (INCI)
Trade names: Lipacide C8CO Al

Aluminum chloride basic
Trade names: Westchlor® 200 Custom Powd. 10;
Westchlor® 200 Impalpable; Westchlor® DM 200
Impalpable

Aluminum chloride hydroxide. *See Aluminum chlorohydrate*

Aluminum chlorohydrate (INCI)
CAS 1327-41-9; 12042-91-0; EINECS 215-477-2
Synonyms: Aluminum chloride hydroxide; Aluminum
chlorohydrol; Aluminum chlorohydroxide
Trade names: Alchlordrate; Aloxicoll® L; Aloxicoll® PC;
Aloxicoll® PF; Aloxicoll® PSF; Aluminum Hydroxy-
chloride 23; Aluminum Hydroxychloride 47;
Chlorhydrol® 50% Sol'n; Chlorhydrol® Granular;
Chlorhydrol, Impalpable; Chlorhydrol® Powd; Dow
Corning® ACH-303; Dow Corning® ACH-323; Dow
Corning® ACH-331; Dow Corning® ACH7-321; Dow
Corning® Q5-7171 AACH Powd; Locron Extra,
Flakes, L, P, P Extra, Powd., S, Sol'n; Macro-
spherical® 95; Micro-Dry®; Micro-Dry® Super-
ultrafine; Micro-Dry® Ultrafine; Reach® 101, 201,
501; Ritachlor 50%; Westchlor® 200

Aluminum chlorohydrex PG (INCI)
Trade names: Rehydrol® II

Aluminum citrate (INCI)
CAS 813-92-3
Synonyms: 2-Hydroxy-1,2,3-propanetricarboxylic acid,
aluminum salt (1:1)
Trade names: Alutrat

Aluminum distearate (INCI)
CAS 300-92-5; EINECS 206-101-8
Trade names: Haro® Chem ALMD-2; Witco® Aluminum
Stearate EA Food Grade

Aluminum formate (INCI)
CAS 7360-53-4; EINECS 230-898-1
Trade names: Altriform S

Aluminum hydroxide (INCI)
CAS 21645-51-2; EINECS 244-492-7
Synonyms: Aluminum oxide trihydrate; Aluminum
trihydrate
Trade names: BB-1; Rehydragel® Compressed Gel;
Rehydragel® Low Visc. Gel; Rehydragel® Thixotro-
pic Gel
Trade names containing: Gilugel R

Aluminum isostearates/laurates/palmitates (INCI)
Trade names containing: Co-Gell® A2/B270

Aluminum/magnesium hydroxide stearate (INCI)
Trade names containing: Gilugel ALM; Gilugel CAO;
Gilugel EUG; Gilugel IPM; Gilugel IPP; Gilugel MIG;
Gilugel MIN; Gilugel OS; Gilugel SIL5

Aluminum oxide. *See Alumina*

Aluminum oxide trihydrate. *See Aluminum hydroxide*

Aluminum PCA (INCI)
CAS 59792-81-3; EINECS 261-931-8
Synonyms: Aluminum, tris (5-oxo-L-prolinato-);
Pyrrolidone carboxylic acid, aluminum salt
Trade names: Aludone®

Aluminumsesquichloride
Trade names: Westchlor® 170 Powd

Aluminum sesquichlorohydrate (INCI)
CAS 11097-68-0
Trade names: Dow Corning® ACH7-308; Westchlor®
170

Aluminum silicate (INCI)
CAS 1327-36-2; 12141-46-7; EINECS 215-475-1
Synonyms: Pyrophyllite
Trade names: Kaopolite® SF; Suspengel Elite;
Suspengel Micro; Suspengel Ultra
Trade names containing: Pad-1

Aluminum starch octenyl succinate (INCI)
CAS 9087-61-0
Synonyms: Starch, octenylbutanedioate, aluminum salt
Trade names: Dry Flo® PC; Fluidamid DF 12

Aluminum stearate
CAS 7047-84-9; 637-12-7
Synonyms: Aluminum, dihydroxy (octadecanoato-o-)
Trade names: Cecavon AL 11; Cecavon AL 12;
Radiastar® 1200; Radiastar® 1208; Synpro® Alumi-
num Stearate USP; Witco® Aluminum Stearate 18
Trade names containing: Base W/O 126; Dehymuls® E;
Dehymuls® F; Dehymuls® K; Hostacerin WO;
Hostacerin WOL; Novogel® ST; Umulse-E

Aluminum sulfate (INCI)
CAS 10043-01-3; EINECS 233-135-0
Synonyms: Alum; Aluminum trisulfate; Cake alum
Trade names: Unichem ALSUL

Aluminum tristearate (INCI)
CAS 637-12-7; EINECS 211-279-5
Trade names: Witco® Aluminum Stearate 132

Aluminum undecylenoyl collagen amino acids (INCI)
Trade names: Lipacid UCO Al

Aluminum zirconium octachlorohydrex GLY (INCI)
Trade names: Westchlor® ZR 82B DM Powd

Aluminum zirconium pentachlorohydrate (INCI)
Trade names: Rezal® 67; Rezal® 67P

Aluminum zirconium pentachlorohydrex GLY (INCI)
Trade names: Westchlor® ZR 80B DM Powd
Trade names containing: Westchlor® A2Z 8106

Aluminum zirconium tetrachlorohydrex GLY (INCI)
Trade names: Dow Corning® AZG-368; Dow Corning®

AZG-369; Dow Corning® AZG-370; Dow Corning® Q5-7155 AAZG Powd; Dow Corning® Q5-7160 AZAG Powd; Dow Corning® Q5-7167 AAZG Powd; Reach® AZP-701, AZP-703; Rezal® 36; Rezal® 36G; Rezal® 36G Conc; Rezal® 36GP; Rezal® 36GP Superultrafine; Westchlor® ZR 35B; Westchlor® ZR 35B DM Powd; Westchlor® ZR 35B Micro Powd; Westchlor® ZR 41; Zirkonal L; Zirkonal P

Aluminum/zirconium trichlorohydrex GLY (INCI)
  Trade names: Reach® AZZ-902; Westchlor® ZR 30B; Westchlor® ZR 30B DM Powd

Amine dodecylbenzene sulfonate
  Trade names: Marlopon® AMS 60; Witconate™ 93S; Witconate™ YLA

Aminoacetic acid. *See Glycine*

p-Aminobenzoic acid. *See PABA*

Amino bispropyl dimethicone (INCI)
  Trade names: ALE-56

2-Amino-1-butanol (INCI)
  CAS 96-20-8; 5856-63-3; EINECS 202-488-2
  Synonyms: 2-Amino-n-butyl alcohol
  Trade names: AB®; BioGir-LAB

Aminobutylene glycol. *See 2-Amino-2-methyl-1,3-propanediol*

1-Amino-1-deoxy-D-glucitol. *See Glucamine*

2-Amino-2-deoxyglucose. *See Glucosamine*

2-Amino-2-ethyl-1,3-propanediol (INCI)
  CAS 115-70-8; EINECS 204-101-2
  Synonyms: AEPD; Aminoamylene glycol
  Trade names: AEPD®

2-Amino-3-hydroxypyridine (INCI)
  CAS 16867-03-1; EINECS 240-886-8
  Synonyms: 2-Amino-3-pyridinol
  Trade names: Rodol 2A3PYR

4-Amino-2-hydroxytoluene (INCI)
  CAS 2835-95-2; EINECS 220-618-6
  Synonyms: 4-Amino-2-hydroxy-1-methylbenzene; 5-Amino-2-methylphenol
  Trade names: Rodol PAOC

2-Amino-2-methyl-1,3-propanediol (INCI)
  CAS 115-69-5; EINECS 204-100-7
  Synonyms: AMPD; Aminobutylene glycol; Butanediolamine; 2-Amino-2-methyl-1,3-propanediol
  Trade names: AMPD

2-Amino-2-methyl-1-propanol (INCI)
  CAS 124-68-5; EINECS 204-709-8
  Synonyms: AMP; Isobutanolamine; Aminomethyl propanol; Isobutanol-2 amine
  Trade names: AMP

2-Amino-3-nitrophenol (INCI)
  CAS 603-85-0; EINECS 210-060-1
  Trade names: Imexine FO

2-Amino-5-nitrophenol (INCI)
  CAS 121-88-0; EINECS 204-503-8
  Synonyms: 5-Nitro-2-aminophenol
  Trade names: Rodol YBA

4-Amino-3-nitrophenol (INCI)
  CAS 610-81-1; EINECS 210-236-8
  Trade names: Imexine FN

m-Aminophenol (INCI)
  CAS 591-27-5; EINECS 209-711-2
  Trade names: Rodol EG
  Trade names containing: Brown GE (Fusion)

o-Aminophenol (INCI)
  CAS 95-55-6; EINECS 202-431-1
  Trade names: Rodol 2G
  Trade names containing: Brown R-36 (Fusion)

p-Aminophenol (INCI)
  CAS 123-30-8; EINECS 204-616-2
  Trade names: Rodol P Base

m-Aminophenol HCl (INCI)
  CAS 51-81-0; EINECS 200-125-2
  Synonyms: 3-Aminophenol hydrochloride
  Trade names: Rodol EGC

m-Aminophenol sulfate (INCI)
  CAS 68239-81-6; EINECS 269-475-1
  Trade names: Rodol EGS

p-Aminophenol sulfate (INCI)
  CAS 63084-98-0; EINECS 263-847-7
  Synonyms: 4-Aminophenol sulfate
  Trade names: Rodol PS

3-Aminopropane sulfonic acid (INCI)
  CAS 3687-18-1; EINECS 222-977-4
  Trade names containing: Capigen CG; Capigen; Capisome

2-Aminopropionic acid. *See Alanine*

Ammonia water
  Trade names containing: Carboset 514H; Carboset 531

Ammonium acrylates/acrylonitrogens copolymer (INCI)
  CAS 123754-28-9
  Trade names: Hypan® SS201

Ammonium acrylates copolymer (INCI)
  Trade names: Dispex GA40
  Trade names containing: Syntran 5130; Syntran 5170; Syntran KL-219

Ammonium alginate (INCI)
  CAS 9005-34-9
  Synonyms: Ammonium polymannuronate; Alginic acid, ammonium salt
  Trade names: Sobalg FD 300 Series; Superloid®
  Trade names containing: Keltose®

Ammonium alum (INCI)
  CAS 7784-25-0; EINECS 232-055-3
  Synonyms: Aluminum ammonium sulfate; Ammonium aluminum sulfate; Sulfuric acid, aluminum ammonium salt (2:1:1), dodecahydrate
  Trade names: Unichem AMAL

Ammonium C12-15 alkyl sulfate (INCI)
  CAS 68815-61-2; EINECS 272-385-5
  Synonyms: Sulfuric acid, mono-C12-15-alkyl esters, ammonium salts; Ammonium C12-15 alcohols sulfate
  Trade names: Standapol® A-215; Unipol A-215

Ammonium C12-15 pareth sulfate (INCI)
  Synonyms: Ammonium pareth-25 sulfate; POE (1–4) C12-15 alcohol ether sulfate
  Trade names: Neodol® 25-3A; Standapol® AP-60; Unipol 230; Unipol AP-60; Witcolate™ AE-3
  Trade names containing: Zetesol AP

Ammonium chloride (INCI)
  CAS 12125-02-9; EINECS 235-186-4
  Synonyms: Sal ammoniac; Salmiac; Ammonium muriate
  Trade names containing: Dermalcare® 1673; Foamtaine CAB-A; Schercotaine CAB-A; Schercotaine SCAB-A

Ammonium cocoyl isethionate
  Trade names: Jordapon® ACI-30

Ammonium cocoyl sarcosinate (INCI)
Synonyms: Amides, coconut oil, with sarcosine, ammonium salts; Glycine, N-methyl-, N-coco amido deriv., ammonium salt; Ammonium N-cocoyl sarcosinate
Trade names: Hamposyl® AC-30

Ammonium cumenesulfonate (INCI)
CAS 37475-88-0; EINECS 253-519-1
Synonyms: Benzenesulfonic acid, (1-methylethyl)-, ammonium salt
Trade names: ACS 60; Eltesol® ACS 60

Ammonium dodecylbenzene sulfonate (INCI)
CAS 1331-61-9; EINECS 215-559-8
Synonyms: Ammonium lauryl benzene sulfonate
Trade names: Ablusol DBM

Ammonium laureth-6 carboxylate (INCI)
Synonyms: PEG-6 lauryl ether carboxylic acid, ammonium salt; Laureth-6 carboxylic acid, ammonium salt; Ammonium POE (6) lauryl ether carboxylate
Trade names: Akypo RLM 45 A

Ammonium laureth sulfate (INCI)
CAS 32612-48-9 (generic); 67762-19-0
Synonyms: Ammonium lauryl ether sulfate
Trade names: Calfoam EA-603; Calfoam NEL-60; Carsonol® SES-A; Empicol® EAA; Empicol® EAA70; Empicol® EAB; Empicol® EAB70; Empicol® EAB/T; Empicol® EAC; Empicol® EAC70; Empicol® EAC/T; Laural EC; Manro ALEC 25; Manro ALEC 27; Manro ALES 60; Neopon LOA; Nikkol SBL-2A-27; Nonasol N4AS; Nutrapon AL 1; Nutrapon AL 2; Nutrapon AL 30; Nutrapon AL 60; Nutrapon AN-3 0481; Rhodapex® EA-2; Sandoz Sulfate 216; Standapol® EA-1; Standapol® EA-2; Standapol® EA-3; Steol® CA-130; Steol® CA-230; Steol® CA-330; Steol® CA-460; Steol® KA-460; Sulfochem EA-1; Sulfochem EA-2; Sulfochem EA-3; Sulfochem EA-60; Sulfochem EA-70; Surfax EKZ; Texapon® EA-1; Texapon® EA-2; Texapon® EA-3; Texapon® PNA-127; Tylorol A; Ungerol AM3-60; Ungerol AM3-75; Unipol EA-1, EA-2, EA-3; Witcolate™ LES-60A; Witcolate™ S1300C; Zoharpon LAEA 253
Trade names containing: Orvus K Liq.; Plantaren® PS-100; Stepanol® AEG; Stepanol® AEM; Surfax CJ; Uniplant PS-100

Ammonium laureth-9 sulfate (INCI)
CAS 32612-48-9 (generic)
Synonyms: PEG-9 lauryl ether sulfate, ammonium salt; Ammonium PEG (450) lauryl ether sulfate; POE (9) lauryl ether sulfate, ammonium salt
Trade names: Geropon® AB/20

Ammonium laureth-12 sulfate (INCI)
CAS 32612-48-9 (generic)
Trade names: Standapol® 230-E; Unipol 230-E
Trade names containing: Equex AEM

Ammonium lauroyl sarcosinate (INCI)
CAS 68003-46-3; EINECS 268-130-2
Synonyms: N-methyl-N-(1-oxododecyl) glycine, ammonium salt
Trade names: Hamposyl® AL-30

Ammonium lauryl benzene sulfonate. See Ammonium dodecylbenzene sulfonate

Ammonium lauryl sulfate (INCI)
CAS 2235-54-3; 68081-96-9; EINECS 218-793-9
Synonyms: Sulfuric acid, monododecyl ester, ammonium salt
Trade names: Akyposal ALS 33; Calfoam ALS-30; Calfoam NLS-30; Carsonol® ALS; Carsonol® ALS-R; Carsonol® ALS-S; Carsonol® ALS Special; Empicol® AL30; Empicol® AL30/T; Empicol® AL70; Manro ALS 25; Manro ALS 30; Marlinat® DFN 30; Neopon LAM; Nikkol ALS-25; Norfox® ALS; Nutrapon HA 3841; Nutrapon PP 3563; Perlankrol® DAF25; Rewopol® ALS 30; Rhodapon® L-22, L-22/C; Rhodapon® L-22HNC; Standapol® A; Standapol® A-HV; Stepanol® AM; Stepanol® AM-V; Sulfochem ALS; Surfax ASD; Surfax NH; Texapon® ALS; Texapon® PNA; Ufarol Am 30; Ufarol Am 70; Unipol A; Witcolate™ NH; Zoharpon LAA
Trade names containing: Empicol® TC34; Empicol® TCR; Plantaren™ PS-300; Stepanol® AEG; Surfax CJ

Ammonium lauryl sulfosuccinate (INCI)
Trade names: Manromate LNT40; Monamate LNT-40

Ammonium muriate. See Ammonium chloride

Ammonium myreth sulfate (INCI)
CAS 27731-61-9
Synonyms: Ammonium myristyl ether sulfate
Trade names: Standapol® EA-40; Texapon® EA-40; Unipol EA-40
Trade names containing: Standapol® 7088; Standapol® EA-K

Ammonium nonoxynol-4 sulfate (INCI)
CAS 9051-57-4; 31691-97-1 (generic); 63351-73-5
Trade names: Rhodapex® CO-436; Rhodapex® HF-433
Trade names containing: Lytron 284; Lytron 288; Lytron 295; Lytron 300; Lytron 305; Lytron 308

Ammonium pareth-25 sulfate. See Ammonium C12-15 pareth sulfate

Ammonium stearate (INCI)
CAS 1002-89-7; EINECS 213-695-2
Synonyms: Octadecanoic acid, ammonium salt
Trade names: Unichem AMST

Ammonium xylenesulfonate (INCI)
CAS 26447-10-9; EINECS 247-710-9
Synonyms: Benzenesulfonic acid, dimethyl-, ammonium salt
Trade names: Eltesol® AX 40; Manrosol AXS40; Witconate™ NXS

Amniotic fluid (INCI)
Trade names: Amniotic Fluid LAS
Trade names containing: Bovine Amniotic Liq.; Diaquasol; Dihydral; Tri-K CMF Complex

Amodimethicone (INCI)
Trade names: GP-4 Silicone Fluid; Wacker Silicone Fluid VP 1653
Trade names containing: Belsil ADM 6042 E; Belsil ADM 6056 E; Belsil ADM 6057 E; Belsil ADM 6059 E; Dow Corning® 929; Dow Corning® 939; E-2153; Sandoperm FE

AMP. See 2-Amino-2-methyl-1-propanol

AMP-acrylates copolymer (INCI)
Trade names: Diahold® A-503

AMP-acrylates/diacetone-acrylamide copolymer (INCI)
Trade names: Plascize L-53P

AMP-coco hydrolyzed soy protein
Trade names: Pro Soy AMP

AMPD. See 2-Amino-2-methyl-1,3-propanediol

AMPD-acrylates/diacetoneacrylamide copolymer (INCI)
Trade names: Plascize L-53D

AMPD-isostearoyl hydrolyzed collagen (INCI)
Trade names: Promois E118D

AMP-isostearoyl gelatin/keratin amino acids/lysine hydroxypropyltrimonium chloride (INCI)
Trade names: Flexiquat AAS-15

AMP isostearoyl hydrolyzed collagen (INCI)
CAS 95032-84-1; 25212-19-5
Synonyms: AMP-isostearoyl hydrolyzed animal protein
Trade names: Crotein AD; Crotein AD Anhyd; Etha-Coll ISO

AMP-isostearoyl hydrolyzed keratin
Trade names: Etha-Keratin™ ISO
Trade names containing: Oleo Keratin™ ISO

AMP-isostearoyl hydrolyzed soy protein (INCI)
Trade names: Etha-Soy™ ISO

AMP isostearoyl hydrolyzed wheat protein (INCI)
Trade names: Crotein ADW

Amygdalin. See Almond oil

Angelica extract (INCI)
CAS 84775-41-7
Synonyms: Angelica archangelica extract; Archangelica officinalis; European angelica extract
Trade names containing: Angelica HS

Animal keratin amino acids. See Keratin amino acids

Animal starch. See Glycogen

Anise extract (INCI)
CAS 84775-42-8; 84650-59-9
Synonyms: Aniseed extract; Pimpinella anisum extract
Trade names containing: Anise LS; Anise Seed Extract HS 2712 G

Anthemis nobilis oil. See Chamomile oil

Aorta extract (INCI)
CAS 90989-47-2
Trade names containing: Epiderm-Complex O

Apple extract (INCI)
Synonyms: Pyrus malus extract
Trade names containing: Apple Extract HS 1806 AT; Apple HS; MFA™ Complex

Apple leaf extract (INCI)
Synonyms: Pyrus malus leaf extract
Trade names containing: Actiphyte of Apple Leaves

Apple pectin extract (INCI)
Synonyms: Pyrus malus pectin extract
Trade names containing: Actiphyte of Apple Pectin

Apricotamide DEA
Trade names: Schercomid SAP

Apricotamidopropyl betaine (CTFA)
CAS 133934-08-4
Synonyms: Qat. ammonium compd., (carboxymethyl)(3-apricotamidopropyl)dimethyl, hydroxide, inner salt; Apricotamidopropyl dimethyl glycine; Apricot amide propylbetaine
Trade names: Schercotaine APAB

Apricotamidopropyl ethyldimonium ethosulfate
CAS 115340-78-8
Trade names: Schercoquat APAS

Apricot extract (INCI)
CAS 68650-44-2; EINECS 272-046-1
Synonyms: Prunus armeniaca extract
Trade names containing: Actiphyte of Apricot Fruit; Apricot Extract HS 2509 G; Apricot Glycolysat; Hormo Fruit Apricot

Apricot kernel oil (INCI)
CAS 72869-69-3
Synonyms: Persic oil; Prunus armeniaca

Trade names: Lipovol P; Nikkol Apricot Kernel Oil; Super Refined™ Apricot Kernel Oil NF
Trade names containing: Carotene Huileux 10000; Lipovol P-S

Apricot kernel oil PEG-6 esters (INCI)
CAS 97488-91-0; 9004-96-0
Trade names: Labrafil® M 1944 CS
Trade names containing: Brillance 515

Apricot leaf extract (INCI)
Synonyms: Prunus armeniaca leaf extract
Trade names containing: Actiphyte of Apricot Leaves

Apricot seed powder (INCI)
Trade names: AP-Grit; Lipo APS 40/60

Arachidonic acid (INCI)
CAS 506-32-1; EINECS 208-033-4
Synonyms: 5,8,11,14-Eicosatetraenoic acid
Trade names containing: Complexe AV.h.; Efaderma; Efadermasterolo; Lipodermol®; Lipotrofina A; Tri-K CMF Complex

Arachidyl alcohol (INCI)
CAS 629-96-9; EINECS 211-119-4
Synonyms: 1-Eicosanol
Trade names: Cachalot® Arachidyl Alcohol AR-20; Nacol® 20-95
Trade names containing: Epal® 1618RT

Arachidyl behenate (INCI)
CAS 42233-14-7; EINECS 255-728-3
Trade names: Waxenol® 822

Arachidyl propionate (INCI)
CAS 65591-14-2; EINECS 265-839-9
Synonyms: Eicosanyl propanoate
Trade names: Waxenol® 801

Arachis oil. See Peanut oil

Arbutus extract (INCI)
CAS 84012-12-4
Synonyms: Arbutus unedo extract; Strawberry tree extract
Trade names containing: Actiphyte of Arbutus

Archangelica officinalis. See Angelica extract

Arginine (INCI)
CAS 74-79-3 (L-form); EINECS 200-811-1
Trade names containing: Endonucleine LS 2143; Omega-CH Activator

Arginine PCA (INCI)
CAS 56265-06-6; EINECS 260-081-5
Synonyms: L-Proline, 5-oxo-, compd. with L-arginine (1:1)
Trade names: Argidone®
Trade names containing: Diaquasol; Dihydral

Arnica extract (INCI)
CAS 8057-65-6
Trade names: Oleosterine Arnica; Unibotan Arnica CLR
Trade names containing: Actiphyte of Arnica; Actiplex™ 745; Arlenfil 4015; Arnica Distillate 2/378370; Arnica Extract HS 2397 G; Arnica HS; Arnica LS; Arnica Oil CLR; Arnica Oil; Arnicaflower Oil PANAROM; Capilotonique HS 245; Cremogen M-I 739001; Dragoplant Arnica 2/034060; Extract Arnica Special; Extrapone Arnica Special 2/032591; Firmogen®; Haircomplex AKS; Herbaliquid Alpine Herbs Special; Herbasol Alpine Herbs Complex; Herbasol Complex A; Herbasol Complex B; Herbasol Stimulant Complex; Herbasol-Extract Arnica; Kalokiros HS 263; Kalokiros LS 663; Leniplex; Regederme HS 236; Regederme LS 636; Tonique HS 290; Tonique LS 690

Arrowroot extract (INCI)
Synonyms: Maranta arundinacea extract
Trade names containing: Actiphyte of Arrowroot

Artichoke extract (INCI)
CAS 84012-14-6
Synonyms: Cynara scolymus extract
Trade names containing: Complex Relax; Complexe AST 1

Ascorbic acid (INCI)
CAS 50-81-7 (L-form); EINECS 200-066-2
Synonyms: 1-Ascorbic acid; Vitamin C
Trade names: Ascorbic Acid Ampul Type No. 604065700; Ascorbic Acid Fine Granular No. 6045655; Ascorbic Acid Ultra-Fine Powd. No. 604565300; Ascorbic Acid USP, FCC Type S No. 604566; Uantox ASCA; Vitazyme® C
Trade names containing: Brookosome® C; Oxynex® K; Oxynex® L

Ascorbyl dipalmitate (INCI)
CAS 28474-90-0
Synonyms: L-Ascorbic acid, dihexadecanoate
Trade names: Nikkol CP

Ascorbyl methylsilanol pectinate (INCI)
Trade names: Ascorbosilane C

Ascorbyl palmitate (INCI)
CAS 137-66-6; EINECS 205-305-4
Trade names: Ascorbyl Palmitate No. 60412; Grindox Ascorbyl Palmitate
Trade names containing: Antioxidant G-2; Brookosome® ACEBC; Controx® VP; Faceur ARL; Oxynex® 2004; Oxynex® K; Oxynex® L; Oxynex® LM

Atelocollagen (INCI)
CAS 9007-34-5
Trade names: Atelo-Collagen; Atelocollagen M; Atelocollagen MS; Atelocollagen SS

ATP. *See Adenosine triphosphate*

Attapulgite (INCI)
CAS 1337-76-4
Synonyms: Fuller's earth; Palygorskite; Dioctrahedral smectite
Trade names: Attasorb RVM Sorbent; Pharmasorb Colloidal Pharmaceutical Grade; Suspentone; Suspentone 1265
Trade names containing: M-P-A® 14; Tektamer® 38 L.V.

Avocadamide DEA (INCI)
Synonyms: Avocado diethanolamide; Avocado fatty acids diethanolamide; Diethanolamine avocado fatty acid condensate
Trade names containing: Avamid 150; Manromid AV150

Avocadamidopropyl dimethylamine (INCI)
Trade names: Incromine AVB-CG

Avocado extract (INCI)
CAS 84695-98-7
Synonyms: Persea americana extract
Trade names containing: Actiphyte of Avocado Fruit; Avocado Extract HS 2384 G; Complex NR

Avocado leaf extract (INCI)
Trade names containing: Actiphyte of Avocado Leaves

Avocado oil (INCI)
CAS 8024-32-6; EINECS 232-428-0
Synonyms: Alligator pear oil; Oils, avocado
Trade names: Avocado Oil CLR; Lipovol A; Natoil AVO; Nikkol Avocado Oil; Super Refined™ Avocado Oil; Tri-Ol AVO
Trade names containing: Avamid 150; L.C.R.E.; Lipovol A-S; Manromid AV150

Avocado oil PEG-11 esters (INCI)
Trade names: Oxypon 365

Avocado oil unsaponifiables (INCI)
Trade names: Crodarom Avocadin
Trade names containing: ASU Complex

Azadirachta indica extract
Trade names: Midecol CF

Babassuamide DEA (INCI)
Synonyms: N,N-Bis(2-hydroxyethyl)babassu fatty acid amide; Diethanolamine babassu fatty acid condensate; Babassu diethanolamide
Trade names: Incromide BAD

Babassamidopropalkonium chloride (INCI)
CAS 124046-05-5
Trade names: Incroquat BA-85

Babassuamidopropylamine oxide (INCI)
Synonyms: N-[3-(Dimethylamino)propyl]babassu amides-N-oxide; Babassu amides, N-[3-(dimethylamino)propyl], N-oxide
Trade names: Incromine Oxide BA

Babassuamidopropyl betaine (INCI)
Trade names: Incronam BA-30

Babassuamidopropyl dimethylamine (INCI)
Trade names: Incromine BAB

Babassu oil (INCI)
Synonyms: Oils, babassu
Trade names: Super Refined™ Babassu Oil

Balm mint extract (INCI)
CAS 84082-61-1
Synonyms: Extract of balm mint; Lemon balm extract; Melissa officinalis extract
Trade names containing: Actiphyte of Balm Mint; Balm Mint HS; Balm Mint Oil Infusion; Epidermin Water-Soluble; Herbasol Alpine Herbs Complex; Herbasol Complex A; Herbasol Complex C; Herbasol Complex D; Herbasol Sedative Complex; Herbasol-Extract Balm Mint; Hexaplant Richter; Sedaplant Richter

Balm mint oil (INCI)
CAS 8014-71-9
Synonyms: Lemon balm; Melissa officinalis oil; Oil of balm
Trade names containing: Cremogen AF; Dragoplant Balm Mint 2/034050; Essentiaderm n.4; Essentiaderm n.6; Essentiaderm n.8

Balsam copaiba (INCI)
CAS 8001-61-4; EINECS 232-288-0
Trade names: EmCon COPA

Barley extract (INCI)
CAS 94349-67-4
Trade names containing: Actiphyte of Malt; Firmogen®; Leniplex

Basic bismuth chloride. *See Bismuth oxychloride*

Basil extract (INCI)
CAS 84775-71-3
Synonyms: Common basil extract; Sweet basil extract; Ocimum basilicum extract
Trade names containing: Actiphyte of Basil

Batyl alcohol (INCI)
CAS 544-62-7; EINECS 208-874-7
Synonyms: Stearyl glyceryl ether; 3-(Octadecyloxy)-1,2-propanediol; Monooctadecyl ether of glycerol
Trade names: Nikkol Batyl Alcohol 100

Batyl isostearate (INCI)
Synonyms: Batyl monoisostearate; Isostearic acid, 2-(octadecyloxy)-3-hydroxypropyl ester

Trade names: Nikkol GM-18IS

Batyl stearate (INCI)
CAS 13232-26-3
Synonyms: Batyl monostearate
Trade names: Nikkol GM-18S

Bayberry wax (INCI)
CAS 8038-77-5
Trade names: Bayberry Wax Stralpitz; Ross Bayberry Wax

Bay laurel extract. *See Laurel extract*

Beeswax (INCI)
CAS 8006-40-4 (white), 8012-89-3 (yellow)
Synonyms: Cera alba
Trade names: Beeswax Commercial SP 1142; Beeswax Semi Bleached SP 752; Beeswax SP 116; Beeswax SP 125; Beeswax SP 139; Beeswax White Refined SP 44; Beeswax White SP 52; Beeswax White Stralpitz; Beeswax Yellow Refined SP 6; Beeswax Yellow SP 57; Bleached Beeswax; Koster Keunen Beeswax; Koster Keunen Beeswax, Filtered; Natural Beeswax; Natwax BEE; Ross Beeswax
Trade names containing: Alcolan® 40; Apicerol 2/014081; Argobase L1; Base WL 2569; Bee's Milk; Cirami No. 1; Cutina® LM; Dehymuls® E; Dehymuls® K; Falba Absorption Base; Hairwax 7686 o.E.; Hostacerin WO; Isobeeswax SP 154; Koster Keunen Beeswax, S&P ISOW; Lanaetex FB; Lanaetex H; Montane 481; Sphingoceryl® Wax LS 2958 B; Tewax TC 81; Umulse-E; Unitina LM

Beeswax, oxidized. *See Oxidized beeswax*

Beeswax, synthetic. *See Synthetic beeswax*

Behenalkonium chloride (INCI)
CAS 16841-14-8; EINECS 240-865-3
Synonyms: Behenyl dimethyl benzyl ammonium chloride; Benzyldocosyldimethylammonium chloride
Trade names: Genamin KDB
Trade names containing: Incroquat B65C; Incroquat Behenyl BDQ/P; Incroquat Behenyl TMC/P

Behenalkonium methosulfate
Trade names containing: Incroquat Behenyl TMS

Behenamidopropyl betaine (INCI)
Synonyms: 1-Propanaminium, N-(carboxymethyl)-N,N-dimethyl-3-[(1-oxobehenyl)amino]-, hydroxide, inner salt; Behenamidopropyl dimethyl glycine; Behenamide propylbetaine
Trade names: Mackam™ BA

Behenamidopropyl dimethylamine (INCI)
CAS 60270-33-9; EINECS 262-134-8
Synonyms: Dimethylaminopropyl behenamide; N-[3-(Dimethylamino)propyl]docosanamide
Trade names: Chemidex B; Incromine BB; Mackine™ 601; Schercodine B

Behenamidopropyl dimethylamine behenate (INCI)
CAS 125804-04-8
Synonyms: Docosanoic acid, compd. with N-[3-(dimethylamino)propyl]docosamide (1:1)
Trade names: Catemol 220-B; Necon BDB

Behenamidopropyl dimethylamine lactate (INCI)
Trade names: Mackalene™ 616

Behenamidopropyl ethyldimonium ethosulfate (INCI)
CAS 68797-65-9; EINECS 258-377-8
Synonyms: 1-Propanaminium, N-ethyl-N,N-dimethyl-1-3-[(1-oxodocosyl)amino]-, ethyl sulfate; N-Behenyl-(3-amidopropyl)-N,N-dimethyl-N-ethyl ammonium ethyl sulfate

Trade names: Foamquat BAS; Schercoquat BAS
Trade names containing: Incroquat BES-35 S

Behenamidopropyl PG-dimonium chloride (INCI)
Trade names: Lexquat® AMG-BEO

Behenamine oxide (INCI)
CAS 26483-35-2; EINECS 247-730-8
Synonyms: N,N-Dimethyl-1-behenamine-N-oxide; N,N-Dimethyl-1-docosanamine-N-oxide; 1-Docosanamine, N,N-dimethyl-, N-oxide
Trade names: Incromine Oxide B; Incromine Oxide B-30P; Incromine Oxide B50

Beheneth-5 (INCI)
Synonyms: PEG-5 behenyl ether; POE (5) behenyl ether
Trade names: Emalex BHA-5; Nikkol BB-5

Beheneth-10 (INCI)
Synonyms: PEG-10 behenyl ether; PEG 500 behenyl ether; POE (10) behenyl ether
Trade names: Emalex BHA-10; Mulsifan CB; Nikkol BB-10

Beheneth-20 (INCI)
Synonyms: PEG-20 behenyl ether; PEG 1000 behenyl ether; POE (20) behenyl ether
Trade names: Emalex BHA-20; Nikkol BB-20

Beheneth-30 (INCI)
Synonyms: PEG-30 behenyl ether; POE (30) behenyl ether
Trade names: Emalex BHA-30; Nikkol BB-30

Behenic acid (INCI)
CAS 112-85-6; EINECS 204-010-8
Synonyms: Docosanoic acid
Trade names: Crodacid B; Hystrene® 7022; Hystrene® 9022; Prifrac 2989

Behenoxy dimethicone (INCI)
Trade names: Abil®-Wax 2440

Behenoyl-PG-trimonium chloride (INCI)
CAS 69537-38-8; EINECS 274-033-6
Synonyms: (3-Behenoyloxy-2-hydroxypropyl) trimethyl ammonium chloride
Trade names: Akypoquat 131; Akypoquat 131 V
Trade names containing: Akypoquat 131 VC

Behentrimonium chloride (INCI)
CAS 17301-53-0; EINECS 241-327-0
Synonyms: Behenyl trimethyl ammonium chloride; 1-Docosanaminium, N,N,N-trimethyl-, chloride
Trade names: Genamin KDM; Genamin KDM-F; Incroquat TMC-80; Incroquat TMC-95; Nikkol CA-2580; Varisoft® BT-85
Trade names containing: Hair-cure 2/011500; Incroquat Behenyl TMC

Behentrimonium methosulfate (INCI)
CAS 81646-13-1
Synonyms: Behenyl trimethyl ammonium methyl sulfate; 1-Docosanaminium, N,N,N-trimethyl-, chloride
Trade names containing: Varisoft® BTMS

Behenyl alcohol (INCI)
CAS 661-19-8; EINECS 211-546-6
Synonyms: 1-Docosanol; Alcohol C_{22}
Trade names: Adol® 60; Cachalot® Behenyl Alcohol BE-22; Lanette® 22 Flakes; Nacol® 22-97; Nikkol Behenyl Alcohol 65, 80; Unihydag Wax 22

Behenyl beeswax (INCI)
CAS 8006-40-4, 144514-52-3
Trade names: Cera Albalate 101; Estol BWB 3640; Koster Keunen Behenyl-Beeswaxate
Trade names containing: Cera Albalate 104

Behenyl behenate (INCI)
CAS 17671-27-1; EINECS 241-646-5
Synonyms: Docosanoic acid, docosyl ester
Trade names: Crodamol BB; Kester Wax® 72; Pelemol
BB

Behenyl betaine (INCI)
CAS 84082-44-0
Synonyms: N-(Carboxymethyl)-N,N-dimethyl-1-
docosanaiminum hydroxide, inner salt; Behen-
amidopropyl betaine
Trade names: Incronam B-40

Behenyl dimethyl benzyl ammonium chloride. *See*
Behenalkonium chloride

Behenyl erucate (INCI)
CAS 18312-32-8; EINECS 242-201-8
Synonyms: Docosyl 13-docosenoate
Trade names: Crodamol BE; Elfacos® BE; Kemester®
BE; Kessco BE; Schercemol BE

Behenyl isostearate (INCI)
Trade names: Pelemol BIS

Behenyl trimethyl ammonium chloride. *See Behen-*
trimonium chloride

Bentonite (INCI)
CAS 1302-78-9; EINECS 215-108-5
Synonyms: Soap clay; Wilkinite; Tonsil L80
Trade names: Albagel 4446; Albagel Premium USP
4444; Albagen 4439; Bentolite H; Bentolite H 4430;
Bentolite L; Bentolite WH; Bentonite USP BC 670;
Korthix H-NF; Polargel® HV; Polargel® NF;
Polargel® T
Trade names containing: Optigel WM

Benzalkonium chloride (INCI)
CAS 8001-54-5; 61789-71-7; 68391-01-5; 68424-85-1;
68989-00-4; 85409-22-9; EINECS 204-479-9; 263-
080-8; 269-919-4; 270-325-2; 287-089-1
Synonyms: Alkyl dimethyl benzyl ammonium chloride
Trade names: Ablumine 18; Alkaquat® DMB-451-50,
DMB-451-80; Arquad® DMMCB-50; Barquat® MB-
50; Barquat® MB-80; BTC® 50 USP; Cathelios CL
50; Cationico SCL; Cequartyl™ A; Empigen®
BAC50; Empigen® BAC50/BP; Empigen® BAC90;
Empigen® BAC/BP; FMB 500-15 Quat U.S.P;
Hyamine® 3500 50%; Kemamine® BQ-6502C;
Maquat LC-12S-50%; Nikkol CA-101; Noramium
DA.50; Swanol CA-101; Unicol 50; Uniquart ADBAC-
50 USP; Variquat® 50MC; Variquat® 60LC;
Variquat® 80MC; Variquat® 80ME
Trade names containing: Arquad® B-100; Variquat®
50AC; Variquat® 50AC; Variquat® 50AE; Variquat®
50AE; Variquat® 50ME; Variquat® 50ME; Variquat®
80AC; Variquat® 80AC; Variquat® 80AE; Variquat®
80AE

Benzenecarboxylic acid. *See Benzoic acid*

1,2-Benzenediol. *See Pyrocatechol*

1,3-Benzenediol. *See Resorcinol*

1,4-Benzenediol. *See Hydroquinone*

1,2,3-Benzenetriol. *See Pyrogallol*

Benzethonium chloride (INCI)
CAS 121-54-0; EINECS 204-479-9
Synonyms: N,N-Dimethyl-N-[2-[2-[4-(1,1,3,3-tetra-
methylbutyl) phenoxy] ethoxy] ethyl] benzene-
methanaminium chloride; Diisobutylphenoxy-
ethoxyethyl dimethyl benzyl ammonium Cl
Trade names: Hyamine® 1622 50%; Hyamine® 1622
Crystals

Benzocaine
CAS 51-05-8
Synonyms: Ethyl-p-aminobenzoate hydrochloride;
Procaine hydrochloride; Anesthesol
Trade names: Unicaine-B

Benzoic acid (INCI)
CAS 65-85-0; EINECS 200-618-2
Synonyms: Benzenecarboxylic acid; Phenylformic acid;
Dracylic acid
Trade names: Benzoic Acid Powd. No. 130; Unisept BZA
Trade names containing: Bee's Milk; Euxyl K 702

Benzoin. *See Gum benzoin*

Benzophenone-1 (INCI)
CAS 131-56-6; EINECS 205-029-4
Synonyms: 2,4-Dihydroxybenzophenone; Benzo-
resorcinol; 4-Benzoyl resorcinol
Trade names: DHBP Quinsorb 010; Uvasorb 20H;
Uvinul® 400

Benzophenone-2 (INCI)
CAS 131-55-5; EINECS 205-028-9
Synonyms: 2,2´,4,4´-Tetrahydroxy benzophenone
Trade names: Uvinul® D 50

Benzophenone-3 (INCI)
CAS 131-57-7; EINECS 205-031-5
Synonyms: 2-Hydroxy-4-methoxybenzophenone; (2-Hy-
droxy-4-methoxyphenyl) phenylmethanone; Oxy-
benzone
Trade names: Escalol® 567; Eusolex® 4360; Marsorb
24; Neo Heliopan, Type BB; Spectra-Sorb® UV 9;
Syntase® 62; Uvasorb MET; Uvinul® M 40

Benzophenone-4 (INCI)
CAS 4065-45-6; EINECS 223-772-2
Synonyms: 2-Hydroxy-4-methoxybenzophenone-5-sul-
fonic acid; Sulisobenzone
Trade names: Syntase® 230; Uvasorb S-5; Uvinul® MS
40

Benzophenone-6 (INCI)
CAS 131-54-4; EINECS 205-027-3
Synonyms: 2,2´-Dihydroxy-4,4´-dimethoxybenzophe-
none; Bis(2-hydroxy-4-methoxyphenyl) methanone
Trade names: Uvinul® D 49

Benzophenone-8 (INCI)
CAS 131-53-3; EINECS 205-026-8
Synonyms: 2,2´-Dihydroxy-4-methoxybenzophenone;
Dioxybenzone
Trade names: Spectra-Sorb® UV 24

Benzophenone-9 (INCI)
CAS 3121-60-6; EINECS 221-498-8
Synonyms: Disodium 2,2´-dihydroxy-4,4´-dimethoxy-
5,5´-disulfobenzophenone
Trade names: Uvinul® DS 49

Benzophenone-11 (INCI)
CAS 1341-54-4
Trade names: Uvinul® M 493

Benzyl alcohol (INCI)
CAS 100-51-6; EINECS 202-859-9
Synonyms: α-Hydroxytoluene; Phenylmethanol;
Phenylcarbinol
Trade names: Unichem BZAL
Trade names containing: Euxyl K 100; Nipaguard® MPA

Benzyl benzoate (INCI)
CAS 120-51-4; EINECS 204-402-9
Trade names: Unichem BZBN

Benzylhemiformal (INCI)
CAS 14548-60-8; EINECS 238-588-8

Trade names: Akyposept B; Preventol D2

3-Benzylidene camphor (INCI)
CAS 15087-24-8; EINECS 239-139-9
Synonyms: 1,7,7-Trimethyl-3-(phenylmethylene)bicyclo [2.2.1]heptan-2-one
Trade names: Unisol S-22
Trade names containing: Unifilter U-41

Benzyl laurate (INCI)
CAS 140-25-0; EINECS 204-405-8
Synonyms: Dodecanoic acid, phenylmethyl ester; Lauric acid, benzyl ester; Phenylmethyl dodecanoate
Trade names: Mazon® EE-1

Benzyl nicotinate (INCI)
CAS 94-44-0; EINECS 202-332-3
Trade names: Benzyl Nicotinate No. 6752

Benzylparaben (INCI)
CAS 94-18-8; EINECS 202-311-9
Synonyms: Benzoic acid, 4-hydroxy-, phenylmethyl ester; Benzyl p-hydroxybenzoate; Phenylmethyl 4-hydroxybenzoate
Trade names: Nipabenzyl; Unisept BZ

Benzyltriethyl ammonium chloride (INCI)
CAS 56-37-1; EINECS 200-270-1
Synonyms: N,N,N-Triethylbenzenemethanaminium chloride
Trade names: Sumquat® 2355

Benzyl trimethyl ammonium chloride
CAS 56-93-9; EINECS 200-300-3
Synonyms: TMBAC; Trimethylbenzylammonium chloride; Benztrimonium chloride
Trade names: Variquat® B200

Bergamot oil (INCI)
CAS 8007-75-8; 85049-52-1
Trade names containing: Essentiaderm n.1; Essentiaderm n.3; Essentiaderm n.4

Beta-carotene. *See Carotene*

Betaine (INCI)
CAS 107-43-7; EINECS 203-490-6
Synonyms: Trimethylglycine
Trade names: Natural Extract AP

Betula alba extract. *See Birch extract*

BHA (INCI)
CAS 5013-16-5, 25013-16-5; EINECS 204-442-7, 246-563-8
Synonyms: Butylated hydroxyanisole; (1,1-Dimethylethyl)-4-methoxyphenol; 3-tert-Butyl-4-hydroxyanisole
Trade names: Sustane® 1-F; Sustane® BHA; Tenox® BHA; Uantox BHA
Trade names containing: Nipanox® Special; Sustane® 3; Tenox® 2; Tenox® 26; Tenox® 4; Tenox® 6; Uantox 3; Uantox HW-4; Uantox W-1; Vyox

BHT (INCI)
CAS 128-37-0; EINECS 204-881-4
Synonyms: DBPC; Butylated hydroxytoluene; 2,6-Di-t-butyl-p-cresol; 2,6-Bis (1,1-dimethylethyl)-4-methylphenol
Trade names: Ionol CP; Sustane® BHT; Tenox® BHT; Uantox BHT; Uninox A 287; Vanox® PCX
Trade names containing: Hydagen® DEO; Oxynex® 2004; Tenox® 25; Tenox® 26; Tenox® 4; Tenox® 4B; Tenox® 6; U-Dagen DEO; Uantox HW-4; Uantox W-1; Vitamin A Palmitate 1.0 BHT in Peanut Oil; Vitamin A Palmitate 1.7 BHT

Bioflavonoids (INCI)

CAS 61788-55-4
Synonyms: Lemon oil flavonoids
Trade names containing: Faceur ARL

Biotin (INCI)
CAS 58-85-5; EINECS 200-399-3
Trade names containing: Asebiol® LS; Soluvit Richter; Trichogen

Birch extract (INCI)
CAS 84012-15-7
Synonyms: Betula alba extract; White birch extract
Trade names containing: Herbasol 7 Herb Complex; Herbasol Complex E

Birch leaf extract (INCI)
Synonyms: Betula verrucosa leaf extract
Trade names containing: Capilotonique HS 220; Cremogen AF

Bisabolol (INCI)
CAS 515-69-5; EINECS 208-205-9
Synonyms: α,4-Dimethyl-α-(4-methyl-3-pentenyl)-3-cyclohexene-1-methanol
Trade names: α-Bisabolol; Dragosantol 2/012681; Hydagen® B; Uhydagen B
Trade names containing: Extrapone Chamomile Special 2/033021

Bis-diglyceryl caprylate/caprate/isostearate/hydroxystearate adipate (INCI)
Trade names: Softisan® 645
Trade names containing: Softisan® Gel

Bis-diglyceryl caprylate/caprate/isostearate/stearate/hydroxystearate adipate (INCI)
Trade names: Softisan® 649

2,6-Bis (1,1-dimethylethyl)-4-methylphenol. *See BHT*

Bishydroxyethyl dihydroxypropyl stearaminium chloride (INCI)
Trade names: Monaquat TG

Bishydroxyethylisodecyloxypropylamine oxide
Trade names: Tomah AO-14-2

Bis 2-hydroxyethyl tallow glycinate
Trade names: Manroteric 1202

Bisisostearamidopropyl ethoxyethyl dimonium chloride
CAS 111381-08-9
Synonyms: N-Ethylether-bis-1,4-(N-isostearylamido-propyl-N,N-dimethyl ammonium chloride)
Trade names: Foamquat 2IAE

Bismuth chloride oxide. *See Bismuth oxychloride*

Bismuth oxychloride (INCI)
CAS 7787-59-9; EINECS 232-122-7
Synonyms: Bismuth chloride oxide; Basic bismuth chloride; Bismuth subchloride
Trade names: Biron®; Biron® B-5; Biron® B-50; Biron® ESQ; Biron® Fines; Biron® HB; Biron® NLD-SP; Mearlite® GBU; Mearlite® GGH; Mearlite® LBU; Pearl I; Pearl II; Pearl-Glo®; Pearl Super Supreme; Pearl Supreme UVS
Trade names containing: Bi-Lite® 20, 1070; Bi-Lite® R, 1051; Bi-Lite® Ultralite 3186; Bi-Lite® Ultrapress 1082; Bi-Lite® Ultrawhite 1084; Bi-Lite® UVR; Bi-Lite®; Bicrona® Carmine; Bicrona® Iron Blue; Biju® BNT; Biju® BTD, BXD; Biju® BWD, BWS; Biju® BWP; Biju® Ultra UNT; Biju® Ultra UTD, UXD; Biju® Ultra UWD, UWS; Biju® Ultra UWP; Biron® B-50 CO; Biron® NLD; Biron® NLY-L-2X AQ; Biron® NLY-L-2X CO; Biron® NLY-L-2X MO; Biron® Silver CO; Bismica 46; Bismica 55; Bismica 596; Bital®; Black 103; Blue 135; Brown 208; Carmine 224; Chroma-

Lite® Aqua 4508; Chroma-Lite® Black 4498; Chroma-Lite® Dark Blue 4501; Chroma-Lite® Magenta 4505; Chroma-Lite® Violet 4507; Chroma-Lite®; Chrome Green 106; Ferric Blue 107; Ferric Blue 114; H Chrome Green 105; M Violet 112; Mearlite® GEH; Mearlite® GEJ; Mearlite® LEM; Mibiron®N-50; Red 119; Red 139; Red 150; Red 219; Shinju® White 100T; Titanium Dioxide 110; U Blue 104; U Pink 113; U Violet 109; Yellow 134; Yellow 201

Bismuth nitrate, basic. *See Bismuth subnitrate*

Bismuth oxynitrate. *See Bismuth subnitrate*

Bismuth subchloride. *See Bismuth oxychloride*

Bismuth subnitrate (INCI)
CAS 1304-85-4; EINECS 215-136-8
Synonyms: Bismuth nitrate, basic; Bismuth oxynitrate.
Trade names containing: Kalixide CT; Kalixide DPG

Bisphenylhexamethicone (INCI)
CAS 18758-91-3
Synonyms: 1,1,1,7,7,7-Hexamethyl-3,5-diphenyl-3,5-bis [(trimethylsilyl) oxy] tetrasiloxane
Trade names: Rhodorsil® Oils 70633 V30

Bispyrithione (INCI)
CAS 3696-28-4; EINECS 223-024-5
Synonyms: Pyridine, 2,2'-dithiobis-, 1,1'-dioxide; 2,2'-Dithiobis (pyridine-1-oxide)
Trade names containing: Omadine® MDS

Bitter almond extract (INCI)
Synonyms: Prunus amygdalus amara extract
Trade names containing: Bitter Almond HS; Bitter Almond LS

Bitter cherry extract (INCI)
CAS 89997-53-5; EINECS 289-688-3
Synonyms: Prunus cerasus extract
Trade names containing: Acerola Extract HS 2855 G

Bitter orange extract (INCI)
Synonyms: Citrus aurantium fruit extract
Trade names containing: Coobato Speciale

Bitter orange oil (INCI)
CAS 68916-04-1
Trade names containing: Essentiaderm n.4; Essentiaderm n.6

Bitter orange peel extract (INCI)
CAS 8028-48-6; EINECS 232-433-8
Synonyms: Citrus aurantium peel extract
Trade names containing: Chinpi Liq.

Blackberry leaf extract (INCI)
Synonyms: Bramble leaf extract; Rubus villosus leaf extract
Trade names containing: Complexe AST 1

Black locust extract (INCI)
Synonyms: Robinia pseudoacacia extract
Trade names containing: Acacia Glycolysat; Acacia Oleat M

Black walnut extract (INCI)
Synonyms: Juglans nigra extract
Trade names containing: Actiphyte of Black Walnut

Bladderwrack extract (INCI)
CAS 84696-13-9
Synonyms: Fucus extract; Fucus vesiculosus extract
Trade names containing: BBC Mineral Complex

Bolus alba. *See Kaolin*

Borage extract (INCI)
CAS 84012-16-8
Synonyms: Borago officinalis extract

Trade names containing: BBC Mineral Complex; BBC Moisture Trol

Borage seed oil (INCI)
Trade names containing: Bio-Oil GLA-10

Borax. *See Sodium borate*

Boron nitride (INCI)
CAS 10043-11-5; EINECS 233-136-6
Trade names: Ceram Blanche

Boswellia carterii resin. *See Olibanum*

Brain extract (INCI)
CAS 90989-78-9
Trade names: Ceraderm S
Trade names containing: Brookosome® ELL; Brookosome® GSL

Brazil wax. *See Carnauba*

5-Bromo-5-nitro-1,3-dioxane (INCI)
CAS 30007-47-7; EINECS 250-001-7
Synonyms: 1,3-Dioxane, 5-bromo-5-nitro-
Trade names: Bronodox L
Trade names containing: Bronidox® L 5; Bronidox® L; Bronodox L-5

2-Bromo-2-nitropropane-1,3-diol (INCI)
CAS 52-51-7; EINECS 200-143-0
Synonyms: 1,3-Propanediol, 2-bromo-2-nitro
Trade names: Bronopol; CoSept BNP; Lexgard® Bronopol; Midpol 97; Midpol 100; Myacide® BT; Tristat BNP
Trade names containing: Midpol 2000; Midpol PHN; Nipaguard® BPX

Broom extract (INCI)
CAS 84696-48-0
Synonyms: Cystisus scoparius extract; Sarothamnus scoparius extract; Scotchbroom extract
Trade names containing: Broom Glycolysat; Broom HS; Broom Oleat M; Broom Tops Extract HS 2645 G

Buckthorn extract (INCI)
CAS 8057-57-6; 84625-48-9; 84929-75-9
Synonyms: Rhamnus frangula extract
Trade names containing: Alder Buckthorn HS

Butane (INCI)
CAS 106-97-8; EINECS 203-448-7
Synonyms: n-Butane; Alkane C_4
Trade names containing: Drivosol®

Butanedioic acid. *See Succinic acid*

1-Butanol. *See Butyl alcohol*

Butcherbroom extract (INCI)
CAS 84012-38-4
Synonyms: Rusco extract; Ruscus aculeatus extract
Trade names containing: Biophytex®; Circulatory Blend HS 318

Butene
CAS 106-98-9
Synonyms: C-4 alpha olefin
Trade names: Ethyl Butene-1; Gulftene® 4

Butoxy diglycol (INCI)
CAS 112-34-5; EINECS 203-961-6
Synonyms: PEG-2 butyl ether; Diethylene glycol butyl ether; 2-(2-Butoxyethoxy) ethanol
Trade names: Butyl Carbitol®; Butyl Dioxitol; Ektasolve® DB

Butoxyethanol (INCI)
CAS 111-76-2; EINECS 203-905-0
Synonyms: 2-Butoxyethanol; Ethylene glycol monobutyl ether; Ethylene glycol butyl ether

Trade names: Butyl Cellosolve®; Butyl Oxitol

Butoxypropanol (INCI)
CAS 5131-66-8; EINECS 225-878-4
Synonyms: 1-Butoxy-2-propanol; Propylene glycol t-butyl ether
Trade names: Butyl Propasol

Buttermilk powder (INCI)
Trade names: Lipo Buttermilk Powd

n-Butyl acetate (INCI)
CAS 123-86-4; EINECS 204-658-1
Synonyms: Acetic acid, butyl ester
Trade names containing: Biju® BNT; Biju® BTD, BXD; Biju® BWD, BWS; Biju® BWP; Biju® Ultra UNT; Biju® Ultra UTD, UXD; Biju® Ultra UWD, UWS; Biju® Ultra UWP; Mearlmaid® CKD; Mearlmaid® CP; Mearlmaid® KN; Mearlmaid® KND; Nagellite® 3050-80; Naturon® CSN-22

Butyl alcohol (INCI)
CAS 71-36-3; EINECS 200-751-6
Synonyms: n-Butyl alcohol; 1-Butanol; Propyl carbinol
Trade names: Nacol® 4-99

Butylated hydroxyanisole. *See BHA*

Butylated hydroxytoluene. *See BHT*

Butylated PVP (INCI)
Synonyms: Butylated polyvinylpyrrolidone
Trade names: Antaron® P-904; Ganex® P-904

2-t-Butylcyclohexyl acetate (INCI)
CAS 88-41-5; EINECS 201-828-7
Trade names: Beldox

Butylene glycol (INCI)
CAS 107-88-0; EINECS 203-529-7
Trade names: Unichem 1-3 BUT-G
Trade names containing: Aloe Extract Vera; Alowcape Liq. B-7; Althea Liq.; Anti-MB; Bactericide MB 2/012582; Benibana Liq.; Biopharco CP-12; Bodaiju Liq.; Emalex FDB-36; Extrapone Arnica Special 2/032591; Extrapone Bio-Tamin Special 2/2032671; Extrapone Chamomile Special 2/033021; Extrapone Hamamelis Super 2/500010; Extrapone Neo-H-Special 2/032441; Extrapone Poly H Special 2/032451; Extrapone Witch Hazel 2/032893; FRS-Diffuser Microreservoir; Gadeneel Liq.; Hamamelis Liq.; Hydro-Diffuser Microreservoir; Ichou Liq.; Isodon Extract; Kamitsure Liq.; Killitol; Koucha Liq.; Lemon Liq.; Mikrokill 300; Nikkol Aquasome EC-5; Nikkol Aquasome VE; Semburi Extract BG; Sohakuhi Extract BG-100; Unipertan VEG 24; Unipertan VEG 242

t-Butyl hydroquinone (INCI)
CAS 1948-33-0; EINECS 217-752-2
Synonyms: TBHQ; Mono-tert-butyl hydroquinone; 1,4-Benzenediol, 2-(1,1-dimethylethyl)-
Trade names: Tenox® TBHQ; Uantox TBHQ
Trade names containing: Stabolec C; Tenox® 20B; Tenox® 22; Tenox® 25; Tenox® 26; Uantox 20; Uantox W-1

3-t-Butyl-4-hydroxyanisole. *See BHA*

Butyl methacrylate (INCI)
CAS 97-88-1; EINECS 202-615-1
Synonyms: Butyl 2-methyl-2-propenoate
Trade names: Rohagum® P-24; Rohasol® P-550
Trade names containing: Rohagum® PM-381; Rohagum® PM-685; Rohasol® PM-560; Rohasol® PM-709

Butyl methoxy dibenzoyl methane (INCI)
CAS 70356-09-1; EINECS 274-581-6

Synonyms: 1-[4-(1,1-Dimethylethyl)phenyl]-3-(4-methoxyphenyl)-1,3-propanedione; Avobenzone
Trade names: Parsol® 1789
Trade names containing: Unifilter U-41

Butyl myristate (INCI)
CAS 110-36-1; EINECS 203-759-8
Synonyms: Butyl n-tetradecanoate
Trade names: Bumyr; Crodamol BM; Nikkol BM; Wickenol® 141

2-Butyl-1-octanol (INCI)
CAS 3913-02-8; EINECS 223-470-0
Trade names: Isofol® 12

Butyl oleate (INCI)
CAS 142-77-8; EINECS 205-559-6
Synonyms: Butyl 9-octadecenoate
Trade names: Kemester® 4000

Butylparaben (INCI)
CAS 94-26-8; EINECS 202-318-7
Synonyms: Butyl p-hydroxybenzoate; 4-Hydroxybenzoic acid butyl ester; n-Butyl p-hydroxybenzoate
Trade names: Butyl Parasept; Butylparaben NF; CoSept B; Lexgard® B; Nipabutyl; Paridol B; Preserval B; Preserval Butylique; Trisept B; Unisept B
Trade names containing: Bactiphen 2506 G; Dekaben; LiquaPar® Oil; Nipastat; Phenonip; Sepicide HB; Sepicide MB; Talcoseptic C; Undebenzofene C; Uniphen P-23

Butyl stearate (INCI)
CAS 123-95-5; EINECS 204-666-5
Synonyms: Butyl octadecanoate; n-Butyl octadecanoate; Octadecanoic acid butyl ester
Trade names: Crodamol BS; Dermol EB; Emerest® 2325; Estol BUS 1550; Kemester® 5410; Kemester® 5510; Kessco® Butyl Stearate; Lasemul 74 NP; Nikkol BS; Norfox® B-54; Radia® 7051; Radia® 7752; Unichem BUTSTE; Witconol™ 2325; Witconol™ 2326
Trade names containing: Lanpro-2; Lexate® TL; Oleo-Coll™ LP; Oleo-Coll™ LP/LF; Prochem 35; Prochem 35A; Protachem 35A; Proto-Lan 8

Butyrolactam. *See 2-Pyrrolidone*

Butyrolactone (INCI)
CAS 96-48-0; EINECS 202-509-5
Synonyms: Dihydro-2(3H)-furanone; γ-Butyrolactone; 4-Hydroxybutyric acid, γ-lactone
Trade names: GBL
Trade names containing: All-Natural Nail Polish Remover

n-Butyroyl tri-n-hexyl citrate (INCI)
CAS 82469-79-2
Trade names: Citroflex B-6

C4 alpha olefin. *See Butene*

C6 alpha olefin. *See 1-Hexene*

C6-10 alcohols
Trade names: Alfol® 610; Alfol® 610 ADE; Alfol® 610 AFC

C6-14 polyolefins
Trade names: Nikkol Syncelane 30

C8 alcohols. *See Caprylic alcohol*

C8 alpha olefin. *See Octene-1*

C8-10 alcohols
CAS 68603-15-5
Trade names: Alfol® 810; Nafol® 810 D

C8-10 pareth-2
Trade names: Novel® N2.2-810

C8-10 pareth-5
Trade names: Novel® N4.9-810

C8-10 pareth-8
Trade names: Novel® N7.7-810

C9-11 alcohols (INCI)
CAS 66455-17-2; 68551-08-6
Synonyms: Alcohols, C9-11
Trade names: Neodol® 91

C9-11 pareth-6 (INCI)
CAS 68439-46-3 (generic)
Synonyms: Pareth-91-6; PEG-6 C9-11 alcohol ether
Trade names: Teric 9A6

C10 alcohol
Trade names: Nafol® 10 D

C10 alpha olefin. *See Decene-1*

C10-11 isoparaffin (INCI)
CAS 64742-48-9
Trade names: Isopar® G

C10-12 alcohols
Trade names: Alfol® 1012 HA

C10-12 pareth-3
Trade names: Alfonic® 1012-2.5; Surfonic® L12-3

C10-12 pareth-6
Trade names: Surfonic® L12-6

C10-12 pareth-8
Trade names: Surfonic® L12-8

C10-13 alkane (INCI)
Trade names: Halpasol 190/240

C10-14 alcohols
Trade names: Alfol® 1014 CDC; Nafol® 1014

C10-18 triglycerides (INCI)
CAS 85665-33-4
Synonyms: Glyceryl tri-C10-18 acids
Trade names: Nesatol

C10-30 cholesterol/lanosterol esters (INCI)
Trade names: Super Sterol Ester
Trade names containing: L.C.R.E.

C11-12 isoparaffin (INCI)
CAS 64742-48-9
Synonyms: Alkanes, C11-12-iso-
Trade names: Isopar® H; Isopar® K

C11-13 isoparaffin (INCI)
CAS 64742-48-9
Synonyms: Alkanes, C11-13-iso-
Trade names: Isopar® L

C11-15 pareth-9 (INCI)
CAS 68131-40-8 (generic)
Synonyms: Pareth-15-9
Trade names containing: Dow Corning® 1669; Dow Corning® X2-1669

C12 alpha olefin. *See Dodecene-1*

C12-13 alcohols (INCI)
CAS 75782-86-4
Synonyms: Alcohols, C12-13
Trade names: Neodol® 23

C12-13 pareth-3 (INCI)
CAS 66455-14-9 (generic)
Synonyms: Pareth-23-3; PEG-3 C12-13 fatty alcohol ether
Trade names: Elfapur® LT 30 SLN; Neodol® 23-3

C12-13 pareth-4 (INCI)
Trade names: Volpo L4

C12-13 pareth-7 (INCI)
CAS 66455-14-9 (generic)
Synonyms: Pareth-23-7; PEG-7 C12–13 fatty alcohol ether
Trade names: Elfapur® LT 65 SLN; Neodol® 23-6.5

C12-13 pareth-9 (INCI)
CAS 66455-14-9 (generic)
Trade names: Elfapur® LT 85/9 SLN

C12-13 pareth-15 (INCI)
CAS 66455-14-9 (generic)
Trade names: Elfapur® LT 150 SLN; Elfapur® LT 150 SN

C12-13 pareth-23 (INCI)
Trade names: Volpo L23

C12-13 pareth-5 carboxylic acid (INCI)
CAS 70750-17-3 (generic)
Synonyms: PEG-5 C12-13 alkyl ether carboxylic acid
Trade names: Akypo 23Q38

C12-14 alcohols
Trade names: Alfol® 1214; Alfol® 1214 GC; Alfol® 1216 CO; Alfol® 1412; CO-1214; Radianol® 1724

C12-14 pareth-2
CAS 68439-50-9
Synonyms: PEG-2 C12-14 alcohol
Trade names: Alfonic® 1214-GC-2; Surfonic® L24-2

C12-14 pareth-3 (INCI)
CAS 68439-50-9
Synonyms: PEG-3 C12-14 alcohol
Trade names: Alfonic® 1412-3; Genapol® 24-L-3; Genapol® 42-L-3; Surfonic® L24-3

C12-14 pareth-7 (INCI)
CAS 68439-50-9
Trade names: Surfonic® L24-7

C12-14 pareth-8
CAS 68439-50-9
Synonyms: PEG-8 C12-14 fatty alcohol
Trade names: Surfonic® L24-9

C12-14 pareth-11
CAS 68439-50-9
Trade names: Surfonic® L24-12

C12-15 alcohols (INCI)
CAS 63393-82-8
Synonyms: Alcohols, C12-15
Trade names: Neodol® 25

C12-15 alkyl benzoate (INCI)
CAS 68411-27-8
Trade names: Crodamol AB; Finsolv® TN
Trade names containing: Bentone® Gel TN; Bentone® Gel TN A-40; Ritaplast TN; Tixogel FTN

C12-15 alkyl lactate (INCI)
Synonyms: C12-15 alcohols lactate
Trade names: Ceraphyl® 41

C12-15 alkyl octanoate (INCI)
Synonyms: C12-15 alcohols octanoate
Trade names: Finester EH-25; Hetester FAO

C12-15 alkyl salicylate (INCI)
Trade names: Dermol NS

C12-15 pareth-2 (INCI)
CAS 68131-39-5
Synonyms: Pareth-25-2
Trade names: Nikkol BD-2

C12-15 pareth-3 (INCI)
CAS 68131-39-5 (generic)
Synonyms: Pareth-25-3; PEG-3 C12–15 fatty alcohol ether

Trade names: Bio-Soft® E-400; Elfapur® LP 25 SL; Neodol® 25-3; Rhodasurf® LA-3; Teric 12A3; Volpo 25 D 3

C12-15 pareth-4 (INCI)
CAS 68131-39-5 (generic)
Synonyms: Pareth-25-4
Trade names: Nikkol BD-4

C12-15 pareth-5 (INCI)
CAS 68131-39-5 (generic)
Synonyms: PEG-5 C12-15 alkyl ether; Pareth-25-5
Trade names: Volpo 25 D 5

C12-15 pareth-7 (INCI)
CAS 68131-39-5 (generic)
Synonyms: Pareth-25-7; PEG-7 C12–15 fatty alcohol ether
Trade names: Bio-Soft® EN 600; Neodol® 25-7; Teric 12A7

C12-15 pareth-9 (INCI)
CAS 68131-39-5 (generic)
Synonyms: Pareth-25-9
Trade names: Neodol® 25-9

C12-15 pareth-10
CAS 68131-39-5
Synonyms: Pareth-25-10
Trade names: Nikkol BD-10; Volpo 25 D 10

C12-15 pareth-11 (INCI)
CAS 68131-39-5 (generic)
Trade names: Elfapur® LP 110 SLN; Elfapur® SP 110 SLN

C12-15 pareth-12 (INCI)
CAS 68131-39-5 (generic)
Synonyms: Pareth 25-12
Trade names: Mulsifan RT 203/80; Neodol® 25-12

C12-15 pareth-15
CAS 68131-39-5
Trade names: Volpo 25 D 15

C12-15 pareth-20
CAS 68131-39-5
Trade names: Volpo 25 D 20

C12-15 pareth-7 carboxylic acid (INCI)
CAS 88497-58-9 (generic)
Synonyms: Pareth-25-7 carboxylic acid; PEG-7 C12-15 alkyl ether carboxylic acid
Trade names: Sandopan® DTC Linear P Acid; Surfine WNT-A

C12-15 pareth-2 phosphate (INCI)
Synonyms: Pareth-25-2 phosphate; PEG-2-C12-15 alcohols phosphate
Trade names: Nikkol TDP-2

C12-16 alcohols (INCI)
CAS 68855-56-1
Trade names: Alfol® 1216; Radianol® 1726

C12-16 pareth-1
CAS 68551-12-2
Trade names: Alfonic® 1216-1.5; Genapol® 26-L-1

C12-16 pareth-2
Trade names: Alfonic® 1216-CO-2; Genapol® 26-L-1.6; Genapol® 26-L-2

C12-16 pareth-3
Synonyms: PEG-3 C12,C14,C16 alcohols
Trade names: Genapol® 26-L-3; Novel® N3.0-1216CO; Tergitol® 26-L-3

C12-16 pareth-5
Trade names: Genapol® 26-L-5

C12-16 pareth-6
Trade names: Genapol® 26-L-45

C12-18 alcohols
CAS 67762-25-8
Trade names: Alfol® 1218 DCBA; Nafol® 1218

C12-20 acid PEG-8 ester (INCI)
Trade names: Xalifin 15

C13-14 isoparaffin (INCI)
CAS 64742-48-9
Synonyms: Alkanes, C13-14-iso-
Trade names: Isopar® M
Trade names containing: Sepigel 305

C13-15 pareth-2
Trade names: Renex® 702

C13-15 pareth-3
Trade names: Renex® 703

C13-15 pareth-7
Trade names: Renex® 707

C13-15 pareth-9
Trade names: Renex® 709

C13-15 pareth-11
Trade names: Renex® 711

C13-15 pareth-20
Trade names: Renex® 720

C13-15 pareth-2 carboxamide MEA. *See Trideceth-2 carboxamide MEA*

C14 alcohol. *See Myristyl alcohol*

C14 alpha olefin. *See Tetradecene-1*

C14-15 alcohols (INCI)
CAS 75782-87-5
Trade names: Neodol® 45

C14-15 pareth-7 (INCI)
CAS 68951-67-7
Synonyms: Pareth 45-7; PEG-7 C14-15 alcohol ether
Trade names: Neodol® 45-7

C14-15 pareth-11 (INCI)
Synonyms: Pareth-45-11
Trade names: Neodol® 45-11

C14-15 pareth-13 (INCI)
Synonyms: Pareth-45-13; PEG-13 C14-15 alcohol ether
Trade names: Neodol® 45-13

C14-15 pareth-8 carboxylic acid (INCI)
Synonyms: PEG-8 C14-15 alkyl ether carboxylic acid; PEG 400 C14-15 alkyl ether carboxylic acid
Trade names: Surfine WNG-A

C14-16 alcohols
Trade names: Alfol® 1416 GC

C14-16 glycol palmitate (INCI)
Trade names: Mexanyl GR

C14-16 pareth-7
Trade names: Surfonic® L46-7

C14-17 alkane
Trade names: Halpasol 240/270

C14-18 alcohols
Trade names: Alfol® 1418 DDB; Alfol® 1418 GBA

C16 alcohol. *See Cetyl alcohol*

C16 alpha olefin. *See Hexadecene-1*

C16-18 alcohols. *See Cetearyl alcohol*

C16-18 pareth-5
Trade names: Novel® N5.1-1618

C18 alpha olefin. *See Octadecene-1*

C18-28 alkyl acetate (INCI)
Trade names: Vybar® 5013

C18-32 alcohols
Trade names containing: Epal® 20+

C18-36 acid (INCI)
Trade names: Syncrowax AW1-C

C18-36 acid glycol ester (INCI)
Trade names: Syncrowax ERL-C

C18-36 acid triglyceride (INCI)
Trade names: Syncrowax HGL-C

C20-24 alcohols
Trade names: Nafol® 20+

C20-24 alpha olefin
CAS 64743-02-8
Trade names: Gulftene® 20-24

C20-40 alcohols (INCI)
Trade names: Unilin® 350 Alcohol; Unilin® 425 Alcohol

C20-40 alkyl behenate (INCI)
Synonyms: C20-40 alcohols behenate
Trade names: Pelemol 300B

C20-40 isoparaffin
Trade names: ESH-C

C20-40 pareth-3 (INCI)
Trade names: Unithox® 420

C20-40 pareth-10 (INCI)
Trade names: Unithox® 450

C20-40 pareth-40 (INCI)
Trade names: Unithox® 480

C24-28 alkyl methicone (INCI)
Trade names: Abil®-Wax 9810

C24-28 alpha olefin
Trade names: Gulftene® 24-28

C24-40 hydrocarbons
Trade names containing: Epal® 20+

C30 alpha olefin
Trade names: Gulftene® 30+

C30-45 alkyl methicone (INCI)
Trade names: Abil®-Wax 9811

C30-50 alcohols (INCI)
Trade names: Unilin® 550 Alcohol

C30-50 pareth-3 (INCI)
Trade names: Unithox® 520

C30-50 pareth-10 (INCI)
Trade names: Unithox® 550

C40-60 alcohols (INCI)
Trade names: Unilin® 700 Alcohol

C40-60 pareth-3 (INCI)
Trade names: Unithox® 720

C40-60 pareth-10 (INCI)
Trade names: Unithox® 750

CA. *See Cellulose acetate*

CAB. *See Cellulose acetate butyrate*

CADG. *See Cocamidopropyl betaine*

Caffeine (INCI)
CAS 58-08-2; EINECS 200-362-1
Synonyms: Theine; Methyltheobromine; 1,3,7-Tri-methylxanthine
Trade names containing: Carnitiline; CoAxel

Caffeine benzoate (INCI)

Trade names containing: Vexel

Cajeputene. *See Dipentene*

Cake alum. *See Aluminum sulfate*

Calcium alginate (INCI)
CAS 9005-35-0
Synonyms: Alginic acid, calcium salt
Trade names: Sobalg FD 460
Trade names containing: Keltose®; Masque Poudre No. 2

Calcium ascorbate
CAS 5743-27-1
Trade names: Calcium Ascorbate FCC No. 60475

Calcium behenate (INCI)
CAS 3578-72-1; EINECS 222-700-7
Synonyms: Calcium docosanoate; Docosanoic acid, calcium salt
Trade names containing: Syncrowax HRS-C

Calcium borogluconate
CAS 5743-34-0
Synonyms: D-Gluconic acid cyclic 4,5-ester with boric acid calcium salt; Calcium diborogluconate
Trade names: Gluconal® CA M B

Calcium carbonate (INCI). *Also see limestone*
CAS 471-34-1; 1317-65-3; EINECS 207-439-9
Synonyms: Carbonic acid, calcium salt; Precipitated calcium carbonate, commercial form; Prepared calcium carbonate, native purified form
Trade names: Camel-WITE®; Unichem CALCARB
Trade names containing: Kalixide LT; Silkall CA

Calcium chloride (INCI)
CAS 10043-52-4; EINECS 233-140-8
Synonyms: Calcium chloride, dihydrate
Trade names: Unichem CALCHLOR

Calcium disodium EDTA (INCI)
CAS 62-33-9; EINECS 200-529-9
Synonyms: Calcium disodium ethylenediamine tetraacetic acid; Edetate calcium disodium
Trade names: Hampene® CaNa$_2$ Pure Crystals; Kelate CDS; Universene CaNa2; Versene CA

Calcium gluconate (INCI)
CAS 299-28-5; EINECS 206-075-8
Synonyms: D-Gluconic acid calcium salt; Calciofon; Glucal
Trade names: Gluconal® CA A; Gluconal® CA M
Trade names containing: Seanamin BD

Calcium hydroxide (INCI)
CAS 1305-62-0; EINECS 215-137-3
Synonyms: Calcium hydrate; Hydrated lime; Slaked lime
Trade names: Calcium Hydroxide USP 802; Unichem CA HYD

Calcium lactate
CAS 814-80-2
Synonyms: 2-Hydroxypropanoic acid, calcium salt
Trade names: Unichem CALAC

Calcium oxide (INCI)
CAS 1305-78-8; EINECS 215-138-9
Synonyms: Lime; Quicklime; Calx
Trade names: Calcium Oxide FCC 801; Unichem CAO

Calcium pantothenate (INCI)
CAS 137-08-6 (D-form); EINECS 205-278-9
Synonyms: Calcium N-(2,4-dihydroxy-3,3-dimethyl-1-oxobutyl-β-alanine; Vitamin B$_5$, calcium salt; Calcium D-pantothenate
Trade names: D-Calcium Pantothenate USP, FCC Type SD No. 63924

Trade names containing: Extrapone Neo-H-Special 2/
032441; Extrapone Poly H Special 2/032451; Hair
Complex 20/70n; Soluvit Richter

Calcium phosphate, dibasic
CAS 7757-93-9
Synonyms: DCP-0; Dicalcium phosphate, anhydr.; Cal-
cium hydrogen orthophosphate
Trade names: Anhydrous Emcompress®

Calcium phosphate, dibasic, dihydrate
CAS 7789-77-7
Synonyms: DCP-2; Dicalcium phosphate, dihydrate;
Calcium hydrogen orthophosphate, dihydrate;
Dicalcium orthophosphate
Trade names: Emcompress®

Calcium propionate (INCI)
CAS 4075-81-4; EINECS 223-795-8
Synonyms: Propionic acid, calcium salt
Trade names: Unistat CALBAN; Unistat CALPRO

Calcium saccharin (INCI)
CAS 6485-34-3; EINECS 229-349-9
Synonyms: 1,2-Benzisothiazol-3(2H)-one, 1,t-dioxide,
calcium salt
Trade names: Unisweet CALSAC

Calcium silicate (INCI)
CAS 1344-95-2, 10101-39-0; EINECS 215-710-8
Synonyms: Silicic acid, calcium salt
Trade names: Hubersorb®; Micro-Cel® C
Trade names containing: Pulvi-Lan

Calcium/sodium PVM/MA copolymer (INCI)
Trade names: Gantrez® MS-955

Calcium stearate (INCI)
CAS 1592-23-0; EINECS 216-472-8
Synonyms: Calcium octadecanoate; Stearic acid, cal-
cium salt
Trade names: Nuodex S-1421 Food Grade; Nuodex S-
1520 Food Grade; Radiastar® 1060; Synpro® Cal-
cium Stearate USP; Unichem CS; Witco® Calcium
Stearate F.P
Trade names containing: B-122

Calcium stearoyl lactylate (INCI)
CAS 5793-94-2; EINECS 227-335-7
Synonyms: Calcium stearoyl-2-lactylate; Calcium
stearyl-2-lactylate; Calcium stelate
Trade names: Artodan CF 40; Crolactil CSL; Pationic®
CSL; Unitolate CSL

Calcium sulfate (anhydrous) (INCI)
CAS 7778-18-9; EINECS 231-900-3
Synonyms: Anhydrite (natural form); Calcium sulfonate;
Anhydrous gypsum
Trade names: Calcium Sulfate Anhydrous NF 164; Etra
Super English Terra Alba; Unichem CS White
Trade names containing: Masque Poudre No. 2

Calcium sulfate (dihydrate)
CAS 10101-41-4
Synonyms: Native calcium sulfate; precipitated calcium
sulfate; Gypsum; Alabaster
Trade names: Compactrol®

Calcium titanate (INCI)
CAS 12049-50-2; EINECS 234-988-1
Synonyms: Perovskite
Trade names containing: Kalixide DPG

Calendula extract (INCI)
CAS 84776-23-8
Synonyms: Calendula officinalis extract; Marigold ex-
tract; Extract of calendula
Trade names: Hydroplastidine Calendula; Unibotan

Calendula CLR
Trade names containing: Actiphyte of Calendula;
Actiphyte of Marigold; Babyderme HS 265;
Babyderme LS 665; Bio-Chelated Derma-Plex I;
Biophytex®; Calendula Oil CLR; Calendula Oil
Monarom; Calendula Oil; Calenfil 3646; Complex
Relax; Crodarom Calendula O; Herbasol-Extract
Calendula; Herbasol-Extract Marigold; Hydrumine
Calendula; Lipoplastidine Calendula; Nutriderme HS
210; Solarium HS 269; Solarium LS 669; Tonique HS
290; Tonique LS 690; Unibotan Vitaplant O CLR;
Vitaplant CLR Oil-Soluble N

Calf skin extract (INCI)
Trade names: Elastobiol
Trade names containing: Epiderm-Complex O; Epiderm-
Complex W; Fibrostimuline P; Lipotrofina M

Calf skin hydrolysate (INCI)
Trade names: Extract From Bovine Foetal Skin Cells

Calx. *See Calcium oxide*

Camellia oil (INCI)
CAS 68916-73-4
Synonyms: Oil of camellia; Thea sinensis oil
Trade names: Camellia Oil; Tri-Ol CAM

Camphor (INCI)
CAS 76-22-2, 464-49-3; EINECS 207-355-2
Synonyms: 1,7,7-Trimethylbicyclo[2.2.1] heptan-2-one;
Gum camphor; 2-Camphanone
Trade names: Unichem CAMP
Trade names containing: Essentiaderm n.7

Candelilla synthetic
CAS 136097-95-5
Trade names: Koster Keunen Synthetic Candelilla;
Koster Keunen Synthetic Candelilla R-4; Koster
Keunen Synthetic Candelilla R-8

Candelilla wax (INCI)
CAS 8006-44-8; EINECS 232-347-0
Trade names: Candelilla Wax Cosmetic Grade Stralpitz;
Koster Keunen Candelilla; Natwax CAN; Ross
Candelilla Wax
Trade names containing: Cirami No. 1; Cutina® LM;
Isobeeswax SP 154; Koster Keunen Beeswax, S&P
ISOW; Ross Beeswax Substitute 628/5; Sphingo-
ceryl® Wax LS 2958 B; Unitina LM

Canolamidopropyl betaine (INCI)
Trade names: Hetaine CLA

Canolamidopropyl ethyldimonium ethosulfate
Synonyms: N-[(Alkyl C16-18)-(3-amidopropyl)]-N-N di-
methyl-N-ethyl ammonium ethyl sulfate
Trade names: Foamquat COAS; Schercoquat COAS

Canola oil (INCI)
CAS 8002-13-9, 120962-03-0
Trade names: Lipex 201; Lipovol CAN

Canola oil glyceride (INCI)
Trade names: Myverol® 18-99

CAP. *See Cellulose acetate propionate*

Capramide DEA (INCI)
CAS 136-26-5; EINECS 205-234-9
Synonyms: Capric acid diethanolamide; N,N-Bis(2-hy-
droxyethyl) decanamide
Trade names: Amidex CP; Comperlan® CD; Hetamide
1069; Mackamide™ CD-10; Monamid® 150-CW;
Monamid® CP-205
Trade names containing: Monamine C-100; Standamid®
CD; Upamide CD; Witcamide® 6544

Capric acid (INCI)
CAS 334-48-5; EINECS 206-376-4
Synonyms: n-Decanoic acid; n-Capric acid; Carboxylic acid C$_{10}$
Trade names: Unifat 10

Caproic acid (INCI)
CAS 142-62-1; EINECS 205-550-7
Synonyms: Carboxylic acid C$_6$; Hexanoic acid
Trade names: Unifat 6

Caprylic acid (INCI)
CAS 124-07-2; EINECS 204-677-5
Synonyms: n-Octanoic acid; Octoic acid
Trade names: Prifrac 2901; Prifrac 2910; Unifat 8
Trade names containing: Antistatique WL 879

Caprylic alcohol (INCI)
CAS 111-87-5; EINECS 203-917-6
Synonyms: n-Octyl alcohol; 1- or n-Octanol; C8 alcohols
Trade names: Nacol® 8-97; Nacol® 8-99

Caprylic/capric diglyceryl succinate (INCI)
Trade names: Miglyol® 829

Caprylic/capric glyceride
Trade names: Unitolate

Caprylic/capric glycerides (INCI)
CAS 26402-26-6
Trade names: Imwitor® 742; Witafrol® 7420

Caprylic/capric/lauric triglyceride (INCI)
CAS 68991-68-4
Trade names: Captex® 350

Caprylic/capric/linoleic triglyceride (INCI)
CAS 67701-28-4
Trade names: Captex® 810A; Captex® 810B; Captex® 810C; Captex® 810D; Miglyol® 818

Caprylic/capric/oleic triglyceride (INCI)
CAS 67701-28-4
Trade names: Captex® 910A; Captex® 910B; Captex® 910C; Captex® 910D

Caprylic/capric/stearic triglyceride (INCI)
Trade names: Emalex SG-37; Softisan® 378

Caprylic/capric triglyceride (INCI)
CAS 65381-09-1, 538-23-8, 85409-09-2; EINECS 265-724-3
Synonyms: Octanoic/decanoic acid triglyceride
Trade names: Aldo® TC; Captex® 300; Captex® 355; Emalex K.T.G; Estasan GT 8-40 3578; Estasan GT 8-60 3575; Estasan GT 8-60 3580; Estasan GT 8-65 3577; Estasan GT 8-65 3581; Estol GTC 3599; Estol GTCC 60 3604; Estol GTCC60 3604; Hodag CC-33; Hodag CC-33-F; Hodag CC-33-L; Hodag CC-33-S; Labrafac® Lipophile WL 1349; Lexol® GT-855; Lexol® GT-865; Liponate GC; Mazol® 1400; Miglyol® 810; Miglyol® 812; Myritol® 312; Myritol® 318; Neobee® M-5; Neobee® O; Protachem CTG; Radia® 7106; Tegosoft® CT; Unitolate 160-K
Trade names containing: Biofloreol Liq. Liposoluble; Camomile Oil Extra; Crodarom Chamomile EO; Crodarom Chamomile O; Gilugel MIG; Miglyol® Gel B; Miglyol® Gel T; Miglyol® Gel; Phosal® 53 MCT

Caprylic/capric triglyceride PEG-4 esters (INCI)
Trade names: Labrafac® Hydro WL 1219

Caprylamphocarboxypropionate. *See Disodium caprylo-amphodipropionate*

Caprylamphodiacetate. *See Disodium capryloamphodi-acetate*

Caprylamphoglycinate. *See Sodium capryloampho-acetate*

Capryloamphopropylsulfonate. *See Sodium caprylo-amphohydroxypropyl sulfonate*

Capryloyl collagen amino acids (INCI)
Synonyms: Capryloyl animal collagen amino acids
Trade names: Lipacide C8CO

Capryloyl glycine (INCI)
CAS 14246-53-8
Trade names: Lipacide C8G

Capryloyl hydrolyzed collagen (INCI)
Synonyms: Capryloyl hydrolyzed animal protein
Trade names: Lipacide CCO

Capryloyl keratin amino acids (INCI)
Synonyms: Capryloyl animal keratin amino acids
Trade names: Lipacide C8K

Caprylyl/capryl glucoside (INCI)
CAS 68515-73-1
Trade names: Oramix CG 110-60; Triton® CG-110

Caprylyl pyrrolidone (INCI)
Synonyms: N-Octyl-2-pyrrolidone
Trade names: Surfadone® LP-100

Capsicum extract (INCI)
CAS 84625-29-6
Trade names: Capsaicin
Trade names containing: Actiphyte of Capsicum; Capilotonique HS 226

Captan (INCI)
CAS 133-06-2; EINECS 205-087-0
Synonyms: N-Trichloromethylthiotetrahydrophthalimide; N-Trichloromethylthio-4-cyclohexene-1,2-dicar-boximide
Trade names: Vancide® 89 RE

Carbamide. *See Urea*

Carbomer (INCI)
CAS 9007-16-3; 9003-01-4; 9007-17-4; 76050-42-5
Trade names: Acrisint 400, 410, 430; Acritamer® 934; Acritamer® 934P; Acritamer® 940; Acritamer® 941; Carbopol® 910; Carbopol® 934P; Carbopol® 940; Carbopol® 941; Carbopol® 954; Carbopol® 980; Carbopol® 981; Carbopol® 2984; Carbopol® 5984; Junlon PW-110; Junlon PW-111
Trade names containing: Antil® 208; Elespher® Almondermin; Elespher® Dermosaccharides GY; Elespher® Dermosaccharides HC; Elespher® Eleseryl SH; Mearlmaid® PLN; Mearlmaid® PLO

Carboxyethyl aminobutyric acid (INCI)
Trade names: Cegaba

Carboxymethylcellulose sodium
CAS 9004-32-4
Synonyms: CMC; Cellulose gum (INCI); Sodium car-boxymethylcellulose; Sodium CMC
Trade names: Akucell CMC; Aqualon® Cellulose Gum; Aquasorb® A250; Blanose 7 Types; Blanose 9 Types; Blanose 12 Types; Dehydazol; Ticalose 15, 30, 75, 150R, 1200, 2000R, 2500, 4000, 4500, 5000R; Tylose® C, CB Series; Tylose® C-p, CB-p
Trade names containing: Avicel RC-591; Lapomer; Optigel WM

Carboxymethyl chitin (INCI)
CAS 52108-64-2
Trade names: Chitin Liq; Chitisol; Chotosolbe

Carboxymethyl chitosan (INCI)
Trade names: Chitoglycan

Carboxymethyl isostearamidopropyl morpholine (INCI)
Trade names: Incronam ISM 30

Carmine (INCI)
CAS 1390-65-4; EINECS 215-724-4
Trade names: Atomergic Carmine; Carmine 5297; Carmine Ultra-fine; Dascolor Carmine
Trade names containing: Bicrona® Carmine; Carmine 224; Chroma-Lite® Magenta 4505; Cloisonné Red; Cloisonné Violet; Colorona® Carmine Red; Dichrona® RB; Dichrona® RG; Dichrona® RY; Duocrome® RB; Gemstone Sunstone CC; Gemtone® Amethyst; Gemtone® Mauve Quartz; Gemtone® Sunstone

Carnauba (INCI)
CAS 8015-86-9; EINECS 232-399-4
Synonyms: Brazil wax
Trade names: Carnauba Wax NC #2 Stralpitz; Carnauba Wax NC #3 Stralpitz; Carnauba Wax SP 8; Koster Keunen Carnauba; Koster Keunen Carnauba No. 1; Koster Keunen Carnauba T-2; Koster Keunen Carnauba T-3; Koster Keunen Carnauba, Micro Granulated; Koster Keunen Carnauba, Powd; Natwax CAR; Ross Brazil Wax; Ross Carnauba Wax
Trade names containing: Cutina® LM; Durawax #1032; Flamenco® Gold CC; Flamenco® Pearl CC; Gemstone Sunstone CC; Gemtone® Tan Opal CC; Isobeeswax SP 154; Koster Keunen Beeswax, S&P ISOW; Soloron Silver Sparkle CO; Sphingoceryl® Wax LS 2958 B; Sterotex® CUnitina LM

Carnauba synthetic
Trade names: Koster Keunen Synthetic Carnauba

Carnitine (INCI)
CAS 541-15-1; EINECS 208-768-0
Synonyms: 3-Carboxy-2-hydroxy-N,N,N-trimethyl-1-propanaminium hydroxide, inner salt
Trade names containing: Carnitiline; CoAxel; Energisome

Carob extract (INCI)
CAS 84961-45-5
Synonyms: Ceratonia siliqua extract; Locust tree extract
Trade names containing: Carob HS

Carob flour. *See Locust bean gum*

Carob seed gum. *See Locust bean gum*

Carotene (INCI)
CAS 7235-40-7; EINECS 230-636-6
Synonyms: β-Carotene; Provitamin A
Trade names: Beta Carotene 30% in Veg. Oil No. 65646; Carotene Standard RR; Crystalline Beta Carotene No. 65638
Trade names containing: Brookosome® ACEBC; Brookosome® BC; Carotene Huileux 10000; Carrot Oil; Carrot Oil CLR

Carrageen. *See Carrageenan*

Carrageenan (INCI)
CAS 9000-07-1; EINECS 232-524-2
Synonyms: Chondrus; Carrageen
Trade names: Aquagel; Aquaron; Aubygel X52; Carraghenate P, Standard, X 2; Gelcarin LA; Genu Carrageenan; Genugel; Genulacta Series; Genuvisco; Seakem 3, LCM; Seaspen PF; Stamere®; Viscarin XLV
Trade names containing: Seanamin BD

Carrageenan extract (INCI)
Synonyms: Chondrus crispus extract; Irish moss extract
Trade names containing: Actiphyte of Irish Moss

Carrot extract (INCI)
CAS 84929-61-3
Synonyms: Daucus carota sativa extract; Extract of carrot

Trade names containing: Carrot Oil CLR; Carrot Oil Extra; Carrot Oil; Carrot Oil; Carrots Extract HS 2597 G; Crodarom Carrot O

Carrot oil (INCI)
CAS 8015-88-1
Synonyms: Carrot seed oil; Oils, carrot seed
Trade names: Daucoil; Unibotan Carrot Oil CLR
Trade names containing: Carrot Oil CLR; Carrot Oil

Carrot seed extract (INCI)
Synonyms: Daucus carota extract
Trade names containing: Babyderme HS 265; Babyderme HS 342; Babyderme LS 642; Babyderme LS 665; Carrot LS; Emollient HS 238; Nutriderme HS 210

Casein. *See Milk protein*

Cassia oil. *See Cinnamon oil*

Castor oil (INCI)
CAS 1323-38-2; 8001-79-4; EINECS 232-293-8
Synonyms: Ricinus oil; Oil of Palma Christi; Tangantangan oil
Trade names: AA USP; Castor Oil USP; Cosmetol® X; Crystal® Crown; Crystal® Crown LP; Crystal® O; Diamond Quality®; EmCon CO; Lanaetex CO; Lipovol CO; Surfactol® 13; Unicast CO; York Krystal Kleer Castor Oil; York USP Castor Oil
Trade names containing: Argonol RIC2; Bentone® Gel CAO; Biron® B-50 CO; Biron® NLY-L-2X CO; Biron® Silver CO; Blanc Covapate W 9765; Blue Covapate W 6763; Castorcet; Cutina® LM; Flamenco® Gold CC; Flamenco® Pearl CC; Gemstone Sunstone CC; Gemtone® Tan Opal CC; Gilugel CAO; Grillocin WE-106; Leniplex; Mearlite® GEH; Mearlite® LEM; Soloron Silver CO; Soloron Silver Fine CO; Soloron Silver Sparkle CO; Sphingoceryl® Wax LS 2958 B; Unitina LM

Castor oil sucroglyceride
Trade names: Mirasoft™ CO 11

Cationic collagen polypeptides
CAS 9007-34-5
Trade names: Cationic Collagen Polypeptides
Trade names containing: Quinta-Pro Conc

Cauliflower unsaponifiables (INCI)
CAS 91771-39-0; EINECS 294-930-6
Trade names containing: Braxicina

Caustic potash. *See Potassium hydroxide*

Caustic soda. *See Sodium hydroxide*

Celandine extract (INCI)
CAS 84603-56-5
Synonyms: Chelidonium majus extract
Trade names containing: Complex Relax

Cellulase
CAS 9012-54-8; EINECS 232-734-4
Trade names: Cellulase 4000; Cellulase Tr Conc; Celluflow C-25; Cellulon; Elcema® F150, G250, P100; Solka-Floc® BW-40; Solka-Floc® BW-100; Solka-Floc® BW-200; Solka-Floc® BW-2030; Solka-Floc® Fine Granular

Cellulose (INCI)
CAS 9004-34-6; EINECS 232-674-9
Synonyms: Wood pulp, bleached; Cotton fiber
Trade names containing: Unispheres G-503; Unispheres R-505; Unispheres U-504; Unispheres YE-501

Cellulose acetate (INCI)
CAS 9004-35-7
Synonyms: CA; Cellulose acetate ester; Acetylcellulose
Trade names: Celluflow TA-25

Cellulose acetate butyrate (INCI)
CAS 9004-36-8
Synonyms: CAB; Cellulose acetobutyrate; Cellulose, acetate butanoate
Trade names: Eastman® CAB

Cellulose acetate propionate (INCI)
CAS 9004-39-1
Synonyms: CAP; Cellulose propionate; Cellulose acetate propionate ester; Cellulose, acetate propanoate
Trade names: Eastman® CAP

Cellulose gum (INCI). See Carboxymethylcellulose sodium

Cellulose methyl ether. See Methylcellulose

Cellulose, nitrate. See Nitrocellulose

Cera alba. See Beeswax

Ceresin (INCI)
CAS 8001-75-0; EINECS 232-290-1
Synonyms: White ozokerite wax; Earth wax; Mineral wax
Trade names: Ceresine Wax Cosmetic Stralpitz; Ceresine Wax SP 84; Koster Keunen Ceresine; Koster Keunen Ceresine 130/135; Koster Keunen Ceresine 140/145; Koster Keunen Ceresine 155; Koster Keunen Ceresine 192; Natwax CER; Ross Ceresine Wax
Trade names containing: Dehymuls® K; PCL SE w/o 2/ 066255

Cetalkonium chloride (INCI)
CAS 122-18-9; EINECS 204-526-3
Synonyms: Cetyl dimethyl benzyl ammonium chloride; Benzylhexadecyldimethylammonium chloride; N-Hexadecyl-N,N-dimethylbenzenemethanaminium chloride
Trade names: Cetol®; Sumquat® 6050

Cetearalkonium bromide (INCI)
Synonyms: Cetyl/stearyl dimethyl benzyl ammonium bromide
Trade names containing: Emulgade® K

Ceteareth-2 (INCI)
CAS 68439-49-6 (generic)
Synonyms: PEG-2 cetyl/stearyl ether; POE (2) cetyl/ stearyl ether; PEG 100 cetyl/stearyl ether
Trade names: Hodag Nonionic CS-2; Lowenol C-279; Macol® CSA-2; Unicol CSA-2

Ceteareth-3 (INCI)
CAS 68439-49-6 (generic)
Synonyms: PEG-3 cetyl/stearyl ether; POE (3) cetyl/ stearyl ether
Trade names: Hostacerin T-3; Procol CS-3; Volpo CS-3
Trade names containing: Almolan AE; Genamin KSE

Ceteareth-4 (INCI)
CAS 68439-49-6 (generic)
Synonyms: PEG-4 cetyl/stearyl ether; POE (4) cetyl/ stearyl ether
Trade names: Hetoxol CS-4; Lipocol SC-4; Macol® CSA-4; Procol CS-4; Prox-onic CSA-1/04; Unicol CSA-4

Ceteareth-5 (INCI)
CAS 68439-49-6 (generic)
Synonyms: PEG-5 cetyl/stearyl ether; POE (5) cetyl/ stearyl ether
Trade names: Hetoxol CS-5; Hodag Nonionic CS-5; Procol CS-5; Unicol CSA-5; Volpo CS-5
Trade names containing: Lanpro-1

Ceteareth-6 (INCI)
CAS 68439-49-6 (generic)
Synonyms: PEG-6 cetyl/stearyl ether; POE (6) cetyl/ stearyl ether

Trade names: Cremophor® A 6; Emulgator B-6; Lipocol SC-6; Marlowet® TA 6; Procol CS-6; Prox-onic CSA-1/06
Trade names containing: Hydro Myristenol 2/014082; Hydro Myristenol 2/014082

Ceteareth-7 (INCI)
CAS 68439-49-6 (generic)
Synonyms: PEG-7 cetyl/stearyl ether
Trade names containing: Cromul EM 0685

Ceteareth-8 (INCI)
CAS 68439-49-6 (generic)
Synonyms: PEG-8 cetyl/stearyl ether; PEG 400 cetyl/ stearyl ether; POE (8) cetyl/stearyl ether
Trade names: Lipocol SC-8; Marlowet® TA 8; Procol CS-8

Ceteareth-9
CAS 68439-49-6 (generic)
Synonyms: PEG-9 cetyl/stearyl ether; POE (9) cetyl/ stearyl ether
Trade names: Hetoxol CS-9; Tewax TC 10

Ceteareth-10 (INCI)
CAS 68439-49-6 (generic)
Synonyms: PEG-10 cetyl/stearyl ether; POE (10) cetyl/ stearyl ether
Trade names: G-4936; Hodag Nonionic CS-10; Lipocol SC-10; Macol® CSA-10; Marlowet® TA 10; Procol CS-10; Prox-onic CSA-1/010; Unicol CSA-10; Volpo CS-10
Trade names containing: Macol® 123; Phoenoxol J

Ceteareth-11 (INCI)
CAS 68439-49-6 (generic)
Synonyms: PEG-11 cetyl/stearyl ether; POE (11) cetyl/ stearyl ether
Trade names: Britex CS 110; Cremophor® A 11; Empilan® KM 11; Marlipal® 1618/11

Ceteareth-12 (INCI)
CAS 68439-49-6 (generic)
Synonyms: PEG-12 cetyl/stearyl ether; POE (12) cetyl/ stearyl ether
Trade names: Eumulgin® B1; G-4822; Incropol CS-12; Lipocol SC-12; Procol CS-12; Unimul-B-1
Trade names containing: Emulgade® K; Emulgade® SE

Ceteareth-13 (INCI)
CAS 68439-49-6
Trade names: Elfapur® T 130 S

Ceteareth-15 (INCI)
CAS 68439-49-6 (generic)
Synonyms: PEG-15 cetyl/stearyl ether; POE (15) cetyl/ stearyl ether
Trade names: Hetoxol 15 CSA; Hetoxol CS-15; Hetoxol CSA-15; Hodag Nonionic CS-15; Lipocol SC-15; Macol® CSA-15; Procol CS-15; Prox-onic CSA-1/ 015; Unicol CSA-15; Volpo CS-15
Trade names containing: Genamin KSE; Homulgator 920 G; Tego® Care 215

Ceteareth-16 (INCI)
CAS 68439-49-6 (generic)
Synonyms: PEG-16 cetyl/stearyl ether; POE (16) cetyl/ stearyl ether
Trade names containing: Simulsol 5719

Ceteareth-17 (INCI)
CAS 68439-49-6 (generic)
Synonyms: PEG-17 cetyl/stearyl ether; POE (17) cetyl/ stearyl ether
Trade names: G-70147; Procol CS-17

Ceteareth-20 (INCI)

CAS 68439-49-6 (generic)
Synonyms: PEG-20 cetyl/stearyl ether; POE (20) cetyl/stearyl ether
Trade names: Acconon W230; Britex CS 200 B; Emthox® 5885; Eumulgin® B2; G-4938; Hetoxol CS-20; Hodag Nonionic CS-20; Incropol CS-20; Lipocol SC-20; Macol® CSA-20; Procol CS-20; Prox-onic CSA-1/020; Rhodasurf® C-20; Ritacet-20; Unicol CSA-20; Unimul-B-2; Varonic® 63 E20; Volpo CS-20
Trade names containing: Brookswax™ C; Brookswax™ D; Brookswax™ G; Brookswax™ J; Brookswax™ Nl; Ceral EF; Ceral EN 6; Ceral G; Ceral PW; Cosmowax J; Cosmowax K; Cosmowax P; Cyclogol Nl; Dermalcare® C-20; Dermalcare® Nl; Dispersen-D; Dispersen-G; Emerwax® 1266; Emulgade® 1000 Nl; Emulgade® SE; Fanwax G; Galenol® 1618 AE; Hetoxol D; Hetoxol G; Hetoxol J; Hodag CSA-103; Isocet; Lexemul® CS-20; Lipowax D; Lipowax G; Macol® 123; Macol® 124; Macol® 125; Maywax D; Phoenoxol T; Procol CS-20-D; Procol ST-20-G; Promulgen® D; Promulgen® G; Ritachol 5000; Ritapro 200; Ritapro 300; Ritapro 300R; Standapol® CAT; Tefose® 70; Teginacid® X SE; Teginacid®; Unimulgade-1000Nl; Varonic® BD; Varonic® BG

Ceteareth-23 (INCI)
CAS 68439-49-6 (generic)
Synonyms: PEG-23 cetyl/stearyl ether; PEG (23) cetyl/stearyl ether; POE (23) cetyl/stearyl ether
Trade names containing: Britex EW/BP

Ceteareth-25 (INCI)
CAS 68439-49-6 (generic)
Synonyms: PEG-25 cetyl/stearyl ether; POE (25) cetyl/stearyl ether
Trade names: Britex CS 250; Cremophor® A 25; Emulgator E 2568; Marlowet® TA 25
Trade names containing: Base O/W 097; Homulgator 920 G; Softisan® 601; Tewax TC 1; Tewax TC 840

Ceteareth-27 (INCI)
CAS 68439-49-6 (generic)
Synonyms: PEG-27 cetyl/stearyl ether; POE (27) cetyl/stearyl ether
Trade names: Procol CS-27

Ceteareth-30 (INCI)
CAS 68439-49-6 (generic)
Synonyms: PEG-30 cetyl/stearyl ether; POE (30) cetyl/stearyl ether
Trade names: Britex CS 300; Eumulgin® B3; G-4940; Hetoxol CS-30; Lipocol SC-30; Procol CS-30; Prox-onic CSA-1/030; Unicol CSA-30; Unimul-B-3
Trade names containing: Emulgator E 2209; Hetoxol L

Ceteareth-33 (INCI)
CAS 68439-49-6
Trade names: Simulsol CS
Trade names containing: Cire De Lanol CTO

Ceteareth-40 (INCI)
CAS 68439-49-6 (generic)
Synonyms: PEG-40 cetyl/stearyl ether; POE (40) cetyl/stearyl ether
Trade names: Hetoxol CS-40; Hetoxol CS-40W; Hodag Nonionic CS-40; Incropol CS-40; Macol® CSA-40; Unicol CSA-40

Ceteareth-50 (INCI)
CAS 68439-49-6 (generic)
Synonyms: PEG-50 cetyl/stearyl ether; POE (50) cetyl/stearyl ether
Trade names: Empilan® KM 50; Hetoxol CS-50; Hetoxol CS-50 Special; Lipocol SC-50; Prox-onic CSA-1/050

Trade names containing: Lipocol F-33B

Ceteareth-60 (INCI)
CAS 68439-49-6 (generic)
Synonyms: PEG-60 cetyl/stearyl ether; POE (60) cetyl/stearyl ether
Trade names: Incropol CS-60

Ceteareth-100 (INCI)
CAS 68439-49-6 (generic)
Synonyms: PEG-100 cetyl/stearyl ether; POE (100) cetyl/stearyl ether
Trade names: Britex CS 1000

Ceteareth-7 carboxylic acid
CAS 68954-89-2
Trade names: Akypo RCS 60

Ceteareth-2 phosphate (INCI)
Trade names: Crodafos CS2 Acid

Ceteareth-5 phosphate (INCI)
Trade names: Crodafos CS5 Acid

Ceteareth-10 phosphate (INCI)
Trade names: Crodafos CS10 Acid

Cetearyl alcohol (INCI)
CAS 8005-44-5; 67762-30-5
Synonyms: Cetostearyl alcohol; Cetyl/stearyl alcohol; C16-18 alcohols
Trade names: Adol® 63; Adol® 64; Adol® 630; Adol® 640; Alfol® 1618; Alfol® 1618 CG; Alfol® 1618 GC; Carsofoam® 1618; Cetax 50; Cetostearyl Alcohol BP; Cetostearyl Alcohol NF; CO-1670; Crodacol CS-50; Hetol CS; Hetoxol CS; Hyfatol CS; Koster Keunen Fatty Alcohol 1618; Lanette® O; Lanol CS; Laurex® 4550; Laurex® CS; Laurex® CS/D; Laurex® CS/W; Mackol 1618; Nafol® 1618 H; Philcohol 1618; Radianol® 1763; Radianol® 1765; Radianol® 1768; Radianol® 1769; TA-1618; Unette-O; Unihydag Wax-O
Trade names containing: Actimulse 250; Almolan AE; Almolan LIS; Amphocerin® E; Amphocerin® K; Amyx ST 3837; Aquabase N.F.; Aquabase; Argobase EUC 2; Argobase L1; Argobase S1; Britex EW/BP; Brookswax™ C; Brookswax™ D; Brookswax™ J; Brookswax™ Nl; Brookswax™ P; Brookswax™ R; Carsoquat® 816-C; Ceral 10; Ceral EF; Ceral EFN; Ceral EN 6; Ceral PW; Cosmowax J; Cosmowax P; Crodacol GP; Crodex A; Crodex C; Crodex N; Cutina® CBS; Cyclochem EM 560; Cyclogol Nl; Dehydag® Wax N; Dehydag® Wax SX; Dehydag® Wax W; Dermalcare® C-20; Dermalcare® Nl; Dermalcare® POL; Dispersen-D; Dispersen-S; Emerwax® 1266; Empiwax SK; Empiwax SK/BP; Emulgade® 1000 Nl; Emulgade® A; Emulgade® CL Special; Emulgade® CL; Emulgade® F Special; Emulgade® F; Emulgade® SE; Fanwax P; Galenol® 1618 AE; Galenol® 1618 CS; Galenol® 1618 DSN; Galenol® 1618 KS; Hetoxol D; Hetoxol J; Hetoxol L; Hodag CSA-101; Hodag CSA-102; Hodag CSA-103; Hostacerin CG; Incroquat Behenyl TMC; Incroquat Behenyl TMS; Incroquat CR Conc; Krim 400; Lanbritol Wax N21; Lanette Wax SX; Lanette® N; Lanette® SX; Lanette® W; Lanette® Wax CAT; Lanette® Wax SX, SXBP; Lexemul® CS-20; Lipowax D; Lipowax Nl; Lipowax P-SPEC; Lipowax P; Lipowax PR; Lipowax; Macol® 123; Macol® 124; Macol® CPS; Maquat SC-1632; Maywax D; Mazawax® 163R; Mazawax® 163SS; Phoenoxol J; Phoenoxol T; Procol NIN; Procol P; Promulgen® D; Quatrex CRC; Relaxer Conc. No. 2; Relaxer Conc. No. 3; Relaxer Conc. No. 4; Ritachol 5000; Ritachol®

1000; Ritachol® 2000; Ritachol® 3000; Ritapro 100; Ritapro 300; Ritapro 300R; Sebase; Standamul® Conc. 1002; Teinowax; Tewax TC 2; Tewax TC 840; Unette-W; Unicol 123; Unicol CPS; Unihydag Wax-SX; Unimul-1002 Conc; Unimulgade-1000NI; Unimulgade-F Special; Unimulgade-F; Upiwax 163; Upiwax 163R; Varisoft® BTMS; Varisoft® C SAC; Varisoft® CRC; Varonic® BD; Zetesap 5165; Zetesap 813A

Cetearyl behenate (INCI)
Trade names: Kester Wax® 62

Cetearyl candelillate (INCI)
CAS 138724-54-6
Trade names: Cera Euphorbia; Koster Keunen Candelilla Ester

Cetearyl glucoside (INCI)
Trade names: Montanol 68

Cetearyl isononanoate (INCI)
Synonyms: Isononanoic acid, cetyl/stearyl ether
Trade names: Cetiol® SN; Tegosoft® CI; Unimul ISN

Cetearyl octanoate (INCI)
CAS 8005-44-5, 59130-69-7, 59130-70-7; EINECS 261-619-1
Synonyms: Cetyl/stearyl 2-ethyl hexanoate; 2-Ethylhexanoic acid, cetyl/stearyl ester
Trade names: Crodamol CAP; Estalan JB; Hest CSO; Lanol 1688; Luvitol® EHO; PCL Liq. 1002/066240; Schercemol 1688; Tegosoft® Liquid
Trade names containing: PCL Liq. 2/066210; PCL Liquid 100; PCL SE w/o 2/066255; PCL-Siccum 2/066215; Pur-Cellin Oil; Tegosoft® Liquid M

Cetearyl palmitate (INCI)
CAS 85341-79-3; 31566-31-1; 11099-07-3; 85666-92-8
Synonyms: Hexadecanoic acid, cetyl/stearyl ether
Trade names: Crodamol CSP

Cetearyl stearate (INCI)
CAS 93820-97-4, 136097-82-0
Synonyms: Cetostearyl stearate
Trade names: Crodamol CSS; Estol 1481; Estol CSS 3709; Kester Wax® 56

Ceteth-2 (INCI)
CAS 9004-95-9 (generic); 5274-61-3
Synonyms: PEG-2 cetyl ether; POE (2) cetyl ether; PEG 100 cetyl ether
Trade names: Brij® 52; Britex C; Britex C 20; Emalex 102; Ethosperse® CA-2; Hetoxol CA-2; Hodag Nonionic C-2; Lanycol-52; Lipocol C-2; Macol® CA-2; Nikkol BC-2; Procol CA-2; Simulsol 52; Unicol CA-2
Trade names containing: Lexate® CRC

Ceteth-3 (INCI)
CAS 9004-95-9 (generic), 4484-59-7
Synonyms: PEG-3 cetyl ether; POE (3) cetyl ether
Trade names: Emalex 103
Trade names containing: Isoxal 5

Ceteth-4 (INCI)
CAS 9004-95-9 (generic), 5274-63-5
Synonyms: PEG-4 cetyl ether; POE (4) cetyl ether
Trade names: Hodag Nonionic C-4; Lipocol C-4; Procol CA-4; Unicol CA-4

Ceteth-5 (INCI)
CAS 9004-95-9 (generic), 4478-97-1
Synonyms: PEG-5 cetyl ether; POE (5) cetyl ether
Trade names: Emalex 105; Emalex 1605
Trade names containing: Cromul EM 0685; Isoxal 12; Solulan® 5

Ceteth-6 (INCI)

CAS 9004-95-9 (generic), 5168-91-2
Synonyms: PEG-6 cetyl ether; POE (6) cetyl ether
Trade names: Nikkol BC-5.5; Procol CA-6

Ceteth-7
CAS 9004-95-9 (generic)
Synonyms: PEG-7 cetyl ether; POE (7) cetyl ether
Trade names: Emalex 107; Nikkol BC-7

Ceteth-10 (INCI)
CAS 9004-95-9 (generic), 14529-40-9
Synonyms: PEG-10 cetyl ether; POE (10) cetyl ether
Trade names: Brij® 56; Britex C 100; Emalex 110; Emalex 1610; Hetoxol CA-10; Hodag Nonionic C-10; Lipocol C-10; Macol® CA-10; Nikkol BC-10TX; Procol CA-10; Simulsol 56; Unicol CA-10
Trade names containing: Isoxal 11

Ceteth-12 (INCI)
CAS 9004-95-9 (generic), 13149-83-2
Synonyms: PEG-12 cetyl ether; POE (12) cetyl ether
Trade names: Emalex 112
Trade names containing: Lanbritol Wax N21

Ceteth-14 (INCI)
CAS 9004-95-9 (generic)
Trade names containing: Aqualose SLT

Ceteth-15 (INCI)
CAS 9004-95-9 (generic)
Synonyms: PEG-15 cetyl ether; POE (15) cetyl ether
Trade names: Emalex 115; Emalex 1615; Nikkol BC-15TX

Ceteth-16 (INCI)
CAS 9004-95-9 (generic)
Synonyms: PEG-16 cetyl ether; POE (16) cetyl ether
Trade names: G-3816
Trade names containing: Lanpro-10; Proto-Lan 20; Proto-Lan 4R; Solulan® 16

Ceteth-17
CAS 9004-95-9 (generic)
Trade names: Emalex 117

Ceteth-20 (INCI)
CAS 9004-95-9 (generic); 68439-49-6
Synonyms: PEG-20 cetyl ether; POE (20) cetyl ether; Cetomacrogol 1000
Trade names: Akyporox RC 200; Brij® 58; Britex C 200; Cetomacrogol 1000 BP; Emalex 120; Emalex 1620; Ethosperse® CA-20; G-3820; Hetoxol CA-20; Hodag Nonionic C-20; Lanycol-58; Lipocol C-20; Nikkol BC-20TX; Procol CA-20; Simulsol 58; Unicol CA-20
Trade names containing: Crodex N; Dermalcare® POL; Emulcire 61 WL 2659; Hetoxol CAWS; Hodag CSA-101; Leniplex; Lipowax NI; Procol NIN; Tefose® 2000; Tefose® 2561; Teginacid® H; Tego® Care 150; Tego® Care 300

Ceteth-23
CAS 9004-95-9 (generic)
Synonyms: PEG-23 cetyl ether; POE (23) cetyl ether
Trade names: Nikkol BC-23

Ceteth-24 (INCI)
CAS 9004-95-9 (generic)
Synonyms: PEG-24 cetyl ether; POE (24) cetyl ether
Trade names containing: Forlan C-24; Ivarlan™ C-24; Solulan® C-24

Ceteth-25 (INCI)
CAS 9004-95-9 (generic)
Synonyms: PEG-25 cetyl ether; POE (25) cetyl ether
Trade names: Emalex 125; Emalex 1625; Nikkol BC-25TX
Trade names containing: Hydrolactol 70; Solulan® 25

Ceteth-30 (INCI)
CAS 9004-95-9 (generic)
Synonyms: PEG-30 cetyl ether; POE (30) cetyl ether
Trade names: Emalex 130; Lipocol C-30; Nikkol BC-30TX; Procol CA-30

Ceteth-40
CAS 9004-95-9 (generic)
Synonyms: PEG-40 cetyl ether; POE (40) cetyl ether
Trade names: Nikkol BC-40TX

Ceteth-3 stearate
PEG-3 cetyl ether stearate
Trade names: Emalex CWS-3

Ceteth-5 stearate
Synonyms: PEG-5 cetyl ether stearate
Trade names: Emalex CWS-5

Ceteth-7 stearate
Trade names: Emalex CWS-7

Ceteth-10 stearate
Trade names: Emalex CWS-10

Cetethyldimonium bromide (INCI)
CAS 124-03-8; EINECS 204-672-8
Synonyms: Cetyl dimethylethyl ammonium bromide; Quaternium-17; N-Ethyl-N,N-dimethyl-1-hexadecanaminium bromide
Trade names: Sumquat® 6020

Cetethyl morpholinium ethosulfate (INCI)
CAS 78-21-7; EINECS 201-094-8
Synonyms: Cetyl ethyl morpholinium ethosulfate;; Quaternium-25; Morpholinium, 4-ethyl-4-hexadecyl, ethyl sulfate
Trade names: Barquat® CME-35

Cetin. *See Cetyl palmitate*

Cetoleth-3
Synonyms: PEG-3 cetyl/oleyl ether; POE (3) cetyl/oleyl ether
Trade names: Ethylan® 172

Cetoleth-4
Trade names: G-3904

Cetoleth-6
Synonyms: PEG-6 cetyl/oleyl ether; POE (6) cetyl/oleyl ether
Trade names: Ethylan® ME

Cetoleth-13
Synonyms: PEG-13 cetyl/oleyl ether; PEG (13) cetyl/oleyl ether
Trade names: Ethylan® OE

Cetoleth-19
Trade names: Ethylan® R

Cetoleth-22
CAS 68920-66-1
Trade names: Britex CO 220

Cetoleth-24 (INCI)
Synonyms: PEG-24 cetyl/oleyl ether; POE (24) cetyl/oleyl ether
Trade names containing: Sandotex A

Cetostearyl alcohol. *See Cetearyl alcohol*

Cetraria islandica extract. *See Iceland moss extract*

Cetrimonium bromide (INCI)
CAS 57-09-0; EINECS 200-311-3
Synonyms: Cetyltrimethylammonium bromide; Hexadecyltrimethylammonium bromide; N,N,N-Trimethyl-1-hexadecanaminium bromide
Trade names: Acetoquat CTAB; Bromat®; Catinal HTB-70; Cetrimide; Cetrimide™ BP; Rhodaquat® M242B/99; Sumquat® 6030; Varisoft® CTB-40
Trade names containing: Crodex C; Lanette® Wax CAT; Miracare® CT100

Cetrimonium chloride (INCI)
CAS 112-02-7; EINECS 203-928-6
Synonyms: Cetyl trimethyl ammonium chloride;; Palmityl trimethyl ammonium chloride;; Hexadecyl trimethyl ammonium chloride
Trade names: Ablumine TMC; Adogen® 444; Ammonyx® CETAC; Ammonyx® CETAC-30; Arquad® 16-25W; Arquad® 16-29; Arquad® 16-29W; Barquat® CT-29; Carsoquat® CT-429; CTAC; Dehyquart® A; Genamin CTAC; Incroquat CTC-30; Incroquat CTC-50; Mackernium™ CTC-30; Nikkol CA-2330; Nikkol CA-2350; Quatrex CTAC; Querton 16Cl-29; Querton 16Cl-50; Radiaquat® 6444; Radiaquat® 6445; Rhodaquat® M242C/29; Tequat BC; Uniquart A; Variquat® E290; Varisoft® 250; Varisoft® 300; Varisoft® 355
Trade names containing: Arquad® 16-25; Arquad® 16-50; Belsil ADM 6057 E; Carsoquat® CB; Dow Corning® 939; Krim 400; Quatrex CT-100

Cetrimonium methosulfate (INCI)
CAS 65060-02-8; EINECS 265-352-1
Synonyms: Cetyltrimethylammonium methosulfate
Trade names: Catigene® CT 70

Cetrimonium tosylate (INCI)
CAS 138-32-9; EINECS 205-324-8
Synonyms: Cetyl trimethyl ammonium p-toluene sulfonate
Trade names: Cetats®

Cetyl acetate (INCI)
CAS 629-70-9; EINECS 211-103-7
Synonyms: Hexadecyl acetate
Trade names: Pelemol CA
Trade names containing: Acelan A; Acetol® 1706; Acetulan®; Argonol ACE 5; Argonol ACE 6; Crodalan AWS; Crodalan LA; Ethoxyol® 1707; Fancol ALA-10; Fancol ALA-15; Fancol ALA; Ivarbase™ 3210; Ivarbase™ 98; Lanaetex-75; Lanalene 97; Lanalene 98; Lanalene AC; Naturon® 2X IPA; Protalan 98; Protalan AC; Ritawax AEO; Ritawax ALA; Solulan® 97; Solulan® 98; Trivent ALA

Cetyl acetyl ricinoleate (INCI)
Trade names: Naturechem® CAR

Cetyl alcohol (INCI)
CAS 36653-82-4; EINECS 253-149-0
Synonyms: Palmityl alcohol; C16 linear primary alcohol; 1-Hexadecanol
Trade names: Adol® 52; Adol® 52 NF; Adol® 520 NF; Alfol® 16; Cachalot® C-50; Cachalot® C-51; Cachalot® C-52; Cetaffine; Cetal; Cetax 16; CO-1695; CoChem CA; Crodacol C-70; Crodacol C-90; Crodacol C-95NF; Epal® 16NF; Fancol CA; Hetol CA; Hyfatol 16-95; Hyfatol 16-98; Lanette® 16; Lanol C; Lipocol C; Mackol 16; Nacol® 16-95; Nacol® 16-98; Philcohol 1600; RITA CA; Unihydag Wax 16
Trade names containing: Akypoquat 131 VC; Amerchol® 400; Base O/W 097; C-Base; Carsoquat® CB; Cutina® LM; Emulcire 61 WL 2659; Emulgade® EO-10; Emulgator E 2209; Epal® 1214; Epal® 1218; Epal® 1416-LD; Epal® 1416; Epal® 1418; Epal® 1618; Epal® 1618RT; Epal® 1618T; Forlan L Conc; Forlan L; Forlan LM; Genamin KSE; Hair-cure 2/011500; Homulgator 920 G; Incroquat B65C; Ivarbase™ 3230; Ivarbase™ 3231; Lamecreme® AOM; Lamecreme® LPM; Lanamol; Monacet; Phos-

Cetyl amine

pholipid SV; Proto-Lan 4R; Relaxer Conc. No. 2; Relaxer Conc. No. 3; Relaxer Conc. No. 4; Ritachol 5000; Ritachol® 3000; Ritachol® 4000; Ross Beeswax Substitute 628/5; Sphingoceryl® Wax LS 2958 B; T-Base; Unitina LM

Cetyl amine. *See Palmitamine*

Cetylamine hydrofluoride (INCI)
CAS 3151-59-5; EINECS 221-588-7
Trade names: Unifluorid H 101

Cetylarachidol (INCI)
CAS 17658-36-8; EINECS 241-637-6
Synonyms: 2-Hexadecyl-1-eicosanol
Trade names: Isofol® 36

Cetyl betaine (INCI)
CAS 693-33-4; EINECS 211-748-4
Synonyms: N-(Carboxymethyl)-N,N-dimethyl-1-hexadecanaminium hydroxide, inner salt
Trade names: Lonzaine® 16S; Lonzaine® 16SP; Mackam™ CET

Cetyl C12-15 pareth-9-carboxylate (INCI)
Synonyms: PEG-9 C12-15 alkyl ether carboxylic acid, cetyl ester; PEG 450 C12-15 alkyl ether carboxylic acid, cetyl ester; POE (9) C12-15 alkyl ether carboxylic acid, cetyl ester
Trade names: Velsan® P8-16

Cetyl caprate
Trade names: Emalex CC-10

Cetyldiethanolaminephosphate
CAS 90388-14-0
Trade names: Crodafos CDP

Cetyl dimethicone (INCI)
Trade names: Abil®-Wax 9801; Abil®-Wax 9814; Dow Corning® 2502 Cosmetic Fluid
Trade names containing: Abil® WS 08

Cetyl dimethicone copolyol (INCI)
Trade names: Abil® B 9806; Abil® EM-90
Trade names containing: Abil® B 9808; Abil® WE 09; Abil® WS 08

Cetyl dimethyl benzyl ammonium chloride. *See Cetalkonium chloride*

Cetyl esters (INCI)
CAS 8002-23-1; CAS 17661-50-6; EINECS 241-640-2
Synonyms: Synthetic spermaceti wax
Trade names: Crodamol SS; Dermalcare® SPS; Espermaceti A; Espermaceti C; Liponate SPS; Protachem MST; Ritaceti; Ross Spermaceti Wax Substitute 573; Spermwax®; Starfol® Wax CG; Unisyn BEE; W.G.S. Synaceti 116 NF/USP
Trade names containing: Cetina; Cyclochem EM 560; Lipowax

Cetyl ethyl... See Cetethyl...

Cetyl glyceryl ether
Trade names: Nikkol Chimyl Alcohol 100

Cetyl hydroxyethyl cellulose (INCI)
Trade names: Natrosol® Plus CS; Natrosol® Plus CS, Grade 330; PolySurf

Cetyl lactate (INCI)
CAS 35274-05-6; EINECS 252-478-7
Synonyms: n-Hexadecyl lactate; 2-Hydroxypropanoic acid hexadecyl ester; 1-Hexadecanol lactate
Trade names: Cegesoft® C 19; Ceraphyl® 28; Cetinol LA; Crodamol CL; Lactabase C16; Lactacet; Liponate CL; Nikkol Cetyl Lactate

Cetyl laurate (INCI)
CAS 20834-06-4; EINECS 244-071-8

Synonyms: Hexadecyl dodecanoate
Trade names: Cetinol LU; Laurate de Cetyle

Cetyl octanoate (INCI)
CAS 59130-69-7; EINECS 261-619-1
Synonyms: Cetyl 2-ethylhexanoate;; n-Hexadecyl 2-ethylhexanoate; Hexanoic acid, 2-ethyl-, hexadecyl ester
Trade names: Bernel® Ester CO; Emalex CC-168; Exceparl HO; Nikkol ClO, ClO-P; Schercemol CO; Tegosoft® CO; Trivent OC-16
Trade names containing: PCL Liquid 100

Cetyl oleate (INCI)
CAS 22393-86-8; EINECS 244-950-6
Trade names: Glicoceride OCS

Cetyl palmitate (INCI)
CAS 540-10-3; EINECS 208-736-6
Synonyms: Hexadecanoic acid, hexadecyl ester; Palmitic acid, hexadecyl ester; Cetin
Trade names: Crodamol CP; Cutina® CP; Elfacos® CP; Emalex CC-16; Estol CEP 3694; Estol CEP-b 3653; Kemester® CP; Kessco® 653; Kessco CP; Nikkol N-SP; Precifac ATO; Radia® 7500; Rewowax CG; Starfol® CP; Trivent CP; Unimul-1616; Unitina CP; W.G.S. Cetyl Palmitate; Waxenol® 815; Waxenol® 816
Trade names containing: Cutina® BW; Cutina® CBS; Emulgade® CL Special; Emulgade® CL; Emulgade® SE; Hairwax 7686 o.E.; Lipocerite Standard; Unitina BW

Cetyl phosphate (INCI)
CAS 3539-43-3; EINECS 222-581-1
Trade names: Crodafos MCA

Cetyl PPG-2 isodeceth-7 carboxylate (INCI)
Synonyms: PEG-7-PPG-isodecyl ether carboxylic acid, cetyl ester; POE (7) POP (2) isodecyl ether carboxylic acid, cetyl ester
Trade names: Velsan® D8P-16

Cetylpyridinium chloride (INCI)
CAS 123-03-5; 6004-24-6; EINECS 204-593-9
Synonyms: 1-Hexadecylpyridinium chloride
Trade names: CPC; CPC Sumquat 6060; Uniquart CPC

Cetyl ricinoleate (INCI)
CAS 10401-55-5; EINECS 233-864-4
Synonyms: Hexadecyl 12-hydroxy-9-octadecenoate; 12-Hydroxy-9-octadecenoic acid ester
Trade names: Liponate CRM; Naturechem® CR; Pelemol CR; Protachem CER

Cetyl stearate (INCI)
CAS 1190-63-2; EINECS 214-724-1
Synonyms: n-Hexadecyl stearate
Trade names: Estol CES 3705
Trade names containing: Lipocerite Standard

Cetyl/stearyl. *See Cetearyl ...*

Cetyl/stearyl dimethyl benzyl ammonium bromide. *See Cetearalkonium bromide*

Cetyl trimethyl ammonium... *See Cetrimonium...*

Chamomile extract (INCI)
CAS 84649-86-5
Trade names: Unibotan Chamomile
Trade names containing: BBC Moisture Trol; BBC Relaxing Complex; Bio-Chelated Sauna-Derm I; Camofil 4064; Chamomile CL 2/033026; Chamomile Distillate 2/380930; Chamomile Extract HS 2779 G; Cremogen Chamomile 739012; Dragoplant Chamomile 2/034010; Glycolysat de camomille; Herbasol Complex A; Herbasol Complex B; Herbasol Complex E;

640

Herbasol Sedative Complex

Chamomile extract, German or Hungarian. *See Matricaria extract*

Chamomile oil (INCI)
CAS 8015-92-7
Synonyms: Anthemis nobilis oil; English chamomile oil; Roman chamomile oil
Trade names containing: Essentiaderm n.3

Chaparral extract (INCI)
CAS 84603-70-3
Synonyms: Creosote bush extract; Larrea divaricata extract; Larrea mexicana extract
Trade names containing: Actiphyte of Chaparral

Cherry pit oil (INCI)
CAS 8022-29-5
Synonyms: Cherry kernel oil
Trade names: Lipovol CP

China clay. *See Kaolin*

Chinese tea extract. *See Thea sinensis extract*

Chinese white. *See Zinc oxide*

Chitin (INCI)
CAS 1398-61-4; EINECS 215-744-3
Synonyms: Poly(N-acetyl-1,4-β-D-glucopyranosamine)
Trade names: Atomergic Chitin; Marine Dew
Trade names containing: Dermosaccharides® SEA

Chitosan (INCI)
CAS 9012-76-4
Trade names: Atomergic Chitosan
Trade names containing: Chitomarine

Chitosan lactate (INCI)
Trade names: Biocelose NC-50; Kytamer® L

Chitosan PCA (INCI)
Trade names: Kytamer® PC

Chlorhexidine digluconate (CTFA)
CAS 18472-51-0; 14007-07-9; EINECS 242-354-0
Synonyms: N,N´-Bis (4-chlorophenyl)-3,12-diimino-2,4,11,13-tetraazatetradecane-diimidamide compd. with D-gluconic acid; Chlorhexidine gluconate
Trade names: Spectradyne® G

1-(3-Chloroallyl)-3,5,7-triaza-1-azoniaadamantane chloride. *See Quaternium-15*

2-Chloro-1,4-benzenediamine sulfate. *See 2-Chloro-p-phenylenediamine sulfate*

4-Chloro-2-benzylphenol. *See Chlorophene*

Chlorobutanol (INCI)
CAS 57-15-8; EINECS 200-317-6
Synonyms: Trichloro-t-butyl alcohol; 1,1-Trichloro-2-methyl-2-propanol; Acetone chloroform
Trade names: Unisept Chlorbut

p-Chloro-m-cresol (INCI)
CAS 59-50-7; EINECS 200-431-6
Synonyms: PCMC; 4-Chloro-3-methyl phenol; Para-chlorometacresol
Trade names containing: Sebase

1-Chloro-1,1-difluoroethane. *See Hydrochlorofluoro-carbon 142B*

Chlorodifluoromethane. *See Hydrochlorofluorocarbon 22*

Chloroethene homopolymer. *See Polyvinyl chloride*

4-Chloro-3-methyl phenol. *See p-Chloro-m-cresol*

Chlorophene (INCI)
CAS 120-32-1; EINECS 204-385-8
Synonyms: 4-Chloro-2-benzylphenol; 5-Chloro-2-hy-

droxydiphenylmethane; Phenol, 4-chloro-2-benzyl-
Trade names: Preventol BP

2-Chloro-p-phenylenediamine sulfate (INCI)
CAS 6219-71-2; EINECS 228-291-1
Synonyms: 2-Chloro-1,4-benzenediamine sulfate
Trade names: Rodol Brown SO

Chlorophyllin-copper complex (INCI)
CAS 11006-34-1; EINECS 234-242-5
Synonyms: Potassium sodium copper chlorophyllin; Chlorophyllin, copper sodium complex; Copper sodium chlorophyllin
Trade names: Dascolor Chlorophyll; Uniphyllin SC
Trade names containing: Unispheres G-503

4-Chlororesorcinol (INCI)
CAS 95-88-5; EINECS 202-462-0
Synonyms: 1,3-Benzenediol, 4-chlor-; 4-Chloro-1,3-benzenediol
Trade names: Rodol CRS

Chloroxylenol (INCI)
CAS 88-04-0; EINECS 201-793-8
Synonyms: p-Chloro-m-xylenol; 4-Chloro-3,5-di-methylphenol; Parachlorometaxylenol
Trade names: Nipacide® MX; Nipacide® PX-R
Trade names containing: Emercide® 1199; Emericide 1199; Mikrokill 2; Phenosept

Chlorphenesin (INCI)
CAS 104-29-0; EINECS 203-192-6
Trade names: Elestab® CPN
Trade names containing: Anti-MB; Killitol

Cholecalciferol (INCI)
CAS 67-97-0; EINECS 200-673-2
Synonyms: 5,7-Cholestadien-3-β-ol; 7-Dehydro-cholesterol; Vitamin D_3
Trade names: Vitazyme® D
Trade names containing: Epiderm-Complex O; Vitamin A and D-3

5,7-Cholestadien-3-β-ol. *See Cholecalciferol*

Cholesterol (INCI)
CAS 57-88-5; EINECS 200-353-2
Synonyms: Cholest-5-en-3β-ol; Cholesteric esters
Trade names: Atomergic Cholesterol; Cholesterol BP; Cholesterol NF; Fancol CH; Liquid Crystal CN/9; Loralan-CH; Unichol
Trade names containing: AFR LS; Almolan LIS; Ceramides LS; Dermatein® GSL; Glycosome; Lanosoluble A; Lipocutin®; Lipodermol®; Lipomicron Vitamin A Palmitate; Lipomicron Vitamin E Acetate; Liposome Anti-Age LS; Liposomes Anti-Age LS; Liquid Crystal (LC) CAPS 122; Nikkol Aquasome LA; Nimlesterol® 1730; Presome Type I; Sphingoceryl® LS; Sphingoceryl® Powd. LS; Sphingoceryl® Wax LS 2958 B; Sphingosomes® AL

Cholesteryl/behenyl/octyldodecyl lauroyl glutamate (INCI)
Trade names: Eldew CL-301

Cholesteryl hydroxystearate (INCI)
CAS 40445-72-5
Trade names: Estemol CHS

Cholesteryl isostearate (INCI)
CAS 83615-24-1
Trade names: IS-CE

Cholesteryl stearate (INCI)
CAS 35602-69-8; EINECS 252-637-0
Synonyms: Cholest-5-en-3-ol, octadecanoate
Trade names: Nikkol CS

Choleth-5
CAS 27321-96-6 (generic)
Trade names: Emalex CS-5

Choleth-10 (INCI)
CAS 27321-96-6 (generic)
Trade names: Emalex CS-10

Choleth-15
CAS 27321-96-6 (generic)
Trade names: Emalex CS-15

Choleth-20 (INCI)
CAS 27321-96-6 (generic)
Trade names: Emalex CS-20

Choleth-24 (INCI)
CAS 27321-96-6 (generic)
Synonyms: PEG-24 cholesteryl ether
Trade names: Emalex CS-24; Ethoxychol-24; Fancol CH-24
Trade names containing: Forlan C-24; Ivarlan™ C-24; Solulan® C-24

Choleth-30
CAS 27321-96-6 (generic)
Trade names: Emalex CS-30

Choleth-20 trioctanoin
Trade names containing: Nikkol Aquasome EC-5

Chondroitin sulfate
CAS 9007-28-7
Synonyms: Chondroitin sulfuric acid
Trade names containing: Brookosome® CS; Cromoist CS

Chondrus. *See Carrageenan*

Chromium hydroxide
Synonyms: Chromium hydrate; Chromic hydroxide; Chromic hydrate
Trade names containing: Chrome Green 106; H Chrome Green 105

Chromium hydroxide green (INCI)
CAS 12001-99-9
Synonyms: Chromic oxide hydrated; Hydrated chromium sesquioxide
Trade names containing: Chroma-Lite® Aqua 4508

Chromium oxide greens (INCI)
CAS 1308-38-9; EINECS 215-160-9
Synonyms: Chromic oxide; Dichromium trioxide
Trade names containing: Colorona® Magestic Green; Gemtone® Emerald

Chromium oxide hydrated
Trade names: Cogilor Emerald

Chrysanthemum extract (INCI)
Synonyms: Chrysanthemum roseum extract
Trade names containing: Actiphyte of Chrysanthemum

Cinchona extract (INCI)
CAS 84929-25-9; 84776-28-3
Synonyms: Peruvian bark extract
Trade names containing: Auxina Tricogena

Cinene. *See Dipentene*

Cinnamon extract (INCI)
CAS 84649-98-9; EINECS 283-479-0
Synonyms: Cinnamomum cassia extract; Cinnamomum zeylanicum extract
Trade names containing: Actiphyte of Cinnamon

Cinnamon oil (INCI)
CAS 8007-80-5
Synonyms: Cassia oil; Cinnamomum cassia oil
Trade names containing: Fitoestesina

Citric acid (INCI)
CAS 77-92-9, 5949-29-1; EINECS 201-069-1
Synonyms: 2-Hydroxy-1,2,3-propanetricarboxylic acid; β-Hydroxytricarballylic acid
Trade names: Anhydrous Citric Acid; Citric Acid USP FCC (Anhyd.) Fine Gran. No. 69941; Citrid Acid USP Fine Granular No. 69941; Unichem CIT-A
Trade names containing: Nipanox® S-1; Nipanox® Special; Oxynex® 2004; Oxynex® K; Oxynex® L; Oxynex® LM; Stabolec C; Sustane® 3; Tenox® 2; Tenox® 20B; Tenox® 22; Tenox® 25; Tenox® 26; Tenox® 6; Uantox 20; Uantox 3; Uantox W-1

Citrulline (INCI)
CAS 372-75-8; EINECS 206-759-6
Synonyms: N~5-(Aminocarbonyl) ornithine
Trade names containing: Hydro-Diffuser Microreservoir

Citrus aurantium fruit extract. *See Bitter orange extract*

Citrus decumana extract. *See Grapefruit extract*

Citrus extract
Trade names containing: MFA™ Complex

Citrus limon extract. *See Lemon extract*

Citrus pectin. *See Pectin*

Citrus sinensis extract. *See Orange extract*

Clary oil (INCI)
CAS 8016-63-5
Trade names containing: Essentiaderm n.3; Essentiaderm n.4

Clove extract (INCI)
Synonyms: Eugenia caryophyllus extract
Trade names containing: Chouji Liq.

Clover blossom extract (INCI)
CAS 85085-25-2
Synonyms: Trifolium extract; Trifolium pratense extract
Trade names containing: BBC Mineral Complex

CMC. *See Carboxymethylcellulose sodium*

Cobalt acetylmethionate (INCI)
CAS 105883-52-1
Trade names: Exsycobalt; Exsymol Cobalt Acetyl-methionate

Cobalt gluconate
Trade names: Gluconal® CO

Cocamide DEA (INCI)
CAS 8051-30-7; 61791-31-9; 68603-42-9; EINECS 263-163-9
Synonyms: Coconut diethanolamide; Cocoyl diethanolamide; N,N-bis (2-hydroxyethyl) coco amides
Trade names: Ablumide CDE; Ablumide CDE-G; Ablumide CKD; Accomid C; Afmide™ C; Alkamide® 2204; Alkamide® CDE; Alkamide® CDM; Alkamide® CDO; Alkamide® CL63; Alkamide® DC-212/S; Alkamide® DC-212/SE; Alkamide® KD; Amidex CE; Amidex KD; Amidex KDO; Aminol COR-4C; Aminol HCA; Aminol KDE; Calamide C; Carsamide® CA; Carsamide® SAC; Chimipal DCL/M; Comperlan® COD; Comperlan® KD; Comperlan® KDO; Comperlan® PD; Comperlan® SD; Comperlan® SDO; Emalex N-83; Emid® 6515; Emid® 6521; Empilan® 2502; Empilan® CDE; Empilan® CDE/FF; Empilan® CDX; Esi-Det CDA; Esi-Terge 10; Esi-Terge S-10; Ethylan® LD; Ethylan® LDA-48; Ethylan® LDG; FMB 128 T; FMB BT; FMB Cocamide DEA; FMB Coco Condensate; Foamid C; Foamid SCE; Hartamide OD; Hetamide DSUC; Hetamide MC; Hetamide MCS; Hetamide RC; Hyamide 1:1; Incromide CA; Karamide 121; Karamide 363; Lauramide 11; Laur-

amide ME; Laurel SD-900M; Lauridit® KD; Lauridit® KDG; Loropan KD; Mackamide™ C; Mackamide™ CD; Mackamide™ CS; Mackamide™ MC; Manro CD; Manro CDS; Manro CDX; Manromid CD; Manromid CDG; Manromid CDS; Marlamid® D 1218; Marlamid® DF 1218; Mazamide® 68; Mazamide® 80; Mazamide® 524; Mazamide® 1281; Mazamide® CCO; Mazamide® CS 148; Mazamide® JT 128; Mazamide® WC Conc; Monamid® 705; Monamid® 759; Monamid® 1159; Monamid® C-305; Monamid® C-310; Monamine ADD-100; Naxonol™ CO; Naxonol™ PN 66; Naxonol™ PO; Ninol® 40-CO; Ninol® 49-CE; Ninol® GR; Norfox® DCS; Norfox® DCSA; Norfox® DOSA; Norfox® KD; Olamida CD; Oramide DL 200 AF; Profan 24 Extra, 128 Extra; Profan 2012E; Protamide CKD; Protamide DCA; Protamide DCAW; Protamide HCA; Purton CFD; Rewomid® DC 212 LS; Rewomid® DC 212 S; Rewomid® DC 212 SE; Rewomid® DC 220 SE; Ritamide C; Rolamid CD; Schercomid SCE; Schercomid SCO-Extra; Stamid HT 3901; Standamid® KD; Standamid® KDO; Standamid® PK-KD; Standamid® PK-KDO; Standamid® PK-KDS; Standamid® PK-SD; Standamid® SD; Standamid® SDO; Synotol CN 60; Synotol CN 80; Synotol CN 90; T-Tergamide 1CD; Tohol N-220; Tohol N-220X; Ufanon K-80; Ufanon KD-S; Unamide® C-72-3; Unamide® D-10; Unamide® LDL; Upamide CA-20; Upamide CS-148; Upamide KD; Varamide® A-10; Varamide® A-12; Varamide® A-2; Varamide® A-80; Varamide® A-83; Varamide® A-84; Varamide® MA-1; Witcamide® 128T; Witcamide® 6404; Witcamide® 6514; Witcamide® 6531; Witcamide® 6625; Witcamide® CD; Witcamide® CDA; Witcamide® GR; Witcamide® LDTS; Witcamide® M-3; Witcamide® S771; Witcamide® S780
Trade names containing: Active #4; Akyposal 2010 S; Alkamide® DC-212; Amide CD 2:1; Aminol COR-2C; Amisol™ 688; Base Nacrante 1100 AD; Base Nacrante 2078; Base Nacrante 9578; Bio-Soft® N-21; Calsuds CD-6; Carsofoam® DEV; Carsofoam® MSP; Carsofoam® SC; Comperlan® LS; Cosmopon BS; Emid® 6530; Emid® 6531; Emid® 6534; Empicol® 0627; Empicol® XC35; Equex AEM; Incromide CAC; Krim CH 25; Mackamide™ CDC; Mackamide™ CDS-80; Manro CD/G; Miracare® NWC; Monamine 779; Monamine AA-100; Monamine AC-100; Monamine CF-100 M; Monaterge 779; Norfox® DC; Orapol DL 210; Perlglanzmittel GM 4175; Rewomid® DL 240; Rewopol® SBV; Schercomid CCD; Schercomid CDA; Schercomid CDO-Extra; Standamid® PD; Standapol® AP Blend; Standapol® BW; Standapol® Conc. 7023; Standapol® DLC; Standapol® EA-K; Stepanol® AEG; Tego®-Pearl B-48; Texapon® IES; Texapon® WW 99; Ufablend MPL; Unipol Conc. 7023; Upamide PD; Witcamide® 5024; Witcamide® 5133; Witcamide® 6533; Witcamide® 6534; Witcamide® 6731; Witcamide® 6731; Witcamide® 82; Witcamide® Coco Condensate. See Witcamide CD; Witcamide® SR200; Zetesol 100

Cocamide MEA (INCI)
CAS 68140-00-1; EINECS 268-770-2
Synonyms: Coconut monoethanolamide; N-(2-hydroxy-ethyl) coco fatty acid amide; Coconut fatty acid monoethanolamide
Trade names: Ablumide CME; Afmide™ CMA; Alkamide® C-212; Alkamide® CME; Amidex CME; Amidex KME; Aminol CM, CM Flakes, CM-C Flakes;

CM-D Flakes; Carsamide® CMEA; Chimipal MC; Comperlan® 100; Comperlan® P 100; Emid® 6500; Empilan® CM/F; Empilan® CME; Foamole M; Hetamide CMA; Hetamide CME; Hetamide CME-CO; Incromide CME; Lauridit® KM; Loropan CME; Loropan KM; Mackamide™ CMA; Mackamide™ LM-Flake; Manro CMEA; Manromid CMEA; Marlamid® M 1218; Mazamide® CFAM; Mazamide® CMEA; Mazamide® CMEA Extra; Monamide; Monamid® CMA; Monamid® CMA-A; Monamid® CMA-A/F; Monamid® CMA-A/M; Monamid® CMA-S; Monamid® CMA-S/F; Monamid® CMA-S/M; Monamid® CMA/F; Monamid® CMA/M; Ninol® CNR; Nissan Stafoam MF; Olamida CM; Oramide ML 115; Phoenamid CMA, CMA-70; Profan AB20; Protamide CME; Rewomid® C 212; Schercomid CME; Standamid® KM; Standamid® SM; Synotol ME 90; Upamide SM; Varamide® C-212; Zoramide CM
Trade names containing: Cycloryl M1; Elfan® SG; Equex STM; Euperlan® MPK 850; Euperlan® PK 771 BENZ; Euperlan® PK 771; Euperlan® PK 776; Euperlan® PK 789; Euperlan® PK 810 AM; Euperlan® PK 810; Genapol® PGL; Genapol® PGM Conc; Genapol® PGM Liq.; Genapol® PGS; Marlamid® PG 20; Miracare® M1; Orvus K Liq.; Perlglanzmittel GM 4006; Perlglanzmittel GM 4175; Standapol® 7088; Standapol® Pearl Conc. 7130; Standapol® S; Stepanol® AEM; Tego®-Pearl B-48; Texapon® EVR; Texapon® SG; Zohar EGMS 771; Zoharpon EGDS-771

Cocamide MIPA (INCI)
CAS 68333-82-4, 68440-05-1; 8039-67-6; EINECS 269-793-0
Synonyms: Coconut monoisopropanolamide
Trade names: Amidex CIPA; Empilan® CIS; Rewomid® IPP 240; Witcamide® PPA

Cocamidopropylamine oxide (INCI)
CAS 68155-09-9; EINECS 268-938-5
Synonyms: Cocamidopropyl dimethylamine oxide; Coco amides, N-[3-(dimethylamino)propyl], N-oxide; N-[3-(Dimethylamino)propyl]coco amides-N-oxide
Trade names: Ablumox CAPO; Afamine™ CAO; Aminoxid WS 35; Ammonyx® CDO; Amyx CDO 3599; Barlox® C; Chemoxide CAW; Chimin CMO; Emcol® CDO; Empigen® OS/A; Empigen® OS/AU; Finamine CO; Foamox CDO; Incromine Oxide C; Incromine Oxide C-35; Mackamine™ CAO; Mazox® CAPA; Mazox® CAPA-37; Monalux CAO-35; Ninox® FCA; Rewominox B 204; Rhodamox® CAPO; Schercamox C-AA; Standamox CAW; Tegamine® Oxide WS-35; Unimox CAW; Varox® 1770; Zoramox
Trade names containing: Amisol™ 634; Anti-Dandruff Usnate AO

Cocamidopropyl betaine (INCI)
CAS 61789-40-0; 70851-07-9; 83138-08-3; 86438-79-1; EINECS 263-058-8; 274-923-4
Synonyms: CADG;; Cocamidopropyl dimethyl glycine
Trade names: Abluter CPB; Afaine™ 35; Afaine™ 35 HP; Amonyl 380 BA; Amonyl 440 NI; Ampholak BCA-30; Ampholan® D197; Ampholyt™ JB 130; Amphosol® CA; Amphosol® CG; Amphoteen BCA-30; Amphotensid B4; Chembetaine C; Chembetaine CGF; Chimin AX; Dehyton® K; Dehyton® PK; Emcol® 6748; Emcol® Coco Betaine; Emcol® DG; Emcol® NA-30; Emery® 6744; Emery® 6748; Empigen® BS; Empigen® BS/AU; Empigen® BS/H; Empigen® BS/P; Enagicol C-30B; FMB CAP B; Foamtaine CAB-G; Genagen CAB; Incronam 30; Lebon 2000; Lexaine® C; Lexaine® CG-30; Lexaine® CS; Lonzaine® C;

Lonzaine® CO; Lowenol C-11034; Mackam™ 35; Mackam™ 35 HP; Mackam™ J; Mackam™ L; Mafo® C; Mafo® CAB; Mafo® CAB 425; Mafo® CAB SP; Mafo® CFA 35; Manroteric CAB; Mirataine® BD-J; Mirataine® BD-R; Mirataine® BET-C-30; Mirataine® BET-W; Mirataine® CAB-A; Mirataine® CAB-O; Mirataine® CB; Mirataine® CB/M; Mirataine® CBC; Mirataine® CBR; Mirataine® CCB; Monateric CAB; Monateric CAB-LC; Monateric CAB-XLC; Monateric COAB; Monateric MCB; Nikkol AM-3130N; Nikkol AM-3130T; Norfox® Coco Betaine; Nutrol Betaine MD 3863; Proteric CAB; Rewoteric® AM B 13; Rewoteric® AM B 14; Rewoteric® AM B-13; Rewoteric® AM B-14; Rewoteric® AM B-14 LS; Rewoteric® AM B-15; Schercotaine CAB; Surfax ACR; Tego®-Betaine C; Tego®-Betaine F; Tego®-Betaine L-5351; Tego®-Betaine L-7; Unibetaine BA-35, BC-35; Unibetaine K; Varion® CADG-HS; Velvetex® BA-35; Velvetex® BK-35

Trade names containing: Base Nacrante 2078; Carsofoam® DEV; Carsofoam® MSP; Dermalcare® 1673; Euperlan® PK 3000 AM; Euperlan® PK 3000 OK; Euperlan® PK 3000 OK; Euperlan® PK 3000; Euperlan® PL 1000; Foamtaine CAB-A; Genapol® PGC; Lumorol K 28; Miracare® BC-10; Miracare® BC-20; Mirasheen® 202; Schercotaine CAB-A; Schercotaine CAB-K; Schercotaine CAB-Z; Standapol® AP Blend; Stepanol® AEG; Tego®-Betaine HS; Tego®-Pearl B-48; Tego®-Pearl S-33; Zetesol 856 T

Cocamidopropyl dimethylamine (INCI)
CAS 68140-01-2; EINECS 268-771-8
Synonyms: N-[3-Dimethylamino)propyl]coco amides
Trade names: Chemidex C; Chemidex WC; Lexamine C-13; Mackine™ 101; Schercodine C; Witcamine® 100
Trade names containing: Teginacid® R

Cocamidopropyl dimethylamine hydrolyzed collagen (INCI)
Synonyms: Cocamidopropyl dimethylamine hydrolyzed animal protein
Trade names: Mackpro™ CHP; Mackpro™ FC
Trade names containing: Mackpro™ FP

Cocamidopropyl dimethylamine lactate (INCI)
CAS 68425-42-3
Synonyms: N-[3-(Dimethylamino)propyl] cocamide lactate
Trade names: Mackalene™ 116

Cocamidopropyl dimethylamine propionate (INCI)
CAS 68425-43-4
Synonyms: N-[3-(Dimethylamino)propyl]coco amides, propionates
Trade names: Afalene™ 117; Foamid 117; Incromate CDP; Mackalene™ 117; Mackam™ CAP

Cocamidopropyl dimethylammonium C8-16 isoalkyl-succinyl lactoglobulin sulfonate (INCI)
Trade names: Monteine LCQ; Polymer SBOCP

N-[3-Cocamido)-propyl]-N,N-dimethyl betaine, potassium salt
Trade names: Schercotaine CAB-KG

Cocamidopropyl dimethyl glycine. *See Cocamidopropyl betaine*

Cocamidopropyldimonium hydroxypropyl hydrolyzed collagen (INCI)
Trade names: Quat-Coll™ CDMA-30QX

Cocamidopropyl ethyldimonium ethosulfate (INCI)
CAS 113492-03-8
Synonyms: 1-Propanaminium, 3-amino-N-ethyl-N,N-di-

methyl-, N-coco acyl derivs., ethyl sulfate; N-Cocoyl-(3-amidopropyl)-N,N-dimethyl-N-ethyl ammonium ethyl sulfate
Trade names: Foamquat CAS; Schercoquat CAS

Cocamidopropyl hydroxysultaine (INCI)
CAS 68139-30-0; 70851-08-0; EINECS 268-761-3
Synonyms: (3-Cocamidopropyl)(2-hydroxy-3-sulfopropyl) dimethyl quaternary ammonium compounds, hydroxides, inner salt
Trade names: Abluter CPS; Amonyl 675 SB; Chembetaine CAS; Crosultaine C-50; Lexaine® CSB-50; Lonzaine® CS; Lonzaine® JS; Mackam™ CBS-50; Mackam™ CBS-50G; Mafo® CSB; Mafo® CSB 50; Mafo® CSB W; Mafo® KCOSB 50; Mirataine® CBS, CBS Mod; Protachem JS; Rewoteric® AM CAS; Rewoteric® AM CAS; Rewoteric® AM CAS-15; Sandobet SC; Schercotaine SCAB; Zohartaine CBS
Trade names containing: Carsofoam® BS-I; Emulmetik™ 310; Foamtaine SCAB-K; Miracare® MS-1; Miracare® MS-2; Miracare® MS-4; Schercotaine SCAB-A; Schercotaine SCAB-KG; Varifoam® SXC

Cocamidopropyl lauryl ether (INCI)
Trade names: Marlamid® KL
Trade names containing: Marlamid® KLP; Perlglanzmittel GM 4006

Cocamidopropyl morpholine (INCI)
Trade names: Incromide CPM

Cocamidopropyl PG-dimonium chloride (INCI)
Synonyms: Cocamidopropyl dimethyl 2,3-dihydroxypropyl ammonium chloride
Trade names: Lexquat® AMG-WC

Cocamidopropyl PG-dimonium chloride phosphate (INCI)
Synonyms: Cocamidopropyl phosphatidyl PG-dimonium chloride
Trade names: Phospholipid PTC

Cocamine (INCI)
CAS 61788-46-3; EINECS 262-977-1
Synonyms: Coconut amine
Trade names: Adogen® 160D; Amine KKD; Armeen® C; Armeen® CD; Kemamine® P-650; Radiamine 6160; Radiamine 6161

Cocamine oxide (INCI)
CAS 61788-90-7, 70592-80-2; EINECS 263-016-9
Synonyms: Coco dimethylamine oxide; Coconut dimethylamine oxide; Dimethyl cocoalkylamine oxide
Trade names: Afamine™ CO; Aminoxid A 4080; Aromox® DMC; Aromox® DMC-W; Barlox® 12; Chemoxide WC; Empigen® OB/AU; Genaminox CS; Genaminox KC; Mackamine™ CO; Naxide™ 1230; Noxamine CA 30; Radiamox® 6800; Schercamox DMC; Synotol C-30
Trade names containing: Aromox® DMCD

Cocaminobutyric acid (INCI)
CAS 68649-05-8; EINECS 272-021-5
Synonyms: Butanoic acid, 3-amino-, N-coco alkyl derivatives; 3-Aminobutanoic acid, n-coco alkyl derivatives
Trade names: Armeen® Z

Cocaminopropionic acid (INCI)
CAS 84812-94-2, 1462-54-0; EINECS 284-219-9
Synonyms: N-coco-2-aminopropionic acid
Trade names: Afoteric™ 151C; Ampholyte KKE-70; Amphoram® CP1; Mackam™ 151C

Coceth-3 (INCI)
CAS 61791-13-7 (generic)

Synonyms: PEG-3 coconut ether; POE (3) cocoyl ether
Trade names containing: Phosal 12WD

Coceth-5 (INCI)
CAS 61791-13-7 (generic)
Synonyms: PEG-5 coconut alcohol; POE (5) coconut ether
Trade names: Genapol® C-050; Marlowet® CA 5

Coceth-8 (INCI)
CAS 61791-13-7 (generic)
Synonyms: PEG-8 coconut alcohol; POE (8) coconut ether; PEG 400 coconut ether
Trade names: Genapol® C-080
Trade names containing: Standapol® S

Coceth-10 (INCI)
CAS 61791-13-7 (generic)
Synonyms: PEG-10 coconut alcohol; POE (10) coconut ether; PEG 500 coconut ether
Trade names: Genapol® C-100; Marlowet® CA 10

Coceth-15
Trade names: Genapol® C-150

Coceth-20
Trade names: Genapol® C-200

Cocoa butter (INCI)
CAS 8002-31-1
Trade names: Atomergic Cocoa Butter; Fancol CB; Fancol CB Extra; Univeg CCB

Cocoalkonium chloride (INCI)
CAS 61789-71-7; EINECS 263-080-8
Synonyms: Coco dimonium chloride; Coco dimethyl benzyl ammonium chloride; Cocoalkyl dimethyl benzyl ammonium chloride
Trade names: Arquad® DNMCB-50; Marlazin® KC 21/50

Cocoamphoacetate. *See Sodium cocoamphoacetate*

Cocoamphocarboxyglycinate. *See Disodium cocoamphodiacetate*

Cocoamphocarboxypropionate. *See Disodium cocoamphodipropionate*

Cocoamphodiacetate. *See Disodium cocoamphodiacetate*

Cocoamphodipropionate. *See Disodium cocoamphodipropionate*

Cocoamphoglycinate. *See Sodium cocoamphoacetate*

Cocoamphohydroxypropylsulfonate. *See Sodium cocoamphohydroxypropyl sulfonate*

Cocoamphopolycarboxyglycinate
CAS 97659-53-5; EINECS 307-458-3
Trade names: Ampholak 7CX; Ampholak 7CX/C

Cocoamphopropionate. *See Sodium cocoamphopropionate*

Cocoamphopropylsulfonate. *See Sodium cocoamphohydroxypropyl sulfonate*

Cocobetainamido amphopropionate (INCI)
CAS 100085-64-1; EINECS 309-206-8
Trade names: Rewoteric® QAM 50

Coco-betaine (INCI)
CAS 68424-94-2, 85409-25-2; EINECS 270-329-4
Synonyms: Quat. ammonium compds., carboxymethyl (coco alkyl) dimethyl hydroxides, inner salts; Coconut betaine; Coco dimethyl glycine
Trade names: Amonyl 265 BA; Ampho B11-34; Ampholan® E210; Amphoteen BCM-30; Chembetaine CB; Dehyton® AB-30; Emcol® CC 37-18; Empigen® BB-AU; Incronam CD-30; Lonzaine® 12C; Mackam™ CB-35; Mafo® CB 40; Protachem

CB 45; Radiateric® 6860; Surfax ACB; Unibetaine AB-30, AB-45; Velvetex® AB-45
Trade names containing: Ampholysat Bois De Panama; Ampholysat Moelle

Coco caprylate/caprate (INCI)
Trade names: Cetiol® LC; Unimul-LC; Unitolate LC
Trade names containing: Copherol® 950LC

Cocodihydroxyethylamine oxide
Synonyms: Coco bis-2-hydroxyethylamine oxide
Trade names: Varox® 743

Coco dimethyl betaine. *See Coco betaine*

Cocodimonium hydroxyethyl cellulose
Synonyms: PG-hydroxyethylcellulose cocodimonium chloride
Trade names: Crodacel QM

Cocodimonium hydroxypropyl hydrolyzed collagen (INCI)
Synonyms: Cocodimonium hydroxypropyl hydrolyzed animal protein; Cocodimonium hydrolyzed collagen; Cocodimonium hydrolyzed animal protein
Trade names: Croquat M; Promois Milk CAQ; Promois W-42 CAQ; Quat-Coll™ CDMA 40

Cocodimonium hydroxypropyl hydrolyzed keratin (INCI)
CAS 68915-25-3
Synonyms: Cocodimonium hydrolyzed keratin; Cocodimonium hydroxypropyl hydrolyzed hair keratin
Trade names: Croquat HH; Croquat WKP; Kera-Quat WKP; Keraquat HK; Quat Keratin™ WKP

Cocodimonium hydroxypropyl hydrolyzed silk (INCI)
Trade names: Promois S-CAQ

Cocodimonium hydroxypropyl hydrolyzed soy protein (INCI)
CAS 977039-11-4, 100684-25-7
Trade names: Quat-Soy™ CDMA-25; Soy-Quat C; Wheat-Quat C

Cocodimonium hydroxypropyl hydrolyzed wheat protein (INCI)
Trade names: Hydrotriticum™ QM; Quat-Wheat™ CDMA-30

Cocodimonium hydroxypropyl silk amino acids (INCI)
Trade names: Crosilkquat

Coco-ethyldimonium ethosulfate (INCI)
CAS 68308-64-5; EINECS 269-662-8
Trade names: Dextrol AS-150

Cocoglycerides (INCI)
Synonyms: Glycerides, coconut, mono-, di-, and tri-
Trade names: Novata® 299, A, AB, B, BBC, BC, BCF, BD, C, D, E; Witarix® 250
Trade names containing: Cutina® CBS; DHA Microspheres

Coco hydrolyzed collagen. *See Cocoyl hydrolyzed collagen*

Cocohydroxyethyl PG-imidazolinium chloride phosphate
Trade names: Phospholipid P-TZ

Coco imidazoline betaine
Trade names: Empigen® CDR30
Trade names containing: Empigen® XDR121; Empigen® XDR123

Cocoiminodipropionate
CAS 97659-50-2; EINECS 307-455-7
Trade names: Ampholak YCE; Ampholan® U 203

Coco morpholine
Trade names: Armeen® N-CMD

Coconut acid (INCI)
CAS 61788-47-4; 67701-05-7, 68937-85-9; EINECS 262-978-7
Synonyms: Coco fatty acids; Coconut oils acids
Trade names: C-108; C-110; Emery® 621; Emery® 622; Emery® 626; Emery® 627; Emery® 629; Industrene® 325; Industrene® 328; Kartacid C 60; Kartacid C 70; Prifrac 5901, 7901; Radiacid® 631
Trade names containing: Emulgade® CL Special; Emulgade® CL; Geropon® AS-200; Geropon® AS-250; Hystrene® 1835; Prifrac 7948

Coconut alcohol (INCI)
CAS 68425-37-6; EINECS 270-351-4
Synonyms: Coconut fatty alcohol
Trade names: CO-618; Radianol® 1728

Coconut extract (INCI)
Synonyms: Cocos nucifera extract
Trade names containing: Actiphyte of Coconut; Extrapone Coco-Nut Special 2/033055

Coconut imidazoline betaine. *See Coco imidazoline betaine*

Coconut oil (INCI)
CAS 8001-31-8; EINECS 232-282-8
Synonyms: Copra oil
Trade names: Coconut Oils® 76, 92, 110; EmCon COCO; Lipovol C-76; Pureco® 76; Univegoil COCO
Trade names containing: Kalixide Grassa; Lipoplastidine Achillea; Lipoplastidine Aesculus; Lipoplastidine Aloe; Lipoplastidine Laminaria

Coconut oil soap
Trade names containing: Mackadet™ WGS

Coconut oil sucroglyceride
Trade names: Mirasoft™ LMO

Coco/oleamidopropyl betaine (CTFA)
CAS 86438-79-1
Trade names: Mirataine® COB

Coco-rapeseedate (INCI)
Trade names: Kester Wax® 59

Cocos nucifera extract. *See Coconut extract*

Cocotrimonium chloride (INCI)
CAS 61789-18-2; EINECS 263-038-9
Synonyms: Coconut trimethyl ammonium chloride; Cocoyl trimethyl ammonium chloride; Quaternary ammonium compds., coco alkyl trimethyl, chlorides
Trade names: Arquad® C-33W; Jet Quat C-50; Kemamine® Q-6503B; Marlazin® KC 30/50; Nikkol CA-2150; Noramium MC 50; Radiaquat® 6460
Trade names containing: Arquad® C-33; Arquad® C-50; Varisoft® 461

Cocoyl glutamic acid (INCI)
Trade names: Amisoft CA

Cocoyl hydrolyzed collagen (INCI)
CAS 68952-15-8
Synonyms: Acid chlorides, coco, reaction prods. with protein hydrolyzates; Coco-hydrolyzed animal protein; Cocoyl hydrolyzed animal protein
Trade names containing: Lanpro-1; Lanpro-2; Oleo-Coll™ LP; Oleo-Coll™ LP/LF; Proto-Lan 4R; Proto-Lan 8

Cocoyl hydrolyzed keratin (INCI)
Trade names containing: Proto-Lan KT

Cocoyl hydrolyzed soy protein (INCI)
Trade names: Oleo-Soy™ C

Cocoyl hydroxyethyl imidazoline (INCI)

CAS 61791-38-6; EINECS 263-170-7
Synonyms: 1H-Imidazole-1-ethanol, 4,5-dihydro-2-norcocoyl-; Cocoyl imidazoline; Coconut hydroxyethyl imidazoline
Trade names: Schercozoline C; Varine C

Cocoyl sarcosinate
Trade names containing: Incromide CAC

Cocoyl sarcosine (INCI)
CAS 68411-97-2; EINECS 270-156-4
Synonyms: N-Cocoyl-N-methyl glycine; N-methyl-N-(1-coconut alkyl) glycine
Trade names: Crodasinic C; Hamposyl® C; Hamposyl® CZ; Vanseal® CS
Trade names containing: Foam-Coll™ 5W; Relaxer Conc. No. 4

Cod liver oil (INCI)
CAS 8001-69-2; EINECS 232-289-6
Synonyms: Oils, cod liver; Morrhua oil
Trade names: Atomergic Cod Liver Oil; EmCon COD

Coffee bean extract (INCI)
CAS 8001-67-0; 84650-00-0; EINECS 283-481-1
Trade names containing: Complex Relax

Coffee extract (INCI)
CAS 84650-00-0; EINECS 283-481-1
Trade names: CMI 321; CMI 324; CMI 400
Trade names containing: CMI 551

Collagen (INCI)
CAS 9007-34-5; EINECS 232-697-4
Synonyms: Collagen fiber; Ossein; Soluble animal collagen
Trade names: Collagen Masks; Collagen Powd; Collagen S.D; Collagene Lyophilized; Lencoll; Polymoist® Mask; Unipro CLR
Trade names containing: Cosiderm Collagen Masks; Cosiderm Masks; Liposome Anti-Age LS; Liposomes Anti-Age LS; Tri-K CMF Complex

Collagen amino acids (INCI)
CAS 9015-54-7
Synonyms: Animal collagen amino acids
Trade names: Amino-Collagen-25, -40; Collagen Amino Acids SF; Collamino™ 25; Collamino™ 40-SF; Crotein CAA/SF; Hycollan; Peptein® CAA
Trade names containing: Aqua-Tein C; Aquaderm; ATP Nucleotides; Collamino™ Complex ESC; Collamino™ Complex L/O; Collamino™ Complex S; Collamino™ Complex; Quinta-Pro Conc; Solu-Coll™ Complex

Collagen hydrolysates. *See Hydrolyzed collagen*

Colloidal sulfur (INCI)
Trade names: Sulcoidal
Trade names containing: Extrapone Neo-H-Special 2/032441

Colophony. *See Rosin*

Colostrum (INCI)
Trade names: Colostrum Clar 101

Colostrum cream (INCI)
Trade names: Clar 120

Colostrum whey (INCI)
Trade names: Clar 142

Coltsfoot extract (INCI)
CAS 84625-50-3
Synonyms: Tussilago farfara extract
Trade names containing: Auxina Tricogena; Cremogen AF; Extrapone Poly H Special 2/032451; Hair Complex Aquosum; Herbalcomplex 1 Special; Herbasol 7

Herb Complex

Comfrey extract (INCI)
CAS 84696-05-9
Trade names containing: Actiphyte of Comfrey; Actiplex™ 745; BBC Moisture Trol; Bio-Chelated Derma-Plex I; Bio-Chelated Sauna-Derm I; GU-61-A; Gu-61-Standard

Common salt. *See Sodium chloride*

Coneflower extract (INCI)
CAS 84696-11-7; 90028-20-9
Synonyms: Echinacea pallida extract; Echinacea purpurea extract; Echinacea root extract
Trade names containing: Unibotan Vitaplant W CLR; Vitaplant CLR Water-Soluble

Connective tissue extract (INCI)
Trade names: Extracellular Matrix CLR

Copper acetylmethionate (INCI)
CAS 105883-51-0
Trade names: Exsycuivre; Exsymol Cupric Acetyl-methionate

Copper acetyl tyrosinate methylsilanol (INCI)
Trade names: Tyrosilane C

Copper gluconate (INCI)
CAS 527-09-3; EINECS 208-408-2
Synonyms: Bis(D-gluconato) copper; Copper, bis(D-gluconato)-
Trade names: Gluconal® CU

Copper glycoproteins
Trade names containing: Brookosome® CU

Copper PCA (INCI)
Trade names: Cuivridone®

Copper PCA methylsilanol (INCI)
Trade names: Silhydrate C

Copra oil. *See Coconut oil*

Coriander extract (INCI)
CAS 84775-50-8
Synonyms: Coriandrum sativum extract
Trade names containing: Actiphyte of Coriander

Coriander oil (INCI)
CAS 8008-52-4
Trade names containing: Essentiaderm n.4; Essentiaderm n.6; Essentiaderm n.8

Corn cob meal (INCI)
Trade names: Beeswing 1/16; Beeswing 3/16; Beeswing 3/32; Cob Flour #4, 6, 100; Cob Grit #1, 2, 3, 8, 150, 3050; Grit-O'Cobs®

Corn cob powd. (INCI)
Trade names: CR Grit

Corn germ extract (INCI)
Synonyms: Zea mays germ extract
Trade names containing: Plant Ceramides

Corn gluten amino acids (INCI)
CAS 65072-01-7
Synonyms: Maize gluten amino acids
Trade names containing: Amino Gluten MG

Corn gluten protein (INCI)
CAS 66071-96-3; 9010-66-6
Trade names containing: Press-Aid™ XF; Press-Aid™

Corn oil (INCI)
CAS 8001-30-7; EINECS 232-281-2
Synonyms: Maize oil; Oils, corn; Zea mays oil
Trade names: Corn Oil, Refined; Lipex 104; Nikkol Corn Germ Oil; Super Refined™ Corn Oil; Univegoil CRN

Trade names containing: Complexe AV.h.; Eglantineol; Microsponge® 5650; Tenox® 25; Tenox® 26; Tenox® 4; Tenox® 4B; Tenox® 6; Tensami 8/09; Uantox HW-4; Uantox W-1

Corn oil PEG-6 esters (INCI)
CAS 85536-08-9; 9004-96-0
Synonyms: Corn oil PEG-6 complex
Trade names: Labrafil® M 2125 CS

Corn oil PEG-8 esters (INCI)
Trade names: Labrafil® WL 2609 BS

Corn oil unsaponifiables (INCI)
Trade names: ETIZM
Trade names containing: Destressine 2000; Liposome Unsapo KM

Corn silk extract (INCI)
Synonyms: Zea mays extract; Stigmata maydis extract
Trade names containing: Actiphyte of Cornsilk; Corn Silk Extract HS 2969 G

Corn starch (INCI)
CAS 9005-25-8; EINECS 232-679-6
Synonyms: Starch, corn
Trade names: Argo Brand Corn Starch; Pure-Dent® B700; Pure-Dent® B810; Purity® 21; 28-1801; Univeg CS
Trade names containing: Zetesap 5165; Zetesap 813A

Corn sugar. *See Glucose*

Corn sugar gum. *See Xanthan gum*

Corn syrup solids
CAS 68131-37-3
Trade names: Maltrin® M200; Maltrin® M250; Maltrin® M365; Maltrin® QD M600

Cotton fiber. *See Cellulose*

Cottonseed glyceride (INCI)
CAS 8029-44-5; EINECS 232-438-5
Synonyms: Cottonseed oil monoglyceride; Glyceryl mono cottonseed oil; Glycerides, cottonseed oil, mono-
Trade names: Myvatex® 7-85; Myverol® 18-85

Cottonseed oil (INCI)
CAS 8001-29-4; EINECS 232-280-7
Trade names: EmCon Cotton; Super Refined™ Cotton-seed Oil; Univegoil COTSD

Cranesbill extract (INCI)
CAS 84650-10-2
Synonyms: Wild geranium extract; Geranium maculatum extract
Trade names containing: Bio-Chelated Derma-Plex I

Creatine. *See Creatinine*

Creatinine (INCI)
Trade names containing: Unimoist U-125

Creosote bush extract. *See Chaparral extract*

Crospovidone
Trade names: Kollidon® CL

Crystallins (INCI)
Trade names containing: Crystallin Protein

Cucumber extract (INCI)
CAS 89998-01-6
Synonyms: Cucumis sativus extract
Trade names containing: Nutriderme HS 210; Uninontan U 34

Cyanocobalamin (INCI)
CAS 68-19-9; EINECS 200-680-0
Synonyms: Vitamin B$_{12}$; Cyanocon(III)alamin; α-(5,6-

Dimethylbenzimidazolyl)cyanocobamide
Trade names: Cyanocobalamin USP (Cryst.)

Cyclamen aldehyde (INCI)
CAS 103-95-7; EINECS 203-161-7
Trade names: Cyclosal

Cycloamylose. *See Cyclodextrin*

Cyclocarboxypropyloleic acid (INCI)
CAS 53980-88-4; EINECS 258-987-1
Trade names: Diacid 1550

Cyclodextrin (INCI)
CAS 7585-39-9; EINECS 231-493-2
Synonyms: Cycloamylose; β-Cycloamylose; Cyclomaltoheptaose
Trade names: Alpha W 6 Pharma Grade; Beta W 7; Cavitron Cyclo-dextrin.™; Dexpearl; Gamma W8; Kleptose; Rhodocap-A, G, N; Ringdex-A, B

Cyclomaltoheptaose. *See Cyclodextrin*

Cyclomethicone (INCI)
CAS 69430-24-6
Synonyms: Cyclic dimethylsiloxane; Cyclic dimethyl polysiloxane with n= 3–6
Trade names: Abil® B 8839; Abil® K 4; Amersil® VS-7158; Amersil® VS-7207; Amersil® VS-7349; Baysilone COM 10,000; Baysilone COM 20,000; Belsil CM 020; Belsil CM 025; Belsil CM 030; Belsil CM 040; Dow Corning® 244 Fluid; Dow Corning® 245 Fluid; Dow Corning® 344 Fluid; Dow Corning® 345 Fluid; KF994; KF9945; Masil® SF-V (4); Masil® SF-V (5); Masil® SF-VL; Masil® SF-VV; Masil® SFV; Rhodorsil® Oils 70045; Rhodorsil® Oils 70045 V2, 70045 V3, 70045 V5; SF1173; SF1202; SF1204; Silatex SF-V; SWS-03314; Unisil SF-V; Volatile Silicone 7158, 7207, 7349
Trade names containing: Abil® OSW 12, OSW 13; Abil® OSW 15; Amersil® ME-358; Arlamol® S3, S7; Belsil CM 1000; Bentone® Gel VS-5 PC; Bentone® Gel VS-5; Dow Corning® 1401 Fluid; Dow Corning® 3225C Formulation Aid; Fancorsil A; Gilugel SIL5; Polytrap® 6035; Polytrap® Q5-6035; Rhodorsil® Oils 71631; Rhodorsil® Oils 71634; Tixogel VSP; Tri-Sil HGC 5000

Cyclopentane carboxylic acid (INCI)
CAS 3400-45-1; EINECS 222-269-5
Trade names: Nikkol Naphthenic Acid

o-Cymen-5-ol (INCI)
CAS 3228-02-2; EINECS 221-761-7
Trade names: Biosol

Cypress extract (INCI)
CAS 84696-07-1
Trade names containing: Circulatory Blend HS 318; Tonique HS 290; Tonique LS 690

Cypress oil (INCI)
CAS 8013-86-3
Trade names containing: Essentiaderm n.3; Essentiaderm n.4

L-Cysteine (INCI)
CAS 52-90-4; EINECS 200-158-2
Synonyms: (+)-2-Amino-3-mercaptopropionic acid; α-Amino-β-thiolpropionic acid
Trade names: Unamino L-CSTE
Trade names containing: Hair Complex 20/70n

Cystine (INCI)
CAS 56-89-3; EINECS 200-296-3
Synonyms: Di(α-amino-β-thiolpropionic acid); β,β'-Dithiobisalanine
Trade names: Unamino L-CSTI

Cytosol extract
Trade names: Plantsol

Dandelion extract (INCI)
CAS 84775-55-3
Synonyms: Taraxacum extract; Taraxacum officinale extract
Trade names containing: Dandelion HS

Daucus carota sativa extract. *See Carrot extract*

DBPC. *See BHT*

D&C Red No. 7 calcium lake (INCI)
Trade names containing: Red 119

D&C Red No. 30 (INCI)
CAS 2379-74-0; EINECS 219-163-6
Trade names containing: Florabeads Micro 28/60 Gypsy Rose

D&C Red No. 30 aluminum lake
Trade names containing: Red 150

D&C Red No. 36 (INCI)
CAS 2814-77-9; EINECS 220-562-2
Trade names containing: Red 219

D&C Yellow No. 5 aluminum lake (INCI)
Trade names containing: Yellow 134

DDBSA. *See Dodecylbenzene sulfonic acid*

DDDM. *See Dichlorophene*

DEA. *See Diethanolamine*

DEA-ceteareth-2 phosphate (INCI)
Trade names: Crodafos CS2N

DEA-cetyl phosphate (INCI)
CAS 61693-41-2
Synonyms: Cetyl DEA phosphate; Bis(2-hydroxyethyl)-ammonium hexadecylphosphate
Trade names: Amphisol®; Brophos™ A
Trade names containing: Monacet; Monamilk

DEA-cocaminopropionate
Trade names containing: Cycloryl XL-M (see Miracare XL)

DEA-coconate
Trade names containing: Mackamide™ CDC

DEA-dodecylbenzene sulfonate (INCI)
CAS 26545-53-9; EINECS 247-784-2
Synonyms: Benzenesulfonic acid, dodecyl-, compd. with 2,2'-iminobis [ethanol] (1:1)
Trade names: Ablusol DBD
Trade names containing: Active #4; Mackamide™ CDS-80

DEA-hydrolyzed lecithin (INCI)
Trade names: Nidaba 318

DEA-lauraminopropionate (INCI)
CAS 65104-36-1; EINECS 265-417-4
Synonyms: β-Alanine, N-dodecyl-, compd. with 2,2'-iminobis [ethanol]
Trade names containing: Carsonol® BDM; Miracare® XL; Standapol® AA-1; Stepanol® LX

DEA-laureth sulfate (INCI)
CAS 58855-36-0; 55353-19-0; 54351-50-7; 81859-24-7
Synonyms: Diethanolamine laureth sulfate
Trade names containing: Monamine 779; Monaterge 779; Standapol® DLC

DEA-lauryl sulfate (INCI)
CAS 143-00-0, 68585-44-4; EINECS 205-577-4
Synonyms: Sulfuric acid, monododecyl ester, compd.

with 2,2´-iminodiethanol (1:1); Diethanolamine lauryl sulfate
Trade names: Carsonol® DLS; Empicol® 0031/T; Empicol® DA; Nutrapon DE 3796; Standapol® DEA; Stepanol® DEA; Sulfochem DLS; Supralate EP; Texapon® DEA; Unipol DEA; Witcolate™ DLS-35; Zoharpon LAD
Trade names containing: Carsofoam® SC; Carsonol® BDM; Miracare® XL; Standapol® AA-1; Standapol® Conc. 7021; Stepanol® LX; Unipol Conc. 7021; Witcamide® 6731; Witcamide® 6731

DEA-myreth sulfate (INCI)
Synonyms: PEG (1-4) myristyl ether sulfate, diethanolamine salt
Trade names containing: Standapol® Conc. 7023; Unipol Conc. 7023

DEA oleate
Trade names containing: Mackamide™ ODM

DEA-oleth-3 phosphate (INCI)
CAS 58855-63-3
Synonyms: Diethanolamine oleth-3 phosphate; Diethanolammonium POE (3) oleyl ether phosphate
Trade names: Brophos™ OL-3N; Chemphos TR-515D; Crodafos N-3 Neutral; Lanafos-N3; Mayphos OL 3N
Trade names containing: Brophos™ OL-3NPG

DEA-oleth-5 phosphate (INCI)
Trade names: Crodafos N5N

DEA-oleth-10 phosphate (INCI)
CAS 58855-63-3
Synonyms: Diethanolamine oleth-10 phosphate; Diethanolammonium POE (10) oletyl ether phosphate
Trade names: Chemphos TR-505D; Crodafos N-10 Neutral; Lanafos-N10

DEA-oleth-20 phosphate (INCI)
Trade names: Crodafos N20A

DEA-styrene/acrylates/DVB copolymer (INCI)
Synonyms: DEA-styrene/acrylates/divinylbenzene copolymer
Trade names containing: Lytron 284; Lytron 288

n-Decanoic acid. *See Capric acid*

1-Decanol. *See n-Decyl alcohol*

Decene-1
CAS 872-05-9
Synonyms: Linear C10 alpha olefin; Decylene
Trade names: Ethyl Decene-1; Gulftene® 10

Deceth-4 (INCI)
CAS 26183-52-8 (generic), 5703-94-6
Synonyms: PEG-4 decyl ether; PEG 200 decyl ether; POE (4) decyl ether
Trade names: Marlipal® 1012/4

n-Decyl alcohol (INCI)
CAS 112-30-1; 68526-85-2; EINECS 203-956-9
Synonyms: Alcohol C-10; Noncarbinol; 1-Decanol
Trade names: Nacol® 10-97; Cachalot® DE-10; Nacol® 10-99

Decylamine oxide (INCI)
CAS 2605-79-0; EINECS 220-020-5
Synonyms: Capric dimethyl amine oxide; Decyl dimethyl amine oxide
Trade names: Barlox® 10S

Decyl dimethyl octyl ammonium chloride. *See Quaternium-24*

Decyl dodecanol
Trade names: Isofol® 24

Decyl glucoside (INCI)
CAS 54549-25-6; EINECS 259-218-1
Trade names: Oramix NS 10

Decyl oleate (INCI)
CAS 3687-46-5; EINECS 222-981-6
Synonyms: Decyl 9-octadecenoate
Trade names: Ceraphyl® 140; Cetiol® V; Crodamol DO; Elfacos® DO; Estalan DO; Estol DCO 3662; Estol DCO-b 3655; Kessco DO; Schercemol DO; Tegosoft® DO; Trivent OL-10; Unimul-CTV; Unitolate V
Trade names containing: Dehymuls® K; Unibiovit B-33

Decyl polyglucose (INCI)
CAS 141464-42-8
Trade names: APG® 300 CS; APG® 325 CS; APG® 350 Glycoside; Plantaren® 2000; Plantaren® 2000 CS/ UP; Plantaren® 2000 UP
Trade names containing: Plantaren™ PS-300; Plantaren® PS-100; Uniplant PS-100

DEET. *See Diethyl toluamide*

DEG. *See Diethylene glycol..., PEG-2...*

Dehydroacetic acid (INCI)
CAS 520-45-6; 771-03-9; EINECS 208-293-9, 212-227-4
Synonyms: DHA; 3-Acetyl-6-methyl-2H-pyran-2,4(3H)-dione, ion(1-),; 2H-Pyran-2,4(3H)-dione, 3-acetyl-6-methyl-; 3-Acetyl-4-hydroxy-6-methyl-2-pyrone
Trade names: Unisept DHA
Trade names containing: Dragocid Forte 2/027045; Euxyl K 702

Denatonium benzoate NF (INCI)
CAS 3734-33-6; EINECS 223-095-2
Synonyms: N-[2-[((2,6-Dimethylphenyl)amino]-2-oxoethyl]-N,N-diethylbenzenemathanaminium benzoate; Benzyldiethyl [(2,6-xylylcarbomoyl)methyl]ammonium benzoate; Lignocaine benzyl benzoate
Trade names: Atomergic Denatonium Benzoate; Bitrex

Denatonium saccharide (INCI)
Trade names: Atomergic Denatonium Saccharide

Deoxyribonucleic acid. *See DNA*

DEP. *See Diethyl phthalate*

Desamido collagen (INCI)
CAS 9007-34-5
Synonyms: Desamido animal collagen
Trade names: Collapuron® DAK; Solu-Coll™ D

DET. *See Diethyl toluamide*

Dexpanthenol. *See Panthenol*

Dextran sulfate (INCI)
CAS 9042-14-2
Synonyms: Sodium dextran sulfate
Trade names containing: BioCare® SA

Dextrin (INCI)
CAS 9004-53-9; EINECS 232-675-4
Synonyms: Dextrine; Starch gum
Trade names: Nadex 360
Trade names containing: Hygroplex HHG

Dextrin palmitate (INCI)
CAS 83271-10-7
Trade names: Rheopearl KL

Dextrose. *See Glucose*

DHA. *See Dehydroacetic acid, Dihydroxyacetone*

2,4-Diaminophenoxyethanol HCl (INCI)
CAS 66422-95-5; EINECS 266-357-1
Trade names: Imexine OAJ

2,6-Diaminopyridine (INCI)
CAS 141-86-6; EINECS 205-507-2
Synonyms: 2,6-Pyridinediamine
Trade names: Rodol 26PYR

Diammonium dimethicone copolyol sulfosuccinate (INCI)
Synonyms: Sulfobutanedioic acid, dimethicone copolyol ester, diammonium salt
Trade names: Mackanate™ DC-30A

Diammonium EDTA (INCI)
CAS 20824-56-0; EINECS 244-063-4
Synonyms: Diammonium edetate; Diammonium ethylene diamine tetraacetate
Trade names: Versene Diammonium EDTA

Diammonium lauryl sulfosuccinate (INCI)
Synonyms: Butanedioic acid, sulfo-, 1-dodecyl ester, diammonium salt; Sulfobutanedioic acid, 1-dodecyl ester, diammonium salt
Trade names: Mackanate™ LA

Diatomaceous earth (INCI)
CAS 7631-86-9; EINECS 231-545-4
Synonyms: Kieselguhr; Diatomite; Infusorial earth
Trade names: Celite® 503; Celite® 512; Celite® 521 AW; Celite® 545; Celite® 550; Celite® 560; Celite® 577; Filter-Cel; Hyflo Super-Cel; Standard Super-Cel; Super Floss
Trade names containing: Masque Poudre No. 2

Diatomite. *See Diatomaceous earth*

Diazolidinyl urea (INCI)
CAS 78491-02-8; EINECS 278-928-2
Synonyms: N-[1,3-Bis(hydroxymethyl)-2,5-dioxo-4-imidazolidinyl]-
Trade names: Germall® II
Trade names containing: Germaben® II-E; Germaben® II

Dibehenyl/diarachidyl dimonium chloride (INCI)
Trade names: Kemamine® Q-1902C; Kemamine® Q-1902X

Dibehenyldimonium methosulfate (INCI)
Trade names: Incroquat DBM-90

Dibehenyl methylamine (INCI)
CAS 61372-91-6; EINECS 262-740-2
Synonyms: N-Docosyl-N-methyl-1-docosamine; Methyl dibehenylamine
Trade names: Kemamine® T-2801

Dibenzylidene sorbitol (INCI)
CAS 32647-67-9; EINECS 251-136-4
Synonyms: Sorbitol acetal; Bis-o-(phenylmethylene)-D-glucitol; D-Glucitol, bis-o-(phenylmethylene)-
Trade names: Disorbene; Millithix® 925

Dibutyl adipate (INCI)
CAS 105-99-7; EINECS 203-350-4
Synonyms: Hexanedioic acid, dibutyl ester
Trade names: Cetiol® B; Unitolate B; Upamate DBA

Dibutyl lauroyl glutamide (INCI)
CAS 63663-21-8; EINECS 264-391-1
Trade names: Gelling Agent GP-1

Dibutyl phthalate (INCI)
CAS 84-74-2; EINECS 201-557-4
Synonyms: 1,2-Benzenedicarboxylic acid, dibutyl ester; Dibutyl-1,2-benzene dicarboxylate; Butyl phthalate
Trade names: Kodaflex® DBP; Uniflex DBP; Uniplex 150
Trade names containing: Blanc Covachip W 9705; Bleu Covachip W 6700

1,2-Dicaproyl-sn-glycero(3) phosphatidylcholine
CAS 3436-44-0

Trade names: Phospholipon® CC

Dicapryl adipate (INCI)
CAS 105-97-5; EINECS 203-349-9
Synonyms: Didecyl hexanedioate; Hexanedioic acid, didecyl ester
Trade names: Hodag DCA; Kessco® DCA

Dicapryloyl cystine (INCI)
CAS 41760-23-0; EINECS 255-537-5
Synonyms: N,N′-Bis(1-oxooctyl)-L-cystine
Trade names: Lipacide C8CY

Diceteareth-10 phosphate (INCI)
Trade names: Marlophor® T10-Acid

Dicetyl dilinoleate
Trade names: Liquiwax™ DC-EFA/SS

Dicetyl dimonium chloride (INCI)
CAS 1812-53-9, 68391-05-9; EINECS 217-325-0
Synonyms: Quaternium-31; N-Hexadecyl-N,N-dimethyl-1-hexadecanaminium chloride; Dicetyl dimethyl ammonium chloride
Trade names: Carsoquat® 868; Carsoquat® 868-E; Carsoquat® 868P; Varisoft® 432-100
Trade names containing: Carsoquat® CB; Varisoft® 432-CG; Varisoft® 432-ET; Varisoft® 432-PPG; Varisoft® CRC

Dicetyl phosphate (INCI)
CAS 2197-63-9, 3539-43-3; EINECS 222-581-1
Synonyms: 1-Hexadecanol, hydrogen phosphate; Phosphoric acid, dihexadecyl ester; Dihexadecyl phosphate
Trade names containing: Lipocutin®

Dichlorobenzyl alcohol (INCI)
CAS 1777-82-8; EINECS 217-210-5
Synonyms: 2,4-Dichlorobenzenemethanol
Trade names: Lexgard® Myacide SP; Midtect TF-60; Myacide® SP; Unikon A-22
Trade names containing: Midtect TFP; Unisuprol S-25

Dichlorophene (INCI)
CAS 97-23-4; EINECS 202-567-1
Synonyms: DDDM; 2,2′-Dihydroxy-5,5′-dichlorodiphenylmethane; Di-(5-chloro-2-hydroxyphenyl) methane; 2,2′-Methylenebis(4-chlorophenol)
Trade names: Preventol GD

Dichlorophenyl imidazoldioxolan (INCI)
CAS 85058-43-1
Trade names: Elubiol

Dicocamine (INCI)
CAS 61789-76-2; EINECS 263-086-0
Synonyms: Dicoco alkyl amine; Amines, dicoco alkyl
Trade names: Armeen® 2C

Dicocodimethylamine dimerate
Trade names: Armocare® E/C 151

Dicocodimonium chloride (INCI)
CAS 61789-77-3; EINECS 263-087-6
Synonyms: Dicoco dimethyl ammonium chloride; Quaternium-34
Trade names: Dodigen 1490; Jet Quat 2C-75; Noramium M2C; Radiaquat® 6462
Trade names containing: Arquad® 2C-75; Arquad® S-2C-50; Arquad® T-2C-50; Variquat® K300; Variquat® K300; Variquat® K375; Variquat® K375; Varisoft® 462

Dicoco methylamine
CAS 61788-62-3
Synonyms: Dicocoalkyl methylamine
Trade names: Armeen® M2C; Jet Amine M2C

Dicocoyl pentaerythrityl distearyl citrate (INCI)
Trade names: Dehymuls® FCE
Trade names containing: Dehymuls® E; Dehymuls® F; Dehymuls® K; Dehymuls® LS

DIDA. *See Diisodecyl adipate*

Didecene (INCI)
Trade names: Ethylflo® 362 NF

Didecylamine
CAS 1120-49-6
Trade names: Armeen® 2-10

Didecyl dimethylamine oxide
CAS 100545-50-4
Trade names: Damox® 1010

Didecyldimonium chloride (INCI)
CAS 7173-51-5; EINECS 230-525-2
Synonyms: Didecyl dimethyl ammonium chloride; N-Decyl-N,N-dimethyl-1-decanaminium chloride; Dimethyl didecyl ammonium chloride
Trade names: Bardac® 2250; BTC® 1010; Maquat 4450-E
Trade names containing: Bardac® 2050

Didecyl methylamine
CAS 7396-58-9; EINECS 230-990-1
Synonyms: Methyl decyl-1-amino decane
Trade names: Armeen® M2-10D

Diethanolamine (INCI)
CAS 111-42-2; EINECS 203-868-0
Synonyms: DEA; 2,2′-Iminobisethanol; Di(2-hydroxyethyl) amine; 2,2′-Iminodiethanol
Trade names: DEA Commercial Grade; DEA Low Freeze Grade; Unichem DEA
Trade names containing: Alkamide® DC-212; Alkamide® DO-280; Amide CD 2:1; Aminol COR-2C; Emid® 6530; Emid® 6531; Emid® 6534; Emid® 6541; Empilan® LDX; Foamid 24; Hetamide DO; Lytron 288; Monamine AA-100; Monamine ACO-100; Monamine ADY-100; Monamine C-100; Monamine CF-100 M; Naetex O-20; Norfox® DC; Orapol DL 210; Protamide N-1918; Protamide OFO; Protamide T; Rewocid® DU 185; Rewomid® DL 203 S; Rewomid® DL 203; Rewomid® DL 240; Rewomid® DO 280; Rewomid® F; Schercomid 1214; Schercomid CCD; Schercomid CDA; Schercomid CDO-Extra; Schercomid LD; Schercomid ODA; Schercomid TO-2; Standamid® CD; Standamid® PD; TEA 85; Upamide CD; Upamide PD; Upamide SS-10; Witcamide® 5024; Witcamide® 5133; Witcamide® 6533; Witcamide® 6534; Witcamide® 6544; Witcamide® 6546; Witcamide® 82; Witcamide CD; Witcamide® SR200

Diethanolaminooleamide DEA (INCI)
Trade names: Witcamide® 5168

Diethylaminoethyl PEG-5 coccoate (INCI)
Trade names: Chimexane CA

Diethylaminoethyl stearate (INCI)
CAS 3179-81-5; EINECS 221-662-9
Synonyms: 2-(Diethylamino) ethyl octadecanoate; Octadecanoic acid, 2-(diethylamino) ethyl ester
Trade names: Cerasynt® 303

N,N-Diethyl-m-aminophenol (INCI)
CAS 91-68-9; EINECS 202-090-9
Synonyms: 3-(Diethylamino) phenol
Trade names: Rodol DEMAP

N,N-Diethyl-m-aminophenol sulfate (INCI)
CAS 68239-84-9; EINECS 269-478-8
Synonyms: 3-(Diethylamino) phenol sulfate

Trade names: Rodol DEMAPS

Diethyl aspartate (INCI)
CAS 43101-48-0; EINECS 256-095-6
Synonyms: Aspartic acid, diethyl ester
Trade names containing: Polyaminon-15; Polyaminon-5

Diethylene glycol... (INCI) *See also PEG-2...*
CAS 111-46-6; EINECS 203-872-2
Synonyms: DEG; Dihydroxydiethyl ether; Diglycol; 2,2′-Oxybisethanol
Trade names: Unichem DEG
Trade names containing: Varisoft® 110 DEG; Varisoft® 110 DEG

Diethylene glycolamine/epichlorohydrin/piperazine copolymer (INCI)
Trade names: Mexomere PL

Diethylene glycol butyl ether. *See Butoxy diglycol*

Diethylene glycol butyl ether acetate
CAS 124-17-4
Trade names: Ektasolve® DB Acetate

Diethylene glycol dibenzoate (INCI)
CAS 120-55-8; EINECS 204-407-6
Synonyms: PEG 100 dibenzoate; POE (2) dibenzoate
Trade names containing: Uniflex 50

Diethylene glycol diisononanoate (INCI)
CAS 106-01-4; EINECS 203-353-0
Synonyms: PEG-2 diisononanoate
Trade names: Dermol 499; Fractalite 499
Trade names containing: Dermol 334; Dermol 489; Dermol MO; Estalan 635

Diethylene glycol diisostearate
Synonyms: PEG-2 diisostearate
Trade names: Emalex DEG-di-IS

Diethylene glycol dioctanoate (INCI)
CAS 72269-52-4; EINECS 276-553-9
Synonyms: PEG-2 dioctanoate
Trade names: Dermol 488
Trade names containing: Dermol 334; Dermol 489; Dermol MO; Estalan 635

Diethylene glycol dioctanoate/diisononanoate (INCI)
Trade names: Estalan 430
Trade names containing: Estalan 560

Diethylene glycol ethyl ether acetate. *See Ethoxydiglycol acetate*

Diethylene glycol methyl ether. *See Methoxydiglycol*

Diethylene glycol propyl ether
CAS 6881-94-3
Synonyms: Diethylene glycol monopropyl ether
Trade names: Ektasolve® DP

Diethylene tricaseinamide (INCI)
Trade names: Hydagen® P

Diethyl glutamate (INCI)
CAS 55895-85-7
Synonyms: Glutamic acid, diethyl ester
Trade names containing: Polyaminon-15; Polyaminon-5

Di-2-ethylhexyl... *See Dioctyl...*

Diethyl phthalate (INCI)
CAS 84-66-2; EINECS 201-550-6
Synonyms: DEP; Ethyl phthalate; Phthalic acid, diethyl ester; Diethyl 1,2-benzenedicarboxylate
Trade names: Estol DEP 3075; Ftalato 2/46; Kodaflex® DEP; Palatinol® A; Uniflex DEP
Trade names containing: Clarax

Diethyl sebacate (INCI)
CAS 110-40-7; EINECS 203-764-5

Diethyl toluamide

Synonyms: Diethyl decanedioate
Trade names: Nikkol DES-SP

Diethyl toluamide (INCI)
CAS 134-62-3; EINECS 205-149-7
Synonyms: DEET; m-Toluic acid diethylamide; N,N-Diethyl-m-toluamide; DET
Trade names containing: Unirep U-18

1,1-Difluoroethane. *See Hydrofluorocarbon 152a*

Diglyceryl caprylate. *See Polyglyceryl-2 caprylate*

Diglyceryl stearate malate (INCI)
Synonyms: Polyglyceryl-2 stearate malate
Trade names: Sunsoft 601

Diglycol. *See Diethylene glycol…, PEG-2…*

Diglycol/CHDM/isophthalates/SIP copolymer (INCI)
Synonyms: Diglycol/cyclohexanedimethanol/iso-phthalates/sulfoisophthalates copolymer
Trade names: Eastman® AQ 38S; Eastman® AQ 55S
Trade names containing: Lipo PE Base G-55; Lipo PE Base GP-55

Dihexyl sodium sulfosuccinate (INCI)
CAS 3006-15-3; 2373-38-8; 6001-97-4; EINECS 221-109-1
Synonyms: Sodium dihexyl sulfosuccinate; Butanedioic acid, sulfo-, 1,4-dihexyl ester, sodium salt
Trade names: Aerosol® MA-80; Monawet MM-80

Dihydroabietyl behenate (INCI)
Synonyms: Behenic acid, dihydroabietyl ester
Trade names: Pelemol HAB

Dihydrocholesteryl octyldecanoate (INCI)
Synonyms: Octyldecanoic acid, dihydrocholesteryl ester
Trade names: Nikkol DCIS

Dihydrocholeth-15 (INCI)
Synonyms: PEG-15 dihydrocholesteryl ether
Trade names: Nikkol DHC-15

Dihydrocholeth-20 (INCI)
Synonyms: PEG-20 dihydrocholesteryl ether
Trade names: Nikkol DHC-20

Dihydrocholeth-30 (INCI)
Synonyms: PEG-30 dihydrocholesteryl ether
Trade names: Nikkol DHC-30

Dihydrogenated tallowamidoethyl hydroxyethylmonium methosulfate (INCI)
Trade names containing: Varisoft® 110-PG; Varisoft® 110; Varisoft® 110

Dihydrogenated tallow benzylmonium chloride (INCI)
CAS 61789-73-9
Synonyms: Dihydrogenated tallow methyl benzyl ammonium chloride; Di(hydrogenated tallow)benzyl methyl ammonium chloride
Trade names: Kemamine® BQ-9701C; Variquat® B343

Dihydrogenated tallow benzylmonium hectorite (INCI)
Trade names: Bentone® SD-3

Dihydrogenated tallow dimonium methosulfate (INCI)
Synonyms: Dimethyl dihydrogenated tallow ammonium methyl sulfate
Trade names containing: Varisoft® 137; Varisoft® 137

Dihydrogenated tallow methylamine (INCI)
CAS 61788-63-4; 67700-99-6; EINECS 262-991-8
Trade names: Amine M2HBG; Armeen® M2HT; Kemamine® T-9701

Dihydrogenated tallow phthalic acid amide (INCI)
CAS 127733-92-0
Trade names: Stepan TAB®-2

Dihydrolanosterol (INCI)
Trade names containing: Isocholesterol EX

Dihydrophytosteryl octyldecanoate (INCI)
Synonyms: Octyldecanoic acid, dihydrophytosteryl ester
Trade names: Nikkol DPIS

Dihydroxyacetone (INCI)
CAS 96-26-4; EINECS 202-494-5
Synonyms: DHA; 1,3-Dihydroxydimethyl ketone; 1,3-Dihydroxy-2-propanone
Trade names: Dihydroxyacetone; Nanospheres 100 Dihydroxyacetone
Trade names containing: Brookosome® DHA; DHA Melanosponge; DHA Microspheres

2,4-Dihydroxybenzophenone. *See Benzophenone-1*

Dihydroxydiethyl ether. *See Diethylene glycol…, PEG-2…*

2,2´-Dihydroxy-4,4´-dimethoxybenzophenone. *See Benzophenone-6*

Dihydroxyethyl C12-15 alkoxypropylamine oxide (INCI)
Trade names: Varox® 185E

Dihydroxyethyl cocamine oxide (INCI)
CAS 61791-47-7; EINECS 263-180-1
Synonyms: N,N (bis (2-hydroxyethyl) cocamine oxide; Coco di(hdyroxyethyl) amine oxide; Ethanol, 2,2´-iminobis, N-coco alkyl, N-oxide
Trade names: Aromox® C/12-W; Schercamox CMA
Trade names containing: Aromox® C/12

Dihydroxyethyl soyamine dioleate (INCI)
Trade names: Lowenol S-216

Dihydroxyethyl tallowamine oleate (INCI)
Trade names: Necon 655

Dihydroxyethyl tallowamine oxide (INCI)
CAS 61791-46-6; EINECS 263-179-6
Synonyms: Bis (2-hydroxyethyl) tallow amine oxide; 2,2´-Iminobisethanol, N-tallow alkyl, N-oxide; Amines, tallow alkyl dihydroxyethyl, oxides
Trade names: Chemoxide T
Trade names containing: Aromox® T/12

Dihydroxyethyl tallow glycinate (INCI)
CAS 61791-45-5, 61791-25-1; 70750-46-8; EINECS 274-845-0
Synonyms: Quaternary ammonium compds., (carboxymethyl)(tallow alkyl)dihydroxyethyl, hydroxides, inner salts; Tallow dihydroxyethyl betaine; Tallow dihydroxyethyl glycine
Trade names: Amphoteen BTH-35; Chembetaine TG; Mackam™ TM; Mirataine® TM; Rewoteric® AM TEG; Tego®-Betaine N-192; Zohartaine TM

Dihydroxyindole (INCI)
CAS 3131-52-0
Synonyms: 5,6-Dihydroxyindole
Trade names: Imexine OAY

2,2´-Dihydroxy-4-methoxybenzophenone. *See Benzophenone-8*

Diiodomethyl p-tolyl sulfone (INCI)
CAS 20018-09-1; EINECS 243-468-3
Trade names: Amical® 48; Amical® Flowable
Trade names containing: Amical® 50

Diisoarachidyl dilinoleate (INCI)
Trade names: Liquiwax™ DIEFA

Diisoarachidyl dodecanedioate (INCI)
Trade names: Liquiwax™ DIADD
Trade names containing: Liquiwax™ DIADD/TiO₂ Disp

Diisocetyl dodecanedioate
Trade names: Liquiwax™ DICDD

Diisodecyl adipate (INCI)
CAS 27178-16-1; EINECS 248-299-9
Synonyms: DIDA; Hexanedioic acid, diisodecyl ester
Trade names: Arlamol® DIDA

Diisononyl adipate (INCI)
CAS 33703-08-1; EINECS 251-646-7
Synonyms: Hexanedioic acid, diisononyl ester; Diisononyl hexanedioate
Trade names: Arlamol® DINA

Diisopropanolamine (INCI)
CAS 110-97-4; EINECS 203-820-9
Synonyms: DIPA; 1,1'-Iminobis-2-propenol
Trade names: DIPA Commercial Grade; DIPA Low Freeze Grade 85; DIPA Low Freeze Grade 90; DIPA NF Grade; Unichem DIPA
Trade names containing: Mearlmaid® PLN; Mearlmaid® PLO

Diisopropyl adipate (INCI)
CAS 6938-94-9; EINECS 248-299-9
Synonyms: Bis(1-methylethyl)hexanedioate; Hexanedioic acid, bis (1-methylethyl) ester
Trade names: Ceraphyl® 230; Crodamol DA; Docoil Dipa; Estalan DIA; Iso-Adipate 2/043700; Nikkol DID; Pelemol DIA; Schercemol DIA; Trivent DIA; Upamate DIPA
Trade names containing: Dragocid Forte 2/027045

Diisopropyl dimer dilinoleate (INCI)
CAS 103213-20-3
Synonyms: Diisopropyl dilinoleate
Trade names: Bernel® Ester DID; Dermol DID; Pripure 3786; Schercemol DID

Diisopropyl sebacate (INCI)
CAS 7491-02-3; EINECS 231-306-4
Synonyms: Bis(1-methylethyl) decanedioate; Decanedioic acid, bis(1-methylethyl) ester
Trade names: Nikkol DIS; Pelemol DIPS; Schercemol DIS
Trade names containing: Myrol-S

Diisostearyl adipate (INCI)
Synonyms: Bis(isooctadecyl)hexanedioate; Hexanedioic acid, diisostearyl ester
Trade names: Salacos 618

Diisostearyl dimer dilinoleate (INCI)
CAS 103213-19-0, 127358-81-0
Synonyms: Diisostearyl dimerate; Dimer acid, diisostearyl ester
Trade names: Dermol DISD; Estalan DISD; Pripure 3785; Schercemol DISD

Diisostearyl fumarate (INCI)
CAS 112385-09-8, 113431-53-1
Trade names: Schercemol DISF

Diisostearyl malate (INCI)
CAS 67763-18-2
Trade names: Bernel® Ester DISM; Cosmol 222

Dilaureth-7 citrate
Trade names: Eucarol B/D

Dilaureth-4 dimonium chloride (INCI)
Trade names: Hoe S 2650

Dilaureth-4 phosphate (INCI)
Trade names: Hostaphat KL 240

Dilaureth-10 phosphate (INCI)
Trade names: Nikkol DLP-10

Dilaurin. *See Glyceryl dilaurate*

1,2-Dilauroyl-sn-glycero(3) phosphocholine
Trade names: Phospholipon® LC

Dilauryl acetyl dimonium chloride (INCI)
CAS 90283-04-8, 129541-39-5
Trade names: Schercoquat ALA

Dilauryldimonium chloride (INCI)
CAS 3401-74-9; EINECS 222-274-2
Trade names: Kemamine® Q-6902C

Dilauryl thiodipropionate (INCI)
CAS 123-28-4; EINECS 204-614-1
Synonyms: Didodecyl 3,3'-thiodipropionate; Thiodipropionic acid, dilauryl ester
Trade names: Argus DLTDP; Evanstab® 12

Dilinoleamidopropyl dimethylamine (INCI)
Trade names: Catemol 360

Dilinoleamidopropyl dimethylamine dimethicone copolyol phosphate (INCI)
CAS 138698-34-7
Trade names containing: Dicopamine DP

Dilinoleic acid (INCI)
CAS 6144-28-1; 61788-89-4
Synonyms: 9,12-Octadecadienoic acid, dimer; Dimer acid
Trade names: Empol® 1008; Empol® 1024

Dilinoleic acid/ethylenediamine copolymer (INCI)
Trade names: Macromelt

Dimer acid. *See Dilinoleic acid*

Dimethicone (INCI)
CAS 9006-65-9; 9016-00-6; 63148-62-9; 68037-74-1 (branched)
Synonyms: PDMS; Dimethyl polysiloxane; Dimethyl silicone; Polydimethylsiloxane
Trade names: Abil® 10-10000; Amersil® L-45 Grades; Amersil® L-45/10; Amersil® L-45/20; Amersil® L-45/50; Amersil® L-45/100; Amersil® L-45/200; Amersil® L-45/350; Amersil® L-45/500; Amersil® L-45/1000; Amersil® L-45/12500; Amersil® L-45/60000; Baysilone Fluid M; Belsil DM 0.65; Belsil DM 35; Belsil DM 100; Belsil DM 350; Belsil DM 100000; DM Fluid 3000; Dow Corning® 200 Fluid; Dow Corning® 225; Dow Corning® Medical Fluid 360; Foamkill® 810F; Foamkill® 830F; Masil® SF 5; Masil® SF 10; Masil® SF 20; Masil® SF 50; Masil® SF 100; Masil® SF 200; Masil® SF 350; Masil® SF 350 FG; Masil® SF 500; Masil® SF 1000; Masil® SF 5000; Masil® SF 10,000; Masil® SF 12,500; Masil® SF 30,000; Masil® SF 60,000; Masil® SF 100,000; Masil® SF 300,000; Masil® SF 500,000; Masil® SF 600,000; Masil® SF 1,000,000; Medical Fluid 360; Rhodorsil® Oils 70047 V2, V5; SF81-50; SF96® (5 cst); SF96® (100 cst); SF96® (350 cst); SF96® (500 cst); SF96® (1000 cst); Silatex SF-50; Silatex SF-300; Silicone L-45; SWS-101; Tri-Sil Wax 105; Ultra Sil™; Viscasil® (10,000 cSt); Viscasil® (12,500 cSt); Wacker Silicone Fluid AKF
Trade names containing: Abil® OSW 12, OSW 13; Abil® OSW 15; Belsil ADM 6056 E; Belsil SDM 6021; Belsil SDM 6022; Dow Corning® 1669; Dow Corning® 593 Fluid; Dow Corning® Q2-1403 Fluid; Dow Corning® QF1-3593A; Dow Corning® X2-1669; Fancorsil A; Gafquat® HSi; Gransil DMG-6; PVP/Si-10; Rhodorsil® Oils 71631; SAG-710, -730; Sericite DNN-2SH; SS-4267; Tektamer® 38 A.D.; Tektamer® 38 L.V.; UV-Titan M260; UV-Titan M262

Dimethicone copolyol (INCI)
CAS 63148-55-0; 64365-23-7; 67762-96-3
Synonyms: Dimethylsiloxane-glycol copolymer
Trade names: Abil® B 8842; Abil® B 8843; Abil® B 8847; Abil® B 8851; Abil® B 8852; Abil® B 8863; Abil® B

8873; Abil® B 88183; Abil® B 88184; Alkasil® NEPCA 250-185; Amersil® DMC-20; Amersil® DMC-287; Amersil® DMC-357; Amersil® DMC-500; Amersil® DMC-604; Belsil DMC 6031; Belsil DMC 6038; Biowax 754; Dow Corning® 190 Surfactant; Dow Corning® 193 Surfactant; Dow Corning® 2501 Cosmetic Wax; Dow Corning® Q2-5220 Resin Modifier; Dow Corning® Q2-5324 Surfactant; Dow Corning® Q2-5434; GP-209 Silicone Polyol Copolymer; GP-215 Silicone Polyol Copolymer; GP-217 Silicone Polyol Copolymer; GP-226; Gransurf 71; Gransurf 72; Gransurf 73; Gransurf 75; Gransurf 76; Gransurf 77; KF353A; KF625A, KF945A; Masil® 280; Masil® 280LP; Masil® 1066C; Masil® 1066D; MFF Series; Rhodorsil® Oils 70646; SF1188; Silatex SF-280; Silwet® L-711; Silwet® L-720; Silwet® L-721; Silwet® L-7000; Silwet® L-7001; Silwet® L-7002; Silwet® L-7004; Silwet® L-7500; Silwet® L-7600; Silwet® L-7602; Silwet® L-7604; Silwet® L-7610; Silwet® L-7614
Trade names containing: Amersil® ME-358; Dow Corning® 3225C Formulation Aid

Dimethicone copolyol acetate (INCI)
Trade names: Belsil DMC 6032; Belsil DMC 6033; Belsil DMC 6035

Dimethicone copolyol adipate (INCI)
Trade names: Fancor Lansil; Fancorsil SLA; Fancorsil SLA-LT

Dimethicone copolyolamine (INCI)
CAS 133779-14-3
Trade names: Silamine 65

Dimethicone copolyol butyl ether (INCI)
Trade names: KF352A; KF354A, KF355A, KF615A

Dimethicone copolyol isostearate (INCI)
CAS 133448-16-5
Trade names: Silwax® WD-IS

Dimethicone copolyol methyl ether (INCI)
CAS 68951-97-3
Synonyms: Siloxanes and silicones, di-me, methoxy terminated
Trade names: KF351A; KF351AS

Dimethicone copolyol phosphate
CAS 132207-31-9
Trade names: Pecosil® PS-100

Dimethicone/mercaptopropyl methicone copolymer (INCI)
Trade names: GP-71-SS Mercapto Modified Silicone Fluid

Dimethicone propylethylenediamine behenate (INCI)
CAS 132207-30-8
Synonyms: Siloxanes and silicones, 3-[(2-aminoethyl amino]propyl, methyl, dimethyl, docosanoates
Trade names: Pecosil® OS-100B

Dimethicone propyl PG-betaine (INCI)
CAS 102523-96-6
Trade names: Abil® B 9950

Dimethicone silylate (INCI)
Trade names: Burst RSD-10; Burst RSD-30

Dimethiconol (INCI)
CAS 31692-79-2
Synonyms: Poly[oxy(dimethylsilylene)], α-hydro-ω-hydroxy-
Trade names: Masil® SFR 70; Mazol® SFR 18,000; Mazol® SFR 50,000; Mazol® SFR 100; Mazol® SFR 150,000; Mazol® SFR 750; Mazol® SFR 2000; Mazol® SFR 3500; Unisil SF-R

Trade names containing: Abil® OSW 12, OSW 13; Abil® OSW 15; Belsil ADM 6056 E; Belsil CM 1000; Dow Corning® 1401 Fluid; Dow Corning® Q2-1403 Fluid; E-2170; Sandoperm FE; SM 2112; Tri-Sil HGC 5000

Dimethiconol arginate
Trade names: Biosil Basics A-30

Dimethiconol cysteinate
Trade names: Biosil Basics L-Cysteine

Dimethiconol fluoroalcohol dilinoleic acid (INCI)
Trade names: Silwax® F

Dimethiconol hydroxystearate (INCI)
Trade names: Silwax® C

Dimethiconol jasminate
Trade names: Biosil Basics Jasmine Wax S

Dimethiconol keratinate
Trade names: Biosil Basics HKP-30

Dimethiconol lysinate
Trade names: Biosil Basics L-30

Dimethiconol panthenate
Trade names: Biosil Basics DL-30

Dimethoxydiglycol (INCI)
CAS 111-96-6; EINECS 203-924-4
Trade names: Diglyme

Dimethoxysilyl ethylene diaminopropyl dimethicone (INCI)
CAS 71750-80-6
Trade names: GP-RA-157 Amine Functional Silicone Fluid

Dimethyl adipate (INCI)
CAS 627-93-0; EINECS 211-020-6
Synonyms: Dimethyl hexanedioate; Methyl adipate
Trade names containing: All-Natural Nail Polish Remover

Dimethylaminoethyl methacrylate (INCI)
CAS 2867-47-2; EINECS 220-688-8
Synonyms: 2-(Dimethylamino)ethyl 2-methyl-2-propenoate
Trade names: Ageflex FM-1

Dimethylaminopropyl behenamide. *See Behenamidopropyl dimethylamine*

Dimethylaminopropyl ricinoleamide benzyl chloride
Trade names containing: ES-1239

Dimethyl aspartic acid (INCI)
CAS 1115-22-6
Trade names: DIMASPA

Dimethyl behenamine (INCI)
CAS 215-42-9; 21542-96-1
Synonyms: Behenyl dimethyl amine; N,N-Dimethyl-1-docosanamine
Trade names: Adogen® MA-112 SF; Kemamine® T-2802D

Dimethyl cocamine (INCI)
CAS 61788-93-0; EINECS 263-020-0
Synonyms: Coco dimethyl amine; Amines, coco alkyl dimethyl; Dimethyl coconut amine
Trade names: Amine 2M1218D; Amine 2MKKD; Armeen® DMCD; Barlene® 12C; Jet Amine DMCD; Kemamine® T-6502; Noram DMC

3,6-Dimethyl-3-cyclohexene-1-carbaldehyde
Trade names: Cyclovertal

2,4-Dimethyl-3-cyclohexene carboxyaldehyde (INCI)
CAS 68039-49-6; EINECS 268-264-1
Synonyms: 3-Cyclohexenene-1-carboxaldehyde, 2,4-dimethyl

Trade names: Belal

Dimethyl decylamine
CAS 1120-24-7
Synonyms: Decyl dimethylamine; C10 alkyl dimethyl-amine; N,N-Dimethyl decylamine
Trade names: Adma® 10
Trade names containing: Adma® WC

Dimethyldiallyl ammonium chloride/acrylic acid copolymer. *See Polyquaternium-22*

Dimethyl diallyl ammonium chloride monomer
CAS 7398-69-8
Synonyms: Diallyl dimethyl ammonium chloride
Trade names: Ageflex mDMDAC

Dimethyl di(hydrogenated tallow)ammonium chloride. *See Quaternium-18*

Dimethyl ether (INCI)
CAS 115-10-6; EINECS 204-065-8
Synonyms: Methane, oxybis-; Oxybismethane; Methyl ether
Trade names: Demeon D; Dymel® A

Dimethyl glutarate (INCI)
CAS 1119-40-0; EINECS 214-277-2
Synonyms: Dimethyl pentanedioate
Trade names containing: All-Natural Nail Polish Remover

Dimethyl hexahydronaphthyl dihydroxymethyl acetal (INCI)
CAS 73979-86-9, 73979-84-7, 73970-38-4, 73970-40-8
Trade names: Bergoxane

Dimethyl hydrogenated tallow amine (INCI)
CAS 61788-95-2; EINECS 263-022-1
Synonyms: Hydrogenated tallow dimethylamine; Hydrogenated tallowalkyl dimethylamine
Trade names: Armeen® DMHTD; Kemamine® T-9702

N,N´-Dimethyl-N-hydroxyethyl-3-nitro-p-phenylenediamine (INCI)
CAS 10228-03-2; EINECS 233-549-1
Trade names: Imexine FD

Dimethylhydroxymethylpyrazole (INCI)
CAS 85264-33-1
Trade names: Busan® 1504

Dimethyl imidazolidinone (INCI)
CAS 80-73-9; EINECS 201-304-8
Synonyms: 1,3-Dimethyl-2-imidazolidinone; 2-Imidazolidinone, 1,3-dimethyl-
Trade names: Nikkol DMI

Dimethyl isosorbide (INCI)
CAS 5306-85-4; EINECS 226-159-8
Synonyms: DMI; Isosorbide dimethyl ether; D-Glucitol, 1,4:3,6-dianhydro-2,5-di-o-methyl
Trade names: Arlasolve® DMI

Dimethyl lauramine (INCI)
CAS 112-18-5; 67700-98-5; EINECS 203-943-8
Synonyms: Lauryl dimethylamine; Dodecyldimethylamine
Trade names: Adma® 12; Adogen® MA-102; Armeen® DM12D; Barlene® 12S; Kemamine® T-6902
Trade names containing: Adma® 1214; Adma® 1416; Adma® 246-451; Adma® 246-621; Adma® WC; Amine 2M1214D

Dimethyl lauramine dimer dilinoleate (INCI)
Trade names: Necon DLD

Dimethyl lauramine isostearate (INCI)
CAS 70729-87-2
Synonyms: Dimethyl laurylamine isostearate
Trade names: Parapel® LIS

Trade names containing: Parapel® HC; Parapel® HC-85; Parapel® HC-99

Dimethyl lauramine oleate (INCI)
Synonyms: Dimethyl laurylamine oleate
Trade names: Lanaetex-LO; Necon A; Necon LO

Dimethyl myristamine (INCI)
CAS 112-75-4; 68439-70-3; EINECS 204-002-4
Synonyms: Dimethyl myristylamine; Myristyl dimethylamine; Tetradecyl dimethylamine
Trade names: Adma® 14; Adogen® MA-104; Amine 2M14D; Armeen® DM14D; Barlene® 14; Barlene® 14S; Kemamine® T-7902
Trade names containing: Adma® 1214; Adma® 1416; Adma® 246-451; Adma® 246-621; Adma® WC; Amine 2M1214D

Z-3,7-Dimethyl-2,6-octadiene-1-al
Trade names: Neral

Dimethyl octylamine
CAS 7378-99-6
Synonyms: DMOA; C8 alkyl dimethylamine; Octyl dimethylamine; N,N-dimethyloctylamine
Trade names: Adma® 8
Trade names containing: Adma® WC

Dimethyl octynediol (INCI)
CAS 1321-87-5; 78-66-0
Synonyms: 3,6-Dimethyl-4-octyne-3,6-diol
Trade names: Surfynol® 82
Trade names containing: Surfynol® 82S

Dimethyl oleamine
CAS 14727-68-5; 28061-69-0
Synonyms: Oleyl dimethylamine
Trade names: Armeen® DMOD; Jet Amine DMOD

Dimethyl oxazolidine (INCI)
CAS 51200-87-4; EINECS 257-048-2
Synonyms: 4,4-Dimethyloxazolidine; Oxazolidine A
Trade names: Nuosept 101 CG; Oxaban®-A

Dimethyl palmitamine (INCI)
CAS 112-69-6; 68037-93-4; EINECS 203-997-2
Synonyms: Palmityl dimethylamine; Hexadecyl dimethylamine; Cetyl dimethylamine
Trade names: Adma® 16; Adogen® MA-106; Amine 2M16D; Armeen® DM16D; Barlene® 16S; Kemamine® T-8902
Trade names containing: Adma® 1416; Adma® 246-451; Adma® 246-621; Adma® WC

N,N-Dimethyl-p-phenylenediamine sulfate (INCI)
CAS 6219-73-4; EINECS 228-292-7
Synonyms: N,N-Dimethyl-1,4-benzenediamine sulfate
Trade names: Rodol Gray DMS

Dimethyl phthalate (INCI)
CAS 131-11-3; EINECS 205-011-6
Synonyms: DMP; Dimethyl 1,2-benzenedicarboxylate; 1,2-Benzenedicarboxylic acid dimethyl ester; Phthalic acid dimethyl ester
Trade names: Kemester® DMP; Kodaflex® DMP; Palatinol® M; Uniplex 110
Trade names containing: Unirep U-18

Dimethylpolysiloxane. *See Dimethicone*

Dimethylsilanol hyaluronate (INCI)
Trade names: D.S.H. C

Dimethylsiloxane. *See Dimethicone*

Dimethylsiloxane-glycol copolymer. *See Dimethicone copolyol*

Dimethyl soyamine (INCI)
CAS 61788-91-8; EINECS 263-017-4

Synonyms: Soya dimethyl amine
Trade names: Armeen® DMSD; Jet Amine DMSD; Kemamine® T-9972

Dimethyl stearamine (INCI)
CAS 124-28-7; EINECS 204-694-8
Synonyms: Stearyl dimethyl amine; Octadecyl dimethylamine; N,N-Dimethyl-1-octadecanamine
Trade names: Adma® 18; Adogen® MA-108; Adogen® MA-108 SF; Amine 2M18D; Armeen® DM18D; Barlene® 18S; Kemamine® T-9902
Trade names containing: Adma® 1416; Adma® WC

Dimethyl succinate (INCI)
CAS 106-65-0; EINECS 203-419-9
Synonyms: Dimethyl butanedioate; Methyl succinate
Trade names containing: All-Natural Nail Polish Remover

Dimethyl tallowamine (INCI)
CAS 68814-69-7
Synonyms: Tallow dimethylamine; Tallow alkyl dimethylamine
Trade names: Armeen® DMTD; Jet Amine DMTD; Kemamine® T-9742

1,2-Dimyristoyl-sn-glycero(3) phosphatidylcholine
CAS 18194-24-6
Trade names: Phospholipon® MC

Dinkum oil. *See Eucalyptus oil*

Dinonoxynol-4 phosphate (CTFA)
Trade names: Nikkol DNPP-4

Dinonyl phenol (INCI)
CAS 1323-65-5; EINECS 215-356-4
Trade names containing: Arlatone® B

Dioctadecylamine
CAS 112-99-2
Synonyms: Distearylamine
Trade names: Armeen® 2-18

Dioctyl adipate (INCI)
CAS 103-23-1; EINECS 203-090-1
Synonyms: DOA; Bis(2-ethylhexyl) hexanedioate; Di(2-ethylhexyl) adipate; Hexanedioic acid, bis (2-ethylhexyl) ester
Trade names: Crodamol DOA; Kodaflex® DOA; Wickenol® 158
Trade names containing: Wickenol® 161; Wickenol® 163

Dioctyl cyclohexane (INCI)
CAS 84753-08-2; 100182-46-5; EINECS 283-854-9
Synonyms: Cyclohexane, 1,3-bis(2-ethylhexyl)-; 1,3 Dioctyl cyclohexane; Cyclohexane, diisooctyl-
Trade names: Cetiol® S

Dioctyl dimer dilinoleate (INCI)
Synonyms: Dioctyl dimerate; Bis(2-ethylhexyl) dimerate; Dimer acid, 2-ethylhexyl ester
Trade names: Kemester® 3681

Dioctyl dimonium chloride
Synonyms: Dioctyl dimethyl ammonium chloride
Trade names containing: Bardac® 2050

Dioctyl dodeceth-2 lauroyl glutamate (INCI)
Trade names: Amiter LGOD-2

Dioctyl dodeceth-5 lauroyl glutamate
Trade names: Amiter LGOD-5

Dioctyl dodecyl fluorocitrate
Trade names: Biosil Basics Fluoro Guerbet 1.0%; Biosil Basics Fluoro Guerbet 3.5%

Dioctyl dodecyl lauroyl glutamate (INCI)
CAS 82204-94-2; EINECS 279-917-5
Synonyms: N-(1-Oxododecyl)-L-glutamic acid, bis(2-

octyldodecyl) ester
Trade names: Amiter LGOD

Di-(2-octyldodecyl) stearoyl glutamate (INCI)
Trade names: Amiter SG-OD

Dioctyl ether
Trade names: Cetiol® OE

Dioctylmalate (INCI)
CAS 15763-02-7, 56235-92-8
Trade names: Ceraphyl® 45

Dioctyl maleate (CTFA)
CAS 142-16-5; 2915-53-9; EINECS 205-524-5
Synonyms: Bis (2-ethylhexyl) maleate; Di-N-octyl maleate; Di-(2-ethylhexyl) maleate
Trade names: Bernel® Ester DOM; Estalan DOM

Dioctyl sebacate (INCI)
CAS 122-62-3, 2432-87-3; EINECS 204-558-8
Synonyms: Di-2-ethylhexyl sebacate; Bis (2-ethylhexyl) decanedioate
Trade names: Docoil DOS; Elfacos® DEHS; Kessco DEHS; Trivent DOS

Dioctyl sodium sulfosuccinate (INCI)
CAS 577-11-7; 1369-66-3; EINECS 209-406-4
Synonyms: DSS; Sodium dioctyl sulfosuccinate; Sodium di(2-ethylhexyl) sulfosuccinate; Docusate sodium
Trade names: Aerosol® OT-75%; Chemax/DOSS-75E; Chimin DOS 70; Emcol® 4500; Gemtex PA-70; Gemtex PA-75E; Gemtex PAX-60; Gemtex SC-75E, SC Powd; Geropon® SBDO; Hodag DOSS-70; Hodag DOSS-75; Marlinat® DF 8; Monawet MO-65-150; Monawet MO-70; Monawet MO-70-150; Monawet MO-70E; Monawet MO-70RP; Nikkol OTP-100; Nikkol OTP-100S; Nikkol OTP-75; Rewopol® SBDO 75; Schercopol DOS-PG-85; Solusol® 75%; Solusol® 100%; Supermontaline SLT65
Trade names containing: Aerosol® OT-70 PG; Aerosol® OT-B; Gemtex PA-70P; Gemtex PA-75; Gemtex PA-85P; Geropon® 99; Midpol 2000; Monawet MO-70R; Monawet MO-70S; Monawet MO-75E; Monawet MO-84R2W; Monawet MO-85P; Schercopol DOS-70; Schercopol DOS-PG-70; Solusol® 85%

Dioctyl succinate (INCI)
CAS 2915-57-3; EINECS 220-836-1
Synonyms: Bis (2-ethylhexyl) butanedioate; Butanedioic acid, bis(2-ethylhexyl) ester; Di(2-ethylhexyl) succinate
Trade names: Crodamol OSU; Wickenol® 159

Dioctyl terephthalate
CAS 422-86-2
Synonyms: DOTP; Di-2-ethylhexyl terephthalate
Trade names: Kodaflex® DOTP

Dioctyl trimonium chloride
Trade names: Nikkol CA-3080

Dioleoyl EDTHP-monium methosulfate (INCI)
Trade names: Hoe S 3121

Dioleyl tocopheryl methylsilanol (INCI)
Trade names: Liposiliol C

1,4-Dioxacyclohexadecane-5,16-dione
CAS 54982-83-1
Trade names: Arova® N

(2,5-Dioxo-4-imidazolidinyl) urea. *See Allantoin*

DIPA. *See Diisopropanolamine*

DIPA-hydrogenated cocoate (INCI)
Trade names containing: Chimexane AC

DIPA-lanolate (INCI)

Trade names containing: Chimexane AC

Dipalmitamine (INCI)
Trade names: Adogen® 216 SF

Dipalmitoylethyl hydroxyethylmonium methosulfate (INCI)
Trade names: Stepanquat® 6585

1,2-Dipalmitoyl-sn-glycero(3) phosphatidylcholine
CAS 2644-64-6
Trade names: Phospholipon® PC

Dipalmitoyl hydroxyproline (INCI)
CAS 41672-81-5; EINECS 255-490-0
Synonyms: L-Proline, 1-(1-oxohexadecyl)-4-[(1-oxohexadecyl)oxy]-, trans-
Trade names: Lipacide DPHP

Dipentaerythrityl hexacaprylate/hexacaprate (INCI)
CAS 68130-24-5
Synonyms: Decanoic acid, ester with 2,2´-[oxybis (methylene)]bis[2-(hydroxymethyl)-1,3-propane-diol]octanoate pentanoate
Trade names: Liponate DPC-6
Trade names containing: Lipovol MOS-130; Lipovol MOS-350

Dipentaerythrityl hexahydroxystearate (INCI)
Trade names: Cosmol 168M

Dipentaerythrityl hexahydroxystearate/isostearate (INCI)
Trade names: Cosmol 168E

Dipentaerythrityl hexahydroxystearate/stearate/rosinate (INCI)
Trade names: Cosmol 168AR

Dipentaerythrityl pentaoctanoate/behenate (INCI)
Trade names: Cosmol 168I

Dipentene (INCI)
CAS 138-86-3; EINECS 205-341-0
Synonyms: Cinene; Limonene, inactive; Cajeputene
Trade names: Dipentene No. 122

Diphenyl dimethicone (INCI)
Synonyms: Diphenyl dimethylsiloxane
Trade names: F-5W-0 100 cs; F-5W-0 300 cs; F-5W-0 1000 cs; F-5W-0 3000 cs; KF54; KF9937

Diphenylmethyl piperazinylbenzimidazole (INCI)
CAS 65215-54-5
Trade names: Iramine

Dipotassium glycyrrhizate (INCI)
CAS 68797-35-3; EINECS 272-296-1
Synonyms: Dipotassium glycyrrhizinate
Trade names: K2 Glycyrrhizinate; Nikkol Dipotassium Glycyrrhizinate; Ritamectant K2

Dipropyl adipate (INCI)
CAS 106-19-4; EINECS 203-371-9
Trade names: Estalan DNPA; Pelemol DNPA

Dipropylene glycol (INCI)
CAS 110-98-5; EINECS 203-821-4
Synonyms: Di-1,2-propylene glycol; 1,1|-Oxybis-2-propanol
Trade names: Adeka Dipropylene Glycol (Cosmetic Grade); Unichem DPG
Trade names containing: Grillocin HY-77; Grillocin® HY 77; Merguard 1190; Nikkol Aquasome LA

Dipropylene glycol dibenzoate (INCI)
CAS 94-51-9, 27138-31-4; EINECS 202-340-7
Synonyms: 3,3´-Oxydyl-1-propanol dibenzoate
Trade names: Uniflex 9-88
Trade names containing: Uniflex 50

Dipropylene glycol salicylate (INCI)
CAS 7491-14-7
Synonyms: POP (2) monosalicylate; PPG-2 salicylate
Trade names: Dipsal

Disodium ascorbyl sulfate (INCI)
Trade names: Nikkol VC-SS

Disodium C12-15 pareth sulfosuccinate (INCI)
CAS 39354-47-5
Synonyms: Disodium pareth-25 sulfosuccinate; Sulfobutanedioic acid, C12-15 pareth ester, disodium salt
Trade names: Emcol® 4300

Disodium capryloamphodiacetate (INCI)
CAS 7702-01-4; 68608-64-0; EINECS 231-721-0; 271-792-5
Synonyms: 1H-Imidazolium, 1-[2-(carboxymethoxy) ethyl]-1-(carboxymethyl)-2-heptyl-4,5-dihydro-, hydroxide, disodium salt; Capryloamphocarboxyglycinate; Capryloamphodiacetate
Trade names: Amphoterge® J-2; Mackam™ 2CY; Schercoteric CY-2; Sochamine A 8955

Disodium capryloamphodipropionate (INCI)
CAS 68815-55-4
Synonyms: Capryloamphocarboxypropionate; Caprylo-amphodipropionate
Trade names: Amphoterge® KJ-2; Mackam™ 2CYSF; Miranol® JBS

Disodium cetearyl sulfosuccinate (INCI)
Synonyms: Disodium cetyl-stearyl sulfosuccinate; Sulfobutanedioic acid, cetyl/stearyl ester, disodium salt
Trade names: Empicol® STT

Disodium cocamido MEA-sulfosuccinate (INCI)
CAS 61791-66-0; 68784-08-7; EINECS 272-219-1
Synonyms: Sulfobutanedioic acid, C-(2-cocamidoethyl) esters, disodium salts; Disodium cocoylmono-ethanolamide sulfosuccinate
Trade names: Emcol® 5315; Emery® 5315; Empicol® SBB; Mackam™ CM-100; Mackanate™ CM; Mackanate™ CM-100; Rewopol® SBC 212; Rewopol® SBC 212 G; Rewopol® SBC 212 P; Schercopol CMA-Na; Schercopol CMS-Na; Surfax SME; Zoharpon SM
Trade names containing: Cosmopon HC

Disodium cocamido MIPA-sulfosuccinate (INCI)
CAS 68515-65-1; EINECS 271-102-2
Synonyms: Sulfobutanedioic acid, 2-cocamido-1-methylethyl esters, disodium salts
Trade names: Afanate™ CP; Mackanate™ CP; Monamate C-1142; Monamate CPA-100; Monamate CPA-40
Trade names containing: Monateric 805

Disodium cocamido PEG-3 sulfopsuccinate (INCI)
Trade names: Elfanol® 850; Empicol® SGG

Disodium cocoamphodiacetate (INCI)
CAS 61791-32-0; 68650-39-5; EINECS 272-043-5
Synonyms: N-Cocamidoethyl-N-2-hydroxyethyl-N-carboxyethylglycine, sodium salt; Cocoamphodiac-etate; Cocoamphocarboxyglycinate
Trade names: Abluter DCM-2; Afoteric™ 2C; Ampholak XCO-30; Amphotensid GB 2009; Amphoterge® W-2; Chimin IMB; Dehyton® G; Dehyton® PG; Dehyton® W; Mackam™ 2C; Manroteric CDX38; Miranol® 2CIB; Miranol® C2M Conc. NP; Miranol® C2M Conc. OP; Miranol® FB-NP; Monateric CDX-38; Monateric CDX-38 Mod; Monateric CLV; Monateric CSH-32; Proteric CDX-38; Rewoteric® AM 2C NM; Rewo-

Disodium cocoamphodipropionate

teric® AM 2C W; Schercoteric MS-2; Sochamine A
7525; Surfax AC 50; Surfax ACI; Unibetaine 2C;
Velvetex® CDC; Zoharteric D; Zoharteric D-SF 70%
Trade names containing: Amphotensid 9M; Cephalipin;
Cycloryl GSC; Empigen® CDR40; Klensoft;
Mackam™ 2CA; Mackam™ 2CAS; Mackam™ 2CT;
Mackam™ 2MCA; Mackam™ 2MCAS; Miracare®
2MCA; Miracare® 2MCAS; Miracare® 2MCT;
Miranol® C2M Conc. NP-PG; Monateric 805;
Monateric CDL; Monateric CDS; Monateric CDTD;
Proteric CDL; Proteric CDTD; Schercoteric MS-2
Modified; Schercoteric MS-2ES Modified; Surfax AC
55; Zoharteric D-2; Zoharteric D.O.; Zoharteric
D.O.T.

Disodium cocoamphodipropionate (INCI)
CAS 86438-35-9; 83138-08-3; 86438-79-1; 68411-57-4;
68604-71-7; 68910-41-5; 68919-40-4; EINECS 270-
131-8; 272-897-9
Synonyms: Cocoamphocarboxypropionate; Cocoam-
phodipropionate
Trade names: Amphoterge® K-2; Mackam™ 2CSF;
Miranol® C2M-SF 70%; Miranol® C2M-SF Conc;
Monateric CEM-38; Nikkol AM-102EX; Rewoteric®
AM 2C SF; Unibetaine 160C; Zoharteric D-SF
Trade names containing: Mackam™ 2CSF-70; Mira-
care® 2MCA-SF

Disodium deceth-5 sulfosuccinate (INCI)
Trade names: Empicol® SFF

Disodium deceth-6 sulfosuccinate (INCI)
CAS 68311-03-5 (generic); 39354-45-5
Synonyms: Sulfobutanedioic acid, deceth-6 ester, diso-
dium salt
Trade names: Aerosol® A-102; Mackanate™ A-102

**Disodium 2,2′-dihydroxy-4,4′-dimethoxy-5,5′-disulfo-
benzophenone.** *See Benzophenone-9*

**Disodium dihydroxyethyl sulfosuccinyl undecylenate
(INCI)**
Trade names: Grillosan DS 7911

Disodium dimethicone copolyol sulfosuccinate (INCI)
Synonyms: Sulfobutanedioic acid, dimethicone copolyol
ester, disodium salt
Trade names: Mackanate™ DC-30; Mackanate™ DC-50

Disodium distyrylbiphenyl disulfonate (INCI)
Trade names: Tinopal® CBS-X

Disodium edetate. *See Disodium EDTA*

Disodium EDTA (INCI)
CAS 139-33-3; EINECS 205-358-3
Synonyms: Disodium edetate; Ethylenediamine-
tetraacetic acid, disodium salt; Edetate disodium
Trade names: BASF Disodium EDTA; Hampene® Na$_2$
Pure Crystals; Nervanaid™ BA2 (BP); Sequestrene®
NA2; Universene Na2; Versene NA
Trade names containing: Hamp-Ene® OH Powd.

Disodium EDTA-copper (CTFA)
CAS 14025-15-1
Synonyms: Copper versenate; Copper disodium EDTA
Trade names: Kelate Cu Liq; Universene Na2 Cu

**Disodium hydrogenated cottonseed glyceride sulfosuc-
cinate (INCI)**
Synonyms: Sulfobutanedioic acid, hydrog. cottonseed
glyceride, disodium salt
Trade names: Emcol® 4072

Disodium hydrogenated tallow glutamate (INCI)
Trade names: Amisoft HS-21

Disodium hydroxydecyl sorbitol citrate (INCI)

Trade names: Eucarol IAS

Disodium isostearamido MIPA-sulfosuccinate (INCI)
Synonyms: Sulfobutanedioic acid, 1-[methyl-2-[(1-
oxoisooctadecyl)amino]ethyl] ester, disodium salt
Trade names: Mackanate™ ISP

Disodium laneth-5 sulfosuccinate (INCI)
CAS 68890-92-6 (generic)
Synonyms: Sulfobutanedioic acid, laneth-5 ester, diso-
dium salt
Trade names: Emery® 5327; Geropon® SB-5; Incrosul
LAFS; Rewolan® 5

Disodium lauramido MEA-sulfosuccinate (INCI)
CAS 25882-44-4; EINECS 247-310-4
Synonyms: Sulfobutanedioic acid, 1-ester with N-(2-
hydroxyethyl) dodecanamide, disodium salt
Trade names: Emcol® 5310; Geropon® SBL-203;
Mackanate™ LM-40; Rewopol® SBL 203; Varsulf®
SBL-203
Trade names containing: Marlinat® SRN 30

Disodium lauraminopropionate
Trade names containing: Miracare® MS-1; Miracare®
MS-2; Miracare® MS-4

Disodium laureth-7 citrate (INCI)
Trade names: Eucarol M

Disodium laureth sulfosuccinate (INCI)
CAS 39354-45-5 (generic); 40754-59-4; 42016-08-0;
58450-52-5; EINECS 255-062-3
Synonyms: Sulfobutanedioic acid, 4-[2-[2-[2-(dodecyl-
oxy)ethoxy]ethoxy]ethyl]ester, disodium salt; Diso-
dium lauryl ether sulfosuccinate
Trade names: Ablusol LAE; Afanate™ EL; Cosmopon
BT; Elfanol® 616; Emcol® 4403; Empicol® SDD;
Genapol® SBE; Geronol ACR/4; Geropon® ACR/4;
Geropon® SBFA-30; Geropon® SS-LA-3; Grillosol
SB3/12; Mackanate™ EL; Marlinat® SL 3/40;
Rewopol® SBFA 30; Rolpon SE 138; Schercopol
LPS; Setacin 103 Spezial; Standapol® SH-124-3;
Stepan-Mild® SL3; Surfagene S 30; Texapon® SB-3;
Varsulf® SBFA-30; Zoharpon SE
Trade names containing: Akypogene HM 12; Akypogene
HM 8; Dermalcare® 1673; Emulmetik™ 310; Lumorol
K 28; Lumorol K 5019; Rewopol® SBV; Stepan-Mild®
LSB; Surfax SLA; Texapon® MG 3; Texapon® SBN

Disodium lauriminodipropionate (INCI)
CAS 3655-00-3; EINECS 222-899-0
Synonyms: Disodium N-lauryl-β-iminodipropionate; Di-
sodium 3,3′-(dodecylimino) dipropionate; N-(2-
Carboxyethyl)-N-dodecyl-β-alanine, disodium salt
Trade names: Deriphat® 160; Monateric 1188M

Disodium lauroamphodiacetate (INCI)
CAS 14350-97-1; 68608-66-2; EINECS 238-306-3
Synonyms: 1H-Imidazolium, 1-[2-(carboxymethoxy)
ethyl]-1-carboxymethyl)-4,5-dihydro-2-undecyl-, hy-
droxide, disodium salt; Lauroamphocarboxy-
glycinate; Lauroamphodiacetate
Trade names: Afoteric™ 2L; Amphoterge® L Special;
Chimin IMZ; Empigen® CDL60; Mackam™ 2L;
Miranol® BM Conc; Miranol® H2M Conc; Monateric
949J; Rewoteric® AM 2L-40; Zoharteric DJ
Trade names containing: Carsofoam® BS-I; Compound
TL; Mackam™ 2LES; Mackam™ 2MHT; Mackam™
LOS; Mackam™ LT; Miracare® 2MHT; Miracare®
BT; Rewoteric® AM CA; Schercoteric LS-2ES MOD;
Schercoteric LS-2TE MOD; Schercoteric LS-2TE;
Velvetex® LTD

Disodium lauroamphodipropionate (INCI)
CAS 68610-43-5; 68929-04-4; 68920-18-3

Synonyms: 1H-Imidazolium,1-[2-(2-carboxyethoxy) ethyl-1-(2-carboxyethyl)-4,5-dihydro-2-undecyl-, hydroxide, disodium salt; Lauroamphocarboxypropionate; Lauroamphodipropionate
Trade names: Mackam™ 2LSF; Miranol® H2M-SF Conc; Zoharteric D-SF/L

Disodium lauryl sulfosuccinate (INCI)
CAS 13192-12-6; 19040-44-9; 26838-05-1; 26838-05-1; 36409-57-1; EINECS 248-030-5; 236-149-5
Synonyms: Sulfobutanedioic acid, 1-dodecyl ester, disodium salt
Trade names: Afanate™ LO; Beaulight SSS; Emcol® 4400-1; Empicol® SCC; Empicol® SLL; Empicol® SLL/P; Geropon® LSS; Geropon® SBF-12; Mackanate™ LO; Mackanate™ LO-100; Mackanate™ LO-Special; Monamate LA-100; Rewopol® SBF 12; Setacin F Spezial Paste; Varsulf® SBF-12; Zoharpon SA
Trade names containing: Monaterge 1164; Rhodaterge® SSB; Zetesap 5165; Zetesap 813A

Disodium malyl tyrosinate (INCI)
CAS 126139-79-5
Trade names: N,L-Malyl-L-Tyrosine

Disodium myristamido MEA-sulfosuccinate (INCI)
CAS 37767-42-3
Synonyms: Sulfobutanedioic acid, 2[(1-oxotetradecyl)amino]ethyl ester, disodium salt; Disodium monomyristamido MEA-sulfosuccinate
Trade names: Emcol® 4100M

Disodium nonoxynol-10 sulfosuccinate (INCI)
CAS 67999-57-9 (generic); 9040-38-4
Synonyms: Sulfobutanedioic acid, nonoxynol-10 ester, disodium salt
Trade names: Aerosol® A-103; Geronol ACR/9; Geropon® ACR/9; Mackanate™ A-103

Disodium oleamido MEA-sulfosuccinate (INCI)
CAS 68479-64-1; 79702-63-0; EINECS 270-864-3
Synonyms: Sulfobutanedioic acid, mono[2-[(1-oxo-9-octadecenyl)amino]ethyl]ester, disodium salt
Trade names: Mackanate™ OM; Rewopol® SBE 280; Schercopol OMS-Na

Disodium oleamido MIPA-sulfosuccinate (INCI)
CAS 43154-85-4; EINECS 256-120-0
Synonyms: Sulfobutanedioic acid, 4-[1-methyl-2-[(1-oxo-9-octadecenyl)amino]ethyl]ester, disodium salt; Disodium oleoyl isopropanolamide sulfosuccinate; Disodium monooleamido MIPA-sulfosuccinate
Trade names: Emcol® 4161L; Fizul MD-318C; Mackanate™ OP; Sole Terge 8

Disodium oleamido PEG-2 sulfosuccinate (INCI)
CAS 56388-43-3; EINECS 260-143-1
Synonyms: Sulfobutanedioic acid, C-[2-[(1-oxo-9-octadecenyl)amino]ethoxy]ethyl]ester, disodium salt; Disodium oleamido diglycol sulfosuccinate
Trade names: Afanate™ OD-28; Anionyx® 12S; Geropon® SBG-280; Mackanate™ OD-35; Monamate OPA-100; Monamate OPA-30; Standapol® SH-100; Standapol® SH-135; Texapon® SH 100; Texapon® SH-135 Special; Unipol SH-100, SH-135
Trade names containing: Mackanate™ NLD; Standapol® SHC-101

Disodium oleoamphodiacetate
CAS 97659-53-5, 70024-77-0; EINECS 307-458-3, 274-269-9
Synonyms: Oleoamphocarboxyglycinate
Trade names: Ampholak XO7

Disodium oleth-3 sulfosuccinate (INCI)

Synonyms: Sulfobutanedioic acid, oleth-3 ester, disodium salt
Trade names: Incrosul OTS

Disodium palmitamido PEG-2 sulfosuccinate (INCI)
Synonyms: Sulfobutanedioic acid, palmitamido PEG-2 ester, disodium salt
Trade names containing: Mackanate™ NLD

Disodium palmitoleamido PEG-2 sulfosuccinate (INCI)
Synonyms: Sulfobutanedioic acid, palmitoleamido PEG-2 ester, disodium salt
Trade names containing: Mackanate™ NLD

Disodium PEG-4 cocamido MIPA sulfosuccinate (INCI)
Trade names: Rewopol® SBZ

Disodium PEG-10 laurylcitrate sulfosuccinate (INCI)
Trade names: Rewopol® SBCS 50

Disodium PEG-8 ricinosuccinate (INCI)
Trade names: Grillosol 8C12
Trade names containing: Grillocin® AT Basis

Disodium ricinoleamido MEA-sulfosuccinate (INCI)
CAS 40754-60-7; 65277-54-5; 67893-42-9; EINECS 267-617-7; 265-672-1
Synonyms: Sulfobutanedioic acid, 1-[2-[(12-hydroxy-1-oxo-9-octadecenyl)amino]ethyl]ester, disodium salt; Disodium ricinoleyl monoethanolamide sulfosuccinate
Trade names: Afanate™ RM; Emcol® 4101; Geropon® SBR-3; Mackanate™ RM; Monamate RMEA-40; Rewoderm® S 1333; Varsulf® S-1333

Disodium sitostereth-14 sulfosuccinate (INCI)
Trade names: Rewoderm® SPS

Disodium stearyl sulfosuccinamate (INCI)
CAS 14481-60-8; EINECS 238-479-5
Synonyms: Sulfobutanedioic acid, monooctadecyl ester, disodium salt; Disodium octadecyl sulfosuccinamate
Trade names: Rewopol® SBF 18

Disodium tallowamido MEA-sulfosuccinate (INCI)
Trade names: Elfan® 510

Disodium tallow amphodiacetate (INCI)
Trade names: Rewoteric® AM 2T

Disodium tallowiminodipropionate (INCI)
CAS 61791-56-8; EINECS 263-190-6
Synonyms: Disodium N-tallow-β iminodipropionate; N-(2-Carboxyethyl)-N-(tallow acyl)-β-alanine
Trade names: Deriphat® 154; Deriphat® 154L; Mirataine® T2C-30

Disodium tridecylsulfosuccinate (INCI)
CAS 83147-64-2; 68133-71-1
Synonyms: Sulfobutanedioic acid, 4-tridecyl ester, disodium slat; Disodium 4-tridecyl sulfobutanedioate
Trade names: Mackanate™ TDS
Trade names containing: Antex-MPD

Disodium undecylenamido MEA-sulfosuccinate (INCI)
CAS 26650-05-5; 37311-67-4; 40839-40-5; 65277-52-3; EINECS 247-873-6
Synonyms: Sulfobutanedioic acid, 4-[2-[(1-oxo-10-undecenyl)amino]ethyl]ester, disodium salt; Disodium undecylenoyl monoethanolamide sulfosuccinate
Trade names: Afanate™ UM; Emcol® 5330; Empicol® SEE; Geropon® SBU-185; Mackanate™ UM-50; Rewocid® SBU 185; Rewocid® SBU 185 P

Disodium wheat germamido PEG-2 sulfosuccinate (INCI)
Synonyms: Sulfobutanedioic acid, C-[2-[2[(wheat germ oil amides)ethoxy]ethyl]ester, disodium salt
Trade names: Afanate™ WGD; Mackanate™ WGD

Disodium wheatgermamphodiacetate (INCI)
Trade names: Mackam™ 2W

Disoyadimonium chloride (INCI)
CAS 61788-92-9
Synonyms: Disoya dimethyl ammonium chloride; Dimethyl soya alkyl ammonium chloride; Disoya alkyl dimethyl ammonium chloride
Trade names: Arquad® 2S-75

Disoyamine (INCI)
CAS 68783-23-3; EINECS 272-190-5
Trade names: Armeen® 2S

Distarch phosphate (INCI)
CAS 55963-33-2
Synonyms: Phosphate cross-linked starch
Trade names: 28-1898

Disteareth-2 lauroyl glutamate (INCI)
Trade names: Amiter LGS-2

Disteareth-5 lauroyl glutamate (INCI)
Trade names: Amiter LGS-5

1,2-Distearoyl-sn-glycero(3) phosphatidylcholine
CAS 816-94-4
Trade names: Phospholipon® SC

Distearyldimethylamine dimerate
Trade names: Armocare® E/C 150

Distearyldimonium chloride (INCI)
CAS 107-64-2; EINECS 203-508-2
Synonyms: Distearyl dimethyl ammonium chloride; Quaternium-5; Dioctadecyl dimethyl ammonium chloride
Trade names: Ablumine DHT75; Arosurf® TA-100; Arosurf® TA-101; Dehyquart® DAM; Genamin DSAC; Kemamine® Q-9902C; Nikkol CA-3475; Protaquat 2HT-75; Sumquat® 6045; Varisoft® TA-100
Trade names containing: Genamin KSE

Distearyl phthalate
CAS 90193-76-3; EINECS 290-580-3
Trade names: Radia® 7505

Distearyl thiodipropionate (INCI)
CAS 693-36-7; EINECS 211-750-5
Synonyms: 3,3'-Thiobispropanoic acid, dioctadecyl ester; 3,3'-Dioctadecyl thiodipropionate; Thiodipropionic acid, distearyl ester
Trade names: Argus DSTDP

Distilled spirits. *See Alcohol*

Ditallowamidoethyl hydroxypropylamine
Trade names: Armocare® PA/11

Ditallowamidoethyl hydroxypropylmonium methosulfate
Trade names: Armocare® PQ/11

Ditallowamine
CAS 68783-24-4
Trade names: Armeen® 2T

Ditallow diamido methosulfate. *See Quaternium-53*

Ditallow dimonium chloride (INCI)
CAS 68153-32-2; 68783-78-8; EINECS 272-207-6
Synonyms: Ditallow dimethyl ammonium chloride; Quaternium-48; Dimethyl ditallow ammonium chloride
Trade names containing: Arquad® 2T; Varisoft® 470

Di-TEA-oleamido PEG-2 sulfosuccinate (INCI)
Trade names: Standapol® SH-300

Ditridecyl adipate (INCI)
CAS 26401-35-4; 16958-92-2; EINECS 247-660-8
Synonyms: Ditridecyl hexanedioate; Hexanedioic acid, ditridecyl ester
Trade names: Kemester® 5654

Ditridecyl dimer dilinoleate (INCI)
CAS 16958-92-2; EINECS 241-029-0
Synonyms: Ditridecyl dimerate; Dimer acid, ditridecyl ester; Ditridecyl dilinoleate
Trade names: Kemester® 3684

Ditridecyl dimonium chloride (INCI)
CAS 68910-56-5
Synonyms: Di (C12-15) alkyl dimethyl ammonium chloride
Trade names: Varisoft® 2TD

Ditridecyl sodium sulfosuccinate (INCI)
CAS 2673-22-5; EINECS 220-219-7
Synonyms: Sodium bistridecyl sulfosuccinate; Sodium ditridecyl sulfosuccinate; Sulfobutanedioic acid, 1,4-ditridecyl ester, sodium salt
Trade names: Hodag DTSS-70

DMAPA acrylates/acrylic acid/acrylonitrogens copolymer (INCI)
Trade names: Hypan® C-100

DMDM hydantoin (INCI)
CAS 6440-58-0; EINECS 229-222-8
Synonyms: 1,3-Dimethylol-5,5-dimethyl hydantoin; 2,4-Imidazolidinedione, 1,3-bis(hydroxymethyl)-5,5-dimethyl-; Dimethylol dimethyl hydantoin
Trade names: Dantoin® DMDMH-55; Dekafald; Glydant®; Glydant® XL-1000; Mackstat® DM; Nipaguard® DMDMH
Trade names containing: Glydant® Plus; Mackstat® DM-PG; Paragon™ II; Paragon™

DMHF (INCI)
CAS 9065-13-8
Synonyms: 2,4-Imidazolidinedione, dimethyl-, polymer with formaldehyde; Dimethyl hydantoin formaldehyde resin
Trade names: Dantoin® DMHF; Dantoin® DMHF-75

DMI. *See Dimethyl isosorbide*

DMOA. *See Dimethyl octylamine*

DMP. *See Dimethyl phthalate*

DNA (INCI)
CAS 9007-49-2
Synonyms: Deoxyribonucleic acid
Trade names: DNA LP; Robeco-DNA
Trade names containing: Brookosome® DNA/RNA; DNA Marine; Endonucleine LS 2143

DNA hydrolysate. *See Hydrolyzed DNA*

DOA. *See Dioctyl adipate*

Docosahexaenoic acid (INCI)
CAS 25167-62-8
Synonyms: 4,7,10,13,16,19-Docosahexaenoic acid
Trade names containing: Destressine 2000; Vitamarine

Docosanoic acid. *See Behenic acid*

1-Docosanol. *See Behenyl alcohol*

n-Dodecanoic acid. *See Lauric acid*

1-Dodecanol. *See Lauryl alcohol*

Dodecene-1
CAS 112-41-4; 6842-15-5; EINECS 203-968-4
Synonyms: C12 alpha olefin; α-Dodecylene; Tetrapropylene
Trade names: Ethyl Dodecene-1; Gulftene® 12
Trade names containing: Ethyl Dodecene-1/Tetradecene-1 Blend

Dodecyl... *See Lauryl...*

Dodecyl alcohol. *See Lauryl alcohol*

Dodecylbenzene sulfonic acid (INCI)
CAS 27176-87-0; 68411-32-5; 68584-22-5; 68608-88-8; 85536-14-7; EINECS 248-289-4
Synonyms: DDBSA
Trade names: Calsoft LAS-99; Lumosäure A; Marlon® AS3; Naxel ™AAS-98S; Reworyl® K; Rueterg SA; Witconate Acide B

Dodecylbenzyltrimonium chloride (INCI)
CAS 1330-85-4; EINECS 215-551-4
Synonyms: 4-Dodecyl-N,N,N-trimethylbenzene-methanaminium chloride; Dodecylbenzyl trimethyl ammonium chloride; Quaternium-28
Trade names containing: Hyamine® 2389

Dodecyl dimethyl ethylbenzyl ammonium chloride. *See Quaternium-14*

Dodecyl gallate (INCI)
CAS 1166-52-5; EINECS 214-620-6
Synonyms: 3,4,5-Trihydroxybenzoic acid, dodecyl ester; Dodecyl-3,4,5-trihydroxybenzoate; Lauryl gallate
Trade names: Progallin® LA

2-Dodecylhexadecanol
CAS 72388-18-2; EINECS 276-627-0
Trade names: Isofol® 28

Dodecylxylylditrimonium chloride (INCI)
Synonyms: Dodecylxylylbis(trimethyl ammonium chloride); Quaternium-29
Trade names containing: Hyamine® 2389

Dodoxynol-6 (INCI)
CAS 9014-92-0 (generic); 26401-47-8 (generic)
Synonyms: PEG-6 dodecyl phenyl ether; POE (6) dodecyl phenyl ether; PEG 300 dodecyl phenyl ether
Trade names: Desonic® 6D; Witconol™ DP60

Dodoxynol-9 (INCI)
CAS 9014-92-0 (generic); 26401-47-8 (generic)
Synonyms: PEG-9 dodecyl phenyl ether; POE (9) dodecyl phenyl ether; PEG 450 dodecyl phenyl ether
Trade names: Desonic® 9D

Dodoxynol-10
CAS 9014-92-0 (generic); 26401-47-8 (generic)
Synonyms: PEG-10 dodecyl phenyl ether; POE (10) dodecyl phenyl ether
Trade names: Desonic® 10D

Dodoxynol-12 (INCI)
CAS 9014-92-0 (generic); 26401-47-8 (generic)
Synonyms: PEG-12 dodecyl phenyl ether; POE (12) dodecyl phenyl ether; PEG 600 dodecyl phenyl ether
Trade names: Desonic® 12D

Domiphen bromide (INCI)
CAS 538-71-6; EINECS 208-702-0
Synonyms: Dodecyldimethyl (2-phenoxyethyl) ammonium bromide; 1-Dodecanaminium, N,N-dimethyl-N-(2-phenoxyethyl)-, bromide
Trade names: Fungitex R

DOTP. *See Dioctyl terephthalate*

Dried egg white. *See Albumen*

Dried egg yolk (INCI)
Trade names: Egg Yolk Solids Type Y-1

DSS. *See Dioctyl sodium sulfosuccinate*

DTPA. *See Pentetic acid*

Earth wax. *See Ceresin*

Echinacin (INCI)
Trade names containing: Lipocare HA/EC

Edathamil. *See Edetic acid*

Edetate sodium. *See Tetrasodium EDTA*

Edetic acid
CAS 60-00-4; EINECS 200-449-4
Synonyms: EDTA (INCI); N,N´-1,2-Ethanediylbis[N-(carboxymethyl) glycine]; Ethylene diamine tetra-acetic acid; Edathamil
Trade names: Hamp-Ene® Acid; Kelate Acid; Sequestrene® AA; Universene ACID; Versene Acid

EDTA (INCI). *See Edetic acid*

EE. *See Ethoxyethanol*

EEA. *See Ethoxyethanol acetate*

EGDS. *See Glycol disterate*

Egg albumin. *See Albumen*

Egg oil (INCI)
CAS 8001-17-0; EINECS 232-271-8
Synonyms: Oil of egg
Trade names: EmCon E-5

Egg yolk extract (INCI)
Trade names containing: Lecithin Ex Ovo; Tensami 8/09

EGMS. *See Glycol stearate*

Eicosanol. *See Arachidyl alcohol*

Eicosanyl propanoate. *See Arachidyl propionate*

Eicosapentaenoic acid (INCI)
CAS 10417-94-4
Synonyms: 5,8,11,14,17-Eicosapentaenoic acid
Trade names containing: Destressine 2000; Vitamarine

5,8,11,14-Eicosatetraenoic acid. *See Arachidonic acid*

Eicosyl erucate
Trade names: Pelemol EE

Elastin (INCI)
Trade names: Bovine Native Insoluble Elastin; Kelisema Bovine Natural Insoluble Elastin; Unipro ELAST CLR

Elastin, hydrolyzed. *See Hydrolyzed elastin*

Elm bark extract (INCI)
Synonyms: Ulmus camperstris extract
Trade names containing: Babyderme HS 342; Babyderme LS 642

Embryo extract (INCI)
Trade names containing: Lipotrofina M

Emulsifying wax NF
CAS 97069-99-0
Trade names: Cera-E; Emerwax® 1257; Emulgade® C; Hetoxol P; Polawax®; Polawax® A31; T-Wax; Uniwax C

English Fullers earth. *See Fullers earth*

Epidermin
Trade names: Unipro Epidermin/Oil Disp; Unipro Epidermin/Water Disp

Epoxidized soybean oil (INCI)
CAS 8013-07-8; EINECS 232-391-0
Synonyms: Soybean oil, epoxidized
Trade names: Epoxyweichmacher LSB

Erucalkonium chloride (INCI)
CAS 90730-68-0
Synonyms: N-13-Docosenyl-N,N-dimethylbenzene-methanaminium chloride
Trade names: Kemamine® BQ-2982B

Erucamidopropyl hydroxysultaine (INCI)
Trade names: Crosultaine E-30

Erucyl erucate (INCI)
CAS 27640-89-7; EINECS 248-587-4

Synonyms: 13-Docosenyl 13-docosenoate; 13-Docosenoic acid, 13-docosenyl ester
Trade names: Kemester® EE
Trade names containing: Scheroba Oil

Erucyl oleate (INCI)
CAS 85617-81-8
Synonyms: 13-Docosenyl 9-octadecenoate; 9-Octadecenoic acid, 13-docosenyl ester
Trade names containing: L.C.R.E.

Erythorbic acid (INCI)
CAS 89-65-6; EINECS 201-928-0
Synonyms: D-Erythro-hex-2-enonic acid, γ-lactone; Isoascorbic acid
Trade names: Uantox EBATE

Esculin (INCI)
CAS 531-75-9; EINECS 208-517-5
Trade names containing: Complexe AV.a.; Extrait No. 30

Ethanoic acid. *See Acetic acid*

Ethanol. *See Alcohol*

Ethene, homopolymer. *See Polyethylene*

Ethiodized oil (INCI)
CAS 8008-53-5
Trade names: Iodorga

Ethoxydiglycol (INCI)
CAS 111-90-0; EINECS 203-919-7
Synonyms: Diethylene glycol monoethyl ether; "Carbitol"; 2-(2-Ethoxyethoxy) ethanol
Trade names: Ektasolve® DE; Solvent APV Spec; Transcutol
Trade names containing: Arlenfil 4015; Biobranil Watersoluble 2/012600; Calenfil 3646; Camofil 4064; Cremogen AF; Cremogen Aloe Vera; Cremogen Camomile Forte; Cremogen Chamomile 739012; Cremogen Hamamelis 739008; Cremogen M-I 739001; Cremogen Pine Needles 739007; Cremogen Yarrow 739017; Dragocid Forte 2/027045; Extract Arnica Special; Extrapone Arnica Special 2/032591; Extrapone Bio-Tamin Special 2/2032671; Extrapone Chamomile Special 2/033021; Extrapone Hamamelis Super 2/500010; Extrapone Neo-H-Special 2/032441; Extrapone Poly H Special 2/032451; Kerafix 620; Lecithin Ex Ovo; Marlowet® RNP/K; Simulsol 5719

Ethoxydiglycol acetate (INCI)
CAS 112-15-2; EINECS 203-940-1
Synonyms: Diethylene glycol monoethyl ether acetate; 2-(2-Ethoxyethoxy)ethanol acetate
Trade names: Carbitol® Acetate; Ektasolve® DE Acetate

Ethoxyethanol (INCI)
CAS 110-80-5; EINECS 203-804-1
Synonyms: EE; Ethylene glycol ethyl ether; 2-Ethoxyethanol; ôCellosolveö
Trade names: Cellosolve®

Ethoxyethanol acetate (INCI)
CAS 111-15-9; EINECS 203-839-2
Synonyms: EEA; Ethylene glycol ethyl ether acetate; 2-Ethoxyethanol acetate; 2-Ethoxyethyl acetate
Trade names: Cellosolve® Acetate

4-Ethoxy-m-phenylenediamine sulfate (INCI)
CAS 68015-98-5; EINECS 268-164-8
Synonyms: 4-Ethoxy-1,3-benzenediamine sulfate; 1,3-Benzenediamine, 4-ethoxy-, sulfate
Trade names: Rodol EOX

Ethyl acrylate
Trade names containing: Rohagum® MB-319

Ethyl alcohol. *See Alcohol*

Ethyl alcohol, undenatured. *See Alcohol*

3-Ethylamino-p-cresol sulfate (INCI)
CAS 68239-79-2; EINECS 269-473-0
Synonyms: 3-(Ethylamino)-4-methyl phenol sulfate (2:1); 2-Hydroxyethyl-2-amino-4-hydroxytoluene sulfate
Trade names: Rodol EACS

Ethyl aspartate (INCI)
CAS 4070-43-3; 21860-85-5; 7361-28-6; EINECS 223-779-0
Synonyms: Aspartic acid, ethyl ester
Trade names containing: Polyaminon-3

p-Ethylbenzaldehyde
CAS 4748-78-1; EINECS 225-268-8
Trade names: Ebal

7-Ethyl bicyclooxazxolidine (INCI)
CAS 7747-35-5; EINECS 231-810-4

Ethyl butylacetylaminopropionate (INCI)
CAS 52304-36-6; EINECS 257-835-0
Trade names: Insect repellent 3535, No. 11887

Ethyl-2-t-butylcyclohexylcarbonate
Trade names: Floramat

Ethyl butyl valerolactone (INCI)
CAS 67770-79-0; EINECS 267-048-4
Trade names: Costaulon
Trade names containing: Costausol

Ethylcellulose (INCI)
CAS 9004-57-3
Synonyms: Cellulose, ethyl ether; Ethocel
Trade names: Ethocel Medium Premium; Ethocel Standard Premium
Trade names containing: Brillance 515

3-Ethyl-2,4-dioxaspiro (5.5) undec-8-ene
Trade names: Spiroflor

Ethylene/acrylic acid copolymer (INCI)
CAS 9010-77-9
Trade names: A-C® 143; A-C® 540, 540A; A-C® 580; A-C® 5120; EA-209

Ethylene alcohol. *See Glycol*

Ethylene bisstearamide. *See Ethylene distearamide*

Ethylene brassylate (INCI)
CAS 105-95-3; EINECS 203-347-8
Synonyms: 1,4-Dioxacycloheptadecane-5,17-dione; Ethylene undecane dicarboxylate
Trade names: Emeressence® 1150

Ethylene/calcium acrylate copolymer (INCI)
CAS 26445-96-5
Trade names: AClyn® 201; AClyn® 201A

Ethylene distearamide (INCI)
CAS 110-30-5, 68955-45-3; EINECS 203-755-6, 273-277-0
Synonyms: N,N´-Ethylene bisstearamide; N,N´-1,2-Ethanediylbisoctadecanamide
Trade names: Kemamide® W-35; Kemamide® W-42; Radia® 7506

Ethylene glycol. *See Glycol*

Ethylene glycol butyl ether. *See Butoxyethanol*

Ethylene glycol ethyl ether. *See Ethoxyethanol*

Ethylene glycol 2-ethylhexyl ether
CAS 1559-35-9
Trade names: Ektasolve® EEH

Ethylene glycol propyl ether
CAS 2807-30-9

Synonyms: Propyl "Cellosolve"; 2-Propoxyethanol; Ethylene glycol monopropyl ether
Trade names: Ektasolve® EP

Ethylene/magnesium acrylate copolymer (INCI)
Trade names: AClyn® 246; AClyn® 246A

Ethylene/propylene copolymer (INCI)
CAS 9010-79-1
Synonyms: Ethene, polymer with 1-propene; 1-Propene, polymer with ethene
Trade names: Petrolite® CP-7; Siltek® L

Ethylene/sodium acrylate copolymer (INCI)
CAS 25750-82-7
Trade names: AClyn® 262A; AClyn® 272, 276, 285; AClyn® 272A; AClyn® 276A; AClyn® 285A

Ethylene/VA copolymer (INCI)
CAS 24937-78-8
Synonyms: EVA copolymer; Ethylene/vinyl acetate copolymer; Acetic acid, ethenyl ester, polymer with ethene
Trade names: A-C® 400; A-C® 400A; A-C® 405M; A-C® 405S; A-C® 405T; A-C® 430; Elvax® 40P

Ethylene/zinc acrylate copolymer (INCI)
Trade names: AClyn® 291, 293, 295; AClyn® 291A; AClyn® 293A; AClyn® 295A

Ethyl ester of hydrolyzed silk. *See Hydrolyzed silk ethyl ester*

Ethyl glutamate (INCI)
CAS 1119-33-1; EINECS 214-274-6
Synonyms: 5-Ethyl-L-glutamate; L-Glutamic acid, 5-ethyl ester
Trade names containing: Polyaminon-3

Ethyl hexanediol (INCI)
CAS 94-96-2; EINECS 202-377-9
Synonyms: Ethohexadiol; 2-Ethyl-1,3-hexanediol; Ethyl hexylene glycol
Trade names containing: Lanoquat® 1756; Lanoquat® 1757; Unirep U-18

2-Ethylhexyl .... *See Octyl ...*

2-Ethylhexylamine
CAS 104-75-6
Synonyms: 2-Ethyl-1-hexylamine; Octylamine
Trade names: Armeen® L8D

2-Ethyl hexyl isostearae
Trade names: Prisorine EHIS 2036

2-Ethylhexyl oleate
Trade names: Radia® 7331

Ethyl hydroxyethyl cellulose. *See Hydroxyethyl ethylcellulose*

Ethyl hydroxymethyl oleyl oxazoline (INCI)
CAS 68140-98-7; 88543-32-2; EINECS 268-820-3
Synonyms: 4-Ethyl-2-(8-heptadecenyl)-4,5-dihydro-4-oxazolemethanol
Trade names: Alkaterge®-E

Ethyl laurate (INCI)
CAS 106-33-2; EINECS 203-386-0
Synonyms: Dodecanoic acid, ethyl ester
Trade names containing: Dermol QE

Ethyl linoleate (INCI)
CAS 544-35-4; EINECS 208-868-4
Synonyms: Linoleic acid ethyl ester; Vitamin F
Trade names: Nikkol VF-E; Safester A-75
Trade names containing: Dermol QE; Safester A 75 WS; Unibiovit B-33; Unibiovit B-332; Univit-F ETHES; Vitamin F Ethyl Ester CLR

Ethyl linolenate (INCI)
CAS 1191-41-9; EINECS 214-734-6
Trade names containing: Vitamin F Ethyl Ester CLR

Ethyl methacrylate (INCI)
CAS 97-63-2; EINECS 202-597-5
Synonyms: Ethyl 2-methyl-2-propenoate; Ethyl-α-methyl acrylate
Trade names: Rohagum® N-742
Trade names containing: Rohagum® N-80

Ethyl morrhuate (INCI)
Synonyms: Cod liver oil, ethyl ester
Trade names: Liponate EM

Ethyl myristate (INCI)
CAS 124-06-1; EINECS 204-675-4
Synonyms: Ethyl tetradecanoate; Tetradecanoic acid, ethyl ester
Trade names containing: Dermol QE

Ethyl oleate (INCI)
CAS 111-62-6, 85049-36-1; EINECS 203-889-5, 285-206-0
Trade names: Elfacos® EO; Estol ETO 3659; Kessco EO; Radia® 7187
Trade names containing: Dermol QE; Univit-F ETHES; Vitamin F Ethyl Ester CLR

Ethyl oliveoleate
Trade names: Nikkol EOO

Ethyl palmitate (INCI)
CAS 628-97-2
Synonyms: Ethyl hexadecanoate; Hexadecanoic acid, ethyl ester
Trade names: Cithrol EP
Trade names containing: Dermol QE

Ethyl panthenol
Trade names: Ethyl Panthenol No. 26100

Ethylparaben (INCI)
CAS 120-47-8; EINECS 204-399-4
Synonyms: Ethyl 4-hydroxybenzoate; Ethyl p-hydroxybenzoate; Ethyl parahydroxybenzoate
Trade names: Aethyl-Steriline; Bentex E; CoSept E; Lexgard® E; Nipagin A; Paridol E; Preserval E; Trisept E; Unisept E
Trade names containing: Bactericide MB 2/012582; Bactiphen 2506 G; Dekaben; Nipastat; Phenonip; Sepicide HB; Sepicide MB; Talcoseptic C; Undebenzofene C; Uniphen P-23

Ethyl PEG-15 cocamine sulfate (INCI)
Trade names: Antaron® PC-37

Ethyl phthalate. *See Diethyl phthalate*

Ethyl serinate (INCI)
CAS 4117-31-1
Trade names containing: Polyaminon-15

Ethyl stearate (INCI)
CAS 111-61-5, 91031-43-5; EINECS 203-887-4, 292-945-2'
Synonyms: Ethyl octadecanoate; Octadecanoic acid, ethyl ester
Trade names: Cithrol ES; Hefti AMS-33; Radia® 7185

Ethyl urocanate (INCI)
CAS 27538-35-8; EINECS 248-515-1
Synonyms: 3-(1H-Imidazol-4-yl)-2-propenoic acid, ethyl ester; 2-Propenoic acid, 3-(1H-imidazol-4-yl)-, ethyl ester
Trade names: Parasonarl Mark II

Ethyl vanillin (INCI)
CAS 121-32-4; EINECS 204-464-7

Synonyms: 3-Ethoxy-4-hydroxybenzaldehyde; Benzaldehyde, 3-ethoxy-4-hydroxy-
Trade names: Unisweet EVAN

Etidronic acid (INCI)
CAS 2809-21-4; EINECS 220-552-8
Synonyms: (1-Hydroxyethylidene) bisphosphonic acid
Trade names: Turpinal® SL; Unitex P

Etocrylene (INCI)
CAS 5232-99-5; EINECS 226-029-0
Synonyms: Ethyl 2-cyano-3,3-diphenylacrylate; Ethyl 2-cyano-3,3-diphenyl-2-propenoate; UV Absorber-2
Trade names: Uvinul® N 35

EtOH. *See Alcohol*

Eucalyptus extract (INCI)
CAS 84625-32-1
Synonyms: Eucalyptus globulus extract
Trade names containing: Actiphyte of Eucalyptus; Blend For Deodorant HS 275; Eucalyptus HS; Eucalyptus Leaves Extract HS 2646 G; Eucalyptus LS; Herbasol-Extract Eucalyptus

Eucalyptus oil (INCI)
CAS 8000-48-4
Synonyms: Dinkum oil
Trade names: EmCon Eucalyptus
Trade names containing: Essentiaderm n.1; Eucalyptus-Extract, Water soluble 4786

EVA copolymer. *See Ethylene/VA copolymer*

Evening primrose oil (INCI)
Synonyms: Oil of Evening Primrose
Trade names: CoPrimrose; E.P.O; Efamol Evening Primrose Oil; Super Refined™ Crossential EPO
Trade names containing: Bio-Oil GLA-10; Brookosome® EPO; Dermasome® EPO

Everlasting extract (INCI)
CAS 90045-56-0
Trade names: Elicrisina

Faba bean extract (INCI)
Synonyms: Vicia faba extract
Trade names containing: Demaquillant LS 687; Nutriderme HS 313; Nutriderme LS 613

Fagus silvatica extract (INCI)
Trade names: Gatuline® R

Farnesol (INCI)
CAS 4602-84-0; EINECS 225-004-1
Synonyms: Trimethyl dodecatrienol
Trade names: Dragoco Farnesol
Trade names containing: Unibiovit B-33; Unibiovit B-332; Unitrienol T-27; Unitrienol T-272

Farnesyl acetate (INCI)
CAS 29548-30-9; EINECS 249-689-1
Synonyms: 2,6,10-Dodecatrien-1-ol, 3,7,11-trimethyl-, acetate; 3,7,11-Trimethyl-2,6,10-dodecatrien-1-ol, acetate
Trade names containing: Unibiovit B-33; Unibiovit B-332; Unitrienol T-27; Unitrienol T-272

FD&C blue no. 1 aluminum lake (INCI)
CAS 53026-57-6; 68921-42-6
Trade names containing: Blue 135

Fennel extract (INCI)
CAS 84625-39-8; 85085-33-2
Synonyms: Extract of fennel; Foeniculum extract; Foeniculum vulgare extract
Trade names: Hydroplastidine Foeniculum
Trade names containing: Bio-Chelated Sauna-Derm I; Hexaplant Richter; Sedaplant Richter

Fenugreek extract (INCI)
CAS 68990-15-8
Synonyms: Trigonella foenungraecum extract
Trade names containing: Blend For Bust Cares HS 201; Capilotonique HS 220; Nutriderme HS 240; Nutriderme HS 243; Nutriderme LS 640

Ferric ammonium ferrocyanide (INCI)
CAS 25869-00-5; 12240-15-2
Synonyms: Iron blue
Trade names containing: Bicrona® Iron Blue; Chroma-Lite® Dark Blue 4501; Ferric Blue 107; Ferric Blue 114

Ferric ferrocyanide (INCI)
CAS 14038-43-8; EINECS 237-875-5
Synonyms: Prussian blue
Trade names: Bleu De Prusse Pur W 745; Cogilor Sapphire
Trade names containing: Bleu Covachip W 6700; Bleu De Prusse Micronise W 6805; Cloisonné Blue; Cloisonné Violet; Colorona® Light Blue; Dichrona® BG; Dichrona® BR; Dichrona® BY; Dichrona® GY; Duocrome® BG; Duocrome® GY; Gemtone® Amethyst; Gemtone® Emerald; Gemtone® Mauve Quartz

Ferrous gluconate
CAS 299-29-6
Synonyms: Iron gluconate; Niconate
Trade names: Gluconal® FE

Fibronectin (INCI)
Trade names: Fibronex
Trade names containing: Bovine Fibronectin Sol'n; Tri-Pronectin

Fibronectin hydrolysate. *See Hydrolyzed fibronectin*

Fischer-Tropsch wax. *See Synthetic wax*

Fish extract (INCI)
CAS 97615-94-6
Trade names containing: Nutrimarine

Fish glycerides (INCI)
CAS 100085-40-3
Trade names containing: Ross Japan Wax Substitute 473; Ross Japan Wax Substitute 525

Flavaxin. *See Riboflavin*

Flaxseed extract. *See Linseed extract*

Formaldehyde ethyl cyclo dodecyl acetal
Trade names: Boisambrene Forte

Fossil wax. *See Ozokerite*

Frankincense. *See Olibanum*

Fructose (INCI)
CAS 57-48-7 (D-form); EINECS 200-333-3
Synonyms: Levulose; D-Fructose
Trade names containing: Aquaderm; Hygroplex HHG; Lactil®; Sweetrex®

Fucus extract
Trade names containing: Brookosome® FIH

Fullers earth (INCI). *See also Attapulgite*
CAS 8031-18-3
Synonyms: English Fullers earth
Trade names: BC

GAG. *See Glycosaminoglycans*

Gallic acid (INCI)
CAS 149-91-7; EINECS 205-749-9
Synonyms: 3,4,5-Trihydroxybenzoic acid
Trade names containing: Ectrait Hamamelis LC 452

Gardenia extract (INCI)
Synonyms: Cape jasmine extract; Gardenia jasminoides extract
Trade names containing: Gadeneel Liq.

Garlic extract (INCI)
CAS 8008-99-9; EINECS 232-371-1
Synonyms: Allium sativum extract
Trade names containing: Actiphyte of Garlic; Garionzet; Garlic Extract HS 2710 G

Gelatin (INCI)
CAS 9000-70-8; EINECS 232-554-6
Synonyms: Gelatine
Trade names: Byco A; Byco C; Byco O; Colla-Gel AC; Cosmetic Gelatin; Crodyne BY-19; HiPure Liq. Gelatin, Cosmetic Grade; Hydrocoll AG-SD; Hydrocoll™ G-40; Hydrocoll™ G-55; Hydrocoll PGA, PGB

Gelatin/keratin amino acids/lysine hydroxypropyltrimonium chloride (INCI)
Trade names: Flexiquat

Gelatin/lysine/polyacrylamide hydroxypropyltrimonium chloride (INCI)
Trade names: Flexiquat B

Gellan gum (INCI)
CAS 71010-52-1
Synonyms: Gum gellan
Trade names: Kelco-Gel® Gellan Gum

Gentian extract (INCI)
CAS 97676-22-7
Synonyms: Gentiana iutea extract; Gentian root extract
Trade names containing: Herbaliquid Alpine Herbs Special; Herbasol Alpine Herbs Complex

Ginger oil (INCI)
CAS 8007-08-7
Trade names: EmCon Ginger
Trade names containing: Fitoestesina

Gingilli oil. *See Sesame oil*

Ginkgo extract (INCI)
CAS 90045-36-6
Synonyms: Ginkgo biloba extract; Maidenhair extract
Trade names containing: Actiplex™ 745; Fancol Gingko Extract; Ichou Liq.

Ginseng extract (INCI)
CAS 90045-38-8
Trade names: Ginseng Vegebios
Trade names containing: Actiphyte of Ginseng; Actiplex™ 745; Bio-Chelated Derma-Plex I; Ginseng Extract HS 2457 G; Ginseng Glycolysat; Ginseng HS; Ginseng LS; Ginseng Oleat M; Glycolysat de ginseng; Guineshing-LV; Herbasol-Extract Ginseng

Glucamine (INCI)
CAS 488-43-7; EINECS 207-677-3
Synonyms: 1-Amino-1-deoxy-D-glucitol; Glycamine
Trade names: Desamina

β-Glucan
Trade names containing: Ritavena™ 5

D-Glucitol. *See Sorbitol*

Glucosamine (INCI)
CAS 3416-24-8; EINECS 222-311-2
Synonyms: 2-Amino-2-deoxyglucose
Trade names containing: Seanamin BD; Seanamin TH

Glucose (INCI)
CAS 50-99-7 (anhydrous), 5996-10-1 (hydrous); EINECS 200-075-1, 207-757-8
Synonyms: Dextrose; Grape sugar; Corn sugar

Trade names: Candex® Plus; Emdex® Plus
Trade names containing: Candex®; Emdex®; Extrapone Chamomile Special 2/033021; Extrapone Hamamelis Super 2/500010; Hydrolyzed NMF; Hygroplex HHG; Myavert C; Sweetrex®; Trichogen

Glucose glutamate (INCI)
Trade names: Wickenol® 545

Glucose oxidase (INCI)
CAS 9001-37-0; EINECS 232-601-0
Synonyms: Oxidase, glucose
Trade names containing: Capigen CG; Myavert C; Sebomine SB12

Glucose tyrosinate
Trade names: Actibronze; Instabronze; Sun-Tanning Bioactivator AMI, VITAMI

L-Glutamic acid (INCI)
CAS 56-86-0; EINECS 200-293-7
Synonyms: L-Glutamic acid; L-2-Aminoglutaric acid; 2-Aminopentanedioic acid
Trade names: Unamino GLUT
Trade names containing: Hydro-Diffuser Microreservoir; Hygroplex HHG; Omega-CH Activator

Glutaral (INCI)
CAS 111-30-8; EINECS 203-856-5
Synonyms: Glutaraldehyde; Glutaric dialdehyde; Pentanedial
Trade names: Ucarcide® 225; Ucarcide® 250

Glutaraldehyde. *See Glutaral*

Glycereth-7 (INCI)
CAS 31694-55-0 (generic)
Synonyms: PEG-7 glyceryl ether; POE (7) glyceryl ether
Trade names: Extan G-7; Hetoxide G-7; Liponic EG-7; Protachem GL-7

Glycereth-12 (INCI)
CAS 31694-55-0 (generic)
Synonyms: PEG-12 glyceryl ether; PEG 600 glyceryl ether; POE (12) glyceryl ether
Trade names: Hodag POE (12) Glycerine; Unipeg-ETG-12

Glycereth-20 (INCI)
CAS 31694-55-0 (generic)
Synonyms: PEG-20 glyceryl ether; PZEG 1000 glyceryl ether; POE (20) glyceryl ether
Trade names: Carbowax® TPEG 990

Glycereth-26 (INCI)
CAS 31694-55-0 (generic)
Synonyms: PEG-26 glyceryl ether; POE (26) glyceryl ether
Trade names: Acconon ETG; Ethosperse® G-26; Extan G-26; Hetoxide G-26; Hodag POE (26) Glycerine; Liponic EG-1; Protachem GL-26; Unipeg-ETG-26

Glycereth-7 benzoate (INCI)
CAS 125804-12-8
Synonyms: PEG-7 glyceryl ether benzoate; POE (7) glyceryl ether benzoate
Trade names: Dermol G-76; Pelemol G7B

Glycereth-7 diisononanoate (INCI)
CAS 125804-15-1
Synonyms: PEG-7 glyceryl ether diisononanoate; POE (7) glyceryl ether diisononanoate
Trade names: Dermol G-7DI
Trade names containing: Dermol MO

Glycereth-7.5 hydroxystearate (INCI)
CAS 138314-11-1
Trade names: Dermolan GLH

Glycereth-5 lactate (INCI)
CAS 125804-13-9
Synonyms: PEG-5 glyceryl ether lactate; POE (5) glyceryl ether lactate
Trade names: Estalan L-45; Pelemol G45L

Glycereth-25 PCA isostearate (INCI)
Synonyms: PEG-25 glyceryl ether PCA isostearate
Trade names: Pyroter GPI-25

Glycereth-26 phosphate (INCI)
Trade names: Crodafos G26A

Glycereth-7 triacetate (INCI)
CAS 57569-76-3
Synonyms: PEG-7 glyceryl ether triacetate; POE (7) glyceryl ether triacetate
Trade names: Dermol GL-7A; Pelemol G7A

Glycerin (INCI)
CAS 56-81-5; EINECS 200-289-5
Synonyms: Glycerol; 1,2,3-Propanetriol; Glycerine
Trade names: Croderol GA 7000; Emery® 912; Emery® 916; Emery® 917; Emery® 918; Glycon® G 100; Glycon® G-300; Kemstrene® 96.0% USP; Kemstrene® 99.7% USP; Optim; Star; Superol; Unichem GLYC
Trade names containing: Amisol™ 406-N; Amisol™ 688; Antex-MP; Antex-MPD; Anti-MB; Bovine Amniotic Liq.; Capigen CG; Capisome; Chronosphere® G; Complexe DM 60; Dermocalmine; Dermosaccharides® GY; Dermosaccharides® HC; Dermosaccharides® SEA; Desaron; DF-100; DNA Marine; EFA-Plexol; Elespher® Dermosaccharides GY; Elespher® Dermosaccharides HC; Endomine NMF; Endonucleine LS 2143; Euperlan® PK 3000 OK; Euperlan® PK 3000 OK; Extrait No. 30; Facteur Hydratant PH; Fibrastil; Fibrostimuline P; Fishlan LS; FRS-Diffuser Microreservoir; Grillocin AT Basis; Grillocin® AT Basis; Hispagel® 100; Hispagel® 200; Hormo Fruit Apricot; Hormo Fruit Pineapple; Hydro-Diffuser Microreservoir; Hydromarine; Hydroviton 2/059353; Keratolan; Killitol; Leniplex; Lipo PE Base G-55; Lipo PE Base GP-55; Lipo-Peptide AME 30; Liposome Centella; Liposome Unsapo KM; Lipostim; Manro CD/G; Microsponge® 5647; Miracare® BC-20; Mirasheen® 202; Nikkol Aquasome LA; Peptidyl; Seanamin FP; Sedermasome; Sphingosomes® AL; Texapon® SG; Thermoplex; Unimoist U-125; UV-Titan M212

Glycerin/oxybutylene copolymer stearyl ether (INCI)
Trade names: Hyglyol S-26

Glycerol. *See Glycerin*

Glycerophosphocholine
CAS 28319-77-9
Trade names: GPC

Glyceryl abietate (INCI)
CAS 1337-89-9
Synonyms: Abietic acid, glyceryl ester
Trade names: Abietate de Glycerol

Glyceryl adipate (INCI)
CAS 26699-71-8; EINECS 247-911-1
Synonyms: Hexanedioic acid, monoester with 1,2,3-propanetriol
Trade names: Trioxene A

Glyceryl alginate (INCI)
Synonyms: Alginic acid, glyceryl ester
Trade names: Karajel

Glyceryl behenate (INCI)
CAS 6916-74-1, 30233-64-8; EINECS 250-097-0

Trade names: Compritol 888 ATO; Glyceryl Behenate WL 251

Glyceryl caprate (INCI)
CAS 26402-22-2; EINECS 247-667-6
Synonyms: Glyceryl monocaprate; Decanoic acid, monoester with 1,2,3-propanetriol
Trade names: Imwitor® 310; Imwitor® 910

Glyceryl caprylate (INCI)
CAS 26402-26-6; EINECS 247-668-1
Synonyms: Glyceryl monocaprylate; Octanoic acid, monoester with 1,2,3-propanetriol; Monooctanoin
Trade names: Imwitor® 308; Imwitor® 908; Imwitor® 988

Glyceryl caprylate/caprate (INCI)
Trade names: Capmul® MCM; Capmul® MCM-90; Estol GMCC 3602; Tegin® 4600 NSE

Glyceryl citrate/lactate/linoleate/oleate (INCI)
Trade names: Imwitor® 375

Glyceryl cocoate (INCI)
CAS 61789-05-7; EINECS 263-027-9
Synonyms: Glycerides, coconut oil mono-; Glycerol mono coconut oil; Glyceryl coconate
Trade names: Imwitor® 928
Trade names containing: Softisan® 601

Glyceryl collagenate (INCI)
CAS 9007-34-5
Trade names: Colla-Moist™ CG

Glyceryl dilaurate (INCI)
CAS 27638-00-2; EINECS 248-586-9
Synonyms: Dilaurin; Dodecanoic acid, diester with 1,2,3-propanetriol
Trade names: Capmul® GDL; Cithrol GDL N/E; Emulsynt® GDL; Kemester® GDL; Kessco® Glycerol Dilaurate; Lexemul® GDL; Liponate GDL
Trade names containing: Isolene

Glyceryl dilaurate SE
Trade names: Cithrol GDL S/E

Glyceryl dimyristate (INCI)
CAS 53563-63-6; EINECS 258-629-3
Trade names containing: Isolene

Glyceryl dioleate (INCI)
CAS 25637-84-7; EINECS 247-144-2
Synonyms: 9-Octadecenoic acid, diester with 1,2,3-propanetriol
Trade names: Cithrol GDO N/E; Kessco® Glycerol Dioleate; Nikkol DGO-80

Glyceryl dioleate SE
Trade names: Cithrol GDO S/E

Glyceryl dipalmitate (INCI)
CAS 26657-95-4; EINECS 247-886-7
Trade names containing: Isolene

Glyceryl distearate (INCI)
CAS 1323-83-7; EINECS 215-359-0
Synonyms: Octadecanoic acid, diester with 1,2,3-propanetriol
Trade names: Cithrol GDS N/E; Estol GDS 3748; Kessco® GDS 386F; Kessco® Glycerol Distearate 386F; Nikkol DGS-80; Unitolate GDS
Trade names containing: Isolene

Glyceryl distearate SE
Trade names: Cithrol GDS S/E

Glyceryl di/tristearate
Trade names: Precirol WL 2155 ATO

Glyceryl erucate (INCI)
CAS 28063-42-5; EINECS 248-812-6

Trade names: Crodamol GE

Glyceryl hydroxystearate (INCI)
CAS 1323-42-8; EINECS 215-355-9
Synonyms: Glyceryl 12-hydroxystearate; Hydroxystearic acid, monoester with glycerol
Trade names: Crodamol GHS; Naturechem® GMHS
Trade names containing: Cutina® BW; Unitina BW

Glyceryl isostearate (INCI)
CAS 32057-14-0; 66085-00-5; 61332-02-3; EINECS 262-710-9, 266-124-4
Synonyms: Glyceryl monoisostearate; Isooctadecanoic acid, monoester with 1,2,3-propanetriol
Trade names: Emalex GWIS-100; Emerest® 2410; Nikkol MGIS; Peceol Isostearique; Prisorine GMIS 2040; Schercemol GMIS; Unitolate ISOST; Witconol™ 2410
Trade names containing: Base PL 1630; Gilugel R; Hydrolactol 70; Hydrolactol 93; Protegin® W; Protegin® WX

Glyceryl lanolate (INCI)
CAS 97404-50-7
Synonyms: Glyceryl monolanolate; Lanolin acid, monoester with 1,2,3-propanetriol
Trade names: Ivarlan™ 3360; Lanesta G

Glyceryl laurate (INCI)
CAS 142-18-7; EINECS 205-526-6
Synonyms: Glyceryl monolaurate; Dodecanoic acid, monoester with 1,2,3-propanetriol; Dodecanoic acid, 2,3-dihydroxypropyl ester
Trade names: Cithrol GML N/E; CPH-34-N; Estol GML 3614; Grillomuls L90; Hodag GML; Imwitor® 312; Kessco® Glycerol Monolaurate; Lauricidin 802, 812, 1012, E; Monomuls® 90-L12; Protachem MLD
Trade names containing: Acconon CON; Crosterol SFA; Lamesoft® LMG; Lamesoft® LMG/NP; Tego®-Betaine HS

Glyceryl laurate/oleate (INCI)
Trade names containing: Trilipidina

Glyceryl laurate SE (INCI)
Trade names: Aldo® MLD; Cithrol GML S/E

Glyceryl linoleate (INCI)
CAS 2277-28-3; EINECS 218-901-4
Synonyms: Monolinolein; 9,12-Octadecadienoic acid, 2,3-dihydroxypropyl ester; 9,12-Octadecadienoic acid, monoester with 1,2,3-propanetriol
Trade names: Dimodan LS Kosher
Trade names containing: Univit-F Glyest CLR; Vitamin F Glyceryl Ester CLR

Glyceryl linolenate (INCI)
CAS 18465-99-1; EINECS 242-347-2
Synonyms: 2,3-Dihydroxypropyl 9,12,15-octadecatrienoate; Glyceryl monolinolenate
Trade names containing: Univit-F Glyest CLR; Vitamin F Glyceryl Ester CLR

Glyceryl mono/dioleate
CAS 25496-72-4
Trade names: Aldo® MO FG

Glyceryl mono/distearate
Trade names: Teginacid® H-SE; Teginacid® SE

Glyceryl myristate (INCI)
CAS 589-68-4; 67701-33-1
Synonyms: Glyceryl monomyristate; Monomyristin; Tetradecanoic acid, monoester with 1,2,3-propanetriol
Trade names: Cithrol GMM; Glyceryl Myristate WL 2130; Hefti GMM-33; Imwitor® 914; Kessco GMN; Nikkol

MGM

Glyceryl oleate (INCI)
CAS 111-03-5; 37220-82-9; EINECS 203-827-7; 253-407-2
Synonyms: Glyceryl monooleate; Monoolein; 9-Octadecenoic acid, monoester with 1,2,3-propanetriol
Trade names: Aldo® MO; Atsurf 594; Capmul® GMO; Cithrol GMO N/E; CPH-31-N; Drewmulse® 85K; Drewmulse® GMO; Dur-Em® 114; Dur-Em® GMO; Elfacos® GMO; Estol 1407; Estol GTOveg 3665; Grillomuls O60; Grillomuls O90; Hodag GMO; Hodag GMO-D; Kemester® 2000; Kessco GMO; Kessco® Glycerol Monoleate; Mazol® 300 K; Mazol® GMO; Mazol® GMO K; Monomuls® 90-O18; Nikkol MGO; Peceol; Radiasurf® 7150; Radiasurf® 7152; Rol MOG; Tegin® O; Unitina GMO; Witconol™ 2421
Trade names containing: Amisol™ 406-N; Arlacel® 186; Atmos 300; Dehymuls® F; Dehymuls® LS; Emulgator BTO; Extan-GO; Oxynex® LM; Protegin® X; Protegin®; Tenox® 25; Tenox® 26; Tenox® 6; Uantox W-1

Glyceryl oleate SE (INCI)
Trade names: Aldo® MOD; Cithrol GMO S/E; Radiasurf® 7151

Glyceryl palmitate (INCI)
CAS 26657-96-5; EINECS 247-887-2
Trade names: Emalex GMS-P; Hodag GMP

Glyceryl palmitate lactate (INCI)
Synonyms: Glyceryl lactopalmitate
Trade names: Lactodan F 15

Glyceryl palmitate/stearate (INCI)
Synonyms: Glyceryl stearate palmitate
Trade names: Imwitor® 940 K; Imwitor® 945
Trade names containing: Imwitor® 965 K; Trilipidina

Glyceryl polyacrylate (INCI)
Trade names containing: Hispagel® 100; Hispagel® 200

Glyceryl polymethacrylate (INCI)
CAS 37310-95-5; 9003-01-4
Trade names: Lubrajel® NP; Lubrajel® Oil; Lubrajel® WA
Trade names containing: Capigen CS; Jeltex; Lubrajel® CG, DV, MS, TW

Glyceryl ricinoleate (INCI)
CAS 141-08-2; EINECS 205-455-0
Synonyms: 12-Hydroxy-9-octadecenoic acid, monoester with 1,2,3-propanetriol; Monoricinolein; Glyceryl monoricinoleate
Trade names: Aldo® MR; Cithrol GMR N/E; CPH-35-N; Flexricin® 13; Hodag GMR; Hodag GMR-D; Mazol® GMR; Radiasurf® 7153; Softigen® 701; Unitina GMRO
Trade names containing: Cutina® LM; Sphingoceryl® Wax LS 2958 B; Unitina LM

Glyceryl ricinoleate SE
Synonyms: Glyceryl triricinoleate SE
Trade names: Cithrol GMR S/E

Glyceryl sorbitan oleo/stearate
Trade names: Tewax TC 80
Trade names containing: Tewax TC 81

Glyceryl stearate (INCI)
CAS 123-94-4; 11099-07-3; 31566-31-1; 85666-92-8; 85251-77-0; EINECS 250-705-4; 234-325-6; 204-664-4; 286-490-9
Synonyms: Monostearin; Glyceryl monostearate; Octadecanoic acid, monoester with 1,2,3-propanetriol

Glyceryl stearate citrate

Trade names: Ablunol GMS; Aldo® HMS; Aldo® MS; Aldo® MS LG; Aldo® MSA; Aldo® MSC; Aldo® MSLG FG; Alkamuls® GMS/C; Arlacel® 129; Atmos 150; Capmul® GMS; Ceral MN; Ceral MNT; Ceral MNX; Cerasynt® GMS; Cerasynt® SD; Chemsperse GMS; Cithrol GMS N/E; CPH-144-N; CPH-53-N; Cutina® GMS; Cutina® MD; Dimodan PM; Drewmulse® 200K; Drewmulse® 900K; Drewmulse® TP; Dur-Em® 117; Edenor GMS; Elfacos® GMS; Emalex GMS-A; Emalex GMS-B; Emerest® 2400; Emerest® 2401; Emuldan FP 40; Emuldan HA 60; Emuldan HLT 40; Estol 1467; Estol 1474; Estol GMS 1473; Estol GMS90 1468; Estol GMSveg 1474; Geleol; Grillomuls S40; Grillomuls S60; Grillomuls S90; Hefti GMS-33; Hefti GMS-99; Hodag GMS; Imwitor® 191; Imwitor® 900; Kemester 5500; Kemester® 6000; Kessco® Glyceryl Monostearate Pure; Kessco GMS; Lanesta 24; Lasemul 92 AE; Lasemul 92 AE/A; Lasemul 92 N 40; Lexemul® 55G; Lexemul® 503; Lexemul® 515; Lipal GMS; Lipo GMS 450; Lipo GMS 600; Mazol® GMS; Mazol® GMS-90; Mazol® GMS-K; Myvaplex® 600P; Nikkol MGS-A; Nikkol MGS-B; Nikkol MGS-C; Nikkol MGS-F20; Nikkol MGS-F40; Nikkol MGS-F50; Nikkol MGS-F75; Nikkol MGS-TG; Nikkol MGS-TGL; Nissan Monogly M; Norfox® 165C; Norfox® GMS; Norfox® GMS-FG; Protachem 26; Protachem G 5509, G 5566; Protachem GMS-450; Protachem HMS; Radiasurf® 7600; Radiasurf® 7900; Rewomul MG; RITA GMS; Schercemol GMS; Sinochem GMS; Sterol GMS; Tegin® 55G VA; Tegin® 90 NSE; Tegin® 515; Tegin® 515 VA; Tegin® 4011; Tegin® 4100 NSE; Tegin® 4480; Tegin® ISO NSE; Tegin® M; Tegin® Spezial; Unitina MD, MD-A; Unitolate GMS; Unitolate GS; Witconol™ 2400; Witconol™ 2401; Witconol™ MST; Zohar GLST

Trade names containing: Actimulse 250; Aldosperse® O-20 FG; Arlacel® 165; Base 4978; Base PL 1630; Carsoquat® CB; Ceral 165; Ceral LE; Ceral ML; Ceral TK; Cerasynt® 945; Cerasynt® WM; Cetax DR; Chemsperse GMS-PS; Ches® 500; Cutina® CBS; Cutina® LE; Dehymuls® LS; Dermalcare® GMS-165; Dracorin 100 SE 2/008479; Drewmulse® HM-100; Elfacos® GMSSE; Emulgade® CL Special; Emulgade® CL; Emulgade® SE; Extan-GMS; Gelot 64®; Gelot WL 3122; GMS-33-SEN; Grillocin WE-106; Hodag GMS-A; Hydrolactol 70; Hydrolactol 93; Kessco® EGAS; Kessco® Glycerol Monostearate SE, Acid Stable; Lexate® TA; Lexate® TL; Lexemul® 561; Lexemul® AR; Lexemul® AS; Lipomulse 165; Mazol® 165C; Myvatex® 40-06S; Myvatex® Texture Lite; Oxynex® 2004; Oxynex® LM; Protachem GMS-165; Ritapro 165; Simulsol 165; Tefose® 2561; Tegacid® Regular VA; Tegacid® Special; Teginacid® H; Teginacid® ML; Teginacid® R; Teginacid® Spezial SE; Teginacid® X SE; Teginacid®; Tego® Care 150; Tego® Care 215; Tego® Care 300; Tewax TC 65; Tewax TC 840; Unitina KD-16; Unitolate 165-C; Zetesap 5165; Zohar GLST SE

Glyceryl stearate citrate (INCI)
CAS 39175-72-9, 91744-38-6
Synonyms: 2-Hydroxy-1,2,3-propanetricarboxylic acid, monoester with 1,2,3-propanetriol monooctadecanoate
Trade names: Imwitor® 370

Glyceryl stearate palmitate. *See Glyceryl palmitate/stearate*

Glyceryl stearate SE (INCI)
CAS 86418-55-5; 31566-31-1; 11099-07-3; 85666-92-8; 977053-96-5

Synonyms: Glyceryl monostearate SE
Trade names: Aldo® MSD; Ceral CK; Ceral MA; Ceral ME; Ceral MET; Ceral MEX; Ceral TG; Ceral TN; Cerasynt® Q; Chemsperse GMS-SE; Cithrol GMS Acid Stable; Cithrol GMS S/E; Cutina® KD16; Dermalcare® GMS/SE; Dracorin GMS SE O/W 2/008475; Dur-Em® 207E; Emalex GMS-10SE; Emalex GMS-15SE; Emalex GMS-20SE; Emalex GMS-25SE; Emalex GMS-45RT; Emalex GMS-50; Emalex GMS-55FD; Emalex GMS-195; Emalex GMS-ASE; Emerest® 2407; Empilan® GMS SE32; Emuldan HA 32/S3; Estol 1461; Estol GMSse 1462; Hefti GMS-33-SES; Hodag GMS-D; Imwitor® 960; Imwitor® 960 K; Kemester® 6000SE; Kessco® Glycerol Monostearate SE; Lamecreme® KSM; Lanesta 40; Lexemul® 55SE; Lexemul® 530; Lexemul® T; Lipal GMS AE; Lipo GMS 470; Mazol® GMS-D; Mazol® GMSDK; Nikkol MGS-150; Nikkol MGS-ASE; Nikkol MGS-BSE-C; Nikkol MGS-DEX; Nikkol MGS-F50SE; Nissan Monogly I; Radiasurf® 7141; Rewomul MG SE; Tegacid® Special VA; Tegin®; Tegin® 4433; Tegin® V; Teginacid® Special; Unitolate GMS-D; Witconol™ 2407; Witconol™ CA; Witconol™ RHT
Trade names containing: Monacet; Tegin® C-1R; Tegin® C-611

Glyceryl triacetate. *See Triacetin*

Glyceryl triacetyl hydroxystearate (INCI)
CAS 27233-00-7; EINECS 248-351-0
Synonyms: Glyceryl (triacetoxystearate); Octadecanoic acid, (acetyloxy)-1,2,3-propanetriyl ester; Octadecanoic acid, 12-hydroxy, 1,2,3-propanetriyl ester
Trade names: Hetester HCA; Naturechem® GTH

Glyceryl triacetyl ricinoleate (INCI)
CAS 101-34-8; EINECS 202-935-1
Synonyms: 9-Octadecenoic acid, 12-(acetyloxy)-, 1,2,3-propanetriol ester; 1,2,3-Propanetriyl 12-(acetyloxy)-9-octadecenoate
Trade names: Naturechem® GTR

Glyceryl tribehenate. *See Tribehenin*

Glyceryl tribenzoate
CAS 614-33-5
Synonyms: Tribenzoin
Trade names: Uniplex 260

Glyceryl tri C8C10
Trade names: Radia® 7108

Glyceryl tricaprate/caprylate
Trade names: Estol GTCC 1527; Crodamol GTCC

Glyceryl triethylhexanoate. *See Trioctanoin*

Glyceryl tri-12-hydroxystearate. *See Trihydroxystearin*

Glyceryl triisostearate. *See Triisostearin*

Glyceryl trilaurate. *See Trilaurin*

Glyceryl trilinoleate. *See Trilinolein*

Glyceryl trilinolenate. *See Trilinolenin*

Glyceryl trimyristate. *See Trimyristin*

Glyceryl trioctanoate. *See Trioctanoin*

Glyceryl trioleate. *See Triolein*

Glyceryl tristearate. *See Tristearin*

Glyceryl undecylenate
Trade names: Pelemol GMU

Glycine (INCI)
CAS 56-40-6; EINECS 200-272-2
Synonyms: Aminoacetic acid; Glycocoll

Trade names: Hampshire® Glycine; Unamino GLCN
Trade names containing: Complexe AV.a.; Hydro-Diffuser Microreservoir; Monteine PRO; Omega-CH Activator; Seanamin TH; Unimoist U-125

Glycogen (INCI)
CAS 9005-79-2; EINECS 232-683-8
Synonyms: Animal starch; Liver starch
Trade names: Pentagen
Trade names containing: Dermosaccharides® GY; Dermosaccharides® HC; Dermosaccharides® SEA; Elespher® Dermosaccharides GY; Elespher® Dermosaccharides HC; Endonucleine LS 2143; Peptidyl; Seanamin AT; Seanamin TH

Glycol (INCI)
CAS 107-21-1; EINECS 203-473-3
Synonyms: Ethylene glycol; 1,2-Ethanediol; Ethylene alcohol
Trade names: Jeffersol DE-75

Glycol dibehenate (INCI)
CAS 79416-55-0, 344-64-8
Synonyms: 1,2-Ethanediyl docosanoate; Ethylene glycol dibehenate
Trade names: Rewopal® PG 340

Glycol dilaurate (INCI)
CAS 624-04-4; EINECS 210-827-0
Synonyms: Ethylene glycol dilaurate; Lauric acid, 1,2-ethanediyl ester; Dodecanoic acid 1,2-ethanediyl ester
Trade names: Emalex EG-di-L; Kemester® EGDL

Glycol dioleate (INCI)
CAS 928-24-5
Synonyms: Ethylene glycol dioleate
Trade names: Emalex EG-di-O

Glycol distearate (INCI)
CAS 627-83-8; EINECS 211-014-3
Synonyms: EGDS; Ethylene glycol distearate; Octadecanoic acid, 1,2-ethanediyl ester
Trade names: Ablunol EGDS; Alkamuls® EGDS; Chemsperse EGDS; CPH-360-N; Cutina® AGS; Elfacos® EGDS; Elfan® L 310; Emalex EG-di-MPS; Emalex EG-di-S; Emalex EG-di-SE; Emerest® 2355; Estol EGDS 3750; Ethylene Glycol Distearate VA; Genapol® PMS; Hest E.G.D.S; Hodag EGDS; Kemester® EGDS; Kessco® Ethylene Glycol Distearate; Lanesta EGD; Lexemul® EGDS; Lipal EGDS; Lipo EGDS; Mackester™ EGDS; Mapeg® EGDS; Nikkol EGDS; Nikkol Estepearl 10, 15; Nikkol Pearl 1222; Pegosperse® 50 DS; Radiasurf® 7269; Radia® 7266; Rewopal® PG 280; RITA EDGS; Secoster® DMS; Tegin® G 1100; Unipeg-EGDS; Witconol™ 2355; Zohar EGDS
Trade names containing: Akyposal 2010 S; Akyposal 2010 SD; Elfan® SG; Euperlan® PK 3000 AM; Euperlan® PK 3000 OK; Euperlan® PK 3000 OK; Euperlan® PK 3000; Euperlan® PK 771 BENZ; Euperlan® PK 771; Euperlan® PK 776; Euperlan® PK 789; Euperlan® PK 810 AM; Euperlan® PK 810; Euperlan® PL 1000; Genapol® PGC; Genapol® PGL; Genapol® PGM Conc; Genapol® PGM Liq.; Genapol® PGS; Lanesta-EO; Lipal MMDG; Standapol® Pearl Conc. 7130; Tego®-Pearl B-48; Tego®-Pearl S-33; Texapon® SG; Zoharpon EGDS-771

Glycol ditallowate (INCI)
Synonyms: Ethylene glycol ditallowate; Tallow fatty acid, 1,2-ethanediyl ester
Trade names containing: Marlamid® PG 20

Glycol hydroxystearate (INCI)
CAS 33907-46-9; EINECS 251-732-4
Synonyms: Ethylene glycol monohydroxystearate; Glycol monohydroxystearate; Hydroxyoctadecanoic acid, 2-hydroxyethyl ester
Trade names: Naturechem® EGHS

Glycol MIPA stearate (CTFA)
Trade names containing: Crodapearl Liq.

Glycol palmitate (INCI)
CAS 4219-49-2; EINECS 224-160-8
Synonyms: Ethylene glycol monopalmitate; Glycol monopalmitate; 2-Hydroxyethyl hexadecanoate
Trade names: Lanol P

Glycol ricinoleate (INCI)
CAS 106-17-2; EINECS 203-369-8
Synonyms: Ethylene glycol monoricinoleate; Glycol monoricinoleate; 2-Hydroxyethyl 12-hydroxy-9-octadecenoate
Trade names: Flexricin® 15

Glycol stearate (INCI)
CAS 111-60-4; 97281-23-7; EINECS 203-886-9; 306-522-8
Synonyms: EGMS; Ethylene glycol monostearate; Glycol monostearate; 2-Hydoxyethyl octadecanoate
Trade names: Ablunol EGMS; Alkamuls® EGMS; Alkamuls® EGMS/C; Alkamuls® SEG; Cerasynt® M; Chemsperse EGMS; CPH-37-NA; Dragil 2/027011; Elfacos® EGMS; Emalex EGS-A; Emalex EGS-B; Emerest® 2350; Empilan® EGMS; Estol EGMS 3749; Ethylene Glycol Monostearate VA; Hodag EGMS; Hodag EGS; Instapearl; Kemester® 5220; Kemester® EGMS; Kessco EGMS; Kessco® Ethylene Glycol Monostearate; Lanesta 35; Lasemul 62 E; Lauramide EG; Lexemul® EGMS; Lipal EGMS; Lipo EGMS; Lonzest® EGMS; Mackester™ EGMS; Mapeg® EGMS; Mapeg® EGMS-K; Monthyle; Nikkol EGMS-70; Nikkol MYS-1EX; Nikkol Pearl 1218; Pegosperse® 50 MS; Protachem EGMS; Radiasurf® 7270; RITA EGMS; Ritasynt IP; Rol GE; Schercemol EGMS; Secoster® EMS; Sterol ST 1; Tegin® G 6100; Unipeg-EGMS; Witconol™ EGMS; Zohar EGMS
Trade names containing: Base Nacrante 1100 AD; Base Nacrante 2078; Base Nacrante 9578; Cerasynt® IP; Cerasynt® LP; Cosmopon HC; Cosmopon MP; Cycloryl M1; Dermalcare® POL; Empicol® 0627; Empicol® XC35; Euperlan® MPK 850; Hodag CSA-101; Krim CH 25; Lexate® CRC; Lipal MMDG; Mackester™ IP; Mackester™ SP; Miracare® M1; Mirasheen® 202; Nutrapon B 1365; Nutrapon TK 3603; Perlglanzmittel GM 4006; Perlglanzmittel GM 4055; Perlglanzmittel GM 4175; Polytex 10M; Sedefos 75®; Standapol® 7092; Standapol® CAT; Standapol® S; Tefose® 63; Texapon® EVR; Trivent EG-18; Unipol 7092; Zohar EGMS 771

Glycol stearate SE (INCI)
CAS 86418-55-5
Synonyms: Ethylene glycol monostearate SE
Trade names: Cerasynt® MN; Monthybase; Tegin® G

Glycoproteins (INCI)
Trade names: Bovine Fetuin; Glyprosol™ 20; Glyprosol™ SD; Musol™ 20

Glycosaminoglycans (INCI)
Synonyms: GAG; Mixed mucopolysaccharides; Mucopolysaccharides
Trade names: Hyalo-Mucopolysaccharides; Hydra-protectol-SM; Nutrex PG
Trade names containing: Ateloglycane; Brookosome®

MPS; Dermasome® MPS; Dermosaccharides® HC; Elespher® Dermosaccharides HC; Glycoderm; Seanamin AT

Glycosphingolipids (INCI)
Trade names containing: AFR LS; Ceramides LS; Dermatein® GSL; Lipodermol®; Sphingoceryl® LS; Sphingoceryl® Powd. LS; Sphingoceryl® Wax LS 2958 B; Sphingosomes® AL

Glycyrrhetinic acid (INCI)
CAS 471-53-4; EINECS 207-444-6
Trade names: Nikkol Glycyrrhetinic Acid
Trade names containing: Antiphlogistic ARO

Glycyrrhetinyl stearate (INCI)
Synonyms: 3-Stearoyloxy glkycyrrhetinic acid
Trade names: Grhetinol-O

Glycyrrhizic acid (INCI)
CAS 1405-86-3; EINECS 215-785-7
Trade names: Nikkol Glycyrrhizic Acid

Gold acetylmethionate (INCI)
CAS 105883-47-4
Trade names: Exsymol Gold Acetylmethionate; Exsymol Silver Acetylmethionate; Exsyor

Golden seal root extract (INCI)
CAS 84603-60-1
Synonyms: Hydrastis canadensis extract
Trade names containing: Actiphyte of Goldenseal

Graham's salt. *See Sodium hexametaphosphate*

Grape extract (INCI)
Synonyms: Vitis vinifera extract
Trade names containing: Blend For Delicate Skins HS 215; Demaquillant LS 658

Grapefruit extract (INCI)
CAS 90045-43-5
Synonyms: Citrus decumana extract
Trade names containing: DF-100

Grapefruit juice (INCI)
Trade names containing: Lipofruit R

Grapefruit seed extract (INCI)
CAS 90045-43-5; EINECS 289-904-6
Trade names containing: DF-100

Grape leaf extract (INCI)
CAS 84929-27-1
Synonyms: Vitis vinifera leaf extract
Trade names containing: Circulatory Blend HS 318

Grape seed extract (INCI)
Synonyms: Vitis vinifera seed extract
Trade names: Leucocyanidins

Grape seed oil (INCI)
CAS 8024-22-4
Synonyms: Oils, grape seed
Trade names: Lipovol G; Nikkol Grapeseed Oil; Super Refined™ Grapeseed Oil

Green tea extract
Trade names containing: MFA™ Complex

Groundnut oil. *See Peanut oil*

Guaiazulene (INCI)
CAS 489-84-9; EINECS 207-701-2
Synonyms: 1,4-Dimethyl-7-(1-methylethyl)azulene
Trade names: Azulene 100% 2/912980
Trade names containing: Azulene 25% WS 2/013000; Azulene 50% 2/012990

Guanidine carbonate (INCI)
CAS 593-85-1; EINECS 209-813-7
Synonyms: Carbonic acid, compd. with guanidine (1:2)

Trade names: Unichem GUADIC

Guanine (INCI)
CAS 73-40-5; EINECS 200-799-8
Synonyms: 2-Amino-1,7-dihydro-6H-purin-6-one; 2-Aminohypoxanthine; 2-Amino-6-hydroxypurine
Trade names: Dew Pearl AH-1; Dew Pearl TS-1
Trade names containing: Mearlmaid® AA; Mearlmaid® CKD; Mearlmaid® CP; Mearlmaid® KN; Mearlmaid® KND; Mearlmaid® OL; Mearlmaid® PLN; Mearlmaid® PLO; Mearlmaid® TR; Naturon® 2X AQ; Naturon® 2X IPA; Naturon® CSN-22

Guar gum (INCI)
CAS 9000-30-0; EINECS 232-536-8
Synonyms: Guar flour; Gum cyamopsis
Trade names: Burtonite V7E; Jaguar® C; Supercol® Guar Gum
Trade names containing: Rhodicare™ SC-225

Guar hydroxypropyltrimonium chloride (INCI)
CAS 65497-29-2
Synonyms: Guar gum, 2-hydroxy-3-(trimethylammonio) propyl ether, chloride; Guar hydroxypropyl trimethyl ammonium chloride
Trade names: Cationic Guar C-261; Chesguar C10, C10R; Chesguar C17; Chesguar C20, C20R; Cosmedia Guar® C-261; Hi-Care® 1000; Jaguar® C-13S; Jaguar® C-14-S; Jaguar® C-17; N-Hance® 3000; Rhaballgum CG-M; Uniquart COSM GUAR

Gum arabic. *See Acacia*

Gum benzoin (INCI)
CAS 9000-05-9; EINECS 232-523-7
Synonyms: Benzoin; Gum sumatra; Siam benzoin; Sumatra benzoin
Trade names containing: Stimulant HS 285

Gum camphor. *See Camphor*

Gum gellan. *See Gellan gum*

Gum rosin. *See Rosin*

Guncotton. *See Nitrocellulose*

Hair keratin amino acids (INCI)
Trade names containing: Crotein HKP Powd.

Harpagophytum extract (INCI)
CAS 84988-65-8
Trade names containing: Rhumacalm HS 328

Hawthorne extract
Trade names: Hawthorn Extract Code 9033

Hazelnut oil (INCI)
Trade names: EmCon Hazelnut; Nikkol Hazel Nut Oil

Heart extract (INCI)
Trade names containing: Lipoliv

Hectorite (INCI)
CAS 12173-47-6; EINECS 235-340-0
Trade names: Bentone® EW; Bentone® MA; Hectabrite® AW; Hectabrite® DP
Trade names containing: Bentone® LT

HEDTA (INCI)
CAS 150-39-0; EINECS 205-759-3
Synonyms: N-[2-Bis(carboxymethyl)amino]ethyl]-N-(2-hydroxyethyl)glycine; Hydroxyethyl ethylenediamine triacetic acid
Trade names: Hamp-Ol® Acid

Hematin (INCI)
Trade names: Growthphyllin

Hemolymph extract (INCI)
Trade names: Seromarine

Henna extract (INCI)
CAS 84929-30-6
Synonyms: Colorless henna; Lawsonia alba extract; Neutral henna
Trade names: Bio-Chelated Neutral Henna Extract
Trade names containing: Actiphyte of Henna

Heparin (INCI)
Trade names containing: Heparinoid HpDI

Heptamethylnonane. *See Isohexadecane*

2-Heptylcyclopentanone (INCI)
CAS 137-03-1; EINECS 205-273-1
Trade names: Frutalone

n-Heptyl p-hydroxybenzoate
Trade names: Nipaheptyl

Heptylundecanol (INCI)
CAS 5333-44-8; EINECS 226-243-4
Trade names: Fine Oxocol

1-Hexadecanol. *See Cetyl alcohol*

Hexadecene-1
CAS 629-73-2
Synonyms: Linear C16 alpha olefin; Cetene
Trade names: Gulftene® 16
Trade names containing: Ethyl Hexadecene-1/Octadecene-1; Ethyl Tetradecene-1/Hexadecene-1

Hexadecyl... *See Cetyl..., Palmityl...*

Hexadecyl eicosanol
Trade names containing: Isofol® 34T

Hexadecyloctadecanol
Trade names containing: Isofol® 34T

Hexadimethrine chloride (INCI)
Trade names: Mexomere PO

Hexahydrohexamethyl cyclopentabenzopyran (INCI)
CAS 1222-05-5; EINECS 214-946-9
Trade names containing: Clarax

Hexahydro-1,3,5-tris (2-hydroxyethyl)-s-triazine
Trade names: Busan® 1506

Hexahydroxy cyclohexane. *See Inositol*

Hexamethyldisilazane
CAS 999-97-3; 68909-20-6; EINECS 213-668-5
Synonyms: HMDS; Bis (trimethylsilyl) amine
Trade names containing: Cab-O-Sil® TS-530

Hexamethyldisiloxane (INCI)
CAS 107-46-0; EINECS 203-492-7
Synonyms: HMDSO; Oxy bis (trimethylsilane); Disiloxane, hexamethyl-
Trade names: Rhodorsil® Oils 70041 VO.65

Hexamidine diisethionate (INCI)
CAS 659-40-5; EINECS 211-533-5
Trade names: Elestab® HP 100

Hexanediol beeswax (INCI)
Trade names: Koster Keunen Hydroxy-Hexanyl-Behenyl-Beeswaxate

Hexanediol behenyl beeswax
CAS 144514-54-5
Trade names: Cera Albalate 103

Hexanetriol beeswax (INCI)
Trade names containing: Cera Albalate 104

1-Hexene
CAS 592-41-6
Synonyms: C6 linear alpha olefin; Hexylene; Butyl ethylene
Trade names: Ethyl Hexene-1; Gulftene® 6

Hexetidine (INCI)
CAS 141-94-6; EINECS 205-513-5
Synonyms: 5-Amino-1,3-bis(2-ethylhexyl)-5-methyl-hexhydropyrimidine; 1,3-Bis(2-ethylhexyl) hexa-hydro-5-methyl-5-pyrimidiamine; Substituted hexa hydropyrimidine
Trade names: Hexetidine 90, 99

Hexyl alcohol (INCI)
CAS 111-27-3; 68526-79-4; EINECS 203-852-3
Synonyms: 1- or n-Hexanol; Pentylcarbinol; Amylcarbinol
Trade names: Nacol® 6-98

2-Hexyl-1-decanol (INCI)
CAS 2425-77-6, 36311-34-9; EINECS 219-370-1
Trade names: Exxal® 16; Isofol® 16

2-Hexyldecyl isostearate
Trade names: Emalex HIS-34

Hexylene glycol (INCI)
CAS 107-41-5; EINECS 203-489-0
Synonyms: 2-Methyl-2,4-pentanediol; 4-Methyl-2,4-pentanediol; a,a,a´-Trimethyltrimethyleneglycol
Trade names containing: Akypoquat 132; Cerasynt® LP; Hygroplex HHG; Klensoft; Mackam™ 2CT; Mackam™ 2LES; Mackam™ 2MCA; Mackam™ 2MHT; Miracare® 2MCA-SF; Miracare® 2MCA; Miracare® 2MCT; Miracare® 2MHT; Rewoteric® AM G 30; Schercoteric LS-2TE MOD; Schercoteric MS-2 Modified; Variquat® K375; Variquat® K375; Zoharteric D.O.; Zoharteric D.O.T.

Hexyl laurate (INCI)
CAS 34316-64-8; EINECS 251-932-1
Synonyms: Dodecanoic acid, hexyl ester
Trade names: Cetiol® A; Rewomul HL; Unimul-CTA; Unitolate A
Trade names containing: Abil® B 9808; Abil® WE 09; Abil® WS 08

Hexyl nicotinate (INCI)
CAS 23597-82-2; EINECS 245-767-4
Synonyms: Hexyl 3-pyridinecarboxylate
Trade names containing: Hygroplex HHG

Hirudinea extract (INCI)
Trade names containing: Dermocalmine

Histidine (INCI)
CAS 71-00-1 (L-form); EINECS 200-745-3
Synonyms: L-Histidine; α-Amino-β-imidazolepropionic acid
Trade names containing: Omega-CH Activator

HMDS. *See Hexamethyldisilazane*

HMDSO. *See Hexamethyldisiloxane*

Homomenthyl salicylate. *See Homosalate*

Homosalate (INCI)
CAS 118-56-9; EINECS 204-260-8
Synonyms: Homomenthyl salicylate; Metahomomenthyl salicylate; 3,3,5-Trimethylcyclohexyl 2-hydroxy-benzoate
Trade names: Homosalate®; Kemester® HMS; Uniderm HOMSAL

Honey (INCI)
CAS 8028-66-8
Trade names: Fancol HON

Honey extract (INCI)
CAS 91052-92-5; EINECS 293-255-4
Trade names: Melhydran®
Trade names containing: Bio-Chelated Derma-Plex I; Liposome Anti-Age LS; Liposomes Anti-Age LS

Honeysuckle extract (INCI)
CAS 84603-62-3; 90045-78-6
Synonyms: Lonicera caprifolium extract
Trade names containing: Actiphyte of Honeysuckle

Hops extract (INCI)
CAS 8016-25-9
Synonyms: Humulus lupulus extract
Trade names containing: Actiphyte of Hops; Blend For Bust Cares HS 201; Glycolysat de Houblon; Herbaliquid Hops Special; Hexaplant Richter; Hops Extract HS 2367 G; Hops HS; Hops LS; Hops Malt Extract HS 2518 G; Hops Oleat M; Nutriderme HS 243; Nutriderme HS 313; Nutriderme LS 613; Regederme HS 236; Regederme HS 330; Regederme LS 630; Regederme LS 636; Relaxant HS 278; Relaxant LS 678; Sedaplant Richter

Horse chestnut extract (INCI)
CAS 90045-79-7
Synonyms: Aesculus hippocastanum extract
Trade names containing: Aftershave HS 292; Aftershave LS 692; Biophytex®; Blend For Chapped Skins HS 361; Brookosome® FIH; Cremogen AF; Extrait No. 30; Lipoplastidine Aesculus; Soluvit Richter; Tonique HS 290; Tonique LS 690

Horsetail extract (INCI)
Synonyms: Dutch rush extract; Equisetum arvense extract; Scouring rush extract
Trade names containing: Aftershave HS 292; Aftershave LS 692; BBC Mineral Complex; BBC Moisture Trol; BBC Relaxing Complex; Bio-Chelated Derma-Plex I; Blend For Bust Cares HS 201; Blend For Elderly Skins HS 296; Brookosome® Herbal; Cremogen AF; Extrapone Poly H Special 2/032451; Hair Complex Aquosum; Haircomplex AKS; Herbaliquid Alpine Herbs Special; Herbasol 7 Herb Complex; Herbasol Complex D; Herbasol Complex E; Kalokiros HS 263; Kalokiros LS 663; Regederme HS 236; Regederme HS 330; Regederme LS 630; Regederme LS 636

HSA. *See Hydroxystearic acid*

Human placental lipids (INCI)
Trade names: Liposoluble Placental Extract E.M.L

Human placental protein (INCI)
Synonyms: Placenta extract, human; Proteins, placental, human
Trade names: Phylderm® Filatov

Humulus lupulus extract. *See Hops extract*

Hyaluronic acid (INCI)
CAS 9004-61-9; EINECS 232-678-0
Trade names: Atomergic Hyaluronic Acid; Biomatrix®; Hyaluronic Acid; Hyladerm®; Hylucare™
Trade names containing: BioCare® Polymer HA-24; BioCare® SA; Complex T-I, T-II; Cromoist HYA; Glyco/Cer HA; Glyco/Cer HALA; Lipocare HA/EC; Polytrix™; Spherica HA

Hybrid safflower oil (INCI)
Synonyms: Safflower oil, hybrid
Trade names: Lipovol SO

Hydrated silica. *See Silica, hydrated*

Hydrochlorofluorocarbon 22 (INCI)
CAS 75-45-6; EINECS 200-871-9
Synonyms: Chlorodifluoromethane; Chlorofluorocarbon 22; Propellant 22
Trade names: Dymel® 22

Hydrochlorofluorocarbon 142B (INCI)
CAS 75-68-3; EINECS 200-891-8
Synonyms: 1-Chloro-1,1-difluoroethane; Chlorofluoro-

carbon 142b; Propellant 142b
Trade names: Dymel® 142b

Hydrocotyl extract (INCI)
CAS 84776-24-9, 84696-21-9
Synonyms: Centella asiatica extract; Fo-ti-tieng extract; Gotu kola extract
Trade names: Hydrocotyl Vegebios
Trade names containing: Biophytex®; Hydrocotyl Glycolysat; Hydrocotyl HS; Hydrocotyl Oleat M; Liposome Centella

Hydrofluorocarbon 152a (INCI)
CAS 75-37-6; EINECS 200-866-1
Synonyms: 1,1-Difluoroethane; Fluorocarbon 152a; Propellant 152a
Trade names: Dymel® 152a; Genetron® 152a

Hydrogenated butylene/ethylene/styrene copolymer (INCI)
Trade names containing: Geahlene

Hydrogenated C12-18 triglycerides (INCI)
Trade names: Lipocerite

Hydrogenated canola oil
Trade names: Lobra

Hydrogenated castor oil (INCI)
CAS 8001-78-3; EINECS 232-292-2
Synonyms: Opalwax; Castorwax; Castor oil, hydrogenated
Trade names: Castorwax® MP-70; Castorwax® MP-80; Castorwax® NF; Cutina® HR; Ross Castor Wax; Unitina HR
Trade names containing: Protegin® W; Protegin® WX; Sterotex® K

Hydrogenated castor oil laurate (INCI)
Trade names: Cetiol® T 1500

Hydrogenated coco-glycerides (INCI)
CAS 977056-87-3
Trade names: Softisan® 100; Softisan® 133; Softisan® 134; Softisan® 138; Softisan® 142; Witepsol® E75; Witepsol® E76; Witepsol® E85; Witepsol® H12; Witepsol® H15; Witepsol® H32; Witepsol® H35; Witepsol® H37; Witepsol® H39; Witepsol® H42; Witepsol® H5; Witepsol® H175; Witepsol® H185; Witepsol® S51; Witepsol® S55; Witepsol® S58; Witepsol® W25; Witepsol® W31; Witepsol® W32; Witepsol® W35; Witepsol® W45

Hydrogenated coconut acid (INCI)
CAS 68938-15-8
Synonyms: Acids, coconut, hydrogenated; Coconut acid, hydrogenated; Fatty acids, coco, hydrogenated
Trade names: Emery® 625; Hystrene® 5012; Industrene® 223

Hydrogenated coconut oil (INCI)
Synonyms: Coconut oil, hydrogenated
Trade names: Hydrobase 32/34; Lipex 401; Pureco® 92; Special Fat 42/44
Trade names containing: Base O/W 097; Forlan L Conc; Forlan L; Forlan LM; New Econa 200 CH; Pureco® 110; Softisan® 601

Hydrogenated cottonseed glyceride (INCI)
CAS 61789-07-9
Synonyms: Glycerides, cottonseed oil, hydrogeanted
Trade names: Myverol® 18-07

Hydrogenated cottonseed oil (INCI)
CAS 68334-00-9; EINECS 269-804-9
Trade names: C-Flakes; Emvelop®; Lipex 109; Lubritab®

Hydrogenated ditallowamine (INCI)
CAS 61789-79-5; EINECS 263-089-7
Synonyms: Dihydrogenated tallow amine; Bis(hydrogenated tallow alkyl) amines; Amines, bis(hydrogenated tallow alkyl)-
Trade names: Adogen® 240 SF; Armeen® 2HT

Hydrogenated ethylene/propylene/styrene copolymer (INCI)
Trade names containing: Geahlene

Hydrogenated jojoba oil (INCI)
CAS 61789-91-1
Synonyms: Jojoba oil, hydrogenated
Trade names: Transjojoba™ 70

Hydrogenated lanolin (INCI)
CAS 8031-44-5; EINECS 232-452-1
Synonyms: Lanolin, hydrogenated
Trade names: Almolan HL; Brooks Hydrogenated Lanolin; Fancol HL; Ivarlan™ HL; Lanaetex-HG; Lanocerina; Lipolan; Lipolan Distilled; Nikkol Wax-500; Super-Sat
Trade names containing: Biofloreol Liposoluble; Forlan LM; Lanpro-1; Proto-Lan 4R

Hydrogenated lecithin (INCI)
CAS 92128-87-5, 97281-48-6; EINECS 295-786-7
Synonyms: Lecithin, hydrogenated
Trade names: Basis LS-60H; Emulmetik™ 320; Emulmetik™ 950; Lipoid S 75-3; Nikkol Lecinol S-10; Nikkol Lecinol S-10E; Nikkol Lecinol S-10EX; Nikkol Lecinol S-10M; Nikkol Lecinol S-30; PhosPho H-00; PhosPho H-150; Phospholipon® 90 H
Trade names containing: Basis LP-20H; Nikkol Aquasome LA; Nikkol Aquasome EC-5; Nikkol Aquasome VE

Hydrogenated lysolecithin
Trade names: Nikkol Lecinol LL-20

Hydrogenated menhaden acid (INCI)
Synonyms: Acids, menhaden, hydrogenated; Menhaden acid, hydrogenated
Trade names: Hystrene® 3022

Hydrogenated menhaden oil (INCI)
CAS 93572-53-3, 68002-72-2
Synonyms: Menhaden oil, hydrogenated; Oils, menhaden, hydrogenated
Trade names: Neustrene® 053

Hydrogenated mink oil (INCI)
Synonyms: Mink oil, hydrogenated; Oils, mink, hydrogenated
Trade names: Visonoil

Hydrogenated orange roughy oil (INCI)
Synonyms: Oils, orange roughy, hydrogenated; Orange roughy oil, hydrogenated
Trade names: Nikkol OR Wax

Hydrogenated palm glyceride (INCI)
CAS 67784-87-6
Synonyms: Palm oil glyceride, hydrogenated; Glycerides, palm oil mono-, hydrogenated
Trade names: Myvatex® 8-16; Myverol® 18-04

Hydrogenated palm glycerides (INCI)
Synonyms: Hydrogenated palm mono-, di- and tri-glycerides; Glycerides, palm oil mono-, di- and tri, hydrogenated
Trade names containing: Lamecreme® AOM; Lamecreme® LPM; Lipocire A; Lipocire CM; Lipocire DM; Massa Estarinum® CM; Suppocire CM

Hydrogenated palm kernel glycerides (INCI)
Trade names containing: Lipocire A; Lipocire CM;

Lipocire DM; Massa Estarinum® CM; Suppocire CM

Hydrogenated palm kernel oil (INCI)
CAS 68990-82-9
Synonyms: Oils, palm kernel, hydrogenated; Palm kernel oil, hydrogenated
Trade names: Witarix® 212

Hydrogenated palm oil (INCI)
CAS 8033-29-2; 68514-74-9
Synonyms: Oils, palm, hydrogenated; Palm oil, hydrogenated
Trade names: Dynasan® P60; P-Flakes; Softisan® 154
Trade names containing: Pureco® 110

Hydrogenated palm/palm kernel oil PEG-6 esters (INCI)
Synonyms: Hydrogeanted palm/palm kernel oil PEG-6 complex
Trade names: Labrafil® M 2130 BS
Trade names containing: Labrafil® M 2130 CS

Hydrogenated peanut oil (INCI)
CAS 68425-36-5; EINECS 270-350-9
Synonyms: Oils, peanut, hydrogenated
Trade names: Witarix® 450
Trade names containing: Amphocerin® E; Amphocerin® K

Hydrogenated polyisobutene (INCI)
CAS 61693-08-1, 68937-10-0
Synonyms: Polyisobutane
Trade names: Panalane® L-14E; Polysynlane; Trisynlane
Trade names containing: Emulzome

Hydrogenated rice bran wax (INCI)
Trade names: Rice Wax RX-100

Hydrogenated shark liver oil (INCI)
Synonyms: Oils, shark liver, hydrogenated; Shark liver oil, hydrogenated
Trade names containing: Robeyl

Hydrogenated soyadimoniumhydroxypropyl polyglucose
Trade names: Brocose Q

Hydrogenated soybean oil (INCI)
CAS 8016-70-4, 68002-71-1; EINECS 232-410-2
Synonyms: Oils, soybean, hydrogenated; Soybean oil, hydrogenated
Trade names: Famous; Lipex 407; Lipovol HS; Neustrene® 064; S-Flakes; Stabland®; Sterotex® HM NF; Witarix® 440
Trade names containing: Ross Japan Wax Substitute 966; Sterotex® C; Sterotex® K

Hydrogenated soy glyceride (INCI)
CAS 61789-08-0; 68002-71-1
Synonyms: Hydrogenated soybean oil monoglyceride; Glycerides, soybean oil, hydrogenated, mono; Hydrogenated soybean glyceride
Trade names: Dimodan PV; Myvatex® 8-06; Myverol® 18-06
Trade names containing: Isobeeswax SP 154; Koster Keunen Beeswax, S&P ISOW

Hydrogenated starch hydrolysate (INCI)
CAS 68425-17-2
Synonyms: Hydrogenated corn syrup; Corn syrup, hydrogenated
Trade names: A-611; Hystar® 3375; Hystar® 4075; Hystar® 5875; Hystar® 6075; Hystar® 7000; Hystar® CG; Hystar® HM-75; Hystar® TPF; Lipo Polyol NC

Hydrogenated tallow (INCI)
CAS 8030-12-4; EINECS 232-442-7
Synonyms: Tallow, hydrogenated

Hydrogenated tallow acid

Trade names: Special Fat 168T

Hydrogenated tallow acid (INCI)
CAS 61790-38-3; EINECS 263-130-9
Synonyms: Acids, tallow, hydrogenated; Tallow acid, hydrogenated
Trade names: Dar-C; Hy-Phi 6001

Hydrogenated tallow alcohol (INCI)
Trade names: Hydrenol® D; Hydrenol® DD
Trade names containing: Tewax TC 1

Hydrogenated tallowalkonium chloride (INCI)
CAS 61789-72-8; EINECS 263-081-3
Synonyms: Hydrogenated tallow dimethyl benzyl ammonium chloride
Trade names: Variquat® B345

Hydrogenated tallowamine (INCI)
CAS 61788-45-2; EINECS 262-976-6
Synonyms: Amines, hydrogenated tallow alkyl; Tallow amine, hydrogenated
Trade names: Amine 2HBG; Armeen® HT; Armeen® HTD; Radiamine 6140; Radiamine 6141

Hydrogenated tallow dimethylamine oxide
CAS 68390-99-8
Trade names: Aromox® DMHT; Aromox® DMHTD

Hydrogenated talloweth-12 (INCI)
Trade names: Elfapur® T 115

Hydrogenated talloweth-25 (INCI)
Trade names: Elfapur® T 250

Hydrogenated talloweth-60 myristyl glycol (INCI)
Trade names: Elfacos® GT 282 L; Elfacos® GT 282 S

Hydrogenated tallow glyceride (INCI)
CAS 61789-09-1; EINECS 263-031-0
Synonyms: Hydrogenated tallow monoglyceride; Glycerides, hydrogenated tallow mono-
Trade names: Monomuls® 90-25
Trade names containing: Lamesoft® 156; Monomuls® 90-25/2, 90-25/5; Ross Synthetic Candelilla Wax

Hydrogenated tallow glyceride citrate (INCI)
CAS 68990-59-0; EINECS 273-613-6
Synonyms: Glycerides, tallow mono-, hydrogenated, citrates
Trade names: Acidan N 12; Lamegin® ZE 30, 60
Trade names containing: Tegin® C-1R; Tegin® C-611

Hydrogenated tallow glyceride lactate (INCI)
CAS 68990-06-7; EINECS 273-576-6
Synonyms: Glycerides, tallow mono-, hydrogenated, lactates
Trade names: Lamegin® GLP 10, 20

Hydrogenated tallow glycerides (INCI)
CAS 68308-54-3, 67701-27-3; EINECS 269-658-6
Synonyms: Hydrogenated tallow mono-, di- and triglycerides; Glycerides, tallow mono-, di- and tri-, hydrogenated
Trade names: Neustrene® 060
Trade names containing: Almolan AE; Lamesoft® 156/NP; Monomuls® 60-25/2; New Econa 200 CH; Ross Beeswax Substitute 628/5; Ross Japan Wax Substitute 930

Hydrogenated tallow glycerides citrate (INCI)
Trade names containing: Controx® KS; Controx® VP

Hydrogenated tallowoyl glutamic acid (INCI)
Trade names: Amisoft HA

Hydrogenated tallowtrimonium chloride (INCI)
CAS 61788-78-1; EINECS 263-005-9
Synonyms: Hydrogenated tallow trimethyl ammonium chloride

Trade names: Arquad® HT-50; Noramium MSH 50

Hydrogenated vegetable glyceride (INCI)
CAS 61789-08-0, 69028-36-0
Synonyms: Glycerides, hydrogenated vegetable mono-; Glycerides, vegetable mono-, hydrogenated
Trade names: Myverol® 18-50

Hydrogenated vegetable glycerides citrate (INCI)
CAS 97593-31-2; EINECS 207-334-9
Trade names: Acidan BC Veg; Acidan N 12 Veg

Hydrogenated vegetable glycerides phosphate (INCI)
CAS 85411-01-4; 25212-19-5
Trade names: Emphos™ F27-85

Hydrogenated vegetable oil (INCI)
CAS 68334-00-9; 68334-28-1; EINECS 269-820-6
Synonyms: Vegetable oil, hydrogenated
Trade names: BBS; Cremeol HF-52, HF-62; Hydrokote® 95; Hydrokote® 97; Hydrokote® 102; Hydrokote® 108; Hydrokote® 112; Hydrokote® 118; Hydrokote® AR, HL; Hydrokote® RM; Lipo SS; Sterotex®; Sterotex® NF; Wecobee® FW; Wecobee® M; Wecobee® S; Wecobee® SS; Wecobee® W

Hydrogen peroxide (INCI)
CAS 7722-84-1; EINECS 231-765-0
Trade names: Albone® 35 CG; Albone® 50 CG; Albone® 70CG

Hydrogen peroxide carbamide. *See Urea peroxide*

Hydrolyzed actin (INCI)
Synonyms: Actin hydrolysate
Trade names containing: Endonucleine LS 2143; Fishlan LS; Seanamin AT; Seanamin BD; Seanamin FP

Hydrolyzed almond protein
Trade names: Gluadin® Almond; Uniglaudin A

Hydrolyzed casein. *See Hydrolyzed milk protein*

Hydrolyzed collagen (INCI)
CAS 9015-54-7
Synonyms: Collagen hydrolysates; Hydrolyzed animal protein; Proteins, collagen, hydrolysate
Trade names: Collagen BIO-5000; Collagen Hydrolysate 30%; Collagen Hydrolyzate Cosmetic 50; Collagen Hydrolyzate Cosmetic 55; Collagen Hydrolyzate Cosmetic N-35; Collagen Hydrolyzate Cosmetic N-55; Collagen Hydrolyzate Cosmetic SD; Collagen P; Collagen Protein WN; Collagen S; Collagenol LS/HC-10; Collagenol LS/HC-50; Collagenon; Crolastin C; Cropepsol 30; Cropepsol 35; Cropepsol 50; Cropepsol SD; Cropeptone 30; Cropeptone 35; Cropeptone 50; Crotein A; Crotein SPA; Crotein SPC; Crotein SPO; Elastovit; Granpro-5; Granpro-40, -50, -55, -100; Hidrolisado de Colageno; Hydrocoll™ AC-30; Hydrocoll AL-50, AL-55, EN-40, EN-55-X, EN-SD-1M, EN-SD-10M; Hydrocoll™ EN-55; Hydrocoll™ EN-SD; Hydrocoll™ HE-35; Hydrocoll™ LE-35; Hydrocoll SS-40, SS-55, T-37, T-55, T-LSN, T-LSN-SD, T-P52; Hydrocoll™ T-LSN; Hydrocolloid 219; Hydrolan; Hydrolyzed Animal Protein SD; Hydrolyzed Animal Protein-55; Lanagen-50, -55, -SD; Lensol; Lexein® X-250; Lexein® X-250HP; Lexein® X-300; Lexein® X-350; Monteine CA; Neptuline® C; Nikkol CCP-40; Nikkol CCP-100; Nikkol CCP-100P; Nutrilan® FPK; Nutrilan® H; Nutrilan® I; Nutrilan® I-50; Nutrilan® I-50/NP; Nutrilan® I Powd; Nutrilan® I-Powd./NP; Nutrilan® L; Nutrilan® L/NP; Nutrilan® M; Peptein® 2000XL; Peptein® 2000®; PF-6®; Polypeptide 10; Polypeptide 12; Polypeptide 37; Polypeptide LSN Anhydrous; Polypeptide SF; Polypro® 5000; Polypro® 15000; Pran H; Pran LIQ;

Prochem 12K; Prochem 100-CG Powd; Prochem SPA; Prolagen C; Promois W-32; Promois W-32LS; Promois W-32R; Promois W-42; Promois W-42CP; Promois W-42K; Promois W-42LS; Promois W-42R; Promois W-52; Promois W-52P; Protein SC; Protein TC; Proteolene H; Tritein-40, -50, -100; Tri-Tein 40N; Tri-Tein 55

Trade names containing: Algogen; Colla-Moist™ WS; Collamino™ Complex SS; Complex T-I, T-II; Cromoist CS; Cromoist HYA; Emulmetik 920; Endomine NMF; Hydrocos; Hydrolyzed NMF; Lactil®; Lanatein-25; Lanotein AWS 30; Lanpro-10; Olamin® K; Olamin® K/NP; Prochem 35A; Prodew 100; Prodew 200; Protachem 35A; Proto-Lan 20; Proto-Lan 30; Quinta-Pro Conc; Unipertan P-2002; Unipertan P-24; Unipertan P-24; Unipertan P-242

Hydrolyzed collagen, ethyl ester (INCI)
CAS 68951-89-3
Synonyms: Ethyl ester of hydrolyzed animal protein
Trade names: Crotein ASC; Etha-Coll AAS-20; Pro-Tein ES-20

Hydrolyzed conchiorin protein (INCI)
Trade names: Promois Pearl P

Hydrolyzed corn protein (INCI)
Synonyms: Corn protein hydrolysate; Proteins, corn, hydrolysate
Trade names: Corn-Pro™ 35; Fractein HCP; Prove HM
Trade names containing: Kerafix 620

Hydrolyzed corn starch (INCI)
Trade names: Nutrex PV

Hydrolyzed DNA (INCI)
Synonyms: DNA hydrolysate
Trade names containing: Bioplex™ RNA

Hydrolyzed elastin (INCI)
CAS 100085-10-7, 73049-73-7; 9007-58-3, 91080-18-1
Synonyms: Elastin, hydrolyzed; Elastin hydrolysate; Hydrolyzed animal elastin
Trade names: Actigen E; Alpha-Elastin; Crolastin; Elastein® 5000; Elastin (Partialhydrolisate) NOVA; Elastin CLR; Elastin H.P.M; Elastin Hydrolysate COS; Elastolan LS HE 20; European Elastin 10; European Elastin 30; European Elastin SD; Exsyproteines 2%, 4%; Hidrolisado de Elastina; Hydrolastan; Hydrolyzed Elastin RE-10 No. 26202; Hydrolyzed Elastin RE-30 No. 26203; Ichtyoelastin; Nutrilan® Elastin E20; Nutrilan® Elastin P; Prolastine; Ritalastin EL-10; Ritalastin EL-30; Solu-Lastin™ 10; Solu-Lastin™ 30; Tri-Lastin 10F
Trade names containing: Brookosome® Elastin; Collamino™ Complex ESC; Elastin PG 2000; Ritacomplex DF 11; Ritacomplex DF 14; Tri-K CMF Complex

Hydrolyzed fibronectin (INCI)
CAS 100085-35-6; EINECS 293-509-4
Synonyms: Fibronectin hydrolysate
Trade names: Cronectin H
Trade names containing: Dermonectin

Hydrolyzed gadidae protein (INCI)
Synonyms: Gadus protein hydrolysate; Hydrolyzed gadus protein
Trade names containing: Ichtyocollagene; Promarine

Hydrolyzed glycosaminoglycans (INCI)
Synonyms: Hydrolyzed mucopolysaccharides
Trade names: Acid Mucopolysaccharides; Actiglow™; Actiglow™ C; Base EAC 20; Cartilage Mucopolysaccharides E.M.A.C; Dermatein® MPS; Dihydral; Esuronammina; Hair Saccharides; Hydrolyzed Mu-

copolysaccharides SD; Ialuramina; Ialuramina 10; Tri-K HMP
Trade names containing: Actiglide™; Actisea™ 100; Carnitiline; Diaquasol; Trichogen; Tri-K CMF Complex

Hydrolyzed golden-pea protein
Trade names: Golden-Pea-Pro™ EN-15

Hydrolyzed hair keratin (INCI)
Trade names: Tri-K KHP

Hydrolyzed hemoglobin (INCI)
Trade names: Cellactin

Hydrolyzed keratin (INCI)
CAS 69430-36-0; EINECS 274-001-1
Synonyms: Hydrolyzed animal keratin; Keratin, hydrolyzed
Trade names: Cheratina 100%; Crotein ASK; Crotein K; Crotein WKP; Cuticulin; Dehydrated Keratine Hydrolysate; Hidrolisado de Queratina; Hydrokeratin™ 100M; Hydrokeratin™ AL-30; Hydrokeratin™ AL-SD; Hydrokeratin™ WKP; Kera-Tein 1000; Kera-Tein 1000 RM SD; Kera-Tein 1000 RM/50; Kera-Tein 1000 SD; Kera-Tein V; Keramois L; Kerapro S; Keratin Hydrolysate; Keratin P; Keratin S; Keratine Hydrolysate H.T.K; Nutrilan® Cashmere W; Nutrilan® Keratin W; Promois WK; Promois WK-H
Trade names containing: Kera-Tein W; Kerasol; Keratolan; Quinta-Pro Conc; Solu-Veg™ Complex #4

Hydrolyzed keratin, ethyl ester (INCI)
Synonyms: Ethyl ester of hydrolyzed keratin
Trade names: Kera-Tein 1000 AS

Hydrolyzed lupine protein (INCI)
Synonyms: Lupine protein hydrolysate
Trade names: Hydrane L

Hydrolyzed marine protein
Trade names: Solu-Mar™ EN-30

Hydrolyzed milk protein (INCI)
CAS 65072-00-6; 92797-39-2; EINECS 265-363-1
Synonyms: Proteins, milk, hydrolysate; Hydrolyzed casein
Trade names: Edamin S; EPCH; Glycoproteins from Milk; Hy Case Amino; Hy Case SF; Hydrolactin 2500; Hydromilk™ EN-20; Lactolan®; Milkpro; Promois Milk; Tri-Tein Milk Polypeptide
Trade names containing: Biophytex®; Hydromilk ENL-SD

Hydrolyzed mucopolysaccharides. *See Hydrolyzed glycosaminoglycans*

Hydrolyzed oat flour
Trade names containing: Ritavena™ 5

Hydrolyzed pea protein (INCI)
CAS 9008-99-8
Trade names: Pea Pro-Tein BK

Hydrolyzed placental protein (INCI)
Trade names: Hidrolisado de Placenta

Hydrolyzed potato protein (INCI)
Trade names: Potato-Pro™ EN-15

Hydrolyzed reticulin (INCI)
Synonyms: Hydrolysate of animal reticulin; Reticulin hydrolysate; Soluble reticulin
Trade names: Reticusol

Hydrolyzed rice protein (INCI)
CAS 97759-33-8
Trade names: Hydrane R; Rice Pro-Tein BK; Rice-Pro™ EN-20

Hydrolyzed RNA (INCI)
Trade names: Lisato RNA
Trade names containing: Bioplex™ RNA

Hydrolyzed serum protein (INCI)
Synonyms: Serum protein, hydrolyzed
Trade names: Eleseryl® SHT; Serumpro™ EN-10
Trade names containing: Asebiol® LS; Brookosome®
Serum; Trichogen

Hydrolyzed silk (INCI)
CAS 96690-41-4
Synonyms: Hydrolyzed silk protein; Silk, hydrolyzed
Trade names: Autolyzed Silk; Autolyzed Silk Protein;
Crosilk 10,000; Crosilk Liq. Complex; Idrolizzato
Della Seta; Promois Silk 700 SP; Promois Silk-1000;
Silk Pro-Tein; Silkpro; Silkpro CM-1000; Silkpro CM-
2000; Solu-Silk™ Protein
Trade names containing: Collamino™ Complex ESC;
Collamino™ Complex SS

Hydrolyzed silk ethyl ester (INCI)
Trade names: Promois Silk A; Silkpro AS

Hydrolyzed soy protein (INCI)
CAS 68607-88-5; 70084-94-5
Synonyms: Soy protein, hydrolyzed
Trade names: Hydrane S; Hydrosoy 2000/SF; Pepsobiol;
Peptein® VgS; Phylderm Vegetal; Promois WS;
Prove HS; Sol-U-Tein 6861; Sol-U-Tein FS-1000;
Sol-U-Tein PS-1000; Sol-U-Tein VG; Solu-Soy™
EN-25; Solu-Tofu EN-10; Soy-Tein NL; Soypro 25;
Tri-K Soypro-25
Trade names containing: Biodermine; Capigen CG;
Capigen CS; Capigen; Capisome; Lipostim;
Oxylastil; Solu-Veg™ Complex #4; Sungen

Hydrolyzed spinal protein (INCI)
Trade names containing: Fibrastil

Hydrolyzed sweet almond protein (INCI)
Synonyms: Sweet almond protein hydrolysate
Trade names: Amanduline

Hydrolyzed vegetable protein (INCI)
CAS 977059-33-8, 100209-45-8
Synonyms: Vegetable protein hydrolysate; Proteins, veg-
etable, hydrolysate
Trade names: Chromoprotulines; Exsymol Chromo-
protuline; Exsymol Protuline; Gunther Pro-Tein 1550;
Hydrosoy 2000; Protulines; Solu-Veg™ EN-35
Trade names containing: Unipertan VEG 24; Unipertan
VEG 242

Hydrolyzed wheat gluten (INCI)
Trade names: Glusol

Hydrolyzed wheat protein (INCI)
CAS 70084-87-6; 100864-25-1; EINECS 309-696-3
Synonyms: Proteins, wheat, hydrolyzed; Wheat protein
hydrolysate
Trade names: Dascare SWP; Fractein HWP; Gluadin®
AGP; Gluadin® Wheat; Granosol 25; Granosol 100;
Hydrane W; Hydrotriticum™; Peptein® VgW;
Promois WG; Prove HT; Uniglaudin W; Vegepro W;
Wheat-Pro™ EN-20; Wheat-Tein NL
Trade names containing: Cropeptide W; Firmogen®;
Ritacomplex DF 15; Solu-Veg™ Complex #4

Hydrolyzed wheat protein polysiloxane copolymer
Trade names: Crodasone W

Hydrolyzed wheat starch (INCI)
Trade names containing: Cropeptide W

Hydrolyzed whole oats
Trade names: Cromoist O-25

Hydrolyzed yeast (INCI)
Synonyms: Yeast hydrolysate
Trade names: Deproteinated Yeasts; Yeast Walls

Hydrolyzed yeast protein (INCI)
CAS 100684-36-4
Trade names: Hydrocell YP-30-P; Hydrocell YP-SD;
Hydrocell™ AYP-30; Hydrocell™ YP-30
Trade names containing: Asebiol® LS; Biophytex®

Hydroquinone (INCI)
CAS 123-31-9; EINECS 204-617-8
Synonyms: 1,4-Benzenediol; p-Dihydroxybenzene;
Hydroquinol
Trade names: Eastman® Hydroquinone; Rodol HQ;
Tecquinol® USP Grade; Uantox HQ

**Hydroxyanthraquinoneaminopropyl methyl morpho-
linium methosulfate (INCI)**
CAS 38866-20-5; EINECS 254-161-9
Trade names: Imexine BD

Hydroxyceteth-60 (INCI)
Trade names: Chimexane NK

Hydroxycetyl hydroxyethyldimonium chloride (INCI)
CAS 84643-53-8
Synonyms: Hydroxyhexadecyl dimethyl hydroxyethyl
ammonium chloride
Trade names: Dehyquart® E; Uniquart E

Hydroxycetyl phosphate (INCI)
Synonyms: Phosphoric acid, hydroxycetyl ester
Trade names: Forlanit® E

2-Hydroxyethyl-2-amino-4-hydroxytoluene sulfate. *See*
3-Ethylamino-p-cresol sulfate

2-Hydroxyethylamino-5-nitroanisole (INCI)
CAS 66095-81-6; EINECS 266-138-0
Trade names: Imexine FM

**Hydroxyethyl carboxymethyl cocamidopropylamine
(INCI)**
Trade names: Chimexane HA

Hydroxyethylcellulose (INCI)
CAS 9004-62-0
Synonyms: Cellulose, 2-hydroxyethyl ether; H.E. cellu-
lose
Trade names: Alcoramnosan; Cellosize® HEC QP
Grades; Cellosize® HEC QP-100M-H; Cellosize®
HEC QP-15,000-H; Cellosize® HEC QP-3-L;
Cellosize® HEC QP-300; Cellosize® HEC QP-40;
Cellosize® HEC QP-4400-H; Cellosize® HEC QP-
52,000-H; Cellosize® HEC WP Grades; Cellosize®
Polymer PCG-10; Idroramnosan; Liporamnosan;
Natrosol® 250; Natrosol® Hydroxyethylcellulose;
Tylose® H Series; Tylose® H-p; Tylose® H-yp;
Viscontran HEC
Trade names containing: Bentone® LT

Hydroxyethyl cetyldimonium phosphate (INCI)
Synonyms: Cetyl dimethyl hydroxyethyl ammonium
phosphate
Trade names: Luviquat® Mono CP

Hydroxyethyl ethylcellulose (INCI)
Synonyms: Cellulose ethyl hydroxyethyl ether; Ethyl
hydroxyethyl cellulose
Trade names: Bermocoll

1-Hydroxyethylidene-1,1-diphosphonic acid
CAS 2809-21-4
Synonyms: HEDPA; Acetodiphosphonic acid
Trade names: Briquest® ADPA-60AW

Hydroxyethyl stearamide-MIPA (INCI)
Trade names containing: Crodapearl NI Liquid

676

Hydroxylated lanolin (INCI)
CAS 68424-66-8; EINECS 270-315-8
Synonyms: Lanolin, hydroxylated
Trade names: Hetlan OH; Hidroxilan; Hydroxylan; Ivarlan™ OH; Landrox; OHlan®; Protalan H; Ritahydrox
Trade names containing: Leniplex

Hydroxylated lecithin (INCI)
CAS 8029-76-3; EINECS 232-440-6
Synonyms: Lecithin, hydroxylated
Trade names: Alcolec® Z-3; Alcolec® Z-7; Centrolene® A, S; Nikkol Lecinol SH; PhosPho 642

Hydroxylated milk glycerides (INCI)
Trade names: Cremerol HMG

2-Hydroxy-4-methoxybenzophenone. *See Benzophenone-3*

2-Hydroxy-4-methoxybenzophenone-5-sulfonic acid.
See Benzophenone-4

Hydroxymethyl dioxoazabicyclooctane (INCI)
CAS 6542-37-6; EINECS 229-457-6
Synonyms: 7-Hydroxymethyl-1,5-dioxo-3-aza-bicyclooctane
Trade names: Zoldine® 55; Zoldine® ZT Oxazolidine

Hydroxyoctacosanyl hydroxystearate (INCI)
Synonyms: 12-Hydroxystearic acid, β-hydroxyoctacosanyl ester
Trade names: Elfacos® C26

Hydroxyproline (INCI)
CAS 51-35-4 (L-form); EINECS 200-091-9
Synonyms: 4-Hydroxy-L-proline; 4-Hydroxy-2-pyrrolidine carboxylic acid
Trade names containing: Monteine PRO

2-Hydroxy-1,2,3-propanetricarboxylic acid. *See Citric acid*

Hydroxypropyl bisisostearamidopropyldimonium chloride (INCI)
CAS 11381-09-0; 111381-08-9
Trade names: Schercoquat 2IAE; Schercoquat 2IAP

Hydroxypropyl bistrimonium diiodide (INCI)
EINECS 204-630-9
Trade names: Iodogene

Hydroxypropylcellulose (INCI)
CAS 9004-64-2
Synonyms: Cellulose, 2-hydroxypropyl ether; Oxypropylated cellulose
Trade names: Klucel® EF; Klucel® ELF, GF, HF, JF, LF, MF

Hydroxypropyl chitosan (INCI)
CAS 84069-44-3
Synonyms: Chitosan, hydroxypropyl
Trade names: Dascare HPCH; HPCH Liq

Hydroxypropyl guar (INCI)
CAS 39421-75-5
Synonyms: Hydroxypropyl guar gum; Guar gum, 2-hydroxypropyl ether; Hydroxypropyl ether guar gum
Trade names: Chesguar HP4; Chesguar HP4R; Chesguar HP6; Jaguar® HP 8; Jaguar® HP 60; Jaguar® HP 120; Jaguar® HP-11; Jaguar® HP-200

Hydroxypropyl guar hydroxypropyl trimonium chloride (INCI)
CAS 71329-50-5
Trade names: Jaguar® C-162

Hydroxypropyl methylcellulose (INCI)
CAS 9004-65-3
Synonyms: Methyl hydroxypropyl cellulose; Cellulose 2-hydroxypropyl methyl ether; Hypromellose
Trade names: Benecel® Hydroxypropyl Methylcellulose; Benecel® MP; Methocel® 40-100; Methocel® 40-101; Methocel® 40-202; Methocel® E3P; Methocel® E4MP; Methocel® E5P; Methocel® E6P; Methocel® E10MP CR; Methocel® E15LVP; Methocel® E50LVP; Methocel® E50P; Methocel® E Premium; Methocel® F Premium; Methocel® J Premium; Methocel® K4MP; Methocel® K4MS; Methocel® K15MP; Methocel® K15MS; Methocel® K35; Methocel® K100LVP; Methocel® K100MP; Methocel® K Premium; Viscontran MHPC
Trade names containing: Unispheres G-503; Unispheres R-505; Unispheres U-504; Unispheres YE-501

Hydroxypropyltrimonium gelatin (INCI)
Trade names: Quat-Coll™ IP10-30

Hydroxypropyltrimonium hydrolyzed casein (INCI)
Trade names: Promois Milk Q

Hydroxypropyltrimonium hydrolyzed collagen (INCI)
CAS 11308-59-1
Trade names: Promois W-42Q; Promois W-42QP; Promois W-52Q; Promois W-52QP

Hydroxypropyltrimonium hydrolyzed keratin (INCI)
Trade names: Promois WK-HQ; Quat Keratin™ QTM-30

Hydroxypropyltrimoniium hydrolyzed silk (INCI)
Trade names: Promois Silk 700 QSP; Promois Silk-1000 Q; Promois Silk-1000 QP; Quat-Silk™ QTM-10

Hydroxypropyltrimonium hydrolyzed soy protein (INCI)
Trade names: Peptein® Qs; Promois WS-Q; Quat-Soy™ QTM-30; Tri-K Soyquat-30

Hydroxypropyltrimonium hydrolyzed vegetable protein (INCI)
Trade names: Quat-Veg™ Q-30

Hydroxypropyltrimonium hydrolyzed wheat protein (INCI)
Trade names: Hydrotriticum™ WQ; Peptein® Qw; Promois WG-Q; Quat-Wheat™ QTM-20

Hydroxy stearamidopropyl trimonium chloride (INCI)
CAS 127312-01-0
Trade names containing: Surfactol® Q2

Hydroxy stearamidopropyl trimonium methosulfate (INCI)
CAS 127312-00-9
Trade names containing: Surfactol® Q3

Hydroxystearic acid (INCI)
CAS 106-14-9; EINECS 203-366-1
Synonyms: HSA; 12-Hydroxyoctadecanoic acid; 12-Hydroxystearic acid; Octadecanoic acid, 12-hydroxy-
Trade names: HSA

α-Hydroxytoluene. *See Benzyl alcohol*

Hydroxyxanthine
Trade names containing: MicroReservoir FRS-Diffuser

Hypericum extract (INCI)
CAS 68917-49-7, 84082-80-4
Synonyms: St. John's wort extract
Trade names containing: Actiphyte of St. John's Wort; Blend For Chapped Skins HS 361; Blend For Delicate Skins HS 215; Crodarom St. John's Wort O; Herbalcomplex 1 Special; Herbasol Complex D; Herbasol-Extract St. John's Wort; Herbasol Stimulant Complex; Hypericum Oil CLR; Solarium HS 269; Solarium HS 270; Solarium LS 669; Solarium LS 670

Iceland moss extract (INCI)
CAS 84776-25-0
Synonyms: Cetraria islandica extract; Lichen islandicus

extract
Trade names containing: Evosina IP 7; Evosina NA 2

Ichthammol (INCI)
CAS 8029-68-3; EINECS 232-439-0
Trade names containing: Antidandruff Agent NOVA

Imidazolidinyl urea (INCI)
CAS 39236-46-9; EINECS 254-372-6
Synonyms: N,N´´-Methylenebis[N´-[1-(hydroxymethyl)-2,5-dioxo-4-imidazolindinyl]urea]
Trade names: Abiol; Atomergic Imidazolidinyl Urea; Biopure 100; Germall® 115; Sepicide CI; Tristat IU; Unicide U-13

Imidurea
Trade names: Unisept IMIDU

Infusorial earth. *See Diatomaceous earth*

Inositol (INCI)
CAS 87-89-8; EINECS 201-781-2
Synonyms: Hexahydroxy cyclohexane; myo-Inositol; meso-Inositol
Trade names: Inositol
Trade names containing: Aquaderm; Extrapone Neo-H-Special 2/032441; Extrapone Poly H Special 2/032451; Hair Complex 20/70n; Hair Complex Aquosum; Lactil®; Soluvit Richter

Iodized corn protein (INCI)
Trade names containing: Jodoprolamina

Iodopropynyl butylcarbamate (INCI)
CAS 55406-53-6
Synonyms: 3-Iodo-2-propynyl butyl carbamate; Butyl-3-iodo-2-propynylcarbamate; Carbamic acid, butyl-3-iodo-2-propynyl ester
Trade names: Glycacil L, S
Trade names containing: Glydant® Plus

IPA. *See Isopropyl alcohol*

IPM. *See Isopropyl myristate*

IPP. *See Isopropyl palmitate*

IR. *See Polyisoprene*

Irish moss extract. *See Carrageenan extract*

Iron blue. *See Ferric ammonium ferrocyanide*

Iron gluconate. *See Ferrous gluconate*

Iron oxides (INCI)
CAS 1309-37-1 (Fe$_2$O$_3$), 1345-25-1 (FeO), 1317-61-9 (Fe$_3$O$_4$); EINECS 215-721-8, 215-168-2, 215-277-5
Trade names: B-3279 Cosmetic Brown; Cogilor Jet; Cogilor Ochre; Cogilor Rouge; Cosmetic Black Iron Oxide 7075; Cosmetic Micro Blend Red Oxide 9268; Jaune Extra W 1800
Trade names containing: B-3389 Cosmetic Umber; Black 103; Black Mica; Brown 208; Chroma-Lite® Black 4498; Cloisonné Gold; Colorona® Bordeaux; Colorona® Bright Gold; Colorona® Copper; Colorona® Sienna; Cosmetic Brown Oxide 7144; Cosmetic Hydrophobic Black Oxide 9333; Dichrona® GY; Dichrona® YB; Dichrona® YG; Dichrona® YR; Duocrome® GY; Duocrome® YR; Flamenco® Twilight Blue; Flonac MX 30 C; Gemstone Sunstone CC; Gemtone® Amber; Gemtone® Sunstone; Gemtone® Tan Opal CC; Jaune Covasop W 1771; Lo-Micron Black Extender B.C. 34-3062-1; Red 139; Sunveil F; Unispheres R-505; Unispheres YE-501; Yellow 201

Isobutane (INCI)
CAS 75-28-5; EINECS 200-857-2
Synonyms: 2-Methylpropane; Propane, 2-methyl-; Isobutane

Trade names containing: Drivosol®

Isobutanolamine. *See 2-Amino-2-methyl-1-propanol*

Isobutylated lanolin oil (INCI)
CAS 85005-47-6
Synonyms: Lanolin oil, isobutylated
Trade names: Argonol 40

p-Isobutylbenzaldehyde
Trade names: Ibbal

Isobutylene/MA copolymer (INCI)
CAS 26426-80-2
Synonyms: Isobutylene/maleic anhydride copolymer; 2-Methyl-1-propene, polymer with 2,5-furandione; 2,5-Furandione, polymer with 2-methyl-1-propene
Trade names: Daxad® 31; Tamol® 731-25%

Isobutyl p-hydroxybenzoate. *See Isobutylparaben*

Isobutyl methacrylate
CAS 97-86-9
Synonyms: Isobutyl-α-methacrylate; 2-Methylpropyl methacrylate
Trade names: Rohagum® P-26; Rohagum® P-28; Rohagum® P-675; Rohagum® PQ-610
Trade names containing: Rohamere® 4885F

Isobutyl oleate
CAS 84988-79-4; EINECS 284-868-8
Trade names: Radia® 7230

Isobutylparaben (INCI)
CAS 4247-02-3; EINECS 224-208-8
Synonyms: Isobutyl p-hydroxybenzoate; 4-Hydroxy-benzoic acid, 2-methylpropyl ester; Isobutyl para-hydroxybenzoate
Trade names containing: LiquaPar® Oil

Isobutyl stearate (INCI)
CAS 646-13-9, 85865-69-6; EINECS 211-466-1, 288-668-1
Synonyms: 2-Methylpropyl octadecanoate; Stearic acid, 2-methylpropyl ester
Trade names: Estol 1476; Estol IBUS 1552; Ibulate; Kemester® 5415; Kessco® Isobutyl Stearate; Radia® 7241; Radia® 7761
Trade names containing: Isolanoate-BS; Tisolate-BS

Isobutyl tallowate (INCI)
CAS 68526-50-1
Synonyms: Fatty acids, tallow, isobutyl esters; Tallow fatty acids, isobutyl esters
Trade names containing: Lacol

Isoceteareth-8 stearate (INCI)
Synonyms: PEG-8 isocetyl/isostearyl ether stearate; PEG 400 isocetyl/isostearyl ether stearate
Trade names: Isoxal E

Isoceteth-20 (INCI)
Synonyms: PEG-20 isocetyl ether; POE (20) isohexa-decyl ether; PEG 1000 isocetyl ether
Trade names: Arlasolve® 200; Arlasolve® 200 Liq

Isoceteth-30 (INCI)
Synonyms: PEG-30 isocetyl ether; POE (30) isocetyl ether
Trade names: Nikkol BH-30

Isoceteth-10 stearate (INCI)
Synonyms: PEG-10 isocetyl ether monostearate
Trade names containing: Isoxal H

Isocetyl alcohol (INCI)
CAS 36311-34-9; EINECS 252-964-9
Synonyms: Isohexadecanol; Isohexadecyl alcohol; Isopalmityl alcohol

Trade names: Ceraphyl® ICA; Eutanol® G16; Michel XO-150-16; Unimul-G-16
Trade names containing: Castorcet

Isocetyl behenate (INCI)
Synonyms: Behenic acid, isocetyl ester; Behenic acid, isohexadecyl ester; Docosanoic acid, isocetyl ester
Trade names: Pelemol ICB

Isocetyl isostearate
Trade names: Nikkol ICIS

Isocetyl myristate (INCI)
CAS 83708-66-1
Synonyms: Myristic acid, isocetyl ester; Tetradecanoic acid, isocetyl ester; Tetradecanoic acid, isohexadecyl ester
Trade names: Nikkol ICM-R

Isocetyl octanoate
Trade names: Bernel® Ester 168

Isocetyl salicylate
CAS 138208-68-1
Trade names: Dermol ICSA

Isocetyl stearate (INCI)
CAS 25339-09-7; EINECS 246-868-6
Trade names: Ceraphyl® 494; Cetiol® G16S; Crodamol ICS; Kemester® 5822; Kessco ICS; Kessco® Isocetyl Stearate; Nikkol ICS-R; Pelemol ICS; Schercemol ICS; Unimul-7061

Isocetyl stearoyl stearate (INCI)
CAS 97338-28-8
Trade names: Ceraphyl® 791; Hetester HSS

Isodeceth-5 (INCI)
Synonyms: PEG-5 isodecyl ether
Trade names: Carsonon® D-5; Hodag Nonionic ID-5; Unicol W-5

Isodecyl citrate (INCI)
CAS 90605-17-7; EINECS 292-416-6
Synonyms: 2-Hydroxy-1,2,3-propanetricarboxylic acid, isodecyl ester
Trade names: Trioxene LV

Isodecyl cocoate (INCI)
Synonyms: Coconut fatty acids, isodecyl ester
Trade names: Trioxene I

Isodecyl isononanoate (INCI)
CAS 41395-89-5
Synonyms: 3,5,5-Trimethylhexanoic acid, isodecyl ester; Hexanoic acid, 3,5,5-trimethyl-, isodecyl ester
Trade names: Dermol 109; Wickenol® 152

Isodecyl laurate (INCI)
CAS 14779-93-2
Synonyms: Dodecanoic acid, dimethyloctyl ester; Dodecanoic acid, isodecyl ester
Trade names: Isostearene

Isodecyl neopentanoate (INCI)
CAS 60209-82-7; EINECS 262-108-6
Synonyms: 2,2-Dimethylpropanoic acid, isodecyl ester
Trade names: Dermol 105; Schercemol 105

Isodecyl octanoate (INCI)
CAS 34962-91-9; 89933-26-6
Synonyms: Isooctanoic acid, isodecyl ester
Trade names: Dermol 108; Pelemol 108
Trade names containing: Dermol 334; Estalan 334

Isodecyl oleate (INCI)
CAS 59231-34-4; EINECS 261-673-6
Synonyms: 9-Octadecenoic acid, isodecyl ester
Trade names: Ceraphyl® 140-A; Estol IDCO 3667;

Pelemol IDO; Schercemol IDO; Trivent OL-10B; Wickenol® 144

Isodecyl salicylate (INCI)
Synonyms: Salicylic acid, isodecyl ester
Trade names: Edesal; Keratoplast

Isodecyl stearate (INCI)
CAS 31565-38-5; EINECS 250-704-9
Trade names: Fractalite IDS

Isododecane (INCI)
CAS 141-70-8, 31807-55-3, 13475-82-6; EINECS 205-495-9
Synonyms: 2,2,6,6-Tetramethyl-4-methyleneheptane
Trade names: Permethyl® 99A
Trade names containing: Bentone® Gel ISD

Isodonis extract (INCI)
Trade names containing: Isodon Extract

Isoeicosane (INCI)
CAS 93685-79-1
Trade names: Permethyl® 102A
Trade names containing: Permethyl® 1082

Isohexadecane (INCI)
CAS 4390-04-9; EINECS 224-506-8
Trade names: Arlamol® HD; Permethyl® 101A

Isohexyl neopentanoate (INCI)
CAS 5434-57-1, 131141-70-3
Synonyms: 2-Ethylbutyl 2,2-dimethylpropanoate
Trade names: Schercemol 65

Isolaureth-6 (INCI)
CAS 60828-78-6
Synonyms: PEG-6 isolauryl ether; POE (6) isolauryl ether; PEG 300 isolauryl ether
Trade names containing: Dow Corning® 7224 Conditioning Agent; Dow Corning® Q2-7224 Conditioning Additive

L-Isoleucine (INCI)
CAS 73-32-5 (L-form); EINECS 200-798-2
Synonyms: 2-Amino-3-methylpentanoic acid
Trade names containing: Omega-CH Activator

Isolongifolene ketone exo (INCI)
CAS 29461-14-1; EINECS 249-649-3
Trade names: Ketosesquine

Isomaltose
Trade names containing: Sweetrex®

Isononyl isononanoate (INCI)
CAS 42131-25-9
Synonyms: 3,5,5-Trimethylhexanoic acid, 3,5,5-trimethylhexyl ester
Trade names: Salacos 99; Wickenol® 151

Isononyl stearate
CAS 91031-57-1
Trade names: Radia® 7510

Isooctyl stearate
CAS 91031-48-0; EINECS 292-951-5
Trade names: Radia® 7131

Isopentyldiol (INCI)
CAS 2568-33-4
Synonyms: 3-Methyl-1,3-butanediol
Trade names: IPG

Isopropanolamine (INCI)
CAS 78-96-6; EINECS 201-162-7
Synonyms: MIPA; 1-Amino-2-propanol; Monoisopropanolamine; 2-Hydroxypropylamine
Trade names containing: Witcamide® 61

Isopropanolamine lanolate (INCI)
Synonyms: 2-Hydroxypropylamine lanolate
Trade names: Lanapol CT

Isopropyl alcohol (INCI)
CAS 67-63-0; EINECS 200-661-7
Synonyms: IPA; Isopropanol; 2-Propanol; Dimethyl carbinol
Trade names containing: Aristoflex A/60% Sol'n; Aromox® C/12; Aromox® DM16; Aromox® DMCD; Aromox® T/12; Arquad® 2C-75; Arquad® 2HT-75; Arquad® 2T; Arquad® 12-33; Arquad® 12-50; Arquad® 16-25; Arquad® 16-50; Arquad® 18-50; Arquad® B-100; Arquad® C-33; Arquad® C-50; Arquad® S-50; Arquad® T-50; Biju® BNT; Biju® BTD, BXD; Biju® BWD, BWS; Biju® BWP; Biju® Ultra UNT; Biju® Ultra UTD, UXD; Biju® Ultra UWD, UWS; Biju® Ultra UWP; Carboset 514A; Carsoquat® SDQ-25; Duoquad® O-50; Duoquad® T-50; Emulmetik™ 310; Emulmetik™ 910; Emulmetik™ 920; Ethoquad® 18/12; Ethoquad® C/12; Ethoquad® C/12 Nitrate; Ethoquad® CB/12; Ethoquad® O/12; Ethoquad® O/12H; Gantrez® ES-335; Gantrez® ES-435; Gemtex PA-75; Lamepon® LPO 30; Mearl-maid® AA; Mearlmaid® CKD; Mearlmaid® CP; Mearlmaid® KN; Mearlmaid® KND; Mearlmaid® OL; Mearlmaid® TR; Naturon® 2X IPA; Naturon® CSN-22; Tauranol ML; Variquat® 50AC; Variquat® 50AC; Variquat® 80AC; Variquat® 80AC; Variquat® 477; Variquat® 477; Variquat® 638; Variquat® K300; Variquat® K300; Variquat® SDC; Varisoft® 110; Varisoft® 137; Varisoft® 222 (75%); Varisoft® 222 (90%); Varisoft® 222 HV (90%); Varisoft® 222 LM (90%); Varisoft® 222 LT (90%); Varisoft® 432-CG; Varisoft® 461; Varisoft® 462; Varisoft® 470; Varisoft® 471; Varisoft® 475; Varisoft® 910; Varisoft® 3690; Varisoft® DHT; Varisoft® OIMS; Varisoft® SDAC

Isopropylamine dodecylbenzenesulfonate (INCI)
CAS 26264-05-1; 68584-24-7; EINECS 247-556-2
Synonyms: Dodecylbenzenesulfonic acid, comp. with 2-propanamine (1:1)
Trade names: Rhodacal® 330

Isopropyl arachidate (INCI)
CAS 26718-90-1; EINECS 247-919-5
Synonyms: Isopropyl eicosanoate; 1-Methylethyl eicosanoate
Trade names containing: Jafaester 2022

Isopropyl behenate (INCI)
CAS 26718-95-6; EINECS 247-922-1
Synonyms: Isopropyl docosanoate; 1-Methylethyl docosanoate
Trade names containing: Jafaester 2022

p-Isopropylbenzaldehyde
CAS 122-03-2; EINECS 204-516-9
Trade names: Cumal

Isopropyl C12-15-pareth-9-carboxylate (INCI)
Synonyms: PEG-9 C12-15 alkyl ether carboxylic acid, isopropyl ester; PEG 450 C12-15 alkyle ther carboxylic acid, isopropyl ester; POE (9) C12-15 alkyl ether carboxylic acid, isopropyl ester
Trade names: Velsan® P8-3

4-Isopropyl-m-cresol
CAS 3228-02-2; EINECS 221-761-7
Synonyms: o-Cymen-5-ol
Trade names: Dekacymen

Isopropyl dibenzoylmethane (INCI)
CAS 63250-25-9; EINECS 264-043-9

Synonyms: 5-Isopropyl-di-benzoylmethane; 1-[4-(1-Methylethyl)phenyl]-3-phenyl-1,3-propanedione
Trade names: Eusolex® 8020

4-Isopropyl-5,5-dimethyl-1,3-dioxane
Trade names: Anthoxan

Isopropyl hydroxycetyl ether (INCI)
Trade names containing: Dragophos S 2/918501

Isopropyl isostearate (INCI)
CAS 31478-84-9, 68171-33-5; EINECS 250-651-1
Trade names: Emerest® 2310; Lanesta 10; Nikkol IPIS; Prisorine IPIS 2021; Schercemol 318; Wickenol® 131; Witconol™ 2310

Isopropyl lanolate (INCI)
CAS 63393-93-1; EINECS 264-119-1
Synonyms: Lanolin fatty acids, isopropyl esters
Trade names: Amerlate® P; Amerlate® W; Fancol IPL; Fancor IPL; Ivarlan™ 3350; Lanesta L; Lanesta S; Lanesta SA-30; Lanisolate; Ritasol
Trade names containing: Ivarbase™ 3240; Rewolan® LP; Ritasol Base 100; Ritasol Base 200

Isopropyl laurate (INCI)
CAS 10233-13-3; EINECS 233-560-1
Synonyms: Dodecanoic acid, 1-methylethyl ester; 1-Methylethyl dodecanoate
Trade names: Crodamol IPL; Estol IPL 1511

Isopropyl linoleate (INCI)
CAS 22882-95-7; EINECS 245-289-6
Synonyms: 1-Methylethyl-9,12-octadecadienoate; 9,12-Octadecadienoic acid, 1-methylethyl ester
Trade names: Ceraphyl® IPL; Nikkol VF-IP

Isopropyl myristate (INCI)
CAS 110-27-0; EINECS 203-751-4
Synonyms: IPM; 1-Methylethyl tetradecanoate; Tetradecanoic acid, 1-methylethyl ester; Myristic acid isopropyl ester
Trade names: Crodamol IPM; Deltyl® Extra; Elfacos® IPM; Emerest® 2314; Estol 1512; Estol 1514; Estol IPM 1508; Estol IPM 1509 (BIO-IPM); Estol IPM 1512; Estol IPM 1514; Estol IPM-b 1509; Isopropylmyristat; Jafaester 14 NF; Jafaester 14-96; Kessco® Isopropyl Myristate; Kessco® Isopropyl Myristate NF; Lanesta 31; Lexol® IPM; Lexol® IPM-NF; Liponate IPM; Nikkol IPM-100; Nikkol IPM-EX; Promyr; Protachem IPM; Radia® 7190; Radia® 7730; Tegosoft® M; Upamate IPM; Wickenol® 101; Witconol™ 2314
Trade names containing: Aloe Extract #104; Aloe Vera Oil 0030X; Arnicaflower Oil PANAROM; Balm Mint Oil Infusion; Bentone® Gel IPM; Carrot Oil Extra; Carrot Oil; Crestalan A; Crestalan B; Crodarom Carrot O; Derma-Vitamincomplex, Oil soluble; Emulgade® CL Special; Evosina IP 7; Fancol ISO; Gilugel IPM; Hydro Myristenol 2/014082; Lexate® TA; Lexein® A240; Lexol® 3975; Lexol® 60; Monacet; Monamilk; Myrol-S; Oleo-Coll™ A240-20; Oleo-Coll™ A240; PCL Liq. 2/066210; PCL SE w/o 2/066255; PCL-Siccum 2/066215; Proto-Lan A240; Pur-Cellin Oil; Tegosoft® Liquid M; Texal-L; Tixogel IPM; Unipherol U-14; Wickenol® 105; Wickenol® 136

Isopropyl oleate (INCI)
CAS 112-11-8, 85116-87-6; EINECS 203-935-4, 285-540-7
Synonyms: 1-Methylethyl-9-octadecenoate; 9-Octadecenoic acid, 1-methylethyl ester
Trade names: Radia® 7231

Isopropyl palmitate (INCI)
CAS 142-91-6; EINECS 205-571-1

Synonyms: IPP; Isopropyl n-hexadecanoate; Hexadecanoic acid, 1-methylethyl ester; 1-Methylethyl hexandecanoate
Trade names: Crodamol IPP; Deltyl® Prime; Elfacos® IPP; Emerest® 2316; Estol 1517; Estol IPP 1517; Estol IPP-b 3651; Isopropyl Palmitate; Jafaester 16 NF; Kessco® Isopropyl Palmitate; Lanesta 23; Lexol® IPP; Lexol® IPP-A; Lexol® IPP-NF; Liponate IPP; Nikkol IPP; Nikkol IPP-EX; Propal; Protachem IPP; Radia® 7200; Radia® 7732; Tegosoft® P; Upamate IPP; Wickenol® 111; Witconol™ 2316
Trade names containing: Aloe Vera Oil 0030X; Apicerol 2/014081; Argonol ISO; Argonol RIC2; Bentone® Gel LOI; Co-Gell® A2/B270; Crestalan CB3910; Cutavit Richter; EFA-Plex; Gilugel IPP; Isopropylan® 33; Isopropylan® 50; Ivarbase™ 3250; Lanalene Liq. 30, 50; Lanalene Liq. 75; Lanapene; Lanosil; Lexol® 3975; Lexol® 60; Oleo Keratin™ ISO; Ritalan® C; Tixogel LAN; Wickenol® 105; Wickenol® 136

Isopropylparaben (INCI)
CAS 4191-73-5; EINECS 224-069-3
Synonyms: Isopropyl p-hydroxybenzoate; 1-Methylethyl-4-hydroxybenzoate; 4-Hydroxybenzoic acid, 1-methylethyl ester
Trade names containing: LiquaPar® Oil

Isopropyl PPG-2-isodeceth-7-carboxylate (INCI)
Synonyms: PEG-7-PPG-2 isodecyl ether carboxylci acid, isopropyl ester; POE(7) POP(2) isodecyl ether carboxylic acid isopropyl ester
Trade names: Velsan® D8P-3

Isopropyl stearate (INCI)
CAS 112-10-7; EINECS 203-934-9
Synonyms: 1-Methylethyl octadecanoate; Octadecanoic acid, 1-methylethyl ester
Trade names: Estol IPS 3702; Kessco IPS; Lasemul 60; Tegosoft® S; Wickenol® 127
Trade names containing: Lexol® 3975; Lexol® 60; Wickenol® 136

Isopropyl titanium triisostearate (INCI)
CAS 61417-49-0; EINECS 262-774-8
Synonyms: Isopropyl triisostearoyl titanate; Tris(isooctadecanoato-O)(2-propanolato) titanium
Trade names: Ken-React® KR TTS

Isosorbide laurate (INCI)
Trade names: Arlamol® ISML

Isostearamide DEA (INCI)
CAS 52794-79-3; EINECS 258-193-4
Synonyms: N,N-Bis(2-hydroxyethyl)isooctadecanamide
Trade names: Afmide™ ISA; Hetamide IS; Mackamide™ ISA; Monamid® 150-IS; Standamid® ID; Witcamide® 5118S

Isostearamidopropylamine oxide (INCI)
Synonyms: N-[3-(Dimethylamino)propyl] isooctadecanamide, N-oxide; Amides, isostearic, N-[3-(dimethylamino)propyl], N-oxide
Trade names: Afamine™ IAO

Isostearamidopropyl betaine (INCI)
CAS 6179-44-8; 63566-37-0; EINECS 228-227-2
Synonyms: N-(Carboxymethyl)-N,N-dimethyl-3-[(1-oxoisooctadecyl)amino]-1-propanaminium hydroxide, inner salt
Trade names: Afaine™ ISA; Lexaine® IS; Mackam™ ISA; Schercotaine IAB

Isostearamidopropyl dimethylamine (INCI)
CAS 67799-04-6; EINECS 267-101-1
Synonyms: N-[3-(Dimethylamino)propyl]isooctadecanamide

Trade names: Chemidex SI; Mackine™ 401; Schercodine I

Isostearamidopropyl dimethylamine gluconate (INCI)
CAS 129541-36-2
Synonyms: Isostearyl amidopropyl dimethylamino gluconate; Isostearyl amidopropyl dimethylaminopentahydroxycaproate
Trade names: Katemul IGU-70

Isostearamidopropyl dimethylamine glycolate (INCI)
CAS 118777-77-8
Synonyms: Isostearyl amidopropyl dimethylamino glycolate
Trade names: Katemul IG-70

Isostearamidopropyl dimethylamine lactate (INCI)
CAS 55852-15-8
Synonyms: Propanoic acid, 2-hydroxy-, compd. with N-[3-(dimethylamino)propyl]-16-methylheptadecanamide (1:1)
Trade names: Afalene™ 416; Emcol® 6613; Mackalene™ 416

Isostearamidopropyl ethyldimonium ethosulfate (INCI)
CAS 67633-63-0; EINECS 266-778-0
Synonyms: N-Ethyl-N,N-dimethyl-3-[(1-oxoisooctadecyl) amino]-1-propanaminium ethyl sulfate; Isostearyl dimethylamidopropyl ethonium ethosulfate
Trade names: Foamquat IAES; M-Quat® 522; Naetex-S; Schercoquat IAS

Isostearamidopropyl laurylacetodimonium chloride (INCI)
CAS 134112-42-8
Synonyms: 1-Propanaminium, N-[2-(dodecyloxy)-2-oxoethyl]-N,N-dimethyl-3-[(1-oxoisooctadecyl) amino]-, chloride; N-Isostearamidopropyl-N,N-dimethyl-N-(dodecyl acetate) ammonium chloride
Trade names: Foamquat IALA; Schercoquat IALA

Isostearamidopropyl morpholine (INCI)
Synonyms: Isooctadecanamide, N-[3-(4-morpholinyl) propyl]-; N-[3-(4-Morpholinyl)propyl]isooctadecanamide
Trade names: Mackine™ 421

Isostearamidopropyl morpholine lactate (INCI)
CAS 72300-24-4; 80145-09-1
Synonyms: Propanoic acid, 2-hydroxy-, compd. with N-[3-(4-morpholinyl)propyl]isooctadecanamide
Trade names: Afalene™ AFC; Emcol® ISML; Incromate ISML; Mackalene™ 426

Isostearamidopropyl morpholine oxide (INCI)
Synonyms: Amides, isostearic, N-[3-(4-morpholinyl)propyl], N-oxide; Isooctadecanamide, N-[3-(4-morpholinyl)propyl]-N-oxide; N-[3-(4-Morpholinyl) propyl]isooctadecanamide-N-oxide
Trade names: Afamine™ ISMO

Isostearamidopropyl PG-dimonium chloride (INCI)
Trade names: Lexquat® AMG-IS

Isosteareth-2 (INCI)
CAS 52292-17-8 (generic)
Synonyms: PEG-2 isostearyl ether; POE (2) isostearyl ether; PEG 100 isostearyl ether
Trade names: Arosurf® 66-E2; Hetoxol IS-2

Isosteareth-3 (INCI)
CAS 52292-17-8 (generic)
Synonyms: PEG-3 isostearyl ether
Trade names: Hetoxol IS-3

Isosteareth-5
Trade names: Emalex 1805

Isosteareth-10 (INCI)
CAS 52292-17-8 (generic)
Synonyms: PEG-10 isostearyl ether; POE (10) isostearyl ether; PEG 500 isostearyl ether
Trade names: Arosurf® 66-E10; Emalex 1810; Hetoxol IS-10

Isosteareth-12 (INCI)
CAS 52292-17-8 (generic)
Trade names: Ethlana 12

Isosteareth-15
Trade names: Emalex 1815

Isosteareth-20 (INCI)
CAS 52292-17-8 (generic)
Synonyms: PEG-20 isostearyl ether; POE (20) isostearyl ether; PEG 1000 isostearyl ether
Trade names: Arosurf® 66-E20; Emalex 1820; Hetoxol IS-20; Lipocol IS-20

Isosteareth-22 (INCI)
CAS 52292-17-8 (generic)
Trade names: Ethlana 22

Isosteareth-25
Trade names: Emalex 1825

Isosteareth-50 (INCI)
CAS 52292-17-8 (generic)
Trade names: Ethlana 50; Ethlana 50-M

Isosteareth-6 carboxylic acid (INCI)
Synonyms: PEG-6 isostearyl ether carboxylic acid; PEG 300 isostearyl ether carboxylic acid
Trade names: Sandopan® TA-10

Isosteareth-11 carboxylic acid (INCI)
Synonyms: PEG-11 isostearyl ether carboxylic acid
Trade names: Sandopan® TA-20

Isosteareth-10 stearate (INCI)
Trade names containing: Isoxal H

Isostearic acid (INCI)
CAS 2724-58-5, 30399-84-9; EINECS 220-336-3
Synonyms: Heptadecanoic acid, 16-methyl-; Isooctadecanoic acid; 16-Methylheptadecanoic acid
Trade names: Emersol® 871; Emersol® 875; Liponate ISA Special; Prisorine 3501; Prisorine 3505; Prisorine ISAC 3505; Unitol ISA
Trade names containing: Grillocin HY-77; Grillocin WE-106; Oleo Keratin™ ISO; Proto-Lan IP; Proto-Lan KT

Isostearic/myristic glycerides (INCI)
Trade names: Exceparl DG-MI

Isostearoyl hydrolyzed collagen (INCI)
Synonyms: Isostearoyl hydrolyzed animal protein; Proteins, hydrolysates, reaction prods. with isostearoyl Cl
Trade names: Crotein IP; Crotein IPX; Oleo-Coll™ ISO
Trade names containing: Proto-Lan IP

Isostearyl alcohol (INCI)
CAS 27458-93-1; 70693-04-8; EINECS 248-470-8
Synonyms: 1-Heptadecanol, 16-methyl-; Isooctadecanol; 16-Methyl-1-heptadecanol
Trade names: Adol® 66; Michel XO-150-1620; Prisorine 3515; Prisorine ISOH 3515
Trade names containing: Celanol A.S.L.; Isocet; Sexadecyl Alcohol, Cosmetic Grade

Isostearyl behenate (INCI)
Synonyms: Docosanoic acid, isooctadecyl ester
Trade names: Fractalite ISB; Pelemol ISB

Isostearyl behenyl beeswax
Trade names: Cera Albalate 102; Koster Keunen Isostearyl-Behenyl Beeswaxate

Isostearyl benzoate (INCI)
CAS 68411-27-8
Synonyms: Benzoic acid, isostearyl ester
Trade names: Finsolv® SB

Isostearyl diglyceryl succinate (INCI)
CAS 66085-00-5
Trade names: Imwitor® 780 K

Isostearyl erucate (INCI)
CAS 977079-10-9
Synonyms: Isooctadecyl 13-docosenoate; 13-Docosenoic acid, isooctadecyl ester
Trade names containing: Scheroba Oil

Isostearyl ethylimidonium ethosulfate (INCI)
CAS 67633-57-2; EINECS 266-778-0
Synonyms: Quaternium-32
Trade names: Monaquat ISIES; Schercoquat IIS

Isostearyl hydroxyethyl imidazoline (INCI)
CAS 68966-38-1; EINECS 273-429-6
Synonyms: Isostearyl imidazoline; 4,5-Dihydro-2-isoheptadecyl-1H-imidazole-1-ethanol
Trade names: Schercozoline I

Isostearyl isostearate (INCI)
CAS 41669-30-1; EINECS 255-485-3
Synonyms: Isooctadecanoic acid, isooctadecyl ester
Trade names: Iso Isotearyle WL 3196; Prisorine ISIS 2039; Rewomul IS; Schercemol 1818

Isostearyl lactate (INCI)
CAS 42131-28-2; EINECS 255-674-0
Synonyms: 2-Hydroxypropanoic acid, isostearyl ester
Trade names: Fractalite ISL; Patlac® IL; Pelemol ISL

Isostearyl myristate (INCI)
CAS 72576-81-9
Synonyms: Tetradecanoic acid, isooctadecyl ester
Trade names: Cosmol 812

Isostearyl neopentanoate (INCI)
CAS 58958-60-4; EINECS 261-521-9
Synonyms: 2,2-Dimethylpropanoic acid, isooctadecyl ester
Trade names: Ceraphyl® 375; Crodamol ISNP; Dermol 185; Schercemol 185

Isostearyl palmitate (INCI)
CAS 72576-80-8; EINECS 276-719-0
Synonyms: Hexadecanoic acid, isooctadecyl ester; Isooctadecyl hexadecanoate
Trade names: Nikkol ISP; Protachem ISP
Trade names containing: Lipocerite Standard

Isostearyl stearoyl stearate (INCI)
CAS 134017-12-2
Trade names: Hetester ISS

Isotridecyl cocoate
Trade names: Trioxene D

Isotridecyl isononanoate (CTFA)
CAS 42131-27-1; 59231-37-7
Synonyms: 3,5,5-Trimethylhexanoic acid, isotridecyl ester; Isononanoic acid, isotridecyl ester
Trade names: Salacos 913; Wickenol® 153

Ivy extract (INCI)
CAS 84082-54-2
Trade names containing: Blend For Greasy Hair HS 312; Blend For Greasy Skin Imperfections HS 315; Blend For Slenderizing Prods. HS 255; Brookosome® FIH; Capilotonique HS 220; Demaquillant HS 287; Demaquillant LS 687; Emollient HS 235; Emollient LS 635; Faceur ARL; Herbasol-Extract Ivy; Stimulant HS 285

Japan wax (INCI)
CAS 8001-39-6, 67701-27-3
Synonyms: Rhus succedanea wax
Trade names: Japan Wax NJ-9002; Japan Wax Stralpitz; Koster Keunen Japan Wax, Synthetic; Koster Keunen Synthetic Japan Wax; Ross Japan Wax

Jasmine extract (INCI)
CAS 90045-94-6, 84776-64-7; EINECS 289-960-1, 283-993-5
Synonyms: White jasmine extract
Trade names: Hydroessential Jasminum

Jewelweed extract
Trade names: Jewelweed Extract Code 9034

Jojoba esters (INCI)
Trade names: Transjojoba™ 15; Transjojoba™ 30; Transjojoba™ 60

Jojoba extract (INCI)
CAS 90045-98-0; EINECS 289-964-3
Synonyms: Simmondsia chinensis extract
Trade names containing: Actiphyte of Jojoba Meal

Jojoba oil (INCI)
CAS 61789-91-1
Synonyms: Oils, jojoba
Trade names: Atomergic Jojoba Oil; Cojoba; Emalex J.J. O-V; Estran™; Estran™-Lite; Estran™-Pure; Estran™-Xtra; Jojoba Oil; Jojoba Oil Cosmetic Grade; Jojoba Oil Pure Grade; Jojoba Oil Refined Grade; Lanaetex Jojoba Oil; Lipovol J; Lipovol J Lite; Nikkol Jojoba Oil S; Simchin® Natural; Simchin® Refined; Wickenol® 139

Jojoba seed powder (INCI)
Trade names: Jojoba Meal 24/60; Jojoba Meal 40; Jojoba Meal 60
Trade names containing: Florabeads JM 28/60

Jojoba wax (INCI)
CAS 66625-78-3
Trade names: Florabeads; Jojoba 28/60 Gypsy Rose; Jojoba 28/60 Jade; Jojoba 28/60 White; Jojoba 40/60 Mandarin; Jojoba 40/60 White; Jojoba 60/100 White; Jojobead Gypsy Rose 40/60; Jojobead Jade 40/60; Jojobead Lapis 40/60; Jojobead White 28/60; Nikkol Jojoba Wax
Trade names containing: Florabeads JM 28/60

Juglans nigra extract. *See Black walnut extract*

Juniper extract (INCI)
CAS 84603-69-0
Synonyms: Juniperus communis extract
Trade names containing: Herbaliquid Alpine Herbs Special; Herbasol Herbes de Provence Complex; Rhumacalm HS 328

Kaolin (INCI)
CAS 1332-58-7; EINECS 296-473-8
Synonyms: Bolus alba; China clay
Trade names: Colloidal Kaolin NF-Bacteria Controlled; Kaopaque 10, 20; Lion English Kaolin; Unimin KA
Trade names containing: Cosmetic Hydrophobic Kaolin 9400; Kalixide AS

Kelp extract (INCI)
Synonyms: Macrocystis pyriferae extract
Trade names containing: Biochelated Sea Kelp Extract

Keratin amino acids (INCI)
CAS 68238-35-7
Synonyms: Animal keratin amino acids; Amino acids, keratin
Trade names: Crotein HKP/SF; Kera-Tein AA; Kera-Tein AA-SD; Kerabiol; Keramino™ 20; Keramino™ 25;

Monteine KL 150
Trade names containing: Kera-Tein H; Kera-Tein W; Keramino™ SD

Kidney bean extract (INCI)
Synonyms: Phaseolus vulgaris extract
Trade names containing: Demaquillant HS 287; Emollient HS 238

Kieselguhr. *See Diatomaceous earth*

Kukui nut oil (INCI)
CAS 8015-80-3
Synonyms: Aleurites moluccana oil; Candlenut oil
Trade names: CoKukui; Nikkol Kukui Nut Oil

Lactamide DGA
Synonyms: Lactamide N-(1-ethoxy-2-hydroxyethyl); Propanamide, 2-hydroxy-N-(1-ethoxy-2-hydroxyethyl)
Trade names: Foamid LM2E
Trade names containing: Foamid LME-75

Lactamide MEA (INCI)
CAS 5422-34-4; EINECS 226-546-1
Synonyms: 2-Hydroxy-N-(2-hydroxyethyl)propanamide; Lactic acid monoethanolamide; Monoethanolamine lactic acid amide
Trade names: Incromectant LMEA; Lipamide LMEA; Mackamide™ LME; Naetex-LAM; Parapel® LAM-100; Schercomid LME; Upamide LACAMEA
Trade names containing: Foamid LME-75; Incromectant LAMEA; Lipomectant AL

Lactamidopropyl trimonium chloride (INCI)
CAS 93507-51-8
Synonyms: (3-Lactamidopropyl)trimethyl ammonium chloride
Trade names: Incromectant LQ

Lactase
CAS 9031-11-2; EINECS 232-864-1
Synonyms: β-Galactosidase
Trade names: Fungal Lactase 100,000; Yeast Lactase L-50,000

Lactic acid (INCI)
CAS 50-21-5; EINECS 200-018-0
Synonyms: 2-Hydroxypropanoic acid; 2-Hydroxy-propionic acid; Milk acid
Trade names: Patlac® LA; Unichem LACA
Trade names containing: Facteur Hydratant PH; Grillocin® HY 77; Hydrolyzed NMF; Hydroviton 2/059353; Lactil®; Moisturizing Factor L

Lactic acid extract
Trade names: BioLac™

Lactoglobuline
Trade names containing: Moisturizing Factor L

Lactoferrin (INCI)
Synonyms: Lactotransferrin
Trade names containing: Capigen CG; FRS-Diffuser Microreservoir; Iniferine; MicroReservoir FRS-Diffuser; Sebomine SB12

Lactoperoxidase (INCI)
CAS 9003-99-0; EINECS 232-668-6
Synonyms: Peroxidase
Trade names containing: Capigen CG; Myavert C; Sebomine SB12

Lactose (INCI)
CAS 63-42-3; EINECS 200-559-2
Synonyms: D-Glucose, 4-O-β-D-galactopyranosyl-; Milk sugar; Saccharum lactis
Trade names: Unisweet L; Unisweet Lactose

Trade names containing: Hydratherm CGI Lyophilized; Hydromilk ENL-SD; Lactofil; Unispheres G-503; Unispheres R-505; Unispheres U-504; Unispheres YE-501

Lactoyl methylsilanol elastinate (INCI)
Trade names: Lasilium C

Lactylic stearate
Trade names containing: Myvatex® 40-06S

Laneth-5 (INCI)
CAS 61791-20-6 (generic)
Synonyms: PEG-5 lanolin ether; POE (5) lanolin ether
Trade names: Aqualose W5; Fancol LA-5; Nikkol BWA-5; Polychol 5; Ritawax 5
Trade names containing: Solulan® 5

Laneth-10 (INCI)
CAS 61791-20-6 (generic)
Synonyms: PEG-10 lanolin ether; POE (10) lanolin ether; PEG 500 lanolin ether
Trade names: Nikkol BWA-10; Ritawax 10

Laneth-15 (INCI)
CAS 61791-20-6 (generic); 84650-19-1
Synonyms: PEG-15 lanolin ether; POE (15) lanolin ether
Trade names: Fancol LA-15; Ivarlan™ 3442; Lanaetex A-15; Polychol 15
Trade names containing: Relaxer Conc. No. 2; Relaxer Conc. No. 3; Relaxer Conc. No. 4

Laneth-16 (INCI)
CAS 61791-20-6 (generic)
Synonyms: PEG-16 lanolin ether; POE (16) lanolin ether
Trade names: Lanaetex-A16; Polychol 16
Trade names containing: Ritachol® 3000; Solulan® 16

Laneth-20 (INCI)
CAS 61791-20-6 (generic)
Synonyms: PEG-20 lanolin ether; POE (20) lanolin ether; PEG 1000 lanolin ether
Trade names: Aqualose W20; Aqualose W20/50; G-1790; Nikkol BWA-20; Ritawax 20
Trade names containing: Aqualose SLW

Laneth-25 (INCI)
CAS 61791-20-6 (generic)
Synonyms: PEG-25 lanolin ether; POE (25) lanolin ether
Trade names containing: Solulan® 25

Laneth-40 (INCI)
CAS 61791-20-6 (generic)
Synonyms: PEG-40 lanolin ether; POE (40) lanolin ether; PEG 2000 lanolin ether
Trade names: Nikkol BWA-40

Laneth-60 (INCI)
CAS 61791-20-6 (generic)
Synonyms: PEG-60 lanolin ether; POE (60) lanolin ether; PEG 3000 lanolin ether
Trade names containing: Relaxer Conc. No. 4

Laneth-10 acetate (INCI)
CAS 65071-98-9 (generic)
Synonyms: Acetylated POE (10) lanolin alcohol; PEG-10 lanolin ether, acetylated; PEG 500 lanolin ether acetate
Trade names: Linsol ETO; Lipolan 98

Lanolic acids. *See Lanolin acid*

Lanolin (INCI)
CAS 8006-54-0 (anhyd.), 8020-84-6 (hyd.); EINECS 232-348-6
Synonyms: Anhydrous lanolin; Wool wax; Wool fat
Trade names: Anhydrous Lanolin Grade 1; Anhydrous Lanolin Grade 2; Anhydrous Lanolin P.80; Anhydrous Lanolin P.95; Anhydrous Lanolin P.95RA; Anhydrous Lanolin Superfine; Anhydrous Lanolin USP; Anhydrous Lanolin USP Cosmetic; Anhydrous Lanolin USP Cosmetic AA; Anhydrous Lanolin USP Cosmetic Grade; Anhydrous Lanolin USP Deodorized AAA; Anhydrous Lanolin USP Pharmaceutical; Anhydrous Lanolin USP Pharmaceutical; Anhydrous Lanolin USP Pharmaceutical Grade; Anhydrous Lanolin USP Pharmaceutical Light Grade; Anhydrous Lanolin USP Superfine; Anhydrous Lanolin USP Ultrafine; Anhydrous Lanolin USP X-tra Deodorized; Corona Lanolin; Corona PNL ; Coronet Lanolin; Cosmetic Lanolin; Cosmetic Lanolin Anhydrous USP; Degras; Emery® 1650; Emery® 1656; Emery® 1660; Emery® HP-2050; Emery® HP-2060; Golden Dawn Grade 1, 2; Ivarlan™ 3000; Ivarlan™ 3001; Ivarlan™ 3006 Light; Ivarlan™ Light; Lanolin Anhydrous USP; Lanolin Cosmetic; Lanolin Extra-Deodorized; Lanolin Pharmaceutical; Lanolin Tech; Lanolin Tech. Grade; Lanolin USP; Pharmaceutical Lanolin USP; RITA Lanolin; Super Corona; Superfine Lanolin Anhydrous USP; Unilan
Trade names containing: Alcolan® 36W; Alcolan® 40; Amerchol® 400; Amerchol® BL; Amerchol® C; Amerchol® H-9; Amphocerin® K; Apicerol 2/014081; Aquaphil K; Argobase L1; Argobase L2; Argobase S1; Cremba; Croda Solid Base; Emery® 1740; Emery® 1747; Falba Absorption Base; Fancol C; Fancol CAB; Forlan 300; Forlan 500; Forlan L Conc; Forlan L; Forlan; Ivarbase™ T; Lanaetex CLC; Lanaetex FB; Lanaetex H; Lanaetex L-15; Lanalan; Lanalene SW; Lanalol; Lanola 90; Lanosoluble A; Lexate® PX; Nimcolan® 1747; PCL SE w/o 2/066255; Protalan SS-100; Rewolan® LP; Ritaderm®; Ritasol Base 200; Tewax TC 840; Unigator B 67

Lanolin acid (INCI)
CAS 68424-43-1; EINECS 270-302-7
Synonyms: Lanolic acids; Lanolin fatty acids; Acids, lanolin
Trade names: Amerlate® LFA; Amerlate® WFA; Argonol LFA Dist; Argowax LFA Distilled; Argowax LFA Standard; Facilan; Fancor LFA; Ritalafa®

Lanolin alcohol (INCI)
CAS 8027-33-6; EINECS 232-430-1
Synonyms: Alcohols, lanolin; Wool wax alcohol
Trade names: Anatol; Argowax Cosmetic Super; Argowax Dist; Argowax Standard; Ceralan®; Dusoran MD; Emery® 1780; Emery® 1795; Emery® HP-2095; Fancol LA; Hartolan; Hartolite; Ivarlan™ 3310; Ritawax; Ritawax Super; Super Hartolan; Unilanal
Trade names containing: Alcolan®; Almolan LIS; Amerchol L-101®; Amerchol® 400; Amerchol® BL; Amerchol® C; Amerchol® CAB; Amerchol® H-9; Amerchol® L-500; Amerchol® L-99; Amerchol® RC; Aquaphil K; Argobase 125; Argobase EU Hydrous; Argobase EU; Argobase EUC 2; Argobase L1; Argobase L2; Argobase S1; Celanol A.S.L.; Cremba; Croda Liq. Base; Croda Solid Base; Crosterol SFA; Emery® 1730; Emery® 1732; Emery® 1747; Falba Absorption Base; Fancol CAB; Fancol LAO; Forlan 200; Forlan 300; Forlan 500; Forlan; Ivarbase™ 101; Ivarbase™ T; Lanaetex CLC; Lanaetex FB; Lanaetex H; Lanaetex L-15; Lanalan; Lanalene ABS; Lanalene SW; Lanalol; Lanion-28; Lanpro-2; Liquid Absorption Base Type A, T; Liquid Absorption Base; Liquid Base; Nimcolan® 1747; Nimlesterol® 1732; Oleo-Coll™ LP; Protalan M-16, M-26; Protalan SS-100; Protegin® X; Protegin®;

Proto-Lan 8; Ritachol®; Stearalchol; Steralchol

Lanolin linoleate (INCI)
Synonyms: 9,12-Octadienoic acid, lanolin alcohol ester
Trade names containing: Polylan®

Lanolin oil (INCI)
CAS 8038-43-5; 70321-63-0; 8006-54-0
Synonyms: Dewaxed lanolin; Oils, lanolin
Trade names: Argonol 50; Argonol 50 Pharmaceutical; Argonol 50 Super; Argonol 60; Fluilan; Ivarlan™ 3100; Lanogene®; Lanoil; Lantrol® 1673; Lantrol® 1674; Lantrol® 1675; Lantrol® HP-2073; Lantrol® HP-2074; Lipolan R; Protalan Oil; Ritalan®; Unilan Oil; Vigilan
Trade names containing: Aloe Extract #103; Aqualose SLT; Aqualose SLW; Argonol ISO; Argonol RIC2; Bentone® Gel LOI; Crestalan A; Crestalan B; Crestalan CB3910; Dermoil; Emery® 1740; Fancol ISO; Isopropylan® 33; Isopropylan® 50; Ivarbase™ 3240; Ivarbase™ 3250; Lanalene Liq. 30, 50; Lanalene Liq. 75; Lanosil; Lanpro-10; Proto-Lan 20; Pulvi-Lan; Ritalan® C; Ritalan® HKS; Ritaplast R; Ritasol Base 100; Tixogel LAN

Lanolin wax (INCI)
CAS 68201-49-0; EINECS 269-220-4
Synonyms: Deoiled lanolin
Trade names: Albalan; Fancor Lanwax; Lanfrax®; Lanfrax® 1776; Lanfrax® 1779; Lanocerin®; Lanowax; Protalan Wax; R.I.T.A. Lanolin Wax; Unilan W
Trade names containing: Argobase L2; Base WL 2569; Juniorlan 1664

Lanosterol (INCI)
CAS 79-63-0; EINECS 201-214-9
Synonyms: Isocholesterol; Lanosta-8,24-dien-3-ol, (3beta)-
Trade names: Croda Lanosterol; Lanosterol
Trade names containing: Isocholesterol EX

Lappa extract (INCI)
CAS 84012-13-5
Synonyms: Arctium lappa extract; Great burdock extract
Trade names containing: Capilotonique HS 220

Lapyrium chloride (INCI)
CAS 6272-74-8; EINECS 228-464-1
Synonyms: 1-(2-Hydroxyethyl)carbamoyl methyl pyridinium chloride laurate; N-(Lauryl colamino formyl methyl) pyridinium chloride
Trade names: Emcol® E-607L

Lard glyceride (INCI)
CAS 61789-10-4; EINECS 263-032-6
Synonyms: Lard monoglyceride; Glycerides, lard mono-
Trade names: Myverol® 18-40

Lauralkonium bromide (INCI)
CAS 7281-04-1; EINECS 230-698-4
Synonyms: Benzenemethanaminium, N-dodecyl-N,N-dimethyl-, bromide; N-Dodecyl-N,N-dimethyl benzenemethanaminium bromide; Lauryl dimethyl benzyl ammonium bromide
Trade names: Amonyl BR 1244

Lauralkonium chloride (INCI)
CAS 139-07-1; EINECS 205-351-5
Synonyms: Lauryl dimethyl benzyl ammonium chloride; N,N-Dimethyl-N-dodecylbenzenemethanaminium chloride
Trade names: Catinal MB-50A; Dehyquart® LDB; Tequat PAN

Lauramide DEA (INCI)
CAS 120-40-1; 52725-64-1; EINECS 204-393-1
Synonyms: Lauric diethanolamide; N,N-Bis(2-hydroxyethyl)dodecanamide; Diethanolamine lauric acid amide
Trade names: Ablumide LDE; Afmide™ LLM; Afmide™ LMD; Alkamide® 327; Alkamide® 1195; Alkamide® DL-203/S; Alkamide® DL-207/S; Alkamide® L9DE; Alkamide® LE; Amidex LD; Amidex LD-8; Aminol LM-30C, LM-30C Special; Carsamide® SAL-7; Carsamide® SAL-82; Carsamide® SAL-9; Chimipal LDA; Comperlan® LD; Comperlan® LDO, LDS; Emid® 6513; Emid® 6519; Empilan® LDE; Empilan® LDE/FF; Ethylan® MLD; Foamid PK; Foamid SL-Extra; Hartamide LDA; Hetamide LL; Hetamide ML; Hetamide MOC; Incromide L90; Incromide LL; Incromide LR; Lauramina; Lipamide LMWC; Loropan LD; Mackamide™ L-10; Mackamide™ L95; Mackamide™ LLM; Mackamide™ LMD; Manromid 1224; Mazamide® 124; Mazamide® 1214; Mazamide® L-298; Mazamide® LM; Mazamide® LM 20; Mazamide® LS 196; Monamid® 31; Monamid® 150-GLT; Monamid® 150-LMWC; Monamid® 150-LWA; Monamid® 716; Monamid® 1034; Monamid® 1224; Monamid® L-350; Monamid® L-355; Monamid® L-360; Monamid® L-365; Monamid® LL-370; Monamid® LM-375; Ninol® 30-LL; Ninol® 55-LL; Ninol® 70-SL; Ninol® 96-SL; Ninol® L-9; Norfox® DLSA; Phoenamid LD, LD Special; Profan AA62; Protamide L-80M, L90, L90A, LM 73, LM 73-L, LM-73 PG, LMAV; Schercomid SL-Extra; Standamid® KDL; Standamid® KDOL; Standamid® KDS; Standamid® LD; Standamid® LDO; Standamid® LDS; Tohol N-230; Tohol N-230X; Upamide LD; Upamide LDS, LM-20, LS-173, LS-196; Varamide® LL-1; Varamide® ML-1; Varamide® ML-4; Witcamide® 5195; Witcamide® 6310; Witcamide® 6510; Witcamide® 6511; Witcamide® 6519; Witcamide® 6590; Witcamide® L-9; Witcamide® LDEA; Witcamide® LL; Witcamide® STD-HP
Trade names containing: Alkamide® L7DE; Bio-Terge® 804; Emid® 6541; Emid® 6590; Empilan® LDX; foamid 24; Foamid SLM; Hetamide LML; Incromide LLA; Loropan LMD; Miracare® ANL; Mirasheen® 202; Monamid® 1007; Monamid® LLN-380; Monamid® R31-42; Monamine ACO-100; Rewomid® DL 203 S; Rewomid® DL 203; Schercomid 1214; Schercomid LD; Schercomid SL-ML; Schercomid SLA; Schercomid SLL; Schercomid SLM-LC; Schercomid SLM-S; Standamid® LD 80/20; Stepanol® 317; Stepanol® 360; Synotol LM 90; Varifoam® SXC

Lauramide/lineamide DEA
Trade names: Naetex-LS

Lauramide/linoleamide DEA
Synonyms: Lauric/linoleic diethanolamide
Trade names: Alkamide® DIN-100

Lauramide MEA (INCI)
CAS 142-78-9; EINECS 205-560-1
Synonyms: Lauric monoethanolamide; N-(2-Hydroxyethyl)dodecanamide; Monoethanolamine lauric acid amide
Trade names: Ablumide LME; Afmide™ LMM; Amidex LMMEA; Comperlan® LMM; Empilan® LME; Hartamide LMEA; Hetamide MML; Lauridit® LM; Loropan LM; Mackamide™ LMM; Manromid LMA; Monamid® LMMA; Ninol® LMP; Phoenamid LMM; Rewomid® L 203; Standamid® LM; Upamide MEA; Varamide® L-203

Lauramide MIPA (INCI)
CAS 142-54-1; EINECS 205-541-8
Synonyms: Lauric monoisopropanolamide; N-(2-Hydroxypropyl)dodecanamide; Monoisopropanolamine lauric acid amide
Trade names: Amidex LIPA; Comperlan® LP; Empilan® LIS; Incromide LI; Incromide LMI; Monamid® LMIPA; Nidaba 3; Profan AD31; Rewomid® IPL 203; Upamide MIPA
Trade names containing: Elfan® SG; Empicol® TCR; Empicol® TLP; Empicol® TLR; Standapol® S; Texapon® EVR

Lauramidopropylamine oxide (INCI)
CAS 61792-31-2; EINECS 263-218-7
Synonyms: Lauramidopropyl dimethylamine oxide; N-[3-(Dimethylamino)propyl]dodecanamide-N-oxide; Amides, lauric, N-[3-(dimethylamino)propyl], N-oxide
Trade names: Chimin LMO; Mackamine™ LAO

Lauramidopropyl betaine (INCI)
CAS 4292-10-8; 86438-78-0; EINECS 224-292-6
Synonyms: N-(Carboxymethyl)N,N-dimethyl-3-[(1-oxododecyl)amino]-1-propanaminium hydroxide, inner salt
Trade names: Afaine™ LMB; Amido Betaine-L; Chembetaine L; Chemoxide L; Chimin LX; Lexaine® LM; Mackam™ LA; Mackam™ LMB; Mackam™ LMB-LS; Mafo® LMAB; Mirataine® BB; Monateric LMAB; Tego®-Betaine L-10 S
Trade names containing: Lexate® BPQ

Lauramidopropyl dimethylamine (INCI)
CAS 3179-80-4; EINECS 221-661-3
Synonyms: N-[3-(Dimethylamino)propyl]dodecanamide; Dimethylaminopropyl lauramide
Trade names: Chemidex L; Lexamine L-13; Mackine™ 801; Schercodine L

Lauramidopropyl dimethylamine propionate (INCI)
Synonyms: Dimethylaminopropyl lauramide propionate
Trade names: Mackam™ LAP

Lauramidopropyl PEG-dimonium chloride phosphate
CAS 83682-78-4
Trade names: Phospholipid PTD

Lauramidopropyl PG-dimonium chloride (INCI)
Trade names: Lexquat® AMG-M

Lauramidopropyl PG-dimonium chloride phosphate
Trade names: Monaquat P-TD. See Phospholipid P-TD

Lauramine (INCI)
CAS 124-22-1; 2016-57-1; EINECS 204-690-6
Synonyms: Lauryl amine; 1-Dodecanamine; Dodecylamine
Trade names: Adogen® 163D; Amine 12; Amine 12-98D; Armeen® 12; Armeen® 12D; Kemamine® P-690; Radiamine 6163; Radiamine 6164

Lauramine oxide (INCI)
CAS 1643-20-5; 70592-80-2; EINECS 216-700-6
Synonyms: Lauryl dimethylamine oxide; N,N-Dimethyl-1-dodecanamine-N-oxide
Trade names: Ablumox LO; Ammonyx® DMCD-40; Ammonyx® LO; Amyx LO 3594; Aromox® DMMC-W; Chemoxide LM-30; Emcol® DMCD-40; Emcol® L; Emcol® LO; Empigen® OB; Incromine Oxide L; Lilaminox M24; Mackamine™ LO; Mazox® LDA; Oxamin LO; Radiamox® 6804; Rewominox L 408; Rhodamox® LO; Schercamox DML; Unimox LO; Varox® 270; Varox® 365; Varox® 375; Zoramox LO
Trade names containing: Standapol® CAT

Lauraminopropionic acid (INCI)

CAS 1462-54-0; 3614-12-8; EINECS 215-968-1
Synonyms: N-Dodecyl-β-alanine; N-Lauryl, myristyl β-aminopropionic acid
Trade names: Afoteric™ 151L; Deriphat® 151C; Mackam™ 151L; Unitex 710-L

Laurdimonium hydroxyethyl cellulose
Synonyms: PG-hydroxyethylcellulose lauryldimonium chloride
Trade names: Crodacel QL

Laurdimonium hydroxypropyl hydrolyzed collagen
Trade names: Croquat L

Laurdimonium hydroxypropyl hydrolyzed soy protein
Trade names: Quat-Soy™ LDMA-30

Laurdimonium hydroxypropyl hydrolyzed wheat protein
Trade names: Hydrotriticum™ QL

Laurel extract (INCI)
CAS 84603-73-6
Synonyms: Bay laurel extract; Grecian laruel extract; Laurus nobilis extract; Sweet bay extract
Trade names containing: Herbasol Herbes de Provence Complex; Relaxant HS 278; Relaxant LS 678; Solarium HS 270; Solarium LS 670

Laureth-1 (INCI)
CAS 4536-30-5; EINECS 224-886-5
Synonyms: PEG-1 lauryl ether; Ethylene glycol monolauryl ether; 2-(Dodecyloxy)ethanol
Trade names: Bio-Soft® E-200; Hetoxol L-1; Lipocol L-1

Laureth-2 (INCI)
CAS 3055-93-4 (generic); 9002-92-0; 68002-97-1; 68439-50-9; EINECS 221-279-7
Synonyms: Diethylene glycol dodecyl ether; PEG-2 lauryl ether; 2-[2-(Dodecyloxy)ethoxy]ethanol
Trade names: Akyporox RLM 22; Arlypon® F; Bio-Soft® E-300; Britex L 20; Carsonon® L-2; Dehydol® LS 2 DEO; Empilan® KB 2; Hetoxol L-2; Lauropal 2; Marlowet® LMA 2; Nikkol BL-2; Oxetal VD 20; Procol LA-2; Prox-onic LA-1/02; Unihydol LS-2
Trade names containing: Comperlan® LS

Laureth-3 (INCI)
CAS 3055-94-5; 9002-92-0 (generic); 68002-97-1; 68439-50-9; EINECS 221-280-2
Synonyms: Triethylene glycol dodecyl ether; 2-[2-[2-(Dodecyloxy)ethoxy]ethoxy]ethanol; PEG-3 lauryl ether
Trade names: Ablunol LA-3; AE-1214/3; Carsonon® L-3; Dehydol® LS 3 DEO; Emalex 703; Empilan® KB 3; Empilan® KC 3; Genapol® L-3; Glicolene; Hetoxol L-3N; Lauropal 3; Oxetal VD 28; Procol LA-3; Rewopal® LA 3; Unihydol LS-3
Trade names containing: Grillocin® CW 90; Isoxal 5; Standapol® CS Paste; Standapol® CS-50; Texapon® WW 99; Unipol CS Paste; Unipol CS-50

Laureth-4 (INCI)
CAS 5274-68-0; 68002-97-1; 68439-50-9; EINECS 226-097-1
Synonyms: PEG-4 lauryl ether; PEG 200 lauryl ether; 3,6,9,12-Tetraoxatetracosan-1-ol
Trade names: Akyporox RLM 40; Brij® 30; Brij® 30SP; Britex L 40; Chemal LA-4; Dehydol® LS 4 DEO; Emthox® 5882; Ethosperse® LA-4; Hetoxol L-4; Hodag Nonionic L-4; Lauropal 4; Lipocol L-4; Macol® LA-4; Marlipal® 124; Marlowet® LA 4; Marlowet® LMA 4; Mulsifan CPA; Nikkol BL-4.2; Procol LA-4; Prox-onic LA-1/04; Rhodasurf® L-4; Simulsol P4; Trycol® 5882; Unicol LA-4; Unihydol LS-4; Witconol™ 5875
Trade names containing: Emulgator BTO; Euperlan® PK

3000 AM; Euperlan® PK 3000 OK; Euperlan® PK 3000 OK; Euperlan® PK 3000; Genapol® PGC; Marlowet® SAF/K; Unigator B 67; Zetesol 100

Laureth-5 (INCI)
CAS 3055-95-6; EINECS 221-281-8
Synonyms: PEG-5 lauryl ether; POE (5) lauryl ether; 3,6,9,12,15-Pentaoxyheptacosan-1-ol
Trade names: Ablunol LA-5; Carsonon® L-5; Emalex 705; Marlowet® LMA 5; Mulsifan RT 23
Trade names containing: Isoxal 12

Laureth-6 (INCI)
CAS 3055-96-7; EINECS 221-282-3
Synonyms: PEG-6 lauryl ether; POE (6) lauryl ether; 3,6,9,12,15,18-Hexaoxatriacontan-1-ol
Trade names: Dehydol® PID 6; Rewopal® LA 6

Laureth-7 (INCI)
CAS 3055-97-8; 9002-92-0 (generic); EINECS 221-283-9
Synonyms: PEG-7 lauryl ether; POE (6) lauryl ether; 3,6,9,12,15,18,21-Heptaoxatritriacontan-1-ol
Trade names: Ablunol LA-7; Emalex 707; Macol® LA-790; Marlipal® MG; Marlowet® LA 7; Procol LA-7; Rhodasurf® L-790
Trade names containing: Sepigel 305

Laureth-8 (INCI)
CAS 3055-98-9; 9002-92-0 (generic)
Synonyms: PEG-8 lauryl ether; POE (8) lauryl ether; 3,6,9,12,15,18,21,24-Octaoxahexatriacontan-1-ol
Trade names: Akyporox RLM 80V
Trade names containing: Elfan® SG

Laureth-9 (INCI)
CAS 3055-99-0; 9002-92-0 (generic); 68439-50-9; EINECS 221-284-4
Synonyms: PEG-9 lauryl ether; POE (9) lauryl ether; 3,6,9,12,15,18,21,24,27-Nonaoxanonatriacontan-1-ol
Trade names: Ablunol LA-9; Britex EMB; Carsonon® L-9; Chemal LA-9; Emalex 709; G-4829; Hetoxol L-9; Hodag Nonionic L-9; Macol® LA-9; Marlipal® 129; Nikkol BL-9EX; Procol LA-9; Prox-onic LA-1/09; Unicol LA-9
Trade names containing: Hetoxol LS-9; Standapol® Pearl Conc. 7130

Laureth-10 (INCI)
CAS 6540-99-4; 9002-92-0 (generic)
Synonyms: PEG-10 lauryl ether; POE (10) lauryl ether; 3,6,9,12,15,18,21,24,27,30-Dexaoxadotetracontan-1-ol
Trade names: Britex L 100; Emalex 710; Marlowet® LMA 10; Procol LA-10; Unihydol 100; Unihydol LS 10
Trade names containing: Emulgade® A; Euperlan® MPK 850; Euperlan® PK 771 BENZ; Euperlan® PK 771; Euperlan® PK 810 AM; Euperlan® PK 810; Isoxal 11; Texapon® CS Paste; Texapon® EVR

Laureth-11 (INCI)
CAS 9002-92-0 (generic)
Synonyms: PEG-11 lauryl ether; POE (11) lauryl ether
Trade names: Remcopal 21411

Laureth-12 (INCI)
CAS 3056-00-6; 9002-92-0 (generic); EINECS 221-286-5
Synonyms: PEG-12 lauryl ether; POE (12) lauryl ether; PEG 600 lauryl ether
Trade names: Ablunol LA-12; Carsonon® L-12; Chemal LA-12; Emalex 712; Emthox® 5967; Ethosperse® LA-12; Hetoxol L-12; Hodag Nonionic L-12; Lipocol L-12; Macol® LA-12; Procol LA-12; Prox-onic LA-1/

012; Trycol® 5967
Trade names containing: Lanette® Wax CAT; Solubilizer L-76

Laureth-15 (INCI)
CAS 9002-92-0 (generic)
Synonyms: PEG-15 lauryl ether; POE (15) lauryl ether
Trade names: Emalex 715; Procol LA-15

Laureth-16 (INCI)
CAS 9002-92-0 (generic)
Synonyms: PEG-16 lauryl ether; POE (16) lauryl ether
Trade names: Ablunol LA-16

Laureth-20 (INCI)
CAS 9002-92-0 (generic)
Synonyms: PEG-20 lauryl ether; POE (20) lauryl ether
Trade names: Emalex 720; Marlowet® LMA 20; Procol LA-20; Sellig LA 1150

Laureth-21
Synonyms: PEG-21 lauryl ether; POE (21) lauryl ether
Trade names: Nikkol BL-21

Laureth-23 (INCI)
CAS 9002-92-0 (generic)
Synonyms: PEG-23 lauryl ether; POE (23) lauryl ether
Trade names: Brij® 35; Britex L 230; Chemal LA-23; Emthox® 5877; Ethosperse® LA-23; Hetoxol L-23; Hodag Nonionic L-23; Lipocol L-23; Macol® LA-23; Procol LA-23; Prox-onic LA-1/023; Rhodasurf® L-25; Ritox 35; Simulsol P23; Trycol® 5964; Unicol LA-23; Witconol™ 5964
Trade names containing: Cerasynt® 945

Laureth-25 (INCI)
CAS 9002-92-0 (generic)
Synonyms: PEG-25 lauryl ether; POE (25) lauryl ether
Trade names: Emalex 725; Nikkol BL-25

Laureth-30 (INCI)
CAS 9002-92-0 (generic)
Synonyms: PEG-30 lauryl ether; POE (30) lauryl ether
Trade names: Emalex 730; Lanycol-30; Marlipal® 24/300; Procol LA-30

Laureth-35
Trade names: Lanycol-35

Laureth-40 (INCI)
CAS 9002-92-0 (generic)
Synonyms: PEG-40 lauryl ether; POE (40) lauryl ether
Trade names: Ablunol LA-40; Procol LA-40

Laureth-50
Trade names: Emalex 750

Laureth-2 acetate (INCI)
Trade names: Estalan 38; Estalan 42; Pelemol L2A
Trade names containing: Lacol

Laureth-2 benzoate (INCI)
Trade names: Dermol 126; Estalan 126
Trade names containing: Estalan 635

Laureth-3 carboxylic acid (INCI)
CAS 20858-24-6; 27306-90-7
Synonyms: PEG-3 lauryl ether carboxylic acid
Trade names: Marlinat® CM 20; Rewopol® CL 30

Laureth-5 carboxylic acid (INCI)
CAS 27306-90-7; 21127-45-7; 68954-89-2
Synonyms: PEG-5 lauryl ether carboxylic acid; POE (5) lauryl ether carboxylic acid
Trade names: Akypo RLM 38; Akypo RLMQ 38; Emcol® CLA-40; Marlinat® CM 40; Sandopan® LA-8

Laureth-6 carboxylic acid (INCI)
CAS 27306-90-7; 20260-64-4; 68954-89-2

Laureth-11 carboxylic acid

Synonyms: PEG-6 lauryl ether carboxylic acid; POE (6) lauryl ether carboxylic acid; PEG 300 lauryl ether carboxylic acid
Trade names: Akypo RLM 45
Trade names containing: Dermalcare® 1673

Laureth-11 carboxylic acid (INCI)
CAS 27306-90-7
Synonyms: PEG-11 lauryl ether carboxylic acid; POE (11) lauryl ether carboxylic acid
Trade names: Akypo RLM 100; Marlinat® CM 100

Laureth-14 carboxylic acid (INCI)
CAS 27306-90-7(; 68954-89-2
Synonyms: PEG-14 lauryl ether carboxylic acid; POE (14) lauryl ether carboxylic acid
Trade names: Akypo RLM 130

Laureth-17 carboxylic acid (INCI)
CAS 27306-90-7; 68954-89-2
Synonyms: PEG-17 lauryl ether carboxylic acid; POE (17) lauryl ether carboxylic acid
Trade names: Akypo RLM 160

Laureth-7 citrate
Trade names: Eucarol B/TA

Laureth-2 octanoate (INCI)
Synonyms: PEG-2 lauryl ether octanoate
Trade names: Estalan 12; Pelemol L2O

Laureth phosphate (CTFA)
Trade names: Abluphat MLP-220

Laureth-3 phosphate (INCI)
CAS 39464-66-9 (generic); 25852-45-3
Synonyms: PEG-3 lauryl ether phosphate; Poly(oxy-1,2-ethanediyl) α-phosphono-ω-(dodecyloxy)-; POE (3) lauryl ether phosphate
Trade names: Elfan® A 913; Hodag PE-1203; Marlophor® MO 3-Acid; Nikkol Phosten HLP-1; urfagene FDD 402

Laureth-4 phosphate (INCI)
CAS 39464-66-9 (generic)
Synonyms: PEG-4 lauryl ether phosphate; PEG 200 lauryl ether phosphate; POE (4) lauryl ether phosphate
Trade names: Chemphos TR-510; Rhodafac® RD-510

Laureth-8 phosphate (INCI)
CAS 39464-66-9 (generic)
Synonyms: PEG-8 lauryl ether phosphate
Trade names: Protaphos SDA

Lauric acid (INCI)
CAS 143-07-7; EINECS 205-582-1
Synonyms: n-Dodecanoic acid; Dodecanoic acid; Dodecoic acid
Trade names: Hystrene® 9512; Kartacid 1299; Kortacid 1295; Unifat 12

Lauroamphoacetate. See Sodium lauroamphoacetate

Lauroamphocarboxyglycinate. See Disodium lauroamphodiacetate

Lauroamphocarboxypropionate. See Disodium lauroamphodipropionate

Lauroamphodiacetate. See Disodium lauroamphodiacetate

Lauroamphodipropionate. See Disodium lauroamphodipropionate

Lauroamphoglycinate. See Sodium lauroamphoacetate

Lauroampho-PG-glycinate phosphate
Trade names: Phospholipid P-TL

Lauroyl collagen amino acids (INCI)
CAS 68920-59-2

Trade names: Lipacide LCO

Lauroyl hydrolyzed collagen (INCI)
CAS 68952-15-8
Synonyms: Lauroyl hydrolyzed animal protein; Proteins, hydrolysates, reaction prod. with lauroyl chloride
Trade names: Collodex
Trade names containing: Lipo-Peptide AME 30; Pro-Tein SA-20

Lauroyl lysine (INCI)
CAS 52315-75-0; EINECS 257-843-4
Synonyms: Lauroyl-1-lysine; Lauroyl-L-lysine
Trade names: Amihope LL-11
Trade names containing: Amilon; Mearlmica® SVA; Sericite WL

Lauroyl PG-trimonium chloride (INCI)
Synonyms: Lauryloxy-2-hydroxypropyl trimethyl ammonium chloride
Trade names containing: Akypoquat 132

Lauroyl sarcosine (INCI)
CAS 97-78-9; EINECS 202-608-3
Synonyms: N-Methyl-N-(1-oxododecyl) glycine
Trade names: Crodasinic L; Hamposyl® L; Nikkol Sarcosinate LH; Oramix L; Sarkosyl® L; Vanseal® LS

Laurtrimonium chloride (INCI)
CAS 112-00-5; EINECS 203-927-0
Synonyms: Lauryl trimethyl ammonium chloride; Dodecyl trimethyl ammonium chloride; N,N,N-Trimethyl-1-dodecanaminium chloride
Trade names: Arquad® 12-37W; Dehyquart® LT; Empigen® 5089; Kemamine® Q-6903B; Laurene; Varisoft® LAC
Trade names containing: Arquad® 12-33; Arquad® 12-50

Lauryl alcohol (INCI)
CAS 112-53-8; 68526-86-3; EINECS 203-982-0
Synonyms: 1-Dodecanol; C12 linear primary alcohol; Dodecyl alcohol
Trade names: Cachalot® L-90; Epal® 12; Laurex® L1; Laurex® NC; Lipocol L; Nacol® 12-96; Nacol® 12-99; Radianol® 1712; Unihydag Wax 12
Trade names containing: Argobase 125; Epal® 12/70; Epal® 12/85; Epal® 1214; Epal® 1218; Epal® 1412

Laurylamine dipropylenediamine (INCI)
CAS 2372-82-9; EINECS 219-145-8
Synonyms: N,N-Bis(3-aminopropyl) dodecylamine; 1,3-Propanediamine, N-(3-aminopropyl)-N-dodecyl
Trade names: Lonzabac-12.100

Lauryl aminopropylglycine (INCI)
CAS 34395-72-7; EINECS 251-993-4
Synonyms: N-[3-(Dodecylamino)propyl]glycine
Trade names containing: Facteur Hydratant PH; Hydroviton 2/059353

Lauryl behenate (INCI)
CAS 42233-07-8
Synonyms: Dodecyl docosanoate
Trade names: Pelemol LB

Lauryl betaine (INCI)
CAS 683-10-3; 11140-78-6; 66455-29-6; EINECS 211-669-5
Synonyms: 1-Dodecanaminium, N-(carboxymethyl)-N,N-dimethyl-, hydroxide, inner salt; Lauryl dimethyl glycine; Lauryl dimethylamine betaine
Trade names: Abluter LDB; Amphoteen 24; Armoteric LB; Arquad® DNHTB-75; Chimin BX; Dehyton® PAB-30; Empigen® BB; LMB; Lonzaine® 14; Nikkol AM-301; Radiateric® 6864; Rewoteric® AM DML; Rewoteric® AM DML-35; Swanol AM-301; Unibetaine LB;

Varion® CDG; Varion® CDG-LS; Zohartaine AB

Lauryl diethylenediaminoglycine (INCI)
CAS 6843-97-6; EINECS 229-930-7
Synonyms: N-[2-[[-(Dodecylamino) ethyl] amino] ethyl] glycine
Trade names containing: Facteur Hydratant PH; Hydroviton 2/059353

Lauryl dimethylamine. See Dimethyl lauramine

Lauryldimethylamine C21 dicarboxylate
Trade names: Armocare® E/C 152

Lauryl dimethylamine oleate
Trade names: Armocare® E/C 100

Lauryl dimethylamine oxide. See Lauramine oxide

Lauryl dimethyl benzyl ammonium chloride. See Lauralkonium chloride

Lauryldimonium hydroxypropyl hydrolyzed collagen (INCI)
Synonyms: Lauryldimonium hydroxypropyl amino hydrolyzed animal protein
Trade names: Lamequat® L; Lamequat® L/NP; Promois Milk LAQ; Promois W-42 LAQ; Uniquart LMQL

Lauryldimonium hydroxypropyl hydrolyzed silk (INCI)
Trade names: Promois S-LAQ

Lauryldimonium hydroxypropyl hydrolyzed soy protein (INCI)
Trade names: Croquat Soya

Lauryl glycol (INCI)
CAS 1119-87-5; EINECS 214-289-8
Synonyms: 1,2-Dodecanediol
Trade names: Mexanyl GU

Lauryl hydroxyethyl imidazoline (INCI)
CAS 136-99-2; EINECS 205-271-0
Synonyms: Lauryl imidazoline; 1H-Imidazole-1-ethanol, 4,5-dihydro-2-undecyl-
Trade names: Schercozoline L

Lauryl hydroxysultaine (INCI)
CAS 13197-76-7; EINECS 236-164-7
Synonyms: Laurylhydroxysulfobetaine
Trade names: Rewoteric® AM HC

Lauryl isostearate (INCI)
Synonyms: Dodecyl isooctadecanoate
Trade names: Isostearene L
Trade names containing: Lipotrofina M

Lauryl lactate (INCI)
CAS 6283-92-7; EINECS 228-504-8
Synonyms: Dodecyl 2-hydroxypropanoate; 2-Hydroxy-propanoic acid, dodecyl ester
Trade names: Alkamuls® LVL; Ceraphyl® 31; Cetinol LL; Crodamol LL; Estalan LL

Lauryl laurate
Trade names: Cetinol 1212

Lauryl menthyl PCA
Trade names: Cryolidone®

Laurylmethicone copolyol (INCI)
Trade names: Dow Corning® Q2-5200

Lauryl methyl gluceth-10 hydroxypropyldimonium chloride (INCI)
Trade names: Glucquat® 100; Glucquat® 125

Lauryl/myristyl dimethylamine oxide
Trade names: Bio-Surf PBC-460

Lauryl oleate (INCI)
CAS 36078-10-1
Trade names: Dermol CV

Lauryl oleyl methylamine
Trade names containing: Collamino™ Complex L/O

Lauryloleylmethylamine soy amino acids
Trade names: Soy-Amino Quat L/O

Lauryl PCA (INCI)
CAS 030657-38-6
Synonyms: Lauryl pyrrolidonecarboxylate; Pyrrolidone carboxylic acid, lauryl ester
Trade names: Laurydone®

Lauryl phosphate (INCI)
CAS 12751-23-4; EINECS 235-798-1
Trade names: Abluphat MLP-200; Crodafos 1214A; Lipophos LMP; Nikkol Phosten HLP

Lauryl polyglucose (INCI)
CAS 110615-47-9
Trade names: APG® 500 Glycoside; APG® 600 CS; APG® 600 SP; APG® 625 CS; Plantaren® 1200; Plantaren® 1200 CS/UP; Plantaren® 1200 UP; Plantaren® 1300
Trade names containing: Euperlan® PL 1000; Plantaren® PS-200; Uniplant PS-200

Lauryl polyglyceryl-6 cetearyl glycol ether (INCI)
Trade names: Chimexane NS

Laurylpyridinium chloride (INCI)
CAS 104-74-5; EINECS 203-232-2
Synonyms: 1-Dodecylpyridinium chloride
Trade names: Dehyquart® C; Dehyquart® C Crystals; Uniquart C

Lauryl pyrrolidone (INCI)
CAS 2687-96-9
Synonyms: N-Dodecyl-2-pyrrolidone
Trade names: Surfadone® LP-300

Lauryl/stearyl thiodipropionate
Trade names: Mark® 5095

Lavender extract (INCI)
CAS 90063-37-9; 84776-65-8
Synonyms: Lavendula officinalis extract
Trade names containing: Actiphyte of Lavender; BBC Relaxing Complex; Herbasol Herbes de Provence Complex; Stimulant HS 280; Stimulant LS 680

Lavender oil (INCI)
CAS 8000-28-0
Synonyms: Lavendula officinalis oil; Lavender flowers oil
Trade names containing: Essentiaderm n.1; Essentiaderm n.2; Essentiaderm n.3; Essentiaderm n.4; Essentiaderm n.6; Essentiaderm n.7; Essentiaderm n.8; Essentiaderm n.9

Lawsone (INCI)
CAS 83-72-7
Synonyms: 2-Hydroxy-1,4-naphthalenedione; 2-Hydroxy-1,4-naphthoquinone
Trade names: Imexine OG

Lead acetate (INCI)
CAS 301-04-2; EINECS 206-104-4
Synonyms: Acetic acid, lead salt; Sugar of lead; Salt of saturn
Trade names: Atomergic Lead Acetate; Unichem PBA; Unichem PBA

Lecithin (INCI)
CAS 8002-43-5; 97281-47-5; EINECS 232-307-2
Trade names: Alcolec® BS; Alcolec® Extra A; Alcolec® F-100; Alcolec® Granules; Alcolec® PG; Alcolec® S; Alcolec® SFG; Asol; Augon 1000; Basis LP-20; Basis LS-60; Centrolex® F; Centrolex® P; Centrophase® C; Centrophase® HR; Centrophase® HR6B;

Centrophil® W; Crolec 4135; Dermasome® MT; Emulmetik™ 100; Emulmetik™ 135; Emulmetik™ 300; Emulmetik™ 970; Lecithin Extract Kosmaflor, Water-Disp.; Lecsoy E; Lecsoy S; Lexin K; Lipoid S 100; Liposome Conc. E-10; Natipide 08010A; Phosal 15; PhosPho E-100; PhosPho F-97; PhosPho LCN-TS; Phospholipon® 25G, 25P, 50; Phospholipon® 80; Phospholipon® 90/90 G; Probiol™ L/N; Unilec S; Unilex, DS, S, SH

Trade names containing: AFR LS; Amisol™ 406-N; Amisol™ 4135; Amisol™ 634; Amisol™ 638; Amisol™ 688; Amisol™ HS-2; Amisol™ HS-3 US; Amisol™ HS-6; Amisol™ MS-10; Amisol™ MS-12 BA; Amisol Nail Strengthener; Antioxidant G-2; Bee's Milk; Brookosome® MSF; Brookosome® SOD; Capisome; Centromix® CPS; Centromix® E; Controx® VP; Dermasome® A; Dermasome® E; Dermasome® EPO; Dermasome® H; Dermasome® MPS; Dermasome® P; Dermasome® RJ; Dermasome® RP; Dermasome® S; Dermasome® SC; Dermasome® SE; Dermasome® SOD; Dermasome® TE; Dermasome® U; Dermasome® V; Emulmetik™ 110; Emulmetik™ 310; Emulmetik 910; Emulmetik 920; FRS-Diffuser Microreservoir; Hydro-Diffuser Microreservoir; Kalixide Grassa; Lanapene; Lanpro-2; Lecithin Water Dispersible CLR; Lipocutin®; Lipophos; Liposome Anti-Age LS; Liposome Centella; Liposome Unsapo KM; Liposomes Anti-Age LS; Lipostim; Lipotrofina A; Myvatex® SSH; Natipide 08010E; Natipide® II PG; Natipide® II; Natipide®; Oleo-Coll™ LP; Oleo-Coll™ LP/LF; Oxynex® LM; Phosal 12WD; Phosal 25 PG; Phosal 35SB; Phosal® 50 SA; Phosal® 53 MCT; Phosal® 60 PG; Phosal® 75 SA; Phosal® NAT-50-PG; Prochem 35; Prochem 35A; Protachem 35A; Proto-Lan 8; Sedermasome; Sericite WL; Sphingosomes® AL; Stabolec C; Tensami 1/05; Unipherol U-14; Vexel

Lemon balm. *See Balm mint oil*

Lemon bioflavonoids extract
Trade names containing: Actiplex™ 745

Lemon extract (INCI)
CAS 8008-56-8; 84929-31-7
Synonyms: Citrus limon extract
Trade names containing: Complexe AST 1; Complexe AV.a.; Lemon Extract HS 2364 G; Lemon HS; Lemon Liq.; Uninontan U 34

Lemongrass extract (INCI)
CAS 89998-14-1; EINECS 289-752-0
Synonyms: Cymbopogon citratus extract
Trade names containing: Biochelated Extract of Lemon Grass

Lemon juice (INCI)
CAS 68916-88-1
Trade names containing: Lipofruit R

Lemon juice extract (INCI)
Synonyms: Citrus limon juice extract
Trade names containing: Actiphyte of Lemon Juice

Lemon oil (INCI)
CAS 8008-56-8
Synonyms: Citrus limon oil
Trade names containing: Essentiaderm n.1; Essentiaderm n.2; Essentiaderm n.4; Essentiaderm n.9

Lemon peel extract (INCI)
Trade names containing: Actiphyte of Lemon Peel

L-Leucine (INCI)
CAS 61-90-5; EINECS 200-522-0
Synonyms: α-Amino-γ-methylvaleric acid; α-Amino-

isocaproic acid
Trade names containing: Omega-CH Activator

Levulinic acid (INCI)
CAS 123-76-2; EINECS 204-649-2
Synonyms: γ-Ketovaleric acid; Acetylpropionic acid; 4-Oxopentanoic acid; Levulic acid
Trade names: Unichem Levula

Levulose. *See Fructose*

Lichen extract (INCI)
CAS 84696-53-7
Synonyms: Usnea barbata extract
Trade names containing: Anti-Dandruff Usnate AO; Deo-Usnate; GU-61-A; Gu-61-Standard

Licorice extract (INCI)
CAS 97676-23-8; 84775-66-6
Synonyms: Glycyrrhiza glabra extract
Trade names containing: Bio-Chelated Sauna-Derm I; Biophytex®; GU-61-A; Gu-61-Standard; Liquiritina; Phytoderm Complex G

Lignite wax. *See Montan wax*

Ligroin. *See Mineral spirits*

Lily extract
Trade names: Clintonia Borealis Extract Code 9035

Lime. *See Calcium oxide*

Lime-tree extract. *See Linden extract*

Linden extract (INCI)
CAS 84929-52-2
Synonyms: Lime-tree extract; Tilia cordata extract
Trade names containing: Bodaiju Liq.

Linoleamide DEA (INCI)
CAS 27883-12-1; 56863-02-6; EINECS 260-410-2
Synonyms: Linoleic diethanolamide; N,N-Bis(2-hydroxyethyl)-9,12-octadecadienamide; Diethanolamine linoleic acid amide
Trade names: Alkamide® DIN-295/S; Amidex LN; Comperlan® F; Foamole A; Hetamide LN; Hetamide LNO; Incromide LA; Mackamide™ LOL; Mazamide® LLD; Mazamide® SS 20; Mazamide® SS-10; Monamid® 15-70W; Monamid® 150-ADY; Monamid® LN-605; Protamide 15W; Protamide LNO; Purton SFD; Schercomid SLE; Standamid® SOMD; Varamide® LO-1; Witcamide® 6540
Trade names containing: Condipon; Hetamide LML; Incromide LLA; Monamid® 1007; Monamid® LLN-380; Monamine AC-100; Monamine ADY-100; Rewomid® F

Linoleamido dimethylamino lactate
CAS 81613-56-1
Synonyms: Lactic acid, compd. with 9,12-octadecadienamide, n-[3-(dimethylamino)propyl] linoleamide; N-Linoleamido-N,N-dimethylamino lactate
Trade names: Necon SOLC

Linoleamidopropalkonium chloride (INCI)
Trade names: Incroquat LI-85

Linoleamidopropyl dimethylamine (INCI)
CAS 81613-56-1
Synonyms: Dimethylaminopropyl linoleamide; N-[3-(Dimethylamino)propyl]-9,12-octadecadienamide
Trade names: Foamine O-80; Naetex O-80

Linoleamidopropyl dimethylamine dimer dilinoleate (INCI)
CAS 125804-10-6
Trade names: Necon LO-80

Linoleamidopropyl dimethylamine lactate (INCI)

Synonyms: Dimethylaminopropyl linoleamide lactate
Trade names: Foamquat VG

Linoleamidopropyl ethyldimonium ethosulfate (INCI)
CAS 99542-23-1
Synonyms: 1-Propanaminium, N-ethyl-N,N-dimethyl-3-
[(1-oxo-9,12-octadecadienyl)amino]-, ethosulfate
Trade names: Foamquat SAQ-90; Naetex-Q
Trade names containing: Foamquat CHP; Parapel® HC-
85; Parapel® HC-99; Parapel® HC

Linoleamidopropyl PG-dimonium chloride phosphate (INCI)
Synonyms: Linoleamidopropyl phosphatidyl PG-dimo-
nium chloride
Trade names: Phospholipid EFA

Linoleic acid (INCI)
CAS 60-33-3; EINECS 200-470-9
Synonyms: 9,12-Octadecadienoic acid; Linolic acid
Trade names: Emersol® 315
Trade names containing: Brookosome® ELL; Complexe
AV.h.; Cutavit Richter; EFA-Liq.; EFA-Plex; EFA-
Plexol; Efaderma; Efadermasterolo; Glyco/Cer
HALA; Lipodermol®; Lipotrofina A; Soluvit Richter;
Tri-K CMF Complex; Univit-F Forte CLR; Vitamin F
Forte CLR; Vitamin F Water-Soluble CLR

Linoleic safflower oil
Trade names: Linoleic Safflower Oil

Linolenic acid (INCI)
CAS 463-40-1; EINECS 207-334-8
Synonyms: 9,12,15-Octadecatrienoic acid; α-Linolenic
acid
Trade names: Univit-F Forte
Trade names containing: Complexe AV.h.; Cutavit Rich-
ter; EFA-Liq.; EFA-Plex; EFA-Plexol; Efaderma;
Efadermasterolo; Lipodermol®; Lipotrofina A; Tri-K
CMF Complex; Univit-F Forte CLR; Vitamin F Forte
CLR; Vitamin F Water-Soluble CLR

Linol linolenic acid
Trade names: Univit-F

Linseed acid (INCI)
CAS 68424-45-3; EINECS 270-304-8
Synonyms: Acids, linseed; Fatty acids, linseed oil; Lin-
seed oil fatty acid
Trade names: Industrene® 20; L-310

Linseed extract (INCI)
Synonyms: Flaxseed extract; Linum usitatissimum ex-
tract
Trade names containing: Actiphyte of Flax Seed;
Almondermin® LS; Elespher® Almondermin

Lipase
CAS 9001-62-1; EINECS 232-619-9
Synonyms: Glycerol ester hydrolase; Triacylglycerol li-
pase
Trade names: Pancreatic Lipase 250

Liquid paraffin. See Mineral oil

Lithium stearate (INCI)
CAS 4485-12-5; EINECS 224-772-5
Synonyms: Lithium octadecanoate; Octadecanoic acid,
lithium salt
Trade names: Witco® Lithium Stearate 306

Liver extract (INCI)
CAS 8002-47-9; EINECS 232-309-3
Trade names: Glycoliv

Liver starch. See Glycogen

Locust bean gum (INCI)
CAS 9000-40-2; EINECS 232-541-5

Synonyms: Carob flour; Carob seed gum; Algaroba
Trade names: Seagel L

Luffa (INCI)
Trade names: Lipo Lufa 30/100

Luffa extract (INCI)
Trade names: Loofah Extract

Lye. See Potassium hydroxide

L-Lysine (INCI)
CAS 56-87-1; EINECS 200-294-2
Synonyms: α, ε-Diaminocaproic acid
Trade names containing: Omega-CH Activator

Lysine aspartate
Trade names: Asparlyne

Lysine carboxymethyl cysteinate (INCI)
Synonyms: Lysine carbocysteinate
Trade names containing: Tiolisina Complex 30

Lysine lauroyl methionate (INCI)
Trade names: Lipacid LML

Lysine thiazolidine carboxylate (INCI)
Trade names containing: Tiolisina Complex 30

Lysolecithin (INCI)
Trade names: Blendmax; Emulmetik™ 120

Macadamia nut oil (INCI)
Trade names: EmCon MAC; Lipovol MAC; Macadamia
Nut Oil; Nikkol Macadamia Nut Oil

Magnesia. See Magnesium oxide

Magnesium acetylmethionate (INCI)
CAS 105883-49-6
Trade names: Exsymagnesium; Exsymol Magnesium
Acetylmethionate

Magnesium aluminum silicate (INCI)
CAS 1327-43-1; 12199-37-0; EINECS 235-374-6
Synonyms: Aluminum magnesium silicate; Aluminosilicic
acid, magnesium salt
Trade names: Gelwhite MAS-H, MAS-L; Magnabrite® F;
Magnabrite® FS; Magnabrite® HS; Magnabrite® HV;
Magnabrite® K; Magnabrite® S; Veegum®;
Veegum® D; Veegum® F; Veegum® HS; Veegum®
HV; Veegum® K; Veegum® Ultra; Veegum® WG

Magnesium ascorbyl phosphate (INCI)
CAS 114040-31-2
Trade names: Nikkol VC-PMG

Magnesium aspartate (INCI)
CAS 18962-61-3; EINECS 242-703-7
Synonyms: Aspartic acid, magnesium salt
Trade names: Oligoidyne Magnesium
Trade names containing: Afron 22; Carbossalina;
Unimoist U-125

Magnesium carbonate (INCI)
CAS 546-93-0; EINECS 208-915-9
Synonyms: Carbonic acid, magnesium salt (1:1); Car-
bonic acid, magnesium salt (2:1)
Trade names: Unichem MC; Unichem MGC
Trade names containing: Pad-1

Magnesium gluconate (INCI)
CAS 3632-91-5; EINECS 222-848-2
Synonyms: Magnesium D-gluconate; D-Gluconic acid
magnesium salt
Trade names: Gluconal® MG

Magnesium hydroxide (INCI)
CAS 1309-42-8; EINECS 215-1703
Synonyms: Magnesium hydrate; Milk of magnesia; Mag-
nesia magma

Magnesium laureth-11 carboxylate

Trade names: Hydro-Magma; Marinco H-USP

Magnesium laureth-11 carboxylate (INCI)
CAS 99330-44-6
Synonyms: PEG-11 lauryl ether carboxylic acid, magnesium salt; Magnesium PEG (11) lauryl ether carboxylate
Trade names: Akypo®-Soft 100 MgV

Magnesium laureth sulfate (INCI)
CAS 62755-21-9; 67702-21-4
Synonyms: Magnesium lauryl ether sulfate
Trade names: Elfan® NS 243 S Mg; Empicol® EGB; Empicol® EGC; Texapon® MG; Tylorol MG; Unipol MGLES; Zoharpon MgES
Trade names containing: Euperlan® MPK 850

Magnesium laureth-8 sulfate (INCI)
Synonyms: Magnesium PEG 400 lauryl ether sulfate
Trade names: Elfan® NS 248 S Mg
Trade names containing: Euperlan® MPK 850; Texapon® ASV

Magnesium laureth-16 sulfate (INCI)
Trade names containing: Akyposal HF 28

Magnesium lauryl hydroxypropyl sulfonate (INCI)
Trade names: Ages 2006/Mg

Magnesium lauryl sulfate (INCI)
CAS 3097-08-3; 68081-97-0; EINECS 221-450-6
Synonyms: Magnesium monododecyl sulfate; Sulfuri acid, monododecyl ester, magnesium salt
Trade names: Akyposal MGLS; Carsonol® MLS; Elfan® 2240 Mg; Empicol® ML 26/F; Empicol® ML30; Rhodapon® LM; Standapol® MG; Stepanol® MG; Sulfetal MG 30; Sulfochem MG; Surfax MG; Texapon® MGLS; Unipol MGLS; Witcolate™ MG-LS; Zoharpon MgS
Trade names containing: Elfan® KM 640 Mg; Lumorol K 28; Texapon® MG 3

Magnesium myreth sulfate (INCI)
Synonyms: Magnesium PEG (1-4) myristyl ether sulfate; Magnesium POE (1-4) myristyl ether sulfate
Trade names containing: Zetesol MS

Magnesium oleth sulfate (INCI)
CAS 87569-97-9
Synonyms: Magnesium PEG (1-4) oleyl ether sulfate; Magnesium POE (1-4) oleyl ether sulfate
Trade names containing: Euperlan® MPK 850; Texapon® ASV; Zetesol OM

Magnesium oxide (INCI)
CAS 1309-48-4; EINECS 215-171-9
Synonyms: Magnesia; Calcined magnesia; Magnesia usta
Trade names: Marinco OH; Marinco OL
Trade names containing: Kalixide CT; White Charcoal MB-15153

Magnesium PEG-3 cocamide sulfate (INCI)
Synonyms: PEG-3 cocamide ether sulfuric acid, magnesium salt
Trade names: Genapol® AMG

Magnesium silicate (INCI)
CAS 1343-88-0; EINECS 215-681-1
Synonyms: Silicic acid, magnesium salt (1:1)
Trade names containing: Kalixide LT

Magnesium stearate (INCI)
CAS 557-04-0; EINECS 209-150-3
Synonyms: Magnesium octadecanoate; Octadecanoic acid, magnesium salt
Trade names: Cecavon MG 51; Nuodex Magnesium Stearate Food Grade; Radiastar® 1100; Synpro®

Magnesium Stearate USP; Unichem MGS; Unichem MS; Witco® Magnesium Stearate N.F
Trade names containing: Base W/O 126; Hostacerin WO; Hostacerin WOL

Magnesium sulfate (INCI)
CAS 7487-88-9; EINECS 231-298-2
Synonyms: Sulfuric acid, magnesium salt (1:1); Trihydrate; Heptahydrate: Bitter salts; epsom salts
Trade names: Unichem EPSAL
Trade names containing: Omadine® MDS

Maidenhair extract. *See Ginkgo extract*

Maize gluten amino acids. *See Corn gluten amino acids*

Maize oil. *See Corn oil*

Maleated soybean oil (INCI)
CAS 68648-66-8
Synonyms: Soybean oil, maleated; Oils, soybean, maleated
Trade names: Ceraphyl® GA; Ceraphyl® GA-D

Mallow extract (INCI)
CAS 84082-57-5
Synonyms: Mallow blossom extract; Malva silvestris extract
Trade names containing: Babyderme HS 342; Babyderme LS 642; Demaquillant LS 658; Emollient HS 235; Emollient LS 635

Maltitol (INCI)
CAS 585-88-6; EINECS 209-567-0
Trade names containing: Nikkol Aquasome LA

Maltodextrin (INCI)
CAS 9050-36-6; EINECS 232-940-4
Trade names: Maltrin® M040; Maltrin® M050; Maltrin® M100; Maltrin® M150; Maltrin® M180; Maltrin® M510; Maltrin® M700; Maltrin® QD M440; Maltrin® QD M500; Maltrin® QD M550; Maltrin® QD M580; Microduct®; Wickenol® 550

Maltose (INCI)
CAS 69-79-4; EINECS 200-716-5
Synonyms: Malt sugar; Maltobiose; r-O-α-D-Glucopyranosyl-D-glucose
Trade names containing: Sweetrex®

Malt sugar. *See Maltose*

Mammary extract (INCI)
Trade names: Extract GLM No. 1
Trade names containing: Epidermin in Oil; Epidermin Water-Soluble

Manganese acetylmethionate (INCI)
CAS 105883-50-9
Trade names: Exsymanganese; Exsymol Manganese Acetylmethionate

Manganese aspartate (INCI)
Synonyms: Aspartic acid, manganese salt
Trade names: Oligoidyne Manganese

Manganese gluconate (INCI)
CAS 6485-39-8; EINECS 229-350-4
Trade names: Gluconal® MN

Manganese violet (INCI)
CAS 10101-66-3; EINECS 233-257-4
Synonyms: Ammonium manganese pyrophosphate; Diphosphoric acid, ammonium manganese (3+) salt (1:1:1); Manganese ammonium pyrophosphate
Trade names: Cogilor Spinel
Trade names containing: Chroma-Lite® Violet 4507; M Violet 112

Mango seed oil (INCI)

Trade names: Lipex 203

Mannide oleate
Trade names: Arlacel® A

Mannitol (INCI)
CAS 69-65-8; EINECS 200-711-8
Trade names: Unisweet MAN
Trade names containing: AFR LS; Dermosaccharides®
SEA; Omega-CH Activator; Seanamin BD

Marigold extract. *See Calendula extract*

Maritime pine extract (INCI)
Trade names containing: Demaquillant LS 658

Matricaria extract (INCI)
Synonyms: Chamomile extract, German or Hungarian;
Matricaria chamomilla extract; Wild chamomile ex-
tract
Trade names: Hydroessential Matricaria; Hydro-
plastidine Matricaria
Trade names containing: Actiphyte of Chamomile;
Aromaphyte of Chamomile; Babyderme HS 265;
Babyderme LS 665; Camomile Oil Extra; Chamomile
Extract HS 2382 G; Chamomile Oil; Coobato
Camomilla; Coobato Speciale; Cremogen AF;
Cremogen Camomile Forte; Cremogen M-I 739001;
Crodarom Chamomile A; Crodarom Chamomile EO;
Crodarom Chamomile O; Extrapone Chamomile
Special 2/033021; Haircomplex AKS; Herbalcomplex
1 Special; Herbaliquid Camomile Special; Hexaplant
Richter; Kamitsure Liq.; Relaxant HS 278; Relaxant
LS 678; Sedaplant Richter

Matricaria oil (INCI)
CAS 8002-66-2
Synonyms: Hungarian chamomile oil; German chamo-
mile oil; Wild chamomile oil
Trade names containing: Aromaphyte of Chamomile;
Essentiaderm n.4; Essentiaderm n.6

MDMH. *See MDM hydantoin*

MDM hydantoin (INCI)
CAS 116-25-6; EINECS 204-132-1
Synonyms: MDMH; 1-(Hydroxymethyl)-5,5-dimethyl hy-
dantoin; Monomethylol dimethyl hydantoin; 1-(Hy-
droxymethyl)-5,5-dimethyl-2,4-imidazolinedione
Trade names: Dantoin® MDMH

Meadowfoam seed oil (INCI)
Trade names: EmCon Limnanthes Alba; Nikkol
Meadowfoam Oil

Meadowsweet extract (INCI)
Synonyms: Drupwort extract; Filipendula ulmaria extract;
Queen of the meadow extract
Trade names containing: Actiphyte of Meadowsweet; IPF
Meadowsweet

MEA-hydrolyzed silk
Trade names containing: Aqua-Tein S

MEA-iodine (INCI)
Trade names: Iodamicid

MEA-laureth sulfate (INCI)
CAS 68184-04-3; 977067-77-8
Synonyms: Monoethanolamine lauryl ether sulfate
Trade names: Akyposal MLES 35; Cosmopon ME;
Empicol® EMB; Surfax ECM; Tylorol LM; Unipol MEA
LES

MEA-lauryl sulfate (INCI)
CAS 4722-98-9; 68908-44-1; EINECS 225-214-3
Synonyms: Sulfuric acid, monododecyl ester, compd.
with 2-aminoethanol (1:1); Monoethanolamine lauryl
sulfate

Trade names: Akyposal MLS 30; Aremsol MA; Aremsol
MR; Cosmopon MO; Elfan® 240M; Elfan® 2240 M;
Empicol® 1220/T; Empicol® LQ33; Empicol® LQ33/
T; Empicol® LQ70; Manro ML 33; Rewopol® MLS 30;
Standapol® MLS; Sulfochem MLS; Surfax MEA;
Texapon® MLS; Unipol MLS; Zoharpon LAM
Trade names containing: Afron 22; Akypogene HM 8;
Cosmopon HC

Medicago sativa extract. *See Alfalfa extract*

Melanin (INCI)
CAS 8049-97-6; 77465-45-3
Trade names: Lipo Melanin
Trade names containing: DHA Melanosponge

Melissa officinalis oil. *See Balm mint oil*

Menadione (INCI)
CAS 58-27-5; EINECS 200-372-6
Synonyms: 2-Methyl-1,4-naphthalenedione; Vitamin K_3
Trade names containing: Extrapone Bio-Tamin Special 2/
2032671

Menhaden oil (INCI)
CAS 8002-50-4; EINECS 232-311-4
Synonyms: Oils, menhaden; Pogy oil; Mossbunker oil
Trade names: Super Refined™ Menhaden Oil

Mentha piperita oil. *See Peppermint oil*

Mentha pulegium extract. *See Pennyroyal extract*

Mentha spicata oil. *See Spearmint oil*

Menthol (INCI)
CAS 89-78-1; EINECS 201-939-0
Synonyms: Hexahydrothymol; 5-Methyl-2-(1-methyl-
ethyl) cyclohexanol; Racemic menthol
Trade names: Fancol Menthol; Nanospheres 100 Men-
thol; Universal MENT
Trade names containing: Leniplex

Menthoxypropanediol (INCI)
CAS 87061-04-9; EINECS 289-296-2
Synonyms: 3-[[5-Methyl-2-(1-methylethyl) cyclo-
hexyl]oxy]-1,2-propanediol
Trade names: Cooling Agent No. 10

Menthyl anthranilate (INCI)
CAS 134-09-8; EINECS 205-129-8
Synonyms: Menthyl o-aminobenzoate; 5-Methyl-2(1-
methylethyl)cyclohexanol-2-aminobenzoate
Trade names: Dermoblock MA; Estalan MA; Neo
Heliopan, Type MA; Trivent MA

Menthyl lactate (INCI)
CAS 59259-38-0; EINECS 261-678-3
Synonyms: Lactic acid menthyl ester
Trade names: Covafresh; Frescolat, Type ML; Frigydil

Meroxapol 105 (INCI)
CAS 9003-11-6 (generic)
Trade names: Hodag Nonionic 5010-R; Pluronic® 10R5

Meroxapol 108 (INCI)
CAS 9003-11-6 (generic)
Trade names: Macol® 16

Meroxapol 171 (INCI)
CAS 9003-11-6 (generic)
Trade names: Hodag Nonionic 1017-R

Meroxapol 172 (INCI)
CAS 9003-11-6 (generic)
Trade names: Hodag Nonionic 2017-R; Pluronic® 17R2

Meroxapol 174 (INCI)
CAS 9003-11-6 (generic)
Trade names: Pluronic® 17R4

Meroxapol 251 (INCI)
CAS 9003-11-6 (generic)
Trade names: Macol® 32

Meroxapol 252 (INCI)
CAS 9003-11-6 (generic)
Trade names: Macol® 40; Pluronic® 25R2

Meroxapol 254 (INCI)
CAS 9003-11-6 (generic)
Trade names: Macol® 34; Pluronic® 25R4

Meroxapol 258 (INCI)
CAS 9003-11-6 (generic)
Trade names: Pluronic® 25R8

Meroxapol 311 (INCI)
CAS 9003-11-6 (generic)
Trade names: Macol® 33; Pluronic® 31R1

Methacryloyl ethyl betaine/methacrylates copolymer (INCI)
Trade names: Diaformer® Z-301; Diaformer® Z-400; Diaformer® Z-A; Diaformer® Z-AT; Diaformer® Z-SM; Diaformer® Z-W

Methenammoniumchloride (INCI)
CAS 76902-90-4
Trade names: Busan® 1500

Methicone (INCI)
CAS 9004-73-3
Synonyms: Hydrogen methyl polysiloxane; Methyl hydrogen polysiloxane; Poly [oxy(methylsilylene)]
Trade names: Dow Corning® 1107 Fluid; Silicone L-31
Trade names containing: Cosmetic Hydrophobic Black Oxide 9333; Cosmetic Hydrophobic Kaolin 9400; Finex-25-020; Luxelen® SS-020; Nylon N-012; Nylon SI-N; Sericite SL-012; Sericite SL-012P; Sericite SLZ-012P; Spheron P-1500-030; Talc Micro-Ace P-2-030; Ti-Sphere AA-1512-030

Methionine (INCI)
CAS 59-51-8; EINECS 200-432-1
Synonyms: 2-Amino-4-(methylthio)butyric acid; 2-Amino-4-(methylmercapto)butyric acid
Trade names containing: Hair Complex 20/70n

Methoxydiglycol (INCI)
CAS 111-77-3; EINECS 203-906-6
Synonyms: Diethylene glycol methyl ether; Ethanol, 2-(2-methoxyethoxy)-; (2-β-methyl "Carbitol"), methoxyethoxy ethanol
Trade names: Ektasolve® DM

N-Methoxyethyl-p-phenyelendiamine HCl (INCI)
Synonyms: 1,4-Benzenediamine, N-methoxyethyl, hydrochloride
Trade names: Imexine OAH

Methoxyisopropanol (INCI)
CAS 107-98-2; EINECS 203-539-1
Synonyms: Monopropylene glycol methyl ether; Propylene glycol methyl ether; 1-Methoxy-2-propanol
Trade names: Solvent PM

Methoxy PEG-17/dodecyl glycol copolymer (INCI)
Trade names: Elfacos® OW-100

Methoxy PEG-22/dodecyl glycol copolymer (INCI)
Trade names: Elfacos® E200

4-Methoxy-m-phenylene diamine (CTFA)
CAS 615-05-4
Synonyms: 4-MMPD; 1,3-Benzenediamine, 4-methoxy; 2,4-Diaminoanisole
Trade names: Rodol BA

2-Methoxy-p-phenylene diamine sulfate (INCI)
CAS 42909-29-5; EINECS 255-999-8

Synonyms: 1,4-Benzenediamine, 2-methoxy-, sulfate; 2-Methoxy-1,4-benzenediamine sulfate
Trade names: Rodol PDAS

Methoxypropanol. See Methoxyisopropanol

Methyl acetyl ricinoleate (INCI)
CAS 140-03-4; EINECS 205-392-9
Synonyms: 12-(Acetyloxy)-9-octadecenoic acid, methyl ester
Trade names: Naturechem® MAR; Pelemol MAR

Methyl acrylate (monomer)
CAS 96-33-3; EINECS 202-500-6
Synonyms: 2-Propenoic acid methyl ester; Acrylic acid methyl ester
Trade names containing: Rohagum® N-80

3-Methylamino-4-nitrophenoxyethanol (INCI)
CAS 59820-63-2; EINECS 261-940-7
Synonyms: 2-[3-(Methylamino)-4-nitrophenoxy]ethanol
Trade names: Imexine FR

p-Methylaminophenol sulfate (INCI)
CAS 55-55-0; EINECS 200-237-1
Synonyms: 4-(Methylamino) phenol sulfate; Metol; Paramethylaminophenol sulfate
Trade names: Rodol PM

Methylbenzene. See Toluene

Methylbenzethonium chloride (INCI)
CAS 25155-18-4; EINECS 246-675-7
Synonyms: Diisobutyl cresoxy ethoxy ethyl dimethyl benzyl ammonium chloride
Trade names: Hyamine® 10X

4-Methylbenzylidene camphor (INCI)
CAS 38102-62-4; 36861-47-9; EINECS 253-242-6
Synonyms: 1,7,7-Trimethyl-3-[(4-methylphenyl)methylene]bicyclo[2.2.1]heptan-2-one; 3-(4-Methylbenzylidene camphor)
Trade names: BioGir-MBC; Eusolex® 6300; Parsol® 5000

Methyl bis (hydrogenated tallow amidoethyl) 2-hydroxyethyl ammonium methosulfate
Trade names containing: Varisoft® 110 DEG; Varisoft® 110 DEG

Methyl bis (2-hydroxyethyl) coco ammonium chloride
Trade names containing: Varisoft® 910; Varisoft® 910

Methyl bis (2-hydroxyethyl) stearmonium chloride
Synonyms: Methyl bis (2-hydroxyethyl) stearyl ammonium chloride
Trade names: Variquat® S-1202

Methyl bis (oleylamidoethyl) 2-hydroxyethyl ammonium methosulfate
Trade names containing: Varisoft® 222 LT (90%); Varisoft® 222 LT (90%)

Methyl bis (tallowamidoethyl) 2-hydroxyethyl ammonium methosulfate
Trade names containing: Varisoft® 222 (75%); Varisoft® 222 (75%); Varisoft® 222 (90%); Varisoft® 222 (90%); Varisoft® 222 HV (90%); Varisoft® 222 HV (90%); Varisoft® 222 LM (90%); Varisoft® 222 LM (90%)

Methyl bis (tallowamidoethyl) 2-hydroxypropyl ammonium methosulfate
Trade names: Varisoft® 238 (90%)

3-Methyl-2-butene-1-ol
Trade names: Prenol

Methyl t-butyl ether
CAS 1634-04-4

Synonyms: Methyl tertiary butyl ether; t-Butyl methyl ether; 2-Methoxy-2-methylpropane
Trade names: Driveron®

2-Methyl-3-(4-t-butylphenyl) propanol
Trade names: Lysmeral®

Methylcellulose (INCI)
CAS 9004-67-5
Synonyms: Cellulose methyl ether
Trade names: Benecel® M; Methocel® A Premium; Methocel® A15-LV; Methocel® A15LVP; Methocel® A4CP; Methocel® A4MP; Viscontran MC
Trade names containing: Mearlmaid® AA; Mearlmaid® PLN; Mearlmaid® PLO; Mearlmaid® TR; Naturon® 2X AQ

Methylchloroform. *See Trichloroethane*

Methylchloroisothiazolinone (INCI)
CAS 26172-55-4; EINECS 247-500-7
Synonyms: 5-Chloro-2-methyl-4-isothiazolin-3-one; 4-Isothiazolin-3-one, 5-chloro-2-methyl-
Trade names containing: Euxyl K 100; Kathon® CG; Kathon® CG II Biocide

Methyl cocoate (INCI)
CAS 61788-59-8; EINECS 262-988-1
Synonyms: Fatty acids, coco, methyl esters
Trade names: CE-618; Radia® 7117

Methylcyclooctylcarbonate
Trade names: Jasmacyclat

Methyldibromo glutaronitrile (INCI)
CAS 35691-65-7; EINECS 252-681-0
Synonyms: 2-Bromo-2-(bromomethyl) glutaronitrile; 2-Bromo-2-(bromomethyl) pentanedinitrile
Trade names: Tektamer® 38
Trade names containing: Euxyl K 400; Merguard 1190; Merguard 1200; Merquat® 2200; Tektamer® 38 A.D.; Tektamer® 38 L.V.

Methyldihydrojasmonate (INCI)
CAS 37172-53-5; EINECS 253-379-1
Synonyms: Methyl (2-amyl-3-ococyclopentyl) acetate; Methyl 2-hexyl-3-oxocyclopentanecarboxylate
Trade names: Hedione

Methylenebis tallow acetamidodimonium chloride (INCI)
Trade names: Chimexane CJ

Methylene casein
Trade names: Plasvita® TSM

Methyl gluceth-10 (INCI)
CAS 68239-42-9
Synonyms: PEG-10 methyl glucose ether; POE (10) methyl glucose ether
Trade names: Glucam® E-10; Grillocam E10; Grillocam E10; Prox-onic MG-010

Methyl gluceth-20 (INCI)
CAS 68239-43-0
Synonyms: PEG-20 methyl glucose ether; POE (20) methyl glucose ether
Trade names: Aloxe MG-20; Glucam® E-20; Grillocam E20; Grillocam E20; Prox-onic MG-020

Methyl gluceth-20 benzoate (INCI)
Trade names: Finsolv® EMG-20

Methyl gluceth-20 distearate
CAS 98073-10-0
Trade names: Glucam® E-20 Distearate

Methyl glucose dioleate (INCI)
CAS 82933-91-3
Trade names: Glucate® DO; Grillocose® DO

Methyl glucose isostearate
Trade names: Grillocose® IS

Methyl glucose laurate (INCI)
Trade names: Glucate® ML

Methyl glucose sesquiisostearate (INCI)
Trade names: Glucate® IS

Methyl glucose sesquistearate (INCI)
CAS 68936-95-8; EINECS 273-049-0
Synonyms: D-Glucopyranoside, methyl, octadecanoate (2:3)
Trade names: Glucate® SS; Grillocose PS

Methyl glucose stearate
Trade names: Grillocose® PS

Methyl hydrogenated rosinate (CTFA)
CAS 8050-13-3
Synonyms: Hydrogenated methyl ester of rosin
Trade names: Hercolyn® D

Methyl (1) hydrogenated tallow amidoethyl (2) hydrogenated tallow imidazolinium methosulfate
Trade names: Varisoft® 445

Methylhydroxy cetyl glucaminium lactate (INCI)
Synonyms: N-Methyl, N-(2-hydroxycetyl) glucaminium lactate
Trade names: Finecat MOGL

2-Methyl-5-hydroxyethylaminophenol (INCI)
CAS 55302-96-0; EINECS 259-583-7
Synonyms: 5-[(2-Hydroxyethyl)amino]-2-methylphenol
Trade names: Imexine OAG

Methyl hydroxyethylcellulose (INCI)
CAS 9032-42-2
Trade names: Benecel® ME; Tylose® MH Grades; Tylose® MH-p, MHB-p; Tylose® MHB

Methyl hydroxypropyl cellulose. *See Hydroxypropyl methylcellulose*

Methyl hydroxystearate (CTFA)
CAS 141-23-1; EINECS 205-471-8
Synonyms: Methyl 12-hydroxyoctadecanoate; Methyl 12-hydroxystearate; 12-Hydroxyoctadecanoic acid, methyl ester
Trade names: Naturechem® MHS

Methyl isostearate (INCI)
CAS 68517-10-2
Synonyms: Methyl isooctadecanoate
Trade names: Prisorine MIS 3760

Methylisothiazolinone (INCI)
CAS 2682-20-4; EINECS 220-239-6
Synonyms: 2-Methyl-4-isothiazolin-3-one; 3(2H)-Isothiazolone, 2-methyl-; 2-Methyl-3(2H)-isothiazolone
Trade names containing: Euxyl K 100; Kathon® CG II Biocide; Kathon® CG

Methyl laurate (INCI)
CAS 111-82-0; 67762-40-7; EINECS 203-911-3
Synonyms: Methyl dodecanoate; Dodecanoic acid, methyl ester
Trade names: CE-1218; CE-1270; CE-1280; CE-1290; CE-1295; Estol MEL 1502; Estol MEL 1507; Kemester® 9012
Trade names containing: Estol ML/M 1519

Methyl methacrylate
(monomer) CAS 80-62-6; EINECS 201-297-1; (polymer) CAS 9011-14-7
Synonyms: (polymer) Acrylite; Methyl methacrylate resin
Trade names: Rohagum® M-345; Rohagum® M-825;

Rohagum® M-890; Rohagum® M-920; Rohamere® 4899F

Trade names containing: Rohagum® M-335; Rohagum® MB-319; Rohagum® PM-381; Rohagum® PM-685; Rohamere® 4885F; Rohasol® PM-560; Rohasol® PM-709

Methyl methacrylate crosspolymer (INCI)
Trade names: Microsphere M-305

2-Methyl-3(4-methylphenyl) propanal
Trade names: Jasmorange®

Methyl myristate (INCI)
CAS 124-10-7; EINECS 204-680-1
Synonyms: Methyl tetradecanoate; Tetradecanoic acid, methyl ester
Trade names: Estol MEM 1518; Estol MYM 3645; Kemester® 9014
Trade names containing: Estol ML/M 1519

N-Methyl-3-nitro-p-phenylenediamine (INCI)
CAS 2973-21-9; EINECS 221-014-5
Synonyms: N-4-Methyl-2-nitro-1,4-benzenediamine
Trade names: Imexine FB

Methyl oleate (INCI)
CAS 112-62-9; 67762-38-3; EINECS 203-992-5; 267-015-4
Synonyms: Methyl 9-octadecenoate; 9-Octadecenoic acid, methyl ester
Trade names: Kemester® 115; Kemester® 8002; Radia® 7060; Witconol™ 2301

Methyl oleylamidoethyl oleyl imidazolinium methosulfate. *See Quaternium-81*

Methyl palmitate (INCI)
CAS 112-39-0; EINECS 203-966-3
Synonyms: Methyl hexadecanoate; Hexadecanoic acid, methyl ester
Trade names: Estol MEP 1503; Kemester® 9016; Radia® 7120

Methylparaben (INCI)
CAS 99-76-3; EINECS 202-785-7
Synonyms: Methyl 4-hydroxybenzoate; 4-Hydroxybenzoic acid, methyl ester; Methyl parahydroxybenzoate
Trade names: Aseptoform; Bentex M; CoSept M; Lexgard® M; Methyl-Steriline; Nipagin M; Paridol M; Preserval M; Trisept M; Unisept M
Trade names containing: Bactericide MB 2/012582; Bactiphen 2506 G; Carsofoam® MSP; Combi-Steriline MP; Dekaben; Dragocid Forte 2/027045; Germaben® II-E; Germaben® II; Killitol; Mikrokill 300; Nipaguard® BPX; Nipaguard® MPA; Nipaguard® MPS; Nipastat; Paragon™ II; Paragon™; Phenonip; Protastat P-211; Sepicide HB; Sepicide MB; Sunveil; Talcoseptic C; Undebenzofene C; Uniphen P-23; Varifoam® SXC

2-Methylpropane. *See Isobutane*

Methyl salicylate (INCI)
CAS 119-36-8; EINECS 204-317-7
Synonyms: Methyl 2-hydroxybenzoate; Sweet birch oil; Oil of wintergreen
Trade names: Unichem METSAL; Unichem METSAL

Methylsilanol acetyltyrosine (INCI)
Trade names: Tyrosilane

Methylsilanol aspartate hydroxyprolinate
Trade names: Hydroxyprolisilane C

Methylsilanol carboxymethyl theophylline alginate (INCI)
Trade names: Theophyllisilane C

Methylsilanol elastinate (INCI)
Trade names: Proteosilane C

Methylsilanol mannuronate (INCI)
Trade names: Algisium-C

Methylsilanol PEG-7 glyceryl cocoate (INCI)
Trade names: Monosiliol

Methylsilanol tri PEG-8 glyceryl cocoate (INCI)
Trade names: Monosiliol C

Methyl stearate (INCI)
CAS 112-61-8; 85586-21-6; EINECS 203-990-4; 287-824-6
Synonyms: Methyl octadecanoate; Octadecanoic acid, methyl ester
Trade names: Kemester® 7018; Kemester® 9718; Radia® 7110

Methylstyrene/vinyltoluene copolymer (INCI)
CAS 9017-27-0
Synonyms: Benzene, ethenylmethyl-, polymer with (1-methylethenyl) benzene
Trade names containing: Durawax #1032

Methyl tallow amidoethyl hydroxyethyl ammonium methosulfate
Trade names containing: Varisoft® 222 PG (90%); Varisoft® 222 PG (90%)

Mica (INCI)
CAS 12001-26-2
Synonyms: Muscovite mica
Trade names: M-102; M-302; Mearlmica® MMCF; Mearlmica® MMSV; Mica PGM-3; Mica PGM-4; Mica PGM-5; Sericite 5, 300S; Sericite DNN; Sericite FSE; Sericite SL; Sericite SLZ; Sericite SP
Trade names containing: Bi-Lite® 20, 1070; Bi-Lite® R, 1051; Bi-Lite® Ultralite 3186; Bi-Lite® Ultrapress 1082; Bi-Lite® Ultrawhite 1084; Bi-Lite® UVR; Bi-Lite®; Bismica 46; Bismica 55; Bismica 596; Black Mica; Cashmir K-II; Chroma-Lite® Aqua 4508; Chroma-Lite® Black 4498; Chroma-Lite® Dark Blue 4501; Chroma-Lite® Magenta 4505; Chroma-Lite® Violet 4507; Chroma-Lite®; Cloisonné Blue; Cloisonné Gold; Cloisonné Red; Cloisonné Violet; Colorona® Bordeaux; Colorona® Bright Gold; Colorona® Carmine Red; Colorona® Copper; Colorona® Light Blue; Colorona® Magestic Green; Colorona® Sienna; Coverleaf PC-2055M; Dichrona® BG; Dichrona® BR; Dichrona® BY; Dichrona® GY; Dichrona® RB; Dichrona® RG; Dichrona® RY; Dichrona® YB; Dichrona® YG; Dichrona® YR; Duocrome® BG; Duocrome® GY; Duocrome® RB; Duocrome® YR; Extender W; Flamenco® Gold CC; Flamenco® Gold; Flamenco® Pearl CC; Flamenco® Pearl; Flamenco® Twilight Blue; Flamenco® Ultra Fine; Flamenco®; Flonac ME 10 C; Flonac MG 30 C; Flonac MI 10 C; Flonac ML 10 C; Flonac MS 10 C; Flonac MS 20 C; Flonac MS 30 C; Flonac MS 33 C; Flonac MS 40 C; Flonac MS 5 C; Flonac MS 60 C; Flonac MS 70 C; Flonac MX 10 C; Flonac MX 30 C; Gemstone Sunstone CC; Gemtone® Amber; Gemtone® Amethyst; Gemtone® Emerald; Gemtone® Mauve Quartz; Gemtone® Sunstone; Gemtone® Tan Opal CC; Lustra-Pearl®; Mearlmica® SVA; Mibiron® N-50; Micronasphere™ M; Nikkol Super Mica D; Sericite DNN-2SH; Sericite SL-012; Sericite SL-012P; Sericite SLZ-012P; Sericite WL; Shinju® White 100T; Soloron Silver CO; Soloron Silver Fine CO; Soloron Silver Fine; Soloron Silver Sparkle CO; Soloron Silver Sparkle; Soloron Silver; Soloron-R-Gold; Spectra-Pearl®; Timiron®; Velvet

Veil 310; Velvet Veil 320; Velvet Veil 620; Velvet Veil 640; Velvet Veil A; Velvetveil X; Velvetveil Y; Velvetveil Z

Microcrystalline cellulose (INCI). *See also Cellulose*
CAS 9004-34-6
Trade names: Acticel™ 12; Acticel™ Plus; Avicel PH-101; Dascare MCCP; Emcocel® 50M; Emcocel® 90M; Emcocel® LM
Trade names containing: Avicel RC-591

Microcrystalline wax (INCI)
CAS 63231-60-7; 64742-42-3; EINECS 264-038-1
Synonyms: Petroleum wax, microcrystalline; Waxes, microcrystalline
Trade names: Be Square® 175; Be Square® 185; Be Square® 195; CS-2080W; Emerwax® 1253; Florabeads Micro 28/60 White; Fortex®; Koster Keunen Microcrystalline Wax 170/180; Koster Keunen Microcrystalline Wax 193/198; Mekon® White; Multiwax® 180-M; Multiwax® 180-W; Multiwax® ML-445; Multiwax® W-445; Multiwax® W-835; Multiwax® X-145A; Permulgin 835; Petrolite® C-1035; Petrolite® C-700; Starwax® 100; Ultraflex®; Victory®
Trade names containing: Cutina® BW; Cutina® LM; Dehymuls® F; Durawax #1032; Florabeads 28/60 Jade; Florabeads Micro 28/60 Gypsy Rose; Florabeads Micro 28/60 Lapis; Gilugel R; Hairwax 7686 o.e.; Hostacerin WO; Lipcare Wax 7782; Ross Japan Wax Substitute 473; Ross Japan Wax Substitute 525; Ross Japan Wax Substitute 930; Sphingoceryl® Wax LS 2958 B; Unitina BW; Unitina LM

Milk acid. *See Lactic acid*

Milk amino acids (INCI)
CAS 65072-00-6
Trade names: Milkamino™ 20

Milk of magnesia. *See Magnesium hydroxide*

Milk protein (INCI)
CAS 9005-46-3, 9000-71-9; EINECS 232-555-1
Synonyms: Casein; Proteins, milk
Trade names: Alacid; Alaren; CMP-1; Cosmetic Grade Casein; Lactobiol; Unipro CAL-CASE, CO-CASE
Trade names containing: Decaprotein; Lactofil; Tensami 3/06

Milk sugar. *See Lactose*

Mimosa bark extract (INCI)
Trade names containing: Tepescohuite AMI Water-soluble; Tepescohuite HG; Tepescohuite HS; Tepescohuite LS

Mineral oil (INCI)
CAS 8012-95-1; 8042-47-5; EINECS 232-384-2; 232-455-8
Synonyms: Heavy or light mineral oil; Paraffin oil; Liquid paraffin
Trade names: Benol®; Blandol®; Britol®; Britol® 6NF; Britol® 7NF; Britol® 9NF; Britol® 20USP; Britol® 24; Britol® 35USP; Britol® 50USP; Carnation®; Crystosol NF 70; Crystosol NF 90; Crystosol USP 200; Crystosol USP 240; Crystosol USP 350; Drakeol 5; Drakeol 6; Drakeol 7; Drakeol 8; Drakeol 9; Drakeol 10; Drakeol 13; Drakeol 15; Drakeol 19; Drakeol 21; Drakeol 32; Drakeol 35; Ervol®; Gloria®; Kaydol®; Klearol®; Orzol®; Peneteck; Protol®; Rudol®; Superla® No. 5; Superla® No. 6; Superla® No. 7; Superla® No. 9; Superla® No. 10; Superla® No. 13; Superla® No. 18; Superla® No. 21; Superla® No. 31;

Superla® No. 35; Uniwhite Oil 55, 70, 85, 130, 185, 205, 350
Trade names containing: Almolan LIS; Amerchol L-101®; Amerchol® BL; Amerchol® L-500; Amerchol® L-99; Amphocerin® K; Antioxidant G-2; Apicerol 2/014081; Argobase 125; Argobase EU Hydrous; Argobase EU; Argobase EUC 2; Argobase L1; Argobase L2; Argobase S1; Azulene 50% 2/012990; Base O/W 097; Bentone® Gel MIO A-40; Bentone® Gel MIO; Biron® NLY-L-2X MO; C-Base; Co-Gell® A2/B270; Cosmetic Hydrophobic Black Oxide 9333; Cosmetic Hydrophobic Kaolin 9400; Cremba; Croda Liq. Base; Crodarom Nut O; Crosterol SFA; Cutina® LM; Dehymuls® K; Dow Corning® Q5-6038 Polymer Beads; Emery® 1730; Emery® 1732; Emery® 1740; Emulzome; Falba Absorption Base; Fancol LAO; Geahlene; Gilugel MIN; Hostacerin WO; Hostacerin WOL; Ivarbase™ 101; Ivarbase™ 3230; Lanaetex FB; Lanalene ABS; Lanamol; Lanpro-1; Lipo-plastidine Calendula; Lipoplastidine Pappa Regalis; Liquid Absorption Base Type A, T; Liquid Absorption Base; Liquid Base; Mearlite® GEJ; Molo-Jel; Nimlesterol® 1732; Novogel® ST; Nylon SI-N; PCL SE w/o 2/066255; Polytrap® Q5-6038 Polymer Beads; Protalan M-16, M-26; Protegin® X; Protegin®; Proto-Lan 4R; Ritachol®; Ritaplast; Salcare SC91; Salcare SC92; Salcare SC95; Sebase; Sericite SL-012P; Sericite SLZ-012P; Sexadecyl Alcohol, Cosmetic Grade; Sphingoceryl® Wax LS 2958 B; Stearalchol; Steralchol; T-Base; Tixogel MIO; Transparent Titanium Dioxide PW Covalim; Unitina LM; Vitamarine

Mineral spirits (INCI)
CAS 8032-32-4; 64475-85-0; EINECS 232-453-7
Synonyms: White spirits; Ligroin; Petroleum spirits
Trade names containing: Monawet MO-70S; Tixogel OMS

Mineral wax. *See Ceresin, Ozokerite*

Minkamidopropyl betaine (INCI)
Synonyms: N-(Carboxymethyl)-N,N-dimethyl-3-[(1-oxomink)amino]-1-propanaminium hydroxide, inner salt; Mink amide propylbetaine; Minkamidopropyl dimethyl glycine
Trade names: Em-U-Taine
Trade names containing: Schercotaine MKAB

Minkamidopropyl dimethylamine (INCI)
CAS 68953-11-7; EINECS 273-187-1
Synonyms: Amides, mink oil, N-[3-(dimethylamine) pro-pyl]-; Dimethylaminopropyl mink fatty acids amide; N-[3-(Dimethylamino)propyl]mink oil amides
Trade names containing: Foamole B; Incromine Mink B

Mink oil (INCI)
Synonyms: Oil of mink
Trade names: Emulan®; Naturol; Super Refined™ Mink Oil
Trade names containing: Dermoil

Mink oil PEG-13 esters (INCI)
Trade names: Oxypon 306

Mink wax (INCI)
Trade names: Emulan® Mink Wax

MIPA. *See Isopropanolamine*

MIPA C12-15 pareth sulfate (INCI)
Trade names: Zetesol 856 D
Trade names containing: Perlglanzmittel GM 4055

MIPA-dodecylbenzenesulfonate (INCI)
CAS 42504-46-1; 54590-52-2; EINECS 255-854-9

Synonyms: Dodecylbenzenesulfonic acid, compd. with 1-amino-2-propanol (1:1); Monoisopropanolamine dodecylbenzenesulfonate
Trade names: Hetsulf IPA

MIPA-laureth sulfate (INCI)
CAS 83016-76-6; 9062-04-8
Synonyms: Poly(oxy-1,2-ethanediyl), α-sulfo-ω-(dodecyloxy)-, compd. with 1-amino-2-propanol; Monoisopropanolamine lauryl ether sulfate
Trade names: Zetesol 856; Zetesol 2056
Trade names containing: Texapon® IES; Texapon® WW 99; Zetesol 100; Zetesol 856 T

MIPA-lauryl sulfate (INCI)
CAS 21142-28-9; EINECS 244-238-5
Synonyms: Sulfuric acid, monododecyl ester, compd. with 1-amino-2-propanol (1:1); Monoisopropanolamine lauryl sulfate; Dodecyl sulfate, compd. with 1-amino-2-propanol (1:1)
Trade names: Empicol® MIPA; Melanol LP 1; Sulfetal CJOT 38; Sulfetal CJOT 60
Trade names containing: Texapon® IES

Mistletoe extract (INCI)
CAS 8031-76-3; 84929-55-5
Synonyms: Viscum alba extract
Trade names containing: Hexaplant Richter; Sedaplant Richter

Mixed isopropanolamines myristate (INCI)
CAS 10525-14-1
Trade names: Lanamine®

4-MMPD. See 4-Methoxy-m-phenylene diamine

Monoethanolamine. See also MEA...
Trade names: MEA Commercial Grade; MEA Electronics Grade; MEA Low Freeze Grade; MEA Low Iron Grade; MEA Low Iron-Low Freeze Grade; MEA NF Grade

Monoisopropanolamine. See also MIPA...
Trade names: MIPA

Monolinolein. See Glyceryl linoleate

Monostearin. See Glyceryl stearate

Montan acid wax (INCI)
CAS 68476-03-9; EINECS 270-664-6
Synonyms: Fatty acids, montan wax; Waxes, montan fatty acids
Trade names: Hoechst Wax E Pharma; Hoechst Wax SW

Montan wax (INCI)
CAS 8002-53-7; EINECS 232-313-5
Synonyms: Lignite wax; Waxes, montan
Trade names: Ross Bleached Montan Wax; Ross Bleached Montan Wax Cosmetic

Montmorillonite (INCI)
CAS 1318-93-0; EINECS 215-288-5
Trade names: Gelwhite GP, H; Gelwhite L; Green Clay

Morpholine (INCI)
CAS 110-91-8; EINECS 203-815-1
Synonyms: Tetrahydro-1,4-oxazine; Tetrahydro-2H-1,4-oxazine; Diethylene oximide
Trade names: Unamine-MORP

Morrhua oil. See Cod liver oil

Mortierella oil (INCI)
Synonyms: Mortierela isabellina oil
Trade names: Bio-EPO

Mother of thyme extract. See Wild thyme extract

MSP. See Sodium phosphate

Mucopolysaccharides. See Glycosaminoglycans

Mulberry root extract (INCI)
Trade names containing: Sohakuhi Extract BG-100; Sohakuhi Extract Ethanol

Muscle extract (INCI)
Trade names containing: Lipotrofina M

Mushroom extract (INCI)
Synonyms: Agaricus bisporus extract; Polyporus extract
Trade names: Cytoplasmine-1
Trade names containing: Extrait No. 30

Mussel extract (INCI)
Trade names containing: Nutrimarine

Myreth-3 (INCI)
CAS 27306-79-2 (generic); 26826-30-2; EINECS 248-016-9
Synonyms: PEG-3 myristyl ether; POE (3) myristyl ether
Trade names: Hetoxol M-3; Witconol™ 5969
Trade names containing: Isoxal 5

Myreth-4 (INCI)
CAS 27306-79-2 (generic); 39034-24-7
Synonyms: PEG-4 myristyl ether; POE (4) myristyl ether; 3,6,9,12-Tetraoxahexacosan-1-ol
Trade names: Lipocol M-4; Procol MA-4
Trade names containing: Homulgator 920 G

Myreth-5 (INCI)
CAS 27306-79-2 (generic); 92669-01-7
Synonyms: PEG-5 myristyl ether; POE (5) myristyl ether
Trade names containing: Isoxal 12

Myreth-10 (INCI)
CAS 27306-79-2 (generic)
Synonyms: PEG-10 myristyl ether; POE (10) myristyl ether; PEG 500 myristyl ether
Trade names containing: Isoxal 11

Myreth-3 caprate (INCI)
Synonyms: Myristyl ethoxy caprate; PEG-3 myristyl ether caprate; POE (3) myristyl ether caprate
Trade names: Unimul-1410

Myreth-3 laurate (INCI)
CAS 84605-13-0,977068-97-5; EINECS 283-390-7
Synonyms: PEG-3 myristyl ether laurate; POE (3) myristyl ether laurate
Trade names: Schercemol MEL-3

Myreth-2 myristate (INCI)
Synonyms: PEG-2 myristyl ether myristate; PEG 100 myristyl ether myristate
Trade names: G-4964

Myreth-3 myristate (INCI)
CAS 59686-68-9
Synonyms: PEG-3 myristyl ether myristate; POE (3) myristyl ether myristate
Trade names: Cetiol® 1414E; Gatarol M 30 M; Lanol 14 M; Liponate 143M; Schercemol MEM-3; Unimul 14E; Unimul-1414EW

Myreth-3 octanoate (INCI)
Synonyms: PEG-3 myristyl ether octanoate
Trade names: Trivent OC-143

Myreth-3 palmitate (INCI)
CAS 84605-14-1; EINECS 293-391-2
Synonyms: PEG-3 myristyl ether palmitate; POE (3) myristyl ether palmitate
Trade names: Schercemol MEP-3

Myristalkonium chloride (INCI)
CAS 139-08-2; EINECS 205-352-0
Synonyms: N,N-Dimethyl-N-tetradecylbenzene-methanaminium chloride; Myristyl dimethyl benzyl ammonium chloride; Tetradecyl dimethyl benzyl am-

monium chloride

Trade names: Arquad® DM14B-90; Barquat® MX-50; Barquat® MX-80; BTC® 824; FMB 451-8 Quat; FMB 551-5 Quat; JAQ Powdered Quat; Kemamine® Q-7903B

Trade names containing: BTC® 2125; BTC® 2125M

Myristamide DEA (INCI)
CAS 7545-23-5; EINECS 231-426-7
Synonyms: Myristic diethanolamide; N,N-Bis(2-hydroxyethyl)myristamide; N,N-Bis(2-hydroxyethyl)tetradecanamide
Trade names: Emalex NN-15; Emalex NN-5; Hetamide M; Miristamina; Monamid® 150-MW; Protamide MRCA
Trade names containing: Alkamide® L7DE; Foamid SLM; Loropan LMD; Schercomid SL-ML; Schercomid SLA; Schercomid SLL; Schercomid SLM-LC; Schercomid SLM-S; Synotol LM 90

Myristamide MEA (INCI)
CAS 142-58-5; EINECS 205-546-5
Synonyms: Myristic monoethanolamide; N-(2-Hydroxyethyl)tetradecanamide; Myristoyl monoethanolamide
Trade names: Hetamide MM; Witcamide® MM

Myristamidopropyl betaine (INCI)
CAS 59272-84-3; EINECS 261-684-6
Synonyms: N-(Carboxymethyl)-N,N-dimethyl-3-[(1-oxotetradecyl)amino]-1-propanaminium hydroxide, inner salt; Myristamidopropyl dimethyl glycine
Trade names: Scherotaine MAB

Myristamidopropyl dimethylamine (INCI)
CAS 45267-19-4; EINECS 256-214-1
Synonyms: Dimethylaminopropyl myristamide; N-[3-(Dimethylamino)propyl]tetradecanamide
Trade names: Chemidex M; Schercodine M

Myristamidopropyl dimethylamine phosphate (INCI)
Trade names: Katemul MP; Miristocor; Myristocor™

Myristamine oxide (INCI)
CAS 3332-27-2; EINECS 222-059-3
Synonyms: Myristyl dimethyl amine oxide; Tetradecyl dimethyl amine oxide; N,N-Dimethyl-1-tetradecanamine-N-oxide
Trade names: Admox® 14-85; Ammonyx® MCO; Ammonyx® MO; Aromox® DM14D-W; Barlox® 14; Emcol® M; Emcol® MO; Empigen® OH25; Incromine Oxide M; Lilaminox M4; Manro AO 25M; Mazox® MDA; Schercamox DMA; Schercamox DMM

Myristic acid (INCI)
CAS 544-63-8; EINECS 208-875-2
Synonyms: Tetradecanoic acid
Trade names: Emery® 655; Kartacid 1495; Kartacid 1498; Prifrac 2940

Myristoyl hydrolyzed collagen (INCI)
CAS 72319-06-3
Synonyms: Proteins, hydrolysates, reaction prods. with myristoyl chloride; Myristoyl hydrolyzed animal protein
Trade names: Etha-Coll 210-20; Lexein® A-200; Lexein® A-210; Pro-Tein SM-20
Trade names containing: Lexein® A-240; Oleo-Coll™ A240-20; Oleo-Coll™ A240; Proto-Lan A240

Myristoyl sarcosine (INCI)
CAS 52558-73-3; EINECS 258-007-1
Synonyms: N-Methyl-N-(1-oxotetradecyl)glycine; Myristoyl N-methylglycine
Trade names: Hamposyl® M; Vanseal® MS

Myristyl alcohol (INCI)

CAS 112-72-1; EINECS 204-000-3
Synonyms: C14 linear primary alcohol; 1-Tetradecanol; Tetradecyl alcohol
Trade names: Cachalot® M-43; Epal® 14; Lanette® 14; Nacol® 14-95; Nacol® 14-98; Unihydag Wax-14
Trade names containing: Cyclochem EM 560; Epal® 12/70; Epal® 12/85; Epal® 1214; Epal® 1218; Epal® 1412; Epal® 1416-LD; Epal® 1416; Epal® 1418; Homulgator 920 G; Lipowax; Texal-L

Myristyl eicosanol. *See Tetradecyleicosanol*

Myristyl eicosyl stearate. *See Tetradecyleicosyl stearate*

Myristyl lactate (INCI)
CAS 1323-03-1; EINECS 215-350-1
Synonyms: 2-Hydroxypropanoic acid, tetradecyl ester; Tetradecyl 2-hydroxypropanoate
Trade names: Cegesoft® C 17; Ceraphyl® 50; Cetinol LM; Crodamol ML; Estalan ML; Lactabase C14; Liponate ML; Nikkol Myristyl Lactate; Schercemol ML; Unimul MYRLAC; Wickenol® 506

Myristyl lignocerate (INCI)
CAS 42233-51-2
Synonyms: Lignoceric acid, myristyl ether; Tetracosanoic acid, tetradecyl ester; Tetradecyl tetracosanoate
Trade names containing: Ross Synthetic Candelilla Wax

Myristyl myristate (INCI)
CAS 3234-85-3; EINECS 221-787-9
Synonyms: Tetradecyl tetradecanoate; Tetradecanoic acid, tetradecyl ester
Trade names: Alkamuls® MM/M; Ceraphyl® 424; Cetinol MM; Cetiol® MM; Crodamol MM; Hefti MYM-33; Kemester® MM; Liponate MM; Nikkol MM; Pelemol MM; Schercemol MM; Unimul 14; Waxenol® 810
Trade names containing: EFA-Plex; Lanpro-1; Oleo Keratin™ ISO; Proto-Lan 4R

Myristyl neopentanoate (INCI)
CAS 116518-82-2
Synonyms: 2,2-Dimethylpropyl tetradecanoate
Trade names: Schercemol 145

Myristyl octanoate (INCI)
Synonyms: 2-Ethylhexanoic acid, myristyl ester
Trade names: Wickenol® 174

Myristyl propionate (INCI)
CAS 6221-95-0; EINECS 226-300-9
Synonyms: 1-Tetradecanol, propanoate
Trade names: Crodamol MP; Lonzest® 143-S; Schercemol MP

Myristyl stearate (INCI)
CAS 17661-50-6; EINECS 241-640-2
Synonyms: Octadecanoic acid, tetradecyl ester
Trade names: Alkamuls® MST; Hest MS; Hetester MS; Kemester® 1418; Pelemol MS

Myristyl trimethyl ammonium bromide. *See Myrtrimonium bromide*

Myrrh extract (INCI)
CAS 100084-96-6
Synonyms: Commiphora extract
Trade names containing: Babyderme HS 265; Babyderme LS 665; Blend For Chapped Skins HS 361; Blend For Deodorant HS 275; Blend For Elderly Skins HS 296; Blend For Greasy Skin Imperfections HS 315; Brookosome® Herbal; Capilotonique HS 220; Nutriderme HS 240; Nutriderme LS 640; Onymyrrhe; Regederme HS 330; Regederme LS 630; Solarium HS 270; Solarium LS 670; Stimulant HS 285

Myrtle extract (INCI)
CAS 84082-67-7

Synonyms: Myrtus communis extract
Trade names containing: Essentiaderm n.2

Myrtrimonium bromide (INCI)
CAS 1119-97-7; EINECS 214-291-9
Synonyms: Myristyl trimethyl ammonium bromide; N,N,N-Trimethyl-1-tetradecanaminium bromide; Tetradonium bromide
Trade names: Mytab®; Rhodaquat® M214B/99; Sumquat® 6110

1,5-Naphthalenediol (INCI)
CAS 83-56-7; EINECS 201-487-4
Synonyms: 1,5-Dihydroxynaphthalene
Trade names: Rodol 15N

2,3-Naphthalenediol (INCI)
CAS 92-44-4; EINECS 202-156-7
Synonyms: 2,3-Dihydroxynaphthalene
Trade names: Rodol 23N

2,7-Naphthalenediol (INCI)
CAS 582-17-2; EINECS 209-478-7
Synonyms: 2,7-Dihydroxynaphthalene
Trade names: Rodol 27N

1-Naphthol (INCI)
CAS 90-15-3; EINECS 201-969-4
Synonyms: Alpha-naphthol; 1-Naphthalenol; 1-Hydroxynaphthalene
Trade names: Rodol ERN

Natto gum (INCI)
Trade names: FSP Liq

Neopentyl dicaprate
Trade names: Bernel® Ester NPDC

Neopentyl glycol
CAS 126-30-7; EINECS 204-781-0
Synonyms: 2,2-Dimethyl-1,3-propanediol
Trade names: NPG® Glycol

Neopentyl glycol dicaprate (INCI)
CAS 27841-06-1
Synonyms: Decanoic acid, 2,2-dimethyl-1,3-propanediol diester
Trade names: Estemol N-01; Schercemol NGDC

Neopentyl glycol dicaprylate/dicaprate (INCI)
CAS 70693-32-2
Synonyms: Decanoic acid, mixed esters with neopentyl glycol and octanoic acid
Trade names: Liponate NPGC-2
Trade names containing: Lipovol MOS-350; Lipovol MOS-70

Neopentyl glycol dicaprylate/dipelargonate/dicaprate (INCI)
Trade names: Liponate NPG-891

Neopentyl glycol dilaurate
Trade names: Schercemol NGDL

Neopentyl glycol dioctanoate
CAS 28510-23-8
Trade names: Cosmol 525; Schercemol NGDO

Nettle extract (INCI)
CAS 84012-40-8
Synonyms: Stinging nettle extract; Urtica dioica extract
Trade names containing: BBC Mineral Complex; Capilotonique HS 226; Capilotonique HS 245; Cremogen AF; Hair Complex Aquosum

Neural extract (INCI)
Trade names containing: Cholecithine

Niacin. *See Nicotinic acid*

Niacinamide (INCI)

CAS 98-92-0; EINECS 202-713-4
Synonyms: Nicotinamide; 3-Pyridinecarboxamide; Nicotinic acid amide
Trade names: Niacinamide USP, FCC No. 69905; Vitazyme® B3
Trade names containing: Aquaderm; Asebiol® LS; Complexe AV.a.; Lactil®; Trichogen

Nickel acetylmethionate (INCI)
CAS 105883-48-5
Trade names: Exsymol Nickel Acetylmethionate; Exsynickel

Niconate. *See Ferrous gluconate*

Nicotinamide. *See Niacinamide*

Nicotinic acid
CAS 59-67-6; EINECS 200-441-0
Synonyms: Niacin; Vitamin B; 3-Picolinic acid; Pyridine-3-carboxylic acid
Trade names: Niacin USP, FCC No. 69902

5-Nitro-2-aminophenol. *See 2-Amino-5-nitrophenol*

2-Nitro-1-butanol
CAS 609-31-4
Trade names: NB

Nitrocellulose (INCI)
CAS 9004-70-0
Synonyms: Cellulose, nitrate; Nitrocotton; Guncotton
Trade names containing: Biju® BNT; Biju® BTD, BXD; Biju® BWD, BWS; Biju® BWP; Biju® Ultra UNT; Biju® Ultra UTD, UXD; Biju® Ultra UWD, UWS; Biju® Ultra UWP; Blanc Covachip W 9705; Bleu Covachip W 6700; Mearlmaid® CKD; Mearlmaid® CP; Mearlmaid® KN; Mearlmaid® KND; Naturon® CSN-22

2-Nitro-2-ethyl-1,3-propanediol
CAS 597-09-1
Trade names: NEPD

2-Nitro-5-glyceryl methylaniline (INCI)
CAS 80062-31-3; EINECS 279-383-3
Trade names: Imexine FT

3-Nitro-p-hydroxyethylaminophenol (INCI)
CAS 65235-31-6; EINECS 265-648-0
Synonyms: 4-[(2-Hydroxyethyl)amino]-3-nitrophenol
Trade names: Imexine FH

2-Nitro-N-hydroxyethyl-p-anisidine (INCI)
CAS 57524-53-5
Synonyms: 2-[(4-Methoxy-2-nitrophenyl)amino]ethanol
Trade names: Imexine FE

Nitromethane (INCI)
CAS 75-52-5; EINECS 200-876-6
Synonyms: Nitrocarbol
Trade names: NM

2-Nitro-p-phenylenediamine (INCI)
CAS 5307-14-2; EINECS 226-164-5
Synonyms: 1,4-Benzenediamine, 2-nitro-; 2-Nitro-1,4-diaminobenzene; o-Nitro-p-phenylenediamine
Trade names: Rodol Brown 2R
Trade names containing: Blonde 90 (Fusion); Blonde R-50 (Fusion)

4-Nitro-m-phenylenediamine (INCI)
CAS 5131-58-8; EINECS 225-876-3
Synonyms: 1,3-Benzenediamine, 4-nitro-; 4-Nitro-1,3-diaminobenzene
Trade names: Rodol LY

4-Nitro-o-phenylenediamine (INCI)
CAS 99-56-9; EINECS 202-766-3

Synonyms: 4-Nitro-1,2-diaminobenzene; 1,2-Benzene-diamine, 4-nitro-
Trade names: Rodol 4J
Trade names containing: Blonde R-50 (Fusion)

4-Nitro-o-phenylenediamine HCl (INCI)
CAS 6219-77-8; EINECS 228-293-2
Synonyms: 4-Nitro-1,2-benzenediamine dihydrochloride
Trade names: Rodol 4GP

6-Nitro-o-toluidine (INCI)
CAS 570-24-1; EINECS 209-329-6
Trade names: Imexine FP

γ-Nonalactone (INCI)
CAS 104-61-0; EINECS 203-219-1
Trade names: Aldehyde C 18 Soc. Coconut (3/010921)

Nonfat dry colostrum (INCI)
Synonyms: Colostrum, nonfat
Trade names: Clar 111

Nonfat dry milk (INCI)
Synonyms: Milk, nonfat dry; Powdered skim milk
Trade names: Cosmerlac
Trade names containing: Ches® 500

Nonoxynol-1 (INCI)
CAS 26027-38-3 (generic); 37205-87-1 (generic); 27986-36-3; EINECS 248-762-5
Synonyms: Ethylene glycol nonyl phenyl ether; PEG-1 nonyl phenyl ether; 2-(Nonylphenoxy) ethanol
Trade names: Alkasurf® NP-1; Desonic® 1.5N; Norfox® NP-1; Prox-onic NP-1.5; Surfonic® N-10; Synperonic NP1

Nonoxynol-2 (INCI)
CAS 26027-38-3 (generic); 37205-87-1 (generic); 27176-93-8 (generic); 9016-45-9 (generic); EINECS 248-291-5
Synonyms: PEG-2 nonyl phenyl ether; POE (2) nonyl phenyl ether; PEG 100 nonyl phenyl ether
Trade names: Carsonon® N-2; Chemax NP-1.5; Emalex NP-2; Hodag Nonionic E-2; Synperonic NP2; Unicol NP-2; Uniterge NP 2

Nonoxynol-3 (INCI)
CAS 27176-95-0 (generic); 84562-92-5 (generic); 51437-95-7 (generic); 9016-45-9 (generic)
Synonyms: PEG-3 nonyl phenyl ether; POE (3) nonyl phenyl ether; 2-[2-[2-(Nonylphenoxy) ethoxy] ethoxy] ethanol
Trade names: Akyporox NP 30; Emalex NP-3; Surfonic® N-31.5

Nonoxynol-4 (INCI)
CAS 7311-27-5; 9016-45-9 (generic); 26027-38-3 (generic); 37205-87-1 (generic); 27176-97-2;; EINECS 230-770-5
Synonyms: PEG-4 nonyl phenyl ether; POE (4) nonyl phenyl ether; PEG 200 nonyl phenyl ether
Trade names: Alkasurf® NP-4; Carsonon® N-4; Chemax NP-4; Desonic® 4N; Hetoxide NP-4; Hodag Nonionic E-4; Igepal® CO-430; Igepal® NP-4; Macol® NP-4; Makon® 4; Naxonic™ NI-40; Norfox® NP-4; Protachem NP-4; Prox-onic NP-04; Remcopal 334; Renex® 647; Surfonic® N-40; Synperonic NP4; Syntopon A 100; Triton® N-42; Unicol NP-4; Uniterge NP 4; Witconol™ NP-40
Trade names containing: Emulsifier 227 G

Nonoxynol-5 (INCI)
CAS 9016-45-9 (generic); 26027-38-3 (generic); 37205-87-1 (generic); 26264-02-8; 20636-48-0; EINECS 247-555-7
Synonyms: PEG-5 nonyl phenyl ether; POE (5) nonyl

phenyl ether; 14-(Nonylphenoxy)-3,6,9,12-tetra-oxatetradecan-1-ol
Trade names: Desonic® 5N; Elfapur® N 50; Emalex NP-5; Hodag Nonionic E-5; Macol® NP-5; Nikkol NP-5; Renex® 648; Synperonic NP5; Synperonic NP5.5; Unicol NP-5; Uniterge NP 5

Nonoxynol-6 (INCI)
CAS 9016-45-9 (generic); 26027-38-3 (generic); 37205-87-1 (generic); 27177-01-1; 27177-05-5
Synonyms: PEG-6 nonyl phenyl ether; POE (6) nonyl phenyl ether; PEG 300 nonyl phenyl ether
Trade names: Alkasurf® NP-6; Chemax NP-6; Desonic® 6N; Hefti NP-55-60; Hetoxide NP-6; Hodag Nonionic E-6; Macol® NP-6; Makon® 6; Naxonic™ NI-60; Norfox® NP-6; Protachem NP-6; Prox-onic NP-06; Renex® 697; Surfonic® N-60; Synperonic NP6; Syntopon A; Unicol NP-6; Uniterge NP 6; Witconol™ NP-60

Nonoxynol-7 (INCI)
CAS 9016-45-9 (generic); 26027-38-3 (generic); 27177-05-5; 37205-87-1 (generic); EINECS 248-292-0
Synonyms: PEG-7 nonyl phenyl ether; POE (7) nonyl phenyl ether
Trade names: Desonic® 7N; Elfapur® N 70; Hodag Nonionic E-7; Synperonic NP7; Unicol NP-7; Uniterge NP 7

Nonoxynol-8 (INCI)
CAS 9016-45-9 (generic); 26027-38-3 (generic); 37205-87-1 (generic); 26571-11-9; 27177-05-5; EINECS 248-293-6; 247-816-5
Synonyms: PEG-8 nonyl phenyl ether; POE (8) nonyl phenyl ether; PEG 400 nonyl phenyl ether
Trade names: Alkasurf® NP-8; Hefti NP-55-80; Hodag Nonionic E-8; Macol® NP-8; Makon® 8; Nikkol NP-7.5; Renex® 688; Surfonic® N-85; Synperonic NP8; Synperonic NP8.5; Synperonic NP8.75; Syntopon B; Unicol NP-8; Uniterge NP 8
Trade names containing: Simulsol 5719

Nonoxynol-9 (INCI)
CAS 9016-45-9 (generic); 26027-38-3 (generic); 26571-11-9; 37205-87-1 (generic); 14409-72-4
Synonyms: PEG-9 nonyl phenyl ether; POE (9) nonyl phenyl ether; PEG 450 nonyl phenyl ether
Trade names: Chemax NP-9; Desonic® 9N; Elfapur® N 90; Empilan® NP9; Ethylan® KEO; Hefti NP-55-90; Hetoxide NP-9; Hodag Nonionic E-9; Igepal® CO-630 Special; Igepal® NP-9; Protachem NP-9; Prox-onic NP-09; Renex® 698; Synperonic NP9; Synperonic NP9.5; Syntopon C; Tergitol® NP-9; Unicol NP-9; Uniterge NP 9; Witconol™ NP-90
Trade names containing: Emulsifier 227 G

Nonoxynol-10 (INCI)
CAS 9016-45-9 (generic); 26027-38-3 (generic); 27177-08-8; 37205-87-1 (generic); 27942-26-3; EINECS 248-294-1
Synonyms: PEG-10 nonyl phenyl ether; POE (10) nonyl phenyl ether; PEG 500 nonyl phenyl ether
Trade names: Chemax NP-10; Emalex NP-10; Hetoxide NP-10; Hodag Nonionic E-10; Makon® 10; Naxonic™ NI-100; Nikkol NP-10; Prox-onic NP-010; Renex® 690; Simulsol 1030 NP; Surfonic® N-100; Surfonic® N-102; Surfonic® N-95; Synperonic NP10; Synperonic NP9.75; Syntopon D; Unicol NP-10; Uniterge NP-10
Trade names containing: Belsil ADM 6057 E; Biofloreol Hydrosoluble; Dow Corning® 929; E-2153; E-2170; Syntran 5002; Syntran 5130; Syntran 5170; Syntran KL-219

Nonoxynol-11 (INCI)
CAS 9016-45-9 (generic); 26027-38-3 (generic); 37205-87-1 (generic)
Synonyms: PEG-11 nonyl phenyl ether; POE (11) nonyl phenyl ether
Trade names: Desonic® 11N; Emalex NP-11; Macol® NP-11; Renex® 670; Witconol™ NP-110

Nonoxynol-12 (INCI)
CAS 9016-45-9 (generic); 26027-38-3 (generic); 37205-87-1 (generic)
Synonyms: PEG-12 nonyl phenyl ether; POE (12) nonyl phenyl ether; PEG 600 nonyl phenyl ether
Trade names: Alkasurf® NP-12; Desonic® 12N; Elfapur® N 120; Emalex NP-12; Hetoxide NP-12; Macol® NP-12; Makon® 12; Renex® 682; Surfonic® N-120; Synperonic NP12; Syntopon D2

Nonoxynol-13 (INCI)
CAS 9016-45-9 (generic); 26027-38-3 (generic); 37205-87-1 (generic)
Synonyms: PEG-13 nonyl phenyl ether; POE (13) nonyl phenyl ether
Trade names: Emalex NP-13; Renex® 679; Surfonic® N-130; Synperonic NP13; Syntopon E; Uniterge NP-13

Nonoxynol-14 (INCI)
CAS 9016-45-9 (generic); 26027-38-3 (generic); 37205-87-1 (generic)
Synonyms: PEG-14 nonyl phenyl ether; POE (14) nonyl phenyl ether
Trade names: Makon® 14

Nonoxynol-15 (INCI)
CAS 9016-45-9 (generic); 26027-38-3 (generic); 37205-87-1 (generic)
Synonyms: PEG-15 nonyl phenyl ether; POE (15) nonyl phenyl ether
Trade names: Alkasurf® NP-15; Chemax NP-15; Desonic® 15N; Elfapur® N 150; Emalex NP-15; Hetoxide NP-15; Macol® NP-15; Nikkol NP-15; Prox-onic NP-015; Renex® 678; Surfonic® N-150; Synperonic NP15; Syntopon F; Triton® N-150; Uniterge NP-15

Nonoxynol-17
Trade names: Synperonic NP17

Nonoxynol-18 (INCI)
CAS 9016-45-9 (generic); 37205-87-1 (generic); 26027-38-3 (generic)
Synonyms: PEG-18 nonyl phenyl ether; POE (18) nonyl phenyl ether
Trade names: Nikkol NP-18TX

Nonoxynol-20 (INCI)
CAS 9016-45-9 (generic); 26027-38-3 (generic); 37205-87-1 (generic)
Synonyms: PEG-20 nonyl phenyl ether; POE (20) nonyl phenyl ether; PEG 1000 nonyl phenyl ether
Trade names: Chemax NP-20; Desonic® 20N; Emalex NP-20; Hodag Nonionic E-20; Macol® NP-20; Macol® NP-20(70); Prox-onic NP-020; Renex® 649; Surfonic® N-200; Synperonic NP20; Syntopon G; Unicol NP-20; Uniterge NP-20

Nonoxynol-23 (INCI)
CAS 9016-45-9 (generic); 26027-38-3 (generic); 37205-87-1 (generic)
Synonyms: PEG-23 nonyl phenyl ether; POE (23) nonyl phenyl ether
Trade names: Emulsogen ELN

Nonoxynol-25
Trade names: Emalex NP-25; Synperonic NP25

Nonoxynol-30 (INCI)
CAS 9016-45-9 (generic); 26027-38-3 (generic); 37205-87-1 (generic)
Synonyms: PEG-30 nonyl phenyl ether; POE (30) nonyl phenyl ether
Trade names: Alkasurf® NP-30, 70%; Carsonon® N-30; Chemax NP-30; Chemax NP-30/70; Desonic® 30N; Desonic® 30N70; Emalex NP-30; Hetoxide NP-30; Hodag Nonionic E-30; Macol® NP-30(70); Makon® 30; Prox-onic NP-030; Prox-onic NP-030/70; Renex® 650; Surfonic® N-300; Surfonic® NB-5; Synperonic NP30; Synperonic NP30/70; Syntopon H; Unicol NP-30; Uniterge NP 30; Witconol™ NP-300; Witconol™ NP-307

Nonoxynol-35 (INCI)
Synonyms: PEG-35 nonyl phenyl ether; POE (35) nonyl phenyl ether
Trade names: Synperonic NP35

Nonoxynol-40 (INCI)
CAS 9016-45-9 (generic); 26027-38-3 (generic); 37205-87-1 (generic)
Synonyms: PEG-40 nonyl phenyl ether; POE (40) nonyl phenyl ether; PEG 2000 nonyl phenyl ether
Trade names: Alkasurf® NP-40, 70%; Carsonon® N-40; Chemax NP-40; Chemax NP-40/70; Desonic® 40N; Desonic® 40N70; Hetoxide NP-40; Hodag Nonionic E-40; Prox-onic NP-040; Prox-onic NP-040/70; Synperonic NP40; Unicol NP-40; Uniterge NP 40

Nonoxynol-44 (INCI)
CAS 9016-45-9 (generic); 26027-38-3 (generic); 37205-87-1 (generic)
Synonyms: PEG-44 nonyl phenyl ether; POE (44) nonyl phenyl ether
Trade names: Uniterge NP-44

Nonoxynol-50 (INCI)
CAS 9016-45-9 (generic); 26027-38-3 (generic); 37205-87-1 (generic)
Synonyms: PEG-50 nonyl phenyl ether; POE (50) nonyl phenyl ether
Trade names: Chemax NP-50; Chemax NP-50/70; Desonic® 50N; Desonic® 50N70; Hetoxide NP-50; Hodag Nonionic E-50; Prox-onic NP-050; Prox-onic NP-050/70; Synperonic NP50; Unicol NP-50; Uniterge NP 50

Nonoxynol-100 (INCI)
CAS 9016-45-9 (generic); 26027-38-3 (generic); 37205-87-1 (generic)
Synonyms: PEG-100 nonyl phenyl ether; POE (100) nonyl phenyl ether
Trade names: Carsonon® N-100; Chemax NP-100; Chemax NP-100/70; Desonic® 100N; Desonic® 100N70; Hodag Nonionic E-100; Macol® NP-100; Prox-onic NP-0100; Prox-onic NP-0100/70; Unicol NP-100; Uniterge NP 100

Nonoxynol-8 carboxylic acid (INCI)
CAS 3115-49-9; 28212-44-4 (generic); 53610-02-9
Synonyms: PEG-8 nonyl phenyl ether carboxylic acid; PEG 400 nonyl phenyl ether carboxylic acid; POE (8) nonyl phenyl ether carboxylic acid
Trade names: Akypo NP 70

Nonoxynol-10 carboxylic acid (INCI)
CAS 28212-44-4 (generic); 53610-02-9
Synonyms: PEG-10 nonyl phenyl ether carboxylic acid; PEG 500 nonyl phenyl ether carboxylic acid; POE (10) nonyl phenyl ether carboxylic acid
Trade names: Surfine AZI-A

Nonoxynol-6 phosphate (INCI)
CAS 51811-79-1; 68412-53-3; 29994-44-3; 51609-41-7

(generic); EINECS 249-992-9
Synonyms: PEG-6 nonyl phenyl ether phosphate; POE (6) nonyl phenyl ether phosphate; PEG 300 nonyl phenyl ether phosphate
Trade names: Emphos™ CS-136

Nonoxynol-10 phosphate (INCI)
CAS 51609-41-7 (generic)
Synonyms: PEG-10 nonyl phenyl ether phosphate; POE (10) nonyl phenyl ether phosphate; PEG 500 nonyl phenyl ether phosphate
Trade names: Emphos™ CS-141; Protaphos P-610

Nonoxynol-20 phosphate
Trade names: Chemphos TC-337

Nonoxynol-4 sulfate
Synonyms: Nonyl phenol ethoxy (4) sulfate
Trade names: Witcolate™ D51-51

Nonoxynol-10 sulfate
Synonyms: Nonyl phenol ethoxy (10) sulfate
Trade names: Witcolate™ D51-53; Witcolate™ D51-53HA

Nonoxynol-30 sulfate
Trade names: Witcolate™ D51-60

Nonoxynol hydroxyethylcellulose (INCI)
Trade names: Amercell® Polymer HM-1500

Nonyl nonoxynol-4
CAS 9014-93-1 (generic)
Synonyms: PEG-4 dinonyl phenyl ether; POE (4) dinonyl phenyl ether
Trade names: Hetoxide DNP-4

Nonyl nonoxynol-5 (INCI)
CAS 9014-93-1 (generic)
Synonyms: PEG-5 dinonyl phenyl ether; POE (5) dinonyl phenyl ether
Trade names: Emalex DNP-5; Hetoxide DNP-5; Macol® DNP-5

Nonyl nonoxynol-10 (INCI)
CAS 9014-93-1 (generic)
Synonyms: PEG-10 dinonyl phenyl ether; POE (10) dinonyl phenyl ether; PEG 500 dinonyl phenyl ether
Trade names: Hetoxide DNP-10; Hetoxide DNP-9.6; Macol® DNP-10

Nonyl nonoxynol-15
Synonyms: PEG-15 dinonyl phenyl ether; POE (15) dinonyl phenyl ether
Trade names: Macol® DNP-15

Nonyl nonoxynol-21
Trade names: Macol® DNP-21

Nonyl nonoxynol-150 (INCI)
CAS 9014-93-1 (generic)
Synonyms: PEG-150 dinonyl phenyl ether; POE (150) dinonyl phenyl ether
Trade names: Igepal® DM-970 FLK

Nonyl nonoxynol-10 phosphate (INCI)
CAS 39464-64-7
Synonyms: PEG-10 dinonyl phenyl ether phosphate; POE (10) dinonyl phenyl ether phosphate; PEG 500 dinonyl phenyl ether phosphate
Trade names: Chemphos TC-341; Rhodafac® RM-510

Nonyl nonoxynol-15 phosphate (INCI)
CAS 39464-64-7
Synonyms: PEG-15 dinonyl phenyl ether phosphate; POE (15) dinonyl phenyl ether phosphate
Trade names: Chemphos TC-349; Rhodafac® RM-710

Norgine. *See Alginic acid*

Nylon
CAS 63428-83-1
Trade names: Orgasol 20030 White 5 Cos

Nylon-6 (INCI)
CAS 25038-54-4
Synonyms: Poly[imino(1-oxo-1,6-hexanediyl)]; Poly (iminocarbonylpentamethylene)
Trade names: Orgasol 1002 D NAT COS; Orgasol 1002 D WHITE 5 COS
Trade names containing: Orgasol 1002 EX D WHITE 10 COS

Nylon-66 (INCI)
CAS 32131-17-2
Synonyms: Poly[imino (1,6-dioxo-1,6-hexanediyl) imino-1,6-hexanediyl; Poly(hexamethyleneadipamide)
Trade names: Standamid® Resin BC-1283; Upamide Resin 1289; Upamide Resin UPC-1283; Versamid® 930
Trade names containing: Nylon N-012; Nylon SI-N

Nylon-12 (INCI)
CAS 25038-74-8; 24937-16-4
Synonyms: Azacyclotridecane-2-one polyamide; Poly(laurolactam)
Trade names: Orgasol 2002 D EXTRA NAT COS; Orgasol 2002 D NAT COS; Orgasol 2002 EX D NAT COS; Orgasol 2002 UD NAT COS; SP-500
Trade names containing: Sphingoceryl® Powd. LS

Oat bran extract (INCI)
Synonyms: Avena sativa bran extract
Trade names containing: Actiphyte of Bran; Actiphyte of Oat Bran

Oat extract (INCI)
CAS 84012-26-0
Synonyms: Arena sativa extract
Trade names: Mircoat™ Oil
Trade names containing: Actiphyte of Oat Flour; BBC Moisture Trol

Oat protein (INCI)
Trade names: Microat™ E

Octacosanyl stearate
Trade names: Kester Wax® 82

n-Octadecanoic acid. *See Stearic acid*

n-Octadecanol. *See Stearyl alcohol*

Octadecene-1
CAS 112-88-9
Synonyms: Linear C18 alpha olefin
Trade names: Gulftene® 18
Trade names containing: Ethyl Hexadecene-1/Octadecene-1

Octamethylcyclotetrasiloxane
CAS 556-67-2; 69430-24-6
Trade names: Arlamol® D4
Trade names containing: Gransil GCM

n-Octanoic acid. *See Caprylic acid*

Octene-1
CAS 111-66-0; EINECS 203-893-7
Synonyms: Linear C8 alpha olefin
Trade names: Ethyl Octene-1; Gulftene® 8

1-Octene-3-ol
Trade names: Morillol®

Octeth-3 carboxylic acid (INCI)
Synonyms: PEG-3 octyl ether carboxylic acid; POE (3) octyl ether carboxylic acid
Trade names: Akypo EH 15

Octocrylene (INCI)
CAS 6197-30-4; EINECS 228-250-8
Synonyms: 2-Ethylhexyl 2-cyano-3,3-diphenylacrylate; 2-Ethylhexyl 2-cyano-3,3-diphenyl-2-propenoate; UV Absorber-3
Trade names: Escalol® 597; Neo Heliopan, Type 303; Uvinul® N 539

Octoxyglyceryl behenate (INCI)
Trade names: Mexanyl GQ

Octoxynol-3 (INCI)
CAS 9002-93-1 (generic); 9004-87-9 (generic); 9036-19-5 (generic); 2315-62-0; 27176-94-9
Synonyms: 2-[2-[2-[p-(1,1,3,3-Tetramethylbutyl) phenoxy]ethoxy]ethoxy]ethanol; PEG-3 octyl phenyl ether; POE (3) octyl phenyl ether
Trade names: Chemax OP-3; Macol® OP-3; Nikkol OP-3; Synperonic OP3

Octoxynol-5 (INCI)
CAS 9002-93-1 (generic); 9036-19-5 (generic); 9004-87-9 (generic); 2315-64-2; 27176-99-4
Synonyms: PEG-5 octyl phenyl ether; POE (5) octyl phenyl ether; 14-(Octylphenoxy)-3,6,9,12-tetra-oxatetradecan-1-ol
Trade names: Chemax OP-5; Emalex OP-5; Macol® OP-5; Synperonic OP4.5

Octoxynol-6
Synonyms: PEG-6 octyl phenyl ether; POE (6) octyl phenyl ether
Trade names: Synperonic OP6

Octoxynol-7 (INCI)
CAS 9002-93-1 (generic); 9004-87-9 (generic); 9036-19-5 (generic); 27177-02-2
Synonyms: PEG-7 octyl phenyl ether; POE (7) octyl phenyl ether; 20-(Octylphenoxy)-3,6,9,12,15,18-hexaoxaeicosan-1-ol
Trade names: Chemax OP-7

Octoxynol-8 (INCI)
CAS 9004-87-9 (generic); 9036-19-5 (generic); 9002-93-1 (generic)
Synonyms: PEG-8 octyl phenyl ether; PEG 400 octyl phenyl ether; POE (8) octyl phenyl ether
Trade names: Emalex OP-8; Macol® OP-8; Synperonic OP7.5

Octoxynol-9 (INCI)
CAS 9002-93-1 (generic); 9004-87-9 (generic); 9010-43-9; 9036-19-5 (generic); 42173-90-0
Synonyms: PEG-9 octyl phenyl ether; POE (9) octyl phenyl ether; PEG 450 octyl phenyl ether
Trade names: Chemax OP-9; Igepal® CA-630; Igepal® OP-9; Lanapeg-15; Remcopal O9; Renex® 759; Syntopon 8 C; Triton® X-100; Witconol™ OP-90
Trade names containing: Lytron 621; Marlowet® RNP/K

Octoxynol-10 (INCI)
CAS 9002-93-1 (generic); 9004-87-9 (generic); 9036-19-5 (generic); 2315-66-4; 27177-07-7
Synonyms: PEG-10 octyl phenyl ether; POE (10) octyl phenyl ether; PEG 500 octyl phenyl ether
Trade names: Emalex OP-10; Macol® OP-10; Macol® OP-10 SP; Nikkol OP-10; Remcopal O11; Renex® 750; Synperonic OP10; Synperonic OP10.5

Octoxynol-11 (INCI)
CAS 9004-87-9 (generic); 9036-19-5 (generic); 9002-93-1 (generic)
Synonyms: PEG-11 octyl phenyl ether; POE (11) octyl phenyl ether
Trade names: Oxypol; Remcopal O12; Synperonic OP11; Syntopon 8 D 1

Trade names containing: Solubilisant γ2420; Solubilisant γ2428

Octoxynol-12 (INCI)
CAS 9002-93-1 (generic); 9036-19-5 (generic); 9004-87-9 (generic)
Synonyms: PEG-12 octyl phenyl ether; POE (12) octyl phenyl ether; PEG 600 octyl phenyl ether
Trade names: Macol® OP-12

Octoxynol-13 (INCI)
CAS 9002-93-1 (generic); 9004-87-9 (generic); 9036-19-5 (generic)
Synonyms: PEG-13 octyl phenyl ether; POE (13) octyl phenyl ether
Trade names: Synperonic OP12.5

Octoxynol-15
Trade names: Emalex OP-15

Octoxynol-16 (INCI)
CAS 9004-87-9 (generic); 9036-19-5 (generic); 9002-93-1 (generic)
Synonyms: PEG-16 octyl phenyl ether; POE (16) octyl phenyl ether
Trade names: Macol® OP-16(75); Synperonic OP16; Synperonic OP16.5

Octoxynol-20 (INCI)
CAS 9002-93-1 (generic); 9036-19-5 (generic); 9004-87-9 (generic)
Synonyms: PEG-20 octyl phenyl ether; POE (20) octyl phenyl ether; PEG 1000 octyl phenyl ether
Trade names: Emalex OP-20; Synperonic OP20

Octoxynol-25 (INCI)
CAS 9002-93-1 (generic); 9036-19-5 (generic); 9004-87-9 (generic)
Synonyms: PEG-25 octyl phenyl ether; POE (25) octyl phenyl ether
Trade names: Akyporox OP 250V; Emalex OP-25; Synperonic OP25

Octoxynol-30 (INCI)
CAS 9004-87-9 (generic); 9036-19-5 (generic); 9002-93-1 (generic)
Synonyms: PEG-30 octyl phenyl ether; POE (30) octyl phenyl ether
Trade names: Chemax OP-30/70; Emalex OP-30; Macol® OP-30(70); Nikkol OP-30; Synperonic OP30

Octoxynol-40 (INCI)
CAS 9002-93-1 (generic); 9004-87-9 (generic); 9036-19-5 (generic)
Synonyms: PEG-40 octyl phenyl ether; POE (40) octyl phenyl ether
Trade names: Chemax OP-40; Chemax OP-40/70; Emalex OP-40; Macol® OP-40(70); Synperonic OP40; Synperonic OP40/70; T-Det® O-407
Trade names containing: Dow Corning® 7224 Conditioning Agent; Dow Corning® Q2-7224 Conditioning Additive

Octoxynol-50
Trade names: Emalex OP-50

Octrizole (INCI)
CAS 3147-75-9; EINECS 221-573-5
Synonyms: 2-(2H-Benzotriazol-2-yl)-4-(1,1,3,3-tetramethylbutyl)phenol; 2-(2´-Hydroxy-5´-t-octylphenyl)benzotriazole; UV Absorber-5
Trade names: Spectra-Sorb® UV 5411

Octylacrylamide/acrylates/butylaminoethyl methacrylate copolymer (INCI)
CAS 70801-07-9
Trade names: Amphomer® 4910; Amphomer® LV-71

Octylacrylamide/acrylates copolymer (CTFA)
Trade names: Versatyl-42

n-Octyl alcohol. *See Caprylic alcohol*

Octyl cocoate (INCI)
CAS 92044-87-6; EINECS 295-366-3
Synonyms: Coconut fatty acids, 2-ethylhexyl ester
Trade names: Crodamol OC; Estol EHC 1540; Trioxene E

2-Octyl-1-decanol (INCI)
CAS 2745-8-931; 45235-48-1
Synonyms: Octyldecyl alcohol; 2-Octyl decanol; 1-Decanol, 2-octyl
Trade names: Exxal® 18

Octyl dimethyl p-aminobenzoate. *See Octyl dimethyl PABA*

Octyl dimethyl PABA (INCI)
CAS 21245-02-3; EINECS 244-289-3
Synonyms: Octyl dimethyl p-aminobenzoate; Padimate O; 2-Ethylhexyl paradimethylaminobenzoate
Trade names: Escalol® 507; Eusolex® 6007; Lipofilter ODP; Padimate O; Solarchem® O

Octyl dodecanol (INCI)
CAS 5333-42-6; EINECS 226-242-9
Synonyms: 2-Octyl dodecanol; 1-Dodecanol, 2-octyl-; Isoeicosyl alcohol
Trade names: Eutanol® G; Exxal® 20; Isofol® 20; Michel XO-150-20; U Tanol G; Unimul-G
Trade names containing: Amerchol® L-500; Argobase 125; Cutina® LM; Gilugel EUG; Lipodermol®; Sphingoceryl® LS; Sphingoceryl® Powd. LS; Sphingoceryl® Wax LS 2958 B; Unitina LM

Octyldodecanol stearate
Trade names: U Tanol GST

Octyldodeceth-5
Trade names: Emalex OD-5

Octyldodeceth-10
Trade names: Emalex OD-10

Octyldodeceth-16 (INCI)
Synonyms: PEG-16 octyldodecyl ether; POE (16) octyldodecyl ether
Trade names: Emalex OD-16; Seodol E-2016

Octyldodeceth-20 (INCI)
Synonyms: PEG-20 octyldodecyl ether; POE (20) octyldodecyl ether; PEG 1000 octyldodecyl ether
Trade names: Emalex OD-20; Seodol E-2020

Octyldodeceth-25 (INCI)
Synonyms: PEG-25 octyldodecyl ether; POE (25) octyldodecyl ether
Trade names: Emalex OD-25; Seodol E-2025

Octyldodecyl behenate (INCI)
Synonyms: Docosanoic acid, 2-octyldodecyl ester
Trade names: Dermol 2022; Pelemol 2022

Octyldodecyl benzoate (INCI)
Synonyms: Benzoic acid, 2-octyldodecyl ester
Trade names: Finsolv® BOD

2-Octyldodecyl erucate (INCI)
CAS 88103-59-7
Trade names: E.O.D

Octyldodecyl lactate (INCI)
Trade names: Cosmol 13

Octyldodecyl myristate (INCI)
CAS 83826-43-1; 22766-83-2
Synonyms: Myristic acid, 2-octyldodecyl ester; Tetradecanoic acid, 2-octyldodecyl ester

Trade names: Bernel® Ester 2014; M.O.D; M.O.D. WL 2949; Nikkol ODM-100; Wickenol® 142
Trade names containing: Enduragloss™

Octyldodecyl N-myristoyl-N-methylalanate
Trade names: Amiema MA-OD

Octyldodecyl neodecanoate (INCI)
Synonyms: Neodecanoic acid, octyldodecyl ester
Trade names: Nikkol N-20; Nikkol Neodecanoate-20

Octyldodecyl neopentanoate (INCI)
Trade names: Elefac™ I-205

Octyldodecyl oleate (INCI)
CAS 22801-45-2; EINECS 245-228-3
Synonyms: 9-Octadecenoic acid, 2-octyldodecyl ester; Oleic acid, octyldodecyl ester
Trade names: O.O.D

2-Octyldodecyl ricinoleate (INCI)
CAS 79490-62-3; 125093-27-8
Trade names: R.O.D

Octyldodecyl stearate (INCI)
CAS 22766-82-1; EINECS 245-204-2
Synonyms: Stearic acid, 2-octyldodecyl ester
Trade names: Starfol® OS

Octyldodecyl stearoyl stearate (INCI)
CAS 58450-52-5; 90052-75-8; EINECS 289-991-0
Synonyms: 12-[(1-Oxooctadecyl)oxy]octadecanoic acid, 2-octyldodecyl ester
Trade names: Ceraphyl® 847; Trivent SS-20

Octyl hydroxystearate (INCI)
CAS 29383-26-4; 29710-25-6
Synonyms: 2-Ethylhexyl oxystearate; 12-Hydroxy-octadecanoic acid, 2-ethylhexyl ester; 2-Ethyl-hexylhydroxystearate
Trade names: Crodamol OHS; Estalan 718; Kessco DHS; Naturechem® OHS; Schercemol OHS; Wickenol® 171

Octyl isononanoate (INCI)
CAS 71566-49-9; EINECS 275-637-2
Synonyms: 2-Ethylhexyl isononanoate; Isononanoic acid, 2-ethylhexyl ester
Trade names: Dermol 89; Isolanoate; Kessco® Octyl Isononanoate; Pelemol 89; Witconol™ 2300
Trade names containing: Dermol 334; Estalan 334; Estalan 560; Estalan 635; Isolanoate-BS; Tisolate-BS

Octyl laurate (INCI)
CAS 20292-08-4; EINECS 243-697-9
Synonyms: 2-Ethylhexyl dodecanoate
Trade names: Estol EHL 3613

Octyl methoxycinnamate (INCI)
CAS 5466-77-3; EINECS 226-775-7
Synonyms: 2-Ethylhexyl methoxycinnamate; 2-Ethyl-hexyl 3-(4-methoxyphenyl)-2-propenoate; Ethyl-hexyl p-methoxycinnamate
Trade names: Escalol® 557; Nanospheres 100 Conc. in O.M.C; Neo Heliopan, Type AV; Parsol® MCX
Trade names containing: Brookosome® UV; Unifilter U-41

Octyl octanoate (INCI)
CAS 7425-14-1; EINECS 231-057-1
Trade names: Dragoxat EH 2/044115; Pelemol 88; Tegosoft® EE

Octyl oxystearate
CAS 29710-25-6
Synonyms: 2-Ethylhexyl 12-hydroxystearate; Octa-decanoic acid, 12-hydroxy, 2-ethylhexyl ester

Trade names: Dermol OO; Estalan OV

Octyl palmitate (INCI)
CAS 29806-73-3; EINECS 249-862-1
Synonyms: 2-Ethylhexyl palmitate; 2-Ethylhexyl hexadecanoate
Trade names: Bernel® Ester EHP; Cegesoft® C 24; Ceraphyl® 368; Crodamol OP; Elfacos® EHP; Estalan 816; Estol 1543; Estol EHP 1543; Estol EHP-b 3652; Kessco EHP; Kessco® Octyl Palmitate; Lexol® EHP; Pelemol OP; Schercemol OP; Tegosoft® OP; Trivent OP; Wickenol® 155
Trade names containing: Aloe Extract #105; Wickenol® 161; Wickenol® 163

Octyl pelargonate (INCI)
CAS 59587-44-9; EINECS 261-819-9
Synonyms: 2-Ethylhexyl pelargonate; Nonanoic acid, 2-ethylhexyl ester
Trade names: Bernel® OPG; Pelemol OPG; Schercemol OPG; Unitolate OPG; Wickenol® 160; Witconol™ 2307

Octyl salicylate (INCI)
CAS 118-60-5; EINECS 204-263-4
Synonyms: 2-Ethylhexyl 2-hydroxybenzoate; 2-Ethylhexyl salicylate; 2-Hydroxybenzoic acid, 2-ethylhexyl ester
Trade names: Dermoblock OS; Escalol® 587; Lanaetex-OS; Neo Heliopan, Type OS; Neotan L; Trivent OS

Octyl stearate (INCI)
CAS 22047-49-0; 26399-02-0; EINECS 244-754-0; 247-655-0
Synonyms: 2-Ethylhexyl stearate; 2-Ethylhexyl octadecanoate; Octadecanoic acid, 2-ethylhexyl ester
Trade names: Cetiol® 868; Estol EHS 1545; Estol EHS-b 3654; Lasemul 130; Radia® 7770; Tegosoft® OS; Unitolate 868; Wickenol® 156
Trade names containing: Emulgade® CL; Gilugel OS; Wickenol® 161; Wickenol® 163

Octyl triazone (INCI)
CAS 88122-99-0
Synonyms: 2,4,6-Trianilino-p-(carbo-2´-ethylhexyl-1´-oxy)-1,3,5-triazine
Trade names: Uvinul® T 150

Olea europaea oil. *See Olive oil*

Olealkonium chloride (INCI)
CAS 37139-99-4; EINECS 253-363-4
Synonyms: Oleyl dimethyl benzyl ammonium chloride; N,N-Dimethyl-N-9-octadecenylbenzenemethanaminium chloride
Trade names: Ammonyx® KP; Ammonyx® LKP; Empigen® BCJ-50; Incroquat O-50; Mackernium™ KP

Oleamide (INCI)
CAS 301-02-0; EINECS 206-103-9
Synonyms: 9-Octadecenamide; Oleyl amide
Trade names: Armid® O

Oleamide DEA (INCI)
CAS 93-83-4; EINECS 202-281-7
Synonyms: Oleic diethanolamide; Diethanolamine oleic acid amide; N,N-Bis(2-hydroxyethyl)9-octadecenamide
Trade names: Alkamide® DO-280/S; Amidex O; Carsamide® O; Chimipal OLD; Comperlan® OD; Crillon ODE; Hetamide OC; Lauridit® OD; Loropan OD; Mackamide™ MO; Mackamide™ NOA; Mackamide™ O; Marlamid® D 1885; Mazamide® O 20; Ninol® 201; Nissan Stafoam DO, DOS;

Rewomid® DO 280 SE; Schercomid SO-A; Upamide O-20; Upamide OD; Varamide® A-7; Witcamide® 5085
Trade names containing: Alkamide® DO-280; Emulmetik™ 110; Hetamide DO; Mackamide™ ODM; Naetex O-20; Protamide OFO; Protamide T; Rewomid® DO 280; Schercomid ODA; Witcamide® 6546

Oleamide MEA (INCI)
CAS 111-58-0; EINECS 203-884-8
Synonyms: Oleic monoethanolamide; N-(2-Hydroxyethyl)-9-octadecenamide; Monoethanolamine oleic acid amide
Trade names: Hetamide MO; Incromide OPM; Schercomid OME

Oleamide MIPA (INCI)
CAS 111-05-7; EINECS 203-828-2
Synonyms: Oleic monoisopropanolamide; N-(2-Hydroxypropyl)-9-octadecenamide; Monoisopropanolamine oleic acid amide
Trade names: Rewomid® IPE 280; Schercomid OMI
Trade names containing: Witcamide® 61

Oleamidopropylamine oxide (INCI)
CAS 25159-40-4; EINECS 246-684-6
Synonyms: 9-Octadecenamide, N-[3-(dimethylamino)propyl]-, N-oxide; Oleamidopropyl dimethylamine oxide; N-[3-(Dimethylamino)propyl]-9-octadecenamide-N-oxide
Trade names: Mackamine™ OAO

Oleamidopropyl betaine (INCI)
CAS 25054-76-6; EINECS 246-584-2
Synonyms: N-(Carboxymethyl)-N,N-dimethyl-3-[(1-oxooctadecenyl)amino]-1-propanaminium hydroxide, inner salt; Oleamidopropyl dimethyl glycine
Trade names: Incronam OP-30; Lexaine® O; Mackam™ HV; Mirataine® BET-O-30

Oleamidopropyl dimethylamine (INCI)
CAS 109-28-4; EINECS 203-661-5
Synonyms: Dimethylaminopropyl oleamide; N-[3-Dimethylamino)propyl]-9-octadecenamide
Trade names: Chemidex O; Incromine OPM; Lexamine O-13; Mackine™ 501; Schercodine O; Unizeen OA

Oleamidopropyl dimethylamine glycolate (INCI)
Synonyms: Dimethylaminopropyl oleamide glycolate
Trade names containing: Foamquat SOAS-MOD

Oleamidopropyl dimethylamine hydrolyzed collagen (INCI)
Synonyms: Oleamidopropyl dimethylamine hydrolyzed animal protein
Trade names: Lexein® CP-125

Oleamidopropyl dimethylamine lactate (INCI)
Synonyms: Dimethylaminopropyl oleamide lactate
Trade names containing: Mackalene™ NLC

Oleamidopropyl dimethylamine propionate (INCI)
Trade names containing: Mackam™ NLB; Mackanate NLP

Oleamidopropyl dimonium hydroxypropyl hydrolyzed collagen (INCI)
Trade names: Mackpro™ OLP

Oleamidopropyl ethyldimonium ethosulfate (INCI)
CAS 90529-57-0?
Trade names: Foamquat ODES
Trade names containing: Foamquat SOAS-MOD

Oleamidopropyl PG-dimonium chloride (INCI)
Synonyms: Oleamidopropyl dimethyl 2,3-dihydroxypropyl ammonium chloride

Trade names: Lexquat® AMG-O
Trade names containing: Lexate® BPQ

Oleamine (INCI)
CAS 112-90-3; EINECS 204-015-5
Synonyms: Oleyl amine; 9-Octadcecen-1-amine
Trade names: Armeen® O; Armeen® OD; Armeen® OL; Armeen® OLD; Kemamine® P-989; Radiamine 6172; Radiamine 6173

Oleamine oxide (INCI)
CAS 14351-50-9; EINECS 238-311-0
Synonyms: Oleyl dimethyl amine oxide; Oleylamine oxide; N,N-Dimethyl-9-octadecen-1-amine-N-oxide
Trade names: Ammonyx® OAO; Chemoxide O; Mackamine™ O2; Mazox® ODA-30; Standamox O1; Unimox OL; Zoramox E

Oleic acid (INCI)
CAS 112-80-1; EINECS 204-007-1
Synonyms: cis-9-Octadecenoic acid; Red oil; Elainic acid; 9-Octadecenoic acid
Trade names: Crodolene LA1020; Emersol® 210; Emersol® 213 NF; Emersol® 221 NF; Emersol® 233 LL; Emersol® 6313 NF; Emersol® 6321 NF; Emersol® 6333 NF; Emersol® 7021; Hy-Phi 1055; Hy-Phi 1088; Hy-Phi 2066; Hy-Phi 2088; Hy-Phi 2102; Industrene® 105; Industrene® 106; Industrene® 206; Priolene 6900; Priolene 6905; Priolene 6906; Priolene 6910; Priolene 6933; Radiacid® 212; Unifat 5L
Trade names containing: EFA-Plex; EFA-Plexol; Prochem 35; Prochem 35A; Protachem 35A; Tri-K CMF Complex

Oleic imidazoline acetate
Trade names: Varine O Acetate

Oleic/linoleic triglyceride (INCI)
Trade names: Special Oil 888

Oleic/palmitic/lauric/myristic/linoleic triglyceride (INCI)
Trade names: Dermol T

Oleic/palmitoleic/linoleic glycerides
Trade names: Lipovol M-SYN

Olein. *See Triolein*

Oleoamphocarboxyglycinate. *See Disodium oleoamphodiacetate*

Oleoamphopropylsulfonate. *See Sodium oleoamphohydroxypropylsulfonate*

Oleostearine (INCI)
Trade names containing: Ross Japan Wax Substitute 473; Ross Japan Wax Substitute 525

Oleoyl hydrolyzed collagen (INCI)
CAS 68458-51-5
Synonyms: Oleoyl hydrolyzed animal protein; Proteins, hydrolysates, reaction prods. with oleoyl chloride
Trade names: Lamepon® LPO
Trade names containing: Lamepon® LPO 30

Oleoyl sarcosine (INCI)
CAS 110-25-8; EINECS 203-749-3
Synonyms: N-Methyl-N-(1-oxo-9-octadecenyl)glycine; Oleyl methylaminoethanoic acid; Oleyl sarcosine
Trade names: Crodasinic O; Hamposyl® O; Nikkol Sarcosinate OH; Oramix O; Vanseal OS
Trade names containing: Lanpro-2; Oleo-Coll™ LP; Oleo-Coll™ LP/LF; Proto-Lan 8

Oleth-2 (INCI)
CAS 9004-98-2 (generic); 5274-65-7
Synonyms: PEG-2 oleyl ether; POE (2) oleyl ether; PEG 100 oleyl ether

Trade names: Ameroxol® OE-2; Brij® 93; Britex O 20; Brox OL-2; Ethosperse® OA-2; Eumulgin® PWM2; Genapol® O-020; Hetoxol OL-2; Hodag Nonionic 1802; Lanycol-92; Lipocol O-2 Special; Macol® OA-2; Marlipal® 1885/2; Nikkol BO-2; Procol OA-2; Ritoleth 2; Simulsol 92; Unicol OA-2

Oleth-3 (INCI)
CAS 9004-98-2 (generic); 5274-66-8
Synonyms: PEG-3 oleyl ether; POE (3) oleyl ether
Trade names: Brox OL-3; Emalex 503; Ethoxol 3; Hetoxol OA-3 Special; Hetoxol OL-3; Lipocol O-3 Special; Procol OA-3; Volpo 3; Volpo N3; Volpo O3

Oleth-4 (INCI)
CAS 9004-98-2 (generic); 5353-26-4
Synonyms: PEG-4 oleyl ether; POE (4) oleyl ether; PEG 200 oleyl ether
Trade names: Brox OL-4; Chemal OA-4; Hetoxol OL-4; Hodag Nonionic 1804; Macol® OA-4; Procol OA-4; Prox-onic OA-1/04; Unicol OA-4

Oleth-5 (INCI)
CAS 9004-98-2 (generic); 5353-27-5
Synonyms: PEG-5 oleyl ether; POE (5) oleyl ether; 3,6,9,12,15-Pentaoxatriacont-24-en-1-ol
Trade names: Ameroxol® OE-5; Brox OL-5; Chemal OA-5; Emulsogen LP; Ethoxol 5; Eumulgin® O5; Eumulgin® PWM5; Genapol® O-050; Hetoxol OA-5 Special; Hetoxol OL-5; Lipocol O-5 Special; Macol® OA-5; Marlowet® OA 5; Procol OA-5; Ritoleth 5; Unimul-05; Volpo 5; Volpo N5; Volpo O5
Trade names containing: Eumulgin® M8; Marlowet® SAF/K; Solulan® 5

Oleth-6 (INCI)
CAS 9004-98-2 (generic)
Synonyms: PEG-6 oleyl ether; POE (6) oleyl ether; PEG 300 oleyl ether
Trade names: Ablunol OA-6; Emalex 506; Empilan® KL 6

Oleth-7 (INCI)
CAS 9004-98-2 (generic)
Synonyms: PEG-7 oleyl ether; POE (7) oleyl ether
Trade names: Ablunol OA-7; Nikkol BO-7

Oleth-8 (INCI)
CAS 9004-98-2 (generic); 27040-03-5
Synonyms: PEG-8 oleyl ether; POE (8) oleyl ether; PEG 400 oleyl ether
Trade names: Emalex 508; G-3908S; Genapol® O-080

Oleth-9 (INCI)
CAS 9004-98-2 (generic)
Synonyms: PEG-9 oleyl ether; POE (9) oleyl ether; PEG 450 oleyl ether
Trade names: Akyporox RO 90; Chemal OA-9; Genapol® O-090; Hodag Nonionic 1809; Prox-onic OA-1/09

Oleth-10 (INCI)
CAS 9004-98-2 (generic); 24871-34-9
Synonyms: PEG-10 oleyl ether; POE (10) oleyl ether; PEG 500 oleyl ether
Trade names: Ameroxol® OE-10; Brij® 97; Britex O 100; Brox OL-10; Chemal OA-10; Emalex 510; Empilan® KL 10; Ethoxol 10; Eumulgin® O10; Eumulgin® PWM10; G-3910; Genapol® O-100; Hetoxol OA-10 Special; Hetoxol OL-10; Hetoxol OL-10H; Hodag Nonionic 1810; Lanycol-96; Lanycol-97; Lipocol O-10; Macol® OA-10; Marlowet® OA 10; Nikkol BO-10TX; Procol OA-10; Ritoleth 10; Simulsol 96; Unicol OA-10; Unimul-10; Volpo 10; Volpo N10; Volpo O10
Trade names containing: Delan 62; Emulgator BTO 2; Ethoxol-CO; Eumulgin® M8

Oleth-12 (INCI)
CAS 9004-98-2 (generic)
Synonyms: PEG-12 oleyl ether; POE (12) oleyl ether;
PEG 600 oleyl ether
Trade names: Emalex 512; Ethoxol 12; Genapol® O-120
Trade names containing: Lanbritol Wax N21

Oleth-15 (INCI)
CAS 9004-98-2 (generic)
Synonyms: PEG-15 oleyl ether; POE (15) oleyl ether
Trade names: Emalex 515; Genapol® O-150; Hetoxol
OCS; Nikkol BO-15TX; Volpo N15; Volpo O15

Oleth-16 (INCI)
CAS 9004-98-2 (generic); 25190-05-0 (generic)
Synonyms: PEG-16 oleyl ether; POE (16) oleyl ether
Trade names containing: Solulan® 16

Oleth-18
Synonyms: PEG-18 oleyl ether; POE (18) oleyl ether
Trade names: Eumulgin® PWM17

Oleth-20 (INCI)
CAS 9004-98-2 (generic)
Synonyms: PEG-20 oleyl ether; POE (20) oleyl ether;
PEG 1000 oleyl ether
Trade names: Ameroxol® OE-20; Arosurf® 32-E20; Brij®
98; Britex O 200; Brox OL-20; Brox OL-20 70% Liq;
Chemal OA-20; Chemal OA-20/70CWS; Chemal OA-
20G; Emalex 520; Empilan® KL 20; Ethosperse®
OA-20; Ethoxol 20; Genapol® O-200; Hetoxol OA-20
Special; Hetoxol OL-20; Hodag Nonionic 1820;
Hostacerin O-20; Lanycol-98; Lanycol-99; Lipocol O-
20; Macol® OA-20; Nikkol BO-20; Nikkol BO-20TX;
Procol OA-20; Prox-onic OA-1/020; Prox-onic OA-2/
020; Rhodasurf® ON-870; Rhodasurf® ON-877;
Ritoleth 20; Simulsol 98; Trycol® 5971; Unicol OA-20;
Varonic® 32-E20; Volpo 20; Volpo N20; Volpo O20

Oleth-23 (INCI)
CAS 9004-98-2 (generic)
Synonyms: PEG-23 oleyl ether; POE (23) oleyl ether
Trade names: Chemal OA-23; Emalex 523; Genapol® O-
230; Hetoxol OL-23; Procol OA-23; Trycol® 5972

Oleth-25 (INCI)
CAS 9004-98-2 (generic)
Synonyms: PEG-25 oleyl ether; POE (25) oleyl ether
Trade names: Lipocol O-25; Procol OA-25
Trade names containing: Emulgade® EO-10; Hydrolactol
70; Solulan® 25

Oleth-30 (INCI)
CAS 9004-98-2 (generic)
Synonyms: PEG-30 oleyl ether; POE (30) oleyl ether
Trade names: Marlowet® OA 30

Oleth-40 (INCI)
CAS 9004-98-2 (generic)
Synonyms: PEG-40 oleyl ether; POE (40) oleyl ether;
PEG 2000 oleyl ether
Trade names: Brox OL-40; Hetoxol OL-40

Oleth-44 (INCI)
CAS 9004-98-2 (generic)
Synonyms: PEG-44 oleyl ether; POE (44) oleyl ether
Trade names: Ethoxol 44
Trade names containing: Ethoxol 44M

Oleth-50 (INCI)
CAS 9004-98-2 (generic)
Synonyms: PEG-50 oleyl ether; POE (50) oleyl ether
Trade names: Emalex 550; Nikkol BO-50

Oleth-2 phosphate (INCI)
CAS 39464-69-2 (generic)
Synonyms: PEG-2 oleyl ether phosphate; POE (2) oleyl

ether phosphate; PEG 100 oleyl ether phosphate
Trade names: Brophos™ OL-2; Crodafos N2A; Crodafos
O2 Acid

Oleth-3 phosphate (INCI)
CAS 39464-69-2 (generic)
Synonyms: PEG-3 oleyl ether phosphate; POE (3) oleyl
ether phosphate; Oleyl triethoxy mono diphosphate
Trade names: Briphos O3D; Brophos-3; Brophos™ OL-
3; Chemphos TR-515; Crafol AP-11; Crodafos N-3
Acid; Empicol® 0216; Hetphos OA-3; Hodag PE-
1803

Oleth-4 phosphate (INCI)
CAS 39464-69-2 (generic)
Synonyms: PEG-4 oleyl ether phosphate; POE (4) oleyl
ether phosphate; PEG 200 oleyl ether phosphate
Trade names: Chemphos TR-541; Protaphos 400-A

Oleth-5 phosphate (INCI)
Synonyms: PEG-5 oleyl ether phosphate; POE (5) oleyl
ether phosphate
Trade names: Crodafos N-5 Acid; Crodafos O5 Acid

Oleth-10 phosphate (INCI)
CAS 39464-69-2 (generic)
Synonyms: PEG-10 oleyl ether phosphate; POE (10)
oleyl ether phosphate; PEG 200 oleyl ether phos-
phate
Trade names: Chemphos TR-505; Crodafos N-10 Acid;
Crodafos O10 Acid; Hodag PE-1810

Oleth-20 phosphate (INCI)
CAS 39464-69-2 (generic)
Synonyms: PEG-20 oleyl ether phosphate; PEG 1000
oleyl ether phosphate; POE (20) oleyl ether phos-
phate
Trade names: Hodag PE-1820

Oleyl acetate (INCI)
CAS 693-80-1
Synonyms: 9-Octadecen-1-yl acetate
Trade names containing: Argonol ACE 6

Oleyl alcohol (INCI)
CAS 143-28-2; EINECS 205-597-3
Synonyms: 9-Octadecen-1-ol; cis-9-Octadecen-1-ol
Trade names: Adol® 80; Adol® 85; Adol® 90; Adol® 90
NF; Cachalot® O-3; Cachalot® O-8; Cachalot® O-
15; Crodacol A-10; Dermaffine; Fancol OA-95; HD
Oleyl Alcohol 70/75; HD Oleyl Alcohol 80/85; HD
Oleyl Alcohol 90/95; HD Oleyl Alcohol CG; HD-
Eutanol®; HD-Ocenol® 90/95; HD-Ocenol® 92/96;
Lancol; Lipocol O; Lipocol O-80; Lipocol O/95; Novol;
U Tanol HD, HD 70/75, HD 80/85, HD 90/95, HD CG;
U Tanol HDL CG
Trade names containing: Argonol ISO; Castorcet; Fancol
ISO; Flamenco® Gold CC; Flamenco® Pearl CC;
Gemstone Sunstone CC; Gemtone® Tan Opal CC;
Ivarbase™ 3240; Monamilk

Oleylamidopropyl dimethylamine ethonium ethosulfate
Trade names: Naetex-CHP

Oleyl betaine (INCI)
CAS 871-37-4; EINECS 212-806-1
Synonyms: N-(Carboxymethyl)-N,N-dimethyl-9-
octadecen-1-aminium hydroxide, inner salt; Oleyl di-
methyl glycine
Trade names: Chembetaine OL; Chembetaine OL-30;
Incronam OD-50; Mackam™ OB-30; Mafo® OB;
Unibetaine OLB-30, OLB-50; Velvetex® OLB-30;
Velvetex® OLB-50

Oleyl dimethylamidopropyl ethonium ethosulfate iso-stearate
Trade names: Naetex-LD

Oleyl dimethylamine. *See Dimethyl oleamine*

Oleyl erucate (INCI)
CAS 17673-56-2; EINECS 241-654-9
Synonyms: 9-Octadecenyl 13-docosenoate; Erucic acid, oleyl ester; 13-Docosenoic acid, 9-octadecenyl ester
Trade names: Cetiol® J600; Crodamol JJ; Dynacerin® 660; Kessco OE; Pelemol OE; Unitolate J600
Trade names containing: Epiderm-Complex O

Oleyl hydroxyethyl imidazoline (INCI)
CAS 95-38-5; 21652-27-7; 27136-73-8; EINECS 248-248-0; 244-501-4; 202-414-9
Synonyms: 2-(8-Heptadecenyl)-4,5-dihydro-1H-imidazole-1-ethanol; 1-Hydroxyethyl-2-oleyl imidazoline; Oleyl imidazoline
Trade names: Schercozoline O; Varine O®

Oleyl lactate (INCI)
CAS 42175-36-0
Synonyms: Oleyl 2-hydroxypropionate
Trade names: Dermol OL; Pelemol OL

Oleyl linoleate (INCI)
CAS 17673-59-3
Synonyms: Linoleic acid, oleyl ester; 9,12-Octadecadienoic acid, 9-octadecenyl ester
Trade names containing: Polylan®

Oleyl N-myristoyl-N-methyl alanate
Trade names: Amiema MA-OL

Oleyl oleate (INCI)
CAS 3687-45-4; EINECS 222-980-4
Synonyms: 9-Octadecenoic acid, 9-octadecenyl ester
Trade names: Cetiol®; Crodamol OO; Schercemol OLO; Unitolate OLOL; Wickenol® 143

Oleyltrimonium chloride
Synonyms: Oleyl trimethyl ammonium chloride
Trade names: Noramium MO 50
Trade names containing: Arquad® S-2C-50

Olibanum (INCI)
CAS 8050-07-5; EINECS 232-474-1
Synonyms: Boswellia carterii resin; Frankincense; Gum olibanum; Resin olibanum; Incense
Trade names: Incense EA; Incense H
Trade names containing: Incense HS; Incense LS; Kalokiros HS 263; Kalokiros LS 663; Stimulant HS 285

Olibanum extract (INCI)
CAS 89957-98-2
Synonyms: Boswellia carterii extract; Boswellia serrata extract; Frankincense extract; Incense extract
Trade names containing: Blend For Bust Cares HS 201; Blend For Delicate Skins HS 215; Regederme HS 236; Regederme LS 636

Olivamide DEA (INCI)
Synonyms: N,N-Bis(2-hydroxyethyl)olive fatty acid amide; Diethanolamine olive fatty acid condensate; Olive oil fatty acid diethanolamide
Trade names: Incromide OLD

Olivamidopropylamine oxide (INCI)
Synonyms: N-[3-(Dimethylamino)propyl]olive amides-N-oxide
Trade names: Incromine Oxide OL

Olivamidopropyl betaine (INCI)
Synonyms: N-(Carboxymethyl-N,N-dimethyl-3-[(1-oxoolive)amino]-1-propanaminium hydroxide, inner salt; Olivamidopropyl dimethyl glycine
Trade names: Incronam OL-30; Incronam OLB

Olivamidopropyl dimethylamine (INCI)

Trade names: Incromine OLB

Olivamidopropyl dimethylamine lactate (INCI)
CAS 124046-31-7
Trade names: Incromate OLL

Olive extract (INCI)
CAS 84012-27-1
Synonyms: Olea europaea extract
Trade names containing: Actiphyte of Olive Leaves

Olive husk oil (INCI)
Trade names containing: Dermoliv; Dermoliv T

Olive oil (INCI)
CAS 8001-25-0; EINECS 232-277-0
Synonyms: Oils, olive; Olea europaea oil
Trade names: EmCon Olive; Lipovol O; Nikkol Olive Oil; Olive Oil, Refined; Super Refined™ Olive Oil; Tri-Ol OLV
Trade names containing: Crodarom St. John's Wort O; Epiderm-Complex O; Hypericum Oil CLR

Olive oil PEG-6 esters (INCI)
CAS 103819-46-1
Trade names: Labrafil® M 1980 CS

Olive oil PEG-10 esters (INCI)
Trade names: Oxypon 288

Olive oil unsaponifiables (INCI)
Synonyms: Unsaponifiable olive oil
Trade names containing: Dermoliv T; Dermoliv; Filagrinol

Opalwax. *See Hydrogenated castor oil*

Orange extract (INCI)
CAS 84012-28-2
Synonyms: Citrus sinensis extract
Trade names containing: Aromaphyte of Orange

Orange flower water (INCI)
CAS 8030-28-2
Synonyms: Eau d'oranger
Trade names containing: BBC Moisture Trol

Orange oil (INCI)
CAS 8008-57-9
Synonyms: Citrus sinensis oil
Trade names: EmCon Orange
Trade names containing: Aromaphyte of Orange

Orange peel extract (INCI)
Trade names containing: Actiphyte of Orange Bioflavonoids; Bio-Chelated Sauna-Derm I

Orange roughy oil (INCI)
Synonyms: Oils, orange roughy
Trade names: EmCon ORO; Super Refined™ Orange Roughy Oil

Orange wax
Trade names: Orange Wax

Origanum majorana oil. *See Sweet marjoram oil*

Origanum vulgare extract. *See Wild marjoarma extract*

Ornithine (INCI)
CAS 70-26-8; EINECS 200-731-7
Trade names containing: Hydro-Diffuser Microreservoir

Oryzanol (INCI)
CAS 11042-64-1
Synonyms: γ-Orizanol
Trade names: Dascare Orizanol; Gamma Oryzanol

Ossein. *See Collagen*

Ovarian extract (INCI)
Trade names containing: Epidermin in Oil; Epidermin Water-Soluble

Oxidized beeswax (INCI)
Synonyms: Beeswax, oxidized
Trade names: Koster Keunen Beeswax AO2535

Oxidized polyethylene. See Polyethylene, oxidized

8-α-12-Oxido-13,14,15,16 tetra-norlabdane
Trade names: Ambroxan

Oxybenzone. See Benzophenone-3

Oyster shell extract (INCI)
Trade names containing: Oligoceane

Ozocerite. See Ozokerite

Ozokerite (INCI)
CAS 8021-55-4
Synonyms: Ozocerite; Mineral wax; Fossil wax
Trade names: Koster Keunen Ozokerite; Koster Keunen
Ozokerite 153/160; Koster Keunen Ozokerite 158/
160; Koster Keunen Ozokerite 160/164; Koster
Keunen Ozokerite 164/170; Koster Keunen Ozoker-
ite 170; Koster Keunen Ozokerite 190; Ross Ozoker-
ite Wax
Trade names containing: Argobase EUC 2; Argobase L2;
Lexate® PX; Protegin® W; Protegin® WX; Protegin®
X; Protegin®

Ozonized jojoba oil (INCI)
Synonyms: Jojoba oil, ozonized
Trade names: Jox 3

PABA (INCI)
CAS 150-13-0; EINECS 205-753-0
Synonyms: Aminobenzoic acid; 4-Aminobenzoic acid; p-
Aminobenzoic acid
Trade names: 4-Aminobenzoic Acid, Pure, No. 102
Trade names containing: Cutavit Richter; Hair Complex
20/70n; Soluvit Richter

Palm glyceride (INCI)
Trade names: Myverol® 18-35

Palmitamide DEA (INCI)
CAS 7545-24-6; EINECS 231-427-2
Synonyms: N,N-Bis(2-hydroxyethyl)hexadecanamide;
N,N-Bis(2-hydroxyethyl)palmitamide; Diethanol-
amine palmitic acid amide
Trade names containing: Schercomid SLA

Palmitamide MEA (INCI)
CAS 544-31-0; EINECS 208-867-9
Synonyms: N-(2-Hydroxyethyl) hexadecanamide; N-(2-
Hydroxyethyl) palmitamide; Monoethanolamine
palmitic acid amide
Trade names: Nikkol PMEA

Palmitamidohexadecanediol (INCI)
CAS 129426-19-3
Trade names: Ceramide II

Palmitamidopropyl betaine (INCI)
CAS 32954-43-1; EINECS 251-306-8
Synonyms: N-(Carboxymethyl)-N,N-dimethyl-3-[(1-
oxohexadecyl)amino]-1-propanaminium hydroxide,
inner salt
Trade names: Schercotaine PAB

Palmitamidopropyl dimethylamine (INCI)
CAS 39669-97-1; EINECS 254-585-4
Synonyms: N-[3-(Dimethylamino)propyl]hexadecan-
amide; Dimethylaminopropyl palmitamide
Trade names: Chemidex P; Schercodine P

Palmitamidopropyl dimethylamine lactate (INCI)
Synonyms: Dimethylaminopropylpalmitamide lactate
Trade names containing: Mackalene™ NLC

Palmitamidopropyl dimethylamine propionate (INCI)

Synonyms: Dimethylaminopropylpalmitamide propi-
onate
Trade names containing: Mackam™ NLB; Mackanate
NLP

Palmitamine (INCI)
CAS 143-27-1; EINECS 205-596-8
Synonyms: Cetyl amine; Palmityl amine; 1-Hexa-
decanamine
Trade names: Amine 16D; Armeen® 16; Armeen® 16D;
Kemamine® P-890

Palmitamine oxide (INCI)
CAS 7128-91-8; EINECS 230-429-0
Synonyms: Cetamine oxide; Cetyl dimethyl amine oxide;
Hexadecyl dimethylamine oxide
Trade names: Ammonyx® CO; Amyx CO 3764; Barlox®
16S; Mazox® CDA
Trade names containing: Aromox® DM16

Palmitic acid (INCI)
CAS 57-10-3; EINECS 200-312-9
Synonyms: Hexadecanoic acid; Cetylic acid; Hexa-
decylic acid
Trade names: Adeka PA Series; Crodacid PD3160;
Edenor L2SM; Emericide 142; Emericide 144;
Emersol® 143; Hystrene® 7016; Hystrene® 9016;
Kartacid 1692; Prifrac 2960; Unifat 16
Trade names containing: Cutina® FS 25 Flakes; Cutina®
FS 45 Flakes

Palmitin. See Tripalmitin

Palmitoleamidopropyl dimethylamine lactate (INCI)
Synonyms: Dimethylaminopropylpalmitoleamide lactate
Trade names containing: Mackalene™ NLC

Palmitoleamidopropyl dimethylamine propionate (INCI)
Synonyms: Dimethylaminopropylpalmitoleamide propi-
onate
Trade names containing: Mackam™ NLB; Mackanate
NLP

Palmito/stearic acid
Trade names containing: Arlatone® SCI-70

Palmitoyl carnitine (INCI)
Trade names containing: Vexel

Palmitoyl collagen amino acids (INCI)
Synonyms: Palmitoyl animal collagen amino acids
Trade names: Lipacide PCO; Monteine PCO

Palmitoyl hydrolyzed milk protein (INCI)
Trade names: Lipacide PCA

Palmitoyl hydrolyzed wheat protein (INCI)
Trade names: Lipacid PVB

Palmitoyl keratin amino acids (INCI)
Trade names: Lipacide PK

Palmityl alcohol. See Cetyl alcohol

Palmityl dimethylamine. See Dimethyl palmitamine

Palm kernel alcohol (INCI)
Synonyms: Alcohols, palm kernel
Trade names: Laurex® PKH

Palm kernelamide DEA (INCI)
CAS 73807-15-5
Synonyms: Palm kernel oil acid diethanolamide; Dietha-
nolamine palm kernel oil acid amide; N,N-Bis(2-
hydroxyethyl)palm kernel oil acid amide
Trade names: Accomid 50; Accomid PK; Afmide™ PK;
Amidex PK; Mackamide™ PK; T-Tergamide 1PD

Palm kernelamide MEA (INCI)
Synonyms: N-(2-Hydroxyethyl) palm kernel oil acid
amide; Monoethanolamine palm kernel oil acid

amide; Palm kernel oil acid monoethanolamide
Trade names: Afmide™ PKM; Mackamide™ PKM

Palm kernel glycerides (INCI)
Synonyms: Glycerides, palm kernel mono-, di- and tri-
Trade names: Cremao CS-33; Cremao CS-34; Cremao CS-36; Emuldan PK 60

Palm kernel oil (INCI)
CAS 8023-79-8; EINECS 232-425-4
Synonyms: Oils, palm kernel
Trade names containing: Labrafil® M 2130 CS

Palm kernel wax (INCI)
Trade names containing: Lipex 402

Palm oil (INCI)
CAS 8002-75-3; EINECS 232-316-1
Synonyms: Oils, palm; Palm butter; Palm grease
Trade names: Lipovol PAL
Trade names containing: Labrafil® M 2130 CS

Palm oil glycerides (CTFA)
Synonyms: Glycerides, palm oil mono-, di- and tri-
Trade names: Imwitor® 940
Trade names containing: Imwitor® 965

Palm oil sucroglyceride
Trade names: Mirasoft™ MSPO 11

Palygorskite. *See Attapulgite*

Pansy extract (INCI)
CAS 84012-42-0
Synonyms: Viola tricolor extract
Trade names: CMI 800
Trade names containing: Herbalcomplex 1 Special

Panthenol (INCI)
CAS 81-13-0 (D-form); 16485-10-2 (DL-form); EINECS 201-327-3 (D-form)
Synonyms: 2,4-Dihydroxy-N-(3-hydroxypropyl)-3,3-dimethylbutanamide; Dexpanthenol; Pantothenyl alcohol; Provitamin B_5
Trade names: Dexpanthenol USP, FCC No. 63909; DL-Panthenol Cosmetic Grade No. 63920; DL-Panthenol USP, FCC No. 63915; Fancol DL; R.I.T.A. d-Panthenol; R.I.T.A. dl-Panthenol; Ritapan D; Ritapan DL
Trade names containing: Antiphlogistic ARO; Asebiol® LS; Biophytex®; Brookosome® P; Dermasome® P; Hair Complex Aquosum; Omega-CH Activator; Trichogen

Panthenolamino dimethicone
Trade names: Biosil Basics Amino DL-30

Panthenyl hydroxypropyl steardimonium chloride (INCI)
CAS 132467-76-6
Trade names: Panthequat®

Panthenyl triacetate (INCI)
CAS 98133-47-2
Trade names: Ritapan TA
Trade names containing: Unitrienol T-27; Unitrienol T-272

Pantothenic acid (INCI)
CAS 79-83-4; EINECS 201-229-0
Synonyms: Vitamin B_5
Trade names: Vitazyme® B5

Paraffin (INCI)
CAS 8002-74-2; EINECS 232-315-6
Synonyms: Paraffin wax; Hard paraffin; Petroleum wax, crystalline
Trade names: CS-2032; CS-2037; CS-2043; CS-2054; Eskar Wax R-25, R-35, R-40, R-45, R-50; Koster Keunen Paraffin Wax 122/128; Koster Keunen Paraffin Wax 130/135; Koster Keunen Paraffin Wax 140/

145; Koster Keunen Paraffin Wax 150/155; Ross Crude Scale Wax; Uniwax PARA
Trade names containing: Argobase EU Hydrous; Argobase EU; Base WL 2569; Falba Absorption Base; Isobeeswax SP 154; Koster Keunen Beeswax, S&P ISOW; Lanaetex FB; Ross Beeswax Substitute 628/5; Ross Japan Wax Substitute 966; Ross Synthetic Candelilla Wax; Zetesap 5165; Zetesap 813A

Paraffin oil. *See Mineral oil*

Parahydroxycinnamic acid
Trade names: Exsymol Parahydroxycinnamic Acid

Pareth 45-7. *See C14-15 pareth-7*

Pareth-15-9. *See C11-15 pareth-9*

Pareth-23-3. *See C12-13 pareth-3*

Pareth-25-2. *See C12-15 pareth-2*

Pareth-91-6. *See C9-11 pareth-6*

Parsley extract (INCI)
CAS 84012-33-9
Synonyms: Petroselinum sativum extract
Trade names containing: BBC Mineral Complex

Passionflower extract (INCI)
CAS 84012-31-7
Synonyms: Passiflora incarnata extract; Passiflora quadrangularis extract
Trade names containing: BBC Relaxing Complex; Complex Relax

PCA (INCI)
CAS 98-79-3; EINECS 202-700-3
Synonyms: Pyrrolidonecarboxylic acid; 5-Oxo-L-proline; L-Pyroglutamic acid
Trade names: Ajidew A-100; Pidolidone®
Trade names containing: Ajidew SP-100; Hydro-Diffuser Microreservoir

PCA ethyl N-cocoyl-L-arginate (INCI)
Synonyms: N^2 Cocoyl-L-arginine ethyl ester DL-pyrrolidone carboxylic acid salt
Trade names: CAE

PCA glyceryl oleate (INCI)
Trade names: Amifat P-30

PCA-Na. *See Sodium PCA*

PCMC. *See p-Chloro-m-cresol*

PDMS. *See Dimethicone*

Peach kernel oil (INCI)
CAS 8023-98-1
Synonyms: Persic oil
Trade names containing: Prochem 35; Prochem 35A; Protachem 35A

Peach pit powder (INCI)
Synonyms: Powdered peach pits
Trade names: Lipo PP

Peanut oil (INCI)
CAS 8002-03-7; EINECS 232-296-4
Synonyms: Arachis oil; Groundnut oil; Katchung oil
Trade names: EmCon Peanut; Lipex 101; Super Refined™ Peanut Oil; Univegoil P-O
Trade names containing: Balm Mint Oil Infusion; Carrot Oil Extra; Crodarom Carrot O; Crodarom Nut O; Lanosoluble A; Vitamin A Palmitate 1.0 BHT in Peanut Oil

Peanut oil PEG-6 esters (INCI)
Trade names: Labrafil® M 1969 CS

Pectin (INCI)
CAS 9000-69-5; EINECS 232-553-0

Synonyms: Citrus pectin
Trade names: Genu Pectins; Mexpectin LA 100 Range; Mexpectin LC 700 Range; Mexpectin XSS 100 Range

Pectinase
CAS 9032-75-1; EINECS 232-885-6
Trade names: Clarex® 5XL; Clarex® L; Pearex® L

PEG-4 (INCI)
CAS 25322-68-3 (generic); 112-60-7; EINECS 203-989-9
Synonyms: PEG 200; POE (4); 2,2´-[Oxybis(2,1-ethanediyloxy)bisethanol
Trade names: Dow E200; Hetoxide PEG-200; Hodag PEG 200; Lipo Polyglycol 200; Lipoxol® 200 MED; Macol® E-200; Pluracol® E200; Poly-G® 200; Teric PEG 200; Unipeg 200; Unipeg-200 X; Upiwax 200

PEG-6 (INCI)
CAS 25322-68-3 (generic); 2615-15-8; EINECS 220-045-1
Synonyms: PEG 300; Hexaethylene glycol; Macrogol 300
Trade names: Carbowax® PEG 300; Carbowax® Sentry® PEG 300; Dow E300 NF; Hetoxide PEG-300; Hodag PEG 300; Lipo Polyglycol 300; Lipoxol® 300 MED; Lutrol® E 300; Macol® E-300; Pluracol® E300; Poly-G® 300; Renex® PEG 300; Teric PEG 300; Upiwax 300
Trade names containing: Carbowax® PEG 540 Blend; Carbowax® Sentry® PEG 540 Blend; Cellulinol; Hodag PEG 540; Labrafil® M 2130 CS; Lanobase SE; Lipoxol® 550 MED; Pluracol® E1500; Unipeg 1500; Unipeg-1500 X; Uniwax 1450

PEG-8 (INCI)
CAS 25322-68-3 (generic); 5117-19-1; EINECS 225-856-4
Synonyms: PEG 400; POE (8); 3,6,9,12,15,18,21-Heptaoxatricosane-1,23-diol
Trade names: Carbowax® PEG 400; Carbowax® Sentry® PEG 400; Dow E400 NF; Emery® 6709; Hodag PEG 400; Lipo Polyglycol 400; Lipoxol® 400 MED; Lutrol® E 400; Macol® E-400; Pluracol® E400; Pluracol® E400 NF; Poly-G® 400; Renex® PEG 400; Rhodasurf® E 400; Teric PEG 400; Unipeg 400; Unipeg-400 X; Upiwax 400
Trade names containing: Afron 22; Carbossalina; Crystallin Protein; Hair Complex Aquosum; Kalixide Idrata; Oxynex® K; Texapon® SG

PEG-9 (INCI)
CAS 25322-68-3 (generic); 3386-18-3; EINECS 222-206-1
Synonyms: PEG 450; POE (9)
Trade names: Rhodasurf® PEG 400

PEG-12 (INCI)
CAS 25322-68-3 (generic); 6790-09-6; EINECS 229-859-1
Synonyms: PEG 600; POE (12); Macrogol 600
Trade names: Carbowax® PEG 600; Carbowax® Sentry® PEG 600; Dow E600 NF; Hodag PEG 600; Lipo Polyglycol 600; Lipoxol® 600 MED; Macol® E-600; Pluracol® E600; Pluracol® E600 NF; Poly-G® 600; Renex® PEG 600; Teric PEG 600; Unipeg-600; Upiwax 600

PEG-14 (INCI)
CAS 25322-68-3 (generic)
Synonyms: POE (14)
Trade names: Rhodasurf® E 600; Rhodasurf® PEG 600

PEG-16 (INCI)

CAS 25322-68-3 (generic)
Synonyms: PEG 800; POE (16)
Trade names: Lipoxol® 800 MED; Teric PEG 800

PEG-20 (INCI)
CAS 25322-68-3 (generic)
Synonyms: PEG 1000; Macrogol 1000; POE (20)
Trade names: Carbowax® PEG 900; Carbowax® PEG 1000; Carbowax® Sentry® PEG 900; Carbowax® Sentry® PEG 1000; Dow E1000 NF; Hodag PEG 1000; Lipo Polyglycol 1000; Lipoxol® 1000 MED; Macol® E-1000; Pluracol® E1000; Poly-G® 1000; Renex® PEG 1000; Teric PEG 1000; Unipeg 1000; Unipeg-1000 X; Upiwax 1000

PEG-32 (INCI)
CAS 25322-68-3 (generic)
Synonyms: PEG 1540; Macrogol 1540; POE (32)
Trade names: Carbowax® PEG 1450; Carbowax® Sentry® PEG 1450; Dow E1450 NF; Hodag PEG 1450; Lipoxol® 1550 MED; Lutrol® E 1500; Lutrol® E1450 NF; Macol® E-1450; Pluracol® E1450; Pluracol® E1450 NF; Protachem 1450 NF; Renex® PEG 1500FL; Unipeg 1540; Unipeg-1540 X
Trade names containing: Carbowax® PEG 540 Blend; Carbowax® Sentry® PEG 540 Blend; Hodag PEG 540; Lanobase SE; Lipoxol® 550 MED; Pluracol® E1500; Unipeg 1500; Unipeg-1500 X; Uniwax 1450

PEG-40 (INCI)
CAS 25322-68-3 (generic)
Synonyms: PEG 2000; POE (40)
Trade names: Lipoxol® 2000 MED; Pluracol® E2000; Poly-G® 2000

PEG-60 (INCI)
CAS 25322-68-3 (generic)
Synonyms: PEG 3000; POE (60)
Trade names: Lipoxol® 3000 MED

PEG-75 (INCI)
CAS 25322-68-3 (generic)
Synonyms: PEG 4000; POE (75)
Trade names: Carbowax® PEG 3350; Carbowax® Sentry® PEG 3350; Dow E3350 NF; Hodag PEG 3350; Lipo Polyglycol 3350; Lipoxol® 4000 MED; Lutrol® E 4000; Macol® E-3350; Pluracol® E4000; Pluracol® E4000 NF; Renex® PEG 4000FL; Teric PEG 4000; Unipeg 4000; Unipeg-4000 X; Upiwax 3350

PEG 100.... *See PEG-2...*

PEG-100 (INCI)
CAS 25322-68-3 (generic)
Synonyms: PEG (100); POE (100)
Trade names: Carbowax® PEG 4600; Carbowax® Sentry® PEG 4600; Dow E4500 NF; Emkapol 5000

PEG-135 (INCI)
CAS 25322-68-3 (generic)
Synonyms: PEG (135); POE (135)
Trade names: Emkapol 6000

PEG-150 (INCI)
CAS 25322-68-3 (generic)
Synonyms: PEG 6000; Macrogol 6000; POE (150)
Trade names: Carbowax® PEG 8000; Carbowax® Sentry® PEG 8000; Dow E8000 NF; Hodag PEG 8000; Lipoxol® 6000 MED; Lutrol® E 6000; Macol® E-8000; Pluracol® E8000; Pluracol® E8000 NF; Renex® PEG 6000FL; Teric PEG 6000; Unipeg 6000; Unipeg-6000 X; Upiwax 8000

PEG 200. *See PEG-4*

PEG-200 (INCI)
CAS 25322-68-3 (generic)

Synonyms: PEG 9000; POE (200)
Trade names: Emkapol 8000; Emkapol 8500

PEG-240 (INCI)
CAS 25322-68-3 (generic)
Synonyms: POE (240)
Trade names: Lipoxol® 12000

PEG 300. *See PEG-6*

Peg-350 (INCI)
Synonyms: PEG 20000; POE (350)
Trade names: Lipoxol® 20000; Upiwax 20000

PEG 400. *See PEG-8*

PEG 450. *See PEG-9*

PEG 500. *See PEG-10*

PEG 600. *See PEG-12*

PEG 800. *See PEG-16*

PEG 1000. *See PEG-20*

PEG 1500. *See PEG-6-32*

PEG 1540. *See PEG-32*

PEG 2000. *See PEG-40*

PEG 3000. *See PEG-60*

PEG 4000. *See PEG-75*

PEG 6000. *See PEG-150*

PEG 9000. *See PEG-200*

PEG-2M (INCI)
CAS 25322-68-3 (generic)
Synonyms: PEG-2000; Polyethylene glycol (2000); POE (2000)
Trade names: Polyox® WSR N-10; Prox-onic PEG-2000

PEG-4M
Trade names: Prox-onic PEG-4000

PEG-5M (INCI)
CAS 25322-68-3 (generic)
Synonyms: PEG-5000; POE (5000)
Trade names: Polyox® WSR 35; Polyox® WSR N-80

PEG-6M
Trade names: Prox-onic PEG-6000

PEG-7M (INCI)
CAS 25322-68-3 (generic)
Synonyms: PEG-7000; POE (7000); PEG 300,000
Trade names: Polyox® WSR N-750

PEG-8M
Trade names: Teric PEG 8000

PEG-9M (INCI)
CAS 25322-68-3 (generic)
Synonyms: PEG-9000; POE (9000)
Trade names: Polyox® WSR 3333

PEG-10M
Trade names: Prox-onic PEG-10,000

PEG-14M (INCI)
CAS 25322-68-3 (generic)
Synonyms: PEG-14000; PEG 600,000; POE (14000)
Trade names: Polyox® WSR 205; Polyox® WSR N-3000

PEG-20M (INCI)
CAS 25322-68-3 (generic)
Synonyms: PEG-20000; POE (20000)
Trade names: Polyox® WSR 1105; Prox-onic PEG-20,000

PEG-23M (INCI)
CAS 25322-68-3 (generic)
Synonyms: PEG-23000; POE (23000)

Trade names: Polyox® WSR N-12K

PEG-35M
Trade names: Prox-onic PEG-35,000

PEG-45M (INCI)
CAS 25322-68-3 (generic)
Synonyms: PEG-45000; POE (45000)
Trade names: Polyox® WSR N-60K

PEG-90M (INCI)
CAS 25322-68-3 (generic)
Synonyms: PEG-90000; POE (90000)
Trade names: Polyox® WSR 301

PEG-115M (INCI)
CAS 25322-68-3 (generic)
Synonyms: PEG-115000; POE (115000)
Trade names: Polyox® Coagulant
Trade names containing: Polytrix™

PEG-20 almond glycerides (INCI)
Synonyms: PEG 1000 almond glycerides; POE (20) almond glycerides
Trade names: Crovol A40

PEG-60 almond glycerides (INCI)
Synonyms: PEG 3000 almond glycerides; POE (60) almond glycerides
Trade names: Crovol A70

PEG-11 avocado glycerides (INCI)
Synonyms: PEG (11) avocado glycerides; POE (11) avocado glycerides
Trade names: Avocado Oil W

PEG-6 beeswax (INCI)
Synonyms: PEG 300 beeswax; POE (6) beeswax
Trade names: Estol 3751; Estol EO3BW 3751

PEG-8 beeswax (INCI)
Synonyms: PEG 400 beeswax; POE (8) beeswax
Trade names: Apifil®; Estol 3752; Estol EO4BW 3752

PEG-12 beeswax (INCI)
Synonyms: PEG 600 beeswax; POE (12) beeswax
Trade names: Estol 3753; Estol EO6BW 3753

PEG-20 beeswax (INCI)
Synonyms: PEG 1000 beeswax; POE (20) beeswax
Trade names: Estol 3754

PEG-8 behenate (INCI)
Synonyms: PEG 400 behenate; POE (8) behenate
Trade names containing: Compritol HD5 ATO

PEG behenyl ether. *See Beheneth series*

PEG-105 behenyl propylenediamine (INCI)
Synonyms: POE (105) behenyl propylenediamine
Trade names: Sandogen NH

PEG-13 betanaphthol ether
Trade names: Hetoxide BN-13

PEG-2 butyl ether. *See Butoxy diglycol*

PEG-6 caprylic/capric glycerides (INCI)
CAS 52504-24-2
Synonyms: PEG 300 caprylic/capric glycerides; POE (6) caprylic/capric glycerides
Trade names: Softigen® 767; Sterol CC 595

PEG-8 caprylic/capric glycerides (INCI)
CAS 57307-99-0
Synonyms: PEG 400 caprylate/caprate glycerides
Trade names: Labrasol; L.A.S.

PEG-2 castor oil (INCI)
CAS 61791-12-6 (generic)
Synonyms: POE (2) castor oil; PEG 100 castor oil
Trade names: Hetoxide C-2

PEG-3 castor oil (INCI)
CAS 61791-12-6 (generic)
Synonyms: POE (3) castor oil
Trade names: Nikkol CO-3

PEG-5 castor oil (INCI)
CAS 61791-12-6 (generic)
Synonyms: POE (5) castor oil
Trade names: Ablunol CO 5; Acconon CA-5; Chemax CO-5; Etocas 5; Prox-onic HR-05; Surfactol® 318

PEG-8 castor oil (INCI)
CAS 61791-12-6 (generic)
Synonyms: POE (8) castor oil; PEG 400 castor oil
Trade names: Hodag Nonionic GR-8; Unipeg-CO-8

PEG-9 castor oil (INCI)
CAS 61791-12-6 (generic)
Synonyms: POE (9) castor oil; PEG 450 castor oil
Trade names: Acconon CA-9; Hetoxide C-9; Protachem CA-9

PEG-10 castor oil (INCI)
CAS 61791-12-6 (generic)
Synonyms: POE (10) castor oil; PEG 500 castor oil
Trade names: Etocas 10; Nikkol CO-10

PEG-11 castor oil (INCI)
CAS 61791-12-6 (generic)
Synonyms: PEG (11) castor oil; POE (11) castor oil
Trade names: Marlowet® R 11/K

PEG-15 castor oil (INCI)
CAS 61791-12-6 (generic)
Synonyms: POE (15) castor oil
Trade names: Ablunol CO 15; Acconon CA-15; Alkamuls® CO-15; Cerex EL 150; Elfapur® R 150; Etocas 15; Hetoxide C-15

PEG-16 castor oil
CAS 61791-12-6 (generic)
Synonyms: POE (16) castor oil
Trade names: Chemax CO-16; Prox-onic HR-016

PEG-17 castor oil
CAS 61791-12-6 (generic)
Synonyms: POE (17) castor oil
Trade names: Servirox OEG 45

PEG-20 castor oil (INCI)
CAS 61791-12-6 (generic)
Synonyms: POE (20) castor oil; PEG 1000 castor oil
Trade names: Emalex C-20; Etocas 20; Nikkol CO-20TX

PEG-25 castor oil (INCI)
CAS 61791-12-6 (generic)
Synonyms: POE (25) castor oil
Trade names: Cerex EL 250; Chemax CO-25; Hetoxide C-25; Hodag Nonionic GR-25; Mapeg® CO-25; Marlowet® R 25/K; Protachem CA-25; Prox-onic HR-025; Ricino Viscoil; Unipeg-CO-25

PEG-26 castor oil (INCI)
CAS 61791-12-6 (generic)
Synonyms: POE (26) castor oil
Trade names: Servirox OEG 55

PEG-28 castor oil
CAS 61791-12-6 (generic)
Synonyms: POE (28) castor oil
Trade names: Chemax CO-28

PEG-29 castor oil (INCI)
Synonyms: POE (29) castor oil
Trade names: Etocas 29

PEG-30 castor oil (INCI)
CAS 61791-12-6 (generic)
Synonyms: POE (30) castor oil

Trade names: Ablunol CO 30; Alkamuls® EL-620; Alkamuls® EL-620L; Cerex EL 300; Chemax CO-30; Desonic® 30C; Emalex C-30; Etocas 30; Fancol CO-30; Hetoxide C-30; Incrocas 30; Mapeg® CO-30; Protachem CA-30; Prox-onic HR-030; Witconol™ 5906

PEG-32 castor oil
CAS 61791-12-6 (generic)
Synonyms: POE (32) castor oil
Trade names: Servirox OEG 65

PEG-33 castor oil (INCI)
CAS 61791-12-6 (generic)
Synonyms: POE (33) castor oil
Trade names: Alkamuls® B; Alkamuls® BR; Emulpon EL 33; Ricinion; Sellig R 3395

PEG-35 castor oil (INCI)
CAS 61791-12-6 (generic)
Synonyms: POE (35) castor oil
Trade names: Cremophor® EL; Etocas 35; Eumulgin® RO 35; Simulsol 5817
Trade names containing: Soluvit Richter

PEG-36 castor oil (INCI)
CAS 61791-12-6 (generic)
Synonyms: POE (36) castor oil; PEG 1800 castor oil
Trade names: Alkamuls® EL-630; Cerex EL 360; Chemax CO-36; Desonic® 36C; Emulsogen EL; Eumulgin® PRT 36; Hodag Nonionic GR-36; Mapeg® CO-36; Prox-onic HR-036; Unipeg-CO-36; Witconol™ 5907
Trade names containing: AFR LS; Safester A 75 WS; Unibiovit B-332; Unitrienol T-272

PEG-40 castor oil (INCI)
CAS 61791-12-6 (generic)
Synonyms: POE (40) castor oil; PEG 2000 castor oil
Trade names: Alkamuls® EL-719; Cerex EL 400; Chemax CO-40; Emalex C-40; Emulpon EL 40; Emulpon EL 40; Etocas 40; Eumulgin® PRT 40; Eumulgin® RO 40; Hetoxide C-40; Hodag Nonionic GR-40; Incrocas 40; Lanaetex C-40; Lanaetex CO-40; Marlowet® R 40; Marlowet® R 40/K; Nikkol CO-40TX; Protachem CA-40; Prox-onic HR-040; Remcopal 40 S3; Simulsol OL 50; Surfactol® 365; Unipeg-CO-40; Witconol™ 5909
Trade names containing: Azulene 25% WS 2/013000; Biobranil Watersoluble 2/012600; Carsoquat® 816-C; Carsoquat® CB; Ceral EFN; Emulgade® F Special; Emulgade® F; Extrapone Bio-Tamin Special 2/2032671; Incroquat CR Conc; Lecithin Water Dispersible CLR; Maquat SC-1632; Marlowet® RNP/K; Quatrex CRC; Unimulgade-F Special; Unimulgade-F; Varisoft® C SAC

PEG-50 castor oil (INCI)
CAS 61791-12-6 (generic)
Synonyms: POE (50) castor oil
Trade names: Emalex C-50; Etocas 50; Nalco® 2395; Nikkol CO-50TX

PEG-52 castor oil
CAS 61791-12-6 (generic)
Synonyms: POE (52) castor oil
Trade names: Hetoxide C-52; Hodag Nonionic GR-52

PEG-54 castor oil (INCI)
CAS 61791-12-6 (generic)
Synonyms: POE (54) castor oil
Trade names: Desonic® 54C

PEG-56 castor oil
Trade names: Eumulgin® PRT 56

PEG-60 castor oil (INCI)
CAS 61791-12-6 (generic)
Synonyms: POE (60) castor oil
Trade names: Etocas 60; Hetoxide C-60; Nikkol CO-60TX; Simulsol 1285

PEG-70 castor oil
Trade names: Marlosol® R70

PEG-75 castor oil (INCI)
Trade names: Ethocas 75

PEG-80 castor oil
CAS 61791-12-6 (generic)
Synonyms: POE (80) castor oil
Trade names: Chemax CO-80; Prox-onic HR-080

PEG-100 castor oil (INCI)
CAS 61791-12-6 (generic)
Synonyms: POE (100) castor oil; PEG (100) castor oil
Trade names: Etocas 100; Protachem CA-100

PEG-180 castor oil
CAS 61791-12-6 (generic)
Synonyms: POE (180) castor oil
Trade names: Servirox OEG 90/50

PEG-200 castor oil (INCI)
CAS 61791-12-6 (generic)
Synonyms: POE (200) castor oil; PEG (200) castor oil
Trade names: Chemax CO-200/50; Etocas 200; Eumulgin® PRT 200; Hetoxide C-200; Hetoxide C-200-50%; Hodag Nonionic GR-200; Mapeg® CO-200; Protachem CA-200; Prox-onic HR-0200; Prox-onic HR-0200/50; Unipeg-CO-200

PEG-18 castor oil dioleate (INCI)
Synonyms: POE (18) castor oil dioleate
Trade names: Marlowet® LVS/K
Trade names containing: Marlowet® LVX/K

PEG cetyl ether. *See Ceteth series*

PEG cetyl/oleyl ether. *See Ceteoleth series*

PEG cetyl/stearyl ethers. *See Ceteareth series*

PEG-2 cocamide
Trade names: Amide CMA-2

PEG-3 cocamide (INCI)
CAS 61791-08-0 (generic)
Synonyms: PEG (3) coconut amide; POE (3) coconut amide
Trade names: Amidox® C-2; Hetoxamide CD-4; Oramide MLM 02; Upamide C-2

PEG-5 cocamide (INCI)
CAS 61791-08-0 (generic)
Synonyms: POE (5) coconut amide
Trade names: Alkamide® C-5; Eumulgin® C4; Genagen CA-050; Hetoxamide C-4

PEG-6 cocamide (INCI)
CAS 61791-08-0 (generic)
Synonyms: POE (6) coconut amide; PEG 300 coconut amide
Trade names: Amidox® C-5; Hetoxamide CD-6; Rewopal® C 6; Unamide® C-5; Upamide C-5

PEG-7 cocamide (INCI)
CAS 61791-08-0 (generic)
Synonyms: POE (7) coconut amide
Trade names: Oramide MLM 06

PEG-11 cocamide (INCI)
CAS 61791-08-0 (generic)
Synonyms: POE (11) coconut amide
Trade names: Oramide MLM 10

PEG-3 cocamide MEA

Trade names: Mazamide® C-2

PEG-6 cocamide MEA
Trade names: Mazamide® C-5

PEG-2 cocamine (INCI)
CAS 61791-14-8 (generic)
Synonyms: PEG 100 coconut amine; POE (2) coconut amine; Bis (2-hydroxyethyl) coco amine
Trade names: Accomeen C2; Chemeen C-2; Ethomeen® C/12; Hetoxamine C-2; Mazeen® C-2; Protox C-2; Unizeen C-2; Varonic® K-202; Varonic® K-202 SF

PEG-3 cocamine (INCI)
CAS 61791-14-8 (generic)
Synonyms: POE (3) coconut amine
Trade names: Lowenol C-243

PEG-5 cocamine (INCI)
CAS 61791-14-8 (generic)
Synonyms: POE (5) coconut amine
Trade names: Accomeen C5; Chemeen C-5; Ethomeen® C/15; Hetoxamine C-5; Mazeen® C-5; Protox C-5; Unizeen C-5; Varonic® K-205; Varonic® K-205 SF

PEG-10 cocamine (INCI)
CAS 61791-14-8 (generic)
Synonyms: POE (10) coconut amine; PEG 500 coconut amine
Trade names: Accomeen C10; Chemeen C-10; Ethomeen® C/20; Ethylan® TN-10; Mazeen® C-10; Protox C-10; Unizeen C-10; Varonic® K-210; Varonic® K-210 SF

PEG-15 cocamine (INCI)
CAS 8051-52-3 (generic); 61791-14-8 (generic)
Synonyms: POE (15) coconut amine
Trade names: Accomeen C15; Chemeen C-15; Ethomeen® C/25; Ethylan® TC; Hetoxamine C-15; Mazeen® C-15; Protox C-15; Varonic® K-215; Varonic® K-215 LC; Varonic® K-215 SF

PEG-15 cocamine oleate/phosphate (INCI)
Synonyms: POE (15) cocamine oleate/phosphate
Trade names: Lanaetex CPS

PEG-75 cocoa butter
Trade names: Unipeg 75 Cocoa Butter

PEG-75 cocoa butter glycerides (INCI)
Synonyms: POE (65) cocoa butter glycerides; PEG 4000 cocoa butter glycerides
Trade names: Emthox® 2730

PEG-2 cocoate
Synonyms: PEG 100 cocoate; POE (2) monococoate; Diglycol coconate
Trade names: Witconol™ RDC-D

PEG-5 cocoate (INCI)
CAS 61791-29-5 (generic)
Synonyms: POE (5) monococoate
Trade names: Ethofat® C/15; Prox-onic CC-05

PEG-9 cocoate
CAS 67762-35-0
Trade names: Prox-onic CC-09

PEG-10 cocoate
CAS 61791-29-5 (generic)
Synonyms: POE (10) monococoate; PEG 500 monococoate
Trade names: Crodet C10

PEG-14 cocoate
Trade names: Prox-onic CC-014

PEG-15 cocoate (INCI)
CAS 61791-29-5 (generic)

Synonyms: POE (15) monococoate
Trade names: Ethofat® C/25

PEG-2 coco-benzonium chloride (INCI)
CAS 61789-68-2
Synonyms: PEG-2 cocobenzyl ammonium chloride; PEG 100 coco-benzonium chloride; POE (2) coco-benzonium chloride
Trade names: Ethoquad® C/12B
Trade names containing: Ethoquad® CB/12

PEG-2 cocomonium chloride (INCI)
CAS 70750-47-9
Synonyms: PEG 100 cocomonium chloride; POE (2) cocomonium chloride; Methyl bis (2-hydroxyethyl) cocammonium chloride
Trade names: Ethoquad® C/25; Variquat® K-1215
Trade names containing: Ethoquad® C/12; Variquat® 638

PEG-15 cocomonium chloride (INCI)
CAS 61791-10-4
Synonyms: POE (15) cocomonium chloride; Methyl-polyoxyethylene (15) coco ammonium chloride; PEG-15 coco methyl ammonium chloride
Trade names containing: SM 2112

PEG-5 cocomonium methosulfate (INCI)
CAS 68989-03-7
Synonyms: POE (5) cocomonium methosulfate; Coconut pentaethoxy methyl ammonium methyl sulfate
Trade names: Rewoquat CPEM

PEG-2 cocomonium nitrate
CAS 71487-00-8
Synonyms: PEG-2 cocomethyl ammonium nitrate
Trade names containing: Ethoquad® C/12 Nitrate

PEG coconut ether. *See Coceth series*

PEG-10 coconut oil esters (INCI)
Trade names: Colan 12
Trade names containing: Delan 62; Ethoxol-CO

PEG-15 cocopolyamine (INCI)
Synonyms: POE (15) coconut polyamine
Trade names: Polyquart® H; Polyquart® H 81
Trade names containing: Polyquart® H 7102; Uniquart 7102

PEG-20 corn glycerides (INCI)
Synonyms: PEG 1000 corn glycerides; POE (20) corn glycerides
Trade names: Crovol M40

PEG-60 corn glycerides (INCI)
Synonyms: PEG 3000 corn glycerides; POE (60) corn glycerides
Trade names: Crovol M70

PEG-crosspolymer (INCI)
Trade names: Cool-Jel

PEG decyl ether. *See Deceth series*

PEG-5 decylpentadecyl ether
Trade names: Emalex 2505

PEG-10 decylpentadecyl ether
Trade names: Emalex 2510

PEG-15 decyl pentadecyl ether
Trade names: Emalex 2515

PEG-20 decyl pentadecyl ether
Trade names: Emalex 2520

PEG-25 decyl pentadecyl ether
Trade names: Emalex 2525

PEG-5 decyl tetradecylether
Trade names: Emalex 2405

PEG-10 decyl tetradecyl ether
Trade names: Emalex 2410

PEG-15 decyl tetradecyl ether
Trade names: Emalex 2415

PEG-20 decyl tetradecyl ether
Trade names: Emalex 2420

PEG-25 decyl tetradecyl ether
Trade names: Emalex 2425

PEG-5 DEDM hydantoin oleate (INCI)
Synonyms: PEG-5 di-(2-hydroxyethyl)-5,5-dimethyl hydantoin oleate; POE (5) DEDM hydantoin oleate
Trade names: Dantosperse® DHE (5) MO

PEG-4 diheptanoate
Trade names: Liponate 2-DH

PEG-2 diisononanoate (INCI)
Synonyms: PEG 100 diisononanoate
Trade names containing: Estalan 334

PEG-3 diisostearate
Trade names: Emalex TEG-di-IS

PEG-4 diisostearate
Trade names: Emalex 200di-IS

PEG-6 diisostearate
Trade names: Emalex 300 di-IS

PEG-8 diisostearate
Trade names: Emalex 400 di-IS

PEG-12 diisostearate
Trade names: Emalex 600 di-IS

PEG-2 dilaurate (CTFA)
CAS 9005-02-1 (generic); 6281-04-5; EINECS 228-486-1
Synonyms: PEG 100 dilaurate; POE (2) dilaurate
Trade names: Emalex DEG-di-L; Protamate 200 DL

PEG-3 dilaurate
Trade names: Emalex TEG-di-L

PEG-4 dilaurate (INCI)
CAS 9005-02-1 (generic)
Synonyms: PEG 200 dilaurate; POE (4) dilaurate
Trade names: Chemax PEG 200 DL; Cithrol 2DL; Emalex 200 di-L; Emerest® 2704; Hetoxamate 200 DL; Hodag 22-L; Kessco® PEG 200 DL; Lexemul® 200 DL; Lexemul® PEG-200 DL; Lipopeg 2-DL; Mapeg® 200 DL; Pegosperse® 200 DL; Protamate 400 DL; Witconol™ 2622

PEG-6 dilaurate (INCI)
CAS 9005-02-1 (generic)
Synonyms: POE (6) dilaurate; PEG 300 dilaurate
Trade names: Emalex 300 di-L; Kessco® PEG 300 DL; Lipopeg 3-DL
Trade names containing: Pegosperse® 1500 DL

PEG-8 dilaurate (INCI)
CAS 9005-02-1 (generic)
Synonyms: POE (8) dilaurate; PEG 400 dilaurate
Trade names: Cithrol 4DL; CPH-361-N; CPH-79-N; Emalex 400 di-L; Hetoxamate 400 DL; Hodag 42-L; Kessco® PEG 400 DL; Lexemul® PEG-400 DL; Lipopeg 4-DL; Mapeg® 400 DL; Pegosperse® 400 DL; Rol DL 40; Unipeg-400 DL

PEG-12 dilaurate (INCI)
CAS 9005-02-1 (generic)
Synonyms: POE (12) dilaurate; PEG 600 dilaurate
Trade names: Cithrol 6DL; Emalex 600 di-L; Kessco® PEG 600 DL; Mapeg® 600 DL

PEG-16 dilaurate
Trade names: Emalex 800 di-L

PEG-20 dilaurate (INCI)
CAS 9005-02-1 (generic)
Synonyms: POE (20) dilaurate; PEG 1000 dilaurate
Trade names: Cithrol 10DL; Emalex 1000 di-L; Kessco®
PEG 1000 DL

PEG-32 dilaurate (INCI)
CAS 9005-02-1 (generic)
Synonyms: POE (32) dilaurate; PEG 1540 dilaurate
Trade names: Kessco® PEG 1540 DL
Trade names containing: Pegosperse® 1500 DL

PEG-75 dilaurate (INCI)
CAS 9005-02-1 (generic)
Synonyms: POE (75) dilaurate; PEG 4000 dilaurate
Trade names: Kessco® PEG 4000 DL

PEG-150 dilaurate (INCI)
CAS 9005-02-1 (generic)
Synonyms: POE (150) dilaurate; PEG 6000 dilaurate
Trade names: Kessco® PEG 6000 DL; Lipopeg 6000-DL

PEG dinonyl phenyl ether. *See Nonyl nonoxynol series*

PEG-2 dioctanoate (INCI)
Trade names containing: Estalan 334

PEG-2 dioleate
CAS 9005-07-6 (generic); 52668-97-0 (generic)
Synonyms: Diethylene glycol dioleate; POE (2) dioleate;
PEG 100 dioleate
Trade names: Emalex DEG-di-O

PEG-3 dioleate
Trade names: Emalex TEG-di-O

PEG-4 dioleate (INCI)
CAS 9005-07-6 (generic); 52688-97-0 (generic); 134141-38-1
Synonyms: POE (4) dioleate; PEG 200 dioleate
Trade names: Cithrol 2DO; Emalex 200 di-O; Hodag 22-O; Kessco® PEG 200 DO; Mapeg® 200 DO

PEG-6 dioleate (INCI)
CAS 9005-07-6 (generic); 52688-97-0 (generic)
Synonyms: POE (6) dioleate; PEG 300 dioleate
Trade names: Emalex 300 di-O; Hodag 32-O; Kessco®
PEG 300 DO

PEG-8 dioleate (INCI)
CAS 9005-07-6 (generic); 52688-97-0 (generic)
Synonyms: POE (8) dioleate; PEG 400 dioleate
Trade names: Alkamuls® 400-DO; Chemax PEG 400
DO; Cithrol 4DO; Emalex 400 di-O; Estol EO4DO
3673; Hodag 42-O; Kessco® PEG 400 DO; Lipopeg
4-DO; Mapeg® 400 DO; Pegosperse® 400 DO;
Protamate 400 DO; Radiasurf® 7443; Rol DO 40;
Unipeg-400 DO; Witconol™ 2648

PEG-12 dioleate (INCI)
CAS 9005-07-6 (generic); 52688-97-0 (generic); 85736-49-8; EINECS 288-459-5
Synonyms: POE (12) dioleate; PEG 600 dioleate
Trade names: Alkamuls® 600-DO; Chemax PEG 600
DO; Cithrol 6DO; CPH-213-N; Emalex 600 di-O; Estol
EO6DO 3675; Hodag 62-O; Kessco® PEG 600 DO;
Mapeg® 600 DO; Marlipal® FS; Marlosol® FS;
Radiasurf® 7444; Unipeg-600 DO
Trade names containing: Marlowet® LVX/K

PEG-20 dioleate (INCI)
CAS 9005-07-6 (generic); 52688-97-0 (generic)
Synonyms: POE (20) dioleate; PEG 1000 dioleate
Trade names: Cithrol 10DO; Kessco® PEG 1000 DO

PEG-32 dioleate (INCI)
CAS 9005-07-6 (generic); 52688-97-0 (generic)
Synonyms: POE (32) dioleate; PEG 1540 dioleate

Trade names: Kessco® PEG 1540 DO

PEG-75 dioleate (INCI)
CAS 9005-07-6 (generic); 52688-97-0 (generic)
Synonyms: POE (75) dioleate; PEG 4000 dioleate
Trade names: Kessco® PEG 4000 DO

PEG-150 dioleate (INCI)
CAS 9005-07-6 (generic); 52688-97-0 (generic)
Synonyms: POE (150) dioleate; PEG 6000 dioleate
Trade names: Kessco® PEG 6000 DO

PEG-2 distearate (INCI)
CAS 109-30-8; 52668-97-0; EINECS 203-663-6
Synonyms: POE (2) distearate; PEG 100 distearate
Trade names: Emalex DEG-di-S

PEG-3 distearate (INCI)
CAS 9005-08-7 (generic); 52668-97-0
Synonyms: Triglycol distearate; Triethylene glycol di-
stearate; POE (3) distearate
Trade names: Cutina® TS; Emalex TEG-di-AS; Emalex
TEG-di-S; Genapol® TS Powd; Nikkol Estepearl 30;
Phoenate 3 DSA; Unipeg 150 DS
Trade names containing: Base Nacrante 6030 CP;
Euperlan® MPK 850; Euperlan® PK 900 BENZ;
Euperlan® PK 900; Genamin KSE; Genapol® TSM

PEG-4 distearate (INCI)
CAS 9005-08-7 (generic); 52668-97-0; 142-20-1
Synonyms: POE (4) distearate; PEG 200 distearate
Trade names: Emalex 200 di-AS; Emalex 200 di-S;
Hodag 22-S; Kessco® PEG 200 DS; Mapeg® 200 DS

PEG-6 distearate (INCI)
CAS 9005-08-7 (generic); 52668-97-0
Synonyms: POE (6) distearate; PEG 300 distearate
Trade names: Alkamuls® PEG 300 DS; Emalex 300 di-
S; Kessco® PEG 300 DS

PEG-8 distearate (INCI)
CAS 9005-08-7 (generic); 52668-97-0
Synonyms: POE (8) distearate; PEG 400 distearate
Trade names: Alkamuls® PEG 400 DS; Cithrol 4DS;
Elfacos® PEG 400 DS; Emalex 400 di-AS; Emalex
400 di-S; Emerest® 2642; Emerest® 2712; Estol
EO4DS 3724; Hefti PGE-400-DS; Hetoxamate 400
DS; Hodag 42-S; Kessco PEG-400 DS-356;
Kessco® PEG 400 DS; Lipal 400 DS; Lipopeg 4-DS;
Mapeg® 400 DS; Pegosperse® 400 DS; Protamate
400 DS; Radiasurf® 7453; Unipeg-400 DS;
Witconol™ 2712

PEG-12 distearate (INCI)
CAS 9005-08-7 (generic); 52668-97-0
Synonyms: POE (12) distearate; PEG 600 distearate
Trade names: Alkamuls® PEG 600 DS; Cithrol 6DS;
Elfacos® PEG 600 DS; Emalex 600 di-AS; Emalex
600 di-S; Estol EO6DS 3726; Hefti PGE-600-DS;
Hetoxamate 600 DS; Hodag 62-S; Kessco® PEG 600
DS; Mapeg® 600 DS; Marlosol® BS; Protamate 600
DS; Radiasurf® 7454; Unipeg-600 DS

PEG-20 distearate (INCI)
CAS 9005-08-7 (generic); 52668-97-0
Synonyms: POE (20) distearate; PEG 1000 distearate
Trade names: Cithrol 10DS; Estol E10DS 3728; Hodag
102-S; Kessco® PEG 1000 DS; Lipopeg 10-DS;
Unipeg 1000 DS

PEG-32 distearate (INCI)
CAS 9005-08-7 (generic); 52668-97-0
Synonyms: POE (32) distearate; PEG 1540 distearate
Trade names: Kessco® PEG 1540 DS; Mapeg® 1540 DS

PEG-75 distearate (INCI)
CAS 9005-08-7 (generic); 52668-97-0

Synonyms: POE (75) distearate; PEG 4000 distearate
Trade names: Kessco® PEG 4000 DS; Unipeg-4000 DS

PEG-120 distearate (INCI)
Synonyms: PEG (120) distearate
Trade names: Cithrol 60DS

PEG-150 distearate (INCI)
CAS 9005-08-7 (generic); 52668-97-0
Synonyms: POE (150) distearate; PEG 6000 distearate
Trade names: Ablunol 6000DS; Algon DS 6000; Emalex 6300 DI-ST; Emulvis®; Estol E60DS 3734; G-1821; Hetoxamate 150 DSA; Hodag 602-S; Kessco PEG 6000DS; Kessco® PEG 6000 DS; Lanoxide-6000DS; Lipal 6000 DS; Lipopeg 6000-DS; Mapeg® 6000 DS; Protamate 6000 DS; Rewopal® PEG 6000 DS; Rol D 600; Unipeg-6000 DS; Witconol™ L3245
Trade names containing: Carsofoam® BS-I; Cycloryl ALC (redesignated Miraspec ALC); Miracare® BC-10; Miracare® BC-20; Miracare® MS-1; Miracare® MS-2; Miracare® MS-4; Viscolene

PEG-4 ditallate
CAS 61791-01-3 (generic)
Synonyms: POE (4) ditallate; PEG 200 ditallate
Trade names: Mapeg® 200 DOT

PEG-8 ditallate (INCI)
CAS 61791-01-3 (generic)
Synonyms: POE (8) ditallate; PEG 400 ditallate
Trade names: Chemax PEG 400 DT; Mapeg® 400 DOT; Pegosperse® 400 DOT

PEG-12 ditallate (INCI)
CAS 61791-01-3 (generic)
Synonyms: POE (12) ditallate; PEG 600 ditallate
Trade names: Chemax PEG 600 DT; Hetoxamate 600 DT; Mapeg® 600 DOT; Pegosperse® 600 DOT

PEG-5 ditridecylmonium chloride (INCI)
Trade names: Varisoft® 5TD

PEG-22/dodecyl glycol copolymer (INCI)
Trade names: Elfacos® S137; Elfacos® ST 37

PEG-45/dodecyl glycol copolymer (INCI)
Trade names: Elfacos® S19; Elfacos® ST 9

PEG dodecyl phenyl ether. *See Dodoxynol series*

PEG-3 ethylhexyl ether
Trade names: Hetoxol CD-3

PEG-4 ethylhexyl ether
Trade names: Hetoxol CD-4

PEG-20 evening primrose glycerides (INCI)
Trade names: Crovol EP-40

PEG-60 evening primrose glycerides (INCI)
Trade names: Crovol EP-70

PEG-7 glyceryl cocoate (INCI)
CAS 66105-29-1; 68201-46-7 (generic)
Synonyms: POE (7) glyceryl monococoate; PEG (7) glyceryl monococoate
Trade names: Cetiol® HE; Estol EO3GC 3606; Extan-PGC; Glycerox HE; Mazol® 159; Rewoderm® ES 90; Tegosoft® GC; Unimul-HE; Unitolate HE
Trade names containing: Grillocin® AT Basis; Rewoderm® LIS 75; Rewoderm® LIS 80

PEG-30 glyceryl cocoate (INCI)
CAS 68201-46-7 (generic)
Synonyms: POE (30) glyceryl monococoate
Trade names: Rewoderm® LI 63; Varonic® LI-63

PEG-40 glyceryl cocoate (INCI)
CAS 68201-46-7 (generic)
Synonyms: POE (40) glyceryl cocoate; PEG 2000 glyceryl cocoate

Trade names containing: Oronal LCG

PEG-78 glyceryl cocoate (INCI)
CAS 68201-46-7 (generic)
Synonyms: POE (78) glyceryl monococoate
Trade names: Rewoderm® LI 67; Rewoderm® LI 67-75; Simulsol CG

PEG-80 glyceryl cocoate (INCI)
CAS 68201-46-7 (generic)
Synonyms: POE (80) glyceryl monococoate
Trade names: Varonic® LI-67; Varonic® LI-67 (75%)

PEG-5 glyceryl dioleate
Trade names: Marlowet® GDO 4

PEG-12 glyceryl dioleate (INCI)
Synonyms: PEG 600 glyceryl dioleate; POE (12) glyceryl dioleate
Trade names: Marlowet® G 12 DO

PEG-4 glyceryl distearate
Trade names: Emalex GWS-204

PEG glyceryl ether. *See Glycereth series*

PEG-18 glyceryl glycol dioleococoate
Trade names: Antil® 171

PEG-3 glyceryl isostearate
Trade names: Emalex GWIS-103

PEG-5 glyceryl isostearate
Trade names: Emalex GWIS-105

PEG-6 glyceryl isostearate
Trade names: Emalex GWIS-106

PEG-8 glyceryl isostearate
Trade names: Emalex GWIS-108

PEG-10 glyceryl isostearate
Trade names: Emalex GWIS-110

PEG-15 glyceryl isostearate (INCI)
Synonyms: POE (15) glyceryl isostearate
Trade names: Emalex GWIS-115; Emalex GWIS-115(M); Oxypon 2145

PEG-20 glyceryl isostearate (INCI)
CAS 69468-44-6
Synonyms: PEG 1000 glyceryl isostearate; POE (20) glyceryl isostearate
Trade names: Emalex GWIS-120

PEG-25 glyceryl isostearate
Trade names: Emalex GWIS-125

PEG-30 glyceryl isostearate (INCI)
CAS 69468-44-6
Synonyms: POE (30) glyceryl isostearate
Trade names: Emalex GWIS-130

PEG-40 glyceryl isostearate
Trade names: Emalex GWIS-140

PEG-50 glyceryl isostearate
Trade names: Emalex GWIS-150

PEG-60 glyceryl isostearate (INCI)
Trade names: Emalex GWIS-160; Emalex GWIS-160N

PEG-7 glyceryl laurate
Trade names: Hodag POE (7) GML

PEG-8 glyceryl laurate (INCI)
Synonyms: POE (8) glyceryl laurate
Trade names: Glycerox L8; Sterol LG 491

PEG-12 glyceryl laurate (INCI)
CAS 59070-56-3 (generic); 51248-32-9
Synonyms: POE (12) glyceryl monolaurate; PEG 600 glyceryl monolaurate
Trade names containing: Safester A 75 WS; Unibiovit B-

332; Unitrienol T-272

PEG-15 glyceryl laurate (INCI)
CAS 59070-56-3 (generic)
Synonyms: POE (15) glyceryl monolaurate
Trade names: Glycerox L15

PEG-20 glyceryl laurate (CTFA)
CAS 59070-56-3 (generic); 51248-32-9
Synonyms: POE (20) glyceryl monolaurate; PEG 1000
glyceryl monolaurate
Trade names: Lamacit® GML 20; Tagat® L2

PEG-23 glyceryl laurate (INCI)
CAS 59070-56-3 (generic); 51248-32-9; 37324-85-9
Synonyms: POE (23) glyceryl laurate
Trade names: Aldosperse® ML-23

PEG-30 glyceryl laurate (INCI)
CAS 59070-56-3 (generic); 51248-32-9
Synonyms: POE (30) glyceryl laurate
Trade names: Glycerox L30; Tagat® L

PEG-40 glyceryl laurate
CAS 59060-56-3 (generic)
Synonyms: POE (40) glyceryl laurate
Trade names: Glycerox L40

PEG-5 glyceryl oleate
Trade names: Nikkol TMGO-5

PEG-10 glyceryl oleate (INCI)
CAS 68889-49-6 (generic)
Synonyms: POE (10) glyceryl monoleate; PEG 500
glyceryl monooleate
Trade names: Nikkol TMGO-10

PEG-15 glyceryl oleate (INCI)
CAS 68889-49-6 (generic)
Synonyms: POE (15) glyceryl monoleate
Trade names: Nikkol TMGO-15

PEG-20 glyceryl oleate (INCI)
CAS 68889-49-6 (generic); 51192-09-7
Synonyms: POE (20) glyceryl oleate; PEG 1000 glyceryl
monooleate
Trade names: Tagat® O2
Trade names containing: Emulgator BTO 2

PEG-30 glyceryl oleate (INCI)
CAS 68889-49-6 (generic); 51192-09-7
Synonyms: POE (30) glyceryl oleate
Trade names: Tagat® O

PEG-20 glyceryl ricinoleate (INCI)
CAS 51142-51-9 (generic)
Synonyms: POE (20) glyceryl monoricinoleate; PEG
1000 glyceryl monoricinoleate
Trade names containing: Lamacit® ER

PEG-1 glyceryl sorbitan isostearate
Trade names: Tewax TC 82

PEG-5 glyceryl stearate (INCI)
CAS 51158-08-8
Synonyms: POE (5) glyceryl monostearate
Trade names: Emalex GM-5; Nikkol TMGS-5; Poem-S-
105; Tewax TC 83

PEG-10 glyceryl stearate (INCI)
Synonyms: PEG 500 glyceryl monostearate; POE (10)
glyceryl monostearate
Trade names: Emalex GM-10

PEG-15 glyceryl stearate
Trade names: Emalex GM-15; Nikkol TMGS-15

PEG-20 glyceryl stearate (INCI)
CAS 68553-11-7; 51158-08-8
Synonyms: PEG 1000 glyceryl monostearate; POE (20)
glyceryl monostearate

Trade names: Aldosperse® MS-20; Capmul® EMG;
Cutina® E24; Emalex GM-20; Eumulgin E-24; Hodag
POE (20) GMS; Mazol® 80 MGK; Tagat® S2; Unitina
E-24; Unitolate 80MG; Varonic® LI-42

PEG-30 glyceryl stearate (INCI)
CAS 51158-08-8
Synonyms: POE (30) glyceryl monostearate
Trade names: Emalex GM-30; Tagat® S

PEG-40 glyceryl stearate (INCI)
Trade names: Emalex GM-40

PEG-60 glyceryl stearate
Trade names: Emalex GM-6000

PEG-200 glyceryl stearate (INCI)
Synonyms: POE (200) glyceryl stearate
Trade names: Alkamuls® VR/50; Simulsol 220 TM;
Soprol VR.50

PEG-80 glyceryl tallowate (INCI)
Synonyms: POE (80) glyceryl monotallowate
Trade names: Rewoderm® LI 48; Rewoderm® LI 48-50;
Varonic® LI-48

PEG-200 glyceryl tallowate (INCI)
Synonyms: POE (200) glyceryl monotallowate
Trade names: Rewoderm® LI 420; Rewoderm® LI 420-
70; Varonic® LI-420; Varonic® LI-420 (70%)
Trade names containing: Rewoderm® LIS 75

PEG-3 glyceryl triisostearate
Trade names: Emalex GWIS-303

PEG-5 glyceryl triisostearate (INCI)
Trade names: Emalex GWIS-305

PEG-10 glyceryl triisostearate
Trade names: Emalex GWIS-310

PEG-20 glyceryl triisostearate
Trade names: Emalex GWIS-320

PEG-30 glyceryl triisostearate
Trade names: Emalex GWIS-330

PEG-40 glyceryl triisostearate
Trade names: Emalex GWIS-340

PEG-50 glyceryl triisostearate
Trade names: Emalex GWIS-350

PEG-60 glyceryl triisostearate
Trade names: Emalex GWIS-360

PEG-3 glyceryl trioleate
Trade names: Emalex GWO-303

PEG-5 glyceryl trioleate
Trade names: Emalex GWO-305

PEG-10 glyceryl trioleate
Trade names: Emalex GWO-310

PEG-20 glyceryl trioleate
Trade names: Emalex GWO-320

PEG-25 glyceryl trioleate (INCI)
CAS 68958-64-5
Synonyms: POE (25) glyceryl trioleate
Trade names: Tagat® TO
Trade names containing: Emulgator BTO

PEG-30 glyceryl trioleate
Trade names: Emalex GWO-330

PEG-40 glyceryl trioleate
Trade names: Emalex GWO-340

PEG-50 glyceryl trioleate
Trade names: Emalex GWO-350

PEG-60 glyceryl trioleate
Trade names: Emalex GWO-360

PEG-3 glyceryl tristearate
Trade names: Emalex GWS-303

PEG-4 glyceryl tristearate
Trade names: Emalex GWS-304

PEG-5 glyceryl tristearate
Trade names: Emalex GWS-305

PEG-6 glyceryl tristearate
Trade names: Emalex GWS-306

PEG-10 glyceryl tristearate
Trade names: Emalex GWS-310

PEG-20 glyceryl tristearate
Trade names: Emalex GWS-320

PEG-5 hydrogenated castor oil (INCI)
CAS 61788-85-0 (generic)
Synonyms: POE (5) hydrogenated castor oil; PEG (5) hydrogenated castor oil
Trade names: Cerex ELS 50; Chemax HCO-5; Emalex HC-5; Nikkol HCO-5; Prox-onic HRH-05

PEG-7 hydrogenated castor oil (INCI)
CAS 61788-85-0 (generic)
Synonyms: POE (7) hydrogenated castor oil
Trade names: Arlacel® 989; Cremophor® WO 7; Croduret 7; Dehymuls® HRE 7; Emalex HC-7; Nikkol HCO-7.5; Remcopal HC 7; Simulsol 989

PEG-10 hydrogenated castor oil
CAS 61788-85-0 (generic)
Synonyms: POE (10) hydrogenated castor oil; PEG 500 hydrogenated castor oil
Trade names: Croduret 10; Emalex HC-10; Nikkol HCO-10

PEG-16 hydrogenated castor oil (INCI)
CAS 61788-85-0 (generic)
Synonyms: POE (16) hydrogenated castor oil
Trade names: Chemax HCO-16; Emthox® 2737; Hetoxide HC-16; Mapeg® CO-16H; Protachem CAH-16; Prox-onic HRH-016; Witconol™ 2737

PEG-20 hydrogenated castor oil (INCI)
CAS 61788-85-0 (generic)
Synonyms: POE (20) hydrogenated castor oil
Trade names: Emalex HC-20; Nikkol HCO-20

PEG-25 hydrogenated castor oil (INCI)
CAS 61788-85-0 (generic)
Synonyms: POE (25) hydrogenated castor oil
Trade names: Arlatone® G; Cerex ELS 250; Chemax HCO-25; Croduret 25; Emthox® 2738; Fancol HCO-25; G-1292; Hetoxide HC-25; Hodag Nonionic GRH-25; Lanaetex CO-25; Mapeg® CO-25H; Protachem CAH-25; Prox-onic HRH-025; Simulsol 1292; Unipeg-CO-25H; Witconol™ 2738

PEG-30 hydrogenated castor oil (INCI)
CAS 61788-85-0 (generic)
Synonyms: POE (30) hydrogenated castor oil
Trade names: Croduret 30; Emalex HC-30; Nikkol HCO-30

PEG-33 hydrogenated castor oil
Trade names: Remcopal HC 33

PEG-35 hydrogenated castor oil (INCI)
CAS 61788-85-0 (generic)
Trade names: Arlatone® 980

PEG-40 hydrogenated castor oil (INCI)
CAS 61788-85-0 (generic)
Synonyms: POE (40) hydrogenated castor oil
Trade names: Akyporox CO 400; Cerex ELS 400; Cremophor® RH 40; Cremophor® RH 410; Croduret 40; Emalex HC-40; Emulsifier 17 P; Eumulgin® HRE 40; Hetoxide HC-40; Hodag Nonionic GRH-40; Lipocol HCO-40; Nikkol HCO-40; Nikkol HCO-40 Pharm; Protachem CAH-40; Remcopal HC 40; Simulsol 1293; Tagat® R40; Unipeg-CO-40H; Witconol™ 2739
Trade names containing: Amyx ST 3837; Chamomile CL 2/033026; Cremophor® RH 455; Emulsifier 2/014160; Hydrocos; Solubilisant γ 2428; Solubiliser LRI; Standamul® Conc. 1002; Unimul-1002 Conc

PEG-45 hydrogenated castor oil (INCI)
CAS 61788-85-0 (generic)
Trade names: Arlatone® 975; Cerex ELS 450

PEG-50 hydrogenated castor oil (INCI)
CAS 61788-85-0 (generic)
Synonyms: POE (50) hydrogenated castor oil
Trade names: Croduret 50; Emalex HC-50; Nikkol HCO-50; Nikkol HCO-50 Pharm

PEG-60 hydrogenated castor oil (INCI)
CAS 61788-85-0 (generic)
Synonyms: POE (60) hydrogenated castor oil
Trade names: Akyporox CO 600; Cremophor® RH 60; Croduret 60; Emalex HC-60; Eumulgin® HRE 60; Hetoxide HC-60; Lipocol HCO-60; Nikkol HCO-60; Nikkol HCO-60 Pharm; Protachem CAH-60; Remcopal HC 60; Simulsol 1294; Tagat® R60
Trade names containing: Extrapone Coco-Nut Special 2/033055; Nikkol Aquasome VE; Tagat® R63

PEG-80 hydrogenated castor oil (INCI)
CAS 61788-85-0 (generic)
Synonyms: POE (80) hydrogenated castor oil
Trade names: Emalex HC-80; Nikkol HCO-80

PEG-100 hydrogenated castor oil (INCI)
CAS 61788-85-0 (generic)
Synonyms: POE (100) hydrogenated castor oil; PEG (100) hydrogenated castor oil
Trade names: Croduret 100; Emalex HC-100; Nikkol HCO-100; Protachem CAH-100
Trade names containing: Nikkol Aquasome EC-5

PEG-200 hydrogenated castor oil (INCI)
CAS 61788-85-0 (generic)
Synonyms: POE (200) hydrogenated castor oil; PEG (200) hydrogenated castor oil
Trade names: Chemax HCO-200/50; Croduret 200; Protachem CAH-200; Prox-onic HRH-0200; Prox-onic HRH-0200/50

PEG-5 hydrogenated castor oil isostearate
Trade names: Emalex RWIS-105

PEG-10 hydrogenated castor oil isostearate
Trade names: Emalex RWIS-110

PEG-15 hydrogenated castor oil isostearate
Trade names: Emalex RWIS-115

PEG-20 hydrogenated castor oil isostearate
Trade names: Emalex RWIS-120

PEG-30 hydrogenated castor oil isostearate
Trade names: Emalex RWIS-130

PEG-40 hydrogenated castor oil isostearate
Trade names: Emalex RWIS-140

PEG-50 hydrogenated castor oil isostearate
Trade names: Emalex RWIS-150

PEG-60 hydrogenated castor oil isostearate
Trade names: Emalex RWIS-160

PEG-20 hydrogenated castor oil laurate
Trade names: Emalex RWL-120

PEG-30 hydrogenated castor oil laurate
Trade names: Emalex RWL-130

PEG-40 hydrogenated castor oil laurate
Trade names: Emalex RWL-140

PEG-50 hydrogenated castor oil laurate
Trade names: Emalex RWL-150

PEG-60 hydrogenated castor oil laurate
Trade names: Emalex RWL-160

PEG-30 hydrogenated castor oil PCA isostearate
Trade names: Pyroter CPI-30

PEG-40 hydrogenated castor oil PCA isostearate (INCI)
Synonyms: PEG-40 hydrogenated castor oil pyroglutamic isostearic diester; PEG 2000 hydrogenated castor oil PCA isostearate
Trade names: Pyroter CPI-40

PEG-60 hydrogenated castor oil PCA isostearate
Trade names: Pyroter CPI-60

PEG-5 hydrogenated castor oil triisostearate
Trade names: Emalex RWIS-305

PEG-10 hydrogenated castor oil triisostearate
Trade names: Emalex RWIS-310

PEG-15 hydrogenated castor oil triisostearate
Trade names: Emalex RWIS-315

PEG-20 hydrogenated castor oil triisostearate
Trade names: Emalex RWIS-320

PEG-30 hydrogenated castor oil triisostearate
Trade names: Emalex RWIS-330

PEG-40 hydrogenated castor oil triisostearate
Trade names: Emalex RWIS-340

PEG-50 hydrogenated castor oil triisostearat
Trade names: Emalex RWIS-350

PEG-60 hydrogenated castor oil triisostearate
Trade names: Emalex RWIS-360

PEG-200 hydrogenated glyceryl palmate (INCI)
Trade names containing: Rewoderm® LIS 80

PEG-20 hydrogenated lanolin (INCI)
CAS 68648-27-1 (generic); CAS 977-55-17-6
Synonyms: POE (20) hydrogenated lanolin; PEG 1000 hydrogenated lanolin
Trade names: Fancol HL-20; Ivarlan™ 3450; Ivarlan™ HL-20; Lanidrol; Lipolan 31-20; Super-Sat AWS-4
Trade names containing: Ritachol 5000

PEG-24 hydrogenated lanolin (INCI)
CAS 68648-27-1 (generic)
Synonyms: POE (24) hydrogenated lanolin
Trade names: Fancol HL-24; Ivarlan™ 3452; Lipolan 31; Super-Sat AWS-24

PEG-20 hydrogenated palm oil glycerides (INCI)
Synonyms: POE (20) hydrogenated palm oil glycerides; PEG 1000 hydrogenated palm oil glycerides
Trade names containing: Lamecreme® AOM

PEG-13 hydrogenated tallow amide (INCI)
CAS 68155-24-8
Synonyms: Ethoxylated (13) hydrogenated tallowamide; POE (13) hydrogenated tallow amide
Trade names: Ethomid® HT/23

PEG-50 hydrogenated tallow amide
CAS 68155-24-8
Trade names: Ethomid® HT/60; Schercomid HT-60

PEG-2 hydrogenated tallow amine (INCI)
CAS 61791-26-2 (generic)
Synonyms: PEG 100 tallow amine; POE (2) tallow amine;

PEG-2 tallow amine
Trade names: Ethomeen® T/12; Hetoxamine T-2; Protox T-2; Unizeen T-2

PEG-5 hydrogenated tallow amine (INCI)
CAS 61791-26-2 (generic)
Synonyms: POE (5) tallow amine
Trade names: Ethomeen® T/15; Hetoxamine T-5; Protox T-5; Unizeen T-5

PEG-15 hydrogenated tallow amine (INCI)
CAS 61791-26-2 (generic)
Synonyms: POE (15) tallow amine
Trade names: Ethomeen® T/25; Hetoxamine T-15; Protox T-15; Unizeen T-15; Varonic® U-215

PEG-20 hydrogenated tallow amine (INCI)
CAS 61791-26-2 (generic)
Synonyms: POE (20) tallow amine; PEG 1000 tallow amine
Trade names: G-3780-A; Hetoxamine T-20; Protox T-20

PEG-30 hydrogenated tallow amine (INCI)
CAS 61791-26-2 (generic)
Synonyms: POE (30) tallow amine
Trade names: Hetoxamine T-30

PEG-40 hydrogenated tallow amine (INCI)
CAS 61791-26-2 (generic)
Synonyms: POE (40) tallow amine; PEG 2000 tallow amine
Trade names: Protox T-40

PEG-50 hydrogenated tallow amine (INCI)
CAS 61791-26-2 (generic); 68783-22-2
Synonyms: POE (50) tallow amine
Trade names: Protox T-50

PEG-15 hydroxystearate (INCI)
Synonyms: POE (15) hydroxystearate
Trade names: G-4972; Solutol® HS 15

PEG isocetyl ether. *See Isoceteth series*

PEG isodecyl ether. *See Isodeceth series*

PEG-6 isolauryl thioether (INCI)
Synonyms: POE (6) isolauryl thioether; PEG 300 isolauryl thioether
Trade names: Sebum Control COS-218/2-A; Sulfocos 2B

PEG-8 isolauryl thioether (INCI)
Synonyms: POE (8) isolauryl thioether; PEG 400 isolauryl thioether
Trade names: Alcodet® SK

PEG-3 isostearate
Trade names: Emalex PEIS-3

PEG-6 isostearate (INCI)
CAS 56002-14-3 (generic)
Synonyms: PEG 300 monoisostearate; POE (6) monoisostearate
Trade names: Emalex PEIS-6; Olepal ISO

PEG-12 isostearate (INCI)
CAS 56002-14-3 (generic)
Synonyms: POE (12) isostearate; PEG 600 mono-isostearate
Trade names: Emalex PEIS-12; Emerest® 2701

PEG-20 isostearate
Trade names: Emalex PEIS-20

PEG isostearyl ether. *See Isosteareth series*

PEG-26 jojoba acid (INCI)
Synonyms: POE (26) jojoba acid
Trade names containing: Oxypon 328

PEG-80 jojoba acid (INCI)
Trade names containing: Jojoba PEG-80

PEG-120 jojoba acid (INCI)
Trade names containing: Jojoba PEG-120

PEG-26 jojoba alcohol (INCI)
Synonyms: POE (26) jojoba alcohol
Trade names containing: Oxypon 328

PEG-80 jojoba alcohol (INCI)
Trade names containing: Jojoba PEG-80

PEG-120 jojoba alcohol (INCI)
Trade names containing: Jojoba PEG-120

PEG-40 jojoba oil
Trade names: Simchin® WS

PEG-2 lactamide (INCI)
Synonyms: Diethylene glycol lactamide
Trade names: Naetex-L

PEG-3 lanolate (INCI)
Synonyms: POE (3) lanolate
Trade names: Agnosol 3

PEG-5 lanolate (INCI)
CAS 68459-50-7 (generic)
Synonyms: PEG-5 lanolin acids; POE (5) lanolate
Trade names: Agnosol 5; Lanpol 5
Trade names containing: Lanpolamide 5

PEG-10 lanolate (INCI)
CAS 68459-50-7 (generic)
Synonyms: POE (10) lanolate; PEG 500 lanolate; PEG-10 lanolin acid
Trade names: Lanpol 10

PEG-20 lanolate (INCI)
CAS 68459-50-7 (generic)
Synonyms: POE (20) lanolate; PEG 1000 lanolate
Trade names: Lanpol 20

PEG-10 lanolin (INCI)
CAS 61790-81-6 (generic)
Synonyms: POE (10) lanolin
Trade names: Nikkol TW-10

PEG-20 lanolin (INCI)
CAS 61790-81-6 (generic)
Synonyms: POE (20) lanolin; PEG 1000 lanolin
Trade names: Nikkol TW-20

PEG-27 lanolin (INCI)
CAS 61790-81-6; 8051-81-8
Synonyms: POE (27) lanolin
Trade names: Lanogel® 21

PEG-30 lanolin (INCI)
CAS 61790-81-6 (generic)
Synonyms: POE (30) lanolin
Trade names: Aqualose L30; Ivarlan™ 3405-L30; Lanalox L 30; Nikkol TW-30; Protalan L-30; Sellig Lano 30
Trade names containing: C-Base; Ivarbase™ 3230; Lanamol; Sebase; T-Base

PEG-40 lanolin (INCI)
CAS 8051-82-9; 61790-81-6 (generic)
Synonyms: POE (40) lanolin
Trade names: Laneto 40; Lanogel® 31

PEG-50 lanolin (INCI)
CAS 61790-81-6 (generic)
Synonyms: POE (50) lanolin
Trade names: Lanolex L-40

PEG-55 lanolin (INCI)
CAS 61790-81-6 (generic)
Synonyms: POE (55) lanolin
Trade names: Solan E

PEG-60 lanolin (INCI)

CAS 61790-81-6 (generic)
Synonyms: POE (60) lanolin
Trade names: Ivarlan™ 3406; Ivarlan™ 3409-60; Laneto 60; Protalan L-60; Solan; Solan 50
Trade names containing: Relaxer Conc. No. 2; Ritachol® 3000; Ritachol® 4000

PEG-70 lanolin
CAS 61790-81-6 (generic)
Synonyms: POE (70) lanolin
Trade names: Teric LAN70

PEG-75 lanolin (INCI)
CAS 8039-09-6; 61790-81-6 (generic)
Synonyms: POE (75) lanolin; PEG 4000 lanolin
Trade names: Aqualose L75; Aqualose L75/50; Brooksgel 41; Ethoxylan® 1685; Ethoxylan® 1686; Hetoxalan 75; Hetoxalan 75-50%; Hetoxolan 75; Hetoxolan 75-50%; Ivarlan™ 3400; Ivarlan™ 3401; Ivarlan™ 3407-E; Ivarlan™ 3408W; Ivarlan™ L575; Lan-Aqua-Sol 50; Lan-Aqua-Sol 100; Laneto 50; Laneto 100; Laneto 100-Flaked; Lanogel® 41; Lanoxal 75; Lantox 55, 110; Protalan L-75; Rewolan® E 50, E 100; Solulan® 75; Solulan® L-575; Super Solan Flaked; Unilaneth 75
Trade names containing: Lanatein-25; Lanion-27; Lanobase SE; Lanpro-10; Proto-Lan 20

PEG-85 lanolin (INCI)
CAS 61790-81-6 (generic)
Synonyms: POE (85) lanolin
Trade names: Brooksgel 61; Ivarlan™ 3410; Lanogel® 61; Protalan 85

PEG-100 lanolin (INCI)
CAS 61790-81-6 (generic)
Synonyms: POE (100) lanolin
Trade names: Aqualose L100; Hetoxalan 100; Hetoxolan 100

PEG-5 lanolinamide (INCI)
Synonyms: POE (5) lanolinamide
Trade names containing: Lanpolamide 5

PEG lanolin ether. *See Laneth series*

PEG-75 lanolin oil (INCI)
CAS 68648-38-4 (generic)
Synonyms: POE (75) lanolin oil; PEG 4000 lanolin oil
Trade names: Lanoil Water/Alcohol Soluble Lanolin; Rewolan® AWS

PEG-3 lauramide (INCI)
CAS 26635-75-6 (generic)
Synonyms: POE (3) lauryl amide; PEG (3) lauryl amide
Trade names: Amidox® L-2; Upamide L-2

PEG-5 lauramide (INCI)
CAS 26635-75-6 (generic)
Synonyms: POE (5) lauryl amide
Trade names: Amidox® L-5

PEG-6 lauramide (INCI)
CAS 26635 76 6 (generic)
Synonyms: POE (6) lauryl amide; PEG 300 lauryl amide
Trade names: Lanidox-5; Upamide L-5

PEG-6 lauramide DEA
Trade names: Mazamide® L-5

PEG-3 lauramine oxide (INCI)
Synonyms: POE (3) lauryl dimethyl amine oxide; PEG (3) lauryl dimethyl amine oxide
Trade names: Empigen® OY

PEG-2 laurate (INCI)
CAS 141-20-8; 9004-81-3; EINECS 205-468-1
Synonyms: Diethylene glycol laurate; Diglycol laurate;

PEG 100 monolaurate
Trade names: Hodag DGL; Kessco® Diglycol Laurate A Neutral; Kessco® Diglycol Laurate ASE; Kessco® Diglycol Laurate N; Kessco® Diglycol Laurate N-Syn; Lipopeg 1-L; Radiasurf® 7420; Unipeg-DGL

PEG-2 laurate SE (INCI)
CAS 141-20-8
Synonyms: Diethylene glycol monolaurate self-emulsifying; PEG 100 monolaurate self-emulsifying; POE (2) monolaurate self-emulsifying
Trade names: Kessco® Diglycol Laurate SE; Lipo DGLS; Pegosperse® 100 L
Trade names containing: Lipocol B

PEG-4 laurate (INCI)
CAS 9004-81-3 (generic); 10108-24-4
Synonyms: POE (4) monolaurate; PEG 200 monolaurate
Trade names: Ablunol 200ML; Algon LA 40; Chemax E-200 ML; Cithrol 2ML; CPH-27-N; Crodet L4; Hetoxamate LA-4; Hodag 20-L; Kessco® PEG 200 ML; Lipopeg 2-L; Mapeg® 200 ML; Pegosperse® 200 ML; Protamate 200 ML; Radiasurf® 7422; Unipeg-200 ML; Witconol™ 2620

PEG-5 laurate
CAS 9004-81-3 (generic)
Synonyms: POE (5) monolaurate
Trade names: Hetoxamate LA-5

PEG-6 laurate (INCI)
CAS 9004-81-3 (generic); 2370-64-1; EINECS 219-136-9
Synonyms: POE (6) monolaurate; PEG 300 monolaurate
Trade names: Kessco® PEG 300 ML
Trade names containing: Amisol™ HS-6

PEG-8 laurate (INCI)
CAS 9004-81-3 (generic); 35179-86-3; 37318-14-2; EINECS 253-458-0
Synonyms: POE (8) monolaurate; PEG 400 monolaurate
Trade names: Ablunol 400ML; Algon LA 80; Alkamuls® PE/400; Chemax E-400 ML; Cithrol 4ML; CPH-30-N; Crodet L8; Elfacos® PEG 400 ML; Hodag 40-L; Karapeg 400-ML; Kessco® PEG 400 ML; Laurate de PEG 400; Lexemul® PEG-400ML; Lipopeg 4-L; Mapeg® 400 ML; Nonisol 100; Pegosperse® 400 ML; Protamate 400 ML; Radiasurf® 7423; Rol L 40; Unipeg-400 ML

PEG-9 laurate (INCI)
CAS 106-08-1; 9004-81-3 (generic); EINECS 203-359-3
Synonyms: POE (9) monolaurate
Trade names: Alkamuls® L-9; Hetoxamate LA-9
Trade names containing: Lipocol B

PEG-10 laurate (INCI)
CAS 9004-81-3 (generic)
Synonyms: PEG 500 monolaurate
Trade names: Nikkol MYL-10

PEG-12 laurate (INCI)
CAS 9004-81-3 (generic)
Synonyms: POE (12) monolaurate; PEG 600 monolaurate
Trade names: Ablunol 600ML; Cithrol 6ML; CPH-43-N; Crodet L12; Hefti PGE-600-ML; Hodag 60-L; Karapeg 600-ML; Kessco® PEG 600 ML; Lipopeg 6-L; Mapeg® 600 ML; Pegosperse® 600 ML; Unipeg-600 ML

PEG-14 laurate (INCI)
CAS 9004-81-3 (generic)
Synonyms: POE (14) monolaurate
Trade names: Chemax E-600 ML

PEG-20 laurate (INCI)
CAS 9004-81-3 (generic)
Synonyms: POE (20) monolaurate; PEG 1000 monolaurate
Trade names: Chemax E-1000 ML; Cithrol 10ML; Kessco® PEG 1000 ML

PEG-24 laurate
CAS 9004-81-3 (generic)
Synonyms: POE (24) monolaurate
Trade names: Crodet L24

PEG-32 laurate (INCI)
CAS 9004-81-3 (generic)
Synonyms: POE (32) monolaurate; PEG 1540 monolaurate
Trade names: Kessco® PEG 1540 ML

PEG-40 laurate
CAS 9004-81-3 (generic)
Synonyms: POE (40) monolaurate
Trade names: Crodet L40

PEG-75 laurate
CAS 9004-81-3 (generic)
Synonyms: POE (75) monolaurate; PEG 4000 monolaurate
Trade names: Kessco® PEG 4000 ML

PEG-100 laurate
CAS 9004-81-3 (generic)
Synonyms: POE (100) monolaurate; PEG (100) monolaurate
Trade names: Crodet L100

PEG-150 laurate (INCI)
CAS 9004-81-3 (generic)
Synonyms: POE (150) monolaurate; PEG 6000 monolaurate
Trade names: Hodag 600-L; Kessco® PEG 6000 ML; Unipeg-6000 ML

PEG-6 laurate/tartarate (INCI)
Trade names: Hydrophore 312

PEG lauryl ether. *See Laureth series*

PEG-2 lauryl ether isostearate
Trade names: Emalex LWIS-2

PEG-5 lauryl ether isostearate
Trade names: Emalex LWIS-5

PEG-8 lauryl ether isostearate
Trade names: Emalex LWIS-8

PEG-10 lauryl ether isostearate
Trade names: Emalex LWIS-10

PEG-3 lauryl ether stearate
Trade names: Emalex LWS-3

PEG-5 lauryl ether stearate
Trade names: Emalex LWS-5

PEG-8 lauryl ether stearate
Trade names: Emalex LWS-8

PEG-10 lauryl ether stearate
Trade names: Emalex LWS-10

PEG-15 lauryl ether stearate
Trade names: Emalex LWS-15

PEG-8 linoleate (INCI)
Synonyms: PEG 400 linoleate
Trade names containing: Efevit S

PEG-8 linolenate (INCI)
Trade names containing: Efevit S

PEG-70 mango glycerides (INCI)
Synonyms: PEG (70 mango glycerides

Trade names: Lipex 20 E-70; Lipex 203 E-70

PEG-6 methyl ether (INCI)
CAS 9004-74-4 (generic)
Synonyms: POE (6) methyl ether; PEG 300 methyl ether;
PEG-6 monomethyl ether
Trade names: Dow MPEG350; Upiwax 350

PEG-10 methyl ether
CAS 9004-74-4 (generic)
Synonyms: POE (10) methyl ether; PEG 500 methyl ether
Trade names: Dow MPEG550

PEG-16 methyl ether
CAS 9004-74-4 (generic)
Synonyms: POE (16) methyl ether
Trade names: Dow MPEG750

PEG-120 methyl glucose dioleate (INCI)
Synonyms: POE (120) methyl glucose dioleate
Trade names: Glucamate® DOE-120

PEG-80 methyl glucose laurate (INCI)
Trade names: Glucamate® MLE-80

PEG-20 methyl glucose sesquistearate (INCI)
CAS 68389-70-8
Synonyms: POE (20) methyl glucose sesquistearate;
PEG 1000 methyl glucose sesquitearate
Trade names: Glucamate® SSE-20; Grillocose PSE-20

PEG-2 milk solids (INCI)
Trade names: Galactene

PEG-13 mink glycerides (INCI)
Synonyms: POE (13) mink glycerides
Trade names: Mink Oil W

PEG-8 myristate (INCI)
Synonyms: PEG 400 myristate; POE (8) myristate
Trade names: Myrlene

PEG-20 myristate (INCI)
Synonyms: POE (20 myristate; PEG 1000 myristate
Trade names containing: Xalidrene

PEG myristyl ether. *See Myreth series*

PEG nonyl phenyl ether. *See Nonoxynol series*

PEG-13 octanoate (INCI)
Synonyms: POE (13) monooctanoate
Trade names: PCL Liq. Watersoluble 2/966213

PEG octyldodecyl ether. *See Octyldodeceth series*

PEG octyl phenyl ether. *See Octoxynol series*

PEG-3 oleamide
CAS 26027-37-2; 31799-71-0
Trade names: Dionil® OC

PEG-4 oleamide (INCI)
Trade names: Dionil® OC/K

PEG-5 oleamide (INCI)
CAS 31799-71-0
Synonyms: POE (5) oleyl amide; PEG (5) oleyl amide
Trade names: Ethomid® O/15

PEG-6 oleamide (INCI)
CAS 26027-37-2
Synonyms: PEG 300 oleyl amide; POE (6) oleyl amide
Trade names: Dionil® SH 100
Trade names containing: Hostacerin CG

PEG-7 oleamide (INCI)
CAS 26027-37-2
Synonyms: Ethoxylated (7) oleamide; POE (7) oleamide
Trade names: Ethomid® O/17

PEG-14 oleamide
Trade names: Dionil® W 100

PEG-5 oleamide dioleate (INCI)
Synonyms: POE (5) oleamide dioleate
Trade names: Lowenol OT-216

PEG-2 oleamine (INCI)
Synonyms: PEG-2 oleyl amine; POE (2) oleyl amine;
PEG 100 oleyl amine
Trade names: Ethomeen® O/12; Hetoxamine O-2;
Protox O-2; Varonic® Q-202; Varonic® Q-202 SF

PEG-5 oleamine (INCI)
Synonyms: POE (5) oleyl amine
Trade names: Ethomeen® O/15; Hetoxamine O-5;
Protox O-5; Varonic® Q-205; Varonic® Q-205 SF

PEG-15 oleamine (INCI)
Synonyms: POE (15) oleyl amine
Trade names: Ethomeen® O/25; Hetoxamine O-15;
Protox O-15

PEG-30 oleamine (INCI)
CAS 58253-49-9
Synonyms: POE (30) oleyl amine
Trade names: Varonic® Q-230; Witcamine® 6622

PEG-2 oleammonium chloride (INCI)
CAS 18448-65-2
Synonyms: PEG 100 oleamonium chloride; POE (2)
oleamonium chloride
Trade names containing: Ethoquad® O/12; Ethoquad®
O/12H

PEG-15 oleammonium chloride (INCI)
CAS 28880-55-9
Synonyms: POE (15) oleamonium chloride
Trade names: Ethoquad® O/25

PEG-2 oleate (INCI)
CAS 106-12-7; EINECS 203-364-0
Synonyms: Diethylene glycol monooleate; Diglycol ole-
ate; POE (2) monooleate
Trade names: Cithrol DEGMO; Emalex 200; Hetoxamate
MO-2; Hodag DGO; Lipopeg 1-O; Nikkol MYO-2;
Radiasurf® 7400; Witconol™ DOSS

PEG-2 oleate SE (INCI)
CAS 106-12-7
Synonyms: Diethylene glycol monooleate self-emulsify-
ing; PEG 100 monooleate self-emulsifying; POE (2)
monooleate self-emulsifying
Trade names: Kessco® Diglycol Oleate L-SE;
Pegosperse® 100 O

PEG-3 oleate (INCI)
CAS 9004-96-0 (generic); 10233-14-4; EINECS 233-561-
7
Trade names: Emalex 218

PEG-4 oleate (INCI)
CAS 9004-96-0 (generic); 10108-25-5; EINECS 233-293-
0
Synonyms: POE (4) monooleate; PEG 200 monooleate
Trade names: Ablunol 200MO; Cithrol 2MO; Crodet O4;
Hetoxamate MO-4; Hodag 20-O; Kessco® PEG 200
MO; Mapeg® 200 MO; Pegosperse® 200 MO;
Protamate 200 OC; Radiasurf® 7402; Remcopal 207;
Unipeg-200 MO

PEG-5 oleate (INCI)
CAS 9004-96-0 (generic); 23336-36-9
Synonyms: POE (5) monooleate
Trade names: Chemax E-200 MO; Ethofat® O/15;
Hetoxamate MO-5; Prox-onic OL-1/05

PEG-6 oleate (INCI)
CAS 9004-96-0 (generic); 60344-26-5
Synonyms: POE (6) monooleate; PEG 300 monooleate
Trade names: Algon OL 60; Crodet O6; Emalex OE-6;

Kessco® PEG 300 MO; Lipopeg 3-O; Nikkol MYO-6; Olepal 1; Pegosperse® 300 MO; Protamate 300 OC; Radiasurf® 7431

PEG-7 oleate (INCI)
CAS 9004-96-0 (generic)
Synonyms: POE (7) monooleate
Trade names: Algon OL 70; G-5507; Marlosol® OL7

PEG-8 oleate (INCI)
CAS 9004-96-0 (generic)
Synonyms: POE (8) monooleate; PEG 400 monooleate
Trade names: Ablunol 400MO; Acconon 400-MO; Cithrol 4MO; Cithrol 4MO; CPH-233-N; CPH-40-N; CPH-46-N; Crodet O8; Elfacos® PEG 400 MO; Estol EO4MO 3672; Hodag 40-O; Kessco® PEG 400 MO; Lipopeg 4-O; Mapeg® 400 MO; Pegosperse® 400 MO; Protamate 400 OC; Radiasurf® 7403; Rol AG; Unipeg-400 MO; Witconol™ H31A

PEG-9 oleate (INCI)
CAS 9004-96-0 (generic)
Synonyms: POE (9) monooleate; PEG 450 monooleate
Trade names: Algon OL 90; Alkamuls® 400-MO; Chemax E-400 MO; Hetoxamate MO-9; Prox-onic OL-1/09

PEG-10 oleate (INCI)
CAS 9004-96-0 (generic)
Synonyms: POE (10) monooleate; PEG 500 monooleate; POE (10) oleic acid
Trade names: Emalex OE-10; Ethofat® O/20; Nikkol MYO-10; Protamate 600 OC

PEG-11 oleate (INCI)
CAS 9004-96-0 (generic)
Trade names: G-5511

PEG-12 oleate (INCI)
CAS 9004-96-0 (generic)
Synonyms: POE (12) monooleate; PEG 600 monooleate
Trade names: Ablunol 600MO; Cithrol 6MO; CPH-41-N; Crodet O12; Estol EO6MO 3674; Hefti PGE-600-MO; Hodag 60-O; Kessco® PEG 600 MO; Lipopeg 6-O; Mapeg® 600 MO; Pegosperse® 600 MO; Radiasurf® 7404; Unipeg-600 MO
Trade names containing: Amisol™ HS-2; Amisol™ HS-3 US; Amisol Nail Strengthener

PEG-14 oleate (INCI)
CAS 9004-96-0 (generic)
Synonyms: POE (14) monooleate
Trade names: Chemax E-600 MO; Hetoxamate MO-14; Prox-onic OL-1/014

PEG-15 oleate (INCI)
CAS 9004-96-0 (generic)
Synonyms: POE (15) monooleate
Trade names: Marlosol® OL15

PEG-20 oleate (INCI)
CAS 9004-96-0 (generic)
Synonyms: POE (20) monooleate; PEG 1000 monooleate
Trade names: Ablunol 1000MO; Chemax E-1000 MO; Cithrol 10MO; Kessco® PEG 1000 MO; Protamate 1000 OC

PEG-23 oleate (INCI)
Trade names: Crodet O23

PEG-24 oleate
Trade names: Crodet O24

PEG-32 oleate (INCI)
CAS 9004-96-0 (generic)
Synonyms: POE (32) monooleate; PEG 1540 monooleate
Trade names: Kessco® PEG 1540 MO

PEG-40 oleate
Trade names: Crodet O40

PEG-75 oleate (INCI)
CAS 9004-96-0 (generic)
Synonyms: POE (75) monooleate; PEG 4000 monooleate
Trade names: Kessco® PEG 4000 MO

PEG-100 oleate
Trade names: Crodet O100

PEG-150 oleate (INCI)
CAS 9004-96-0 (generic)
Synonyms: POE (150) monooleate; PEG 6000 monooleate
Trade names: Kessco® PEG 6000 MO

PEG oleyl ether. *See Oleth series*

PEG-2 oleyl/stearyl amine
Trade names: Rhodameen® OS-12

PEG-6 olive oil
CAS 103819-46-1
Trade names: Cerex U 60

PEG-25 PABA (INCI)
CAS 15716-30-0; 113010-52-9
Synonyms: POE (25) PABA; 4-Bis(polyethoxy)-p-aminobenzoic acid polyethoxyethyl ester
Trade names: Unipabol U-17; Uvinul® P 25

PEG-20 palmitate (INCI)
CAS 9004-94-8 (generic)
Synonyms: POE (20) monopalmitate; PEG 1000 monopalmitate
Trade names containing: Xalidrene

PEG-8 palmitostearate
Trade names: Stearate 400 WL 817

PEG-150 palmitostearate
Trade names: Stearate 6000 WL 1644

PEG-12 palm kernel glycerides (INCI)
Synonyms: PEG 600 palm kernel glycerides; POE (12) palm kernel gycerides
Trade names: Crovol PK40

PEG-45 palm kernel glycerides (INCI)
Synonyms: POE (45) palm kernel glycerides
Trade names: Crovol PK70

PEG-5 pentaerythrityl ether (INCI)
Synonyms: POE (5) pentaerythritol ether
Trade names containing: Lanolide; Seboside

PEG-5 phytosterol
Trade names: Nikkol BPS-5

PEG-10 phytosterol
Trade names: Nikkol BPS-10

PEG-20 phytosterol
Trade names: Nikkol BPS-20

PEG-25 phytosterol (INCI)
Trade names: Nikkol BPSH-25

PEG-30 phytosterol
Trade names: Nikkol BPS-30

PEG-10 polyglyceryl-2 laurate (INCI)
Synonyms: POE (10) polyglyceryl-2 laurate; PEG 500 polyglyceryl-2 laurate
Trade names: Hostacerin DGL

PEG-4 polyglyceryl-2 stearate (INCI)
Trade names: Lamecreme® DGE-18

PEG/PPG-17/6 copolymer (INCI)
CAS 9003-11-6 (generic)

Trade names: Ucon® 75-H-450

PEG/PPG-35/9 copolymer (INCI)
CAS 9003-11-6 (generic)
Trade names: Ucon® 75-H-1400

PEG/PPG-125/30 copolymer (INCI)
CAS 9003-11-6 (generic)
Trade names: Ucon® 75-H-90000

PEG-20-PPG-10 glyceryl stearate (INCI)
Trade names: Acconon TGH

PEG-6 PPG-3 tridecylether
Trade names: Hetoxol TDEP-63

PEG-10 PPG-15 tridecyl ether
Trade names: Hetoxol TDEP-15

PEG-4 proline linoleate (INCI)
Synonyms: PEG 200 proline linoleate
Trade names containing: Aminoefaderma

PEG-4 proline linolenate (INCI)
Synonyms: PEG 200 proline linolenate
Trade names containing: Aminoefaderma

PEG-10 propylene glycol (INCI)
Synonyms: POE (10) propylene glycol; PEG 500 propylene glycol
Trade names containing: Acconon CON

PEG-8 propylene glycol cocoate (INCI)
Synonyms: POE (8) propylene glycol cocoate; PEG 400 propylene glycol cocoate
Trade names containing: Emulsynt® 1055

PEG-55 propylene glycol oleate (INCI)
Synonyms: POE (55) propylene glycol oleate
Trade names containing: Antil® 141 Liq.

PEG-25 propylene glycol stearate (INCI)
Synonyms: POE (25) propylene glycol monostearate
Trade names: G-2162; Simulsol PS20

PEG-4 rapeseedamide (INCI)
CAS 85536-23-8
Synonyms: POE (4) rapeseedamide; PEG 200 rapeseedamide
Trade names: Aminol N

PEG-2 rapeseedamine
Trade names: Amide RMA-2

PEG-7 ricinoleate (INCI)
CAS 9004-97-1 (generic)
Synonyms: POE (7) ricinoleate; POE (7) ricinoleate
Trade names containing: Grillocin WE-106

PEG-8 ricinoleate (INCI)
CAS 9004-97-1 (generic)
Synonyms: PEG 400 ricinoleate; POE (8) ricinoleate
Trade names: Hodag 40-R

PEG-9 ricinoleate (INCI)
CAS 9004-97-1 (generic)
Synonyms: PEG 450 ricinoleate; POE (9) ricinoleate
Trade names: Cerex EL 429; G-4929

PEG-8 sesquioleate (INCI)
Synonyms: PEG 400 sesquioleate; POE (8) sesquioleate
Trade names: Unipeg-400 SO

PEG-50 shea butter
Trade names: Shebu® WS

PEG-75 shea butter glycerides (INCI)
Trade names: Lipex 102 E-75

PEG-75 shorea butter glycerides (INCI)
Trade names: Lipex 106 E-75

PEG-6 sorbitan beeswax (INCI)

CAS 8051-15-8
Synonyms: PEG 300 sorbitan beeswax; POE (6) sorbitol beeswax
Trade names: G-1702; Nikkol GBW-25

PEG-8 sorbitan beeswax (INCI)
Synonyms: POE (8) sorbitol beeswax; PEG 400 sorbitan beeswax
Trade names: Nikkol GBW-8

PEG-20 sorbitan beeswax (INCI)
CAS 8051-73-8
Synonyms: POE (20) sorbitol beeswax; PEG 1000 sorbitan beeswax
Trade names: G-1726; Nikkol GBW-125

PEG-40 sorbitan diisostearate (INCI)
Synonyms: POE (40) sorbitan diisostearate
Trade names: Emsorb® 2726

PEG-40 sorbitan hexaoleate (CTFA)
CAS 57171-56-9
Synonyms: PEG-40 sorbitol hexaoleate; POE (40) sorbitol hexaoleate; PEG 2000 sorbitol hexaoleate
Trade names: Trylox® 6746

PEG-50 sorbitan hexaoleate (CTFA)
CAS 57171-56-9
Synonyms: PEG-50 sorbitol hexaoleate; POE (50) sorbitol hexaoleate
Trade names: G-1096

PEG-40 sorbitan hexatallate
Trade names: Glycosperse® HTO-40

PEG-5 sorbitan isostearate (INCI)
CAS 66794-58-9 (generic)
Synonyms: POE (5) sorbitan isostearate
Trade names: Montanox 71

PEG-20 sorbitan isostearate (INCI)
CAS 66794-58-9 (generic)
Synonyms: PEG 1000 sorbitan monoisostearate; POE (20) sorbitan monoisostearate; Polysorbate 120
Trade names: Crillet 6; Isoixol 6; Montanox 70; Nikkol TI-10; Sorbilene ISM

PEG-20 sorbitan lanolate
Synonyms: POE (20) sorbitol lanolate; PEG 1000 sorbitan lanolate
Trade names: G-1425

PEG-40 sorbitan lanolate (INCI)
CAS 8036-77-9
Synonyms: POE (40) sorbitol lanolate; PEG 2000 sorbitan lanolate
Trade names: G-1441

PEG-4 sorbitan laurate. *See Polysorbate 21*

PEG-5 sorbitan laurate
Synonyms: POE (5) sorbitan monolaurate
Trade names: Montanox 21

PEG-6 sorbitan laurate
Trade names: Nikkol GL-1

PEG-10 sorbitan laurate (INCI)
CAS 9005-64-5 (generic)
Synonyms: POE (10) sorbitan monolaurate; PEG 500 sorbitan monolaurate
Trade names: Glycosperse® L-10; Hetsorb L-10; Liposorb L-10

PEG-20 sorbitan laurate. *See Polysorbate 20*

PEG-44 sorbitan laurate (INCI)
CAS 9005-64-5 (generic)
Trade names: Hetsorb L-44

PEG-80 sorbitan laurate (INCI)

CAS 9005-64-5 (generic)
Synonyms: POE (80) sorbitan monolaurate
Trade names: Emsorb® 2721; G-4280; Hetsorb L-80-72%; Hodag PSML-80; Laxan-S; T-Maz® 28; Unisorb 80L
Trade names containing: Carsofoam® BS-I; Cycloryl ALC (redesignated Miraspec ALC); Miracare® BC-10; Miracare® BC-20; Miracare® MS-1; Miracare® MS-2; Miracare® MS-4

PEG-3 sorbitan oleate (INCI)
CAS 9005-65-6 (generic)
Trade names: Emalex EG-2854-OL

PEG-5 sorbitan oleate. *See Polysorbate 81*

PEG-6 sorbitan oleate (INCI)
CAS 9005-65-6 (generic)
Synonyms: POE (6) sorbitan oleate; PEG 300 sorbitan monooleate
Trade names: Nikkol TO-106

PEG-20 sorbitan oleate. *See Polysorbate 80*

PEG-40 sorbitan oleate
Trade names: Emalex ET-8040

PEG-80 sorbitan palmitate (INCI)
CAS 9005-66-7 (generic)
Synonyms: PEG (80) sorbitan monopalmitate; POE (80) sorbitan monopalmitate
Trade names: G-4252

PEG-40 sorbitan peroleate (INCI)
Synonyms: POE (40) sorbitan peroleate; PEG 2000 sorbitan peroleate; POE (40) sorbitol septaoleate
Trade names: Arlatone® T

PEG-20 sorbitan resinolate
Trade names: Montanox 90

PEG-4 sorbitan stearate. *See Polysorbate 61*

PEG-6 sorbitan stearate (INCI)
CAS 9005-67-8 (generic)
Synonyms: POE (6) sorbitan monostearate; PEG 300 sorbitan monostearate
Trade names: Nikkol TS-106

PEG-20 sorbitan stearate. *See Polysorbate 60*

PEG-20 sorbitan tallate
Trade names: T-Maz® 90

PEG-4 sorbitan tetraoleate
Trade names: Emalex EG-2854-O

PEG-6 sorbitan tetraoleate
Trade names: Nikkol GO-4

PEG-30 sorbitan tetraoleate (INCI)
Synonyms: POE (30) sorbitan tetraoleate
Trade names: Nikkol GO-430

PEG-40 sorbitan tetraoleate (INCI)
CAS 9003-11-6
Synonyms: POE (40) sorbitan tetraoleate; PEG 2000 sorbitan tetraoleate
Trade names: Nikkol GO-440; Rheodol 440

PEG-60 sorbitan tetraoleate (INCI)
Synonyms: POE (60) sorbitan tetraoleate
Trade names: Nikkol GO-460; Rheodol 460

PEG-60 sorbitan tetrastearate (INCI)
Synonyms: POE (60) sorbitan tetrastearate; Sorbeth-60 tetrastearate
Trade names: Nikkol GS-460

PEG-4 sorbitan triisostearate
Trade names: Emalex EG-2854-IS

PEG-17 sorbitan trioleate

Trade names: Hefti TO-55-EL

PEG-18 sorbitan trioleate
CAS 9005-70-3
Trade names: Hefti TO-55-E

PEG-20 sorbitan trioleate. *See Polysorbate 85*

PEG-4 sorbitan tristearate
Trade names: Emalex EG-2854-S

PEG-20 sorbitan tristearate. *See Polysorbate 65*

PEG-20 sorbitan tritallate
Trade names: T-Maz® 95

PEG sorbitol ethers. *See Sorbeth series*

PEG-30 sorbitol tetraoleate laurate (INCI)
Trade names: G-1144

PEG-2 soyamine (INCI)
CAS 61791-24-0 (generic)
Synonyms: POE (2) soya amine; PEG 100 soya amine; Bis (2-hydroxyethyl) soya amine
Trade names: Accomeen S2; Ethomeen® S/12; Hetoxamine S-2; Mazeen® S-2; Protox S-2

PEG-5 soyamine (INCI)
CAS 61791-24-0 (generic)
Synonyms: POE (5) soya amine
Trade names: Ethomeen® S/15; Hetoxamine S-5; Mazeen® S-5; Protox S-5

PEG-10 soyamine (INCI)
CAS 61791-24-0 (generic)
Synonyms: POE (10) soya amine; PEG 500 soya amine
Trade names: Accomeen S10; Ethomeen® S/20; Mazeen® S-10; Protox S-10; Unizeen S-10

PEG-15 soyamine (INCI)
CAS 61791-24-0 (generic)
Synonyms: POE (15) soya amine
Trade names: Accomeen S15; Ethomeen® S/25; Hetoxamine S-15; Mazeen® S-15; Protox S-15; Unizeen S-15

PEG-5 soya sterol (INCI)
Synonyms: POE (5) soya sterol
Trade names: Generol® 122E5; Genurol 122 E-5
Trade names containing: Dehymuls® LS

PEG-10 soya sterol (INCI)
Synonyms: POE (10) soya sterol
Trade names: Generol® 122E10; Genurol 122 E-10

PEG-16 soya sterol (INCI)
Synonyms: POE (16) soya sterol
Trade names: Generol® 122E16

PEG-25 soya sterol (INCI)
Synonyms: POE (25) soya sterol
Trade names: Generol® 122E25; Genurol 122 E-25

PEG-30 soya sterol (INCI)
Trade names containing: Ivarbase™ 3231

PEG-4 stearamide (INCI)
Synonyms: POE (4) stearyl amide; POE (4) stearamide; PEG 200 stearamide
Trade names: Nikkol TAMDS-4

PEG-9 stearamide carboxylic acid (INCI)
CAS 90453-59-1
Synonyms: POE (9) stearamide carboxylic acid; PEG 450 stearamide carboxylic acid
Trade names: Akypo®-Muls 400

PEG-2 stearamine (INCI)
CAS 10213-78-2; EINECS 233-520-3
Synonyms: 2,2´-(Octadecylimino)bisethanol; Bis-2-hydroxyethyl stearamine; PEG 100 stearyl amine; POE

(2) stearyl amine
Trade names: Chemeen 18-2; Ethomeen® 18/12; Hetoxamine ST-2; Protox HTA-2; Varonic® S-202; Varonic® S-202 SF

PEG-5 stearamine (INCI)
CAS 26635-92-7
Synonyms: POE (5) stearyl amine
Trade names: Chemeen 18-5; Ethomeen® 18/15; Hetoxamine ST-5

PEG-10 stearamine (INCI)
CAS 26635-92-7
Synonyms: POE (10) stearyl amine; PEG 500 stearyl amine
Trade names: Ethomeen® 18/20; Protox HTA-10

PEG-15 stearamine (INCI)
CAS 26635-92-7
Synonyms: POE (15) stearyl amine
Trade names: Ethomeen® 18/25; Hetoxamine ST-15; Protox HTA-15

PEG-50 stearamine (INCI)
CAS 26635-92-7
Synonyms: POE (50) stearyl amine; Ethoxylated 1-aminooctadecane
Trade names: Chemeen 18-50; Ethomeen® 18/60; Hetoxamine ST-50; Protox HTA-50

PEG-1 stearate. *See Glycol stearate*

PEG-2 stearate (INCI)
CAS 106-11-6; 9004-99-3 (generic); 85116-97-8; EINECS 203-363-5; 285-550-1
Synonyms: Diethylene glycol stearate; Diglycol stearate; PEG 100 monostearate
Trade names: Ablunol DEGMS; Alkamuls® SDG; Cithrol DGMS N/E; Emalex DEG-m-S; Estol DEMS 3710; Glicosterina DPG; Hefti DMS-33; Hodag DGS; Hodag DGS-N; Hydrine; Karapeg DEG-MS; Kemester® 5221; Kessco® Diethylene Glycol Monostearate; Kessco® Diglycol Stearate Neutral; Lipal DGMS; Lipopeg 1-S; Nikkol DEGS; Nikkol MYS-2; Nopalcol 1-S; Protachem DGS; Protachem DGS-C; Radiasurf® 7410; Rol DGE; Sterol ST 2; Tegin® D 6100; Witconol™ CAD
Trade names containing: Base PL 1630; Kessco Diglycol Stearate; Monamilk; Ritapro 165; Sedefos 75®; Tefose® 70

PEG-2 stearate SE (INCI)
CAS 106-11-6
Synonyms: POE (2) monostearate self-emulsifying; Diethylene glycol monostearate self-emulsifying; PEG 100 monostearate self-emulsifying
Trade names: Cithrol DGMS S/E; CPH-104-DC-SE; CPH-104-DG-SE; Estol DEMS-se 3711; Hodag DGS-C; Kemester® 5221SE; Pegosperse® 100-S; Radiasurf® 7411
Trade names containing: Base O/W 097; Kessco Diglycol Stearate SE

PEG-3 stearate (INCI)
CAS 10233-24-6; 9004-99-3 (generic); EINECS 233-562-2
Synonyms: POE (3) stearate; 2-[2-(2-Hydroxyethoxy)ethoxy]ethyl octadecanoate
Trade names: Emalex 400A; Emalex 400B; Marlosol® 183; Tegin® D 1102

PEG-4 stearate (INCI)
CAS 106-07-0; 9004-99-3 (generic); EINECS 203-358-8
Synonyms: POE (4) stearate; PEG 200 monostearate
Trade names: Ablunol 200MS; Acconon 200-MS; Cithrol 2MS; Crodet S4; Ethofat® 18/14; Hodag 20-S;

Kessco® PEG 200 MS; Lipopeg 2-S; Mapeg® 200 MS; Nikkol MYS-4; Pegosperse® 200 MS; Protamate 200 DPS; Unipeg-200 MS

PEG-5 stearate (INCI)
CAS 9004-99-3 (generic)
Synonyms: POE (5) stearate
Trade names: Algon ST 50; Chemax E-200 MS; Emalex 805; Ethofat® 60/15; Hetoxamate SA-5; Prox-onic ST-05

PEG-6 stearate (INCI)
CAS 9004-99-3 (generic); 10108-28-8
Synonyms: POE (6) stearate; PEG 300 monostearate
Trade names: Alkamuls® S-6; Cithrol 3MS; Hetoxamate SA-6; Kessco® PEG 300 MS; Lipopeg 3-S; Polystate C; Protamate 300 DPS; Radiasurf® 7432; Super-polystate
Trade names containing: Gelot WL 3122; Tefose® 2000; Tefose® 2561

PEG-6-32 stearate (CTFA)
CAS 9004-99-3 (generic)
Synonyms: PEG 1500 monostearate; POE 1500 monostearate
Trade names: Hodag 150-S; Lipopeg 15-S; Mapeg® 1500 MS; Pegosperse® 1500 MS; Protamate 1500 DPS; Tefose® 1500
Trade names containing: Tefose® 63

PEG-7 stearate (INCI)
CAS 9004-99-3 (generic)
Synonyms: POE (7) stearate
Trade names: Hetoxamate SA-7

PEG-8 stearate (INCI)
CAS 9004-99-3 (generic); 70802-40-3
Synonyms: POE (8) stearate; PEG 400 monostearate
Trade names: Ablunol 400MS; Acconon 400-MS; Algon ST 80; Cithrol 4MS; CPH-50-N; Cremophor® S 9; Crodet S8; Elfacos® PEG 400 MS; Emerest® 2711; Estol EO4MS 3723; Eumulgin® ST-8; Hefti PGE-400-MS; Hetoxamate SA-8; Hodag 40-S; Kessco® PEG 400 MS; Lasemul 400 E; Lipal 400 S; Lipopeg 4-S; Mapeg® 400 MS; Marlosol® 188; Myrj® 45; Pegosperse® 400 MS; Protamate 400 DPS; Radiasurf® 7413; Radiasurf® 7473; Rol 400; Simulsol M 45; Unipeg-400 MS; Witconol™ 2711
Trade names containing: Cetax DR; Lanola 90

PEG-9 stearate (INCI)
CAS 9004-99-3 (generic); 5349-52-0; EINECS 226-312-9
Synonyms: POE (9) stearate
Trade names: Chemax E-400 MS; Hetoxamate SA-9; Prox-onic ST-09; Serdox NSG 400
Trade names containing: Lipocol B

PEG-10 stearate (INCI)
CAS 9004-99-3 (generic)
Synonyms: POE (10) stearate; PEG 500 monostearate
Trade names: Algon ST 100; Emalex 810; Ethofat® 60/20; Nikkol MYS-10

PEG-12 stearate (INCI)
CAS 9004-99-3 (generic)
Synonyms: POE (12) stearate; PEG 600 monostearate
Trade names: Ablunol 600MS; Cithrol 6MS; Crodet S12; Elfacos® PEG 600 MS; Emerest® 2662; Estol EO6MS 3725; Hefti PGE-600-MS; Hetoxamate SA-12; Hetoxamate SA-13; Hodag 60-S; Kessco® PEG 600 MS; Lipopeg 6-S; Mapeg® 600 MS; Protamate 600 DPS; Radiasurf® 7414; Unipeg-600 MS
Trade names containing: Upiwax 163

PEG-14 stearate (INCI)

CAS 9004-99-3 (generic); 10289-94-8; EINECS 233-641-1
Synonyms: POE (14) stearate
Trade names: Chemax E-600 MS; Prox-onic ST-014

PEG-20 stearate (INCI)
CAS 9004-99-3 (generic)
Synonyms: POE (20) stearate; PEG 1000 monostearate
Trade names: Ablunol 1000MS; Algon ST 200; Cerasynt® 840; Chemax E-1000 MS; Cithrol 10MS; CPH-90-N; Elfacos® PEG 1000 MS; Emalex 820; Estol E10MS 3727; Hetoxamate SA-20; Hetoxamate SA-23; Hodag 100-S; Kessco® PEG 1000 MS; Lipopeg 10-S; Mapeg® 1000 MS; Marlosol® 1820; Myrj® 49; Protamate 1000 DPS; Simulsol M 49; Unipeg-1000 MS; Witconol™ 2713
Trade names containing: Aquabase

PEG-21 stearate
Trade names: Stearate PEG 1000

PEG-23 stearate
CAS 9004-99-3 (generic)
Synonyms: POE (23) stearate
Trade names: Prox-onic ST-023

PEG-24 stearate
CAS 9004-99-3 (generic)
Synonyms: POE (24) stearate
Trade names: Crodet S24

PEG-25 stearate (INCI)
CAS 9004-99-3 (generic)
Synonyms: POE (25) stearate
Trade names: Hetoxamate SA-25; Nikkol MYS-25

PEG-30 stearate (INCI)
CAS 9004-99-3 (generic)
Synonyms: POE (30) stearate
Trade names: Emalex 830; G-2151; Myrj® 51; Simulsol M 51

PEG-32 stearate (INCI)
CAS 9004-99-3 (generic)
Synonyms: PEG 1540 stearate
Trade names: Hodag 154-S; Kessco® PEG 1540 MS; Protamate 1540 DPS; Unipeg-1540 MS

PEG-35 stearate (INCI)
CAS 9004-99-3 (generic)
Synonyms: POE (35) stearate
Trade names: Hetoxamate SA-35; Lipopeg 16-S

PEG-40 stearate (INCI)
CAS 9004-99-3 (generic); 31791-00-2
Synonyms: POE (40) stearate; PEG 2000 monostearate
Trade names: Algon ST 400; Alkamuls® ST-40; Crodet S40; Emalex 840; Emerest® 2715; Hefti RS-55-40; Hetoxamate SA-40; Hodag POE (40) MS; Lanoxide-52; Lipopeg 39-S; Mapeg® S-40; Mapeg® S-40K; Myrj® 52; Myrj® 52S; Nikkol MYS-40; Pegosperse® 1750 MS; Pegosperse® 1750 MS K Spec; Protamate 2000 DPS; Ritox 52; Rol 52; Simulsol M 52; Unipeg-S-40
Trade names containing: Ceral ML; Drewmulse® HM-100; Ritachol 5000; Teginacid® ML

PEG-45 stearate (INCI)
CAS 9004-99-3 (generic)
Synonyms: POE (45) stearate
Trade names: Lipopeg 20-S; Nikkol MYS-45

PEG-50 stearate (INCI)
CAS 9004-99-3 (generic)
Synonyms: POE (50) stearate
Trade names: Algon ST 500; Crodet S50; G-2153; Lanoxide-53; Myrj® 53; Ritox 53; Rol 53; Simulsol M 53

PEG-55 stearate
CAS 9004-99-3 (generic)
Synonyms: POE (55) stearate
Trade names: Nikkol MYS-55

PEG-69 stearate
Trade names containing: Actimulse 250

PEG-75 stearate (INCI)
CAS 9004-99-3 (generic)
Synonyms: POE (75) stearate; PEG 4000 monostearate
Trade names: Cithrol 40MS; Kessco® PEG 4000 MS; Protamate 4000 DPS; Unipeg-4000 MS
Trade names containing: Gelot 64®

PEG-90 stearate (INCI)
CAS 9004-99-3 (generic)
Synonyms: POE (90) stearate
Trade names: Hetoxamate SA-90; Hetoxamate SA-90F

PEG-100 stearate (INCI)
CAS 9004-99-3 (generic)
Synonyms: POE (100) stearate; PEG (100) monostearate
Trade names: Algon ST 1000; Crodet S100; Emerest® 2717; Hefti RS-55-100; Hetoxamate 100S; Hetoxamate SA-100; Lanoxide-59; Lipopeg 100-S; Mapeg® S-100; Myrj® 59; Protamate 4400 DPS; Ritox 59; Rol 59; Simulsol M 59
Trade names containing: Arlacel® 165; Ceral 165; Chemsperse GMS-PS; Dermalcare® GMS-165; Dracorin 100 SE 2/008479; Elfacos® GMSSE; Extan-GMS; Hodag GMS-A; Kessco® Glycerol Monostearate SE, Acid Stable; Lexemul® 561; Lipomulse 165; Mazol® 165C; Protachem GMS-165; Simulsol 165; Tewax TC 60; Tewax TC 65; Unitolate 165-C

PEG-150 stearate (INCI)
CAS 9004-99-3 (generic)
Synonyms: POE (150) stearate; PEG 6000 monostearate
Trade names: Emalex 6300 M-ST; Estol E60MS 3733; Hodag 600-S; Kessco® PEG 6000 MS; Mapeg® S-150; Ritapeg 150 DS; Unipeg-6000 MS
Trade names containing: Brookswax® R; Crodacol GP; Hodag CSA-102; Lipowax PR; Macol® CPS; Procol P; Relaxer Conc. No. 2; Relaxer Conc. No. 3; Ritachol 5000; Ritachol® 1000; Ritachol® 3000; Teinowax; Unicol CPS; Viscolene

PEG-1500 stearate
Trade names: Radiasurf® 7417

PEG-45 stearate phosphate (INCI)
Trade names: Emulgator DMR

PEG-2 stearmonium chloride (INCI)
CAS 60687-87-8; 3010-24-0
Synonyms: N,N-Bis(2-hydroxyethyl)-N-methylocta-decanaminium chloride; PEG 100 stearmonium chloride; POE (2) stearmonium chloride
Trade names containing: Ethoquad® 18/12

PEG-5 stearmonium chloride (CTFA)
Synonyms: N,N-Bis[2-(2-hydroxyethoxy)ethyl]-N-(2-hydroxyethyl)octadecanaminium chloride; Quaternium-36
Trade names: Genamin KS 5

PEG-15 stearmonium chloride (INCI)
CAS 28724-32-5
Synonyms: POE (15) stearmonium chloride
Trade names: Ethoquad® 18/25

PEG-5 stearyl ammonium lactate (INCI)
Synonyms: POE (5) stearyl ammonium lactate
Trade names: Genamin KSL

PEG stearyl ether. *See Steareth series*

PEG-4 stearyl ether stearate
  Trade names: Emalex SWS-4

PEG-6 stearyl ether stearate
  Trade names: Emalex SWS-6

PEG-9 stearyl ether stearate
  Trade names: Emalex SWS-9

PEG-10 stearyl ether stearate
  Trade names: Emalex SWS-10

PEG-12 stearyl ether stearate
  Trade names: Emalex SWS-12

PEG-8 stearyl stearate
  Trade names: Sterol SES

PEG-4 tallate (INCI)
  CAS 61791-00-2 (generic)
  Synonyms: POE (4) monotallate; PEG 200 monotallate
  Trade names: Hetoxamate FA 2-5; Mapeg® 200 MOT; Protamate 200 T

PEG-5 tallate (INCI)
  CAS 61791-00-2 (generic)
  Synonyms: POE (5) monotallate
  Trade names: Hetoxamate FA-5

PEG-8 tallate (INCI)
  CAS 61791-00-2 (generic)
  Synonyms: POE (8) monotallate; PEG 400 monotallate
  Trade names: Chemax E-400 MT; Hodag 40-T (redesignated Hodag WA-56); Mapeg® 400 MOT; Protamate 400 T; Unipeg-400 MOT

PEG-12 tallate (INCI)
  CAS 61791-00-2 (generic)
  Synonyms: POE (12) monotallate; PEG 600 monotallate
  Trade names: Mapeg® 600 MOT; Protamate 600 T

PEG-14 tallate
  Trade names: Sellig T 14 100

PEG-15 tallate
  CAS 61791-00-2 (generic); 65071-95-6
  Synonyms: POE (15) monotallate; POE (15) tall oil acid
  Trade names: Ethofat® 242/25; Ethofat® 433

PEG-16 tallate (INCI)
  CAS 61791-00-2 (generic)
  Synonyms: POE (16) monotallate
  Trade names: Renex® 20

PEG-20 tallate (INCI)
  CAS 61791-00-2 (generic)
  Synonyms: POE (20) monotallate; PEG 1000 monotallate
  Trade names: Hetoxamate FA-20; Protamate 1000 T

PEG-660 tallate
  Trade names: Mapeg® TAO-15

PEG-50 tallow amide (CTFA)
  CAS 8051-63-6
  Synonyms: POE (50) hydrogenated tallow amide
  Trade names: Methomid 60

PEG-2 tallowamine
  CAS 61791-44-4
  Synonyms: Bis (2-hydroxyethyl) tallow amine
  Trade names: Accomeen T2; Desomeen® TA-2; Hodag CSA-86; Mazeen® T-2; Varonic® T-202; Varonic® T-202 SF; Varonic® T-202 SR

PEG-5 tallowamine
  CAS 61791-44-4
  Trade names: Accomeen T5; Desomeen® TA-5; Mazeen® T-5; Varonic® T-205; Varonic® T-205 SF

PEG-8 tallowamine
  Trade names: Lowenol 1985; Varonic® 2271

PEG-10 tallowamine
  Trade names: Mazeen® T-10; Varonic® T-210; Varonic® T-210 SF

PEG-15 tallow amine
  Trade names: Accomeen T15; Desomeen® TA-15; Ethylan® TT-15; Mazeen® T-15; Varonic® T-215; Varonic® T-215 SF; Varonic® T-215LC; Witcamine® 6606

PEG-20 tallowamine
  Trade names: Desomeen® TA-20; Varonic® T-220

PEG-50 tallowamine
  Trade names: Ethomeen® T/60; Hetoxamine T-50; Hetoxamine T-50-70%; Varonic® T-250

PEG-3 tallow aminopropylamine (INCI)
  CAS 61790-85-0
  Synonyms: POE (3) tallow aminopropylamine; PEG-3 N-tallow-1,3-diaminopropane
  Trade names: Ethoduomeen® T/13

PEG-10 tallow aminopropylamine (INCI)
  CAS 61790-85-0 (generic)
  Synonyms: POE (10) tallow aminopropylamine; PEG 500 tallow aminopropylamine; PEG-10 N-tallow-1,3-di-aminopropane
  Trade names: Ethoduomeen® T/20

PEG-15 tallow aminopropylamine (INCI)
  CAS 61790-85-0 (generic)
  Synonyms: POE (15) tallow aminopropylamine; PEG-15 N-tallow-1,3-diaminopropane
  Trade names: Ethoduomeen® T/25

PEG-2 tallowate
  CAS 68153-64-0 (generic)
  Synonyms: Diethylene glycol monotallowate; POE (2) tallowate; PEG-2 tallow acid ester
  Trade names: Nopalcol 1-TW

PEG tallow ether. *See Talloweth series*

PEG-2 tallowmonium chloride
  CAS 67784-77-4
  Trade names containing: Ethoquad® T/12

PEG-15 tallow polyamine (INCI)
  CAS 63601-33-2; 37220-82-9
  Synonyms: POE (15) tallow polyamine
  Trade names: Uniquart H

PEG-3 tallow propylenedimonium dimethosulfate (INCI)
  CAS 93572-63-5; EINECS 297-495-0
  Synonyms: N-Tallowalkyl-N,N′0dimethyl-N,N′-polyethyleneglycol-propylenebis-ammonium-bis-methosulfate; POE (3) tallow propylenedimonium dimethosulfate
  Trade names: Rewoquat DQ 35

PEG-5 tricaprylyl citrate (INCI)
  Synonyms: POE (5) caprylyl tricitrate
  Trade names containing: Trioxene L

PEG-5 tricetyl citrate (INCI)
  Synonyms: POE (5) cetyl tricitrate
  Trade names containing: Trioxene S

PEG-5 tridecyl citrate (INCI)
  Synonyms: POE (5) decyl tricitrate
  Trade names containing: Trioxene L

PEG tridecyl ether. *See Trideceth series*

PEG-66 trihydroxystearin (INCI)
  CAS 61788-85-0
  Synonyms: POE (66) trihydroxystearin

Trade names: Lipocol HCO-66; Surfactol® 575

PEG-200 trihydroxystearin (INCI)
Synonyms: POE (200) trihydroxystearin
Trade names: Naturechem® THS-200; Surfactol® 590

PEG-5 trilauryl citrate (INCI)
Synonyms: POE (5) lauryl tricitrate
Trade names containing: Trioxene L

PEG-3 trimethylolpropane distearate
Trade names: Emalex TPS-203

PEG-4 trimethylolpropane distearate
Trade names: Emalex TPS-204

PEG-5 trimethylolpropane distearate
Trade names: Emalex TPS-205

PEG-3 trimethylolpropane triisostearate
Trade names: Emalex TPIS-303

PEG-20 trimethylolpropane triisostearate
Trade names: Emalex TPIS-320

PEG-25 trimethylolpropane triisostearate
Trade names: Emalex TPIS-325

PEG-30 trimethylolpropane triisostearate
Trade names: Emalex TPIS-330

PEG-40 trimethylolpropane triisostearate
Trade names: Emalex TPIS-340

PEG-50 trimethylolpropane triisostearate
Trade names: Emalex TPIS-350

PEG-3 trimethylolpropane trimyristate
Trade names: Emalex TPM-303

PEG-5 trimethylolpropane trimyristate (INCI)
Trade names: Emalex TPM-305

PEG-8 trimethylolpropane trimyristate
Trade names: Emalex TPM-308

PEG-20 trimethylolpropane trimyristate
Trade names: Emalex TPM-320

PEG-25 trimethylolpropane trimyristate
Trade names: Emalex TPM-325

PEG-30 trimethylolpropane trimyristate
Trade names: Emalex TPM-330

PEG-3 trimethylolpropane tristearate
Trade names: Emalex TPS-303

PEG-5 trimethylolpropane tristearate
Trade names: Emalex TPS-305

PEG-8 trimethylolpropane tristearate
Trade names: Emalex TPS-308

PEG-10 trimethylolpropane tristearate
Trade names: Emalex TPS-310

PEG-5 trimyristyl citrate (INCI)
Synonyms: POE (5) myristyl tricitrate
Trade names containing: Trioxene S

PEG-5 tristearyl citrate (INCI)
Synonyms: POE (5) stearyl tricitrate
Trade names containing: Trioxene S

PEG-6 undecylenate (INCI)
Trade names: Undelene

PEI-10 (INCI)
CAS 25987-06-8
Synonyms: Polyethylenimine 10
Trade names: Polymin® FG SG

PEI-15 (INCI)
CAS 9002-98-6 (generic)
Synonyms: Polyethylenimine 15
Trade names: Epomin SP-006

PEI-30 (INCI)
CAS 9002-98-6 (generic)
Synonyms: Polyethylenimine 30
Trade names: Epomin SP-012

PEI-35 (INCI)
Synonyms: Polyethylenimine 35
Trade names: Polymin® G-35 SG

PEI-45 (INCI)
CAS 9002-98-6 (generic)
Synonyms: Polyethylenimine 45
Trade names: Epomin SP-018

PEI-250 (INCI)
Synonyms: Polyethylenimine 250
Trade names: Polymin® Waterfree SG

PEI-1400 (INCI)
CAS 9002-98-6 (generic)
Synonyms: Polyethylenimine 1400
Trade names: Nalco® 634

PEI-1500 (INCI)
CAS 9002-98-6 (generic); 68130-97-2
Synonyms: Polyethylenimine 1500
Trade names: Polymin® P SG; Polymin® PS SG

PEI-1750 (INCI)
CAS 9002-98-6 (generic)
Synonyms: Polyethylenimine 1750
Trade names: Epomin P-1000

Pellitory extract (INCI)
CAS 84012-32-8
Synonyms: Parietary extract
Trade names containing: Babyderme HS 342; Baby-
derme LS 642; Demaquillant HS 287; Demaquillant
LS 687; Emollient HS 235; Emollient LS 635

Pennyroyal extract (INCI)
CAS 90064-00-9
Synonyms: Mentha pulegium extract
Trade names containing: Actiphyte of Pennyroyal

Pentadecalactone (INCI)
CAS 106-02-5; EINECS 203-354-6
Synonyms: Oxacyclohexadecan-2-one
Trade names: Exaltex; Exaltolide

Pentadecyl alcohol (INCI)
CAS 629-76-5
Synonyms: 1-Pentadecanol; C15 linear primary alcohol
Trade names: Neodol® 5

Pentadoxynol-200 (INCI)
CAS 40160-92-7 (generic); 39346-74-2 (generic)
Synonyms: PEG-200 pentadecyl phenyl ether
Trade names: Applichem PDP-200

Pentaerythrityl oleate
Trade names: Radiasurf® 7156

Pentaerythrityl stearate
CAS 85116-93-4; EINECS 285-547-5
Trade names: Radiasurf® 7175

Pentaerythrityl tetrabehenate (CTFA)
CAS 61682-73-3; 84539-90-2; EINECS 262-895-6; 283-
078-0
Synonyms: 2,2-Bis[[(1-oxodocosyl)oxy]methyl]1,3-pro-
panediyl docosanoate; Pentaerythritol tetrabehenate
Trade names: Liponate PB-4; Radia® 7514

Pentaerythrityltetracapratecaprylate
CAS 3008-50-2
Trade names: Lonzest® 163-S

Pentaerythrityl tetracaprylate/caprate (INCI)
CAS 68441-68-9; 69226-96-6; EINECS 270-474-3

Pentaerythrityl tetraisononanoate
Trade names: Crodamol PTC; Lipo PE 810; Liponate PE-810; Radia® 7178

Pentaerythrityl tetraisononanoate (INCI)
CAS 93803-89-5; EINECS 298-364-0
Synonyms: 2,2-Bis[[(1-oxoisononyl)oxy]methyl]-1,3-propanediyl isononanoate
Trade names: Pelemol P-49

Pentaerythrityl tetraisostearate (INCI)
Trade names: Crodamol PTIS; Kessco PTIS

Pentaerythrityl tetralaurate (INCI)
CAS 13057-50-6; EINECS 235-946-5
Synonyms: Dodecanoic acid, 2,2-bis[[(1-oxododecyl)oxy]methyl] 1,3-propanediyl ester
Trade names: Pelemol PTL

Pentaerythrityl tetraoctanoate (INCI)
CAS 7299-99-2; EINECS 230-743-8; 221-123-8
Synonyms: 2-Ethylhexanoic acid, 2,2-bis[[(1-oxo-2-ethylhexyl)oxy]methyl]-1,3-propanediyl ester
Trade names: Nikkol Pentarate 408; Trivent PE-48

Pentaerythrityl tetraoleate (INCI)
CAS 19321-40-5; 68604-44-4; EINECS 242-960-5; 271-694-2
Synonyms: Pentaerythritol tetraoleate
Trade names: Liponate PO-4; Pelemol PTO; Radia® 7171

Pentaerythrityl tetrapelargonate (INCI)
CAS 14450-05-6; EINECS 238-430-8
Synonyms: Nonanoic acid, 2,2-bis[[(1-oxononyl)oxy]methyl]1,3-propanediyl ester; Pentaerythritol tetrapelargonate
Trade names: Emerest® 2486; Unitolate PTP

Pentaerythrityl tetrastearate (INCI)
CAS 115-83-3; 91050-82-7; EINECS 204-110-1; 293-029-5
Synonyms: Pentaerythritol tetrastearate
Trade names: Alkamuls® PETS; Crodamol PETS; Kessco PTS; Liponate PS-4; Radia® 7176

N,N,N´,N´,N´-Pentamethyl-N-octadecenyl-1,3-diammonium dichloride
CAS 68310-73-6
Trade names containing: Duoquad® O-50

Pentasodium DTPA. See Pentasodium pentetate

Pentasodium pentetate (INCI)
CAS 140-01-2; EINECS 205-391-3
Synonyms: DTPANa$_5$; Pentasodium diethylene triamine pentaacetate; Pentasodium DTPA
Trade names: Hamp-Ex® 80; Mayoquest 300; Versenex 80
Trade names containing: Mayoquest 1545M

Pentetic acid (INCI)
CAS 67-43-6; EINECS 200-652-8
Synonyms: DTPA; N,N-Bis[2-[bis(carboxymethyl)amino]ethyl]glycine; Diethylene triamine pentaacetic acid; Pentacarboxymethyl diethylenetriamine
Trade names: Chel DTPA; Hamp-Ex® Acid

Peppermint extract (INCI)
CAS 84082-70-2
Synonyms: Mentha piperita extract
Trade names containing: Actiphyte of Peppermint; Aromaphyte of Peppermint; BBC Moisture Trol; BBC Relaxing Complex; Herbasol-Extract Peppermint

Peppermint oil (INCI)
CAS 8006-90-4
Synonyms: Mentha piperita oil
Trade names containing: Aromaphyte of Peppermint;

Essentiaderm n.1; Essentiaderm n.6; Essentiaderm n.8

Perfluoropolymethyl isopropyl ether (INCI)
Trade names: Fomblin® HC/04, HC/25, HC/R
Trade names containing: Brookosome® F; Fomblin® HC/P-04, HC/P-25, HC/P-R

Perovskite. See Calcium titanate

Persea americana extract. See Avocado extract

Persic oil. See Apricot kernel oil, Peach kernel oil

Peruvian bark extract. See Cinchona extract

Petrolatum (INCI)
CAS 8009-03-8 (NF); 8027-32-5 (USP); EINECS 232-373-2
Synonyms: Petroleum jelly; Petrolatum amber; Petrolatum white
Trade names: Amojell Petrolatum Amber, Dark, Snow White; Fonoline® White; Fonoline® Yellow; Mineral Jelly No. 5; Mineral Jelly No. 10; Mineral Jelly No. 10; Mineral Jelly No. 14; Mineral Jelly No. 15; Mineral Jelly No. 17; Mineral Jelly No. 20; Mineral Jelly No. 25; Ointment Base No. 3; Ointment Base No. 4; Ointment Base No. 6; Penreco Amber; Penreco Blond; Penreco Cream; Penreco Lily; Penreco Regent; Penreco Royal; Penreco Snow; Penreco Super; Penreco Ultima; Perfecta® USP; Protopet® Alba; Protopet® White 1S; Protopet® White 2L; Protopet® White 3C; Protopet® Yellow 2A; Snow White Petrolatum; Sono Jell® No. 4; Sono Jell® No. 9; Super White Fonoline®; Super White Protopet®; Unipet
Trade names containing: Alcolan® 36W; Alcolan® 40; Alcolan®; Aloe Extract #102; Amerchol® 400; Amerchol® C; Amerchol® CAB; Amerchol® H-9; Amerchol® RC; Amphocerin® K; Apicerol 2/014081; Argobase EU Hydrous; Argobase EU; Argobase EUC 2; Argobase L2; Cremba; Croda Solid Base; Crosterol SFA; Dehymuls® K; Emery® 1740; Emery® 1747; Fancol C; Fancol CAB; Forlan 200; Forlan 300; Forlan 500; Forlan L Conc; Forlan L; Forlan LM; Forlan; Ivarbase™ T; Lanaetex CLC; Lanaetex H; Lanaetex L-15; Lanalene SW; Lanalol; Leniplex; Lexate® PX; Molo-Jel; Nimcolan® 1747; Protalan SS-100; Protegin® W; Protegin® WX; Protegin® X; Protegin®; Ritaderm®; Sphingoceryl® Wax LS 2958 B; Unigator B 67

Petroleum distillates (INCI)
CAS 8002-05-9; 64742-14-9; 64742-47-8; EINECS 232-298-5
Trade names: Halpasol 230 W; Penreco 2251 Oil; Penreco 2263 Oil
Trade names containing: Bentone® Gel SS71

Petroleum jelly. See Petrolatum

Petroleum spirits. See Mineral spirits

Petroleum wax, crystalline. See Paraffin

Petroleum wax, microcrystalline. See Microcrystalline wax

Phenethyl alcohol (INCI)
CAS 60-12-8; EINECS 200-456-2
Synonyms: Benzeneethanol; 2-Phenylethanol; Phenylethyl alcohol
Trade names: Etaphen

Phenol sulfonic acid
CAS 98-67-9; 1333-39-7
Synonyms: p-Phenolsulfonic acid; 4-Hydroxybenzenesulfonic acid; Sulfocarbolic acid
Trade names: Eltesol® PSA 65

Phenoxyethanol (INCI)

CAS 122-99-6; EINECS 204-589-7
Synonyms: 2-Phenoxyethanol; Phenoxytol; Ethylene glycol monophenyl ether
Trade names: Cephene™; Emeressence® 1160 Rose Ether; Emthox® 6705; K-Preserve Liq; Phenoxen; Phenoxetol; Phenoxyethanol O; Rewopal® MPG 10; Sepicide LD; Unisept POE
Trade names containing: Bactiphen 2506 G; Dekaben; Emercide® 1199; Emericide 1199; Euxyl K 400; Euxyl K 702; Merguard 1200; Merquat® 2200; Midpol PHN; Midtect TFP; Nipaguard® BPX; Phenonip; Sepicide HB; Sepicide MB; Talcoseptic C; Undebenzofene C; Uniphen P-23; Unisuprol S-25

Phenoxyethylparaben (INCI)
Trade names containing: Undebenzofene

Phenoxyisopropanol (INCI)
CAS 4169-04-4; EINECS 224-027-4
Synonyms: 1-Phenoxy-2-propanol
Trade names: Propylene Phenoxetol
Trade names containing: Phenosept

Phenoxytol. *See Phenoxyethanol*

L-Phenylalanine (INCI)
CAS 63-91-2; EINECS 200-568-1
Trade names containing: Omega-CH Activator

Phenylbenzimidazole sulfonic acid (INCI)
CAS 27503-81-7
Synonyms: 2-Phenylbenzimidazole-5-sulfonic acid
Trade names: BioGir-PISA; Eusolex® 232; Neo Heliopan, Type Hydro; Parsol® HS

Phenylcarbinol. *See Benzyl alcohol*

Phenyl dimethicone (INCI)
CAS 9005-12-3; 2116-84-9; 63148-58-3
Synonyms: Methyl phenyl polysilocane; Polyphenylmethyl siloxane
Trade names: Belsil PDM 20; Belsil PDM 200; Belsil PDM 1000
Trade names containing: Rhodorsil® Oils 71634

m-Phenylenediamine (INCI)
CAS 108-45-2; EINECS 203-584-7
Synonyms: 1,3-Benzenediamine; 1,3-Phenylenediamine; 3-Aminoaniline
Trade names: Rodol MPD

p-Phenylenediamine (INCI)
CAS 106-50-3; EINECS 203-404-7
Synonyms: 1,4-Benzenediamine; 1,4-Phenylenediamine
Trade names: Rodol D
Trade names containing: Blonde 90 (Fusion); Blonde R-50 (Fusion); Brown GE (Fusion); Brown R-36 (Fusion)

m-Phenylenediamine sulfate (INCI)
CAS 541-70-8; EINECS 208-791-6
Synonyms: 1,3-Phenylenediamine sulfate
Trade names: Rodol MPDS

p-Phenylenediamine sulfate (INCI)
CAS 16245-77-5; EINECS 240-357-1
Synonyms: 1,4-Benzenediamine sulfate (1:1)
Trade names: Rodol DS

Phenylformic acid. *See Benzoic acid*

Phenylmethanol. *See Benzyl alcohol*

o-Phenylphenol (INCI)
CAS 90-43-7; EINECS 201-993-5
Synonyms: (1,1´-Biphenyl)-2-ol; 2-Phenyl phenol
Trade names: Dowicide 1

N-Phenyl-p-phenylenediamine (INCI)
CAS 101-54-2; EINECS 202-951-9
Synonyms: 4-Aminodiphenylamine; p-Aminodiphenylamine; N-Phenyl-1,4-benzenediamine
Trade names: Rodol Gray B Base

N-Phenyl-p-phenylenediamine sulfate (INCI)
CAS 4698-29-7; EINECS 225-173-1
Synonyms: p-Aminodiphenylamine sulfate; N-Phenyl-1,4-benzenediamine sulfate
Trade names: Rodol Gray BS

Phenyl salicylate (INCI)
CAS 118-55-8; EINECS 204-259-2
Synonyms: Phenyl-2-hydroxybenzoate
Trade names containing: Leniplex

Phenyl trimethicone (INCI)
CAS 2116-84-9; EINECS 218-320-6
Synonyms: Methyl phenyl polysiloxane; Polyphenylmethyl siloxane
Trade names: Abil® AV 20-1000; Abil® AV 8853; Baysilone Fluid PD 5; Baysilone Fluid PK 20; Dow Corning® 556 Fluid; Emalex MTS-30E; KF56, KF58; Masil® 556; Rhodorsil® Oils 70641 V 200

Phosphatides. *See Phospholipids*

Phosphatidylcholine (INCI)
CAS 97281-47-5
Trade names: Emulmetik™ 930; Phosal 25 SB; Phosal 25 SB; Phosal® 50 PG; Phospholipon® 90/90G; Phospholipon® 100; Phospholipon® 100 H

Phosphoglyco proteins
Trade names containing: Brookosome® Biophos

Phospholipids (INCI)
Synonyms: Phosphatides; Phospholipin
Trade names: Brookosome® MT; Ceramax
Trade names containing: Brookosome® A-Plus; Brookosome® A; Brookosome® ACEBC; Brookosome® ANE; Brookosome® BC; Brookosome® Biophos; Brookosome® C; Brookosome® CS; Brookosome® CU; Brookosome® DHA; Brookosome® DNA/RNA; Brookosome® E; Brookosome® Elastin; Brookosome® ELL; Brookosome® EPO; Brookosome® F; Brookosome® FIH; Brookosome® GSL; Brookosome® H; Brookosome® Herbal; Brookosome® MPS; Brookosome® P; Brookosome® RJ; Brookosome® RP; Brookosome® S; Brookosome® SC; Brookosome® SE; Brookosome® Serum; Brookosome® TE; Brookosome® TYE; Brookosome® U; Brookosome® UV; Brookosome® V; Ceramides LS; Dermatein® GSL; Glyco/Cer HA; Glyco/Cer HALA; Glyco/Cer; Glycoderm; Glycosome; Lipodermol®; Lipomicron Vitamin A Palmitate; Lipomicron Vitamin E Acetate; Liposomes CLR; Presome Type I; Sphingoceryl® LS; Sphingoceryl® Powd. LS; Sphingoceryl® Wax LS 2958 B

Phosphoric acid (INCI)
CAS 7664-38-2; EINECS 231-633-2
Synonyms: Orthophosphoric acid
Trade names containing: Hydrocos

Phytosterols
Trade names containing: Chronosphere® Planell®

PIB. *See Polybutene*

Pigskin extract (INCI)
Trade names containing: Epidermin in Oil; Epidermin Water-Soluble; Unibotan Vitaplant O CLR; Vitaplant CLR Oil-Soluble N

Pimpinella anisum extract. *See Anise extract*

Pineapple extract

Pineapple extract (INCI)
Synonyms: Ananas comosus extract
Trade names containing: Ritacomplex DF 26

Pineapple juice (INCI)
Trade names containing: Hormo Fruit Pineapple; Lipofruit R

Pine needle extract (INCI)
CAS 84012-35-1
Trade names containing: Cremogen Pine Needles 739007; Herbaliquid Alpine Herbs Special

Pine oil (INCI)
CAS 8002-09-3
Synonyms: Oils, pine; Yarmor
Trade names containing: Essentiaderm n.2; Essentiaderm n.7; Essentiaderm n.9

Piroctone olamine (INCI)
CAS 68890-66-4; EINECS 272-574-2
Trade names containing: Antidandruff Agent NOVA

Placental lipids (INCI)
Synonyms: Lipids, placental
Trade names: Lipotrofina Placentare; Placentaliquid Oil-Soluble; Unipro Placenta Liq./OS
Trade names containing: Epidermin in Oil; Epidermin Water-Soluble; Lipotrofina M

Placental protein (INCI)
Trade names: Dascare Bovine Placenta; Placentaliquid Water-Soluble; Unipro Placenta Liq./WS
Trade names containing: Biopharco CP-12; Diaquasol; Dihydral; Epiderm-Complex O; Epiderm-Complex W; Glycolysat de placenta bovin; Hair Complex 20/70n; Trichogen

Plantain extract (INCI)
CAS 85085-64-9; 84929-43-1
Synonyms: English plantain extract
Trade names containing: Bio-Chelated Derma-Plex I

POE . See PEG

Pollen extract (INCI)
Trade names containing: Actiphyte of Bee Pollen; Biofloreol Hydrosoluble; Biofloreol Liposoluble; Biofloreol Liq. Liposoluble; Filagrinol

Poloxamer 101 (INCI)
CAS 9003-11-6 (generic)
Synonyms: Methyl oxirane polymers (generic); Polyethylenepolypropylene glycols, polymers (generic)
Trade names: Hodag Nonionic 1031-L; Macol® 46

Poloxamer 105 (INCI)
CAS 9003-11-6 (generic)
Trade names: Hodag Nonionic 1035-L; Macol® 35; Pluronic® L35; Synperonic PE/L35

Poloxamer 108 (INCI)
CAS 9003-11-6 (generic)
Trade names: Hodag Nonionic 1038-F; Pluronic® F38

Poloxamer 122 (INCI)
CAS 9003-11-6 (generic)
Trade names: Hodag Nonionic 1042-L; Macol® 42

Poloxamer 123 (INCI)
CAS 9003-11-6 (generic)
Trade names: Hodag Nonionic 1043-L; Pluronic® L43

Poloxamer 124 (INCI)
CAS 9003-11-6 (generic)
Trade names: Hodag Nonionic 1044-L; Macol® 44; Pluronic® L44

Poloxamer 181 (INCI)

CAS 9003-11-6 (generic)
Trade names: Chemal BP 261; Dow EP530; Hodag Nonionic 1061-L; Macol® 1; Pluronic® L61

Poloxamer 182 (INCI)
CAS 9003-11-6 (generic)
Trade names: Chemal BP-262; Hodag Nonionic 1062-L; Macol® 2; Pluronic® L62

Poloxamer 183 (INCI)
CAS 9003-11-6 (generic)
Trade names: Hodag Nonionic 1063-L

Poloxamer 184 (INCI)
CAS 9003-11-6 (generic)
Trade names: Antarox® L-64; Hodag Nonionic 1064-L; Macol® 4; Pluracare® L64; Pluronic® L64

Poloxamer 185 (INCI)
CAS 9003-11-6 (generic)
Trade names: Hodag Nonionic 1065-P; Pluracare® P65; Pluronic® P65

Poloxamer 188 (INCI)
CAS 9003-11-6 (generic)
Trade names: Hodag Nonionic 1068-F; Macol® 8; Pluracare® F68; Pluronic® F68; Synperonic PE/F68
Trade names containing: Unigator B 67

Poloxamer 212 (INCI)
CAS 9003-11-6 (generic)
Trade names: Hodag Nonionic 1072-L; Macol® 72

Poloxamer 215 (INCI)
CAS 9003-11-6 (generic)
Trade names: Hodag Nonionic 1075-P

Poloxamer 217 (INCI)
CAS 9003-11-6 (generic)
Trade names: Hodag Nonionic 1077-F; Macol® 77; Pluracare® F77; Pluronic® F77

Poloxamer 231 (INCI)
CAS 9003-11-6 (generic)
Trade names: Hodag Nonionic 1081-L; Pluronic® L81

Poloxamer 234 (INCI)
CAS 9003-11-6 (generic)
Trade names: Hodag Nonionic 1084-P; Pluronic® P84

Poloxamer 235 (INCI)
CAS 9003-11-6 (generic)
Trade names: Hodag Nonionic 1085-P; Macol® 85; Pluronic® P85; Synperonic PE/P85

Poloxamer 237 (INCI)
CAS 9003-11-6 (generic)
Trade names: Antarox® PGP 23-7; Hodag Nonionic 1087-F; Pluronic® F87; Synperonic PE/F87

Poloxamer 238 (INCI)
CAS 9003-11-6 (generic)
Trade names: Hodag Nonionic 1088-F; Pluronic® F88

Poloxamer 282 (INCI)
CAS 9003-11-6 (generic)
Trade names: Hodag Nonionic 1092-L; Pluronic® L92

Poloxamer 284 (INCI)
CAS 9003-11-6 (generic)
Trade names: Hodag Nonionic 1094-P

Poloxamer 288 (INCI)
CAS 9003-11-6 (generic)
Trade names: Hodag Nonionic 1098-F; Pluronic® F98

Poloxamer 331 (INCI)
CAS 9003-11-6 (generic)
Trade names: Chemal BP-2101; Hodag Nonionic 1101-L; Macol® 101; Pluronic® L101

Poloxamer 333 (INCI)
CAS 9003-11-6 (generic)
Trade names: Hodag Nonionic 1103-P; Pluronic® P103

Poloxamer 334 (INCI)
CAS 9003-11-6 (generic)
Trade names: Hodag Nonionic 1104-P; Pluronic® P104

Poloxamer 335 (INCI)
CAS 9003-11-6 (generic)
Trade names: Hodag Nonionic 1105-P; Pluronic® P105

Poloxamer 338 (INCI)
CAS 9003-11-6 (generic)
Trade names: Hodag Nonionic 1108-F; Macol® 108; Pluracare® F108; Pluronic® F108

Poloxamer 401 (INCI)
CAS 9003-11-6 (generic)
Trade names: Hodag Nonionic 1121-L; Pluronic® L121

Poloxamer 402 (INCI)
CAS 9003-11-6 (generic)
Trade names: Hodag Nonionic 1122-L; Pluronic® L122

Poloxamer 403 (INCI)
CAS 9003-11-6 (generic)
Trade names: Hodag Nonionic 1123-P; Macol® 23; Pluronic® P123

Poloxamer 407 (INCI)
CAS 9003-11-6 (generic)
Trade names: Hodag Nonionic 1127-F; Macol® 27; Pluracare® F127; Pluronic® F127; Synperonic PE/ F127

Poloxamer 105 benzoate
Trade names: Finsolv® PL-355

Poloxamer 182 benzoate
Trade names: Finsolv® PL-62

Poloxamine 304 (INCI)
CAS 11111-34-5 (generic)
Trade names: Tetronic® 304

Poloxamine 701 (INCI)
CAS 11111-34-5 (generic)
Trade names: Tetronic® 701

Poloxamine 704 (INCI)
CAS 11111-34-5 (generic)
Trade names: Tetronic® 704

Poloxamine 901 (INCI)
CAS 11111-34-5 (generic)
Trade names: Tetronic® 901

Poloxamine 904 (INCI)
CAS 11111-34-5 (generic)
Trade names: Tetronic® 904

Poloxamine 908 (INCI)
CAS 11111-34-5 (generic)
Trade names: Tetronic® 908

Poloxamine 1301 (INCI)
CAS 11111-34-5 (generic)
Trade names: Synperonic T/1301

Poloxamine 1302 (INCI)
CAS 11111-34-5 (generic)
Trade names: Synperonic T/1302

Poloxamine 1307 (INCI)
CAS 11111-34-5 (generic)
Trade names: Tetronic® 1307

Polyacrylamide (INCI)
CAS 9003-05-8
Synonyms: 2-Propenamide, homopolymer
Trade names containing: Sepigel 305

Polyacrylamidomethylpropane sulfonic acid (INCI)
CAS 27119-07-9
Trade names: Cosmedia® Polymer HSP 1180; Unipoly HSP 1180

Polyacrylic acid (INCI)
CAS 9003-01-4
Synonyms: 2-Propenoic acid, homopolymer; Acrylic acid polymers
Trade names: Acrysol® A-1; Carbopol® 907; Covacryl IIO, III

Polyaminopropyl biguanide (INCI)
CAS 27083-27-8
Trade names: Cosmocil CQ; Mikrokill 20
Trade names containing: Mikrokill 2; Mikrokill 300

Polyamino sugar condensate (INCI)
CAS 120022-92-6
Trade names containing: Aqualizer EJ; Croderm MF

Polybutene (INCI)
CAS 9003-28-5
Synonyms: PIB; Polybutylene; 1-Butene, homopolymer
Trade names containing: Ritalan® HKS

Polybutylene. *See Polybutene*

Polydecene (INCI)
CAS 37309-58-3
Synonyms: Decene, homopolymer
Trade names: Ethylflo® 364 NF; Ethylflo® 366 NF

PolyDMDAAC. *See Polyquaternium-6*

Polyethylene (INCI)
CAS 9002-88-4; EINECS 200-815-3
Synonyms: Ethene, homopolymer
Trade names: A-O® 6; A-C® 6A; A-C® 7, 7A; A-C® 8, 8A; A-C® 9, 9A, 9F; A-C® 15; A-C® 16; A-C® 617, 617A; A-C® 617G; A-C® 1702; ACumist™ A-12; ACumist™ A-18; ACumist™ B-6; ACumist™ B-9; ACumist™ B-12; ACumist™ B-18; ACumist™ C-5; ACumist™ C-9; ACumist™ C-12; ACumist™ C-18; ACumist™ D-9; ACuscrub® 41; ACuscrub® 42; ACuscrub® 43; ACuscrub® 44; ACuscrub® 52; Micropoly 520; Micropoly 524; Micropoly 524-XF; Microthene® MN-714, MN-722; Polyethylene 1000 HE; Polyspend™; Polywax® 500; Polywax® 655; Polywax® 850; Polywax® 1000; Polywax® 2000; Polywax® 3000; Siltek® GR; Siltek® M; Siltek® M Super; Siltek® PL
Trade names containing: ACuscrub® 40; Lipcare Wax 7782; Micropoly 2001; Ritaplast R; Ritaplast TN; Ritaplast

Polyethylene, oxidized (INCI)
CAS 68441-17-8
Synonyms: Oxidized polyethylene; Ethene, homopolymer, oxidized
Trade names: A-C® 316, 316A; A-C® 395, 395A; A-C® 629, 629A; A-C® 655; A-C® 656; A-C® 6702; ACuscrub® 31; ACuscrub® 32; ACuscrub® 51
Trade names containing: ACuscrub® 30; ACuscrub® 50

Polyethylenimine . *See PEI series*

Polyglyceryl-3 beeswax (INCI)
CAS 136097-93-3
Synonyms: Polyglycerol-3 beeswax; PG-3 beeswax
Trade names: Cera Bellina®

Polyglyceryl-2 caprylate (INCI)
Synonyms: Diglyceryl caprylate
Trade names: Imwitor® 708

Polyglyceryl-3 cetyl ether (INCI)
CAS 128895-87-4

Synonyms: Triglycerol, monohexadecyl ether; Triglyceryl cetyl ether
Trade names: Chimexane NL

Polyglyceryl-10 decaisostearate
Synonyms: Decaglycerin decaisostearate
Trade names: Nikkol Decaglyn 10-IS

Polyglyceryl-10 decaoleate (INCI)
CAS 11094-60-3; EINECS 234-316-7
Synonyms: Decaglycerol decaoleate; Decaglyceryl decaoleate
Trade names: Caprol® 10G10O; Drewmulse® 10-10-O; Drewpol® 10-10-O; Hodag PGO-1010; Nikkol Decaglyn 10-O; Santone® 10-10-O; Unitolate PGO-1010

Polyglyceryl-10 decastearate (INCI)
CAS 39529-26-5; EINECS 254-495-5
Synonyms: Decaglycerol decastearate; Decaglyceryl decastearate; Octadecanoic acid, decaester with decaglycerol
Trade names: Caprol® 10G10S; Nikkol Decaglyn 10-S

Polyglyceryl-3 decyltetradecanol (INCI)
Synonyms: Triglyceryl decyltetradecyl ether
Trade names: Chimexane NR

Polyglyceryl-2 diisostearate (INCI)
CAS 67938-21-0; EINECS 267-821-6
Synonyms: Diglyceryl diisostearate; Isooctadecanoic acid, diester with diglycerol
Trade names: Cosmol 42; Dermol DGDIS; Emalex DISG-2

Polyglyceryl-3 diisostearate (INCI)
CAS 66082-42-6; 85404-84-8; 31566-31-1; 11099-07-3; 85666-92-8
Synonyms: Triglyceryl diisostearate
Trade names: Emalex DISG-3; Emerest® 2452; Lameform® TGI; Unimul LAM-TGI

Polyglyceryl-5 diisostearate
Trade names: Emalex DISG-5

Polyglyceryl-10 diisostearate (INCI)
CAS 102033-55-6
Synonyms: Decaglyceryl diisostearate
Trade names: Emalex DISG-10; Nikkol Decaglyn 2-IS

Polyglyceryl-2 dioleate (INCI)
CAS 67965-56-4; 60219-68-3
Synonyms: Diglyceryl dioleate
Trade names: Nikkol DGDO

Polyglyceryl-3 dioleate (INCI)
CAS 79665-94-4
Synonyms: Triglyceryl dioleate; 9-Octadecenoic acid, diester with triglycerol
Trade names: Cremophor® GO32

Polyglyceryl-6 dioleate (INCI)
CAS 76009-37-5
Synonyms: Hexaglycerol dioleate; Hexaglyceryl dioleate
Trade names: Caprol® 6G2O; Plurol Oleique WL 1173

Polyglyceryl-10 dioleate (INCI)
CAS 33940-99-7
Synonyms: Decaglycerol dioleate; Decaglycerin dioleate; Decaglyceryl dioleate
Trade names: Caprol® 10G2O; Nikkol Decaglyn 2-O

Polyglyceryl-2 distearate
Trade names: Emalex DSG-2

Polyglyceryl-3 distearate (INCI)
CAS 94423-19-5
Synonyms: Triglyceryl distearate
Trade names: Cremophor® GS32; Emalex DSG-3

Polyglyceryl-5 distearate
Trade names: Emalex DSG-5

Polyglyceryl-6 distearate (INCI)
CAS 34424-97-0
Synonyms: Hexaglycerol distearate; Hexaglyceryl distearate
Trade names: Caprol® 6G2S; Plurol Stearique WL 1009

Polyglyceryl-10 distearate (INCI)
CAS 12764-60-2
Synonyms: Decaglycerin distearate; Decaglyceryl distearate
Trade names: Emalex DSG-10; Nihon Polyglyceryl-10 Distearate; Nikkol Decaglyn 2-S

Polyglyceryl-10 heptaisostearate
Synonyms: Decaglycerin heptaisostearate; Decaglyceryl heptaisostearate
Trade names: Nikkol Decaglyn 7-IS

Polyglyceryl-10 heptaoleate (INCI)
CAS 103175-09-3
Synonyms: Decaglycerin heptaoleate; Decaglyceryl heptaoleate
Trade names: Nikkol Decaglyn 7-O

Polyglyceryl-10 heptastearate (INCI)
CAS 99126-54-2
Synonyms: Decaglycerin heptastearate; Decaglyceryl heptastearate
Trade names: Nikkol Decaglyn 7-S

Polyglyceryl-3 hydroxylauryl ether (INCI)
Synonyms: Triglyceryl hydroxylauryl ether; Triglyceryl monohydroxylauryl ether
Trade names: Chimexane NF

Polyglyceryl-2 isostearate (INCI)
CAS 73296-86-3; 81752-33-2
Synonyms: Diglyceryl isostearate
Trade names: Apifac; Cosmol 41; Nikkol DGMIS

Polyglyceryl-3 isostearate (INCI)
CAS 127512-63-4
Synonyms: Triglyceryl monoisostearate
Trade names: Isolan® GI 34

Polyglyceryl-4 isostearate (INCI)
CAS 91824-88-3
Synonyms: Tetraglyceryl monoisostearate; Isooctanoic acid, monoester with tetraglycerol
Trade names: Witconol™ 18L
Trade names containing: Abil® WE 09

Polyglyceryl-6 isostearate (INCI)
CAS 126928-07-2
Trade names: Plurol Isostearique

Polyglyceryl-10 isostearate (INCI)
CAS 133738-23-5
Synonyms: Decaglycerin monoisostearate; Decaglyceryl monoisostearate
Trade names: Nikkol Decaglyn 1-IS

Polyglyceryl isostearostearate
Trade names: Lafil WL 3254

Polyglyceryl-2 lanolin alcohol ether (INCI)
Synonyms: Diglyceryl monolanolin ether; Polyglyceryl-2 lanolin ether
Trade names: Chimexane NH

Polyglyceryl-6 laurate (INCI)
CAS 51033-38-6
Synonyms: Hexaglycerin monolaurate; Hexaglyceryl monolaurate
Trade names: Nikkol Hexaglyn 1-L

Polyglyceryl-10 laurate (INCI)
CAS 34406-66-1
Synonyms: Decaglycerin monolaurate; Decaglyceryl monolaurate
Trade names: Nikkol Decaglyn 1-L

Polyglyceryl-10 linoleate
Synonyms: Decaglycerin monolinoleate
Trade names: Nikkol Decaglyn 1-LN

Polyglycerylmethacrylate. *See Glyceryl polymethacrylate*

Polyglyceryl methyl glucose distearate
Trade names: Tego® Care 450

Polyglyceryl-6 myristate
Trade names: Nikkol Hexaglyn 1-M

Polyglyceryl-10 myristate (INCI)
CAS 87390-32-7
Synonyms: Decaglycerin monomyristate
Trade names: Nikkol Decaglyn 1-M

Polyglyceryl-2 oleate (INCI)
CAS 9007-48-1 (generic); 49553-76-6
Synonyms: Diglyceryl monooleate
Trade names: Cosmol O-42T; Nikkol DGMO-90; Nikkol DGMO-C

Polyglyceryl-3 oleate (INCI)
CAS 9007-48-1 (generic); 33940-98-6
Synonyms: Triglyceryl oleate
Trade names: Caprol® 3GO; Drewpol® 3-1-O; Isolan® GO 33; Mazol® PGO-31 K
Trade names containing: Abil® WS 08; Protegin® W; Protegin® WX

Polyglyceryl-4 oleate (INCI)
CAS 9007-48-1 (generic); 71012-10-7
Synonyms: Tetraglyceryl monooleate
Trade names: Nikkol Tetraglyn 1-O; Protachem 100
Trade names containing: Emulsynt® 1055

Polyglyceryl-6 oleate (INCI)
CAS 9007-48-1 (generic); 79665-92-2
Synonyms: Hexaglycerin monooleate; Hexaglyceryl oleate
Trade names: Drewpol® 6-1-O; Nikkol Hexaglyn 1-O

Polyglyceryl-10 oleate (INCI)
CAS 9007-48-1 (generic); 79665-93-3
Synonyms: Decaglycerin monooleate; Decaglyceryl monooleate
Trade names: Nikkol Decaglyn 1-O

Polyglyceryl-4 PEG-2 cocamide (INCI)
Synonyms: Tetraglyceryl PEG-2 cocamide
Trade names: Chimexane NJ

Polyglyceryl-2-PEG-4 stearate (INCI)
Synonyms: Diglyceryl PEG-4 stearate
Trade names: Hostacerin DGS; Hostacerin DGSB

Polyglyceryl-10 pentaisostearate
Synonyms: Decaglyceryl pentaiosostearate
Trade names: Nikkol Decaglyn 5-IS

Polyglyceryl-4 pentaoleate
Synonyms: Tetraglyceryl pentaoleate
Trade names: Nikkol Tetraglyn 5-O

Polyglyceryl-6 pentaoleate (INCI)
CAS 104934-17-0
Synonyms: Hexaglyceryl pentaoleate
Trade names: Nikkol Hexaglyn 5-O

Polyglyceryl-10 pentaoleate (INCI)
CAS 86637-84-5
Synonyms: Decaglycerin pentaoleate
Trade names: Nikkol Decaglyn 5-O

Polyglyceryl-4 pentastearate
Synonyms: Tetraglyceryl pentastearate
Trade names: Nikkol Tetraglyn 5-S

Polyglyceryl-6 pentastearate (INCI)
CAS 99734-30-2
Synonyms: Hexaglyceryl pentastearate
Trade names: Nikkol Hexaglyn 5-S

Polyglyceryl-10 pentastearate (INCI)
CAS 95461-64-6
Synonyms: Decaglycerin pentastearate; Decaglyceryl pentastearate
Trade names: Nikkol Decaglyn 5-S

Polyglyceryl-6 polyricinoleate
Synonyms: Hexaglyceryl polyricinoleate
Trade names: Nikkol Hexaglyn PR-15

Polyglyceryl-2 sesquiisostearate (INCI)
Synonyms: Diglyceryl sesquiisostearate
Trade names: Hoe S 2721; Hostacerin DGI
Trade names containing: Hostacerin WO; Hostacerin WOL

Polyglyceryl-2 sesquioleate (INCI)
Synonyms: Diglyceryl sesquioleate
Trade names containing: Apicerol 2/014081

Polyglyceryl-2 stearate (INCI)
CAS 12694-22-3; EINECS 235-777-7
Synonyms: Diglyceryl monostearate
Trade names: Emalex MSG-2; Emalex MSG-2MA; Emalex MSG-2MB; Emalex MSG-2ME; Emalex MSG-2ML; Nikkol DGMS

Polyglyceryl-3 stearate (INCI)
CAS 37349-34-1 (generic); 27321-72-8; 26855-43-6; EINECS 248-403-2
Synonyms: Triglyceryl stearate
Trade names: Caprol® 3GS; Hefti GMS-333

Polyglyceryl-4 stearate (INCI)
CAS 37349-34-1 (generic); 68004-11-5; 26855-44-7
Synonyms: Tetraglyceryl monostearate; Octadecanoic acid, monoester with tetraglycerol
Trade names: Nikkol Tetraglyn 1-S

Polyglyceryl-6 stearate
Synonyms: Hexaglycerol stearate; Hexaglyceryl stearate
Trade names: Nikkol Hexaglyn 1-S

Polyglyceryl-10 stearate (INCI)
CAS 79777-30-3
Synonyms: Decaglycerin monostearate; Decaglyceryl monostearate; Octadecanoic acid, monoester with decaglycerol
Trade names: Nikkol Decaglyn 1-S

Polyglyceryl-2 tetraisostearate (INCI)
CAS 121440-30-0
Synonyms: Diglyceryl tetraisostearate; Isooctadecanoic acid, tetraester with diglycerol
Trade names: Cosmol 44

Polyglyceryl-10 tetraoleate (INCI)
CAS 34424-98-1; EINECS 252-011-7
Synonyms: Decaglyceryl tetraoleate; 9-Octadecenoic acid, tetraester with decaglycerol
Trade names: Caprol® 10G4O; Drewpol® 10-4-O; Mazol® PGO-104

Polyglyceryl-2 tetrastearate (INCI)
CAS 72347-89-8
Synonyms: Diglycerol tetrastearate; Diglyceryl tetrastearate; Octadecanoic acid, tetraester with diglycerol
Trade names: Caprol® 2G4S

Polyglyceryl-2 triisostearate (INCI)
CAS 120486-24-0
Synonyms: Diglyceryl triisostearate; Isooctadecanoic acid, triester with diglycerol
Trade names: Cosmol 43; Emalex TISG-2

Polyglyceryl-10 triisostearate
Trade names: Nikkol Decaglyn 3-IS

Polyglyceryl-10 trioleate (INCI)
CAS 102051-00-3
Synonyms: Decaglycerin trioleate; Decaglyceryl trioleate
Trade names: Nikkol Decaglyn 3-O

Polyglyceryl-4 tristearate
Synonyms: Tetraglyceryl tristearate
Trade names: Nikkol Tetraglyn 3-S

Polyglyceryl-6 tristearate (INCI)
CAS 71185-87-0
Synonyms: Hexaglycerin tristearate
Trade names: Nikkol Hexaglyn 3-S

Polyglyceryl-10 tristearate (INCI)
CAS 12709-64-7
Synonyms: Decaglycerin tristearate; Decaglyceryl tristearate
Trade names: Nikkol Decaglyn 3-S

Polygonum extract
Trade names containing: Fo-Ti 5:1 PG

Polyisobutene (INCI)
CAS 9003-27-4; 9003-29-6
Synonyms: Polyisobutylene; 2-Methyl-1-propene, homopolymer
Trade names: Permethyl® 104A; Permethyl® 106A; Permethyl® 108A
Trade names containing: Permethyl® 1082

Polyisoprene (INCI)
CAS 9006-04-6; 9003-31-0
Synonyms: IR; Isoprene rubber; 2-Methyl-1,3-butadiene, homopolymer; cis-1,4-Polyisoprene rubber
Trade names: Syntesqual
Trade names containing: Sebopessina

Polylysine (INCI)
Trade names: CPC Peptide

Polymethacrylamidopropyl trimonium chloride (INCI)
CAS 68039-13-4
Synonyms: Polydimethylaminopropyl methacrylamide methylchloride quaternium
Trade names: Lexquat® 2240; Nalquat 2240; Polycare® 133

Polymethacrylic acid (INCI)
CAS 25087-26-7
Trade names: Coatex 9065 C

Polymethoxy bicyclic oxazolidine (INCI)
CAS 56709-13-8
Synonyms: 5-Hydroxypoly[methyleneoxy]methyl-1-aza-3,7-dioxabicyclo-3,3-octane
Trade names: Nuosept C

Polymethyl methacrylate (INCI)
CAS 9011-14-7
Synonyms: 2-Propenoic acid, 2-methyl-, methyl ester, homopolymer
Trade names: BPA-500; Jurymer; Jurymer MB-1; Microma-100; Micropearl M100; Microsphere M-100; PMMA Beads; Rohadon® M-449; Rohadon® M-527; Rohadon® MW-235; Rohadon® MW-332; Rohadon® MW-422; Rohagum® M-914; Rohamere® 8744F

Poly[oxyethylene(dimethyliminio)ethylene(dimethyliminio)
ethylene dichloride]
Trade names: Busan® 1507

Polyoxypropylene . *See* PPG

Polypentene (INCI)
Synonyms: Pentene, homopolymer
Trade names: Escorez 1271 U

Polypropylene (INCI)
CAS 9003-07-0; 9010-79-1 (nucleated)
Synonyms: PP; 1-Propene, homopolymer; Propylene polymer; Polypropene
Trade names: Hoechst Wax PP 690

Polyquaternium-2 (INCI)
CAS 63451-27-4; 68555-36-2
Trade names: Mirapol® A-15

Polyquaternium-4 (INCI)
Synonyms: Diallyldimonium chloride/hydroxyethylcellulose copolymer
Trade names: Celquat® H-100; Celquat® L-200

Polyquaternium-6 (INCI)
CAS 26062-79-3
Synonyms: PolyDMDAAC; N,N-Dimethyl-N-2-propenyl-2-propen-1-aminium chloride, homopolymer; Poly (dimethyl diallyl ammonium chloride); Quaternium-40
Trade names: Agequat 400; Conditioner P6; Genamin PDAC; M-Quat® 40; Mackernium™ 006; Merquat® 100; Mirapol® CP40; Salcare SC30

Polyquaternium-7 (INCI)
CAS 26590-05-6
Synonyms: N,N-Dimethyl-N-2-propenyl-2-propen-1-aminium chloride, polymer with 2-propenamide; Quaternium-41
Trade names: Agequat 500, -5008; Conditioner P7; Mackernium™ 007; Merquat® 550; Merquat® S; Mirapol® 550; Salcare SC10
Trade names containing: Merquat® 2200

Polyquaternium-10 (INCI)
CAS 53568-66-4; 55353-19-0; 54351-50-7; 68610-92-4; 81859-24-7
Synonyms: Quaternium-19
Trade names: Celquat® SC-230M; Celquat® SC-240; Celquat® SC-240C, 28-6804; Leogard GP; Ucare® Polymer JR-30M, JR-125, JR-400; Ucare® Polymer LK; Ucare® Polymer LR 30M, LR 400; Ucare® Polymer SR-10

Polyquaternium-11 (INCI)
CAS 53633-54-8
Synonyms: Vinylpyrrolidone/dimethylaminoethyl methacrylate copolymer/diethyl sulfate reaction product; Quaternium-23
Trade names: Gafquat® 734; Gafquat® 755; Gafquat® 755N
Trade names containing: Condipon

Polyquaternium-16 (INCI)
CAS 29297-55-0
Synonyms: Vinylpyrrolidone/vinyl imidazolinium methochloride copolymer
Trade names: Luviquat® FC 370; Luviquat® FC 550; Luviquat® FC 905; Luviquat® HM 552

Polyquaternium-17 (INCI)
CAS 90624-75-2
Trade names: Mirapol® AD-1

Polyquaternium-22 (INCI)
CAS 53694-17-0
Synonyms: Dimethyldiallyl ammonium chloride/acrylic acid copolymer
Trade names: Merquat® 280

Polyquaternium-24 (INCI)
CAS 107987-23-5
Trade names: Quatrisoft® Polymer LM-200
Trade names containing: BioCare® Polymer HA-24

Polyquaternium-28 (INCI)
Synonyms: Vinylpyrrolidone/methacrylamidopropyl-trimethyl ammonium chloride copolymer
Trade names: Gafquat® HS-100
Trade names containing: Gafquat® HSi

Polyquaternium-29
Trade names: Kytamer® KC; Lexquat® CH

Polyquaternium-31 (INCI)
CAS 136505-02-7
Trade names: Hypan® QT100

Polyquaternium-32 (INCI)
CAS 35429-19-7
Synonyms: Ethanaminium, N,N,N-trimethyl-2-[(2-methyl-1-oxo-2-propenyl)oxy]-, chloride, polymer with 2-propenamide
Trade names containing: Salcare SC92

Polyquaternium-37 (INCI)
CAS 26161-33-1
Trade names containing: Salcare SC95

Polysorbate 20 (INCI)
CAS 9005-64-5 (generic)
Synonyms: POE (20) sorbitan monolaurate; PEG-20 sorbitan laurate; Sorbimacrogol laurate 300
Trade names: Alkamuls® PSML-20; Alkamuls® T-20; Armotan® PML 20; Capmul® POE-L; Crillet 1; Drewmulse® POE-SML; Durfax® 20; Emalex ET-2020; Emsorb® 2720; Emsorb® 6915; Estol SML20 3618; Ethylan® GEL2; Eumulgin® SML 20; Glycosperse® L-20; Hefti ML-55-F; Hetsorb L-20; Hodag PSML-20; Ionet T-20 C; Ixol 2; Laxan-ESL; Liposorb L-20; Lonzest® SML-20; Montanox 20; Montanox 20 DF; Mulsifan RT 141; Nikkol TL-10, TL-10EX; Nissan Nonion LT-221; Norfox® Sorbo T-20; Protasorb L-20; Prox-onic SML-020; Ritabate 20; Sorbax PML-20; Sorbilene L; Sorbilene LH; Sorbon T-20; T-Maz® 20; Tween® 20; Unisorb 20; Witconol™ 2720
Trade names containing: Aldosperse® L L-20; Amisol™ 4135; Amisol™ MS-12 BA; Biron® NLD; Biron® NLY-L-2X AQ; Epidermin Water-Soluble; Eucalyptus-Extract, Water soluble 4786; Herbaliquid Watercress Special; Onymyrrhe; Solubilisant γ2420; Solubilisant γ2428; Soluvit Richter; Vitamin F Water-Soluble CLR

Polysorbate 21 (INCI)
CAS 9005-64-5 (generic)
Synonyms: POE (4) sorbitan monolaurate; PEG-4 sorbitan laurate
Trade names: Crillet 11; Hefti ML-55-F-4; Hetsorb L-4; Hodag PSML-4; Protasorb L-5; Sorbilene L 4; Tween® 21; Unisorb 21
Trade names containing: Amisol™ MS-10

Polysorbate 40 (INCI)
CAS 9005-66-7
Synonyms: POE (20) sorbitan monopalmitate; Sorbimacrogol palmitate 300; Sorbitan, mono-hexadecanoate, poly(oxy-1,2-ethaneidyl) derivs.
Trade names: Crillet 2; Glycosperse® P-20; Hetsorb P-20; Hodag PSMP-20; Ixol 4; Laxan-ESP; Liposorb P-20; Lonzest® SMP-20; Montanox 40; Montanox 40 DF; Nikkol TP-10; Protasorb P-20; Prox-onic SMP-020; Ritabate 40; Sorbax PMP-20; Sorbilene P; T-Maz® 40; Tween® 40; Unisorb 40

Polysorbate 60 (INCI)

CAS 9005-67-8 (generic)
Synonyms: POE (20) sorbitan monostearate; PEG-20 sorbitan stearate; Sorbimacrogol stearate 300
Trade names: Alkamuls® PSMS-20; Alkamuls® T-60; Capmul® POE-S; Crillet 3; Drewmulse® POE-SMS; Durfax® 60; Emsorb® 2728; Estol SMS20 3716; Ethylan® GES6; Eumulgin® SMS 20; Glycosperse® S-20; Hefti MS-55-F; Hetsorb S-20; Hodag PSMS-20; Ixol 6; Laxan-ESS; Liposorb S-20; Lonzest® SMS-20; Montanox 60; Montanox 60 DF; Nikkol TS-10; Protasorb S-20; Prox-onic SMS-020; Ritabate 60; Sorbax PMS-20; Sorbilene S; T-Maz® 60; T-Maz® 60K; Tween® 60; Unisorb 60; Witconol™ 2728
Trade names containing: Amisol™ MS-12 BA; Aquabase N.F.; Brookswax™ P; Brookswax™ R; Crodacol GP; Dispersen-S; Fanwax P; Hodag CSA-102; Lipowax P-SPEC; Lipowax P; Lipowax PR; Macol® CPS; Mazawax® 163R; Mazawax® 163SS; Procol P; Relaxer Conc. No. 2; Relaxer Conc. No. 3; Relaxer Conc. No. 4; Ritachol 5000; Ritachol® 1000; Ritachol® 2000; Ritachol® 3000; Teinowax; Upiwax 163R

Polysorbate 61 (INCI)
CAS 9005-67-8 (generic)
Synonyms: POE (4) sorbitan monostearate; PEG-4 sorbitan stearate
Trade names: Crillet 31; Hetsorb S-4; Hodag PSMS-4; Laxan-ESE; Liposorb S-4; Montanox 61; Sorbilene S 4; T-Maz® 61; Tween® 61; Unisorb 61

Polysorbate 65 (INCI)
CAS 9005-71-4
Synonyms: POE (20) sorbitan tristearate; PEG-20 sorbitan tristearate; Sorbimacrogol tristearate 300
Trade names: Crillet 35; Drewmulse® POE-STS; Glycosperse® TS-20; Hetsorb TS-20; Hodag PSTS-20; Laxan-ESR; Liposorb TS-20; Lonzest® STS-20; Montanox 65; Nikkol TS-30; Prox-onic STS-020; Sorbax PTS-20; Sorbilene TS; T-Maz® 65; Tween® 65; Unisorb 65; Witconol™ 6907

Polysorbate 80 (INCI)
CAS 9005-65-6 (generic); 37200-49-0; 61790-86-1
Synonyms: POE (20) sorbitan monooleate; PEG-20 sorbitan oleate; Sorbimacrogol oleate 300
Trade names: Alkamuls® PSMO-20; Armotan® PMO 20; Crillet 4; Drewmulse® POE-SMO; Durfax® 80; Emalex ET-8020; Emsorb® 2722; Emsorb® 2725; Emsorb® 6900; Estol SMO20 3686; Ethylan® GEO8; Eumulgin® SMO 20; Glycosperse® O-20; Hefti MO-55-F; Hetsorb O-20; Hodag PSMO-20; Incrosorb O-80; Ixol 8; Laxan-ESO; Liposorb O-20; Lonzest® SMO-20; Montanox 80; Montanox 80 DF; Mulsifan RT 146; Nikkol TO-10; Nikkol TO-10M; Norfox® Sorbo T-80; Protasorb O-20; Prox-onic SMO-020; Ritabate 80; Sorbax PMO-20; Sorbilene O; T-Maz® 80; T-Maz® 80K; T-Maz® 80KLM; Tween® 80; Tween® 80K; Unisorb 80; Witconol™ 2722
Trade names containing: Aldosperse® O-20 FG; Base W/O 126; Biosulphur Fluid CLR; Centromix® CPS; Crodalan AWS; Emulmetik 910; Ethoxyol® 1707; Fancol ALA-10; Fancol ALA-15; Ivarbase™ 98; Lanalene 98; Mearlmaid® OL; Myvatex® MSPS; Naturon® 2X IPA; Protalan 98; Ritawax AEO; Solulan® 98

Polysorbate 81 (INCI)
CAS 9005-65-5 (generic)
Synonyms: POE (5) sorbitan monooleate; PEG-5 sorbitan oleate
Trade names: Alkamuls® PSMO-5; Crillet 41; Ethylan®

GEO81; Glycosperse® O-5; Hetsorb O-5; Hodag PSMO-5; Laxan-ESM; Liposorb O-5; Montanox 81; Protasorb O-5; Prox-onic SMO-05; Sorbax PMO-5; Sorbilene O 5; T-Maz® 81; Tween® 81
Trade names containing: Alcolan® 40

Polysorbate 85 (INCI)
CAS 9005-70-3
Synonyms: POE (20) sorbitan trioleate; PEG-20 sorbitan trioleate; Sorbimacrogol trioleate 300
Trade names: Alkamuls® PSTO-20; Alkamuls® T-85; Crillet 45; Ethylan® GPS85; Glycosperse® TO-20; Hefti TO-55-F; Hetsorb TO-20; Hodag PSTO-20; Laxan-EST; Liposorb TO-20; Lonzest® STO-20; Montanox 85; Nikkol TO-30; Protasorb TO-20; Prox-onic STO-020; Sorbanox CO; Sorbax PTO-20; Sorbilene TO; T-Maz® 85; Tween® 85; Unisorb 85; Witconol™ 6903
Trade names containing: Arlatone® B; Carsoquat® CB; Ritaderm®

Polysorbate 80 acetate (INCI)
Synonyms: POE (20) sorbitan monooleate acetate
Trade names containing: Lanalene 97; Solulan® 97

Polystyrene (INCI)
CAS 9003-53-6
Synonyms: PS; Styrene polymer; Ethenylbenzene, homopolymer; Benzene, ethenyl-, homopolymer
Trade names: Lytron 614 Latex
Trade names containing: Polysphere 3000 SP

Polytetrafluoroethylene
CAS 9002-84-0
Synonyms: PTFE, TFE; Tetrafluoroethene homopolymer; Tetrafluoroethylene polymer; Polytetrafluoroethylene resin
Trade names: PTFE-20
Trade names containing: Fomblin® HC/P-04, HC/P-25, HC/P-R; Micropoly 2001; PTFE-19

Polyurethane/acrylate copolymer
Trade names containing: Chronosphere® G; Chronosphere® Planell®; Chronosphere® SAL; Chronosphere® V-AE

Polyurethane prepolymer
Trade names: Hypol® 2000; Hypol® 2002; Hypol® 3000; Hypol® 4000; Hypol® 5000

Polyvinyl acetate (homopolymer) (INCI)
CAS 9003-20-7
Synonyms: PVAc; Acetic acid, ethenyl ester, homopolymer; Acetic acid vinyl ester polymers; Ethenyl acetate, homopolymer
Trade names: Resyn® 28-3307; Vinac® 880

Polyvinyl alcohol (INCI)
CAS 9002-89-5 (super and fully hydrolyzed); EINECS 209-183-3
Synonyms: PVA; PVAL; Ethenol, homopolymer; PVOH
Trade names: Elvanol® 71-30; Elvanol® 75-15; Elvanol® 85–82; Elvanol® 90-50; Elvanol® HV; Vinol 523, 540

Polyvinyl chloride
CAS 9002-86-2; EINECS 208-750-2
Synonyms: PVC; Chloroethene homopolymer; Chloroethylene polymer
Trade names containing: Rohagum® M-335

Polyvinyl laurate (INCI)
Trade names: Mexomere PP

Polyvinylpyrrolidone. *See PVP*

Potash. *See Potassium carbonate*

Potassium
CAS 7440-09-7; EINECS 231-119-8

Trade names containing: Foamtaine SCAB-K

Potassium abietoyl hydrolyzed collagen (INCI)
CAS 68918-77-4
Synonyms: Proteins hydrolyzates reaction prod. with abietoyl chloride, compds. with potassium
Trade names: Lamepon® PA-K; Lamepon® PA-K/NP

Potassium alginate (INCI)
CAS 9005-36-1
Synonyms: Potassium polymannuronate; Alginic acid, potassium salt
Trade names: Kelmar®; Kelmar® Improved; Sobalg FD 200 Series

Potassium ascorbyl tocopheryl phosphate (INCI)
Trade names: EPC-K

Potassium butyl paraben (INCI)
CAS 38566-94-8
Synonyms: Butylparaben, potassium salt; n-Butyl-4-hydroxybenzoate potassium salt
Trade names: Nipabutyl Potassium

Potassium carbonate (INCI)
CAS 584-08-7; EINECS 209-529-3
Synonyms: Carbonic acid, dipotassium salt; Dipotassium carbonate; Potash
Trade names: Unichem POCARB

Potassium caroate (INCI)
Synonyms: Caro's acid, potassium salt
Trade names: Caroat

Potassium caseinate (INCI)
CAS 68131-54-4
Synonyms: Casein, potassium salt
Trade names: Alanate 351

Potassium cetyl phosphate (INCI)
CAS 19035-79-1; EINECS 242-769-1
Synonyms: Phosphoric acid, cetyl ester, potassium salt
Trade names: Amphisol® K; Crodafos CKP

Potassium chloride (INCI)
CAS 7447-40-7; EINECS 231-211-8
Trade names: Unichem KCL; Unichem POCHLOR
Trade names containing: Schercotaine CAB-K; Schercotaine SCAB-KG

Potassium cocamidopropyl hydroxysultaine
Trade names containing: Schercotaine SCAB-K

Potassium cocoate (INCI)
CAS 61789-30-8; EINECS 263-049-9
Synonyms: Potassium coconate; Coconut acid, potassium salt; Fatty acids, coconut oil, potassium salts
Trade names: Mackadet™ 40K; Norfox® 1101; Protachem LP-40
Trade names containing: Akypogene ZA 97 SP; Collagen-CCK-Complex; Emulgade® CL Special; Emulgade® CL; Kelisema Collagen-CCK Complex

Potassium coconate
Trade names: Afdet™ KCS
Trade names containing: Afdet™ WGS

Potassium cocoyl glutamate (INCI)
Trade names: Amisoft CK-11

Potassium cocoyl hydrolyzed collagen (INCI)
CAS 68920-65-0
Synonyms: Acid chlorides, coco, reaction prods. with protein hydrolyzates, potassium salts; Potassium cocoyl hydrolyzed animal protein; Potassium coco-hydrolyzed animal protein
Trade names: Collagen-Cocoate-Complex V 2037; Foam-Coll™ 4C; Lamepon® 4SK; Lamepon® S; Lamepon® S/NP; Liprot CK; May-Tein C; Maypon

4C; Monteine LCK-32; Nikkol CCK-40; Peptein® KC; Promois ECP; Promois ECP-C; Promois ECP-P; Rewotein CPK; Texatein C; Unipro LAN-S
Trade names containing: Foam-Coll™ 5; Lamesoft® 156; Lamesoft® 156/NP; Lamesoft® LMG; Lamesoft® LMG/NP; Olamin® K; Olamin® K/NP

Potassium cocoyl hydrolyzed keratin (INCI)
Trade names: May-Tein KK

Potassium cyanate (INCI)
CAS 590-28-3; EINECS 209-677-9
Trade names containing: Capigen CG

Potassium dimethicone copolyol phosphate (INCI)
Trade names: Pecosil® PS-100K

Potassium DNA (INCI)
Synonyms: DNA, potassium salt
Trade names: Robeco-DNA-K

Potassium ethylparaben (INCI)
CAS 36457-19-9
Synonyms: Ethylparaben, potassium salt; Ethyl-4-hydroxybenzoate potassium salt
Trade names: Nipagin A Potassium

Potassium D-gluconate
CAS 299-27-4; EINECS 206-074-2
Synonyms: D-Gluconic acid potassium salt
Trade names: Gluconal® K

Potassium hydroxide (INCI)
CAS 1310-58-3; EINECS 215-181-3
Synonyms: Caustic potash; Potassium hydrate; Lye
Trade names: Unichem KOHYD

Potassium iodate
CAS 7758-05-6; EINECS 231-831-9
Trade names: Unichem KIO3

Potassium iodide (INCI)
CAS 7681-11-0; EINECS 231-659-4
Trade names: Unichem KI; Unichem KI

Potassium lauroyl collagen amino acids (INCI)
Trade names: Aminofoam C Potassium Salt

Potassium lauroyl hydrolyzed soy protein (INCI)
Trade names: Aminofoam Soya

Potassium lauroyl sarcosinate
Trade names: Nikkol Sarcosinate LK-30

Potassium lauryl hydroxypropyl sulfonate (INCI)
Trade names: Ages 2006K

Potassium lauryl sulfate (INCI)
CAS 4706-78-9; EINECS 225-190-4
Synonyms: Sulfuric acid, monododecyl ester, potassium salt
Trade names: Nikkol KLS; Sulfochem K

Potassium metabisulfite (INCI)
CAS 16731-55-8; EINECS 240-795-3
Synonyms: Disulfurous acid, dipotassium salt; Potassium pyrosulfite; Dipotassium disulfite
Trade names: Uantox PMBS; Uantox POMEBIS

Potassium methylparaben (INCI)
CAS 26112-07-2; EINECS 247-464-2
Synonyms: 4-Hydroxybenzoic acid, methyl ester, potassium salt; Methylparaben, potassium salt
Trade names: Nipagin M Potassium

Potassium octoxynol-12 phosphate (INCI)
CAS 68891-73-6
Trade names containing: Syntran 5002; Syntran 5130; Syntran 5170

Potassium oleate (INCI)
CAS 143-18-0; EINECS 205-590-5

Synonyms: Potassium 9-octadecenoate; Oleic acid, potassium salt
Trade names: Norfox® KO

Potassium PCA (INCI)
CAS 4810-50-8; EINECS 225-373-9
Synonyms: L-Proline, 5-oxo-, monopotassium salt
Trade names: Kalidone®

Potassium phosphate (INCI)
CAS 7778-77-0; EINECS 231-913-4
Synonyms: Potassium phosphate, monobasic
Trade names containing: Afron 22

Potassium propylparaben (INCI)
CAS 84930-16-5
Synonyms: Propylparaben, potassium salt; n-Propyl-4-hydroxybenzoate potassium salt
Trade names: Nipasol M Potassium

Potassium sodium tartrate (INCI)
CAS 6381-59-5; EINECS 206-156-8
Synonyms: Potassium sodium tartrate tetrahydrate; Rochelle salt; Seignette salt
Trade names: Unichem ROSAL

Potassium sorbate (INCI)
CAS 590-00-1; EINECS 246-376-1
Synonyms: 2,4-Hexadienoic acid, potassium salt; Sorbic acid, potassium salt; Potassium 2,4-hexadienoate
Trade names: Tristat K; Unistat K
Trade names containing: Myvatex® 40-06S; Protastat P-211

Potassium stearate (INCI)
CAS 593-29-3; EINECS 209-786-1
Synonyms: Octadecanoic acid, potassium salt; Stearic acid, potassium salt
Trade names: Witco® Potassium Stearate
Trade names containing: Ceral TK; Emulgade® CL Special; Emulgade® CL; Imwitor® 965 K; Imwitor® 965

Potassium tallate (INCI)
CAS 61790-44-1
Synonyms: Tall oil acid, potassium salt
Trade names containing: Akypogene ZA 97 SP

Potassium thiocyanate (INCI)
CAS 333-20-0; EINECS 206-370-1
Synonyms: Thiocyanic acid, potassium salt
Trade names containing: Sebomine SB12

Potassium undecylenoyl hydrolyzed collagen (INCI)
CAS 68951-92-8
Synonyms: Proteins, hydrolsates, reaction prods. with 10-undecenoyl chloride, potassium salts; Potassium undecylenoyl hydrolyzed animal protein
Trade names: Lamepon® UD/NP; Liprot UK; Maypon UD; Promois EUP

Potassium xylene sulfonate (INCI)
Synonyms: Xylene sulfonic acid, potassium salt
Trade names containing: Akypogene ZA 97 SP

Povidone. *See PVP*

PP. *See Polypropylene*

PPG-5
Trade names containing: Hetoxol CAWS

PPG-9 (INCI)
CAS 25322-69-4 (generic)
Synonyms: Polyoxypropylene (9); Polypropylene glycol (9); PPG 400
Trade names: Dow P425; Hodag PPG-400; Unicol P-400; Witconol™ PPG 400

PPG-17 (INCI)
CAS 25322-69-4 (generic)

Synonyms: Polyoxypropylene (17); Polypropylene glycol (12)
Trade names: Dow P1000TB

PPG-20 (INCI)
CAS 25322-69-4 (generic)
Synonyms: Polyoxypropylene (20); Polypropylene glycol (20); PPG 1200
Trade names: Dow P1200; Hodag PPG-1200; Macol® P-1200; Unicol 1200

PPG-26 (INCI)
CAS 25322-69-4 (generic)
Synonyms: Polyoxypropylene (26); Polypropylene glycol (26); PPG 2000
Trade names: Dow P2000; Hodag PPG-2000; Jeffox PPG-2000; Macol® P-2000; Unicol P-2000

PPG-30 (INCI)
CAS 25322-69-4 (generic)
Synonyms: Polyoxypropylene (30); Polypropylene glycol (30); PPG 4000
Trade names: Dow P4000; Hodag PPG-4000; Macol® P-4000; Unicol P-4000

PPG-34 (INCI)
CAS 25322-69-4 (generic)
Synonyms: Polyoxypropylene (34); Polypropylene glycol (34)
Trade names: Witconol™ CD-17

PPG-10 butanediol (INCI)
Trade names: Macol® 57; Probutyl DB-10

PPG-2-buteth-3 (INCI)
CAS 9038-95-3 (generic); 9065-63-8 (generic)
Synonyms: POE (3) POP (2) monobutyl ether; POP (2) POE (3) monobuty ether; Oxirane, methyl, polymer and oxibane, butyl ether
Trade names: Hodag Polyglycol 5055; Ucon® 50-HB-55

PPG-3-buteth-5 (INCI)
CAS 9038-95-3 (generic); 9065-63-8 (generic)
Synonyms: POE (5) POP (3) monobutyl ether; POP (3) POE (5) monobutyl ether
Trade names: Ucon® 50-HB-100

PPG-5-buteth-7 (INCI)
CAS 9038-95-3 (generic); 9065-63-8 (generic); 74623-31-7
Synonyms: POE (7) POP (5) monobutyl ether; POP (5) POE (6) monobutyl ether
Trade names: Ucon® 50-HB-170

PPG-7-buteth-10 (INCI)
CAS 9038-95-3 (generic); 9065-63-8 (generic)
Trade names: Ucon® 50-HB-260

PPG-9-buteth-12 (INCI)
CAS 9038-95-3 (generic); 9065-63-8 (generic)
Synonyms: POE (12) POP (9) monobutyl ether; POP (9) POE (12) monobutyl ether
Trade names: Ucon® 50-HB-400

PPG-12-buteth-16 (INCI)
CAS 9038-95-3 (generic); 9065-63-8 (generic); 74623-31-7
Synonyms: POE (16) POP (12) monobutyl ether; POP (12) POE (16) monobutyl ether
Trade names: Hodag Polyglycol 5066; Ucon® 50-HB-660

PPG-20-buteth-30 (INCI)
CAS 9038-95-3 (generic); 9065-63-8 (generic)
Synonyms: POE (30) POP (20) monobutyl ether; POP (20) POE (30) monobutyl ether
Trade names: Ucon® 50-HB-2000

PPG-26 buteth-26 (INCI)
CAS 9038-95-3 (generic); 9065-63-8 (generic)
Synonyms: POE (26) POP (26) monobutyl ether; POP (26) POE (26) monobutyl ether
Trade names: Witconol™ APEB
Trade names containing: Solubiliser LRI

PPG-28-buteth-35 (INCI)
CAS 9038-95-3 (generic); 9065-63-8 (generic)
Synonyms: POE (35) POP (28) monobutyl ether; POP (28) POE (35) monobutyl ether
Trade names: Hodag Polyglycol 5035; Pluracol® W3520N; Ucon® 50-HB-3520

PPG-33-buteth-45 (INCI)
CAS 9038-95-3 (generic); 9065-63-8 (generic)
Synonyms: POE (45) POP (33) monobutyl ether; POP (33) POE (45) monobutyl ether
Trade names: Hodag Polyglycol 5051; Pluracol® W5100N; Ucon® 50-HB-5100

PPG-3 butyl ether
Trade names: Nissan Unilube MB-38

PPG-5 butyl ether (INCI)
CAS 9003-13-8 (generic)
Synonyms: POP (5) butyl ether
Trade names: Ucon® LB-65

PPG-9 butyl ether (INCI)
CAS 9003-13-8 (generic)
Synonyms: POP (9) butyl ether
Trade names: Ucon® LB-135

PPG-14 butyl ether (INCI)
CAS 9003-13-8 (generic)
Synonyms: POP (14) butyl ether
Trade names: Dow L910; Fluid AP; Probutyl 14; Ucon® Fluid AP; Witconol™ APB

PPG-15 butyl ether (INCI)
CAS 9003-13-8 (generic)
Synonyms: POP (15) butyl ether
Trade names: Hodag PB-285; Ucon® LB-285

PPG-16 butyl ether (INCI)
CAS 9003-13-8 (generic)
Synonyms: POP (16) butyl ether
Trade names: Hodag PB-300

PPG-18 butyl ether (INCI)
CAS 9003-13-8 (generic)
Synonyms: POP (18) butyl ether; PPG (18) butyl ether
Trade names: Dow L1150; Ucon® LB-385

PPG-22 butyl ether (INCI)
CAS 9003-13-8 (generic)
Synonyms: POP (22) butyl ether
Trade names: Ucon® LB-525

PPG-24 butyl ether (INCI)
CAS 9003-13-8 (generic)
Synonyms: POP (24) butyl ether; PPG (24) butyl ether
Trade names: Hodag PB-625; Ucon® LB-625

PPG-33 butyl ether (INCI)
CAS 9003-13-8 (generic)
Synonyms: POP (33) butyl ether; PPG (33) butyl ether
Trade names: Ucon® LB-1145

PPG-40 butyl ether (INCI)
CAS 9003-13-8 (generic)
Synonyms: POP (40) butyl ether; PPG (40) butyl ether
Trade names: Hodag PB-1715; Ucon® LB-1715; Unilube MB-370

PPG-53 butyl ether (INCI)
CAS 9003-13-8 (generic)
Synonyms: POP (53) butyl ether; PPG (53) butyl ether

Trade names: Ucon® LB-3000

PPG-2-ceteareth-9 (INCI)
Synonyms: POE (9) POP (2) cetyl/stearyl ether; POP (2) POE (9) cetyl/stearyl ether
Trade names: Eumulgin® L; Unichol EUM-L

PPG-4 ceteth-1 (INCI)
CAS 9087-53-0 (generic); 37311-01-6 (generic)
Synonyms: POE (1) POP (4) cetyl ether; POP (4) POE (1) cetyl ether
Trade names: Nikkol PBC-31

PPG-4-ceteth-10 (INCI)
CAS 9087-53-0 (generic); 37311-01-6 (generic)
Synonyms: POE (10) POP (4) cethyl ether
Trade names: Nikkol PBC-33

PPG-4-ceteth-20 (INCI)
CAS 9087-53-0 (generic); 37311-01-6 (generic)
Synonyms: POE (20) POP (4) cetyl ether
Trade names: Nikkol PBC-34

PPG-5-ceteth-20 (INCI)
CAS 9087-53-0 (generic); 37311-01-6 (generic)
Synonyms: POE (20) POP (5) cetyl ether; POP (5) POE (20) cetyl ether
Trade names: Brox AWS; Procetyl AWS
Trade names containing: Crodapearl NI Liquid

PPG-8-ceteth-1 (INCI)
CAS 9087-53-0 (generic); 37311-01-6 (generic)
Synonyms: POE (1) POP (8) cetyl ether; POP (8) POE (1) cetyl ether
Trade names: Nikkol PBC-41

PPG-8-ceteth-20 (INCI)
CAS 9087-53-0 (generic); 37311-01-6 (generic)
Synonyms: POE (20) POP (8) cetyl ether; POP (8) POE (20) cetyl ether
Trade names: Nikkol PBC-44

PPG-5 ceteth-10 phosphate (INCI)
CAS 50643-20-4
Synonyms: POE (10) POP (5) cetyl ether phosphate; POP (5) POE (10) cetyl ether phosphate
Trade names: Brophos™ 5C10; Crodafos SG; Hetphos SG; Mayphos 5C10

PPG-10 cetyl ether (INCI)
CAS 9035-85-2 (generic)
Synonyms: POP (10) cetyl ether; PPG (10) cetyl ether
Trade names: Acconon CA 10; Carsonon® 169-P; Procetyl 10

PPG-30 cetyl ether (INCI)
CAS 9035-85-2 (generic)
Synonyms: POP (30) cetyl ether; PPG (30) cetyl ether
Trade names: Fancol 707; Macol® CA 30P; Procetyl 30; Wickenol® 707

PPG-50 cetyl ether (INCI)
CAS 9035-85-2 (generic)
Synonyms: POP (50) cetyl ether; PPG (50) cetyl ether
Trade names: Procetyl 50

PPG-10 cetyl ether phosphate (INCI)
CAS 111019-03-5
Synonyms: POP (10) cetyl ether phosphate
Trade names: Crodafos CAP

PPG-4 deceth-4 (INCI)
Trade names containing: Genapol® PGL

PPG-6-decyltetradeceth-12 (INCI)
Synonyms: POE (12) POP (6) decyltetradecyl ether; POP (6) POE (12) decyltetradecyl ether
Trade names: Nikkol PEN-4612

PPG-6-decyltetradeceth-20 (INCI)
Synonyms: POE (20) POP (6) decyltetradecyl ether; POP (6) POE (20) decyltetradecyl ether
Trade names: Nikkol PEN-4620

PPG-6-decyltetradeceth-30 (INCI)
Synonyms: POE (30) POP (6) decyltetradecyl ether; POP (6) POE (30) decyltetradecyl ether
Trade names: Nikkol PEN-4630

PPG-20-decyltetradeceth-10 (INCI)
Synonyms: POE (10) POP (20) decyltetradecyl ether; POP (20) POE (10) decyltetradecyl ether
Trade names: S-Safe 2010

PPG-9 diethylmonium chloride (INCI)
CAS 9042-76-6
Synonyms: POP (9) methyl diethyl ammonium chloride; Quaternium-6
Trade names: Emcol® CC-9

PPG-25 diethylmonium chloride (INCI)
Synonyms: POP (25) methyl diethyl ammonium chloride; Quaternium-20
Trade names: Emcol® CC-36

PPG-40 diethylmonium chloride (INCI)
CAS 9076-43-1
Synonyms: POP (40) methyl diethyl ammonium chloride; Quaternium-21
Trade names: Emcol® CC-42

PPG-17 dioleate (INCI)
CAS 26571-49-3 (generic)
Synonyms: POP (17) dioleate
Trade names: CPH-327-N

PPG-24-glycereth-24 (INCI)
CAS 51258-15-2 (generic); 9082-00-2
Synonyms: PEG/PPG-24/24 glycerin; POE (24) POP (24) glyceryl ether; POP (24) POE (24) glyceryl ether
Trade names: Adeka GH-200; Dow 15-200

PPG-66-glycereth-12 (INCI)
CAS 51258-15-2 (generic)
Trade names: Dow 112-2

PPG-10 glyceryl ether (INCI)
CAS 25791-96-2
Trade names: Dow PT700

PPG-27 glyceryl ether (INCI)
CAS 25791-96-2 (generic); EINECS 247-144-2
Trade names: Witconol™ CD-18

PPG-55 glyceryl ether (INCI)
CAS 25791-96-2 (generic)
Synonyms: POP (55) glyceryl ether
Trade names: Dow PT3000; Witconol™ CC-43

PPG-3 hydrogenated castor oil (INCI)
Synonyms: POP (3) hydrogenated castor oil
Trade names: Hetester HCP

PPG-2 isoceteth-20 acetate (INCI)
CAS 110332-91-7
Synonyms: Dipropylene glycol isoceteth-20 acetate
Trade names: CUPL® PIC

PPG-3-isosteareth-9 (INCI)
Synonyms: POE (9) POP (3) isostearyl ether; POP (3) POE (9) isostearyl ether; PEG-9-PPG-3 isostearyl ether
Trade names: Arosurf® 66-PE12

PPG-2 lanolin alcohol ether (INCI)
CAS 68439-53-2 (generic)
Synonyms: POP (2) lanolin ether; PPG (2) lanolin ether; PPG-2 lanolin ether

Trade names: Solulan® PB-2

PPG-5 lanolin alcohol ether (INCI)
CAS 68439-53-2 (generic)
Synonyms: POP (5) lanolin ether; PPG (5) lanolin ether;
PPG-5 lanolin ether
Trade names: Solulan® PB-5

PPG-10 lanolin alcohol ether (INCI)
CAS 68439-53-2 (generic)
Synonyms: POP (10) lanolin ether; PPG (10) lanolin
ether; PPG-10 lanolin ether
Trade names: Solulan® PB-10

PPG-20 lanolin alcohol ether (INCI)
CAS 68439-53-2 (generic)
Synonyms: POP (20) lanolin ether; PPG (20) lanolin
ether; PPG-20 lanolin ether
Trade names: Solulan® PB-20

PPG-30 lanolin alcohol ether (INCI)
CAS 68439-53-2 (generic)
Synonyms: POP (30) lanolin ether; PPG (30) lanolin
ether; PPG-30 lanolin ether
Trade names: Hetoxol PLA; Wickenol® 727

PPG-5 lanolin wax (INCI)
Synonyms: POP (5) lanolin wax
Trade names: Unicol Propox 1695

PPG-5 lanolin wax glyceride (INCI)
Synonyms: POP (5) lanolin wax glyceride
Trade names: Propoxyol® 1695

PPG-3-laureth-9 (INCI)
Synonyms: POE (9) POP (3) lauryl ether; POP (3) POE
(9) lauryl ether
Trade names: Acconon 1300

PPG-5-laureth-5 (INCI)
Synonyms: POE (5) POP (5) lauryl ether; POP (5) POE
(5) lauryl ether
Trade names: Aethoxal® B; Unicol AETH-8

PPG-25-laureth-25 (INCI)
CAS 37311-00-5
Synonyms: POE (25) POP (25) lauryl ether; POP (25)
POE (25) lauryl ether
Trade names: ADF Oleile

PPG-10 methyl glucose ether (INCI)
CAS 61849-72-7
Synonyms: POP (10) methyl glucose ether; PPG (10)
methyl glucose ether
Trade names: Glucam® P-10

PPG-20 methyl glucose ether (INCI)
CAS 61849-72-7
Synonyms: POP (20) methyl glucose ether; PPG (20)
methyl glucose ether
Trade names: Glucam® P-20; Prox-onic MG-020 P

PPG-20 methyl glucose ether distearate (INCI)
Synonyms: PPG-20 methyl glucoside distearate; POP
(20) methyl glucose ether distearate; PPG (20) methyl glucose ether distearate
Trade names: Glucam® P-20 Distearate

PPG-3-myreth-3 (INCI)
CAS 37311-04-9 (generic)
Trade names: Witconol™ APEM

PPG-3 myristyl ether (INCI)
CAS 63793-60-2 (generic)
Synonyms: Tripropylene glycol myristyl ether; POP (3)
myristyl ether; PPG (3) myristyl ether
Trade names: Acconon MA3; Carsonon® 144-P; Hetoxol
MP-3; Procol PMA-3; Promyristyl PM-3; Witconol™
APM

PPG-2 myristyl ether propionate (INCI)
Synonyms: POP (2) myristyl ether propionate; PPG (2)
myristyl ether propionate
Trade names: Crodamol PMP

PPG-26 oleate (INCI)
CAS 31394-71-5 (generic)
Synonyms: POP (26) monooleate; PPG (26) monooleate
Trade names: Hodag CSA-80; Lutrol® OP 2000

PPG-36 oleate (INCI)
CAS 31394-71-5 (generic)
Synonyms: POP (36) monooleate; PPG (36) monooleate
Trade names: Witconol™ F2646

PPG-10 oleyl ether (INCI)
CAS 52581-71-2 (generic)
Synonyms: POP (10) oleyl ether; PPG (10) oleyl ether
Trade names: Hodag CSA-91

PPG-50 oleyl ether (INCI)
CAS 52581-71-2 (generic)
Synonyms: POP (50) oleyl ether; PPG (50) oleyl ether
Trade names: Provol 50

PPG-2-PEG-6 coconut oil esters (INCI)
Trade names: Colan 32

PPG-12-PEG-50 lanolin (INCI)
CAS 68458-88-8 (generic)
Synonyms: POE (50) POP (12) lanolin; POP (12) POE
(50) lanolin
Trade names: Hetlan AWS; Ivarlan™ 3420; Laneto AWS;
Lanexol AWS; Lanoil AWS

PPG-12-PEG-65 lanolin oil (INCI)
CAS 68458-58-8 (generic)
Synonyms: POE (65) POP (12) lanolin oil; POP (12) POE
(65) lanolin oil
Trade names: Fluilan AWS; Ivarlan™ AWS; Lantrol®
AWS 1692; Ritalan® AWS; Unilaneth PPG-12-PEG-
65; Vigilan AWS
Trade names containing: Colla-Moist™ WS; Lanotein
AWS 30; Proto-Lan 30

PPG-40-PEG-60 lanolin oil (INCI)
Synonyms: POE (60) POP (40) lanolin oil; POP (40) POE
(60) lanolin oil
Trade names: Aqualose LL100

PPG-24-PEG-21 tallowaminopropylamine (INCI)
Trade names: Cartafix U

PPG-5 pentaerythrityl ether (INCI)
Synonyms: POP (5) pentaerythritol ether; POP (5) pen-
taerythrityl ether
Trade names: PME
Trade names containing: Lanolide; Seboside

PPG-2 salicylate. See *Dipropylene glycol salicylate*

PPG-12/SMDI copolymer (INCI)
CAS 9042-82-4
Synonyms: Poly[oxy(methyl-1,2-ethanediyl)], α-hydro-
ω-hydroxy-, polymer with 1,1′-methylenebis[4-
isocyanatocyclohexane]
Trade names: Polyolprepolymer-2

PPG-9-steareth-3 (INCI)
CAS 9038-43-1 (generic)
Synonyms: POE (3) POP (9) stearyl ether; POP (9) POE
(3) stearyl ether
Trade names: Witconol™ APES

PPG-11 stearyl ether (INCI)
CAS 25231-21-4 (generic)
Synonyms: POP (11) stearyl ether; PPG (11) stearyl
ether
Trade names: Arlamol® F; Hodag CSA-70; Procol PSA-

11; Witconol™ APS

PPG-15 stearyl ether (INCI)
CAS 25231-21-4 (generic)
Synonyms: POP (15) stearyl ether; PPG (15) stearyl ether
Trade names: Acconon E; Arlamol® E; Fancol SA-15; Hetoxol SP-15; Hodag CSA-75; Procol PSA-15
Trade names containing: Arlamol® S3, S7

PPG-15 stearyl ether benzoate (INCI)
Synonyms: POP (15) stearyl ether benzoate
Trade names: Finsolv® P

PPG-7/succinic acid copolymer (INCI)
Trade names: Cosmol 102

PPG-1 trideceth-6 (INCI)
Trade names containing: Salcare SC91; Salcare SC95

Precipitated silica. *See Silica, hydrated*

Procollagen (INCI)
Trade names: Solu-Coll™ P

Proline (INCI)
CAS 147-85-3 (L-form); EINECS 205-702-2
Synonyms: L-Proline; 2-Pyrrolidine carboxylic acid
Trade names containing: Hydro-Diffuser Microreservoir; Monteine PRO; Prodew 100; Prodew 200

Propane (INCI)
CAS 74-98-6; EINECS 200-827-9
Synonyms: Dimethylmethane; Propyl hydride
Trade names containing: Drivosol®

Propionic acid
CAS 79-09-4; EINECS 201-176-3
Synonyms: Methylacetic acid; Propanoic acid; Ethylformic acid
Trade names containing: Myvatex® SSH

Propionyl collagen amino acids (INCI)
Trade names: Lipacide C3CO

Propyl carbinol. *See Butyl alcohol*

Propylene alginate
Trade names: Unigum PGA

Propylene carbonate (INCI)
CAS 108-32-7; EINECS 203-572-1
Synonyms: 1,3-Dioxolan-2-one, 4-methyl; 4-Methyl-1,3-dioxolan-2-one; Carbonic acid, 1,2-propylene glycol ester
Trade names containing: Bentone® Gel CAO; Bentone® Gel IPM; Bentone® Gel ISD; Bentone® Gel LOI; Bentone® Gel M20; Bentone® Gel MIO; Bentone® Gel SS71; Bentone® Gel TN; Bentone® Gel VS-5 PC; Miglyol® 840 Gel B; Miglyol® 840 Gel T; Miglyol® Gel B; Miglyol® Gel T; Softisan® Gel; Tixogel FTN; Tixogel IPM; Tixogel LAN; Tixogel OMS; Tixogel VSP

Propylene glycol (INCI)
CAS 57-55-6; EINECS 200-338-0
Synonyms: 1,2-Propanediol; 1,2-Dihydroxypropane; Methyl glycol
Trade names: Adeka Propylene Glycol (P); Unichem PROP-G
Trade names containing: Acacia Flower Extract HS 2744 G; Acacia Glycolysat; Acerola Extract HS 2855 G; Actiphyte of Acacia; Actiphyte of Alfalfa; Actiphyte of Almond; Actiphyte of Aloe Vera 10-Fold; Actiphyte of Aloe Vera 20-Fold; Actiphyte of Aloe Vera 40-Fold; Actiphyte of Aloe Vera; Actiphyte of Apple Leaves; Actiphyte of Apple Pectin; Actiphyte of Apricot Fruit; Actiphyte of Apricot Leaves; Actiphyte of Arbutus; Actiphyte of Arnica; Actiphyte of Arrowroot; Actiphyte of Avocado Fruit; Actiphyte of Avocado Leaves;

Actiphyte of Balm Mint; Actiphyte of Basil; Actiphyte of Bee Pollen; Actiphyte of Black Walnut; Actiphyte of Bran; Actiphyte of Calendula; Actiphyte of Capsicum; Actiphyte of Chamomile; Actiphyte of Chaparral; Actiphyte of Chrysanthemum; Actiphyte of Cinnamon; Actiphyte of Coconut; Actiphyte of Comfrey; Actiphyte of Coriander; Actiphyte of Cornsilk; Actiphyte of Eucalyptus; Actiphyte of Flax Seed; Actiphyte of Garlic; Actiphyte of Ginseng; Actiphyte of Goldenseal; Actiphyte of Henna; Actiphyte of Honeysuckle; Actiphyte of Hops; Actiphyte of Irish Moss; Actiphyte of Jojoba Meal; Actiphyte of Lavender; Actiphyte of Lemon Juice; Actiphyte of Lemon Peel; Actiphyte of Malt; Actiphyte of Marigold; Actiphyte of Meadowsweet; Actiphyte of Oat Bran; Actiphyte of Oat Flour; Actiphyte of Olive Leaves; Actiphyte of Orange Bioflavonoids; Actiphyte of Pennyroyal; Actiphyte of Peppermint; Actiphyte of Rice Bran; Actiphyte of Rose Hips; Actiphyte of Rose; Actiphyte of Royal Jelly; Actiphyte of St. John's Wort; Actiphyte of Tansy; Actiphyte of Wheat Germ; Actiphyte of Wheat; Actiphyte of Wintergreen; Actiphyte of Witch Hazel; Aerosol® OT-70 PG; Aftershave HS 292; Agave Extract HS 2817 G; Alder Buckthorn HS; Alfalfa Herb Extract HS 2967 G; Aloe Extract HS 2386 G; Aloe Extract Special; Aloe Flower Extract PG; Aloe HS; Aminoefaderma; Amisol™ 406-N; Amisol™ HS-2; Amisol™ HS-3 US; Amisol™ HS-6; Amisol Nail Strengthener; Angelica HS; Anise Seed Extract HS 2712 G; Antex-MP; Antex-MPD; Antil® 141 Liq.; Antil® 208; Antiphlogistic ARO; Apple Extract HS 1806 AT; Apple HS; Apricot Extract HS 2509 G; Apricot Glycolysat; Aqua-Tein S; Arlacel® 186; Arnica Extract HS 2397 G; Arnica HS; Aromaphyte of Almond; Aromaphyte of Chamomile; Aromaphyte of Orange; Aromaphyte of Peppermint; Asebiol® LS; Atmos 300; ATP Nucleotides; Avocado Extract HS 2384 G; Awapuhi Extract; Babyderme HS 265; Babyderme HS 342; Balm Mint HS; Biobranil Watersoluble 2/012600; Biodermine; Biophytex®; Bioplex™ RNA; Bitter Almond HS; Blanc Covasop W 9775; Blend For Bust Cares HS 201; Blend For Chapped Skins HS 361; Blend For Delicate Skins HS 215; Blend For Deodorant HS 275; Blend For Elderly Skins HS 296; Blend For Greasy Hair HS 312; Blend For Greasy Skin Imperfections HS 315; Blend For Slenderizing Prods. HS 255; Bleu Covasop W 6776; Bovine Amniotic Liq.; Bronidox® L 5; Bronidox® L; Bronodox L-5; Broom Glycolysat; Broom HS; Broom Tops Extract HS 2645 G; Brophos™ OL-3NPG; Capigen CS; Capilotonique HS 220; Capilotonique HS 226; Capilotonique HS 245; Capisome; Carob HS; Carrots Extract HS 2597 G; Cellulinol; Ceraphyl® 70; Ceraphyl® 85; Chamomile Extract HS 2382 G; Chamomile Extract HS 2779 G; Chitomarine; Circulatory Blend HS 318; Colla-Moist™ WS; Collamino™ Complex ESC; Collamino™ Complex S; Collamino™ Complex SS; Collamino™ Complex; Complex GT; Complex NR; Complex Relax; Complexe AST 1; Complexe AV.a.; Coobato Camomilla; Coobato Hamamelis; Coobato Speciale; Corn Silk Extract HS 2969 G; Cremogen AF; Cremogen Aloe Vera; Cremogen Camomile Forte; Cremogen Chamomile 739012; Cremogen Hamamelis 739008; Cremogen M-I 739001; Cremogen Pine Needles 739007; Cremogen Yarrow 739017; Cremophor® RH 455; Crodarom Chamomile A; Crystallin Protein; Dandelion HS; Dehymuls® F; Delan 62; Demaquillant HS 287; Deo-Usnate; Dermascreen; Dermonectin; Dicopamine DP; DNA Marine; Dow Corning® 7224

Conditioning Agent; Dow Corning® Q2-7224 Conditioning Additive; Elastin PG 2000; Emid® 6590; Emollient HS 235; Emollient HS 238; Emulmetik™ 310; Endonucleine LS 2143; ES-1239; Ethoxol 44M; Eucalyptus HS; Eucalyptus Leaves Extract HS 2646 G; Euperlan® PL 1000; Extan-GO; Extract Arnica Special; Extrapone Arnica Special 2/032591; Extrapone Bio-Tamin Special 2/2032671; Extrapone Chamomile Special 2/033021; Extrapone Coco-Nut Special 2/033055; Extrapone Hamamelis Super 2/500010; Extrapone Poly H Special 2/032451; Fancol Gingko Extract; Fo-Ti 5:1 PG; Foamquat CHP; Fondix G Bis; Garlic Extract HS 2710 G; Gemtex PA-70P; Gemtex PA-85P; Germaben® II; Germaben® II-E; Geropon® 99; Ginseng Extract HS 2457 G; Ginseng Glycolysat; Ginseng HS; Glycolysat de camomille; Glycolysat de ginseng; Glycolysat de Houblon; Glycolysat de placenta bovin; Granoliq. Wheat Germ Extract, Water soluble; Grillocin® AT Basis; Grillocin® CW 90; GU-61-A; Gu-61-Standard; Haircomplex AKS; Hamamelis Extract HS 2456 G; Herbalcomplex 1 Special; Herbalcomplex 2 Special; Herbaliquid Alpine Herbs Special; Herbaliquid Camomile Special; Herbaliquid Hops Special; Herbaliquid Rosemary Special; Herbaliquid Watercress Special; Herbasol 7 Herb Complex; Herbasol Alpine Herbs Complex; Herbasol Complex A; Herbasol Complex B; Herbasol Complex C; Herbasol Complex D; Herbasol Complex E; Herbasol Extract Walnut Shell Water-Sol; Herbasol Herbes de Provence Complex; Herbasol Sedative Complex; Herbasol Stimulant Complex; Herbasol-Extract Algae; Herbasol-Extract Almond; Herbasol-Extract Aloe; Herbasol-Extract Arnica; Herbasol-Extract Balm Mint; Herbasol-Extract Calendula; Herbasol-Extract Eucalyptus; Herbasol-Extract Ginseng; Herbasol-Extract Hamemelis; Herbasol-Extract Ivy; Herbasol-Extract Marigold; Herbasol-Extract Peppermint; Herbasol-Extract St. John's Wort; Herbasol-Extract Yarrow; Hops Extract HS 2367 G; Hops HS; Hops Malt Extract HS 2518 G; Hydratherm CGI Glycolic; Hydrocotyl Glycolysat; Hydrocotyl HS; Hydromarine; Hydrumine Calendula; Hydrumine Witchazel; Ichtyocollagene; Incense HS; Incroquat Behenyl BDQ/P; Incroquat Behenyl TMC/P; Jaune Covasop W 1771; Jeltex; Jodoprolamina; Kalokiros HS 263; Laminarina; Lanotein AWS 30; Lanpro-10; Lemon Extract HS 2364 G; Lemon HS; Lipo PE Base GP-55; Liposome Centella; Liposome Unsapo KM; Lipostim; Lubrajel® CG, DV, MS, TW; Mackam™ 2CSF-70; Mackam™ 2MCAS; Mackstat® DM-PG; Miracare® 2MCAS; Miracare® XL; Miranol® C2M Conc. NP-PG; Monamid® R31-42; Monawet MO-70R; Monawet MO-84R2W; Natipide® II PG; Nipaguard® MPS; Nipanox® S-1; Nipanox® Special; Nutriderme HS 210; Nutriderme HS 240; Nutriderme HS 243; Nutriderme HS 313; Nutrimarine; Oligoceane; Oxylastil; Oxynex® 2004; Paragon™ II; Paragon™; Perlglanzmittel GM 4175; Phosal 25 PG; Phosal® 60 PG; Phosal® NAT-50-PG; Phytoderm Complex G; Promarine; Proto-Lan 20; Proto-Lan 30; Regederme HS 236; Regederme HS 330; Relaxant HS 278; Rhodaterge® SSB; Rhumacalm HS 328; Schercopol DOS-70; Schercopol DOS-PG-70; Sedermasome; Solarium HS 269; Solarium HS 270; Stabolec C; Standamid® LD 80/20; Standapol® CAT; Standapol® Pearl Conc. 7130; Stimulant HS 280; Stimulant HS 285; Surfactol® Q1; Surfactol® Q2; Surfactol® Q3; Sustane® 3; Syntran 5002; Syntran 5130; Syntran 5170; Syntran KL-219; Tagat® R63; Tenox® 2; Tenox® 20B; Tenox® 22; Tenox® 25;

Tenox® 26; Tenox® 6; Tepescohuite AMI Water-soluble; Tepescohuite HG; Tepescohuite HS; Tonique HS 290; Transparent Titanium Dioxide PW Covasop; Trichogen; Uantox 20; Uantox 3; Uantox W-1; Uninontan U 34; Varisoft® 110-PG; Varisoft® 222 PG (90%); Varisoft® 222 PG (90%); Varisoft® 432-PPG; Varisoft® PIMS; Westchlor® A2Z 8106; Zetesol AP

Propylene glycol alginate (INCI)
CAS 9005-37-2
Synonyms: Hydroxypropyl alginate; Alginic acid, ester with 1,2-propanediol
Trade names: Kelcoloid® D; Kelcoloid® DH, DO, DSF; Kelcoloid® HVF, LVF, O, S
Trade names containing: Ches® 500

Propylene glycol caprylate (INCI)
CAS 31565-12-5
Synonyms: Caprylic acid, monoester with 1,2-propanediol
Trade names: Imwitor® 408; Nikkol Sefsol 218

Propylene glycol ceteth-3 acetate (INCI)
CAS 93385-03-6
Synonyms: Propylene glycol PEG (3) cetyl ether acetate
Trade names: Hetester PCA

Propylene glycol ceteth-3 propionate (INCI)
Synonyms: Propylene glycol PEG (3) cetyl ether propionate
Trade names: Hetester PCP

Propylene glycol citrate (INCI)
Trade names containing: Arrectosina

Propylene glycol dicaprylate (INCI)
CAS 7384-98-7; EINECS 230-962-9
Synonyms: Octanoic acid, 1-methyl-1,2-ethanediyl ester
Trade names: Crodamol PC; Nikkol Sefsol 228

Propylene glycol dicaprylate/dicaprate (INCI)
CAS 9062-04-8; 58748-27-9; 68583-51-7; 68988-72-7
Synonyms: Decanoic acid, 1-methyl-1,2-ethanediyl ester mixed with 1-methyl-1,2-ethanediyl dioctanoate
Trade names: Aldo® DC; Captex® 200; Edenol 302; Estol 1526; Estol PDCC 1526; Hodag CC-22; Hodag CC-22-S; Lexol® PG-855; Lexol® PG-865; Liponate PC; Miglyol® 840; Myritol® PC; Neobee® 20; Neobee® M-20; Unitolate 302; Unitolate 380
Trade names containing: Acacia Oleat M; Bentone® Gel M20; Broom Oleat M; Ginseng Oleat M; Hops Oleat M; Hydrocotyl Oleat M; Miglyol® 840 Gel B; Miglyol® 840 Gel T; Miglyol® 840 Gel

Propylene glycol didecanoate
Trade names: Nikkol PDD

Propylene glycol diisononanoate (INCI)
Synonyms: Isononanoic acid, 1-methyl-1,2-ethanediyl ester
Trade names: Liponate L

Propylene glycol diisostearate (INCI)
Synonyms: Isooctadecanoic acid, 1,3-propanediyl ester
Trade names: Emalex PG-di-IS; Prisorine PDIS 2035

Propylene glycol dilaurate (INCI)
CAS 22788-19-8; EINECS 245-217-3
Trade names: Emalex PG-di-L

Propylene glycol dioctanoate (INCI)
CAS 7384-98-7; 56519-71-2
Synonyms: 2-Ethylhexanoic acid, 1-methyl-1,2-ethanediyl ester; Octanoic acid, 1,3-propanediyl ester
Trade names: Captex® 800; Lexol® PG-800

Propylene glycol dioleate (INCI)
CAS 105-62-4; 85049-34-9; EINECS 203-315-3; 285-203-4
Trade names: Cithrol PGDO; Emalex PG-di-O; Radia® 7204

Propylene glycol dipelargonate (INCI)
CAS 41395-83-9; EINECS 255-350-9
Synonyms: Propylene glycol dinonanoate; Nonanoic acid, 1-methyl-1,2-ethanediyl ester
Trade names: D.P.P.G; Emerest® 2388; Estol PDP 3601; Lexol® PG-900; Schercemol PGDP; Unitolate PG/DPG

Propylene glycol distearate (INCI)
CAS 6182-11-2; EINECS 228-229-3
Synonyms: Octadecanoic acid, 1-methyl-1,2-ethanediyl ester
Trade names: Emalex PG-di-S

Propylene glycol hydroxystearate (INCI)
CAS 33907-47-0; EINECS 251-734-5
Synonyms: Octadecanoic acid, 12-hydroxy-, monoester with 1,2-propanediol
Trade names: Naturechem® PGHS

Propylene glycol isoceteth-3 acetate (INCI)
CAS 93385-13-8
Synonyms: Propylene glycol PEG (3) isocetyl ether acetate
Trade names: Hetester PHA

Propylene glycol isostearate (INCI)
CAS 68171-38-0; EINECS 269-027-5
Synonyms: Propylene glycol monoisostearate; Isooctadecanoic acid, monoester with 1,2-propanediol
Trade names: Emerest® 2384; Emerest® 2389; Hydrophilol ISO; Prisorine PMIS 2034; Unitolate PGIST; Witconol™ 2384
Trade names containing: Hydrolactol 70; Hydrolactol 93

Propylene glycol laurate (INCI)
CAS 142-55-2; 27194-74-7; EINECS 205-542-3
Synonyms: Dodecanoic acid, 2-hydroxypropyl ester; Dodecanoic acid, monoester with 1,2-propanediol; Propylene glycol monolaurate
Trade names: Cithrol PGML N/E; Emalex PGML; Hodag PGML; Imwitor® 412; Kessco PGML-X533; Kessco® PGML-X533; Kessco® Propylene Glycol Monolaurate E; Laurate de Propylene Glycol; Lauroglycol; Rol LP; Schercemol PGML; Unipeg-PGML
Trade names containing: Amisol™ 4135

Propylene glycol laurate SE
Trade names: Cithrol PGML S/E

Propylene glycol linoleate (INCI)
Synonyms: Linoleic acid, monoester with 1,2-propanediol
Trade names containing: Efevit E

Propylene glycol linolenate (INCI)
Trade names containing: Efevit E

Propylene glycol methyl ether. See Methoxyisopropanol

Propylene glycol methyl ether acetate
CAS 108-65-6
Synonyms: PM acetate
Trade names: Ektasolve® PM Acetate

Propylene glycol myristate (INCI)
CAS 29059-24-3; EINECS 249-395-3
Synonyms: Propylene glycol monomyristate; Tetradecanoic acid, monoester with 1,2-propanediol
Trade names: Cithrol PGMM; Kessco PGNM; Radiasurf® 7196

Propylene glycol myristyl ether acetate (INCI)
Synonyms: PPG-1 myristyl ether acetate
Trade names: Hetester PMA

Propylene glycol oleate (INCI)
CAS 1330-80-9; EINECS 215-549-3
Synonyms: 9-Octadecenoic acid, monoester with 1,2-propanediol
Trade names: Cithrol PGMO N/E; CPH-3-SE; Emalex PGO; Radiasurf® 7206

Propylene glycol oleate SE (INCI)
Trade names: Cithrol PGMO S/E

Propylene glycol oleth-5 (INCI)
Synonyms: Propylene glycol PEG (5) oleyl ether
Trade names: Marlowet® OA 4/1

Propylene glycol palmitate (INCI)
Trade names: Hodag PGMP

Propylene glycol palmito/stearate (INCI)
Trade names: Monosteol

Propylene glycol ricinoleate (INCI)
CAS 26402-31-3; EINECS 247-669-7
Synonyms: 12-Hydroxy-9-octadecenoic acid, monoester with 1,2-propanediol; Propylene glycol mono-ricinoleate
Trade names: Cithrol PGMR N/E; Flexricin® 9; Naturechem® PGR; Rol RP

Propylene glycol ricinoleate SE
Trade names: Cithrol PGMR S/E

Propylene glycol soyate (INCI)
CAS 67784-79-6; EINECS 267-054-7
Trade names: Kessco® 3283

Propylene glycol stearate (INCI)
CAS 1323-39-3; EINECS 215-354-3
Synonyms: Propylene glycol monostearate; Octadecanoic acid, monoester with 1,2-propanediol
Trade names: Capmul® PGMS; Ceral P; Cerasynt® PA; Cithrol PGMS N/E; Elfacos® PGMS; Emalex PGMS; Emalex PGS; Emerest® 2380; Estol PMS 3737; Hefti PMS-33; Hodag PGMS; Kessco PGMS; Kessco PGMS-R; Kessco PGMS-X534F; Kessco® Propylene Glycol Monostearate Pure; Lipal PGMS; Lipo PGMS; Mazol® PGMSK; Myverol® P-06; Nikkol PMS-1C; Nikkol PMS-FR; Pegosperse® PMS CG; Radiasurf® 7201; Schercemol PGMS; Unipeg-PGMS; Unitolate PGMS; Witconol™ 2380
Trade names containing: Amisol™ 4135; Cetasal; Hydrolactol 70; Hydrolactol 93; Myvatex® 40-06S; Myvatex® Texture Lite

Propylene glycol stearate SE (INCI)
Trade names: Ceral PA; Ceral TP; Cithrol PGMS S/E; CPH-52-SE; Kessco PGMS-8615; Kessco PGMS-X174; Lexemul® P; Nikkol PMS-1CSE; Tegin® P; Tesal; Witconol™ 2381; Witconol™ RHP

Propyl gallate (INCI)
CAS 121-79-9; EINECS 204-498-2
Synonyms: 3,4,5-Trihydroxybenzoic acid, propyl ester; n-Propyl 3,4,5-trihydroxybenzoate; Gallic acid, propyl ester
Trade names: Atomergic Propyl Gallate; Progallin® P; Tenox® PG; Uantox PG
Trade names containing: Nipanox® S-1; Nipanox® Special; Sustane® 3; Tenox® 2; Tenox® 6; Uantox 3

Propyl p-hydroxybenzoate. See Propylparaben

Propylparaben (INCI)
CAS 94-13-3; EINECS 202-307-7
Synonyms: Propyl p-hydroxybenzoate; 4-Hydroxy-

benzoic acid, propyl ester; Propyl parahydroxy-
benzoate
Trade names: Bentex P; CoSept P; Lexgard® P; Nipasol
M; Paridol P; Preserval P; Propyl-Steriline; Trisept P;
Unisept P; Unisept PNA
Trade names containing: Bactericide MB 2/012582;
Bactiphen 2506 G; Bentone® Gel LOI; Combi-
Steriline MP; Dekaben; Dragocid Forte 2/027045;
Germaben® II-E; Germaben® II; Mikrokill 300;
Nipaguard® BPX; Nipaguard® MPA; Nipaguard®
MPS; Nipastat; Paragon™ II; Phenonip; Protastat P-
211; Sepicide HB; Sepicide MB; Talcoseptic C;
Undebenzofene C; Uniphen P-23

Propyltrimonium hydrolyzed collagen (INCI)
Synonyms: Propyltrimonium hyrolyzed animal protein
Trade names: Protectein™

Protease
CAS9014-01-1; EINECS 232-752-2
Trade names: Bromelain 1:10; Bromelain Conc; Fungal
Protease 31,000; Fungal Protease 60,000; Fungal
Protease 500,000; Fungal Protease Conc; Papain
16,000; Papain 30,000; Papain Conc

Prunus amygdalus dulcis extract. *See Sweet almond extract*

Prunus armeniaca. *See Apricot kernel oil*

Prussian blue. *See Ferric ferrocyanide*

PS. *See Polystyrene*

PTFE. *See Polytetrafluoroethylene*

PVA. *See Polyvinyl alcohol*

PVAc. *See Polyvinyl acetate (homopolymer)*

PVAL. *See Polyvinyl alcohol*

PVC. *See Polyvinyl chloride*

PVM/MA copolymer (INCI)
CAS 9011-16-9
Synonyms: Methyl vinyl ether/maleic anhydride copoly-
mer; Poly(methyl vinyl ether/maleic anhydride); 2,5-
Furandione, polymer with methoxyethylene
Trade names: Gantrez® AN; Luviform® FA 119

PVM/MA copolymer, butyl ester (INCI)
CAS 54018-18-7; 54578-91-5; 53200-28-5
Synonyms: Poly(methylvinyl ether/maleic acid) butyl es-
ter; Butyl ester of PVM/MA copolymer (CTFA); 2-
Butenedioic acid, polymer with methoxyethene, butyl
ester
Trade names containing: Gantrez® ES-425; Gantrez®
ES-435; Gantrez® V-425

PVM/MA copolymer, ethyl ester (INCI)
CAS 50935-57-4; 67724-93-0; 54578-90-4
Trade names: Gantrez® SP-215
Trade names containing: Gantrez® ES-225; Gantrez® V-
215; Gantrez® V-225

PVM/MA copolymer, isopropyl ester (INCI)
CAS 54578-88-0; 54077-45-1; 56091-51-1
Synonyms: Poly(methylvinyl ether/maleic acid) isopropyl
ester
Trade names containing: Gantrez® ES-335

PVM/MA decadiene crosspolymer (INCI)
Trade names: Gantrez® XL-80; Stabileze™ 06

PVOH. *See Polyvinyl alcohol*

PVP (INCI)
CAS 9003-39-8; EINECS 201-800-4
Synonyms: Polyvinylpyrrolidone; Povidone; 1-Ethenyl-2-
pyrrolidinone, homopolymer

Trade names: H₂old™ EP-1; Kollidon®; Luviskol® K17;
Luviskol® K30; Luviskol® K60; Luviskol® K80;
Luviskol® K90; Luviskol® LD-9025; Plasdone® C-
15; Plasdone® C-30; Plasdone® K-25, K-90;
Plasdone® K-26/28, K-29/32; PVP K-15; PVP K-30
Trade names containing: Kerafix 620; PVP/Si-10

PVP/decene copolymer (INCI)
Synonyms: Polyvinylpyrrolidone/decene copolymer
Trade names: Antaron® ET-201; Ganex® Et-201

PVP/dimethiconylacrylate/polycarbamyl/polyglycol es-ter (INCI)
Trade names: Pecogel S-1120

PVP/dimethylaminoethylmethacrylate copolymer (INCI)
CAS 30581-59-0
Synonyms: 2-Propenoic acid, 2-methyl-, 2-(dimethyl-
amino) ethyl ester, polymer with 1-ethenyl-2-
pyrrolidinone; Vinylpyrrolidone/dimethylaminoethyl
methacrylate copolymer
Trade names: Copolymer 845; Copolymer 937
Trade names containing: Copolymer 958

PVP/dimethylaminoethyl methacrylate/polycarbamyl polyglycol ester (INCI)
Trade names: Pecogel GC-310, GC-1110

PVP/eicosene copolymer (INCI)
CAS 28211-18-9
Synonyms: 1-Ethenyl-2-pyrrolidinone, polymer with 1-
eicosene; 1-Eicosene, polymer with 1-ethenyl-2-
pyrrolidinone
Trade names: Antaron® V-220; Ganex® V-220; Unimer
U-15

PVP/hexadecene copolymer (INCI)
CAS 32440-50-9
Synonyms: Polyvinylpyrrolidone/hexadecene copolymer
Trade names: Antaron® V-216; Ganex® V-216; Unimer
U-151

PVP-iodine (INCI)
CAS 25655-41-8
Synonyms: Polyvinylpyrrolidone-iodine complex;
Povidone-iodine; 2-Pyrrolidinone, 1-ethenyl-, ho-
mopolymer, compd. with iodine
Trade names: PVP-Iodine 17/12, 30/06

PVP/polycarbamyl polyglycol ester (INCI)
Trade names: Pecogel A-12; Pecogel H-12, H-115, H-
1220

PVP/VA copolymer (INCI)
CAS 25086-89-9
Synonyms: 1-Ethenyl-2-pyrrolidinone, polymer with ace-
tic acid ethenyl ester; Polyvinylpyrrolidone/vinyl ace-
tate copolymer; Vinylpyrrolidone/vinyl acetate co-
polymer
Trade names: Luviskol® VA28E; Luviskol® VA28I;
Luviskol® VA37E; Luviskol® VA37I; Luviskol®
VA55E; Luviskol® VA55I; Luviskol® VA64; Luviskol®
VA64E; Luviskol® VA64W; Luviskol® VA73E;
Luviskol® VA73I; Luviskol® VA73W; Nasuna® B;
PVP/VA E-335, E-535, E-635; PVP/VA S-630
Trade names containing: PVP/VA E-735

PVP/VA/vinyl propionate copolymer (INCI)
Synonyms: PVP/VA/vinyl propionate terpolymer
Trade names: Luviskol® VAP343 E; Luviskol® VAP343 I

Pyridoxine (INCI)
CAS 65-23-6; EINECS 200-603-0
Synonyms: 5-Hydroxy-6-methyl-3,4-pyridinedimethanol
Trade names containing: Asebiol® LS; Complexe AV.a.;
Trichogen

Pyridoxine dicaprylate (INCI)
CAS 106483-04-9
Trade names: Nikkol DK

Pyridoxine dilaurate (INCI)
Synonyms: Dodecanoic acid, diester with pyridoxol; Vitamin B6 dilaurate
Trade names: Nikkol DL

Pyridoxine dipalmitate (INCI)
CAS 635-38-1
Synonyms: Palmitic acid, diester with pyridoxol; Vitamin B6 dipalmitate
Trade names: Nikkol DP

Pyrocatechol (INCI)
CAS 120-80-9; EINECS 204-427-5
Synonyms: 1,2-Benzenediol; Pyrocatechin; 1,2-Dihydroxybenzene
Trade names: Rodol C

Pyrogallol (INCI)
CAS 87-66-1; EINECS 201-762-9
Synonyms: 1,2,3-Benzenetriol; Pyrogallic acid; 1,2,3-Trihydroxybenzene
Trade names: Rodol PG

L-Pyroglutamic acid. *See PCA*

Pyrophyllite. *See Aluminum silicate*

2-Pyrrolidone
CAS 616-45-5; EINECS 204-648-7
Synonyms: Butyrolactam; Pyrrolidone-2
Trade names: Soluphor® P

Pyrus malus extract. *See Apple extract*

Quaterinum-2. *See Soyaethyl morpholinium ethosulfate*

Quaternium-5. *See Distearyldimonium chloride*

Quaternium-6. *See PPG-9 diethylmonium chloride*

Quaternium-9. *See Soytrimonium chloride*

Quaternium-14 (INCI)
CAS 27479-28-3; EINECS 248-486-5
Synonyms: Dodecyl dimethyl ethylbenzyl ammonium chloride; N-Dodecyl-ar-ethyl-N,N-dimethylbenzene-methanaminium chloride
Trade names containing: BTC® 2125; BTC® 2125M

Quaternium-15 (INCI)
CAS 51229-78-8; 4080-31-3; EINECS 223-805-0
Synonyms: 1-(3-Chloroallyl)-3,5,7-triaza-1-azoniaada-mantane chloride; N-(3-Chloroallyl)hexaminium chloride; Chlorallyl methenamine chloride
Trade names: CoSept 200; Dowicil® 200

Quaternium-17. *See Cetethyldimonium bromide*

Quaternium-18 (INCI)
CAS 61789-80-8, 68002-59-5; EINECS 263-090-2
Synonyms: Dimethyl di(hydrogenated tallow)ammonium chloride; Dihydrogenated tallow dimethyl ammonium chloride; Ditallowalkonium chloride
Trade names: Arquad® HC; Noramium M2SH; Querton 442; Querton 442-11; Querton 442-82; Querton 442E; Querton 442H; Radiaquat® 6442; Varisoft® 442-100P
Trade names containing: Arquad® 2HT-75; Varisoft® DHT

Quaternium-19. *See Polyquaternium-10*

Quaternium-20. *See PPG-25 diethylmonium chloride*

Quaternium-21. *See PPG-40 diethylmonium chloride*

Quaternium-22 (INCI)
CAS 51812-80-7; 82970-95-4; EINECS 257-440-3
Synonyms: 1-Propanaminium, 3-(D-gluconoylamino)-N-(2-hydroxyethyl)-N,N-dimethyl-, chloride; γ-Gluconamidopropyl dimethyl 2-hydroxyethyl ammonium Cl
Trade names: Ceraphyl® 60

Quaternium-23. *See Polyquaternium-11*

Quaternium-24 (INCI)
CAS 32426-11-2; EINECS 251-035-5
Synonyms: Decyl dimethyl octyl ammonium chloride; Octyl decyl dimethyl ammonium chloride
Trade names containing: Bardac® 2050

Quaternium-25. *See Cetethyl morpholinium ethosulfate*

Quaternium-26 (INCI)
CAS 68953-64-0; EINECS 273-222-0
Synonyms: Quaternary ammonium compds., (hydroxy-ethyl)dimethyl(3-mink oil amidopropyl), chlorides; Minkamidopropyl dimethyl 2-hydroxyethyl ammonium chloride
Trade names: Ceraphyl® 65; Incroquat 26

Quaternium-27 (INCI)
CAS 86088-85-9, 68122-86-1
Synonyms: Methyl-1-tallow amido ethyl-2-tallow imidazolinium methyl sulfate; Tallow imidazolinium methosulfate
Trade names: Incrosoft S-90; Rewoquat W 75; Rewoquat W 75 PG; Unisoft 475; Unsoft 475; Varisoft® TIMS
Trade names containing: Varisoft® 475; Varisoft® PIMS

Quaternium-28. *See Dodecylbenzyltrimonium chloride*

Quaternium-29. *See Dodecylxylylditrimonium chloride*

Quaternium-31. *See Dicetyl dimonium chloride*

Quaternium-32. *See Isostearyl ethylimidonium ethosulfate*

Quaternium-33 (INCI)
Trade names containing: Lanoquat® 1756; Lanoquat® 1757

Quaternium-34. *See Dicocodimonium chloride*

Quaternium-36. *See PEG-5 stearmonium chloride*

Quaternium-40. *See Polyquaternium-6*

Quaternium-41. *See Polyquaternium-7*

Quaternium-45 (INCI)
CAS 21034-17-3; EINECS 244-158-0
Trade names: Luminex

Quaternium-48. *See Ditallow dimonium chloride*

Quaternium-51 (INCI)
CAS 1463-95-2; EINECS 215-976-5
Synonyms: 6-[2-[(5-Bromo-2-pyridyl)amino]vinyl]-1-ethyl-2-picolinium iodide
Trade names: Takanal

Quaternium-52 (INCI)
CAS 58069-11-7
Trade names: Dehyquart® SP; Uniquart SP
Trade names containing: Condipon

Quaternium-53 (INCI)
CAS 68410-69-5; 130124-24-2
Synonyms: Ditallow diamido methosulfate
Trade names: Incrosoft T-90; Rewoquat W 222 PG

Quaternium-61 (INCI)
CAS 111905-55-6
Synonyms: Dimer acid, bis[amidopropyl-N,N-dimethyl-N-ethyl ammonium ethosulfate]
Trade names: Schercoquat DAS

Quaternium-62 (INCI)
Synonyms: N-(3-Isostearylamidopropyl)-N,N-dimethyl, N-(2,3-epoxypropyl) ammonium choloride

Trade names: Schercoquat IEP

Quaternium-70 (INCI)
CAS 68921-83-5; EINECS 272-964-2
Synonyms: Stearamidopropyl dimethyl (myristyl acetate) ammonium chloride
Trade names containing: Ceraphyl® 70

Quaternium-73 (INCI)
Synonyms: 2-[2-(3-Heptyl-4-methyl-2-thiazolin-2-ylidene)methene]-3-heptyl-4-methyl thiazolinium iodide
Trade names: Kankoh SO 201

Quaternium-75 (INCI)
Trade names: Finquat CT

Quaternium-77 (INCI)
Trade names containing: Finsoft HCM-100

Quaternium-78 (INCI)
Trade names containing: Finsoft HCM-100

Quaternium-80 (INCI)
CAS 134737-05-6
Trade names: Abil®-Quat 3270; Abil®-Quat 3272; Silquat Q-100

Quaternium-81 (INCI)
Synonyms: Methyl-1-oleyl amido ethyl-2-oleyl imidazolinium methyl sulfate
Trade names: Varisoft® 3690N (90%)
Trade names containing: Varisoft® 3690; Varisoft® OIMS

Quaternium-82 (INCI)
Trade names: Amonyl DM

Quaternium-84 (INCI)
Trade names: Mackernium™ NLE

Quaternium-18 bentonite (INCI)
CAS 68953-58-2; EINECS 273-219-4
Synonyms: Quaternary ammonium compounds, bis(hydrog. tallow alkyl) dimethyl, chlorides, reaction products with bentonite
Trade names: Bentone® 34; Claytone 34; Claytone 40; Claytone XL; Tixogel VP
Trade names containing: Tixogel MIO; Tixogel OMS; Tixogel VSP

Quaternium-18 benzalkoniumbentonite
Trade names: Claytone GR; Claytone HT; Claytone PS

Quaternium-18 hectorite (INCI)
CAS 12001-31-9; 71011-27-3; EINECS 234-406-6
Synonyms: Quaternary ammonium compounds, bis(hydrog. tallow alkyl) dimethyl, chlorides, reaction products with hectorite
Trade names: Bentone® 38
Trade names containing: Bentone® Gel ISD; Bentone® Gel M20; Bentone® Gel MIO A-40; Bentone® Gel MIO; Bentone® Gel SS71; Bentone® Gel VS-5 PC; Bentone® Gel VS-5; M-P-A® 14

Quaternium-76 hydrolyzed collagen (INCI)
Synonyms: Quaternium-76 hydrolyzed animal protein
Trade names: Lexein® QX-3000

Quaternium-79 hydrolyzed collagen (INCI)
Trade names: Mackpro™ NLP

Quaternium-79 hydrolyzed keratin (INCI)
Trade names: Mackpro™ KLP

Quaternium-79 hydrolyzed milk protein (INCI)
Trade names: Mackpro™ MLP

Quaternium-79 hydrolyzed silk (INCI)
Trade names: Mackpro™ NSP

Quaternium-79 hydrolyzed soy protein (INCI)
Trade names: Mackpro™ SLP

Quaternium-79 hydrolyzed wheat protein (INCI)
Trade names: Mackpro™ NLW

Queen bee jelly. *See Royal jelly*

Queen of the meadow extract. *See Meadowsweet extract*

Quicklime. See Calcium oxide

Quillaja extract (INCI)
Synonyms: Panama wood extract; Quillaja saponaria extract
Trade names containing: Ampholysat Bois De Panama

Rapeseedamidopropyl epoxypropyl dimonium chloride (INCI)
CAS 112324-11-5
Synonyms: Rapeseedamidopropyl dimethyl epoxypropyl ammonium chloride
Trade names: Schercoquat ROEP

Rapeseedamidopropyl ethyldimonium ethosulfate (INCI)
CAS 94552-41-7
Trade names: Schercoquat ROAS

Red raspberry leaf extract (INCI)
CAS 84929-76-0
Trade names containing: BBC Mineral Complex

Resorcinol (INCI)
CAS 108-46-3; EINECS 203-585-2
Synonyms: 1,3-Benzenediol; m-Dihydroxybenzene; Resorcin
Trade names: Rodol RS; Unichem RSC; Unichem RSC
Trade names containing: Blonde 90 (Fusion); Blonde R-50 (Fusion); Brown R-36 (Fusion)

Retinol (INCI)
CAS 68-26-8; 11103-57-4; EINECS 234-328-2; 200-683-7
Synonyms: Vitamin A
Trade names: Vitazyme® A-Plus
Trade names containing: Complexe AV.h.; Lipodermol®

Retinyl acetate (INCI)
CAS 127-47-9; EINECS 204-844-2
Synonyms: Acetic acid, retinyl ester; Vitamin A acetate
Trade names: Nanospheres 100 Vitamin A Acetate

Retinyl palmitate (INCI)
CAS 79-81-2; EINECS 201-228-5
Synonyms: Retinol, hexadecanoate; Vitamin A palmitate
Trade names: Aquapalm No. 63841; Vitamin A Palmitate Type P1.7; Vitamin A Palmitate Type P1.7/BHT; Vitamin A Palmitate Type PIMO/BH
Trade names containing: Brookosome® ACEBC; Brookosome® ANE; Brookosome® ELL; Brookosome® RP; Chronosphere® V-AE; Cutavit Richter; Derma-Vitamincomplex, Oil soluble; Dermasome® RP; Epiderm-Complex O; Extrapone Bio-Tamin Special 2/2032671; Faceur ARL; L.C.R.E.; Lipomicron Vitamin A Palmitate; ; Microsponge® 5650; Soluvit Richter; Vitamin A and D-3; Vitamin A Palmitate 1.0 BHT in Peanut Oil; Vitamin A Palmitate 1.7 BHT

Retinyl palmitate polypeptide
Trade names containing: Brookosome® A-Plus

Rhus succedanea wax. *See Japan wax*

Riboflavin (INCI)
CAS 83-88-5; EINECS 201-507-1
Synonyms: Vitamin B₂; 7,8-Dimethyl-10-(1|d-ribityl) isoalloxazine; Flavaxin; Lactoflavin; Vitamin G
Trade names: Riboflavin USP, FCC Type S; Riboflavin-5′-Phosphate Sodium USP, FCC
Trade names containing: Unipertan P-2002; Unipertan P-24; Unipertan P-24; Unipertan VEG 24

Ribonucleic acid. *See RNA*

Ribose nucleic acid. *See RNA*

Rice bran extract (INCI)
  Trade names: Gamma Oryzanol
  Trade names containing: Actiphyte of Rice Bran

Rice bran oil (INCI)
  CAS 68553-81-1; 84696-37-7; EINECS 271-397-8
  Synonyms: Oils, rice bran; Rice oil
  Trade names: Dascare Oryza-Oil; EmCon Rice Bran;
    Natoil RBO; Rice Bran Oil; Rice Bran Oil SO; Tri-Ol
    RBO

Rice bran wax (INCI)
  CAS 8016-60-2; EINECS 232-409-7
  Synonyms: Waxes, rice bran
  Trade names: Natwax RB; Rice Wax No. 1; Rose Rice
    Bran Wax

Rice starch (INCI)
  CAS 9005-25-8
  Trade names: Dascare Micropearl

Ricinoleamide DEA (INCI)
  CAS 40716-42-5; EINECS 255-051-3
  Synonyms: N,N-Bis(2-hydroxyethyl)ricinoleamide; Di-
    ethanolamine ricinoleic acid amide; 12-Hydroxy-N,N-
    bis(2-hydroxyethyl)-9-octadecenamide
  Trade names: Afmide™ R; Amidex RC; Aminol CA-2;
    Mackamide™ R; Olamida RD; Protamide CA
  Trade names containing: Lamacit® ER

Ricinoleamide MEA (INCI)
  CAS 106-16-1; EINECS 203-368-2
  Synonyms: Ricinoleoyl monoethanolamide; N-(2-Hy-
    droxyethyl)-12-hydroxy-9-octadecenamide; Mono-
    ethanolamine ricinoleic acid amide
  Trade names: Emid® 6573; Rewomid® R 280

Ricinoleamidopropyl betaine (INCI)
  CAS 71850-81-2; 86089-12-5
  Synonyms: N-(Carboxymethyl)-N,N-dimethyl-3[(1-
    oxoricinoleyl)amino]-1-propanaminium hydroxide,
    inner salt; Ricinoleamidopropyl dimethyl glycine
  Trade names: Rewoteric® AM R40; Varion® AM-R40

Ricinoleamidopropyl dimethylamine (INCI)
  CAS 20457-75-4; 977010-66-4; EINECS 243-835-8
  Synonyms: N-[3-(Dimethylamino)propyl]ricinoleamide;
    Ricinoleamide, N-[3-(dimethylamino)propyl]-
  Trade names: Chemidex R; Mackine™ 201

Ricinoleamidopropyl dimethylamine lactate (INCI)
  CAS 977012-91-1
  Synonyms: N-[3-(Dimethylamino)propyl]ricinoleamide
    lactate
  Trade names: Afalene™ 216; Emcol® 3555; Macka-
    lene™ 216

Ricinoleamidopropyl ethyldimonium ethosulfate (INCI)
  CAS 112324-16-0
  Synonyms: N-Ethyl-N,N-dimethyl-3-[(1-oxoricin-
    oleyl)amino]-1-propanaminium ethosulfate; Ricinole-
    amidopropyl ethyl dimethyl ammonium ethyl sulfate
  Trade names: Lipoquat R; Surfactol® Q4

Ricinoleamidopropyl trimonium chloride (INCI)
  CAS 127311-98-2
  Synonyms: Ricinoleamidopropyl trimethyl ammonium
    chloride
  Trade names containing: Surfactol® Q1

Ricinoleamidopropyl trimonium methosulfate (INCI)
  CAS 85508-38-9; EINECS 287-462-9
  Synonyms: Ricinoleamidopropyl trimethylammonium
    methyl sulfate

Trade names: Rewoquat RTM 50

Ricinoleic acid (INCI)
  CAS 141-22-0; EINECS 205-470-2
  Synonyms: 12-Hydroxy-9-octadecenoic acid; 9-
    Octadecenoic acid, 12-hydroxy-; d-12-Hydroxyoleic
    acid
  Trade names containing: Grillocin WE-106

Ricinoleth-40 (INCI)
  Synonyms: PEG-40 ricinoleyl ether; PEG 2000 ricinoleyl
    ether; POE (40) ricinoleyl ether
  Trade names: Poliglicoleum

Ricinus oil. *See Castor oil*

RNA (INCI)
  CAS 63231-63-0
  Synonyms: Ribonucleic acid; Ribose nucleic acid
  Trade names: Atomergic Ribonucleic Acid
  Trade names containing: Brookosome® DNA/RNA;
    Endonucleine LS 2143

Rocket extract (INCI)
  CAS 90028-42-5
  Synonyms: Eruca sativa extract
  Trade names containing: Blend For Greasy Hair HS 312;
    Blend For Greasy Skin Imperfections HS 315

Rock salt. *See Sodium chloride*

Rose extract (INCI)
  CAS 84696-47-9; EINECS 283-652-0
  Synonyms: Rosa canina extract
  Trade names containing: Actiphyte of Rose; BBC Mois-
    ture Trol; BBC Relaxing Complex; Coobato Speciale

Rose fruit extract
  Trade names: Eijitsu Extract BG

Rose hips extract (INCI)
  CAS 84696-47-9
  Trade names containing: Actiphyte of Rose Hips; Blend
    For Delicate Skins HS 215; Eglantineol

Rose hips oil (INCI)
  CAS 84603-93-0
  Trade names: Nikkol Rose Hip Oil

Rosemary extract (INCI)
  CAS 84604-14-8
  Synonyms: Extract of rosemary; Rosmarinum officinalis
    extract
  Trade names: Amiox; Uantox ROSM
  Trade names containing: Capilotonique HS 226;
    Capilotonique HS 245; Cremogen AF; Herbaliquid
    Rosemary Special; Herbasol 7 Herb Complex;
    Herbasol Alpine Herbs Complex; Herbasol Herbes de
    Provence Complex; Herbasol Stimulant Complex;
    Stimulant HS 280; Stimulant LS 680

Rosemary oil (INCI)
  CAS 8000-25-7
  Trade names containing: Essentiaderm n.2; Essen-
    tiaderm n.7; Essentiaderm n.9

Rose oil (INCI)
  CAS 8007-01-0; 84603-93-0
  Trade names: EmCon Rose

Rosin (INCI)
  CAS 8050-09-7; 8052-10-6; EINECS 232-475-7
  Synonyms: Colophony; Gum rosin; Rosin gum
  Trade names containing: Enduragloss™

Rosin acrylate (INCI)
  Synonyms: Acrylic acid, rosin ester
  Trade names: Hairspray Additive S

Royal jelly (INCI)
  CAS 8031-67-2

Royal jelly extract

Synonyms: Queen bee jelly
Trade names: Atomergic Royal Jelly
Trade names containing: Brookosome® RJ; Derma-some® RJ

Royal jelly extract (INCI)
Trade names containing: Actiphyte of Royal Jelly; Lipoplastidine Pappa Regalis

Royal jelly powder (INCI)
Trade names: Dascare Royal Jelly Powd

Saccharide hydrolysate
Trade names containing: Unimoist U-125

Saccharide isomerate (INCI)
Trade names: Pentavitin®

Saccharin (INCI)
CAS 81-07-2; EINECS 201-321-0; 220-120-9
Synonyms: Saccharin, insoluble; 1,1-Dioxide-1,2-benzisothiazol-3(2H)-one; 1,2-Benzothiazol-3(2H)-one 1,1-dioxide
Trade names: Unisweet SAC

Saccharose. *See Sucrose*

Saccharose distearate
CAS 25168-73-4
Trade names: Sucro Ester 7

Saccharose mono/distearate
Trade names: Sucro Ester 11

Saccharose palmitate
CAS 25168-73-4
Trade names: Sucro Ester 15

Saffloweramidopropyl ethyldimonium ethosulfate (INCI)
CAS 113492-04-9
Synonyms: Saffloweramidopropyl dimethylethyl ammonium ethyl sulfate
Trade names: Schercoquat FOAS

Safflower extract (INCI)
Synonyms: Carthamus tinctorius extract
Trade names containing: Benibana Liq.

Safflower oil (INCI)
CAS 8001-23-8; EINECS 232-276-5
Synonyms: Carthamus tinctorious oil; Oils, safflower
Trade names: Lipovol SAF; Natoil SAF; Neobee® 18; Nikkol Safflower Oil; Super Refined™ Safflower Oil USP; Tri-Ol SAF
Trade names containing: Aloe Vera Oil 0040X; Phosal® 50 SA; Phosal® 75 SA

Sage extract (INCI)
CAS 84082-79-1
Trade names containing: Bio-Chelated Derma-Plex I; Blend For Deodorant HS 275; Capilotonique HS 226; Capilotonique HS 245; Cremogen AF; Herbalcomplex 1 Special; Herbalcomplex 2 Special; Herbasol Alpine Herbs Complex; Herbasol Complex A; Herbasol Complex C; Herbasol Herbes de Provence Complex; Herbasol Stimulant Complex; Stimulant HS 280; Stimulant LS 680

Saint John's wort extract. *See Hypericum extract*

Saint John's wort oil
Trade names: Unibotan St. Johns Wort Oil

Sal ammoniac. *See Ammonium chloride*

Salicylic acid (INCI)
CAS 69-72-7; EINECS 200-712-3
Synonyms: 2-Hydroxybenzoic acid; o-Hydroxybenzoic acid; Benzoic acid, 2-hydroxy-
Trade names: Unichem SALAC
Trade names containing: Chronosphere® SAL

Salmiac. *See Ammonium chloride*

Salt. *See Sodium chloride*

Sambucus extract (INCI)
CAS 84603-58-7
Synonyms: Elder flower extract; Sambucus nigra extract
Trade names containing: Babyderme HS 265; Bio-Chelated Derma-Plex I; Emollient HS 235; Emollient LS 635

Sapogenin glycosides. *See Saponins*

Saponins (INCI)
CAS 11006-75-0
Synonyms: Sapogenin glycosides
Trade names containing: Tensami 10/06

Sasanqua oil
Trade names: Nikkol Sasanqua Oil

Sclerotium gum (INCI)
Synonyms: Gums, sclerotium
Trade names: Amigel

SD alcohol 39C (INCI)
Trade names containing: Almondermin® LS; Chamomile Distillate 2/380930

SD alcohol 40 (INCI)
Trade names containing: Bentone® Gel MIO A-40; Bentone® Gel TN A-40; Bentone® Gel VS-5; Schercoteric LS-2ES MOD

SD alcohol 40-B (INCI)
Trade names containing: Equex AEM; Orvus K Liq.

SDS. *See Sodium lauryl sulfate*

Sea salt (INCI)
Trade names: Afrosalt; Dacriosalt

Sea silt extract (INCI)
Trade names containing: Oligoceane

Selachyl alcohol
Trade names: Nikkol Selachyl Alcohol

Selenium aspartate (INCI)
Trade names: Oligoidyne Selenium

Sericite
Trade names: Nikkol Sericite; S-100; S-152; S-SM; SS-88
Trade names containing: Coverleaf PC-2035

L-Serine (INCI)
CAS 56-45-1; EINECS 200-274-3
Synonyms: 2-Amino-3-hydroxypropionic acid
Trade names containing: Facteur Hydratant PH; Hydro-Diffuser Microreservoir; Hydroviton 2/059353

Serum albumin (INCI)
CAS 9048-46-8; EINECS 232-936-2
Synonyms: Albumin from blood; Albuminate (obsolete); Serum proteins
Trade names: Bovinal-20; Bovine Serum Albumin Sol'n; Bovinol 30
Trade names containing: Hydagen® BP1

Serum protein (INCI)
Trade names: Eleseryl® SH; Fibrostimuline S
Trade names containing: Elespher® Eleseryl SH; Leniplex; Liposome Anti-Age LS; Liposomes Anti-Age LS; Peptidyl

Sesame oil (INCI)
CAS 8008-74-0; EINECS 232-370-6
Synonyms: Gingilli oil; Oils, sesame
Trade names: Hy-SES; Lipovol SES; Sesame Oil USP/NF 16; Super Refined™ Sesame Oil; Tri-Ol SES; Uniderm SSME

Trade names containing: Bee's Milk; Epidermin in Oil; Lanpro-2; Lipovol SES-S; Oleo-Coll™ LP; Oleo-Coll™ LP/LF; Proto-Lan 8; Unibotan Vitaplant O CLR; Vitaplant CLR Oil-Soluble N

Sesamide DEA (INCI)
CAS 124046-35-1
Trade names: Incromide SED

Sesamidopropyl betaine (INCI)
Synonyms: N-(Carboxymethyl)-N,N-dimethyl-3-[(1-oxosesame)amino]-1-propanaminium hydroxide, inner salt; Sesame amide propylbetaine; Sesamidopropyl dimethyl glycine
Trade names: Incronam SE-30

Sesamidopropyl dimthylamine (INCI)
Synonyms: N-[3-(Dimethylamino)propyl]sesame amides
Trade names: Incromine SEB

Shark liver oil (INCI)
CAS 68990-63-6; EINECS 273-616-2
Synonyms: Oils, shark liver
Trade names: Dermane SLO; Super Refined™ Shark Liver Oil

Shea butter (INCI)
CAS 68424-60-2
Trade names: Cetiol® SB45; Fancol Karite Butter; Karite Butter; Kelisema Natural Pure Shea Butter; Lipex 102; Lipex 202; Lipex 205; Shea Butter; Shebu® Refined; Unimulse
Trade names containing: Cirami No. 1

Shea butter extract (INCI)
CAS 68424-59-9
Trade names: Fancol Karite Extract

Shea butter unsaponifiables (INCI)
Synonyms: Unsaponifiable shea butter
Trade names: Karite Nonsaponifiable; Shea Unsaponifiable Conc
Trade names containing: Destressine 2000; Liposome Unsapo KM; Sungen

Shellac wax (INCI)
Trade names: Ross Bleached Refined Shellac Wax; Ross Bleached Refined Shellac Wax Cosmetic Grade

SHMP. See Sodium hexametaphosphate

Shorea butter (INCI)
Trade names: Cremeol SH; Lipex 106

Silica (INCI)
CAS 7631-86-9; 112945-52-5
Synonyms: Silicon dioxide, fumed; Silicon dioxide; Silicic anhydride
Trade names: Aerosil® 130; Aerosil® 200; Aerosil® 255; Aerosil® 300; Aerosil® 380; Aerosil® R812; Aerosil® R972; Bubble Breaker® 3056A; Cab-O-Sil® HS-5; Cab-O-Sil® L-90; H-40; SB-150; SB-700; Sident® 15; Sident® 22LS; Sident® 22S; Spherica; Spheron L-1500; Spheron P-1000; Spheron P-1500; Tullanox HM-250; Wacker HDK® H20; Wacker HDK® N20; Wacker HDK® V15
Trade names containing: Amilon; Cab-O-Sil® TS-530; Cashmir K-II; DHA Microspheres; Dow Corning® MDX-4-4210; Dow Corning® Q7-4840; Kalixide AS; Luxelen® SS-020; Luxelen® SS; Micronasphere™ M; PCL-Siccum 2/066215; SAG-710, -730; Spherica HA; Spheron P-1500-030; Sphingoceryl® Powd. LS; Surfynol® 82S; Ti-Sphere AB-15155A; Velvet Veil 310; Velvet Veil 320; Velvet Veil 620; Velvet Veil 640; Velvet Veil A; Velvetveil X; Velvetveil Y; Velvetveil Z; White Charcoal MB-15153

Silica, amorphous. See Silica

Silica, hydrated (INCI)
CAS 1343-98-2 (silicic acid); 112926-00-8; EINECS 215-68-32
Synonyms: Silicic acid; Silica gel; Precipitated silica
Trade names: Elfadent SM 500; FK 500LS; Quso® G27, G29, G35, G38, WR55, WR83; Quso® WR55-FG; Sipernat® 22; Sipernat® 22LS; Sipernat® 22S; Sipernat® 50; Sipernat® 50S; Tixosil 38AB, 43, 53, 63, 73, 83, 93; Tixosil 331; Tixosil 333, 343; Zeo® 49; Zeodent® 113; Zeodent® 115, 119, 163, 173, 177; Zeofree® 80; Zeofree® 153; Zeosyl® 110SD; Zeosyl® 200; Zeothix® 95; Zeothix® 265

Silicic acid. See Silica, hydrated

Silicon dioxide. See Silica

Silicon dioxide, fumed. See Silica

Silicone
Synonyms: Organosiloxane
Trade names: Dow Corning® Q5-0158A Wax; Silwax® F-D; Silwax® S; Silwax® WD-S; Silwax® WS

Silicone emulsions and compounds. See also Dimethicone, Cyclomethicone, Polysiloxane
Trade names: Dow Corning® Antifoam 1520-US; Nikkol NET SG-60A; Nikkol NET-HO; Silicone Emulsion E-130; Silicone Emulsion E-131; Silicone Emulsion E-133; SWS-231; SWS-232

Silicone quaternium-2 (INCI)
Trade names: Silquat AM

Silk (INCI)
Trade names: Silkall 100
Trade names containing: Silkall CA; Silkall TI; Silkall TL; Silkall ZN

Silk amino acids (INCI)
CAS 977077-71-6
Trade names: Amino-Silk SF; Crosilk Liq; Solu-Silk™ 25; Solu-Silk™ SF; Tri-Tein Silk AA
Trade names containing: Collamino™ Complex S

Silk powder (INCI)
CAS 9009-99-8
Trade names: Crosilk Powder; Fibro-Silk™ Powd; Uniderm SILPOW

Silver aluminum magnesium phosphate. See Silver magnesium aluminum phosphate

Silver borosilicate (INCI)
Trade names: Ionpure Type A

Silver magnesium aluminum phosphate (INCI)
Trade names: Ionpure Type B

Simethicone (INCI)
CAS 8050-81-5
Trade names: Amersil® Simethicone EM; Dow Corning® Antifoam A; Dow Corning® Medical Antifoam A Compound; Dow Corning® Medical Antifoam AF Emulsion; Dow Corning® Medical Antifoam C Emulsion; Hodag Antifoam F-1; Mazu® DF 200SP; Rhodorsil® AF 70414, 70416, 70426 R, 70452; Unisil DF-200S, DF-200SP; Unisil SF; Wacker Silicone Antifoam Agent S 184; Wacker Silicone Antifoam Emulsion SE 6; Wacker Silicone Antifoam Emulsion SE 9

Sisal extract (INCI)
Synonyms: Agave sisalona extract
Trade names containing: Agave Extract HS 2817 G

Slaked lime. See Calcium hydroxide

Slippery elm bark (INCI)
Synonyms: Ulmus fulva bark

Trade names containing: BBC Moisture Trol

SMO. *See Sorbitan oleate*

SMS. *See Sorbitan stearate*

Soap clay. *See Bentonite*

Sodium acetate (INCI)
CAS 127-09-3; EINECS 204-823-8
Synonyms: Sodium acetate anhydrous; Acetic acid sodium salt anhydrous
Trade names: Unichem SODAC

Sodium alginate. *See Algin*

Sodium alpha olefin sulfonate
CAS 68188-45-5; 68439-57-6
Trade names: Nikkol OS-14

Sodium aluminum chlorohydroxy lactate (INCI)
CAS 8038-93-5
Trade names: Chloracel® 40% Sol'n; Chloracel® Solid

Sodium ascorbate (INCI)
CAS 134-03-2; EINECS 205-126-1
Synonyms: L(+)-Ascorbic acid sodium salt; Vitamin C sodium salt
Trade names: Sodium Ascorbate USP, FCC Fine Powd. No. 6047708; Uantox SODASC

Sodium behenoyl lactylate
Trade names: Pationic® SBL

Sodium bentonite
Trade names: Geltone; Geltone 1665; Geltone II; Volclay NF-ID; Volclay® NF-BC

Sodium benzoate (INCI)
CAS 532-32-1; EINECS 208-534-8
Synonyms: Benzoic acid, sodium salt
Trade names: Unisept SB
Trade names containing: Aerosol® OT-B; Lactil®; Monawet MO-85P; Solusol® 85%

Sodium bicarbonate (INCI)
CAS 144-55-8; EINECS 205-633-8
Synonyms: Baking soda; Sodium hydrogen carbonate; Bicarbonate of soda; Carbonic acid, monosodium salt
Trade names: Unichem BICARB-S; Unichem BICARB-S

Sodium bischlorophenyl sulfamine (INCI)
CAS 58727-01-8
Trade names: Eucoriol

Sodium bisglycol ricinosulfosuccinate (INCI)
Trade names: Grillosol 8C

Sodium bisulfite (INCI)
CAS 7631-90-5; EINECS 231-548-0
Synonyms: Sodium acid sulfite; Sulfurous acid, monosodium salt; Sodium hydrogen sulfite
Trade names: Uantox SBS

Sodium borate (INCI)
CAS 1303-96-4, 1330-43-4
Synonyms: Sodium tetraborate; Sodium pyroborate; Borax
Trade names: Unichem SOBOR

Sodium bromate (INCI)
CAS 7789-38-0; EINECS 232-160-4
Synonyms: Bromic acid, sodium salt
Trade names: Unineut SOBROM

Sodium butoxynol-12 sulfate (INCI)
Synonyms: PEG-12 butyl phenyl ether sulfate, sodium salt
Trade names: Akyposal TBP 120

Sodium butylparaben (INCI)
CAS 36457-20-2

Synonyms: Butylparaben, sodium salt; Sodium n-butyl-4-hydroxybenzoate; Sodium butyl-p-hydroxybenzoate
Trade names: Nipabutyl Sodium; Unisept BNA

Sodium C4-12 olefin/maleic acid copolymer (INCI)
Trade names: Demol EP

Sodium C8-16 isoalkylsuccinyl lactoglobulin sulfonate (INCI)
Trade names: Bio-Pol® EA; Bio-Pol® OE; Bio-Pol® OE/SD

Sodium C9-22 alkyl sec sulfonate (INCI)
CAS 68188-18-1
Trade names: Mersolat H 95

Sodium C12-13 pareth sulfate (INCI)
CAS 68957-18-6
Synonyms: Sodium pareth-23 sulfate
Trade names: Akyposal 23 ST 70; Akyposal DS 56; Elfan® NS 213 SL Conc; Elfan® NS 232 S Conc
Trade names containing: Akypogene HM 12

Sodium C12-14 olefin sulfonate (INCI)
Trade names containing: Marlinat® SRN 30

Sodium C12-15 alkoxypropyl iminodipropionate (INCI)
Trade names: Amphoteric N

Sodium C12-15 alkyl sulfate (INCI)
Synonyms: Sodium C12-15 alcohols sulfate
Trade names: Standapol® WAQ-115; Unipol WAQ-115
Trade names containing: Lanette® Wax SX, SXBP

Sodium C12-15 pareth-6 carboxylate (INCI)
CAS 70632-06-3 (generic)
Synonyms: PEG-6 C12-15 alkyl ether carboxylic acid, sodium salt; PEG 300 C12-15 alkyl ether carboxylic acid, sodium salt
Trade names: Sandopan® DTC Linear P

Sodium C12-15 pareth-7 carboxylate (INCI)
CAS 70632-06-3 (generic)
Synonyms: PEG-7 C12-15 alkyl ether carboxylic acid, sodium salt; POE (7) C12-15 alkyl ether carboxylic acid, sodium salt; Sodium pareth-25-7 carboxylate
Trade names: Surfine WNT Gel; Surfine WNT LC; Surfine WNT-LS

Sodium C12-15 pareth sulfate (INCI)
Synonyms: Sodium pareth-25 sulfate; POE (1–4) C12–15 fatty alcohol ether sulfated, sodium salt
Trade names: Elfan® NS 252 S; Elfan® NS 252 S Conc; Elfan® NS 252 SL Conc; Neodol® 25-3S; Standapol® SP-60; Unipol SP-60; Witcolate™ 1050; Witcolate™ SE-5
Trade names containing: Elfan® KM 730

Sodium C12-15 pareth-3 sulfonate (INCI)
Trade names: Avanel® S-30

Sodium C12-15 pareth-7 sulfonate (INCI)
Trade names: Avanel® S-70

Sodium C12-15 pareth-9 sulfonate
Trade names: Avanel® S-90

Sodium C12-15 pareth-15 sulfonate (INCI)
Trade names: Avanel® S-150

Sodium C12-18 alkyl sulfate (INCI)
Synonyms: Sodium C12-18 alcohols sulfate
Trade names: Stokopol LO
Trade names containing: Galenol® 1618 KS

Sodium C13-17 alkane sulfonate (INCI)
Trade names: Marlon® PS 30; Marlon® PS 60; Marlon® PS 65
Trade names containing: Marlon® PF 40

Sodium C14-16 olefin sulfonate (INCI)

CAS 68439-57-6; EINECS 270-407-8
Trade names: Bio-Terge® AS-40; Calsoft AOS-40; Carsonol® AOS; Elfan® OS 46; Norfox® ALPHA XL; Rhodacal® 301-10F; Rhodacal® A-246 LX; Rhodacal® A-246L; Witconate™ AOK; Witconate™ AOS; Witconate™ AOS-EP; Witconate™ AOS-PC
Trade names containing: Bio-Terge® 804; Compound 3143F; Elfan® KM 640 Mg; Elfan® KM 730; Elfan® SG; Mackam™ LOS; Miracare® ANL; Tego®-Pearl S-33

Sodium C14-17 alkyl sec sulfonate (INCI)
CAS 68037-49-0; EINECS 268-213-3
Synonyms: Sodium C14-17 sec alcohol sulfonate; Sodium C14-17 alcohol sulfonate; Sodium C14-17 sec alkane sulfonate
Trade names: Hostapur SAS 30; Hostapur SAS 60; Hostapur SAS 93
Trade names containing: Hostacerin CG; Olamin® K; Olamin®/NP

Sodium caproamphoacetate (INCI)
CAS 14350-94-8; 68647-46-1; 25704-59-0; 68608-61-7; EINECS 271-951-9; 238-303-7
Synonyms: 1H-Imidazolium, 1-(carboxymethyl)-4,5-dihydro-1-(2-hydroxyethyl)-2-nonyl-, hydroxide, sodium salt; Caproamphoglycinate
Trade names: Mackam™ 1CY; Miranol® SM Conc

Sodium caproyl lactylate (INCI)
CAS 29051-57-8
Synonyms: Sodium capryl lactylate
Trade names: Pationic® 122A

Sodium capryloamphoacetate (INCI)
CAS 13039-35-5; EINECS 235-907-2
Synonyms: Capryloamphoglycinate; Capryloamphoacetate
Trade names: Emery® 5418

Sodium capryloamphohydroxypropyl sulfonate (INCI)
CAS 68610-39-9
Synonyms: Capryloamphopropylsulfonate
Trade names: Mackam™ JS

Sodium carboxymethylcellulose. *See Carboxymethylcellulose sodium*

Sodium carboxymethyl chitin (INCI)
Synonyms: Chitin, carboxymethyl, sodium salt
Trade names: Atomergic Carboxymethyl Chitin; Atomergic Water Soluble Chitin; Dascare Chitin Liq

Sodium carboxymethyl oleyl polypropylamine (INCI)
CAS 97659-53-5; EINECS 307-458-3
Synonyms: Oleoamphopolycarboxyglycinate
Trade names: Ampholak XO7/C

Sodium carboxymethyl tallow polypropylamine (INCI)
CAS 97659-53-5; EINECS 307-458-3
Synonyms: Tallowamphopolycarboxyglycinate
Trade names: Ampholak 7TX; Ampholak 7TX-SD 55; Ampholak 7TX-T; Ampholak 7TX/C

Sodium carrageenan (INCI)
CAS 9061-82-9; 60616-95-7
Synonyms: Carrageenan, sodium salt; Sodium carrageenate
Trade names: Viscarin

Sodium caseinate (INCI)
CAS 9005-46-3; 9004-36-3
Synonyms: Casein, sodium salt
Trade names: Alanate 110; Unipro SO-CASE

Sodium cetearyl sulfate (INCI)
CAS 59186-41-3; 68955-20-4
Synonyms: Sodium cetostearyl sulfate; Sodium cetyl/ stearyl sulfate
Trade names: Empicol® TAS30; Lanette® E; Rhodapon® EC111; Unihydag Wax E
Trade names containing: Cutina® LE; Dehydag® Wax N; Emulgade® F; Galenol® 1618 CS; Lanette® N; Unimulgade-F

Sodium ceteth-13 carboxylate (INCI)
CAS 33939-65-0 (generic)
Synonyms: Ceteth-13 carboxylic acid, sodium salt; PEG-13 cetyl ether carboxylic acid, sodium salt
Trade names: Sandopan® KST-A

Sodium cetyl sulfate (INCI)
CAS 1120-01-0; EINECS 214-292-4
Synonyms: 1-Hexadecanol, hydrogen sulfate, sodium salt
Trade names: Nikkol SCS
Trade names containing: Standapol® CS Paste; Standapol® CS-50; Texapon® CS Paste; Unipol CS Paste; Unipol CS-50

Sodium chloride (INCI)
CAS 7647-14-5; EINECS 231-598-3
Synonyms: Rock salt; Salt; Common salt
Trade names: Alberger®
Trade names containing: Amino Gluten MG; Crotein HKP Powd.; Elfan® SG; Hydroviton 2/059353; Kera-Tein H; Keramino™ SD; Kerasol; Schercotaine MKAB; Seanamin BD; Tektamer® 38 A.D.

Sodium chondroitin sulfate (INCI)
CAS 9007-28-7; 9082-07-9; EINECS 232-696-9
Trade names: Atomergic Sodium Chondroitin Sulfate; Chondroitin Sulfate A
Trade names containing: Complex T-I, T-II; Heparinoid HpDI; Hydromarine

Sodium citrate (INCI)
CAS 68-04-2; EINECS 200-675-3
Synonyms: Sodium citrate dihydrate; Trisodium citrate; Citric acid trisodium salt dihydrate
Trade names: Sodium Citrate USP, FCC (Dihydrate) Fine Gran. No. 69975; Unichem SODCIT
Trade names containing: Uninontan U 34

Sodium CMC. *See Carboxymethylcellulose sodium*

Sodium coceth sulfate (INCI)
Synonyms: Sodium PEG (1-4) coconut ether sulfate; Sodium POE (1-4) coconut ether sulfate
Trade names containing: Base Nacrante 6030 CP; Oronal LCG

Sodium cocoamphoacetate (INCI)
CAS 68334-21-4; 68608-65-1; 68390-66-9; 68647-53-0; EINECS 269-819-0, 271-793-0
Synonyms: Cocoamphoacetate; Cocoamphoglycinate
Trade names: Afoteric™ 1C; Ampholak XCO-40; Amphoterge® W; Emcol® CMCD; Emery® 5412; Empigen® CDR60; Kelisema Collagen-IMZ Complex; Mackam™ 1C; Miranol® CM Conc. NP; Monateric CM-36S; Proteric CM-36 S; Schercoteric MS; Standapol® CIM-40; Unibetaine CDC; Unibetaine GC-88; Unipol CIM-40; Velvetex® GC-88; Zoharteric M
Trade names containing: Collagen-IMZ Complex; Empigen® CDR40; Empigen® XDR302

Sodium cocoamphohydroxypropyl sulfonate (INCI)
CAS 68604-73-9; EINECS 271-705-0
Synonyms: Cocoamphopropylsulfonate; Cocoamphohydroxypropylsulfonate
Trade names: Amphoterge® SB; Mackam™ CS; Miranol® CS Conc; Sandoteric CFL; Schercoteric MS-EP

Sodium cocoamphopropionate (INCI)
CAS 68919-41-5; 93820-52-1
Synonyms: Coconut fattyacid amidoethyl-N-2-hydroxyethylaminopropionate; Cocoamphopropionate
Trade names: Amphoterge® K; Mackam™ CSF; Miranol® CM-SF Conc; Monateric CA-35; Rewoteric® AM KSF-40; Sochamine A 7527
Trade names containing: Compound 3143F

Sodium cocoate (INCI)
CAS 61789-31-9; EINECS 263-050-4
Synonyms: Coconut oil fatty acid, sodium salt; Fatty acids, coconut oil, sodium salts; Sodium coconut oil soap
Trade names: Norfox® Coco Powder
Trade names containing: Emulgade® CL Special; Emulgade® CL; Ivory Beads

Sodium coco/hydrogenated tallow sulfate (INCI)
Trade names: Elfan® KT 550

Sodium cocomonoglyceride sulfate (INCI)
CAS 61789-04-6; EINECS 263-026-3
Synonyms: Sodium coconut monoglyceride sulfate
Trade names: Nikkol SGC-80N; Poem-LS-90

Sodium coco-sulfate (INCI)
Synonyms: Sodium coconut sulfate; Sulfuric acid, monococoyl ester, sodium salt
Trade names: Elfan® 280
Trade names containing: Marlinat® KT 50

Sodium cocoyl collagen amino acids (INCI)
Trade names containing: Foam-Coll™ 5W

Sodium cocoyl glutamate (INCI)
CAS 68187-32-6; EINECS 269-087-2
Synonyms: Monosodium N-cocoyl-L-glutamate; L-Glutamic acid, N-coco acyl derivs., monosodium salts; Sodium N-cocoyl-L-glutamate
Trade names: Amisoft CS-11; Hostapon KCG
Trade names containing: Acylglutamate GS-11; Amisoft GS-11

Sodium cocoyl hydrolyzed collagen (INCI)
CAS 68188-38-5
Synonyms: Acid chlorides, coco, reaction prod. with protein hydrolyzates, sodium salts; Sodium cocoyl hydrolyzed animal protein; Sodium coco-hydrolyzed animal protein
Trade names: Bio-Pol® NCHAP; Foam-Coll™ SK; Geliderm 3000 P; Geliderm 3000 S; Hostapon SCHC; Hostapon SCHC-Powd; May-Tein SK; Monteine LCS 30; Nikkol CCN-40; Promois ECS

Sodium cocoyl hydrolyzed keratin (INCI)
Trade names: May-Tein KT

Sodium cocoyl hydrolyzed rice protein (INCI)
Trade names containing: Supro-Tein R

Sodium cocoyl hydrolyzed soy protein (INCI)
Trade names: Foam-Soy™ C; Pro Soy CO; Proteol VS22
Trade names containing: Supro-Tein S

Sodium cocoyl hydrolyzed wheat protein
Trade names: Foam-Wheat C; Pro Wheat CO

Sodium cocoyl isethionate (INCI)
CAS 61789-32-0; 58969-27-0; EINECS 263-052-5
Synonyms: Fatty acids, coconut oil, sulfoethyl esters, sodium salts
Trade names: Arlatone® SCI; Elfan® AT 84; Elfan® AT 84 G; Hostapon KA Powd; Hostapon SCI; Hostapon SCID; Jordapon® CI Disp; Jordapon® CI Powd; Jordapon® CI Prill; Jordapon® CI-UP; Tauranol I-78; Tauranol I-78 Flakes; Tauranol I-78-3; Tauranol I-78-

6; Tauranol I-78E, I-78E Flakes
Trade names containing: Arlatone® SCI-70; Geropon® AS-200; Geropon® AS-250; Jordapon® CI 60; Jordapon® CI 65; Jordapon® CI 75; Jordapon® CI-60; Tauranol I-78/80; Zetesap 5165

Sodium cocoyl lactylate
Trade names: Pationic® SCL

Sodium cocoyl sarcosinate (INCI)
CAS 61791-59-1; EINECS 263-193-2
Synonyms: Amides, coconut oil, with sarcosine, sodium salts; Sodium N-cocoyl sarcosinate
Trade names: Closyl 30 2089; Crodasinic CS; Hamposyl® C-30; Medialan KA; Nikkol Sarcosinate CN-30; Vanseal® NACS-30

Sodium cumenesulfonate (CTFA)
CAS 32073-22-6; EINECS 250-913-5; 248-938-7
Synonyms: (1-Methylethyl)benzene, monosulfo deriv., sodium salt
Trade names: SCS 40; Witconate™ SCS 45%; Witconate™ SCS 93%

Sodium cyclodextrin sulfate (INCI)
CAS 37191-69-8
Trade names: Cavitron Cyclodextrin-Sulfated

Sodium cyclopentane carboxylate (INCI)
Synonyms: Cyclopentane carboxylic acid, sodium salt
Trade names: Nikkol Sodium Naphthenate

Sodium deceth sulfate (INCI)
Synonyms: Sodium decyl ether sulfate
Trade names: Witcolate™ 7093

Sodium decylbenzene sulfonate (INCI)
CAS 1322-98-1; EINECS 215-347-5
Synonyms: Decylbenzenesulfonic acid, sodium salt
Trade names: Witconate™ DS

Sodium decyl sulfate (CTFA)
CAS 142-87-0; 84501-49-5
Trade names: Empicol® 0758

Sodium dehydroacetate (INCI)
CAS 4418-26-2; EINECS 224-580-1
Synonyms: 3-Acetyl-6-methyl-2H-pyran-2,4(3H)-dione, ion(1-), sodium salt
Trade names: Fongasel; Trisept SDHA; Tristat SDHA; Unisept DSA
Trade names containing: Fondix G Bis

Sodium dermatan sulfate (INCI)
Trade names: Dermatan Sulfate
Trade names containing: Heparinoid HpDI

Sodium dicarboxyethyl cocophosphoethyl imidazoline (INCI)
Trade names: Phosphoteric® T-C6

Sodium diceteareth-10 phosphate (INCI)
Trade names: Marlophor® T10-Sodium Salt

Sodium diethylaminopropyl cocoaspartamide (INCI)
Trade names: Chimexane HB

Sodium dihexyl sulfosuccinate. *See Dihexyl sodium sulfosuccinate*

Sodium dihydroxycetyl phosphate (INCI)
Trade names containing: Dragophos S 2/918501

Sodium dihydroxyethylglycinate (INCI)
CAS 139-41-3; EINECS 205-360-4
Synonyms: Sodium N,N-bis-2-hydroxyethyl glycinate; N,N-Bis(2-hydroxyethyl)glycine, monosodium salt
Trade names: Hampshire® DEG
Trade names containing: Kelene 77

Sodium dilaureth-7 citrate (INCI)

Trade names: Eucarol D
Trade names containing: Eucarol LS

Sodium 1,2-dimyristoyl-sn-glycero(3)phosphatidyl-choline
Trade names: Phospholipon® MG Na

Sodium dioctyl sulfosuccinate. *See Dioctyl sodium sulfo-succinate*

Sodium dioleth-8 phosphate (INCI)
Trade names: Nikkol DOP-8N

Sodium 1,2-dipalmitoyl-sn-glycero(3)phosphatidyl-choline
Trade names: Phospholipon® PG Na

Sodium 1,2-distearoyl-sn-glycero(3)phosphatidyl-choline
Trade names: Phospholipon® SG Na

Sodium DNA (INCI)
Synonyms: DNA, sodium salt
Trade names: Robeco-DNA-Na

Sodium dodecylbenzenesulfonate (INCI)
CAS 25155-30-0; 68081-81-2; 85117-50-6; EINECS 246-680-4
Synonyms: Sodium lauryl benzene sulfonate; Dodecyl-benzenesulfonic acid, sodium salt; Dodecylbenzene sodium sulfonate
Trade names: Bio-Soft® D-60; Calsoft F-90; Calsoft L-40; Calsoft L-60; Hartofol 40; Hetsulf Acid; Marlon® AFR; Nacconol® 35SL; Naxel™ AAS-40S; Naxel™ AAS-45S; Sul-fon-ate AA-10; Ufasan 35; Witconate™ 30DS; Witconate™ 45BX; Witconate™ 60B; Witconate™ 90F H; Witconate™ 1238; Witconate™ 1240; Witconate™ 1250; Witconate™ C50H; Witconate™ DS Dense; Witconate™ SK
Trade names containing: Olamin® K; Olamin® K/NP; Witconate™ 1260; Witconate™ 45 Liq.; Witconate™ 45LX; Witconate™ LX F; Witconate™ LX Powd.

Sodium erythorbate (INCI)
CAS 6381-77-7; EINECS 228-973-9
Synonyms: D-Erythro-hex-2-enonic acid, γ-lactone, monosodium salt; Sodium isoascorbate
Trade names: Uantox SEBATE; Uantox SODERT

Sodium ethylparaben (INCI)
CAS 35285-68-8; EINECS 252-487-6
Synonyms: 4-Hydroxybenzoic acid, ethyl ester, sodium salt; Ethylparaben, sodium salt
Trade names: Nipagin A Sodium
Trade names containing: Nipasept Sodium

Sodium ethyl 2-sulfolaurate (INCI)
CAS 7381-01-3
Synonyms: Dodecanoic acid, 2-sulfoethyl ester, sodium salt; Sodium 2-sulfoethyldodecanoate
Trade names containing: Alpha-Step® ML-40

Sodium gluconate (INCI)
CAS 527-07-1; EINECS 208-407-7
Synonyms: D-Gluconic acid, monosodium salt; Gluconic acid sodium salt
Trade names: Gluconal® NA
Trade names containing: Seanamin AT

Sodium glucuronate (INCI)
Trade names containing: Seanamin BD

Sodium glyceryl oleate phosphate (INCI)
Trade names: Emphos™ D70-30C
Trade names containing: Ches® 500

Sodium glyceryl trioleate sulfate
Trade names: Actrasol EO

Sodium glycyrrhizinate
Trade names: Unisweet SODGLYCRZ

Sodium hectorite
Trade names: Hectalite® 200

Sodium heparin (INCI)
CAS 9041-08-1 (generic)
Trade names containing: Heparinoid HpDI

Sodium hexametaphosphate (INCI)
CAS 10124-56-8; EINECS 233-343-1
Synonyms: SHMP; Metaphosphoric acid, hexasodium salt; Graham's salt; Sodium phosphate glass
Trade names: Calgon

Sodium hyaluronate (INCI)
CAS 9067-32-7
Trade names: Actimoist™; Actimoist™ Bio-2; Avian Sodium Hyaluronate Powd; Avian Sodium Hyaluro-nate Sol'n; Hyala-Dew; Hyaluronic Acid; Hyaluronic Acid AH-602; Hyaluronic Acid-BT; Hyaluronic Acid (Na); Hyasol; Hyasol-BT; Jaluronid; Kelisema Sodium Hyaluronate Bio; Nikkol Bio-Sodium Hyaluro-nate Powd. and 1% Sol'n; Nikkol Sodium Hyaluro-nate; Pronova™; RITA HA C-1-C; Saccaluronate CC; Saccaluronate CW; Saccaluronate LC; Sodium Hyaluronate RCC-1 No. 26228
Trade names containing: Actiglide™; Brookosome® H; Dermasome® H; Desaron; Ritacomplex DF 12, DF 13; Ritacomplex DF 14; Ritacomplex DF 15; Ritacomplex DF 26

Sodium hyaluronate dimethylsilanol (INCI)
CAS 57601-56-6
Trade names: DSH

Sodium hydrogenated tallow glutamate (INCI)
CAS 38517-23-6
Synonyms: Sodium hydrogenated tallowyl glutamate; Sodium N-hydrog. tallowyl-L-glutamate
Trade names: Amisoft HS-11
Trade names containing: Acylglutamate GS-11; Amisoft GS-11

Sodium hydroxide (INCI)
CAS 1310-73-2; EINECS 215-185-5
Synonyms: Caustic soda; Sodium hydrate; White caustic
Trade names: Unichem SOHYD
Trade names containing: Elespher® Almondermin; Elespher® Dermosaccharides GY; Elespher® Dermosaccharides HC; Elespher® Eleseryl SH

Sodium hydroxymethylglycinate (INCI)
CAS 70161-44-3; EINECS 274-357-8
Trade names: Suttocide® A

Sodium iodate (INCI)
CAS 7681-55-2; EINECS 231-672-5
Trade names: Unichem SODIOD

Sodium isethionate (INCI)
CAS 1562-00-1; EINECS 216-343-6
Synonyms: Sodium 2-hydroxyethanesulfonic acid; 2-Hydroxyethanesulfonic acid, sodium salt
Trade names: Witconate™ NIS

Sodium isosteareth-6 carboxylate (INCI)
Synonyms: Isosteareth-6 carboxylic acid, sodium salt; PEG-6 isostearyl ether carboxylic acid, sodium salt; PEG 300 isostearyl ether carboxylic acid, sodium salt
Trade names: Sandopan® TS-10

Sodium isosteareth-11 carboxylate (INCI)
Synonyms: Isosteareth-11 carboxylic acid, sodium salt; PEG-11 isostearyl ether carboxylic acid, sodium salt; POE (11) isostearyl ether carboxylic acid, sodium salt
Trade names: Sandopan® TS-20

Sodium isostearoamphopropionate (INCI)
CAS 68630-96-6; EINECS 271-929-9
Synonyms: 1H-Imidazolium, 1-(2-carboxyethyl)-4,5-dihydro-3-(2-hydroxyethyl)-2-isoheptadeceyl-, hydroxide, inner salt; Isostearoamphopropionate
Trade names: Monateric ISA-35; Schercoteric I-AA

Sodium isostearoyl lactylate (INCI)
CAS 66988-04-3; EINECS 266-533-8
Trade names: Crolactil SISL; Pationic® ISL

Sodium lactate (INCI)
CAS 72-17-3; EINECS 200-772-0
Synonyms: 2-Hydroxypropanoic acid, monosodium salt; Lacolin
Trade names: Patlac® NAL; Unichem SOLAC
Trade names containing: Aquaderm; Croderm MF; Endomine NMF; Facteur Hydratant PH; Grillocin HY-77; Hydrocos; Hydroviton 2/059353; Lactil®; Prodew 100; Prodew 200

Sodium lactate methylsilanol (INCI)
Trade names: Lasilium

Sodium lauramido MEA-sulfosuccinate
Trade names: Geropon® SS-L9ME

Sodium lauraminopropionate (INCI)
CAS 3546-96-1; EINECS 222-597-9
Synonyms: N-Dodecyl-β-alanine, monosodium salt
Trade names containing: Carsonol® BDM; Miracare® XL; Standapol® AA-1; Stepanol® LX

Sodium laureth-5 carboxylate (INCI)
CAS 33939-64-9 (generic); 38975-03-0
Synonyms: PEG-5 lauryl ether carboxylic acid, sodium salt; Sodium POE (5) lauryl ether carboxylate; Laureth-5 carboxylic acid, sodium salt
Trade names: Marlinat® CM 45; Nikkol Akypo RLM 45 NV; Sandopan® LA-8-HC

Sodium laureth-6 carboxylate (INCI)
CAS 33939-64-9 (generic); 53610-02-9
Synonyms: PEG-6 lauryl ether carboxylic acid, sodium salt; Sodium POE (6) lauryl ether carboxylate; Laureth-6 carboxylic acid, sodium salt
Trade names: Akypo RLM 45 N; Akypo®-Soft 45 NV

Sodium laureth-11 carboxylate (INCI)
CAS 33939-64-9 (generic); 53610-02-9; 68987-89-3
Synonyms: PEG-11 lauryl ether carboxylic acid, sodium salt; Sodium POE (11) lauryl ether carboxylate; Laureth-11 carboxylic acid, sodium salt
Trade names: Akypo RLM 100 NV; Akypo®-Soft 100 NV; Marlinat® CM 105; Rewopol® CLN 100

Sodium laureth-13 carboxylate (INCI)
CAS 33939-64-9 (generic); 70632-06-3
Synonyms: PEG-13 lauryl ether carboxylic acid, sodium salt; POE (13) lauryl ether carboxylic acid, sodium salt; Laureth-13 carboxylic acid, sodium salt
Trade names: Miranate® LEC; Sandopan® LS-24; Surfine WLL
Trade names containing: Carsofoam® BS-I; Miracare® BC-10; Miracare® BC-20; Miracare® MS-1; Miracare® MS-2; Miracare® MS-4

Sodium laureth-14 carboxylate (INCI)
CAS 33939-64-9 (generic); 68987-89-3
Synonyms: PEG-14 lauryl ether carboxylic acid, sodium salt; POE (14) lauryl ether carboxylic acid, sodium salt; Laureth-14 carboxylic acid, sodium salt
Trade names: Akypo®-Soft 130 NV

Sodium laureth-17 carboxylate (INCI)
CAS 33939-64-9 (generic); 68987-89-3
Synonyms: PEG-17 lauryl ether carboxylic acid, sodium salt; POE (17) lauryl ether carboxylic acid, sodium salt; Laureth-17 carboxylic acid, sodium salt
Trade names: Akypo RLM 160 N; Akypo Soft 160 NV; Akypo®-Soft 160 NV

Sodium laureth-4 phosphate (INCI)
CAS 42612-52-2 (generic)
Synonyms: Sodium POE (4) lauryl ether phosphate; Sodium PEG 200 lauryl ether phosphate
Trade names: Chemphos TR-510S; Rhodafac® MC-470

Sodium laureth sulfate (INCI)
CAS 1335-72-4; 3088-31-1; 9004-82-4 (generic); 13150-00-0; 15826-16-1; 68891-38-3; EINECS 221-416-0
Synonyms: Sodium lauryl ether sulfate (n=104); PEG (1-4) lauryl ether sulfate, sodium salt
Trade names: Akyposal DS 28; Akyposal EO 20; Akyposal EO 20 MW; Akyposal EO 2067; Berol 452; Calfoam ES-30; Calfoam ES-303; Calfoam ES-603; Calfoam SEL-60; Carsonol® SES-S; Carsonol® SLES; Carsonol® SLES-2; Carsonol® SLES-3; Carsonol® SLES-4; Chemsalan RLM 28; Chemsalan RLM 56; Chemsalan RLM 70; Cosmopon LE 50; Elfan® NS 242; Elfan® NS 242 A; Elfan® NS 242 Conc; Elfan® NS 243 S; Elfan® NS 243 S Conc; Empicol® 0251/70; Empicol® ESA; Empicol® ESA70; Empicol® ESB; Empicol® ESB3; Empicol® ESB3/D; Empicol® ESB3/M; Empicol® ESB70; Empicol® ESB70-AU; Empicol® ESC/AU; Empicol® ESC3; Empicol® ESC70; Empicol® ESC70/AU; Empimin® KSN70; Genapol® ARO Paste; Genapol® LRO Liq., Paste; Genapol® ZRO Liq., Paste; Laural LS; Manro BEC 28; Manro BEC 70; Manro BES 27; Manro BES 60; Manro BES 70; Manro NEC 28; Manro NEC 28H; Manro NEC 28L; Manro NEC 70; Marlinat® 242/28; Marlinat® 242/70; Marlinat® 242/70 S; Marlinat® 243/28; Marlinat® 243/70; Neopon LOS 2 N 70; Neopon LOS 3 N 70; Neopon LOS 70; Neopon LOS/NF; Nikkol SBL-2N-27; Nikkol SBL-3N-27; Nikkol SBL-4N; Nonasol N4SS; Norfox® SLES-02; Norfox® SLES-03; Norfox® SLES-60; Nutrapon BM 3960; Nutrapon ES-2 3677; Nutrapon ES-60 3568; Nutrapon ESY 2299; Nutrapon KF 3846; Nutrapon KPC 0156; Oronal BLD; Perlankrol® ADP3; Perlankrol® ASC2; Perlankrol® ASC38; Perlankrol® ASC49; Perlankrol® ASC82; Rewopol® NL 2-28; Rewopol® NL 3; Rewopol® NL 3-28; Rewopol® NL 3-70; Rhodapex® ES; Rhodapex® ES-12; Rhodapex® ES-2; Rhodapex® ESY; Rolpon 24/230; Rolpon 24/270; Rolpon 24/330 N; Sandet EN; Sandoz Sulfate 219; Sandoz Sulfate 219 Special; Standapol® ES-1; Standapol® ES-2; Standapol® ES-250; Standapol® ES-3; Standapol® ES-350; Steol® 4N; Steol® CS-130; Steol® CS-230; Steol® CS-330; Steol® CS-460; Steol® KS-460; Sulfochem ES-1; Sulfochem ES-2; Sulfochem ES-3; Sulfochem ES-60; Sulfochem ES-70; Surfax EAD; Surfax EVE; Tensagex DLM 927; Tensagex DLM 970; Tensagex EOC 628; Tensagex EOC 670; Texapon® ES-1; Texapon® ES-2; Texapon® ES-250; Texapon® ES-3; Texapon® ES-40; Texapon® LT-327; Texapon® N 70; Texapon® NC 70; Texapon® NSO; Texapon® PLT-227; Texapon® PN-235; Texapon® PN-254; Texapon® QLV; Tylorol 2S, 2S/25; Tylorol 3S; Tylorol BS; Tylorol S; Ungerol LES 2-28; Ungerol LES 2-70; Ungerol LES 3-28; Ungerol LES 3-70; Ungerol N2-28; Ungerol N2-70; Ungerol N3-28; Ungerol N3-70; Unipol ES; Unipol ES-1, ES-2, ES-3; Witcolate™ ES-1; Witcolate™ ES-2; Witcolate™ ES-3; Witcolate™ LES-60C; Witcolate™ OME; Witcolate™ S1285C; Witcolate™ SE-2; Zetesol NL; Zoharpon ETA 27;

Zoharpon ETA 70; Zoharpon ETA 270 (OXO); Zoharpon ETA 271; Zoharpon ETA 273; Zoharpon ETA 603; Zoharpon ETA 700 (OXO); Zoharpon ETA 703

Trade names containing: Akyposal 2010 S; Akyposal HF 28; Amphotensid 9M; Base Nacrante 1100 AD; Base Nacrante 9578; Bio-Terge® 804; Carsofoam® DEV; Carsofoam® SC; Cerasynt® LP; Cosmopon BS; Cosmopon MP; Crodapearl Liq.; Cycloryl GSC; Cycloryl M1; Dermalcare® 1673; Elfan® SG; Empicol® 0627; Empicol® XC35; Empigen® XDR121; Empigen® XDR123; Euperlan® MPK 850; Euperlan® PK 771 BENZ; Euperlan® PK 771; Euperlan® PK 776; Euperlan® PK 789; Euperlan® PK 810 AM; Euperlan® PK 810; Euperlan® PK 900 BENZ; Euperlan® PK 900; Genapol® PGM Conc; Genapol® PGM Liq.; Genapol® PGS; Genapol® TSM; Krim CH 25; Mackam™ 2CAS; Mackam™ 2MCAS; Marlamid® KLP; Marlon® PF 40; Miracare® 2MCAS; Miracare® ANL; Miracare® NWC; Monateric CDL; Olamin® K; Olamin® K/NP; Perlglanzmittel GM 4006; Perlglanzmittel GM 4175; Plantaren® PS-200; Proteric CDL; Rewopol® SBV; Rewoteric® AM CA; Schercoteric LS-2ES MOD; Schercoteric MS-2ES Modified; Standapol® 7092; Standapol® AP Blend; Standapol® Pearl Conc. 7130; Standapol® S; Surfax SLA; Syntran 5130; Syntran KL-219; Texapon® ASV-70 Spec; Texapon® ASV; Texapon® EVR; Texapon® SBN; Texapon® SG; Ufablend MPL; Unette-W; Uniplant PS-200; Unipol 7092; Zetesol MS; Zetesol OM; Zohar EGMS 771; Zoharpon EGDS-771; Zoharpon ETA 35; Zoharteric D-2; Zoharteric D-3; Zoharteric D.O.T.; Zoharteric M-2; Zoharteric M-3

Sodium laureth-8 sulfate (CTFA)
CAS 9004-82-4 (generic)
Synonyms: PEG (8) lauryl ether sulfate, sodium salt; PEG 400 lauryl ether sulfate, sodium salt; Sodium POE (8) lauryl ether sulfate
Trade names containing: Euperlan® MPK 850; Texapon® ASV-70 Spec; Texapon® ASV

Sodium laureth-12 sulfate (INCI)
CAS 9004-82-4 (generic); 66161-57-7
Synonyms: PEG (12) lauryl ether sulfate, sodium salt; PEG 600 lauryl ether sulfate, sodium salt; Sodium POE (12) lauryl ether sulfate
Trade names: Disponil FES 92E; Standapol® 125-E; Standapol® 130-E; Unipol 125-E, 130-E; Unipol ES-40

Sodium laureth sulfosuccinate
Trade names: Secosol® ALL40

Sodium laureth-7 tartrate (INCI)
Synonyms: PEG-7 lauryl ether tartrate, sodium salt
Trade names: Eucarol TA

Sodium lauriminodipropionate (INCI)
CAS 14960-06-6; 26256-79-1; EINECS 239-032-7
Synonyms: Sodium N-lauryl-β-iminodipropionate; N-(2-Carboxyethyl)-N-dodecyl-β-alanine, monosodium salt
Trade names: Afoteric™ 160C; Deriphat® 160C; Mackam™ 160C-30; Mirataine® H2C-HA; Rewoteric® AM LP; Unibetaine 160; Unitex 610-L

Sodium lauroamphoacetate (INCI)
CAS 14350-96-0; 68647-44-9; 26837-33-2; 68298-21-5; 68608-66-2; EINECS 271-949-8; 269-547-2; 238-305-8
Synonyms: 1H-Imidazolium, 1-(carboxymethyl)-4,5-dihydro-1-(2-hydroxyethyl)-2-undecyl-, hydroxide,

sodium salt; Lauroamphoacetate; Lauroamphoglycinate
Trade names: Afoteric™ 1L; Ampholyt™ JA 140; Dehyton® PLG; Dehyton® PMG; Mackam™ 1L; Mackam™ 1L-30; Miranol® HM Conc; Monateric LMM-30; Unibetaine G-20
Trade names containing: Mackam™ MLT; Miracare® BC-10; Miracare® BC-20; Miracare® MHT; Monateric 985A; Rewoteric® AM G 30

Sodium lauroyl glutamate (INCI)
CAS 29923-31-7 (L-form); 29923-34-0 (DL-form); 42926-22-7 (L-form); 98984-78-2; EINECS 249-958-3
Synonyms: N-Dodecyl-L-glutamic acid, monosodium salt; N-(1-Oxodecyl)glutamic acid, monosodium salt; Sodium N-lauroyl-L-glutamate
Trade names: Amisoft LS-11
Trade names containing: Emalex FDB-36

Sodium lauroyl hydrolyzed silk
Trade names: Promois EFLS

Sodium lauroyl lactylate (INCI)
CAS 13557-75-0; EINECS 236-942-6
Synonyms: Dodecanoic acid, 2-(1-carboxyethoxy)-1-methyl-2-oxoethyl ester, sodium salt
Trade names: Pationic® 138C

Sodium lauroyl methylaminopropionate (INCI)
Synonyms: N-Sodium N-lauroyl-N-methyl alaninate
Trade names: Enagicol L-30AN; Nikkol Alaninate LN-30

Sodium lauroyl sarcosinate (INCI)
CAS 137-16-6; EINECS 205-281-5
Synonyms: N-Methyl-N-(1-oxododecyl)glycine, sodium salt; N-Lauroylsarcosine sodium salt; Sodium-N-dodecanoyl-N-methylglycinate
Trade names: Chimin L; Closyl LA 3584; Crodasinic LS30; Crodasinic LS35; Hamposyl® L-30; Hamposyl® L-95; Maprosyl® 30; Medialan LD; Nikkol Sarcosinate LN; Nikkol Sarcosinate LN-30; Oramix L30; Secosyl; Unipol LAUROYLSAR; Vanseal® NALS-30; Vanseal® NALS-95; Zoharsyl L-30

Sodium lauroyl taurate (INCI)
CAS 70609-66-4; EINECS 274-695-6
Synonyms: Sodium 2-[(1-oxododecyl) amino] ethanesulfonate
Trade names: Hostapon KTW

Sodium lauryl/cetearyl sulfate
Synonyms: Sodium lauryl/cetostearyl sulfate
Trade names: Empicol® 0775; Empicol® 0775/55

Sodium lauryl phosphate (INCI)
Trade names: Nikkol Phosten HLP-N; Nikkol SLP-N

Sodium lauryl sulfate (INCI)
CAS 151-21-3; 68585-47-7; 68955-19-1; EINECS 205-788-1
Synonyms: SDS; Sulfuric acid, monododecyl ester, sodium salt; Sodium dodecyl sulfate
Trade names: Akyporox SAL SAS; Akyposal NLS; Alscoap LN-40, LN-90; Calfoam SLS-30; Carsonol® SLS; Carsonol® SLS Paste B; Carsonol® SLS Special; Carsonol® SLS-R; Carsonol® SLS-S; Chemsalan NLS 30; Cosmopon 35; Elfadent SM 514; Elfan® 240; Empicol® 0045; Empicol® 0045V; Empicol® 0185; Empicol® 0303; Empicol® 0303V; Empicol® LM45; Empicol® LS30B; Empicol® LS30P; Empicol® LX; Empicol® LX100; Empicol® LX28; Empicol® LXS95; Empicol® LXV; Empicol® LXV/D; Empicol® LXV100; Empicol® LZ; Empicol® LZ/D; Empicol® LZV; Empicol® LZV/D; Empicol® WAK; Gardinol WA Paste; Manro SLS 28; Marlinat® DFK 30; Naxolate™ WA Special; Naxolate™ WA-97;

Naxolate™ WAG; Neopon LS/NF; Nikkol SLS; Nikkol SLS-30; Norfox® SLS; Nutrapon DL 3891; Nutrapon W 1367; Nutrapon WAC 3005; Nutrapon WAQ; Nutrapon WAQE 2364; Perlankrol® DSA; Rewopol® NLS 28; Rewopol® NLS 90; Rhodapon® LSB, LSB/CT; Rhodapon® SB-8208/S; Rhodapon® SM Special; Rolpon LSX; Standapol® WA-AC; Standapol® WAQ Special; Standapol® WAQ-LC; Stepanol® ME Dry; Stepanol® WA Extra; Stepanol® WA Paste; Stepanol® WA Special; Stepanol® WA-100; Stepanol® WAC; Stepanol® WAQ; Sulfochem SAC; Sulfochem SLC; Sulfochem SLN; Sulfochem SLP; Sulfochem SLP-95; Sulfochem SLS; Sulfopon® 101 Special; Sulfopon® 103; Sulfopon® P-40; Sulfopon® WA 3; Sulfopon® WAQ LCX; Sulfopon® WAQ Special; Supralate C; Supralate QC; Supralate WA Paste; Surfax 100; Surfax 100 AG; Surfax CN; Texapon® K-12 Needles; Texapon® K-12 Powd; Texapon® K-1296; Texapon® L-100; Texapon® LS 100 F; Texapon® LS Highly Conc. Needles; Texapon® OT Highly Conc. Needles; Texapon® VHC Needles; Texapon® Z; Texapon® ZHC Needles; Texapon® ZHC Powder; Ufarol Na-30; Unipol SLS; Unipol WA-AC; Unipol WAC Special; Unipol WAQ-LC; Unipon K12, K1296, L-100, ZHC Needles, ZHC Powd; Unipon ZHC Needles; Witcolate™ A Powder; Witcolate™ C; Witcolate™ LCP; Witcolate™ SL-1; Witcolate™ WAC; Witcolate™ WAC-GL; Witcolate™ WAC-LA; Zoharpon LAS; Zoharpon LAS 70%; Zoharpon LAS Special; Zoharpon LAS Spray Dried
Trade names containing: Amisol™ 638; Ceral 10; Ceral EF; Ceral EFN; Ceral LE; Cerasynt® WM; Collagen-LSS Complex; Cosmopon BS; Crodex A; Cyclochem EM 560; Dehydag® Wax SX; Dehydag® Wax W; Empigen® XDR302; Empiwax SK; Empiwax SK/BP; Emulmetik™ 310; Equex STM; Eucarol LS; Galenol® 1618 DSN; Kelisema Collagen-LSS Complex; Klensoft; Lanette® SX; Lanette® W; Lexemul® AS; Lytron 621; Mackam™ 2CA; Mackam™ 2CAS; Mackam™ 2MCA; Mackam™ 2MCAS; Miracare® 2MCA-SF; Miracare® 2MCA; Miracare® 2MCAS; Miracare® M1; Monaterge 1164; Monateric CDS; Nutrapon B 1365; Nutrapon TK 3603; Nutrapon TW 3987; Proteric CDL; Rewoteric® AM G 30; Rhodaterge® SSB; Schercoteric MS-2 Modified; Standapol® BW; Standapol® CS Paste; Standapol® CS-50; Standapol® S; Standapol® SHC-101; Stepanol® 360; Surfax AC 55; Tegacid® Special; Teginacid® Spezial SE; Texapon® CS Paste; Texapon® EVR; Unihydag Wax-SX; Unipol CS Paste; Unipol CS-50; Zetesap 813A; Zoharteric D.O.

Sodium lauryl sulfoacetate (INCI)
CAS 1847-58-1; EINECS 217-431-7
Synonyms: Acetic acid, sulfo-, 1-dodecyl ester, sodium salt; Sulfoacetic acid, 1-dodecyl ester, sodium salt
Trade names: Lathanol® LAL; Nikkol LSA
Trade names containing: Lumorol K 5019; Stepan-Mild® LSB

Sodium lauryl sulfosuccinate (CTFA)
Trade names: Secosol® AL 959

Sodium/magnesium laureth sulfate
Trade names: Empicol® BSD 52

Sodium/magnesium laureth sulfonate
Trade names: Empicol® BSD

Sodium magnesium silicate (INCI)
CAS 53320-86-8; EINECS 258-476-2
Trade names: Laponite® D; Laponite® XLG
Trade names containing: Lapomer; Laponite® XLS

Sodium mannuronate methylsilanol (INCI)
CAS 23732-95-8
Trade names: Algisium

Sodium/MEA laureth-2 sulfosuccinate (INCI)
Trade names: Empicol® SHH

Sodium metabisulfite (INCI)
CAS 7681-57-4; EINECS 231-673-0
Synonyms: Disulfurous acid, disodium salt; Sodium pyrosulfite; Sodium bisulfite
Trade names: Uantox SMBS

Sodium methyl cocoyl taurate (INCI)
CAS 12765-39-8; 61791-42-2
Synonyms: Sodium cocoyl methyl taurate; Sodium N-cocoyl-N-methyl taurate; Sodium N-methyl-N-cocoyl taurate
Trade names: Adinol CT95; Geropon® TC-42; Hostapon CT Paste; Nikkol CMT-30; Protapon 24A; Somepon T25; Tauranol WS H.P; Tauranol WS, WS Conc; Tauranol WSP

Sodium methyl lauroyl taurate (INCI)
CAS 4337-75-1; EINECS 224-388-8
Synonyms: Sodium lauroyl methyl taurate; Sodiun N-lauroyl methyl taurate; Sodium N-methyl-N-lauroyl taurate
Trade names: Nikkol LMT; Zoharpon LMT42

Sodium methyl myristoyl taurate (INCI)
CAS 18469-44-8; EINECS 242-349-3
Synonyms: Sodium myristoyl methyl taurate; Sodium N-methyl-N-myristoyl taurate; Sodium N-myristoyl methyl taurate
Trade names: Nikkol MMT

Sodium methyl oleoyl taurate (INCI)
CAS 137-20-2; EINECS 205-285-7
Synonyms: Sodium N-oleoyl-N-methyl taurate; Oleyl methyl tauride; Sodium N-methyl-N-oleoyl taurate
Trade names: Adinol OT16; Geropon® T-77; Hostapon SO; Hostapon T Paste 33; Hostapon T Powd. Highly Conc; Protapon 33; Tauranol M-35; Tauranol MS; Tauranol T-Gel
Trade names containing: Tauranol ML

Sodium methyl palmitoyl taurate (INCI)
CAS 3737-55-1; EINECS 223-114-4
Synonyms: Sodium palmitoyl methyl taurate; Sodium N-methyl-N-palmitoyl taurate; Sodium N-palmitoyl methyl taurate
Trade names: Nikkol PMT

Sodium methylparaben (INCI)
CAS 5026-62-0; EINECS 225-714-1
Synonyms: 4-Hydroxybenzoic acid, methyl ester, sodium salt; Methylparaben, sodium salt
Trade names: Nipagin M Sodium; Unisept M NA
Trade names containing: Fondix G Bis; Nipasept Sodium

Sodium methyl stearoyl taurate (INCI)
CAS 149-39-3; EINECS 205-738-9; 205-713-2
Synonyms: Sodium stearoyl methyl taurate; Sodium N-methyl-N-stearoyl taurate; Sodium N-stearoyl-N-methyl taurate
Trade names: Hostapon STT Paste; Nikkol SMT

Sodium methyl 2-sulfolaurate (INCI)
Trade names containing: Alpha-Step® ML-40

Sodium methyl tallow taurate
Trade names: Nissan Diapon T

Sodium myreth sulfate (INCI)
CAS 25446-80-4; 68891-38-3; EINECS 246-986-8
Synonyms: Sodium myristyl ether sulfate; PEG (1-4) myristyl ether sulfate, sodium salt

Trade names: Elfan® NS 423 SH; Standapol® ES-40; Standapol® ES-50; Texapon® K-14S 70 Special; Texapon® K-14S Spec

Sodium myristoyl glutamate (INCI)
CAS 38517-37-2; 71368-20-2; EINECS 253-981-4
Synonyms: N-(1-Oxotetradecyl)glutamic acid, monosodium salt
Trade names: Amisoft MS-11

Sodium myristoyl sarcosinate (INCI)
CAS 30364-51-3; EINECS 250-151-3
Synonyms: N-Methyl-N-(1-oxotetradecyl)glycine, sodium salt
Trade names: Crodasinic MS; Hamposyl® M-30; Nikkol Sarcosinate MN; Vanseal® NAMS-30

Sodium myristyl sulfate (INCI)
CAS 1191-50-0; 139-88-8; EINECS 214-737-2
Synonyms: Sodium tetradecyl sulfate; Sulfuric acid, monotetradecyl ester, sodium salt
Trade names: Niaproof® Anionic Surfactant 4; Nikkol SMS
Trade names containing: Texapon® CS Paste

Sodium nonoxynol-9 phosphate (INCI)
Synonyms: PEG-9 nonyl phenyl ether phosphate, sodium salt; PEG 450 nonyl phenyl ether phosphate, sodium salt; Sodium PEG-9 nonyl phenyl ether phosphate
Trade names: Chemphos TC-231S; Emphos™ CS-1361

Sodium nonoxynol-4 sulfate (INCI)
CAS 9014-90-8 (generic); 68891-39-4
Synonyms: PEG-4 nonyl phenyl ether sulfate, sodium salt; PEG 200 nonyl phenyl ether sulfate, sodium salt; Sodium PEG-4 nonyl phenyl ether sulfate
Trade names: Nikkol SNP-4N; Rhodapex® CO-433; Witcolate™ D51-51EP

Sodium nonoxynol-8 sulfate (INCI)
CAS 9014-90-8 (generic)
Synonyms: PEG-8 nonyl phenyl ether sulfate, sodium salt; PEG 400 nonyl phenyl ether sulfate, sodium salt; POE (8) nonyl phenyl ether sulfate, sodium salt
Trade names: Elfan® NS 98 N

Sodium octoxynol-2 ethane sulfonate (INCI)
CAS 2917-94-4; 67923-87-9; EINECS 267-791-4; 220-851-3
Synonyms: 2-[2-[2-Octylphenoxy)ethoxy]ethoxy]ethanesulfonic acid, sodium salt; Entsufon
Trade names: Avanel® S-35

Sodium octyl sulfate (INCI)
CAS 126-92-1; 142-31-4; EINECS 204-812-8
Synonyms: Sodium 2-ethylhexyl sulfate; Sulfuric acid, mono (2-ethylhexyl) ester, sodium salt
Trade names: Cosmopon SES; Empicol® 0585/A; Niaproof® Anionic Surfactant 08; Witcolate™ D-510

Sodium oleoamphohydroxypropylsulfonate (INCI)
CAS 68610-38-8
Synonyms: Oleoamphopropylsulfonate; Oleoamphohydroxypropylsulfonate
Trade names: Mackam™ OS; Sandopan® TFL Conc; Sandoteric TFL Conc

Sodium oleth sulfate (INCI)
CAS 27233-34-7
Synonyms: Sodium PEG (1-4) oleyl ether sulfate; Sodium POE (1-4) oleyl ether sulfate; PEG (1-4) oleyl ether sulfate, sodium salt
Trade names containing: Euperlan® MPK 850; Texapon® ASV-70 Spec; Texapon® ASV

Sodium oleyl/cetyl sulfate

Trade names: Elfan® 680

Sodium oleyl phosphate
Trade names: Nikkol TOP-O

Sodium palmitoyl sarcosinate
Trade names: Nikkol Sarcosinate PN

Sodium PCA (INCI)
CAS 28874-51-3; 54571-67-4; EINECS 249-277-1
Synonyms: PCA-Na; PCA Soda; 5-Oxo-DL-proline, sodium salt; Sodium pyroglutamate
Trade names: Ajidew N-50; Dermidrol; Nalidone®; Ritamectant PCA
Trade names containing: Ajidew SP-100; Aquaderm; Croderm MF; Endomine NMF; Hydrolyzed NMF; Lactil®; Prodew 100; Prodew 200; Ritaderm®

Sodium PEG-6 cocamide carboxylate (INCI)
CAS 107628-03-5
Synonyms: PEG-6 cocamide ether carboxylic acid, sodium salt; POE (6) cocamide ether carboxylic acid, sodium salt; PEG 300 cocamide ether carboxylic acid, sodium salt
Trade names: Akypo®-Soft KA 250 BVC
Trade names containing: Akypo®-Soft KA 250 BV; Akypogene HM 12; Akypogene HM 8; Akyposal 2010 SD

Sodium PEG-3 lauramide carboxylate (INCI)
Synonyms: PEG-3 lauramide ether carboxylic acid, sodium salt; POE (3) lauramide ether carboxylic acid, sodium salt
Trade names: Akypo AD 100 SPC

Sodium PG-propyl thiosulfate dimethicone (INCI)
Trade names: Abil® S201; Abil® S255

Sodium o-phenylphenate (CTFA)
CAS 132-27-4; EINECS 205-055-6
Synonyms: o-Phenylphenol sodium salt; (1,1´-Biphenyl)-2-ol, sodium salt; Sodium o-phenylphenolate
Trade names: Dowicide A

Sodium phosphate (INCI)
CAS 7558-80-7; EINECS 231-449-2
Synonyms: MSP; Sodium phosphate, monobasic; Monosodium dihydrogen phosphate; Sodium biphosphate
Trade names containing: Bovine Fibronectin Sol'n

Sodium polyacrylate (INCI)
CAS 9003-04-7
Synonyms: Polyacrylic acid, sodium salt
Trade names containing: Salcare SC91

Sodium polyacrylate starch (INCI)
Trade names: Sanwet® COS-905; Sanwet® COS-915; Sanwet® COS-960; Sanwet® COS-965

Sodium polydimethylglycinophenolsulfonate (INCI)
Trade names: Hamplex DPS

Sodium polyglutamate (INCI)
CAS 28829-38-1
Trade names: Ajicoat SPG

Sodium polymannuronate. *See Algin*

Sodium polymethacrylate (INCI)
CAS 25086-62-8; 54193-36-1
Synonyms: 2-Propenoic acid, 2-methyl-, homopolymer, sodium salt
Trade names: Daxad® 30

Sodium polynaphthalene sulfonate (INCI)
CAS 9084-06-4
Synonyms: Sodium naphthalene-formaldehyde sulfonate
Trade names: Petro® 11

Sodium polystyrene sulfonate (INCI)
CAS 9003-59-2; 25704-18-1
Synonyms: Ethenylbenzenesulfonic acid, sodium salt, homopolymer
Trade names: Flexan® 130

Sodium potassium aluminosilicate
Synonyms: Nepheline syenite
Trade names: Abscents® Deodorizing Powd

Sodium propionate (INCI)
CAS 137-40-6; EINECS 205-290-4
Synonyms: Propanoic acid, sodium salt
Trade names: Unistat SOBAN

Sodium propylparaben (INCI)
CAS 35285-69-9; EINECS 252-488-1
Synonyms: 4-Hydroxybenzoic acid, propyl ester, sodium salt; Propyl-4-hydroxybenzoate, sodium salt; Propylparaben, sodium salt
Trade names: Nipasol M Sodium
Trade names containing: Nipasept Sodium

Sodium pyrithione (INCI)
CAS 3811-73-2; EINECS 223-296-5
Synonyms: Sodium 2-pyridinethiol-1-oxide; Sodium (2-pyridylthio)-N-oxide; 2-Pyridinethiol, 1-oxide, sodium salt
Trade names: Sodium Omadine®, 40% Aq. Sol'n

Sodium pyroglutamate. *See Sodium PCA*

Sodium saccharin (INCI)
CAS 128-44-9; EINECS 204-886-1
Synonyms: 1,1-Dioxide-1,2-benzisothiazol-3(2H)-one, sodium salt
Trade names: Unisweet SOSAC

Sodium sesquicarbonate (INCI)
CAS 533-96-0; EINECS 208-580-9
Synonyms: Carbonic acid, sodium salt (2:3)
Trade names: Snow Fine; Snow Flake

Sodium silicate (INCI)
CAS 1344-09-8; EINECS 215-687-4
Synonyms: Silicic acid, sodium salt; Water glass; Soluble glass
Trade names: Britesil; O Silicate

Sodium silicoaluminate (INCI)
CAS 1344-00-9; EINECS 215-684-8
Synonyms: Sodium aluminosilicate; Sodium silico-aluminate; Sodium aluminum silicate
Trade names: Valfor® Zeolite Na-A; Zeolex® 7; Zeolex® 23A

Sodium starch glycolate
CAS 9063-38-1
Trade names: Explotab®

Sodium stearate (INCI)
CAS 822-16-2; EINECS 212-490-5
Synonyms: Sodium octadecanoate; Octadecanoic acid, sodium salt; Stearic acid, sodium salt
Trade names: Cecavon NA 61; Norfox® B; Sodium Stéarate C7L; Unichem SS; Witco® Sodium Stearate C-1; Witco® Sodium Stearate C-7
Trade names containing: Alcolite; Emulgade® CL Special; Emulgade® CL; Monomuls® 60-25/2; Monomuls® 90-25/2, 90-25/5; Zohar GLST SE

Sodium stearoamphoacetate (INCI)
CAS 30473-39-3; 68608-63-9; EINECS 250-215-0
Synonyms: 1H-Imidazolium, 1-(carboxymethyl)-2-heptadecyl-4,5-dihydro-1-(2-hydroxyethyl)-, hydroxide, disodium salt; Stearoamphoacetate; Stearoamphoglycinate
Trade names: Amphoterge® S; Miranol® DM; Miranol®

DM Conc. 45%

Sodium stearoyl lactylate (INCI)
CAS 25383-99-7; EINECS 246-929-7
Synonyms: Octadecanoic acid, 2-(1-carboxyethoxy)-1-methyl-2-oxoethyl ester, sodium salt; Sodium stearyl-2-lactylate
Trade names: Artodan SP 55 Kosher; Crolactil SSL; Pationic® SSL; Unitolate SSL
Trade names containing: Myvatex® Texture Lite

Sodium stearyl fumarate
CAS 4070-80-8
Trade names: Pruv™

Sodium stearyl sulfate (INCI)
CAS 1120-04-3; EINECS 214-295-0
Synonyms: Sulfuric acid, monooctadecyl ester, sodium salt
Trade names: Nikkol SSS
Trade names containing: Texapon® CS Paste

Sodium styrene/acrylates/divinylbenzene copolymer (INCI)
Trade names containing: Lytron 295

Sodium styrene/acrylates/PEG-10 dimaleate copolymer (INCI)
Trade names containing: Lytron 300

Sodium styrene/PEG-10 maleate/nonoxynol-10 maleate/acrylates copolymer (INCI)
Trade names containing: Lytron 305

Sodium tallamphodipropionate
Trade names: Miranol® TBS

Sodium tallowate (INCI)
CAS 8052-48-0; EINECS 232-491-4
Synonyms: Tallow, sodium salt
Trade names: Norfox® XXX Granules
Trade names containing: Ivory Beads

Sodium tallow sulfate (INCI)
CAS 8052-50-4; 68140-10-3; 68955-20-4; EINECS 232-494-0
Synonyms: Sodium tallow alcohol sulfate; Sulfuric acid, monotallow alkyl esters, sodium salts
Trade names containing: Marlinat® KT 50

Sodium tauride acrylates/acrylic acid/acrylonitrogens copolymer (INCI)
Trade names: Hypan® TC-200

Sodium/TEA-lauroyl collagen amino acids (INCI)
Synonyms: Proteins, hydrolysate, reaction prod. with lauroyl chloride, compds. with sodium and triethanol-amine; Sodium/TEA-lauroyl animal collagen amino acids
Trade names: Silflex A22

Sodium/TEA-lauroyl hydrolyzed collagen (INCI)
Synonyms: Sodium/TEA-lauroyl hydrolyzed animal protein
Trade names: Foam-Keratin LK

Sodium/TEA-lauroyl hydrolyzed collagen amino acid
Trade names: Lipoproteol LCO

Sodium/TEA-lauroyl hydrolyzed keratin (INCI)
Trade names: May-Tein KTS

Sodium/TEA-lauroyl hydrolyzed keratin amino acids (INCI)
Trade names: Lipoproteol LK

Sodium/TEA-undecenoyl collagen amino acids (INCI)
Synonyms: Sodium/TEA-undecylenoyl animal collagen amino acids
Trade names: Lipoproteol UCO

Sodium toluenesulfonate (INCI)
CAS 657-84-1; 12068-03-0; EINECS 235-088-1
Synonyms: Methylbenzenesulfonic acid, sodium salt
Trade names: Eltesol® ST 34; Eltesol® ST 40; Witconate™ STS

Sodium trideceth-3 carboxylate (INCI)
CAS 68891-17-8 (generic); 61757-59-3 (generic)
Synonyms: PEG-3 tridecyl ether carboxylic acid, sodium salt; Sodium POE (3) tridecyl ether carboxylate
Trade names: Nikkol ECT-3NEX, ECTD-3NEX

Sodium trideceth-6 carboxylate (INCI)
CAS 68891-17-8 (generic); 61757-59-3 (generic)
Synonyms: PEG-6 tridecyl ether carboxylic acid, sodium salt; Sodium POE (6) tridecyl ether carboxylate
Trade names: Nikkol ECTD-6NEX

Sodium trideceth-7 carboxylate (INCI)
CAS 68891-17-8 (generic); 61757-59-3 (generic)
Synonyms: PEG-7 tridecyl ether carboxylic acid, sodium salt; POE (7) tridecyl ether carboxylic acid, sodium salt
Trade names: Rolpon C 200; Sandopan® DTC; Sandopan® DTC-100

Sodium trideceth sulfate (INCI)
CAS 25446-78-0 (n=3); 66161-58-8 (n=4); EINECS 246-985-2
Synonyms: Sodium tridecyl ether sulfate; Sodium POE tridecyl sulfate
Trade names: Cedepal TD-403; Cedepal TD-407; Cedepal TD-484; Liposurf EST-30; Rhodapex® 674/C; Rhodapex® EST-30; Tensagex DLM 627; Tensagex DLM 670; Tensagex DLS 670; Tensagex DLS 970
Trade names containing: Carsofoam® BS-I; Compound TL; Mackam™ 2CT; Mackam™ 2LES; Mackam™ 2MHT; Mackam™ MLT; Miracare® 2MCT; Miracare® 2MHT; Miracare® BC-10; Miracare® BC-20; Miracare® BT; Miracare® MHT; Miracare® MS-1; Miracare® MS-2; Miracare® MS-4; Miraspec ALC; Monateric 985A; Monateric CDTD; Proteric CDTD; Schercoteric LS-2TE MOD; Schercoteric LS-2TE; Velvetex® LTD

Sodium trideceth sulfonate
Trade names containing: Mackam™ LT

Sodium tridecylbenzene sulfonate (INCI)
CAS 26248-24-8; EINECS 247-536-3
Synonyms: Tridecylbenzenesulfonic acid, sodium salt
Trade names: Witconate™ TDB

Sodium tridecyl sulfate (INCI)
CAS 3026-63-9; EINECS 221-188-2
Synonyms: 1-Tridecanol, hydrogen sulfate, sodium salt
Trade names: Rhodapon® TDS

Sodium tripolyphosphate
CAS 7758-29-4; 13573-18-7; EINECS 231-694-5
Synonyms: STFF; Sodium triphosphate, tripoly; Pentasodium triphosphate
Trade names: Uniphos STPP

Sodium undecylenate (INCI)
CAS 3398-33-2; EINECS 222-264-8
Synonyms: 10-Undecenoic acid, sodium salt
Trade names: Undenat

Sodium wheat germamphoacetate (INCI)
Trade names: Mackam™ 1W

Sodium xylenesulfonate (INCI)
CAS 1300-72-7; EINECS 215-090-9
Synonyms: Dimethylbenzene sulfonic acid, sodium salt
Trade names: Carsosulf SXS; Eltesol® SX 30; Eltesol®

SX 93; Manrosol SXS30; Manrosol SXS40; SXS 40; Witconate™ SXS 40%; Witconate™ SXS 90%
Trade names containing: Witconate™ 1260; Witconate™ 45 Liq.; Witconate™ 45LX; Witconate™ LX F; Witconate™ LX Powd.

Soluble almond protein
Trade names: Unihypro GLADIN A

Soluble animal collagen. *See Soluble collagen*

Soluble collagen (INCI)
CAS 9007-34-5; EINECS 232-697-4
Synonyms: Soluble animal collagen; Soluble native collagen
Trade names: Actigen C; Ateco; Clearcol; Colladerm Procollagene SC; Collagen; Collagen CLR; Collagen Nativ 1%; Collagen Native Extra 1%; Collagene SPO; Collapuron N; Collapur®; Collasol; Dermacol; Desamidocollagen K 1.0; Desamidocollagen K 1.5; Grancol SP-01; Hydracol®; Kollagen KD; Kollagen S; Kollaplex 0.3; Kollaplex 1.0; Kollaron; Liquid Animal Collagen; Maricol CLR; Oceagen®; Pancogene® S; Ritacollagen BA-1; Ritacollagen S-1; Sollagen® EC; Sollagen® LA; Soluble Native Collagen RA-1 No. 26206; Soluble Native Collagen RS-1 No. 26205; Solu-Coll™; Solu-Coll™ C, CLR; Solu-Coll™ Complex VY; Solu-Coll™ Native; Trillagene®; Unihypro LAN
Trade names containing: Ateloglycane; Brookosome® SC; Collagen-CCK-Complex; Collagen-IMZ Complex; Collagen-LSS Complex; Collapurol® E 1; Cosiderm Collagen Masks; Cosiderm Masks; Dermasome® SC; Desaron; Elastin PG 2000; Elastosol; Hydagen® BP1; Kelisema Collagen-CCK Complex; Kelisema Collagen-IMZ Complex; Kelisema Collagen-LSS Complex; Ritacomplex DF 10; Ritacomplex DF 11; Ritacomplex DF 12, DF 13; Ritacomplex DF 14; Solu-Coll™ Complex; Thermoplex; Tri-Pronectin

Soluble elastin
Trade names: Granlastin 10%
Trade names containing: Elastosol; Ritacomplex DF 10

Soluble keratin
Trade names: Solu Kera-Tein M

Soluble proteoglycan (INCI)
Trade names: Proteodermin CLR

Soluble wheat protein
Trade names: Tritisol™; Unihypro GLADIN W

Sorbeth-6 (INCI)
Synonyms: PEG-6 sorbitol ether; PEG 300 sorbitol ether
Trade names: G-2240

Sorbeth-20 (INCI)
CAS 53694-15-8
Synonyms: PEG-20 sorbitol ether; POE (20) sorbitol ether; PEG 1000 sorbitol ether
Trade names: Ethosperse® SL-20; G-2320; Liponic SO-20; Trylox® 6753

Sorbeth-30 (INCI)
Synonyms: PEG-30 sorbitol ether
Trade names: G-2330

Sorbeth-40 (INCI)
Synonyms: PEG-40 sorbitol ether; PEG 2000 sorbitol; POE (40) sorbitol
Trade names: Witconol™ SE-40

Sorbeth-6 hexastearate (INCI)
CAS 66828-20-4
Trade names: Nikkol GS-6

Sorbic acid (INCI)
CAS 110-44-1; 22500-92-1; EINECS 203-768-7
Synonyms: 2,4-Hexadienoic acid
Trade names: Tristat; Unistat; Unistat SORBA
Trade names containing: Dragocid Forte 2/027045; Fondix G Bis

Sorbitan caprylate
Trade names: Nissan Nonion CP-08R

Sorbitan dioleate (INCI)
CAS 29116-98-1; EINECS 249-448-0
Synonyms: Sorbide dioleate; Sorbitan, di-9-octadecenoate; Anhydrosorbitol dioleate
Trade names: Hefti DO-33-F

Sorbitan distearate (INCI)
CAS 36521-89-8
Synonyms: Anhydrosorbitol distearate; Sorbitan dioctadecanoate
Trade names: Sorbon S-66

Sorbitan isostearate (INCI)
CAS 54392-26-6; 71902-01-7
Synonyms: Anhydrosorbitol monoisostearate; 1,4-Anhydro-D-glucitol, 6-isooctadecanoate; Sorbitan monoisooctadecanoate
Trade names: Arlacel® 987; Crill 6; Emalex SPIS-100; Montane 70; Nikkol SI-10R; Nikkol SI-10T; Nikkol SI-15T; Sorbirol ISM

Sorbitan laurate (INCI)
CAS 1338-39-2; 5959-89-7; EINECS 215-663-3; 227-729-9
Synonyms: Sorbitan monolaurate; Anhydrosorbitol monolaurate; Sorbitan monododecanoate
Trade names: Ablunol S-20; Alkamuls® SML; Arlacel® 20; Armotan® ML; Crill 1; Dehymuls® SML; Drewmulse® SML; Durtan® 20; Emsorb® 2515; Estol SML 3617; Ethylan® GL20; Extan-LT; Glycomul® L; Hefti ML-33-F; Hetan SL; Hodag SML; Ionet S-20; Ixolene 2; Kemester® S20; Liposorb L; Montane 20; Nikkol SL-10; Nissan Nonion LP-20R, LP-20RS; Protachem SML; Prote-sorb SML; Radiasurf® 7125; S-Maz® 20; Sorbax SML; Sorbitol L; Sorbon S-20; Sorgen 90; Span® 20; Unitan-L; Witconol™ 2515
Trade names containing: Aldosperse® L L-20; Amisol™ 4135; Amisol™ MS-12 BA; Tego®-Pearl S-33

Sorbitan myristate
Trade names: Nissan Nonion MP-30R

Sorbitan oleate (INCI)
CAS 1338-43-8; 5938-38-5; EINECS 215-665-4
Synonyms: SMO; Sorbitan monooleate; Sorbitan mono-9-octadecenoate; Anhydrosorbitol monooleate
Trade names: Ablunol S-80; Alkamuls® SMO; Arlacel® 80; Armotan® MO; Crill 4; Crill 50; Dehymuls® SMO; Drewmulse® SMO; Emalex SPO-100; Emsorb® 2500; Estol SMO 3685; Ethylan® GO80; Extan-OT; Famodan SMO; Glycomul® O; Hefti MO-33-F; Hetan SO; Hodag SMO; Ionet S-80; Ixolene 8; Kemester® S80; Liposorb O; Montane 80; Montane 80 SP; Nikkol SO-10; Nikkol SO-10R; Nissan Nonion OP-80R; Protachem SMO; Prote-sorb SMO; S-Maz® 80; S-Maz® 80K; Sorban AO; Sorbax SMO; Sorbirol O; Sorbon S-80; Sorgen 40; Sorgen S-40-H; Span® 80; Unitan-O; Witconol™ 2500
Trade names containing: Arlacel® 1689; Base W/O 126; Lexein® A-240; Montane 481; Oleo-Coll™ A240-20; Oleo-Coll™ A240; Proto-Lan A240; Proto-Lan KT

Sorbitan palmitate (INCI)
CAS 26266-57-9; EINECS 247-568-8

Synonyms: Sorbitan monopalmitate; 1,4-Anhydro-D-glucitol, 6-hexadecanoate
Trade names: Ablunol S-40; Arlacel® 40; Armotan® MP; Armotan® NP; Crill 2; Emsorb® 2510; Extan-PT; Glycomul® P; Hefti MP-33-F; Hodag SMP; Ixolene 4; Kemester® S40; Liposorb P; Montane 40; Nikkol SP-10; Nissan Nonion PP-40R; Protachem SMP; Prote-sorb SMP; S-Maz® 40; Sorbax SMP; Sorbirol P; Sorbon S-40; Span® 40; Unitan-P; Witconol™ 2510

Sorbitan sesquiisostearate (INCI)
Synonyms: Sorbitan, monohexadecanoate
Trade names: Emalex SPIS-150; Montane 73; Nikkol SI-15R; Protachem SQI

Sorbitan sesquioleate (INCI)
CAS 8007-43-0; EINECS 232-360-1
Synonyms: Anhydrosorbitol sesquioleate; Anhydrohexitol sesquioleate; Sorbitan, 9-octadecenoate (2:3)
Trade names: Arlacel® 83; Arlacel® C; Crill 43; Dehymuls® SSO; Emalex SPO-150; Emsorb® 2502; Extan-SOT; Glycomul® SOC; Hefti QO-33-F; Hodag SSO; Liposorb SQO; Montane 83; Nikkol SO-15; Nikkol SO-15EX; Nikkol SO-15R; Nissan Nonion OP-83RAT; Protachem SOC; S-Maz® 83R; Sorbirol SQ; Sorgen 30; Sorgen S-30-H; Witconol™ 2502
Trade names containing: Alcolan® 36W; Alcolan® 40; Alcolan®; Dehymuls® E; Dehymuls® K; Forlan L Conc; Forlan L; Forlan LM; Lanaetex H; PCL SE w/o 2/066255; Umulse-E

Sorbitan sesquistearate (INCI)
Synonyms: Anhydrosorbitol sesquistearate
Trade names: Emalex SPE-150S; Nikkol SS-15

Sorbitan stearate (INCI)
CAS 1338-41-6; EINECS 215-664-9
Synonyms: SMS; Sorbitan monostearate; Sorbitan monooctadecanoate; Anhydrosorbitol monostearate
Trade names: Ablunol S-60; Alkamuls® SMS; Arlacel® 60; Armotan® MS; Crill 3; Dehymuls® SMS; Drewmulse® SMS; Emalex SPE-100S; Emsorb® 2505; Emultex SMS; Estol SMS 3715; Ethylan® GS60; Extan-ST; Glycomul® S; Glycomul® S FG; Glycomul® S KFG; Hefti MS-33-F; Hetan SS; Hodag SMS; Ionet S-60 C; Ixolene 6; Kemester® S60; Liposorb S; Liposorb SC; Montane 60; Nikkol SS-10; Nissan Nonion SP-60R; Protachem SMS; Prote-sorb SMS; S-Maz® 60; S-Maz® 60K; S-Maz® 60KHM; Sorban AST; Sorbax SMS; Sorbirol S; Sorbon S-60; Sorgen 50; Span® 60 VS; Span® 60, 60K; Unitan-S; Witconol™ 2505
Trade names containing: Arlatone® 2121

Sorbitan tallate
Trade names: S-Maz® 90

Sorbitan trioleate (INCI)
CAS 26266-58-0; 85186-88-5; EINECS 247-569-3; 286-074-7
Synonyms: STO; Anhydrosorbitol trioleate; Sorbitan tri-9-octadecenoate
Trade names: Ablunol S-85; Arlacel® 85; Crill 45; Emsorb® 2503; Ethylan® GT85; Glycomul® TO; Hefti TO-33-F; Hodag STO; Ionet S-85; Kemester® S85; Liposorb TO; Montane 85; Nikkol SO-30; Nikkol SO-30R; Nissan Nonion OP-85R; Protachem STO; Prote-sorb STO; Radia® 7355; S-Maz® 85; S-Maz® 85K; Sorbax STO; Sorbirol TO; Span® 85; Unitan-TRIOL; Witconol™ 2503

Sorbitan tristearate (INCI)
CAS 26658-19-5; 72869-62-6; EINECS 247-891-4; 276-951-2

Synonyms: STS; Anhydrosorbitol tristearate; Sorbitan trioctadecanoate
Trade names: Crill 35; Crill 41; Drewmulse® STS; Emsorb® 2507; Glycomul® TS; Glycomul® TS KFG; Hefti TS-33-F; Hodag STS; Kemester® S65; Liposorb TS; Montane 65; Nikkol SS-30; Protachem STS; Prote-sorb STS; Radia® 7345; S-Maz® 65K; Sorbax STS; Sorbirol TS; Span® 65; Unitan-TRIST; Witconol™ 2507
Trade names containing: Lipex 402

Sorbitan tritallate
Trade names: S-Maz® 95

Sorbitol (INCI)
CAS 50-70-4; EINECS 200-061-5
Synonyms: D-Glucitol; D-Sorbitol; D-Sorbite
Trade names: A-641; Arlex; Fancol SORB; Hefti Sorbex-R; Hefti Sorbex-RP; Hydex® 100 Gran. 206; Hydex® Coarse Powd; Hydex® Powd. 60; Hydex® Tablet Grade; Liponic 70-NC; Liponic 76-NC; Liponic 83-NC; Liposorb 70; Sorbelite™ C; Sorbelite™ FG; Sorbo®; Unisweet 70; Unisweet 70/CONC; Unisweet CONC
Trade names containing: Antistatique WL 879; Bleu Covasorb W 6783 A; Facteur Hydratant PH; Foam-Coll™ 5; Foam-Coll™ 5W; Hydrocos; Hydroviton 2/059353; Lexein® S620S/Superpro 5A; Liprot CTS; Monteine V; Nikkol Aquasome LA; Ormagel AC-400; Ormagel SH; Ormagel XPU; Pro-Lan V; Prodew 100; Prodew 200; Seanamin AT; Seanamin BD; Seanamin SU; Seanamin TH; Superpro 5A; Supro-Tein S; Supro-Tein V; Tripro-5

Soy acid (INCI)
CAS 68308-53-2; 67701-08-0; EINECS 269-657-0
Synonyms: Acids, soy; Fatty acids, soya
Trade names: S-210

Soya dimethyl amine. *See Dimethyl soyamine*

Soya dimonium hydrolyzed wheat protein
Trade names: Quat-Wheat™ SDMA-25

Soyaethyl morpholinium ethosulfate (INCI)
CAS 61791-34-2; EINECS 263-167-0
Synonyms: N-Soya-N-ethyl morpholinium ethosulfate; Quaterinum-2
Trade names: Forestall

Soyamide DEA (INCI)
CAS 68425-47-8; EINECS 270-355-6
Synonyms: Soya diethanolamide; N,N-Bis(hydroxyethyl)soya amides
Trade names: Afmide™ S; Alkamide® SDO; Amidex S; Comperlan® VOD; Empigen® 2125-AU; Empilan® 2125-AU; Mackamide™ S; Mackamide™ SD; Manromid 150-ADY; Marlamid® DF 1818; Schercomid SLS; Stamid LS 5487; Witcamide® SSA
Trade names containing: Upamide SS-10

Soyamidopropalkonium chloride (INCI)
Trade names: Quatrex S

Soyamidopropyl betaine (INCI)
Synonyms: Soy amide propylbetaine; Soyamidopropyl dimethyl glycine
Trade names: Chembetaine S

Soyamidopropyl dimethylamine (INCI)
CAS 68188-30-7
Synonyms: N-[3-(Dimethylamino)propyl]soya amides; Dimethylaminopropyl soyamide
Trade names: Chemidex SO; Mackine™ 901

Soyamidopropyl dimethylamino gluconate (CTFA)
CAS 129541-36-2

Synonyms: D-Gluconic acid, compd. with n-[3-(dimethylamine)propyl] soyamide; Soya-(3-amidopropyl)-N,N-dimethylamino gluconate
Trade names: Necon SOGU

Soyamidopropyl dimethylamino glycolate (CTFA)
CAS 118777-77-8
Synonyms: Acetic acid, hydroxy-, compd. with N-[3-(dimethylamine)propyl]soyamide; Soya-(3-amidopropyl)-N,N-dimethylamine glycolate
Trade names: Necon SOG

Soyamidopropyl ethyldimonium ethosulfate (INCI)
CAS 90529-57-0; EINECS 291-990-5
Synonyms: 1-Propanaminium, 3-amino-N-ethyl-N,N-dimethyl-, N-soya acyl derivs., ethyl sulfates; N-Alkyl-(3-amidopropyl)-N,N-dimethyl-N-ethyl ammonium ethyl sulfate
Trade names: Foamquat SOAS; Schercoquat SOAS

Soyamine (INCI)
CAS 61790-18-9; EINECS 263-112-0
Synonyms: Soya primary amine; Amines, soya alkyl; Soyaalkylamine
Trade names: Armeen® S; Armeen® SD; Kemamine® P-997

Soybean oil (INCI)
CAS 8001-22-7; EINECS 232-274-4
Synonyms: Oils, soybean; Soya oil
Trade names: EmCon Soya; Lipovol SOY; Super Refined™ Soybean Oil USP
Trade names containing: Arnica Oil CLR; Arnicaflower Oil PANAROM; Braxicina; Calendula Oil CLR; Calendula Oil Monarom; Carrot Oil CLR; Crodarom Calendula O; Efadermasterolo; Emulmetik™ 110; Gilugel R; Lipophos; Lipoplastidine Soja; Lipotrofina A; Lipotrofina M; Phosal 12WD; Tocopherol Oil CLR; Unibotan Vitaplant O CLR; Vitaplant CLR Oil-Soluble N

Soybean oil unsaponifiables (INCI)
Synonyms: Unsaponifiable soybean oil
Trade names containing: ASU Complex; Efadermasterolo; Filagrinol

Soyethyldimonium ethosulfate (INCI)
CAS 68308-67-8
Synonyms: Soya dimethyl ethyl ammonium ethyl sulfate; Soyaethyldimonium ethosulfate
Trade names: M-Quat® 1033

Soy flour (INCI)
CAS 68513-95-1
Synonyms: Flour, soy
Trade names: Centex; Emcosoy®

Soy germ extract (INCI)
CAS 84776-91-0
Trade names containing: Complex NR; Lipoplastidine Soja

Soy glyceride
Synonyms: Glyceryl mono soya oil; Glyceryl mono-soyate; Soybean oil glyceride
Trade names containing: Myvatex® MSPS; Myvatex® SSH

Soy protein (INCI)
CAS 68153-28-6
Synonyms: Proteins, soy
Trade names: Dascare FSP Liq; Octaprotein; Tofupro-U
Trade names containing: Decaprotein; Tensami 4/07

Soy sterol (INCI)
Synonyms: Soy sterol
Trade names: Generol® 122; Sitostene

Trade names containing: Lanolide; Lipotrofina A; Sebopessina; Seboside

Soy sterol acetate (INCI)
Trade names: Dermol PSA

Soytrimonium chloride (INCI)
CAS 61790-41-8; EINECS 263-134-0
Synonyms: Soya trimethyl ammonium chloride; Quaternium-9; N-(Soya alkyl)-N,N,N-trimethyl ammonium chloride
Trade names: Jet Quat S-50; Kemamine® Q-9973B
Trade names containing: Arquad® S-50

Spearmint oil (INCI)
CAS 8008-79-5
Synonyms: Mentha spicata oil
Trade names: EmCon Spearmint

Sphingolipids (INCI)
Trade names: Sphingolipid CB-1
Trade names containing: Glyco/Cer HA; Glyco/Cer HALA; Glyco/Cer; Glycoderm; Glycosome; Liposomes CLR

Spinal cord extract (INCI)
Trade names containing: Ampholysat Moelle

Spiraea extract (INCI)
Trade names containing: Blend For Slenderizing Prods. HS 255; Relaxant HS 278; Relaxant LS 678; Rhumacalm HS 328

Spirulina extract (INCI)
Trade names: Spirulina Extract COS

Spleen extract (INCI)
Trade names: Nutrex RT; Tri-Derm SE
Trade names containing: Brookosome® SE; Dermasome® SE; Epiderm-Complex W; Fibrastil

Squalane (INCI)
CAS 111-01-3; EINECS 203-825-6
Synonyms: Dodecahydrosqualene; Spinacane; 2,6,10,15, 19,23-Hexamethyltetracosane; Perhydrosqualene
Trade names: Carolane; Cosbiol; Dermane; Fitoderm; Nikkol Squalane; Prisorine SQS 3758; Robane®
Trade names containing: Brookosome® S; Chronosphere® Planell®; Dermasome® S; L.C.R.E.; Lipoliv; Polysphere 3000 SP

Squalene (INCI)
CAS 111-02-4; EINECS 203-826-1
Synonyms: 2,6,10,15,19,23-Hexamethyl-2,6,10, 14,18,22-tetracosahexaene
Trade names: Dermene; Nikkol Squalene EX; Squatol S; Supraene®
Trade names containing: Chronosphere® Planell®; Robeyl; Transparent Titanium Dioxide PW Squatol S

Starch/acrylates/acrylamide copolymer (INCI)
Trade names: Water Lock® A-100

Starch, corn. *See Corn starch*

Starch gum. *See Dextrin*

Steapyrium chloride (INCI)
CAS 1341-08-8; 14492-68-3; 42566-92-7; EINECS 238-501-3
Synonyms: 1-[2-Oxo-2-[[(1-oxooctadecyl)oxy]ethyl] amino]ethyl]pyridinium chloride; Quaternium-7; N-(Stearoyl colamino formyl methyl) pyridinium chloride
Trade names: Emcol® E-607S

Stearalkonium bentonite (INCI)
Trade names: Claytone AF; Claytone APA; Tixogel LG; Tixogel VZ

Trade names containing: Miglyol® 840 Gel T; Miglyol® Gel T; Tixogel FTN; Tixogel IPM; Tixogel LAN

Stearalkonium chloride (INCI)
CAS 122-19-0; EINECS 204-527-9
Synonyms: Stearyl dimethyl benzyl ammonium chloride; Octadecyl dimethyl benzyl ammonium chloride; N,N-Dimethyl-N-octadecylbenzenemethanaminium chloride
Trade names: Ablumine 1618; Ammonyx® 4; Ammonyx® 4B; Ammonyx® 485; Ammonyx® 4002; Ammonyx® CA-Special; Amyx A-25-S 0040; Carsoquat® SDQ-85; Catinal OB-80E; Emcol® 4; Hetquat S-20; Incroquat S-85; Incroquat SDQ-25; M-Quat® B-25; M-Quat® JS-25; Mackernium™ SDC-25; Mackernium™ SDC-85; Maquat SC-18; Miracare® SCS; Nikkol CA-1485; Quatrex STC-25; Quatrex STC-85; Rhodaquat® M270C/18; Stedbac®; Sumquat® 6210; Unisoft SAC; Varisoft® SDAC-W; Zoharquat 25; Zoharquat 75
Trade names containing: Amyx ST 3837; Carsoquat® 816-C; Carsoquat® SDQ-25; Incroquat CR Conc; Lanion-27; Lanion-28; Maquat SC-1632; Polyquart® H 7102; Quatrex CRC; Standamul® Conc. 1002; Unimul-1002 Conc; Uniquart 7102; Variquat® SDC; Variquat® SDC; Varisoft® C SAC; Varisoft® SDAC; Varisoft® SDC-85

Stearalkonium hectorite (INCI)
CAS 94891-33-5; 12691-60-0
Trade names: Bentone® 27
Trade names containing: Bentone® Gel CAO; Bentone® Gel IPM; Bentone® Gel LOI; Bentone® Gel TN; Bentone® Gel TN A-40; Biju® BNT; Biju® BTD, BXD; Biju® Ultra UNT; Biju® Ultra UTD, UXD; Miglyol® 840 Gel B; Miglyol® 840 Gel; Miglyol® Gel B; Miglyol® Gel; Softisan® Gel

Stearamide (INCI)
CAS 124-26-5; EINECS 204-693-2
Synonyms: Octadecanamide; Stearic acid amide; Amide C_{18}
Trade names: Armid® 18

Stearamide AMP (INCI)
CAS 36284-86-3
Synonyms: N-(2-Hydroxy-1,1-dimethylethyl) octadecanamide
Trade names containing: Kessco® EGAS; Polytex 10M; Trivent EG-18

Stearamide DEA (INCI)
CAS 93-82-3; EINECS 202-280-1
Synonyms: Stearic acid diethanolamide; Stearoyl diethanolamide; N,N-bis(2-hydroxyethyl) octadecanamide
Trade names: Alkamide® DS-280/S; Alkamide® HTDE; Amidex SE; Hetamide DS; Lipamide S; Monamid® 718; Olamida ED; Protamide SA; Upamide SD
Trade names containing: Cetina; Protamide N-1918

Stearamide DIBA-stearate (INCI)
Trade names: Paramul® SAS

Stearamide MEA (INCI)
CAS 111-57-9; EINECS 203-883-2
Synonyms: Stearic acid monoethanolamide; Stearoyl monoethanolamide; N-(2-hydroxyethyl) octadecanamide
Trade names: Ablumide SME; Alkamide® S-280; Amidex SME; CPH-380-N; Hetamide MS; Incromide SM; Mackamide™ SMA; Mazamide® SMEA; Monamid® S; Monamid® S/M; Olamida SM; Phoenamid SM; Rewomid® S 280; Upamide SME-M; Witcamide® 70; Witcamide® 6507

Trade names containing: Mackester™ SP; Miracare® M1

Stearamide MEA-stearate (INCI)
CAS 14351-40-7; EINECS 238-310-5
Synonyms: Octadecanoic acid, 2-[(1-oxooctadecyl) amino]ethyl ester; Stearic monoethanolamide stearate; 2-[(1-Oxooctadecyl)amino]ethyl octadecanoate
Trade names: Cerasynt® D; Witcamide® MAS

Stearamidoethyl diethylamine (INCI)
CAS 16889-14-8; EINECS 240-924-3
Synonyms: Diethylaminoethyl stearamide; N-[2-Diethylamino)ethyl]octadecanamide
Trade names: Chemical Base 6532; Lexamine 22; Nikkol Amidoamine S; Swanol Amidoamine S
Trade names containing: Lexemul® AR; Tegacid® Regular VA

Stearamidoethyl dimethylamine
Trade names: Chemidex SE

Stearamidoethyl ethanolamine (INCI)
CAS 141-21-9; EINECS 205-469-7
Synonyms: Ethanolaminoethyl stearamide; N-[2-[(2-Hydroxyethyl)amino]ethyl]octadecanamide
Trade names: Catemol 18SA; Chemical 39 Base

Stearamidoethyl ethanolamine phosphate (INCI)
Trade names containing: Sandotex A

Stearamidopropalkonium chloride (INCI)
CAS 65694-10-2; EINECS 265-880-2
Synonyms: N,N-Dimethyl-N-[3-[(1-oxooctadecyl)amino] propyl] benzenemethanaminium chloride; Stearamidopropyl dimethyl benzyl ammonium chloride; Stearamidopropyl benzyldimonium chloride
Trade names: Incroquat SBQ 75P

Stearamidopropylamine oxide (INCI)
CAS 25066-20-0; EINECS 246-598-9
Synonyms: N-[3-(Dimethylamino)propyl]octadecanamide-N-oxide
Trade names: Chemoxide SAO

Stearamidopropyl cetearyl dimonium tosylate (INCI)
Synonyms: Stearamidopropyl dimethyl cetearyl ammonium tosylate
Trade names containing: Ceraphyl® 85

Stearamidopropyl dimethylamine (INCI)
CAS 7651-02-7; EINECS 231-609-1
Synonyms: Dimethylaminopropyl stearamide; N-[3-(Dimethylamino)propyl]octadecanamide
Trade names: Adogen® S-18 V; Chemidex S; Incromine SB; Lexamine S-13; Lipamine SPA; Mackine™ 301; Miramine® SODI; Schercodine S; Tegamine® 18; Tego®-Amid S 18; Unizeen SA
Trade names containing: Lexate® CRC; Varisoft® CRC

Stearamidopropyl dimethylamine lactate (INCI)
CAS 55819-53-9; EINECS 259-837-7
Synonyms: Propanoic acid, 2-hydroxy-, compd. with N-[3-(dimethylamino)propyl]octadecanamide
Trade names: Hetamine 5L-25; Incromate SDL; Lexamine S-13 Lactate; Mackalene™ 316; Protachem SDM

Stearamidopropyl dimethylamine stearate (INCI)
Trade names: Catemol 180-S

Stearamidopropyl ethyldimonium ethosulfate (INCI)
CAS 67846-16-6; EINECS 267-360-0
Synonyms: N-Ethyl-N,N-dimethyl-3-[(1-oxooctadecyl) amino]-1-propanaminium ethyl sulfate; Stearamidopropyl ethyl dimonium ethyl sulfate; Stearamidopropyl dimethyl ethyl ammonium ethyl sulfate
Trade names: Schercoquat SAS

Stearamidopropyl morpholine (INCI)
CAS 55852-13-6
Synonyms: N-[3-(4-Morpholinyl)propyl]octadecanamide
Trade names: Mackine™ 321

Stearamidopropyl morpholine lactate (INCI)
CAS 55852-14-7; EINECS 259-860-2
Synonyms: Propanoic acid, 2-hydroxy-, compd. with N-[3-(4-morpholinyl)propyl]octadecanamide
Trade names: Emcol® SML; Mackalene™ 326

Stearamidopropyl PG-dimonium chloride phosphate (INCI)
Trade names: Phospholipid P-TS
Trade names containing: Phospholipid SV

Stearamidopropyl trimonium methosulfate (INCI)
CAS 19277-88-4; EINECS 242-930-1
Synonyms: N,N,N-Trimethyl-3-[(1-oxooctadecyl)amino]-1-propanaminium methyl sulfate
Trade names: Catigene® SA 70

Stearamine (INCI)
CAS 124-30-1; EINECS 204-695-3
Synonyms: Stearyl amine; Octadecylamine; 1-Octadecanamine
Trade names: Adogen® 140D; Amine 18-90; Amine 18-90 D; Amine 18-95; Armeen® 18; Armeen® 18D

Stearamine oxide (INCI)
CAS 2571-88-2; EINECS 219-919-5
Synonyms: Stearyl dimethylamine oxide; Octadecyl dimethylamine oxide; N,N-Dimethyl-1-octadecanamine-N-oxide
Trade names: Admox® 18-85; Ammonyx® SO; Amyx SO 3734; Annonyx SO; Barlox® 18S; Chemoxide ST; Emcol® SO; Incromine Oxide S; Mackamine™ SO; Mazox® SDA; Rewominox S 300; Schercamox DMS; Standamox PS; Unimox SO

Steardimonium hydroxyethyl cellulose
Synonyms: PG-hydroxyethylcellulose stearyldimonium chloride
Trade names: Crodacel QS

Steardimonium hydroxypropyl hydrolyzed collagen (INCI)
Synonyms: Steardimonium hydrolyzed collagen; Steardimonium hydrolyzed animal protein
Trade names: Croquat S; Promois Milk SAQ; Promois W-42 SAQ

Steardimonium hydroxypropyl hydrolyzed silk (INCI)
Trade names: Promois S-SAQ

Steardimonium hydroxypropyl hydrolyzed wheat protein (INCI)
Trade names: Hydrotriticum™ QS

Steareth-2 (INCI)
CAS 9005-00-9 (generic); 16057-43-5
Synonyms: PEG-2 stearyl ether; POE (2) stearyl ether; PEG 100 stearyl ether
Trade names: Brij® 72; Britex S 20; Brox S-2; Emalex 602; Hetoxol STA-2; Hodag Nonionic S-2; Lanycol-72; Lipocol S-2; Macol® SA-2; Nikkol BS-2; Procol SA-2; Rhodasurf® S-2; Simulsol 72; Unicol SA-2; Volpo S-2

Steareth-3 (INCI)
CAS 9005-00-9 (generic); 4439-32-1
Synonyms: PEG-3 stearyl ether; POE (3) stearyl ether
Trade names: Emalex 603
Trade names containing: Isoxal 5

Steareth-4 (INCI)
CAS 9005-00-9 (generic); 59970-10-4
Synonyms: PEG-4 stearyl ether; POE (4) stearyl ether;

3,6,9,12-Tetraoxatriacontan-1-ol
Trade names: Nikkol BS-4; Procol SA-4

Steareth-5 (INCI)
CAS 9005-00-9 (generic); 71093-13-5
Synonyms: PEG-5 stearyl ether; POE (5) stearyl ether
Trade names: Emalex 605; Macol® SA-5
Trade names containing: Isoxal 12; Solulan® 5

Steareth-6 (INCI)
CAS 2420-29-3; 9005-00-9 (generic)
Trade names: Emalex 606

Steareth-7 (INCI)
CAS 9005-00-9 (generic); 66146-84-7
Synonyms: PEG-7 stearyl ether; POE (7) stearyl ether;
3,6,9,12,15,18,21-Heptaoxanonatriacontan-1-ol
Trade names: Ablunol SA-7
Trade names containing: Emulgator E 2149; Emulgator E 2155; Lamecreme® AOM

Steareth-8
CAS 9005-00-9 (generic)
Trade names: Emalex 608; Tewax TC 72

Steareth-9
Trade names containing: Hetoxol LS-9

Steareth-10 (INCI)
CAS 9005-00-9 (generic); 13149-86-5
Synonyms: PEG-10 stearyl ether; POE (10) stearyl ether; PEG 500 stearyl ether
Trade names: Brij® 76; Britex S 100; Hetoxol STA-10; Hodag Nonionic S-10; Lipocol S-10; Macol® SA-10; Procol SA-10; Simulsol 76; Unicol SA-10; Volpo S-10
Trade names containing: Cosmowax; Emulgator E 2155; Isoxal 11; Ritapro 100; Unicol 123

Steareth-11 (INCI)
CAS 9005-00-9 (generic)
Synonyms: PEG-11 stearyl ether; POE (11) stearyl ether
Trade names: Emalex 611

Steareth-13 (INCI)
CAS 9005-00-9 (generic)
Synonyms: PEG-13 stearyl ether; POE (13) stearyl ether
Trade names: Hodag Nonionic S-13; Unicol SA-13

Steareth-14 (INCI)
CAS 9005-00-9 (generic)
Trade names containing: Aqualose SLT

Steareth-15 (INCI)
CAS 9005-00-9 (generic)
Synonyms: PEG-15 stearyl ether; POE (15) stearyl ether
Trade names: Emalex 615; Macol® SA-15; Unicol SA-15

Steareth-16 (INCI)
CAS 9005-00-9 (generic)
Synonyms: PEG-16 stearyl ether; POE (16) stearyl ether
Trade names containing: Solulan® 16

Steareth-20 (INCI)
CAS 9005-00-9 (generic)
Synonyms: PEG-20 stearyl ether; POE (20) stearyl ether; PEG 1000 stearyl ether
Trade names: Brij® 78; Britex S 200; Brox S-20; Emalex 620; Hetoxol STA-20; Hodag Nonionic S-20; Lanycol-78; Lipocol S-20; Macol® SA-20; Nikkol BS-20; Procol SA-20; Rhodasurf® S-20; Simulsol 7; Simulsol 78; Unicol SA-20; Volpo S-20
Trade names containing: Brookswax™ R; Cosmowax; Crodacol GP; Emulcire 61 WL 2659; Hodag CSA-102; Lipowax PR; Macol® CPS; Procol P; Relaxer Conc. No. 2; Relaxer Conc. No. 3; Ritachol® 1000; Ritachol® 3000; Ritachol® 4000; Ritapro 100; Tefose® 2000; Teinowax; Unicol CPS

Steareth-21 (INCI)
CAS 9005-00-9 (generic)
Synonyms: PEG-21 stearyl ether; POE (21) stearyl ether
Trade names: Brij® 721; Brij® 721S; Cromul EM 1207; Lanycol-79

Steareth-25 (INCI)
CAS 9005-00-9 (generic)
Synonyms: PEG-25 stearyl ether; POE (25) stearyl ether
Trade names: Emalex 625
Trade names containing: Solulan® 25; Tego® Care 150; Tego® Care 300

Steareth-27 (INCI)
CAS 9005-00-9 (generic)
Trade names: Brox HLB-13

Steareth-30 (INCI)
CAS 9005-00-9 (generic)
Synonyms: PEG-30 stearyl ether; POE (30) stearyl ether
Trade names: Brox S-30; Emalex 630; Hetoxol STA-30

Steareth-40 (INCI)
CAS 9005-00-9 (generic)
Synonyms: PEG-40 stearyl ether; POE (40) stearyl ether; PEG 2000 stearyl ether
Trade names: Emalex 640; Hodag Nonionic S-40; Macol® SA-40; Unicol SA-40

Steareth-100 (INCI)
CAS 9005-00-9 (generic)
Synonyms: PEG-100 stearyl ether; POE (100) stearyl ether
Trade names: Brij® 700; Brij® 700S; Lanycol-700

Steareth-10 allyl ether/acrylates copolymer (INCI)
Trade names: Salcare SC90

Steareth-7 carboxylic acid
CAS 68954-89-2; 59559-30-7
Trade names: Akypo RS 60

Steareth-11 carboxylic acid
Trade names: Akypo RS 100

Steareth-2 phosphate (INCI)
Trade names: Crodafos S2A

Stearic acid (INCI)
CAS 57-11-4; EINECS 200-313-4
Synonyms: n-Octadecanoic acid; Carboxylic acid C_{18}
Trade names: Cetax TP; Crosterene SA4310; Emersol® 110; Emersol® 120; Emersol® 132 NF Lily®; Emersol® 150; Emersol® 6320; Emersol® 6332 NF; Emersol® 6349; Emersol® 6351; Hy-Phi 1199; Hy-Phi 1303; Hy-Phi 1401; Hystrene® 4516; Hystrene® 5016 NF; Hystrene® 9718 NF; Industrene® 9018; Kartacid 1890; Koster Keunen Stearic Acid XXX; Prifrac 2980; Prifrac 2981; Pristerene 4904; Pristerene 4905; Pristerene 4910; Pristerene 4911; Pristerene 4915; Pristerene 4921; Radiacid® 152; Radiacid® 416; Radiacid® 423; Radiacid® 427; Radiacid® 428; Radiacid® 464; Unifat 54; Unifat 55L
Trade names containing: Alcolite; B-122; Base 4978; Basis LP-20H; Cetasal; Cutina® FS 25 Flakes; Cutina® FS 45 Flakes; DHA Microspheres; Emulgade® CL Special; Emulgade® CL; Geropon® AS-200; Geropon® AS-250; Isobeeswax SP 154; Jordapon® Cl 60; Jordapon® Cl 65; Jordapon® Cl 75; Jordapon® Cl-60; Kessco Diglycol Stearate SE; Kessco Diglycol Stearate; Koster Keunen Beeswax; S&P ISOW; Montane 481; Ross Beeswax Substitute 628/5; Ross Synthetic Candelilla Wax; Tauranol I-78/80

Stearone (INCI)
CAS 504-53-0; EINECS 207-993-1

Synonyms: Diheptadecyl ketone; 18-Pentatriacontanone
Trade names containing: Amerchol® 400; Amerchol® RC

Stearoxy dimethicone (INCI)
CAS 68554-53-0
Synonyms: Dimethyl siloxy stearoxy siloxane polymer; Poly(dimethylsiloxy)stearoxysiloxane
Trade names: Abil®-Wax 2434
Trade names containing: Belsil SDM 6021; Belsil SDM 6022

Stearoxymethicone/dimethicone copolymer (INCI)
Trade names: Masilwax 135

Stearoxytrimethylsilane (INCI)
CAS 18748-91-9; EINECS 242-553-2
Trade names containing: Dow Corning® 580 Wax

Stearoyl sarcosine (INCI)
CAS 142-48-3; EINECS 205-539-7
Synonyms: Stearoyl N-methylglycine; Stearoyl N-methylaminoacetic acid; N-Methyl-N-(1-oxo-octadecyl)glycine
Trade names: Crodasinic S; Hamposyl® S

Steartrimonium chloride (INCI)
CAS 112-03-8; EINECS 203-929-1
Synonyms: Stearyl trimethyl ammonium chloride; Octadecyl trimethyl ammonium chloride; N,N,N-Tri-methyl-1-octadecanaminium chloride
Trade names: Ablumine TMS; Genamin STAC; Kemamine® Q-9903B; Nikkol CA-2450; Nikkol CA-2465; Varisoft® ST-50; Varisoft® TSC
Trade names containing: Arquad® 18-50; Varisoft® TS-50

Steartrimonium hydroxyethyl hydrolyzed collagen (INCI)
CAS 111174-62-0
Synonyms: Stearyltrimonium hydroxyethyl hydrolyzed collagen
Trade names: Crotein Q; Granquat S; Pran QC; Quat-Coll™ QS; Quat-Pro S; Quat-Pro S 30; Quatex S; Tri-Quat-S

Steartrimonium methosulfate (INCI)
CAS 18684-11-2
Synonyms: Stearyl trimethyl ammonium methyl sulfate; N,N,N-Trimethyl-1-cotadecanaminium methyl sulfate
Trade names: Catigene® ST 70; Empigen® CM

Stearyl alcohol (INCI)
CAS 112-92-5; EINECS 204-017-6
Synonyms: n-Octadecanol; 1-Octadecanol; C18 linear alcohol
Trade names: Adol® 61; Adol® 61 NF; Adol® 62 NF; Adol® 620 NF; Alfol® 18; Cachalot® S-54; Cachalot® S-56; Cetax 18; CO-1895; Crodacol S-70; Crodacol S-95NF; Epal® 18NF; Fancol SA; Hetoxol SA; Hyfatol 18-95; Hyfatol 18-98; Lanette® 18; Lanette® 18 DEO; Lanol S; Lipocol S; Mackol 18; Nacol® 18-94; Nacol® 18-98; Nikkol Stearyl Alcohol; Philcohol 1800; Radianol® 1898; RITA SA; Stearal; Steraffine; Unihydag Wax-18
Trade names containing: Amerchol® RC; Brookswax™ G; Carsoquat® SDQ-25; Ceral G; Cerasynt® WM; Cosmowax K; Cosmowax; Dispersen-G; Dow Corning® 580 Wax; Emulgator E 2149; Emulgator E 2155; Epal® 1218; Epal® 1418; Epal® 1618; Epal® 1618RT; Epal® 1618T; Fanwax G; Forlan L Conc; Forlan L; Forlan LM; Hetoxol G; Homulgator 920 G; Incroquat BES-35 S; Lipowax G; Macol® 125; Miracare® CT100; Promulgen® G; Quatrex CT-100; Ritapro 200; Tego® Care 150; Tewax TC 60; Varisoft® SDC-85; Varonic® BG

Stearyl/aminopropyl methicone copolymer (INCI)
CAS 110720-64-4
Trade names: EXP-61

Stearyl behenate (INCI)
CAS 24271-12-3; EINECS 246-115-1
Synonyms: Docosanoic acid, octadecyl ester
Trade names: Pelemol SB

Stearyl benzoate (INCI)
CAS 10578-34-4; EINECS 234-169-9
Synonyms: Octadecyl benzoate
Trade names: Finsolv® 116

Stearyl betaine (INCI)
CAS 820-66-6; EINECS 212-470-6
Synonyms: N-(Carboxymethyl)-N,N-dimethyl-1-octadecanaminium hydroxide, inner salt; Stearyl di-methyl glycine
Trade names: Lonzaine® 18S; Varion® SDG

Stearyl caprylate (INCI)
CAS 18312-31-7; EINECS 242-200-2
Synonyms: Octanoic acid, octadecyl ester
Trade names containing: Pur-Cellin Wax

Stearyl dimethicone (INCI)
Trade names: Abil®-Wax 9800; Dow Corning® 2503 Cosmetic Wax; Dow Corning® 2504 Cosmetic Fluid

Stearyl dimethyl amine. See Dimethyl stearamine

Stearyl glycyrrhetinate (INCI)
CAS 13832-70-7
Trade names: Co-Grhetinol; Nikkol Stearyl Glycyrrheti-nate

Stearyl heptanoate (INCI)
CAS 66009-41-4
Synonyms: Heptanoic acid, octadecyl ester
Trade names: Crodamol W; Tegosoft® SH
Trade names containing: Emulzome; PCL SE w/o 2/066255; PCL-Siccum 2/066215; Pur-Cellin Wax

Stearyl lactate (INCI)
CAS 35230-14-9; EINECS 252-447-8
Synonyms: Octadecyl lactate; Octadecyl 2-hydroxy-propanoate
Trade names: Lactabase C18

Stearyl methicone (INCI)
CAS 68607-75-0
Synonyms: Polyoctadecylmethylsiloxane
Trade names: Abil®-Wax 9809

Stearyl octyldimonium chloride (INCI)
Synonyms: Quaternary ammonium compds., (stearyl, 2-ethylhexyl) dimethyl, chlorides
Trade names: Arquad® HTL8-Cl

Stearyl octyldimonium methosulfate (INCI)
Synonyms: Quaternary ammonium compds., (stearyl, 2-ethylhexyl) dimethyl, ethyl sulfates
Trade names: Arquad® HTL8-MS

Stearyl stearate (INCI)
CAS 2778-96-3; 85536-04-5; EINECS 220-476-5; 287-484-9
Synonyms: Octadecanoic acid, octadecyl ester
Trade names: Alkamuls® SS; Cetinol EE; Emalex CC-18; Estol STST 3706; Hetester 412; Lexol® SS; Liponate SS; Radia® 7501; Ritachol SS; Unimul 1818
Trade names containing: Lexate® TA; Lexate® TL; Lipocerite Standard

Stearyl stearoyl stearate (INCI)
Trade names: Hetester SSS

STFF. See Sodium tripolyphosphate

Stinging nettle extract
  Trade names containing: Herbasol 7 Herb Complex; Herbasol Complex E

STO. *See Sorbitan trioleate*

STS. *See Sorbitan tristearate*

Styrene/acrylamide copolymer (INCI)
  CAS 24981-13-3
  Synonyms: Ethenylbenzene, polymer with 2-propenamide; 2-Propenamide, polymer with ethenylbenzene
  Trade names: Esi-Cryl 12
  Trade names containing: Lytron 308

Styrene/acrylates/acrylonitrile copolymer (INCI)
  Trade names: NeoCryl B-1000

Styrene/acrylates/ammonium methacrylate copolymer (INCI)
  Trade names containing: Syntran 5002

Styrene/acrylates copolymer (INCI)
  Synonyms: Styrene/acrylate copolymer
  Trade names: Esi-Cryl 11
  Trade names containing: Lytron 621

Styrene-divinylbenzene copolymer. *See Styrene/DVB copolymer*

Styrene/DVB copolymer (INCI)
  CAS 9003-70-7
  Synonyms: Styrene-divinylbenzene copolymer
  Trade names: Microsponge®; Nikkol Plastic Powder FP-SQ

Styrene/PVP copolymer (INCI)
  CAS 25086-29-7
  Synonyms: 1-Ethenyl-2-pyrroldinone, polymer with ethenylbenzene; Vinylpyrrolidone/styrene copolymer; PVP/styrene copolymer
  Trade names: Polectron® 430

Succinic acid (INCI)
  CAS 110-15-6; EINECS 203-740-4
  Synonyms: Butanedioic acid; Amber acid; Ethylene succinic acid
  Trade names containing: Grillocin WE-106

Sucrose (INCI)
  CAS 57-50-1; EINECS 200-334-9
  Synonyms: β-D-Fructofuranosyl-α-D-glucopyranoside; Saccharose; Sugar
  Trade names containing: Hygroplex HHG; Sugartab®

Sucrose cocoate (INCI)
  CAS 91031-88-8
  Trade names: Crodesta SL-40; Grilloten® LSE 65 K; Grilloten® LSE 65 K Soft; Grilloten® LSE 87 K; Grilloten® LSE 87 K Soft
  Trade names containing: Arlatone® 2121

Sucrose dilaurate (INCI)
  Trade names: Ryoto Sugar Ester L-595

Sucrose distearate (INCI)
  CAS 27195-16-0; EINECS 248-317-5
  Synonyms: α-D-Glucopyranoside, β-D-fructofuranosyl, dioctadecanoate
  Trade names: Crodesta DKS F10; Crodesta DKS F20; Crodesta DKS F50; Crodesta DKS F70; Crodesta F-10; Crodesta F-50; Crodesta F-140; Ryoto Sugar Ester S-570; Ryoto Sugar Ester S-770; Ryoto Sugar Ester S-970
  Trade names containing: Crodesta F-110

Sucrose laurate (INCI)
  CAS 25339-99-5; EINECS 246-873-3

Synonyms: α-D-Glucopyranoside, β-D-fructofuranosyl, monododecanoate
  Trade names: Grilloten LSE 65; Grilloten LSE 65 Soft; Grilloten LSE 87; Grilloten LSE 87 Soft; Ryoto Sugar Ester L-1570; Ryoto Sugar Ester L-1695

Sucrose myristate (INCI)
  Trade names: Ryoto Sugar Ester M-1695

Sucrose oleate (INCI)
  Trade names: Ryoto Sugar Ester O-1570; Ryoto Sugar Ester OWA-1570

Sucrose palmitate (INCI)
  CAS 26446-38-8; EINECS 247-706-7
  Trade names: Ryoto Sugar Ester P-1570; Ryoto Sugar Ester P-1570S; Ryoto Sugar Ester P-1670

Sucrose polylaurate (INCI)
  Trade names: Ryoto Sugar Ester L-195

Sucrose polylinoleate (INCI)
  Trade names: Ryoto Sugar Ester LN-195

Sucrose polyoleate (INCI)
  Trade names: Ryoto Sugar Ester 0-170

Sucrose polystearate (INCI)
  Synonyms: Sucrose mono/distearate
  Trade names: Ryoto Sugar Ester S-070; Ryoto Sugar Ester S-170; Ryoto Sugar Ester S-270

Sucrose stearate (INCI)
  CAS 25168-73-4; EINECS 246-705-9
  Synonyms: α-D-Glucopyranoside, β-D-fructofuranosyl, monooctadecanoate
  Trade names: Crodesta DKS F110; Crodesta F-160; Grilloten PSE 141G; Grilloten® PSE 141 G Pellets; Ryoto Sugar Ester S-1170; Ryoto Sugar Ester S-1170S; Ryoto Sugar Ester S-1570; Ryoto Sugar Ester S-1670; Ryoto Sugar Ester S-1670S
  Trade names containing: Crodesta F-110; Crodesta F-140

Sucrose tetrastearate triacetate (INCI)
  Trade names: Ryoto Sugar Ester S-170 Ac

Sucrose tribehenate (INCI)
  Trade names: Ryoto Sugar Ester B-370

Sucrose tristearate (INCI)
  Trade names: Ryoto Sugar Ester S-370; Ryoto Sugar Ester S-370F

Sugar cane extract
  Trade names containing: MFA™ Complex

Sulfated castor oil (INCI)
  CAS 8002-33-3; EINECS 232-306-7
  Synonyms: Castor oil sulfated; Sulfonated castor oil; Turkey-red oil
  Trade names: Haroil SCO-50; Laurel R-50; Nopcocastor; Standapol® SCO; Turkey Red Oil 100%; Türkischrotöl 100%; Unipol SCO
  Trade names containing: Amisol™ HS-2; Amisol™ HS-3 US; Amisol Nail Strengthener; Celasal

Sulfocarbolic acid. *See Phenol sulfonic acid*

α-Sulfo methyl laurate
  Trade names: Calester

Sulfonic acid
  Trade names containing: Eltesol® TA 65

Sulfur (INCI)
  CAS 7704-34-9; EINECS 231-722-6
  Synonyms: Brimstone; Sulphur
  Trade names: Biosulphur Powder; Unisulcoidal
  Trade names containing: Biosulphur Fluid CLR

Sunflower oil
Trade names containing: Herbasol Extract Walnut Shell Oil-Sol; Tepescohuite LS

Sunflower seed extract (INCI)
CAS 84776-03-4
Trade names containing: Blend For Elderly Skins HS 296; Brookosome® Herbal; Demaquillant HS 287; Demaquillant LS 687; Kalokiros HS 263; Kalokiros LS 663; Nutriderme HS 240; Nutriderme HS 243; Nutriderme HS 313; Nutriderme LS 613; Nutriderme LS 640

Sunflower seed oil (INCI)
CAS 8001-21-6; EINECS 232-273-9
Synonyms: Oils, sunflower seed
Trade names: Florasun™-90; Lipex 103; Lipovol SUN; Nikkol Sunflower Oil; Super Refined™ Sunflower Oil; Tri-K Sunflower Oil; Tri-Ol SUN; Univegoil SUNFL
Trade names containing: Aftershave LS 692; Alkanet LS; Anise LS; Arnica LS; Arnica Oil; Babyderme LS 642; Babyderme LS 665; BBC Moisture Trol; Bio-Oil GLA-10; Bitter Almond LS; Calendula Oil; Carrot LS; Carrot Oil; Carrot Oil; Chamomile Oil; Demaquillant LS 658; Demaquillant LS 687; Emollient LS 635; Eucalyptus LS; Ginseng LS; Hops LS; Incense LS; Kalokiros LS 663; Nutriderme LS 613; Nutriderme LS 640; Phosal 35SB; Regederme LS 630; Regederme LS 636; Relaxant LS 678; Solarium LS 669; Solarium LS 670; Stimulant LS 680; Tonique LS 690

Sunflower seed oil glyceride (INCI)
Synonyms: Glycerides, sunflower seed mono-
Trade names: Myverol® 18-92

Superoxide dismutase (INCI)
Trade names: Biocell S.O.D; Dascare S.O.D
Trade names containing: Brookosome® SOD; Dermasome® SOD

Sweet almond extract (INCI)
Synonyms: Prunus amygdalus dulcis extract
Trade names containing: Actiphyte of Almond; Almondermin® LS; Aromaphyte of Almond; Elespher® Almondermin; Herbasol-Extract Almond

Sweet almond oil (INCI)
CAS 8007-69-0
Synonyms: Oil of sweet almond; Almond oil, sweet
Trade names: Lipovol ALM; Nikkol Sweet Almond Oil; Tri-Ol ALM
Trade names containing: Aromaphyte of Almond; Eglantineol; Gilugel ALM; Lipovol ALM-S

Sweet basil extract. See Basil extract

Sweet marjoram oil (INCI)
CAS 8015-01-8
Synonyms: Origanum majorana oil
Trade names containing: Essentiaderm n.2; Essentiaderm n.7; Essentiaderm n.9

Swertia extract (INCI)
CAS 97766-44-4
Trade names containing: Semburi Extract BG; Semburi Extract Ethanol

Sylvic acid. See Abietic acid

Synthetic beeswax (INCI)
CAS 71243-51-1; EINECS 275-286-5
Trade names: Abesin E; Abesin NE; Beeswax Synthetic Stralpitz; Cyclochem EM 326A; Koster Keunen Synthetic Beeswax; Lipobee 102; Lipowax 6138G; Permulgin CSB; Permulgin RWB; Ross Beeswax Synthetic; Ross Beeswax Synthetic Cosmetic Grade; Syncrowax BB-4; Upiwax Synbee; Waxenol® 821

Synthetic jojoba oil (INCI)
Trade names: Dermol Jojoba E

Synthetic spermaceti wax. See Cetyl esters

Synthetic wax (INCI)
CAS 8002-74-2
Synonyms: Fischer-Tropsch wax; Fischer-Tropsch wax, oxidized
Trade names: Microfine 2, 2F, 2FS, 8, 8F; Press-Aid™ SP; Press-Aid™ XP; PT-0602; Uniwax AW-1060; Vybar® 103; Vybar® 260; Vybar® 825
Trade names containing: Micropoly 2001; Press-Aid™ XF; Press-Aid™

Talc (INCI)
CAS 14807-96-6; EINECS 238-877-9
Synonyms: Hydrous magnesium silicate; Industrial, cosmetic, or platy talc; Talcum
Trade names: Act II 500 USP; AGI Talc, BC 1615; Alphafil 200 USP; Alphafil 500 USP; Alpine Talc USP BC 127; Altalc 200 USP; Altalc 400 USP; Altalc 500 USP; Brillante; Dover 50 A; J-13; J-24; J-46; J-68; J-80; Lo-Micron Talc 1; Olympic; PT-46; Purtalc USP; Rose Talc; SteriLine 200; SteriLine 665; Supra A; Supra EF; Supra EF A; Suprafino A; Suprafino SMD; Supreme USP; Talc LCW; Talc Micro-Ace P-2; Talc Micro-Ace P-4; Talc OOC; Ultrafino; Vertal CO+
Trade names containing: B-3389 Cosmetic Umber; Bital®; Bleu De Prusse Micronise W 6805; Cosmetic Brown Oxide 7144; Coverleaf PC-2055T; Ferric Blue 114; Grillocin P-176; Grillocin® P 176; Kalixide AS; Kalixide Grassa; Kalixide Idrata; Lo-Micron Black Extender B.C& 34-3062-1; Silkall TL; Talc Micro-Ace P-2-030; Talcoseptic C

Tallamide DEA (INCI)
CAS 68155-20-4; EINECS 268-949-5
Synonyms: Diethanolamine tall oil acid amide; Tall oil acid diethanolamide; Tall oil diethanolamide
Trade names: Hetamide DT; Schercomid SO-T
Trade names containing: Schercomid TO-2

Tallamidopropyl dimethylamine
CAS 68650-79-3
Trade names: Schercodine T

Tall oil acid (INCI)
CAS 61790-12-3; EINECS 263-107-3
Synonyms: Acids, tall oil; Fatty acids, tall oil
Trade names: Acintol® 2122; Acintol® 7002; Pamak 4

Tall oil hydroxyethyl imidazoline (INCI)
CAS 61791-39-7; EINECS 263-171-2
Synonyms: 1-Hydroxyethyl-2-tall oil imidazoline; Tall oil imidazoline; 4,5-Dihydro-7-nortall oil-1H-imidazole-1-ethanol
Trade names: Varine T

Tallow acid (INCI)
CAS 61790-37-2; 67701-06-8; EINECS 263-129-3
Synonyms: Fatty acids, tallow; Acids, tallow
Trade names: Hy-Phi 4204; Prifac 7920; Prifac 7935; T-11; T-18; T-20; T-22
Trade names containing: Hystrene® 1835; Prifrac 7948

Tallow alcohol (INCI)
Synonyms: Alcohols, tallow
Trade names containing: Emulgade® K

Tallow amide (INCI)
Trade names: Kemamide® S-65

Tallowamide MEA (INCI)
CAS 68153-63-9; 68440-25-5
Synonyms: N-(2-Hydroxyethyl) tallow acid amide; Tallow

acid monoethanolamide; Monoethanolamine tallow acid amide
Trade names: Marlamid® M 1618

Tallowamido-polyamino-polyglycinate
Trade names: Ampholak XTP

Tallowamidopropylamine oxide (INCI)
CAS 68647-77-8; EINECS 271-972-3
Synonyms: Amides, tallow, N-[3-(dimethylamino)propyl]-N-oxides; N-3-(Dimethylamino)propyl tallow amide, N-oxide
Trade names: Chemoxide TAO

Tallowamidopropyl dimethylamine (INCI)
CAS 68425-50-3; EINECS 270-356-1
Synonyms: Dimethylaminopropyl tallow amide; N-[3-(Dimethylamino)propyl] tallow amides
Trade names: Chemidex T

Tallowamidopropyl hydroxysultaine (INCI)
Synonyms: Quaternary ammonium compds., (3-tallowamidopropyl)(2-hydroxy-3-sulfopropyl) dimethyl, hydroxide, inner salt
Trade names: Crosultaine T-30

Tallow amine (INCI)
CAS 61790-33-8; EINECS 263-125-1
Synonyms: Amines, tallow alkyl; Tallowamine; Tallowalkylamine
Trade names: Adogen® 170D; Armeen® T; Armeen® TD; Kemamine® P-974; Radiamine 6170; Radiamine 6171

Tallowamine oxide (INCI)
Synonyms: Tallow dimethylamine oxide; Amines, tallow alkyl dimethyl, oxides
Trade names: Mackamine™ TAO

Tallowamphopolycarboxyglycinate. *See Sodium carboxymethyl tallow polypropylamine*

Tallowamphopolycarboxypropionic acid
CAS 97488-62-5; EINECS 306-998-7
Trade names: Ampholak 7TY

Tallow bis hydroxyethyl methyl ammonium chloride
Synonyms: Methyl bis (2-hydroxyethyl) tallow ammonium chloride
Trade names: Varisoft® 920

Tallow dimethylamine. *See Dimethyl tallowamine*

Tallowdimonium propyltrimonium dichloride (INCI)
CAS 68607-29-4; EINECS 271-762-1
Synonyms: N,N,N′,N′,N′-Pentamethyl-N-tallow alkyl-1,3-propanediammonium dichloride; N-Tallow pentamethyl propane diammonium dichloride
Trade names containing: Duoquad® T-50

Talloweth-6 (INCI)
CAS 61791-28-4 (generic)
Synonyms: PEG-6 tallow ether; PEG 300 tallow ether; POE (6) tallow ether
Trade names: Hetoxol TA-6

Talloweth-7 carboxylic acid
Trade names: Akypo RT 60

Tallow glyceride (INCI)
CAS 61789-13-7; EINECS 263-035-2
Synonyms: Tallow monoglyceride; Glycerides, tallow mono-
Trade names: Myverol® 18-30

Tallow glycerides (INCI)
CAS 67701-27-3
Synonyms: Tallow mono, di and tri glycerides; Glycerides, tallow mono-, di- and tri-

Trade names: Koster Keunen Tallow Glyceride
Trade names containing: Ross Japan Wax Substitute 473; Ross Japan Wax Substitute 525; Unitina KD-16

N-Tallow pentamethyl propane diammonium dichloride
Trade names containing: Variquat® 477; Variquat® 477

Tallowtrimonium chloride (INCI)
CAS 8030-78-2; 7491-05-2; 68002-61-9; EINECS 232-447-4
Synonyms: Quaternary ammonium compds., tallow alkyl trimethyl, chlorides; Tallow trimethyl ammonium chloride
Trade names: Arquad® T-30; Jet Quat T-27W; Jet Quat T-50; Kemamine® Q-9703B; Nikkol CA-2450T; Noramium MS 50; Radiaquat® 6471
Trade names containing: Arquad® T-27W; Arquad® T-2C-50; Arquad® T-50; Dow Corning® 1669; Dow Corning® 929; Dow Corning® X2-1669; E-2153; Varisoft® 471

Tannic acid (INCI)
CAS 1401-55-4; EINECS 215-753-2
Trade names: Atomergic Tannic Acid; Unichem TANAC

Tansy extract (INCI)
CAS 84961-64-8; EINECS 284-653-9
Synonyms: Tanacetum vulgare extract
Trade names containing: Actiphyte of Tansy

Tartaric acid (INCI)
CAS 87-69-4 (L-form); 147-71-7 (D-form); 133-37-9 (dl-α); EINECS 205-695-6; 205-105-7; 201-766-0
Synonyms: DL-Tartaric acid anhydrous; Dihydroxysuccinic acid
Trade names: Unichem TAR AC

TBAB. *See Tetrabutyl ammonium bromide*

TBHQ. *See t-Butyl hydroquinone*

TEA. *See Triethanolamine*

TEA-abietoyl hydrolyzed collagen (INCI)
CAS 68918-77-4
Synonyms: Proteins, hydrolysates, reaction prods. with abietoyl chloride, compd. with triethanolamine; Triethanolamine abietoyl hydrolyzed animal protein; TEA-abietoyl hydrolyzed animal protein
Trade names: Lamepon® PA-TR; Lamepon® PA-TR/NP; Lexein® A-520; Uniprolam PAJR

TEA-acrylates/acrylonitrogens copolymer (INCI)
Trade names: Hypan® SS500W

TEA-C12-15 alkyl sulfate (INCI)
Synonyms: TEA-C12-15 alcohols sulfate; Triethanolamine C12-15 alcohols sulfate
Trade names: Elfan® 250 TS; Standapol® T-315; Unipol T-315

TEA cocoate (INCI)
CAS 61790-64-5; EINECS 263-155-5
Synonyms: Fatty acids, coconut oil, triethanolamine salts; Triethanolamine coconut acid
Trade names: Akypogene FP 35 T

TEA-cocoyl-glutamate (INCI)
CAS 68187-29-1; EINECS 269-084-6
Synonyms: L-Glutamic acid, N-coco acyl derivs., compds. with triethanolamine; Triethanolamine cocoyl glutamate
Trade names: Amisoft CT-12

TEA-cocoyl hydrolyzed collagen (INCI)
CAS 68952-16-9
Synonyms: TEA-coco-hydrolyzed animal protein; TEA-cocoyl hydrolyzed animal protein
Trade names: Bio-Soft® MT 40; Foam-Coll™ 4CT;

Granpro-10; Lamepon® S-TR/NP; Lamepon® ST 40/ NP; Lexein® S620TA; Liprot CT; May-Tein CT; Maypon 4CT; Monteine LCT; Peptein® TEAC; Promois ECT; Promois ECT-C; Rewotein CPT; Texatein CT; Uniprolam ST-40
Trade names containing: Lexate® BPQ; Lexein® S620S/ Superpro 5A; Liprot CTS; Monteine V; Pro-Lan V; Relaxer Conc. No. 2; Superpro 5A; Supro-Tein V; Tripro-5

TEA-cocoyl hydrolyzed soy protein
Trade names: May-Tein SY

TEA-cocoyl sarcosinate (INCI)
CAS 68411-96-1
Synonyms: N-Methylglycine, N-coco acyl derivs., compds. with triethanolamine; Triethanolamine cocoyl sarcosinate
Trade names containing: Hamposyl® TOC-30

TEA-dodecylbenzenesulfonate (INCI)
CAS 27323-41-7; 68411-31-4; 29381-93-9; EINECS 248-406-9
Synonyms: Dodecylbenzenesulfonic acid, compd. with 2,2´,2´´-nitrilotris[ethanol] (1:1); Triethanolamine dodecylbenzene sulfonate
Trade names: Ablusol DBT; Bio-Soft® N-300; Calsoft T-60; Carosulf T-60-L; Carsofoam® T-60-L; Elfan® WAT; Hartofol 60T; Hexaryl D 60 L; Manro TDBS 60; Marlopon® AT; Marlopon® AT 50; Marlopon® CA; Mazon® 60T; Naxel™ AAS-60S; Norfox® T-60; Rhodacal® DDB 60T; Witconate™ 60T; Witconate™ 79S; Witconate™ LXH; Witconate™ S-1280; Witconate™ TAB
Trade names containing: Bio-Soft® N-21; Lecithin Water Dispersible CLR; Stepanol® 317

Tea extract. *See Thea sinensis extract*

TEA hydrochloride (INCI)
CAS 637-39-8; EINECS 211-284-2
Synonyms: Triethanolamine hydrochloride; 2,2´,2´´-Nitrilotris[ethanol], hydrochloride
Trade names containing: Hamp-Ene® OH Powd.

TEA-hydrogenated tallow glutamate (INCI)
Synonyms: Triethanolamine hydrogenated tallowyl glutamate; Triethanolamine hydrogenated tallow glutamate
Trade names: Amisoft HT-12

TEA hydro-iodide (INCI)
Synonyms: Triethanolamine iodohydrate
Trade names: Iodobio 45; Iodotrat

TEA-isostearoyl hydrolyzed collagen (INCI)
Synonyms: TEA-isostearoyl hydrolyzed animal protein
Trade names containing: Lamecreme® LPM

TEA-lactate (INCI)
CAS 20475-12-1; EINECS 243-846-8
Synonyms: Triethanolamine lactate
Trade names containing: Facteur Hydratant PH; Hydroviton 2/059353

TEA-laureth sulfate (INCI)
CAS 27028-82-6
Synonyms: Triethanolamine lauryl ether sulfate
Trade names: Alscoap TA-40; Empicol® ETB; Montelane LT 4088; Neopon LOT/NF; Nikkol SBL-2T-36; Nikkol SBL-4T; Surfax EDT; Tylorol LT50; Zoharpon LAET
Trade names containing: Stepanol® 317

TEA-lauroyl collagen amino acids (INCI)
Synonyms: TEA-lauroyl animal collagen amino acids
Trade names: Aminofoam C; Foamamino 40CT

TEA-lauroyl glutamate (INCI)

CAS 53576-49-1; 31955-67-6; EINECS 258-636-1
Synonyms: L-Glutamic acid, N-lauryl and 2,2´,2´´-nitrilotriethanol (1:1); Triethanolamine lauroyl glutamate
Trade names: Amisoft LT-12

TEA-lauroyl keratin amino acids (INCI)
Synonyms: TEA-lauroyl animal keratin amino acids
Trade names: Aminofoam K

TEA lauroyl sarcosinate (INCI)
CAS 2224-49-9; 16693-53-1; EINECS 240-736-1
Synonyms: Glycine, N-methyl-N-(oxododecyl)-, compd. with 2,2´,2´´-nitrilotris[ethanol] (1:1); Triethanolamine lauroyl sarcosinate
Trade names: Crodasinic LT40; Hamposyl® TL-40

TEA-lauryl sulfate (INCI)
CAS 139-96-8; 68908-44-1; EINECS 205-388-7
Synonyms: Sulfuric acid, monododecyl ester, compd. with 2,2´,2´´-nitrilotris[ethanol] (1:1); Triethanolammonium lauryl sulfate; Triethanolamine lauryl sulfate
Trade names: Akyposal TLS 42; Aremsol TA; Berol 480; Calfoam TLS-40; Carsonol® TLS; Cosmopon TR; Elfan® 240T; Empicol® TA40; Empicol® TA40A; Empicol® TL40; Empicol® TL40/T; Genapol® CRT 40; Genapol® LRT 40; Laural D; Manro TL 40; Marlinat® DFL 40; Neopon LT/NF; Nikkol TEALS; Nikkol TEALS-42; Norfox® TLS; Nutrapon TLS-500; Perlankrol® ATL40; Rewopol® TLS 40; Rhodapon® LT-6; Sandoz Sulfate TL; Standapol® T; Stepanol® WAT; Sulfetal KT 400; Sulfochem TLS; Sunnol LM-1140T; Surfax 40; Texapon® T; Texapon® T 42; Ufarol TA-40; Unipol T; Witcolate™ T; Witcolate™ TLS-500; Zoharpon LAT
Trade names containing: Carsofoam® MSP; Empicol® TC34; Empicol® TCR; Empicol® TLP; Empicol® TLR; Equex STM; Mearlmaid® TR; Miracare® NWC; Nutrapon TW 3987; Standapol® Conc. 7021; Standapol® SHC-301; Unipol Conc. 7021; Varifoam® SXC

TEA-myristoyl hydrolyzed collagen (INCI)
CAS 69430-23-5
Synonyms: TEA-myristoyl hydrolyzed animal protein; Triethanolamine myristoyl hydrolyzed animal protein
Trade names: Lexein® A-220

TEA nonoxynol-4 sulfate
Trade names: Nikkol SNP-4T

TEA-oleamido PEG-2 sulfosuccinate (CTFA)
Synonyms: Triethanolamine monooleamido PEG-2 sulfosuccinate
Trade names: Unipol SH-300
Trade names containing: Standapol® SHC-301

TEA oleoyl sarcosinate (INCI)
CAS 17736-08-2; EINECS 241-727-5
Synonyms: Sarcosine, N-oleoyl-, compd. with 2,2´,2´´-nitrilotris[ethanol] (1:1); Triethanolamine oleoyl sarcosinate
Trade names containing: Hamposyl® TOC-30

TEA-palm kernel sarcosinate (INCI)
Synonyms: Triethanolamine palm kernel sarcosinate
Trade names: Medialan KF

TEA-PEG-3 cocamide sulfate (INCI)
Trade names: Genapol® AMS

TEA-salicylate (INCI)
CAS 2174-16-5; EINECS 218-531-3
Synonyms: 2-Hydroxybenzoic acid, compd. with 2,2´,2´´-Nitrilotris[ethanol] (1:1)

Trade names: Neotan W
Trade names containing: Cellulinol

TEA-stearate (INCI)
CAS 4568-28-9; EINECS 224-945-5
Synonyms: Triethanolamine stearate
Trade names containing: Cetasal

Tea tree oil (INCI)
CAS 68647-73-4
Trade names: EmCon Tea Tree

TEA-undecenoyl hydrolyzed collagen (INCI)
CAS 68951-91-7
Synonyms: Proteins, hydrolysates, reaction prods. with 10-undecenoyl chloride, compds. with triethanol-amine; TEA-undecylenoyl hydrolyzed animal protein; Triethanolamine undecylenoyl hydrolyzed animal protein
Trade names: Liprot UT; Promois EUT

TEA-wheat germ oil soap
Trade names containing: Afdet™ WGS

Terminalia sericea extract (INCI)
Trade names: Sericoside Phytosome®

Testicular extract (INCI)
Trade names containing: Complexe DM 60; Epidermin in Oil; Epidermin Water-Soluble

Tetraammonium EDTA
Trade names: Versene Tetraammonium EDTA

Tetrabromo-o-cresol
CAS 576-55-6
Synonyms: 3,4,5,6-Tetrabromocresol; 2-Methyl-3,4,5,6-tetrabromophenol
Trade names: Deodorant Richter/K

Tetrabutoxypropyl methicone
Trade names: Masil® 756

Tetrabutyl ammonium bromide (INCI)
CAS 1643-19-2; EINECS 216-699-2
Synonyms: TBAB; Tetra-N-butylammonium bromide
Trade names: TBAB

Tetradecanoic acid. *See Myristic acid*

Tetradecene-1
CAS 1120-36-1
Synonyms: Linear C14 alpha olefin
Trade names: Ethyl Tetradecene-1; Gulftene® 14
Trade names containing: Ethyl Dodecene-1/Tetrade-cene-1 Blend; Ethyl Tetradecene-1/Hexadecene-1

Tetradecyl... *See Myristyl...*

Tetradecyleicosanol (INCI)
Synonyms: Myristyl eicosanol
Trade names: Eutanol® G 32/36; Unimul-G-32/36
Trade names containing: Isofol® 34T

Tetradecyleicosyl stearate (INCI)
Synonyms: Myristyleicosyl stearate
Trade names: Hetester 3236S; Unimul-7115

2-Tetradecyloctadecanol (INCI)
CAS 32582-32-4; EINECS 251-110-2
Synonyms: Myristyloctadecanol; 2-Tetradecylocta-decanol
Trade names: Isofol® 32
Trade names containing: Isofol® 34T

2,2´,4,4´-Tetrahydroxy benzophenone. *See Benzophe-none-2*

Tetrahydroxypropyl ethylenediamine (INCI)
CAS 102-60-3; EINECS 203-041-4
Trade names: Mazeen® 173; Mazeen® 174; Mazeen®

174-75; Neutrol® TE
Trade names containing: Grillocin® CW 90

2,2,5,5-Tetramethyl-4-isopropyl-1,3-dioxane
Trade names: Verdoxan

Tetrapotassium pyrophosphate (INCI)
CAS 7320-34-5; EINECS 230-785-7
Synonyms: TKPP; Diphosphoric acid, tetrapotassium salt; Potassium pyrophosphate
Trade names: Empiphos 4KP

Tetrasodium dicarboxyethyl stearyl sulfosuccinamate (INCI)
CAS 3401-73-8; 37767-39-8; 38916-42-6; EINECS 222-273-7
Synonyms: Tetrasodium dicarboxyethyl octadecyl sulfo-succinamate
Trade names: Monawet SNO-35

Tetrasodium EDTA (INCI)
CAS 64-02-8; EINECS 200-573-9
Synonyms: EDTA Na$_4$; Edetate sodium; Tetrasodium edetate; Ethylene diamine tetraacetic acid, sodium salt
Trade names: Chelon 100; Hamp-Ene® 100; Hamp-Ene® 220; Hamp-Ene® Na$_4$; Kelate 220; Seques-trene® 220; Universene Na4; Versene 100; Versene 100 EP; Versene 100 LS; Versene 100 SRG; Versene 100 XL; Versene 220
Trade names containing: Fondix G Bis

Tetrasodium etidronate (INCI)
CAS 3794-83-0; EINECS 223-267-7
Synonyms: Tetrasodium 1-hydroxyethane-1,1-diphos-phonate; (1-Hydroxyethylidene)bisphosphonic acid, tetrasodium salt
Trade names: Mayoquest 1530; Turpinal® 4 NL; Universene AC
Trade names containing: Mayoquest 1545M

Tetrasodium pyrophosphate (INCI)
CAS 7722-88-5; EINECS 231-767-1
Synonyms: TSPP; Tetrasodium diphosphate; Diphos-phoric acid, tetrasodium salt; Sodium pyrophosphate
Trade names containing: Laponite® XLS; Masque Poudre No. 2

THAM. *See Tris (hydroxymethyl) aminomethane*

Thea sinensis extract (INCI)
CAS 84650-60-2
Synonyms: Camellia sinensis extract; Chinese tea ex-tract; Tea extract
Trade names containing: Koucha Liq.

Thea sinensis oil. *See Camellia oil*

Theine. *See Caffeine*

Thenoyl methionine (INCI)
CAS 60752-63-8
Synonyms: 2-Thenoylamino 4-methylthio butanoic acid; N-(2-Thienylcarbonyl)-L-methionine
Trade names: T.A.M

Theophylline (INCI)
CAS 58-55-9; EINECS 200-385-7
Trade names containing: Nanospheres 100 Lipo Plus

Theophyllisilane
Trade names containing: Nanospheres 100 Lipo Plus

Thiamine HCl (INCI)
CAS 67-03-8; EINECS 200-641-8
Synonyms: Thiamine dichloride; Vitamin B$_1$; Aneurine hydrochloride
Trade names containing: Extrapone Bio-Tamin Special 2/ 2032671

Thioglycerin (INCI)
CAS 96-27-5; EINECS 202-495-0
Synonyms: 3-Mercapto-1,2-propanediol; Mono-thioglycerol; Thioglycerol
Trade names: Thiovanol®

Thioglycolic acid (INCI)
CAS 68-11-1; EINECS 200-677-4
Synonyms: 2-Mercaptoacetic acid
Trade names: Thiovanic® Acid

Thioxanthine (INCI)
CAS 261-31-4; EINECS 205-972-1
Trade names containing: FRS-Diffuser Microreservoir; Iniferine

Thyme extract (INCI)
CAS 84929-51-1
Trade names: Hydroessential Thymus
Trade names containing: Aftershave HS 292; Aftershave LS 692; Stimulant HS 280; Stimulant LS 680

Thyme oil (INCI)
CAS 8007-46-3
Trade names containing: Essentiaderm n.1; Essentiaderm n.7; Fitoestesina

Thymol (INCI)
CAS 89-83-8; EINECS 201-944-8
Synonyms: 5-Methyl-2-(1-methylethyl) phenol; 6-Isopropyl-m-cresol; 2-Isopropyl-5-methylphenol
Trade names: Unichem THYMOL

Thymus extract (INCI)
Trade names containing: Brookosome® TE; Brookosome® TYE; Dermasome® TE; Epidermin in Oil; Epidermin Water-Soluble

Thymus hydrolysate (INCI)
Trade names: Nutrex TM
Trade names containing: Fibrastil

Tin oxide (ic) (INCI)
CAS 1317-45-9; 18282-10-5; EINECS 242-159-0
Synonyms: Tin dioxide; Stannic oxide; Cassiterite
Trade names containing: Soloron Silver CO; Soloron Silver Fine CO; Soloron Silver Fine; Soloron Silver Sparkle CO; Soloron Silver Sparkle; Soloron Silver; Soloron-R-Gold

TIPA. *See Triisopropanolamine*

TIPA-laureth sulfate (INCI)
CAS 107600-36-2
Synonyms: Triisopropanolamine lauryl ether sulfate
Trade names: Akyposal 100 DAL

TIPA-lauryl sulfate (INCI)
CAS 66161-60-2
Synonyms: Sulfuric acid, monododecyl ester, compd. with 1,1′,1″-nitrilotris[2-propanol]; Triisopropanolamine lauryl sulfate
Trade names: Akyposal TIPA 45; Rewopol® TLS 90 L

Titanium dioxide (INCI)
CAS 13463-67-7; EINECS 236-675-5
Synonyms: Titanic anhydride; Titanic acid anhydride; Titanium oxide
Trade names: Atlas White Titanium Dioxide; Kowet Titanium Dioxide; Kronos® 1025; Luxelen® D; MTD-25; Solar Shield™; Spherititan; Sunveil 6010; Sunveil 6030; Ti-Sphere AA-1512-LL; Ti-Sphere AA-1515; Titanium Dioxide P25; Titanium Dioxide SPA; Transparent Titanium Dioxide PW Covafluor; Transparent Titanium Dioxide PW Covasil S; Transparent Titanium Dioxide PW Powd; Uniwhite AO; Uniwhite KO
Trade names containing: Bi-Lite® Ultrawhite 1084; Black

Mica; Blanc Covachip W 9705; Blanc Covanail W 9737; Blanc Covapate W 9765; Blanc Covasop W 9775; Cloisonné Blue; Cloisonné Gold; Cloisonné Red; Cloisonné Violet; Colorona® Bright Gold; Colorona® Carmine Red; Colorona® Light Blue; Colorona® Magestic Green; Coverleaf PC-2035; Coverleaf PC-2055M; Coverleaf PC-2055T; Dichrona® BG; Dichrona® BR; Dichrona® BY; Dichrona® GY; Dichrona® RB; Dichrona® RG; Dichrona® RY; Dichrona® YB; Dichrona® YG; Dichrona® YR; Duocrome® BG; Duocrome® GY; Duocrome® RB; Duocrome® YR; Extender W; Flamenco® Gold CC; Flamenco® Gold; Flamenco® Pearl CC; Flamenco® Pearl; Flamenco® Twilight Blue; Flamenco® Ultra Fine; Flamenco®; Flonac ME 10 C; Flonac MG 30 C; Flonac MI 10 C; Flonac ML 10 C; Flonac MS 10 C; Flonac MS 20 C; Flonac MS 30 C; Flonac MS 33 C; Flonac MS 40 C; Flonac MS 5 C; Flonac MS 60 C; Flonac MS 70 C; Flonac MX 10 C; Flonac MX 30 C; Gemstone Sunstone CC; Gemtone® Amber; Gemtone® Amethyst; Gemtone® Emerald; Gemtone® Mauve Quartz; Gemtone® Sunstone; Gemtone® Tan Opal CC; Kalixide CT; Liquiwax™ DIADD/TiO$_2$ Disp; Lustra-Pearl®; Luxelen® SS-020; Luxelen® SS; Nikkol Super Mica D; Orgasol 1002 EX D WHITE 10 COS; PTFE-19; Silkall Tl; Soloron Silver CO; Soloron Silver Fine CO; Soloron Silver Fine; Soloron Silver Sparkle CO; Soloron Silver Sparkle; Soloron Silver; Soloron-R-Gold; Spectra-Pearl®; Sunveil F; Sunveil; Ti-Sphere AA-1512-030; Ti-Sphere AB-15155A; Timiron®; Titanium Dioxide 110; Transparent Titanium Dioxide PW Covalim; Transparent Titanium Dioxide PW Covasop; Transparent Titanium Dioxide PW Squatol S; UV-Titan M210; UV-Titan M212; UV-Titan M260; UV-Titan M262; Zetesap 5165; Zetesap 813A

TKPP. *See Tetrapotassium pyrophosphate*

TME. *See Trimethylolethane*

Tocopherol (INCI)
CAS 1406-18-4; 59-02-9 (d-α), 10191-41-0 (dl-α); EINECS 215-798-8; 200-412-2
Synonyms: Vitamin E; D-α tocopherol; DL-α tocopherol
Trade names: Copherol® F-1300; Covi-Ox® T-30P; Covi-Ox® T-50; Covi-Ox® T-70; Covitol 80/20M; Covitol F-1000; Covitol F-350M; Covitol F-600; Eastman® Vitamin E 4-50; Eastman® Vitamin E 4-80; Eastman® Vitamin E 5-40; Eastman® Vitamin E 5-67; Tenox® GT-1, GT-2; dl-α-Tocopherol; Unatox; Vitamin E USP Tocopherol; Vitazyme® E
Trade names containing: Arnica Oil CLR; Arnicaflower Oil PANAROM; Balm Mint Oil Infusion; Bio-Oil GLA-10; Biobranil Watersoluble 2/012600; Brookosome® ACEBC; Calendula Oil CLR; Calendula Oil Monarom; Carrot Oil CLR; Carrot Oil Extra; Chronosphere® Planell®; Complexe AV.h.; Controx® KS; Controx® VP; Copherol® 950LC; Crodarom Calendula O; Crodarom Carrot O; Cutavit Richter; Derma-Vitamincomplex, Oil soluble; EFA-Glycerides; EFA-Liq.; EFA-Plex; EFA-Plexol; Grillocin HY-77; Hypericum Oil CLR; Lipodermol®; Lipotrofina A; MicroReservoir FRS-Diffuser; Oxynex® K; Oxynex® L; Oxynex® LM; Soluvit Richter; Tocopherol Oil CLR; Unibotan Vitaplant O CLR; Unipherol U-14; Vitaplant CLR Oil-Soluble N; Vyox

Tocophersolan (INCI)
CAS 9002-96-4; 30999-06-5
Trade names: Eastman® Vitamin E TPGS; Glycol 1000 Succinate

Tocopheryl acetate (INCI)
CAS 1406-70-8; 7695-91-2 (d-α); EINECS 231-710-0
Synonyms: D-α Tocopheryl acetate; DL-α Tocopheryl acetate; Vitamin E acetate
Trade names: Copherol® 1250; Covitol 1100; Covitol 1360; Eastman® Vitamin E 6-100; Eastman® Vitamin E 6-40; Eastman® Vitamin E 6-81; Eastman® Vitamin E 700; Nanospheres 100 Vitamine E Acetate; dl-α-Tocopheryl Acetate, Cosmetic Grade No. 60574; Uantox 1250; Univit-E Acetate; Vitamin E Acetate Cosmetic Oil; Vitamin E Acetate USP Oil
Trade names containing: AFR LS; Antioxidant G-2; Brookosome® ANE; Brookosome® E; Brookosome® ELL; Chronosphere® V-AE; Dermasome® E; Destressine 2000; Epiderm-Complex O; Faceur ARL; L.C.R.E.; Lipoliv; Lipomicron Vitamin E Acetate; Midpol 2000; Nikkol Aquasome EC-5; Nikkol Aquasome VE; Tri-K CMF Complex; Unisphères YE-501

Tocopheryl linoleate (INCI)
CAS 36148-84-2
Synonyms: D-α Tocopheryl linoleate; DL-α Tocopheryl linoleate; Vitamin E linoleate
Trade names: Linoleate de Tocopherol; dl-α-Tocopheryl Linoleate No. 26364

Tocopheryl nicotinate (INCI)
CAS 16676-75-8
Synonyms: D-α Tocopheryl nicotinate; DL-α Tocopheryl nicotinate; Vitamin E nicotinate
Trade names: Vitamin E Nicotinate

Tocopheryl succinate (INCI)
CAS 4345-03-3 (d-α); 17407-37-3; EINECS 224-403-8
Synonyms: D-α Tocopheryl succinate; DL-α Tocopheryl succinate; Vitamin E acid succinate
Trade names: Covitol 1185; Covitol 1210; Eastman® Vitamin E Succinate

p-Tolualdehyde
CAS 104-87-0; EINECS 203-246-9
Trade names: PTAL

Toluene (INCI)
CAS 108-88-3; EINECS 203-625-9
Synonyms: Methylbenzene; Phenylmethane; Toluol
Trade names containing: Biju® BTD, BXD; Biju® BWD, BWS; Biju® BWP; Biju® Ultra UTD, UXD; Biju® Ultra UWD, UWS; Biju® Ultra UWP

Toluene-2,5-diamine sulfate (INCI)
CAS 615-50-9; EINECS 210-431-8
Synonyms: 2-Methyl-1,4-benzenediamine sulfate; 2,5-Diaminotoluene sulfate; p-Toluenediamine sulfate
Trade names: Rodol BLFX

Toluenesulfonamide/formaldehyde resin. *See Tosylamide/formaldehyde resin*

Toluene sulfonic acid (INCI)
CAS 104-15-4; 70788-37-3; EINECS 203-180-0
Synonyms: 4-Methylbenzenesulfonic acid
Trade names: Eltesol® TSX; Eltesol® TSX/A; Eltesol® TSX/SF; Witconate™ TX Acid
Trade names containing: Eltesol® TA 65

Tormentil extract (INCI)
CAS 90083-09-3; 85085-66-1
Synonyms: Potentilla erecta extract
Trade names containing: Herbalcomplex 2 Special; Stimulant HS 285

Tosylamide/epoxy resin (INCI)
Synonyms: Toluenesulfonamide/epoxy resin
Trade names: Decoset-Z; Lustrabrite® S; Nagellite®

3050
Trade names containing: Nagellite® 3050-80

Tosylamide/formaldehyde resin (INCI)
CAS 25035-71-6; 1338-51-8
Synonyms: Benzenesulfonamide, 4-methyl-, polymer with formaldehyde; Toluenesulfonamide/formaldehyde resin
Trade names: Ketjenflex® MH; Ketjenflex® MS-80

TOTM. *See Trioctyl trimellitate*

Trachea hydrolysate (INCI)
Synonyms: Hydrolyzed trachea
Trade names: Complex T-I, T-II

Triacetin (INCI)
CAS 102-76-1; EINECS 203-051-9
Synonyms: Glyceryl triacetate; 1,2,3-Propanetriol triacetate; Triacetyl glycerol
Trade names: Priacetin; Unitolate GTA

Tribehenin (INCI)
CAS 18641-57-1; EINECS 242-471-7
Synonyms: Glyceryl tribehenate; 1,2,3-Propanetriol tridocosanoate
Trade names: Compritol 888; Compritol WL 3241; Lipovol GTB; Pelemol GTB; Syncrowax HR-C
Trade names containing: Compritol HD5 ATO; Syncrowax HRS-C

Tribenzoin. *See Glyceryl tribenzoate*

Tributyl citrate (INCI)
CAS 77-94-1; EINECS 201-071-2
Synonyms: 2-Hydroxy-1,2,3-propanetricarboxylic acid, tributyl ester
Trade names: Crodamol TBC; TBC; Uniflex TBC

Tricaprin (INCI)
CAS 621-71-6; EINECS 210-702-0
Synonyms: 1,2,3-Propanol tridecanoate
Trade names: Dynasan® 110

Tricaprylin (INCI)
CAS 538-23-8; EINECS 208-686-5
Synonyms: Glyceryl tricaprylate; Caprylic acid, 1,2,3-propanetriyl ester; Octanoic acid, 1,2,3-propanetriyl ester; 1,2,3-Propanetriol trioctanoate
Trade names: Captex® 8000; Estol GTC 1803; Miglyol® 808

Triceteareth-4 phosphate (INCI)
Trade names: Hostaphat KW 340 N
Trade names containing: Hostacerin CG

Triceteth-5 phosphate (INCI)
Trade names: Nikkol TCP-5

Tricetylmonium chloride (INCI)
CAS 52467-63-7
Synonyms: Tricetyl monomethyl ammonium chloride
Trade names: Arquad® 316; Varisoft® TC-90

Tricetyl phosphate (INCI)
CAS 56827-95-3; 68814-13-1; EINECS 272-336-8
Synonyms: 1-Hexadecanol, phosphate (3:1)
Trade names: Nikkol Wax-600

Trichloro-t-butyl alcohol. *See Chlorobutanol*

Trichloroethane (INCI)
CAS 71-55-6; EINECS 200-756-3; 201-166-9
Synonyms: 1,1,1-Trichloroethane; Ethane, 1,1,1-trichloro-; Methylchloroform
Trade names: Aerothene TT; Solvent 111

N-Trichloromethylthiotetrahydrophthalimide. *See Captan*

Triclosan (INCI)

CAS 3380-34-5; EINECS 222-182-2
Synonyms: 2,4,4´-Trichloro-2´-hydroxydiphenyl ether; 5-Chloro-2(2,4-dichlorophenoxy)phenol
Trade names: Irgasan DP300

Tricontanyl PVP (INCI)
Synonyms: 2-Pyrrolidone, 1-ethenyl polymer with 1-triacontane
Trade names: Antaron® WP-660; Ganex® WP-660

Trideceth-2 (INCI)
CAS 678213-23-0
Synonyms: PEG 100 tridecyl ether; POE (2) tridecyl ether
Trade names: Synperonic A2

Trideceth-3 (INCI)
CAS 4403-12-7; 24938-91-8 (generic); EINECS 224-540-3
Synonyms: PEG-3 tridecyl ether; PEG (3) tridecyl ether; POE (3) tridecyl ether
Trade names: Bio-Soft® TD 400; Chemal TDA-3; Hetoxol TD-3; Lipocol TD-3; Macol® TD-3; Procol TDA-3; Synperonic A3; Volpo T-3

Trideceth-5 (INCI)
CAS 24938-91-8 (generic)
Synonyms: PEG-5 tridecyl ether; POE (5) tridecyl ether
Trade names: Volpo T-5
Trade names containing: Belsil ADM 6056 E; Belsil ADM 6059 E

Trideceth-6 (INCI)
CAS 24938-91-8 (generic); 78330-21-9
Synonyms: PEG-6 tridecyl ether; PEG 300 tridecyl ether; POE (6) tridecyl ether
Trade names: Britex TR 60; Chemal TDA-6; Desonic® 6T; Hetoxol TD-6; Hodag Nonionic TD-6; Lipocol TD-6; Macol® TD-610; Procol TDA-6; Renex® 36; Witconol™ TD-60
Trade names containing: Belsil ADM 6041 E; Belsil ADM 6042 E

Trideceth-7 (INCI)
CAS 24938-91-8 (generic); 78330-21-9; 68213-23-0
Synonyms: PEG-7 tridecyl ether; POE (7) tridecyl ether
Trade names: Flo-Mo® AJ-100; Flo-Mo® AJ-100; Flo-Mo® AJ-85; Flo-Mo® AJ-85; Synperonic A7

Trideceth-8 (INCI)
CAS 24938-91-8 (generic)
Synonyms: PEG-8 tridecyl ether; POE (8) tridecyl ether
Trade names: Bio-Soft® TD 630; Macol® TD-8

Trideceth-9 (INCI)
CAS 24938-91-8 (generic)
Synonyms: PEG-9 tridecyl ether; PEG 450 tridecyl ether; POE (9) tridecyl ether
Trade names: Chemal TDA-9; Desonic® 9T; Hetoxol TD-9; Rhodasurf® TD-9; Synperonic A9
Trade names containing: Chamomile CL 2/033026; Emulsifier 2/014160

Trideceth-10 (INCI)
CAS 24938-91-8 (generic); 78330-21-9
Synonyms: PEG-10 tridecyl ether; PEG 500 tridecyl ether; POE (10) tridecyl ether
Trade names: Macol® TD-10; Volpo T-10; Witconol™ TD-100
Trade names containing: Belsil ADM 6059 E

Trideceth-11 (INCI)
CAS 24938-91-8 (generic)
Synonyms: PEG-11 tridecyl ether; POE (11) tridecyl ether
Trade names: Synperonic A11

Trideceth-12 (INCI)
CAS 24938-91-8 (generic)

Synonyms: PEG-12 tridecyl ether; PEG 600 tridecyl ether; POE (12) tridecyl ether
Trade names: Britex TR 120; Chemal TDA-12; Desonic® 12T; Hetoxol TD-12; Hodag Nonionic TD-12; Lipocol PT-400; Lipocol TD-12; Macol® TD-12; Procol TDA-12; Renex® 30; Unicol 12
Trade names containing: Dow Corning® 939; Solubilizer L-76

Trideceth-15 (INCI)
CAS 24938-91-8 (generic); 78330-21-9
Synonyms: PEG-15 tridecyl ether; POE (15) tridecyl ether
Trade names: Chemal TDA-15; Desonic® 15T; Hodag Nonionic TD-15; Macol® TD-15; Procol TDA-15; Unicol 15; Unicol TD-15; Volpo T-15
Trade names containing: Belsil ADM 6056 E

Trideceth-18
CAS 24938-91-8 (generic)
Synonyms: PEG-18 tridecyl ether; POE (18) tridecyl ether
Trade names: Chemal TDA-18; Hetoxol TD-18

Trideceth-20 (INCI)
CAS 24938-91-8 (generic)
Synonyms: PEG-20 tridecyl ether; PEG 1000 tridecyl ether; POE (20) tridecyl ether
Trade names: Synperonic A20; Volpo T-20

Trideceth-25
CAS 24938-91-8 (generic)
Synonyms: PEG-25 tridecyl ether; POE (25) tridecyl ether
Trade names: Hetoxol TD-25

Trideceth-50 (INCI)
CAS 24938-91-8 (generic)
Synonyms: POE (50) tridecyl ether
Trade names: Synperonic A50

Trideceth-100
CAS 24938-91-8 (generic)
Synonyms: PEG-100 tridecyl ether; POE (100) tridecyl ether
Trade names: Macol® TD-100

Trideceth-2 carboxamide MEA (INCI)
CAS 107628-04-6
Trade names: Aminol A-15
Trade names containing: Akypogene HM 12

Trideceth-3 carboxylic acid (INCI)
CAS 24938-91-8 (generic); 68412-55-5 (generic)
Synonyms: POE (3) tridecyl ether carboxylic acid
Trade names: Nikkol ECT-3

Trideceth-7 carboxylic acid (INCI)
CAS 56388-96-6 (generic); 68412-55-5 (generic); 24938-91-8 (generic)
Synonyms: PEG-7 tridecyl ether carboxylic acid; POE (7) tridecyl ether carboxylic acid
Trade names: Emcol® CBA60; Incrodet TD7-C; Liposurf TD-7C; Nikkol ECT-7; Rewopol® CT 65; Sandopan® DTC-Acid; Surfine T-A

Trideceth-19 carboxylic acid (INCI)
CAS 24938-91-8 (generic); 68412-55-5 (generic)
Synonyms: POE (19) tridecyl ether carboxylic acid
Trade names: Sandopan® JA-36

Trideceth-2 phosphate
CAS 9046-01-9 (generic)
Synonyms: PEG-2 tridecyl ether phosphate
Trade names: Crodafos T2 Acid

Trideceth-5 phosphate
CAS 9046-01-9 (generic)
Synonyms: PEG-5 tridecyl ether phosphate; POE (5) tridecyl ether phosphate
Trade names: Crodafos T5 Acid

Trideceth-10 phosphate
CAS 9046-01-9 (generic)
Synonyms: PEG-10 tridecyl ether phosphate; POE (10) tridecyl ether phosphate
Trade names: Crodafos T10 Acid

Tridecyl behenate (INCI)
Synonyms: Docosanoic acid, tridecyl ester
Trade names: Trivent BE-13

Tridecyl erucate (INCI)
CAS 131154-74-0
Synonyms: 13-Docosenoic acid, tridecyl ester
Trade names: Pelemol TDE

Tridecyl isononanoate (INCI)
CAS 125804-18-4
Synonyms: 3,5,5-Trimethylhexanoic acid, tridecyl ester; Isononanoic acid, tridecyl ester
Trade names: Dermol 139

Tridecyl neopentanoate (INCI)
CAS 106436-39-9
Synonyms: Neopentanoic acid, tridecyl ester
Trade names: Ceraphyl® 55; Trivent NP-13

Tridecyl octanoate (INCI)
Synonyms: 2-Ethylhexanoic acid, tridecyl ester
Trade names: Dermol 138; Trivent OC-13

Tridecyl salicylate (INCI)
Synonyms: 2-Hydroxybenzoic acid, tridecyl ester
Trade names: BTN

Tridecyl stearate (INCI)
CAS 31556-45-3; EINECS 250-696-7
Synonyms: Octadecanoic acid, tridecyl ester
Trade names: Kemester® 5721; Liponate TDS
Trade names containing: Lipovol MOS-130; Lipovol MOS-350; Lipovol MOS-70

Tridecyl stearoyl stearate (INCI)
Trade names: Trivent SS-13

Tridecyl trimellitate (INCI)
CAS 70225-05-7
Synonyms: 1,2,4-Benzenetricarboxylic acid, branched tridecyl isodecyl esters
Trade names: Liponate TDTM
Trade names containing: Lipovol MOS-130; Lipovol MOS-350; Lipovol MOS-70

Triethanolamine (INCI)
CAS 102-71-6; EINECS 203-049-8
Synonyms: TEA; 2,2´,2´´-Nitrilotris(ethanol); Trolamine; Trihydroxytriethylamine
Trade names: Alkanolamine 144; Alkanolamine 244; Alkanolamine 244 Low Freeze Grade; TEA 85 Low Freeze Grade; TEA 99 Low Freeze Grade; TEA 99 Standard Grade; Trolamine 85 NF Grade; Trolamine 99 NF Grade; Unichem TEA
Trade names containing: Argobase L1; Grillocin® AT Basis; Grillocin® HY 77; Hydroviton 2/059353; TEA 85

Triethonium hydrolyzed collagen ethosulfate (INCI)
CAS 111174-64-2
Synonyms: Triethonium hydrolyzed animal protein ethosulfate
Trade names: Quat-Pro E
Trade names containing: Quinta-Pro Conc

Triethyl citrate (INCI)
CAS 77-93-0; EINECS 201-070-7
Synonyms: 2-Hydroxy-1,2,3-propanetricarboxylic acid, triethyl ester; Ethyl citrate
Trade names: Crodamol TC; Hydagen® C.A.T; TEC; Uniflex TEC

Trade names containing: Costausol; Hydagen® DEO; U-Dagen DEO; Vyox

Triethylene glycol (INCI. *See also PEG-3...*
CAS 112-27-6; EINECS 203-953-2
Synonyms: 2,2´-[1,2-Ethanediylbis(oxy)]bisethanol
Trade names containing: Unisuprol S-25

Trifluoromethyl C1-4 alkyl dimethicone (INCI)
Trade names: Gransil DM-100

Trifolium extract. *See Clover blossom extract*

Trigonella foenungraecum extract. *See Fenugreek extract*

Triheptanoin (INCI)
Synonyms: Glyceryl triheptanoate; Heptanoic acid, 1,2,3-propanetriyl ester; 1,2,3-Propanetriol triheptanoate
Trade names: Kessco GTM

Trihexadecylamine
CAS 67701-00-2
Trade names: Armeen® 3-16

1,2,4-Trihydroxybenzene (INCI)
CAS 533-73-3; EINECS 208-575-1
Synonyms: 1,2,4-Benzenetriol
Trade names: Imexine OAM

3,4,5-Trihydroxybenzoic acid. *See Gallic acid*

Trihydroxy methoxystearin (INCI)
Trade names: Cetiol® R

Trihydroxypalmitamidohydroxypropyl myristyl ether (INCI)
Trade names: Ceramide HO3

Trihydroxystearin (INCI)
CAS 8001-78-3; 139-44-6
Synonyms: Glyceryl tri(12-hydroxystearate); 12-Hydroxyoctadecanoic acid, 1,2,3-propanetriyl ester
Trade names: Flowtone R; Rol TR; Thixcin® R
Trade names containing: Cutina® BW; PCL SE w/o 2/066255; Unitina BW

Triisocetyl citrate (INCI)
Trade names: Citmol™ 316; Hetester TICC

Triisononanoin (INCI)
Synonyms: 1,2,3-Propanetriol triisononoate
Trade names: Isodragol 2/050300

Triisopropanolamine (INCI)
CAS 122-20-3; EINECS 204-528-4
Synonyms: TIPA; 1,1´,1´´-Nitrilotris-2-propanol; Tris(2-hydroxypropyl)amine
Trade names: TIPA 99; TIPA 101; TIPA Low Freeze Grade; Unichem TIPA

Triisostearin (INCI)
Synonyms: Glyceryl triisostearate; 1,2,3-Propenetriol triisooctadecanoate
Trade names: Prisorine GTIS 2041; Special Oil 619; Sun Espol G-318

Triisostearin PEG-6 esters (INCI)
Trade names: Labrafil® Isostearlque

Triisostearyl citrate (INCI)
CAS 113431-54-2
Synonyms: Citric acid, triisostearyl ester
Trade names: Schercemol TISC

Triisostearyl trilinoleate (INCI)
CAS 103213-22-5
Synonyms: Triisostearyl trimerate; Trimer acid, octadecyl triester; Triiosoctadecyl trimerate
Trade names: Schercemol TIST

Trilaneth-4 phosphate (INCI)
Synonyms: PEG-4 lanolin ether triphosphate

Trade names containing: Sedefos 75®

Trilaureth-8 citrate
Trade names: Eucarol T

Trilaureth-4 phosphate (INCI)
Trade names: Hostaphat KL 340N; Nikkol TLP-4

Trilaurin (INCI)
CAS 538-24-9; EINECS 208-687-0
Synonyms: Glyceryl trilaurate; Dodecanoic acid, 1,2,3-propanetriyl ester; 1,2,3-Propanetriol tridodecanoate
Trade names: Dynasan® 112; Lipo 320; Massa Estarinum® AM

Trilaurylamine (INCI)
CAS 102-87-4; EINECS 203-063-4
Synonyms: Trilauramine; Tridodecyl amine; N,N-Didodecyl-1-dodecanamine
Trade names: Armeen® 3-12

Trilauryl phosphate (INCI)
Synonyms: Phosphoric acid, trilauryl ester
Trade names: Marlophor® LN-Acid

Trilinoleic acid (INCI)
CAS 7049-66-3; 68939-90-6
Synonyms: Trimer acid; Fatty acids, C18, unsaturated, trimers; 9,12-Octadecadienoic acid, trimer
Trade names: Empol® 1045

Trilinolein (INCI)
CAS 537-40-6; EINECS 208-666-6
Synonyms: Glyceryl trilinoleate; 1,2,3-Propanetriol trilinoleate; 1,2,3-Propenetriol tri(9,12-octadecaienoate)
Trade names: Efaderma-F
Trade names containing: EFA-Glycerides; Lacol

Trilinolenin (INCI)
CAS 14465-68-0; EINECS 238-457-5
Synonyms: Glyceryl trilinolenate; 1,2,3-Propanetriyl linolenate; 1,2,3-Propanetriyl-9,12,15-octadecatrienoate
Trade names containing: EFA-Glycerides

Trimer acid. *See Trilinoleic acid*

N-(3-Trimethylammonio-2-hydroxypropyl) hydrolyzed silk
Trade names: Silkpro-Q

N-(3-Trimethylammonio-2-hydroxypropyl) hydrolyzed casein
Trade names: Milkpro-Q

Trimethyldodecatrieneol
Trade names: Nerolidol

Trimethyl dodecatrienol. *See Farnesol*

Trimethylglycine. *See Betaine*

Trimethylolethane
CAS 77-85-0
Synonyms: TME; Pentaglycerine; Methyltrimethylolmethane; 1,1,1-Tris(hydroxymethyl) ethane
Trade names containing: UV-Titan M210

Trimethylol propane tricaprate/caprylate
CAS 4826-87-3
Trade names: Lonzest® 153-S

Trimethylolpropane tricaprylate/tricaprate (INCI)
CAS 68956-08-1; 68130-52-9; EINECS 268-595-1
Synonyms: 2-Ethyl-2-[[(oxo-octyl/decyl)oxy]methyl]-1,3-propanediyl octanoate/decanoate; Trimethylolpropane tricaprylate/caprate
Trade names: Estamol TR 8-60

Trimethylolpropane triisostearate (CTFA)
CAS 68541-50-4; EINECS 271-347-5

Synonyms: 2-Ethyl-2-[[(Oxoisooctadecyl)oxy]methyl]-1,3-proapnediyl isooctadecanoate
Trade names: Nikkol Trialan 318; Salacos 6318

Trimethylolpropane trioctanoate (INCI)
CAS 4826-87-3; EINECS 225-404-6
Synonyms: 2-Ethyl-2-[[(oxo-2-ethylhexyl)oxy]methyl]-1,3-propanediyl 2-ethylhexanoate
Trade names: Nikkol Trialan 308

2,2,4-Trimethyl-1,3-pentanediol
CAS 144-19-4
Trade names: TMPD® Glycol

Trimethyl-1,3-pentanediol, 2,2,4- diisobutyrate
CAS 6846-50-0
Trade names: Kodaflex® TXIB

Trimethylpentanediol/isophthalic acid/trimellitic anhydride copolymer (INCI)
Trade names: Liporez NEP-Special

Trimethylpropane trioleate
CAS 68002-79-9; EINECS 268-093-2
Trade names: Radia® 7370

Trimethylsiloxysilicate (INCI)
Trade names containing: Dow Corning® 593 Fluid; Dow Corning® QF1-3593A; SS-4267

Trimethylsilylamodimethicone (INCI)
Trade names: Dow Corning® Q2-8220 Conditioning Additive
Trade names containing: Belsil ADM 6041 E; Dow Corning® 7224 Conditioning Agent; Dow Corning® Q2-7224 Conditioning Additive

Trimyristin (INCI)
CAS 555-45-3; EINECS 209-099-7
Synonyms: Glyceryl trimyristate; 1,2,3-Propanetriol tritetradecanoate; Myristin
Trade names: Dynasan® 114"anoin (INCI)
CAS 538-23-8; 7360-38-5; EINECS 230-896-0
Synonyms: Glyceryl tri(2-ethylhexanoate); Glyceryl trioctanoate
Trade names: Emalex O.T.G; Estol GTEH 3609; Nikkol Trifat S-308; Pelemol GTO; Trivent OC-G

Trioctyl citrate (CTFA)
CAS 7147-34-4; EINECS 230-457-3
Synonyms: 2-Hydroxy-1,2,3-propanetricarboxylic acid, tris(2-ethylhexyl) ester
Trade names: Bernel® Ester TOC; Estalan TC

Trioctyldodecyl borate (INCI)
Synonyms: Boric acid, trioctyldodecyl ester
Trade names: Guerbo

Trioctyldodecyl citrate (INCI)
CAS 126121-35-5
Synonyms: 2-Hydroxy-1,2,3-propanetricarboxylic acid, tris(2-octyldodecyl) ester
Trade names: CE-2000; Citmol 320; Pelemol TGC; Trimol CE 2000

Trioctyl trimellitate
CAS 3319-31-1
Synonyms: TOTM; Tri (2-ethylhexyl) trimellitate
Trade names: Kodaflex® TOTM

Triolein (INCI)
CAS 122-32-7; 67701-30-8; EINECS 204-534-7; 266-948-4
Synonyms: Glyceryl trioleate; Olein; 9-Octadecenoic acid, 1,2,3-propanetriyl ester
Trade names: Cithrol GTO; CPH-399-N; Emerest® 2423; Emery® 2423; Hodag GTO; Kemester® 1000; Radia® 7363; Witconol™ 2423

Trade names containing: EFA-Glycerides; Juniorlan 1664

Triolein PEG-6 esters (INCI)
Synonyms: Triolein PEG-6 complex
Trade names: Labrafil® M 2735 CS
Trade names containing: Arlenfil 4015; Calenfil 3646; Camofil 4064

Trioleth-8 phosphate (INCI)
Trade names: Hostaphat KO 380

Trioleyl phosphate (INCI)
Trade names: Hostaphat KO 300

Tripalmitin (INCI)
CAS 555-44-2; EINECS 209-098-1
Synonyms: Glyceryl tripalmitate; Palmitin; Hexadecanoic acid, 1,2,3-propanetriyl ester
Trade names: Dynasan® 116
Trade names containing: Precirol ATO 5

Tripropylene glycol citrate (INCI)
Trade names: Dodecalene

Tris (hydroxymethyl) aminomethane
CAS 77-86-1; EINECS 201-064-4
Synonyms: THAM; Tromethamine (INCI); 2-Amino-2-(hydroxymethyl)-1,3-propanediol; Tris Buffer
Trade names: Tris Amino®
Trade names containing: Omega-CH Activator

Tris (hydroxymethyl) nitromethane (INCI)
CAS 126-11-4; EINECS 204-769-5
Synonyms: (2-Hydroxymethyl) 2-nitro-1,3-propanediol; Trimethylolnitromethane; 2-Nitro-2-(hydroxymethyl)-1,3-propanediol
Trade names: Tris Nitro®

Trishydroxy nitromethane
Trade names containing: Midpol 2000

Trisodium EDTA (INCI)
CAS 150-38-9; EINECS 205-758-8
Synonyms: Edetate trisodium; Trisodium ethylene-diamine tetraacetate; Trisodium hydrogen ethylene diaminetetraacetate
Trade names: Hamp-Ene® Na₃T; Sequestrene® NA3; Universene Na3

Trisodium HEDTA (INCI)
CAS 139-89-9; EINECS 205-381-9
Synonyms: HEDTANa₃; N-[2-[Bis(carboxymethyl)amino] ethyl]-N-(2-hydroxyethyl)glycine, trisodium salt; Tri-sodium hydroxyethyl ethylenediaminetriacetate
Trade names: Chel DM-41; Hamp-Ol® 120; Hamp-Ol® Crystals; Versenol 120
Trade names containing: Kelene 77

Trisodium lauroampho PG-acetate phosphate chloride (INCI)
Trade names: Phosphoteric® QL38

Tristearin (INCI)
CAS 555-43-1; EINECS 209-097-6
Synonyms: Glyceryl tristearate; 1,2,3-Propanetriol trioctadecanoate; Octadecanoic acid, 1,2,3-propanetriyl ester
Trade names: Aldo® TS; Dynasan® 118
Trade names containing: Precirol ATO 5

Tristearyl citrate (INCI)
CAS 7775-50-0; EINECS 231-896-3
Synonyms: 2-Hydroxy-1,2,3-propanetricarboxylic acid, trioctadecyl este; Citric acid, triethyl ester; Citric acid, tributyl ester
Trade names: Crodamol TSC

Triticum aestivum extract. *See Wheat extract*

Triundecanoin (INCI)
CAS 13552-80-2; EINECS 236-935-8
Trade names: Captex® 8227; Dermol M-27

Trolamine. *See Triethanolamine*

Tromethamine (INCI). *See Tris (hydroxymethyl) amino-methane*

Tromethamine acrylates/acrylonitrogens copolymer (INCI)
Trade names: Hypan® SS500V

Tromethamine magnesium aluminum silicate (INCI)
Trade names: Veegum® PRO

DL-α-Tryptophan (INCI)
CAS 54-12-6; EINECS 200-194-9
Synonyms: Indole-α-aminopropionic acid; 1-α-Amino-3-indolepropionic acid
Trade names containing: Hair Complex 20/70n

TSPP. *See Tetrasodium pyrophosphate*

Turkey-red oil. *See Sulfated castor oil*

Tyrosine (INCI)
CAS 60-18-4 (L-); 556-03-6 (DL-α); 556-02-5 (D-); EINECS 200-460-4(L);209-113-1(DL);209-112-6(D)
Synonyms: β-p-Hydroxyphenylalanine; α-Amino-β-p-hydroxyphenylpropionic acid
Trade names: Chemodyne Tyrosine
Trade names containing: Omega-CH Activator; Unipertan P-24; Unipertan P-24

Ubiquinone
Trade names containing: Energisome

Udder extract (INCI)
Trade names containing: Epiderm-Complex W

Ultramarine blue. *See also Ultramarines*
CAS 1317-97-1
Trade names: Cogilor Aquamarine
Trade names containing: Florabeads Micro 28/60 Lapis; U Blue 104

Ultramarine pink. *See also Ultramarines*
CAS 977058-55-1
Trade names: Cogilor Rose
Trade names containing: U Pink 113

Ultramarines (INCI)
CAS 1317-97-1 (blue); 1345-00-2; 12769-96-9 (violet); EINECS 235-811-0; 215-711-3
Trade names: Bleu D'Outremer Special
Trade names containing: Bleu Covasop W 6776; Bleu Covasorb W 6783 A; Blue Covapate W 6763; Unispheres U-504

Ultramarine violet. *See also Ultramarines*
CAS 12769-96-9
Trade names: Cogilor Amethyst
Trade names containing: U Violet 109

γ-Undecalactone (INCI)
CAS 104-67-6; EINECS 203-225-4
Synonyms: 5-Heptyldihydro-2(3H)-furanone
Trade names: Aldehyde C 14 Soc. Peach (3/010811)

Undecyl alcohol (INCI)
CAS 112-42-5; EINECS 203-970-5
Synonyms: Alcohol, undecyl; C11 primary alcohol; Alcohols, C11
Trade names: Neodol® 1

Undecylenamide DEA (INCI)
CAS 25377-64-1; 60239-68-1; EINECS 246-914-5
Synonyms: Undecylenoyl diethanolamide; N,N-Bis(2-hydroxyethyl)undecenamide
Trade names: Fungicide DA 2/938070; Olamida UD;

Olamida UD 21; Undamide
Trade names containing: Rewocid® DU 185

Undecylenamide MEA (INCI)
CAS 20545-92-0; 25377-63-3; EINECS 243-870-9
Synonyms: Undecylenoyl monoethanolamide; N-(2-Hydroxyethyl)undecenamide
Trade names: Fungicide UMA 2/938080; Incromide UM; Rewocid® U 185; Witcamide® 6570

Undecylenamidopropyl betaine (INCI)
CAS 133798-12-6
Synonyms: N-(Carboxymethyl)-N,N-dimethyl-3-[(1-oxoundecylenyl)amino]-1-propanaminium hydroxide, inner salt; Bis(undecylenic amidopropyl dimethyl glycinate)
Trade names: Schercotaine UAB

Undecylenamidopropyl trimonium methosulfate (INCI)
Synonyms: Undecylenamidopropyl trimethylammonium methyl sulfate
Trade names: Rewocid® UTM 185

Undecylenic acid (INCI)
CAS 112-38-9; EINECS 203-965-8
Synonyms: 10-Undecenoic acid; Undecenoic acid; 11-Undecenoic acid
Trade names containing: Ivex® 10

Undecylenoyl collagen amino acids (INCI)
Synonyms: Undecylenoyl animal collagen amino acids
Trade names: Lipacide UCO

Undecylenoyl PEG-5 paraben (INCI)
Trade names containing: Undebenzofene

Undecylpentadecanol (INCI)
CAS 68444-33-7; 70693-05-9; EINECS 270-593-0
Synonyms: Isohexacosanol
Trade names: Exxal® 26

Urea (INCI)
CAS 57-13-6; EINECS 200-315-5
Synonyms: Carbamide; Carbonyldiamide
Trade names: Unichem UREA
Trade names containing: Antiphlogistic ARO; Aquaderm; Aqualizer EJ; Bovine Fibronectin Sol'n; Brookosome® U; Dermasome® U; Endomine NMF; Facteur Hydratant PH; Hydrocos; Hydroviton 2/059353; Hygroplex HHG; Lactil®; Sedaplant Richter; Unimoist U-125

Urea-D-glucuronic acid (INCI)
Trade names: Glucuron

Urea peroxide (INCI)
CAS 124-43-6; EINECS 204-701-4
Synonyms: Hydrogen peroxide carbamide; Urea hydrogen peroxide
Trade names: Unichem UREA-P

Uric acid (INCI)
CAS 69-93-2; EINECS 200-720-7
Synonyms: 2,6,8-Trihydroxypurine; 2,6,8-Trioxypurine; Lithic acid; Uric oxide
Trade names containing: FRS-Diffuser Microreservoir; Iniferine

Usnic acid (INCI)
CAS 125-46-2; EINECS 204-740-7
Synonyms: 2,6-Diacetyl-7,9-dihydroxy-8,9b-dimethyl-1,3(2H,9bH)-dibenzofurandione
Trade names: Phytoderm Complex U

VA/butyl maleate/isobornyl acrylate copolymer (INCI)
Synonyms: Vinyl acetate/butyl maleate/isobornyl acrylate copolymer
Trade names containing: Advantage CP; Advantage V

VA/crotonates copolymer (INCI)
CAS 25609-89-6
Synonyms: Vinyl acetate/crotonic acid copolymer; Vinyl acetate/crotonates copolymer; 2-Butenoic acid, polymer with ethenyl acetate
Trade names: Aristoflex A; Luviset® CA66; Resyn® 28-1310
Trade names containing: Aristoflex A/60% Sol'n

VA/crotonates/vinyl neodecanoate copolymer (INCI)
CAS 55353-21-4
Synonyms: Vinyl acetate/crotonic acid/vinyl neodecanoate copolymer
Trade names: Resyn® 28-2913; Resyn® 28-2930

VA/crotonates/vinyl propionate copolymer (INCI)
Synonyms: Vinyl acetate/crotonic acid/vinyl propionate copolymer
Trade names: Luviset® CAP

VA/isobutyl maleate/vinyl neodecanoate copolymer (INCI)
Synonyms: Vinyl acetate/isobutyl maleate/vinyl neodecanoate copolymer
Trade names: Polycare® 509

Valerian extract (INCI)
CAS 8057-49-6; EINECS 232-501-7
Trade names containing: Herbasol Sedative Complex

Valine
CAS 72-18-4 (L-form); 516-06-3 (DL-α); 640-68-6 (D-form); EINECS 200-773-6
Synonyms: α-Aminoisovaleric acid
Trade names containing: Omega-CH Activator

Vanillin (INCI)
CAS 121-33-5; EINECS 204-465-2
Synonyms: Benzaldehyde, 4-hydroxy-3-methoxy-; 4-Hydroxy-3-methoxybenzaldehyde
Trade names: Unisweet VAN

Vaseline
Trade names: Vaseline 335 G; Vaseline 7702; Vaseline 8332; Vaseline 10049 BL; Vaseline A

Vegetable amino acids
Trade names: Vegamino™ 30-SF

Vegetable oil (INCI)
CAS 68956-68-3; EINECS 273-313-5
Synonyms: Oils, vegetable
Trade names containing: Amphocerin® K; Lipovol A-S; Lipovol ALM-S; Lipovol P-S; Lipovol SES-S; Oxynex® L

Vicia faba extract. *See Faba bean extract*

Vinegar acid. *See Acetic acid*

Vinyl acetate.... *See VA...*

Vinyl caprolactam/PVP/dimethylaminoethyl methacrylate copolymer (INCI)
Synonyms: Vinylcaprolactam/vinyl pyrrolidone/dimethylaminoethyl methacrylate terpolymer
Trade names: Copolymer VC-713
Trade names containing: Gaffix® VC-713

Vinyldimethicone (INCI)
Synonyms: Dimethicone, vinyl functional
Trade names containing: Dow Corning® MDX-4-4210; Dow Corning® Q7-4840

Vinylpyrrolidone/vinyl imidazolinium methochloride copolymer. *See Polyquaternium-16*

Viola tricolor extract. *See Pansy extract*

Vitamin A. *See Retinol*

Vitamin A acetate. *See Retinyl acetate*

Vitamin A palmitate. *See Retinyl palmitate*

Vitamin B. *See Nicotinic acid*

Vitamin B₁. *See Thiamine HCl*

Vitamin B₂. *See Riboflavin*

Vitamin B₅. *See Pantothenic acid*

Vitamin B₆
Synonyms: Pyridoxine hydrochloride
Trade names: Pyridoxine Hydrochloride USP

Vitamin B₁₂. *See Cyanocobalamin*

Vitamin C. *See Ascorbic acid*

Vitamin D₃. *See Cholecalciferol*

Vitamin E. *See Tocopherol*

Vitamin E acetate. *See Tocopheryl acetate*

Vitamin F. *See Ethyl linoleate*

Vitamin K₃. *See Menadione*

Vitis vinifera extract. *See Grape extract*

Walnut extract (INCI)
CAS 84012-43-1
Synonyms: Juglans regia extract
Trade names containing: Crodarom Nut O

Walnut oil (INCI)
CAS 8024-09-7; 84604-00-2
Synonyms: Oils, walnut
Trade names: EmCon Walnut; Lipovol W

Walnut shell powder (INCI)
Trade names: Lipo WSF 35/60, 60/100
Trade names containing: Herbasol Extract Walnut Shell
Oil-Sol; Herbasol Extract Walnut Shell Water-Sol

Watercress extract (INCI)
CAS 84775-70-2
Synonyms: Nasturtium officinalis extract
Trade names containing: Blend For Greasy Hair HS 312;
Blend For Greasy Skin Imperfections HS 315;
Capilotonique HS 245; Emollient HS 238; Herbaliquid
Watercress Special; Nutriderme HS 210; Nutriderme
HS 243

Wheat amino acids (INCI)
Synonyms: Amino acids, wheat
Trade names: Hydrotriticum™ WAA

Wheat bran lipids (INCI)
Trade names: Biobranil 2/948100
Trade names containing: Biobranil Watersoluble 2/
012600; Hair-cure 2/011500

Wheat extract (INCI)
CAS 84012-44-2; EINECS 281-689-7
Synonyms: Triticum aestivum extract
Trade names containing: Actiphyte of Wheat

Wheat germ acid (INCI)
Trade names containing: Foam-Coll™ 5W

Wheat germamide DEA (INCI)
CAS 124046-39-5
Trade names: Incromide WGD; Schercomid SWG

Wheat germamide PEG-2
Trade names: Afmide™ WGA

Wheat germamidopropalkonium chloride (INCI)
CAS 124046-09-9
Trade names: Incroquat WG-85

Wheat germamidopropylamine oxide (INCI)
Synonyms: Wheat germ oil amides, N-[3-(dimethylamino)propyl]-, N-oxide; N-[3-(Dimethylamino) pro-
pyl] wheat germ oil amides, N-oxide

Trade names: Afamine™ WGO; Incromine Oxide WG;
Mackamine™ WGO; Mackanate™ WGO

Wheat germamidopropyl betaine (INCI)
CAS 133934-09-5
Synonyms: N-(Carboxymethyl)-N,N-dimethyl-3-[(1-
oxowheat germ alkyl)amino]-1-propanaminium
hyroxides, inner salts; Wheat germ oil amido betaine
Trade names: Afaine™ WGB; Incronam WG-30;
Mackam™ WGB; Schercotaine WOAB

Wheat germamidopropyl dimethylamine (INCI)
Synonyms: Dimethylaminopropyl wheat germamide
Trade names: Mackine™ 701

**Wheatgermamidopropyl dimethylamine hydrolyzed col-
lagen (INCI)**
Trade names containing: Mackpro™ FP

**Wheatgermamidopropyl dimethylamine hydrolyzed
wheat protein (INCI)**
Trade names: Afpro™ WWP; Mackpro™ WWP

Wheat germamidopropyl dimethylamine lactate (INCI)
CAS 124046-40-8
Synonyms: N-[3-(Dimethylamino)propyl] wheat
germamide lactate
Trade names: Afalene™ 716; Incromate WGL;
Mackalene™ 716

**Wheat germamidopropyldimonium hydroxypropyl hy-
drolyzed wheat protein (INCI)**
Trade names: Mackpro™ WLW

**Wheatgermamidopropyl ethyldimonium ethosulfate
(INCI)**
CAS 115340-80-2
Trade names: Schercoquat WOAS

**Wheat germamidopropyl silk hydroxypropyl dimonium
chloride**
Trade names: Afpro™ WLP

Wheat germamphodiacetate
Trade names: Afoteric™ 2W

Wheat germ extract (INCI)
CAS 84012-44-2; EINECS 281-689-7
Synonyms: Triticum aestivum germ extract
Trade names containing: Actiphyte of Wheat Germ; Blend
For Elderly Skins HS 296; Brookosome® Herbal;
Complex GT; Emollient HS 238; Granoliq. Wheat
Germ Extract, Water soluble; Kalokiros HS 263;
Kalokiros LS 663; Nutriderme HS 313; Nutriderme LS
613; Plant Ceramides; Regederme HS 330;
Regederme LS 630; Solarium HS 269; Solarium LS
669

Wheat germ glycerides (INCI)
CAS 68990-07-8; 8046-25-1
Synonyms: Wheat germ oil mono-, di-, and triglycerides;
Glycerides, wheat germ oil mono-, di- and tri-
Trade names: Vita-Cos; Wickenol® 535

Wheat germ oil (INCI)
CAS 8006-95-9
Synonyms: Oil of wheat germ; Triticum aestivum germ oil
Trade names: EmCon W; Lipovol WGO; Super Refined™
Wheat Germ Oil; Tri-Ol WG; Uniderm WGO; Wheat
Germ Oil; Wheat Germ Oil; Wheat Germ Oil CLR
Trade names containing: Cephalipin; Foam-Coll™ 5W;
L.C.R.E.; Mackadet™ WGS

Wheat germ oil unsaponifiables (INCI)
Trade names containing: Filagrinol

Wheat lipid epoxide
Trade names: Mackernium™ WLE

Whey protein (INCI)
CAS 84082-51-9
Trade names: Alacen; Alatal

White caustic. *See Sodium hydroxide*

White ginger extract (INCI)
Synonyms: Hawaiian white ginger extract; Hedycium coronarium koenig extract
Trade names containing: Awapuhi Extract

White lily extract (INCI)
CAS 84776-67-0
Synonyms: Lilium album extract; Lilium candidum extract
Trade names containing: Complex NR

White ozokerite wax. *See Ceresin*

White spirits. *See Mineral spirits*

Wild chamomile oil. *See Matricaria oil*

Wild marjoram extract (INCI)
Synonyms: Origanum vulgare extract
Trade names containing: Stimulant HS 285

Wild pansy extract
Trade names: CMI 800
Trade names containing: CMI 551

Wild thyme extract (INCI)
CAS 84776-98-7
Synonyms: Mother of thyme extract; Thymus serpyllum extract
Trade names containing: Herbalcomplex 2 Special; Herbasol 7 Herb Complex; Herbasol Alpine Herbs Complex; Herbasol Herbes de Provence Complex

Wilkinite. *See Bentonite*

Wintergreen extract (INCI)
CAS 90045-28-6; EINECS 289-888-0
Synonyms: Gaultheria procumbens extract
Trade names containing: Actiphyte of Wintergreen

Witch hazel distillate (INCI)
Trade names: Cremogen Hamamelis Dest. 1841 739022
Trade names containing: Cremogen M-I 739001

Witch hazel extract (INCI)
CAS 84696-19-5; 68916-39-2
Trade names: Hamamelitannin Conc. 250A; Hamamelitannin Conc. 250M; Unibotan Witch Hazel
Trade names containing: Actiphyte of Witch Hazel; Aftershave HS 292; Aftershave LS 692; Circulatory Blend HS 318; Coobato Hamamelis; Coobato Speciale; Cremogen Hamamelis 739008; Dragoplant Witch Hazel 2/034020; Ectrait Hamamelis LC 452; Extrapone Hamamelis Super 2/500010; Extrapone Witch Hazel 2/032893; Hamamelis Extract HS 2456 G; Hamamelis Liq.; Herbalcomplex 2 Special; Herbasol Complex D; Herbasol-Extract Hamemelis; Hydrumine Witchazel

Wood pulp, bleached. *See Cellulose*

Wool fat. *See Lanolin*

Xanthan gum (INCI)
CAS 11138-66-2; EINECS 234-394-2
Synonyms: Corn sugar gum; Xanthan
Trade names: Biozan; Gomme Xanthane; Kelgum CG; Keltrol CG; Keltrol CG 1000; Keltrol CG BT; Keltrol CG F; Keltrol CG GM; Keltrol CG RD; Keltrol CG SF; Keltrol CG T; Keltrol CG TF; Keltrol®; Keltrol® F; Merezan® 8; Merezan® 20; Rhodicare™ D; Rhodicare™ H; Rhodicare™ S; Rhodicare™ XC; Rhodigel®; Rhodigel® 23; Rhodigel® 200; Rhodigel® EZ; Rhodopol® SC; Unigum XAN; Xanthan XP

Trade names containing: Almondermin® LS; Ches® 500; Elespher® Almondermin; Rhodicare™ SC-225; Tektamer® 38 A.D.; Tektamer® 38 L.V.; Tensami 1/05; Tensami 10/06; Tensami 3/06; Tensami 4/07

Xanthophyll (INCI)
CAS 127-40-2; EINECS 204-840-0
Trade names: Fitoxantina

Yarrow extract (INCI)
CAS 84082-83-7
Synonyms: Achillea millefolium extract; Extract of yarrow; Milfoil extract
Trade names: Hydroplastidine Achillea
Trade names containing: Auxina Tricogena; Bio-Chelated Sauna-Derm I; Cremogen M-I 739001; Cremogen Yarrow 739017; Herbalcomplex 1 Special; Herbasol Complex A; Herbasol 7 Herb Complex; Herbasol Complex D; Herbasol-Extract Yarrow; Hexaplant Richter; Leniplex; Lipoplastidine Achillea; Sedaplant Richter

Yeast betaglucan (INCI)
Trade names containing: Brookosome® MSF

Yeast extract (INCI)
CAS 8013-01-2
Synonyms: Extract of yeast
Trade names: Cytoplasmine-2; Vitacell LS; Vitamin B Complex CLR; Yeast Extract SC
Trade names containing: Trichogen

Yogurt filtrate (INCI)
Trade names containing: FM Extract

Yucca glauca extract
Trade names: Yucca Glauca Extract Code 9030

Zea mays extract. *See Corn silk extract*

Zea mays oil. *See Corn oil*

Zedoary oil (INCI)
Trade names containing: Fitoestesina

Zeolite (INCI)
Trade names: Abscents 1000; Abscents 2000; Abscents 5000

Zinc acetylmethionate (INCI)
CAS 102868-96-2
Trade names: Exsymol Zinc Acetylmethionate; Exsyzinc

Zinc aspartate (INCI)
CAS 546-46-3; EINECS 208-901-2; 286-541-5
Synonyms: Aspartic acid, zinc salt
Trade names: Oligoidyne Zincum

Zinc chloride (INCI)
CAS 7646-85-7; EINECS 231-592-0
Trade names containing: Schercotaine CAB-Z

Zinc citrate (INCI)
CAS 546-46-3; EINECS 208-901-2; 286-541-5
Synonyms: Citric acid, zinc salt; 2-Hydroxy-1,2,3-propanetricarboxylic acid, zinc salt
Trade names containing: Arrectosina

Zinc gluconate (INCI)
CAS 4468-02-4
Trade names: Gluconal® ZN

Zinc glycinate
Trade names containing: Westchlor® A2Z 8106

Zinc hydrolyzed collagen (INCI)
Synonyms: Zinc hydrolyzed animal protein
Trade names: Collamoist ZN

Zinc oxide (INCI)
CAS 1314-13-2; EINECS 215-222-5

Synonyms: Chinese white; Zinc white; Flowers of zinc
Trade names: Finex-25; MZO-25; UFZO; Unichem ZO; USP-1; USP-2; Z-Cote®; Zinc Oxide USP 66
Trade names containing: Finex-25-020; Kalixide DPG; Silkall ZN

Zinc PCA (INCI)
CAS 15454-75-8
Synonyms: PCA, zinc salt
Trade names: Zincidone®

Zinc pentadecene tricarboxylate (INCI)
Trade names: Grilloderm L 60

Zinc phenolsulfonate (INCI)
CAS 127-82-2; EINECS 204-867-8
Synonyms: 4-Hydroxybenzenesulfonic acid (2:1); Zinc sulfocarbolate
Trade names: Unichem ZPS; Universal ZPS

Zinc pyrithione (INCI)
CAS 13463-41-7; EINECS 236-671-3
Synonyms: Bis[1-hydroxy-2(1H)-pyridinethinato-O,S]-(T-4) zinc; Zinc 2-pyridinethiol-1-oxide; Pyrithione zinc
Trade names: Atomergic Zinc Pyrithione; Zinc Omadine® 48% Disp; Zinc Omadine® Powd; Zink Pyrion

Zinc ricinoleate (INCI)
CAS 13040-19-2; EINECS 235-911-4
Synonyms: 12-Hydroxy-9-octadecenoic acid, zinc salt; 9-Octadecenoic acid, 12-hydroxy-, zinc salt
Trade names: Grillocin CW-90; Grillocin® PY 88 Pellets;

Grillocin® PY 88 Pulver/Powd; Grillocin® S 803/7; Grillocin S-803/12
Trade names containing: Grillocin AT Basis; Grillocin HY-77; Grillocin P-176; Grillocin WE-106; Grillocin® AT Basis; Grillocin® CW 90; Grillocin® HY 77; Grillocin® P 176

Zinc rosinate (INCI)
CAS 9010-69-9; EINECS 232-723-4
Synonyms: Resin acid, zinc salt; Zinc resinate
Trade names containing: Grillocin HY-77

Zinc stearate (INCI)
CAS 557-05-1; EINECS 209-151-9
Synonyms: Zinc octadecanoate; Octadecanoic acid, zinc salt
Trade names: Cecavon ZN 70; Cecavon ZN 71; Cecavon ZN 72; Cecavon ZN 73; Cecavon ZN 735; Radiastar® 1170; Synpro® Zinc Stearate USP; Unichem ZS; Witco® Zinc Stearate U.S.P.-D

Zinc undecylenate (INCI)
CAS 557-08-4; EINECS 209-155-0
Synonyms: 10-Undecenoic acid, zinc salt; Zinc undecenoate
Trade names: Undezin

Zinc yeast derivative (INCI)
Trade names: Biomin® Z/P/C

Zirconium dioxide (INCI)
CAS 1314-23-4
Trade names: Dascare Zirconia

Part IV
Manufacturers Directory

Manufacturers Directory

Aarhus Oliefabrik A/S
Postboks 50, Bruunsgade 27
DK-8100 Aarhus C
Denmark
Tel.: 86-12 60 00
Telefax: 86-18 38 39
Telex: 64341

Aceto Chemical Co., Inc.
1 Hollow Lane, Suite 201
Lake Success, NY 11042-1215
USA
Tel.: 516-627-6000
Telefax: 516-627-6093
Telex: FTCC 824609

Active Organics, Inc.
7715 Densmore Ave.
Van Nuys, CA 91406
USA
Tel.: 818-786-3310
Telefax: 818-786-3313

Advanced Polymer Systems, Inc.
3696 Haven Ave.
Redwood City, CA 94063
USA
Tel.: 415-366-2626
Telefax: 415-365-6490
Telex: 361-290 aps incud

Agro-Mar, Inc.
3901 N. Kings Hwy., Suite 15
Myrtle Beach, SC 29577
USA
Tel.: 803-449-2895
Telefax: 803-449-7967

Air Products and Chemicals, Inc.
7201 Hamilton Blvd.
Allentown, PA 18195
USA
Tel.: 215-481-4911; 800-345-3148
Telefax: 215-481-5900
Telex: 847416

Air Products Nederland B.V.
Herculesplein 359, PO Box 85075
NL 3508 AB Utrecht
The Netherlands
Tel.: 30-511828

Ajinomoto Co., Inc.
15-1, Kyobashi 1-chome
Chuo-ku
Tokyo, 104
Japan

Tel.: (03) 5250-8111
Telex: J22690

Ajinomoto USA, Inc.
Glenpointe Centre West, 500 Frank W. Burr Blvd.
Teaneck, NJ 07666-6894
USA
Tel.: 201-488-1212
Telefax: 201-488-6472
Telex: 275425 (AJNJ)

Akzo Chemicals Inc./Chemicals Div.
300 S. Riverside Plaza
Chicago, IL 60606
USA
Tel.: 312-906-7500; 800-257-8292
Telefax: 312-906-7680
Telex: 25-3233

Akzo Chemicals Ltd.
100 University Ave., Suite 906
Toronto, Ontario MSJ IV6
Canada

Akzo Chemie UK Ltd
1-5, Queens Road, Hersham
Walton-on-Thames
Surrey KT12 5NL
UK
Tel.: 0932-247891
Telefax: 0932-231204
Telex: 21997

Akzo Chemie
Postfach 100146, Kreuzauer Strasse 46
DW 5160 Duren-Niederau
Germany
Tel.: 02421-5951
Telefax: 02421-595380

Akzo Chemie BV
Div of Akzo NV
Postbus 975
Stationsstraat 48
3800 AZ Amerfoort
The Netherlands
Tel.: 33-643454
Telefax: 33-637448
Telex: 79276

Akzo België NV
Div of Akzo NV
Marnixlaan 13
B-1050 Bruxelles
Belgium
Tel.: 2-518 04 07
Telex: 22071 ORGABE B

Akzo Chemie GmbH
Div of Akzo NV
Postfach 100132
Phillippstrasse 27
W-5160 Düren
Germany
Tel.: 2421-492261
Telefax: 2421-492487
Telex: 833911

Akzo Chemie Italia SpA
Div of Akzo NV
Via E Vismara 80
I-20020 Arese
Italy
Tel.: 2-938 08 71
Telefax: 2-938 08 16
Telex: 332526

Akzo Japan Ltd.
Godo Kaikan Bldg., 3-27 Kioi-cho, Chiyoda-Ku
Tokyo, 102
Japan

Akzo Salt Co.
Abington Executive Park
Clarks Summit, PA 18411
USA
Tel.: 717-587-5131
Telefax: 717-586-6278
Telex: 756470

Alban Muller Int'l.
212, rue de Rosny
93100 Montreuil
France
Tel.: 1-48-58-30-25
Telefax: 1-48-58-03-71
Telex: 236030 F

Albright & Wilson Ltd., European Hdqtrs.
PO Box 3, 210-222 Hagley Rd. West, Oldbury, Warley
West Midlands B68 0NN
UK
Tel.: 21-429-4942
Telefax: 21-420-5151
Telex: 336291

Albright & Wilson Americas
PO Box 26229
Richmond, VA 23260-6229
USA
Tel.: 804-550-4300; 800-446-3700
Telefax: 804-550-4385

Albright & Wilson Am. (Canada)
2 Gibbs Rd.
Islington, Ontario M9B 1R1
Canada
Tel.: 416-234-7000; 800-268-2520
Telefax: 416-237-1064

Marchon France SA
BP 19, Han sur Meuse
F-55300, St Mihiel
France
Tel.: 29-91 7300
Telefax: 29-91 7399

Albright & Wilson (Australia) Ltd.
PO Box 20
Yarraville, Victoria
Australia
Tel.: 3-688-7777

Telefax: 3-688-7788

Albright & Wilson Ltd. Japan
No. 2 Okamotoya Bldg. 6 Fl.
1-24, Toranomon 1-chome, Minato-ku
Tokyo, 105
Japan
Tel.: (03) 3508-9461
Telefax: (03) 3591-0733

Alcoa Industrial Chemicals Div.
PO Box 300
Bauxite, AR 72011
USA
Tel.: 501-776-4981; 800-643-8771
Telefax: 501-776-4685
Telex: 536447

Allied Colloids Inc.
2301 Wilroy Rd.
PO Box 820
Suffolk, VA 23439-0820
USA
Tel.: 804-538-3700
Telefax: 804-538-0204

Allied Colloids Ltd
Div of Allied Colloids Group plc
PO Box 38, Low Moor, Bradford
West Yorkshire BD12 0JZ
UK
Tel.: 0274-671267
Telefax: 0274-606499
Telex: 51646

Allied-Signal Inc
PO Box 1053
Columbia Rd. & Park Ave.
Morristown, NJ 07960
USA
Tel.: 201-455-2000; 800-526-0717
Telefax: 201-455-3198
Telex: 136410

Allied-Signal Inc/A-C® Performance Additives
PO Box 2332R
101 Columbia Rd.
Morristown, NJ 07962-2332
USA
Tel.: 201-455-2145; 800-222-0094
Telefax: 201-455-6154
Telex: 990433

Allied Corp. Int'l. NV-SA
International House, Bickenhill Lane
Birmingham B37 7HQ
UK

**Allied-Signal Int'l. NV-SA/
A-C Performance Additives**
Haasrode Research Park
Grauwmeer
B-3001 Heverlee (Leuven)
Belgium
Tel.: 32-16-39 12 11
Telefax: 32-16-400-039
Telex: 26283 ALCHEM B

Alma Chimica S.R.L.
Va Scalabrini, 9/A
22073 Fino Mornasco Como
Italy
Tel.: (031) 928383

Aloecorp
910 Houston St., Suite 500
Fort Worth, TX 76102-6227
USA
Tel.: 800-458-ALOE
Telefax: 817-336-1507

Alzo Inc.
6 Gulfstream Blvd.
Matawan, NJ 07747
USA
Tel.: 908-254-1901
Telefax: 908-254-4423

Amerchol Corp.
PO Box 4051
136 Talmadge Rd.
Edison, NJ 08818-4051
USA
Tel.: 908-248-6000; 800-367-3534
Telefax: 908-287-4186
Telex: 833472

Amerchol, D.F. Anstead Ltd.
Victoria House, Radford Way
Bellericay
Essex CM12 0DE
UK
Tel.: 0277-630063
Telefax: 0277 631356
Telex: 851-99410 ANSTED G

Amerchol Europe
Havenstraat 86
B-1800 Vilvoorde
Belgium
Tel.: 2-252-4012
Telefax: 2-252-4909
Telex: 846-69105 AMRCHL B

American Casein Co.
109 Elbow Lane
Burlington, NJ 08016
USA
Tel.: 609-387-3130
Telefax: 609-387-7204

American Colloid Co.
Highway 212 West
PO Box 160
Belle Fourche, SD 57717
USA
Tel.: 605-892-2591; 800-535-1935
Telefax: 605-892-4880

American Cyanamid/Corporate Headquarters
One Cyanamid Plaza
Wayne, NJ 07470
USA
Tel.: 201-831-3339; 800-922-0187
Telefax: 201-831-2637

Cyanamid Canada Inc./Carbide Products Div.
88 McNabb St.
Markham, Ontario L3R 6E6
Canada
Tel.: 416-470-3600
Telefax: 416-470-3852
Telex: 06-966602

Cyanamid BV
Postbus 1523
NL 3000 BM Rotterdam
The Netherlands

Tel.: 010-4116340
Telefax: 010-4136788
Telex: 23554

American Ingredients Co.
14622 S. Lakeside Ave.
Dolton, IL 60419
USA
Tel.: 708-849-8590; 800-821-2250
Telefax: 816-561-0422

American Lecithin Co.   *See under Rhone-Poulenc*

American Maize Products Co./Amaizo
1100 Indianapolis Blvd.
Hammond, IN 46320-1094
USA
Tel.: 219-659-2000; 800-348-9896
Telefax: 219-473-6601

Amoco Chemical Co.
200 East Randolph Dr., Mail code 4106
Chicago, IL 60601
USA
Tel.: 800-621-4567
Telefax: 312-856-4151
Telex: 25-3731

Amoco Chemical (Europe) SA
Div of Amoco Corp
15, Rue Rothschild
CH-1211 Geneva 21
Switzerland
Tel.: 22-31-02-81
Telex: 422787

Amoco Performance Products, Japan Ltd.
10th Floor, Tonichi Bldg.
2-31 Roppongi 6-Chome, Mianto Ku
Tokyo, 106
Japan

Amoco Lubricants Business Unit
MC 1102, 200 East Randolph Dr.
Chicago, IL 60601
USA
Tel.: 312-856-4599

The Andersons
PO Box 119
Maumee, OH 43537
USA
Tel.: 419-893-5050; 800-537-3370
Telefax: 419-891-6539

Angus Chemical Co.
1500 E. Lake Cook Rd.
Buffalo Grove, IL 60089
USA
Tel.: 708-215-8600; 800-362-2580
Telefax: 708-215-8626
Telex: 275422 ANGUS UR

Angus Chemie GmbH
19, Moorgate St.
Rotherham, Yorkshire S60 2DA
UK
Tel.: 0709-377743
Telefax: 0709-370596
Telex: 547159 ANGUK G

Angus Chemie GmbH
Huyssenallee 5
W-4300 Essen 1,
Germany
Tel.: 201-233531
Telefax: 201-238661
Telex: 8571563 ANGE D

Angus Chemie GmbH
Le Bonaparte, Centre d'Affaires Paris-Nord
F-93153 Le Blanc Mesnil, Paris
France
Tel.: 1-48-65-73-40
Telefax: 1-48-65-73-20
Telex: ANGUS 232089 F

Angus Chemical (Singapore) Pte. Ltd.
Blk 265, Serangoon Central Dr., #04-263
1955
Singapore
Tel.: 382-4468
Telefax: 286-0739
Telex: RS 28521 ANGUS

Application Chemicals, Inc.
555 South Broad St.
Glen Rock, NJ 07452
USA
Tel.: 201-612-0897
Telefax: 201-670-7368

Apree, Inc.
11220 Grader St., Suite 800
Dallas, TX 75238
USA
Tel.: 214-341-4949
Telefax: 214-343-8850

Aqualon Co
A Hercules Inc Co
1313 North Market St.
Wilmington, DE 19899
USA
Tel.: 302-594-6000; 800-345-8104
Telefax: 302-594-6660
Telex: 4761123

Aqualon Canada Inc.
5407 Eglinton Ave. West, Suite 103
Etobicoke
Ontario M9C 5K6
Canada
Tel.: 416-620-5400

Aqualon (UK) Ltd.
Genesis Centre, Garrett Field, Birchwood
Warrington
Cheshire WA3 7BH
UK
Tel.: 925-830077

Aqualon GmbH
PO Box 130125, Paul Thomas Strasse 58
D-4000 Düsseldorf 13
Germany
Tel.: 0211-7491-0

Aqualon France
44, Ave. de Chatou
F-92508 Rueil Malmaison Cedex
France
Tel.: 1-4751-2919

Aquatec Quimica SA
Rua Sampaio Viana, 425
CEP 0400 Postal 4885
Sao Paulo
Brazil
Tel.: 011-884-4466 ext.329
Telefax: 11-884-0747
Telex: 1121312

Arco Chemical/Headquarters, Research & Engineering Center
3801 West Chester Pike
Newtown Sq., PA 19073
USA
Tel.: 215-359-2000; 800-345-0252

Arco Chemical Canada Inc.
100 Consilium Pl., Suite 306
Scarborough
Ontario M1H 3E3
Canada

Arco Chemical Europe Inc.
Bridge Ave., Maidenhead
Berkshire SL6 1YP
UK
Tel.: 628-775000

Arco Chemical Asia/Pacific Ltd.
Toranomon 37 Mori Bldg., 5th Floor
5-1 Toranomon 3-Chome, Minato-Ku
Tokyo, 105
Japan

Argeville SA
2, Place du Port
CH-1204 Geneva
Switzerland
Tel.: 022-312-1707
Telefax: 022-312-1789
Telex: 427-441 ALAC CH

Arista Industries, Inc.
1082 Post Rd.
Darien, CT 06820
USA
Tel.: 203-655-0881; 800-255-6457
Telefax: 203-655-0881
Telex: 996493

Arizona Chemical Co
Div. of International Paper
1001 E. Business Hwy. 98
Panama City, FL 32401
USA
Tel.: 904-785-6700; 800-526-5294
Telefax: 904-785-2203
Telex: 441695

Arol Chemical Products Co.
649 Ferry St.
Newark, NJ 07105
USA
Tel.: 201-344-1510
Telefax: 201-344-7127

Aruba Aloe Balm N.V.
Sabana Blanco 41
Aruba, Dutch Carib.
Tel.: 011/2978-31928
Telefax: 011/2978-26081

Asahi Denka Kogyo K.K.
Furukawa Bldg. 3-14, Nihonbashi Muro-machi 2-chome
Chuo-ku
Tokyo, 103
Japan
Tel.: (03) 5255-9017
Telefax: (03) 3270-2463
Telex: 222-2407 TOKADK

Assessa-Industria Comercio and Exportacao, Ltd.
Rua Cardoso Quintao, 110-CEP 21 381
Rio de Janeiro
Brazil
Tel.: 021-591-4345
Telex: 21-39602 SESX-BR

Astor Wax Corp.
200 Piedmont Ct.
Doraville, GA 30340
USA
Tel.: 404-448-8083
Telefax: 404-840-0954

Atlas Refinery, Inc.
142 Lockwood St.
Newark, NJ 07105
USA
Tel.: 201-589-2002
Telefax: 201-589-7377
Telex: 138-425 ATLASOIL

Atochem. *See Elf Atochem*

Atomergic Chemetals Corp.
222 Sherwood Ave.
Farmingdale, NY 11735-1718
USA
Tel.: 516-694-9000
Telefax: 516-694-9177
Telex: 6852289

Auschem SpA
Via Cavriana, 14
20134 Milano
Italy
Tel.: 0039-2-70140259
Telefax: 0039-2-70140201
Telex: 312093 AUSCHEM 1

Ausimont USA Inc.
44 Whippany Rd.
Morristown, NJ 07962-1838
USA
Tel.: 201-292-6250; 800-323-AUSI
Telefax: 201-292-0886

Aventura Industries, Inc.
PO Box 1966
Hallandale, FL 33008-1966
USA
Tel.: 305-456-6878
Telefax: 305-456-5167

Bärlocher GmbH, Otto
Riesstrasse 16
8000 München 50
Germany
Tel.: 089-1488-0
Telefax: 089-1488-312
Telex: 5215701

Barnet Products Corp.
560 Sylvan Ave.
Englewood Cliffs, NJ 07632
USA
Tel.: 201-569-6622
Telefax: 201-569-8847

BASF AG
ESA/WA-H 201
D-6700 Ludwigshafen
Germany
Tel.: 0621-60-99603
Telefax: 0621-60-41787
Telex: 469499-0 BAS D

BASF Corp.
100 Cherry Hill Rd.
Parsippany, NJ 07054
USA
Tel.: 201-316-3000; 800-669-BASF
Telefax: 201-397-2737

BASF Canada Ltd.
PO Box 430
Montreal, Quebec H4L 4V8
Canada

BASF plc
PO Box 4, Earl Road
Cheadle Hulme, Cheadle
Cheshire SK8 6QG
UK
Tel.: 061-485-6222
Telefax: 061-486-0891
Telex: 669211 BASFCH G

BASF Belgium S.A.
Ave. Hamoir-laan 14
B-1180 Brussels
Belgium

BASF S.A. Compagnie Francaise
MC-NT, 140, Rue Jules Guesde
92303 Levallois-Perret
France

BASF India, Ltd.
Maybaker House, S.K. Ahire Marg.
PO Box 19108
Bombay 400 025
India

BASF Japan Ltd.
3-3, Kioicho, Chiyoda-ku
Tokyo, 102
Japan
Tel.: (03) 3238-2300
Telex: 222-2130 BASFTK

Bayer AG
Bayerwerk
5090 Leverkusen
Germany
Tel.: (0214)30-1
Telefax: (0214)30 6 51 36
Telex: 85103-0 byd

Bayer plc
Bayer House, Strawberry Hill
Newbury, Berkshire RG13 1JA
UK
Tel.: 0635-39000
Telefax: 0635-563393
Telex: 847205 BAYNEW G

Bayer Antwerpen NV
Kanaaldok 1
B-2040 Antwerp 4
Belgium
Tel.: 3-540 30 11
Telefax: 3-541 69 36
Telex: 71175 BAYANT B

Bell Flavors & Fragrances, Inc.
500 Academy Dr.
Northbrook, IL
USA
Tel.: 708-291-8300; 800-323-4387
Telefax: 708-291-1217
Telex: 910-686-0653

Belmay, Inc.
200 Corporate Blvd. South
Yonkers, NY 10701
USA
Tel.: 914-376-1515
Telefax: 914-376-1784

Bernel Chemical Co., Inc.
174 Grand Ave.
Englewood, NJ 07631
USA
Tel.: 201-569-8934
Telefax: 201-569-1741

Berol Nobel AB
Box 11536
S-10061 Stockholm
Sweden
Tel.: 8-743-4000
Telefax: 8-644-3955
Telex: 10513 benobl s

Berol Nobel Inc.
Meritt 8 Corporate Park
99 Hawley Lane
Stratford, CT 06497
USA
Tel.: 203-378-0500
Telefax: 203-378-5960

Berol Nobel SA
Rue Gachard 88, Bte 9
B-1050 Bruxelles
Belgium
Tel.: 2-640-5065
Telefax: 2-640-6997
Telex: 62812

Bio-Botanica, Inc.
75 Commerce Dr.
Hauppauge, NY 11788
USA
Tel.: 516-231-5522; 800-645-5720
Telefax: 516-231-7332

Biodev
71 Ave. de Limoges
87270 Couzeix
France
Tel.: 55 36 47 70
Telefax: 55 36 48 37
Telex: F 580-915 A70

Bioiberica S.A.
Pligono Industrial de Palafolls
Ctra. N.II, Km. 680
08389 Palafolls, Barcelona
Spain

Tel.: 34/3 764 05 01
Telefax: 34/3764 02 86

Henley Chemicals, Inc., distributor
50 Chestnut Ridge Rd.
Montvale, NJ 07645
USA
Tel.: 201-307-0422; 800-635-3558
Telefax: 201-307-0424
Telex: 232210

Biomex France
B.P. 123-Les Algorithmes-Pythagore
Sophia Antipolis
06561 Valbonne Cedex
France
Tel.: 93/267091
Telex: 461 175

Biosil Technologies, Inc.
88 West Sheffield Ave.
Englewood, NJ 07631
USA
Tel.: 201-871-9797
Telefax: 201-871-3697

Blew Chemical Co.
PO Box 501
Palos Heights, IL 60463
USA
Tel.: 708-448-5780
Telefax: 708-448-5781

Boliden Intertrade Inc.
3400 Peachtree Rd. NE, Suite 401
Atlanta, GA 30326
USA
Tel.: 404-239-6700; 800-241-1912
Telefax: 404-239-6701
Telex: 981036

The Boots Co plc
D110 Main Office, Beeston, Nottingham
Nottinghamshire NG2 3AA
UK
Tel.: 0602 591 7642
Telefax: 0602 591 680

Boots Microcheck
Nottingham NG2 3AA
UK
Tel.: 0602-592584
Telefax: 0602-595508

Bretagne Chimie Fine SA
Div of Guyomarc'h, Diana Div
Boisel
F-56140 Pleucadeuc
France
Tel.: 97 26 91 21
Telefax: 97 26 90 46
Telex: 951084 BCFF

Brooks Industries Inc.
70 Tyler Place
South Plainfield, NJ 07080
USA
Tel.: 908-561-5200
Telefax: 908-561-9174

Buckman Labs Int'l., Inc.
1256 North McLean Blvd.
Memphis, TN 38108
USA

Tel.: 901-278-0330; 800-727-2772
Telex: 68-28020

Burlington Chemical Co., Inc.
PO Box 111
Burlington, NC 27216
USA
Tel.: 919-584-0111; 800-672-5888
Telefax: 919-584-3548
Telex: 9102502503

Cabot Corp./Cab-O-Sil Div.
PO Box 188
Tuscola, IL 61953
USA
Tel.: 217-253-3370; 800-222-6745
Telefax: 217-253-4334
Telex: 910-663-2542

Cabot GmbH/Cab-O-Sil Div.
PO Box 1766
D-7888 Rheinfelden
Germany
Tel.: 7623-9090
Telefax: 7623-90932
Telex: 773451

Calgene Chemical Inc
7247 North Central Park Ave.
Skokie, IL 60076-4093
USA
Tel.: 708-675-3950; 800-432-7187
Telefax: 708-675-3013
Telex: 72-4417

Calgon Corp.
PO Box 717
Pittsburgh, PA 15230-0717
USA
Tel.: 412-787-6700; 800-4-CARBON
Telefax: 4412-787-6713
Telex: 671183CCC

Carroll Co.
2900 W. Kingsley
Garland, TX 75041
USA
Tel.: 214-278-1304; 800-527-5722
Telefax: 214-840-0678

CasChem Inc.
40 Ave. A
Bayonne, NJ 07002
USA
Tel.: 201-858-7900; 800-CASCHEM
Telefax: 201-437-2728
Telex: 710-729-4466

Ceca SA
Div of Atochem
22, place de l'Iris, La Défense 2
Cedex 54
92062 Paris-La Défense
France
Tel.: 147-96-9090
Telefax: 147-96-9234
Telex: 611444 ckd

Celanese. *See under Hoechst-Celanese*

Celite Corp.
PO Box 519
Lompoc, CA 93438-0519
USA

Tel.: 805-735-7791
Telefax: 805-735-5699
Telex: 62776493 ESL UD

Celite Corp
9 rue du Colonel de Rochebrune
BP 240
F-92500 Rueil Malmaison
France
Tel.: 1-47 49 05 60
Telefax: 1-47 08 30 25
Telex: 631969 CELITE F

Central Soya Co., Inc./Chemurgy Div.
PO Box 2507
Fort Wayne, IN 46801-2507
USA
Tel.: 219-425-5432; 800-348-0960
Telefax: 219-425-5301
Telex: 49609682

Central Soya
PO Box 5063
3008 AB Rotterdam
Netherlands
Tel.: 10-42-39-600
Telefax: 10-42-30-897
Telex: 20041 CNSOY NL

C.E.P., Centre D'Etudes de Physiologie D'Hygeniene et de Cosmetologie
87 Ave. de l'Epinette, B.P. 560
77332 Meaux Cedex
France
Tel.: 1/64-33-17-71
Telefax: 1/60-25-25-31
Telex: 690446 F

CGI-Universal Flavors
Viale f.lli Casiraghi 508
20099 Sesto San Giovani, Milan
Italy
Tel.: 02/2627651
Telefax: 02/2620373
Telex: 311044 CURT I

Chemax, Inc.
PO Box 6067, Highway 25 South
Greenville, SC 29606
USA
Tel.: 803-277-7000; 800-334-6234
Telefax: 803-277-7807
Telex: 570412 IPM15SC

Chemie Linz GmbH
Div of Chemie Holding AG
St Peter-Strasse 25
A-4021 Linz
Austria
Tel.: 732-59160
Telefax: 732-5916155
Telex: 21324 LINZ A

Chemie Linz UK Ltd
Div of Chemie Linz GmbH
12 The Green, Richmond
Surrey TW9 1PX
UK
Tel.: 081-948 6966
Telefax: 081-332 2516
Telex: 924941

Chemie Linz North America, Inc
65 Challenger Rd
Ridgefield Park, NJ 07660
USA
Tel.: 201-641-6410
Telefax: 201-641-2323
Telex: 853211 Chemie Linz

Chemie Research & Manufacturing Co., Inc.
160 Concord Drive
PO Box 181279
Casselberry, FL 32718-1279
USA
Tel.: 407-831-4519
Telefax: 407-830-6037

Chemische Laboratorium Dr. Kurt Richter GmbH. *See under Richter*

ChemMark Development Inc.
70 Tyler Place
South Plainfield, NJ 07080
USA
Tel.: 908-561-5200
Telefax: 908-561-9174

Chemodyne S.A.
7 Ave. Krieg
CH-1208 Geneva
Switzerland
Tel.: 41/22/347 52 22
Telefax: 41/22/347 08 73
Telex: 423137 cdyn ch

Chemplex Chemicals, Inc.
201 Route 17 #300
Rutherford, NJ 07070
USA
Tel.: 201-935-8903
Telefax: 201-935-9051

Chemron Corp.
PO Box 2299
Paso Robles, CA 93447
USA
Tel.: 805-239-1550
Telefax: 805-239-8551

Chemsal Chemicals & Co. KG
Joint venture of Chem-Y GmbH and Salim
Kupferstrasse 1, PO Box 100262
D-4240 Emmerich 1
Germany
Tel.: 02822 711-0
Telefax: 02822 18294
Telex: 8125124

Chem-Y GmbH
Kupferstrasse 1
Postfach 10 02 62
D46446 Emmerich
Germany
Tel.: 2822/7110
Telefax: 2822/18294
Telex: 81251124 cyem

Chevron Chemical Co./Olefin & Derivs.
PO Box 3766
Houston, TX 77253
USA
Tel.: 713-754-2000; 800-231-3260
Telex: 762799

Chiba Flour Milling Co. Ltd.
17, Sinminato, Chiba-shi
Chiba-ken
Japan
Tel.: (472) 41-0111
Telefax: (472)47-8282

Chimex
16 rue Maurice-Berteaux
Le Thillay, 95500
Gonesse
France
Tel.: 39-88 00 55
Telefax: 39 88 28 08
Telex: 605784

Charles B. Chrystal Co. Inc.
30 Vesey St.
New York, NY 10007
USA
Tel.: 212-227-2151
Telefax: 212-233-7916
Telex: 420803 CBCC

Ciba-Geigy AG
CH-4002
Basel
Switzerland
Tel.: 061 223 1341
Telefax: 061 231 7422
Telex: 668083

Ciba-Geigy Corp.
444 Saw Mill River Rd.
Ardsley, NY 10502
USA
Tel.: 914-478-3131; 800-431-1874
Telefax: 914-478-3480

Ciba-Geigy Corp./Dyestuffs & Chemicals Div.
PO Box 18300
Greensboro, NC 27419
USA
Tel.: 919-632-2964; 800-334-9481
Telefax: 919-632-7008
Telex: 131411

Ciba-Geigy Marienberg GmbH
Div of Ciba-Geigy AG
Postfach 1253
D-6140 Bensheim 1
Germany
Tel.: 6254 79 0
Telefax: 6254 79505
Telex: 468141

Ciba-Geigy (Japan) Ltd.
10-66, Miyuki-cho
Takarazuka-shi
Hyogo, 665
Japan
Tel.: (0797) 74-2472
Telefax: (0797) 74-2472
Telex: 5645684 CIGYTZ J

Cimbar Performance Minerals
25 Old River Rd. S.E.
PO Box 250
Cartersville, GA 30120
USA
Tel.: 404-387-0319; 800-852-6868
Telefax: 404-386-6785

Clar S.A.R.L.
Domaine de Radinghem
Radinghem 62310 Fruges
France
Tel.: 33-21 41 40 62
Telefax: 33-21 03 74 19

Clark Chemical Inc.
25 Trammel St.
Marietta, GA 30064
USA
Tel.: 404-514-8909
Telefax: 404-514-8906

Clark Colors
Warner-Jenkinson Co Div of Universal Foods Corp
155 Helen St.
PO Box 705
South Planfield, NJ 07080
USA
Tel.: 201-757-4500
Telefax: 201-757-3170

Climax Fluids Additives
Div of Climax Performance
7666 West 63rd St.
Summit, IL 60501
USA
Tel.: 708-458-8450
Telefax: 708-458-0286

Clough Chemical Co., Ltd.
178 St. Pierre
PO Box 1017
St-Jean-sur-Richelieu
Quebec, J3B 7B5
Canada
Tel.: 514-346-6848; 800-363-9284
Telefax: 514-346-7263

Coatex
35 Rue Aper/Zi Lyon Nord
F 69730 Genay
France
Tel.: 33-72 008 20 00
Telefax: 33-72-08 20 30

Collaborative Labs
3 Technology Dr.
E. Setauket, NY 11733
Tel.: 516-689-0200
Telefax: 516-689-0205

Condea Chemie GmbH
Überseering 40
2000 Hamburg 60
Germany
Tel.: 40 6375-0
Telefax: 40 6375 3595
Telex: 215166 conh d

Condea Chimie Sarl
125 Rue de Saussure
B.P. 89-11
75813 Paris Cedex 17
France
Tel.: 01-47 662424
Telefax: 01-47662425
Telex: 650386 condea f

Condea Vista Japan Inc.
PO Box 110
Kasumigaseki Bldg., 25th Floor, Chiyoda-ku

Tokyo 110
Japan
Tel.: 3593-0611
Telefax: 3593-0615
Telex: J 29368 VISTACHM

Corn Products/Unit of CPC Int'l.
6500 Archer Rd.
Summit-Argo, IL 60501
USA
Tel.: 708-563-2400
Telefax: 708-563-6852
Telex: 708-563-6763

Cosmetochem USA, Inc.
Industrial West
Clifton, NJ 07012
USA
Tel.: 201-471-8301
Telefax: 201-471-3783
Telex: 642643

Costec, Inc.
PO Box 693
Palatine, IL 60013
USA
Tel.: 708-359-5713
Telefax: 708-359-5887

CPS Chemical Co Inc
PO Box 162
Old Bridge, NJ 08857
USA
Tel.: 908-727-3100
Telefax: 908-727-2260
Telex: 844532-CPSOLDB

Croda Chemicals Ltd
Div of Croda International plc
Cowick Hall, Snaith Goole
North Humberside DN14 9AA
UK
Tel.: 0405-8605551
Telefax: 0405-860205
Telex: 57601

Croda Surfactants Ltd.
Cowick Hall, Snaith, Goole
North Humberside DN14 9AA
UK
Tel.: 0405 860551
Telefax: 0405 860205
Telex: 57601

Croda Universal Ltd.
Div of Croda International plc
Cowick Hall, Snaith, Goole
North Humberside , DN14 9AA
UK
Tel.: 0405 860551
Telefax: 0405 860205
Telex: 57601

Croda Inc
7 Century Dr.
Parsippany, NJ 07054-4698
USA
Tel.: 201-644-4900
Telefax: 201-644-9222

Croda Canada Ltd.
78 Tisdale Ave.
Toronto, Ontario M4A 1Y7
Canada

Tel.: 416-751-3571
Telefax: 416-751-9611

Croda do Brazil Ltda
Rua Croda 230 Distrito Industrial
CEP 13.053
Campinas/SP-C.P. 1098
Brazil

Croda Italiana Srl
Via Grocco
N917 27036
Mortara (PV)
Italy

Croda Chemicals Group Pty. Ltd.
PO Box 1012
Richmond, North Victoria 3121
Australia

Croda Japan KK
Aceman Bldg.
1-10, Tokuicho 1-chome, Chuo-ku
Osaka 540
Japan
Tel.: (06) 942-1791
Telefax: (06) 942-1790
Telex: 5233117

Crompton & Knowles Corp./Dyes & Chems. Div.
PO Box 33188
Charlotte, NC 28233
USA
Tel.: 704-372-5890; 800-438-4122
Telefax: 704-372-1522

Crompton & Knowles Tertre SA
Div of Crompton & Knowles Corp
141 ave de la Reine
B-1210 Brussels
Belgium
Tel.: 2-216 2045
Telefax: 2-242 84 83
Telex: 24595 CKBR B

Crucible Chemical Co Inc
PO Box 6786, Donaldson Center
Greenville, SC 29606
USA
Tel.: 803-277-1284; 800-845-8873
Telefax: 803-299-1192

Crystal, Inc./H & S Chemical
A Huntington Company
970 E. Tipton St.
Huntington, IN 46750
USA
Tel.: 219-356-7073
Telefax: 219-356-6485

Dai-ichi Kogyo Seiyaku Co., Ltd.
New Kyoto Center Bldg.
614, Higashishiokoji-cho, Shimokyo-ku
Kyoto 600
Japan
Tel.: (075) 343-1181
Telefax: (075) 343-1421

Darling & Co.
1251 W. 46th St.
Chicago, IL 60609
USA
Tel.: 312-927-3000

Dasco
60 Sunfield Ave.
Annadale, NY 10312
USA
Tel.: 718-984-3600
Telefax: 718-984-5333
Telex: 275757 Dasco UR

Decorative Industries, Inc.
PO Box 138
Sloatsburg, NY 10974
USA
Tel.: 914-753-2796
Telefax: 914-753-5107

Degussa AG
Postfach 1345
D-6450 Hanau 1
Germany
Tel.: 6181-59-3983
Telefax: 6181-59-4309
Telex: 415200-25 dwd

Degussa Corp.
65 Challenger Rd.
Ridgefield Park, NJ 07660
USA
Tel.: 201-641-6100
Telefax: 201-807-3183
Telex: 221420 degus ur

Degussa Ltd
Div of Degussa AG
Winterton House
Winterton Way, Macclesfield
Cheshire SK11 0LP
UK
Tel.: 061-4866211
Telefax: 0625 502096

Jan Dekker BV
Postbus 10
NL-1520 AA Wormerveer
The Netherlands
Tel.: 75-2782 78
Telefax: 75-21 38 83
Telex: 19273

Desert King Jojoba Corp.
1550 E. Missouri Ave., Suite 201
Phoenix, AZ 85014
USA
Tel.: 602-263-8350
Telefax: 602-263-8276

Dexter Chemical Corp.
845 Edgewater Rd.
Bronx, NY 10474
USA
Tel.: 718-542-7700
Telefax: 718-991-7684
Telex: 127061

Dextran Products, Ltd.
Div of Polydex Pharmaceuticals
415-421 Comstock Rd.
Scarborough, Ontario MIL 2H5
Canada
Tel.: 416-755-2231
Telefax: 416-755-0334
Telex: 06-963599

DGF Stoess, Inc.
520 Speedwell Ave.
PO Box 226
Morris Plains, NJ 07950-0226
USA
Tel.: 201-540-1696
Telefax: 201-984-8031

The E.E. Dickinson Co.
PO Box 990
Railroad Ave.
Essex, CT 06426
USA
Tel.: 203-767-8261
Telefax: 203-767-0721

Dow Chemical U.S.A.
2020 W.H. Dow Center
Midland, MI 48674
USA
Tel.: 517-636-1000; 800-441-4DOW

Dow Chemical Co Ltd
Div of The Dow Chemical Co
Lakeside House, Stockley Park
Uxbridge, Middlesex UB10 1BE
UK
Tel.: 081-848-8688
Telefax: 081-848-5400
Telex: 934626

Dow Europe SA
Bachtobelstrasse 3
CH-8810 Horgen
Switzerland
Tel.: 1-728-2111
Telefax: 1-728-2935
Telex: 826940

Dow Chemical Pacific ltd.
39th Floor, Sun Hung Kai Centre
30 Harbour Rd., Wanchai, PO Box 711
Hong Kong

Dow Corning Corp.
2200 W. Salzburg Rd.
Midland, MI 48686-0994
USA
Tel.: 517-496-6000; 800-248-2481
Telefax: 517-496-5324
Telex: 227450

Dow Corning Ltd
Div of Dow Corning Corp
Kings Court, 185 Kings Rd
Reading, Berkshire RG1 4EX
UK
Tel.: 0736-507251
Telefax: 0736-575051

Dow Corning France SA
Div of Dow Corning Corp
Le Britannia A10, 20 Bid E Deruelle
69432 Lyon Cedex 03
France
Tel.: 78 60 51 48
Telefax: 78 62 78 98
Telex: 300537

Dow Corning Kabushiki Kaisha
507-1, Kishi Yamakita-cho
Ashigarakami-gun
Kanagawa 258-01
Japan

Tel.: (0465) 76-3108
Telefax: (0465) 75-1064

Dragoco Inc.
10 Gordon Dr.
Totowa, NJ 07512
USA
Tel.: 201-256-3850
Telefax: 201-256-6420
Telex: 130449

Dragoco Japan Ltd.
Kokusai Higashinihonbashi Bldg., 5F.,
7-2, Higashinihonbashi 2-chome, Chuo-ku
Tokyo 103
Japan
Tel.: (03) 3851-5120
Telefax: (03) 3851-5130
Telex: DRANP J 2524306

Drew Industrial Div., Ashland Chemical Inc.
One Drew Plaza
Boonton, NJ 07005
USA
Tel.: 201-263-7800; 800-526-1015 x7800
Telefax: 201-263-4483
Telex: DREWCHEMS BOON

DS Industries APS
Islands Brygge 24
DK-2300 Copenhagen S
Denmark
Tel.: 45/31546600
Telefax: 45/31577657
Telex: 31313 dasoy dk

Duphar BV. *See Solvay Duphar BV*

E.I. DuPont de Nemours & Co., Inc.
1007 Market St.
Wilmington, DE 19898
USA
Tel.: 302-774-7573; 800-441-7515
Telefax: 302-774-7573
Telex: 302-774-7573

DuPont Canada Inc.
Box 2200, Streetsville
Mississauga, Ontario L5M 2H3
Canada
Tel.: 416-821-5612

DuPont (UK) Ltd
Div of E I Du Pont de Nemours & Co
Wedgewood Way
Stevenage, Hertsfordshire SG1 4QN
UK
Tel.: 0438 734000
Telefax: 0438 734154
Telex: 825591 DUPONT G

DuPont de Nemours (France) S.A.
137 rue de L'Université
F-75334 Paris
France
Tel.: 45 50 65 50
Telefax: 47 53 09 65
Telex: 206772

DuPont Far East Inc.
Kowa Bldg. No. 2
11-39 Akasaka 1-Chome, Minato-Ku
Tokyo 107
Japan
Tel.: 585-5511

Eastern Color & Chemical Co.
35 Livingston St.
PO Box 6161
Providence, RI 02904
USA
Tel.: 401-331-9000
Telefax: 401-331-2155

Eastman Chemical Co.
PO Box 431
Kingsport, TN 37662
USA
Tel.: 615-229-2318; 800-EASTMAN
Telefax: 615-229-1196
Telex: 6715569

Eastman Chemical (UK) Ltd.
Hemel Hempstead, PO Box 66
Kodak House, Station Road
Herts HP1 1JU
UK
Tel.: 0442-241171
Telefax: 0442 241177
Telex: 826502

Eastman Chemical International AG
Hertizentrum 6
CH-6300 Zug 6
Switzerland
Tel.: 042 23 25 25
Telefax: 042 21 12 52
Telex: 868 824

Eastman Japan Ltd.
Nishi-Shinbashi Mitsui Bldg.
1-24-14 Nishi-Shinbashi, Minato-Ku
Tokyo 105
Japan

Efamol Ltd.
Efamol House, Woodbridge Meadows
Guildford, Surrey GU1 1BA
UK
Tel.: 483/57 80 60
Telefax: 483 50 66 82

Elf Atochem S.A.
4, cours Michelet
La Défense 10
F-92091 Paris Cedex 42
France
Tel.: 49-00-8080
Telefax: 49-00-7447
Telex: 611922 ATO F

Elf Atochem North America Inc.
Three Parkway
Philadelphia, PA 19102
USA
Tel.: 215-587-7000; 800-225-7788
Telefax: 215-587-7591

Elf Atochem Canada
PO Box 278
Oakville
Ontario L6J 5A3
Canada
Tel.: 416-827-9841
Telefax: 416-827-7913

Elf Atochem UK Ltd
Colthrop Lane, Thatcham, Newbury
Berkshire RG13 4LW
UK

Tel.: 0635-70000
Telefax: 0635-61212
Telex: 847689 ATOKEM G

Atochem Deutschland GmbH
Niederlassung Düsseldorf
Uerdiger Strasse 5, Postfach 30 01 52
D-4000 Düsseldorf 30
Germany
Tel.: 0211-4552-0
Telefax: 0211-14552-112
Telex: 8584682

Ellis & Everard Personal Care
D.F. Anstead
Radford House, Radford Way
Billericay, Essex
UK
Tel.: 0277 630063
Telefax: 2077 631356

Emulan Inc.
3726 Roosevelt Rd., PO Box 582
Kenosha, WI 53141
USA
Tel.: 414-654-0734
Telefax: 414-654-3410

Emulsion Systems Inc.
70 East Sunrise Hwy.
Valley Stream, NY 11581-1233
USA
Tel.: 516-825-3232; 800-ESI-CRYL
Telefax: 516-825-3233

Engelhard Corp./Performance Minerals Group
101 Wood Ave., CN 770
Iselin, NJ 08830-0770
USA
Tel.: 908-205-5000; 800-631-9505
Telefax: 908-205-6711
Telex: 219984 ENGL UR

Enterprise Chemical Corp.
4 Parkview Dr.
Dover, OH 44622
USA
Tel.: 216-343-8861
Telefax: 216-343-8853

Esperis SpA
Via Ambrogio Binda, 29
I-20143 Milan
Italy
Tel.: 2-891-22219-27-36
Telefax: 02-891-22257
Telex: 310-485

Ethox Chemicals, Inc.
PO Box 5094, Sta. B
Greenville, SC 29606
USA
Tel.: 803-277-1620
Telefax: 803-277-8981

Ethyl Corp.
451 Florida Blvd.
Baton Rouge, LA 70801
USA
Tel.: 504-388-7040; 800-535-3030
Telefax: 504-388-7686
Telex: 586441, 586431

Ethyl Canada, Inc.
350 Burnhamthorpe Rd. West
Suite 600
Mississauga, Ontario L5B 3JI
Canada
Tel.: 416-566-9222
Telefax: 416-566-99962

Ethyl SA
London Rd
Bracknell, Berkshire RG12 2UW
UK
Tel.: 0344 780378
Telefax: 0344 778360
Telex: 848291

Ethyl SA
523 Ave. Louise, Box 19
B-1050 Brussels
Belgium
Tel.: 2-642-4411
Telefax: 2-648-4336
Telex: 22549

Ethyl Japan
Christy Bldg. 2/F
1-22 Moto Azabu 3-Chome, Minato-Ku
Tokyo 106
Japan

Evans Chemetics. *See under W.R. Grace*

Expanchimie
77, Blvd de la Mission-Marchand
92400 Courbevoie
France
Tel.: 1/43 34 31 11
Telefax: 1/43 33 99 37
Telex: 620727 F

Exsymol
4 Ave. Prince Hereditaire Albert, Zone F-Bloc C
MC 98000
Monaco
Tel.: 93-30-13-08
Telefax: 93-50-43-47
Telex: 479625 MC

Biosil Technologies, Inc., distributor
88 West Sheffield Ave.
Englewood, NJ 07631
USA
Tel.: 201-871-9797
Telefax: 201-871-3697

Exxon Chemical Co.
PO Box 3272
Houston, TX 77253-3272
USA
Tel.: 713-870-6000; 800-526-0749
Telefax: 713-870-6661
Telex: 794588

Exxon Chemical Co./Application Chemicals Div., Tomah Products
1012 Terra Dr., PO Box 388
Milton, WI 53563
USA
Tel.: 608-868-6811; 800-441-0708
Telefax: 608-868-6810
Telex: 910-280-1401

Exxon Chemical Ltd
4600 Parkway, Solent Business Park
Whiteley, Fareham
Hampshire PO15 7AZ
UK
Tel.: 0489-884400
Telex: 47437

Exxon Chemical Holland BV
Div of Exxon Corp
's Gravelandse 298
NL-3125 BK Schiedam
The Netherlands
Tel.: 10-488 19 11
Telefax: 10-488 13 88
Telex: 22402 ECSCH NL

Exxon Chemical Belgium
Div of Exxon Corp
Vorstlaan 280
B-1160 Brussels
Belgium
Tel.: 2-674 41 11
Telefax: 2-674 41 29
Telex: 22364

Exxon Chemical Mediterranea SpA
Via Paleocapa 7
I-20121 Milano
Italy
Tel.: 2 88031
Telefax: 2 8803231
Telex: 311561 ESSOCH I

Exxon Chemical Japan Ltd.
TBS Kaikan Bldg.
3-3, Akasaka 5-Chome, Minato-Ku
Tokyo 107
Japan
Tel.: (03) 582-9243
Telex: 22846

Fabriquimica S.R.L.
Calle 32 No. 3313
San Martin 1650
Argentina
Tel.: 1-755-7290
Telefax: 54-1-755-7290

The Fanning Corp.
1775 W. Diversity Pkwy.
Chicago, IL 60614-1009
USA
Tel.: 312-248-5700
Telefax: 312-248-6810
Telex: 910-221-1335

Fanwood
219 Martine Ave. North
PO Box 159
Fanwood, NJ 07023
USA
Tel.: 201-322-8440

Fina Chemicals
Div of Petrofina SA
Nijverheldsstraat
52 Rue de l'Industrie
B-1040 Brussels
Belgium
Tel.: 2-288-9111
Telefax: 32-2-288-3388
Telex: 21 556 PFINA B

Fina Oil and Chemical Co.
8350 North Central Expressway
PO Box 2159
Dallas, TX 75221
USA
Tel.: 214-750-2400; 800-344-FINA

Finetex Inc.
418 Falmouth Ave.
PO Box 216
Elmwood Park, NJ 07407
USA
Tel.: 201-797-4686
Telefax: 201-797-6558
Telex: 710-988-2239

Firmenich, Inc.
PO Box 5880
Princeton, NJ 08543-5880
USA
Tel.: 609-452-1000; 800-257-9591
Telefax: 609-921-0719
Telex: 21-99-15

Firmenich SA
PO Box 239
CH-1211 Geneva 8
Switzerland
Tel.: 22-42 42 00
Telefax: 22-43 73 22
Telex: 423181 FICO CH

Florida Food Prods., Inc./Aloe Div.
2231 W. Hwy. 44
PO Box 1300
Eustis, FL 32727-1300
USA
Tel.: 904-357-4141; 800-874-2331
Telefax: 904-483-3192

Fluka Chemical Corp
980 South Second St.
Ronkonkoma, NY 11779
USA
Tel.: 516-467-0980; 800-FLUKA-US
Telefax: 800-441-8841
Telex: 96-7807

Fluka Chemicals Ltd
Peakdale Rd
Glossop, Derbyshire SK13 9XE
UK
Tel.: 0457 862518
Telex: 669960

Fluka Sarl
BP 1114
68052 Mulhouse Cedex
France
Tel.: 89 61 87 47
Telex: 881236 F

Fluka Chemie AG
Industriestrasse 25
CH-9470 Buchs
Switzerland
Tel.: 41/85 69511
Telefax: 41/85 654459
Telex: 855 282

FMC Corp./Chemical Products Group
1735 Market St.
Philadelphia, PA 19103
USA

Tel.: 215-299-6000; 800-346-5101
Telefax: 215-299-6291
Telex: 685-1326

Fractal Laboratories, Inc.
6 Bayview Ave.
Northport, NY 11768
USA
Tel.: 516-261-9800
Telefax: 516-261-9802

Freeman Chemical Corp.
217 Freeman Dr.
Port Washington, WI 53074
USA
Tel.: 414-284-5541

Gattefosse SA
36 Chemin de Genas, BP 603
F 69804 Saint Priest
France
Tel.: 72 22 98 00
Telefax: 78 90 45 67
Telex: 340 240 F

Gattefosse Corp.
189 Kinderkamack Rd.
Westwood, NJ 07675
USA
Tel.: 201-573-1700
Telefax: 201-573-9671

General Electric Co./Silicone Products Div.
260 Hudson River Rd.
Waterford, NY 12188
USA
Tel.: 518-237-3330; 800-255-8886
Telefax: 518-233-3931

GE Silicones
Old Hall Rd, Sale
Cheshire M33 2HG
UK
Tel.: 061-905 5000
Telefax: 061-905 5022

GE Silicones Europe
Postbus 117
Plasticslaan 1
NL-4600 AC Bergen op Zoom
The Netherlands
Tel.: 1640-32291
Telefax: 1640-32708
Telex: 78421

Genesee Polymers Corp.
G-5251 Fenton Rd., PO Box 7047
Flint, MI 48507-0047
USA
Tel.: 313-238-4966
Telefax: 313-767-3016

Genstar Stone Products Co.
Executive Plaza IV
11350 McCormick Rd.
Hunt Valley, MD 21031
USA
Tel.: 301-527-4000
Telefax: 301-527-4535

Genzyme Fine Chemicals
Hollands Rd., Haverhill
Suffolk CB9 8PU
UK

Tel.: 0440 703522
Telefax: 0440 707783
Telex: 81333 GENFIN

Lipo Chemicals Inc., distributor
207 19th Ave.
Paterson, NJ 07504
USA
Tel.: 201-345-8600

Girindus Chemie GmbH & Co. KG
Buchenallee 20
PO Box 100 259
D-51402 Bergisch
Germany
Tel.: 0-2204-6-30-52
Telefax: 0-2204-6-34-14
Telex: 8874555 GIR D

Giulini Corp.
105 East Union Ave.
Bound Brook, NJ 08805
USA
Tel.: 908-469-6504
Telefax: 908-469-8418
Telex: 700179

Givaudan-Roure Corp.
100 Delawanna Ave.
Clifton, NJ 07015
USA
Tel.: 201-365-8000
Telefax: 201-777-9304
Telex: 219259 givc ur

Givaudan-Roure SA
5 Chemin de la Perfumiere
CH-1214 Vernier-Geneva
Switzerland
Tel.: 22-780 91 11
Telefax: 22-780 91 50

Global United Industries, Inc.
13609 Industrial Rd., Suite 117
Houston, TX 77015
USA
Tel.: 713-453-2400
Telefax: 713-451-5005
Telex: 798465

Th. Goldschmidt AG
Goldschmidtstrasse 100, Postfach 101461
D-4300 Essen 1
Germany
Tel.: 0201-173-2947
Telefax: 201-173-2160
Telex: 857170

Goldschmidt Chemical Corp.
914 E. Randolph Rd., PO Box 1299
Hopewell, VA 23860
USA
Tel.: 804-541-8658; 800-446-1809
Telefax: 804-541-2783
Telex: 710-958-1350

Goldschmidt Ltd
Tego House, Victoria Road
Ruislip, Middlesex HA4 0YL
UK
Tel.: 081-422 7788
Telefax: 081-864 8159
Telex: 923146

Goldschmidt Japan KK, Th.
Rm. 1113, Shuwa Kioi-cho TBR Bldg. No. 7
5-Chome, Koji-machi, Chiyoda-ku
Tokyo 102
Japan

Goo Chemical Industries Co., Ltd.
Ijiri-58, Iseda-Cho, Uji-shi
Kyoto
Japan
Tel.: 0774-46-7777
Telefax: 0774-43-3552
Telex: 5453-643 GOOJ

BFGoodrich Co./Specialty Polymers & Chem. Div.
9921 Brecksville Rd.
Brecksville, OH 44141
USA
Tel.: 216-447-5000; 800-331-1144
Telefax: 216-447-5720
Telex: 4996831

BFGoodrich (UK) Ltd
The Lawn, 100 Lampton Road
Hounslow, Middlesex TW3 4EB
UK
Tel.: 081-570 4700
Telefax: 081-570 0850

BFGoodrich Canada
195 Columbia St. West
Waterloo, Ontario N2J 4N9
Canada

BFGoodrich Chemical (Deutschland) GmbH
Goerlitzer Str. 1
4040 Neuss 1
Germany

W.R. Grace/Organic Chemicals Div.
55 Hayden Ave.
Lexington, MA 02173
USA
Tel.: 617-861-6600; 800-232-6100
Telefax: 617-862-3869
Telex: 200076

W.R. Grace Ltd
Northdale House, North Circular Road
London NW10 7UH
UK
Tel.: 081-965-0611
Telex: 25139

Evans Chemetics Div.
55 Hayden Ave.
Lexington, MA 02173
USA
Tel.: 617-861-6600 x2331
Telefax: 617-862-3869
Telex: 200076 GRLX UR

Evans Chemetics
Griffin Lane, Aylesbury
Bucks HP19 3BP
UK
Tel.: 0296 84877
Telefax: 0296 393122

Graden Chemical Co., Inc.
426 Bryan St.
Havertown, PA 19083
USA
Tel.: 215-449-3808

Grain Processing Corp.
1600 Oregon St.
Muscatine, IA 52761
USA
Tel.: 319-264-4265
Telefax: 319-264-4289
Telex: 46-8497

Grant Industries Inc.
PO Box 360, 125 Main St.
Elmwood Park, NJ 07407
USA
Tel.: 201-791-6700
Telefax: 201-791-0038

Grau Aromatics GmbH & Co. KG
Bismarckstrasse 4
D-707 Schwabisch Gmünd
Germany
Tel.: 07171/63094
Telefax: 07171/68140
Telex: 7248807

J. Manheimer, U.S. distributor
47-22 Pearson Pl.
Long Island City, NY 11101
Tel.: 212-392-7800

R.W. Greeff & Co Inc
777 West Putnam Ave
Greenwich, CT 06830
USA
Tel.: 203-532-2900
Telefax: 203-532-2980
Telex: 996609

Grillo-Werke AG
Sparte Chemie, Postfach 11 02 65
Weseler Strasse 1
D-4100 Duisburg 11
Germany
Tel.: 02 03/55 57-332
Telefax: 02 03/55 57-473
Telex: 8 551 525 gllo d

R.I.T.A., U.S. distributor
1725 Kilkenny Court
PO Box 585
Woodstock, IL 60098
USA
Tel.: 815-337-2500; 800-426-7759
Telefax: 815-337-2522
Telex: 72-2438

Grindsted Products A/S
Edwin Rahrs Vej 38
DK-8220 Brabrand
Denmark
Tel.: 06-25-3366
Telefax: 06-25-1077
Telex: 64177

Grindsted Products Inc.
201 Industrial Pkwy., PO Box 26
Industrial Airport, KS 66031
USA
Tel.: 913-764-8100; 800-255-6837
Telefax: 913-764-5407
Telex: 4-37295

Grindsted do Brazil
Ind. Ecom Ltda., Rodovia Regisé Bitten Court
KM 275, 5 Cx. Postal 172
06800 Embú S.P.
Brazil

Grindsted Products Ltd.
Northern Way, Bury St. Edmunds
Suffolk IP32 6NP
UK
Tel.: 284769631

Grindstedvaerket GmbH
Roberts-Bosch Strabe
D-2085 Quickborn, Deutschland
Germany

Grinsted France S.A.R.L.
Parc D'Activités de Tissaloup
Ave. Jean D'Alembert
F-78190 Trappes
France

Grünau, Chemische Fabrick Grünau GmbH
A Henkel Group Co.
Robert-Hansen Str. 1, Postfach 1063
W-7918 Illertissen, Bavaria
Germany
Tel.: (07303)13-0
Telefax: (07303)13206
Telex: 719114 gruea-d

Guardian Laboratories
Div. of United-Guardian, Inc
PO Box 2500
Smithtown, NY 11787
USA
Tel.: 516-273-0900; 800-645-5566
Telefax: 516-273-0858
Telex: 497-4275 GCCHAVP

Haarmann & Reimer GmbH
Postfach 1253
D-3450 Holzminden
Germany
Tel.: 0 55 31/7011
Telefax: 055 31/7016 49
Telex: 965 330

Haarmann & Reimer Corp.
PO Box 175
70 Diamond Road
Springfield, NJ 07081
USA
Tel.: 201-467-5600; 800-422-1559
Telefax: 201-912-0499
Telex: 219134 HAR UR

Haarmann & Reimer Ltd
Fieldhouse Lane
Marlow, Buckinghamshire SL7 1NA
UK
Tel.: 0628 472051
Telefax: 06288 472238
Telex: 848 859

C P Hall Co.
7300 South Central Ave.
Chicago, IL 60638-0428
USA
Tel.: 708-594-6000; 800-321-8242
Telefax: 708-458-0428

Haltermann GmbH
Ferdinand Strasse 55-57
D-2000 Hamburg 1
Germany
Tel.: 040-3338280
Telefax: 040 3338214
Telex: 2165425 jhlt d

Hampshire Chemical Corp.
55 Hayden Ave.
Lexington, MA 02173
USA
Tel.: 617-861-9700
Telefax: 617-861-0135
Telex: 200076 GRLX UR

Harcros Chemicals UK Ltd./Specialty Chemicals Div.
Lankro House
PO Box 1, Eccles
Manchester M30 0BH
UK
Tel.: 061-789-7300
Telefax: 061-788-7886
Telex: 667725

Harcros Chemicals Inc.
5200 Speaker Rd., PO Box 2930
Kansas City, KS 66106-1095
USA
Tel.: 913-321-3131
Telefax: 913-621-7718
Telex: 477266

Harcros Chemicals France Sarl
BP 40, 441220 St. Laurent
Nouan
France

Harcros Chemicals BV
Haagen House, PO Box 44
6040 AA Roermond
The Netherlands
Tel.: 04750-9-1777
Telefax: 04750-1-7489

Harcros Chemicals Scandia ApS
Vesterbrogade 14A
1620 Copenhagen V
Denmark
Tel.: 31 21 42 00
Telefax: 31 21 42 27
Telex: 16 152 LANKRO DK

Hart Chemicals Ltd.
256 Victoria Rd. South
Guelph, Ontario N1H 6K8
Canada
Tel.: 519-824-3280
Telefax: 519-824-0755
Telex: 06956537

Hart Products Corp.
173 Sussex St.
Jersey City, NJ 07302
USA
Tel.: 201-433-6632

Hefti Ltd. Chemical Products
PO Box 1623
CH-8048 Zurich
Switzerland
Tel.: 01-432-1340
Telefax: 01-432-2940
Telex: 822225 hexa ch

Henkel Corp./Cospha
300 Brookside Ave.
Ambler, PA 19002
USA
Tel.: 215-628-1476; 800-531-0815 (sales)
Telefax: 215-628-1450

Henkel Corp./Functional Products
300 Brookside Ave.
Ambler, PA 19002
USA
Tel.: 215-628-1466; 800-654-7588
Telefax: 215-628-1155

Henkel Corp./Organic Products Div.
300 Brookside Ave.
Ambler, PA 19022
USA
Tel.: 215-628-1000; 800-922-0605
Telefax: 215-628-1200
Telex: 6851092

Henkel Corp./Textile Chemicals
11709 Fruehauf Dr.
Charlotte, NC 28273-6507
USA
Tel.: 800-634-2436
Telefax: 704-587-3804

Henkel Canada Ltd.
2290 Argentia Rd.
Mississauga, Ontario L5N 6H9
Canada
Tel.: 416-542-7550
Telefax: 416-542-7588

Henkel Ltd
Div of Henkel KG
Henkel House
292-308 Southbury Road
Enfield, Middlesex
EN1 1TS
UK
Tel.: 081-804 3343
Telefax: 081-805 0398
Telex: 922708 HENKEL G

Henkel KGaA/Cospha
Postfach 101100
D-40191, Düsseldorf
Germany
Tel.: 0211-797-1
Telefax: 0211-798-7696
Telex: 085817-0

Henkel France SA
Div of Henkel KG
BP 309
150 rue Gallieni
F-92102 Boulogne Billancourt
France
Tel.: 46 84 90 00
Telefax: 46 84 90 90
Telex: 633177 HENKEL F

Henkel-Nopco SA/Process Chem. Div.
185 Ave. de Fontainebleau, 77310 St. Fargeau
Ponthierry
France
Tel.: 60-65-9090
Telefax: 60-65-7880
Telex: 692027

Henkel Belgium NV
Div of Henkel KG
66 ave du Port
B-1210 Brussels
Belgium
Tel.: 2-423 17 11
Telefax: 2-428 34 67
Telex: 21294 HENKEL B

Henkel Corp./Emery Group
11501 Northlake Dr.
Cincinnati, OH 45249
USA
Tel.: 513-530-7300; 800-543-7370
Telefax: 513-530-7581
Telex: 4333016

Henkel Corp./Emery Group/OPG
3300 Westinghouse Blvd.
Charlotte, NC 28217
USA
Tel.: 800-634-2436

Henley Chemicals, Inc.
Div of Boehringer Ingelheim
50 Chestnut Ridge Rd.
Montvale, NJ 07645
USA
Tel.: 201-307-0422; 800-635-3558
Telefax: 201-307-0424
Telex: 232210

Henningsen Foods, Inc.
2 Corporate Park Drive
White Plains, NY 10604
USA
Tel.: 914-694-1000
Telefax: 914-694-1221
Telex: 221819 Heno UR

Hercules Inc.
Hercules Plaza-6205SW
Wilmington, DE 19894
USA
Tel.: 302-594-6500; 800-247-4372
Telefax: 302-594-5400
Telex: 835-479

Hercules Ltd
Div of Hercules Inc
31 London Road
Reigate, Surrey RH2 9YA
UK
Tel.: 0737-242434
Telefax: 0737-224288
Telex: 25803

Hercules BV
8 Veraartlaan, PO Box 5822
2280 HV Rijswijk
The Netherlands
Tel.: 070-150-000
Telex: 31172

Hercules Inc./PFW Aroma Chemicals
33 Sprague Ave.
Middletown, NY 10940
USA
Tel.: 914-343-1000
Telefax: 914-343-8794
Telex: 283303

Herstellung von Naturextrakten GmbH
Strassburg 16
6948 Wald-Michelbach
Tel.: (06207) 7007
Telefax: (06207) 1276

Lipo Chemicals Inc., distributor
207 19th Ave.
Paterson, NJ 07504
USA
Tel.: 201-345-8600

Heterene Chemical Co., Inc.
PO Box 247
795 Vreeland Ave.
Paterson, NJ 07543
USA
Tel.: 201-278-2000
Telefax: 201-278-7512
Telex: 883358

Hickson Danchem Corp.
1975 Richmond Blvd.
Danville, VA 24540
USA
Tel.: 804-797-8105
Telefax: 804-799-2814
Telex: 940103 WU PUBTLXBSN

Hickson Manro Ltd.
Bridge St., Stalybridge
Cheshire SK15 1PH
UK
Tel.: 061-338-5511
Telefax: 061-303-2991
Telex: 668442

Hilton Davis Chemical Co.
2235 Langdon Farm Rd.
Cincinnati, OH 45237
USA
Tel.: 513-841-4000; 800-477-1022
Telefax: 800-477-4565

Hispano Quimica s.a.
P° Zona Franca 61-67
08004 Barcelona
Spain

Centerchem Inc., distributor
225 High Ridge Rd.
Stamford, CT 06905
USA
Tel.: 203-975-9800
Telefax: 203-975-8777

HK Color Group
Warner-Jenkinson Co
155 Helen St.
South Plainfield, NJ 07080-1301
USA
Tel.: 201-769-1122
Telefax: 201-757-3170

Hoechst Celanese/Int'l. Headqtrs.
26 Main St.
Chatham, NJ 07928
USA
Tel.: 201-635-2600; 800-235-2637
Telefax: 201-635-4330
Telex: 136346

Hoechst Celanese/Colorants & Surfactants Div.
5200 77 Center Dr.
Charlotte, NC 28217
USA
Tel.: 704-599-4000; 800-255-6189
Telefax: 704-559-6323

Hoechst Celanese/Specialty Chem. /Polymer Additives Group
77 Center Dr., Bldg. 5200
PO Box 1026
Charlotte, NC 28201-1026
USA

Tel.: 704-559-6027
Telefax: 704-559-6780

Hoechst Canada Inc
Div of Hoechst AG
800 Blvd Rene Levesque O
Montreal, Quebec PQH38121
Canada
Tel.: 514-871-5511

Hoechst Chemicals (UK) Ltd
Div of Hoechst AG
Hoechst House, Salisbury Road
Hounslow, Middlesex TW4 6JH
UK
Tel.: 081-570 7712
Telefax: 081-577 1854
Telex: 22284

Hoechst AG
Entwicklung TH 1
D-6230 Frankfurt am Main 80
Germany
Tel.: 069-305-2298
Telefax: 069-318435
Telex: 6990936

Geo. A. Hormel & Co.
501 16th Ave. NE, Box 933
Austin, MN 55912
USA
Tel.: 507-437-5676
Telefax: 507-437-5120

J.M. Huber Corp./Chemicals Div.
PO Box 310
Revolution St.
Havre de Grace, MD 21078
USA
Tel.: 410-939-3500
Telefax: 410-939-0394

Hüls AG
Postfach 1320
D-4370 Marl 1
Germany
Tel.: 02365-49-1
Telefax: 02365-49-2000
Telex: 829211-0

Hüls America Inc.
PO Box 365, 80 Centennial Ave.
Piscataway, NJ 08855-0456
USA
Tel.: 908-980-6800; 800-631-5275
Telefax: 908-980-6970
Telex: 279977 nuodex ur

Hüls Canada, Inc.
235 Orenda Rd.
Brampton, Ontario L6T 1E6
Canada
Tel.: 416-451-3810
Telefax: 416-451-4469
Telex: 0697557

Hüls (UK) Ltd
Edinburgh House
43-51 Windsor Rd., Slough
Berkshire SL1 2HL
UK
Tel.: 0753-71851
Telefax: 0753-820480
Telex: 848243 huels g

Hüls France SA
49-51 Quai de Dion Bouton
F-92815 Puteaux Cedex
France
Tel.: 1 49 06 55 00
Telefax: 1 47 73 97 65
Telex: 611868 huels f

Hüls Japan Ltd.
4-28, Mita 1-cho, Minato-Ku
Tokyo 108
Japan
Tel.: (03) 4551981
Telefax: (03) 4533233
Telex: 2422288 huels jp j

Hydrolabs, Inc.
2028 Kingsley Dr.
PO Box 610
Albemarle, NC 28002
USA
Tel.: 704-983-4136
Telefax: 704-983-3969

Hysan Corp.
4309 S. Morgan St.
Chicago, IL 60609
USA
Tel.: 312-376-8981

Ichimaru Pharcos Co., Ltd.
337 Takatomi Takatomi-Cho
Yamagata-Gun
Gifu-Pref.
Japan
Tel.: 581/22-2551
Telefax: 581/22-3076
Telex: 4722232 Pharco J

ICI plc
9 Millbank
London SW1 3JF
UK
Tel.: 071 834 4444
Telefax: 071 834 2040

ICI Americas, Inc.
Subsidiary of ICI plc
New Murphy Rd. & Concord Pike
Wilmington, DE 19897
USA
Tel.: 302-886-3000; 800-456-3669
Telefax: 302-886-2972
Telex: 4945649

ICI Specialty Chemicals
Concord Pike & New Murphy Rd.
Wilmington, DE 19897
USA
Tel.: 302-886-3000; 800-822-8215
Telefax: 302-886-2972

ICI Surfactants
Wilmington, DE 19897
USA
Tel.: 302-886-3000; 800-822-8215
Telefax: 302-887-3525
Telex: 4945649

ICI Surfactants Ltd. (UK)
PO Box 90
Wilton Centre
Middlesbrough, Cleveland TS6 8JE
UK

Tel.: (0642) 454144
Telefax: (0642) 437374
Telex: 587461

ICI Deutsche GmbH
Postfach 500728
Emil-von-Behring-Strasse 2
W-6000 Frankfurt am Main
Germany
Tel.: 69-5801-00
Telefax: 69-6802345
Telex: 416974 ICI D

ICI Belgium SA
Everslaan 45
B-3078 Everberg
Belgium
Tel.: 2-758 92 11
Telefax: 2-759 77 22
Telex: 21332 ICIEVB B

ICI Surfactants (Belgium)
Everslaan 45
B-3078 Everberg
Belgium
Tel.: 02-758-9211
Telefax: 02-758-9652
Telex: 26151

ICI Moscow
Krasnopresnenskaya Naberezhnaya 12
Moscow
Russia
Tel.: 95-253 2056
Telefax: 95-230 2044
Telex: 413241 ICIMO SU

**ICI Australia Operations Pty. Ltd./
   ICI Surfactants Australia**
ICI House, 1 Nicholson St.
Melbourne
300
Australia
Tel.: 3-665-7111
Telefax: 61-03-665-7009
Telex: 30192

ICI Japan Ltd.
Osaka Green Bldg.
1,3-Chome Kitahama, Higashi-Ku
Osaka
541
Japan

ICI Surfactants Asia Pacific (ICI (China) Ltd.)
PO Box 107
1, Pacific Pl., 14th Floor
HK-88 Queensway
Hong Kong
Tel.: 8434888
Telefax: 8685282
Telex: 73248

ICI Resins US
730 Main St.
Wilmington, MA 01887-0677
USA
Tel.: 508-658-6600; 800-225-0947
Telefax: 508-657-7978

ICN Pharmaceuticals Inc
ICN Plaza
3300 Hyland Ave
Costa Mesa, CA 92626
USA

Tel.: 714-545-0100; 800-556-1937

IGI Petroleum Specialities
164 Sheridan St.
Perth Amboy, NJ 08861
USA
Tel.: 201-826-0140
Telefax: 201-826-0641

Ikeda Corp.
New Tokyo Bldg., 3-1-Marunouchi, 3-Chome
Chiyoda-ku
Tokyo 100
Japan
Tel.: (03) 212-8791
Telefax: (03) 215-5069
Telex: J26370

Indena Gruppo Inverni Della Beffa
Via Ripamonti, 99
20141 Milano
Italy
Tel.: (02) 574961
Telefax: (02) 57404620
Telex: 312535 Idebef I

Lipo Chemicals Inc., distributor
207 19th Ave.
Paterson, NJ 07504
USA
Tel.: 201-345-8600
Telefax: 201-345-8365

Induchem AG
Lagerstrasse 14
CH-8600 Dübendorf 1
Switzerland
Tel.: 1/820-11 61
Telefax: 1/820 21 13
Telex: 828-455

Lipo Chemicals Inc., distributor
207 19th Ave.
Paterson, NJ 07504
USA
Tel.: 201-345-8600
Telefax: 201-345-8365

Industrial Quimica Lasem, S.A.
Avda. Del Valles, 69
08228 Terrassa, Barcelona
Spain
Tel.: 34-3-786-1111
Telefax: 34-3-731-0091

Innovachem, Inc.
555 S. Broad St.
Glen Rock, NJ 07452
USA
Tel.: 201-670-6990

Tri-K Industries, distributor
27 Bland St.
PO Box 312
Emerson, NJ 07630
USA
Tel.: 201-261-2800; 800-526-0372
Telefax: 201-261-1432
Telex: 215085 TRIK UR

Inolex Chemical Co.
Jackson & Swanson Sts.
Philadelphia, PA 19148-3497
USA

Tel.: 215-289-9065; 800-521-9891
Telefax: 215-271-2621
Telex: 834617

Intergen Company
Two Manhattanville Rd.
Purchase, NY 10577
USA
Tel.: 914-694-1700; 800-431-4505
Telefax: 914-694-1429
Telex: 426973

International Bio-Synthetics Inc.
PO Box 241068
Charlotte, NC 28224
USA
Tel.: 704-527-9000; 800-438-1361
Telefax: 704-527-8184

International Biosynthetics Ltd
Hale Bank
Widnes, Cheshire WA8 8NS
UK
Tel.: 051-424 3671
Telefax: 051-420 1301
Telex: 629491 WBCHEM

International Flora Technologies, Inc.
FloraTech Am.
2295 S. Coconino Dr.
Apache Junction, AZ 85220
USA
Tel.: 602-983-7909
Telefax: 602-982-4183

International Sourcing Inc.
121 Pleasant Ave.
Upper Saddle River, NJ 07458
USA
Tel.: 201-934-8900; 800-772-7672
Telefax: 201-934-8291
Telex: 697-2957 INSOURC

Interpolymer Corp.
220 Dan Rd.
Canton, MA 02021
USA
Tel.: 617-828-7120; 800-262-1281
Telefax: 617-821-2485
Telex: 6974364

Intex Chemical, Inc
Div. of EZE Prods., Inc.
603 High Tech Court
Greenville, SC 29650
USA
Tel.: 803-877-5747; 800-845-1668
Telefax: 803-879-7196

ISP, International Specialty Products, World Headquarters
1361 Alps Rd.
Wayne, NJ 07470-3688
USA
Tel.: 201-628-4000; 800-622-4423
Telefax: 201-628-4117
Telex: 219264

ISP (Canada) Inc.
1075 The Queensway East
Unit 16
Mississauga, Ontario L4Y 4C1
Canada

Tel.: 416-277-0381
Telefax: 416-272-0552
Telex: 06961186

ISP Europe
40 Alan Turing Rd.
Surrey Research Park, Guildford
Surrey GU2 5YF
UK
Tel.: 0483-301757
Telefax: 0483 302175
Telex: 859142

ISP Global Technologies Deutschland GmbH
Rudolf-Diesel-Strasse 25
Postfach 1380
5020 Frechen
Germany
Tel.: 02234 105-0
Telefax: 02234 105-211
Telex: 889931

ISP (Australasia) Pty. Ltd.
73-75 Derby St.
Silverwater, N.S.W. 2144
Australia
Tel.: Sydney (02) 648-5177
Telefax: (02) 647-1608
Telex: 73711

ISP (Japan) Ltd.
Shinkawa Iwade Bldg. 8F
26-9, Shinkawa 1-Chome, Chuo-Ku
Tokyo 104
Japan
Tel.: (03) 3555-1571
Telefax: (03) 3555-1660
Telex: 23568

ISP Asia Pacific Pte. Ltd.
200 Cantonment Rd.
Hex 06-05 Southpoint 0208
Singapore
Tel.: 224-9406
Telefax: 226-0853
Telex: 25071

ISP Van Dyk, Inc
Member of the ISP Group
Main & William Sts.
Belleville, NJ 07109
USA
Tel.: 201-450-7724
Telefax: 201-751-2047
Telex: 710-995-4928

Ivax Corp.
8800 Northwest 36th St.
Miami, FL 33178-2404
USA
Tel.: 305-590-2200
Telefax: 305-590-2252

James River Corp./Berlin-Gorham Group
650 Main St.
Berlin, NH 03570
USA
Tel.: 603-752-4600

Janssen Research Foundation
Turnhoutseweg 30
B-2340 Beersee
Belgium
Tel.: 32-14-602111
Telefax: 32-14-602841

Japanese Research Institute
Nishiki 564-176, Fujita
Okayama-shi
Japan
Tel.: 862/96-7012
Telefax: 862/96-7040

Jetco Chemicals, Inc.
PO Box 1898
Corsicana, TX 75110
USA
Tel.: 903-872-3011; 800-477-5353
Telefax: 903-872-4216
Telex: 75110

Kahl & Co./Wax Refiners & Chemical Manufacturers
Otto-Hahn-Strasse 2
D-2077 Trittau
Germany
Tel.: 014154-3011
Telefax: 04154-81508

Kao Corp.
14-10, Nihonbashi, Kayabacho 1-chome
Chuo-ku
Tokyo
103
Japan
Tel.: (03) 3660-7351
Telefax: 03-660-7949
Telex: KAOTYO A J24816

Kao Corp. S.A.
Puig dels Tudons, 10
08210 Barbera Del Valles
Barcelona
Spain
Tel.: 3-729-0000
Telefax: 3-718-9829
Telex: 59749

Kaopolite, Inc.
2444 Morris Ave.
Union, NJ 07083
USA
Tel.: 908-789-0609
Telefax: 908-851-2974

Karlshamns Lipids for Care
S-374 82
Karlshamn
Sweden
Tel.: 454-823-00
Telefax: 454-129-11
Telex: 4500 fopart s

Karlshamns Lipids for Care
525 W. First Ave.
PO Box 569
Columbus, OH 43216
USA
Tel.: 614-299-3131; 800-848-1340
Telefax: 614-299-2584
Telex: 245494 capctyprdcol

Kawasaki Steel Corp.
HIbiya Kokusai Bldg., 2-3 Uchisaiwaicho
2-Chome, Chiyoda-ku
Tokyo 100
Japan
Tel.: (03) 3597-4622

Telefax: (03) 3597-3633
Telex: 0222-3673 KWST TJ

Kelco, Div of Merck & Co Inc
8355 Aero Drive
PO Box 23576
San Diego, CA 92123-1718
USA
Tel.: 619-292-4900; 800-535-2656
Telefax: 619-467 6520
Telex: WUD 695228

Kelco International Ltd
Westminster Tower
3 Albert Embankment
London SE1 7RZ
UK
Tel.: 071-735-0333
Telefax: 071-735-1363
Telex: 23815 KAILIL G

Kelisema Srl/G.F. Secchi
Via Urago 13/B
22038 Tavernerio/Como
Italy
Tel.: 031-427746
Telefax: 031-427745

Kemira Oy
Vuorikemia
SF-28840 Pori
Finland
Tel.: 358-39-341000
Telefax: 358-39-341 919
Telex: 66248 kepom sf

Kempen, Elektrochemische Fabrik Kempen GmbH
Postfach 100 260
D-4152 Kempen 1
Germany

Kenrich Petrochemicals, Inc.
140 E. 22nd St., PO Box 32
Bayonne, NJ 07002-0032
USA
Tel.: 201-823-9000; 800-LICA KPI
Telefax: 201-823-0691
Telex: 12-5023

Kingston Technologies, Inc.
2235-B Route 130
Dayton, NJ 08810
USA
Tel.: 908-274-2288
Telefax: 908-274-2426

Kobo Prods., Inc.
607 Montrose Ave.
South Plainfield, NJ 07080
USA
Tel.: 908-757-0033
Telefax: 908-757-0905
Telex: 405609 KOBO UD

Koken Co., Ltd.
3-14-3 Mejiro, Toshima-ku
Tokyo 171
Japan
Tel.: 03/3950-6600
Telefax: 03/3950-6602
Telex: 02723296 MKOKENJ

Kolmar Laboratories, Inc.
123 Pike St.
PO Box 1111
Port Jervis, NY 12771
USA
Tel.: 914-856-5311
Telefax: 914-856-5507
Telex: 230-646260

Koshiro Co., Ltd.
Doshomachi 2-5-8, Chu-ku
Osaka 541
Japan
Tel.: 6/231-1803
Telefax: 6/2270187

Koster Keunen, Inc.
90 Bourne Blvd.
PO Box 447
Sayville, NY 11782
USA
Tel.: 516-589-0456
Telefax: 516-589-0120

Koster Keunen Holland BV
Postbus 53
5530 AB Bladel
The Netherlands
Tel.: 4977-2929
Telex: 51422 KOKEU NL

Koyo Chemical Co., Ltd.
Iidabashi, Hitown-Bldg. 2-28
Shimomiyabi-cho, Shinzyuku-ku
Tokyo 162
Japan
Tel.: 03/268-1717
Telefax: 03/268-1723

Kronos, Inc.
PO Box 60087
3000 N. Sam Houston Pkwy. East
Houston, TX 77205
USA
Tel.: 713-987-6300; 800-866-5600
Telefax: 713-987-6358

Kronos Ltd
St Ann's House, Wilmslow
Cheshire SK9 1HG
UK
Tel.: 0625 529511
Telefax: 0625 533123
Telex: 669055

Kuraray Co. Ltd.
Shuwa Higashi Yaesu Bldg., 10th Fl.
9-1-2 Chome, Hacchobori, Chuo-ku
Tokyo 104
Japan
Tel.: 33297-9013
Telefax: 33297-9494
Telex: 222-2272 Kurart J

Robeco Chemicals Inc., distributor
99 Park Ave.
New York, NY 10016
USA
Tel.: 212-986-6410
Telefax: 212-986-6419
Telex: 23-3053 A (RCA)

Laboratoires Prod'Hyg
Z.O. des Marais, 16, rue des osiers
78310 Coignieres
France
Tel.: 3461-7757
Telefax: 3461-2387
Telex: 699-007-F

Laboratoires Seporga
50 Boulevard Jean-Baptiste
Verany-06300 Nice
France
Tel.: 93 55 59 45
Telefax: 93 26 77 73

Laboratoires Sérobiologiques S.A.
3, Rue de Seichamps
F-54420 Pulnoy
France
Tel.: 83 29 08 02
Telefax: 83 29 18 04
Telex: LABSERO 961 008 F

Laboratoires Sérobiologiques, Inc.
161 Chambers Brook Rd.
Somerville, NJ 08876
USA
Tel.: 908-218-0330
Telefax: 908-218-0333
Telex: 709485 LABSEBIO

Lanaetex Products, Inc.
151-157 Third Ave.
PO Box 52 Station A
Elizabeth, NJ 07206
USA
Tel.: 908-351-9700
Telefax: 908-351-8753
Telex: 3792268 TLAP1

Laporte Inc., Southern Clay Prods. Inc.
PO Box 44
Gonzales, TX 78629
USA
Tel.: 210-672-2891; 800-324-2891
Telefax: 512-672-3930

Laserson SA
BP 57, Zone Industrielle
91151 Etampes Cedex
France
Tel.: 64 94 31 24
Telefax: 64 94 98 97
Telex: 601532 LASAROM

Laserson & Sabetay Ets. *See Laserson SA*

Lauricidin, Inc.
4841 Southbridge Rd.
Toledo, OH 43623
USA
Tel.: 419-841-1821

Lensfield Prods. Ltd.
Maulden Rd.-Flitwick
Bedford, MK 45 5
UK

Les Colorants Wackherr
7 Rue de l'Industrie
95310 St-Ouen l'Aumone
France
Tel.: 34/64 94 15
Telefax: 34/64 44 40

Lever Industriel
103 Rue DeParis
9300 Bobigny
France

Lion Corp.
3-7, Honjo 1-chome
Sumida-ku
Tokyo 130
Japan
Tel.: (03) 3621-6211
Telefax: (03) 3621-6048
Telex: 262-2114 LIOCOR J

Lipo Chemicals, Inc.
207 19th Ave.
Paterson, NJ 07504
USA
Tel.: 201-345-8600
Telefax: 201-345-8365
Telex: 130117

Lipo do Brasil Ltda.
Rua Roque Petrella, 376
04581 Sao Paulo
SP Brasil
Tel.: (11) 533-2354
Telefax: (11) 533-8997

Adina Chemicals Ltd., representative
Chapman House, Chapman Way
North Farm Rd., Tunbridge Wells
Kent TN2 3EF
UK
Tel.: (892) 517585
Telefax: (892) 517565

Lipoid KG
Frigenstrasse 4
W-6700 Ludwigshafen 24
Germany
Tel.: 0621/553018
Telefax: 0621/553559

Lonza Inc.
17-17 Route 208
Fair Lawn, NJ 07410
USA
Tel.: 201-794-2400; 800-777-1875 (tech.)
Telefax: 201-703-2028
Telex: 4754539 LONZAF

Lonza (UK) Ltd
Imperial House
Lypiatt Road, Cheltenham
Gloucestershire GL50 2QJ
UK
Tel.: 242 513211
Telefax: 242 222294
Telex: 43152

Lonza France SARL
Div of Alusuisse
10-12 rue des Trois Fontanot
F-92000 Nanterre
France
Tel.: 47 75 87 08
Telefax: 47 78 06 27
Telex: 613647

Luzenac America, Inc
9000 E. Nichols Ave.
Englewood, CO 80112
USA

Tel.: 303-643-0400; 800-325-0299
Telefax: 303-643-0444

Macfarlan Smith Ltd
Wheatfield Road
Midlothian, Edinburgh EH11 2QA
Scotland
Tel.: 031-337 2434
Telefax: 031-337 9813
Telex: 727271

Dr. Madis Labs Inc.
375 Huyler St.
South Hackensack, NJ 07606
USA
Tel.: 201-440-5000
Telefax: 201-342-8000
Telex: 134-200

Manchem Inc.
77 Maple Dr.
Hudson, OH 44238
USA

Marine Colloids
Div of FMC Corp.
1735 Market St.
Philadelphia, PA 19103
USA
Tel.: 215-299-6199

Marine Magnesium Co.
995 Beaver Grade Rd.
Coraopolis, PA 15108
USA
Tel.: 412-264-0200
Telefax: 412-264-9020

Maruzen Fine Chemicals Inc.
Div of Maruzen Kasei Co Ltd
525 Yale Ave
Pitman, NJ 08071
USA
Tel.: 609-589-4042
Telefax: 609-582-8894
Telex: 333812 MARFINE

Mason Chemical Co
721 West Algonquin Rd.
Arlington Heights, IL 60005
USA
Tel.: 708-290-1621; 800-362-1855
Telefax: 708-290-1625

Matsumoto Yushi-Seiyaku Co., Ltd.
1-3, Shibukawa-cho 2-chome
Yao-shi
Osaka 581
Japan
Tel.: (0729) 91-1001
Telefax: (0729) 94-8812
Telex: 5353-556 MATUCOJ

Maybrook Inc.
570 Broadway
PO Box 68
Lawrence, MA 01842
USA
Tel.: 508-682-1853
Telefax: 508-682-2544

Mayo Chemical Co., Inc.
5544 Oakdale Rd., South East
Smyrna, GA 30082
USA

Tel.: 404-696-6711; 800-962-6296
Telefax: 404-696-7463

M-CAP Technologies Int'l.
PO Box 7136
Wilmington, DE 19803-0136
USA
Tel.: 302-695-5616
Telefax: 302-695-5681

McIntyre Chemical Co., Ltd.
1000 Governors Hwy.
University Park, IL 60466
USA
Tel.: 708-534-6200
Telefax: 708-534-6216

Mearl Corp.
217 North Highland Ave., PO Box 960
Ossining, NY 10562
USA
Tel.: 914-941-7450
Telefax: 914-941-7858

Meer Corp.
PO Box 9006
9500 Railroad Ave.
N. Bergen, NJ 07047-1206
USA
Tel.: 201-861-9500
Telefax: 201-861-9267
Telex: 219130

Edward Mendell Co., Inc.
A Penwest Company
2981 Rt. 22
Patterson, NY 12563-9970
USA
Tel.: 914-878-3414; 800-431-2457
Telefax: 914-878-3484
Telex: 4971034

E. Merck
Postfach 4119
Frankfurter Strasse 250
D-6100 Darmstadt 1
Germany
Tel.: 06151-72-0
Telefax: 06151-72-3684
Telex: 419328-0 em d

Lucas Meyer GmbH & Co.
PO Box 261665
D-2000 Hamburg 26
Germany
Tel.: 40-789-550
Telefax: 40-789-8329
Telex: 2163220 myer d

M. Michel & Co., Inc
90 Broad St.
New York, NY 10004
USA
Tel.: 212-344-3878
Telefax: 212-344-3880
Telex: 421468

Microbial Systems Int'l. Ltd.
Gothic House, Barker Gate
Nottingham NG1 1JU
UK
Tel.: 0602 521181
Telefax: 0602 521281

Tri-K Industries, distributor
27 Bland St.
PO Box 312
Emerson, NJ 07630
USA
Tel.: 201-261-2800; 800-526-0372
Telefax: 201-261-1432
Telex: 215085 TRIK UR

Microfluidics Corp
Subsid. of Biotechnology Development Corp
90 Oak St.
PO Box 9101
Newton, MA 02164-9101
USA
Tel.: 617-969-5452; 800-370-5452
Telefax: 617-965-1213

Miles Inc./Organic Products Div.
Bldg. 14, Mobay Rd.
Pittsburgh, PA 15205-9741
USA
Tel.: 412-777-2000; 800-662-2927
Telefax: 412-777-7840
Telex: 1561261

Miles Inc
One Mellon Center
500 Grant Street
Pittsburgh, PA 15219-2502
USA
Tel.: 412-394 5500
Telefax: 412-394 5578

Milliken Chemicals
PO Box 1927
Spartanburg, SC 29304
USA
Tel.: 803-573-2625
Telefax: 803-573-2430
Telex: 810-282-2580

Mitsubishi Gas Chemical Co., Inc.
Mitsubishi Bldg., 2-5-2, Marunouchi 2-chome
Chiyoda-ku
Tokyo 100
Japan
Tel.: (03) 3283-4799
Telefax: (03)3214-0938
Telex: 222-2624 MGCHO J

Mitsubishi Kasei Corp.
Mitsubishi Bldg., 5-2, Marunouchi 2-chome
Chiyoda-ku
Tokyo 100
Japan
Tel.: (03) 3283-6254
Telex: BISICH J 24901

Mitsubishi-Kasei Foods Corp.
Ichikawa Bldg., 13-3, Ginza 5-chome
Chuo-ku
Tokyo 104
Japan
Tel.: (03) 3542-6525
Telefax: (03) 3545-4860
Telex: BISICHJ 24901 AH.MFC

Mitsubishi Petrochemical Co., Ltd.
Mitsubishi Bldg., 5-2, Marunouchi 2-chome
Chiyoda-ku
Tokyo 100
Japan

Tel.: (03) 3283-5700
Telefax: (03) 3283-5472
Telex: 222-3172

Mona Industries Inc.
PO Box 425, 76 E. 24th St.
Paterson, NJ 07544
USA
Tel.: 201-345-8220; 800-553-6662
Telefax: 201-345-3527
Telex: 130308

Montana Talc Co.
28769 Sappington Rd.
Three Forks, MT 59752
USA
Tel.: 406-285-3286
Telefax: 406-285-3530

Morflex, Inc.
2110 High Point Rd.
Greensboro, NC 27403
USA
Tel.: 910-292-1781
Telefax: 910-854-4058
Telex: 910240 7846

Morton International Inc
100 N Riverside Plaza
Randolph Street
Chicago, IL 60606-1598
USA
Tel.: 312-807-2562
Telefax: 312-807-2899
Telex: 25-4433

Morton International Ltd./
Specialty Chem., Ind. Chem. & Addit.
7900-A Taschereau Blvd., Suite 106
Brossard, Quebec J4X 1C2
Canada
Tel.: 514-466-7764
Telefax: 514-466-7771

Morton International Ltd
Greville House
Hibernia Road, Hounslow
Greater London TW3 3RX
UK
Tel.: 081-570 7766
Telefax: 081-570 6943
Telex: 262002

Morton International NV SA
Chaussee de la Hulpe 130, Boite 5
B-1050 Brussels
Belgium
Tel.: 2-6602909
Telefax: 2-6604702
Telex: 23708

Mt. Pulaski Products, Inc.
PO Box 110
904 North Vine
Mt. Pulaski, IL 62548
USA
Tel.: 217-792-3211
Telefax: 217-792-5040

Nalco Chemical Co.
One Nalco Center
Naperville, IL 60563-1198
USA

Tel.: 708-305-1000; 800-527-7753
Telefax: 708-305-2900

Natural Oils International, Inc.
12350 Montague St., Unit C & D
Pacoima, CA 91331
USA
Tel.: 818-897-0536
Telefax: 818-896-4277
Telex: 371-0352

Nepera, Inc.
A Cambrex Co.
Route 17
Harriman, NY 10926
USA
Tel.: 914-782-1202
Telefax: 914-782-2418
Telex: 510-249-4847

New Zealand Milk Prods., Inc.
3637 Westwind Blvd.
Santa Rosa, CA 95403
USA
Tel.: 707-524-6600
Telefax: 707-524-6666

Niacet Corp.
PO Box 258
400 47th St.
Niagara Falls, NY 14304
USA
Tel.: 716-285-1474; 800-828-1207
Telefax: 716-285-1497
Telex: 6730170

Nihon Emulsion Co., Ltd.
Minami 5-32-7, Koenji
Suginami-ku
Tokyo
Japan
Tel.: (03) 314-3211
Telefax: (03) 312-7207
Telex: 2322358 EMALEX J

Nihon Junyaku Co., Ltd.
1-13, Nihonbashi Hon-cho 4-chome
Chuo-ku
Tokyo 103
Japan
Tel.: (03) 3242-1731
Telefax: (03) 3242-1734

Nihon Surfactants Kogyo KK
3-24-3 Hasune, Itabashi-Ku
Tokyo
Japan
Tel.: (03) 966-7331

Nikko Chemicals Co., Ltd.
4-8, Nihonbashi, Bakuro-cho 1-chome
Chuo-ku
Tokyo 103
Japan
Tel.: (03) 3661-1677
Telefax: (03) 3664-8620
Telex: 2522744 NIKKOL J

Chesham Chemicals Ltd., representative
Cunningham House
Westfield Lane
Harrow HA3 9ED
UK

Tel.: 081-907 7779
Telefax: 081-909 1053
Telex: 8811603

Nipa Laboratories, Inc.
3411 Silverside Rd.
104 Hagley Bldg.
Wilmington, DE 19810
USA
Tel.: 302-478-1522
Telefax: 302-478-4097
Telex: 905030

Nippon Chemical Co., Ltd.
3-1 Iwamoto-cho, 2-Chome
Chiyoda-ku
Tokyo
Japan
Tel.: 03-861-2291

Nippon Oils & Fats Co., Ltd. (NOF Corp.)
Yurakucho Bldg., 10-1, Yarakucho 1-chome
Chiyoda-Ku
Tokyo 100
Japan
Tel.: (03) 3283-7295
Telefax: (03) 3283-7178
Telex: 222-2041 NIPOIL J

Nissan Chemical Industries, Ltd.
Kowa-Hitotsubashi Bldg.
7-1, Kanda-Nishiki-cho 3-chome
Chiyoda-ku
Tokyo 101
Japan
Tel.: (03) 3296-8111
Telefax: (03) 3296-8360
Telex: 222-3071

Nisshin Oil Mills, Ltd.
23-1 1-Chome, Shinkawa, Chuo-Ku
Tokyo 104
Japan
Tel.: 03-3206-5113
Telefax: 03-3206-6456

Norland Products Inc.
695 Joyce Kilmer Ave.
New Brunswick, NJ 08902
USA
Tel.: 908-545-7828
Telefax: 908-545-9542

Norman, Fox & Co.
5511 S. Boyle Ave., PO Box 58727
Vernon, CA 90058
USA
Tel.: 213-583-0016; 800-632-1777
Telefax: 213-583-9769

Nova Molecular Technologies, Inc.
1 Parker Place, Suite 495
Janesville, WI 53545
USA
Tel.: 608-754-NOVA
Telefax: 608-654-6878

Novarom GmbH
Postfach 1309
D-3450 Holzminden 1
Germany
Tel.: 49/5531-8537
Telefax: 49/5531-80492
Telex: 965315 nova d

Nurture, Inc.
5840 Expressway
Missoula, MT 59802
USA
Tel.: 406-728-0260
Telefax: 406-728-0261

Olin Chemicals
120 Long Ridge Rd., PO Box 1355
Stamford, CT 06904
USA
Tel.: 203-356-3036; 800-243-9171
Telefax: 203-356-3273
Telex: 420202

Olin Brasil Limitada
Rua Galeno de Castro, 165
Jurubatuba, Santo Amaro
04696 Sao Paulo, SP
Brazil
Tel.: 5511-548-7566
Telex: 11-25034

Olin U.K. Ltd
42 High St.
Guildford, Surrey
UK
Tel.: (44483) 64726
Telex: 859391

Olin Europe SA
90 Ave. des Champs Elysees
75008 Paris
France
Tel.: (331) 562-32-10
Telex: 650769

Olin Chemicals Pty., Ltd.
1-3 Atchison St.
PO Box 141
St. Leonards 2065, N.S.W.
Australia
Tel.: 612-439-6222
Telex: 26328

Olin Japan Inc.
Shiozaki Bldg.
7-1 Hirakawa-Cho 2-Chome, Chiyoda-ku
Tokyo 102
Japan
Tel.: (813) 263-4615
Telex: 023-24031

Onyx Chemical Co
Millmaster Onyx Group
Jersey City, NJ 07302
USA

Osaka Kasei Co., Ltd.
6-11 Nakajima 2-Chome
Nishiyodogawa-ku
Osaka 555
Japan
Tel.: 06/474-3621
Telefax: 06/476-2260

OSi Specialties, Inc.
39 Old Ridgebury Rd.
Danbury, CT 06810-5121
USA
Tel.: 800-523-2862

OSi Specialties Canada, Inc.
1210 Sheppard Ave. East, Suite 210
Box 38

Willowdale, Ontario M2K 1E3
Canada
Tel.: 416-490-0466

OSi Specialties S.A.
7 Rue de Pre-Bouvier
Meyrin
CH-1217 Geneva
Switzerland
Tel.: 41-22-989-2111

OSi Specialties Singapore PTE, Ltd.
22-01 Treasury Bldg.
8 Shenton Way
0106
Singapore
Tel.: 65-322-9922

Penederm, Inc.
320 Lakeside Dr., Suite A
Foster City, CA 94404
USA
Tel.: 415-358-0100
Telefax: 415-358-0101

Penn-Squire Ltd.
2075 Parkview Drive
Lansdale, PA 19446
USA
Tel.: 215-855-6323

Penreco
Div of Pennzoil Prods. Co.
RD 2, Box 1
Kars City, PA 16041
USA
Tel.: 412-756-0110; 800-245-3952
Telefax: 412-756-1050
Telex: 1561596

Pentapharm Ltd
Engelgasse 109
CH-4002 Basel
Switzerland
Tel.: 061-312-9680
Telefax: 061-311-2049
Telex: 963 473 pefa ch

Centerchem, Inc., distributor
225 High Ridge Rd
Stamford, CT 06905-3036
USA
Tel.: 203-975-9800
Telefax: 203-975-8777

Petrolite Corp./Industrial Chemicals Div.
369 Marshall Ave
St. Louis, MO 63119
USA

Pfaltz & Bauer Inc.
172 E. Aurora St.
Waterbury, CT 06708
USA
Tel.: 203-574-0075; 800-225-5172
Telefax: 203-574-3181
Telex: 996471

Phoenix Chemical, Inc.
322 Courtyard Dr.
Somerville, NJ 08876
USA
Tel.: 908-707-0232
Telefax: 908-707-0186

Pilot Chemical Co.
11756 Burke St.
Santa Fe Springs, CA 90670
USA
Tel.: 213-723-0036
Telefax: 213-945-1877
Telex: 4991200 PILOT

PPG Industries, Inc./Specialty Chemicals
3938 Porett Dr.
Gurnee, IL 60031
USA
Tel.: 708-244-3410; 800-323-0856
Telefax: 708-244-9633
Telex: 25-3310

PPG Canada Inc./Specialty Chem.
2 Robert Speck Pkwy., Suite 750
Mississauga, Ontario L4Z 1H8
Canada
Tel.: 416-848-2500
Telefax: 416-848-2501
Telex: 06960351 canbiz miss

PPG Industrial do Brazil Ltda.
Edificio Grande Avenida, Paulista Ave. 1754, Suite 153
Sao Paulo
Brazil 01310
Tel.: 011-2840433
Telefax: 011-2892105
Telex: 391-1139104ppgbrazil

PPG Industries (UK) Ltd./Specialty Chem.
Carrington Business Park, Carrington, Urmston
Manchester M31 4DD
UK
Tel.: 061-777-9203
Telefax: 061-777-9064
Telex: 851-94014896 mazu g

PPG Industries (France) SA
BP 377, Écluse Folien
F-59307 Valenciennes
France
Tel.: 27 14 46 00
Telefax: 27 29 36 34

PPG Industries/Asia/Pacific Ltd.
Takanawa Court, 5th floor
12-1 Takanawa 3-Chome, Minato-Ku
Tokyo 108
Japan
Tel.: (03) 3280-2911
Telefax: (03) 3280-2920
Telex: 02-42719 PPGPACJ

PQ Corp.
PO Box 840
Valley Forge, PA 19482
USA
Tel.: 215-293-7200; 800-944-7411
Telefax: 215-688-3835
Telex: 476 1129 PQCO VAF

Presperse Inc.
601 Hadley Rd.
South Plainfield, NJ 07080
USA
Tel.: 908-756-2023
Telefax: 908-756-8754
Telex: (910)2409388

Proalan S.A.
Apartado de Correos 301
08400 Granollers, Barcelona
Spain
Tel.: 93/849-53-99
Telefax: 93/849-10-18
Telex: 94129GNSA

Procter & Gamble Co/Chemicals Div
PO Box 599
Cincinnati, OH 45201
USA
Tel.: 513-983-3928; 800-543-1580
Telefax: 513-983-1436
Telex: 21-4185, P&GCIN

Prod'Hyg. *See Laboratoires Prod'Hyg*

Pronova Olechemicals
PO Box 2051
N-3202 Sandefjord
Norway
Tel.: 47 34/74-700
Telefax: 47 34/74-720
Telex: 8320351

Protameen Chemicals, Inc.
375 Minnisink Rd.
PO Box 166
Totowa, NJ 07511
USA
Tel.: 201-256-4374
Telefax: 201-256-6764
Telex: 130125

Protan Biopolymer A/S
Postboks 494
N-3002 Drammen
Norway
Tel.: 47-3-837300
Telefax: 47-3-833488
Telex: 76594 prota n

Protex
6 Rue Barbes
92305 Levallois
France

Provital
Centro Industrial Santiaga
Talleres 6, no. 15, Apartado Correos 78
Barcelona
Spain
Tel.: 93-718-80-12
Telefax: 93-718-38-30
Telex: 98476 DITT E

Pulcra SA
Sector E C/42
Barcelona
08040
Spain
Tel.: 3-323-5914
Telefax: 3-323-6760
Telex: 98301

Quantum Chemical Corp./USI Div.
11500 Northlake Dr., PO Box 429550
Cincinnati, OH 45249
USA
Tel.: 513-530-6556; 800-543-7900
Telefax: 513-530-6562
Telex: 155116

Quest International Fragrances USA, Inc.
400 International Dr.
Mt. Olive, NJ 07828
USA
Tel.: 201-691-7100
Telefax: 201-691-7479
Telex: 6714933

Quest International UK Ltd
Kennington Road
Ashford, Kent TN24 0LT
UK
Tel.: 0233-644444
Telefax: 0233-644146
Telex: 96369

Quest International Deutschland GmbH
Postfach 650170
Poppenbütteler Chaussee 36
W-2000 Hamburg 65
Germany
Tel.: 40-607970
Telefax: 40-6079710
Telex: 215196

Quest International
Lindtsedijk 8
3336 le Zwijndrecht
The Netherlands
Tel.: 78-128511
Telefax: 78-195279
Telex: 29477

Quimigal-Quimica de Portugal E.P.
Av. Infante Santo No. 2
1300 Lisboa
Portugal
Tel.: 1-604040
Telex: 12301

Reheis Inc.
PO Box 609
235 Snyder Ave.
Berkeley Heights, NJ 07922
USA
Tel.: 908-464-1500
Telefax: 908-464-8094
Telex: 219463 RCCA UR

Reheis Ireland
Kilbarrack Rd.
Dublin, 5
Irish Republic
Tel.: 1-322621
Telefax: 1-392205
Telex: 32532 REHI EI

Reilly-Whiteman Inc.
801 Washington St.
Conshohocken, PA 19428
USA
Tel.: 215-828-3800; 800-533-4514
Telefax: 215-834-7855
Telex: 5106608845

Research Corp. of Am.
4 Warehouse Lane
Elmsford, NY 10523
USA
Tel.: 914-592-9405

Rewo. *See under Witco*

Rheox Inc

PO Box 700
Wyckoffs Mill Road
Hightstown, NJ 08520
USA
Tel.: 609-443-2500; 800-866-6800
Telefax: 609-443-2422
Telex: 642240

Rheox Inc.

31 rue de l'Hôpital
B-1000 Brussels
Belgium
Tel.: 02-512-0048
Telefax: 02-513 24 25
Telex: 24662 EUR B

Rhone-Poulenc S.A.

18, ave. d'Alsace
92400 Courbevoie, Paris
France

Rhone-Poulenc, Inc./Surfactants & Specialties

CN 7500, Prospect Plains Rd.
Cranberry, NJ 08512-7500
USA
Tel.: 609-860-8300; 800-922-2189
Telefax: 609-860-7626

Rhone-Poulenc Surfactants & Specialties Canada

2000 Argentia Rd.
Plaza 3, Suite 400
Mississauga, Ontario LSN 1V9
Canada
Tel.: 416-821-4450
Telefax: 416-821-9339

Rhone-Poulenc Chemicals Ltd, Perf. Prods. Group

Div of Rhone-Poulenc SA
Poleacre Lane
Woodley, Stockport
Cheshire SK6 1PQ
UK
Tel.: 061-430-4391
Telefax: 061-430-4364
Telex: 667835

Rhone-Poulenc Chimie

Div of Rhone-Poulenc SA
25 Quai Paul Doumer
F-92408 Courbevoie Cedex
France
Tel.: 47 68 1234
Telefax: 47 68 23 00
Telex: 610500

Rhone-Poulenc Chimie (France)/Secteur Specialites Chimiques

Cedex 29
F-92097 Paris La Défense
France
Tel.: 47-68 02 01
Telefax: 47-68 13 31

Rhone-Poulenc NV

Kuhlmannkaai
B-9020 Ghent
Belgium
Tel.: 091 44 8891
Telex: 11275 RPCHEM B

Rhone-Poulenc Geronazzo SpA

Div of Rhone-Poulenc SA
Via Milano 78
Ospiate Di Bollate
I-20021 Milano
Italy
Tel.: 2-350-3212
Telefax: 2-350-1770
Telex: 331547 GERO I

Rhone-Poulenc, Inc./Chemicals Div.

Box 125
Monmouth Junction, NJ 08852
USA
Tel.: 201-297-0100
Telefax: 201-297-1597

Rhone-Poulenc Basic Chemical Co.

One Corporate Dr., Box 881
Shelton, CT 06484
USA
Tel.: 203-925-3300; 800-642-4200
Telefax: 203-925-3627

Rhone-Poulenc Food Ingredients

CN 7500, Prospect Plains Rd.
Cranbury, NJ 08512
USA
Tel.: 609-860-4600; 800-253-5052

Rhone-Poulenc, Inc./Water Soluble Polymers

CN 7500, Prospect Plains Rd.
Cranberry, NJ 08512-7500
USA
Tel.: 800-288-1175

Rhone-Poulenc Rorer Pharmaceuticals Inc.

500 Arcola Road
Collegeville, PA 19426-2911
USA
Tel.: 215-454-8000

Rhone-Poulenc Rorer Ltd

Div of Rhone-Poulenc SA
Rainham Rd South
Dagenham, Essex RM10 7XS
UK
Tel.: 081 592 3060
Telefax: 081-593 2140
Telex: 28691 MBDAGN G

American Lecithin Co.

Div of Rhone-Poulenc Rorer/Nattermann
33 Turner Rd.
Danbury, CT 06813-1908
USA
Tel.: 203-790-2700
Telefax: 203-790-2705

Dr. Kurt Richter GmbH, Chemische Laboratorium

PO Box 410480
Bennigsenstrasse 25
D-1000 Berlin 41
Germany
Tel.: 30-852-70-75
Telefax: 30-851-18-22
Telex: 184626 clr d

Riken Vitamin Oil Co., Ltd.

TDC Bldg., 9-18, Misaki-Cho 2-chome
Chiyoda-Ku
Tokyo 101
Japan

Tel.: (03) 5275-5111
Telefax: (03) 3261-2628
Telex: 2322783

Ringdex
16 Rue Ballu
F-75009 Paris
France
Tel.: 33/1 40 82 35 95
Telefax: 33/1 42 85 17 17
Telex: 650847 F

RITA Corp.
1725 Kilkenny Court
PO Box 585
Woodstock, IL 60098
USA
Tel.: 815-337-2500; 800-426-7759
Telefax: 815-337-2522
Telex: 72-2438

Robeco Chemicals Inc.
99 Park Ave.
New York, NY 10016
USA
Tel.: 212-986-6410
Telefax: 212-986-6419
Telex: 23-3053 A (RCA)

Roche Chem. Div.
Div. of Hoffman-La Roche Inc
340 Kingsland St.
Nutley, NJ 07110-1199
USA
Tel.: 201-235-5000
Telefax: 201-535-7606

Phillip Rockley, Inc.
20505 Dag Hammarskjold Plaza
76 9th Ave.
New York, NY 10011
USA
Tel.: 212-355-5770
Telefax: 212-355-5771

Rohm & Haas Co.
Independence Mall West
Philadelphia, PA 19105
USA
Tel.: 215-592-3000; 800-323-4165
Telefax: 215-592-2285
Telex: 845-247

Rohm & Haas Canada Inc.
2 Manse Rd.
West Hill, Ontario M1E 3T9
Canada

Rohm & Haas Co. European Operations
Chesterfield House, Bloomsbury Way 15-19
London WC1A 2TP
UK
Tel.: 071 242 4455
Telefax: 071 404 4126
Telex: 24139

Rohm & Haas (UK) Ltd
Lennig House, 2 Mason's Avenue
Croydon CR9 3NB
UK
Tel.: 081-686-8844
Telefax: 081-686 8329
Telex: 917266

Röhm GmbH Chemische Fabrik
Kirschenallee, Postfach 4242
D-6100 Darmstadt
Germany
Tel.: 6151 18 01
Telefax: 6151 184007

Rohm & Haas (Australia) Pty. Ltd.
969 Burke Rd., PO Box 11
Camberwell, Victoria 3124
Australia

Rohm & Haas Asia Ltd.
Kaisei Bldg.
8-10 Azabudai 1-Chome, Minato-ku
Tokyo 106
Japan

Rohm Tech Inc.
83 Authority Dr.
Fitchburg, MA 01420
USA
Tel.: 508-342-5831
Telefax: 508-345-1971

Rona
Div of EM Industries, Inc.
5 Skyline Dr.
Hawthorne, NY 10532
USA
Tel.: 914-592-4660
Telefax: 914-592-9469
Telex: 17-8993

Ronsheim & Moore Ltd.
Div of Hickson & Welch Ltd
Wheldon Road, Castleford
West Yorkshire WF10 2JT
UK
Tel.: 0977-556565
Telefax: 0977-518058
Telex: 55378

Roquette Corp.
1550 Northwestern Ave.
Gurnee, IL 60031
USA
Tel.: 312-249-5950; 800-223-5305
Telefax: 708-578-1027
Telex: 687 1679 ROQ ILL

Roquette (UK) Ltd
Pantiles House, 2 Nevill Street
Tunbridge Wells, Kent TN2 5TT
UK
Tel.: 0892-540188
Telefax: 0892-510872
Telex: 957558 G

Ross Chemical, Inc.
303 Dale Dr.
PO Box 458
Fountain Inn, SC 29644
USA
Tel.: 803-862-4474; 800-521-8246
Telefax: 803-862-2912

Frank B. Ross Co., Inc.
22 Halladay St., PO Box 4085
Jersey City, NJ 07304-0085
USA
Tel.: 201-433-4512
Telefax: 201-332-3555

Ruetgers-Nease Chemical Co., Inc.
Subsid of Rütgerswerke AG
201 Struble Rd.
State College, PA 16801
USA
Tel.: 814-238-2424
Telefax: 814-238-1567

L.A. Salomon Inc.
150 River Rd., Suite A-4
Montville, NJ 07045
USA
Tel.: 201-335-8300
Telefax: 201-335-1236
Telex: 96-1470

Sandoz Chemicals Corp.
4000 Monroe Rd.
Charlotte, NC 28205
USA
Tel.: 704-331-7000; 800-631-8077
Telefax: 704-372-5787
Telex: 704-216-922

Sandoz Chemicals (UK) Ltd
Div of Sandoz AG
Calverley Lane, Horsforth
Leeds, West Yorkshire LS18 4RP
UK
Tel.: 0532 584646
Telefax: 0532 390063
Telex: 557114

Sandoz Nutrition
5320 West 23rd St.
Minneapolis, MN 55416
USA
Tel.: 612-593-2163
Telefax: 612-593-2087

Sanyo Chemical Industries, Ltd.
11-1, Ikkyo Nomoto-cho
Higashiyama-ku
Kyoto 605
Japan
Tel.: (075) 541-4311
Telefax: (075) 551-2557
Telex: 05422110

Scher Chemicals, Inc.
Industrial West & Styertowne Rd.
PO Box 4317
Clifton, NJ 07012
USA
Tel.: 201-471-1300
Telefax: 201-471-3783
Telex: 642643 Scherclif

Schülke & Mayr GmbH
Robert-Koch-Strasse 2
D-22840 Norderstedt
Germany
Tel.: 040/521-00-0
Telefax: 040/521-00-577
Telex: 215-486 sagro d

G.F. Secchi. See Kelisema Srl

Sederma
29 Rue Du Chemin Vert
78610 Le Perray En Yvelines
France
Tel.: (1)34 84 10 10

Telefax: (1)34 84 11 30
Telex: 689728

Sederma Inc.
7110 Fort Hamilton Pkwy.
Brooklyn, NY 11228
USA
Tel.: 718-833-1046
Telefax: 718-833-7028

Seiwa Kasei Co., Ltd.
1-2-14 Nunoichi-cho
Higashi-osaka
Osaka 579
Japan
Tel.: 0729 87-2626
Telefax: 0729-87-2072

R.I.T.A., U.S. distributor
1725 Kilkenny Court
PO Box 585
Woodstock, IL 60098
USA
Tel.: 815-337-2500; 800-426-7759
Telefax: 815-337-2522
Telex: 72-2438

Senju Pharmaceutical Co., Ltd.
2-5-8, Hiranomachi, Chuo-ku
Osaka
Japan
Tel.: 06/201-9620
Telefax: 06/229-3293

Seporga. See Laboratoires Seporga

Seppic
Div of L'Air Liquide
75 Quai d'Orsay
F-75321 Paris Cedex 07
France
Tel.: 40 62 55 55
Telefax: 40 62 52 53
Telex: 202901 SEPPI F

Seppic Inc
30 Two Bridges Rd., Suite 370
Fairfield, NJ 07004
USA
Tel.: 201-882-5597
Telefax: 201-882-5178

Servo Delden B.V.
Postbus 1
NL-7490 AA Delden
The Netherlands
Tel.: 5407-63535
Telefax: 5407-64125
Telex: 44347

Sheffield Prods.
Div of Quest Int'l.
Woods Corners
Norwich, NY 13815
USA
Tel.: 607-334-9951
Telefax: 607-334-5022
Telex: 646056

Shell Chemical Co.
PO Box 2463
One Shell Plaza, Suite 1866 OSP
Houston, TX 77252-2463
USA

Tel.: 713-241-6161
Telefax: 713-241-4043
Telex: 762248

Pecten Chemicals, Inc.
representing for Int'l. sales
One Shell Plaza
Houston, TX 77252-9932
USA
Tel.: 713-241-6161

Shell Chemicals UK Ltd
Shell-Mex House
Strand
London WC2R0DX
UK
Tel.: 071-257 40000
Telefax: 071-257 1336
Telex: 21795

Shell Chimie SA
BP 319
23-25 ave de Republique
7539 Paris Cedex 08
F-92506 Rueil-Malmaison
France
Tel.: 47 52 27 00
Telefax: 47 52 28 02
Telex: 632051 SHELL F

Shell Nederland Chemie B.V.
PO Box 187
2501 CD The Hague
The Netherlands

Shin-Etsu Silicones of America, Inc.
431 Amapola Ave.
Torrance, CA 90501
USA
Tel.: 213-533-6961
Telefax: 213-533-8936

Shiseido Co., Ltd.
Shiseido Am. Technocenter
100 Tokeneke Rd., Suite A
Darien, CT 06820
USA
Tel.: 203-656-7999
Telefax: 203-656-7995

Siegmar Laboratori Ricerca S.R.L.
27028 San Martino Siccomario
Via Brodolini, 5/7
Italy
Tel.: 0382499 451

3V-Sigma
1500 Harbor Blvd.
Weehawken, NJ 07087
USA
Tel.: 201-865-3600
Telefax: 201-865-1892

Silab/Societe Industrielle Limousine D'Applications Biologiques
6 Rue Charles Brun, B.P. 213
19108 Brive
France
Tel.: 55 87 75 46
Telefax: 55 87 68 80

Siltech Inc.
4437 Park Dr., Suite E
Norcross, GA 30093
USA

Tel.: 404-279-8601
Telefax: 404-279-8535

Sinerga Srl
Via Pitagora, 11
20016 Pero, Milan
Italy
Tel.: 011 39 2 3538635
Telefax: 011 39 2 33910183

Trivent Chemical Co., U.S. distributor
45 Ridge Rd.
PO Box 597
South River, NJ 08882
Tel.: 908-251-1116
Telefax: 908-251-0967

Sino-Japan Chemical Co.
3 fl. 237 Sec. 1, Chien Kuo South Rd.
Taipei, Hsien
Taiwan, R.O.C.
Tel.: 886-2-700-1422
Telefax: 886-2-707-3921

Werner G Smith, Inc
1730 Train Ave.
Cleveland, OH 44113
USA
Tel.: 216-861-3676; 800-535-8343
Telefax: 216-861-3680

Solabia
29 Rue Delizy
93500 Pantin
France
Tel.: 148 91 02 32
Telefax: 148 91 18 77
Telex: 230 827 BIOSOR

Barnet Prods. Corp., distributor
560 Sylvan Ave.
Englewood Cliffs, NJ 07632
USA
Tel.: 201-569-6622
Telefax: 201-569-8847

Solvay SA
33 rue du Prince Albert
B-1050 Brussels
Belgium
Tel.: 2-509-6111
Telefax: 2-509-6617
Telex: 21337

Solvay Chemicals Ltd.
Unit 1, Grovelands Business Centre
Boundary Way, Hemel Hempstead
Herts HP2 7TE
UK
Tel.: 0442-236555

**Solvay Deutschland GmbH/
  Solvay Catalysts GmbH**
Postfach 220
W-3000 Hannover-1
Germany
Tel.: 511-857-0
Telefax: 511-282126
Telex: 922-755

Solvay Duphar BV
Postbus 900
1380 DA Weesp
The Netherlands

Tel.: 2940-77711
Telefax: 2940-80253
Telex: 14232

Solvay Enzymes, Inc.
PO Box 4859
1230 Randolph St.
Elkhart, IN 46514-0859
USA
Tel.: 219-523-3700; 800-342-2097
Telefax: 219-523-3800

Solvay Enzymes GmbH & Co KG
Div of Solvay & Cie SA
Postfach 690307
Hans Böckler Allee 20
W-3000 Hannover 1
Germany
Tel.: 511-8570
Telefax: 511-8572371
Telex: 922755

Southern Clay Prods. *See Laporte Inc.*

A.E. Staley Manufacturing Co.
2200 E. Eldorado St.
Decatur, IL 62525
USA
Tel.: 217-423-4411
Telefax: 217-421-2936

Stepan Co
22 West Frontage Rd.
Northfield, IL 60093
USA
Tel.: 708-446-7500; 800-745-7837
Telefax: 708-501-2443

Stepan Canada
90 Matheson Blvd. W., Suite 201
Mississauga, Ontario L5R 3P3
Canada
Tel.: 416-507-1631
Telefax: 416-507-1633

Stepan Europe
BP127
38340 Voreppe
France
Tel.: 7650-8133
Telefax: 7656-7165
Telex: 320511 F

Stepan Co./PVO Dept.
100 West Hunter Ave.
Maywood, NJ 07607
USA
Tel.: 201-845-3030
Telefax: 201-845-6754
Telex: 710-990-5170

Stevenson Brothers & Co Inc
PO Box 38349
1039 West Venango St.
Philadelphia, PA 19140
USA
Tel.: 215-223-2600
Telefax: 215-223-3597

Stockhausen, Inc.
2408 Doyle St.
Greensboro, NC 27406
USA
Tel.: 919-333-3500

Telefax: 919-333-3545
Telex: 574405

Strahl & Pitsch, Inc.
PO box 1098
230 Great E. Neck Rd.
W. Babylon, NY 11704
USA
Tel.: 516-587-9000
Telefax: 516-587-9120
Telex: 221636 STRALUR

Sun Chemical Corp./Colors Group
441 Tompkins Ave.
Staten Island, NY 10305
USA
Tel.: 718-981-1600
Telefax: 718-816-8289
Telex: 125063

SunSmart Inc.
PO Box 1451
Wainscott, NY 11975
USA
Tel.: 516-324-8061
Telefax: 516-324-9752

Sutton Laboratories, Inc
Member of the ISP Inc Group
116 Summit Ave., PO Box 837
Chatham, NJ 07928-0837
USA
Tel.: 201-635-1551
Telefax: 201-635-4964
Telex: 710-999-5607

Swastik Household & Industrial Products Ltd.
Shahibag House, 13 Walchand Hirachand Marg
Ballard Estate
Bombay 400 038
India

Syntex Corporation
3401 Hillview Ave
Palo Alto, CA 94304
USA
Tel.: 415-855-5050

Synthelabo-Pharmacie
30/38 Ave. Gustave Eiffel
B.P. 0166
37001 Tours Cedex
France

International Sourcing, distributor
121 Pleasant Ave.
Upper Saddle River, NJ 07458
Tel.: 201-934-8900; 800-772-7672
Telefax: 201-934-8291
Telex: 697-2957 INSOURC

Synthetic Products Co.
Subsid of Cookson America Inc
1000 Wayside Rd.
Cleveland, OH 44110
USA
Tel.: 216-531-6010; 800-321-4236
Telefax: 216-486-6638

Taiwan Surfactant Corp.
No. 106, 8-1 Floor, Sec. 2
Chung An E. Rd.
Taipei
Taiwan, R.O.C.

Tel.: 886-2-507-9155
Telefax: 886-2-507-7011
Telex: 27568 surfact

Taiyo Kagaku Co., Ltd.
9-5, Akahori-shinmachi
Yokkaichi-shi
Mie 510
Japan
Tel.: (0593) 52-2555
Telefax: (0593) 52-9312

Takasago International Corp.
19-22, Takanawa 3-chome
Minato-ku
Tokyo 108
Japan
Tel.: (03) 3442-1211
Telefax: (03) 3442-1285
Telex: TAKAS A J32508

Takasago International Corp.
11 Volvo Dr.
Rockleigh, NJ 07647
USA
Tel.: 201-767-9001
Telefax: 201-767-8062
Telex: 685-3936

Telechemische Inc.
222 Dupont Ave., #14
Newburgh, NY 12550
USA
Tel.: 914-561-3237
Telefax: 914-561-3622
Telex: 62954502 WU

Tenneco Chemicals, Inc.
Turner Place, PO Box 365
Piscataway, NJ 08854
USA
Tel.: 201-981-5000

Terry Laboratories
390 Wickham Rd. N.
Melbourne, FL 32932
USA
Tel.: 407-259-1630; 800-367-2563
Telefax: 407-242-0625

La Tessilchimica SpA. See Auschem SpA

Texaco Chemical Co
PO Box 27707
Houston, TX 77227
USA
Tel.: 713-961-3711; 800-231-3107
Telex: 227-031

Texaco Ltd
1 Knightsbrige Green
London SW1X 7QJ
UK
Tel.: 071-584 5000
Telefax: 071-584 6999
Telex: 8956681 TEXACO G

Texaco Chemical Deutschland GmbH
Baumwall 5
2000 Hamburg 11
Germany
Tel.: 011-49-40-36-3737

Texaco France S.A.
5, rue Bellini, Tour Arago
F-92806 Puteaux Cedex
France
Tel.: 011-33-1-47-78-1655

SA Texaco Belgium N.V.
Int'l. Congress Center, Citadel Park
B-900 Ghent
Belgium
Tel.: 011-32-91-41-5920

Texaco Olie Matschappij BV
Weena 170
NL-3012 CR Rotterdam
The Netherlands
Tel.: 614471
Telex: 31542

TIC Gums, Inc.
4609 Richlynn Dr.
Belcamp, MD 21017
USA
Tel.: 301-273-7300
Telefax: 301-273-6469
Telex: 221049

Toho Chemical Industry Co., Ltd.
No. 1-2-5, Ningyo-cho
Nihonbashi, Chuo-ku
Tokyo 103
Japan
Tel.: (03) 3668-2271
Telefax: (03) 3668-2278
Telex: 252-2332 TOHO K J

Tomah Div. See under Exxon

Tomen America Inc.
1800 Cross Beam Dr.
Charlotte, NC 28217
USA
Tel.: 704-357-0050
Telefax: 704-357-0057
Telex: WU800567

Tosoh Corp.
7-7 Akasaka 1-chome
Minato-ku
Tokyo 107
Japan
Tel.: (03) 3585-6707
Telefax: (03) 3582-7846
Telex: J24475tosoh

Tosoh USA Inc.
1100 Circle 75 Pkwy., Suite 600
Atlanta, GA 30339
USA
Tel.: 404-956-1100
Telefax: 404-956-7368
Telex: 542272 tosoh atl

Tosoh Canada Ltd.
1200 Sheppard Ave. East, Suite 511
Willowdale, Ontario M2K 2S5
Canada
Tel.: 416-756-2226
Telefax: 416-756-2750

Tosoh Europe BV
World Trade Centre Amsterdam, Tower C, Floor 13
Strawinskylaan 1351
1077 XX Amsterdam
The Netherlands

Tel.: 020-644026
020-623412
Telex: 18573tosoh nl

Thomas Triantaphyllou SA
405 Tatoiou Ave., TK 136 71, Acharnes
Athens
Greece
Tel.: 1-807-6413
Telex: 216370

Tri-K Industries, Inc.
27 Bland St.
PO Box 312
Emerson, NJ 07630
USA
Tel.: 201-261-2800; 800-526-0372
Telefax: 201-261-1432
Telex: 215085 TRIK UR

Trivent Chemical Co., Inc.
45 Ridge Rd.
PO Box 597
South River, NJ 08882
USA
Tel.: 908-251-1116
Telefax: 908-251-0967

Tsuno Rice Fine Chemicals Co., Ltd.
94 Shinden
Katsuragi-cho, Ito-gun
Wakayama-Ken
Japan
Tel.: 81-736-22-0061

Tulco, Inc.
9 Bishop Rd.
Ayer, MA 01432
USA
Tel.: 508-772-4412
Telefax: 508-772-1751

UCIB/Usines Chimiques D'Ivry-La-Bataille
Route D'Oulins
28260 Anet
France
Tel.: (33) 37 62 82 00
Telefax: (33) 37 41 91 32

Barnet Products, distributor
560 Sylvan Ave.
Englewood Cliffs, NJ 07632
USA
Tel.: 201-569-6622
Telefax: 201-569-8847

SST Corp., distributor
635 Brighton Rd.
PO Box 1649
Clifton, NJ 07015
USA
Tel.: 201-473-4300
Telefax: 201-473-4326
Telex: RCA 219149

Unger Fabrikker AS
PO Boks 254
N-1601 Fredrikstad
Norway
Tel.: 9-32-0020
Telefax: 9-32-3775
Telex: 76382 unger n

Unichema International
Postbus 309
NL-2800 AH Gouda
The Netherlands
Tel.: 1820-42933
Telefax: 1820-26877

Unichema North America
4650 S. Racine Ave.
Chicago, IL 60609
USA
Tel.: 312-376-9000; 800-833-2864
Telefax: 312-376-0095
Telex: 176068

Unichema Chemicals Ltd
Bebington
Wirral, Merseycide L62 4UF
UK
Tel.: 051-645-2020
Telefax: 051-645-9197
Telex: 629408

Unichema Chemie GmbH
Postfach 1280
Steintor 9
D-4240 Emmerich
Germany
Tel.: 2822-720
Telefax: 2822-72276
Telex: 8125113

Unichema France SA
148 Boulevard Haussemann
75008 Paris
France
Tel.: 1 45630863
Telefax: 1 42563188
Telex: 643217

Unichema Chemie BV
Postbus 2
NL-2800 AA Gouda
The Netherlands
Tel.: 1820-42911
Telefax: 1820-42250

Unichema Japan
Sankei Bldg. 7F 708
4-9, Umeda 2-chome, Kita-ku
Osaka 530
Japan
Tel.: 6341-7221
Telefax: 6341-7725

Union Camp Corp.
1600 Valley Rd.
Wayne, NJ 07470
USA
Tel.: 201-628-2680; 800-628-9220
Telex: 130735

Union Carbide Chem. & Plastics Co. Inc./ Specialty Chem. Div.
39 Old Ridgebury Rd. H2375
Danbury, CT 06817-0001
USA
Tel.: 203-794-2000; 800-568-4000

Union Carbide Specialty Powders
1555 Main St.
PO Box 24184
Indianapolis, IN 46224
USA

Tel.: 317-240-2187
Telefax: 317-240-2225
Telex: 27413 SPZ

Union Carbide Canada Ltd.
10455 Metropolitan E.
Montreal East
Quebec
H1B 1A1
Canada
Tel.: 514-493-2610

Union Carbide (UK) Ltd/Chemicals & Plastics
93/95 High Street
Rickmansworth
Herts WD3 1RB
UK
Tel.: 0923-720 366
Telefax: 0923-896721

Union Carbide Europe S.A.
15 Chemin Louis-Dunant
CH-1211 Geneve 20
Switzerland
Tel.: 22-739-6111
Telefax: 22-739-6545
Telex: 419207

Union Carbide Japan KK
Toranomon 45 Mori Bldg.
1-5 Toranomon, 5-Chome Minato-Ku
Tokyo 105
Japan
Tel.: 3431-7281

United Catalysts Inc.
PO Box 32370
Louisville, KY 40232
USA
Tel.: 502-634-7500; 800-468-7210
Telefax: 502-637-3732
Telex: 204190, 204239

United Coconut Chemicals, Inc./Cocochem
UCPB Bldg., 17th Fl., Makat Ave., Makati
Metro Manila
Philippines
Tel.: 818-8361
Telefax: (00632) 817-2251
Telex: 66928 COCOCHEM PN

Unitex Chemical Corp.
PO Box 16344
520 Broome Rd.
Greensboro, NC 27406
USA
Tel.: 919-378-0965
Telefax: 919-272-4312

Unitex Ltd
Halfpenny Lane
Knaresborough
North Yorkshire HG5 0PP
UK
Tel.: 0423-862677
Telefax: 0423-868340
Telex: 57884

U. S. Cosmetics
313 Lake Rd.
PO Box 859
Dayville, CT 06241
USA
Tel.: 203-779-3990; 800-752-0490
Telefax: 203-779-3994

Universal Preserv-A-Chem Inc/UPI
297 North 7th St.
Brooklyn, NY 11211
USA
Tel.: 718-782-7429

UOP
777 Old Saw Mill River Rd.
Tarrytown, NY 10591-6799
USA
Tel.: 914-789-2246
Telefax: 914-789-2279

UPI. *See Universal Preserv-A-Chem, Inc.*

Ursa-Chemie GmbH
Am Alten Galgen 14
56410 Montabaur
Germany
Tel.: 02602-92160
Telefax: 02602-921624

Van Den Bergh Foods Co.
2200 Cabot Dr.
Lisle, IL 60532
USA
Tel.: 708-955-5276; 800-325-7286
Telefax: 708-955-5497

R.T. Vanderbilt Co Inc
30 Winfield St
PO Box 5150
Norwalk, CT 06856
USA
Tel.: 203-853-1400; 800-243-6064
Telefax: 203-853-1452
Telex: 6813581 RTVAN

Van Dyk. *See ISP Van Dyk*

Van Schuppen Chemie. *See Solvay Duphar BV*

Variati & Co., S.p.A.
Via Pestalozza 16
20131 Milano
Italy
Tel.: 02/2663755
Telefax: 02/2663294

Vevy Europe SpA
Via P. Semeria 18
PO Box 716
I-16131 Genova
Italy
Tel.: 010-5221212
Telefax: 010-5221530
Telex: 281257 Vevy-1

Vevy
366 N. Broadway, Suite 310
Jericho, NY 11753
USA
Tel.: 516-333-9554
Telefax: 516-333-3976

Vista Chemical Co.
900 Threadneedle
PO Box 19029
Houston, TX 77224-9029
USA
Tel.: 713-588-3000; 800-231-8216
Telefax: 713-588-3236
Telex: 794557

Vista Chemical Europe
Hilton Tower, Blvd. de Waterloo #39
B-81000 Brussels
Belgium
Tel.: 2-513-7490

Vitamins, Inc.
200 E. Randolph Dr.
Chicago, IL 60601
USA
Tel.: 312-861-0700
Telefax: 312-861-0708
Telex: 25 4717

Vulcan Materials Co./Chemicals Div.
PO Box 530390
Birmingham, AL 35253-0390
USA
Tel.: 205-877-3000
Telefax: 205-877-3448

Wacker-Chemie GmbH
Div S, Hanns-Seidel-Platz 4
D-81737 München
Germany
Tel.: (089) 62 79 01
Telefax: (089) 62791771
Telex: 52912156

Wacker Chemicals (USA) Inc.
535 Connecticut Ave.
Norwalk, CT 06854
USA
Tel.: 203-866-9400
Telefax: 203-866-9427
Telex: 643 444

Wacker Silicones Corp.
Subsid of Wacker-Chemie
3301 Sutton Rd.
Adrian, MI 49221-9397
USA
Tel.: 517-264-8500; 800-248-0063
Telefax: 517-264-8246
Telex: 510-450-2700 sadrnud

Wacker Química do Brasil Ltda.
Avenida Adolfo Pinheiro
2056-9° Andar, Santo Amaro
04734-003 Sao Paulo-SP
Brazil
Tel.: (011) 548 81 33
Telefax: (011) 2 46 99 75
Telex: 1 156 946 wack br

Wacker Chemicals Ltd
The Clock Tower, Mount Felix
Bridge Street, Walton-on-Thames
Surrey KT12 1AS
UK
Tel.: 0932-246111
Telefax: 0932-240141
Telex: 28 391 wacker g

Wacker Quimica Ibérica SA
Div of Wacker-Chemie GmbH
Corcega, 303-2° 3a
E-08008 Barcelona
Spain
Tel.: (93)-217 59 00
Telefax: (93)-217 57 66
Telex: 97801 wqsa e

Wacker Chemie Danmark A/S
Hovedvejen 91
DK-2600 Glostrop
Denmark
Tel.: (43) 43 03 00
Telefax: (43) 43 03 16

Wacker Chemicals Australia Pty. Ltd.
PO Box 4337
Melbourne, Victoria 3004
Australia
Tel.: (03) 525 16 00
Telefax: (03) 521 27 43
Telex: 30 367 hoechst aa

Wacker Chemicals East Asia Ltd.
Thoma Nishi-Waseda Bldg.
2-14-1, Nishi Waseda, Shinjuku-ku
Tokyo 169
Japan
Tel.: (03)52 72 31 21
Telefax: (03) 52 72 31 40

Wackherr. *See Les Colorants Wackherr*

Waitaki Int'l. Biosciences
Tri-K Industries, Inc., distributor
27 Bland St.
PO Box 312
Emerson, NJ 07630
USA
Tel.: 201-261-2800; 800-526-0372
Telefax: 201-261-1432
Telex: 215085 TRIK UR

Warren Laboratories, Inc.
12603 Executive Dr., Suite 806
Stafford, TX 77477
USA
Tel.: 713-240-2563

Westbrook Lanolin Co.
Argonaut Works, Laisterdyke
Bradford, West Yorkshire BD4 8AU
UK
Tel.: 0274-663331
Telefax: 0274-667665
Telex: 51502

Westvaco Chemical Div.
PO Box 70848
Charleston Hts., SC 29415-0848
USA
Tel.: 803-740-2300; 800-336-2211
Telefax: 803-747-2270
Telex: 4611159

Westwood Chemical Corp.
46 Tower Dr.
Middletown, NY 10940
USA
Tel.: 914-692-6721
Telefax: 914-695-1906

Weyerhaeuser Co.
STC 1K39
Tacoma, WA 98477
USA
Tel.: 206-924-4330
Telefax: 206-924-4395

Whittaker, Clark & Daniels
1000 Coolidge St.
South Plainfield, NJ 07080
USA
Tel.: 908-561-6100; 800-833-8139
Telefax: 908-757-3488
Telex: 221478

Will & Baumer, Inc.
PO Box 4880
Syracuse, NY 13221
USA
Tel.: 315-451-1000
Telefax: 315-451-0120

Witco Corp/Household, Industrial, Personal Care
520 Madison Ave.
New York, NY 10022
USA
Tel.: 212-605-3680
Telefax: 212-486-4198

Witco Canada Ltd
2 Lansing Sq., Suite 1200
Willowdale, Ontario M2J 4Z4
Canada
Tel.: 416-497-9991

Witco Chemical Ltd (UK)
Union Lane, Droitwich
Worcester WR9 9BB
UK

Witco BV
1 Canalside
Lowesmoor Wharf
Worcester, Worcestershire WR1 2RS
UK
Tel.: 0905-21521
Telefax: 0905-611593

Rewo Chemische Werke GmbH
Postfach 1160, 36392 Steinau an der Strasse
Max Wolf Strasse 7, Industriegebiet West
W-6497 Steinau
Germany
Tel.: 06663-540
Telefax: 06663-54-129
Telex: 493589

Witco SA
10 Rue Cambaceres
75008 Paris
France
Tel.: 42-65-99-03
Telefax: 42-65-67-61
Telex: 290233

Witco BV
PO Box 5
NL-1540 LZ Koog aan de Zaan
The Netherlands
Tel.: 75-283854
Telefax: 75-210811
Telex: 19270

Witco Ltd
PO Box 10245
26112 Haifa Bay
Israel

Tel.: 04-469-111
Telefax: 04-469-137
Telex: 45198

Witco Corp/Argus Chem. Div.
Bussey Rd., PO Box 1439
Marshall, TX 75671-1439
USA
Tel.: 903-938-5141; 800-431-1413
Telefax: 903-938-2647

Witco Corp/Petroleum Specialty
520 Madison Ave.
New York, NY 10022-4236
USA
Tel.: 212-605-3972
Telefax: 212-754-5676
Telex: 62470

Zeeland Chemicals, Inc
A Cambrex Co.
215 N. Centennial St.
Zeeland, MI 49464
USA
Tel.: 616-772-2193; 800-223-0453
Telefax: 616-772-7344
Telex: 226375

Zinc Corp. of America
300 Frankfort Rd.
Monaca, PA 15061
USA
Tel.: 412-774-1020; 800-962-7500
Telefax: 412-773-2269

Zohar Detergent Factory
PO Box 11 300
Tel-Aviv 61 112
Israel
Tel.: 03-528-7236
Telefax: 03-5287239
Telex: 33557 zohar il

Zschimmer & Schwarz GmbH & Co.
Postfach 2179
D-5420 Lahnstein/Rhein
Germany
Tel.: 2621 121
Telefax: 2621-12407
Telex: 869816 ZSO D

Zschimmer & Schwarz SARL
10 rue Saint-Marc
F-75002 Paris
France
Tel.: 42 33 10 33
Telefax: 40 26 23 81
Telex: 670465 ZS F

Zschimmer & Schwarz Italiana SpA
Casella Postale 1
I-13038 Tricerro (Vc)
Italy
Tel.: 161-82 14 21
Telex: 200313 ZSI I

Zschimmer & Schwarz Argentina S.A.
Bdo. de Irigoyen 556-5 B
Buenos Aires
Argentina

Appendices

Appendices

CAS Number-to-Trade Name
Cross-Reference

CAS numbers reference specific chemicals or chemical groups. Trade name products are associated with CAS numbers through their major chemical constituent.

CAS 50-21-5	Patlac® LA	CAS 56-81-5	Glycon® G 100
CAS 50-21-5	Unichem LACA	CAS 56-81-5	Glycon® G-300
CAS 50-70-4	A-641	CAS 56-81-5	Kemstrene® 96.0% USP
CAS 50-70-4	Arlex	CAS 56-81-5	Kemstrene® 99.7% USP
CAS 50-70-4	Fancol SORB	CAS 56-81-5	Optim
CAS 50-70-4	Hefti Sorbex-R	CAS 56-81-5	Star
CAS 50-70-4	Hefti Sorbex-RP	CAS 56-81-5	Superol
CAS 50-70-4	Hydex® 100 Gran. 206	CAS 56-81-5	Unichem GLYC
CAS 50-70-4	Hydex® Coarse Powd.	CAS 56-86-0	Unamino GLUT
CAS 50-70-4	Hydex® Powd. 60	CAS 56-89-3	Unamino L-CSTI
CAS 50-70-4	Hydex® Tablet Grade	CAS 57-09-0	Acetoquat CTAB
CAS 50-70-4	Liponic 70-NC	CAS 57-09-0	Bromat®
CAS 50-70-4	Liponic 76-NC	CAS 57-09-0	Catinal HTB-70
CAS 50-70-4	Liponic 83-NC	CAS 57-09-0	Cetrimide
CAS 50-70-4	Liposorb 70	CAS 57-09-0	Cetrimide™ BP
CAS 50-70-4	Sorbelite™ C	CAS 57-09-0	Rhodaquat® M242B/99
CAS 50-70-4	Sorbelite™ FG	CAS 57-09-0	Sumquat® 6030
CAS 50-70-4	Sorbo®	CAS 57-09-0	Varisoft® CTB-40
CAS 50-70-4	Unisweet 70	CAS 57-10-3	Adeka PA Series
CAS 50-70-4	Unisweet 70/CONC.	CAS 57-10-3	Crodacid PD3160
CAS 50-70-4	Unisweet CONC.	CAS 57-10-3	Edenor L2SM
CAS 50-81-7	Ascorbic Acid Ampul Type No. 604065700	CAS 57-10-3	Emersol® 142
		CAS 57-10-3	Emersol® 143
CAS 50-81-7	Ascorbic Acid Fine Granular No. 6045655	CAS 57-10-3	Emersol® 144
		CAS 57-10-3	Hystrene® 7016
CAS 50-81-7	Ascorbic Acid Ultra-Fine Powd. No. 604565300	CAS 57-10-3	Hystrene® 9016
		CAS 57-10-3	Kartacid 1692
CAS 50-81-7	Ascorbic Acid USP, FCC Type S No. 604566	CAS 57-10-3	Prifrac 2960
		CAS 57-10-3	Unifat 16
CAS 50-81-7	Uantox ASCA	CAS 57-11-4	Cetax TP
CAS 50-81-7	Vitazyme® C	CAS 57-11-4	Crosterene SA4310
CAS 50-99-7	Candex® Plus	CAS 57-11-4	Emersol® 110
CAS 50-99-7	Emdex® Plus	CAS 57-11-4	Emersol® 120
CAS 51-05-8	Unicaine-B	CAS 57-11-4	Emersol® 132 NF Lily®
CAS 51-81-0	Rodol EGC	CAS 57-11-4	Emersol® 150
CAS 52-51-7	Bronopol	CAS 57-11-4	Emersol® 6320
CAS 52-51-7	CoSept BNP	CAS 57-11-4	Emersol® 6332 NF
CAS 52-51-7	Lexgard® Bronopol	CAS 57-11-4	Emersol® 6349
CAS 52-51-7	Midpol 97	CAS 57-11-4	Emersol® 6351
CAS 52-51-7	Midpol 100	CAS 57-11-4	Hy-Phi 1199
CAS 52-51-7	Myacide® BT	CAS 57-11-4	Hy-Phi 1303
CAS 52-51-7	Tristat BNP	CAS 57-11-4	Hy-Phi 1401
CAS 52-90-4	Unamino L-CSTE	CAS 57-11-4	Hystrene® 4516
CAS 55-55-0	Rodol PM	CAS 57-11-4	Hystrene® 5016 NF
CAS 56-37-1	Sumquat® 2355	CAS 57-11-4	Hystrene® 9718 NF
CAS 56-40-6	Hampshire® Glycine	CAS 57-11-4	Industrene® 9018
CAS 56-40-6	Unamino GLCN	CAS 57-11-4	Kartacid 1890
CAS 56-81-5	Croderol GA 7000	CAS 57-11-4	Koster Keunen Stearic Acid XXX
CAS 56-81-5	Emery® 912	CAS 57-11-4	Prifrac 2980
CAS 56-81-5	Emery® 916	CAS 57-11-4	Prifrac 2981
CAS 56-81-5	Emery® 917	CAS 57-11-4	Pristerene 4904
CAS 56-81-5	Emery® 918	CAS 57-11-4	Pristerene 4905

CAS 57-11-4	Pristerene 4910	CAS 75-37-6	Dymel® 152a
CAS 57-11-4	Pristerene 4911	CAS 75-37-6	Genetron® 152a
CAS 57-11-4	Pristerene 4915	CAS 75-45-6	Dymel® 22
CAS 57-11-4	Pristerene 4921	CAS 75-52-5	NM
CAS 57-11-4	Radiacid® 152	CAS 75-68-3	Dymel® 142b
CAS 57-11-4	Radiacid® 416	CAS 76-22-2	Unichem CAMP
CAS 57-11-4	Radiacid® 423	CAS 77-86-1	Tris Amino®
CAS 57-11-4	Radiacid® 427	CAS 77-89-4	ATEC
CAS 57-11-4	Radiacid® 428	CAS 77-90-7	ATBC
CAS 57-11-4	Radiacid® 464	CAS 77-90-7	Citroflex A-4
CAS 57-11-4	Unifat 54	CAS 77-90-7	Uniplex 84
CAS 57-11-4	Unifat 55L	CAS 77-92-9	Anhydrous Citric Acid
CAS 57-13-6	Unichem UREA	CAS 77-92-9	Citric Acid USP FCC (Anhyd.) Fine
CAS 57-15-8	Unisept Chlorbut		Gran. No. 69941
CAS 57-55-6	Adeka Propylene Glycol (P)	CAS 77-92-9	Citrid Acid USP Fine Granular No.
CAS 57-55-6	Unichem PROP-G		69941
CAS 57-88-5	Atomergic Cholesterol	CAS 77-92-9	Unichem CIT-A
CAS 57-88-5	Cholesterol	CAS 77-93-0	Crodamol TC
CAS 57-88-5	Cholesterol BP	CAS 77-93-0	Hydagen® C.A.T
CAS 57-88-5	Cholesterol NF	CAS 77-93-0	TEC
CAS 57-88-5	Fancol CH	CAS 77-93-0	Uniflex TEC
CAS 57-88-5	Liquid Crystal CN/9	CAS 77-94-1	Crodamol TBC
CAS 57-88-5	Loralan-CH	CAS 77-94-1	TBC
CAS 57-88-5	Unichol	CAS 77-94-1	Uniflex TBC
CAS 59-02-9	Eastman® Vitamin E 5-40	CAS 78-21-7	Barquat® CME-35
CAS 59-02-9	Eastman® Vitamin E 5-67	CAS 78-66-0	Surfynol® 82
CAS 59-67-6	Niacin USP, FCC No. 69902	CAS 79-63-0	Croda Lanosterol
CAS 60-00-4	Hamp-Ene® Acid	CAS 79-63-0	Lanosterol
CAS 60-00-4	Kelate Acid	CAS 79-81-2	Aquapalm No. 63841
CAS 60-00-4	Sequestrene® AA	CAS 80-73-9	Nikkol DMI
CAS 60-00-4	Universene ACID	CAS 81-07-2	Unisweet SAC
CAS 60-00-4	Versene Acid	CAS 81-13-0	Ritapan D
CAS 60-12-8	Etaphen	CAS 81-13-0	R.I.T.A. d-Panthenol
CAS 60-33-3	Emersol® 315	CAS 84-66-2	Estol DEP 3075
CAS 62-33-9	Hampene® CaNa₂ Pure Crystals	CAS 84-66-2	Ftalato 2/46
CAS 62-33-9	Kelate CDS	CAS 84-66-2	Kodaflex® DEP
CAS 62-33-9	Universene CaNa2	CAS 84-66-2	Palatinol® A
CAS 62-33-9	Versene CA	CAS 84-66-2	Uniflex DEP
CAS 63-42-3	Unisweet L	CAS 84-74-2	Kodaflex® DBP
CAS 63-42-3	Unisweet Lactose	CAS 84-74-2	Uniflex DBP
CAS 64-02-8	Chelon 100	CAS 84-74-2	Uniplex 150
CAS 64-02-8	Hamp-Ene® 100	CAS 87-66-1	Rodol PG
CAS 64-02-8	Hamp-Ene® 220	CAS 87-89-8	Inositol
CAS 64-02-8	Hamp-Ene® Na₄	CAS 88-04-0	Nipacide® MX
CAS 64-02-8	Kelate 220	CAS 88-04-0	Nipacide® PX-R
CAS 64-02-8	Sequestrene® 220	CAS 88-41-5	Beldox
CAS 64-02-8	Universene Na4	CAS 89-65-6	Uantox EBATE
CAS 64-02-8	Versene 100	CAS 89-78-1	Fancol Menthol
CAS 64-02-8	Versene 100 EP	CAS 89-78-1	Nanospheres 100 Menthol
CAS 64-02-8	Versene 100 LS	CAS 89-78-1	Universal MENT
CAS 64-02-8	Versene 100 SRG	CAS 89-83-8	Unichem THYMOL
CAS 64-02-8	Versene 100 XL	CAS 90-43-7	Dowicide 1
CAS 64-02-8	Versene 220	CAS 91-68-9	Rodol DEMAP
CAS 64-19-7	Unichem ACETA	CAS 92-44-4	Rodol 23N
CAS 65-85-0	Benzoic Acid Powd. No. 130	CAS 93-82-3	Alkamide® DS-280/S
CAS 65-85-0	Unisept BZA	CAS 93-82-3	Alkamide® HTDE
CAS 67-43-6	Chel DTPA	CAS 93-82-3	Amidox SE
CAS 67-43-6	Hamp-Ex® Acid	CAS 93-82-3	Hetamide DS
CAS 68-04-2	Sodium Citrate USP, FCC	CAS 93-82-3	Lipamide S
	(Dihydrate) Fine Gran. No. 69975	CAS 93-82-3	Monamid® 718
CAS 68-04-2	Unichem SODCIT	CAS 93-82-3	Olamida ED
CAS 68-11-1	Thiovanic® Acid	CAS 93-82-3	Protamide SA
CAS 69-65-8	Unisweet MAN	CAS 93-82-3	Upamide SD
CAS 69-72-7	Unichem SALAC	CAS 93-83-4	Alkamide® DO-280/S
CAS 71-36-3	Nacol® 4-99	CAS 93-83-4	Amidex O
CAS 71-55-6	Aerothene TT	CAS 93-83-4	Carsamide® O
CAS 71-55-6	Solvent 111	CAS 93-83-4	Chimipal OLD
CAS 72-17-3	Patlac® NAL	CAS 93-83-4	Comperlan® OD
CAS 72-17-3	Unichem SOLAC	CAS 93-83-4	Crillon ODE
CAS 73-40-5	Dew Pearl TS-1	CAS 93-83-4	Hetamide OC

CAS 93-83-4	Lauridit® OD
CAS 93-83-4	Loropan OD
CAS 93-83-4	Mackamide™ MO
CAS 93-83-4	Mackamide™ NOA
CAS 93-83-4	Mackamide™ O
CAS 93-83-4	Marlamid® D 1885
CAS 93-83-4	Mazamide® O 20
CAS 93-83-4	Ninol® 201
CAS 93-83-4	Nissan Stafoam DO, DOS
CAS 93-83-4	Rewomid® DO 280 SE
CAS 93-83-4	Schercomid SO-A
CAS 93-83-4	Upamide O-20
CAS 93-83-4	Upamide OD
CAS 93-83-4	Varamide® A-7
CAS 93-83-4	Witcamide® 5085
CAS 94-13-3	Bentex P
CAS 94-13-3	CoSept P
CAS 94-13-3	Lexgard® P
CAS 94-13-3	Nipasol M
CAS 94-13-3	Paridol P
CAS 94-13-3	Preserval P
CAS 94-13-3	Propyl-Steriline
CAS 94-13-3	Trisept P
CAS 94-13-3	Unisept P
CAS 94-13-3	Unisept PNA
CAS 94-18-8	Nipabenzyl
CAS 94-18-8	Unisept BZ
CAS 94-26-8	Butylparaben NF
CAS 94-26-8	Butyl Parasept
CAS 94-26-8	CoSept B
CAS 94-26-8	Lexgard® B
CAS 94-26-8	Nipabutyl
CAS 94-26-8	Paridol B
CAS 94-26-8	Preserval B
CAS 94-26-8	Preserval Butylique
CAS 94-26-8	Trisept B
CAS 94-26-8	Unisept B
CAS 94-44-0	Benzyl Nicotinate No. 6752
CAS 94-51-9	Uniflex 9-88
CAS 95-38-5	Schercozoline O
CAS 95-55-6	Rodol 2G
CAS 95-88-5	Rodol CRS
CAS 96-20-8	AB®
CAS 96-26-4	Dihydroxyacetone
CAS 96-26-4	Nanospheres 100 Dihydroxy-acetone
CAS 96-27-5	Thiovanol®
CAS 96-48-0	GBL
CAS 97-23-4	Preventol GD
CAS 97-59-6	Allantoin
CAS 97-59-6	Allantoin Powd. No. 1015
CAS 97-59-6	Atomergic Allantoin
CAS 97-59-6	Chemie Linz Allantoin
CAS 97-59-6	Fancol TOIN
CAS 97-59-6	Tri-K Allantoin
CAS 97-59-6	Uniderm A
CAS 97-63-2	Rohagum® N-742
CAS 97-78-9	Crodasinic L
CAS 97-78-9	Hamposyl® L
CAS 97-78-9	Nikkol Sarcosinate LH
CAS 97-78-9	Oramix L
CAS 97-78-9	Sarkosyl® L
CAS 97-78-9	Vanseal® LS
CAS 97-86-9	Rohagum® P-26
CAS 97-86-9	Rohagum® P-28
CAS 97-86-9	Rohagum® P-675
CAS 97-86-9	Rohagum® PQ-610
CAS 97-88-1	Rohagum® P-24
CAS 97-88-1	Rohasol® P-550
CAS 98-79-3	Ajidew A-100
CAS 98-79-3	Pidolidone®
CAS 98-92-0	Niacinamide USP, FCC No. 69905
CAS 98-92-0	Vitazyme® B3
CAS 99-56-9	Rodol 4J
CAS 99-76-3	Aseptoform
CAS 99-76-3	Bentex M
CAS 99-76-3	CoSept M
CAS 99-76-3	Lexgard® M
CAS 99-76-3	Methyl-Steriline
CAS 99-76-3	Nipagin M
CAS 99-76-3	Paridol M
CAS 99-76-3	Preserval M
CAS 99-76-3	Trisept M
CAS 99-76-3	Unisept M
CAS 100-51-6	Unichem BZAL
CAS 101-34-8	Naturechem® GTR
CAS 101-54-2	Rodol Gray B Base
CAS 102-60-3	Mazeen® 173
CAS 102-60-3	Mazeen® 174
CAS 102-60-3	Mazeen® 174-75
CAS 102-60-3	Neutrol® TE
CAS 102-71-6	Alkanolamine 144
CAS 102-71-6	Alkanolamine 244
CAS 102-71-6	Alkanolamine 244 Low Freeze Grade
CAS 102-71-6	TEA 85 Low Freeze Grade
CAS 102-71-6	TEA 99 Low Freeze Grade
CAS 102-71-6	TEA 99 Standard Grade
CAS 102-71-6	Trolamine 85 NF Grade
CAS 102-71-6	Trolamine 99 NF Grade
CAS 102-71-6	Unichem TEA
CAS 102-76-1	Priacetin
CAS 102-76-1	Unitolate GTA
CAS 102-87-4	Armeen® 3-12
CAS 103-23-1	Crodamol DOA
CAS 103-23-1	Kodaflex® DOA
CAS 103-23-1	Wickenol® 158
CAS 103-95-7	Cyclosal
CAS 104-15-4	Eltesol® TSX/A
CAS 104-15-4	Eltesol® TSX/SF
CAS 104-15-4	Witconate™ TX Acid
CAS 104-29-0	Elestab® CPN
CAS 104-67-6	Aldehyde C 14 Soc. Peach (3/010811)
CAS 104-74-5	Dehyquart® C
CAS 104-74-5	Dehyquart® C Crystals
CAS 104-74-5	Uniquart C
CAS 104-75-6	Armeen® L8D
CAS 105-62-4	Cithrol PGDO
CAS 105-62-4	Emalex PG-di-O
CAS 105-95-3	Emeressence® 1150
CAS 105-97-5	Hodag DCA
CAS 105-97-5	Kessco® DCA
CAS 105-99-7	Cetiol® B
CAS 105-99-7	Unitolate B
CAS 105-99-7	Upamate DBA
CAS 106-01-4	Dermol 499
CAS 106-01-4	Fractalite 499
CAS 106-11-6	Alkamuls® SDG
CAS 106-11-6	Emalex DEG-m-S
CAS 106-11-6	Estol DEMS 3710
CAS 106-11-6	Glicosterina DPG
CAS 106-11-6	Hefti DMS-33
CAS 106-11-6	Hodag DGS-N
CAS 106-11-6	Kemester® 5221
CAS 106-11-6	Kessco® Diethylene Glycol Monostearate
CAS 106-11-6	Kessco® Diglycol Stearate Neutral
CAS 106-11-6	Lipopeg 1-S
CAS 106-11-6	Nikkol DEGS

CAS 106-11-6	Nikkol MYS-2
CAS 106-11-6	Pegosperse® 100-S
CAS 106-11-6	Protachem DGS
CAS 106-11-6	Protachem DGS-C
CAS 106-11-6	Rol DGE
CAS 106-11-6	Witconol™ CAD
CAS 106-12-7	Cithrol DEGMO
CAS 106-12-7	Emalex 200
CAS 106-12-7	Hetoxamate MO-2
CAS 106-12-7	Hodag DGO
CAS 106-12-7	Lipopeg 1-O
CAS 106-12-7	Nikkol MYO-2
CAS 106-12-7	Pegosperse® 100 O
CAS 106-12-7	Witconol™ DOSS
CAS 106-14-9	HSA
CAS 106-16-1	Emid® 6573
CAS 106-16-1	Rewomid® R 280
CAS 106-17-2	Flexricin® 15
CAS 106-19-4	Estalan DNPA
CAS 106-19-4	Pelemol DNPA
CAS 106-50-3	Rodol D
CAS 106-98-9	Ethyl Butene-1
CAS 106-98-9	Gulftene® 4
CAS 107-21-1	Jeffersol DE-75
CAS 107-46-0	Rhodorsil® Oils 70041 VO.65
CAS 107-64-2	Ablumine DHT75
CAS 107-64-2	Arosurf® TA-100
CAS 107-64-2	Arosurf® TA-101
CAS 107-64-2	Dehyquart® DAM
CAS 107-64-2	Genamin DSAC
CAS 107-64-2	Kemamine® Q-9902C
CAS 107-64-2	Nikkol CA-3475
CAS 107-64-2	Protaquat 2HT-75
CAS 107-64-2	Sumquat® 6045
CAS 107-64-2	Varisoft® TA-100
CAS 108-46-3	Rodol RS
CAS 108-46-3	Unichem RSC
CAS 108-65-6	Ektasolve® PM Acetate
CAS 109-28-4	Chemidex O
CAS 109-28-4	Incromine OPM
CAS 109-28-4	Lexamine O-13
CAS 109-28-4	Mackine™ 501
CAS 109-28-4	Schercodine O
CAS 109-28-4	Unizeen OA
CAS 109-30-8	Emalex DEG-di-S
CAS 110-25-8	Crodasinic O
CAS 110-25-8	Hamposyl® O
CAS 110-25-8	Nikkol Sarcosinate OH
CAS 110-25-8	Oramix O
CAS 110-25-8	Vanseal OS
CAS 110-27-0	Crodamol IPM
CAS 110-27-0	Deltyl® Extra
CAS 110-27-0	Elfacos® IPM
CAS 110-27-0	Emerest® 2314
CAS 110-27-0	Estol 1512
CAS 110-27-0	Estol 1514
CAS 110-27-0	Estol IPM 1508
CAS 110-27-0	Estol IPM 1509 (BIO-IPM)
CAS 110-27-0	Estol IPM 1512
CAS 110-27-0	Estol IPM 1514
CAS 110-27-0	Estol IPM-b 1509
CAS 110-27-0	Isopropylmyristat
CAS 110-27-0	Jafaester 14-96
CAS 110-27-0	Jafaester 14 NF
CAS 110-27-0	Kessco® Isopropyl Myristate
CAS 110-27-0	Kessco® Isopropyl Myristate NF
CAS 110-27-0	Lanesta 31
CAS 110-27-0	Lexol® IPM
CAS 110-27-0	Lexol® IPM-NF
CAS 110-27-0	Liponate IPM
CAS 110-27-0	Nikkol IPM-100
CAS 110-27-0	Nikkol IPM-EX
CAS 110-27-0	Promyr
CAS 110-27-0	Protachem IPM
CAS 110-27-0	Radia® 7190
CAS 110-27-0	Radia® 7730
CAS 110-27-0	Tegosoft® M
CAS 110-27-0	Upamate IPM
CAS 110-27-0	Wickenol® 101
CAS 110-27-0	Witconol™ 2314
CAS 110-30-5	Kemamide® W-35
CAS 110-30-5	Kemamide® W-42
CAS 110-36-1	Bumyr
CAS 110-36-1	Crodamol BM
CAS 110-36-1	Nikkol BM
CAS 110-36-1	Wickenol® 141
CAS 110-40-7	Nikkol DES-SP
CAS 110-44-1	Tristat
CAS 110-44-1	Unistat
CAS 110-44-1	Unistat SORBA
CAS 110-80-5	Cellosolve®
CAS 110-91-8	Unamine-MORP
CAS 110-97-4	DIPA Commercial Grade
CAS 110-97-4	DIPA Low Freeze Grade 85
CAS 110-97-4	DIPA Low Freeze Grade 90
CAS 110-97-4	DIPA NF Grade
CAS 110-97-4	Unichem DIPA
CAS 111-01-3	Carolane
CAS 111-01-3	Cosbiol
CAS 111-01-3	Dermane
CAS 111-01-3	Fitoderm
CAS 111-01-3	Nikkol Squalane
CAS 111-01-3	Prisorine SQS 3758
CAS 111-01-3	Robane®
CAS 111-02-4	Dermene
CAS 111-02-4	Nikkol Squalene EX
CAS 111-02-4	Squatol S
CAS 111-02-4	Supraene®
CAS 111-03-5	Aldo® MO
CAS 111-03-5	Capmul® GMO
CAS 111-03-5	Cithrol GMO N/E
CAS 111-03-5	Kemester® 2000
CAS 111-03-5	Kessco® Glycerol Monoleate
CAS 111-03-5	Mazol® 300 K
CAS 111-03-5	Mazol® GMO
CAS 111-03-5	Mazol® GMO K
CAS 111-03-5	Monomuls® 90-O18
CAS 111-03-5	Radiasurf® 7152
CAS 111-03-5	Witconol™ 2421
CAS 111-05-7	Rewomid® IPE 280
CAS 111-05-7	Schercomid OMI
CAS 111-15-9	Cellosolve® Acetate
CAS 111-27-3	Nacol® 6-98
CAS 111-30-8	Ucarcide® 225
CAS 111-30-8	Ucarcide® 250
CAS 111-42-2	DEA Commercial Grade
CAS 111-42-2	DEA Low Freeze Grade
CAS 111-42-2	Unichem DEA
CAS 111-46-6	Unichem DEG
CAS 111-57-9	Ablumide SME
CAS 111-57-9	Alkamide® S-280
CAS 111-57-9	Amidex SME
CAS 111-57-9	CPH-380-N
CAS 111-57-9	Hetamide MS
CAS 111-57-9	Incromide SM
CAS 111-57-9	Mackamide™ SMA
CAS 111-57-9	Mazamide® SMEA
CAS 111-57-9	Monamid® S
CAS 111-57-9	Monamid® S/M
CAS 111-57-9	Olamida SM

CAS 111-57-9	Phoenamid SM
CAS 111-57-9	Rewomid® S 280
CAS 111-57-9	Upamide SME-M
CAS 111-57-9	Witcamide® 70
CAS 111-57-9	Witcamide® 6507
CAS 111-58-0	Hetamide MO
CAS 111-58-0	Incromide OPM
CAS 111-58-0	Schercomid OME
CAS 111-60-4	Ablunol EGMS
CAS 111-60-4	Alkamuls® EGMS
CAS 111-60-4	Alkamuls® EGMS/C
CAS 111-60-4	Alkamuls® SEG
CAS 111-60-4	Cerasynt® M
CAS 111-60-4	Chemsperse EGMS
CAS 111-60-4	CPH-37-NA
CAS 111-60-4	Dragil 2/027011
CAS 111-60-4	Elfacos® EGMS
CAS 111-60-4	Emalex EGS-A
CAS 111-60-4	Emalex EGS-B
CAS 111-60-4	Emerest® 2350
CAS 111-60-4	Empilan® EGMS
CAS 111-60-4	Estol EGMS 3749
CAS 111-60-4	Ethylene Glycol Monostearate VA
CAS 111-60-4	Hodag EGMS
CAS 111-60-4	Hodag EGS
CAS 111-60-4	Instapearl
CAS 111-60-4	Kemester® 5220
CAS 111-60-4	Kemester® EGMS
CAS 111-60-4	Kessco EGMS
CAS 111-60-4	Kessco® Ethylene Glycol Monostearate
CAS 111-60-4	Lanesta 35
CAS 111-60-4	Lasemul 62 E
CAS 111-60-4	Lauramide EG
CAS 111-60-4	Lexemul® EGMS
CAS 111-60-4	Lipal EGMS
CAS 111-60-4	Lipo EGMS
CAS 111-60-4	Lonzest® EGMS
CAS 111-60-4	Mackester™ EGMS
CAS 111-60-4	Mapeg® EGMS
CAS 111-60-4	Mapeg® EGMS-K
CAS 111-60-4	Monthyle
CAS 111-60-4	Nikkol EGMS-70
CAS 111-60-4	Nikkol Pearl 1218
CAS 111-60-4	Pegosperse® 50 MS
CAS 111-60-4	Protachem EGMS
CAS 111-60-4	RITA EGMS
CAS 111-60-4	Ritasynt IP
CAS 111-60-4	Rol GE
CAS 111-60-4	Schercemol EGMS
CAS 111-60-4	Secoster® EMS
CAS 111-60-4	Sterol ST 1
CAS 111-60-4	Tegin® G 6100
CAS 111-60-4	Unipeg-EGMS
CAS 111-60-4	Witconol™ EGMS
CAS 111-60-4	Zohar EGMS
CAS 111-61-5	Cithrol ES
CAS 111-61-5	Hefti AMS-33
CAS 111-62-6	Elfacos® EO
CAS 111-62-6	Estol ETO 3659
CAS 111-62-6	Kessco EO
CAS 111-66-0	Ethyl Octene-1
CAS 111-66-0	Gulftene® 8
CAS 111-76-2	Butyl Cellosolve®
CAS 111-76-2	Butyl Oxitol
CAS 111-77-3	Ektasolve® DM
CAS 111-82-0	CE-1218
CAS 111-82-0	CE-1270
CAS 111-82-0	CE-1280
CAS 111-82-0	CE-1290
CAS 111-82-0	CE-1295
CAS 111-82-0	Estol MEL 1502
CAS 111-82-0	Estol MEL 1507
CAS 111-82-0	Kemester® 9012
CAS 111-87-5	Nacol® 8-97
CAS 111-87-5	Nacol® 8-99
CAS 111-90-0	Ektasolve® DE
CAS 111-90-0	Solvent APV Spec
CAS 111-90-0	Transcutol
CAS 111-96-6	Diglyme
CAS 112-00-5	Arquad® 12-37W
CAS 112-00-5	Dehyquart® LT
CAS 112-00-5	Empigen® 5089
CAS 112-00-5	Kemamine® Q-6903B
CAS 112-00-5	Laurene
CAS 112-00-5	Varisoft® LAC
CAS 112-02-7	Ablumine TMC
CAS 112-02-7	Adogen® 444
CAS 112-02-7	Ammonyx® CETAC
CAS 112-02-7	Ammonyx® CETAC-30
CAS 112-02-7	Arquad® 16-25W
CAS 112-02-7	Arquad® 16-29
CAS 112-02-7	Arquad® 16-29W
CAS 112-02-7	Barquat® CT-29
CAS 112-02-7	Carsoquat® CT-429
CAS 112-02-7	CTAC
CAS 112-02-7	Dehyquart® A
CAS 112-02-7	Genamin CTAC
CAS 112-02-7	Incroquat CTC-30
CAS 112-02-7	Incroquat CTC-50
CAS 112-02-7	Mackernium™ CTC-30
CAS 112-02-7	Nikkol CA-2330
CAS 112-02-7	Nikkol CA-2350
CAS 112-02-7	Quatrex CTAC
CAS 112-02-7	Querton 16Cl-29
CAS 112-02-7	Querton 16Cl-50
CAS 112-02-7	Radiaquat® 6444
CAS 112-02-7	Radiaquat® 6445
CAS 112-02-7	Rhodaquat® M242C/29
CAS 112-02-7	Tequat BC
CAS 112-02-7	Uniquart A
CAS 112-02-7	Variquat® E290
CAS 112-02-7	Varisoft® 250
CAS 112-02-7	Varisoft® 300
CAS 112-02-7	Varisoft® 355
CAS 112-03-8	Ablumine TMS
CAS 112-03-8	Genamin STAC
CAS 112-03-8	Kemamine® Q-9903B
CAS 112-03-8	Nikkol CA-2450
CAS 112-03-8	Nikkol CA-2465
CAS 112-03-8	Varisoft® ST-50
CAS 112-03-8	Varisoft® TSC
CAS 112-10-7	Estol IPS 3702
CAS 112-10-7	Kessco IPS
CAS 112-10-7	Lasemul 60
CAS 112-10-7	Tegosoft® S
CAS 112-10-7	Wickenol® 127
CAS 112-15-2	Carbitol® Acetate
CAS 112-15-2	Ektasolve® DE Acetate
CAS 112-18-5	Adma® 12
CAS 112-18-5	Adogen® MA-102
CAS 112-18-5	Armeen® DM12D
CAS 112-18-5	Barlene® 12S
CAS 112-18-5	Kemamine® T-6902
CAS 112-30-1	Cachalot® DE-10
CAS 112-30-1	Nacol® 10-97
CAS 112-30-1	Nacol® 10-99
CAS 112-34-5	Butyl Carbitol®
CAS 112-34-5	Butyl Dioxitol
CAS 112-34-5	Ektasolve® DB

CAS 112-39-0	Estol MEP 1503	CAS 112-90-3	Radiamine 6172
CAS 112-39-0	Kemester® 9016	CAS 112-90-3	Radiamine 6173
CAS 112-39-0	Radia® 7120	CAS 112-92-5	Adol® 61
CAS 112-41-4;	Gulftene® 12	CAS 112-92-5	Adol® 61 NF
CAS 112-42-5	Neodol® 1	CAS 112-92-5	Adol® 62 NF
CAS 112-53-8	Cachalot® L-90	CAS 112-92-5	Adol® 620 NF
CAS 112-53-8	Epal® 12	CAS 112-92-5	Alfol® 18
CAS 112-53-8	Laurex® L1	CAS 112-92-5	Cachalot® S-54
CAS 112-53-8	Laurex® NC	CAS 112-92-5	Cachalot® S-56
CAS 112-53-8	Lipocol L	CAS 112-92-5	Cetax 18
CAS 112-53-8	Nacol® 12-96	CAS 112-92-5	CO-1895
CAS 112-53-8	Nacol® 12-99	CAS 112-92-5	Crodacol S-70
CAS 112-53-8	Radianol® 1712	CAS 112-92-5	Crodacol S-95NF
CAS 112-53-8	Unihydag Wax 12	CAS 112-92-5	Epal® 18NF
CAS 112-61-8	Kemester® 7018	CAS 112-92-5	Fancol SA
CAS 112-61-8	Kemester® 9718	CAS 112-92-5	Hetoxol SA
CAS 112-62-9	Kemester® 115	CAS 112-92-5	Hyfatol 18-95
CAS 112-62-9	Kemester® 8002	CAS 112-92-5	Hyfatol 18-98
CAS 112-62-9	Witconol™ 2301	CAS 112-92-5	Lanette® 18
CAS 112-69-6	Adma® 16	CAS 112-92-5	Lanette® 18 DEO
CAS 112-69-6	Adogen® MA-106	CAS 112-92-5	Lanol S
CAS 112-69-6	Armeen® DM16D	CAS 112-92-5	Lipocol S
CAS 112-69-6	Barlene® 16S	CAS 112-92-5	Mackol 18
CAS 112-69-6	Kemamine® T-8902	CAS 112-92-5	Nacol® 18-94
CAS 112-72-1	Cachalot® M-43	CAS 112-92-5	Nacol® 18-98
CAS 112-72-1	Epal® 14	CAS 112-92-5	Nikkol Stearyl Alcohol
CAS 112-72-1	Lanette® 14	CAS 112-92-5	Philcohol 1800
CAS 112-72-1	Nacol® 14-95	CAS 112-92-5	Radianol® 1898
CAS 112-72-1	Nacol® 14-98	CAS 112-92-5	RITA SA
CAS 112-72-1	Unihydag Wax-14	CAS 112-92-5	Stearal
CAS 112-75-4	Adma® 14	CAS 112-92-5	Steraffine
CAS 112-75-4	Adogen® MA-104	CAS 112-92-5	Unihydag Wax-18
CAS 112-75-4	Armeen® DM14D	CAS 112-99-2	Armeen® 2-18
CAS 112-75-4	Barlene® 14	CAS 115-10-6	Demeon D
CAS 112-75-4	Barlene® 14S	CAS 115-10-6	Dymel® A
CAS 112-75-4	Kemamine® T-7902	CAS 115-69-5	AMPD
CAS 112-80-1	Crodolene LA1020	CAS 115-70-8	AEPD®
CAS 112-80-1	Emersol® 210	CAS 115-83-3	Alkamuls® PETS
CAS 112-80-1	Emersol® 213 NF	CAS 115-83-3	Crodamol PETS
CAS 112-80-1	Emersol® 221 NF	CAS 115-83-3	Kessco PTS
CAS 112-80-1	Emersol® 233 LL	CAS 115-83-3	Liponate PS-4
CAS 112-80-1	Emersol® 6313 NF	CAS 116-25-6	Dantoin® MDMH
CAS 112-80-1	Emersol® 6321 NF	CAS 118-56-9	Homosalate®
CAS 112-80-1	Emersol® 6333 NF	CAS 118-56-9	Kemester® HMS
CAS 112-80-1	Emersol® 7021	CAS 118-56-9	Uniderm HOMSAL
CAS 112-80-1	Hy-Phi 1055	CAS 118-60-5	Dermoblock OS
CAS 112-80-1	Hy-Phi 1088	CAS 118-60-5	Escalol® 587
CAS 112-80-1	Hy-Phi 2066	CAS 118-60-5	Lanaetex-OS
CAS 112-80-1	Hy-Phi 2088	CAS 118-60-5	Neo Heliopan, Type OS
CAS 112-80-1	Hy-Phi 2102	CAS 118-60-5	Neotan L
CAS 112-80-1	Industrene® 105	CAS 118-60-5	Trivent OS
CAS 112-80-1	Industrene® 106	CAS 119-36-8	Unichem METSAL
CAS 112-80-1	Industrene® 206	CAS 120-32-1	Preventol BP
CAS 112-80-1	Priolene 6900	CAS 120-40-1	Ablumide LDE
CAS 112-80-1	Priolene 6905	CAS 120-40-1	Afmide™ LLM
CAS 112-80-1	Priolene 6906	CAS 120-40-1	Afmide™ LMD
CAS 112-80-1	Priolene 6910	CAS 120-40-1	Alkamide® 327
CAS 112-80-1	Priolene 6933	CAS 120-40-1	Alkamide® 1195
CAS 112-80-1	Radiacid® 212	CAS 120-40-1	Alkamide® DL-203/S
CAS 112-80-1	Unifat 5L	CAS 120-40-1	Alkamide® DL-207/S
CAS 112-85-6	Crodacid B	CAS 120-40-1	Alkamide® L9DE
CAS 112-85-6	Hystrene® 7022	CAS 120-40-1	Alkamide® LE
CAS 112-85-6	Hystrene® 9022	CAS 120-40-1	Amidex LD
CAS 112-85-6	Prifrac 2989	CAS 120-40-1	Amidex LD-8
CAS 112-88-9	Gulftene® 18	CAS 120-40-1	Aminol LM-30C, LM-30C Special
CAS 112-90-3	Armeen® O	CAS 120-40-1	Carsamide® SAL-7
CAS 112-90-3	Armeen® OD	CAS 120-40-1	Carsamide® SAL-9
CAS 112-90-3	Armeen® OL	CAS 120-40-1	Carsamide® SAL-82
CAS 112-90-3	Armeen® OLD	CAS 120-40-1	Chimipal LDA
CAS 112-90-3	Kemamine® P-989	CAS 120-40-1	Comperlan® LD

CAS 120-40-1	Comperlan® LDO, LDS	CAS 120-40-1	Witcamide® 6511
CAS 120-40-1	Emid® 6513	CAS 120-40-1	Witcamide® 6519
CAS 120-40-1	Emid® 6519	CAS 120-40-1	Witcamide® 6590
CAS 120-40-1	Empilan® LDE	CAS 120-40-1	Witcamide® L-9
CAS 120-40-1	Empilan® LDE/FF	CAS 120-40-1	Witcamide® LDEA
CAS 120-40-1	Ethylan® MLD	CAS 120-40-1	Witcamide® LL
CAS 120-40-1	Foamid PK	CAS 120-40-1	Witcamide® STD-HP
CAS 120-40-1	Foamid SL-Extra	CAS 120-47-8	Aethyl-Steriline
CAS 120-40-1	Hartamide LDA	CAS 120-47-8	Bentex E
CAS 120-40-1	Hetamide LL	CAS 120-47-8	CoSept E
CAS 120-40-1	Hetamide ML	CAS 120-47-8	Lexgard® E
CAS 120-40-1	Hetamide MOC	CAS 120-47-8	Nipagin A
CAS 120-40-1	Incromide L90	CAS 120-47-8	Paridol E
CAS 120-40-1	Incromide LL	CAS 120-47-8	Preserval E
CAS 120-40-1	Incromide LR	CAS 120-47-8	Trisept E
CAS 120-40-1	Lauramina	CAS 120-47-8	Unisept E
CAS 120-40-1	Lipamide LMWC	CAS 120-51-4	Unichem BZBN
CAS 120-40-1	Loropan LD	CAS 120-80-9	Rodol C
CAS 120-40-1	Mackamide™ L-10	CAS 121-32-4	Unisweet EVAN
CAS 120-40-1	Mackamide™ L95	CAS 121-33-5	Unisweet VAN
CAS 120-40-1	Mackamide™ LLM	CAS 121-54-0	Hyamine® 1622 50%
CAS 120-40-1	Mackamide™ LMD	CAS 121-54-0	Hyamine® 1622 Crystals
CAS 120-40-1	Manromid 1224	CAS 121-79-9	Atomergic Propyl Gallate
CAS 120-40-1	Mazamide® 124	CAS 121-79-9	Progallin® P
CAS 120-40-1	Mazamide® 1214	CAS 121-79-9	Tenox® PG
CAS 120-40-1	Mazamide® L-298	CAS 121-79-9	Uantox PG
CAS 120-40-1	Mazamide® LM	CAS 121-88-0	Rodol YBA
CAS 120-40-1	Mazamide® LM 20	CAS 122-03-2	Cumal
CAS 120-40-1	Mazamide® LS 196	CAS 122-18-9	Cetol®
CAS 120-40-1	Monamid® 31	CAS 122-18-9	Sumquat® 6050
CAS 120-40-1	Monamid® 150-GLT	CAS 122-19-0	Ablumine 1618
CAS 120-40-1	Monamid® 150-LMWC	CAS 122-19-0	Ammonyx® 4
CAS 120-40-1	Monamid® 150-LWA	CAS 122-19-0	Ammonyx® 4B
CAS 120-40-1	Monamid® 716	CAS 122-19-0	Ammonyx® 485
CAS 120-40-1	Monamid® 1034	CAS 122-19-0	Ammonyx® 4002
CAS 120-40-1	Monamid® 1224	CAS 122-19-0	Ammonyx® CA-Special
CAS 120-40-1	Monamid® L-350	CAS 122-19-0	Amyx A-25-S 0040
CAS 120-40-1	Monamid® L-355	CAS 122-19-0	Carsoquat® SDQ-85
CAS 120-40-1	Monamid® L-360	CAS 122-19-0	Catinal OB-80E
CAS 120-40-1	Monamid® L-365	CAS 122-19-0	Emcol® 4
CAS 120-40-1	Monamid® LL-370	CAS 122-19-0	Hetquat S-20
CAS 120-40-1	Monamid® LM-375	CAS 122-19-0	Incroquat S-85
CAS 120-40-1	Ninol® 30-LL	CAS 122-19-0	Incroquat SDQ-25
CAS 120-40-1	Ninol® 55-LL	CAS 122-19-0	Mackernium™ SDC-25
CAS 120-40-1	Ninol® 70-SL	CAS 122-19-0	Mackernium™ SDC-85
CAS 120-40-1	Ninol® 96-SL	CAS 122-19-0	Maquat SC-18
CAS 120-40-1	Ninol® L-9	CAS 122-19-0	Miracare® SCS
CAS 120-40-1	Norfox® DLSA	CAS 122-19-0	M-Quat® B-25
CAS 120-40-1	Phoenamid LD, LD Special	CAS 122-19-0	M-Quat® JS-25
CAS 120-40-1	Profan AA62	CAS 122-19-0	Nikkol CA-1485
CAS 120-40-1	Protamide L-80M, L90, L90A, LM	CAS 122-19-0	Quatrex STC-25
	73, LM 73-L, LM-73 PG, LMAV	CAS 122-19-0	Quatrex STC-85
CAS 120-40-1	Schercomid SL-Extra	CAS 122-19-0	Rhodaquat® M270C/18
CAS 120-40-1	Standamid® KDL	CAS 122-19-0	Stedbac®
CAS 120-40-1	Standamid® KDOL	CAS 122-19-0	Sumquat® 6210
CAS 120-40-1	Standamid® KDS	CAS 122-19-0	Unisoft SAC
CAS 120-40-1	Standamid® LD	CAS 122-19-0	Varisoft® SDAC-W
CAS 120-40-1	Standamid® LDO	CAS 122-19-0	Zoharquat 25
CAS 120-40-1	Standamid® LDS	CAS 122-19-0	Zoharquat 75
CAS 120-40-1	Tohol N-230	CAS 122-20-3	TIPA 99
CAS 120-40-1	Tohol N-230X	CAS 122-20-3	TIPA 101
CAS 120-40-1	Upamide LD	CAS 122-20-3	TIPA Low Freeze Grade
CAS 120-40-1	Upamide LDS, LM-20, LS-173,	CAS 122-20-3	Unichem TIPA
	LS-196	CAS 122-32-7	Cithrol GTO
CAS 120-40-1	Varamide® LL-1	CAS 122-32-7	CPH-399-N
CAS 120-40-1	Varamide® ML-1	CAS 122-32-7	Emerest® 2423
CAS 120-40-1	Varamide® ML-4	CAS 122-32-7	Emery® 2423
CAS 120-40-1	Witcamide® 5195	CAS 122-32-7	Hodag GTO
CAS 120-40-1	Witcamide® 6310	CAS 122-32-7	Kemester® 1000
CAS 120-40-1	Witcamide® 6510	CAS 122-32-7	Witconol™ 2423

CAS 122-62-3	Docoil DOS		CAS 124-43-6	Unichem UREA-P
CAS 122-62-3	Elfacos® DEHS		CAS 124-68-5	AMP
CAS 122-62-3	Kessco DEHS		CAS 126-11-4	Tris Nitro®
CAS 122-62-3	Trivent DOS		CAS 126-30-7	NPG® Glycol
CAS 122-99-6	Cephene™		CAS 126-92-1	Cosmopon SES
CAS 122-99-6	Emeressence® 1160 Rose Ether		CAS 126-92-1	Empicol® 0585/A
CAS 122-99-6	Emthox® 6705		CAS 126-92-1	Niaproof® Anionic Surfactant 08
CAS 122-99-6	K-Preserve Liq		CAS 126-92-1	Witcolate™ D-510
CAS 122-99-6	Phenoxen		CAS 127-09-3	Unichem SODAC
CAS 122-99-6	Phenoxetol		CAS 127-82-2	Unichem ZPS
CAS 122-99-6	Phenoxyethanol O		CAS 127-82-2	Universal ZPS
CAS 122-99-6	Rewopal® MPG 10		CAS 128-37-0	Ionol CP
CAS 122-99-6	Sepicide LD		CAS 128-37-0	Sustane® BHT
CAS 122-99-6	Unisept POE		CAS 128-37-0	Tenox® BHT
CAS 123-03-5	CPC		CAS 128-37-0	Uantox BHT
CAS 123-03-5	CPC Sumquat 6060		CAS 128-37-0	Uninox A 287
CAS 123-03-5	Uniquart CPC		CAS 128-37-0	Vanox® PCX
CAS 123-28-4	Argus DLTDP		CAS 128-44-9	Unisweet SOSAC
CAS 123-28-4	Evanstab® 12		CAS 131-11-3	Kemester® DMP
CAS 123-30-8	Rodol P Base		CAS 131-11-3	Kodaflex® DMP
CAS 123-31-9	Eastman® Hydroquinone		CAS 131-11-3	Palatinol® M
CAS 123-31-9	Rodol HQ		CAS 131-11-3	Uniplex 110
CAS 123-31-9	Tecquinol® USP Grade		CAS 131-53-3	Spectra-Sorb® UV 24
CAS 123-31-9	Uantox HQ		CAS 131-54-4	Uvinul® D 49
CAS 123-76-2	Unichem Levula		CAS 131-55-5	Uvinul® D 50
CAS 123-94-4	Aldo® HMS		CAS 131-56-6	DHBP Quinsorb 010
CAS 123-94-4	Aldo® MS		CAS 131-56-6	Uvasorb 20H
CAS 123-94-4	Aldo® MSA		CAS 131-56-6	Uvinul® 400
CAS 123-94-4	Aldo® MSD		CAS 131-57-7	Escalol® 567
CAS 123-94-4	Aldo® MS LG		CAS 131-57-7	Eusolex® 4360
CAS 123-95-5	Crodamol BS		CAS 131-57-7	Marsorb 24
CAS 123-95-5	Dermol EB		CAS 131-57-7	Neo Heliopan, Type BB
CAS 123-95-5	Emerest® 2325		CAS 131-57-7	Spectra-Sorb® UV 9
CAS 123-95-5	Estol BUS 1550		CAS 131-57-7	Syntase® 62
CAS 123-95-5	Kemester® 5410		CAS 131-57-7	Uvasorb MET
CAS 123-95-5	Kemester® 5510		CAS 131-57-7	Uvinul® M 40
CAS 123-95-5	Kessco® Butyl Stearate		CAS 132-27-4	Dowicide A
CAS 123-95-5	Lasemul 74 NP		CAS 133-06-2	Vancide® 89 RE
CAS 123-95-5	Nikkol BS		CAS 134-03-2	Sodium Ascorbate USP, FCC Fine
CAS 123-95-5	Norfox® B-54			Powd. No. 6047708
CAS 123-95-5	Radia® 7752		CAS 134-03-2	Uantox SODASC
CAS 123-95-5	Unichem BUTSTE		CAS 134-09-8	Dermoblock MA
CAS 123-95-5	Witconol™ 2326		CAS 134-09-8	Estalan MA
CAS 124-03-8	Sumquat® 6020		CAS 134-09-8	Neo Heliopan, Type MA
CAS 124-07-2	Prifrac 2901		CAS 134-09-8	Trivent MA
CAS 124-07-2	Prifrac 2910		CAS 136-26-5	Amidex CP
CAS 124-07-2	Unifat 8		CAS 136-26-5	Comperlan® CD
CAS 124-10-7	Estol MEM 1518		CAS 136-26-5	Hetamide 1069
CAS 124-10-7	Estol MYM 3645		CAS 136-26-5	Mackamide™ CD-10
CAS 124-10-7	Kemester® 9014		CAS 136-26-5	Monamid® 150-CW
CAS 124-17-4	Ektasolve® DB Acetate		CAS 136-26-5	Monamid® CP-205
CAS 124-22-1	Adogen® 163D		CAS 136-99-2	Schercozoline L
CAS 124-22-1	Armeen® 12		CAS 137-08-6	D-Calcium Pantothenate USP,
CAS 124-22-1	Armeen® 12D			FCC Type SD No. 63924
CAS 124-22-1	Kemamine® P-690		CAS 137-16-6	Chimin L
CAS 124-22-1	Radiamine 6163		CAS 137-16-6	Closyl LA 3584
CAS 124-22-1	Radiamine 6164		CAS 137-16-6	Crodasinic LS30
CAS 124-26-5	Armid® 18		CAS 137-16-6	Crodasinic LS35
CAS 124-28-7	Adma® 18		CAS 137-16-6	Hamposyl® L-30
CAS 124-28-7	Adogen® MA-108		CAS 137-16-6	Hamposyl® L-95
CAS 124-28-7	Adogen® MA-108 SF		CAS 137-16-6	Maprosyl® 30
CAS 124-28-7	Amine 2M18D		CAS 137-16-6	Medialan LD
CAS 124-28-7	Armeen® DM18D		CAS 137-16-6	Nikkol Sarcosinate LN
CAS 124-28-7	Barlene® 18S		CAS 137-16-6	Nikkol Sarcosinate LN-30
CAS 124-28-7	Kemamine® T-9902		CAS 137-16-6	Oramix L30
CAS 124-30-1	Amine 18-90		CAS 137-16-6	Secosyl
CAS 124-30-1	Amine 18-90 D		CAS 137-16-6	Unipol LAUROYLSAR
CAS 124-30-1	Amine 18-95		CAS 137-16-6	Vanseal® NALS-30
CAS 124-30-1	Armeen® 18		CAS 137-16-6	Vanseal® NALS-95
CAS 124-30-1	Armeen® 18D		CAS 137-16-6	Zoharsyl L-30

CAS 137-20-2	Adinol OT16
CAS 137-20-2	Geropon® T-77
CAS 137-20-2	Hostapon SO
CAS 137-20-2	Hostapon T Paste 33
CAS 137-20-2	Hostapon T Powd. Highly Conc.
CAS 137-20-2	Protapon 33
CAS 137-20-2	Tauranol M-35
CAS 137-20-2	Tauranol MS
CAS 137-20-2	Tauranol T-Gel
CAS 137-40-6	Unistat SOBAN
CAS 137-66-6	Ascorbyl Palmitate No. 60412
CAS 137-66-6	Grindox Ascorbyl Palmitate
CAS 138-32-9	Cetats®
CAS 138-86-3	Dipentene No. 122
CAS 139-07-1	Catinal MB-50A
CAS 139-07-1	Dehyquart® LDB
CAS 139-07-1	Tequat PAN
CAS 139-08-2	Arquad® DM14B-90
CAS 139-08-2	Barquat® MX-50
CAS 139-08-2	Barquat® MX-80
CAS 139-08-2	BTC® 824
CAS 139-08-2	FMB 451-8 Quat
CAS 139-08-2	FMB 551-5 Quat
CAS 139-08-2	JAQ Powdered Quat
CAS 139-08-2	Kemamine® Q-7903B
CAS 139-33-3	BASF Disodium EDTA
CAS 139-33-3	Hampene® Na$_2$ Pure Crystals
CAS 139-33-3	Nervanaid™ BA2 (BP)
CAS 139-33-3	Sequestrene® NA2
CAS 139-33-3	Universene Na2
CAS 139-33-3	Versene NA
CAS 139-41-3	Hampshire® DEG
CAS 139-88-8	Niaproof® Anionic Surfactant 4
CAS 139-89-9	Chel DM-41
CAS 139-89-9	Hamp-Ol® 120
CAS 139-89-9	Hamp-Ol® Crystals
CAS 139-89-9	Versenol 120
CAS 139-96-8	Akyposal TLS 42
CAS 139-96-8	Aremsol TA
CAS 139-96-8	Berol 480
CAS 139-96-8	Calfoam TLS-40
CAS 139-96-8	Carsonol® TLS
CAS 139-96-8	Cosmopon TR
CAS 139-96-8	Elfan® 240T
CAS 139-96-8	Empicol® TA40A
CAS 139-96-8	Empicol® TL40
CAS 139-96-8	Genapol® CRT 40
CAS 139-96-8	Genapol® LRT 40
CAS 139-96-8	Laural D
CAS 139-96-8	Manro TL 40
CAS 139-96-8	Marlinat® DFL 40
CAS 139-96-8	Neopon LT/NF
CAS 139-96-8	Nikkol TEALS
CAS 139-96-8	Nikkol TEALS-42
CAS 139-96-8	Norfox® TLS
CAS 139-96-8	Nutrapon TLS-500
CAS 139-96-8	Perlankrol® ATL40
CAS 139-96-8	Rewopol® TLS 40
CAS 139-96-8	Rhodapon® LT-6
CAS 139-96-8	Sandoz Sulfate TL
CAS 139-96-8	Standapol® T
CAS 139-96-8	Stepanol® WAT
CAS 139-96-8	Sulfetal KT 400
CAS 139-96-8	Sulfochem TLS
CAS 139-96-8	Sunnol LM-1140T
CAS 139-96-8	Surfax 40
CAS 139-96-8	Texapon® T
CAS 139-96-8	Texapon® T 42
CAS 139-96-8	Ufarol TA-40
CAS 139-96-8	Unipol T

CAS 139-96-8	Witcolate™ T
CAS 139-96-8	Witcolate™ TLS-500
CAS 139-96-8	Zoharpon LAT
CAS 139-96-8	Empicol® TL40/T
CAS 140-01-2	Hamp-Ex® 80
CAS 140-01-2	Mayoquest 300
CAS 140-01-2	Versenex 80
CAS 140-03-4	Naturechem® MAR
CAS 140-03-4	Pelemol MAR
CAS 140-25-0	Mazon® EE-1
CAS 140-87-0	PTAL
CAS 141-08-2	Aldo® MR
CAS 141-08-2	Cithrol GMR N/E
CAS 141-08-2	CPH-35-N
CAS 141-08-2	Flexricin® 13
CAS 141-08-2	Hodag GMR
CAS 141-08-2	Hodag GMR-D
CAS 141-08-2	Mazol® GMR
CAS 141-08-2	Radiasurf® 7153
CAS 141-08-2	Softigen® 701
CAS 141-08-2	Unitina GMRO
CAS 141-20-8	Kessco® Diglycol Laurate A Neutral
CAS 141-20-8	Kessco® Diglycol Laurate ASE
CAS 141-20-8	Kessco® Diglycol Laurate N
CAS 141-20-8	Kessco® Diglycol Laurate N-Syn
CAS 141-20-8	Lipopeg 1-L
CAS 141-20-8	Unipeg-DGL
CAS 141-21-9	Catemol 18SA
CAS 141-21-9	Chemical 39 Base
CAS 141-23-1	Naturechem® MHS
CAS 141-86-6	Rodol 26PYR
CAS 141-94-6	Hexetidine 90, 99
CAS 142-18-7	Cithrol GML N/E
CAS 142-18-7	CPH-34-N
CAS 142-18-7	Estol GML 3614
CAS 142-18-7	Grillomuls L90
CAS 142-18-7	Hodag GML
CAS 142-18-7	Imwitor® 312
CAS 142-18-7	Kessco® Glycerol Monolaurate
CAS 142-18-7	Lauricidin 802, 812, 1012, E
CAS 142-18-7	Monomuls® 90-L12
CAS 142-18-7	Protachem MLD
CAS 142-26-7	Amidex AME
CAS 142-26-7	Carsamide® AMEA
CAS 142-26-7	Foamid AME-70
CAS 142-26-7	Foamid AME-75
CAS 142-26-7	Foamid AME-100
CAS 142-26-7	Hetamide MA
CAS 142-26-7	Incromectant AMEA-70
CAS 142-26-7	Incromectant AMEA-100
CAS 142-26-7	Lipamide MEAA
CAS 142-26-7	Mackamide™ AME-75, AME-100
CAS 142-26-7	Schercomid AME
CAS 142-26-7	Upamide ACMEA
CAS 142-26-7	Witcamide® CMEA
CAS 142-48-3	Crodasinic S
CAS 142-48-3	Hamposyl® S
CAS 142-54-1	Amidex LIPA
CAS 142-54-1	Comperlan® LP
CAS 142-54-1	Empilan® LIS
CAS 142-54-1	Incromide LI
CAS 142-54-1	Incromide LMI
CAS 142-54-1	Monamid® LMIPA
CAS 142-54-1	Nidaba 3
CAS 142-54-1	Profan AD31
CAS 142-54-1	Rewomid® IPL 203
CAS 142-54-1	Upamide MIPA
CAS 142-55-2	Cithrol PGML N/E
CAS 142-55-2	Emalex PGML

CAS 142-55-2	Hodag PGML
CAS 142-55-2	Imwitor® 412
CAS 142-55-2	Kessco® PGML-X533
CAS 142-55-2	Kessco® Propylene Glycol Monolaurate E
CAS 142-55-2	Lauroglycol
CAS 142-55-2	Rol LP
CAS 142-55-2	Unipeg-PGML
CAS 142-58-5	Hetamide MM
CAS 142-58-5	Witcamide® MM
CAS 142-62-1	Unifat 6
CAS 142-77-8	Kemester® 4000
CAS 142-78-9	Ablumide LME
CAS 142-78-9	Afmide™ LMM
CAS 142-78-9	Amidex LMMEA
CAS 142-78-9	Comperlan® LMM
CAS 142-78-9	Empilan® LME
CAS 142-78-9	Hartamide LMEA
CAS 142-78-9	Hetamide MML
CAS 142-78-9	Lauridit® LM
CAS 142-78-9	Loropan LM
CAS 142-78-9	Mackamide™ LMM
CAS 142-78-9	Manromid LMA
CAS 142-78-9	Monamid® LMMA
CAS 142-78-9	Ninol® LMP
CAS 142-78-9	Phoenamid LMM
CAS 142-78-9	Rewomid® L 203
CAS 142-78-9	Standamid® LM
CAS 142-78-9	Upamide MEA
CAS 142-78-9	Varamide® L-203
CAS 142-87-0	Akyporox SAL SAS
CAS 142-91-6	Crodamol IPP
CAS 142-91-6	Deltyl® Prime
CAS 142-91-6	Elfacos® IPP
CAS 142-91-6	Emerest® 2316
CAS 142-91-6	Estol 1517
CAS 142-91-6	Estol IPP 1517
CAS 142-91-6	Estol IPP-b 3651
CAS 142-91-6	Isopropyl Palmitate
CAS 142-91-6	Jafaester 16 NF
CAS 142-91-6	Kessco® Isopropyl Palmitate
CAS 142-91-6	Lanesta 23
CAS 142-91-6	Lexol® IPP
CAS 142-91-6	Lexol® IPP-A
CAS 142-91-6	Lexol® IPP-NF
CAS 142-91-6	Liponate IPP
CAS 142-91-6	Nikkol IPP
CAS 142-91-6	Nikkol IPP-EX
CAS 142-91-6	Propal
CAS 142-91-6	Protachem IPP
CAS 142-91-6	Radia® 7200
CAS 142-91-6	Radia® 7732
CAS 142-91-6	Tegosoft® P
CAS 142-91-6	Upamate IPP
CAS 142-91-6	Wickenol® 111
CAS 142-91-6	Witconol™ 2316
CAS 143-00-0	Carsonol® DLS
CAS 143-00-0	Nutrapon DE 3796
CAS 143-00-0	Standapol® DEA
CAS 143-00-0	Stepanol® DEA
CAS 143-00-0	Sulfochem DLS
CAS 143-00-0	Supralate EP
CAS 143-00-0	Texapon® DEA
CAS 143-00-0	Unipol DEA
CAS 143-00-0	Witcolate™ DLS-35
CAS 143-00-0	Zoharpon LAD
CAS 143-07-7	Hystrene® 9512
CAS 143-07-7	Kartacid 1299
CAS 143-07-7	Kortacid 1295
CAS 143-07-7	Unifat 12
CAS 143-18-0	Norfox® KO
CAS 143-27-1	Amine 16D
CAS 143-27-1	Armeen® 16
CAS 143-27-1	Armeen® 16D
CAS 143-27-1	Kemamine® P-890
CAS 143-28-2	Adol® 80
CAS 143-28-2	Adol® 85
CAS 143-28-2	Adol® 90
CAS 143-28-2	Adol® 90 NF
CAS 143-28-2	Cachalot® O-3
CAS 143-28-2	Cachalot® O-8
CAS 143-28-2	Cachalot® O-15
CAS 143-28-2	Crodacol A-10
CAS 143-28-2	Dermaffine
CAS 143-28-2	Fancol OA-95
CAS 143-28-2	HD-Eutanol®
CAS 143-28-2	HD-Ocenol® 90/95
CAS 143-28-2	HD-Ocenol® 92/96
CAS 143-28-2	HD Oleyl Alcohol 70/75
CAS 143-28-2	HD Oleyl Alcohol 80/85
CAS 143-28-2	HD Oleyl Alcohol 90/95
CAS 143-28-2	HD Oleyl Alcohol CG
CAS 143-28-2	Lancol
CAS 143-28-2	Lipocol O
CAS 143-28-2	Lipocol O-80
CAS 143-28-2	Lipocol O/95
CAS 143-28-2	Novol
CAS 143-28-2	U Tanol HD, HD 70/75, HD 80/85, HD 90/95, HD CG
CAS 143-28-2	U Tanol HDL CG
CAS 144-19-4	TMPD® Glycol
CAS 144-55-8	Unichem BICARB-S
CAS 149-39-3	Hostapon STT Paste
CAS 149-39-3	Nikkol SMT
CAS 150-39-0	Hamp-Ol® Acid
CAS 151-21-3	Akyposal NLS
CAS 151-21-3	Alscoap LN-40, LN-90
CAS 151-21-3	Calfoam SLS-30
CAS 151-21-3	Carsonol® SLS
CAS 151-21-3	Carsonol® SLS Paste B
CAS 151-21-3	Carsonol® SLS-R
CAS 151-21-3	Carsonol® SLS-S
CAS 151-21-3	Carsonol® SLS Special
CAS 151-21-3	Chemsalan NLS 30
CAS 151-21-3	Cosmopon 35
CAS 151-21-3	Elfadent SM 514
CAS 151-21-3	Elfan® 240
CAS 151-21-3	Empicol® 0045
CAS 151-21-3	Empicol® 0045V
CAS 151-21-3	Empicol® 0185
CAS 151-21-3	Empicol® 0303
CAS 151-21-3	Empicol® 0303V
CAS 151-21-3	Empicol® LM45
CAS 151-21-3	Empicol® LS30B
CAS 151-21-3	Empicol® LX28
CAS 151-21-3	Empicol® LX100
CAS 151-21-3	Empicol® LXS95
CAS 151-21-3	Empicol® LXV
CAS 151-21-3	Empicol® LXV100
CAS 151-21-3	Empicol® LXV/D
CAS 151-21-3	Empicol® LZV/D
CAS 151-21-3	Empicol® WAK
CAS 151-21-3	Gardinol WA Paste
CAS 151-21-3	Manro SLS 28
CAS 151-21-3	Marlinat® DFK 30
CAS 151-21-3	Naxolate™ WA-97
CAS 151-21-3	Naxolate™ WAG
CAS 151-21-3	Naxolate™ WA Special
CAS 151-21-3	Neopon LS/NF
CAS 151-21-3	Nikkol SLS

CAS 151-21-3	Nikkol SLS-30	CAS 151-21-3	Zoharpon LAS Spray Dried
CAS 151-21-3	Norfox® SLS	CAS 215-42-9	Adogen® MA-112 SF
CAS 151-21-3	Nutrapon DL 3891	CAS 215-42-9	Kemamine® T-2802D
CAS 151-21-3	Nutrapon W 1367	CAS 299-27-4	Gluconal® K
CAS 151-21-3	Nutrapon WAC 3005	CAS 299-28-5	Gluconal® CA A
CAS 151-21-3	Nutrapon WAQ	CAS 299-28-5	Gluconal® CA M
CAS 151-21-3	Nutrapon WAQE 2364	CAS 299-29-6	Gluconal® FE
CAS 151-21-3	Perlankrol® DSA	CAS 300-92-5	Haro® Chem ALMD-2
CAS 151-21-3	Rewopol® NLS 28	CAS 300-92-5	Witco® Aluminum Stearate EA
CAS 151-21-3	Rewopol® NLS 90		Food Grade
CAS 151-21-3	Rhodapon® LSB, LSB/CT	CAS 301-02-0	Armid® O
CAS 151-21-3	Rhodapon® SB-8208/S	CAS 301-04-2	Atomergic Lead Acetate
CAS 151-21-3	Rhodapon® SM Special	CAS 301-04-2	Unichem PBA
CAS 151-21-3	Rolpon LSX	CAS 334-48-5	Unifat 10
CAS 151-21-3	Standapol® WA-AC	CAS 422-86-2	Kodaflex® DOTP
CAS 151-21-3	Standapol® WAQ-LC	CAS 463-40-1	Univit-F Forte
CAS 151-21-3	Standapol® WAQ Special	CAS 471-34-1	Camel-WITE®
CAS 151-21-3	Stepanol® ME Dry	CAS 471-34-1	Unichem CALCARB
CAS 151-21-3	Stepanol® WA-100	CAS 471-53-4	Nikkol Glycyrrhetinic Acid
CAS 151-21-3	Stepanol® WAC	CAS 488-43-7	Desamina
CAS 151-21-3	Stepanol® WA Extra	CAS 489-84-9	Azulene 100% 2/912980
CAS 151-21-3	Stepanol® WA Paste	CAS 515-69-5	α-Bisabolol
CAS 151-21-3	Stepanol® WAQ	CAS 515-69-5	Dragosantol 2/012681
CAS 151-21-3	Stepanol® WA Special	CAS 515-69-5	Hydagen® B
CAS 151-21-3	Sulfochem SAC	CAS 515-69-5	Uhydagen B
CAS 151-21-3	Sulfochem SLC	CAS 520-45-6	Unisept DHA
CAS 151-21-3	Sulfochem SLN	CAS 527-07-1	Gluconal® NA
CAS 151-21-3	Sulfochem SLP	CAS 527-09-3	Gluconal® CU
CAS 151-21-3	Sulfochem SLP-95	CAS 532-32-1	Unisept SB
CAS 151-21-3	Sulfochem SLS	CAS 533-73-3	Imexine OAM
CAS 151-21-3	Sulfopon® 101 Special	CAS 533-96-0	Snow Fine
CAS 151-21-3	Sulfopon® 103	CAS 533-96-0	Snow Flake
CAS 151-21-3	Sulfopon® P-40	CAS 537-55-3	Chemodyne N-Acetyltyrosine
CAS 151-21-3	Sulfopon® WA 3	CAS 538-23-8	Aldo® TC
CAS 151-21-3	Sulfopon® WAQ LCX	CAS 538-23-8	Captex® 8000
CAS 151-21-3	Sulfopon® WAQ Special	CAS 538-23-8	Emalex O.T.G
CAS 151-21-3	Supralate C	CAS 538-23-8	Estol GTC 1803
CAS 151-21-3	Supralate QC	CAS 538-23-8	Estol GTEH 3609
CAS 151-21-3	Supralate WA Paste	CAS 538-23-8	Miglyol® 808
CAS 151-21-3	Surfax 100	CAS 538-23-8	Nikkol Trifat S-308
CAS 151-21-3	Surfax 100 AG	CAS 538-23-8	Pelemol GTO
CAS 151-21-3	Surfax CN	CAS 538-23-8	Trivent OC-G
CAS 151-21-3	Texapon® K-12 Needles	CAS 538-24-9	Dynasan® 112
CAS 151-21-3	Texapon® K-12 Powd.	CAS 538-24-9	Lipo 320
CAS 151-21-3	Texapon® K-1296	CAS 538-24-9	Massa Estarinum® AM
CAS 151-21-3	Texapon® L-100	CAS 538-71-6	Fungitex R
CAS 151-21-3	Texapon® LS 100 F	CAS 540-10-3	Crodamol CP
CAS 151-21-3	Texapon® OT Highly Conc.	CAS 540-10-3	Elfacos® CP
	Needles	CAS 540-10-3	Emalex CC-16
CAS 151-21-3	Texapon® VHC Needles	CAS 540-10-3	Estol CEP 3694
CAS 151-21-3	Texapon® Z	CAS 540-10-3	Estol CEP-b 3653
CAS 151-21-3	Texapon® ZHC Powder	CAS 540-10-3	Kemester® CP
CAS 151-21-3	Ufarol Na-30	CAS 540-10-3	Kessco® 653
CAS 151-21-3	Unipol SLS	CAS 540-10-3	Kessco® CP
CAS 151-21-3	Unipol WA-AC	CAS 540-10-3	Nikkol N-SP
CAS 151-21-3	Unipol WAC Special	CAS 540-10-3	Precifac ATO
CAS 151-21-3	Unipol WAQ-LC	CAS 540-10-3	Rewowax CG
CAS 151-21-3	Unipon K12, K1296, L-100, ZHC	CAS 540-10-3	Starfol® CP
	Needles, ZHC Powd.	CAS 540-10-3	Trivent CP
CAS 151-21-3	Unipon ZHC Needles	CAS 540-10-3	Unimul-1616
CAS 151-21-3	Witcolate™ A Powder	CAS 540-10-3	Unitina CP
CAS 151-21-3	Witcolate™ C	CAS 540-10-3	Waxenol® 815
CAS 151-21-3	Witcolate™ LCP	CAS 540-10-3	Waxenol® 816
CAS 151-21-3	Witcolate™ SL-1	CAS 540-10-3	W.G.S. Cetyl Palmitate
CAS 151-21-3	Witcolate™ WAC	CAS 541-70-8	Rodol MPDS
CAS 151-21-3	Witcolate™ WAC-GL	CAS 544-31-0	Nikkol PMEA
CAS 151-21-3	Witcolate™ WAC-LA	CAS 544-35-4	Nikkol VF-E
CAS 151-21-3	Zoharpon LAS	CAS 544-35-4	Safester A-75
CAS 151-21-3	Zoharpon LAS 70%	CAS 544-62-7	Nikkol Batyl Alcohol 100, EX
CAS 151-21-3	Zoharpon LAS Special	CAS 544-63-8	Emery® 655

CAS 544-63-8	Kartacid 1495
CAS 544-63-8	Kartacid 1498
CAS 544-63-8	Prifrac 2940
CAS 546-93-0	Unichem MC
CAS 546-93-0	Unichem MGC
CAS 555-43-1	Aldo® TS
CAS 555-43-1	Dynasan® 118
CAS 555-44-2	Dynasan® 116
CAS 555-45-3	Dynasan® 114
CAS 557-04-0	Cecavon MG 51
CAS 557-04-0	Nuodex Magnesium Stearate Food Grade
CAS 557-04-0	Radiastar® 1100
CAS 557-04-0	Synpro® Magnesium Stearate USP
CAS 557-04-0	Unichem MGS
CAS 557-04-0	Unichem MS
CAS 557-04-0	Witco® Magnesium Stearate N.F
CAS 557-05-1	Cecavon ZN 70
CAS 557-05-1	Cecavon ZN 71
CAS 557-05-1	Cecavon ZN 72
CAS 557-05-1	Cecavon ZN 73
CAS 557-05-1	Cecavon ZN 735
CAS 557-05-1	Radiastar® 1170
CAS 557-05-1	Synpro® Zinc Stearate USP
CAS 557-05-1	Unichem ZS
CAS 557-05-1	Witco® Zinc Stearate U.S.P.-D
CAS 557-08-4	Undezin
CAS 570-24-1	Imexine FP
CAS 575-44-6	Rodol 15N
CAS 577-11-7	Aerosol® OT-75%
CAS 577-11-7	Chemax/DOSS-75E
CAS 577-11-7	Chimin DOS 70
CAS 577-11-7	Emcol® 4500
CAS 577-11-7	Gemtex PA-70
CAS 577-11-7	Gemtex PA-75E
CAS 577-11-7	Gemtex PAX-60
CAS 577-11-7	Gemtex SC-75E, SC Powd.
CAS 577-11-7	Geropon® SBDO
CAS 577-11-7	Hodag DOSS-70
CAS 577-11-7	Hodag DOSS-75
CAS 577-11-7	Marlinat® DF 8
CAS 577-11-7	Monawet MO-65-150
CAS 577-11-7	Monawet MO-70
CAS 577-11-7	Monawet MO-70-150
CAS 577-11-7	Monawet MO-70E
CAS 577-11-7	Monawet MO-70RP
CAS 577-11-7	Nikkol OTP-75
CAS 577-11-7	Nikkol OTP-100
CAS 577-11-7	Nikkol OTP-100S
CAS 577-11-7	Rewopol® SBDO 75
CAS 577-11-7	Schercopol DOS-PG-85
CAS 577-11-7	Solusol® 75%
CAS 577-11-7	Solusol® 100%
CAS 577-11-7	Supermontaline SLT65
CAS 582-17-2	Rodol 27N
CAS 584-08-7	Unichem POCARB
CAS 589-68-4	Cithrol GMM
CAS 589-68-4	Glyceryl Myristate WL 2130
CAS 589-68-4	Imwitor® 914
CAS 589-68-4	Kessco GMN
CAS 589-68-4	Nikkol MGM
CAS 590-00-1	Tristat K
CAS 590-00-1	Unistat K
CAS 591-27-5	Rodol EG
CAS 592-41-6	Ethyl Hexene-1
CAS 592-41-6	Gulftene® 6
CAS 593-29-3	Witco® Potassium Stearate
CAS 597-09-1	NEPD
CAS 603-85-0	Imexine FO
CAS 609-31-4	NB
CAS 610-81-1	Imexine FN
CAS 614-33-5	Uniplex 260
CAS 615-05-4	Rodol BA
CAS 615-50-9	Rodol BLFX
CAS 621-71-6	Dynasan® 110
CAS 624-04-4	Emalex EG-di-L
CAS 624-04-4	Kemester® EGDL
CAS 627-83-8	Ablunol EGDS
CAS 627-83-8	Alkamuls® EGDS
CAS 627-83-8	Chemsperse EGDS
CAS 627-83-8	CPH-360-N
CAS 627-83-8	Cutina® AGS
CAS 627-83-8	Elfacos® EGDS
CAS 627-83-8	Elfan® L 310
CAS 627-83-8	Emalex EG-di-MPS
CAS 627-83-8	Emalex EG-di-S
CAS 627-83-8	Emalex EG-di-SE
CAS 627-83-8	Emerest® 2355
CAS 627-83-8	Estol EGDS 3750
CAS 627-83-8	Ethylene Glycol Distearate VA
CAS 627-83-8	Genapol® PMS
CAS 627-83-8	Hest E.G.D.S
CAS 627-83-8	Hodag EGDS
CAS 627-83-8	Kemester® EGDS
CAS 627-83-8	Kessco® Ethylene Glycol Distearate
CAS 627-83-8	Lanesta EGD
CAS 627-83-8	Lexemul® EGDS
CAS 627-83-8	Lipal EGDS
CAS 627-83-8	Lipo EGDS
CAS 627-83-8	Mackester™ EGDS
CAS 627-83-8	Mapeg® EGDS
CAS 627-83-8	Nikkol EGDS
CAS 627-83-8	Nikkol Estepearl 10, 15
CAS 627-83-8	Nikkol Pearl 1222
CAS 627-83-8	Pegosperse® 50 DS
CAS 627-83-8	Radiasurf® 7269
CAS 627-83-8	Rewopal® PG 280
CAS 627-83-8	RITA EDGS
CAS 627-83-8	Secoster® DMS
CAS 627-83-8	Tegin® G 1100
CAS 627-83-8	Unipeg-EGDS
CAS 627-83-8	Witconol™ 2355
CAS 627-83-8	Zohar EGDS
CAS 629-70-9	Pelemol CA
CAS 629-73-2	Gulftene® 16
CAS 629-76-5	Neodol® 5
CAS 629-82-3	Cetiol® OE
CAS 629-96-9	Cachalot® Arachidyl Alcohol AR-20
CAS 629-96-9	Nacol® 20-95
CAS 635-38-1	Nikkol DP
CAS 637-12-7	Witco® Aluminum Stearate 132
CAS 646-13-9	Estol 1476
CAS 646-13-9	Estol IBUS 1552
CAS 646-13-9	Ibulate
CAS 646-13-9	Kemester® 5415
CAS 646-13-9	Kessco® Isobutyl Stearate
CAS 646-13-9	Radia 7761
CAS 657-84-1	Eltesol® ST 34
CAS 657-84-1	Eltesol® ST 40
CAS 659-40-5	Elestab® HP 100
CAS 661-19-8	Adol® 60
CAS 661-19-8	Cachalot® Behenyl Alcohol BE-22
CAS 661-19-8	Nacol® 22-97
CAS 661-19-8	Nikkol Behenyl Alcohol 65, 80
CAS 661-19-8	Unihydag Wax 22
CAS 683-10-3	Abluter LDB
CAS 683-10-3	Amphoteen 24

CAS Number	Trade Name
CAS 683-10-3	Armoteric LB
CAS 683-10-3	Arquad® DNHTB-75
CAS 683-10-3	Chimin BX
CAS 683-10-3	Dehyton® PAB-30
CAS 683-10-3	LMB
CAS 683-10-3	Lonzaine® 14
CAS 683-10-3	Nikkol AM-301
CAS 683-10-3	Radiateric® 6864
CAS 683-10-3	Rewoteric® AM DML
CAS 683-10-3	Swanol AM-301
CAS 683-10-3	Unibetaine LB
CAS 683-10-3	Varion® CDG
CAS 683-10-3	Varion® CDG-LS
CAS 683-10-3	Zohartaine AB
CAS 693-33-4	Lonzaine® 16S
CAS 693-33-4	Lonzaine® 16SP
CAS 693-33-4	Mackam™ CET
CAS 693-36-7	Argus DSTDP
CAS 813-92-3	Alutrat
CAS 816-94-4	Phospholipon® SC
CAS 820-66-6	Lonzaine® 18S
CAS 820-66-6	Varion® SDG
CAS 822-16-2	Cecavon NA 61
CAS 822-16-2	Norfox® B
CAS 822-16-2	Sodium Stéarate C7L
CAS 822-16-2	Unichem SS
CAS 822-16-2	Witco® Sodium Stearate C-1
CAS 822-16-2	Witco® Sodium Stearate C-7
CAS 871-37-4	Chembetaine OL
CAS 871-37-4	Chembetaine OL-30
CAS 871-37-4	Incronam OD-50
CAS 871-37-4	Mackam™ OB-30
CAS 871-37-4	Mafo® OB
CAS 871-37-4	Unibetaine OLB-30, OLB-50
CAS 871-37-4	Velvetex® OLB-30
CAS 871-37-4	Velvetex® OLB-50
CAS 872-05-9	Gulftene® 10
CAS 928-24-5	Emalex EG-di-O
CAS 1002-89-7	Unichem AMST
CAS 1115-22-6	DIMASPA
CAS 1119-87-5	Mexanyl GU
CAS 1119-97-7	Mytab®
CAS 1119-97-7	Rhodaquat® M214B/99
CAS 1119-97-7	Sumquat® 6110
CAS 1120-01-0	Nikkol SCS
CAS 1120-04-3	Nikkol SSS
CAS 1120-24-7	Adma® 10
CAS 1120-36-1	Gulftene® 14
CAS 1120-49-6	Armeen® 2-10
CAS 1166-52-5	Progallin® LA
CAS 1190-63-2	Estol CES 3705
CAS 1191-50-0	Nikkol SMS
CAS 1300-72-7	Carsosulf SXS
CAS 1300-72-7	Eltesol® SX 30
CAS 1300-72-7	Eltesol® SX 93
CAS 1300-72-7	Manrosol SXS30
CAS 1300-72-7	Manrosol SXS40
CAS 1300-72-7	SXS 40
CAS 1300-72-7	Witconate™ SXS 40%
CAS 1300-72-7	Witconate™ SXS 90%
CAS 1302-78-9	Albagel 4446
CAS 1302-78-9	Albagel Premium USP 4444
CAS 1302-78-9	Albagen 4439
CAS 1302-78-9	Bentolite H
CAS 1302-78-9	Bentolite H 4430
CAS 1302-78-9	Bentolite L
CAS 1302-78-9	Bentolite WH
CAS 1302-78-9	Bentonite USP BC 670
CAS 1302-78-9	Korthix H-NF
CAS 1302-78-9	Polargel® HV
CAS 1302-78-9	Polargel® NF
CAS 1302-78-9	Polargel® T
CAS 1303-96-4	Unichem SOBOR
CAS 1305-62-0	Calcium Hydroxide USP 802
CAS 1305-62-0	Unichem CA HYD
CAS 1305-78-8	Calcium Oxide FCC 801
CAS 1305-78-8	Unichem CAO
CAS 1309-42-8	Hydro-Magma
CAS 1309-42-8	Marinco H-USP
CAS 1309-48-4	Marinco OH
CAS 1309-48-4	Marinco OL
CAS 1310-58-3	Unichem KOHYD
CAS 1310-73-2	Unichem SOHYD
CAS 1314-13-2	Finex-25
CAS 1314-13-2	MZO-25
CAS 1314-13-2	UFZO
CAS 1314-13-2	Unichem ZO
CAS 1314-13-2	USP-1
CAS 1314-13-2	USP-2
CAS 1314-13-2	Z-Cote®
CAS 1314-13-2	Zinc Oxide USP 66
CAS 1314-23-4	Dascare Zirconia
CAS 1318-93-0	Gelwhite GP, H
CAS 1318-93-0	Gelwhite L
CAS 1318-93-0	Green Clay
CAS 1322-98-1	Witconate™ DS
CAS 1323-03-1	Cegesoft® C 17
CAS 1323-03-1	Ceraphyl® 50
CAS 1323-03-1	Cetinol LM
CAS 1323-03-1	Crodamol ML
CAS 1323-03-1	Estalan ML
CAS 1323-03-1	Lactabase C14
CAS 1323-03-1	Liponate ML
CAS 1323-03-1	Nikkol Myristyl Lactate
CAS 1323-03-1	Schercemol ML
CAS 1323-03-1	Unimul MYRLAC
CAS 1323-03-1	Wickenol® 506
CAS 1323-38-2	Surfactol® 13
CAS 1323-39-3	Capmul® PGMS
CAS 1323-39-3	Ceral P
CAS 1323-39-3	Cerasynt® PA
CAS 1323-39-3	Cithrol PGMS N/E
CAS 1323-39-3	Elfacos® PGMS
CAS 1323-39-3	Emalex PGMS
CAS 1323-39-3	Emalex PGS
CAS 1323-39-3	Emerest® 2380
CAS 1323-39-3	Estol PMS 3737
CAS 1323-39-3	Hefti PMS-33
CAS 1323-39-3	Hodag PGMS
CAS 1323-39-3	Kessco PGMS
CAS 1323-39-3	Kessco PGMS-R
CAS 1323-39-3	Kessco PGMS-X534F
CAS 1323-39-3	Kessco® Propylene Glycol Monostearate Pure
CAS 1323-39-3	Lipal PGMS
CAS 1323-39-3	Lipo PGMS
CAS 1323-39-3	Mazol® PGMSK
CAS 1323-39-3	Myverol® P-06
CAS 1323-39-3	Nikkol PMS-1C
CAS 1323-39-3	Nikkol PMS-FR
CAS 1323-39-3	Pegosperse® PMS CG
CAS 1323-39-3	Radiasurf® 7201
CAS 1323-39-3	Schercemol PGMS
CAS 1323-39-3	Unipeg-PGMS
CAS 1323-39-3	Unitolate PGMS
CAS 1323-39-3	Witconol™ 2380
CAS 1323-42-8	Crodamol GHS
CAS 1323-42-8	Naturechem® GMHS
CAS 1323-83-7	Cithrol GDS N/E
CAS 1323-83-7	Estol GDS 3748

CAS 1323-83-7	Kessco® GDS 386F	CAS 1338-39-2	S-Maz® 20
CAS 1323-83-7	Kessco® Glycerol Distearate 386F	CAS 1338-39-2	Sorbax SML
CAS 1323-83-7	Nikkol DGS-80	CAS 1338-39-2	Sorbitol L
CAS 1323-83-7	Unitolate GDS	CAS 1338-39-2	Sorbon S-20
CAS 1327-36-2	Kaopolite® SF	CAS 1338-39-2	Span® 20
CAS 1327-36-2	Suspengel Elite	CAS 1338-41-6	Ablunol S-60
CAS 1327-36-2	Suspengel Micro	CAS 1338-41-6	Alkamuls® SMS
CAS 1327-36-2	Suspengel Ultra	CAS 1338-41-6	Arlacel® 60
CAS 1327-41-9	Alchlordrate	CAS 1338-41-6	Armotan® MS
CAS 1327-41-9	Aloxicoll® L	CAS 1338-41-6	Crill 3
CAS 1327-41-9	Aloxicoll® PC	CAS 1338-41-6	Dehymuls® SMS
CAS 1327-41-9	Aloxicoll® PF	CAS 1338-41-6	Drewmulse® SMS
CAS 1327-41-9	Aloxicoll® PSF	CAS 1338-41-6	Emalex SPE-100S
CAS 1327-41-9	Aluminum Hydroxychloride 23	CAS 1338-41-6	Emsorb® 2505
CAS 1327-41-9	Aluminum Hydroxychloride 47	CAS 1338-41-6	Emultex SMS
CAS 1327-41-9	Chlorhydrol® 50% Sol'n.	CAS 1338-41-6	Estol SMS 3715
CAS 1327-41-9	Chlorhydrol® Granular	CAS 1338-41-6	Ethylan® GS60
CAS 1327-41-9	Chlorhydrol, Impalpable	CAS 1338-41-6	Extan-ST
CAS 1327-41-9	Chlorhydrol® Powd.	CAS 1338-41-6	Glycomul® S
CAS 1327-41-9	Dow Corning® ACH-303	CAS 1338-41-6	Glycomul® S FG
CAS 1327-41-9	Dow Corning® ACH-323	CAS 1338-41-6	Glycomul® S KFG
CAS 1327-41-9	Dow Corning® ACH-331	CAS 1338-41-6	Hefti MS-33-F
CAS 1327-41-9	Dow Corning® ACH7-321	CAS 1338-41-6	Hetan SS
CAS 1327-41-9	Dow Corning® Q5-7171 AACH Powd.	CAS 1338-41-6	Hodag SMS
		CAS 1338-41-6	Ionet S-60 C
CAS 1327-41-9	Locron Extra, Flakes, L, P, P Extra, Powd., S, Sol'n.	CAS 1338-41-6	Ixolene 6
		CAS 1338-41-6	Kemester® S60
CAS 1327-41-9	Macrospherical® 95	CAS 1338-41-6	Liposorb S
CAS 1327-41-9	Micro-Dry®	CAS 1338-41-6	Liposorb SC
CAS 1327-41-9	Micro-Dry® Superultrafine	CAS 1338-41-6	Montane 60
CAS 1327-41-9	Micro-Dry® Ultrafine	CAS 1338-41-6	Nikkol SS-10
CAS 1327-41-9	Reach® 101, 201, 501	CAS 1338-41-6	Nissan Nonion SP-60R
CAS 1327-41-9	Ritachlor 50%	CAS 1338-41-6	Protachem SMS
CAS 1327-41-9	Westchlor® 200	CAS 1338-41-6	Prote-sorb SMS
CAS 1330-80-9	Cithrol PGMO N/E	CAS 1338-41-6	S-Maz® 60
CAS 1330-80-9	CPH-3-SE	CAS 1338-41-6	S-Maz® 60K
CAS 1330-80-9	Emalex PGO	CAS 1338-41-6	S-Maz® 60KHM
CAS 1330-80-9	Radiasurf® 7206	CAS 1338-41-6	Sorban AST
CAS 1331-61-9	Ablusol DBM	CAS 1338-41-6	Sorbax SMS
CAS 1332-58-7	Colloidal Kaolin NF-Bacteria Controlled	CAS 1338-41-6	Sorbirol S
		CAS 1338-41-6	Sorbon S-60
CAS 1332-58-7	Kaopaque 10, 20	CAS 1338-41-6	Sorgen 50
CAS 1332-58-7	Lion English Kaolin	CAS 1338-41-6	Span® 60, 60K
CAS 1332-58-7	Unimin KA	CAS 1338-41-6	Span® 60 VS
CAS 1333-39-7	Eltesol® PSA 65	CAS 1338-41-6	Unitan-S
CAS 1335-72-4	Neopon LOS 70	CAS 1338-41-6	Witconol™ 2505
CAS 1335-72-4	Neopon LOS/NF	CAS 1338-43-8	Ablunol S-80
CAS 1337-76-4	Attasorb RVM Sorbent	CAS 1338-43-8	Alkamuls® SMO
CAS 1337-76-4	Pharmasorb Colloidal Pharmaceutical Grade	CAS 1338-43-8	Arlacel® 80
		CAS 1338-43-8	Armotan® MO
CAS 1337-76-4	Suspentone	CAS 1338-43-8	Crill 4
CAS 1337-76-4	Suspentone 1265	CAS 1338-43-8	Crill 50
CAS 1337-89-9	Abietate de Glycerol	CAS 1338-43-8	Dehymuls® SMO
CAS 1338-39-2	Ablunol S-20	CAS 1338-43-8	Drewmulse® SMO
CAS 1338-39-2	Alkamuls® SML	CAS 1338-43-8	Emalex SPO-100
CAS 1338-39-2	Armotan® ML	CAS 1338-43-8	Emsorb® 2500
CAS 1338-39-2	Crill 1	CAS 1338-43-8	Estol SMO 3685
CAS 1338-39-2	Drewmulse® SML	CAS 1338-43-8	Ethylan® GO80
CAS 1338-39-2	Durtan® 20	CAS 1338-43-8	Extan-OT
CAS 1338-39-2	Emsorb® 2515	CAS 1338-43-8	Famodan SMO
CAS 1338-39-2	Ethylan® GL20	CAS 1338-43-8	Glycomul® O
CAS 1338-39-2	Glycomul® L	CAS 1338-43-8	Hefti MO-33-F
CAS 1338-39-2	Hefti ML-33-F	CAS 1338-43-8	Hetan SO
CAS 1338-39-2	Hetan SL	CAS 1338-43-8	Hodag SMO
CAS 1338-39-2	Hodag SML	CAS 1338-43-8	Ionet S-80
CAS 1338-39-2	Ionet S-20	CAS 1338-43-8	Ixolene 8
CAS 1338-39-2	Liposorb L	CAS 1338-43-8	Kemester® S80
CAS 1338-39-2	Montane 20	CAS 1338-43-8	Liposorb O
CAS 1338-39-2	Nissan Nonion LP-20R, LP-20RS	CAS 1338-43-8	Montane 80
CAS 1338-39-2	Prote-sorb SML	CAS 1338-43-8	Montane 80 SP

CAS 1338-43-8	Nikkol SO-10
CAS 1338-43-8	Nikkol SO-10R
CAS 1338-43-8	Nissan Nonion OP-80R
CAS 1338-43-8	Protachem SMO
CAS 1338-43-8	Prote-sorb SMO
CAS 1338-43-8	S-Maz® 80
CAS 1338-43-8	S-Maz® 80K
CAS 1338-43-8	Sorban AO
CAS 1338-43-8	Sorbax SMO
CAS 1338-43-8	Sorbirol O
CAS 1338-43-8	Sorbon S-80
CAS 1338-43-8	Sorgen 40
CAS 1338-43-8	Sorgen S-40-H
CAS 1338-43-8	Span® 80
CAS 1338-43-8	Unitan-O
CAS 1338-43-8	Witconol™ 2500
CAS 1341-54-4	Uvinul® M 493
CAS 1344-00-9	Valfor® Zeolite Na-A
CAS 1344-00-9	Zeolex® 7
CAS 1344-00-9	Zeolex® 23A
CAS 1344-09-8	Britesil
CAS 1344-09-8	O Silicate
CAS 1344-95-2	Hubersorb®
CAS 1344-95-2	Micro-Cel® C
CAS 1390-65-4	Atomergic Carmine
CAS 1390-65-4	Carmine 5297
CAS 1390-65-4	Carmine Ultra-fine
CAS 1390-65-4	Dascolor Carmine
CAS 1398-61-4	Atomergic Chitin
CAS 1398-61-4	Marine Dew
CAS 1401-55-4	Atomergic Tannic Acid
CAS 1401-55-4	Unichem TANAC
CAS 1405-86-3	Nikkol Glycyrrhizic Acid
CAS 1462-54-0	Afoteric™ 151L
CAS 1462-54-0	Amphoram® CP1
CAS 1462-54-0	Deriphat® 151C
CAS 1462-54-0	Mackam™ 151L
CAS 1462-54-0	Unitex 710-L
CAS 1463-95-2	Takanal
CAS 1559-35-9	Ektasolve® EEH
CAS 1562-00-1	Witconate™ NIS
CAS 1592-23-0	Nuodex S-1421 Food Grade
CAS 1592-23-0	Nuodex S-1520 Food Grade
CAS 1592-23-0	Radiastar® 1060
CAS 1592-23-0	Synpro® Calcium Stearate USP
CAS 1592-23-0	Unichem CS
CAS 1592-23-0	Witco® Calcium Stearate F.P
CAS 1643-19-2	TBAB
CAS 1643-20-5	Ablumox LO
CAS 1643-20-5	Ammonyx® DMCD-40
CAS 1643-20-5	Ammonyx® LO
CAS 1643-20-5	Amyx LO 3594
CAS 1643-20-5	Aromox® DMMC-W
CAS 1643-20-5	Chemoxide LM-30
CAS 1643-20-5	Emcol® DMCD-40
CAS 1643-20-5	Emcol® L
CAS 1643-20-5	Emcol® LO
CAS 1643-20-5	Empigen® OB
CAS 1643-20-5	Incromine Oxide L
CAS 1643-20-5	Lilaminox M24
CAS 1643-20-5	Mackamine™ LO
CAS 1643-20-5	Mazox® LDA
CAS 1643-20-5	Oxamin LO
CAS 1643-20-5	Radiamox® 6804
CAS 1643-20-5	Rewominox L 408
CAS 1643-20-5	Rhodamox® LO
CAS 1643-20-5	Schercamox DML
CAS 1643-20-5	Unimox LO
CAS 1643-20-5	Varox® 270
CAS 1643-20-5	Varox® 365
CAS 1643-20-5	Varox® 375
CAS 1643-20-5	Zoramox LO
CAS 1777-82-8	Lexgard® Myacide SP
CAS 1777-82-8	Midtect TF-60
CAS 1777-82-8	Myacide® SP
CAS 1777-82-8	Unikon A-22
CAS 1812-53-9	Carsoquat® 868
CAS 1812-53-9	Carsoquat® 868-E
CAS 1812-53-9	Carsoquat® 868P
CAS 1812-53-9	Varisoft® 432-100
CAS 1847-55-8	Nikkol TOP-O
CAS 1847-58-1	Lathanol® LAL
CAS 1847-58-1	Nikkol LSA
CAS 1948-33-0	Tenox® TBHQ
CAS 1948-33-0	Uantox TBHQ
CAS 2016-57-1	Amine 12
CAS 2016-57-1	Amine 12-98D
CAS 2116-84-9	Abil® AV 20-1000
CAS 2116-84-9	Abil® AV 8853
CAS 2116-84-9	Baysilone Fluid PD 5
CAS 2116-84-9	Baysilone Fluid PK 20
CAS 2116-84-9	Dow Corning® 556 Fluid
CAS 2116-84-9	Emalex MTS-30E
CAS 2116-84-9	KF56, KF58
CAS 2116-84-9	Masil® 556
CAS 2116-84-9	Rhodorsil® Oils 70641 V 200
CAS 2174-16-5	Neotan W
CAS 2235-54-3	Akyposal ALS 33
CAS 2235-54-3	Calfoam ALS-30
CAS 2235-54-3	Calfoam NLS-30
CAS 2235-54-3	Carsonol® ALS
CAS 2235-54-3	Carsonol® ALS-R
CAS 2235-54-3	Carsonol® ALS-S
CAS 2235-54-3	Carsonol® ALS Special
CAS 2235-54-3	Empicol® AL30/T
CAS 2235-54-3	Manro ALS 25
CAS 2235-54-3	Manro ALS 30
CAS 2235-54-3	Marlinat® DFN 30
CAS 2235-54-3	Neopon LAM
CAS 2235-54-3	Nikkol ALS-25
CAS 2235-54-3	Norfox® ALS
CAS 2235-54-3	Nutrapon HA 3841
CAS 2235-54-3	Nutrapon PP 3563
CAS 2235-54-3	Perlankrol® DAF25
CAS 2235-54-3	Rewopol® ALS 30
CAS 2235-54-3	Rhodapon® L-22, L-22/C
CAS 2235-54-3	Rhodapon® L-22HNC
CAS 2235-54-3	Standapol® A
CAS 2235-54-3	Standapol® A-HV
CAS 2235-54-3	Stepanol® AM
CAS 2235-54-3	Stepanol® AM-V
CAS 2235-54-3	Sulfochem ALS
CAS 2235-54-3	Surfax ASD
CAS 2235-54-3	Surfax NH
CAS 2235-54-3	Texapon® ALS
CAS 2235-54-3	Texapon® PNA
CAS 2235-54-3	Ufarol Am 30
CAS 2235-54-3	Ufarol Am 70
CAS 2235-54-3	Unipol A
CAS 2235-54-3	Witcolate™ NH
CAS 2235-54-3	Zoharpon LAA
CAS 2277-28-3	Dimodan LS Kosher
CAS 2372-82-9	Lonzabac-12.100
CAS 2425-77-6	Isofol® 16
CAS 2568-33-4	IPG
CAS 2571-88-2	Admox® 18-85
CAS 2571-88-2	Ammonyx® SO
CAS 2571-88-2	Amyx SO 3734
CAS 2571-88-2	Annonyx SO
CAS 2571-88-2	Barlox® 18S

CAS 2571-88-2	Chemoxide ST	CAS 3055-97-8	Ablunol LA-7
CAS 2571-88-2	Emcol® SO	CAS 3055-97-8	Emalex 707
CAS 2571-88-2	Incromine Oxide S	CAS 3055-97-8	Macol® LA-790
CAS 2571-88-2	Mackamine™ SO	CAS 3055-97-8	Marlowet® LA 7
CAS 2571-88-2	Mazox® SDA	CAS 3055-97-8	Procol LA-7
CAS 2571-88-2	Rewominox S 300	CAS 3055-98-9	Akyporox RLM 80V
CAS 2571-88-2	Schercamox DMS	CAS 3055-99-0	Ablunol LA-9
CAS 2571-88-2	Standamox PS	CAS 3055-99-0	Britex EMB
CAS 2571-88-2	Unimox SO	CAS 3055-99-0	Carsonon® L-9
CAS 2605-79-0	Barlox® 10S	CAS 3055-99-0	Chemal LA-9
CAS 2644-64-6	Phospholipon® PC	CAS 3055-99-0	Emalex 709
CAS 2673-22-5	Hodag DTSS-70	CAS 3055-99-0	G-4829
CAS 2724-58-5	Liponate ISA Special	CAS 3055-99-0	Hetoxol L-9
CAS 2724-58-5	Prisorine 3501	CAS 3055-99-0	Hodag Nonionic L-9
CAS 2724-58-5	Prisorine 3505	CAS 3055-99-0	Macol® LA-9
CAS 2724-58-5	Prisorine ISAC 3505	CAS 3055-99-0	Marlipal® 129
CAS 2724-58-5	Unitol ISA	CAS 3055-99-0	Nikkol BL-9EX
CAS 2745-8-931	Exxal® 18	CAS 3055-99-0	Procol LA-9
CAS 2778-96-3	Alkamuls® SS	CAS 3055-99-0	Prox-onic LA-1/09
CAS 2778-96-3	Cetinol EE	CAS 3055-99-0	Unicol LA-9
CAS 2778-96-3	Emalex CC-18	CAS 3056-00-6	Ablunol LA-12
CAS 2778-96-3	Estol STST 3706	CAS 3056-00-6	Carsonon® L-12
CAS 2778-96-3	Hetester 412	CAS 3056-00-6	Chemal LA-12
CAS 2778-96-3	Lexol® SS	CAS 3056-00-6	Emalex 712
CAS 2778-96-3	Liponate SS	CAS 3056-00-6	Emthox® 5967
CAS 2778-96-3	Ritachol SS	CAS 3056-00-6	Hetoxol L-12
CAS 2778-96-3	Unimul 1818	CAS 3056-00-6	Hodag Nonionic L-12
CAS 2807-30-9	Ektasolve® EP	CAS 3056-00-6	Lipocol L-12
CAS 2809-21-4	Turpinal® SL	CAS 3056-00-6	Macol® LA-12
CAS 2809-21-4	Unitex P	CAS 3056-00-6	Procol LA-12
CAS 2835-95-2	Rodol PAOC	CAS 3056-00-6	Prox-onic LA-1/012
CAS 2867-47-2	Ageflex FM-1	CAS 3088-31-1	Surfax EVE
CAS 2915-57-3	Crodamol OSU	CAS 3097-08-3	Akyposal MGLS
CAS 2915-57-3	Wickenol® 159	CAS 3097-08-3	Carsonol® MLS
CAS 2973-21-9	Imexine FB	CAS 3097-08-3	Elfan® 2240 Mg
CAS 3006-15-3	Aerosol® MA-80	CAS 3097-08-3	Empicol® ML30
CAS 3006-15-3	Monawet MM-80	CAS 3097-08-3	Rhodapon® LM
CAS 3008-50-2	Lonzest® 163-S	CAS 3097-08-3	Standapol® MG
CAS 3026-63-9	Rhodapon® TDS	CAS 3097-08-3	Stepanol® MG
CAS 3055-93-4	Akyporox RLM 22	CAS 3097-08-3	Sulfetal MG 30
CAS 3055-93-4	Arlypon® F	CAS 3097-08-3	Sulfochem MG
CAS 3055-93-4	Bio-Soft® E-300	CAS 3097-08-3	Surfax MG
CAS 3055-93-4	Carsonon® L-2	CAS 3097-08-3	Texapon® MGLS
CAS 3055-93-4	Hetoxol L-2	CAS 3097-08-3	Unipol MGLS
CAS 3055-93-4	Lauropal 2	CAS 3097-08-3	Witcolate™ MG-LS
CAS 3055-93-4	Marlowet® LMA 2	CAS 3097-08-3	Zoharpon MgS
CAS 3055-93-4	Nikkol BL-2	CAS 3115-49-9	Akypo NP 70
CAS 3055-93-4	Oxetal VD 20	CAS 3121-60-6	Uvinul® DS 49
CAS 3055-93-4	Procol LA-2	CAS 3131-52-0	Imexine OAY
CAS 3055-93-4	Prox-onic LA-1/02	CAS 3147-75-9	Spectra-Sorb® UV 5411
CAS 3055-93-4	Unihydol LS-2	CAS 3151-59-5	Unifluorid H 101
CAS 3055-94-5	Ablunol LA-3	CAS 3179-80-4	Chemidex L
CAS 3055-94-5	AE-1214/3	CAS 3179-80-4	Lexamine L-13
CAS 3055-94-5	Carsonon® L-3	CAS 3179-80-4	Mackine™ 801
CAS 3055-94-5	Emalex 703	CAS 3179-80-4	Schercodine L
CAS 3055-94-5	Empilan® KC 3	CAS 3179-81-5	Cerasynt® 303
CAS 3055-94-5	Genapol® L-3	CAS 3228-02-2	Biosol
CAS 3055-94-5	Glicolene	CAS 3228-02-2	Dekacymen
CAS 3055-94-5	Hetoxol L-3N	CAS 3234-85-3	Alkamuls® MM/M
CAS 3055-94-5	Lauropal 3	CAS 3234-85-3	Ceraphyl® 424
CAS 3055-94-5	Oxetal VD 28	CAS 3234-85-3	Cetinol MM
CAS 3055-94-5	Procol LA-3	CAS 3234-85-3	Cetiol® MM
CAS 3055-94-5	Rewopal® LA 3	CAS 3234-85-3	Crodamol MM
CAS 3055-94-5	Unihydol LS-3	CAS 3234-85-3	Hefti MYM-33
CAS 3055-95-6	Ablunol LA-5	CAS 3234-85-3	Kemester® MM
CAS 3055-95-6	Carsonon® L-5	CAS 3234-85-3	Liponate MM
CAS 3055-95-6	Emalex 705	CAS 3234-85-3	Nikkol MM
CAS 3055-95-6	Marlowet® LMA 5	CAS 3234-85-3	Pelemol MM
CAS 3055-95-6	Mulsifan RT 23	CAS 3234-85-3	Schercemol MM
CAS 3055-96-7	Rewopal® LA 6	CAS 3234-85-3	Unimul 14

CAS 3234-85-3	Waxenol® 810
CAS 3319-31-1	Kodaflex® TOTM
CAS 3332-27-2	Admox® 14-85
CAS 3332-27-2	Ammonyx® MCO
CAS 3332-27-2	Ammonyx® MO
CAS 3332-27-2	Aromox® DM14D-W
CAS 3332-27-2	Barlox® 14
CAS 3332-27-2	Emcol® M
CAS 3332-27-2	Emcol® MO
CAS 3332-27-2	Empigen® OH25
CAS 3332-27-2	Incromine Oxide M
CAS 3332-27-2	Lilaminox M4
CAS 3332-27-2	Manro AO 25M
CAS 3332-27-2	Mazox® MDA
CAS 3332-27-2	Schercamox DMA
CAS 3332-27-2	Schercamox DMM
CAS 3380-34-5	Irgasan DP300
CAS 3398-33-2	Undenat
CAS 3400-45-1	Nikkol Naphthenic Acid
CAS 3401-73-8	Monawet SNO-35
CAS 3401-74-9	Kemamine® Q-6902C
CAS 3436-44-0	Phospholipon® CC
CAS 3539-43-3	Crodafos MCA
CAS 3632-91-5	Gluconal® MG
CAS 3655-00-3	Deriphat® 160
CAS 3655-00-3	Monateric 1188M
CAS 3687-45-4	Cetiol®
CAS 3687-45-4	Crodamol OO
CAS 3687-45-4	Schercemol OLO
CAS 3687-45-4	Unitolate OLOL
CAS 3687-45-4	Wickenol® 143
CAS 3687-46-5	Cetiol® V
CAS 3687-46-5	Crodamol DO
CAS 3687-46-5	Elfacos® DO
CAS 3687-46-5	Estalan DO
CAS 3687-46-5	Estol DCO 3662
CAS 3687-46-5	Estol DCO-b 3655
CAS 3687-46-5	Kessco DO
CAS 3687-46-5	Schercemol DO
CAS 3687-46-5	Tegosoft® DO
CAS 3687-46-5	Trivent OL-10
CAS 3687-46-5	Unimul-CTV
CAS 3687-46-5	Unitolate V
CAS 3734-33-6	Atomergic Denatonium Benzoate
CAS 3734-33-6	Bitrex
CAS 3737-55-1	Nikkol PMT
CAS 3794-83-0	Mayoquest 1530
CAS 3794-83-0	Turpinal® 4 NL
CAS 3794-83-0	Universene AC
CAS 3811-73-2	Sodium Omadine®, 40% Aq. Sol'n.
CAS 3913-02-8	Isofol® 12
CAS 4065-45-6	Syntase® 230
CAS 4065-45-6	Uvasorb S-5
CAS 4065-45-6	Uvinul® MS 40
CAS 4070-80-8	Pruv™
CAS 4075-81-4	Unistat CALBAN
CAS 4075-81-4	Unistat CALPRO
CAS 4169-04-4	Propylene Phenoxetol
CAS 4207-40-3	Tri-K Allantoin Acetyl Methionine
CAS 4219-49-2	Lanol P
CAS 4292-10-8	Chimin LX
CAS 4292-10-8	Lexaine® LM
CAS 4337-75-1	Nikkol LMT
CAS 4337-75-1	Zoharpon LMT42
CAS 4345-03-3	Covitol 1185
CAS 4345-03-3	Covitol 1210
CAS 4345-03-3	Eastman® Vitamin E Succinate
CAS 4390-04-9	Arlamol® HD
CAS 4390-04-9	Permethyl® 101A
CAS 4403-12-7	Bio-Soft® TD 400
CAS 4403-12-7	Chemal TDA-3
CAS 4403-12-7	Hetoxol TD-3
CAS 4403-12-7	Lipocol TD-3
CAS 4403-12-7	Macol® TD-3
CAS 4403-12-7	Procol TDA-3
CAS 4403-12-7	Synperonic A3
CAS 4403-12-7	Volpo T-3
CAS 4418-26-2	Fongasel
CAS 4418-26-2	Trisept SDHA
CAS 4418-26-2	Tristat SDHA
CAS 4418-26-2	Unisept DSA
CAS 4468-02-4	Gluconal® ZN
CAS 4485-12-5	Witco® Lithium Stearate 306
CAS 4536-30-5	Bio-Soft® E-200
CAS 4536-30-5	Hetoxol L-1
CAS 4536-30-5	Lipocol L-1
CAS 4602-84-0	Dragoco Farnesol
CAS 4698-29-7	Rodol Gray BS
CAS 4706-78-9	Nikkol KLS
CAS 4706-78-9	Sulfochem K
CAS 4722-98-9	Akyposal MLS 30
CAS 4722-98-9	Aremsol MA
CAS 4722-98-9	Aremsol MR
CAS 4722-98-9	Cosmopon MO
CAS 4722-98-9	Elfan® 240M
CAS 4722-98-9	Elfan® 2240 M
CAS 4722-98-9	Empicol® 1220/T
CAS 4722-98-9	Empicol® LQ33/T
CAS 4722-98-9	Empicol® LQ70
CAS 4722-98-9	Manro ML 33
CAS 4722-98-9	Rewopol® MLS 30
CAS 4722-98-9	Standapol® MLS
CAS 4722-98-9	Sulfochem MLS
CAS 4722-98-9	Surfax MEA
CAS 4722-98-9	Texapon® MLS
CAS 4722-98-9	Unipol MLS
CAS 4722-98-9	Zoharpon LAM
CAS 4748-78-1	Ebal
CAS 4810-50-8	Kalidone®
CAS 4826-87-3	Lonzest® 153-S
CAS 4826-87-3	Nikkol Trialan 308
CAS 5013-16-5	Tenox® BHA
CAS 5026-62-0	Nipagin M Sodium
CAS 5026-62-0	Unisept M NA
CAS 5131-66-8	Butyl Propasol
CAS 5232-99-5	Uvinul® N 35
CAS 5274-68-0	Akyporox RLM 40
CAS 5274-68-0	Brij® 30
CAS 5274-68-0	Brij® 30SP
CAS 5274-68-0	Chemal LA-4
CAS 5274-68-0	Emthox® 5882
CAS 5274-68-0	Hetoxol L-4
CAS 5274-68-0	Hodag Nonionic L-4
CAS 5274-68-0	Lipocol L-4
CAS 5274-68-0	Macol® LA-4
CAS 5274-68-0	Marlowet® LA 4
CAS 5274-68-0	Marlowet® LMA 4
CAS 5274-68-0	Mulsifan CPA
CAS 5274-68-0	Nikkol BL-4.2
CAS 5274-68-0	Procol LA-4
CAS 5274-68-0	Prox-onic LA-1/04
CAS 5274-68-0	Simulsol P4
CAS 5274-68-0	Trycol® 5882
CAS 5274-68-0	Unicol LA-4
CAS 5274-68-0	Unihydol LS-4
CAS 5274-68-0	Witconol™ 5875
CAS 5306-85-4	Arlasolve® DMI
CAS 5333-42-6	Eutanol® G
CAS 5333-42-6	Exxal® 20

CAS 5333-42-6	Isofol® 20
CAS 5333-42-6	Michel XO-150-20
CAS 5333-42-6	Unimul-G
CAS 5333-42-6	U Tanol G
CAS 5422-34-4	Incromectant LMEA
CAS 5422-34-4	Lipamide LMEA
CAS 5422-34-4	Mackamide™ LME
CAS 5422-34-4	Naetex-ŁAM
CAS 5422-34-4	Parapel® LAM-100
CAS 5422-34-4	Schercomid LME
CAS 5422-34-4	Upamide LACAMEA
CAS 5434-57-1	Schercemol 65
CAS 5466-77-3	Escalol® 557
CAS 5466-77-3	Nanospheres 100 Conc. in O.M.C
CAS 5466-77-3	Neo Heliopan, Type AV
CAS 5466-77-3	Parsol® MCX
CAS 5793-94-2	Artodan CF 40
CAS 5793-94-2	Crolactil CSL
CAS 5793-94-2	Pationic® CSL
CAS 5793-94-2	Unitolate CSL
CAS 6144-28-1	Empol® 1024
CAS 6179-44-8	Schercotaine IAB
CAS 6182-11-2	Emalex PG-di-S
CAS 6197-30-4	Escalol® 597
CAS 6197-30-4	Neo Heliopan, Type 303
CAS 6197-30-4	Uvinul® N 539
CAS 6219-71-2	Rodol Brown SO
CAS 6219-73-4	Rodol Gray DMS
CAS 6219-77-8	Rodol 4GP
CAS 6221-95-0	Crodamol MP
CAS 6221-95-0	Lonzest® 143-S
CAS 6221-95-0	Schercemol MP
CAS 6272-74-8	Emcol® E-607L
CAS 6283-92-7	Alkamuls® LVL
CAS 6283-92-7	Ceraphyl® 31
CAS 6283-92-7	Cetinol 1212
CAS 6283-92-7	Cetinol LL
CAS 6283-92-7	Crodamol LL
CAS 6283-92-7	Estalan LL
CAS 6381-59-5	Unichem ROSAL
CAS 6381-77-7	Uantox SEBATE
CAS 6381-77-7	Uantox SODERT
CAS 6440-58-0	Dekafald
CAS 6440-58-0	Glydant®
CAS 6440-58-0	Glydant® XL-1000
CAS 6440-58-0	Mackstat® DM
CAS 6440-58-0	Nipaguard® DMDMH
CAS 6485-34-3	Unisweet CALSAC
CAS 6485-39-8	Gluconal® MN
CAS 6540-99-4	Emalex 710
CAS 6540-99-4	Marlowet® LMA 10
CAS 6540-99-4	Procol LA-10
CAS 6540-99-4	Unihydol 100
CAS 6540-99-4	Unihydol LS 10
CAS 6542-37-6	Zoldine® ZT-55
CAS 6542-37-6	Zoldine® ZT Oxazolidine
CAS 6846-50-0	Kodaflex® TXIB
CAS 6881-94-3	Ektasolve® DP
CAS 6938-94-9	Ceraphyl® 230
CAS 6938-94-9	Crodamol DA
CAS 6938-94-9	Docoil Dipa
CAS 6938-94-9	Estalan DIA
CAS 6938-94-9	Iso-Adipate 2/043700
CAS 6938-94-9	Nikkol DID
CAS 6938-94-9	Pelemol DIA
CAS 6938-94-9	Schercemol DIA
CAS 6938-94-9	Trivent DIA
CAS 6938-94-9	Upamate DIPA
CAS 7128-91-8	Ammonyx® CO
CAS 7128-91-8	Amyx CO 3764

CAS 7128-91-8	Barlox® 16S
CAS 7128-91-8	Mazox® CDA
CAS 7173-51-5	Bardac® 2250
CAS 7173-51-5	BTC® 1010
CAS 7173-51-5	Maquat 4450-E
CAS 7235-40-7	Beta Carotene 30% in Veg. Oil No. 65646
CAS 7235-40-7	Carotene Standard RR
CAS 7235-40-7	Crystalline Beta Carotene No. 65638
CAS 7281-04-1	Amonyl BR 1244
CAS 7299-99-2	Nikkol Pentarate 408
CAS 7299-99-2	Trivent PE-48
CAS 73-40-5	Dew Pearl AH-1
CAS 7320-34-5	Empiphos 4KP
CAS 7360-53-4	Altriform S
CAS 7378-99-6	Adma® 8
CAS 7384-98-7	Captex® 800
CAS 7384-98-7	Crodamol PC
CAS 7384-98-7	Nikkol Sefsol 228
CAS 7396-58-9	Armeen® M2-10D
CAS 7398-69-8	Ageflex mDMDAC
CAS 7425-14-1	Dragoxat EH 2/044115
CAS 7425-14-1	Pelemol 88
CAS 7425-14-1	Tegosoft® EE
CAS 7447-40-7	Unichem KCL
CAS 7447-40-7	Unichem POCHLOR
CAS 7487-88-9	Unichem EPSAL
CAS 7491-02-3	Schercemol DIS
CAS 7491-14-7	Dipsal
CAS 7491-92-3	Nikkol DIS
CAS 7491-92-3	Pelemol DIPS
CAS 7545-23-5	Emalex NN-5
CAS 7545-23-5	Emalex NN-15
CAS 7545-23-5	Hetamide M
CAS 7545-23-5	Miristamina
CAS 7545-23-5	Monamid® 150-MW
CAS 7545-23-5	Protamide MRCA
CAS 7585-39-9	Alpha W 6 Pharma Grade
CAS 7585-39-9	Beta W 7
CAS 7585-39-9	Cavitron Cyclo-dextrin™
CAS 7585-39-9	Dexpearl
CAS 7585-39-9	Gamma W8
CAS 7585-39-9	Kleptose
CAS 7585-39-9	Rhodocap-A, G, N
CAS 7585-39-9	Ringdex-A, B
CAS 7631-86-9	Celite® 503
CAS 7631-86-9	Celite® 512
CAS 7631-86-9	Celite® 521 AW
CAS 7631-86-9	Celite® 545
CAS 7631-86-9	Celite® 550
CAS 7631-86-9	Celite® 560
CAS 7631-86-9	Celite® 577
CAS 7631-86-9	Filter-Cel
CAS 7631-86-9	Hyflo Super-Cel
CAS 7631-86-9	Spheron L-1500
CAS 7631-86-9	Spheron P-1000
CAS 7631-86-9	Spheron P-1500
CAS 7631-86-9	Standard Super-Cel
CAS 7631-86-9	Super Floss
CAS 7631-90-5	Uantox SBS
CAS 7651-02-7	Adogen® S-18 V
CAS 7651-02-7	Chemidex S
CAS 7651-02-7	Incromine SB
CAS 7651-02-7	Lexamine S-13
CAS 7651-02-7	Lipamine SPA
CAS 7651-02-7	Mackine™ 301
CAS 7651-02-7	Miramine® SODI
CAS 7651-02-7	Schercodine S
CAS 7651-02-7	Tegamine® 18

CAS 7651-02-7	Tego®-Amid S 18	CAS 8001-25-0	Nikkol Olive Oil
CAS 7651-02-7	Unizeen SA	CAS 8001-25-0	Olive Oil, Refined
CAS 7681-11-0	Unichem KI	CAS 8001-25-0	Super Refined™ Olive Oil
CAS 7681-55-2	Unichem SODIOD	CAS 8001-25-0	Tri-Ol OLV
CAS 7681-57-4	Uantox SMBS	CAS 8001-29-4	EmCon Cotton
CAS 7695-91-2	Eastman® Vitamin E 6-40	CAS 8001-29-4	Super Refined™ Cottonseed Oil
CAS 7695-91-2	Eastman® Vitamin E 6-81	CAS 8001-29-4	Univegoil COTSD
CAS 7695-91-2	Eastman® Vitamin E 6-100	CAS 8001-30-7	Corn Oil, Refined
CAS 7695-91-2	Eastman® Vitamin E 700	CAS 8001-30-7	Lipex 104
CAS 7695-91-2	Nanospheres 100 Vitamine E Acetate	CAS 8001-30-7	Nikkol Corn Germ Oil
		CAS 8001-30-7	Super Refined™ Corn Oil
CAS 7695-91-2	Uantox 1250	CAS 8001-30-7	Univegoil CRN
CAS 7702-01-4	Amphoterge® J-2	CAS 8001-31-8	Coconut Oils® 76, 92, 110
CAS 7702-01-4	Mackam™ 2CY	CAS 8001-31-8	EmCon COCO
CAS 7702-01-4	Schercoteric CY-2	CAS 8001-31-8	Lipovol C-76
CAS 7702-01-4	Sochamine A 8955	CAS 8001-31-8	Pureco® 76
CAS 7704-34-9	Biosulphur Powder	CAS 8001-31-8	Univegoil COCO
CAS 7704-34-9	Unisulcoidal	CAS 8001-39-6	Japan Wax NJ-9002
CAS 7722-84-1	Albone® 35 CG	CAS 8001-39-6	Japan Wax Stralpitz
CAS 7722-84-1	Albone® 50 CG	CAS 8001-39-6	Ross Japan Wax
CAS 7722-84-1	Albone® 70CG	CAS 8001-54-5	Noramium DA.50
CAS 7747-35-5	Oxaban®-E	CAS 8001-61-4	EmCon COPA
CAS 7757-93-9	Anhydrous Emcompress®	CAS 8001-69-2	Atomergic Cod Liver Oil
CAS 7758-05-6	Unichem KIO3	CAS 8001-69-2	EmCon COD
CAS 7775-50-0	Crodamol TSC	CAS 8001-75-0	Ceresine Wax Cosmetic Stralpitz
CAS 7778-18-9	Calcium Sulfate Anhydrous NF 164	CAS 8001-75-0	Ceresine Wax SP 84
		CAS 8001-75-0	Koster Keunen Ceresine
CAS 7778-18-9	Etra Super English Terra Alba	CAS 8001-75-0	Koster Keunen Ceresine 130/135
CAS 7778-18-9	Unichem CS White	CAS 8001-75-0	Koster Keunen Ceresine 140/145
CAS 7784-25-0	Unichem AMAL	CAS 8001-75-0	Koster Keunen Ceresine 155
CAS 7787-59-9	Biron®	CAS 8001-75-0	Koster Keunen Ceresine 192
CAS 7787-59-9	Biron® B-5	CAS 8001-75-0	Natwax CER
CAS 7787-59-9	Biron® B-50	CAS 8001-75-0	Ross Ceresine Wax
CAS 7787-59-9	Biron® ESQ	CAS 8001-78-3	Castorwax® MP-70
CAS 7787-59-9	Biron® Fines	CAS 8001-78-3	Castorwax® MP-80
CAS 7787-59-9	Biron® HB	CAS 8001-78-3	Castorwax® NF
CAS 7787-59-9	Biron® NLD-SP	CAS 8001-78-3	Cutina® HR
CAS 7787-59-9	Mearlite® GBU	CAS 8001-78-3	Flowtone R
CAS 7787-59-9	Mearlite® GGH	CAS 8001-78-3	Rol TR
CAS 7787-59-9	Mearlite® LBU	CAS 8001-78-3	Ross Castor Wax
CAS 7787-59-9	Pearl I	CAS 8001-78-3	Thixcin® R
CAS 7787-59-9	Pearl II	CAS 8001-78-3	Unitina HR
CAS 7787-59-9	Pearl-Glo®	CAS 8001-79-4	AA USP
CAS 7787-59-9	Pearl Super Supreme	CAS 8001-79-4	Castor Oil USP
CAS 7787-59-9	Pearl Supreme UVS	CAS 8001-79-4	Cosmetol® X
CAS 7789-38-0	Unineut SOBROM	CAS 8001-79-4	Crystal® O
CAS 7789-77-7	Emcompress®	CAS 8001-79-4	Crystal® Crown
CAS 8000-48-4	EmCon Eucalyptus	CAS 8001-79-4	Crystal® Crown LP
CAS 8001-17-0	EmCon E-5	CAS 8001-79-4	Diamond Quality®
CAS 8001-21-6	Florasun™-90	CAS 8001-79-4	EmCon CO
CAS 8001-21-6	Lipex 103	CAS 8001-79-4	Lanaetex CO
CAS 8001-21-6	Lipovol SUN	CAS 8001-79-4	Lipovol CO
CAS 8001-21-6	Nikkol Sunflower Oil	CAS 8001-79-4	Unicast CO
CAS 8001-21-6	Super Refined™ Sunflower Oil	CAS 8001-79-4	York Krystal Kleer Castor Oil
CAS 8001-21-6	Tri-K Sunflower Oil	CAS 8001-79-4	York USP Castor Oil
CAS 8001-21-6	Tri-Ol SUN	CAS 8001-97-6	Aloe Vera Whole Leaf Dried Powd.
CAS 8001-21-6	Univegoil SUNFL	CAS 8002-03-7	EmCon Peanut
CAS 8001-22-7	EmCon Soya	CAS 8002-03-7	Lipex 101
CAS 8001-22-7	Lipovol SOY	CAS 8002-03-7	Super Refined™ Peanut Oil
CAS 8001-22-7	Super Refined™ Soybean Oil USP	CAS 8002-03-7	Univegoil P-O
CAS 8001-23-8	Linoleic Safflower Oil	CAS 8002-31-1	Atomergic Cocoa Butter
CAS 8001-23-8	Lipovol SAF	CAS 8002-31-1	Fancol CB
CAS 8001-23-8	Natoil SAF	CAS 8002-31-1	Fancol CB Extra
CAS 8001-23-8	Neobee® 18	CAS 8002-31-1	Univeg CCB
CAS 8001-23-8	Nikkol Safflower Oil	CAS 8002-33-3	Haroil SCO-50
CAS 8001-23-8	Super Refined™ Safflower Oil USP	CAS 8002-33-3	Laurel R-50
		CAS 8002-33-3	Nopcocastor
CAS 8001-23-8	Tri-Ol SAF	CAS 8002-33-3	Standapol® SCO
CAS 8001-25-0	EmCon Olive	CAS 8002-33-3	Turkey Red Oil 100%
CAS 8001-25-0	Lipovol O	CAS 8002-33-3	Türkischrotöl 100%

CAS 8002-33-3	Unipol SCO
CAS 8002-43-5	Alcolec® BS
CAS 8002-43-5	Alcolec® Extra A
CAS 8002-43-5	Alcolec® F-100
CAS 8002-43-5	Alcolec® Granules
CAS 8002-43-5	Alcolec® PG
CAS 8002-43-5	Alcolec® S
CAS 8002-43-5	Alcolec® SFG
CAS 8002-43-5	Asol
CAS 8002-43-5	Augon 1000
CAS 8002-43-5	Basis LP-20
CAS 8002-43-5	Basis LS-60
CAS 8002-43-5	Centrolex® F
CAS 8002-43-5	Centrolex® P
CAS 8002-43-5	Centrophase® C
CAS 8002-43-5	Centrophase® HR
CAS 8002-43-5	Centrophase® HR6B
CAS 8002-43-5	Centrophil® W
CAS 8002-43-5	Crolec 4135
CAS 8002-43-5	Dermasome® MT
CAS 8002-43-5	Emulmetik™ 100
CAS 8002-43-5	Emulmetik™ 135
CAS 8002-43-5	Emulmetik™ 300
CAS 8002-43-5	Emulmetik™ 970
CAS 8002-43-5	Lecithin Extract Kosmaflor, Water-Disp.
CAS 8002-43-5	Lecsoy E
CAS 8002-43-5	Lecsoy S
CAS 8002-43-5	Lexin K
CAS 8002-43-5	Lipoid S 100
CAS 8002-43-5	Liposome Conc. E-10
CAS 8002-43-5	Natipide 08010A
CAS 8002-43-5	Phosal 15
CAS 8002-43-5	PhosPho E-100
CAS 8002-43-5	PhosPho F-97
CAS 8002-43-5	PhosPho LCN-TS
CAS 8002-43-5	Phospholipon® 25G, 25P, 50
CAS 8002-43-5	Phospholipon® 80
CAS 8002-43-5	Probiol™ L/N
CAS 8002-43-5	Unilec S
CAS 8002-43-5	Unilex, DS, S, SH
CAS 8002-50-4	Super Refined™ Menhaden Oil
CAS 8002-53-7	Ross Bleached Montan Wax
CAS 8002-53-7	Ross Bleached Montan Wax Cosmetic
CAS 8002-74-2	CS-2032
CAS 8002-74-2	CS-2037
CAS 8002-74-2	CS-2043
CAS 8002-74-2	CS-2054
CAS 8002-74-2	Eskar Wax R-25, R-35, R-40, R-45, R-50
CAS 8002-74-2	Koster Keunen Paraffin Wax
CAS 8002-74-2	Koster Keunen Paraffin Wax 122/128
CAS 8002-74-2	Koster Keunen Paraffin Wax 130/135
CAS 8002-74-2	Koster Keunen Paraffin Wax 140/145
CAS 8002-74-2	Koster Keunen Paraffin Wax 150/155
CAS 8002-74-2	Microfine 2, 2F, 2FS, 8, 8F
CAS 8002-74-2	Press-Aid™ SP
CAS 8002-74-2	Press-Aid™ XP
CAS 8002-74-2	PT-0602
CAS 8002-74-2	Ross Crude Scale Wax
CAS 8002-74-2	Uniwax AW-1060
CAS 8002-74-2	Uniwax PARA
CAS 8002-74-2	Vybar® 103
CAS 8002-74-2	Vybar® 260
CAS 8002-74-2	Vybar® 825
CAS 8002-75-3	Lipovol PAL
CAS 8005-44-5	Cetax 50
CAS 8005-44-5	Koster Keunen Fatty Alcohol 1618
CAS 8006-44-8	Candelilla Wax Cosmetic Grade Stralpitz
CAS 8006-44-8	Koster Keunen Candelilla
CAS 8006-44-8	Natwax CAN
CAS 8006-44-8	Ross Candelilla Wax
CAS 8006-54-0	Anhydrous Lanolin Grade 1
CAS 8006-54-0	Anhydrous Lanolin Grade 2
CAS 8006-54-0	Anhydrous Lanolin P.80
CAS 8006-54-0	Anhydrous Lanolin P.95
CAS 8006-54-0	Anhydrous Lanolin P.95RA
CAS 8006-54-0	Anhydrous Lanolin Superfine
CAS 8006-54-0	Anhydrous Lanolin USP
CAS 8006-54-0	Anhydrous Lanolin USP Cosmetic
CAS 8006-54-0	Anhydrous Lanolin USP Cosmetic AA
CAS 8006-54-0	Anhydrous Lanolin USP Cosmetic Grade
CAS 8006-54-0	Anhydrous Lanolin USP Deodorized AAA
CAS 8006-54-0	Anhydrous Lanolin USP Pharmaceutical
CAS 8006-54-0	Anhydrous Lanolin USP Pharmaceutical Grade
CAS 8006-54-0	Anhydrous Lanolin USP Pharmaceutical Light Grade
CAS 8006-54-0	Anhydrous Lanolin USP Superfine
CAS 8006-54-0	Anhydrous Lanolin USP Ultrafine
CAS 8006-54-0	Anhydrous Lanolin USP X-tra Deodorized
CAS 8006-54-0	Corona Lanolin
CAS 8006-54-0	Coronet Lanolin
CAS 8006-54-0	Cosmetic Lanolin
CAS 8006-54-0	Cosmetic Lanolin Anhydrous USP
CAS 8006-54-0	Emery® 1650
CAS 8006-54-0	Emery® 1656
CAS 8006-54-0	Emery® 1660
CAS 8006-54-0	Emery® HP-2050
CAS 8006-54-0	Emery® HP-2060
CAS 8006-54-0	Fluilan
CAS 8006-54-0	Golden Dawn Grade 1, 2
CAS 8006-54-0	Ivarlan™ 3000
CAS 8006-54-0	Ivarlan™ 3001
CAS 8006-54-0	Ivarlan™ 3006 Light
CAS 8006-54-0	Ivarlan™ Light
CAS 8006-54-0	Lanolin Anhydrous USP
CAS 8006-54-0	Lanolin Cosmetic
CAS 8006-54-0	Lanolin Extra-Deodorized
CAS 8006-54-0	Lanolin Pharmaceutical
CAS 8006-54-0	Lanolin Tech
CAS 8006-54-0	Lanolin Tech. Grade
CAS 8006-54-0	Lanolin U.S.P
CAS 8006-54-0	Lantrol® HP-2073
CAS 8006-54-0	Pharmaceutical Lanolin USP
CAS 8006-54-0	RITA Lanolin
CAS 8006-54-0	Super Corona
CAS 8006-54-0	Superfine Lanolin Anhydrous USP
CAS 8006-54-0	Unilan
CAS 8006-95-9	EmCon W
CAS 8006-95-9	Lipovol WGO
CAS 8006-95-9	Super Refined™ Wheat Germ Oil
CAS 8006-95-9	Tri-Ol WG
CAS 8006-95-9	Uniderm WGO
CAS 8006-95-9	Wheat Germ Oil
CAS 8006-95-9	Wheat Germ Oil CLR
CAS 8007-08-7	EmCon Ginger
CAS 8007-43-0	Arlacel® 83
CAS 8007-43-0	Arlacel® C

CAS 8007-43-0	Crill 43	CAS 8021-55-4	Ross Ozokerite Wax
CAS 8007-43-0	Dehymuls® SSO	CAS 8022-29-5	Lipovol CP
CAS 8007-43-0	Emalex SPO-150	CAS 8024-09-7	EmCon Walnut
CAS 8007-43-0	Emsorb® 2502	CAS 8024-22-4	Lipovol G
CAS 8007-43-0	Extan-SOT	CAS 8024-22-4	Nikkol Grapeseed Oil
CAS 8007-43-0	Glycomul® SOC	CAS 8024-22-4	Super Refined™ Grapeseed Oil
CAS 8007-43-0	Hefti QO-33-F	CAS 8024-32-6	Avocado Oil
CAS 8007-43-0	Hodag SSO	CAS 8024-32-6	Avocado Oil CLR
CAS 8007-43-0	Liposorb SQO	CAS 8024-32-6	Lipovol A
CAS 8007-43-0	Montane 83	CAS 8024-32-6	Natoil AVO
CAS 8007-43-0	Nikkol SO-15	CAS 8024-32-6	Nikkol Avocado Oil
CAS 8007-43-0	Nikkol SO-15EX	CAS 8024-32-6	Super Refined™ Avocado Oil
CAS 8007-43-0	Nikkol SO-15R	CAS 8024-32-6	Tri-Ol AVO
CAS 8007-43-0	Nissan Nonion OP-83RAT	CAS 8027-32-5	Fonoline® White
CAS 8007-43-0	Protachem SOC	CAS 8027-32-5	Fonoline® Yellow
CAS 8007-43-0	S-Maz® 83R	CAS 8027-32-5	Ointment Base No. 3
CAS 8007-43-0	Sorbirol SQ	CAS 8027-32-5	Ointment Base No. 4
CAS 8007-43-0	Sorgen 30	CAS 8027-32-5	Ointment Base No. 6
CAS 8007-43-0	Sorgen S-30-H	CAS 8027-32-5	Penreco Amber
CAS 8007-43-0	Witconol™ 2502	CAS 8027-32-5	Penreco Blond
CAS 8008-53-5	Iodorga	CAS 8027-32-5	Penreco Cream
CAS 8008-57-9	EmCon Orange	CAS 8027-32-5	Penreco Lily
CAS 8008-74-0	Hy-SES	CAS 8027-32-5	Penreco Regent
CAS 8008-74-0	Lipovol SES	CAS 8027-32-5	Penreco Royal
CAS 8008-74-0	Sesame Oil USP/NF 16	CAS 8027-32-5	Penreco Snow
CAS 8008-74-0	Super Refined™ Sesame Oil	CAS 8027-32-5	Penreco Super
CAS 8008-74-0	Tri-Ol SES	CAS 8027-32-5	Penreco Ultima
CAS 8008-74-0	Uniderm SSME	CAS 8027-32-5	Perfecta® USP
CAS 8008-79-5	EmCon Spearmint	CAS 8027-32-5	Protopet® Alba
CAS 8009-03-8	Mineral Jelly No. 5	CAS 8027-32-5	Protopet® White 1S
CAS 8009-03-8	Mineral Jelly No. 10	CAS 8027-32-5	Protopet® White 2L
CAS 8009-03-8	Mineral Jelly No. 14	CAS 8027-32-5	Protopet® White 3C
CAS 8009-03-8	Mineral Jelly No. 15	CAS 8027-32-5	Protopet® Yellow 2A
CAS 8009-03-8	Mineral Jelly No. 17	CAS 8027-32-5	Super White Fonoline®
CAS 8009-03-8	Mineral Jelly No. 20	CAS 8027-32-5	Super White Protopet®
CAS 8009-03-8	Mineral Jelly No. 25	CAS 8027-33-6	Anatol
CAS 8012-89-3	Koster Keunen Beeswax, Filtered	CAS 8027-33-6	Argowax Cosmetic Super
CAS 8013-07-8	Epoxyweichmacher LSB	CAS 8027-33-6	Argowax Dist.
CAS 8015-86-9	Carnauba Wax NC #2 Stralpitz	CAS 8027-33-6	Argowax Standard
CAS 8015-86-9	Carnauba Wax NC #3 Stralpitz	CAS 8027-33-6	Ceralan®
CAS 8015-86-9	Carnauba Wax SP 8	CAS 8027-33-6	Dusoran MD
CAS 8015-86-9	Koster Keunen Carnauba	CAS 8027-33-6	Emery® 1780
CAS 8015-86-9	Koster Keunen Carnauba, Micro	CAS 8027-33-6	Emery® 1795
	Granulated	CAS 8027-33-6	Emery® HP-2095
CAS 8015-86-9	Koster Keunen Carnauba No. 1	CAS 8027-33-6	Fancol LA
CAS 8015-86-9	Koster Keunen Carnauba, Powd.	CAS 8027-33-6	Hartolan
CAS 8015-86-9	Koster Keunen Carnauba T-2	CAS 8027-33-6	Hartolite
CAS 8015-86-9	Koster Keunen Carnauba T-3	CAS 8027-33-6	Ivarlan™ 3310
CAS 8015-86-9	Natwax CAR	CAS 8027-33-6	Ritawax
CAS 8015-86-9	Ross Brazil Wax	CAS 8027-33-6	Ritawax Super
CAS 8015-86-9	Ross Carnauba Wax	CAS 8027-33-6	Super Hartolan
CAS 8015-88-1	Daucoil	CAS 8027-33-6	Unilanal
CAS 8015-88-1	Unibotan Carrot Oil CLR	CAS 8028-66-8	Fancol HON
CAS 8016-60-2	Natwax RB	CAS 8029-44-5	Myvatex® 7-85
CAS 8016-60-2	Rice Wax No. 1	CAS 8029-44-5	Myverol® 18-85
CAS 8016-60-2	Rose Rice Bran Wax	CAS 8029-76-3	Alcolec® Z-3
CAS 8016-70-4	Famous	CAS 8029-76-3	Alcolec® Z-7
CAS 8016-70-4	Lipex 407	CAS 8029-76-3	Centrolene® A, S
CAS 8016-70-4	Lipovol HS	CAS 8029-76-3	Nikkol Lecinol SH
CAS 8016-70-4	S-Flakes	CAS 8029-76-3	PhosPho 642
CAS 8016-70-4	Stabland®	CAS 8030-12-4	Special Fat 168T
CAS 8016-70-4	Sterotex® HM NF	CAS 8030-78-2	Arquad® T-30
CAS 8016-70-4	Witarix® 440	CAS 8030-78-2	Jet Quat T-27W
CAS 8021-55-4	Koster Keunen Ozokerite	CAS 8030-78-2	Jet Quat T-50
CAS 8021-55-4	Koster Keunen Ozokerite 153/160	CAS 8030-78-2	Kemamine® Q-9703B
CAS 8021-55-4	Koster Keunen Ozokerite 158/160	CAS 8030-78-2	Nikkol CA-2450T
CAS 8021-55-4	Koster Keunen Ozokerite 160/164	CAS 8030-78-2	Noramium MS 50
CAS 8021-55-4	Koster Keunen Ozokerite 164/170	CAS 8031-44-5	Almolan HL
CAS 8021-55-4	Koster Keunen Ozokerite 170	CAS 8031-44-5	Brooks Hydrogenated Lanolin
CAS 8021-55-4	Koster Keunen Ozokerite 190	CAS 8031-44-5	Fancol HL

CAS 8031-44-5	Ivarlan™ HL
CAS 8031-44-5	Lanaetex-HG
CAS 8031-44-5	Lanocerina
CAS 8031-44-5	Lipolan
CAS 8031-44-5	Lipolan Distilled
CAS 8031-44-5	Nikkol Wax-500
CAS 8031-44-5	Super-Sat
CAS 8031-67-2	Atomergic Royal Jelly
CAS 8038-43-5	Vigilan
CAS 8038-77-5	Bayberry Wax Stralpitz
CAS 8038-77-5	Ross Bayberry Wax
CAS 8038-93-5	Chloracel® 40% Sol'n.
CAS 8038-93-5	Chloracel® Solid
CAS 8039-09-6	Lan-Aqua-Sol 50
CAS 8039-09-6	Lan-Aqua-Sol 100
CAS 8039-09-6	Laneto 50
CAS 8042-47-5	Drakeol 5
CAS 8042-47-5	Drakeol 6
CAS 8042-47-5	Drakeol 7
CAS 8042-47-5	Drakeol 9
CAS 8042-47-5	Drakeol 13
CAS 8042-47-5	Drakeol 15
CAS 8042-47-5	Drakeol 19
CAS 8042-47-5	Drakeol 21
CAS 8042-47-5	Drakeol 32
CAS 8042-47-5	Drakeol 35
CAS 8042-47-5	Peneteck
CAS 8050-07-5	Incense EA
CAS 8050-07-5	Incense H
CAS 8051-15-8	G-1702
CAS 8051-15-8	Nikkol GBW-25
CAS 8051-30-7	Empilan® 2502
CAS 8051-73-8	G-1726
CAS 8051-73-8	Nikkol GBW-125
CAS 8052-48-0	Norfox® XXX Granules
CAS 8057-65-6	Oleosterine Arnica
CAS 8057-65-6	Unibotan Arnica CLR
CAS 8067-32-1	Precirol WL 2155 ATO
CAS 8103-01-2	Cytoplasmine-2
CAS 8103-01-2	Vitacell LS
CAS 8103-01-2	Vitamin B Complex CLR
CAS 8103-01-2	Yeast Extract SC
CAS 9000-01-5	Spray Dried Gum Arabic NF Type CSP
CAS 9000-07-1	Aquagel
CAS 9000-07-1	Aquaron
CAS 9000-07-1	Aubygel X52
CAS 9000-07-1	Carraghenate P, Standard, X 2
CAS 9000-07-1	Gelcarin LA
CAS 9000-07-1	Genu Carrageenan
CAS 9000-07-1	Genugel
CAS 9000-07-1	Genulacta Series
CAS 9000-07-1	Genuvisco
CAS 9000-07-1	Seakem 3, LCM
CAS 9000-07-1	Seaspen PF
CAS 9000-07-1	Stamere®
CAS 9000-07-1	Viscarin XLV
CAS 9000-30-0	Burtonite V7E
CAS 9000-30-0	Jaguar® C
CAS 9000-30-0	Supercol® Guar Gum
CAS 9000-40-2	Seagel L
CAS 9000-69-5	Genu Pectins
CAS 9000-69-5	Mexpectin LA 100 Range
CAS 9000-69-5	Mexpectin LC 700 Range
CAS 9000-69-5	Mexpectin XSS 100 Range
CAS 9000-70-8	Byco A
CAS 9000-70-8	Byco C
CAS 9000-70-8	Byco O
CAS 9000-70-8	Colla-Gel AC
CAS 9000-70-8	Cosmetic Gelatin

CAS 9000-70-8	Crodyne BY-19
CAS 9000-70-8	HiPure Liq. Gelatin, Cosmetic Grade
CAS 9000-70-8	Hydrocoll AG-SD
CAS 9000-70-8	Hydrocoll™ G-40
CAS 9000-70-8	Hydrocoll™ G-55
CAS 9000-70-8	Hydrocoll PGA, PGB
CAS 9000-71-9	Alacid
CAS 9000-71-9	Alaren
CAS 9000-71-9	CMP-I
CAS 9000-71-9	Cosmetic Grade Casein
CAS 9000-71-9	Lactobiol
CAS 9000-71-9	Unipro CAL-CASE, CO-CASE
CAS 9002-84-0	PTFE-20
CAS 9002-88-4	A-C® 6
CAS 9002-88-4	A-C® 6A
CAS 9002-88-4	A-C® 7, 7A
CAS 9002-88-4	A-C® 8, 8A
CAS 9002-88-4	A-C® 9, 9A, 9F
CAS 9002-88-4	A-C® 15
CAS 9002-88-4	A-C® 16
CAS 9002-88-4	A-C® 617, 617A
CAS 9002-88-4	A-C® 617G
CAS 9002-88-4	A-C® 1702
CAS 9002-88-4	ACumist™ A-12
CAS 9002-88-4	ACumist™ A-18
CAS 9002-88-4	ACumist™ B-6
CAS 9002-88-4	ACumist™ B-9
CAS 9002-88-4	ACumist™ B-12
CAS 9002-88-4	ACumist™ B-18
CAS 9002-88-4	ACumist™ C-5
CAS 9002-88-4	ACumist™ C-9
CAS 9002-88-4	ACumist™ C-12
CAS 9002-88-4	ACumist™ C-18
CAS 9002-88-4	ACumist™ D-9
CAS 9002-88-4	ACuscrub® 41
CAS 9002-88-4	ACuscrub® 42
CAS 9002-88-4	ACuscrub® 43
CAS 9002-88-4	ACuscrub® 44
CAS 9002-88-4	ACuscrub® 52
CAS 9002-88-4	Micropoly 520
CAS 9002-88-4	Micropoly 524
CAS 9002-88-4	Micropoly 524-XF
CAS 9002-88-4	Microthene® MN-714, MN-722
CAS 9002-88-4	Polyethylene 1000 HE
CAS 9002-88-4	Polyspend™
CAS 9002-88-4	Polywax® 500
CAS 9002-88-4	Polywax® 655
CAS 9002-88-4	Polywax® 850
CAS 9002-88-4	Polywax® 1000
CAS 9002-88-4	Polywax® 2000
CAS 9002-88-4	Polywax® 3000
CAS 9002-88-4	Siltek® GR
CAS 9002-88-4	Siltek® M
CAS 9002-88-4	Siltek® M Super
CAS 9002-88-4	Siltek® PL
CAS 9002-89-5	Elvanol® 71-30
CAS 9002-89-5	Elvanol® 75-15
CAS 9002-89-5	Elvanol® 85–82
CAS 9002-89-5	Elvanol® 90-50
CAS 9002-89-5	Elvanol® HV
CAS 9002-89-5	Vinol 523, 540
CAS 9002-92-0	Ablunol LA-16
CAS 9002-92-0	Ablunol LA-40
CAS 9002-92-0	Brij® 35
CAS 9002-92-0	Britex L 20
CAS 9002-92-0	Britex L 40
CAS 9002-92-0	Britex L 100
CAS 9002-92-0	Britex L 230
CAS 9002-92-0	Chemal LA-23

CAS 9002-92-0	Emalex 715
CAS 9002-92-0	Emalex 720
CAS 9002-92-0	Emalex 725
CAS 9002-92-0	Emalex 730
CAS 9002-92-0	Emalex 750
CAS 9002-92-0	Emthox® 5877
CAS 9002-92-0	Ethosperse® LA-4
CAS 9002-92-0	Ethosperse® LA-12
CAS 9002-92-0	Ethosperse® LA-23
CAS 9002-92-0	Hetoxol L-23
CAS 9002-92-0	Hodag Nonionic L-23
CAS 9002-92-0	Lanycol-30
CAS 9002-92-0	Lanycol-35
CAS 9002-92-0	Lauropal 4
CAS 9002-92-0	Lipocol L-23
CAS 9002-92-0	Macol® LA-23
CAS 9002-92-0	Marlipal® 24/300
CAS 9002-92-0	Marlipal® 124
CAS 9002-92-0	Marlipal® MG
CAS 9002-92-0	Marlowet® LMA 20
CAS 9002-92-0	Nikkol BL-25
CAS 9002-92-0	Procol LA-15
CAS 9002-92-0	Procol LA-20
CAS 9002-92-0	Procol LA-23
CAS 9002-92-0	Procol LA-30
CAS 9002-92-0	Procol LA-40
CAS 9002-92-0	Prox-onic LA-1/023
CAS 9002-92-0	Remcopal 21411
CAS 9002-92-0	Rhodasurf® L-25
CAS 9002-92-0	Rhodasurf® L-790
CAS 9002-92-0	Ritox 35
CAS 9002-92-0	Sellig LA 1150
CAS 9002-92-0	Simulsol P23
CAS 9002-92-0	Trycol® 5964
CAS 9002-92-0	Trycol® 5967
CAS 9002-92-0	Unicol LA-23
CAS 9002-92-0	Volpo L4
CAS 9002-92-0	Volpo L23
CAS 9002-92-0	Witconol™ 5964
CAS 9002-93-1	Akyporox OP 250V
CAS 9002-93-1	Chemax OP-3
CAS 9002-93-1	Chemax OP-5
CAS 9002-93-1	Chemax OP-7
CAS 9002-93-1	Chemax OP-9
CAS 9002-93-1	Chemax OP-30/70
CAS 9002-93-1	Chemax OP-40
CAS 9002-93-1	Chemax OP-40/70
CAS 9002-93-1	Emalex OP-5
CAS 9002-93-1	Emalex OP-8
CAS 9002-93-1	Emalex OP-10
CAS 9002-93-1	Emalex OP-15
CAS 9002-93-1	Emalex OP-20
CAS 9002-93-1	Emalex OP-25
CAS 9002-93-1	Emalex OP-30
CAS 9002-93-1	Emalex OP-40
CAS 9002-93-1	Emalex OP-50
CAS 9002-93-1	Igepal® CA-630
CAS 9002-93-1	Igepal® OP-9
CAS 9002-93-1	Lanapeg-15
CAS 9002-93-1	Macol® OP-3
CAS 9002-93-1	Macol® OP-5
CAS 9002-93-1	Macol® OP-8
CAS 9002-93-1	Macol® OP-10
CAS 9002-93-1	Macol® OP-10 SP
CAS 9002-93-1	Macol® OP-12
CAS 9002-93-1	Macol® OP-16(75)
CAS 9002-93-1	Macol® OP-30(70)
CAS 9002-93-1	Macol® OP-40(70)
CAS 9002-93-1	Nikkol OP-3
CAS 9002-93-1	Nikkol OP-10
CAS 9002-93-1	Nikkol OP-30
CAS 9002-93-1	Oxypol
CAS 9002-93-1	Remcopal O9
CAS 9002-93-1	Remcopal O11
CAS 9002-93-1	Remcopal O12
CAS 9002-93-1	Renex® 750
CAS 9002-93-1	Renex® 759
CAS 9002-93-1	Synperonic OP3
CAS 9002-93-1	Synperonic OP4.5
CAS 9002-93-1	Synperonic OP6
CAS 9002-93-1	Synperonic OP7.5
CAS 9002-93-1	Synperonic OP10
CAS 9002-93-1	Synperonic OP10.5
CAS 9002-93-1	Synperonic OP11
CAS 9002-93-1	Synperonic OP12.5
CAS 9002-93-1	Synperonic OP16
CAS 9002-93-1	Synperonic OP16.5
CAS 9002-93-1	Synperonic OP20
CAS 9002-93-1	Synperonic OP25
CAS 9002-93-1	Synperonic OP30
CAS 9002-93-1	Synperonic OP40
CAS 9002-93-1	Synperonic OP40/70
CAS 9002-93-1	Syntopon 8 C
CAS 9002-93-1	Syntopon 8 D 1
CAS 9002-93-1	T-Det® O-407
CAS 9002-93-1	Triton® X-100
CAS 9002-93-1	Witconol™ OP-90
CAS 9002-96-4	Eastman® Vitamin E TPGS
CAS 9002-96-4	Glycol 1000 Succinate
CAS 9002-98-6	Epomin P-1000
CAS 9002-98-6	Epomin SP-006
CAS 9002-98-6	Epomin SP-012
CAS 9002-98-6	Epomin SP-018
CAS 9002-98-6	Nalco® 634
CAS 9002-98-6	Polymin® G-35 SG
CAS 9002-98-6	Polymin® Waterfree SG
CAS 9003-01-4	Acrysol® A-1
CAS 9003-01-4	Carbopol® 907
CAS 9003-01-4	Covacryl IIO, III
CAS 9003-01-4	Lubrajel® NP
CAS 9003-01-4	Lubrajel® Oil
CAS 9003-01-4	Lubrajel® WA
CAS 9003-07-0	Hoechst Wax PP 690
CAS 9003-11-6	Antarox® L-64
CAS 9003-11-6	Antarox® PGP 23-7
CAS 9003-11-6	Chemal BP 261
CAS 9003-11-6	Chemal BP-262
CAS 9003-11-6	Chemal BP-2101
CAS 9003-11-6	Hodag Nonionic 1017-R
CAS 9003-11-6	Hodag Nonionic 1031-L
CAS 9003-11-6	Hodag Nonionic 1035-L
CAS 9003-11-6	Hodag Nonionic 1038-F
CAS 9003-11-6	Hodag Nonionic 1042-L
CAS 9003-11-6	Hodag Nonionic 1043-L
CAS 9003-11-6	Hodag Nonionic 1044-L
CAS 9003-11-6	Hodag Nonionic 1061-L
CAS 9003-11-6	Hodag Nonionic 1062-L
CAS 9003-11-6	Hodag Nonionic 1063-L
CAS 9003-11-6	Hodag Nonionic 1064-L
CAS 9003-11-6	Hodag Nonionic 1065-P
CAS 9003-11-6	Hodag Nonionic 1068-F
CAS 9003-11-6	Hodag Nonionic 1072-L
CAS 9003-11-6	Hodag Nonionic 1075-P
CAS 9003-11-6	Hodag Nonionic 1077-F
CAS 9003-11-6	Hodag Nonionic 1081-L
CAS 9003-11-6	Hodag Nonionic 1084-P
CAS 9003-11-6	Hodag Nonionic 1085-P
CAS 9003-11-6	Hodag Nonionic 1087-F
CAS 9003-11-6	Hodag Nonionic 1088-F
CAS 9003-11-6	Hodag Nonionic 1092-L

CAS 9003-11-6	Hodag Nonionic 1094-P	CAS 9003-11-6	Pluronic® P104
CAS 9003-11-6	Hodag Nonionic 1098-F	CAS 9003-11-6	Pluronic® P105
CAS 9003-11-6	Hodag Nonionic 1101-L	CAS 9003-11-6	Pluronic® P123
CAS 9003-11-6	Hodag Nonionic 1103-P	CAS 9003-11-6	Rheodol 440
CAS 9003-11-6	Hodag Nonionic 1104-P	CAS 9003-11-6	Synperonic PE/F68
CAS 9003-11-6	Hodag Nonionic 1105-P	CAS 9003-11-6	Synperonic PE/F87
CAS 9003-11-6	Hodag Nonionic 1108-F	CAS 9003-11-6	Synperonic PE/F127
CAS 9003-11-6	Hodag Nonionic 1121-L	CAS 9003-11-6	Synperonic PE/L35
CAS 9003-11-6	Hodag Nonionic 1122-L	CAS 9003-11-6	Synperonic PE/P85
CAS 9003-11-6	Hodag Nonionic 1123-P	CAS 9003-11-6	Ucon® 75-H-450
CAS 9003-11-6	Hodag Nonionic 1127-F	CAS 9003-11-6	Ucon® 75-H-1400
CAS 9003-11-6	Hodag Nonionic 2017-R	CAS 9003-11-6	Ucon® 75-H-90000
CAS 9003-11-6	Hodag Nonionic 5010-R	CAS 9003-13-8	Dow L910
CAS 9003-11-6	Macol® 1	CAS 9003-13-8	Dow L1150
CAS 9003-11-6	Macol® 2	CAS 9003-13-8	Fluid AP
CAS 9003-11-6	Macol® 4	CAS 9003-13-8	Hodag PB-285
CAS 9003-11-6	Macol® 8	CAS 9003-13-8	Hodag PB-300
CAS 9003-11-6	Macol® 16	CAS 9003-13-8	Hodag PB-625
CAS 9003-11-6	Macol® 23	CAS 9003-13-8	Hodag PB-1715
CAS 9003-11-6	Macol® 27	CAS 9003-13-8	Probutyl 14
CAS 9003-11-6	Macol® 32	CAS 9003-13-8	Ucon® Fluid AP
CAS 9003-11-6	Macol® 33	CAS 9003-13-8	Ucon® LB-65
CAS 9003-11-6	Macol® 34	CAS 9003-13-8	Ucon® LB-135
CAS 9003-11-6	Macol® 35	CAS 9003-13-8	Ucon® LB-285
CAS 9003-11-6	Macol® 40	CAS 9003-13-8	Ucon® LB-385
CAS 9003-11-6	Macol® 42	CAS 9003-13-8	Ucon® LB-525
CAS 9003-11-6	Macol® 44	CAS 9003-13-8	Ucon® LB-625
CAS 9003-11-6	Macol® 46	CAS 9003-13-8	Ucon® LB-1145
CAS 9003-11-6	Macol® 72	CAS 9003-13-8	Ucon® LB-1715
CAS 9003-11-6	Macol® 77	CAS 9003-13-8	Ucon® LB-3000
CAS 9003-11-6	Macol® 85	CAS 9003-13-8	Unilube MB-370
CAS 9003-11-6	Macol® 101	CAS 9003-13-8	Witconol™ APB
CAS 9003-11-6	Macol® 108	CAS 9003-27-4	Permethyl® 108A
CAS 9003-11-6	Nikkol GO-440	CAS 9003-29-6	Permethyl® 104A
CAS 9003-11-6	Pluracare® F68	CAS 9003-29-6	Permethyl® 106A
CAS 9003-11-6	Pluracare® F77	CAS 9003-31-0	Syntesqual
CAS 9003-11-6	Pluracare® F108	CAS 9003-39-8	H₂old™ EP-1
CAS 9003-11-6	Pluracare® F127	CAS 9003-39-8	Kollidon®
CAS 9003-11-6	Pluracare® L64	CAS 9003-39-8	Luviskol® K17
CAS 9003-11-6	Pluracare® P65	CAS 9003-39-8	Luviskol® K30
CAS 9003-11-6	Pluronic® 10R5	CAS 9003-39-8	Luviskol® K60
CAS 9003-11-6	Pluronic® 17R2	CAS 9003-39-8	Luviskol® K80
CAS 9003-11-6	Pluronic® 17R4	CAS 9003-39-8	Luviskol® K90
CAS 9003-11-6	Pluronic® 25R2	CAS 9003-39-8	Luviskol® LD-9025
CAS 9003-11-6	Pluronic® 25R4	CAS 9003-39-8	Plasdone® C-15
CAS 9003-11-6	Pluronic® 25R8	CAS 9003-39-8	Plasdone® C-30
CAS 9003-11-6	Pluronic® 31R1	CAS 9003-39-8	Plasdone® K-25, K-90
CAS 9003-11-6	Pluronic® F38	CAS 9003-39-8	Plasdone® K-26/28, K-29/32
CAS 9003-11-6	Pluronic® F68	CAS 9003-39-8	PVP K-15
CAS 9003-11-6	Pluronic® F77	CAS 9003-39-8	PVP K-30
CAS 9003-11-6	Pluronic® F87	CAS 9003-53-6	Lytron 614 Latex
CAS 9003-11-6	Pluronic® F88	CAS 9003-59-2	Flexan® 130
CAS 9003-11-6	Pluronic® F98	CAS 9004-00-9	Britex S 20
CAS 9003-11-6	Pluronic® F108	CAS 9004-00-9	Britex S 100
CAS 9003-11-6	Pluronic® F127	CAS 9004-00-9	Britex S 200
CAS 9003-11-6	Pluronic® L35	CAS 9004-32-4	Aqualon® Cellulose Gum
CAS 9003-11-6	Pluronic® L43	CAS 9004-32-4	Aquasorb® A250
CAS 9003-11-6	Pluronic® L44	CAS 9004-32-4	Ticalose 15, 30, 75, 150R, 1200,
CAS 9003-11-6	Pluronic® L61		2000R, 2500, 4000, 4500, 5000R
CAS 9003-11-6	Pluronic® L62	CAS 9004-32-4	Tylose® C, CB Series
CAS 9003-11-6	Pluronic® L64	CAS 9004-32-4	Tylose® C-p, CB-p
CAS 9003-11-6	Pluronic® L81	CAS 9004-34-6	Acticel™ 12
CAS 9003-11-6	Pluronic® L92	CAS 9004-34-6	Acticel™ Plus
CAS 9003-11-6	Pluronic® L101	CAS 9004-34-6	Avicel PH-101
CAS 9003-11-6	Pluronic® L121	CAS 9004-34-6	Celluflow C-25
CAS 9003-11-6	Pluronic® L122	CAS 9004-34-6	Cellulon
CAS 9003-11-6	Pluronic® P65	CAS 9004-34-6	Dascare MCCP
CAS 9003-11-6	Pluronic® P84	CAS 9004-34-6	Elcema® F150, G250, P100
CAS 9003-11-6	Pluronic® P85	CAS 9004-34-6	Emcocel® 50M
CAS 9003-11-6	Pluronic® P103	CAS 9004-34-6	Emcocel® 90M

CAS Number	Trade Name	CAS Number	Trade Name
CAS 9004-34-6	Emcocel® LM	CAS 9004-67-5	Viscontran MC
CAS 9004-34-6	Solka-Floc® BW-40	CAS 9004-73-3	Dow Corning® 1107 Fluid
CAS 9004-34-6	Solka-Floc® BW-100	CAS 9004-73-3	Silicone L-31
CAS 9004-34-6	Solka-Floc® BW-200	CAS 9004-74-4	Dow MPEG350
CAS 9004-34-6	Solka-Floc® BW-2030	CAS 9004-74-4	Dow MPEG550
CAS 9004-34-6	Solka-Floc® Fine Granular	CAS 9004-74-4	Dow MPEG750
CAS 9004-35-7	Celluflow TA-25	CAS 9004-74-4	Upiwax 350
CAS 9004-36-8	Eastman® CAB	CAS 9004-81-3	Ablunol 200ML
CAS 9004-53-9	Nadex 360	CAS 9004-81-3	Ablunol 400ML
CAS 9004-57-3	Ethocel Medium Premium	CAS 9004-81-3	Ablunol 600ML
CAS 9004-57-3	Ethocel Standard Premium	CAS 9004-81-3	Algon LA 40
CAS 9004-61-9	Atomergic Hyaluronic Acid	CAS 9004-81-3	Algon LA 80
CAS 9004-61-9	Biomatrix®	CAS 9004-81-3	Alkamuls® L-9
CAS 9004-61-9	Hyaluronic Acid	CAS 9004-81-3	Alkamuls® PE/400
CAS 9004-61-9	Hyaderm®	CAS 9004-81-3	Chemax E-200 ML
CAS 9004-61-9	Hylucare™	CAS 9004-81-3	Chemax E-400 ML
CAS 9004-62-0	Alcoramnosan	CAS 9004-81-3	Chemax E-600 ML
CAS 9004-62-0	Cellosize® HEC QP Grades	CAS 9004-81-3	Chemax E-1000 ML
CAS 9004-62-0	Cellosize® HEC QP-3-L	CAS 9004-81-3	Cithrol 2ML
CAS 9004-62-0	Cellosize® HEC QP-40	CAS 9004-81-3	Cithrol 4ML
CAS 9004-62-0	Cellosize® HEC QP-100M-H	CAS 9004-81-3	Cithrol 6ML
CAS 9004-62-0	Cellosize® HEC QP-300	CAS 9004-81-3	Cithrol 10ML
CAS 9004-62-0	Cellosize® HEC QP-4400-H	CAS 9004-81-3	CPH-27-N
CAS 9004-62-0	Cellosize® HEC QP-15,000-H	CAS 9004-81-3	CPH-30-N
CAS 9004-62-0	Cellosize® HEC QP-52,000-H	CAS 9004-81-3	CPH-43-N
CAS 9004-62-0	Cellosize® HEC WP Grades	CAS 9004-81-3	Crodet L4
CAS 9004-62-0	Cellosize® Polymer PCG-10	CAS 9004-81-3	Crodet L8
CAS 9004-62-0	Idroramnosan	CAS 9004-81-3	Crodet L12
CAS 9004-62-0	Liporamnosan	CAS 9004-81-3	Crodet L24
CAS 9004-62-0	Natrosol® 250	CAS 9004-81-3	Crodet L40
CAS 9004-62-0	Natrosol® Hydroxyethylcellulose	CAS 9004-81-3	Crodet L100
CAS 9004-62-0	Tylose® H Series	CAS 9004-81-3	Elfacos® PEG 400 ML
CAS 9004-62-0	Tylose® H-p	CAS 9004-81-3	Hefti PGE-600-ML
CAS 9004-62-0	Tylose® H-yp	CAS 9004-81-3	Hetoxamate LA-4
CAS 9004-62-0	Viscontran HEC	CAS 9004-81-3	Hetoxamate LA-5
CAS 9004-64-2	Klucel® EF	CAS 9004-81-3	Hetoxamate LA-9
CAS 9004-64-2	Klucel® ELF, GF, HF, JF, LF, MF	CAS 9004-81-3	Hodag 20-L
CAS 9004-65-3	Benecel® Hydroxypropyl Methylcellulose	CAS 9004-81-3	Hodag 40-L
		CAS 9004-81-3	Hodag 60-L
CAS 9004-65-3	Benecel® MP	CAS 9004-81-3	Hodag 600-L
CAS 9004-65-3	Methocel® 40-100	CAS 9004-81-3	Hodag DGL
CAS 9004-65-3	Methocel® 40-101	CAS 9004-81-3	Karapeg 400-ML
CAS 9004-65-3	Methocel® 40-202	CAS 9004-81-3	Karapeg 600-ML
CAS 9004-65-3	Methocel® E3P	CAS 9004-81-3	Kessco® PEG 200 ML
CAS 9004-65-3	Methocel® E4MP	CAS 9004-81-3	Kessco® PEG 300 ML
CAS 9004-65-3	Methocel® E5P	CAS 9004-81-3	Kessco® PEG 400 ML
CAS 9004-65-3	Methocel® E6P	CAS 9004-81-3	Kessco® PEG 600 ML
CAS 9004-65-3	Methocel® E10MP CR	CAS 9004-81-3	Kessco® PEG 1000 ML
CAS 9004-65-3	Methocel® E15LVP	CAS 9004-81-3	Kessco® PEG 1540 ML
CAS 9004-65-3	Methocel® E50LVP	CAS 9004-81-3	Kessco® PEG 4000 ML
CAS 9004-65-3	Methocel® E50P	CAS 9004-81-3	Kessco® PEG 6000 ML
CAS 9004-65-3	Methocel® E Premium	CAS 9004-81-3	Laurate de PEG 400
CAS 9004-65-3	Methocel® F Premium	CAS 9004-81-3	Lexemul® PEG-400ML
CAS 9004-65-3	Methocel® J Premium	CAS 9004-81-3	Lipo DGLS
CAS 9004-65-3	Methocel® K3P	CAS 9004-81-3	Lipopeg 2-L
CAS 9004-65-3	Methocel® K4MP	CAS 9004-81-3	Lipopeg 4-L
CAS 9004-65-3	Methocel® K4MS	CAS 9004-81-3	Lipopeg 6-L
CAS 9004-65-3	Methocel® K15MP	CAS 9004-81-3	Mapeg® 200 ML
CAS 9004-65-3	Methocel® K15MS	CAS 9004-81-3	Mapeg® 400 ML
CAS 9004-65-3	Methocel® K35	CAS 9004-81-3	Mapeg® 600 ML
CAS 9004-65-3	Methocel® K100LVP	CAS 9004-81-3	Nikkol MYL-10
CAS 9004-65-3	Methocel® K100MP	CAS 9004-81-3	Nonisol 100
CAS 9004-65-3	Methocel® K Premium	CAS 9004-81-3	Pegosperse® 200 ML
CAS 9004-65-3	Viscontran MHPC	CAS 9004-81-3	Pegosperse® 400 ML
CAS 9004-67-5	Benecel® M	CAS 9004-81-3	Pegosperse® 600 ML
CAS 9004-67-5	Methocel® A4CP	CAS 9004-81-3	Protamate 200 ML
CAS 9004-67-5	Methocel® A4MP	CAS 9004-81-3	Protamate 400 ML
CAS 9004-67-5	Methocel® A15-LV	CAS 9004-81-3	Radiasurf® 7420
CAS 9004-67-5	Methocel® A15LVP	CAS 9004-81-3	Radiasurf® 7422
CAS 9004-67-5	Methocel® A Premium	CAS 9004-81-3	Rol L 40

CAS 9004-81-3	Unipeg-200 ML	CAS 9004-82-4	Ungerol N2-28
CAS 9004-81-3	Unipeg-400 ML	CAS 9004-82-4	Ungerol N2-70
CAS 9004-81-3	Unipeg-600 ML	CAS 9004-82-4	Ungerol N3-28
CAS 9004-81-3	Unipeg-6000 ML	CAS 9004-82-4	Ungerol N3-70
CAS 9004-81-3	Witconol™ 2620	CAS 9004-82-4	Unipol 125-E, 130-E
CAS 9004-82-4	Akyposal EO 20 MW	CAS 9004-82-4	Unipol ES-40
CAS 9004-82-4	Akyposal EO 2067	CAS 9004-82-4	Witcolate™ ES-2
CAS 9004-82-4	Calfoam ES-30	CAS 9004-82-4	Witcolate™ ES-3
CAS 9004-82-4	Calfoam SEL-60	CAS 9004-82-4	Witcolate™ LES-60C
CAS 9004-82-4	Carsonol® SES-S	CAS 9004-82-4	Witcolate™ OME
CAS 9004-82-4	Carsonol® SLES	CAS 9004-82-4	Witcolate™ S1285C
CAS 9004-82-4	Chemsalan RLM 28	CAS 9004-82-4	Zetesol NL
CAS 9004-82-4	Chemsalan RLM 56	CAS 9004-82-4	Zoharpon ETA 27
CAS 9004-82-4	Chemsalan RLM 70	CAS 9004-82-4	Zoharpon ETA 70
CAS 9004-82-4	Cosmopon LE 50	CAS 9004-82-4	Zoharpon ETA 270 (OXO)
CAS 9004-82-4	Disponil FES 92E	CAS 9004-82-4	Zoharpon ETA 271
CAS 9004-82-4	Elfan® NS 242	CAS 9004-82-4	Zoharpon ETA 273
CAS 9004-82-4	Elfan® NS 242 Conc.	CAS 9004-82-4	Zoharpon ETA 603
CAS 9004-82-4	Elfan® NS 243 S	CAS 9004-82-4	Zoharpon ETA 700 (OXO)
CAS 9004-82-4	Elfan® NS 243 S Conc.	CAS 9004-82-4	Zoharpon ETA 703
CAS 9004-82-4	Empicol® ESB	CAS 9004-83-5	Alcodet® SK
CAS 9004-82-4	Empicol® ESB3	CAS 9004-92-2	Hetoxol OL-2
CAS 9004-82-4	Empimin® KSN70	CAS 9004-95-9	Akyporox RC 200
CAS 9004-82-4	Genapol® ARO Paste	CAS 9004-95-9	Brij® 52
CAS 9004-82-4	Genapol® LRO Liq., Paste	CAS 9004-95-9	Brij® 56
CAS 9004-82-4	Genapol® ZRO Liq., Paste	CAS 9004-95-9	Brij® 58
CAS 9004-82-4	Laural LS	CAS 9004-95-9	Britex C
CAS 9004-82-4	Manro BES 27	CAS 9004-95-9	Britex C 20
CAS 9004-82-4	Manro BES 60	CAS 9004-95-9	Britex C 100
CAS 9004-82-4	Manro BES 70	CAS 9004-95-9	Britex C 200
CAS 9004-82-4	Marlinat® 242/28	CAS 9004-95-9	Cetomacrogol 1000 BP
CAS 9004-82-4	Marlinat® 242/70	CAS 9004-95-9	Emalex 102
CAS 9004-82-4	Marlinat® 242/70 S	CAS 9004-95-9	Emalex 103
CAS 9004-82-4	Marlinat® 243/28	CAS 9004-95-9	Emalex 105
CAS 9004-82-4	Marlinat® 243/70	CAS 9004-95-9	Emalex 107
CAS 9004-82-4	Nonasol N4SS	CAS 9004-95-9	Emalex 110
CAS 9004-82-4	Norfox® SLES-02	CAS 9004-95-9	Emalex 112
CAS 9004-82-4	Norfox® SLES-03	CAS 9004-95-9	Emalex 115
CAS 9004-82-4	Norfox® SLES-60	CAS 9004-95-9	Emalex 117
CAS 9004-82-4	Nutrapon ES-60 3568	CAS 9004-95-9	Emalex 120
CAS 9004-82-4	Nutrapon KPC 0156	CAS 9004-95-9	Emalex 125
CAS 9004-82-4	Rewopol® NL 2-28	CAS 9004-95-9	Emalex 130
CAS 9004-82-4	Rewopol® NL 3	CAS 9004-95-9	Emalex 1605
CAS 9004-82-4	Rewopol® NL 3-28	CAS 9004-95-9	Emalex 1610
CAS 9004-82-4	Rewopol® NL 3-70	CAS 9004-95-9	Emalex 1615
CAS 9004-82-4	Rhodapex® ES	CAS 9004-95-9	Emalex 1620
CAS 9004-82-4	Rolpon 24/230	CAS 9004-95-9	Emalex 1625
CAS 9004-82-4	Rolpon 24/270	CAS 9004-95-9	Ethosperse® CA-2
CAS 9004-82-4	Rolpon 24/330 N	CAS 9004-95-9	Ethosperse® CA-20
CAS 9004-82-4	Sandet EN	CAS 9004-95-9	G-3816
CAS 9004-82-4	Sandoz Sulfate 219	CAS 9004-95-9	G-3820
CAS 9004-82-4	Standapol® 125-E	CAS 9004-95-9	Hetoxol CA-2
CAS 9004-82-4	Standapol® 130-E	CAS 9004-95-9	Hetoxol CA-10
CAS 9004-82-4	Standapol® ES-250	CAS 9004-95-9	Hetoxol CA-20
CAS 9004-82-4	Standapol® ES-350	CAS 9004-95-9	Hodag Nonionic C-2
CAS 9004-82-4	Steol® 4N	CAS 9004-95-9	Hodag Nonionic C-4
CAS 9004-82-4	Steol® CS-460	CAS 9004-95-9	Hodag Nonionic C-10
CAS 9004-82-4	Sulfochem ES-2	CAS 9004-95-9	Hodag Nonionic C-20
CAS 9004-82-4	Sulfochem ES-70	CAS 9004-95-9	Lanycol-52
CAS 9004-82-4	Texapon® LT-327	CAS 9004-95-9	Lanycol-58
CAS 9004-82-4	Texapon® N 70	CAS 9004-95-9	Lipocol C-2
CAS 9004-82-4	Texapon® NC 70	CAS 9004-95-9	Lipocol C-4
CAS 9004-82-4	Texapon® NSO	CAS 9004-95-9	Lipocol C-10
CAS 9004-82-4	Texapon® PN-235	CAS 9004-95-9	Lipocol C-20
CAS 9004-82-4	Texapon® PN-254	CAS 9004-95-9	Lipocol C-30
CAS 9004-82-4	Texapon® PLT-227	CAS 9004-95-9	Macol® CA-2
CAS 9004-82-4	Ungerol LES 2-28	CAS 9004-95-9	Macol® CA-10
CAS 9004-82-4	Ungerol LES 2-70	CAS 9004-95-9	Nikkol BC-2
CAS 9004-82-4	Ungerol LES 3-28	CAS 9004-95-9	Nikkol BC-5.5
CAS 9004-82-4	Ungerol LES 3-70	CAS 9004-95-9	Nikkol BC-7

CAS 9004-95-9	Nikkol BC-10TX	CAS 9004-96-0	Kessco® PEG 600 MO
CAS 9004-95-9	Nikkol BC-15TX	CAS 9004-96-0	Kessco® PEG 1000 MO
CAS 9004-95-9	Nikkol BC-20TX	CAS 9004-96-0	Kessco® PEG 1540 MO
CAS 9004-95-9	Nikkol BC-23	CAS 9004-96-0	Kessco® PEG 4000 MO
CAS 9004-95-9	Nikkol BC-25TX	CAS 9004-96-0	Kessco® PEG 6000 MO
CAS 9004-95-9	Nikkol BC-30TX	CAS 9004-96-0	Lipopeg 3-O
CAS 9004-95-9	Nikkol BC-40TX	CAS 9004-96-0	Lipopeg 4-O
CAS 9004-95-9	Procol CA-2	CAS 9004-96-0	Lipopeg 6-O
CAS 9004-95-9	Procol CA-4	CAS 9004-96-0	Mapeg® 200 MO
CAS 9004-95-9	Procol CA-6	CAS 9004-96-0	Mapeg® 400 MO
CAS 9004-95-9	Procol CA-10	CAS 9004-96-0	Mapeg® 600 MO
CAS 9004-95-9	Procol CA-20	CAS 9004-96-0	Marlosol® OL7
CAS 9004-95-9	Procol CA-30	CAS 9004-96-0	Marlosol® OL15
CAS 9004-95-9	Simulsol 52	CAS 9004-96-0	Nikkol MYO-6
CAS 9004-95-9	Simulsol 56	CAS 9004-96-0	Nikkol MYO-10
CAS 9004-95-9	Simulsol 58	CAS 9004-96-0	Olepal 1
CAS 9004-95-9	Unicol CA-2	CAS 9004-96-0	Pegosperse® 200 MO
CAS 9004-95-9	Unicol CA-4	CAS 9004-96-0	Pegosperse® 300 MO
CAS 9004-95-9	Unicol CA-10	CAS 9004-96-0	Pegosperse® 400 MO
CAS 9004-95-9	Unicol CA-20	CAS 9004-96-0	Pegosperse® 600 MO
CAS 9004-96-0	Ablunol 200MO	CAS 9004-96-0	Protamate 200 OC
CAS 9004-96-0	Ablunol 400MO	CAS 9004-96-0	Protamate 300 OC
CAS 9004-96-0	Ablunol 600MO	CAS 9004-96-0	Protamate 400 OC
CAS 9004-96-0	Ablunol 1000MO	CAS 9004-96-0	Protamate 600 OC
CAS 9004-96-0	Acconon 400-MO	CAS 9004-96-0	Protamate 1000 OC
CAS 9004-96-0	Algon OL 60	CAS 9004-96-0	Prox-onic OL-1/05
CAS 9004-96-0	Algon OL 70	CAS 9004-96-0	Prox-onic OL-1/09
CAS 9004-96-0	Algon OL 90	CAS 9004-96-0	Prox-onic OL-1/014
CAS 9004-96-0	Alkamuls® 400-MO	CAS 9004-96-0	Radiasurf® 7431
CAS 9004-96-0	Chemax E-200 MO	CAS 9004-96-0	Remcopal 207
CAS 9004-96-0	Chemax E-400 MO	CAS 9004-96-0	Rol AG
CAS 9004-96-0	Chemax E-600 MO	CAS 9004-96-0	Unipeg-200 MO
CAS 9004-96-0	Chemax E-1000 MO	CAS 9004-96-0	Unipeg-400 MO
CAS 9004-96-0	Cithrol 2MO	CAS 9004-96-0	Unipeg-600 MO
CAS 9004-96-0	Cithrol 4MO	CAS 9004-96-0	Witconol™ H31A
CAS 9004-96-0	Cithrol 6MO	CAS 9004-97-1	Cerex EL 429
CAS 9004-96-0	Cithrol 10MO	CAS 9004-97-1	G-4929
CAS 9004-96-0	CPH-40-N	CAS 9004-97-1	Hodag 40-R
CAS 9004-96-0	CPH-41-N	CAS 9004-98-2	Ablunol OA-6
CAS 9004-96-0	CPH-46-N	CAS 9004-98-2	Ablunol OA-7
CAS 9004-96-0	CPH-233-N	CAS 9004-98-2	Akyporox RO 90
CAS 9004-96-0	Crodet O4	CAS 9004-98-2	Ameroxol® OE-2
CAS 9004-96-0	Crodet O6	CAS 9004-98-2	Ameroxol® OE-5
CAS 9004-96-0	Crodet O8	CAS 9004-98-2	Ameroxol® OE-10
CAS 9004-96-0	Crodet O12	CAS 9004-98-2	Ameroxol® OE-20
CAS 9004-96-0	Crodet O23	CAS 9004-98-2	Arosurf® 32-E20
CAS 9004-96-0	Crodet O24	CAS 9004-98-2	Brij® 93
CAS 9004-96-0	Crodet O40	CAS 9004-98-2	Brij® 97
CAS 9004-96-0	Crodet O100	CAS 9004-98-2	Brij® 98
CAS 9004-96-0	Elfacos® PEG 400 MO	CAS 9004-98-2	Britex O 20
CAS 9004-96-0	Emalex 218	CAS 9004-98-2	Britex O 100
CAS 9004-96-0	Emalex OE-6	CAS 9004-98-2	Britex O 200
CAS 9004-96-0	Emalex OE-10	CAS 9004-98-2	Brox OL-2
CAS 9004-96-0	Estol EO4MO 3672	CAS 9004-98-2	Brox OL-3
CAS 9004-96-0	Estol EO6MO 3674	CAS 9004-98-2	Brox OL-4
CAS 9004-96-0	Ethofat® O/15	CAS 9004-98-2	Brox OL-5
CAS 9004-96-0	Ethofat® O/20	CAS 9004-98-2	Brox OL-10
CAS 9004-96-0	G-5507	CAS 9004-98-2	Brox OL-20
CAS 9004-96-0	G-5511	CAS 9004-98-2	Brox OL-20 70% Liq
CAS 9004-96-0	Hefti PGE-600-MO	CAS 9004-98-2	Brox OL-40
CAS 9004-96-0	Hetoxamate MO-4	CAS 9004-98-2	Chemal OA-4
CAS 9004-96-0	Hetoxamate MO-5	CAS 9004-98-2	Chemal OA-5
CAS 9004-96-0	Hetoxamate MO-9	CAS 9004-98-2	Chemal OA-9
CAS 9004-96-0	Hetoxamate MO-14	CAS 9004-98-2	Chemal OA-10
CAS 9004-96-0	Hodag 20-O	CAS 9004-98-2	Chemal OA-20
CAS 9004-96-0	Hodag 40-O	CAS 9004-98-2	Chemal OA-20/70CWS
CAS 9004-96-0	Hodag 60-O	CAS 9004-98-2	Chemal OA-20G
CAS 9004-96-0	Kessco® PEG 200 MO	CAS 9004-98-2	Chemal OA-23
CAS 9004-96-0	Kessco® PEG 300 MO	CAS 9004-98-2	Emalex 503
CAS 9004-96-0	Kessco® PEG 400 MO	CAS 9004-98-2	Emalex 506

CAS 9004-98-2	Emalex 508	CAS 9004-98-2	Macol® OA-20
CAS 9004-98-2	Emalex 510	CAS 9004-98-2	Marlipal® 1885/2
CAS 9004-98-2	Emalex 512	CAS 9004-98-2	Marlowet® OA 5
CAS 9004-98-2	Emalex 515	CAS 9004-98-2	Marlowet® OA 10
CAS 9004-98-2	Emalex 520	CAS 9004-98-2	Marlowet® OA 30
CAS 9004-98-2	Emalex 523	CAS 9004-98-2	Nikkol BO-2
CAS 9004-98-2	Emalex 550	CAS 9004-98-2	Nikkol BO-7
CAS 9004-98-2	Empilan® KL 6	CAS 9004-98-2	Nikkol BO-10TX
CAS 9004-98-2	Empilan® KL 10	CAS 9004-98-2	Nikkol BO-15TX
CAS 9004-98-2	Empilan® KL 20	CAS 9004-98-2	Nikkol BO-20
CAS 9004-98-2	Emulsogen LP	CAS 9004-98-2	Nikkol BO-20TX
CAS 9004-98-2	Ethosperse® OA-2	CAS 9004-98-2	Nikkol BO-50
CAS 9004-98-2	Ethosperse® OA-20	CAS 9004-98-2	Procol OA-2
CAS 9004-98-2	Ethoxol 3	CAS 9004-98-2	Procol OA-3
CAS 9004-98-2	Ethoxol 5	CAS 9004-98-2	Procol OA-4
CAS 9004-98-2	Ethoxol 10	CAS 9004-98-2	Procol OA-5
CAS 9004-98-2	Ethoxol 12	CAS 9004-98-2	Procol OA-10
CAS 9004-98-2	Ethoxol 20	CAS 9004-98-2	Procol OA-20
CAS 9004-98-2	Ethoxol 44	CAS 9004-98-2	Procol OA-23
CAS 9004-98-2	Eumulgin® O5	CAS 9004-98-2	Procol OA-25
CAS 9004-98-2	Eumulgin® O10	CAS 9004-98-2	Prox-onic OA-1/04
CAS 9004-98-2	Eumulgin® PWM2	CAS 9004-98-2	Prox-onic OA-1/09
CAS 9004-98-2	Eumulgin® PWM5	CAS 9004-98-2	Prox-onic OA-1/020
CAS 9004-98-2	Eumulgin® PWM10	CAS 9004-98-2	Prox-onic OA-2/020
CAS 9004-98-2	Eumulgin® PWM17	CAS 9004-98-2	Rhodasurf® ON-870
CAS 9004-98-2	G-3908S	CAS 9004-98-2	Rhodasurf® ON-877
CAS 9004-98-2	G-3910	CAS 9004-98-2	Ritoleth 2
CAS 9004-98-2	Genapol® O-020	CAS 9004-98-2	Ritoleth 5
CAS 9004-98-2	Genapol® O-050	CAS 9004-98-2	Ritoleth 10
CAS 9004-98-2	Genapol® O-080	CAS 9004-98-2	Ritoleth 20
CAS 9004-98-2	Genapol® O-090	CAS 9004-98-2	Simulsol 92
CAS 9004-98-2	Genapol® O-100	CAS 9004-98-2	Simulsol 96
CAS 9004-98-2	Genapol® O-120	CAS 9004-98-2	Simulsol 98
CAS 9004-98-2	Genapol® O-150	CAS 9004-98-2	Trycol® 5971
CAS 9004-98-2	Genapol® O-200	CAS 9004-98-2	Trycol® 5972
CAS 9004-98-2	Genapol® O-230	CAS 9004-98-2	Unicol OA-2
CAS 9004-98-2	Hetoxol OA-3 Special	CAS 9004-98-2	Unicol OA-4
CAS 9004-98-2	Hetoxol OA-5 Special	CAS 9004-98-2	Unicol OA-10
CAS 9004-98-2	Hetoxol OA-10 Special	CAS 9004-98-2	Unicol OA-20
CAS 9004-98-2	Hetoxol OA-20 Special	CAS 9004-98-2	Unimul-05
CAS 9004-98-2	Hetoxol OCS	CAS 9004-98-2	Unimul-10
CAS 9004-98-2	Hetoxol OL-3	CAS 9004-98-2	Varonic® 32-E20
CAS 9004-98-2	Hetoxol OL-4	CAS 9004-98-2	Volpo 3
CAS 9004-98-2	Hetoxol OL-5	CAS 9004-98-2	Volpo 5
CAS 9004-98-2	Hetoxol OL-10	CAS 9004-98-2	Volpo 10
CAS 9004-98-2	Hetoxol OL-10H	CAS 9004-98-2	Volpo 20
CAS 9004-98-2	Hetoxol OL-20	CAS 9004-98-2	Volpo N3
CAS 9004-98-2	Hetoxol OL-23	CAS 9004-98-2	Volpo N5
CAS 9004-98-2	Hetoxol OL-40	CAS 9004-98-2	Volpo N10
CAS 9004-98-2	Hodag Nonionic 1802	CAS 9004-98-2	Volpo N15
CAS 9004-98-2	Hodag Nonionic 1804	CAS 9004-98-2	Volpo N20
CAS 9004-98-2	Hodag Nonionic 1809	CAS 9004-98-2	Volpo O3
CAS 9004-98-2	Hodag Nonionic 1810	CAS 9004-98-2	Volpo O5
CAS 9004-98-2	Hodag Nonionic 1820	CAS 9004-98-2	Volpo O10
CAS 9004-98-2	Hostacerin O-20	CAS 9004-98-2	Volpo O15
CAS 9004-98-2	Lanycol-92	CAS 9004-98-2	Volpo O20
CAS 9004-98-2	Lanycol-96	CAS 9004-99-3	Ablunol 200MS
CAS 9004-98-2	Lanycol-97	CAS 9004-99-3	Ablunol 400MS
CAS 9004-98-2	Lanycol-98	CAS 9004-99-3	Ablunol 600MS
CAS 9004-98-2	Lanycol-99	CAS 9004-99-3	Ablunol 1000MS
CAS 9004-98-2	Lipocol O-2 Special	CAS 9004-99-3	Ablunol DEGMS
CAS 9004-98-2	Lipocol O-3 Special	CAS 9004-99-3	Acconon 200-MS
CAS 9004-98-2	Lipocol O-5 Special	CAS 9004-99-3	Acconon 400-MS
CAS 9004-98-2	Lipocol O-10	CAS 9004-99-3	Algon ST 50
CAS 9004-98-2	Lipocol O-20	CAS 9004-99-3	Algon ST 80
CAS 9004-98-2	Lipocol O-25	CAS 9004-99-3	Algon ST 100
CAS 9004-98-2	Macol® OA-2	CAS 9004-99-3	Algon ST 200
CAS 9004-98-2	Macol® OA-4	CAS 9004-99-3	Algon ST 400
CAS 9004-98-2	Macol® OA-5	CAS 9004-99-3	Algon ST 500
CAS 9004-98-2	Macol® OA-10	CAS 9004-99-3	Algon ST 1000

CAS 9004-99-3	Alkamuls® S-6		CAS 9004-99-3	Hetoxamate SA-90
CAS 9004-99-3	Alkamuls® ST-40		CAS 9004-99-3	Hetoxamate SA-90F
CAS 9004-99-3	Cerasynt® 840		CAS 9004-99-3	Hetoxamate SA-100
CAS 9004-99-3	Chemax E-200 MS		CAS 9004-99-3	Hodag 20-S
CAS 9004-99-3	Chemax E-400 MS		CAS 9004-99-3	Hodag 40-S
CAS 9004-99-3	Chemax E-600 MS		CAS 9004-99-3	Hodag 60-S
CAS 9004-99-3	Chemax E-1000 MS		CAS 9004-99-3	Hodag 100-S
CAS 9004-99-3	Cithrol 2MS		CAS 9004-99-3	Hodag 150-S
CAS 9004-99-3	Cithrol 3MS		CAS 9004-99-3	Hodag 154-S
CAS 9004-99-3	Cithrol 4MS		CAS 9004-99-3	Hodag 600-S
CAS 9004-99-3	Cithrol 6MS		CAS 9004-99-3	Hodag DGS
CAS 9004-99-3	Cithrol 10MS		CAS 9004-99-3	Hodag DGS-C
CAS 9004-99-3	Cithrol 40MS		CAS 9004-99-3	Hodag POE (40) MS
CAS 9004-99-3	Cithrol DGMS N/E		CAS 9004-99-3	Hydrine
CAS 9004-99-3	Cithrol DGMS S/E		CAS 9004-99-3	Karapeg DEG-MS
CAS 9004-99-3	CPH-50-N		CAS 9004-99-3	Kemester® 5221SE
CAS 9004-99-3	CPH-90-N		CAS 9004-99-3	Kessco® PEG 200 MS
CAS 9004-99-3	CPH-104-DC-SE		CAS 9004-99-3	Kessco® PEG 300 MS
CAS 9004-99-3	CPH-104-DG-SE		CAS 9004-99-3	Kessco® PEG 400 MS
CAS 9004-99-3	Cremophor® S 9		CAS 9004-99-3	Kessco® PEG 600 MS
CAS 9004-99-3	Crodet S4		CAS 9004-99-3	Kessco® PEG 1000 MS
CAS 9004-99-3	Crodet S8		CAS 9004-99-3	Kessco® PEG 1540 MS
CAS 9004-99-3	Crodet S12		CAS 9004-99-3	Kessco® PEG 4000 MS
CAS 9004-99-3	Crodet S24		CAS 9004-99-3	Kessco® PEG 6000 MS
CAS 9004-99-3	Crodet S40		CAS 9004-99-3	Lanoxide-52
CAS 9004-99-3	Crodet S50		CAS 9004-99-3	Lanoxide-53
CAS 9004-99-3	Crodet S100		CAS 9004-99-3	Lanoxide-59
CAS 9004-99-3	Elfacos® PEG 400 MS		CAS 9004-99-3	Lasemul 400 E
CAS 9004-99-3	Elfacos® PEG 600 MS		CAS 9004-99-3	Lipal DGMS
CAS 9004-99-3	Elfacos® PEG 1000 MS		CAS 9004-99-3	Lipopeg 2-S
CAS 9004-99-3	Emalex 400A		CAS 9004-99-3	Lipopeg 3-S
CAS 9004-99-3	Emalex 400B		CAS 9004-99-3	Lipopeg 4-S
CAS 9004-99-3	Emalex 805		CAS 9004-99-3	Lipopeg 6-S
CAS 9004-99-3	Emalex 810		CAS 9004-99-3	Lipopeg 10-S
CAS 9004-99-3	Emalex 820		CAS 9004-99-3	Lipopeg 15-S
CAS 9004-99-3	Emalex 830		CAS 9004-99-3	Lipopeg 16-S
CAS 9004-99-3	Emalex 840		CAS 9004-99-3	Lipopeg 20-S
CAS 9004-99-3	Emalex 6300 M-ST		CAS 9004-99-3	Lipopeg 39-S
CAS 9004-99-3	Emerest® 2662		CAS 9004-99-3	Lipopeg 100-S
CAS 9004-99-3	Emerest® 2711		CAS 9004-99-3	Mapeg® 200 MS
CAS 9004-99-3	Emerest® 2715		CAS 9004-99-3	Mapeg® 400 MS
CAS 9004-99-3	Emerest® 2717		CAS 9004-99-3	Mapeg® 600 MS
CAS 9004-99-3	Estol DEMS-se 3711		CAS 9004-99-3	Mapeg® 1000 MS
CAS 9004-99-3	Estol E04MS 3723		CAS 9004-99-3	Mapeg® 1500 MS
CAS 9004-99-3	Estol E06MS 3725		CAS 9004-99-3	Mapeg® S-40
CAS 9004-99-3	Estol E10MS 3727		CAS 9004-99-3	Mapeg® S-40K
CAS 9004-99-3	Estol E60MS 3733		CAS 9004-99-3	Mapeg® S-100
CAS 9004-99-3	Ethofat® 18/14		CAS 9004-99-3	Mapeg® S-150
CAS 9004-99-3	Ethofat® 60/15		CAS 9004-99-3	Marlosol® 183
CAS 9004-99-3	Ethofat® 60/20		CAS 9004-99-3	Marlosol® 188
CAS 9004-99-3	Eumulgin® ST-8		CAS 9004-99-3	Marlosol® 1820
CAS 9004-99-3	G-2151		CAS 9004-99-3	Myrj® 45
CAS 9004-99-3	G-2153		CAS 9004-99-3	Myrj® 49
CAS 9004-99-3	Hefti PGE-400-MS		CAS 9004-99-3	Myrj® 51
CAS 9004-99-3	Hefti PGE-600-MS		CAS 9004-99-3	Myrj® 52
CAS 9004-99-3	Hefti RS-55-40		CAS 9004-99-3	Myrj® 52S
CAS 9004-99-3	Hefti RS-55-100		CAS 9004-99-3	Myrj® 53
CAS 9004-99-3	Hetoxamate 100S		CAS 9004-99-3	Myrj® 59
CAS 9004-99-3	Hetoxamate SA-5		CAS 9004-99-3	Nikkol MYS-4
CAS 9004-99-3	Hetoxamate SA-6		CAS 9004-99-3	Nikkol MYS-10
CAS 9004-99-3	Hetoxamate SA-7		CAS 9004-99-3	Nikkol MYS-25
CAS 9004-99-3	Hetoxamate SA-8		CAS 9004-99-3	Nikkol MYS-40
CAS 9004-99-3	Hetoxamate SA-9		CAS 9004-99-3	Nikkol MYS-45
CAS 9004-99-3	Hetoxamate SA-12		CAS 9004-99-3	Nikkol MYS-55
CAS 9004-99-3	Hetoxamate SA-13		CAS 9004-99-3	Nopalcol 1-S
CAS 9004-99-3	Hetoxamate SA-20		CAS 9004-99-3	Pegosperse® 200 MS
CAS 9004-99-3	Hetoxamate SA-23		CAS 9004-99-3	Pegosperse® 400 MS
CAS 9004-99-3	Hetoxamate SA-25		CAS 9004-99-3	Pegosperse® 1500 MS
CAS 9004-99-3	Hetoxamate SA-35		CAS 9004-99-3	Pegosperse® 1750 MS
CAS 9004-99-3	Hetoxamate SA-40		CAS 9004-99-3	Pegosperse® 1750 MS K Spec

CAS 9004-99-3	Polystate C	CAS 9005-00-9	Emalex 625
CAS 9004-99-3	Protamate 200 DPS	CAS 9005-00-9	Emalex 630
CAS 9004-99-3	Protamate 300 DPS	CAS 9005-00-9	Emalex 640
CAS 9004-99-3	Protamate 400 DPS	CAS 9005-00-9	Hetoxol STA-2
CAS 9004-99-3	Protamate 600 DPS	CAS 9005-00-9	Hetoxol STA-10
CAS 9004-99-3	Protamate 1000 DPS	CAS 9005-00-9	Hetoxol STA-20
CAS 9004-99-3	Protamate 1500 DPS	CAS 9005-00-9	Hetoxol STA-30
CAS 9004-99-3	Protamate 1540 DPS	CAS 9005-00-9	Hodag Nonionic S-2
CAS 9004-99-3	Protamate 2000 DPS	CAS 9005-00-9	Hodag Nonionic S-10
CAS 9004-99-3	Protamate 4000 DPS	CAS 9005-00-9	Hodag Nonionic S-13
CAS 9004-99-3	Protamate 4400 DPS	CAS 9005-00-9	Hodag Nonionic S-20
CAS 9004-99-3	Prox-onic ST-05	CAS 9005-00-9	Hodag Nonionic S-40
CAS 9004-99-3	Prox-onic ST-09	CAS 9005-00-9	Lanycol-72
CAS 9004-99-3	Prox-onic ST-014	CAS 9005-00-9	Lanycol-78
CAS 9004-99-3	Prox-onic ST-023	CAS 9005-00-9	Lanycol-79
CAS 9004-99-3	Radiasurf® 7411	CAS 9005-00-9	Lanycol-700
CAS 9004-99-3	Radiasurf® 7413	CAS 9005-00-9	Lipocol S-2
CAS 9004-99-3	Radiasurf® 7432	CAS 9005-00-9	Lipocol S-10
CAS 9004-99-3	Ritapeg 150 DS	CAS 9005-00-9	Lipocol S-20
CAS 9004-99-3	Ritox 52	CAS 9005-00-9	Macol® SA-2
CAS 9004-99-3	Ritox 53	CAS 9005-00-9	Macol® SA-5
CAS 9004-99-3	Ritox 59	CAS 9005-00-9	Macol® SA-10
CAS 9004-99-3	Rol 52	CAS 9005-00-9	Macol® SA-15
CAS 9004-99-3	Rol 53	CAS 9005-00-9	Macol® SA-20
CAS 9004-99-3	Rol 59	CAS 9005-00-9	Macol® SA-40
CAS 9004-99-3	Rol 400	CAS 9005-00-9	Nikkol BS-2
CAS 9004-99-3	Serdox NSG 400	CAS 9005-00-9	Nikkol BS-4
CAS 9004-99-3	Simulsol M 45	CAS 9005-00-9	Nikkol BS-20
CAS 9004-99-3	Simulsol M 49	CAS 9005-00-9	Procol SA-2
CAS 9004-99-3	Simulsol M 51	CAS 9005-00-9	Procol SA-4
CAS 9004-99-3	Simulsol M 52	CAS 9005-00-9	Procol SA-10
CAS 9004-99-3	Simulsol M 53	CAS 9005-00-9	Procol SA-20
CAS 9004-99-3	Simulsol M 59	CAS 9005-00-9	Rhodasurf® S-2
CAS 9004-99-3	Stearate PEG 1000	CAS 9005-00-9	Rhodasurf® S-20
CAS 9004-99-3	Sterol ST 2	CAS 9005-00-9	Simulsol 7
CAS 9004-99-3	Superpolystate	CAS 9005-00-9	Simulsol 72
CAS 9004-99-3	Tefose® 1500	CAS 9005-00-9	Simulsol 76
CAS 9004-99-3	Tegin® D 1102	CAS 9005-00-9	Simulsol 78
CAS 9004-99-3	Tegin® D 6100	CAS 9005-00-9	Tewax TC 72
CAS 9004-99-3	Unipeg-200 MS	CAS 9005-00-9	Unicol SA-2
CAS 9004-99-3	Unipeg-400 MS	CAS 9005-00-9	Unicol SA-10
CAS 9004-99-3	Unipeg-600 MS	CAS 9005-00-9	Unicol SA-13
CAS 9004-99-3	Unipeg-1000 MS	CAS 9005-00-9	Unicol SA-15
CAS 9004-99-3	Unipeg-1540 MS	CAS 9005-00-9	Unicol SA-20
CAS 9004-99-3	Unipeg-4000 MS	CAS 9005-00-9	Unicol SA-40
CAS 9004-99-3	Unipeg-6000 MS	CAS 9005-00-9	Volpo S-2
CAS 9004-99-3	Unipeg-S-40	CAS 9005-00-9	Volpo S-10
CAS 9004-99-3	Witconol™ 2711	CAS 9005-00-9	Volpo S-20
CAS 9004-99-3	Witconol™ 2713	CAS 9005-02-1	Chemax PEG 200 DL
CAS 9005-00-9	Ablunol SA-7	CAS 9005-02-1	Cithrol 2DL
CAS 9005-00-9	Brij® 72	CAS 9005-02-1	Cithrol 4DL
CAS 9005-00-9	Brij® 76	CAS 9005-02-1	Cithrol 6DL
CAS 9005-00-9	Brij® 78	CAS 9005-02-1	Cithrol 10DL
CAS 9005-00-9	Brij® 700	CAS 9005-02-1	CPH-79-N
CAS 9005-00-9	Brij® 700S	CAS 9005-02-1	CPH-361-N
CAS 9005-00-9	Brij® 721	CAS 9005-02-1	Emalex 200 di-L
CAS 9005-00-9	Brij® 721S	CAS 9005-02-1	Emalex 300 di-L
CAS 9005-00-9	Brox HLB-13	CAS 9005-02-1	Emalex 400 di-L
CAS 9005-00-9	Brox S-2	CAS 9005-02-1	Emalex 600 di-L
CAS 9005-00-9	Brox S-20	CAS 9005-02-1	Emalex 800 di-L
CAS 9005-00-9	Brox S-30	CAS 9005-02-1	Emalex 1000 di-L
CAS 9005-00-9	Cromul EM 1207	CAS 9005-02-1	Emalex DEG-di-L
CAS 9005-00-9	Emalex 602	CAS 9005-02-1	Emalex TEG-di-L
CAS 9005-00-9	Emalex 603	CAS 9005-02-1	Emerest® 2704
CAS 9005-00-9	Emalex 605	CAS 9005-02-1	Hetoxamate 200 DL
CAS 9005-00-9	Emalex 606	CAS 9005-02-1	Hetoxamate 400 DL
CAS 9005-00-9	Emalex 608	CAS 9005-02-1	Hodag 22-L
CAS 9005-00-9	Emalex 611	CAS 9005-02-1	Hodag 42-L
CAS 9005-00-9	Emalex 615	CAS 9005-02-1	Kessco® PEG 200 DL
CAS 9005-00-9	Emalex 620	CAS 9005-02-1	Kessco® PEG 300 DL

CAS 9005-02-1	Kessco® PEG 400 DL
CAS 9005-02-1	Kessco® PEG 600 DL
CAS 9005-02-1	Kessco® PEG 1000 DL
CAS 9005-02-1	Kessco® PEG 1540 DL
CAS 9005-02-1	Kessco® PEG 4000 DL
CAS 9005-02-1	Kessco® PEG 6000 DL
CAS 9005-02-1	Lexemul® 200 DL
CAS 9005-02-1	Lexemul® PEG-200 DL
CAS 9005-02-1	Lexemul® PEG-400 DL
CAS 9005-02-1	Lipopeg 2-DL
CAS 9005-02-1	Lipopeg 3-DL
CAS 9005-02-1	Lipopeg 4-DL
CAS 9005-02-1	Lipopeg 6000-DL
CAS 9005-02-1	Mapeg® 200 DL
CAS 9005-02-1	Mapeg® 400 DL
CAS 9005-02-1	Mapeg® 600 DL
CAS 9005-02-1	Pegosperse® 200 DL
CAS 9005-02-1	Pegosperse® 400 DL
CAS 9005-02-1	Protamate 200 DL
CAS 9005-02-1	Protamate 400 DL
CAS 9005-02-1	Rol DL 40
CAS 9005-02-1	Unipeg-400 DL
CAS 9005-02-1	Witconol™ 2622
CAS 9005-07-6	Alkamuls® 400-DO
CAS 9005-07-6	Alkamuls® 600-DO
CAS 9005-07-6	Chemax PEG 400 DO
CAS 9005-07-6	Chemax PEG 600 DO
CAS 9005-07-6	Cithrol 2DO
CAS 9005-07-6	Cithrol 4DO
CAS 9005-07-6	Cithrol 6DO
CAS 9005-07-6	Cithrol 10DO
CAS 9005-07-6	CPH-213-N
CAS 9005-07-6	Emalex 200 di-O
CAS 9005-07-6	Emalex 300 di-O
CAS 9005-07-6	Emalex 400 di-O
CAS 9005-07-6	Emalex 600 di-O
CAS 9005-07-6	Estol EO4DO 3673
CAS 9005-07-6	Estol EO6DO 3675
CAS 9005-07-6	Hodag 22-O
CAS 9005-07-6	Hodag 32-O
CAS 9005-07-6	Hodag 42-O
CAS 9005-07-6	Hodag 62-O
CAS 9005-07-6	Kessco® PEG 200 DO
CAS 9005-07-6	Kessco® PEG 300 DO
CAS 9005-07-6	Kessco® PEG 400 DO
CAS 9005-07-6	Kessco® PEG 600 DO
CAS 9005-07-6	Kessco® PEG 1000 DO
CAS 9005-07-6	Kessco® PEG 1540 DO
CAS 9005-07-6	Kessco® PEG 4000 DO
CAS 9005-07-6	Kessco® PEG 6000 DO
CAS 9005-07-6	Lipopeg 4-DO
CAS 9005-07-6	Mapeg® 200 DO
CAS 9005-07-6	Mapeg® 400 DO
CAS 9005-07-6	Mapeg® 600 DO
CAS 9005-07-6	Marlipal® FS
CAS 9005-07-6	Marlosol® FS
CAS 9005-07-6	Pegosperse® 400 DO
CAS 9005-07-6	Protamate 400 DO
CAS 9005-07-6	Rol DO 40
CAS 9005-07-6	Unipeg-400 DO
CAS 9005-07-6	Unipeg-600 DO
CAS 9005-07-6	Witconol™ 2648
CAS 9005-08-7	Ablunol 6000DS
CAS 9005-08-7	Algon DS 6000
CAS 9005-08-7	Alkamuls® PEG 300 DS
CAS 9005-08-7	Alkamuls® PEG 400 DS
CAS 9005-08-7	Alkamuls® PEG 600 DS
CAS 9005-08-7	Cithrol 4DS
CAS 9005-08-7	Cithrol 6DS
CAS 9005-08-7	Cithrol 10DS
CAS 9005-08-7	Cithrol 60DS
CAS 9005-08-7	Cutina® TS
CAS 9005-08-7	Elfacos® PEG 400 DS
CAS 9005-08-7	Elfacos® PEG 600 DS
CAS 9005-08-7	Emalex 200 di-AS
CAS 9005-08-7	Emalex 200 di-S
CAS 9005-08-7	Emalex 300 di-S
CAS 9005-08-7	Emalex 400 di-AS
CAS 9005-08-7	Emalex 400 di-S
CAS 9005-08-7	Emalex 600 di-AS
CAS 9005-08-7	Emalex 600 di-S
CAS 9005-08-7	Emalex 6300 DI-ST
CAS 9005-08-7	Emalex TEG-di-AS
CAS 9005-08-7	Emalex TEG-di-S
CAS 9005-08-7	Emerest® 2642
CAS 9005-08-7	Emerest® 2712
CAS 9005-08-7	Emulvis®
CAS 9005-08-7	Estol E04DS 3724
CAS 9005-08-7	Estol E06DS 3726
CAS 9005-08-7	Estol E10DS 3728
CAS 9005-08-7	Estol E60DS 3734
CAS 9005-08-7	G-1821
CAS 9005-08-7	Genapol® TS Powd.
CAS 9005-08-7	Hefti PGE-400-DS
CAS 9005-08-7	Hefti PGE-600-DS
CAS 9005-08-7	Hetoxamate 150 DSA
CAS 9005-08-7	Hetoxamate 400 DS
CAS 9005-08-7	Hetoxamate 600 DS
CAS 9005-08-7	Hodag 22-S
CAS 9005-08-7	Hodag 42-S
CAS 9005-08-7	Hodag 62-S
CAS 9005-08-7	Hodag 102-S
CAS 9005-08-7	Hodag 602-S
CAS 9005-08-7	Kessco® PEG 200 DS
CAS 9005-08-7	Kessco® PEG 300 DS
CAS 9005-08-7	Kessco PEG-400 DS-356
CAS 9005-08-7	Kessco® PEG 400 DS
CAS 9005-08-7	Kessco® PEG 600 DS
CAS 9005-08-7	Kessco® PEG 1000 DS
CAS 9005-08-7	Kessco® PEG 1540 DS
CAS 9005-08-7	Kessco® PEG 4000 DS
CAS 9005-08-7	Kessco PEG 6000DS
CAS 9005-08-7	Kessco® PEG 6000 DS
CAS 9005-08-7	Lanoxide-6000DS
CAS 9005-08-7	Lipopeg 4-DS
CAS 9005-08-7	Lipopeg 10-DS
CAS 9005-08-7	Lipopeg 6000-DS
CAS 9005-08-7	Mapeg® 200 DS
CAS 9005-08-7	Mapeg® 400 DS
CAS 9005-08-7	Mapeg® 600 DS
CAS 9005-08-7	Mapeg® 1540 DS
CAS 9005-08-7	Mapeg® 6000 DS
CAS 9005-08-7	Marlosol® BS
CAS 9005-08-7	Nikkol Estepearl 30
CAS 9005-08-7	Pegosperse® 400 DS
CAS 9005-08-7	Phoenate 3 DSA
CAS 9005-08-7	Protamate 400 DS
CAS 9005-08-7	Protamate 600 DS
CAS 9005-08-7	Protamate 6000 DS
CAS 9005-08-7	Rewopal® PEG 6000 DS
CAS 9005-08-7	Rol D 600
CAS 9005-08-7	Unipeg 150 DS
CAS 9005-08-7	Unipeg-400 DS
CAS 9005-08-7	Unipeg-600 DS
CAS 9005-08-7	Unipeg 1000 DS
CAS 9005-08-7	Unipeg-4000 DS
CAS 9005-08-7	Unipeg-6000 DS
CAS 9005-08-7	Witconol™ 2712
CAS 9005-08-7	Witconol™ L3245
CAS 9005-25-8	Argo Brand Corn Starch

CAS 9005-25-8	Dascare Micropearl	CAS 9005-64-5	Prox-onic SML-020
CAS 9005-25-8	Pure-Dent® B700	CAS 9005-64-5	Ritabate 20
CAS 9005-25-8	Pure-Dent® B810	CAS 9005-64-5	Sorbax PML-20
CAS 9005-25-8	Purity® 21	CAS 9005-64-5	Sorbilene L
CAS 9005-25-8	28-1801	CAS 9005-64-5	Sorbilene L 4
CAS 9005-25-8	Univeg CS	CAS 9005-64-5	Sorbilene LH
CAS 9005-32-7	Alginic Acid FCC	CAS 9005-64-5	Sorbon T-20
CAS 9005-32-7	Kelacid®	CAS 9005-64-5	T-Maz® 20
CAS 9005-32-7	Satialgine™ H8	CAS 9005-64-5	T-Maz® 28
CAS 9005-34-9	Sobalg FD 300 Series	CAS 9005-64-5	Tween® 20
CAS 9005-34-9	Superloid®	CAS 9005-64-5	Tween® 21
CAS 9005-35-0	Sobalg FD 460	CAS 9005-64-5	Unisorb 20
CAS 9005-36-1	Kelmar®	CAS 9005-64-5	Unisorb 21
CAS 9005-36-1	Kelmar® Improved	CAS 9005-64-5	Unisorb 80L
CAS 9005-36-1	Sobalg FD 200 Series	CAS 9005-64-5	Witconol™ 2720
CAS 9005-38-3	Dariloid® QH	CAS 9005-65-6	Alkamuls® PSMO-5
CAS 9005-38-3	Kelco® HV	CAS 9005-65-6	Alkamuls® PSMO-20
CAS 9005-38-3	Kelco® LV	CAS 9005-65-6	Armotan® PMO 20
CAS 9005-38-3	Kelcosol®	CAS 9005-65-6	Crillet 4
CAS 9005-38-3	Kelgin® F	CAS 9005-65-6	Crillet 41
CAS 9005-38-3	Kelgin® HV	CAS 9005-65-6	Drewmulse® POE-SMO
CAS 9005-38-3	Kelgin® LV, MV	CAS 9005-65-6	Durfax® 80
CAS 9005-38-3	Kelgin® QL	CAS 9005-65-6	Emalex ET-8020
CAS 9005-38-3	Kelgin® XL	CAS 9005-65-6	Emsorb® 2722
CAS 9005-38-3	Keltone	CAS 9005-65-6	Emsorb® 2725
CAS 9005-46-3	Alanate 110	CAS 9005-65-6	Emsorb® 6900
CAS 9005-46-3	Unipro SO-CASE	CAS 9005-65-6	Estol SMO20 3686
CAS 9005-64-5	Alkamuls® PSML-20	CAS 9005-65-6	Ethylan® GEO8
CAS 9005-64-5	Alkamuls® T-20	CAS 9005-65-6	Ethylan® GEO81
CAS 9005-64-5	Armotan® PML 20	CAS 9005-65-6	Eumulgin® SMO 20
CAS 9005-64-5	Capmul® POE-L	CAS 9005-65-6	Glycosperse® O-5
CAS 9005-64-5	Crillet 1	CAS 9005-65-6	Glycosperse® O-20
CAS 9005-64-5	Crillet 11	CAS 9005-65-6	Hetsorb O-5
CAS 9005-64-5	Drewmulse® POE-SML	CAS 9005-65-6	Hetsorb O-20
CAS 9005-64-5	Durfax® 20	CAS 9005-65-6	Hodag PSMO-5
CAS 9005-64-5	Emalex ET-2020	CAS 9005-65-6	Hodag PSMO-20
CAS 9005-64-5	Emsorb® 2720	CAS 9005-65-6	Incrosorb O-80
CAS 9005-64-5	Emsorb® 2721	CAS 9005-65-6	Ixol 8
CAS 9005-64-5	Emsorb® 6915	CAS 9005-65-6	Laxan-ESM
CAS 9005-64-5	Estol SML20 3618	CAS 9005-65-6	Laxan-ESO
CAS 9005-64-5	Ethylan® GEL2	CAS 9005-65-6	Liposorb O-5
CAS 9005-64-5	Eumulgin® SML 20	CAS 9005-65-6	Liposorb O-20
CAS 9005-64-5	G-4280	CAS 9005-65-6	Lonzest® SMO-20
CAS 9005-64-5	Glycosperse® L-10	CAS 9005-65-6	Montanox 80
CAS 9005-64-5	Glycosperse® L-20	CAS 9005-65-6	Montanox 80 DF
CAS 9005-64-5	Hefti ML-55-F	CAS 9005-65-6	Montanox 81
CAS 9005-64-5	Hefti ML-55-F-4	CAS 9005-65-6	Mulsifan RT 146
CAS 9005-64-5	Hetsorb L-4	CAS 9005-65-6	Nikkol TO-10
CAS 9005-64-5	Hetsorb L-10	CAS 9005-65-6	Nikkol TO-10M
CAS 9005-64-5	Hetsorb L-20	CAS 9005-65-6	Norfox® Sorbo T-80
CAS 9005-64-5	Hetsorb L-44	CAS 9005-65-6	Protasorb O-5
CAS 9005-64-5	Hetsorb L-80-72%	CAS 9005-65-6	Protasorb O-20
CAS 9005-64-5	Hodag PSML-4	CAS 9005-65-6	Prox-onic SMO-05
CAS 9005-64-5	Hodag PSML-20	CAS 9005-65-6	Prox-onic SMO-020
CAS 9005-64-5	Hodag PSML-80	CAS 9005-65-6	Ritabate 80
CAS 9005-64-5	Ionet T-20 C	CAS 9005-65-6	Sorbax PMO-5
CAS 9005-64-5	Ixol 2	CAS 9005-65-6	Sorbax PMO-20
CAS 9005-64-5	Laxan-ESL	CAS 9005-65-6	Sorbilene O
CAS 9005-64-5	Laxan-S	CAS 9005-65-6	Sorbilene O 5
CAS 9005-64-5	Liposorb L-10	CAS 9005-65-6	T-Maz® 80
CAS 9005-64-5	Liposorb L-20	CAS 9005-65-6	T-Maz® 80K
CAS 9005-64-5	Lonzest® SML-20	CAS 9005-65-6	T-Maz® 80KLM
CAS 9005-64-5	Montanox 20	CAS 9005-65-6	T-Maz® 81
CAS 9005-64-5	Montanox 20 DF	CAS 9005-65-6	Tween® 80
CAS 9005-64-5	Mulsifan RT 141	CAS 9005-65-6	Tween® 80K
CAS 9005-64-5	Nikkol TL-10, TL-10EX	CAS 9005-65-6	Tween® 81
CAS 9005-64-5	Nissan Nonion LT-221	CAS 9005-65-6	Unisorb 80
CAS 9005-64-5	Norfox® Sorbo T-20	CAS 9005-65-6	Witconol™ 2722
CAS 9005-64-5	Protasorb L-5	CAS 9005-66-7	Crillet 2
CAS 9005-64-5	Protasorb L-20	CAS 9005-66-7	G-4252

CAS 9005-66-7	Glycosperse® P-20		CAS 9005-70-3	Laxan-EST
CAS 9005-66-7	Hetsorb P-20		CAS 9005-70-3	Liposorb TO-20
CAS 9005-66-7	Hodag PSMP-20		CAS 9005-70-3	Lonzest® STO-20
CAS 9005-66-7	Ixol 4		CAS 9005-70-3	Montanox 85
CAS 9005-66-7	Laxan-ESP		CAS 9005-70-3	Nikkol TO-30
CAS 9005-66-7	Liposorb P-20		CAS 9005-70-3	Protasorb TO-20
CAS 9005-66-7	Lonzest® SMP-20		CAS 9005-70-3	Prox-onic STO-020
CAS 9005-66-7	Montanox 40		CAS 9005-70-3	Sorbanox CO
CAS 9005-66-7	Montanox 40 DF		CAS 9005-70-3	Sorbax PTO-20
CAS 9005-66-7	Nikkol TP-10		CAS 9005-70-3	Sorbilene TO
CAS 9005-66-7	Protasorb P-20		CAS 9005-70-3	T-Maz® 85
CAS 9005-66-7	Prox-onic SMP-020		CAS 9005-70-3	Tween® 85
CAS 9005-66-7	Ritabate 40		CAS 9005-70-3	Unisorb 85
CAS 9005-66-7	Sorbax PMP-20		CAS 9005-70-3	Witconol™ 6903
CAS 9005-66-7	Sorbilene P		CAS 9005-71-4	Crillet 35
CAS 9005-66-7	T-Maz® 40		CAS 9005-71-4	Drewmulse® POE-STS
CAS 9005-66-7	Tween® 40		CAS 9005-71-4	Glycosperse® TS-20
CAS 9005-66-7	Unisorb 40		CAS 9005-71-4	Hetsorb TS-20
CAS 9005-67-8	Alkamuls® PSMS-20		CAS 9005-71-4	Hodag PSTS-20
CAS 9005-67-8	Alkamuls® T-60		CAS 9005-71-4	Laxan-ESR
CAS 9005-67-8	Capmul® POE-S		CAS 9005-71-4	Liposorb TS-20
CAS 9005-67-8	Crillet 3		CAS 9005-71-4	Lonzest® STS-20
CAS 9005-67-8	Crillet 31		CAS 9005-71-4	Montanox 65
CAS 9005-67-8	Drewmulse® POE-SMS		CAS 9005-71-4	Nikkol TS-30
CAS 9005-67-8	Durfax® 60		CAS 9005-71-4	Prox-onic STS-020
CAS 9005-67-8	Emsorb® 2728		CAS 9005-71-4	Sorbax PTS-20
CAS 9005-67-8	Estol SMS20 3716		CAS 9005-71-4	Sorbilene TS
CAS 9005-67-8	Ethylan® GES6		CAS 9005-71-4	T-Maz® 65
CAS 9005-67-8	Eumulgin® SMS 20		CAS 9005-71-4	Tween® 65
CAS 9005-67-8	Glycosperse® S-20		CAS 9005-71-4	Unisorb 65
CAS 9005-67-8	Hefti MS-55-F		CAS 9005-71-4	Witconol™ 6907
CAS 9005-67-8	Hetsorb S-4		CAS 9005-79-2	Pentagen
CAS 9005-67-8	Hetsorb S-20		CAS 9006-50-2	Egg White Solids Type P-20
CAS 9005-67-8	Hodag PSMS-4		CAS 9006-50-2	Granular Hennegg Albumen Type G-1
CAS 9005-67-8	Hodag PSMS-20			
CAS 9005-67-8	Ixol 6		CAS 9006-50-2	Instant Egg White Solids Type P-600
CAS 9005-67-8	Laxan-ESE			
CAS 9005-67-8	Laxan-ESS		CAS 9007-34-5	Actigen C
CAS 9005-67-8	Liposorb S-4		CAS 9007-34-5	Ateco
CAS 9005-67-8	Liposorb S-20		CAS 9007-34-5	Atelo-Collagen
CAS 9005-67-8	Lonzest® SMS-20		CAS 9007-34-5	Atelocollagen M
CAS 9005-67-8	Montanox 60		CAS 9007-34-5	Atelocollagen MS
CAS 9005-67-8	Montanox 60 DF		CAS 9007-34-5	Atelocollagen SS
CAS 9005-67-8	Montanox 61		CAS 9007-34-5	Cationic Collagen Polypeptides
CAS 9005-67-8	Nikkol TS-10		CAS 9007-34-5	Clearcol
CAS 9005-67-8	Nikkol TS-106		CAS 9007-34-5	Colladerm Procollagene SC
CAS 9005-67-8	Protasorb S-20		CAS 9007-34-5	Collagen
CAS 9005-67-8	Prox-onic SMS-020		CAS 9007-34-5	Collagen CLR
CAS 9005-67-8	Ritabate 60		CAS 9007-34-5	Collagen S.D
CAS 9005-67-8	Sorbax PMS-20		CAS 9007-34-5	Collagene SPO
CAS 9005-67-8	Sorbilene S		CAS 9007-34-5	Collagene Lyophilized
CAS 9005-67-8	Sorbilene S 4		CAS 9007-34-5	Collagen Masks
CAS 9005-67-8	T-Maz® 60		CAS 9007-34-5	Collagen Nativ 1%
CAS 9005-67-8	T-Maz® 60K		CAS 9007-34-5	Collagen Native Extra 1%
CAS 9005-67-8	T-Maz® 61		CAS 9007-34-5	Collagen Powd.
CAS 9005-67-8	Tween® 60		CAS 9007-34-5	Collapur®
CAS 9005-67-8	Tween® 61		CAS 9007-34-5	Collapuron® DAK
CAS 9005-67-8	Unisorb 60		CAS 9007-34-5	Collapuron N
CAS 9005-67-8	Unisorb 61		CAS 9007-34-5	Collasol
CAS 9005-67-8	Witconol™ 2728		CAS 9007-34-5	Dermacol
CAS 9005-70-3	Alkamuls® PSTO-20		CAS 9007-34-5	Desamidocollagen K 1.0
CAS 9005-70-3	Alkamuls® T-85		CAS 9007-34-5	Desamidocollagen K 1.5
CAS 9005-70-3	Crillet 45		CAS 9007-34-5	Grancol SP-01
CAS 9005-70-3	Ethylan® GPS85		CAS 9007-34-5	Hydracol®
CAS 9005-70-3	Glycosperse® TO-20		CAS 9007-34-5	Kollagen KD
CAS 9005-70-3	Hefti TO-55-E		CAS 9007-34-5	Kollagen S
CAS 9005-70-3	Hefti TO-55-EL		CAS 9007-34-5	Kollaplex 0.3
CAS 9005-70-3	Hefti TO-55-F		CAS 9007-34-5	Kollaplex 1.0
CAS 9005-70-3	Hetsorb TO-20		CAS 9007-34-5	Kollaron
CAS 9005-70-3	Hodag PSTO-20		CAS 9007-34-5	Lencoll

CAS 9007-34-5	Liquid Animal Collagen
CAS 9007-34-5	Maricol CLR
CAS 9007-34-5	Oceagen®
CAS 9007-34-5	Pancogene® S
CAS 9007-34-5	Polymoist® Mask
CAS 9007-34-5	Ritacollagen BA-1
CAS 9007-34-5	Ritacollagen S-1
CAS 9007-34-5	Sollagen® EC
CAS 9007-34-5	Sollagen® LA
CAS 9007-34-5	Soluble Native Collagen RA-1 No. 26206
CAS 9007-34-5	Soluble Native Collagen RS-1 No. 26205
CAS 9007-34-5	Solu-Coll™
CAS 9007-34-5	Solu-Coll™ C, CLR
CAS 9007-34-5	Solu-Coll™ Complex VY
CAS 9007-34-5	Solu-Coll™ Native
CAS 9007-34-5	Trillagene®
CAS 9007-34-5	Unihypro LAN
CAS 9007-34-5	Unipro CLR
CAS 9007-48-1	Caprol® 3GO
CAS 9007-48-1	Cosmol O-42T
CAS 9007-48-1	Drewpol® 3-1-O
CAS 9007-48-1	Drewpol® 6-1-O
CAS 9007-48-1	Isolan® GO 33
CAS 9007-48-1	Mazol® PGO-31 K
CAS 9007-48-1	Nikkol DGMO-90
CAS 9007-48-1	Nikkol DGMO-C
CAS 9007-48-1	Nikkol Decaglyn 1-O
CAS 9007-48-1	Nikkol Hexaglyn 1-O
CAS 9007-48-1	Nikkol Tetraglyn 1-O
CAS 9007-48-1	Protachem 100
CAS 9007-49-2	DNA LP
CAS 9007-49-2	Robeco-DNA
CAS 9007-58-3	Exsyproteines 2%, 4%
CAS 9008-99-8	Pea Pro-Tein BK
CAS 9009-99-8	Crosilk Powder
CAS 9009-99-8	Fibro-Silk™ Powd.
CAS 9009-99-8	Uniderm SILPOW
CAS 9010-77-9	A-C® 143
CAS 9010-77-9	A-C® 540, 540A
CAS 9010-77-9	A-C® 580
CAS 9010-77-9	A-C® 5120
CAS 9010-77-9	EA-209
CAS 9010-79-1	Petrolite® CP-7
CAS 9010-79-1	Siltek® L
CAS 9011-14-7	BPA-500
CAS 9011-14-7	Jurymer
CAS 9011-14-7	Jurymer MB-1
CAS 9011-14-7	Microma-100
CAS 9011-14-7	Micropearl M100
CAS 9011-14-7	Microsphere M-100
CAS 9011-14-7	PMMA Beads
CAS 9011-14-7	Rohadon® M-449
CAS 9011-14-7	Rohadon® M-527
CAS 9011-14-7	Rohadon® MW-235
CAS 9011-14-7	Rohadon® MW-332
CAS 9011-14-7	Rohadon® MW-422
CAS 9011-14-7	Rohagum® M-914
CAS 9011-14-7	Rohamere® 8744F
CAS 9011-16-9	Gantrez® AN
CAS 9011-16-9	Luviform® FA 119
CAS 9012-54-8	Cellulase 4000
CAS 9012-54-8	Cellulase Tr Conc.
CAS 9012-76-4	Atomergic Chitosan
CAS 9014-90-8	Elfan® NS 98 N
CAS 9014-90-8	Nikkol SNP-4N
CAS 9014-90-8	Witcolate™ D51-51EP
CAS 9014-93-1	Emalex DNP-5
CAS 9014-93-1	Hetoxide DNP-4

CAS 9014-93-1	Hetoxide DNP-5
CAS 9014-93-1	Hetoxide DNP-9.6
CAS 9014-93-1	Hetoxide DNP-10
CAS 9014-93-1	Igepal® DM-970 FLK
CAS 9014-93-1	Macol® DNP-5
CAS 9014-93-1	Macol® DNP-10
CAS 9014-93-1	Macol® DNP-15
CAS 9014-93-1	Macol® DNP-21
CAS 9015-54-7	Collagen BIO-5000
CAS 9015-54-7	Collagen P
CAS 9015-54-7	Collagen S
CAS 9015-54-7	Collagen Hydrolysate 30%
CAS 9015-54-7	Collagen Hydrolyzate Cosmetic 50
CAS 9015-54-7	Collagen Hydrolyzate Cosmetic 55
CAS 9015-54-7	Collagen Hydrolyzate Cosmetic N-35
CAS 9015-54-7	Collagen Hydrolyzate Cosmetic N-55
CAS 9015-54-7	Collagen Hydrolyzate Cosmetic SD
CAS 9015-54-7	Collagenol LS/HC-10
CAS 9015-54-7	Collagenol LS/HC-50
CAS 9015-54-7	Collagenon
CAS 9015-54-7	Collagen Protein WN
CAS 9015-54-7	Crolastin C
CAS 9015-54-7	Cropepsol 30
CAS 9015-54-7	Cropepsol 35
CAS 9015-54-7	Cropepsol 50
CAS 9015-54-7	Cropepsol SD
CAS 9015-54-7	Cropeptone 30
CAS 9015-54-7	Cropeptone 35
CAS 9015-54-7	Cropeptone 50
CAS 9015-54-7	Crotein A
CAS 9015-54-7	Crotein SPA
CAS 9015-54-7	Crotein SPC
CAS 9015-54-7	Crotein SPO
CAS 9015-54-7	Elastovit
CAS 9015-54-7	Granpro-5
CAS 9015-54-7	Granpro-40, -50, -55, -100
CAS 9015-54-7	Hidrolisado de Colageno
CAS 9015-54-7	Hydrocoll™ AC-30
CAS 9015-54-7	Hydrocoll AL-50, AL-55, EN-40, EN-55-X, EN-SD-1M, EN-SD-10M
CAS 9015-54-7	Hydrocoll™ EN-55
CAS 9015-54-7	Hydrocoll™ EN-SD
CAS 9015-54-7	Hydrocoll™ HE-35
CAS 9015-54-7	Hydrocoll™ LE-35
CAS 9015-54-7	Hydrocoll SS-40, SS-55, T-37, T-55, T-LSN, T-LSN-SD, T-P52
CAS 9015-54-7	Hydrocoll™ T-LSN
CAS 9015-54-7	Hydrocolloid 219
CAS 9015-54-7	Hydrolan
CAS 9015-54-7	Hydrolyzed Animal Protein-55
CAS 9015-54-7	Hydrolyzed Animal Protein SD
CAS 9015-54-7	Lanagen-50, -55, -SD
CAS 9015-54-7	Lensol
CAS 9015-54-7	Lexein® X-250
CAS 9015-54-7	Lexein® X-250HP
CAS 9015-54-7	Lexein® X-300
CAS 9015-54-7	Lexein® X-350
CAS 9015-54-7	Monteine CA
CAS 9015-54-7	Neptuline® C
CAS 9015-54-7	Nikkol CCP-40
CAS 9015-54-7	Nikkol CCP-100
CAS 9015-54-7	Nikkol CCP-100P
CAS 9015-54-7	Nutrilan® FPK
CAS 9015-54-7	Nutrilan® H
CAS 9015-54-7	Nutrilan® I
CAS 9015-54-7	Nutrilan® I-50
CAS 9015-54-7	Nutrilan® I-50/NP

CAS 9015-54-7	Nutrilan® I Powd.	CAS 9016-45-9	Desonic® 12N
CAS 9015-54-7	Nutrilan® I-Powd./NP	CAS 9016-45-9	Desonic® 15N
CAS 9015-54-7	Nutrilan® L	CAS 9016-45-9	Desonic® 20N
CAS 9015-54-7	Nutrilan® L/NP	CAS 9016-45-9	Desonic® 30N
CAS 9015-54-7	Nutrilan® M	CAS 9016-45-9	Desonic® 30N70
CAS 9015-54-7	Peptein® 2000®	CAS 9016-45-9	Desonic® 40N
CAS 9015-54-7	Peptein® 2000XL	CAS 9016-45-9	Desonic® 40N70
CAS 9015-54-7	PF-6®	CAS 9016-45-9	Desonic® 50N
CAS 9015-54-7	Polypeptide 10	CAS 9016-45-9	Desonic® 50N70
CAS 9015-54-7	Polypeptide 12	CAS 9016-45-9	Desonic® 100N
CAS 9015-54-7	Polypeptide 37	CAS 9016-45-9	Desonic® 100N70
CAS 9015-54-7	Polypeptide LSN Anhydrous	CAS 9016-45-9	Elfapur® N 50
CAS 9015-54-7	Polypeptide SF	CAS 9016-45-9	Elfapur® N 70
CAS 9015-54-7	Polypro® 5000	CAS 9016-45-9	Elfapur® N 90
CAS 9015-54-7	Polypro® 15000	CAS 9016-45-9	Elfapur® N 120
CAS 9015-54-7	Pran H	CAS 9016-45-9	Elfapur® N 150
CAS 9015-54-7	Pran LIQ	CAS 9016-45-9	Emalex NP-3
CAS 9015-54-7	Prochem 12K	CAS 9016-45-9	Emalex NP-5
CAS 9015-54-7	Prochem 100-CG Powd.	CAS 9016-45-9	Emalex NP-10
CAS 9015-54-7	Prochem SPA	CAS 9016-45-9	Emalex NP-11
CAS 9015-54-7	Prolagen C	CAS 9016-45-9	Emalex NP-12
CAS 9015-54-7	Promois W-32	CAS 9016-45-9	Emalex NP-13
CAS 9015-54-7	Promois W-32LS	CAS 9016-45-9	Emalex NP-15
CAS 9015-54-7	Promois W-32R	CAS 9016-45-9	Emalex NP-20
CAS 9015-54-7	Promois W-42	CAS 9016-45-9	Emalex NP-25
CAS 9015-54-7	Promois W-42CP	CAS 9016-45-9	Emalex NP-30
CAS 9015-54-7	Promois W-42K	CAS 9016-45-9	Empilan® NP9
CAS 9015-54-7	Promois W-42LS	CAS 9016-45-9	Emulsogen ELN
CAS 9015-54-7	Promois W-42R	CAS 9016-45-9	Ethylan® KEO
CAS 9015-54-7	Promois W-52	CAS 9016-45-9	Hefti NP-55-60
CAS 9015-54-7	Promois W-52P	CAS 9016-45-9	Hefti NP-55-80
CAS 9015-54-7	Protein SC	CAS 9016-45-9	Hefti NP-55-90
CAS 9015-54-7	Protein TC	CAS 9016-45-9	Hetoxide NP-4
CAS 9015-54-7	Proteolene H	CAS 9016-45-9	Hetoxide NP-6
CAS 9015-54-7	Tritein-40, -50, -100	CAS 9016-45-9	Hetoxide NP-9
CAS 9015-54-7	Tri-Tein 40N	CAS 9016-45-9	Hetoxide NP-10
CAS 9015-54-7	Tri-Tein 55	CAS 9016-45-9	Hetoxide NP-12
CAS 9016-45-9	Akyporox NP 30	CAS 9016-45-9	Hetoxide NP-15
CAS 9016-45-9	Alkasurf® NP-4	CAS 9016-45-9	Hetoxide NP-30
CAS 9016-45-9	Alkasurf® NP-6	CAS 9016-45-9	Hetoxide NP-40
CAS 9016-45-9	Alkasurf® NP-8	CAS 9016-45-9	Hetoxide NP-50
CAS 9016-45-9	Alkasurf® NP-12	CAS 9016-45-9	Hodag Nonionic E-4
CAS 9016-45-9	Alkasurf® NP-15	CAS 9016-45-9	Hodag Nonionic E-5
CAS 9016-45-9	Alkasurf® NP-30, 70%	CAS 9016-45-9	Hodag Nonionic E-6
CAS 9016-45-9	Alkasurf® NP-40, 70%	CAS 9016-45-9	Hodag Nonionic E-7
CAS 9016-45-9	Carsonon® N-4	CAS 9016-45-9	Hodag Nonionic E-8
CAS 9016-45-9	Carsonon® N-30	CAS 9016-45-9	Hodag Nonionic E-9
CAS 9016-45-9	Carsonon® N-40	CAS 9016-45-9	Hodag Nonionic E-10
CAS 9016-45-9	Carsonon® N-100	CAS 9016-45-9	Hodag Nonionic E-20
CAS 9016-45-9	Chemax NP-1.5	CAS 9016-45-9	Hodag Nonionic E-30
CAS 9016-45-9	Chemax NP-4	CAS 9016-45-9	Hodag Nonionic E-40
CAS 9016-45-9	Chemax NP-6	CAS 9016-45-9	Hodag Nonionic E-50
CAS 9016-45-9	Chemax NP-9	CAS 9016-45-9	Hodag Nonionic E-100
CAS 9016-45-9	Chemax NP-10	CAS 9016-45-9	Igepal® CO-430
CAS 9016-45-9	Chemax NP-15	CAS 9016-45-9	Igepal® CO-630 Special
CAS 9016-45-9	Chemax NP-20	CAS 9016-45-9	Igepal® NP-4
CAS 9016-45-9	Chemax NP-30	CAS 9016-45-9	Igepal® NP-9
CAS 9016-45-9	Chemax NP-30/70	CAS 9016-45-9	Macol® NP-4
CAS 9016-45-9	Chemax NP-40	CAS 9016-45-9	Macol® NP-5
CAS 9016-45-9	Chemax NP-40/70	CAS 9016-45-9	Macol® NP-6
CAS 9016-45-9	Chemax NP-50	CAS 9016-45-9	Macol® NP-8
CAS 9016-45-9	Chemax NP-50/70	CAS 9016-45-9	Macol® NP-11
CAS 9016-45-9	Chemax NP-100	CAS 9016-45-9	Macol® NP-12
CAS 9016-45-9	Chemax NP-100/70	CAS 9016-45-9	Macol® NP-15
CAS 9016-45-9	Desonic® 4N	CAS 9016-45-9	Macol® NP-20
CAS 9016-45-9	Desonic® 5N	CAS 9016-45-9	Macol® NP-20(70)
CAS 9016-45-9	Desonic® 6N	CAS 9016-45-9	Macol® NP-30(70)
CAS 9016-45-9	Desonic® 7N	CAS 9016-45-9	Macol® NP-100
CAS 9016-45-9	Desonic® 9N	CAS 9016-45-9	Makon® 4
CAS 9016-45-9	Desonic® 11N	CAS 9016-45-9	Makon® 6

CAS 9016-45-9	Makon® 8	CAS 9016-45-9	Synperonic NP10
CAS 9016-45-9	Makon® 10	CAS 9016-45-9	Synperonic NP12
CAS 9016-45-9	Makon® 12	CAS 9016-45-9	Synperonic NP13
CAS 9016-45-9	Makon® 14	CAS 9016-45-9	Synperonic NP15
CAS 9016-45-9	Makon® 30	CAS 9016-45-9	Synperonic NP17
CAS 9016-45-9	Naxonic™ NI-40	CAS 9016-45-9	Synperonic NP20
CAS 9016-45-9	Naxonic™ NI-60	CAS 9016-45-9	Synperonic NP25
CAS 9016-45-9	Naxonic™ NI-100	CAS 9016-45-9	Synperonic NP30
CAS 9016-45-9	Nikkol NP-5	CAS 9016-45-9	Synperonic NP30/70
CAS 9016-45-9	Nikkol NP-7.5	CAS 9016-45-9	Synperonic NP35
CAS 9016-45-9	Nikkol NP-10	CAS 9016-45-9	Synperonic NP40
CAS 9016-45-9	Nikkol NP-15	CAS 9016-45-9	Synperonic NP50
CAS 9016-45-9	Nikkol NP-18TX	CAS 9016-45-9	Syntopon A
CAS 9016-45-9	Norfox® NP-4	CAS 9016-45-9	Syntopon A 100
CAS 9016-45-9	Norfox® NP-6	CAS 9016-45-9	Syntopon B
CAS 9016-45-9	Protachem NP-4	CAS 9016-45-9	Syntopon C
CAS 9016-45-9	Protachem NP-6	CAS 9016-45-9	Syntopon D
CAS 9016-45-9	Protachem NP-9	CAS 9016-45-9	Syntopon D2
CAS 9016-45-9	Prox-onic NP-04	CAS 9016-45-9	Syntopon E
CAS 9016-45-9	Prox-onic NP-06	CAS 9016-45-9	Syntopon F
CAS 9016-45-9	Prox-onic NP-09	CAS 9016-45-9	Syntopon G
CAS 9016-45-9	Prox-onic NP-010	CAS 9016-45-9	Syntopon H
CAS 9016-45-9	Prox-onic NP-015	CAS 9016-45-9	Tergitol® NP-9
CAS 9016-45-9	Prox-onic NP-020	CAS 9016-45-9	Triton® N-42
CAS 9016-45-9	Prox-onic NP-030	CAS 9016-45-9	Triton® N-150
CAS 9016-45-9	Prox-onic NP-030/70	CAS 9016-45-9	Unicol NP-4
CAS 9016-45-9	Prox-onic NP-040	CAS 9016-45-9	Unicol NP-5
CAS 9016-45-9	Prox-onic NP-040/70	CAS 9016-45-9	Unicol NP-6
CAS 9016-45-9	Prox-onic NP-050	CAS 9016-45-9	Unicol NP-7
CAS 9016-45-9	Prox-onic NP-050/70	CAS 9016-45-9	Unicol NP-8
CAS 9016-45-9	Prox-onic NP-0100	CAS 9016-45-9	Unicol NP-9
CAS 9016-45-9	Prox-onic NP-0100/70	CAS 9016-45-9	Unicol NP-10
CAS 9016-45-9	Remcopal 334	CAS 9016-45-9	Unicol NP-20
CAS 9016-45-9	Renex® 647	CAS 9016-45-9	Unicol NP-30
CAS 9016-45-9	Renex® 648	CAS 9016-45-9	Unicol NP-40
CAS 9016-45-9	Renex® 649	CAS 9016-45-9	Unicol NP-50
CAS 9016-45-9	Renex® 650	CAS 9016-45-9	Unicol NP-100
CAS 9016-45-9	Renex® 670	CAS 9016-45-9	Uniterge NP 4
CAS 9016-45-9	Renex® 678	CAS 9016-45-9	Uniterge NP 5
CAS 9016-45-9	Renex® 679	CAS 9016-45-9	Uniterge NP 6
CAS 9016-45-9	Renex® 682	CAS 9016-45-9	Uniterge NP 7
CAS 9016-45-9	Renex® 688	CAS 9016-45-9	Uniterge NP 8
CAS 9016-45-9	Renex® 690	CAS 9016-45-9	Uniterge NP 9
CAS 9016-45-9	Renex® 697	CAS 9016-45-9	Uniterge NP-10
CAS 9016-45-9	Renex® 698	CAS 9016-45-9	Uniterge NP-13
CAS 9016-45-9	Simulsol 1030 NP	CAS 9016-45-9	Uniterge NP-15
CAS 9016-45-9	Surfonic® N-31.5	CAS 9016-45-9	Uniterge NP-20
CAS 9016-45-9	Surfonic® N-40	CAS 9016-45-9	Uniterge NP 30
CAS 9016-45-9	Surfonic® N-60	CAS 9016-45-9	Uniterge NP 40
CAS 9016-45-9	Surfonic® N-85	CAS 9016-45-9	Uniterge NP-44
CAS 9016-45-9	Surfonic® N-95	CAS 9016-45-9	Uniterge NP 50
CAS 9016-45-9	Surfonic® N-100	CAS 9016-45-9	Uniterge NP 100
CAS 9016-45-9	Surfonic® N-102	CAS 9016-45-9	Witconol™ NP-40
CAS 9016-45-9	Surfonic® N-120	CAS 9016-45-9	Witconol™ NP-60
CAS 9016-45-9	Surfonic® N-130	CAS 9016-45-9	Witconol™ NP-90
CAS 9016-45-9	Surfonic® N-150	CAS 9016-45-9	Witconol™ NP-110
CAS 9016-45-9	Surfonic® N-200	CAS 9016-45-9	Witconol™ NP-300
CAS 9016-45-9	Surfonic® N-300	CAS 9016-45-9	Witconol™ NP-307
CAS 9016-45-9	Surfonic® NB-5	CAS 9032-42-2	Benecel® ME
CAS 9016-45-9	Synperonic NP4	CAS 9032-42-2	Tylose® MH Grades
CAS 9016-45-9	Synperonic NP5	CAS 9032-42-2	Tylose® MHB
CAS 9016-45-9	Synperonic NP5.5	CAS 9032-42-2	Tylose® MH-p, MHB-p
CAS 9016-45-9	Synperonic NP6	CAS 9032-75-1	Clarex® 5XL
CAS 9016-45-9	Synperonic NP7	CAS 9032-75-1	Clarex® L
CAS 9016-45-9	Synperonic NP8	CAS 9032-75-1	Pearex® L
CAS 9016-45-9	Synperonic NP8.5	CAS 9035-85-2	Acconon CA 10
CAS 9016-45-9	Synperonic NP8.75	CAS 9035-85-2	Carsonon® 169-P
CAS 9016-45-9	Synperonic NP9	CAS 9035-85-2	Fancol 707
CAS 9016-45-9	Synperonic NP9.5	CAS 9035-85-2	Macol® CA 30P
CAS 9016-45-9	Synperonic NP9.75	CAS 9035-85-2	Procetyl 10

CAS 9035-85-2	Procetyl 30	CAS 10101-66-3	Cogilor Spinel
CAS 9035-85-2	Procetyl 50	CAS 10124-56-8	Calgon
CAS 9035-85-2	Wickenol® 707	CAS 10213-78-2	Chemeen 18-2
CAS 9038-43-1	Witconol™ APES	CAS 10213-78-2	Ethomeen® 18/12
CAS 9038-95-3	Pluracol® W3520N	CAS 10213-78-2	Hetoxamine ST-2
CAS 9040-38-4	Aerosol® A-103	CAS 10213-78-2	Protox HTA-2
CAS 9042-76-6	Emcol® CC-9	CAS 10213-78-2	Varonic® S-202
CAS 9042-82-4	Polyolprepolymer-2	CAS 10213-78-2	Varonic® S-202 SF
CAS 9046-01-9	Crodafos T2 Acid	CAS 10228-03-2	Imexine FD
CAS 9046-01-9	Crodafos T5 Acid	CAS 10233-13-3	Crodamol IPL
CAS 9046-01-9	Crodafos T10 Acid	CAS 10233-13-3	Estol IPL 1511
CAS 9050-36-6	Maltrin® M040	CAS 10401-55-5	Liponate CRM
CAS 9050-36-6	Maltrin® M050	CAS 10401-55-5	Naturechem® CR
CAS 9050-36-6	Maltrin® M100	CAS 10401-55-5	Pelemol CR
CAS 9050-36-6	Maltrin® M150	CAS 10401-55-5	Protachem CER
CAS 9050-36-6	Maltrin® M180	CAS 10578-34-4	Finsolv® 116
CAS 9050-36-6	Maltrin® M510	CAS 11006-34-1	Dascolor Chlorophyll
CAS 9050-36-6	Maltrin® M700	CAS 11006-34-1	Uniphyllin SC
CAS 9050-36-6	Maltrin® QD M440	CAS 11042-64-1	Dascare Orizanol
CAS 9050-36-6	Maltrin® QD M500	CAS 11042-64-1	Gamma Oryzanol
CAS 9050-36-6	Maltrin® QD M550	CAS 11094-60-3	Caprol® 10G10O
CAS 9050-36-6	Maltrin® QD M580	CAS 11094-60-3	Drewmulse® 10-10-O
CAS 9050-36-6	Microduct®	CAS 11094-60-3	Drewpol® 10-10-O
CAS 9050-36-6	Wickenol® 550	CAS 11094-60-3	Hodag PGO-1010
CAS 9051-57-4	Rhodapex® CO-436	CAS 11094-60-3	Nikkol Decaglyn 10-O
CAS 9063-38-1	Explotab®	CAS 11094-60-3	Santone® 10-10-O
CAS 9065-13-8	Dantoin® DMHF	CAS 11094-60-3	Unitolate PGO-1010
CAS 9065-13-8	Dantoin® DMHF-75	CAS 11097-68-0	Westchlor® 170
CAS 9065-63-8	Witconol™ APEB	CAS 11111-34-5	Synperonic T/1301
CAS 9067-32-7	Actimoist™	CAS 11111-34-5	Synperonic T/1302
CAS 9067-32-7	Actimoist™ Bio-2	CAS 11111-34-5	Tetronic® 304
CAS 9067-32-7	Avian Sodium Hyaluronate Powd.	CAS 11111-34-5	Tetronic® 701
CAS 9067-32-7	Avian Sodium Hyaluronate Sol'n.	CAS 11111-34-5	Tetronic® 704
CAS 9067-32-7	Hyala-Dew	CAS 11111-34-5	Tetronic® 901
CAS 9067-32-7	Hyaluronic Acid	CAS 11111-34-5	Tetronic® 904
CAS 9067-32-7	Hyaluronic Acid AH-602	CAS 11111-34-5	Tetronic® 908
CAS 9067-32-7	Hyaluronic Acid-BT	CAS 11111-34-5	Tetronic® 1307
CAS 9067-32-7	Hyaluronic Acid (Na)	CAS 11138-66-2	Biozan
CAS 9067-32-7	Hyasol	CAS 11138-66-2	Fitoxantina
CAS 9067-32-7	Hyasol-BT	CAS 11138-66-2	Gomme Xanthane
CAS 9067-32-7	Jaluronid	CAS 11138-66-2	Kelgum CG
CAS 9067-32-7	Kelisema Sodium Hyaluronate Bio	CAS 11138-66-2	Keltrol®
CAS 9067-32-7	Nikkol Bio-Sodium Hyaluronate Powd. and 1% Sol'n.	CAS 11138-66-2	Keltrol CG
		CAS 11138-66-2	Keltrol CG 1000
CAS 9067-32-7	Nikkol Sodium Hyaluronate	CAS 11138-66-2	Keltrol CG BT
CAS 9067-32-7	Pronova™	CAS 11138-66-2	Keltrol CG F
CAS 9067-32-7	RITA HA C-1-C	CAS 11138-66-2	Keltrol CG GM
CAS 9067-32-7	Saccaluronate CC	CAS 11138-66-2	Keltrol CG RD
CAS 9067-32-7	Saccaluronate CW	CAS 11138-66-2	Keltrol CG SF
CAS 9067-32-7	Saccaluronate LC	CAS 11138-66-2	Keltrol CG T
CAS 9067-32-7	Sodium Hyaluronate RCC-1 No. 26228	CAS 11138-66-2	Keltrol CG TF
		CAS 11138-66-2	Keltrol® F
CAS 9076-43-1	Emcol® CC-42	CAS 11138-66-2	Merezan® 8
CAS 9082-00-2	Dow 15-200	CAS 11138-66-2	Merezan® 20
CAS 9082-00-2	Dow 112-2	CAS 11138-66-2	Rhodicare™ D
CAS 9084-06-4	Petro® 11	CAS 11138-66-2	Rhodicare™ H
CAS 9087-53-0	Procetyl AWS	CAS 11138-66-2	Rhodicare™ S
CAS 9087-61-0	Dry Flo® PC	CAS 11138-66-2	Rhodicare™ XC
CAS 9087-61-0	Fluidamid DF 12	CAS 11138-66-2	Rhodigel®
CAS 9105-54-7	Amino-Collagen-25, -40	CAS 11138-66-2	Rhodigel® 23
CAS 9105-54-7	Collagen Amino Acids SF	CAS 11138-66-2	Rhodigel® 200
CAS 9105-54-7	Collamino™ 25	CAS 11138-66-2	Rhodigel® EZ
CAS 9105-54-7	Collamino™ 40-SF	CAS 11138-66-2	Rhodopol® SC
CAS 9105-54-7	Crotein CAA/SF	CAS 11138-66-2	Unigum XAN
CAS 9105-54-7	Hycollan	CAS 11138-66-2	Xanthan XP
CAS 9105-54-7	Peptein® CAA	CAS 11140-78-6	Rewoteric® AM DML-35
CAS 10043-01-3	Unichem ALSUL	CAS 11308-59-1	Promois W-42Q
CAS 10043-11-5	Ceram Blanche	CAS 11308-59-1	Promois W-42QP
CAS 10043-52-4	Unichem CALCHLOR	CAS 11308-59-1	Promois W-52Q
CAS 10101-41-4	Compactrol®	CAS 11308-59-1	Promois W-52QP

CAS 12001-26-2	M-102
CAS 12001-26-2	M-302
CAS 12001-26-2	Mearlmica® MMCF
CAS 12001-26-2	Mearlmica® MMSV
CAS 12001-26-2	Mica PGM-3
CAS 12001-26-2	Mica PGM-4
CAS 12001-26-2	Mica PGM-5
CAS 12001-26-2	Sericite 5, 300S
CAS 12001-26-2	Sericite DNN
CAS 12001-26-2	Sericite FSE
CAS 12001-26-2	Sericite SL
CAS 12001-26-2	Sericite SLZ
CAS 12001-26-2	Sericite SP
CAS 12001-31-9	Bentone® 38
CAS 12068-03-0	Witconate™ STS
CAS 12173-47-6	Bentone® EW
CAS 12173-47-6	Bentone® MA
CAS 12173-47-6	Hectabrite® AW
CAS 12173-47-6	Hectabrite® DP
CAS 12199-37-0	Gelwhite MAS-H, MAS-L
CAS 12199-37-0	Magnabrite® F
CAS 12199-37-0	Magnabrite® FS
CAS 12199-37-0	Magnabrite® HS
CAS 12199-37-0	Magnabrite® HV
CAS 12199-37-0	Magnabrite® K
CAS 12199-37-0	Magnabrite® S
CAS 12199-37-0	Veegum®
CAS 12199-37-0	Veegum® D
CAS 12199-37-0	Veegum® F
CAS 12199-37-0	Veegum® HS
CAS 12199-37-0	Veegum® HV
CAS 12199-37-0	Veegum® K
CAS 12199-37-0	Veegum® Ultra
CAS 12199-37-0	Veegum® WG
CAS 12694-22-3	Emalex MSG-2
CAS 12694-22-3	Emalex MSG-2MA
CAS 12694-22-3	Emalex MSG-2MB
CAS 12694-22-3	Emalex MSG-2ME
CAS 12694-22-3	Emalex MSG-2ML
CAS 12694-22-3	Nikkol DGMS
CAS 12709-64-7	Nikkol Decaglyn 3-S
CAS 12751-23-4	Abluphat MLP-200
CAS 12751-23-4	Crodafos 1214A
CAS 12751-23-4	Lipophos LMP
CAS 12751-23-4	Nikkol Phosten HLP
CAS 12764-60-2	Emalex DSG-10
CAS 12764-60-2	Nihon Polyglyceryl-10 Distearate
CAS 12764-60-2	Nikkol Decaglyn 2-S
CAS 13039-35-5	Emery® 5418
CAS 13040-19-2	Grillocin CW-90
CAS 13040-19-2	Grillocin® PY 88 Pellets
CAS 13040-19-2	Grillocin® PY 88 Pulver/Powd.
CAS 13040-19-2	Grillocin® S 803/7
CAS 13040-19-2	Grillocin S-803/12
CAS 13057-50-6	Pelemol PTL
CAS 13192-12-6	Beaulight SSS
CAS 13197-76-7	Rewoteric® AM HC
CAS 13232-26-3	Nikkol GM-18S
CAS 13463-41-7	Atomergic Zinc Pyrithione
CAS 13463-41-7	Zinc Omadine® 48% Disp.
CAS 13463-41-7	Zinc Omadine® Powd.
CAS 13463-41-7	Zink Pyrion
CAS 13463-67-7	Atlas White Titanium Dioxide
CAS 13463-67-7	Kowet Titanium Dioxide
CAS 13463-67-7	Kronos® 1025
CAS 13463-67-7	Luxelen® D
CAS 13463-67-7	MTD-25
CAS 13463-67-7	Solar Shield™
CAS 13463-67-7	Spherititan
CAS 13463-67-7	Sunveil 6010
CAS 13463-67-7	Sunveil 6030
CAS 13463-67-7	Ti-Sphere AA-1512-LL
CAS 13463-67-7	Ti-Sphere AA-1515
CAS 13463-67-7	Titanium Dioxide P25
CAS 13463-67-7	Titanium Dioxide SPA
CAS 13463-67-7	Transparent Titanium Dioxide PW Covafluor
CAS 13463-67-7	Transparent Titanium Dioxide PW Covasil S
CAS 13463-67-7	Transparent Titanium Dioxide PW Powd.
CAS 13463-67-7	Uniwhite AO
CAS 13463-67-7	Uniwhite KO
CAS 13475-82-6	Permethyl® 99A
CAS 13552-80-2	Captex® 8227
CAS 13552-80-2	Dermol M-27
CAS 13557-75-0	Pationic® 138C
CAS 13832-70-7	Co-Grhetinol
CAS 13832-70-7	Nikkol Stearyl Glycyrrhetinate
CAS 14025-15-1	Kelate Cu Liq.
CAS 14025-15-1	Universene Na2 Cu
CAS 14246-53-8	Lipacide C8G
CAS 14350-96-0	Dehyton® PLG
CAS 14350-96-0	Dehyton® PMG
CAS 14350-97-1	Amphoterge® L Special
CAS 14350-97-1	Chimin IMZ
CAS 14350-97-1	Mackam™ 2L
CAS 14350-97-1	Monateric 949J
CAS 14350-97-1	Rewoteric® AM 2L-40
CAS 14350-97-1	Zoharteric DJ
CAS 14351-40-7	Cerasynt® D
CAS 14351-40-7	Witcamide® MAS
CAS 14351-50-9	Ammonyx® OAO
CAS 14351-50-9	Chemoxide O
CAS 14351-50-9	Mackamine™ O2
CAS 14351-50-9	Mazox® ODA-30
CAS 14351-50-9	Standamox O1
CAS 14351-50-9	Unimox OL
CAS 14351-50-9	Zoramox E
CAS 14450-05-6	Emerest® 2486
CAS 14450-05-6	Unitolate PTP
CAS 14481-60-8	Rewopol® SBF 18
CAS 14548-60-8	Akyposept B
CAS 14548-60-8	Preventol D2
CAS 14727-68-5;	Jet Amine DMOD
CAS 14779-93-2	Isostearene
CAS 14807-96-6	Act II 500 USP
CAS 14807-96-6	AGI Talc, BC 1615
CAS 14807-96-6	Alphafil 200 USP
CAS 14807-96-6	Alphafil 500 USP
CAS 14807-96-6	Alpine Talc USP BC 127
CAS 14807-96-6	Altalc 200 USP
CAS 14807-96-6	Altalc 400 USP
CAS 14807-96-6	Altalc 500 USP
CAS 14807-96-6	Brillante
CAS 14807-96-6	Dover 50 A
CAS 14807-96-6	J-13
CAS 14807-96-6	J-24
CAS 14807-96-6	J-46
CAS 14807-96-6	J-68
CAS 14807-96-6	J-80
CAS 14807-96-6	Lo-Micron Talc 1
CAS 14807-96-6	Olympic
CAS 14807-96-6	PT-46
CAS 14807-96-6	Purtalc USP
CAS 14807-96-6	Rose Talc
CAS 14807-96-6	SteriLine 200
CAS 14807-96-6	SteriLine 665
CAS 14807-96-6	Supra A
CAS 14807-96-6	Supra EF

866

CAS 14807-96-6	Supra EF A	CAS 18962-61-3	Oligoidyne Magnesium
CAS 14807-96-6	Suprafino A	CAS 19035-79-1	Amphisol® K
CAS 14807-96-6	Suprafino SMD	CAS 19035-79-1	Crodafos CKP
CAS 14807-96-6	Supreme USP	CAS 19321-40-5	Liponate PO-4
CAS 14807-96-6	Talc LCW	CAS 19321-40-5	Pelemol PTO
CAS 14807-96-6	Talc OOC	CAS 20018-09-1	Amical® Flowable
CAS 14807-96-6	Talc Micro-Ace P-2	CAS 20292-08-4	Estol EHL 3613
CAS 14807-96-6	Talc Micro-Ace P-4	CAS 20457-75-4	Chemidex R
CAS 14807-96-6	Ultrafino	CAS 20457-75-4	Mackine™ 201
CAS 14807-96-6	Vertal CO+	CAS 20545-92-0	Fungicide UMA 2/938080
CAS 14960-06-6	Afoteric™ 160C	CAS 20545-92-0	Incromide UM
CAS 14960-06-6	Mackam™ 160C-30	CAS 20545-92-0	Rewocid® U 185
CAS 14960-06-6	Mirataine® H2C-HA	CAS 20545-92-0	Witcamide® 6570
CAS 14960-06-6	Rewoteric® AM LP	CAS 20824-56-0	Versene Diammonium EDTA
CAS 14960-06-6	Unibetaine 160	CAS 20834-06-4	Cetinol LU
CAS 14960-06-6	Unitex 610-L	CAS 20834-06-4	Laurate de Cetyle
CAS 15087-24-8	Unisol S-22	CAS 21034-17-3	Luminex
CAS 15454-75-8	Zincidone®	CAS 21142-28-9	Empicol® MIPA
CAS 16245-77-5	Rodol DS	CAS 21142-28-9	Melanol LP 1
CAS 16485-10-2	Fancol DL	CAS 21142-28-9	Sulfetal CJOT 38
CAS 16693-53-1	Crodasinic LT40	CAS 21142-28-9	Sulfetal CJOT 60
CAS 16693-53-1	Hamposyl® TL-40	CAS 21245-02-3	Escalol® 507
CAS 16731-55-8	Uantox PMBS	CAS 21245-02-3	Eusolex® 6007
CAS 16731-55-8	Uantox POMEBIS	CAS 21245-02-3	Lipofilter ODP
CAS 16841-14-8	Genamin KDB	CAS 21245-02-3	Padimate O
CAS 16867-03-1	Rodol 2A3PYR	CAS 21245-02-3	Solarchem® O
CAS 16889-14-8	Chemical Base 6532	CAS 21645-51-2	BB-1
CAS 16889-14-8	Lexamine 22	CAS 21645-51-2	Rehydragel® Compressed Gel
CAS 16889-14-8	Nikkol Amidoamine S	CAS 21645-51-2	Rehydragel® Low Visc. Gel
CAS 16889-14-8	Swanol Amidoamine S	CAS 21645-51-2	Rehydragel® Thixotropic Gel
CAS 16958-92-2	Kemester® 3684	CAS 22393-86-8	Glicoceride OCS
CAS 17301-53-0	Genamin KDM	CAS 22766-82-1	Starfol® OS
CAS 17301-53-0	Genamin KDM-F	CAS 22788-19-8	Emalex PG-di-L
CAS 17301-53-0	Incroquat TMC-80	CAS 22801-45-2	O.O.D
CAS 17301-53-0	Incroquat TMC-95	CAS 22882-95-7	Ceraphyl® IPL
CAS 17301-53-0	Nikkol CA-2580	CAS 22882-95-7	Nikkol VF-IP
CAS 17301-53-0	Varisoft® BT-85	CAS 24817-92-3	Citroflex A-6
CAS 17658-36-8	Isofol® 36	CAS 24937-78-8	A-C® 400
CAS 17661-50-6	Alkamuls® MST	CAS 24937-78-8	A-C® 400A
CAS 17661-50-6	Hest MS	CAS 24937-78-8	A-C® 405M
CAS 17661-50-6	Hetester MS	CAS 24937-78-8	A-C® 405S
CAS 17661-50-6	Kemester® 1418	CAS 24937-78-8	A-C® 405T
CAS 17661-50-6	Pelemol MS	CAS 24937-78-8	A-C® 430
CAS 17661-50-6	Spermwax®	CAS 24937-78-8	Elvax® 40P
CAS 17671-27-1	Crodamol BB	CAS 24938-91-8	Bio-Soft® TD 630
CAS 17671-27-1	Kester Wax® 72	CAS 24938-91-8	Britex TR 120
CAS 17671-27-1	Pelemol BB	CAS 24938-91-8	Britex TR 60
CAS 17673-56-2	Cetiol® J600	CAS 24938-91-8	Chemal TDA-6
CAS 17673-56-2	Crodamol JJ	CAS 24938-91-8	Chemal TDA-9
CAS 17673-56-2	Dynacerin® 660	CAS 24938-91-8	Chemal TDA-12
CAS 17673-56-2	Kessco OE	CAS 24938-91-8	Chemal TDA-15
CAS 17673-56-2	Pelemol OE	CAS 24938-91-8	Chemal TDA-18
CAS 17673-56-2	Unitolate J600	CAS 24938-91-8	Desonic® 6T
CAS 18194-24-6	Phospholipon® MC	CAS 24938-91-8	Desonic® 9T
CAS 18285-71-7	Phospholipon® LC	CAS 24938-91-8	Desonic® 12T
CAS 18312-32-8	Crodamol BE	CAS 24938-91-8	Desonic® 15T
CAS 18312-32-8	Elfacos® BE	CAS 24938-91-8	Flo-Mo® AJ-85
CAS 18312-32-8	Kemester® BE	CAS 24938-91-8	Flo-Mo® AJ-100
CAS 18312-32-8	Kessco BE	CAS 24938-91-8	Hetoxol TD-6
CAS 18312-32-8	Schercemol BE	CAS 24938-91-8	Hetoxol TD-9
CAS 18469-44-8	Nikkol MMT	CAS 24938-91-8	Hetoxol TD-12
CAS 18472-51-0	Spectradyne® G	CAS 24938-91-8	Hetoxol TD-18
CAS 18641-57-1	Compritol 888	CAS 24938-91-8	Hetoxol TD-25
CAS 18641-57-1	Compritol WL 3241	CAS 24938-91-8	Hodag Nonionic TD-6
CAS 18641-57-1	Lipovol GTB	CAS 24938-91-8	Hodag Nonionic TD-12
CAS 18641-57-1	Pelemol GTB	CAS 24938-91-8	Hodag Nonionic TD-15
CAS 18641-57-1	Syncrowax HR-C	CAS 24938-91-8	Lipocol PT-400
CAS 18684-11-2	Catigene® ST 70	CAS 24938-91-8	Lipocol TD-6
CAS 18684-11-2	Empigen® CM	CAS 24938-91-8	Lipocol TD-12
CAS 18758-91-3	Rhodorsil® Oils 70633 V30	CAS 24938-91-8	Macol® TD-8

CAS 24938-91-8	Macol® TD-10	CAS 25155-30-0	Witconate™ 30DS
CAS 24938-91-8	Macol® TD-12	CAS 25155-30-0	Witconate™ 45BX
CAS 24938-91-8	Macol® TD-15	CAS 25155-30-0	Witconate™ 60B
CAS 24938-91-8	Macol® TD-100	CAS 25155-30-0	Witconate™ 90F H
CAS 24938-91-8	Macol® TD-610	CAS 25155-30-0	Witconate™ 1238
CAS 24938-91-8	Procol TDA-6	CAS 25155-30-0	Witconate™ 1240
CAS 24938-91-8	Procol TDA-12	CAS 25155-30-0	Witconate™ 1250
CAS 24938-91-8	Procol TDA-15	CAS 25155-30-0	Witconate™ C50H
CAS 24938-91-8	Renex® 30	CAS 25155-30-0	Witconate™ DS Dense
CAS 24938-91-8	Renex® 36	CAS 25155-30-0	Witconate™ SK
CAS 24938-91-8	Rhodasurf® TD-9	CAS 25159-40-4	Mackamine™ OAO
CAS 24938-91-8	Synperonic A7	CAS 25168-73-4	Crodesta DKS F110
CAS 24938-91-8	Synperonic A9	CAS 25168-73-4	Crodesta F-160
CAS 24938-91-8	Synperonic A11	CAS 25168-73-4	Grilloten PSE 141G
CAS 24938-91-8	Synperonic A20	CAS 25168-73-4	Ryoto Sugar Ester S-1170
CAS 24938-91-8	Synperonic A50	CAS 25168-73-4	Ryoto Sugar Ester S-1170S
CAS 24938-91-8	Unicol 12	CAS 25168-73-4	Ryoto Sugar Ester S-1570
CAS 24938-91-8	Unicol 15	CAS 25168-73-4	Ryoto Sugar Ester S-1670
CAS 24938-91-8	Unicol TD-15	CAS 25168-73-4	Ryoto Sugar Ester S-1670S
CAS 24938-91-8	Volpo T-5	CAS 25168-73-4	Sucro Ester 7
CAS 24938-91-8	Volpo T-10	CAS 25168-73-4	Sucro Ester 11
CAS 24938-91-8	Volpo T-15	CAS 25168-73-4	Sucro Ester 15
CAS 24938-91-8	Volpo T-20	CAS 25231-21-4	Acconon E
CAS 24938-91-8	Witconol™ TD-60	CAS 25231-21-4	Arlamol® E
CAS 24938-91-8	Witconol™ TD-100	CAS 25231-21-4	Arlamol® F
CAS 25013-16-5	Sustane® 1-F	CAS 25231-21-4	Fancol SA-15
CAS 25013-16-5	Sustane® BHA	CAS 25231-21-4	Hetoxol SP-15
CAS 25013-16-5	Uantox BHA	CAS 25231-21-4	Hodag CSA-70
CAS 25038-54-4	Orgasol 1002 D NAT COS	CAS 25231-21-4	Hodag CSA-75
CAS 25038-54-4	Orgasol 1002 D WHITE 5 COS	CAS 25231-21-4	Procol PSA-11
CAS 25038-74-8	Orgasol 2002 D EXTRA NAT COS	CAS 25231-21-4	Procol PSA-15
CAS 25038-74-8	Orgasol 2002 D NAT COS	CAS 25231-21-4	Witconol™ APS
CAS 25038-74-8	Orgasol 2002 EX D NAT COS	CAS 25322-68-3	Carbowax® PEG 300
CAS 25038-74-8	Orgasol 2002 UD NAT COS	CAS 25322-68-3	Carbowax® PEG 400
CAS 25038-74-8	SP-500	CAS 25322-68-3	Carbowax® PEG 600
CAS 25054-76-6	Incronam OP-30	CAS 25322-68-3	Carbowax® PEG 900
CAS 25054-76-6	Lexaine® O	CAS 25322-68-3	Carbowax® PEG 1000
CAS 25054-76-6	Mackam™ HV	CAS 25322-68-3	Carbowax® PEG 1450
CAS 25054-76-6	Mirataine® BET-O-30	CAS 25322-68-3	Carbowax® PEG 3350
CAS 25066-20-0	Chemoxide SAO	CAS 25322-68-3	Carbowax® PEG 4600
CAS 25085-02-3	Hostacerin PN 73	CAS 25322-68-3	Carbowax® PEG 8000
CAS 25086-62-8	Daxad® 30	CAS 25322-68-3	Carbowax® Sentry® PEG 300
CAS 25086-89-9	Luviskol® VA28E	CAS 25322-68-3	Carbowax® Sentry® PEG 400
CAS 25086-89-9	Luviskol® VA28I	CAS 25322-68-3	Carbowax® Sentry® PEG 600
CAS 25086-89-9	Luviskol® VA37E	CAS 25322-68-3	Carbowax® Sentry® PEG 900
CAS 25086-89-9	Luviskol® VA37I	CAS 25322-68-3	Carbowax® Sentry® PEG 1000
CAS 25086-89-9	Luviskol® VA55E	CAS 25322-68-3	Carbowax® Sentry® PEG 1450
CAS 25086-89-9	Luviskol® VA55I	CAS 25322-68-3	Carbowax® Sentry® PEG 3350
CAS 25086-89-9	Luviskol® VA64	CAS 25322-68-3	Carbowax® Sentry® PEG 4600
CAS 25086-89-9	Luviskol® VA64E	CAS 25322-68-3	Carbowax® Sentry® PEG 8000
CAS 25086-89-9	Luviskol® VA64W	CAS 25322-68-3	Dow E200
CAS 25086-89-9	Luviskol® VA73E	CAS 25322-68-3	Dow E300 NF
CAS 25086-89-9	Luviskol® VA73I	CAS 25322-68-3	Dow E400 NF
CAS 25086-89-9	Luviskol® VA73W	CAS 25322-68-3	Dow E600 NF
CAS 25086-89-9	Nasuna® B	CAS 25322-68-3	Dow E1000 NF
CAS 25086-89-9	PVP/VA E-335, E-535, E-635	CAS 25322-68-3	Dow E1450 NF
CAS 25086-89-9	PVP/VA S-630	CAS 25322-68-3	Dow E3350 NF
CAS 25155-18-4	Hyamine® 10X	CAS 25322-68-3	Dow E4500 NF
CAS 25155-30-0	Bio-Soft® D-60	CAS 25322-68-3	Dow E8000 NF
CAS 25155-30-0	Calsoft F-90	CAS 25322-68-3	Emery® 6709
CAS 25155-30-0	Calsoft L-40	CAS 25322-68-3	Emkapol 5000
CAS 25155-30-0	Calsoft L-60	CAS 25322-68-3	Emkapol 8000
CAS 25155-30-0	Hartofol 40	CAS 25322-68-3	Emkapol 8500
CAS 25155-30-0	Hetsulf Acid	CAS 25322-68-3	Hetoxide PEG-200
CAS 25155-30-0	Marlon® AFR	CAS 25322-68-3	Hetoxide PEG-300
CAS 25155-30-0	Nacconol® 35SL	CAS 25322-68-3	Hodag PEG 200
CAS 25155-30-0	Naxel™ AAS-40S	CAS 25322-68-3	Hodag PEG 300
CAS 25155-30-0	Naxel™ AAS-45S	CAS 25322-68-3	Hodag PEG 400
CAS 25155-30-0	Sul-fon-ate AA-10	CAS 25322-68-3	Hodag PEG 600
CAS 25155-30-0	Ufasan 35	CAS 25322-68-3	Hodag PEG 1000

CAS 25322-68-3	Hodag PEG 1450
CAS 25322-68-3	Hodag PEG 3350
CAS 25322-68-3	Hodag PEG 8000
CAS 25322-68-3	Lipo Polyglycol 200
CAS 25322-68-3	Lipo Polyglycol 300
CAS 25322-68-3	Lipo Polyglycol 400
CAS 25322-68-3	Lipo Polyglycol 600
CAS 25322-68-3	Lipo Polyglycol 1000
CAS 25322-68-3	Lipo Polyglycol 3350
CAS 25322-68-3	Lipoxol® 200 MED
CAS 25322-68-3	Lipoxol® 300 MED
CAS 25322-68-3	Lipoxol® 400 MED
CAS 25322-68-3	Lipoxol® 600 MED
CAS 25322-68-3	Lipoxol® 800 MED
CAS 25322-68-3	Lipoxol® 1000 MED
CAS 25322-68-3	Lipoxol® 1550 MED
CAS 25322-68-3	Lipoxol® 2000 MED
CAS 25322-68-3	Lipoxol® 3000 MED
CAS 25322-68-3	Lipoxol® 4000 MED
CAS 25322-68-3	Lipoxol® 6000 MED
CAS 25322-68-3	Lipoxol® 12000
CAS 25322-68-3	Lutrol® E 300
CAS 25322-68-3	Lutrol® E 400
CAS 25322-68-3	Lutrol® E1450 NF
CAS 25322-68-3	Lutrol® E 1500
CAS 25322-68-3	Lutrol® E 4000
CAS 25322-68-3	Lutrol® E 6000
CAS 25322-68-3	Macol® E-200
CAS 25322-68-3	Macol® E-300
CAS 25322-68-3	Macol® E-400
CAS 25322-68-3	Macol® E-600
CAS 25322-68-3	Macol® E-1000
CAS 25322-68-3	Macol® E-1450
CAS 25322-68-3	Macol® E-3350
CAS 25322-68-3	Macol® E-8000
CAS 25322-68-3	Pluracol® E200
CAS 25322-68-3	Pluracol® E300
CAS 25322-68-3	Pluracol® E400
CAS 25322-68-3	Pluracol® E400 NF
CAS 25322-68-3	Pluracol® E600
CAS 25322-68-3	Pluracol® E600 NF
CAS 25322-68-3	Pluracol® E1000
CAS 25322-68-3	Pluracol® E1450
CAS 25322-68-3	Pluracol® E1450 NF
CAS 25322-68-3	Pluracol® E2000
CAS 25322-68-3	Pluracol® E4000
CAS 25322-68-3	Pluracol® E4000 NF
CAS 25322-68-3	Pluracol® E8000
CAS 25322-68-3	Pluracol® E8000 NF
CAS 25322-68-3	Poly-G® 200
CAS 25322-68-3	Poly-G® 300
CAS 25322-68-3	Poly-G® 400
CAS 25322-68-3	Poly-G® 600
CAS 25322-68-3	Poly-G® 1000
CAS 25322-68-3	Poly-G® 2000
CAS 25322-68-3	Polyox® WSR 35
CAS 25322-68-3	Polyox® WSR 205
CAS 25322-68-3	Polyox® WSR 301
CAS 25322-68-3	Polyox® WSR 1105
CAS 25322-68-3	Polyox® WSR 3333
CAS 25322-68-3	Polyox® WSR N-10
CAS 25322-68-3	Polyox® WSR N-12K
CAS 25322-68-3	Polyox® WSR N-60K
CAS 25322-68-3	Polyox® WSR N-80
CAS 25322-68-3	Polyox® WSR N-750
CAS 25322-68-3	Polyox® WSR N-3000
CAS 25322-68-3	Protachem 1450 NF
CAS 25322-68-3	Prox-onic PEG-2000
CAS 25322-68-3	Prox-onic PEG-6000
CAS 25322-68-3	Prox-onic PEG-20,000
CAS 25322-68-3	Renex® PEG 300
CAS 25322-68-3	Renex® PEG 400
CAS 25322-68-3	Renex® PEG 600
CAS 25322-68-3	Renex® PEG 1000
CAS 25322-68-3	Renex® PEG 1500FL
CAS 25322-68-3	Renex® PEG 4000FL
CAS 25322-68-3	Renex® PEG 6000FL
CAS 25322-68-3	Rhodasurf® E 400
CAS 25322-68-3	Rhodasurf® E 600
CAS 25322-68-3	Rhodasurf® PEG 400
CAS 25322-68-3	Rhodasurf® PEG 600
CAS 25322-68-3	Teric PEG 200
CAS 25322-68-3	Teric PEG 300
CAS 25322-68-3	Teric PEG 400
CAS 25322-68-3	Teric PEG 600
CAS 25322-68-3	Teric PEG 800
CAS 25322-68-3	Teric PEG 1000
CAS 25322-68-3	Teric PEG 4000
CAS 25322-68-3	Teric PEG 6000
CAS 25322-68-3	Teric PEG 8000
CAS 25322-68-3	Unipeg 200
CAS 25322-68-3	Unipeg-200 X
CAS 25322-68-3	Unipeg 400
CAS 25322-68-3	Unipeg-400 X
CAS 25322-68-3	Unipeg-600
CAS 25322-68-3	Unipeg 1000
CAS 25322-68-3	Unipeg-1000 X
CAS 25322-68-3	Unipeg 1500
CAS 25322-68-3	Unipeg 1540
CAS 25322-68-3	Unipeg-1540 X
CAS 25322-68-3	Unipeg 4000
CAS 25322-68-3	Unipeg-4000 X
CAS 25322-68-3	Unipeg 6000
CAS 25322-68-3	Unipeg-6000 X
CAS 25322-68-3	Upiwax 200
CAS 25322-68-3	Upiwax 300
CAS 25322-68-3	Upiwax 400
CAS 25322-68-3	Upiwax 600
CAS 25322-68-3	Upiwax 1000
CAS 25322-68-3	Upiwax 3350
CAS 25322-68-3	Upiwax 8000
CAS 25322-69-4	Dow P425
CAS 25322-69-4	Dow P1000TB
CAS 25322-69-4	Dow P1200
CAS 25322-69-4	Dow P2000
CAS 25322-69-4	Dow P4000
CAS 25322-69-4	Hodag PPG-400
CAS 25322-69-4	Hodag PPG-1200
CAS 25322-69-4	Hodag PPG-2000
CAS 25322-69-4	Hodag PPG-4000
CAS 25322-69-4	Jeffox PPG-2000
CAS 25322-69-4	Macol® P-1200
CAS 25322-69-4	Macol® P-2000
CAS 25322-69-4	Macol® P-4000
CAS 25322-69-4	Unicol 1200
CAS 25322-69-4	Unicol P-400
CAS 25322-69-4	Unicol P-2000
CAS 25322-69-4	Unicol P-4000
CAS 25322-69-4	Witconol™ CD-17
CAS 25322-69-4	Witconol™ PPG 400
CAS 25339-09-7	Ceraphyl® 494
CAS 25339-09-7	Cetiol® G16S
CAS 25339-09-7	Crodamol ICS
CAS 25339-09-7	Kemester® 5822
CAS 25339-09-7	Kessco ICS
CAS 25339-09-7	Kessco® Isocetyl Stearate
CAS 25339-09-7	Nikkol ICS-R
CAS 25339-09-7	Pelemol ICS
CAS 25339-09-7	Schercemol ICS
CAS 25339-09-7	Unimul-7061

CAS 25339-99-5	Grilloten LSE 65	CAS 26266-57-9	Montane 40
CAS 25339-99-5	Grilloten LSE 65 Soft	CAS 26266-57-9	Nikkol SP-10
CAS 25339-99-5	Grilloten LSE 87	CAS 26266-57-9	Nissan Nonion PP-40R
CAS 25339-99-5	Grilloten LSE 87 Soft	CAS 26266-57-9	Protachem SMP
CAS 25339-99-5	Ryoto Sugar Ester L-1570	CAS 26266-57-9	Prote-sorb SMP
CAS 25339-99-5	Ryoto Sugar Ester L-1695	CAS 26266-57-9	S-Maz® 40
CAS 25383-99-7	Artodan SP 55 Kosher	CAS 26266-57-9	Sorbax SMP
CAS 25383-99-7	Crolactil SSL	CAS 26266-57-9	Sorbirol P
CAS 25383-99-7	Pationic® SSL	CAS 26266-57-9	Sorbon S-40
CAS 25383-99-7	Unitolate SSL	CAS 26266-57-9	Span® 40
CAS 25446-78-0	Rhodapex® 674/C	CAS 26266-57-9	Unitan-P
CAS 25446-78-0	Rhodapex® EST-30	CAS 26266-57-9	Witconol™ 2510
CAS 25446-80-4	Elfan® NS 423 SH	CAS 26266-58-0	Ablunol S-85
CAS 25446-80-4	Standapol® ES-40	CAS 26266-58-0	Arlacel® 85
CAS 25446-80-4	Standapol® ES-50	CAS 26266-58-0	Crill 45
CAS 25446-80-4	Texapon® K-14S Spec	CAS 26266-58-0	Emsorb® 2503
CAS 25496-72-4	Tegin® O	CAS 26266-58-0	Ethylan® GT85
CAS 25609-89-6	Aristoflex A	CAS 26266-58-0	Glycomul® TO
CAS 25609-89-6	Luviset® CA66	CAS 26266-58-0	Hefti TO-33-F
CAS 25609-89-6	Resyn® 28-1310	CAS 26266-58-0	Hodag STO
CAS 25637-84-7	Cithrol GDO N/E	CAS 26266-58-0	Ionet S-85
CAS 25637-84-7	Kessco® Glycerol Dioleate	CAS 26266-58-0	Kemester® S85
CAS 25637-84-7	Nikkol DGO-80	CAS 26266-58-0	Liposorb TO
CAS 25655-41-8	PVP-Iodine 17/12, 30/06	CAS 26266-58-0	Montane 85
CAS 25750-82-7	AClyn® 262A	CAS 26266-58-0	Nikkol SO-30
CAS 25750-82-7	AClyn® 272, 276, 285	CAS 26266-58-0	Nikkol SO-30R
CAS 25750-82-7	AClyn® 272A	CAS 26266-58-0	Nissan Nonion OP-85R
CAS 25750-82-7	AClyn® 276A	CAS 26266-58-0	Protachem STO
CAS 25750-82-7	AClyn® 285A	CAS 26266-58-0	Prote-sorb STO
CAS 25791-96-2	Dow PT700	CAS 26266-58-0	S-Maz® 85
CAS 25791-96-2	Dow PT3000	CAS 26266-58-0	S-Maz® 85K
CAS 25791-96-2	Witconol™ CC-43	CAS 26266-58-0	Sorbax STO
CAS 25791-96-2	Witconol™ CD-18	CAS 26266-58-0	Sorbirol TO
CAS 25869-00-5	Bleu De Prusse Pur W 745	CAS 26266-58-0	Span® 85
CAS 25869-00-5	Cogilor Sapphire	CAS 26266-58-0	Unitan-TRIOL
CAS 25882-44-4	Emcol® 5310	CAS 26266-58-0	Witconol™ 2503
CAS 25882-44-4	Geropon® SBL-203	CAS 26402-22-2	Imwitor® 310
CAS 25882-44-4	Mackanate™ LM-40	CAS 26402-22-2	Imwitor® 910
CAS 25882-44-4	Rewopol® SBL 203	CAS 26402-26-6	Imwitor® 308
CAS 25882-44-4	Varsulf® SBL-203	CAS 26402-26-6	Imwitor® 742
CAS 25987-06-8	Polymin® FG SG	CAS 26402-26-6	Imwitor® 908
CAS 26027-37-2	Dionil® OC	CAS 26402-26-6	Imwitor® 988
CAS 26027-37-2	Dionil® SH 100	CAS 26402-26-6	Witafrol® 7420
CAS 26027-37-2	Dionil® W 100	CAS 26402-31-3	Cithrol PGMR N/E
CAS 26027-37-2	Ethomid® O/17	CAS 26402-31-3	Flexricin® 9
CAS 26062-79-3	Agequat 400	CAS 26402-31-3	Naturechem® PGR
CAS 26062-79-3	Conditioner P6	CAS 26402-31-3	Rol RP
CAS 26062-79-3	Genamin PDAC	CAS 26426-80-2	Daxad® 31
CAS 26062-79-3	Mackernium™ 006	CAS 26426-80-2	Tamol® 731-25%
CAS 26062-79-3	Merquat® 100	CAS 26445-96-5	AClyn® 201
CAS 26062-79-3	Mirapol® CP40	CAS 26445-96-5	AClyn® 201A
CAS 26062-79-3	M-Quat® 40	CAS 26446-38-8	Ryoto Sugar Ester P-1570
CAS 26062-79-3	Salcare SC30	CAS 26446-38-8	Ryoto Sugar Ester P-1570S
CAS 26112-07-2	Nipagin M Potassium	CAS 26446-38-8	Ryoto Sugar Ester P-1670
CAS 26248-24-8	Witconate™ TDB	CAS 26447-10-9	Eltesol® AX 40
CAS 26256-79-1	Deriphat® 160C	CAS 26447-10-9	Manrosol AXS40
CAS 26264-05-1	Rhodacal® 330	CAS 26447-10-9	Witconate™ NXS
CAS 26266-57-9	Ablunol S-40	CAS 26483-35-2	Incromine Oxide B
CAS 26266-57-9	Arlacel® 40	CAS 26483-35-2	Incromine Oxide B-30P
CAS 26266-57-9	Armotan® MP	CAS 26483-35-2	Incromine Oxide B50
CAS 26266-57-9	Armotan® NP	CAS 26545-53-9	Ablusol DBD
CAS 26266-57-9	Crill 2	CAS 26589-26-4	Luviflex® VBM 35
CAS 26266-57-9	Emsorb® 2510	CAS 26589-26-4	Stepanhold® Extra
CAS 26266-57-9	Extan-PT	CAS 26589-26-4	Stepanhold® R-1
CAS 26266-57-9	Glycomul® P	CAS 26590-05-6	Agequat 500, -5008
CAS 26266-57-9	Hefti MP-33-F	CAS 26590-05-6	Conditioner P7
CAS 26266-57-9	Hodag SMP	CAS 26590-05-6	Mackernium™ 007
CAS 26266-57-9	Ixolene 4	CAS 26590-05-6	Merquat® 550
CAS 26266-57-9	Kemester® S40	CAS 26590-05-6	Merquat® S
CAS 26266-57-9	Liposorb P	CAS 26590-05-6	Mirapol® 550

CAS 26590-05-6	Salcare SC10	CAS 27306-79-2	Lipocol M-4
CAS 26635-75-6	Amidox® L-2	CAS 27306-79-2	Procol MA-4
CAS 26635-75-6	Amidox® L-5	CAS 27306-79-2	Witconol™ 5969
CAS 26635-75-6	Lanidox-5	CAS 27306-90-7	Akypo RLM 100
CAS 26635-75-6	Upamide L-2	CAS 27306-90-7	Akypo RLM 160
CAS 26635-75-6	Upamide L-5	CAS 27306-90-7	Marlinat® CM 100
CAS 26635-92-7	Chemeen 18-5	CAS 27321-96-6	Emalex CS-10
CAS 26635-92-7	Chemeen 18-50	CAS 27321-96-6	Emalex CS-15
CAS 26635-92-7	Ethomeen® 18/15	CAS 27321-96-6	Emalex CS-20
CAS 26635-92-7	Ethomeen® 18/20	CAS 27321-96-6	Emalex CS-24
CAS 26635-92-7	Ethomeen® 18/25	CAS 27321-96-6	Emalex CS-30
CAS 26635-92-7	Ethomeen® 18/60	CAS 27321-96-6	Ethoxychol-24
CAS 26635-92-7	Hetoxamine ST-5	CAS 27321-96-6	Fancol CH-24
CAS 26635-92-7	Hetoxamine ST-15	CAS 27323-41-7	Ablusol DBT
CAS 26635-92-7	Hetoxamine ST-50	CAS 27323-41-7	Bio-Soft® N-300
CAS 26635-92-7	Protox HTA-10	CAS 27323-41-7	Calsoft T-60
CAS 26635-92-7	Protox HTA-15	CAS 27323-41-7	Carosulf T-60-L
CAS 26635-92-7	Protox HTA-50	CAS 27323-41-7	Carsofoam® T-60-L
CAS 26658-19-5	Crill 35	CAS 27323-41-7	Elfan® WAT
CAS 26658-19-5	Crill 41	CAS 27323-41-7	Hartofol 60T
CAS 26658-19-5	Drewmulse® STS	CAS 27323-41-7	Hexaryl D 60 L
CAS 26658-19-5	Emsorb® 2507	CAS 27323-41-7	Manro TDBS 60
CAS 26658-19-5	Glycomul® TS	CAS 27323-41-7	Marlopon® CA
CAS 26658-19-5	Glycomul® TS KFG	CAS 27323-41-7	Mazon® 60T
CAS 26658-19-5	Hefti TS-33-F	CAS 27323-41-7	Naxel™ AAS-60S
CAS 26658-19-5	Hodag STS	CAS 27323-41-7	Norfox® T-60
CAS 26658-19-5	Kemester® S65	CAS 27323-41-7	Rhodacal® DDB 60T
CAS 26658-19-5	Liposorb TS	CAS 27323-41-7	Witconate™ 60T
CAS 26658-19-5	Montane 65	CAS 27323-41-7	Witconate™ 79S
CAS 26658-19-5	Nikkol SS-30	CAS 27323-41-7	Witconate™ LXH
CAS 26658-19-5	Protachem STS	CAS 27323-41-7	Witconate™ S-1280
CAS 26658-19-5	Prote-sorb STS	CAS 27323-41-7	Witconate™ TAB
CAS 26658-19-5	S-Maz® 65K	CAS 27458-93-1	Adol® 66
CAS 26658-19-5	Sorbax STS	CAS 27458-93-1	Prisorine 3515
CAS 26658-19-5	Sorbirol TS	CAS 27458-93-1	Prisorine ISOH 3515
CAS 26658-19-5	Span® 65	CAS 27503-81-7	BioGir-PISA
CAS 26658-19-5	Unitan-TRIST	CAS 27503-81-7	Eusolex® 232
CAS 26658-19-5	Witconol™ 2507	CAS 27503-81-7	Neo Heliopan, Type Hydro
CAS 26699-71-8	Trioxene A	CAS 27503-81-7	Parsol® HS
CAS 27028-82-6	Alscoap TA-40	CAS 27538-35-8	Parasonarl Mark II
CAS 27028-82-6	Empicol® ETB	CAS 27638-00-2	Capmul® GDL
CAS 27028-82-6	Montelane LT 4088	CAS 27638-00-2	Cithrol GDL N/E
CAS 27028-82-6	Neopon LOT/NF	CAS 27638-00-2	Emulsynt® GDL
CAS 27028-82-6	Nikkol SBL-2T-36	CAS 27638-00-2	Kemester® GDL
CAS 27028-82-6	Nikkol SBL-4T	CAS 27638-00-2	Kessco® Glycerol Dilaurate
CAS 27028-82-6	Surfax EDT	CAS 27638-00-2	Lexemul® GDL
CAS 27028-82-6	Tylorol LT50	CAS 27638-00-2	Liponate GDL
CAS 27028-82-6	Zoharpon LAET	CAS 27640-89-7	Kemester® EE
CAS 27083-27-8	Cosmocil CQ	CAS 27731-61-9	Standapol® EA-40
CAS 27083-27-8	Mikrokill 20	CAS 27731-61-9	Texapon® EA-40
CAS 27176-87-0	Calsoft LAS-99	CAS 27731-61-9	Unipol EA-40
CAS 27176-87-0	Lumosäure A	CAS 27841-06-1	Estemol N-01
CAS 27176-87-0	Naxel ™AAS-98S	CAS 27841-06-1	Schercemol NGDC
CAS 27176-87-0	Reworyl® K	CAS 28061-69-0	Armeen® DMOD
CAS 27176-87-0	Rueterg SA	CAS 28063-42-5	Crodamol GE
CAS 27176-87-0	Witconate Acide B	CAS 28211-18-9	Antaron® V-220
CAS 27178-16-1	Arlamol® DIDA	CAS 28211-18-9	Ganex® V-220
CAS 27194-74-7	Schercemol PGML	CAS 28211-18-9	Unimer U-15
CAS 27195-16-0	Crodesta DKS F10	CAS 28319-77-9	GPC
CAS 27195-16-0	Crodesta DKS F20	CAS 28474-90-0	Nikkol CP
CAS 27195-16-0	Crodesta DKS F50	CAS 28510-23-8	Cosmol 525
CAS 27195-16-0	Crodesta DKS F70	CAS 28510-23-8	Schercemol NGDO
CAS 27195-16-0	Crodesta F-10	CAS 28724-32-5	Ethoquad® 18/25
CAS 27195-16-0	Crodesta F-50	CAS 28829-38-1	Ajicoat SPG
CAS 27195-16-0	Ryoto Sugar Ester S-570	CAS 28874-51-3	Ajidew N-50
CAS 27195-16-0	Ryoto Sugar Ester S-770	CAS 28874-51-3	Dermidrol
CAS 27195-16-0	Ryoto Sugar Ester S-970	CAS 28874-51-3	Nalidone®
CAS 27233-00-7	Hetester HCA	CAS 28874-51-3	Ritamectant PCA
CAS 27233-00-7	Naturechem® GTH	CAS 29059-24-3	Cithrol PGMM
CAS 27306-79-2	Hetoxol M-3	CAS 29059-24-3	Kessco PGNM

CAS 29059-24-3	Radiasurf® 7196	CAS 31692-79-2	Mazol® SFR 18,000
CAS 29116-98-1	Hefti DO-33-F	CAS 31692-79-2	Mazol® SFR 50,000
CAS 29297-55-0	Luviquat® FC 370	CAS 31692-79-2	Mazol® SFR 150,000
CAS 29297-55-0	Luviquat® FC 550	CAS 31692-79-2	Unisil SF-R
CAS 29297-55-0	Luviquat® FC 905	CAS 31694-55-0	Acconon ETG
CAS 29297-55-0	Luviquat® HM 552	CAS 31694-55-0	Carbowax® TPEG 990
CAS 29381-93-9	Marlopon® AT	CAS 31694-55-0	Ethosperse® G-26
CAS 29383-26-4	Crodamol OHS	CAS 31694-55-0	Extan G-7
CAS 29383-26-4	Estalan 718	CAS 31694-55-0	Extan G-26
CAS 29383-26-4	Kessco DHS	CAS 31694-55-0	Hetoxide G-7
CAS 29383-26-4	Naturechem® OHS	CAS 31694-55-0	Hetoxide G-26
CAS 29383-26-4	Schercemol OHS	CAS 31694-55-0	Hodag POE (12) Glycerine
CAS 29383-26-4	Wickenol® 171	CAS 31694-55-0	Hodag POE (26) Glycerine
CAS 29461-14-1	Ketosesquine	CAS 31694-55-0	Liponic EG-1
CAS 29710-25-6	Dermol OO	CAS 31694-55-0	Liponic EG-7
CAS 29710-25-6	Estalan OV	CAS 31694-55-0	Protachem GL-7
CAS 29806-73-3	Bernel® Ester EHP	CAS 31694-55-0	Protachem GL-26
CAS 29806-73-3	Cegesoft® C 24	CAS 31694-55-0	Unipeg-ETG-12
CAS 29806-73-3	Ceraphyl® 368	CAS 31694-55-0	Unipeg-ETG-26
CAS 29806-73-3	Crodamol OP	CAS 31799-71-0	Ethomid® O/15
CAS 29806-73-3	Elfacos® EHP	CAS 32057-14-0	Peceol Isostearique
CAS 29806-73-3	Estalan 816	CAS 32073-22-6	SCS 40
CAS 29806-73-3	Estol 1543	CAS 32073-22-6	Witconate™ SCS 45%
CAS 29806-73-3	Estol EHP 1543	CAS 32073-22-6	Witconate™ SCS 93%
CAS 29806-73-3	Estol EHP-b 3652	CAS 32131-17-2	Standamid® Resin BC-1283
CAS 29806-73-3	Kessco EHP	CAS 32131-17-2	Upamide Resin 1289
CAS 29806-73-3	Kessco® Octyl Palmitate	CAS 32131-17-2	Upamide Resin UPC-1283
CAS 29806-73-3	Lexol® EHP	CAS 32131-17-2	Versamid® 930
CAS 29806-73-3	Pelemol OP	CAS 32440-50-9	Antaron® V-216
CAS 29806-73-3	Schercemol OP	CAS 32440-50-9	Ganex® V-216
CAS 29806-73-3	Tegosoft® OP	CAS 32440-50-9	Unimer U-151
CAS 29806-73-3	Trivent OP	CAS 32582-32-4	Isofol® 32
CAS 29806-73-3	Wickenol® 155	CAS 32612-48-9	Calfoam EA-603
CAS 29923-31-7	Amisoft LS-11	CAS 32612-48-9	Calfoam NEL-60
CAS 30007-47-7	Bronodox L	CAS 32612-48-9	Carsonol® SES-A
CAS 30364-51-3	Crodasinic MS	CAS 32612-48-9	Empicol® EAA
CAS 30364-51-3	Hamposyl® M-30	CAS 32612-48-9	Empicol® EAB/T
CAS 30364-51-3	Nikkol Sarcosinate MN	CAS 32612-48-9	Empicol® EAC
CAS 30364-51-3	Vanseal® NAMS-30	CAS 32612-48-9	Empicol® EAC70
CAS 30399-84-9	Emersol® 871	CAS 32612-48-9	Empicol® EAC/T
CAS 30399-84-9	Emersol® 875	CAS 32612-48-9	Laural EC
CAS 30473-39-3	Amphoterge® S	CAS 32612-48-9	Manro ALEC 25
CAS 30581-59-0	Copolymer 845	CAS 32612-48-9	Manro ALEC 27
CAS 30581-59-0	Copolymer 937	CAS 32612-48-9	Manro ALES 60
CAS 30657-38-6	Laurydone®	CAS 32612-48-9	Neopon LOA
CAS 31394-71-5	Hodag CSA-80	CAS 32612-48-9	Nikkol SBL-2A-27
CAS 31394-71-5	Lutrol® OP 2000	CAS 32612-48-9	Nonasol N4AS
CAS 31394-71-5	Witconol™ F2646	CAS 32612-48-9	Nutrapon AL 1
CAS 31556-45-3	Kemester® 5721	CAS 32612-48-9	Nutrapon AL 2
CAS 31556-45-3	Liponate TDS	CAS 32612-48-9	Nutrapon AL 30
CAS 31565-12-5	Imwitor® 408	CAS 32612-48-9	Nutrapon AL 60
CAS 31565-12-5	Nikkol Sefsol 218	CAS 32612-48-9	Nutrapon AN-3 0481
CAS 31565-38-5	Fractalite IDS	CAS 32612-48-9	Sandoz Sulfate 216
CAS 31566-31-1	Aldo® MSC	CAS 32612-48-9	Standapol® EA-1
CAS 31566-31-1	Aldo® MSLG FG	CAS 32612-48-9	Standapol® EA-2
CAS 31566-31-1	Alkamuls® GMS/C	CAS 32612-48-9	Standapol® EA-3
CAS 31566-31-1	Cithrol GMS Acid Stable	CAS 32612-48-9	Steol® CA-130
CAS 31566-31-1	Cithrol GMS N/E	CAS 32612-48-9	Steol® CA-230
CAS 31566-31-1	Cithrol GMS S/E	CAS 32612-48-9	Steol® CA-330
CAS 31566-31-1	Geleol	CAS 32612-48-9	Steol® CA-460
CAS 31566-31-1	Imwitor® 191	CAS 32612-48-9	Steol® KA-460
CAS 31566-31-1	Lipal GMS	CAS 32612-48-9	Sulfochem EA-1
CAS 31566-31-1	Sterol GMS	CAS 32612-48-9	Sulfochem EA-2
CAS 31566-31-1	Tegin® 4011	CAS 32612-48-9	Sulfochem EA-3
CAS 31566-31-1	Tegin® 4100 NSE	CAS 32612-48-9	Sulfochem EA-60
CAS 31692-79-2	Masil SFR 70	CAS 32612-48-9	Sulfochem EA-70
CAS 31692-79-2	Mazol® SFR 100	CAS 32612-48-9	Surfax EKZ
CAS 31692-79-2	Mazol® SFR 750	CAS 32612-48-9	Texapon® EA-1
CAS 31692-79-2	Mazol® SFR 2000	CAS 32612-48-9	Texapon® EA-2
CAS 31692-79-2	Mazol® SFR 3500	CAS 32612-48-9	Texapon® EA-3

CAS 32612-48-9	Texapon® PNA-127	CAS 36653-82-4	Adol® 52 NF
CAS 32612-48-9	Tylorol A	CAS 36653-82-4	Adol® 520 NF
CAS 32612-48-9	Ungerol AM3-60	CAS 36653-82-4	ppend
CAS 32612-48-9	Ungerol AM3-75	CAS 36653-82-4	Cachalot® C-50
CAS 32612-48-9	Unipol EA-1, EA-2, EA-3	CAS 36653-82-4	Cachalot® C-51
CAS 32612-48-9	Witcolate™ LES-60A	CAS 36653-82-4	Cachalot® C-52
CAS 32612-48-9	Witcolate™ S1300C	CAS 36653-82-4	Cetaffine
CAS 32612-48-9	Zoharpon LAEA 253	CAS 36653-82-4	Cetal
CAS 32647-67-9	Disorbene	CAS 36653-82-4	Cetax 16
CAS 32647-67-9	Millithix® 925	CAS 36653-82-4	CO-1695
CAS 32954-43-1	Schercotaine PAB	CAS 36653-82-4	Crodacol C-70
CAS 33703-08-1	Arlamol® DINA	CAS 36653-82-4	Crodacol C-90
CAS 33907-46-9	Naturechem® EGHS	CAS 36653-82-4	Crodacol C-95NF
CAS 33907-47-0	Naturechem® PGHS	CAS 36653-82-4	Epal® 16NF
CAS 33939-64-9	Akypo RLM 45 N	CAS 36653-82-4	Fancol CA
CAS 33939-64-9	Akypo RLM 100 NV	CAS 36653-82-4	Hetol CA
CAS 33939-64-9	Akypo RLM 160 N	CAS 36653-82-4	Hyfatol 16-95
CAS 33939-64-9	Akypo®-Soft 45 NV	CAS 36653-82-4	Hyfatol 16-98
CAS 33939-64-9	Akypo®-Soft 160 NV	CAS 36653-82-4	Lanette® 16
CAS 33939-64-9	Marlinat® CM 45	CAS 36653-82-4	Lanol C
CAS 33939-64-9	Marlinat® CM 105	CAS 36653-82-4	Lipocol C
CAS 33939-64-9	Nikkol Akypo RLM 45 NV	CAS 36653-82-4	Mackol 16
CAS 33939-64-9	Rewopol® CLN 100	CAS 36653-82-4	Nacol® 16-95
CAS 33939-64-9	Sandopan® LA-8-HC	CAS 36653-82-4	Nacol® 16-98
CAS 33939-64-9	Sandopan® LS-24	CAS 36653-82-4	Philcohol 1600
CAS 33939-64-9	Surfine WLL	CAS 36653-82-4	RITA CA
CAS 33939-65-0	Sandopan® KST-A	CAS 36653-82-4	Unihydag Wax 16
CAS 33940-99-7	Caprol® 10G2O	CAS 36861-47-9	Parsol® 5000
CAS 33940-99-7	Nikkol Decaglyn 2-O	CAS 37139-99-4	Ammonyx® KP
CAS 34316-64-8	Cetiol® A	CAS 37139-99-4	Ammonyx® LKP
CAS 34316-64-8	Rewomul HL	CAS 37139-99-4	Empigen® BCJ-50
CAS 34316-64-8	Unimul-CTA	CAS 37139-99-4	Incroquat O-50
CAS 34316-64-8	Unitolate A	CAS 37139-99-4	Mackernium™ KP
CAS 34406-66-1	Nikkol Decaglyn 1-L	CAS 37172-53-5	Hedione
CAS 34424-97-0	Caprol® 6G2S	CAS 37191-69-8	Cavitron Cyclodextrin-Sulfated
CAS 34424-97-0	Plurol Stearique WL 1009	CAS 37309-58-3	Ethylflo® 364 NF
CAS 34424-98-1	Caprol® 10G4O	CAS 37309-58-3	Ethylflo® 366 NF
CAS 34424-98-1	Drewpol® 10-4-O	CAS 37311-00-5	ADF Oleile
CAS 34424-98-1	Mazol® PGO-104	CAS 37318-14-2	Radiasurf® 7423
CAS 34938-91-8	Dehydol® PID 6	CAS 37318-31-3	Grilloten® PSE 141 G Pellets
CAS 34962-91-9	Dermol 108	CAS 37324-85-9	Aldosperse® ML-23
CAS 35274-05-6	Cegesoft® C 19	CAS 37354-45-5	Empicol® SDD
CAS 35274-05-6	Ceraphyl® 28	CAS 37475-88-0	ACS 60
CAS 35274-05-6	Cetinol LA	CAS 37475-88-0	Eltesol® ACS 60
CAS 35274-05-6	Crodamol CL	CAS 38102-62-4	BioGir-MBC
CAS 35274-05-6	Lactabase C16	CAS 38102-62-4	Eusolex® 6300
CAS 35274-05-6	Lactacet	CAS 38517-23-6	Amisoft HS-11
CAS 35274-05-6	Liponate CL	CAS 38566-94-8	Nipabutyl Potassium
CAS 35274-05-6	Nikkol Cetyl Lactate	CAS 38866-20-5	Imexine BD
CAS 35285-68-8	Nipagin A Sodium	CAS 39236-46-9	Abiol
CAS 35285-69-9	Nipasol M Sodium	CAS 39236-46-9	Atomergic Imidazolidinyl Urea
CAS 35545-57-4	Hetoxide BN-13	CAS 39236-46-9	Biopure 100
CAS 35602-69-8	Nikkol CS	CAS 39236-46-9	Germall® 115
CAS 35691-65-7	Tektamer® 38	CAS 39236-46-9	Sepicide CI
CAS 36148-84-2	Linoleate de Tocopherol	CAS 39236-46-9	Tristat IU
CAS 36148-84-2	dl-α-Tocopheryl Linoleate No.	CAS 39236-46-9	Unicide U-13
	26364	CAS 39354-45-5	Aerosol® A-102
CAS 36311-34-9	Ceraphyl® ICA	CAS 39354-45-5	Cosmopon BT
CAS 36311-34-9	Eutanol® G16	CAS 39354-45-5	Rolpon SE 138
CAS 36311-34-9	Exxal® 16	CAS 39354-45-5	Schercopol LPS
CAS 36311-34-9	Michel XO-150-16	CAS 39354-45-5	Surfagene S 30
CAS 36311-34-9	Unimul-G-16	CAS 39421-75-5	Chesguar HP4
CAS 36409-57-1	Empicol® SLL	CAS 39421-75-5	Chesguar HP4R
CAS 36409-57-1	Empicol® SLL/P	CAS 39421-75-5	Chesguar HP6
CAS 36409-57-1	Geropon® LSS	CAS 39421-75-5	Jaguar® HP 8
CAS 36457-19-9	Nipagin A Potassium	CAS 39421-75-5	Jaguar® HP-11
CAS 36457-20-2	Nipabutyl Sodium	CAS 39421-75-5	Jaguar® HP 60
CAS 36457-20-2	Unisept BNA	CAS 39421-75-5	Jaguar® HP 120
CAS 36521-89-8	Sorbon S-66	CAS 39421-75-5	Jaguar® HP-200
CAS 36653-82-4	Adol® 52	CAS 39464-64-7	Chemphos TC-341

CAS 39464-64-7	Chemphos TC-349	CAS 42909-29-5	Rodol PDAS
CAS 39464-64-7	Rhodafac® RM-510	CAS 43154-85-4	Emcol® 4161L
CAS 39464-64-7	Rhodafac® RM-710	CAS 43154-85-4	Fizul MD-318C
CAS 39464-66-9	Chemphos TR-510	CAS 43154-85-4	Mackanate™ OP
CAS 39464-66-9	Elfan® A 913	CAS 43154-85-4	Sole Terge 8
CAS 39464-66-9	Hodag PE-1203	CAS 45267-19-4	Chemidex M
CAS 39464-66-9	Marlophor® MO 3-Acid	CAS 45267-19-4	Schercodine M
CAS 39464-66-9	Protaphos SDA	CAS 50643-20-4	Brophos™ 5C10
CAS 39464-66-9	Rhodafac® RD-510	CAS 50643-20-4	Crodafos SG
CAS 39464-66-9	Surfagene FDD 402	CAS 50643-20-4	Hetphos SG
CAS 39464-69-2	Briphos O3D	CAS 50643-20-4	Mayphos 5C10
CAS 39464-69-2	Brophos-3	CAS 51033-38-6	Nikkol Hexaglyn 1-L
CAS 39464-69-2	Brophos™ OL-2	CAS 51158-08-8	Aldosperse® MS-20
CAS 39464-69-2	Brophos™ OL-3	CAS 51158-08-8	Tagat® S
CAS 39464-69-2	Chemphos TR-505	CAS 51158-08-8	Tagat® S2
CAS 39464-69-2	Chemphos TR-515	CAS 51158-08-8	Tewax TC 83
CAS 39464-69-2	Chemphos TR-541	CAS 51192-09-7	Tagat® O
CAS 39464-69-2	Crafol AP-11	CAS 51192-09-7	Tagat® O2
CAS 39464-69-2	Crodafos N2A	CAS 51200-87-4	Nuosept 101 CG
CAS 39464-69-2	Crodafos N-3 Acid	CAS 51200-87-4	Oxaban®-A
CAS 39464-69-2	Crodafos N-5 Acid	CAS 51229-78-8	CoSept 200
CAS 39464-69-2	Crodafos N-10 Acid	CAS 51229-78-8	Dowicil® 200
CAS 39464-69-2	Crodafos O2 Acid	CAS 51248-32-9	Lamacit® GML 20
CAS 39464-69-2	Crodafos O5 Acid	CAS 51248-32-9	Tagat® L
CAS 39464-69-2	Crodafos O10 Acid	CAS 51248-32-9	Tagat® L2
CAS 39464-69-2	Empicol® 0216	CAS 51258-15-2	Adeka GH-200
CAS 39464-69-2	Hetphos OA-3	CAS 51609-41-7	Emphos™ CS-141
CAS 39464-69-2	Hodag PE-1803	CAS 51609-41-7	Protaphos P-610
CAS 39464-69-2	Hodag PE-1810	CAS 51812-80-7	Ceraphyl® 60
CAS 39464-69-2	Hodag PE-1820	CAS 52108-64-2	Chitin Liq.
CAS 39464-69-2	Protaphos 400-A	CAS 52108-64-2	Chitisol
CAS 39529-26-5	Caprol® 10G10S	CAS 52108-64-2	Chotosolbe
CAS 39529-26-5	Nikkol Decaglyn 10-S	CAS 52292-17-8	Arosurf® 66-E2
CAS 39669-97-1	Chemidex P	CAS 52292-17-8	Arosurf® 66-E10
CAS 39669-97-1	Schercodine P	CAS 52292-17-8	Arosurf® 66-E20
CAS 40160-92-7	Applichem PDP-200	CAS 52292-17-8	Emalex 1805
CAS 40445-72-5	Estemol CHS	CAS 52292-17-8	Emalex 1810
CAS 40716-42-5	Afmide™ R	CAS 52292-17-8	Emalex 1815
CAS 40716-42-5	Amidex RC	CAS 52292-17-8	Emalex 1820
CAS 40716-42-5	Aminol CA-2	CAS 52292-17-8	Emalex 1825
CAS 40716-42-5	Mackamide™ R	CAS 52292-17-8	Ethlana 12
CAS 40716-42-5	Olamida RD	CAS 52292-17-8	Ethlana 22
CAS 40716-42-5	Protamide CA	CAS 52292-17-8	Ethlana 50
CAS 40754-60-7	Geropon® SBR-3	CAS 52292-17-8	Ethlana 50-M
CAS 41395-83-9	D.P.P.G	CAS 52292-17-8	Hetoxol IS-2
CAS 41395-83-9	Emerest® 2388	CAS 52292-17-8	Hetoxol IS-3
CAS 41395-83-9	Estol PDP 3601	CAS 52292-17-8	Hetoxol IS-10
CAS 41395-83-9	Lexol® PG-900	CAS 52292-17-8	Hetoxol IS-20
CAS 41395-83-9	Schercemol PGDP	CAS 52292-17-8	Lipocol IS-20
CAS 41395-83-9	Unitolate PG/DPG	CAS 52304-36-6	Insect Repellent 3535, No. 11887
CAS 41395-89-5	Dermol 109	CAS 52315-75-0	Amihope LL-11
CAS 41395-89-5	Wickenol® 152	CAS 52467-63-7	Arquad® 316
CAS 41669-30-1	Iso Isotearyle WL 3196	CAS 52467-63-7	Varisoft® TC-90
CAS 41669-30-1	Prisorine ISIS 2039	CAS 52504-24-2	Softigen® 767
CAS 41669-30-1	Rewomul IS	CAS 52504-24-2	Sterol CC 595
CAS 41669-30-1	Schercemol 1818	CAS 52558-73-3	Hamposyl® M
CAS 41672-81-5	Lipacide DPHP	CAS 52558-73-3	Vanseal® MS
CAS 41760-23-0	Lipacide C8CY	CAS 52581-71-2	Hodag CSA-91
CAS 42131-25-9	Salacos 99	CAS 52581-71-2	Provol 50
CAS 42131-25-9	Wickenol® 151	CAS 52794-79-3	Afmide™ ISA
CAS 42131-28-2	Fractalite ISL	CAS 52794-79-3	Hetamide IS
CAS 42131-28-2	Patlac® IL	CAS 52794-79-3	Mackamide™ ISA
CAS 42131-28-2	Pelemol ISL	CAS 52794-79-3	Monamid® 150-IS
CAS 42175-36-0	Dermol OL	CAS 52794-79-3	Standamid® ID
CAS 42175-36-0	Pelemol OL	CAS 52794-79-3	Witcamide® 5118S
CAS 42233-07-8	Pelemol LB	CAS 53320-86-8	Laponite® D
CAS 42233-14-7	Waxenol® 822	CAS 53320-86-8	Laponite® XLG
CAS 42504-46-1	Hetsulf IPA	CAS 53610-02-9	Surfine AZI-A
CAS 42612-52-2	Chemphos TR-510S	CAS 53633-54-8	Gafquat® 734
CAS 42612-52-2	Rhodafac® MC-470	CAS 53633-54-8	Gafquat® 755

CAS 53633-54-8	Gafquat® 755N
CAS 53637-25-5	Dow EP530
CAS 53694-15-8	Ethosperse® SL-20
CAS 53694-17-0	Merquat® 280
CAS 53980-88-4	Diacid 1550
CAS 54392-26-6	Arlacel® 987
CAS 54392-26-6	Emalex SPIS-100
CAS 54392-26-6	Nikkol SI-10R
CAS 54392-26-6	Nikkol SI-10T
CAS 54392-26-6	Nikkol SI-15T
CAS 54392-26-6	Sorbirol ISM
CAS 54549-25-6	Oramix NS 10
CAS 54982-83-1	Arova® N
CAS 55353-21-4	Resyn® 28-2913
CAS 55353-21-4	Resyn® 28-2930
CAS 55406-53-6	Glycacil L, S
CAS 55819-53-9	Hetamine 5L-25
CAS 55819-53-9	Incromate SDL
CAS 55819-53-9	Lexamine S-13 Lactate
CAS 55819-53-9	Mackalene™ 316
CAS 55819-53-9	Protachem SDM
CAS 55852-13-6	Mackine™ 321
CAS 55852-14-7	Emcol® SML
CAS 55852-14-7	Mackalene™ 326
CAS 55852-15-8	Afalene™ 416
CAS 55852-15-8	Emcol® 6613
CAS 55852-15-8	Mackalene™ 416
CAS 55963-33-2	28-1898
CAS 56002-14-3	Emalex PEIS-3
CAS 56002-14-3	Emalex PEIS-6
CAS 56002-14-3	Emalex PEIS-12
CAS 56002-14-3	Emalex PEIS-20
CAS 56002-14-3	Emerest® 2701
CAS 56002-14-3	Olepal ISO
CAS 56235-92-8	Ceraphyl® 45
CAS 56265-06-6	Argidone®
CAS 56388-43-3	Afanate™ OD-28
CAS 56388-43-3	Anionyx® 12S
CAS 56388-43-3	Geropon® SBG-280
CAS 56388-43-3	Mackanate™ OD-35
CAS 56388-43-3	Monamate OPA-30
CAS 56388-43-3	Monamate OPA-100
CAS 56388-43-3	Standapol® SH-100
CAS 56388-43-3	Standapol® SH-135
CAS 56388-43-3	Texapon® SH 100
CAS 56388-43-3	Texapon® SH-135 Special
CAS 56388-43-3	Unipol SH-100, SH-135
CAS 56519-71-2	Lexol® PG-800
CAS 56709-13-8	Nuosept C
CAS 56863-02-6	Amidex LN
CAS 56863-02-6	Comperlan® F
CAS 56863-02-6	Foamole A
CAS 56863-02-6	Hetamide LN
CAS 56863-02-6	Hetamide LNO
CAS 56863-02-6	Incromide LA
CAS 56863-02-6	Mackamide™ LOL
CAS 56863-02-6	Mazamide® LLD
CAS 56863-02-6	Mazamide® SS-10
CAS 56863-02-6	Mazamide® SS 20
CAS 56863-02-6	Monamid® 15-70W
CAS 56863-02-6	Monamid® 150-ADY
CAS 56863-02-6	Monamid® LN-605
CAS 56863-02-6	Protamide 15W
CAS 56863-02-6	Protamide LNO
CAS 56863-02-6	Purton SFD
CAS 56863-02-6	Schercomid SLE
CAS 56863-02-6	Standamid® SOMD
CAS 56863-02-6	Varamide® LO-1
CAS 56863-02-6	Witcamide® 6540
CAS 57171-56-9	G-1096
CAS 57171-56-9	Trylox® 6746
CAS 57524-53-5	Imexine FE
CAS 57569-76-3	Dermol GL-7A
CAS 57569-76-3	Pelemol G7A
CAS 58069-11-7	Dehyquart® SP
CAS 58069-11-7	Uniquart SP
CAS 58450-52-5	Trivent SS-20
CAS 58855-63-3	Crodafos N-3 Neutral
CAS 58855-63-3	Crodafos N-10 Neutral
CAS 58958-60-4	Ceraphyl® 375
CAS 58958-60-4	Crodamol ISNP
CAS 58958-60-4	Dermol 185
CAS 58958-60-4	Schercemol 185
CAS 59070-56-3	Glycerox L15
CAS 59070-56-3	Glycerox L30
CAS 59130-69-7	Bernel® Ester CO
CAS 59130-69-7	Emalex CC-168
CAS 59130-69-7	Exceparl HO
CAS 59130-69-7	Nikkol CIO, CIO-P
CAS 59130-69-7	Schercemol 1688
CAS 59130-69-7	Schercemol CO
CAS 59130-69-7	Tegosoft® CO
CAS 59130-69-7	Trivent OC-16
CAS 59186-41-3	Rhodapon® EC111
CAS 59186-41-3	Unihydag Wax E
CAS 59231-34-4	Ceraphyl® 140
CAS 59231-34-4	Ceraphyl® 140-A
CAS 59231-34-4	Estol IDCO 3667
CAS 59231-34-4	Pelemol IDO
CAS 59231-34-4	Schercemol IDO
CAS 59231-34-4	Trivent OL-10B
CAS 59231-34-4	Wickenol® 144
CAS 59259-38-0	Covafresh
CAS 59259-38-0	Frescolat, Type ML
CAS 59259-38-0	Frigydil
CAS 59272-84-3	Schercotaine MAB
CAS 59355-61-2	Empigen® OY
CAS 59587-44-9	Bernel® OPG
CAS 59587-44-9	Pelemol OPG
CAS 59587-44-9	Schercemol OPG
CAS 59587-44-9	Unitolate OPG
CAS 59587-44-9	Wickenol® 160
CAS 59587-44-9	Witconol™ 2307
CAS 59686-68-9	Cetiol® 1414E
CAS 59686-68-9	Gatarol M 30 M
CAS 59686-68-9	Lanol 14 M
CAS 59686-68-9	Liponate 143M
CAS 59686-68-9	Schercemol MEM-3
CAS 59686-68-9	Unimil 14E
CAS 59686-68-9	Unimul-1414EW
CAS 59792-81-3	Aludone®
CAS 60209-82-7	Dermol 105
CAS 60209-82-7	Schercemol 105
CAS 60239-68-1	Fungicide DA 2/938070
CAS 60239-68-1	Olamida UD
CAS 60239-68-1	Olamida UD 21
CAS 60239-68-1	Undamide
CAS 60270-33-9	Chemidex B
CAS 60270-33-9	Incromine BB
CAS 60270-33-9	Mackine™ 601
CAS 60270-33-9	Schercodine B
CAS 61372-91-6	Kemamine® T-2801
CAS 61417-49-0	Ken-React® KR TTS
CAS 61682-73-3	Liponate PB-4
CAS 61693-41-2	Amphisol®
CAS 61693-41-2	Brophos™ A
CAS 61731-12-6	Emulpon EL 40
CAS 61731-12-6	Emulpon EL 40
CAS 61731-31-9	Witcamide® LDTS
CAS 61788-40-7	Hypan® SA100H

CAS 61788-45-2	Amine 2HBG
CAS 61788-45-2	Armeen® HT
CAS 61788-45-2	Armeen® HTD
CAS 61788-45-2	Radiamine 6140
CAS 61788-45-2	Radiamine 6141
CAS 61788-46-3	Adogen® 160D
CAS 61788-46-3	Amine KKD
CAS 61788-46-3	Armeen® C
CAS 61788-46-3	Armeen® CD
CAS 61788-46-3	Kemamine® P-650
CAS 61788-46-3	Radiamine 6160
CAS 61788-46-3	Radiamine 6161
CAS 61788-47-4	Emery® 621
CAS 61788-47-4	Emery® 622
CAS 61788-47-4	Industrene® 325
CAS 61788-47-4	Industrene® 328
CAS 61788-48-5	Acelan L
CAS 61788-48-5	Acetadeps
CAS 61788-48-5	Acylan
CAS 61788-48-5	Fancol Acel
CAS 61788-48-5	Ivarlan™ 3300
CAS 61788-48-5	Lanacet® 1705
CAS 61788-48-5	Lanolin A.C
CAS 61788-48-5	Modulan®
CAS 61788-48-5	Ritacetyl®
CAS 61788-48-5	Unilan Acetyl
CAS 61788-49-6	Hetlan AC
CAS 61788-49-6	Protalan MOD
CAS 61788-59-8	CE-618
CAS 61788-59-8	Radia® 7117
CAS 61788-62-3	Armeen® M2C
CAS 61788-62-3;	Jet Amine M2C
CAS 61788-63-4	Amine M2HBG
CAS 61788-63-4	Armeen® M2HT
CAS 61788-63-4	Kemamine® T-9701
CAS 61788-78-1	Arquad® HT-50
CAS 61788-78-1	Noramium MSH 50
CAS 61788-85-0	Akyporox CO 400
CAS 61788-85-0	Akyporox CO 600
CAS 61788-85-0	Arlacel® 989
CAS 61788-85-0	Arlatone® 975
CAS 61788-85-0	Arlatone® 980
CAS 61788-85-0	Arlatone® G
CAS 61788-85-0	Cerex ELS 50
CAS 61788-85-0	Cerex ELS 250
CAS 61788-85-0	Cerex ELS 400
CAS 61788-85-0	Cerex ELS 450
CAS 61788-85-0	Chemax HCO-5
CAS 61788-85-0	Chemax HCO-16
CAS 61788-85-0	Chemax HCO-25
CAS 61788-85-0	Chemax HCO-200/50
CAS 61788-85-0	Cremophor® RH 40
CAS 61788-85-0	Cremophor® RH 60
CAS 61788-85-0	Cremophor® RH 410
CAS 61788-85-0	Cremophor® WO 7
CAS 61788-85-0	Croduret 7
CAS 61788-85-0	Croduret 10
CAS 61788-85-0	Croduret 25
CAS 61788-85-0	Croduret 30
CAS 61788-85-0	Croduret 40
CAS 61788-85-0	Croduret 50
CAS 61788-85-0	Croduret 60
CAS 61788-85-0	Croduret 100
CAS 61788-85-0	Croduret 200
CAS 61788-85-0	Dehymuls® HRE 7
CAS 61788-85-0	Emalex HC-5
CAS 61788-85-0	Emalex HC-7
CAS 61788-85-0	Emalex HC-10
CAS 61788-85-0	Emalex HC-20
CAS 61788-85-0	Emalex HC-30
CAS 61788-85-0	Emalex HC-40
CAS 61788-85-0	Emalex HC-50
CAS 61788-85-0	Emalex HC-60
CAS 61788-85-0	Emalex HC-80
CAS 61788-85-0	Emalex HC-100
CAS 61788-85-0	Emthox® 2737
CAS 61788-85-0	Emthox® 2738
CAS 61788-85-0	Emulsifier 17 P
CAS 61788-85-0	Eumulgin® HRE 40
CAS 61788-85-0	Eumulgin® HRE 60
CAS 61788-85-0	Fancol HCO-25
CAS 61788-85-0	G-1292
CAS 61788-85-0	Hetoxide HC-16
CAS 61788-85-0	Hetoxide HC-25
CAS 61788-85-0	Hetoxide HC-40
CAS 61788-85-0	Hetoxide HC-60
CAS 61788-85-0	Hodag Nonionic GRH-25
CAS 61788-85-0	Hodag Nonionic GRH-40
CAS 61788-85-0	Lanaetex CO-25
CAS 61788-85-0	Lipocol HCO-40
CAS 61788-85-0	Lipocol HCO-60
CAS 61788-85-0	Lipocol HCO-66
CAS 61788-85-0	Mapeg® CO-16H
CAS 61788-85-0	Mapeg® CO-25H
CAS 61788-85-0	Naturechem® THS-200
CAS 61788-85-0	Nikkol HCO-5
CAS 61788-85-0	Nikkol HCO-7.5
CAS 61788-85-0	Nikkol HCO-10
CAS 61788-85-0	Nikkol HCO-20
CAS 61788-85-0	Nikkol HCO-30
CAS 61788-85-0	Nikkol HCO-40
CAS 61788-85-0	Nikkol HCO-40 Pharm
CAS 61788-85-0	Nikkol HCO-50
CAS 61788-85-0	Nikkol HCO-50 Pharm
CAS 61788-85-0	Nikkol HCO-60
CAS 61788-85-0	Nikkol HCO-60 Pharm
CAS 61788-85-0	Nikkol HCO-80
CAS 61788-85-0	Nikkol HCO-100
CAS 61788-85-0	Protachem CAH-16
CAS 61788-85-0	Protachem CAH-25
CAS 61788-85-0	Protachem CAH-40
CAS 61788-85-0	Protachem CAH-60
CAS 61788-85-0	Protachem CAH-100
CAS 61788-85-0	Protachem CAH-200
CAS 61788-85-0	Prox-onic HRH-05
CAS 61788-85-0	Prox-onic HRH-016
CAS 61788-85-0	Prox-onic HRH-025
CAS 61788-85-0	Prox-onic HRH-0200
CAS 61788-85-0	Prox-onic HRH-0200/50
CAS 61788-85-0	Remcopal HC 7
CAS 61788-85-0	Remcopal HC 33
CAS 61788-85-0	Remcopal HC 40
CAS 61788-85-0	Remcopal HC 60
CAS 61788-85-0	Simulsol 989
CAS 61788-85-0	Simulsol 1292
CAS 61788-85-0	Simulsol 1293
CAS 61788-85-0	Simulsol 1294
CAS 61788-85-0	Surfactol® 575
CAS 61788-85-0	Surfactol® 590
CAS 61788-85-0	Tagat® R40
CAS 61788-85-0	Tagat® R60
CAS 61788-85-0	Unipeg-CO-25H
CAS 61788-85-0	Unipeg-CO-40H
CAS 61788-85-0	Witconol™ 2737
CAS 61788-85-0	Witconol™ 2738
CAS 61788-85-0	Witconol™ 2739
CAS 61788-90-7	Afamine™ CO
CAS 61788-90-7	Aminoxid A 4080
CAS 61788-90-7	Aromox® DMC
CAS 61788-90-7	Aromox® DMC-W

CAS 61788-90-7	Barlox® 12		CAS 61789-77-3	Radiaquat® 6462
CAS 61788-90-7	Chemoxide WC		CAS 61789-79-5	Adogen® 240 SF
CAS 61788-90-7	Genaminox CS		CAS 61789-79-5	Armeen® 2HT
CAS 61788-90-7	Genaminox KC		CAS 61789-80-8	Arquad® HC
CAS 61788-90-7	Mackamine™ CO		CAS 61789-80-8	Noramium M2SH
CAS 61788-90-7	Naxide™ 1230		CAS 61789-80-8	Querton 442
CAS 61788-90-7	Noxamine CA 30		CAS 61789-80-8	Querton 442-11
CAS 61788-90-7	Radiamox® 6800		CAS 61789-80-8	Querton 442-82
CAS 61788-90-7	Schercamox DMC		CAS 61789-80-8	Querton 442E
CAS 61788-90-7	Synotol C-30		CAS 61789-80-8	Querton 442H
CAS 61788-91-8	Armeen® DMSD		CAS 61789-80-8	Radiaquat® 6442
CAS 61788-91-8	Jet Amine DMSD		CAS 61789-80-8	Varisoft® 442-100P
CAS 61788-91-8	Kemamine® T-9972		CAS 61789-91-1	Atomergic Jojoba Oil
CAS 61788-93-0	Amine 2M1218D		CAS 61789-91-1	Cojoba
CAS 61788-93-0	Amine 2MKKD		CAS 61789-91-1	Emalex J.J. O-V
CAS 61788-93-0	Armeen® DMCD		CAS 61789-91-1	Estran™
CAS 61788-93-0	Barlene® 12C		CAS 61789-91-1	Estran™-Lite
CAS 61788-93-0	Jet Amine DMCD		CAS 61789-91-1	Estran™-Pure
CAS 61788-93-0	Kemamine® T-6502		CAS 61789-91-1	Estran™-Xtra
CAS 61788-93-0	Noram DMC		CAS 61789-91-1	Jojoba Oil
CAS 61788-95-2	Armeen® DMHTD		CAS 61789-91-1	Jojoba Oil Cosmetic Grade
CAS 61788-95-2	Kemamine® T-9702		CAS 61789-91-1	Jojoba Oil Pure Grade
CAS 61789-04-6	Nikkol SGC-80N		CAS 61789-91-1	Jojoba Oil Refined Grade
CAS 61789-04-6	Poem-LS-90		CAS 61789-91-1	Lanaetex Jojoba Oil
CAS 61789-05-7	Imwitor® 928		CAS 61789-91-1	Lipovol J
CAS 61789-07-9	Myverol® 18-07		CAS 61789-91-1	Lipovol J Lite
CAS 61789-08-0	Myvaplex® 600P		CAS 61789-91-1	Nikkol Jojoba Oil S
CAS 61789-08-0	Myverol® 18-06		CAS 61789-91-1	Simchin® Natural
CAS 61789-09-1	Monomuls® 90-25		CAS 61789-91-1	Simchin® Refined
CAS 61789-10-4	Myverol® 18-40		CAS 61789-91-1	Transjojoba™ 70
CAS 61789-13-7	Myverol® 18-30		CAS 61789-91-1	Wickenol® 139
CAS 61789-18-2	Arquad® C-33W		CAS 61790-12-3	Acintol® 2122
CAS 61789-18-2	Jet Quat C-50		CAS 61790-12-3	Acintol® 7002
CAS 61789-18-2	Kemamine® Q-6503B		CAS 61790-12-3	Pamak 4
CAS 61789-18-2	Marlazin® KC 30/50		CAS 61790-18-9	Armeen® S
CAS 61789-18-2	Nikkol CA-2150		CAS 61790-18-9	Kemamine® P-997
CAS 61789-18-2	Noramium MC 50		CAS 61790-33-8	Adogen® 170D
CAS 61789-18-2	Radiaquat® 6460		CAS 61790-33-8	Armeen® T
CAS 61789-30-8	Mackadet™ 40K		CAS 61790-33-8	Armeen® TD
CAS 61789-30-8	Norfox® 1101		CAS 61790-33-8	Kemamine® P-974
CAS 61789-30-8	Protachem LP-40		CAS 61790-33-8	Radiamine 6170
CAS 61789-31-9	Norfox® Coco Powder		CAS 61790-33-8	Radiamine 6171
CAS 61789-40-0	Chimin AX		CAS 61790-37-2	Hy-Phi 4204
CAS 61789-40-0	Dehyton® K		CAS 61790-37-2	Prifac 7920
CAS 61789-40-0	Dehyton® PK		CAS 61790-37-2	Prifac 7935
CAS 61789-40-0	Empigen® BS/AU		CAS 61790-38-3	Dar-C
CAS 61789-40-0	Empigen® BS/P		CAS 61790-38-3	Hy-Phi 6001
CAS 61789-40-0	Foamtaine CAB-G		CAS 61790-41-8	Jet Quat S-50
CAS 61789-40-0	Incronam 30		CAS 61790-41-8	Kemamine® Q-9973B
CAS 61789-40-0	Mirataine® BET-W		CAS 61790-63-4	Marlamid® DF 1218
CAS 61789-40-0	Mirataine® CAB-A		CAS 61790-64-5	Akypogene FP 35 T
CAS 61789-40-0	Mirataine® CAB-O		CAS 61790-81-6	Aqualose L30
CAS 61789-40-0	Rewoteric® AM B-13		CAS 61790-81-6	Aqualose L75
CAS 61789-40-0	Rewoteric® AM B-14		CAS 61790-81-6	Aqualose L75/50
CAS 61789-40-0	Schercotaine CAB		CAS 61790-81-6	Aqualose L100
CAS 61789-40-0	Surfax ACR		CAS 61790-81-6	Brooksgel 41
CAS 61789-40-0	Tego®-Betaine C		CAS 61790-81-6	Brooksgel 61
CAS 61789-40-0	Tego®-Betaine F		CAS 61790-81-6	Ethoxylan® 1685
CAS 61789-40-0	Tego®-Betaine L-7		CAS 61790-81-6	Ethoxylan® 1686
CAS 61789-40-0	Tego®-Betaine L-5351		CAS 61790-81-6	Hetoxalan 75
CAS 61789-68-2	Ethoquad® C/12B		CAS 61790-81-6	Hetoxalan 75-50%
CAS 61789-71-7	Alkaquat® DMB-451-50,		CAS 61790-81-6	Hetoxalan 100
	DMB-451-80		CAS 61790-81-6	Ivarlan™ 3400
CAS 61789-71-7	Arquad® DNMCB-50		CAS 61790-81-6	Ivarlan™ 3401
CAS 61789-71-7	Marlazin® KC 21/50		CAS 61790-81-6	Ivarlan™ 3405-L30
CAS 61789-72-8	Variquat® B345		CAS 61790-81-6	Ivarlan™ 3406
CAS 61789-76-2	Armeen® 2C		CAS 61790-81-6	Ivarlan™ 3407-E
CAS 61789-77-3	Dodigen 1490		CAS 61790-81-6	Ivarlan™ 3408W
CAS 61789-77-3	Jet Quat 2C-75		CAS 61790-81-6	Ivarlan™ 3409-60
CAS 61789-77-3	Noramium M2C		CAS 61790-81-6	Ivarlan™ 3410

CAS 61790-81-6	Ivarlan™ L575	CAS 61791-08-0	Oramide MLM 06
CAS 61790-81-6	Lanalox L 30	CAS 61791-08-0	Oramide MLM 10
CAS 61790-81-6	Laneto 40	CAS 61791-08-0	Rewopal® C 6
CAS 61790-81-6	Laneto 60	CAS 61791-08-0	Unamide® C-5
CAS 61790-81-6	Laneto 100	CAS 61791-08-0	Upamide C-2
CAS 61790-81-6	Laneto 100-Flaked	CAS 61791-08-0	Upamide C-5
CAS 61790-81-6	Lanogel® 21	CAS 61791-10-4	Ethoquad® C/25
CAS 61790-81-6	Lanogel® 31	CAS 61791-10-4	Variquat® K-1215
CAS 61790-81-6	Lanogel® 41	CAS 61791-12-6	Ablunol CO 5
CAS 61790-81-6	Lanogel® 61	CAS 61791-12-6	Ablunol CO 15
CAS 61790-81-6	Lanolex L-40	CAS 61791-12-6	Ablunol CO 30
CAS 61790-81-6	Lanoxal 75	CAS 61791-12-6	Acconon CA-5
CAS 61790-81-6	Lantox 55, 110	CAS 61791-12-6	Acconon CA-9
CAS 61790-81-6	Nikkol TW-10	CAS 61791-12-6	Acconon CA-15
CAS 61790-81-6	Nikkol TW-20	CAS 61791-12-6	Alkamuls® B
CAS 61790-81-6	Nikkol TW-30	CAS 61791-12-6	Alkamuls® BR
CAS 61790-81-6	Protalan 85	CAS 61791-12-6	Alkamuls® CO-15
CAS 61790-81-6	Protalan L-30	CAS 61791-12-6	Alkamuls® EL-620
CAS 61790-81-6	Protalan L-60	CAS 61791-12-6	Alkamuls® EL-620L
CAS 61790-81-6	Protalan L-75	CAS 61791-12-6	Alkamuls® EL-630
CAS 61790-81-6	Rewolan® E 50, E 100	CAS 61791-12-6	Alkamuls® EL-719
CAS 61790-81-6	Sellig Lano 30	CAS 61791-12-6	Cerex EL 150
CAS 61790-81-6	Solan	CAS 61791-12-6	Cerex EL 250
CAS 61790-81-6	Solan 50	CAS 61791-12-6	Cerex EL 300
CAS 61790-81-6	Solan E	CAS 61791-12-6	Cerex EL 360
CAS 61790-81-6	Solulan® 75	CAS 61791-12-6	Cerex EL 400
CAS 61790-81-6	Solulan® L-575	CAS 61791-12-6	Chemax CO-5
CAS 61790-81-6	Super Solan Flaked	CAS 61791-12-6	Chemax CO-16
CAS 61790-81-6	Teric LAN70	CAS 61791-12-6	Chemax CO-25
CAS 61790-81-6	Unilaneth 75	CAS 61791-12-6	Chemax CO-28
CAS 61790-85-0	Ethoduomeen® T/13	CAS 61791-12-6	Chemax CO-30
CAS 61790-85-0	Ethoduomeen® T/20	CAS 61791-12-6	Chemax CO-36
CAS 61790-85-0	Ethoduomeen® T/25	CAS 61791-12-6	Chemax CO-40
CAS 61790-86-1	Hefti MO-55-F	CAS 61791-12-6	Chemax CO-80
CAS 61790-95-2	Hefti GMS-333	CAS 61791-12-6	Chemax CO-200/50
CAS 61791-00-2	Chemax E-400 MT	CAS 61791-12-6	Cremophor® EL
CAS 61791-00-2	Ethofat® 242/25	CAS 61791-12-6	Desonic® 30C
CAS 61791-00-2	Ethofat® 433	CAS 61791-12-6	Desonic® 36C
CAS 61791-00-2	Hetoxamate FA 2-5	CAS 61791-12-6	Desonic® 54C
CAS 61791-00-2	Hetoxamate FA-5	CAS 61791-12-6	Elfapur® R 150
CAS 61791-00-2	Hetoxamate FA-20	CAS 61791-12-6	Emalex C-20
CAS 61791-00-2	Hodag WA-56	CAS 61791-12-6	Emalex C-30
CAS 61791-00-2	Mapeg® 200 MOT	CAS 61791-12-6	Emalex C-40
CAS 61791-00-2	Mapeg® 400 MOT	CAS 61791-12-6	Emalex C-50
CAS 61791-00-2	Mapeg® 600 MOT	CAS 61791-12-6	Emulpon EL 33
CAS 61791-00-2	Mapeg® TAO-15	CAS 61791-12-6	Emulsogen EL
CAS 61791-00-2	Protamate 200 T	CAS 61791-12-6	Etocas 5
CAS 61791-00-2	Protamate 400 T	CAS 61791-12-6	Etocas 10
CAS 61791-00-2	Protamate 600 T	CAS 61791-12-6	Etocas 15
CAS 61791-00-2	Protamate 1000 T	CAS 61791-12-6	Etocas 20
CAS 61791-00-2	Renex® 20	CAS 61791-12-6	Etocas 29
CAS 61791-00-2	Sellig T 14 100	CAS 61791-12-6	Etocas 30
CAS 61791-00-2	Unipeg-400 MOT	CAS 61791-12-6	Etocas 35
CAS 61791-01-3	Chemax PEG 400 DT	CAS 61791-12-6	Etocas 40
CAS 61791-01-3	Chemax PEG 600 DT	CAS 61791-12-6	Etocas 50
CAS 61791-01-3	Hetoxamate 600 DT	CAS 61791-12-6	Etocas 60
CAS 61791-01-3	Mapeg® 200 DOT	CAS 61791-12-6	Ethocas 75
CAS 61791-01-3	Mapeg® 400 DOT	CAS 61791-12-6	Etocas 100
CAS 61791-01-3	Mapeg® 600 DOT	CAS 61791-12-6	Etocas 200
CAS 61791-01-3	Pegosperse® 400 DOT	CAS 61791-12-6	Eumulgin® PRT 36
CAS 61791-01-3	Pegosperse® 600 DOT	CAS 61791-12-6	Eumulgin® PRT 40
CAS 61791-08-0	Alkamide® C-5	CAS 61791-12-6	Eumulgin® PRT 56
CAS 61791-08-0	Amidox® C-2	CAS 61791-12-6	Eumulgin® PRT 200
CAS 61791-08-0	Amidox® C-5	CAS 61791-12-6	Eumulgin® RO 35
CAS 61791-08-0	Eumulgin® C4	CAS 61791-12-6	Eumulgin® RO 40
CAS 61791-08-0	Genagen CA-050	CAS 61791-12-6	Fancol CO-30
CAS 61791-08-0	Hetoxamide C-4	CAS 61791-12-6	Hetoxide C-2
CAS 61791-08-0	Hetoxamide CD-4	CAS 61791-12-6	Hetoxide C-9
CAS 61791-08-0	Hetoxamide CD-6	CAS 61791-12-6	Hetoxide C-15
CAS 61791-08-0	Oramide MLM 02	CAS 61791-12-6	Hetoxide C-25

CAS 61791-12-6	Hetoxide C-30
CAS 61791-12-6	Hetoxide C-40
CAS 61791-12-6	Hetoxide C-52
CAS 61791-12-6	Hetoxide C-60
CAS 61791-12-6	Hetoxide C-200
CAS 61791-12-6	Hetoxide C-200-50%
CAS 61791-12-6	Hodag Nonionic GR-8
CAS 61791-12-6	Hodag Nonionic GR-25
CAS 61791-12-6	Hodag Nonionic GR-36
CAS 61791-12-6	Hodag Nonionic GR-40
CAS 61791-12-6	Hodag Nonionic GR-52
CAS 61791-12-6	Hodag Nonionic GR-200
CAS 61791-12-6	Incrocas 30
CAS 61791-12-6	Incrocas 40
CAS 61791-12-6	Lanaetex C-40
CAS 61791-12-6	Lanaetex CO-40
CAS 61791-12-6	Mapeg® CO-25
CAS 61791-12-6	Mapeg® CO-30
CAS 61791-12-6	Mapeg® CO-36
CAS 61791-12-6	Mapeg® CO-200
CAS 61791-12-6	Marlosol® R70
CAS 61791-12-6	Marlowet® R 11/K
CAS 61791-12-6	Marlowet® R 25/K
CAS 61791-12-6	Marlowet® R 40
CAS 61791-12-6	Marlowet® R 40/K
CAS 61791-12-6	Nalco® 2395
CAS 61791-12-6	Nikkol CO-3
CAS 61791-12-6	Nikkol CO-10
CAS 61791-12-6	Nikkol CO-20TX
CAS 61791-12-6	Nikkol CO-40TX
CAS 61791-12-6	Nikkol CO-50TX
CAS 61791-12-6	Nikkol CO-60TX
CAS 61791-12-6	Protachem CA-9
CAS 61791-12-6	Protachem CA-25
CAS 61791-12-6	Protachem CA-30
CAS 61791-12-6	Protachem CA-40
CAS 61791-12-6	Protachem CA-100
CAS 61791-12-6	Protachem CA-200
CAS 61791-12-6	Prox-onic HR-05
CAS 61791-12-6	Prox-onic HR-016
CAS 61791-12-6	Prox-onic HR-025
CAS 61791-12-6	Prox-onic HR-030
CAS 61791-12-6	Prox-onic HR-036
CAS 61791-12-6	Prox-onic HR-040
CAS 61791-12-6	Prox-onic HR-080
CAS 61791-12-6	Prox-onic HR-0200
CAS 61791-12-6	Prox-onic HR-0200/50
CAS 61791-12-6	Remcopal 40 S3
CAS 61791-12-6	Ricinion
CAS 61791-12-6	Ricino Viscoil
CAS 61791-12-6	Sellig R 3395
CAS 61791-12-6	Servirox OEG 45
CAS 61791-12-6	Servirox OEG 55
CAS 61791-12-6	Servirox OEG 65
CAS 61791-12-6	Servirox OEG 90/50
CAS 61791-12-6	Simulsol 1285
CAS 61791-12-6	Simulsol 5817
CAS 61791-12-6	Simulsol OL 50
CAS 61791-12-6	Surfactol® 318
CAS 61791-12-6	Surfactol® 365
CAS 61791-12-6	Unipeg-CO-8
CAS 61791-12-6	Unipeg-CO-25
CAS 61791-12-6	Unipeg-CO-36
CAS 61791-12-6	Unipeg-CO-40
CAS 61791-12-6	Unipeg-CO-200
CAS 61791-12-6	Witconol™ 5906
CAS 61791-12-6	Witconol™ 5907
CAS 61791-12-6	Witconol™ 5909
CAS 61791-13-7	Genapol® C-050
CAS 61791-13-7	Genapol® C-080
CAS 61791-13-7	Genapol® C-100
CAS 61791-13-7	Genapol® C-150
CAS 61791-13-7	Genapol® C-200
CAS 61791-13-7	Marlowet® CA 5
CAS 61791-13-7	Marlowet® CA 10
CAS 61791-14-8	Accomeen C2
CAS 61791-14-8	Accomeen C5
CAS 61791-14-8	Accomeen C10
CAS 61791-14-8	Accomeen C15
CAS 61791-14-8	Chemeen C-2
CAS 61791-14-8	Chemeen C-5
CAS 61791-14-8	Chemeen C-10
CAS 61791-14-8	Chemeen C-15
CAS 61791-14-8	Ethomeen® C/12
CAS 61791-14-8	Ethomeen® C/15
CAS 61791-14-8	Ethomeen® C/20
CAS 61791-14-8	Ethomeen® C/25
CAS 61791-14-8	Ethylan® TC
CAS 61791-14-8	Ethylan® TN-10
CAS 61791-14-8	Hetoxamine C-2
CAS 61791-14-8	Hetoxamine C-5
CAS 61791-14-8	Hetoxamine C-15
CAS 61791-14-8	Lowenol C-243
CAS 61791-14-8	Mazeen® C-2
CAS 61791-14-8	Mazeen® C-5
CAS 61791-14-8	Mazeen® C-10
CAS 61791-14-8	Mazeen® C-15
CAS 61791-14-8	Protox C-2
CAS 61791-14-8	Protox C-5
CAS 61791-14-8	Protox C-10
CAS 61791-14-8	Protox C-15
CAS 61791-14-8	Unizeen C-2
CAS 61791-14-8	Unizeen C-5
CAS 61791-14-8	Unizeen C-10
CAS 61791-14-8	Varonic® K-202
CAS 61791-14-8	Varonic® K-202 SF
CAS 61791-14-8	Varonic® K-205
CAS 61791-14-8	Varonic® K-205 SF
CAS 61791-14-8	Varonic® K-210
CAS 61791-14-8	Varonic® K-210 SF
CAS 61791-14-8	Varonic® K-215
CAS 61791-14-8	Varonic® K-215 LC
CAS 61791-14-8	Varonic® K-215 SF
CAS 61791-20-6	Aqualose W5
CAS 61791-20-6	Aqualose W20
CAS 61791-20-6	Aqualose W20/50
CAS 61791-20-6	Fancol LA-5
CAS 61791-20-6	Fancol LA-15
CAS 61791-20-6	G-1790
CAS 61791-20-6	Ivarlan™ 3442
CAS 61791-20-6	Lanaetex A-15
CAS 61791-20-6	Lanaetex-A16
CAS 61791-20-6	Nikkol BWA-5
CAS 61791-20-6	Nikkol BWA-10
CAS 61791-20-6	Nikkol BWA-20
CAS 61791-20-6	Nikkol BWA-40
CAS 61791-20-6	Polychol 5
CAS 61791-20-6	Polychol 15
CAS 61791-20-6	Polychol 16
CAS 61791-20-6	Ritawax 5
CAS 61791-20-6	Ritawax 10
CAS 61791-20-6	Ritawax 20
CAS 61791-24-0	Accomeen S2
CAS 61791-24-0	Accomeen S10
CAS 61791-24-0	Accomeen S15
CAS 61791-24-0	Ethomeen® S/12
CAS 61791-24-0	Ethomeen® S/15
CAS 61791-24-0	Ethomeen® S/20
CAS 61791-24-0	Ethomeen® S/25
CAS 61791-24-0	Hetoxamine S-2

CAS 61791-24-0	Hetoxamine S-5	CAS 61791-31-9	Esi-Terge S-10
CAS 61791-24-0	Hetoxamine S-15	CAS 61791-31-9	Ethylan® LD
CAS 61791-24-0	Mazeen® S-2	CAS 61791-31-9	Ethylan® LDA-48
CAS 61791-24-0	Mazeen® S-5	CAS 61791-31-9	Ethylan® LDG
CAS 61791-24-0	Mazeen® S-10	CAS 61791-31-9	FMB 128 T
CAS 61791-24-0	Mazeen® S-15	CAS 61791-31-9	FMB BT
CAS 61791-24-0	Protox S-2	CAS 61791-31-9	FMB Cocamide DEA
CAS 61791-24-0	Protox S-5	CAS 61791-31-9	FMB Coco Condensate
CAS 61791-24-0	Protox S-10	CAS 61791-31-9	Hartamide OD
CAS 61791-24-0	Protox S-15	CAS 61791-31-9	Hetamide DSUC
CAS 61791-24-0	Unizeen S-10	CAS 61791-31-9	Hetamide MC
CAS 61791-24-0	Unizeen S-15	CAS 61791-31-9	Hetamide MCS
CAS 61791-25-1	Amphoteen BTH-35	CAS 61791-31-9	Hetamide RC
CAS 61791-25-1	Mirataine® TM	CAS 61791-31-9	Hyamide 1:1
CAS 61791-25-1	Rewoteric® AM TEG	CAS 61791-31-9	Incromide CA
CAS 61791-25-1	Tego®-Betaine N-192	CAS 61791-31-9	Karamide 121
CAS 61791-26-2	Ethomeen® T/12	CAS 61791-31-9	Karamide 363
CAS 61791-26-2	Ethomeen® T/15	CAS 61791-31-9	Lauramide 11
CAS 61791-26-2	Ethomeen® T/25	CAS 61791-31-9	Lauramide ME
CAS 61791-26-2	G-3780-A	CAS 61791-31-9	Laurel SD-900M
CAS 61791-26-2	Hetoxamine T-2	CAS 61791-31-9	Lauridit® KD
CAS 61791-26-2	Hetoxamine T-5	CAS 61791-31-9	Lauridit® KDG
CAS 61791-26-2	Hetoxamine T-15	CAS 61791-31-9	Loropan KD
CAS 61791-26-2	Hetoxamine T-20	CAS 61791-31-9	Mackamide™ C
CAS 61791-26-2	Hetoxamine T-30	CAS 61791-31-9	Mackamide™ CD
CAS 61791-26-2	Protox T-2	CAS 61791-31-9	Mackamide™ CS
CAS 61791-26-2	Protox T-5	CAS 61791-31-9	Mackamide™ MC
CAS 61791-26-2	Protox T-15	CAS 61791-31-9	Manro CD
CAS 61791-26-2	Protox T-20	CAS 61791-31-9	Manro CDS
CAS 61791-26-2	Protox T-40	CAS 61791-31-9	Manro CDX
CAS 61791-26-2	Protox T-50	CAS 61791-31-9	Manromid CD
CAS 61791-26-2	Unizeen T-2	CAS 61791-31-9	Manromid CDG
CAS 61791-26-2	Unizeen T-5	CAS 61791-31-9	Manromid CDS
CAS 61791-26-2	Unizeen T-15	CAS 61791-31-9	Marlamid® D 1218
CAS 61791-26-2	Varonic® U-215	CAS 61791-31-9	Mazamide® 68
CAS 61791-28-4	Hetoxol TA-6	CAS 61791-31-9	Mazamide® 80
CAS 61791-29-5	Crodet C10	CAS 61791-31-9	Mazamide® 524
CAS 61791-29-5	Ethofat® C/15	CAS 61791-31-9	Mazamide® 1281
CAS 61791-29-5	Ethofat® C/25	CAS 61791-31-9	Mazamide® CCO
CAS 61791-29-5	Prox-onic CC-05	CAS 61791-31-9	Mazamide® CS 148
CAS 61791-29-5	Prox-onic CC-09	CAS 61791-31-9	Mazamide® JT 128
CAS 61791-29-5	Prox-onic CC-014	CAS 61791-31-9	Mazamide® WC Conc.
CAS 61791-31-9	Ablumide CDE	CAS 61791-31-9	Monamid® 705
CAS 61791-31-9	Ablumide CDE-G	CAS 61791-31-9	Monamid® 759
CAS 61791-31-9	Ablumide CKD	CAS 61791-31-9	Monamid® 1159
CAS 61791-31-9	Accomid C	CAS 61791-31-9	Monamid® C-305
CAS 61791-31-9	Afmide™ C	CAS 61791-31-9	Monamid® C-310
CAS 61791-31-9	Alkamide® 2204	CAS 61791-31-9	Monamine ADD-100
CAS 61791-31-9	Alkamide® CL63	CAS 61791-31-9	Naxonol™ CO
CAS 61791-31-9	Amidex CE	CAS 61791-31-9	Naxonol™ PN 66
CAS 61791-31-9	Amidex KD	CAS 61791-31-9	Naxonol™ PO
CAS 61791-31-9	Amidex KDO	CAS 61791-31-9	Ninol® 40-CO
CAS 61791-31-9	Aminol COR-4C	CAS 61791-31-9	Ninol® 49-CE
CAS 61791-31-9	Aminol HCA	CAS 61791-31-9	Ninol® GR
CAS 61791-31-9	Calamide C	CAS 61791-31-9	Norfox® DCS
CAS 61791-31-9	Carsamide® CA	CAS 61791-31-9	Norfox® DCSA
CAS 61791-31-9	Carsamide® CAO	CAS 61791-31-9	Norfox® DOSA
CAS 61791-31-9	Comperlan® COD	CAS 61791-31-9	Norfox® KD
CAS 61791-31-9	Comperlan® KD	CAS 61791-31-9	Olamida CD
CAS 61791-31-9	Comperlan® KDO	CAS 61791-31-9	Oramide DL 200 AF
CAS 61791-31-9	Comperlan® PD	CAS 61791-31-9	Profan 2012E
CAS 61791-31-9	Comperlan® SD	CAS 61791-31-9	Profan 24 Extra, 128 Extra
CAS 61791-31-9	Comperlan® SDO	CAS 61791-31-9	Protamide CKD
CAS 61791-31-9	Emalex N-83	CAS 61791-31-9	Protamide DCA
CAS 61791-31-9	Emid® 6515	CAS 61791-31-9	Protamide DCAW
CAS 61791-31-9	Emid® 6521	CAS 61791-31-9	Protamide HCA
CAS 61791-31-9	Empilan® CDE	CAS 61791-31-9	Purton CFD
CAS 61791-31-9	Empilan® CDE/FF	CAS 61791-31-9	Rewomid® DC 212 LS
CAS 61791-31-9	Esi-Det CDA	CAS 61791-31-9	Rewomid® DC 212 S
CAS 61791-31-9	Esi-Terge 10	CAS 61791-31-9	Rewomid® DC 212 SE

CAS 61791-31-9	Rewomid® DC 220 SE	CAS 61791-59-1	Hamposyl® C-30
CAS 61791-31-9	Ritamide C	CAS 61791-59-1	Medialan KA
CAS 61791-31-9	Rolamid CD	CAS 61791-59-1	Nikkol Sarcosinate CN-30
CAS 61791-31-9	Stamid HT 3901	CAS 61791-59-1	Vanseal® NACS-30
CAS 61791-31-9	Standamid® KD	CAS 61792-31-2	Chimin LMO
CAS 61791-31-9	Standamid® KDO	CAS 61792-31-2	Mackamine™ LAO
CAS 61791-31-9	Standamid® PK-KD	CAS 61970-18-9	Armeen® SD
CAS 61791-31-9	Standamid® PK-KDO	CAS 62755-21-9	Elfan® NS 243 S Mg
CAS 61791-31-9	Standamid® PK-KDS	CAS 62755-21-9	Empicol® EGC
CAS 61791-31-9	Standamid® PK-SD	CAS 62755-21-9	Texapon® MG
CAS 61791-31-9	Standamid® SD	CAS 62755-21-9	Tylorol MG
CAS 61791-31-9	Standamid® SDO	CAS 62755-21-9	Unipol MGLES
CAS 61791-31-9	Synotol CN 80	CAS 62755-21-9	Zoharpon MgES
CAS 61791-31-9	Synotol CN 90	CAS 63084-98-0	Rodol PS
CAS 61791-31-9	Tohol N-220	CAS 63231-60-7	Be Square® 175
CAS 61791-31-9	Tohol N-220X	CAS 63231-60-7	Be Square® 185
CAS 61791-31-9	T-Tergamide 1CD	CAS 63231-60-7	Be Square® 195
CAS 61791-31-9	Ufanon K-80	CAS 63231-60-7	CS-2080W
CAS 61791-31-9	Ufanon KD-S	CAS 63231-60-7	Emerwax® 1253
CAS 61791-31-9	Unamide® C-72-3	CAS 63231-60-7	Florabeads Micro 28/60 White
CAS 61791-31-9	Unamide® D-10	CAS 63231-60-7	Fortex®
CAS 61791-31-9	Unamide® LDL	CAS 63231-60-7	Koster Keunen Microcrystalline
CAS 61791-31-9	Upamide CA-20		Wax 170/180
CAS 61791-31-9	Upamide CS-148	CAS 63231-60-7	Mekon® White
CAS 61791-31-9	Upamide KD	CAS 63231-60-7	Multiwax® 180-M
CAS 61791-31-9	Varamide® A-2	CAS 63231-60-7	Multiwax® 180-W
CAS 61791-31-9	Varamide® A-10	CAS 63231-60-7	Multiwax® ML-445
CAS 61791-31-9	Varamide® A-12	CAS 63231-60-7	Multiwax® W-445
CAS 61791-31-9	Varamide® A-80	CAS 63231-60-7	Multiwax® W-835
CAS 61791-31-9	Varamide® A-83	CAS 63231-60-7	Multiwax® X-145A
CAS 61791-31-9	Varamide® A-84	CAS 63231-60-7	Permulgin 835
CAS 61791-31-9	Varamide® MA-1	CAS 63231-60-7	Petrolite® C-700
CAS 61791-31-9	Witcamide® 128T	CAS 63231-60-7	Petrolite® C-1035
CAS 61791-31-9	Witcamide® 6404	CAS 63231-60-7	Starwax® 100
CAS 61791-31-9	Witcamide® 6514	CAS 63231-60-7	Ultraflex®
CAS 61791-31-9	Witcamide® 6531	CAS 63231-60-7	Victory®
CAS 61791-31-9	Witcamide® 6625	CAS 63231-63-0	Atomergic Ribonucleic Acid
CAS 61791-31-9	Witcamide® CD	CAS 63250-25-9	Eusolex® 8020
CAS 61791-31-9	Witcamide® CDA	CAS 63393-82-8	Neodol® 25
CAS 61791-31-9	Witcamide® GR	CAS 63393-93-1	Amerlate® P
CAS 61791-31-9	Witcamide® M-3	CAS 63393-93-1	Amerlate® W
CAS 61791-31-9	Witcamide® S771	CAS 63393-93-1	Fancol IPL
CAS 61791-31-9	Witcamide® S780	CAS 63393-93-1	Fancor IPL
CAS 61791-32-0	Rewoteric® AM 2C NM	CAS 63393-93-1	Ivarlan™ 3350
CAS 61791-34-2	Forestall	CAS 63393-93-1	Lanesta L
CAS 61791-38-6	Schercozoline C	CAS 63393-93-1	Lanesta S
CAS 61791-38-6	Varine C	CAS 63393-93-1	Lanesta SA-30
CAS 61791-39-7	Varine T	CAS 63393-93-1	Lanisolate
CAS 61791-42-2	Adinol CT95	CAS 63393-93-1	Ritasol
CAS 61791-42-2	Geropon® TC-42	CAS 63663-21-8	Gelling Agent GP-1
CAS 61791-44-4	Accomeen T2	CAS 63793-60-2	Acconon MA3
CAS 61791-44-4	Accomeen T5	CAS 63793-60-2	Carsonon® 144-P
CAS 61791-44-4	Desomeen® TA-2	CAS 63793-60-2	Hetoxol MP-3
CAS 61791-44-4	Desomeen® TA-5	CAS 63793-60-2	Procol PMA-3
CAS 61791-44-4	Hodag CSA-86	CAS 63793-60-2	Promyristyl PM-3
CAS 61791-44-4	Mazeen® T-2	CAS 63793-60-2	Witconol™ APM
CAS 61791-44-4	Mazeen® T-5	CAS 64742-14-9	Penreco 2251 Oil
CAS 61791-44-4	Varonic® T-202	CAS 64742-42-3	Koster Keunen Microcrystalline
CAS 61791-44-4	Varonic® T-202 SF		Wax 193/198
CAS 61791-44-4	Varonic® T-202 SR	CAS 64742-42-3	Koster Keunen Microcrystalline
CAS 61791-44-4	Varonic® T-205		Waxes
CAS 61791-44-4	Varonic® T-205 SF	CAS 64742-47-8	Isopar® M
CAS 61791-46-6	Chemoxide T	CAS 64742-47-8	Penreco 2263 Oil
CAS 61791-47-7	Aromox® C/12-W	CAS 64742-48-9	Isopar® G
CAS 61791-47-7	Schercamox CMA	CAS 64742-48-9	Isopar® H
CAS 61791-56-8	Deriphat® 154	CAS 64742-48-9	Isopar® K
CAS 61791-56-8	Deriphat® 154L	CAS 64742-48-9	Isopar® L
CAS 61791-56-8	Mirataine® T2C-30	CAS 65060-02-8	Catigene® CT 70
CAS 61791-59-1	Closyl 30 2089	CAS 65072-00-6	Edamin S
CAS 61791-59-1	Crodasinic CS	CAS 65072-00-6	EPCH

CAS 65072-00-6	Glycoproteins from Milk
CAS 65072-00-6	Hy Case Amino
CAS 65072-00-6	Hy Case SF
CAS 65072-00-6	Hydromilk™ EN-20
CAS 65072-00-6	Milkamino™ 20
CAS 65072-00-6	Milkpro
CAS 65072-00-6	Promois Milk
CAS 65215-54-5	Iramine
CAS 65235-31-6	Imexine FH
CAS 65381-09-1	Captex® 300
CAS 65381-09-1	Captex® 355
CAS 65381-09-1	Emalex K.T.G
CAS 65381-09-1	Estasan GT 8-40 3578
CAS 65381-09-1	Estasan GT 8-60 3575
CAS 65381-09-1	Estasan GT 8-60 3580
CAS 65381-09-1	Estasan GT 8-65 3577
CAS 65381-09-1	Estasan GT 8-65 3581
CAS 65381-09-1	Estol GTC 3599
CAS 65381-09-1	Estol GTCC 60 3604
CAS 65381-09-1	Hodag CC-33
CAS 65381-09-1	Hodag CC-33-F
CAS 65381-09-1	Hodag CC-33-L
CAS 65381-09-1	Hodag CC-33-S
CAS 65381-09-1	Labrafac® Lipophile WL 1349
CAS 65381-09-1	Lexol® GT-855
CAS 65381-09-1	Lexol® GT-865
CAS 65381-09-1	Liponate GC
CAS 65381-09-1	Mazol® 1400
CAS 65381-09-1	Miglyol® 810
CAS 65381-09-1	Miglyol® 812
CAS 65381-09-1	Neobee® M-5
CAS 65381-09-1	Neobee® O
CAS 65381-09-1	Protachem CTG
CAS 65381-09-1	Radia® 7106
CAS 65381-09-1	Tegosoft® CT
CAS 65381-09-1	Unitolate 160-K
CAS 65497-29-2	Cationic Guar C-261
CAS 65497-29-2	Chesguar C10, C10R
CAS 65497-29-2	Chesguar C17
CAS 65497-29-2	Chesguar C20, C20R
CAS 65497-29-2	Cosmedia Guar® C-261
CAS 65497-29-2	Hi-Care® 1000
CAS 65497-29-2	Jaguar® C-13S
CAS 65497-29-2	Jaguar® C-14-S
CAS 65497-29-2	Jaguar® C-17
CAS 65497-29-2	N-Hance® 3000
CAS 65497-29-2	Rhaballgum CG-M
CAS 65497-29-2	Uniquart COSM GUAR
CAS 65591-14-2	Waxenol® 801
CAS 65694-10-2	Incroquat SBQ 75P
CAS 66009-41-4	Crodamol W
CAS 66009-41-4	Tegosoft® SH
CAS 66082-42-6	Emalex DISG-3
CAS 66082-42-6	Emerest® 2452
CAS 66082-42-6	Lameform® TGI
CAS 66082-42-6	Unimul LAM-TGI
CAS 66085-00-5	Imwitor® 780 K
CAS 66085-00-5	Schercemol GMIS
CAS 66095-81-6	Imexine FM
CAS 66161-60-2	Akyposal TIPA 45
CAS 66161-60-2	Rewopol® TLS 90 L
CAS 66422-95-5	Imexine OAJ
CAS 66455-14-9	Elfapur® LT 30 SLN
CAS 66455-14-9	Elfapur® LT 65 SLN
CAS 66455-14-9	Elfapur® LT 85/9 SLN
CAS 66455-14-9	Elfapur® LT 150 SLN
CAS 66455-14-9	Elfapur® LT 150 SN
CAS 66455-14-9	Neodol® 23-3
CAS 66455-14-9	Neodol® 23-6.5
CAS 66455-17-2;	Neodol® 91
CAS 66455-29-6	Empigen® BB
CAS 66455-29-6	Empigen® BB-AU
CAS 66625-78-3	Florabeads
CAS 66625-78-3	Jojoba 28/60 Gypsy Rose
CAS 66625-78-3	Jojoba 28/60 Jade
CAS 66625-78-3	Jojoba 28/60 White
CAS 66625-78-3	Jojoba 40/60 Mandarin
CAS 66625-78-3	Jojoba 40/60 White
CAS 66625-78-3	Jojoba 60/100 White
CAS 66625-78-3	Jojobead Gypsy Rose 40/60
CAS 66625-78-3	Jojobead Jade 40/60
CAS 66625-78-3	Jojobead Lapis 40/60
CAS 66625-78-3	Jojobead White 28/60
CAS 66625-78-3	Nikkol Jojoba Wax
CAS 66794-58-9	Crillet 6
CAS 66794-58-9	Isoixol 6
CAS 66794-58-9	Montanox 70
CAS 66794-58-9	Montanox 71
CAS 66794-58-9	Nikkol TI-10
CAS 66794-58-9	Sorbilene ISM
CAS 66828-20-4	Nikkol GS-6
CAS 66988-04-3	Crolactil SISL
CAS 66988-04-3	Pationic® ISL
CAS 67633-57-2	Monaquat ISIES
CAS 67633-57-2	Schercoquat IIS
CAS 67633-63-0	Foamquat IAES
CAS 67633-63-0	M-Quat® 522
CAS 67633-63-0	Naetex-S
CAS 67633-63-0	Schercoquat IAS
CAS 67701-00-2	Armeen® 3-16
CAS 67701-05-7;	C-108
CAS 67701-05-7;	C-110
CAS 67701-06-8	T-11
CAS 67701-06-8	T-18
CAS 67701-06-8	T-20
CAS 67701-06-8	T-22
CAS 67701-08-0	S-210
CAS 67701-27-3	Koster Keunen Japan Wax, Synthetic
CAS 67701-27-3	Koster Keunen Synthetic Japan Wax
CAS 67701-27-3	Koster Keunen Tallow Glyceride
CAS 67701-27-3	Neustrene® 060
CAS 67701-28-4	Captex® 810A
CAS 67701-28-4	Captex® 810B
CAS 67701-28-4	Captex® 810C
CAS 67701-28-4	Captex® 810D
CAS 67701-28-4	Captex® 910A
CAS 67701-28-4	Captex® 910B
CAS 67701-28-4	Captex® 910C
CAS 67701-28-4	Captex® 910D
CAS 67701-28-4	Miglyol® 818
CAS 67701-30-8	Radia® 7363
CAS 67701-33-1	Cutina® GMS
CAS 67701-33-1	Hefti GMM-33
CAS 67702-21-4	Empicol® EGB
CAS 67762-19-0	Empicol® EAA70
CAS 67762-19-0	Empicol® EAB
CAS 67762-19-0	Empicol® EAB70
CAS 67762-19-0	Rhodapex® EA-2
CAS 67762-27-0	Lanette® O
CAS 67762-30-5	TA-1618
CAS 67762-38-3	Radia® 7060
CAS 67762-41-8	CO-1214
CAS 67762-85-0	Silwet® L-7001
CAS 67762-87-2	Silwet® L-7002
CAS 67763-18-2	Bernel® Ester DISM
CAS 67763-18-2	Cosmol 222
CAS 67770-79-0	Costaulon
CAS 67784-79-6	Kessco® 3283

CAS 67784-87-6	Myvatex® 8-16	CAS 68139-30-0	Mafo® CSB W
CAS 67784-87-6	Myverol® 18-04	CAS 68139-30-0	Mafo® KCOSB 50
CAS 67799-04-6	Chemidex SI	CAS 68139-30-0	Protachem JS
CAS 67799-04-6	Mackine™ 401	CAS 68139-30-0	Rewoteric® AM CAS
CAS 67799-04-6	Schercodine I	CAS 68139-30-0	Rewoteric® AM CAS
CAS 67846-16-6	Schercoquat SAS	CAS 68139-30-0	Rewoteric® AM CAS-15
CAS 67999-57-9	Geronol ACR/9	CAS 68139-30-0	Sandobet SC
CAS 67999-57-9	Geropon® ACR/9	CAS 68139-30-0	Schercotaine SCAB
CAS 67999-57-9	Mackanate™ A-103	CAS 68139-30-0	Zohartaine CBS
CAS 68002-61-9	Radiaquat® 6471	CAS 68140-00-1	Ablumide CME
CAS 68002-71-1	Neustrene® 064	CAS 68140-00-1	Afmide™ CMA
CAS 68002-72-2	Neustrene® 053	CAS 68140-00-1	Alkamide® C-212
CAS 68002-79-9	Radia® 7370	CAS 68140-00-1	Alkamide® CME
CAS 68002-97-1	Empilan® KB 2	CAS 68140-00-1	Amidex CME
CAS 68002-97-1	Empilan® KB 3	CAS 68140-00-1	Amidex KME
CAS 68002-97-1	Rhodasurf® L-4	CAS 68140-00-1	Aminol CM, CM Flakes, CM-C
CAS 68003-46-3	Hamposyl® AL-30		Flakes, CM-D Flakes
CAS 68015-98-5	Rodol EOX	CAS 68140-00-1	Carsamide® CMEA
CAS 68037-49-0	Hostapur SAS 30	CAS 68140-00-1	Chimipal MC
CAS 68037-49-0	Hostapur SAS 60	CAS 68140-00-1	Comperlan® 100
CAS 68037-49-0	Hostapur SAS 93	CAS 68140-00-1	Comperlan® P 100
CAS 68037-93-4	Amine 2M16D	CAS 68140-00-1	Emid® 6500
CAS 68039-13-4	Lexquat® 2240	CAS 68140-00-1	Empilan® CME
CAS 68039-13-4	Nalquat 2240	CAS 68140-00-1	Empilan® CM/F
CAS 68039-13-4	Polycare® 133	CAS 68140-00-1	Foamole M
CAS 68039-49-6	Belal	CAS 68140-00-1	Hetamide CMA
CAS 68081-96-9	Empicol® AL30	CAS 68140-00-1	Hetamide CME
CAS 68081-96-9	Empicol® AL70	CAS 68140-00-1	Hetamide CME-CO
CAS 68081-97-0	Empicol® ML 26/F	CAS 68140-00-1	Incromide CME
CAS 68122-86-1	Varisoft® TIMS	CAS 68140-00-1	Lauridit® KM
CAS 68130-24-5	Liponate DPC-6	CAS 68140-00-1	Loropan CME
CAS 68130-97-2	Polymin® P SG	CAS 68140-00-1	Loropan KM
CAS 68130-97-2	Polymin® PS SG	CAS 68140-00-1	Mackamide™ CMA
CAS 68131-37-3	Maltrin® M200	CAS 68140-00-1	Mackamide™ LM-Flake
CAS 68131-37-3	Maltrin® M250	CAS 68140-00-1	Manro CMEA
CAS 68131-37-3	Maltrin® M365	CAS 68140-00-1	Manromid CMEA
CAS 68131-37-3	Maltrin® QD M600	CAS 68140-00-1	Marlamid® M 1218
CAS 68131-39-5	Bio-Soft® E-400	CAS 68140-00-1	Mazamide® CFAM
CAS 68131-39-5	Bio-Soft® EN 600	CAS 68140-00-1	Mazamide® CMEA
CAS 68131-39-5	Elfapur® LP 25 SL	CAS 68140-00-1	Mazamide® CMEA Extra
CAS 68131-39-5	Elfapur® LP 110 SLN	CAS 68140-00-1	Monamid® CMA
CAS 68131-39-5	Elfapur® SP 110 SLN	CAS 68140-00-1	Monamid® CMA-A
CAS 68131-39-5	Mulsifan RT 203/80	CAS 68140-00-1	Monamid® CMA-A/F
CAS 68131-39-5	Neodol® 25-3	CAS 68140-00-1	Monamid® CMA-A/M
CAS 68131-39-5	Neodol® 25-7	CAS 68140-00-1	Monamid® CMA/F
CAS 68131-39-5	Neodol® 25-9	CAS 68140-00-1	Monamid® CMA/M
CAS 68131-39-5	Neodol® 25-12	CAS 68140-00-1	Monamid® CMA-S
CAS 68131-39-5	Nikkol BD-2	CAS 68140-00-1	Monamid® CMA-S/F
CAS 68131-39-5	Nikkol BD-4	CAS 68140-00-1	Monamid® CMA-S/M
CAS 68131-39-5	Nikkol BD-10	CAS 68140-00-1	Monamide
CAS 68131-39-5	Rhodasurf® LA-3	CAS 68140-00-1	Ninol® CNR
CAS 68131-39-5	Teric 12A3	CAS 68140-00-1	Nissan Stafoam MF
CAS 68131-39-5	Teric 12A7	CAS 68140-00-1	Olamida CM
CAS 68131-39-5	Volpo 25 D 3	CAS 68140-00-1	Oramide ML 115
CAS 68131-39-5	Volpo 25 D 5	CAS 68140-00-1	Phoenamid CMA, CMA-70
CAS 68131-39-5	Volpo 25 D 10	CAS 68140-00-1	Profan AB20
CAS 68131-39-5	Volpo 25 D 15	CAS 68140-00-1	Protamide CME
CAS 68131-39-5	Volpo 25 D 20	CAS 68140-00-1	Rewomid® C 212
CAS 68131-54-4	Alanate 351	CAS 68140-00-1	Schercomid CME
CAS 68139-30-0	Abluter CPS	CAS 68140-00-1	Standamid® KM
CAS 68139-30-0	Amonyl 675 SB	CAS 68140-00-1	Standamid® SM
CAS 68139-30-0	Chembetaine CAS	CAS 68140-00-1	Synotol ME 90
CAS 68139-30-0	Crosultaine C-50	CAS 68140-00-1	Upamide SM
CAS 68139-30-0	Lexaine® CSB-50	CAS 68140-00-1	Varamide® C-212
CAS 68139-30-0	Lonzaine® CS	CAS 68140-00-1	Zoramide CM
CAS 68139-30-0	Lonzaine® JS	CAS 68140-01-2	Chemidex C
CAS 68139-30-0	Mackam™ CBS-50	CAS 68140-01-2	Chemidex WC
CAS 68139-30-0	Mackam™ CBS-50G	CAS 68140-01-2	Lexamine C-13
CAS 68139-30-0	Mafo® CSB	CAS 68140-01-2	Mackine™ 101
CAS 68139-30-0	Mafo® CSB 50	CAS 68140-01-2	Schercodine C

CAS 68140-01-2	Witcamine® 100	CAS 68201-49-0	Protalan Wax
CAS 68140-98-7	Alkaterge®-E	CAS 68201-49-0	R.I.T.A. Lanolin Wax
CAS 68153-28-6	Dascare FSP Liq.	CAS 68201-49-0	Unilan W
CAS 68153-28-6	Octaprotein	CAS 68238-35-1	Kera-Tein AA-SD
CAS 68153-28-6	Tofupro-U	CAS 68238-35-7	Crotein HKP/SF
CAS 68153-63-9	Marlamid® M 1618	CAS 68238-35-7	Kerabiol
CAS 68154-36-9	Radiasurf® 7125	CAS 68238-35-7	Keramino™ 20
CAS 68155-09-9	Ablumox CAPO	CAS 68238-35-7	Keramino™ 25
CAS 68155-09-9	Afamine™ CAO	CAS 68238-35-7	Kera-Tein AA
CAS 68155-09-9	Aminoxid WS 35	CAS 68238-35-7	Monteine KL 150
CAS 68155-09-9	Ammonyx® CDO	CAS 68239-42-9	Glucam® E-10
CAS 68155-09-9	Amyx CDO 3599	CAS 68239-42-9	Grillocam E10
CAS 68155-09-9	Barlox® C	CAS 68239-42-9	Prox-onic MG-010
CAS 68155-09-9	Chemoxide CAW	CAS 68239-43-0	Aloxe MG-20
CAS 68155-09-9	Chimin CMO	CAS 68239-43-0	Glucam® E-20
CAS 68155-09-9	Emcol® CDO	CAS 68239-43-0	Grillocam E20
CAS 68155-09-9	Empigen® OS/A	CAS 68239-43-0	Prox-onic MG-020
CAS 68155-09-9	Empigen® OS/AU	CAS 68239-81-6	Rodol EGS
CAS 68155-09-9	Finamine CO	CAS 68239-84-9	Rodol DEMAPS
CAS 68155-09-9	Foamox CDO	CAS 68308-64-5	Dextrol AS-150
CAS 68155-09-9	Incromine Oxide C	CAS 68311-03-5	Mackanate™ A-102
CAS 68155-09-9	Incromine Oxide C-35	CAS 68333-82-4	Amidex CIPA
CAS 68155-09-9	Mackamine™ CAO	CAS 68333-82-4	Rewomid® IPP 240
CAS 68155-09-9	Mazox® CAPA	CAS 68333-82-4	Witcamide® PPA
CAS 68155-09-9	Mazox® CAPA-37	CAS 68334-00-9	C-Flakes
CAS 68155-09-9	Monalux CAO-35	CAS 68334-00-9	Emvelop®
CAS 68155-09-9	Ninox® FCA	CAS 68334-00-9	Lipex 109
CAS 68155-09-9	Rewominox B 204	CAS 68334-00-9	Lubritab®
CAS 68155-09-9	Rhodamox® CAPO	CAS 68334-00-9	Sterotex® NF
CAS 68155-09-9	Schercamox C-AA	CAS 68334-21-4	Empigen® CDR60
CAS 68155-09-9	Standamox CAW	CAS 68334-21-4	Schercoteric MS
CAS 68155-09-9	Tegamine® Oxide WS-35	CAS 68334-28-1	BBS
CAS 68155-09-9	Unimox CAW	CAS 68334-28-1	Cremeol HF-52, HF-62
CAS 68155-09-9	Varox® 1770	CAS 68334-28-1	Hydrokote® 95
CAS 68155-09-9	Zoramox	CAS 68334-28-1	Hydrokote® 97
CAS 68155-20-4	Hetamide DT	CAS 68334-28-1	Hydrokote® 102
CAS 68155-20-4	Schercomid SO-T	CAS 68334-28-1	Hydrokote® 108
CAS 68155-24-8	Ethomid® HT/23	CAS 68334-28-1	Hydrokote® 112
CAS 68155-24-8	Ethomid® HT/60	CAS 68334-28-1	Hydrokote® 118
CAS 68171-33-5	Schercemol 318	CAS 68334-28-1	Hydrokote® AR, HL
CAS 68171-38-0	Emerest® 2384	CAS 68334-28-1	Hydrokote® RM
CAS 68171-38-0	Emerest® 2389	CAS 68334-28-1	Lipo SS
CAS 68171-38-0	Hydrophilol ISO	CAS 68334-28-1	Sterotex®
CAS 68171-38-0	Prisorine PMIS 2034	CAS 68334-28-1	Wecobee® FW
CAS 68171-38-0	Unitolate PGIST	CAS 68334-28-1	Wecobee® M
CAS 68171-38-0	Witconol™ 2384	CAS 68334-28-1	Wecobee® S
CAS 68184-04-3	Akyposal MLES 35	CAS 68334-28-1	Wecobee® SS
CAS 68187-29-1	Amisoft CT-12	CAS 68334-28-1	Wecobee® W
CAS 68187-32-6	Amisoft CS-11	CAS 68389-70-8	Glucamate® SSE-20
CAS 68187-32-6	Hostapon KCG	CAS 68389-70-8	Grillocose PSE-20
CAS 68188-18-1	Mersolat H 95	CAS 68390-99-8	Aromox® DMHT
CAS 68188-30-7	Chemidex SO	CAS 68390-99-8	Aromox® DMHTD
CAS 68188-30-7	Mackine™ 901	CAS 68410-69-5	Rewoquat W 222 PG
CAS 68188-38-5	Bio-Pol® NCHAP	CAS 68411-27-8	Crodamol AB
CAS 68188-38-5	Foam-Coll™ SK	CAS 68411-27-8	Finsolv® TN
CAS 68188-38-5	Geliderm 3000 P	CAS 68411-31-4	Marlopon® AT 50
CAS 68188-38-5	Geliderm 3000 S	CAS 68411-97-2	Crodasinic C
CAS 68188-38-5	Hostapon SCHC	CAS 68411-97-2	Hamposyl® C
CAS 68188-38-5	Hostapon SCHC-Powd.	CAS 68411-97-2	Hamposyl® CZ
CAS 68188-38-5	May-Tein SK	CAS 68411-97-2	Vanseal® CS
CAS 68188-38-5	Monteine LCS 30	CAS 68424-43-1	Amerlate® LFA
CAS 68188-38-5	Nikkol CCN-40	CAS 68424-43-1	Amerlate® WFA
CAS 68188-38-5	Promois ECS	CAS 68424-43-1	Argonol LFA Dist.
CAS 68201-49-0	Albalan	CAS 68424-43-1	Argowax LFA Distilled
CAS 68201-49-0	Fancor Lanwax	CAS 68424-43-1	Argowax LFA Standard
CAS 68201-49-0	Lanfrax®	CAS 68424-43-1	Facilan
CAS 68201-49-0	Lanfrax® 1776	CAS 68424-43-1	Fancor LFA
CAS 68201-49-0	Lanfrax® 1779	CAS 68424-43-1	Ritalafa®
CAS 68201-49-0	Lanocerin®	CAS 68424-45-3	Industrene® 20
CAS 68201-49-0	Lanowax	CAS 68424-45-3	L-310

CAS 68424-59-9	Fancol Karite Extract	CAS 68425-47-8	Witcamide® SSA
CAS 68424-60-2	Cetiol® SB45	CAS 68425-50-3	Chemidex T
CAS 68424-60-2	Fancol Karite Butter	CAS 68439-46-3	Teric 9A6
CAS 68424-60-2	Karite Butter	CAS 68439-49-6	Acconon W230
CAS 68424-60-2	Kelisema Natural Pure Shea Butter	CAS 68439-49-6	Britex CS 110
		CAS 68439-49-6	Britex CS 200 B
CAS 68424-60-2	Lipex 102	CAS 68439-49-6	Britex CS 250
CAS 68424-60-2	Lipex 202	CAS 68439-49-6	Britex CS 300
CAS 68424-60-2	Lipex 205	CAS 68439-49-6	Britex CS 1000
CAS 68424-60-2	Shea Butter	CAS 68439-49-6	Cremophor® A 6
CAS 68424-60-2	Shebu® Refined	CAS 68439-49-6	Cremophor® A 11
CAS 68424-60-2	Unimulse	CAS 68439-49-6	Cremophor® A 25
CAS 68424-61-3	Radiasurf® 7150	CAS 68439-49-6	Elfapur® T 130 S
CAS 68424-66-8	Hetlan OH	CAS 68439-49-6	Empilan® KM 11
CAS 68424-66-8	Hidroxilan	CAS 68439-49-6	Empilan® KM 50
CAS 68424-66-8	Hydroxylan	CAS 68439-49-6	Emthox® 5885
CAS 68424-66-8	Ivarlan™ OH	CAS 68439-49-6	Emulgator B-6
CAS 68424-66-8	Landrox	CAS 68439-49-6	Emulgator E 2568
CAS 68424-66-8	OHlan®	CAS 68439-49-6	Eumulgin® B1
CAS 68424-66-8	Protalan H	CAS 68439-49-6	Eumulgin® B2
CAS 68424-66-8	Ritahydrox	CAS 68439-49-6	Eumulgin® B3
CAS 68424-85-1	Hyamine® 3500 50%	CAS 68439-49-6	G-4822
CAS 68424-94-2	Amonyl 265 BA	CAS 68439-49-6	G-4936
CAS 68424-94-2	Ampho B11-34	CAS 68439-49-6	G-4938
CAS 68424-94-2	Ampholan® E210	CAS 68439-49-6	G-4940
CAS 68424-94-2	Amphoteen BCM-30	CAS 68439-49-6	G-70147
CAS 68424-94-2	Chembetaine CB	CAS 68439-49-6	Hetoxol 15 CSA
CAS 68424-94-2	Dehyton® AB-30	CAS 68439-49-6	Hetoxol CS-4
CAS 68424-94-2	Emcol® CC 37-18	CAS 68439-49-6	Hetoxol CS-5
CAS 68424-94-2	Incronam CD-30	CAS 68439-49-6	Hetoxol CS-9
CAS 68424-94-2	Lonzaine® 12C	CAS 68439-49-6	Hetoxol CS-15
CAS 68424-94-2	Mackam™ CB-35	CAS 68439-49-6	Hetoxol CS-20
CAS 68424-94-2	Mafo® CB 40	CAS 68439-49-6	Hetoxol CS-30
CAS 68424-94-2	Protachem CB 45	CAS 68439-49-6	Hetoxol CS-40
CAS 68424-94-2	Radiateric® 6860	CAS 68439-49-6	Hetoxol CS-40W
CAS 68424-94-2	Surfax ACB	CAS 68439-49-6	Hetoxol CS-50
CAS 68424-94-2	Unibetaine AB-30, AB-45	CAS 68439-49-6	Hetoxol CS-50 Special
CAS 68424-94-2	Velvetex® AB-45	CAS 68439-49-6	Hetoxol CSA-15
CAS 68425-17-2	A-611	CAS 68439-49-6	Hodag Nonionic CS-2
CAS 68425-17-2	Hystar® 3375	CAS 68439-49-6	Hodag Nonionic CS-5
CAS 68425-17-2	Hystar® 4075	CAS 68439-49-6	Hodag Nonionic CS-10
CAS 68425-17-2	Hystar® 5875	CAS 68439-49-6	Hodag Nonionic CS-15
CAS 68425-17-2	Hystar® 6075	CAS 68439-49-6	Hodag Nonionic CS-20
CAS 68425-17-2	Hystar® 7000	CAS 68439-49-6	Hodag Nonionic CS-40
CAS 68425-17-2	Hystar® CG	CAS 68439-49-6	Hostacerin T-3
CAS 68425-17-2	Hystar® HM-75	CAS 68439-49-6	Incropol CS-12
CAS 68425-17-2	Hystar® TPF	CAS 68439-49-6	Incropol CS-20
CAS 68425-17-2	Lipo Polyol NC	CAS 68439-49-6	Incropol CS-40
CAS 68425-36-5	Witarix® 450	CAS 68439-49-6	Incropol CS-60
CAS 68425-37-6	CO-618	CAS 68439-49-6	Lipocol SC-4
CAS 68425-37-6	Radianol® 1728	CAS 68439-49-6	Lipocol SC-6
CAS 68425-42-3	Mackalene™ 116	CAS 68439-49-6	Lipocol SC-8
CAS 68425-43-4	Afalene™ 117	CAS 68439-49-6	Lipocol SC-10
CAS 68425-43-4	Foamid 117	CAS 68439-49-6	Lipocol SC-12
CAS 68425-43-4	Incromate CDP	CAS 68439-49-6	Lipocol SC-15
CAS 68425-43-4	Mackalene™ 117	CAS 68439-49-6	Lipocol SC-20
CAS 68425-43-4	Mackam™ CAP	CAS 68439-49-6	Lipocol SC-30
CAS 68425-47-8	Afmide™ S	CAS 68439-49-6	Lowenol C-279
CAS 68425-47-8	Alkamide® DIN-295/S	CAS 68439-49-6	Macol® CSA-2
CAS 68425-47-8	Alkamide® SDO	CAS 68439-49-6	Macol® CSA-4
CAS 68425-47-8	Amidex S	CAS 68439-49-6	Macol® CSA-10
CAS 68425-47-8	Comperlan® VOD	CAS 68439-49-6	Macol® CSA-15
CAS 68425-47-8	Empigen® 2125-AU	CAS 68439-49-6	Macol® CSA-20
CAS 68425-47-8	Empilan® 2125-AU	CAS 68439-49-6	Macol® CSA-40
CAS 68425-47-8	Mackamide™ S	CAS 68439-49-6	Marlipal® 1618/11
CAS 68425-47-8	Mackamide™ SD	CAS 68439-49-6	Marlowet® TA 6
CAS 68425-47-8	Manromid 150-ADY	CAS 68439-49-6	Marlowet® TA 8
CAS 68425-47-8	Marlamid® DF 1818	CAS 68439-49-6	Marlowet® TA 10
CAS 68425-47-8	Schercomid SLS	CAS 68439-49-6	Marlowet® TA 25
CAS 68425-47-8	Stamid LS 5487	CAS 68439-49-6	Procol CS-3

CAS 68439-49-6	Procol CS-4	CAS 68441-17-8	A-C® 395, 395A
CAS 68439-49-6	Procol CS-5	CAS 68441-17-8	A-C® 629, 629A
CAS 68439-49-6	Procol CS-6	CAS 68441-17-8	A-C® 655
CAS 68439-49-6	Procol CS-8	CAS 68441-17-8	A-C® 656
CAS 68439-49-6	Procol CS-10	CAS 68441-17-8	A-C® 6702
CAS 68439-49-6	Procol CS-12	CAS 68441-17-8	ACuscrub® 31
CAS 68439-49-6	Procol CS-15	CAS 68441-17-8	ACuscrub® 32
CAS 68439-49-6	Procol CS-17	CAS 68441-17-8	ACuscrub® 51
CAS 68439-49-6	Procol CS-20	CAS 68441-68-9	Crodamol PTC
CAS 68439-49-6	Procol CS-27	CAS 68441-68-9	Lipo PE 810
CAS 68439-49-6	Procol CS-30	CAS 68441-68-9	Liponate PE-810
CAS 68439-49-6	Prox-onic CSA-1/04	CAS 68441-68-9	Radia® 7178
CAS 68439-49-6	Prox-onic CSA-1/06	CAS 68458-51-5	Lamepon® LPO
CAS 68439-49-6	Prox-onic CSA-1/010	CAS 68458-58-8	Fluilan AWS
CAS 68439-49-6	Prox-onic CSA-1/015	CAS 68458-58-8	Ivarlan™ AWS
CAS 68439-49-6	Prox-onic CSA-1/020	CAS 68458-58-8	Lantrol® AWS 1692
CAS 68439-49-6	Prox-onic CSA-1/030	CAS 68458-58-8	Ritalan® AWS
CAS 68439-49-6	Prox-onic CSA-1/050	CAS 68458-58-8	Unilaneth PPG-12-PEG-65
CAS 68439-49-6	Rhodasurf® C-20	CAS 68458-58-8	Vigilan AWS
CAS 68439-49-6	Ritacet-20	CAS 68458-88-8	Hetlan AWS
CAS 68439-49-6	Simulsol CS	CAS 68458-88-8	Ivarlan™ 3420
CAS 68439-49-6	Tewax TC 10	CAS 68458-88-8	Laneto AWS
CAS 68439-49-6	Unicol CSA-2	CAS 68458-88-8	Lanexol AWS
CAS 68439-49-6	Unicol CSA-4	CAS 68458-88-8	Lanoil AWS
CAS 68439-49-6	Unicol CSA-5	CAS 68459-50-7	Agnosol 3
CAS 68439-49-6	Unicol CSA-10	CAS 68459-50-7	Agnosol 5
CAS 68439-49-6	Unicol CSA-15	CAS 68459-50-7	Lanpol 5
CAS 68439-49-6	Unicol CSA-20	CAS 68459-50-7	Lanpol 10
CAS 68439-49-6	Unicol CSA-30	CAS 68459-50-7	Lanpol 20
CAS 68439-49-6	Unicol CSA-40	CAS 68476-03-9	Hoechst Wax E Pharma
CAS 68439-49-6	Unimul-B-1	CAS 68476-03-9	Hoechst Wax SW
CAS 68439-49-6	Unimul-B-2	CAS 68479-64-1	Schercopol OMS-Na
CAS 68439-49-6	Unimul-B-3	CAS 68513-95-1	Centex
CAS 68439-49-6	Varonic® 63 E20	CAS 68513-95-1	Emcosoy®
CAS 68439-49-6	Volpo CS-3	CAS 68515-65-1	Afanate™ CP
CAS 68439-49-6	Volpo CS-5	CAS 68515-65-1	Mackanate™ CP
CAS 68439-49-6	Volpo CS-10	CAS 68515-65-1	Monamate C-1142
CAS 68439-49-6	Volpo CS-15	CAS 68515-65-1	Monamate CPA-40
CAS 68439-49-6	Volpo CS-20	CAS 68515-65-1	Monamate CPA-100
CAS 68439-50-9	Alfonic® 1412-3	CAS 68515-73-1	Oramix CG 110-60
CAS 68439-50-9	Dehydol® LS 2 DEO	CAS 68515-73-1	Triton® CG-110
CAS 68439-50-9	Dehydol® LS 3 DEO	CAS 68517-10-2	Prisorine MIS 3760
CAS 68439-50-9	Dehydol® LS 4 DEO	CAS 68541-50-4	Nikkol Trialan 318
CAS 68439-50-9	Genapol® 24-L-3	CAS 68541-50-4	Salacos 6318
CAS 68439-50-9	Genapol® 42-L-3	CAS 68551-12-2	Alfonic® 1216-1.5
CAS 68439-50-9	Surfonic® L24-3	CAS 68551-12-2	Genapol® 26-L-1
CAS 68439-50-9	Surfonic® L24-7	CAS 68553-81-1	EmCon Rice Bran
CAS 68439-51-0	Aethoxal® B	CAS 68554-53-0	Abil®-Wax 2434
CAS 68439-53-2	Hetoxol PLA	CAS 68554-65-4	Silwet® L-720
CAS 68439-53-2	Solulan® PB-2	CAS 68555-36-2	Mirapol® A-15
CAS 68439-53-2	Solulan® PB-5	CAS 68583-51-7	Captex® 200
CAS 68439-53-2	Solulan® PB-10	CAS 68583-51-7	Myritol® PC
CAS 68439-53-2	Solulan® PB-20	CAS 68585-34-2	Empicol® ESA
CAS 68439-53-2	Wickenol® 727	CAS 68585-34-2	Empicol® ESA70
CAS 68439-57-6	Bio-Terge® AS-40	CAS 68585-34-2	Empicol® ESB70
CAS 68439-57-6	Calsoft AOS-40	CAS 68585-34-2	Empicol® ESC/AU
CAS 68439-57-6	Carsonol® AOS	CAS 68585-34-2	Empicol® ESC3
CAS 68439-57-6	Elfan® OS 46	CAS 68585-34-2	Rhodapex® ES-2
CAS 68439-57-6	Norfox® ALPHA XL	CAS 68585-34-2	Rhodapex® ESY
CAS 68439-57-6	Rhodacal® 301-10F	CAS 68585-34-2	Tensagex EOC 628
CAS 68439-57-6	Rhodacal® A-246L	CAS 68585-34-2	Tensagex EOC 670
CAS 68439-57-6	Rhodacal® A-246 LX	CAS 68585-44-4	Empicol® 0031/T
CAS 68439-57-6	Witconate™ AOK	CAS 68585-44-4	Empicol® DA
CAS 68439-57-6	Witconate™ AOS	CAS 68585-47-4	Empicol® LX
CAS 68439-57-6	Witconate™ AOS-EP	CAS 68585-47-7	Empicol® LS30P
CAS 68439-57-6	Witconate™ AOS-PC	CAS 68603-42-9	Alkamide® CDE
CAS 68439-70-3	Amine 2M14D	CAS 68603-42-9	Alkamide® CDM
CAS 68440-05-1	Empilan® CIS	CAS 68603-42-9	Alkamide® CDO
CAS 68440-66-4	Silwet® L-7500	CAS 68603-42-9	Alkamide® DC-212/S
CAS 68441-17-8	A-C® 316, 316A	CAS 68603-42-9	Alkamide® DC-212/SE

CAS 68603-42-9	Alkamide® KD
CAS 68603-42-9	Aminol KDE
CAS 68603-42-9	Chimipal DCL/M
CAS 68603-42-9	Empilan® CDX
CAS 68603-42-9	Foamid C
CAS 68603-42-9	Foamid SCE
CAS 68603-42-9	Schercomid SCE
CAS 68603-42-9	Schercomid SCO-Extra
CAS 68603-42-9	Synotol CN 60
CAS 68604-44-4	Radia® 7171
CAS 68604-71-7	Miranol® C2M-SF 70%
CAS 68604-71-7	Miranol® C2M-SF Conc.
CAS 68604-73-9	Amphoterge® SB
CAS 68604-73-9	Mackam™ CS
CAS 68604-73-9	Miranol® CS Conc.
CAS 68604-73-9	Sandoteric CFL
CAS 68604-73-9	Schercoteric MS-EP
CAS 68607-75-0	Abil®-Wax 9809
CAS 68607-88-5	Hydrane S
CAS 68607-88-5	Hydrosoy 2000/SF
CAS 68607-88-5	Pepsobiol
CAS 68607-88-5	Peptein® VgS
CAS 68607-88-5	Phylderm Vegetal
CAS 68607-88-5	Promois WS
CAS 68607-88-5	Prove HS
CAS 68607-88-5	Solu-Soy™ EN-25
CAS 68607-88-5	Sol-U-Tein 6861
CAS 68607-88-5	Sol-U-Tein FS-1000
CAS 68607-88-5	Sol-U-Tein PS-1000
CAS 68607-88-5	Sol-U-Tein VG
CAS 68607-88-5	Solu-Tofu EN-10
CAS 68607-88-5	Soypro 25
CAS 68607-88-5	Tri-K Soypro-25
CAS 68608-61-7	Miranol® SM Conc.
CAS 68608-63-9	Miranol® DM
CAS 68608-63-9	Miranol® DM Conc. 45%
CAS 68608-65-1	Ampholak XCO-40
CAS 68608-65-1	Miranol® CM Conc. NP
CAS 68608-66-2	Empigen® CDL60
CAS 68608-66-2	Miranol® BM Conc.
CAS 68608-66-2	Miranol® H2M Conc.
CAS 68608-66-2	Miranol® HM Conc.
CAS 68610-38-8	Mackam™ OS
CAS 68610-38-8	Sandopan® TFL Conc.
CAS 68610-38-8	Sandoteric TFL Conc.
CAS 68610-39-9	Mackam™ JS
CAS 68610-43-5	Miranol® H2M-SF Conc.
CAS 68630-96-6	Monateric ISA-35
CAS 68630-96-6	Schercoteric I-AA
CAS 68647-53-0	Dehyton® G
CAS 68647-53-0	Miranol® 2CIB
CAS 68647-73-4	EmCon Tea Tree
CAS 68647-77-8	Chemoxide TAO
CAS 68648-27-1	Fancol HL-20
CAS 68648-27-1	Fancol HL-24
CAS 68648-27-1	Ivarlan™ 3450
CAS 68648-27-1	Ivarlan™ 3452
CAS 68648-27-1	Ivarlan™ HL-20
CAS 68648-27-1	Lanidrol
CAS 68648-27-1	Lipolan 31
CAS 68648-27-1	Lipolan 31-20
CAS 68648-38-4	Lanoil Water/Alcohol Soluble Lanolin
CAS 68648-38-4	Rewolan® AWS
CAS 68648-66-8	Ceraphyl® GA
CAS 68648-66-8	Ceraphyl® GA-D
CAS 68649-05-8	Armeen® Z
CAS 68650-39-5	Abluter DCM-2
CAS 68650-39-5	Afoteric™ 2C
CAS 68650-39-5	Ampholak XCO-30
CAS 68650-39-5	Amphotensid GB 2009
CAS 68650-39-5	Amphoterge® W-2
CAS 68650-39-5	Chimin IMB
CAS 68650-39-5	Dehyton® PG
CAS 68650-39-5	Dehyton® W
CAS 68650-39-5	Mackam™ 2C
CAS 68650-39-5	Manroteric CDX38
CAS 68650-39-5	Miranol® C2M Conc. NP
CAS 68650-39-5	Miranol® C2M Conc. OP
CAS 68650-39-5	Miranol® FB-NP
CAS 68650-39-5	Monateric CDX-38
CAS 68650-39-5	Monateric CDX-38 Mod
CAS 68650-39-5	Monateric CLV
CAS 68650-39-5	Monateric CSH-32
CAS 68650-39-5	Proteric CDX-38
CAS 68650-39-5	Rewoteric® AM 2C W
CAS 68650-39-5	Schercoteric MS-2
CAS 68650-39-5	Sochamine A 7525
CAS 68650-39-5	Surfax AC 50
CAS 68650-39-5	Surfax ACl
CAS 68650-39-5	Unibetaine 2C
CAS 68650-39-5	Velvetex® CDC
CAS 68650-39-5	Zoharteric D
CAS 68650-39-5	Zoharteric D-SF 70%
CAS 68650-79-3	Schercodine T
CAS 68783-22-2	Schercomid HT-60
CAS 68783-24-4	Armeen® 2T
CAS 68783-41-5	Empol® 1008
CAS 68784-08-7	Schercopol CMS-Na
CAS 68797-35-3	K2 Glycyrrhizinate
CAS 68797-35-3	Nikkol Dipotassium Glycyrrhizinate
CAS 68797-35-3	Ritamectant K2
CAS 68797-65-9	Foamquat BAS
CAS 68797-65-9	Schercoquat BAS
CAS 68814-69-7	Armeen® DMTD
CAS 68814-69-7	Jet Amine DMTD
CAS 68814-69-7	Kemamine® T-9742
CAS 68815-55-4	Miranol® JBS
CAS 68815-56-5	Geropon® SBFA-30
CAS 68815-61-2	Standapol® A-215
CAS 68815-61-2	Unipol A-215
CAS 68855-56-1	Alfol® 1216
CAS 68855-56-1	Radianol® 1726
CAS 68889-49-6	Nikkol TMGO-10
CAS 68889-49-6	Nikkol TMGO-15
CAS 68890-92-6	Emery® 5327
CAS 68891-38-3	Berol 452
CAS 68891-38-3	Texapon® K-14S 70 Special
CAS 68891-39-4	Rhodapex® CO-433
CAS 68908-44-1	Empicol® LQ33
CAS 68908-44-1	Empicol® TA40
CAS 68910-56-5	Varisoft® 2TD
CAS 68915-25-3	Croquat HH
CAS 68915-25-3	Croquat WKP
CAS 68915-25-3	Keraquat HK
CAS 68915-25-3	Kera-Quat WKP
CAS 68915-25-3	Quat Keratin™ WKP
CAS 68918-77-4	Lamepon® PA-K
CAS 68918-77-4	Lamepon® PA-K/NP
CAS 68918-77-4	Lamepon® PA-TR
CAS 68918-77-4	Lamepon® PA-TR/NP
CAS 68918-77-4	Lexein® A-520
CAS 68918-77-4	Uniprolam PAJR
CAS 68919-41-5	Amphoterge® K
CAS 68919-41-5	Mackam™ CSF
CAS 68919-41-5	Miranol® CM-SF Conc.
CAS 68920-65-0	Collagen-Cocoate-Complex V 2037
CAS 68920-65-0	Foam-Coll™ 4C
CAS 68920-65-0	Lamepon® 4SK

CAS 68920-65-0	Lamepon® S	CAS 68954-89-2	Akypo RS 60
CAS 68920-65-0	Lamepon® S/NP	CAS 68954-89-2	Akypo RS 100
CAS 68920-65-0	Liprot CK	CAS 68954-89-2	Akypo RT 60
CAS 68920-65-0	Maypon 4C	CAS 68955-19-1	Empicol® LZ
CAS 68920-65-0	May-Tein C	CAS 68955-19-1	Empicol® LZ/D
CAS 68920-65-0	Monteine LCK-32	CAS 68955-19-1	Empicol® LZV
CAS 68920-65-0	Nikkol CCK-40	CAS 68955-19-1	Texapon® ZHC Needles
CAS 68920-65-0	Peptein® KC	CAS 68955-20-4	Empicol® TAS30
CAS 68920-65-0	Promois ECP	CAS 68955-20-4	Lanette® E
CAS 68920-65-0	Promois ECP-C	CAS 68955-45-3	Radia® 7506
CAS 68920-65-0	Promois ECP-P	CAS 68957-18-6	Akyposal DS 28
CAS 68920-65-0	Rewotein CPK	CAS 68957-18-6	Akyposal DS 56
CAS 68920-65-0	Texatein C	CAS 68958-48-5	Tegin® ISO NSE
CAS 68920-65-0	Unipro LAN-S	CAS 68958-64-5	Tagat® TO
CAS 68920-66-1	Britex CO 220	CAS 68966-38-1	Schercozoline I
CAS 68936-95-8	Glucate® SS	CAS 68987-89-3	Akypo®-Soft 100 NV
CAS 68936-95-8	Grillocose PS	CAS 68987-89-3	Akypo®-Soft 130 NV
CAS 68937-54-2	Silwet® L-7604	CAS 68989-03-7	Rewoquat CPEM
CAS 68937-55-3	Abil® B 8851	CAS 68990-06-7	Lamegin® GLP 10, 20
CAS 68937-55-3	Abil® B 8852	CAS 68990-07-8	Vita-Cos
CAS 68937-55-3	Abil® B 8843	CAS 68990-07-8	Wickenol® 535
CAS 68937-55-3	Abil® B 88183	CAS 68990-58-9	Lamegin® EE
CAS 68937-55-3	Abil® B 88184	CAS 68990-59-0	Acidan N 12
CAS 68937-85-9	Emery® 627	CAS 68990-59-0	Lamegin® ZE 30, 60
CAS 68937-90-6	Empol® 1045	CAS 68990-63-6	Dermane SLO
CAS 68938-15-8	Emery® 625	CAS 68990-63-6	Super Refined™ Shark Liver Oil
CAS 68938-15-8	Emery® 626	CAS 68990-82-9	Witarix® 212
CAS 68938-15-8	Hystrene® 5012	CAS 68991-68-4	Captex® 350
CAS 68938-15-8	Industrene® 223	CAS 68991-88-8	Miranol® TBS
CAS 68938-54-5	Silwet® L-7600	CAS 69028-36-0	Myverol® 18-50
CAS 68938-54-5	Silwet® L-7602	CAS 69430-24-6	Abil® B 8839
CAS 68951-67-7	Neodol® 45-7	CAS 69430-24-6	Abil® K 4
CAS 68951-89-3	Crotein ASC	CAS 69430-24-6	Amersil® VS-7158
CAS 68951-89-3	Pro-Tein ES-20	CAS 69430-24-6	Amersil® VS-7207
CAS 68951-91-7	Liprot UT	CAS 69430-24-6	Amersil® VS-7349
CAS 68951-91-7	Promois EUT	CAS 69430-24-6	Baysilone COM 10,000
CAS 68951-92-8	Lamepon® UD/NP	CAS 69430-24-6	Baysilone COM 20,000
CAS 68951-92-8	Liprot UK	CAS 69430-24-6	Belsil CM 020
CAS 68951-92-8	Maypon UD	CAS 69430-24-6	Belsil CM 025
CAS 68951-92-8	Promois EUP	CAS 69430-24-6	Belsil CM 030
CAS 68951-97-3	KF351A	CAS 69430-24-6	Belsil CM 040
CAS 68951-97-3	KF351AS	CAS 69430-24-6	Dow Corning® 244 Fluid
CAS 68952-16-9	Bio-Soft® MT 40	CAS 69430-24-6	Dow Corning® 245 Fluid
CAS 68952-16-9	Foam-Coll™ 4CT	CAS 69430-24-6	Dow Corning® 344 Fluid
CAS 68952-16-9	Granpro-10	CAS 69430-24-6	Dow Corning® 345 Fluid
CAS 68952-16-9	Lamepon® ST 40/NP	CAS 69430-24-6	KF994
CAS 68952-16-9	Lamepon® S-TR/NP	CAS 69430-24-6	KF9945
CAS 68952-16-9	Lexein® S620TA	CAS 69430-24-6	Masil® SFV
CAS 68952-16-9	Liprot CT	CAS 69430-24-6	Masil® SF-V (4)
CAS 68952-16-9	Maypon 4CT	CAS 69430-24-6	Masil® SF-V (5)
CAS 68952-16-9	May-Tein CT	CAS 69430-24-6	Masil® SF-VL
CAS 68952-16-9	Monteine LCT	CAS 69430-24-6	Masil® SF-VV
CAS 68952-16-9	Peptein® TEAC	CAS 69430-24-6	Rhodorsil® Oils 70045
CAS 68952-16-9	Promois ECT	CAS 69430-24-6	Rhodorsil® Oils 70045 V2, 70045
CAS 68952-16-9	Promois ECT-C		V3, 70045 V5
CAS 68952-16-9	Rewotein CPT	CAS 69430-24-6	SF1173
CAS 68952-16-9	Texatein CT	CAS 69430-24-6	SF1202
CAS 68953-11-7	Foamole B	CAS 69430-24-6	SF1204
CAS 68953-11-7	Incromine Mink B	CAS 69430-24-6	Silatex SF-V
CAS 68953-58-2	Bentone® 34	CAS 69430-24-6	SWS-03314
CAS 68953-58-2	Claytone 34	CAS 69430-24-6	Unisil SF-V
CAS 68953-58-2	Claytone 40	CAS 69430-24-6	Volatile Silicone 7158, 7207, 7349
CAS 68953-58-2	Claytone XL	CAS 69430-36-0	Crotein ASK
CAS 68953-58-2	Tixogel VP	CAS 69430-36-0	Crotein K
CAS 68953-64-0	Ceraphyl® 65	CAS 69430-36-0	Crotein WKP
CAS 68953-64-0	Incroquat 26	CAS 69430-36-0	Dehydrated Keratine Hydrolysate
CAS 68954-89-2	Akypo RCS 60	CAS 69430-36-0	Hidrolisado de Queratina
CAS 68954-89-2	Akypo RLM 45	CAS 69430-36-0	Hydrokeratin™ 100M
CAS 68954-89-2	Akypo RLM 130	CAS 69430-36-0	Hydrokeratin™ AL-30
CAS 68954-89-2	Akypo RLMQ 38	CAS 69430-36-0	Hydrokeratin™ AL-SD

CAS 69430-36-0	Hydrokeratin™ WKP
CAS 69430-36-0	Keramois L
CAS 69430-36-0	Kerapro S
CAS 69430-36-0	Kera-Tein 1000
CAS 69430-36-0	Kera-Tein 1000 RM/50
CAS 69430-36-0	Kera-Tein 1000 RM SD
CAS 69430-36-0	Kera-Tein 1000 SD
CAS 69430-36-0	Kera-Tein V
CAS 69430-36-0	Keratin P
CAS 69430-36-0	Keratin S
CAS 69430-36-0	Keratine Hydrolysate H.T.K
CAS 69430-36-0	Keratin Hydrolysate
CAS 69430-36-0	Nutrilan® Cashmere W
CAS 69430-36-0	Nutrilan® Keratin W
CAS 69430-36-0	Promois WK
CAS 69430-36-0	Promois WK-H
CAS 69468-44-6	Emalex GWIS-120
CAS 69468-44-6	Emalex GWIS-130
CAS 69468-44-6	Emalex GWIS-160N
CAS 69537-38-8	Akypoquat 131
CAS 69537-38-8	Akypoquat 131 V
CAS 70084-87-6	Dascare SWP
CAS 70084-87-6	Fractein HWP
CAS 70084-87-6	Granosol 25
CAS 70084-87-6	Granosol 100
CAS 70084-87-6	Hydrane W
CAS 70084-87-6	Hydrotriticum™
CAS 70084-87-6	Peptein® VgW
CAS 70084-87-6	Promois WG
CAS 70084-87-6	Prove HT
CAS 70084-87-6	Uniglaudin W
CAS 70084-87-6	Vegepro W
CAS 70084-87-6	Wheat-Pro™ EN-20
CAS 70084-94-5	Soy-Tein NL
CAS 70161-44-3	Suttocide® A
CAS 70225-05-7	Liponate TDTM
CAS 70356-09-1	Parsol® 1789
CAS 70592-80-2	Empigen® OB/AU
CAS 70609-66-4	Hostapon KTW
CAS 70632-06-3	Miranate® LEC
CAS 70632-06-3	Sandopan® DTC Linear P
CAS 70632-06-3	Surfine WNT Gel
CAS 70632-06-3	Surfine WNT LC
CAS 70632-06-3	Surfine WNT-LS
CAS 70693-04-8	Michel XO-150-1620
CAS 70693-05-9	Exxal® 26
CAS 70693-32-2	Liponate NPGC-2
CAS 70729-87-2	Parapel® LIS
CAS 70750-17-3	Akypo 23Q38
CAS 70788-37-3	Eltesol® TSX
CAS 70801-07-9	Amphomer® 4910
CAS 70801-07-9	Amphomer® LV-71
CAS 70851-07-9	Ampholak BCA-30
CAS 70851-07-9	Amphoteen BCA-30
CAS 70851-07-9	Enagicol C-30B
CAS 70851-07-9	Mirataine® BD-J
CAS 70851-07-9	Mirataine® BD-R
CAS 70851-07-9	Mirataine® BET-C-30
CAS 70851-07-9	Mirataine® CB
CAS 70851-07-9	Mirataine® CBC
CAS 70851-07-9	Mirataine® CBR
CAS 70851-07-9	Mirataine® CCB
CAS 70851-08-0	Mirataine® CBS, CBS Mod
CAS 71185-87-0	Nikkol Hexaglyn 3-S
CAS 71243-51-1	Permulgin CSB
CAS 71243-51-1	Permulgin RWB
CAS 71329-50-5	Jaguar® C-162
CAS 71566-49-9	Dermol 89
CAS 71566-49-9	Isolanoate
CAS 71566-49-9	Kessco® Octyl Isononanoate
CAS 71566-49-9	Pelemol 89
CAS 71566-49-9	Witconol™ 2300
CAS 71750-80-6	GP-RA-157 Amine Functional Silicone Fluid
CAS 71850-81-2	Varion® AM-R40
CAS 71902-01-7	Crill 6
CAS 71902-01-7	Montane 70
CAS 72319-06-3	Etha-Coll 210-20
CAS 72319-06-3	Lexein® A-200
CAS 72319-06-3	Lexein® A-210
CAS 72319-06-3	Pro-Tein SM-20
CAS 72347-89-8	Caprol® 2G4S
CAS 72388-18-2	Isofol® 28
CAS 72576-80-8	Nikkol ISP
CAS 72576-80-8	Protachem ISP
CAS 72576-81-9	Cosmol 812
CAS 72869-62-6	Radia® 7345
CAS 72869-69-3	Lipovol P
CAS 72869-69-3	Nikkol Apricot Kernel Oil
CAS 72869-69-3	Super Refined™ Apricot Kernel Oil NF
CAS 73049-73-7	European Elastin 10
CAS 73049-73-7	European Elastin 30
CAS 73049-73-7	European Elastin SD
CAS 73807-15-5	Accomid 50
CAS 73807-15-5	Accomid PK
CAS 73807-15-5	Afmide™ PK
CAS 73807-15-5	Amidex PK
CAS 73807-15-5	Mackamide™ PK
CAS 73807-15-5	T-Tergamide 1PD
CAS 74623-31-7	Pluracol® W5100N
CAS 75782-86-4;	Neodol® 23
CAS 75782-87-5;	Neodol® 45
CAS 76009-37-5	Caprol® 6G2O
CAS 76009-37-5	Plurol Oleique WL 1173
CAS 76902-90-4	Busan® 1500
CAS 78491-02-8	Germall® II
CAS 79416-55-0	Rewopal® PG 340
CAS 79665-94-4	Cremophor® GO32
CAS 79777-30-3	Nikkol Decaglyn 1-S
CAS 80062-31-3	Imexine FT
CAS 81613-56-1	Foamine O-80
CAS 81613-56-1	Naetex O-80
CAS 81613-56-1	Necon SOLC
CAS 82204-94-2	Amiter LGOD
CAS 82469-79-2	Citroflex B-6
CAS 83271-10-7	Rheopearl KL
CAS 83615-24-1	IS-CE
CAS 83682-78-4	Phospholipid PTD
CAS 83708-66-1	Nikkol ICM-R
CAS 83933-91-3	Glucate® DO
CAS 83933-91-3	Grillocose® DO
CAS 83933-91-3	Grillocose DO
CAS 84012-26-0	Mircoat™ Oil
CAS 84012-42-0	CMI 800
CAS 84069-44-3	Dascare HPCH
CAS 84069-44-3	HPCH Liq.
CAS 84082-44-0	Incronam B-40
CAS 84082-51-9	Alacen
CAS 84082-51-9	Alatal
CAS 84082-83-7	Hydroplastidine Achillea
CAS 84539-90-2	Radia® 7514
CAS 84605-13-0	Schercemol MEL-3
CAS 84605-14-1	Schercemol MEP-3
CAS 84605-15-2	Schercoquat IEP
CAS 84643-53-8	Dehyquart® E
CAS 84643-53-8	Uniquart E
CAS 84649-86-5	Unibotan Chamomile
CAS 84650-00-0	CMI 321
CAS 84650-00-0	CMI 324

CAS 84650-00-0	CMI 400	CAS 90283-04-8	Schercoquat ALA
CAS 84696-25-3	Midecol CF	CAS 90388-14-0	Crodafos CDP
CAS 84776-23-8	Hydroplastidine Calendula	CAS 90453-59-1	Akypo®-Muls 400
CAS 84776-23-8	Unibotan Calendula CLR	CAS 90529-57-0	Foamquat SOAS
CAS 84812-94-2	Afoteric™ 151C	CAS 90529-57-0	Schercoquat SOAS
CAS 84812-94-2	Ampholyte KKE-70	CAS 90605-17-7	Trioxene LV
CAS 84812-94-2	Mackam™ 151C	CAS 90624-75-2	Mirapol® AD-1
CAS 84930-16-5	Nipasol M Potassium	CAS 90730-68-0	Kemamine® BQ-2982B
CAS 84988-79-4	Radia® 7230	CAS 90989-78-9	Ceraderm S
CAS 85005-47-6	Argonol 40	CAS 91031-31-1	Radia® 7266
CAS 85049-34-9	Radia® 7204	CAS 91031-43-5	Radia® 7185
CAS 85049-36-1	Radia® 7187	CAS 91031-48-0	Cetiol® 868
CAS 85049-37-2	Radia® 7331	CAS 91031-48-0	Radia® 7131
CAS 85058-43-1	Elubiol	CAS 91031-57-1	Radia® 7510
CAS 85116-87-6	Radia® 7231	CAS 91031-88-8	Crodesta SL-40
CAS 85116-93-4	Radiasurf® 7175	CAS 91031-88-8	Grilloten® LSE 65 K
CAS 85116-97-8	Radiasurf® 7410	CAS 91031-88-8	Grilloten® LSE 65 K Soft
CAS 85186-88-5	Radia® 7355	CAS 91031-88-8	Grilloten® LSE 87 K
CAS 85251-77-0	Radiasurf® 7600	CAS 91031-88-8	Grilloten® LSE 87 K Soft
CAS 85264-33-1	Busan® 1504	CAS 91050-82-7	Radia® 7176
CAS 85341-79-3	Crodamol CSP	CAS 91052-47-0	Radiasurf® 7900
CAS 85408-76-0	Radia® 7051	CAS 91052-92-5	Melhydran®
CAS 85409-09-2	Myritol® 312	CAS 91053-41-7	Lipocerina
CAS 85409-09-2	Myritol® 318	CAS 91080-18-1	Nutrilan® Elastin E20
CAS 85409-09-2	Radia® 7108	CAS 91080-18-1	Nutrilan® Elastin P
CAS 85411-01-4	Emphos™ F27-85	CAS 91744-38-6	Imwitor® 370
CAS 85507-69-3	Activera™ 106 LIPO M	CAS 91824-88-3	Witconol™ 18L
CAS 85507-69-3	Activera™ 107 LIPO C	CAS 92044-87-6	Crodamol OC
CAS 85507-69-3	Aloe Extract #101	CAS 92044-87-6	Estol EHC 1540
CAS 85507-69-3	Aloe Vera Aqueous Extract Conc.	CAS 92044-87-6	Trioxene E
CAS 85507-69-3	Aloe Vera Lipo-Quinone Extract	CAS 92128-87-5	Basis LS-60H
CAS 85507-69-3	Aloe Vera Polysaccharide #0179121B01	CAS 92128-87-5	Emulmetik™ 320
		CAS 92128-87-5	Emulmetik™ 950
CAS 85507-69-3	Veragel® Aq. Conc. 1:10	CAS 92128-87-5	Lipoid S 75-3
CAS 85507-69-3	Veragel® Lipoid	CAS 92128-87-5	Nikkol Lecinol S-10
CAS 85508-38-9	Rewoquat RTM 50	CAS 92128-87-5	Nikkol Lecinol S-10E
CAS 85536-04-5	Radia® 7501	CAS 92128-87-5	Nikkol Lecinol S-10EX
CAS 85536-07-8	Labrasol	CAS 92128-87-5	Nikkol Lecinol S-10M
CAS 85536-07-8	L.A.S	CAS 92128-87-5	Nikkol Lecinol S-30
CAS 85536-08-9	Labrafil® M 2125 CS	CAS 92128-87-5	PhosPho H-00
CAS 85536-14-7	Marlon® AS3	CAS 92128-87-5	PhosPho H-150
CAS 85536-23-8	Aminol N	CAS 92797-39-2	Hydrolactin 2500
CAS 85586-07-8	Texapon® LS Highly Conc. Needles	CAS 92797-39-2	Lactolan®
		CAS 92797-39-2	Tri-Tein Milk Polypeptide
CAS 85586-21-6	Radia® 7110	CAS 93385-03-6	Hetester PCA
CAS 85665-33-4	Nesatol	CAS 93385-13-8	Hetester PHA
CAS 85711-45-1	Radiasurf® 7156	CAS 93455-78-8	Radiasurf® 7400
CAS 85736-49-8	Radiasurf® 7402	CAS 93572-63-5	Rewoquat DQ 35
CAS 85736-49-8	Radiasurf® 7403	CAS 93685-79-1	Permethyl® 102A
CAS 85736-49-8	Radiasurf® 7404	CAS 93803-89-5	Pelemol P-49
CAS 85736-49-8	Radiasurf® 7443	CAS 93820-52-1	Rewoteric® AM KSF-40
CAS 85736-49-8	Radiasurf® 7444	CAS 93820-97-4	Crodamol CSS
CAS 85865-69-6	Radia® 7241	CAS 93820-97-4	Estol 1481
CAS 86088-85-9	Incrosoft S-90	CAS 93820-97-4	Estol CSS 3709
CAS 86089-12-5	Rewoteric® AM R40	CAS 94423-19-5	Cremophor® GS32
CAS 86418-55-5	Cerasynt® MN	CAS 94423-19-5	Emalex DSG-3
CAS 86418-55-5	Monthybase	CAS 94552-41-7	Schercoquat ROAS
CAS 86418-55-5	Tegin® G	CAS 95032-84-1	Crotein AD
CAS 86438-78-0	Mirataine® BB	CAS 95032-84-1	Crotein AD Anhyd
CAS 86438-79-1	Mirataine® COB	CAS 95032-84-1	Etha-Coll ISO
CAS 86637-84-5	Nikkol Decaglyn 5-O	CAS 95912-87-1	Cutina® CP
CAS 88103-59-7	E.O.D	CAS 96690-41-4	Autolyzed Silk
CAS 88122-99-0	Uvinul® T 150	CAS 96690-41-4	Autolyzed Silk Protein
CAS 88497-58-9	Sandopan® DTC Linear P Acid	CAS 96690-41-4	Crosilk 10,000
CAS 88497-58-9	Surfine WNT-A	CAS 96690-41-4	Crosilk Liq. Complex
CAS 89933-26-6	Pelemol 108	CAS 96690-41-4	Idrolizzato Della Seta
CAS 90045-38-8	Ginseng Vegebios	CAS 96690-41-4	Promois Silk 700 SP
CAS 90045-56-0	Elicrisina	CAS 96690-41-4	Promois Silk-1000
CAS 90052-75-8	Ceraphyl® 847	CAS 96690-41-4	Silkpro
CAS 90193-76-3	Radia® 7505	CAS 96690-41-4	Silkpro CM-1000

CAS 96690-41-4	Silkpro CM-2000		CAS 100085-64-1	Rewoteric® QAM 50
CAS 96690-41-4	Silk Pro-Tein		CAS 100209-19-6	Gluadin® Almond
CAS 96690-41-4	Solu-Silk™ Protein		CAS 100209-45-8	Chromoprotulines
CAS 97026-94-0	Koster Keunen Synthetic Beeswax		CAS 100209-45-8	Exsymol Chromoprotuline
CAS 97069-99-0	Cera-E		CAS 100209-45-8	Exsymol Protuline
CAS 97281-23-7	Radiasurf® 7270		CAS 100209-45-8	Gunther Pro-Tein 1550
CAS 97281-23-7	Radiasurf® 7414		CAS 100209-45-8	Hydrosoy 2000
CAS 97281-23-7	Radiasurf® 7417		CAS 100209-45-8	Protulines
CAS 97281-23-7	Radiasurf® 7453		CAS 100209-45-8	Solu-Veg™ EN-35
CAS 97281-23-7	Radiasurf® 7454		CAS 100684-25-1	Gluadin® AGP
CAS 97281-23-7	Radiasurf® 7473		CAS 100684-25-1	Gluadin® Wheat
CAS 97281-47-5	Phospholipon® 90/90 G		CAS 100684-25-7	Wheat-Quat C
CAS 97281-47-5	Phospholipon® 100		CAS 100684-36-4	Hydrocell™ AYP-30
CAS 97281-48-6	Phospholipon® 90 H		CAS 100684-36-4	Hydrocell™ YP-30
CAS 97281-48-6	Phospholipon® 100 H		CAS 100684-36-4	Hydrocell YP-30-P
CAS 97338-28-8	Ceraphyl® 791		CAS 100684-36-4	Hydrocell YP-SD
CAS 97338-28-8	Hetester HSS		CAS 100864-25-1	Wheat-Tein NL
CAS 97404-33-6	Radia® 7500		CAS 102033-55-6	Emalex DISG-10
CAS 97404-50-7	Ivarlan™ 3360		CAS 102033-55-6	Nikkol Decaglyn 2-IS
CAS 97404-50-7	Lanesta G		CAS 102051-00-3	Nikkol Decaglyn 3-O
CAS 97488-62-5	Ampholak 7TY		CAS 102523-96-6	Abil® B 9950
CAS 97488-91-0	Labrafil® M 1944 CS		CAS 102868-96-2	Exsymol Zinc Acetylmethionate
CAS 97552-91-5	Lanette® 22 Flakes		CAS 102868-96-2	Exsyzinc
CAS 97593-31-2	Acidan BC Veg		CAS 103175-09-3	Nikkol Decaglyn 7-O
CAS 97593-31-2	Acidan N 12 Veg		CAS 103213-19-0	Schercemol DISD
CAS 97659-50-2	Ampholak YCE		CAS 103213-20-3	Schercemol DID
CAS 97659-50-2	Ampholan® U 203		CAS 103213-22-5	Schercemol TIST
CAS 97659-53-5	Ampholak 7CX		CAS 103819-46-1	Cerex U 60
CAS 97659-53-5	Ampholak 7CX/C		CAS 103819-46-1	Labrafil® M 1980 CS
CAS 97659-53-5	Ampholak 7TX		CAS 104934-17-0	Nikkol Hexaglyn 5-O
CAS 97659-53-5	Ampholak 7TX/C		CAS 105883-46-3	Exsymol Silver Acetylmethionate
CAS 97659-53-5	Ampholak 7TX-SD 55		CAS 105883-46-3	Exsyor
CAS 97659-53-5	Ampholak 7TX-T		CAS 105883-47-4	Exsymol Gold Acetylmethionate
CAS 97659-53-5	Ampholak XO7		CAS 105883-48-5	Exsymol Nickel Acetylmethionate
CAS 97659-53-5	Ampholak XO7/C		CAS 105883-48-5	Exsynickel
CAS 97759-33-8	Hydrane R		CAS 105883-49-6	Exsymagnesium
CAS 97759-33-8	Rice-Pro™ EN-20		CAS 105883-49-6	Exsymol Magnesium Acetyl-methionate
CAS 97759-33-8	Rice Pro-Tein BK		CAS 105883-50-9	Exsymanganese
CAS 98073-10-0	Glucam® E-20 Distearate		CAS 105883-50-9	Exsymol Manganese Acetyl-methionate
CAS 98133-47-2	Ritapan TA			
CAS 99126-54-2	Nikkol Decaglyn 7-S		CAS 105883-51-0	Exsycuivre
CAS 99330-44-6	Akypo®-Soft 100 MgV		CAS 105883-51-0	Exsymol Cupric Acetylmethionate
CAS 99542-23-1	Foamquat SAQ-90		CAS 105883-52-1	Exsycobalt
CAS 99542-23-1	Naetex-Q		CAS 105883-52-1	Exsymol Cobalt Acetylmethionate
CAS 99734-30-2	Nikkol Hexaglyn 5-S		CAS 106436-39-9	Ceraphyl® 55
CAS 100085-10-7	Actigen E		CAS 106436-39-9	Trivent NP-13
CAS 100085-10-7	Alpha-Elastin		CAS 106483-04-9	Nikkol DK
CAS 100085-10-7	Crolastin		CAS 107600-36-2	Akyposal 100 DAL
CAS 100085-10-7	Elastein® 5000		CAS 107628-03-5	Akypo®-Soft KA 250 BVC
CAS 100085-10-7	Elastin		CAS 107987-23-5	Quatrisoft® Polymer LM-200
CAS 100085-10-7	Elastin 5000		CAS 110332-91-7	CUPL® PIC
CAS 100085-10-7	Elastin CLR		CAS 110615-47-9	APG® 500 Glycoside
CAS 100085-10-7	Elastin H.P.M		CAS 110615-47-9	APG® 600 SP
CAS 100085-10-7	Elastin Hydrolysate COS		CAS 110615-47-9	Plantaren® 1200
CAS 100085-10-7	Elastin (Partialhydrolisate) NOVA		CAS 110615-47-9	Plantaren® 1200 CS/UP
CAS 100085-10-7	Elastolan LS HE 20		CAS 110615-47-9	Plantaren® 1200 UP
CAS 100085-10-7	Hidrolisado de Elastina		CAS 110615-47-9	Plantaren® 1300
CAS 100085-10-7	Hydrolastan		CAS 111019-03-5	Crodafos CAP
CAS 100085-10-7	Hydrolyzed Elastin RE-10 No. 26202		CAS 111174-62-0	Crotein Q
			CAS 111174-62-0	Granquat S
CAS 100085-10-7	Hydrolyzed Elastin RE-30 No. 26203		CAS 111174-62-0	Pran QC
			CAS 111174-62-0	Quat-Coll™ QS
CAS 100085-10-7	Ichtyoelastin		CAS 111174-62-0	Quatex S
CAS 100085-10-7	Prolastine		CAS 111174-62-0	Quat-Pro S
CAS 100085-10-7	Ritalastin EL-10		CAS 111174-62-0	Quat-Pro S 30
CAS 100085-10-7	Ritalastin EL-30		CAS 111174-62-0	Tri-Quat-S
CAS 100085-10-7	Solu-Lastin™ 10		CAS 111174-64-2	Quat-Pro E
CAS 100085-10-7	Solu-Lastin™ 30		CAS 111381-08-9	Foamquat 2IAE
CAS 100085-10-7	Tri-Lastin 10F		CAS 111905-55-6	Schercoquat DAS
CAS 100085-35-6	Cronectin H			

CAS 112324-11-5	Schercoquat ROEP	CAS 134017-12-2	Hetester ISS
CAS 112324-16-0	Lipoquat R	CAS 134112-42-8	Foamquat IALA
CAS 112324-16-0	Surfactol® Q4	CAS 134112-42-8	Schercoquat IALA
CAS 112926-00-8	Sident® 22S	CAS 134737-05-6	Abil®-Quat 3270
CAS 112926-00-8	Sipernat® 22	CAS 134737-05-6	Abil®-Quat 3272
CAS 112926-00-8	Sipernat® 22S	CAS 134737-05-6	Silquat Q-100
CAS 112926-00-8	Sipernat® 50	CAS 136097-81-9	Kester Wax® 62
CAS 112926-00-8	Sipernat® 50S	CAS 136097-82-0	Kester Wax® 56
CAS 112945-52-5	Cab-O-Sil® L-90	CAS 136097-93-3	Cera Bellina®
CAS 113010-52-9	Uvinul® P 25	CAS 136097-94-4	Kester Wax® 59
CAS 113431-53-1	Schercemol DISF	CAS 136097-95-5	Koster Keunen Synthetic Candelilla
CAS 113431-54-2	Schercemol TISC		
CAS 113492-03-8	Foamquat CAS	CAS 136097-95-5	Koster Keunen Synthetic Candelilla R-4
CAS 113492-03-8	Schercoquat CAS		
CAS 113492-04-9	Schercoquat FOAS	CAS 136097-95-5	Koster Keunen Synthetic Candelilla R-8
CAS 114040-31-2	Nikkol VC-PMG		
CAS 115340-78-8	Schercoquat APAS	CAS 136097-96-6	Kester Wax® 82
CAS 115340-80-2	Schercoquat WOAS	CAS 136097-96-6	Koster Keunen Synthetic Carnauba
CAS 116518-82-2	Schercemol 145		
CAS 116870-30-5	Phospholipon® MG Na	CAS 136505-00-5	Hypan® SR150H
CAS 116870-31-6	Phospholipon® PG Na	CAS 138208-68-1	Dermol ICSA
CAS 118441-80-8	Lamequat® L	CAS 138314-11-1	Dermolan GLH
CAS 118441-80-8	Lamequat® L/NP	CAS 138724-54-6	Cera Euphorbia
CAS 118777-77-8	Katemul IG-70	CAS 138724-54-6	Koster Keunen Candelilla Ester
CAS 118777-77-8	Necon SOG	CAS 138724-55-7	Koster Keunen Beeswax AO2535
CAS 120486-24-0	Cosmol 43	CAS 141464-42-8	Plantaren® 2000 CS/UP
CAS 120486-24-0	Emalex TISG-2	CAS 141464-42-8	Plantaren® 2000 UP
CAS 121440-30-0	Cosmol 44	CAS 144514-51-2	Orange Wax
CAS 123754-28-9	Hypan® SS201	CAS 144514-52-3	Cera Albalate 101
CAS 124046-05-5	Incroquat BA-85	CAS 144514-53-4	Cera Albalate 102
CAS 124046-09-9	Incroquat WG-85	CAS 144514-54-5	Cera Albalate 103
CAS 124046-31-7	Incromate OLL	CAS 144514-54-5	Koster Keunen Hydroxy-Hexanyl-Behenyl-Beeswaxate
CAS 124046-35-1	Incromide SED		
CAS 124046-39-5	Incromide WGD	CAS 678213-23-0	Synperonic A2
CAS 124046-39-5	Schercomid SWG	CAS 977000-98-8	Sol-U-Tein EA
CAS 124046-40-8	Afalene™ 716	CAS 977012-91-1	Afalene™ 216
CAS 124046-40-8	Incromate WGL	CAS 977012-91-1	Emcol® 3555
CAS 124046-40-8	Mackalene™ 716	CAS 977012-91-1	Mackalene™ 216
CAS 125804-04-8	Catemol 220-B	CAS 977013-38-9	Myverol® 18-35
CAS 125804-04-8	Necon BDB	CAS 977039-11-4	Soy-Quat C
CAS 125804-10-6	Necon LO-80	CAS 977053-29-4	Lipal 400 DS
CAS 125804-12-8	Dermol G-76	CAS 977053-96-5	Lipal GMS AE
CAS 125804-13-9	Estalan L-45	CAS 977053-96-5	Rewomul MG SE
CAS 125804-13-9	Pelemol G45L	CAS 977055-17-6	Super-Sat AWS-4
CAS 125804-15-1	Dermol G-7DI	CAS 977055-17-6	Super-Sat AWS-24
CAS 125804-18-4	Dermol 139	CAS 977055-39-2	Lipal 400 S
CAS 126121-35-5	CE-2000	CAS 977055-48-3	Lipal 6000 DS
CAS 126121-35-5	Citmol 320	CAS 977055-83-6	Myvacet® 5-07
CAS 126121-35-5	Pelemol TGC	CAS 977056-87-3	Softisan® 100
CAS 126121-35-5	Trimol CE 2000	CAS 977056-87-3	Softisan® 133
CAS 126928-07-2	Plurol Isostearique	CAS 977056-87-3	Softisan® 134
CAS 127358-81-0	Dermol DISD	CAS 977056-87-3	Softisan® 138
CAS 127512-63-4	Isolan® GI 34	CAS 977056-87-3	Softisan® 142
CAS 127733-92-0	Stepan TAB®-2	CAS 977056-87-3	Witepsol® E75
CAS 129426-19-3	Ceramide II	CAS 977056-87-3	Witepsol® E76
CAS 129541-36-2	Katemul IGU-70	CAS 977056-87-3	Witepsol® E85
CAS 129541-36-2	Necon SOGU	CAS 977056-87-3	Witepsol® H5
CAS 130124-24-2	Incrosoft T-90	CAS 977056-87-3	Witepsol® H12
CAS 131154-74-0	Pelemol TDE	CAS 977056-87-3	Witepsol® H15
CAS 132207-31-9	Pecosil® PS-100	CAS 977056-87-3	Witepsol® H32
CAS 132467-76-6	Panthequat®	CAS 977056-87-3	Witepsol® H35
CAS 133448-12-1	Pecosil® OS-100B	CAS 977056-87-3	Witepsol® H37
CAS 133448-16-5	Silwax® WD-IS	CAS 977056-87-3	Witepsol® H39
CAS 133738-23-5	Nikkol Decaglyn 1-IS	CAS 977056-87-3	Witepsol® H42
CAS 133798-12-6	Schercotaine UAB	CAS 977056-87-3	Witepsol® H175
CAS 133934-08-4	Schercotaine APAB	CAS 977056-87-3	Witepsol® H185
CAS 133934-09-5	Afaine™ WGB	CAS 977056-87-3	Witepsol® S51
CAS 133934-09-5	Incronam WG-30	CAS 977056-87-3	Witepsol® S55
CAS 133934-09-5	Mackam™ WGB	CAS 977056-87-3	Witepsol® S58
CAS 133934-09-5	Schercotaine WOAB	CAS 977056-87-3	Witepsol® W25

CAS 977056-87-3	Witepsol® W31		CAS 977077-71-6	Amino-Silk SF
CAS 977056-87-3	Witepsol® W32		CAS 977077-71-6	Crosilk Liq
CAS 977056-87-3	Witepsol® W35		CAS 977077-71-6	Solu-Silk™ 25
CAS 977056-87-3	Witepsol® W45		CAS 977077-71-6	Solu-Silk™ SF
CAS 977060-94-8	Mayphos OL 3N		CAS 977077-71-6	Tri-Tein Silk AA
CAS 977067-77-8	Surfax ECM			

CAS Number-to-Chemical
Cross-Reference

CAS 50-21-5	Lactic acid	CAS 67-63-0	Isopropyl alcohol
CAS 50-70-4	Sorbitol	CAS 67-97-0	Cholecalciferol
CAS 50-81-7	L-Ascorbic acid	CAS 68-04-2	Sodium citrate
CAS 50-99-7	Glucose (anhydrous)	CAS 68-11-1	Thioglycolic acid
CAS 51-05-8	Benzocaine	CAS 68-19-9	Cyanocobalamin
CAS 51-35-4	L-Hydroxyproline	CAS 68-26-8	Retinol
CAS 51-81-0	m-Aminophenol HCl	CAS 69-65-8	Mannitol
CAS 52-51-7	2-Bromo-2-nitropropane-1,3-diol	CAS 69-72-7	Salicylic acid
CAS 52-90-4	L-Cysteine	CAS 69-79-4	Maltose
CAS 54-12-6	DL-α-Tryptophan	CAS 69-93-2	Uric acid
CAS 55-55-0	p-Methylaminophenol sulfate	CAS 70-26-8	Ornithine
CAS 56-37-1	Benzyltriethyl ammonium chloride	CAS 71-00-1	L-Histidine
CAS 56-40-6	Glycine	CAS 71-36-3	Butyl alcohol
CAS 56-41-7	L-Alanine	CAS 71-55-6	Trichloroethane
CAS 56-45-1	L-Serine	CAS 72-17-3	Sodium lactate
CAS 56-65-5	Adenosine triphosphate	CAS 72-18-4	L-Valine
CAS 56-81-5	Glycerin	CAS 73-32-5	L-Isoleucine
CAS 56-86-0	L-Glutamic acid	CAS 73-40-5	Guanine
CAS 56-87-1	L-Lysine	CAS 74-79-3	L-Arginine
CAS 56-89-3	Cystine	CAS 74-98-6	Propane
CAS 56-93-9	Benzyl trimethyl ammonium chloride	CAS 75-28-5	Isobutane
		CAS 75-37-6	Hydrofluorocarbon 152a
CAS 57-09-0	Cetrimonium bromide	CAS 75-45-6	Hydrochlorofluorocarbon 22
CAS 57-10-3	Palmitic acid	CAS 75-52-5	Nitromethane
CAS 57-11-4	Stearic acid	CAS 75-68-3	Hydrochlorofluorocarbon 142B
CAS 57-13-6	Urea	CAS 76-22-2	Camphor
CAS 57-15-8	Chlorobutanol	CAS 77-85-0	Trimethylolethane
CAS 57-48-7	D-Fructose	CAS 77-86-1	Tris (hydroxymethyl) amino-methane
CAS 57-50-1	Sucrose		
CAS 57-55-6	Propylene glycol	CAS 77-89-4	Acetyl triethyl citrate
CAS 57-88-5	Cholesterol	CAS 77-90-7	Acetyl tributyl citrate
CAS 58-08-2	Caffeine	CAS 77-92-9	Citric acid
CAS 58-27-5	Menadione	CAS 77-93-0	Triethyl citrate
CAS 58-55-9	Theophylline	CAS 77-94-1	Tributyl citrate
CAS 58-85-5	Biotin	CAS 78-21-7	Cetethyl morpholinium ethosulfate
CAS 59-02-9	d-α-Tocopherol	CAS 78-66-0	Dimethyl octynediol
CAS 59-50-7	p-Chloro-m-cresol	CAS 78-96-6	Isopropanolamine
CAS 59-51-8	Methionine	CAS 79-09-4	Propionic acid
CAS 59-67-6	Nicotinic acid	CAS 79-63-0	Lanosterol
CAS 60-00-4	Edetic acid	CAS 79-81-2	Retinyl palmitate
CAS 60-12-8	Phenethyl alcohol	CAS 79-83-4	Pantothenic acid
CAS 60-18-4	L-Tyrosine	CAS 80-62-6	Methyl methacrylate (monomer)
CAS 60-33-3	Linoleic acid	CAS 80-73-9	Dimethyl imidazolidinone
CAS 61-90-5	L-Leucine	CAS 81-07-2	Saccharin
CAS 62-33-9	Calcium disodium EDTA	CAS 81-13-0	D-Panthenol
CAS 63-42-3	Lactose	CAS 83-56-7	1,5-Naphthalenediol
CAS 63-91-2	L-Phenylalanine	CAS 83-72-7	Lawsone
CAS 64-02-8	Tetrasodium EDTA	CAS 83-88-5	Riboflavin
CAS 64-17-5	Alcohol	CAS 84-66-2	Diethyl phthalate
CAS 64-19-7	Acetic acid	CAS 84-74-2	Dibutyl phthalate
CAS 65-23-6	Pyridoxine	CAS 87-66-1	Pyrogallol
CAS 65-85-0	Benzoic acid	CAS 87-69-4	L-Tartaric acid
CAS 67-03-8	Thiamine HCl	CAS 87-89-8	Inositol
CAS 67-43-6	Pentetic acid	CAS 88-04-0	Chloroxylenol

CAS 88-41-5	2-t-Butylcyclohexyl acetate
CAS 89-65-6	Erythorbic acid
CAS 89-78-1	Menthol
CAS 89-83-8	Thymol
CAS 90-15-3	1-Naphthol
CAS 90-43-7	o-Phenylphenol
CAS 91-68-9	N,N-Diethyl-m-aminophenol
CAS 92-44-4	2,3-Naphthalenediol
CAS 93-82-3	Stearamide DEA
CAS 93-83-4	Oleamide DEA
CAS 94-13-3	Propylparaben
CAS 94-18-8	Benzylparaben
CAS 94-26-8	Butylparaben
CAS 94-44-0	Benzyl nicotinate
CAS 94-51-9	Dipropylene glycol dibenzoate
CAS 94-96-2	Ethyl hexanediol
CAS 95-38-5	Oleyl hydroxyethyl imidazoline
CAS 95-55-6	o-Aminophenol
CAS 95-88-5	4-Chlororesorcinol
CAS 96-20-8	2-Amino-1-butanol
CAS 96-26-4	Dihydroxyacetone
CAS 96-27-5	Thioglycerin
CAS 96-33-3	Methyl acrylate (monomer)
CAS 96-48-0	Butyrolactone
CAS 97-23-4	Dichlorophene
CAS 97-59-6	Allantoin
CAS 97-63-2	Ethyl methacrylate
CAS 97-78-9	Lauroyl sarcosine
CAS 97-86-9	Isobutyl methacrylate
CAS 97-88-1	Butyl methacrylate
CAS 98-67-9	Phenol sulfonic acid
CAS 98-79-3	PCA
CAS 98-92-0	Niacinamide
CAS 99-56-9	4-Nitro-o-phenylenediamine
CAS 99-76-3	Methylparaben
CAS 100-51-6	Benzyl alcohol
CAS 101-34-8	Glyceryl triacetyl ricinoleate
CAS 101-54-2	N-Phenyl-p-phenylenediamine
CAS 102-60-3	Tetrahydroxypropyl ethylene-diamine
CAS 102-71-6	Triethanolamine
CAS 102-76-1	Triacetin
CAS 102-87-4	Trilaurylamine
CAS 103-23-1	Dioctyl adipate
CAS 103-95-7	Cyclamen aldehyde
CAS 104-15-4	Toluene sulfonic acid
CAS 104-29-0	Chlorphenesin
CAS 104-61-0	γ-Nonalactone
CAS 104-67-6	γ-Undecalactone
CAS 104-74-5	Laurylpyridinium chloride
CAS 104-75-6	2-Ethylhexylamine
CAS 104-87-0	p-Tolualdehyde
CAS 105-62-4	Propylene glycol dioleate
CAS 105-95-3	Ethylene brassylate
CAS 105-97-5	Dicapryl adipate
CAS 105-99-7	Dibutyl adipate
CAS 106-01-4	Diethylene glycol diisononanoate
CAS 106-02-5	Pentadecalactone
CAS 106-07-0	PEG-4 stearate
CAS 106-08-1	PEG-9 laurate
CAS 106-11-6	PEG-2 stearate
CAS 106-11-6	PEG-2 stearate SE
CAS 106-12-7	PEG-2 oleate
CAS 106-12-7	PEG-2 oleate SE
CAS 106-14-9	Hydroxystearic acid
CAS 106-16-1	Ricinoleamide MEA
CAS 106-17-2	Glycol ricinoleate
CAS 106-19-4	Dipropyl adipate
CAS 106-33-2	Ethyl laurate
CAS 106-50-3	p-Phenylenediamine
CAS 106-65-0	Dimethyl succinate
CAS 106-97-8	Butane
CAS 106-98-9	Butene
CAS 107-21-1	Glycol
CAS 107-41-5	Hexylene glycol
CAS 107-43-7	Betaine
CAS 107-46-0	Hexamethyldisiloxane
CAS 107-64-2	Distearyldimonium chloride
CAS 107-88-0	Butylene glycol
CAS 107-98-2	Methoxyisopropanol
CAS 108-32-7	Propylene carbonate
CAS 108-45-2	m-Phenylenediamine
CAS 108-46-3	Resorcinol
CAS 108-65-6	Propylene glycol methyl ether acetate
CAS 108-88-3	Toluene
CAS 109-28-4	Oleamidopropyl dimethylamine
CAS 109-30-8	PEG-2 distearate
CAS 110-15-6	Succinic acid
CAS 110-25-8	Oleoyl sarcosine
CAS 110-27-0	Isopropyl myristate
CAS 110-30-5	Ethylene distearamide
CAS 110-36-1	Butyl myristate
CAS 110-40-7	Diethyl sebacate
CAS 110-44-1	Sorbic acid
CAS 110-80-5	Ethoxyethanol
CAS 110-91-8	Morpholine
CAS 110-97-4	Diisopropanolamine
CAS 110-98-5	Dipropylene glycol
CAS 111-01-3	Squalane
CAS 111-02-4	Squalene
CAS 111-03-5	Glyceryl oleate
CAS 111-05-7	Oleamide MIPA
CAS 111-15-9	Ethoxyethanol acetate
CAS 111-27-3	Hexyl alcohol
CAS 111-30-8	Glutaral
CAS 111-42-2	Diethanolamine
CAS 111-46-6	Diethylene glycol
CAS 111-57-9	Stearamide MEA
CAS 111-58-0	Oleamide MEA
CAS 111-60-4	Glycol stearate
CAS 111-61-5	Ethyl stearate
CAS 111-62-6	Ethyl oleate
CAS 111-66-0	Octene-1
CAS 111-76-2	Butoxyethanol
CAS 111-77-3	Methoxydiglycol
CAS 111-82-0	Methyl laurate
CAS 111-87-5	Caprylic alcohol
CAS 111-90-0	Ethoxydiglycol
CAS 111-96-6	Dimethoxydiglycol
CAS 112-00-5	Laurtrimonium chloride
CAS 112-02-7	Cetrimonium chloride
CAS 112-03-8	Steartrimonium chloride
CAS 112-10-7	Isopropyl stearate
CAS 112-11-8	Isopropyl oleate
CAS 112-15-2	Ethoxydiglycol acetate
CAS 112-18-5	Dimethyl lauramine
CAS 112-27-6	Triethylene glycol
CAS 112-30-1	n-Decyl alcohol
CAS 112-34-5	Butoxy diglycol
CAS 112-38-9	Undecylenic acid
CAS 112-39-0	Methyl palmitate
CAS 112-41-4	Dodecene-1
CAS 112-42-5	Undecyl alcohol
CAS 112-53-8	Lauryl alcohol
CAS 112-60-7	PEG-4
CAS 112-61-8	Methyl stearate
CAS 112-62-9	Methyl oleate
CAS 112-69-6	Dimethyl palmitamine
CAS 112-72-1	Myristyl alcohol

CAS 112-75-4	Dimethyl myristamine	CAS 132-27-4	Sodium o-phenylphenate
CAS 112-80-1	Oleic acid	CAS 133-06-2	Captan
CAS 112-85-6	Behenic acid	CAS 133-37-9	dl-α-Tartaric acid
CAS 112-88-9	Octadecene-1	CAS 134-03-2	Sodium ascorbate
CAS 112-90-3	Oleamine	CAS 134-09-8	Menthyl anthranilate
CAS 112-92-5	Stearyl alcohol	CAS 134-62-3	Diethyl toluamide
CAS 112-99-2	Dioctadecylamine	CAS 136-26-5	Capramide DEA
CAS 115-10-6	Dimethyl ether	CAS 136-99-2	Lauryl hydroxyethyl imidazoline
CAS 115-69-5	2-Amino-2-methyl-1,3-propanediol	CAS 137-03-1	2-Heptylcyclopentanone
CAS 115-70-8	2-Amino-2-ethyl-1,3-propanediol	CAS 137-08-6	D-Calcium pantothenate
CAS 115-83-3	Pentaerythrityl tetrastearate	CAS 137-16-6	Sodium lauroyl sarcosinate
CAS 116-25-6	MDM hydantoin	CAS 137-20-2	Sodium methyl oleoyl taurate
CAS 118-55-8	Phenyl salicylate	CAS 137-40-6	Sodium propionate
CAS 118-56-9	Homosalate	CAS 137-66-6	Ascorbyl palmitate
CAS 118-60-5	Octyl salicylate	CAS 138-32-9	Cetrimonium tosylate
CAS 119-36-8	Methyl salicylate	CAS 138-86-3	Dipentene
CAS 120-32-1	Chlorophene	CAS 139-07-1	Lauralkonium chloride
CAS 120-40-1	Lauramide DEA	CAS 139-08-2	Myristalkonium chloride
CAS 120-47-8	Ethylparaben	CAS 139-33-3	Disodium EDTA
CAS 120-51-4	Benzyl benzoate	CAS 139-41-3	Sodium dihydroxyethylglycinate
CAS 120-55-8	Diethylene glycol dibenzoate	CAS 139-44-6	Trihydroxystearin
CAS 120-80-9	Pyrocatechol	CAS 139-88-8	Sodium myristyl sulfate
CAS 121-32-4	Ethyl vanillin	CAS 139-89-9	Trisodium HEDTA
CAS 121-33-5	Vanillin	CAS 139-96-8	TEA-lauryl sulfate
CAS 121-54-0	Benzethonium chloride	CAS 140-01-2	Pentasodium pentetate
CAS 121-79-9	Propyl gallate	CAS 140-03-4	Methyl acetyl ricinoleate
CAS 121-88-0	2-Amino-5-nitrophenol	CAS 140-25-0	Benzyl laurate
CAS 122-03-2	p-Isopropylbenzaldehyde	CAS 141-08-2	Glyceryl ricinoleate
CAS 122-18-9	Cetalkonium chloride	CAS 141-20-8	PEG-2 laurate
CAS 122-19-0	Stearalkonium chloride	CAS 141-20-8	PEG-2 laurate SE
CAS 122-20-3	Triisopropanolamine	CAS 141-21-9	Stearamidoethyl ethanolamine
CAS 122-32-7	Triolein	CAS 141-22-0	Ricinoleic acid
CAS 122-62-3	Dioctyl sebacate	CAS 141-23-1	Methyl hydroxystearate
CAS 122-99-6	Phenoxyethanol	CAS 141-70-8	Isododecane
CAS 123-03-5	Cetylpyridinium chloride	CAS 141-86-6	2,6-Diaminopyridine
CAS 123-28-4	Dilauryl thiodipropionate	CAS 141-94-6	Hexetidine
CAS 123-30-8	p-Aminophenol	CAS 142-16-5	Dioctyl maleate
CAS 123-31-9	Hydroquinone	CAS 142-18-7	Glyceryl laurate
CAS 123-76-2	Levulinic acid	CAS 142-20-1	PEG-4 distearate
CAS 123-86-4	n-Butyl acetate	CAS 142-26-7	Acetamide MEA
CAS 123-94-4	Glyceryl stearate	CAS 142-31-4	Sodium octyl sulfate
CAS 123-95-5	Butyl stearate	CAS 142-48-3	Stearoyl sarcosine
CAS 124-03-8	Cetethyldimonium bromide	CAS 142-54-1	Lauramide MIPA
CAS 124-06-1	Ethyl myristate	CAS 142-55-2	Propylene glycol laurate
CAS 124-07-2	Caprylic acid	CAS 142-58-5	Myristamide MEA
CAS 124-10-7	Methyl myristate	CAS 142-62-1	Caproic acid
CAS 124-17-4	Diethylene glycol butyl ether acetate	CAS 142-77-8	Butyl oleate
		CAS 142-78-9	Lauramide MEA
CAS 124-22-1	Lauramine	CAS 142-87-0	Sodium decyl sulfate
CAS 124-26-5	Stearamide	CAS 142-91-6	Isopropyl palmitate
CAS 124-28-7	Dimethyl stearamine	CAS 143-00-0	DEA-lauryl sulfate
CAS 124-30-1	Stearamine	CAS 143-07-7	Lauric acid
CAS 124-43-6	Urea peroxide	CAS 143-18-0	Potassium oleate
CAS 124-68-5	2-Amino-2-methyl-1-propanol	CAS 143-27-1	Palmitamine
CAS 125-46-2	Usnic acid	CAS 143-28-2	Oleyl alcohol
CAS 126-11-4	Tris (hydroxymethyl) nitromethane	CAS 144-19-4	2,2,4-Trimethyl-1,3-pentanediol
CAS 126-30-7	Noopontyl glyool	CAS 144-55-8	Sodium bicarbonate
CAS 126-92-1	Sodium octyl sulfate	CAS 147-71-7	D-Tartaric acid
CAS 127-09-3	Sodium acetate	CAS 147-85-3	L-Proline
CAS 127-40-2	Xanthophyll	CAS 149-39-3	Sodium methyl stearoyl taurate
CAS 127-47-9	Retinyl acetate	CAS 149-91-7	Gallic acid
CAS 127-82-2	Zinc phenolsulfonate	CAS 150-13-0	PABA
CAS 128-37-0	BHT	CAS 150-38-9	Trisodium EDTA
CAS 128-44-9	Sodium saccharin	CAS 150-39-0	HEDTA
CAS 131-11-3	Dimethyl phthalate	CAS 151-21-3	Sodium lauryl sulfate
CAS 131-53-3	Benzophenone-8	CAS 215-42-9	Dimethyl behenamine
CAS 131-54-4	Benzophenone-6	CAS 261-31-4	Thioxanthine
CAS 131-55-5	Benzophenone-2	CAS 299-27-4	Potassium D-gluconate
CAS 131-56-6	Benzophenone-1	CAS 299-28-5	Calcium gluconate
CAS 131-57-7	Benzophenone-3	CAS 299-29-6	Ferrous gluconate

CAS 300-92-5	Aluminum distearate
CAS 301-02-0	Oleamide
CAS 301-04-2	Lead acetate
CAS 333-20-0	Potassium thiocyanate
CAS 334-48-5	Capric acid
CAS 344-64-8	Glycol dibehenate
CAS 372-75-8	Citrulline
CAS 422-86-2	Dioctyl terephthalate
CAS 439-32-1	Steareth-3
CAS 463-40-1	Linolenic acid
CAS 471-34-1	Calcium carbonate
CAS 471-53-4	Glycyrrhetinic acid
CAS 488-43-7	Glucamine
CAS 489-84-9	Guaiazulene
CAS 504-53-0	Stearone
CAS 506-32-1	Arachidonic acid
CAS 514-10-3	Abietic acid
CAS 515-69-5	Bisabolol
CAS 516-06-3	DL-α-Valine
CAS 520-45-6	Dehydroacetic acid
CAS 527-07-1	Sodium gluconate
CAS 527-09-3	Copper gluconate
CAS 531-75-9	Esculin
CAS 532-32-1	Sodium benzoate
CAS 533-73-3	1,2,4-Trihydroxybenzene
CAS 533-96-0	Sodium sesquicarbonate
CAS 537-40-6	Trilinolein
CAS 537-55-3	Acetyltyrosine
CAS 538-23-8	Tricaprylin
CAS 538-24-9	Trilaurin
CAS 538-71-6	Domiphen bromide
CAS 540-10-3	Cetyl palmitate
CAS 541-15-1	Carnitine
CAS 541-70-8	m-Phenylenediamine sulfate
CAS 544-31-0	Palmitamide MEA
CAS 544-35-4	Ethyl linoleate
CAS 544-62-7	Batyl alcohol
CAS 544-63-8	Myristic acid
CAS 546-46-3	Zinc citrate
CAS 546-93-0	Magnesium carbonate
CAS 555-43-1	Tristearin
CAS 555-44-2	Tripalmitin
CAS 555-45-3	Trimyristin
CAS 556-02-5	D-Tyrosine
CAS 556-03-6	DL-α-Tyrosine
CAS 556-67-2	Octamethylcyclotetrasiloxane
CAS 557-04-0	Magnesium stearate
CAS 557-05-1	Zinc stearate
CAS 557-08-4	Zinc undecylenate
CAS 570-24-1	6-Nitro-o-toluidine
CAS 575-44-6	1,6-Naphthalenediol
CAS 576-55-6	Tetrabromo-o-cresol
CAS 577-11-7	Dioctyl sodium sulfosuccinate
CAS 582-17-2	2,7-Naphthalenediol
CAS 584-08-7	Potassium carbonate
CAS 585-88-6	Maltitol
CAS 589-68-4	Glyceryl myristate
CAS 590-00-1	Potassium sorbate
CAS 590-28-3	Potassium cyanate
CAS 591-27-5	m-Aminophenol
CAS 592-41-6	1-Hexene
CAS 593-29-3	Potassium stearate
CAS 593-85-1	Guanidine carbonate
CAS 597-09-1	2-Nitro-2-ethyl-1,3-propanediol
CAS 603-85-0	2-Amino-3-nitrophenol
CAS 609-31-4	2-Nitro-1-butanol
CAS 610-81-1	4-Amino-3-nitrophenol
CAS 614-33-5	Glyceryl tribenzoate
CAS 615-05-4	4-Methoxy-m-phenylene diamine
CAS 615-50-9	Toluene-2,5-diamine sulfate

CAS 616-45-5	2-Pyrrolidone
CAS 621-71-6	Tricaprin
CAS 624-04-4	Glycol dilaurate
CAS 627-83-8	Glycol distearate
CAS 627-93-0	Dimethyl adipate
CAS 628-97-2	Ethyl palmitate
CAS 629-70-9	Cetyl acetate
CAS 629-73-2	Hexadecene-1
CAS 629-76-5	Pentadecyl alcohol
CAS 629-96-9	Arachidyl alcohol
CAS 635-38-1	Pyridoxine dipalmitate
CAS 637-12-7	Aluminum stearate
CAS 637-12-7	Aluminum tristearate
CAS 637-39-8	TEA hydrochloride
CAS 640-68-6	D-Valine
CAS 646-13-9	Isobutyl stearate
CAS 657-84-1	Sodium toluenesulfonate
CAS 659-40-5	Hexamidine diisethionate
CAS 661-19-8	Behenyl alcohol
CAS 683-10-3	Lauryl betaine
CAS 693-33-4	Cetyl betaine
CAS 693-36-7	Distearyl thiodipropionate
CAS 693-80-1	Oleyl acetate
CAS 771-03-9	Dehydroacetic acid
CAS 813-92-3	Aluminum citrate
CAS 816-94-4	1,2-Distearoyl-sn-glycero(3) phosphatidylcholine
CAS 820-66-6	Stearyl betaine
CAS 822-16-2	Sodium stearate
CAS 871-37-4	Oleyl betaine
CAS 872-05-9	Decene-1
CAS 928-24-5	Glycol dioleate
CAS 999-97-3	Hexamethyldisilazane
CAS 1002-89-7	Ammonium stearate
CAS 1093-13-5	Steareth-5
CAS 1115-22-6	Dimethyl aspartic acid
CAS 1119-33-1	Ethyl glutamate
CAS 1119-40-0	Dimethyl glutarate
CAS 1119-87-5	Lauryl glycol
CAS 1119-97-7	Myrtrimonium bromide
CAS 1120-01-0	Sodium cetyl sulfate
CAS 1120-04-3	Sodium stearyl sulfate
CAS 1120-24-7	Dimethyl decylamine
CAS 1120-36-1	Tetradecene-1
CAS 1120-49-6	Didecylamine
CAS 1166-52-5	Dodecyl gallate
CAS 1190-63-2	Cetyl stearate
CAS 1191-41-9	Ethyl linolenate
CAS 1191-50-0	Sodium myristyl sulfate
CAS 1222-05-5	Hexahydrohexamethyl cyclo-pentabenzopyran
CAS 1300-72-7	Sodium xylenesulfonate
CAS 1302-78-9	Bentonite
CAS 1303-96-4	Sodium borate
CAS 1304-85-4	Bismuth subnitrate
CAS 1305-62-0	Calcium hydroxide
CAS 1305-78-8	Calcium oxide
CAS 1308-38-9	Chromium oxide greens
CAS 1309-37-1	Iron oxides (Fe_2O_3)
CAS 1309-42-8	Magnesium hydroxide
CAS 1309-48-4	Magnesium oxide
CAS 1310-58-3	Potassium hydroxide
CAS 1310-73-2	Sodium hydroxide
CAS 1314-13-2	Zinc oxide
CAS 1314-23-4	Zirconium dioxide
CAS 1317-45-9	Tin oxide (ic)
CAS 1317-61-9	Iron oxides (Fe_3O_4)
CAS 1317-65-3	Calcium carbonate
CAS 1317-97-1	Ultramarine blue
CAS 1318-93-0	Montmorillonite

CAS 1321-87-5	Dimethyl octynediol	CAS 2420-29-3	Steareth-6
CAS 1322-98-1	Sodium decylbenzene sulfonate	CAS 2425-77-6	2-Hexyl-1-decanol
CAS 1323-03-1	Myristyl lactate	CAS 2432-87-3	Dioctyl sebacate
CAS 1323-38-2	Castor oil	CAS 2568-33-4	Isopentyldiol
CAS 1323-39-3	Propylene glycol stearate	CAS 2571-88-2	Stearamine oxide
CAS 1323-42-8	Glyceryl hydroxystearate	CAS 2605-79-0	Decylamine oxide
CAS 1323-65-5	Dinonyl phenol	CAS 2615-15-8	PEG-6
CAS 1323-83-7	Glyceryl distearate	CAS 2644-64-6	1,2-Dipalmitoyl-sn-glycero(3)
CAS 1327-36-2	Aluminum silicate		phosphatidylcholine
CAS 1327-41-9	Aluminum chlorohydrate	CAS 2673-22-5	Ditridecyl sodium sulfosuccinate
CAS 1327-43-1	Magnesium aluminum silicate	CAS 2682-20-4	Methylisothiazolinone
CAS 1330-43-4	Sodium borate	CAS 2687-96-9	Lauryl pyrrolidone
CAS 1330-80-9	Propylene glycol oleate	CAS 2724-58-5	Isostearic acid
CAS 1330-85-4	Dodecylbenzyltrimonium chloride	CAS 2778-96-3	Stearyl stearate
CAS 1331-61-9	Ammonium dodecylbenzene	CAS 2807-30-9	Ethylene glycol propyl ether
	sulfonate	CAS 2809-21-4	Etidronic acid
CAS 1332-58-7	Kaolin	CAS 2814-77-9	D&C Red No. 36
CAS 1333-39-7	Phenol sulfonic acid	CAS 2835-95-2	4-Amino-2-hydroxytoluene
CAS 1333-84-2	Alumina, hydrate	CAS 2867-47-2	Dimethylaminoethyl methacrylate
CAS 1335-72-4	Sodium laureth sulfate	CAS 2915-53-9	Dioctyl maleate
CAS 1337-76-4	Attapulgite	CAS 2915-57-3	Dioctyl succinate
CAS 1337-89-9	Glyceryl abietate	CAS 2917-94-4	Sodium octoxynol-2 ethane
CAS 1338-39-2	Sorbitan laurate		sulfonate
CAS 1338-41-6	Sorbitan stearate	CAS 2973-21-9	N-Methyl-3-nitro-p-phenylenedi-
CAS 1338-43-8	Sorbitan oleate		amine
CAS 1338-51-8	Tosylamide/formaldehyde resin	CAS 3006-15-3	Dihexyl sodium sulfosuccinate
CAS 1341-08-8	Steapyrium chloride	CAS 3008-50-2	Pentaerythrityl tetracaprate-
CAS 1341-54-4	Benzophenone-11		caprylate
CAS 1343-88-0	Magnesium silicate	CAS 3010-24-0	PEG-2 stearmonium chloride
CAS 1343-98-2	Silicic acid	CAS 3026-63-9	Sodium tridecyl sulfate
CAS 1344-00-9	Sodium silicoaluminate	CAS 3055-93-4	Laureth-2
CAS 1344-09-8	Sodium silicate	CAS 3055-94-5	Laureth-3
CAS 1344-28-1	Alumina	CAS 3055-95-6	Laureth-5
CAS 1344-95-2	Calcium silicate	CAS 3055-96-7	Laureth-6
CAS 1345-00-2	Ultramarines	CAS 3055-97-8	Laureth-7
CAS 1345-25-1	Iron oxides (FeO)	CAS 3055-98-9	Laureth-8
CAS 1369-66-3	Dioctyl sodium sulfosuccinate	CAS 3055-99-0	Laureth-9
CAS 1390-65-4	Carmine	CAS 3056-00-6	Laureth-12
CAS 1398-61-4	Chitin	CAS 3088-31-1	Sodium laureth sulfate
CAS 1401-55-4	Tannic acid	CAS 3097-08-3	Magnesium lauryl sulfate
CAS 1405-86-3	Glycyrrhizic acid	CAS 3115-49-9	Nonoxynol-8 carboxylic acid
CAS 1406-18-4	Tocopherol	CAS 3121-60-6	Benzophenone-9
CAS 1406-70-8	Tocopheryl acetate	CAS 3131-52-0	Dihydroxyindole
CAS 1462-54-0	Lauraminopropionic acid	CAS 3147-75-9	Octrizole
CAS 1463-95-2	Quaternium-51	CAS 3149-86-5	Steareth-10
CAS 1506-02-1	Acetyl hexamethyl tetralin	CAS 3151-59-5	Cetylamine hydrofluoride
CAS 1559-35-9	Ethylene glycol 2-ethylhexyl ether	CAS 3179-80-4	Lauramidopropyl dimethylamine
CAS 1562-00-1	Sodium isethionate	CAS 3179-81-5	Diethylaminoethyl stearate
CAS 1592-23-0	Calcium stearate	CAS 3228-02-2	4-Isopropyl-m-cresol
CAS 1634-04-4	Methyl t-butyl ether	CAS 3234-85-3	Myristyl myristate
CAS 1643-19-2	Tetrabutyl ammonium bromide	CAS 3319-31-1	Trioctyl trimellitate
CAS 1643-20-5	Lauramine oxide	CAS 3332-27-2	Myristamine oxide
CAS 1777-82-8	Dichlorobenzyl alcohol	CAS 3380-34-5	Triclosan
CAS 1812-53-9	Dicetyl dimonium chloride	CAS 3386-18-3	PEG-9
CAS 1847-58-1	Sodium lauryl sulfoacetate	CAS 3398-33-2	Sodium undecylenate
CAS 1948-33-0	t-Butyl hydroquinone	CAS 3400-45-1	Cyclopentane carboxylic acid
CAS 2016-57-1	Lauramine	CAS 3401-73-8	Tetrasodium dicarboxyethyl stearyl
CAS 2116-84-9	Phenyl trimethicone		sulfosuccinamate
CAS 2174-16-5	TEA-salicylate	CAS 3401-74-9	Dilauryldimonium chloride
CAS 2197-63-9	Dicetyl phosphate	CAS 3416-24-8	Glucosamine
CAS 2224-49-9	TEA lauroyl sarcosinate	CAS 3436-44-0	1,2-Dicaproyl-sn-glycero(3)
CAS 2235-54-3	Ammonium lauryl sulfate		phosphatidylcholine
CAS 2277-28-3	Glyceryl linoleate	CAS 3539-43-3	Cetyl phosphate
CAS 2315-62-0	Octoxynol-3	CAS 3546-96-1	Sodium lauraminopropionate
CAS 2315-64-2	Octoxynol-5	CAS 3578-72-1	Calcium behenate
CAS 2315-66-4	Octoxynol-10	CAS 3614-12-8	Lauraminopropionic acid
CAS 2370-64-1	PEG-6 laurate	CAS 3632-91-5	Magnesium gluconate
CAS 2372-82-9	Laurylamine dipropylenediamine	CAS 3655-00-3	Disodium lauriminodipropionate
CAS 2373-38-8	Dihexyl sodium sulfosuccinate	CAS 3687-18-1	3-Aminopropane sulfonic acid
CAS 2379-74-0	D&C Red No. 30	CAS 3687-45-4	Oleyl oleate

CAS 3687-46-5	Decyl oleate	CAS 6050-42-5	Carbomer
CAS 3696-28-4	Bispyrithione	CAS 6057-43-5	Steareth-2
CAS 3734-33-6	Denatonium benzoate NF	CAS 6144-28-1	Dilinoleic acid
CAS 3737-55-1	Sodium methyl palmitoyl taurate	CAS 6146-84-7	Steareth-7
CAS 3794-83-0	Tetrasodium etidronate	CAS 6179-44-8	Isostearamidopropyl betaine
CAS 3811-73-2	Sodium pyrithione	CAS 6182-11-2	Propylene glycol distearate
CAS 3913-02-8	2-Butyl-1-octanol	CAS 6197-30-4	Octocrylene
CAS 4065-45-6	Benzophenone-4	CAS 6219-71-2	2-Chloro-p-phenylenediamine sulfate
CAS 4070-43-3	Ethyl aspartate		
CAS 4070-80-8	Sodium stearyl fumarate	CAS 6219-73-4	N,N-Dimethyl-p-phenylenediamine sulfate
CAS 4075-81-4	Calcium propionate		
CAS 4080-31-3	Quaternium-15	CAS 6219-77-8	4-Nitro-o-phenylenediamine HCl
CAS 4117-31-1	Ethyl serinate	CAS 6221-95-0	Myristyl propionate
CAS 4169-04-4	Phenoxyisopropanol	CAS 6272-74-8	Lapyrium chloride
CAS 4191-73-5	Isopropylparaben	CAS 6281-04-5	PEG-2 dilaurate
CAS 4207-40-3	Allantoin acetyl methionine	CAS 6283-92-7	Lauryl lactate
CAS 4219-49-2	Glycol palmitate	CAS 6381-59-5	Potassium sodium tartrate
CAS 4247-02-3	Isobutylparaben	CAS 6381-77-7	Sodium erythorbate
CAS 4292-10-8	Lauramidopropyl betaine	CAS 6440-58-0	DMDM hydantoin
CAS 4337-75-1	Sodium methyl lauroyl taurate	CAS 6485-34-3	Calcium saccharin
CAS 4345-03-3	d-α-Tocopheryl succinate	CAS 6485-39-8	Manganese gluconate
CAS 4390-04-9	Isohexadecane	CAS 6540-99-4	Laureth-10
CAS 4403-12-7	Trideceth-3	CAS 6542-37-6	Hydroxymethyl dioxoaza-bicyclooctane
CAS 4418-26-2	Sodium dehydroacetate		
CAS 4468-02-4	Zinc gluconate	CAS 6790-09-6	PEG-12
CAS 4478-97-1	Ceteth-5	CAS 6842-15-5	Dodecene-1
CAS 4484-59-7	Ceteth-3	CAS 6843-97-6	Lauryl diethylenediaminoglycine
CAS 4485-12-5	Lithium stearate	CAS 6846-50-0	Trimethyl-1,3-pentanediol, 2,2,4-diisobutyrate
CAS 4536-30-5	Laureth-1		
CAS 4568-28-9	TEA-stearate	CAS 6881-94-3	Diethylene glycol propyl ether
CAS 4602-84-0	Farnesol	CAS 6916-74-1	Glyceryl behenate
CAS 4698-29-7	N-Phenyl-p-phenylenediamine sulfate	CAS 6938-94-9	Diisopropyl adipate
		CAS 7047-84-9	Aluminum stearate
CAS 4706-78-9	Potassium lauryl sulfate	CAS 7049-66-3	Trilinoleic acid
CAS 4722-98-9	MEA-lauryl sulfate	CAS 7128-91-8	Palmitamine oxide
CAS 4748-78-1	p-Ethylbenzaldehyde	CAS 7147-34-4	Trioctyl citrate
CAS 4810-50-8	Potassium PCA	CAS 7173-51-5	Didecyldimonium chloride
CAS 4826-87-3	Trimethylolpropane trioctanoate	CAS 7177-05-5	Nonoxynol-7
CAS 5013-16-5	BHA	CAS 7177-08-8	Nonoxynol-10
CAS 5026-62-0	Sodium methylparaben	CAS 7205-87-1	Nonoxynol-11
CAS 5117-19-1	PEG-8	CAS 7235-40-7	Carotene
CAS 5131-58-8	4-Nitro-m-phenylenediamine	CAS 7281-04-1	Lauralkonium bromide
CAS 5131-66-8	Butoxypropanol	CAS 7299-99-2	Pentaerythrityl tetraoctanoate
CAS 5168-91-2	Ceteth-6	CAS 7311-27-5	Nonoxynol-4
CAS 5232-99-5	Etocrylene	CAS 7320-34-5	Tetrapotassium pyrophosphate
CAS 5274-61-3	Ceteth-2	CAS 7360-38-5	Trioctanoin
CAS 5274-63-5	Ceteth-4	CAS 7360-53-4	Aluminum formate
CAS 5274-65-7	Oleth-2	CAS 7361-28-6	Ethyl aspartate
CAS 5274-66-8	Oleth-3	CAS 7378-99-6	Dimethyl octylamine
CAS 5274-68-0	Laureth-4	CAS 7381-01-3	Sodium ethyl 2-sulfolaurate
CAS 5306-85-4	Dimethyl isosorbide	CAS 7384-98-7	Propylene glycol dicaprylate
CAS 5307-14-2	2-Nitro-p-phenylenediamine	CAS 7396-58-9	Didecyl methylamine
CAS 5333-42-6	Octyl dodecanol	CAS 7398-69-8	Dimethyl diallyl ammonium chloride monomer
CAS 5333-44-8	Heptylundecanol		
CAS 5349-52-0	PEG-9 stearate	CAS 7425-14-1	Octyl octanoate
CAS 5353-26-4	Oleth-4	CAS 7440-09-7	Potassium
CAS 5353-27-5	Oleth-5	CAS 7447-40-7	Potassium chloride
CAS 5422-34-4	Lactamide MEA	CAS 7487-88-9	Magnesium sulfate
CAS 5434-57-1	Isohexyl neopentanoate	CAS 7491-02-3	Diisopropyl sebacate
CAS 5466-77-3	Octyl methoxycinnamate	CAS 7491-05-2	Tallowtrimonium chloride
CAS 5703-94-6	Deceth-4	CAS 7491-14-7	Dipropylene glycol salicylate
CAS 5743-34-0	Calcium borogluconate	CAS 7545-23-5	Myristamide DEA
CAS 5793-94-2	Calcium stearoyl lactylate	CAS 7545-24-6	Palmitamide DEA
CAS 5856-63-3	2-Amino-1-butanol	CAS 7558-80-7	Sodium phosphate
CAS 5938-38-5	Sorbitan oleate	CAS 7585-39-9	Cyclodextrin
CAS 5949-29-1	Citric acid	CAS 7631-86-9	Diatomaceous earth
CAS 5959-89-7	Sorbitan laurate	CAS 7631-86-9	Silica
CAS 5996-10-1	Glucose (hydrous)	CAS 7631-90-5	Sodium bisulfite
CAS 6001-97-4	Dihexyl sodium sulfosuccinate	CAS 7646-85-7	Zinc chloride
CAS 6004-24-6	Cetylpyridinium chloride	CAS 7647-14-5	Sodium chloride

CAS 7651-02-7	Stearamidopropyl dimethylamine	CAS 8007-69-0	Sweet almond oil
CAS 7664-38-2	Phosphoric acid	CAS 8007-75-8	Bergamot oil
CAS 7681-11-0	Potassium iodide	CAS 8007-80-5	Cinnamon oil
CAS 7681-55-2	Sodium iodate	CAS 8008-52-4	Coriander oil
CAS 7681-57-4	Sodium metabisulfite	CAS 8008-53-5	Ethiodized oil
CAS 7695-91-2	d-α-Tocopheryl acetate	CAS 8008-56-8	Lemon extract
CAS 7702-01-4	Disodium capryloamphodiacetate	CAS 8008-56-8	Lemon oil
CAS 7704-34-9	Sulfur	CAS 8008-57-9	Orange oil
CAS 7722-84-1	Hydrogen peroxide	CAS 8008-74-0	Sesame oil
CAS 7722-88-5	Tetrasodium pyrophosphate	CAS 8008-79-5	Spearmint oil
CAS 7747-35-5	7-Ethyl bicyclooxazolidine	CAS 8008-99-9	Garlic extract
CAS 7757-93-9	Calcium phosphate, dibasic	CAS 8009-03-8	Petrolatum NF
CAS 7758-05-6	Potassium iodate	CAS 8012-89-3	Yellow beeswax
CAS 7758-29-4	Sodium tripolyphosphate	CAS 8012-95-1	Mineral oil
CAS 7775-50-0	Tristearyl citrate	CAS 8013-01-2	Yeast extract
CAS 7778-18-9	Calcium sulfate (anhydrous)	CAS 8013-07-8	Epoxidized soybean oil
CAS 7778-77-0	Potassium phosphate	CAS 8013-86-3	Cypress oil
CAS 7784-25-0	Ammonium alum	CAS 8014-71-9	Balm mint oil
CAS 7787-59-9	Bismuth oxychloride	CAS 8015-01-8	Sweet marjoram oil
CAS 7789-38-0	Sodium bromate	CAS 8015-80-3	Kukui nut oil
CAS 7789-77-7	Calcium phosphate, dibasic, dihydrate	CAS 8015-86-9	Carnauba
		CAS 8015-88-1	Carrot oil
CAS 8000-25-7	Rosemary oil	CAS 8015-92-7	Chamomile oil
CAS 8000-28-0	Lavender oil	CAS 8016-25-9	Hops extract
CAS 8000-48-4	Eucalyptus oil	CAS 8016-60-2	Rice bran wax
CAS 8001-17-0	Egg oil	CAS 8016-63-5	Clary oil
CAS 8001-21-6	Sunflower seed oil	CAS 8016-70-4	Hydrogenated soybean oil
CAS 8001-22-7	Soybean oil	CAS 8020-84-6	Lanolin (hydrous)
CAS 8001-23-8	Safflower oil	CAS 8021-55-4	Ozokerite
CAS 8001-25-0	Olive oil	CAS 8022-29-5	Cherry pit oil
CAS 8001-29-4	Cottonseed oil	CAS 8023-79-8	Palm kernel oil
CAS 8001-30-7	Corn oil	CAS 8023-98-1	Peach kernel oil
CAS 8001-31-8	Coconut oil	CAS 8024-09-7	Walnut oil
CAS 8001-39-6	Japan wax	CAS 8024-22-4	Grape seed oil
CAS 8001-54-5	Benzalkonium chloride	CAS 8024-32-6	Avocado oil
CAS 8001-61-4	Balsam copaiba	CAS 8027-32-5	Petrolatum USP
CAS 8001-67-0	Coffee bean extract	CAS 8027-33-6	Lanolin alcohol
CAS 8001-69-2	Cod liver oil	CAS 8028-48-6	Bitter orange peel extract
CAS 8001-75-0	Ceresin	CAS 8028-66-8	Honey
CAS 8001-78-3	Hydrogenated castor oil	CAS 8029-44-5	Cottonseed glyceride
CAS 8001-78-3	Trihydroxystearin	CAS 8029-68-3	Ichthammol
CAS 8001-79-4	Castor oil	CAS 8029-76-3	Hydroxylated lecithin
CAS 8001-97-6	Aloe	CAS 8030-12-4	Hydrogenated tallow
CAS 8002-03-7	Peanut oil	CAS 8030-28-2	Orange flower water
CAS 8002-05-9	Petroleum distillates	CAS 8030-78-2	Tallowtrimonium chloride
CAS 8002-09-3	Pine oil	CAS 8031-18-3	Fullers earth. See also Attapulgite
CAS 8002-13-9	Canola oil	CAS 8031-44-5	Hydrogenated lanolin
CAS 8002-23-1	Cetyl esters	CAS 8031-67-2	Royal jelly
CAS 8002-31-1	Cocoa butter	CAS 8031-76-3	Mistletoe extract
CAS 8002-33-3	Sulfated castor oil	CAS 8032-32-4	Mineral spirits
CAS 8002-43-5	Lecithin	CAS 8033-29-2	Hydrogenated palm oil
CAS 8002-47-9	Liver extract	CAS 8036-77-9	PEG-40 sorbitan lanolate
CAS 8002-50-4	Menhaden oil	CAS 8038-43-5	Lanolin oil
CAS 8002-53-7	Montan wax	CAS 8038-77-5	Bayberry wax
CAS 8002-66-2	Matricaria oil	CAS 8038-93-5	Sodium aluminum chlorohydroxy lactate
CAS 8002-74-2	Paraffin		
CAS 8002-74-2	Synthetic wax	CAS 8039-09-6	PEG-75 lanolin
CAS 8002-75-3	Palm oil	CAS 8039-67-6	Cocamide MIPA
CAS 8005-44-5	Cetearyl alcohol	CAS 8042-47-5	Mineral oil
CAS 8006-40-4	Behenylbeeswax	CAS 8046-25-1	Wheat germ glycerides
CAS 8006-40-4	White beeswax	CAS 8049-97-6	Melanin
CAS 8006-44-8	Candelilla wax	CAS 8050-07-5	Olibanum
CAS 8006-54-0	Lanolin (anhydrous)	CAS 8050-09-7	Rosin
CAS 8006-54-0	Lanolin oil	CAS 8050-13-3	Methyl hydrogenated rosinate
CAS 8006-90-4	Peppermint oil	CAS 8050-81-5	Simethicone
CAS 8006-95-9	Wheat germ oil	CAS 8051-15-8	PEG-6 sorbitan beeswax
CAS 8007-01-0	Rose oil	CAS 8051-30-7	Cocamide DEA
CAS 8007-08-7	Ginger oil	CAS 8051-52-3	PEG-15 cocamine
CAS 8007-43-0	Sorbitan sesquioleate	CAS 8051-63-6	PEG-50 tallow amide
CAS 8007-46-3	Thyme oil	CAS 8051-73-8	PEG-20 sorbitan beeswax

CAS 8051-81-8	PEG-27 lanolin	CAS 9004-87-9	Octoxynol series
CAS 8051-82-9	PEG-40 lanolin	CAS 9004-94-8	PEG-20 palmitate
CAS 8052-10-6	Rosin	CAS 9004-95-9	Ceteth series
CAS 8052-48-0	Sodium tallowate	CAS 9004-96-0	PEG oleate series
CAS 8052-50-4	Sodium tallow sulfate	CAS 9004-97-1	PEG ricinoleate series
CAS 8057-49-6	Valerian extract	CAS 9004-98-2	Oleth series
CAS 8057-57-6	Buckthorn extract	CAS 9004-99-3	PEG stearate series
CAS 8057-65-6	Arnica extract	CAS 9005-00-9	Steareth series
CAS 9000-01-5	Acacia	CAS 9005-02-1	PEG dilaurate series
CAS 9000-05-9	Gum benzoin	CAS 9005-07-6	PEG dioleate series
CAS 9000-07-1	Carrageenan	CAS 9005-08-7	PEG distearate series
CAS 9000-30-0	Guar gum	CAS 9005-12-3	Phenyl dimethicone
CAS 9000-40-2	Locust bean gum	CAS 9005-25-8	Corn starch
CAS 9000-69-5	Pectin	CAS 9005-25-8	Rice starch
CAS 9000-70-8	Gelatin	CAS 9005-32-7	Alginic acid
CAS 9000-71-9	Milk protein	CAS 9005-34-9	Ammonium alginate
CAS 9001-37-0	Glucose oxidase	CAS 9005-35-0	Calcium alginate
CAS 9001-62-1	Lipase	CAS 9005-36-1	Potassium alginate
CAS 9002-84-0	Polytetrafluoroethylene	CAS 9005-37-2	Propylene glycol alginate
CAS 9002-86-2	Polyvinyl chloride	CAS 9005-38-3	Algin
CAS 9002-88-4	Polyethylene	CAS 9005-46-3	Sodium caseinate
CAS 9002-89-5	Polyvinyl alcohol (super and fully hydrolyzed)	CAS 9005-64-5	PEG sorbitan laurate series
		CAS 9005-64-5	Polysorbate 20
CAS 9002-92-0	Laureth series	CAS 9005-64-5	Polysorbate 21
CAS 9002-93-1	Acrylates/octylacrylamide copolymer	CAS 9005-65-5	Polysorbate 81
		CAS 9005-65-6	PEG sorbitan oleate series
CAS 9002-93-1	Octoxynol series	CAS 9005-65-6	Polysorbate 80
CAS 9002-96-4	Tocophersolan	CAS 9005-66-7	PEG-80 sorbitan palmitate
CAS 9002-98-6	PEI series	CAS 9005-66-7	Polysorbate 40
CAS 9003-01-4	Carbomer	CAS 9005-67-8	PEG sorbitan stearate series
CAS 9003-01-4	Glyceryl polymethacrylate	CAS 9005-67-8	Polysorbate 60
CAS 9003-01-4	Polyacrylic acid	CAS 9005-67-8	Polysorbate 61
CAS 9003-04-7	Sodium polyacrylate	CAS 9005-70-3	PEG-18 sorbitan trioleate
CAS 9003-05-8	Polyacrylamide	CAS 9005-70-3	Polysorbate 85
CAS 9003-07-0	Polypropylene	CAS 9005-71-4	Polysorbate 65
CAS 9003-11-6	Meroxapol series	CAS 9005-79-2	Glycogen
CAS 9003-11-6	PEG/PPG copolymers	CAS 9006-04-6	Polyisoprene
CAS 9003-11-6	Poloxamer series	CAS 9006-50-2	Albumen
CAS 9003-13-8	PPG butyl ethers	CAS 9006-65-9	Dimethicone
CAS 9003-20-7	Polyvinyl acetate (homopolymer)	CAS 9007-16-3	Carbomer
CAS 9003-27-4	Polyisobutene	CAS 9007-17-4	Carbomer
CAS 9003-28-5	Polybutene	CAS 9007-28-7	Chondroitin sulfate
CAS 9003-29-6	Polyisobutene	CAS 9007-28-7	Sodium chondroitin sulfate
CAS 9003-31-0	Polyisoprene	CAS 9007-34-5	Atelocollagen
CAS 9003-39-8	PVP	CAS 9007-34-5	Cationic collagen polypeptides
CAS 9003-53-6	Polystyrene	CAS 9007-34-5	Collagen
CAS 9003-59-2	Sodium polystyrene sulfonate	CAS 9007-34-5	Desamido collagen
CAS 9003-70-7	Styrene/DVB copolymer	CAS 9007-34-5	Glyceryl collagenate
CAS 9003-99-0	Lactoperoxidase	CAS 9007-34-5	Soluble collagen
CAS 9004-32-4	Carboxymethylcellulose sodium	CAS 9007-48-1	Polyglyceryl oleate series
CAS 9004-34-6	Cellulose	CAS 9007-49-2	DNA
CAS 9004-34-6	Microcrystalline cellulose	CAS 9007-58-3	Hydrolyzed elastin
CAS 9004-35-7	Cellulose acetate	CAS 9008-99-8	Hydrolyzed pea protein
CAS 9004-36-3	Sodium caseinate	CAS 9009-99-8	Silk powder
CAS 9004-36-8	Cellulose acetate butyrate	CAS 9010-43-9	Octoxynol-9
CAS 9004-39-1	Cellulose acetate propionate	CAS 9010-66-6	Corn gluten protein
CAS 9004-53-9	Dextrin	CAS 9010-69-9	Zinc rosinate
CAS 9004-57-3	Ethylcellulose	CAS 9010-77-9	Ethylene/acrylic acid copolymer
CAS 9004-61-9	Hyaluronic acid	CAS 9010-79-1	Ethylene/propylene copolymer
CAS 9004-62-0	Hydroxyethylcellulose	CAS 9010-79-1	Polypropylene (nucleated)
CAS 9004-64-2	Hydroxypropylcellulose	CAS 9011-14-7	Methyl methacrylate polymer
CAS 9004-65-3	Hydroxypropyl methylcellulose	CAS 9011-14-7	Polymethyl methacrylate
CAS 9004-67-5	Methylcellulose	CAS 9011-16-9	PVM/MA copolymer
CAS 9004-70-0	Nitrocellulose	CAS 9012-54-8	Cellulase
CAS 9004-73-3	Methicone	CAS 9012-76-4	Chitosan
CAS 9004-74-4	PEG methyl ethers	CAS 9014-01-1	Protease
CAS 9004-81-1	PEG laurate series	CAS 9014-90-8	Sodium nonoxynol sulfate series
CAS 9004-82-4	Sodium laureth sulfate	CAS 9014-92-0	Dodoxynol series
CAS 9004-87-9	Acrylates/octylacrylamide copolymer	CAS 9014-93-1	Nonyl nonoxynol series
		CAS 9015-54-7	Collagen amino acids

CAS 9015-54-7	Hydrolyzed collagen	CAS 11138-66-2	Xanthan gum
CAS 9016-00-6	Dimethicone	CAS 11140-78-6	Lauryl betaine
CAS 9016-45-9	Nonoxynol series	CAS 11308-59-1	Hydroxypropyltrimonium
CAS 9017-27-0	Methylstyrene/vinyltoluene		hydrolyzed collagen
	copolymer	CAS 11381-09-0	Hydroxypropyl bisisostearamido-
CAS 9032-42-2	Methyl hydroxyethylcellulose		propyldimonium chloride
CAS 9032-75-1	Pectinase	CAS 12001-26-2	Mica
CAS 9035-85-2	PPG cetyl ether series	CAS 12001-31-9	Quaternium-18 hectorite
CAS 9036-19-5	Acrylates/octylacrylamide	CAS 12001-99-9	Chromium hydroxide green
	copolymer	CAS 12042-91-0	Aluminum chlorohydrate
CAS 9036-19-5	Octoxynol series	CAS 12049-50-2	Calcium titanate
CAS 9038-43-1	PPG-9-steareth-3	CAS 12068-03-0	Sodium toluenesulfonate
CAS 9038-95-3	PPG buteth series	CAS 12125-02-9	Ammonium chloride
CAS 9040-38-4	Disodium nonoxynol-10	CAS 12141-46-7	Aluminum silicate
	sulfosuccinate	CAS 12173-47-6	Hectorite
CAS 9041-08-1	Sodium heparin	CAS 12199-37-0	Magnesium aluminum silicate
CAS 9042-14-2	Dextran sulfate	CAS 12240-15-2	Ferric ammonium ferrocyanide
CAS 9042-76-6	PPG-9 diethylmonium chloride	CAS 12691-60-0	Stearalkonium hectorite
CAS 9042-82-4	PPG-12/SMDI copolymer	CAS 12694-22-3	Polyglyceryl-2 stearate
CAS 9046-01-9	Trideceth phosphate series	CAS 12709-64-7	Polyglyceryl-10 tristearate
CAS 9048-46-8	Serum albumin	CAS 12751-23-4	Lauryl phosphate
CAS 9050-36-6	Maltodextrin	CAS 12764-60-2	Polyglyceryl-10 distearate
CAS 9051-57-4	Ammonium nonoxynol-4 sulfate	CAS 12765-39-8	Sodium methyl cocoyl taurate
CAS 9061-82-9	Sodium carrageenan	CAS 12769-96-9	Ultramarine violet
CAS 9062-04-8	MIPA-laureth sulfate	CAS 13039-35-5	Sodium capryloamphoacetate
CAS 9062-04-8	Propylene glycol dicaprylate/	CAS 13040-19-2	Zinc ricinoleate
	dicaprate	CAS 13057-50-6	Pentaerythrityl tetralaurate
CAS 9063-38-1	Sodium starch glycolate	CAS 13149-83-2	Ceteth-12
CAS 9065-13-8	DMHF	CAS 13150-00-0	Sodium laureth sulfate
CAS 9065-63-8	PPG buteth series	CAS 13192-12-6	Disodium lauryl sulfosuccinate
CAS 9067-32-7	Sodium hyaluronate	CAS 13197-76-7	Lauryl hydroxysultaine
CAS 9076-43-1	PPG-40 diethylmonium chloride	CAS 13232-26-3	Batyl stearate
CAS 9082-00-2	PPG-24-glycereth-24	CAS 13463-41-7	Zinc pyrithione
CAS 9082-07-9	Sodium chondroitin sulfate	CAS 13463-67-7	Titanium dioxide
CAS 9084-06-4	Sodium polynaphthalene sulfonate	CAS 13475-82-6	Isododecane
CAS 9087-53-0	PPG ceteth series	CAS 13552-80-2	Triundecanoin
CAS 9087-61-0	Aluminum starch octenyl succinate	CAS 13557-75-0	Sodium lauroyl lactylate
CAS 9970-10-4	Steareth-4	CAS 13573-18-7	Sodium tripolyphosphate
CAS 10043-01-3	Aluminum sulfate	CAS 13832-70-7	Stearyl glycyrrhetinate
CAS 10043-11-5	Boron nitride	CAS 14007-07-9	Chlorhexidine digluconate
CAS 10043-52-4	Calcium chloride	CAS 14025-15-1	Disodium EDTA-copper
CAS 10101-39-0	Calcium silicate	CAS 14038-43-8	Ferric ferrocyanide
CAS 10101-41-4	Calcium sulfate (dihydrate)	CAS 14246-53-8	Caployl glycine
CAS 10101-66-3	Manganese violet	CAS 14350-94-8	Sodium caproamphoacetate
CAS 10108-24-4	PEG-4 laurate	CAS 14350-96-0	Sodium lauroamphoacetate
CAS 10108-25-5	PEG-4 oleate	CAS 14350-97-1	Disodium lauroamphodiacetate
CAS 10108-28-8	PEG-6 stearate	CAS 14351-40-7	Stearamide MEA-stearate
CAS 10124-56-8	Sodium hexametaphosphate	CAS 14351-50-9	Oleamine oxide
CAS 10191-41-0	dl-α-Tocopherol	CAS 14409-72-4	Nonoxynol-9
CAS 10213-78-2	PEG-2 stearamine	CAS 14450-05-6	Pentaerythrityl tetrapelargonate
CAS 10228-03-2	N,N´-Dimethyl-N-hydroxyethyl-3-	CAS 14465-68-0	Trilinolenin
	nitro-p-phenylenediamine	CAS 14481-60-8	Disodium stearyl sulfosuccinamate
CAS 10233-13-3	Isopropyl laurate	CAS 14492-68-3	Steapyrium chloride
CAS 10233-14-4	PEG-3 oleate	CAS 14529-40-9	Ceteth-10
CAS 10233-24-6	PEG-3 stearate	CAS 14548-60-8	Benzylhemiformal
CAS 10289-94-8	PEG-14 stearate	CAS 14727-68-5	Dimethyl oleamine
CAS 10401-55-5	Cetyl ricinoleate	CAS 14779-93-2	Isodecyl laurate
CAS 10417-94-4	Eicosapentaenoic acid	CAS 14807-96-6	Talc
CAS 10525-14-1	Mixed isopropanolamines	CAS 14960-06-6	Sodium lauriminodipropionate
	myristate	CAS 15087-24-8	3-Benzylidene camphor
CAS 10578-34-4	Stearyl benzoate	CAS 15323-35-0	Acetyl hexamethyl indan
CAS 11006-34-1	Chlorophyllin-copper complex	CAS 15454-75-8	Zinc PCA
CAS 11006-75-0	Saponins	CAS 15716-30-0	PEG-25 PABA
CAS 11042-64-1	Oryzanol	CAS 15763-02-7	Dioctylmalate
CAS 11094-60-3	Polyglyceryl-10 decaoleate	CAS 16245-77-5	p-Phenylenediamine sulfate
CAS 11097-68-0	Aluminum sesquichlorohydrate	CAS 16485-10-2	DL-Panthenol
CAS 11099-07-3	Glyceryl stearate	CAS 16676-75-8	Tocopheryl nicotinate
CAS 11099-07-3	Glyceryl stearate SE	CAS 16693-53-1	TEA lauroyl sarcosinate
CAS 11103-57-4	Retinol	CAS 16731-55-8	Potassium metabisulfite
CAS 11111-34-5	Poloxamine series	CAS 16841-14-8	Behenalkonium chloride

CAS 16867-03-1	2-Amino-3-hydroxypyridine
CAS 16889-14-8	Stearamidoethyl diethylamine
CAS 16958-92-2	Ditridecyl adipate
CAS 16958-92-2	Ditridecyl dimer dilinoleate
CAS 17301-53-0	Behentrimonium chloride
CAS 17407-37-3	Tocopheryl succinate
CAS 17658-36-8	Cetylarachidol
CAS 17661-50-6	Cetyl esters
CAS 17661-50-6	Myristyl stearate
CAS 17671-27-1	Behenyl behenate
CAS 17673-56-2	Oleyl erucate
CAS 17673-59-3	Oleyl linoleate
CAS 17736-08-2	TEA oleoyl sarcosinate
CAS 18194-24-6	1,2-Dimyristoyl-sn-glycero(3) phosphatidylcholine
CAS 18282-10-5	Tin oxide (ic)
CAS 18312-31-7	Stearyl caprylate
CAS 18312-32-8	Behenyl erucate
CAS 18448-65-2	PEG-2 oleammonium chloride
CAS 18465-99-1	Glyceryl linolenate
CAS 18469-44-8	Sodium methyl myristoyl taurate
CAS 18472-51-0	Chlorhexidine digluconate
CAS 18641-57-1	Tribehenin
CAS 18684-11-2	Steartrimonium methosulfate
CAS 18748-91-9	Stearoxytrimethylsilane
CAS 18758-91-3	Bisphenylhexamethicone
CAS 18962-61-3	Magnesium aspartate
CAS 19035-79-1	Potassium cetyl phosphate
CAS 19040-44-9	Disodium lauryl sulfosuccinate
CAS 19277-88-4	Stearamidopropyl trimonium methosulfate
CAS 19321-40-5	Pentaerythrityl tetraoleate
CAS 20018-09-1	Diiodomethyl p-tolyl sulfone
CAS 20260-64-4	Laureth-6 carboxylic acid
CAS 20292-08-4	Octyl laurate
CAS 20457-75-4	Ricinoleamidopropyl dimethyl-amine
CAS 20475-12-1	TEA-lactate
CAS 20545-92-0	Undecylenamide MEA
CAS 20636-48-0	Nonoxynol-5
CAS 20824-56-0	Diammonium EDTA
CAS 20834-06-4	Cetyl laurate
CAS 20858-24-6	Laureth-3 carboxylic acid
CAS 21034-17-3	Quaternium-45
CAS 21127-45-7	Laureth-5 carboxylic acid
CAS 21142-28-9	MIPA-lauryl sulfate
CAS 21245-02-3	Octyl dimethyl PABA
CAS 21542-96-1	Dimethyl behenamine
CAS 21645-51-2	Alumina, hydrate
CAS 21645-51-2	Aluminum hydroxide
CAS 21652-27-7	Oleyl hydroxyethyl imidazoline
CAS 21860-85-5	Ethyl aspartate
CAS 22047-49-0	Octyl stearate
CAS 22393-86-8	Cetyl oleate
CAS 22500-92-1	Sorbic acid
CAS 22766-82-1	Octyldodecyl stearate
CAS 22766-83-2	Octyldodecyl myristate
CAS 22788-19-8	Propylene glycol dilaurate
CAS 22801-45-2	Octyldodecyl oleate
CAS 22882-95-7	Isopropyl linoleate
CAS 23336-36-9	PEG-5 oleate
CAS 23597-82-2	Hexyl nicotinate
CAS 23732-95-8	Sodium mannuronate methyl-silanol
CAS 24271-12-3	Stearyl behenate
CAS 24817-92-3	Acetyl tri-n-hexyl citrate
CAS 24871-34-9	Oleth-10
CAS 24937-16-4	Nylon-12
CAS 24937-78-8	Ethylene/VA copolymer
CAS 24938-91-8	Trideceth series
CAS 24938-91-8	Trideceth-7 carboxylic acid
CAS 24981-13-3	Styrene/acrylamide copolymer
CAS 25013-16-5	BHA
CAS 25035-71-6	Tosylamide/formaldehyde resin
CAS 25038-54-4	Nylon-6
CAS 25038-74-8	Nylon-12
CAS 25054-76-6	Oleamidopropyl betaine
CAS 25066-20-0	Stearamidopropylamine oxide
CAS 25085-02-3	Acrylamide/sodium acrylate copolymer
CAS 25086-29-7	Styrene/PVP copolymer
CAS 25086-62-8	Sodium polymethacrylate
CAS 25086-89-9	PVP/VA copolymer
CAS 25087-26-7	Polymethacrylic acid
CAS 25155-18-4	Methylbenzethonium chloride
CAS 25155-30-0	Sodium dodecylbenzenesulfonate
CAS 25159-40-4	Oleamidopropylamine oxide
CAS 25167-62-8	Docosahexaenoic acid
CAS 25168-73-4	Saccharose distearate
CAS 25168-73-4	Saccharose palmitate
CAS 25168-73-4	Sucrose stearate
CAS 25190-05-0	Oleth-16
CAS 25212-19-5	Adipic acid/epoxypropyl diethylenetriamine copolymer
CAS 25212-19-5	AMP isostearoyl hydrolyzed collagen
CAS 25212-19-5	Hydrogenated vegetable glycerides phosphate
CAS 25231-21-4	PPG stearyl ether series
CAS 25322-68-3	PEG series
CAS 25322-69-4	PPG series
CAS 25339-09-7	Isocetyl stearate
CAS 25339-99-5	Sucrose laurate
CAS 25377-63-3	Undecylenamide MEA
CAS 25377-64-1	Undecylenamide DEA
CAS 25383-99-7	Sodium stearoyl lactylate
CAS 25446-78-0	Sodium trideceth sulfate (n = 3)
CAS 25446-80-4	Sodium myreth sulfate
CAS 25496-72-4	Glyceryl mono/dioleate
CAS 25609-89-6	VA/crotonates copolymer
CAS 25637-84-7	Glyceryl dioleate
CAS 25655-41-8	PVP-iodine
CAS 25704-18-1	Sodium polystyrene sulfonate
CAS 25704-59-0	Sodium caproamphoacetate
CAS 25750-82-7	Ethylene/sodium acrylate copolymer
CAS 25791-96-2	PPG glyceryl ether series
CAS 25869-00-5	Ferric ammonium ferrocyanide
CAS 25882-44-4	Disodium lauramido MEA-sulfosuccinate
CAS 25987-06-8	PEI-10
CAS 26027-37-2	PEG oleamide series
CAS 26027-38-3	Nonoxynol series
CAS 26062-79-3	Polyquaternium-6
CAS 26112-07-2	Potassium methylparaben
CAS 26161-33-1	Polyquaternium-37
CAS 26172-55-4	Methylchloroisothiazolinone
CAS 26183-52-8	Deceth-4
CAS 26248-24-8	Sodium tridecylbenzene sulfonate
CAS 26256-79-1	Sodium lauriminodipropionate
CAS 26264-02-8	Nonoxynol-5
CAS 26264-05-1	Isopropylamine dodecylbenzene-sulfonate
CAS 26266-57-9	Sorbitan palmitate
CAS 26266-58-0	Sorbitan trioleate
CAS 26399-02-0	Octyl stearate
CAS 26401-35-4	Ditridecyl adipate
CAS 26401-47-8	Dodoxynol series
CAS 26402-22-2	Glyceryl caprate
CAS 26402-26-6	Caprylic/capric glycerides

CAS 26402-26-6	Glyceryl caprylate	CAS 28319-77-9	Glycerophosphocholine
CAS 26402-31-3	Propylene glycol ricinoleate	CAS 28474-90-0	Ascorbyl dipalmitate
CAS 26426-80-2	Isobutylene/MA copolymer	CAS 28510-23-8	Neopentyl glycol dioctanoate
CAS 26445-96-5	Ethylene/calcium acrylate copolymer	CAS 28724-32-5	PEG-15 stearmonium chloride
		CAS 28829-38-1	Sodium polyglutamate
CAS 26446-38-8	Sucrose palmitate	CAS 28874-51-3	Sodium PCA
CAS 26447-10-9	Ammonium xylenesulfonate	CAS 28880-55-9	PEG-15 oleammonium chloride
CAS 26483-35-2	Behenamine oxide	CAS 29051-57-8	Sodium caproyl lactylate
CAS 26545-53-9	DEA-dodecylbenzene sulfonate	CAS 29059-24-3	Propylene glycol myristate
CAS 26571-11-9	Nonoxynol series	CAS 29116-98-1	Sorbitan dioleate
CAS 26571-49-3	PPG dioleate series	CAS 29297-55-0	Polyquaternium-16
CAS 26589-26-4	Acrylates/PVP copolymer	CAS 29381-93-9	TEA-dodecylbenzenesulfonate
CAS 26590-05-6	Polyquaternium-7	CAS 29383-26-4	Octyl hydroxystearate
CAS 26635-75-6	PEG lauramide series	CAS 29461-14-1	Isolongifolene ketone exo
CAS 26635-92-7	PEG stearamine series	CAS 29548-30-9	Farnesyl acetate
CAS 26650-05-5	Disodium undecylenamido MEA-sulfosuccinate	CAS 29710-25-6	Octyl hydroxystearate
		CAS 29710-25-6	Octyl oxystearate
CAS 26657-95-4	Glyceryl dipalmitate	CAS 29806-73-3	Octyl palmitate
CAS 26657-96-5	Glyceryl palmitate	CAS 29923-31-7	L-Sodium lauroyl glutamate
CAS 26658-19-5	Sorbitan tristearate	CAS 29923-34-0	DL-Sodium lauroyl glutamate
CAS 26699-71-8	Glyceryl adipate	CAS 29994-44-3	Nonoxynol-6 phosphate
CAS 26718-90-1	Isopropyl arachidate	CAS 30007-47-7	5-Bromo-5-nitro-1,3-dioxane
CAS 26718-95-6	Isopropyl behenate	CAS 30233-64-8	Glyceryl behenate
CAS 26826-30-2	Myreth-3	CAS 30364-51-3	Sodium myristoyl sarcosinate
CAS 26837-33-2	Sodium lauroamphoacetate	CAS 30399-84-9	Isostearic acid
CAS 26838-05-1	Disodium lauryl sulfosuccinate	CAS 30473-39-3	Sodium stearoamphoacetate
CAS 26855-43-6	Polyglyceryl-3 stearate	CAS 30581-59-0	PVP/dimethylaminoethyl-methacrylate copolymer
CAS 26855-44-7	Polyglyceryl-4 stearate		
CAS 27028-82-6	TEA-laureth sulfate	CAS 30657-38-6	Lauryl PCA
CAS 27040-03-5	Oleth-8	CAS 30999-06-5	Tocophersolan
CAS 27083-27-8	Polyaminopropyl biguanide	CAS 31394-71-5	PPG oleate series
CAS 27119-07-9	Polyacrylamidomethylpropane sulfonic acid	CAS 31478-84-9	Isopropyl isostearate
		CAS 31556-45-3	Tridecyl stearate
CAS 27136-73-8	Oleyl hydroxyethyl imidazoline	CAS 31565-12-5	Propylene glycol caprylate
CAS 27138-31-4	Dipropylene glycol dibenzoate	CAS 31565-38-5	Isodecyl stearate
CAS 27176-87-0	Dodecylbenzene sulfonic acid	CAS 31566-31-1	Glyceryl stearate
CAS 27176-93-8	Nonoxynol-2	CAS 31566-31-1	Glyceryl stearate SE
CAS 27176-94-9	Octoxynol-3	CAS 31691-97-1	Ammonium nonoxynol sulfate series
CAS 27176-95-0	Nonoxynol-3		
CAS 27176-97-2	Nonoxynol-4	CAS 31692-79-2	Dimethiconol
CAS 27176-99-4	Octoxynol-5	CAS 31694-55-0	Glycereth series
CAS 27177-01-1	Nonoxynol-6	CAS 31791-00-2	PEG-40 stearate
CAS 27177-02-2	Octoxynol-7	CAS 31799-71-0	PEG oleamide series
CAS 27177-05-5	Nonoxynol series	CAS 31807-55-3	Isododecane
CAS 27177-07-7	Octoxynol-10	CAS 31955-67-6	TEA-lauroyl glutamate
CAS 27178-16-1	Diisodecyl adipate	CAS 32057-14-0	Glyceryl isostearate
CAS 27194-74-7	Propylene glycol laurate	CAS 32073-22-6	Sodium cumenesulfonate
CAS 27195-16-0	Sucrose distearate	CAS 32131-17-2	Nylon-66
CAS 27233-00-7	Glyceryl triacetyl hydroxystearate	CAS 32426-11-2	Quaternium-24
CAS 27233-34-7	Sodium oleth sulfate	CAS 32440-50-9	PVP/hexadecene copolymer
CAS 27306-79-2	Myreth series	CAS 32582-32-4	2-Tetradecyloctadecanol
CAS 27306-90-7	Laureth carboxylic acid series	CAS 32612-48-9	Ammonium laureth sulfate series
CAS 27321-72-8	Polyglyceryl-3 stearate	CAS 32647-67-9	Dibenzylidene sorbitol
CAS 27321-96-6	Choleth series	CAS 32954-43-1	Palmitamidopropyl betaine
CAS 27323-41-7	TEA-dodecylbenzenesulfonate	CAS 33703-08-1	Diisononyl adipate
CAS 27458-93-1	Isostearyl alcohol	CAS 33907-46-9	Glycol hydroxystearate
CAS 27479-28-3	Quaternium-14	CAS 33907-47-0	Propylene glycol hydroxystearate
CAS 27503-81-7	Phenylbenzimidazole sulfonic acid	CAS 33939-64-9	Sodium laureth-13 carboxylate
CAS 27538-35-8	Ethyl urocanate	CAS 33939-65-0	Sodium ceteth-13 carboxylate
CAS 27638-00-2	Glyceryl dilaurate	CAS 33940-98-6	Polyglyceryl-3 oleate
CAS 27640-89-7	Erucyl erucate	CAS 33940-99-7	Polyglyceryl-10 dioleate
CAS 27731-61-9	Ammonium myreth sulfate	CAS 34316-64-8	Hexyl laurate
CAS 27841-06-1	Neopentyl glycol dicaprate	CAS 34395-72-7	Lauryl aminopropylglycine
CAS 27883-12-1	Linoleamide DEA	CAS 34406-66-1	Polyglyceryl-10 laurate
CAS 27942-26-3	Nonoxynol-10	CAS 34424-97-0	Polyglyceryl-6 distearate
CAS 27986-36-3	Nonoxynol-1	CAS 34424-98-1	Polyglyceryl-10 tetraoleate
CAS 28061-69-0	Dimethyl oleamine	CAS 34962-91-9	Isodecyl octanoate
CAS 28063-42-5	Glyceryl erucate	CAS 35179-86-3	PEG-8 laurate
CAS 28211-18-9	PVP/eicosene copolymer	CAS 35230-14-9	Stearyl lactate
CAS 28212-44-4	Nonoxynol carboxylic acid series	CAS 35274-05-6	Cetyl lactate

CAS 35285-68-8	Sodium ethylparaben
CAS 35285-69-9	Sodium propylparaben
CAS 35429-19-7	Polyquaternium-32
CAS 35602-69-8	Cholesteryl stearate
CAS 35691-65-7	Methyldibromo glutaronitrile
CAS 36078-10-1	Lauryl oleate
CAS 36148-84-2	Tocopheryl linoleate
CAS 36284-86-3	Stearamide AMP
CAS 36311-34-9	Isocetyl alcohol
CAS 36409-57-1	Disodium lauryl sulfosuccinate
CAS 36457-19-9	Potassium ethylparaben
CAS 36457-20-2	Sodium butylparaben
CAS 36521-89-8	Sorbitan distearate
CAS 36653-82-4	Cetyl alcohol
CAS 36861-47-9	4-Methylbenzylidene camphor
CAS 37139-99-4	Olealkonium chloride
CAS 37172-53-5	Methyldihydrojasmonate
CAS 37191-69-8	Sodium cyclodextrin sulfate
CAS 37200-49-0	Polysorbate 80
CAS 37205-87-1	Nonoxynol series
CAS 37220-82-9	Glyceryl oleate
CAS 37220-82-9	PEG-15 tallow polyamine
CAS 37309-58-3	Polydecene
CAS 37310-95-5	Glyceryl polymethacrylate
CAS 37311-00-5	PPG-25-laureth-25
CAS 37311-01-6	PPG ceteth series
CAS 37311-04-9	PPG-3-myreth-3
CAS 37311-67-4	Disodium undecylenamido MEA-sulfosuccinate
CAS 37318-14-2	PEG-8 laurate
CAS 37324-85-9	PEG-23 glyceryl laurate
CAS 37349-34-1	Polyglyceryl stearate series
CAS 37475-88-0	Ammonium cumenesulfonate
CAS 37767-39-8	Tetrasodium dicarboxyethyl stearyl sulfosuccinamate
CAS 37767-42-3	Disodium myristamido MEA-sulfosuccinate
CAS 38102-62-4	4-Methylbenzylidene camphor
CAS 38517-23-6	Sodium hydrogenated tallow glutamate
CAS 38517-37-2	Sodium myristoyl glutamate
CAS 38566-94-8	Potassium butyl paraben
CAS 38866-20-5	Hydroxyanthraquinoneaminopropyl methyl morpholinium methosulfate
CAS 38916-42-6	Tetrasodium dicarboxyethyl stearyl sulfosuccinamate
CAS 39034-24-7	Myreth-4
CAS 39175-72-9	Glyceryl stearate citrate
CAS 39236-46-9	Imidazolidinyl urea
CAS 39346-74-2	Pentadoxynol series
CAS 39354-45-5	Disodium laureth sulfosuccinate
CAS 39354-47-5	Disodium C12-15 pareth sulfosuccinate
CAS 39421-75-5	Hydroxypropyl guar
CAS 39464-64-7	Nonyl nonoxynol phosphate series
CAS 39464-66-9	Laureth phosphate series
CAS 39464-69-2	Oleth phosphate series
CAS 39529-26-5	Polyglyceryl-10 decastearate
CAS 39669-97-1	Palmitamidopropyl dimethylamine
CAS 40160-92-7	Pentadoxynol-200
CAS 40445-72-5	Cholesteryl hydroxystearate
CAS 40716-42-5	Ricinoleamide DEA
CAS 40754-59-4	Disodium laureth sulfosuccinate
CAS 40754-60-7	Disodium ricinoleamido MEA-sulfosuccinate
CAS 40839-40-5	Disodium undecylenamido MEA-sulfosuccinate
CAS 41395-83-9	Propylene glycol dipelargonate
CAS 41395-89-5	Isodecyl isononanoate
CAS 41669-30-1	Isostearyl isostearate
CAS 41672-81-5	Dipalmitoyl hydroxyproline
CAS 41760-23-0	Dicaprylyol cystine
CAS 42016-08-0	Disodium laureth sulfosuccinate
CAS 42131-25-9	Isononyl isononanoate
CAS 42131-27-1	Isotridecyl isononanoate
CAS 42131-28-2	Isostearyl lactate
CAS 42173-90-0	Octoxynol-9
CAS 42175-36-0	Oleyl lactate
CAS 42233-07-8	Lauryl behenate
CAS 42233-14-7	Arachidyl behenate
CAS 42233-51-2	Myristyl lignocerate
CAS 42504-46-1	MIPA-dodecylbenzenesulfonate
CAS 42566-92-7	Steapyrium chloride
CAS 42612-52-2	Sodium laureth-4 phosphate
CAS 42909-29-5	2-Methoxy-p-phenylene diamine sulfate
CAS 42926-22-7	L-Sodium lauroyl glutamate
CAS 43101-48-0	Diethyl aspartate
CAS 43154-85-4	Disodium oleamido MIPA-sulfosuccinate
CAS 45235-48-1	2-Octyl-1-decanol
CAS 45267-19-4	Myristamidopropyl dimethylamine
CAS 49553-76-6	Polyglyceryl-2 oleate
CAS 50643-20-4	PPG-5 ceteth-10 phosphate
CAS 50935-57-4	PVM/MA copolymer, ethyl ester
CAS 51033-38-6	Polyglyceryl-6 laurate
CAS 51142-51-9	PEG-20 glyceryl ricinoleate
CAS 51158-08-8	PEG glyceryl stearate series
CAS 51200-87-4	Dimethyl oxazolidine
CAS 51229-78-8	Quaternium-15
CAS 51248-32-9	PEG glyceryl laurate series
CAS 51258-15-2	PPG glycereth series
CAS 51437-95-7	Nonoxynol-3
CAS 51609-41-7	Nonoxynol phosphate series
CAS 51811-79-1	Nonoxynol-6 phosphate
CAS 51812-80-7	Quaternium-22
CAS 51218-64-2	Carboxymethyl chitin
CAS 52292-17-8	Isosteareth series
CAS 52304-36-6	Ethyl butylacetylaminopropionate
CAS 52315-75-0	Lauroyl lysine
CAS 52467-63-7	Tricetylmonium chloride
CAS 52504-24-2	PEG-6 caprylic/capric glycerides
CAS 52558-73-3	Myristoyl sarcosine
CAS 52581-71-2	PPG oleyl ether series
CAS 52668-97-0	PEG dioleate series
CAS 52668-97-0	PEG distearate series
CAS 52725-64-1	Lauramide DEA
CAS 52794-79-3	Isostearamide DEA
CAS 52932-31-7	Adipic acid/epoxypropyl diethylenetriamine copolymer
CAS 53026-57-6	FD&C blue no. 1 aluminum lake
CAS 53200-28-5	PVM/MA copolymer, butyl ester
CAS 53320-86-8	Sodium magnesium silicate
CAS 53563-63-6	Glyceryl dimyristate
CAS 53568-66-4	Polyquaternium-10
CAS 53576-49-1	TEA-lauroyl glutamate
CAS 53610-02-9	Nonoxynol-8 carboxylic acid
CAS 53633-54-8	Polyquaternium-11
CAS 53694-15-8	Sorbeth-20
CAS 53694-17-0	Polyquaternium-22
CAS 53980-88-4	Cyclocarboxypropyloleic acid
CAS 54018-18-7	PVM/MA copolymer, butyl ester
CAS 54077-45-1	PVM/MA copolymer, isopropyl ester
CAS 54193-36-1	Sodium polymethacrylate
CAS 54351-50-7	DEA-laureth sulfate
CAS 54351-50-7	Polyquaternium-10
CAS 54392-26-6	Sorbitan isostearate
CAS 54549-25-6	Decyl glucoside
CAS 54571-67-4	Sodium PCA

CAS 54578-88-0	PVM/MA copolymer, isopropyl ester	CAS 60270-33-9	Behenamidopropyl dimethylamine
		CAS 60344-26-5	PEG-6 oleate
CAS 54578-90-4	PVM/MA copolymer, ethyl ester	CAS 60616-95-7	Sodium carrageenan
CAS 54578-91-5	PVM/MA copolymer, butyl ester	CAS 60687-87-8	PEG-2 stearmonium chloride
CAS 54590-52-2	MIPA-dodecylbenzenesulfonate	CAS 60752-63-8	Thenoyl methionine
CAS 54982-83-1	1,4-Dioxacyclohexadecane-5,16-dione	CAS 60828-78-6	Isolaureth-6
		CAS 61332-02-3	Glyceryl isostearate
CAS 55302-96-0	2-Methyl-5-hydroxyethyl-aminophenol	CAS 61372-91-6	Dibehenyl methylamine
		CAS 61417-49-0	Isopropyl titanium triisostearate
CAS 55353-19-0	DEA-laureth sulfate	CAS 61682-73-3	Pentaerythrityl tetrabehenate
CAS 55353-19-0	Polyquaternium-10	CAS 61693-08-1	Hydrogenated polyisobutene
CAS 55353-21-4	VA/crotonates/vinyl neodecanoate copolymer	CAS 61693-41-2	DEA-cetyl phosphate
		CAS 61757-59-3	Sodium trideceth carboxylate series
CAS 55406-53-6	Iodopropynyl butylcarbamate		
CAS 55819-53-9	Stearamidopropyl dimethylamine lactate	CAS 61788-40-7	Acrylic acid/acrylonitrogens copolymer
CAS 55852-13-6	Stearamidopropyl morpholine	CAS 61788-45-2	Hydrogenated tallowamine
CAS 55852-14-7	Stearamidopropyl morpholine lactate	CAS 61788-46-3	Cocamine
		CAS 61788-47-4	Coconut acid
CAS 55852-15-8	Isostearamidopropyl dimethyl-amine lactate	CAS 61788-48-5	Acetylated lanolin
		CAS 61788-49-6	Acetylated lanolin alcohol
CAS 55895-85-7	Diethyl glutamate	CAS 61788-55-4	Bioflavonoids
CAS 55963-33-2	Distarch phosphate	CAS 61788-59-8	Methyl cocoate
CAS 56002-14-3	PEG isostearate series	CAS 61788-62-3	Dicoco methylamine
CAS 56091-51-1	PVM/MA copolymer, isopropyl ester	CAS 61788-63-4	Dihydrogenated tallow methy-lamine
CAS 56235-92-8	Dioctylmalate	CAS 61788-78-1	Hydrogenated tallowtrimonium chloride
CAS 56265-06-6	Arginine PCA		
CAS 56388-43-3	Disodium oleamido PEG-2 sulfosuccinate	CAS 61788-85-0	PEG hydrogenated castor oil series
CAS 56388-96-6	Trideceth-7 carboxylic acid	CAS 61788-85-0	PEG-66 trihydroxystearin
CAS 56519-71-2	Propylene glycol dioctanoate	CAS 61788-89-4	Dilinoleic acid
CAS 56709-13-8	Polymethoxy bicyclic oxazolidine	CAS 61788-90-7	Cocamine oxide
CAS 56827-95-3	Tricetyl phosphate	CAS 61788-91-8	Dimethyl soyamine
CAS 56863-02-6	Linoleamide DEA	CAS 61788-92-9	Disoyadimonium chloride
CAS 57171-56-9	PEG sorbitan hexaoleate series	CAS 61788-93-0	Dimethyl cocamine
CAS 57307-99-0	PEG-8 caprylic/capric glycerides	CAS 61788-95-2	Dimethyl hydrogenated tallow amine
CAS 57524-53-5	2-Nitro-N-hydroxyethyl-p-anisidine		
CAS 57569-76-3	Glycereth-7 triacetate	CAS 61789-04-6	Sodium cocomonoglyceride sulfate
CAS 57601-56-6	Sodium hyaluronate dimethyl-silanol	CAS 61789-05-7	Glyceryl cocoate
		CAS 61789-07-9	Hydrogenated cottonseed glyceride
CAS 58069-11-7	Quaternium-52		
CAS 58253-49-9	PEG-30 oleamine	CAS 61789-08-0	Hydrogenated soy glyceride
CAS 58450-52-5	Disodium laureth sulfosuccinate	CAS 61789-08-0	Hydrogenated vegetable glyceride
CAS 58450-52-5	Octyldodecyl stearoyl stearate	CAS 61789-09-1	Hydrogenated tallow glyceride
CAS 58727-01-8	Sodium bischlorophenyl sulfamine	CAS 61789-10-4	Lard glyceride
CAS 58748-27-9	Propylene glycol dicaprylate/dicaprate	CAS 61789-13-7	Tallow glyceride
		CAS 61789-18-2	Cocotrimonium chloride
CAS 58855-36-0	DEA-laureth sulfate	CAS 61789-30-8	Potassium cocoate
CAS 58855-63-3	DEA-oleth phosphate series	CAS 61789-31-9	Sodium cocoate
CAS 58958-60-4	Isostearyl neopentanoate	CAS 61789-32-0	Sodium cocoyl isethionate
CAS 59060-56-3	PEG glyceryl laurate series	CAS 61789-40-0	Cocamidopropyl betaine
CAS 59130-69-7	Cetyl octanoate	CAS 61789-68-2	PEG-2 coco-benzonium chloride
CAS 59130-70-7	Cetearyl octanoate	CAS 61789-71-7	Benzalkonium chloride
CAS 59186-41-3	Sodium cetearyl sulfate	CAS 61789-72-8	Hydrogenated tallowalkonium chloride
CAS 59231-34-4	Isodecyl oleate		
CAS 59231-37-7	Isotridecyl isononanoate	CAS 61789-73-9	Dihydrogenated tallow benzyl-monium chloride
CAS 59259-38-0	Menthyl lactate		
CAS 59272-84-3	Myristamidopropyl betaine	CAS 61789-76-2	Dicocamine
CAS 59559-30-7	Steareth-7 carboxylic acid	CAS 61789-77-3	Dicocodimonium chloride
CAS 59587-44-9	Octyl pelargonate	CAS 61789-79-5	Hydrogenated ditallowamine
CAS 59686-68-9	Myreth-3 myristate	CAS 61789-80-8	Quaternium-18
CAS 59792-81-3	Aluminum PCA	CAS 61789-91-1	Hydrogenated jojoba oil
CAS 59820-63-2	3-Methylamino-4-nitrophen-oxyethanol	CAS 61789-91-1	Jojoba oil
		CAS 61790-12-3	Tall oil acid
CAS 51192-09-7	PEG glyceryl oleate series	CAS 61790-18-9	Soyamine
CAS 58969-27-0	Sodium cocoyl isethionate	CAS 61790-33-8	Tallow amine
CAS 60209-82-7	Isodecyl neopentanoate	CAS 61790-37-2	Tallow acid
CAS 60219-68-3	Polyglyceryl-2 dioleate	CAS 61790-38-3	Hydrogenated tallow acid
CAS 60239-68-1	Undecylenamide DEA	CAS 61790-41-8	Soytrimonium chloride

CAS 61790-44-1	Potassium tallate	CAS 65072-00-6	Hydrolyzed milk protein
CAS 61790-64-5	TEA cocoate	CAS 65072-00-6	Milk amino acids
CAS 61790-81-6	PEG lanolin series	CAS 65072-01-7	Corn gluten amino acids
CAS 61790-85-0	PEG tallow aminopropylamine series	CAS 65104-36-1	DEA-lauraminopropionate
		CAS 65215-54-5	Diphenylmethyl piperazinyl-benzimidazole
CAS 61790-86-1	Polysorbate 80		
CAS 61791-00-2	PEG tallate series	CAS 65235-31-6	3-Nitro-p-hydroxyethyl-aminophenol
CAS 61791-01-3	PEG ditallate series		
CAS 61791-08-0	PEG cocamide series	CAS 65277-52-3	Disodium undecylenamido MEA-sulfosuccinate
CAS 61791-10-4	PEG-15 cocomonium chloride		
CAS 61791-12-6	PEG castor oil series	CAS 65277-54-5	Disodium ricinoleamido MEA-sulfosuccinate
CAS 61791-13-7	Coceth series		
CAS 61791-14-8	PEG cocamine series	CAS 65381-09-1	Caprylic/capric triglyceride
CAS 61791-20-6	Laneth series	CAS 65497-29-2	Guar hydroxypropyltrimonium chloride
CAS 61791-24-0	PEG soyamine series		
CAS 61791-25-1	Dihydroxyethyl tallow glycinate	CAS 65591-14-2	Arachidyl propionate
CAS 61791-26-2	PEG hydrogenated tallow amine series	CAS 65694-10-2	Stearamidopropalkonium chloride
		CAS 66009-41-4	Stearyl heptanoate
CAS 61791-28-4	Talloweth-6	CAS 66071-96-3	Corn gluten protein
CAS 61791-29-5	PEG cocoate series	CAS 66082-42-6	Polyglyceryl-3 diisostearate
CAS 61791-31-9	Cocamide DEA	CAS 66085-00-5	Glyceryl isostearate
CAS 61791-32-0	Disodium cocoamphodiacetate	CAS 66085-00-5	Isostearyl diglyceryl succinate
CAS 61791-34-2	Soyaethyl morpholinium ethosulfate	CAS 66095-81-6	2-Hydroxyethylamino-5-nitroanisole
CAS 61791-38-6	Cocoyl hydroxyethyl imidazoline	CAS 66105-29-1	PEG-7 glyceryl cocoate
CAS 61791-39-7	Tall oil hydroxyethyl imidazoline	CAS 66161-57-7	Sodium laureth-12 sulfate
CAS 61791-42-2	Sodium methyl cocoyl taurate	CAS 66161-58-8	Sodium trideceth sulfate (n = 4)
CAS 61791-44-4	PEG tallowamine series	CAS 66161-60-2	TIPA-lauryl sulfate
CAS 61791-45-5	Dihydroxyethyl tallow glycinate	CAS 66422-95-5	2,4-Diaminophenoxyethanol HCl
CAS 61791-46-6	Dihydroxyethyl tallowamine oxide	CAS 66455-14-9	C12-13 pareth series
CAS 61791-47-7	Dihydroxyethyl cocamine oxide	CAS 66455-17-2	C9-11 alcohols
CAS 61791-56-8	Disodium tallowiminodipropionate	CAS 66455-29-6	Lauryl betaine
CAS 61791-59-1	Sodium cocoyl sarcosinate	CAS 66625-78-3	Jojoba wax
CAS 61791-66-0	Disodium cocamido MEA-sulfosuccinate	CAS 66794-58-9	PEG sorbitan isostearate series
		CAS 66828-20-4	Sorbeth-6 hexastearate
CAS 61792-31-2	Lauramidopropylamine oxide	CAS 66988-04-3	Sodium isostearoyl lactylate
CAS 61840-27-5	Adipic acid/dimethylaminohydroxy-propyl diethylenetriamine copolymer	CAS 67633-57-2	Isostearyl ethylimidonium ethosulfate
		CAS 67633-63-0	Isostearamidopropyl ethyldimo-nium ethosulfate
CAS 61849-72-7	PPG methyl glucose ether series		
CAS 62755-21-9	Magnesium laureth sulfate	CAS 67700-98-5	Dimethyl lauramine
CAS 63084-98-0	p-Aminophenol sulfate	CAS 67700-99-6	Dihydrogenated tallow methyl-amine
CAS 63148-55-0	Dimethicone copolyol		
CAS 63148-58-3	Phenyl dimethicone	CAS 67701-00-2	Trihexadecylamine
CAS 63148-62-9	Dimethicone	CAS 67701-05-7	Coconut acid
CAS 63231-60-7	Microcrystalline wax	CAS 67701-06-8	Tallow acid
CAS 63231-63-0	RNA	CAS 67701-08-0	Soy acid
CAS 63250-25-9	Isopropyl dibenzoylmethane	CAS 67701-27-3	Hydrogenated tallow glycerides
CAS 63351-73-5	Ammonium nonoxynol-4 sulfate	CAS 67701-27-3	Japan wax
CAS 63393-82-8	C12-15 alcohols	CAS 67701-27-3	Tallow glycerides
CAS 63393-93-1	Isopropyl lanolate	CAS 67701-28-4	Caprylic/capric/linoleic triglyceride
CAS 63428-83-1	Nylon	CAS 67701-28-4	Caprylic/capric/oleic triglyceride
CAS 63451-27-4	Polyquaternium-2	CAS 67701-30-8	Triolein
CAS 63566-37-0	Isostearamidopropyl betaine	CAS 67701-33-1	Glyceryl myristate
CAS 63601-33-2	PEG-15 tallow polyamine	CAS 67702-21-4	Magnesium laureth sulfate
CAS 63663-21-8	Dibutyl lauroyl glutamide	CAS 67724-93-0	PVM/MA copolymer, ethyl ester
CAS 63793-60-2	PPG-3 myristyl ether	CAS 67762-19-0	Ammonium laureth sulfate
CAS 64365-23-7	Dimethicone copolyol	CAS 67762-25-8	C12-18 alcohols
CAS 64475-85-0	Mineral spirits	CAS 67762-27-5	Cetearyl alcohol
CAS 64742-14-9	Petroleum distillates	CAS 67762-35-0	PEG-9 cocoate
CAS 64742-42-3	Microcrystalline wax	CAS 67762-38-3	Methyl oleate
CAS 64742-47-8	Petroleum distillates	CAS 67762-40-7	Methyl laurate
CAS 64742-48-9	C10-11 isoparaffin	CAS 67762-96-3	Dimethicone copolyol
CAS 64742-48-9	C11-12 isoparaffin	CAS 67763-18-2	Diisostearyl malate
CAS 64742-48-9	C11-13 isoparaffin	CAS 67770-79-0	Ethyl butyl valerolactone
CAS 64742-48-9	C13-14 isoparaffin	CAS 67784-77-4	PEG-2 tallowmonium chloride
CAS 64743-02-8	C20-24 alpha olefin	CAS 67784-79-6	Propylene glycol soyate
CAS 65060-02-8	Cetrimonium methosulfate	CAS 67784-87-6	Hydrogenated palm glyceride
CAS 65071-95-6	PEG-15 tallate	CAS 67799-04-6	Isostearamidopropyl dimethyl-amine
CAS 65071-98-9	Laneth-10 acetate		

CAS 67846-16-6	Stearamidopropyl ethyldimonium ethosulfate		CAS 68239-42-9	Methyl gluceth-10
CAS 67893-42-9	Disodium ricinoleamido MEA-sulfosuccinate		CAS 68239-43-0	Methyl gluceth-20
			CAS 68239-79-2	3-Ethylamino-p-cresol sulfate
CAS 67923-87-9	Sodium octoxynol-2 ethane sulfonate		CAS 68239-81-6	m-Aminophenol sulfate
			CAS 68239-84-9	N,N-Diethyl-m-aminophenol sulfate
CAS 67938-21-0	Polyglyceryl-2 diisostearate			
CAS 67965-56-4	Polyglyceryl-2 dioleate		CAS 68298-21-5	Sodium lauroamphoacetate
CAS 67999-57-9	Disodium nonoxynol-10 sulfosuccinate		CAS 68308-53-2	Soy acid
			CAS 68308-54-3	Hydrogenated tallow glycerides
CAS 68002-59-5	Quaternium-18		CAS 68308-64-5	Coco-ethyldimonium ethosulfate
CAS 68002-61-9	Tallowtrimonium chloride		CAS 68308-67-8	Soyethyldimonium ethosulfate
CAS 68002-71-1	Hydrogenated soy glyceride		CAS 68310-73-6	N,N,N´,N´,N´-Pentamethyl-N-octadecenyl-1,3-diammonium dichloride
CAS 68002-71-1	Hydrogenated soybean oil			
CAS 68002-72-2	Hydrogenated menhaden oil			
CAS 68002-79-9	Trimethylpropane trioleate		CAS 68311-03-5	Disodium deceth-6 sulfosuccinate
CAS 68002-97-1	Laureth series		CAS 68333-82-4	Cocamide MIPA
CAS 68003-46-3	Ammonium lauroyl sarcosinate		CAS 68334-00-9	Hydrogenated cottonseed oil
CAS 68004-11-5	Polyglyceryl-4 stearate		CAS 68334-00-9	Hydrogenated vegetable oil
CAS 68015-98-5	4-Ethoxy-m-phenylenediamine sulfate		CAS 68334-21-4	Sodium cocoamphoacetate
			CAS 68334-28-1	Hydrogenated vegetable oil
CAS 68037-49-0	Sodium C14-17 alkyl sec sulfonate		CAS 68389-70-8	PEG-20 methyl glucose sesquistearate
CAS 68037-74-1	Dimethicone (branched)			
CAS 68037-93-4	Dimethyl palmitamine		CAS 68390-66-9	Sodium cocoamphoacetate
CAS 68039-13-4	Polymethacrylamidopropyl trimonium chloride		CAS 68390-99-8	Hydrogenated tallow dimethyl-amine oxide
CAS 68039-49-6	2,4-Dimethyl-3-cyclohexene carboxyaldehyde		CAS 68391-01-5	Benzalkonium chloride
			CAS 68391-05-9	Dicetyl dimonium chloride
CAS 68081-81-2	Sodium dodecylbenzenesulfonate		CAS 68410-69-5	Quaternium-53
CAS 68081-96-9	Ammonium lauryl sulfate		CAS 68411-27-8	C12-15 alkyl benzoate
CAS 68081-97-0	Magnesium lauryl sulfate		CAS 68411-27-8	Isostearyl benzoate
CAS 68122-86-1	Quaternium-27		CAS 68411-31-4	TEA-dodecylbenzenesulfonate
CAS 68130-24-5	Dipentaerythrityl hexacaprylate/ hexacaprate		CAS 68411-32-5	Dodecylbenzene sulfonic acid
			CAS 68411-57-4	Disodium cocoamphodipropionate
CAS 68130-52-9	Trimethylolpropane tricaprylate/ tricaprate		CAS 68411-96-1	TEA-cocoyl sarcosinate
			CAS 68411-97-2	Cocoyl sarcosine
CAS 68130-97-2	PEI-1500		CAS 68412-53-3	Nonoxynol-6 phosphate
CAS 68131-37-3	Corn syrup solids		CAS 68412-55-5	Trideceth carboxylic acid series
CAS 68131-39-5	C12-15 pareth series		CAS 68424-43-1	Lanolin acid
CAS 68131-40-8	C11-15 pareth series		CAS 68424-45-3	Linseed acid
CAS 68131-54-4	Potassium caseinate		CAS 68424-59-9	Shea butter extract
CAS 68133-71-1	Disodium tridecylsulfosuccinate		CAS 68424-60-2	Shea butter
CAS 68139-30-0	Cocamidopropyl hydroxysultaine		CAS 68424-66-8	Hydroxylated lanolin
CAS 68140-00-1	Cocamide MEA		CAS 68424-85-1	Benzalkonium chloride
CAS 68140-01-2	Cocamidopropyl dimethylamine		CAS 68424-94-2	Coco-betaine
CAS 68140-10-3	Sodium tallow sulfate		CAS 68425-17-2	Hydrogenated starch hydrolysate
CAS 68140-98-7	Ethyl hydroxymethyl oleyl oxazoline		CAS 68425-36-5	Hydrogenated peanut oil
			CAS 68425-37-6	Coconut alcohol
CAS 68153-28-6	Soy protein		CAS 68425-42-3	Cocamidopropyl dimethylamine lactate
CAS 68153-32-2	Ditallow dimonium chloride			
CAS 68153-63-9	Tallowamide MEA		CAS 68425-43-4	Cocamidopropyl dimethylamine propionate
CAS 68153-64-0	PEG tallowate series			
CAS 68155-09-9	Cocamidopropylamine oxide		CAS 68425-47-8	Soyamide DEA
CAS 68155-20-4	Tallamide DEA		CAS 68425-50-3	Tallowamidopropyl dimethylamine
CAS 68155-24-8	PEG hydrogenated tallow amide series		CAS 68439-46-3	C9-11 pareth series
			CAS 68439-49-6	Ceteareth series
			CAS 68439-50-9	C12-14 pareth series
CAS 68171-33-5	Isopropyl isostearate		CAS 68439-50-9	Laureth series
CAS 68171-38-0	Propylene glycol isostearate		CAS 68439-53-2	PPG lanolin alcohol ether series
CAS 68184-04-3	MEA-laureth sulfate		CAS 68439-57-6	Sodium C14-16 olefin sulfonate
CAS 68187-29-1	TEA-cocoyl-glutamate		CAS 68439-70-3	Dimethyl myristamine
CAS 68187-32-6	Sodium cocoyl glutamate		CAS 68440-05-1	Cocamide MIPA
CAS 68188-18-1	Sodium C9-22 alkyl sec sulfonate		CAS 68440-25-5	Tallowamide MEA
CAS 68188-30-7	Soyamidopropyl dimethylamine		CAS 68441-17-8	Polyethylene, oxidized
CAS 68188-38-5	Sodium cocoyl hydrolyzed collagen		CAS 68441-68-9	Pentaerythrityl tetracaprylate/ caprate
CAS 68188-45-5	Sodium alpha olefin sulfonate		CAS 68444-33-7	Undecylpentadecanol
CAS 68201-46-7	PEG glyceryl cocoate series		CAS 68458-51-5	Oleoyl hydrolyzed collagen
CAS 68201-49-0	Lanolin wax		CAS 68458-58-8	PPG-PEG lanolin oil series
CAS 68213-23-0	Trideceth-7		CAS 68458-88-8	PPG-PEG lanolin series
CAS 68238-35-7	Keratin amino acids		CAS 68459-50-7	PEG lanolate series

CAS 68476-03-9	Montan acid wax
CAS 68479-64-1	Disodium oleamido MEA-sulfosuccinate
CAS 68513-95-1	Soy flour
CAS 68514-74-9	Hydrogenated palm oil
CAS 68515-65-1	Disodium cocamido MIPA-sulfosuccinate
CAS 68515-73-1	Caprylyl/capryl glucoside
CAS 68517-10-2	Methyl isostearate
CAS 68526-50-1	Isobutyl tallowate
CAS 68526-79-4	Hexyl alcohol
CAS 68526-85-2	n-Decyl alcohol
CAS 68526-86-3	Lauryl alcohol
CAS 68541-50-4	Trimethylolpropane triisostearate
CAS 68551-08-6	C9-11 alcohols
CAS 68551-12-2	C12-16 pareth-1
CAS 68553-11-7	PEG-20 glyceryl stearate
CAS 68553-81-1	Rice bran oil
CAS 68554-53-0	Stearoxy dimethicone
CAS 68555-36-2	Polyquaternium-2
CAS 68583-51-7	Propylene glycol dicaprylate/dicaprate
CAS 68584-22-5	Dodecylbenzene sulfonic acid
CAS 68584-24-7	Isopropylamine dodecylbenzene-sulfonate
CAS 68585-44-4	DEA-lauryl sulfate
CAS 68585-47-7	Sodium lauryl sulfate
CAS 68603-15-5	C8-10 alcohols
CAS 68603-42-9	Cocamide DEA
CAS 68604-44-4	Pentaerythrityl tetraoleate
CAS 68604-71-7	Disodium cocoamphodipropionate
CAS 68604-73-9	Sodium cocoamphohydroxypropyl sulfonate
CAS 68607-29-4	Tallowdimonium propyltrimonium dichloride
CAS 68607-75-0	Stearyl methicone
CAS 68607-88-5	Hydrolyzed soy protein
CAS 68608-61-7	Sodium caproamphoacetate
CAS 68608-63-9	Sodium stearoamphoacetate
CAS 68608-64-0	Disodium caprylamphodiacetate
CAS 68608-65-1	Sodium cocoamphoacetate
CAS 68608-66-2	Disodium lauroamphodiacetate
CAS 68608-66-2	Sodium lauroamphoacetate
CAS 68608-88-8	Dodecylbenzene sulfonic acid
CAS 68610-38-8	Sodium oleoamphohydroxypropyl-sulfonate
CAS 68610-39-9	Sodium capryloamphohydroxy-propyl sulfonate
CAS 68610-43-5	Disodium lauroamphodipropionate
CAS 68610-92-4	Polyquaternium-10
CAS 68630-96-6	Sodium isostearoamphopropionate
CAS 68647-44-9	Sodium lauroamphoacetate
CAS 68647-46-1	Sodium caproamphoacetate
CAS 68647-53-0	Sodium cocoamphoacetate
CAS 68647-73-4	Tea tree oil
CAS 68647-77-8	Tallowamidopropylamine oxide
CAS 68648-27-1	PEG hydrogenated lanolin series
CAS 68648-38-4	PEG-75 lanolin oil
CAS 68648-66-8	Maleated soybean oil
CAS 68649-05-8	Cocaminobutyric acid
CAS 68650-39-5	Disodium cocoamphodiacetate
CAS 68650-44-2	Apricot extract
CAS 68650-79-3	Tallamidopropyl dimethylamine
CAS 68783-22-2	PEG-50 hydrogenated tallow amine
CAS 68783-23-3	Disoyamine
CAS 68783-24-4	Ditallowamine
CAS 68783-78-8	Ditallow dimonium chloride
CAS 68784-08-7	Disodium cocamido MEA-sulfosuccinate

CAS 68797-35-3	Dipotassium glycyrrhizate
CAS 68797-65-9	Behenamidopropyl ethyldimonium ethosulfate
CAS 68814-13-1	Tricetyl phosphate
CAS 68814-69-7	Dimethyl tallowamine
CAS 68815-55-4	Disodium capryloamphodipropio-nate
CAS 68815-61-2	Ammonium C12-15 alkyl sulfate
CAS 68855-56-1	C12-16 alcohols
CAS 68889-49-6	PEG glyceryl oleate series
CAS 68890-66-4	Piroctone olamine
CAS 68890-92-6	Disodium laneth-5 sulfosuccinate
CAS 68891-17-8	Sodium trideceth carboxylate series
CAS 68891-38-3	Sodium laureth sulfate
CAS 68891-38-3	Sodium myreth sulfate
CAS 68891-39-4	Sodium nonoxynol-4 sulfate
CAS 68891-73-6	Potassium octoxynol-12 phosphate
CAS 68908-44-1	MEA-lauryl sulfate
CAS 68908-44-1	TEA-lauryl sulfate
CAS 68909-20-6	Hexamethyldisilazane
CAS 68910-41-5	Disodium cocoamphodipropionate
CAS 68910-56-5	Ditridecyl dimonium chloride
CAS 68915-25-3	Cocodimonium hydroxypropyl hydrolyzed keratin
CAS 68916-04-1	Bitter orange oil
CAS 68916-39-2	Witch hazel extract
CAS 68916-73-4	Camellia oil
CAS 68916-88-1	Lemon juice
CAS 68917-49-7	Hypericum extract
CAS 68917-51-1	Algae extract
CAS 68918-77-4	Potassium abietoyl hydrolyzed collagen
CAS 68918-77-4	TEA-abietoyl hydrolyzed collagen
CAS 68919-40-4	Disodium cocoamphodipropionate
CAS 68919-41-5	Sodium cocoamphopropionate
CAS 68920-18-3	Disodium lauroamphodipropionate
CAS 68920-59-2	Lauroyl collagen amino acids
CAS 68920-65-0	Potassium cocoyl hydrolyzed collagen
CAS 68920-66-1	Cetoleth-22
CAS 68921-42-6	FD&C blue no. 1 aluminum lake
CAS 68921-83-5	Quaternium-70
CAS 68929-04-4	Disodium lauroamphodipropionate
CAS 68936-95-8	Methyl glucose sesquistearate
CAS 68937-10-0	Hydrogenated polyisobutene
CAS 68937-85-9	Coconut acid
CAS 68938-15-8	Hydrogenated coconut acid
CAS 68939-90-6	Trilinoleic acid
CAS 68951-67-7	C14-15 pareth-7
CAS 68951-89-3	Hydrolyzed collagen, ethyl ester
CAS 68951-91-7	TEA-undecenoyl hydrolyzed collagen
CAS 68951-92-8	Potassium undecylenoyl hydrolyzed collagen
CAS 68951-97-3	Dimethicone copolyol methyl ether
CAS 68952-15-8	Cocoyl hydrolyzed collagen
CAS 68952-15-8	Lauroyl hydrolyzed collagen
CAS 68952-16-9	TEA-cocoyl hydrolyzed collagen
CAS 68953-11-7	Minkamidopropyl dimethylamine
CAS 68953-58-2	Quaternium-18 bentonite
CAS 68953-64-0	Quaternium-26
CAS 68954-89-2	Ceteareth-7 carboxylic acid
CAS 68954-89-2	Laureth carboxylic acid series
CAS 68954-89-2	Steareth-7 carboxylic acid
CAS 68955-19-1	Sodium lauryl sulfate
CAS 68955-20-4	Sodium cetearyl sulfate
CAS 68955-20-4	Sodium tallow sulfate
CAS 68955-45-3	Ethylene distearamide

CAS 68956-08-1	Trimethylolpropane tricaprylate/ tricaprate			diaminopropyl dimethicone
CAS 68956-68-3	Vegetable oil	CAS 71850-81-2	Ricinoleamidopropyl betaine
CAS 68957-18-6	Sodium C12-13 pareth sulfate	CAS 71902-01-7	Sorbitan isostearate
CAS 68958-64-5	PEG-25 glyceryl trioleate	CAS 72269-52-4	Diethylene glycol dioctanoate
CAS 68966-38-1	Isostearyl hydroxyethyl imidazoline	CAS 72300-24-4	Isostearamidopropyl morpholine lactate
CAS 68987-89-3	Sodium laureth-11 carboxylate	CAS 72319-06-3	Myristoyl hydrolyzed collagen
CAS 68988-72-7	Propylene glycol dicaprylate/ dicaprate	CAS 72347-89-8	Polyglyceryl-2 tetrastearate
		CAS 72388-18-2	2-Dodecylhexadecanol
CAS 68989-00-4	Benzalkonium chloride	CAS 72576-80-8	Isostearyl palmitate
CAS 68989-03-7	PEG-5 cocomonium methosulfate	CAS 72576-81-9	Isostearyl myristate
CAS 68990-06-7	Hydrogenated tallow glyceride lactate	CAS 72869-62-6	Sorbitan tristearate
		CAS 72869-69-3	Apricot kernel oil
CAS 68990-07-8	Wheat germ glycerides	CAS 73049-73-7	Hydrolyzed elastin
CAS 68990-15-8	Fenugreek extract	CAS 73296-86-3	Polyglyceryl-2 isostearate
CAS 68990-58-9	Acetylated hydrogenated tallow glyceride	CAS 73807-15-5	Palm kernelamide DEA
		CAS 73970-38-4	Dimethyl hexahydronaphthyl dihydroxymethyl acetal
CAS 68990-59-0	Hydrogenated tallow glyceride citrate	CAS 73970-40-8	Dimethyl hexahydronaphthyl dihydroxymethyl acetal
CAS 68990-63-6	Shark liver oil	CAS 73979-84-7	Dimethyl hexahydronaphthyl dihydroxymethyl acetal
CAS 68990-82-9	Hydrogenated palm kernel oil		
CAS 68991-68-4	Caprylic/capric/lauric triglyceride	CAS 73979-86-9	Dimethyl hexahydronaphthyl dihydroxymethyl acetal
CAS 69028-36-0	Hydrogenated vegetable glyceride		
CAS 69226-96-6	Pentaerythrityl tetracaprylate/ caprate	CAS 74623-31-7	PPG buteth series
CAS 69430-23-5	TEA-myristoyl hydrolyzed collagen	CAS 75782-86-4	C12-13 alcohols
CAS 69430-24-6	Cyclomethicone	CAS 75782-87-5	C14-15 alcohols
CAS 69430-24-6	Octamethylcyclotetrasiloxane	CAS 76009-37-5	Polyglyceryl-6 dioleate
CAS 69430-36-0	Hydrolyzed keratin	CAS 76902-90-4	Methenammoniumchloride
CAS 69468-44-6	PEG glyceryl isostearate series	CAS 77465-45-3	Melanin
CAS 69537-38-8	Behenoyl-PG-trimonium chloride	CAS 78330-21-9	Trideceth series
CAS 70024-77-0	Disodium oleoamphodiacetate	CAS 78491-02-8	Diazolidinyl urea
CAS 70084-87-6	Hydrolyzed wheat protein	CAS 79416-55-0	Glycol dibehenate
CAS 70084-94-5	Hydrolyzed soy protein	CAS 79490-62-3	2-Octyldodecyl ricinoleate
CAS 70161-44-3	Sodium hydroxymethylglycinate	CAS 79665-92-2	Polyglyceryl-6 oleate
CAS 70225-05-7	Tridecyl trimellitate	CAS 79665-93-3	Polyglyceryl-10 oleate
CAS 70321-63-0	Lanolin oil	CAS 79665-94-4	Polyglyceryl-3 dioleate
CAS 70356-09-1	Butyl methoxy dibenzoyl methane	CAS 79702-63-0	Disodium oleamido MEA- sulfosuccinate
CAS 70592-80-2	Cocamine oxide		
CAS 70592-80-2	Lauramine oxide	CAS 79777-30-3	Polyglyceryl-10 stearate
CAS 70609-66-4	Sodium lauroyl taurate	CAS 80062-31-3	2-Nitro-5-glyceryl methylaniline
CAS 70632-06-3	Sodium C12-15 pareth carboxylate series	CAS 80145-09-1	Isostearamidopropyl morpholine lactate
CAS 70632-06-3	Sodium laureth-13 carboxylate	CAS 81613-56-1	Linoleamidopropyl dimethylamine
CAS 70693-04-8	Isostearyl alcohol	CAS 81646-13-1	Behentrimonium methosulfate
CAS 70693-05-9	Undecylpentadecanol	CAS 81752-33-2	Polyglyceryl-2 isostearate
CAS 70693-32-2	Neopentyl glycol dicaprylate/ dicaprate	CAS 81859-24-7	DEA-laureth sulfate
		CAS 81859-24-7	Polyquaternium-10
CAS 70729-87-2	Dimethyl lauramine isostearate	CAS 82204-94-2	Dioctyldodecyl lauroyl glutamate
CAS 70750-17-3	C12-13 pareth-5 carboxylic acid	CAS 82469-79-2	n-Butyroyl tri-n-hexyl citrate
CAS 70750-46-8	Dihydroxyethyl tallow glycinate	CAS 82933-91-3	Methyl glucose dioleate
CAS 70750-47-9	PEG-2 cocomonium chloride	CAS 82970-95-4	Quaternium-22
CAS 70788-37-3	Toluene sulfonic acid	CAS 83016-76-6	MIPA-laureth sulfate
CAS 70801-07-9	Octylacrylamide/acrylates/ butylaminoethyl methacrylate copolymer	CAS 83138-08-3	Disodium cocoamphodipropionate
		CAS 83138-08-3	Cocamidopropyl betaine
		CAS 83147-64-2	Disodium tridecylsulfosuccinate
CAS 70802-40-3	PEG-8 stearate	CAS 83271-10-7	Dextrin palmitate
CAS 70851-07-9	Cocamidopropyl betaine	CAS 83615-24-1	Cholesteryl isostearate
CAS 70851-08-0	Cocamidopropyl hydroxysultaine	CAS 83682-78-4	Lauramidopropyl PEG-dimonium chloride phosphate
CAS 71010-52-1	Gellan gum		
CAS 71011-27-3	Quaternium-18 hectorite	CAS 83708-66-1	Isocetyl myristate
CAS 71012-10-7	Polyglyceryl-4 oleate	CAS 83826-43-1	Octyldodecyl myristate
CAS 71185-87-0	Polyglyceryl-6 tristearate	CAS 84012-12-4	Arbutus extract
CAS 71243-51-1	Synthetic beeswax	CAS 84012-13-5	Lappa extract
CAS 71329-50-5	Hydroxypropyl guar hydroxypropyl trimonium chloride	CAS 84012-14-6	Artichoke extract
		CAS 84012-15-7	Birch extract
CAS 71368-20-2	Sodium myristoyl glutamate	CAS 84012-16-8	Borage extract
CAS 71487-00-8	PEG-2 cocomonium nitrate	CAS 84012-26-0	Oat extract
CAS 71566-49-9	Octyl isononanoate	CAS 84012-27-1	Olive extract
CAS 71750-80-6	Dimethoxysilyl ethylene	CAS 84012-28-2	Orange extract

CAS 84012-31-7	Passionflower extract
CAS 84012-32-8	Pellitory extract
CAS 84012-33-9	Parsley extract
CAS 84012-35-1	Pine needle extract
CAS 84012-38-4	Butcherbroom extract
CAS 84012-40-8	Nettle extract
CAS 84012-42-0	Pansy extract
CAS 84012-43-1	Walnut extract
CAS 84012-44-2	Wheat extract
CAS 84012-44-2	Wheat germ extract
CAS 84069-44-3	Hydroxypropyl chitosan
CAS 84082-36-0	Alfalfa extract
CAS 84082-44-0	Behenyl betaine
CAS 84082-51-9	Whey protein
CAS 84082-54-2	Ivy extract
CAS 84082-57-5	Mallow extract
CAS 84082-61-1	Balm mint extract
CAS 84082-67-7	Myrtle extract
CAS 84082-70-2	Peppermint extract
CAS 84082-79-1	Sage extract
CAS 84082-80-4	Hypericum extract
CAS 84082-83-7	Yarrow extract
CAS 84501-49-5	Sodium decyl sulfate
CAS 84539-90-2	Pentaerythrityl tetrabehenate
CAS 84562-92-5	Nonoxynol-3
CAS 84603-56-5	Celandine extract
CAS 84603-58-7	Sambucus extract
CAS 84603-60-1	Golden seal root extract
CAS 84603-62-3	Honeysuckle extract
CAS 84603-69-0	Juniper extract
CAS 84603-70-3	Chaparral extract
CAS 84603-73-6	Laurel extract
CAS 84603-93-0	Rose hips oil
CAS 84603-93-0	Rose oil
CAS 84604-00-2	Walnut oil
CAS 84604-14-8	Rosemary extract
CAS 84605-13-0	Myreth-3 laurate
CAS 84605-14-1	Myreth-3 palmitate
CAS 84625-29-6	Capsicum extract
CAS 84625-32-1	Eucalyptus extract
CAS 84625-39-8	Fennel extract
CAS 84625-50-3	Coltsfoot extract
CAS 84643-53-8	Hydroxycetyl hydroxyethyl-dimonium chloride
CAS 84649-86-5	Chamomile extract
CAS 84649-98-9	Cinnamon extract
CAS 84650-00-0	Coffee bean extract
CAS 84650-00-0	Coffee extract
CAS 84650-10-2	Cranesbill extract
CAS 84650-19-1	Laneth-15
CAS 84650-59-9	Anise extract
CAS 84650-60-2	Thea sinensis extract
CAS 84695-98-7	Avocado extract
CAS 84696-05-9	Comfrey extract
CAS 84696-07-1	Cypress extract
CAS 84696-11-7	Coneflower extract
CAS 84696-13-9	Bladderwrack extract
CAS 84696-19-5	Witch hazel extract
CAS 84696-21-9	Hydrocotyl extract
CAS 84696-37-7	Rice bran oil
CAS 84696-47-9	Rose extract
CAS 84696-47-9	Rose hips extract
CAS 84696-48-0	Broom extract
CAS 84696-53-7	Lichen extract
CAS 84753-08-2	Dioctyl cyclohexane
CAS 84775-41-7	Angelica extract
CAS 84775-42-8	Anise extract
CAS 84775-50-8	Coriander extract
CAS 84775-55-3	Dandelion extract
CAS 84775-66-6	Licorice extract
CAS 84775-70-2	Watercress extract
CAS 84775-71-3	Basil extract
CAS 84776-03-4	Sunflower seed extract
CAS 84776-23-8	Calendula extract
CAS 84776-24-9	Hydrocotyl extract
CAS 84776-25-0	Iceland moss extract
CAS 84776-28-3	Cinchona extract
CAS 84776-64-7	Jasmine extract
CAS 84776-65-8	Lavender extract
CAS 84776-67-0	White lily extract
CAS 84776-91-0	Soy germ extract
CAS 84776-98-7	Wild thyme extract
CAS 84812-94-2	Cocaminopropionic acid
CAS 84929-25-9	Cinchona extract
CAS 84929-27-1	Grape leaf extract
CAS 84929-30-6	Henna extract
CAS 84929-31-7	Lemon extract
CAS 84929-43-1	Plantain extract
CAS 84929-51-1	Thyme extract
CAS 84929-52-2	Linden extract
CAS 84929-61-3	Carrot extract
CAS 84929-76-0	Red raspberry leaf extract
CAS 84930-16-5	Potassium propylparaben
CAS 84961-45-5	Carob extract
CAS 84961-64-8	Tansy extract
CAS 84988-65-8	Harpagophytum extract
CAS 84988-79-4	Isobutyl oleate
CAS 85005-47-6	Isobutylated lanolin oil
CAS 85049-34-9	Propylene glycol dioleate
CAS 85049-36-1	Ethyl oleate
CAS 85049-52-1	Bergamot oil
CAS 85058-43-1	Dichlorophenyl imidazoldioxolan
CAS 85085-25-2	Clover blossom extract
CAS 85085-33-2	Fennel extract
CAS 85085-64-9	Plantain extract
CAS 85085-66-1	Tormentil extract
CAS 85116-87-6	Isopropyl oleate
CAS 85116-93-4	Pentaerythrityl stearate
CAS 85116-97-8	PEG-2 stearate
CAS 85117-50-6	Sodium dodecylbenzenesulfonate
CAS 85186-88-5	Sorbitan trioleate
CAS 85251-77-0	Glyceryl stearate
CAS 85264-33-1	Dimethylhydroxymethylpyrazole
CAS 85341-79-3	Cetearyl palmitate
CAS 85404-84-8	Polyglyceryl-3 diisostearate
CAS 85409-09-2	Caprylic/capric triglyceride
CAS 85409-22-9	Benzalkonium chloride
CAS 85409-25-2	Coco-betaine
CAS 85411-01-4	Hydrogenated vegetable glycerides phosphate
CAS 85507-69-3	Aloe extract
CAS 85508-38-9	Ricinoleamidopropyl trimonium methosulfate
CAS 85536-04-5	Stearyl stearate
CAS 85536-08-9	Corn oil PEG-6 esters
CAS 85536-14-7	Dodecylbenzene sulfonic acid
CAS 85536-23-8	PEG-4 rapeseedamide
CAS 85586-21-6	Methyl stearate
CAS 85617-81-8	Erucyl oleate
CAS 85665-33-4	C10-18 triglycerides
CAS 85666-92-8	Glyceryl stearate SE
CAS 85736-49-8	PEG-12 dioleate
CAS 85865-69-6	Isobutyl stearate
CAS 86088-85-9	Quaternium-27
CAS 86089-12-5	Ricinoleamidopropyl betaine
CAS 86418-55-5	Glycol stearate SE
CAS 86438-35-9	Disodium cocoamphodipropionate
CAS 86438-78-0	Lauramidopropyl betaine
CAS 86438-79-1	Cocamidopropyl betaine
CAS 86438-79-1	Coco/oleamidopropyl betaine

CAS 86438-79-1	Disodium cocoamphodipropionate
CAS 86637-84-5	Polyglyceryl-10 pentaoleate
CAS 87061-04-9	Menthoxypropanediol
CAS 87390-32-7	Polyglyceryl-10 myristate
CAS 87569-97-9	Magnesium oleth sulfate
CAS 88103-59-7	2-Octyldodecyl erucate
CAS 88122-99-0	Octyl triazone
CAS 88497-58-9	C12-15 pareth-7 carboxylic acid
CAS 88543-32-2	Ethyl hydroxymethyl oleyl oxazoline
CAS 89933-26-6	Isodecyl octanoate
CAS 89957-98-2	Olibanum extract
CAS 89997-53-5	Bitter cherry extract
CAS 89998-01-6	Cucumber extract
CAS 89998-14-1	Lemongrass extract
CAS 90028-20-9	Coneflower extract
CAS 90028-42-5	Rocket extract
CAS 90045-28-6	Wintergreen extract
CAS 90045-36-6	Ginkgo extract
CAS 90045-38-8	Ginseng extract
CAS 90045-43-5	Grapefruit extract
CAS 90045-43-5	Grapefruit seed extract
CAS 90045-56-0	Everlasting extract
CAS 90045-78-6	Honeysuckle extract
CAS 90045-79-7	Horse chestnut extract
CAS 90045-94-6	Jasmine extract
CAS 90045-98-0	Jojoba extract
CAS 90052-75-8	Octyldodecyl stearoyl stearate
CAS 90063-37-9	Lavender extract
CAS 90064-00-9	Pennyroyal extract
CAS 90083-09-3	Tormentil extract
CAS 90193-76-3	Distearyl phthalate
CAS 90283-04-8	Dilauryl acetyl dimonium chloride
CAS 90388-14-0	Cetyldiethanolaminephosphate
CAS 90453-59-1	PEG-9 stearamide carboxylic acid
CAS 90529-57-0	Soyamidopropyl ethyldimonium ethosulfate
CAS 90529-57-0	Oleamidopropyl ethyldimonium ethosulfate
CAS 90605-17-7	Isodecyl citrate
CAS 90624-75-2	Polyquaternium-17
CAS 90730-68-0	Erucalkonium chloride
CAS 90989-47-2	Aorta extract
CAS 90989-78-9	Brain extract
CAS 91031-43-5	Ethyl stearate
CAS 91031-48-0	Isooctyl stearate
CAS 91031-57-1	Isononyl stearate
CAS 91031-88-8	Sucrose cocoate
CAS 91050-82-7	Pentaerythrityl tetrastearate
CAS 91052-92-5	Honey extract
CAS 91053-41-7	Acetylated hydrogenated lanolin
CAS 91080-18-1	Hydrolyzed elastin
CAS 91771-39-0	Cauliflower unsaponifiables
CAS 91824-88-3	Polyglyceryl-4 isostearate
CAS 92044-87-6	Octyl cocoate
CAS 92128-82-0	Algae extract
CAS 92128-87-5	Hydrogenated lecithin
CAS 92669-01-7	Myreth-5
CAS 92797-39-2	Hydrolyzed milk protein
CAS 93385-03-6	Propylene glycol ceteth-3 acetate
CAS 93385-13-8	Propylene glycol isoceteth-3 acetate
CAS 93507-51-8	Lactamidopropyl trimonium chloride
CAS 93572-53-3	Hydrogenated menhaden oil
CAS 93572-63-5	PEG-3 tallow propylenedimonium dimethosulfate
CAS 93685-79-1	Isoeicosane
CAS 93803-89-5	Pentaerythrityl tetraisononanoate
CAS 93820-52-1	Sodium cocoamphopropionate

CAS 93820-97-4	Cetearyl stearate
CAS 94349-67-4	Barley extract
CAS 94423-19-5	Polyglyceryl-3 distearate
CAS 94552-41-7	Rapeseedamidopropyl ethyldimonium ethosulfate
CAS 94891-33-5	Stearalkonium hectorite
CAS 95032-84-1	AMP isostearoyl hydrolyzed collagen
CAS 95461-64-6	Polyglyceryl-10 pentastearate
CAS 96690-41-4	Hydrolyzed silk
CAS 97069-99-0	Emulsifying wax NF
CAS 97281-23-7	Glycol stearate
CAS 97281-47-5	Lecithin
CAS 97281-47-5	Phosphatidylcholine
CAS 97281-48-6	Hydrogenated lecithin
CAS 97338-28-8	Isocetyl stearoyl stearate
CAS 97404-50-7	Glyceryl lanolate
CAS 97488-62-5	Tallowamphopolycarboxypropionic acid
CAS 97488-91-0	Apricot kernel oil PEG-6 esters
CAS 97593-31-2	Hydrogenated vegetable glycerides citrate
CAS 97615-94-6	Fish extract
CAS 97659-50-2	Cocoiminodipropionate
CAS 97659-53-5	Cocoamphopolycarboxyglycinate
CAS 97659-53-5	Sodium carboxymethyl oleyl polypropylamine
CAS 97659-53-5	Sodium carboxymethyl tallow polypropylamine
CAS 97659-53-5	Disodium oleoamphodiacetate
CAS 97676-22-7	Gentian extract
CAS 97676-23-8	Licorice extract
CAS 97676-24-9	Althea extract
CAS 97755-17-6	PEG-20 hydrogenated lanolin
CAS 97759-33-8	Hydrolyzed rice protein
CAS 97766-44-4	Swertia extract
CAS 98073-10-0	Methyl gluceth-20 distearate
CAS 98133-47-2	Panthenyl triacetate
CAS 98984-78-2	Sodium lauroyl glutamate
CAS 99126-54-2	Polyglyceryl-10 heptastearate
CAS 99330-44-6	Magnesium laureth-11 carboxylate
CAS 99542-23-1	Linoleamidopropyl ethyldimonium ethosulfate
CAS 99734-30-2	Polyglyceryl-6 pentastearate
CAS 100084-96-6	Myrrh extract
CAS 100085-10-7	Hydrolyzed elastin
CAS 100085-35-6	Hydrolyzed fibronectin
CAS 100085-40-3	Fish glycerides
CAS 100085-64-1	Cocobetainamido amphopropionate
CAS 100182-46-5	Dioctyl cyclohexane
CAS 100209-45-8	Hydrolyzed vegetable protein
CAS 100545-50-4	Didecyl dimethylamine oxide
CAS 100684-25-7	Cocodimonium hydroxypropyl hydrolyzed soy protein
CAS 100684-36-4	Hydrolyzed yeast protein
CAS 100864-25-1	Hydrolyzed wheat protein
CAS 102033-55-6	Polyglyceryl-10 diisostearate
CAS 102051-00-3	Polyglyceryl-10 trioleate
CAS 102523-96-2	Dimethicone propyl PG-betaine
CAS 102868-96-2	Zinc acetylmethionate
CAS 103175-09-3	Polyglyceryl-10 heptaoleate
CAS 103213-19-0	Diisostearyl dimer dilinoleate
CAS 103213-20-3	Diisopropyl dimer dilinoleate
CAS 103213-22-5	Triisostearyl trilinoleate
CAS 103819-46-1	Olive oil PEG-6 esters
CAS 104934-17-0	Polyglyceryl-6 pentaoleate
CAS 105883-47-4	Gold acetylmethionate
CAS 105883-48-5	Nickel acetylmethionate
CAS 105883-49-6	Magnesium acetylmethionate

CAS 105883-50-9	Manganese acetylmethionate
CAS 105883-51-0	Copper acetylmethionate
CAS 105883-52-1	Cobalt acetylmethionate
CAS 106436-39-9	Tridecyl neopentanoate
CAS 106483-04-9	Pyridoxine dicaprylate
CAS 107600-36-2	TIPA-laureth sulfate
CAS 107628-03-5	Sodium PEG-6 cocamide carboxylate
CAS 107628-04-6	Trideceth-2 carboxamide MEA
CAS 107987-23-5	Polyquaternium-24
CAS 110332-91-7	PPG-2 isoceteth-20 acetate
CAS 110615-47-9	Lauryl polyglucose
CAS 110720-64-4	Stearyl/aminopropyl methicone copolymer
CAS 111019-03-5	PPG-10 cetyl ether phosphate
CAS 111174-62-0	Steartrimonium hydroxyethyl hydrolyzed collagen
CAS 111174-64-2	Triethonium hydrolyzed collagen ethosulfate
CAS 111381-08-9	Bisisostearamidopropyl ethoxyethyl dimonium chloride
CAS 111381-08-9	Hydroxypropyl bisisostearamido-propyldimonium chloride
CAS 111905-55-6	Quaternium-61
CAS 112324-11-5	Rapeseedamidopropyl epoxy-propyl dimonium chloride
CAS 112324-16-0	Ricinoleamidopropyl ethyldimo-nium ethosulfate
CAS 112385-09-8,	Diisostearyl fumarate
CAS 112926-00-8	Silica, hydrated
CAS 112945-52-5	Silica
CAS 113010-52-9	PEG-25 PABA
CAS 113431-53-1	Diisostearyl fumarate
CAS 113431-54-2	Triisostearyl citrate
CAS 113492-03-8	Cocamidopropyl ethyldimonium ethosulfate
CAS 113492-04-9	Saffloweramidopropyl ethyldimo-nium ethosulfate
CAS 114040-31-2	Magnesium ascorbyl phosphate
CAS 115340-78-8	Apricotamidopropyl ethyldimonium ethosulfate
CAS 115340-80-2	Wheatgermamidopropyl ethyldimonium ethosulfate
CAS 116518-82-2	Myristyl neopentanoate
CAS 118777-77-8	Isostearamidopropyl dimethyl-amine glycolate
CAS 118777-77-8	Soyamidopropyl dimethylamino glycolate
CAS 120022-92-6	Polyamino sugar condensate
CAS 120486-24-0	Polyglyceryl-2 triisostearate
CAS 120962-03-0	Canola oil
CAS 121440-30-0	Polyglyceryl-2 tetraisostearate
CAS 123754-28-9	Ammonium acrylates/acrylo-nitrogens copolymer
CAS 123776-56-7	Acetamidopropyl trimonium chloride
CAS 124046-05-5	Babassamidopropalkonium chloride
CAS 124046-09-9	Wheat germamidopropalkonium chloride
CAS 124046-31-7	Olivamidopropyl dimethylamine lactate
CAS 124046-35-1	Sesamide DEA
CAS 124046-39-5	Wheat germamide DEA
CAS 124046-40-8	Wheat germamidopropyl dimethylamine lactate
CAS 125093-27-8	2-Octyldodecyl ricinoleate
CAS 125804-04-8	Behenamidopropyl dimethylamine behenate
CAS 125804-10-6	Linoleamidopropyl dimethylamine

	dimer dilinoleate
CAS 125804-12-8	Glycereth-7 benzoate
CAS 125804-13-9	Glycereth-5 lactate
CAS 125804-15-1	Glycereth-7 diisononanoate
CAS 125804-18-4	Tridecyl isononanoate
CAS 126121-35-5	Trioctyldodecyl citrate
CAS 126139-79-5	Disodium malyl tyrosinate
CAS 126928-07-2	Polyglyceryl-6 isostearate
CAS 127311-98-2	Ricinoleamidopropyl trimonium chloride
CAS 127312-00-9	Hydroxy stearamidopropyl trimonium methosulfate
CAS 127312-01-0	Hydroxy stearamidopropyl trimonium chloride
CAS 127358-81-0	Diisostearyl dimer dilinoleate
CAS 127512-63-4	Polyglyceryl-3 isostearate
CAS 127733-92-0	Dihydrogenated tallow phthalic acid amide
CAS 128895-87-4	Polyglyceryl-3 cetyl ether
CAS 129426-19-3	Palmitamidohexadecanediol
CAS 129541-36-2	Isostearamidopropyl dimethyl-amine gluconate
CAS 129541-36-2	Soyamidopropyl dimethylamino gluconate
CAS 129541-39-5	Dilauryl acetyl dimonium chloride
CAS 130124-24-2	Quaternium-53
CAS 131141-70-3	Isohexyl neopentanoate
CAS 131154-74-0	Tridecyl erucate
CAS 132207-30-8	Dimethicone propylethylene-diamine behenate
CAS 132207-31-9	Dimethicone copolyol phosphate
CAS 132467-76-6	Panthenyl hydroxypropyl steardimonium chloride
CAS 133448-16-5	Dimethicone copolyol isostearate
CAS 133738-23-5	Polyglyceryl-10 isostearate
CAS 133779-14-3	Dimethicone copolyolamine
CAS 133798-12-6	Undecylenamidopropyl betaine
CAS 133934-08-4	Apricotamidopropyl betaine
CAS 133934-09-5	Wheat germamidopropyl betaine
CAS 134017-12-2	Isostearyl stearoyl stearate
CAS 134112-42-8	Isostearamidopropyl laurylaceto-dimonium chloride
CAS 134141-38-1	PEG-4 dioleate
CAS 134737-05-6	Quaternium-80
CAS 136097-82-0	Cetearyl stearate
CAS 136097-93-3	Polyglyceryl-3 beeswax
CAS 136097-95-5	Candelilla synthetic
CAS 136505-00-5	Acrylic acid/acrylonitrogens copolymer
CAS 136505-01-6	Acrylic acid/acrylonitrogens copolymer
CAS 136505-02-7	Polyquaternium-31
CAS 138208-68-1	Isocetyl salicylate
CAS 138314-11-1	Glycereth-7.5 hydroxystearate
CAS 138698-34-7	Dilinoleamidopropyl dimethylamine dimethicone copolyol phosphate
CAS 138724-54-6	Cetearyl candelillate
CAS 141464-42-8	Decyl polyglucose
CAS 144514-52-3	Behenylbeeswax
CAS 144514-54-5	Hexanediol behenyl beeswax
CAS 678213-23-0	Trideceth-2
CAS 977012-91-1	Ricinoleamidopropyl dimethyl-amine lactate
CAS 977039-11-4	Cocodimonium hydroxypropyl hydrolyzed soy protein
CAS 977053-96-5	Glyceryl stearate SE
CAS 977055-83-6	Acetylated hydrogenated cottonseed glyceride
CAS 977056-87-3	Hydrogenated coco-glycerides
CAS 977058-55-1	Ultramarine pink

CAS 977059-33-8	Hydrolyzed vegetable protein	CAS 977077-71-6	Silk amino acids
CAS 977068-97-5	Myreth-3 laurate	CAS 977079-10-9	Isostearyl erucate

EINECS Number-to-Trade Name Cross-Reference

EINECS	Trade name	EINECS	Trade name	EINECS	Trade name
200-018-0	Patlac® LA	200-289-5	Emery® 917	200-313-4	Prifrac 2981
200-018-0	Unichem LACA	200-289-5	Emery® 918	200-313-4	Pristerene 4904
200-061-5	A-641	200-289-5	Glycon® G 100	200-313-4	Pristerene 4905
200-061-5	Arlex	200-289-5	Glycon® G-300	200-313-4	Pristerene 4910
200-061-5	Fancol SORB	200-289-5	Kemstrene® 96.0%	200-313-4	Pristerene 4911
200-061-5	Hefti Sorbex-R		USP	200-313-4	Pristerene 4915
200-061-5	Hefti Sorbex-RP	200-289-5	Kemstrene® 99.7%	200-313-4	Pristerene 4921
200-061-5	Hydex® 100 Gran. 206		USP	200-313-4	Radiacid® 152
200-061-5	Hydex® Coarse Powd.	200-289-5	Optim	200-313-4	Radiacid® 416
200-061-5	Hydex® Powd. 60	200-289-5	Star	200-313-4	Radiacid® 423
200-061-5	Hydex® Tablet Grade	200-289-5	Superol	200-313-4	Radiacid® 427
200-061-5	Liponic 70-NC	200-293-7	Unamino GLUT	200-313-4	Radiacid® 428
200-061-5	Liponic 76-NC	200-296-3	Unamino L-CSTI	200-313-4	Radiacid® 464
200-061-5	Liponic 83-NC	200-311-3	Acetoquat CTAB	200-313-4	Unifat 54
200-061-5	Liposorb 70	200-311-3	Bromat®	200-313-4	Unifat 55L
200-061-5	Sorbelite™ C	200-311-3	Catinal HTB-70	200-315-5	Unichem UREA
200-061-5	Sorbelite™ FG	200-311-3	Cetrimide	200-317-6	Unisept Chlorbut
200-061-5	Sorbo®	200-311-3	Cetrimide™ BP	200-334-9	Sugartab®
200-061-5	Unisweet 70	200-311-3	Rhodaquat® M242B/99	200-338-0	Adeka Propylene Glycol
200-061-5	Unisweet 70/CONC	200-311-3	Sumquat® 6030		(P)
200-061-5	Unisweet CONC	200-311-3	Varisoft® CTB-40	200-338-0	Unichem PROP-G
200-066-2	Ascorbic Acid Ampul	200-312-9	Adeka PA Series	200-353-2	Atomergic Cholesterol
	Type No. 604065700	200-312-9	Crodacid PD3160	200-353-2	Cholesterol
200-066-2	Ascorbic Acid Fine	200-312-9	Edenor L2SM	200-353-2	Cholesterol BP
	Granular No. 6045655	200-312-9	Emersol® 142	200-353-2	Cholesterol NF
200-066-2	Ascorbic Acid Ultra-	200-312-9	Emersol® 143	200-353-2	Fancol CH
	Fine Powd. No.	200-312-9	Emersol® 144	200-353-2	Liquid Crystal CN/9
	604565300	200-312-9	Hystrene® 7016	200-353-2	Loralan-CH
200-066-2	Ascorbic Acid USP,	200-312-9	Hystrene® 9016	200-353-2	Unichol
	FCC Type S No.	200-312-9	Kartacid 1692	200-449-4	Hamp-Ene® Acid
	604566	200-312-9	Prifrac 2960	200-449-4	Kelate Acid
200-066-2	Uantox ASCA	200-312-9	Unifat 16	200-449-4	Sequestrene® AA
200-066-2	Vitazyme® C	200-313-4	Cetax TP	200-449-4	Universene ACID
200-075-1	Candex®	200-313-4	Crosterene SA4310	200-449-4	Versene Acid
200-075-1	Candex® Plus	200-313-4	Emersol® 110	200-456-2	Etaphen
200-075-1	Emdex®	200-313-4	Emersol® 120	200-470-9	Emersol® 315
200-075-1	Emdex® Plus	200-313-4	Emersol® 132 NF Lily®	200-529-9	Hampene® CaNa₂ Pure
200-125-2	Rodol EGC	200-313-4	Emersol® 150		Crystals
200-143-0	Bronopol	200-313-4	Emersol® 6320	200-529-9	Kelate CDS
200-143-0	CoSept BNP	200-313-4	Emersol® 6332 NF	200-529-9	Universene CaNa2
200-143-0	Lexgard® Bronopol	200-313-4	Emersol® 6349	200-529-9	Versene CA
200-143-0	Midpol 97	200-313-4	Emersol® 6351	200-573-9	Chelon 100
200-143-0	Midpol 100	200-313-4	Hy-Phi 1199	200-573-9	Hamp-Ene® 100
200-143-0	Myacide® BT	200-313-4	Hy-Phi 1303	200-573-9	Hamp-Ene® 220
200-143-0	Tristat BNP	200-313-4	Hy-Phi 1401	200-573-9	Hamp-Ene® Na₄
200-158-2	Unamino L-CSTE	200-313-4	Hystrene® 4516	200-573-9	Kelate 220
200-237-1	Rodol PM	200-313-4	Hystrene® 5016 NF	200-573-9	Sequestrene® 220
200-270-1	Sumquat® 2355	200-313-4	Hystrene® 9718 NF	200-573-9	Universene Na4
200-272-2	Hampshire® Glycine	200-313-4	Industrene® 9018	200-573-9	Versene 100
200-272-2	Unamino GLCN	200-313-4	Kartacid 1890	200-573-9	Versene 100 EP
200-289-5	Croderol GA 7000	200-313-4	Koster Keunen Stearic	200-573-9	Versene 100 LS
200-289-5	Emery® 912		Acid XXX	200-573-9	Versene 100 SRG
200-289-5	Emery® 916	200-313-4	Prifrac 2980	200-573-9	Versene 100 XL

915

EINECS	Trade name	EINECS	Trade name	EINECS	Trade name
202-592-8	Atomergic Allantoin	203-315-3	Emalex PG-di-O	203-508-2	Arosurf® TA-100
202-592-8	Chemie Linz Allantoin	203-347-8	Emeressence® 1150	203-508-2	Arosurf® TA-101
202-592-8	Fancol TOIN	203-349-9	Hodag DCA	203-508-2	Dehyquart® DAM
202-592-8	Tri-K Allantoin	203-349-9	Kessco® DCA	203-508-2	Genamin DSAC
202-592-8	Uniderm A	203-350-4	Cetiol® B	203-508-2	Kemamine® Q-9902C
202-597-5	Rohagum® N-742	203-350-4	Unitolate B	203-508-2	Nikkol CA-3475
202-608-3	Crodasinic L	203-350-4	Upamate DBA	203-508-2	Protaquat 2HT-75
202-608-3	Hamposyl® L	203-353-0	Dermol 499	203-508-2	Sumquat® 6045
202-608-3	Nikkol Sarcosinate LH	203-353-0	Fractalite 499	203-508-2	Varisoft® TA-100
202-608-3	Oramix L	203-358-8	Ablunol 200MS	203-585-2	Rodol RS
202-608-3	Sarkosyl® L	203-358-8	Acconon 200-MS	203-585-2	Unichem RSC
202-608-3	Vanseal® LS	203-358-8	Cithrol 2MS	203-661-5	Chemidex O
202-615-1	Rohagum® P-24	203-358-8	Crodet S4	203-661-5	Incromine OPM
202-615-1	Rohasol® P-550	203-358-8	Ethofat® 18/14	203-661-5	Lexamine O-13
202-700-3	Ajidew A-100	203-358-8	Hodag 20-S	203-661-5	Mackine™ 501
202-700-3	Pidolidone®	203-358-8	Kessco® PEG 200 MS	203-661-5	Schercodine O
202-713-4	Niacinamide USP, FCC No. 69905	203-358-8	Lipopeg 2-S	203-661-5	Unizeen OA
		203-358-8	Mapeg® 200 MS	203-663-6	Emalex DEG-di-S
202-713-4	Vitazyme® B3	203-358-8	Nikkol MYS-4	203-749-3	Crodasinic O
202-766-3	Rodol 4J	203-358-8	Pegosperse® 200 MS	203-749-3	Hamposyl® O
202-785-7	Aseptoform	203-358-8	Protamate 200 DPS	203-749-3	Nikkol Sarcosinate OH
202-785-7	Bentex M	203-358-8	Unipeg-200 MS	203-749-3	Oramix O
202-785-7	CoSept M	203-359-3	Alkamuls® L-9	203-749-3	Vanseal OS
202-785-7	Lexgard® M	203-363-5	Ablunol DEGMS	203-751-4	Crodamol IPM
202-785-7	Methyl-Steriline	203-363-5	Alkamuls® SDG	203-751-4	Deltyl® Extra
202-785-7	Nipagin M	203-363-5	Cithrol DGMS N/E	203-751-4	Elfacos® IPM
202-785-7	Paridol M	203-363-5	Emalex DEG-m-S	203-751-4	Emerest® 2314
202-785-7	Preserval M	203-363-5	Estol DEMS 3710	203-751-4	Estol 1512
202-785-7	Trisept M	203-363-5	Glicosterina DPG	203-751-4	Estol 1514
202-785-7	Unisept M	203-363-5	Hefti DMS-33	203-751-4	Estol IPM 1508
202-859-9	Unichem BZAL	203-363-5	Hodag DGS	203-751-4	Estol IPM 1509 (BIO-IPM)
202-935-1	Naturechem® GTR	203-363-5	Hodag DGS-N		
202-951-9	Rodol Gray B Base	203-363-5	Hydrine	203-751-4	Estol IPM 1512
203-041-4	Mazeen® 173	203-363-5	Karapeg DEG-MS	203-751-4	Estol IPM 1514
203-041-4	Mazeen® 174	203-363-5	Kemester® 5221	203-751-4	Estol IPM-b 1509
203-041-4	Mazeen® 174-75	203-363-5	Kessco® Diethylene Glycol Monostearate	203-751-4	Isopropylmyristat
203-041-4	Neutrol® TE			203-751-4	Jafaester 14-96
203-049-8	Alkanolamine 144	203-363-5	Kessco® Diglycol Stearate Neutral	203-751-4	Jafaester 14 NF
203-049-8	Alkanolamine 244			203-751-4	Kessco® Isopropyl Myristate
203-049-8	Alkanolamine 244 Low Freeze Grade	203-363-5	Lipal DGMS		
		203-363-5	Lipopeg 1-S	203-751-4	Kessco® Isopropyl Myristate NF
203-049-8	TEA 85 Low Freeze Grade	203-363-5	Nikkol DEGS		
		203-363-5	Nikkol MYS-2	203-751-4	Lanesta 31
203-049-8	TEA 99 Low Freeze Grade	203-363-5	Nopalcol 1-S	203-751-4	Lexol® IPM
		203-363-5	Protachem DGS	203-751-4	Lexol® IPM-NF
203-049-8	TEA 99 Standard Grade	203-363-5	Protachem DGS-C	203-751-4	Liponate IPM
		203-363-5	Rol DGE	203-751-4	Nikkol IPM-100
203-049-8	Trolamine 85 NF Grade	203-363-5	Sterol ST 2	203-751-4	Nikkol IPM-EX
203-049-8	Trolamine 99 NF Grade	203-363-5	Tegin® D 6100	203-751-4	Promyr
203-049-8	Unichem TEA	203-363-5	Witconol™ CAD	203-751-4	Radia® 7190
203-051-9	Priacetin	203-364-0	Cithrol DEGMO	203-751-4	Radia® 7730
203-051-9	Unitolate GTA	203-364-0	Emalex 200	203-751-4	Tegosoft® M
203-063-4	Armeen® 3-12	203-364-0	Hetoxamate MO-2	203-751-4	Upamate IPM
203-090-1	Crodamol DOA	203-364-0	Hodag DGO	203-751-4	Wickenol® 101
203-090-1	Kodaflex® DOA	203-364-0	Lipopeg 1-O	203-751-4	Witconol™ 2314
203-090-1	Wickenol® 158	203-364-0	Nikkol MYO-2	203-751-4'	Protachem IPM
203-161-7	Cyclosal	203-364-0	Witconol™ DOSS	203-755-6	Kemamide® W-35
203-180-0	Eltesol® TSX/A	203-366-1	HSA	203-755-6	Kemamide® W-42
203-180-0	Eltesol® TSX/SF	203-368-2	Emid® 6573	203-759-8	Bumyr
203-180-0	Witconate™ TX Acid	203-368-2	Rewomid® R 280	203-759-8	Crodamol BM
203-192-6	Elestab® CPN	203-369-8	Flexricin® 15	203-759-8	Nikkol BM
203-225-4	Aldehyde C 14 Soc. Peach (3/010811)	203-371-9	Estalan DNPA	203-759-8	Wickenol® 141
		203-371-9	Pelemol DNPA	203-764-5	Nikkol DES-SP
203-232-2	Dehyquart® C	203-404-7	Rodol D	203-768-7	Tristat
203-232-2	Dehyquart® C Crystals	203-473-3	Jeffersol DE-75	203-768-7	Unistat
203-232-2	Uniquart C	203-492-7	Rhodorsil® Oils 70041 VO.65	203-768-7	Unistat SORBA
203-246-9	PTAL			203-804-1	Cellosolve®
203-315-3	Cithrol PGDO	203-508-2	Ablumine DHT75	203-815-1	Unamine-MORP

EINECS	Trade name	EINECS	Trade name	EINECS	Trade name
203-820-9	DIPA Commercial Grade	203-886-9	Instapearl	203-928-6	Arquad® 16-25W
203-820-9	DIPA Low Freeze Grade 85	203-886-9	Kemester® 5220	203-928-6	Arquad® 16-29
		203-886-9	Kemester® EGMS	203-928-6	Arquad® 16-29W
		203-886-9	Kessco EGMS	203-928-6	Arquad® 16-50
203-820-9	DIPA Low Freeze Grade 90	203-886-9	Kessco® Ethylene Glycol Monostearate	203-928-6	Barquat® CT-29
				203-928-6	Carsoquat® CT-429
203-820-9	DIPA NF Grade	203-886-9	Lanesta 35	203-928-6	CTAC
203-820-9	Unichem DIPA	203-886-9	Lasemul 62 E	203-928-6	Dehyquart® A
203-825-6	Carolane	203-886-9	Lauramide EG	203-928-6	Genamin CTAC
203-825-6	Cosbiol	203-886-9	Lexemul® EGMS	203-928-6	Incroquat CTC-30
203-825-6	Dermane	203-886-9	Lipal EGMS	203-928-6	Incroquat CTC-50
203-825-6	Fitoderm	203-886-9	Lipo EGMS	203-928-6	Mackernium™ CTC-30
203-825-6	Nikkol Squalane	203-886-9	Lonzest® EGMS	203-928-6	Nikkol CA-2330
203-825-6	Prisorine SQS 3758	203-886-9	Mackester™ EGMS	203-928-6	Nikkol CA-2350
203-825-6	Robane®	203-886-9	Mackester™ IP	203-928-6	Quatrex CTAC
203-826-1	Dermene	203-886-9	Mapeg® EGMS	203-928-6	Querton 16Cl-29
203-826-1	Nikkol Squalene EX	203-886-9	Mapeg® EGMS-K	203-928-6	Radiaquat® 6444
203-826-1	Squatol S	203-886-9	Monthyle	203-928-6	Radiaquat® 6445
203-826-1	Supraene®	203-886-9	Nikkol EGMS-70	203-928-6	Rhodaquat® M242C/29
203-828-2	Rewomid® IPE 280	203-886-9	Nikkol Pearl 1218	203-928-6	Tequat BC
203-828-2	Schercomid OMI	203-886-9	Pegosperse® 50 MS	203-928-6	Uniquart A
203-839-2	Cellosolve® Acetate	203-886-9	Protachem EGMS	203-928-6	Variquat® E290
203-852-3	Nacol® 6-98	203-886-9	RITA EGMS	203-928-6	Varisoft® 250
203-856-5	Ucarcide® 225	203-886-9	Ritasynt IP	203-928-6	Varisoft® 300
203-856-5	Ucarcide® 250	203-886-9	Rol GE	203-928-6	Varisoft® 355
203-868-0	DEA Commercial Grade	203-886-9	Schercemol EGMS	203-929-1	Ablumine TMS
		203-886-9	Secoster® EMS	203-929-1	Arquad® 18-50
203-868-0	DEA Low Freeze Grade	203-886-9	Sterol ST 1	203-929-1	Genamin STAC
203-868-0	Unichem DEA	203-886-9	Tegin® G 6100	203-929-1	Kemamine® Q-9903B
203-872-2	Unichem DEG	203-886-9	Unipeg-EGMS	203-929-1	Nikkol CA-2450
203-883-2	Ablumide SME	203-886-9	Witconol™ EGMS	203-929-1	Nikkol CA-2465
203-883-2	Alkamide® S-280	203-886-9	Zohar EGMS	203-929-1	Varisoft® ST-50
203-883-2	Amidex SME	203-887-4	Cithrol ES	203-929-1	Varisoft® TS-50
203-883-2	CPH-380-N	203-887-4	Hefti AMS-33	203-929-1	Varisoft® TSC
203-883-2	Hetamide MS	203-889-5	Elfacos® EO	203-934-9	Estol IPS 3702
203-883-2	Incromide SM	203-889-5	Estol ETO 3659	203-934-9	Kessco IPS
203-883-2	Mackamide™ SMA	203-889-5	Kessco EO	203-934-9	Lasemul 60
203-883-2	Mazamide® SMEA	203-893-7	Ethyl Octene-1	203-934-9	Tegosoft® S
203-883-2	Monamid® S	203-905-0	Butyl Cellosolve®	203-934-9	Wickenol® 127
203-883-2	Monamid® S/M	203-905-0	Butyl Oxitol	203-940-1	Carbitol® Acetate
203-883-2	Olamida SM	203-906-6	Ektasolve® DM	203-943-8	Adma® 12
203-883-2	Phoenamid SM	203-911-3	CE-1218	203-943-8	Adogen® MA-102
203-883-2	Rewomid® S 280	203-911-3	CE-1270	203-943-8	Armeen® DM12D
203-883-2	Upamide SME-M	203-911-3	CE-1280	203-943-8	Barlene® 12S
203-883-2	Witcamide® 70	203-911-3	CE-1290	203-943-8	Kemamine® T-6902
203-883-2	Witcamide® 6507	203-911-3	CE-1295	203-956-9	Cachalot® DE-10
203-884-8	Hetamide MO	203-911-3	Estol MEL 1502	203-956-9	Nacol® 10-97
203-884-8	Incromide OPM	203-911-3	Estol MEL 1507	203-956-9	Nacol® 10-99
203-884-8	Schercomid OME	203-911-3	Kemester® 9012	203-961-6	Butyl Carbitol®
203-886-9	Ablunol EGMS	203-917-6	Nacol® 8-97	203-961-6	Butyl Dioxitol
203-886-9	Alkamuls® EGMS	203-917-6	Nacol® 8-99	203-961-6	Ektasolve® DB
203-886-9	Alkamuls® EGMS/C	203-919-7	Ektasolve® DE	203-966-3	Estol MEP 1503
203-886-9	Alkamuls® SEG	203-919-7	Solvent APV Spec	203-966-3	Kemester® 9016
203-886-9	Cerasynt® IP	203-919-7	Transcutol	203-966-3	Radia® 7120
203-886-9	Cerasynt® M	203-924-4	Diglyme	203-982-0	Cachalot® L-90
203-886-9	Chemsperse EGMS	203-927-0	Arquad® 12-33	203-982-0	Epal® 12
203-886-9	CPH-37-NA	203-927-0	Arquad® 12-37W	203-982-0	Laurex® L1
203-886-9	Dragil 2/027011	203-927-0	Arquad® 12-50	203-982-0	Laurex® NC
203-886-9	Elfacos® EGMS	203-927-0	Dehyquart® LT	203-982-0	Lipocol L
203-886-9	Emalex EGS-A	203-927-0	Empigen® 5089	203-982-0	Nacol® 12-96
203-886-9	Emalex EGS-B	203-927-0	Kemamine® Q-6903B	203-982-0	Nacol® 12-99
203-886-9	Emerest® 2350	203-927-0	Laurene	203-982-0	Radianol® 1712
203-886-9	Empilan® EGMS	203-927-0	Varisoft® LAC	203-982-0	Unihydag Wax 12
203-886-9	Estol EGMS 3749	203-928-6	Ablumine TMC	203-989-9	Dow E200
203-886-9	Ethylene Glycol Monostearate VA	203-928-6	Adogen® 444	203-989-9	Hetoxide PEG-200
		203-928-6	Ammonyx® CETAC	203-989-9	Hodag PEG 200
203-886-9	Hodag EGMS	203-928-6	Ammonyx® CETAC-30	203-989-9	Lipo Polyglycol 200
203-886-9	Hodag EGS	203-928-6	Arquad® 16-25	203-989-9	Lipoxol® 200 MED

EINECS	Trade name	EINECS	Trade name	EINECS	Trade name
203-989-9	Macol® E-200	204-017-6	Alfol® 18	204-393-1	Empilan® LDE/FF
203-989-9	Pluracol® E200	204-017-6	Cachalot® S-54	204-393-1	Ethylan® MLD
203-989-9	Poly-G® 200	204-017-6	Cachalot® S-56	204-393-1	Foamid PK
203-989-9	Teric PEG 200	204-017-6	Cetax 18	204-393-1	Foamid SL-Extra
203-989-9	Unipeg 200	204-017-6	CO-1895	204-393-1	Hartamide LDA
203-989-9	Unipeg-200 X	204-017-6	Crodacol S-70	204-393-1	Hetamide LL
203-989-9	Upiwax 200	204-017-6	Crodacol S-95NF	204-393-1	Hetamide ML
203-990-4	Kemester® 7018	204-017-6	Epal® 18NF	204-393-1	Hetamide MOC
203-990-4	Kemester® 9718	204-017-6	Fancol SA	204-393-1	Incromide L90
203-992-5	Kemester® 115	204-017-6	Hetoxol SA	204-393-1	Incromide LL
203-992-5	Kemester® 8002	204-017-6	Hyfatol 18-95	204-393-1	Incromide LR
203-992-5	Witconol™ 2301	204-017-6	Hyfatol 18-98	204-393-1	Lauramina
203-997-2	Adma® 16	204-017-6	Lanette® 18	204-393-1	Lipamide LMWC
203-997-2	Adogen® MA-106	204-017-6	Lanette® 18 DEO	204-393-1	Loropan LD
203-997-2	Armeen® DM16D	204-017-6	Lanol S	204-393-1	Mackamide™ L-10
203-997-2	Barlene® 16S	204-017-6	Lipocol S	204-393-1	Mackamide™ L95
203-997-2	Kemamine® T-8902	204-017-6	Mackol 18	204-393-1	Mackamide™ LLM
204-000-3	Cachalot® M-43	204-017-6	Nacol® 18-94	204-393-1	Mackamide™ LMD
204-000-3	Epal® 14	204-017-6	Nacol® 18-98	204-393-1	Manromid 1224
204-000-3	Lanette® 14	204-017-6	Nikkol Stearyl Alcohol	204-393-1	Mazamide® 124
204-000-3	Nacol® 14-95	204-017-6	Philcohol 1800	204-393-1	Mazamide® 1214
204-000-3	Nacol® 14-98	204-017-6	Radianol® 1898	204-393-1	Mazamide® L-298
204-000-3	Unihydag Wax-14	204-017-6	RITA SA	204-393-1	Mazamide® LM
204-002-4	Adma® 14	204-017-6	Stearal	204-393-1	Mazamide® LM 20
204-002-4	Adogen® MA-104	204-017-6	Steraffine	204-393-1	Mazamide® LS 196
204-002-4	Armeen® DM14D	204-017-6	Unihydag Wax-18	204-393-1	Monamid® 31
204-002-4	Barlene® 14	204-065-8	Demeon D	204-393-1	Monamid® 150-GLT
204-002-4	Barlene® 14S	204-065-8	Dymel® A	204-393-1	Monamid® 150-LMWC
204-002-4	Kemamine® T-7902	204-100-7	AMPD	204-393-1	Monamid® 150-LWA
204-007-1	Crodolene LA1020	204-101-2	AEPD®	204-393-1	Monamid® 716
204-007-1	Emersol® 210	204-110-1	Alkamuls® PETS	204-393-1	Monamid® 1034
204-007-1	Emersol® 213 NF	204-110-1	Crodamol PETS	204-393-1	Monamid® 1224
204-007-1	Emersol® 221 NF	204-110-1	Kessco PTS	204-393-1	Monamid® L-350
204-007-1	Emersol® 233 LL	204-110-1	Liponate PS-4	204-393-1	Monamid® L-355
204-007-1	Emersol® 6313 NF	204-132-1	Dantoin® MDMH	204-393-1	Monamid® L-360
204-007-1	Emersol® 6321 NF	204-260-8	Homosalate®	204-393-1	Monamid® L-365
204-007-1	Emersol® 6333 NF	204-260-8	Kemester® HMS	204-393-1	Monamid® LL-370
204-007-1	Emersol® 7021	204-260-8	Uniderm HOMSAL	204-393-1	Monamid® LM-375
204-007-1	Hy-Phi 1055	204-263-4	Dermoblock OS	204-393-1	Ninol® 30-LL
204-007-1	Hy-Phi 1088	204-263-4	Escalol® 587	204-393-1	Ninol® 55-LL
204-007-1	Hy-Phi 2066	204-263-4	Lanaetex-OS	204-393-1	Ninol® 70-SL
204-007-1	Hy-Phi 2088	204-263-4	Neo Heliopan, Type OS	204-393-1	Ninol® 96-SL
204-007-1	Hy-Phi 2102	204-263-4	Neotan L	204-393-1	Ninol® L-9
204-007-1	Industrene® 105	204-263-4	Trivent OS	204-393-1	Norfox® DLSA
204-007-1	Industrene® 106	204-317-7	Unichem METSAL	204-393-1	Phoenamid LD, LD
204-007-1	Industrene® 206	204-385-8	Preventol BP		Special
204-007-1	Priolene 6900	204-393-1	Ablumide LDE	204-393-1	Profan AA62
204-007-1	Priolene 6905	204-393-1	Afmide™ LLM	204-393-1	Protamide L-80M, L90,
204-007-1	Priolene 6906	204-393-1	Afmide™ LMD		L90A, LM 73, LM 73-L,
204-007-1	Priolene 6910	204-393-1	Alkamide® 327		LM-73 PG, LMAV
204-007-1	Priolene 6933	204-393-1	Alkamide® 1195	204-393-1	Schercomid SL-Extra
204-007-1	Radiacid® 212	204-393-1	Alkamide® DL-203/S	204-393-1	Schercomid SLM-S
204-007-1	Unifat 5L	204-393-1	Alkamide® DL-207/S	204-393-1	Standamid® KDL
204-010-8	Crodacid B	204-393-1	Alkamide® L9DE	204-393-1	Standamid® KDOL
204-010-8	Hystrene® 7022	204-393-1	Alkamide® LE	204-393-1	Standamid® KDS
204-010-8	Hystrene® 9022	204-393-1	Amidex LD	204-393-1	Standamid® LD
204-010-8	Prifrac 2989	204-393-1	Amidex LD-8	204-393-1	Standamid® LDO
204-015-5	Armeen® O	204-393-1	Aminol LM-30C, LM-	204-393-1	Standamid® LDS
204-015-5	Armeen® OD		30C Special	204-393-1	Tohol N-230
204-015-5	Armeen® OL	204-393-1	Carsamide® SAL-7	204-393-1	Tohol N-230X
204-015-5	Armeen® OLD	204-393-1	Carsamide® SAL-9	204-393-1	Upamide LD
204-015-5	Kemamine® P-989	204-393-1	Carsamide® SAL-82	204-393-1	Upamide LDS, LM-20,
204-015-5	Radiamine 6172	204-393-1	Chimipal LDA		LS-173, LS-196
204-015-5	Radiamine 6173	204-393-1	Comperlan® LD	204-393-1	Varamide® LL-1
204-017-6	Adol® 61	204-393-1	Comperlan® LDO, LDS	204-393-1	Varamide® ML-1
204-017-6	Adol® 61 NF	204-393-1	Emid® 6513	204-393-1	Varamide® ML-4
204-017-6	Adol® 62 NF	204-393-1	Emid® 6519	204-393-1	Witcamide® 5195
204-017-6	Adol® 620 NF	204-393-1	Empilan® LDE	204-393-1	Witcamide® 6310

EINECS	Trade name	EINECS	Trade name	EINECS	Trade name
204-393-1	Witcamide® 6510		Grade	204-694-8	Adogen® MA-108
204-393-1	Witcamide® 6511	204-528-4	Unichem TIPA	204-694-8	Adogen® MA-108 SF
204-393-1	Witcamide® 6519	204-534-7	Cithrol GTO	204-694-8	Amine 2M18D
204-393-1	Witcamide® 6590	204-534-7	CPH-399-N	204-694-8	Armeen® DM18D
204-393-1	Witcamide® L-9	204-534-7	Emerest® 2423	204-694-8	Barlene® 18S
204-393-1	Witcamide® LDEA	204-534-7	Emery® 2423	204-694-8	Kemamine® T-9902
204-393-1	Witcamide® LL	204-534-7	Hodag GTO	204-695-3	Amine 18-90
204-393-1	Witcamide® STD-HP	204-534-7	Kemester® 1000	204-695-3	Amine 18-90 D
204-399-4	Aethyl-Steriline	204-534-7	Witconol™ 2423	204-695-3	Amine 18-95
204-399-4	Bentex E	204-558-8	Docoil DOS	204-695-3	Armeen® 18
204-399-4	CoSept E	204-558-8	Elfacos® DEHS	204-695-3	Armeen® 18D
204-399-4	Lexgard® E	204-558-8	Kessco DEHS	204-701-4	Unichem UREA-P
204-399-4	Nipagin A	204-558-8	Trivent DOS	204-709-8	AMP
204-399-4	Paridol E	204-589-7	Cephene™	204-769-5	Tris Nitro®
204-399-4	Preserval E	204-589-7	Emeressence® 1160	204-781-0	NPG® Glycol
204-399-4	Trisept E		Rose Ether	204-812-8	Cosmopon SES
204-399-4	Unisept E	204-589-7	Emthox® 6705	204-812-8	Empicol® 0585/A
204-402-9	Unichem BZBN	204-589-7	K-Preserve Liq.	204-812-8	Niaproof® Anionic
204-405-8	Mazon® EE-1	204-589-7	Phenoxen		Surfactant 08
204-427-5	Rodol C	204-589-7	Phenoxetol	204-812-8	Witcolate™ D-510
204-464-7	Unisweet EVAN	204-589-7	Phenoxyethanol O	204-823-8	Unichem SODAC
204-465-2	Unisweet VAN	204-589-7	Rewopal® MPG 10	204-867-8	Unichem ZPS
204-479-9	Hyamine® 1622 50%	204-589-7	Sepicide LD	204-867-8	Universal ZPS
204-479-9	Hyamine® 1622	204-589-7	Unisept POE	204-881-4	Ionol CP
	Crystals	204-593-9	CPC	204-881-4	Sustane® BHT
204-498-2	Atomergic Propyl	204-593-9	CPC Sumquat 6060	204-881-4	Tenox® BHT
	Gallate	204-593-9	Uniquart CPC	204-881-4	Uantox BHT
204-498-2	Progallin® P	204-614-1	Argus DLTDP	204-881-4	Uninox A 287
204-498-2	Tenox® PG	204-614-1	Evanstab® 12	204-881-4	Vanox® PCX
204-498-2	Uantox PG	204-616-2	Rodol P Base	204-886-1	Unisweet SOSAC
204-503-8	Rodol YBA	204-617-8	Eastman® Hydroqui-	205-011-6	Kemester® DMP
204-516-9	Cumal		none	205-011-6	Kodaflex® DMP
204-526-3	Cetol®	204-617-8	Rodol HQ	205-011-6	Palatinol® M
204-526-3	Sumquat® 6050	204-617-8	Tecquinol® USP Grade	205-011-6	Uniplex 110
204-527-9	Ablumine 1618	204-617-8	Uantox HQ	205-026-8	Spectra-Sorb® UV 24
204-527-9	Ammonyx® 4	204-630-9	Iodogene	205-027-3	Uvinul® D 49
204-527-9	Ammonyx® 4B	204-649-2	Unichem Levula	205-028-9	Uvinul® D 50
204-527-9	Ammonyx® 485	204-666-5	Crodamol BS	205-029-4	DHBP Quinsorb 010
204-527-9	Ammonyx® 4002	204-666-5	Dermol EB	205-029-4	Uvasorb 20H
204-527-9	Ammonyx® CA-Special	204-666-5	Emerest® 2325	205-029-4	Uvinul® 400
204-527-9	Amyx A-25-S 0040	204-666-5	Estol BUS 1550	205-031-5	Escalol® 567
204-527-9	Carsoquat® SDQ-85	204-666-5	Kemester® 5410	205-031-5	Eusolex® 4360
204-527-9	Catinal OB-80E	204-666-5	Kemester® 5510	205-031-5	Marsorb 24
204-527-9	Emcol® 4	204-666-5	Kessco® Butyl Stearate	205-031-5	Neo Heliopan, Type BB
204-527-9	Hetquat S-20	204-666-5	Lasemul 74 NP	205-031-5	Spectra-Sorb® UV 9
204-527-9	Incroquat S-85	204-666-5	Nikkol BS	205-031-5	Syntase® 62
204-527-9	Incroquat SDQ-25	204-666-5	Norfox® B-54	205-031-5	Uvasorb MET
204-527-9	Mackernium™ SDC-25	204-666-5	Radia® 7752	205-031-5	Uvinul® M 40
204-527-9	Mackernium™ SDC-85	204-666-5	Unichem BUTSTE	205-055-6	Dowicide A
204-527-9	Maquat SC-18	204-666-5	Witconol™ 2326	205-087-0	Vancide® 89 RE
204-527-9	Miracare® SCS	204-672-8	Bretol®	205-126-1	Sodium Ascorbate
204-527-9	M-Quat® B-25	204-672-8	Sumquat® 6020		USP, FCC Fine Powd.
204-527-9	M-Quat® JS-25	204-677-5	Prifrac 2901		No. 6047708
204-527-9	Nikkol CA-1485	204-677-5	Prifrac 2910	205-126-1	Uantox SODASC
204-527-9	Quatrex STC-25	204-677-5	Unifat 8	205-129-8	Dermoblock MA
204-527-9	Quatrex STC-85	204-680-1	Estol MEM 1518	205-129-8	Estalan MA
204-527-9	Rhodaquat® M270C/18	204-680-1	Estol MYM 3645	205-129-8	Neo Heliopan, Type MA
204-527-9	Stedbac®	204-680-1	Kemester® 9014	205-129-8	Trivent MA
204-527-9	Sumquat® 6210	204-690-6	Adogen® 163D	205-234-9	Amidex CP
204-527-9	Unisoft SAC	204-690-6	Amine 12	205-234-9	Comperlan® CD
204-527-9	Variquat® SDC	204-690-6	Amine 12-98D	205-234-9	Hetamide 1069
204-527-9	Varisoft® SDAC	204-690-6	Armeen® 12	205-234-9	Mackamide™ CD-10
204-527-9	Varisoft® SDAC-W	204-690-6	Armeen® 12D	205-234-9	Monamid® 150-CW
204-527-9	Zoharquat 25	204-690-6	Kemamine® P-690	205-234-9	Monamid® CP-205
204-527-9	Zoharquat 75	204-690-6	Radiamine 6163	205-234-9	Monamine C-100
204-528-4	TIPA 99	204-690-6	Radiamine 6164	205-234-9	Standamid® CD
204-528-4	TIPA 101	204-693-2	Armid® 18	205-234-9	Upamide CD
204-528-4	TIPA Low Freeze	204-694-8	Adma® 18	205-234-9	Witcamide® 6544

EINECS	Trade name	EINECS	Trade name	EINECS	Trade name
205-271-0	Schercozoline L	205-388-7	Elfan® 240T		Monolaurate
205-278-9	D-Calcium Pantothen-ate USP, FCC Type SD No. 63924	205-388-7	Empicol® TA40A	205-526-6	Lauricidin 802, 812, 1012, E
		205-388-7	Empicol® TL40		
		205-388-7	Empicol® TL40/T	205-526-6	Monomuls® 90-L12
205-281-5	Chimin L	205-388-7	Genapol® CRT 40	205-526-6	Protachem MLD
205-281-5	Closyl LA 3584	205-388-7	Genapol® LRT 40	205-530-8	Amidex AME
205-281-5	Crodasinic LS30	205-388-7	Laural D	205-530-8	Carsamide® AMEA
205-281-5	Crodasinic LS35	205-388-7	Manro TL 40	205-530-8	Foamid AME-70
205-281-5	Hamposyl® L-30	205-388-7	Marlinat® DFL 40	205-530-8	Foamid AME-75
205-281-5	Hamposyl® L-95	205-388-7	Neopon LT/NF	205-530-8	Foamid AME-100
205-281-5	Maprosyl® 30	205-388-7	Nikkol TEALS	205-530-8	Hetamide MA
205-281-5	Medialan LD	205-388-7	Nikkol TEALS-42	205-530-8	Incromectant AMEA-70
205-281-5	Nikkol Sarcosinate LN	205-388-7	Norfox® TLS	205-530-8	Incromectant AMEA-100
205-281-5	Nikkol Sarcosinate LN-30	205-388-7	Nutrapon TLS-500		
		205-388-7	Perlankrol® ATL40	205-530-8	Lipamide MEAA
205-281-5	Oramix L30	205-388-7	Rewopol® TLS 40	205-530-8	Mackamide™ AME-75, AME-100
205-281-5	Secosyl	205-388-7	Rhodapon® LT-6		
205-281-5	Unipol LAUROYLSAR	205-388-7	Sandoz Sulfate TL	205-530-8	Schercomid AME
205-281-5	Vanseal® NALS-30	205-388-7	Standapol® T	205-530-8	Upamide ACMEA
205-281-5	Vanseal® NALS-95	205-388-7	Stepanol® WAT	205-530-8	Witcamide® CMEA
205-281-5	Zoharsyl L-30	205-388-7	Sulfetal KT 400	205-539-7	Crodasinic S
205-285-7	Adinol OT16	205-388-7	Sulfochem TLS	205-539-7	Hamposyl® S
205-285-7	Geropon® T-77	205-388-7	Sunnol LM-1140T	205-541-8	Amidex LIPA
205-285-7	Hostapon SO	205-388-7	Surfax 40	205-541-8	Comperlan® LP
205-285-7	Hostapon T Paste 33	205-388-7	Texapon® T	205-541-8	Empilan® LIS
205-285-7	Hostapon T Powd. Highly Conc.	205-388-7	Texapon® T 42	205-541-8	Incromide LI
		205-388-7	Ufarol TA-40	205-541-8	Incromide LMI
205-285-7	Protapon 33	205-388-7	Unipol T	205-541-8	Monamid® LMIPA
205-285-7	Tauranol M-35	205-388-7	Witcolate™ T	205-541-8	Nidaba 3
205-285-7	Tauranol ML	205-388-7	Witcolate™ TLS-500	205-541-8	Profan AD31
205-285-7	Tauranol MS	205-388-7	Zoharpon LAT	205-541-8	Rewomid® IPL 203
205-285-7	Tauranol T-Gel	205-391-3	Hamp-Ex® 80	205-541-8	Upamide MIPA
205-290-4	Unistat SOBAN	205-391-3	Mayoquest 300	205-542-3	Cithrol PGML N/E
205-305-4	Ascorbyl Palmitate No. 60412	205-391-3	Versenex 80	205-542-3	Emalex PGML
		205-392-9	Naturechem® MAR	205-542-3	Hodag PGML
205-305-4	Grindox Ascorbyl Palmitate	205-392-9	Pelemol MAR	205-542-3	Imwitor® 412
		205-455-0	Aldo® MR	205-542-3	Kessco® PGML-X533
205-324-8	Cetats®	205-455-0	Cithrol GMR N/E	205-542-3	Kessco® Propylene Glycol Monolaurate E
205-341-0	Dipentene No. 122	205-455-0	CPH-35-N		
205-351-5	Catinal MB-50A	205-455-0	Flexricin® 13	205-542-3	Lauroglycol
205-351-5	Dehyquart® LDB	205-455-0	Hodag GMR	205-542-3	Rol LP
205-351-5	Tequat PAN	205-455-0	Hodag GMR-D	205-542-3	Schercemol PGML
205-352-0	Arquad® DM14B-90	205-455-0	Mazol® GMR	205-542-3	Unipeg-PGML
205-352-0	Barquat® MX-50	205-455-0	Radiasurf® 7153	205-546-5	Hetamide MM
205-352-0	Barquat® MX-80	205-455-0	Softigen® 701	205-546-5	Witcamide® MM
205-352-0	BTC® 824	205-455-0	Unitina GMRO	205-550-7	Unifat 6
205-352-0	FMB 451-8 Quat	205-468-1	Kessco® Diglycol Laurate A Neutral	205-559-6	Kemester® 4000
205-352-0	FMB 551-5 Quat			205-560-1	Ablumide LME
205-352-0	JAQ Powdered Quat	205-468-1	Kessco® Diglycol Laurate ASE	205-560-1	Afmide™ LMM
205-352-0	Kemamine® Q-7903B			205-560-1	Amidex LMMEA
205-358-3	BASF Disodium EDTA	205-468-1	Kessco® Diglycol Laurate N	205-560-1	Comperlan® LMM
205-358-3	Hampene® Na₂ Pure Crystals			205-560-1	Empilan® LME
		205-468-1	Kessco® Diglycol Laurate N-Syn	205-560-1	Hartamide LMEA
205-358-3	Nervanaid™ BA2 (BP)			205-560-1	Hetamide MML
205-358-3	Sequestrene® NA2	205-468-1	Lipopeg 1-L	205-560-1	Lauridit® LM
205-358-3	Universene Na2	205-468-1	Unipeg-DGL	205-560-1	Loropan LM
205-358-3	Versene NA	205-469-7	Catemol 18SA	205-560-1	Mackamide™ LMM
205-360-4	Hampshire® DEG	205-469-7	Chemical 39 Base	205-560-1	Manromid LMA
205-381-9	Chel DM-41	205-471-8	Naturechem® MHS	205-560-1	Monamid® LMMA
205-381-9	Hamp-Ol® 120	205-507-2	Rodol 26PYR	205-560-1	Ninol® LMP
205-381-9	Hamp-Ol® Crystals	205-513-5	Hexetidine 90, 99	205-560-1	Phoenamid LMM
205-381-9	Versenol 120	205-526-6	Cithrol GML N/E	205-560-1	Rewomid® L 203
205-388-7	Akyposal TLS 42	205-526-6	CPH-34-N	205-560-1	Standamid® LM
205-388-7	Aremsol TA	205-526-6	Estol GML 3614	205-560-1	Upamide MEA
205-388-7	Berol 480	205-526-6	Grillomuls L90	205-560-1	Varamide® L-203
205-388-7	Calfoam TLS-40	205-526-6	Hodag GML	205-571-1	Crodamol IPP
205-388-7	Carsonol® TLS	205-526-6	Imwitor® 312	205-571-1	Deltyl® Prime
205-388-7	Cosmopon TR	205-526-6	Kessco® Glycerol	205-571-1	Elfacos® IPP

EINECS	Trade name	EINECS	Trade name	EINECS	Trade name
205-571-1	Emerest® 2316	205-633-8	Unichem BICARB-S	205-788-1	Sulfochem SLP
205-571-1	Estol 1517	205-759-3	Hamp-Ol® Acid	205-788-1	Sulfochem SLP-95
205-571-1	Estol IPP 1517	205-788-1	Akyposal NLS	205-788-1	Sulfochem SLS
205-571-1	Estol IPP-b 3651	205-788-1	Alscoap LN-40, LN-90	205-788-1	Sulfopon® 101 Special
205-571-1	Isopropyl Palmitate	205-788-1	Calfoam SLS-30	205-788-1	Sulfopon® 103
205-571-1	Jafaester 16 NF	205-788-1	Carsonol® SLS	205-788-1	Sulfopon® P-40
205-571-1	Kessco® Isopropyl Palmitate	205-788-1	Carsonol® SLS Paste B	205-788-1	Sulfopon® WA 3
				205-788-1	Sulfopon® WAQ LCX
205-571-1	Lanesta 23	205-788-1	Carsonol® SLS-R	205-788-1	Sulfopon® WAQ Special
205-571-1	Lexol® IPP	205-788-1	Carsonol® SLS-S		
205-571-1	Lexol® IPP-A	205-788-1	Carsonol® SLS Special	205-788-1	Supralate C
205-571-1	Lexol® IPP-NF	205-788-1	Chemsalan NLS 30	205-788-1	Supralate QC
205-571-1	Liponate IPP	205-788-1	Cosmopon 35	205-788-1	Supralate WA Paste
205-571-1	Nikkol IPP	205-788-1	Elfadent SM 514	205-788-1	Surfax 100
205-571-1	Nikkol IPP-EX	205-788-1	Elfan® 240	205-788-1	Surfax 100 AG
205-571-1	Propal	205-788-1	Empicol® 0045	205-788-1	Surfax CN
205-571-1	Protachem IPP	205-788-1	Empicol® 0045V	205-788-1	Texapon® K-12 Needles
205-571-1	Radia® 7200	205-788-1	Empicol® 0185		
205-571-1	Radia® 7732	205-788-1	Empicol® 0303	205-788-1	Texapon® K-12 Powd.
205-571-1	Tegosoft® P	205-788-1	Empicol® 0303V	205-788-1	Texapon® K-1296
205-571-1	Upamate IPP	205-788-1	Empicol® LM45	205-788-1	Texapon® L-100
205-571-1	Wickenol® 111	205-788-1	Empicol® LS30B	205-788-1	Texapon® LS 100 F
205-571-1	Witconol™ 2316	205-788-1	Empicol® LX28	205-788-1	Texapon® OT Highly Conc. Needles
205-577-4	Carsonol® DLS	205-788-1	Empicol® LX100		
205-577-4	Nutrapon DE 3796	205-788-1	Empicol® LXS95	205-788-1	Texapon® VHC Needles
205-577-4	Standapol® DEA	205-788-1	Empicol® LXV		
205-577-4	Stepanol® DEA	205-788-1	Empicol® LXV100	205-788-1	Texapon® Z
205-577-4	Sulfochem DLS	205-788-1	Empicol® LXV/D	205-788-1	Texapon® ZHC Powder
205-577-4	Supralate EP	205-788-1	Empicol® LZV/D	205-788-1	Ufarol Na-30
205-577-4	Texapon® DEA	205-788-1	Empicol® WAK	205-788-1	Unipol SLS
205-577-4	Unipol DEA	205-788-1	Gardinol WA Paste	205-788-1	Unipol WA-AC
205-577-4	Witcolate™ DLS-35	205-788-1	Manro SLS 28	205-788-1	Unipol WAC Special
205-577-4	Zoharpon LAD	205-788-1	Marlinat® DFK 30	205-788-1	Unipol WAQ-LC
205-582-1	Hystrene® 9512	205-788-1	Naxolate™ WA-97	205-788-1	Unipon K12, K1296, L-100, ZHC Needles, ZHC Powd.
205-582-1	Kartacid 1299	205-788-1	Naxolate™ WAG		
205-582-1	Kortacid 1295	205-788-1	Naxolate™ WA Special		
205-582-1	Unifat 12	205-788-1	Neopon LS/NF		
205-590-5	Norfox® KO	205-788-1	Nikkol SLS	205-788-1	Unipon ZHC Needles
205-596-8	Amine 16D	205-788-1	Nikkol SLS-30	205-788-1	Witcolate™ A Powder
205-596-8	Armeen® 16	205-788-1	Norfox® SLS	205-788-1	Witcolate™ C
205-596-8	Armeen® 16D	205-788-1	Nutrapon DL 3891	205-788-1	Witcolate™ LCP
205-596-8	Kemamine® P-890	205-788-1	Nutrapon W 1367	205-788-1	Witcolate™ SL-1
205-597-3	Adol® 80	205-788-1	Nutrapon WAC 3005	205-788-1	Witcolate™ WAC
205-597-3	Adol® 85	205-788-1	Nutrapon WAQ	205-788-1	Witcolate™ WAC-GL
205-597-3	Adol® 90	205-788-1	Nutrapon WAQE 2364	205-788-1	Witcolate™ WAC-LA
205-597-3	Adol® 90 NF	205-788-1	Perlankrol® DSA	205-788-1	Zoharpon LAS
205-597-3	Cachalot® O-3	205-788-1	Rewopol® NLS 28	205-788-1	Zoharpon LAS 70%
205-597-3	Cachalot® O-8	205-788-1	Rewopol® NLS 90	205-788-1	Zoharpon LAS Special
205-597-3	Cachalot® O-15	205-788-1	Rhodapon® LSB, LSB/CT	205-788-1	Zoharpon LAS Spray Dried
205-597-3	Crodacol A-10				
205-597-3	Dermaffine	205-788-1	Rhodapon® SB-8208/S	206-074-2	Gluconal® K
205-597-3	Fancol OA-95	205-788-1	Rhodapon® SM Special	206-075-8	Gluconal® CA A
205-597-3	HD-Eutanol®			206-075-8	Gluconal® CA M
205-597-3	HD-Ocenol® 90/95	205-788-1	Rolpon LSX	206-101-8	Haro® Chem ALMD-2
205-597-3	HD-Ocenol® 92/96	205-788-1	Standapol® WA-AC	206-101-8	Witco® Aluminum Stearate EA Food Grade
205-597-3	HD Oleyl Alcohol 70/75	205-788-1	Standapol® WAQ-LC		
205-597-3	HD Oleyl Alcohol 80/85	205-788-1	Standapol® WAQ Special		
205-597-3	HD Oleyl Alcohol 90/95			206-103-9	Armid® O
205-597-3	HD Oleyl Alcohol CG	205-788-1	Stepanol® ME Dry	206-104-4	Atomergic Lead Acetate
205-597-3	Lancol	205-788-1	Stepanol® WA-100	206-104-4	Unichem PBA
205-597-3	Lipocol O	205-788-1	Stepanol® WAC	206-156-8	Unichem ROSAL
205-597-3	Lipocol O-80	205-788-1	Stepanol® WA Extra	206-376-4	Unifat 10
205-597-3	Lipocol O/95	205-788-1	Stepanol® WA Paste	207-334-9	Univit-F Forte
205-597-3	Novol	205-788-1	Stepanol® WAQ	207-334-9	Acidan BC Veg
205-597-3	U Tanol HD, HD 70/75, HD 80/85, HD 90/95, HD CG	205-788-1	Stepanol® WA Special	207-334-9	Acidan N 12 Veg
		205-788-1	Sulfochem SAC	207-355-2	Unichem CAMP
		205-788-1	Sulfochem SLC	207-439-9	Camel-WITE®
205-597-3	U Tanol HDL CG	205-788-1	Sulfochem SLN	207-439-9	Unichem CALCARB
				207-444-6	Nikkol Glycyrrhetinic

EINECS NUMBER-TO-TRADE NAME CROSS-REFERENCE

EINECS	Trade name	EINECS	Trade name	EINECS	Trade name
	Acid	209-150-3	Synpro® Magnesium	211-014-3	Alkamuls® EGDS
207-677-3	Desamina		Stearate USP	211-014-3	Chemsperse EGDS
207-701-2	Azulene 100%	209-150-3	Unichem MGS	211-014-3	CPH-360-N
	2/912980	209-150-3	Unichem MS	211-014-3	Cutina® AGS
208-205-9	α-Bisabolol	209-150-3	Witco® Magnesium	211-014-3	Elfacos® EGDS
208-205-9	Dragosantol 2/012681		Stearate N.F	211-014-3	Elfan® L 310
208-205-9	Hydagen® B	209-151-9	Cecavon ZN 70	211-014-3	Emalex EG-di-MPS
208-205-9	Uhydagen B	209-151-9	Cecavon ZN 71	211-014-3	Emalex EG-di-S
208-293-9	Unisept DHA	209-151-9	Cecavon ZN 72	211-014-3	Emalex EG-di-SE
208-407-7	Gluconal® NA	209-151-9	Cecavon ZN 73	211-014-3	Emerest® 2355
208-408-2	Gluconal® CU	209-151-9	Cecavon ZN 735	211-014-3	Estol EGDS 3750
208-534-8	Unisept SB	209-151-9	Radiastar® 1170	211-014-3	Ethylene Glycol
208-575-1	Imexine OAM	209-151-9	Synpro® Zinc Stearate		Distearate VA
208-580-9	Snow Fine		USP	211-014-3	Genapol® PMS
208-580-9	Snow Flake	209-151-9	Unichem ZS	211-014-3	Hest E.G.D.S
208-671-3	Chemodyne N-	209-151-9	Witco® Zinc Stearate	211-014-3	Hodag EGDS
	Acetyltyrosine		U.S.P.-D	211-014-3	Kemester® EGDS
208-686-5	Captex® 8000	209-155-0	Undezin	211-014-3	Kessco® Ethylene
208-686-5	Emalex O.T.G	209-329-6	Imexine FP		Glycol Distearate
208-686-5	Estol GTC 1803	209-386-7	Rodol 15N	211-014-3	Lanesta EGD
208-686-5	Estol GTEH 3609	209-406-4	Aerosol® OT-70 PG	211-014-3	Lanesta-EO
208-686-5	Miglyol® 808	209-406-4	Aerosol® OT-75%	211-014-3	Lexemul® EGDS
208-686-5	Nikkol Trifat S-308	209-406-4	Chemax/DOSS-75E	211-014-3	Lipal EGDS
208-686-5	Pelemol GTO	209-406-4	Chimin DOS 70	211-014-3	Lipo EGDS
208-686-5	Trivent OC-G	209-406-4	Emcol® 4500	211-014-3	Mackester™ EGDS
208-687-0	Dynasan® 112	209-406-4	Gemtex PA-70	211-014-3	Mapeg® EGDS
208-687-0	Lipo 320	209-406-4	Gemtex PA-70P	211-014-3	Nikkol EGDS
208-687-0	Massa Estarinum® AM	209-406-4	Gemtex PA-75	211-014-3	Nikkol Estepearl 10, 15
208-702-0	Fungitex R	209-406-4	Gemtex PA-75E	211-014-3	Nikkol Pearl 1222
208-736-6	Crodamol CP	209-406-4	Gemtex PA-85P	211-014-3	Pegosperse® 50 DS
208-736-6	Cutina® CP	209-406-4	Gemtex PAX-60	211-014-3	Radiasurf® 7269
208-736-6	Elfacos® CP	209-406-4	Gemtex SC-75E, SC	211-014-3	Rewopal® PG 280
208-736-6	Emalex CC-16		Powd.	211-014-3	RITA EDGS
208-736-6	Estol CEP 3694	209-406-4	Geropon® 99	211-014-3	Secoster® DMS
208-736-6	Estol CEP-b 3653	209-406-4	Geropon® SBDO	211-014-3	Tegin® G 1100
208-736-6	Kemester® CP	209-406-4	Hodag DOSS-70	211-014-3	Unipeg-EGDS
208-736-6	Kessco® 653	209-406-4	Hodag DOSS-75	211-014-3	Witconol™ 2355
208-736-6	Kessco CP	209-406-4	Marlinat® DF 8	211-014-3	Zohar EGDS
208-736-6	Nikkol N-SP	209-406-4	Monawet MO-65-150	211-103-7	Pelemol CA
208-736-6	Precifac ATO	209-406-4	Monawet MO-70	211-119-4	Cachalot® Arachidyl
208-736-6	Rewowax CG	209-406-4	Monawet MO-70-150		Alcohol AR-20
208-736-6	Starfol® CP	209-406-4	Monawet MO-70E	211-279-5	Witco® Aluminum
208-736-6	Trivent CP	209-406-4	Monawet MO-70R		Stearate 132
208-736-6	Unimul-1616	209-406-4	Monawet MO-70RP	211-466-1	Estol 1476
208-736-6	Unitina CP	209-406-4	Monawet MO-70S	211-466-1	Estol IBUS 1552
208-736-6	Waxenol® 815	209-406-4	Monawet MO-75E	211-466-1	Ibulate
208-736-6	Waxenol® 816	209-406-4	Nikkol OTP-75	211-466-1	Kemester® 5415
208-736-6	W.G.S. Cetyl Palmitate	209-406-4	Nikkol OTP-100	211-466-1	Kessco® Isobutyl
208-791-6	Rodol MPDS	209-406-4	Nikkol OTP-100S		Stearate
208-867-9	Nikkol PMEA	209-406-4	Rewopol® SBDO 75	211-466-1	Radia® 7761
208-868-4	Nikkol VF-E	209-406-4	Schercopol DOS-70	211-533-5	Elestab® HP 100
208-868-4	Safester A-75	209-406-4	Schercopol DOS-PG-70	211-546-6	Adol® 60
208-874-7	Nikkol Batyl Alcohol	209-406-4	Schercopol DOS-PG-85	211-546-6	Cachalot® Behenyl
	100, EX	209-406-4	Solusol® 75%		Alcohol BE-22
208-875-2	Emery® 655	209-406-4	Solusol® 100%	211-546-6	Lanette® 22 Flakes
208-875-2	Kartacid 1495	209-406-4	Supermontaline SLT65	211-546-6	Nacol® 22-97
208-875-2	Kartacid 1498	209-478-7	Rodol 27N	211-546-6	Nikkol Behenyl Alcohol
208-875-2	Prifrac 2940	209-529-3	Unichem POCARB		65, 80
208-915-9	Unichem MC	209-711-2	Rodol EG	211-546-6	Unihydag Wax 22
208-915-9	Unichem MGC	209-786-1	Witco® Potassium	211-669-5	Abluter LDB
209-097-6	Aldo® TS		Stearate	211-669-5	Amphoteen 24
209-097-6	Dynasan® 118	210-060-1	Imexine FO	211-669-5	Armoteric LB
209-098-1	Dynasan® 116	210-236-8	Imexine FN	211-669-5	Arquad® DNHTB-75
209-099-7	Dynasan® 114	210-431-8	Rodol BLFX	211-669-5	Chimin BX
209-150-3	Cecavon MG 51	210-702-0	Dynasan® 110	211-669-5	Dehyton® PAB-30
209-150-3	Nuodex Magnesium	210-827-0	Emalex EG-di-L	211-669-5	LMB
	Stearate Food Grade	210-827-0	Kemester® EGDL	211-669-5	Lonzaine® 14
209-150-3	Radiastar® 1100	211-014-3	Ablunol EGDS	211-669-5	Nikkol AM-301

EINECS	Trade name	EINECS	Trade name	EINECS	Trade name
211-669-5	Radiateric® 6864	215-170-3	Marinco H-USP	215-475-1	Suspengel Micro
211-669-5	Rewoteric® AM DML	215-171-9	Marinco OH	215-475-1	Suspengel Ultra
211-669-5	Swanol AM-301	215-171-9	Marinco OL	215-477-2	Alchlordrate
211-669-5	Unibetaine LB	215-181-3	Unichem KOHYD	215-477-2	Aloxicoll® L
211-669-5	Varion® CDG	215-185-5	Unichem SOHYD	215-477-2	Aloxicoll® PC
211-669-5	Varion® CDG-LS	215-222-5	Finex-25	215-477-2	Aloxicoll® PF
211-669-5	Zohartaine AB	215-222-5	MZO-25	215-477-2	Aloxicoll® PSF
211-748-4	Lonzaine® 16S	215-222-5	UFZO	215-477-2	Aluminum Hydroxy-chloride 23
211-748-4	Lonzaine® 16SP	215-222-5	Unichem ZO		
211-748-4	Mackam™ CET	215-222-5	USP-1	215-477-2	Aluminum Hydroxy-chloride 47
211-750-5	Argus DSTDP	215-222-5	USP-2		
212-470-6	Lonzaine® 18S	215-222-5	Z-Cote®	215-477-2	Chlorhydrol® 50% Sol'n.
212-470-6	Varion® SDG	215-222-5	Zinc Oxide USP 66		
212-490-5	Cecavon NA 61	215-288-5	Gelwhite GP, H	215-477-2	Chlorhydrol® Granular
212-490-5	Norfox® B	215-288-5	Gelwhite L	215-477-2	Chlorhydrol, Impalpable
212-490-5	Sodium Stéarate C7L	215-288-5	Green Clay	215-477-2	Chlorhydrol® Powd.
212-490-5	Unichem SS	215-347-5	Witconate™ DS	215-477-2	Dow Corning® ACH-303
212-490-5	Witco® Sodium Stearate C-1	215-350-1	Cegesoft® C 17		
		215-350-1	Ceraphyl® 50	215-477-2	Dow Corning® ACH-323
212-490-5	Witco® Sodium Stearate C-7	215-350-1	Cetinol LM		
		215-350-1	Crodamol ML	215-477-2	Dow Corning® ACH-331
212-806-1	Chembetaine OL	215-350-1	Estalan ML		
212-806-1	Chembetaine OL-30	215-350-1	Lactabase C14	215-477-2	Dow Corning® ACH7-321
212-806-1	Incronam OD-50	215-350-1	Liponate ML		
212-806-1	Mackam™ OB-30	215-350-1	Nikkol Myristyl Lactate	215-477-2	Dow Corning® Q5-7171 AACH Powd.
212-806-1	Mafo® OB	215-350-1	Schercemol ML		
212-806-1	Unibetaine OLB-30, OLB-50	215-350-1	Unimul MYRLAC	215-477-2	Locron Extra, Flakes, L, P, P Extra, Powd., S, Sol'n.
		215-350-1	Wickenol® 506		
212-806-1	Velvetex® OLB-30	215-354-3	Capmul® PGMS	215-477-2	Macrospherical® 95
212-806-1	Velvetex® OLB-50	215-354-3	Ceral P	215-477-2	Micro-Dry®
213-695-2	Unichem AMST	215-354-3	Cerasynt® PA	215-477-2	Micro-Dry® Super-ultrafine
214-289-8	Mexanyl GU	215-354-3	Cithrol PGMS N/E		
214-291-9	Mytab®	215-354-3	Elfacos® PGMS	215-477-2	Micro-Dry® Ultrafine
214-291-9	Rhodaquat® M214B/99	215-354-3	Emalex PGMS	215-477-2	Reach® 101, 201, 501
214-291-9	Sumquat® 6110	215-354-3	Emalex PGS	215-477-2	Ritachlor 50%
214-292-4	Nikkol SCS	215-354-3	Emerest® 2380	215-477-2	Westchlor® 200
214-295-0	Nikkol SSS	215-354-3	Estol PMS 3737	215-549-3	Cithrol PGMO N/E
214-620-6	Progallin® LA	215-354-3	Hefti PMS-33	215-549-3	CPH-3-SE
214-724-1	Estol CES 3705	215-354-3	Hodag PGMS	215-549-3	Emalex PGO
214-737-2	Nikkol SMS	215-354-3	Kessco PGMS	215-549-3	Radiasurf® 7206
215-090-9	Carsosulf SXS	215-354-3	Kessco PGMS-R	215-559-8	Ablusol DBM
215-090-9	Eltesol® SX 30	215-354-3	Kessco PGMS-X534F	215-663-3	Montane 20
215-090-9	Eltesol® SX 93	215-354-3	Kessco® Propylene Glycol Monostearate Pure	215-664-9	Ablunol S-60
215-090-9	Manrosol SXS30			215-664-9	Alkamuls® SMS
215-090-9	Manrosol SXS40			215-664-9	Arlacel® 60
215-090-9	SXS 40	215-354-3	Lipal PGMS	215-664-9	Armotan® MS
215-090-9	Witconate™ SXS 40%	215-354-3	Lipo PGMS	215-664-9	Crill 3
215-090-9	Witconate™ SXS 90%	215-354-3	Mazol® PGMSK	215-664-9	Dehymuls® SMS
215-108-5	Albagel 4446	215-354-3	Myverol® P-06	215-664-9	Drewmulse® SMS
215-108-5	Albagel Premium USP 4444	215-354-3	Nikkol PMS-1C	215-664-9	Emalex SPE-100S
		215-354-3	Nikkol PMS-FR	215-664-9	Emsorb® 2505
215-108-5	Albagen 4439	215-354-3	Pegosperse® PMS CG	215-664-9	Emultex SMS
215-108-5	Bentolite H	215-354-3	Radiasurf® 7201	215-664-9	Estol SMS 3715
215-108-5	Bentolite H 4430	215-354-3	Schercemol PGMS	215-664-9	Ethylan® GS60
215-108-5	Bentolite L	215-354-3	Unipeg-PGMS	215-664-9	Extan-ST
215-108-5	Bentolite WH	215-354-3	Unitolate PGMS	215-664-9	Glycomul® S
215-108-5	Bentonite USP BC 670	215-354-3	Witconol™ 2380	215-664-9	Glycomul® S FG
215-108-5	Korthix H-NF	215-355-9	Crodamol GHS	215-664-9	Glycomul® S KFG
215-108-5	Polargel® HV	215-355-9	Naturechem® GMHS	215-664-9	Hefti MS-33-F
215-108-5	Polargel® NF	215-359-0	Cithrol GDS N/E	215-664-9	Hetan SS
215-108-5	Polargel® T	215-359-0	Estol GDS 3748	215-664-9	Hodag SMS
215-137-3	Calcium Hydroxide USP 802	215-359-0	Kessco® GDS 386F	215-664-9	Ionet S-60 C
		215-359-0	Kessco® Glycerol Distearate 386F	215-664-9	Ixolene 6
215-137-3	Unichem CA HYD			215-664-9	Kemester® S60
215-138-9	Calcium Oxide FCC 801	215-359-0	Nikkol DGS-80	215-664-9	Liposorb S
		215-359-0	Unitolate GDS	215-664-9	Liposorb SC
215-138-9	Unichem CAO	215-475-1	Kaopolite® SF	215-664-9	Montane 60
215-170-3	Hydro-Magma	215-475-1	Suspengel Elite		

EINECS	Trade name	EINECS	Trade name	EINECS	Trade name
215-664-9	Nikkol SS-10	215-744-3	Atomergic Chitin	218-320-6	Rhodorsil® Oils 70641
215-664-9	Nissan Nonion SP-60R	215-744-3	Marine Dew		V 200
215-664-9	Protachem SMS	215-753-2	Atomergic Tannic Acid	218-531-3	Neotan W
215-664-9	Prote-sorb SMS	215-753-2	Unichem TANAC	218-793-9	Akyposal ALS 33
215-664-9	S-Maz® 60	215-785-7	Nikkol Glycyrrhizic Acid	218-793-9	Calfoam ALS-30
215-664-9	S-Maz® 60K	215-968-1	Afoteric™ 151L	218-793-9	Calfoam NLS-30
215-664-9	S-Maz® 60KHM	215-968-1	Deriphat® 151C	218-793-9	Carsonol® ALS
215-664-9	Sorban AST	215-968-1	Mackam™ 151L	218-793-9	Carsonol® ALS-R
215-664-9	Sorbax SMS	215-968-1	Unitex 710-L	218-793-9	Carsonol® ALS-S
215-664-9	Sorbirol S	215-976-5	Takanal	218-793-9	Carsonol® ALS Special
215-664-9	Sorbon S-60	216-343-6	Witconate™ NIS	218-793-9	Empicol® AL30
215-664-9	Sorgen 50	216-472-8	Nuodex S-1421 Food	218-793-9	Empicol® AL30/T
215-664-9	Span® 60, 60K		Grade	218-793-9	Empicol® AL70
215-664-9	Span® 60 VS	216-472-8	Nuodex S-1520 Food	218-793-9	Manro ALS 25
215-664-9	Unitan-S		Grade	218-793-9	Manro ALS 30
215-664-9	Witconol™ 2505	216-472-8	Radiastar® 1060	218-793-9	Marlinat® DFN 30
215-665-4	Ablunol S-80	216-472-8	Synpro® Calcium	218-793-9	Neopon LAM
215-665-4	Alkamuls® SMO		Stearate USP	218-793-9	Nikkol ALS-25
215-665-4	Arlacel® 80	216-472-8	Unichem CS	218-793-9	Norfox® ALS
215-665-4	Armotan® MO	216-472-8	Witco® Calcium	218-793-9	Nutrapon HA 3841
215-665-4	Crill 4		Stearate F.P	218-793-9	Nutrapon PP 3563
215-665-4	Crill 50	216-699-2	TBAB	218-793-9	Perlankrol® DAF25
215-665-4	Dehymuls® SMO	216-700-6	Ablumox LO	218-793-9	Rewopol® ALS 30
215-665-4	Drewmulse® SMO	216-700-6	Ammonyx® DMCD-40	218-793-9	Rhodapon® L-22, L-22/
215-665-4	Emalex SPO-100	216-700-6	Ammonyx® LO		C
215-665-4	Emsorb® 2500	216-700-6	Amyx LO 3594	218-793-9	Rhodapon® L-22HNC
215-665-4	Estol SMO 3685	216-700-6	Aromox® DMMC-W	218-793-9	Standapol® A
215-665-4	Ethylan® GO80	216-700-6	Chemoxide LM-30	218-793-9	Standapol® A-HV
215-665-4	Extan-OT	216-700-6	Emcol® DMCD-40	218-793-9	Stepanol® AM
215-665-4	Famodan SMO	216-700-6	Emcol® L	218-793-9	Stepanol® AM-V
215-665-4	Glycomul® O	216-700-6	Emcol® LO	218-793-9	Sulfochem ALS
215-665-4	Hefti MO-33-F	216-700-6	Empigen® OB	218-793-9	Surfax ASD
215-665-4	Hetan SO	216-700-6	Incromine Oxide L	218-793-9	Surfax NH
215-665-4	Hodag SMO	216-700-6	Lilaminox M24	218-793-9	Texapon® ALS
215-665-4	Ionet S-80	216-700-6	Mackamine™ LO	218-793-9	Texapon® PNA
215-665-4	Ixolene 8	216-700-6	Mazox® LDA	218-793-9	Ufarol Am 30
215-665-4	Kemester® S80	216-700-6	Oxamin LO	218-793-9	Ufarol Am 70
215-665-4	Liposorb O	216-700-6	Radiamox® 6804	218-793-9	Unipol A
215-665-4	Montane 80	216-700-6	Rewominox L 408	218-793-9	Witcolate™ NH
215-665-4	Montane 80 SP	216-700-6	Rhodamox® LO	218-793-9	Zoharpon LAA
215-665-4	Nikkol SO-10	216-700-6	Schercamox DML	218-901-4	Dimodan LS Kosher
215-665-4	Nikkol SO-10R	216-700-6	Unimox LO	219-136-9	Kessco® PEG 300 ML
215-665-4	Nissan Nonion OP-80R	216-700-6	Varox® 270	219-145-8	Lonzabac-12.100
215-665-4	Protachem SMO	216-700-6	Varox® 365	219-370-1	Isofol® 16
215-665-4	Prote-sorb SMO	216-700-6	Varox® 375	219-919-5	Admox® 18-85
215-665-4	S-Maz® 80	216-700-6	Zoramox LO	219-919-5	Ammonyx® SO
215-665-4	S-Maz® 80K	217-210-5	Lexgard® Myacide SP	219-919-5	Amyx SO 3734
215-665-4	Sorban AO	217-210-5	Midtect TF-60	219-919-5	Annonyx SO
215-665-4	Sorbax SMO	217-210-5	Myacide® SP	219-919-5	Barlox® 18S
215-665-4	Sorbirol O	217-210-5	Unikon A-22	219-919-5	Chemoxide ST
215-665-4	Sorbon S-80	217-325-0	Carsoquat® 868	219-919-5	Emcol® SO
215-665-4	Sorgen 40	217-325-0	Carsoquat® 868-E	219-919-5	Incromine Oxide S
215-665-4	Sorgen S-40-H	217-325-0	Carsoquat® 868P	219-919-5	Mackamine™ SO
215-665-4	Span® 80	217-325-0	Varisoft® 432-100	219-919-5	Mazox® SDA
215-665-4	Unitan-O	217-430-1	Nikkol TOP-O	219-919-5	Rewominox S 300
215-665-4	Witconol™ 2500	217-431-7	Lathanol® LAL	219-919-5	Schercamox DMS
215-683-2	Elfadent SM 500	217-431-7	Nikkol LSA	219-919-5	Standamox PS
215-684-8	Valfor® Zeolite Na-A	217-752-2	Tenox® TBHQ	219-919-5	Unimox SO
215-684-8	Zeolex® 7	217-752-2	Uantox TBHQ	220-020-5	Barlox® 10S
215-684-8	Zeolex® 23A	218-320-6	Abil® AV 20-1000	220-045-1	Carbowax® PEG 300
215-687-4	Britesil	218-320-6	Abil® AV 8853	220-045-1	Carbowax® Sentry®
215-687-4	O Silicate	218-320-6	Baysilone Fluid PD 5		PEG 300
215-710-8	Hubersorb®	218-320-6	Baysilone Fluid PK 20	220-045-1	Dow E300 NF
215-710-8	Micro-Cel® C	218-320-6	Dow Corning® 556	220-045-1	Hetoxide PEG-300
215-724-4	Atomergic Carmine		Fluid	220-045-1	Hodag PEG 300
215-724-4	Carmine 5297	218-320-6	Emalex MTS-30E	220-045-1	Lipo Polyglycol 300
215-724-4	Carmine Ultra-fine	218-320-6	KF56, KF58	220-045-1	Lipoxol® 300 MED
215-724-4	Dascolor Carmine	218-320-6	Masil® 556	220-045-1	Lutrol® E 300

EINECS	Trade name	EINECS	Trade name	EINECS	Trade name
220-045-1	Macol® E-300	221-282-3	Rewopal® LA 6	221-787-9	Nikkol MM
220-045-1	Pluracol® E300	221-283-9	Ablunol LA-7	221-787-9	Pelemol MM
220-045-1	Poly-G® 300	221-283-9	Emalex 707	221-787-9	Schercemol MM
220-045-1	Renex® PEG 300	221-283-9	Macol® LA-790	221-787-9	Unimul 14
220-045-1	Teric PEG 300	221-283-9	Marlipal® MG	221-787-9	Waxenol® 810
220-045-1	Upiwax 300	221-283-9	Marlowet® LA 7	222-059-3	Admox® 14-85
220-219-7	Hodag DTSS-70	221-283-9	Procol LA-7	222-059-3	Ammonyx® MCO
220-336-3	Liponate ISA Special	221-283-9	Rhodasurf® L-790	222-059-3	Ammonyx® MO
220-336-3	Prisorine 3501	221-284-4	Ablunol LA-9	222-059-3	Aromox® DM14D-W
220-336-3	Prisorine 3505	221-284-4	Britex EMB	222-059-3	Barlox® 14
220-336-3	Prisorine ISAC 3505	221-284-4	Carsonon® L-9	222-059-3	Emcol® M
220-336-3	Unitol ISA	221-284-4	Chemal LA-9	222-059-3	Emcol® MO
220-476-5	Alkamuls® SS	221-284-4	Emalex 709	222-059-3	Empigen® OH25
220-476-5	Cetinol EE	221-284-4	G-4829	222-059-3	Incromine Oxide M
220-476-5	Emalex CC-18	221-284-4	Hetoxol L-9	222-059-3	Lilaminox M4
220-476-5	Estol STST 3706	221-284-4	Hodag Nonionic L-9	222-059-3	Manro AO 25M
220-476-5	Hetester 412	221-284-4	Macol® LA-9	222-059-3	Mazox® MDA
220-476-5	Lexol® SS	221-284-4	Marlipal® 129	222-059-3	Schercamox DMA
220-476-5	Liponate SS	221-284-4	Nikkol BL-9EX	222-059-3	Schercamox DMM
220-476-5	Ritachol SS	221-284-4	Procol LA-9	222-182-2	Irgasan DP300
220-476-5	Unimul 1818	221-284-4	Prox-onic LA-1/09	222-206-1	Rhodasurf® PEG 400
220-552-8	Turpinal® SL	221-284-4	Unicol LA-9	222-264-8	Undenat
220-552-8	Unitex P	221-286-5	Ablunol LA-12	222-269-5	Nikkol Naphthenic Acid
220-618-6	Rodol PAOC	221-286-5	Carsonon® L-12	222-273-7	Monawet SNO-35
220-688-8	Ageflex FM-1	221-286-5	Chemal LA-12	222-274-2	Kemamine® Q-6902C
220-836-1	Crodamol OSU	221-286-5	Emalex 712	222-581-1	Crodafos MCA
220-836-1	Wickenol® 159	221-286-5	Emthox® 5967	222-848-2	Gluconal® MG
221-014-5	Imexine FB	221-286-5	Ethosperse® LA-12	222-899-0	Deriphat® 160
221-109-1	Aerosol® MA-80	221-286-5	Hetoxol L-12	222-899-0	Monateric 1188M
221-109-1	Monawet MM-80	221-286-5	Hodag Nonionic L-12	222-980-4	Cetiol®
221-123-8	Trivent PE-48	221-286-5	Lipocol L-12	222-980-4	Crodamol OO
221-188-2	Rhodapon® TDS	221-286-5	Macol® LA-12	222-980-4	Schercemol OLO
221-279-7	Akyporox RLM 22	221-286-5	Procol LA-12	222-980-4	Unitolate OLOL
221-279-7	Arlypon® F	221-286-5	Prox-onic LA-1/012	222-980-4	Wickenol® 143
221-279-7	Bio-Soft® E-300	221-286-5	Trycol® 5967	222-981-6	Cetiol® V
221-279-7	Britex L 20	221-450-6	Akyposal MGLS	222-981-6	Crodamol DO
221-279-7	Carsonon® L-2	221-450-6	Carsonol® MLS	222-981-6	Elfacos® DO
221-279-7	Dehydol® LS 2 DEO	221-450-6	Elfan® 2240 Mg	222-981-6	Estalan DO
221-279-7	Empilan® KB 2	221-450-6	Empicol® ML30	222-981-6	Estol DCO 3662
221-279-7	Hetoxol L-2	221-450-6	Rhodapon® LM	222-981-6	Estol DCO-b 3655
221-279-7	Lauropal 2	221-450-6	Standapol® MG	222-981-6	Kessco DO
221-279-7	Marlowet® LMA 2	221-450-6	Stepanol® MG	222-981-6	Schercemol DO
221-279-7	Nikkol BL-2	221-450-6	Sulfetal MG 30	222-981-6	Tegosoft® DO
221-279-7	Oxetal VD 20	221-450-6	Sulfochem MG	222-981-6	Trivent OL-10
221-279-7	Procol LA-2	221-450-6	Surfax MG	222-981-6	Unimul-CTV
221-279-7	Prox-onic LA-1/02	221-450-6	Texapon® MGLS	222-981-6	Unitolate V
221-279-7	Unihydol LS-2	221-450-6	Unipol MGLS	223-095-2	Atomergic Denatonium
221-280-2	Ablunol LA-3	221-450-6	Witcolate™ MG-LS		Benzoate
221-280-2	AE-1214/3	221-450-6	Zoharpon MgS	223-095-2	Bitrex
221-280-2	Carsonon® L-3	221-498-8	Uvinul® DS 49	223-114-4	Nikkol PMT
221-280-2	Dehydol® LS 3 DEO	221-573-5	Spectra-Sorb® UV	223-267-7	Mayoquest 1530
221-280-2	Emalex 703		5411	223-267-7	Turpinal® 4 NL
221-280-2	Empilan® KB 3	221-588-7	Unifluorid H 101	223-267-7	Universene AC
221-280-2	Empilan® KC 3	221-661-3	Chemidex L	223-296-5	Sodium Omadine®,
221-280-2	Genapol® L-3	221-661-3	Lexamine L-13		40% Aq. Sol'n.
221-280-2	Glicolene	221-661-3	Mackine™ 801	223-470-0	Isofol® 12
221-280-2	Hetoxol L-3N	221-661-3	Schercodine L	223-772-2	Syntase® 230
221-280-2	Lauropal 3	221-662-9	Cerasynt® 303	223-772-2	Uvasorb S-5
221-280-2	Oxetal VD 28	221-761-7	Biosol	223-772-2	Uvinul® MS 40
221-280-2	Procol LA-3	221-761-7	Dekacymen	223-795-8	Unistat CALBAN
221-280-2	Rewopal® LA 3	221-787-9	Alkamuls® MM/M	223-795-8	Unistat CALPRO
221-280-2	Unihydol LS-3	221-787-9	Ceraphyl® 424	223-805-0	CoSept 200
221-281-8	Ablunol LA-5	221-787-9	Cetinol MM	223-805-0	Dowicil® 200
221-281-8	Carsonon® L-5	221-787-9	Cetiol® MM	224-126-2	Tri-K Allantoin Acetyl
221-281-8	Emalex 705	221-787-9	Crodamol MM		Methionine
221-281-8	Marlowet® LMA 5	221-787-9	Hefti MYM-33	224-160-8	Lanol P
221-281-8	Mulsifan RT 23	221-787-9	Kemester® MM	224-292-6	Afaine™ LMB
221-282-3	Dehydol® PID 6	221-787-9	Liponate MM	224-292-6	Amido Betaine-L

EINECS	Trade name	EINECS	Trade name	EINECS	Trade name
224-292-6	Chembetaine L	225-856-4	Emery® 6709	227-335-7	Artodan CF 40
224-292-6	Chemoxide L	225-856-4	Hodag PEG 400	227-335-7	Crolactil CSL
224-292-6	Chimin LX	225-856-4	Lipo Polyglycol 400	227-335-7	Pationic® CSL
224-292-6	Lexaine® LM	225-856-4	Lipoxol® 400 MED	227-335-7	Unitolate CSL
224-292-6	Mackam™ LA	225-856-4	Lutrol® E 400	228-227-2	Schercotaine IAB
224-292-6	Mackam™ LMB	225-856-4	Macol® E-400	228-229-3	Emalex PG-di-S
224-292-6	Mackam™ LMB-LS	225-856-4	Pluracol® E400	228-250-8	Escalol® 597
224-292-6	Mafo® LMAB	225-856-4	Pluracol® E400 NF	228-250-8	Neo Heliopan, Type
224-292-6	Mirataine® BB	225-856-4	Poly-G® 400		303
224-292-6	Monateric LMAB	225-856-4	Renex® PEG 400	228-250-8	Uvinul® N 539
224-292-6	Tego®-Betaine L-10 S	225-856-4	Rhodasurf® E 400	228-291-1	Rodol Brown SO
224-388-8	Nikkol LMT	225-856-4	Teric PEG 400	228-292-7	Rodol Gray DMS
224-388-8	Zoharpon LMT42	225-856-4	Unipeg 400	228-293-2	Rodol 4GP
224-403-8	Covitol 1185	225-856-4	Unipeg-400 X	228-464-1	Emcol® E-607L
224-403-8	Covitol 1210	225-856-4	Upiwax 400	228-486-1	Emalex DEG-di-L
224-403-8	Eastman® Vitamin E	225-878-4	Butyl Propasol	228-486-1	Protamate 200 DL
	Succinate	226-029-0	Uvinul® N 35	228-504-8	Alkamuls® LVL
224-506-8	Arlamol® HD	226-097-1	Akyporox RLM 40	228-504-8	Ceraphyl® 31
224-506-8	Permethyl® 101A	226-097-1	Brij® 30	228-504-8	Cetinol 1212
224-540-3	Bio-Soft® TD 400	226-097-1	Brij® 30SP	228-504-8	Cetinol LL
224-540-3	Chemal TDA-3	226-097-1	Britex L 40	228-504-8	Crodamol LL
224-540-3	Hetoxol TD-3	226-097-1	Chemal LA-4	228-504-8	Estalan LL
224-540-3	Lipocol TD-3	226-097-1	Dehydol® LS 4 DEO	228-973-9	Uantox SEBATE
224-540-3	Macol® TD-3	226-097-1	Emthox® 5882	228-973-9	Uantox SODERT
224-540-3	Procol TDA-3	226-097-1	Ethosperse® LA-4	229-222-8	Dekafald
224-540-3	Synperonic A3	226-097-1	Hetoxol L-4	229-222-8	Glydant®
224-540-3	Volpo T-3	226-097-1	Hodag Nonionic L-4	229-222-8	Glydant® XL-1000
224-580-1	Fongasel	226-097-1	Lauropal 4	229-222-8	Mackstat® DM
224-580-1	Trisept SDHA	226-097-1	Lipocol L-4	229-222-8	Nipaguard® DMDMH
224-580-1	Tristat SDHA	226-097-1	Macol® LA-4	229-349-9	Unisweet CALSAC
224-580-1	Unisept DSA	226-097-1	Marlipal® 124	229-350-4	Gluconal® MN
224-772-5	Witco® Lithium	226-097-1	Marlowet® LA 4	229-457-6	Zoldine® ZT-55
	Stearate 306	226-097-1	Marlowet® LMA 4	229-457-6	Zoldine® ZT
224-886-5	Bio-Soft® E-200	226-097-1	Mulsifan CPA		Oxazolidine
224-886-5	Hetoxol L-1	226-097-1	Nikkol BL-4.2	229-859-1	Carbowax® PEG 600
224-886-5	Lipocol L-1	226-097-1	Procol LA-4	229-859-1	Carbowax® Sentry®
2240-27-4	Propylene Phenoxetol	226-097-1	Prox-onic LA-1/04		PEG 600
225-004-1	Dragoco Farnesol	226-097-1	Rhodasurf® L-4	229-859-1	Dow E600 NF
225-173-1	Rodol Gray BS	226-097-1	Simulsol P4	229-859-1	Hodag PEG 600
225-190-4	Nikkol KLS	226-097-1	Trycol® 5882	229-859-1	Lipo Polyglycol 600
225-190-4	Sulfochem K	226-097-1	Unicol LA-4	229-859-1	Lipoxol® 600 MED
225-214-3	Akyposal MLS 30	226-097-1	Unihydol LS-4	229-859-1	Macol® E-600
225-214-3	Aremsol MA	226-097-1	Witconol™ 5875	229-859-1	Pluracol® E600
225-214-3	Aremsol MR	226-159-8	Arlasolve® DMI	229-859-1	Pluracol® E600 NF
225-214-3	Cosmopon MO	226-242-9	Eutanol® G	229-859-1	Poly-G® 600
225-214-3	Elfan® 240M	226-242-9	Exxal® 20	229-859-1	Renex® PEG 600
225-214-3	Elfan® 2240 M	226-242-9	Isofol® 20	229-859-1	Teric PEG 600
225-214-3	Empicol® 1220/T	226-242-9	Michel XO-150-20	229-859-1	Unipeg-600
225-214-3	Empicol® LQ33	226-242-9	Unimul-G	229-859-1	Upiwax 600
225-214-3	Empicol® LQ33/T	226-242-9	U Tanol G	230-429-0	Ammonyx® CO
225-214-3	Empicol® LQ70	226-300-9	Crodamol MP	230-429-0	Amyx CO 3764
225-214-3	Manro ML 33	226-300-9	Lonzest® 143-S	230-429-0	Aromox® DM16
225-214-3	Rewopol® MLS 30	226-300-9	Schercemol MP	230-429-0	Barlox® 16S
225-214-3	Standapol® MLS	226-312-9	Hetoxamate SA-9	230-429-0	Mazox® CDA
225-214-3	Sulfochem MLS	226-312-9	Prox-onic ST-09	230-525-2	Bardac® 2250
225-214-3	Surfax MEA	226-312-9	Serdox NSG 400	230-525-2	BTC® 1010
225-214-3	Texapon® MLS	226-546-1	Incromectant LMEA	230-525-2	Maquat 4450-E
225-214-3	Unipol MLS	226-546-1	Lipamide LMEA	230-636-6	Beta Carotene 30% in
225-214-3	Zoharpon LAM	226-546-1	Mackamide™ LME		Veg. Oil No. 65646
225-268-8	Ebal	226-546-1	Naetex-LAM	230-636-6	Carotene Standard RR
225-373-9	Kalidone®	226-546-1	Parapel® LAM-100	230-636-6	Crystalline Beta
225-404-6	Nikkol Trialan 308	226-546-1	Schercomid LME		Carotene No. 65638
225-714-1	Nipagin M Sodium	226-546-1	Upamide LACAMEA	230-698-4	Amonyl BR 1244
225-714-1	Unisept M NA	226-775-7	Escalol® 557	230-743-8	Nikkol Pentarate 408
225-856-4	Carbowax® PEG 400	226-775-7	Nanospheres 100	230-785-7	Empiphos 4KP
225-856-4	Carbowax® Sentry®		Conc. in O.M.C	230-898-1	Altriform S
	PEG 400	226-775-7	Neo Heliopan, Type AV	230-962-9	Crodamol PC
225-856-4	Dow E400 NF	226-775-7	Parsol® MCX	230-962-9	Nikkol Sefsol 228

EINECS	Trade name	EINECS	Trade name	EINECS	Trade name
230-990-1	Armeen® M2-10D	231-765-0	Albone® 35 CG	232-282-8	EmCon COCO
231-057-1	Dragoxat EH 2/044115	231-765-0	Albone® 50 CG	232-282-8	Lipovol C-76
231-057-1	Pelemol 88	231-765-0	Albone® 70CG	232-282-8	Pureco® 76
231-057-1	Tegosoft® EE	231-810-4	Oxaban®-E	232-282-8	Univegoil COCO
231-211-8	Unichem KCL	231-831-9	Unichem KIO3	232-288-0	EmCon COPA
231-211-8	Unichem POCHLOR	231-896-3	Crodamol TSC	232-289-6	Atomergic Cod Liver Oil
231-298-2	Unichem EPSAL	231-900-3	Calcium Sulfate	232-289-6	EmCon COD
231-306-4	Nikkol DIS		Anhydrous NF 164	232-290-1	Ceresine Wax
231-306-4	Pelemol DIPS	231-900-3	Etra Super English		Cosmetic Stralpitz
231-306-4	Schercemol DIS		Terra Alba	232-290-1	Ceresine Wax SP 84
231-426-7	Emalex NN-5	231-900-3	Unichem CS White	232-290-1	Koster Keunen
231-426-7	Emalex NN-15	232-055-3	Unichem AMAL		Ceresine
231-426-7	Hetamide M	232-122-7	Biron®	232-290-1	Koster Keunen
231-426-7	Miristamina	232-122-7	Biron® B-5		Ceresine 130/135
231-426-7	Monamid® 150-MW	232-122-7	Biron® B-50	232-290-1	Koster Keunen
231-426-7	Protamide MRCA	232-122-7	Biron® ESQ		Ceresine 140/145
231-493-2	Alpha W 6 Pharma	232-122-7	Biron® Fines	232-290-1	Koster Keunen
	Grade	232-122-7	Biron® HB		Ceresine 155
231-493-2	Beta W 7	232-122-7	Biron® NLD-SP	232-290-1	Koster Keunen
231-493-2	Cavitron Cyclodextrin™	232-122-7	Mearlite® GBU		Ceresine 192
231-493-2	Dexpearl	232-122-7	Mearlite® GGH	232-290-1	Natwax CER
231-493-2	Gamma W8	232-122-7	Mearlite® LBU	232-290-1	Ross Ceresine Wax
231-493-2	Kleptose	232-122-7	Pearl I	232-292-2	Castorwax® MP-70
231-493-2	Rhodocap-A, G, N	232-122-7	Pearl II	232-292-2	Castorwax® MP-80
231-493-2	Ringdex-A, B	232-122-7	Pearl-Glo®	232-292-2	Castorwax® NF
231-545-4	Celite® 503	232-122-7	Pearl Super Supreme	232-292-2	Cutina® HR
231-545-4	Celite® 512	232-122-7	Pearl Supreme UVS	232-292-2	Ross Castor Wax
231-545-4	Celite® 521 AW	232-160-4	Unineut SOBROM	232-292-2	Unitina HR
231-545-4	Celite® 545	232-271-8	EmCon E-5	232-293-8	AA USP
231-545-4	Celite® 550	232-273-9	Florasun™-90	232-293-8	Castor Oil USP
231-545-4	Celite® 560	232-273-9	Lipex 103	232-293-8	Cosmetol® X
231-545-4	Celite® 577	232-273-9	Lipovol SUN	232-293-8	Crystal® O
231-545-4	Filter-Cel	232-273-9	Nikkol Sunflower Oil	232-293-8	Crystal® Crown
231-545-4	Hyflo Super-Cel	232-273-9	Super Refined™	232-293-8	Crystal® Crown LP
231-545-4	Standard Super-Cel		Sunflower Oil	232-293-8	Diamond Quality®
231-545-4	Super Floss	232-273-9	Tri-K Sunflower Oil	232-293-8	EmCon CO
231-548-0	Uantox SBS	232-273-9	Tri-Ol SUN	232-293-8	Lanaetex CO
231-609-1	Adogen® S-18 V	232-273-9	Univegoil SUNFL	232-293-8	Lipovol CO
231-609-1	Chemidex S	232-274-4	EmCon Soya	232-293-8	Unicast CO
231-609-1	Incromine SB	232-274-4	Lipovol SOY	232-293-8	York Krystal Kleer
231-609-1	Lexamine S-13	232-274-4	Super Refined™		Castor Oil
231-609-1	Lipamine SPA		Soybean Oil USP	232-293-8	York USP Castor Oil
231-609-1	Mackine™ 301	232-276-5	Lipovol SAF	232-296-4	EmCon Peanut
231-609-1	Miramine® SODI	232-276-5	Natoil SAF	232-296-4	Lipex 101
231-609-1	Schercodine S	232-276-5	Neobee® 18	232-296-4	Super Refined™
231-609-1	Tegamine® 18	232-276-5	Nikkol Safflower Oil		Peanut Oil
231-609-1	Tego®-Amid S 18	232-276-5	Super Refined™	232-296-4	Univegoil P-O
231-609-1	Unizeen SA		Safflower Oil USP	232-306-7	Haroil SCO-50
231-659-4	Unichem KI	232-276-5	Tri-Ol SAF	232-306-7	Laurel R-50
231-672-5	Unichem SODIOD	232-277-0	EmCon Olive	232-306-7	Nopcocastor
231-673-0	Uantox SMBS	232-277-0	Lipovol O	232-306-7	Standapol® SCO
231-710-0	Eastman® Vitamin E	232-277-0	Nikkol Olive Oil	232-306-7	Turkey Red Oil 100%
	6-40	232-277-0	Olive Oil, Refined	232-306-7	Türkischrotöl 100%
231-710-0	Eastman® Vitamin E	232-277-0	Super Refined™ Olive	232-306-7	Unipol SCO
	6-81		Oil	232-307-2	Alcolec® BS
231-710-0	Eastman® Vitamin E	232-277-0	Tri-Ol OLV	232-307-2	Alcolec® Extra A
	6-100	232-280-7	EmCon Cotton	232-307-2	Alcolec® F-100
231-710-0	Eastman® Vitamin E	232-280-7	Super Refined™	232-307-2	Alcolec® Granules
	700		Cottonseed Oil	232-307-2	Alcolec® PG
231-710-0	Nanospheres 100	232-280-7	Univegoil COTSD	232-307-2	Alcolec® S
	Vitamine E Acetate	232-281-2	Corn Oil, Refined	232-307-2	Alcolec® SFG
231-710-0	Uantox 1250	232-281-2	Lipex 104	232-307-2	Asol
231-721-0	Amphoterge® J-2	232-281-2	Nikkol Corn Germ Oil	232-307-2	Augon 1000
231-721-0	Mackam™ 2CY	232-281-2	Super Refined™ Corn	232-307-2	Basis LP-20
231-721-0	Schercoteric CY-2		Oil	232-307-2	Basis LS-60
231-721-0	Sochamine A 8955	232-281-2	Univegoil CRN	232-307-2	Centrolex® F
231-722-6	Biosulphur Powder	232-282-8	Coconut Oils® 76, 92,	232-307-2	Centrolex® P
231-722-6	Unisulcoidal		110	232-307-2	Centromix® E

EINECS	Trade name	EINECS	Trade name	EINECS	Trade name
232-307-2	Centrophase® C	232-348-6	Anhydrous Lanolin	232-360-1	Montane 83
232-307-2	Centrophase® HR		Superfine	232-360-1	Nikkol SO-15
232-307-2	Centrophase® HR6B	232-348-6	Anhydrous Lanolin USP	232-360-1	Nikkol SO-15EX
232-307-2	Centrophil® W	232-348-6	Anhydrous Lanolin USP	232-360-1	Nikkol SO-15R
232-307-2	Crolec 4135		Cosmetic	232-360-1	Nissan Nonion OP-
232-307-2	Dermasome® MT	232-348-6	Anhydrous Lanolin USP		83RAT
232-307-2	Emulmetik™ 100		Cosmetic AA	232-360-1	Protachem SOC
232-307-2	Emulmetik™ 135	232-348-6	Anhydrous Lanolin USP	232-360-1	S-Maz® 83R
232-307-2	Emulmetik™ 300		Cosmetic Grade	232-360-1	Sorbirol SQ
232-307-2	Emulmetik™ 970	232-348-6	Anhydrous Lanolin USP	232-360-1	Sorgen 30
232-307-2	Lecithin Extract		Deodorized AAA	232-360-1	Sorgen S-30-H
	Kosmaflor, Water-Disp	232-348-6	Anhydrous Lanolin USP	232-360-1	Witconol™ 2502
232-307-2	Lecsoy E		Pharmaceutical	232-370-6	Hy-SES
232-307-2	Lecsoy S	232-348-6	Anhydrous Lanolin USP	232-370-6	Lipovol SES
232-307-2	Lexin K		Pharmaceutical Grade	232-370-6	Sesame Oil USP/NF 16
232-307-2	Lipoid S 100	232-348-6	Anhydrous Lanolin USP	232-370-6	Super Refined™
232-307-2	Liposome Conc. E-10		Pharmaceutical Light		Sesame Oil
232-307-2	Natipide 08010A		Grade	232-370-6	Tri-Ol SES
232-307-2	Phosal 15	232-348-6	Anhydrous Lanolin USP	232-370-6	Uniderm SSME
232-307-2	PhosPho E-100		Superfine	232-373-2	Amojell Petrolatum
232-307-2	PhosPho F-97	232-348-6	Anhydrous Lanolin USP	232-373-2	Amber, Dark, Snow
232-307-2	PhosPho LCN-TS		Ultrafine		White
232-307-2	Phospholipon® 25G,	232-348-6	Anhydrous Lanolin USP	232-373-2	Fonoline® White
	25P, 50		X-tra Deodorized	232-373-2	Fonoline® Yellow
232-307-2	Phospholipon® 80	232-348-6	Corona Lanolin	232-373-2	Mineral Jelly No. 5
232-307-2	Probiol™ L/N	232-348-6	Coronet Lanolin	232-373-2	Mineral Jelly No. 10
232-307-2	Unilec S	232-348-6	Cosmetic Lanolin	232-373-2	Mineral Jelly No. 14
232-307-2	Unilex, DS, S, SH	232-348-6	Cosmetic Lanolin	232-373-2	Mineral Jelly No. 15
232-311-4	Super Refined™		Anhydrous USP	232-373-2	Mineral Jelly No. 17
	Menhaden Oil	232-348-6	Cosmetic Lanolin	232-373-2	Mineral Jelly No. 20
232-313-5	Ross Bleached Montan		Anhydrous USP	232-373-2	Mineral Jelly No. 25
	Wax	232-348-6	Emery® 1650	232-373-2	Ointment Base No. 3
232-313-5	Ross Bleached Montan	232-348-6	Emery® 1656	232-373-2	Ointment Base No. 4
	Wax Cosmetic	232-348-6	Emery® 1660	232-373-2	Ointment Base No. 6
232-315-6	CS-2032	232-348-6	Emery® HP-2050	232-373-2	Penreco Amber
232-315-6	CS-2037	232-348-6	Emery® HP-2060	232-373-2	Penreco Blond
232-315-6	CS-2043	232-348-6	Golden Dawn Grade 1,	232-373-2	Penreco Cream
232-315-6	CS-2054		2	232-373-2	Penreco Lily
232-315-6	Eskar Wax R-25, R-35,	232-348-6	Ivarlan™ 3000	232-373-2	Penreco Regent
	R-40, R-45, R-50	232-348-6	Ivarlan™ 3001	232-373-2	Penreco Royal
232-315-6	Koster Keunen Paraffin	232-348-6	Ivarlan™ 3006 Light	232-373-2	Penreco Snow
	Wax	232-348-6	Ivarlan™ Light	232-373-2	Penreco Super
232-315-6	Koster Keunen Paraffin	232-348-6	Lanolin Anhydrous USP	232-373-2	Penreco Ultima
	Wax 122/128	232-348-6	Lanolin Cosmetic	232-373-2	Perfecta® USP
232-315-6	Koster Keunen Paraffin	232-348-6	Lanolin Extra-	232-373-2	Protopet® Alba
	Wax 130/135		Deodorized	232-373-2	Protopet® White 1S
232-315-6	Koster Keunen Paraffin	232-348-6	Lanolin Pharmaceutical	232-373-2	Protopet® White 2L
	Wax 140/145	232-348-6	Lanolin Tech	232-373-2	Protopet® White 3C
232-315-6	Koster Keunen Paraffin	232-348-6	Lanolin Tech. Grade	232-373-2	Protopet® Yellow 2A
	Wax 150/155	232-348-6	Lanolin U.S.P	232-373-2	Snow White Petrolatum
232-315-6	Ross Crude Scale Wax	232-348-6	Pharmaceutical Lanolin	232-373-2	Sono Jell® No. 4
232-315-6	Uniwax PARA		USP	232-373-2	Sono Jell® No. 9
232-316-1	Lipovol PAL	232-348-6	RITA Lanolin	232-373-2	Super White Fonoline®
232-347-0	Candelilla Wax	232-348-6	Super Corona	232-373-2	Super White Protopet®
	Cosmetic Grade	232-348-6	Superfine Lanolin	232-373-2	Unipet
	Stralpitz		Anhydrous USP	232-391-0	Epoxyweichmacher
232-347-0	Koster Keunen	232-348-6	Unilan		LSB
	Candelilla	232-360-1	Arlacel® 83	232-399-4	Carnauba Wax NC #2
232-347-0	Natwax CAN	232-360-1	Arlacel® C		Stralpitz
232-347-0	Ross Candelilla Wax	232-360-1	Crill 43	232-399-4	Carnauba Wax NC #3
232-348-6	Anhydrous Lanolin	232-360-1	Dehymuls® SSO		Stralpitz
	Grade 1	232-360-1	Emalex SPO-150	232-399-4	Carnauba Wax SP 8
232-348-6	Anhydrous Lanolin	232-360-1	Emsorb® 2502	232-399-4	Koster Keunen
	Grade 2	232-360-1	Extan-SOT		Carnauba
232-348-6	Anhydrous Lanolin P.80	232-360-1	Glycomul® SOC	232-399-4	Koster Keunen
232-348-6	Anhydrous Lanolin P.95	232-360-1	Hefti QO-33-F		Carnauba, Micro
232-348-6	Anhydrous Lanolin	232-360-1	Hodag SSO		Granulated
	P.95RA	232-360-1	Liposorb SQO	232-399-4	Koster Keunen

EINECS	Trade name	EINECS	Trade name	EINECS	Trade name
	Carnauba No. 1	232-452-1	Lipolan	232-679-6	Argo Brand Corn Starch
232-399-4	Koster Keunen	232-452-1	Lipolan Distilled	232-679-6	Pure-Dent® B700
	Carnauba, Powd.	232-452-1	Nikkol Wax-500	232-679-6	Pure-Dent® B810
232-399-4	Koster Keunen	232-452-1	Super-Sat	232-679-6	Purity® 21
	Carnauba T-2	232-474-1	Incense EA	232-679-6	28-1801
232-399-4	Koster Keunen	232-474-1	Incense H	232-680-1	Alginic Acid FCC
	Carnauba T-3	232-491-4	Norfox® XXX Granules	232-680-1	Kelacid®
232-399-4	Ross Brazil Wax	232-519-5	Spray Dried Gum	232-680-1	Satialgine™ H8
232-409-7	Natwax RB		Arabic NF Type CSP	232-683-8	Pentagen
232-409-7	Rice Wax No. 1	232-524-2	Aquagel	232-696-9	Atomergic Sodium
232-409-7	Rose Rice Bran Wax	232-524-2	Aquaron		Chondroitin Sulfate
232-410-2	Famous	232-524-2	Aubygel X52	232-696-9	Chondroitin Sulfate A
232-410-2	Lipex 407	232-524-2	Carraghenate P,	232-697-4	Actigen C
232-410-2	Lipovol HS		Standard, X 2	232-697-4	Ateco
232-410-2	S-Flakes	232-524-2	Gelcarin LA	232-697-4	Clearcol
232-410-2	Stabland®	232-524-2	Genu Carrageenan	232-697-4	Colladerm Procollagene
232-410-2	Sterotex® HM NF	232-524-2	Genugel		SC
232-410-2	Witarix® 440	232-524-2	Genulacta Series	232-697-4	Collagen
232-428-0	Avocado Oil	232-524-2	Genuvisco	232-697-4	Collagen CLR
232-428-0	Avocado Oil CLR	232-524-2	Seakem 3, LCM	232-697-4	Collagen S.D
232-428-0	Lipovol A	232-524-2	Seaspen PF	232-697-4	Collagene SPO
232-428-0	Natoil AVO	232-524-2	Stamere®	232-697-4	Collagene Lyophilized
232-428-0	Nikkol Avocado Oil	232-524-2	Viscarin XLV	232-697-4	Collagen Masks
232-428-0	Super Refined™	232-536-8	Burtonite V7E	232-697-4	Collagen Nativ 1%
	Avocado Oil	232-536-8	Jaguar® C	232-697-4	Collagen Native Extra
232-428-0	Tri-Ol AVO	232-536-8	Supercol® Guar Gum		1%
232-430-1	Anatol	232-541-5	Seagel L	232-697-4	Collagen Powd.
232-430-1	Argowax Cosmetic	232-553-0	Genu Pectins	232-697-4	Collapur®
	Super	232-553-0	Mexpectin LA 100	232-697-4	Collapuron N
232-430-1	Argowax Dist		Range	232-697-4	Collasol
232-430-1	Argowax Standard	232-553-0	Mexpectin LC 700	232-697-4	Dermacol
232-430-1	Ceralan®		Range	232-697-4	Desamidocollagen K
232-430-1	Dusoran MD	232-553-0	Mexpectin XSS 100		1.0
232-430-1	Emery® 1780		Range	232-697-4	Desamidocollagen K
232-430-1	Emery® 1795	232-554-6	Byco A		1.5
232-430-1	Emery® HP-2095	232-554-6	Byco C	232-697-4	Grancol SP-01
232-430-1	Fancol LA	232-554-6	Byco O	232-697-4	Hydracol®
232-430-1	Hartolan	232-554-6	Colla-Gel AC	232-697-4	Kollagen KD
232-430-1	Hartolite	232-554-6	Cosmetic Gelatin	232-697-4	Kollagen S
232-430-1	Ivarlan™ 3310	232-554-6	Crodyne BY-19	232-697-4	Kollaplex 0.3
232-430-1	Ritawax	232-554-6	HiPure Liq. Gelatin,	232-697-4	Kollaplex 1.0
232-430-1	Ritawax Super		Cosmetic Grade	232-697-4	Kollaron
232-430-1	Super Hartolan	232-554-6	Hydrocoll AG-SD	232-697-4	Lencoll
232-430-1	Unilanal	232-554-6	Hydrocoll™ G-40	232-697-4	Liquid Animal Collagen
232-438-5	Myvatex® 7-85	232-554-6	Hydrocoll™ G-55	232-697-4	Maricol CLR
232-438-5	Myverol® 18-85	232-554-6	Hydrocoll PGA, PGB	232-697-4	Oceagen®
232-440-6	Alcolec® Z-3	232-555-1	Alacid	232-697-4	Pancogene® S
232-440-6	Alcolec® Z-7	232-555-1	Alaren	232-697-4	Polymoist® Mask
232-440-6	Centrolene® A, S	232-555-1	Cosmetic Grade Casein	232-697-4	Ritacollagen BA-1
232-440-6	Nikkol Lecinol SH	232-555-1	Unipro CAL-CASE, CO-	232-697-4	Ritacollagen S-1
232-440-6	PhosPho 642		CASE	232-697-4	Sollagen® EC
232-442-7	Special Fat 168T	232-674-9	Celluflow C-25	232-697-4	Sollagen® LA
232-447-4	Arquad® T-27W	232-674-9	Cellulon	232-697-4	Soluble Native Collagen
232-447-4	Arquad® T-30	232-674-9	Elcema® F150, G250,		RA-1 No. 26206
232-447-4	Arquad® T-50		P100	232-697-4	Soluble Native Collagen
232-447-4	Jet Quat T-27W	232-674-9	Solka-Floc® BW-40		RS-1 No. 26205
232-447-4	Jet Quat T-50	232-674-9	Solka-Floc® BW-100	232-697-4	Solu-Coll™
232-447-4	Kemamine® Q-9703B	232-674-9	Solka-Floc® BW-200	232-697-4	Solu-Coll™ C, CLR
232-447-4	Nikkol CA-2450T	232-674-9	Solka-Floc® BW-2030	232-697-4	Solu-Coll™ Complex
232-447-4	Noramium MS 50	232-674-9	Solka-Floc® Fine		VY
232-447-4	Varisoft® 471		Granular	232-697-4	Solu-Coll™ Native
232-452-1	Almolan HL	232-675-4	Nadex 360	232-697-4	Trillagene®
232-452-1	Brooks Hydrogenated	232-678-0	Atomergic Hyaluronic	232-697-4	Unihypro LAN
	Lanolin		Acid	232-697-4	Unipro CLR
232-452-1	Fancol HL	232-678-0	Biomatrix®	232-734-4	Cellulase 4000
232-452-1	Ivarlan™ HL	232-678-0	Hyaluronic Acid	232-734-4	Cellulase Tr Conc.
232-452-1	Lanaetex-HG	232-678-0	Hyladerm®	232-885-6	Clarex® 5XL
232-452-1	Lanocerina	232-678-0	Hylucare™	232-885-6	Clarex® L

EINECS	Trade name	EINECS	Trade name	EINECS	Trade name
232-885-6	Pearex® L	234-394-2	Keltrol CG F		Dioxide
232-940-4	Maltrin® M040	234-394-2	Keltrol CG GM	236-675-5	Kowet Titanium Dioxide
232-940-4	Maltrin® M050	234-394-2	Keltrol CG RD	236-675-5	Kronos® 1025
232-940-4	Maltrin® M100	234-394-2	Keltrol CG SF	236-675-5	Luxelen® D
232-940-4	Maltrin® M150	234-394-2	Keltrol CG T	236-675-5	MTD-25
232-940-4	Maltrin® M180	234-394-2	Keltrol CG TF	236-675-5	Solar Shield™
232-940-4	Maltrin® M510	234-394-2	Keltrol® F	236-675-5	Spherititan
232-940-4	Maltrin® M700	234-394-2	Merezan® 8	236-675-5	Sunveil 6010
232-940-4	Maltrin® QD M440	234-394-2	Merezan® 20	236-675-5	Sunveil 6030
232-940-4	Maltrin® QD M500	234-394-2	Rhodicare™ D	236-675-5	Ti-Sphere AA-1512-LL
232-940-4	Maltrin® QD M550	234-394-2	Rhodicare™ H	236-675-5	Ti-Sphere AA-1515
232-940-4	Maltrin® QD M580	234-394-2	Rhodicare™ S	236-675-5	Titanium Dioxide P25
232-940-4	Microduct®	234-394-2	Rhodicare™ XC	236-675-5	Titanium Dioxide SPA
232-940-4	Wickenol® 550	234-394-2	Rhodigel®	236-675-5	Transparent Titanium
233-135-0	Unichem ALSUL	234-394-2	Rhodigel® 23		Dioxide PW Covafluor
233-136-6	Ceram Blanche	234-394-2	Rhodigel® 200	236-675-5	Transparent Titanium
233-140-8	Unichem CALCHLOR	234-394-2	Rhodigel® EZ		Dioxide PW Covasil S
233-257-4	Cogilor Spinel	234-394-2	Rhodopol® SC	236-675-5	Transparent Titanium
233-293-0	Ablunol 200MO	234-394-2	Unigum XAN		Dioxide PW Powd.
233-293-0	Cithrol 2MO	234-394-2	Xanthan XP	236-675-5	Uniwhite AO
233-293-0	Crodet O4	234-406-6	Bentone® 38	236-675-5	Uniwhite KO
233-293-0	Hetoxamate MO-4	235-088-1	Witconate™ STS	236-935-8	Captex® 8227
233-293-0	Hodag 20-O	235-340-0	Bentone® EW	236-935-8	Dermol M-27
233-293-0	Kessco® PEG 200 MO	235-340-0	Bentone® MA	236-942-6	Pationic® 138C
233-293-0	Mapeg® 200 MO	235-340-0	Hectabrite® AW	238-306-3	Amphoterge® L Special
233-293-0	Pegosperse® 200 MO	235-340-0	Hectabrite® DP	238-306-3	Chimin IMZ
233-293-0	Protamate 200 OC	235-374-6	Gelwhite MAS-H,	238-306-3	Mackam™ 2L
233-293-0	Remcopal 207		MAS-L	238-306-3	Monateric 949J
233-293-0	Unipeg-200 MO	235-374-6	Magnabrite® F	238-306-3	Rewoteric® AM 2L-40
233-343-1	Calgon	235-374-6	Magnabrite® FS	238-306-3	Zoharteric DJ
233-520-3	Chemeen 18-2	235-374-6	Magnabrite® HS	238-310-5	Cerasynt® D
233-520-3	Ethomeen® 18/12	235-374-6	Magnabrite® HV	238-310-5	Witcamide® MAS
233-520-3	Hetoxamine ST-2	235-374-6	Magnabrite® K	238-311-0	Ammonyx® OAO
233-520-3	Protox HTA-2	235-374-6	Magnabrite® S	238-311-0	Chemoxide O
233-520-3	Varonic® S-202	235-374-6	Veegum®	238-311-0	Mackamine™ O2
233-520-3	Varonic® S-202 SF	235-374-6	Veegum® D	238-311-0	Mazox® ODA-30
233-549-1	Imexine FD	235-374-6	Veegum® F	238-311-0	Standamox O1
233-560-1	Crodamol IPL	235-374-6	Veegum® HS	238-311-0	Unimox OL
233-560-1	Estol IPL 1511	235-374-6	Veegum® HV	238-311-0	Zoramox E
233-561-7	Emalex 218	235-374-6	Veegum® K	238-430-8	Emerest® 2486
233-562-2	Emalex 400A	235-374-6	Veegum® Ultra	238-430-8	Unitolate PTP
233-562-2	Emalex 400B	235-374-6	Veegum® WG	238-479-5	Rewopol® SBF 18
233-562-2	Marlosol® 183	235-777-7	Emalex MSG-2	238-588-8	Akyposept B
233-562-2	Tegin® D 1102	235-777-7	Emalex MSG-2MA	238-588-8	Preventol D2
233-641-1	Chemax E-600 MS	235-777-7	Emalex MSG-2MB	238-877-9	Act II 500 USP
233-641-1	Prox-onic ST-014	235-777-7	Emalex MSG-2ME	238-877-9	AGI Talc, BC 1615
233-864-4	Liponate CRM	235-777-7	Emalex MSG-2ML	238-877-9	Alphafil 200 USP
233-864-4	Naturechem® CR	235-777-7	Nikkol DGMS	238-877-9	Alphafil 500 USP
233-864-4	Pelemol CR	235-798-1	Abluphat MLP-200	238-877-9	Alpine Talc USP BC
233-864-4	Protachem CER	235-798-1	Crodafos 1214A		127
234-169-9	Finsolv® 116	235-798-1	Lipophos LMP	238-877-9	Altalc 200 USP
234-242-5	Dascolor Chlorophyll	235-798-1	Nikkol Phosten HLP	238-877-9	Altalc 400 USP
234-242-5	Uniphyllin SC	235-907-2	Emery® 5418	238-877-9	Altalc 500 USP
234-316-7	Caprol® 10G10O	235-911-4	Grillocin CW-90	238-877-9	Brillante
234-316-7	Drewmulse® 10-10-O	235-911-4	Grillocin® PY 88 Pellets	238-877-9	Dover 50 A
234-316-7	Drewpol® 10-10-O	235-911-4	Grillocin® PY 88	238-877-9	J-13
234-316-7	Hodag PGO-1010		Pulver/Powd.	238-877-9	J-24
234-316-7	Nikkol Decaglyn 10-O	235-911-4	Grillocin® S 803/7	238-877-9	J-46
234-316-7	Santone® 10-10-O	235-911-4	Grillocin S-803/12	238-877-9	J-68
234-316-7	Unitolate PGO-1010	235-946-5	Pelemol PTL	238-877-9	J-80
234-394-2	Biozan	236-164-7	Rewoteric® AM HC	238-877-9	Lo-Micron Talc 1
234-394-2	Fitoxantina	236-671-3	Atomergic Zinc	238-877-9	Olympic
234-394-2	Gomme Xanthane		Pyrithione	238-877-9	PT-46
234-394-2	Kelgum CG	236-671-3	Zinc Omadine® 48%	238-877-9	Purtalc USP
234-394-2	Keltrol®		Disp	238-877-9	Rose Talc
234-394-2	Keltrol CG	236-671-3	Zinc Omadine® Powd.	238-877-9	SteriLine 200
234-394-2	Keltrol CG 1000	236-671-3	Zink Pyrion	238-877-9	SteriLine 665
234-394-2	Keltrol CG BT	236-675-5	Atlas White Titanium	238-877-9	Supra A

EINECS	Trade name	EINECS	Trade name	EINECS	Trade name
238-877-9	Supra EF	242-960-5	Pelemol PTO	246-680-4	Witconate™ 1250
238-877-9	Supra EF A	243-468-3	Amical® Flowable	246-680-4	Witconate™ C50H
238-877-9	Suprafino A	243-697-9	Estol EHL 3613	246-680-4	Witconate™ DS Dense
238-877-9	Suprafino SMD	243-835-8	Chemidex R	246-680-4	Witconate™ SK
238-877-9	Supreme USP	243-835-8	Mackine™ 201	246-684-6	Mackamine™ OAO
238-877-9	Talc LCW	243-870-9	Fungicide UMA 2/	246-705-9	Crodesta DKS F110
238-877-9	Talc OOC		938080	246-705-9	Crodesta DKS F160
238-877-9	Talc Micro-Ace P-2	243-870-9	Incromide UM	246-705-9	Crodesta F-160
238-877-9	Talc Micro-Ace P-4	243-870-9	Rewocid® U 185	246-705-9	Grilloten PSE 141G
238-877-9	Ultrafino	243-870-9	Witcamide® 6570	246-705-9	Grilloten® PSE 141 G
238-877-9	Vertal CO+	244-063-4	Versene Diammonium		Pellets
239-032-7	Afoteric™ 160C		EDTA	246-705-9	Ryoto Sugar Ester S-
239-032-7	Mackam™ 160C-30	244-071-8	Cetinol LU		1170
239-032-7	Mirataine® H2C-HA	244-071-8	Laurate de Cetyle	246-705-9	Ryoto Sugar Ester S-
239-032-7	Rewoteric® AM LP	244-158-0	Luminex		1170S
239-032-7	Unibetaine 160	244-238-5	Empicol® MIPA	246-705-9	Ryoto Sugar Ester S-
239-032-7	Unitex 610-L	244-238-5	Melanol LP 1		1570
239-139-9	Unisol S-22	244-238-5	Sulfetal CJOT 38	246-705-9	Ryoto Sugar Ester S-
240-357-1	Rodol DS	244-238-5	Sulfetal CJOT 60		1670
240-736-1	Crodasinic LT40	244-289-3	Escalol® 507	246-705-9	Ryoto Sugar Ester S-
240-736-1	Hamposyl® TL-40	244-289-3	Eusolex® 6007		1670S
240-795-3	Uantox PMBS	244-289-3	Lipofilter ODP	246-868-6	Ceraphyl® 494
240-795-3	Uantox POMEBIS	244-289-3	Padimate O	246-868-6	Cetiol® G16S
240-865-3	Genamin KDB	244-289-3	Solarchem® O	246-868-6	Crodamol ICS
240-886-8	Rodol 2A3PYR	244-492-7	BB-1	246-868-6	Kemester® 5822
240-924-3	Chemical Base 6532	244-492-7	Rehydragel®	246-868-6	Kessco ICS
240-924-3	Lexamine 22		Compressed Gel	246-868-6	Kessco® Isocetyl
240-924-3	Nikkol Amidoamine S	244-492-7	Rehydragel® Low Visc.		Stearate
240-924-3	Swanol Amidoamine S		Gel	246-868-6	Nikkol ICS-R
241-029-0	Kemester® 3684	244-492-7	Rehydragel®	246-868-6	Pelemol ICS
241-327-0	Genamin KDM		Thixotropic Gel	246-868-6	Schercemol ICS
241-327-0	Genamin KDM-F	244-950-6	Glicoceride OCS	246-868-6	Unimul-7061
241-327-0	Incroquat TMC-80	245-204-2	Starfol® OS	246-873-3	Grilloten LSE 65
241-327-0	Incroquat TMC-95	245-205-8	Isofol® 20 Myristat	246-873-3	Grilloten LSE 65 Soft
241-327-0	Nikkol CA-2580	245-217-3	Emalex PG-di-L	246-873-3	Grilloten LSE 87
241-327-0	Varisoft® BT-85	245-228-3	Isofol® 20 Oleat	246-873-3	Grilloten LSE 87 Soft
241-637-6	Isofol® 36	245-228-3	O.O.D	246-873-3	Ryoto Sugar Ester L-
241-640-2	Alkamuls® MST	245-289-6	Ceraphyl® IPL		1570
241-640-2	Hest MS	245-289-6	Nikkol VF-IP	246-873-3	Ryoto Sugar Ester L-
241-640-2	Hetester MS	246-376-1	Tristat K		1695
241-640-2	Kemester® 1418	246-376-1	Unistat K	246-914-5	Fungicide DA 2/938070
241-640-2	Pelemol MS	246-563-8	Sustane® 1-F	246-914-5	Olamida UD
241-640-2	Spermwax®	246-563-8	Sustane® BHA	246-914-5	Olamida UD 21
241-646-5	Crodamol BB	246-563-8	Uantox BHA	246-914-5	Undamide
241-646-5	Kester Wax® 72	246-584-2	Incronam OP-30	246-929-7	Artodan SP 55 Kosher
241-646-5	Pelemol BB	246-584-2	Lexaine® O	246-929-7	Crolactil SSL
241-654-9	Cetiol® J600	246-584-2	Mackam™ HV	246-929-7	Pationic® SSL
241-654-9	Crodamol JJ	246-584-2	Mirataine® BET-O-30	246-929-7	Unitolate SSL
241-654-9	Dynacerin® 660	246-598-9	Chemoxide SAO	246-986-8	Elfan® NS 423 SH
241-654-9	Kessco OE	246-675-7	Hyamine® 10X	246-986-8	Standapol® ES-40
241-654-9	Pelemol OE	246-680-4	Bio-Soft® D-60	246-986-8	Standapol® ES-50
241-654-9	Unitolate J600	246-680-4	Calsoft F-90	246-986-8	Texapon® K-14S Spec
242-201-8	Crodamol BE	246-680-4	Calsoft L-40	247-144-2	Cithrol GDO N/E
242-201-8	Elfacos® BE	246-680-4	Calsoft L-60	247-144-2	Kessco® Glycerol
242-201-8	Kemester® BE	246-680-4	Hartofol 40		Dioleate
242-201-8	Kessco BE	246-680-4	Hotsulf Acid	247-144-2	Nikkol DGO-80
242-201-8	Schercemol BE	246-680-4	Marlon® AFR	247-144-2	Witconol™ CD-18
242-349-3	Nikkol MMT	246-680-4	Nacconol® 35SL	247-310-4	Emcol® 5310
242-354-0	Spectradyne® G	246-680-4	Naxel™ AAS-40S	247-310-4	Geropon® SBL-203
242-471-7	Compritol 888	246-680-4	Naxel™ AAS-45S	247-310-4	Mackanate™ LM-40
242-471-7	Compritol WL 3241	246-680-4	Sul-fon-ate AA-10	247-310-4	Rewopol® SBL 203
242-471-7	Lipovol GTB	246-680-4	Ufasan 35	247-310-4	Varsulf® SBL-203
242-471-7	Pelemol GTB	246-680-4	Witconate™ 30DS	247-464-2	Nipagin M Potassium
242-471-7	Syncrowax HR-C	246-680-4	Witconate™ 45BX	247-536-3	Witconate™ TDB
242-703-7	Oligoidyne Magnesium	246-680-4	Witconate™ 60B	247-556-2	Rhodacal® 330
242-769-1	Amphisol® K	246-680-4	Witconate™ 90F H	247-568-8	Ablunol S-40
242-769-1	Crodafos CKP	246-680-4	Witconate™ 1238	247-568-8	Arlacel® 40
242-960-5	Liponate PO-4	246-680-4	Witconate™ 1240	247-568-8	Armotan® MP

EINECS	Trade name	EINECS	Trade name	EINECS	Trade name
247-568-8	Armotan® NP	247-891-4	Crill 35	248-299-9	Nikkol DID
247-568-8	Crill 2	247-891-4	Crill 41	248-299-9	Pelemol DIA
247-568-8	Emsorb® 2510	247-891-4	Drewmulse® STS	248-299-9	Schercemol DIA
247-568-8	Extan-PT	247-891-4	Emsorb® 2507	248-299-9	Trivent DIA
247-568-8	Glycomul® P	247-891-4	Glycomul® TS	248-299-9	Upamate DIPA
247-568-8	Hefti MP-33-F	247-891-4	Glycomul® TS KFG	248-317-5	Crodesta DKS F10
247-568-8	Hodag SMP	247-891-4	Hefti TS-33-F	248-317-5	Crodesta DKS F20
247-568-8	Ixolene 4	247-891-4	Hodag STS	248-317-5	Crodesta DKS F50
247-568-8	Kemester® S40	247-891-4	Kemester® S65	248-317-5	Crodesta DKS F70
247-568-8	Liposorb P	247-891-4	Liposorb TS	248-317-5	Crodesta F-10
247-568-8	Montane 40	247-891-4	Montane 65	248-317-5	Crodesta F-50
247-568-8	Nikkol SP-10	247-891-4	Nikkol SS-30	248-317-5	Ryoto Sugar Ester S-570
247-568-8	Nissan Nonion PP-40R	247-891-4	Protachem STS		
247-568-8	Protachem SMP	247-891-4	Prote-sorb STS	248-317-5	Ryoto Sugar Ester S-770
247-568-8	Prote-sorb SMP	247-891-4	S-Maz® 65K		
247-568-8	S-Maz® 40	247-891-4	Sorbax STS	248-317-5	Ryoto Sugar Ester S-970
247-568-8	Sorbax SMP	247-891-4	Sorbirol TS		
247-568-8	Sorbirol P	247-891-4	Span® 65	248-351-0	Hetester HCA
247-568-8	Sorbon S-40	247-891-4	Unitan-TRIST	248-351-0	Naturechem® GTH
247-568-8	Span® 40	247-891-4	Witconol™ 2507	248-403-2	Caprol® 3GS
247-568-8	Unitan-P	247-911-1	Trioxene A	248-403-2	Hefti GMS-333
247-568-8	Witconol™ 2510	248-016-9	Hetoxol M-3	248-406-9	Ablusol DBT
247-569-3	Ablunol S-85	248-016-9	Witconol™ 5969	248-406-9	Bio-Soft® N-300
247-569-3	Arlacel® 85	248-248-0	Schercozoline O	248-406-9	Calsoft T-60
247-569-3	Crill 45	248-289-4	Calsoft LAS-99	248-406-9	Carosulf T-60-L
247-569-3	Emsorb® 2503	248-289-4	Lumosäure A	248-406-9	Carsofoam® T-60-L
247-569-3	Ethylan® GT85	248-289-4	Naxel ™AAS-98S	248-406-9	Elfan® WAT
247-569-3	Glycomul® TO	248-289-4	Reworyl® K	248-406-9	Hartofol 60T
247-569-3	Hefti TO-33-F	248-289-4	Rueterg SA	248-406-9	Hexaryl D 60 L
247-569-3	Hodag STO	248-289-4	Witconate Acide B	248-406-9	Manro TDBS 60
247-569-3	Ionet S-85	248-291-5	Carsonon® N-2	248-406-9	Marlopon® CA
247-569-3	Kemester® S85	248-291-5	Chemax NP-1.5	248-406-9	Mazon® 60T
247-569-3	Liposorb TO	248-291-5	Emalex NP-2	248-406-9	Naxel™ AAS-60S
247-569-3	Montane 85	248-291-5	Hodag Nonionic E-2	248-406-9	Norfox® T-60
247-569-3	Nikkol SO-30	248-291-5	Nikkol NP-2	248-406-9	Rhodacal® DDB 60T
247-569-3	Nikkol SO-30R	248-291-5	Synperonic NP2	248-406-9	Witconate™ 60T
247-569-3	Nissan Nonion OP-85R	248-291-5	Unicol NP-2	248-406-9	Witconate™ 79S
247-569-3	Protachem STO	248-291-5	Uniterge NP 2	248-406-9	Witconate™ LXH
247-569-3	Prote-sorb STO	248-292-0	Desonic® 7N	248-406-9	Witconate™ S-1280
247-569-3	S-Maz® 85	248-292-0	Elfapur® N 70	248-406-9	Witconate™ TAB
247-569-3	S-Maz® 85K	248-292-0	Hodag Nonionic E-7	248-470-8	Adol® 66
247-569-3	Sorbax STO	248-292-0	Synperonic NP7	248-470-8	Prisorine 3515
247-569-3	Sorbirol TO	248-292-0	Unicol NP-7	248-470-8	Prisorine ISOH 3515
247-569-3	Span® 85	248-292-0	Uniterge NP 7	248-515-1	Parasonarl Mark II
247-569-3	Unitan-TRIOL	248-294-1	Chemax NP-10	248-586-9	Capmul® GDL
247-569-3	Witconol™ 2503	248-294-1	Emalex NP-10	248-586-9	Cithrol GDL N/E
247-667-6	Imwitor® 310	248-294-1	Hetoxide NP-10	248-586-9	Emulsynt® GDL
247-667-6	Imwitor® 910	248-294-1	Hodag Nonionic E-10	248-586-9	Kemester® GDL
247-668-1	Imwitor® 308	248-294-1	Makon® 10	248-586-9	Kessco® Glycerol Dilaurate
247-668-1	Imwitor® 908	248-294-1	Naxonic™ NI-100		
247-668-1	Imwitor® 988	248-294-1	Nikkol NP-10	248-586-9	Lexemul® GDL
247-669-7	Cithrol PGMR N/E	248-294-1	Prox-onic NP-010	248-586-9	Liponate GDL
247-669-7	Flexricin® 9	248-294-1	Renex® 690	248-587-4	Kemester® EE
247-669-7	Naturechem® PGR	248-294-1	Simulsol 1030 NP	248-762-5	Alkasurf® NP-1
247-669-7	Rol RP	248-294-1	Surfonic® N-95	248-762-5	Desonic® 1.5N
247-706-7	Ryoto Sugar Ester P-1570	248-294-1	Surfonic® N-100	248-762-5	Norfox® NP-1
		248-294-1	Surfonic® N-102	248-762-5	Prox-onic NP-1.5
247-706-7	Ryoto Sugar Ester P-1570S	248-294-1	Synperonic NP9.75	248-762-5	Surfonic® N-10
		248-294-1	Synperonic NP10	248-762-5	Synperonic NP1
247-706-7	Ryoto Sugar Ester P-1670	248-294-1	Syntopon D	248-812-6	Crodamol GE
		248-294-1	Unicol NP-10	249-277-1	Ajidew N-50
247-710-9	Eltesol® AX 40	248-294-1	Uniterge NP-10	249-277-1	Dermidrol
247-710-9	Manrosol AXS40	248-299-9	Arlamol® DIDA	249-277-1	Nalidone®
247-710-9	Witconate™ NXS	248-299-9	Ceraphyl® 230	249-277-1	Ritamectant PCA
247-730-8	Incromine Oxide B	248-299-9	Crodamol DA	249-395-3	Cithrol PGMM
247-730-8	Incromine Oxide B-30P	248-299-9	Docoil Dipa	249-395-3	Kessco PGNM
247-730-8	Incromine Oxide B50	248-299-9	Estalan DIA	249-395-3	Radiasurf® 7196
247-784-2	Ablusol DBD	248-299-9	Iso-Adipate 2/043700	249-448-0	Hefti DO-33-F

EINECS	Trade name	EINECS	Trade name	EINECS	Trade name
249-649-3	Ketosesquine	252-964-9	Eutanol® G16	255-485-3	Iso Isotearyle WL 3196
249-862-1	Bernel® Ester EHP	252-964-9	Michel XO-150-16	255-485-3	Prisorine ISIS 2039
249-862-1	Cegesoft® C 24	252-964-9	Unimul-G-16	255-485-3	Rewomul IS
249-862-1	Ceraphyl® 368	253-149-0	Adol 52	255-485-3	Schercemol 1818
249-862-1	Crodamol OP	253-149-0	Adol® 52 NF	255-490-0	Lipacide DPHP
249-862-1	Elfacos® EHP	253-149-0	Adol® 520 NF	255-537-5	Lipacide C8CY
249-862-1	Estalan 816	253-149-0	ppend	255-674-0	Fractalite ISL
249-862-1	Estol 1543	253-149-0	Cachalot® C-50	255-674-0	Patlac® IL
249-862-1	Estol EHP 1543	253-149-0	Cachalot® C-51	255-674-0	Pelemol ISL
249-862-1	Estol EHP-b 3652	253-149-0	Cachalot® C-52	255-728-3	Waxenol® 822
249-862-1	Kessco EHP	253-149-0	Cetaffine	255-854-9	Hetsulf IPA
249-862-1	Kessco® Octyl	253-149-0	Cetal	255-999-8	Rodol PDAS
	Palmitate	253-149-0	Cetax 16	256-120-0	Emcol® 4161L
249-862-1	Lexol® EHP	253-149-0	CO-1695	256-120-0	Fizul MD-318C
249-862-1	Pelemol OP	253-149-0	Crodacol C-70	256-120-0	Mackanate™ OP
249-862-1	Schercemol OP	253-149-0	Crodacol C-90	256-120-0	Sole Terge 8
249-862-1	Tegosoft® OP	253-149-0	Crodacol C-95NF	256-214-1	Chemidex M
249-862-1	Trivent OP	253-149-0	Epal® 16NF	256-214-1	Schercodine M
249-862-1	Wickenol® 155	253-149-0	Fancol CA	257-048-2	Nuosept 101 CG
250-001-7	Bronidox® L	253-149-0	Hetol CA	257-048-2	Oxaban®-A
250-001-7	Bronidox® L 5	253-149-0	Hyfatol 16-95	257-440-3	Ceraphyl® 60
250-001-7	Bronodox L	253-149-0	Hyfatol 16-98	257-835-0	Insect Repellent 3535,
250-001-7	Bronodox L-5	253-149-0	Lanette® 16		No. 11887
250-151-3	Crodasinic MS	253-149-0	Lanol C	257-843-4	Amihope LL-11
250-151-3	Hamposyl® M-30	253-149-0	Lipocol C	258-007-1	Hamposyl® M
250-151-3	Nikkol Sarcosinate MN	253-149-0	Mackol 16	258-007-1	Vanseal® MS
250-151-3	Vanseal® NAMS-30	253-149-0	Nacol 16-95	258-193-4	Afmide™ ISA
250-215-0	Amphoterge® S	253-149-0	Nacol® 16-98	258-193-4	Hetamide IS
250-651-1	Emerest® 2310	253-149-0	Philcohol 1600	258-193-4	Mackamide™ ISA
250-651-1	Lanesta 10	253-149-0	RITA CA	258-193-4	Monamid® 150-IS
250-651-1	Nikkol IPIS	253-149-0	Unihydag Wax 16	258-193-4	Standamid® ID
250-651-1	Prisorine IPIS 2021	253-242-6	Parsol® 5000	258-193-4	Witcamide® 5118S
250-651-1	Schercemol 318	253-363-4	Ammonyx® KP	258-377-8	Foamquat BAS
250-651-1	Wickenol® 131	253-363-4	Ammonyx® LKP	258-377-8	Schercoquat BAS
250-651-1	Witconol™ 2310	253-363-4	Empigen® BCJ-50	258-476-2	Laponite® D
250-696-7	Kemester® 5721	253-363-4	Incroquat O-50	258-476-2	Laponite® XLG
250-696-7	Liponate TDS	253-363-4	Mackernium™ KP	258-636-1	Amisoft LT-12
250-704-9	Fractalite IDS	253-379-1	Hedione	258-987-1	Diacid 1550
250-913-5	SCS 40	253-458-0	Radiasurf® 7423	259-218-1	Oramix NS 10
250-913-5	Witconate™ SCS 45%	253-519-1	ACS 60	259-627-5	Glycacil L, S
250-913-5	Witconate™ SCS 93%	253-519-1	Eltesol® ACS 60	259-837-7	Hetamine 5L-25
251-110-2	Isofol® 32	253-981-4	Amisoft MS-11	259-837-7	Incromate SDL
251-136-4	Disorbene	254-161-9	Imexine BD	259-837-7	Lexamine S-13 Lactate
251-136-4	Millithix® 925	254-372-6	Abiol	259-837-7	Mackalene™ 316
251-306-8	Schercotaine PAB	254-372-6	Atomergic Imidazoli-	259-837-7	Protachem SDM
251-646-7	Arlamol® DINA		dinyl Urea	259-860-2	Emcol® SML
251-732-4	Naturechem® EGHS	254-372-6	Biopure 100	259-860-2	Mackalene™ 326
251-734-5	Naturechem® PGHS	254-372-6	Germall® 115	260-081-5	Argidone®
251-932-1	Cetiol® A	254-372-6	Sepicide CI	260-143-1	Afanate™ OD-28
251-932-1	Rewomul HL	254-372-6	Tristat IU	260-143-1	Anionyx® 12S
251-932-1	Unimul-CTA	254-372-6	Unicide U-13	260-143-1	Geropon® SBG-280
251-932-1	Unitolate A	254-495-5	Caprol® 10G10S	260-143-1	Mackanate™ OD-35
251-959-9	Isofol® 16 Laurat	254-495-5	Nikkol Decaglyn 10-S	260-143-1	Monamate OPA-30
252-011-7	Caprol® 10G4O	254-585-4	Chemidex P	260-143-1	Monamate OPA-100
252-011-7	Drewpol® 10-4-O	254-585-4	Schercodine P	260-143-1	Standapol® SH-100
252-011-7	Mazol® PGO-104	255-051-3	Afmide™ R	260-143-1	Standapol® SH-135
252-478-7	Cegesoft® C 19	255-051-3	Amidex RC	260-143-1	Texapon® SH 100
252-478-7	Ceraphyl® 28	255-051-3	Aminol CA-2	260-143-1	Texapon® SH-135
252-478-7	Cetinol LA	255-051-3	Mackamide™ R		Special
252-478-7	Crodamol CL	255-051-3	Olamida RD	260-143-1	Unipol SH-100, SH-135
252-478-7	Lactabase C16	255-051-3	Protamide CA	260-410-2	Amidex LN
252-478-7	Lactacet	255-062-3	Schercopol LPS	260-410-2	Comperlan® F
252-478-7	Liponate CL	255-350-9	D.P.P.G	260-410-2	Foamole A
252-478-7	Nikkol Cetyl Lactate	255-350-9	Emerest® 2388	260-410-2	Hetamide LN
252-487-6	Nipagin A Sodium	255-350-9	Estol PDP 3601	260-410-2	Hetamide LNO
252-637-0	Nikkol CS	255-350-9	Lexol® PG-900	260-410-2	Incromide LA
252-681-0	Tektamer® 38	255-350-9	Schercemol PGDP	260-410-2	Mackamide™ LOL
252-964-9	Ceraphyl® ICA	255-350-9	Unitolate PG/DPG	260-410-2	Mazamide™ LLD

EINECS	Trade name	EINECS	Trade name	EINECS	Trade name
260-410-2	Mazamide® SS-10	262-979-2	Acylan	263-052-5	Hostapon SCID
260-410-2	Mazamide® SS 20	262-979-2	Fancol Acel	263-052-5	Jordapon® CI Disp
260-410-2	Monamid® 15-70W	262-979-2	Ivarlan™ 3300	263-052-5	Jordapon® CI Powd.
260-410-2	Monamid® 150-ADY	262-979-2	Lanacet® 1705	263-052-5	Jordapon® CI Prill
260-410-2	Monamid® LN-605	262-979-2	Lanolin A.C	263-052-5	Jordapon® CI-UP
260-410-2	Protamide 15W	262-979-2	Modulan®	263-052-5	Tauranol I-78
260-410-2	Protamide LNO	262-979-2	Ritacetyl®	263-052-5	Tauranol I-78 Flakes
260-410-2	Purton SFD	262-979-2	Unilan Acetyl	263-052-5	Tauranol I-78-3
260-410-2	Schercomid SLE	262-980-8	Hetlan AC	263-052-5	Tauranol I-78-6
260-410-2	Standamid® SOMD	262-980-8	Protalan MOD	263-052-5	Tauranol I-78E, I-78E
260-410-2	Varamide® LO-1	262-988-1	CE-618		Flakes
260-410-2	Witcamide® 6540	262-988-1	Radia® 7117	263-058-8	Foamtaine CAB-G
261-521-9	Ceraphyl® 375	262-991-8	Amine M2HBG	263-058-8	Schercotaine CAB
261-521-9	Crodamol ISNP	262-991-8	Armeen® M2HT	263-080-8	Arquad® DNMCB-50
261-521-9	Dermol 185	262-991-8	Kemamine® T-9701	263-080-8	Marlazin® KC 21/50
261-521-9	Schercemol 185	263-005-9	Arquad® HT-50	263-081-3	Variquat® B345
261-619-1	Bernel® Ester CO	263-005-9	Noramium MSH 50	263-086-0	Armeen® 2C
261-619-1	Emalex CC-168	263-016-9	Afamine™ CO	263-087-6	Arquad® 2C-75
261-619-1	Exceparl HO	263-016-9	Aminoxid A 4080	263-087-6	Dodigen 1490
261-619-1	Nikkol CIO, CIO-P	263-016-9	Aromox® DMC	263-087-6	Jet Quat 2C-75
261-619-1	Schercemol 1688	263-016-9	Aromox® DMCD	263-087-6	Noramium M2C
261-619-1	Schercemol CO	263-016-9	Aromox® DMC-W	263-087-6	Radiaquat® 6462
261-619-1	Tegosoft® CO	263-016-9	Barlox® 12	263-087-6	Variquat® K300
261-619-1	Trivent OC-16	263-016-9	Chemoxide WC	263-087-6	Variquat® K375
261-673-6	Ceraphyl® 140-A	263-016-9	Genaminox CS	263-087-6	Varisoft® 462
261-673-6	Estol IDCO 3667	263-016-9	Genaminox KC	263-089-7	Adogen® 240 SF
261-673-6	Pelemol IDO	263-016-9	Mackamine™ CO	263-089-7	Armeen® 2HT
261-673-6	Schercemol IDO	263-016-9	Naxide™ 1230	263-090-2	Arquad® HC
261-673-6	Trivent OL-10B	263-016-9	Noxamine CA 30	263-090-2	Noramium M2SH
261-673-6	Wickenol® 144	263-016-9	Radiamox® 6800	263-090-2	Querton 442
261-678-3	Covafresh	263-016-9	Schercamox DMC	263-090-2	Querton 442-11
261-678-3	Frescolat, Type ML	263-016-9	Synotol C-30	263-090-2	Querton 442-82
261-678-3	Frigydil	263-017-4	Armeen® DMSD	263-090-2	Querton 442E
261-684-6	Schercotaine MAB	263-017-4	Jet Amine DMSD	263-090-2	Querton 442H
261-819-9	Bernel® OPG	263-017-4	Kemamine® T-9972	263-090-2	Radiaquat® 6442
261-819-9	Pelemol OPG	263-020-0	Amine 2M1218D	263-090-2	Varisoft® 442-100P
261-819-9	Schercemol OPG	263-020-0	Amine 2MKKD	263-107-3	Acintol® 2122
261-819-9	Unitolate OPG	263-020-0	Armeen® DMCD	263-107-3	Acintol® 7002
261-819-9	Wickenol® 160	263-020-0	Barlene® 12C	263-107-3	Pamak 4
261-819-9	Witconol™ 2307	263-020-0	Jet Amine DMCD	263-112-0	Armeen® S
261-931-8	Aludone®	263-020-0	Kemamine® T-6502	263-112-0	Armeen® SD
262-108-6	Dermol 105	263-020-0	Noram DMC	263-112-0	Kemamine® P-997
262-108-6	Schercemol 105	263-022-1	Armeen® DMHTD	263-125-1	Adogen® 170D
262-134-8	Chemidex B	263-022-1	Kemamine® T-9702	263-125-1	Armeen® T
262-134-8	Incromine BB	263-026-3	Nikkol SGC-80N	263-125-1	Armeen® TD
262-134-8	Mackine™ 601	263-026-3	Poem-LS-90	263-125-1	Kemamine® P-974
262-134-8	Schercodine B	263-027-9	Imwitor® 928	263-125-1	Radiamine 6170
262-740-2	Kemamine® T-2801	263-031-0	Monomuls® 90-25	263-125-1	Radiamine 6171
262-774-8	Ken-React® KR TTS	263-032-6	Myverol® 18-40	263-129-3	Hy-Phi 4204
262-895-6	Liponate PB-4	263-035-2	Myverol® 18-30	263-129-3	Prifac 7920
262-976-6	Amine 2HBG	263-038-9	Arquad® C-33W	263-129-3	Prifac 7935
262-976-6	Armeen® HT	263-038-9	Arquad® C-50	263-130-9	Dar-C
262-976-6	Armeen® HTD	263-038-9	Jet Quat C-50	263-130-9	Hy-Phi 6001
262-976-6	Radiamine 6140	263-038-9	Kemamine® Q-6503B	263-134-0	Arquad® S-50
262-976-6	Radiamine 6141	263-038-9	Marlazin® KC 30/50	263-134-0	Jet Quat S-50
262-977-1	Adogen® 160D	263-038-9	Nikkol CA-2150	263-134-0	Kemamine® Q-9973B
262-977-1	Amine KKD	263-038-9	Noramium MC 50	263-155-5	Akypogene FP 35 T
262-977-1	Armeen® C	263-038-9	Radiaquat® 6460	263-163-9	Ablumide CDE
262-977-1	Armeen® CD	263-038-9	Varisoft® 461	263-163-9	Ablumide CDE-G
262-977-1	Kemamine® P-650	263-049-9	Mackadet™ 40K	263-163-9	Ablumide CKD
262-977-1	Radiamine 6160	263-049-9	Norfox® 1101	263-163-9	Accomid C
262-977-1	Radiamine 6161	263-049-9	Protachem LP-40	263-163-9	Afmide™ C
262-978-7	Emery® 621	263-050-4	Norfox® Coco Powder	263-163-9	Alkamide® 2204
262-978-7	Emery® 622	263-052-5	Arlatone® SCI	263-163-9	Alkamide® CDE
262-978-7	Industrene® 325	263-052-5	Elfan® AT 84	263-163-9	Alkamide® CDM
262-978-7	Industrene® 328	263-052-5	Elfan® AT 84 G	263-163-9	Alkamide® CDO
262-979-2	Acelan L	263-052-5	Hostapon KA Powd.	263-163-9	Alkamide® CL63
262-979-2	Acetadeps	263-052-5	Hostapon SCI	263-163-9	Alkamide® DC-212/S

EINECS	Trade name	EINECS	Trade name	EINECS	Trade name
263-163-9	Alkamide® DC-212/SE	263-163-9	Mazamide® CCO	263-163-9	Varamide® A-84
263-163-9	Alkamide® KD	263-163-9	Mazamide® CS 148	263-163-9	Varamide® MA-1
263-163-9	Amidex CE	263-163-9	Mazamide® JT 128	263-163-9	Witcamide® 128T
263-163-9	Amidex KD	263-163-9	Mazamide® WC Conc.	263-163-9	Witcamide® 6404
263-163-9	Amidex KDO	263-163-9	Monamid® 705	263-163-9	Witcamide® 6514
263-163-9	Aminol COR-4C	263-163-9	Monamid® 759	263-163-9	Witcamide® 6531
263-163-9	Aminol HCA	263-163-9	Monamid® 1159	263-163-9	Witcamide® 6625
263-163-9	Aminol KDE	263-163-9	Monamid® C-305	263-163-9	Witcamide® CD
263-163-9	Calamide C	263-163-9	Monamid® C-310	263-163-9	Witcamide® CDA
263-163-9	Carsamide® CA	263-163-9	Monamine ADD-100	263-163-9	Witcamide® GR
263-163-9	Carsamide® SAC	263-163-9	Naxonol™ CO	263-163-9	Witcamide® LDTS
263-163-9	Chimipal DCL/M	263-163-9	Naxonol™ PN 66	263-163-9	Witcamide® M-3
263-163-9	Comperlan® COD	263-163-9	Naxonol™ PO	263-163-9	Witcamide® S771
263-163-9	Comperlan® KD	263-163-9	Ninol® 40-CO	263-163-9	Witcamide® S780
263-163-9	Comperlan® KDO	263-163-9	Ninol® 49-CE	263-167-0	Forestall
263-163-9	Comperlan® PD	263-163-9	Ninol® GR	263-170-7	Schercozoline C
263-163-9	Comperlan® SD	263-163-9	Norfox® DCS	263-170-7	Varine C
263-163-9	Comperlan® SDO	263-163-9	Norfox® DCSA	263-171-2	Varine T
263-163-9	Emalex N-83	263-163-9	Norfox® DOSA	263-179-6	Aromox® T/12
263-163-9	Emid® 6515	263-163-9	Norfox® KD	263-179-6	Chemoxide T
263-163-9	Emid® 6521	263-163-9	Olamida CD	263-180-1	Aromox® C/12
263-163-9	Empilan® 2502	263-163-9	Oramide DL 200 AF	263-180-1	Aromox® C/12-W
263-163-9	Empilan® CDE	263-163-9	Profan 2012E	263-180-1	Schercamox CMA
263-163-9	Empilan® CDE/FF	263-163-9	Profan 24 Extra, 128	263-190-6	Deriphat® 154
263-163-9	Empilan® CDX		Extra	263-190-6	Deriphat® 154L
263-163-9	Esi-Det CDA	263-163-9	Protamide CKD	263-190-6	Mirataine® T2C-30
263-163-9	Esi-Terge 10	263-163-9	Protamide DCA	263-193-2	Closyl 30 2089
263-163-9	Esi-Terge S-10	263-163-9	Protamide DCAW	263-193-2	Crodasinic CS
263-163-9	Ethylan® LD	263-163-9	Protamide HCA	263-193-2	Hamposyl® C-30
263-163-9	Ethylan® LDA-48	263-163-9	Purton CFD	263-193-2	Medialan KA
263-163-9	Ethylan® LDG	263-163-9	Rewomid® DC 212 LS	263-193-2	Nikkol Sarcosinate CN-30
263-163-9	FMB 128 T	263-163-9	Rewomid® DC 212 S		
263-163-9	FMB BT	263-163-9	Rewomid® DC 212 SE	263-193-2	Vanseal® NACS-30
263-163-9	FMB Cocamide DEA	263-163-9	Rewomid® DC 220 SE	263-218-7	Chimin LMO
263-163-9	FMB Coco Condensate	263-163-9	Ritamide C	263-218-7	Mackamine™ LAO
263-163-9	Foamid C	263-163-9	Rolamid CD	263-847-7	Rodol PS
263-163-9	Foamid SCE	263-163-9	Schercomid CCD	264-038-1	Be Square® 175
263-163-9	Hartamide OD	263-163-9	Schercomid CDO-Extra	264-038-1	Be Square® 185
263-163-9	Hetamide DSUC	263-163-9	Schercomid SCE	264-038-1	Be Square® 195
263-163-9	Hetamide MC	263-163-9	Schercomid SCO-Extra	264-038-1	CS-2080W
263-163-9	Hetamide MCS	263-163-9	Stamid HT 3901	264-038-1	Emerwax® 1253
263-163-9	Hetamide RC	263-163-9	Standamid® KD	264-038-1	Florabeads Micro 28/60 White
263-163-9	Hyamide 1:1	263-163-9	Standamid® KDO		
263-163-9	Incromide CA	263-163-9	Standamid® PK-KD	264-038-1	Fortex®
263-163-9	Karamide 121	263-163-9	Standamid® PK-KDO	264-038-1	Koster Keunen
263-163-9	Karamide 363	263-163-9	Standamid® PK-KDS		Microcrystalline Wax
263-163-9	Lauramide 11	263-163-9	Standamid® PK-SD		170/180
263-163-9	Lauramide ME	263-163-9	Standamid® SD	264-038-1	Mekon® White
263-163-9	Laurel SD-900M	263-163-9	Standamid® SDO	264-038-1	Multiwax® 180-M
263-163-9	Lauridit® KD	263-163-9	Synotol CN 60	264-038-1	Multiwax® 180-W
263-163-9	Lauridit® KDG	263-163-9	Synotol CN 80	264-038-1	Multiwax® ML-445
263-163-9	Loropan KD	263-163-9	Synotol CN 90	264-038-1	Multiwax® W-445
263-163-9	Mackamide™ C	263-163-9	Tohol N-220	264-038-1	Multiwax® W-835
263-163-9	Mackamide™ CD	263-163-9	Tohol N-220X	264-038-1	Multiwax® X-145A
263-163-9	Mackamide™ CS	263-163-9	T-Tergamide 1CD	264-038-1	Permulgin 835
263-163-9	Mackamide™ MC	263-163-9	Ufanon K-80	264-038-1	Petrolite® C-700
263-163-9	Manro CD	263-163-9	Ufanon KD-S	264-038-1	Petrolite® C-1035
263-163-9	Manro CDS	263-163-9	Unamide® C-72-3	264-038-1	Starwax® 100
263-163-9	Manro CDX	263-163-9	Unamide® D-10	264-038-1	Ultraflex®
263-163-9	Manromid CD	263-163-9	Unamide® LDL	264-038-1	Victory®
263-163-9	Manromid CDG	263-163-9	Upamide CA-20	264-043-9	Eusolex® 8020
263-163-9	Manromid CDS	263-163-9	Upamide CS-148	264-119-1	Amerlate® P
263-163-9	Marlamid® D 1218	263-163-9	Upamide KD	264-119-1	Amerlate® W
263-163-9	Marlamid® DF 1218	263-163-9	Varamide® A-2	264-119-1	Fancol IPL
263-163-9	Mazamide® 68	263-163-9	Varamide® A-10	264-119-1	Fancor IPL
263-163-9	Mazamide® 80	263-163-9	Varamide® A-12	264-119-1	Ivarlan™ 3350
263-163-9	Mazamide® 524	263-163-9	Varamide® A-80	264-119-1	Lanesta L
263-163-9	Mazamide® 1281	263-163-9	Varamide® A-83	264-119-1	Lanesta P

EINECS	Trade name	EINECS	Trade name	EINECS	Trade name
264-119-1	Lanesta S	268-761-3	Mirataine® CBS, CBS	268-770-2	Zoramide CM
264-119-1	Lanesta SA-30		Mod	268-771-8	Chemidex C
264-119-1	Lanisolate	268-761-3	Protachem JS	268-771-8	Chemidex WC
264-119-1	Ritasol	268-761-3	Rewoteric® AM CAS	268-771-8	Lexamine C-13
264-391-1	Gelling Agent GP-1	268-761-3	Rewoteric® AM CAS	268-771-8	Mackine™ 101
265-352-1	Catigene® CT 70	268-761-3	Rewoteric® AM CAS-	268-771-8	Schercodine C
265-363-1	Edamin S		15	268-771-8	Witcamine® 100
265-363-1	EPCH	268-761-3	Sandobet SC	268-820-3	Alkaterge®-E
265-363-1	Glycoproteins from Milk	268-761-3	Schercotaine SCAB	268-910-2	Radiasurf® 7125
265-363-1	Hy Case SF	268-761-3	Zohartaine CBS	268-938-5	Ablumox CAPO
265-363-1	Hy Case Amino	268-770-2	Ablumide CME	268-938-5	Afamine™ CAO
265-363-1	Hydromilk™ EN-20	268-770-2	Afmide™ CMA	268-938-5	Aminoxid WS 35
265-363-1	Milkpro	268-770-2	Alkamide® C-212	268-938-5	Ammonyx® CDO
265-363-1	Promois Milk	268-770-2	Alkamide® CME	268-938-5	Amyx CDO 3599
265-648-0	Imexine FH	268-770-2	Amidex CME	268-938-5	Barlox® C
265-724-3	Estasan GT 8-60 3575	268-770-2	Amidex KME	268-938-5	Chemoxide CAW
265-839-9	Waxenol® 801	268-770-2	Aminol CM, CM Flakes,	268-938-5	Chimin CMO
265-880-2	Incroquat SBQ 75P		CM-C Flakes, CM-D	268-938-5	Emcol® CDO
266-124-4	Schercemol GMIS		Flakes	268-938-5	Empigen® OS/A
266-138-0	Imexine FM	268-770-2	Carsamide® CMEA	268-938-5	Empigen® OS/AU
266-357-1	Imexine OAJ	268-770-2	Chimipal MC	268-938-5	Finamine CO
266-533-8	Crolactil SISL	268-770-2	Comperlan® 100	268-938-5	Foamox CDO
266-533-8	Pationic® ISL	268-770-2	Comperlan® P 100	268-938-5	Incromine Oxide C
266-778-0	Foamquat IAES	268-770-2	Emid® 6500	268-938-5	Incromine Oxide C-35
266-778-0	Monaquat ISIES	268-770-2	Empilan® CME	268-938-5	Mackamine™ CAO
266-778-0	M-Quat® 522	268-770-2	Empilan® CM/F	268-938-5	Mazox® CAPA
266-778-0	Naetex-S	268-770-2	Foamole M	268-938-5	Mazox® CAPA-37
266-778-0	Schercoquat IAS	268-770-2	Hetamide CMA	268-938-5	Monalux CAO-35
266-778-0	Schercoquat IIS	268-770-2	Hetamide CME	268-938-5	Ninox® FCA
266-948-4	Radia® 7363	268-770-2	Hetamide CME-CO	268-938-5	Rewominox B 204
267-006-5	Epal® 1218	268-770-2	Incromide CME	268-938-5	Rhodamox® CAPO
267-008-6	Epal® 1618	268-770-2	Lauridit® KM	268-938-5	Schercamox C-AA
267-008-6	Epal® 1618RT	268-770-2	Loropan CME	268-938-5	Standamox CAW
267-008-6	Epal® 1618T	268-770-2	Loropan KM	268-938-5	Tegamine® Oxide WS-
267-009-1	Epal® 1418	268-770-2	Mackamide™ CMA		35
267-015-4	Radia® 7060	268-770-2	Mackamide™ LM-Flake	268-938-5	Unimox CAW
267-019-6	Epal® 12/70	268-770-2	Manro CMEA	268-938-5	Varox® 1770
267-019-6	Epal® 12/85	268-770-2	Manromid CMEA	268-938-5	Zoramox
267-019-6	Epal® 1214	268-770-2	Marlamid® M 1218	268-949-5	Hetamide DT
267-019-6	Epal® 1412	268-770-2	Mazamide® CFAM	268-949-5	Schercomid SO-T
267-048-4	Costaulon	268-770-2	Mazamide® CMEA	268-949-5	Schercomid TO-2
267-054-7	Kessco® 3283	268-770-2	Mazamide® CMEA	269-027-5	Emerest® 2384
267-101-1	Chemidex SI		Extra	269-027-5	Emerest® 2389
267-101-1	Mackine™ 401	268-770-2	Monamid® CMA	269-027-5	Hydrophilol ISO
267-101-1	Schercodine I	268-770-2	Monamid® CMA-A	269-027-5	Prisorine PMIS 2034
267-360-0	Schercoquat SAS	268-770-2	Monamid® CMA-A/F	269-027-5	Unitolate PGIST
2679-790-4	Epal® 1416-LD	268-770-2	Monamid® CMA-A/M	269-027-5	Witconol™ 2384
268-093-2	Radia® 7370	268-770-2	Monamid® CMA/F	269-084-6	Amisoft CT-12
268-093-2	Radia® 7371	268-770-2	Monamid® CMA/M	269-087-2	Amisoft CS-11
268-130-2	Hamposyl® AL-30	268-770-2	Monamid® CMA-S	269-087-2	Hostapon KCG
268-164-8	Rodol EOX	268-770-2	Monamid® CMA-S/F	269-131-0	Isofol® 34T
268-213-3	Hostapur SAS 30	268-770-2	Monamid® CMA-S/M	269-220-4	Albalan
268-213-3	Hostapur SAS 60	268-770-2	Monamide	269-220-4	Fancor Lanwax
268-213-3	Hostapur SAS 93	268-770-2	Ninol® CNR	269-220-4	Lanfrax®
268-264-1	Belal	268-770-2	Nissan Stafoam MF	269-220-4	Lanfrax® 1776
268-761-3	Abluter CPS	268-770-2	Olamida CM	269-220-4	Lanfrax® 1779
268-761-3	Amonyl 675 SB	268-770-2	Oramide ML 115	269-220-4	Lanocerin®
268-761-3	Chembetaine CAS	268-770-2	Phoenamid CMA, CMA-	269-220-4	Lanowax
268-761-3	Crosultaine C-50		70	269-220-4	Protalan Wax
268-761-3	Lexaine® CSB-50	268-770-2	Profan AB20	269-220-4	R.I.T.A. Lanolin Wax
268-761-3	Lonzaine® CS	268-770-2	Protamide CME	269-220-4	Unilan W
268-761-3	Lonzaine® JS	268-770-2	Rewomid® C 212	269-475-1	Rodol EGS
268-761-3	Mackam™ CBS-50	268-770-2	Schercomid CME	269-478-8	Rodol DEMAPS
268-761-3	Mackam™ CBS-50G	268-770-2	Standamid® KM	269-662-8	Dextrol AS-150
268-761-3	Mafo® CSB	268-770-2	Standamid® SM	269-790-4	Epal® 1416
268-761-3	Mafo® CSB 50	268-770-2	Synotol ME 90	269-793-0	Amidex CIPA
268-761-3	Mafo® CSB W	268-770-2	Upamide SM	269-793-0	Empilan® CIS
268-761-3	Mafo® KCOSB 50	268-770-2	Varamide® C-212	269-793-0	Rewomid® IPP 240

EINECS	Trade name	EINECS	Trade name	EINECS	Trade name
269-793-0	Witcamide® PPA	270-355-6	Afmide™ S	272-043-5	Dehyton® W
269-804-9	C-Flakes	270-355-6	Alkamide® SDO	272-043-5	Mackam™ 2C
269-804-9	Emvelop®	270-355-6	Amidex S	272-043-5	Manroteric CDX38
269-804-9	Lipex 109	270-355-6	Comperlan® VOD	272-043-5	Miranol® C2M Conc.
269-804-9	Lubritab®	270-355-6	Empigen® 2125-AU		NP
269-819-0	Schercoteric MS	270-355-6	Empilan® 2125-AU	272-043-5	Miranol® C2M Conc.
269-820-6	BBS	270-355-6	Mackamide™ S		OP
269-820-6	Cremeol HF-52, HF-62	270-355-6	Mackamide™ SD	272-043-5	Miranol® FB-NP
269-820-6	Hydrokote® 95	270-355-6	Manromid 150-ADY	272-043-5	Monateric CDX-38
269-820-6	Hydrokote® 97	270-355-6	Marlamid® DF 1818	272-043-5	Monateric CDX-38 Mod
269-820-6	Hydrokote® 102	270-355-6	Schercomid SLS	272-043-5	Monateric CLV
269-820-6	Hydrokote® 108	270-355-6	Stamid LS 5487	272-043-5	Monateric CSH-32
269-820-6	Hydrokote® 112	270-355-6	Witcamide® SSA	272-043-5	Proteric CDX-38
269-820-6	Hydrokote® 118	270-356-1	Chemidex T	272-043-5	Rewoteric® AM 2C W
269-820-6	Hydrokote® AR, HL	270-407-8	Bio-Terge® AS-40	272-043-5	Schercoteric MS-2
269-820-6	Hydrokote® RM	270-407-8	Calsoft AOS-40	272-043-5	Sochamine A 7525
269-820-6	Lipo SS	270-407-8	Carsonol® AOS	272-043-5	Surfax AC 50
269-820-6	Sterotex®	270-407-8	Elfan® OS 46	272-043-5	Surfax ACI
269-820-6	Sterotex® NF	270-407-8	Norfox® ALPHA XL	272-043-5	Unibetaine 2C
269-820-6	Wecobee® FS	270-407-8	Rhodacal® 301-10F	272-043-5	Velvetex® CDC
269-820-6	Wecobee® FW	270-407-8	Rhodacal® A-246L	272-043-5	Zoharteric D
269-820-6	Wecobee® M	270-407-8	Rhodacal® A-246 LX	272-043-5	Zoharteric D-SF 70%
269-820-6	Wecobee® S	270-407-8	Witconate™ AOK	272-219-1	Schercopol CMS-Na
269-820-6	Wecobee® SS	270-407-8	Witconate™ AOS	272-296-1	K2 Glycyrrhizinate
269-820-6	Wecobee® W	270-407-8	Witconate™ AOS-EP	272-296-1	Nikkol Dipotassium
270-156-4	Crodasinic C	270-407-8	Witconate™ AOS-PC		Glycyrrhizinate
270-156-4	Hamposyl® C	270-474-3	Crodamol PTC	272-296-1	Ritamectant K2
270-156-4	Hamposyl® CZ	270-474-3	Lipo PE 810	272-385-5	Standapol® A-215
270-156-4	Vanseal® CS	270-474-3	Liponate PE-810	272-385-5	Unipol A-215
270-302-7	Amerlate® LFA	270-474-3	Radia® 7178	272-778-1	Epal® 20+
270-302-7	Amerlate® WFA	270-664-6	Hoechst Wax E Pharma	273-049-0	Glucate® SS
270-302-7	Argonol LFA Dist	270-664-6	Hoechst Wax SW	273-049-0	Grillocose PS
270-302-7	Argowax LFA Distilled	270-864-3	Schercopol OMS-Na	273-187-1	Foamole B
270-302-7	Argowax LFA Standard	271-064-7	Querton 442P	273-187-1	Incromine Mink B
270-302-7	Facilan	271-064-7	Querton 442P-11	273-219-4	Bentone® 34
270-302-7	Fancor LFA	271-102-2	Afanate™ CP	273-219-4	Claytone 34
270-302-7	Ritalafa®	271-102-2	Mackanate™ CP	273-219-4	Claytone 40
270-304-8	Industrene® 20	271-102-2	Monamate C-1142	273-219-4	Claytone XL
270-304-8	L-310	271-102-2	Monamate CPA-40	273-219-4	Tixogel VP
270-312-1	Radiasurf® 7150	271-102-2	Monamate CPA-100	273-222-0	Ceraphyl® 65
270-315-8	Hetlan OH	271-347-5	Nikkol Trialan 318	273-222-0	Incroquat 26
270-315-8	Hidroxilan	271-347-5	Salacos 6318	273-277-0	Radia® 7506
270-315-8	Hydroxylan	271-397-8	Dascare Oryza-Oil	273-429-6	Schercozoline I
270-315-8	Ivarlan™ OH	271-397-8	EmCon Rice Bran	273-576-6	Lamegin® GLP 10, 20
270-315-8	Landrox	271-397-8	Natoil RBO	273-612-0	Lamegin® EE
270-315-8	OHlan®	271-397-8	Rice Bran Oil	273-613-6	Acidan N 12
270-315-8	Protalan H	271-397-8	Rice Bran Oil SO	273-613-6	Lamegin® ZE 30, 60
270-315-8	Ritahydrox	271-397-8	Tri-Ol RBO	273-616-2	Dermane SLO
270-329-4	Amonyl 265 BA	271-649-2	Radia® 7171	273-616-2	Super Refined™ Shark
270-329-4	Ampho B11-34	271-705-0	Amphoterge® SB		Liver Oil
270-329-4	Ampholan® E210	271-705-0	Mackam™ CS	273-942-5	Isofol® 16 Palmitat
270-329-4	Amphoteen BCM-30	271-705-0	Miranol® CS Conc.	274-001-1	Crotein ASK
270-329-4	Chembetaine CB	271-705-0	Sandoteric CFL	274-001-1	Crotein K
270-329-4	Dehyton® AB-30	271-705-0	Schercoteric MS-EP	274-001-1	Crotein WKP
270-329-4	Emcol® CC 37-18	271-762-1	Duoquad® T-50	274-001-1	Dehydrated Keratine
270-320-4	Inoronam CD 30	271-793-0	Ampholak XCO-40		Hydrolysate
270-329-4	Lonzaine® 12C	271-929-9	Monateric ISA-35	274-001-1	Hidrolisado de
270-329-4	Mackam™ CB-35	271-929-9	Schercoteric I-AA		Queratina
270-329-4	Mafo® CB 40	271-957-1	Dehyton® G	274-001-1	Hydrokeratin™ 100M
270-329-4	Protachem CB 45	271-972-3	Chemoxide TAO	274-001-1	Hydrokeratin™ AL-30
270-329-4	Radiateric® 6860	272-021-5	Armeen® Z	274-001-1	Hydrokeratin™ AL-SD
270-329-4	Surfax ACB	272-043-5	Abluter DCM-2	274-001-1	Hydrokeratin™ WKP
270-329-4	Unibetaine AB-30, AB-	272-043-5	Afoteric™ 2C	274-001-1	Keramois L
	45	272-043-5	Ampholak XCO-30	274-001-1	Kerapro S
270-329-4	Velvetex® AB-45	272-043-5	Amphotensid GB 2009	274-001-1	Kera-Tein 1000
270-350-9	Witarix® 450	272-043-5	Amphoterge® W-2	274-001-1	Kera-Tein 1000 RM/50
270-351-4	CO-618	272-043-5	Chimin IMB	274-001-1	Kera-Tein 1000 RM SD
270-351-4	Radianol® 1728	272-043-5	Dehyton® PG	274-001-1	Kera-Tein 1000 SD

EINECS	Trade name	EINECS	Trade name	EINECS	Trade name
274-001-1	Kera-Tein V	285-203-4	Radia® 7204	295-786-7	Emulmetik™ 320
274-001-1	Keratin P	285-206-0	Radia® 7187	295-786-7	Emulmetik™ 950
274-001-1	Keratin S	285-207-6	Radia® 7331	295-786-7	Lipoid S 75-3
274-001-1	Keratine Hydrolysate	285-540-7	Radia® 7231	295-786-7	Nikkol Lecinol S-10
	H.T.K	285-547-5	Radiasurf® 7175	295-786-7	Nikkol Lecinol S-10E
274-001-1	Keratin Hydrolysate	285-550-1	Radiasurf® 7410	295-786-7	Nikkol Lecinol S-10EX
274-001-1	Nutrilan® Cashmere W	286-074-7	Radia® 7355	295-786-7	Nikkol Lecinol S-10M
274-001-1	Nutrilan® Keratin W	286-490-9	Radiasurf® 7600	295-786-7	Nikkol Lecinol S-30
274-001-1	Promois WK	287-039-9	Radia® 7051	295-786-7	PhosPho H-00
274-001-1	Promois WK-H	287-075-5	Radia® 7108	295-786-7	PhosPho H-150
274-033-6	Akypoquat 131	287-462-9	Rewoquat RTM 50	296-473-8	Colloidal Kaolin NF-
274-033-6	Akypoquat 131 V	287-484-9	Radia® 7501		Bacteria Controlled
274-357-8	Suttocide® A	287-824-6	Radia® 7110	296-473-8	Kaopaque 10, 20
274-695-6	Hostapon KTW	288-305-7	Radiasurf® 7156	296-473-8	Lion English Kaolin
274-845-0	Amphoteen BTH-35	288-459-5	Radiasurf® 7402	296-473-8	Unimin KA
274-845-0	Mirataine® TM	288-459-5	Radiasurf® 7403	297-364-8	Radiasurf® 7400
274-845-0	Rewoteric® AM TEG	288-459-5	Radiasurf® 7404	297-495-0	Rewoquat DQ 35
274-845-0	Tego®-Betaine N-192	288-459-5	Radiasurf® 7443	298-104-6	Isofol® 16 Caprylat
274-923-4	Amphoteen BCA-30	288-459-5	Radiasurf® 7444	298-364-0	Pelemol P-49
275-637-2	Dermol 89	288-668-1	Radia® 7241	302-928-6	Querton 16Cl-50
275-637-2	Isolanoate	289-991-0	Ceraphyl® 847	304-693-3	Isofol® 16 Oleat
275-637-2	Kessco® Octyl	289-991-0	Trivent SS-20	306-522-8	Radiasurf® 7270
	Isononanoate	290-580-3	Radia® 7505	306-522-8	Radiasurf® 7414
275-637-2	Pelemol 89	291-990-5	Foamquat SOAS	306-522-8	Radiasurf® 7417
275-637-2	Witconol™ 2300	291-990-5	Schercoquat SOAS	306-522-8	Radiasurf® 7453
276-627-0	Isofol® 28	292-416-6	Trioxene LV	306-522-8	Radiasurf® 7454
276-719-0	Nikkol ISP	292-932-1	Radia® 7266	306-522-8	Radiasurf® 7473
276-719-0	Protachem ISP	292-945-2	Radia® 7185	306-797-4	Radia® 7500
276-951-2	Radia® 7345	292-951-5	Radia® 7131	306-998-7	Ampholak 7TY
278-928-2	Germall® II	292-960-4	Radia® 7510	307-455-7	Ampholak YCE
279-383-3	Imexine FT	293-029-5	Radia® 7176	307-455-7	Ampholan® U 203
279-917-5	Amiter LGOD	293-208-8	Radiasurf® 7900	307-458-3	Ampholak 7CX
283-078-0	Radia® 7514	293-255-4	Melhydran®	307-458-3	Ampholak 7CX/C
283-390-7	Schercemol MEL-3	293-306-0	Lipocerina	307-458-3	Ampholak 7TX
283-481-1	CMI 321	293-391-2	Schercemol MEP-3	307-458-3	Ampholak 7TX/C
283-481-1	CMI 324	293-509-4	Cronectin H	307-458-3	Ampholak 7TX-SD 55
283-481-1	CMI 400	293-509-4	Nutrilan® Elastin E20	307-458-3	Ampholak 7TX-T
283-644-7	Midecol CF	293-509-4	Nutrilan® Elastin P	307-458-3	Ampholak XO7
284-219-9	Afoteric™ 151C	295-366-3	Crodamol OC	307-458-3	Ampholak XO7/C
284-219-9	Ampholyte KKE-70	295-366-3	Estol EHC 1540	309-206-8	Rewoteric® QAM 50
284-219-9	Mackam™ 151C	295-366-3	Trioxene E	309-327-6	Gluadin® Almond
284-868-8	Radia® 7230	295-786-7	Basis LS-60H	309-696-3	Gluadin® AGP

EINECS Number-to-Chemical Cross-Reference

EINECS	Chemical	EINECS	Chemical	EINECS	Chemical
200-018-0	Lactic acid	200-603-0	Pyridoxine	201-327-3	D-Panthenol
200-061-5	Sorbitol	200-618-2	Benzoic acid	201-487-4	1,5-Naphthalenediol
200-066-2	Ascorbic acid	200-641-8	Thiamine HCl	201-507-1	Riboflavin
200-075-1	Glucose	200-652-8	Pentetic acid	201-550-6	Diethyl phthalate
200-091-9	Hydroxyproline	200-661-7	Isopropyl alcohol	201-557-4	Dibutyl phthalate
200-125-2	m-Aminophenol HCl	200-673-2	Cholecalciferol	201-762-9	Pyrogallol
200-143-0	2-Bromo-2-nitropro-	200-675-3	Sodium citrate	201-766-0	Tartaric acid
	pane-1,3-diol	200-677-4	Thioglycolic acid	201-781-2	Inositol
200-158-2	L-Cysteine	200-680-0	Cyanocobalamin	201-793-8	Chloroxylenol
200-194-9	DL-α-Tryptophan	200-683-7	Retinol	201-800-4	PVP
200-237-1	p-Methylaminophenol	200-711-8	Mannitol	201-828-7	2-t-Butylcyclohexyl
	sulfate	200-712-3	Salicylic acid		acetate
200-270-1	Benzyltriethyl	200-716-5	Maltose	201-928-0	Erythorbic acid
	ammonium chloride	200-720-7	Uric acid	201-939-0	Menthol
200-272-2	Glycine	200-731-7	Ornithine	201-944-8	Thymol
200-273-8	Alanine	200-745-3	Histidine	201-969-4	1-Naphthol
200-274-3	L-Serine	200-751-6	Butyl alcohol	201-993-5	o-Phenylphenol
200-283-2	Adenosine triphosphate	200-756-3	Trichloroethane	202-090-9	N,N-Diethyl-m-
200-289-5	Glycerin	200-772-0	Sodium lactate		aminophenol
200-293-7	L-Glutamic acid	200-773-6	Valine	202-156-7	2,3-Naphthalenediol
200-294-2	L-Lysine	200-798-2	L-Isoleucine	202-280-1	Stearamide DEA
200-296-3	Cystine	200-799-8	Guanine	202-281-7	Oleamide DEA
200-300-3	Benzyl trimethyl	200-811-1	Arginine	202-307-7	Propylparaben
	ammonium chloride	200-815-3	Polyethylene	202-311-9	Benzylparaben
200-311-3	Cetrimonium bromide	200-827-9	Propane	202-318-7	Butylparaben
200-312-9	Palmitic acid	200-857-2	Isobutane	202-332-3	Benzyl nicotinate
200-313-4	Stearic acid	200-866-1	Hydrofluorocarbon	202-340-7	Dipropylene glycol
200-315-5	Urea		152a		dibenzoate
200-317-6	Chlorobutanol	200-871-4	Hydrochlorofluoro-	202-377-9	Ethyl hexanediol
200-333-3	Fructose		carbon 22	202-414-9	Oleyl hydroxyethyl
200-334-9	Sucrose	200-876-6	Nitromethane		imidazoline
200-338-0	Propylene glycol	200-891-8	Hydrochlorofluoro-	202-431-1	o-Aminophenol
200-353-2	Cholesterol		carbon 142B	202-462-0	4-Chlororesorcinol
200-362-1	Caffeine	201-064-4	Tris (hydroxymethyl)	202-488-2	2-Amino-1-butanol
200-372-6	Menadione		aminomethane	202-494-5	Dihydroxyacetone
200-385-7	Theophylline	201-066-5	Acetyl triethyl citrate	202-495-0	Thioglycerin
200-399-3	Biotin	201-067-0	Acetyl tributyl citrate	202-500-6	Methyl acrylate
200-412-2	Tocopherol	201-069-1	Citric acid		(monomer)
200-431-6	p-Chloro-m-cresol	201-070-7	Triethyl citrate	202-509-5	Butyrolactone
200-432-1	Methionine	201-071-2	Tributyl citrate	202-567-1	Dichlorophene
200-441-0	Nicotinic acid	201-094-8	Cetethyl morpholinium	202-592-8	Allantoin
200-449-4	Edetic acid		ethosulfate	202-597-5	Ethyl methacrylate
200-456-2	Phenethyl alcohol	201-162-7	Isopropanolamine	202-608-3	Lauroyl sarcosine
200-460-4	L-Tyrosine	201-166-9	Trichloroethane	202-615-1	Butyl methacrylate
200-470-9	Linoleic acid	201-176-3	Propionic acid	202-700-3	PCA
200-522-0	L-Leucine	201-214-9	Lanosterol	202-713-4	Niacinamide
200-529-9	Calcium disodium	201-228-5	Retinyl palmitate	202-766-3	4-Nitro-o-phenylenedi-
	EDTA	201-229-0	Pantothenic acid		amine
200-559-2	Lactose	201-297-1	Methyl methacrylate	202-785-7	Methylparaben
200-568-1	L-Phenylalanine		(monomer)	202-859-9	Benzyl alcohol
200-573-9	Tetrasodium EDTA	201-304-8	Dimethyl imidazoli-	202-935-1	Glyceryl triacetyl
200-578-6	Alcohol		dinone		ricinoleate
200-580-7	Acetic acid	201-321-0	Saccharin	202-951-9	N-Phenyl-p-

EINECS	Chemical	EINECS	Chemical	EINECS	Chemical
	phenylenediamine	203-868-0	Diethanolamine	204-526-3	Cetalkonium chloride
203-041-4	Tetrahydroxypropyl	203-872-2	Diethylene glycol	204-527-9	Stearalkonium chloride
	ethylenediamine	203-883-2	Stearamide MEA	204-528-4	Triisopropanolamine
203-049-8	Triethanolamine	203-884-8	Oleamide MEA	204-534-7	Triolein
203-051-9	Triacetin	203-886-9	Glycol stearate	204-558-8	Dioctyl sebacate
203-063-4	Trilaurylamine	203-887-4	Ethyl stearate	204-589-7	Phenoxyethanol
203-090-1	Dioctyl adipate	203-889-5	Ethyl oleate	204-593-9	Cetylpyridinium chloride
203-161-7	Cyclamen aldehyde	203-893-7	Octene-1	204-614-1	Dilauryl thiodipropio-
203-180-0	Toluene sulfonic acid	203-905-0	Butoxyethanol		nate
203-192-6	Chlorphenesin	203-906-6	Methoxydiglycol	204-616-2	p-Aminophenol
203-219-1	γ-Nonalactone	203-911-3	Methyl laurate	204-617-8	Hydroquinone
203-225-4	γ-Undecalactone	203-917-6	Caprylic alcohol	204-630-9	Hydroxypropyl
203-232-2	Laurylpyridinium	203-919-7	Ethoxydiglycol		bistrimonium diiodide
	chloride	203-924-4	Dimethoxydiglycol	204-648-7	2-Pyrrolidone
203-246-9	p-Tolualdehyde	203-927-0	Laurtrimonium chloride	204-649-2	Levulinic acid
203-315-3	Propylene glycol	203-928-6	Cetrimonium chloride	204-658-1	n-Butyl acetate
	dioleate	203-929-1	Steartrimonium chloride	204-664-4	Glyceryl stearate
203-347-8	Ethylene brassylate	203-934-9	Isopropyl stearate	204-666-5	Butyl stearate
203-349-9	Dicapryl adipate	203-935-4	Isopropyl oleate	204-672-8	Cetethyldimonium
203-350-4	Dibutyl adipate	203-940-1	Ethoxydiglycol acetate		bromide
203-353-0	Diethylene glycol	203-943-8	Dimethyl lauramine	204-675-4	Ethyl myristate
	diisononanoate	203-953-2	Triethylene glycol	204-677-5	Caprylic acid
203-354-6	Pentadecalactone	203-956-9	n-Decyl alcohol	204-680-1	Methyl myristate
203-358-8	PEG-4 stearate	203-961-6	Butoxy diglycol	204-690-6	Lauramine
203-359-3	PEG-9 laurate	203-965-8	Undecylenic acid	204-693-2	Stearamide
203-363-5	PEG-2 stearate	203-966-3	Methyl palmitate	204-694-8	Dimethyl stearamine
203-364-0	PEG-2 oleate	203-968-4	Dodecene-1	204-695-3	Stearamine
203-366-1	Hydroxystearic acid	203-970-5	Undecyl alcohol	204-701-4	Urea peroxide
203-368-2	Ricinoleamide MEA	203-982-0	Lauryl alcohol	204-709-8	2-Amino-2-methyl-1-
203-369-8	Glycol ricinoleate	203-989-9	PEG-4		propanol
203-371-9	Dipropyl adipate	203-990-4	Methyl stearate	204-740-7	Usnic acid
203-386-0	Ethyl laurate	203-992-5	Methyl oleate	204-769-5	Tris (hydroxymethyl)
203-404-7	p-Phenylenediamine	203-997-2	Dimethyl palmitamine		nitromethane
203-419-9	Dimethyl succinate	204-000-3	Myristyl alcohol	204-781-0	Neopentyl glycol
203-448-7	Butane	204-002-4	Dimethyl myristamine	204-812-8	Sodium octyl sulfate
203-473-3	Glycol	204-007-1	Oleic acid	204-823-8	Sodium acetate
203-489-0	Hexylene glycol	204-010-8	Behenic acid	204-840-0	Xanthophyll
203-490-6	Betaine	204-015-5	Oleamine	204-844-2	Retinyl acetate
203-492-7	Hexamethyldisiloxane	204-017-6	Stearyl alcohol	204-867-8	Zinc phenolsulfonate
203-508-2	Distearyldimonium	204-065-8	Dimethyl ether	204-881-4	BHT
	chloride	204-100-7	2-Amino-2-methyl-1,3-	204-886-1	Sodium saccharin
203-529-7	Butylene glycol		propanediol	205-011-6	Dimethyl phthalate
203-539-1	Methoxyisopropanol	204-101-2	2-Amino-2-ethyl-1,3-	205-026-8	Benzophenone-8
203-572-1	Propylene carbonate		propanediol	205-027-3	Benzophenone-6
203-584-7	m-Phenylenediamine	204-110-1	Pentaerythrityl	205-028-9	Benzophenone-2
203-585-2	Resorcinol		tetrastearate	205-029-4	Benzophenone-1
203-625-9	Toluene	204-132-1	MDM hydantoin	205-031-5	Benzophenone-3
203-661-5	Oleamidopropyl	204-259-2	Phenyl salicylate	205-055-6	Sodium o-phenyl-
	dimethylamine	204-260-8	Homosalate		phenate
203-663-6	PEG-2 distearate	204-263-4	Octyl salicylate	205-087-0	Captan
203-740-4	Succinic acid	204-317-7	Methyl salicylate	205-105-7	Tartaric acid
203-749-3	Oleoyl sarcosine	204-385-8	Chlorophene	205-126-1	Sodium ascorbate
203-751-4	Isopropyl myristate	204-393-1	Lauramide DEA	205-129-8	Menthyl anthranilate
203-755-6	Ethylene distearamide	204-399-4	Ethylparaben	205-149-7	Diethyl toluamide
203-759-8	Butyl myristate	204-402-9	Benzyl benzoate	205-234-9	Capramide DEA
203-764-5	Diethyl sebacate	204-405-8	Benzyl laurate	205-271-0	Lauryl hydroxyethyl
203-768-7	Sorbic acid	204-407-6	Diethylene glycol		imidazoline
203-804-1	Ethoxyethanol		dibenzoate	205-273-1	2-Heptylcyclo-
203-815-1	Morpholine	204-427-5	Pyrocatechol		pentanone
203-820-9	Diisopropanolamine	204-442-7	BHA	205-278-9	Calcium pantothenate
203-821-4	Dipropylene glycol	204-464-7	Ethyl vanillin	205-281-5	Sodium lauroyl
203-825-6	Squalane	204-465-2	Vanillin		sarcosinate
203-826-1	Squalane	204-479-9	Benzalkonium chloride	205-285-7	Sodium methyl oleoyl
203-827-7	Glyceryl oleate	204-479-9	Benzethonium chloride		taurate
203-828-2	Oleamide MIPA	204-498-2	Propyl gallate	205-290-4	Sodium propionate
203-839-2	Ethoxyethanol acetate	204-503-8	2-Amino-5-nitrophenol	205-305-4	Ascorbyl palmitate
203-852-3	Hexyl alcohol	204-516-9	p-Isopropylbenz-	205-324-8	Cetrimonium tosylate
203-856-5	Glutaral		aldehyde	205-341-0	Dipentene

EINECS	Chemical	EINECS	Chemical	EINECS	Chemical
205-351-5	Lauralkonium chloride	208-033-4	Arachidonic acid	212-227-4	Dehydroacetic acid
205-352-0	Myristalkonium chloride	208-178-3	Abietic acid	212-470-6	Stearyl betaine
205-358-3	Disodium EDTA	208-205-9	Bisabolol	212-490-5	Sodium stearate
205-360-4	Sodium dihydroxyethyl-glycinate	208-293-9	Dehydroacetic acid	212-806-1	Oleyl betaine
		208-407-7	Sodium gluconate	213-668-5	Hexamethyldisilazane
205-381-9	Trisodium HEDTA	208-408-2	Copper gluconate	213-695-2	Ammonium stearate
205-388-7	TEA-lauryl sulfate	208-517-5	Esculin	214-274-6	Ethyl glutamate
205-391-3	Pentasodium pentetate	208-534-8	Sodium benzoate	214-277-2	Dimethyl glutarate
205-392-9	Methyl acetyl ricinoleate	208-575-1	1,2,4-Trihydroxy-benzene	214-289-8	Lauryl glycol
205-455-0	Glyceryl ricinoleate			214-291-9	Myrtrimonium bromide
205-468-1	PEG-2 laurate	208-580-9	Sodium sesquicarbon-ate	214-292-4	Sodium cetyl sulfate
205-469-7	Stearamidoethyl ethanolamine	208-666-6	Trilinolein	214-295-0	Sodium stearyl sulfate
205-470-2	Ricinoleic acid	208-671-3	Acetyltyrosine	214-620-6	Dodecyl gallate
205-471-8	Methyl hydroxystearate	208-686-5	Tricaprylin	214-724-1	Cetyl stearate
205-495-9	Isododecane	208-687-0	Trilaurin	214-734-6	Ethyl linolenate
205-507-2	2,6-Diaminopyridine	208-702-0	Domiphen bromide	214-737-2	Sodium myristyl sulfate
205-513-5	Hexetidine	208-736-6	Cetyl palmitate	214-946-9	Hexahydrohexamethyl cyclopentabenzopyran
205-524-5	Dioctyl maleate	208-750-2	Polyvinyl chloride	215-090-9	Sodium xylenesulfonate
205-526-6	Glyceryl laurate	208-768-0	Carnitine	215-108-5	Bentonite
205-530-8	Acetamide MEA	208-791-6	m-Phenylenediamine sulfate	215-136-8	Bismuth subnitrate
205-539-7	Stearoyl sarcosine			215-137-3	Calcium hydroxide
205-541-8	Lauramide MIPA	208-867-9	Palmitamide MEA	215-138-9	Calcium oxide
205-542-3	Propylene glycol laurate	208-868-4	Ethyl linoleate	215-160-9	Chromium oxide greens
205-546-5	Myristamide MEA	208-874-7	Batyl alcohol	215-168-2	Iron oxides
205-550-7	Caproic acid	208-875-2	Myristic acid	215-170-3	Magnesium hydroxide
205-559-6	Butyl oleate	208-901-2	Zinc citrate	215-171-9	Magnesium oxide
205-560-1	Lauramide MEA	208-915-9	Magnesium carbonate	215-181-3	Potassium hydroxide
205-571-1	Isopropyl palmitate	209-097-6	Tristearin	215-185-5	Sodium hydroxide
205-577-4	DEA-lauryl sulfate	209-098-1	Tripalmitin	215-222-5	Zinc oxide
205-582-1	Lauric acid	209-099-7	Trimyristin	215-277-5	Iron oxides
205-590-5	Potassium oleate	209-112-6	D-Tyrosine	215-288-5	Montmorillonite
205-596-8	Palmitamine	209-113-1	DL-Tyrosine	215-347-5	Sodium decylbenzene sulfonate
205-597-3	Oleyl alcohol	209-150-3	Magnesium stearate		
205-633-8	Sodium bicarbonate	209-151-9	Zinc stearate	215-350-1	Myristyl lactate
205-695-6	Tartaric acid	209-155-0	Zinc undecylenate	215-354-3	Propylene glycol stearate
205-702-2	Proline	209-183-3	Polyvinyl alcohol		
205-713-2	Sodium methyl stearoyl taurate	209-329-6	6-Nitro-o-toluidine	215-355-9	Glyceryl hydroxystear-ate
		209-386-7	1,6-Naphthalenediol		
205-738-9	Sodium methyl stearoyl taurate	209-406-4	Dioctyl sodium sulfosuccinate	215-356-4	Dinonyl phenol
				215-359-0	Glyceryl distearate
205-749-9	Gallic acid	209-478-7	2,7-Naphthalenediol	215-475-1	Aluminum silicate
205-753-0	PABA	209-529-3	Potassium carbonate	215-477-2	Aluminum chloro-hydrate
205-758-8	Trisodium EDTA	209-567-0	Maltitol		
205-759-3	HEDTA	209-677-9	Potassium cyanate	215-549-3	Propylene glycol oleate
205-788-1	Sodium lauryl sulfate	209-711-2	m-Aminophenol	215-551-4	Dodecylbenzyl-trimonium chloride
205-972-1	Thioxanthine	209-786-1	Potassium stearate		
206-074-2	Potassium D-gluconate	209-813-7	Guanidine carbonate	215-559-8	Ammonium dodecyl-benzene sulfonate
206-075-8	Calcium gluconate	210-060-1	2-Amino-3-nitrophenol		
206-101-8	Aluminum distearate	210-236-8	4-Amino-3-nitrophenol	215-663-3	Sorbitan laurate
206-103-9	Oleamide	210-431-8	Toluene-2,5-diamine sulfate	215-664-9	Sorbitan stearate
206-104-4	Lead acetate			215-665-4	Sorbitan oleate
206-156-8	Potassium sodium tartrate	210-702-0	Tricaprin	215-68-32	Silica, hydrated
		210-827-0	Glycol dilaurate	215-681-1	Magnesium silicate
206-370-1	Potassium thiocyanate	211-014-3	Glycol distearate	215-684-8	Sodium silicoaluminate
206-376-4	Capric acid	211-020-6	Dimethyl adipate	215-687-4	Sodium silicate
206-759-6	Citrulline	211-103-7	Cetyl acetate	215-691-6	Alumina
207-334-8	Linolenic acid	211-119-4	Arachidyl alcohol	215-710-8	Calcium silicate
207-334-9	Hydrogenated vegetable glycerides citrate	211-279-5	Aluminum tristearate	215-711-3	Ultramarines
		211-284-2	TEA hydrochloride	215-721-8	Iron oxides
		211-466-1	Isobutyl stearate	215-724-4	Carmine
207-355-2	Camphor	211-533-5	Hexamidine diisethionate	215-744-3	Chitin
207-439-9	Calcium carbonate			215-753-2	Tannic acid
207-444-6	Glycyrrhetinic acid	211-546-6	Behenyl alcohol	215-785-7	Glycyrrhizic acid
207-677-3	Glucamine	211-669-5	Lauryl betaine	215-798-8	Tocopherol
207-701-2	Guaiazulene	211-748-4	Cetyl betaine	215-968-1	Lauraminopropionic acid
207-757-8	Glucose	211-750-5	Distearyl thiodipropio-nate		
207-993-1	Stearone			215-976-5	Quaternium-51

EINECS	Chemical	EINECS	Chemical	EINECS	Chemical
216-133-4	Acetyl hexamethyl tetralin	222-059-3	Myristamine oxide	226-097-1	Laureth-4
216-343-6	Sodium isethionate	222-182-2	Triclosan	226-159-8	Dimethyl isosorbide
216-472-8	Calcium stearate	222-206-1	PEG-9	226-164-5	2-Nitro-p-phenylenediamine
216-699-2	Tetrabutyl ammonium bromide	222-264-8	Sodium undecylenate	226-242-9	Octyl dodecanol
		222-269-5	Cyclopentane carboxylic acid	226-243-4	Heptylundecanol
216-700-6	Lauramine oxide	222-273-7	Tetrasodium dicarboxyethyl stearyl sulfosuccinamate	226-300-9	Myristyl propionate
217-210-5	Dichlorobenzyl alcohol			226-312-9	PEG-9 stearate
217-325-0	Dicetyl dimonium chloride			226-546-1	Lactamide MEA
217-431-7	Sodium lauryl sulfoacetate	222-274-2	Dilauryldimonium chloride	226-775-7	Octyl methoxycinnamate
217-752-2	t-Butyl hydroquinone	222-311-2	Glucosamine	227-335-7	Calcium stearoyl lactylate
218-320-6	Phenyl trimethicone	222-581-1	Cetyl phosphate	227-729-9	Sorbitan laurate
218-531-3	TEA-salicylate	222-597-9	Sodium lauraminopropionate	228-227-2	Isostearamidopropyl betaine
218-793-9	Ammonium lauryl sulfate	222-700-7	Calcium behenate	228-229-3	Propylene glycol distearate
218-901-4	Glyceryl linoleate	222-848-2	Magnesium gluconate	228-250-8	Octocrylene
219-136-9	PEG-6 laurate	222-899-0	Disodium lauriminodipropionate	228-291-1	2-Chloro-p-phenylenediamine sulfate
219-145-8	Laurylamine dipropylenediamine	222-977-4	3-Aminopropane sulfonic acid	228-292-7	N,N-Dimethyl-p-phenylenediamine sulfate
219-163-6	D&C Red No. 30	222-980-4	Oleyl oleate		
219-370-1	2-Hexyl-1-decanol	222-981-6	Decyl oleate	228-293-2	4-Nitro-o-phenylenediamine HCl
219-919-5	Stearamine oxide	223-024-5	Bispyrithione		
220-020-5	Decylamine oxide	223-095-2	Denatonium benzoate NF	228-464-1	Lapyrium chloride
220-045-1	PEG-6			228-486-1	PEG-2 dilaurate
220-120-9	Saccharin	223-114-4	Sodium methyl palmitoyl taurate	228-504-8	Lauryl lactate
220-219-7	Ditridecyl sodium sulfosuccinate	223-267-7	Tetrasodium etidronate	228-973-9	Sodium erythorbate
220-239-6	Methylisothiazolinone	223-296-5	Sodium pyrithione	229-222-8	DMDM hydantoin
220-336-3	Isostearic acid	223-470-0	2-Butyl-1-octanol	229-349-9	Calcium saccharin
220-476-5	Stearyl stearate	223-772-2	Benzophenone-4	229-350-4	Manganese gluconate
220-552-8	Etidronic acid	223-779-0	Ethyl aspartate	229-457-6	Hydroxymethyl dioxoazabicyclooctane
220-562-2	D&C Red No. 36	223-795-8	Calcium propionate		
220-618-6	4-Amino-2-hydroxytoluene	223-805-0	Quaternium-15	229-859-1	PEG-12
		224-027-4	Phenoxyisopropanol	229-930-7	Lauryl diethylenediaminoglycine
220-688-8	Dimethylaminoethyl methacrylate	224-069-3	Isopropylparaben		
		224-126-2	Allantoin acetyl methionine	230-429-0	Palmitamine oxide
220-836-1	Dioctyl succinate	224-160-8	Glycol palmitate	230-457-3	Trioctyl citrate
220-851-3	Sodium octoxynol-2 ethane sulfonate	224-208-8	Isobutylparaben	230-525-2	Didecyldimonium chloride
221-014-5	N-Methyl-3-nitro-p-phenylenediamine	224-292-6	Lauramidopropyl betaine	230-636-6	Carotene
221-109-1	Dihexyl sodium sulfosuccinate	224-388-8	Sodium methyl lauroyl taurate	230-698-4	Lauralkonium bromide
		224-403-8	Tocopheryl succinate	230-743-8	Pentaerythrityl tetraoctanoate
221-123-8	Pentaerythrityl tetraoctanoate	224-506-8	Isohexadecane		
221-188-2	Sodium tridecyl sulfate	224-540-3	Trideceth-3	230-770-5	Nonoxynol-4
221-279-7	Laureth-2	224-580-1	Sodium dehydroacetate	230-785-7	Tetrapotassium pyrophosphate
221-280-2	Laureth-3	224-772-5	Lithium stearate		
221-281-8	Laureth-5	224-886-5	Laureth-1	230-896-0	Trioctanoin
221-282-3	Laureth-6	224-945-5	TEA-stearate	230-898-1	Aluminum formate
221-283-9	Laureth-7	225-004-1	Farnesol	230-962-9	Propylene glycol dicaprylate
221-284-4	Laureth-9	225-173-1	N-Phenyl-p-phenylenediamine sulfate		
221-286-5	Laureth-12			230-990-1	Didecyl methylamine
221-416-0	Sodium laureth sulfate			231-057-1	Octyl octanoate
221-450-6	Magnesium lauryl sulfate	225-190-4	Potassium lauryl sulfate	231-119-8	Potassium
		225-214-3	MEA-lauryl sulfate	231-211-8	Potassium chloride
221-498-8	Benzophenone-9	225-268-8	p-Ethylbenzaldehyde	231-298-2	Magnesium sulfate
221-573-5	Octrizole	225-373-9	Potassium PCA	231-306-4	Diisopropyl sebacate
221-588-7	Cetylamine hydrofluoride	225-404-6	Trimethylolpropane trioctanoate	231-426-7	Myristamide DEA
				231-427-2	Palmitamide DEA
221-661-3	Lauramidopropyl dimethylamine	225-714-1	Sodium methylparaben	231-449-2	Sodium phosphate
		225-856-4	PEG-8	231-493-2	Cyclodextrin
221-662-9	Diethylaminoethyl stearate	225-876-3	4-Nitro-m-phenylenediamine	231-545-4	Diatomaceous earth
				231-548-0	Sodium bisulfite
221-761-7	4-Isopropyl-m-cresol	225-878-4	Butoxypropanol	231-592-0	Zinc chloride
221-787-9	Myristyl myristate	226-029-0	Etocrylene	231-598-3	Sodium chloride
				231-609-1	Stearamidopropyl

EINECS	Chemical	EINECS	Chemical	EINECS	Chemical
	dimethylamine		chloride		silicate
231-633-2	Phosphoric acid	232-452-1	Hydrogenated lanolin	235-777-7	Polyglyceryl-2 stearate
231-659-4	Potassium iodide	232-453-7	Mineral spirits	235-798-1	Lauryl phosphate
231-672-5	Sodium iodate	232-455-8	Mineral oil	235-811-0	Ultramarines
231-673-0	Sodium metabisulfite	232-474-1	Olibanum	235-907-2	Sodium capryloampho-
231-694-5	Sodium tripolyphos-	232-475-7	Rosin		acetate
	phate	232-491-4	Sodium tallowate	235-911-4	Zinc ricinoleate
231-710-0	Tocopheryl acetate	232-494-0	Sodium tallow sulfate	235-946-5	Pentaerythrityl
231-721-0	Disodium capryloam-	232-501-7	Valerian extract		tetralaurate
	phodiacetate	232-519-5	Acacia	236-149-5	Disodium lauryl
231-722-6	Sulfur	232-523-7	Gum benzoin		sulfosuccinate
231-765-0	Hydrogen peroxide	232-524-2	Carrageenan	236-164-7	Lauryl hydroxysultaine
231-767-1	Tetrasodium	232-536-8	Guar gum	236-671-3	Zinc pyrithione
	pyrophosphate	232-541-5	Locust bean gum	236-675-5	Titanium dioxide
231-810-4	7-Ethyl bicyclo-	232-553-0	Pectin	236-935-8	Triundecanoin
	oxazolidine	232-554-6	Gelatin	236-942-6	Sodium lauroyl lactylate
231-831-9	Potassium iodate	232-555-1	Milk protein	237-875-5	Ferric ferrocyanide
231-896-3	Tristearyl citrate	232-601-0	Glucose oxidase	238-303-7	Sodium caproampho-
231-900-3	Calcium sulfate	232-619-9	Lipase		acetate
	(anhydrous)	232-668-6	Lactoperoxidase	238-305-8	Sodium lauroamphoac-
231-913-4	Potassium phosphate	232-674-9	Cellulose		etate
232-055-3	Ammonium alum	232-675-4	Dextrin	238-306-3	Disodium lauroampho-
232-122-7	Bismuth oxychloride	232-678-0	Hyaluronic acid		diacetate
232-160-4	Sodium bromate	232-679-6	Corn starch	238-310-5	Stearamide MEA-
232-271-8	Egg oil	232-680-1	Alginic acid		stearate
232-273-9	Sunflower seed oil	232-683-8	Glycogen	238-311-0	Oleamine oxide
232-274-4	Soybean oil	232-696-9	Sodium chondroitin	238-430-8	Pentaerythrityl
232-276-5	Safflower oil		sulfate		tetrapelargonate
232-277-0	Olive oil	232-697-4	Collagen	238-457-5	Trilinolenin
232-280-7	Cottonseed oil	232-697-4	Soluble collagen	238-479-5	Disodium stearyl
232-281-2	Corn oil	232-723-4	Zinc rosinate		sulfosuccinamate
232-282-8	Coconut oil	232-734-4	Cellulase	238-501-3	Steapyrium chloride
232-288-0	Balsam copaiba	232-752-2	Protease	238-588-8	Benzylhemiformal
232-289-6	Cod liver oil	232-885-6	Pectinase	238-877-9	Talc
232-290-1	Ceresin	232-936-2	Serum albumin	239-032-7	Sodium lauriminodipro-
232-292-2	Hydrogenated castor oil	232-940-4	Maltodextrin		pionate
232-293-8	Castor oil	233-135-0	Aluminum sulfate	239-139-9	3-Benzylidene camphor
232-296-4	Peanut oil	233-136-6	Boron nitride	239-360-0	Acetyl hexamethyl
232-298-5	Petroleum distillates	233-140-8	Calcium chloride		indan
232-306-7	Sulfated castor oil	233-257-4	Manganese violet	240-357-1	p-Phenylenediamine
232-307-2	Lecithin	233-293-0	PEG-4 oleate		sulfate
232-309-3	Liver extract	233-343-1	Sodium hexametaphos-	240-736-1	TEA lauroyl sarcosinate
232-311-4	Menhaden oil		phate	240-795-3	Potassium metabisulfite
232-313-5	Montan wax	233-520-3	PEG-2 stearamine	240-865-3	Behenalkonium chloride
232-315-6	Paraffin	233-549-1	N,N´-Dimethyl-N-	240-886-8	2-Amino-3-hydroxy-
232-316-1	Palm oil		hydroxyethyl-3-nitro-p-		pyridine
232-347-0	Candelilla wax		phenylenediamine	240-924-3	Stearamidoethyl
232-348-6	Lanolin	233-560-1	Isopropyl laurate		diethylamine
232-360-1	Sorbitan sesquioleate	233-561-7	PEG-3 oleate	241-029-0	Ditridecyl dimer
232-370-6	Sesame oil	233-562-2	PEG-3 stearate		dilinoleate
232-371-1	Garlic extract	233-641-1	PEG-14 stearate	241-327-0	Behentrimonium
232-373-2	Petrolatum	233-864-4	Cetyl ricinoleate		chloride
232-384-2	Mineral oil	234-169-9	Stearyl benzoate	241-637-6	Cetylarachidol
232-391-0	Epoxidized soybean oil	234-242-5	Chlorophyllin-copper	241-640-2	Cetyl esters
232-399-4	Carnauba		complex	241-640-2	Myristyl stearate
232-409-7	Rice bran wax	234-316-7	Polyglyceryl-10	241-646-5	Behenyl behenate
232-410-2	Hydrogenated soybean		decaoleate	241-654-9	Oleyl erucate
	oil	234-325-6	Glyceryl stearate	241-727-5	TEA oleoyl sarcosinate
232-425-4	Palm kernel oil	234-328-2	Retinol	242-159-0	Tin oxide (ic)
232-428-0	Avocado oil	234-394-2	Xanthan gum	242-200-2	Stearyl caprylate
232-430-1	Lanolin alcohol	234-406-6	Quaternium-18	242-201-8	Behenyl erucate
232-433-8	Bitter orange peel		hectorite	242-347-2	Glyceryl linolenate
	extract	234-988-1	Calcium titanate	242-349-3	Sodium methyl
232-438-5	Cottonseed glyceride	235-088-1	Sodium toluenesulfo-		myristoyl taurate
232-439-0	Ichthammol		nate	242-354-0	Chlorhexidine
232-440-6	Hydroxylated lecithin	235-186-4	Ammonium chloride		digluconate
232-442-7	Hydrogenated tallow	235-340-0	Hectorite	242-471-7	Tribehenin
232-447-4	Tallowtrimonium	235-374-6	Magnesium aluminum	242-553-2	Stearoxytrimethylsilane

EINECS	Chemical	EINECS	Chemical	EINECS	Chemical
242-703-7	Magnesium aspartate	247-660-8	Ditridecyl adipate	250-696-7	Tridecyl stearate
242-769-1	Potassium cetyl phosphate	247-667-6	Glyceryl caprate	250-704-9	Isodecyl stearate
		247-668-1	Glyceryl caprylate	250-705-4	Glyceryl stearate
242-930-1	Stearamidopropyl trimonium methosulfate	247-669-7	Propylene glycol ricinoleate	250-913-5	Sodium cumenesulfonate
242-960-5	Pentaerythrityl tetraoleate	247-706-7	Sucrose palmitate	251-035-5	Quaternium-24
		247-710-9	Ammonium xylenesulfonate	251-110-2	2-Tetradecyloctadecanol
243-468-3	Diiodomethyl p-tolyl sulfone	247-730-8	Behenamine oxide	251-136-4	Dibenzylidene sorbitol
243-697-9	Octyl laurate	247-784-2	DEA-dodecylbenzene sulfonate	251-306-8	Palmitamidopropyl betaine
243-835-8	Ricinoleamidopropyl dimethylamine	247-816-5	Nonoxynol-8	251-646-7	Diisononyl adipate
243-846-8	TEA-lactate	247-873-6	Disodium undecylenamido MEA-sulfosuccinate	251-732-4	Glycol hydroxystearate
243-870-9	Undecylenamide MEA			251-734-5	Propylene glycol hydroxystearate
244-063-4	Diammonium EDTA				
244-071-8	Cetyl laurate	247-886-7	Glyceryl dipalmitate	251-932-1	Hexyl laurate
244-158-0	Quaternium-45	247-887-2	Glyceryl palmitate	251-993-4	Lauryl aminopropylglycine
244-238-5	MIPA-lauryl sulfate	247-891-4	Sorbitan tristearate		
244-289-3	Octyl dimethyl PABA	247-911-1	Glyceryl adipate	252-011-7	Polyglyceryl-10 tetraoleate
244-492-7	Aluminum hydroxide	247-919-5	Isopropyl arachidate		
244-501-4	Oleyl hydroxyethyl imidazoline	247-922-1	Isopropyl behenate	252-447-8	Stearyl lactate
		248-016-9	Myreth-3	252-478-7	Cetyl lactate
244-754-0	Octyl stearate	248-030-5	Disodium lauryl sulfosuccinate	252-487-6	Sodium ethylparaben
244-950-6	Cetyl oleate			252-488-1	Sodium propylparaben
245-204-2	Octyldodecyl stearate	248-248-0	Oleyl hydroxyethyl imidazoline	252-637-0	Cholesteryl stearate
245-217-3	Propylene glycol dilaurate	248-289-4	Dodecylbenzene sulfonic acid	252-681-0	Methyldibromo glutaronitrile
245-228-3	Octyldodecyl oleate	248-291-5	Nonoxynol-2	252-964-9	Isocetyl alcohol
245-289-6	Isopropyl linoleate	248-292-0	Nonoxynol-7	253-149-0	Cetyl alcohol
245-767-4	Hexyl nicotinate	248-293-6	Nonoxynol-8	253-242-6	4-Methylbenzylidene camphor
246-115-1	Stearyl behenate	248-294-1	Nonoxynol-10		
246-376-1	Potassium sorbate	248-299-9	Diisodecyl adipate	253-363-4	Olealkonium chloride
246-563-8	BHA	248-299-9	Diisopropyl adipate	253-379-1	Methyldihydrojasmonate
246-584-2	Oleamidopropyl betaine	248-317-5	Sucrose distearate		
246-598-9	Stearamidopropylamine oxide	248-351-0	Glyceryl triacetyl hydroxystearate	253-407-2	Glyceryl oleate
				253-458-0	PEG-8 laurate
246-675-7	Methylbenzethonium chloride	248-403-2	Polyglyceryl-3 stearate	253-519-1	Ammonium cumenesulfonate
246-680-4	Sodium dodecylbenzenesulfonate	248-406-9	TEA-dodecylbenzenesulfonate	253-981-4	Sodium myristoyl glutamate
246-684-6	Oleamidopropylamine oxide	248-470-8	Isostearyl alcohol	254-161-9	Hydroxyanthraquinoneaminopropyl methyl morpholinium methosulfate
		248-486-5	Quaternium-14		
246-705-9	Sucrose stearate	248-515-1	Ethyl urocanate		
246-868-6	Isocetyl stearate	248-586-9	Glyceryl dilaurate		
246-873-3	Sucrose laurate	248-587-4	Erucyl erucate	254-372-6	Imidazolidinyl urea
246-914-5	Undecylenamide DEA	248-762-5	Nonoxynol-1	254-495-5	Polyglyceryl-10 decastearate
246-929-7	Sodium stearoyl lactylate	248-812-6	Glyceryl erucate		
		248-938-7	Sodium cumenesulfonate	254-585-4	Palmitamidopropyl dimethylamine
246-985-2	Sodium trideceth sulfate	249-277-1	Sodium PCA	255-051-3	Ricinoleamide DEA
246-986-8	Sodium myreth sulfate	249-395-3	Propylene glycol myristate	255-062-3	Disodium laureth sulfosuccinate
247-144-2	Glyceryl dioleate				
247-144-2	PPG-27 glyceryl ether	249-448-0	Sorbitan dioleate	255-350-9	Propylene glycol dipelargonate
247-310-4	Disodium lauramido MEA-sulfosuccinate	249-649-3	Isolongifolene ketone exo	255-485-3	Isostearyl isostearate
				255-490-0	Dipalmitoyl hydroxyproline
247-464-2	Potassium methylparaben	249-689-1	Farnesyl acetate		
		249-862-1	Octyl palmitate	255-537-5	Dicapryloyl cystine
247-500-7	Methylchloroisothiazolinone	249-958-3	Sodium lauroyl glutamate	255-674-0	Isostearyl lactate
				255-728-3	Arachidyl behenate
247-536-3	Sodium tridecylbenzene sulfonate	249-992-9	Nonoxynol-6 phosphate	255-854-3	MIPA-dodecylbenzenesulfonate
		250-001-7	5-Bromo-5-nitro-1,3-dioxane		
247-555-7	Nonoxynol-5			255-999-8	2-Methoxy-p-phenylene diamine sulfate
247-556-2	Isopropylamine dodecylbenzenesulfonate	250-097-0	Glyceryl behenate		
		250-151-3	Sodium myristoyl sarcosinate	256-095-6	Diethyl aspartate
247-568-8	Sorbitan palmitate	250-215-0	Sodium stearoamphoacetate	256-120-0	Disodium oleamido MIPA-sulfosuccinate
247-569-3	Sorbitan trioleate				
247-655-0	Octyl stearate	250-651-1	Isopropyl isostearate	256-214-1	Myristamidopropyl

EINECS	Chemical	EINECS	Chemical	EINECS	Chemical
	dimethylamine		glyceride sulfate	266-124-4	Glyceryl isostearate
257-048-2	Dimethyl oxazolidine	263-027-9	Glyceryl cocoate	266-138-0	2-Hydroxyethylamino-5-
257-440-3	Quaternium-22	263-031-0	Hydrogenated tallow		nitroanisole
257-835-0	Ethyl butylacetylamino-		glyceride	266-357-1	2,4-Diaminophenoxy-
	propionate	263-032-6	Lard glyceride		ethanol HCl
257-843-4	Lauroyl lysine	263-035-2	Tallow glyceride	266-533-8	Sodium isostearoyl
258-007-1	Myristoyl sarcosine	263-038-9	Cocotrimonium chloride		lactylate
258-193-4	Isostearamide DEA	263-049-9	Potassium cocoate	266-778-0	Isostearamidopropyl
258-377-8	Behenamidopropyl	263-050-4	Sodium cocoate		ethyldimonium
	ethyldimonium	263-052-5	Sodium cocoyl		ethosulfate
	ethosulfate		isethionate	266-778-0	Isostearyl ethyl-
258-476-2	Sodium magnesium	263-058-8	Cocamidopropyl		imidonium ethosulfate
	silicate		betaine	266-948-4	Triolein
258-629-3	Glyceryl dimyristate	263-080-8	Benzalkonium chloride	267-015-4	Methyl oleate
258-636-1	TEA-lauroyl glutamate	263-081-3	Hydrogenated	267-048-4	Ethyl butyl valero-
258-987-1	Cyclocarboxypropyl-		tallowalkonium chloride		lactone
	oleic acid	263-086-0	Dicocamine	267-054-7	Propylene glycol soyate
259-218-1	Decyl glucoside	263-087-6	Dicocodimonium	267-101-1	Isostearamidopropyl
259-583-7	2-Methyl-5-hydroxy-		chloride		dimethylamine
	ethylaminophenol	263-089-7	Hydrogenated	267-360-0	Stearamidopropyl
259-837-7	Stearamidopropyl		ditallowamine		ethyldimonium
	dimethylamine lactate	263-090-2	Quaternium-18		ethosulfate
259-860-2	Stearamidopropyl	263-107-3	Tall oil acid	267-617-7	Disodium ricinoleamido
	morpholine lactate	263-112-0	Soyamine		MEA-sulfosuccinate
260-081-5	Arginine PCA	263-125-1	Tallow amine	267-791-4	Sodium octoxynol-2
260-143-1	Disodium oleamido	263-129-3	Tallow acid		ethane sulfonate
	PEG-2 sulfosuccinate	263-130-9	Hydrogenated tallow	267-821-6	Polyglyceryl-2
260-410-2	Linoleamide DEA		acid		diisostearate
261-521-9	Isostearyl neo-	263-134-0	Soytrimonium chloride	268-093-2	Trimethylpropane
	pentanoate	263-155-5	TEA cocoate		trioleate
261-619-1	Cetearyl octanoate	263-163-9	Cocamide DEA	268-130-2	Ammonium lauroyl
261-619-1	Cetyl octanoate	263-167-0	Soyaethyl morpholinium		sarcosinate
261-673-6	Isodecyl oleate		ethosulfate	268-164-8	4-Ethoxy-m-
261-678-3	Menthyl lactate	263-170-7	Cocoyl hydroxyethyl		phenylenediamine
261-684-6	Myristamidopropyl		imidazoline		sulfate
	betaine	263-171-2	Tall oil hydroxyethyl	268-213-3	Sodium C14-17 alkyl
261-819-9	Octyl pelargonate		imidazoline		sec sulfonate
261-931-8	Aluminum PCA	263-179-6	Dihydroxyethyl	268-264-1	2,4-Dimethyl-3-
261-940-7	3-Methylamino-4-		tallowamine oxide		cyclohexene
	nitrophenoxyethanol	263-180-1	Dihydroxyethyl		carboxyaldehyde
262-108-6	Isodecyl neopentanoate		cocamine oxide	268-595-1	Trimethylolpropane
262-134-8	Behenamidopropyl	263-190-6	Disodium tallowimino-		tricaprylate/tricaprate
	dimethylamine		dipropionate	268-761-3	Cocamidopropyl
262-710-9	Glyceryl isostearate	263-193-2	Sodium cocoyl		hydroxysultaine
262-740-2	Dibehenyl methylamine		sarcosinate	268-770-2	Cocamide MEA
262-774-8	Isopropyl titanium	263-218-7	Lauramidopropylamine	268-771-8	Cocamidopropyl
	triisostearate		oxide		dimethylamine
262-895-6	Pentaerythrityl	263-847-7	p-Aminophenol sulfate	268-820-3	Ethyl hydroxymethyl
	tetrabehenate	264-038-1	Microcrystalline wax		oleyl oxazoline
262-976-6	Hydrogenated	264-043-9	Isopropyl dibenzoyl-	268-938-5	Cocamidopropylamine
	tallowamine		methane		oxide
262-977-1	Cocamine	264-119-1	Isopropyl lanolate	268-949-5	Tallamide DEA
262-978-7	Coconut acid	264-391-1	Dibutyl lauroyl	269-027-5	Propylene glycol
262-979-2	Acetylated lanolin		glutamate		isostearate
262-980-8	Acetylated lanolin	265-352-1	Cetrimonium	269-084-6	TEA-cocoyl-glutamate
	alcohol		methosulfate	269-087-2	Sodium cocoyl
262-988-1	Methyl cocoate	265-363-1	Hydrolyzed milk protein		glutamate
262-991-8	Dihydrogenated tallow	265-417-4	DEA-lauramino-	269-220-4	Lanolin wax
	methylamine		propionate	269-473-0	3-Ethylamino-p-cresol
263-005-9	Hydrogenated	265-648-0	3-Nitro-p-hydroxyethyl-		sulfate
	tallowtrimonium		aminophenol	269-475-1	m-Aminophenol sulfate
	chloride	265-672-1	Disodium ricinoleamido	269-478-8	N,N-Diethyl-m-
263-016-9	Cocamine oxide		MEA-sulfosuccinate		aminophenol sulfate
263-017-4	Dimethyl soyamine	265-724-3	Caprylic/capric	269-547-2	Sodium lauroampho-
263-020-0	Dimethyl cocamine		triglyceride		acetate
263-022-1	Dimethyl hydrogenated	265-839-9	Arachidyl propionate	269-657-0	Soy acid
	tallow amine	265-880-2	Stearamidopropal-	269-658-6	Hydrogenated tallow
263-026-3	Sodium cocomono-		konium chloride		glycerides

EINECS	Chemical	EINECS	Chemical	EINECS	Chemical
269-662-8	Coco-ethyldimonium ethosulfate		glycyrrhizate	285-203-4	Propylene glycol dioleate
269-793-0	Cocamide MIPA	272-336-8	Tricetyl phosphate	285-206-0	Ethyl oleate
269-804-9	Hydrogenated cottonseed oil	272-385-5	Ammonium C12-15 alkyl sulfate	285-540-7	Isopropyl oleate
269-819-0	Sodium cocoamphoac-etate	272-574-2	Piroctone olamine	285-547-5	Pentaerythrityl stearate
		272-897-9	Disodium cocoampho-dipropionate	285-550-1	PEG-2 stearate
269-820-6	Hydrogenated vegetable oil	272-964-2	Quaternium-70	286-074-7	Sorbitan trioleate
269-919-4	Benzalkonium chloride	273-049-0	Methyl glucose sesquistearate	286-490-9	Glyceryl stearate
270-131-8	Disodium cocoampho-dipropionate			286-541-5	Zinc citrate
270-156-4	Cocoyl sarcosine	273-187-1	Minkamidopropyl dimethylamine	287-089-1	Benzalkonium chloride
270-302-7	Lanolin acid	273-219-4	Quaternium-18 bentonite	287-462-9	Ricinoleamidopropyl trimonium methosulfate
270-304-8	Linseed acid			287-484-9	Stearyl stearate
270-315-8	Hydroxylated lanolin	273-222-0	Quaternium-26	287-824-6	Methyl stearate
270-325-2	Benzalkonium chloride	273-277-0	Ethylene distearamide	288-459-5	PEG-12 dioleate
270-329-4	Coco-betaine	273-313-5	Vegetable oil	288-668-1	Isobutyl stearate
270-350-9	Hydrogenated peanut oil	273-429-6	Isostearyl hydroxyethyl imidazoline	289-296-2	Menthoxypropanediol
				289-688-3	Bitter cherry extract
270-351-4	Coconut alcohol	273-576-6	Hydrogenated tallow glyceride lactate	289-752-0	Lemongrass extract
270-355-6	Soyamide DEA			289-888-0	Wintergreen extract
270-356-1	Tallowamidopropyl dimethylamine	273-612-0	Acetylated hydroge-nated tallow glyceride	289-904-6	Grapefruit seed extract
270-407-8	Sodium C14-16 olefin sulfonate	273-613-6	Hydrogenated tallow glyceride citrate	289-960-1	Jasmine extract
				289-964-3	Jojoba extract
270-474-3	Pentaerythrityl tetracaprylate/caprate	273-616-2	Shark liver oil	289-991-0	Octyldodecyl stearoyl stearate
270-593-0	Undecylpentadecanol	274-001-1	Hydrolyzed keratin	290-580-3	Distearyl phthalate
270-664-6	Montan acid wax	274-033-6	Behenoyl-PG-trimonium chloride	291-990-5	Soyamidopropyl ethyldimonium ethosulfate
270-864-3	Disodium oleamido MEA-sulfosuccinate	274-269-9	Disodium oleoampho-diacetate		
271-102-2	Disodium cocamido MIPA-sulfosuccinate	274-357-8	Sodium hydroxymethyl-glycinate	292-416-6	Isodecyl citrate
				292-945-2	Ethyl stearate
271-347-5	Trimethylolpropane triisostearate	274-581-6	Butyl methoxy dibenzoyl methane	292-951-5	Isooctyl stearate
				293-029-5	Pentaerythrityl tetrastearate
271-397-8	Rice bran oil	274-695-6	Sodium lauroyl taurate	293-255-4	Honey extract
271-694-2	Pentaerythrityl tetraoleate	274-845-0	Dihydroxyethyl tallow glycinate	293-306-0	Acetylated hydroge-nated lanolin
271-705-0	Sodium cocoamphohy-droxypropyl sulfonate	274-923-4	Cocamidopropyl betaine	293-391-2	Myreth-3 palmitate
				293-509-4	Hydrolyzed fibronectin
271-762-1	Tallowdimonium propyltrimonium dichloride	275-286-5	Synthetic beeswax	294-930-6	Cauliflower unsaponifiables
		275-637-2	Octyl isononanoate	295-366-3	Octyl cocoate
		276-553-9	Diethylene glycol dioctanoate	295-786-7	Hydrogenated lecithin
271-792-5	Disodium capryloam-phodiacetate	276-627-0	2-Dodecylhexadecanol	296-473-8	Kaolin
		276-719-0	Isostearyl palmitate	297-495-0	PEG-3 tallow propylenedimonium dimethosulfate
271-793-0	Sodium cocoampho-acetate	276-951-2	Sorbitan tristearate		
271-929-9	Sodium isostearo-amphopropionate	278-928-2	Diazolidinyl urea	298-364-0	Pentaerythrityl tetraisononanoate
		279-383-3	2-Nitro-5-glyceryl methylaniline	306-522-8	Glycol stearate
271-949-8	Sodium lauroamphoac-etate	279-917-5	Dioctyldodecyl lauroyl glutamate	306-998-7	Tallowamphopoly-carboxypropionic acid
271-951-9	Sodium caproampho-acetate	281-689-7	Wheat extract	307-455-7	Cocoiminodipropionate
		281-689-7	Wheat germ extract	307-458-3	Cocoamphopolycarbox-yglycinate
271-972-3	Tallowamidopropyl-amine oxide	283-078-0	Pentaerythrityl tetrabehenate	307-458-3	Disodium oleoampho-diacetate
272-021-5	Cocaminobutyric acid	283-390-7	Myreth-3 laurate		
272-043-5	Disodium cocoampho-diacetate	283-479-0	Cinnamon extract	307-458-3	Sodium carboxymethyl oleyl polypropylamine
		283-481-1	Coffee bean extract		
272-046-1	Apricot extract	283-481-1	Coffee extract	307-458-3	Sodium carboxymethyl tallow polypropylamine
272-190-5	Disoyamine	283-652-0	Rose extract		
272-207-6	Ditallow dimonium chloride	283-854-9	Dioctyl cyclohexane	309-206-8	Cocobetainamido amphopropionate
		283-993-5	Jasmine extract		
272-219-1	Disodium cocamido MEA-sulfosuccinate	284-219-9	Cocaminopropionic acid	309-696-3	Hydrolyzed wheat protein
		284-653-9	Tansy extract		
272-296-1	Dipotassium	284-868-8	Isobutyl oleate		

Trade Name Status Reference

Abil® 281. [Goldschmidt] Polysiloxane polyether copolymer.†

Abil® B 8. [Goldschmidt] Polysiloxane polyether copolymer.†

Abil® B 9800, B 9801. [Goldschmidt] Polysiloxane polyalkylene copolymer.†

Abil® B 9905, B 9907, B 9908, B 9909. [Goldschmidt] Polysiloxane polydimethyl dimethylammonium acetate copolymer.†

Abil® K 520. [Goldschmidt] Hexamethyldisiloxane.*

Ablumine 280. [Taiwan Surf.] Stearyl dimethyl benzyl ammonium chloride.†

Accobetaine CL. [Karlshamns] Complex coco betaine.†

Acconon 200-DL. [Karlshamns] PEG-4 dilaurate.†

Acconon 300-MO. [Karlshamns] PEG 300 oleate.†

Acconon 400-DO. [Karlshamns] PEG-8 dioleate.†

Acconon 400-ML. [Karlshamns] PEG-8 laurate.†

Acconon CA-8. [Karlshamns] PEG-8 castor oil.†

Acconon CA-25. [Karlshamns] PEG-25 castor oil.†

Acconon GTO. [Karlshamns] Glyceryl trioleate.†

Acylglutamate CS-11. [Ajinomoto] Sodium cocoyl glutamate.†

Acylglutamate CS-21. [Ajinomoto] Disodium cocoyl glutamate.†

Acylglutamate CT-12. [Ajinomoto] TEA N-cocoyl-L-glutamate.†

Acylglutamate GS-11. [Ajinomoto] Sodium hydrogenated tallow glutamate, sodium cocoyl glutamate.†

Acylglutamate GS-21. [Ajinomoto] Disodium cocoyl/tallowyl glutamate.†

Acylglutamate HS-11. [Ajinomoto] Sodium hydrogeanted tallow glutamate.†

Acylglutamate HS-21. [Ajinomoto] Disodium stearoyl glutamate.†

Acylglutamate LS-11. [Ajinomoto] Sodium lauroyl glutamate.†

Acylglutamate LT-12. [Ajinomoto] TEA lauroyl glutamate.†

Acylglutamate MS-11. [Ajinomoto] Sodium myristoyl glutamate.†

AHP. [Henkel] Disodium azacycloheptane diphosphonate.*

Akypo RLM 100 MGV. [Chem-Y GmbH] Fatty alcohol polyglycol ether carboxylic acid, magnesium salt.†

Akypo RLM 130 NV. [Chem-Y GmbH] Fatty alcohol polyglycol ether carboxylate, Na salt.†

Akypo RLM 160 NV. [Chem-Y GmbH] Fatty alcohol polyglycol ether carboxylate, sodium salt.†

Alcodet® 218. [Rhone-Poulenc Surf. & Spec.] PEG-10 isolauryl thioether.*

Alconate® CPA. [Rhone-Poulenc Surf. & Spec.] Disodium cocamido MIPA sulfosuccinate.*

Alconate® SB-5. [Rhone-Poulenc Surf. & Spec.] Disodium laneth-5 sulfosuccinate.*

Alconate® SBFA 30. (redesignated Geropon® SBFA 30) [Rhone-Poulenc Surf. & Spec.] Disodium laureth sulfosuccinate.*

Alconate® SBG-280. [Rhone-Poulenc Surf. & Spec.] Disodium oleamido MEA-sulfosuccinate.*

Alconate® SBR-3. (redesignated Geropon® SBR-3) [Rhone-Poulenc Surf. & Spec.] .*

Aldo® ML. [Lonza] Glyceryl monodilaurate.†

Aldo® MOD FG. [Lonza] Glyceryl monodioleate, disp.†

Aldo® MS-20 FG. [Lonza] PEG-20 glyceryl stearate.†

Aldo® PMS. [Lonza] Propylene glycol stearate.†

Algogen. [Grant Industries] Water, algae extract, hydrolyzed collagen from marine sources.*

Alipal® CO-433. (redesignated Rhodapex® CO-433) [Rhone-Poulenc Surf. & Spec.] .*

Alipal® CO-436. (redesignated Rhodapex® CO-436) [Rhone-Poulenc Surf. & Spec.] .*

Alkamide® 101 CG. [Rhone-Poulenc Surf. & Spec.] Cocamide DEA, DEA.*

Alkamide® 1002. [Rhone-Poulenc Surf. & Spec.] 2:1 Cocamide DEA.*

Alkamide® 1182. [Rhone-Poulenc Surf. & Spec.] Lauramide DEA, modified.*

Alkamide® 1188. [Rhone-Poulenc Surf. & Spec.] Lauramide DEA.*

Alkamide® 2124. [Rhone-Poulenc Surf. & Spec.] 2:1 Lauramide DEA.*

Alkamide® CAA. [Rhone-Poulenc Surf. & Spec.] Cocamidopropyl dimethylamine.*

Alkamide® CMO. [Rhone-Poulenc Surf. & Spec.] Cocamide MEA.*

Alkamide® DL-203. [Rhone-Poulenc Surf. & Spec.] 2:1 Lauric diethanolamide.*

Alkamide® HTME. (see Alkamide® S-280) [Rhone-Poulenc Surf. & Spec.] Stearamide MEA.*

Alkamide® IS-DEA. [Rhone-Poulenc Surf. & Spec.] Isostearamide DEA.*

Alkamide® IS-MEA. [Rhone-Poulenc Surf. & Spec.] Linoleamide MEA.*

Alkamide® L7DE-BT. [Rhone-Poulenc Surf. & Spec.] Lauramide DEA.*

Alkamide® L7DE-PG. [Rhone-Poulenc Surf. & Spec.] Lauramide DEA.*

Alkamide® L7ME. (see Alkamide® L-203) [Rhone-Poulenc Surf. & Spec.] Lauramide MEA.*

Alkamide® L9ME. (see Alkamide® L-203) [Rhone-Poulenc Surf. & Spec.] Lauramide MEA.*

Alkamide® LIPA. (see Alkamide® LIPA/C) [Rhone-Poulenc Surf. & Spec.] Lauramide MIPA.*

Alkamox® CAPO. (redesignated Rhodamox® CAPO) [Rhone-Poulenc Surf. & Spec.] Cocamidopropylamine oxide.*

---

* Discontinued or redesignated   † Unverified   ‡ No longer standard

Alkamox® L20. [Rhone-Poulenc Surf. & Spec.] Lauramine oxide.*

Alkamox® LO. (redesignated Rhodamox® LO) [Rhone-Poulenc Surf. & Spec.] Lauramine oxide.*

Alkamuls® 200-DL. [Rhone-Poulenc Surf. & Spec.] PEG-4 dilaurate.*

Alkamuls® 200-DO. [Rhone-Poulenc Surf. & Spec.] PEG-4 dioleate.*

Alkamuls® 200-DS. [Rhone-Poulenc Surf. & Spec.] PEG-4 distearate.*

Alkamuls® 400-DL. [Rhone-Poulenc Surf. & Spec.] PEG-8 dilaurate.*

Alkamuls® 400-DS. [Rhone-Poulenc Surf. & Spec.] PEG-8 distearate.*

Alkamuls® 400-ML. [Rhone-Poulenc Surf. & Spec.] PEG-8 laurate.*

Alkamuls® 400-MS. [Rhone-Poulenc Surf. & Spec.] PEG-8 stearate.*

Alkamuls® 600-DL. [Rhone-Poulenc Surf. & Spec.] PEG-12 dilaurate.*

Alkamuls® 600-DS. [Rhone-Poulenc Surf. & Spec.] PEG-12 distearate.*

Alkamuls® 600-GML. [Rhone-Poulenc Surf. & Spec.] PEG-12 laurate.*

Alkamuls® 600-ML. [Rhone-Poulenc Surf. & Spec.] PEG-12 laurate.*

Alkamuls® 600-MO. [Rhone-Poulenc Surf. & Spec.] PEG-12 oleate.*

Alkamuls® 6000-DS. [Rhone-Poulenc Surf. & Spec.] PEG-150 distearate.*

Alkamuls® EPS. (see Rhodaterge EPS) [Rhone-Poulenc Surf. & Spec.] Modified alkylphenol ethoxylate.*

Alkamuls® GMO. [Rhone-Poulenc Surf. & Spec.] Glyceryl oleate.*

Alkamuls® GMO-45LG. [Rhone-Poulenc Surf. & Spec.] Glyceryl oleate.*

Alkamuls® MS-40. [Rhone-Poulenc Surf. & Spec.] Ethoxylated fatty acids.*

Alkamuls® PSMS-4. [Rhone-Poulenc Surf. & Spec.] Polysorbate 61.*

Alkamuls® PSTS-20. [Rhone-Poulenc Surf. & Spec.] Polysorbate 65.*

Alkamuls® STS. [Rhone-Poulenc Surf. & Spec.] Sorbitan tristearate.*

Alkapol PEG 300. [Rhone-Poulenc Surf. & Spec.] PEG-6.*

Alkapol PEG 400. (redesignated Rhodasurf® PEG 400) [Rhone-Poulenc Surf. & Spec.] PEG-9.*

Alkaquat® DMB-ST, 25%. (redesignated Rhodaquat® DMB-ST-25) [Rhone-Poulenc Surf. & Spec.] Stearalkonium chloride.*

Alkasurf® CA-2. [Rhone-Poulenc Surf. & Spec.] Ceteareth-2.*

Alkasurf® CA-4. [Rhone-Poulenc Surf. & Spec.] Ceteareth-4.*

Alkasurf® CA-20. [Rhone-Poulenc Surf. & Spec.] Ceteareth-20.*

Alkasurf® L-9. (redesignated Alkamuls® L-9) [Rhone-Poulenc Surf. & Spec.] PEG-9 laurate.*

Alkasurf® L-14. [Rhone-Poulenc Surf. & Spec.] PEG-14 laurate.*

Alkasurf® LAN-1. [Rhone-Poulenc Surf. & Spec.] Laureth-1.*

Alkasurf® LAN-12. [Rhone-Poulenc Surf. & Spec.] Laureth-12.*

Alkasurf® OP-1. (see Igepal® CA-210) [Rhone-Poulenc Surf. & Spec.] Octoxynol-1.*

Alkasurf® SA-20. [Rhone-Poulenc Surf. & Spec.] Steareth-20.*

Alkasurf® SS-L7DE. (redesignated Geropon® SS-L7DE) [Rhone-Poulenc Surf. & Spec.] .*

Alkasurf® SS-L9ME. (redesignated Geropon® SS-L9ME) [Rhone-Poulenc Surf. & Spec.] Disodium lauramido MEA-sulfosuccinate.*

Alkasurf® SS-LA-3. (see Geropon® SBFA-30) [Rhone-Poulenc Surf. & Spec.] Disodium laureth sulfosuccinate.*

Alkasurf® ST-40. [Rhone-Poulenc Surf. & Spec.] PEG-40 stearate.*

Alkasurf® T [Rhone-Poulenc Surf. & Spec.] TEA-dodecyl-benzene sulfonate, cosmetic grade.*

Alkasurf® TDA-10. [Rhone-Poulenc Surf. & Spec.] Trideceth-10.*

Alkasurf® TDA-12. [Rhone-Poulenc Surf. & Spec.] Trideceth-12.*

Alkasurf® TLS. [Rhone-Poulenc Surf. & Spec.] TEA-lauryl sulfate.*

Alkateric® 2CIB. (redesignated Miranol® 2CIB) [Rhone-Poulenc Surf. & Spec.] .*

Alkateric® CAB-A. (redesignated Mirataine® CAB-A) [Rhone-Poulenc Surf. & Spec.] .*

Alkateric® CB. (redesignated Mirataine® CB/M) [Rhone-Poulenc Surf. & Spec.] .*

Alkateric® CIB. [Rhone-Poulenc Surf. & Spec.] Sodium cocoamphoacetate.*

Alkateric® LAB. (see Mirataine® BB) [Rhone-Poulenc Surf. & Spec.] .*

Alkateric® PB. [Rhone-Poulenc Surf. & Spec.] Cetyl betaine.*

Aloe Powd. 1-200. [Apree] Aloe.*

Aloe Vera Conc. 1-40. [Apree] Aloe vera gel.*

Ameroxol® LE-4. [Amerchol; Amerchol Europe] Laureth-4.*

Ameroxol® LE-23. [Amerchol; Amerchol Europe] Laureth-23.*

Amfotex FV-10. [Pulcra SA] Dicarboxylic coconut deriv., sodium salt.†

Amfotex FV-16. [Pulcra SA] Monocarboxylic lauric deriv., sodium salt.†

Amfotex FV-28. [Pulcra SA] Cocamido betaine.†

Amifat P-21. [Ajinomoto; Ajinomoto USA] PCA glyceryl stearate.*

Amino Acid Gelatinization Agent. [Ajinomoto] N-Acyl glutamic acid diamide.†

Aminol LNO. [Finetex] Linoleamide DEA.*

Aminol OF. [Finetex] Oleamide DEA.†

Amisol™ 329. [Lucas Meyer] Lecithin.*

Ampholan® B-171. [Harcros UK] Betaine.†

Anhydrous Lanolin HP-2050. [Henkel/Cospha; Henkel Canada] Lanolin.†

Antarox® PGP 18-2D. [Rhone-Poulenc Surf. & Spec.] Ethoxylated propoxylated glycol.*

Antarox® PGP 18-4 .(see Antarox L-64) [Rhone-Poulenc Surf. & Spec.] Ethoxylated propoxylated glycol.*

Antarox® PGP 33-8. [Rhone-Poulenc Surf. & Spec.] Ethoxylated propoxylated glycol.*

Aquasol 104. [Apree] Aloe vera gel.*

Aquasol 105. [Apree] Aloe extract.*

Aremsol A. [Ronsheim & Moore] Cocamidopropyl betaine.†

Aremsol P Lotion. [Ronsheim & Moore] Pearly shampoo conc.†

Arlatone® 507. [ICI Spec. Chem.] Octyl dimethyl PABA.*

Arlatone® B. [ICI Spec. Chem.; ICI Surf. Am.] Polysorbate 85 and dinonyl phenol.*

Arlatone® UVB. [ICI Surf. UK] Octyl dimethyl PABA.*

Armotan® PMD 20. [Akzo Italia] Polysorbate 80.*

Arquad® C-33. [Akzo] Cocotrimonium chloride, IPA.†

Arquad® DM18B-90. [Akzo] Octadecyl-dimethylbenzyl ammonium chloride.†

Arquad® S-2C-50. [Akzo BV] 1:1 mixt. of oleyltrimethyl ammonium chloride and dicocodimethyl ammonium chloride.*

Arquad® T-2C-50. [Akzo BV] 1:1 mixt. of tallow trimonium chloride and dicoco dimonium chloride.*

Atlas G-271. (redesignated Forestall) [ICI Am.; ICI Surf. UK] Soya ethyl morpholinium ethosulfate.*

Avicel PH-102. [FMC] Microcryst. cellulose NF.†

Avicel PH-103. [FMC] Microcryst. cellulose NF.†

Avicel PH-105. [FMC] Microcryst. cellulose NF.†

Avirol® 300. [Henkel/Functional Prods.] TEA lauryl sulfate.†

Axol® E 61. [Goldschmidt AG] Acetylated hydrog. lard glyceride.*

Axol® E 66. [Goldschmidt AG] Acetic acid ester of mono/diglycerides.*

Bentone® 500. [Rheox] Org. deriv. of a montmorillonite clay.†

Bina QAT-43. [Ciba-Geigy] Lauramidopropyl acetamidodimonium chloride.†

Brij® 92. [ICI Spec. Chem.; ICI Surf. Am.; ICI Surf. Belgium] Oleth-2 with preservatives.*

Brij® 96. [ICI Spec. Chem.; ICI Surf. Am.; ICI Surf. Belgium] Oleth-10 with antioxidants.*

Brij® 98G. [ICI Spec. Chem.] Oleth-20 with preservatives.*

Brij® 99. [ICI Spec. Chem.; ICI Surf. Am.; ICI Surf. UK] Oleth-20 with preservatives.*

Camilol. [Maybrook] α-Bisabolol.*

Capmul® POE-O. [Karlshamns] Polysorbate 80.*

Carbopol® 1706. [BFGoodrich] High m.w. polyacrylic acids, crosslinked with polyalkenyl polyether.†

Carbopol® 1720. [BFGoodrich] High m.w. polyacrylic acids, crosslinked with polyalkenyl polyether.†

Carboset 514A. [BFGoodrich] Acrylic resin, IPA.†

Carboset 514H. [BFGoodrich] Acrylic resin, ammonia water.†

Carboset 531. [BFGoodrich] Acrylic resin, ammonia water.†

Carboset XL-11. [BFGoodrich] Acrylic resin.†

Carboset XL-19. [BFGoodrich] Acrylic resin.†

Carmine 40. [R.I.T.A.] Carmine.*

Carmisol-50. [Presperse] Carmine.*

Carsofoam® MS Conc. [Lonza] †

Carsofoam® PS-1, PS-3. [Lonza] †

Carsofoam® SC. [Lonza] Sodium laureth sulfate, cocamide DEA, DEA lauryl sulfate.†

Carsonol® ANS. [Lonza] Sulfated nonylphenol ethoxylate, aluminum salt.†

Carsonol® BD. [Lonza] Blend of carboxybetaine, sulfate and amine groups.†

Carsonol® ILS. [Lonza] Mixed isopropanolamines lauryl sulfate.†

Carsoquat® CTM-29. [Lonza] Cetyl trimethyl ammonium chloride.†

Carsoquat® CTM-429. [Lonza] Cetyl trimethyl ammonium chloride.†

Catinal LQ-75. [Toho Chem. Industry] Alkyl isoquinolinium bromide.†

Cation G-40. [Sanyo Chem. Industries] Benzalkonium chloride.†

Cation S. [Sanyo Chem. Industries] Stearyl dimethyl benzyl ammonium chloride.†

Cedepon LA-30. [Stepan Canada] Ammonium lauryl sulfate.†

Cedepon® LS-30PM. [Rhone-Poulenc Surf. & Spec.] Sodium lauryl sulfate.*

Cedepon LT-40. [Stepan Canada] TEA lauryl sulfate.†

Cegesoft® C 25. [Henkel KGaA/Cospha] 2-Ethyl hexyl palmitate.†

Ceramol. [Aceto] Partially sulfonated fatty alcohol from hydrog. veg. oil.†

Ceranine HC Hi Conc. [Sandoz] †

Cetiol® G20S. [Henkel] Octadodecanol stearate.†

Cithrol 40MO. [Croda Chem. Ltd.] PEG-75 oleate.†

Cithrol 60ML. [Croda Chem. Ltd.] PEG 6000 laurate.†

Cithrol 60MO. [Croda Chem. Ltd.] PEG 6000 oleate.†

Cithrol GMS A/S ES 0743. [Croda Chem. Ltd.] Glyceryl stearate.†

Clearlan® 1650. [Henkel/Emery] Lanolin anhydrous, USP.†

Clearlan® K50. [Henkel/Emery] Anhydrous lanolin, USP.†

Cobee 76. [Stepan/PVO] Refined, bleached, deodorized coconut oil.†

Cobee 92. [Stepan/PVO] Refined, bleached, deodorized, hydrog. coconut oil.†

Cobee 110. [Stepan/PVO] Refined, bleached, deodorized, hydrog. coconut oil.†

Collagen Complex. [Maybrook] Soluble collagen.*

Collone™ NI. (redesignated Dermalcare® NI) [Rhone-Poulenc Surf. & Spec.] Cetomacrogol emulsifying wax BP.*

Colorin 102, 104, 202. [Sanyo Chem. Industries] Polyether polyol.†

Comperlan® HS. [Henkel KGaA/Cospha] Stearamide MEA.*

Comperlan® ID. [Henkel] 1:1 Isostearamide DEA.†

Comperlan® KM. [Henkel KGaA/Cospha] Cocamide MEA.*

Comperlan® LD 9. [Henkel] Distearyldimonium chloride.†

Comperlan® LM. [Henkel KGaA/Cospha] Lauramide MEA.*

Comperlan® LMD. [Henkel KGaA/Cospha] Lauramide DEA.*

Comperlan® SM. [Henkel] Cocamide MEA.†

Comperlan® UDM. [Henkel] Undecylenamide MEA.†

Cosiderm Collagen Masks. [Maybrook] Soluble collagen and collagen.*

Cosmedia Guar® U. [Henkel] Guar gum.†

Cosmowax. [Croda Inc.] Stearyl alcohol, steareth-20, steareth-10.†

Covitol 544. [Henkel] Tocopheryl acetate.†

Covitol 700C. [Henkel] d-α-Tocopheryl acetate.†

Cralane KR-13, -14. [Pulcra SA] Ethoxylated lanolin.†

Cralane LR-10. [Pulcra SA] Ethoxylated lanolin (75 EO).†

Cralane LR-11. [Pulcra SA] Ethoxylated lanolin.†

Crapol FU-25. [Pulcra SA] Dimethyl dihydrog. tallow ammonium chloride.†

Cremba. [Croda Inc.] Min. oil, petrolatum, lanolin alcohol, and lanolin.‡

Cremophor® NP 10. [BASF AG] Nonoxynol-10.*

Cremophor® NP 14. [BASF AG] Nonoxynol-14.*

Crestalans. [Croda Chem. Ltd.] Fractionated liq. lanolin and isopropyl ester deriv.†

Crillon LME. [Croda Chem. Ltd.] Lauramide MEA.†

Crodacol C-NF. [Croda Inc.] Cetyl alcohol.‡

Crodacol S-USP. [Croda Inc.] Stearyl alcohol.‡

Crodasinic OS35. [Croda Chem. Ltd.] Sodium N-oleoyl sarcosinate.†

Croderol G7000. [Croda Chem. Ltd.] Glycerin.†

Crodesta A10. [Croda Inc.] Acetylated sucrose distearate†

Crolastin 10. [Croda Inc.] Partially hydrolyzed elastin.‡

Crolastin 30. [Croda Inc.; Croda Chem. Ltd.] Partially hydrolyzed elastin.‡

Cronectin. [Croda Chem. Ltd.] Hydrolyzed fibronectin.†

Croquat K. [Croda Inc.] Quat. deriv. of hydrolyzed keratin.‡

Crossential EPO, Super Refined. [Croda Inc.] Evening primrose oil.‡

---

* Discontinued or redesignated   † Unverified   ‡ No longer standard

Crotein ADX. [Croda Inc.] AMP-isostearic hydrolyzed animal protein†

Crotein BTA. [Croda Inc.] Benzyl trimethyl ammonium hydrolyzed animal protein†

Crotein O. [Croda Inc.; Croda Chem. Ltd.] Hydrolyzed collagen.‡

Crotein SPA 55. [Croda Inc.] Hydrolyzed collagen.‡

Cutina® CP-A. [Henkel] Cetyl palmitate.†

Cutina® EGMS. [Henkel] Ethylene glycol stearate.†

Cutina® LE. [Henkel/Cospha; Henkel KGaA/Cospha] Glyceryl stearate, sodium cetearyl sulfate.*

Cutina® MD-A. [Henkel/Cospha; Henkel KGaA/Cospha] Glyceryl stearate.*

Cyclochem® EGMS. (redesignated Alkamuls® EGMS/C) [Rhone-Poulenc Surf. & Spec.] .*

Cyclochem® GMO. [Rhone-Poulenc Surf. & Spec.] Glyceryl oleate.*

Cyclochem® LVL. [Rhone-Poulenc Surf. & Spec.] Lauryl lactate.*

Cyclochem® MM/M. (redesignated Alkamuls® MM/M) [Rhone-Poulenc Surf. & Spec.] .*

Cyclochem® NI. (redesignated Dermalcare® NI) [Rhone-Poulenc Surf. & Spec.] .*

Cyclochem® PEG 200DS. [Rhone-Poulenc Surf. & Spec.] PEG-4 distearate.*

Cyclochem® PEG 400 DS. [Rhone-Poulenc Surf. & Spec.] PEG-8 distearate.*

Cyclochem® PEG 600DS. [Rhone-Poulenc Surf. & Spec.] PEG-12 distearate.*

Cyclochem® PEG 6000DS. [Rhone-Poulenc Surf. & Spec.] PEG-150 distearate.*

Cyclochem® PETS. [Rhone-Poulenc Surf. & Spec.] Pentaerythritol tetrastearate.*

Cyclochem® POL. (redesignated Dermalcare® POL) [Rhone-Poulenc Surf. & Spec.] .*

Cyclochem® SEG. (redesignated Alkamuls® SEG) [Rhone-Poulenc Surf. & Spec.] .*

Cyclochem® SS. (redesignated Alkamuls® SS) [Rhone-Poulenc Surf. & Spec.] .*

Cyclomox® L. (redesignated Rhodamox® LO) [Rhone-Poulenc Surf. & Spec.] .*

Cyclomox® SO. [Rhone-Poulenc Surf. & Spec.] Stearamidopropylamine oxide.*

Cycloryl ALC. (redesignated Miraspec ALC) [Rhone-Poulenc Surf. & Spec.] PEG-80 sorbitan laurate, sodium trideceth sulfate, PEG-150 distearate blend.*

Cycloryl DCA. (redesignated Rhodaterge® DCA) [Rhone-Poulenc Surf. & Spec.] .*

Cycloryl GSC. [Rhone-Poulenc Surf. & Spec.] Disodium cocoamphodiacetate, sodium laureth sulfate.*

Cycloryl NWC. (redesignated Miracare® NWC) [Rhone-Poulenc Surf. & Spec.] .*

Cycloryl XL-M. (see Miracare XL) [Rhone-Poulenc Surf. & Spec.] DEA-lauryl sulfate and DEA cocaminopropionate.*

Cyclosheen 202. (redesignated Mirasheen 202) [Rhone-Poulenc Surf. & Spec.] .*

Cycloteric BET-C-30. (redesignated Mirataine® BET-C-30) [Rhone-Poulenc Surf. & Spec.] .*

Cycloteric BET-C41. (see Mirataine® CB/M) [Rhone-Poulenc Surf. & Spec.] Coco betaine.*

Cycloteric BET-CB. (see Mirataine® CB) [Rhone-Poulenc Surf. & Spec.] Cocamidopropyl betaine, cosmetic grade, glycerin-free.*

Cycloteric BET-L31 [Rhone-Poulenc Surf. & Spec.] Lauryl betaine.*

Cycloteric BET-O30. (redesignated Mirataine® BET-O-30) [Rhone-Poulenc Surf. & Spec.] .*

Cycloteric BET-OB50. [Rhone-Poulenc Surf. & Spec.] Oleyl betaine.*

Cycloteric BET-T2 40. (see Mirataine® TM) [Rhone-Poulenc Surf. & Spec.] †

Cycloteric CAPA. [Rhone-Poulenc Surf. & Spec.] Cocaminopropionic acid.*

Cycloteric SLIP. [Rhone-Poulenc Surf. & Spec.] Sodium lauriminodipropionate.*

Cycloton® 7LUF. [Rhone-Poulenc Surf. & Spec.] Oleakonium chloride.*

Cycloton® D261C/70. [Rhone-Poulenc Surf. & Spec.] Ditallowalkonium chloride (Quaternium 18).*

Cycloton® M270C/18. [Rhone-Poulenc Surf. & Spec.] Stearalkonium chloride.*

Cycloton® M270C/85. [Rhone-Poulenc Surf. & Spec.] Stearalkonium chloride.*

Cyncal®. [Hilton-Davis] Myristalkonium chloride.*

D-400. [Olin] PPG diol.†

D-1000. [Olin] PPG diol.†

D-1200. [Olin] PPG diol.†

D-1300. [Olin] PPG diol.†

D-2000. [Olin] PPG diol.†

D-3000. [Olin] PPG diol.†

D-4000. [Olin] PPG diol.†

Dantoin® DMHF Refined. [Lonza] Dimethyl hydantoin formaldehyde, refined grade.†

Dar Chem-11. [Unichema] Single pressed stearic acid.†

Dar Chem-12. [Unichema] Double pressed stearic acid.†

Dastar. [Croda Chem. Ltd.] Cholesterol.†

Dehydag® Wax 14. [Henkel] Myristyl alcohol.†

Dehydag® Wax 16. [Henkel] Cetyl alcohol.†

Dehydag® Wax 18. [Henkel] Stearyl alcohol.†

Dehydag® Wax 22 (Lanette) [Henkel] Behenyl alcohol.†

Dehydag® Wax E. [Henkel] Sodium cetearyl sulfate.†

Dehydag® Wax N. [Henkel] Cetearyl alcohol and sodium cetearyl sulfate.†

Dehydag® Wax O. [Henkel] Cetearyl alcohol.†

Dehydag® Wax SX. [Henkel] Cetearyl alcohol, sodium lauryl sulfate (90:10 ratio).†

Dehydag® Wax W. [Henkel] Cetearyl alcohol and sodium lauryl sulfate (90:10 ratio).†

Dehyquart® STC-25. [Henkel] Stearalkonium chloride.†

Dehyton® G-SF. [Henkel KGaA/Cospha] Sodium cocoamphopropionate.*

Demelan CB-28. [Pulcra SA] Alkylbenzene sulfonate blend.†

Demelan FB-12. [Pulcra SA] Alkylbenzene sulfonate blend.†

Depasol AS-26. [Pulcra SA] Monoalkyl sulfosuccinate.†

Dermalcare® 326A. [Rhone-Poulenc Surf. & Spec.] Syn. beeswax.*

Dermalcare® C-20. [Rhone-Poulenc Surf. & Spec.] Cetearyl alcohol and cetearath-20.*

Dermalcare® EGMS/SE. [Rhone-Poulenc Surf. & Spec.] Glycol stearate SE.*

Dermalcare® GMS. (redesignated Alkamuls® GMS/C) [Rhone-Poulenc Surf. & Spec.] .*

Dermalcare® GTIS. [Rhone-Poulenc Surf. & Spec.] Triisostearin.*

Dermalcare® HL. [Rhone-Poulenc Surf. & Spec.] Hexyl laurate.*

Dermalcare® LVL. [Rhone-Poulenc Surf. & Spec.] Lauryl lactate.*

Dermalcare® MM/M. (redesignated Alkamuls® MM/M) [Rhone-Poulenc Surf. & Spec.] .*

Dermalcare® MST. [Rhone-Poulenc Surf. & Spec.] Myristyl stearate.*

---

* Discontinued or redesignated   † Unverified   ‡ No longer standard

Dermalcare® PGMS. [Rhone-Poulenc Surf. & Spec.] Propylene glycol stearate.*

Dermalcare® SDG. (redesignated Alkamuls® SDG) [Rhone-Poulenc Surf. & Spec.] .*

Dermalcare® SS. (redesignated Alkamuls® SS) [Rhone-Poulenc Surf. & Spec.] .*

Desadipol AX Extra. [Seppic] Alkylpolyethoxyether.†

Desamidocollagen. [Henkel/Cospha; Henkel Canada] Soluble collagen.†

DeSonate AOS. [Witco/H-I-P] Sodium alpha olefin sulfonate.*

DeSonate AUS. [Witco/H-I-P] Sodium C14-C16 alpha olefin sulfonate.*

DeSonol A. . (redesignated Witcolate 6431) [Witco/H-I-P] Ammonium lauryl sulfate.*

DeSonol AE. (redesignated Witcolate AE) [Witco/H-I-P] Ammonium laureth sulfate.*

DeSonol AES. [Witco/H-I-P] Ammonium laureth sulfate.*

DeSonol S. (redesignated Witcolate S) [Witco/H-I-P] Sodium lauryl sulfate.*

DeSonol SE. (redesignated Witcolate SE) [Witco/H-I-P] Sodium laureth sulfate.*

DeSonol SE-2. [Witco/H-I-P] Sodium laureth-2 sulfate.*

DeSonol T. (redesignated Witcolate 6434) [Witco/H-I-P] TEA lauryl sulfate.*

Diadol 13. [Mitsubishi Kasei] Higher alcohol.†

Diadol 18G. [Mitsubishi Kasei] Isostearyl alcohol.†

Diaion® HP 10. [Mitsubishi Kasei] †

Diaion® WK10. [Mitsubishi Kasei] †

Diaion® WK20. [Mitsubishi Kasei] †

Dihydroxy-acetone. [Int'l. Bio-Synthetics] Dihydroxyacetone.†

Distilled Lipolan. [Lipo] Hydrog. lanolin.†

Dow Corning® 1315 Surfactant. [Dow Corning] Silicone glycol copolymer.†

Dow Corning® 5103 Surfactant. [Dow Corning] Silicone glycol copolymer.†

Drewfax® 0007. [Drew Ind. Div.] Sodium dioctyl sulfosuccinate.†

Drewmulse® 3-1-O. [Stepan/PVO] Triglyceryl oleate.†

Drewmulse® 3-1-S. [Stepan/PVO] Triglyceryl stearate.†

Drewmulse® 6-2-S. [Stepan/PVO] Hexaglyceryl distearate.†

Drewmulse® 10-10-S. [Stepan/PVO] Decaglyceryl decastearate.†

Drewmulse® 10-4-O. [Stepan/PVO] Decaglyceryl tetraoleate.†

Drewmulse® 10-8-O. [Stepan/PVO] Decaglyceryl octaoleate.†

Drewmulse® DGMS. [Aquatec Quimica SA] Diethylene glycol stearate.†

Drewmulse® EGDS. [Aquatec Quimica SA] Ethylene glycol distearate.†

Drewmulse® EGMS. [Aquatec Quimica SA] Ethylene glycol stearate.†

Drewmulse® GMRO. [Aquatec Quimica SA] Glyceryl ricinoleate.†

Drewmulse® GMS. [Aquatec Quimica SA] Glyceryl stearate.†

Drewmulse® GMS-AE. [Aquatec Quimica SA] Glyceryl stearate.†

Drewmulse® PGMS. [Aquatec Quimica SA] Propylene glycol stearate.†

Drewmulse® V. [Stepan/PVO] Glyceryl stearate (veg.).†

Drewmulse® V-SE. [Stepan/PVO] Glyceryl stearate SE.†

Dulectin. [Duphar] De-oiled soybean lecithin.†

Elas-Tein AS-20. [Maybrook] Elastin, ethyl ester in ethanol.*

Elastinhydrolysate, Liq. [Henkel/Cospha; Henkel Canada] Hydrolyzed animal elastin.†

Elastinhydrolysate, Powd. [Henkel/Cospha; Henkel Canada] Hydrolyzed animal elastin.†

Elastosol. [Croda Inc.; Croda Chem. Ltd.] Soluble elastin and soluble collagen.‡

Elfan® 200. [Akzo BV] Sodium lauryl sulfate.*

Elfan® 240 TS. [Akzo BV] TEA-lauryl sulfate†

Elfan® 260 S. [Akzo] Sodium lauryl sulfate.†

Elfan® 280 Powd. [Akzo BV] Sulfated coconut fatty alcohol, sodium salt.*

Elfan® A. [Akzo] Betaine-type surfactant.†

Elfan® A 432. [Akzo BV] Betaine type from lauric-myristic acid.*

Elfan® KM 730. [Akzo BV] Sodium C14-16 olefin sulfonate and sodium C12-15 pareth sulfate.*

Elfan® OS. [Akzo] Olefin sulfonates.†

Elfan® SP 325. [Akzo BV] Blend.*

Elfanol® 510. [Akzo; Akzo BV] Sulfosuccinic acid monoester of tallow fatty acid monoethanolamide, sodium salt.*

Elfanol® 883. [Akzo BV] Sodium dioctyl sulfosuccinate.*

Elfapur® KA 45. [Akzo; Akzo BV] PEG-5 cocamide.*

Elfapur® LM 20. [Akzo BV] Laureth-2.*

Elfapur® LM 25. [Akzo BV] C12-14 lauryl alcohol polyglycol ether.*

Elfapur® LM 30 S. [Akzo BV] Laureth-3.*

Elfapur® LM 75 S. [Akzo BV] Laureth-8.*

Elfapur® LP 25 S. [Akzo BV] C12-15 pareth-3.*

Elfapur® LT. [Akzo BV] Syn. fatty alcohol ethoxylate.*

Elfapur® T 110. [Akzo BV] Tallow fatty alcohol polyglycol ether.*

Elvanol® 20-25. [DuPont] Fully hydrolyzed polyvinyl alcohol.*

Elvanol® 85-50. [DuPont] PVAL.*

Emal 20C. [Kao Corp. SA] Sodium POE alkyl ether sulfate.†

Emal E-25C, -70C. [Kao Corp. SA] Sodium POE alkyl ether sulfate.†

Emal NC-35. [Kao Corp. SA] Sodium POE alkylaryl ether sulfate.†

Emanon 3199, 3299R. [Kao Corp. SA] PEG fatty acid esters.†

Emanon 4110. [Kao Corp. SA] PEG fatty acid ester.†

Emasol L-106. [Kao Corp. SA] PEG-4 sorbitan laurate.†

Emasol L-120. [Kao Corp. SA] PEG-20 sorbitan laurate.†

Emasol P-120. [Kao Corp. SA] PEG-20 sorbitan palmitate.†

Emcol® 5430. (see Emcol NA-30) [Witco/H-I-P] Cocamidopropyl betaine.*

Emerest® 1723. [Henkel/Emery] Isopropyl ester of lanolic acids.†

Emerest® 2381. [Henkel/Emery] Propylene glycol stearate SE.†

Emerest® 2421 (see Witconol 2421) [Henkel/Emery; Henkel/Cospha; Henkel Canada] Glyceryl oleate.*

Emerest® 11723. [Henkel/Emery] Isopropyl ester of lanolic acids.†

Emery® 1720. [Henkel/Emery] Lanolin oil/isopropyl ester blend.†

Emery® 1781. [Henkel/Emery] Lanolin acids.†

Emery® 6752. [Henkel/Emery] Monocarboxylate coconut imidazolinium deriv.†

Emid® 6510. [Henkel/Emery] Lauramide DEA.†

Emid® 6518. [Henkel/Emery] Lauramide DEA.†

Emid® 6531. [Henkel/Emery] Cocamide DEA and diethanolamine.†

Emid® 6534. [Henkel/Emery] Cocamide DEA, diethanolamine.†

Empicol® 0344. [Albright & Wilson UK] Sodium lauryl

---

* Discontinued or redesignated † Unverified ‡ No longer standard

sulfate.*

Empicol® 0384. [Albright & Wilson UK] MEA-lauryl sulfate.*

Empicol® 0627. [Albright & Wilson UK] Sodium laureth sulfate, glycol stearate, and cocamide DEA.*

Empicol® 0919. [Albright & Wilson UK] Sodium lauryl sulfate.*

Empicol® DLS. [Albright & Wilson UK] DEA-lauryl sulfate.*

Empicol® EL. [Albright & Wilson UK] MEA-lauryl sulfate.*

Empicol® EMD. [Albright & Wilson UK] Blend of natural, straight chain fatty alcohol.*

Empicol® ESB3/S. [Albright & Wilson UK] Sodium laureth sulfate.*

Empicol® ESB3GA. [Albright & Wilson UK] Sodium laureth sulfate.*

Empicol® ESB30. [Albright & Wilson UK] Sodium laureth sulfate.*

Empicol® ESB50. [Albright & Wilson UK] Sodium laureth sulfate.*

Empicol® HL25. [Albright & Wilson UK] Lithium lauryl sulfate.*

Empicol® LM. [Albright & Wilson UK] Sodium lauryl sulfate.*

Empicol® LM/T. [Albright & Wilson UK] Sodium lauryl sulfate.*

Empicol® LMV. [Albright & Wilson UK] Sodium lauryl sulfate.*

Empicol® LMV/T. [Albright & Wilson UK] Sodium lauryl sulfate.*

Empicol® LZP. [Albright & Wilson UK] Sodium lauryl sulfate.*

Empicol® MD. [Albright & Wilson UK] Alkyl ether sulfate.*

Empicol® TC30/T. [Albright & Wilson UK] TEA-ammonium lauryl sulfate.*

Empicol® TC34. [Albright & Wilson UK] Ammonium lauryl sulfate and TEA-lauryl sulfate.*

Empicol® TCR. [Albright & Wilson UK] Ammonium lauryl sulfate, TEA-lauryl sulfate and lauramide MIPA.*

Empicol® TCR/T. [Albright & Wilson UK] Mixed ammonium/ TEA lauryl sulfate.*

Empicol® TDL 75. [Albright & Wilson UK] TEA-lauryl sulfate.*

Empicol® TL40/S. [Albright & Wilson UK] TEA salt of sulfated fatty alcohol.*

Empicol® TLP. [Albright & Wilson UK] TEA-lauryl sulfate and lauramide MIPA.*

Empicol® TLP/T. [Albright & Wilson UK] TEA-lauryl sulfate.*

Empicol® TLR. [Albright & Wilson UK] TEA-lauryl sulfate and lauramide MIPA.*

Empicol® TLR/T. [Albright & Wilson UK] TEA-lauryl sulfate.*

Empicol® XC35/S. [Albright & Wilson UK] Blend of anionic and nonionic components.*

Empicol® XDB. [Albright & Wilson UK] Detergent complex.*

Empicol® XT 45. [Albright & Wilson UK] MEA-lauryl sulfate.*

Empigen® 5073. [Albright & Wilson UK] Tert. amine.*

Empigen® 5083. [Albright & Wilson UK] Coco dimethylamine oxide.*

Empigen® BAC80. [Albright & Wilson UK] Benzalkonium chloride.*

Empigen® BCM75, BCM75/A. [Albright & Wilson UK] Hydrog.-tallow dimethyl benzyl ammonium chloride.*

Empigen® BCP/25. [Albright & Wilson UK] Stearyl dimethyl benzyl ammonium chloride.*

Empigen® BT. [Albright & Wilson UK] Alkyl amido propyl dimethyl amine betaine.*

Empigen® CDL10. [Albright & Wilson UK] Lauric imidazoline betaine.*

Empigen® CDR10. [Albright & Wilson UK] Coconut imidazoline betaine.*

Empigen® CHB. [Albright & Wilson UK] Myrtrimonium bromide.*

Empigen® CMC. [Albright & Wilson UK] Alkyl trimethyl ammonium chloride.*

Empigen® CSC. [Albright & Wilson UK] Cocamidopropyltrimonium chloride.*

Empigen® FKH75L. [Albright & Wilson UK] Dialkyl diamido amine lactate.*

Empigen® XDR112. [Albright & Wilson UK] Coconut imidazoline betaine binary deriv.*

Empigen® XDR121. [Albright & Wilson UK] Coconut imidazoline betaine with sodium lauryl ethoxy sulfate.*

Empigen® XDR123. [Albright & Wilson UK] Coconut imidazoline betaine with sodium lauryl ethoxy sulfate.*

Empigen® XDR302. [Albright & Wilson UK] Sodium cocoamphoacetate with sodium lauryl sulfate.*

Empilan® 7132. [Albright & Wilson UK] Fatty amine alkoxylate.*

Empilan® CDEY. [Albright & Wilson UK] Cocamide DEA.*

Empilan® CM. [Albright & Wilson Australia] Cocamide MEA.*

Empilan® FD. [Albright & Wilson Australia] Cocamide DEA.*

Empilan® FE. [Albright & Wilson UK] Cocamide DEA.*

Empilan® GMS SE40. [Albright & Wilson UK] Glyceryl stearate SE.*

Emsorb® 2729. [Henkel/Emery] Polysorbate 65 NF.†

Emsorb® 6905. [Henkel/Emery] PEG-20 sorbitan stearate.†

Emthox® 5940. [Henkel/Emery] Trideceth-6.†

Emthox® 5941. [Henkel/Emery] Trideceth-9.†

Emthox® 5942. [Henkel/Emery] Trideceth-11.†

Emthox® 5943. [Henkel/Emery] Trideceth-12.†

Emthox® 5964. [Henkel/Emery] Laureth-23.†

Emthox® 6957. [Henkel/Emery] Nonoxynol-40.†

Emthox® 6961. [Henkel/Emery] Nonoxynol-4.†

Emthox® 6962. [Henkel/Emery] Nonoxynol-6.†

Emthox® 6964. [Henkel/Emery] Nonoxynol-9.†

Emthox® 6965. [Henkel/Emery] Nonoxynol-11.†

Emthox® 6967. [Henkel/Emery] Nonoxynol-20.†

Emthox® 6968. [Henkel/Emery] Nonoxynol-30.†

Emthox® 6970. [Henkel/Emery] Nonoxynol-40.†

Emthox® 6971. [Henkel/Emery] Nonoxynol-40.†

Emthox® 6972. [Henkel/Emery] Nonoxynol-50.†

Emthox® 6984. [Henkel/Emery] Octoxynol-40.†

Emulgade® A. [Henkel KGaA/Cospha] Cetearyl alcohol and laureth-10.*

Emulgade® CRC. [Henkel] †

Emulgade® F Special. [Henkel/Cospha; Henkel Canada; Henkel KGaA/Cospha] Cetearyl alcohol and PEG-40 castor oil.*

Emulgade® K. [Henkel; Henkel KGaA/Cospha] Tallow alcohol, cetearalkonium bromide, and ceteareth-12.*

Emulphor® EL-620. (redesignated Alkamuls® EL-620) [Rhone-Poulenc Surf. & Spec.] .*

Emulphor® EL-620L. (redesignated Alkamuls® EL-620L) [Rhone-Poulenc Surf. & Spec.] .*

Emulphor® EL-719. (redesignated Alkamuls® EL-719) [Rhone-Poulenc Surf. & Spec.] .*

Emulphor® EL-719L. (redesignated Alkamuls® EL-719L) [Rhone-Poulenc Surf. & Spec.] .*

Emulphor® ON-877. (redesignated Rhodasurf® ON-877) [Rhone-Poulenc Surf. & Spec.] .*

Emulphor® VN-430. [Rhone-Poulenc Surf. & Spec.] PEG-5 oleate.*

Epal® 618. [Ethyl] C16-C18 linear primary alcohol.†

Equex AEM. [Procter & Gamble] Ammonium laureth-12 sulfate, cocamide DEA and SD alcohol 40-B.†

Equex S. [Procter & Gamble] Sodium lauryl sulfate.†

Equex STM. [Procter & Gamble] Sodium lauryl sulfate, cocamide MEA and TEA-lauryl sulfate.†
Equex SW. [Procter & Gamble] Sodium lauryl sulfate.†
Equex T. [Procter & Gamble] TEA-lauryl sulfate.†
ES-1239. [CasChem] Dimethylaminopropyl ricinolamide benzyl chloride, propylene glycol.†
Espesilor AC Series. [Pulcra SA] Fatty acid DEAs.†
Espesilor AC-43. [Pulcra SA] Linoleic alkanolamide.†
Espesilor AC-50. [Pulcra SA] Alkanolamide.†
Estol 1406. [Unichema] Isopropyl oleate.†
Estol 1414. [Unichema] Isobutyl oleate.†
Estol 1427. [Unichema] Trimethylolpropane trioleate.†
Estol 1445. [Unichema] Pentaerythrityl tetraoleate.†
Estol 1502. [Unichema] Methyl laurate.†
Estol 1574. [Unichema] Ethylene glycol diacetate.†
Estol 1579. [Unichema] Triacetin.†
Estol 1583. [Unichema] Glyceryl diacetate.†
Estol 1593. [Unichema] Triethylene glycol diacetate.†
Ethofat® 60/25. [Akzo] PEG-15 stearate.†
Ethofat® 142/20. [Akzo] PEG-10 glycol tallate.†
Ethosperse® TDA-6. [Lonza] Trideceth-6.†
Ethylan® CL. [Harcros UK] Alkylolamide EO condensate.†
Ethylan® GEP4. [Harcros UK] Polysorbate 40.†
Ethylan® GLE-21. [Harcros UK] Polysorbate 21.†
Ethylan® GOE-21. [Harcros UK] Polysorbate 81.†
Ethylan® HBI-TG. [Harcros UK] 2-Phenoxyethanol.†
Ethylan® L10. [Harcros UK] PEG 1000 laurate.†
Ethylan® LDS. [Harcros UK] Cocamide DEA.†
Ethylan® TCO. [Harcros UK] Complex amine oxide.†
Etocas 9. [Croda Chem. Ltd.] PEG-9 castor oil.*
Eumulgin® EP 2L. [Henkel KGaA/Cospha] Ethoxylated oleyl/cetyl alcohol.*
Eumulgin® KP92. [Henkel KGaA/Cospha] Mixt. of fatty acid polyglycol esters.*
Eumulgin® TI 60. [Henkel KGaA/Cospha] Fatty acid polyglycol ester.*
Eumulgin® TL 30. [Henkel KGaA/Cospha] Fatty acid polyglycol ester.*
Eumulgin® TL 55. [Henkel KGaA/Cospha] Fatty acid polyglycol ester.*
Euperlan® K 771. [Henkel] †
Eureka 102-WK. [Atlas Refinery] Sulfated castor oil.†
Exceparl IPM. [Kao Corp. SA] IPM.†
Exceparl IPP. [Kao Corp. SA] IPP.†
Exceparl OD-M. [Kao Corp. SA] Octyldodecyl myristate.†
Exceparl OD-OL. [Kao Corp. SA] Octyldodecyl oleate.†
Exceparl TGO. [Kao Corp. SA] 2-Ethylhexyl triglyceride.†
Extrakt ZS 8590. [Zschimmer & Schwarz] MIPA-ammonium fatty alcohol sulfate, modified.†
Ferric Blue 107. [Presperse] Ferric ammonium ferrocyanide (90%), bismuthoxychloride (10%).*
Ferric Blue 114. [Presperse] Ferric ammonium ferrocyanide, talc, bismuthoxychloride.*
Finex-25-020. [Presperse] Zinc oxide, methicone.*
Five Star Lanolin Anhyd. USP. [Maybrook] Lanolin.*
Foamkill® 30 Series. [Crucible] Org. and organo-silicone conc.†
Foamkill® 80J Series. [Crucible] Silicone compd.†
Foamkill® 618 Series. [Crucible] Org. and organo-silicone conc.†
Foamkill® 634 Series. [Crucible] Org. and organo-silicone conc.†
Foamkill® 634B-HP. [Crucible] Org. and organo-silicone conc.†
Foamkill® 634D-HP. [Crucible] Org. and organo-silicone conc.†
Foamkill® 634F-HP. [Crucible] Org. and organo-silicone

conc.†
Foamkill® 644 Series. [Crucible] Org. and organo-silicone conc.†
Foamkill® 652H. [Crucible] Org. and organo-silicone conc.†
Foamkill® 652-HF. [Crucible] Org. and organo-silicone conc.†
Foamkill® 684 Series. [Crucible] Org. and organo-silicone conc.†
Foamkill® 836A. [Crucible] Silicone emulsions.†
Foamkill® 1001 Series. [Crucible] Org. and organo-silicone conc.†
Foamkill® GCP Series. [Crucible] Silicone fluid.†
Foamkill® RP. [Crucible] Org. and organo-silicone conc.†
Forlan 100. (see Ritachol) [R.I.T.A.] Min. oil, lanolin alcohol.*
G-100. (redesignated Arlasolve DMI) [ICI Am.; ICI Surf. UK] Dimethylisosorbide.*
G-1795. [ICI Am.] PEG-50 lanolin deriv.†
Gafac® MC-470. (redesignated Rhodafac® MC-470) [Rhone-Poulenc Surf. & Spec.] .*
Gafac® RD-510. (redesignated Rhodafac® RD-510) [Rhone-Poulenc Surf. & Spec.] .*
Gafac® RE-877. [Rhone-Poulenc Surf. & Spec.] Aromatic phosphate ester.*
Gafac® RM-510. (redesignated Rhodafac® RM-510) [Rhone-Poulenc Surf. & Spec.] .*
Gafac® RM-710. (redesignated Rhodafac® RM-710) [Rhone-Poulenc Surf. & Spec.] .*
Genamine C-050. [Hoechst Celanese] Coconut fatty amine oxethylate.†
Genamine C-080. [Hoechst Celanese] Coconut fatty amine oxethylate.†
Genamine C-100. [Hoechst Celanese] Coconut fatty amine oxethylate.†
Genamine C-150. [Hoechst Celanese] Coconut fatty amine oxethylate.†
Genamine C-200. [Hoechst Celanese] Coconut fatty amine oxethylate.†
Genamine C-250. [Hoechst Celanese] Coconut fatty amine oxethylate.†
Genamine O-020. [Hoechst Celanese] Oleylamine oxethylate.†
Genamine O-050. [Hoechst Celanese] Oleylamine oxethylate.†
Genamine O-080. [Hoechst Celanese] Oleylamine oxethylate.†
Genamine O-100. [Hoechst Celanese] Oleylamine oxethylate.†
Genamine O-150. [Hoechst Celanese] Oleylamine oxethylate.†
Genamine O-200. [Hoechst Celanese] Oleylamine oxethylate.†
Genamine O-250. [Hoechst Celanese] Oleylamine oxethylate.†
Genamine S-020. [Hoechst Celanese] Stearylamine oxethylate.†
Genamine S-050. [Hoechst Celanese] Stearylamine oxethylate.†
Genamine S-080. [Hoechst Celanese] Stearylamine oxethylate.†
Genamine S-100. [Hoechst Celanese] Stearylamine oxethylate.†
Genamine S-150. [Hoechst Celanese] Stearylamine oxethylate.†
Genamine S-200. [Hoechst Celanese] Stearylamine oxethylate.†
Genamine S-250. [Hoechst Celanese] Stearylamine oxethylate.†

---

* Discontinued or redesignated   † Unverified   ‡ No longer standard

12

Genapol® CRO. [Hoechst Celanese/Colorants & Surf.] Sodium myreth sulfate.*

Genapol® PGL. [Hoechst Celanese/Colorants & Surf.] Glycol distearate, cocamide MEA, PPG-4 deceth-4.*

Genapol® PGS. [Hoechst Celanese/Colorants & Surf.] Sodium laureth sulfate, glycol distearate, cocamide MEA.*

Genapol® S-020. [Hoechst Celanese/Colorants & Surf.] Stearyl alcohol polyglycol ether.†

Genapol® S-050. [Hoechst Celanese/Colorants & Surf.] Stearyl alcohol polyglycol ether.†

Genapol® S-080. [Hoechst Celanese/Colorants & Surf.] Stearyl alcohol polyglycol ether.†

Genapol® S-100. [Hoechst Celanese/Colorants & Surf.] Stearyl alcohol polyglycol ether.†

Genapol® S-150. [Hoechst Celanese/Colorants & Surf.] Stearyl alcohol polyglycol ether.†

Genapol® S-200. [Hoechst Celanese/Colorants & Surf.] Stearyl alcohol polyglycol ether.†

Genapol® S-250. [Hoechst Celanese/Colorants & Surf.] Stearyl alcohol polyglycol ether.†

Geropon® AC-78. [Rhone-Poulenc Surf. & Spec.] Sodium cocoyl isethionate.*

Geropon® SS-L7DE. [Rhone-Poulenc Surf. & Spec.] Sodium lauramido DEA sulfosuccinate.*

Geropon® SS-TA. [Rhone-Poulenc Surf. & Spec.] Sodium N-octadecyl sulfosuccinamate.*

Glo-Mul 780. [Global United Industries] Sorbitan monooleate.*

Glo-Mul 781. [Global United Industries] PEG-400 dioleate.*

Glo-Mul 782. [Global United Industries] PEG-400 oleate.*

Glo-Mul 783. [Global United Industries] PEG-400 stearate.*

Glo-Mul 789. [Global United Industries] Glyceryl monostearate.*

Glo-Mul 4001. [Global United Industries] Sodium dialkylsulfosuccinate.*

Glo-Mul 4007. [Global United Industries] Disodium alkylsulfosuccinate.*

Glycomul® LC. [Lonza] Sorbitan laurate, cosmetic grade.†

Glycomul® MA. [Lonza] Sorbitan ester mixed fatty acids.†

Glycomul® TAO. [Lonza] Sorbitan ester mixed resin and fatty acids.†

Glycon® DP. [Lonza] Stearic acid.*

Glycosperse® O-20 Veg. [Lonza] Polysorbate 80, veg. grade.†

Glycosperse® O-20X. [Lonza] Polysorbate 80, anhyd.†

Glycowax® S 932. [Lonza] Triester wax.†

Golden Dawn Superfine. [Westbrook Lanolin] Anhyd. lanolin.†

Golden Fleece DF. [Westbrook Lanolin] Extra refined anhyd. lanolin (detergent-free).†

Golden Fleece Lanolin. [Westbrook Lanolin] Anhyd. lanolin, purified.†

Golden Fleece P-80. [Westbrook Lanolin] Anhyd. lanolin (trace pesticides reduced by 80%).†

Golden Fleece P-95. [Westbrook Lanolin] Anhyd. lanolin (trace pesticides reduced by 95%, low in natural free alcohols).†

Golden Fleece RA. [Westbrook Lanolin] Anhyd. lanolin (detergent-free and low in natural free alcohols).†

Grancol-1, -10. [Grant Industries] Soluble collagen.*

Granlastin 20, 30, 100. [Grant Industries] Hydrolyzed elastin.*

Grilloten ZT-40. [R.I.T.A.] Sucrose ricinoleate.*

Grilloten ZT-80. [R.I.T.A.] Sucrose ricinoleate.*

Grindtek LA 15. [Grindsted Prods.] Glyceryl palmitate lactate.†

Grindtek LA 30. [Grindsted Prods.] Glyceryl stearate lactate.†

Grindtek ML 90. [Grindsted Prods.] Glyceryl laurate.*

Grindtek MM 90. [Grindsted Prods.] Glyceryl myristate.*

Grindtek MOL 90. (see Dimodan LS Kosher) [Grindsted Prods.] Glyceryl linoleate.†

Grindtek MOP 90. [Grindsted Prods.] Lard glyceride.†

Grindtek MSP 32-6. [Grindsted Prods.] Glyceryl stearate SE.†

Grindtek MSP 40. [Grindsted Prods.] Glyceryl stearate.†

Grindtek MSP 40F. [Grindsted Prods.] Glyceryl stearate.†

Grindtek MSP 52. [Grindsted Prods.] Glyceryl stearate.†

Grindtek MSP 90. [Grindsted Prods.] Glyceryl stearate.†

Grindtek PK 60. [Grindsted Prods.] Palm kernel glycerides.†

Haroil SCO-65, -7525. [Graden] Sulfated castor oil.†

H Chrome Green 105. [Presperse] Chromium hydroxide, bismuthoxychloride.*

Herbavert. [Henkel] 3,3,5-Trimethylcyclohexylethyl ether.†

Hetamide LA. [Heterene] Lauric acid.†

Hetamide MMC, OC. [Heterene] Mixed fatty acids.†

Hetoxamate MO-15. [Heterene] PEG-15 oleate.†

Hetoxide BP-3. [Heterene] Modified butanol ethoxylate.†

Hetoxide BY-3. [Heterene] PEG-3 butynediol.†

Hetoxol L-4N. [Heterene] Laureth-4.†

Hetoxol L-9N. [Heterene] Laureth-9.†

Hetsulf 60T. [Heterene] Amine dodecylbenzene sulfonate.†

Hi-Care® 200. [Rhone-Poulenc Surf. & Spec.] Polymethacrylamidopropyltrimonium chloride.*

HiStyle 133. [Rhone-Poulenc Surf. & Spec.] Polymethacrylamidopropyltrimonium chloride.*

Hoe S 2568. [Hoechst Celanese/Colorants & Surf.] Aminopropyl laurylglutamine.*

Hoe S 2793. [Hoechst Celanese/Colorants & Surf.] Acrylamide/sodium acrylate copolymer.*

Hoe S 3495. [Hoechst Celanese/Colorants & Surf.] PEG-10 polyglyceryl-2 laurate.*

Hoe S 3654. [Hoechst Celanese/Colorants & Surf.] Polyquaternium-6.*

Hoe S 3924. [Hoechst Celanese/Colorants & Surf.] Laureth-3.*

Hoechst Wax W. [Hoechst Celanese] Montan wax.*

Hostacerin DGO. [Hoechst Celanese/Colorants & Surf.; Hoechst AG] Polyglyceryl-2 sesquioleate.*

Hostacerin O-3. [Hoechst Celanese/Colorants & Surf.] Oleth-3.*

Hostacerin O-5. [Hoechst Celanese/Colorants & Surf.] Oleth-5.*

Humectant SD-35. [Presperse] Panthenyl ethyl ether.*

Hyamine® 2389. [Lonza] Dodecylbenzyl trimonium chloride (80%), dodecylxylyldimonium chloride (20%).†

Hyamine® 3500-NF. [Lonza] Benzalkonium chloride.†

Hydagen® BP1. [Henkel/Cospha; Henkel Canada] Soluble collagen and low molecular serum components.†

Hydagen® F. [Henkel] Sodium acrylate/vinyl alcohol copolymer.*

Hydrofol Acid 1655NF. [Procter & Gamble] Stearic acid, triple pressed.†

Hydrofol Acid 1690. [Procter & Gamble] Palmitic acid (90%).†

Hydrofol Acid 1855. [Procter & Gamble] Stearic acid (55%), double pressed.†

Hydrokote® 25. [Karlshamns] Hydrog. veg. oil.†

Hydrokote® 27. [Karlshamns] Hydrog. veg. oil.†

Hydrokote® 79. [Karlshamns] Hydrog. veg. oil.†

Hydrokote® 711. [Karlshamns] Hydrog. veg. oil.†

Hydrokote® S-7. [Karlshamns] Hydrog. veg. oil.†

Hydrokote® SP. [Karlshamns] Hydrog. veg. oil.†

Hydromond. [Croda Chem. Ltd] Hydrolyzed almond protein.†

Hydrotriticum™ Powd. [Croda Inc.] Hydrolyzed whole wheat protein.‡
Hypol® X6100. [W.R. Grace/Organics] PU prepolymer derived from isophorone diisocyanate.†
Hystar® 7570. [Lonza] Sorbitol.*
Igepal® CA-630G. [Rhone-Poulenc Surf. & Spec.] Octoxynol-9 USP-NF.*
Igepon® AC-78. (redesignated Geropon® AC-78) [Rhone-Poulenc Surf. & Spec.] .*
Igepon® TC-42. (redesignated Geropon® TC-42) [Rhone-Poulenc Surf. & Spec.] .*
Imwitor® 900 K. [Hüls Am.] Glyceryl stearate.†
Imwitor® 965 K. [Hüls Am.] Glyceryl stearate/palmitate and potassium stearate.†
Incromate ALL. [Croda Inc.] Almondamidopropyl dimethylamine lactate.‡
Incromate BAL. [Croda Inc.] Babassamidopropyl dimethylamine lactate.‡
Incromate CDL. [Croda Inc.] Cocamidopropyl dimethylamine lactate.‡
Incromate IDL. [Croda Inc.] Isostearamidopropyl dimethylamine lactate.‡
Incromate Mink L. [Croda Inc.] Minkamidopropyl dimethylamine lactate.‡
Incromate SEL. [Croda Inc.] Sesamidopropyl dimethylamine lactate.‡
Incromide BED. [Croda Inc.] Behenamide DEA (1:1).‡
Incromide BEM. [Croda Inc.] Behenamide MEA (1:1).‡
Incromide CM. [Croda Inc.] Cocamide MEA.‡
Incromide LCL. [Croda Inc.] Lauramide MEA.‡
Incromide LM-70. [Croda Inc.] Lauramide DEA.‡
Incromide Mink D. [Croda Inc.] Minkamide DEA.‡
Incromide OD. [Croda Inc.] Oleamide DEA (1:1).‡
Incromine CB. [Croda Inc.] Cocamidopropyl dimethylamine.‡
Incromine OPB. [Croda Inc.] Oleamidopropyl dimethylamine.‡
Incromine PB. [Croda Inc.] Palmitamidopropyl dimethylamine.‡
Incromine Oxide AL. [Croda Inc.] Almondamidopropylamine oxide.‡
Incromine Oxide I. [Croda Inc.; Croda Surf. Ltd.] Isostearamidopropylamine oxide.‡
Incromine Oxide ISMO. [Croda Inc.] Isostearamidopropyl morpholine oxide.‡
Incromine Oxide L-40. [Croda Inc.] Lauramine oxide.‡
Incromine Oxide MC. [Croda Inc.] Myristyl/cetyl amine oxide.‡
Incromine Oxide Mink. [Croda Inc.] Minkamidopropylamine oxide.‡
Incromine Oxide O. [Croda Inc.; Croda Surf. Ltd.] Oleamidopropylamine oxide.‡
Incromine Oxide OD-50. [Croda Inc.; Croda Surf. Ltd.] Oleyl dimethylamine oxide.‡
Incromine Oxide SE. [Croda Inc.] Sesamidopropylamine oxide.‡
Incronam I-30. [Croda Inc.; Croda Surf. Ltd.] Isostearamidopropyl betaine.‡
Incronam Mink 30. [Croda Inc.] Minkamidopropyl betaine.‡
Incropol CS-50. [Croda Inc.] Ceteareth-50.‡
Incropol L-23. [Croda Inc.] Laureth-23.‡
Incroquat 100. [Croda Inc.] Methyl bis (hydrogenated tallow amidoethyl) 2-hydroxyethyl ammonium chloride.‡
Incroquat 248. [Croda Inc.] Quaternium-72.‡
Incroquat AL-85. [Croda Inc.] Almondamidopropalkonium chloride.‡
Incroquat I-85. [Croda Inc.] Isostearaminopropalkonium chloride.‡
Incroquat Mink-85. [Croda Inc.] Minkamidopropalkonium chloride.‡
Incroquat OL-85. [Croda Inc.] Olivamidopropalkonium chloride.‡
Incroquat S-75CG. [Croda Inc.] Quaternium-27.‡
Incroquat SE-85. [Croda Inc.] Sesamidopropalkonium chloride.‡
Incroquat Behenyl TMC. [Croda Inc.; Croda Surf. Ltd.] Cetearyl alcohol, behentrimonium chloride.‡
Incrosul LMA. [Croda Inc.] Diammonium lauramido-MEA sulfosuccinate.‡
Incrosul LMS. [Croda Inc.] Disodium lauramido MEA-sulfosuccinate.‡
Incrosul LS. [Croda Inc.] Disodium lauryl sulfosuccinate.‡
Incrosul LSA. [Croda Inc.] Diammonium lauryl sulfosuccinate.‡
Incrosul LTS. [Croda Inc.] Disodium laureth sulfosuccinate.‡
Incrosul OMS. [Croda Inc.] Disodium oleamido MEA-sulfosuccinate.‡
Incrosul TS. [Croda Inc.] Disodium tridecyl sulfosuccinate.‡
Intravon® AN. [Crompton & Knowles] Fatty acid deriv.†
Iscolan. [Croda Chem. Ltd.] Lanolin ester.†
Isopropylan® 50. [Amerchol] Isopropyl palmitate, lanolin oil.*
Jaguar® HP-79. [Rhone-Poulenc/Water Soluble Polymers] Hydroxypropyl guar.*
Juniorlan 1664. [Henkel/Organic Prods.] Lanolin wax and triolein.*
Kalcohl 68. [Kao Corp. SA] Cetyl stearyl alcohol.†
Kalcohl 80. [Kao Corp. SA] Stearyl alcohol.†
Katemul IB-70. [Scher] N-(3-Isostearamidopropyl)-N,N-dimethylamino glycolate.†
Katioran® AF. [BASF AG] Fatty acid hydroxylalkylamide and ethoxylated fatty alcohol.*
Kelate DS. [Tri-K Industries] Disodium EDTA.*
Kessco® GMC-8. [Stepan; Stepan Canada] Glyceryl caprylate/caprate.*
Kessco® GML. [Stepan; Stepan Canada] Glyceryl laurate.*
Kessco PEG 400DS. [Akzo BV] PEG-8 distearate.*
Lamacit® ER. [Grünau] PEG-20 glyceryl ricinoleate and ricinoleamide DEA.†
Lamacit® GML 12. [Grünau] PEG-12 glyceryl laurate.†
Lamacit® GMO 25. [Grünau] PEG-25 glyceryl oleate.†
Lamecerin 50-80. [Grünau] POE glycol lanolin derivate.†
Lamecreme® SA 7. [Grünau] POE stearoylether.†
Lamegin® NSL. [Grünau] Sodium stearoyl lactylate.†
Lamepon® ST40. [Henkel/Cospha; Henkel Canada; Henkel KGaA/Cospha; Grünau] TEA-coco-hydrolyzed collagen.*
Lamepon® S-TR. [Henkel KGaA/Cospha; Grünau] TEA-coco-hydrolyzed collagen.*
Lamepon® UD. [Henkel/Cospha; Henkel Canada; Henkel KGaA/Cospha; Grünau] Potassium undecylenoyl hydrolyzed collagen.*
Lanalene 97. [Maybrook] Polysorbate 80 acetate, cetyl acetate, acetylated lanolin alcohol.*
Lanalene 98. [Maybrook] Polysorbate 80, cetyl acetate, acetylated lanolin alcohol.*
Lanalene ABS. [Maybrook] Min. oil, lanolin alcohol.*
Lanalene AC. [Maybrook] Cetyl acetate, acetylated lanolin alcohol.*
Lanalene Liq. 30, 50. [Maybrook] Isopropyl palmitate, lanolin oil.*
Lanalene Liq. 75. [Maybrook] Lanolin oil, isopropyl palmitate.*
Lanalene Liq. Super. [Maybrook] Lanolin oil.*

Lanalene S. [Maybrook] Isopropyl lanolate.*
Lanalene SW. [Maybrook] Petrolatum, lanolin, and lanolin alcohol.*
Lanalene Wax. [Maybrook] Lanolin wax.*
Lanalol Distilled, Standard. [Maybrook] Lanolin alcohol.*
Lanalox HL 20. [Maybrook] PEG-20 hydrog. lanolin.*
Lanalox L75/50. [Maybrook] PEG-75 lanolin.*
Lanamol. [Maybrook] Min. oil, PEG-30 lanolin, cetyl alcohol.*
Lancare. [Henkel-Nopco] †
Lanethyl. [Croda Chem. Ltd.] Alcohol extract of lanolin alcohols.†
Laneto 20. [R.I.T.A.] PEG-20 lanolin.*
Laneto 27. [R.I.T.A.] PEG-27 lanolin.*
Laneto 30. [R.I.T.A.] PEG-30 lanolin.*
Laneto 49. [R.I.T.A.] PEG-50 lanolin.*
Laneto 85. [R.I.T.A.] PEG-85 lanolin.*
Laneto 99. [R.I.T.A.] PEG-100 lanolin.*
Lanette® 18-22. [Henkel] Fatty alcohol C18-C22.†
Lanette® Wax B.P. [Henkel] SE wax.†
Lanette® Wax CAT. [Henkel] Cetearyl alcohol, cetrimonium bromide, and laureth-12.†
Lanex. [Croda Chem. Ltd.] Alcohol extract of pure lanolin.†
Lanexol. [Croda Chem. Ltd.] Alkoxylated liq. lanolin.†
Lanfrax® 1694. [Henkel/Organic Prods.] PEG-75 lanolin wax.*
Lanfrax® 1777 Deodorized. [Henkel/Emery] Specially deodorized lanolin wax fraction.†
Lanfrax® WS 55. [Henkel/Emery] PEG-75 lanolin wax.†
Lankropearl™ T. [Harcros UK] Blend of pearlizing agents in an anionic base.*
Lanogen 1500. [Hoechst AG] PEG mixt.†
Lanolic Acid. [Croda Chem. Ltd.] Lanolin acid.†
Lanolin Anhydrous USP Grade 1. [Maybrook] Lanolin.*
Lanolin Anhydrous USP Super Fine. [Maybrook] Lanolin.*
Lanolox AWS. [Maybrook] PPG-12-PEG-50 lanolin.*
Lanotex 730. [Tessilchimica] Lanolin, ethoxylated.†
Lanpol 520 [Croda Chem. Ltd.] POE lanolin acid.†
Lanpolamide 5. [Croda Inc.] PEG-5 lanolinamide, PEG-5 lanolate.‡
Lantrol® [Henkel/Emery] Lanolin oil.†
Lantrol® AWS. [Henkel/Emery] Ethoxylated lanolin.†
Laurex® CH. [Albright & Wilson UK] Coconut alcohol.*
Lauridit® LMI. [Akzo BV] LauramideMIPA.*
Lauridit® PPD. [Akzo BV] Palm kernelamide DEA.*
Lauridit® SDG. [Akzo BV] Soyamide DEA.*
Leoguard G. [Lion] Cellulosic resin.†
Leoguard GP. [Lion] Cellulosic resin.†
Lipacide SH-V. [Seppic] Lipoaminoacid complex.†
Lipal EB. [Aquatec Quimica SA] Butyl stearate.†
Lipal LC. [Aquatec Quimica SA] Cetyl lactate.†
Lipal ST. [Aquatec Quimica SA] Isopropyl stearate.†
Lipo DGS-SE. [Lipo] Diethylene glycol stearate SE.†
Lipocol. [Croda Chem. Ltd.] Lanolin-derived base.†
Lipolan 1400. [Lion] α-Olefin sulfonate.†
Lipolan S. [Lipo] Hydrog. lanolin.†
Lipovol ALM-S. [Lipo] Veg. oil, sweet almond oil.†
Lipovol A-S. [Lipo] Veg. oil, avocado oil.†
Lipovol P-S. [Lipo] Veg. oil, apricot kernel oil.†
Liquester. [Robeco] Ester C30–46 piscine oil.†
Liquid Base. [Croda Inc.] Min. oil and lanolin alcohol.‡
Liquid Crystal (LC) CAPS 122. [Presperse] Cholesteric esters, acacia, gum arabic.*
Lomar® PWC. [Henkel/Organic Prods.] Sodium polynaphthalenesulfonate.*
Lonzest® PEG 4-L. [Lonza] PEG-8 laurate.†
Lonzest® PEG 4-O. [Lonza] PEG-8 oleate.†
Lutavit® Calpan. [BASF AG] Calcium D-pantothenate.*

Lutavit® Niacin. [BASF AG] Nicotinic acid.*
Lutensit® AS 2230, 2270. [BASF AG] Sulfated natural alcohol polyglycol ether, sodium salt.†
Lutensit® AS 3330. [BASF AG] Sodium salt of sulfated oxoalcohol polyglycol ether.†
Lutensit® AS 3334. [BASF AG] Sodium salt of sulfated fatty alcohol polyglycol ether.†
Lutensol® FA 12. [BASF AG] Oleyl amine ethoxylate.*
Lutrol® E 8000. [BASF AG] PEG-150.*
Lutrol® W-3520. [BASF] PPG-28-buteth-35.*
Luviflex® D 430 I, D 455 I. [BASF AG] Vinylpyrrolidone/vinyl acetate/alkylaminoacrylate terpolymer.†
Luviform® ES 22. [BASF AG] Ethyl ester of PVM/MA copolymer.*
Luviform® ES 42. [BASF AG] Butyl ester of PVM/MA copolymer.*
Luviset® CAP X. [BASF] Crotonic acid/vinyl acetate/vinyl propionate terpolymer.†
Luviskol® K12. [BASF; BASF AG] PVP.*
Luviskol® VA64I. [BASF; BASF AG] PVP/VA copolymer (60:40 ratio) isopropanol sol'n.*
Luvitol® HP. [BASF] Hydrog. polyisobutene.*
Luxelen® Silk D. [Presperse] Anatase titanium dioxide.*
Mackadet™ TLC-45. [McIntyre] Sulfosuccinate blend.*
Mackalene™ NLC. [McIntyre] Oleamidopropyl dimethylamine lactate, palmitamidopropyl dimethylamine lactate, palmitoleamidopropyl dimethylamine lactate.*
Mackam™ 1C-SF. [McIntyre] Coco imidazoline carboxylate.*
Mackam™ 2C-75. [McIntyre] Disodium cocoamphodiacetate.*
Mackam™ CB-LS. [McIntyre] Coco betaine, low salt.*
Mackam™ ISP. [McIntyre] Isostearamido dimethylaminopropionate.*
Mackam™ OB. [McIntyre] Oleyl betaine.†
Mackam™ RA. [McIntyre] Ricinoleamidopropyl betaine.*
Mackamate WGD. [McIntyre] Disodium wheat germamido PEG-2 sulfosuccinate.†
Mackamide™ 100-A. [McIntyre] Cocamide DEA.†
Mackamide™ AN55. [McIntyre] Alkylolamide DEA.†
Mackamide™ CDC. [McIntyre] Cocamide DEA, DEA coconate.*
Mackamide™ EC. [McIntyre] Cocamide DEA.†
Mackamide™ OP. [McIntyre] Oleamide MIPA.*
Mackamine™ BAO. [McIntyre] Behenamido propylamine oxide.†
Mackamine™ IAO. [McIntyre] Isostearamidopropylamine oxide.*
Mackamine™ ISMO. [McIntyre] Isostearamidopropyl morpholine oxide.*
Mackamine™ SAO. [McIntyre] Stearamidopropylamine oxide.*
Mackanate™ DG30. [McIntyre] Disodium silicone polyol sulfosuccinate.†
Mackanate™ IM. [McIntyre] Disodium isostearamido MEA sulfosuccinate.†
Mackanate™ L-1, L-2. [McIntyre] Disodium laureth sulfosuccinate.*
Mackanate™ MM. [McIntyre] Disodium myristamido MEA-sulfosuccinate.†
Mackanate™ O-3. [McIntyre] Disodium oleth sulfosuccinate.*
Mackanate™ OD. [McIntyre] Disodium oleamide PEG-2 sulfosuccinate.†
Mackanate™ OD-2. [McIntyre] Sulfosuccinate sulfate blend.*
Mackanate™ ODT. [McIntyre] TEA-oleamido PEG-2 sulfo-

---

succinate.†

Mackanate™ ODT-2. [McIntyre] Sulfosuccinate sulfate.†

Mackanate™ OL. [McIntyre] Sulfosuccinate.†

Mackanate™ UD. [McIntyre] Undecylenic sulfosuccinate.†

Mackanate™ WG. [McIntyre] Disodium wheat germamido MEA sulfosuccinate.†

Mackernium™ SDC-50. [McIntyre] Stearalkonium chloride.†

Mackester™ IDO. [McIntyre] Isodecyl oleate.*

Mackester™ TD-88. [McIntyre] Triethylene glycol dioctoate.*

Mackpearl LV. [McIntyre] †

Macol® CSA-50. [PPG/Specialty Chem.] Ceteareth-50.*

Manoxol OT/P. [Manchem] Dioctyl sodium sulfosuccinate.†

Mapeg® CO-16. [PPG/Specialty Chem.] PEG-16 castor oil.*

Marinco CH, CL. [Marine Magnesium] Magnesium carbonate.*

Marlinat® DRL 40. [Hüls Am.] TEA-lauryl sulfate.*

Marlinat® HA 12. [Hüls AG] Sodium salt of lauric acid monoethanolamide sulfosuccinate.†

Marlipal® 1885/5. [Hüls Am.] Oleth-5.*

Marlipal® BS. [Hüls Am.] Fatty acid polyglycol ester.†

Marlowet® CA 12. [Hüls Am.] Laureth-12.*

Marlowet® LMA 3. [Hüls Am.; Hüls AG] Laureth-3.*

Marlowet® LMA 7. [Hüls Am.; Hüls AG] Laureth-7.*

Marlowet® TA 18. [Hüls Am.] Ceteareth-18.*

May-Tein R. [Maybrook] Potassium cocoyl hydroylzed rice protein.*

Mazamide® 62. [PPG/Specialty Chem.] Lauramide DEA.*

Mearlmaid® KN. [Mearl] Butyl acetate, guanine, nitrocellulose, isopropyl alcohol.*

Mearlmaid® PLO. [Mearl] Water, carbomer, guanine, methylcellulose, diisopropanolamine.*

Meyprofix® 509. (redesignated Polycare® 509) [Rhone-Poulenc Surf. & Spec.] Vinyl acetate/isobutyl maleate/ vinyl neodecanoate copolymer.*

Meypro-Guar™ CASA M-225. [Rhone-Poulenc Surf. & Spec.] Guar gum.*

Miglyol® 840 Gel. [Hüls Am.] Propylene glycol dicaprylate/ dicaprate and stearalkonium hectorite.†

Miglyol® Gel. [Hüls Am.] Caprylic/capric triglyceride and stearalkonium hectorite.†

Mikrokill. [Brooks Industries] Polyaminopropyl biguanide.*

Mikrokill 300. [Brooks Industries] Butylene glycol, methylparaben, polyaminopropyl biguanide, propylparaben.*

Milvex 1000. [Henkel] Nylon-66.*

Miramine® CODI. [Rhone-Poulenc Surf. & Spec.] Cocamidopropyl dimethylamine.*

Miramine® SC. [Rhone-Poulenc Surf. & Spec.] Soya hydroxyethyl imidazoline.*

Miranate® LSS. (redesignated Geropon® LSS) [Rhone-Poulenc Surf. & Spec.] .*

Miranol® 2MCA. (redesignated Miracare® 2 MCA) [Rhone-Poulenc Surf. & Spec.] †

Miranol® 2MCAS. (redesignated Miracare® 2MCAS) [Rhone-Poulenc Surf. & Spec.] .*

Miranol® 2MCT. (redesignated Miracare® 2MCT) [Rhone-Poulenc Surf. & Spec.] .*

Miranol® 2MHT. (redesignated Miracare® 2MHT) [Rhone-Poulenc Surf. & Spec.] .*

Miranol® BT. (redesignated Miracare® BT) [Rhone-Poulenc Surf. & Spec.] .*

Miranol® Ester PO-LM4. [Rhone-Poulenc Surf. & Spec.] Pentaerythrityl tetralaurate.*

Miranol® H2M Anhyd. Acid. [Rhone-Poulenc Surf. & Spec.] Lauroamphodipropionic acid.*

Miranol® H2M-SF 70%. (see Miranol® H2M-SF Conc.) [Rhone-Poulenc Surf. & Spec.] Disodium lauroamphodipropionate.*

Miranol® HM Special, HM Special Conc. [Rhone-Poulenc Surf. & Spec.] Disodium lauroamphodiacetate.*

Miranol® OM. [Rhone-Poulenc Surf. & Spec.] Sodium oleoamphoacetate.*

Miranol® OM-SF Conc. [Rhone-Poulenc Surf. & Spec.] Sodium oleoamphopropionate.*

Miranol® OS-D. [Rhone-Poulenc Surf. & Spec.] Sodium oleoamphohydroxypropylsulfonate.*

Miranol® S2M Conc. [Rhone-Poulenc Surf. & Spec.] Disodium caproamphodiacetate.*

Miranol® S2M-SF Conc. [Rhone-Poulenc Surf. & Spec.] Disodium caproamphodipropionate.*

Miranol® SM-SF Conc. [Rhone-Poulenc Surf. & Spec.] Sodium caproamphopropionate.*

Mirapol® 9, 95, 175. [Rhone-Poulenc Surf. & Spec.] Polyquaternium-27.*

Mirapol® 1941. (see Sipothix 1941) [Rhone-Poulenc Surf. & Spec.] Acrylates/steareth-20 methylacrylate copolymer.*

Mirapol® AZ-1. [Rhone-Poulenc Surf. & Spec.] Polyquaternium-18.*

Mirataine® AP-C. [Rhone-Poulenc Surf. & Spec.] N-Coco beta aminopropionic acid.*

Mirataine® BET-CS. (see Mirataine® CBS) [Rhone-Poulenc Surf. & Spec.] Cocamidopropyl hydroxysultaine.*

Mirataine® BET-P-30. [Rhone-Poulenc Surf. & Spec.] Cetyl betaine.*

Mirataine® H2C. (see Mirataine® H2C-HA) [Rhone-Poulenc Surf. & Spec.] Disodium lauriminodipropionate.*

Mirataine® HC-Acid. [Rhone-Poulenc Surf. & Spec.] Lauraminopropionic acid.*

Mirataine® HC-HA. [Rhone-Poulenc Surf. & Spec.] Lauraminopropionic acid.*

Mirataine® ODMB-35. [Rhone-Poulenc Surf. & Spec.] Oleyl betaine.*

Mirataine® XL. (redesignated Miracare® XL) [Rhone-Poulenc Surf. & Spec.] .*

Monamid® 770. [Mona Industries] Modified cocamide DEA (1:1).*

Monaquat P-TC. (see Phospholipid P-TC) [Mona Industries] Cocamidopropyl PG-dimonium chloride phosphate.*

Monaquat P-TD. (see Phospholipid P-TD) [Mona Industries] Lauramidopropyl PG-dimonium chloride phosphate.*

Monaquat P-TL. (see Phospholipid P-TL) [Mona Industries] Lauroampho PG-glycinate phosphate.*

Monaquat P-TS. (see Phospholipid P-TS) [Mona Industries] Stearamidopropyl PG-dimonium chloride phosphate.*

Monaquat P-TZ. (see Phospholipid P-TZ) [Mona Industries] Cocohydroxyethyl PG-imidazolinium chloride phosphate.*

Monateric 805. [Mona Industries] Cocoamphodiacetate, disodium cocamido MIPA-sulfosuccinate.*

Monateric 810-A-50. [Mona Industries] Caprylic/capric carboxylic propionate, imidazoline-derived, salt-free.*

Monateric 951A. [Mona Industries] Disodium lauroamphodiacetate.*

Monateric 1202. [Mona Industries] Dihydroxyethyl tallow glycinate.*

Monateric 1203. [Mona Industries] Sodium hydrog. tallow dimethyl glycinate.*

Monateric ADFA. [Mona Industries] Cocamidopropyl betaine.*

Monateric CDS. [Mona Industries] Disodium cocoamphodiacetate, sodium lauryl sulfate.*

Monateric CDTD. [Mona Industries] Disodium cocoampho-

---

diacetate, sodium trideceth sulfate.*

Monateric CEM-38CG. [Mona Industries] Disodium coco-amphodipropionate.*

Monateric CyMM-40. [Mona Industries] Caprylic dicarboxylic propionate, imidazoline-derived, salt-free.*

Monateric TA-35. [Mona Industries] Sodium tallamphopropionate.*

Monawet DL-30. [Mona Industries] Disodium deceth-6 sulfosuccinate.*

Monawet TD-30. [Mona Industries] Disodium deceth-6 sulfosuccinate.†

Monolan® PPG440, PPG1100, PPG2200. [Harcros UK] PPG.†

Monomuls® 60-10. [Henkel] Lard glycerides.†

Monomuls® 60-15. [Henkel] Hydrog. lard glycerides.†

Monomuls® 60-20. [Henkel] Tallow glycerides.†

Monomuls® 60-25. [Henkel; Grünau] Hydrog. tallow glycerides.*

Monomuls® 60-25/2. [Henkel] Hydrog. tallow glycerides with 2% sodium stearate.†

Monomuls® 60-30. [Henkel] Palm oil glycerides.†

Monomuls® 60-35. [Henkel] Hydrog. palm oil glycerides.*

Monomuls® 60-40. [Henkel] Sunflower seed oil glycerides.†

Monomuls® 60-45. [Henkel] Hydrog. soybean oil glycerides.†

Monomuls® 90-10. [Henkel] Dist. lard glyceride.†

Monomuls® 90-15. [Henkel] Dist. hydrog. lard glyceride.†

Monomuls® 90-20. [Henkel] Dist. tallow glyceride.†

Monomuls® 90-25/2, 90-25/5. [Henkel] Dist. hydrog. tallow glyceride with 2% and 5% sodium stearate resp.†

Monomuls® 90-30. [Henkel] Dist. palm oil glyceride.†

Monomuls® 90-35. [Henkel; Grünau] Dist. hydrog. palm oil glyceride.*

Monomuls® 90-40. [Henkel] Dist. sunflower seed oil glyceride.†

Monomuls® 90-45. [Henkel] Dist. hydrog. soybean oil glyceride.†

Montosol IF-21. [Pulcra SA] Sodium laureth-12 sulfate.†

Montosol IL-13. [Pulcra SA] IPA laureth-2.7 sulfate.†

Montosol IL-17. [Pulcra SA] Magnesium laureth-2.7 sulfate.†

Montosol PF-10. [Pulcra SA] Sodium laureth-2.8 sulfate.†

Montosol PF-14. [Pulcra SA] Sodium laureth-2 sulfate.†

Montosol PF-16, -18. [Pulcra SA] Ammonium laureth-1.5 sulfate.†

Montosol PF-26, PG-10. [Pulcra SA] Sodium laureth-2.4 sulfate.†

Montosol PG-12. [Pulcra SA] Ammonium laureth sulfate.†

Montosol PG-17. [Pulcra SA] MEA laureth sulfate.†

Montosol PL-14. [Pulcra SA] TEA laureth-2 sulfate.†

Montosol PL-16. [Pulcra SA] Sodium laureth-2.4 sulfate.†

Montosol PQ-11, -15. [Pulcra SA] Ammonium laureth-3 sulfate.†

Montosol PQ-17. [Pulcra SA] Sodium laureth-3 sulfate.†

Montosol TQ-11. [Pulcra SA] Ammonium laureth-2.4 sulfate.†

Montovol GF-15. [Pulcra SA] DEA lauryl sulfate.†

Montovol RF-10. [Pulcra SA] Sodium lauryl sulfate.†

Montovol RF-11. [Pulcra SA] TEA lauryl sulfate.†

Montovol RF-12. [Pulcra SA] Ammonium lauryl sulfate.†

Montovol RF-13. [Pulcra SA] Isopropanolamine lauryl sulfate.†

Montovol RL-10. [Pulcra SA] TEA lauryl sulfate.†

Montovol RQ-10. [Pulcra SA] Ammonium fatty alcohol sulfate.†

M-Quat® Dimer 18 PG. [PPG/Specialty Chem.] Hydroxypropyl bisstearyldimonium chloride.*

M-Quat® Dimer JB-25. [PPG/Specialty Chem.] Stearalkonium chloride.*

M-Quat® Dimer JN. [PPG/Specialty Chem.] Ricinolamidopropyl ethyldimonium ethosulfate.*

M-Quat® Dimer S-50 PG. [PPG/Specialty Chem.] Hydroxypropyl bisoleyldimonium chloride.*

M-Quat® JO-50. [PPG/Specialty Chem.] Olealkonium chloride.*

M-Quat® JS-25 SP. [PPG/Specialty Chem.] Stearalkonium chloride.*

Mulsifan RT 69. [Zschimmer & Schwarz] PEG-40 castor oil.†

Mulsifan RT 302. [Zschimmer & Schwarz] Ethoxylated hydrog. castor oil.†

Myvatem® 06K. [Eastman] Diacetyl tartaric acid ester of dist. monoglycerides (from hydrog. soybean oil).†

Myvatem® 92K. [Eastman] Diacetyl tartaric acid ester of dist. monoglycerides (from refined sunflower oil).†

Nansa® HS55. [Albright & Wilson UK] Sodium dodecylbenzene sulfonate.*

Natipide®. [Rhone-Poulenc Surf. & Spec.] Water, lecithin, and alcohol.*

Neustrene® 045. [Witco/H-I-P] Hydrog. menhaden oil.*

Nikkol BEG-1630. [Nikko Chem. Co. Ltd.] Isoceteth-30.†

Nikkol BPS-15. [Nikko Chem. Co. Ltd.] PEG-15 phytosterol.†

Nikkol BPS-25. [Nikko Chem. Co. Ltd.] PEG-25 phytosterol.†

Nikkol PEMS. [Nikko Chem. Co. Ltd.] Pentaerythritol stearate.†

Nikkol Jojoba Oil N. [Nikko Chem. Co. Ltd.] Jojoba oil.†

Nimco® 1780. [Henkel/Emery] Lanolin alcohols.†

Nimcolan® 1747. [Henkel/Emery] Petrolatum, lanolin and lanolin alcohol.†

Nimlesterol® 1730. [Henkel/Emery] Fractionated blend of cholesterol and related sterols.†

Niox EO-10. [Pulcra SA] Cetyl alcohol blend.†

Niox EO-26. [Pulcra SA] Cetearyl alcohol blend.†

Niox EO-33. [Pulcra SA] PEG diester.†

Niox KG-11. [Pulcra SA] Linear fatty alcohol ethoxylate.†

Niox KI Series. [Pulcra SA] Ethoxylated castor oil.†

Niox KI-29. [Pulcra SA] Ethoxylated castor oil.†

Niox KJ-10. [Pulcra SA] Ethoxylated oleyl alcohol.†

Niox KJ-72. [Pulcra SA] Linear fatty alcohol ethoxylated sat.†

Niox KP-62, -63, -67. [Pulcra SA] Isotridecanol, ethoxylated.†

Niox KS Series. [Pulcra SA] PEGs.†

Nissan Anon BL. [Nippon Oils & Fats] Dimethyl dodecyl betaine.†

Nissan Stafoam DF-1, DF-2. [Nippon Oils & Fats] Cocamide DEA.†

Noiox KJ Series. [Pulcra SA] PEG unsat. fatty alcohols.†

Noiox KJ-12. [Pulcra SA] Oleth-18.†

Noiox KJ-15. [Pulcra SA] Oleth-10.†

Noiox KS-10, -12, -13, -14, -16. [Pulcra SA] PEG.†

Nonisol 300. [Ciba-Geigy] PEG-8 stearate.†

Nopalcol Series. [Henkel/Functional Prods.] PEG fatty esters.†

Noramium S 75. [Ceca SA] Tallow dimethyl benzyl ammonium chloride.†

Norfox® DESA. [Norman, Fox] Cocamide DEA.†

Norfox® EGMS. [Norman, Fox] Glycol stearate.†

Nutrilan® Angora W. [Henkel] Hydrolyzed keratin.*

Nutrilan® Mohair W. [Henkel] Hydrolyzed keratin.*

Obazoline CS-65. [Toho Chem. Industry] Imidazoline deriv.†

Ogtac-85. [Chem-Y GmbH] Glycidyl trimethyl ammonium chloride.†

Onyxol® 42. [Onyx] Stearamide DEA.†
Onyxol® 336. [Onyx] Lauramide DEA.†
Onyxol® SD. (redesignated Ninol 49CE) [Stepan] Laur-amide DEA.†
Paricin® 1. [CasChem] Methyl hydroxystearate.†
Paricin® 9. [CasChem] Propylene glycol hydroxystearate.†
Paricin® 13. [CasChem] Glyceryl hydroxystearate.†
Paricin® 15. [CasChem] Ethylene glycol hydroxystearate.†
Pationic® 145A. [R.I.T.A.] Sodium stearoyl-1-lactylate.†
PCL-Siccum 2/066215. [Dragoco] Cetearyl octanoate, silica, stearyl heptanoate, isopropyl myristate.*
PCL Solid 2/066220. [Dragoco] Stearyl heptanoate.*
Pearl III. [Presperse] Bismuth oxychloride.*
Pearl Luster Agent MS. [Hoechst Celanese] Glycol disteararate.*
Pearl Supreme. [Presperse] Bismuth oxychloride.*
Pegol® F-68LF. [Rhone-Poulenc Surf. & Spec.] EO/PO block copolymer.*
Pegol® F-87. (see Antarox® PGP-23-7) [Rhone-Poulenc Surf. & Spec.] EO/PO block copolymer.*
Pegol® F-88. (redesignated Antarox® F88) [Rhone-Poulenc Surf. & Spec.] .*
Pegol® L-43. [Rhone-Poulenc Surf. & Spec.] EO/PO block copolymer.*
Pegol® L-44. [Rhone-Poulenc Surf. & Spec.] EO/PO block copolymer.*
Pegol® L-62. (redesignated Antarox® L-62) [Rhone-Poulenc Surf. & Spec.] .*
Pegol® L-62D [Rhone-Poulenc Surf. & Spec.] .*
Pegol® L-62LF. (redesignated Antarox® L-62 LF) [Rhone-Poulenc Surf. & Spec.] .*
Pegol® L-64. (redesignated Antarox® L-64) [Rhone-Poulenc Surf. & Spec.] .*
Pegol® L-72. [Rhone-Poulenc Surf. & Spec.] EO/PO block copolymer.*
Pegol® L-92. [Rhone-Poulenc Surf. & Spec.] EO/PO block copolymer.*
Pegol® P-65. [Rhone-Poulenc Surf. & Spec.] EO/PO block copolymer.*
Pegol® P-75. [Rhone-Poulenc Surf. & Spec.] EO/PO block copolymer.*
Pegol® P-85. [Rhone-Poulenc Surf. & Spec.] EO/PO block copolymer.*
Pegol® P-400. [Rhone-Poulenc Surf. & Spec.] PPG.*
Pegol® P-700. [Rhone-Poulenc Surf. & Spec.] PPG.*
Pegol® P-1000. [Rhone-Poulenc Surf. & Spec.] PPG.*
Pegol® P-2000. [Rhone-Poulenc Surf. & Spec.] PPG.*
Pegosperse® 350 MS. [Lonza] PEG-7 stearate.*
Pegosperse® 4000 DO. [Lonza] PEG-75 dioleate.*
Pegosperse® 6000 DS. [Lonza] PEG-150 distearate.†
Pegosperse® EGMS-70. [Lonza] Glycol stearate.†
Perglanzmittel GM 4006. [Zschimmer & Schwarz] Nonionics and fatty alcohol ether sulfate.†
Perlankrol® ACM2. [Harcros UK] Sodium fatty alkylolamide ether sulfate.†
Perlatum® 400. [IGI Petroleum Spec.] Wh. petrolatum USP†
Perlatum® 410. [IGI Petroleum Spec.] Wh. petrolatum USP†
Perlatum® 410 CG. [IGI Petroleum Spec.] Wh. petrolatum USP†
Perlatum® 415. [IGI Petroleum Spec.] Petrolatum USP.†
Perlatum® 415 CG. [IGI Petroleum Spec.] Petrolatum USP†
Perlatum® 420. [IGI Petroleum Spec.] Wh. petrolatum USP†
Perlatum® 425. [IGI Petroleum Spec.] Petrolatum USP†
Perlatum® 510. [IGI Petroleum Spec.] Wh. petrolatum USP.†
Perlglanz-Konzentrat B-30. [Goldschmidt AG] Cocamide DEA.†

Perlglanz-Konzentrat B-48. [Goldschmidt AG] Cocamide DEA.†
P & G Amide No. 27. [Procter & Gamble] Cocamide MEA.†
Pluracol® E1500. [BASF] PEG-6-32.†
Pluracol® E4500. [BASF] PEG.*
Pluracol® E6000. [BASF] PEG-150.†
Pluracol® W170. [BASF] PPG-5-buteth-7.*
Pluracol® W260. [BASF] Polyalkoxylated polyether.*
Pluracol® W660. [BASF] PPG-12-buteth-16.*
Pluracol® W2000. [BASF] PPG-20-buteth-30.*
Pluracol® W3520N-RL. [BASF] PPG.*
Pluracol® WD1400. [BASF] Polyalkoxylated polyether.*
Pluriol® E 1500. [BASF AG] PEG.†
Pluronic® 10R8. [BASF] Meroxapol 108.*
Pluronic® 12R3. [BASF] PO/EO block copolymer.*
Pluronic® 17R1. [BASF] Meroxapol 171.*
Pluronic® 17R8. [BASF] Meroxapol 178.*
Pluronic® 22R4. [BASF] Block copolymer.*
Pluronic® 25R1. [BASF] Meroxapol 251.*
Pluronic® 25R5. [BASF] Meroxapol 255.*
Pluronic® 31R2. [BASF] Meroxapol 312.*
Pluronic® 31R4. [BASF] Meroxapol 314.*
Pluronic® F68LF. [BASF] Poloxamer 108.*
Pluronic® L10. [BASF] PO/EO block copolymer.*
Pluronic® L42. [BASF] Poloxamer 122.*
Pluronic® L62D. [BASF] Poloxamer 108.*
Pluronic® L62LF. [BASF] Poloxamer 108.*
Pluronic® L63. [BASF] Poloxamer 183.*
Pluronic® L72. [BASF] Poloxamer 212.*
Pluronic® P75. [BASF] Poloxamer 215.*
Pluronic® P94. [BASF] Poloxamer 284.†
Polyaldo® DGHO. [Lonza] Polyglyceryl-10 hexaoleate.†
Polychol 10. [Croda Inc.; Croda Chem. Ltd.] Laneth-10.‡
Polychol 20. [Croda Inc.; Croda Chem. Ltd.] Laneth-20.‡
Polychol 40. [Croda Inc.; Croda Chem. Ltd.] Laneth-40.‡
Poly-DAC 40. [Rhone-Poulenc Surf. & Spec.] Polyquaternium-6.*
Polylan®. [Amerchol; Amerchol Europe] Oleyl linoleate, lanolin linoleate.*
Polymer Additive GH. [BASF] Polyoxyisobutylene/methylene urea copolymer.*
Polysphere 3000 SP. [Presperse] Polystyrene, squalane.*
Product DDN. [DuPont] Lauryl betaine.*
Produkt B 2045. [Croda Chem. Ltd.] Alkenyl succinic anhydride.†
Produkt GM 4055. [Zschimmer & Schwarz] Fatty acid glycol ester and fatty alcohol ether sulfate.†
Produkt GS 5001. [Zschimmer & Schwarz] Fatty acid DEA, modified.†
Produkt RT 275. [Zschimmer & Schwarz] Abietic acid polyglycol ester.†
Produkt RT 288. [Zschimmer & Schwarz] Olive oil ethoxylate.†
Progacyl® COS-1. [Rhone-Poulenc] Guar gum.*
Progacyl® COS-10. [Rhone-Poulenc] Carboxymethyl guar.*
Progacyl® COS-20, -70. [Rhone-Poulenc] Hydroxypropyl guar.*
Prostearyl 15. [Croda Inc.; Croda Chem. Ltd.] PPG-15 stearyl ether.‡
Proto-Lan A240. [Maybrook] Isopropyl myristate, sorbitan oleate, myristoyl hydrolyzed collagen.*
Provol 10. [Croda Inc.] PPG-10 oleyl ether.‡
Provol 30. [Croda Inc.] PPG-30 oleyl ether.‡
PTFE-19. [Presperse] PTFE, titanium dioxide.*
Puxol CB-22. [Pulcra SA] TEA dodecylbenzene sulfonate.†
Pyridine 1°. [Nepera] Pyridine.†

---

* Discontinued or redesignated   † Unverified   ‡ No longer standard

Quartamin 86W. [Kao Corp. SA] Stearyl trimethyl ammonium chloride.†

Quinta-Pro Conc. [Maybrook] Hydrolyzed collagen, triethonium hydrolyzed collagen ethosulfate, cationic collagen polypeptides, hydrolyzed keratin, collagen amino acids.*

Radianol® 7106. [Fina Chemicals] Glyceryl tricaprate/caprylate.†

Radiasurf® 7000. [Fina Chemicals] PEG-20 glyceryl stearate.†

Relaxer Conc. No. 3. [Brooks Industries] Cetearyl aclohol, polysorbate 60, laneth-15, cetyl alcohol, steareth-20, PEG-150 stearate.*

Relaxer Conc. No. 4. [Brooks Industries] Cetearyl alcohol, cetyl alcohol, polysorbate 60, laneth-15, laneth-60, cocoyl sarcosine.*

Remanol 1300. [Kempen] Collagen protein hydrolysate.†

Remanol 1300/35. [Kempen] Collagen protein hydrolysate.†

Rewomat B 2003. [Rewo GmbH] Tetrasodium (1,2-dicarboxyethyl)-N-alkyl sulfosuccinamide.†

Rewomid® 203/S. [Rewo GmbH] Lauramide DEA.†

Rewomid® DL 203. [Rewo GmbH] Lauramide DEA and diethanolamine.†

Rewominoxid B 204. [Rewo GmbH] Cocamidopropylamine oxide.†

Rewopal® CSF 11. [Rewo GmbH] Ceteareth-11.†

Rewopol® MLS 35. [Rewo GmbH] MEA-lauryl sulfate.†

Rewopol® SBDO 70. [Rewo GmbH] Dioctyl sodium sulfosuccinate.†

Rewopol® SBR 12-Powder. [Rewo GmbH] Disodium lauryl sulfosuccinate.†

Rewopon® AM-2C. [Rewo GmbH] Coconut-based ampholyte.†

Rewopon® AM-2L. [Rewo GmbH] Imidazoline-based ampholyte.†

Rewopon® AM-B 13. [Rewo GmbH] Alkyl amido betaine.†

Rewopon® AM-CA. [Rewo GmbH] Coconut-based ampholyte.†

Rewoquat QA 100. [Rewo GmbH] Myristalkonium saccharinate.†

Rewoquat UTM 185. [Rewo GmbH] Undecylenic quat. ammonium methosulfate.†

Rewoquat W 7500 H. [Rewo GmbH] Quat. dialkyl imidazolinium methosulfate, hydrog.†

Rheodol 430, 450. [Kao Corp. SA] POE polyol fatty acid ester.†

Rheodol AO-10. [Kao Corp. SA] Sorbitan oleate.†

Rheodol AO-15. [Kao Corp. SA] Sorbitan sesquioleate.†

Rheodol AS-10. [Kao Corp. SA] Sorbitan stearate.†

Rheodol MO-60. [Kao Corp. SA] Glyceryl oleate.†

Rheodol MS-50, MS-60, SEM. [Kao Corp. SA] Glyceryl stearate.†

Rheodol SP-L10. [Kao Corp. SA] Sorbitan laurate.†

Rheodol SP-P10. [Kao Corp. SA] Sorbitan palmitate.†

Rheodol TW-L106, -L120. [Kao Corp. SA] POE sorbitan laurate.†

Rheodol TW-P120. [Kao Corp. SA] PEG-20 sorbitan palmitate.†

Rhodacal® LA Acid. [Rhone-Poulenc Surf. & Spec.] Dodecylbenzene sulfonic acid.*

Rhodacal® T. [Rhone-Poulenc Surf. & Spec.] TEA dodecylbenzene sulfonate.*

Rhodafac® RE-870. [Rhone-Poulenc Surf. & Spec.] Free acid of complex org. phosphate ester.*

Rhodapex® EAY. [Rhone-Poulenc Surf. & Spec.] Ammonium laureth sulfate.*

Rhodapex® N 70. (see Rhodapex ES-2) [Rhone-Poulenc

Surf. & Spec.] Sodium laureth sulfate.*

Rhodasurf® C-2. [Rhone-Poulenc Surf. & Spec.] Ceteareth-2.*

Rhodasurf® LAN-3 .(see Rhodasurf® A-24) [Rhone-Poulenc Surf. & Spec.] .*

Rhodasurf® LAN-23-75%. [Rhone-Poulenc Surf. & Spec.] Laureth-23.*

Rhodialux™ A. [Rhone-Poulenc Surf. & Spec.] Benzophenone-3.*

Rhodialux™ D. [Rhone-Poulenc Surf. & Spec.] Benzophenone-1.*

Rhodialux™ S. [Rhone-Poulenc Surf. & Spec.] Benzophenone-4.*

Rhodiasurf B. (redesignated Alkamuls® B) [Rhone-Poulenc].*

Rhodiasurf O. (redesignated Igepal® O) [Rhone-Poulenc] .*

RITA AZ. [R.I.T.A.] Guay-azulene sodium sulfonate.*

RITA KA. [R.I.T.A.] Kojic acid.*

Ritacetin. [R.I.T.A.] Quercetin.*

Ritalafa® 5. [R.I.T.A.] PEG-5 lanolate.*

Ritalafa® 10. [R.I.T.A.] PEG-10 lanolate.*

Ritalan® HKS. [R.I.T.A.] Polybutene, lanolin oil.*

Ritalanine. [R.I.T.A.] Σb-Alanine.*

Ritapan CAP. [R.I.T.A.] Calcium pantothenate.*

Ritapan NAP. [R.I.T.A.] Sodium pantothenate.*

Ritapeg 100 DS. [R.I.T.A.] Ethoxylated distearic acid ester.*

Ritapeg 400 DS. [R.I.T.A.] PEG-8 distearate.*

Ritaphenone 3. [R.I.T.A.] Benzophenone-3.*

Ritaplast R. [R.I.T.A.] Lanolin oil, polyethylene.*

Ritaplast TN. [R.I.T.A.] C12-15 alcohols benzoate and polyethylene.*

Ritapro 300K. [R.I.T.A.] Ethoxylated fatty alcohol ether.*

Ritapro 300R. [R.I.T.A.] Cetearyl alcohol, ceteareth-20.*

Ritaquat Q. [R.I.T.A.] Steartrimonium hydrolyzed animal protein.*

Ritasilk. [R.I.T.A.] Hydrolyzed silk protein.*

Ritasilk Powd. [R.I.T.A.] Silk powd.*

Ritasol Base 100. [R.I.T.A.] Isopropyl lanolate, lanolin oil.*

Ritasol Base 200. [R.I.T.A.] Lanolin, isopropyl lanolate.*

Ritatin. [R.I.T.A.] Biotin.*

Ritawax 15. [R.I.T.A.] Laneth-15.*

Ritawax 40. [R.I.T.A.] Laneth-40.*

Ritox 721. [R.I.T.A.] Steareth-21.*

Robecote. [Robeco] Shark liver oil.†

Robeyl. [Robeco] Squalene, hydrog. shark liver oil.†

Sactol 2 OS 2. [Lever Industriel] Sodium laureth sulfate.†

Sactol 2 OS 28. [Lever Industriel] Sodium laureth sulfate.†

Sactol 2 OT. [Lever Industriel] TEA laureth sulfate.†

Sactol 2 S 3. [Lever Industriel] Sodium lauryl sulfate.†

Sactol 2 T. [Lever Industriel] TEA lauryl sulfate.†

Sandoz Amide NT. [Sandoz] Alkanolamide.†

Sandoz Amide PE. [Sandoz] Lauryl alkanolamide (1:1).†

Sandoz Amide PL. [Sandoz] Lauryl alkanolamide (2:1).†

Sandoz Amide PO. [Sandoz] Coconut alkanolamide (1:1).†

Sandoz Amine Oxide XA-C. [Sandoz] Cetyl amine oxide.†

Sandoz Amine Oxide XA-L. [Sandoz] Lauryl amine oxide.†

Sandoz Amine Oxide XA-M. [Sandoz] Myristyl amine oxide.†

Sandoz Sulfate A. [Sandoz] Ammonium lauryl sulfate.†

Sandoz Sulfate EP. [Sandoz] DEA-lauryl sulfate.†

Sandoz Sulfate ES-3. [Sandoz] Sodium laureth sulfate (3 EO).†

Sandoz Sulfate K. [Sandoz] Ammonium mixed alkyl sulfate.†

Sandoz Sulfate WA-9. [Sandoz] Sodium lauryl sulfate.†

Sandoz Sulfate WA Dry. [Sandoz] Sodium lauryl sulfate.†

Sandoz Sulfate WA Special. [Sandoz] Sodium lauryl

sulfate.†
Sandoz Sulfate WAG. [Sandoz] Sodium lauryl sulfate.†
Sandoz Sulfate WAS. [Sandoz] Sodium lauryl sulfate.†
Sandoz Sulfate WE. [Sandoz] Sodium laureth sulfate (3.5 EO).†
Sandoz Sulfonate AAS 60S. [Sandoz] Linear alkyl (C12) benzene sulfonate, TEA salt.†
Sanisol C. [Kao Corp. SA] Benzalkonium chloride.†
Sanisol CPR, CR, CR-80%. [Kao Corp. SA] Benzalkonium chloride.†
Sanisol HTPR. [Kao Corp. SA] Benzalkonium chloride.†
Sanisol OPR, TPR. [Kao Corp. SA] Benzalkonium chloride.†
Sarkosine KA Conc. [Hoechst Celanese] Sodium cocoyl sarcosinate.*
Sarkosine KF. [Hoechst Celanese] TEA-palm kernel sarcosinate.*
Sarkosine LD. [Hoechst Celanese] Sodium lauroyl sarcosinate.*
Sarkosyl® LC. [Ciba-Geigy AG] Cocoyl sarcosine.†
Sarkosyl® NL-30. [Ciba-Geigy AG] Sodium lauroyl sarcosinate.†
Sarkosyl® O. [Ciba-Geigy AG] Oleoyl sarcosine.†
Satexlan 20. [Croda Inc.; Croda Chem. Ltd.] PEG-20 hydrog. lanolin.‡
Satulan. [Croda Inc.; Croda Chem. Ltd.] Hydrog. lanolin.‡
Schercamox T-12. [Scher] Dihydroxyethyl tallowamine oxide.†
Schercemol 85. [Scher] Octyl neopentanoate.*
Schercemol CM. [Scher] Cetyl myristate.*
Schercemol CP. [Scher] Cetyl palmitate.*
Schercemol CS. [Scher] Cetyl stearate.*
Schercemol DED. [Scher] Ethyl dimerate.†
Schercemol DEGMS. [Scher] PEG-2 stearate.*
Schercemol DEIS. [Scher] Decyl isostearate.†
Schercemol DICA. [Scher] Diisocetyl adipate.*
Schercemol EE. [Scher] Erucyl erucate.*
Schercemol IPM. [Scher] IPM.†
Schercemol IPO. [Scher] Isopropyl oleate.†
Schercemol ISE. [Scher] Isostearyl erucate.*
Schercemol SE. [Scher] Stearyl erucate.*
Schercemol TT. [Scher] Triisopropyl trilinoleate.†
Schercomid 1-102. [Scher] Cocamide DEA.†
Schercomid AME-70. [Scher] Acetamide MEA.†
Schercomid CDA-H. [Scher] Cocamide DEA.†
Schercomid CMI. [Scher] Cocamide MIPA.*
Schercomid ID. [Scher] Isostearamide DEA.†
Schercomid IMI. [Scher] Isostearamide MIPA.†
Schercomid LD. [Scher] Lauramide DEA and diethanolamine.†
Schercomid M. [Scher] Isostearamide DEA.†
Schercomid MD-Extra. [Scher] Myristamide DEA.†
Schercomid MME. [Scher] Myristamide MEA.†
Schercomid SD-DS. [Scher] Stearamide DEA disterate.†
Schercomid SI-M. [Scher] Isostearamide DEA.†
Schercomid SLA. [Scher] Lauric/myristic/palmitic DEA.†
Schercomid SLL. [Scher] Lauric/myristic super DEA.†
Schercomid SLM. [Scher] Lauramide DEA.†
Schercomid SLMC-75. [Scher] Lauramide DEA.*
Schercomid SM. [Scher] Myristamide DEA.†
Schercomid SME-A. [Scher] Stearamide MEA.†
Schercomid SME-M. [Scher] Stearamide MEA (1:1).†
Schercomid SME-S. [Scher] Stearamide MEA stearate.†
Schercopearl EA-100. [Scher] Stearamide MEA.†
Schercopol CMIS-Na. [Scher] Disodium cocamido MIPA-sulfosuccinate.*
Schercopol OMES-A. [Scher] Diammonium oleamido PEG-2 sulfosuccinate.*

Schercopol OMES-Na. [Scher] Disodium oleamido PEG-2 sulfosuccinate.*
Schercopol OMIS-Na. [Scher] Disodium oleamido MIPA-sulfosuccinate.*
Schercopol RMS-Na. [Scher] Disodium ricinoleamido MEA-sulfosuccinate.*
Schercoquat IAS-LC. [Scher] N-(3-isostearylamidopropyl), N-N dimethyl, N-ethyl ammonium ethyl sulfate.*
Schercoquat IB. [Scher] Isostearamidopropalkonium chloride.†
Schercoquat IIB. [Scher] Isostearyl benzylimidonium chloride.†
Schercoquat IIS-R. [Scher] Isostearyl ethyl imidonium ethosulfate.†
Schercoquat IIS-RD. [Scher] 2-Isoalkyl (C14-C20), 1-hydroxyethyl, 1-ethyl imidazolinium ethyl sulfate.†
Schercoquat ROAB. [Scher] Rapeseedamidopropyl benzyldimonium chloride.†
Schercoquat SOAB. [Scher] Soyamidopropyl benzyl-dimonium chloride.†
Schercoquat WOAB. [Scher] Wheat germamidopropyl betaine.*
Schercotaine CAB-G. [Scher] Cocoamidopropyl betaine.†
Schercotaine CAB-Z. [Scher] Cocamidopropyl betaine, zinc chloride.*
Schercotaine LAB. [Scher] Lauramidopropyl betaine.*
Schercotaine OAB. [Scher] Oleamidopropyl betaine.*
Schercotaine OB. [Scher] Oleyl betaine.*
Schercoteric LS. [Scher] Lauroamphoacetate.*
Schercoteric LS-2. [Scher] Lauroamphodiacetate.†
Schercoteric LS-2ES MOD. [Scher] Lauroamphodiacetate, sodium laureth sulfate, SD alcohol 40.†
Schercoteric LS-2TE. [Scher] Lauroamphocarboxy-glycinate, sodium trideceth sulfate.†
Schercoteric LS-2TE MOD. [Scher] Lauroamphocarboxy-glycinate, sodium trideceth sulfate, hexylene glycol.†
Schercoteric LS-EP. [Scher] Lauroamphohydroxypropyl-sulfonate.†
Schercoteric LS-SF, LS-SF Conc. [Scher] Lauroampho-propionate.†
Schercoteric LS-SF-2. [Scher] Lauroamphodipropionate.†
Schercoteric LS-SF-2 Conc. [Scher] Lauric imidazolinium deriv. dicarboxylate.†
Schercoteric LS-SF-2 Super Conc. [Scher] Lauric imidazolinium deriv. dicarboxylate.†
Schercoteric MS-2ES Modified. [Scher] Disodium cocoam-phodiacetate, sodium laureth sulfate.*
Schercoteric MS-2 Modified. [Scher] Disodium cocoam-phodiacetate, sodium lauryl sulfate, hexylene glycol.*
Schercoteric MS-SF-2 (70%). [Scher] Disodium cocoam-phodipropionate.†
Schercoteric MS-SF-2 Super Conc. [Scher] Coco imidazolinium deriv. dicarboxylate.†
Schercoteric MS-SF (38%). [Scher] Coco imidazolinium deriv. monocarboxylate.†
Schercoteric MS-SF (70%). [Scher] Coco imidazolinium deriv. monocarboxylate.†
Schercoteric OS-SF. [Scher] Oleoamphopropionate.†
Schercoteric STS. [Scher] Stearoamphodiacetate.†
Schercozoline B. [Scher] Behenyl hydroxyethyl imidazo-line.†
Schercozoline S. [Scher] Stearyl imidazoline.†
Scheroba Oil. [Scher] Isostearyl erucate and erucyl erucate.*
SD-35. [Presperse] Panthenyl ethyl ether.*
Secosol® EA/40. [Stepan Europe] Sodium mono alkylethanolamide sulfosuccinate.†

Sentry Simethicone NF. [Union Carbide] Simethicone.*

Sequestrene® NA4. [Ciba-Geigy/Dyestuffs] Tetrasodium EDTA.†

Serdet DCK 3/70. [Servo Delden BV] Sodium laureth sulfate (2 EO).†

Serdet DCK 30. [Servo Delden BV] Sodium laureth sulfate (3 EO).†

Serdet DCN 30. [Servo Delden BV] Ammonium C12–C14 alkyl ether sulfate (3 EO).†

Serdet DFK 40. [Servo Delden BV] Sodium lauryl sulfate.†

Serdet DFL 40. [Servo Delden BV] TEA-lauryl sulfate.†

Serdet DFM 33. [Servo Delden BV] MEA-lauryl sulfate.†

Serdet DFN 30. [Servo Delden BV] Ammonium lauryl sulfate.†

Serdet DMK 75. [Servo Delden BV] Sodium dodecylbenzene sulfonate.†

Serdet DML 45. [Servo Delden BV] Triethanolammonium dodecylbenzene sulfonate.†

Serdet DPK 3/70. [Servo Delden BV] Sodium C12–15 alkyl ether sulfate (3 EO).†

Serdet DPK 30. [Servo Delden BV] Sodium C12–15 pareth sulfate.†

Serdet NZ 60. [Servo Delden BV] Lauryl ether sulfate and alkylolamide.†

Serdolamide POF 61. [Servo Delden BV] Oleic acid polydiethanolamide.†

Serdolamide PYF 77. [Servo Delden BV] Fatty acid DEA.†

Servo Amfolyt JA 110. [Servo Delden BV] Imidazoline, modified.†

Servo Amfolyt JA 140. [Servo Delden BV] Imidazoline, modified.†

Servoxyl VLB 1123. [Servo Delden BV] Sodium monoalkyl polyglycol ether sulfosuccinate.†

Servoxyl VPGZ 7/100. [Servo Delden BV] Cetyl oleyl ether phosphate, acid form (7 EO).†

Servoxyl VPIZ 100. [Servo Delden BV] Acid butyl phosphate.†

Servoxyl VPNZ 10/100. [Servo Delden BV] Nonylphenol ether phosphate, acid form (10 EO).†

Servoxyl VPQZ 9/100. [Servo Delden BV] Dinonylphenol polyglycol ether phosphate, acid form (9 EO).†

Servoxyl VPTZ 100. [Servo Delden BV] 2-Ethylhexyl phosphate, acid form.†

Servoxyl VPTZ 3/100. [Servo Delden BV] 2-Ethylhexyl polyglycol ether phosphate, acid form.†

Servoxyl VPUZ. [Servo Delden BV] Acid methyl phosphate.†

Servoxyl VPYZ 500. [Servo Delden BV] Acid phosphate ester, modified.†

SF1214. [GE Silicones] Silicone fluid.†

SGP 502S Absorbent Polymer. [Henkel/Emery/OPG] Corn starch/acrylamide/sodium acrylate copolymer.*

Silbione™ Antifoam 70414, 70416, 70426R, 70452. (see Rhodorsil) [Rhone-Poulenc] Simethicone.*

Silbione™ Oils 70041 VO.65. (see Rhodorsil) [Rhone-Poulenc] Hexamethyldisiloxane.*

Silbione™ Oils 70045. (see Rhodorsil) [Rhone-Poulenc] Cyclomethicone.*

Silbione™ Oils 70641 V200. (see Rhodorsil) [Rhone-Poulenc] Diphenyl dimethicone.*

Silk Protein Complex. [Croda Chem. Ltd.] Hydrolyzed silk protein.†

Sipex® 280. (see Rhodapex® CO-436) [Rhone-Poulenc Surf. & Spec.] .*

Sipex® EC-111. (redesignated Rhodapon® EC111) [Rhone-Poulenc Surf. & Spec.] .*

Sipex® EST-75. (see Rhodapex® EST-30) [Rhone-Poulenc Surf. & Spec.] Sodium trideceth sulfate.*

Sipon® 101-10. (see Rhodapon SB-8208/S) [Rhone-Poulenc Surf. & Spec.] Sodium lauryl sulfate.*

Sipon® EA. (redesignated Rhodapex® EA) [Rhone-Poulenc Surf. & Spec.] Ammonium laureth sulfate.*

Sipon® EAY. (redesignated Rhodapex® EAY) [Rhone-Poulenc Surf. & Spec.] Ammonium laureth sulfate.*

Sipon® ES. (redesignated Rhodapex® ES) [Rhone-Poulenc Surf. & Spec.] .*

Sipon® ES-2. (redesignated Rhodapex® ES-2) [Rhone-Poulenc Surf. & Spec.] .*

Sipon® ES-7. [Rhone-Poulenc Surf. & Spec.] Sodium laureth sulfate (7 EO).*

Sipon® ESY. (redesignated Rhodapex® ESY) [Rhone-Poulenc Surf. & Spec.] .*

Sipon® L-22. (redesignated Rhodapon® L-22) [Rhone-Poulenc Surf. & Spec.] .*

Sipon® LD. [Rhone-Poulenc Surf. & Spec.] DEA-lauryl sulfate.*

Sipon® LM. (redesignated Rhodapon® LM) [Rhone-Poulenc Surf. & Spec.] .*

Sipon® LSB. (redesignated Rhodapon® LSB) [Rhone-Poulenc Surf. & Spec.] .*

Sipon® LT-6. (redesignated Rhodapon® LT-6) [Rhone-Poulenc Surf. & Spec.] .*

Siponate® 301-10. (redesignated Rhodacal® 301-10) [Rhone-Poulenc Surf. & Spec.] .*

Siponate® 301-10F. (redesignated Rhodacal 301-10F) [Rhone-Poulenc Surf. & Spec.] Sodium C14–16 olefin sulfonate.*

Siponate® A-246 L. (redesignated Rhodacal® A-246 L) [Rhone-Poulenc Surf. & Spec.] .*

Siponic® 260. (redesignated Alcodet® 260) [Rhone-Poulenc Surf. & Spec.] .*

Siponic® E-2. [Rhone-Poulenc Surf. & Spec.] Ceteareth-4.*

Siponic® E-3. [Rhone-Poulenc Surf. & Spec.] Ceteareth-6.*

Siponic® E-5. [Rhone-Poulenc Surf. & Spec.] Ceteareth-10.*

Siponic® E-7. [Rhone-Poulenc Surf. & Spec.] Ceteareth-14.*

Siponic® E-10. [Rhone-Poulenc Surf. & Spec.] Ceteareth-20.*

Siponic® E-15. [Rhone-Poulenc Surf. & Spec.] Ceteareth-30.*

Siponic® F-160. [Rhone-Poulenc Surf. & Spec.] Octoxynol-16.*

Siponic® F-300. (see Igepal® CA-887) [Rhone-Poulenc Surf. & Spec.] Octoxynol-30.*

Siponic® F-400. (see Igepal® CA-897) [Rhone-Poulenc Surf. & Spec.] Octoxynol-40.*

Siponic® F-707. [Rhone-Poulenc Surf. & Spec.] Octoxynol-70.*

Siponic® L-3 . (see Rhodasurf LA-3) [Rhone-Poulenc Surf. & Spec.] Laureth-3.*

Siponic® L-4. (redesignated Rhodasurf® L-4) [Rhone-Poulenc Surf. & Spec.] .*

Siponic® L-7-90. (redesignated Rhodasurf® L-790) [Rhone-Poulenc Surf. & Spec.] .*

Siponic® L-12. (see Rhodasurf® LA-12) [Rhone-Poulenc Surf. & Spec.] Laureth-12.*

Siponic® L-25. (redesignated Rhodasurf® L-25) [Rhone-Poulenc Surf. & Spec.] .*

Siponic® NP-7. [Rhone-Poulenc Surf. & Spec.] Nonoxynol-7.*

Siponic® NP-8. (see Alkasurf® NP-8) [Rhone-Poulenc Surf. & Spec.] Nonoxynol-8.*

Siponic® NP-9.5. (see Igepal® CO-630) [Rhone-Poulenc

---

* Discontinued or redesignated   † Unverified   ‡ No longer standard

Surf. & Spec.] Nonoxynol-9.5.*

Siponic® NP-10 .(see Igepal® CO-660) [Rhone-Poulenc Surf. & Spec.] Nonoxynol-10.*

Siponic® NP-13. (see Igepal® CO-720) [Rhone-Poulenc Surf. & Spec.] Nonoxynol-13.*

Siponic® NP-407. (see Igepal® CO-897) [Rhone-Poulenc Surf. & Spec.] Nonoxynol-40.*

Siponic® S-2. (redesignated Rhodasurf® S-2) [Rhone-Poulenc Surf. & Spec.] .*

Siponic® S-20. (redesignated Rhodasurf® S-20) [Rhone-Poulenc Surf. & Spec.] .*

Siponic® SK. (redesignated Alcodet® SK) [Rhone-Poulenc Surf. & Spec.] PEG-8 isolauryl thioether.*

Siponic® TD-3. (see Rhodasurf® BC-420) [Rhone-Poulenc Surf. & Spec.] Trideceth-3.*

Siponic® TD-12. [Rhone-Poulenc Surf. & Spec.] Trideceth-12.*

Siponic® Y500-70. (see Rhodasurf® ON-877) [Rhone-Poulenc Surf. & Spec.] Oleth-25.*

Sipothix® H-65. [Rhone-Poulenc Surf. & Spec.] Ethylacrylate/methylacrylic acid copolymer.*

Skliro Distilled. [Croda Inc.] Lanolin acid.‡

Solangel 401. [Croda Inc.] PEG-75 lanolin.‡

Solidester. [Robeco] Ester-hydrog. piscine oil.†

Solwax C-24. [Van Schuppen] Polyethoxylated cholesterol.†

Solwax L20. [Van Schuppen] Alkoxylated deriv. of pharmaceutical lanolin.†

Solwax LG 35. [Van Schuppen] Alkoxylated deriv. of lanolin alcohols.†

Sorba. [Croda Chem. Ltd.] Lanolin.†

Spheron PL-700. [Presperse] Silica.*

Spinomar NaSS. [Tosoh] Sodium p-styrenesulfonate.†

Stafoam DF-1. [Nippon Oils & Fats] Cocamide DEA (1:1).†

Stafoam DF-4. [Nippon Oils & Fats] Cocamide DEA (1:1).†

Stafoam DL. [Nippon Oils & Fats] Lauramide DEA (1:1).†

Standamid® 100. [Henkel] Cocamide MEA.†

Standamid® CMG. [Henkel] Cocamide MEA.†

Standamid® KDM. [Henkel] Cocamide DEA (1:2).†

Standamid® LDM. [Henkel] Lauramide DEA, modified.†

Standamid® LP. [Henkel] Lauramide MIPA.†

Standamox C 30. [Henkel] Coco amido amine oxide.†

Standamul® 302. [Henkel] Propylene glycol dicaprylate/dicaprate.†

Standamul® 318. [Henkel] Caprylic/capric triglyceride.†

Standamul® 1414-E. [Henkel] Myreth-3 myristate.†

Standamul® 1616. [Henkel] Cetyl palmitate.†

Standamul® 7061. [Henkel] Isocetyl stearate.†

Standamul® 7063. [Henkel] Octyl dodecyl stearate.†

Standamul® 7105. [Henkel] Caprylic/capric triglyceride.†

Standamul® 7115. [Henkel] Myristyleicosyl stearate.*

Standamul® B-1. [Henkel] Ceteareth-12.†

Standamul® B-2. [Henkel] Ceteareth-20.†

Standamul® B-3. [Henkel] Ceteareth-30.†

Standamul® CTA. [Henkel] Hexyl laurate.†

Standamul® CTV. [Henkel] Decyl oleate.†

Standamul® G. [Henkel] Octyl dodecanol.†

Standamul® G-16. [Henkel] Isocetyl alcohol.†

Standamul® G-32/36. [Henkel] Myristyl eicosanol.†

Standamul® G-32/36 Stearate. [Henkel] Myristyl eicosyl stearate.†

Standamul® GT-3236. [Henkel] Myristyl eicosanol.†

Standamul® GTO-26. [Henkel] Undecylpentadecanol.*

Standamul® HE. [Henkel] PEG-7 glyceryl cocoate.†

Standamul® LC. [Henkel] Coco caprylate/caprate.†

Standamul® M-8. [Henkel] Oleyl and cetyl alcohol PEG ether.†

Standamul® O-5. [Henkel] Oleth-5.†

Standamul® O-10. [Henkel] Oleth-10.†

Standamul® O-20. [Henkel] Oleth-20.†

Standamul® OXL. [Henkel] PPG-10 ceteareth-20.†

Standamul® STC-25. [Henkel] Stearalkonium chloride.†

Standapol® AB-45. [Henkel] Coco betaine.†

Standapol® AL-60. [Henkel] Ammonium laureth sulfate.†

Standapol® AMS-100. [Henkel] Ammonium lauryl sulfate.†

Standapol® BAW. [Henkel] Cocamidopropyl betaine.†

Standapol® BC-35. [Henkel] Cocamidopropyl betaine.†

Standapol® ES-7099. [Henkel] Sodium laureth sulfate.†

Standapol® OLB-30. [Henkel] Oleyl betaine.†

Standapol® OLB-50. [Henkel] Oleyl betaine.†

Standapol® SH-200. [Henkel] Ammonium oleamido PEG-2 sulfosuccinate.†

Standapol® SHC-301. [Henkel] TEA oleamido PEG-2 sulfosuccinate and TEA lauryl sulfate.†

Standapol® SL-60. [Henkel] Sodium laureth sulfate.†

Standapol® TS-100. [Henkel] TEA-lauryl sulfate.†

Standapol® WAS-100. [Henkel] Sodium lauryl sulfate.†

Sulfetal CA 30. [Zschimmer & Schwarz] Ammonium lauryl sulfate.†

Sul-fon-ate AA-9. [Boliden Intertrade] Sodium dodecylbenzene sulfonate.†

Sul-fon-ate LA-10. [Boliden Intertrade] Sodium dodecylbenzene sulfonate.†

Sulfopon® WA 30. [Henkel Canada] Sodium lauryl sulfate.†

Sulfostat KNT. [Zschimmer & Schwarz] Amido alkylamine acetate.†

Sulfotex DOS. [Henkel Canada] Disodium oleamido PEG sulfosuccinate.†

Sulfotex WA. [Henkel Canada] Sodium lauryl sulfate.†

Sulfotex WAT. [Henkel] TEA lauryl sulfate.†

Sulphonated 'Lorol' Liquid MA, MR. [Ronsheim & Moore] MEA-lauryl sulfate.†

Sulphonated 'Lorol' Liquid NH. [Ronsheim & Moore] Ammonium lauryl sulfate.†

Sulphonated 'Lorol' Liquid TA, TN, TNR. [Ronsheim & Moore] TEA-lauryl sulfate.†

Sulphonated 'Lorol' Paste. [Ronsheim & Moore] Sodium lauryl sulfate.†

Sunnol LBN. [Lion] POE lauryl ether sulfate.†

Sunnol LDF-110. [Lion] Alcohol sulfate.†

Sunnol LL-103. [Lion] Alcohol sulfate.†

Sunnol LST. [Lion] TEA lauryl sulfate.†

Super Refined™ Coconut Oil. [Croda Inc.; Croda Surf. Ltd.] Coconut oil.‡

Supro-Tein R. [Maybrook] Sodium cocoyl hydrolyzed rice protein, sorbitol.*

Surfine WCT-Gel. [Finetex] Sodium C11–15 pareth-7 carboxylate.†

Surfine WNT Liq. [Finetex] Sodium C12-15 pareth-7 carboxylate.*

Swascol L-327. [Swastik] Sodium laureth sulfate.†

Sykanol DKM 45, 80. [Henkel KGaA/Cospha] Sulfated castor oil.†

Synoquart P 50. [Aquatec Quimica SA] Cetrimonium chloride.†

Synotol 119 N. [Aquatec Quimica SA] Cocamide DEA.†

Synotol CN 20. [Aquatec Quimica SA] Cocamide DEA.†

Synotol L 60. [Aquatec Quimica SA] Lauramide DEA.†

Synotol L 90. [Aquatec Quimica SA] Lauramide DEA.†

Synotol LM 60. [Aquatec Quimica SA] Lauramide DEA.†

Synotol LM 90. [Aquatec Quimica SA] Lauric/myristic acid DEA.†

Synotol Detergent E. [Aquatec Quimica SA] Cocamide DEA.†

---

* Discontinued or redesignated   † Unverified   ‡ No longer standard

Synperonic 3S25. [ICI plc] Syn. primary alcohol ethoxylate sulfate, sodium salt.†

Synperonic 3S27S. [ICI plc] Syn. primary alcohol ethylene oxide condensate, sodium salt.†

Synperonic 3S70. [ICI plc] Syn. primary alcohol ethoxylate.†

Synperonic A6. [ICI Am.] Syn. primary alcohol ethoxylate.†

Synprolam 35DMO. [ICI plc] C13-15 alkyl dimethyl amine oxide.†

Synprolam 35MX1/O. [ICI plc] C13–15 alkyl methyl hydroxyethyl amine oxide.†

Synprolam 35X2/O. [ICI plc] C13-15 alkyl bis (2-hydroxyethyl) amine oxide.†

Syntofor A03, A04, AB03, AB04, AL3, AL4, B03, B04. [Witco/H-I-P] Polyglycol fatty ester.†

Syntran KL-219. [Interpolymer] Ammonium acrylates copolymer, propylene glycol, sodium laureth sulfate, nonoxynol-10.*

Tagat® I. [Goldschmidt; Goldschmidt AG] PEG-30 glyceryl isostearate.*

Tagat® I2. [Goldschmidt; Goldschmidt AG] PEG-20 glyceryl isostearate.*

Tagat® RI. [Goldschmidt AG] PEG-15 glyceryl ricinoleate.*

Talc MS. [Presperse] Talc.*

Tauranol M. [Finetex] Sodium methyl oleoyl taurate.†

Tegamine® P-7. [Goldschmidt] Cocamidopropyl dimethylamine.†

Tegin® A-412. [Goldschmidt] Propylene glycol stearate.†

Tegin® A-422. [Goldschmidt] Diethylene glycol stearate.†

Tegin® C-1R. [Goldschmidt] Glyceryl stearate SE and hydrog. tallow glyceride citrate.†

Tegin® C-61. [Goldschmidt] Hydrog. tallow glyceride citrate.*

Tegin® C-62 SE. [Goldschmidt AG] Hydrog. tallow glyceride citrate.*

Tegin® C-63. [Goldschmidt] Monodiglyceride citric acid ester.†

Tegin® C-63 SE. [Goldschmidt] Hydrog. tallow glyceride citrate.†

Tegin® C-64. [Goldschmidt] Hydrog. tallow glyceride citrate.*

Tegin® C-611. [Goldschmidt] Glyceryl stearate SE and hydrog. tallow glyceride citrate.*

Tegin® DGS. [Goldschmidt] Diglycol stearate.†

Tegin® E-41. [Goldschmidt] Acetylated hydrog. tallow glyceride.*

Tegin® E-41 NSE. [Goldschmidt] Acetylated hydrog. tallow glycerides.†

Tegin® E-61. [Goldschmidt] Acetylated hydrog. lard glyceride.*

Tegin® E-61 NSE. [Goldschmidt] Acetylated hydrog. lard glyceride.†

Tegin® E-66. [Goldschmidt] Acetylated lard glyceride.*

Tegin® E-66 NSE. [Goldschmidt] Acetylated lard glyceride.†

Tegin® GO. [Goldschmidt] Ethylene glycol oleate.†

Tegin® GRB. [Goldschmidt] Glyceryl stearate.*

Tegin® GRB NSE. [Goldschmidt] Glyceryl stearate.†

Tegin® L 61, L 62. [Goldschmidt] Hydrog. tallow glyceride lactate.*

Tegin® MAV. [Goldschmidt] Glyceryl stearate.*

Tegin® M NSE. [Goldschmidt] Glycerol stearate.*

Tegin® O NSE. [Goldschmidt AG] Glyceryl oleate.*

Tegin® P-411. [Goldschmidt] Propylene glycol stearate.*

Tegin® P-411 SE. [Goldschmidt] Propylene glycol stearate SE.†

Tegin® P-SE. [Goldschmidt] Propylene glycol stearate SE.†

Tegin® PL. [Goldschmidt] Propylene glycol laurate.†

Tegin® RZ. [Goldschmidt] Glyceryl ricinoleate.*

Tegin® RZ NSE. [Goldschmidt] Glyceryl ricinoleate.†

Tegin® SE. [Goldschmidt AG] Glyceryl stearate SE.*

Tegin® T 4753. [Goldschmidt] Polyglyceryl-4 isostearate.*

Tegin® VA. [Goldschmidt] Glyceryl stearate SE.*

Tegin® VA 55G. [Goldschmidt] Glyceryl stearate.†

Tegin® VA 515. [Goldschmidt] Glyceryl stearate.†

Teginacid® ML. [Goldschmidt] Glyceryl stearate and PEG-40 stearate.*

Teginacid® R. [Goldschmidt] Glyceryl stearate and cocamidopropyl dimethylamine.†

Teginacid® R-SE. [Goldschmidt] Glyceryl monodistearate.†

Tego®-Amid D 5040. [Goldschmidt] Cocamidopropyl dimethylamine.*

Tego®-Amid O 18. [Goldschmidt] Oleamidopropyl dimethylamine.*

Tego®-Betaine L-90. [Goldschmidt] Lauramidopropyl betaine.*

Tego®-Betaine L-5290. [Goldschmidt AG] Ricinoleamidopropyl betaine.*

Tego®-Betaine S. [Goldschmidt] Cocamidopropyl betaine.*

Tego®-Betaine T. [Goldschmidt AG] Cocamidopropyl betaine.*

Tego®-Pearl S-33. [Goldschmidt AG] Sodium C14-16 olefin sulfonate, glycol distearate, cocamidopropyl betaine, sorbitan laurate.*

Tegosipon®. [Goldschmidt] Silicone.*

Tegosoft® 168. [Goldschmidt] Cetyl isononanoate.*

Tegosoft® 189. [Goldschmidt] Isostearyl isononanoate.*

Tegotain L 7. [Goldschmidt AG] Cocamidopropyl betaine.*

Tegotain S. [Goldschmidt AG] Cocamidopropyl betaine.*

Tetronic® 50R1. [BASF] EO/PO ethylene diamine block copolymer.*

Tetronic® 50R4. [BASF] EO/PO ethylene diamine block copolymer.*

Tetronic® 50R8. [BASF] EO/PO ethylene diamine block copolymer.*

Tetronic® 70R1. [BASF] EO/PO ethylene diamine block copolymer.*

Tetronic® 70R2. [BASF] EO/PO ethylene diamine block copolymer.*

Tetronic® 70R4. [BASF] EO/PO ethylene diamine block copolymer.*

Tetronic® 90R1. [BASF] EO/PO ethylene diamine block copolymer.*

Tetronic® 90R4. [BASF] EO/PO ethylene diamine block copolymer.*

Tetronic® 90R8. [BASF] EO/PO ethylene diamine block copolymer.*

Tetronic® 110R1. [BASF] EO/PO ethylene diamine block copolymer.*

Tetronic® 110R2. [BASF] EO/PO ethylene diamine block copolymer.*

Tetronic® 110R7. [BASF] EO/PO ethylene diamine block copolymer.*

Tetronic® 130R1. [BASF] EO/PO ethylene diamine block copolymer.*

Tetronic® 130R2. [BASF] EO/PO ethylene diamine block copolymer.*

Tetronic® 150R1. [BASF] EO/PO ethylene diamine block copolymer.*

Tetronic® 150R4. [BASF] EO/PO ethylene diamine block copolymer.*

Tetronic® 150R8. [BASF] EO/PO ethylene diamine block copolymer.*

Tetronic® 504. [BASF] Poloxamine 504.*

Tetronic® 702. [BASF] Poloxamine 702.*

Tetronic® 707. [BASF] Poloxamine 707.*

---

* Discontinued or redesignated   † Unverified   ‡ No longer standard

Tetronic® 909. [BASF] EO/PO ethylene diamine block copolymer.*
Tetronic® 1101. [BASF] Poloxamine 1101.*
Tetronic® 1102. [BASF] Poloxamine 1102.*
Tetronic® 1104. [BASF] Poloxamine 1104.*
Tetronic® 1107. [BASF] Poloxamine 1107.*
Tetronic® 1301. [BASF] Poloxamine 1301.*
Tetronic® 1302. [BASF] Poloxamine 1302.*
Tetronic® 1304. [BASF] Poloxamine 1304.*
Tetronic® 1501. [BASF] Poloxamine 1501.*
Tetronic® 1502. [BASF] Poloxamine 1502.*
Tetronic® 1504. [BASF] Poloxamine 1504.*
Tetronic® 1508. [BASF] Poloxamine 1508.*
Texapon® A. [Henkel/Cospha; Henkel Canada; Henkel KGaA/Cospha] Ammonium lauryl sulfate.*
Texapon® A 400. [Henkel/Cospha; Henkel KGaA/Cospha] Ammonium lauryl sulfate.*
Texapon® ASV-70 Spec. [Henkel KGaA/Cospha] Sodium laureth sulfate, sodium laureth-8 sulfate, sodium oleth sulfate.*
Texapon® CS Paste. [Henkel/Cospha; Henkel Canada; Henkel KGaA/Cospha] Sodium lauryl sulfate, sodium myristyl sulfate, sodium cetyl sulfate, sodium stearyl sulfate, laureth-10.*
Texapon® IES. [Henkel KGaA/Cospha] MIPA-laureth sulfate, MIPA-lauryl sulfate, and cocamide DEA.*
Texapon® K-12 Granules. [Henkel/Cospha; Henkel KGaA/Cospha] Sodium lauryl sulfate.*
Texapon® K-1294. [Henkel] Sodium lauryl sulfate (C12).†
Texapon® MG 3. [Henkel KGaA/Cospha] Magnesium lauryl sulfate and disodium laureth sulfosuccinate.*
Texapon® MGS. [Henkel KGaA/Cospha] Magnesium lauryl sulfate.*
Texapon® N 25. [Henkel KGaA/Cospha; Pulcra SA] Sodium laureth (2) sulfate.*
Texapon® N 40. [Henkel KGaA/Cospha; Pulcra SA] Sodium laureth (2) sulfate.*
Texapon® N 42. [Henkel] TEA-lauryl sulfate.†
Texapon® N 70-88. [Henkel] Fatty alcohol ether sulfate.†
Texapon® N 70 N. [Henkel] Sodium laureth sulfate.†
Texapon® N 103. [Henkel KGaA/Cospha] Sodium laureth sulfate (3 EO).*
Texapon® NA. [Henkel KGaA/Cospha] Ammonium laureth sulfate.*
Texapon® NC 70 LS. [Henkel/Cospha; Henkel KGaA/Cospha] Sodium laureth sulfate.*
Texapon® N Conc. [Henkel] Sodium lauryl ether sulfate.†
Texapon® NT. [Henkel KGaA/Cospha] TEA-laureth sulfate.*
Texapon® SBN. [Henkel KGaA/Cospha] Sodium laureth sulfate and disodium laureth sulfosuccinate.*
Texapon® SG. [Henkel KGaA/Cospha] Sodium laureth sulfate, PEG-8, cocamide MEA, glycol distearate, and glycerin.*
Texapon® Special. [Henkel] Ammonium lauryl sulfate.†
Texapon® TH. [Henkel KGaA/Cospha] TEA-lauryl sulfate.*
Texapon® VHC Powd. [Henkel/Cospha; Henkel KGaA/Cospha] Sodium lauryl sulfate.*
Texapon® WW 99. [Henkel KGaA/Cospha] MIPA-laureth sulfate, laureth-3, and cocamide DEA.*
Texapon® Z Granules. [Henkel KGaA/Cospha] Sodium lauryl sulfate C12-C14.*
Tri-K 30. [Tri-K Industries] PVP.*
Trilane. [Tri-K Industries] Squalane.*
Trisolan 1720. [Henkel/Emery] Lanolin-isopropyl ester.†
Trycol® 5878. [Henkel/Emery] Ethoxylated fatty alcohol ethers.†
Trydet LA-5. [Henkel/Emery] PEG-5 laurate.†

Trydet SA-23. [Henkel/Emery] PEG-23 stearate.†
Trydet SA-40. [Henkel/Emery] PEG-40 stearate.†
Tween® 20 SD. [ICI Spec. Chem.] POE sorbitan monolaurate.†
Tylopur MH, MHB. [Hoechst Celanese] Methyl hydroxyethylcellulose.*
Ultra Anhydrous Lanolin HP-2060. [Henkel/Cospha; Henkel Canada] Lanolin.†
Ultra Lantrol® HP-2074. [Henkel/Cospha; Henkel Canada] Lanolin oil.†
Ultra Sulfate SE-5. [Witco/H-I-P] Sodium alcohol ether sulfate.†
Ultra Sulfate SL-1. [Witco/H-I-P] Sodium lauryl sulfate.†
Unamide® C-2. [Lonza] PEG-3 cocamide.†
Unamide® CDX. [Lonza] Cocamide DEA.†
Unamide® CMX. [Lonza] 1:1 Cocamide MEA.†
Unamide® J-56. [Lonza] Lauramide DEA.†
Unamide® L-2. [Lonza] PEG-3 lauramide.†
Unamide® L-5. [Lonza] PEG-6 lauramide.†
Unamide® LDX. [Lonza] Lauramide DEA.†
Unamide® LMDX. [Lonza] Lauramide DEA.†
Unamide® N-72-3. [Lonza] Cocamide DEA.*
Unamide® S. [Lonza] Stearamide DEA.*
Unamine® OZ. [Lonza] Ethyl hydroxymethyl oleyl oxazoline.*
Ungerol CG27. [Unger Fabrikker AS] Sodium laureth sulfate.†
Ungerol LES 3-54. [Unger Fabrikker AS] Sodium laureth sulfate.†
Unimate® BYS. [Union Camp] n-Butyl stearate.†
Unimate® DBS. [Union Camp] Di-n-butyl sebacate.†
Unimate® DCA. [Union Camp] Dicapryl adipate.†
Unimate® DIPA. [Union Camp] Diisopropyl adipate.†
Unimate® DIPS. [Union Camp] Diisopropyl sebacate.†
Unimate® DOS. [Union Camp] Di-2-ethylhexyl sebacate.†
Unimate® EHP. [Union Camp] 2-Ethylhexyl palmitate.†
Unimate® IPM. [Union Camp] IPM.†
Unimate® IPP. [Union Camp] IPP.†
Unimate® IPPM. [Union Camp] Isopropyl palmitate/myristate.†
Union Carbide® L-45 Series. [Union Carbide] Dimethylpolysiloxane polymers.†
Union Carbide® LE-45. [Union Carbide] Dimethylpolysiloxane emulsion.†
UV Absorber DHB. [Fanwood] Benzophenone-1.*
UV Absorber HMB. [Fanwood] Benzophenone-3.*
UV Absorber HMBS. [Fanwood] Benzophenone-4.*
UV Absorber HOB. [Fanwood] Benzophenone-12.*
Uvinul® O 18. [BASF] Octyl salicylate.*
Vanate Acid. [R.T. Vanderbilt] EDTA.*
Vanate PSPA. [R.T. Vanderbilt] Pentasodium diethylene triamine pentaacetate sol'n.*
Vanate TS. [R.T. Vanderbilt] Tetrasodium EDTA.*
Vanate TSD. [R.T. Vanderbilt] Tetrasodium EDTA, dihydrate.*
Vanate TSHE. [R.T. Vanderbilt] Trisodium N-hydroxyethylene diamine triacetate sol'n.*
Vanate TS-N. [R.T. Vanderbilt] Tetrasodium EDTA.*
Vanate TST. [R.T. Vanderbilt] Tetrasodium EDTA, tetrahydrate.*
Varion® 2C. (see Rewoteric AM 2C-W) [Witco/H-I-P] Disodium cocoamphodiacetate.*
Varion® 2L. (see Rewoteric AM 2L-40) [Witco/H-I-P] Disodium lauroamphodiacetate.*
Varion® AM-B14. (see Rewoteric AM B-14) [Witco/H-I-P] Cocamidopropyl betaine.*

---

* Discontinued or redesignated   † Unverified   ‡ No longer standard

Varion® AM-KSF-40. (see Rewoteric AM KSF-40) [Witco/H-I-P] Disodium cocoamphodipropionate.*
Varion® AM-KSF-40. (see Rewoteric AM KSF-40) [Witco/H-I-P] Disodium cocoamphodipropionate.*
Varion® AM-V. (see Rewoteric AM V.) [Witco/H-I-P] Caprylic glycinate.*
Varion® CADG-LS. (see Rewoteric AM B-14 LS) [Witco/H-I-P] Cocamidopropyl betaine.*
Varion® CADG-W. (see Rewoteric AM B-14) [Witco/H-I-P] Cocamidopropyl betaine.*
Varion® CAS. (see Rewoteric AM CAS-15) [Witco/H-I-P] Cocamidopropyl hydroxysultaine.*
Varion® CAS-W. (see Rewoteric AM CAS) [Witco/H-I-P] Cocamidopropyl hydroxysultaine.*
Varion® HC. (see Rewoteric AM HC) [Witco/H-I-P] Lauryl hydroxysultaine.*
Varion® LP. (see Rewoteric AM LP) [Witco/H-I-P] Sodium lauryliminodipropionate.*
Varion® TEG. (see Rewoteric AM TEG) [Witco/H-I-P] Dihydroxyethyl tallow glycinate.*
Varion® TEG-40%. (see Rewoteric AM TEG-40) [Witco/H-I-P] Dihydroxyethyl tallow glycinate.*
Velvetex® 610L. [Henkel Canada] Sodium lauriminodipropionate.†
Velvetex® 710L. [Henkel] Lauraminopropionic acid.†
Velvetex® BC. [Henkel] Coco betaine.†
Velvetex® BC-35. [Henkel] Cocamidopropyl betaine.†
Velvet Veil 320. [Presperse] Mica (80%), silica beads (20%).*
Velvet Veil 620. [Presperse] Mica (80%), silica beads (20%).*
Velvet Veil 640. [Presperse] Mica (60%), silica beads (40%).*
Verajuice-Cold Processed. [Apree] Aloe vera gel.*
Versilan MX167. [Harcros UK] Alcohol ether sulfate.†
Vifcoll CCN-40, CCN-40 Powd. [Nikko Chem. Co. Ltd.] N-Cocoyl collagen peptide, sodium salt.†
White Swan. [Croda Chem. Ltd.] Lanolin BP, anhyd.†
Witcamide® 6515. (see Witcamide 128T) [Witco/H-I-P] Cocamide DEA.*
Witcamide® Coco Condensate. (see Witcamide CD) [Witco/H-I-P] Cocamide DEA, diethanolamine.*
Witcolate™ 6400. [Witco/H-I-P] Sodium lauryl sulfate.*
Witcolate™ 6430. [Witco/H-I-P] Ammonium lauryl sulfate.*
Witcolate™ 6431. [Witco/H-I-P] Ammonium lauryl sulfate.*
Witcolate™ 6434. (see Witcolate TLS-500) [Witco/H-I-P] TEA-lauryl sulfate.*
Witcolate™ 6450. (see Witcolate ES-1) [Witco/H-I-P] Sodium laureth (1) sulfate.*

Witcolate™ 6453. (see Witcolate ES-3) [Witco/H-I-P] Sodium laureth sulfate.*
Witcolate™ 6455. (see Witcolate ES-2) [Witco/H-I-P] Sodium laureth (2) sulfate.*
Witcolate™ 6465. (see Witcolate D-510) [Witco/H-I-P] Sodium 2-ethylhexyl sulfate.*
Witcolate™ A. [Witco/H-I-P] Sodium lauryl sulfate.*
Witcolate™ AE. (see Witcolate AE-3) [Witco/H-I-P] Ammonium laureth sulfate.*
Witcolate™ AM. [Witco/H-I-P] Ammonium lauryl sulfate.*
Witcolate™ S. [Witco/H-I-P] Sodium lauryl sulfate.*
Witcolate™ SE. (see Witcolate SE-5) [Witco/H-I-P] Sodium laureth sulfate.*
Witconate 40RA. [Witco/H-I-P] Linear alkylaryl sodium sulfonate.†
Witconate™ 45DS. (see Witconate 45 Liq.) [Witco/H-I-P] Sodium dodecylbenzene sulfonate.*
Witconate 85. [Witco/H-I-P] Linear alkylaryl sodium sulfonate.†
Witconate 90. [Witco/H-I-P] Linear alkylaryl sodium sulfonate.†
Witconate 1245. [Witco/H-I-P] Linear alkylaryl sodium sulfonate.†
Witconate 1288. [Witco/H-I-P] Linear alkylaryl sulfonic acid.†
Witconate 1298. [Witco/H-I-P] Linear alkylaryl sulfonic acid.†
Witconate 1388. [Witco/H-I-P] Linear alkylaryl sulfonic acid.†
Witconate™ K. (see Witconate 90F) [Witco/H-I-P] Sodium dodecylbenzenesulfonate.*
Witconate™ K Dense. (see Witconate 90 Dense) [Witco/H-I-P] Sodium dodecylbenzene sulfonate.*
Witconate™ KX. (see Witconate LX F) [Witco/H-I-P] Sodium dodecylbenzene sulfonate.*
Witconol™ 2640. (see Witconol 2711) [Witco/H-I-P] PEG-8 stearate.*
Witconol™ 2642. (see Witconol 2712) [Witco/H-I-P] PEG-8 distearate.*
Yeoman. [Croda Chem. Ltd.] Anhyd. lanolin BP.†
Zetesol 2210. [Zschimmer & Schwarz] Lauryl alcohol ether sulfate, MEA salt.†
Zetesol SE 35. [Zschimmer & Schwarz] MIPA fatty alcohol ether sulfate with pearlescent and fatty acid amido alkyl betaine.†

---

* Discontinued or redesignated   † Unverified   ‡ No longer standard

Manufacturer Successors

Former	Present
Alcolac	Rhone-Poulenc Surfactants & Specialties
Alkaril	Rhone-Poulenc Surfactants & Specialties
Allied Corp.	Allied-Signal
American Hoechst	Hoechst Celanese
Amico	Lucas Meyer
Armak	Akzo
Berol	Berol Nobel
Berol Kemi AB	Berol Nobel AB
Bofors Lakeway	Rhone-Poulenc
Capital City	Karlshamns
Chemetic	Apree, Inc.
CLE	Apree, Inc.
Clintwood	Rhone-Poulenc Surfactants & Specialties
Colloids Inc.	Rhone-Poulenc Surfactants & Specialties
Conoco Chem.	Vista
Continental Oil Co.	Vista
Cyclo	Rhone-Poulenc Surfactants & Specialties
Cyprus Industrial Minerals	Luzenac Am.
Darling & Co.	Unichema Chemicals
DeSoto	Witco/H-I-P
Diamond Shamrock	Henkel
Drew Produtos Quimicos Ltds.	Aquatec Quimica S/A
Duphar	Solvay Duphar BV
Durkee	Van Den Bergh Foods
Dynamit Nobel	Hüls
Emery	Henkel/Emery
GAF	ISP
GAF Surfactants	Rhone-Poulenc Surfactants & Specialties
Geronazzo SpA	Rhone-Poulenc Geronazzo SpA
Gist-Brocades USA	Int'l. Bio-Synthetics Inc.
Givaudan	Givaudan-Roure Corp.
Glyco	Lonza
W.R. Grace/Hampshire Div.	Hampshire Chemical Corp.
Hexcel	Zeeland Chemicals Inc.
Hodag	Calgene Chem. Inc.
Hunt Chem. Corp., Philip A./Org. Div.	Olin Corp.
ICI United States	ICI Americas Inc.
Jojoba Growers & Processors	International Flora Technologies, Inc.
Jordan Chem. Co.	PPG Specialty Chem.
Kenobel SA	Berol Nobel
Lankro Chem. Ltd.	Harcros Chem. UK Ltd.
Laserson & Sebetay	Laserson SA
Manro Products Ltd.	Hickson Manro Ltd.
Manville	Celite
Mars	Rhone-Poulenc Surfactants & Specialties
Mazer	PPG Specialty Chem.
Miles/Biotech	Solvay Enzymes
Miranol	Rhone-Poulenc Surfactants & Specialties
Mobay	Miles
Morton Thiokol	Morton Int'l.
Nease	Ruetgers-Nease
NJ Zinc	Zinc Corp. of America
NL Treating	Rheox

MANUFACTURER SUCCESSORS

North Am. Silica Co. (NASILCO) .... Degussa
Oleofina .... Fina Chemicals
Patco .... Am. Ingredients
Pearsall .... Witco/Argus
Petrarch .... Hüls
PPF Int'l. .... Quest Int'l.
PPG Mazer .... PPG Specialty Chem.
PVO Int'l. .... Stepan Co./PVO Dept.
Quantum Chem. Corp./Emery Div. .... Henkel/Emery
Rhone-Poulenc SpA .... Rhone-Poulenc Geronazzo SpA
Rilsan .... Dai-ichi Kogyo Seiyaku
Rona Pearl .... Rona
Sherex .... Witco/H-I-P
Sinor Kao SA .... KAO Corp. S.A.
Synfina-Oleofin .... Fina Chemicals
Tessilchimica .... Auschem SpA
Thompson-Hayward Chem. Co. .... Harcros Chem.
U.S. Peroxygen .... Witco/Argus
Union Carbide OrganoSilicon Prods. .... OSi Specialties, Inc.
USI Chemicals Co. .... Quantum Chem. Corp./USI Div.
Van Dyk .... ISP Van Dyk
Van Schuppen .... Solvay Duphar BV
Witco/Organics .... Witco/H-I-P

Gardner's Chemical Synonyms and Trade Names
Tenth Edition

Executive Editors Michael and Irene Ash

Nine previous editions over 65 years have established GARDNER'S as a standard source of reference for industrial chemists, the libraries of large industrial and commercial organizations, and registrars of patents and trademarks worldwide. The Tenth Edition represents a total revision of all existing entries, many of which have been edited, expanded, or deleted, and the addition of thousands more. New and greatly expanded subject coverage includes: adhesives, insecticides, pesticides, leading pharmaceuticals, petrochemicals, fillers, fibres, coatings, plastics, polymers and synthetics.

Key features of the Tenth Edition include:
* Over 40,000 trade names and chemicals covered: 18,000 new to this edition
* 13,500 entries now include CAS (Chemical Abstract Service) and/or EINECS (European Inventory of Existing Commercial Chemical Substances) numbers
* Nearly 3,000 manufacturers listed – more than twice those in the 9th Edition
* Historical synonyms and obsolete chemicals have been retained as GARDNER'S remains one of the key references in this area

Entries give descriptions, classification, chemical formulas/applications, and manufacturers. Trade entries have been obtained direct from manufacturers worldwide, supplemented by a research programme.

1994   1,312 pages   0 566 07491 5

Gower

Handbook of Industrial Surfactants

Compiled by Michael and Irene Ash

Over 16,000 tradename surface-active agents for industrial applications, manufactured worldwide, are contained in this new reference. General-use surfactants, such as emulsifiers, wetting agents, foaming agents, detergents, dispersants, and solubilizers are included, as well as detergent raw materials, defoamers, and antifoaming agents.

The types and quantities of surfactants available commercially are numerous and the difficulty in making choices between products is becoming overwhelming. It is the purpose of this reference book to guide those who are involved in the selection of these materials through the process of identifying, classifying, and selecting the most appropriate products for their requirements. It is therefore organized so that the user can search for and locate products based on a variety of essential distinguishing attributes.

Another important feature of the book is that products that have been discontinued by companies have been noted; products with name changes are cross referenced to the new tradename; and a list of companies that have been acquired by other chemical manufacturers is included in the Appendix. Full addresses are given for listed manufacturers.

1993   928 pages   0 566 07457 5

Gower